T0340711

Blackwell's Five-Minute Veterinary Consult: Canine and Feline

Seventh Edition

BLACKWELL'S FIVE-MINUTE VETERINARY CONSULT

Canine and Feline

Seventh Edition

Edited by

Larry P. Tilley, DVM
Diplomate, American College of Veterinary Internal Medicine
(Small Animal Internal Medicine)
President, VetMed Consultants, Inc.
Santa Fe, New Mexico
USA

Francis W.K. Smith, Jr., DVM
Diplomate, American College of Veterinary Internal Medicine
(Small Animal Internal Medicine and Cardiology)
Vice-President, VetMed Consultant, Inc.
Lexington, Massachusetts
USA

Meg M. Sleeper, VMD
Diplomate, American College of Veterinary Internal Medicine
(Cardiology)
Professor of Clinical Cardiology
College of Veterinary Medicine
University of Florida, Florida
USA

Benjamin M. Brainard, VMD
Diplomate, American College of Veterinary
Anesthesia and Analgesia and
American College of Veterinary Emergency and
Critical Care
Edward H. Gunst
Professor of Small Animal Critical Care
College of Veterinary Medicine
University of Georgia
Athens, Georgia
USA

WILEY Blackwell

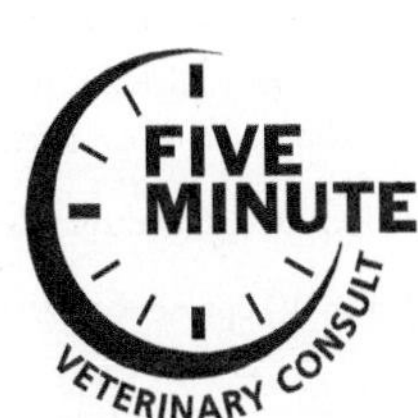

Edition History
First Edition 1997 © Lippincott Williams & Wilkins
Second Edition 2000 © Lippincott Williams & Wilkins
Third edition 2004 © Lippincott Williams & Wilkins
Fourth Edition 2007 © Blackwell Publishing Professional
Fifth edition 2011 © John Wiley & Sons, Inc.
Sixth Edition 2016 © John Wiley & Sons, Inc.

Blackwell Publishing was acquired by John Wiley & Sons in February 2007. Blackwell's publishing program has been merged with Wiley's global Scientific, Technical and Medical business to form Wiley-Blackwell.

Registered Office
John Wiley & Sons, Inc., 111 River Street, Hoboken, NJ 07030, USA

Editorial Office
111 River Street, Hoboken, NJ 07030, USA
For details of our global editorial offices, customer services, and more information about Wiley products visit us at www.wiley.com.

Wiley also publishes its books in a variety of electronic formats and by print-on-demand. Some content that appears in standard print versions of this book may not be available in other formats.

Library of Congress Cataloging-in-Publication Data

Names: Tilley, Lawrence P., editor. | Smith, Francis W. K., Jr., editor. | Sleeper, Meg M., editor. | Brainard, Benjamin, editor.
Title: Blackwell's five-minute veterinary consult. Canine and feline / edited by Larry P. Tilley, Francis W.K. Smith, Jr., Margaret M. Sleeper, Benjamin Brainard.
Other titles: Five-minute veterinary consult. Canine and feline
Description: Seventh edition. | Hoboken, NJ : Wiley-Blackwell, 2021. | Includes bibliographical references and index.
Identifiers: LCCN 2020025494 (print) | LCCN 2020025495 (ebook) | ISBN 9781119513179 (hardback) | ISBN 9781119513155 (adobe pdf) | ISBN 9781119513162 (epub)
Subjects: MESH: Dog Diseases–diagnosis | Cat Diseases–diagnosis | Dog Diseases–therapy | Cat Diseases–therapy | Veterinary Medicine–methods | Handbook
Classification: LCC SF991 (print) | LCC SF991 (ebook) | NLM SF 991 | DDC 636.7/0896–dc23
LC record available at https://lccn.loc.gov/2020025494
LC ebook record available at https://lccn.loc.gov/2020025495

Cover Design and Images: Wiley

Set in 9/10pt AdobeGarmondPro by SPi Global, Pondicherry, India

SKY10069259_030824

To my love and joy in life, Ellen Lefkowitz, my son Kyle, and grandson Tucker.
To my late mother Dorothy, who instilled values that have helped me throughout life.
To family and animals who represent the purity of life.

Larry P. Tilley

To my wife, May, my son, Ben, and my daughter, Jade, who are a constant source of inspiration, love, and joy. To my late father, Frank, who was my perfect role model. To Kaylee (dog) and Centie (cat) who remind me each day to make time for play.

Francis W.K. Smith, Jr.

To my parents and sister for their stalwart support and to the many animals who have touched my life and made me a better person.

Meg M. Sleeper

To my family, my mentors, my colleagues; to colleagues and friends who are no longer with us. "Keep cool, but care"—Thomas Pynchon.

Benjamin M. Brainard

CONTENTS

TOPIC	

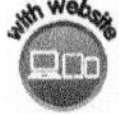

331 client education handouts are available at www.fiveminutevet.com/canineandfeline7th for you to download and use in practice

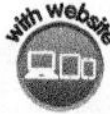

331 client education handouts are available at www.fiveminutevet.com/canineandfeline7th for you to download and use in practice

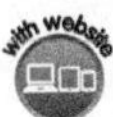

331 client education handouts are available at www.fiveminutevet.com/canineandfeline7th for you to download and use in practice

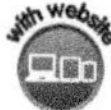

331 client education handouts are available at www.fiveminutevet.com/canineandfeline7th for you to download and use in practice

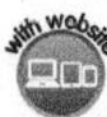

331 client education handouts are available at www.fiveminutevet.com/canineandfeline7th for you to download and use in practice

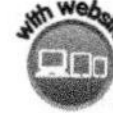

331 client education handouts are available at www.fiveminutevet.com/canineandfeline7th for you to download and use in practice

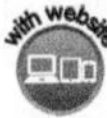

331 client education handouts are available at www.fiveminutevet.com/canineandfeline7th for you to download and use in practice

331 client education handouts are available at www.fiveminutevet.com/canineandfeline7th for you to download and use in practice

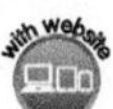

331 client education handouts are available at www.fiveminutevet.com/canineandfeline7th for you to download and use in practice

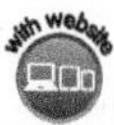

331 client education handouts are available at www.fiveminutevet.com/canineandfeline7th for you to download and use in practice

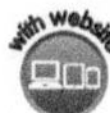

331 client education handouts are available at www.fiveminutevet.com/canineandfeline7th for you to download and use in practice

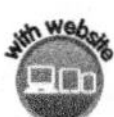

331 client education handouts are available at www.fiveminutevet.com/canineandfeline7th for you to download and use in practice

331 client education handouts are available at www.fiveminutevet.com/canineandfeline7th for you to download and use in practice

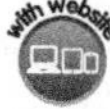

331 client education handouts are available at www.fiveminutevet.com/canineandfeline7th for you to download and use in practice

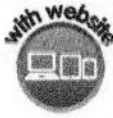

331 client education handouts are available at www.fiveminutevet.com/canineandfeline7th for you to download and use in practice

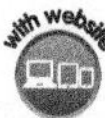

331 client education handouts are available at www.fiveminutevet.com/canineandfeline7th for you to download and use in practice

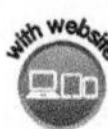

331 client education handouts are available at www.fiveminutevet.com/canineandfeline7th for you to download and use in practice

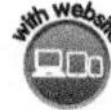

331 client education handouts are available at www.fiveminutevet.com/canineandfeline7th for you to download and use in practice

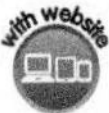

331 client education handouts are available at www.fiveminutevet.com/canineandfeline7th for you to download and use in practice

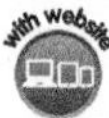

331 client education handouts are available at www.fiveminutevet.com/canineandfeline7th for you to download and use in practice

331 client education handouts are available at www.fiveminutevet.com/canineandfeline7th for you to download and use in practice

CONTENTS *by Subject*

TOPIC

APPENDICES

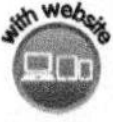

331 client education handouts are available at www.fiveminutevet.com/canineandfeline7th for you to download and use in practice

Behavior

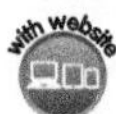

331 client education handouts are available at www.fiveminutevet.com/canineandfeline7th for you to download and use in practice

CARDIOLOGY

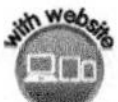

331 client education handouts are available at www.fiveminutevet.com/canineandfeline7th for you to download and use in practice

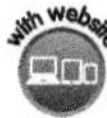

331 client education handouts are available at www.fiveminutevet.com/canineandfeline7th for you to download and use in practice

DENTISTRY

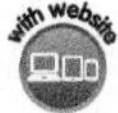

331 client education handouts are available at www.fiveminutevet.com/canineandfeline7th for you to download and use in practice

DERMATOLOGY

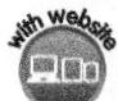

331 client education handouts are available at www.fiveminutevet.com/canineandfeline7th for you to download and use in practice

ENDOCRINOLOGY AND METABOLISM

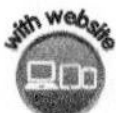

331 client education handouts are available at www.fiveminutevet.com/canineandfeline7th for you to download and use in practice

Gastroenterology

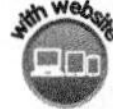

331 client education handouts are available at www.fiveminutevet.com/canineandfeline7th for you to download and use in practice

HEMATOLOGY/ IMMUNOLOGY

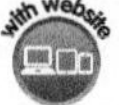

331 client education handouts are available at www.fiveminutevet.com/canineandfeline7th for you to download and use in practice

HEPATOLOGY

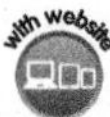

331 client education handouts are available at www.fiveminutevet.com/canineandfeline7th for you to download and use in practice

Infectious Diseases

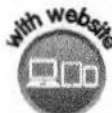

331 client education handouts are available at www.fiveminutevet.com/canineandfeline7th for you to download and use in practice

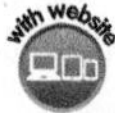

331 client education handouts are available at www.fiveminutevet.com/canineandfeline7th for you to download and use in practice

MUSCULOSKELETAL

NEPHROLOGY/ UROLOGY

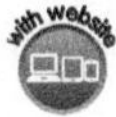

331 client education handouts are available at www.fiveminutevet.com/canineandfeline7th for you to download and use in practice

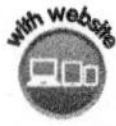

331 client education handouts are available at www.fiveminutevet.com/canineandfeline7th for you to download and use in practice

NEUROLOGY

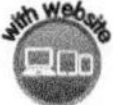

331 client education handouts are available at www.fiveminutevet.com/canineandfeline7th for you to download and use in practice

ONCOLOGY

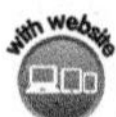

331 client education handouts are available at www.fiveminutevet.com/canineandfeline7th for you to download and use in practice

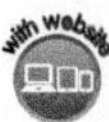

331 client education handouts are available at www.fiveminutevet.com/canineandfeline7th for you to download and use in practice

OPHTHALMOLOGY

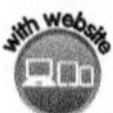

331 client education handouts are available at www.fiveminutevet.com/canineandfeline7th for you to download and use in practice

RESPIRATORY

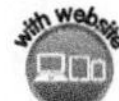

331 client education handouts are available at www.fiveminutevet.com/canineandfeline7th for you to download and use in practice

THERIOGENOLOGY

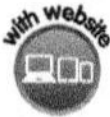

331 client education handouts are available at www.fiveminutevet.com/canineandfeline7th for you to download and use in practice

TOXICOLOGY

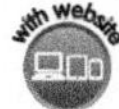

331 client education handouts are available at www.fiveminutevet.com/canineandfeline7th for you to download and use in practice

331 client education handouts are available at www.fiveminutevet.com/canineandfeline7th for you to download and use in practice

PREFACE

Keeping abreast of advances in veterinary internal medicine is extremely difficult, especially for the busy general practitioner. To keep current with all the veterinary journals while practicing medicine is impossible. The veterinarian in practice can be overwhelmed by all of the findings and conclusions of thousands of studies conducted by veterinary specialists. *Blackwell's Five-Minute Veterinary Consult* is designed to provide the busy veterinary practitioner and student of veterinary medicine with concise practical reviews of almost all the diseases and clinical problems in dogs and cats. Our goal in creating this textbook was also to provide up-to-date information in an easy-to-use format. Emphasis is placed on diagnosis and treatment of problems and diseases likely to be seen by veterinarians.

Our fondest dream was realized when the first six editions of this book were chosen as a comprehensive reference source for canine and feline medicine by veterinary students, practicing veterinarians, and board-certified specialists. The format has proven easy to use and very popular with busy practitioners. The scope of the book and the number of Consulting Editors and authors have been expanded. We have also increased the number of authors from outside North America, to provide the best advice in the world. The number of topics has been increased, and every topic has been updated to provide you with the most current information possible in a textbook. The appendixes have also been expanded to include more useful tables.

Several good veterinary internal medicine textbooks are available. The uniqueness and value of *Blackwell's Five-Minute Veterinary Consult* as a quick reference is the consistency of presentation, the breadth of coverage, the contribution of large numbers of experts, and the timely preparation of the manuscript. The format of every topic is identical, making it easy to find information. An extensive list of topic headings ensures complete coverage of each topic.

As the title implies, one objective of this book is to make information quickly available. To this end, we have organized topics alphabetically from A to Z. Most topics can be found without using the index. A table of contents broken out by organ system and a detailed index are provided. Large volumes of useful information are summarized in charts in the appendixes. Included in the appendixes are normal laboratory values, endocrine testing protocols, common procedures and testing protocols, toxicology tables, pain management tables, Rx for Osteoarthritis, disease-modifying drugs table, an epilepsy classification table, conversion tables, and other information pages with important resources for veterinarians. For this new edition, an appendix has been added to include common procedures and testing protocols used in veterinary medicine.

We are delighted and privileged to have had the assistance of numerous experts in veterinary internal medicine from around the world. More than 450 veterinary specialists contributed to this text, allowing each chapter to be written by an expert on the subject. In addition to providing outstanding information, this large pool of experts allowed us to publish this major text in a timely manner.

Many large textbooks take several years to write, making some of the information outdated by the time the book is published. We are indebted to the many contributors and Consulting Editors whose hard work allowed us to write, edit, and publish this work in 3 years, with most chapters completed within a year of publication. Our goal is to revise the text every 3–4 years, so that the contents will always be current.

Blackwell's Five-Minute Veterinary Consult: Canine and Feline, Seventh Edition is available in a variety of digital formats. Visit www.wiley.com/go/5MVC for more information. This edition also includes Client Education Handouts based on the content of *Blackwell's Five-Minute Veterinary Consult.* The complimentary Client Education Handouts are available on a companion website at www.fiveminutevet.com/canineandfeline featuring 331 Client Education Handouts for you to customize and use in practice. These Handouts can be edited to reflect your practice preferences and then printed on your letterhead to distribute to your clients.

The book will also be published as an e-book, in downloadable ePub/ePDF formats. Now veterinarians can quickly access information about necessary clinical skills and new developments in diagnosis and treatment on their computers or mobile versions. The electronic versions offer fast, affordable access to much of the accumulated wisdom in veterinary medicine. This technology brings to the clinic examination room and doctor's office an easy-to-use resource that will markedly improve the quality of continuing education and clinical practice, and a companion website offers client education handouts to be downloaded and used in practice.

The seventh edition of this textbook constitutes an important, up-to-date medical reference source for your practice and clinical education. We strived to make it complete yet practical and easy to use. Our dreams are realized if this text helps you to quickly locate and use the "momentarily important" information that is essential to the practice of high-quality veterinary medicine. We would appreciate your input so that we can make future editions even more useful. If you would like to see any changes in content or format, additions, or deletions, please let us know. Send comments to the following:

Drs. Tilley, Smith, Sleeper and Brainard
c/o John Wiley & Sons
1606 Golden Aspen Dr Ste 104
Ames, IA 50010, USA

ACKNOWLEDGMENTS

The completion of this textbook provides a welcome opportunity to recognize in writing the many individuals who have helped along the way. The Editors gratefully acknowledge the Consulting Editors and the contributors who, by their expertise, have so unmistakably enhanced the quality of this textbook.

We would also like to acknowledge and thank our families for their support of this project and the sacrifices they made to allow us the time to complete the book.

In addition to thanking veterinarians who have referred patients to us, we would like to express our gratitude to all the veterinary students, interns, and residents who we have had the privilege to teach. Their curiosity and intellectual stimulation have enabled us to grow and have prompted us to undertake the task of writing this book.

Finally, a special acknowledgment goes to everyone at Wiley Blackwell. The marketing and sales departments also must be acknowledged for generating such an interest in this book. They are all meticulous workers and kind people who have made the final stages of preparing this book both inspiring and fun. We would also like to thank copy-editors Sally Osborn and Harriet Stewart-Jones, and Erica Judisch, Executive Editor. A special thank you goes to Mirjana Misina, Editorial Project Manager, who spent hours and days keeping track of all the contributors and the deadline dates for manuscripts. This edition would not have taken place without her. An important life goal of ours has been fulfilled: to provide expertise in small animal internal medicine worldwide and to teach the principles contained in this textbook to veterinarians and students everywhere.

Larry P. Tilley, Francis W.K. Smith, Jr.,
Meg M. Sleeper and Benjamin M. Brainard

Consulting Editors

MICHAEL AHERNE, MVB, GradDipVetStud, MS, MANZCVS (Small Animal Surgery)
Diplomate ACVIM (Cardiology)
Clinical Assistant Professor
Department of Small Animal Clinical Sciences
College of Veterinary Medicine
University of Florida
Gainesville, Florida, USA
Subject: Cardiology

MELINDA S. CAMUS, DVM
Diplomate ACVP (Clinical Pathology)
Associate Professor
Department of Pathology
College of Veterinary Medicine
University of Georgia
Athens, Georgia, USA
Subject: Hematology/Immunology

TIMOTHY M. FAN, DVM, PhD
Diplomate ACVIM (Small Animal Internal Medicine, Oncology)
Professor
Department of Veterinary Clinical Medicine
College of Veterinary Medicine
University of Illinois at Urbana-Champaign
Urbana, Illinois, USA
Subject: Oncology

J.D. FOSTER, VMD
Diplomate ACVIM (Small Animal Internal Medicine)
Nephrology/Urology & Internal Medicine
Friendship Hospital for Animals
Washington, DC, USA
Subject: Nephrology

MATHIEU M. GLASSMAN, VMD
Diplomate ACVS
Chief of Surgery
Friendship Surgical Specialists
Friendship Hospital for Animals
Washington, DC, USA
Subject: Musculoskeletal

KATE HOLAN, BS, DVM
Diplomate ACVIM (Small Animal Internal Medicine)
Assistant Professor and Head
Small Animal Internal Medicine
Department of Small Animal Clinical Sciences
Michigan State University
East Lansing, Michigan, USA
Subject: Hepatology

LYNN R. HOVDA, RPH, DVM, MS
Diplomate ACVIM (Large Animal Internal Medicine)
Director of Veterinary Medicine
SafetyCall International & Pet Poison Helpline
Bloomington, Minnesota;
Assistant Adjunct Professor
Department of Veterinary Biomedical Sciences
College of Veterinary Medicine
University of Minnesota
St. Paul, Minnesota, USA
Subject: Toxicology

AMIE KOENIG, DVM
Diplomate ACVIM (Small Animal Internal Medicine), Diplomate ACVECC
Professor of Emergency and Critical Care
Department of Small Animal Medicine and Surgery
College of Veterinary Medicine
University of Georgia
Athens, Georgia, USA
Subject: Infectious Diseases

GARY M. LANDSBERG, BSc, DVM
Diplomate ACVB, ECAWBM
Veterinary Behaviourist
Vice-President
CanCog Incorporated
Fergus, Ontario;
Head
Fear Free Research
Canada
Subject: Behavior

PATTY A. LATHAN, VMD, MS
Diplomate ACVIM (Small Animal Internal Medicine)
Associate Professor
Department of Clinical Sciences
Mississippi State University
Mississippi State, Mississippi, USA
Subject: Endocrinology/Metabolism

HEIDI B. LOBPRISE, DVM
Diplomate AVDC (Dentistry)
Main Street Veterinary Dental Clinic
Flower Mound, Texas, USA
Subject: Dentistry

KATHERN E. MYRNA, DVM, MS
Diplomate ACVO
Associate Professor of Ophthalmology
Department of Small Animal Medicine and Surgery
College of Veterinary Medicine
University of Georgia
Athens, Georgia, USA
Subject: Ophthalmology

MARK P. RONDEAU, DVM
Diplomate ACVIM (Small Animal Internal Medicine)
Professor of Clinical Medicine
Department of Clinical Sciences and Advanced Medicine
School of Veterinary Medicine
University of Pennsylvania
Philadelphia, Pennsylvania, USA
Subject: Gastroenterology

ELIZABETH ROZANSKI, DVM
Diplomate ACVECC
Diplomate DACVIM (Small Animal Internal Medicine)
Associate Professor
Department of Clinical Science
Cummings School of Veterinary Medicine
Tufts University
North Grafton, Massachusetts, USA
Subject: Respiratory

ERIN E. RUNCAN, DVM
Diplomate ACT
Associate Professor—Clinical
Theriogenology and Reproductive Medicine
Department of Veterinary Clinical Sciences
The Ohio State University
College of Veterinary Medicine
Columbus, Ohio, USA
Subject: Theriogenology

ALEXANDER H. WERNER RESNICK, VMD
Diplomate ACVD
Staff Dermatologist
Animal Dermatology Center
Studio City & Westlake Village
California, USA
Subject: Dermatology

Acknowledgment

The Book Editors acknowledge the prior contribution of the following Consulting Editors:

Stephen C. Barr (Infectious Diseases)
Deborah S. Greco (Endocrinology)
Sara K. Lyle (Theriogenology)
Stanley L. Marks (Gastroenterology)
Paul E. Miller (Ophthalmology)
Joane M. Parent (Neurology)
Carl A. Osborne (Nephrology/Urology)
Alan H. Rebar (Hematology/Immunology)
Walter C. Renberg (Musculoskeletal)

CONTRIBUTORS

JONATHAN A. ABBOTT, DVM
Diplomate ACVIM (Cardiology)
Associate Professor
Department of Small Animal Clinical Sciences
College of Veterinary Medicine
University of Tennessee
Knoxville, Tennessee
USA

ANTHONY C.G. ABRAMS-OGG, DVM, DVSc
Diplomate ACVIM (Small Animal Internal Medicine)
Professor
Department of Clinical Studies
University of Guelph
Ontario Veterinary College
Guelph, Ontario
Canada

LARRY G. ADAMS, DVM, PhD
Diplomate ACVIM (Small Animal Internal Medicine)
Professor of Small Animal Internal Medicine
Department of Veterinary Clinical Sciences
College of Veterinary Medicine
Purdue University
West Lafayette, Indiana
USA

DARCY B. ADIN, DVM
Diplomate ACVIM (Cardiology)
Clinical Associate Professor
College of Veterinary Medicine
Department of Large Animal Clinical Sciences
University of Florida
Gainesville, Florida
USA

MICHAEL AHERNE, MVB, GradDipVetStud, MS, MANZCVS (Small Animal Surgery)
Diplomate ACVIM (Cardiology)
Clinical Assistant Professor
Department of Small Animal Clinical Sciences
College of Veterinary Medicine
University of Florida
Gainesville, Florida
USA

HASAN ALBASAN, DVM, MS, PhD
Associate Veterinarian
Nephrology & Urology
Veterinary Care Specialists
Milford, Michigan
USA

RACHEL A. ALLBAUGH, DVM, MS
Diplomate ACVO (Ophthalmology)
Associate Professor
Department of Veterinary Clinical Sciences
College of Veterinary Medicine
Iowa State University
Ames, Iowa
USA

KARIN ALLENSPACH, Dr.med.vet, PhD, FHEA, AGAF
Diplomate ECVIM-CA
Professor
Department of Clinical Sciences
College of Veterinary Medicine
Iowa State University
Ames, Iowa
USA

COLLEEN M. ALMGREN, DVM, PhD
Diplomate DABT
Diplomate DABVT
Veterinary Toxicologist
Pet Poison Helpline/SafetyCall International
Bloomington, Minnesota
USA

SARAH R. ALPERT, DVM
Diplomate ABT
Consulting Veterinarian, Clinical Toxicology
Pet Poison Helpline & SafetyCall International
Bloomington, Minnesota
USA

SOPHIE ASCHENBROICH, DVM, PhD
Diplomate ACVP (Anatomic Pathology)
Assistant Professor
Department of Pathobiological Sciences
School of Veterinary Medicine
University of Wisconsin-Madison
Madison, Wisconsin
USA

GENNA ATIEE, DVM
Diplomate ACVIM (Small Animal Internal Medicine)
Interventional Radiology Fellow
College of Veterinary Medicine
University of Georgia
Veterinary Medical Center
Athens, Georgia
USA

MELISSA J. BAIN, DVM, MS
Diplomate ACVB (Behavior)
Diplomate ACAW (Welfare)
Professor, Clinical Animal Behavior
Department of Veterinary Medicine and Epidemiology
School of Veterinary Medicine
University of California, Davis
Davis, California
USA

TOMAS W. BAKER
Pound Sound Consulting
Three Rivers, California
USA

CHERYL E. BALKMAN, DVM
Diplomate ACVIM (Small Animal Internal Medicine, Oncology)
Senior Lecturer
Department of Clinical Sciences
College of Veterinary Medicine
Cornell University
Ithaca, New York
USA

GAD BANETH, DVM, PhD
Diplomate ECVCP
Professor
Koret School of Veterinary Medicine
The Hebrew University
Rehovot
Israel

KRISTIN M. BANNON, DVM, FAVD
Diplomate AVDC
Veterinary Dentistry and Oral Surgery of New Mexico, LLC
Algodones, New Mexico
USA

RENEE BARBER, DVM, PhD
Diplomate ACVIM (Neurology)
Assistant Professor of Neurology and Neurosurgery
Department of Small Animal Medicine and Surgery
College of Veterinary Medicine
University of Georgia
Athens, Georgia
USA

LAURA A. BARBUR, DVM
Diplomate ACVS (Small Animal)
Small Animal Surgeon
Department of Surgery
Friendship Hospital for Animals
Washington, DC
USA

ADRIENNE M. BARCHARD COUTS, DVM
Resident ACVECC (SA)
Westford Veterinary Emergency and Referral Center
Westford, Massachusetts
USA

HEIDI L. BARNES HELLER, DVM
Diplomate ACVIM (Neurology)
Clinical Associate Professor, Neurology/ Neurosurgery
School of Veterinary Medicine
University of Wisconsin-Madison
Madison, Wisconsin
USA

MARGARET C. BARR, DVM, PhD
Associate Dean for Academic Affairs
Professor of Virology and Immunology
College of Veterinary Medicine
Western University of Health Sciences
Pomona, California
USA

CARLA BARSTOW, DVM, MS
Diplomate ACT (Theriogenology)
Highland Pet Hospital
Lakeland, Florida
USA

JOSEPH W. BARTGES, DVM, PhD
Diplomate ACVIM (Small Animal Internal Medicine)
Diplomate ACVN
Professor of Medicine and Nutrition
Department of Small Animal Medicine and Surgery
College of Veterinary Medicine
The University of Georgia
Athens, Georgia
USA

KRISTEN BARTHOLOMEW, DVM
Emergency Clinician
Veterinary Referral Center
Malvern, Pennsylvania
USA

FIONA L. BATEMAN, BVSc
Diplomate ACVD
Assistant Professor of Dermatology
Department of Small Animal Medicine and Surgery
College of Veterinary Medicine
University of Georgia
Athens, Georgia
USA

REBECCA M. BATES, DVM
Cardiology Resident
Department of Small Animal Medicine and Surgery
College of Veterinary Medicine
University of Georgia
Athens, Georgia
USA

ADRIENNE C. BAUTISTA, DVM, PhD
Diplomate ABVT
Scientific Services Veterinarian
Royal Canin
Davis, California
USA

ASHLEY E. BAVA, BVetMed (Hons)
Emergency Clinician
Garden State Veterinary Specialists
Tinton Falls, New Jersey
USA

SARAH S.K. BEATTY, DVM
Diplomate ACVP (Clincial Pathology)
Clinical Assistant Professor
Department of Comparative, Diagnostic, and
Population Medicine
College of Veterinary Medicine
University of Florida
Gainesville, Florida
USA

JAN BELLOWS, DVM
Diplomate AVDC
Diplomate ABVP
All Pets Dental
Weston, Florida
USA

ELSA BELTRAN, Ldo Vet, PGDipVetEd, MRCVS
Diplomate ECVN
Associate Professor in Veterinary Neurology & Neurosurgery
Department of Clinical Science & Services
The Royal Veterinary College
University of London
North Mymms
Hatfield, Herts
United Kingdom

MARIAN E. BENITEZ, DVM, MS
Diplomate ACVS-SA
Surgeon/Owner
Dogwood Veterinary Surgical Care, PLLC
Huntersville, North Carolina
USA

KIA BENSON, DVM
Associate Veterinarian, Clinical Toxicology
SafetyCall International & Pet Poison Helpline
Bloomington, Minnesota
USA

ELLISON BENTLEY, DVM
Diplomate ACVO
Clinical Professor, Comparative Ophthalmology
Department of Surgical Sciences
School of Veterinary Medicine
University of Wisconsin-Madison
Madison, Wisconsin
USA

ALLYSON BERENT, DVM, DACVIM
Director, Interventional Endoscopy Services
Staff Internal Medicine Specialist
Animal Medical Center
New York, NY
USA

JEANNINE BERGER, DVM, CAWA
Diplomate ACVB (Behavior)
Diplomate ACAW (Welfare)
Senior VP of Rescue and Welfare
The Society for Prevention of Cruelty to Animals (SPCA)
San Francisco, California
USA

MATTHEW R. BERRY, DVM
Medical Oncology Resident
Department of Veterinary Clinical Medicine;
PhD Candidate
Department of Pathobiology
University of Illinois at Urbana-Champaign
Urbana, Illinois
USA

CHRISTINE F. BERTHELIN-BAKER, DVM
Diplomate ACVIM (Neurology)
Diplomate ECVN
Neurologist
Atlanta, Georgia
USA

JEAN M. BETKOWSKI, VMD
Diplomate ACVIM (Cardiology)
Staff Cardiologist
Cape Cod Veterinary Specialists
S. Dennis, Massachusetts
USA

ADAM J. BIRKENHEUER, DVM, PhD
Diplomate ACVIM
Professor of Internal Medicine
Department of Clinical Medicine
North Carolina State University
Raleigh, North Carolina
USA

KARYN BISCHOFF, DVM, MS
Diplomate ABVT
Diagnostic Toxicologist
New York State Animal Health Diagnostic Laboratory
Department of Population Medicine and Diagnostic Sciences
College of Veterinary Medicine
Cornell University
Ithaca, New York
USA

MARIE-CLAUDE BLAIS, DVM
Diplomate ACVIM (Small Animal Internal Medicine)
Associate Professor
Department of Clinical Sciences
Faculty of Veterinary Medicine
Université de Montréal
St-Hyacinthe, Quebec
Canada

APRIL E. BLONG, DVM
Diplomate ACVECC
Assistant Professor
Department of Veterinary Clinical Sciences
College of Veterinary Medicine
Iowa State University
Ames, Iowa
USA

JOHN D. BONAGURA, DVM, MS
Diplomate ACVIM (Cardiology, Internal Medicine)
Department of Clinical Sciences
College of Veterinary Medicine
North Carolina State University
Raleigh, North Carolina;
Professor Emeritus of Veterinary Clinical Sciences
The Ohio State University
Columbus, Ohio
USA

LINDSAY BOOZER, DVM
Diplomate ACVIM (Neurology)
Staff Neurologist
Friendship Hospital for Animals
Washington, DC
USA

DWIGHT D. BOWMAN, MS, PhD
Diplomate ACVM (Parasitology, Honorary)
Professor
Department of Microbiology and Immunology
College of Veterinary Medicine
Cornell University
Ithaca, New York
USA

SØREN BOYSEN, DVM
Diplomate ACVECC
Professor
Veterinary Emergency and Critical Care
Department of Veterinary Clinical and Diagnostic Sciences
Faculty of Veterinary Medicine
University of Calgary
Calgary, Alberta
Canada

BENJAMIN M. BRAINARD, VMD
Diplomate ACVAA and ACVECC
Edward H. Gunst Professor of Small Animal Critical Care
Department of Small Animal Medicine and Surgery
College of Veterinary Medicine
University of Georgia
Athens, Georgia
USA

RANDI BRANNAN, DVM, FAVD
Diplomate AVDC (Dentistry)
Animal Dental Clinic
Portland, Oregon
USA

MATT BREWER, DVM, PhD
Diplomate ACVM (Parasitology)
Associate Professor
Department of Veterinary Pathology
College of Veterinary Medicine
Iowa State University
Ames, Iowa
USA

ALYSSA J. BROOKER, DVM
Resident, Clinical Pathology
Department of Pathology
College of Veterinary Medicine
University of Georgia
Athens, Georgia
USA

MARJORY B. BROOKS, DVM
Diplomate ACVIM (Small Animal)
Director
Comparative Coagulation Section, Animal Health Diagnostic Laboratory
Department of Population Medicine and Diagnostic Sciences
Cornell University
Ithaca, New York
USA

AHNA G. BRUTLAG, DVM, MS
Diplomate ABT
Diplomate ABVT
Director, Veterinary Services & Senior Veterinary Toxicologist
Pet Poison Helpline & SafetyCall International
Bloomington, Minnesota;
Adjunct Assistant Professor
Department of Veterinary and Biomedical Sciences
College of Veterinary Medicine
University of Minnesota
St. Paul, Minnesota
USA

JÖRG BUCHELER, DVM, PhD, FTA
Diplomate ACVIM (IM)
Diplomate ECVIM-CA
Veterinary Specialty Hospital of Palm Beach Gardens
Palm Beach Gardens, Florida
USA

ANDREW C. BUGBEE, DVM
Diplomate ACVIM (Small Animal Internal Medicine)
Associate Clinical Professor of IM
Department of Small Animal Medicine & Surgery
College of Veterinary Medicine
University of Georgia
Athens, Georgia
USA

ANNE E. BUGLIONE, DVM
Postdoctoral Associate
Department of Neurobiology and Behavior
Cornell University
Ithaca, New York
USA

KARAH BURNS DEMARLE, DVM
Staff Internist, Small Animal Internal Medicine
Northstar VETS
Robbinsville, New Jersey
USA

JENNA H. BURTON, DVM, MS
Diplomate ACVIM (Oncology)
Associate Professor Clinical Oncology
Department of Surgical and Radiological Sciences
School of Veterinary Medicine
University of California, Davis
Davis, California
USA

JULIE K. BYRON, DVM, MS
Diplomate ACVIM (Small Animal Medicine)
Professor—Clinical
Department of Veterinary Clinical Sciences
College of Veterinary Medicine
The Ohio State University
Columbus, Ohio
USA

LAURA CAGLE, DVM
Diplomate ACVECC
PhD Candidate – Integrative Pathobiology
School of Veterinary Medicine
University of California, Davis
Davis, California
USA

KAREN L. CAMPBELL, DVM, MS
Diplomate ACVIM (Small Animal Internal Medicine)
Diplomate ACVD
Professor Emerita
University of Illinois;
Clinical Professor
Department of Veterinary Sciences
College of Veterinary Medicine
University of Missouri
Veterinary Health Center-Wentzville
Wentzville, Missouri
USA

MELINDA S. CAMUS, DVM
Diplomate ACVP (Clinical Pathology)
Associate Professor
Department of Pathology
College of Veterinary Medicine
University of Georgia
Athens, Georgia
USA

RENEE T. CARTER, DVM
Diplomate ACVO
Associate Professor, Ophthalmology
Department of Veterinary Clinical Sciences
School of Veterinary Medicine
Louisiana State University
Baton Rouge, Louisiana
USA

AUDE M.H. CASTEL, DV, MSc
Diplomate ACVIM (Neurology)
Assistant Professor, Neurology and Neurosurgery
Department of Clinical Sciences
Faculty of Veterinary Medicine
University of Montreal
St-Hyacinthe, Quebec
Canada

MEGAN N. CAUDILL, DVM, MS
Diplomate ACVP (Clinical Pathology)
Department of Comparative, Diagnostic, and Population Medicine
College of Veterinary Medicine
University of Florida
Gainesville, Florida

JULIE T. CECERE, DVM, MS, DACT
Clinical Associate Professor, Theriogenology
Department of Small Animal Clinical Sciences
Virginia-Maryland College of Veterinary Medicine
Blacksburg, Virginia
USA

SHARON A. CENTER, DVM
Diplomate ACVIM (Small Animal Internal Medicine)
Professor
Department of Clinical Sciences
Cornell University
Cornell University Hospital for Animals
Ithaca, New York
USA

SERGE CHALHOUB, DVM
Diplomate ACVIM (Small Animal Internal Medicine)
Senior Instructor, Small Animal Internal Medicine
Department of Veterinary Clinical and Diagnostic Sciences
Faculty of Veterinary Medicine
University of Calgary
Calgary, Alberta
Canada

GEORGINA CHILD, BVSc
Diplomate ACVIM (Neurology)
Consultant
Small Animal Specialist Hospital
North Ryde;
Senior Lecturer
School of Veterinary Science
University of Sydney
Sydney, NSW
Australia

BRUCE W. CHRISTENSEN, DVM, MS
Diplomate ACT
Kokopelli Assisted Reproductive Services
Franklin Ranch Pet Hospital
Elk Grove, California
USA

E'LISE CHRISTENSEN BELL
Diplomate ACVB
Owner
Behavior Vets
New York and Colorado
USA

JOHN A. CHRISTIAN, DVM, PhD
Associate Professor of Clinical Pathology
Department of Comparative Pathobiology
College of Veterinary Medicine
Purdue University
West Lafayette, Indiana
USA

RUTHANNE CHUN, DVM
Diplomate ACVIM (Oncology)
Clinical Professor
Department of Medical Sciences
University of Wisconsin School of Veterinary Medicine
Madison, Wisconsin
USA

DAVID B. CHURCH, BVSc, PhD, MACVSc, FHEA, MRCVS
Professor of Small Animal Studies and Deputy Principal
The Royal Veterinary College
Hatfield, Herts
United Kingdom

JOHN J. CIRIBASSI, DVM
Diplomate ACVB
Chicagoland Veterinary Behavior Consultants
Schererville, Indiana
USA

CÉCILE CLERCX, DVM, PhD
Diplomate ECVIM-CA
Professor
Department of Companion Animal Clinical Sciences
Faculty of Veterinary Medicine
University of Liège
Belgium

ANDREANNE CLEROUX
Diplomate ACVIM (Small Animal Internal Medicine)
Lecturer in Internal Medicine & Interventional Radiology
Department of Clinical Sciences & Advanced Medicine
School of Veterinary Medicine
University of Pennsylvania
Philadelphia, Pennsylvania
USA

CRAIG A. CLIFFORD, DVM, MS
Diplomate ACVIM (Oncology)
Medical Oncologist
Director of Clinical Trials
Hope Veterinary Specialists
Malvern, Pennsylvania
USA

JOAN R. COATES, BS, DVM, MS
Diplomate ACVIM (Neurology)
Professor of Veterinary Neurology & Neurosurgery
Department of Veterinary Medicine and Surgery
College of Veterinary Medicine
University of Missouri
Columbia, Missouri
USA

SUSAN M. COCHRANE, BSc, MSc, DVM, DVSc
Diplomate ACVIM (Neurology)
Veterinary Emergency Clinic and Referral Centre
Toronto, Ontario
Canada

STEVEN M. COGAR, DVM
Diplomate ACVS-SA
Carolina Veterinary Specialists
Winston-Salem, North Carolina
USA

WILLIAM M. COLE, DVM
Small Animal Internal Medicine
Metropolitan Animal Specialty Hospital
Los Angeles, California
USA

AMANDA E. COLEMAN, DVM, DACVIM (Cardiology)
Associate Professor of Cardiology
Department of Small Animal Medicine and Surgery
University of Georgia College of Veterinary Medicine
Athens, Georgia
USA

HEATHER E. CONNALLY, DVM, MS
Diplomate ACVECC
Veterinary Specialty Center on Tucson (retired)
Associate Veterinarian
Tucson, Arizona
USA

FRANCISCO O. CONRADO, DVM, MSc
Diplomate ACVP (Clinical Pathology)
Assistant Professor
Department of Biomedical Sciences
Cummings School of Veterinary Medicine
Tufts University
North Grafton, Massachusetts
USA

AUDREY K. COOK, BVM&S, MSc VetEd, MRCVS
Diplomate ACVIM (Small Animal Internal Medicine)
Diplomate ECVIM-CA
Diplomate ABVP (Feline Practice)
Professor, Small Animal Internal Medicine
Department of Small Animal Clinical Sciences
College of Veterinary Medicine and Biomedical Sciences
Texas A&M University
College Station, Texas
USA

LESLIE LARSON COOPER, DVM
Diplomate ACVB
Animal Behavior Counseling and Therapy
Davis, California
USA

EDWARD S. COOPER, VMD, MS
Diplomate ACVECC
Professor—Clinical
Department of Veterinary Clinical Sciences
College of Veterinary Medicine
Ohio State University
Columbus, Ohio
USA

RHIAN COPE, BVSc, BSc(Hon1), PhD, FACTRA
Diplomate ABT
Diplomate ABVT
Principal Toxicologist
Australian Pesticides and Veterinary Medicines Authority
Symonston
Australia

JOHN M. CRANDELL, DVM
Diplomate ACVIM (Small Animal Internal Medicine)
Veterinary Internist
MedVet Akron
Akron, Ohio
USA

SIGNE E. CREMER, DVM, PhD
Associate Professor, Clinical Pathology
Department of Veterinary Clinical Sciences
Faculty of Health and Medical Sciences
University of Copenhagen
Frederiksberg
Denmark

SUZANNE M. CUNNINGHAM, DVM
Diplomate ACVIM (Cardiology)
Associate Professor
Department of Clinical Sciences
Cummings School of Veterinary Medicine
Tufts University
North Grafton, Massachusetts
USA

ELIZABETH A. CURRY-GALVIN, DVM
Barrington Hills, Illinois
USA

TERRY MARIE CURTIS, DVM, MS
Diplomate ACVB
Veterinary Behaviorist
St. Augustine, Florida
USA

SARAH L. CZERWINSKI, BSc, DVM
Diplomate ACVO
Clinical Assistant Professor
Department of Small Animal Medicine and Surgery
College of Veterinary Medicine
University of Georgia
Athens, Georgia
USA

RONALDO CASIMIRO DA COSTA, DMV, MSc, PhD
Diplomate ACVIM (Neurology)
Professor and Service Head, Neurology and Neurosurgery
Department of Veterinary Clinical Sciences
College of Veterinary Medicine
The Ohio State University
Columbus, Ohio
USA

AUTUMN P. DAVIDSON, DVM, MS
Diplomate ACVIM (Small Animal Internal Medicine)
Clinical Professor
VMTH
School of Veterinary Medicine
University of California
Davis, California
USA

THOMAS K. DAY, DVM, MS
Diplomate ACVAA
Diplomate ACVECC
Emergency and Critical Care Specialist
Anesthesiology and Pain Management Specialist
VCA Veterinary Emergency Service and Specialty Center
Middleton, Wisconsin
USA

ALEXANDER DE LAHUNTA, DVM, PhD
Retired Professor of Veterinary Anatomy at Cornell University
Ithaca, New York
USA

HELIO S. AUTRAN DE MORAIS, DVM, PhD
Diplomate ACVIM (Internal Medicine and Cardiology)
Director
Lois Bates Acheson Veterinary Teaching Hospital
College of Veterinary Medicine
Oregon State University
Corvallis, Oregon
USA

JONATHAN D. DEAR, DVM, MAS
Diplomate ACVIM (Small Animal Internal Medicine)
Assistant Professor of Clinical Internal Medicine
Department of Medicine and Epidemiology
School of Veterinary Medicine
University of California, Davis
Davis, California
USA

TERESA C. DEFRANCESCO, DVM
Diplomate ACVIM (Cardiology), ACVECC
Department of Clinical Sciences
College of Veterinary Medicine
North Carolina State University
Raleigh, North Carolina
USA

VICTORIA A. DEMELLO, DVM
Nashville Veterinary Specialists
Nashville, Tennessee
USA

SAGI DENENBERG, DVM, MRCVS
Veterinary Psychiatrist
Diplomate ACVB
Diplomate ECAWBM
RCVS Recognized Specialist in Veterinary Behavioural Medicine
North Toronto Veterinary Behaviour Specialty Clinic
Thornhill, Ontario
Canada

THERESA L. DEPORTER, BSc, DVM, MRCVS
Diplomate DECAWBM
Diplomate ACVB (Behavior)
Veterinary Behaviorist
Behavioral Medicine Department
Oakland Veterinary Referral Services
Bloomfield Hills, Michigan
USA

NICK DERVISIS, DVM, PhD
DACVIM (Oncology)
Medical Oncology
Associate Professor
Department of Small Animal Clinical Sciences;
Associate Professor
Faculty of Health Sciences
VA-MD College of Veterinary Medicine
DSACS, Phase II
Blacksburg, Virginia
USA

IAN DESTEFANO, DVM
Resident, Emergency & Critical Care
Foster Hospital for Small Animals
Tufts University
North Grafton, Massachusetts
USA

SHARON M. DIAL, DVM, PhD
Diplomate ACVP (Clinical and Anatomic Pathology)
Research Scientist
College of Veterinary Medicine
University of Arizona
Tucson, Arizona
USA

STEPHEN P. DIBARTOLA, DVM
Diplomate ACVIM (Small Animal Internal Medicine)
Professor Emeritus of Internal Medicine
Department of Veterinary Clinical Sciences
College of Veterinary Medicine
Ohio State University
Columbus, Ohio
USA

DAVID C. DORMAN, DVM, PhD
Diplomate ABVT
Diplomate ABT
Professor of Toxicology
Department of Molecular Biomedical Sciences
College of Veterinary Medicine
North Carolina State University
Raleigh, North Carolina
USA

ELIZABETH R. DRAKE, DVM
Diplomate ACVD
Associate Professor
Department of Small Animal Clinical Sciences
College of Veterinary Medicine
University of Tennessee
Knoxville, Tennessee
USA

EDWARD J. DUBOVI, PhD
Professor of Virology
Department of Population Medicine and Diagnostic Sciences
Animal Health Diagnostic Center
College of Veterinary Medicine
Cornell University
Ithaca, New York
USA

DAVID D. DUCLOS, DVM
Diplomate ACVD
Clinical Dermatologist—Animal Skin & Allergy Clinic
Lynnwood, Washington
USA

CEDRIC P. DUFAYET, DVM
Associate Veterinarian
Advanced Urinary Disease and Extracorporeal Therapies Service
University of California Veterinary Medicine Center
San Diego, California
USA

STÉPHANIE DUGAS, DVM, MSc
Diplomate ACVIM (Neurology)
Medical Neurologist
BluePearl Specialty & Emergency Hospital
Irvine, California
USA

ERIC K. DUNAYER, MS, VMD
Diplomate ABT
Diplomate ABVT
Senior Toxicologist
ASPCA Animal Poison Control Center
Urbana, Illinois
USA

CAROLINA DUQUE, DVM, MSc, DVSc
Diplomate ACVIM (Neurology)
Mississauga Oakville Emergency Hospital and Referral Group
Oakville, Ontario
Canada

DAVID DYCUS, DVM, MS, CCRP
Diplomate ACVS (Small Animal)
Chief of Orthopedics
Nexus Veterinary Bone & Joint Center
Medical Director
Nexus Veterinary Specialists
Baltimore, Maryland
USA

HEATHER D. EDGINTON, DVM
Diplomate ACVD
Animal Medical Center of Seattle
Shoreline, Washington
USA

MELISSA N.C. EISENSCHENK, DVM, MS
Diplomate ACVD
Owner, Veterinary Dermatologist
Pet Dermatology Clinic
Maple Grove, Minnesota
USA

MARC ELIE, DVM
Diplomate ACVIM (Internal Medicine)
Staff Internist
Small Animal Internal Medicine
BluePearl Veterinary Partners
Southfield, Michigan
USA

ROBYN ELLERBROCK, DVM, PhD
Diplomate ACT
Assistant Professor
Department of Large Animal Medicine
College of Veterinary Medicine
University of Georgia
Athens, Georgia
USA

NAHVID M. ETEDALI, DVM
Diplomate ACVIM (Small Animal Internal Medicine)
Staff Internist
Head of Hemodialysis and Extracorporeal Therapies
Animal Medical Center
New York, New York
USA

TIMOTHY M. FAN, DVM, PhD
Diplomate ACVIM (Small Animal Internal Medicine, Oncology)
Professor
Department of Veterinary Clinical Medicine
College of Veterinary Medicine
University of Illinois at Urbana-Champaign
Urbana, Illinois
USA

JUSTIN FARRIS, DVM
Clinical Pathology Resident
Department of Pathology
College of Veterinary Medicine
University of Georgia
Athens, Georgia
USA

RICHARD A. FAYRER-HOSKEN, BVSc, PhD
Diplomate ACT (Theriogenology)
Diplomate ECAR
Research Scientist
Institute for Conservation Research
San Diego Zoo Global
Escondido, California
USA

LEAH FERGUSON, DVM, MS
Diplomate ACVIM (Internal Medicine)
Veterinary Internist
VCA Great Lakes Veterinary Specialists
Warrensville Heights, Ohio
USA

LLUÍS FERRER, BVSc, PhD
Diplomate ECVD
Professor
Department of Animal Medicine and Surgery
Veterinary School
Universitat Autònoma de Barcelona,
Bellaterra, Barcelona
Spain

MARIA SOLEDAD FERRER, DVM, MS
Diplomate DACT (Theriogenology)
Associate Professor
Department of Large Animal Medicine
College of Veterinary Medicine
University of Georgia
Athens, Georgia
USA

TESSA FIAMENGO, DVM, MS
Diplomate ACT
Slade Veterinary Hospital
Framingham, Massachusetts
USA

ANDREA M. FINNEN, DVM, DES, MSc
Diplomate ACVIM (Neurology)
Mississauga Oakville Veterinary Emergency Hospital
Neurology Service
Oakville, Ontario
Canada

ANDREA FISCHER, DVM, Dr.med.vet., Dr. habil.
Diplomate ACVIM (Neurology)
Diplomate ECVN
Professor
Centre for Clinical Veterinary Medicine
LMU University of Munich
Munich
Germany

GERRARD FLANNIGAN, DVM, MSc
Diplomate ACVB
Kernersville, North Carolina
USA

LINDA M. FLEEMAN, BVSc, PhD, MANZCVS
Animal Diabetes Australia
Melbourne, Victoria
Australia

CHARLOTTE FLINT, DVM, DABT
Senior Consulting Veterinarian, Clinical Toxicology
Pet Poison Helpline & SafetyCall International
Bloomington, Minnesota
USA

J.D. FOSTER, VMD
Diplomate ACVIM (Small Animal Internal Medicine)
Nephrology/Urology & Internal Medicine
Friendship Hospital for Animals
Washington, DC
USA

DANIEL S. FOY, MS, DVM
Diplomate ACVIM (Small Animal Internal Medicine)
Diplomate ACVECC
Clinical Assistant Professor
College of Veterinary Medicine
Midwestern University
Glendale, Arizona
USA

LINDA A. FRANK, MS, DVM
Diplomate ACVD
Professor
Department of Small Animal Clinical Sciences
College of Veterinary Medicine
University of Tennessee
Knoxville, Tennessee
USA

JONI L. FRESHMAN, DVM MS CVA
Diplomate ACVIM (Internal Medicine)
Owner
Canine Consultations
Peyton, Colorado
USA

CANNY FUNG, DVM
Surgery Intern
Southwest Veterinary Surgical Service
Phoenix Arizona
USA

EVA FURROW, VMD, PhD
Diplomate ACVIM (Small Animal Internal Medicine)
Associate Professor
Department of Veterinary Clinical Sciences
College of Veterinary Medicine
University of Minnesota
St. Paul, Minnesota
USA

LUIS GAITERO, DVM
Diplomate ECVN
Associate Professor and Head Neurology and Neurosurgery Service
HSC Chief Medical Officer
Department of Clinical Studies
Ontario Veterinary College
University of Guelph
Guelph, Ontario
Canada

JOAO FELIPE DE BRITO GALVAO, MV, MS
Diplomate ACVIM (Small Animal Internal Medicine)
Internal Medicine Specialist
VCA Arboretum View Animal Hospital
Downers Grove, Illinois;
Adjunct Assistant Professor
The Ohio State University
Columbus, Ohio
USA

BRIDGET C. GARNER, DVM, PhD
Diplomate ACVP (Clinical Pathology)
Associate Professor
Department of Pathology
College of Veterinary Medicine
University of Georgia
Athens, Georgia
USA

LAURENT GAROSI, DVM, FRCVS
Diplomate ECVN
RCVS and EBVS®
European Specialist in Veterinary Neurology
Clinical Director Vet Oracle Teleneurology
Bedford
United Kingdom

LAURA D. GARRETT, DVM
Diplomate ACVIM (Oncology)
Clinical Professor
Department of Veterinary Clinical Medicine
College of Veterinary Medicine
University of Illinois
Urbana, Illinois
USA

CATHY J. GARTLEY, DVM, DVSc
Diplomate ACT
Assistant Professor
Department of Population Medicine
Ontario Veterinary College
University of Guelph
Guelph, Ontario
Canada

ANNA R.M. GELZER, Dr.med.vet., PhD
Diplomate ACVIM
Diplomate ECVIM-CA-Cardiology
Professor of Cardiology
Department of Clinical Sciences & Advanced Medicine
School of Veterinary Medicine
University of Pennsylvania
Philadelphia, Pennsylvania
USA

ANNE J. GEMENSKY METZLER, DVM, MS
Diplomate ACVO
Professor—Clinical
Department of Veterinary Clinical Sciences
College of Veterinary Medicine
The Ohio State University
Columbus, Ohio
USA

KATHERINE GERKEN, DVM, MS
Diplomate ACVECC
Assistant Clinical Professor
Small Animal Emergency and Critical Care
Department of Clinical Sciences
Bailey Small Animal Teaching Hospital
College of Veterinary Medicine
Auburn University
Auburn, Alabama
USA

VIRGINIA L. GILL, DVM
Diplomate DACVIM (Oncology)
Medical Director
Maine Veterinary Medical Center
Scarborough, Maine
USA

MARGI A. GILMOUR, DVM
Diplomate ACVO
Professor
Department of Veterinary Clinical Sciences
College of Veterinary Medicine
Oklahoma State University
Stillwater, Oklahoma
USA

ERIC N. GLASS, MS, DVM
Diplomate ACVIM (Neurology)
Section Head, Neurology and Neurosurgery
Red Bank Veterinary Hospital
Tinton Falls, New Jersey;
Chief of Neurology and Neurosurgery
Compassion First Pet Hospital
Tinton Falls, New Jersey
USA

MATHIEU M. GLASSMAN, VMD
Diplomate ACVS
Chief of Surgery
Friendship Surgical Specialists
Friendship Hospital for Animals
Washington, DC
USA

RITA GONÇALVES, DVM, MVM, FHEA, MRCVS
Diplomate ECVN
European and RCVS Recognized Specialist in Veterinary Neurology
Senior Lecturer in Veterinary Neurology
Small Animal Clinical Science
University of Liverpool
Neston, Cheshire
United Kingdom

SARA E. GONZALEZ, DVM, MS
Clinical Assistant Professor of Community Practice
Department of Small Animal Medicine and Surgery
University of Georgia College of Veterinary Medicine
Athens, Georgia
USA

JENNIFER GOOD, DVM
Diplomate ACVECC (Emergency and Critical Care)
Assistant Clinical Professor
Department of Emergency and Critical Care
College of Veterinary Medicine
University of Georgia
Athens, Georgia
USA

SHARON FOOSHEE GRACE, M Agric, MS, DVM
Diplomate ACVIM (Small Animal)
Diplomate ABVP (Canine/Feline)
Clinical Professor
Department of Clinical Sciences
College of Veterinary Medicine
Mississippi State University
Mississippi State, Mississippi
USA

W. DUNBAR GRAM, DVM, MRCVS
Diplomate ACVD
Clinical Associate Professor and Dermatology Service Chief
Small Animal Clinical Sciences, University of Florida
Gainesville, Florida
USA

JENNIFER L. GRANICK, DVM, PhD
Diplomate ACVIM (Small Animal Internal Medicine)
Associate Professor
Department of Veterinary Clinical Sciences
College of Veterinary Medicine
University of Minnesota
St. Paul, Minnesota
USA

GREGORY F. GRAUER, DVM, MS
Diplomate ACVIM (Small Animal Internal Medicine)
Professor Emeritus
Department of Clinical Sciences
College of Veterinary Medicine
Kansas State University
Manhattan, Kansas
USA

SARAH L. GRAY, DVM
Diplomate ACVECC (Emergency and Critical Care)
Horizon Veterinary Specialist
Ventura, California
USA

KURT A. GRIMM, DVM, MS, PhD
Diplomate ACVCP
Diplomate ACVAA
Owner
Veterinary Specialist Services, PC
Conifer, Colorado
USA

AMY M. GROOTERS, DVM
Diplomate ACVIM (Small Animal Internal Medicine)
Professor, Companion Animal Medicine
Veterinary Clinical Sciences
Louisiana State University
Baton Rouge, Louisiana
USA

MARGARET E. GRUEN, DVM, PhD
Diplomate ACVB
Assistant Professor, Behavioral Medicine
Department of Clinical Sciences
College of Veterinary Medicine
North Carolina State University
Raleigh, North Carolina
USA

SOPHIE A. GRUNDY, BVSc (Hons), MANZCVS (Small Animal Internal Medicine)
Diplomate ACVIM (Small Animal Internal Medicine)
Internal Medicine Consultant
IDEXX Laboratories, Inc.
Westbrook, Maine
USA

REBEKAH G. GUNN-CHRISTIE, DVM
Diplomate ACVP (Clinical Pathology)
Veterinary Clinical Pathologist
Antech Diagnostics
Cary, North Carolina
USA

TALIA GUTTIN, VMD
Diplomate ACVIM (Small Animal Internal Medicine)
Assistant Professor
Small Animal Medicine and Surgery Department
School of Veterinary Medicine
St. George's University
True Blue Campus
St. George, Grenada
West Indies

SHARON GWALTNEY-BRANT, DVM, PhD
Diplomate ABVT
Diplomate ABT
Consultant
Veterinary Information Network
Mahomet, Illinois
USA

TIMOTHY B. HACKETT, DVM, MS
Diplomate ACVECC
Professor
Department of Clinical Sciences
College of Veterinary Medicine and Biomedical Sciences
Colorado State University
Fort Collins, Colorado
USA

DEBORAH J. HADLOCK, VMD
Diplomate ABVP (Canine and Feline)
Certified Veterinary Acupuncturist—CVA (IVAS)
Certified Veterinary Spinal Manipulative Therapist—CVSMT (HOWC)
Owner
Hadlock Integrative Veterinary Consulting
Salt Lake City, Utah
USA

JENS HÄGGSTRÖM, DVM, PhD
Diplomate ECVIM-CA (Cardiology)
Professor
Department of Clinical Sciences
Faculty of Veterinary Medicine and Animal Science
Swedish University of Agricultural Sciences
Uppsala
Sweden

FRASER A. HALE, DVM, FAVD
Diplomate AVC
Hale Veterinary Clinic
Guelph, Ontario
Canada

EDWARD J. HALL, MA, VetMB, PhD, FRCVS
Diplomate ECVIM-CA
Emeritus Professor of Small Animal Internal Medicine
Langford Vets
Bristol Veterinary School
University of Bristol
Langford
United Kingdom

STEVEN R. HANSEN, DVM, MS, MBA
Diplomate ACAW
Diplomate ABVT
President and CEO
Arizona Humane Society
Phoenix, Arizona
USA

TISHA A.M. HARPER, DVM, MS, CCRP
Diplomate ACVS-SA
Diplomate ACVSMR
Clinical Associate Professor
Department of Veterinary Clinical Medicine
University of Illinois College of Veterinary Medicine
Urbana, Illinois
USA

JOHN W. HARVEY, DVM, PhD
Diplomate ACVP (Clinical Pathology)
Professor Emeritus
Department of Physiological Sciences
College of Veterinary Medicine
University of Florida
Gainesville, Florida
USA

LORE I. HAUG, DVM, MS
Diplomate ACVB
Texas Veterinary Behavior Services
Sugar Land, Texas
USA

ELEANOR C. HAWKINS, DVM
Diplomate ACVIM (Small Animal Internal Medicine)
Professor
Department of Clinical Sciences
College of Veterinary Medicine
North Carolina State University
Raleigh, North Carolina
USA

CRISTINE L. HAYES, DVM
Diplomate ABVT
Diplomate ABT
Medical Director
ASPCA Animal Poison Control Center
Urbana, Illinois
USA

IAN P. HERRING, DVM, MS
Diplomate ACVO (Ophthalmology)
Associate Professor
VA-MD Regional College of Veterinary Medicine
Virginia Tech
Blacksburg, Virginia
USA

MEGHAN E. HERRON, DVM
Diplomate ACVB
Senior Director Behavioral Medicine, Education, and Outreach
Gigi's (Shelter for Dogs)
Canal Winchester, Ohio
USA

MILAN HESS, DVM, MS
Diplomate ACT (Theriogenology)
Colorado Veterinary Specialty Group
Littleton, Colorado
USA

STEVE HILL, DVM, MS
Diplomate ACVIM (Small Animal Internal Medicine)
Small Animal Internal Medicine Consultant
Flagstaff Veterinary Internal Medicine Consulting
Flagstaff, Arizona
USA

TRACY HILL, DVM PhD
Diplomate ACVIM (Small Animal Internal Medicine)
Assistant Professor
Department of Small Animal Medicine and Sur gery
College of Veterinary Medicine
University of Georgia
Athens, Georgia
USA

LORA S. HITCHCOCK, DVM
Diplomate ACVIM (Cardiology)
Clinical Cardiologist
Ohio Veterinary Cardiology, Ltd
Metropolitan Veterinary Hospital
Akron, Ohio
USA

KATE HOLAN, BS, DVM
Diplomate ACVIM (Small Animal Internal Medicine)
Assistant Professor and Head
Small Animal Internal Medicine
Department of Small Animal Clinical Sciences
Michigan State University
East Lansing, Michigan
USA

MASON HOLLAND, VMD
Diplomate ACVR
Staff Radiologist
Port City Veterinary Referral Hospital
Portsmouth, New Hampshire
USA

SUSAN HOLLAND, DVM
Associate Veterinarian, Clinical Toxicology
Pet Poison Helpline
Bloomington, Minnesota
USA

FIONA HOLLINSHEAD, BVSc (Hons), PhD, MANZCVS
Diplomate ACT (Theriogenology)
Registered Specialist in Small Animal Reproduction
Glenbred, Matamata Veterinary Services Ltd
Matamata
New Zealand

STEPHEN B. HOOSER, DVM, PhD
Diplomate ABVT
Professor of Veterinary Toxicology & Head Toxicology Section
Department of Comparative Pathobiology & ADDL
College of Veterinary Medicine
Purdue University
West Lafayette, Indiana
USA

KATE HOPPER, BVSc, PhD
Diplomate ACVECC
Associated Professor, Small Animal Emergency & Critical Care
Department of Veterinary Surgical & Radiological Sciences
School of Veterinary Medicine
University of California, Davis
Davis, California
USA

DEBRA F. HORWITZ, DVM
Diplomate ACVB
Veterinary Behavior Consultations
St. Louis, Missouri
USA

LYNN R. HOVDA, RPH, DVM, MS
Diplomate ACVIM (Large Animal Internal Medicine)
Director of Veterinary Medicine
SafetyCall International & Pet Poison Helpline
Bloomington, Minnesota;
Assistant Adjunct Professor
Department of Veterinary and Biomedical Sciences
College of Veterinary Medicine
University of Minnesota
St. Paul, Minnesota
USA

TYNE HOVDA, DVM
Anesthesia Intern
College of Veterinary Medicine
North Carolina State University
Raleigh, North Carolina
USA

JUNE C. HUANG, DVM, PhD
Diplomate ACVP (Clinical Pathology)
Veterinary Clinical Pathologist
ANTECH Diagnostics
Atlanta, Georgia
USA

WAYNE HUNTHAUSEN, DVM
Director
Animal Behavior Consultations
Westwood, Kansas
USA

CASSANDRA O. JANSON, DVM
Diplomate ACVECC
Staff Criticalist
Mount Laurel Animal Hospital
Mount Laurel, New Jersey
USA

NICK D. JEFFERY, BVSc, PhD, MSc, FRCVS
Diplomate ECVS
Diplomate ECVN
Professor, Neurology & Neurosurgery
Department of Small Animal Clinical Sciences
College of Veterinary Medicine
Texas A&M University
College Station, Texas
USA

ALBERT E. JERGENS, DVM, PhD, AGAF
Diplomate ACVIM (Small Animal Internal Medicine)
Professor, Associate Chair for Research and Graduate Studies and Donn E. and Beth M. Bacon Professor in Small Animal Medicine and Surgery
Department of Veterinary Clinical Sciences
College of Veterinary Medicine
Iowa State University
Ames, Iowa
USA

JEBA R.J. JESUDOSS CHELLADURAI, BVSc, MS, PhD
Diplomate ACVM (Parasitology)
Postdoctoral Associate
Department of Veterinary Pathology
College of Veterinary Medicine
Iowa State University
Ames, Iowa
USA

AIME K. JOHNSON, DVM
Diplomate American College of Theriogenology
Associate Professor
Department of Clinical Sciences
Auburn University College of Veterinary Medicine
Auburn, Alabama
USA

JESSICA JOHNSON, DVM
Senior Dental & Oral Surgery Resident
Elevate Your Small Animal Dental Team, LLC
Main Street Veterinary Hospital & Dental Clinic
Dallas, Texas
USA

LYNELLE R. JOHNSON, DVM, MS, PhD
Diplomate ACVIM (Small Animal Internal Medicine)
Professor
Department of Medicine and Epidemiology
University of California, Davis
Davis, California
USA

SPENCER A. JOHNSTON, VMD
Diplomate ACVS
James and Marjorie Waggoner Professor
Head
Department of Small Animal Medicine and Surgery
College of Veterinary Medicine
University of Georgia
Athens, Georgia
USA

RICHARD J. JOSEPH, DVM
Diplomate ACVIM (Neurology)
Founder, CEO
AnimalMR.com
VetsOnCall.org
Katonah, New York
USA

RONNIE KAUFMANN, BSc, DVM
Diplomate ECVD (Dermatology)
Head of Dermatology Service
The Veterinary Teaching Hospital
Koret School of Veterinary Medicine
The Hebrew University of Jerusalem
Israel

BRUCE W. KEENE, DVM, MSc
Diplomate ACVIM (Cardiology)
Jane Lewis Seaks Distinguished Professor of Companion Animal Medicine
Department of Clinical Sciences
College of Veterinary Medicine
North Carolina State University
Raleigh, North Carolina
USA

LISA S. KELLY, DVM, PhD
Diplomate ACVP (Clinical Pathology)
Veterinary Clinical Pathologist
Antech Diagnostics
Atlanta, Georgia
USA

DANIEL E. KEYLER, BS, PharmD, FAACT
Senior Clinical Toxicologist
SafetyCall International
Bloomington, Minnesota;
Adjunct Professor
Experimental & Clinical Pharmacology
University of Minnesota
Minneapolis, Minnesota
USA

YUNJEONG KIM, DVM, PhD
Diplomate ACVM (Immunology)
Associate Professor
Department of Diagnostic Medicine and Pathobiology
College of Veterinary Medicine
Kansas State University
Manhattan, Kansas
USA

SHAWNA L. KLAHN, DVM
Diplomate ACVIM (Oncology)
Associate Professor
Department of Small Animal Clinical Sciences
Virginia-Maryland College of Veterinary Medicine
Virginia Tech
Blacksburg, Virginia
USA

MARY P. KLINCK, DVM, PhD
Diplomate ACVB
Veterinary Behavioural Medicine Consultant
Sainte-Anne-de-Bellevue, Quebec
Canada

MARGUERITE F. KNIPE, DVM
Diplomate ACVIM (Neurology)
Health Sciences Associate Clinical Professor, Neurology/Neurosurgery
Department of Surgical and Radiological Sciences
UC Davis School of Veterinary Medicine
Davis, California
USA

JOYCE S. KNOLL, VMD, PhD
Diplomate ACVP (Clinical Pathology)
Associate Professor and Interim Chair
Department of Biomedical Sciences
Cummings School of Veterinary Medicine
Tufts University
North Grafton, Massachusetts
USA

AMIE KOENIG, DVM
Diplomate ACVIM (Small Animal Internal Medicine)
Diplomate ACVECC
Professor of Emergency and Critical Care
Department of Small Animal Medicine and Surgery
College of Veterinary Medicine
University of Georgia
Athens, Georgia
USA

CASEY J. KOHEN, DVM
Diplomate ACVECC
Emergency and Critical Care Specialist
MarQueen Veterinary Emergency and Specialty
Roseville, California
USA

BARBARA KOHN, Prof. Dr. med. vet
Diplomate ECVIM-CA
Clinic for Small Animals
Faculty of Veterinary Medicine
Freie Universität Berlin
Germany

MARC S. KRAUS, DVM
Professor of Clinical Cardiology
Diplomate ACVIM (Cardiology, Internal Medicine)
Diplomate ECVIM-CA (Cardiology)
University of Pennsylvania
Department of Clinical Sciences and Advanced Medicine
Philadelphia, Pennsylvania
USA

NATALI KREKELER, Dr. med. vet., PhD
Diplomate ACT
Senior Lecturer in Veterinary Reproduction
Melbourne Veterinary School
The University of Melbourne
Werribee, Victoria
Australia

ERIKA L. KRICK, VMD
Diplomate ACVIM (Oncology)
Medical Oncologist and Oncology Department Head
Mount Laurel Animal Hospital
Mount Laurel, New Jersey
USA

PAULA M. KRIMER, DVM, DVSc
Diplomate ACVP (Clinical Pathology)
Professor & Outreach Services Chief
Athens Veterinary Diagnostic Laboratory and Department of Pathology
College of Veterinary Medicine
University of Georgia
Athens, Georgia
USA

ANNEMARIE T. KRISTENSEN, DVM, PhD
Diplomate ACVIM (Small Animal)
Diplomate ECVIM-CA & Oncology
Professor, Companion Animal Clinical Oncology
Department of Veterinary Clinical Sciences
Faculty of Health and Medical Sciences
University of Copenhagen
Frederiksberg
Denmark

JOHN M. KRUGER, DVM, PhD
Diplomate ACVIM- SAIM
Professor and Carrigan Chair in Feline Health
Department of Small Animal Clinical Sciences
College of Veterinary Medicine
Michigan State University
East Lansing, Michigan
USA

STEPHANIE KUBE, DVM, CCRT, CVPP
Diplomate ACVIM (Neurology)
Veterinary Neurology and Pain Management Center of New England
Walpole, Massachusetts
USA

KAREN A. KUHL, DVM
Diplomate ACVD
Midwest Veterinary Dermatology Center
Veterinary Specialty Center
Buffalo Grove, Illinois
USA

LEIGH A. LAMONT, DVM, MS
Diplomate ACVAA
Associate Dean of Academic and Student Affairs
Atlantic Veterinary College
University of Prince Edward Island
Charlottetown, Prince Edward Island
Canada

GARY M. LANDSBERG, BSc, DVM
Diplomate ACVB, ECAWBM
Veterinary Behaviorist
Vice-President
CanCog Incorporated
Fergus, Ontario;
Head
Fear Free Research
Canada

SELENA LANE, DVM
Diplomate ACVECC
Clinical Assistant Professor of Small Animal Emergency and Critical Care
Small Animal Medicine and Surgery
University of Georgia College of Veterinary Medicine
Athens, Georgia
USA

CATHY E. LANGSTON, DVM
Diplomate ACVIM (Small Animal Internal Medicine)
Professor - Clinical
Veterinary Medical Center
College of Veterinary Medicine
The Ohio State University
Columbus, Ohio
USA

PATTY A. LATHAN, VMD, MS
Diplomate ACVIM (Small Animal Internal Medicine)
Associate Professor
Department of Clinical Sciences
Mississippi State University
Mississippi State, Mississippi
USA

KENNETH S. LATIMER, DVM, PhD
Diplomate ACVP (Clinical Pathology)
Lanexa Veterinary & Consulting Services, LLC
Toano, Virginia
USA

ROBIN LAZARO, RVT, VTS(ECC)
ICU Supervisor
North Carolina State Veterinary Hospital
College of Veterinary Medicine
Raleigh, North Carolina
USA

AMY LEARN, VMD
Resident in Clinical Behavior Medicine
Animal Behavior Wellness Center
Richmond, Virginia
USA

MYLÈNE-KIM LECLERC, DMV
Diplomate ACVIM (Neurology)
Head of the Neurology Service
Centre Veterinaire Rive Sud
Brossard, Quebec
Canada

RICHARD A. LECOUTEUR, BVSc, PhD
Diplomate ACVIM (Neurology)
Diplomate ECVN
Professor Emeritus
Department of Surgical & Radiological Sciences
School of Veterinary Medicine
University of California, Davis
Davis, California
USA

MICHAEL S. LEIB, DVM, MS
Diplomate ACVIM (Small Animal Internal Medicine)
Emeritus Professor of Internal Medicine
Department of Small Animal Clinical Sciences
Virginia-Maryland College of Veterinary Medicine
Virginia Tech
Blacksburg, Virginia
USA

MATTHEW S. LEMMONS, DVM
Diplomate AVDC
Dentistry and Oral Surgery
MedVet
Carmel, Indiana
USA

JOSE A. LEN, DVM, MS, PhD
Diplomate ACT
Assistant Professor, Theriogenology
College of Veterinary Medicine
North Carolina State University
Raleigh, North Carolina
USA

SOPHIE LE PODER, DVM, MS, PhD
Professor in Virology
Unity of Bacteriology, Immunology and Virology
Ecole Nationale Vétérinaire d'Alfort
Maisons-Alfort
France

JOHN R. LEWIS, VMD, FAVD
Diplomate AVDC
Veterinary Dentistry Specialists
Silo Academy Education Center
Chadds Ford, Pennsylvania
USA

ELLEN M. LINDELL, VMD
Diplomate ACVB
Veterinary Behaviorist
Central Hospital for Veterinary Medicine
North Haven, Connecticut
USA

MERYL P. LITTMAN, VMD
Diplomate ACVIM (Small Animal Internal Medicine)
Professor Emerita of Medicine
Department of Clinical Sciences & Advanced Medicine
School of Veterinary Medicine
University of Pennsylvania
Philadelphia, Pennsylvania
USA

INGRID LJUNGVALL, DVM, PhD
Diplomate ECVIM-CA (Cardiology)
Associate Professor
Department of Clinical Sciences
Faculty of Veterinary Medicine
Swedish University of Agricultural Sciences
Uppsala
Sweden

HEIDI B. LOBPRISE, DVM
Diplomate AVDC (Dentistry)
Main Street Veterinary Dental Clinic
Flower Mound, Texas
USA

JOHN P. LOFTUS, PhD, DVM
Diplomate ACVIM (Small Animal Internal Medicine)
Assistant Professor
Department of Clinical Sciences
College of Veterinary Medicine
Cornell University
Ithaca, New York
USA

DAWN E. LOGAS, DVM
Diplomate ACVD
Owner/Staff Dermatologist
Veterinary Dermatology Center
Maitland, Florida
USA

JAYME S. LOOPER, DVM
Diplomate ACVR (Radiation Oncology)
Associate Professor
Department of Veterinary Clinical Sciences
School of Veterinary Medicine
Louisiana State University
Baton Rouge, Louisiana
USA

CHERYL LOPATE, MS, DVM
Diplomate ACT
Veterinarian and Owner
Reproductive Revolutions and Wilsonville Veterinary Clinic
Wilsonville, Oregon
USA

BIANCA N. LOURENÇO, DVM, MSc, PhD
Diplomate ACVIM (Small Animal Internal Medicine)
Assistant Professor
Department of Small Animal and Surgery
College of Veterinary Medicine
University of Georgia
Athens, Georgia
USA

VIRGINIA LUIS FUENTES, MA, VetMB, PhD, CertVR, DVC, MRCVS
Diplomate ACVIM (Cardiology)
Diplomate ECVIM-CA (Cardiology)
Professor
Department of Veterinary Clinical Science and Services
Royal Veterinary College
North Mymms
United Kingdom

JODY P. LULICH, DVM, PhD
Diplomate ACVIM (Internal Medicine)
Professor
Department of Veterinary Clinical Sciences
Director of the Minnesota Urolith Center
College of Veterinary Medicine
University of Minnesota
St. Paul, Minnesota
USA

ALYCEN P. LUNDBERG, DVM
Diplomate ACVIM (Oncology)
Assistant Professor
Department of Veterinary Clinical Medicine
College of Veterinary Medicine
University of Illinois at Urbana-Champaign
Urbana, Illinois
USA

CANDACE C. LYMAN, DVM
Diplomate DACT (Theriogenology)
Associate Professor
Department of Clinical Sciences
College of Veterinary Medicine
Auburn University
Auburn, Alabama
USA

KASEY E. MABRY, DVM
Resident, Small Animal Internal Medicine
Department of Small Animal Medicine and Surgery
College of Veterinary Medicine
University of Georgia
Athens, Georgia
USA

CATRIONA M. MACPHAIL, DVM, PhD
Diplomate ACVS
ACVS Founding Fellow, Surgical Oncology
Professor, Small Animal Surgery
Department of Clinical Sciences
Colorado State University
Fort Collins, Colorado
USA

ORLA MAHONY, MVB
Diplomate ACVIM (Internal Medicine)
Diplomate ECVIM
Clinical Assistant Professor
Department of Clinical Sciences
Cummings School of Veterinary Medicine at Tufts University
North Grafton, Massachusetts
USA

SEAN B. MAJOY, DVM, MS
Diplomate ACVECC
Clinical Assistant Professor
Department of Clinical Sciences
Cummings School of Veterinary Medicine at Tufts University
North Grafton, Massachusetts
USA

GUILLERMINA MANIGOT, DMV UBA
Diplomate CPMV (Dermatology)
Dermlink Buenos Aires
Buenos Aires
Argentina

KATIA MARIONI-HENRY, DMV, PhD, MRCVS
Diplomate ACVIM (Neurology) and ECVN
EBVS® European Veterinary Specialist in Small Animal Neurology
RCVS Specialist in Veterinary Neurology;
Senior Lecturer
Neurology/Neurosurgery Service
Hospital for Small Animals
Royal (Dick) School of Veterinary Studies
University of Edinburgh
Roslin, Midlothian
United Kingdom

STANLEY L. MARKS, BVSc, PhD
Diplomate ACVIM (Internal Medicine, Oncology)
Diplomate ACVN
Professor
Department of Medicine & Epidemiology
University of California, Davis
School of Veterinary Medicine
Davis, California
USA

STEVEN L. MARKS, BVSc, MS, MRCVS
Diplomate ACVIM (Small Animal Internal Medicine)
Associate Dean, Director of Veterinary Medical Services
College of Veterinary Medicine
NC State University
Raleigh, North Carolina
USA

SINA MARSILIO, Dr.med.vet., PhD
Diplomate ACVIM (Small Animal Internal Medicine)
Diplomate ECVIM-CA
Assistant Professor
University of California, Davis School of Veterinary Medicine
Department of Veterinary Medicine and Epidemiology
Davis, California
USA

DEBBIE MARTIN, LVT, VTS (Behavior)
Veterinary Technician Specialist (Behavior)
TEAM Education in Animal Behavior, LLC
Veterinary Behavior Consultations, LLC
Spicewood, Texas
USA

KATY A. MARTIN, DVM, MPH
USDA Resident in Veterinary Parasitology
Graduate Research Assistant
Department of Veterinary Pathology
College of Veterinary Medicine
Iowa State University
Ames, Iowa
USA

KENNETH M. MARTIN, DVM
Diplomate ACVB (Veterinary Behaviorists)
TEAM Education in Animal Behavior, LLC
Veterinary Behavior Consultations, LLC
Spicewood, Texas
USA

PAULA MARTÍN VAQUERO, DVM, PhD
Diplomate ACVIM (Neurology)
FCB Health Europe
FCB Health Madrid
Madrid
Spain

KENNETH V. MASON, BSc, MVSc, FACVSc
Veterinary Dermatologist
Managing Director
Dermcare-Vet Pty Ltd
Springwood, Queensland
Australia

PHILIPP D. MAYHEW, BVM&S, MRCVS
Diplomate ACVS
Professor, Small Animal Surgery
Department of Surgical and Radiological Sciences
University of California, Davis
Davis, California
USA

TERRI L. MCCALLA, DVM, MS
Diplomate ACVO
Animal HealthQuest Solutions LLC
Bellingham, Washington
USA

MEGAN MCCLOSKY, DVM
Clinical Assistant Professor
Small Animal Internal Medicine
Department of Clinical Sciences and Advanced Medicine
University of Pennsylvania School of Veterinary Medicine
Philadelphia, Pennsylvania
USA

PATRICK L. MCDONOUGH, MS, PhD
Atkinson Center for a Sustainable Future Faculty Fellow
Professor Emeritus of Veterinary Microbiology
Animal Health Diagnostic Center
Department of Population Medicine and Diagnostic Sciences
College of Veterinary Medicine
Cornell University
Ithaca, New York
USA

KATHRYN M. MCGONIGLE, MPH DVM
Diplomate ACVIM (Internal Medicine)
Assistant Professor
Clinical Small Animal Internal Medicine
Department of Clinical Sciences and Advanced Medicine
University of Pennsylvania School of Veterinary Medicine
Philadelphia, Pennsylvania
USA

ANNA K. MCMANAMEY, DVM
Cardiology Resident
North Carolina State University Veterinary Hospital
Raleigh, North Carolina
USA

STEPHEN MEHLER, DVM
Diplomate ACVS
Chief Medical Officer
Veterinarian Recommended Solutions
Blue Bell, Pennsylvania
USA

KRISTINA MEICHNER, DVM
Diplomate ECVIM-CA (Oncology)
Diplomate ACVP (Clinical Pathology)
Assistant Professor
Department of Pathology
College of Veterinary Medicine
University of Georgia
Athens, Georgia
USA

KATHRYN M. MEURS, DVM, PhD
Diplomate ACVIM (Cardiology)
Professor
Department of Clinical Sciences
North Carolina State University College of Veterinary Medicine
Raleigh, North Carolina
USA

LYNDA M.J. MILLER, DVM, PhD
Diplomate ACT
Director of Large Animal Clinical Skills
Associate Professor of Theriogenology
Lincoln Memorial University
College of Veterinary Medicine
Harrogate, Tennessee
USA

MATTHEW W. MILLER, DVM, MS
Diplomate ACVIM (Cardiology)
Staff Cardiologist and Cardiology Section Head
VetMed Emergency and Specialty Care
Phoenix, Arizona
USA

PAUL E. MILLER, DVM
Diplomate ACVO
Clinical Professor of Comparative Ophthalmology
Department of Surgical Sciences
School of Veterinary Medicine
University of Wisconsin-Madison
Madison, Wisconsin
USA

MELISSA L. MILLIGAN, VMD
Resident in Internal Medicine
The Animal Medical Center
New York, New York
USA

KELLY MOFFAT, DVM
Diplomate ACVB (Behavior)
Medical Director
VCA Mesa Animal Hospital
Mesa, Arizona
USA

SARAH A. MOORE, DVM
Diplomate ACVIM (Neurology)
Professor
Department of Veterinary Clinical Sciences
College of Veterinary Medicine
The Ohio State University
Columbus, Ohio
USA

ANDREW R. MOORHEAD, DVM, MS, PhD
Diplomate ACVM (Parasitology)
Assistant Professor
Department of Infectious Diseases
University of Georgia
College of Veterinary Medicine
Athens, Georgia
USA

DANIEL O. MORRIS, DVM, MPH
Diplomate ACVD
Professor of Dermatology & Allergy
Department of Clinical Studies
School of Veterinary Medicine
University of Pennsylvania
Philadelphia, Pennsylvania
USA

BRADLEY L. MOSES, DVM
Diplomate ACVIM (Cardiology)
Staff Clinician
VCA Roberts Animal Hospital and
VCA South Shore Animal Hospital
South Weymouth, Massachusetts
USA

JOCELYN MOTT, DVM
Diplomate ACVIM (Small Animal Internal Medicine)
VCA TLC Pasadena Veterinary Specialty and Emergency
South Pasadena, California
USA

CHRISTINE MULLIN, VMD
Diplomate ACVIM (Oncology)
Medical Oncologist
Hope Veterinary Specialists
Malvern, Pennsylvania
USA

JENNIFER M. MULZ, DVM
Diplomate ACVIM (Cardiology)
BluePearl Veterinary Partners
Sarasota, Florida
USA

KAREN R. MUÑANA, DVM, MS
Diplomate ACVIM (Neurology)
Professor, Neurology
Department of Clinical Sciences
College of Veterinary Medicine
North Carolina State University
Raleigh, North Carolina
USA

LISA A. MURPHY, VMD
Diplomate ABT
Associate Professor of Toxicology
Department of Pathobiology
University of Pennsylvania
School of Veterinary Medicine
PADLS New Bolton Center Toxicology Laboratory
Kennett Square, Pennsylvania
USA

ANTHONY J. MUTSAERS, DVM, PhD
Diplomate ACVIM (Oncology)
Associate Professor
Department of Clinical Studies
Department of Biomedical Sciences
Ontario Veterinary College
University of Guelph
Guelph, Ontario
Canada

KATHERN E. MYRNA, DVM, MS
Diplomate ACVO
Associate Professor of Ophthalmology
Department of Small Animal Medicine and Surgery
College of Veterinary Medicine
University of Georgia
Athens, Georgia
USA

GEORGINA M. NEWBOLD, DVM
Diplomate ACVO
Assistant Professor- Ophthalmology
Department of Veterinary Clinical Sciences
College of Veterinary Medicine
The Ohio State University
Columbus, Ohio
USA

REBECCA G. NEWMAN, DVM, MS
Diplomate ACVIM (Oncology)
Medical Oncologist
Pittsburgh Veterinary Medical Specialist and Emergency Center
Pittsburgh, Pennsylvania
USA

DENNIS P. O'BRIEN, DVM, PhD
Diplomate ACVIM (Neurology)
Professor Emeritus
Department of Veterinary Medicine and Surgery
College of Veterinary Medicine
University of Missouri
Columbia, Missouri
USA

LINDA K. OKONKOWSKI, DVM
Internal Medicine Resident, ACVIM (Small Animal Internal Medicine)
Small Animal Clinical Sciences
Michigan State University
College of Veterinary Medicine
East Lansing, Michigan
USA

NATASHA J. OLBY, Vet MB, PhD, MRCVS
Diplomate ACVIM (Neurology)
Professor of Neurology/Neurosurgery
Dr. Kady M. Gjessing and Rahna M. Davidson Distinguished Chair in Gerontology
Department of Clinical Sciences
Member of the Comparative Medicine Institute
North Carolina State CVM
Raleigh, North Carolina
USA

GAVIN L. OLSEN, DVM
Diplomate ACVIM (Small Animal Internal Medicine)
Staff Internist
Carolina Veterinary Specialists
Greensboro, North Carolina
USA

JENNIFER L. OWEN, DVM, PhD
Diplomate ACVP (Clinical Pathology)
Assistant Professor
Department of Physiological Sciences
College of Veterinary Medicine
University of Florida
Gainesville, Florida
USA

JOANE M. PARENT, DVM, MVetSc
ACVIM Neurology
Professor
Centre Hospitalier Universitaire Vétérinaire
Faculté de Médecine Vétérinaire
Université de Montréal
Montréal
Canada

VALERIE J. PARKER, DVM
Diplomate ACVIM
Diplomate ACVN
Associate Professor, Clinical
Department of Veterinary Clinical Sciences
College of Veterinary Medicine
The Ohio State University
Columbus, Ohio
USA

THOMAS PARMENTIER, DVM
Diplomate ACVIM (Neurology)
PhD Candidate
Department of Biomedical Sciences
Ontario Veterinary College
University of Guelph
Guelph, Ontario
Canada

R. MICHAEL PEAK, DVM
Diplomate AVCD
The Pet Dentist at Tampa Bay
Largo, Florida
USA

KATHERINE L. PETERSON, DVM
Diplomate ACVECC
Diplomate ABT
Emergency and Critical Care Specialist
Pet Poison Helpline & SafetyCall International
Bloomington, Minnesota
USA

MICHAEL E. PETERSON, DVM, MS
Gem Veterinary Clinic
Emmett, Idaho
USA

JASON PIEPER, DVM, MS
Diplomate ACVD
Assistant Professor
Department of Veterinary Clinical Medicine
University of Illinois at Urbana-Champaign
Urbana, Illinois
USA

SARAH B. PIERARD, BVSc, PgCertVS, MVS
Animal Diabetes Australia
Melbourne, Victoria
Australia

AMY L. PIKE, DVM
Diplomate ACVB
Owner, Animal Behavior Wellness Center
Fairfax, Virginia
USA

KATHRYN A. PITT, DVM, MS
Diplomate ACVS-SA
Assistant Professor of Small Animal Soft Tissue Surgery
Small Animal Clinical Sciences
Michigan State University
East Lansing, Michigan
Bloomington, Minnesota
USA

AMANDA L. POLDOSKI, DVM
Senior Consulting Veterinarian, Clinical Toxicology
Associate Manager of Veterinary & Regulatory Affairs
Pet Poison Helpline & SafetyCall International
Bloomington, Minnesota
USA

DAVID J. POLZIN, DVM, PhD
Diplomate ACVIM (Internal Medicine)
Professor and Chief of Small Animal Internal Medicine
University of Minnesota
College of Veterinary Medicine
Department of Veterinary Clinical Sciences
St. Paul, Minnesota
USA

JILL S. POMRANTZ, DVM
Diplomate ACVIM (Small Animal Internal Medicine)
Small Animal Internal Medicine Consultant
IDEXX Laboratories, Inc.
Westbrook, Maine
USA

ERIC R. POPE, DVM, MS
Diplomate ACVS
Professor of Surgery
Department of Clinical Sciences
Ross University School of Veterinary Medicine
Basseterre
St Kitts

ROBERT H. POPPENGA, DVM, PhD
Diplomate ABVT
Head, Toxicology Section
California Animal Health and Food Safety Laboratory
School of Veterinary Medicine
University of California
Davis, California
USA

SIMON A. POT, DVM
Diplomate ACVO
Diplomate ECVO
Associate Professor of Ophthalmology
Equine Department
Vetsuisse Faculty
University of Zurich
Zurich
Switzerland

SILVIA G. PRYOR, DVM
Diplomate ACVO
Ophthalmology Service
BluePearl Emergency and Specialty Hospital-Irvine
Irvine, California
USA

DAVID A. PUERTO, DVM
Diplomate ACVS
Chief of Surgery
Center for Animal Referral and Emergency Services
Langhorne, Pennsylvania
USA

BIRGIT PUSCHNER, DVM, PhD
Diplomate ABVT
Dean and Professor
College of Veterinary Medicine
Michigan State University
East Lansing, Michigan
USA

ANDHIKA PUTRA, DVM, MS
Dermatology Specialty Intern
Department of Small Animal Medicine and Surgery
University of Georgia
Athens, Georgia
USA

BARBARA QUROLLO, MS, DVM
Associate Research Professor
Department of Clinical Sciences-CVM
North Carolina State University
Raleigh, North Carolina
USA

MARYANN G. RADLINSKY, DVM, MS
Diplomate ACVS
Founding Fellow
Minimally Invasive Surgery, Small Animal Soft Tissue Surgeon
Salt River Veterinary Specialists
Scottsdale, Arizona
USA

LISA RADOSTA, DVM
Diplomate ACVB
Florida Veterinary Behavior Service
West Palm Beach, Florida
USA

ELEANOR RAFFAN, BVM&S, PhD, CertSAM, MRCVS
Diplomate ECVIM-CA
University Lecturer in Systems Physiology
Department of Physiology, Development and Neuroscience
University of Cambridge
Cambridge
United Kingdom

MERL F. RAISBECK, DVM, MS, PhD
Diplomate ABVT
Emeritus Professor
Department Veterinary Sciences
University of Wyoming
Laramie, Wyoming
USA

LAURA RAYHEL, DVM
Assistant Professor
Department of Medicine
College of Veterinary Medicine
Midwestern University
Glendale, Arizona
USA

JONJO REECE, DVM, ECFVG, BSc
Small Animal Internal Medicine Resident
Department of Clinical Sciences
Cummings School of Veterinary Medicine
Tufts University
North Grafton, Massachusetts
USA

TABATHA J. REGEHR, DVM
Consulting Veterinarian, Clinical Toxicology
SafetyCall International & Pet Poison Helpline
Bloomington, Minnesota
USA

MARSHA R. REICH, DVM
Diplomate ACVB
Veterinary Behaviorist
Maryland-Virginia Veterinary Behavioral Consulting
Silver Spring, Maryland
USA

JENNIFER M. REINHART, DVM, PhD
Diplomate ACVIM (Small Animal Internal Medicine)
Diplomate ACVCP
Assistant Professor
Department of Veterinary Clinical Medicine
College of Veterinary Medicine
University of Illinois Urbana-Champaign
Urbana, Illinois
USA

ILANA R. REISNER, DVM, PhD
Diplomate ACVB (Behavior)
Reisner Veterinary Behavior Services, LLC
Wallingford, Pennsylvania
USA

ALEXANDER M. REITER, Dipl.Tzt., Dr.med.vet
Diplomate AVDC, Diplomate EVDC
Professor of Dentistry and Oral Surgery
Department of Clinical Sciences and Advanced Medicine
School of Veterinary Medicine
University of Pennsylvania
Philadelphia, Pennsylvania
USA

LISA RESTINE, DVM
Associate Veterinarian
Alamo Feline Health Center
San Antonio, Texas
USA

AUSTIN RICHMAN, DVM
Diplomate ACVD
Los Angeles, California
USA

SHARON L. RIPPEL, DVM
Diplomate ABVT
Diplomate ABT
Clinical Toxicologist
Pet Poison Helpline
Bloomington, Minnesota
USA

WESLEY J. ROACH, DVM
Diplomate ACVS
Head of Surgery Department
Nashville Veterinary Specialists
Nashville, Tennessee
USA

TRACIE D. ROMSLAND, DVM, MS
Diplomate ACVP (Clinical Pathology)
Staff Clinical Pathologist
Friendship Hospital for Animals
Washington, DC
USA

KATHRYN A. ROOK, VMD
Diplomate ACVD
Assistant Professor of Clinical Dermatology
Department of Clinical Sciences and Advanced Medicine
School of Veterinary Medicine
University of Pennsylvania
Philadelphia, Pennsylvania
USA

SHERI ROSS, BSc, DVM, PhD
Diplomate ACVIM (Internal Medicine)
Coordinator
Advanced Urinary Disease and Extracorporeal Therapies Service
University of California Veterinary Medical Center - San Diego
San Diego, California
USA

JAMES K. ROUSH, DVM, MS
Diplomate ACVS
Doughman Chair Professor
Department of Clinical Sciences
College of Veterinary Medicine
Kansas State University
Manhattan, Kansas
USA

ELIZABETH ROZANSKI, DVM
Diplomate ACVECC
Diplomate DACVIM (Small Animal Internal Medicine)
Associate Professor
Department of Clinical Science
Cummings School of Veterinary Medicine
Tufts University
North Grafton, Massachusetts
USA

RENEE RUCINSKY, DVM
Diplomate ABVP (Feline Practice)
Medical Director
Mid Atlantic Cat Hospital
Mid Atlantic Feline Thyroid Center
Queenstown, Maryland
USA

ELKE RUDLOFF, DVM, CVMA
Diplomate ACVECC
Clinical Specialist
Emergency and Critical Care
Lakeshore Veterinary Specialists
Glendale, Wisconsin
USA

HÉLÈNE L.M. RUEL, DVM, DES, MSc
Diplomate ACVIM (Neurology)
PhD Candidate
Department of Clinical Sciences
Faculty of Veterinary Medicine
Université de Montréal
Saint-Hyacinthe, Québec
Canada

WILSON K. RUMBEIHA, BVM, PhD, ATS
Diplomate ABT
Diplomate ABVT
Professor of One Environmental Health Toxicology
Department of Molecular Biosciences
School of Veterinary Medicine
University of California, Davis
Davis, California
USA

ERIN E. RUNCAN, DVM
Diplomate ACT
Associate Professor, Clinical Theriogenology and Reproductive Medicine
Department of Veterinary Clinical Sciences
The Ohio State University
College of Veterinary Medicine
Columbus, Ohio
USA

CLARE RUSBRIDGE, BVMS, PhD, FRCVS
Diplomate ECVN
Professor in Veterinary Neurology
University of Surrey
School of Veterinary Medicine
Faculty of Health & Medical Sciences
Guildford, Surrey
United Kingdom

JOHN E. RUSH, DVM, MS
Diplomate ACVIM (Cardiology)
Diplomate ACVECC
Professor
Department of Clinical Sciences
Tufts University
Cummings School of Veterinary Medicine
North Grafton, Massachusetts
USA

KAREN E. RUSSELL, DVM, PhD
Diplomate ACVP (Clinical Pathology)
Professor and Associate Department Head for Clinical Services and Residency Programs
Department of Veterinary Pathobiology
College of Veterinary Medicine & Biomedical Sciences
Texas A&M University
College Station, Texas
USA

SHERISSE A. SAKALS, DVM
Diplomate ACVS-SA
VCA Vancouver Animal Emergency & Referral Center
Vancouver, WA
Canada

CARL D. SAMMARCO, BVSc MRCVS
Diplomate ACVIM (Cardiology)
Head of Cardiology
Red Bank Veterinary Hospital
Tinton Falls, New Jersey
USA

SHERRY LYNN SANDERSON, BS, DVM, PhD
Diplomate ACVIM (Small Animal Internal Medicine)
Diplomate ACVN
Associate Professor
Department of Veterinary Biosciences and Diagnostic Imaging
College of Veterinary Medicine
The University of Georgia
Athens, Georgia
USA

DOMENICO SANTORO, DVM, MS, DrSc, PhD
Diplomate ACVD
Diplomate ECVD
Diplomate ACVM (Bacteriology/Mycology/Immunology)
Assistant Professor
Department of Small Animal Clinical Sciences
College of Veterinary Medicine
University of Florida
Gainesville, Florida
USA

ASHLEY B. SAUNDERS, DVM
Diplomate ACVIM (Cardiology)
Professor of Cardiology
Department of Veterinary Small Animal Clinical Sciences
College of Veterinary Medicine & Biomedical Sciences
Texas A&M University
College Station, Texas
USA

BRIAN A. SCANSEN, DVM, MS
Diplomate ACVIM (Cardiology)
Associate Professor and Service Head, Cardiology & Cardiac Surgery
Department of Clinical Sciences
Colorado State University
Fort Collins, Colorado
USA

MICHAEL SCHAER, DVM
Diplomate ACVIM (Small Animal Internal Medicine)
Diplomate ACVECC
Emeritus Professor
Adjunct Professor, Emergency and Critical Care Medicine
University of Florida
College of Veterinary Medicine
Gainesville, Florida
USA

THOMAS SCHERMERHORN, VMD
Diplomate ACVIM (Small Animal Internal Medicine)
Professor and Jarvis Chair
Department of Clinical Sciences
College of Veterinary Medicine
Kansas State University
Manhattan, Kansas
USA

PHILIP SCHISSLER, DVM
Diplomate ACVIM (Neurology)
Staff Neurologist/Neurosurgeon
Veterinary Neurology Center
Tustin, California
USA

RENEE D. SCHMID, DVM
Diplomate ABVT
Diplomate ABT
Senior Consulting Veterinarian, Clinical Toxicology
Pet Poison Helpline & SafetyCall International
Bloomington, Minnesota
USA

KARSTEN E. SCHOBER, DVM, MS, PhD
Diplomate ECVIM-CA (Cardiology)
Professor
Head, Cardiology and Interventional Medicine
Department of Veterinary Clinical Sciences
College of Veterinary Medicine
The Ohio State University
Columbus, Ohio
USA

GRETCHEN L. SCHOEFFLER, DVM
Diplomate ACVECC
Chief, Emergency and Critical Care
Department of Clinical Sciences
College of Veterinary Medicine
Cornell University
Ithaca, New York
USA

JOHAN P. SCHOEMAN, BVSc, MMedVet(Med)(Pretoria), PhD(Cantab), DSAM(RCVS-UK)
Diplomate ECVIM-CA
EBVS® European Veterinary Specialist in Internal Medicine
RCVS Recognized Specialist in Small Animal Medicine;
Professor
Department of Companion Animal Clinical Studies
Chair, Pathobiology Research
Faculty of Veterinary Science
University of Pretoria
Onderstepoort
South Africa

DONALD P. SCHROPE, DVM
Diplomate ACVIM (Cardiology)
Department of Cardiology
Oradell Animal Hospital
Paramus, New Jersey
USA

ERIN M. SCOTT, VMD
Diplomate ACVO
Department of Small Animal Clinical Sciences
College of Veterinary Medicine
Texas A&M University
College Station, Texas
USA

CHRISTOPHER J. SCUDDER, BVSc, MVetMed, PhD, MRCVS
Diplomate ACVIM-SAIM
Diplomate ECVIM-CA
Head of Internal Medicine
Southfields Veterinary Specialists
Essex
United Kingdom

LYNNE M. SEIBERT, DVM, MS, PhD
Diplomate ACVB
Veterinary Behavior Consultants LLC
Lawrenceville, Georgia
USA

ASHLEIGH SEIGNEUR, DVM, MVSc
Diplomate ACVIM
Associate Veterinarian
Internal Medicine Department
South Carolina Veterinary Specialists and Emergency Care
Columbia, South Carolina
USA

KIM A. SELTING, DVM, MS
Diplomate ACVIM (Oncology)
Diplomate ACVR (Radiation Oncology)
Associate Professor
Department of Veterinary Clinical Medicine
College of Veterinary Medicine
University of Illinois at Urbana-Champaign
Urbana, Illinois
USA

LINDA G. SHELL, DVM
Diplomate ACVIM (Neurology)
Veterinary Neurology Education and Consulting
Pilot, Virginia
USA

BARBARA L. SHERMAN, MS, PhD, DVM
Diplomate ACVB (Behavior) & ACAW (Animal Welfare)
Clinical Professor Emerita
Department of Clinical Sciences
College of Veterinary Medicine
North Carolina State University
Raleigh, North Carolina
USA

TRACI A. SHREYER, MA
Applied Animal Behaviorist
Consultant
Department of Comparative Pathobiology
Purdue University
West Lafayette, Indiana
USA

DEBORAH C. SILVERSTEIN, DVM
Diplomate ACVECC
Professor of Critical Care
Department of Clinical Sciences and Advanced Medicine
University of Pennsylvania
School of Veterinary Medicine
Philadelphia, Pennsylvania
USA

LESLIE SINN, DVM
Diplomate ACVB
Specialist in Behavior
Behavior Solutions
Hamilton, Virginia
USA

KIM SLENSKY, DVM
Diplomate ACVECC
Assistant Professor of Clinical Emergency and Critical Care
Department of Clinical Sciences and Advanced Medicine
School of Veterinary Medicine
University of Pennsylvania
Philadelphia, Pennsylvania
USA

FRANCIS W.K. SMITH, JR., DVM
Diplomate, ACVIM (Small Animal Internal Medicine and Cardiology)
Vice-President
VetMed Consultants, Inc.
Lexington, Massachusetts
USA

MARK M. SMITH, VMD
Diplomate ACVS
Diplomate AVDC
Founding Fellow, ACVS Oral & Maxillofacial Surgery
Founding Fellow, AVDC Oral & Maxillofacial Surgery
Center for Veterinary Dentistry and Oral Surgery
Gaithersburg, Maryland
USA

PATRICIA J. SMITH, MS, DVM, PhD
Diplomate ACVO
PJSmith Animal Eye Consulting
Adjunct Ophthalmologist Animal Eye Care
Milpitas, California
USA

CHRISTOPHER J. SNYDER, DVM
Diplomate AVDC
Clinical Associate Professor
Dentistry and Oral Surgery, Department of Surgical Sciences
University of Wisconsin-Madison
School of Veterinary Medicine
Madison, Wisconsin
USA

PAUL W. SNYDER, DVM, PhD
Diplomate ACVP (Anatomical Pathology)
Fellow, International Academy Toxicologic Pathologists
Senior Pathologist
Experimental Pathology Laboratories, Inc.
Bonita Springs, Florida
USA

LAIA SOLANO-GALLEGO, DVM, PhD
Diplomate ECVCP
Professora Agregada (Associate Professor)
Departament de Medicina i Cirurgia Animals
Facultat de Veterinària
Universitat Autònoma de Barcelona
Barcelona
Spain

MITCHELL D. SONG, DVM
Diplomate ACVD
Animal Dermatology, PC
Phoenix, Arizona;
Adjunct Assistant Clinical Professor
Midwestern University
College of Veterinary Medicine
Glendale, Arizona
USA

JASON W. SOUKUP, DVM
Diplomate AVDC
Founding Fellow, AVDC Oral & Maxillofacial Surgery
Clinical Associate Professor
Dentistry and Oromaxillofacial Surgery
Department of Surgical Sciences
School of Veterinary Medicine
University of Wisconsin-Madison
Madison, Wisconsin
USA

SAMANTHA B. SOUTHER, DVM
Diplomate ACT
Associate Veterinarian, Theriogenology
Mohnacky Animal Hospitals
Carlsbad, California
USA

CLARISSA P. SOUZA, DVM, MS, PhD
Diplomate ACVD
Assistant Professor of Dermatology and Otology
Department of Veterinary Clinical Medicine
College of Veterinary Medicine
University of Illinois
Urbana-Champaign, Illinois
USA

JÖRG M. STEINER, MedVet, DrVetMed, PhD, AGAF
Diplomate ACVIM
Diplomate ECVIM-CA
University Distinguished Professor
Dr. Mark Morris Chair in Small Animal Gastroenterology and Nutrition
Director, Gastrointestinal Laboratory
Department of Small Animal Clinical Sciences
College of Veterinary Medicine and Biomedical Sciences
Texas A&M University
College Station, Texas
USA

KEVIN S. STEPANIUK, DVM, FAVD
Diplomate AVDC
Veterinary Dentistry Education and Consulting Services
Ridgefield, Washington
USA

JOSHUA A. STERN, DVM, PhD
Diplomate ACVIM (Cardiology)
Associate Professor
Department of Medicine & Epidemiology
School of Veterinary Medicine
University of California, Davis
Davis, California
USA

VICTOR J. STORA, DVM
Postdoctoral Fellow Transgenesis & Large Animal Model Creation
Vite Lab, Referral Center for Animal Models
Department of Clinical Sciences and Advanced Medicine
School of Veterinary Medicine
University of Pennsylvania
Philadelphia, Pennsylvania
USA

JAN S. SUCHODOLSKI, MedVet, DrVetMed, PhD, AGAF
Diplomate ACVM (Immunology)
Associate Professor
Small Animal Medicine
Associate Director for Research
Head of Microbiome Sciences
Gastrointestinal Laboratory
Texas A&M University
College of Veterinary Medicine
Department of Small Animal Clinical Sciences
College Station, Texas
USA

ALYSSA M. SULLIVANT, DVM, MS
Diplomate ACVIM (Small Animal Internal Medicine)
Assistant Professor
Department of Clinical Sciences
College of Veterinary Medicine
Mississippi State University
Mississippi State, Mississipi
USA

ANNIKA SUNDBY, DVM
Rotating Intern
Nashville Veterinary Specialists
Nashville, Tennessee
USA

WAILANI SUNG, MS, PhD, DVM
Diplomate ACVB
Veterinary Behaviorist
Behavior Service
The San Francisco Society for the Prevention of Cruelty to Animals (SPCA)
San Francisco, California
USA

STEVEN E. SUTER, VMD, MS, PhD
Diplomate ACVIM (Oncology)
Professor
Department of Clinical Sciences
North Carolina State University College of Veterinary Medicine
Raleigh, North Carolina
USA

JANE E. SYKES, BVSc(Hons), PhD
Diplomate ACVIM (Small Animal Internal Medicine)
Professor of Small Animal Internal Medicine
Department of Medicine & Epidemiology
University of California, Davis
Davis, California
USA

JOSEPH TABOADA, DVM
Diplomate ACVIM
Professor and Associate Dean
Department of Veterinary Clinical Sciences
School of Veterinary Medicine
Louisiana State University
Baton Rouge, Louisiana
USA

LAUREN TALARICO, BS, DVM
Diplomate ACVIM (Neurology)
Section Head Neurology/Neurosurgery
VCA Southpaws Veterinary Specialty & Emergency Center
Fairfax, Virginia
USA

PATRICIA A. TALCOTT, MS, DVM, PhD
Diplomate ABVT
Professor
Department of Integrative Physiology and Neuroscience
College of Veterinary Medicine
Washington State University
Pullman, Washington
USA

KENDALL TANEY, DVM
Diplomate AVDC
Center for Veterinary Dentistry and Oral Surgery
Gaithersburg, Maryland
USA

JAIME L. TARIGO, DVM, PhD
Diplomate ACVP (Clinical Pathology)
Associate Professor
Department of Pathology
College of Veterinary Medicine
University of Georgia
Athens, Georgia
USA

DOMINIC A. TAUER, DVM
Diplomate ABT
Consulting Veterinarian in Clinical Toxicology
Pet Poison Helpline and SafetyCall International, PLLC
Bloomington, Minnesota
USA

SUSAN M. TAYLOR, DVM
Diplomate ACVIM
Professor Emeritus
Department of Small Animal Clinical Sciences
Western College of Veterinary Medicine
University of Saskatchewan
Saskatoon, Saskatchewan
Canada

MICHELLE C. TENSLEY, DVM, MS
Diplomate ACVIM (Neurology)
Associate Neurologist
The Animal Neurology and Imaging Center
Algodones, New Mexico
USA

VINCENT J. THAWLEY, VMD
Diplomate ACVECC
Clinical Assistant Professor
Emergency and Critical Care Medicine
Department of Clinical Sciences and Advanced Medicine
School of Veterinary Medicine
University of Pennsylvania
Philadelphia, Pennsylvania
USA

JUSTIN D. THOMASON, DVM
Diplomate ACVIM (Cardiology; SAIM)
Clinical Associate Professor
Department of Clinical Sciences
College of Veterinary Medicine
Kansas State University
Manhattan, Kansas
USA

CRAIG A. THOMPSON, DVM
Diplomate ACVP
Clinical Associate Professor - Clinical Pathology
Department of Comparative Pathobiology
Purdue University- College of Veterinary Medicine
West Lafayette, Indiana
USA

JERRY A. THORNHILL, DVM
Diplomate ACVIM
Director, Nephrology & Dialysis
Division of Internal Medicine
Veterinary Specialty Center
Buffalo Grove, Illinois
USA

MARY ANNA THRALL, BA, DVM, MS
Diplomate ACVP (Clinical Pathology)
Professor
Department of Biomedical Sciences
Ross University School of Veterinary Medicine
Basseterre, St. Kitts
West Indies

LARRY P. TILLEY, DVM
Diplomate ACVIM (Small Animal Internal Medicine)
President
VetMed Consultants, Inc.
Santa Fe, New Mexico
USA

ANDREA TIPOLD, DVM
Diplomate ECVN (Veterinary Neurology)
Department of Small Animal Medicine and Surgery
University of Veterinary Medicine Hannover
Hannover
Germany

SHEILA M.F. TORRES, DVM, MS, PhD
Diplomate ACVD (Dermatology)
Professor
Department of Veterinary Clinical Sciences
College of Veterinary Medicine
University of Minnesota
St. Paul, Minnesota
USA

SANDRA P. TOU, DVM
Diplomate ACVIM (Cardiology and Internal Medicine)
Clinical Assistant Professor of Cardiology
Department of Clinical Sciences
North Carolina State University
College of Veterinary Medicine
Raleigh, North Carolina
USA

WILLIAM J. TRANQUILLI, Bs in Ed, Ms, DVM
Diplomate ACVAA
Professor Emeritus
Departments of Clinical Science, Biological Sciences, and Pathobiology
University of Illinois-Urbana
Illinois
USA

VALARIE V. TYNES, DVM
Diplomate ACVB (Veterinary Behavior)
Diplomate ACAW (Animal Welfare)
Veterinary Services Specialist
Ceva Animal Health
Lenexa, Kansas
USA

YU UEDA, DVM, PhD
Clinical Assistant Professor
Small Animal Emergency and Critical Care
Department of Clinical Sciences
College of Veterinary Medicine
North Carolina State University
Raleigh, North Carolina
USA

STEFAN UNTERER, Dr.med.vet., Dr. habil.
Diplomate ECVIM
Head of Gastroenterology Service
Clinic of Small Animal Internal Medicine
Ludwig-Maximilians-University
Munich
Germany

SHELLY VADEN, DVM, PhD
Diplomate ACVIM (Internal Medicine)
Professor, Small Animal Nephrology and Urology
Department of Clinical Sciences
College of Veterinary Medicine
North Carolina State University
Raleigh, North Carolina
USA

SUZY Y.M. VALENTIN, DVM, MS
Diplomate ACVIM
Diplomate ECVIM-CA (Internal Medicine)
Internal Medicine Specialist
Internal Medicine Service
Centre Hospitalier Vétérinaire Pommery
Reims
France

MEGHAN VAUGHT, DVM
Diplomate ACVECC
Staff Criticalist;
ECC Medical Director
Maine Veterinary Medicine Center
Scarborough, Maine
USA

GUILHERME G. VEROCAI, DVM, MSc, PhD
Diplomate ACVM (Parasitology)
Clinical Assistant Professor
Director Parasitology Diagnostic Laboratory
Department of Veterinary Pathobiology
College of Veterinary Medicine and Biomedical Sciences
Texas A&M University
College Station, Texas
USA

MARIA VIANNA, DVM
Diplomate DACVS
Veterinary Specialty Hospital of Palm Beach Gardens
Palm Beach Gardens, Florida
USA

ALYSHA VINCENT, DVM
Internal Medicine Resident (Small Animal Internal Medicine)
Department of Small Animal Clinical Sciences
College of Veterinary Medicine
Michigan State University
East Lansing, Michigan
USA

KAREN A. VON DOLLEN, DVM, MS
Diplomate ACT
Hagyard Equine Medical Institute
Lexington, Kentucky
USA

DIRSKO J.F. VON PFEIL, Dr.med.vet, DVM
Diplomate ACVS
Diplomate ECVS
Diplomate ACVSMR
Sirius Veterinary Orthopedic Center
Omaha, Nebraska;
Small Animal Surgery Locum, PLLC
Dallas, Texas
USA

LORI S. WADDELL, DVM
Diplomate ACVECC
Professor, Clinical Critical Care
Department of Clinical Studies and Advancement of Medicine
School of Veterinary Medicine
University of Pennsylvania
Philadelphia, Pennsylvania
USA

LIORA WALDMAN, BVM&S, MRCVS
CertSAD
Dermatology and Allergy Clinic
Haifa
Israel

JULIE M. WALKER, DVM
Diplomate ACVECC
Clinical Associate Professor
Department of Medical Sciences
School of Veterinary Medicine
University of Wisconsin-Madison
Madison, Wisconsin
USA

REBECCA A.L. WALTON, DVM
Diplomate ACVECC
Clinical Assistant Professor
Department of Veterinary Clinical Sciences
College of Veterinary Medicine
Iowa State University
Ames, Iowa
USA

STUART A. WALTON, BVSc, BScAgr
MANZCVS (Small Animal Internal Medicine)
Diplomate ACVIM (Small Animal Internal Medicine)
Clinical Assistant Professor
Department of Small Animal Clinical Sciences
College of Veterinary Medicine
University of Florida
Gainesville, Florida
USA

ANDREA WANG MUNK, MA, DVM
Diplomate ACVIM (Small Animal Internal Medicine)
Small Animal Internal Medicine Consultant
IDEXX Laboratories, Inc.
Westbrook, Maine
USA

KIRSTEN E. WARATUKE, DVM
Diplomate ABT
Toxicologist
ASPCA Animal Poison Control Center
Urbana, Illinois
USA

BRETT A. WASIK, DVM
Diplomate ACVIM (Small Animal Internal Medicine)
Antech Diagnostics - Internal Medicine/ Endocrinology Consultant
Veterinary Information Network - Internal Medicine/Endocrinology Consultant
UC Davis Endocrinology Post-doctorate
Allen, Texas
USA

NICOLE M. WEINSTEIN, DVM
Diplomate ACVP (Clinical Pathology)
Associate Professor
Department of Pathobiology
School of Veterinary Medicine
University of Pennsylvania
Philadelphia, Pennsylvania
USA

GLADE WEISER, DVM
Diplomate ACVP Emeritus
Clinical Pathologist
Loveland, Colorado
USA

SARA A. WENNOGLE, DVM, PhD
Diplomate ACVIM-SAIM
Assistant Professor
Small Animal Clinical Sciences
Michigan State University
East Lansing, Michigan
USA

MICHAEL D. WILLARD, DVM, MS
Diplomate ACVIM (Small Animal)
Senior Professor
Department of Small Animal Clinical Sciences
College of Veterinary Medicine
Texas A&M University
College Station, Texas
USA

LAUREL E. WILLIAMS, DVM
Diplomate ACVIM (Oncology)
Adjunct Professor
Department of Clinical Sciences
College of Veterinary Medicine
North Carolina State University
Raleigh, North Carolina;
Oncologist, Medical Director
Veterinary Specialty Center of Seattle
Lynwood, Washington
USA

HEATHER M. WILSON-ROBLES, DVM
Diplomate ACVIM (Oncology)
Professor
Department of Veterinary Small Animal Clinical Sciences
College of Veterinary Medicine
Texas A&M University
College Station, Texas
USA

TINA WISMER, DVM, MS
Diplomate ABVT
Diplomate ABT
Medical Director
ASPCA Animal Poison Control Center
Urbana, Illinois
USA

EWAN D.S. WOLFF, PhD, DVM
Diplomate ACVIM
Small Animal Internist
BluePearl - Affiliated Veterinary Specialists
USA

MICHAEL W. WOOD, DVM, PhD
Diplomate ACVIM (Small Animal Internal Medicine)
Assistant Professor
Department of Medical Sciences
School of Veterinary Medicine
University of Wisconsin-Madison
Madison, Wisconsin
USA

R. DARREN WOOD, DVM, DVSc
Diplomate ACVP (Clinical Pathology)
Associate Professor
Department of Pathobiology
Ontario Veterinary College
University of Guelph
Guelph, Ontario
Canada

J. PAUL WOODS, DVM, MS
Diplomate ACVIM (Internal Medicine, Oncology)
Professor of Internal Medicine and Oncology
Department of Clinical Studies
Ontario Veterinary College;
Co-Director
Institute for Comparative Cancer Investigation
University of Guelph
Guelph, Ontario
Canada

CORRY K. YEUROUKIS, DVM, MS
Diplomate ACVP (Clinical)
Clinical Pathologist
ANTECH Diagnostics
Annapolis, Maryland
USA

HANY YOUSSEF, BVSc, MS, DVM
Diplomate ABT
Diplomate ABVT
Watseka Animal Hospital
Watseka, Illinois;
Iroquois County Animal Control Director
Watseka, Illinois
USA

DANIELLE ZWUESTE, DVM
Diplomate ACVIM (Neurology)
Vancouver Animal Emergency and Referral Centre
Vancouver
British Columbia
Canada

About the Companion Website

This book is accompanied by a companion website:

www.fiveminutevet.com/canineandfeline7th

The website includes:

- Videos
- Images
- Client Education Handouts
- Additional references and internet resources

The password for the companion website: pl58ez690xle

5-FLUOROURACIL (5-FU) TOXICOSIS

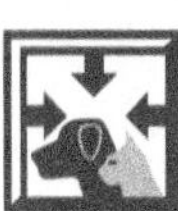

BASICS

OVERVIEW

- Antimetabolite, antineoplastic agent; it is metabolized to thymidine, which blocks the methylation reaction of deoxyuridylic and thymidylic acids, resulting in thymine deficiency; thymine is critical for DNA and to a lesser extent RNA replication; the result is cell death due to interruption of normal DNA and RNA synthesis; this mechanism targets rapidly growing cells like bone marrow and intestinal crypts; 5-FU has various active metabolites resulting in delayed clearance from bone marrow and γ-aminobutyric acid (GABA) depletion in the brain.
- Labeled for human use only.
- Topical preparation for actinic and solar keratoses: Efudex® (5% cream, 2% and 5% solution), Carac® (0.5% cream), Fluoroplex® (1% cream), Tolak® (4% cream).
- IV preparation used for a variety of neoplastic conditions: Adrucil® (50 mg/m: IV solution).
- Causes acute and severe gastroenteritis and seizures; seizures can develop within 30 minutes to 6 hours post exposure; bone marrow suppression occurs 7–21 days after acute presentation.
- Patients may survive acute toxicity to succumb to bone marrow suppression later.
- Any suspected exposure in animals warrants immediate veterinary evaluation.

SIGNALMENT

- No species or breed predilection.

SIGNS

- Cardiovascular—hypotension, myocardial ischemia, arrhythmias.
- Immune—bone marrow suppression of all cell lines.
- Gastrointestinal (GI)—nausea, salivation, profuse vomiting, hematemesis, diarrhea, hematochezia, abdominal pain, stomatitis.
- Nervous—lethargy, ataxia, depression, disorientation, tremors, seizures (often refractory to treatment), death.
- Ophthalmic—blindness (cats).
- Reproductive—teratogenic, embryotoxic.
- Respiratory—noncardiogenic pulmonary edema, dyspnea, cyanosis, tachypnea.

CAUSES & RISK FACTORS

- Access to topical preparations in the home.
- Cats and small dogs may be exposed by licking pet owner.
- Pets in geographic locations of high human UV exposure due to increased human use.

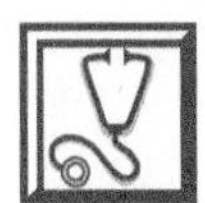

DIAGNOSIS

DIFFERENTIAL DIAGNOSIS

- Other toxins—bromethalin, castor bean, cycad palms (*Cycas* and *Zamia* spp.), disulfoton, iron, metaldehyde, mushrooms (*Amanita*, *Galerina*, and *Lepiota* spp.), sodium fluoroacetate (Compound 1080), strychnine.
- Metabolic—hepatic failure, hepatic encephalopathy.
- Nervous—idiopathic epilepsy, meningitis, neoplasia.

CBC/BIOCHEMISTRY/URINALYSIS

- CBC—baseline, then continue to monitor q3–4 days post exposure for 21 days; monitor for echinocytes; leukopenia develops by day 7 and continues to day 13; thrombocytopenia develops by day 7 and can continue for 21 days; acute anemia due to blood loss can be secondary to bone marrow suppression by day 9, persisting until day 21.
- Chemistry—baseline; hepatic values may increase.
- Electrolytes—baseline; recheck PRN based on GI losses.

OTHER LABORATORY TESTS

- Blood gases—metabolic acidosis can occur; monitor PRN.
- Packed cell volume (PCV)/total protein (TP) q6–24h.
- Blood glucose q2–4h.

IMAGING

N/A

DIAGNOSTIC PROCEDURES

N/A

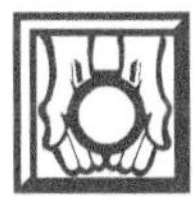

TREATMENT

- Emesis—not typically indicated due to rapid onset of seizures.
- Single dose activated charcoal with sorbitol in asymptomatic patients; seizures may develop before opportunity to administer charcoal.
- Gastric lavage can be performed in patients with recent exposure; a single dose of activated charcoal with a cathartic (AC/C) can be administered, recovering patient with endotracheal tube in place.
- Balanced crystalloid IVF to maintain hydration, aid in elimination, and maintain perfusion.
- Monitor blood pressure q4–6h.

MEDICATIONS

DRUG(S) OF CHOICE

- Anticonvulsant—levetiracetam 60 mg/kg IV loading dose, 20 mg/kg IV q8h; propofol 4–6 mg/kg IV bolus followed by 0.6 mg/kg/minute CRI; inhalant anesthesia; valium is typically ineffective; phenobarbital and pentobarbital have unpredictable efficacy, but can be attempted, phenobarbital 5–8 mg/kg IV slowly to effect.
- Antiemetic—maropitant 1 mg/kg IV, SC q24h; ondansetron 0.1–0.2 mg/kg IV q6–12h; metoclopramide 0.1–0.5 mg/kg IV, SC q6–8h.
- GI protection—proton pump inhibitors, H2 blockers, sucralfate.
- Analgesia—buprenorphine 0.005–0.03 mg/kg IM or IV q6–12h, butorphanol 0.1–0.5 mg/kg SC, IV, or IM.
- Antibiotic—broad-spectrum antibiotic therapy if total white blood cell count is below 2000.
- Bone marrow stimulation—filgrastim (Neupogen®) 4–6 μg/kg SQ q24h.
- Transfusion therapy may be indicated if PCV <20%.
- 20% intravenous fat emulsion (IFE) unlikely to be effective.
- Antidote—uridine triacetate has not been used in veterinary medicine; must be instituted prior to development of CNS signs; cost prohibitive.

CONTRAINDICATIONS/POSSIBLE INTERACTIONS

- Avoid nonsteroidal anti-inflammatory drugs (NSAIDs) and CNS depressants.

FOLLOW-UP

- CBC q3–4 days for 21 days or more.

MISCELLANEOUS

ABBREVIATIONS

- 5-FU = 5-fluorouracil.
- AC/C = activated charcoal with a cathartic.
- GABA = γ-aminobutyric acid.
- GI = gastrointestinal.
- IFE = intravenous fat emulsion.
- NSAID = nonsteroidal anti-inflammatory drug.
- PCV = packed cell volume.
- TP = total protein.

Suggested Reading

Sayre RS, Barr JW, Bailey EM. Accidental and experimentally induced 5-fluorouracil toxicity in dogs. J Vet Emerg Crit Care 2012; 22(3):545–549.

Author Tabatha J. Regehr

Consulting Editor Lynn R. Hovda

ABORTION, SPONTANEOUS (EARLY PREGNANCY LOSS)—CATS

BASICS

DEFINITION

• Abortion: loss of a pregnancy at any time prior to the fetus's ability to survive outside the uterus. • Early pregnancy loss: loss of a pregnancy and death of conceptus within the first half of gestation

PATHOPHYSIOLOGY

• Noninfectious causes—more common. • Infectious causes—direct infection of embryo, uterus, placenta, or fetuses, or indirectly by systemic infection.

SYSTEMS AFFECTED

• Reproductive. • Endocrine. • Other systems resulting in debilitating illness.

GENETICS

Higher incidence in purebred or closed research catteries with closely related individuals; heritability of susceptibility to feline infectious peritonitis virus (FIPV) suspected to be high.

INCIDENCE/PREVALENCE

Difficult to determine, as pregnancy may not be diagnosed early. Loss or resorption of one or two conceptus within a litter is not uncommon.

GEOGRAPHIC DISTRIBUTION

N/A

SIGNALMENT

Increased incidence in queens >5 years old; increased risk in purebred cats with high inbreeding.

SIGNS

General Comments

Frequently no clinical symptoms other than lack of pregnancy or reduced litter size.

Historical Findings

Failure to deliver kittens at expected due date, return to estrus sooner than expected (approximately 45 days), discovery of fetal tissues or placenta, behavior change, systemic illness.

Physical Examination Findings

Signs range from normal to dehydration, fever, abdominal straining, and discomfort to presence of purulent, mucoid, watery, or sanguineous vaginal discharge.

CAUSES

Infectious

• Bacterial—organisms implicated in causing abortion via ascending infection through the vaginal vault and cervix include *E. coli*, *Staphylococcus* spp., *Streptococcus* spp., *Chlamydia* spp., *Pasteurella* spp., *Klebsiella* spp., *Pseudomonas* spp., *Salmonella* spp., *Mycoplasma* spp., and *Ureaplasma* spp. • Protozoal—*Toxoplasma gondii*. • Viral— feline leukemia virus (FeLV), feline herpesvirus 1 (FHV-1), FIP, feline immunodeficiency virus (FIV), feline panleukopenia virus (FPLV).

Noninfectious

• Uterine—cystic endometrial hyperplasia, endometritis, pyometra, anatomic abnormalities of uterus (e.g., adhesions or strictures), uterine trauma. • Ovarian—primary hypoluteoidism is rare in cats, but secondary hypoluteoidism may result from prostaglandin exposure, prolonged stress, and uterine inflammation. • Fetal—chromosomal abnormalities resulting in abnormal or arrested development and embryonic or fetal death. • Systemic—malnutrition or nutritional disorders (e.g., taurine deficiency, vitamin A deficiency or toxicity), severe nonreproductive illness, exposure to exogenous estrogens, glucocorticoids, chemotherapeutic agents, antifungal agents, some antibiotics (trimethoprim–sulfonamides, tetracyclines, gentamicin), modified live vaccines.

RISK FACTORS

• Cats with high coefficient of inbreeding (COI). • Previous pregnancy loss. • Previous history of reduced litter size. • Evidence of cystic endometrial hyperplasia (CEH) on ultrasound. • Concurrent systemic disease or recent trauma. • Older queens (over 6 years). • Malnourishment. • Unsanitary housing conditions. • Raw diets.

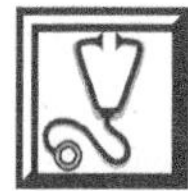

DIAGNOSIS

DIFFERENTIAL DIAGNOSIS

• Early pregnancy loss—failure to ovulate, failure to conceive, chromosomal disorder, or disorder of sexual development. • Vaginal discharge—pyometra, uterine stump pyometra, mucometra, vaginitis, neoplasia, cystitis, active labor or impending abortion, trauma to urogenital tract. • Mass or tissue from vaginal vault—dystocia, neoplasia, hemorrhage/blood clot, uterine prolapse.

CBC/BIOCHEMISTRY/URINALYSIS

• Generally normal. • Inflammatory leukogram with infection or systemic disease. • Anemia of pregnancy; hemoconcentration and azotemia may be seen with dehydration or hypovolemia.

OTHER LABORATORY TESTS

Infectious Causes

• Cytology and bacterial culture of vaginal discharge, fetus, fetal membranes, or uterine contents (aerobic and mycoplasma). • FeLV—test for antigens in queens using ELISA or indirect fluorescent antibody (IFA). • FHV-1—IFA or PCR from corneal or conjunctival swabs, viral isolation from conjunctival, nasal, or pharyngeal swabs. • FIP—submit fetal tissue for histopathology and immunohistochemistry. • FIV—ELISA: confirm positive results with Western blot. • FPLV—viral isolation from fetuses submitted for necropsy; document seroconversion in queen.

Noninfectious Causes

• To rule out anovulatory cycle, confirm progesterone >2 ng/mL one week following mating. • Hypoluteoidism—serum progesterone level <1.0 ng/mL prior to abortion indicates luteal failure. • Disorder of sexual development—evaluate external genitalia, karyotype, and histopathology of reproductive tract and gonads.

IMAGING

• Abdominal ultrasound—most specific; pregnancy confirmed after 25 days. Re-ultrasound every 1–2 weeks for high-risk queens. Confirm fetal heart rates and assess fetal fluids and placenta in late gestation (normal fetal heart rates >200 bpm). Visualization of fetal kidney and intestinal peristalsis indicates fetal maturity. • Abdominal radiographs—after 45 days, can evaluate fetal number, relative size, and position; also assess fetal death (gas pockets) or fetal malformation.

DIAGNOSTIC PROCEDURES

• Submit aborted, stillborn, mummified fetuses and fetal membranes (fresh or refrigerated on ice) for gross necropsy, histopathology, cultures, and viral isolation. Submit culture of reproductive tract or entire tract if removed (uterus, ovaries, oviducts). Submit samples from aborted and stillborn fetus for karyotyping. • Pedigree analysis—evaluate COI. • Evaluate cattery management for vaccination protocols, feeding regime, sanitation procedures, and quarantine procedures. • Nutrition—nutritional analysis of diet: of particular importance when queen is fed homemade and/or raw diet.

PATHOLOGIC FINDINGS

Variable with etiology.

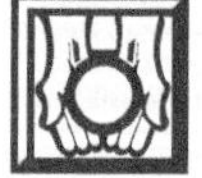

TREATMENT

APPROPRIATE HEALTH CARE

None, for noninfectious, stable queens; primary hypoluteoidism—managed on outpatient basis.

NURSING CARE

Inpatient management if systemically ill, debilitated, severely dehydrated, or for medical management of ongoing fetal loss or pyometra.

ACTIVITY

• Isolation for queens with infectious disease. • No activity restrictions for most; restrict activity as indicated if due to trauma.

DIET

• Feed commercially available diet labeled for use in pregnancy. • Correct diets with inappropriate taurine or vitamin A concentrations. • Avoid feeding raw meats or allowing queens to hunt during pregnancy to reduce risk for ingestion of pathogenic bacteria and *T. gondii.*

CLIENT EDUCATION

• Infectious diseases—verify vaccination status (vaccinate prior to pregnancy) and disease surveillance measures; ensure use of quarantine facilities for pregnant queens and new arrivals. • Breeding management—keep detailed records of reproductive performance, pedigree analysis, and social behavior of queens (including when not receptive to male). • Nutrition—advise feeding commercial cat food during pregnancy. • Genetic disease—discuss COI and value of introducing new genetics. • Discuss risk of zoonotic disease from *T. gondii.*

SURGICAL CONSIDERATIONS

Ovariohysterectomy (OHE) may be considered if queen is systemically ill from uterine infection or deceased fetuses. If valuable breeding animal, Cesarean section can be performed to remove deceased fetuses.

MEDICATIONS

DRUG(S) OF CHOICE

• Depends on etiology. • Amoxicillin–clavulanic acid 13.75 mg/kg PO q12h—safe for pregnancy. • Enrofloxacin 5 mg/kg/day PO—excellent penetration to uterus; contraindicated if live fetuses present. • Prostaglandin $F_{2\alpha}$ ($PGF_{2\alpha}$; dinoprost/Lutalyse®) 80–100 µg/kg IM q8–12h—promotes uterine contractions, loss of corpus luteum, and cervical opening to expulse aborted materials. • Tocolytics—prevent uterine contractions: terbutaline 0.03–1.0 mg PO as needed based on tocodynamometry (www.whelpwise.com); 0.03 mg/kg PO q8h if tocodynamometry not available. • Hypoluteoidism—oral progestogene (altrenogest) 0.088 mg/kg PO q24h to maintain pregnancy; can monitor queen's progesterone, as altrenogest will not interfere with progesterone assay.

CONTRAINDICATIONS

• Terbutaline—cardiac disease, pyometra, infectious disease, hypertension.
• Altrenogest—contaminated uterus with systemically ill queen. • Prostaglandin-cats with previously diagnosed respiratory disease.

PRECAUTIONS

• Use of tocolytics requires accurate breeding dates to know when to stop treatment; most successful in combination with tocodynamometry. • Terbutaline can cause hypertension leading to hemorrhage from placental sites during parturition or at time of Cesarean section. • Altrenogest can cause agalactia and failure of parturition, leading to death of litter; discontinue use 2 days before due date. • Caution with use of altrenogest with infectious processes or necrotic fetuses in uterus; may keep infection within uterus, causing metritis and systemic illness; monitor pregnancy often with ultrasound. • $PGF_{2\alpha}$—side effects vomiting, hypersalivation, defecation, urination, and tachypnea; dose dependent and self-limiting.

POSSIBLE INTERACTIONS

• Progesterone administration during pregnancy associated with masculinization of female fetuses; do not administer in first half of pregnancy and use with informed consent thereafter. • Tocolytics associated with increased risk of dystocia, failure of placental separation, lack of milk production, and poor maternal behavior for first days postpartum.

ALTERNATIVE DRUG(S)

Dopamine agonists (e.g., cabergoline 5 µg/kg PO q24h) can be used to lower progesterone and facilitate uterine emptying. Use in conjunction with low dose of $PGF_{2\alpha}$.

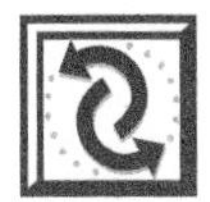

FOLLOW-UP

PATIENT MONITORING

• Serial ultrasound—follow pregnancy loss, uterine emptying, or viability of remaining fetuses; initially daily; decrease frequency when stable, continue until birth (with partial loss) or uterus is free of fluid (complete abortion). • Monitor health and attitude of queen. • If live fetuses are present—delayed parturition my occur with progesterone or terbutaline treatment; Cesarean section may be necessary.

PREVENTION/AVOIDANCE

• Institute infectious disease prevention, control, and surveillance. • Replace subfertile queens with more reproductively fit individuals. • Avoid exposure to abortifacient, teratogenic, or fetotoxic drugs. • Serial progesterone assays and fetal ultrasound during next pregnancy.

POSSIBLE COMPLICATIONS

• Loss of entire litter. • Metritis, chronic endometritis, uterine rupture, sepsis, shock.
• Uterine pathology. • Masculinization of female fetuses with progesterone therapy.

EXPECTED COURSE AND PROGNOSIS

• Poor prognosis for live kittens for current litter, even with aggressive monitoring and treatment. • May recur in future pregnancies depending on cause and treatment. • Poor prognosis for normal pregnancy with severe CEH. • Fair prognosis for successful pregnancy with treatment for primary hypoluteoidism; significant monitoring required for good outcome. • Pregnancy loss due to genetic abnormalities likely to recur if queen is bred to tom with similar pedigree.

MISCELLANEOUS

ASSOCIATED CONDITIONS

Severe systemic disease otf any kind, malnutrition.

AGE-RELATED FACTORS

Queens >6 years old—higher incidence of lower litter size and infertility.

ZOONOTIC POTENTIAL

T. gondii.

PREGNANCY/FERTILITY/BREEDING

Queens with previous pregnancy loss are at higher risk of subsequent pregnancy loss or infertility and should be monitored intensively.

SYNONYMS

• Pregnancy loss. • Abortion. • Fetal mummification. • Early embryonic loss.

SEE ALSO

• Breeding, Timing.
• Sexual Development Disorders.

ABBREVIATIONS

• CEH = cystic endometrial hyperplasia.
• COI = coefficient of inbreeding.
• FeLV = feline leukemia virus.
• FHV-1 = feline herpesvirus 1.
• FIPV = feline infectious peritonitis virus.
• FIV = feline immunodeficiency virus.
• FPLV = feline panleukopenia virus.
• IFA = indirect fluorescent antibody.
• OHE = ovariohysterectomy.
• $PGF_{2\alpha}$ = prostaglandin $F_{2\alpha}$.

Suggested Reading

Lamm CG. Clinical approach to abortion, stillbirth, and neonatal death in dogs and cats. Vet Clin North Am Small Anim Pract 2012, (42)3:501–513.

Verstegen J, Dhaliwal G, Verstegen-Onclin K. Canine and feline pregnancy loss due to viral and non-infectious causes: a review. Theriogenology 2008, 70(3):304–319.

Author Aime K. Johnson

Consulting Editor Erin E. Runcan

Acknowledgment The author and editors acknowledge the prior contribution of Milan Hess.

Client Education Handout available online

A

ABORTION, SPONTANEOUS (EARLY PREGNANCY LOSS)—DOGS

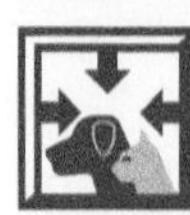

BASICS

DEFINITION

Loss of a fetus because of resorption in early stages or expulsion in later stages of pregnancy.

PATHOPHYSIOLOGY

- Direct—congenital abnormality, infectious disease, trauma.
- Indirect—infectious placentitis, abnormal ovarian function, abnormal uterine environment.

SYSTEMS AFFECTED

- Reproductive.
- Any major body system dysfunction can adversely affect pregnancy.

GENETICS

- No genetic basis for most causes.
- Lymphocytic hypothyroidism—single-gene recessive trait in Borzois.

INCIDENCE/PREVALENCE

- True incidence unknown.
- Resorption estimated between 11% and 13%, up to 30% (at least one resorption).
- Incidence of stillbirth 2.2–4.4%; with dystocia up to 22.3%.

SIGNALMENT

Species

Dog

Breed Predilections

- Familial lymphocytic hypothyroidism (Borzoi)—prolonged interestrus interval, poor conception rate, mid-gestation abortion, stillbirths.
- Many breeds at risk for hypothyroidism, although evidence of role in abortion unclear.

Mean Age and Range

- Infectious causes, pharmacologic agents causing abortion, fetal defects—all ages.
- Cystic endometrial hyperplasia—usually >6 years old.

Predominant Sex

Intact bitches.

SIGNS

Historical Findings

- Failure to whelp on time.
- Expulsion of recognizable fetuses or placental tissues.
- Decrease in abdominal size; weight loss.
- Anorexia, vomiting, diarrhea.
- Behavioral changes.

Physical Examination Findings

- Sanguineous or purulent vulvar discharge.
- Disappearance of previously documented vesicles or fetuses.
- Abdominal straining, discomfort.
- Depression.
- Dehydration.
- Fever.

CAUSES

Infectious

- *Brucella canis*.
- Canine herpesvirus.
- *Toxoplasma gondii, Neospora caninum*.
- *Mycoplasma* and *Ureaplasma*.
- Bacteria—*Escherichia coli, Streptococcus, Campylobacter, Salmonella*.
- Viruses—distemper, parvovirus, adenovirus.

Uterine

- Cystic endometrial hyperplasia and pyometra.
- Trauma—acute and chronic.
- Neoplasia.

Ovarian

- Hypoluteoidism—abnormal luteal function in absence of fetal, uterine, or placental disease: progesterone concentrations <1–2 ng/mL, most commonly 40–45 days' gestation.

Exogenous Administration

- Embryotoxic drugs.
- Chemotherapeutic agents.
- Estrogens.
- Glucocorticoids.
- Prostaglandins—lysis of corpora lutea.
- Dopamine agonists—lysis of corpora lutea via suppression of prolactin; bromocriptine, cabergoline.

Hormonal Dysfunction

- Hypothyroidism (less common).
- Hyperadrenocorticism.
- Endocrine-disrupting contaminants documented in human and wildlife fetal loss.

Fetal Defects

- Lethal chromosomal abnormality or organ defects.

RISK FACTORS

- Exposure of brood bitch to carrier animals.
- Old age.
- Hereditary factors.

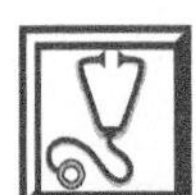

DIAGNOSIS

DIFFERENTIAL DIAGNOSIS

- Differentiate infectious from noninfectious causes—*B. canis* immediate and zoonotic concern.
- Differentiate resorption from infertility—helped by early diagnosis of pregnancy.
- History of drug use during pregnancy—particularly during first trimester, or use of drugs (e.g., dexamethasone, prostaglandins, ketoconazole, griseofulvin, doxycycline, tetracycline, dantrolene) known to cause fetal death.
- Vulvar discharge during diestrus—may mimic abortion; evaluate discharge and origin to differentiate uterine from distal reproductive tract disease.
- Necropsy of aborted fetus, stillborn puppies, and placenta(s)—enhance chances of definitive diagnosis.
- Systemic or endocrine disease—problems with maternal environment.

CBC/BIOCHEMISTRY/URINALYSIS

- Usually normal.
- Systemic disease, uterine infection, viral infection, or endocrine abnormalities—may produce changes in CBC, biochemistries, or urinalysis.

OTHER LABORATORY TESTS

- Serologic testing—*B. canis*, canine herpesvirus, *Toxoplasma*, *Neospora*; collect serum as soon as possible after abortion; repeat testing for paired titers for canine herpesvirus, *Toxoplasma*, *Neospora*.
- *B. canis*—
  - Slide test (D-Tec CB®, Zoetis) very sensitive; negative results reliable; prevalence of false positives as high as 60%.
  - PCR best to use on abortive discharge (Kansas State Veterinary Diagnostic Laboratory).
  - Definitive diagnosis made via culture of abortive discharge or dam serum.
  - Tube agglutination—titers >1 : 200 considered positive; titers 1 : 50–1 : 200 suspicious.
  - Agar gel immunodiffusion—differentiates between false positives and true positives in agglutination tests; detects cytoplasmic and cell surface antigens.
- Baseline T_4 serum concentration—hypothyroidism possible cause for fetal wastage; role in pregnancy loss unclear.
- Serum progesterone concentration (hypoluteoidism; if no infectious cause); dogs depend on ovarian progesterone production throughout gestation (minimum of 2 ng/mL required to maintain pregnancy); determine as soon as possible after abortion; in subsequent pregnancies, start weekly monitoring at week 3 (may be before pregnancy documented with ultrasound); start biweekly sampling around gestational age of prior loss. Pregnancy loss typically occurs during seventh week of gestation (see Premature Labor).
- Vaginal culture—*B. canis* with positive serologic test; *Mycoplasma*, *Ureaplasma*, other bacterial agents; all except *B. canis* can be normal flora, so diagnosis difficult from vaginal culture alone; limited benefit unless heavy growth of single organism; *Salmonella* associated with systemic illness.

IMAGING

- Radiography—identifies fetal structures after 45 days of gestation; earlier determines uterine enlargement but not uterine contents.
- Ultrasonography—identify uterine size and contents; assess fluid and its consistency; assess fetal viability (heartbeats: normal, >200 bpm; stress, <150 or >280 bpm).

(CONTINUED) ABORTION, SPONTANEOUS (EARLY PREGNANCY LOSS)—DOGS

DIAGNOSTIC PROCEDURES

- Vaginoscopy—identify source of vulvar discharge and vaginal lesions; use scope of sufficient length (16–20 cm) to examine entire length of vagina.
- Cytologic examination, bacterial culture—may reveal inflammatory process (e.g., uterine infection): use guarded swab to ensure anterior sample (distal reproductive tract is heavily contaminated with bacteria), or collect secretions by transcervical catheterization.

PATHOLOGIC FINDINGS

Histopathologic examination and culture of fetal and placental tissue—may reveal infectious organisms; tissue culture, particularly of stomach contents, may identify infectious bacteria.

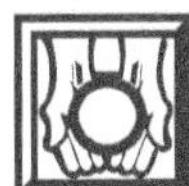

TREATMENT

APPROPRIATE HEALTH CARE

- Most bitches should be isolated pending diagnosis.
- Hospitalization of infectious patients preferred.
- *B. canis*—highly infective; shed in high numbers during abortion; suspected dogs should be isolated.
- Outpatient—medically stable patients with noninfectious pregnancy loss.
- Partial abortion—attempt to salvage live fetuses; antibiotics indicated if bacterial component.

NURSING CARE

Dehydration—isotonic crystalloid fluids, electrolyte supplementation as indicated.

ACTIVITY

Partial abortion—cage rest, but effect on reducing further abortion unknown.

DIET

No special considerations; abortions have been associated with raw diets.

CLIENT EDUCATION

- Critical for *B. canis*—if confirmed, euthanasia recommended due to lack of successful treatment and to prevent spread; may try ovariohysterectomy (OHE) and long-term antibiotics with surveillance program for kennel situations (monthly serology, culling any positive animals until three consecutive negative tests are obtained); discuss zoonotic potential.
- Primary uterine disease—OHE is indicated in nonbreeding patients; cystic endometrial hyperplasia (CEH) is irreversible.
- Infertility or pregnancy loss—may recur in subsequent estrous cycles despite successful immediate treatment; pedigree analysis may be beneficial in highly linebred animals if pregnancy loss and small litter size due to inbreeding depression.
- Prostaglandin treatment—discuss side effects (e.g., abortion).
- Infectious disease—establish surveillance and control measures.

SURGICAL CONSIDERATIONS

OHE preferred for stable nonbreeding patients.

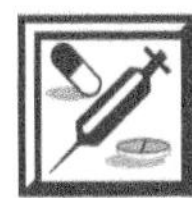

MEDICATIONS

DRUG(S) OF CHOICE

- Prostaglandin F2α ($PGF_{2\alpha}$; Lutalyse®, dinoprost tromethamine)—uterine evacuation after abortion; 0.05–0.1 mg/kg SC q8–24h; cloprostenol (Estrumate®, cloprostenol)—1–5 μg/kg SC q24h; not approved for use in dogs, but adequate documentation for use; use only if all living fetuses expelled.
- Antibiotics—broad-spectrum agent appropriate pending culture and sensitivity of vaginal tissue or fetus.
- Progesterone (altrenogest) at 0.088 mg/kg (1 mL/25 kg PO q24h); progesterone in oil at 2 mg/kg IM q48–72h; progesterone (Prometrium®; 10 mg/kg PO q24h, adjust daily dosage based on serum progesterone)—for documented hypoluteoidism only to maintain pregnancy; must have accurate due date to know when to discontinue therapy; inadvertently prolonging gestation results in fetal death.

CONTRAINDICATIONS

Progestogen supplementation contraindicated with endometrial or mammary gland disease.

PRECAUTIONS

- $PGF_{2\alpha}$—dose-related side effects related to smooth muscle contraction, diminish with each injection; panting, salivation, vomiting, and defecation common; caution in brachycephalics; dosing critical (LD_{50} for dinoprost—5 mg/kg).
- Progesterone supplementation will prevent whelping—administration needs to be discontinued before 2–3 days prior to due date; risk of masculinization of female fetuses if used before day 45 of gestation.

ALTERNATIVE DRUG(S)

Oxytocin—1 U/5 kg SC q6–24h for uterine evacuation; consider only where uterine evacuation solely through uterine contraction desired.

FOLLOW-UP

PATIENT MONITORING

- Partial abortion—monitor viability of remaining fetuses with ultrasonography; monitor systemic health of dam for rest of pregnancy.
- Vulvar discharges—daily; for decreasing amount, odor, and inflammatory component; for consistency (increasing mucoid content prognostically good).
- $PGF_{2\alpha}$—continued for 5 days or until most of discharge ceases (range 3–15 days).
- *B. canis*—monitor after neutering and antibiotic therapy; yearly serologic testing (identify recrudescence).
- Hypothyroidism—see Hypothyroidism.

PREVENTION/AVOIDANCE

- Brucellosis, other infectious agents—surveillance programs to prevent spread to kennel.
- OHE—for nonbreeding bitches.
- Use of modified-live vaccines (e.g., some distemper, parvovirus), currently unavailable in United States.

POSSIBLE COMPLICATIONS

- Untreated pyometra—septicemia, death.
- Brucellosis—discospondylitis, endophthalmitis, uveitis, zoonotic.

EXPECTED COURSE AND PROGNOSIS

- Pyometra—recurrence during subsequent cycle likely (up to 70%) unless pregnant.
- CEH—recovery of fertility unlikely; pyometra common complication.
- Hormonal dysfunction—manageable; heritability should be considered.
- Brucellosis—guarded; extremely difficult to eliminate infection even with neutering.

MISCELLANEOUS

AGE-RELATED FACTORS

Older bitches more likely to have CEH.

ZOONOTIC POTENTIAL

B. canis—can be transmitted to humans (especially if immunosuppressed), particularly when handling bitch and expelled tissues. Notify pathologists if *B. canis* is suspected.

SEE ALSO

- Brucellosis.
- Hypothyroidism.
- Infertility, Female—Dogs.
- Premature Labor.
- Pyometra.

ABBREVIATIONS

- CEH = cystic endometrial hyperplasia.
- OHE = ovariohysterectomy.
- $PGF_{2\alpha}$ = prostaglandin $F_{2\alpha}$.

Suggested Reading

Verstegen J, Dhaliwal G, Verstegen-Onclin K. Canine and feline pregnancy loss due to viral and non-infectious causes: a review. Theriogenology 2008, 70(3):304–319.

Author Julie T. Cecere

Consulting Editor Erin E. Runcan

Client Education Handout available online

ABORTION, TERMINATION OF PREGNANCY

BASICS

DEFINITION

Termination of an unwanted pregnancy. May be accomplished by drugs that alter embryo transport in the oviduct, impeding establishment of a pregnancy, and/or cause luteal regression, terminating an established pregnancy. Due to their possible side effects (cystic endometrial hyperplasia, aplastic anemia, and bone marrow suppression), drugs that impair embryonic transit through the oviduct (estrogens) are not commonly used or recommended.

PATHOPHYSIOLOGY

After fertilization the embryo travels the oviduct in a timely manner before entering the uterus. Impaired embryo transport through the oviduct leads to embryonic degeneration and implantation abnormalities. In the dog and cat, pregnancy maintenance is dependent on progesterone production from the corpora lutea. In dogs and cats, maintenance of the corpora lutea during the second half of gestation is also supported by prolactin (PRL). Drugs that cause luteal regression, antagonize PRL, and/or compete with progesterone receptors will terminate pregnancy.

SYSTEMS AFFECTED

- Cardiovascular.
- Digestive.
- Neurologic (caused by drugs used for treatment).
- Reproductive.
- Respiratory.

GENETICS

N/A

INCIDENCE/PREVALENCE

N/A

GEOGRAPHIC DISTRIBUTION

N/A

SIGNALMENT

Species

Dog and cat.

Breed Predilections

N/A

Mean Age and Range

Postpubertal bitch and queen.

Predominant Sex

Female

SIGNS

- Depends on stage of gestation:
  - None.
  - Vaginal discharge.
  - Fetal expulsion.

CAUSES

- Impaired oviductal transport.
- Luteal regression.
- Progesterone receptor antagonism.

RISK FACTORS

N/A

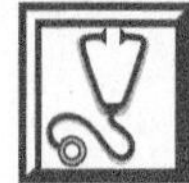

DIAGNOSIS

- Confirm pregnancy first, ~60% of mismated bitches do not become pregnant:
  - Abdominal palpation—bitch: 31–33 days after luteinizing hormone (LH) surge; queen: 21–25 days after breeding.
  - Transabdominal ultrasound—bitch: >25 days after LH surge; queen: >16 days after breeding.
  - Abdominal radiographs—bitch: >45 days after LH surge; queen: >38 days after breeding.
  - Serum relaxin concentration in the bitch (>28 days after LH surge; Witness® Relaxin, Synbiotics/Zoetis).

DIFFERENTIAL DIAGNOSIS

- Hydrometra.
- Mucometra.
- Hematometra.
- Pyometra.
- Pseudopregnancy.

CBC/BIOCHEMISTRY/URINALYSIS

- Within normal limits during first half of pregnancy in healthy patients.
- Decrease in hematocrit during second half of pregnancy in bitches and queens is normal.
- Recommended as screening tests prior to treatment in patients with suspected underlying disease.

OTHER LABORATORY TESTS

- Vaginal cytology—determines stage of estrous cycle and presence of sperm (absence does not rule out previous breeding).
- Serum progesterone concentration determines if female in diestrus and monitors luteal regression during treatment.

IMAGING

- Transabdominal ultrasound (method of choice)—diagnose pregnancy and monitor uterine evacuation during treatment.
- Abdominal radiographs.

DIAGNOSTIC PROCEDURES

N/A

PATHOLOGIC FINDINGS

N/A

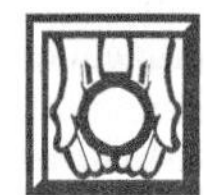

TREATMENT

APPROPRIATE HEALTH CARE

- Physical examination before initiation of treatment.
- Monitor 30–60 minutes after treatment for side effects (vomiting, defecation, hypersalivation, hyperpnea, micturition, tachycardia).
- Pregnancy status in early diestrus is unknown; ultrasound confirmation of pregnancy not possible until ~4 weeks after breeding.
- Treatment on day 6–10 of diestrus—may have reduced efficacy compared to mid-gestation, but can be less distasteful to client (less discharge and recognizable fetuses are not passed).
- Multimodal treatment improves efficacy of drugs given alone.

NURSING CARE

N/A

ACTIVITY

Normal

DIET

Avoid feeding prior to each treatment and for 1–2 hours after treatments (reduces nausea and vomiting).

CLIENT EDUCATION

- Discuss patient's reproductive future with owner. If no litters are desired, then ovario-hysterectomy (OHE) is the best option.
- Discuss with client potential side effects of treatment options; reach mutual agreement on treatment plan.

SURGICAL CONSIDERATIONS

OHE recommended for patients with no reproductive value or when owners do not desire future litters.

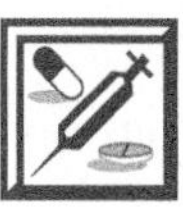

MEDICATIONS

DRUG(S) OF CHOICE

- Confirmation of pregnancy before initiating any of treatment protocols suggested below is recommended. Duration of suggested treatment may vary; treatments should be continued until abortion is complete.
- Prostaglandin $F_{2\alpha}$ ($PGF_{2\alpha}$)—causes luteal regression with subsequent decline in progesterone concentration, cervical relaxation, and uterine contractions. Higher doses necessary prior to day 28 of gestation.
  - Bitch low dose protocol—10 µg/kg SC q6h for 7–10 days or until pregnancy termination.
  - Bitch standard dose protocol—100 µg/kg SC q8h for 2 days, then 200 µg/kg SC q8h until pregnancy termination.
  - Queen low dose protocol—25 µg/kg SC q6h for 1–2 days, then 50 µg/kg SC q6h for 3–4 days (queen more resistant to luteolytic effects of $PGF_{2\alpha}$ than bitches; often higher doses for longer periods are required).
  - Queen standard protocol—0.5–1 mg/kg SC q12h every other day (>day 40), or 2 mg/cat SC q24h for 5 days (>day 33).
- Cloprostenol (prostaglandin analogue):
  - Bitch—2.5 µg/kg SC q8–12h every 48 hours until pregnancy termination (~6 days after start of treatment).
- Dexamethasone—mode of action unknown:
  - Bitch—0.2 mg/kg PO q8–12h for 5 days, then decreasing incrementally from

0.16 to 0.02 mg/kg over last 5 days; treatment failures not uncommon.

- Cabergoline (PRL antagonist)—causes luteal regression:
    - Bitch—1.65 µg/kg SC q24h for 5 days or 5 µg/kg PO q24h for 5 days (>day 40).
    - Queen—1.65 µg/kg SC for 5 days (>day 30) or 5 µg/kg PO q24h for 5 days (>day 35).
- Bromocriptine (PRL antagonist)—causes luteal regression:
    - Bitch—50–100 µg/kg IM/PO q12h for 4–7 days >day 35 (50% effective); common side effect vomiting; reduce dose and give with meal.
- Cloprostenol and cabergoline combination:
    - Bitch—cabergoline 5 µg/kg PO q24h for 10 days plus cloprostenol 2.5 µg/kg SC at start of treatment or 1 µg/kg SC at start of treatment and at day 5 of treatment; treatment should be initiated >28 days post-LH surge.
    - Queen—cabergoline 5 µg/kg PO q24h plus cloprostenol 5 µg/kg SC q48h (>30 days after breeding) until abortion complete (~9 days).
- Cloprostenol and bromocriptine combination:
    - Bitch—bromocriptine 30 µg/kg PO q8h for 10 days plus cloprostenol 2.5 µg/kg SC or 1 µg/kg SC at start of treatment and at day 5 of treatment; treatment should be initiated >28 days post-LH surge.

CONTRAINDICATIONS

- $PGF_{2\alpha}$ and analogues—animals with respiratory disease (bronchoconstriction); do not administer intravenously. Use with caution in brachycephalic breeds.
- Cabergoline and bromocriptine—avoid administration in animals hypersensitive to ergot alkaloids; use with caution in patients with impaired liver function.
- Estrogens may cause cystic endometrial hyperplasia (CEH), pyometra, and bone marrow suppression leading to pancytopenia.

PRECAUTIONS

- $PGF_{2\alpha}$ and analogues—side effects dose dependent and include vomiting, defecation, dyspnea, tachycardia, salivation, restlessness, and anxiety; side effects subside within 60 minutes; use extreme caution in dogs and cats with preexisting cardiopulmonary, liver, and renal diseases.
- Dexamethasone—polydipsia, polyuria, and polyphagia are reported side effects; long-term administration can result in signs of hyperadrenocorticism.
- Cabergoline and bromocriptine—should be administered with caution in patients with impaired liver function; side effects may include vomiting and anorexia; prolonged use (>2 weeks) may cause coat color changes.

POSSIBLE INTERACTIONS

- $PGF_{2\alpha}$ and analogues—effect may be reduced by concomitant administration of progestins; use may enhance effects of oxytocin.
- Cabergoline and bromocriptine—cabergoline effects may be reduced with concomitant treatment with dopamine (D_2) antagonists; avoid concomitant treatment with drugs causing hypotension.

ALTERNATIVE DRUG(S)

- The following drugs are recommended for use in bitches but are not readily available in the United States:
    - Aglepristone (progestin and glucocorticoid receptors antagonist)—10 mg/kg SC q24h for 2 days >14 days post-LH surge; highly effective in preventing pregnancy (>95% treatment efficacy); abdominal ultrasound at 28–30 days essential to insure treatment success; if pregnancy still present, repeat injection protocol. Mild reactions at injection site have been reported; mild vaginal discharge may be observed; slight risk (3.4%) of development of pyometra in field studies.
    - Aglepristone and cloprostenol combination—aglepristone (10 mg/kg SC) combined with cloprostenol (1 µg/kg SC) q24h for 2 days >25 days' pregnancy; pregnancy terminated within 6 days. Side effects after treatment include vomiting and diarrhea; vaginal discharge may be observed.
    - Aglepristone (10 mg/kg SC q24h for 2 days) with intravaginal misoprostol (200–400 µg depending on body size) daily until abortion complete; abortion complete within 7 days. Vomiting, diarrhea, polydipsia, anorexia not observed with this regimen.

FOLLOW-UP

PATIENT MONITORING

In animals treated with luteolytic drugs (prostaglandins and PRL antagonists), progesterone assays and transabdominal ultrasound examinations should be performed to monitor decrease of serum progesterone concentration and complete evacuation of uterine contents. In patients treated with progesterone receptor antagonist drugs, transabdominal ultrasound examinations are recommended to monitor complete evacuation of the uterus.

PREVENTION/AVOIDANCE

- OHE for bitches and queens not intended for breeding.
- Estrus suppression or confinement of bitches and queens intended for breeding during a later cycle to avoid mismating.

POSSIBLE COMPLICATIONS

Pregnancy termination may not be achieved after one treatment protocol and continuation or change in treatment protocol may be necessary.

EXPECTED COURSE AND PROGNOSIS

- Interestrous interval in bitches treated with prostaglandins and PRL inhibitors may be shortened (~1 month). Queens may resume estrous behavior 7–10 days after pregnancy termination.
- Subsequent estrus fertility not affected.

MISCELLANEOUS

ASSOCIATED CONDITIONS

N/A

AGE-RELATED FACTORS

N/A

ZOONOTIC POTENTIAL

N/A

PREGNANCY/FERTILITY/BREEDING

N/A

SYNONYMS

Induced abortion.

SEE ALSO

Breeding, Timing.

ABBREVIATIONS

- CEH = cystic endometrial hyperplasia.
- LH = luteinizing hormone.
- OHE = ovariohysterectomy.
- $PGF_{2\alpha}$ = prostaglandin $F_{2\alpha}$.
- PRL = prolactin.

Suggested Reading

Eilts BE. Pregnancy termination in the bitch and queen. Clin Tech Small Anim Pract 2002, 17:116–123.

Fieni F, Dumon C, Tainturier D, Bruyas JF. Clinical protocol for pregnancy termination in bitches using prostaglandin $F_{2\alpha}$. J Reprod Fertil Suppl 1997, 51:245–250.

Author Jose A. Len

Consulting Editor Erin E. Runcan

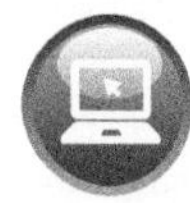

Client Education Handout available online

A

ABSCESSATION

BASICS

DEFINITION

An abscess is a focal collection of purulent exudate within a confined tissue space or cavity.

PATHOPHYSIOLOGY

- Bacterial organisms may enter tissue by penetrating trauma, spread from another source of infection (hematogenous or adjacent infected tissues), or migration of a contaminated object (e.g., plant awn).
- Most often, bacteria are inoculated under the skin via puncture or bite wounds.
- When bacteria or foreign objects persist in tissue, purulent exudate accumulates.
- If exudate not quickly resorbed or drained, fibrous capsule forms to "wall off" infection; abscess may eventually rupture.
- With fibrous capsule—to heal, the cavity must fill with granulation tissue from which causative agent may not be totally eliminated; may lead to chronic or intermittent discharge of exudate from a draining tract.
- Sterile abscesses can occur when irritants (injectable medications, venom) or inflammatory processes (pancreatitis, immune mediated, decreased blood supply) lead to local collection of purulent exudate.

SYSTEMS AFFECTED

- Skin/exocrine—percutaneous (cats > dogs); anal sac (dogs > cats).
- Reproductive—prostate gland (dogs > cats); mammary gland.
- Ophthalmic—periorbital tissues.
- Hepatobiliary—liver parenchyma.
- Gastrointestinal—pancreas (dogs > cats).
- Respiratory—pulmonary parenchyma.

GENETICS

N/A

INCIDENCE/PREVALENCE

N/A

GEOGRAPHIC DISTRIBUTION

N/A

SIGNALMENT

Species

Cat and dog.

Breed Predilections

N/A

Mean Age and Range

N/A

Predominant Sex

Mammary glands (female); prostate gland (male).

SIGNS

General Comments

- Determined by organ system and/or tissue affected.
- Associated with combination of inflammation (pain, swelling, redness, heat, and loss of function), tissue destruction, and/or organ system dysfunction caused by accumulation of exudates.

Historical Findings

- Often nonspecific signs (e.g., lethargy, anorexia).
- History of trauma or prior infection.
- Rapidly appearing painful swelling with or without discharge, if affected area is visible.

Physical Examination Findings

- Determined by organ system or tissue affected.
- Classic signs of inflammation (heat, pain, swelling, and loss of function) associated with specific anatomic location of abscess.
- Inflammation and discharge from fistulous tract may be visible if abscess has ruptured to an external surface.
- Variably sized, painful mass of fluctuant to firm consistency attached to surrounding tissues.
- Fever common, but may be absent if abscess has ruptured.
- Sepsis or infection of body cavity (e.g., pyothorax) may be seen if abscess ruptures internally.

CAUSES

- Foreign objects.
- Pyogenic bacteria—*Staphylococcus* spp., *Escherichia coli*, β-hemolytic *Streptococcus* spp., *Pseudomonas*, *Mycoplasma* and *Mycoplasma*-like organisms (l-forms), *Pasteurella multocida*, *Corynebacterium*, *Actinomyces* spp., *Nocardia*, *Bartonella*.
- Obligate anaerobes—*Bacteroides* spp., *Clostridium* spp., *Peptostreptococcus*, *Fusobacterium*.
- Noninfectious—pancreatitis, suture reaction, vaccination, other injectable drug administration, stinging insects, snake envenomation, immune-mediated panniculitis, dermatitis, neoplasia (especially when blood supply outgrown).

RISK FACTORS

- Anal sac—impaction, anal sacculitis.
- Brain—otitis interna, sinusitis, oral infection.
- Liver—omphalophlebitis, sepsis.
- Lung—foreign object aspiration or migration, bacterial pneumonia.
- Mammary gland—mastitis.
- Periorbital—dental disease, chewing of wood or other plant material.
- Percutaneous—fighting, trauma, or surgery.
- Prostate gland—bacterial prostatitis.
- Immunosuppression—feline leukemia virus (FeLV) or feline immunodeficiency virus (FIV) infection, immunosuppressive chemotherapy, acquired or inherited immune system dysfunctions, underlying predisposing disease (e.g., diabetes mellitus, chronic renal failure, hyperadrenocorticism).

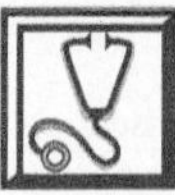

DIAGNOSIS

DIFFERENTIAL DIAGNOSIS

Mass Lesions

- Cyst—transiently painful, slower growing, no overt signs of inflammation.
- Fibrous scar tissue—firm, nonpainful.
- Granuloma—less painful, slower growing, firmer without fluctuant center.
- Hematoma/seroma—variable pain, nonencapsulated, rapid initial growth but slows once full size attained, fluctuant initially, may become more firm over time.
- Neoplasia—variable growth, variable pain.

Draining Tracts

- Fungal infection—blastomycosis, coccidioidomycosis, cryptococcosis, histoplasmosis, sporotrichosis.
- Mycobacterial disease.
- Mycetoma—botryomycosis, actinomycotic mycetoma, eumycotic mycetoma.
- Neoplasia.
- Phaeohyphomycosis.

CBC/BIOCHEMISTRY/URINALYSIS

- CBC—normal, neutrophilia with or without left shift, neutropenia and degenerative left shift (severe infection).
- Serum chemistry profile—depends on severity, system affected. Signs of cholestasis if pancreatic abscess causes obstruction, hyperglycemia if diabetes mellitus, etc.
- Urinalysis—pyuria (prostatic abscess).

OTHER LABORATORY TESTS

- FeLV, FIV testing—recurrent or slow-healing abscesses (cats).
- Cerebrospinal fluid evaluation—increased cellularity and protein with brain abscess.
- Adrenal function—hyperadrenocorticism.

IMAGING

- Radiography—soft-tissue density mass in affected area, may reveal foreign material.
- Ultrasonography—determine if mass is fluid filled; may reveal foreign object; echogenic fluid suggests purulent exudate.
- Echocardiography—pericardial abscess, endocarditis.
- CT or MRI—pulmonary or brain abscess.

DIAGNOSTIC PROCEDURES

Fine-Needle Aspiration

- Red, white, yellow, or greenish liquid.
- Protein content >2.5–3.0 g/dL.
- Nucleated cell count—3,000–100,000 (or more) cells/μL; primarily degenerate neutrophils, fewer macrophages, lymphocytes.
- Bacteria—intra- and extracellular:
    - Gram stain to classify organism for empiric therapy.
    - If causative agent not readily identified with a Romanowsky-type stain, acid-fast

stain to detect mycobacteria or *Nocardia* and periodic acid-Schiff stain to detect fungus.

Biopsy

- Sample should contain both normal and abnormal tissue.
- Impression smears.
- Tissue—for histopathologic examination and culture.
- Necessary to confirm nodular panniculitis.

Culture and Susceptibility Testing

- Affected tissue and/or exudate—aerobic and anaerobic bacterial and fungal.
- Blood and/or urine if systemic disease.

PATHOLOGIC FINDINGS

- Exudate-containing mass lesion accompanied by inflammation.
- Causative agent may be detectable.

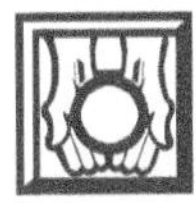

TREATMENT

APPROPRIATE HEALTH CARE

- Establish and maintain adequate drainage.
- Surgical removal of nidus of infection or foreign object(s) if necessary.
- Initiate appropriate antimicrobial therapy.
- Outpatient—minor abscesses, localized infection, nodular panniculitis.
- Inpatient—sepsis or systemic inflammation, extensive surgical procedures, treatment requiring hospitalization.

NURSING CARE

- Depends on location of abscess.
- Apply hot packs to inflamed area as needed.
- Use protective bandaging, Elizabethan collar as needed.
- Accumulated exudate—surgical drainage, debridement of necrotic tissue.
- Sepsis, peritonitis, pyothorax—fluid therapy, antimicrobial therapy, intensive care.

ACTIVITY

Restrict until abscess has resolved and adequate healing occurs.

DIET

N/A

CLIENT EDUCATION

- Correct or prevent risk factors.
- Maintain adequate drainage and continue antimicrobial therapy for adequate period of time.

SURGICAL CONSIDERATIONS

- Appropriate debridement and drainage—may need to leave wound open to external surface; may need drain placement.
  - Penrose drains must exit ventrally to encourage drainage; may be bandaged, if bandage is changed regularly.
  - If no ventral drainage, use active drains (e.g., Jackson-Pratt drain).
- Early drainage—to prevent further tissue damage and abscess wall formation.
- Remove foreign objects(s), necrotic tissue, nidus of infection.
- Complications to discuss include progressive tissue damage, necrosis, dehiscence of wound, prolonged healing times in high-motion areas (axillary, inguinal).

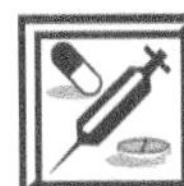

MEDICATIONS

DRUG(S) OF CHOICE

- Antimicrobial drugs that are effective against infectious agent and penetrate site of infection.
- Broad-spectrum agent—bactericidal with both aerobic and anaerobic activity until results of culture and sensitivity are known; Gram stain of exudate may guide therapy.
  - Dogs and cats—amoxicillin (22 mg/kg PO q12h); amoxicillin–clavulanic acid (22 mg/kg PO q12h); clindamycin (5–10 mg/kg PO q12h); trimethoprim–sulfadiazine (15 mg/kg PO q12h).
  - Cats only—pradofloxacin (7.5 mg/kg PO q24 for 7 days).
  - Cats with *Mycoplasma* and L-forms—doxycycline (5 mg/kg PO q12h).
- Aggressive IV antimicrobial therapy—sepsis, peritonitis, pyothorax.
- Antimicrobials not required for confirmed sterile abscesses.

CONTRAINDICATIONS

N/A

PRECAUTIONS

N/A

POSSIBLE INTERACTIONS

N/A

ALTERNATIVE DRUG(S)

Sterile nodular panniculitis—corticosteroids.

FOLLOW-UP

PATIENT MONITORING

Monitor for progressive decrease in drainage, resolution of inflammation, and improvement of clinical signs.

PREVENTION/AVOIDANCE

- Percutaneous abscesses—prevent fighting; consider castration to reduce roaming or aggressive behavior.
- Anal sac abscesses—prevent impaction; consider anal saculectomy for recurrent cases.
- Prostatic abscesses—consider castration.
- Mastitis—prevent lactation (spay).
- Periorbital abscesses—do not allow chewing on foreign objects.

POSSIBLE COMPLICATIONS

- Sepsis.
- Peritonitis/pleuritis if intra-abdominal or intrathoracic abscess ruptures.
- Compromise of organ function.
- Delayed evacuation may lead to chronic, draining fistulous tracts.

EXPECTED COURSE AND PROGNOSIS

Depends on cause, organ system involved, and amount of tissue destruction.

MISCELLANEOUS

ASSOCIATED CONDITIONS

- FeLV or FIV infection.
- Immunosuppression.

AGE-RELATED FACTORS

N/A

ZOONOTIC POTENTIAL

- Mycobacteria and systemic fungal infections carry some potential.
- If prostatitis secondary to *Brucella canis*.

PREGNANCY/FERTILITY/BREEDING

N/A

SEE ALSO

- Actinomycosis and Nocardia.
- Anaerobic Infections.
- Colibacillosis.
- Mycoplasmosis.
- Nocardiosis/Actinomycosis—Cutaneous.
- Sepsis and Bacteremia.

ABBREVIATIONS

- FeLV = feline leukemia virus.
- FIV = feline immunodeficiency virus.

Suggested Reading

Green CE, Goldstein EJC. Bite wound infections. In: Greene CE, ed., Infectious Diseases of the Dog and Cat, 4th ed. St. Louis, MO: Elsevier Saunders, 2012, pp. 528–542.

Singh A, Scott Weese J. Wound infections and antimicrobial use. In: Johnston SA, Tobias KM, eds., Veterinary Surgery Small Animal, 2nd ed. St. Louis, MO: Elsevier, 2018, pp. 148–155.

Author Selena Lane

Consulting Editor Amie Koenig

Acknowledgment The author and editors acknowledge the prior contribution of Adam J. Birkenheuer.

Client Education Handout available online

ACETAMINOPHEN (APAP) TOXICOSIS

BASICS

DEFINITION

Results from accidental animal ingestion or owner administration of over-the-counter acetaminophen-containing analgesic and antipyretic medications.

PATHOPHYSIOLOGY

When the normal biotransformation mechanisms for detoxification (glucuronidation and sulfation) are saturated, cytochrome P450–mediated oxidation produces a toxic metabolite (*N*-acetyl-p-benzoquinone imine) that is electrophilic, conjugates with glutathione, and binds to sulfhydryl groups, leading to hepatic necrosis.

Dogs

- Liver is most susceptible to toxicity.
- Signs commonly observed at exposures >75–100 mg/kg.
- Methemoglobinemia may develop at doses >200 mg/kg.

Cats

- Cannot effectively glucuronidate; more limited capacity for acetaminophen elimination than dogs.
- Saturate glucuronidation and sulfation biotransformation routes.
- Red blood cells (RBCs) are most susceptible to oxidative injury following glutathione depletion.
- Develop toxic cytochrome P450 metabolite at much lower doses than dogs.
- Poisoned by as little as 50–60 mg/kg (often as little as one half tablet); deacetylation of acetaminophen to p-aminophenol (PAP) causes oxidative damage to RBCs, rapidly producing methemoglobinemia by binding to sulfhydryl groups on hemoglobin.
- Slower-developing hepatotoxicosis may not be fully expressed before development of fatal methemoglobinemia.

SYSTEMS AFFECTED

- Hemic/lymph/immune—RBCs damaged by glutathione depletion, allowing oxidation of hemoglobin to methemoglobin.
- Hepatobiliary—liver necrosis (more common in dogs).
- Cardiovascular (primarily cats)—edema of face, paws, and (to lesser degree) forelimbs through undefined mechanism.

GENETICS

Cats—genetic deficiency in the glucuronide conjugation pathway makes them vulnerable.

INCIDENCE/PREVALENCE

Common drug toxicity in cats; less frequent in dogs.

GEOGRAPHIC DISTRIBUTION

N/A

SIGNALMENT

Species

Cats more often than dogs.

SIGNS

General Comments

Relatively common—owing to widespread human use.

Historical Findings

- Depression.
- Hyperventilation.
- Darkened mucous membranes.
- Signs may develop 1–4 hours after dosing.

Physical Examination Findings

- Progressive depression.
- Salivation.
- Vomiting.
- Abdominal pain.
- Tachypnea and cyanosis or muddy mucous membranes—reflect methemoglobinemia.
- Edema—face, paws, and possibly forelimbs; after several hours.
- Chocolate-colored urine—hematuria and methemoglobinuria; especially in cats.
- Icterus.
- Hypothermia.
- Shock.
- Death.

CAUSES

Acetaminophen toxicosis.

RISK FACTORS

- Nutritional deficiencies of glucose and/or sulfate.
- Simultaneous administration of other glutathione-depressing drugs.

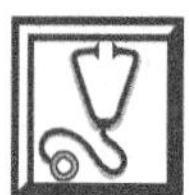

DIAGNOSIS

DIFFERENTIAL DIAGNOSIS

Other Causes of Liver Injury

- Hepatotoxic mushrooms.
- Blue-green algae.
- Aflatoxins.
- Iron, copper, zinc.
- Xylitol.
- Cycad palms.
- Nonsteroidal anti-inflammatory drugs (NSAIDs).

Other Causes of Methemoglobinemia

- Onions/garlic.
- Naphthalene.
- Chlorates.
- Nitrites.
- Sulfites.
- Phenol.
- Benzocaine.
- Propylene glycol (cats).

CBC/BIOCHEMISTRY/URINALYSIS

- Methemoglobinemia and progressively rising serum concentrations of liver enzymes (alanine aminotransferase [ALT], aspartate transaminase [AST])—characteristic.
- As hepatic function becomes impaired—decreased blood urea nitrogen (BUN), cholesterol, and albumin, and increased serum bilirubin.
- Heinz bodies (cats)—prominent in RBCs within 72 hours.
- Anemia, hemoglobinemia, and hemoglobinuria or hematuria.

OTHER LABORATORY TESTS

Acetaminophen plasma, serum, or urine concentrations.

IMAGING

N/A

DIAGNOSTIC PROCEDURES

N/A

PATHOLOGIC FINDINGS

- Methemoglobinemia.
- Pulmonary edema.
- Centrilobular necrosis and congestion of the liver.
- Renal tubular edema and degeneration with proteinaceous tubular casts.

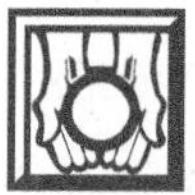

TREATMENT

APPROPRIATE HEALTH CARE

- With methemoglobinemia—must evaluate promptly.
- With dark or bloody colored urine or icterus—inpatient.

NURSING CARE

- Gentle handling—imperative for clinically affected patients.
- Induced emesis and gastric lavage—useful within 4–6 hours of ingestion.
- Anemia, hematuria, or hemoglobinuria—may require whole blood transfusion.
- Fluid therapy—maintain hydration and electrolyte balance.
- Oxygen therapy may be needed.
- Drinking water—available at all times.
- Food—offered 24 hours after initiation of treatment.

ACTIVITY

Restricted

DIET

N/A

CLIENT EDUCATION

- Warn client that treatment in clinically affected patients may be prolonged and expensive.
- Inform client that patients with liver injury may require prolonged and costly management.

SURGICAL CONSIDERATIONS

N/A

MEDICATIONS

DRUG(S) OF CHOICE

- Activated charcoal 1–2 g/kg PO with a cathartic; immediately after completion of emesis or gastric lavage.
- *N*-acetylcysteine (Mucomyst®) 140 mg/kg diluted in 5% dextrose injection (D5W) as loading dose PO/IV; then 70 mg/kg diluted in D5W PO/IV q6h for 7 additional treatments. Large overdoses may require up to 17 treatments.
- S-adenosylmethionine (SAMe) as a glutathione donor; 40 mg/kg PO × 1 dose, then 20 mg/kg q24h PO × 7 days.
- Added benefit of using methylene blue, cimetidine, and/or ascorbic acid is controversial.

CONTRAINDICATIONS

Drugs that contribute to methemoglobinemia or hepatotoxicity.

PRECAUTIONS

Drugs requiring extensive liver metabolism or biotransformation—use with caution; expect their half-lives to be extended.

POSSIBLE INTERACTIONS

Drugs requiring activation or metabolism by the liver have reduced effectiveness.

FOLLOW-UP

PATIENT MONITORING

- Continual clinical monitoring of methemoglobinemia—vital for effective management; laboratory determination of methemoglobin percentage every 2–3 hours.
- Serum liver enzyme activities (ALT, ALP) every 12 hours; monitor liver damage.

PREVENTION/AVOIDANCE

- Never give acetaminophen to cats.
- Give careful attention to acetaminophen dose in dogs.

POSSIBLE COMPLICATIONS

Liver necrosis and resulting fibrosis—may compromise long-term liver function in recovered patients.

EXPECTED COURSE AND PROGNOSIS

- Rapidly progressive methemoglobinemia—serious sign.
- Methemoglobin concentrations ≥50%—grave prognosis.
- Progressively rising serum liver enzymes 12–24 hours after ingestion—serious concern.
- Expect clinical signs to persist 12–48 hours; death owing to methemoglobinemia possible at any time.
- Dogs and cats receiving prompt treatment that reverses methemoglobinemia and prevents excessive liver necrosis—may recover fully.
- Dogs—death as a result of liver necrosis may occur within 72 hours.
- Cats—death as a result of methemoglobinemia occurs 18–36 hours after ingestion.

MISCELLANEOUS

ASSOCIATED CONDITIONS

Keratoconjunctivitis sicca may develop in small-breed dogs as a sequela.

AGE-RELATED FACTORS

Young and small dogs and cats—greater risk from owner-given single-dose acetaminophen medications.

PREGNANCY/FERTILITY/BREEDING

Imposes additional stress and higher risk on exposed animals.

SYNONYMS

- Paracetamol.
- Tylenol®.

SEE ALSO

Poisoning (Intoxication) Therapy.

ABBREVIATIONS

- ALT = alanine aminotransferase.
- AST = aspartate transaminase.
- BUN = blood urea nitrogen.
- D5W = 5% dextrose injection.
- NSAID = nonsteroidal anti-inflammatory drug.
- PAP = p-aminophenol.
- RBC = red blood cell.
- SAMe = S-adenosylmethionine.

INTERNET RESOURCES

https://www.aspca.org/pet-care/animal-poison-control

Suggested Reading

Plumb DC. Acetaminophen. In: Plumb DC, ed., Plumb's Veterinary Drug Handbook, 9th ed. Ames, IA: Wiley-Blackwell, 2018, pp. 6–8.

Plumlee KH. Hematic system. In: Plumlee KH, ed., Clinical Veterinary Toxicology. St. Louis, MO: Mosby, 2004, p. 59.

Schell MM, Gwaltney-Brant S. OTC drugs. In: Poppenga RH, Gwaltney-Brant SM, eds., Small Animal Toxicology Essentials. Chichester: Wiley-Blackwell, 2011, pp. 231–233.

Sellon RK. Acetaminophen. In: Peterson ME, Talcott PA, eds. Small Animal Toxicology, 3rd ed. St. Louis, MO: Elsevier, 2013, pp. 423–429.

Stockham SL, Scott MA. Fundamentals of Veterinary Clinical Pathology, 2nd ed. Oxford: Blackwell, 2008, p. 186.

Author Lisa A. Murphy

Consulting Editor Lynn R. Hovda

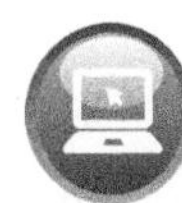

Client Education Handout available online

A

ACIDOSIS, METABOLIC

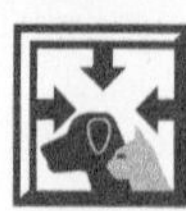

BASICS

DEFINITION

A process in the body that leads to a decrease in pH below the reference interval. A decline in blood pH is specifically termed acidemia. Associated with a decrease in plasma bicarbonate concentration (HCO_3^- ; dogs, <18 mEq/L; cats, <16 mEq/L) and base excess (BE; –4 mmol/L) with a compensatory decrease in carbon dioxide tension (PCO_2).

PATHOPHYSIOLOGY

- Metabolic acidosis may develop either from a *loss of* HCO_3^- (hyperchloremic acidosis) or a *gain in acid* (high anion gap [AG] acidosis). It is usually secondary to an accumulation of metabolically produced strong anions (strong ion gap or high anion gap acidosis), accumulation of weak acids (hyperphosphatemia), corrected hyperchloremia (hyperchloremic acidosis), or as a compensatory mechanism for respiratory alkalosis.
- *High anion gap* acidosis—increase in the concentration of other strong anions through addition (e.g., ethylene glycol toxicity), excessive production (e.g., lactate produced by prolonged anaerobic metabolism), or renal retention (e.g., renal failure) of strong anions other than Cl^- causes metabolic acidosis without increasing Cl^- concentration (so-called normochloremic or high AG metabolic acidosis).
- *Hyperphosphatemic* acidosis—increase in plasma weak acids (e.g., inorganic phosphate) is associated with metabolic acidosis and increased AG. At a pH of 7.4, a 1 mg/dL increase in phosphate concentration is associated with a 0.58 mEq/L decrease in HCO_3^- and a 0.58 mEq/L increase in AG. Hyperphosphatemia commonly develops with decreased renal phosphorus excretion (e.g., renal failure, hypoparathyroidism), cellular lysis (e.g., tumor lysis syndrome, trauma, rhabdomyolysis), bone neoplasms (increased bone resorption), and hypervitaminosis D.
- *Hyperchloremic* acidosis—may be caused by Cl^- retention (e.g., renal failure, renal tubular acidosis) that typically occurs in response to HCO_3^- loss. Cl^- and HCO_3^- are reciprocally related; loss of HCO_3^- generally results in retention of Cl^-. Other mechanisms for hyperchloremic acidosis include excessive loss of Na^+ relative to Cl^- (e.g., diarrhea, Addison's) and administration of substances containing more Cl^- than Na^+ compared with normal extracellular fluid composition (e.g., administration of KCl, 0.9% NaCl). Acidemia is usually not severe in patients with hyperchloremic acidosis.

SYSTEMS AFFECTED

- Cardiovascular—fall in pH results in increase in sympathetic discharge, but simultaneously causes decrease in responsiveness of cardiac myocytes and vascular smooth muscle to effects of catecholamines. In mildly acidemic conditions (pH >7.2), effects of increased sympathetic stimulation predominate and result in mild increase in heart rate and cardiac output. More severe acidemia (pH <7.1), especially if acute, may decrease cardiac contractility and predispose heart to ventricular arrhythmias and ventricular fibrillation.
- Respiratory—increased hydrogen ion [H^+] stimulates peripheral and central chemoreceptors to increase alveolar ventilation; hyperventilation decreases PCO_2, which counters effects of low plasma HCO_3^- on pH. In dogs, a decrease of approximately 1 mmHg in PCO_2 is expected for each 1 mEq/L decrease in plasma HCO_3^-. Little known about compensation in cats, but appears to be almost nonexistent.
- Renal/urologic—kidneys increase net acid excretion, primarily by increasing excretion of NH_4^+ and Cl^-. This compensatory mechanism not very effective in cats.

SIGNALMENT

Any breed, age, or sex of dog and cat.

SIGNS

Historical Findings

Chronic disease processes that lead to metabolic acidosis (e.g., renal failure, diabetes mellitus, and hypoadrenocorticism), acute circulatory shock (hemorrhagic), exposure to toxins (e.g., ethylene glycol, salicylate, and paraldehyde), diarrhea, administration of carbonic anhydrase inhibitors (e.g., acetazolamide and dichlorphenamide).

PHYSICAL EXAMINATION FINDINGS

- Generally relate to underlying disease.
- Depression, stupor, seizures, and/or generalized muscle weakness in severely acidotic patients.
- Tachypnea in some patients results from compensatory increase in ventilation.
- Kussmaul's respiration, typically seen in human beings with metabolic acidosis, not commonly observed in dogs and cats.
- Vomiting and/or diarrhea.

CAUSES

Associated with Hyperchloremia (Hyperchloremic Metabolic Acidosis)

- Renal—renal tubular acidosis; carbonic anhydrase inhibitors.
- Gastrointestinal—diarrhea.
- Other: Cl^--rich fluids (e.g., 0.9% NaCl, KCl supplementation); total parenteral nutrition with cationic amino acids: lysine, arginine, and histidine; rapid correction of hypocapnia (chronic respiratory alkalosis); NH_4Cl or HCl.

Associated with Normochloremia (High Anion Gap Metabolic Acidosis)

- Renal—uremic acidosis, acute renal failure.
- Ketoacidosis—diabetic ketoacidosis, starvation, liver disease.
- Lactic acidosis—impaired perfusion, impaired carbohydrate metabolism.
- Toxins—ethylene glycol, salicylate, paraldehyde, methanol intoxication.
- Hyperphosphatemia (see Hyperphosphatemia)—raises AG. At a pH of 7.4, each 1 mg/dL increase in phosphate concentration is associated with a 0.58 mEq/L increase in AG.

RISK FACTORS

- Chronic renal failure, diabetes mellitus, and hypoadrenocorticism.
- Poor tissue perfusion or hypoxia—lactic acidosis.
- Tumor lysis syndrome or osteosarcoma—hyperphosphatemia.
- Trauma, snake envenomation, or malignant hyperthermia—rhabdomyolysis.

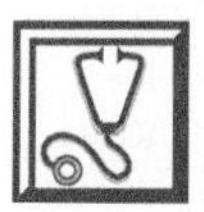

DIAGNOSIS

DIFFERENTIAL DIAGNOSIS

Low plasma HCO_3^- and hyperchloremia may also be compensatory in animals with chronic respiratory alkalosis, in which PCO_2 is low and pH is high or near normal, despite decreased HCO_3^- and increase in Cl^- concentration. Blood gas determination is required to differentiate.

LABORATORY FINDINGS

Drugs That May Alter Laboratory Results

Potassium bromide measured as Cl^- in most analyzers; administration artificially decreases AG.

Disorders That May Alter Laboratory Results

- Too much heparin (>10% of sample) decreases HCO_3^-.
- Blood samples stored at room temperature for >15 minutes have low pH because of increased PCO_2.
- Hypoalbuminemia lowers AG; negative charges of albumin are main component of AG.

Valid if Run in Human Laboratory?

Yes

CBC/BIOCHEMISTRY/URINALYSIS

- Low total CO_2—total CO_2 in serum samples handled aerobically closely approximates serum HCO_3^- concentration; unfortunately, patients with chronic respiratory alkalosis also have low total CO_2, and distinction cannot be made without blood gas analysis.
- Metabolic acidoses traditionally divided into hyperchloremic and high AG by means of AG. Anion gap, the difference between the measured cations and the measured anions, is calculated as AG = $[Na^+] - (HCO_3^- + [Cl^-])$ or AG = $([Na^+] + [K^+]) - (HCO_3^- + [Cl^-])$, depending on preference of clinician or laboratory. Normal values with potassium included in calculation usually 12–24 mEq/L

in dogs and 13–27 mEq/L in cats. Negative charges of albumin are major contributors to normal AG; this should be taken into account when evaluating AG in patients with hypoalbuminemia. At pH 7.4 in dogs, decrease of 1 g/dL in albumin associated with decrease of 4.1 mEq/L in AG.

- Normal AG (i.e., hyperchloremic metabolic acidosis).
- High AG (i.e., normochloremic metabolic acidosis).
- Hyperglycemia.
- Azotemia.
- Hyperphosphatemia.
- High lactate concentration.
- Hyperkalemia (*formulas to adjust potassium concentration based on pH changes should not be used*).

OTHER LABORATORY TESTS

Blood gas analysis reveals low HCO_3^-, low PCO_2, and low pH.

DIAGNOSTIC PROCEDURES

None

TREATMENT

- Acid-base disturbances are secondary phenomena; successful resolution depends on diagnosis and treatment of underlying disease process.
- Restore blood volume and perfusion deficits before considering sodium bicarbonate ($NaHCO_3$).
- Treat patients with blood pH ≤7.1 aggressively while pursuing definitive diagnosis.
- Discontinue drugs that may cause metabolic acidosis.
- Nursing care—isotonic, *buffered* electrolyte solution is fluid of choice for patients with mild metabolic acidosis and normal liver function.

MEDICATIONS

DRUG(S) OF CHOICE

- $NaHCO_3$ may help patients with hyperchloremic, hyperhosphatemic, or uremic acidosis, but not patients with lactic acidosis or diabetic ketoacidosis.
- $NaHCO_3$ may be considered for alkaline diuresis in salicylate toxicity. ◦ Estimation of HCO_3^- dose—dogs, 0.3 × body weight (kg) × (21 – patient HCO_3^-); cats, 0.3 × body weight (kg) × (19 – patient HCO_3^-). Give half of this dose slowly IV and reevaluate blood gases before deciding on need for additional administration. Empirical dose of 1–2 mEq/kg followed by reevaluation of blood gas status is safe in most patients. ◦ Potential complications of $NaHCO_3$ administration—volume overload resulting from administered Na^+, tetany from low ionized calcium concentration, increased affinity of hemoglobin for oxygen, paradoxical CNS acidosis, overshoot metabolic alkalosis, hypokalemia.
- Hyperchloremic acidosis—$NaHCO_3$ may be effective and considered whenever pH <7.1.
- Uremic acidosis—efficacy of $NaHCO_3$ in acute therapy of uremic acidosis is related to shift of phosphate inside cells and consequent amelioration of hyperphosphatemic acidosis.
- Lactic acidosis—$NaHCO_3$ increases lactate production and is of little to no value in lactic acidosis. Therapy should be directed at augmenting oxygen delivery to tissues and reestablishing cardiac output. Small titrated doses of $NaHCO_3$ can be used as temporizing measure to maintain HCO_3^- above 5 mEq/L, if needed.
- Diabetic ketoacidosis—$NaHCO_3$ adversely affects outcome in humans with diabetic ketoacidosis even when pH is <7.0. Administration of $NaHCO_3$ to ketoacidotic patients cannot be recommended at any pH. Therapy should be direct at insulin and fluid administration. Reestablishing plasma volume and renal perfusion will allow kidneys to excrete ketoanions, replacing them with Cl^-.

CONTRAINDICATIONS

- Avoid $NaHCO_3$ in patients with respiratory acidosis because it generates CO_2.
- Patients with respiratory acidosis cannot adequately excrete CO_2, and increased PCO_2 will further decrease pH.
- Avoid diuretics that act in distal nephron (e.g., spironolactone).
- Avoid carbonic anhydrase inhibitors (e.g., acetazolamide, dichlorphenamide).
- Avoid $NaHCO_3$ in acute (<10 mins) cardiac arrest as it may impair tissue oxygen unloading.

PRECAUTIONS

Use $NaHCO_3$ cautiously in patients with congestive heart failure because Na^+ load may cause decompensation of heart failure.

POSSIBLE INTERACTIONS

None

ALTERNATIVE DRUG(S)

None

FOLLOW-UP

PATIENT MONITORING

Recheck acid-base status; frequency dictated by underlying disease and patient response to treatment.

POSSIBLE COMPLICATIONS

- Hyperkalemia in acute hyperchloremic acidosis.
- Myocardial depression and ventricular arrhythmias.

MISCELLANEOUS

ASSOCIATED CONDITIONS

- Hyperkalemia.
- Hyperchloremia.

AGE-RELATED FACTORS

None

PREGNANCY/FERTILITY/BREEDING

N/A

SYNONYMS

- Dilutional acidosis—metabolic acidosis resulting from increased free water in plasma.
- Hyperchloremic acidosis—normal anion gap acidosis.
- Hyperphosphatemic acidosis—metabolic acidosis resulting from high phosphate concentration.
- Nonrespiratory acidosis.
- Normochloremic acidosis—high anion gap acidosis.
- Organic acidosis—metabolic acidosis resulting from accumulation of organic anions (e.g., ketoacidosis, uremic acidosis, and lactic acidosis).

SEE ALSO

- Azotemia and Uremia.
- Diabetes Mellitus With Ketoacidosis.
- Hyperchloremia.
- Hyperkalemia.
- Hyperphosphatemia.
- Lactic Acidosis (Hyperlactatemia).

ABBREVIATIONS

- AG= anion gap.
- BE = base excess.
- H^+ = hydrogen ion.
- HCO_3^- = bicarbonate.
- $NaHCO_3$ = sodium bicarbonate.
- PCO_2 = carbon dioxide tension.

Suggested Reading

de Morais HA, Constable PD. Strong ion approach to acid-base disorders. In: DiBartola SP, ed., Fluid, Electrolyte and Acid-Base Disorders, 4th ed. St. Louis, MO: Saunders, 2012, pp. 316–330.

de Morais HA, Leisewitz AL. Mixed acid-base disorders. In: DiBartola SP, ed., Fluid, Electrolyte and Acid-Base Disorders, 4th ed. St. Louis, MO: Saunders, 2012, pp. 302–315.

DiBartola SP. Metabolic acid-base disorders. In: DiBartola SP, ed., Fluid, Electrolyte and Acid-Base Disorders, 4th ed. St. Louis, MO: Saunders, 2012, pp. 271–280.

Hopper K. Traditional acid-base analysis. In: Silverstein DC, Hopper K, eds., Small Animal Critical Care Medicine, 2nd ed. St. Louis, MO: Elsevier, 2015, pp. 289–299.

Author Helio S. Autran de Morais

Consulting Editor J.D. Foster

Acknowledgment The author and book editor acknowledge the prior contribution of Lee E. Palmer.

ACNE—CATS

BASICS

OVERVIEW

• Inflammatory dermatitis affecting the chin and lips.
• Symptoms may be recurrent or persistent.

SIGNALMENT

• Cats.
• Prevalence for sex, age, or breed not reported.

SIGNS

• Cats may have a single episode, a life-long recurrent problem, or a continual disease.
• Frequency and severity of each occurrence vary with the individual.
• Comedones, mild erythematous papules, serous crusts, and dark keratin debris develop on the chin and less commonly on the lips.
• Swelling of the chin.
• Severe cases—nodules, hemorrhagic crusts, pustules, cysts, fistulae, severe erythema, alopecia, and pain.
• Pain often associated with bacterial furunculosis.

CAUSES & RISK FACTORS

Precise etiology unknown; often is associated with allergic skin diseases; may be a disorder of keratinization, poor grooming, abnormal sebum production, immunosuppression, viral infection, or stress.

DIAGNOSIS

DIFFERENTIAL DIAGNOSIS

• Hypersensitivity (atopy, flea bite, food, contact).
• Bacterial folliculitis.
• Demodicosis.
• *Malassezia* infection.
• Dermatophytosis.
• Neoplasia of sebaceous or apocrine glands.
• Eosinophilic granuloma.

CBC/BIOCHEMISTRY/URINALYSIS

N/A

OTHER LABORATORY TESTS

N/A

IMAGING

N/A

DIAGNOSTIC PROCEDURES

• Skin scrapings—demodicosis.
• Bacterial culture—resistant infection.
• Fungal culture—dermatophytosis.
• Cytology—bacteria, *Malassezia*.
• Biopsy—rarely needed; necessary in selected cases to characterize changes such as cystic follicles, to differentiate acne from other diseases such as demodicosis, infections (bacterial, yeast, or dermatophytes), or to diagnose neoplasia.

PATHOLOGIC FINDINGS

• Mild disease—follicular distention with keratin (comedo), hyperkeratosis, and follicular plugging, most often associated with allergic dermatitis.
• Severe disease—mild to severe folliculitis and perifolliculitis with follicular pustule formation leading to furunculosis and pyogranulomatous dermatitis.
• Bacteria and *Malassezia* in these lesions are considered secondary invaders and not causative agents.
• *Demodex* mites can be primary agents of this disease.

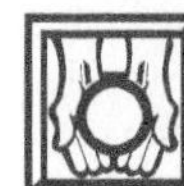

TREATMENT

• Initial treatment—gentle clipping and soakings to soften crusts.
• Food elimination diet.
• Intradermal allergy testing.
• Continue one or a combination of the therapies listed below until all lesions have resolved.
• Discontinue treatment by tapering medication over a 2- to 3-week period.
• Recurrent episodes—once the recurrence rate is determined, an appropriate maintenance protocol can be designed for each individual.
• Continual episodes—life-long maintenance treatment necessary.

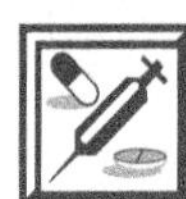

MEDICATIONS

DRUG(S) OF CHOICE

Topical

• Shampoo—once or twice weekly with antiseborrheic (sulfur-salicylic acid, benzoyl peroxide, or ethyl lactate).
• Cleansing agents—benzoyl peroxide, salicylic acid, chlorhexidinephytosphingosine.
• Medicated wipes.
• Antibiotic ointment—mupirocin 2%.
• Other topicals—clindamycin or erythromycin solution or ointment.
• Combination topicals—benzoyl peroxide-antibiotic gels (e.g., Benzamycin).
• Topical retinoids—tretinoin (e.g., Retin-A® 0.01%): gel more effective because of better penetration.
• In severe inflammatory periods 10–14 days of oral prednisolone (1–2 mg/kg q24h) may help to reduce scar tissue formation.

Systemic

• Antibiotics—amoxicillin with clavulanate, cephalosporin, or fluoroquinolone.
• Severe cases may warrant treatment with isotretinoin (Accutane) or cyclosporine, modified (Atopica®).
• Demodicosis—isoxazoline parasiticides.

CONTRAINDICATIONS/POSSIBLE INTERACTIONS

• Benzoyl peroxide and salicylic acids—can be irritating.
• Some wipes contain alcohols that can be irritating.
• Systemic isotretinoin—use with caution, if animal will not allow application of topical medications; potential deleterious side effects in human beings (drug interactions and teratogenicity); container should be labeled for animal use only and kept separate from human medications to avoid accidental use; currently difficult to obtain for animal patients.

FOLLOW-UP

• Monitor for relapses.
• Maintenance cleansing programs can be used to reduce relapses; affected cats are likely to have variable numbers of comedones life-long, which often are just cosmetic, and treatment is not necessary.

MISCELLANEOUS

PREGNANCY/FERTILITY/BREEDING

Systemic isotretinoin should not be used on breeding animals.

Suggested Reading

Jazic E, Coyner KS, Loeffler DG, Lewis TP. An evaluation of the clinical, cytological, infectious and histopathological features of feline acne. Vet Dermatol 2006, 17(2):134–140.

Miller WH, Griffin CE, Campbell KL. Acne. In: Muller & Kirk's Small Animal Dermatology, 7th ed. St. Louis, MO: Elsevier, 2013, pp. 640–642.

Rosencrantz WS. The pathogenesis, diagnosis, and management of feline acne. Vet Med 1993, 5:504–512.

Werner AH, Power HT. Retinoids in veterinary dermatology. Clin Dermatol 1994, 12(4):579–586.

White SD. Feline acne and results of treatment with mupirocin in an open clinical trial: 25 cases (1994–96). Vet Dermatol 1997, 8:157.

Author David D. Duclos

Consulting Editor Alexander H. Werner Resnick

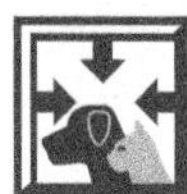

BASICS

OVERVIEW

- Also (more correctly) muzzle folliculitis and furunculosis.
- Chronic inflammatory disorder of the chin and lips of mostly young animals.
- Characterized by folliculitis and furunculosis; almost never comedogenic as seen in "true acneiform" lesions of human beings.
- Recognized almost exclusively in short-coated breeds.
- Genetic predisposition, local trauma, and allergic disease often play a role.

SIGNALMENT

- Dogs, often younger, sometimes puppies.
- Predisposed short-coated breeds—boxer, Doberman pinscher, English bulldog, Great Dane, Weimaraner, mastiff, Rottweiler, German shorthaired pointer, pit bull terrier.

SIGNS

- Ventral chin and lip margins may have few to numerous erythematous papules and sometimes bullae. These may coalesce to form plaques.
- Initial lesions are inflammatory and sterile; bacteria may not be isolated and lesions may not respond to antibiotics.
- Advanced lesions may contain pus or blood, indicating secondary deep bacterial folliculitis and furunculosis.
- Lesions may be pruritic, some are painful on palpation, but most are nonpainful and nonpruritic.
- Chronic and pruritic lesions may become hyperpigmented, lichenified, scarred, and alopecic.

CAUSES & RISK FACTORS

Several short-coated breeds appear to be genetically predisposed to acne. Lesions may be worse in allergic individuals.

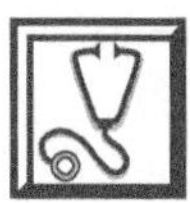

DIAGNOSIS

DIFFERENTIAL DIAGNOSIS

- Dermatophytosis.
- Demodicosis.
- Juvenile cellulitis.
- Contact dermatitis.
- With other symptoms, consider allergic/atopic disease as playing a role.

CBC/BIOCHEMISTRY/URINALYSIS

N/A

OTHER LABORATORY TESTS

N/A

IMAGING

N/A

DIAGNOSTIC PROCEDURES

- Impression cytology will help determine if bacteria or yeast are present.
- Skin scrape—demodicosis.
- Dermatophyte culture—dermatophytosis.
- Bacterial culture and sensitivity testing—in patients with suppurative folliculitis and furunculosis that are nonresponsive to initial antibiotic selection.
- Biopsy—histologic confirmation for cases in which diagnosis is in question.

PATHOLOGIC FINDINGS

- Clinical signs and histopathologic findings are diagnostic.
- Characterized histopathologically by folliculitis and furunculosis.
- Bacteria—not always isolated from lesions in early stages.
- As disease progresses, papules enlarge and rupture, promoting a suppurative folliculitis and furunculosis.

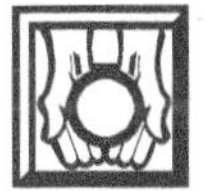

TREATMENT

- Reduce behavioral trauma to the chin (e.g., rubbing on the carpet, chewing bones that increase salivation).
- Frequent cleaning with chlorhexidine-containing pads, shampoos, or solutions can be helpful, but instruct owners not to scrub at the area.
- Gentamicin/steroid-containing ointments for the ears work well on the chin when applied twice daily.
- If topicals are not helpful by themselves, add oral antibiotics based on positive cytology and culture and sensitivity testing.
- Severe cases may necessitate short courses of oral steroids.
- Evaluate for underlying allergic/atopic disease and institute proper therapy for diagnosis and control of these diseases; control of allergic disease may permit resolution of muzzle folliculitis and furunculosis.
- Instruct owners to avoid squeezing the lesions; trauma may make inflammation worse.

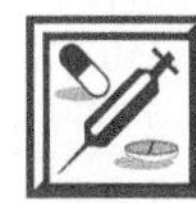

MEDICATIONS

DRUG(S)

Topical

- Daily cleaning with chlorhexidine-containing pads, shampoos, or solutions can be helpful; instruct owners not to scrub at the areas.
- Gentamicin/steroid-containing ointments for the ears can be applied to localized lesions twice daily; most useful for lesions on the chin, as the pet cannot lick this area. Constant long-term use over months may cause alopecia and cutaneous atrophy: limit frequency and duration of application.

Systemic

- Antibiotics based on culture and sensitivity—when indicated (e.g., cephalexin, 22–30 mg/kg PO q12h for 2–4 weeks).
- Oral corticosteroids: tapering dosages of prednisolone (initial 0.5 mg/kg/day) to reduce significant inflammation; not for continued use.
- Evaluate for and manage concurrent allergic/atopic skin disease.

CONTRAINDICATIONS/POSSIBLE INTERACTIONS

- Topical steroids—may cause adrenal suppression and thinning of skin with frequent or constant use.

FOLLOW-UP

PATIENT MONITORING

- Continue antibiotics until lesions have healed.
- Repeat bacterial culture/sensitivity if lesions worsen.
- Discontinue topical corticosteroids when possible.

EXPECTED COURSE AND PROGNOSIS

- Long-term topical treatment may be required.
- Chronic scarring may be prevented by early and aggressive therapy.

MISCELLANEOUS

ASSOCIATED CONDITIONS

Allergic/atopic disease may cause and exacerbate this condition.

Suggested Reading

Miller WH, Griffin CE, Campbell KL. Muzzle folliculitis and furunculosis. In: Muller & Kirk's Small Animal Dermatology, 7th ed. St. Louis, MO: Elsevier, 2013, pp. 201, 640.

Author Melissa N.C. Eisenschenk

Consulting Editor Alexander H. Werner Resnick

Acknowledgment The author and editors acknowledge the prior contribution of Karen Helton Rhodes.

A

ACRAL LICK DERMATITIS

BASICS

OVERVIEW

- Compulsion to lick limb/s resulting in plaque formation.
- Skin/exocrine affected.

SIGNALMENT

- Dogs.
- Most common in large breeds—Labrador retrievers, Doberman pinschers, Great Danes, Irish setters, golden retrievers, German shepherd dogs, boxers, and Weimaraners.
- Median age 4 yrs, range 1–12 yrs; no sex predilection.

SIGNS

- Excessive licking of affected area.
- Alopecic, eroded/ulcerated, thickened, and raised firm plaques with scabs and exudation, usually located on dorsal aspect of carpus, metacarpus, tarsus, or metatarsus.
- Single or multiple lesions.

CAUSES & RISK FACTORS

- Anything causing local irritation or lesion may initiate lick–itch cycle.
- Associated diseases: staphylococcal furunculosis, hypersensitivity, endocrinopathy, demodicosis, dermatophytosis, foreign body reaction, neoplasia, underlying joint disease or arthritis, trauma, neuropathy, psychogenic, or sensory nerve dysfunction.

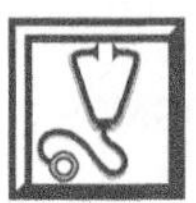

DIAGNOSIS

DIFFERENTIAL DIAGNOSIS

- Neoplasia.
- Bacterial furunculosis.
- Focal demodicosis.
- Focal dermatophytosis.

CBC/BIOCHEMISTRY/URINALYSIS

Usually normal.

OTHER LABORATORY TESTS

Endocrinopathy—total T_4/free T_4/thyroid-stimulating hormone (TSH); adrenocorticotropin hormone (ACTH) stimulation test or low-dose dexamethasone suppression test (LDDST).

IMAGING

Radiology (entire limb +/– neck/lumbar region)—neoplasia; local trauma; radiopaque foreign bodies; bony proliferation may be seen secondary to chronic irritation; evidence of underlying arthritis if over a joint.

DIAGNOSTIC PROCEDURES

- Skin scrapings—demodicosis.
- Dermatophyte PCR and/or culture—fungal infection.
- Epidermal cytology—bacterial infection.
- Bacterial culture and sensitivity—tissue cultures may differ from surface culture.
- Food elimination diet—determine food allergy.
- Intradermal allergy testing—atopy.
- Biopsy—to rule out neoplasia, other infections.
- Behavioral history (additional behavioral signs typical).
- Neurologic and orthopedic evaluation.

PATHOLOGIC FINDINGS

Histopathology—epidermal hyperplasia, plasmacytic dermal inflammation, folliculitis, furunculosis, perihidradenitis, hidradenitis, epitrichial gland dilation/rupture, vertical streaking fibrosis.

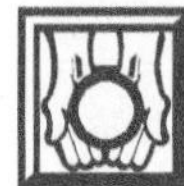

TREATMENT

- Rule in/out bacterial, fungal, ectoparasitic, endocrine causes and treat accordingly along with pruritus control.
- If infection resolves and pruritus and/or lesions persist, consider biopsy, allergy workup, neurologic/orthopedic exam, radiographs, behavioral modification.
- Physical restraints—to permit healing.
- Limited research to support effectiveness: radiation, acupuncture, CO_2 laser, cryosurgery, standard surgery.
- Difficult to treat, especially if no underlying cause found; warn owner that patience and time are necessary.

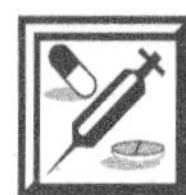

MEDICATIONS

DRUG(S) OF CHOICE

Antibiotics

Based on bacterial culture/susceptibility. Administer until resolution of infection plus 2 weeks.

Systemic

- Pruritus—antihistamines (2 weeks for response typically), e.g., hydroxyzine (2.2 mg/kg PO q8h); chlorpheniramine (4–8 mg/dog PO q8–12h; maximum of 0.5 mg/kg q12h); amitriptyline (1–2 mg/kg PO q12h), also tricyclic antidepressant (TCA); corticosteroids, e.g., prednisolone 1 mg/kg PO q24h and taper based on response (or other steroid equivalent).
- Behavioral—selective serotonin reuptake inhibitors (SSRIs), e.g., fluoxetine (1 mg/kg PO q24h); TCAs, e.g., amitriptyline (1–2 mg/kg PO q12h, also antihistamine); doxepin (3–5 mg/kg PO q12h; maximum 150 mg q12h); clomipramine (2–4 mg/kg PO q24h); dopamine antagonists, e.g., naltrexone (2.2 mg/kg PO q24h).
- Combine/withdraw administration of these medications carefully.

Topical

Pruritus—flunixin meglumine and fluocinolone in dimethyl sulfoxide (combined), topical capsaicin products; intralesional corticosteroids rarely helpful; wear gloves when applying; prevent licking of area for 10–15 minutes.

CONTRAINDICATIONS/POSSIBLE INTERACTIONS

- Doxepin—caution using with monoamine oxidase inhibitors, clonidine, anticonvulsants, oral anticoagulants, steroid hormones, antihistamines, or aspirin.
- Antihistamines—may cause sedation.
- Psychotropic medications should be combined and/or withdrawn carefully.
- Cardiotoxicity and hepatoxicity—rare cases in animals on TCAs. Routine monitoring recommended.

FOLLOW-UP

- Monitor level of licking and chewing closely.
- Treat underlying disease to prevent recurrence.
- If no underlying disease detected, psychogenic causes possible (compulsive or self-mutilation disorder); prognosis is guarded.

MISCELLANEOUS

AGE-RELATED FACTORS

Dogs <5 years old—strongly consider allergy.

ZOONOTIC POTENTIAL

Dermatophytosis (rare) and methicillin-resistant *Staphylococcus aureus* may have zoonotic implications.

ABBREVIATIONS

- ACTH = adrenocorticotropin hormone.
- LDDST = low-dose dexamethasone suppression test.
- SSRI = selective serotonin reuptake inhibitor.
- TCA = tricyclic antidepressant.
- TSH = thyroid-stimulating hormone.

Suggested Reading

Shumaker AK. Diagnosis and treatment of canine acral lick dermatitis. Vet Clin North Am Small Anim Pract. 2019, 49:105–123.

Author Heather D. Edginton

Consulting Editor Alexander H. Werner Resnick

Acknowledgment The author acknowledges the prior contribution of Alexander H. Werner Resnick.

Actinomycosis and Nocardia

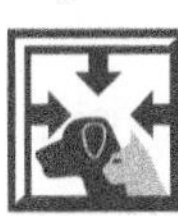

BASICS

OVERVIEW

- Opportunistic bacterial infections caused by branching Gram-positive bacteria that cause clinically similar suppurative-to-granulomatous inflammation:
  - *Actinomyces* spp. (anaerobic-to-microaerophilic, normal flora of mucous membranes, gastrointestinal and urogenital tracts).
  - *Nocardia* spp. (aerobic soil saprophytes).
- Organ systems affected may include:
  - Skin and subcutaneous.
  - Respiratory.
  - Cardiovascular.
  - Musculoskeletal.
  - Nervous.
  - Disseminated (*Nocardia*).

SIGNALMENT

- Dogs and cats (uncommon).
- Dogs with outdoor access (*Actinomyces*); young dogs (*Nocardia*); male cats (both).

SIGNS

- Depends on whether infection is localized or disseminated (*Nocardia*) and on organ systems involved.
- Cutaneous and subcutaneous swellings (cervicofacial—*Actinomyces*), abscesses, or nonhealing wounds with draining tracts; localized draining cutaneous lesions are common in cats.
- Poor body condition, pain, fever, weight loss.
- Exudative pleural or peritoneal effusions.
- Cough, dyspnea, decreased ventral lung sounds (empyema).
- Lameness due to osteomyelitis.
- Motor and sensory deficits.
- Retroperitonitis (*Actinomyces*)—lumbar pain, rear limb paresis or paralysis.

CAUSES & RISK FACTORS

Scratches and bite wounds, traumatic inoculation, foreign body migration (e.g., grass awn), immunosuppression (*Nocardia*).

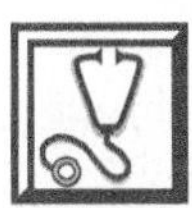

DIAGNOSIS

DIFFERENTIAL DIAGNOSIS

- *Actinomyces* and *Nocardia* appear similar and are not reliably distinguished by Gram staining, cytology, or clinical signs. *Actinomyces* is usually accompanied by multiple other coinfective bacteria.
- Other causes of similar clinical signs must be considered, including other bacterial or fungal infections, neoplasia, and other diseases that cause effusions.

CBC/BIOCHEMISTRY/URINALYSIS

- Nonregenerative anemia.
- Leukocytosis with a left shift and monocytosis.
- Hyperglobulinemia.
- Ionized hypercalcemia (nocardiosis).

OTHER LABORATORY TESTS

N/A

IMAGING

- Dependent on systems affected.
- Thoracic radiographs—alveolar and interstitial lung pattern with possible alveolar disease, pleural effusion (pyothorax), pericardial effusion, subcutaneous masses.
- Abdominal radiographs—peritoneal effusion, abdominal mass effect.
- Radiographs of infected bone—periosteal new bone, reactive osteosclerosis, osteolysis.

DIAGNOSTIC PROCEDURES

- Gram staining, cytology, and acid-fast staining are helpful, but do not preclude the need for culture; acid-fast stain—*Actinomyces* negative, *Nocardia* variable; sulfur granules suggest *Actinomyces*.
- Exudates or osteolytic bone fragments submitted in aerobic and anaerobic specimen containers for culture can provide a definitive diagnosis (see Anaerobic Infections).
- Nocardia may require speciation if not responding to empiric therapy.

PATHOLOGIC FINDINGS

Histopathologic examination—pyogranulomatous or granulomatous cellulitis with colonies of filamentous bacteria; special stains may enhance visualization. Sulfur granules are a useful diagnostic tool, but can be difficult to find.

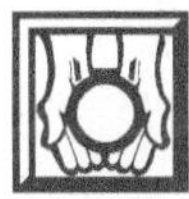

TREATMENT

- Prolonged antimicrobial therapy is required.
- Surgical debridement or excision of infected tissue (e.g., lung lobe, body wall mass) may improve outcome.
- Exudative fluid (thorax, abdomen, subcutaneous tissue) should be drained and the infected cavity lavaged.
- A thoracostomy tube with intermittent or continuous drainage is usually needed for cats with pyothorax; dogs may benefit from surgical exploration of thorax prior to thoracostomy tube placement to attempt foreign body removal.

MEDICATIONS

DRUG(S) OF CHOICE

- Important to distinguish between *Actinomyces* and *Nocardia* for appropriate antimicrobial selection.
- Antibiotics—protracted course of therapy (weeks to months) usually required; continue for several weeks after resolution of all signs.
- Actinomycosis—penicillins considered drug of choice; amoxicillin: 20–40 mg/kg PO q8h.
- Nocardiosis—potentiated sulfonamides at 15–30 mg/kg PO q12h are usually first choice.

CONTRAINDICATIONS/POSSIBLE INTERACTIONS

- Dogs can develop toxic or hypersensitivity adverse reactions to sulfonamides.
- Metronidazole and aminoglycosides are ineffective against *Actinomyces* spp.

FOLLOW-UP

PATIENT MONITORING

Monitor closely for recurrence after therapy discontinued.

PREVENTION/AVOIDANCE

Avoid areas with grass awns; prevent bites and scratches.

POSSIBLE COMPLICATIONS

Difficult to fully clear infection.

EXPECTED COURSE AND PROGNOSIS

- Redevelopment of infection after discontinuation of antibiotics is possible.
- *Actinomyces*—up to 90% cure reported in dogs after appropriate therapy.
- *Nocardia*—up to 50% mortality reported.

MISCELLANEOUS

AGE-RELATED FACTORS

Young outdoor dogs.

ZOONOTIC POTENTIAL

No reports of humans being infected by either organism through direct contact. Bite and scratch wounds can cause human disease.

SEE ALSO

Anaerobic Infections.

Suggested Reading

Sykes JE. Actinomycosis and nocardiosis. In: Greene CE, ed., Infectious Diseases of the Dog and Cat, 4th ed. St. Louis, MO: Saunders Elsevier, 2011, pp. 484–495.

Author Sharon Fooshee Grace

Consulting Editor Amie Koenig

A

ACUTE ABDOMEN

BASICS

DEFINITION

An emergency condition characterized by historical and physical examination findings of a tense, painful abdomen. May represent a life-threatening condition.

PATHOPHYSIOLOGY

- An affected patient has pain associated with either distention of an organ, inflammation, traction on the mesentery or peritoneum, or ischemia.
- Abdominal viscera are sparsely innervated, and diffuse involvement is often necessary to elicit pain; nerve endings also exist in the submucosa-muscularis of the intestinal wall.
- Inflammation produces abdominal pain by releasing vasoactive substances that directly stimulate nerve endings.

SYSTEMS AFFECTED

- Behavioral—trembling, inappetence, vocalizing, lethargy, and abnormal postural changes such as the praying position to achieve comfort.
- Cardiovascular—ischemia, severe inflammation, systemic inflammatory response syndrome and sepsis may lead to shock. Tachycardia or other arrhythmia may affect capillary refill time and mucous membrane color. Pain may cause arrhythmias.
- Gastrointestinal (GI)—vomiting, diarrhea, inappetence, generalized functional ileus; pancreatic inflammation, necrosis, and abscesses may lead to cranial abdominal pain, vomiting, and ileus.
- Hepatobiliary—jaundice associated with cholestasis from biliary obstruction (including pancreatitis) or bile peritonitis. Hyperbilirubinemia may occur secondary to sepsis.
- Renal/urologic—azotemia due to prerenal (dehydration, hypovolemia, and shock), renal (acute pyelonephritis and acute kidney injury), and postrenal causes (ureteral obstruction, urethral obstruction, and uroperitoneum from bladder rupture).
- Respiratory—increased respiratory rate due to pain or metabolic/acid-base disturbances.

SIGNALMENT

Species

- Dogs and cats.
- Dogs more commonly; often challenging to identify abdominal pain in feline patients.

Breed Predilections

- Male Dalmatians have a higher risk of urethral obstruction because of the high incidence of urate urolithiasis.
- German shepherds with pancreatic atrophy have a higher risk of mesenteric volvulus.

Mean Age and Range

Any

Predominant Sex

Male cats and dogs are at higher risk for urethral obstruction.

SIGNS

General Comments

Clinical signs vary greatly, depending on type and severity of underlying disease.

Historical Findings

- Trembling, reluctance to move, inappetence, vomiting, diarrhea, vocalizing, and abnormal postures (tucked up or praying position).
- Question owner carefully to ascertain what system is affected; for example, melena with a history of nonsteroidal anti-inflammatory drug (NSAID) treatment may suggest GI mucosal ulceration.

Physical Examination Findings

- Abdominal pain, splinting of abdominal musculature, gas- or fluid-filled abdominal organs, abdominal mass, ascites, pyrexia or hypothermia, tachycardia, and tachypnea.
- Pain may be localizable to cranial, middle, or caudal abdomen.
- Perform rectal examination to evaluate colon, pelvic bones, urethra, and prostate, as well as for presence of melena.
- Rule out extra-abdominal causes of pain by careful palpation of kidneys and thoracolumbar vertebrae.
- Pain associated with intervertebral disc disease often causes referred abdominal guarding and may be mistaken for true abdominal pain. Renal pain can be associated with pyelonephritis.

CAUSES

GI

- Stomach—gastritis, ulceration, perforation, foreign body, gastric dilatation-volvulus.
- Intestine—obstruction (foreign body, intussusception, mass, etc.), enteritis, ulceration, perforation.
- Rupture after obstruction, ulceration, or blunt or penetrating trauma, or due to tumor growth.
- Vascular compromise from infarction, mesenteric volvulus, or torsion.

Pancreas

- Inflammation, abscess, ischemia.
- Mass or inflammation obstructing common bile duct may cause jaundice.

Hepatic and Biliary System

- Acute hepatitis—rapid distention of the liver and its capsule can cause pain.
- Biliary obstruction, rupture, or necrosis may lead to bile leakage and peritonitis.
- Gallbladder mucocele.
- Hepatic abscess.

Spleen

Torsion, mass, thrombus, abscess.

Urinary Tract

- Distention is main cause of pain in urinary tract.
- Obstruction due to tumors of trigone area of bladder or urethra, urinary calculi, or granulomatous urethritis.
- Traumatic rupture of ureters or bladder.
- Urethral tear associated with pelvic fractures from acute trauma.
- Uroabdomen leads to chemical peritonitis.
- Acute pyelonephritis, acute kidney injury, nephroliths, and ureteroliths are uncommon causes of acute abdomen.

Genital Tract

- Prostatitis and prostatic abscess, pyometra; a ruptured pyometra or prostatic abscess can cause endotoxemia, sepsis, and cardiovascular collapse.
- Uncommon—rupture of gravid uterus after blunt abdominal trauma, uterine torsion, ovarian tumor or torsion, and intra-abdominal testicular torsion (cryptorchid).

Abdominal Wall/Diaphragm

- Umbilical, inguinal, scrotal, abdominal, or peritoneal hernia with strangulated viscera.
- Organ displacement or entrapment in hernia will lead to abdominal pain if vascular supply of organ(s) involved becomes impaired or ischemic.

RISK FACTORS

- Exposure to NSAIDs or corticosteroid treatment (increased risk when used concurrently)—gastric, duodenal, or colonic ulcers.
- Garbage or fatty food ingestion—pancreatitis.
- Foreign body ingestion—intestinal obstruction.
- Abdominal trauma—hollow viscus rupture.
- Hernia—intestinal obstruction/strangulation.

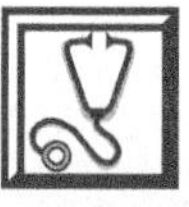

DIAGNOSIS

DIFFERENTIAL DIAGNOSIS

- Renal-associated pain, retroperitoneal pain, spinal or paraspinal pain, and disorders causing diffuse muscle pain may mimic abdominal pain; careful history and physical examination are essential in pursuing the appropriate problem.
- Parvoviral enteritis can present similarly to intestinal obstructive disease; fecal parvoviral antigen assay and CBC (leukopenia) are helpful differentiating diagnostic tests.

CBC/BIOCHEMISTRY/URINALYSIS

- Inflammation or infection may be associated with leukocytosis or leukopenia.
- Active inflammation may be characterized by a neutrophilic left shift.
- Anemia may be seen with blood loss associated with GI ulceration.

• Azotemia is associated with prerenal, renal, and postrenal causes.
• Electrolyte abnormalities can help to evaluate GI disease (i.e., hypochloremic metabolic alkalosis with gastric outflow obstruction) and renal disease (i.e., hyperkalemia with acute kidney injury or postrenal obstruction).
• Hyperbilirubinemia and increased hepatic enzyme activity help localize a problem to liver or biliary system.
• Urine specific gravity (before fluid therapy) is needed to help differentiate prerenal, renal, and postrenal azotemia.
• Urine sediment may be helpful in acute kidney injury, ethylene glycol intoxication, and pyelonephritis.

OTHER LABORATORY TESTS

• Venous blood gas analysis including lactate concentration may indicate acid-base abnormalities, and increased lactate may be associated with hypoperfusion.
• Canine and feline pancreatic lipase immunoreactivity can be useful in evaluating pancreatitis.

IMAGING

Abdominal Radiography

• May see abdominal mass or changes in shape or shifting of abdominal organs.
• Loss of abdominal detail suggests abdominal fluid accumulation.
• Free abdominal gas suggests ruptured GI viscus or infection with gas-producing bacteria and is indication for emergency surgery.
• Use caution when interpreting radiographs following abdominocentesis with an open needle. Free gas may be introduced with this technique.
• Use caution when evaluating postoperative radiographs; free gas is a normal postoperative finding.
• Diffuse GI distension is a consistent finding with peritonitis.
• Foreign bodies may be radiopaque.
• Upper GI barium contrast radiographs are useful in evaluating the GI tract, particularly for determination of GI obstruction.
• Loss of contrast or radiographic detail in the area of the pancreas can be observed with pancreatic inflammation.

Abdominal Ultrasound

• A sensitive diagnostic tool for detection of GI obstruction, pancreatitis, abdominal masses, abdominal fluid, abscesses, cysts, lymphadenopathy, and biliary or urinary calculi.
• Focused Assessment with Sonography in Trauma (FAST) may be used for rapid assessment.

Abdominal CT

May provide superior information to ultrasound in large patients; useful when surgeon requires additional information.

DIAGNOSTIC PROCEDURES

Abdominocentesis/Abdominal Fluid Analysis

• Perform abdominocentesis on all patients presenting with acute abdomen. Four-quadrant approach may improve yield. Fluid can often be obtained for diagnostic evaluation, even when only a small amount of free abdominal fluid exists, well before detectable radiographically. Ultrasound is much more sensitive than radiography for detection of fluid and can be used to direct abdominocentesis. Blind abdominocentesis can be performed safely without ultrasound guidance. Abdominal fluid analysis with elevated white blood cell (WBC) count, degenerate neutrophils, and intracellular bacteria is consistent with septic peritonitis and is an indication for immediate surgery.
• Diagnostic peritoneal lavage can be performed by introducing sterile saline (10–20 mL/kg) and performing abdominocentesis, with or without ultrasound guidance.
• Measurement of glucose concentration in abdominal effusion in comparison with peripheral blood may aid in diagnosis of septic abdomen. A blood-to-abdominal fluid glucose difference of >20 mg/dL is consistent with septic effusion.
• Pancreatitis patients may have abdominal effusion characterized as nonseptic (sterile) peritonitis.
• Creatinine concentration higher in abdominal fluid than in serum indicates urinary tract leakage.
• Similarly, higher bilirubin concentration in abdominal fluid than in serum indicates bile peritonitis.

Sedation and Abdominal Palpation

Because of abdominal splinting associated with pain, thorough abdominal palpation is often not possible without sedation; this is particularly useful for detecting intestinal foreign bodies that do not appear on survey radiographs.

Exploratory Laparotomy

Surgery may be useful diagnostically (as well as therapeutically) when ultrasonography (or other advanced imaging) is not available, or when no definitive cause of acute abdomen has been established with appropriate diagnostics.

PATHOLOGIC FINDINGS

Varies with underlying disease.

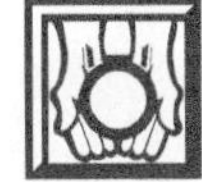

TREATMENT

APPROPRIATE HEALTH CARE

• Inpatient management with supportive care until decision about whether problem to be treated medically or surgically. Early intervention with surgery is important when indicated.
• Aggressive therapy and prompt identification of underlying cause are very important.
• Many causes of acute abdominal pain require emergency surgical intervention.

NURSING CARE

• Keep patient NPO if vomiting, until a definitive cause is determined and addressed.
• Intravenous fluid therapy usually required because of large fluid loss associated with acute abdomen; goal is to restore normal circulating blood volume.
• If shock exists, supplement initially with isotonic crystalloid fluids (up to 90 mL/kg, dogs; 70 mL/kg, cats) to restore volume; hypertonic fluids or colloids may also be beneficial if refractory to isotonic crystalloids or hypoproteinemic.
• Evaluate hydration and electrolytes (with appropriate treatment adjustments) frequently after commencement of treatment.

ACTIVITY

N/A

DIET

Early nutritional support is important. Nutritional support can be enteral (oral, nasoesophageal, esophageal tube, gastrostomy tube, enterostomy tube) or parenteral.

CLIENT EDUCATION

Acute abdomen may represent a life-threatening condition. Prompt diagnosis and appropriate treatment essential to a favorable outcome.

SURGICAL CONSIDERATIONS

• Many different causes of acute abdomen exist; make definitive diagnosis whenever possible prior to surgical intervention.
• Definitive diagnosis prior to surgery can prevent both potentially unnecessary and expensive surgical procedures and associated morbidity and mortality.
• Also allows surgeon to prepare for task and educate owner on prognosis and financial investment.

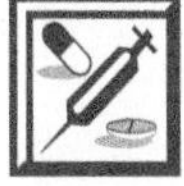

MEDICATIONS

DRUG(S) OF CHOICE

Analgesics

• Pain medication may be indicated for control of abdominal discomfort.
• Opioids are good choices.
  ◦ Fentanyl—2–5 μg/kg as initial IV bolus, 2–10 μg/kg/h as CRI.
  ◦ Hydromorphone—0.05–0.2 mg/kg SC/IM/IV q4–6h.
  ◦ Morphine—0.5–2 mg/kg SC/IM, q4–6h.
  ◦ Buprenorphine—0.01–0.02 mg/kg SC/IM/IV q4–6h.
  ◦ Methadone—0.1–0.4 mg/kg SC/IM/IV q6h.

A

ACUTE ABDOMEN (CONTINUED)

Histamine H2 Antagonists

- Reduce gastric acid production.
- Famotidine 0.5–1 mg/kg IV/SC/IM q12h.
- Ranitidine 2 mg/kg IV q12h.

Proton Pump Inhibitor

Pantoprazole 0.5 mg/kg IV q12h or 0.05–0.1 mg/kg/hr as CRI.

Protectants

Sucralfate 0.25–1 g PO q8h.

Antiemetics

- Metoclopramide 0.2–0.4 mg/kg IV q6–8h (or 24-hour CRI at 1–2 mg/kg/24h).
- Maropitant: dogs 2–4 months of age, 1 mg/kg SC q 24h; dogs >4 months of age and cats, 1 mg/kg SC/IV q24h.
- Ondansetron 0.2–0.5 mg/kg IV slowly q6–12h.

Antibiotics

- Antibiotics may be indicated if signs of infection are seen or hemorrhagic diarrhea is present.
- Broad-spectrum coverage pending culture results.
- Obtain cultures prior to treatment if possible, but do not delay intervention if indicated.

CONTRAINDICATIONS

- Do not use metoclopramide if GI obstruction is suspected.
- Do not use barium if GI perforation is suspected; use iodinated contrast agent instead.

PRECAUTIONS

- Gentamicin and NSAIDs can be nephrotoxic and should be avoided in hypovolemic patients and those with renal impairment.
- NSAIDs may also cause GI complications.

POSSIBLE INTERACTIONS

N/A

ALTERNATIVE DRUGS

N/A

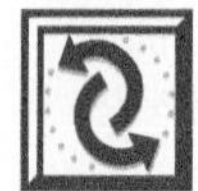

FOLLOW-UP

PATIENT MONITORING

Patients usually require intensive medical care and frequent evaluation of vital signs and laboratory parameters.

PREVENTION/AVOIDANCE

Avoidance of indiscriminate eating may prevent GI foreign body obstruction and decrease incidence of pancreatitis.

POSSIBLE COMPLICATIONS

Varies with underlying cause.

EXPECTED COURSE AND PROGNOSIS

Varies with underlying cause; guarded until this is determined.

MISCELLANEOUS

AGE-RELATED FACTORS

Younger animals have higher incidence of trauma-related problems, intussusceptions, and acquired diet- and infection-related diseases; older animals have higher incidence of malignancies.

SYNONYMS

Colic

SEE ALSO

- Gastric Dilation and Volvulus Syndrome.
- Gastroduodenal Ulceration/Erosion.
- Gastrointestinal Obstruction.
- Intussusception.
- Pancreatitis—Cats.
- Pancreatitis—Dogs.
- Prostatitis and Prostatic Abscess.
- Pyelonephritis.
- Urinary Tract Obstruction.

ABBREVIATIONS

- FAST = Focused Assessment with Sonography in Trauma.
- GI = gastrointestinal.
- NSAID = nonsteroidal anti-inflammatory drug.
- WBC = white blood cell.

Suggested Reading

Beal MW. Approach to the acute abdomen. Vet Clin North Am Small Anim Pract 2005, 35:375–396.

Heeren V, Edwards L, Mazzaferro EM. Acute abdomen: diagnosis. Compend Contin Educ Pract Vet 2004, 26:350–363.

Heeren V, Edwards L, Mazzaferro EM. Acute abdomen: treatment. Compend Contin Educ Pract Vet 2004, 26:3566–3673.

Author Steven L. Marks

Consulting Editor Mark P. Rondeau

ACUTE DIARRHEA

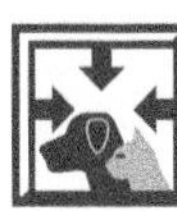

BASICS

DEFINITION

Nonepisodic diarrhea of fewer than 7 days' duration.

PATHOPHYSIOLOGY

Excess water and/or solid content of feces is caused by five main mechanisms:
• Osmotic—from maldigestion, ingestion of poorly absorbable compounds, toxins.
• Decreased absorption—mucosal damage causing loss of absorptive cells from infection, inflammation, or toxins. • Increased secretion (secretory)—mediated by toxins, inflammation, parasympathetic stimulation.
• Increased permeability/exudative—severe mucosal, lacteal, and vessel damage, due to inflammation, ulceration, or direct damage.
• Dysmotility—increased or decreased motility alters digestion, absorption, secretion, and therefore water regulation.

SYSTEMS AFFECTED

• Cardiovascular—fluid losses can be significant, with progressive dehydration to hypovolemia.
• Gastrointestinal (GI)—colitis can develop secondary to orad causes of diarrhea.
• Immune—with enterocyte loss, the mucosal barrier can be compromised, leading to translocation of GI bacteria and sepsis. • Metabolic—electrolyte losses, especially bicarbonate and potassium. Hypokalemia is common with concurrent hyporexia. • Vascular—albumin and globulin losses via increased permeability can be significant and lead to hypoalbuminemia, decreased vascular oncotic pressure, and edema or cavitary effusion.

GENETICS

N/A

INCIDENCE/PREVALENCE

Increased incidence due to dietary indiscretion or infectious etiologies in young patients.

GEOGRAPHIC DISTRIBUTION

Some infectious etiologies have specific geographic distributions.

SIGNALMENT

• Species—dog and cat. • Breed predilections—none. • Mean age and range—common in puppies and kittens due to dietary indiscretion and infectious etiologies.
• Predominant sex—N/A.

SIGNS

General Comments

• Acute diarrhea common, and usually self-limiting. Most animals stable, and require minimal diagnostics/treatment. • In patients that are unstable, with cardiovascular or metabolic compromise, more aggressive diagnostic and treatment approach is warranted.

Historical Findings

• Dietary history, dietary indiscretion, medication/toxin history, and general husbandry should be investigated. ○ Special care should be taken to identify potentially contagious causes of diarrhea, and isolate these patients early. ○ Patients that should be isolated for further diagnostics include unvaccinated, raw diet consumption, housing with many other cats/dogs, or multiple cats/dogs from same household affected.
• Varying activity levels can be seen, from normal to lethargic. • Character of diarrhea can help localize etiology: ○ Small intestinal diarrhea characteristics: large volume, normal frequency, concurrent weight loss and/or vomiting. ○ Melena, if present, points to gastric or upper small intestinal bleed.
○ Steatorrhea, if present, points to maldigestive disorder like exocrine pancreatic insufficiency (EPI). ○ Large intestinal diarrhea characteristics—small volume, increased frequency, tenesmus, mucus, hematochezia.

Physical Examination Findings

• Patients can vary from stable to unstable.
• Common findings—dehydration, hypovolemia, abdominal pain, nausea, fluid–gas interface on intestinal palpation, increased borborygmi. • Rectal examination may reveal melena, hematochezia, steatorrhea.

CAUSES

• Extra-GI causes: ○ Common—hepatobiliary disease, pancreatitis, neoplasia (non-GI).
○ Uncommon—endocrine (hypoadrenocorticism, hyperthyroidism), peritonitis, sepsis.
• Intra-GI causes: ○ Infectious—bacterial: *Campylobacter* spp., *E. coli*, *Salmonella* spp., Clostridial enterotoxins; parasitic: many species of ascarids, cestodes, hookworms, whipworms; protozoal: giardiasis, tritrichomoniasis, coccidiosis; viral: parvovirus, canine distemper virus, corona virus; rickettsial: salmon poisoning (*Neorickettsia*); fungal: histoplasmosis, mycotoxins. ○ Inflammatory (most common cause)—acute enteritis/enterocolitis due to dietary indiscretion or sudden diet change, acute hemorrhagic diarrhea syndrome.
○ Medications/toxins—antibiotics, chemotherapeutic agents, methimazole, nonsteroidal anti-inflammatory drugs (NSAIDS), toxins (corrosive, heavy metals). ○ Motility—obstructive or nonobstructive foreign bodies, intussusception, mesenteric torsion. ○ Neoplasia—primary neoplasia including adenocarcinoma, lymphoma (small cell and large cell) leiomyoma/leiomyosarcoma, mast cell tumor (cats), metastatic.

RISK FACTORS

• Dietary—abrupt diet change or dietary indiscretion. • Medications—many medications can cause acute diarrhea (see Causes).
• Infectious—geographic distribution effect.

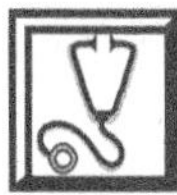

DIAGNOSIS

DIFFERENTIAL DIAGNOSIS

Unlikely to be confused with other conditions; however, rarely intestinal bleeding or expulsion of liquid in constipated patient can mimic acute diarrhea.

CBC/BIOCHEMISTRY/URINALYSIS

• Extra-GI etiologies—may reflect etiology:
○ Increased hepatic enzyme activity in hepatobiliary diseases. ○ Increased hepatic enzyme activity, hypoalbuminemia, inflammatory leukogram in pancreatitis.
○ Hypoalbuminemia, decreased Na : K ratio in hypoadrenocorticism. • Intra-GI causes of diarrhea—often normal. • Parvoviral enteritis causes significant neutropenia.
• As result of diarrhea, following may be present: ○ Hemoconcentration. ○ Prerenal azotemia. ○ Hypokalemia. ○ Hypoalbuminemia, hypocholesterolemia. ○ Hypoglycemia—toy breed puppies with GI signs predisposed.

OTHER LABORATORY TESTS

• Extra-GI interrogation: ○ Baseline cortisol or adrenocorticotropic hormone (ACTH) stimulation test in dogs. ○ T_4 in cats.
○ Quantitative pancreatic lipase immunoreactivity. ○ Trypsin-like immunoreactivity if EPI suspected. • Intra-GI interrogation:
○ Parvovirus ELISA should be immediately performed in any suspect so isolation protocols may be initiated as soon as possible.
○ Fecal flotation, fecal direct smear cytology, *Giardia* ELISA. ○ Diarrhea PCR panel may be useful for specific pathogens (i.e., *Salmonella*), but note there is controversy about some bacteria on this panel causing clinical signs.

IMAGING

Abdominal Radiography

• Survey abdominal radiographs interrogate mainly extra-GI causes of diarrhea. • Acute enteritis/enterocolitis—mild gas and/or fluid dilation of stomach/intestine. • Pancreatitis—widened gastroduodenal angle, focal decreased serosal detail at proximal duodenal flexure.

Abdominal Ultrasonography

• Abdominal ultrasonography may be useful in interrogation of intra- and extra-GI causes of diarrhea, such as pancreatitis. • Emergency cage-side focused ultrasonographic examination of abdomen is indicated in patients with acute abdominal pain, to evaluate for etiologies that are surgical emergencies, such as septic or bile peritonitis. • If peritoneal effusion is seen, abdominocentesis and immediate in-house cytology are indicated (+/– culture).

DIAGNOSTIC PROCEDURES

Endoscopy rarely indicated in acute diarrhea, except for patients with melena where gastroduodenal ulceration is suspected.

ACUTE DIARRHEA (CONTINUED)

PATHOLOGIC FINDINGS

Dependent on underlying etiology.

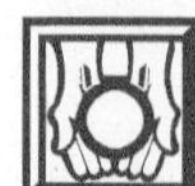

TREATMENT

APPROPRIATE HEALTH CARE

• Stable patients, mild diarrhea—outpatient medical care. Careful assessment of young patients should be made, as they can become unstable with mild signs. • Unstable patients, hypovolemic or acute abdominal pain—inpatient medical care.

NURSING CARE

• Isolation protocols should be instituted immediately for any patient that may have a contagious etiology of diarrhea, i.e., patients that are unvaccinated, fed raw diets, come from housing situations with many other animals, or if multiple animals in same household are exhibiting same clinical signs.
• Fluid therapy as mandated by hydration/perfusion status and ongoing losses. • Most hyporexic patients with dehydration/hypovolemia need isotonic crystalloids to replenish losses and provide maintenance. • Potassium supplementation may be needed.

ACTIVITY

Activity restriction only required in postoperative care of surgical patients.

DIET

Feeding bland, highly digestible diet is indicated for 3–5 days, then gradual reintroduction of patient's routine diet.

CLIENT EDUCATION

Client education on dietary indiscretion, gradual diet changes, routine deworming, and vaccination may be appropriate.

SURGICAL CONSIDERATIONS

Surgery rarely may be indicated to treat etiology, such as mechanical obstruction.

MEDICATIONS

DRUG(S) OF CHOICE

• In acute diarrhea caused by stress or antibiotics, veterinary-grade probiotics may be useful. • Antibiotics not indicated in acute diarrhea patients, and should be avoided in accordance with antibiotic stewardship, unless specifically indicated with known bacterial etiology, or in cases where bacterial translocation and sepsis are of concern (e.g., parvoviral enteritis with neutropenia). Gastric antacids not indicated unless concurrent vomiting and/or regurgitation. • Anti-diarrheal medications like loperamide not indicated in acute diarrhea, as usually self-limiting; if diarrhea persists beyond 5–7 days, further etiologic investigation and appropriate treatment are warranted. • Anthelmintics (e.g., fenbendazole 50 mg/kg PO q24h for 5 days) are recommended for empiric treatment of parasitic enteritis. • Antiprotozoal or coccidiostatic medication should be used if fecal analysis warrants.

CONTRAINDICATIONS

• Prokinetic medications should not be given to patients with diarrhea. • Anti-diarrheal medications like loperamide should not be given to breeds with possible ABCB-1/MDR-1 mutation.

PRECAUTIONS

• For puppies and kittens, see manufacturer's instructions regarding age and safety labeling.
• Many drugs such as antibiotics and anti-diarrheal medications can perpetuate diarrhea.
• Metronidazole can cause neurologic toxic effects with high dose and/or chronic use.

POSSIBLE INTERACTIONS

N/A

ALTERNATIVE DRUG(S)

N/A

FOLLOW-UP

PATIENT MONITORING

• Continuation of diarrhea for 3–5 days is to be expected, but should be continual improvement in signs. • If diarrhea not improving, or getting more severe, further diagnostics are warranted. • If diarrhea persists beyond 7 days or recurs despite appropriate therapy, consider chronic diarrhea etiologies.

PREVENTION/AVOIDANCE

Avoid rapid diet changes and dietary indiscretion, and institute prophylactic deworming and vaccinations.

POSSIBLE COMPLICATIONS

• Dehydration and hypovolemia.
• Hypoalbuminemia and subsequent cavitary effusion.

EXPECTED COURSE AND PROGNOSIS

• Mild acute diarrhea usually self-limiting.
• Other prognoses etiology dependent.

MISCELLANEOUS

ASSOCIATED CONDITIONS

• Acute vomiting. • Hyporexia.

AGE-RELATED FACTORS

Younger patients more likely to have infectious etiologies.

ZOONOTIC POTENTIAL

Parasitic, protozoal, and bacterial etiologies (e.g., *Ancylostoma, Campylobacter, Giardia, Salmonella*).

PREGNANCY/FERTILITY/BREEDING

Varies with treatment.

SYNONYMS

N/A

SEE ALSO

• Acute Vomiting. • Diarrhea, Chronic—Cats. • Diarrhea, Chronic—Dogs.
• Gastroenteritis, Acute Hemorrhagic Diarrhea Syndrome. • Pancreatitis—Cats.
• Pancreatitis—Dogs.

ABBREVIATIONS

• ACTH = adrenocorticotropic hormone.
• EPI = exocrine pancreatic insufficiency.
• GI = gastrointestinal. • NSAID = nonsteroidal anti-inflammatory.

INTERNET RESOURCES

• https://www.avma.org/practicemanagement/clientmaterials/pages/default.aspx • https://veterinarypartner.vin.com

Suggested Reading

Hall J. Physiology of gastrointestinal disorders. In: Hall J, ed., Guyton and Hall's Textbook of Medical Physiology, 13th ed. Philadelphia, PA: Elsevier, 2016, 843–852.

Marks SL, Kook PH, Papich MG, et al. ACVIM consensus statement: Support for rational administration of gastrointestinal protectants to dogs and cats. J Vet Intern Med 2018, 32:1823–1840.

Marks SL, Rankin SC, Byrne BA, Weese JS. Enteropathogenic bacteria in dogs and cats: diagnosis, epidemiology, treatment, and control. J Vet Intern Med 2011, 25: 1195–1208.

Weese JS, Giguère S, Guardabassi L, et al. ACVIM consensus statement on therapeutic antimicrobial use in animals and antimicrobial resistance. J Vet Intern Med 2015, 29:487–498.

Willard MD. Diarrhea. In: Ettinger SJ, ed., Textbook of Veterinary Internal Medicine, 8th ed. St. Louis, MO: Elsevier, 2017, pp. 164–166.

Author Talia Guttin
Consulting Editor Mark P. Rondeau
Acknowledgment The author and editor acknowledge the prior contribution of Erin Portillo.

Client Education Handout available online

BASICS

DEFINITION

- Acute kidney injury (AKI) represents a continuum of renal injury, from mild, clinically inapparent, nephron loss to severe acute renal failure.
- AKI is likely underrecognized. Any increase in serum creatinine >0.3 mg/dL from hydrated baseline is considered an AKI.
- The spectrum of injury is highly variable and may range from mild subclinical to severe damage, requiring renal replacement therapy.
- Patients with AKI have the potential for recovery of renal function.

PATHOPHYSIOLOGY

- AKI may be categorized as prerenal, intrinsic renal, or postrenal based on underlying etiology. Pre- and postrenal causes may progress to intrinsic renal damage.
- Patients with preexisting chronic kidney disease (CKD) are very predisposed to development of clinical AKI due to decreased renal reserve. Special care must be taken in patients with existing CKD to minimize predisposing factors: volume depletion, nephrotoxic medications, etc.

SYSTEMS AFFECTED

- Renal/urologic.
- Uremia may affect all body systems.

INCIDENCE/PREVALENCE

- Prevalence is lower than for CKD.
- Prevalence may increase in environments that support *Leptospira*.
- Ureteral obstruction is most common cause of severe acute uremia in cats.

SIGNALMENT

Species

Dog and cat.

Breed Predilections

None

Mean Age and Range

- 6–8 years peak prevalence.
- Older animals at greater risk due to decreased renal reserve (AKI on CKD).

SIGNS

Historical Findings

Sudden onset of anorexia, listlessness, depression, vomiting or diarrhea (± blood), halitosis, ataxia, seizures, known toxin or drug exposure, recent medical or surgical procedure.

Physical Examination Findings

Normal body condition and hair coat, depression, dehydration (or iatrogenic overhydration), scleral injection, oral ulceration, necrosis of tongue, uremic breath, hypothermia, fever, tachypnea, bradycardia, nonpalpable urinary bladder, and asymmetric, enlarged, painful, or firm kidneys.

CAUSES

Hemodynamic/Hypoperfusion

Shock, trauma, thromboembolism (e.g., disseminated intravascular coagulation [DIC]), vasculitis, transfusion reaction), heatstroke, excessive vasoconstriction (e.g., administration of nonsteroidal anti-inflammatory drugs [NSAIDs]), adrenal insufficiency, excessive vasodilation (e.g., angiotensin-converting enzyme inhibitors [ACEIs] or antihypertensive drugs), prolonged anesthesia, significant hypertension, heart failure.

Nephrotoxic

Grape or raisin ingestion (dogs), lily ingestion (cats), ethylene glycol, aminoglycoside, amphotericin B, chemotherapeutic agents, NSAIDs, radiographic contrast agents, heavy metals, insect or snake venom, heme pigment, and many others. Patients with ethylene glycol toxicity may be exposed from other sources than antifreeze, such as some paints, freezer packs, catering heat sources, etc.

Intrinsic and Systemic Disease

Leptospirosis, immune-mediated glomerulonephritis, pancreatitis, septicemia, DIC, hepatic failure, heat stroke, transfusion reaction, bacterial endocarditis, pyelonephritis, lymphoma, and ureteral obstruction.

RISK FACTORS

- Endogenous—preexisting CKD, pancreatitis, dehydration, sepsis, hypovolemia, hypotension, advanced age, concurrent disease.
- Exogenous—drugs, prolonged anesthesia, trauma, multiple organ disease, high environmental temperature.

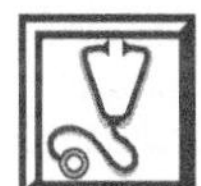

DIAGNOSIS

DIFFERENTIAL DIAGNOSIS

- Prerenal azotemia—oliguria correctable with fluid repletion. Typically hypersthenuric, but consider ability to concentrate urine: preexisting kidney disease, endocrine disorders, medications, and diet may all affect concentrating ability.
- Postrenal azotemia—anuria, dysuria, stranguria, painful or asymmetric kidneys, ureteral/urethral obstruction, enlarged prostate, urethral tear, uroperitoneum.
- CKD—polyuria, polydipsia, history of chronic illness, loss of body condition, anemia.
- Hypoadrenocorticism—hyponatremia, hyperkalemia, low serum cortisol.
- Pancreatitis—cranial abdominal pain, hyperbilirubinemia, increase in liver enzyme activity.

CBC/BIOCHEMISTRY/URINALYSIS

- Variable packed cell volume (PCV), leukocytosis, or lymphopenia.
- Variable increases in blood urea nitrogen (BUN), creatinine, phosphorus, potassium, and glucose; and variably low bicarbonate and calcium.
- Urine specific gravity (USG) ≤1.020, mild to moderate proteinuria, glucosuria, casts, pyuria, hematuria, and tubular epithelial cells; variable bacteriuria and crystalluria.

OTHER LABORATORY TESTS

- Metabolic acidosis—mixed disorders may occur.
- Leptospirosis testing.
- Ethylene glycol testing.
- Canine pancreatic lipase immunoreactivity (cPLI) for pancreatitis.

IMAGING

- Survey and contrast radiography—kidneys normal to large with smooth contours; asymmetric in cats ("big kidney–little kidney" syndrome) with ureteral obstruction, uroliths may be seen.
- Antegrade nephropyelography for ureteral obstruction.
- Ultrasonography—evidence of pancreatitis, marked cortical hyperechogenicity may suggest ethylene glycol toxicity. Moderate cortical hyperechogenicity suggests glomerulonephritis or nephrosis. Pelvic and/or ureteral dilation may suggest outflow obstruction.

DIAGNOSTIC PROCEDURES

- Monitor urine output (UOP): anuria (≤0.25 mL/kg/h), oliguria, polyuria (≥2 mL/kg/h). Avoid urinary catheterization due to infection risk. Assess UOP with serial body weights, ultrasound bladder assessment, weigh bedding, etc.
- Fine-needle aspiration may diagnose lymphoma.
- Renal biopsy may help identify underlying cause and prognosticate recovery.

PATHOLOGIC FINDINGS

Nephrosis or nephritis, glomerulonephritis, calcium oxalate crystals, interstitial edema, and lack of interstitial fibrosis, variable tubular regeneration.

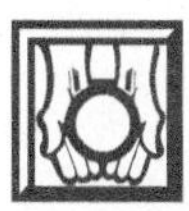

TREATMENT

APPROPRIATE HEALTH CARE

Inpatient management—eliminate inciting causes; discontinue nephrotoxic drugs; maintain hemodynamic stability; ameliorate life-threatening fluid imbalances, biochemical abnormalities, and uremic complications.

NURSING CARE

- Hypovolemia—correct estimated fluid deficits with balanced isotonic solution within 2–4 hours if patient condition permits; once hydrated, ongoing fluid requirements are provided by 5% dextrose for insensible losses (~20–25 mL/kg/day) and balanced electrolyte solution equal to sensible losses; avoid overhydration.
- Hypervolemia—stop fluid administration and eliminate excess fluid by diuretics or dialysis.

ACUTE KIDNEY INJURY (CONTINUED)

• Monitor body weight and blood pressure several times daily and adjust fluids to maintain stable weight once rehydrated.

DIET

• Nutritional support should be provided within 3 days using moderately protein-restricted diets.
• Caloric and protein requirements supplied by blended renal diets, liquid enteral solutions, or formulated diets delivered by enteral feeding tube. Parenteral nutrition may be needed in some cases.

CLIENT EDUCATION

• Depending on inciting cause, prognosis for recovery of renal function is variable. Average recovery for all causes of AKI is 50%. Likelihood of some degree of persistent kidney damage.
• Potential for complications of treatment (e.g., fluid overload, pancreatitis, sepsis, and multiple organ failure); expense of prolonged hospitalization; options for continued care if conventional medical management fails (hemodialysis, peritoneal dialysis); zoonotic potential of leptospirosis.

SURGICAL CONSIDERATIONS

• See Ureterolithiasis.
• Renal transplantation may provide long-term survival for cats with severe, nonrecovered AKI.

Peritoneal or Hemodialysis

• Dialysis can stabilize the patient to allow time for renal recovery. Without, most oliguric patients die before sufficient renal repair occurs.
• Indications—oliguria or anuria, life-threatening fluid overload or acid-base/electrolyte disturbances, BUN ≥100 mg/dL, serum creatinine ≥5 mg/dL, clinical course refractory to conservative treatment, perioperative stabilization, and poisoning/overdosage with dialyzable toxin/drug.

MEDICATIONS

DRUG(S) OF CHOICE

Inadequate Urine Production

• Avoid overhydration. Once fluid replete, administer diuretics.
• Hypertonic mannitol (20%)—0.5 g/kg IV over 15–30 minutes; if effective, continue IV bolus q6h.
• Furosemide—1–4 mg/kg IV; if effective, continue at 0.5 mg/kg/h or 2 mg/kg q6h.
• Dopamine—potential side effects and lack of efficacy contraindicate its use except for pressor control. Fenoldopam may be more efficacious.
• Dialysis for refractory cases.

Metabolic Disorders, Acid-Base Disorders

Administer bicarbonate if serum bicarbonate ≤16 mEq/L; bicarbonate replacement: mEq = bicarbonate deficit × body weight (kg) × 0.3; give half IV over 30 minutes and remainder over 2–4 hours, then reassess.

Hyperkalemia

• Correct dehydration with potassium-free fluids.
• Minimize potassium intake.
• Discontinue medications that promote hyperkalemia.
• Loop diuretics—furosemide 1–2 mg/kg IV.
• Sodium bicarbonate—correct bicarbonate deficit, if bicarbonate status unknown 1–2 mEq/kg IV.
• Dextrose ± insulin—1–2 mL/kg of 50% dextrose diluted to 25% IV or regular insulin 0.1–0.2 U/kg IV bolus followed by 1–2 g dextrose/unit insulin.
• Calcium gluconate 10%—0.5–1.0 mL/kg IV over 10–15 minutes (cardioprotective, does not alter serum potassium).
• Refractory hyperkalemia—dialysis.

Vomiting

• Reduce gastric acid production—pantoprazole (1 mg/kg IV q12h), famotidine CRI.
• Mucosal protectant for gastrointestinal (GI) ulceration—sucralfate (0.25–1 g PO q6–8h).
• Antiemetics—maropitant (1 mg/kg SC/IV q24h); ondansetron (0.2–1 mg/kg IV q8–12h).

PRECAUTIONS

Modify dosages of drugs requiring renal metabolism or elimination.

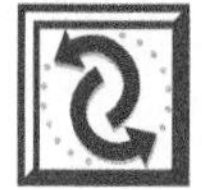

FOLLOW-UP

PATIENT MONITORING

Fluid, electrolyte, and acid-base balances; body weight; blood pressure; UOP; and clinical status.

PREVENTION/AVOIDANCE

• Anticipate AKI in aged patients or those with systemic disease, sepsis, trauma, hemodynamic instability, receiving nephrotoxic drugs, multiple organ failure, or undergoing prolonged anesthesia.
• Monitor urine production, BUN, and creatinine in high-risk patients.

POSSIBLE COMPLICATIONS

Seizures, coma, cardiac arrhythmias, hypo- or hypertension, congestive heart failure, pulmonary edema, uremic pneumonitis, GI bleeding, sepsis, cardiopulmonary arrest, and death.

EXPECTED COURSE AND PROGNOSIS

• Prognosis depends on underlying cause, extent of renal injury, concomitant disease or organ failure, and response to therapy.
• Survival rate ~50%, but depends on cause: <20% for advanced ethylene glycol toxicosis, >80% for acute leptospirosis.
• Polyuric AKI—typically milder than oliguric; recovery may occur over 2–6 weeks, but prognosis remains guarded.
• Oliguric AKI—extensive kidney injury, difficult to manage, and has poor prognosis for recovery without dialysis; recovery may be signaled by sudden (and often excessive) polyuria and sluggish and possibly incomplete return of renal function over 4–12 weeks; dialysis extends potential for renal regeneration and repair.
• Anuric AKI—poor prognosis without dialysis. Anuria is not prognostic and does not impact ability for renal recovery, if hemodialysis is available to maintain patient during recovery period.

MISCELLANEOUS

ZOONOTIC POTENTIAL

Leptospirosis

PREGNANCY/FERTILITY/BREEDING

A rare complication of pregnancy; promoted by acute metritis, pyometra, and postpartum sepsis or hemorrhage.

SYNONYMS

• Acute renal failure.
• Acute tubular necrosis.
• Acute uremia.

SEE ALSO

• Azotemia and Uremia.
• Hyperkalemia.
• Hypertension, Systemic Arterial.
• Leptospirosis.
• Ureterolithiasis.

ABBREVIATIONS

• ACEI = angiotensin-converting enzyme inhibitors.
• AKI = acute kidney injury.
• BUN = blood urea nitrogen.
• CKD = chronic kidney disease.
• cPLI = canine pancreatic lipase immunoreactivity.
• DIC = disseminated intravascular coagulation.
• GI = gastrointestinal.
• NSAID = nonsteroidal anti-inflammatory drug.
• PCV = packed cell volume.
• UOP = urine output.
• USG = urine specific gravity.

Suggested Reading

Cowgill LD, Langston C. Acute kidney insufficiency. In: Bartges J, Polzin DJ, eds., Nephrology and Urology of Small Animals. Ames, IA: Wiley-Blackwell, 2011, pp. 472–523.
Sykes JE, Hartmann K, Lunn KF, et al. 2010 ACVIM small animal consensus statement on leptospirosis: diagnosis, epidemiology, treatment, and prevention. J Vet Intern Med 2011, 25(1):1–13.

Authors Sheri Ross and Cedric P. Dufayet
Consulting Editor J.D. Foster

Client Education Handout available online

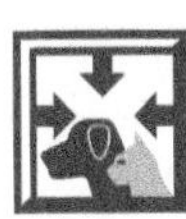

BASICS

DEFINITION

• Acute respiratory distress syndrome (ARDS) is a syndrome of acute onset of respiratory failure typified by diffuse bilateral pulmonary infiltrates on a dorsoventral thoracic radiograph, with no clinical evidence of left atrial hypertension or volume overload. ARDS results from an overwhelming inflammatory reaction in the alveolocapillary membrane in response to a systemic or pulmonary inflammatory insult. The end result is increased vascular permeability leading to edema. • The 2012 Berlin Definition of ARDS defines three categories of severity based on PaO_2/FiO_2 (PF) ratio and level of positive end-expiratory pressure (PEEP) employed during ventilation, with mild ARDS defined by a PF ratio of 200–300 mmHg with PEEP ≥5 mmHg, moderate ARDS as a PF ratio of 100–200 mmHg with PEEP ≥5 mmHg, and severe ARDS as a PF ratio <100 mmHg with PEEP ≥5 mmHg.

PATHOPHYSIOLOGY

• ARDS is due to a diffuse inflammatory insult that causes widespread damage to alveolar endothelial and epithelial cells, resulting in thickening of the membrane and impaired gas exchange. This inflammatory insult can be triggered by primary pulmonary disease or it can be of nonpulmonary origin, and leads to exudative, proliferative, and fibrotic changes within the lung. • First, excessive accumulation and activation of neutrophils, monocytes, and platelets in the pulmonary microvasculature lead to increased alveolar endothelial permeability. This causes protein-rich edema fluid and inflammatory cells to leak into the interstitial and alveolar spaces. • Alveolar epithelial injury results from release of cytokines and other inflammatory mediators from leukocytes and platelets. • Epithelial injury involves both type I and type II alveolar epithelial cells, and results in alveolar flooding and surfactant dysfunction. This causes collapse and consolidation of alveoli with development of severe hypoxemia, and hyaline membrane formation in the alveolar spaces.
• Microthrombi in the pulmonary vasculature, hypoxic pulmonary vasoconstriction, and release of endogenous vasoconstrictors lead to pulmonary arterial hypertension, which can lead to right-sided heart failure. • Proliferation of type 2 alveolar epithelial cells and pulmonary fibrosis occurs in the late stages of ARDS.

SYSTEMS AFFECTED

• Respiratory. • Cardiovascular—right-sided heart failure secondary to pulmonary hypertension; hemodynamic compromise may be associated with aggressive mechanical ventilator settings.

GENETICS

Certain humans are more prone to developing ARDS than others due to specific gene polymorphisms. This has not been investigated in the veterinary population.

INCIDENCE/PREVALENCE

Unknown

SIGNALMENT

Species

Dog and cat.

Breed Predilections

A familial form of ARDS has been reported in a group of related Dalmatian dogs; it is clinically indistinguishable from ARDS.

Mean Age and Range

Unknown

SIGNS

Historical Findings

• Acute onset of respiratory distress in patient with significant underlying disease or exposure to known risk factors. • Patient often hospitalized for primary disease when develops ARDS.

Physical Examination Findings

• Severe respiratory distress. • Crackles (if present) heard bilaterally on auscultation.
• Fever—depends on underlying disease.
• Cyanosis in more severe cases. • Signs relevant to primary disease process.

CAUSES

Primary Pulmonary Causes

• Aspiration pneumonia. • Pneumonia.
• Pulmonary contusion. • Near drowning.
• Chemical or smoke inhalation. • Idiopathic form of ARDS associated with acute interstitial pneumonia or idiopathic pulmonary fibrosis has been reported in humans and dogs.

Nonpulmonary Causes

• Systemic inflammatory response syndrome (SIRS). • Sepsis. • Neoplasia. • Pancreatitis.
• Severe trauma and shock. • Severe bee sting envenomation.

RISK FACTORS

• SIRS. • Sepsis. • Severity of illness. • Multiple transfusions.

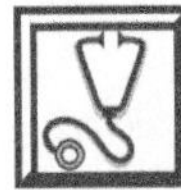

DIAGNOSIS

DIFFERENTIAL DIAGNOSIS

• Left-sided congestive heart failure. • Fluid overload. • Diffuse pneumonia. • Pulmonary hemorrhage.

CBC/BIOCHEMISTRY/URINALYSIS

• Leukocytosis or leukopenia. • Other changes dependent on underlying disease process.

OTHER LABORATORY TESTS

• Arterial blood gases—low PF ratio (where PaO_2 is measured in mmHg and FiO_2 is 0.21–1.0). Normal PF ratio = 500; comparison of this ratio allows evaluation of severity of lung disease and direct comparison of blood gases taken at different FiO_2. $PaCO_2$ is often low; hypercapnia tends to be late (preterminal) development. • Total protein of airway edema fluid compared with serum total protein—ratio of edema fluid to serum total protein <0.5 supportive of low-protein hydrostatic pressure pulmonary edema (e.g., heart failure, fluid overload); edema fluid/serum total protein ratio >0.7 suggests high-protein, increased permeability pulmonary edema such as ARDS and pneumonia. • Coagulation panel may reveal hypocoagulable state supportive of disseminated intravascular coagulation (DIC) or cause of pulmonary hemorrhage.

IMAGING

Thoracic Radiographs

• Bilateral/diffuse pulmonary infiltrates.
• Severity of radiographic signs can lag behind clinical disease by 12–24 hours. • Can be difficult to distinguish from cardiogenic edema; cardiac silhouette and pulmonary vascular size usually normal in ARDS.

Echocardiography

• Attempt to rule out cardiogenic cause for pulmonary edema. • May be able to estimate degree of pulmonary hypertension.

DIAGNOSTIC PROCEDURES

Pulmonary artery catheter to measure pulmonary artery occlusion pressure can be used to rule out cardiogenic cause for edema; by definition, ARDS is associated with pulmonary artery occlusion pressure (PAOP) ≤18 mmHg.

PATHOLOGIC FINDINGS

Gross Pathology

Lungs are dark, heavy, and ooze fluid when cut.

Histopathology

• Acute phase—pulmonary vascular congestion with edema fluid and inflammatory cell accumulation in interstitium and alveoli; epithelial cell damage, hyaline membrane formation, microthrombi, microatelectasis.
• Proliferative phase—hyperplasia of type 2 pneumocytes, interstitial mononuclear infiltration, organization of hyaline membranes, and fibroproliferation.

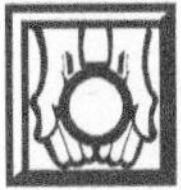

TREATMENT

APPROPRIATE HEALTH CARE

• No specific therapy; general aims to maintain tissue oxygenation and minimize iatrogenic lung injury while treating underlying disease.
• Oxygen therapy—no more than required to maintain PaO_2 >60–80 mmHg to minimize oxygen toxicity. • Positive-pressure ventilation (PPV) essential in management of ARDS patients; indicated in patients that are hypoxemic despite

ACUTE RESPIRATORY DISTRESS SYNDROME (CONTINUED)

oxygen therapy, patients requiring high levels of inspired oxygen for prolonged periods, or patients working so hard to breathe that at risk of exhaustion. • ARDS thought to be exacerbated by ventilator-induced lung injury associated with alveolar overdistension compounded by cyclic opening and collapse of atelectatic alveoli; therefore, lung-protective strategies of PPV with moderate to high PEEP, low tidal volumes, and permissive hypercapnia recommended to minimize ventilator-induced lung injury; tidal volumes of 6 mL/kg have been found to increase survival significantly in human ARDS patients compared to tidal volumes of 12 mL/kg. • Recruitment maneuvers and high levels of PEEP can both cause significant hemodynamic compromise and patients should have constant direct arterial blood pressure monitoring. • Intensive supportive care of cardiovascular system and other organ systems is vital, as these patients at high risk for development of multiple organ dysfunction.

NURSING CARE

• Monitor temperature closely, especially if using an oxygen cage, as animals with excessive work of breathing can easily become hyperthermic. • Ventilator patients require frequent position changes and physical therapy; regular oral care with dilute chlorhexidine solution is important to reduce oral colonization with bacteria as source of sepsis, and frequent endotracheal tube suctioning needed to prevent occlusion; inflate cuff carefully and change endotracheal cuff position regularly to prevent tracheal damage. • Blood pressure monitoring, as septic patients prone to hypotension. • Fluid therapy important to support cardiovascular system and maintain normovolemia while avoiding fluid overload, as this will negatively affect lung function.

ACTIVITY

If not anesthetized for ventilation, strict cage confinement.

DIET

Nutritional support important but challenging. Enteral feeding desired over parenteral nutrition, but must consider high risk of regurgitation and aspiration in recumbent patient.

CLIENT EDUCATION

Clients need to be aware of the guarded prognosis and high costs of therapy.

SURGICAL CONSIDERATIONS

Underlying disease may require surgery.

MEDICATIONS

DRUG(S) OF CHOICE

• No specific drug therapy. • Antibiotics for underlying disease where indicated. • Vasoactive drugs to maintain blood pressure. • Anesthetic drugs to allow PPV. • Analgesia as appropriate. • Low-dose corticosteroid—use remains controversial, with conflicting reports of efficacy for low-dose steroids in early or late ARDS.

ALTERNATIVE DRUG(S)

Furosemide may produce pulmonary venous dilation and improve lung function, as intermittent bolus of 1 mg/kg IV q6–12h or as CRI of 0.2 mg/kg/h IV. Beware dehydration and effects on organ function.

FOLLOW-UP

PATIENT MONITORING

Arterial blood gases, pulse oximetry, end-tidal carbon dioxide, thoracic radiographs, arterial blood pressure, ECG, temperature, urine output, CBC, coagulation profiles, serum chemistry, blood cultures, monitoring for other organ dysfunction.

PREVENTION/AVOIDANCE

• Appropriate therapy of primary disease processes to reduce inflammatory insult to lung. • Intensive cardiovascular monitoring and support of critically ill animals to ensure adequate tissue perfusion. • Careful management of recumbent animals to reduce chance of aspiration, especially if patient has neurologic disease or upper airway disorders that reduce ability to protect airway. • Judicious use of blood products in patients with inflammatory or severe systemic disease.

POSSIBLE COMPLICATIONS

• Multiorgan dysfunction syndrome—acute kidney injury, DIC, and gastrointestinal disease are more common forms of organ dysfunction seen. • Barotrauma—can result in pneumothorax; incidence thought to be less with lower tidal volume ventilation strategies. • Ventilator-associated pneumonia—patients on PPV have increased risk of pneumonia that may be difficult to differentiate from worsening of initial lung injury; airway cultures should be considered in deteriorating patients. • Oxygen toxicity may be unavoidable due to severity of hypoxemia in spite of PPV; oxygen toxicity indistinguishable from ARDS on histopathology, making incidence of this problem impossible to determine.

EXPECTED COURSE AND PROGNOSIS

• Mortality in human patients remains at 40–60%. • Mortality in veterinary patients is likely greater than 90%.

MISCELLANEOUS

ASSOCIATED CONDITIONS

SIRS, multiple organ dysfunction syndrome, sepsis.

SYNONYMS

• Acute hypoxemic respiratory failure. • Acute interstitial pneumonia. • Adult respiratory distress syndrome. • High-protein pulmonary edema. • Shock lung.

SEE ALSO

• Dyspnea and Respiratory Distress. • Panting and Tachypnea. • Pulmonary Edema, Noncardiogenic. • Sepsis and Bacteremia.

ABBREVIATIONS

• ARDS = acute respiratory distress syndrome.
• DIC = disseminated intravascular coagulation.
• PAOP = pulmonary artery occlusion pressure (formerly pulmonary capillary wedge pressure).
• PEEP = positive end-expiratory pressure.
• PF ratio = PaO_2/FiO_2 ratio. • PPV = positive-pressure ventilation. • SIRS = systemic inflammatory response syndrome.

INTERNET RESOURCES

www.ardsnet.org

Suggested Reading

ARDS Definition Task Force, Ranieri VM, Rubenfeld GD, et al. Acute respiratory distress syndrome: the Berlin Definition. J Am Med Assoc 2012, 307(23):2526–2533.

Balakrishnan A, Drobatz KJ, Silverstein DC. Retrospective evaluation of the prevalence, risk factors, management, outcome, and necropsy findings of acute lung injury and acute respiratory distress syndrome in dogs and cats: 29 cases (2011–2013). J Vet Emerg Crit Care 2017, 27(6):662–673.

Matthay MA, Ware LB, Zimmerman GA. The acute respiratory distress syndrome. J Clin Invest 2012, 122(8):2731–2740.

Parent C, King LG, Van Winkle TJ, Walker LM. Respiratory function and treatment in dogs with acute respiratory distress syndrome: 19 cases (1985–1993). J Am Vet Med Assoc 1996, 208:1428–1433.

Ware LB, Matthay MA. The acute respiratory distress syndrome. N Engl J Med 2000, 342:1334–1349.

Wilkins PA, Otto CM, Baumgardner JE, et al. Acute lung injury and acute respiratory distress syndromes in veterinary medicine: consensus definitions: The Dorothy Russell Havemeyer Working Group on ALI and ARDS in Veterinary Medicine. J Vet Emerg Crit Care (San Antonio) 2007, 17(4):333–339.

Author Casey J. Kohen
Consulting Editor Elizabeth Rozanski

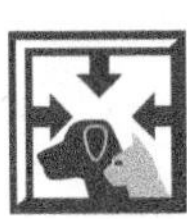

BASICS

DEFINITION

Vomiting of fewer than 7 days' duration.

PATHOPHYSIOLOGY

• Vomiting is a reflex initiated by the vomiting center in the medulla, triggered by three major mechanisms—gastric/duodenal mucosal irritation, gastric/duodenal distention, or the chemoreceptor trigger zone (CRTZ). • Mucosal irritation or gastric/duodenal distention signal the vomiting center via sympathetic and vagal afferent innervation. Anti-peristaltic waves force intestinal contents back to the duodenum, then distention becomes the main trigger for the vomiting reflex. • The CRTZ can directly trigger the vomiting center via receptor activation or vestibular input; known receptors are α_2, D_2, H1, M1, NK_1, $5HT_3$. • Cerebral cortex and vestibular apparatus can also directly stimulate the vomiting center. • The vomiting center initiates an autonomic motor reaction via spinal nerves to diaphragmatic and abdominal muscles, and cranial nerves 5, 7, 9, 10, and 12 to the upper gastrointestinal (GI) tract. • The reflex involves a deep breath, opening the upper esophageal sphincter, closing the glottis, strong diaphragmatic and abdominal muscle contractions, and lower esophageal sphincter relaxation, leading to expulsion of contents.

SYSTEMS AFFECTED

• Cardiovascular—fluid losses can be significant, with progressive dehydration to hypovolemia; vagal stimulation can lead to bradycardia, and rarely syncope. • GI—esophagitis. • Metabolic—vomiting of mixed small intestinal and gastric contents results in isotonic electrolyte losses; pyloric obstruction results in metabolic alkalosis; hypokalemia is common with concurrent hyporexia. • Respiratory—aspiration pneumonitis/pneumonia.

GENETICS

N/A

INCIDENCE/PREVALENCE

Increased incidence of infectious causes and dietary indiscretion in young patients.

GEOGRAPHIC DISTRIBUTION

Some infectious etiologies have specific geographic distributions.

SIGNALMENT

• Species—dog and cat. • No breed, age, or sex predilections.

SIGNS

Historical Findings

• Care should be taken to differentiate vomiting from regurgitation. • Dietary indiscretion, foreign body, and medication/toxin history should be investigated. • Nausea and hypersalivation. • Varying amounts, frequency, and severity of vomiting. • Varying activity levels can be seen, from normal to lethargic. • Hematemesis may be seen.

Physical Examination Findings

• Dehydration/hypovolemia, cranial abdominal pain, nausea, fluid–gas interface on intestinal palpation, increased borborygmi. • Careful sublingual examination for anchored linear foreign bodies. • Careful abdominal palpation for mechanical obstruction. • Rectal examination for melena or concurrent diarrhea.

CAUSES

• Extra-GI causes: ○ Common—hepatobiliary disease, kidney disease, pancreatitis, neoplasia (non-GI). ○ Uncommon—CNS, cardiac, endocrine (hypoadrenocorticism, hyperthyroidism, diabetic ketoacidosis), respiratory disease, peritonitis, sepsis. ○ Intra-GI causes: ○ Congenital/genetic—hiatal hernia. ○ Infectious—parasitic, protozoal, viral (parvovirus, canine distemper virus, corona virus), fungal, bacterial (*Campylobacter*, *Salmonella*). ○ Inflammatory (most common cause)—acute gastritis/gastroenteritis due to dietary indiscretion or sudden diet change, acute hemorrhagic diarrhea syndrome. ○ Mechanical obstruction—foreign body, intussusception, obstructive mass (granuloma, neoplasia, pyloric hypertrophy, trichobezoar), torsion/volvulus (gastric, mesenteric). ○ Medications/toxins—α_2 agonists, antibiotics, apomorphine, chemotherapeutic agents, methimazole, nonsteroidal anti-inflammatory drugs (NSAIDS), opioids, toxins (corrosive, heavy metals). ○ Neoplasia—primary such as adenocarcinoma, lymphoma, leiomyoma/leiomyosarcoma, gastrointestinal stromal tumor, mast cell tumor (cats), metastatic. ○ Ulcers—gastric and/or duodenal ulceration is usually secondary: NSAIDS, neoplasia (primary GI, mast cell tumor, gastrinoma), hypoadrenocorticism, uremia, infectious (controversial—*Helicobacter*), stress.

RISK FACTORS

• Dietary—abrupt diet change or dietary indiscretion. • Medications—many medications can cause acute vomiting. • Infectious—geographic distribution effect.

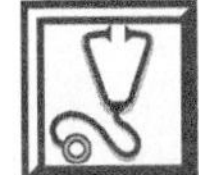

DIAGNOSIS

DIFFERENTIAL DIAGNOSIS

• Vomiting can be mistaken for regurgitation. ○ Vomiting—prodromal nausea (hypersalivation), retching, abdominal contractions. ○ Regurgitation—no prodromal nausea, passive expulsion of fluid/food. ○ Vomiting can lead to regurgitation via esophagitis, so if both signs are present, it is important to establish chronology. • In cats, vomiting can be mistaken for coughing. ○ Coughing involves extension of neck and elbows. ○ Physical exam findings may differentiate. ○ Videos can be helpful to differentiate.

CBC/BIOCHEMISTRY/URINALYSIS

• Extra-GI causes: ○ Increased hepatic enzyme activity in hepatobiliary diseases. ○ Renal azotemia in kidney disease. ○ Increased hepatic enzyme activity, hypoalbuminemia, inflammatory leukogram in pancreatitis. ○ Hypoalbuminemia, decreased Na : K ratio in hypoadrenocorticism. • Intra-GI causes—often normal. • As result of vomiting, following may be present: ○ Hemoconcentration. ○ Prerenal azotemia. ○ Hypokalemia, hypochloremia. ○ Hypoalbuminemia, hypocholesterolemia. ○ Hypoglycemia—toy-breed puppies predisposed.

OTHER LABORATORY TESTS

• Extra-GI interrogation—baseline cortisol or adrenocorticotropic hormone (ACTH) stimulation test in dogs, T_4 in cats, quantitative pancreatic lipase immunoreactivity. • Intra-GI interrogation—fecal flotation, fecal direct smear cytology.

IMAGING

Abdominal Radiography

• Survey abdominal radiographs indicated in most acutely vomiting patients to evaluate potential surgical emergencies, like mechanical obstructions and sepsis. Survey abdominal radiographs also interrogate many extra-GI causes of vomiting. • Acute gastritis/gastroenteritis—mild gas and/or fluid dilation of stomach/intestine. • Mechanical obstruction—foreign body may be radiopaque, or two populations of bowel may be seen, one distended orad to the obstruction, and one normal aborad to the obstruction. • If foreign body is suspected, but no radiographic evidence, serial radiographs every 6 hours or contrast radiography may be considered. • Gastric dilatation and volvulus—malpositioned pylorus on right lateral radiograph. • Pancreatitis—widened gastroduodenal angle, focal decreased serosal detail at proximal duodenal flexure.

Abdominal Ultrasonography

• Abdominal ultrasonography may be useful in interrogation of intra- and extra-GI causes of vomiting, such as pancreatitis and intussusception. • Emergency cage-side focused ultrasonographic examination of abdomen is indicated in patients with acute abdominal pain, to evaluate for etiologies that are surgical emergencies, such as septic or bile peritonitis. • If peritoneal effusion seen, abdominocentesis and immediate in-house cytology are indicated (+/- culture).

A

ACUTE VOMITING (CONTINUED)

DIAGNOSTIC PROCEDURES

• Endoscopy rarely indicated in acute vomiting, except for gastric foreign bodies or gastric ulceration. • Exploratory celiotomy may be considered with high suspicion for mechanical obstruction, even when not confirmed with imaging.

PATHOLOGIC FINDINGS

Dependent on underlying etiology.

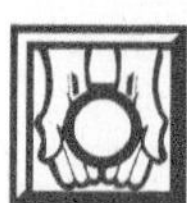

TREATMENT

APPROPRIATE HEALTH CARE

• Stable patients, mild vomiting—outpatient medical care. Careful assessment of young patients should be made, as they can become unstable with mild signs. • Unstable patients, hypovolemic or acute abdominal pain—inpatient medical care. • Emergency surgery may be indicated—mechanical obstruction, septic or bile peritonitis, volvulus.

NURSING CARE

• Fluid therapy as mandated by hydration/perfusion status. • Most patients with dehydration/hypovolemia need isotonic crystalloids to replenish losses and provide maintenance. • Nothing PO—only indicated in patients with mechanical obstruction, severe intractable vomiting, or patients with high risk of aspiration.

ACTIVITY

Activity restriction only required in postoperative care of surgical patients.

DIET

Once vomiting resolves, gradual reintroduction of small amounts of water, then small, frequent meals of bland, highly digestible diet is indicated for 3–5 days, then gradual reintroduction of patient's routine diet and feeding schedule.

CLIENT EDUCATION

Client education on dietary indiscretion, gradual diet changes, and foreign body avoidance may be appropriate.

SURGICAL CONSIDERATIONS

Surgery may be indicated to treat etiology, such as mechanical obstruction.

MEDICATIONS

DRUG(S) OF CHOICE

• Anti-emetics not usually needed for mild acute vomiting, but may be needed in more severe cases—$5HT_3$ antagonists such as ondansetron (0.2–1 mg/kg SC/IV q8h), NK_1 antagonist maropitant (1 mg/kg SC q24h or 2 mg/kg PO q24h), dopamine antagonist and prokinetic metoclopramide (0.2–0.5 mg/kg SC/PO q6–8h, or 1–2 mg/kg/day as CRI), phenothiazine derivative chlorpromazine (0.5 mg/kg SC q8h). • Refractory vomiting patients (i.e., pancreatitis) may need multimodal anti-emetics that act on different receptors. • Gastric/duodenal ulcers—proton pump inhibitor such as pantoprazole IV or omeprazole PO (1 mg/kg IV/PO q12h) is preferred treatment. Sucralfate, while used conventionally in ulcers, has only been shown to help cats with esophagitis, and due to impaired absorption of concurrently given medications, and q8 dosing, is of questionable efficacy. • NSAID-induced ulceration—consider misoprostol. • Vestibular mediated—H_1 antagonist like diphenhydramine (2–4 mg/kg PO/IM q6–8h).

CONTRAINDICATIONS

• Prokinetic medications should not be given to patients with mechanical obstruction.
• Phenothiazine derivatives—caution in patients with seizures or hypovolemia/hypotension.
• Anticholinergics should not be given, as exacerbation of signs from ileus can result.

PRECAUTIONS

Anti-emetic medications should not be given to patient receiving outpatient care, unless mechanical obstruction has been ruled out.

POSSIBLE INTERACTIONS

Ondansetron IV can react with other medications and precipitate.

ALTERNATIVE DRUGS

Dolasetron, famotidine.

FOLLOW-UP

PATIENT MONITORING

• If patient receives anti-emetic with outpatient medical care, and continues to vomit—hospitalize for further diagnostics and inpatient medical care. • If vomiting not improving, or getting more severe, further diagnostics are warranted. • If vomiting persists beyond 7 days or recurs despite appropriate therapy, consider chronic vomiting etiologies.

PREVENTION/AVOIDANCE

Avoid rapid diet changes and dietary indiscretion, and institute prophylactic deworming and vaccinations.

POSSIBLE COMPLICATIONS

• Aspiration pneumonia. • Esophagitis.
• Dehydration and hypovolemia.

EXPECTED COURSE AND PROGNOSIS

• Mild acute vomiting from acute gastritis/gastroenteritis usually self-limiting.
• Mechanical obstruction from foreign bodies has good prognosis with rapid recognition and treatment. • Other prognoses etiology dependent.

MISCELLANEOUS

ASSOCIATED CONDITIONS

Acute diarrhea, hyporexia.

AGE-RELATED FACTORS

Younger patients more likely to have ingested foreign body or have infectious etiologies.

ZOONOTIC POTENTIAL

Parasitic, protozoal, and bacterial etiologies (*Ancylostoma, Campylobacter, Giardia, Salmonella*).

PREGNANCY/FERTILITY/BREEDING

Misoprostol for treatment of NSAID-induced ulcers is contraindicated in pregnant animals and humans.

SYNONYMS

Emesis

SEE ALSO

• Acute Diarrhea. • Gastroduodenal Ulceration/Erosion. • Gastroenteritis, Acute Hemorrhagic Diarrhea Syndrome.
• Pancreatitis – Cats. • Pancreatitis – Dogs.
• Vomiting, Chronic.

ABBREVIATIONS

• ACTH = adrenocorticotropic hormone.
• CRTZ = chemoreceptor trigger zone.
• GI = gastrointestinal. • NSAID = nonsteroidal anti-inflammatory drug.

INTERNET RESOURCES

• https://www.avma.org/practicemanagement/clientmaterials/pages/default.aspx • https://veterinarypartner.vin.com

Suggested Reading

Gallagher A. Vomiting and regurgitation. In: Ettinger SJ, ed., Textbook of Veterinary Internal Medicine, 8th ed. St. Louis, MO: Elsevier, 2017, pp. 158–164.

Hall J. Physiology of gastrointestinal disorders. In: Hall J, ed., Guyton and Hall's Textbook of Medical Physiology, 13th ed. Philadelphia, PA: Elsevier, 2016, 843–852.

Marks SL, Kook PH, Papich MG, et al. ACVIM consensus statement: support for rational administration of gastrointestinal protectants to dogs and cats. J Vet Intern Med 2018, 32:1823–1840.

Unterer S, Busch K, Leipig M, et al. Endoscopically visualized lesions, histologic findings, and bacterial invasion in the gastrointestinal mucosa of dogs with acute hemorrhagic diarrhea syndrome. J Vet Intern Med 2014, 28:52–58.

Author Talia Guttin

Consulting Editor Mark P. Rondeau

Acknowledgment The author and editor acknowledge the prior contribution of Erin Portillo.

Client Education Handout available online

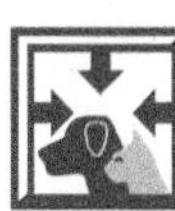

BASICS

DEFINITION

Malignant neoplasm derived from the apocrine glands of the anal sac.

PATHOPHYSIOLOGY

- Locally invasive.
- High metastatic rate (~50–80% at diagnosis), often to locoregional lymph nodes including medial iliac (MILN), internal iliac, sacral, less frequently to distant sites including liver, spleen, or lungs.
- Frequently associated with hypercalcemia, secondary to parathyroid hormone–related peptide (PTH-rP) secretion.
- Prognosis good to guarded with appropriate treatment intervention.

SYSTEMS AFFECTED

- Gastrointestinal.
- Endocrine/metabolic.
- Hemic/lymphatic/immune.

GENETICS

English cocker spaniels significantly over-represented, springer and Cavalier King Charles spaniels also overrepresented.

INCIDENCE/PREVALENCE

Relatively uncommon—17% of perianal tumors, 2% of all skin/subcutaneous tumors.

SIGNALMENT

- Older dogs; extremely rare in cats.
- Females overrepresented in some studies.
- Breed predilection as stated above.

SIGNS

Historical Findings

Signs may be due to physical presence of primary tumor (visible mass near anus, tenesmus, scooting behaviors) or lymph nodes enlarged due to metastasis (tenesmus, obstipation, stranguria), or systemic manifestations due to hypercalcemia (polyuria/polydipsia, anorexia).

Physical Examination Findings

- Mass associated with anal sac; may be quite small relative to significant metastatic disease burdens.
- Caudal abdominal lymphadenopathy—on rectal or abdominal palpation.

CAUSES & RISK FACTORS

None definitively identified.

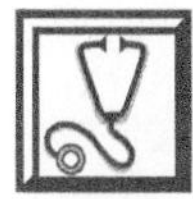

DIAGNOSIS

DIFFERENTIAL DIAGNOSIS

- Anal sac abscess.
- Perianal adenoma/adenocarcinoma.
- Mast cell tumor.
- Melanoma.
- Lymphoma.
- Squamous cell carcinoma.
- Perineal hernias.

CBC/BIOCHEMISTRY/URINALYSIS

- Hypercalcemia—15–30% of cases; associated hyposthenuria.
- Secondary renal failure may develop with longstanding and severe hypercalcemia. Beware of interpreting urine specific gravity to differentiate prerenal versus renal azotemia in hypercalcemic patients. Hypercalcemia inhibits concentrating abilities of kidneys, thus azotemia with dilute urine may be seen with both prerenal and renal azotemia. Treatment of disease to resolve hypercalcemia and fluid therapy is needed to determine if underlying renal pathology is present.

OTHER LABORATORY TESTS

If hypercalcemia is present, and tumor cannot be identified, parathyroid hormone and PTHrP levels can be assessed—high PTHrP supports neoplasia as cause of hypercalcemia. This ancillary screening test is not commonly required, as anal gland tumors are easily palpable.

IMAGING

- Abdominal radiography—to evaluate medial iliac lymph nodes and lumbar and pelvic bones.
- Thoracic radiography—to evaluate for pulmonary metastasis.
- Abdominal ultrasonography—may identify enlarged locoregional lymph nodes not visible radiographically, and also metastatic lesions involving visceral organs (liver/spleen).
- CT scan—identifies lymphadenopathy with greater sensitivity than ultrasound. In one study ultrasound found all affected lymph nodes in only 30.8% of cases where CT identified multiple nodes involved.

DIAGNOSTIC PROCEDURES

- Fine-needle aspiration and cytology of anal sac mass to rule out conditions other than adenocarcinoma; while differentiation of benign versus malignant neoplasm of perianal masses is difficult, apocrine gland adenocarcinoma of anal sac will have neuroendocrine appearance and can be differentiated from perianal gland tumors.
- Fine-needle aspiration and cytology of enlarged lymph nodes, liver, or splenic nodules to confirm metastasis.
- Histopathology required for definitive diagnosis. Incisional biopsy can be considered, but excisional biopsy appropriate if location of mass and cytology supportive of anal sac neoplasia.

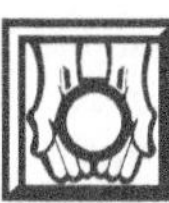

TREATMENT

- Surgical resection is treatment of choice.
- Resection of primary tumor and enlarged lymph nodes prolongs survival—both at initial diagnosis and upon relapse.
- If mass is large and locally invasive at diagnosis, surgery will be palliative, not curative.
- Debulking all disease present may control hypercalcemia until tumor recurrence.
- Surgery may not be possible if primary mass is very large.
- Adjuvant radiation for microscopic disease may help delay local recurrence and evidence of lymph node metastases.
- Hypofractionated radiation can provide benefit in cases of advanced or inoperable disease, with about one-third of dogs showing partial response to radiation, and about two-thirds of dogs having improvement or resolution of their clinical signs.

MEDICATIONS

DRUG(S) OF CHOICE

- Saline diuresis (200–300 mL/kg/day) preoperatively if hypercalcemia is severe. Also can consider bisphosphonate (zoledronate, pamidronate) or low-dose (0.25 mg/kg BID) prednisone to increase calciuresis, if corticosteroids not contraindicated.
- Low-dose prednisone can also be used to manage hypercalcemia palliatively in dogs that are not receiving any other therapy.
- No controlled studies showing improved outcomes with adjuvant chemotherapy postoperatively; however, such studies fraught with challenges, including range of stages of presenting dogs and retrospective nature of most publications. Theoretically, systemic therapy needed to address the highly metastatic biologic behavior of this tumor.
- Limited reports of partial responses to platinum compounds in dogs—cisplatin (70 mg/m^2 IV with 6h saline diuresis—18.3 mL/kg/h), carboplatin (300 mg/m^2 IV as slow bolus) every 3 weeks.
- Mitoxantrone (5 mg/m^2 IV every 3 weeks for five treatments) in combination with radiation therapy used in one small case series.
- Possible role for melphalan after debulking surgery (7 mg/m^2 PO q24h for 5 days every 3 weeks).
- Toceranib phosphate reported to have some benefit (partial response or stable disease) in 28 dogs with measurable tumor. In 15 dogs with stage 4 (distant metastasis) disease,

ADENOCARCINOMA, ANAL SAC (CONTINUED)

toceranib phosphate led to stable disease and modest improvement in clinical signs in 13 dogs, with median progression-free interval and survival time of 1 year.

• Phase 1 trial combining carboplatin and toceranib phosphate in 11 dogs, 4 of which had apocrine adenocarcinoma of anal sac, identified combination of carboplatin (200 mg/m^2 IV every 3 weeks) and toceranib phosphate (~2.75 mg/kg PO every other day) to be well tolerated. Neutropenia was dose-limiting toxicity. All dogs with anal sac tumors responded, with 1 partial response and 3 stable disease. Further studies are warranted.

CONTRAINDICATIONS/POSSIBLE INTERACTIONS

• Use caution with platinum chemotherapeutic agents in dogs with renal insufficiency.
• Do not use cisplatin in cats.

FOLLOW-UP

PATIENT MONITORING

• If complete resection was achieved—physical examination, thoracic radiography, abdominal ultrasonography, or abdominal +/– thoracic CT and serum biochemistry at 3, 6, 9, and 12 months postoperatively, then every 6 months thereafter.
• Incomplete resection—frequency of and modalities for monitoring dependent on ancillary treatments selected. If further therapies declined, at minimum monitor tumor size, blood calcium, and renal values. If using adjuvant therapy, monitor based on specifics of therapy.

EXPECTED COURSE AND PROGNOSIS

• Wide ranges of survivals reported. Many dogs do well with multiple surgeries with or without adjuvant therapies (chemotherapy, radiation therapy). Long-term prognosis is fair, with both local progression and metastasis occurring.
• Cures may occur if tumor is found early and treated aggressively—median survival time for nonmetastatic tumors <3.2 cm in largest diameter was 1,237 days.
• Growth of tumor may be slow and debulking lymph node metastatic disease burdens may significantly prolong survival.
• Hypercalcemia variably associated with poor prognosis, with some studies showing it as negative factor.
• Four papers (involving 200 dogs) showed median survival times of 6–20 months, depending on stage and treatment.
• Dogs with lymph node metastasis lived significantly longer if nodes were extirpated.
• Ultimately, dogs that cannot have their tumors excised completely succumb to hypercalcemia-related complications or mass effect from primary tumor or regional nodal metastases.

MISCELLANEOUS

ASSOCIATED CONDITIONS

Hypercalcemia as paraneoplastic syndrome.

ABBREVIATIONS

• MILN = medial iliac.
• PTHrP = parathyroid hormone-related peptide.

Suggested Reading

Barnes DC, Demetriou JL. Surgical management of primary, metastatic and recurrent anal sac adenocarcinoma in the dog: 52 cases. J Small Anim Pract 2017; 58:263–268.

Elliott JW. Response and outcome following toceranib phosphate treatment for stage four anal sac apocrine gland adenocarcinoma in dogs: 15 cases (2013–2017). J Am Vet Med Assoc 2019; 254:960–966.

McQuown B, Keyerleber MA, Rosen K, et al. Treatment of advanced canine anal sac adenocarcinoma with hypofractionated radiation therapy: 77 cases (1999–2013). Vet Comp Oncol 2017; 15:840–851.

Palladino S, Keyerleber MA, King RG, et al. Utility of computed tomography versus abdominal ultrasound examination to identify iliosacral lymphadenomegaly in dogs with apocrine gland adenocarcinoma of the anal sac. J Vet Intern Med 2016; 30:1858–1863.

Pradel J, Berlato D, Dobromylskyj M, et al. Prognostic significance of histopathology in canine anal sac gland adenocarcinomas: preliminary results in a retrospective study of 39 cases. Vet Comp Oncol 2018; 16:518–528.

Author Laura D. Garrett
Consulting Editor Timothy M. Fan

Client Education Handout available online

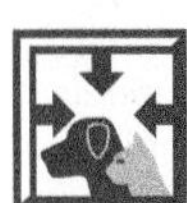

BASICS

OVERVIEW

• Comprises >75% of primary pulmonary tumors in dogs and cats. • Strongest predictors of outcome: tumor grade, node involvement, clinical signs. • May metastasize. • May be associated with hypertrophic osteopathy.

SIGNALMENT

Dogs

• 1% of all tumors. • Mean age of affected animals 10 yrs. • No sex predilection, though more females in some reports. • Medium to large breeds overrepresented.

Cats

• Rarer than in dogs. • Mean age of affected animals 11 yrs. • No breed predilection.

SIGNS

Historical Findings

• Related to presence of lung mass: ○ Nonproductive cough (>50% dogs, ~40% cats). ○ Dyspnea (may be related to pneumothorax or pleural effusion). ○ Tachypnea. ○ Hemoptysis. • Paraneoplastic signs: ○ Lameness—bone metastasis or hypertrophic osteopathy (dogs or cats), weight-bearing lytic digit metastasis (cats). ○ Polyuria or polydipsia—hypercalcemia or hyperadrenocorticism from ectopic production of adrenocorticotrophic hormone (ACTH). ○ Fever.

Physical Examination Findings

• May be asymptomatic or lack respiratory signs (~25% dogs, 9% cats). • Tachypnea, dyspnea. • Fever. • Limb swelling. • Ascites, pleural effusion.

CAUSES & RISK FACTORS

Some (controversial) evidence correlates risk to urban environment; secondhand environmental tobacco smoke not definitively linked to primary lung cancer in dogs, though weak association seen in dogs with short and medium-length noses.

DIAGNOSIS

• Cytology of mass aspirate. • Tissue biopsy/definitive resection.

DIFFERENTIAL DIAGNOSIS

• Granulomatous lesion (fungal, foreign body, parasitic). • Pulmonary abscess. • Other primary lung tumor: ○ Squamous cell carcinoma. ○ Sarcomas (osteo-, chondro-, lipo-). • Metastatic lung tumor. • Pneumonia. • Asthma. • Pulmonary thromboembolism. • Congenital cyst. • Lung torsion/hematoma.

CBC/BIOCHEMISTRY/URINALYSIS

No specific abnormalities.

OTHER LABORATORY TESTS

N/A

IMAGING

• Thoracic radiography—usually demonstrates focal, solitary, well-circumscribed mass in dogs, often in caudal lung lobes; caudal lobes most common in cats, though radiographic patterns vary more and can include diffuse interstitial disease; radiographs must be performed in cats presenting with multiple digit tumors to screen for primary lung tumor (lung-digit syndrome). • Ultrasonography—to obtain aspirate or biopsy specimen if mass in contact with chest wall, or evaluate abdomen for primary tumor. • CT—to assess surgical feasibility, lymphadenopathy (93% accuracy), metastatic disease; can see cavitated areas, irregular margins, bronchial invasion.

DIAGNOSTIC PROCEDURES

• Thoracocentesis with cytologic examination (for pleural effusion). • Cytology—transthoracic fine-needle aspiration (83% agreement with histopathology). • Percutaneous tissue biopsy—use Tru-Cut instrument, not commonly performed. • Open lung biopsy—via thoracotomy, or minimally invasive thoracoscopy.

PATHOLOGIC FINDINGS

• Adenocarcinoma—classified by location (bronchial, bronchiolar, bronchiolar-alveolar, or alveolar) and degree of differentiation. • Immunohistochemistry on biopsy for thyroid transcription factor-1 (TTF-1), surfactant protein A, and napsin A to confirm pulmonary carcinoma, especially adenocarcinoma. TTF-1 and napsin A can also be seen in thyroid tumors. • Cats tend to have less differentiated tumors, corresponding to more aggressive behavior.

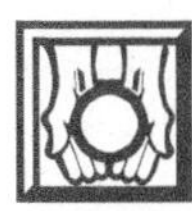

TREATMENT

• Surgery—mainstay of treatment: partial or complete lobectomy with tracheobronchial lymph node biopsy or removal; thoracoscopic removal possible at limited centers and offers less postoperative morbidity. • Radiotherapy—reports anecdotal, but certain patients may benefit. • Chemotherapy should be considered following surgery for tumors that are high grade, undifferentiated, and/or have nodal involvement, though no benefit confirmed. Intracavitary chemotherapy can be used to treat malignant pleural effusion.

MEDICATIONS

DRUG(S) OF CHOICE

• Chemotherapy—vinorelbine concentrates in lungs and responses have been seen. ○ Doxorubicin, cisplatin, carboplatin, mitoxantrone, vinorelbine, and/or vindesine: rational choices for primary or adjuvant therapy. ○ Platinum-based or gemcitabine chemotherapy may be superior. ○ Toceranib phosphate (Palladia) has shown some anecdotal success. • Chemotherapy can be toxic; seek advice if unfamiliar with cytotoxic drugs.

CONTRAINDICATIONS/POSSIBLE INTERACTIONS

• Doxorubicin—cardiotoxic, avoid in dogs with myocardial disease (arrhythmias); nephrotoxic in cats. • Cisplatin—do not give to cats (fatal); do not use in dogs with preexisting renal disease; never use without appropriate and concurrent diuresis.

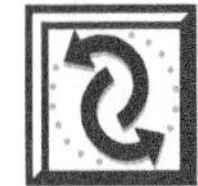

FOLLOW-UP

PATIENT MONITORING

• Serial thoracic radiographs—every 3 mths; administer minimum two cycles of chemotherapy before evaluating response. • Perform CBC (with any chemotherapy), biochemical analysis (cisplatin), and urinalysis (cisplatin) before each chemotherapy.

POSSIBLE COMPLICATIONS

• Following diagnostic procedures or thoracotomy—pneumo- or hemothorax. • Resulting from chemotherapy—myelosuppression, fever, sepsis, nausea.

EXPECTED COURSE AND PROGNOSIS

• Metastasis to tracheobronchial lymph nodes—single best prognostic indicator; median survival without metastasis approaches 1 yr and with metastasis, 60 days. More common (75%) in cats. • Postoperative survival around 2 yrs in both cats and dogs if positive prognostic factors present, and ~1 yr overall in dogs, 4 mths overall in cats. • Other patient, tumor, and treatment factors positively influencing prognosis—complete surgical excision; size of primary tumor (<5 cm); lack of metastasis; well-differentiated cellular morphology on histopathology, lack of clinical signs prior to surgery. • Poor prognosis for cats with lung-digit syndrome poor (~1 mth).

MISCELLANEOUS

PREGNANCY/FERTILITY/BREEDING

Chemotherapy not advised in pregnant animals.

ABBREVIATIONS

• ACTH = adrenocorticotrophic hormone.
• TTF-1 = thyroid transcription factor-1.

Suggested Reading

Rissetto KC, Lucas P, Fan TM. An update on diagnosing and treating primary lung tumors. Vet Med 2008, 103(3):154.

Author Kim A. Selting
Consulting Editor Timothy M. Fan

ADENOCARCINOMA, NASAL

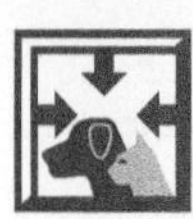

BASICS

DEFINITION

Malignant neoplasm involving the nasal cavity and paranasal sinuses.

PATHOPHYSIOLOGY

Progressive local and regional invasion of the nasal cavity, paranasal sinuses, and surrounding tissues by neoplastic epithelial and glandular epithelial cells.

SYSTEMS AFFECTED

- Respiratory—congestion, epistaxis, mucopurulent nasal discharge, obstruction, dyspnea.
- Ophthalmic—exophthalmos, epiphora.
- Musculoskeletal—facial deformity.
- Nervous—seizures, altered mentation.

INCIDENCE/PREVALENCE

- In dogs, less than 2% of all tumors are nasal tumors.
- In dogs, adenocarcinoma more common than squamous cell carcinoma, chondrosarcoma, and other histologies, comprising 31.5% of all nasal tumors.
- In cats, nasal tumors comprise <1% of all tumors. In cats, adenocarcinoma and lymphoma are most common.

GEOGRAPHIC DISTRIBUTION

Nasal adenocarcinomas are more commonly reported in urban areas.

SIGNALMENT

- Dog and cat.
- Median age in dogs is 10 years and in cats is 13 years.
- In dogs, medium to large breeds affected more commonly, with possible overrepresentation of mesocephalic and dolichocephalic breeds.

SIGNS

Historical Findings

- Intermittent and progressive history of unilateral to bilateral epistaxis and/or mucopurulent discharge that initially responds to antibiotic therapy (median duration 3 months).
- Sneezing and increased upper respiratory noises, including reverse sneezing.
- Open-mouth breathing.
- Halitosis.
- Anorexia (more frequent in cats).
- Seizures (rare—secondary to invasion of cranial vault).

Physical Examination Findings

- Nasal discharge (blood, mucopurulent).
- Decreased or absent airflow in nasal passages (unilateral or bilateral).
- Facial deformity, exophthalmos, epiphora.
- Pain upon nasal or paranasal sinus palpation or upon opening mouth.
- Regional lymphadenomegaly (rare).
- Abnormal mentation or other neurologic findings (rare).

CAUSES

Dolichocephalic morphology, p53 mutations, and cyclooxygenase-2 (COX-2) overexpression may all play a role.

RISK FACTORS

Urban environment and secondhand smoke may be risk factors.

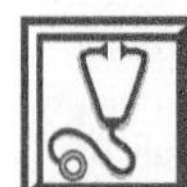

DIAGNOSIS

DIFFERENTIAL DIAGNOSIS

- Other sinonasal tumors (e.g., squamous cell carcinoma, lymphoma, sarcomas, olfactory neuroblastoma).
- Intracranial neoplasia (in dogs or cats with neurologic signs).
- Viral infection—cats.
- Fungal infections, including aspergillosis (dogs) and cryptococcosis (cats).
- Bacterial sinusitis.
- Parasites (e.g., nasal mites).
- Foreign body.
- Trauma.
- Tooth root abscess and oronasal fistula.
- Coagulopathies (nasal tumors most often tend to be unilateral epistaxis; coagulopathy tends to be bilateral epistaxis).
- Systemic hypertension (nasal tumors most often tend to be unilateral epistaxis; hypertension tends to be bilateral epistaxis).

CBC/BIOCHEMISTRY/URINALYSIS

- Usually normal.
- Occasional blood loss anemia.

OTHER LABORATORY TESTS

- Cytologic examination—occasionally helpful (e.g., aspirates of subcutaneous mass if facial deformity).
- Coagulation profile to rule out coagulopathy.
- Blood pressure to rule out systemic hypertension.

IMAGING

- Survey skull radiography—not sensitive; may show asymmetric destruction of turbinates accompanied by soft tissue mass effect; may see fluid density in frontal sinuses secondary to outflow obstruction.
- Thoracic radiography—evaluate for lung metastasis (uncommon).
- CT or MRI best imaging method for local staging and observing integrity of cribriform plate or orbital invasion; also used for therapeutic planning.

DIAGNOSTIC PROCEDURES

- Oral examination under anesthesia.
- Rhinoscopy may permit visual observation of mass and aid biopsy.
- Tissue biopsy necessary for definitive diagnosis—biopsies may be performed blind, following advanced imaging, using pinch biopsy instrument including retroflex rhinoscopic biopsy of nasopharynx, cannula (closed suction), or hydropulsion techniques.
- Cytologic evaluation of regional lymph nodes to detect regional metastatic disease.

PATHOLOGIC FINDINGS

- Bilateral involvement and osteolysis common.
- Regional lymph node metastasis <10% at time of diagnosis, but up to 45% at necropsy.

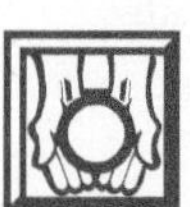

TREATMENT

APPROPRIATE HEALTH CARE

- Radiation therapy is standard of care.
- Radiation therapy can be administered with curative intent (conventional definitive or stereotactic radiotherapy) or for palliation of clinical signs.
- Conventional definitive radiation involves multiple fractions for high total dose; usually 10–20 fractions to allow normal tissue recovery with goal of minimizing risk of late permanent radiation side effects.
- Stereotactic radiation therapy is newer technique that allows more conformal treatment than conventional techniques to avoid toxicity to normal tissue without sacrificing tumor control; comparable dose delivered over much shorter time than with conventional techniques; stereotactic radiotherapy involves 1–5 consecutive daily fractions.
- Palliative radiation involves much lower total dose than definitive to minimize toxicity while improving quality of life through reduction of tumor size; usually 4–6 fractions.
- Combining radiation therapy with novel drug therapy (toceranib phosphate—Palladia®, and others) appears safe and well tolerated.
- Radiation therapy followed by surgery to debulk residual mass may improve local control time, but results in higher rate of complications.
- Surgery alone considered ineffective, with most tumors relapsing within 6 months.

NURSING CARE

- During radiation therapy, supportive care for radiation-related mucositis may involve softening food; rinsing mouth with "magic mouthwash" (topical anesthetic), saline, or dilute black tea; and administration of medications to control discomfort.
- These side effects temporary, but may cause discomfort for 10–14 days.

ACTIVITY

- Limit activity to minimize risk of epistaxis and dyspnea.
- Using harness instead of collar during walks may help minimize epistaxis.

DIET

- Soften food if needed during radiation therapy.

• Avoid extremes of temperatures and salty foods with radiation therapy–related mucositis.

CLIENT EDUCATION

• Nasal adenocarcinoma may be painful even though pet not showing visible signs of pain.
• Consider use of medications for discomfort, epistaxis, and congestion.
• Radiation therapy most effective option and well tolerated using modern radiotherapy techniques, with fewer side effects than previously reported.
• Radiation side effects may impact patient's quality of life during treatment, but most pets enjoy relatively normal quality of life following treatment.
• Intermittent congestion, nasal discharge, and sneezing may occur post therapy due to increased sensitivity from tumor's destruction of nasal turbinates.

SURGICAL CONSIDERATIONS

Anesthetic recovery—ensure airway is maintained until animal is sternal and alert, to prevent apnea in patients with bilateral nasal obstruction.

MEDICATIONS

DRUG(S) OF CHOICE

• Chemotherapy is considered ineffective for durable tumor control, but may benefit some patients if radiation therapy is not viable option. Various drugs have been described, including cisplatin (dogs only), carboplatin, doxorubicin, and piroxicam. Toceranib phosphate (Palladia) exerts therapeutic activity against nasal carcinoma.
• Consult with oncologist for more details.
• Adequate analgesic therapy should be employed as needed in patients suffering from invasive disease with bone destruction, signs of pain, or radiation therapy side effects.

CONTRAINDICATIONS

Cisplatin—never use in cats.

PRECAUTIONS

• Most chemotherapeutics have risk of gastrointestinal, hematologic, and other potential side effects, and should be administered and monitored by an oncologist.
• Piroxicam can cause gastric ulceration, so careful monitoring of appetite, vomiting, and stool color (melena) is recommended.

POSSIBLE INTERACTIONS

Concurrent radiation therapy and chemotherapy will increase risk of side effects, but have not shown to significantly improve tumor control.

ALTERNATIVE DRUG(S)

• Palladia, a tyrosine kinase inhibitor, may have anticancer activity in some carcinomas, including nasal adenocarcinomas. It is currently being investigated alone and in combination with radiation therapy.
• Objective responses have been documented with use of Palladia alone.
• Yunnan Baiyao, a Chinese herbal medication, is often prescribed for epistaxis.

FOLLOW-UP

PATIENT MONITORING

• Clinical response is usually observed within 2–3 weeks from start of radiation therapy. Reductions in epistaxis, nasal discharge, congestion, and sneezing are expected.
• CT or MRI is needed to assess objective tumor response to therapy and is recommended 2–3 months post radiation treatment.
• Other staging tests, including thoracic imaging (radiography or CT) and lymph node evaluation, are generally recommended at 3-month intervals during/following therapy.
• Routine staging with CT/MRI and monitoring of recurrent clinical signs can detect early recurrence.

POSSIBLE COMPLICATIONS

• Pain.
• Dyspnea.
• Epistaxis.
• Secondary infections.
• Weight loss.
• Anorexia.
• Chemotherapy or radiation toxicity.

EXPECTED COURSE AND PROGNOSIS

• Untreated—median survival around 2–6 months.
• Definitive conventional and stereotactic radiation therapy—median survival times reported at 12–18 months in dogs and 12–20 months in cats; 1-year survival rate 20–57% (dogs and cats); 2-year survival rate 20–48% (dogs and cats).
• Presence of cribriform lysis, brain involvement, or metastatic disease (advanced stage) are poor prognostic indicators.
• Ophthalmic complications of radiation therapy—more likely in dogs than cats.
• Incidence and severity of ophthalmic toxicity have dramatically decreased with advanced radiation therapy techniques now commonly used.
• Chronic rhinitis is possible following radiation therapy for sinonasal tumors and may require periodic symptomatic therapy.

MISCELLANEOUS

PREGNANCY/FERTILITY/BREEDING

Chemotherapeutic drugs and general anesthesia are a risk to the fetus and would not be recommended in pregnant animals.

SYNONYMS

• Nasal carcinoma.
• Nasal tumor.

SEE ALSO

• Chondrosarcoma, Nasal and Paranasal Sinus.
• Squamous Cell Carcinoma, Nasal and Paranasal Sinus.
• Squamous Cell Carcinoma, Nasal Planum.

ABBREVIATIONS

• COX-2 = cyclooxygenase-2.

INTERNET RESOURCES

• https://veterinarymedicine.dvm360.com/vetmed/Medicine/Canine-and-feline-nasaltumors/ArticleStandard/Article/detail/735167
• https://www.ncbi.nlm.nih.gov/pubmed?term=dog+nasal+carcinoma+radiotherapy&cmd=DetailsSearch

Suggested Reading

Adams WA, Bjorling DE, McAnulty JF, et al. Outcome of accelerated radiotherapy alone or accelerated radiotherapy followed by exenteration of the nasal cavity in dogs with intranasal neoplasia: 53 cases (1990–2002). J Am Vet Med Assoc 2005, 227:936–941.
Adams WA, Kleiter MM, Thrall DE, et al. Prognostic significance of tumor histology and computed tomographic staging for radiation treatment response of canine nasal tumors. Vet Radiol Ultrasound 2009, 50(3):330–335.
Geiger TL, Nolan MW. Linac-based stereotactic radiation therapy for canine non-lymphomatous nasal tumors: 29 cases (2013–2016). Vet Comp Oncol 2018, 16:E68–E75.
Henry CJ, Brewer WG, Tyler JW, et al. Survival in dogs with nasal adenocarcinoma: 64 cases (1981–1995). J Vet Intern Med 1998, 12:436–439.
LaDue TA, Dodge R, Page RL, et al. Factors influencing survival after radiotherapy of nasal tumors in 130 dogs. Vet Radiol Ultrasound 1999, 40:312–317.

Author Jayme S. Looper
Consulting Editor Timothy M. Fan

ADENOCARCINOMA, PANCREAS

BASICS

OVERVIEW

• Malignant tumor of ductal or acinar origin arising from the exocrine pancreas.
• Usually metastatic by the time of diagnosis, affecting regional lymph nodes and visceral abdominal organs (liver) and associated peritoneal cavity.

SIGNALMENT

• Rare in dogs—0.5–1.8% of all tumors.
• Rare in cats—2.8% of all tumors.
• Older female dogs and Airedale terriers at higher risk than others.
• Median age (dogs)—9.2 years.
• Mean age (cats)—11.6 years.

SIGNS

• Nonspecific—fever; vomiting; weakness; anorexia; icterus; malabsorption syndrome; weight loss.
• Abdominal pain—variable.
• Abdominal effusion—malignant.
• Metastasis to bone and soft tissue common.
• Pathologic fractures secondary to metastasis reported.
• Palpable abdominal mass (cats).
• Paraneoplastic syndromes of epidermal necrosis, hyperinsulinemia, and hyperglucagonemia may be present.
• Average duration of clinical signs (cats): 41 days, range 2–180 days.

CAUSES & RISK FACTORS

Unknown

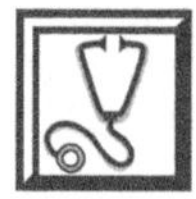

DIAGNOSIS

DIFFERENTIAL DIAGNOSIS

• Primary pancreatitis; may be concurrent and complicate or delay early diagnosis.
• Pancreatic pseudocyst.
• Pancreatic nodular hyperplasia.
• Hepatic neoplasia.
• Other causes of vomiting and icterus.
• Peritoneal carcinomatosis.
• Other causes of abdominal effusion in cats.

CBC/BIOCHEMISTRY/URINALYSIS

• Usually nonspecific changes (e.g., mild anemia and neutrophilia).
• Hyperamylasemia less reliable than hyperlipasemia.
• Lipase concentrations are often markedly elevated and may serve as a noninvasive biochemical marker of neoplasia in dogs.

OTHER LABORATORY TESTS

Rarely there may be significant metabolic alterations that affect glucagon, insulin, and amino acid concentrations.

IMAGING

• Abdominal radiographs may reveal a mass or loss of serosal detail associated with concurrent pancreatitis or peritoneal effusion.
• Ultrasonography may reveal one or more masses or concurrent pancreatitis (mixed echogenicity, large pancreas, hyperechoic peripancreatic fat). Pancreatic thickening, abdominal effusion, and single to multiple nodules of varying size may be identified. Sonographic findings may be impossible to distinguish from pancreatic nodular hyperplasia. Rarely the ultrasound of the pancreas may appear normal except for dilation of the pancreatic duct.
• Abdominal CT will allow for therapeutic decisions regarding surgical resectability and approach, which can affect the owner's willingness to treat.

DIAGNOSTIC PROCEDURES

• Surgical biopsy—definitive.
• Fine-needle aspirate cytology—supportive. In many cases, where the tumor is not resectable, the fine-needle aspirates may provide strong enough evidence to start medical treatment.

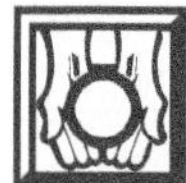

TREATMENT

• None reported curative.
• Palliation of pain with aggressive analgesic combinations is necessary.
• Surgical intervention to alleviate intestinal and biliary obstruction, if necessary.
• Surgery is typically not a good option in many cases, due to the extent of the disease at the time of diagnosis.
• If surgery is an option, partial or total pancreatectomy may prolong survival. A Whipple procedure (pancreaticoduodenectomy) and/or partial colon resection may be required for tumor resection. This can influence the perisurgical morbidity and mortality risk.
• Treat concurrent pancreatitis.
• Antiemetics and supportive care (hydration and caloric requirements).

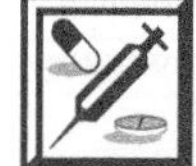

MEDICATIONS

DRUG(S) OF CHOICE

• Gemcitabine is used in humans for the treatment of pancreatic carcinoma, and while used in dogs with cancer, it has not been established as the standard of care for dogs with pancreatic adenocarcinoma.
• Always consult a veterinary oncologist for updates in treating this rare neoplasm.

CONTRAINDICATIONS/POSSIBLE INTERACTIONS

N/A

FOLLOW-UP

POSSIBLE COMPLICATIONS

• Intestinal obstruction
• Biliary obstruction
• Pancreatic abscess
• Peritonitis
• Metastasis

EXPECTED COURSE AND PROGNOSIS

Progression to death is often rapid given that there is no successful curative treatment available. Despite the grave prognosis, individual patients treated with complete resection of their tumor and chemotherapy, in the absence of systemic metastasis, may have prolonged survival.

MISCELLANEOUS

ASSOCIATED CONDITIONS

Gastrin-secreting pancreatic carcinoma (gastrinoma) has been reported in dogs and cats. Clinical signs are associated with hypergastrinemia, which results in inappropriate hydrochloric acid secretion by the stomach, leading to gastroduodenitis.

Suggested Reading

Cave T, Evans H, Hargreavest J, et al. Metabolic epidermal necrosis in a dog associated with pancreatic adenocarcinoma, hyperglucagonaemia, hyperinsulinaemia, and hypoaminoacidaemia. J Small Anim Pract 2007, 48:522–526.

Hecht S, Penninck DG, Keating JH. Imaging findings in pancreatic neoplasia and nodular hyperplasia in 19 cats. Vet Radiol Ultrasound 2006, 48:45–50.

Linderman MJ, Brodsky EM, de Lorimier LP, et al. Feline exocrine pancreatic carcinoma: a retrospective study of 34 cases. Vet Comp Oncol 2013, 11(3):208–218.

Author Nick Dervisis

Consulting Editor Timothy M. Fan

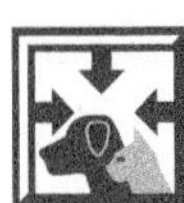

BASICS

OVERVIEW

- Prostatic adenocarcinoma (PAC) is a malignant tumor that occurs in both neutered and intact male dogs.
- Although this neoplasm represents <1% of all canine malignancies, it is the most common prostatic disorder in neutered male dogs.
- Metastases to regional lymph nodes, lungs, and the lumbosacral skeleton are common.

SIGNALMENT

- Dogs and rarely cats.
- Medium- to large-breed intact or neutered male dogs.
- Median age of 9–10 years.

SIGNS

Historical Findings

- Tenesmus (with the production of ribbon-like stool).
- Weight loss.
- Stranguria and dysuria.
- Rear limb lameness.
- Lethargy.
- Exercise intolerance.

Physical Examination Findings

- A firm, asymmetric, and immobile prostate gland.
- Prostatomegaly is common, but is not always present.
- Pain may be elicited in response to abdominal or rectal palpation.
- Caudal abdominal mass, cachexia, pyrexia, and dyspnea may also be identified.

CAUSES & RISK FACTORS

Neutered males are at increased risk for prostatic neoplasia.

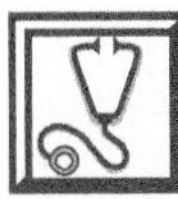

DIAGNOSIS

DIFFERENTIAL DIAGNOSIS

- Other primary neoplasia (i.e., squamous cell carcinoma, transitional cell carcinoma).
- Metastatic or locally invasive neoplasia (i.e., transitional cell carcinoma).
- Acute or chronic prostatitis, benign prostatic hypertrophy, and prostatic cysts are possible differentials in intact male dogs, but are highly unlikely in neutered dogs.

CBC/BIOCHEMISTRY/URINALYSIS

- Inflammatory leukogram possible.
- Alkaline phosphatase may be high.
- Postrenal azotemia may be present if urethral obstruction exists.
- It is prudent to evaluate urine samples via cystocentesis and free-catch techniques, as hematuria, pyuria, and malignant epithelial cells may be observed in free-catch samples, but are unusual in samples obtained by cystocentesis.

OTHER LABORATORY TESTS

Serum and seminal plasma markers such as acid phosphatase, prostate-specific antigen, and canine prostate-specific esterase are not elevated in dogs with PAC.

IMAGING

- Thoracic radiography—metastases may appear as pulmonary nodules or increased interstitial markings.
- Abdominal radiography—sublumbar lymphadenomegaly, mineralization of the prostate, and lytic lesions to the lumbar vertebrae or pelvis may be seen.
- Abdominal ultrasonography—focal to multifocal hyperechogenicity with asymmetry and irregular prostatic outline, ± prostatic mineralization.
- Contrast cystography may help differentiate prostatic from urinary bladder disease.

DIAGNOSTIC PROCEDURES

- Prostatic aspirate (percutaneous or trans-rectal).
- Prostatic wash.
- Prostatic biopsy performed percutaneously or surgically.
- Percutaneous biopsy has been associated with tumor seeding along the biopsy tract.

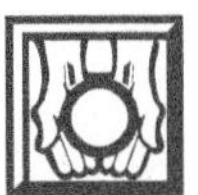

TREATMENT

- Prostatectomy if local disease (success of this procedure depends on skill of surgeon and extent of disease).
- Radiation therapy may palliate signs and prolong survival.
- Neutering—however, most tumors are not androgen responsive.
- Stenting of the prostatic urethra will resolve urinary outflow obstruction and thereby prolong survival.

MEDICATIONS

DRUG(S) OF CHOICE

- Chemotherapy—carboplatin, cisplatin, or doxorubicin; may offer short-term benefit.
- Pain relief with nonsteroidal anti-inflammatory drugs (NSAIDs), morphine-derived drugs.
- Stool softeners to relieve tenesmus.

CONTRAINDICATIONS/POSSIBLE INTERACTIONS

N/A

FOLLOW-UP

PATIENT MONITORING

Ability to urinate and defecate, pain secondary to skeletal metastases, quality of life.

PREVENTION/AVOIDANCE

Keeping dogs sexually intact may decrease risk.

POSSIBLE COMPLICATIONS

- Urethral obstruction.
- Metastasis to regional lymph nodes, skeleton, and lungs.

EXPECTED COURSE AND PROGNOSIS

Guarded to poor, survival of 2–6 months depending upon presenting clinical symptoms.

MISCELLANEOUS

ZOONOTIC POTENTIAL

None

PREGNANCY/FERTILITY/BREEDING

N/A

ABBREVIATIONS

- NSAID = nonsteroidal anti-inflammatory drug.
- PAC = prostatic adenocarcinoma.

Suggested Reading

Axiak SM, Bigio A. Canine prostatic carcinoma. Compend Contin Educ Vet 2012, 34(10):E1–E4.

Author Ruthanne Chun
Consulting Editor Timothy M. Fan

A

ADENOCARCINOMA, RENAL

BASICS

OVERVIEW

- Accounts for <1% of all reported neoplasms in dogs.
- Renal tumors tend to be highly metastatic, locally invasive, and often bilateral.
- Renal cystadenocarcinoma, a rare heritable syndrome with a less aggressive behavior and better long-term prognosis than renal adenocarcinoma, has been described in German shepherd dogs.

SIGNALMENT

- Adenocarcinoma—older (8–9 years) dogs, 1.6 : 1 male-to-female ratio, no breed predilection.
- Cystadenocarcinoma—German shepherd dogs, often female.

SIGNS

- Adenocarcinoma—insidious, nonspecific signs such as weight loss, inappetance, lethargy, hematuria, and pale mucous membranes.
- Cystadenocarcinoma—may present for nodular dermatofibrosis, a syndrome of painless, firm, fibrous lesions of the skin and subcutaneous tissues.

CAUSES & RISK FACTORS

- Adenocarcinoma—unknown.
- Cystadenocarcinoma—heritable in German shepherd dogs.

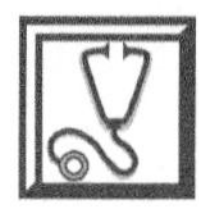

DIAGNOSIS

DIFFERENTIAL DIAGNOSIS

- Other primary neoplasia (i.e., lymphoma, nephroblastoma).
- Metastatic neoplasia (i.e., hemangiosarcoma).
- Renal adenoma or cyst.
- Pyelonephritis.

CBC/BIOCHEMISTRY/URINALYSIS

- CBC may show paraneoplastic polycythemia or leukocytosis, or anemia.
- Biochemistry may be normal, or may reveal azotemia. Marked gamma-glutamyltransferase (GGT) elevation may be prognostic.
- Urinalysis may show hematuria, proteinuria, bacteriuria, or casts.

OTHER LABORATORY TESTS

Urine culture and sensitivity.

IMAGING

- Thoracic radiographs—metastatic disease reported in up to 16% of patients.
- Abdominal radiographs—mass visualized in 81% of patients.
- Abdominal ultrasonography, CT, or contrast radiography—useful in identifying and staging the disease.

DIAGNOSTIC PROCEDURES

- Renal biopsy (ultrasound guided or surgical) for definitive diagnosis.
- Mitotic index found to be prognostic in 70 dogs treated with nephrectomy.

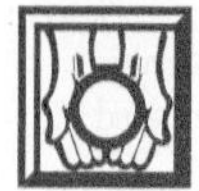

TREATMENT

- Aggressive surgical excision is the treatment of choice for unilateral disease.
- Successful chemotherapeutic management of either disease has not been described.
- Supportive management for patients in renal failure may be necessary.

MEDICATIONS

DRUG(S) OF CHOICE

None

CONTRAINDICATIONS/POSSIBLE INTERACTIONS

N/A

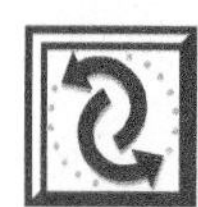

FOLLOW-UP

PATIENT MONITORING

- Renal failure—measure serum urea nitrogen and creatinine; urinalysis.
- Quality of life if bilateral or otherwise nonsurgical disease.

PREVENTION/AVOIDANCE

N/A

POSSIBLE COMPLICATIONS

- Renal failure.
- Metastatic disease.
- Invasion of local vital structures (vena cava, aorta).

EXPECTED COURSE AND PROGNOSIS

- Adenocarcinoma—median reported survival of 49 dogs was 16 months (range 0–59).
- Cystadenocarcinoma—few large studies of this rare disease, reported median survival of 12+ months with no definitive therapy.
- Based on mitotic index: >30 mitotic figures/10 high-power fields (hpf; median survival of 187 days) vs. 10–30/10 hpf (median survival of 452 days) vs. <10/hpf (median survival of 1184 days).

MISCELLANEOUS

ASSOCIATED CONDITIONS

- The paraneoplastic syndromes of hypertrophic osteopathy, polycythemia, and a neutrophilic leukocytosis have been reported in isolated cases.
- Renal failure.
- Nodular dermatofibrosis and uterine leiomyomas are commonly associated with cystadenocarcinoma.

ABBREVIATIONS

- GGT = gamma-glutamyltransferase.
- hpf = high-power field.

Suggested Reading

Bryan JN, Henry CJ, Turnquist SE, et al. Primary renal neoplasia of dogs. J Vet Intern Med 2006, 20:1155–1160.

De Lorimier LP, Bernard S. Marked serum GGT elevations in two dogs with renal carcinoma. Letter to the Editor. J Small Anim Pract 2017, 58:187.

Edmondson EF, Hess AM, Powers BE. Prognostic significance of histologic features in canine renal cell carcinomas: 70 nephrectomies. Vet Pathol 2015, 52:260–268.

Knapp DW. Tumors of the urinary system. In: Withrow SJ, Vail DM, eds., Small Animal Clinical Oncology, 4th ed. Philadelphia, PA: Saunders, 2007, pp. 649–658.

Author Ruthanne Chun

Consulting Editor Timothy M. Fan

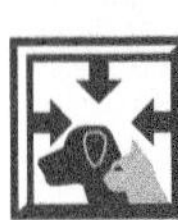

BASICS

OVERVIEW

• Tumor arising from major (e.g., parotid, mandibular, sublingual, or zygomatic) or minor salivary glands.
• Mandibular or parotid glands constitute 80% of cases.
• Mandibular gland most frequently affected in dogs.
• Parotid gland most frequently affected in cats.
• Locally invasive.
• Cats typically have more advanced disease than dogs at time of diagnosis.
• Metastasis—regional lymph node in 39% of cats and 17% of dogs at diagnosis; distant metastasis reported in 16% of cats and 8% of dogs at diagnosis, but may be slow to develop.
• Epithelial malignancies—constitute roughly 85% of salivary gland tumors.
• Adenomas comprise only 5% of salivary tumors.

SIGNALMENT

• Dogs and cats.
• Mean age, 10–12 years.
• Siamese cats may be at relatively higher risk.
• Male cats affected twice as often as female cats.
• No other breed or sex predilection has been determined.

SIGNS

• Unilateral, firm, painless swelling of the upper neck (mandibular and sublingual), ear base (parotid), upper lip or maxilla (zygomatic), or mucous membrane of lip (accessory or minor salivary tissue).
• Other signs may include halitosis, weight loss, anorexia, dysphagia, exophthalmus, Horner's syndrome, sneezing, and dysphonia.

CAUSES & RISK FACTORS

Unknown

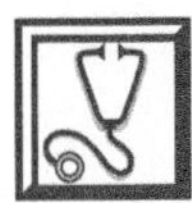

DIAGNOSIS

DIFFERENTIAL DIAGNOSIS

• Squamous cell carcinoma.
• Mucocele.
• Abscess.
• Soft tissue sarcoma, e.g., fibrosarcoma.
• Lymphoma.

CBC/BIOCHEMISTRY/URINALYSIS

Results often normal.

OTHER LABORATORY TESTS

N/A

IMAGING

• Regional radiographs usually are normal; may see periosteal reaction on adjacent bones or displacement of surrounding structures.
• MRI or CT imaging allows superior discrimination of tumor for surgery and/or radiation treatment planning.
• Thoracic radiographs indicated to check for lung metastases.

DIAGNOSTIC PROCEDURES

• Cytologic examination of aspirate may differentiate salivary adenocarcinoma from mucocele and abscess.
• Biopsy for histopathology is required for definitive diagnosis.

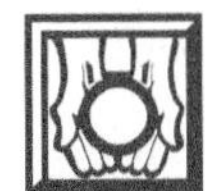

TREATMENT

• Aggressive surgical resection—when possible; most are invasive and difficult to excise completely.
• Radiotherapy—good local control and prolonged survival may be possible.
• Aggressive local resection (usually histologically incomplete) followed by adjuvant radiation can achieve local control and long-term survival in some cases, but further studies are needed to determine the most effective treatment, including the possible role for chemotherapy.

MEDICATIONS

DRUG(S) OF CHOICE

Chemotherapy efficacy is largely unreported; however, it may be indicated for treatment/palliation of metastatic disease.

CONTRAINDICATIONS/POSSIBLE INTERACTIONS

N/A

FOLLOW-UP

PATIENT MONITORING

Evaluations—physical examination and thoracic radiographs every 3 months reasonable if aggressive surgery and/or radiation therapy employed.

POSSIBLE COMPLICATIONS

Temporary acute side effects (e.g., moist dermatitis and alopecia) expected with radiation therapy. Consultation with a radiation oncologist is recommended regarding specific, anatomic site–related side effects associated with planned dose and field size.

EXPECTED COURSE AND PROGNOSIS

• Improved survival time in dogs without evidence of nodal or distant metastasis at diagnosis; clinical stage not prognostic for cats.
• Median survival 550 days for dogs and 516 days for cats in retrospective study.
• Local control obtained through radiation and/or surgery is critical to outcome.

MISCELLANEOUS

Suggested Reading

Hammer A, Getzy D, Ogilvie G, et al. Salivary gland neoplasia in the dog and cat: survival times and prognostic factors. JAAHA 2001, 37:478–482.

Blackwood L, Harper A, Elliot J, Gramar I. External beam radiotherapy for the treatment of feline salivary gland carcinoma: six new cases and a review of the literature. J Feline Med Surg 2019, 21(2):186–194.

Author Anthony J. Mutsaers
Consulting Editor Timothy M. Fan

ADENOCARCINOMA, SKIN (SWEAT GLAND, SEBACEOUS)

BASICS

OVERVIEW

• Malignant growth originating from sebaceous or apocrine sweat glands of the skin.
• Approximately 2% of all skin tumors in dogs.

SIGNALMENT

• Apocrine sweat gland—rare in dogs, uncommon in cats.
• Sebaceous gland—rare in both dogs and cats.
• Middle-aged to older pets.
• Male intact dogs overrepresented for sebaceous gland adenocarcinomas.
• Female dogs overrepresented for apocrine adenocarcinoma in one study.

SIGNS

• May appear as solid, firm, raised, superficial skin lesions.
• May be ulcerated and bleeding and accompanied by inflammation of the surrounding tissue.
• Apocrine sweat gland—often poorly circumscribed, ulcerated and potentially purple in color; very invasive into underlying tissue; may occur anywhere on the body, frequently affecting the limbs and trunk in dogs and head, limbs, and abdomen in cats.
• Sebaceous gland—often nodular, ulcerated and inflamed, moderate risk of lymph node involvement; frequently found on head and neck in dogs and on the head, thorax, and perineum in cats.
• Dermal and lymphatic tracking can be observed early in disease course.

CAUSES & RISK FACTORS

Unknown

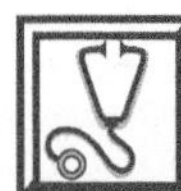

DIAGNOSIS

DIFFERENTIAL DIAGNOSIS

• Other more frequent skin tumors.
• Cutaneous histiocytic diseases.
• Immune-mediated skin diseases.
• Deep bacterial/fungal infections.

CBC/BIOCHEMISTRY/URINALYSIS

Normal

OTHER LABORATORY TESTS

N/A

IMAGING

Thoracic radiographs recommended at time of diagnosis to assess for distant metastases.

DIAGNOSTIC PROCEDURES

• Biopsy for histopathology and definitive diagnosis.
• Cytologic examination or biopsy of draining lymph nodes.

PATHOLOGIC FINDINGS

• Apocrine gland adenocarcinomas are divided into multiple subtypes based on the anatomic location they arise in. They typically are invasive into the underlying stroma and blood vessels, and often show poorly demarcated borders and a high mitotic index.
• Sebaceous gland adenocarcinomas often reveal lymphatic vessel invasion.

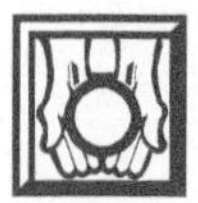

TREATMENT

• Aggressive *en bloc* surgical excision, including resection of draining lymph node, recommended for both types. Histopathologic analysis of lymph nodes assists with determining prognosis and establishing adjuvant treatment plan.
• Margins of entire tissue specimen must be evaluated histologically to assess completeness of resection.
• Radiation therapy may be recommended for treatment of draining lymph nodes after resection to prevent recurrence and development of regional metastasis; radiation therapy of primary tumor site recommended when wide and complete resection not possible.

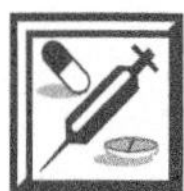

MEDICATIONS

DRUG(S) OF CHOICE

• Chemotherapy has been used anecdotally for the treatment of both tumor types, in both species.
• Contact a veterinary oncologist for any updated treatments that may be available.
• Nonsteroidal anti-inflammatory drugs and other analgesics are recommended, as indicated, for pain control.

CONTRAINDICATIONS/POSSIBLE INTERACTIONS

None

FOLLOW-UP

• Sebaceous gland adenocarcinoma—little is known about the metastatic potential of this malignancy, but it may be rapidly metastatic to regional lymph nodes in some patients; long-term prognosis is anecdotally good with multimodal therapy combining aggressive surgery, chemotherapy, and radiation therapy.
• Apocrine gland adenocarcinoma—fair to good long-term prognosis; the histologic finding of vascular invasion is a negative prognostic factor predicting systemic metastases; aggressive surgical resection (local and regional tumor control) followed by adjuvant chemotherapy is recommended to improve survival. A study reported a postexcisional median survival time of 30 months in dogs.

MISCELLANEOUS

Suggested Reading

Carpenter JL, Andrews LK, Holzworth J. Tumors and tumor like lesions. In: Holzworth J, ed. Diseases of the Cat: Medicine and Surgery. Philadelphia, PA: Saunders, 1987, pp. 406–596.

Hauck ML. Tumors of the skin and subcutaneous tissues. In: Withrow SJ, Vail DM, Page RL, eds., Small Animal Clinical Oncology, 5th ed. St. Louis, MO: Elsevier Saunders, 2013, pp. 305–320.

Haziroglu R, Haligur M, Keles H. Histopathological and immunohistochemical studies of apocrine sweat gland adenocarcinomas in cats. Vet Comp Oncol 2014, 12(1):85–90.

Kycko A, Jasik A, Bocian L, et al. Epidemiological and histopathological analysis of 40 apocrine sweat gland carcinomas in dogs: a retrospective study. J Vet Res 2016, 61:331–337.

Pakhrin B, Kang MS, Bae IH, et al. Retrospective study of canine cutaneous tumors in Korea. J Vet Sci 2007, 8:229–236.

Simko E, Wilcock BP, Yager JA. A retrospective study of 44 canine apocrine sweat gland adenocarcinomas. Can Vet J 2003, 44(1):38–42.

Author Jason Pieper

Consulting Editor Timothy M. Fan

Acknowledgment The author and book editor acknowledge the prior contribution of Louis-Philippe de Lorimier.

ADENOCARCINOMA, STOMACH, SMALL AND LARGE INTESTINE, RECTAL

BASICS

OVERVIEW

• Uncommon tumor arising from the epithelial lining of the gastrointestinal tract.
• Prognosis guarded to poor.

SIGNALMENT

• Dog more commonly affected than cat.
• Middle-aged to older (>6 years) animals; age range 3–13 years.
• No breed predisposition.
• Possible male predisposition.

SIGNS

Historical Findings

• Stomach—vomiting, anorexia, weight loss, hematemesis, and melena.
• Small intestine—vomiting, weight loss, borborygmus, flatulence, and melena.
• Large intestine and rectum—mucus, blood-tinged feces, and tenesmus.

Physical Examination Findings

• Stomach—nonspecific, melena on rectal exam.
• Small intestine—may feel mid-abdominal mass; distended, painful loops of small bowel.
• Large intestine and rectum—palpable mass per rectum, may form annular ring, may have multiple nodular lesions protruding into the colon; bright red blood on rectal exam.

CAUSES & RISK FACTORS

• Unknown.
• Possible genetic cause—gastric adenocarcinomas in related Belgian shepherds and Dutch Tervuren shepherds.

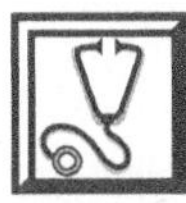

DIAGNOSIS

DIFFERENTIAL DIAGNOSIS

• Foreign body.
• Inflammatory bowel disease.
• Lymphoma.
• Parasites.
• Leiomyoma.
• Leiomyosarcoma.
• Pancreatitis.

CBC/BIOCHEMISTRY/URINALYSIS

• Stomach and small intestine—may see microcytic, hypochromic, nonregenerative anemia (iron-deficiency anemia). Mild and persistent elevations in blood urea nitrogen in the face of normal creatinine can support GI protein or blood loss.
• Large intestine and rectum—no characteristic changes.

OTHER LABORATORY TESTS

Fecal occult blood may be positive; diet affects results—can recheck to confirm after 3 days of non-meat diet.

IMAGING

• Ultrasound—may reveal a thickened stomach or bowel wall; may see mass in the gastrointestinal tract, enlarged lymph nodes.
• Positive contrast radiography—filling defect (stomach); intraluminal space-occupying or annular constriction (small bowel); gastric neoplasm most often found in distal two-thirds of stomach.
• Double contrast radiography—large intestine and rectum; polypoid or annular space-occupying masses.
• Advanced imaging with contrast CT can provide highest-quality images of gastrointestinal tract and assessment for presence and extent of lymphadenopathy.

DIAGNOSTIC PROCEDURES

• Ultrasound-guided fine-needle aspirate of bowel mass or enlarged lymph node may provide definitive cytologic diagnosis.
• Endoscopic biopsy may be nondiagnostic because tumors are frequently deep to the mucosal surface; thus surgical biopsy often required.
• Presence of signet ring cells and/or cytoplasmic microvacuolation on cytologic evaluation of gastric biopsy squash prep samples correlated well with diagnosis of gastric adenocarcinoma in one study.

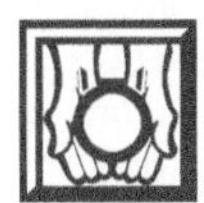

TREATMENT

• Surgical resection—treatment of choice; seldom curative.
• Gastric—usually nonresectable.
• Small intestine—remove by resection and anastomosis; metastasis to regional lymph nodes and liver common.
• Large intestine and rectal—may occasionally be resected via pull-through surgical procedure; metastasis common; transcolonic debulking may provide palliation of obstruction.

MEDICATIONS

DRUG(S) OF CHOICE

• Chemotherapy—only anecdotal reports, usually unsuccessful.
• Piroxicam 0.3 mg/kg PO q24h can provide palliation for large intestinal and rectal tumors.

CONTRAINDICATIONS/POSSIBLE INTERACTIONS

Seek advice before initiating treatment with cytotoxic drugs.

FOLLOW-UP

Physical examination, thoracic radiographs, and abdominal ultrasound—at 1, 3, 6, 9, and 12 months post surgery.

EXPECTED COURSE AND PROGNOSIS

Dogs

• Overall poor; pedunculated rectal tumors do best; most cases recur locally, develop metastasis, or do both rapidly.
• Median survival gastric—2 months.
• Median survival small intestinal—10 months.
• Mean survival large intestinal—annular 1.6 months vs. pedunculated 32 months.

Cats

• Guarded.
• Few reported cases, but may have prolonged survival (>1 year).

MISCELLANEOUS

Suggested Reading

Crawshaw J, Berg J, Sardinas JC, et al. Prognosis for dogs with nonlymphomatous small intestinal tumors treated by surgical excision. J Am Anim Hosp Assoc 1998, 34:451–456.

Riondato F, Miniscalco B, Berio E, et al. Diagnosis of canine gastric adenocarcinoma using squash preparation cytology. Vet J 2014, 201(3):390–394.

Seim-Wikse T, Jorundsson E, Nodtvedt A, et al. Breed predisposition to canine gastric carcinoma: a study based on the Norwegian canine cancer register. Acta Vet Scand 2013, 55:25.

Swann HM, Holt DE. Canine gastric adenocarcinoma and leiomyosarcoma: a retrospective study of 21 cases (1986–1999) and literature review. J Am Anim Hosp Assoc 2002, 38:157–164.

von Babo V, Eberle N, Mischke R, et al. Canine non-hematopoietic gastric neoplasia: epidemiologic and diagnostic characteristics in 38 dogs with post-surgical outcome of five cases. Tierarztl Prax Ausg K Kleintiere Heimtiere 2012, 40(4):243–249.

Author Laura D. Garrett
Consulting Editor Timothy M. Fan

ADENOCARCINOMA, THYROID—DOGS

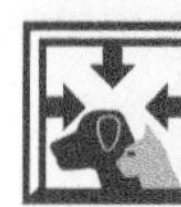

BASICS

DEFINITION

A malignant tumor arising from the follicular or parafollicular cells (medullary/C-cells) of the thyroid gland.

PATHOPHYSIOLOGY

• About 60% of patients are euthyroid, 30% hypothyroid, and 10% hyperthyroid.
• Typically very invasive tumors with high rate of metastasis (lungs, retropharyngeal lymph nodes, liver), with up to 35–40% of dogs having metastasis at time of diagnosis.
• Animals with bilateral tumors have a 16 times greater risk of developing metastatic disease than animal with unilateral tumors.

SYSTEMS AFFECTED

• Cardiovascular—hyperthyroid dogs are usually tachycardic and may have systemic hypertension. • Endocrine/metabolic—affected dogs may be hypothyroid, euthyroid, or hyperthyroid; hypercalcemia may be seen as a paraneoplastic syndrome or secondary to concurrent parathyroid hyperplasia or parathyroid adenocarcinoma. • Respiratory—dogs may be dyspneic owing to a space-occupying mass adjacent to the trachea; metastasis to the lungs common. Large compressive masses can result in caval syndrome manifested as facial edema. Compression and/or deviation of the trachea can lead to nonproductive cough.

GENETICS

Unknown

INCIDENCE/PREVALENCE

Accounts for 1.2–3.8% of all canine tumors and represents 10–15% of all primary head and neck tumors.

GEOGRAPHIC DISTRIBUTION

May be more common in iodine-deficient areas.

SIGNALMENT

Species

Dog

Breed Predilections

Boxers, golden retrievers, Siberian huskies, and beagles at increased risk, but seen in any breed.

Mean Age and Range

Older dogs (median 9–15 years; range 4–18 years).

Predominant Sex

No sex predilection.

SIGNS

General Comments

• Usually not diagnosed until a large mass is palpable. • Approximately 65% are unilateral, 35% are bilateral.

Historical Findings

• Palpable mass/swelling in cervical neck, coughing, dyspnea, dysphagia, dysphonia, facial edema, neck pain. • If functional thyroid tumor—may see polyuria, polydipsia, polyphagia, weight loss, restless behavior, diarrhea (symptoms associated with hyperthyroidism). • If hypothyroid—may see poor hair coat, weight gain, lethargy.

Physical Examination Findings

• Freely movable or fixed cervical mass, unilateral or bilateral. • Rarely may see Horner's syndrome, or cranial vena cava syndrome. • If hyperthyroid—cardiac arrhythmias or murmurs.

CAUSES

Unknown

RISK FACTORS

• Breed predilection.
• Iodine deficiency.

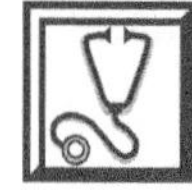

DIAGNOSIS

DIFFERENTIAL DIAGNOSIS

• Other primary neoplasms—lymphoma; soft tissue sarcoma; salivary gland adenocarcinoma; parathyroid carcinoma; carotid body tumor. • Secondary tumors—metastatic oral/tonsillar squamous cell carcinoma; oral melanoma. • Inflammatory—abscess or granuloma. • Salivary mucocele.

CBC/BIOCHEMISTRY/URINALYSIS

• Usually normal. • May see nonregenerative normocytic normochromic anemia of chronic disease, leukocytosis. • Rare—hypercalcemia; isosthenuria.

OTHER LABORATORY TESTS

Thyroid hormone (T_4 and/or free T_4 levels) and endogenous thyroid-stimulating hormone (TSH) levels.

IMAGING

• Thoracic radiography (three-view)—evaluation of lungs and other thoracic structures for metastasis. • Cervical ultrasonography, CT, and MRI—evaluation of tissue of origin, vascularity, invasion, and cervical lymph nodes. • Technetium-99m scintigraphy to evaluate for ectopic and functional thyroid tissue or metastatic lesions. • Radioiodine studies—may provide information about the tumor's ability to produce thyroid hormone.

DIAGNOSTIC PROCEDURES

Biopsy

Tru-Cut® not recommended owing to high risk of severe hemorrhage; open biopsy usually required and allows for controlled hemostasis in the event of bleeding.

Cytology

• Examination of fine-needle aspirates from tumor and palpable regional lymph nodes.
• Specimen almost always heavily contaminated with blood owing to highly vascular nature of tumor. • Homogeneous population of epithelial cells, sometimes with colloid and/or tyrosine-containing granules. Often, cell fragility leads to cell rupture and free nuclei. • Unable to differentiate malignant from benign thyroid cells; but almost all thyroid neoplasms in dogs are malignant.

PATHOLOGIC FINDINGS

Gross

• Characterized by high vascularity with areas of hemorrhage and necrosis. • Usually poorly encapsulated; often invade adjacent tissues (e.g., trachea and esophagus, and surrounding vasculature); may adhere to jugular vein, carotid artery, and vagosympathetic trunk.

Histopathology

• Thyroid follicular carcinomas are subclassified as well differentiated (follicular, compact, follicular–compact, or papillary), poorly differentiated, or undifferentiated—with follicular–compact and compact tumors most common in dogs. • C-cell (e.g., parafollicular, medullary) carcinomas less common. May need special stains to differentiate between C-cell and follicular carcinomas.

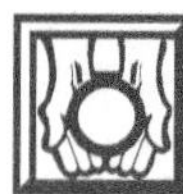

TREATMENT

APPROPRIATE HEALTH CARE

• Definitive treatment dependent on tumor stage (tumor size, mobility, and evidence of metastatic disease). • Complete surgical excision recommended for freely movable thyroid tumors. • Full course external beam radiation therapy recommended preoperatively for large tumors, as sole therapy for nonresectable tumors, or postoperatively for incompletely surgically removed tumors.
• Palliative radiation and/or chemotherapy recommended for tumors that are metastatic at presentation. • Functional thyroid carcinomas can be treated with iodine-131, but doses are very large (60–100 mCi) and therefore there are limited facilities that offer this therapy. • Toceranib phosphate (Palladia®) can exert cytoreductive activity. • Isotretinoin 9-cis postoperatively may improve median survival time (MST) in follicular–compact and compact thyroid carcinoma.

NURSING CARE

Varies with signs on examination.

ACTIVITY

Restrict activity if dyspneic.

CLIENT EDUCATION

• Warn owners of importance of controlling heart rate and rhythm in hyperthyroid patients and of possibility of episodes of collapse. • Warn owners of possible postoperative laryngeal paralysis and intraoperative hemorrhage. • Warn owners of acute radiation therapy toxicities—moist desquamation, laryngitis, tracheitis, esophagitis.

SURGICAL CONSIDERATIONS

See Appropriate Health Care.

Risks

• Marked hemorrhage—tumors highly vascular and invasive into surrounding structures, including vasculature; may need blood transfusion and intensive postoperative care. • Laryngeal paralysis—owing to trauma to recurrent laryngeal nerve. • Damaged parathyroid glands—may occur during surgery.

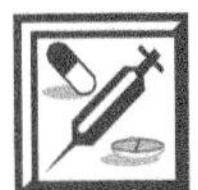

MEDICATIONS

DRUG(S) OF CHOICE

• Chemotherapeutic agents: ∘ Chemotherapy recommended as sole therapy, or possibly in combination with surgery and/or radiation therapy. ∘ Cisplatin (60 mg/m^2 every 3 weeks), carboplatin (300 mg/m^2 every 3 weeks), or doxorubicin (30 mg/m^2 every 3 weeks)—reported to effect partial remission in approximately 50% of cases. ∘ Toceranib (2.5–3 mg/kg 3 times a week)—had biologic activity in 80% of cases (26% partial remission, 53% stable disease). ∘ Isotretinoin 9-cis (2 mg/kg/day)—potentially difficult to obtain in United States due to prescribing restrictions. • Thyroid management: ∘ Thyroxine—maintenance doses to decrease TSH production have been recommended; some tumors contain TSH receptors; value of hormone replacement therapy in affected dogs not determined. ∘ Methimazole 5 mg PO q8h for medium to large dogs; may be beneficial for hyperthyroid patients. ∘ Beta blockers—may be indicated for tachycardia or hypertension in hyperthyroid patients.

CONTRAINDICATIONS

• Doxorubicin is cumulatively toxic to cardiac myocytes, causing decreased myocardial function; do not give to animals with poor cardiac function or dilated cardiomyopathy. • Cisplatin is nephrotoxic; do not give to animals with renal disease.

PRECAUTIONS

Chemotherapy can cause gastrointestinal, bone marrow, cardiac, and other toxicities—seek advice from medical oncologist if unfamiliar with cytotoxic drugs.

POSSIBLE INTERACTIONS

Verapamil—may potentiate doxorubicin-induced cardiotoxicity.

ALTERNATIVE DRUG(S)

N/A

FOLLOW-UP

PATIENT MONITORING

• Serum calcium concentration—if bilateral thyroidectomy was performed; signs of hypocalcemia (agitation, panting, muscle tremors, tetany, and seizures) may be observed. ∘ Treat with 10% calcium gluconate (1–1.5 mL/kg IV over 10–20 minutes). ∘ Maintain serum calcium with dihydrotachysterol (vitamin D) orally and/or oral calcium supplementation if necessary. • Thyroid hormone—supplementation with thyroxine may be necessary after bilateral thyroidectomy. • TSH concentration—a goal of thyroxin supplementation is to downregulate the body's secretion of TSH. • Site of primary tumor—physical examination and cervical ultrasound; thoracic radiographs every 3 months to detect pulmonary metastasis.

PREVENTION/AVOIDANCE

Unknown

POSSIBLE COMPLICATIONS

• Tumor—anemia; thrombocytopenia; hypercalcemia; respiratory distress. • Chemotherapy—dilated cardiomyopathy; renal failure; pancreatitis; sepsis; gastrointestinal upset. • Surgery—hemorrhage; hypothyroidism; hypoparathyroidism leading to hypocalcemia; laryngeal paralysis. • Radiotherapy—acute side effects: moist desquamation, pharyngeal mucositis, esophagitis, tracheitis; late side effects: hypothyroidism, alopecia, and skin or coat color change (at radiation site).

EXPECTED COURSE AND PROGNOSIS

• Prognosis—related to grade and stage of disease (tumor size, mobility, and evidence of metastatic disease) with small, low-grade, nonattached unilateral, nonmetastatic tumors having best prognosis. • MST after surgical removal of unilateral thyroid tumors is 1,462 days vs. 365 days for patients undergoing bilateral thyroidectomy. • For animals treated with full course external beam radiation therapy—progression-free survival at 1 year 80% and 72% at 3 years in one study, and in another study MST 24.5 months. • Palliative radiation therapy in 13 dogs—MST 24 months vs. 170 days in dogs with advanced disease. • ^{131}I therapy in combination with surgery—MST 34 months, or ^{131}I alone MST 30 months. • Animals treated with cisplatin alone (13 dogs)—overall response rate 53%, median progression-free interval for responders 202 days, and overall MST 98 days.

MISCELLANEOUS

ASSOCIATED CONDITIONS

• Nonthyroidal malignancies common.
• Multiple endocrine neoplasia reported.

AGE-RELATED FACTORS

None

PREGNANCY/FERTILITY/BREEDING

It is not recommended to breed animals with cancer. Chemotherapy is teratogenic—do not give to pregnant animals.

SYNONYMS

Thyroid carcinoma.

ABBREVIATIONS

• MST = median survival time.
• TSH = thyroid stimulating hormone.

Suggested Reading

Lunn KF, Page RL. Tumors of the endocrine system. In: Withrow SJ, Vail DM, Page RL, eds., Small Animal Clinical Oncology, 5th ed. Philadelphia, PA: Saunders, 2013, pp. 513–515.

Nadeau ME, Kitchell BE. Evaluation of the use of chemotherapy and other prognostic variables for surgically excised canine thyroid carcinoma with and without metastasis. Can Vet J 2011, 52(9):994–998.

Pack L, Roberts RE, Davson SD, Dookwah HD. Definitive radiation therapy for infiltrative thyroid carcinoma in dogs. Vet Radiol Ultrasound 2001, 42:471–474.

Author Rebecca G. Newman
Consulting Editor Timothy M. Fan

AGGRESSION—BETWEEN DOGS IN THE HOUSEHOLD

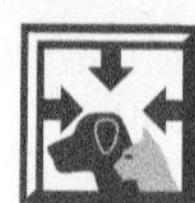

BASICS

OVERVIEW

• Aggression toward other dog(s) within a household or with dogs that are familiar and spend time together regularly. • Dogs can form stable social relationships quickly, sometimes within minutes of being introduced. Aggression usually revolves around resources (e.g., food, toys, owner attention, resting places), but may be fear related or can occur at times of excitement/arousal (e.g., visitors or other dogs on the property). • Usually within the range of normal behavior, but may be excessive, abnormal, or related to underlying medical conditions.

SYSTEMS AFFECTED

Behavioral

INCIDENCE/PREVALENCE

Approximately 11%.

SIGNALMENT

Breed Predilections

• No breed or sex predilection. • Although genetic factors contribute, environment may play a stronger role in degree of aggression exhibited.

Mean Age and Range

Signs usually develop at social maturity (approximately 18–36 months of age).

Predominant Sex

May be more common/intense between intact males and females.

SIGNS

• Barking, growling, lip-lifting, snarling, snapping, lunging, biting, directed toward other dogs in the home. • Subtle communication signals between dogs may include blocking access to rooms or other resources, hard stare, taller stance, tail elevated, ears perked forward, and approaching/direct contact with other dog. • May be accompanied by fearful/submissive body postures/facial expressions (e.g., crouching, backing away, ears back, tail tucked, looking away, lip-licking). • Dogs fighting in a household may get along well except in specific trigger situations, especially resources, access to passageways/doorways, and at times of arousal. • Predictors of aggression—presence of owner; access to resources such as food, toys, spaces, and beds; periods of high arousal such as people entering the house.

CAUSES & RISK FACTORS

• Underlying medical conditions including pain, endocrinopathies, neurologic, and sensory decline. • May be normal canine behavior; can be strongly influenced by previous experience (e.g., early socialization, previous aggressive encounters with other dogs, inappropriate punishment) and other behavioral disorders such as anxiety; in some cases, one dog may not read or respond appropriately to other dog's body language. • Aggression likely to be more severe between dogs of equal size, age, and sex. • Owner's inability to read early signs of conflict between household dogs. • Owner's failure to create or maintain social stability and predictability in dogs' interactions and relationship with each other.

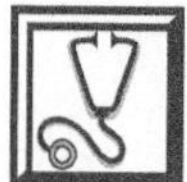

DIAGNOSIS

DIFFERENTIAL DIAGNOSIS

• Status-related aggression. • Conflict-related aggression. • Play behavior/nonaggressive arousal. • Possessive aggression. • Protective aggression. • Fear aggression. • Pain-related aggression. • Irritable aggression. • Generalized anxiety disorder.

CBC/BIOCHEMISTRY/URINALYSIS

To rule out underlying medical conditions and as baseline prior to drug use.

OTHER LABORATORY TESTS

As needed to rule out underlying medical conditions; thyroid screening.

IMAGING

As needed to rule out underlying medical conditions, (e.g., pain); MRI if CNS disease suspected.

DIAGNOSTIC PROCEDURES

N/A

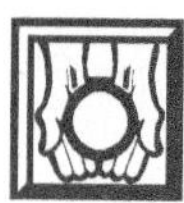

TREATMENT

CLIENT EDUCATION

General Comments

• Treatment requires a multifaceted approach, including immediate management to ensure safety and prevent recurrence, behavior modification, and medication (if indicated). • Successful treatment requires owner understanding of canine social behavior and communication, identification of all aggression-eliciting stimuli, risks involved in living with an aggressive dog(s), willingness and ability to follow safety and management recommendations, and effective implementation of reward-based behavior modification. • Realistic expectation is for managing triggers, most often for rest of dog's life and gradually improving, not resolving. • Owners must be aware that the only way to entirely prevent future injuries may be to continually separate dogs when no one is home, remove one of the dogs from the home, or use of safety equipment and constant supervision to safely manage when dogs are in same space. • Positive punishment and dominance-based training can lead to increased aggression, fear, and injuries, and must be avoided.

Safety Recommendations

• *Never* allow dogs to "fight it out," as serious injuries may occur. • Owners must ensure safety by identifying and avoiding all situations that may trigger aggressive interactions, such as when dogs are walking past each other in a confined space or being given attention or high-valued treats; the dogs may at least initially need to be kept physically separated to prevent agonistic encounters. • Owners must be instructed in methods of safely breaking up fights by never reaching toward the dogs' heads or necks to physically pull them apart; preferred methods include physical barrier deterrent (e.g., noise distractor, water, or deterrent spray) or leashes left constantly attached when dogs are together. • Owners should be advised of their liability for bites. • For treatment to be effective, aggression-provoking stimuli should be prevented prior to behavior modification. • At any time or place an aggression-evoking situation could arise (e.g., around food/valued resources), dogs must be confined away from each other or under direct physical control of a responsible adult; dogs can be separated by placing in separate rooms, with pet gates, exercise pens, or crates, or securely tethered short term to hooks installed in walls. • Tools for safety and management include head halters, basket muzzles, or harnesses with leashes attached for prevention, and to safely remove dogs from situations that may elicit aggression. • If safety cannot be ensured, it may be necessary to rehome dog to a single-dog household, where all triggers can be avoided.

Behavior Therapy

• Structured interaction programs (such as "Learn to earn" or "Say please by sitting"), where dog is taught to consistently perform a desired behavior (e.g., sit) before receiving anything it values (e.g., attention, food), give the dog control of its resources by being calm, provide structure and predictability in all interactions, teach impulse control, and train dog using positive interactions (e.g., good things happen by sitting calmly). • Separately, teach each dog behaviors that will serve as a foundation for management and control when together including sit and relax, down-settle, go to mat or crate, focus on owner (e.g., watch/look), and leave it; private sessions with force-free trainer can be the best option for achieving success. • Once each dog can reliably perform foundation and relaxation exercises, then owners can work with dogs together, separated by distance to ensure both dogs can remain focused or engaged in desirable behaviors (e.g., mat) that can be reinforced. • During times together, close supervision is needed; owners must be able to recognize body language and be vigilant for stimuli that might incite aggression; verbal cues should be used to prevent or interrupt undesirable behaviors and teach what is desirable; use of a leash attached to each dog with head halter or while wearing basket muzzle will increase safety when dogs are in close proximity. • Use positive reinforcement (e.g., treats, toys, petting) to teach behaviors incompatible with those that lead to aggression (e.g., response substitution, differential reinforcement of alternative behavior). • Systematic desensitization and counter-conditioning to triggers—desensitization is a process by which dogs will be exposed to their triggers under their threshold; food, toys, verbal praise, or physical attention (e.g., petting) can be used to reward calm behavior. Counter-conditioning is a process in which positive associations are paired with each stimulus exposure, (e.g., most-valued treats); dogs should be exposed to each other under control of handlers and at distance at which they can remain calm and focused on their handlers while performing cued behaviors for rewards; gradually dogs can be moved closer in proximity to each other and in varied situations while focusing on handlers.

SURGICAL CONSIDERATIONS

Castration reduced intermale aggression in 62% of dogs.

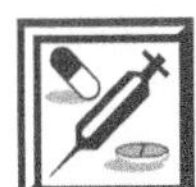

MEDICATIONS

DRUG(S) OF CHOICE

- No medications licensed for treatment of canine aggression; owners must have informed consent of potential side effects and risks, and that use is off-label. • Owners need to understand that medication will not ensure safety and to follow all safety procedures.
- Medications may be indicated for moderate to intense fear and anxiety, impulsivity, and reactivity. • Proper diagnosis with behavioral modification plan, including appropriate selection of behavioral drugs, leads to most successful outcomes.

Selective Serotonin Reuptake Inhibitors (SSRIs)

- Fluoxetine 0.5–2 mg/kg PO q24h.
- Paroxetine 0.5–1 mg/kg PO q24h.
- Sertraline 1–3 mg/kg PO q24h. • Side effects—sedation, irritability, gastrointestinal tract (GIT) effects, agitation; decreased appetite common and usually transient.

Tricyclic Antidepressants (TCAs)

- Clomipramine 1–3 mg/kg q12h (label-restricted for aggression). • Side effects—sedation, GIT effects, anticholinergic effects, cardiac conduction disturbances if predisposed, agitation.

For Situational or Adjunctive Use

Alpha-2 Agonists

- Clonidine 0.01–0.05 mg/kg PO PRN 1.5–2 hours before eliciting trigger, up to q8–12h. • Side effects—transient hyperglycemia, anticholinergic, hypotension, collapse, bradycardia, and agitation.

Serotonin 2a Antagonist/Reuptake Inhibitors

- Trazodone 2–5 mg/kg PO PRN prior to eliciting trigger, up to q8h—may titrate up to 8–10 mg/kg if no adverse effects; use cautiously at higher doses and when combining with other drugs that increase serotonin due to risk of serotonin syndrome. • Side effects—sedation, anorexia, ataxia, GIT effects, cardiac conduction disturbances, agitation.

Benzodiazepines

- Might be used to reduce anxiety prior to eliciting trigger. • Side effects—sedation, lethargy, ataxia, paradoxical excitement; may disinhibit aggression.

CONTRAINDICATIONS

Corticosteroids may cause or contribute to polyphagia, increased food guarding, and irritability.

PRECAUTIONS

Use caution, as any psychotropic medication may cause undesirable changes in behavior, including increased irritability and aggression.

POSSIBLE INTERACTIONS

Do not combine SSRIs, TCAs, or monoamine oxidase (MAO) inhibitors (e.g., amitraz, selegiline) and use cautiously or avoid with opioids, tramadol, or other medications that increase serotonin—can result in serotonin syndrome.

ALTERNATIVE DRUG(S)

Natural products—dog-appeasing pheromones, supplements containing alpha-casozepine or l-theanine, or a calming probiotic might be considered for mild to moderate anxiety or used adjunctively.

FOLLOW-UP

PATIENT MONITORING

- Clients will need ongoing assistance and should receive at least one follow-up within first 1–3 weeks after consultation. Provisions for further follow-up should be made at that time. • Drugs should only be prescribed under direct supervision and monitoring of veterinarian.

PREVENTION/AVOIDANCE

Safety and management recommendations are lifelong.

POSSIBLE COMPLICATIONS

Injuries to dogs and humans.

EXPECTED COURSE AND PROGNOSIS

- Lifelong management likely necessary.
- Prognosis for improvement depends on severity of aggression; motivation; whether triggers can be identified, avoided, and safely managed; and owner compliance; prognosis more favorable if triggers are predictable and preventable, and aggression occurs at low intensity. • Aggression may recur with change in routine, housing, or health, and increasing age.

MISCELLANEOUS

ASSOCIATED CONDITIONS

Other fear- or anxiety-related conditions; possessive, redirected, and territorial aggression.

ZOONOTIC POTENTIAL

Human injury/bite wounds.

PREGNANCY/FERTILITY/BREEDING

Do not breed dogs that exhibit aggressive behavior.

SEE ALSO

- Aggression, Food and Resource Guarding—Dogs.
- Aggression, Overview—Dogs.
- Fears, Phobias, and Anxieties—Dogs.

ABBREVIATIONS

- GIT = gastrointestinal tract.
- MAO = monoamine oxidase.
- SSRI = selective serotonin reuptake inhibitor.
- TCA = tricyclic antidepressant.

Suggested Reading

Herron ME, Shofer SS, Reisner IR. Survey of the use and outcome of confrontational and non-confrontational training methods in client-owned dogs showing undesired behaviors. Appl Anim Behav Sci 2009, 117:47–54.

Landsberg G, Hunthausen W, Ackerman L. Behavior Problems of the Dog and Cat, 3rd ed. St. Louis, MO: Saunders Elsevier, 2013, pp. 320–324.

Pike A. Managing canine aggression in the home. Vet Clin N Am Small Anim Pract 2018, 48:387–402.

Authors Jeannine Berger and Wailani Sung

Consulting Editor Gary M. Landsberg

Acknowledgment The authors and editors acknowledge the prior contributions of Meredith E. Stepita and Laurie Bergman.

AGGRESSION TO UNFAMILIAR PEOPLE AND UNFAMILIAR DOGS—DOGS

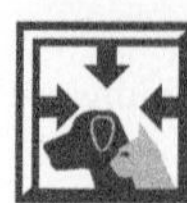

BASICS

OVERVIEW

• Aggression directed toward person or dog that does not live in the household. • Variety of motivations including fear, territoriality, conflict, and possessiveness. • Usually within range of normal behavior, but may be excessive or abnormal due to learning, early experiences, genetics, or underlying medical conditions.

SYSTEMS AFFECTED

Behavioral

INCIDENCE/PREVALENCE

Stranger-directed aggression represents 32.5% of canine behavioral referral caseload. May be skewed as many cases may go unreported.

SIGNALMENT

Breed Predilections

None

Mean Age and Range

• Any age. • Signs may begin to emerge as primary socialization wanes (12–16 weeks of age) or may arise or intensify at social maturity (18–36 months). • Genetic concerns and more guarded prognosis when signs arise before 12 weeks.

Predominant Sex

• May be overrepresented in males.
• Territorial aggression more common in intact males—initial signs usually present by 1 year.

SIGNS

• Barking, growling, lip-lifting, snarling, snapping, lunging, biting, directed toward other dogs or people. • Subtle communication signals may include blocking access to resources, hard stare, taller stance, tail elevated, ears perked forward, and approaching or direct contact. • May be accompanied by fearful/submissive body postures/facial expressions (e.g., crouching, backing away, ears back, tail tucked, looking away, lip-licking).
• Territorial aggression arises in familiar locations or spaces (e.g., home, yard, car) with confident body language. • Fear aggression more likely when dog is cornered or cannot escape. • May be more frequent or severe on- than off-leash, on own property, or when behind barrier (e.g., fence, pet gate, crate).

CAUSES & RISK FACTORS

• Underlying medical conditions, including pain, endocrinopathies, neurologic, sensory decline. • May be normal canine behavior. Strongly influenced by previous experience, (e.g., socialization, unpleasant outcomes/ associations) such as previous fear-evoking or aggressive encounters with dogs or people, punishment, and other behavior disorders including fear, anxiety, and reactivity. • May begin as unruly or exuberant behavior or during leash (walk) training. Owner responses including leash corrections, verbal and/or physical punishment may increase fear, anxiety, and arousal, and condition further negative associations. • Owner's inability to read early signs of fear or conflict. • Owner's failure to create or maintain predictable pattern of positive interactions with unfamiliar people and dogs. • Fear of strangers.

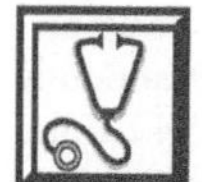

DIAGNOSIS

DIFFERENTIAL DIAGNOSIS

• Fear aggression. • Territorial aggression.
• Possessive aggression. • Protective aggression. • Conflict-related aggression.
• Generalized anxiety disorder. • Pain-related aggression. • Irritable aggression.

CBC/BIOCHEMISTRY/URINALYSIS

To rule out underlying medical conditions and as baseline prior to any drug use.

OTHER LABORATORY TESTS

As needed to rule out underlying medical conditions, including thyroid screening.

IMAGING

As needed to rule out underlying medical conditions, (e.g., pain); MRI if CNS disease suspected.

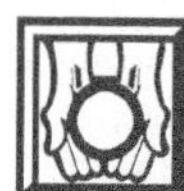

TREATMENT

CLIENT EDUCATION

General Comments

• Treatment requires a multifaceted approach including management to ensure safety and prevent recurrence, behavior modification, and medication. • Treatment must focus on managing the problem and gradually modifying behavior to reduce fear, anxiety, and aggression, not cure/full resolution. • Successful treatment requires owner understanding of canine social behavior and communication, risks, identification of all aggression-eliciting stimuli, how to implement safe management, and effective implementation of reward-based behavior modification. • Owners must be aware that the only certain way to prevent future injuries is avoidance of stimuli.
• Educate owners that use of physical or verbal punishment, confrontation, or establishing dominance (such as alpha rolls), and corrections with choke chains or prong collars, can lead to human injury, further negative associations with stimuli, increased fear, anxiety, and aggression, and disruption of human–animal bond.

Safety Recommendations

• Preventing or avoiding stimuli/triggers that evoke fear, anxiety, or aggression is essential to ensure safety, prevent further repetition and potential intensification of the problem, address pet welfare, and provide an environment in which pet can learn and desired outcomes can be achieved, prior to implementing behavior modification.
• Decrease or avoid visitors and unfamiliar dogs to the home. • Avoid walks at times or in locations where stimulus exposure might occur. On walks, maintain a 15 ft distance from other people and dogs. • Confine dog away from potential targets; stay below threshold, (e.g., distance, location); and ensure direct physical control of adult together with safety products if any possible exposure. • Confine territorial dogs to where they cannot see/hear visitors approaching territory before they become alerted or aggressive. Confine dogs for duration of visitor's stay inside house. • Safety measures include training dogs to wear a basket muzzle, use of head collars or harnesses with leashes attached, and confinement training (e.g., safe haven, closed doors, barricades) away from potential triggers. • Owners should be advised of their liability for bites. • Ensure that dog cannot escape through fencing or unlatched gates or doors. • If safety cannot be ensured, dog should be removed from household.

Behavior Therapy

• Structured interaction programs (such as "Learn to earn" or "Say please by sitting"), where dog is taught to consistently perform desired behavior (e.g., to sit) before receiving anything it values (e.g., attention, petting, feeding, going for a walk), give dog control of its resources for being calm, provide structure and predictability in all interactions, teach impulse control, and train dog using positive interactions (e.g., good things happen by sitting calmly). • Use positive reinforcement to train alternative desirable behaviors (e.g., response substitution) that can be used during stimulus exposure. • Train each behavior in neutral situations with most motivating rewards (e.g., treats, food, toys, petting) to achieve outcomes immediately and successfully in absence of stimuli, including a calm sit; go to bed or crate to settle; walk on loose leash; focus on owner for guidance using eye contact (e.g., watch, look); find it (e.g., move away for a reward); and hand target (e.g., touch nose to owner's hand). • Private sessions with force-free trainer are often recommended to achieve foundation basics before any exposure. • Behavior modification—desensitization (DS) is process by which dogs will be exposed to their triggers under their threshold and rewarded if remain calm. Counter-conditioning (CC) is process in which trigger or stimulus is paired with positive outcomes with each exposure.
• When owner can effectively keep dog calm and under control, and get desirable outcomes on cue in absence of stimuli, begin exposure by determining limit (e.g., distance, location,

person, dog) at which dog will orient but not yet react. Pair highest-value rewards with each exposure. • Gradually (baby steps) increase stimulus intensity, staying below threshold that will result in fear and/or aggression by decreasing distance, increasing distractions, or moving to more challenging environments.
• Progress is slow (typically weeks to months). Carefully monitor body language to avoid setbacks. • Owners must always be vigilant for approach of stimuli that might incite fear or aggression. • Discuss whether referral to veterinary behavior specialist is recommended for counseling on risk assessment, prognosis, behavioral management, behavior modification, and medication use.

SURGICAL CONSIDERATIONS

Castration reduced aggression by at least 50% toward unfamiliar dogs in <20% of dogs and toward human territorial intruders in <10% of dogs. Castration reduced intermale aggression in 62% of dogs.

MEDICATIONS

DRUG(S) OF CHOICE

• No medications licensed for treatment of canine aggression. Owners must have informed consent of risks, potential side effects, and that medication use is off-label.
• Medications may be indicated for moderate to intense fear, anxiety, impulsivity, and reactivity. • Ensure that owners understand risks of owning aggressive dog, that medication will not ensure safety, and that they follow safety procedures. • Proper diagnosis with behavioral modification plan, including appropriate selection of behavioral drugs, leads to most successful outcome.

For Ongoing Use

Selective Serotonin Reuptake Inhibitors

• Fluoxetine 0.5–2 mg/kg PO q24h.
• Paroxetine 0.5–1 mg/kg PO q24h.
• Sertraline 1–3 mg/kg PO q24h. • Side effects—sedation, irritability, gastrointestinal tract (GIT) effects, agitation; decreased appetite common and usually transient.

Tricyclic Antidepressants

• Clomipramine 1–3 mg/kg q12h (label-restricted for aggression). • Side effects—sedation, GIT effects, anticholinergic effects, cardiac conduction disturbances if predisposed, and increased agitation.

For Situational or Adjunctive Use

Alpha-2 Agonists

• Clonidine 0.01–0.05 mg/kg PO PRN 1.5–2 hours before eliciting trigger, up to q8–12h. • Side effects—transient hyperglycemia, anticholinergic, hypotension, bradycardia, and agitation.

Serotonin 2a Antagonist/Reuptake Inhibitors

• Trazodone 2–5 mg/kg PO PRN prior to eliciting trigger, up to q8h—may titrate up to 8–10 mg/kg if no adverse effects. Use cautiously at higher doses and when combining with other drugs that increase serotonin due to risk of serotonin syndrome. • Side effects—sedation, anorexia, ataxia, GIT effects, cardiac conduction disturbances, agitation.

Benzodiazepines

• May be used to reduce anxiety prior to eliciting trigger. • Side effects—sedation, lethargy, ataxia, paradoxical excitement, may disinhibit aggression.

CONTRAINDICATIONS

Corticosteroids can be contraindicated in food-aggressive dogs; could cause or contribute to polyphagia, resource guarding, and irritability.

PRECAUTIONS

Use caution—any psychotropic medication may cause undesirable changes in behavior, including increased irritability or aggression.

POSSIBLE INTERACTIONS

Do not combine selective serotonin reuptake inhibitors (SSRIs), tricyclic antidepressants (TCAs), and monoamine oxidase (MAO) inhibitors (e.g., amitraz, selegiline) and use cautiously or avoid with opioids, tramadol, and other medications that increase serotonin—can result in serotonin syndrome.

ALTERNATIVE DRUG(S)

Natural products—dog-appeasing pheromones, supplements containing alpha-casozepine or l-theanine, or a calming probiotic might be considered for mild to moderate anxiety or used adjunctively.

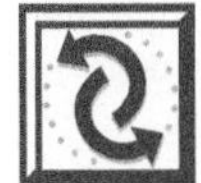

FOLLOW-UP

PATIENT MONITORING

• Clients will need ongoing assistance with at least one follow-up within the first 1–3 weeks after consultation. Provisions for further follow-up should be made at that time.
• Drugs should only be prescribed under the supervision and monitoring of a veterinarian.

PREVENTION/AVOIDANCE

Safety and management recommendations are lifelong.

POSSIBLE COMPLICATIONS

Injuries to dogs and humans.

EXPECTED COURSE AND PROGNOSIS

• Resolution may not be achievable and lifelong management may be necessary.
• Prognosis based on whether triggers can be avoided to ensure safety and prevent recurrence, and whether improvement can be achieved with behavior modification and medication.
• Prognosis more favorable if aggression occurs at low intensity and in predictable situations.
• Prognosis dependent on owner compliance.
• Approximately 75% of dogs aggressive toward unfamiliar dogs could be around other dogs on leash after treatment.

MISCELLANEOUS

ASSOCIATED CONDITIONS

Other fear- or anxiety-related conditions; possessive, redirected, and territorial aggression.

ZOONOTIC POTENTIAL

Human/dog injury and bite wounds.

PREGNANCY/FERTILITY/BREEDING

Do not breed dogs that exhibit aggressive behavior.

SEE ALSO

• Aggression, Food and Resource Guarding—Dogs.
• Aggression, Overview—Dogs.
• Fear and Aggression in Veterinary Visits—Dogs.
• Fears, Phobias, and Anxieties—Dogs.

ABBREVIATIONS

• GIT = gastrointestinal tract.
• MAO = monoamine oxidase.
• SSRI = selective serotonin reuptake inhibitor.
• TCA = tricyclic antidepressant.

Suggested Reading

Herron ME, Shofer SS, Reisner IR. Survey of the use and outcome of confrontational and non-confrontational training methods in client-owned dogs showing undesired behaviors. Appl Anim Behav Sci 2009, 177:47–54.

Horwitz D, ed. Blackwell's 5 Minute Consult Clinical Companion: Canine and Feline Behavior, 2nd ed. Hoboken, NJ: Wiley-Blackwell, 2018, pp. 58–69, 89–99.

Landsberg G, Hunthausen W, Ackerman L. Behavior Problems of the Dog and Cat, 3rd ed. St. Louis, MO: Saunders Elsevier, 2013, pp. 320–324.

Authors Jeannine Berger and Wailani Sung

Consulting Editor Gary M. Landsberg

Acknowledgment The authors and editors acknowledge the prior contributions of Meredith E. Stepita and Laurie Bergman.

A

AGGRESSION TOWARD CHILDREN—DOGS

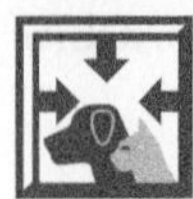

BASICS

OVERVIEW

Children are the most frequently reported victims of dog bites and tend to be injured more severely than adults.

SIGNALMENT

Dogs of any breed, age, sex, and neuter status.

Breed

• Breeds vary with demographics. Breed identification may be unreliable. • Breeds most commonly presenting to a behavior referral service that had bitten a child include English springer spaniel, German shepherd, Labrador retriever, Golden retriever, and American cocker spaniel.
• Most fatal attacks (rare) are attributed to Rottweilers, pit bulls, and their mixes.
• Larger dogs may be more likely to inflict severe injury. • Smaller breeds can also be dangerous and may invite inappropriate handling by children.

Sex

• More frequent in males than females.
• Unneutered males are overrepresented in severe bites. • Neutering will not significantly reduce the risk.

Age

• Any age, but more frequent at or beyond social maturity (2+ years). • Risk may increase in geriatric dogs because of pain, sensory impairment, or cognitive decline.

SIGNS

Aggression

CAUSES & RISK FACTORS

Clinical Categories/Motivation

• Fear related. • Pain related. • Play related.
• Conflict related. • Predatory behavior.
• Territorial. • Resource guarding.

Dog-Associated Risk Factors

• Disease and associated irritability.
• Pain-related aggression and resource guarding are the most common reasons for bites to familiar children <6 years old.
• Anxiety. • Fear. • Dog lying down, particularly under or on furniture. • Parent/littermate aggression. • History of growling, snapping, biting.

Environmental/Social Risk Factors

• Younger children most likely bitten by the family pet or other familiar dogs. • Presence of infants (risk of predatory attacks).
• Presence of young children. • Presence of food, edible toys. • Punishment-based training triggering defensiveness. • Inadequate supervision by parents/caregivers. • Hugging, kissing, or bending over anxious, fearful, conflict-aggressive, or resource-guarding dogs.

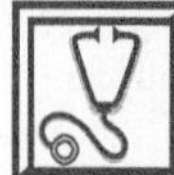

DIAGNOSIS

DIFFERENTIAL DIAGNOSIS

See Causes & Risk Factors.

CBC/BIOCHEMISTRY/URINALYSIS

To rule out medical contributing factors.

OTHER LABORATORY TESTS

Anecdotal evidence correlates hypothyroidism with increased aggression; however, no data-based evidence exists.

IMAGING

N/A

DIAGNOSTIC PROCEDURES

• Detailed history of the bite event and the behavior of both dog and child to determine motivation or trigger. • Pain assessment.

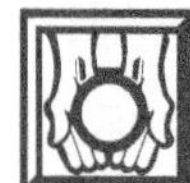

TREATMENT

SAFETY WITH FAMILIAR DOGS

• Never leave infants or young children unsupervised with dogs. Securely separate infants from dogs when alone, even if both asleep. • If one adult is present, separate dog from young children. • If more than one adult is present, assign responsibility for one adult to dog, and one to child. • Educate owners to read and recognize canine communication signals and triggers. • Do not allow child to approach or interact with dog when dog is lying down or in possession of resources. • Separate dog when eating or chewing valued items. • Do not allow child to hug, kiss, bend over, or lie down beside dog.

SAFETY WITH UNFAMILIAR DOGS

• Do not tether unsupervised. • Do not allow young children to interact with unfamiliar dogs. • Securely lock gates in yards. • Avoid underground electric fences that do not prevent entry of children into yard or escape of dogs.

BEHAVIOR MODIFICATION

• Establish secure, separate "safe haven" for dog.
• Restrict fearful or reactive dog on lead and offer food at safe distance from children, to turn a negative situation into a positive one. • Do not rely on training alone; safety requires prevention.
• Redirect dog's attention: teach "look" or "touch" cues. • Consider positive conditioning to basket muzzle; however, supervised interactions are still essential, as muzzles do not insure safety. • Avoid punishment, which may increase anxiety and aggression.

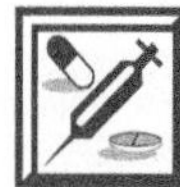

MEDICATIONS

DRUG(S) OF CHOICE

May be indicated for dogs with generalized or situational anxiety or fearful behavior.

Selective Serotonin Reuptake Inhibitors (SSRIs)

• Fluoxetine 0.5–2.0 mg/kg q24h.
• Sertraline 0.5–4 mg/kg q24h or divided q12h. • Paroxetine 0.5–1.5 mg/kg q24h.

Tricyclic Antidepressants (TCAs)

• Clomipramine 1–3 mg/kg q12h.
Natural products containing alpha-casozepine, l-theanine, calming probiotic, or a dog-appeasing pheromone may aid in reducing anxiety.

CONTRAINDICATIONS/POSSIBLE INTERACTIONS

• Psychotropic medication can increase agitation and anxiety or disinhibit aggression. Use with safety recommendations to prevent bites. • Avoid SSRI or TCA in combination.
◦ Use cautiously or avoid with any drugs that increase serotonin. ◦ Avoid use of SSRI or TCA + monoamine oxidase inhibitor (MAOI), including amitraz.

FOLLOW-UP

PREVENTION/AVOIDANCE

• Do not rely on training alone to eliminate aggression. • Preventive measures are most important in management of aggression to children. • Even well-trained, socialized dogs may bite.

POSSIBLE COMPLICATIONS

• Family may not recognize or acknowledge risks. • Disease may aggravate aggression.
• Family may not be compliant. • Psychotropic drug may be unrealistically relied upon or ineffective. • Access of young children to dog may be difficult to control.

EXPECTED COURSE AND PROGNOSIS

• Aggressive behavior can often be reduced and controlled, but not "cured." Lifetime compliance is needed. • Prognosis is poor if social/physical environment cannot be controlled. • In some cases it may be necessary to rehome or euthanize dog, while in some dogs behavior may improve as child grows older.

MISCELLANEOUS

ABBREVIATIONS

• MAOI = monoamine oxidase inhibitor.
• SSRI = selective serotonin reuptake inhibitor. • TCA = tricyclic antidepressant.

Suggested Reading

Reisner IR, Shofer FS, Nance ML. Behavioral assessment of child-directed canine aggression. Inj Prev 2007, 13:348–351.

Author Ilana R. Reisner
Consulting Editor Gary M. Landsberg

AGGRESSION TOWARD FAMILIAR PEOPLE—DOGS

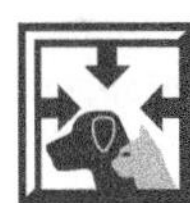

BASICS

OVERVIEW

• Aggression directed toward household members or people with an established relationship with the dog, often in situations when they are handling or attempting to interact with the dog, or involving access to certain resources. • Variety of motivations including fear, protective, conflict, and possessiveness. • Usually within range of normal behavior, but may be excessive, abnormal, or related to underlying medical conditions.

SYSTEMS AFFECTED

Behavioral

INCIDENCE/PREVALENCE

• Approximately 7%. • Represents 20–44% of behavioral referral caseloads may be skewed as many cases unreported. • Bites from larger dogs may require medical attention, therefore more likely documented.

SIGNALMENT

Breed Predilections

• Behavior is a result of interplay between ontogeny and phylogeny. • Environmental stimuli may play a more critical role in aggression. • May be increased occurrence in related dogs. • May be genetic factors associated with impulse dyscontrol in English springer spaniel and English cocker spaniel; more common in conformation lineage than field lineage in English springer spaniels. • In other breeds, dogs bred for show may be associated with less aggression.

Mean Age and Range

• Usually manifested by social maturity (12–36 months of age). • Genetic concerns and poorer prognosis if signs arise before 12 weeks.

Predominant Sex

May be overrepresented in males (castrated and intact).

SIGNS

• Barking, growling, lip-lifting, snarling, snapping, lunging, biting, directed toward familiar people. • Subtle communication signals may include blocking access to resources, hard stare, taller stance, tail elevated, ears perked forward, and approaching or direct contact. • May be accompanied by fearful/submissive body postures/facial expressions (e.g., crouching, backing away, ears back, tail tucked, looking away, lip-licking). • May be more frequent when handled or approached when resting, avoiding, or hiding (e.g., under furniture) or grabbing (e.g., collar). • Protective or possessive aggression arises in vicinity of highly valued objects/space or people. • Fear aggression can be defensive or offensive and more likely to occur when cornered or cannot escape.

CAUSES & RISK FACTORS

• Underlying medical conditions including pain, endocrinopathies, neurologic, and sensory decline. • May be normal canine behavior; can be strongly influenced by previous experience (e.g., socialization, early development, unpleasant outcomes including previous aggressive encounters, punishment), and other behavioral disorders such as fear, anxiety, and impulsivity. • Owner's inability to read early signs of fear or conflict. • Owner's failure to create or maintain predictable pattern of positive interactions.

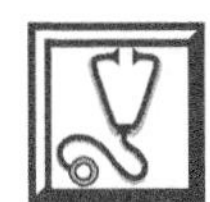

DIAGNOSIS

DIFFERENTIAL DIAGNOSIS

• Fear/defensive aggression. • Territorial aggression. • Possessive aggression. • Protective aggression. • Conflict-related aggression. • Generalized anxiety disorder. • Pain-related aggression. • Irritable aggression.

CBC/BIOCHEMISTRY/URINALYSIS

To rule out underlying medical conditions and as baseline prior to drug use.

OTHER LABORATORY TESTS

As needed to rule out underlying medical conditions; thyroid screening.

IMAGING

As needed to rule out underlying medical conditions (e.g., pain); MRI if CNS disease suspected.

DIAGNOSTIC PROCEDURES

N/A

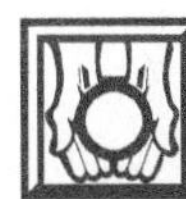

TREATMENT

CLIENT EDUCATION

General Comments

• Treatment requires multifaceted approach, including immediate management to ensure safety and prevent recurrence, behavior modification, and medication (where indicated). • Realistic expectation is for managing triggers, most often for rest of dog's life, and gradually improving, not resolving, the problem. • Successful treatment requires owner understanding of canine social behavior and communication, identification of all aggression-eliciting stimuli, willingness and ability to follow safety and management recommendations, and effective implementation of reward-based behavior modification. • Educate owners that use of physical or verbal punishment, confrontation, or establishing dominance such as with alpha rolls, and corrections with choke chains or prong collars, can lead to human injury, further negative associations with the stimuli, increased fear, anxiety and aggression, and disruption of human–animal bond.

Safety Recommendations

• Owners must ensure safety by identifying and avoiding situations that may evoke fearful or aggressive response; identification and avoidance of triggers is essential to ensure safety, for pet welfare, and to provide environment in which pet can learn and desired outcomes be achieved, prior to implementing behavior modification. • Safety measures include training to wear a basket muzzle, use of head collars or harnesses with leashes attached, and use of confinement training and barriers (e.g., safe haven, gates, closed doors) to keep dog from triggers and triggers from dog. • Owners should be advised of their liability for bites. • Treatment more likely to be successful if aggression-provoking stimuli can be effectively prevented prior to behavior modification. • Common triggers include handling or moving dog when on furniture or resting, use of physical punishment, touching painful areas, and removing valued items; this can be managed by keeping dog away from areas/furniture, when using physical punishment, using pain control and taking dog to veterinarian for uncomfortable procedures, and not to give (or confine when giving) valued items. • If safety cannot be ensured, dogs should be removed from household and euthanasia considered if prognosis poor for safe rehoming.

Behavior Therapy

• Structured interaction programs (such as "Learn to earn" or "Say please by sitting") where dog is consistently taught to perform a desired behavior (e.g., sit) before receiving anything it values (e.g., attention, petting, feeding, toys) give dog control of its resources for being calm, provide structure and predictability in all interactions, teach impulse control, and train dog using positive interactions (e.g., good things happen by sitting calmly). • Use positive reinforcement to teach alternative desirable behaviors that are incompatible (e.g., response substitution) with those that have resulted in aggression. • Teach each behavior in neutral situations using most motivating rewards (e.g., food, toys, play, attention), including sit and relax on verbal cue; down-settle; go to bed or crate; focus on owner (e.g., watch/look), and hand targeting (e.g., touch nose to owner's hand). Private sessions with force-free trainer often recommended to achieve foundation basics before any exposure. • Behavior modification—desensitization is process by which dogs are exposed to triggers under their threshold; rewards should be given when calm (e.g., food, toys, verbal praise, or physical attention); counter-conditioning is process in which positive associations paired with exposure to stimulus, (e.g., most valued treats); operant counter-conditioning or response substitution is process in which acceptable alternative behaviors that are incompatible with undesirable behavior are reinforced. • Reinforce your dog for being calm as family members approach or beyond threshold distance when in a location or in possession of an item that might trigger aggression; always use nonconfrontational techniques; start handling in nonpainful/sensitive areas. • Start by staying below threshold that would result in fear and/or aggression, then gradually (baby steps) increase stimulus intensity by decreasing distance, increasing distractions, or moving to more challenging environments. • Progress is slow (typically months); however, immediate safety and welfare can be achieved if triggers can be identified and prevented or avoided; owners should be counselled on reading and monitoring body language to identify thresholds and avoid setbacks. • Owners must always be vigilant for stimuli that might incite fear or aggression. • Discuss whether referral to veterinary behavior specialist is recommended for counseling on risk assessment, prognosis, behavioral management, behavior modification, and medication.

SURGICAL CONSIDERATIONS

Aggression may be lower in neutered animals, but opposite has also been reported.

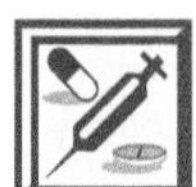

MEDICATIONS

DRUG(S) OF CHOICE

• No medications licensed for treatment of canine aggression; owners must give informed consent that use is off-label and be advised of potential side effects and risks. • Medications are likely indicated for moderately intense fear and anxiety, impulsivity, and reactivity.
• Ensure that owners understand risks in owning an aggressive dog, that medication will not ensure safety, and that they must follow safety procedures. • Proper diagnosis with behavioral modification plan, together with appropriate selection of behavioral drugs, leads to most successful outcome.

Selective Serotonin Reuptake Inhibitors

• Fluoxetine 0.5–2 mg/kg PO q24h.
• Paroxetine 0.5–1 mg/kg PO q24h.
• Sertraline 1–3 mg/kg PO q24h. • Side effects—sedation, irritability, gastrointestinal tract (GIT) effects, agitation; decreased appetite is common and usually transient.

Tricyclic Antidepressants

• Clomipramine 1–3 mg/kg q12h (label-restricted for aggression). • Side effects—sedation, GIT effects, anticholinergic effects, cardiac conduction disturbances if predisposed, agitation.

For Situational or Adjunctive Use

Alpha-2 Agonists

• Clonidine 0.01–0.05 mg/kg PO PRN 1.5–2 hours before eliciting trigger, up to q8–12h. • Side effects—transient hyperglycemia, anticholinergic, hypotension, collapse, bradycardia, agitation.

Serotonin 2a Antagonist/Reuptake Inhibitors

• Trazodone 2–5 mg/kg PO PRN prior to eliciting trigger, up to q8h—may titrate up to 8–10 mg/kg if no adverse effects. Use cautiously at higher doses and when combining with other drugs that increase serotonin due to risk of serotonin syndrome. • Side effects—sedation, anorexia, ataxia, GIT effects, cardiac conduction disturbances, agitation.

Benzodiazepines

• Might be used to reduce anxiety prior to eliciting triggers. • Side effects—sedation, lethargy, ataxia, paradoxical excitement, may disinhibit aggression.

CONTRAINDICATIONS

Corticosteroids may contribute to polyphagia, increased food guarding, and irritability.

PRECAUTIONS

Use caution, as any psychotropic medication may cause undesirable changes in behavior, including increased irritability or aggression.

POSSIBLE INTERACTIONS

Do not combine selective serotonin reuptake inhibitors (SSRIs), tricyclic antidepressants (TCAs), or monoamine oxidase (MAO) inhibitors (e.g., amitraz, selegiline), and use cautiously or avoid with opioids, tramadol, or other medications that increase serotonin—can result in serotonin syndrome.

ALTERNATIVE DRUGS

Natural products—dog-appeasing pheromones, supplements containing alpha-casozepine or l-theanine, or a calming probiotic might be considered for mild to moderate anxiety or used adjunctively.

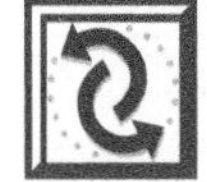

FOLLOW-UP

PATIENT MONITORING

• Clients will need ongoing assistance and should receive at least one follow-up within first 1–3 weeks after the consultation. Provisions for further follow-up should be made at that time. • Drugs should only be prescribed under supervision and monitoring of veterinarian.

PREVENTION/AVOIDANCE

Safety and management recommendations are lifelong.

POSSIBLE COMPLICATIONS

Injuries to humans.

EXPECTED COURSE AND PROGNOSIS

• Lifelong management is necessary.
• Prognosis for improvement determined by severity of aggression; motivation; whether triggers can be identified, avoided, and safely managed; owner compliance; and level that might be achieved with behavior modification and medication. • Prognosis more favorable if aggression occurs at low intensity and in predictable situations.

MISCELLANEOUS

ASSOCIATED CONDITIONS

Other fear- or anxiety-related conditions; possessive and redirected aggression, impulsivity, reactivity.

ZOONOTIC POTENTIAL

Human injury/bite wounds.

PREGNANCY/FERTILITY/BREEDING

Do not breed dogs that exhibit aggressive behavior.

SEE ALSO

• Aggression, Food and Resource Guarding—Dogs. • Aggression, Overview—Dogs.
• Fears, Phobias, and Anxieties—Dogs.

ABBREVIATIONS

• GIT = gastrointestinal tract. • MAO = monoamine oxidase. • SSRI = selective serotonin reuptake inhibitor. • TCA = tricyclic antidepressant.

Suggested Reading

Herron ME, Shofer SS, Reisner IR. Survey of the use and outcome of confrontational and non-confrontational training methods in client-owned dogs showing undesired behaviors. Appl Anim Behav Sci 2009, 177:47–54.

Horwitz D, ed. Blackwell's 5 Minute Consult Clinical Companion: Canine and Feline Behavior, 2nd ed. Hoboken, NJ: Wiley-Blackwell, 2018, pp. 45–57.

Sueda KL, Malamed R. Aggression toward people—a guide for practitioners. Vet Clin N Am 2014, 14:599–628.

Authors Wailani Sung and Jeannine Berger

Consulting Editor Gary M. Landsberg

Acknowledgment The authors and editors acknowledge the prior contributions of Meredith E. Stepita and Laurie Bergman.

Client Education Handout available online

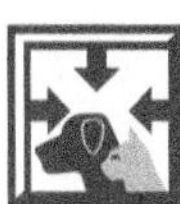

BASICS

DEFINITION

Human-directed aggression in cats.

PATHOPHYSIOLOGY

- Most common causes for human-directed aggression in cats include play, fear/pain-related, redirected, maternal, and petting intolerance.
- Context contributes greatly when making correct diagnosis. For example, play aggression is likely to be seen in young, solitary cat, while pain-related/fear aggression is common behavior seen in clinic setting.

SYSTEMS AFFECTED

- Behavioral.
- Gastrointestinal—decreased appetite if fear and/or pain related.
- Hemic/lymphatic/immune—chronic stress effects on immune function.
- Ophthalmic—dilated pupils in response to autonomic nervous system stimulation.
- Skin/exocrine—may show displacement behaviors such as overgrooming.

GENETICS

No known genetic basis.

INCIDENCE/PREVALENCE

Aggression is second to inappropriate elimination for feline cases seen by veterinary behavior specialists.

GEOGRAPHIC DISTRIBUTION

None

SIGNALMENT

- Cats of any age, sex/neuter status, breed can be affected.
- Play-motivated aggression more likely in juvenile, solitary cat.

SIGNS

- Play motivated—cat approaches its "victim," crouches in wait, stalks and chases; tail is twitching and ears are forward. Typically will attack moving target.
- Fear/pain related—ears back, body and tail lowered, piloerection, pupils dilated; may hiss and growl. Avoidance of person(s) who elicit aggression. Attacks if approached and/or cornered. Extreme cases: expression of anal glands, urination, and/or defecation. Hiding behavior.
- Redirected—cat highly aroused by stimulus and seeks out alternate target. Aggression can be very severe given cat's level of arousal.
- Maternal—usually predictable and self-limiting. Queen will act to protect her kittens.
- Petting intolerance—cat signals its "displeasure" by twitching its tail and skin when being petted in an undesired location and/or for too long. Ears usually back; mydriasis; may hiss and growl before turning to bite person.

CAUSES & RISK FACTORS

- Play motivated—lacking in opportunities for normal play: solitary cat, insufficient and/or inappropriate toys; history of owner using hands/feet to play with kitten and/or playing roughly with kitten.
- Fear—poor socialization with humans and/or feral living, aversive event associated with a person, or people in general.
- Pain related—medical/physical condition such as abscess, especially in indoor/outdoor cat.
- Redirected—occurs during interference in, or interruption of, situations that have caused cat to become aggressively aroused, such as cat fight (between familiar household cats), presence of a cat outside, or noise.
- Maternal—recent birth of litter.
- Petting intolerance—etiology unknown. Cats tend to groom each other on head/neck, so human petting of cat in other locations may contribute to aggressive reaction.

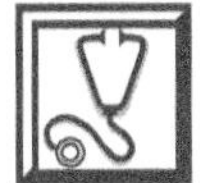

DIAGNOSIS

DIFFERENTIAL DIAGNOSIS

See Causes & Risk Factors.

CBC/BIOCHEMISTRY/URINALYSIS

- To rule out contributing medical conditions and screening prior to drug use.
- Urinalysis if concurrent inappropriate elimination or marking.

OTHER LABORATORY TESTS

Middle age/senior cats—thyroid profile.

IMAGING

If indicated based on clinical examination and/or suspected pain.

DIAGNOSTIC PROCEDURES

Thorough behavioral history, including description of cat's postures during aggression and injuries inflicted, context, presence of outside cats, early historical information, litter box use, food consumption, and hiding behaviors.

PATHOLOGIC FINDINGS

N/A

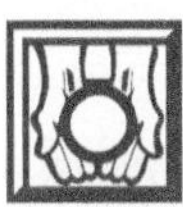

TREATMENT

APPROPRIATE HEALTH CARE

Only if health/medical issue diagnosed.

NURSING CARE

Only if health/medical issue diagnosed.

ACTIVITY

- Play motivated—cat should be provided with increased opportunity for appropriate play, either in the form of toys, human interaction, or additional housemate.
- Redirected—cat should be denied access to windows where outside cats can be seen.

DIET

Potential anxiolytic effects of "calming" diets (see Supplements).

CLIENT EDUCATION

- Play motivated—normal play behavior and importance of opportunities for appropriate play.
- Fear—avoidance of fear-inducing situations: ongoing exposure may worsen signs, cause severe stress, and compromise welfare.
- Redirected—addressing primary stimuli, such as outside cats.
- Maternal—normal maternal and kitten-protective behavior; same as for fear-motivated aggression.
- Petting intolerance—normal feline grooming patterns; observation of cat's warnings so that behavior does not escalate.

Behavior Modification Exercises

Desensitization and Counter-Conditioning (DS&CC)

- Desensitization—exposing cat to fear-inducing stimulus (scary person) at a low level so cat does *not* react fearfully or aggressively. Over time, intensity of stimulus is increased (i.e., distance between cat and stimulus is decreased) without causing fearful responses.
- Operant conditioning (response substitution)—rewarding cat with special treat, toy, grooming, petting, for relaxation.

Classical Conditioning (CC)

Classical counter-conditioning conditioning—pairing threatening stimulus (e.g., a person) with tasty treat, toy, petting; example: scary person = tuna fish.

MEDICATIONS

Short-term use of medication may be necessary to decrease overall levels of anxiety and reactivity in more severe cases.

DRUG(S) OF CHOICE

Azapirones

- Buspirone 0.5–1.0 mg/kg PO q12h.
- Most useful for fearful and withdrawn cats; decreases anxiety and may increase "self-confidence."
- Anecdotal reports of "increase in affection," therefore might be useful in severe cases of petting intolerance.
- Response noted in 1–2 weeks.

Selective Serotonin Reuptake Inhibitors (SSRIs)

- Fluoxetine, paroxetine, sertraline 0.5–1.5 mg/kg PO q24h.
- SSRIs must be given daily; may take 4–8 weeks to reach peak effects.

Tricyclic Antidepressants (TCAs)

- Amitriptyline 0.5–2.0 mg/kg PO q12–24h.
- Clomipramine 0.25–1.0 mg/kg PO q24h.

AGGRESSION TOWARD HUMANS—CATS (CONTINUED)

- TCAs must be given daily; may take 4–8 weeks to reach peak effects.

Benzodiazepines

- Alprazolam 0.125–0.25 mg/cat PO q8–24h.
- Diazepam 0.1–1.0 mg/kg PO q12–24h (rarely used due to potential hepatopathies).
- Can be given "as needed" for specific encounters with people inducing fear response and during DS&CC and CC sessions.
- Can be used in conjunction with azapirones, SSRIs, and TCAs.

CONTRAINDICATIONS/PRECAUTIONS/ POSSIBLE INTERACTIONS

- None of drugs listed are approved for use in cats.
- All medications to be administered orally, as have not been shown to reach therapeutic levels by transdermal dosing.
- Azapirones—side effects uncommon, but occasional excitement noted; should not be given in combination with monoamine oxidase (MAO) inhibitor; avoid use in the aggressor cat as may increase any "bully" behavior.
- Neither SSRIs nor TCAs should be given with each other, nor in combination with MAOIs.
- SSRIs—side effects include mild sedation and decreased appetite, constipation, and urinary retention; competitive inhibition of cytochrome P450 liver enzymes; when administered concurrently with medication utilizing P450 enzymes, elevated plasma levels of medications may increase.
- TCAs—side effects include sedation, constipation, diarrhea, urinary retention, appetite changes, ataxia, decreased tear production, mydriasis, cardiac arrhythmias, tachycardia, and changes in blood pressure.
- Benzodiazepines—side effects include sedation, ataxia, muscle relaxation, increased appetite, paradoxical excitation, and increased friendliness; idiopathic hepatic necrosis has been reported in cats following treatment with diazepam.
- Specific recommendations for the use of diazepam—baseline physical exam, CBC, and blood chemistries to confirm good health; repeat the blood chemistries at 3–5 days; if elevated alanine aminotransferase (ALT) or aspartate aminotransferase (AST), discontinue medication.

ALTERNATIVE DRUG(S)

Pheromones

- Used alone or concurrently with drugs.
- F3 facial pheromone (Feliway®) diffuser, spray, and wipes.
- Maternal pheromone—Feliway MultiCat (Friends) diffuser for feline social conflict.
- Maternal pheromone collar (NurtureCALM 24/7).

Supplements

Used alone or concurrently with drugs: L-theanine (Anxitane®); alpha-casozepine (Zylkene®); combination products also containing thiamine, whey protein, and calming plant extracts (Solliquin®); or diets supplemented with alpha-casozepine and l-tryptophan (Multifunction Urinary + Calm Diet, Royal Canin®).

FOLLOW-UP

PATIENT MONITORING

- Weekly follow-up recommended in early stages of treatment.
- For cats on medication, follow-up blood testing recommended every 6–12 months.

PREVENTION/AVOIDANCE

- Play motivated—provide opportunities for appropriate play.
- Fear—avoidance of fear-inciting stimuli; early socialization to people and events may help prevent some occurrences of fear-related responses to people.
- Pain—treat underlying conditions.
- Redirected—address possible arousing stimuli, indoors and outdoors.
- Maternal—as for fear.
- Petting intolerance—limit amount of time petting cat; DS&CC to petting.

POSSIBLE COMPLICATIONS

Potential human injury, especially if cat is approached, cornered, and/or highly aroused.

EXPECTED COURSE AND PROGNOSIS

- Progress occurs slowly; relearning is a process and each case is individual.
- If medications are indicated, begin at low dose and titrate up as necessary.
- To discontinue medication, wait until new behavior is stable (8–12 weeks) and wean off slowly, usually over weeks.
- If aggressive behavior recurs, return to lowest effective dose.

MISCELLANEOUS

ASSOCIATED CONDITIONS

N/A

AGE-RELATED FACTORS

Play motivated—typically seen in young, solitary cat in household.

ZOONOTIC POTENTIAL

People injured during aggressive attack should seek prompt medical attention; infection by *Bartonella henselae* can result from cat scratch or bite.

PREGNANCY/FERTILITY/BREEDING

Avoid medications in breeding/nursing cats.

SYNONYMS

N/A

SEE ALSO

- Aggression, Overview—Cats.
- Fears, Phobias, and Anxieties—Cats.

ABBREVIATIONS

- ALT = alanine aminotransferase.
- AST = aspartate aminotransferase.
- CC = classical conditioning.
- DS & CC = desensitization and counter-conditioning.
- MAO = monoamine oxidase.
- SSRI = selective serotonin reuptake inhibitor.
- TCA = tricyclic antidepressant.

Suggested Reading

Bradshaw J, Ellis S. The Trainable Cat: A Practical Guide to Making Life Happier for You and Your Cat. New York: Basic Books, 2016.

Horwitz D, ed. Blackwell's 5 Minute Consult Clinical Companion: Canine and Feline Behavior, 2nd ed. Hoboken, NJ: Wiley-Blackwell, 2018, pp. 143–250.

Landsberg GM, Hunthausen W, Ackerman L. Behavior Problems of the Dog and Cat, 3rd ed. St. Louis, MO: Saunders Elsevier, 2013, pp. 327–343.

Overall K. Manual of Clinical Behavioral Medicine for Dogs and Cats. St. Louis, MO: Mosby, 2013, pp. 390–426.

Seksel K. Behavior problems. In: Little SE, ed., The Cat: Clinical Medicine and Management. St. Louis, MO: Saunders, 2012, pp. 219–224.

Author Terry Marie Curtis

Consulting Editor Gary M. Landsberg

AGGRESSION, FOOD AND RESOURCE GUARDING—DOGS

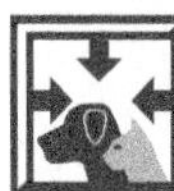

BASICS

OVERVIEW

• Aggression displayed while guarding food (e.g., in food bowl, dog "chews"), scavenged items, objects (e.g., toys, stolen objects), resting locations (e.g., bed, couch), or people. Usually within the range of normal behavior, but may be excessive or abnormal due to early experience, learning, genetic factors, or underlying medical conditions.

SYSTEM AFFECTED

Behavioral.

SIGNALMENT

No breed or sex predilections.

SIGNS

• Barking, growling, lip-lifting, snarling, snapping, lunging, biting, directed toward other dogs or people.
• Subtle communication signals may include blocking access to resources, hard stare, taller stance, tail elevated, and ears perked forward when in possession of valued resource.
• May be accompanied by fearful/submissive body postures/facial expressions (e.g., crouching, backing away, ears back, tail tucked, looking away, lip licking).
• Can be motivated by fear—defensive or offensive.
• Most common near valued resources (e.g., food), stolen items (e.g., tissues, owner clothing), scavenged items (e.g., garbage), and lasting items (e.g., chews).

CAUSES & RISK FACTORS

• Underlying medical conditions, especially pain, endocrinopathies, gastrointestinal disease, or those causing changes in appetite.
• May be a normal canine behavior, influenced by previous negative experience (e.g., lack of socialization, physically removing resources, punishment or confrontation) or other behavioral disorders, such as anxiety.
• Owner's inability to read and recognize signs of fear or conflict.

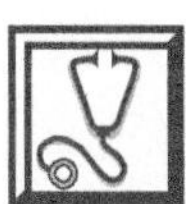

DIAGNOSIS

DIFFERENTIAL DIAGNOSIS

• Fear aggression.
• Social status aggression.
• Conflict-related aggression.
• Generalized anxiety disorder.
• Pain-related aggression.
• Irritable aggression.

CBC/BIOCHEMISTRY/URINALYSIS

To rule out underlying contributing medical conditions.

OTHER LABORATORY TESTS

As needed to rule out underlying medical conditions, particularly if signs of polyphagia; thyroid screen.

IMAGING

As needed to rule out underlying medical conditions, (e.g., pain); MRI if CNS disease suspected.

DIAGNOSTIC PROCEDURES

Gastrointestinal diagnostics.

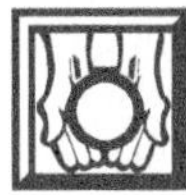

TREATMENT

GENERAL COMMENTS

• Treatment consists of a multifaceted approach including management to ensure safety and prevent recurrence, behavior modification, and medication (if indicated).
• A realistic expectation is for successful management, not full resolution. In most cases, owners will need to manage triggers for the rest of the dog's life.
• Successful treatment depends on the owner's understanding of canine social behavior and communication, identifying and preventing all aggression-eliciting stimuli (e.g., situations, people, resources), willingness and ability to follow safety recommendations, and effective implementation of reward-based behavior modification.
• Owners must be educated about the risks of using physical punishment and training techniques that use "dominating," such as alpha rolls, corrections with choke chains or prong collars, verbal punishment, and of physically taking away resources that can lead to increased aggression, anxiety, and resource guarding, and disruption of the human–animal bond.

SAFETY RECOMMENDATIONS

• Prevention/avoidance is essential to ensure safety, address the pet's welfare, and prevent further repetition and potential intensification of the problem.
• Safety measures include training dogs to wear a basket muzzle, placing head collars or harnesses with leashes attached, and the use of pet gates and confinement training to prevent access to resources that might be guarded.
• Confine the dog away from potential victims and items and/or keep people away from the dog when it is in possession of resources that might be guarded; alternately, the dog must be under direct physical control, (e.g., with leash attached), of a responsible adult.
• Identify and prevent or avoid any situation that might trigger aggression. Never forcibly remove objects in the dog's possession. Wait until the dog is finished with the resource and will walk away, or cue and reward the dog for an alternative behavior, (e.g., drop, touch) (see training below).
• If the dog is in possession of an object that must be removed for safety, offer a reward (e.g., treat, toy, walk) of higher value or use a stimulus (e.g., doorbell) that will move the dog away.
• If safety cannot be ensured, the dog should be removed from the household.

BEHAVIOR THERAPY

• Structured interaction programs where the dog is taught to consistently perform a desired behavior (e.g., sit) before receiving anything it values (e.g., attention, petting, treats, going for a walk) give the dog control of its resources for being calm, provide structure and predictability in all interactions, teach impulse control, and train the dog using positive interactions (e.g., good things happen by sitting calmly).
• Provide sufficient outlets for play, chew, and feeding, such as in food-filled toys in locations and at times where the dog can be left alone or physically confined, (e.g., to a room, behind a barrier, or in a safe haven (pen, crate)) until the dog finishes with the resource, will walk away, or can be cued away and rewarded.
• Training—focus on teaching behaviors in neutral situations using positive reinforcement (e.g., food, toys, play, petting) that can be used to:
  ◦ Keep the dog away from resources, (e.g., leave it, go to bed or crate, or watch).
  ◦ Move the dog away from resources, (e.g., touch (hand target), find it).
  ◦ Release the object (e.g., drop).
• Private sessions with a force-free trainer may provide the best guidance for successful training.
• Behavior modification—desensitization (DS) is the process by which dogs are exposed to their triggers under their threshold (e.g., distance, low-value resource). Food, toys, verbal praise, or attention/petting can be used as rewards for calm responses. Counter-conditioning (CC) is the process in which favored rewards are paired with the stimulus to change the emotional response to one that is positive.
• Gradually (baby steps) increase stimulus intensity, staying below the threshold that would result in fear and/or aggression, (e.g., decreasing distance, increasing resource value, changing environments).
• The owner can toss treats when walking by the food bowl at sufficient distance that the pet associates approach with a positive outcome in association with the food bowl and toys.
• Progress is slow (typically months). Carefully monitor body language to avoid setbacks.
• Owners must be vigilant to prevent approach in situations where dog might guard.

AGGRESSION, FOOD AND RESOURCE GUARDING—DOGS (CONTINUED)

• Discuss referral to a veterinary behavior specialist where recommended for assessment and counseling.

MEDICATIONS

DRUG(S) OF CHOICE

• Medications are generally not indicated for resource guarding.
• May be indicated for moderate to marked fear or anxiety, or when behavior is abnormal in intensity, reactivity, or impulsivity.
• Owners must receive informed consent of potential risks and side effects, that the use of a medication is off-label, and that medication does not insure safety.
• For ongoing medication, a selective serotonin reuptake inhibitor (SSRI; e.g., fluoxetine, paroxetine, sertraline) or clomipramine might be indicated.
• For situational or as needed use, trazodone, clonidine, or benzodiazepines might be considered alone or in conjunction with an ongoing medication.
• For doses, side effects, precautions, and contraindications, see Aggression toward Familiar People—Dogs.

CONTRAINDICATIONS/POSSIBLE INTERACTIONS

• Use caution, as any psychotropic medication might cause undesirable changes in behavior, including increased irritability and aggression. Drugs that increase appetite (e.g., psychotropic drugs, steroids) may increase resource guarding.
• Corticosteroids can be contraindicated in food-aggressive dogs; could cause or contribute to polyphagia, resource guarding, and irritability.

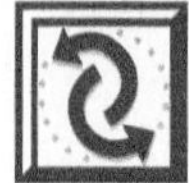

FOLLOW-UP

PATIENT MONITORING

In most cases, follow-up should be within the first 1–3 weeks after consultation. Provisions for further follow-up should be made at that time.

PREVENTION/AVOIDANCE

Owner should receive counseling from first visit on socialization, making positive associations with handling, reward-based training to cues (including touch and drop), and never forcing a pet to relinquish resources.

POSSIBLE COMPLICATIONS

Injuries to dogs and humans.

EXPECTED COURSE AND PROGNOSIS

• Resolution may not be achievable and lifelong management is usually necessary.
• Prognosis for improvement depends on severity of aggression, number and type of resources guarded, and whether they can be effectively identified and prevented.
• Prognosis is highly dependent on owner compliance.

MISCELLANEOUS

ASSOCIATED CONDITIONS

Other fear- or anxiety-related conditions.

ZOONOTIC POTENTIAL

Human injury and bite wounds.

PREGNANCY/FERTILITY/BREEDING

Do not breed dogs that exhibit aggressive behavior.

SEE ALSO

• Aggression to Unfamiliar People and Unfamiliar Dogs—Dogs.
• Aggression toward Familiar People—Dogs.
• Aggression, Overview—Dogs.

ABBREVIATIONS

• CC = counter-conditioning.
• DS = desensitization.
• SSRI = selective serotonin reuptake inhibitor.

Suggested Reading

Horwitz D, ed. Blackwell's 5 Minute Consult Clinical Companion: Canine and Feline Behavior, 2nd ed. Hoboken, NJ: Wiley-Blackwell, 2018, pp. 100–109.

Authors Jeannine Berger and Wailani Sung
Consulting Editor Gary M. Landsberg
Acknowledgment The authors and editors acknowledge the prior contribution of Meredith E. Stepita and Laurie Bergman.

AGGRESSION, INTERCAT AGGRESSION

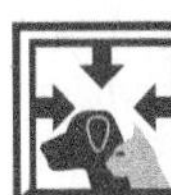

BASICS

DEFINITION

Intercat aggression—offensive or defensive aggression between cats consisting of staring, displacing, vocalizing (growling, yowling, shrieking), spitting, hissing, swatting, lunging, chasing/stalking, and/or biting other cats.

PATHOPHYSIOLOGY

• May be normal behavior or abnormal.
• May be caused by underlying medical disease (e.g., CNS) or concurrent medical disease that may lower the threshold for irritable responses (e.g., pain, hyperthyroid).
• May be multiple motivations including predatory/play, disputes over territory, sexual, fear, anxiety, and redirected, fear, anxiety, non-recognition, and redirected.

SYSTEMS AFFECTED

• Behavioral. • Skin/exocrine—secondary to traumatic injury. • Immune—chronic stress may alter the immune response. • Secondary infection (cat bite abscesses) is not uncommon.
• Nervous.

GENETICS

None. However, friendliness may be mostly related to paternal effects.

INCIDENCE/PREVALENCE

Unknown

SIGNALMENT

Breed Predilections

None

Mean Age and Range

• Can occur at any age due to changes in social environment or be redirected. • Previously stable relationships can deteriorate as cats reach social maturity (2–4 years of age).

Sex

• Intact males more likely to initiate intercat aggression (related to territory, and/or proximity to females). • Females will defend their young from unfamiliar individuals.
• Male kittens more likely to initiate intercat aggression related to predatory components of play.

SIGNS

Historical Findings

• May arise spontaneously and vary in frequency and intensity. • Owners most likely to seek behavioral intervention if there are physical injuries, the welfare of the aggressor and/or victim is compromised, or fighting becomes sufficiently distressing. • Human attempts to interrupt fighting may trigger human-directed aggression/injury.

Aggressor (Usually Offensive)

• Covert signs—staring, displacing other cats, stiff body language/movements while approaching other cat. • Overt signs—growling, yowling, spitting, hissing, swatting, lunging, chasing/stalking, and/or biting other cats, dilated pupils, may be accompanied by body language of fear (e.g., classic Halloween cat stance: piloerection, back arched, tail up) or more offensive body language (tense muscles, tail head elevated but rest of tail down, back straight or slightly slanted toward head, ears forward or to the side), excessive facial marking, and perhaps urine marking.

Victim (Usually Defensive)

• Covert—avoidance of aggressor, hiding, change in grooming and eating habits, hypervigilance, dilated pupils. • Overt—hissing, swatting, running, vocalizing (including growling), Halloween cat stance, may escalate to defensive attack if cornered.

Elimination Outside of Litter Box

• Aggressors may block access to litter box area, forcing victims to choose alternative locations; secondary substrate and/or location preferences and aversions can develop. • Both victims and aggressors may urine mark.
• Extremely fearful cats may urinate or defecate in midst of aggressive events.

Physical Examination

• Normal, except injury from fights or if underlying medical issues. • Stress may affect eating and self-grooming (increased or decreased).

CAUSES

• Lack of appropriate socialization to other cats prior to 7 weeks of age. • May be component of normal social behavior. • Social and environmental instability such as addition of new cat, loss of resident cat, odor stimuli (return of cat from veterinarian or giving one cat a bath), aging or illness of one or both cats, cats reaching social maturity. • Household change, e.g., moving, changing furniture or resting areas. • Genetically unrelated cats and cats that have recently moved in together are more likely to show aggressive behaviors toward each other. • Resident cats commonly need prolonged exposure to new cats before accepting them into group. • Resource limitation, e.g., vertical and/or horizontal space, hiding/resting areas, food, water, and litter boxes in multicat households. • Exposure to arousing stimuli (cats in yard, visitors, noises, scents, etc.) can cause redirected aggression, after which aggression might persist. • Medical problems including CNS disorders, hyperthyroidism, or any disorder that causes pain and/or increased irritability.

RISK FACTORS

• Singleton and/or bottle-raised kittens.
• Lack of socialization exposure and experience with conspecifics during socialization period (2–7 weeks) and beyond. • Male intact cats. • Postpartum females with kittens.
• Separating and returning housemate (e.g., following veterinary visit, groomer). • Changes in social group such as addition of "new" cat. • Scratching and biting during first introduction. • Access to outdoors and/or intrusion of unfamiliar cats onto territory. • Crowding or lack of adequate social space and access to resources.

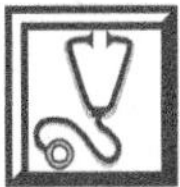

DIAGNOSIS

DIFFERENTIAL DIAGNOSIS

Behavioral Differentials

• Fear-related aggression—cat may hiss, spit, arch the back, display piloerection, and attempt to flee unless escape is thwarted; pupil dilation will accompany a fear response.
• Status-related aggression—may occur with change or instability of social hierarchy and control of access to resources; it is undecided if cats have dominance hierarchies or if conflict is better explained by territorial defense. • Territorial aggression—in response to threat to territory; boundaries marked with urine, feces, or scent glands. • Redirected aggression—exposure to agitating stimuli (cats in yard, visitors, noises, scents, etc.), with aggression directed toward target other than stimulus. • Failure of recognition—aggression between feline housemates after returning from separation (e.g., veterinary visit, grooming); most likely due to change in odor, visual cues, or stress of returning cat.
• Maternal aggression—aggression during periparturient period; females guard kittens and nesting sites. • Intermale aggression—between males in response to territorial disputes, hierarchical status, or mates; may be more pronounced at social maturity. • Sexual aggression—male typical behavior of chasing, pouncing, biting on nape of neck, and mounting. • Predatory/play-related aggression—predatory components of play directed toward another cat; recipient often older cat that is not interested in playing.

Medical Differentials

• Any illness causing malaise, pain, or increased irritability. • Endocrine—e.g., hyperthyroidism. • Neurologic—e.g., neoplasia, seizures, cognitive decline.
• Infectious—e.g., toxoplasmosis, feline immunodeficiency virus (FIV), feline leukemia virus (FeLV). • Iatrogenic—medications that increase irritability or disinhibit aggression (e.g., mirtazapine, benzodiazepines, buspirone). • Toxins—lead, illicit substances.

CBC/BIOCHEMISTRY/URINALYSIS

To rule out medical causes and as baseline if drug therapy indicated.

OTHER LABORATORY TESTS

• FeLV/FIV. • Total thyroxine (T_4) in cats >6 years.

IMAGING

As indicated based on history and physical signs.

DIAGNOSTIC PROCEDURES

• Detailed behavioral and medical history. • Identify if there is a clear aggressor and/or victim and if aggression is overt or covert. • If multiple cats, determine which cats spend time together and mutually groom, and which avoid each other. • Identify preferred core areas of each cat for feeding, play, and resting, and locations of any house soiling or marking. • Identify number, location, types of litter boxes, and their management. • Videos, photographs, and/or drawn floor plans can provide spatial details and information regarding body language during social interactions. • Note any other changes in demeanor, routine, eating, and grooming.

PATHOLOGIC FINDINGS

None unless concurrent medical diseases.

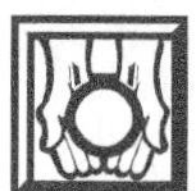

TREATMENT

APPROPRIATE HEALTH CARE

Treat as outpatient.

NURSING CARE

Supportive care if any injuries.

ACTIVITY

• May need to be restricted if confinement required to prevent perpetuation of aggression and negative emotional responses. • Provide sufficient alternate outlets for each cat during confinement and during release.

CLIENT EDUCATION

For chronic, severe cases or for aggression that does not respond to treatment, may require permanent separation, either by rehoming one of the cats or by confining them in separate parts of the home.

Cases with Low Frequency of Intense, Injurious Aggressive Outbursts

• Separate cats when they cannot be supervised (create "safe zones"). • Either keep separate in same areas each day in effort to form separate core territories for each cat, or "time share" space between cats. • Confine newly introduced cat or aggressor to smaller, less familiar area. • For multiple cats, separate by stability of relationship between cats. Any despotic/bully cats should be confined alone. • Consider "artificial allomarking" to form communal scent between cats that are fighting; a towel (facecloth) may be rubbed (cephalocaudally) to obtain scent of one cat and then rubbed onto other cat, and vice versa. • Towels should be left in environment to allow for habituation to each other's scent, especially if cats are kept separated. • Reward cats with food, play, and/or attention for being in same room together without having aggressive events. Cats should stay at a distance that allows for calm participation. • Engage cats in daily sessions of pleasurable activities (e.g., play, training, eating delectable food treats) at distances that do not incite aggression. Gradually move fun sessions closer to each other, making sure to stay at a distance that does not trigger overt/covert aggression. • Teach cats a "come and/or go to place" cue using positive reinforcement at times, in situations, and with sufficient rewards that cats are most able to learn. • Interrupt or redirect cats by cueing to come or go to their place, or by luring one or both cats to their safe zones with food, treats, wand toys, tossed toys, or laser pointers before aggression starts or as initial signs are seen (e.g., staring, tail twitching, pupil dilation). • Aversives and/or punishers can increase aggressive behavior and increase negative associations with other cats, so must be avoided. • Goal of management and safety is to prevent aggressive events. In an emergency, use of laundry basket or blanket placed between or over cats can stop aggression, and direct cat to its safe area until calm, but should not be considered as a standalone treatment. • Bell the aggressor (using quick release or safety collar) so both owners and victim can quickly identify his or her location. • Increase number of resources and locations (e.g., food, water, scratching, perching, bedding, play and feeding toys) throughout the residence, including each cat's core area. Efficacy of multimodal environmental enrichment should not be underestimated. • Increase litter boxes to number of cats plus one divided among multiple locations, so that one cat cannot keep another from accessing boxes; locations with more than one exit/entry are ideal. • Increase number of hiding and resting areas, especially by increasing vertical space (e.g., shelves, window sills). • No new cats should be added to the house.

Cases Where Cats Cannot be in Same Room without Immediately Becoming Agitated

• Separate cats completely when unsupervised. • Meet each cat's needs for play, litter boxes, food, water, perching, resting, and attention. • Large wire dog kennel or vertically oriented wire cat cage (with shelving) may be better tolerated than smaller cat kennels and can be used for controlled exposure. • Cats may be taught to tolerate harnesses and leashes so that they can be used during training and controlled reintroduction. This is especially valuable for the aggressor. • Set up desensitization and counter-conditioning sessions daily; initially utilize physical and visual barriers (e.g., opposite sides of solid door). • Proceed to controlled visual introduction, across glass or screen door, in their kennels, or on leash and harness, insuring they are at a distance that prevents overt/covert aggression. Feed cats or engage in play for classical counter-conditioning. • Over many sessions gradually reduce distance between cats, being careful to stay far enough apart during each session that no overt or covert behavioral signs of aggression and/or fear are seen. Start and end all sessions on successful note. • Teach each cat a "come and/or go to place" cue using operant counter-conditioning and positive reinforcement at times when cats are not stressed. Practice several times daily so each cat learns to respond reliably. • When ready to allow cats more freedom with each other, follow instructions for less severe intercat aggression (above).

SURGICAL CONSIDERATIONS

Neutering reduces roaming, intercat aggression, and urine spraying in approximately 90% of intact males. Neutering/spaying reduces mounting and sexual behavior.

MEDICATIONS

DRUG(S) OF CHOICE

As all medications are extra-label, insure client is informed, and review target desirable outcomes and potential adverse effects.

For Aggressor and/or Victim

Selective Serotonin Reuptake Inhibitors (SSRIs)

• Fluoxetine or paroxetine 0.5–1 mg/kg PO q24h. • Drugs of choice for aggression, anxiety, and/or urine marking; may decrease impulsivity. • Side effects may include gastrointestinal upset, decreased appetite, sedation, urinary retention, constipation, lowered seizure threshold, and increased agitation/irritability.

Tricyclic Antidepressants (TCAs)

• Clomipramine 0.25–0.5 mg/kg PO q24h—serotonin selective tricyclic, for anxiety and aggression. • Side effects include gastrointestinal upset, sedation, urinary retention, constipation, and lowered seizure threshold. Do not use in patients with arrhythmias or cardiomyopathies.

Pheromones

• Feliway® Multicat/Friends (Ceva)—synthetic feline mammary gland pheromone that may be helpful for reducing intercat social conflicts when combined with a multimodal plan. • Feliway Classic (Ceva)—synthetic feline facial pheromone that may be helpful in reducing stress and associated marking behavior.

For Victim

Azapirone

• Buspirone 0.5–1 mg/kg PO q8–24h—reserved for victims to increase social confidence. • Side effects rare; may include decreased sociability and increased agitation/irritability; victim may be more confident and fight back.

Benzodiazepines

• Lorazepam 0.125–0.25 mg/CAT PO up to q12–24h or oxazepam 0.2–0.5 mg/kg PO q12–24h for anxious or fearfully aggressive cats and as an appetite stimulant, helping to facilitate classical counter-conditioning; may be used as needed, with peak effects seen within 1 hour. • Side effects may include increased appetite, ataxia, inhibited learning, and disinhibition of aggression.
• Note: controlled substance; dependence can develop; should be gradually weaned if used consistently for longer than 2 weeks.

CONTRAINDICATIONS

• Benzodiazepines should be used cautiously or avoided in cats with hepatopathies. • SSRIs and TCAs may produce anticholinergic side effects. • SSRIs and TCAs should be used with caution in patients with cardiac abnormalities, seizures, and liver disease.

PRECAUTIONS

• Any behavioral drug may produce paradoxical reactions, including fear, anxiety, hyperexcitability, and/or aggression.
• Medications that alter serotonin levels have the potential to produce serotonin syndrome.

POSSIBLE INTERACTIONS

• Avoid concurrent use of SSRIs and TCAs; avoid using monoamine oxidase inhibitors (MAOIs, such as selegiline) with SSRIs and TCAs; use SSRIs and TCAs cautiously or avoid with buspirone, tramadol, and tryptophan due to possible serotonin syndrome. • Caution with concurrent medications considered substrates of cytochrome P450.

ALTERNATIVE DRUG(S)

• Amitriptyline (TCA) 0.5–1 mg/kg PO q12–24h—for anxious cats, especially if comorbid recurrent feline idiopathic cystitis/feline lower urinary tract disease (FIC/FLUTD); not selective for serotonin reuptake inhibition and likely less effective for aggressor. Side effects include sedation, decreased grooming, and increased weight.
• Dietary supplementation with l-theanine (Anxitane, Virbac), or with alpha-casozepine (Zylkene®, Vetoquinol), Royal Canin Veterinary Diet Calm® (contains alpha-casezopine, l-tryptophan, and nicotinamide), or Hill's Prescription Diet® Multicare Feline Urinary Stress (contains l-tryptophan and milk protein hydrolysate).

FOLLOW-UP

PATIENT MONITORING

• Monitor patients 2 weeks after treatment initiation and monthly for first few months; follow-up visit should be scheduled 4–8 weeks into treatment if drugs dispensed to assess response and adjust dose if necessary.
• Benzodiazepines may rarely cause cases of fatal hepatopathies; patients should be rechecked immediately if any adverse events occur, including anorexia. • Medication should be used for at least 4–6 weeks after resolution of signs, then gradually weaned by reducing dosage no faster than 25% per day on weekly basis. • Some patients require long-term medication; recheck laboratory work every 6 months to 1 year, depending on health and age.

PREVENTION/AVOIDANCE

• Proper socialization through 2–7 weeks of age and ongoing. • Gradual introduction more closely resembles natural process through which new cats enter existing group at the periphery and may be accepted over time.
• Negative initial encounter often associated with future intercat aggression. • Related and familiar cats less likely to have intense intercat aggression. • In stable multicat households, avoid adding additional cats. • Avoid reintroduction aggression by avoiding separating cats when possible.

POSSIBLE COMPLICATIONS

Abrupt withdrawal of behavioral medications may result in aggression and rebound anxiety.

EXPECTED COURSE AND PROGNOSIS

• Prognosis for most cases is fair; complicated by prolonged duration, high intensity, underlying medical conditions, and incomplete owner compliance. In one study 62% were considered cured and 37% not cured (rehomed, euthanized, or permanently separated). • Recent and mild cases may have better long-term outcomes.

MISCELLANEOUS

ASSOCIATED CONDITIONS

• Urine marking/spraying. • House soiling.
• Excessive grooming. • Fearful/anxiety-related behavior. • Human-directed or interspecies aggression.

AGE-RELATED FACTORS

Predatory/play-related aggression more common in young active and playful cats housed indoors with more sedentary or aged individuals.

ZOONOTIC POTENTIAL

Human intervention may lead to bite or scratch injuries.

PREGNANCY/FERTILITY/BREEDING

Most behavioral medications are contraindicated in breeding animals.

SYNONYMS

Feline intraspecies aggression.

SEE ALSO

• Aggression, Overview—Cats.
• Kitten Behavior Problems.

ABBREVIATIONS

• FeLV = feline leukemia virus.
• FIC/FLUTD = feline idiopathic cystitis/feline lower urinary tract disease.
• FIV = feline immunodeficiency virus.
• MAOI = monoamine oxidase inhibitor.
• SSRI = selective serotonin reuptake inhibitor.
• T_4 = thyroxine.
• TCA = tricyclic antidepressant.

INTERNET RESOURCES

• https://indoorpet.osu.edu/cats • https://catvets.com

Suggested Reading

Heath S. Feline aggression. In: Horwitz DF, Mills D, eds. BSAVA Manual of Canine and Feline Behavioural Medicine, 2nd ed. Gloucester: BSAVA, 2009, pp. 223–235.

Landsberg G, Hunthausen W, Ackerman L. Feline aggression. In: Behavior Problems of the Dog and Cat, 3rd ed. Philadelphia, PA: Elsevier Saunders, 2013, pp. 327–343.

Pachel CL. Intercat aggression: restoring harmony in the home. A guide for practitioners. Vet Clin North Am 2014, 44:565–579.

Authors E'Lise Christensen Bell and Kenneth M. Martin

Consulting Editor Gary M. Landsberg

AGGRESSION, OVERVIEW—CATS

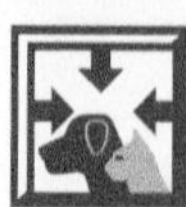

BASICS

DEFINITION

• Aggression is a behavioral strategy used to manage aversive situations. • May be normal and appropriate in certain contexts. • May be abnormal with deleterious effects on cat's physical and emotional well-being. • Aggressive—describes both mood and temperament traits relating to propensity to show aggression when environmental circumstances dictate.

Play Aggression (toward People)

• Typically refers to cat who scratches and bites owners during play. • Not true aggression, but overzealous play without proper impulse control due to lack of training or proper intraspecific social feedback. • Cat's intent is not to harm the person. • Behavior encouraged and rewarded by owners through rough play with kitten; when larger and stronger, becomes perceived as aggression rather than overzealous play.

Predatory Aggression (toward People or Other Animals)

• Cats have innate drive to "hunt" or show predation, which includes stalk, hide, and pounce. • Predatory behavior is not a direct function of hunger. • Typically stimulated by fast movements and can progress to cat hiding and waiting for animal or person to walk by. • Play is way for young cats to perfect predation skills; play aggression and predatory aggression may overlap.

Redirected Aggression (toward People or Other Animals)

• Cats who see, hear, or smell a trigger and direct aggressive behavior toward the closest bystander. • In some cases, one person or animal in the home becomes designated victim, and cat may bypass a nearby individual and attack preferred target. • Cats may remain aroused for 24–72 hours after triggering event. • Common triggers inciting redirected aggression are seeing another cat or wildlife outside or loud noises.

Fear/Defensive Aggression (toward People or Other Animals)

• Cat will show body postures indicative of fear/anxiety and may use aggression as strategy to manage that aversive situation. • Typical behaviors include combination of any of the following: hissing, spitting, piloerection, arched back, turning away, running away, cowering, rolling on back, and pawing (defensive) if cornered. • With learning and repetition, may display more offensive signs.

Territorial Aggression (toward People or Other Animals)

• Some cats, particularly males, show territorial behavior in domestic home settings due to perceived need to defend multiple resources (e.g., people, food, resting areas, feeding areas, elimination sites, etc.). • Territorial behaviors include marking with urine and/or feces, bunting (rubbing of cheeks on surfaces to deposit pheromones), and scratching (also deposits pheromones and leaves visual mark) that may be associated with aggression. • In severe cases, aggressor may seek out the other individual and attack. • Body posture with territorial aggression is assertive and confident.

Pain Aggression (toward People and Animals)

Cats in pain may show aggression (hiss, growl, scratch, bite) when physically handled or immediately prior to or after activity such as jumping on or off a piece of furniture.

Maternal Aggression

Female cat may show aggressive behavior toward individuals approaching her kittens.

Impulse Control Aggression

Cats who show intense aggressive responses to mild stimuli without much or any warning may have impulse control disorder arising from dysfunctional serotonin neural circuits.

Frustration-Induced Aggression (to People and Other Animals)

Some cats with very outgoing, social personalities may exhibit aggression if restricted life indoors does not meet their behavioral needs.

Contact-Induced/Petting Aggression (toward People)

• Cats may show early signs of aversion during petting and handling with ears going back and tail swishing. • If physical contact continues, they may bite. • Owners often miss early warning signs. • When cats groom one another, they typically limit grooming to the head region. • Some cats appear to be particularly sensitive to being stroked along the dorsum.

Intercat Aggression within Home

• After introducing new cat to home, 50% of cat owners report fighting (scratching and biting). • Number of cats, sex, and age are not significant factors in predicting which cats will show aggression toward each other. • Any of the above categories of aggression are all possibilities for fights between or among cats. • Fear/anxiety is most common cause of intraspecific aggression. • Learning—consequences/outcome (reinforcement, punishment) further compound the problem.

PATHOPHYSIOLOGY

Behavior problems are typically multifactorial in cause. Figure 1 illustrates some of the common components that need to be evaluated to accurately diagnose and treat aggression cases.

SYSTEMS AFFECTED

• Behavioral—vary with type of aggression, occur alone or in combination: tail swishing/twitching, ears turned sideways or flattened, stiffening of shoulders/legs, crouching, dilation of pupils, hissing, spitting, growling, piloerection, staring, chasing, stalking, pawing, lunging. • Cardiovascular—signs associated with sympathetic activation and hypothalamic-pituitary-adrenal (HPA) activation. • Endocrine/metabolic—long-term aggression associated with fear/stress/anxiety, symptoms associated with long-term activation of HPA system. • Gastrointestinal (GI)—with chronic HPA stimulation: may see cat more prone to anorexia and GI ulcers; with acute fear aggression: evacuation of bowel and possible diarrhea; inflammatory bowel disease (IBD) possible in chronic stress. • Hemic/lymphatic/immune—decreased immune response with chronic HPA stimulation; stress leukogram. • Both victim and aggressor may suffer injuries; with chronic activation of HPA, muscle wasting may occur. • Nervous—increased reactivity up to 72 hours following aggressive event; may see increase in aggression with decreased provocation as synapses in amygdala become sensitized; in some animals may be associated with decreased serotonin, causing aggressive outbursts; may see ritualized motor patterns, shaking, or trembling. • Ophthalmic—dilated pupils with sympathetic stimulation. • Renal/urologic—may see spraying or small amounts of urine on horizontal surfaces; stress may be contributor to feline interstitial cystitis. • Respiratory—tachypnea in acute cases or when stressed. • Skin/exocrine—damage due to fights or to excessive grooming associated with fear/anxiety/distress.

SIGNALMENT

• Preliminary evidence that behavioral traits in cats vary by breed and sex. • Males more likely to show aggression toward other cats, while females more likely to show aggression toward owners. • Abyssinian, Russian blue, Somali, Siamese, and chinchilla breeds showed more aggression. • Maine Coon, ragdoll, and Scottish folds showed least aggressiveness.

SIGNS

• May appear at social maturity (2–4 years of age) except for play-related and should occur in specific social contexts/interactions. If onset occurs in older cat, medical causes should be ruled out first. • General comments—most owners able to detect overt signs of aggression (biting, hissing, growling), but may miss more subtle signs of aggression that typically occur between cats (staring) and resulting anxious behaviors that can result in aggression (meatloaf position, averting gaze, etc.). Videotapes of intercat interactions allow clinician to assess behavior.

CAUSES

• Underlying medical issues can cause aggression. • Temperament/behavior influenced by genetics, rearing, socialization, environment in which cat lives, and types of interactions cat has with people.

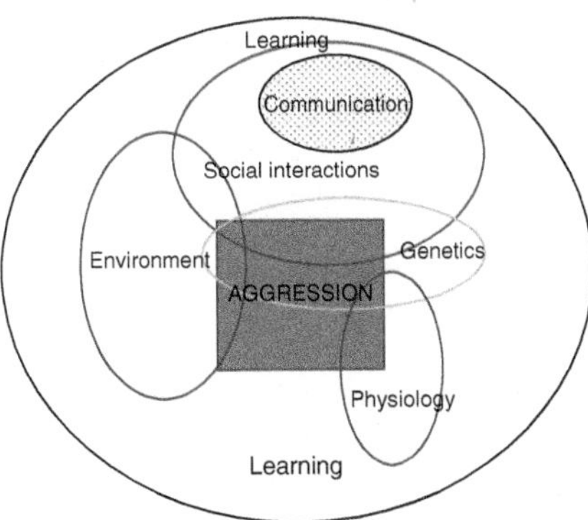

Figure 1.

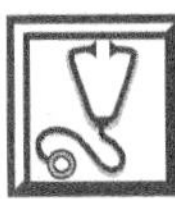

DIAGNOSIS

DIFFERENTIAL DIAGNOSIS

• CNS diseases (e.g., infections, toxins, tumors, partial seizures, focal seizures). • Hyperthyroid. • Hepatic encephalopathy. • Any condition causing pain (e.g., arthritis, pancreatitis, dental disease, anal sacculitis, diabetic neuropathy). • Lead poisoning.

CBC/CHEMISTRY/URINALYSIS

Physical examination, baseline blood, and urine screening followed by additional diagnostics as indicated based on history, examination, and laboratory results.

OTHER LABORATORY TESTS

• Discuss *Bartonella* testing in any cat that bites or scratches people. • Thyroid levels. • Urinalysis ± culture if house soiling. • Feline serology—feline calicivirus (FCV), feline leukemia virus (FeLV), female immunodeficiency virus (FIV).

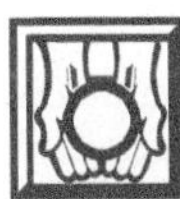

TREATMENT

• Never use physical correction/punishment; may escalate aggression. • Never try to physically handle or manipulate a cat in an aggressive state. • Avoid known triggers. • Identify triggers and desensitize and counter-condition to triggers. • Implement safety measures (nail caps, wearing long pants/long sleeves, keep flattened cardboard boxes around home to place between target and cat, redirect behavior in early arousal phase). • Behavior modifications to redirect cat and reduce arousal (specific plans dependent upon specifics of each case). • Train cat to commands such as "sit," "go to place," etc. • Environmental enrichment and meeting behavioral needs. • Teach owners to identify early signs of arousal so cat can be redirected or so they can avoid cat. • After aggressive outburst, keep aggressor isolated in a room for at least 24 hours (as long as cat remains aroused after attack). • Pheromones. • Medications.

MEDICATIONS

DRUG(S) OF CHOICE

• Selective serotonin reuptake inhibitors (SSRIs)—fluoxetine or paroxetine 0.5 mg/kg PO q24h. • Tricyclic antidepressants (TCAs)—clomipramine 0.25–1.0 mg/kg PO q24h. • Buspirone at 0.5–1.0 mg/kg q8–24h, benzodiazepines such as oxazepam at 0.2–0.5 mg/kg q12–24h, or lorazepam 0.125–0.25 mg/cat might reduce fear and build confidence and support counter-conditioning in fearful cat that avoids or retreats.

CONTRAINDICATIONS

• Cats with renal or hepatic disease. • Caution with TCAs and SSRIs in diabetics. • TCAs in patients with cardiac abnormalities.

POSSIBLE INTERACTIONS

• TCAs and SSRIs should not be used together. • Mirtazapine should be used cautiously in combination with TCA or SSRI. • Practitioner should evaluate all drugs and natural supplements administered to verify safety in combination.

ALTERNATIVE DRUG(S)

• Amitriptyline 0.5–1.0 mg/kg PO q12–24h. • S-adenosyl-L-methionine-tosylate disulfate (SAMe) 100 mg PO q24h. • Alpha-casozepine 75 mg (15 mg/kg or greater) PO q24h. • l-theanine 25 mg PO q24h. • Cat-appeasing pheromone (Feliway® Multicat or Friends). • F3 cheek gland pheromone (Feliway). • Calming and stress diets containing alpha-casozepine and l-tryptophan.

FOLLOW-UP

PATIENT MONITORING

• Call owners once every 1–2 weeks for first 2 months after treatment plan has been recommended; determine implementation of safety recommendations and behavioral plan. • If medication dispensed, dose should be reevaluated every 3–4 weeks. • Frequency of follow-up will be dictated by severity of case and owner compliance. • CBC, chemistry, T_4 prior to medication; recheck liver and kidney values 2–3 weeks after starting medication; recheck bloodwork annually in young healthy patients, semiannually in older patients. • Repeat physical exams in older patients semiannually, as painful conditions may exacerbate aggression.

EXPECTED COURSE AND PROGNOSIS

• Depends on type of aggression and compliance of clients with suggested behavior plan. • Most cases need combination of behavioral modification, environmental modification, training, and, when necessary, medication. • Some types of aggression can resolve or improve within a few weeks, whereas others may take several months or longer. • Some forms of aggression have poor prognosis.

MISCELLANEOUS

AGE-RELATED FACTORS

• Older cats—cognitive decline, CNS disease, arthritis, meningioma, other medical conditions. • Age 2–4 years—social maturity, when cats may start to show certain kinds of aggression.

SEE ALSO

• Aggression, Intercat Aggression. • Aggression Toward Humans—Cats.

ABBREVIATIONS

• FCV = feline calicivirus. • FeLV = feline leukemia virus. • FIV = feline immunodeficiency virus. • GI = gastrointestinal. • HPA = hypothalamic-pituitary-adrenal. • IBD = inflammatory bowel disease. • SAMe = S-adenosyl-L-methionine-tosylate disulfate. • SSRI = selective serotonin reuptake inhibitor. • TCA = tricyclic antidepressant.

Suggested Reading

Bain M. Feline aggression toward family members: a guide for practitioners. Vet Clin North Am Small Anim Pract 2014, 44:581–594.

Crowell-Davis SL, Murray T, Dantas L. Veterinary Psychopharmacology, 2nd ed. Hoboken, NJ: Wiley, 2018.

Levine ED, Perry P, Scarlett J, et al. Intercat aggression in households following the introduction of a new cat. Appl Anim Behav Sci 2004, 90:325–336.

Pachel C. Intercat aggression: restoring harmony in the home: a guide for practitioners. Vet Clin North Am Small Anim Pract 2014, 44:565–579.

Author Leslie Sinn

Consulting Editor Gary M. Landsberg

Acknowledgment The author and editors acknowledge the prior contribution of Emily D. Levine.

Client Education Handout available online

AGGRESSION, OVERVIEW—DOGS

BASICS

DEFINITION

• Action by one dog directed against another organism with the result of limiting, depriving, or harming. Aggression refers to any behavior along an aggression continuum, from a stare to immobility (freeze), growl, snarl, lunge, air snap, single bite, multiple bite, multiple attacks, and chase and attack.
• Numerous functional types have been posited. Here, aggression is classified on the basis of (1) affective aggression, (2) predatory aggression, and (3) play-related aggression. Affective states, such as fear and arousal, and motivational factors, such as hunger and sexual drive, influence the probability of overt aggression, such as biting. Affective aggression may be human-directed or dog-directed. Within these contexts, there may be additional specificity, such as human-directed aggression toward unfamiliar persons, or human-directed aggression toward familiar persons. Often dogs display aggression in a single context.
• Human-directed aggression toward familiar persons in response to controlling gestures was historically called dominance aggression, although newer terminology, such as conflict aggression, may be used to avoid erroneous semantic assumptions inherent in the term "dominance."
• Human- or animal-directed aggression, generally toward unfamiliar individuals and specific to home location, is called territorial aggression. Location is commonly at door of entry, but may also involve defense of special favored locations such as beds.
• Predatory aggression refers to behaviors associated with chasing and hunting prey. It is often considered nonaffective and may be socially facilitated by other dogs. Predatory behaviors may be triggered by movement or high-pitched sounds, and may be redirected to humans or objects.
• Play-related aggression involves aggressive gestures, such as growling and biting, in the context of play and is commonly displayed toward other dogs or humans. It is often initiated by signs of play, such as the play bow.
• In all cases, medical factors that might contribute to aggression (including pain) must be evaluated.

PATHOPHYSIOLOGY

• Affective aggression involves arousal of the sympathetic nervous system. Some pathologic conditions are associated with an increase in aggression because of CNS effects such as pain or irritability.
• Abnormalities in the CNS serotonin neurotransmitter system have been implicated in one type of impulsive human-directed aggression, colloquially called "rage," directed toward familiar persons and triggered by controlling gestures.
• Aggression generally has a learned component, whereby dogs learn to use aggression to manage distance from fearful stimuli or control resources, as this behavior is often effective as a distance-increasing technique.

SYSTEMS AFFECTED

• Behavior.
• Other, if there is an underlying medical etiology.

GENETICS

• In some breeding programs, aggressive tendencies and bite styles have been selected for (or against).
• Behavioral genetics is an active area of research, with several genes identified that may be associated with fear and aggression in dogs.
• One study in the United States linked English springer spaniels that display human-directed dominance aggression to one breeding sire, implicating a heritable component.
• One study of human-directed dominance aggression among English cocker spaniels reported that males were more aggressive than females, and dogs with solid coat color were more aggressive than those with parti coat color.

INCIDENCE/PREVALENCE

• Reported problem by approximately 30% of owners.
• Most common diagnostic category seen by board-certified veterinary behaviorists in North America.
• According to Centers for Disease Control and Prevention, about 4.7 million people bitten by dogs each year in United States, although this number considered an underestimation as majority of dog bites not reported.
• In United States, estimated that one in five of those bitten require medical attention for dog bite–related injuries.
• Among children and adults, males more likely than females to be bitten.
• Based on emergency room data in United States, rate of dog bite–related injuries highest for children aged 5–9 years.
• In majority of cases, people are bitten by dogs that are known to them; this is not the case for dog injury–related fatalities.

GEOGRAPHIC DISTRIBUTION

Worldwide

SIGNALMENT

Species

Dog

Breed Predispositions

Any breed or breed mix.

Mean Age and Range

Any age, although some forms of aggression may arise more commonly at sexual or social maturity, while medical causes increasingly more likely in adult- or senior-onset aggression.

Predominant Sex

• Either sex.
• Males—intact or castrated, most commonly implicated in cases of human-directed "dominance"-type aggression. Intact males overrepresented in dog-bite fatalities, but covariables, such as owner management, are present.
• Females—spayed most commonly implicated in aggression to other female dogs in the home. In some studies, spayed females less likely than males to display human-directed aggression.

SIGNS

General Comments

• Any dog can display aggression. Many factors, including temperament, experience, and situational factors, influence propensity to bite.
• Dogs may display behavioral signals as warnings, including immobility, growls, snarls, or air snaps, which may provide time to avoid overt aggression. These signs should not be punished, as this might decrease the probability of warning signs without affecting the underlying risk, or may further intensify the aggressive (defensive) response. Instead, the animal should be safely removed from the situation and the underlying triggers for the affective state addressed.

Historical Findings

• Variable.
• Basis for risk analysis and details of treatment program. Important questions: Who/what was the target? Who was present to manage the dog? How severe were the resulting injuries? What are the circumstances (including location, time) in which aggression occurred? Are there any reliable triggers for aggressive behavior? Abnormalities in mentation or awareness might indicate a medical cause.

Physical Examination Findings

• Usually unremarkable.
• Use extreme care when handling aggressive dogs.
• A comfortable, well-fitting basket muzzle recommended prior to examination of any dog with history of human-directed aggression. Desensitize and countercondition to muzzle application and use. Basket-style muzzles allow dogs to pant.
• Abnormalities on physical or neurologic examination may suggest organic disease process (e.g., neurologic, pain, blindness). Dogs can display aggression during preictal, ictal, or postictal periods. Dogs with underlying

pain typically display defensive (body-protective) aggression.

CAUSES

- Part of normal range of behavior; strongly influenced by individual temperament, experience, early socialization (before 12 weeks), and other variables.
- Harsh handling and confrontational responses can escalate aggression and should be avoided.
- May be manifestation of organic condition, such as hepatic encephalopathy or pain.
- In all cases, evaluate medical causes of aggression.

RISK FACTORS

- Inadequate socialization during canine critical period (3–12 weeks).
- Traumatic/fearful/negative experience(s).
- Predisposing environmental conditions—lack of training, inadequate restraint, harsh handling.
- Inability of owner to safely confine or manage the dog in order to prevent future incidents. Helpful devices include barrier fence, muzzle, collar or head halter, leash.
- Previous aggression/bite history (number of incidents, number of bites per incident, target, severity of injury); legal citation for biting.
- Unpredictability of aggressive behaviors, lack of warning signals.
- Presence of children, elderly people, or other humans or animals at high risk living in or visiting household.

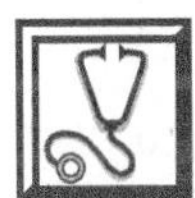

DIAGNOSIS

DIFFERENTIAL DIAGNOSIS

- Thorough medical evaluation should be conducted on all cases of aggression.
- Identify pathologic conditions associated with aggression before making purely behavioral diagnosis.
- Rule out developmental abnormalities (e.g., hepatic shunts), metabolic disorders (e.g., hepatic encephalopathy), endocrinopathies (e.g., hypothyroidism, hyperadrenocorticism), dermatopathy, neurologic conditions (intracranial neoplasm, seizures), toxins, inflammatory diseases, cognitive dysfunction, acute or chronic pain, and iatrogenic causes, such as glucocorticoid administration.

CBC/BIOCHEMISTRY/URINALYSIS

- Usually no significant findings unless underlying medical etiology.
- Indicated to evaluate dog as candidate for behavioral medications.

OTHER LABORATORY TESTS

- Thyroid testing.
- Others as indicated by history and physical exam.

IMAGING

- May be indicated to identify sources of pain or disease.
- MRI or CT—particularly if cerebral disease/neoplasia suspected.

DIAGNOSTIC PROCEDURES

- Collection of thorough behavioral history and evaluation of medical concerns.
- Postmortem fluorescent antibody test indicated for any aggressive dog for which rabies is differential diagnosis.

PATHOLOGIC FINDINGS

None

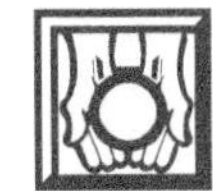

TREATMENT

APPROPRIATE HEALTH CARE

- Manage any underlying medical conditions.
- Management success—combination of multiple modalities: safe environmental control, behavior modification to teach animals appropriate behavior, and pharmacotherapy.
- Consult veterinarian with experience and training in aggression management.
- Euthanasia should be discussed or recommended when risk of injury is high. Note recommendation in medical record.
- Rehoming aggressive dogs may put those involved at liability risk.

NURSING CARE

A boarding facility able to safely manage the dog might be used until a safe management plan can be implemented, or until an outcome decision can be made.

ACTIVITY

Since frustration and arousal may increase incidence of aggression, appropriate and safe exercise regime should be incorporated into treatment program.

DIET

There is minimal evidence that a low-protein diet may reduce territorial aggression in dogs, an effect that might be enhanced with tryptophan supplementation.

CLIENT EDUCATION

- Safe practices should dictate all decisions. These practices include safe confinement, physical barriers, head halters, leash control, muzzle use, and supervision by a competent adult.
- Situations that have led to aggression in the past should be listed and a specific plan developed to avoid these situations and associated locations in the future, and a long-term management plan developed.
- The dog should calmly be removed from aggression-provoking situations.
- Safe, nonconfrontational techniques that manage resources and use positive reinforcement to teach the dog appropriate responses should be employed.
- Confrontational management techniques, such as roll-overs, or even verbal discipline increase the probability of a defensive aggressive response, may lead to human injury, and should be strictly avoided.
- Management ("dominance") techniques including punishment are associated with defensive fear responses by the dog and an increased risk of human-directed aggression. These should be avoided and replaced with positive management techniques.
- The client should be advised to consider personal and legal liability risks of keeping the dog. Human injury, bite-related lawsuits, and homeowner's insurance claims can result from canine aggression. Such risk assessment may help the client objectively evaluate the situation.
- Euthanasia should be considered if safe management cannot be employed, or when the risk of injury is high.

SURGICAL CONSIDERATIONS

Castration of males may reduce the incidence of intermale aggression.

MEDICATIONS

DRUG(S) OF CHOICE

- None approved by FDA for treatment of aggression.
- No drug will eliminate probability of aggression.
- Use drugs only when safe management plan has been implemented.
- Inform client of extra-label nature of medication and risk involved; document in medical record; obtain signed informed consent.
- Drugs that increase serotonin may be helpful to reduce anxiety, arousal, and impulsivity.
- Treatment duration—minimum 4 months, maximum lifetime.
- See Table 1 for drugs used to facilitate management of aggression in combination with safe management plan.

CONTRAINDICATIONS

- Fluoxetine should be used cautiously in cases of seizures.
- Clomipramine contraindicated in cases of cardiac conduction disturbances or seizures; in one open trial, clomipramine was no more effective than control in cases of human-directed aggression.

AGGRESSION, OVERVIEW—DOGS (CONTINUED)

Table 1

Drugs and dosages used to manage canine aggression.

Drug	*Drug Class*	*Oral Dosage in Dogs*	*Frequency*	*Side Effects—Usually Transient*
Fluoxetine	SSRI	1.0–2.0 mg/kg	q24h	Decreased appetite, sleepiness
Paroxetine	SSRI	1.0–2.0 mg/kg	q24h	Constipation
Sertraline	SSRI	2.0–4.0 mg/kg	q24h	Sleepiness
Clomipramine	TCA	1.0–3.0 mg/kg	q12h	Sleepiness, vomiting

PRECAUTIONS

Benzodiazepines (e.g., diazepam) may contribute to behavioral disinhibition. Aggression may increase when dogs lose their fear of the repercussions of biting.

POSSIBLE INTERACTIONS

Do not use selective serotonin reuptake inhibitors (SSRIs) or tricyclic antidepressants (TCAs) with monoamine oxidase inhibitors, including amitraz and selegiline, or with each other because of risk of serotonin syndrome. Caution when combining SSRI or TCA with any drug that might increase serotonin, including trazodone.

ALTERNATIVE DRUG(S)

- Trazodone (4–10 mg/kg PO q12h or PRN) may be used with drugs listed in Table 1 to reduce anxiety and arousal.
- Clonidine (0.01–0.05 mg/kg PO q12h or PRN) may be used with drugs listed in Table 1 to reduce anxiety and arousal.
- Natural products that may aid in reducing anxiety—l-tryptophan (10 mg/kg PO bid); alpha-casozepine (15 mg/kg or higher daily) alone or in diet combined with l-tryptophan; l-theanine alone (2.5–5 mg/kg bid) or in combination with products containing whey protein, *Phellodendron amurense*, and *Magnolia officinalis*; "calming" probiotic supplement; or dog-appeasing pheromone.

FOLLOW-UP

PATIENT MONITORING

Weekly to biweekly contact recommended in initial phases to guide clients with behavior modification plans and medication management.

PREVENTION/AVOIDANCE

- To prevent aggressive incidents, avoid all situations that have led to aggression in the past, using safe confinement, gates, halters, collars, leashes, muzzles.
- Reduce risk of aggression in young dogs (3–12 weeks) with positive socialization program; avoid intimidation techniques and negative, fear-inducing situations.

POSSIBLE COMPLICATIONS

- Injury to humans or animals.
- Liability to client, veterinarian.
- In cases of dog-directed aggression, although not the intended target, humans who interfere are often seriously injured, either by accident or by redirected aggression; owners should not reach for fighting dogs—pull apart with leashes.
- Aggressive dogs are at risk for relinquishment or euthanasia.

EXPECTED COURSE AND PROGNOSIS

- Aggressive dogs weighing over 18.5 kg are at increased risk for behavioral euthanasia.
- Aggressive dogs may be successfully managed, but should not be considered "cured."
- Prognosis is case dependent due to risk factors and management features of each situation.

MISCELLANEOUS

AGE-RELATED FACTORS

Onset of aggression in mature dogs suggests medical cause; carefully evaluate sensory acuity, sources of pain, endocrinopathy, cognitive function.

ZOONOTIC POTENTIAL

- Dog bites are significant public health risk.
- Rabies is potential cause of aggression.

PREGNANCY/FERTILITY/BREEDING

TCAs and trazodone are contraindicated in breeding males and pregnant females.

SYNONYMS

Biting

SEE ALSO

- Aggression—Between Dogs in the Household.
- Aggression, Food and Resource Guarding—Dogs.
- Aggression to Unfamiliar People and Unfamiliar Dogs—Dogs.
- Aggression Toward Children—Dogs.
- Aggression Toward Familiar People—Dogs.

ABBREVIATIONS

- SSRI = selective serotonin reuptake inhibitor.
- TCA = tricyclic antidepressant.

INTERNET RESOURCES

- https://www.avma.org/resources-tools/pet-owners/dog-bite-prevention
- https://www.cdph.ca.gov/Programs/CID/DCDC/CDPH%20Document%20Library/DontLettheDogsBiteActivityBook.pdf

Suggested Reading

Casey RA, Loftus B, Bolster C, et al. Human directed aggression in domestic dogs (*Canis familiaris*): occurrence in different contexts and risk factors. Appl Anim Behav Sci 2014, 152:52–63.

deKeuster T, Jung H. Aggression toward familiar people and animals. In: Horwitz DF, Mills D, eds. BSAVA Manual of Canine and Feline Behavioural Medicine, 2nd ed. Gloucester: BSAVA, 2009, pp. 182–210.

Landsberg G. Canine aggression. In: Landsberg G, Hunthausen W, Ackerman L, eds. Behavior Problems of the Dog and Cat, 3rd ed. New York: Saunders/Elsevier, 2013, pp. 197–326.

Pike A. Managing canine aggression in the home. Vet Clin North Am Small Anim Pract 2018, 48:387–402.

Authors Margaret E. Gruen and Barbara L. Sherman

Consulting Editor Gary M. Landsberg

Client Education Handout available online

ALKALINE HYPERPHOSPHATASEMIA IN DOGS

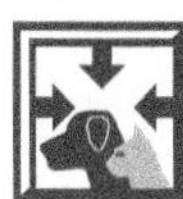

BASICS

DEFINITION

Increase in serum alkaline phosphatase (ALP) activity above reference interval.

PATHOPHYSIOLOGY

• ALPs are heterogeneous group of isoenzymes that catalyze hydrolysis of organic phosphate esters in extracellular space. • Membrane-bound enzymes present in liver, bone, placenta, intestine, and kidney. • Total serum ALP attributed to liver (L-ALP), bone (B-ALP), and glucocorticoid-induced (G-ALP) isoenzymes; proportion of each isoenzyme changes with age in normal dogs. • Serum ALP activity increases with cholestatic, necroinflammatory, and neoplastic injury; many hepatic and nonhepatic causes; affected dogs often asymptomatic. • Anticonvulsants (phenobarbital, primidone, phenytoin) and steroids can induce L-ALP synthesis; steroids, inflammation, and chronic disease can induce G-ALP synthesis. • ALP has high sensitivity but poor specificity for hepatobiliary disease; reflects common induction of enzyme synthesis due to nonhepatic causes, i.e., "reactive hepatopathy." • Increased ALP activity with concurrent increase in GGT activity increases specificity for hepatobiliary disease.

SYSTEMS AFFECTED

• Multiple organ systems can influence ALP synthesis. • Increased ALP activity does not cause direct damage to other organ systems.

GENETICS

• Benign familial alkaline hyperphosphatasemia in Siberian huskies—presumed autosomal. • Vacuolar hepatopathy of Scottish terriers—breed relationship.

INCIDENCE/PREVALENCE

Increased ALP activity is common biochemical abnormality in dogs.

SIGNALMENT

• Any age, breed, or sex. • Young dogs, <1 year of age—increased B-ALP activity. • Siberian huskies and Scottish terriers. • Older dogs—conditions causing increased L-ALP, G-ALP, and/or B-ALP activity.

SIGNS

General Comments

• Many dogs with increased ALP activity are asymptomatic. • Dogs with hepatic or nonhepatic disorders causing increased ALP may be asymptomatic or have clinical signs related to underlying disorder. • Dogs with drug-induced elevations of ALP may have clinical signs related to drug side effects.

Historical Findings

• Dependent on cause. • Medication history important, including exposure to topical/ocular medications used by humans.

Physical Examination Findings

• Highly variable depending on cause; often normal. • Hepatomegaly or microhepatica. • Jaundice. • Abdominal pain. • Musculoskeletal—pendulous abdomen, muscle atrophy, lameness, difficulty walking, palpable bony swelling. • Dermatologic—alopecia, cutaneous hyperpigmentation, comedones, thin skin, pyoderma, calcinosis cutis.

CAUSES

• Age and breed (see Signalment). • Drug induced. • Bone-related disorders—neoplasia, osteomyelitis, hyperparathyroidism (primary or secondary), healing fractures. • Chronic stress, acute-phase response (endogenous cortisol). • Endocrinopathies (hyperadrenocorticism, diabetes mellitus, hypothyroidism). • Primary hepatobiliary disorders. • Extrahepatic disorders—extrahepatic biliary obstruction (EHBO), pancreatic/intestinal/other inflammation, neoplasia. • Infection—Leptospirosis, sepsis, viral. • Systemic inflammation/infection causing ischemic injury/cholestasis. • Hepatic or nonhepatic neoplasia (e.g., benign or malignant mammary tumors).

RISK FACTORS

• Age (young). • Breed—Siberian husky, Scottish terrier. • Breed association to conditions causing alkaline hyperphosphatasemia (e.g., Shetland sheepdog predisposition to gallbladder mucocele).

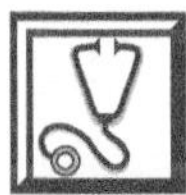

DIAGNOSIS

LABORATORY FINDINGS

Drugs That May Alter Laboratory Results

Corticosteroids, certain anticonvulsants.

Disorders That May Alter Laboratory Results

• Severe hemolysis (>500 hemolysis index) can falsely elevate ALP. • Lipemia and icterus have no significant effect on ALP.

CBC/BIOCHEMISTRY/URINALYSIS

• Thrombocytosis possible with hyperadrenocorticism and pancreatic, gastrointestinal disease. • Thrombocytopenia possible with leptospirosis, hepatic failure, neoplasia. • Leukocytosis or leukopenia with left shift, monocytosis with sepsis, systemic inflammation. • Stress leukogram with hyperadrenocorticism. • Concurrent elevation of other liver enzyme activities including alanine aminotransferase (ALT), aspartate aminotransferase (AST), and/or gamma glutamyltransferase (GGT), depending on underlying cause. • ± markers of hepatic synthetic dysfunction (hypoalbuminemia, hypoglycemia, hypocholesterolemia, decreased blood urea nitrogen [BUN]); many primary hepatic disorders. • Hyperbilirubinemia in EHBO, end-stage chronic hepatopathies, acute hepatic toxicities, infections. • Hypercholesterolemia with many causes of cholestasis, endocrinopathies. • Urinalysis—proteinuria with hyperadrenocorticism, other liver disorders; dilute urine, bacteriuria, pyuria with endocrinopathies; glucosuria with diabetes mellitus, copper-associated hepatopathy; ammonium biurate crystalluria with portosystemic vascular anomaly (PSVA; young dogs). • Conditions with often sole increase in serum ALP include idiopathic vacuolar hepatopathy, hepatic nodular hyperplasia, drug-induction breed-related disorders, some hepatic neoplasias, sudden acquired retinal degeneration (SARDS). • Hyperphosphatemia, hypercalcemia (young growing dogs, usually mild). • Hyperglycemia—mild with hyperadrenocorticism. • Azotemia—prerenal or renal with pancreatitis, pyelonephritis, Leptospirosis.

OTHER LABORATORY TESTS

• Serum bile acids; redundant test if hepatic hyperbilirubinemia. • Testing for endocrine disorders—hypothyroidism or hyperadrenocorticism based on clinical signs, physical exam findings, and associated laboratory abnormalities. • Infectious disease testing—leptospirosis PCR, microagglutination test (MAT), immunoglobulin (Ig) M; urine, bile cultures; tick-borne disease screening. • Blood pressure measurement. • Urine protein qualitative; quantitative with protein; creatinine if inactive sediment and culture negative.

IMAGING

• Radiographs—for liver most useful for hepatomegaly, microhepatica; nonhepatic findings may also be identified (pancreatitis, ascites, cystoliths, pyometra, pleural effusion). • Sonographic evaluation for hepatic parenchymal abnormalities (hyper- or hypoechoic nodules, heterogeneity, hyper- or hypoechoic hepatic echogenicity; changes in echodensity, echotexture; microhepatica, hepatomegaly, hepatic masses), biliary tract (gallbladder mucocele, gallbladder wall abnormalities, cholelithiasis, choledochitis, biliary tract neoplasia), pancreas, adrenal enlargement, neoplasia. • Abdominal CT ± angiography may be useful if suspicion of pancreatitis, gallbladder disease, or hepatic vascular disorders.

DIAGNOSTIC PROCEDURES

• Hepatic fine-needle aspirate (FNA) for cytology; caution as cytologic and histologic agreement may be as low as 30%; cytology is not diagnostic for many hepatobiliary conditions. • FNA of liver tends to agree with histology in cases of vacuolar hepatopathy, hepatic lipidosis, and some neoplasias (e.g., lymphoma). • If primary hepatobiliary

ALKALINE HYPERPHOSPHATASEMIA IN DOGS (CONTINUED)

disease suspected after elimination of other causes, hepatic biopsy may be warranted; biopsy at least three liver lobes; laparoscopic or wedge samples preferred; Tru-Cut® needle biopsy may be too small, use 14–16G needle.

PATHOLOGIC FINDINGS

Variable depending on cause; see specific chapters for pathologic findings.

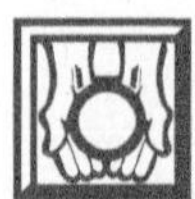

TREATMENT

APPROPRIATE HEALTH CARE

- Dictated by underlying disorder.
- Asymptomatic dogs often do not require any specific treatment.

NURSING CARE

Variable as above.

ACTIVITY

Alteration of activity typically unnecessary.

DIET

- Dietary alteration unnecessary in most cases. • Dietary fat restriction in some cases (pancreatitis, hypertriglyceridemia, obesity, chronic EHBO). • Commercial liver diets *rarely* indicated (see Portosystemic Vascular Anomaly, Congenital; Hepatic Encephalopathy).

CLIENT EDUCATION

- Dictated by underlying disorder. • Clients with asymptomatic dogs should be counseled on potential for subsequent development of endocrine disease, neoplasia (Scottish terriers), other causes. • Liver biopsy necessary for definitive diagnosis if other underlying causes are ruled out and/or if ALP value continues to elevate; rarely pursued initially in asymptomatic dogs without other underlying disorder.

SURGICAL CONSIDERATIONS

- Refractory hypotension is common peri- and postoperative complication in dogs with obstructive cholestasis (see EHBO). • Dogs with end-stage hepatic disease (cirrhosis) may have alterations of coagulation and/or higher anesthetic risk.

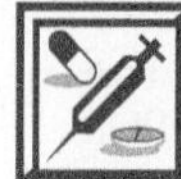

MEDICATIONS

DRUG(S) OF CHOICE

- Specific for underlying cause. • Certain drugs/supplements have general hepatobiliary protective effects; see Hepatosupportive Therapies.

CONTRAINDICATIONS

Depending on cause, drugs requiring hepatic metabolism or capable of causing hepatotoxicity should be limited or avoided when possible.

PRECAUTIONS

Drugs known to induce elevation of ALP may confuse monitoring of underlying condition.

FOLLOW-UP

PATIENT MONITORING

- Dependent on the underlying cause.
- Suspected benign causes of ALP elevation can be monitored for elevations in other serum liver enzyme activities, further elevation in ALP, and/or synthetic hepatic function tests.

EXPECTED COURSE AND PROGNOSIS

- Dependent on underlying cause.
- Increased ALP activity for which underlying cause cannot be found after complete diagnostic evaluation may be benign.

MISCELLANEOUS

ASSOCIATED CONDITIONS

Elevation of other serum liver enzymes, hyperbilirubinemia, alterations in hepatic synthetic function tests.

AGE-RELATED FACTORS

Young dogs (see Signalment).

ZOONOTIC POTENTIAL

Leptospirosis has high zoonotic potential; see Leptospirosis.

PREGNANCY/FERTILITY/BREEDING

Placental ALP can increase in late-term pregnant cats; not reported in dogs.

SYNONYMS

- Elevated ALP. • Serum alkaline phosphatase (SAP).

SEE ALSO

- Bile Duct Obstruction (Extrahepatic).
- Cholangitis/Cholangiohepatitis Syndrome.
- Cholecystitis and Choledochitis.
- Cholelithiasis.
- Copper Associated Hepatology.
- Glycogen-Type Vacuolar Hepatopathy
- Hepatic Failure, Acute.
- Hepatic Nodular Hyperplasia and Dysplastic Hyperplasia.
- Hepatitis, Chronic.
- Hyperadrenocorticism (Cushing's Syndrome)—Dogs.
- Leptospirosis.
- Pancreatitis—Dogs.

ABBREVIATIONS

- ALP = alkaline phosphatase.
- ALT = alanine aminotransferase.
- AST = aspartate aminotransferase.
- B-ALP = bone isoform.
- BUN = blood urea nitrogen.
- G-ALP = glucocorticoid isoform.
- EHBO = extrahepatic biliary obstruction.
- FNA = fine-needle aspirate.
- GGT = gamma glutamyltransferase.
- Ig = immunoglobulin.
- L-ALP = liver isoform.
- MAT = microagglutination test.
- PSVA = portosystemic vascular anomaly.
- SAP = serum alkaline phosphatase.
- SARDS = sudden acquired retinal degeneration.

Suggested Reading

Cortright CC, Center SA, Randolph JF, et al. Clinical features of progressive vacuolar hepatopathy in Scottish Terriers with and without hepatocellular carcinoma: 114 cases (1980–2013). J Vet Intern Med 2014, 245:797–788.

Lidbury JA, Steiner JM. Diagnostic evaluation of the liver. In: Washabau RJ, Day MJ, eds., Canine and Feline Gastroenterology. St. Louis, MO: Elsevier, 2013, pp. 863–875.

Author Sara A. Wennogle

Consulting Editor Kate Holan

BASICS

DEFINITION

A process in the body that leads to an increase in pH above the reference interval. An increase in blood pH is specifically termed alkalemia. Associated with an increase in plasma bicarbonate concentration (HCO_3^-; dogs, >24 mEq/L; cats, >22 mEq/L) and base excess (BE; >4 mmol/L) with a compensatory increase in carbon dioxide tension (PCO_2).

PATHOPHYSIOLOGY

• Metabolic alkalosis may develop from either a *gain of bicarbonate* or a *loss of acid*: ○ *Bicarbonate gain* subsequent to: contraction alkalosis due to free water deficit; iatrogenic administration of alkalinizing therapy (e.g., $NaHCO_3$); metabolism of organic ions (lactate, citrate, acetate, and ketones); hypokalemia; and renal ammoniagenesis. ○ *Acid loss* subsequent to: gastric or renal acid loss (loop or thiazide diuretic); mineralocorticoid excess; presence of nonreabsorbable anions; decreased weak acids (hypoalbuminemia, hypophosphatemia). ○ Renal HCO_3^- excretion very efficient in eliminating an excess HCO_3^- load, but hindered by decreased effective circulating volume; hypokalemia, hypochloremia, and hyperaldosteronism; metabolic alkalosis persists only if renal excretion of HCO_3^- is impaired, which primarily occurs from continued high rate of alkali administration, or some stimulus for kidneys to retain Na^+ in presence of a relative Cl^- deficit. • *Hypochloremic (corrected)* metabolic alkalosis results from loss of fluid rich in Cl^- and hydrogen ion (H^+), primarily from alimentary tract or kidneys; loss of Cl^- and H^+ associated with increase in plasma HCO_3^- concentration; with Cl^- loss and volume depletion, kidneys reabsorb Na^+ with HCO_3^- instead of Cl^-, perpetuating metabolic alkalosis. Hypochloremic alkalosis divided into *chloride-responsive* and *chloride-resistant*: ○ *Chloride-responsive* results primarily from loss of Cl^- rich fluid and characterized by decreased extracellular fluid volume, hypochloremia, and low urinary Cl^- concentration; this type of alkalosis responds to administration of chloride salt. ○ *Chloride-resistant* characterized by excessive mineralocorticoid leading to increased effective circulating volume and is not responsive to chloride salt. • *Hypokalemia* may contribute to metabolic alkalosis by shifting H^+ intracellularly; stimulating apical H^+/K^+ ATPase in collecting duct; stimulating renal ammoniagenesis; impairing Cl^- reabsorption in distal nephron; and reducing glomerular filtration rate (GFR), which decreases filtered load of HCO_3^- and, in presence of volume depletion, impairs renal excretion of excess HCO_3^-. • *Hypoalbuminemic* alkalosis is due to decrease in plasma albumin concentration; plasma albumin is a weak acid. • *Compensatory* metabolic alkalosis occurs in response to respiratory acidosis; this is associated with low pH and increased PCO_2.

SYSTEMS AFFECTED

• Nervous—muscle twitching and seizures occur rarely in dogs. Metabolic alkalosis and associated hypokalemia may precipitate hepatic encephalopathy in patients with liver failure.
• Urinary—kidneys rapidly and effectively excrete excessive alkali. In patients with Cl^- deficiency and volume depletion, kidneys cannot excrete excess alkali. Therefore, metabolic alkalosis is maintained. In these patients, Cl^- administration is required for renal compensation to occur. Volume expansion will hasten compensation. Patients with mineralocorticoid excess have excessive Cl^- loss. Therefore, Cl^- administration does not lead to hyperchloremia and correction of metabolic alkalosis (so-called chloride-resistant metabolic alkalosis). • Respiratory—low [H^+] (increased pH) decreases alveolar ventilation. Hypoventilation increases PCO_2 and helps offset the effects of high plasma HCO_3^- on pH. In dogs, for each 1 mEq/L increase in plasma HCO_3^- there is an expected increase of approximately 0.7 mmHg in PCO_2. Limited data available for cats, but degree of respiratory compensation appears to be similar.

SIGNALMENT

Any breed, age, or sex of dog and cat.

SIGNS

Historical Findings

• Administration of loop diuretics (e.g., furosemide) or thiazides. • Vomiting.

Physical Examination Findings

• Signs related to underlying disease or accompanying potassium depletion (e.g., weakness, cardiac arrhythmias, ileus).
• Muscle twitching caused by low ionized calcium concentration. • Dehydration in volume-depleted patients. • Muscle twitching and seizures in patients with neurologic involvement (rare).

CAUSES

• *Chloride-responsive*—gastrointestinal losses (e.g., gastric vomiting, nasogastric tube suctioning); renal losses (diuretic therapy); and rapid correction of chronic hypercapnia (respiratory acidosis). • *Chloride-resistant*—hyperadrenocorticism and primary hyperaldosteronism. • *Oral administration of alkalinizing agents*—sodium bicarbonate or other organic anions with Na^+ (e.g., lactate, acetate, gluconate); administration of cation-exchange resin with nonabsorbable alkali (e.g., phosphorus binders).
• *Hypoalbuminemia*—liver disease, protein-losing nephropathy, protein-losing enteropathy.
• *Free water deficit*—diabetes insipidus; water deprivation; postobstructive diuresis; polyuric renal failure. • *Hypokalemia.*

RISK FACTORS

• Administration of loop or thiazide diuretics.
• Vomiting. • Stomach drainage. • Diseases associated with hypoalbuminemia (e.g., protein-losing nephropathy, liver failure).

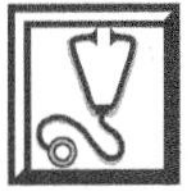

DIAGNOSIS

DIFFERENTIAL DIAGNOSIS

High plasma HCO_3^- and hypochloremia may also occur in animals compensating for chronic respiratory acidosis, in which PCO_2 is high and pH is low despite high HCO_3^- and low Cl^- concentration; blood gas determination is required to differentiate.

LABORATORY FINDINGS

Drugs That May Alter Laboratory Results

None

Disorders That May Alter Laboratory Results

• Too much heparin (>10% of sample) decreases pH, PCO_2, and HCO_3^-. • Blood samples stored at room temperature for more than 15 minutes have low pH because of increased PCO_2. • Exposure to room air decreases PCO_2. • Venous samples may have pH 0.5–1 unit lower and PCO_2 5–10 mmHg higher than arterial sample.

Valid if Run in Human Laboratory?

Yes

CBC/BIOCHEMISTRY/URINALYSIS

• High total CO_2 (total CO_2 in samples handled aerobically closely approximates HCO_3^-). • Low blood ionized calcium concentration. • Serum electrolyte abnormalities vary with underlying cause.
• Hypochloremia—consider hypochloremic metabolic alkalosis, the most common reason for metabolic alkalosis in dogs and cats, which usually results from diuretic administration or vomiting of stomach contents. • High Na^+ but normal Cl^- concentration—consider chloride-resistant metabolic alkalosis (e.g., hyperadrenocorticism or primary hyperaldosteronism) or administration of alkali. • Hypoalbuminemia—consider hypoalbuminemic metabolic alkalosis (e.g., liver failure, protein-losing enteropathy, and protein-losing nephropathy). In vitro, a 1 g/dL decrease in albumin concentration is associated with an increase in pH of 0.093 in cats and 0.047 in dogs. • Hypokalemia—likely results from intracellular potassium shifting due to metabolic alkalosis or underlying problem (e.g., vomiting of stomach contents or loop diuretic administration). • Urinary Cl^- concentrations—chloride-responsive metabolic alkalosis characterized by urine Cl^- concentrations <10 mEq/L, whereas

A

ALKALOSIS, METABOLIC (CONTINUED)

chloride-resistant metabolic alkalosis associated with urine Cl^- concentrations >20 mEq/L.

OTHER LABORATORY TESTS

Blood gas analysis reveals high HCO_3^-, PCO_2, pH, and BE. Unlike HCO3-, BE is independent of changes in metabolic acid-base status, and is thus more reliable measure of metabolic acid-base changes.

IMAGING

None

DIAGNOSTIC PROCEDURES

• Blood pressure—combination of hypertension, hypernatremia, and hypokalemia with metabolic alkalosis may indicate presence of hyperaldosteronism. • Diagnostic testing for hyperadrenocorticism or primary hyperaldosteronism (e.g., plasma renin activity and aldosterone concentration).

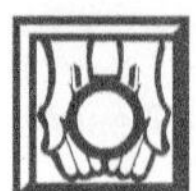

TREATMENT

• Acid-base disturbances are secondary phenomena; diagnosis and treatment of underlying disease process are essential to successful resolution of acid-base disorders.
• Severe alkalemia is uncommon, but may be life-threatening. Patients with chronic respiratory disease and respiratory alkalosis are at risk of developing severe alkalemia if they start vomiting or receive diuretics.
• Discontinue drugs that may cause metabolic alkalosis. • *Chloride-responsive*—fluid of choice for patients with volume depletion is 0.9% saline or balanced isotonic replacement fluid supplemented with KCl; patients with hypokalemia may require large amounts of KCl (see Hypokalemia).
• *Chloride-resistant* metabolic alkalosis can only be corrected by resolution of underlying disease; metabolic alkalosis usually mild in these patients. • If metabolic alkalosis associated with hypokalemia and total body potassium deficits, correcting deficit with KCl is particularly effective way to reverse alkalosis.

NURSING CARE

Supportive care to maintain normal hydration, plasma volume, and adequate nutrition.

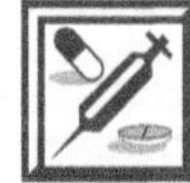

MEDICATIONS

DRUG(S) OF CHOICE

Hypochloremic Alkalosis

• If chloride-responsive alkalosis occurs during edematous state (e.g., congestive heart failure), oral administration of compounds containing Cl^- without Na^+ is recommended to correct alkalosis; if diuresis needed due to volume overload, carbonic anhydrase inhibitor (e.g., acetazolamide) or potassium-sparing diuretic (e.g., spironolactone, amiloride) can be used to correct alkalosis.
• H2-blocking agents such as famotidine decrease gastric acid secretion and may be considered as adjunctive therapy if gastric losses are ongoing. • Antiemetics may help prevent further gastric acid loss.

Hypoalbuminemic Alkalosis

• Treatment for hypoalbuminemic alkalosis should be directed at underlying cause and decreased colloid oncotic pressure. • Enteral nutrition will facilitate endogenous albumin production. • Consider species-specific plasma or albumin (e.g., canine albumin) therapy.

CONTRAINDICATIONS

• Avoid chloride-free fluids—they may correct volume depletion, but will not correct hypochloremic alkalosis. • Avoid using salts of potassium without Cl^- (e.g., potassium phosphate)—potassium will be excreted in urine and will correct neither alkalosis nor potassium deficit.

PRECAUTIONS

Do not use distal-acting, potassium-sparing diuretics (e.g., spironolactone) in volume-depleted patients.

POSSIBLE INTERACTIONS

None

ALTERNATIVE DRUG(S)

None

FOLLOW-UP

PATIENT MONITORING

Acid-base status—frequency dictated by underlying disease and patient response to treatment.

POSSIBLE COMPLICATIONS

• Hypokalemia. • Neurologic signs.

MISCELLANEOUS

ASSOCIATED CONDITIONS

• Hypokalemia. • Hypochloremia.

AGE-RELATED FACTORS

None

PREGNANCY/FERTILITY/BREEDING

N/A

SYNONYMS

• Nonrespiratory alkalosis. • Chloride-responsive metabolic alkalosis—metabolic alkalosis that responds to Cl^- administration.
• Chloride-resistant alkalosis—metabolic alkalosis secondary to increased mineralocorticoid activity that does not respond to Cl^- administration. • Hypochloremic alkalosis—metabolic alkalosis caused by low Cl^- concentration. • Hypoalbuminemic alkalosis—metabolic alkalosis caused by low albumin concentration. • Concentration alkalosis—metabolic alkalosis resulting from decreased free water in plasma. • Contraction alkalosis—metabolic alkalosis formerly attributed to volume contraction, but now known to be caused by Cl^- depletion; volume depletion is common but not essential feature.

SEE ALSO

• Hypochloremia.
• Hypokalemia.

ABBREVIATIONS

• BE = base excess.
• GFR = glomerular filtration rate.
• H^+ = hydrogen ion.
• HCO_3^- = bicarbonate.
• PCO_2 = carbon dioxide tension.

Suggested Reading

de Morais HA. Chloride ion in small animal practice: the forgotten ion. J Vet Emerg Crit Care 1992, 2:11–24.

de Morais HA, Constable PD. Strong ion approach to acid-base disorders. In: DiBartola SP, ed., Fluid, Electrolyte and Acid-Base Disorders, 4th ed. St. Louis, MO: Saunders, 2012, pp, pp. 316–330.

de Morais HA, Leisewitz AL. Mixed acid-base disorders. In: DiBartola SP, ed., Fluid, Electrolyte and Acid-Base Disorders, 4th ed. St. Louis, MO: Saunders, 2012, pp. 302–315.

DiBartola SP. Metabolic acid-base disorders. In: DiBartola SP, ed., Fluid, Electrolyte and Acid-Base Disorders, 4th ed. St. Louis, MO: Saunders, 2012, pp. 271–280.

Hopper K. Traditional acid-base analysis. In: Silverstein DC, Hopper K, eds. Small Animal Critical Care Medicine, 2nd ed. St. Louis, MO: Elsevier, 2015, pp. 289–299.

Robinson EP, Hardy RM. Clinical signs, diagnosis, and treatment of alkalemia in dogs: 20 cases (1982–1984). J Am Vet Med Assoc 1988, 192:943–949.

Authors Helio S. Autran de Morais and Stephen P. DiBartola

Consulting Editor J.D. Foster

Acknowledgment The authors and editors acknowledge the prior contribution of Lee E. Palmer.

BASICS

DEFINITION

Common problem, seen as abnormal lack of hair coat.

PATHOPHYSIOLOGY

Specific and unique for each cause.

SYSTEMS AFFECTED

- Endocrine/metabolic.
- Hemic/lymphatic/immune.
- Skin/exocrine.

SIGNALMENT

- Age, breed, or sex predilections specific to each condition.
- Neoplastic- and paraneoplastic-associated alopecias generally recognized in older cats.

SIGNS

Depends on specific diagnosis. Knowing whether cat is pruritic is a very important part of workup for alopecia.

CAUSES

- Infectious—dermatophytosis, parasitic (mites, fleas), superficial and deep bacterial infections, viral: herpesvirus, papillomaviral plaques, feline immunodeficiency virus (FIV)– and feline leukemia virus (FeLV)–associated giant cell dermatosis.
- Hypersensitivity—atopy/allergy, oral medication reaction, topical medication reaction.
- Disorders of hair follicle cycling—telogen effluvium, Cushing's (iatrogenic and hyperadrenocorticism), hypothyroidism (iatrogenic).
- Congenital—hair follicle dystrophy, alopecia universalis (normal in sphynx cats), feline hypotrichosis (Siamese and Rex cats), pinnal hypotrichosis.
- Environmental—solar damage, burns, frostbite, scarring.
- Ischemic—post matting alopecia, post traumatic.
- Autoimmune—alopecia areata, pemphigus foliaceus.
- Neoplastic—epitheliotropic lymphoma, mastocytosis, squamous cell carcinoma in situ.
- Manifestation of internal disease—sebaceous adenitis (thymoma-associated exfoliative dermatitis), paraneoplastic alopecia, mural lymphocytic folliculitis, hyperthyroidism, hyperadrenocorticism, diabetes.
- Psychogenic—compulsive disorder.

RISK FACTORS

FeLV/FIV—reported risk for demodicosis (not all cases associated with viral infection).

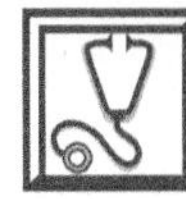

DIAGNOSIS

DIFFERENTIAL DIAGNOSIS

Infectious

- Dermatophytosis.
- Parasites
  - Mites—*Demodex gatoi*, *cheyletiella*, *notoedres* are often pruritic and scaly; *Demodex cati* cause hair loss with minimal inflammatory change in many cases.
  - Fleas can cause alopecia if patient is hypersensitive and pruritic; severe on caudal dorsum, abdomen, and around ears.
  - Tick attachment sites can cause alopecic granuloma.
- Bacterial:
  - Alopecia secondary to deep bacterial infection.
  - Superficial bacterial infections secondary to underlying cause.
- Viral:
  - Herpesvirus can cause neuralgia, pruritus, alopecia, and ulcerated eosinophilic skin lesions, most commonly on the face.
  - FIV- and FeLV-associated giant cell dermatosis.
  - Papillomaviral plaques in older cats may transform to squamous cell carcinoma.

Hypersensitivities

- Food, flea bites, or environmental allergens (atopy)—ears, face, and abdomen are most affected.
- Oral medication reactions—severe facial pruritus caused by methimazole: symptoms resolve when medication discontinued.
- Topical parasite preventives—rare cause of alopecia at site of application; usually temporary.

Disorders of Hair Follicle Cycling

- Telogen effluvium:
  - Caused by severe stressful situation or hormonal change such as anesthesia/surgery, parturition, severe illness, drugs.
  - Sudden onset of large symmetric areas of hair thinning or alopecia.
  - Hair regrows over weeks.
- Cushing's syndrome:
  - Long-term (months) corticosteroid administration, oral or injectable.
  - Megestrol acetate administration.
  - Hyperadrenocorticism from adrenal tumor or pituitary tumor.
  - Causes symmetric alopecic and atrophic/thin skin, sometimes skin fragility/tearing, ear tips droop.
- Hypothyroidism—iatrogenic is most common cause, due to treatment of hyperthyroidism.

Congenital

- Hair follicle dystrophy/sebaceous gland dystrophy can cause thin hair diffusely or waxy accumulations on the hairs.
- Alopecia universalis (normal in sphynx cats):
  - Hereditary, complete absence of primary hairs; decreased secondary hairs.
  - Sebaceous and apocrine ducts open onto skin surface; oily feel to skin.
  - Wrinkled foreheads; gold eyes; no whiskers; downy fur on paws, tip of tail, and scrotum.
  - Comedones with or without secondary folliculitis.
- Feline hypotrichosis:
  - Siamese and Devon Rex cats (autosomal recessive alopecia).
  - Poorly developed primary telogen hair follicles.
  - Born with normal coat, which becomes thin and sparse as young adult.

Environmental

- Solar damage—skin can be damaged with prolonged sun exposure; most common in outdoor light-colored cats. Areas with thin hair most affected: ears, eyes, and nose; early signs alopecia, scaling, and erythema; can transform to squamous cell carcinoma.
- Burns/frostbite—burns are location dependent' sometimes have a drip-like pattern if caused by hot liquid; affect pressure points if due to heating pad. Third-degree burns will have permanent scars. Frostbite commonly affects ear tips and causes alopecia and necrosis.
- Scarring is loss of hair follicles and usually pigment from area of skin.

Ischemic

- Post matting/traction—caused by loss of blood supply to hair follicle due to tight prolonged matting or pulling of hair; usually hair regrows with time.
- Post traumatic—rare, alopecia with little inflammation can be seen with injuries where nerve or blood supply interrupted to the skin.

Autoimmune

- Alopecia areata—rare, alopecia with little outward inflammation, most common on face and head.
- Pemphigus foliaceus—crusting and alopecia on ears, sometimes nose, feet, and other areas; pruritus variable.

Neoplastic

- Epitheliotropic lymphoma—scaly alopecia, eventually plaques and nodules.
- Squamous cell carcinoma in situ—papillomaviral plaques: in older cats, scaly, crusty, often pigmented, multifocal, sometimes pruritic.

Manifestation of Internal Disease

- Thymoma-associated exfoliative dermatitis:
  - Nonpruritic dramatic scaling dermatitis that starts on head and neck.
  - Surgical removal of thymoma resolves dermatitis over 4–5 months.

ALOPECIA—CATS (CONTINUED)

- Paraneoplastic alopecia:
  - Most cases associated with pancreatic adenocarcinomas, bile duct carcinomas.
  - Nonpruritic alopecia has acute onset, progresses rapidly; bilaterally symmetric, ventrally distributed (also located along bridge of nose and periocular); hair epilates easily; dry fissuring footpads; skin often thin and hypotonic; rapid weight loss.
- Mural lymphocytic folliculitis—sometimes paraneoplastic: alopecia of face, eyelids, muzzle; skin has thick, waxy feel; histologic lymphocytic invasion of follicular outer root sheath and epidermis.
- Hyperthyroidism—alopecia due to self-barbering; can see weight loss as well.
- Hyperadrenocorticism—symmetric, nonpruritic; older cat if natural, any age if iatrogenic; can have severe skin fragility.
- Diabetes—unkempt and unhealthy coat, skin infections.

Psychogenic

Although anxiety may make overgrooming worse from any underlying condition, a pure compulsive disorder is very rare; all other causes of alopecia must be ruled out prior to considering.

CBC/BIOCHEMISTRY/URINALYSIS

Abnormalities may be noted with diabetes mellitus, hyperadrenocorticism, and hyperthyroidism.

OTHER LABORATORY TESTS

- FeLV and FIV—risk factors for demodicosis and other infections.
- Thyroid hormones—document hyperthyroidism/hypothyroidism.

IMAGING

- Abdominal ultrasound—assess adrenals in hyperadrenocorticism and look for neoplasia in animals with paraneoplastic syndrome.
- Chest radiographs/ultrasound to rule out thymoma.
- CT scan—look for pituitary or other neoplasia tumors in animals with hyperadrenocorticism.

DIAGNOSTIC PROCEDURES

- Skin scrapes.
- Dermatophyte culture.
- Parasite treatment trials, since negative skin scrapes do not rule out all parasites.
- Skin biopsy.
- Shirts/collar to prove self-trauma if pruritus is questioned.
- Food elimination trials if parasites and dermatophytes are ruled out.
- Intradermal allergy testing.

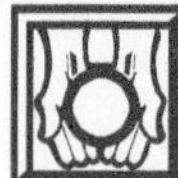

TREATMENT

- See specific chapters for full list of medications, doses, and other therapies.
- If pet is compliant, shampoo and topical therapy may relieve secondary problems such as hyperkeratosis, crusting, or secondary bacterial infections.

MEDICATIONS

DRUG(S) OF CHOICE

- Demodicosis—fluralaner topically as per label every 3 months; lime sulfur dips at weekly intervals for six dips; other mites and fleas also respond to appropriate topical or oral treatments.
- Allergic dermatitis—antihistamines only rarely helpful; novel restricted-ingredient diet; corticosteroids; cyclosporine (5–7 mg/kg/day initially); allergen-specific immunotherapy; ectoparasite control.
- Hyperthyroidism—methimazole, thyroidectomy, or radioactive iodine therapy.
- Diabetes mellitus—regulation of glucose levels (insulin, weight loss, diet).
- Hyperadrenocorticism—discontinue glucocorticoids if iatrogenic; if natural, trilostane, mitotane, and surgery are options.
- Paraneoplastic alopecia—surgical excision of neoplasia; but neoplasia often fatal.
- Epitheliotropic lymphoma—corticosteroids, lomustine.
- Sebaceous adenitis—surgical removal of thymoma, corticosteroids, cyclosporine.
- Squamous cell carcinoma in situ—surgical excision, retinoids (topical and oral), topical imiquimod cream.

PRECAUTIONS

Toxicity with griseofulvin and itraconazole (see Dermatophytosis).

FOLLOW-UP

PATIENT MONITORING

Determined by specific diagnosis.

PREVENTION/AVOIDANCE

Determined by specific diagnosis.

POSSIBLE COMPLICATIONS

Determined by specific diagnosis.

EXPECTED COURSE AND PROGNOSIS

Determined by specific diagnosis.

MISCELLANEOUS

ZOONOTIC POTENTIAL

- Dermatophytosis—can cause skin lesions in humans.
- Cheyletiellosis—can cause irritation in humans.

SEE ALSO

- Cheyletiellosis.
- Demodicosis.
- Dermatophytosis.
- Diabetes Mellitus Without Complication—Cats.
- Feline Paraneoplastic Alopecia.
- Flea Bite Hypersensitivity and Flea Control.
- Hyperadrenocorticism (Cushing's Syndrome)—Cats.
- Hyperthyroidism.
- Lymphoma, Cutaneous Epitheliotropic.
- Pemphigus.
- Sebaceous Adenitis, Granulomatous.
- Squamous Cell Carcinoma, Skin.
- Thymoma.

ABBREVIATIONS

- FeLV = feline leukemia virus.
- FIV = feline immunodeficiency virus.

Suggested Reading

Backel K, Cain C. Skin as a marker of general feline health: cutaneous manifestations of infectious disease. J Feline Med Surg, 2017, 19(11):1149–1165.

Diesel A. Cutaneous hypersensitivity dermatoses in the feline patient: a review of allergic skin disease in cats. Vet Sci, 2017, 4(2):25.

Mecklenburg L, Linek M, Tobin DJ. Hair Loss Disorders in Domestic Animals. Chichester: Wiley, 2009.

Vogelnest LJ. Skin as a marker of general feline health: cutaneous manifestations of systemic disease. J Feline Med Surg, 2017, 19(9):948–960.

Author Melissa N.C. Eisenschenk

Consulting Editor Alexander H. Werner Resnick

Acknowledgment The author and editors acknowledge the prior contribution of Karen Helton Rhodes.

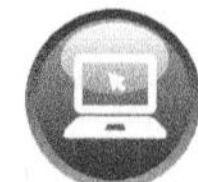

Client Education Handout available online

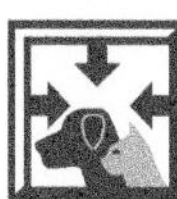

BASICS

DEFINITION

- Common disorder.
- Characterized by complete or partial loss of hair in areas where it is normally present.
- May be associated with multiple causes, be the primary problem, or be secondary to an underlying cause.

PATHOPHYSIOLOGY

- Multiple causes.
- Represents removal of hair or disruption in the growth of the hair from hypersensitivity, infection, genetic abnormality, trauma, immunologic attack, mechanical "plugging," endocrine abnormalities, neoplasia, drug reaction, and/or blockage of receptor sites for stimulation of hair growth cycle.

SYSTEMS AFFECTED

- Endocrine/metabolic.
- Hemic/lymphatic/immune.
- Skin/exocrine.

SIGNALMENT

Age, breed, and sex predilections are specific to each cause listed.

SIGNS

- May be acute in onset or slowly progressive.
- Multifocal patches of alopecia are associated with folliculitis caused by demodicosis, dermatophytosis, or, most commonly, staphylococcus infection.
- Large, more diffuse areas of alopecia may indicate follicular dysplasia or metabolic component.
- Pattern and degree of hair loss, along with presence of pruritus, are important for establishing differential diagnoses.

CAUSES

- Infectious—dermatophytosis, parasitic (mites, fleas), superficial and deep bacterial infections.
- Hypersensitivity/reaction—atopy/allergy, oral medication reaction, topical medication reaction.
- Disorders of hair follicle cycling—telogen effluvium, Cushing's (iatrogenic and hyper-adrenocorticism), hypothyroidism (iatrogenic), alopecia X, seasonal flank alopecia.
- Congenital—hair follicle dystrophy.
- Environmental—solar damage, burns, frostbite, scarring.
- Ischemic—post-matting alopecia, barrette or rubber band too tight, dermatomyositis, post vaccine, vasculitis.
- Autoimmune—alopecia areata, pemphigus foliaceus, sebaceous adenitis, vasculitis.
- Neoplastic—epitheliotropic lymphoma.
- Manifestation of internal disease—hypo-thyroidism, hyperadrenocorticism.

RISK FACTORS

Chronic corticosteroid use causes hair cycle arrest with other signs of iatrogenic Cushing's.

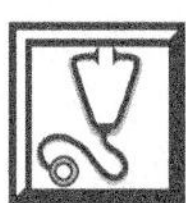

DIAGNOSIS

DIFFERENTIAL DIAGNOSIS

Multifocal Alopecia

- Demodicosis—partial to complete alopecia with erythema, comedones, and mild scaling; lesions may become inflamed and crusted.
- Dermatophytosis—partial to complete alopecia with scaling, with or without erythema, not usually ring-like.
- Staphylococcal folliculitis—circular patterns of alopecia with epidermal collarettes, erythema, crusting, and hyperpigmented macules.
- Injection/topical medication reactions—inflammation with alopecia and/or cutaneous atrophy from scarring.
- Rabies vaccine vasculitis—well-demarcated patch of alopecia observed 1–3 months post vaccination. Small-breed dogs more predisposed.
- Alopecia areata—noninflammatory areas of complete alopecia.
- Sebaceous adenitis of short-coated breeds—annular to polycyclic areas of alopecia and scaling.

Symmetric Alopecia

- Hyperadrenocorticism—truncal alopecia associated with atrophic skin, comedones, and pyoderma, as well as other systemic signs.
- Hypothyroidism—thinning of truncal haircoat; generalized alopecia is uncommon presentation; alopecic "rat" tail.
- Noninflammatory alopecia (alopecia X)—symmetric truncal alopecia associated with hyperpigmentation; alopecia often starts along collar area of neck; Pomeranian, chow chow, Akita, Samoyed, Keeshonden, Alaskan Malamute, and Siberian husky.
- Hyperestrogenism (females)—symmetric alopecia of flanks and perineal and inguinal regions with enlarged vulva and mammary glands; may also be associated with exogenous hormone exposure.
- Male feminization from Sertoli cell tumor—alopecia of perineum and genital region with gynecomastia.
- Seasonal/cyclic/flank alopecia—common, serpiginous flank alopecia with hyperpig-mentation; boxer, English bulldog, Airedale terrier.
- Color mutant/dilution alopecia—brittle or coarse hair, thinning of blue or fawn-colored hair coat, and secondary folliculitis; other colors of hair normal.
- Follicular dysplasia—slowly progressive alopecia affecting one color of hair.
- Anagen defluxion and telogen defluxion—acute onset of alopecia due to stressful event.
- Epitheliotropic lymphoma—diffuse, generalized truncal alopecia with scaling and intense erythema; later nodule and plaque formation.
- Pemphigus foliaceus—hair loss associated with scale and crust formation.
- Sebaceous adenitis—hair straightening, thinning, with dry hyperkeratosis; standard poodles and crosses, Havanese, other breeds.
- Allergic dermatitis with secondary infections and self-trauma due to pruritus.

Specific Locations

- Pinnal alopecia/pattern baldness—miniaturization of hairs and progressive alopecia; dachshund, greyhound, American water spaniel, Portuguese water spaniel, Boston terrier, Manchester terrier, whippet, Italian greyhound, Chihuahua.
- Pinnal alopecia with crusting or necrosis—consider vasculitis, which can have many triggers.
- Traction alopecia—hair loss secondary to having barrettes or rubber bands applied to the hair, or prolonged tight matting of the hair.
- Post-clipping alopecia—failure to regrow after clipping associated with slow or arrested hair cycle.
- Melanoderma (alopecia of Yorkshire terriers)—symmetric alopecia of pinnae, bridge of nose, tail, and feet.
- Seasonal/cyclic/canine flank alopecia—serpiginous flank alopecia with hyperpig-mentation; boxer, English bulldog, Airedale terrier.
- Black hair follicular dysplasia—alopecia of black-haired areas only.
- Dermatomyositis—alopecia of face, tip of ears, tail, and digits; associated with scale crusting and scarring.

Breed-Related Alopecia

- Alopecic breeds—Chinese crested, Mexican hairless, Inca hairless, Peruvian Inca orchid, American hairless terrier (often associated with comedones, folliculitis, and furunculosis).
- Congenital hypotrichosis—cocker spaniel, Belgian shepherd, poodle, whippet, beagle, French bulldog, Yorkshire terrier, Labrador retriever, bichon frise, Lhasa apso, basset hound.
- Color dilution alopecia—blue or fawn Doberman pinscher, silver Labrador, cream chow chow, blond Irish setter, blue pit bull terrier, other breeds with dilute coat colors.
- Melanoderma with alopecia—Yorkshire terrier.
- Seasonal/cyclic/canine flank alopecia—serpiginous flank alopecia with hyperpig-mentation; boxer, English bulldog, Airedale terrier.
- Pinnal alopecia/pattern baldness—miniaturization of hairs and progressive alopecia; dachshund, greyhound, American water spaniel, Portuguese water spaniel, Boston

terrier, Manchester terrier, whippet, Italian greyhound, Chihuahua.
- Noninflammatory alopecia (alopecia X)—symmetric truncal alopecia associated with hyperpigmentation; alopecia often starts along collar area of neck; Pomeranian, chow chow, Akita, Samoyed, keeshond, Alaskan Malamute, Siberian husky.

CBC/BIOCHEMISTRY/URINALYSIS

Rule out metabolic causes such as hyperadrenocorticism.

OTHER LABORATORY TESTS

- Thyroid panel—do not rely on low T_4 (total thyroxine) alone); diagnose hypothyroidism.
- Adrenocorticotropic hormone (ACTH)-response test, low-dose dexamethasone-suppression test (LDDST), and high-dose dexamethasone-suppression test (HDDST)—evaluate for hyperadrenocorticism.
- Sex hormone profiles (questionable validity, often not useful for diagnosis or therapy).

IMAGING

Ultrasonography—evaluate adrenal glands for evidence of hyperadrenocorticism.

DIAGNOSTIC PROCEDURES

- Cytology.
- Skin scraping.
- Fungal culture.
- Skin biopsy—very useful to evaluate status of follicle/hair growth as well as epidermal changes associated with specific conditions.

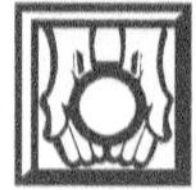

TREATMENT

- Treatments depend on the underlying causes of alopecia; see specific chapters for each condition.
- Bathing can be useful as adjunctive therapy for many conditions.

MEDICATIONS

DRUG(S) OF CHOICE

- Demodicosis or other external parasites — isoxazoline antiparasitics as per label.
- Dermatophytosis—terbinafine, ketoconazole, fluconazole, itraconazole, lime sulfur dips, griseofulvin.
- Staphylococcal folliculitis—investigate and treat underlying cause, shampoo and antibiotic therapy.
- Sebaceous adenitis—topical therapy, essential fatty acid supplementation, cyclosporine.
- Iatrogenic Cushing's—stop all glucocorticoids.
- Natural hyperadrenocorticism—trilostane, mitotane, surgical removal of tumor.
- Hypothyroidism—levothyroxine supplementation.
- Follicular dysplasia—control concurrent allergies and infections.
- Alopecia X and seasonal flank alopecia—sometimes responds to melatonin.
- Ischemic lesions—consider pentoxifylline.

CONTRAINDICATIONS

N/A

POSSIBLE INTERACTIONS

None

ALTERNATIVE DRUG(S)

None

FOLLOW-UP

PATIENT MONITORING

Determined by cause.

POSSIBLE COMPLICATIONS

N/A

MISCELLANEOUS

ASSOCIATED CONDITIONS

N/A

AGE-RELATED FACTORS

N/A

ZOONOTIC POTENTIAL

Dermatophytosis can cause skin lesions in humans.

PREGNANCY/FERTILITY/BREEDING

Avoid retinoids and griseofulvin in pregnant animals.

SEE ALSO

- Demodicosis.
- Dermatophytosis.
- Flea Bite Hypersensitivity and Flea Control.
- Hyperadrenocorticism (Cushing's Syndrome)—Dogs.
- Hypothyroidism.
- Lymphoma, Cutaneous Epitheliotropic.
- Pemphigus.
- Sebaceous Adenitis, Granulomatous.
- Sertoli Cell Tumor.

ABBREVIATIONS

- ACTH = adrenocorticotropic hormone.
- HDDST = high-dose dexamethasone-suppression test.
- LDDST = low-dose dexamethasone-suppression test.
- T_4 = Total thyroxine.

Suggested Reading

Behrend EN, Kooistra HS, Nelson R, et al. Diagnosis of spontaneous canine hyperadrenocorticism: 2012 ACVIM consensus statement (small animal). J Vet Intern Med, 2013 27(6):1292–1304.

Mecklenburg L, Linek M, Tobin DJ. Hair Loss Disorders in Domestic Animals. Chichester: Wiley, 2009.

Moriello KA, Coyner K, Paterson S, Mignon B. Diagnosis and treatment of dermatophytosis in dogs and cats: clinical consensus guidelines of the World Association for Veterinary Dermatology. Vet Dermatol, 2017, 28(3):266–e68.

Morris DO. Ischemic dermatopathies. Vet Clin North Am Small Anim Pract, 2013, 43(1):99–111.

Vandenabeele S, Declercq J, De Cock H, Daminet S. Canine recurrent flank alopecia: a synthesis of theory and practice. Vlaams Diergeneeskd Tijdschr, 2014, 83(6):275–283.

Author Melissa N.C. Eisenschenk

Consulting Editor Alexander H. Werner Resnick

Acknowledgment The author and editor acknowledge the prior contribution of Karen Helton Rhodes.

Client Education Handout available online

ALOPECIA, NONINFLAMMATORY—DOGS

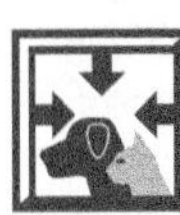

BASICS

DEFINITION

• Uncommon alopecic disorders that are associated with abnormal hair follicle cycling. • Both endocrine and nonendocrine diseases can be associated with alopecia. • Definitive diagnosis often requires ruling out the more common endocrine alopecias.

PATHOPHYSIOLOGY

• Many factors affect the hair cycle, both hormonal and nonhormonal. • Increased sex hormones can affect the hair cycle. Estrogen is a known inhibitor of anagen, the growth phase of the hair follicle. • The mechanism by which alopecia X influences the hair cycle is not known. • Exposure to human exogenous hormone replacement therapy.

SYSTEMS AFFECTED

• Behavioral. • Endocrine/metabolic. • Hemic/lymphatic/immune. • Skin/exocrine.

GENETICS

Breed predispositions exist for alopecia X; however, the mode of inheritance is unknown.

INCIDENCE/PREVALENCE

• Hyperestrogenism and hyperandrogenism are uncommon to rare causes of alopecia.
• Alopecia X is relatively common in predisposed breeds.

GEOGRAPHIC DISTRIBUTION

None

SIGNALMENT

Species

Dogs

Breed Predilections

• Hyperestrogenism and hyperandrogenism—no breed predilections. • Alopecia X—miniature poodle and plush-coated breeds such as Pomeranian, chow chow, Akita, Samoyed, keeshond, Alaskan Malamute, and Siberian husky; recently described in Schipperke breed.

Mean Age and Range

• Hyperestrogenism and hyperandrogenism—middle-aged to old intact dogs. • Alopecia X—1–5 years of age; however, older dogs may develop the condition.

Predominant Sex

• Hyperandrogenism, primarily intact males.
• Hyperestrogenism, primarily intact females or males. • Alopecia X, neutered or intact dogs of either sex.

SIGNS

Historical Findings

• Overall change in hair coat—dry or bleached because hairs not being replaced; lack of normal shed. • Males with hyperestrogenism may attract other male dogs.

Physical Examination Findings

• Alopecia—usually diffuse and bilaterally symmetric truncal alopecia sparing the head and distal extremities; uncommon with hyperandrogenism. • Hair coat—may be dry or bleached. • Secondary seborrhea, pruritus, pyoderma, comedones, ceruminous otitis externa, and hyperpigmentation—variable.
• Enlargement of nipples, mammary glands, vulva, prepuce—may be associated with hyperestrogenism. • Macular melanosis and linear preputial dermatitis—may be associated with hyperestrogenism. • Abnormal-sized or different-sized testicles—may be associated with hyperestrogenism or hyperandrogenism. • Testicles may also appear normal in size. • Tail gland hyperplasia and perianal gland hyperplasia—usually associated with hyperandrogenism.
• Systemic signs (polyuria/polydipsia [PU/PD]/polyphagia) are usually *not* present.

CAUSES

Hyperestrogenism—Females

Estrogen excess associated with cystic ovaries, ovarian tumors (rare), exogenous estrogen supplementation, or exposure to human topical hormone replacement.

Hyperestrogenism—Males

• Estrogen excess due to Sertoli cell tumor (most common), seminoma, or interstitial cell tumor (rare), or exposure to human topical hormone replacement. • Associated with male pseudohermaphrodism in miniature schnauzers.

Hyperandrogenism—Males

Androgen-producing testicular tumors (especially interstitial cell tumors).

Alopecia X

Hairs fail to cycle, but underlying endocrine cause has not been identified.

RISK FACTORS

• Intact male and female dogs at increased risk for developing testicular tumors and ovarian cysts/tumors, respectively.
• Cryptorchid males at increased risk for developing testicular tumors. • Exogenous estrogen supplementation. • Exposure to human exogenous hormone replacement therapy. • No known risk factors for alopecia X other than breed predisposition.

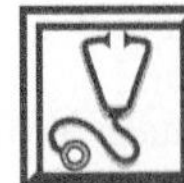

DIAGNOSIS

DIFFERENTIAL DIAGNOSIS

• Inflammatory causes of alopecia (pyoderma, demodicosis, and dermatophytosis)—usually cause patchy rather than diffuse pattern of alopecia. • Sebaceous adenitis—inflammatory cause of alopecia more common in specific breeds (Samoyed, Akita). • Hypothyroidism and hyperadrenocorticism—may cause very similar pattern of diffuse alopecia associated with lack of hair follicle cycling. • Follicular dysplasia including color dilution alopecia and black hair follicular dysplasia—alopecia should be color restricted. • Patterned alopecia of various breeds (dachshund, Boston terrier, greyhound, water spaniel, and others)—breed-specific alopecia of unknown cause. • Seasonal/cyclic/canine flank alopecia—alopecia of flank and dorsum, often serpiginous patterns with hyperpigmentation, more often in short-coated breeds (boxer, English bulldog, Airedale) and may recur seasonally.
• Postclipping alopecia—hair fails to regrow following clipping; however, hair regrowth occurs within one year. • Telogen defluxion—alopecia occurs 1–2 months following illness or severe stressful episode and usually more sudden in onset, with relative ease of epilation.

CBC/BIOCHEMISTRY/URINALYSIS

• Usually unremarkable. • Anemia, hypercholesterolemia associated with severe hypothyroidism. • Anemia and/or bone marrow hypoplasia or aplasia can be associated with hyperestrogenism.

OTHER LABORATORY TESTS

• Serum sex hormone concentrations—often normal, treat according to suspected diagnosis based on clinical signs and ruling out other disorders. • Serum estradiol concentrations—sometimes elevated in male dogs with testicular tumors or female dogs with cystic ovaries; however, normal fluctuation of estradiol occurs throughout the day, making interpretation of estradiol concentrations difficult. • Adrenal sex hormone panel not useful for diagnosis of alopecia X.

IMAGING

Radiography, ultrasonography, and laparoscopy—identify cystic ovaries, ovarian tumors, testicular tumors (scrotal or abdominal), adrenal tumors, sublumbar lymphadenopathy, and possible thoracic metastases of malignant tumors.

DIAGNOSTIC PROCEDURES

• Preputial cytology—may demonstrate cornification of cells in males with hyperestrogenism (similar to bitch in estrus).
• Skin biopsy.

PATHOLOGIC FINDINGS

Histologic changes associated with endocrine dermatoses (telogen hairs, follicular keratoses, hyperkeratosis, excess trichilemmal keratinization [flame follicles], thin epidermis, and thin dermis) may also be seen with noninflammatory alopecias including

ALOPECIA, NONINFLAMMATORY—DOGS (CONTINUED)

hyperestrogenism and alopecia X. Histopathology will help rule out inflammatory causes of alopecia (pyoderma, demodicosis, dermatophytosis, sebaceous adenitis) and some of the other differentials listed above.

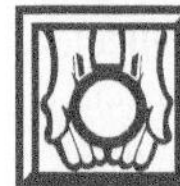

TREATMENT

DIET

None

CLIENT EDUCATION

Alopecia X is a cosmetic condition resulting in coat loss only and there is no definitive cure for the hair loss. The risk of treatment should be emphasized. Hair regrowth will only occur in a portion of dogs regardless of treatment chosen, and hair loss may recur months to years later in spite of continued treatment.

SURGICAL CONSIDERATIONS

Hyperestrogenism/Hyperandrogenism

• Castration—scrotal testicular tumors.
• Exploratory laparotomy—diagnosis and surgical removal (ovariohysterectomy and castration) for ovarian cysts and tumors and abdominal testicular tumors.

Alopecia X

• Neuter intact animals—a certain number will regrow hair following neutering; hair regrowth may take up to 3 months to become evident. • Microneedling technique may induce hair regrowth.

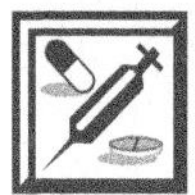

MEDICATIONS

DRUG(S) OF CHOICE

General Treatments

• Topical antiseborrheic shampoos—for comedones and seborrhea associated with alopecia. • Antibiotics and topical antimicrobial shampoos—for secondary skin infections associated with alopecia.

Alopecia X

• Melatonin—implants (8 mg or 18 mg every 4–6 months) or oral (3 mg q12h for small breeds and 6–12 mg q12h for large breeds); evidence of hair regrowth may take up to 3 months. Effective in approximately 40% of cases. Because this treatment is benign, it is considered the treatment of choice following neutering. Once hair regrowth has occurred, discontinue treatment. • Medroxyprogesterone acetate—5–10 mg/kg SC q4 weeks for 4 treatments. Hair regrowth can take up to 6 months. Effective in approximately 40–50% of cases.

CONTRAINDICATIONS

None

PRECAUTIONS

• Melatonin at high doses can cause insulin resistance. Use caution in treating dogs with diabetes mellitus. • Medroxyprogesterone acetate can cause mammary nodules and cystic endometrial hyperplasia with long-term use. Diabetes mellitus has been reported in a few dogs.

POSSIBLE INTERACTIONS

None

ALTERNATIVE DRUG(S)

• Mitotane—15–25 mg/kg once daily as induction for 5–7 days, followed by twice weekly maintenance; hair regrowth occurs in portion of dogs treated and can take up to 3 months to become evident. Use of this drug can result in an Addisonian crisis and other side effects, as for treatment of Cushing's syndrome. • Trilostane—dosages as described for treatment of Cushing's syndrome; hair regrowth occurs in a portion of dogs treated and can take up to 3 months to become evident. Use of this drug can result in an Addisonian crisis and other side effects, as for treatment of Cushing's syndrome.

FOLLOW-UP

PATIENT MONITORING

• Medroxyprogesterone acetate—complete physical examination and chemistry panel regularly. • Mitotane—electrolytes and cortisol with adrenocorticotropic hormone (ACTH) stimulation testing regularly.
• Trilostane—electrolytes and cortisol with ACTH stimulation testing regularly.

PREVENTION/AVOIDANCE

None

POSSIBLE COMPLICATIONS

None

EXPECTED COURSE AND PROGNOSIS

• Estrogen- and androgen-secreting tumors—resolution of signs should occur within 3–6 months after castration or ovariohysterectomy. • Alopecia X—hair regrowth will occur in only a portion of dogs regardless of treatment chosen and hair loss may recur in spite of continued treatment. Therefore, if hair regrowth occurs, discontinue treatment to preserve treatment for future recurrence of alopecia. Risk of treatment should be weighed with the fact that this is a cosmetic disease.

MISCELLANEOUS

ASSOCIATED CONDITIONS

• Pyoderma, seborrhea, comedones may be associated with alopecia. • Behavioral changes associated with hyperestrogenism or hyper-androgenism.

AGE-RELATED FACTORS

None

ZOONOTIC POTENTIAL

None

PREGNANCY/FERTILITY/BREEDING

N/A—neutering usually recommended for managing these conditions.

SYNONYMS

Alopecia X—growth hormone-responsive alopecia, castration-responsive alopecia, adrenal hyperplasia-like syndrome, adrenal sex hormone imbalance of plush-coated breeds, among others.

ABBREVIATIONS

• ACTH = adrenocorticotropic hormone.
• PU/PD = polyuria/polydipsia.

INTERNET RESOURCES

https://vetmed.tennessee.edu/vmc/SmallAnimalHospital/Dermatology

Suggested Reading

Frank LA. Endocrine and metabolic diseases. In: Miller WH, Griffin CE, Campbell KL, eds., Muller and Kirk's Small Animal Dermatology, 7th ed. Philadelphia, PA: W.B. Saunders, 2013, pp. 501–553.

Frank LA. Alopecia X in a Pomeranian. Clinicians Brief, 2017, Nov:26–30.

Stroll S, Dietlin C, Nett-Mettler CS. Microneedling as a successful treatment for alopecia X in two Pomeranian siblings. Vet Dermatol 2015, 26:387–390.

Author Linda A. Frank

Consulting Editor Alexander H. Werner Resnick

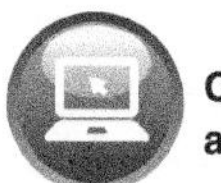

Client Education Handout available online

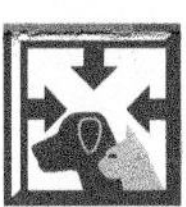

BASICS

OVERVIEW

• Common oral tumor of odontogenic (tooth structure) ectoderm origin.
• Biologically these tumors are benign histologically, but possess locally invasive properties.
• Tumors may arise anywhere within the dental arcade.
• Several histologic subtypes exist with similar invasive behavior.

SIGNALMENT

• Middle-aged and old dogs.
• Rare in cats.

SIGNS

• Dogs may present with a smooth, firm, gingival mass that is usually nonulcerated.
• May be incidental finding during dental prophylaxis/procedures. If involving rostral dental arcade, incisor teeth can be displaced and enveloped by proliferative tissue.

CAUSES & RISK FACTORS

N/A

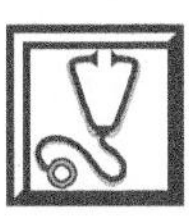

DIAGNOSIS

DIFFERENTIAL DIAGNOSIS

• Epulis.
• Gingival hyperplasia.
• Squamous cell carcinoma.
• Amelanotic melanoma.
• Plasma cell tumor.
• Other tumors related to the odontogenic apparatus.

CBC/BIOCHEMISTRY/URINALYSIS

Unaffected

OTHER LABORATORY TESTS

N/A

IMAGING

• Dental radiographs may show bone lysis deep to the superficial mass. Not particularly useful for diagnostic or treatment planning.
• Regional and distant metastasis has not been described.
• CT is ideal for planning surgery or radiation therapy, especially in large or caudal tumors.

DIAGNOSTIC PROCEDURES

• Deep tissue biopsies are necessary and recommended for definitive diagnosis.
• Squamous cell carcinoma may be misdiagnosed as ameloblastoma.

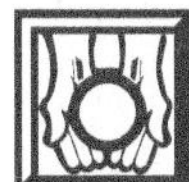

TREATMENT

• Surgical excision such as hemi- or total mandibulectomy or maxillectomy with >1–2 cm margins is recommended as a curative treatment option. Always submit resected tissue for histopathology, in order to confirm the original diagnosis, and evaluate soft tissue and bone margins.
• Radiation therapy may provide long-term control in large tumors, or when owners decline surgery.
• Intralesional chemotherapy with bleomycin has been reported, but results are generally inferior to those of surgery or radiation.

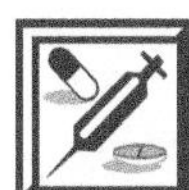

MEDICATIONS

DRUG(S) OF CHOICE

N/A

CONTRAINDICATIONS/POSSIBLE INTERACTIONS

N/A

FOLLOW-UP

Careful oral examination at 1, 3, 6, 9, and 12 months after definitive treatment is recommended to monitor for local recurrence.

MISCELLANEOUS

Suggested Reading

Amory JT, Reetz JA, Sanchez MD, et al. Computed tomographic characteristics of odontogenic neoplasms in dogs. Vet Radiol Ultrasound 2014, 55(2):147–158.

Fiani N, Verstraete FJ, Kass PH, Cox DP. Clinicopathologic characterization of odontogenic tumors and focal fibrous hyperplasia in dogs: 152 cases (1995–2005). J Am Vet Med Assoc 2011, 238(4):495–500.

Goldschmidt SL, Bell CM, Hetzel S, Soukup J. Clinical characterization of canine acanthomatous ameloblastoma (CAA) in 263 dogs and the influence of postsurgical histopathological margin on local recurrence. J Vet Dent 2017, 34(4):241–247.

Author Nick Dervisis
Consulting Editor Timothy M. Fan

AMPHETAMINE AND ADD/ADHD MEDICATION TOXICOSIS

BASICS

DEFINITION

Acute neurologic, neuromuscular, and cardiac toxicosis as the result of excessive consumption of amphetamine or a derivative. May be due to ingestion of prescription medications or illegal drugs.

PATHOPHYSIOLOGY

- Amphetamine and its derivatives belong to the CNS stimulant class phenylethylamines. Various substitutions of the basic phenylethylamine structure account for many pharmaceutical and illicit compounds found today.
- Amphetamine is a sympathomimetic that is structurally related to norepinephrine.
- Central action—stimulates cortical centers including cerebral cortex, medullary respiratory center, and reticular activating systems.
- Peripheral action—directly stimulates alpha and beta receptors and stimulates release of norepinephrine from stores in adrenergic nerve terminals.
- Amphetamine may slow catecholamine metabolism by inhibition of monoamine oxidase.
- Several different product formulations, including immediate and extended release and topical patch.
- Amphetamines are well absorbed orally; peak plasma levels are generally reached in 1–3 hours; this may be delayed with extended release formulations.
- Metabolism is minimal.
- The half-life, which varies from 7 to 34 hours, and rate of excretion of unchanged amphetamine in the urine are both dependent upon urine pH, with shorter half-lives associated with more acidic urine.
- Clinical signs may be seen at doses below 1 mg/kg.
- Oral lethal dose in dogs for most amphetamines ranges from 10 mg/kg to 23 mg/kg and for methamphetamine sulfate it is 9–11 mg/kg. Oral lethal dose for amphetamine sulfate is 20–27 mg/kg.
- Amphetamine and its derivatives are used in humans to treat attention deficit disorder (ADD)/attention deficit hyperactivity disorder (ADHD), narcolepsy, and obesity.
- Illicit use of amphetamines in humans is also prevalent.

SYSTEMS AFFECTED

- Cardiovascular—stimulation most common: tachycardia and hypertension.
- Nervous—stimulation most common, depression uncommon.
- Neuromuscular—stimulation: muscle tremors and seizures.
- Respiratory—stimulation, tachypnea.
- Ophthalmic—mydriasis.
- Gastrointestinal (GI)—anorexia, vomiting, diarrhea.

INCIDENCE/PREVALENCE

N/A

SIGNALMENT

Species

Dogs and cats, although more prevalent in dogs.

Breed Predilections

N/A

Mean Age and Range

N/A

Predominant Sex

N/A

SIGNS

Historical Findings

- Abnormal behavior—usually hyperactivity, anxiety or pacing, anorexia, fast heart rate, panting; observed or evidence of exposure by owner/caretaker.
- Onset of signs typically begins within 30 minutes to 6 hours post ingestion; depends on product formulation.

Physical Examination Findings

- Nervous—hyperactivity, agitation, restlessness, head bobbing, pacing, circling, vocalization, disorientation, hyperesthesia, ataxia, lethargy or depression (less common).
- Cardiovascular—tachycardia or bradycardia (less common, may be reflexive), hypertension.
- Neuromuscular—muscle fasciculation or tremors, seizures.
- Gastrointestinal—vomiting, diarrhea, anorexia, excessive salivation.
- Respiratory—tachypnea.
- Ophthalmic—mydriasis with possibly poor to unresponsive pupillary light response.
- Other—hyperthermia.

CAUSES

Accidental ingestion or administration, malicious poisoning.

RISK FACTORS

Households with children or adults currently taking prescription or illicit amphetamine or derivative.

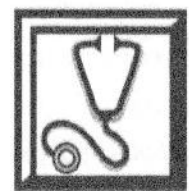

DIAGNOSIS

DIFFERENTIAL DIAGNOSIS

- Strychnine.
- Organochlorine insecticides.
- Methylxanthine.
- 4-aminopyridine.
- Metaldehyde.
- Phenylpropanolamine.
- Albuterol.
- Nicotine.
- Tremorgenic mycotoxins.
- Hypernatremia.
- Pseudoephedrine, phenylephrine.
- 5-fluorouracil.
- Ma huang, guarana, or ephedra.

CBC/BIOCHEMISTRY/URINALYSIS

- CBC—generally normal with mild to moderate intoxications; disseminated intravascular coagulopathy secondary to severe hyperthermia (rare).
- Chemistry—generally normal with mild to moderate intoxications.
- Azotemia—prerenal: secondary to dehydration; renal: secondary to rhabdomyolysis and myoglobinuria (rare).
- Elevated liver enzymes—secondary to seizures and/or hyperthermia (rare).
- Hypoglycemia.
- Urinalysis—evidence of myoglobinuria, urine specific gravity (high: prerenal azotemia; isosthenuria: renal failure).

OTHER LABORATORY TESTS

- Electrolytes—imbalances secondary to GI effects.
- Acid-base status—acidosis may occur.
- Over-the-counter urine drug screens—watch for false positive or negative; consult user handbook for further information.
- Amphetamines are present in blood, urine, and saliva; consult with local veterinary diagnostic lab or human hospital for availability and proper sample submission.

IMAGING

N/A

DIAGNOSTIC PROCEDURES

- ECG for presence of any tachyarrhythmia or less commonly bradyarrhythmia.
- Blood pressure—identification of hypertension.

PATHOLOGIC FINDINGS

On necropsy presence of amphetamines may be found in gastric contents, urine, plasma, liver, kidney, or muscle.

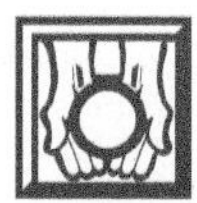

TREATMENT

APPROPRIATE HEALTH CARE

Majority of cases require emergency inpatient intensive care management.

NURSING CARE

- Intravenous fluid therapy to correct dehydration and electrolyte imbalances as well as support renal function and promote excretion of amphetamines; use blood pressure to help guide fluid rate.
- Cool intravenous fluids, fans, cool water baths for hyperthermia.

ACTIVITY

Minimize activity and stimuli.

DIET

Withhold food if moderately to severely affected. Bland diet for few days post exposure if significant GI signs were noted.

CLIENT EDUCATION

In case of exposure, owner should contact local veterinarian or veterinary poison center immediately.

SURGICAL CONSIDERATIONS

N/A

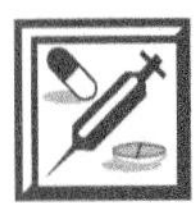

MEDICATIONS

DRUG(S) OF CHOICE

Decontamination

- Induce emesis—if recent exposure and pet is not already symptomatic.
- Apomorphine—0.04 mg/kg IV, subconjunctival.
- Hydrogen peroxide 3%—2.2 mL/kg, maximum dose 45 mL.
- Gastric lavage if extremely large ingestion or patient is already symptomatic.
- Activated charcoal with cathartic.

CNS Signs of Stimulation

- Acepromazine 0.05–1.0 mg/kg IV/IM, start low and titrate to effect.
- Chlorpromazine 0.5 mg/kg IV, titrate up as needed.
- Cyproheptadine (serotonin antagonist)—dogs, 1.1 mg/kg orally or rectally, may be repeated q8h as needed for signs consistent with serotonin syndrome; cats, 2–4 mg/cat, may repeat q12h as needed for signs consistent with serotonin syndrome.
- Methocarbamol (for muscle tremors)—50–220 mg/kg IV, titrate to effect; do not exceed 330 mg/kg/day.

Cardiovascular Signs

- Tachyarrhythmia—beta blockers such as propranolol 0.02–0.04 mg/kg IV or esmolol or metoprolol; caution using propranolol in significantly hypertensive patient.
- Ventricular premature contractions—lidocaine: dogs at 2–4 mg/kg IV (to maximum of 8 mg/kg over 10-minute period); cats: start with 0.1–0.4 mg/kg and increase cautiously to 0.25–0.75 mg/kg IV slowly if no response; cats are reportedly very sensitive to lidocaine, so monitor carefully if used.

Promote Elimination

Ascorbic acid or ammonium chloride—for urinary acidification to promote elimination; however, only use if can measure acid-base status.

CONTRAINDICATIONS

- While diazepam has been successfully used to treat amphetamine exposures, there is evidence that benzodiazepines may intensify neurologic signs.
- Urinary acidification if unable to monitor acid-base status or if myoglobinuria is present.
- Inducing emesis in symptomatic patient.

PRECAUTIONS

N/A

POSSIBLE INTERACTIONS

- Amphetamines inhibit metabolism of adrenergic blockers (doxazosin, phenoxybenzamine, prazosin, terazosin), phenobarbital, and phenytoin.
- Amphetamines potentiate metabolism of coumarin anticoagulants, monoamine oxidase inhibitors, opioid analgesics, and tricyclic antidepressants.

ALTERNATIVE DRUG(S)

Phenobarbital, pentobarbital, and propofol for CNS stimulatory signs.

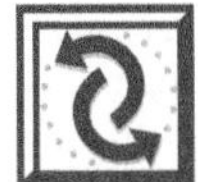

FOLLOW-UP

PATIENT MONITORING

- Monitor in hospital until resolution of clinical signs.
- If severely affected, monitor liver and kidney values every 24 hours for 72 hours or until resolution.

PREVENTION/AVOIDANCE

All medications and illicit drugs should be kept out of pets' reach at all times.

POSSIBLE COMPLICATIONS

Acute renal failure secondary to myoglobinuria or disseminated intravascular coagulation (DIC; rare).

EXPECTED COURSE AND PROGNOSIS

- Expected course of clinical signs is 12–72 hours, depending on dose, product formulation, effectiveness of decontamination and treatment, and rate of elimination.
- Prognosis—most patients do well with prompt and appropriate veterinary care. Seizures or severe hyperthermia may be poor prognostic indicator.

MISCELLANEOUS

ASSOCIATED CONDITIONS

N/A

AGE-RELATED FACTORS

N/A

ZOONOTIC POTENTIAL

Pets exposed to human waste products from those taking amphetamines or derivatives could become symptomatic.

PREGNANCY/FERTILITY/BREEDING

Amphetamines are a known teratogen in humans. They have been found to cross the placenta in animals and may also be found in milk.

SYNONYMS

- Common brand names of prescription amphetamine drugs and their active ingredient—Adderall® (amphetamine and dextroamphetamine); Ritalin®, Metadate®, and Concerta® (methylphenidate); Daytrana® (methylphenidate transdermal patch); Focalin® (dexmethylphenidate); Vyvanse® (lisdexamfetamine); Cylert® (pemoline); Adipex-P® (phentermine); Dexedrine® (dextroamphetamine).
- Illicit drug street names—ice, glass, crank, speed, uppers, ecstasy, meth, and many others.

SEE ALSO

- Antidepressant Toxicosis—SSRIs and SNRIs.
- Antidepressant Toxicosis—Tricyclics.
- Pseudoephedrine/Phenylephrine Toxicosis.

ABBREVIATIONS

- ADD = attention deficit disorder.
- ADHD = attention deficit hyperactivity disorder.
- DIC = disseminated intravascular coagulation.
- GI = gastrointestinal.

INTERNET RESOURCES

- https://www.aspcapro.org/animal-health/toxicology-poison-control
- http://www.petpoisonhelpline.com

Suggested Reading

Stern LA, Schell M. Management of attention-deficit disorder and attention-deficit/hyperactivity disorder drug intoxication in dogs and cats. Vet Clin North Am Small Anim Pract 2012, 42(2):279–287.

Teitler JB. Evaluation of a human on-site urine multi drug test for emergency use with dogs. J Am Anim Hosp Assoc 2009, 45(2):59–66.

Volmer PA. Human drugs of abuse. In: Bonagua JD, Twedt DC, eds., Current Veterinary Therapy XIV. St. Louis, MO: Elsevier, 2009, pp. 144–145.

Volmer PA. "Recreational" drugs. In: Peterson ME, Talcott PA, eds., Small Animal Toxicology, 3rd ed. St. Louis, MO: Elsevier, 2013, pp. 309–334.

Wismer T. Amphetamines. In: Osweiler GD, Hovda LR, Brutlag AG, Lee JL, eds. Blackwell's Five-Minute Veterinary Consult Clinical Companion Small Animal Toxicology. Ames, IA: Wiley-Blackwell, 2011, pp. 125–130.

Author Kirsten E. Waratuke

Consulting Editor Lynn R. Hovda

A

AMYLOIDOSIS

BASICS

DEFINITION

Group of conditions of diverse causes in which extracellular deposition of insoluble fibrillar proteins (amyloid) in various organs and tissues compromises normal function.

PATHOPHYSIOLOGY

• Patients usually affected by reactive (secondary) amyloidosis; tissue deposits contain amyloid A protein (AA), fragment of acute-phase reactant protein called serum amyloid A protein (SAA). • Macrophage-derived cytokines, e.g., IL-1 and IL-6, stimulate hepatocytes to synthesize SAA. • Cellular and extracellular components involved in formation and deposition of AA. • Specific pathophysiology varies among different species and breeds; reactive amyloidosis occurs as familial disease in Chinese Shar-Pei dog and Abyssinian cat. • Chinese Shar-Pei dog—mutation involving overexpression of *HAS2* results in overproduction of hyaluronic acid, which acts as danger signal activating inflammasome pathway and IL-1 production; this mutation linked to increased likelihood of developing shar-pei autoinflammatory disease (SPAID), and also responsible for breed's meat-mouth phenotype; amyloid deposition occurs in medulla of all dogs, with majority of dogs also having glomerular involvement. • Non-shar-pei dogs—amyloid deposits found more commonly in glomeruli than medulla. • Abyssinian cat—amyloid deposits usually found in medulla, but may occur in glomeruli. • Siamese and oriental shorthair cats with familial amyloidosis—amyloid deposition occurs in liver. • Pancreatic islet amyloid polypeptide, or amylin, deposits in pancreas of old cats; amylin secreted with insulin by pancreatic beta cells; chronic increased stimulus for secretion of amylin by beta cells (e.g., states of insulin resistance) leads to pancreatic islet cell amyloidosis.

SYSTEMS AFFECTED

• Renal/urologic—predilection for renal AA deposition. • Liver, spleen, adrenal glands, pancreas, tracheobronchial tree, gastrointestinal tract also may be affected.

GENETICS

• Familial amyloidosis occurs in Chinese Shar-Pei, English foxhound, and beagle dogs, and in Abyssinian, oriental shorthair, and Siamese cats. • A genetic mutation that increases likelihood of SPAID in shar-pei dogs has been identified; chronic inflammatory episodes in SPAID result in renal amyloid deposition.

INCIDENCE/PREVALENCE

Uncommon, occurs mostly in dogs; rare in cats, except Abyssinian, Siamese, and oriental shorthair.

SIGNALMENT

Species

Dog and cat.

Breed Predilections

• Dog—Chinese Shar-Pei, beagle, English foxhound, Walker hound, collies. • Cat—Abyssinian, Siamese, oriental shorthair.

Mean Age and Range

• Cats—mean age at diagnosis 7 years; range 1–17 years; Abyssinian cats with familial renal amyloidosis usually die by 5 years of age; Siamese cats with familial amyloidosis of liver and thyroid gland usually develop signs of liver disease when 1–4 years old. • Dogs—mean age at diagnosis 9 years; range 1–15 years; Chinese Shar-Pei affected younger, with median age at diagnosis of 5 years, range 3.6–17 years. • Prevalence increases with age.

Predominant Sex

None

SIGNS

General Comments

Clinical signs depend on organs affected; usually caused by kidney involvement.

Historical Findings

• No clear history of predisposing disorder in most cases. • Anorexia, lethargy, polyuria/polydipsia, weight loss, vomiting. • Owners may appreciate ascites and peripheral edema in animals with glomerular amyloidosis. • Chinese Shar-Pei dogs may have history of previous episodic joint swelling and high fever that resolves spontaneously within few days (SPAID). • Siamese and oriental shorthair cats may present with acute collapse and hemoabdomen due to spontaneous hepatic fracture.

Physical Examination Findings

• Related to primary inflammatory or neoplastic disease process. • Animals with renal disease may have muscle wasting, abnormal renal palpation, uremic ulceration, hypertensive fundic lesions. • Fluid retention may be present (ascites, peripheral edema). • Chinese Shar-Pei dogs may have evidence of SPAID if present during active flare-up (joint effusion and pain, fever). • Signs of thromboembolic disease may be present in up to 40% of dogs with renal amyloidosis (dyspnea with pulmonary embolism, caudal paresis with aortic embolism). • Siamese and oriental shorthair cats with hepatic dysfunction may have jaundice; pallor and abdominal fluid wave may be present with hepatic fracture and hemoabdomen.

CAUSES

• Neoplasia and chronic infectious and noninfectious inflammatory conditions can be found in 30–50% of dogs with reactive amyloidosis. • Chronic inflammation—systemic mycoses, chronic bacterial infections, parasitic infections (dirofilariasis, leishmaniasis, hepatozoonosis), inflammatory and immune-mediated diseases (SPAID, systemic lupus erythematosus, juvenile polyarteritis of beagle); amyloid deposits can be found in up to 35% of feline immunodeficiency virus (FIV)-positive cats. • Neoplasia (lymphoma, plasmacytoma, multiple myeloma, mammary tumors, testicular tumors). • Familial—Chinese Shar-Pei, English foxhound, and beagle dogs; Abyssinian, Siamese, and oriental shorthair cats. • Other—cyclic hematopoiesis in gray collies.

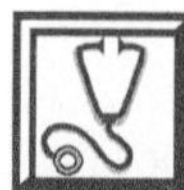

DIAGNOSIS

DIFFERENTIAL DIAGNOSIS

• Depends on organ affected. • Renal (glomerular) amyloidosis—immune-complex glomerulonephritis (GN; e.g., membranoproliferative GN [MPGN], membranous GN [MGN]), non-immune-complex GN, glomerulosclerosis, focal segmental glomerulosclerosis, other glomerulopathies. • Renal (medullary) amyloidosis—other causes of medullary renal disease (e.g., pyelonephritis, chronic interstitial nephritis). • Hepatic amyloidosis—other causes of hepatic dysfunction (e.g., infectious, inflammatory, portosystemic shunt, neoplasia); in animals with hepatic fracture and hemoabdomen, consider other causes of hemoabdomen (e.g., hemangiosarcoma, hematoma).

CBC/BIOCHEMISTRY/URINALYSIS

• CBC—nonregenerative anemia found in some dogs and cats. • Chemistry profile—changes reflect distribution of amyloid deposition; with renal medullary amyloidosis, azotemia, hyperphosphatemia, metabolic acidosis may be seen; hypoalbuminemia common with glomerular amyloidosis; hyperglobulinemia may be seen due to underlying inflammatory condition resulting in reactive amyloidosis. • Urinalysis—isosthenuria, proteinuria, cylindruria common with renal amyloidosis; proteinuria may be mild or absent in patients without glomerular amyloidosis; isosthenuria may not be present in patients without medullary involvement.

OTHER LABORATORY TESTS

• Urine protein–creatinine ratio (UPC) should be performed for quantification of proteinuria. • Urine sodium dodecyl sulfate–polyacrylamide gel electrophoresis (SDS-PAGE)—can differentiate between high and low molecular weight proteinuria; high molecular weight proteinuria expected with glomerular disease.

IMAGING

Abdominal Radiographic Findings

Kidneys—usually small in affected cats; small, normal size, or large in affected dogs.

Abdominal Ultrasonographic Findings

• Renal size, shape, and architecture variable; kidneys usually hyperechoic and small in affected cats; may be small, normal size, or large in affected dogs. • Echogenic effusion may be present in cats with hepatic amyloidosis, due to hepatic fracture and hemoabdomen.

DIAGNOSTIC PROCEDURES

Renal biopsy—histopathology required for definitive diagnosis, and to rule out other causes of GN; ultrasound-guided sampling preferred over surgical methods; samples should be assessed under dissecting microscope to ensure glomeruli present; risk factors for hemorrhage include body weight <5 kg, serum creatinine >5 mg/dL.

PATHOLOGIC FINDINGS

• Amyloid deposits appear homogeneous and eosinophilic when stained by hematoxylin and eosin and viewed by conventional light microscopy. • Demonstrate green birefringence after Congo red staining when viewed under polarized light; AA amyloid loses Congo red affinity after permanganate oxidation.
• Ultrastructurally, fibrils are 9–11 nm in diameter, nonbranching, haphazardly arranged.

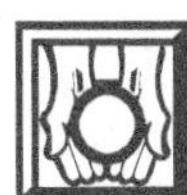

TREATMENT

APPROPRIATE HEALTH CARE

• Identify underlying inflammatory and neoplastic processes and treat if possible.
• Animals symptomatic from uremia or clinically dehydrated may require hospitalization.
• Stable, euhydrated animals can be managed as outpatients with standard therapy for proteinuria.

DIET

• Low-protein, low-phosphorous renal diets recommended for animals with proteinuria and/or renal dysfunction. • Esophageal feeding tube placement should be considered for enteral hydration and nutritional support.

CLIENT EDUCATION

• Discuss progression of disease and potential for underlying primary disease process.
• Discuss familial predisposition in susceptible breeds.

MEDICATIONS

DRUG(S) OF CHOICE

Management of Proteinuria

• Animals with proteinuria should be treated with standard therapy for proteinuria (see Glomerulonephritis and Proteinuria).
• Patients with evidence of active thromboembolic disease require antiplatelet drugs (clopidogrel or aspirin) and/or anticoagulant therapy (heparin, low molecular weight heparin, or factor Xa inhibitors).

Management of Renal Insufficiency and Hypertension

• As indicated by IRIS guidelines for stage of renal disease. • Amlodipine (0.3–0.8 mg/kg PO SID) as first-line therapy for management of hypertension.

Management of Amyloid Deposition

• Dimethylsulfoxide (DMSO; dogs—90% DMSO diluted 1 : 4 with sterile water subcutaneously at dosage of 90 mg/kg 3 times per week) may help patients by solubilizing amyloid fibrils, reducing serum concentration of SAA, and reducing interstitial inflammation and fibrosis in affected kidneys, though benefit of DMSO is controversial. • Colchicine (dogs—0.01–0.04 mg/kg PO q24h) impairs release of SAA from hepatocytes, and used for amyloidosis in humans with familial Mediterranean fever (familial amyloidosis similar in pathology to SPAID); no evidence for benefit once patient develops renal amyloidosis and dysfunction; colchicine used particularly in shar-pei dogs with episodic fever or polyarthritis before development of renal failure.

PRECAUTIONS

• Dose reduction of drugs may be needed in patients with renal insufficiency. • Use of nonsteroidal anti-inflammatory drugs (NSAIDs) should be avoided in patients with renal insufficiency; SPAID flare-ups usually resolve on their own, do not require NSAIDs.
• Animals with glomerular disease are prone to overhydration due to abnormal renal sodium handling; fluid therapy should be used judiciously, only to correct dehydration; even patients with mild hypoalbuminemia can become significantly overhydrated from inappropriate fluid therapy.

FOLLOW-UP

PATIENT MONITORING

BUN, creatinine, albumin, electrolyte concentrations, 3-day pooled UPC, and blood pressure 1 month following medication changes, and every 3-4 months in stable patients.

PREVENTION/AVOIDANCE

Do not breed affected animals.

POSSIBLE COMPLICATIONS

• Renal insufficiency and progressive chronic kidney disease. • Nephrotic syndrome and fluid overload. • Thromboembolic disease occurs in up to 40% of dogs, but uncommon in cats. • Hepatic rupture causing hemoabdomen (hepatic amyloidosis). • Otic and airway hemorrhage (vascular amyloidosis) reported.

EXPECTED COURSE AND PROGNOSIS

• Disease is progressive and usually advanced at time of diagnosis. In one study, median survival time for all dogs with renal amyloidosis 5 days (range: 0–443 days), shorter in Chinese Shar-Pei dogs (2 days, range: 0–368 days).
• Serum creatinine concentration has significant negative association with survival. • Cats with renal insufficiency because of amyloidosis usually survive <1 year; cats with systemic amyloidosis (i.e., liver, vascular) have grave prognosis due to complications such as hepatic fracture and pulmonary hemorrhage.

MISCELLANEOUS

ASSOCIATED CONDITIONS

• Shar-pei autoinflammatory disease.
• Juvenile polyarteritis in beagles.

SEE ALSO

• Chronic Kidney Disease.
• Glomerulonephritis.
• Proteinuria.

ABBREVIATIONS

• AA = amyloid A protein. • BUN = blood urea nitrogen. • DMSO = dimethylsulfoxide.
• FIV = feline immunodeficiency virus.
• GN = glomerulonephritis.
• MGN = membranous GN.
• MPGN = membranoproliferative GN.
• NSAID = nonsteroidal anti-inflammatory drug. • SAA = serum amyloid A protein.
• SDS-PAGE = sodium dodecyl sulfate–polyacrylamide gel electrophoresis.
• SPAID = shar-pei autoinflammatory disease.
• UPC = urine protein–creatinine ratio.

Suggested Reading

Bartges J, Wall J. Amyloidosis. In Bartges J, Polzin DJ. Nephrology and Urology of Small Animals. Oxford: Wiley-Blackwell, 2011, pp. 547–554.

Olsson M, Meadows JRS, Truvé K, et al. A novel unstable duplication upstream of HAS2 predisposes to a breed-defining skin phenotype and a periodic fever syndrome in Chinese Shar-Pei dogs. PLoS Genet 2011, 7:e1001332.

Segev G, Cowgill LD, Jessen S et al. Renal amyloidosis in dogs: a retrospective study of 91 cases with comparison of the disease between Shar-Pei and non-Shar-Pei dogs. J Vet Intern Med 2012, 26:259–268.

Author Nahvid M. Etedali

Consulting Editor J.D. Foster

Acknowledgment The author and book editors acknowledge the prior contributions of Helio S. Autran de Morais and Stephen P. DiBartola.

Client Education Handout available online

ANAEROBIC INFECTIONS

BASICS

OVERVIEW

- Anaerobic bacteria require low oxygen tension to live, and constitute a large portion of the normal flora.
- May be Gram-positive or Gram-negative cocci or rods, and individual organisms vary in potential to withstand oxygen exposure.
- Most common genera—*Bacteroides, Fusobacterium, Actinomyces, Propionibacterium, Peptostreptococcus* (enteric *Streptococcus*), *Porphyromonas*, and *Clostridium*.
- Most anaerobic infections are polymicrobial and can contain anaerobes admixed with facultative anaerobes or aerobic bacteria (especially *E. coli*).
- Injurious toxins and enzymes elaborated by the organisms may allow extension of infection into adjacent, healthy tissue.

SIGNALMENT

Dog and cat.

SIGNS

General Comments

- Depend on body system involved.
- Areas associated with mucous membranes are more commonly associated with anaerobic infection.
- It is possible to overlook anaerobes in an infectious process, leading to confusion in interpreting culture results and selection of antimicrobials.

Physical Examination Findings

- Foul odor associated with wound or exudative discharge.
- Gas in the tissue or exudates.
- Discolored tissue.
- Ascites (peritonitis), pleural effusion (pyothorax), or signs of pyometra (vaginal discharge, palpable structure in caudal abdomen).
- Dental disease.
- Wounds or deep abscesses that do not heal as anticipated.

CAUSES & RISK FACTORS

- Usually caused by normal flora; break in protective barriers allows bacterial invasion.
- Predisposing factors—immunosuppression, bite wounds, dental disease, open fractures, abdominal surgery, migrating foreign bodies.

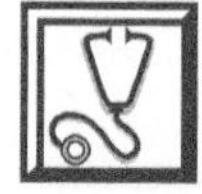

DIAGNOSIS

DIFFERENTIAL DIAGNOSIS

- Infection with aerobic or fungal organisms—culture recommended.
- Necrosis due to trauma or hypoperfusion.
- Neoplasia.

CBC/BIOCHEMISTRY/URINALYSIS

- Neutrophilic leukocytosis, monocytosis.
- Biochemical abnormalities depend on specific organ involvement.
- Sepsis suggested by leukocytosis/leukopenia, hypoglycemia, hypoalbuminemia.

OTHER LABORATORY TESTS

- Anaerobic bacterial culture often unrewarding because of fastidious growth requirements and errors in sample handling.
  - Appropriate media and containers should be available prior to sample collection.
  - Samples should not be refrigerated.
  - Suitable samples for culture include fluid or tissue.

IMAGING

As indicated for individual patient; gas may be apparent radiographically.

DIAGNOSTIC PROCEDURES

- Cytologic inspection of fluid or tissue reveals degenerate neutrophils with morphologically diverse intracellular and extracellular bacteria; presence of large filamentous bacteria is suggestive.
- Gram staining should be performed on sample.

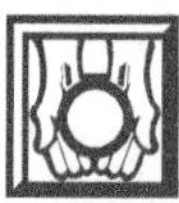

TREATMENT

- Wound drainage/debridement should be established as soon as possible—including placement of drains or thoracostomy tubes, as indicated.
  - Combine with systemic antimicrobial therapy.
  - Devitalized tissue should be aggressively debrided.
  - Improves local blood flow and increases tissue oxygen tension.
- Exploratory surgery indicated when anaerobic organisms complicate osteomyelitis or intraabdominal disease (e.g., pyometra, peritonitis).

MEDICATIONS

DRUG(S) OF CHOICE

- Antimicrobial therapy alone is unlikely to be successful without debridement or drainage.
  - Antibiotic selection—largely empiric (difficult to isolate anaerobes).
  - Because most anaerobic infections are polymicrobial, therapy targeted against both anaerobes *and* aerobic organisms is indicated.
- Amoxicillin with clavulanate (22–30 mg/kg PO q12h)—antibiotic of choice; clavulanate improves activity against *Bacteroides*. Injectable potentiated beta-lactams include ampicillin/sulbactam, ticarcillin/clavulanate, and piperacillin/tazobactam.
- Cefoxitin (30 mg/kg IV/IM q6–8h)—reliable activity against anaerobes.
- Clindamycin (11–33 mg/kg PO q12–24h; 10 mg/kg IV q12h)—useful for respiratory tract infections.
- Chloramphenicol (25–50 mg/kg PO q8h, dogs only)—good tissue penetration but bacteriostatic; concern for human exposure.
- Metronidazole (10 mg/kg IV/PO q12h)—useful against all clinically significant anaerobes except *Actinomyces*.
- Cefovecin (8 mg/kg SC)—infections originating from the periodontal cavity, skin, or urinary tract.
- Imipenem—significant activity against serious, resistant infections, not first-line choice.
- Quinolones—newer third-generation quinolones (e.g., pradofloxacin) have some activity against anaerobes; others ineffective.

CONTRAINDICATIONS/POSSIBLE INTERACTIONS

N/A

FOLLOW-UP

PATIENT MONITORING

Varies with the circumstances of each patient.

POSSIBLE COMPLICATIONS

Localized infection may progress to systemic infection if not appropriately identified and treated.

EXPECTED COURSE AND PROGNOSIS

Dependent upon identification and resolution of the underlying cause; long-term antibiotic therapy may be required.

MISCELLANEOUS

ASSOCIATED CONDITIONS

See Causes & Risk Factors.

Suggested Reading

Greene CE, Jang SS. Anaerobic infections. In: Greene CE, ed., Infectious Diseases of the Dog and Cat, 4th ed. St. Louis, MO: Saunders Elsevier, 2011, pp. 411–416.

Author Sharon Fooshee Grace

Consulting Editor Amie Koenig

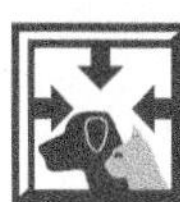

BASICS

OVERVIEW

• Anal sacs are reservoirs for secretions normally evacuated by compression during defecation. • Normal gland secretions vary widely in consistency and color. • Disorders include impaction, infection/sacculitis, and neoplasia. • Treatment options include manual expression, flushing, antibiotics, and surgical excision.

SIGNALMENT

Impaction/Infection

• Dogs and cats (rarely)—no age or sex predisposition. • Breeds predisposed (impaction)—smaller breeds (miniature/toy poodle, Chihuahua, American cocker and English springer spaniel).

Neoplasia

• Adenocarcinoma—English cocker spaniel most commonly reported.

SIGNS

Impaction/Infection

• Anal/perianal pruritus—often manifested by "scooting." • Hesitancy to defecate. • Tenesmus. • Tail chasing. • Foul-smelling, nonfeces anal discharge. • Refusal to sit and/or lift tail. • Cats—excessive licking of the ventral abdomen and tail head. • Abscess—often unilateral; localized pain and discharge.

Neoplasia

• Mass or swelling in perianal region.
• Tenesmus, constipation, polyuria/polydipsia (due to hypercalcemia with adenocarcinoma).
• L4-Cd myelopathy reported in one cat (adenocarcinoma).

CAUSES & RISK FACTORS

Impaction/Infection

• Predisposing factors—changes in muscle tone, fecal form (soft stool/diarrhea), secretion character/volume leading to decreased/lack of expression; intestinal disease, obesity, endocrine disease. • Infection/abscess—chronic or recurrent impactions.

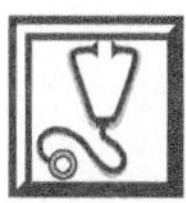

DIAGNOSIS

DIFFERENTIAL DIAGNOSIS

Impaction/Infection/Neoplasia

• Hypersensitivity (flea, atopy, food).
• Tapeworm infestation. • Tail fold bacterial folliculitis. • Malassezia dermatitis. • Compulsive disorder (anal licking). • Colitis or other intestinal disorder. • Keratinization disorder. • Anal sac neoplasia (adenocarcinoma, squamous cell carcinoma, melanoma). • Perianal adenoma, adenocarcinoma. • Perianal fistulae.

CBC/BIOCHEMISTRY/URINALYSIS

Impaction/Infection

Usually normal.

Neoplasia

Hypercalcemia—anal sac adenocarcinoma.

OTHER LABORATORY TESTS

None unless indicated by an underlying cause.

IMAGING

None unless indicated by an underlying cause.

DIAGNOSTIC PROCEDURES

• Digital palpation of anal sacs—should not be palpable externally. • Expression of anal sac contents—varies widely in gross appearance and microscopic characteristics. • Cytology (normal dogs/cats)—one study reports Gram-positive cocci/rods, Gram-negative cocci/rods, yeast, nondegenerate neutrophils without phagocytosis, mononuclear cells, and corneocytes; erythrocytes uncommonly found in dogs, rare in cats. Another study had similar findings but with intracellular bacteria in clinically normal dog anal sacs.

Impaction/Infection

• Cytology—no statistically significant difference in bacterial counts or inflammatory cells found between normal dogs and those with clinical signs of anal sac disease. • Bacterial culture and susceptibility—*Bacillus, Escherichia coli, Micrococcus, Proteus mirabilis, Streptococcus* spp., others possible.

Neoplasia

• Surgical excision with histopathology.

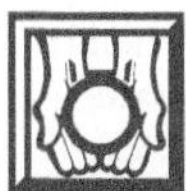

TREATMENT

Impaction/Infection

• Gentle manual expression and/or flushing of contents. Sedation may be necessary to flush severely impacted or painful anal sacs.
• Feeding high-fiber diets may help natural expression of anal sacs. • Identification of underlying causes of predisposing disease.
• Chronic disease—anal sac excision.
• Infection—infusion of antibiotic and/or corticosteroid medications directly into the anal sacs, drainage of abscesses, use of appropriate oral antibiotics and/or antiyeast medication.

Neoplasia

• Surgical excision and staging; combine with chemotherapy.

MEDICATIONS

DRUG(S) OF CHOICE

Infection

Use of appropriate oral antibiotics: cephalexin (dog, 22–30 mg/kg q12h), amoxicillin trihydrate–clavulanate potassium (dog, 13.75 mg/kg q12h; cat, 62.5 mg/cat q12h), clindamycin (dog, 11–22 mg/kg q24h; cat, 11–30 mg/kg q24h), trimethoprim–sulfamethoxasole (dog, 15 mg/kg q12h); metronidazole (dog, 15–25 mg/kg q12–24h); enrofloxacin (dog, 10–20 mg/kg q24h), orbifloxacin (dog/cat, 5 mg/kg q24h).

CONTRAINDICATIONS/POSSIBLE INTERACTIONS

Trimethoprim–sulfamethoxasole—Dobermans highly susceptible to type III hypersensitivity reactions.

FOLLOW-UP

Impaction/Infection

• Reassess patients weekly initially, then as necessary to monitor healing. • Manually express anal sac contents and/or flush contents until sacs empty without intervention.
• Trimethoprim–sulfamethoxasole—monitor tear production, liver function; affects thyroid serum values.

MISCELLANEOUS

SEE ALSO

• Adenocarcinoma, Anal Sac
• Perianal Fistula

Suggested Reading

Helton Rhodes KA, Werner A. Blackwell's Five-Minute Veterinary Consult: Clinical Companion: Small Animal Dermatology, 3rd ed. Hoboken, NJ: Wiley-Blackwell, 2018.

James DJ, Griffin CE, Polissar NL, Neradilek MB. Comparison of anal sac cytological findings and behaviour in clinically normal dogs and those affected with anal sac disease. Vet Derm 2010, 22:80–87.

Author Heather D. Edginton

Consulting Editor Alexander H. Werner Resnick

Acknowledgment The author acknowledges the prior contribution of Alexander H. Werner Resnick.

A

ANAPHYLAXIS

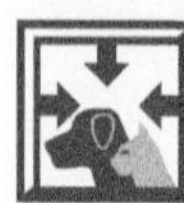

BASICS

DEFINITION

• Acute manifestation of a type I hypersensitivity reaction mediated through the introduction of an antigen into a host having antigen-specific antibodies of the immunoglobulin (Ig) E subclass.
• Binding of antigen to mast cells sensitized with IgE results in the release of preformed and newly synthesized chemical mediators.
• Anaphylactic reactions may be localized (atopy) or systemic (anaphylactic shock).
• Anaphylaxis not mediated by IgE is designated an anaphylactoid (nonimmunologic) reaction and will not be discussed; however, the treatment is the same for either reaction.

PATHOPHYSIOLOGY

• First exposure of the patient to a particular antigen (allergen) causes a humoral response and results in production of IgE, which binds to the surface of mast cells. The patient is then considered to be sensitized to that antigen.
• Second exposure to the antigen results in cross-linking of two or more IgE molecules on the cell surface, resulting in mast cell degranulation and activation. Release of mast cell granules initiates an anaphylactic reaction.
• Major mast cell–derived mediators include histamine, eosinophilic chemotactic factor, arachidonic acid and metabolites (e.g., prostaglandins, leukotrienes, and thromboxanes), platelet-activating factor, and proteases. Release of these mediators causes an inflammatory response characterized by increased vascular permeability, smooth muscle contraction, inflammatory cell influx, and tissue damage.
• Clinical manifestations depend on the route of antigen exposure, the dose of antigen, and the level and specificity of the IgE response.

SYSTEMS AFFECTED

• Gastrointestinal—salivation, vomiting, and diarrhea.
• Cardiovascular—hypotension, cardiac arrhythmias, shock.
• Respiratory—dyspnea, cyanosis/hypoxemia.
• Skin/exocrine—pruritus, urticaria, and edema.
• Hepatobiliary (dogs)—portal hypertension, vasoconstriction, ascites.

GENETICS

Familial basis reported for type I hypersensitivity reaction in dogs.

INCIDENCE/PREVALENCE

• Localized type I hypersensitivity reactions not uncommon.
• Systemic type I hypersensitivity reactions rare.

GEOGRAPHIC DISTRIBUTION

None

SIGNALMENT

Species

Dog and cat.

Breed Predilections

• Dogs—numerous breeds documented as having a predilection for developing atopy.
• Cats—no breeds documented as having predilection for atopy.

Mean Age and Range

• Dogs—age of clinical onset ranges from 3 months to several years; most affected animals 1–3 years old.
• Cats—age of clinical onset ranges from 6 months to 2 years.

Predominant Sex

• Dogs—atopy more common in females, no predilection for acute anaphylaxis.
• Cats—no reported sex predilection.

SIGNS

General Comments

• Initial clinical signs vary depending on the route of exposure to the inciting antigen (allergen).
• Shock—a severe anaphylactic reaction attributable to cardiovascular collapse and impaired oxygen delivery.
• May be localized to the site of exposure, but may progress to a systemic reaction.

Historical Findings

• Onset of signs usually within minutes, history of exposure to insects or medications.
• Dogs—pruritus, urticaria, vomiting, defecation, urination, collapse if severe.
• Cats—intense pruritus about the head, dyspnea, salivation, vomiting, collapse if severe.

Physical Examination Findings

• Localized cutaneous edema and erythemia at the site of exposure, macropapular rash.
• Dyspnea, cyanosis, respiratory wheezes.
• Tachycardia, hypotension (poor pulses), pale or muddy mucous membranes in animals with shock.
• Conjunctivitis, lacrimation.
• Painful abdomen, hepatomegaly (dogs).
• Hyperexcitability possible in early stages, altered mentation from hypoperfusion in systemic anaphylaxis.

CAUSES

Virtually any agent; those commonly reported include venoms (bees, wasps and hornets, fire ants, etc.), blood-based products (including antivenom and other animal-derived products), vaccines, medications, and foods.

RISK FACTORS

Previous exposure (sensitization) increases the chance of the animal developing a reaction.

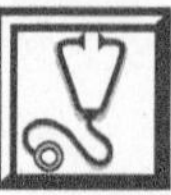

DIAGNOSIS

DIFFERENTIAL DIAGNOSIS

• Other types of shock.
• Asthma.
• Depends on the major organ system involved or if reaction is localized; diagnosis can be made largely based on history and clinical signs.

CBC/BIOCHEMISTRY/URINALYSIS

Because of the acute onset of disease, no tests reliably predict individual susceptibility.

OTHER LABORATORY TESTS

• In heartworm-endemic areas, a positive heartworm test may indicate a worm embolus as a cause for anaphylaxis.
• If ascites is present, abdominocentesis may reveal hemoperitoneum.
• Intradermal skin testing to identify allergens.
• Radioallergosorbent test to quantify the concentration of serum IgE specific for a particular antigen.

IMAGING

• Radiographic findings—if hemoperitoneum is present, ascites may be apparent in abdominal radiographs.
• Ultrasonographic findings—may show presence of edema in the gall bladder wall ("halo sign") or peritoneal effusion.

DIAGNOSTIC PROCEDURES

Limited, because a severely allergic animal can develop an anaphylactic reaction when exposed to even small quantities of antigen.

PATHOLOGIC FINDINGS

• Lesions vary, depending on severity of reaction, from localized cutaneous edema to severe pulmonary edema (in cats) and visceral pooling of blood (in dogs).
• Other nonspecific findings vary and are characteristic of shock.
• Nonspecific characteristics of localized reactions include edema, vasculitis, and thromboembolism.

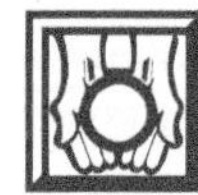

TREATMENT

APPROPRIATE HEALTH CARE

In an acutely affected animal, the reaction is considered a medical emergency requiring hospitalization and intensive care.

NURSING CARE

Elimination of inciting antigen, if possible.

Systemic Anaphylaxis

• Goal—emergency life support through the maintenance of an open airway, treating circulatory collapse, and reestablishing physiologic parameters.

• Administer fluids (isotonic crystalloids and/or colloids) intravenously to counteract hypotension; in severely affected animals, pressor agents (e.g., pinephrine) may be necessary to support blood pressure.
• In coagulopathic animals, transfusion with fresh frozen plasma or red blood cell–containing products may be indicated.

Localized Anaphylaxis

Goal—limit the reaction and prevent progression to a systemic reaction.

ACTIVITY

N/A

DIET

If a food-based allergen is suspected (uncommon), avoid foods associated with hypersensitivity reaction.

CLIENT EDUCATION

• Discuss the unpredictable nature of the disease.
• Discuss the need to recognize that the animal has an allergic condition that may require immediate medical care.

SURGICAL CONSIDERATIONS

None

MEDICATIONS

DRUG(S) OF CHOICE

Systemic Anaphylaxis

• Epinephrine hydrochloride (5–10 µg/kg [0.005–0.01 mg/kg] IV/IM).
• Corticosteroids—dexamethasone sodium phosphate (0.1–0.5 mg/kg IV), methylprednisolone sodium succinate (30 mg/kg IV).
• Isotonic crystalloid fluids (20–30 mL/kg IV over 15–20 minutes, followed by reassessment and additional boluses if necessary, targeting a maximum of 90 mL/kg in dogs and 60 mL/kg in cats) to treat hypotension and relative hypovolemia.
• Atropine (0.02–0.04 mg/kg IV) to treat symptomatic bradycardia.
• Bronchodilators—aminophylline (10 mg/kg IM or slowly IV) in severely dyspneic patients; albuterol inhalers (90 µg/actuation, via inhalation).
• Oxygen should be administered to hypoxemic patients, either by mask or a cage with an elevated oxygen content (targeting a 40% fraction of inspired oxygen [FiO_2]).
• Norepinephrine (0.5–3 µg/kg/min IV).

Localized Anaphylaxis

• Antihistamines—diphenhydramine hydrochloride (0.5–1.0 mg/kg IV/IM/PO); famotidine (0.5–1.0 mg/kg IV); ranitidine (0.5–2.5 mg/kg IV).
• Prednisolone (1–2 mg/kg PO).
• If shock develops, initiate treatment for a systemic anaphylaxis.

CONTRAINDICATIONS

None

PRECAUTIONS

Localized reaction can develop into systemic reaction.

POSSIBLE INTERACTIONS

N/A

ALTERNATIVE DRUG(S)

N/A

FOLLOW-UP

PATIENT MONITORING

• Closely monitor hospitalized patients for 24–48 hours.
• In patients with systemic anaphylaxis, monitoring should focus on normalization and monitoring of blood pressure, heart rate and rhythm, urine output, coagulation status, and oxygenation.
• If patients have continued fluid loss (e.g., due to diarrhea or vomiting), fluid administration rates should be adjusted accordingly.

PREVENTION/AVOIDANCE

If inciting antigen (allergen) can be identified, eliminate or reduce exposure.

POSSIBLE COMPLICATIONS

None

EXPECTED COURSE AND PROGNOSIS

• If localized reaction is treated early, prognosis is good.
• Some patients with systemic anaphylaxis that respond initially can have a recurrence of shock, usually within 12 hours of initial presentation.
• If the animal is in shock on presentation, prognosis is guarded.

MISCELLANEOUS

ASSOCIATED CONDITIONS

None

AGE-RELATED FACTORS

None

ZOONOTIC POTENTIAL

None

PREGNANCY/FERTILITY/BREEDING

N/A

SEE ALSO

Shock, hypovolemic.

ABBREVIATIONS

• FiO_2 = fraction of inspired oxygen.
• Ig = immunoglobulin.

Suggested Reading

Shmuel DL, Cortes Y. Anaphylaxis in dogs and cats. J Vet Emerg Crit Care 2013, 23(4):377–394.

Author Paul W. Snyder
Consulting Editor Melinda S. Camus

Client Education Handout available online

ANEMIA OF CHRONIC KIDNEY DISEASE

BASICS

OVERVIEW

- Progressive decrease in packed cell volume (PCV), red blood cell (RBC) count, and hemoglobin, and hypoplasia of erythroid elements of bone marrow are predictable features of chronic kidney disease (CKD).
- Anemia is normocytic, normochromic, nonregenerative, and proportional to stage of CKD; underlying cause of anemia is multifactorial.
- Gastrointestinal (GI) blood loss, reduced RBC survival, deficiencies in iron and/or folate, cytokines, and inflammatory mediators may be involved; however, primary cause of anemia in CKD is inadequate production of erythropoietin (EPO) by the kidneys.
- EPO is hormone that regulates bone marrow RBC generation and is produced in peritubular interstitial cells in response to decreased tissue oxygen.

SIGNALMENT

Any patient with advanced CKD—juvenile or acquired.

SIGNS

- Anemia contributes to anorexia, weight loss, fatigue, lethargy, depression, weakness, and behavior changes characterizing CKD.
- Pallor.
- Tachypnea.
- Tachycardia.
- Systolic murmur.

CAUSES & RISK FACTORS

- All inherited, congenital, and acquired forms of CKD.
- Exacerbated by iron deficiency, inflammatory or neoplastic disease, GI bleeding, hemolysis, and myeloproliferative disorders.

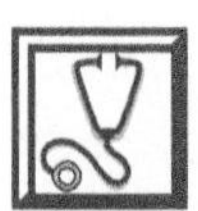

DIAGNOSIS

DIFFERENTIAL DIAGNOSIS

- Anemia of chronic infectious, inflammatory, or neoplastic disease; myeloproliferative disease; chronic blood loss; aplastic anemia; endocrine disease; drug reaction; chronic immune-mediated, toxic, viral, rickettsial, or parasitic anemia; hemodilution.
- Regenerative anemia excludes diagnosis of anemia of CKD.

CBC/BIOCHEMISTRY/URINALYSIS

- Normocytic, normochromic, hypoproliferative anemia.
- Reticulocytes—low corrected indices and absolute counts (≤10,000/µL).
- Typically, IRIS stage 3 or greater CKD.
- High blood urea nitrogen (BUN) : creatinine ratio may predict concurrent GI bleeding.

OTHER LABORATORY TESTS

- Serum iron—normal or variably low.
- Transferrin saturation—normal or variably low (<20%).
- Feline leukemia virus (FeLV), feline immunodeficiency virus (FIV), mycoplasma, or rickettsial testing to exclude infection-induced myelodyscrasia.
- Serum EPO—inappropriately normal or low.

IMAGING

- Small, irregular kidneys with loss or disruption of renal architecture often seen.
- Less commonly enlarged, polycystic, hydronephrotic, infiltrative.

DIAGNOSTIC PROCEDURES

Bone marrow cytology—erythroid hypoplasia; myeloid : erythroid ratio normal or high; stainable iron normal or low.

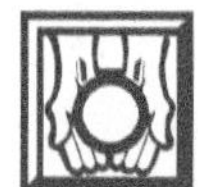

TREATMENT

- Stabilize azotemia in patients with uremic crisis.
- Ensure adequate nutrition.
- Stabilize any metabolic derangement (e.g., acidosis) that could contribute to shortened RBC lifespan.
- Minimize micronutrient deficiencies that could reduce RBC production.
- Identify and manage GI bleeding.
- Parenteral iron supplementation if needed.
- Correct systemic hypertension.

MEDICATIONS

DRUG(S) OF CHOICE

Blood Transfusion

- Short-term, rapid correction needed if hypoxic distress (typically PCV ≤15%)—give compatible packed RBCs.
- May transfuse intermittently for prolonged management, although compatibility issues are likely to occur.
- Preferred treatment is EPO support for progressive or symptomatic anemia.

EPO Replacement

- Darbepoetin alfa (Aranesp®)—an analogue of recombinant human EPO (r-HuEPO) with prolonged half-life and sustained effects; very effective with less tendency for antibody induction; should be used preferentially to epoetin alfa.
- Target PCV—dogs, 30–35%; cats, 30%.
- Dosage—0.8–1.0 µg/kg SC once weekly until PCV reaches low end of target, then decrease to q2-4 weeks as needed to maintain target; check PCV first to avoid overtreatment.
- If PCV exceeds target, discontinue until upper target range is achieved, then increase dosing interval.
- Iron dextran (5–10 mg/kg IM) should be administered as needed to normalize serum iron and transferrin saturation before initiating and during EPO treatment; injectable iron more effective than oral preparations.
- r-HuEPO—original synthetic erythropoiesis-stimulating protein, replica of human EPO (Epogen® and Procrit®); higher potential for anti-r-HuEPO antibody production and pure red cell aplasia (PRCA); use no longer recommended,

Anabolic Steroids

Not indicated.

FOLLOW-UP

PATIENT MONITORING

- PCV and blood pressure.
- Iron and transferrin saturation—at 1, 3, and 6 months, then semiannually.
- Discontinue EPO if patient develops evidence of polycythemia, local or systemic sensitivity, PRCA, or refractory hypertension.

POSSIBLE COMPLICATIONS

EPO Related

- Development of polycythemia, seizures, hypertension, iron depletion, injection pain, and mucocutaneous reactions.
- Development of PRCA during epoetin alfa treatment suggests formation of anti-r-HuEPO antibodies, which neutralize r-HuEPO and native EPO, causing severe anemia in 20–30% of animals; often reversible with cessation of treatment.
- Development of anti-r-HuEPO antibodies occurs in <10% of patients receiving darbepoetin alfa.
- Signs associated with production of anti-r-HuEPO antibodies include decreasing PCV, erythroid hypoplasia, reticulocyte count nearing zero, and myeloid : erythroid ratio ≥8.
- EPO replacements should be used cautiously or withheld if hypertension or iron deficiency develops; treatment can be reinstituted once hypertension or iron deficiency is corrected.

Transfusion Related

- Incompatibility reaction.
- Circulatory or iron overload.
- Systemic hypertension.
- Transmissible infection.

EXPECTED COURSE AND PROGNOSIS

- Correction of anemia increases appetite, activity, and quality of life.

- Use of EPO replacement agents requires careful assessment of risks and benefits.
- Short-term prognosis depends on severity of CKD.
- Long-term prognosis is guarded to poor because of underlying CKD.

MISCELLANEOUS

ABBREVIATIONS

- BUN = blood urea nitrogen.
- CKD = chronic kidney disease.
- EPO = erythropoietin.
- FeLV = feline leukemia virus.
- FIV = feline immunodeficiency virus.
- GI = gastrointestinal.
- PCV = packed cell volume.
- PRCA = pure red cell aplasia.
- RBC = red blood cell.
- r-HuEPO = recombinant human erythropoietin.

Suggested Reading

Chalhoub S, Langston C, Eatroff A. Anemia of renal disease: what it is, what to do, and what's new. J Feline Med Surg 2011, 13:629–640.

Chalhoub S, Langston C, Farrely J. The use of Darbepoetin to stimulate erythropoiesis in anemia of chronic kidney disease. J Vet Intern Med 2012; 26:363–369.

Cowgill LD, James KM, Lew JK, et al. Use of recombinant human erythropoietin for management of anemia in dogs and cats with renal failure. J Am Vet Med Assoc 1998, 212:521–528.

Fiocchi EH, Cowgill LD, Brown DC, et al. The use of Darbepoetin to stimulate erythropoiesis in the treatment of anemia of chronic kidney disease in dogs. J Vet Intern Med 2017, 31:476–485.

Authors Sheri Ross and Cedric P. Dufayet

Consulting Editor J.D. Foster

Acknowledgment The authors and book editors acknowledge the prior contribution of Ilaria Lippi.

ANEMIA, APLASTIC

BASICS

OVERVIEW

• A disorder of hematopoietic precursor cells characterized by replacement of normal bone marrow with adipose tissue. There is decreased production of granulocytes, erythrocytes, and platelets, resulting in pancytopenia in the peripheral blood. The disease is sometimes also referred to as aplastic pancytopenia. • In the acute form, neutropenia and thrombocytopenia predominate because of the shorter life spans of these cells; in the chronic form, nonregenerative anemia also occurs. In both forms, the bone marrow exhibits variable degrees of panhypoplasia. • Precipitating causes can include infectious diseases, drug or toxin exposure, and starvation; immune-mediated mechanisms are often suspected.
• Hemic/lymphatic/immune systems affected.

SIGNALMENT

Dogs and cats, no apparent breed or sex predilection. In one study, the mean age of nine affected dogs was 3 years.

SIGNS

• Acute form—fever, petechial hemorrhages, epistaxis, hematuria, melena; i.e., signs due to neutropenia and thrombocytopenia. • Chronic form—pale mucous membranes, weakness, lethargy; i.e., signs due to anemia, in addition to signs observed in acute forms.

CAUSES & RISK FACTORS

Often not identified.

Infectious Agents

• Feline leukemia virus (FeLV), feline immunodeficiency virus (FIV). • Canine and feline parvovirus. • Rickettsial organisms (e.g., *Ehrlichia* spp.)

Drugs and Chemicals

• Estrogen (exogenous administration, Sertoli and interstitial cell tumors). • Methimazole (cats). • Chemotherapeutic drugs, including azathioprine, cyclophosphamide, cytosine arabinoside, doxorubicin, vinblastine, and hydroxyurea. • Antibiotics, including trimethoprim–sulfadiazine, cephalosporins, and chloramphenicol. • Griseofulvin.
• Nonsteroidal anti-inflammatory drugs (NSAIDs), including phenylbutazone and meclofenamic acid. • Fenbendazole, albendazole. • Captopril. • Quinidine.
• Thiacetarsamide. • Ionizing radiation.
• Mycotoxins (cats).

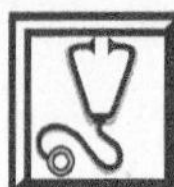

DIAGNOSIS

DIFFERENTIAL DIAGNOSIS

Causes of pancytopenia with normal to increased bone marrow cellularity (e.g., myelodysplastic syndromes, leukemias, myelofibrosis).

CBC/BIOCHEMISTRY/URINALYSIS

• Leukopenia characterized by neutropenia with or without lymphopenia. • Normocytic, normochromic, nonregenerative anemia.
• Thrombocytopenia.

OTHER LABORATORY TESTS

• Immunologic tests for infectious diseases, e.g., serologic titers, ELISA, immunofluorescent antibody (IFA).
• PCR for infectious agents. • Positive tests for antierythrocyte antibodies (Coombs' test) and/or antinuclear antibody (ANA) may indicate immune-mediated mechanisms.

IMAGING

N/A

DIAGNOSTIC PROCEDURES

• Bone marrow aspiration—frequently an inadequate or fatty sample is obtained because of decreased hematopoietic tissue and replacement by adipocytes. • Bone marrow core biopsy—permits an evaluation of architecture and reveals hypoplasia of cell lines and replacement by adipose tissue.

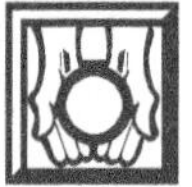

TREATMENT

Supportive treatment, antibiotics, blood component therapy, as dictated by clinical condition and results of infectious disease testing.

MEDICATIONS

DRUG(S) OF CHOICE

• Cyclosporine A—10–25 mg/kg PO q12h (dogs), 4–5 mg/kg PO q12h (cats).
• Mycophenolate mofetil—10 mg/kg PO/IV q12h. • Recombinant hematopoietic growth factors, e.g., recombinant human granulocyte colony-stimulating factor (rhG-CSF) 5 µg/kg/day SC. • Androgen and corticosteroid administration have been largely unsuccessful.

Other Drugs

• Antibiotics to treat secondary infections if fever and neutropenia present. • Whole or component blood transfusion if indicated.

CONTRAINDICATIONS/POSSIBLE INTERACTIONS

N/A

FOLLOW-UP

PATIENT MONITORING

• Daily physical examination. • CBC every 3–5 days. • Repeat bone marrow evaluation if necessary.

PREVENTION/AVOIDANCE

• Castration of cryptorchid males (to prevent development of Sertoli or interstitial cell tumors). • Vaccination for infectious diseases.
• Frequent monitoring of CBC in cancer patients receiving chemotherapy or radiation.

POSSIBLE COMPLICATIONS

• Sepsis. • Hemorrhage.

EXPECTED COURSE AND PROGNOSIS

• Guarded to poor. • Recovery of hematopoiesis may take weeks to months, if it occurs at all. • Spontaneous recovery occasionally occurs, especially in younger animals.

MISCELLANEOUS

SEE ALSO

Pancytopenia.

ABBREVIATIONS

• ANA = antinuclear antibody.
• FeLV = feline leukemia virus.
• FIV = feline immunodeficiency virus.
• IFA = immunofluorescent antibody (test).
• NSAID = nonsteroidal anti-inflammatory drug.
• rhG-CSF = recombinant human granulocyte colony-stimulating factor.

Suggested Reading

Brazzell JL, Weiss DJ. A retrospective study of aplastic pancytopenia in the dog: 9 cases (1996–2003). Vet Clin Path 2006, 35:413–417.

Weiss DJ. Aplastic anemia. In: Weiss DJ, Wardrop KJ, eds., Schalm's Veterinary Hematology, 6th ed. Ames, IA: Blackwell, 2010, pp. 256–260.

Author R. Darren Wood

Consulting Editor Melinda S. Camus

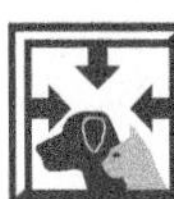

BASICS

OVERVIEW

• Heinz bodies occur in red blood cells (RBCs) following damage from chemical or dietary oxidants, can cause hemolytic anemia. • When oxidants overwhelm protective reductive pathways in RBCs, denaturation of hemoglobin (Hb) causes precipitation and attachment to cell membrane. • RBCs with Heinz bodies are removed by splenic macrophages, and occasionally undergo intravascular lysis, forming ghost cells. • The spleen may occasionally remove Heinz bodies, resulting in spherocytes. • Cats more susceptible to Heinz body formation because have less reductive enzymatic capacity and closed splenic circulation, preventing macrophages from removing Heinz bodies. • Healthy cats may have low numbers of Heinz bodies without anemia. • Heinz bodies reported in patients with hyperthyroidism, lymphoma, and diabetes mellitus. • Heinz bodies may be accompanied by methemoglobinemia (Hb containing Fe^{3+}) and/or eccentrocytes (indicating oxidative damage to RBC membranes).

SIGNALMENT

No species, sex, breed, or age disposition.

SIGNS

Historical Findings

• Oxidant exposure. • Sudden onset of weakness, lethargy, or anorexia secondary to anemia. • Signs related to underlying disease if present.

Physical Examination Findings

• Pale, occasionally icteric mucous membranes, dark or chocolate-colored if methemoglobinemia. • Tachypnea, tachycardia.

CAUSES & RISK FACTORS

• Dietary—onions (raw, cooked, dehydrated, powdered), garlic, propylene glycol (cats).
• Drugs—acetaminophen, phenacetin (cats), phenazopyridine (cats), methylene blue, vitamin K1 or K3 (dogs), DL-methionine (cats), benzocaine, phenylhydrazine (dogs), propofol (cats). • Miscellaneous—zinc (bolts, pennies minted after 1982, dermatologic or sun creams), naphthalene (mothballs), skunk musk.

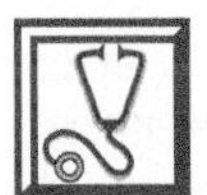

DIAGNOSIS

DIFFERENTIAL DIAGNOSIS

Immune-mediated or hemoparasitic hemolysis.

CBC/BIOCHEMISTRY/URINALYSIS

• Diagnosis of Heinz body anemia requires regenerative anemia, evidence of hemolytic process, presence of Heinz bodies in peripheral blood, and elimination of other causes of hemolysis or blood loss. • Regenerative anemia; severity depends on dose and duration of oxidant exposure. • Hb concentration and mean corpuscular hemoglobin concentration (MCHC) may be falsely increased due to Heinz body interference with measurement. • Heinz bodies on routinely stained blood smear appear as small, nonstaining to pale red, round inclusions that may protrude from RBC surface. • Single, small (<0.5 µm) Heinz bodies may be found in cats without anemia, but large or multiple Heinz bodies in anemic cat suggest hemolytic anemia. • Dogs may have concurrent eccentrocytosis.
• Hyperbilirubinemia, bilirubinuria, hemoglobinemia, and hemoglobinuria possible with intravascular hemolysis.

OTHER LABORATORY TESTS

• New methylene blue stains Heinz bodies blue, making them easy to identify and quantify on a blood smear. • Measure methemoglobin or perform spot test if blood is dark or chocolate-colored. • Serum zinc concentration.

IMAGING

Abdominal radiographs may reveal metallic foreign bodies contributing to zinc toxicity.

DIAGNOSTIC PROCEDURES

N/A

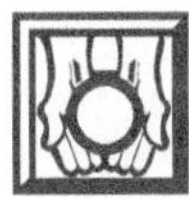

TREATMENT

• Immediate identification and removal of oxidant may be sufficient, though often takes several days after exposure for severity of anemia to reach nadir. • Treatment depends on severity and may include IV fluids, RBC transfusions, oxygen, and restricted activity.
• Endoscopy or surgery to remove metallic items in gastrointestinal tract.

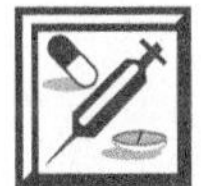

MEDICATIONS

DRUG(S) OF CHOICE

• Acetaminophen toxicity in cats—N-acetylcysteine (Mucomyst®) 140 mg/kg PO/IV, followed by seven additional treatments of 70 mg/kg PO/IV q8h). • Ascorbic acid (vitamin C) 30 mg/kg PO q6-12h, to reduce methemoglobin concentrations.

Alternative Drug(s)

Use of dietary antioxidants (e.g., bioflavonoids) is controversial, but may help prevent further formation of Heinz bodies.

CONTRAINDICATIONS/POSSIBLE INTERACTIONS

Administration of methylene blue to treat methemoglobinemia may exacerbate Heinz body formation.

FOLLOW-UP

PATIENT MONITORING

Serial CBCs and review of blood smears to assess RBC regeneration and disappearance of Heinz bodies.

PREVENTION/AVOIDANCE

Counsel clients about identifying and preventing exposure to oxidant compounds.

POSSIBLE COMPLICATIONS

Without proper treatment and removal of oxidant, condition can be fatal.

EXPECTED COURSE AND PROGNOSIS

Prognosis is good with removal of oxidant and supportive care once hemolytic crisis is over.

MISCELLANEOUS

SEE ALSO

- Acetaminophen (APAP) Toxicosis.
- Methemoglobinemia.
- Zinc Toxicosis.

ABBREVIATIONS

- Hb = hemoglobin.
- MCHC = mean corpuscular hemoglobin concentration.
- RBC = red blood cell.

Suggested Reading

Andrews D. Disorders of red blood cells. In: Handbook of Small Animal Practice, 5th ed. St. Louis, MO: Saunders, 2008, pp. 632–635.

Desnoyers M. Anemias associated with oxidative injury. In: Schalm's Veterinary Hematology, 6th ed. Ames, IA: Blackwell, 2010, pp. 239–245.

Author Melinda S. Camus

Consulting Editor Melinda S. Camus

Acknowledgment The author and book editors acknowledge the prior contribution of Jennifer S. Thomas.

A

ANEMIA, IMMUNE-MEDIATED

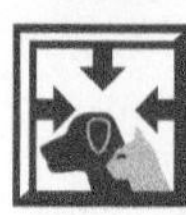

BASICS

DEFINITION

Accelerated removal or hemolysis of red blood cells (RBCs) due to a type II hypersensitivity reaction.

PATHOPHYSIOLOGY

• Antibodies form against endogenous RBC antigens (primary/nonassociative immune-mediated hemolytic anemia [IMHA]), or RBC membrane antigens, or antigens altered by infectious organisms, drugs, or neoplasia (secondary/associative IMHA).
• Immunoglobulin deposited on RBC membrane, causing either direct intravascular hemolysis or accelerated extravascular removal by monocyte/macrophage system. • Intravascular hemolysis occurs when adsorbed antibodies (especially immunoglobulin [Ig] M) activate complement. • Extravascular removal of RBCs occurs when RBCs coated with antibodies (especially IgG) are engulfed by splenic macrophages. • RBC agglutination occurs when IgM or high titers of IgG causes RBC bridging. • Nonregenerative IMHA caused by immune-mediated destruction of RBC precursors in bone marrow.

SYSTEMS AFFECTED

• Hemic/lymphatic/immune—destruction of RBCs, release of proinflammatory mediators, disseminated intravascular coagulation (DIC).
• Cardiovascular—signs of anemia, thromboembolism. • Hepatobiliary—hyperbilirubinemia, icterus, bilirubinuria; centrilobular necrosis. • Respiratory—tachypnea (secondary to anemia or inflammation), hypoxemia (pulmonary thromboembolism [PTE]). • Integument—rare: cold-type IMHA causes necrosis of extremities and ear tips.

GENETICS

Cocker spaniels are at increased risk.

INCIDENCE/PREVALENCE

Most common hemolytic anemia of dogs, relatively rare in cats.

GEOGRAPHIC DISTRIBUTION

Secondary IMHA may have higher prevalence where associated infectious diseases endemic; incidence may vary seasonally.

SIGNALMENT

Species

Dog and cat.

Breed Predilections

• Cocker spaniel, English springer spaniel, Old English sheepdog, Doberman pinscher, collie, bichon frise, miniature pinscher, Finnish spitz. • Domestic shorthair cats.

Mean Age and Range

• Dogs—mean age 5–6 years (range: 1–13 years). • Cats—mean age 2 years (range: 0.5–9 years).

Predominant Sex

• Female dogs at higher risk. • Male cats overrepresented.

SIGNS

Historical Findings

• Lethargy/weakness/collapse. • Anorexia.
• Dyspnea, tachypnea. • Vomiting and/or diarrhea. • Pigmenturia. • Pica (cats).

Physical Examination Findings

• Pale mucous membranes, tachycardia, tachypnea. • Splenomegaly/hepatomegaly.
• Icterus and pigmenturia (hemoglobin or bilirubin). • Fever/lymphadenopathy.
• Systolic heart murmur. • Petechiae, ecchymoses, or melena (if concurrent thrombocytopenia or DIC). • Other findings possible (e.g., joint pain) when IMHA is component of systemic lupus erythematosus (SLE). • Necrosis of extremities and ear tips in cold-type IMHA (rare).

CAUSES & RISK FACTORS

Primary IMHA

Poorly characterized immune dysregulation.

Secondary IMHA

• Infectious causes—hemotrophic *Mycoplasma* spp., *Ehrlichia* spp., *Anaplasma phagocytophilum*, *Anaplasma platys*, *Babesia* spp., *Leishmaniasis*, *Dirofilaria immitis*, feline leukemia virus (FeLV), feline immunodeficiency virus (FIV), chronic bacterial infection. • Neoplasia—lymphoma, lymphoid leukemia, hemangiosarcoma, hemophagic histiocytic sarcoma. • Drugs—penicillins, cephalosporins, propylthiouracil, methimazole, sulfonamides. • SLE.
• Neonatal isoerythrolysis. • Dog erythrocyte antigen (DEA) incompatible blood transfusion.
• Vaccination, surgery, hormonal changes, or other stressful events hypothesized as potential triggers.

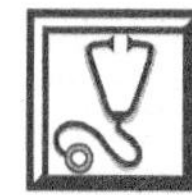

DIAGNOSIS

DIFFERENTIAL DIAGNOSIS

Dogs

• Toxicity (zinc, onions, garlic, naphthalene, skunk musk). • Snake/spider envenomation (coral snakes, recluse spiders). • Severe hypophosphatemia. • Anemia due to hemorrhage, hemoperitoneum.
• Microangiopathic anemia due to splenic neoplasia or torsion. • Pyruvate kinase or phosphofructokinase deficiency.

Cats

• Toxicity (acetaminophen, zinc, onions, garlic). • Severe hypophosphatemia.
• Congenital feline porphyria. • Increased osmotic fragility (Abyssinian, Somali).

CBC/BIOCHEMISTRY/URINALYSIS

• CBC—anemia, normal to high mean cell volume (MCV), spherocytosis, polychromasia, ghost cells, leukocytosis with neutrophilia and left shift, monocytosis; anemia nonregenerative in 30% of dogs and 50% of cats. • Serum biochemistry—hyperbilirubinemia, high alanine aminotransferase (ALT). • Urinalysis—hemoglobinuria, bilirubinuria.

OTHER LABORATORY TESTS

• Positive saline agglutination test. • Direct antiglobulin (Coombs') test—positive in up to 75% of animals with IMHA.
• Reticulocytosis if regenerative.
• Thrombocytopenia—60% of dogs.
• Prolonged activated partial thromboplastin time (APTT), ± prolonged prothrombin time (PT), increased fibrin degradation products (FDP) and d-dimer, decreased antithrombin in animals with DIC. • Blood smear—evidence of hematologic parasites.
• Infectious disease testing—especially *Babesia* spp. (serology, PCR), *Mycoplasma hemofelis* (PCR), other vector-borne pathogens.

IMAGING

Abdominal radiography, ultrasonography—hepatomegaly/splenomegaly, neoplasia.

DIAGNOSTIC PROCEDURES

Bone marrow aspirate to identify nonregenerative (RBC precursor-directed) IMHA or myelofibrosis in chronic cases.

PATHOLOGIC FINDINGS

• Hepatosplenomegaly, centrilobular hepatic necrosis. • Splenic and hepatic extramedullary hematopoiesis. • PTE and DIC.

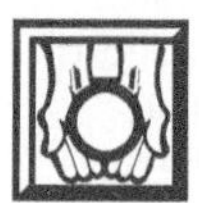

TREATMENT

APPROPRIATE HEALTH CARE

• Inpatient intensive care during acute hemolytic crisis and if complications such as DIC, PTE, thrombocytopenia, gastrointestinal (GI) bleeding, or need for multiple transfusions occur.
• Outpatient when PCV stable, hemolysis controlled, and clinical signs of anemia resolved.

NURSING CARE

• Fluid therapy as needed. • Packed RBCs (or whole blood), fresh frozen plasma (FFP) if coagulopathic. • Oxygen therapy as needed.
• Monitor for complications.

ACTIVITY

Cage rest.

DIET

N/A

CLIENT EDUCATION

• IMHA can be fatal and difficult to treat, with guarded prognosis. • Lifelong maintenance therapy may be needed; side effects may be severe. • Disease may recur.

SURGICAL CONSIDERATIONS

Splenectomy can be considered if medical management fails.

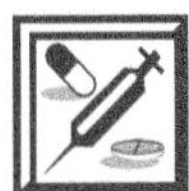

MEDICATIONS

DRUG(S) OF CHOICE

• Corticosteroids—prednisone 2–3 mg/kg/day PO; dexamethasone sodium phosphate (0.2–0.4 mg/kg IV q24h) can be used in patients unable to take oral medication.
• Adjunctive immunosuppressants (if poor response to corticosteroids or to avoid side effects of prednisone)—cyclosporine 5 mg/kg PO q12h, cats: 0.5–3 mg/kg PO q12h; mycophenolate mofetil 8–12 mg/kg PO/IV q12h; azathioprine 2 mg/kg PO q24h, can decrease to 0.5–1.0 mg/kg PO q48h after 3 weeks or if bone marrow suppression occurs, monitor for side effects; *do not use in cats.*
• Once PCV above 30%, decrease prednisone dosage to 1 mg/kg PO q12h; then taper by maximum rate of 25–50% per month over 3–6-month period, depending upon PCV and severity of side effects; additional immunosuppressant drugs may be tapered as well. • For prevention of thromboembolism consider unfractionated heparin 150–300 U/kg SC q6–8h (dose adjusted based on APTT prolongation or measurement of anti-Xa activity) and/or clopidogrel 1–2 mg/kg PO q24h; low molecular weight heparins (enoxaparin 0.8 mg/kg SC q6–8h or dalteparin 150 U/kg SC q8h) or rivaroxaban (0.5–1.0 mg/kg PO q24h) may be considered in lieu of unfractionated heparin. • Address underlying cause (secondary IMHA).
• Therapeutic plasma exchange/plasmapheresis may be useful adjunctive therapy.

CONTRAINDICATIONS

Anticoagulant medications should be used cautiously in patients with thrombocytopenia (<40,000 platelets/µL).

PRECAUTIONS

• Prednisone/prednisolone can cause signs of hyperadrenocorticism and may increase risk of PTE, pancreatitis, diabetes mellitus, secondary infection, gastric ulcers (consider gastric protectants). • Immunosuppressive drugs can cause bone marrow suppression, secondary infection, pancreatitis (azathioprine), GI upset (cyclosporine, azathioprine, mycophenolate mofetil), gingival hyperplasia, papillomatosis (cyclosporine), infertility.

ALTERNATIVE DRUG(S)

• Chlorambucil—for cats, 0.1–0.2 mg/kg PO q24h initially, then q48h. • Human IV immunoglobulin (hIVIG; 0.5–1 g/kg IV) in dogs not responding to other therapies.

FOLLOW-UP

PATIENT MONITORING

• Monitor heart rate, respiratory rate, body temperature frequently. • Monitor for adverse reactions to treatment. • If PTE suspected, CT angiography indicated for diagnosis; oxygenation can be assessed with pulse oximetry or arterial blood gas analysis.
• Initially, check packed cell volume (PCV) daily until stable, then every 1–2 weeks for 2 months; if still stable, recheck monthly for 6 months, then 2–4 times/year. • CBC and reticulocyte count at least monthly; if neutrophil count falls <3,000 cells/µL, discontinue cytotoxic drugs until count recovers; reinstitute at lower dosage.

PREVENTION/AVOIDANCE

Consider need for vaccination on case-by-case basis in dogs with IMHA; measurement of titers prior to elective vaccinations may be indicated.

POSSIBLE COMPLICATIONS

• Pulmonary/multiorgan thromboembolism.
• DIC. • Centrilobular hepatic necrosis and renal tubular necrosis secondary to hypoxia.
• Infection secondary to immunosuppressive therapy. • GI ulceration due to high-dose glucocorticoids. • Iatrogenic hyperadrenocorticism.

EXPECTED COURSE AND PROGNOSIS

• Mortality—30–70% (dog), 24% (cat).
• Hyperbilirubinemia >5 mg/dL, autoagglutination, intravascular hemolysis, severe thrombocytopenia, hypoalbuminemia associated with poorer prognosis. • Response to treatment may take weeks to months; nonregenerative IMHA may have more gradual onset than typical IMHA and be slower to respond to treatment. Most patients receive immunosuppressive therapy for 4–8 months.

MISCELLANEOUS

ASSOCIATED CONDITIONS

See above.

ZOONOTIC POTENTIAL

None

SYNONYMS

• Autoimmune hemolytic anemia.
• Immune-mediated anemia.

SEE ALSO

• Anemia, Regenerative.
• Cold Agglutinin Disease.

ABBREVIATIONS

• ALT = alanine aminotransferase.
• APTT = activated partial thromboplastin time.
• DEA = dog erythrocyte antigen.
• DIC = disseminated intravascular coagulation.
• FDP = fibrin degradation products.
• FeLV = feline leukemia virus.
• FFP = fresh frozen plasma.
• FIV = feline immunodeficiency virus.
• GI = gastrointestinal.
• hIVIG = human IV immunoglobulin.
• Ig = immunoglobulin.
• IMHA = immune-mediated hemolytic anemia.
• MCV = mean cell volume.
• PCV = packed cell volume.
• PT = prothrombin time.
• PTE = pulmonary thromboembolism.
• RBC = red blood cell.
• SLE = systemic lupus erythematosus.

Suggested Reading

Garden OA, Kidd L, Mexas AM, et al. ACVIM consensus statement on the diagnosis of immune-mediated hemolytic anemia in dogs and cats. J Vet Intern Med 2019, 33(2):313–334.

Kohn B, Weingart C, Eckmann V, et al. Primary immune-mediated hemolytic anemia in 19 cats: diagnosis, therapy, and outcome (1998–2004). J Vet Intern Med 2006, 20:159–166.

Swann JW, Garden OA, Fellman CL, et al. ACVIM consensus statement on the treatment of immune-mediated hemolytic anemia in dogs. J Vet Intern Med 2019, 33(3):1141–1172.

Author Bridget C. Garner

Consulting Editor Melinda S. Camus

Acknowledgment The author and book editors acknowledge the prior contribution of J. Catharine R. Scott-Moncrieff.

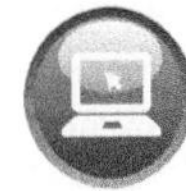

Client Education Handout available online

ANEMIA, IRON-DEFICIENCY

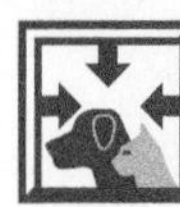

BASICS

OVERVIEW

Caused by chronic external blood loss or iron-limited erythropoiesis.

SIGNALMENT

- Fairly common in adult dogs, rare in adult cats.
- Transient neonatal iron-deficiency anemia may occur at 5–10 weeks of age in kittens.

SIGNS

- Signs of anemia (e.g., lethargy, weakness, tachypnea, pale mucous membranes).
- Cardiovascular—bounding pulses, tachycardia, systolic heart murmur.
- Gastrointestinal—intermittent melena or hematochezia, diarrhea.
- Integumentary—heavy hematophagous parasite burden (e.g., fleas), wounds.

CAUSES & RISK FACTORS

- Chronic external blood loss.
- Gastrointestinal—hookworms, lymphoma or other neoplasia, ulceration (related to medications, [e.g., non-steroidal anti-inflammatories] or disease [e.g., renal disease]).
- Less common—severe flea infestation, urinary tract hemorrhage.
- Iatrogenic—blood donor overuse, excessive diagnostic blood sampling.
- Inappropriate home-cooked diet (low dietary iron).

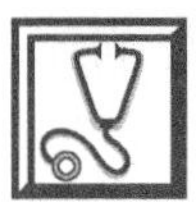

DIAGNOSIS

DIFFERENTIAL DIAGNOSIS

- Any cause of anemia, especially hemorrhage.
- Microcytic anemia in portosystemic shunt disease may or may not be due to iron deficiency.
- Anemia of inflammatory disease—iron-limited erythropoiesis.

CBC/BIOCHEMISTRY/URINALYSIS

- Packed cell volume (PCV) variably decreased; may be within reference interval.
- Regenerative or nonregenerative anemia.
- Microcytosis—low normal or low mean cell volume (MCV), low mean reticulocyte volume (MCVr), anisocytosis, widened erythrocyte histogram, or increased red cell distribution width (RDW). Decreased mean cell hemoglobin concentration (MCHC) not sensitive or specific.
- Red blood cell (RBC) morphology—microcytosis, hypochromia, keratocyte (indicating oxidative damage), and schistocyte formation.
- Reticulocyte indices reticulocyte corpuscular hemoglobin concentration mean (CHCMr), reticulocyte hemoglobin content (CHr), hypochromic reticulocyte RBCs (%HYPOr), and %LowCHr are sensitive for detecting iron-limited erythropoiesis, but not specific.
- Lab tests indicating iron-limited erythropoiesis do not differentiate true from functional iron deficiency. Clinical findings of inflammatory disease are required to differentiate iron-limited erythropoiesis. Inflammatory disease and true iron deficiency may also occur concurrently.
- Thrombocytosis due to chronic blood loss.
- Hypoproteinemia—from blood loss.

OTHER LABORATORY TESTS

- Hypoferremia (serum iron <70 μg/dL) and transferrin saturation <15% support diagnosis.
- Serum iron values may be normal during iron repletion if blood loss is intermittent.
- Fecal exam for hookworms.
- Fecal examination for occult blood or melena.

IMAGING

Abdominal radiography, ultrasonography—abnormalities in gastrointestinal tract causing blood loss.

DIAGNOSTIC PROCEDURES

- Bone marrow aspirate, staining with Prussian blue (dogs only) to indicate body iron stores.
- Gastrointestinal endoscopy to identify sites of gastrointestinal blood loss.

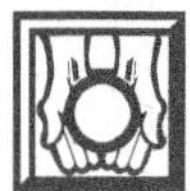

TREATMENT

- Identify/correct cause of blood loss, treat underlying disease.
- Administer iron until hematologic features of iron deficiency resolve.
- If severe anemia (i.e., PCV <15%), transfusion may be required, using whole blood (10–30 mL/kg IV) or packed RBC (10 mL/kg IV).

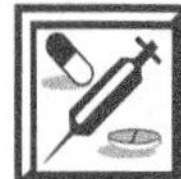

MEDICATIONS

DRUG(S) OF CHOICE

Parenteral Iron Supplementation

- Iron therapy should begin with injectable iron.
- Iron dextran—10–20 mg/kg IM (dog), 50 mg IM (cat), followed by oral supplementation.

Oral Iron Supplementation—Dogs Only

- Animals with severe iron deficiency may have impaired intestinal iron absorption, making oral therapy of little value until partial iron repletion has occurred.
- Oral iron supplementation should continue 1–2 months, or until resolved.
- Ferrous sulfate powder—place in food or drinking water, 100–300 mg PO q24h.
- Ferrous gluconate—325 mg PO q24h.

CONTRAINDICATIONS/POSSIBLE INTERACTIONS

- Oral iron is associated with unexplained death in kittens and should be avoided.
- Kittens undergo spontaneous iron replection beginning at 5–6 weeks of age.

FOLLOW-UP

- Monitor CBC every 1–4 weeks, more frequently as needed.
- Effective treatment associated with an increase in MCV and reticulocyte volume.
- Erythrocyte histogram—effective treatment reduces microcytic subpopulation over time (2–3 months).

MISCELLANEOUS

ABBREVIATIONS

- CHCMr = mean reticulocyte corpuscular hemoglobin concentration.
- CHr = reticulocyte hemoglobin content.
- HYPOr = hypochromic reticulocyte RBCs.
- MCHC = mean cell hemoglobin concentration.
- MCV = mean cell volume.
- MCVr = mean reticulocyte volume.
- PCV = packed cell volume.
- RBC = red blood cell.
- RDW = red cell distribution width.

Suggested Reading

Fry MM, Kirk CA. Reticulocyte indices in a canine model of nutritional iron deficiency. Vet Clin Pathol 2006, 35:172–181.

Radakovich LB, Santangelo KS, Olver CS. Reticulocyte hemoglobin content (CHr) does not differentiate true from functional iron deficiency in dogs. Vet Clin Pathol 2015, 44:511–518.

Schaefer DM, Stokol T. The utility of reticulocyte indices in distinguishing iron deficiency anemia from anemia of inflammatory disease, portosystemic shunting, and breed-associated microcytosis in dogs. Vet Clin Pathol 2015, 44:109–119.

Authors Glade Weiser and Melinda S. Camus
Consulting Editor Melinda S. Camus

ANEMIA, NONREGENERATIVE

BASICS

DEFINITION

Low red blood cell (RBC) mass due to low erythroid production, without evidence of polychromasia or reticulocytosis in peripheral blood. Anemia with reticulocyte counts <80 × 10^3/µL (dog) or 60 × 10^3/µL (cat) considered nonregenerative. Caused by altered erythropoiesis or bone marrow injury.

PATHOPHYSIOLOGY

• Alterations in erythropoiesis include deficient erythropoietin (EPO) production, nutritional deficiency, cytokine-mediated iron sequestration, disturbed metabolism in or destruction of RBC precursors (e.g., immune-mediated).
• Bone marrow injury usually caused by toxins, infection, or infiltrative processes.
• Anemia of inflammatory disease results from increased hepcidin production and release of cytokines from white blood cells (WBCs) leading to iron sequestration and decreased iron absorption. Low serum iron and transferrin, increased ferritin, decreased EPO production, shortened RBC lifespan result in anemia.

SYSTEMS AFFECTED

• Cardiovascular—shock from decreased systemic oxygen delivery.
• Hemic/lymph/immune.
• Hepatobiliary—from hypoxic injury.

SIGNALMENT

• Nonregenerative immune-mediated hemolytic anemia (IMHA)—middle-aged female dogs and male cats <3 years old.
• Congenital cobalamin malabsorption reported in Komondor, beagle, giant schnauzer, Australian shepherd, border collie, shar-pei.

SIGNS

General Comments

Usually secondary; signs associated with primary disease often precede signs of anemia.

Historical Findings

• Lethargy, exercise intolerance, inappetence, pica.
• Other findings reflect primary condition—polyuria/polydipsia (chronic kidney disease [CKD]), old paint exposure (lead poisoning), estrogen therapy or feminization in male dogs, failure to thrive (hereditary cobalamin malabsorption).

Physical Examination Findings

• Pallor, heart murmur (due to anemia), tachycardia, tachypnea, shock.
• Digital rectal examination may reveal melena if gastrointestinal (GI) blood loss.
• Signs reflecting primary condition—oral ulcerations (CKD), cachexia, organomegaly, GI or nervous system abnormalities (cobalamin malabsorption, lead poisoning), symmetric alopecia (hypothyroidism, hyperestrogenism).

CAUSES

Nonregenerative Anemia without Other Cytopenias

• Anemia of inflammatory disease (AID)—most common cause of mild nonregenerative anemia (also anemia of chronic disease).
• CKD—decreased EPO production by kidneys; uremic toxins shorten RBC lifespan and impair bone marrow response to EPO.
• Chronic liver disease—shortened RBC survival due to changes in RBC membrane lipids; functional iron deficiency due to decreased transferrin synthesis and impaired mobilization of hepatic iron.
• Hypothyroidism, hypoadrenocorticism—thyroid hormones and cortisol stimulate erythropoiesis.
• Immune-mediated destruction of precursors—spectrum from nonregenerative IMHA to pure red cell aplasia.

Nutritional or Mineral Deficiency/Toxicity

• Iron deficiency—usually due to chronic external blood loss.
• Copper deficiency—secondary to chelation therapy.
• Cobalamin (vitamin B_{12}) and/or folate deficiency—rare; can be caused by dietary insufficiency, malabsorption, congenital defects in cobalamin absorption.
• Disruption of precursor metabolism—chronic lead toxicity and possibly high concentrations of aluminum, arsenic, and cadmium inhibit heme synthesis; cadmium and lead cause renal toxicity, impaired EPO production.

Nonregenerative Anemia with Other Cytopenias

• Toxicities—drugs or chemicals, hormones (e.g., estrogen).
• Infections—feline leukemia virus (FeLV), feline immunodeficiency virus (FIV), ehrlichiosis, babesiosis, *Cytauxzoon felis*, parvovirus (occasionally just erythroid line affected).
• Infiltrative processes—myelodysplasia, myeloproliferative and lymphoproliferative diseases, histiocytic sarcoma, metastatic neoplasia, myelofibrosis, osteosclerosis.

RISK FACTORS

• CKD.
• Inflammatory or chronic disease.
• Multicat household/cattery (infectious disease risk).
• Daily exposure to toxins (e.g., old homes with lead paint, environmental pollution).

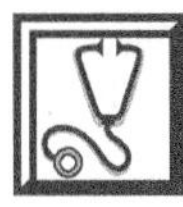

DIAGNOSIS

DIFFERENTIAL DIAGNOSIS

Regenerative anemia can initially appear nonregenerative (especially in cats); exacerbation of chronic condition may produce appearance of acute onset.

CBC/BIOCHEMISTRY/URINALYSIS

CBC and Blood Smear

• Packed cell volume (PCV), hematocrit (HCT), RBC count, and hemoglobin concentration low.
• Anemia usually normocytic, normochromic, with normal mean cell volume (MCV) and mean corpuscular hemoglobin concentration (MCHC); occasionally severe vitamin B_{12} deficiency; characteristic large erythrocytes can be masked by presence of misshapen and/or small RBCs, giving normal MCV but widened red cell distribution.
• Macrocytosis (high MCV)—without polychromasia suggests nuclear maturation defect; seen in cats with FeLV.
• Microcytosis suggests maturation complete; iron deficiency most common cause; in late stages concurrent hypochromasia common in dogs.
• Characteristic RBC morphologies—schistocytes ± hypochromic RBCs common with iron deficiency; acanthocytes with liver disease; target cells with iron deficiency, liver disease, hypothyroidism.
• Inflammatory leukogram supports AID.
• Thrombocytosis common in iron deficiency.
• High number of nucleated red blood cells (NRBCs) without polychromasia or disproportionate to degree of anemia and polychromasia seen with lead toxicity, extramedullary hematopoiesis (EMH), heat stroke, bone marrow injury.
• RBC or WBC precursors in peripheral blood without orderly progression to more mature forms suggest myelodysplasia or myeloproliferative disease.
• Cobalamin malabsorption characterized by normocytic anemia, neutropenia, hypersegmented neutrophils; megaloblastic changes possible in marrow.
• RBC inclusions may be visible on blood smear with some infectious diseases (e.g., *C. felis*).

Serum Biochemistry and Urinalysis

• CKD—azotemia with isosthenuria, possible proteinuria, hypokalemia.
• Liver disease—elevated alanine aminotransferase (ALT) ± alkaline phosphatase (ALP) activities, elevated total bilirubin, bile acids, ammonia concentrations, hypoglycemia, hypoalbuminemia.
• Hypothyroidism—hypercholesterolemia (>500 mg/dL).

- Hypoadrenocorticism—hyponatremia, hyperkalemia, lymphocytosis, eosinophilia.

OTHER LABORATORY TESTS

- Reticulocyte count.
- Spherocytosis, autoagglutination, or positive Coombs' test supports immune-mediated destruction of erythroid precursors.
- Serum iron profile—with iron deficiency both serum iron and ferritin low, while total iron-binding capacity varies; with AID, serum iron low but serum ferritin high.
- Serum lead—indicated when NRBCs present; >30 µL/dL (0.3 ppm) strongly supports lead intoxication.
- Serologic testing—FeLV, FIV in cats; *Ehrlichia canis*, *Anaplasma phagocytophilia* in dogs, particularly if anemia with thrombocytopenia.
- Endocrine testing—adrenocorticotropic hormone (ACTH) stimulation test or thyroid function testing to rule out hypoadrenocorticism or hypothyroidism, respectively.
- Serum cobalamin, homocysteine, methylmalonic acid ± urine methylmalonic acid concentrations—to diagnose hereditary cobalamin malabsorption.

DIAGNOSTIC PROCEDURES

Cytologic Examination of Bone Marrow and Core Biopsy

- Cytologic examination of bone marrow aspirate indicated in all patients unless primary cause apparent, and bone marrow core biopsy useful in evaluation of bone marrow architecture and overall cellularity.
- Erythroid hypoplasia or aplasia confirms pure red cell aplasia; erythroid hyperplasia suggests IMHA; increased erythrophagia or incomplete maturation sequence suggests immune-mediated or toxic injury to specific maturation stage, or incomplete recovery from previous injury.
- Expanded erythron and high numbers of metarubricytes suggest iron deficiency; absence of iron stores supportive in dogs, but not cats.
- Disorderly maturation and atypical cellular morphology suggest myelodysplastic syndrome.
- Hypercellular marrow with increased blast cells consistent with hematopoietic neoplasia; immunophenotyping can identify affected cell line.
- Hypocellular sample can suggest aplastic marrow or myelofibrosis.

Abdominal Radiographs, Ultrasound

As part of evaluation for underlying causes such as neoplasia, CKD, or GI blood loss.

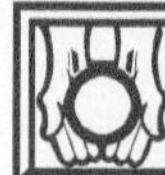

TREATMENT

- Anemia usually resolves with resolution of underlying disease.
- Conditions associated with severe anemia or pancytopenia often carry guarded to poor prognosis and may involve long-term treatment with incomplete resolution.
- Mild to moderate anemia (PCV >20%) generally requires no immediate supportive intervention.
- Patients with severe anemia (PCV <12–15%) require transfusion for stabilization (e.g., 6–10 mL/kg packed RBCs or 10–20 mL/kg whole blood).
- Determine blood type prior to transfusion (imperative for cats, ideal for dogs).
- If blood volume and tissue perfusion compromised by concurrent blood loss or shock, administer isotonic crystalloid solution (10–20 mL/kg IV, repeat as necessary) or isotonic colloid solution (2–5 mL/kg IV, to total 20 mL/kg/24h). See Shock, Hypovolemic.
- With chronic anemia, animals may be hypervolemic, and volume overload may be a concern during blood and fluid therapy.

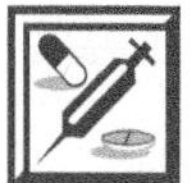

MEDICATIONS

DRUG(S) OF CHOICE

- EPO or darbopoetin in patients with anemia of CKD.
- Iron supplementation in patients with iron deficiency anemia.
- Immunosuppressive drugs.
- May supplement with cobalamin (vitamin B_{12}) at rate of 100–200 mg PO q24h (dogs) or 50–100 mg PO q24h (cats); parenteral cyanocobalamin administration (50 µg/kg SC/IM weekly to monthly) needed in dogs with inherited cobalamin malabsorption.

PRECAUTIONS

Monitor for transfusion reactions.

FOLLOW-UP

PATIENT MONITORING

- With severe anemia—serial physical examinations, PCV/CBC, blood smear examination every 1–2 days.
- Stable animals with chronic or slowly improving disease course—reevaluate every 1–2 weeks.

MISCELLANEOUS

PREGNANCY/FERTILITY/BREEDING

Pregnant animals have mildly low PCV.

SEE ALSO

- Anemia, Immune-Mediated.
- Anemia, Iron-Deficiency.
- Blood Transfusion Reactions.
- Shock, Hypovolemic.

ABBREVIATIONS

- ACTH = adrenocorticotropic hormone.
- AID = anemia of inflammatory disease.
- ALP = alkaline phosphatase.
- ALT = alanine aminotransferase.
- CKD = chronic kidney disease.
- EMH = extramedullary hematopoiesis.
- EPO = erythropoietin.
- FeLV = feline leukemia virus.
- FIV = feline immunodeficiency virus.
- GI = gastrointestinal.
- HCT = hematocrit.
- IMHA = immune-mediated hemolytic anemia.
- MCHC = mean corpuscular hemoglobin concentration.
- MCV = mean cell volume.
- NRBC = nucleated red blood cell.
- PCV = packed cell volume.
- RBC = red blood cell.
- WBC = white blood cell.

Suggested Reading

Hohenhaus, AE, Winzelberg SE. Nonregenerative anemia. In: Ettinger SJ, Feldman EC, eds., Textbook of Veterinary Internal Medicine: Diseases of the Dog and Cat, 8th ed. St. Louis, MO: Elsevier Saunders, 2017, pp. 838–843.

Rebar AH, MacWilliams PS, Feldman BF, et al. Erythrocytes: overview, morphology, quantity. In: A Guide to Hematology in Dogs and Cats, Jackson, WY: Teton NewMedia. http://www.ivis.org/advances/Rebar/Chap4/chapter.asp?LA=1

Author Joyce S. Knoll

Consulting Editor Melinda S. Camus

ANEMIA, NUCLEAR MATURATION DEFECTS (ANEMIA, MEGALOBLASTIC)

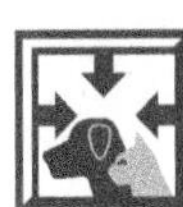

BASICS

OVERVIEW

- Nonregenerative anemia characterized by impaired DNA synthesis in red blood cell (RBC) precursors (nuclear : cytoplasmic asynchrony).
- Affected RBC precursors fail to divide normally and thus are larger than corresponding normal precursors; their nuclei are deficient in chromatin with open and stippled appearance; these giant precursors with atypical nuclei are known as megaloblasts. Hemoglobin content in these precursors is normal.
- Asynchronous changes most prominent in RBC precursors, but white blood cell (WBC) and platelet precursors similarly affected.

SIGNALMENT

- Cats—often associated with feline leukemia virus (FeLV) infection.
- Dogs—usually acquired, but may be inherited.
- Breed predilection for inherited cobalamin malabsorption—giant schnauzers, Australian shepherds, Komondorok, and beagles—present as young as 8–12 weeks; border collies as young adults.
- Familial macrocytosis and megaloblastic change in toy/miniature poodles.

SIGNS

- In dogs, anemia often not symptomatic. For cobalamin deficiency, clinical signs include gastrointestinal signs and failure to thrive. Affected poodles usually not anemic.
- In cats, anemia may be mild to marked, if FeLV positive.

CAUSES & RISK FACTORS

- Infectious—FeLV most common cause in cats. Feline immunodeficiency virus (FIV) infrequently reported as causative agent.
- Nutritional—folic acid and cobalamin deficiencies, primarily in dogs with inherited cobalamin malabsorption (uncommon with other causes of cobalamin deficiency).
- Toxic—many drugs such as immunomodulators, chemotherapeutic agents, anticonvulsants, antibiotics.
- Congenital—toy/miniature poodles.

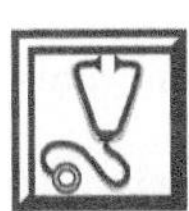

DIAGNOSIS

DIFFERENTIAL DIAGNOSIS

- In dogs, all other mild to moderate nonregenerative anemias, including anemia of inflammatory disease and lead poisoning.
- Differentiation based on distinctive CBC and bone marrow findings.
- In cats, FeLV infection is primary differential.

CBC/BIOCHEMISTRY/URINALYSIS

- Classically, anemia macrocytic and normochromic, but often normocytic.
- Large, fully hemoglobinized RBC; few to many nucleated RBC precursors, no polychromasia.
- In dogs, mild to moderate anemia; may see neutropenia with hypersegmented neutrophils.
- In cats, mild to marked anemia.
- In cats with FeLV, anemia may occur with myelodysplastic syndrome or leukemia.
- In dogs with inherited cobalamin malabsorption, can see proteinuria and variable biochemistry derangements.

OTHER LABORATORY TESTS

- FeLV in blood and bone marrow.
- Genetic tests for dogs with inherited cobalamin malabsorption (available at University of Pennsylvania, PennGen).
- Serum cobalamin.
- Methylmalonic acid (MMA) in serum or urine (increase caused by inhibited cobalamin-dependent enzyme).

IMAGING

N/A

DIAGNOSTIC PROCEDURES

Bone Marrow Biopsy

- In dogs, usually hyperplastic; may be hypocellular with hemosiderosis.
- In cats, may be hypo- or hyperplastic.
- Maturation arrest with nuclear : cytoplasmic asynchrony possible in all cell lines.
- Megaloblastic RBC precursors.
- Macrophage hyperplasia with phagocytosis of nucleated RBCs.

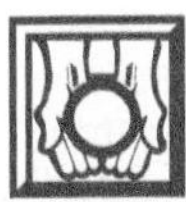

TREATMENT

- Anemia often mild and does not need specific therapy. FeLV-positive cats may require blood transfusion for stabilization.
- Target underlying cause and address concurrent signs.

MEDICATIONS

DRUG(S) OF CHOICE

- In animals with drug toxicity, discontinue offending drug.
- In animals with hypocobalaminemia, supplement with vitamin B_{12} (0.25–1 mg cyanocobalamin SC weekly to monthly or hydroxycobalamin IM every few months; oral may be effective in some patients—dogs, 250–1000 µg/day PO; cats, 250 µg/day PO).

CONTRAINDICATIONS/POSSIBLE INTERACTIONS

Avoid drugs known to cause megaloblastic anemia in patients whose condition results from other causes.

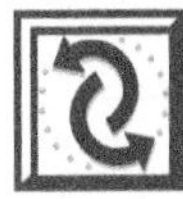

FOLLOW-UP

- Monitor response to treatment by CBC (weekly to every few months).
- Closely monitor FeLV-positive cats for disease progression.
- Prognosis depends on underlying cause; in FeLV-positive cats, prognosis poor; with drug-induced anemia, prognosis good if drug discontinued; inherited cobalamin malabsorption has good prognosis, with lifelong cobalamin supplementation.

MISCELLANEOUS

SEE ALSO

- Anemia, Nonregenerative.
- Feline Leukemia Virus (FeLV) Infection.

ABBREVIATIONS

- FeLV = feline leukemia virus.
- FIV = feline immunodeficiency virus.
- MMA = methylmalonic acid.
- RBC = red blood cell.
- WBC = white blood cell.

Suggested Reading

Harvey JW. Veterinary Hematology: A Diagnostic Guide and Color Atlas. Beijing: Elsevier, 2012, pp. 273–275.

Rebar AH, MacWilliams PS, Feldman BF, et al. A Guide to Hematology in Dogs and Cats. Jackson, WY: Teton NewMedia, 2002, pp. 57–58.

Weiss, DJ. Congenital dyserythropoiesis. In: Weiss DJ, Wardrop KJ, eds., Schalm's Veterinary Hematology, 6th ed. Ames, IA: Wiley-Blackwell, 2010, pp. 196–198.

Author Lisa S. Kelly

Consulting Editor Melinda S. Camus

Acknowledgment The author and book editors acknowledge the prior contribution of Alan H. Rebar.

ANEMIA, REGENERATIVE

BASICS

DEFINITION

Decreased circulating red blood cell (RBC) mass (indicated by low packed cell volume [PCV] or hematocrit [HCT], hemoglobin, and total RBC count) accompanied by appropriate, compensatory increase in RBC production by the bone marrow.

PATHOPHYSIOLOGY

- Caused by blood loss or hemolysis.
- Hemolysis—caused by intrinsic RBC defects (e.g., congenital RBC membrane defects or enzyme deficiencies) or extrinsic factors (e.g., RBC parasites, oxidative injury, hemolysins, osmotic changes, immune-mediated RBC destruction, hemophagocytic neoplasia, heat stroke, and severe hypophosphatemia).

SYSTEMS AFFECTED

- Cardiovascular—murmurs with marked anemia; tachycardia.
- Hemic/lymph/immune—erythroid hyperplasia in bone marrow; splenic extramedullary hematopoiesis (EMH).
- Hepatic—decreased oxygen delivery causes centrilobular degeneration of liver.
- Renal—severe intravascular hemolysis rarely leads to pigmentary nephropathy and acute renal failure.
- Musculoskeletal—progressive osteoclerosis seen in pyruvate kinase (PK)-deficient dogs.

SIGNALMENT

- PK deficiency—basenji, beagle, cairn terrier, Chihuahua, dachshund, Labrador retriever, labradoodle, miniature poodle, pug, West Highland white terrier, and American Eskimo; Somali, Abyssinian, domestic shorthair cats.
- PFK deficiency—Australian labradoodle, English springer spaniel, American cocker spaniel, cockapoo, English cocker spaniel, whippet, wachtelhund, and mixed breed dogs with spaniel parentage.
- Marked RBC osmotic fragility—English springer spaniel; Abyssinian, Somali, Siamese, and domestic shorthair cats.
- Feline congenital porphyria—Siamese and domestic shorthair cats.
- Heritable coagulopathies (e.g., factor VIII or IX deficiency), von Willebrand disease.
- Immune-mediated hemolytic anemia (IMHA)—middle-aged female dogs, especially American cocker spaniels, English springer spaniels, Irish setters, Old English sheepdogs, poodles, and Shetland sheepdogs.
- Hemophagocytic histiocytic sarcoma—Bernese mountain dog, Rottweiler, golden retriever, and flat-coated retriever.

SIGNS

- Pallor.
- Weakness, exercise intolerance, collapse.
- Anorexia.
- Possible heart murmur, tachycardia, bounding pulses (unless hemorrhage is present).
- Possible jaundice and hemoglobinuria.
- Petechiae, epistaxis, melena suggest blood loss due to vasculitis or thrombopathia.
- Hematomas or cavity bleeds suggest coagulation factor inhibition or deficiency.
- Clinical signs depend on degree of anemia and rapidity of onset.
- Rapid loss of 15–25% blood volume or acute hemolysis results in shock.
- With chronic anemia, compensatory increases in heart rate, and eventually heart size, occur; hemoglobin can drop to as low as 50% of minimum normal value without overt signs of shock or decreased oxygen delivery.

CAUSES

- Immune-mediated (IMHA).
- RBC toxins—snake venom and bee stings may cause RBC hemolysis; oxidants can cause Heinz body formation.
- Erythrocyte parasites—cats: *Mycoplasma* spp., *Cytauxzoon felis* (may be nonregenerative); dogs: *Mycoplasma haemocanis*, *Babesia* spp.
- Mechanical RBC fragmentation—caused by vasculitis, thromboembolic disease, or disease of any vascular organ; rare cause of significant anemia unless accompanied by hemorrhage.
- Inherited RBC abnormalities:
  - PK deficiency.
  - Phosphofructokinase (PFK) deficiency.
  - Increased RBC osmotic fragility (unknown RBC defect), leads to recurrent severe anemia and splenomegaly.
  - Feline congenital porphyria—enzyme deficiency in heme synthetic pathway leads to accumulation of heme precursors, hemolytic anemia, and brown-red discoloration of teeth and bones; Siamese tend to have severe hemolytic anemia, while domestic shorthair cats have less severe autosomal dominant trait that causes mild anemia.
- Hypophosphatemia—severe hypophosphatemia impairs adenosine triphosphate (ATP) production, leading to increased erythrocyte fragility and hemolysis; seen with refeeding syndrome and insulin administration.
- Blood loss:
  - Trauma.
  - Bleeding neoplasms.
  - Coagulopathies (e.g., warfarin toxicity, hemophilia, thrombocytopenia).
  - Blood-feeding parasites.
  - Gastrointestinal ulcers.

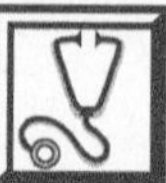

DIAGNOSIS

DIFFERENTIAL DIAGNOSIS

Differentiated from nonregenerative anemia by a reticulocyte count above the regenerative threshold for that species, generally above $80 \times 10^3/\mu L$ in dogs and $60 \times 10^3/\mu L$ in cats.

LABORATORY FINDINGS

Disorders That May Alter Laboratory Results

- Lipemia can cause mild in vitro hemolysis, without appreciable anemia, and may falsely elevate mean corpuscular hemoglobin concentration (MCHC).
- Autoagglutination may falsely decrease RBC count and increase MCV.
- Exercise and excitement can increase RBC count, PCV, and reticulocyte count through splenic contraction, masking severity of anemia.

Valid If Run in Human Laboratory?

- Dogs—yes.
- Cats—yes, if hematology instrument uses species-specific parameters; instruments designed for analysis of human specimens may undercount small feline RBCs and be unable to distinguish between erythrocytes and platelets.

CBC/BIOCHEMISTRY/URINALYSIS

- PCV, RBC count, and hemoglobin are below the reference interval.
- Total protein is often low with blood loss anemia and may be the only sign with acute blood loss due to splenic contraction, which elevates the circulating RBC count.
- RBC indices vary depending on the cause of anemia and degree of regenerative response:
  - Mean cell volume (MCV) is normal to high with regeneration, but low with iron deficiency.
  - MCHC is normal to low in most patients, low with iron deficiency, and artificially high with hemolysis.
- Specific RBC morphologies may suggest the cause of hemolysis:
  - Marked spherocytosis suggests immune-mediated disease in dogs.
  - Heinz bodies or eccentrocytes suggest oxidant injury.
  - Numerous schistocytes suggest microangiopathy.
  - RBC parasites may be found on or within RBC.
- Agglutinated RBCs indicate anemia is immune mediated; distinguish autoagglutination from rouleaux by saline agglutination test (see Appendix X).
- Hemolysis is often accompanied by an inflammatory leukogram.

• Animals with IMHA often have a concurrent thrombocytopenia, while iron deficiency is often accompanied by thrombocytosis.
• Hyperbilirubinemia and bilirubinuria accompany marked hemolysis; hemoglobinemia and hemoglobinuria can be seen following intravascular hemolysis.

OTHER LABORATORY TESTS

• Reticulocytosis may be absent in the first 3–5 days after onset of blood loss or hemolysis.
• Direct antiglobulin test (Coombs' test) is indicated when IMHA is suspected, in the absence of agglutination; a positive test is confirmatory.
• The rapid osmotic fragility test detects erythrocyte membrane defects and can help to discriminate hemolytic from nonhemolytic conditions.
• Coagulation testing may be indicated in cases of blood loss.
• PCR is more sensitive for diagnosis of *Babesia* and hemotropic *Mycoplasma* than microscopic blood smear exam; can differentiate between species.
• PCR for PK deficiency.
• PCR for PFK deficiency.

DIAGNOSTIC PROCEDURES

Fine-needle aspiration and cytologic exam of abnormal spleen, lung, or lymph nodes may help to diagnose hemophagocytic histiocytic sarcoma.

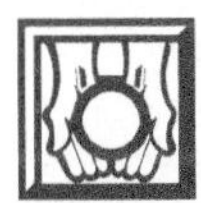

TREATMENT

• Emergency if anemia is severe or has developed rapidly.
• Massive hemorrhage leads to hypovolemic shock and decreased oxygen delivery to tissues; acute hemolysis also leads to decreased oxygen content in the blood.
• In cases of massive hemorrhage, crystalloid fluids can rapidly correct hypovolemia and restore circulation, but RBC replacement (and resolving the source of hemorrhage) is necessary for definitive therapy.
• RBC replacement (packed RBCs or whole blood) indicated with severe anemia (PCV <15%) or rapid drops (>15%) in HCT. Initial dosage depends on product selected; 1 mL/kg of packed RBCs will raise the HCT by approximately 1%; 3 mL/kg of whole blood will raise the PCV by approximately 1%, both depending on the PCV of the donor product.
• In cases of hemorrhage or coagulopathy, fresh whole blood will also provide volume expansion and coagulation factor replacement, compared to packed RBCs.
• Determine blood type prior to transfusion, especially in cats (who have preexisting autoantibodies to opposite blood types). Cross-match against donor blood if blood typing reagents not available, or if patient requires second transfusion more than 4 days after first transfusion.
• Animals with chronic blood loss or hemolytic anemias are generally normovolemic with increased cardiac output, therefore attention should be paid to transfusion volumes and rates.

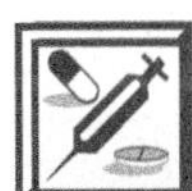

MEDICATIONS

DRUG(S) OF CHOICE

• Iron may benefit animals with chronic blood-loss anemia (see Anemia, Iron-Deficiency).
• Hemolytic anemias—varies with cause of hemolysis.

FOLLOW-UP

PATIENT MONITORING

• Initially, monitor PCV and morphologic features of RBCs on a blood smear every 24 hours to evaluate effectiveness of treatment and bone marrow responsiveness; polychromasia may be seen as regenerative response starts.
• As regeneration becomes apparent, recheck every 3–5 days.
• During and following transfusion, monitor for transfusion reactions (see Blood Transfusion Reactions).

MISCELLANEOUS

SEE ALSO

• Anemia, Heinz Body.
• Anemia, Immune-Mediated.
• Anemia, Iron-Deficiency.
• Babesiosis.
• Bartonellosis.
• Blood Transfusion Reactions.
• Cytauxzoonosis.
• Phosphofructokinase Deficiency.
• Pyruvate Kinase Deficiency.
• Von Willebrand Disease.
• Zinc Toxicosis.

ABBREVIATIONS

• ATP = adenosine triphosphate.
• EMH = extramedullary hematopoiesis.
• HCT = hematocrit.
• IMHA = immune-mediated hemolytic anemia.
• MCHC = mean corpuscular hemoglobin concentration.
• MCV = mean cell volume.
• PCV = packed cell volume.
• PFK = phosphofructokinase.
• PK = pyruvate kinase.
• RBC = red blood cell.

Suggested Reading

Piek C. Immune-mediated haemolytic anemia and other regenerative anemias. In: Ettinger SJ, Feldman EC, eds., Textbook of Veterinary Internal Medicine: Diseases of the Dog and Cat, 8th ed. St. Louis, MO: Elsevier Saunders, 2017, pp. 829–837.

Rebar AH, MacWilliams PS, Feldman BF, et al. Erythrocytes: overview, morphology, quantity. In: A Guide to Hematology in Dogs and Cats, Jackson, WY: Teton NewMedia. http://www.ivis.org/advances/Rebar/Chap4/chapter.asp?LA=1

Author Joyce S. Knoll
Consulting Editor Melinda S. Camus

A

ANISOCORIA

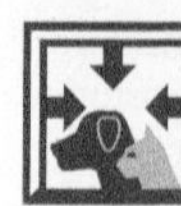

BASICS

DEFINITION

Asymmetric pupils.

PATHOPHYSIOLOGY

- Disruption of sympathetic (causing miosis) or parasympathetic (causing mydriasis) innervation to the eye.
- Ocular disease—numerous causes.

SYSTEMS AFFECTED

- Nervous.
- Ophthalmic.

GENETICS

None

INCIDENCE/PREVALENCE

Common

GEOGRAPHIC DISTRIBUTION

None

SIGNALMENT

- Dog and cat.
- All ages affected.
- No gender predisposition.

SIGNS

Unequal pupil size.

CAUSES

Neurologic

See Table 1.

Ocular

See Table 2.

RISK FACTORS

N/A

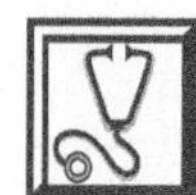

DIAGNOSIS

DIFFERENTIAL DIAGNOSIS

- Must determine which pupil is abnormal—see Figure 1 and Tables 1 and 2.
- Distinguish between neurologic and ocular causes.

CBC/BIOCHEMISTRY/URINALYSIS

N/A

OTHER LABORATORY TESTS

N/A

IMAGING

- See Table 1.
- Ultrasound—use to identify ocular, retrobulbar, or jugular groove lesions.
- MRI—use to identify CNS lesions.
- CT—use to identify tympanic bulla lesions.

DIAGNOSTIC PROCEDURES

- See Table 1.
- Cerebral spinal fluid (CSF) tap—evaluate for CNS inflammation/infection.
- ERG—evaluate retinal function.
- Pharmacologic testing—see Figure 1; postganglionic lesions cause denervation supersensitivity, resulting in more rapid constriction or dilation with application of

Table 1

Neurologic lesions causing anisocoria.

Sign	Pupillary Light Reflex (PLR)	Lesion Localization	Differential List	Diagnostic Test
Mydriasis—inability to constrict the pupil	No direct, present indirect	Ipsilateral optic nerve/chiasm	Neuritis, neoplasia	MRI/CSF tap/ERG
			Encephalitis, neoplasia, trauma, retrobulbar mass	MRI/CSF tap
				Ultrasound orbit
Miosis—inability to dilate the pupil	Present	Brainstem	Encephalitis, neoplasia, trauma	MRI/CSF tap
		C1-T2 myelopathy or C6-T3 brachial plexus	Trauma, myelitis, neoplasia, intervertebral disc herniation (IVDH; rare)	MRI/myelogram/CT
				MRI/ultrasound
		Vagosympathetic trunk	Jugular venipuncture, trauma	MRI/CT
		Tympanic bulla	Otitis media, neoplasia, trauma	MRI
		Trigeminal nerve	Neuritis, neoplasia	

Table 2

Ocular diseases causing anisocoria.

Lesion	Associated Signs	Causes
Anterior uveitis	Miosis, aqueous flare, corneal edema, conjunctival hyperemia	Infectious/inflammatory disease, trauma, neoplasia
Glaucoma	Mydriasis Sluggish/absent PLR, increased intraocular pressure, corneal edema	Primary glaucoma, secondary glaucoma
Neoplasm	Miosis/mydriasis, iris color change	Lymphoma, melanoma
Posterior synechia	Variable pupil shape, sluggish/absent PLR, anterior uveitis	Secondary to anterior uveitis
Iris atrophy	Variable pupil shape, iridal thinning, sluggish PLR	Old age change
Iris hypoplasia	Sluggish/absent PLR, irregular pupil margin, other ocular abnormalities	Congenital
Pharmacologic blockade	Mydriasis Absent direct/consensual PLR Normal vision	Atropine
Spastic pupil syndrome	Miosis, normal vision	Feline leukemia virus

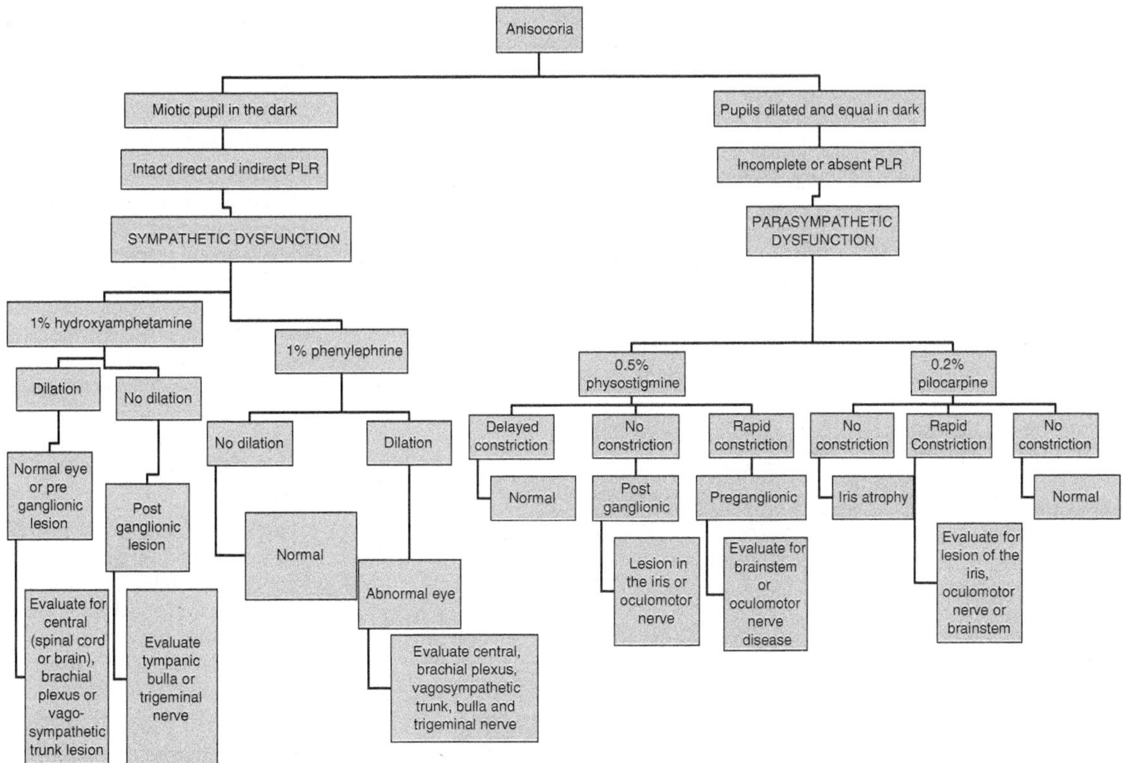

Figure 1.

pharmacologic agents. Differentiation of pre- or postganglionic lesions can be difficult if based solely on pharmacologic testing.

PATHOLOGIC FINDINGS

Dependent on underlying diagnosis.

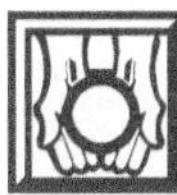

TREATMENT

Dependent on underlying disease.

MEDICATIONS

DRUG(S) OF CHOICE

Dependent on underlying disease.

CONTRAINDICATIONS

N/A

PRECAUTIONS

N/A

POSSIBLE INTERACTIONS

N/A

ALTERNATIVE DRUG(S)

N/A

FOLLOW-UP

PATIENT MONITORING

N/A

PREVENTION/AVOIDANCE

N/A

POSSIBLE COMPLICATIONS

N/A

EXPECTED COURSE AND PROGNOSIS

Depends on underlying disease.

MISCELLANEOUS

ASSOCIATED CONDITIONS

N/A

AGE-RELATED FACTORS

N/A

ZOONOTIC POTENTIAL

N/A

PREGNANCY/FERTILITY/BREEDING

N/A

SYNONYMS

None

SEE ALSO

- Anterior Uveitis—Cats.
- Anterior Uveitis—Dogs.
- Glaucoma.
- Horner's Syndrome.
- Iris Atrophy.
- Optic Neuritis and Papilledema.

ABBREVIATIONS

- CSF = cerebrospinal fluid.
- IVDH = intervertebral disc herniation.
- PLR = pupillary light reflex.

Suggested Reading

Cottrill NB. Differential diagnosis of anisocoria. In: Bonagura J, Twedt D, eds., Kirk's Current Veterinary Therapy, 14th ed. St. Louis, MO: Saunders, 2009, pp. 1168–1174.

Lorenz MD, Kornegay JN. Blindness, anisocoria and abnormal eye movements. In: Lorenz MD, Kornegay, JN, eds., Handbook of Veterinary Neurology, 4th ed. St. Louis, MO: Saunders, 2004, pp. 283–295.

Author Heidi L. Barnes Heller
Consulting Editor Kathern E. Myrna

Client Education Handout available online

A

ANOREXIA

BASICS

DEFINITION

Anorexia is the lack or loss of appetite for food. Hyporexia is a reduction in appetite, while dysrexia is a change in appetite or lack of consistent appetite. Anorexia results in decreased food intake, which then leads to weight loss, dehydration, nutritional deficiencies, and/or sarcopenia.

PATHOPHYSIOLOGY

• The control of appetite is a complex interaction between the central nervous system, the environment, and the gastrointestinal (GI) tract. • The hypothalamus and brainstem contain feeding-regulatory neurons that act as input stations for sensory and metabolic signals. These cell populations project to several brain regions and interconnect extensively. • Sensory signals that affect appetite include the odor, taste, texture, and temperature of food, as well as gastric and duodenal distention. • Metabolic signals for hunger and satiety include a variety of peptides and hormones released during the fasting and fed states, as well as plasma concentrations of glucose, amino acids, and fatty acids. • Insulin, glucagon, somatostatin, cholecystokinin, peptide tyrosine tyrosine (PYY), and pancreatic peptide decrease hunger centrally. • Leptin, produced primarily by adipocytes, acts on specific hypothalamic receptors to increase metabolism and decrease appetite. • Neuropeptide Y, released from the GI tract after food restriction, induces hunger and decreases energy expenditure. • Ghrelin, produced by the stomach, is a prokinetic and increases appetite; it decreases leptin and increases neuropeptide Y production.
• Serotonin is an important central mediator and acts via a serotonergic tract that passes near the ventromedial hypothalamic nuclei (satiety center). • Dopaminergic tracts in the hypothalamus help regulate food intake and are closely associated with the lateral hypothalamic nuclei (feeding center). • Environmental factors including the location and timing of meals, as well as learned behaviors and circadian rhythms, modulate appetite. • Brain lesions that affect the hypothalamus can decrease or increase appetite; any disorder that decreases cerebral arousal will potentially decrease food intake. • Inflammatory and neoplastic diseases can cause hyporexia by the release of proinflammatory cytokines. • The expected upregulation of dietary intake in response to increased energy expenditure is frequently absent in patients with neoplastic and advanced cardiac diseases.
• Exogenous and endogenous toxins (e.g., renal and liver failure) cause hyporexia. • Neoplasia, metabolic disorders, pancreatitis, and primary GI diseases are associated with hyporexia.
• Fear, pain, and stress may decrease appetite.

SYSTEMS AFFECTED

All body systems.

GENETICS

N/A

INCIDENCE/PREVALENCE

Unknown

GEOGRAPHIC DISTRIBUTION

N/A

SIGNALMENT

Species

Dog and cat.

Breed Predilections

N/A

Mean Age and Range

N/A

Predominant Sex

N/A

SIGNS

Historical Findings

• Refusal to eat is a common presenting complaint and causes owners significant distress. • Weight loss may be reported.

Physical Examination Findings

• Findings vary depending on the underlying cause. • Low body condition score and muscle wasting may be evident depending upon the duration of decreased food intake.
• Pseudoanorectic patients commonly display halitosis, excessive drooling, difficulty with prehension or mastication, and odynophagia (painful swallowing).

CAUSES

Anorexia/Hyporexia/Dysrexia

• Possible manifestations of a myriad of systemic disorders. • Psychological—food aversion, stress, alterations in routine or environment. • Pain.
• Toxicities and drug adverse effects. • GI and pancreatic diseases. • Acid-base disorders.
• Organ failure—e.g., cardiac, renal, hepatic.
• Endocrine and metabolic diseases. • Neoplasia.
• Infectious diseases. • Immune-mediated diseases. • Respiratory diseases. • Musculoskeletal diseases. • Neurologic diseases.
• Miscellaneous (e.g., motion sickness, high environmental temperature).

Pseudoanorexia

Any disease causing painful or dysfunctional prehension, mastication, or swallowing.

RISK FACTORS

N/A

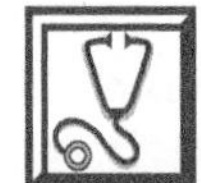

DIAGNOSIS

DIFFERENTIAL DIAGNOSIS

• Pseudoanorexia is a term describing patients who are hungry but are unable to eat due to disorders causing dysfunction or pain of the face, neck, oropharynx, and esophagus.
• Animals lacking a sense of smell (anosmia) often show a lack of interest in food.

CBC/BIOCHEMISTRY/URINALYSIS

• Abnormalities vary with different underlying diseases. • May be normal.

OTHER LABORATORY TESTS

• Additional diagnostic tests may be necessary to investigate specific diseases suggested by history, physical examination, and preliminary tests. • Heartworm serology, tick serology, retrovirus serology, thyroid level, and histologic/cytologic examination of tissue/cell samples may be required to make a definitive diagnosis.
• A baseline cortisol or an adrenocorticotropic hormone (ACTH) stimulation test to rule out hypoadrenocorticism is warranted even when there are no significant laboratory changes.

IMAGING

• Thoracic and abdominal imaging (radiographs and ultrasound) studies are often included in the minimum database to detect anatomic or functional abnormalities.
• Videofluoroscopy and endoscopy may be indicated to specifically evaluate pharyngeal, esophageal, and GI function and appearance.

DIAGNOSTIC PROCEDURES

• Perform a nutritional assessment; collect a thorough dietary history, evaluate food intake, and obtain body and muscle condition scores.
• Elicit a thorough history regarding the patient's environment, changes in routine, people, or other pets, to help identify potential sources of psychologic stress.
• Observe the patient's interest in food and ability to prehend, masticate, and swallow food. • Complete a thorough physical examination including ophthalmic, oropharyngeal, neurologic, orthopedic, thoracic, abdominal, and rectal exam to determine the presence of disease.

PATHOLOGIC FINDINGS

Dependent on underlying disease.

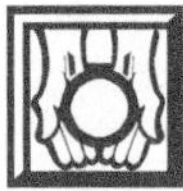

TREATMENT

APPROPRIATE HEALTH CARE

• Assisted feeding (enteral and/or parenteral feeding) should be considered immediately for significantly malnourished patients (≥10% body weight loss, hypoalbuminemia, poor body condition score, evidence of muscle wasting, and/or chronic disease processes). In well-conditioned patients with decreased appetite, assisted feeding should be considered if food consumption is less than the resting energy requirement [RER = 70 x (body $weight_{kg}^{0.75}$)] for 3–5 days without trends toward improvement. • Force feeding should be avoided, particularly in cats, considering the association with conditioned food aversions.

NURSING CARE

• Medications the patient is receiving should be reviewed for possible side effects leading to reduced appetite. • Provide comfort and nutrition to the patient while efforts are directed at identifying and correcting the underlying disease so that more specific treatment can be provided. • Symptomatic therapy includes correcting fluid deficits and electrolyte derangements, control of pain and/or nausea, reduction in environmental stressors, and modification of the diet to improve palatability.

ACTIVITY

N/A

DIET

• Palatability can be improved by adding flavored toppings such as low-sodium broth, increasing the moisture, fat, or protein content of the food, and warming the food to body temperature. • When learned food aversion is suspected, food should be removed immediately at the first signs of aversion.

CLIENT EDUCATION

Depends on specific diagnosis.

SURGICAL CONSIDERATIONS

N/A

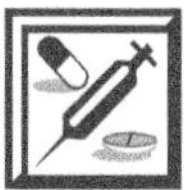

MEDICATIONS

DRUG(S) OF CHOICE

• Pharmacologic interventions aimed at improving appetite should not replace diagnostic efforts to identify the specific cause(s) of decreased appetite. • Mirtazapine antagonizes inhibitory, presynaptic, α2-adrenergic receptors, facilitating release of norepinephrine and serotonin (5-HT). It is also a 5-HT2 and 5-HT3 antagonist on the postsynaptic neuron. Stimulation of 5-HT1 produces antidepressant effects, while inhibition of 5-HT2 and 5-HT3 produces anti-emetic and appetite-stimulating effects. Canine dosing is 0.5 mg/kg q24h. Mirataz® is FDA approved for use in cats, with a recommended dose of a 1.5 in. strip applied to the inner pinna once daily for 14 days. Alternatively, 1.88 mg/cat PO q24–48h (for cats with chronic kidney disease) can be given to stimulate appetite. • Capromorelin is a ghrelin receptor agonist that stimulates appetite centrally in the hypothalamus. Entyce® is capromorelin, approved by the FDA for dogs as an appetite stimulant. A trial in healthy laboratory beagles demonstrated significant increases in food consumption and weight compared to placebo, and a clinical field trial in inappetent client-owned dogs demonstrated increases in appetite and body weight compared to placebo. Dosing at 3 mg/kg PO q24h is safe for long-term administration. Capromorelin is not approved for cats, though a safety trial has been published and clinical trials are underway. • Diazepam (0.1 mg/kg IV q24h) is a short-acting appetite stimulant with sedative properties. Oral diazepam should be avoided in cats due to possible idiosyncratic hepatotoxicosis. • Cyproheptadine (0.2–0.4 mg/kg PO, 10–20 minutes prior to feeding), an antihistamine with antiserotonergic properties, has been used as an appetite stimulant with mixed success. • Prokinetics such as metoclopramide (0.2–0.4 mg/kg SC/PO q8–12h), ranitidine (2 mg/kg SC/IV/PO q12h), or erythromycin (0.5–1 mg/kg PO q8–12h) are useful if anorexia is associated with ileus. • Antiemetics are useful in decreasing nausea or vomiting, but are not appetite stimulants. Ondansetron (0.5–1.0 mg/kg SC/IV/PO q12h) and dolasetron (0.6–1.0 mg/kg SC/IV/PO q24h) are potent antiemetics as 5-HT3 antagonists. Maropitant is a substance P analogue, which binds neurokinin-1 receptors in the chemoreceptor trigger zone (CRTZ) and vomiting center, inhibiting vomiting. Cerenia® is maropitant, approved by the FDA for dogs and cats as an antiemetic (dogs: 1 mg/kg SC/IV or 2 mg/kg PO q24h; cats: 1 mg/kg SC/IV/PO q24h). • Omega-3 fatty acids can reduce inflammatory cytokines and have modest benefit for appetite.

CONTRAINDICATIONS

Avoid antiemetics and prokinetics if GI obstruction is present or suspected.

PRECAUTIONS

N/A

POSSIBLE INTERACTIONS

Mirtazapine should not be combined with drugs that interact with or affect serotoninergic systems including monoamine oxidase inhibitors (MAOIs), tricyclic antidepressants (TCAs), and selective serotonin reuptake inhibitors (SSRIs). Ondansetron and dolasetron, as well as metoclopramide, are 5-HT3 antagonists, and care should be used with combining these drugs with mirtazapine.

ALTERNATIVE DRUG(S)

N/A

FOLLOW-UP

PATIENT MONITORING

• Body weight, body and muscle condition score, and hydration assessment. • Monitor caloric intake to ensure return of appetite is sufficient to meet nutritional needs.

PREVENTION/AVOIDANCE

N/A

POSSIBLE COMPLICATIONS

• Dehydration, malnutrition, cachexia, and sarcopenia are sequelae of prolonged anorexia/hyporexia/dysrexia; these exacerbate the underlying disease. • A loss of more than 25–30% of body protein compromises the immune system and muscle strength, and death results from infection and/or cardiopulmonary failure. • Hepatic lipidosis is a possible complication of anorexia, particularly in cats. • Breakdown of the intestinal mucosal barrier further compromises debilitated patients.

EXPECTED COURSE AND PROGNOSIS

Depends on the underlying cause(s).

MISCELLANEOUS

ASSOCIATED CONDITIONS

N/A

AGE-RELATED FACTORS

Nutritional support and glucose-containing fluids may be necessary to treat or prevent hypoglycemia in anorectic puppies and kittens.

ZOONOTIC POTENTIAL

N/A

PREGNANCY/FERTILITY/BREEDING

N/A

SYNONYMS

N/A

SEE ALSO

Weight Loss and Cachexia.

ABBREVIATIONS

• 5-HT = 5-hydroxytryptamine (serotonin).
• ACTH = adrenocorticotropic hormone.
• CRTZ = chemoreceptor trigger zone.
• GI = gastrointestinal. • MAOI = monoamine oxidase inhibitor. • PYY = peptide tyrosine tyrosine. • RER = resting energy requirement.
• SSRI = selective serotonin reuptake inhibitor.
• TCA = tricyclic antidepressant.

INTERNET RESOURCES

https://entyce.aratana.com/resources/clinical-references

Suggested Reading

Forman MA. Anorexia. In: Ettinger SJ, Feldman EC, Côté E, eds. Textbook of Veterinary Internal Medicine, 8th ed. St. Louis, MO: Elsevier Saunders, 2017, pp. 97–100.

Quimby JM, Lunn KF. Mirtazapine as an appetite stimulant and anti-emetic in cats with chronic kidney disease: a masked placebo-controlled crossover clinical trial. Vet J 2013, 197(3):651–655.

Schermerhorn T. Gastrointestinal endocrinology. In: Ettinger SJ, Feldman EC, Côté E, eds., Textbook of Veterinary Internal Medicine, 8th ed. St. Louis, MO: Elsevier Saunders, 2017, pp. 1833–1838.

Wofford JA, Zollers B, Rhodes L, et al. Evaluation of the safety of daily administration of capromorelin in cats. J Vet Pharmacol Ther 2018, 41(2):324–333.

Author Andrea Wang Munk
Consulting Editor Mark P. Rondeau
Acknowledgment The author and book editors acknowledge the prior contribution of Kathryn E. Michel.

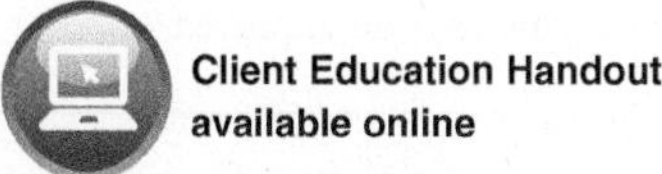

ANTEBRACHIAL GROWTH DEFORMITIES

BASICS

DEFINITION

Abnormally shaped antebrachium and distal part of the thoracic limb, and/or malalignments of the elbow or antebrachiocarpal joints that result from maldevelopment of the radius or ulna in the growing animal.

PATHOPHYSIOLOGY

- Antebrachium—predisposed to deformities resulting from growth of one bone after premature growth cessation or growth retardation of the paired bone.
- Decreased rate of elongation in one bone behaves as a retarding strap; the growing paired bone must twist and curve around the short bone or overgrow at the elbow or carpus; causes joint malalignment.
- Normal growth—bones elongate through the process of endochondral ossification, which occurs in the physis; physis closure occurs when the germinal cell layer stops producing new cartilage and the existing cartilage hypertrophies, ossifies, and is remodeled into bone.
- Hereditary—may be a component of common elbow joint malalignment in many chondrodysplastic breeds (e.g., basset hound and Lhasa apso).
- Osteochondrosis (OC) or dietary oversupplementation—possibly associated with retardation of endochondral ossification (retained cartilaginous cores) in giant-breed dogs.
- Hypertrophic osteodystrophy (HOD)—juvenile growth syndrome with physeal and periosteal inflammation that may impede growth.
- Trauma—most common cause; if germinal cell layer of the physis is damaged, new cartilage production and bone elongation are stopped. Commonly occurs with injury (fractures or crushing injuries) involving the distal ulnar or radial growth plates.

SYSTEMS AFFECTED

Musculoskeletal

GENETICS

- Skye terriers—reported as a recessive inheritable trait.
- Chondrodysplastic breeds (dogs)—disturbed endochondral ossification results in asynchronous growth of the paired bone system, resulting in altered growth, angular deformity, and possible elbow malalignment.

INCIDENCE/PREVALENCE

- Traumatic—may occur in up to 10% of actively growing dogs that sustain injuries of the antebrachium; uncommon in cats.
- Elbow malalignment syndrome ± angular deformity (chondrodysplastic dog breeds)—fairly common and can be bilateral; clinical abnormality in affected individuals is variable.
- Nutritionally induced—incidence decreasing as nutritional standards are improved.
- Congenital agenesis of the radius (cats and rarely dogs)—occurs infrequently; results in severely bowed antebrachium and carpal subluxation.

SIGNALMENT

Species

Dog and cat.

Breed Predilections

- Skye terrier—recessive inheritable form.
- Chondrodysplastic and toy breeds (especially basset hound, dachshund, Lhasa apso, Pekingese, Jack Russell terrier)—may be predisposed to elbow malalignment and incongruity.
- Giant breeds (e.g., Great Dane, wolfhound)—may be induced by rapid growth owing to excessive or unbalanced nutrition, OC, or HOD.

Mean Age and Range

- Traumatic—any time during the active growth phase.
- Elbow malarticulations—during growth; may not be recognized until secondary arthritic changes become severe, occasionally at several years of age.

Predominant Sex

N/A

SIGNS

General Comments

- Longer-limbed dogs—angular deformities generally more common.
- Shorter-limbed dogs—tend to develop more severe joint malalignments.
- Age at time of premature closure—affects relative degree of deformity and joint malarticulation; dogs with more growth potential remaining tend to develop more severe deformity.

Historical Findings

- Traumatic—progressive limb angulation or lameness noticed 3–4 weeks after injury; owner may not be aware of causative event.
- Developmental elbow malalignments—insidious onset of lameness in one or both thoracic limbs; most apparent after exercise.

Physical Examination Findings

Premature Distal Ulnar Closure

- Results in three deformities of the distal radius—lateral deviation (valgus), cranial bowing (procurvatum), and external torsion resulting in supination of the manus.
- Relative shortening of limb length—if unilateral can compare to the contralateral normal limb.
- Caudolateral subluxation of the radiocarpal joint and malarticulation of the elbow joint—may occur; causes lameness and painful joint restriction.

Premature Radial Physeal Closure

- Affected limb—significantly shorter than the normal contralateral limb.
- Severity of lameness—depends on degree of joint malarticulation.
- Complete symmetric closure of distal physis—may note straight limb with a widened radiocarpal or radiohumeral joint space; may note caudal bow (recurvatum) to radius and ulna.
- Asymmetric closure of medial aspect of distal radial physis—varus angular deformity; occasionally internal torsion and pronation.
- Closure of lateral aspect of distal radial physis—valgus angular deformity; external torsion and supination.
- Closure of proximal radial physis with continued ulnar growth—malarticulation of the elbow joint; widened radiohumeral space; and proximal subluxation of the humeroulnar joint (increased humerus to anconeal process space).

CAUSES

- Trauma.
- Developmental basis.
- Nutritional basis.

RISK FACTORS

- Thoracic limb trauma.
- Excessive dietary supplementation.

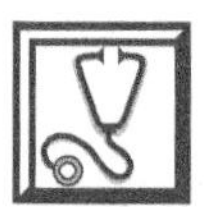

DIAGNOSIS

DIFFERENTIAL DIAGNOSIS

- Elbow dysplasia.
- Fragmented medial coronoid process (FMCP).
- Ununited anconeal process (UAP).
- Panosteitis.
- Flexor tendon contracture.
- HOD.

CBC/BIOCHEMISTRY/URINALYSIS

N/A

OTHER LABORATORY TESTS

N/A

IMAGING

- Damage to growth potential of the physis—commonly cannot be seen at the time of trauma; usually 2–4 weeks before radiographically apparent.
- Craniocaudal and mediolateral radiographic views—include both entire elbow and carpal joints; compare with normal contralateral limb.
- Degree of angular deformities and relative shortening—determined by comparing relative lengths of radius and ulna within the deformed pair to the normal contralateral pair.
- Degree of torsional deformity—cross-sectional imaging and creation of models using stereolithography is most useful for full appreciation of torsional deformity.
- Elbow and carpal joints—evaluate for malalignment and degenerative change; presence of degenerative change is associated with less optimal outcome following surgical treatment.
- Elbow joint—evaluate for associated UAP and FMCP.

DIAGNOSTIC PROCEDURES

N/A

PATHOLOGIC FINDINGS

Cartilage of abnormal growth plate often replaced with bone. Angular deformity can occur due to retained cartilage core (OC) of the distal ulnar physis.

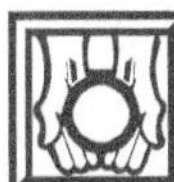

TREATMENT

APPROPRIATE HEALTH CARE

- Genetic predisposition—do not breed.
- Traumatic physeal damage—not seen at time of injury; revealed 2–4 weeks later.
- In young (<6 months) animals, surgical treatment is generally recommended as soon as possible following diagnosis; treatment may require multiple surgical procedures.

NURSING CARE

N/A

ACTIVITY

Exercise restriction—reduces joint malalignment damage; slows arthritic progression.

DIET

- Decrease nutritional supplementation in giant-breed dogs—slows rapid growth; may reduce incidence.
- Avoid excess weight—helps control arthritic pain resulting from joint malalignment and overuse.

CLIENT EDUCATION

- Discuss heritability in chondrodysplastic breeds.
- Explain that damage to physeal growth potential is not apparent at time of trauma and that the diagnosis is often made 2–4 weeks following an injury.
- Discuss the importance of joint malalignment and resultant osteoarthritis as primary causes of lameness.
- Emphasize that early surgical treatment leads to a better prognosis.
- Depending on the patient's age, treatment may involve multiple procedures.

SURGICAL CONSIDERATIONS

- Premature closure of the distal ulnar physis in a patient <5–6 months of age (significant amount of radial growth potential remaining)—treated with partial ulnar ostectomy; valgus deformities ≤25° may improve and may not require additional surgery; young patients and those with more severe deformities often require a second definitive correction after maturity.
- Radial or ulnar physeal closure in a mature patient (limited or no growth potential) requires definitive deformity correction, joint realignment, or both.
- Deformity (torsional and angular) correction—may be accomplished with a variety of osteotomy techniques; may be stabilized with several different internal or external fixation devices.
- Joint malalignment (particularly elbow)—must correct to minimize arthritis development (primary cause of lameness); typically performed via dynamic proximal ulnar osteotomy (use triceps brachii muscle traction and joint pressure) or shortening longer bone (radial or ulnar ostectomy).
- Significant limb length discrepancies—distraction osteogenesis; osteotomy of the shortened bone is progressively distracted at the rate of 1 mm/day with an external fixator system to create new bone length.

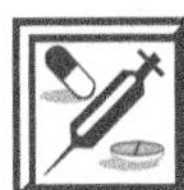

MEDICATIONS

DRUG(S) OF CHOICE

Anti-inflammatory drugs—symptomatic treatment of osteoarthritis.

CONTRAINDICATIONS

Corticosteroids—do not use owing to potential systemic side effects and cartilage damage seen with long-term use.

PRECAUTIONS

Nonsteroidal anti-inflammatory drugs (NSAIDs)—gastrointestinal irritation or renal/hepatic toxicity may preclude use in some patients.

POSSIBLE INTERACTIONS

N/A

ALTERNATIVE DRUG(S)

N/A

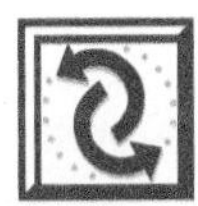

FOLLOW-UP

PATIENT MONITORING

- Postoperative—depends on surgical treatment.
- Periodic checkups—evaluate arthritic status and anti-inflammatory therapy.

PREVENTION/AVOIDANCE

- Selective breeding of susceptible breeds.
- Avoid dietary oversupplementation in rapidly growing giant-breed dogs.

POSSIBLE COMPLICATIONS

Routinely seen with various osteotomy fixation techniques (e.g., infection, nonunion of osteotomy, fixator pin tract inflammation, undercorrection).

EXPECTED COURSE AND PROGNOSIS

- Best results seen with early diagnosis and surgical treatment—minimizes osteoarthritis.
- Premature ulnar closure—easier to manage than premature closure of the radial growth plates; prognosis dependent on severity of the deformity, joint congruity, and presence of degenerative joint disease; prognosis worsens with increasing severity.
- Limb lengthening by distraction osteogenesis—requires extensive postoperative management by the veterinarian and owner; high rate of complications.

MISCELLANEOUS

ASSOCIATED CONDITIONS

- OC.
- HOD.
- UAP.

AGE-RELATED FACTORS

The younger the patient at the time of traumatically induced physeal closure, the more severe the deformity and malarticulation.

ZOONOTIC POTENTIAL

N/A

PREGNANCY/FERTILITY/BREEDING

N/A

SYNONYMS

Radius curvus.

ABBREVIATIONS

- FMCP = fragmented medial coronoid process.
- HOD = hypertrophic osteodystrophy.
- NSAID = nonsteroidal anti-inflammatory drug.
- OC = osteochondrosis.
- UAP = ununited anconeal process.

Suggested Reading

Fox DB. Radius and ulna. In Johnston SA, Tobias KM, eds. Veterinary Surgery Small Animal, 2nd ed. St. Louis, MO: Elsevier Saunders, 2018, pp. 896–920.

Fox DB, Tomlinson JL. Principles of angular limb deformity correction. In Johnston SA, Tobias KM, eds. Veterinary Surgery Small Animal, 2nd ed. St. Louis, MO: Elsevier Saunders, 2018, pp. 762–774.

Author Spencer A. Johnston

Consulting Editor Mathieu M. Glassman

Client Education Handout available online

ANTERIOR UVEITIS—CATS

BASICS

DEFINITION

• Inflammation of the anterior uveal tissues, including iris (iritis), ciliary body (cyclitis), or both (iridocyclitis). • May be associated with concurrent posterior uveal and retinal inflammation (choroiditis; chorioretinitis). • Unilateral or bilateral.

PATHOPHYSIOLOGY

• Increased permeability of the blood–aqueous barrier due to infectious, immune-mediated, neoplastic, traumatic, or other causes; plasma proteins and blood cells enter aqueous humor. • Disruption of blood–aqueous barrier initiated and maintained by chemical mediators.

SYSTEMS AFFECTED

• Ophthalmic. • Other systems if underlying disease.

INCIDENCE/PREVALENCE

• Relatively common. • True incidence/prevalence unknown.

GEOGRAPHIC DISTRIBUTION

Geographic location may affect incidence of certain infections.

SIGNALMENT

Species

Cat

Mean Age and Range

• Mean age 7–9 years. • Any age may be affected.

Predominant Sex

Males more commonly affected than females.

SIGNS

Historical Findings

• Cloudy eye—corneal edema, aqueous flare, hypopyon. • Painful eye—blepharospasm, photophobia, or rubbing eye; usually less severe than dogs. • Red eye—conjunctival hyperemia and ciliary flush; usually less severe than dogs. • Vision loss—variable.

Physical Examination Findings

A thorough physical examination is crucial.

Ophthalmic Findings

• Ocular discomfort—manifest by blepharospasm and photophobia. • Ocular discharge—usually serous; sometimes mucoid to mucopurulent. • Conjunctival hyperemia—bulbar and palpebral conjunctiva affected.
• Corneal edema—diffuse; mild to severe.
• Keratic precipitates—multifocal aggregates of inflammatory cells adherent to corneal endothelium; most notable ventrally.
• Aqueous flare—cloudiness of aqueous humor due to increased protein content and cellular debris; visualized with a bright, narrow beam of light shone through anterior chamber. • Ciliary flush—injection of deep perilimbal anterior ciliary vessels. • Deep corneal vascularization—circumcorneal distribution (brush border). • Miosis or resistance to pharmacologic dilation. • Iridal swelling—may be generalized or nodular.
• Reduced intraocular pressure (IOP) consistent with anterior uveitis, but not uniform finding. • Posterior synechia—adhesions between posterior iris and anterior lens surface. • Fibrin in anterior chamber.
• Hypopyon or hyphema—accumulations of white or red blood cells, respectively, in anterior chamber; usually settle in ventral aspect of chamber, but may be diffuse.
• Chronic changes may include rubeosis iridis, iridal hyperpigmentation, secondary cataract, lens luxation, pupillary seclusion, iris bombé, secondary glaucoma, and phthisis bulbi.

CAUSES

• Infectious—mycotic (*Blastomyces* spp., *Cryptococcus neoformans, Coccidiodes immitis, Histoplasma capsulatum*); protozoal (*Toxoplasma gondii, Leishmania infantum*); bacterial (*Bartonella* spp., *Mycobacterium* spp., or other bacteria); viral (feline immunodeficiency virus [FIV], feline leukemia virus [FeLV], feline coronavirus [FCoV], feline herpesvirus type 1 [FHV-1]); parasitic (ophthalmomyiasis, ocular nematodiasis).
• Idiopathic—lymphocytic-plasmacytic uveitis. • Immune-mediated—reaction to lens proteins (due to cataract or lens trauma/rupture). • Neoplastic—primary ocular tumors, metastasis to uveal tract. • Metabolic—hyperlipidemia, hyperviscosity, systemic hypertension. • Miscellaneous—trauma (blunt or penetrating), ulcerative keratitis, corneal stromal abscess, toxemia.

RISK FACTORS

Immune suppression and geographic location may increase risk for certain infectious causes of uveitis.

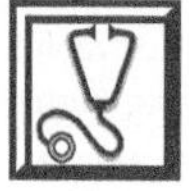

DIAGNOSIS

DIFFERENTIAL DIAGNOSIS

• Conjunctivitis—redness limited to conjunctival hyperemia (no ciliary flush); discharge thicker and more copious than uveitis; discomfort alleviated by topical anesthetic. • Glaucoma—elevated IOP, dilated pupil, Haab's striae, and buphthalmos.
• Ulcerative keratitis—corneal fluorescein staining detects ulcers; corneal edema is either localized to or most severe at site of ulcer; ocular discharge thicker and more copious than uveitis; discomfort alleviated by topical anesthetic. • Horner's syndrome—miosis, enophthalmos, and nictitans protrusion are similar, but Horner's is nonpainful without ocular discharge; ptosis with Horner's is not blepharospasm, as the latter is an active process; minor conjunctival hyperemia may be noted with Horner's, but cornea and anterior chamber are clear; clinical signs resolve with topical ophthalmic 1–10% phenylephrine.

CBC/BIOCHEMISTRY/URINALYSIS

• CBC—normal, or reflects underlying disease.
• Biochemistry—most common abnormality is elevated serum proteins (usually due to polyclonal gammopathy). • Urinalysis—normal, or reflects underlying disease.

OTHER LABORATORY TESTS

• Serum titers for FeLV, FIV, and FCoV; FCoV titers not specific for feline infectious peritonitis (FIP), but very high titers may increase the index of suspicion; reverse transcription polymerase chain reaction (RT-PCR) testing can help support diagnosis, but not definitive. • *Toxoplasma gondii* serum immunoglobulin (Ig) M and IgG titers and/or PCR performed on serum and/or aqueous humor. • *Bartonella* spp. serology, PCR (serum or aqueous humor).

IMAGING

• Thoracic radiography—may show evidence of metastatic or infectious disease. • Ocular ultrasound—if opacity of ocular media precludes direct examination; may reveal intraocular neoplasm or retinal detachment.

DIAGNOSTIC PROCEDURES

• Tonometry—low IOP consistent with uveitis; elevated IOP indicates glaucoma (primary or secondary to uveitis). • Ocular centesis—if retinal detachment is present, cytology of subretinal aspirate may reveal causative agents; anterior chamber centesis for cytology, titers, or FCoV immunocytochemistry.

PATHOLOGIC FINDINGS

• Lymphoplasmacytic infiltrate of iris and ciliary body (either diffuse or nodular) is most common histopathologic finding.
• Histopathologic—may observe corneal edema, peripheral corneal deep stromal vascularization, keratic precipitates, preiridal fibrovascular membrane, anterior or posterior synechia, entropion or ectropion uveae. Leukocyte accumulation in iris, ciliary body, sclera, choroid (lymphocytic, plasmacytic, suppurative, or granulomatous infiltrates, depending on etiology), secondary cataract, cyclitic membrane, vitreal traction bands, and retinal detachment.

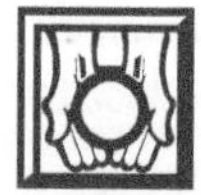

TREATMENT

APPROPRIATE HEALTH CARE

Outpatient

ACTIVITY

No changes.

DIET

No changes.

CLIENT EDUCATION

• Systemic disease may cause ophthalmic signs; emphasize importance of appropriate diagnostic testing. • In addition to symptomatic treatment, treatment of underlying disease (when possible) is paramount. • Inform of potential complications and emphasize compliance with treatment and follow-up recommendations to reduce likelihood of complications.

SURGICAL CONSIDERATIONS

• None in most cases. • Specific instances include removal of ruptured lenses and surgical management of secondary glaucoma. • Chronic uveitis leading to secondary glaucoma commonly requires enucleation of the eye. • Enucleation is recommended in cats with uveitis related to diffuse iris melanoma or other intraocular tumors.

MEDICATIONS

DRUG(S) OF CHOICE

Corticosteroids

Topical

• Prednisolone acetate 1% or dexamethasone 0.1%—apply 2–8 times daily, depending on severity of disease; taper as condition resolves.
• Stopping topical corticosteroids abruptly may result in rebound ocular inflammation.

Subconjunctival

• Often not required; indicated only in severe cases as one-time injection. • Triamcinolone acetonide—4 mg by subconjunctival injection.
• Methylprednisolone—4 mg by subconjunctival injection.

Systemic

• Prednisone—1–3 mg/kg/day PO initially; taper dose after 7–10 days. • Only if infectious causes of uveitis have been ruled out.

Nonsteroidal Anti-inflammatory Drugs (NSAIDs)

Topical

• Flurbiprofen—apply 2–4 times daily, depending on severity of disease.
• Diclofenac or ketorolac—apply 2–4 times daily, depending on severity of disease.

Systemic

• Meloxicam—0.3 mg/kg SC once.
• Robenacoxib—1 mg/kg PO once daily; limit duration of use to 3 days.

Topical Mydriatic/Cycloplegic

Atropine sulfate 1%—apply 1–4 times daily, depending on severity of disease. Use lowest frequency adequate to maintain dilated pupil; taper medication as condition resolves. Ointment in cats causes less salivation.

CONTRAINDICATIONS

• Avoid the use of miotic medications, including topical prostaglandins (e.g., latanoprost), in the presence of uveitis.
• Topical and subconjunctival corticosteroids are contraindicated with ulcerative keratitis.
• Corticosteroids (especially systemic) should be avoided in cats with systemic hypertension. • Avoid systemic nonsteroidal anti-inflammatory drugs (NSAIDs) in cats with renal disease and in combination with corticosteroids.

PRECAUTIONS

Owing to concern for secondary glaucoma, topical atropine should be used judiciously and IOP monitored periodically.

POSSIBLE INTERACTIONS

Systemic corticosteroids and NSAIDs should not be used concurrently.

FOLLOW-UP

PATIENT MONITORING

Recheck in 3–7 days, depending on severity of disease. IOP should be monitored to detect secondary glaucoma. Frequency of subsequent rechecks dictated by severity of disease and response to treatment.

POSSIBLE COMPLICATIONS

• Secondary glaucoma—common complication of chronic uveitis in cats.
• Secondary cataract. • Lens luxation.
• Retinal detachment. • Phthisis bulbi.

EXPECTED COURSE AND PROGNOSIS

• Guarded prognosis for affected eyes; depends on underlying disease and response to treatment. • Cats with treatable underlying disease (e.g., toxoplasmosis) are more likely to have a favorable ophthalmic outcome than those with idiopathic lymphoplasmacytic uveitis or untreatable underlying condition (e.g., FIP, FIV).

MISCELLANEOUS

AGE-RELATED FACTORS

• Younger cats more likely to be diagnosed with infectious uveitis. • Older cats at higher risk of idiopathic lymphocytic-plasmacytic uveitis and intraocular neoplasia.

ZOONOTIC POTENTIAL

• None in most cases. • Some systemic infections causing uveitis may pose a risk to immunocompromised owners.

PREGNANCY/FERTILITY/BREEDING

Avoid systemic corticosteroids. Because of systemic absorption, topical corticosteroids may also pose a risk, especially with frequent application.

SYNONYMS

Iridocyclitis

SEE ALSO

• Horner's Syndrome.
• Red Eye.

ABBREVIATIONS

• FCoV = Feline coronavirus.
• FeLV = feline leukemia virus.
• FHV-1 = feline herpesvirus type 1.
• FIP = feline infectious peritonitis.
• FIV = feline immunodeficiency virus.
• Ig = immunoglobulin.
• IOP = intraocular pressure.
• NSAID = nonsteroidal anti-inflammatory drug.
• RT-PCR = reverse transcription polymerase chain reaction.

Suggested Reading

Cullen C, Webb A. Ocular manifestations of systemic diseases. Part 2: The cat. In: Gelatt KN, ed., Veterinary Ophthalmology, 5th ed. Ames, IA: Wiley-Blackwell, 2013, pp. 1978–2036.

Miller P. Diseases of the uvea. In: Maggs DJ, Miller PE, Ofri R, eds., Slatter's Fundamentals of Veterinary Ophthalmology, 6th ed. St. Louis, MO: Elsevier Saunders, 2018, pp. 254–276.

Pickett JP. Anterior uvea and anterior chamber. In: Martin C, Pickett J, Spiess B, eds., Ophthalmic Disease in Veterinary Medicine. Boca Raton, FL: CRC Press, 2018, pp. 411–474.

Stiles J. Feline ophthalmology. In: Gelatt KN, ed., Veterinary Ophthalmology, 5th ed. Ames, IA: Wiley-Blackwell, 2013, pp. 1477–1559.

Author Ian P. Herring
Consulting Editor Kathern E. Myrna

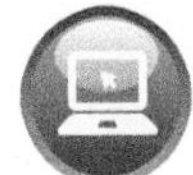

Client Education Handout available online

A

ANTERIOR UVEITIS—DOGS

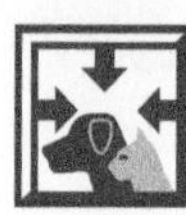

BASICS

DEFINITION

• Inflammation of anterior uvea, including iris (iritis), ciliary body (cyclitis), or both (iridocyclitis). • May be associated with posterior uveal and retinal inflammation (choroiditis; chorioretinitis). • Unilateral or bilateral.

PATHOPHYSIOLOGY

• Increased permeability of blood–aqueous barrier due to infectious, immune-mediated, traumatic, or other causes allows plasma proteins and blood cells to enter aqueous humor. • Disruption of blood–aqueous barrier is initiated and maintained by numerous mediators.

SYSTEMS AFFECTED

• Ophthalmic. • Other systems if systemic disease.

INCIDENCE/PREVALENCE

• Relatively common. • True incidence/prevalence unknown.

GEOGRAPHIC DISTRIBUTION

Geographic location may affect incidence of certain infections.

SIGNALMENT

Species

Dog

Breed Predilections

• None for most causes. • Uveitis associated with iridociliary cysts in golden retriever (golden retriever pigmentary uveitis) and Great Dane. • Increased incidence of uveodermatologic syndrome in Siberian husky, Akita, Samoyed, and Shetland sheepdog.

Mean Age and Range

• Any age. • Uveodermatologic syndrome—mean 2.8 years. • Golden retriever pigmentary uveitis—mean 8.6 years.

SIGNS

Historical Findings

• Red eye (conjunctival hyperemia, ciliary flush). • Cloudy eye (corneal edema, aqueous flare, hypopyon). • Painful eye (blepharospasm, photophobia, or rubbing eye). • Vision loss—variable.

Physical Examination Findings

Thorough physical examination is critical.

Ophthalmic Findings

• Ocular discomfort—blepharospasm, photophobia, and rubbing eye. • Ocular discharge—usually serous; sometimes mucoid to mucopurulent. • Conjunctival hyperemia—bulbar and palpebral conjunctiva affected. • Corneal edema—diffuse; mild to severe. • Keratic precipitates—aggregates of inflammatory cells adherent to corneal endothelium. • Aqueous flare—cloudiness of aqueous humor due to increased protein content and cellular debris; best seen with a bright, narrow beam of light shone through anterior chamber. • Ciliary flush—injection of deep perilimbal anterior ciliary vessels. • Deep corneal vascularization—circumcorneal distribution. • Miosis and/or resistance to pharmacologic dilation. • Iridal swelling. • Reduced intraocular pressure (IOP) is consistent with uveitis, but not a uniform finding. • Posterior synechia—adhesions between posterior iris and anterior lens surface. • Fibrin in anterior chamber. • Hypopyon or hyphema—accumulation of white or red blood cells, respectively, in anterior chamber; usually settles horizontally in ventral aspect of chamber, but may be diffuse. • Chronic changes may include rubeosis iridis, iridal hyperpigmentation, secondary cataract, lens luxation, pupillary seclusion, iris bombé, secondary glaucoma, and phthisis bulbi.

CAUSES

• Infectious—fungal (*Blastomyces dermatitidis, Cryptococcus neoformans, Coccidioides immitis, Histoplasma capsulatum, Candida* spp., *Aspergillus* spp., *Encephalitozoon cuniculi*), protozoal (*Toxoplasma gondii, Neospora caninum, Leishmania donovani*), rickettsial (*Ehrlichia canis, Rickettsia rickettsii*), bacterial (*Leptospira* spp., *Bartonella* spp., *Brucella canis, Borrelia burgdorferi*, and others), algal (*Prototheca* spp.), viral (adenovirus, distemper, rabies, herpes), parasitic (ocular filariasis, ocular nematodiasis, ophthalmomyiasis). • Immune-mediated—reaction to lens proteins (due to cataract or lens trauma), uveodermatologic syndrome, postvaccinal reaction to canine adenovirus vaccine, vasculitis. • Neoplastic—primary ocular tumors (uveal melanoma, iridociliary adenoma/adenocarcinoma), metastasis to uveal tract (e.g., lymphosarcoma). • Metabolic—hyperlipidemia, hyperviscosity, systemic hypertension. • Miscellaneous—idiopathic, trauma, golden retriever pigmentary uveitis, ulcerative keratitis, corneal stromal abscess, scleritis, lens instability/luxation.

RISK FACTORS

Immune suppression and geographic location may increase risk for infectious causes of uveitis; consider breed predispositions.

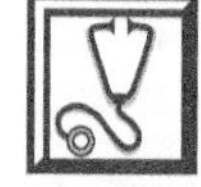

DIAGNOSIS

DIFFERENTIAL DIAGNOSIS

• Conjunctivitis—redness limited to conjunctival hyperemia (i.e., no ciliary flush); discharge usually thicker and more copious; discomfort alleviated with topical anesthetic. • Glaucoma—elevated IOP, diffuse corneal edema, dilated pupil, Haab's striae, buphthalmos. • Lens luxation—corneal edema may be localized to site of lens contact with endothelium or diffuse as a result of secondary uveitis and/or glaucoma; breed associated. • Ulcerative keratitis—corneal fluorescein stain detects ulcers; corneal edema localized to, or most severe at, site of ulcer; discomfort alleviated by topical anesthetic. • Corneal endothelial dystrophy or degeneration—diffuse corneal edema with normal IOP; conjunctival hyperemia and ocular discomfort generally absent. • Horner's syndrome—miosis, enophthalmos, and nictitans protrusion in both conditions, but Horner's is nonpainful without ocular discharge; ptosis with Horner's is distinguished from blepharospasm as the latter is an active process; minor conjunctival hyperemia may be noted, but cornea and anterior chamber are clear; clinical signs of Horner's syndrome resolve with topical ophthalmic 1–10% phenylephrine.

CBC/BIOCHEMISTRY/URINALYSIS

Normal, or reflect underlying disease.

OTHER LABORATORY TESTS

Serology for infectious diseases may be indicated, especially in patients with signs of systemic illness.

IMAGING

• Thoracic radiography and abdominal ultrasound may be warranted for systemic disease. • Ocular ultrasound is indicated if ocular media opacity precludes direct examination.

DIAGNOSTIC PROCEDURES

• Tonometry—low IOP consistent with uveitis; elevated IOP indicates glaucoma (primary disease or secondary to uveitis). • Ocular centesis—if retinal detachment is present, cytology of subretinal aspirate may reveal causative agents; anterior chamber centesis unrewarding, except in cases of lymphoma.

PATHOLOGIC FINDINGS

Histopathologic—may observe corneal edema, peripheral corneal deep stromal vascularization, keratic precipitates, preiridal fibrovascular membrane, anterior or posterior synechia, entropion or ectropion uveae. Leukocyte accumulation in iris, ciliary body, sclera, choroid may be lymphocytic, plasmacytic, suppurative, or granulomatous, depending on etiology. Secondary cataract, cyclitic membrane, vitreal traction bands, and retinal detachment may be present.

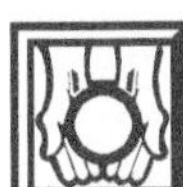

TREATMENT

APPROPRIATE HEALTH CARE

Outpatient

ACTIVITY

• No changes in most cases. • Reduced exposure to bright light may alleviate discomfort.

DIET

No changes.

CLIENT EDUCATION

• Systemic disease may cause ophthalmic signs; emphasize importance of appropriate diagnostic testing. • In addition to symptomatic uveitis treatment, treatment of underlying disease (when possible) is paramount. • Inform of potential complications and emphasize compliance with treatment and follow-up recommendations to reduce likelihood of complications.

SURGICAL CONSIDERATIONS

• None (most cases). • Specific instances include removal of ruptured lenses, removal of cataracts causing uveitis (if prognosis is otherwise favorable), surgical management of corneal disease causing uveitis, and surgical management of secondary glaucoma.

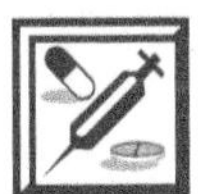

MEDICATIONS

DRUG(S) OF CHOICE

Corticosteroids

Topical

• Prednisolone acetate 1% or dexamethasone 0.1%—apply 2–8 times daily, depending on severity of disease; taper as condition resolves.
• Stopping topical corticosteroids abruptly may result in rebound ocular inflammation.

Subconjunctival

• Often not required; indicated only in severe cases as one-time injection. • Triamcinolone acetonide—4–6 mg, subconjunctival injection.
• Methylprednisolone—3–10 mg, subconjunctival injection.

Systemic

• Prednisone—0.5–2.2 mg/kg/day PO initially; taper dose after 7–10 days. Long-term treatment with immunosuppressive medication may be warranted for immune-mediated uveitis.
• Use only if systemic infectious causes of uveitis have been ruled out.

Nonsteroidal Anti-inflammatory Drugs (NSAIDs)

Topical

• Less effective than topical corticosteroids; can be combined with topical steroids.
• Flurbiprofen, diclofenac, ketorolac—apply 2–4 times daily, depending on severity of disease.

Systemic

• Do not use concurrently with systemic corticosteroids; avoid in presence of hyphema.
• Carprofen—2.2 mg/kg PO q12h or 4.4 mg/kg PO q24h. • Meloxicam—0.2 mg/kg on day 1, followed by 0.1 mg/kg PO q24h. • Deracoxib—1–2 mg/kg PO q24h. • Firocoxib—5 mg/kg PO q24h.

Topical Mydriatic/Cycloplegic

Atropine sulfate 1%—apply 1–4 times daily, depending on severity of disease; use lowest frequency adequate to maintain dilated pupil and ocular comfort; taper medication as condition resolves.

CONTRAINDICATIONS

• Avoid topical miotic medications (e.g., pilocarpine), including topical prostaglandins (e.g., latanoprost), in presence of uveitis.
• Avoid topical atropine in cases of uveitis with secondary glaucoma. • Topical and subconjunctival corticosteroids are contraindicated with ulcerative keratitis. • Avoid systemic corticosteroids in dogs with systemic infection.

PRECAUTIONS

Out of concern for secondary glaucoma, topical atropine should be used judiciously and IOP should be monitored periodically.

POSSIBLE INTERACTIONS

Systemic corticosteroids and NSAIDs should not be used concurrently.

ALTERNATIVE DRUG(S)

N/A

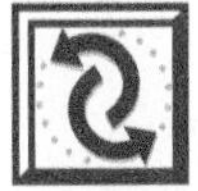

FOLLOW-UP

PATIENT MONITORING

Recheck in 3–7 days, depending on severity of disease. IOP should be monitored to detect secondary glaucoma. Frequency of subsequent rechecks dictated by severity of disease and response to treatment.

POSSIBLE COMPLICATIONS

• Many systemic complications, including death, may occur due to systemic etiology of uveitis. • Ophthalmic complications include secondary cataract, secondary glaucoma, lens luxation, retinal detachment, phthisis bulbi.

EXPECTED COURSE AND PROGNOSIS

Extremely variable; depends on underlying disease and response to treatment.

MISCELLANEOUS

ZOONOTIC POTENTIAL

None in most cases. Some etiologies of systemic infection may pose a risk to immune-compromised owners.

PREGNANCY/FERTILITY/BREEDING

Avoid systemic corticosteroids. Because of possibility of systemic absorption, topical corticosteroids may also pose risk, especially with frequent application in small dogs.

SYNONYMS

Iridocyclitis

SEE ALSO

Red Eye.

ABBREVIATIONS

• IOP = intraocular pressure.
• NSAID = nonsteroidal anti-inflammatory drug.

Suggested Reading

Cullen C, Webb A. Ocular manifestations of systemic diseases. Part 1: The dog. In: Gelatt KN, ed., Veterinary Ophthalmology, 5th ed. Ames, IA: Wiley-Blackwell, 2013, pp. 1897–1977.

Hendrix D. Diseases and surgery of the canine anterior uvea. In: Gelatt KN, ed., Veterinary Ophthalmology, 5th ed. Ames, IA: Wiley-Blackwell, 2013, pp. 1146–1198.

Miller P. Diseases of the uvea. In: Maggs DJ, Miller PE, Ofri R, eds., Slatter's Fundamentals of Veterinary Ophthalmology, 6th ed. St. Louis, MO: Elsevier Saunders, 2018, pp. 254–276.

Pickett JP. Anterior uvea and anterior chamber. In: Martin C, Pickett J, Spiess B, eds., Ophthalmic Disease in Veterinary Medicine. Boca Raton, FL: CRC Press, 2018, pp. 411–474.

Author Ian P. Herring

Consulting Editor Kathern E. Myrna

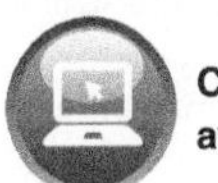

Client Education Handout available online

ANTIDEPRESSANT TOXICOSIS—SSRIs AND SNRIs

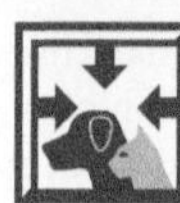

BASICS

DEFINITION

- Toxicity secondary to the overdose of a selective serotonin reuptake inhibitor (SSRI), serotonin and norepinephrine reuptake inhibitor (SNRI), or coingestion of two types of serotonergic drugs.
- SSRIs include citalopram (Celexa®), escitalopram (Lexapro®), fluoxetine (Prozac®), fluvoxamine (Luvox®), paroxetine (Paxil®), sertraline (Zoloft®), vilazodone (Viibryd®), and vortioxetine (Brintellix®). SNRIs include desvenlafaxine (Pristiq®), duloxetine (Cymbalta®), levomilnacipran (Fetzima®), milnacipran (Ixel®, Savella®), tofenacin (Elamol®, Tofacine®), and venlafaxine (Effexor®).

PATHOPHYSIOLOGY

- SSRIs and SNRIs are antidepressants that inhibit reuptake of serotonin, a neurotransmitter involved in aggression, anxiety, appetite, depression, migraine, pain, and sleep. Antidepressant effects are secondary to inhibition of reuptake of serotonin into serotonergic neurons via binding to the serotonin transporter, resulting in increased synaptic availability of serotonin. SNRIs also inhibit the reuptake of norepinephrine by the same mechanism.
- Excessive stimulation of serotonin receptors can occur by enhanced serotonin synthesis, increased presynaptic serotonin release, inhibition of serotonin uptake into the presynaptic neuron, inhibition of serotonin metabolism, or serotonin agonism. Ingesting too much of one medication or a combination of medications that increase serotonin via different methods can lead to serotonin syndrome.
- Serotonin syndrome is characterized in humans as a combination of symptoms that include at least three of the following: myoclonus, mental aberration, agitation, hyperreflexia, tremors, diarrhea, ataxia, or hyperthermia.
- Toxic dosage varies widely among commonly available SSRIs and SNRIs and is not well defined in veterinary medicine.

SYSTEMS AFFECTED

- Cardiovascular—decreased vascular tone (hypotension), increased heart rate and stroke volume (tachycardia).
- Gastrointestinal—increased smooth muscle contractility (vomiting, diarrhea).
- Nervous—stimulation (agitation, restlessness, seizures) and altered mental status (vocalization, disorientation).
- Neuromuscular—autonomic dysfunction (hyperactivity) and neuromuscular hyperactivity (hyperreflexia, myoclonus, tremors).
- Ophthalmic—increased autonomic function (mydriasis).
- Respiratory—increased bronchial smooth muscle contraction (dyspnea).

INCIDENCE/PREVALENCE

Second most common human prescription medication toxicosis (after cardiac medications).

SIGNALMENT

Species

Dogs and cats.

Mean Age and Range

Any age can be affected.

SIGNS

Historical Findings

- Agitation or lethargy.
- Dilated pupils.
- Vomiting.
- Tremors.
- Hypersalivation.
- Diarrhea.
- Seizures.
- Nystagmus.

Physical Examination Findings

- Agitation.
- Ataxia.
- Mydriasis.
- Tremors.
- Vomiting.
- Disorientation.
- Hyperthermia.
- Vocalization.
- Depression.
- Tachycardia.
- Hypotension.
- Diarrhea.
- Blindness.
- Seizures.
- Hypersalivation.
- Death.

CAUSES

- SSRI/SNRI overdose—accidental exposure, inappropriate administration, or therapeutic use.
- Ingestion of an SSRI/SNRI along with another class of medications that increases serotonin (tricyclic antidepressants [TCAs], monoamine oxidase inhibitors [MAOIs], novel antidepressants, tramadol, fentanyl, meperidine, amphetamines, cocaine, dextromethorphan, 5-hydroxytryptophan [5-HTP], buspirone, bupropion, triptans, LSD).

RISK FACTORS

- Animals on a serotonergic drug.
- Underlying liver or kidney disease; cats are attracted to venlafaxine and will eat multiple capsules.

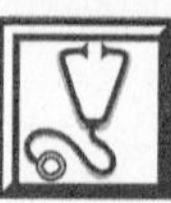

DIAGNOSIS

DIFFERENTIAL DIAGNOSIS

- Toxicologic—TCAs, MAOIs, metaldehyde, lead, ethylene glycol, hops, anticholinergics, antihistamines.
- Nontoxicologic—meningitis (e.g., rabies, canine distemper), neoplasia, heat stroke, malignant hyperthermia.

CBC/BIOCHEMISTRY/URINALYSIS

- CBC/biochemistry—no direct changes are expected, but creatine kinase (CK) may be elevated secondary to tremors.
- Urinalysis—myoglobinuria secondary to rhabdomyolysis may be seen.

OTHER LABORATORY TESTS

- Blood gas—metabolic acidosis may be seen.
- Testing for SSRIs/SNRIs can be performed, but the tests are not clinically useful.
- Note: venlafaxine will give a false positive for phencyclidine (PCP; angel dust) on many urine drug screens.

DIAGNOSTIC PROCEDURES

There are no diagnostic tests to confirm serotonin syndrome.

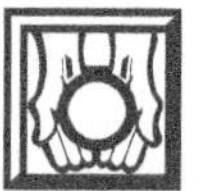

TREATMENT

APPROPRIATE HEALTH CARE

- Emesis (if asymptomatic and recent ingestion) or gastric lavage (if large number of pills ingested).
- Activated charcoal with cathartic (if severe signs are expected, may need to repeat due to long half-life).

NURSING CARE

IV fluids to help maintain blood pressure and body temperature, and to protect kidneys from myoglobinuria.

CLIENT EDUCATION

If animal appears blind, sight should return.

MEDICATIONS

DRUG(S) OF CHOICE

- Agitation:
  - Phenothiazines (acepromazine 0.025–0.05 mg/kg IV, titrate up as needed).
  - Cyproheptadine (dog, 1.1 mg/kg; cat, 2–4 mg PO q4–6h or can be given rectally if vomiting).
  - Benzodiazepines (diazepam 0.5–2 mg/kg IV; see Precautions).
  - Tremors—methocarbamol (50–150 mg/kg IV, titrate up as needed).

CONTRAINDICATIONS

- High risk of serotonin syndrome—other SSRIs, SNRIs, MAOIs, TCAs, amphetamines, 5-HTP, clarithromycin, dextromethorphan, lithium, St. John's wort.
- Low risk of serotonin syndrome—tramadol, fentanyl, amantadine, bupropion, carbamazepine, codeine.

PRECAUTIONS

Benzodiazepines (e.g., diazepam) are reported by some sources to exacerbate serotonin syndrome and their use for SSRI/SNRI toxicosis is not universally recommended.

POSSIBLE INTERACTIONS

- Decreased metabolism of SSRIs/SNRIs—cimetidine, diuretics, quinidine, lithium.
- Increased levels of medications (decreased metabolism)—theophylline, coumadin, digoxin.

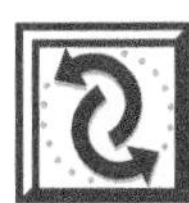

FOLLOW-UP

PATIENT MONITORING

Blood pressure, heart rate, urine color—monitor hourly, then less frequently as the animal remains stable.

PREVENTION/AVOIDANCE

- Keep medications out of the reach of animals.
- Follow label directions when giving serotonergic drugs to animals.

POSSIBLE COMPLICATIONS

Renal failure secondary to myoglobinuria from rhabdomyolysis; disseminated intravascular coagulation (DIC) secondary to hyperthermia.

EXPECTED COURSE AND PROGNOSIS

- Prognosis is good in most cases, with recovery in 12–24 hours.
- Patients that present in status epilepticus or with severe hyperthermia have a guarded prognosis.

MISCELLANEOUS

AGE-RELATED FACTORS

Young and elderly animals are more at risk for developing serious toxicosis.

PREGNANCY/FERTILITY/BREEDING

SSRIs and SNRIs can cause increased litter mortality and possible birth defects.

ABBREVIATIONS

- 5-HTP = 5-hydroxytryptophan.
- CK = creatine kinase.
- DIC = disseminated intravascular coagulation.
- MAOI = monoamine oxidase inhibitor.
- PCP = phencyclidine (angel dust).
- SNRI = serotonin and norepinephrine reuptake inhibitor.
- SSRI = selective serotonin reuptake inhibitor.
- TCA = tricyclic antidepressant.

Suggested Reading

Pugh CM, Sweeney JT, Bloch CP, et al. Selective serotonin reuptake inhibitor (SSRI) toxicosis in cats: 33 cases (2004–2010). J Vet Emerg Crit Care 2013, 23(5):565–570.

Thomas DE, Lee JA, Hovda LR. Retrospective evaluation of toxicosis from selective serotonin reuptake inhibitor antidepressants: 313 dogs (2005–2010). J Vet Emerg Crit Care 2012, 22(6):674–681.

Wismer TA. Antidepressant drug overdoses in dogs. Vet Med 2000, 95(7):520–525.

Author Tina Wismer

Consulting Editor Lynn R. Hovda

ANTIDEPRESSANT TOXICOSIS—TRICYCLIC

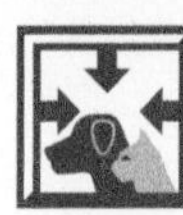

BASICS

DEFINITION

• Toxicity secondary to the acute or chronic ingestion of a tricyclic antidepressant (TCA).
• TCA medications include amitriptyline, amoxapine, clomipramine, desipramine, doxepin, imipramine, maprotiline (tetracyclic antidepressant), nortriptyline, protriptyline, trimipramine, and many others.

PATHOPHYSIOLOGY

• TCAs block the reuptake of norepinephrine, dopamine, and serotonin at the neuronal membrane. They also have anticholinergic activity and are thought to have membrane-stabilizing effects on the myocardium (particularly inhibiting fast sodium channels in the ventricular myocardium). They can also have slight alpha-adrenergic blocking activity and antihistaminic effects.
• TCAs are rapidly and well absorbed across the digestive tract. They can decrease GI motility and delay gastric emptying, resulting in delayed drug absorption.
• Lipophilic, protein bound, and well distributed across all tissues.
• They are metabolized by the liver and undergo enterohepatic recirculation. The inactive metabolites are eliminated in the urine.

SYSTEMS AFFECTED

• Nervous—increased dopamine, serotonin, and norepinephrine levels in the CNS contribute to CNS signs.
• Cardiovascular—anticholinergic effects and inhibition of norepinephrine reuptake contribute to tachycardia; alpha adrenergic blockade, cardiac membrane stabilization, and decreased cardiac contractility contribute to hypotension and arrhythmias.
• Gastrointestinal (GI)—anticholinergic effects may cause ileus and delayed gastric emptying.
• Ophthalmic—anticholinergic effects can cause pupillary dilation.
• Renal/urologic—anticholinergic effects may cause urinary retention.

GENETICS

Species and individual differences in absorption, metabolism, and elimination can be significant.

INCIDENCE/PREVALENCE

Incidence is unknown.

SIGNALMENT

Species

Dogs and cats.

Breed Predilections

None

Mean Age and Range

None

SIGNS

General Comments

• Signs can occur at therapeutic doses.
• Signs of toxicosis can occur within 30–60 minutes or be delayed by several hours.

Historical Findings

• Evidence of accidental consumption of the owner's or another pet's medication.
• CNS depression (lethargy, ataxia).
• Vocalization.
• Vomiting or hypersalivation.
• Panting.
• Agitation or restlessness.
• Tachypnea or dyspnea.
• Tremors.
• Seizures.

Physical Examination Findings

• CNS depression or stimulation.
• Tachycardia.
• Ataxia.
• Mydriasis.
• Hypothermia.
• Hypertension.
• Pallor.
• Cyanosis.
• Hyperthermia.
• Arrhythmias.
• Hypotension.
• Urinary retention.
• Constipation.

CAUSES

Accidental exposure, inappropriate administration, or therapeutic use.

RISK FACTORS

• Concurrent use of other antipsychotic medication.
• Preexisting cardiac disease.

DIAGNOSIS

DIFFERENTIAL DIAGNOSIS

• Toxicity caused by other antipsychotic medication, stimulant substances (e.g., amphetamines, cocaine, methylxanthines, or pseudoephedrine), or substances capable of causing cardiac arrhythmias (e.g., quinidine, propranolol, albuterol, digoxin).
• Nontoxicologic differentials include hyperkalemia, cardiac ischemia, cardiomyopathy, and other diseases of cardiac conduction.

CBC/BIOCHEMISTRY/URINALYSIS

Expected to be normal.

OTHER LABORATORY TESTS

• Blood gases—metabolic acidosis may be noted.
• Over-the-counter (OTC) urine drug screen for TCAs—can be used to determine if exposure has occurred; not useful in determining degree of toxicity.
• Serum TCA levels—can be used to determine if exposure has occurred.

IMAGING

N/A

DIAGNOSTIC PROCEDURES

• ECG to monitor for arrhythmias.
• Blood pressure monitoring.

PATHOLOGIC FINDINGS

No specific lesions expected.

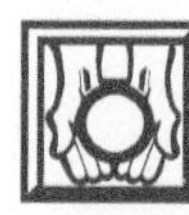

TREATMENT

APPROPRIATE HEALTH CARE

• Outpatient—not recommended for symptomatic patients, patients with cardiac disease, or patients ingesting greater than a therapeutic dose of TCAs.
• Inpatient—asymptomatic:
  ◦ Decontamination with emesis (less than 15 minutes of exposure time), gastric lavage in large exposures, and activated charcoal.
  ◦ Monitor at a clinic for a minimum of 6 hours after exposure.
• Inpatient—symptomatic: stabilize the cardiovascular (CV) system and CNS and provide supportive care.

NURSING CARE

• Fluid therapy—restore hydration due to vomiting, regulate blood pressure when hypotension is noted.
• Thermoregulation as needed.
• Enema with warm water if not defecating within 6–12 hours.

ACTIVITY

N/A

DIET

NPO if vomiting.

CLIENT EDUCATION

• With a prescribed TCA, instruct client to monitor for adverse or idiosyncratic effects, and to stop the medication and contact the clinic if they occur.
• Prevent exposure to nonprescribed medication.

SURGICAL CONSIDERATIONS

N/A

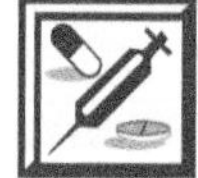

MEDICATIONS

DRUG(S) OF CHOICE

Decontamination

• Emesis within 15 minutes of ingestion *only if asymptomatic*; induce emesis with either hydrogen peroxide (dog, 1–2 mL/kg PO),

apomorphine (dog, 0.03–0.05 mg/kg IV/IM, or 0.1 mg/kg SC, or 0.25 mg instilled in conjunctiva of eye), or dexmedetomidine (cat, 7 μg/kg IM or 3.5 μg/kg IV).
- Gastric lavage under anesthesia may be considered with large exposures.
- After emesis (or if >15 min of exposure), administer activated charcoal (1–2 g/kg PO) with a cathartic such as sorbitol (70% sorbitol at 3 mL/kg) or sodium sulfate (0.25 tsp/5 kg) if no diarrhea.
- Repeat one-half dose of activated charcoal in 4–6 hours if patient is still symptomatic.

Other

- Cyproheptadine—dogs, 1.1 mg/kg q8h PO or rectally; cats, 2–4 mg/cat q12–24h PO or rectally; used for treatment of serotonin syndrome.
- 20% intravenous lipid emulsion—prevents lipophilic TCAs from reaching site of action by acting as sequestrant in expanded plasma lipid phase; 1.5 mL/kg IV bolus followed by 0.25 mL/kg/min IV CRI for 1 hour. Can repeat bolus and CRI in 4–6 hours if serum is not lipemic and a poor response to treatment is seen.
- Sodium bicarbonate—used to maintain blood pH at 7.55; if not monitoring acid-base status, start with 2–3 mEq/kg IV over 15–30 minutes in a symptomatic patient.
- Diazepam—0.5–1 mg/kg IV, repeat if necessary; for agitation or seizures.
- Acepromazine—0.02 mg/kg IV, repeat if necessary; for agitation or mild hypertension.
- Phenobarbital—as needed for seizure control.

CONTRAINDICATIONS

- Atropine should not be used, because TCAs have anticholinergic effects that are exacerbated by atropine.
- Trazodone should not be used, because it can result in serotonin syndrome when given concurrently.
- Magnesium sulfate should not be used as a cathartic. Ileus or reduced GI motility will enhance absorption of magnesium and may result in magnesium toxicity.
- Beta blockers (e.g., propranolol, atenolol) should not be used for tachycardia because of their potential to exacerbate hypotension.
- Do not induce emesis in a patient already showing clinical signs.

PRECAUTIONS

N/A

POSSIBLE INTERACTIONS

- TCAs increase risk of hyperthermia, seizures, and death with use of monoamine oxidase inhibitors (MAOIs).
- Sympathomimetic and anticholinergic medications increase the risk for arrhythmias or cardiac effects from TCAs.
- Levothyroxine increases the risk for arrhythmias when used with TCAs.

ALTERNATIVE DRUG(S)

N/A

FOLLOW-UP

PATIENT MONITORING

- Acid-base status—monitor for acidosis and if implementing sodium bicarbonate therapy.
- Blood pressure—monitor until asymptomatic.
- ECG—monitor until asymptomatic.

PREVENTION/AVOIDANCE

Keep medications out of reach of pets.

POSSIBLE COMPLICATIONS

Pulmonary edema can occur secondary to aggressive fluid therapy.

EXPECTED COURSE AND PROGNOSIS

- Due to the variable half-lives of the different TCAs, signs can last 24 hours or longer.
- Prognosis is generally good in patients exhibiting mild to moderate signs.
- Prognosis is guarded in patients exhibiting severe signs such as seizures, arrhythmias, or hypotension that are poorly responsive to therapy.

MISCELLANEOUS

ASSOCIATED CONDITIONS

Serotonin syndrome may occur as a result of TCA ingestion.

AGE-RELATED FACTORS

None

PREGNANCY/FERTILITY/BREEDING

TCAs cross the placenta and can be found in breast milk; the significance of this is not known at this time.

SEE ALSO

- Antidepressant Toxicosis—SSRIs and SNRIs.
- Poisoning (Intoxication) Therapy.

ABBREVIATIONS

- CV = cardiovascular.
- GI = gastrointestinal.
- MAOI = monoamine oxidase inhibitor.
- OTC = over-the-counter.
- TCA = tricyclic antidepressant.

INTERNET RESOURCES

- http://www.aspcapro.org/poison
- http://www.petpoisonhelpline.com

Suggested Reading

Gwaltney-Brant S. Antidepressants: tricyclic antidepressants. In: Plumlee KH, ed., Clinical Veterinary Toxicology. St. Louis, MO: Mosby, 2004, pp. 286–288.

Gwaltney-Brant S, Meadows I. Use of intravenous lipid emulsions in veterinary clinical toxicology. Vet Clin North Am Small Anim Pract 2018, 48:933–942.

Johnson LR. Tricyclic antidepressant toxicosis. Vet Clin North Am Small Anim Pract 1990, 20:393–403.

Volmer PA. Recreational drugs: tricyclic antidepressants. In: Peterson ME, Talcott PA, eds., Small Animal Toxicology, 3rd ed. St. Louis, MO: Elsevier Saunders, 2013, pp. 328–330.

Wismer TA. Antidepressant drug overdoses in dogs. Vet Med 2000, 95:520–525.

Author Cristine L. Hayes

Consulting Editor Lynn R. Hovda

AORTIC STENOSIS

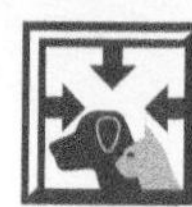

BASICS

DEFINITION

• A narrowing of the left ventricular outflow tract (LVOT) that restricts blood flow leaving the ventricle; most commonly congenital, often heritable. • Lesion is most commonly subvalvular in dogs, but may be valvular or supravalvular (more often in cats).
• Subvalvular aortic stenosis (SAS) in dogs is caused by fibrous tissue manifested as nodules, a ridge, a ring, or a tunnel-like lesion. SAS may be associated with other defects, including mitral valve dysplasia.

PATHOPHYSIOLOGY

• Restriction to outflow generates pressure overload of left ventricle (LV). • Degree of obstruction is related to severity of secondary changes. • LV pressure overload causes thickened LV walls, resulting in diminished blood supply relative to muscle demand and myocardial ischemia; this may result in arrhythmogenesis and, if severe or infarction occurs, mechanical dysfunction. • Restriction to blood flow causes high-velocity, turbulent flow across valve, which may cause endothelial damage, lead to aortic insufficiency (AI), and predispose to endocarditis. • SAS may lead to chamber enlargement, distortion of the mitral valve annulus, and mitral regurgitation, with possible sequela of left-sided congestive heart failure (CHF). • Sudden death is common with severe SAS and may be secondary to arrhythmias or infarction.

SYSTEMS AFFECTED

• Cardiovascular—LV pressure overload leading to arrhythmias, syncope, sudden death, heart failure, endocarditis. • Respiratory—possible pulmonary edema with CHF.
• Multisystemic—possible due to low cardiac output or endocarditis.

GENETICS

• SAS inherited in the Newfoundland, golden retriever, Rottweiler, bullmastiff, and dogue de Bordeaux. • Mutation in phosphatidylinositol-binding clathrin assembly protein gene (PICALM) reported in Newfoundlands; screening test is available. • Dominant inheritance patterns proposed for Newfoundlands with incomplete penetrance responsible for disease appearing to skip generations. • More than one gene or modifying genes may be involved. • Golden retrievers, Rottweilers, and bullmastiffs appear to inherit SAS in autosomal recessive pattern, but no associated mutation yet identified.

INCIDENCE/PREVALENCE

• SAS is one of most common congenital heart defects of dogs; it is reported as second most common, but difficulty in diagnosing mild disease may underestimate true prevalence.
• Aortic stenosis reported as small contributor of feline congenital heart disease, about 6%; approximately 2 out of 1,000 dogs and 0.2 per 1,000 cats evaluated at veterinary teaching hospitals are diagnosed with aortic stenosis, SAS most often in dogs and supravalvular aortic stenosis most often in cats.

GEOGRAPHIC DISTRIBUTION

N/A

SIGNALMENT

Species

Dog and cat.

Breed Predilections

• Newfoundland, bullmastiff, golden retriever, Rottweiler, bouvier des Flandres, dogue de Bordeaux, German shepherd, and boxer have highest incidence of SAS and familial component or heritability is reported.
• No breed predilection reported for cats.

Mean Age and Range

• Clinical signs may be seen at any age.
• Although often inherited, SAS becomes identifiable during first few weeks to months of life as subvalvular lesion progresses. • Full phenotype is appreciated by 1 year of age.

Predominant Sex

N/A

SIGNS

Historical Findings

• Many dogs show no clinical signs and have no relevant historical findings. • Historical findings related to disease severity and may include syncope, exercise intolerance, sudden death, and signs due to CHF such as respiratory distress and/or coughing if severe.

Physical Examination Findings

• Systolic left basilar ejection murmur; may radiate to apex, right side of thorax, include carotid arteries, and if very loud the cranium; precordial thrill may be palpable; murmur intensity loosely correlated to severity; as disease worsens during early life, some may have absence of or quiet murmur that develops to more characteristic finding by 1 year. • Diastolic murmur may be present with significant AI; combination of this diastolic murmur with systolic ejection murmur is to-and-fro murmur. • Arrhythmias may be ausculted. • Pulse deficits may be appreciated, often associated with ventricular arrhythmias.
• Weak pulses may be appreciated that are late or slow to rise with severe SAS (pulsus parvus et tardus). • Tachypnea, respiratory distress, and crackles may occur with CHF.

General Comments

• Boxers have relatively small aorta compared to other breeds, which can be difficult to distinguish from mild SAS. • Bull terriers overrepresented for combined mitral valve dysplasia and SAS. • Newfoundland dogs overrepresented for combined patent ductus arteriosus (PDA) and SAS. • Volume overload of PDA can cause relative aortic stenosis and be difficult to distinguish from PDA with mild SAS.

CAUSES

• Congenital heart disease. • Secondary to valvular change, as with aortic valve endocarditis or calcification. • Component of complex congenital heart disease, as with some cases of mitral valve dysplasia.

RISK FACTORS

• Familial history of SAS. • SAS predisposes to aortic valve endocarditis. • Aortic valve endocarditis predisposes to valvar aortic stenosis.

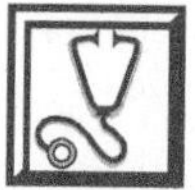

DIAGNOSIS

DIFFERENTIAL DIAGNOSIS

• Systolic murmur must be differentiated from other causes of similar murmurs.
• Innocent or physiologic murmurs commonly ausculted in athletic dogs, or with anemia, fever, stress, or excitement.
• Pulmonic stenosis and tetralogy of Fallot cause similar murmur. • Weak pulses may also occur with conditions that reduce cardiac output, such as heart failure, cardiomyopathy, and severe pulmonic stenosis. • Other obstruction to flow may cause reduced pulse quality, such as aortic thromboembolism, or rarely aortic coarctation/tubular hypoplasia.

CBC/BIOCHEMISTRY/URINALYSIS

Typically within normal limits.

OTHER LABORATORY TESTS

Genetic testing for mutation associated with Newfoundland SAS is breeding tool to reduce frequency in this breed.

IMAGING

Thoracic Radiography

• Mild disease may be radiographically silent.
• LV hypertrophy may be subtle, as pressure overload causes concentric hypertrophy. • Left heart enlargement. • Prominent aortic root and/or widened mediastinum. • Lung fields typically normal unless CHF with pulmonary venous distention and interstitial to alveolar infiltrates.

Echocardiography

• Findings variably present and associated with disease severity. • Ridge, ring, nodule, or tunnel-like narrowing below aortic valve with SAS. • Thickened LV free wall or interventricular septum. • Aortic valve thickening and increased echogenicity with valvar stenosis.
• Mitral regurgitation and thickening of valve leaflets possible. • Poststenotic aortic dilation.
• Hyperechoic myocardium associated with ischemia. • AI with secondary LV chamber enlargement and volume overload if significant.
• Left atrial enlargement may be seen with significant mitral valve regurgitation. • Elevated

LVOT flow velocity (>2.4 m/s), with acceleration proximal to stenosis and turbulent flow distal to obstruction and valve.
• Transvalvular pressure gradient estimated by LVOT flow velocity (4 × flow velocity^2); estimated gradients of 25–49 mmHg considered mild, 50–79 mmHg moderate, and ≥80 mmHg severe. • With myocardial failure, estimated pressure gradient may be falsely low.
• Effective valve orifice, if calculated, is reduced.

DIAGNOSTIC PROCEDURES

• ECG may show changes consistent with LV hypertrophy (tall R waves, widened QRS complexes, left axis deviation); signs of myocardial ischemia (ST segment deviation or slurring); ventricular arrhythmias may occur and contribute to syncope or sudden death.
• Holter monitoring may be used to quantify arrhythmia severity and therapeutic response.

PATHOLOGIC FINDINGS

• Findings vary with severity, but typically include LV concentric or mixed (if significant AI) hypertrophy. • Variable subvalvular lesion of dense fibrous tissue is seen. • Myocardial ischemia, necrosis, and replacement fibrosis may be evident. • Poststenotic dilation of aorta, associated valvular endothelial damage, and sometimes left atrial enlargement are reported.

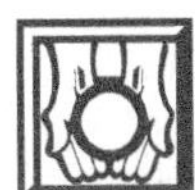

TREATMENT

APPROPRIATE HEALTH CARE

Therapy limited prior to onset of complications and aimed at preventing clinical signs.

NURSING CARE

Aimed at relieving symptoms and complications such as arrhythmias, syncope, and CHF.

ACTIVITY

Restriction warranted with severe disease; exertion may increase incidence of arrhythmias, syncope, and therefore risk of sudden death.

DIET

Modest salt restriction with CHF.

CLIENT EDUCATION

• SAS considered inherited disease; affected animals should not be bred. • Owners should be counseled on risk of endocarditis and appropriate antibiotics for any wounds, infections, or surgical procedures. • Alert owners to risks of sudden death, CHF, and increased anesthetic risk.

SURGICAL CONSIDERATIONS

• No surgical or interventional technique has been shown to extend life beyond medical therapy. • Balloon valvuloplasty or combined cutting and traditional balloon valvuloplasty may acutely reduce pressure gradient and temporarily alleviate some clinical signs; however, effects not yet shown to be beneficial beyond those achieved with beta blockers. • Currently, data does not support surgery or intervention, but this remains area of continued research.

MEDICATIONS

DRUG(S) OF CHOICE

• Beta adrenergic blockers advocated with moderate to severe SAS, particularly with ventricular arrhythmias, syncope, or ECG evidence of ischemia; may reduce myocardial oxygen demand, eliminate or protect against ventricular arrhythmias, and reduce heart rate; atenolol is most common (dogs, 0.5–1.5 mg/kg PO q12h; cats, 6.25 mg/cat PO q12–24h). • Therapy for ventricular arrhythmias, CHF, atrial fibrillation, or endocarditis may be required.

CONTRAINDICATIONS

• Beta blockers contraindicated in animals with bronchoconstriction such as asthmatic cats. • Starting beta blockers with CHF contraindicated and continued use in patients that develop CHF is controversial.

PRECAUTIONS

• Beta blockers negatively impact cardiac output and starting low doses with gradual up-titration warranted. • Positive inotropes may worsen fixed obstruction and are used with caution when treating CHF. • Anesthetic drugs that cause hypotension, arrhythmias, or cardiac depression should be avoided with severe SAS.

POSSIBLE INTERACTIONS

N/A

ALTERNATIVE DRUG(S)

• Carvedilol (dogs, 0.5–1.5 mg/kg PO q12h).
• Metoprolol tartrate (dogs, 0.5–1.5 mg/kg PO q12h).

FOLLOW-UP

PATIENT MONITORING

• Monitor by ECG, Holter monitor, thoracic radiography, and echocardiography.
• Treatment of complications such as CHF and arrhythmias may necessitate additional monitoring for renal/electrolyte, blood pressure, and rhythm disturbances.

PREVENTION/AVOIDANCE

N/A

POSSIBLE COMPLICATIONS

Ventricular arrhythmias, syncope, myocardial infarction, sudden death, AI, mitral regurgitation, endocarditis.

EXPECTED COURSE AND PROGNOSIS

• Mildly affected dogs may have normal lifespan and quality without therapy.
• Severely affected dogs have limited lifespans and typically succumb to sudden death or CHF; in one study average lifespan for dogs with severe SAS on atenolol was about 4.5 years.

MISCELLANEOUS

ASSOCIATED CONDITIONS

Increased risk of infective endocarditis.

AGE-RELATED FACTORS

SAS may not be immediately apparent at birth, but appears over first few weeks to months of life.

PREGNANCY/FERTILITY/BREEDING

Contraindicated

SYNONYMS

Subaortic stenosis, discrete subaortic stenosis.

SEE ALSO

• Cardiomyopathy, Hypertrophic—Cats.
• Cardiomyopathy, Hypertrophic—Dogs.
• Congestive Heart Failure, Left-Sided.
• Endocarditis, Infective.

ABBREVIATIONS

• AI = aortic insufficiency. • CHF = congestive heart failure. • LV = left ventricle. • LVOT = left ventricular outflow tract. • PDA = patent ductus arteriosus. • SAS = subvalvular aortic stenosis.

Suggested Reading

Caivano D, Dickson D, Martin M, et al. Murmur intensity in adult dogs with pulmonic and subaortic stenosis reflects disease severity. J Small Anim Pract 2018, 59(3):161–166.

Kienle RD, Thomas WP, Pion PD. The natural clinical history of canine congenital subaortic stenosis. J Vet Intern Med 1994, 8(6):423–431.

Meurs KM, Lehmkuhl LB, Bonagura JD. Survival times in dogs with severe subvalvular aortic stenosis treated with balloon valvuloplasty or atenolol. J Am Vet Med Assoc 2005, 227(3):420–424.

Ontiveros ES, Fousse SL, Crofton AE, et al. Congenital cardiac outflow tract abnormalities in dogs: prevalence and pattern of inheritance from 2008 to 2017. Front Vet Sci 2019, 6(52), doi: 10.3389/fvets.2019.00052.

Stern JA, White SN, Lehmkuhl LB, et al. A single codon insertion in PICALM is associated with development of familial subvalvular aortic stenosis in Newfoundland dogs. Hum Genet 2014, 133(9):1139–1148.

Author Joshua A. Stern
Consulting Editor Michael Aherne

Client Education Handout available online

A

AORTIC THROMBOEMBOLISM

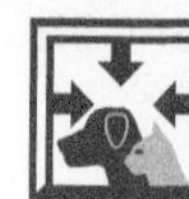

BASICS

DEFINITION

A thrombus or blood clot that is dislodged within the aorta, causing severe ischemia to the tissues served by that segment of aorta.

PATHOPHYSIOLOGY

- Aortic thromboembolism (ATE) is commonly associated with myocardial disease in cats, most commonly hypertrophic cardiomyopathy (HCM). It is theorized that abnormal blood flow (stasis) and a hypercoagulable state contribute to thrombus formation within the left atrium. The thrombus then embolizes distally to the aorta. The most common site of embolization is the caudal aortic trifurcation (hind legs). Other less common sites include the front legs, kidneys, gastrointestinal tract, or cerebrum.
- ATE in dogs typically is associated with neoplasia, sepsis, infectious endocarditis, Cushing's disease, protein-losing nephropathy and enteropathy, or other hypercoagulable states. However, in one recent retrospective study, no concurrent condition was identified in 58% of dogs.

SYSTEMS AFFECTED

- Cardiovascular—most affected cats have advanced heart disease and left heart failure.
- Nervous/musculoskeletal—severe ischemia to muscles and nerves served by segment of occluded aorta causes variable pain and paresis. Gait abnormality or paralysis results in leg or legs involved.

GENETICS

HCM, a common associated disease, is likely heritable. Additionally, a family of domestic shorthair cats with remodeled HCM who all died of ATE has been reported.

INCIDENCE/PREVALENCE

- In a recent observation study of over 1000 asymptomatic cats with HCM, nearly 12% developed ATE within 10 years after initial diagnosis. In two previous smaller case series of cats with clinical and preclinical HCM, 12–16% presented with signs of ATE; only 11–25% of cats had evidence of previously known heart disease.
- Rare in dogs.

GEOGRAPHIC DISTRIBUTION

N/A

SIGNALMENT

Species

Cat, rarely dog.

Breed Predilections

Mixed-breed cats most commonly affected. Abyssians, Birmans, and ragdolls overrepresented in one study. In dogs, no breed predilection identified in United States; European study suggested cavalier King Charles spaniels may be overrepresented.

Mean Age and Range

Age range—1–20 years. Median age—approximately 8–9 years (cats); 8–10 years (dogs).

Predominant Sex

Cats—males > females (2 : 1). Dogs—no sex predilection in United States; European study suggested male predilection.

SIGNS

Presence of 5 "Ps" is helpful to remember classic clinical signs associated with ATE—Pain, Paralysis or Paresis, Pulselessness, Pallor, and Poikilothermic (cold).

Historical Findings

- Acute onset paralysis and pain—most common in cats. Vocalization and anxiety also common.
- Lameness or gait abnormality, typically of several weeks' duration, more common in dogs.
- Tachypnea or respiratory distress common in cats.
- About 15% of cats may vomit prior to ATE.

Physical Examination Findings

- Usually paraparesis or paralysis of rear legs with signs of lower motor neuron injury. Less commonly, monoparesis of a front leg. In dogs, majority are paretic and ambulatory.
- Absent or diminished femoral pulses.
- Pain upon palpation of legs.
- Gastrocnemius muscle often becomes firm several hours after embolization.
- Cyanotic or pale nail beds and foot pads.
- Tachypnea/dyspnea and hypothermia are common in cats.
- Since commonly associated with heart disease in cats, cardiac murmur, arrhythmias, or gallop sound may be present.

CAUSES

- Cardiomyopathy (all types).
- Hyperthyroidism.
- Neoplasia.
- Sepsis (dogs).
- Hyperadrenocorticism (dogs).
- Protein-losing nephropathy and enteropathy (dogs).

RISK FACTORS

- In cats, cardiomyopathy, male sex, and gallop sound on exam are risk factors. Echocardiographic risk factors include enlarged left atrium, decreased left atrial function and left atrial appendage velocity, presence of spontaneous echocardiographic contrast (smoke) or left atrial thrombus, and restrictive left ventricular filling pattern.
- In dogs, hypercoagulable conditions, such as neoplasia, sepsis, endocarditis, protein-losing nephropathies/enteropathies, and hyperadrenocorticism are risk factors.

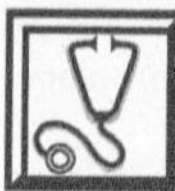

DIAGNOSIS

DIFFERENTIAL DIAGNOSIS

Hind limb paresis secondary to spinal neoplasia, trauma, myelitis, fibrocartilaginous infarction, or intervertebral disc protrusion. These conditions resulting in spinal cord injury present with signs of upper motor neuron disease, whereas ATE patients present with signs of lower motor neuron disease.

CBC/BIOCHEMISTRY/URINALYSIS

- High creatine kinase due to muscle injury.
- Higher blood lactate and lower blood glucose in affected limbs compared to normal limbs.
- High aspartate aminotransferase and alanine aminotransferase due to muscle and liver injury.
- Stress hyperglycemia.
- High blood urea nitrogen and creatinine due to low cardiac output and possible renal emboli.
- Electrolyte derangements, due to low output and muscle damage, such as hypocalcemia, hyponatremia, hyperphosphatemia, and hyperkalemia, are not uncommon.
- Nonspecific CBC and urinalysis changes.

OTHER LABORATORY TESTS

Routinely available coagulation profiles typically do not reveal significant abnormalities because hypercoagulability results from hyperaggregable platelets. In dogs, thromboelastrography may suggest hypercoagulable state with clot strength (increased maximum amplitude) or shortened clotting time (decreased R).

IMAGING

Radiography

- Cardiomegaly is common in cats.
- Pulmonary edema and/or pleural effusion in approximately 50% of cats.
- Rarely, a mass is seen in the lungs, suggestive of neoplasia.

Echocardiography

- In cats, changes consistent with cardiomyopathy. HCM is most common, followed by restrictive or unclassified cardiomyopathy, and then dilated cardiomyopathy.
- Most cases have severe left atrial enlargement (i.e., left atrial to aortic ratio of ≥2). Decreased left atrial function (fractional shortening) and decreased left atrial appendage velocity (<0.2 m/s).
- Left atrial thrombus or spontaneous echocardiographic contrast (smoke) may be seen.

Abdominal Ultrasonography

- May be able to identify the thrombus and visualize lack of blood flow in the caudal aorta.

• Typically unnecessary to reach a diagnosis in cats, but often needed to reach a diagnosis in dogs.

DIAGNOSTIC PROCEDURES

ECG

• Sinus rhythm and sinus tachycardia most common. Less common rhythms include atrial fibrillation, ventricular arrhythmias, supraventricular arrhythmias, and sinus bradycardia.
• Left ventricular enlargement pattern and left ventricular conduction disturbances (left anterior fascicular block) are common.

Doppler Blood Pressure

No or diminished audible blood flow in affected limbs.

PATHOLOGIC FINDINGS

• Thrombus typically identified at caudal aortic trifurcation.
• Occasionally, left atrial thrombus seen.
• Emboli of kidneys, gastrointestinal tract, cerebrum, and other organs also may be seen.

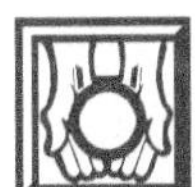

TREATMENT

APPROPRIATE HEALTH CARE

Initially, cats with ATE should be treated as inpatients, as many have concurrent congestive heart failure (CHF) and require injectable drugs, in addition to being in considerable pain and distress.

NURSING CARE

• Fluid therapy is cautiously used, as most cats have advanced myocardial disease. If in CHF, IV fluids may not be necessary.
• Supplemental oxygen or thoracocentesis may be beneficial if in CHF.
• Initially, minimally handle affected legs. However, as reperfusion occurs, physical therapy (passive extension and flexion) may speed full recovery.
• Do not perform venipuncture on affected legs.
• Animals may have difficulty posturing to urinate and may need bladder expression to prevent overdistention or urine scald.

ACTIVITY

Restrict activity and stress.

DIET

Initially, most cats are anorexic; tempt with any type of diet to keep them eating and avoid hepatic lipidosis.

CLIENT EDUCATION

• Short- and long-term prognosis is poor in both dogs and cats.
• Many cats do not survive their initial episode of ATE; if they survive, the cat will often reembolize or die of CHF within a few months to one year. Most cats that survive an initial episode will be on some type of anticoagulant and heart failure medications that may require frequent reevaluation and an indoor lifestyle.
• Most cats that survive an initial episode will recover complete function to the legs; however, if ischemia is severe and prolonged, sloughing of parts of the distal extremities or persistent neurologic deficits may result. In one study, approximately 15% of cats had permanent neuromucscular abnormalities after surviving the initial ATE.
• Prognosis in dogs is generally poor, but may be better in dogs presenting with chronic (vs. acute) lameness and dogs treated appropriately with warfarin.

SURGICAL CONSIDERATIONS

• Surgical embolectomy typically not recommended, since patients are high risk due to severe heart disease.
• Rheolytic thrombectomy has been used with limited success in a small number of cats with ATE.

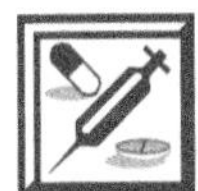

MEDICATIONS

DRUG(S) OF CHOICE

Medical management focuses on (1) the thrombus, (2) analgesia, and (3) heart failure treatments (if needed).

Management of Thrombus

• Thrombolytic therapy (e.g., tissue plasminogen activator [TPA]) is used extensively in humans and infrequently in animals. These drugs are expensive and carry a significant risk for bleeding complications; to date, improved treatment efficacy is unproven and thus they are rarely used in general practice. TPA is theorized to be more beneficial if given early, ideally within the first few hours of the ATE.
• Unfractionated heparin is the preferred anticoagulant in general practice for initial management of feline ATE. Heparin has no effect on the established clot; however, it prevents further activation of the coagulation cascade. In either cat or dog, use an initial dose of 100–200 units/kg IV and then 200–300 units/kg SC q8h. Alternatively, heparin can be continued as a constant rate infusion, at a dose of 25–35 units/kg/h. Some advocate titrating the dose to prolong the activated partial thromboplastin time (APTT) approximately twofold.
• Clopidogrel is an antiplatelet aggregation drug. A loading dose may be chosen for treatment of an acute ATE. The loading dose in the cat is 75 mg/cat PO once, and then a maintenance dose of 18.75 mg/cat (one-fourth of a 75 mg tablet) PO q24h. The loading dose in the dog is approximately 10 mg/kg once, and then a maintenance dose of 1 mg/kg q24h. Compared to aspirin, clopidogrel was superior in preventing reembolization, resulting in improved survival times in cats that had survived an ATE. The combination of unfractionated heparin and clopidogrel is commonly used for the management of ATE in cats.

Other Options

• Aspirin is theoretically beneficial during and after an ATE event due to its antiplatelet effects. The dose in cats is an 81 mg tablet PO q48–72h. Vomiting and diarrhea are not uncommon. Some specialists advocate a mini dose of 5 mg/cat q72h. Antithrombotic dose recommendations for dogs range from 0.5 to 2 mg/kg q24h. Always give aspirin with food.
• Warfarin, a vitamin K antagonist, is the anticoagulant most widely used in humans and has been proposed for prevention of reembolization in cats surviving an initial episode. The initial dose is 0.25–0.5 mg/cat PO q24h, or 0.05–0.2 mg/kg PO q24h in the dog. Overlap with heparin therapy for 3 days. The dose is then adjusted to prolong the prothrombin time (PT) approximately twice its baseline value, or to attain an international normalized ratio (INR) of 2 to 3. Long-term management with warfarin can be challenging because of frequent monitoring and dose adjustments in addition to bleeding complications. In one study, dogs treated appropriately with warfarin had a better clinical outcome.
• Low molecular weight heparin (LMWH) has recently been proposed for the long-term prevention of feline ATE. LMWH has a more predictable relationship between dose and response than warfarin and does not need monitoring or dose adjustments. It also has a lower risk of bleeding complications. The main disadvantages are high drug cost and the injectable route of administration. The two LMWHs that have been used in feline ATE are dalteparin (100–150 units/kg SC q8–24h) and enoxaparin (1 mg/kg SC q12–24h). The best dose is unknown. LMWH is usually started q24h due to cost. Some studies suggest q6h dosing is necessary for stable blood levels, but may increase bleeding risk. LMWH can be used as an adjunctive anticoagulant combined with clopidogrel.
• Rivaroxaban, a newer anticoagulant drug, is an inhibitor of activated clotting factor X and prothrombinase activity that has shown promise for treatment and prevention of arterial thromboembolism in both dogs and cats. Rivaroxaban has a more predictable anticoagulant effect than warfarin and does not require any monitoring or dose adjustments. The cat dose is 1.25 mg/cat PO q24h. The dose recommended in dogs is 0.5–1 mg/kg PO q24h. The main disadvantage of rivaroxaban is its high cost at the time of this writing. However, it has the advantage of a shorter half-time than clopidogrel if there is a

AORTIC THROMBOEMBOLISM

need to discontinue the medication because of a bleeding complication or need to perform an invasive procedure. A clinical trial is currently ongoing to compare rivaroxaban and clopidogrel in cats that have survived an ATE.

Analgesics

• Buprenorphine in the cat is a useful and widely available drug for analgesia and sedation at a dose of 5–20 µg/kg IV, SC, or in cheek pouch q6–8h. For stronger analgesia, use fentanyl or hydromorphone. Butorphanol, while a good sedative, does not provide sufficient analgesia.
• Acepromazine may be cautiously used for its sedative and vasodilatory properties at a dose of 0.01–0.02 mg SC q8–12h. However, vasodilatory effects are mixed and therefore results are often variable.

CONTRAINDICATIONS

N/A

PRECAUTIONS

• Anticoagulant therapy with heparin, warfarin, or thrombolytics may cause bleeding complications.
• Avoid a nonselective beta blocker such as propranolol as it may enhance peripheral vasoconstriction.

POSSIBLE INTERACTIONS

Warfarin may interact with other drugs, which may enhance its anticoagulant effects.

ALTERNATIVE DRUG(S)

N/A

FOLLOW-UP

PATIENT MONITORING

• ECG monitoring while cat in hospital is helpful to detect reperfusion injury and hyperkalemia-related ECG changes. Look for loss of P-waves and widening of QRS complexes.
• Monitoring electrolytes and renal parameters periodically may be helpful to optimize management of cardiac disease.
• Examine legs frequently to assess clinical response. Initially, APTT should be performed once daily to titrate heparin dose.
• If warfarin used, PT or INR is measured approximately 3 days after initiation of therapy and then weekly until desired anticoagulant effect reached. Thereafter, measure 3–4 times yearly or when drug regimen is altered.

PREVENTION/AVOIDANCE

Because of high rate of reembolization, prevention with either clopidogrel, aspirin, warfarin, or LMWH is strongly recommended.

POSSIBLE COMPLICATIONS

• Bleeding with anticoagulant therapy.
• Permanent neurologic deficits or muscular abnormalities in hind limbs may arise with prolonged ischemia.
• Recurrent CHF or sudden death.
• Reperfusion injury and death usually associated with hyperkalemic arrhythmias.

EXPECTED COURSE AND PROGNOSIS

• Expected course is days to weeks for full recovery of function to legs.
• Prognosis, both short and long term, is poor in cats.
• In two large studies, ~60% of cats were euthanized or died during initial thromboembolic episode. Long-term prognosis varies between 2 months and several years; however, average is a few months with treatment. Predictors of poorer prognosis include hypothermia (<99 °F) and CHF. One study demonstrated median survival time of 77 days in cats with CHF and 223 days in cats without CHF. Predictors of better prognosis include normothermia, single leg affected, and presence of motor function on initial exam.
• In dogs, the disease is rare and prognosis in general is also poor. One study suggested a better prognosis if the dog had chronic clinical signs and if treated with warfarin.
• Recurrence of ATE is common.

MISCELLANEOUS

ASSOCIATED CONDITIONS

See Causes & Risk Factors.

AGE-RELATED FACTORS

N/A

ZOONOTIC POTENTIAL

None

PREGNANCY/FERTILITY/BREEDING

N/A

SYNONYMS

• Saddle thromboembolism.
• Systemic thromboembolism.

SEE ALSO

• Cardiomyopathy, Dilated—Cats.
• Cardiomyopathy, Hypertrophic—Cats.
• Cardiomyopathy, Restrictive—Cats.

ABBREVIATIONS

• APTT = activated partial thromboplastin time.
• ATE = aortic thromboembolism.
• CHF = congestive heart failure.
• HCM = hypertrophic cardiomyopathy.
• INR = international normalized ratio.
• LMWH = low molecular weight heparin.
• PT = prothrombin time.
• TPA = tissue plasminogen activator.

Suggested Reading

Luis Fuentes V. Arterial thromboembolism: risks, realities and a rational first-line approach. J Feline Med Surg 2012, 14(7):459–470.

Winter RL, Sedacca CD, Adams A, Orton EC. Aortic thrombosis in dogs: presentation, therapy, and outcome in 26 cases. J Vet Cardiol 2012, 14:333–342.

Author Teresa C. DeFrancesco
Consulting Editor Michael Aherne

Client Education Handout available online

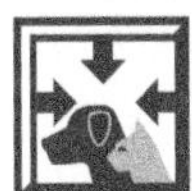

BASICS

OVERVIEW

• Tumors of endocrine cells that are capable of amine precursor uptake and decarboxylation (APUD) and secretion of peptide hormones. • APUD cells are generally found in gastrointestinal tract and CNS. • Hypergastrinemia from gastrin-secreting tumors (gastrinomas) causes gastritis and duodenal hyperacidity, which can cause gastric ulceration, gastric mucosal hypertrophy, esophageal dysfunction (chronic reflux), and intestinal villous atrophy.
• Polypeptide-secreting tumors (polypeptidomas) may not cause clinical signs, but high concentration of pancreatic polypeptide may cause gastric hyperacidity and gastrointestinal ulceration.

SIGNALMENT

• Gastrinoma—rare in dogs, very rare in cats; age range 3–12 years, mean 7.5 years (dogs).
• Pancreatic polypeptidoma—extremely rare in dogs.

SIGNS

• Vomiting. • Weight loss. • Anorexia.
• Diarrhea. • Lethargy, depression.
• Melena. • Abdominal pain. • Hematemesis, hematochezia. • Fever. • Polydipsia.
• Polypeptidomas may not cause any clinical signs.

CAUSES & RISK FACTORS

Unknown

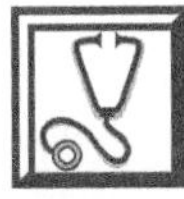

DIAGNOSIS

DIFFERENTIAL DIAGNOSIS

• Conditions associated with hypergastrinemia, gastric hyperacidity, and gastrointestinal ulceration: ○ Uremia. ○ Hepatic failure.
○ Drug-induced ulceration, e.g., nonsteroidal anti-inflammatory drugs (NSAIDs) or steroids. ○ Inflammatory gastritis. ○ Stress-induced ulceration. ○ Mast cell disease.

CBC/BIOCHEMISTRY/URINALYSIS

• Normal or reflective of chronic disease or iron-deficiency anemia due to chronic gastrointestinal bleeding. • Regenerative anemia. • Increased blood urea nitrogen (BUN). • Hypoproteinemia. • Electrolyte abnormalities.

OTHER LABORATORY TESTS

• Serum gastrin concentration—normal or high normal if gastrinoma. Antacid treatment increases serum gastrin, resulting in false-positive diagnosis of gastrinoma; withdrawal of drugs for at least 7 days returns gastrin concentrations to baseline in dogs without gastrinoma. • Induced gastrin secretion—increased gastrin concentration after IV calcium gluconate or secretin suggests gastrinoma; rarely reported in veterinary medicine.

IMAGING

Abdominal ultrasound may demonstrate pancreatic mass or evidence of gastrointestinal ulceration/thickened gastric wall; frequently, the primary mass is too small to be detected.

DIAGNOSTIC PROCEDURES

• CT or MRI to identify pancreatic masses and/or metastatic lesions. • Endoscopy with gastric and duodenal biopsy. • Aspirate any detectable masses (rule out mast cell disease).

PATHOLOGIC FINDINGS

• Endoscopic biopsy—gastrointestinal ulceration. • Histopathology of pancreatic tumors—islet cell tumor (not specific for hormone type). • Immunocytochemical staining can aid specific diagnosis. • Liver and regional lymph node biopsies may reveal metastasis.

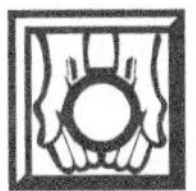

TREATMENT

• Most apudomas are malignant and have metastasized by the time of diagnosis; long-term control is difficult. • Aggressive medical management can palliate signs for months to years. • Surgical exploration and excisional biopsy/surgical debulking of a pancreatic mass are important both diagnostically and therapeutically. • Medical management for gastric hyperacidity.

MEDICATIONS

DRUG(S) OF CHOICE

• Omeprazole—proton pump inhibitor; potent inhibitor of gastric acid secretion; preferred.
• Histamine H_2-receptor antagonists—cimetidine, ranitidine, famotidine; decrease acid secretion by gastric parietal cells. • Sucralfate—adheres to ulcerated gastric mucosa and protects from acid; promotes healing by binding pepsin and bile acids and stimulating local prostaglandins. • Octreotide–somatostatin analog—used successfully in 2 dogs and 1 cat with gastrinoma.

CONTRAINDICATIONS/POSSIBLE INTERACTIONS

Because sucralfate may be less effective in an alkaline environment and may reduce absorption of other drugs, it should be given as a suspension, 1–2 hours prior to antacid drugs.

FOLLOW-UP

PATIENT MONITORING

• Physical examination and clinical signs are most useful measures of treatment effectiveness and disease progression. • Gastroscopy can monitor progression of gastritis, but is not necessary. • Abdominal radiography or ultrasound may detect development of abdominal masses. • Monitoring of CBC and serum protein levels may aid in assessing gastrointestinal hemorrhage.

POTENTIAL COMPLICATIONS

Gastrointestinal perforations may occur with severe ulceration.

EXPECTED COURSE AND PROGNOSIS

Survival time for gastrinoma ranges from weeks to years.

MISCELLANEOUS

SEE ALSO

Gastroduodenal Ulceration/Erosion.

ABBREVIATIONS

• APUD = amine precursor uptake and decarboxylation.
• BUN = blood urea nitrogen.
• NSAID = nonsteroidal anti-inflammatory drug.

Suggested Reading

Hughes SM. Canine gastrinoma: a case study and literature review of therapeutic options. N Z Vet J 2006, 54(5):242–247.

Lane M, Larson J, Hecht S, Tolbert MK. Medical management of gastrinoma in a cat. JFMS Open Rep 2016, 2(1):2055116916646389.

Author Alyssa M. Sullivant

Consulting Editor Patty A. Lathan

Acknowledgment The author and editor acknowledge the prior contribution of Thomas K. Graves.

ARTERIOVENOUS FISTULA AND ARTERIOVENOUS MALFORMATION

BASICS

OVERVIEW

- Abnormal, low-resistance connections between an artery and a vein (systemic or portal) that bypass a capillary bed.
- Arteriovenous malformation (AVM)—typically congenital, involving a vascular nidus, or complex network of communicating vessels.
- Arteriovenous fistula (AVF)—often acquired, direct, and singular connections.
- Large lesions cause marked drop in systemic vascular resistance and compensatory increase in cardiac output; this may cause circulatory volume overload and congestive heart failure (CHF).
- Variable location:
  - AVM most often reported in liver of dogs (termed arterioportal malformations/fistulas).
  - AVF more often in limbs or at sites of previous surgery/trauma.

SIGNALMENT

- Dog and cat (rare in both).
- No specific age, breed, or sex—AVMs typically in younger animals; 15% of hepatic AVMs found in Labrador retrievers in a recent multicenter study.

SIGNS

Historical Findings

- Depends on the lesion location (e.g., ascites with hepatic AVM).
- Often prior trauma to affected area with AVF.
- Warm, nonpainful swelling at site may be noted.
- Shunt may cause local organ dysfunction.

Physical Examination Findings

- Vary and depend on location.
- Signs of CHF (e.g., tachypnea, cough, exercise intolerance) may develop with chronic disease and high blood flow.
- Bounding pulses may be present due to high ejection volume and rapid runoff through AVM/AVF.
- Continuous murmur (bruit) at the site.
- Cautious compression of the artery proximal to the lesion abolishes the bruit. When blood flow is high, this may also elicit an immediate reflex decrease in heart rate (Branham's sign).
- Edema, ischemia, and congestion of organs and tissues caused by high venous pressure in proximity of lesion.
- If the lesion is on a limb, pitting edema, lameness, ulceration, scabbing, and gangrene may result.
- Lesions near vital organs may cause signs associated with organ failure, e.g., ascites (liver), seizures (brain), paresis (spinal cord).

CAUSES & RISK FACTORS

- AVM is rare; frequently congenital.
- Acquired AVF typically results from local vascular damage via trauma, surgery, venipuncture, perivascular injection, or neoplasia.

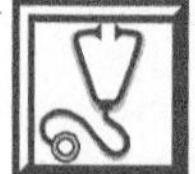

DIAGNOSIS

DIFFERENTIAL DIAGNOSIS

- Peripheral lesions (limb, ear) may look like a mass.
- Vascular aneurysm or pseudoaneurysm.
- Atypical clinical findings, depending on location, may suggest other disease processes; AVF/AVM may be a late diagnostic consideration.

CBC/BIOCHEMISTRY/URINALYSIS

May reflect damage to systems in vicinity of lesion, i.e., hepatic, renal, or other organ dysfunction.

OTHER LABORATORY TESTS

N/A

IMAGING

Thoracic Radiography

Cardiomegaly and pulmonary overcirculation with hemodynamically significant lesions. Microhepatica and loss of abdominal detail in hepatic AVMs.

Ultrasonography

- Lesions appear as cavernous, often tortuous, vascular structures.
- May observe high-velocity, turbulent flow on Doppler ultrasound.
- Hepatofugal flow in portal vein (away from the liver) nearly always apparent in hepatic AVM.
- Echocardiography may show four-chamber dilation and functional atrioventricular valve regurgitation due to increased circulating blood volume.

Cross-sectional Imaging

CT or MRI can aid in diagnosis, particularly when contrast is timed to highlight vascular anatomy.

Angiography

Selective angiography is the optimal test and is performed at time of intervention, if transcatheter therapy is pursued; digital subtraction angiography can improve visualization.

DIAGNOSTIC PROCEDURES

N/A

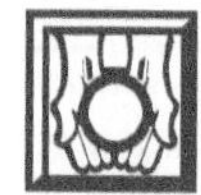

TREATMENT

- Surgery can be difficult, labor-intensive, and may require blood transfusion. Ligation or division of an AVF is often curative; *en bloc* resection of an AVM is necessary for cure.
- Transcatheter therapies with coils, devices, or glue are newer treatment options; potential advantages include less invasive therapy and intravascular access to remote lesions. Coils or occlusive devices are often sufficient for treatment of AVF; AVMs have been terminated by glue embolization of the arterial nidus, and more recently by embolization or ligation of the dominant outflow vein, which appears to limit shunt flow.
- Lesions may recur. In some cases, staged procedures or surgical removal of the affected limb or organ (e.g., amputation, liver lobectomy) may be necessary.

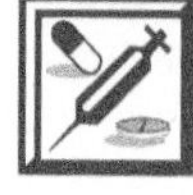

MEDICATIONS

DRUG(S) OF CHOICE

- Depend on site of lesion and secondary clinical features.
- Medical treatment for CHF or other organ dysfunction may be required before surgery.

CONTRAINDICATIONS/POSSIBLE INTERACTIONS

Avoid excessive fluid administration; patients are often volume overloaded and in a high cardiac output state.

FOLLOW-UP

Postoperative reevaluation and imaging needed to determine whether the lesion has recurred and if organ dysfunction has resolved.

MISCELLANEOUS

SEE ALSO

Congestive Heart Failure, Left-Sided.

ABBREVIATIONS

- AVF = arteriovenous fistula.
- AVM = arteriovenous malformation.
- CHF = congestive heart failure.

Suggested Reading

Weisse C, Berent A, eds. Veterinary Image-Guided Interventions. Ames, IA: Wiley-Blackwell, 2015.

Author Brian A. Scansen
Consulting Editor Michael Aherne

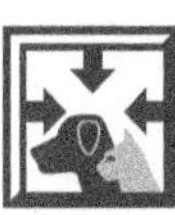

BASIC

OVERVIEW

- Intrahepatic arteriovenous (AV) malformations (also referred to as AV fistulae) are communications between proper hepatic arteries and intrahepatic portal veins; this anatomic union results in hepatofugal (away from the liver) splanchnic circulation.
- Blood flows directly from a hepatic artery into portal vasculature retrograde into the vena cava through multiple acquired portosystemic shunts (APSS).
- Associated with ascites.
- Uncommon, usually congenital, but may be acquired (surgical injury, trauma, neoplasia).

SIGNALMENT

- Dogs, less common in cats.
- Age-related presentation (congenital): <2 years.
- No sex or breed predilection.

SIGNS

General Comments

Vague or acute illness; present for signs caused by portal hypertension and APSS—ascites and hepatic encephalopathy (HE).

Historical Findings

- Dogs may have a normal transition to growth foods, unlike portosystemic vascular anomalies (PSVA) that demonstrate HE.
- May have an acute onset of ascites or HE.
- Vague signs include lethargy, anorexia, vomiting, diarrhea, weight loss, polydipsia, dementia, abdominal distention, and uroliths causing obstructive uropathy.

Physical Examination Findings

- Lethargic, poor body condition, ascites; enlarged liver lobe containing the AV malformation; rarely palpated on initial examination.
- Rarely, bruit auscultated over AV malformation.

CAUSES & RISK FACTORS

- Usually congenital vascular malformations (single or multiple vessels) reflecting failed differentiation of common embryologic anlage.
- Rare—secondary to abdominal trauma, inflammation, neoplasia, surgical interventions, or diagnostic procedures (e.g., liver biopsy).
- Portal hypertension—reflects arterialization of valveless portal system—establishing APSS.

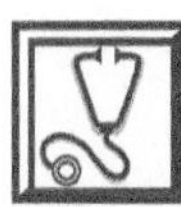

DIAGNOSIS

DIFFERENTIAL DIAGNOSIS

- CNS signs—infectious disorders (e.g., distemper); toxicity (e.g., lead); hydrocephalus; idiopathic epilepsy; metabolic disorders (e.g., hypoglycemia, hypokalemia, or hyperkalemia); HE (e.g., acquired liver disease or PSVA).
- Abdominal effusion—pure transudate (ascites; protein-losing nephropathy, protein-losing enteropathy, liver disease); modified transudate (congenital cardiac malformations, right-sided heart failure, pericardial tamponade, supradiaphragmatic vena caval obstruction, neoplasia, portal vein thrombosis); hemorrhage.
- Portal hypertension—chronic hepatic disease, ductal plate malformations/ congenital hepatic fibrosis, noncirrhotic or idiopathic portal hypertension, cirrhosis, portal thrombi.

CBC/BIOCHEMISTRY/URINALYSIS

- Erythrocyte microcytosis (APSS), target cells.
- Hypoalbuminemia with normal or low serum globulins; alkaline phosphatase (ALP) and alanine aminotransferase (ALT) activity normal or moderately increased; variable low blood urea nitrogen (BUN); hypocholesterolemia; anicteric.
- Hyposthenuria or isosthenuria.
- Ammonium biurate crystalluria.

OTHER LABORATORY TESTS

- Coagulation tests—variable, may be normal; low protein C activity reflects APSS.
- Total serum bile acids—preprandial values variable, postprandial values increased; classic shunting pattern.
- Plasma ammonia—usually increased, inferred by ammonium biurate crystalluria.
- Peritoneal fluid—pure transudate (total protein <2.5 g/dL) or modified transudate.

IMAGING

Radiography

- Abdominal effusion.
- Microhepatia or normal-sized liver due to enlarged lobe with AV malformation.
- Renomegaly.
- Normal thorax.

Abdominal Ultrasonography

- Abdominal effusion.
- Liver lobe with AV malformation—large compared to most other liver lobes that are atrophied due to portal hypoperfusion.
- Tortuous anechoic tubules represent AV structure with unidirectional pulsating or turbulent flow on color-flow Doppler.
- Hepatic artery and/or portal vein branches may appear tortuous.
- Hepatofugal portal flow (away from the liver)—through APSS.
- Renomegaly.
- Urolithiasis—urinary bladder or renal pelvis.
- Rule out portal thrombosis (luminal filling defect, abrupt blood flow termination).

Radiographic Contrast Angiography

- Not indicated in most cases.
- Venous portography—only confirms APSS.
- Hepatic arteriography—required to confirm AV communication (celiac trunk or anterior mesenteric artery contrast injection).

Multisector CT

Noninvasive contrast imaging of hepatic vasculature; arterial and venous phases; three-dimensional reconstruction illustrates AV malformation, large liver lobe, atrophied liver.

Echocardiography

Rule out right-sided heart disease, pericardial disease, and vena caval occlusion.

DIAGNOSTIC PROCEDURES

- Multisector CT and exploratory laparotomy.
- Liver biopsy—collect samples from *affected* and *unaffected* liver lobes; "normal" liver often demonstrates severe vascular arterialization (more severe than associated with PSVA).

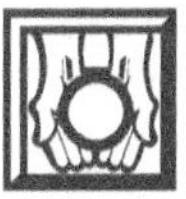

TREATMENT

APPROPRIATE HEALTH CARE

Inpatient—treat HE and ascites prior to surgical approach or percutaneous selective acrylamide embolization.

NURSING CARE

- *Diet*—restrict nitrogen intake to ameliorate HE and hyperammonemia; restrict sodium to attenuate ascites formation.
- *HE*—resolve endoparasitism, electrolyte and hydration disturbances, treat infections, initiate treatments to alter enteric uptake and formation of HE toxins (see Hepatic Encephalopathy).
- *Ascites*—mobilize by restricting activity and sodium intake and instituting dual diuretic therapy (furosemide and spironolactone); reserve therapeutic abdominocentesis for tense ascites impairing ventilation, nutrition, sleep, or recumbent posture (see Hypertension, Portal; Portosystemic Shunting, Acquired; and below).

SURGICAL CONSIDERATIONS

- Resection of liver lobe containing AV malformation is complicated by coexistence of additional hepatic vascular malformations; clinical cure possible but unlikely.
- Percutaneous selective acrylamide vascular embolization; complicated by risk of thromboembolism of additional vasculature; temporary improvement, but treatment may be curative.
- Multiple microscopic vascular malformations continue portal hypertension and APSS.
- Do not ligate APSS nor band the vena cava.

ARTERIOVENOUS MALFORMATION OF THE LIVER (CONTINUED)

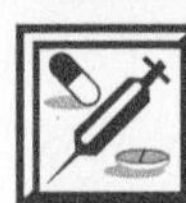

MEDICATIONS

DRUG(S) OF CHOICE

Hepatic Encephalopathy

See Hepatic Encephalopathy

Ascites

- Restrict sodium intake.
- Furosemide (0.5–2 mg/kg PO IM or IV q12–24h)—combine with spironolactone.
- Spironolactone (0.5–2 mg/kg PO q12h)—double initial dose as loading dose once.
- Chronic diuretic therapy—individualized to response, 4- to 7-day assessment intervals used to titrate dose to response, avoiding hydration, electrolyte, and HE complications.
- Diuretic-resistant ascites—may require therapeutic abdominocentesis; to initiate diuresis.
- Vasopressin V_2 receptor antagonists newly available may control ascites accumulation. (See Portosystemic Shunting, Acquired.)

Bleeding Tendencies

See Coagulopathy of Liver Disease.

Gastrointestinal Hemorrhage

- *Histamine type-2 receptor antagonists* (famotidine 0.5–2.0 mg/kg PO, IV, or SC q12–24h); or *HCl pump inhibitors* (omeprazole 1.0 mg/kg/24h PO or pantoprazole 1.0 mg/kg/24h IV; omeprazole may induce p450 cytochrome-associated drug interactions and may have a 24–48h delayed onset of action; some clinicians recommend chronic treatment to minimize GI bleeding and ulceration that may be chronic problems).
- *Gastroprotectant*—sucralfate: 0.25–1.0 g/10 kg PO q8–12h; titrate to effect, beware of drug interactions as sucralfate may bind other medications, reducing bioavailability.
- *Eliminate endoparasitism.*

CONTRAINDICATIONS/POSSIBLE INTERACTIONS

Avoid drugs dependent on hepatic biotransformation or first-pass hepatic extraction (reduced by APSS) or that react with γ-aminobutyric acid (GABA)-benzodiazepine receptors because of propensity for HE.

FOLLOW-UP

PATIENT MONITORING

Biochemistry—initially monthly until stabilized after surgery or AV malformation embolization, thereafter quarterly; monitor for hypoalbuminemia, infection, optimization of HE management, and control of ammonium biurate crystalluria.

EXPECTED COURSE AND PROGNOSIS

- Prognosis fair if patient survives surgical resection of AV malformation or embolization.
- Most patients require indefinite nutritional and medical management (HE, ascites) because of coexisting microscopic vascular malformations across the liver; APSS persists requiring continued management of HE.

MISCELLANEOUS

SEE ALSO

- Ascites.
- Coagulopathy of Liver Disease.
- Hepatic Encephalopathy.
- Hypertension, Portal.
- Portosystemic Shunting, Acquired.
- Portosystemic Vascular Anomaly, Congenital.

ABBREVIATIONS

- ALP = alkaline phosphatase.
- ALT = alanine aminotransferase.
- APSS = acquired portosystemic shunt.
- AV = arteriovenous.
- BUN = blood urea nitrogen.
- GABA = γ-aminobutyric acid.
- HE = hepatic encephalopathy.
- PSVA = portosystemic vascular anomalies.

Author Sharon A. Center
Consulting Editor Kate Holan

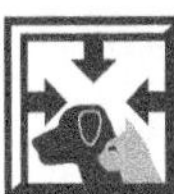

BASICS

DEFINITION

Osteoarthritis (OA) or degenerative joint disease is a chronic and progressive disease that leads to loss of articular cartilage and ultimately failure of the joint. OA is characterized as a noninfectious disorder of diarthrodial (synovial) joints, such that the disease process involves the entire joint, not just the articular cartilage. It is due to both primary (idiopathic) and secondary causes.

PATHOPHYSIOLOGY

- Ebb and flow characterization with periods of calmness followed by periods of exacerbation of clinical signs (flare-ups).
- OA initiated by mechanical stress—traumatic injury, instability, abnormal conformation, abnormal activity, etc.
- Inflammatory mediators and free radicals such as metalloproteinases, serine proteases, cysteine protease enzymes, and reactive oxygen species are released from damaged chondrocytes and synovium, resulting in breakdown of extracellular matrix of articular cartilage, causing collagen degradation and loss of collagen cross-linking.
- Collagen synthesis is altered, resulting in decreased collagen/proteoglycan interaction and reduced hydrophilic matrix properties.
- Extracellular matrix further compromised by increased breakdown of proteoglycans along with manufacture of poorer-quality proteoglycans.
- Nitric oxide released along with other free radicals, which mediates cartilage breakdown and supports chronic inflammation. Chondrocyte apoptosis facilitated by cyclooxygenase-2 enzymes and oxidative stress.
- Synovitis is driving force of the inflammatory cascade in OA, in addition to resulting in decreased viscosity of synovial fluid, reducing lubrication.
- Poorer-quality synovial fluid reduces oxygen and nutrient supply to chondrocytes as well as waste removal.
- Subchondral bone becomes sclerotic, worsening loading qualities of bone and overlying cartilage.
- Pain of OA results from distention of the joint capsule and stimulation of pain receptors, inflammation of synovium, increased mechanical loading of subchondral bone, alteration of function of surrounding tendons and ligaments, as well as development of periarticular fibrosis.
- The result of these processes is progressive cartilage degradation ranging from fibrillation to deep fissuring of cartilage. Full-thickness cartilage loss can eventually occur.
- Periarticular fibrosis occurs, resulting in a reduction of joint motion (and pain), leading to poorer vascularity of synovial membrane as well as lack of functionality of synovium due to lack of motion in joint.
- Osteophytes and enthesiophytes develop around and within joint to increase load-bearing surface area.
- These changes reduce functionality and may eventually lead to ankylosis.

SYSTEMS AFFECTED

Musculoskeletal—diarthrodial joints.

GENETICS

- Primary OA rare, occurring more commonly in cats or in smaller (manus, pes) joints of dogs.
- Dogs—causes of secondary OA are varied, including hip and elbow dysplasia, osteochondritis dessicans (OCD), patellar luxations, congenital shoulder luxation, Legg-Perthes, cranial cruciate ligament rupture, intra-articular fractures, obesity, as well as many other causes.
- Cats—causes of secondary OA are patellar luxation, hip dysplasia, obesity, and arthropathy.

INCIDENCE/PREVALENCE

- Dog—very common; 20% of dogs older than 1 year have some degree of OA.
- Cat—90% of cats over 12 years of age had evidence of OA on radiographs.
- Clinical problems are more prevalent in larger, overweight, and very active animals.
- Primary OA is rare.

SIGNALMENT

Species

Dog and cat.

Mean Age and Range

- Secondary OA due to congenital disorders (OCD, hip dysplasia) seen in immature animals; some present with OA signs when mature (hip and elbow dysplasia).
- Secondary to trauma—any age.

SIGNS

Historical Findings

- Dogs—decreased activity level, unwilling to perform certain tasks; intermittent lameness or stiff gait that slowly progresses; possible history of joint trauma, OCD, or developmental disorders; may be exacerbated by exercise, long periods of recumbency, and cold weather.
- Cats—overt lameness may not be seen. Reduction in activity, reluctance to jump, unkempt appearance, difficulty accessing litter box, and increased irritability.

Physical Examination Findings

- Stiff-legged or altered gait or nonuse of leg.
- Decreased range of motion.
- Crepitus.
- Joint swelling (effusion and/or thickening of the joint capsule).
- Joint pain.
- Joint instability.

CAUSES

- Primary—no known cause.
- Secondary—results from initiating cause: abnormal wear on normal cartilage (e.g., joint instability, joint incongruity, trauma to cartilage or supporting soft tissues, obesity) or normal wear on abnormal cartilage (e.g., osteochondral defects).

RISK FACTORS

- Working, athletic, and obese dogs place more stress on their joints.
- Dogs with disorders that affect collagen or cartilage (Cushing's disease, diabetes mellitus, hypothyroidism, hyperlaxity, prolonged steroid use).

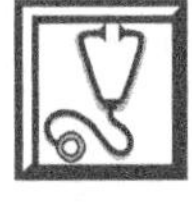

DIAGNOSIS

DIFFERENTIAL DIAGNOSIS

- Neoplastic (synovial sarcoma; rarely, chondrosarcoma; osteosarcoma).
- Septic arthritis (caused by bacteria; spirochetes; L forms in cats; *Mycoplasma*; *Rickettsia*; *Ehrlichia*; viruses such as feline calicivirus; fungi and protozoa).
- Immune-mediated arthritis (erosive vs. nonerosive).
- Other musculoskeletal conditions that cause lameness.
- Neurologic conditions causing lameness or decreased activity/weakness.

OTHER LABORATORY TESTS

- Coombs' test, antinuclear antibody (ANA), and rheumatoid factor may help to rule out immune-mediated arthritis.
- Serum titers for *Borrelia*, *Ehrlichia*, and *Rickettsia* to evaluate for infectious arthritis.

IMAGING

- Radiographic changes—include joint capsular distention, osteophytosis, enthesophytosis, soft-tissue thickening, and narrowed joint spaces. In severely affected patients: subchondral sclerosis and intra-articular calcified bodies (joint mice).
- Radiographic severity often does not correlate with clinical severity.
- Stress radiography may identify underlying instability and accentuate joint incongruity (e.g., distraction index, passive hip laxity of coxofemoral joint is predictive of hip OA).
- Bone nuclear scintigraphy can assist in localizing subtle OA.
- Arthroscopy can allow direct observation of cartilage and characterization by Modified Outerbridge Score.

DIAGNOSTIC PROCEDURES

- Arthrocentesis and synovial fluid analysis—cell counts are normal or slightly increased (<2,000–5,000 cells/mL) predominantly

A

ARTHRITIS (OSTEOARTHRITIS) (CONTINUED)

mononuclear (macrophages) and occasional synovial lining cells.
• Bacterial culture of synovial fluid or synovium—negative.
• Biopsy of synovial tissue to rule out neoplasia or immune-mediated arthropathy (lymphocytic plasmacytic synovitis, systemic lupus erythematosus).

PATHOLOGIC FINDINGS

• Fibrillation or erosion of articular cartilage.
• Eburnation and sclerosis of subchondral bone.
• Thickening and fibrosis of joint capsule.
• Synovial fluid can be grossly normal to thin and watery, usually increased volume.
• Synovial villous hypertrophy and hyperplasia.
• Osteophytes and enthesiophytes at joint capsule attachments and adjacent to the joint.
• Neovascularization or pannus in severe cases over joint surfaces.

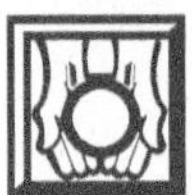

TREATMENT

APPROPRIATE HEALTH CARE

• Medical—usually tried initially.
• Surgical options—to improve joint geometry or remove bone-on-bone contact areas through total joint arthroplasty, ostectomy, or joint fusion.

NURSING CARE

• Physical rehabilitation—very beneficial during periods of flare-ups.
• Maintaining or increasing joint motion—active and passive range of motion exercises, stretching, massage, therapeutic exercises, and hydrotherapy.
• Pain management—cold and heat therapy, transcutaneous electrical stimulation (TENS), and acupuncture.
• Muscle tone/strengthening—daily leash walking, incorporation of inclines/declines, stair ascent and stair descent, walking on uneven terrain, open water swimming, underwater and land treadmill.
• Maintenance of a lean body weight through both diet and daily exercise.

ACTIVITY

• During periods of calmness, daily leash walks to work up to twice-daily level flat ground for 20 minutes before incorporation of increased time or terrain.
• Limitation of daily activity that minimizes aggravation of clinical signs during periods of flare-up (avoidance of running, chasing, jumping, and playing).

DIET

• Weight reduction for obese patients—decreases stress placed on arthritic joints. Begin by feeding 60% of calories needed to maintain current body weight.
• Omega n-3 fatty acids decrease production of certain prostaglandins and modulate inflammation. Dosage should be 150–175 mg/kg DHA/EPA daily.

CLIENT EDUCATION

• Medical therapy is palliative and the condition is likely to progress.
• Describe identifying signs of flare-ups and importance of getting it under control quickly.
• Discuss management options, daily exercise, activity level, and diet.

SURGICAL CONSIDERATIONS

• Arthrotomy—used to remove aggravating causes (e.g., fragmented coronoid process, ununited anconeal process, osteochondral flaps).
• Arthroscopy—used to diagnose and remove aggravating causes.
• Reconstructive procedures—used to eliminate joint instability and correct anatomic problems (cruciate ligament rupture, patella luxation, angular deformity).
• Joint removal—femoral head and neck ostectomy, temperomandibular joint arthroplasty.
• Joint replacement—total hip replacement is widely used, total elbow and stifle replacement are used with less frequency, total ankle and shoulder replacment are experimental and used infrequently at this time.
• Joint fusion (arthrodesis)—in selected chronic cases and for joint instability, complete or partial; carpus, hock: generally excellent outcome; shoulder, elbow, stifle: less predictable outcome.

MEDICATIONS

DRUG(S) OF CHOICE

Nonsteroidal Anti-inflammatory Drugs (NSAIDs)

• Inhibit prostaglandin synthesis through cyclooxygenase enzymes.
• Deracoxib (3–4 mg/kg PO q24h, chewable).
• Carprofen (2.2 mg/kg PO q12h or q24h).
• Meloxicam (load 0.2 mg/kg PO, then 0.1 mg/kg PO q24h, liquid).
• Tepoxalin (load 20 mg/kg, then 10 mg/kg PO q24h).
• Cats—meloxicam (0.1 mg/kg PO q24h, liquid) or robenacoxib (1 mg/kg PO q24h for 3 days).
• Inhibit prostaglandin synthesis at receptor specific sites.
• Grapiprant (2.0 mg/kg PO q24h, chewable).

Disease-Modifying Osteoarthritis Agents (DMOAs)

• Host of products, many with little production oversight so effects vary widely. Supply polysulfated glycosaminoglycan (PSGAG) molecules to repair and regenerate cartilage.
• Adequan®—clinical study in dogs with hip dysplasia; 4.4 mg/kg IM every 3–5 days for 8 injections had positive, temporary effect.
• Glucosamine and chondroitin sulfate—oral Cosequin®, oral methylsulfonylmethane (MSM), mixtures with MSM, or other supplements (e.g., Dasuquin® Advanced, GlycoFlex® 2, Synflex).

CONTRAINDICATIONS

• NSAIDs must not be given with steroids.
• Acetaminophen must not be given to cats.

PRECAUTIONS

• NSAIDs may cause gastric ulceration.
• Cyclooxygenase-2 (COX-2)-selective drugs may interfere with liver function when used outside of dosage range
• When switching NSAIDs—wait 3 days for washout before starting new drug.

POSSIBLE INTERACTIONS

Steroids with NSAIDS.

ALTERNATIVE DRUG(S)

• Free-radical scavengers.
• Amantadine (3–5 mg/kg PO q24h)—best used in combination with another analgesic such as NSAID. Only analgesic (other than NSAID) with scientific evidence for usage with OA.
• Gabapentin (5–10 mg/kg PO q8-12h)—no scientific evidence for usage with OA.
• Codeine (1–2 mg/kg PO q 8–12h)—no scientific evidence for usage with OA; suggested for short-term use during flare-ups.
• Glucocorticoids—inhibit inflammatory mediators and cytokines; however, chronic use delays healing and initiates damage to articular cartilage; potential systemic side effects documented; goal is low dose (dogs, 0.5–2 mg/kg; cats, 2–4 mg/kg) q48h.
• Prednisone—initial dose 1–2 mg/kg PO q24h for dogs and 4 mg/kg PO q24h for cats.
• Triamcinolone hexacetonide—intra-articular injection of 5 mg in dogs showed a protective and therapeutic effect in one model.
• Hyaluronic acid—intra-articular injection (15–30 mg/joint) used as a series of 3 separated by 1 week or in combination with an intra-articular steroid.
• Platelet-rich plasma—intra-articular injection to decrease inflammatory mediators; many patients need more than 1 injection separated by 2 weeks; weak scientific evidence for efficacy.

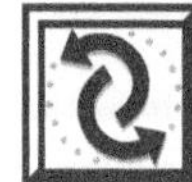

FOLLOW-UP

PATIENT MONITORING

• During flare-up recheck 2 weeks later; pain should be better controlled at this time; then recheck every 4–6 weeks until flare-up under control.
• Recheck OA patients every 4–6 months for life.
• Any clinical deterioration could indicate a flare-up—need to change drug selection or dosage; may indicate need for intra-articular

injection, formal rehabilitation therapy, or surgical intervention.

PREVENTION/AVOIDANCE

Early identification of predisposing causes and prompt treatment to help reduce progression of secondary conditions, e.g., surgical removal of osteochondral lesions.

EXPECTED COURSE AND PROGNOSIS

- Slow progression of disease likely.
- Some form of medical or surgical treatment usually allows a good quality of life when managed appropriately and aggressively.

MISCELLANEOUS

SYNONYMS

- Degenerative arthritis.
- Degenerative joint disease.
- Osteoarthritis.
- Osteoarthrosis.

ABBREVIATIONS

- ANA = antinuclear antibody.
- COX-2 = cyclooxygenase-2.
- DMOA = disease-modifying osteoarthritis agent.
- MSM = methylsulfonylmethane.
- NSAID = nonsteroidal anti-inflammatory drug.
- OA = osteoarthritis.
- OCD = osteochondritis dessicans.
- PSGAG = polysulfated glycosaminoglycan.

Suggested Reading

Aragon CL, Hofmeister EH, Budsberg SC. Systematic review of clinical trials of treatments for osteoarthritis in dogs. J Am Vet Med Assoc 2007, 230(4):514–521.

Baime MJ. Glucosamine and chondroitin sulphate did not improve pain in osteoarthritis of the knee. Evid Based Med 2006, 11(4):115.

Budsberg SC, Bartges JW. Nutrition and osteoarthritis in dogs: does it help? Vet Clin North Am Small Anim Pract 2006, 36(6):1307–1323.

Glass GG. Osteoarthritis. Dis Mon 2006, 52(9):343–362 (human review).

Hampton T. Efficacy still uncertain for widely used supplements for arthritis. J Am Med Assoc 2007 297(4):351–352.

Herrero-Beaumont G, Ivorra JA, Del Carmen Trabado M, et al. Glucosamine sulfate in the treatment of knee osteoarthritis symptoms: a randomized, double-blind, placebo-controlled study using acetaminophen as a side comparator. Arthritis Rheum 2007, 56(2):555–567.

Johnston SJ. Osteoarthritis joint anatomy, physiology and pathobiology. Vet Clin North Am 1997, 27:699–723.

Mlacnik E, Bockstahler BA, Muller M, et al. Effects of caloric restriction and a moderate or intense physiotherapy program for treatment of lameness in overweight dogs with osteoarthritis. J Am Vet Med Assoc 2006, 229(11):1756–1760.

Van Der Kraan PM, Van Den Berg WB. Osteophytes: relevance and biology. Osteoarthritis Cartilage 2007, 15(3):237–244.

Author David Dycus

Consulting Editor Mathieu M. Glassman

Acknowledgment The author and book editors acknowledge the prior contribution of Walter C. Renberg.

Client Education Handout available online

ARTHRITIS, SEPTIC

BASICS

DEFINITION

Pathogenic microorganisms within the closed space of one or more synovial joints.

PATHOPHYSIOLOGY

• Usually caused by contamination associated with traumatic injury (e.g., a direct penetrating injury such as bite, gunshot wound, foreign object), a sequela to surgery, arthrocentesis or joint injection, hematogenous spread of microorganisms from a distant septic focus, or less commonly the extension of primary osteomyelitis. • Primary sources of hematogenous infection—urogenital, integumentary (including ears and anal sacs), respiratory, cardiac, and gastrointestinal systems.

SYSTEMS AFFECTED

Musculoskeletal—usually affects one joint.

GENETICS

N/A

INCIDENCE/PREVALENCE

Relatively uncommon cause of monoarticular arthritis in dogs and cats.

GEOGRAPHIC DISTRIBUTION

May be an increased incidence in areas with endemic Lyme disease.

SIGNALMENT

Species

• Most common in dogs. • Rare in cats.

Breed Predilections

Any; medium to large breeds—most commonly German shepherds, Dobermans, and Labrador retrievers.

Mean Age and Range

Any age; usually between 4 and 7 years. Hematogenous—more common in immature animals.

Predominant Sex

Male

SIGNS

General Comments

Always consider the diagnosis in patients with acute, monoarticular lameness associated with soft tissue swelling, heat, and pain.

Historical Findings

• Lameness—acute onset most common, but can present as chronic lameness. • Lethargy. • Anorexia. • May report previous trauma—dog bite, penetrating injury, prior surgery or other invasive procedure of the joint.

Physical Examination Findings

• Monoarticular lameness, rarely polyarticular. • Joint pain and effusion—commonly carpus, stifle, hock, shoulder, or cubital joint. • Localized joint heat. • Decreased range of motion. • Local lymphadenopathy. • Pyrexia.

CAUSES

• Aerobic bacterial organisms—most common: staphylococci, streptococci, coliforms, and *Pasteurella*. • Anaerobic organisms—most common: *Propionibacterium*, *Peptostreptococcus*, *Fusobacterium*, and *Bacteroides*. • Spirochete—*Borrelia burgdorferi*. • *Mycoplasma*. • Fungal agents—*Blastomyces*, *Cryptococcus*, and *Coccidioides*. • *Rickettsial—Anaplasma*, *Ehrlichia*, *Rickettsia*. • *Leishmania*. • Feline calicivirus.

RISK FACTORS

• Predisposing factors for hematogenous infection—diabetes mellitus, hypoadrenocorticism (Addison's disease), immunosuppression. • Penetrating trauma to the joint including surgery. • Existing osteoarthritis or other joint damage. • Intra-articular injection, particularly if steroid injected.

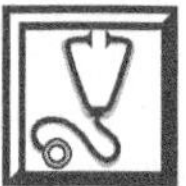

DIAGNOSIS

DIFFERENTIAL DIAGNOSIS

• Osteoarthritis. • Trauma. • Immune-mediated arthropathy. • Postvaccinal transient polyarthritis. • Greyhound polyarthritis. • Feline progressive polyarthritis. • Crystal-induced joint disease. • Synovial sarcoma.

CBC/BIOCHEMISTRY/URINALYSIS

• Hemogram—inflammatory left shift in some cases. • Other results normal.

OTHER LABORATORY TESTS

Serologic testing for specific pathogens.

IMAGING

Radiography

• Early disease—may reveal thickened and dense periarticular tissues; may see evidence of synovial effusion. Often difficult to diagnose early disease radiographically. • Late disease—reveals bone destruction, osteolysis, irregular joint space, discrete erosions, and periarticular osteophytosis.

DIAGNOSTIC PROCEDURES

Synovial Fluid Analysis

• Increased volume. • Turbid fluid. • Decreased viscosity. • Decreased mucin clot reaction. • Make slides immediately; if additional fluid is obtained, place in EDTA tube. • Elevated white blood cell (WBC) count—i.e., >80% neutrophils with >40,000/mm^3 (normal joint fluid <10% neutrophils and <3,000/mm^3) • Neutrophils may show degenerative changes (chromatolysis, vacuolation, nuclear swelling, loss of segmentation). • Neutrophils with phagocytosed bacteria—definitive diagnosis or bacteria in the synovial fluid.

Synovial Fluid Culture

• Positive culture is definitive but not necessary for diagnosis; negative culture does not rule out infection. • Must be collected aseptically; requires heavy sedation or general anesthesia. • Place fluid sample in aerobic and anaerobic culturettes and in blood culture medium. • Use 1 : 9 dilution of synovial fluid to blood culture media. • Culturette samples—cultured immediately upon arrival at the laboratory. • Blood culture medium—reculturing after 24 hours of incubation increases accuracy by 50% and is the preferred method. • *Mycoplasma*, bacterial L-forms, and protozoa require specific culture procedures—contact laboratory prior to sample collection.

Other

• Synovial biopsy—to rule out immune-mediated joint disease; no more effective than incubated blood culture medium for growing bacterial organisms. • Blood and urine cultures if hematogenous source is suspected.

PATHOLOGIC FINDINGS

• Synovium—thickened; discolored; often very proliferative. • Histology—evidence of hyperplastic synoviocytes. • Increased numbers of neutrophils, macrophages, and fibrinous debris. • Cartilage—loss of proteoglycan, destruction of articular surface, pannus formation.

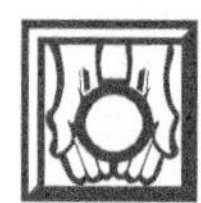

TREATMENT

APPROPRIATE HEALTH CARE

• Inpatient—initial stabilization; initiate systemic antibiotic therapy as soon as fluid is obtained for bacterial culture; consider joint drainage/lavage as soon as possible to minimize intra-articular injury. • Analgesia with anti-inflammatory medications if appropriate, and intravenous opioid. • Identify and treat source if hematogenous spread is suspected. • Outpatient—long-term management.

NURSING CARE

Alternating heat and cold packing—beneficial in promoting increased blood flow and decreased swelling.

ACTIVITY

Restricted until resolution of symptoms.

DIET

N/A

CLIENT EDUCATION

• Discuss probable cause. • Warn client about the need for long-term antibiotics and the likelihood of residual degenerative joint disease.

SURGICAL CONSIDERATIONS

• Acute disease with minimal radiographic changes—joint drainage and lavage via needle arthrocentesis, arthroscopic lavage, or arthrotomy; an irrigation catheter (ingress/egress) can be placed in larger joints. • Chronic disease—may require open arthrotomy with debridement of the synovium and copious lavage; if appropriate, an irrigation catheter (ingress/egress) may be placed to lavage the joint postoperatively. • Lavage—use warmed physiologic saline or lactated Ringer's solution (2–4 mL/kg q8h) until effluent is clear; do not add povidone/iodine or chlorhexidine to lavage fluid. • Effluent fluid—cytologically monitored daily for existence and character of bacteria and neutrophils. • Removal of catheters—when effluent fluid has no bacteria and the neutrophils are cytologically healthy. • Arthroscopy allows for visual assessment of articular cartilage, lavage, and biopsy, and is a less invasive method of thorough joint lavage than arthrotomy. • Recent reports suggest there may be no difference between combined medical and surgical management and medical management alone.

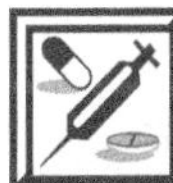

MEDICATIONS

DRUG(S) OF CHOICE

• Pending culture susceptibility data—bactericidal antibiotics, such as first-generation cephalosporin or amoxicillin–clavulanic acid, preferred. • Choice of antimicrobial drugs—primarily depends on in vitro determination of susceptibility of microorganisms; toxicity, frequency, route of administration, and expense also considered; most penetrate the synovium well; need to be given for a minimum of 4–8 weeks. • Nonsteroidal anti-inflammatory drugs (NSAIDs)—may help decrease pain and inflammation.

CONTRAINDICATIONS

Avoid fluorinated quinolones in pediatric patients, as their use has induced cartilage lesions experimentally.

PRECAUTIONS

Failure to respond to conventional antibiotic therapy—may indicate anaerobic disease, other unusual cause (fungal, spirochete), or aseptic arthritides.

POSSIBLE INTERACTIONS

N/A

ALTERNATIVE DRUG(S)

N/A

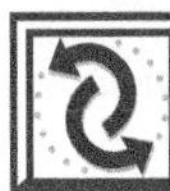

FOLLOW-UP

PATIENT MONITORING

• If drainage and irrigation catheters have been placed—may be removed after 4–6 days or after reassessment of synovial fluid cytology. • Duration of antibiotic therapy—2 weeks following resolution of clinical signs; total treatment may be 4–8 weeks or longer, depending on clinical signs and pathogenic organism. • Persistent synovial inflammation without viable bacterial organisms (dogs)—may be caused by antigenic bacterial fragments or antigen antibody deposition. • Systemic corticosteroid therapy (after joint sepsis has been resolved) and aggressive physical therapy—may be needed to maximize normal joint dynamics.

PREVENTION/AVOIDANCE

If clinical signs recur, early (within 24–48 hours) treatment provides the greatest benefit.

POSSIBLE COMPLICATIONS

• Chronic disease—severe degenerative joint disease. • Recurrence of infection. • Limited range of joint motion. • Generalized sepsis. • Osteomyelitis.

EXPECTED COURSE AND PROGNOSIS

• Acutely diagnosed disease (within 24–48 hours) responds well to antibiotic therapy. • Delayed diagnosis or resistant or highly virulent organisms—guarded to poor prognosis.

MISCELLANEOUS

ASSOCIATED CONDITIONS

N/A

AGE-RELATED FACTORS

N/A

ZOONOTIC POTENTIAL

N/A

PREGNANCY/FERTILITY/BREEDING

N/A

SYNONYMS

• Infectious arthritis. • Joint ill.

SEE ALSO

• Osteomyelitis.
• Polyarthritis, Erosive, Immune-Mediated.

ABBREVIATIONS

• NSAID = nonsteroidal anti-inflammatory drug.
• WBC = white blood cell.

Suggested Reading

Benzioni H, Shahar R, Yudelevitch S, Milgram J. Bacterial infective arthritis of the coxofemoral joint in dogs with hip dysplasia. Vet Comp Orthop Traumatol 2008, 21:262–266.

Clements DN, Owen MR, Mosely JR, et al. Retrospective study of bacterial infective arthritis in 31 dogs. J Small Anim Pract 2005, 46:171–176.

Ellison RS. The cytologic examination of synovial fluid. Semin Vet Med Surg Small Anim 1988, 3:133–139.

Fitch RB, Hogan TC, Kudnig ST. Hematogenous septic arthritis in the dog: results of five patients treated nonsurgically with antibiotics. J Am Anim Hosp Assoc 2003, 39:563–566.

Luther JF, Cook JL, Stoll MR. Arthroscopic exploration and biopsy for diagnosis of septic arthritis and osteomyelitis of the coxofemoral joint in a dog. Vet Comp Orthop Traumatol 2005, 18:47–51.

Machevsky AM, Read RA. Bacterial septic arthritis in 19 dogs. Aust Vet J 1999, 77:233–237.

MacWilliams PS, Friedrichs KR. Laboratory evaluation and interpretation of synovial fluid. Vet Clin Small Anim 2003, 33:153–178.

Mielko B, Comerford E, English K, et al. Spontaneous septic arthritis of canine elbows: twenty-one cases. Vet Comp Orthop Traumatol 2018, 31:488–493.

Montgomery RD, Long IR, Milton JL. Comparison of aerobic culturette, synovial membrane biopsy, and blood culture medium in detection of canine bacterial arthritis. Vet Surg 1989, 18:300–303.

Scharf VF, Lewis ST, Wellehan JF, et al. Retrospective evaluation of the efficacy of isolating bacteria from synovial fluid in dogs with suspected septic arthritis. Aust Vet J 2015, 93:200–203.

Author Sherisse A. Sakals
Consulting Editor Mathieu M. Glassman

Client Education Handout available online

A

ASCITES

BASICS

DEFINITION

The escape of fluid, either transudate or exudate, into the abdominal cavity between the parietal and visceral peritoneum.

PATHOPHYSIOLOGY

- Ascites can be caused by the following:
  - Congestive heart failure (CHF) and associated interference in venous return.
  - Depletion of plasma proteins associated with inappropriate loss of protein from renal or gastrointestinal disease—protein-losing nephropathy or enteropathy, respectively.
  - Obstruction of the vena cava or portal vein, or lymphatic drainage due to neoplastic occlusion.
  - Overt neoplastic effusion.
  - Peritonitis—infective or inflammatory.
  - Electrolyte imbalance, especially hypernatremia.
  - Liver cirrhosis.

SYSTEMS AFFECTED

- Cardiovascular.
- Gastrointestinal.
- Hemic/lymph/immune.
- Renal/urologic.

SIGNALMENT

- Dog and cat.
- No species or breed predisposition.

SIGNS

- Episodic weakness.
- Lethargy.
- Abdominal fullness.
- Abdominal discomfort when palpated.
- Dyspnea from abdominal distension or associated pleural effusion.
- Anorexia.
- Vomiting.
- Weight gain.
- Scrotal or preputial edema.
- Groaning when lying down.

CAUSES

- Nephrotic syndrome.
- Cirrhosis of liver.
- Right-sided CHF.
- Hypoproteinemia.
- Ruptured bladder.
- Peritonitis.
- Abdominal neoplasia.
- Abdominal hemorrhage.

RISK FACTORS

N/A

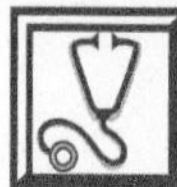

DIAGNOSIS

DIFFERENTIAL DIAGNOSIS

Differentiating Abdominal Distension without Effusion

- Organomegaly—hepatomegaly, splenomegaly, renomegaly, and hydrometra.
- Abdominal neoplasia.
- Pregnancy.
- Bladder distension.
- Obesity.
- Gastric dilatation.

Differentiating Diseases

- Transudate—nephrotic syndrome, cirrhosis of liver, right-sided CHF, hypoproteinemia, and ruptured bladder.
- Exudate—peritonitis, abdominal neoplasia, and hemorrhage.

CBC/BIOCHEMISTRY/URINALYSIS

- Neutrophilic leukocytosis occurs in patients with systemic infection.
- Albumin is low in patients with impaired liver synthesis, gastrointestinal loss, or renal loss.
- Cholesterol is low in patients with impaired liver synthesis.

Liver Enzymes

- Low to normal in patients with impaired liver synthesis.
- High in patients with liver inflammation, hyperadrenocorticism, gallbladder obstruction, and chronic passive congestion.

Total and Direct Bilirubin

- Low to normal in patients with impaired liver synthesis.
- High in patients with biliary obstruction caused by tumor, gallbladder distension, or obstruction.

Blood Urea Nitrogen (BUN) and Creatinine

- High in patients with renal failure.
- BUN low in patients with impaired liver synthesis or hyperadrenocorticism.

Glucose

Low in patients with impaired liver synthesis.

OTHER LABORATORY TESTS

- To detect hypoproteinemia—protein electrophoresis and immune profile.
- To detect proteinuria—urinary protein : creatinine ratio (normal <0.5 : 1).
- To detect liver ascites—analysis of serum ascites albumin gradient.

IMAGING

- Thoracic and abdominal radiography is sometimes helpful.
- Ultrasonography of the liver, spleen, pancreas, kidney, bladder, and abdomen can often determine cause.
- Stages of ascites:
  - Stage I—minimal ascites: detected by ultrasound only.
  - Stage II—moderate ascites: abdominal distention visible and/or noted on ballottement.
  - Stage III—significant ascites: marked abdominal distention; patient uncomfortable, possibly with labored breathing.

DIAGNOSTIC PROCEDURES

Ascitic Fluid Evaluation

Exfoliative cytologic examination and bacterial culture and antibiotic sensitivity—remove approximately 3–5 mL of abdominal fluid via aseptic technique.

Transudate

- Clear and colorless.
- Protein <2.5 g/dL.
- Specific gravity <1.018.
- Cells <1,000/mm^3—neutrophils and mesothelial cells.

Modified Transudate

- Red or pink; may be slightly cloudy.
- Protein 2.5–5 g/dL.
- Specific gravity >1.018.
- Cells <5,000/mm^3—neutrophils, mesothelial cells, erythrocytes, and lymphocytes.

Exudate (Nonseptic)

- Pink or white; cloudy.
- Protein 2.5–5 g/dL.
- Specific gravity >1.018.
- Cells 5,000–50,000/mm^3—neutrophils, mesothelial cells, macrophages, erythrocytes, and lymphocytes.

Exudate (Septic)

- Red, white, or yellow; cloudy.
- Protein >4.0 g/dL.
- Specific gravity >1.018.
- Cells 5,000–100,000/mm^3—neutrophils, mesothelial cells, macrophages, erythrocytes, lymphocytes, and bacteria.

Hemorrhage

- Red; spun supernatant clear and sediment red.
- Protein >5.5 g/dL.
- Specific gravity 1.007–1.027.
- Cells consistent with peripheral blood.
- Does not clot.

Chyle

- Pink, straw, or white.
- Protein 2.5–7 g/dL.
- Specific gravity 1.007–1.040 and above.
- Cells <10,000/mm^3—neutrophils, mesothelial cells, and large population of small lymphocytes.

• Other—fluid in tube separates into cream-like layer when refrigerated; fat droplets stain with Sudan III.

Pseudochyle

• White.
• Protein >2.5 g/dL.
• Specific gravity 1.007–1.040.
• Cells <10,000/mm^3—neutrophils, mesothelial cells, and small lymphocytes.
• Other—fluid in tube does not separate into cream-like layer when refrigerated; does not stain with Sudan III.

Urine

• Clear to pale yellow.
• Protein >2.5 g/dL.
• Specific gravity 1–1.040 and above.
• Cells 5,000–50,000/mm^3—neutrophils, erythrocytes, lymphocytes, and macrophages.
• Other—if the urinary bladder ruptured <12 hours before, urinary glucose and protein could be negative; if bladder ruptured >12 hours before, urine becomes a dialysis medium with ultrafiltrate of plasma, and urine contains glucose and protein.

Bile

• Slightly cloudy and yellow.
• Protein >2.5 g/dL.
• Specific gravity >1.018.
• Cells 5,000–750,000/mm^3—neutrophils, erythrocytes, macrophages, and lymphocytes.
• Other—bilirubin confirmed by urine dipstick; nonicteric patient may have gallbladder rupture, biliary tree leakage, or rupture in the proximal bowel.

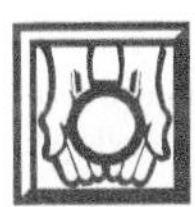

TREATMENT

• Can design treatment on an outpatient basis, with follow-up or inpatient care, depending on physical condition and underlying cause.
• If patients are markedly uncomfortable when lying down or become more dyspneic with stress, consider removing enough ascites to reverse these signs.
• Dietary salt restriction may help control transudate fluid accumulation due to CHF, cirrhosis, or hypoproteinemia.
• For exudate ascites control, address the underlying cause; corrective surgery is often indicated, followed by specific therapeutic management (e.g., patient with splenic tumor: tumor removed, abdominal bleeding controlled, blood transfusion administered).

Large-Volume Paracentesis

• Stage III treatment.
• Pretreat patient with hetastarch (6%) @ 1–2 mL/kg for 2 hours.
• Abdominal tap (paracentesis), until drainage slows.
• Post-treat patient with hetastarch (6%) @ 1–2 mL/kg for 4 hours.

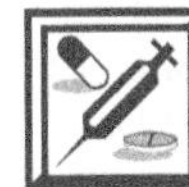

MEDICATIONS

DRUG(S) OF CHOICE

• Patients with liver insufficiency or CHF—restrict sodium and give a diuretic combination of furosemide (1–2 mg/kg q8h PO) and spironolactone (1–2 mg/kg q12h PO); if control is inadequate, hydrochlorothiazide (1–4 mg/kg q12h PO) can be added (*cautiously*); must monitor serum potassium concentration to prevent potassium imbalances.
• Additionally for patients in CHF—pimobendan (0.3 mg/kg q12h PO) and an angiotensin-converting-enzyme inhibitor (e.g., enalapril 0.25-0.5 mg/kg q12h PO).
• Patients with hypoproteinemia, nephrotic syndrome, and associated ascitic fluid accumulation—can treat as above with the addition of hetastarch (6% hetastarch in 0.9% NaCl); administer an IV bolus (dogs, 20 mL/kg; cats, 10–15 mL/kg) slowly over ~1 hour; hetastarch increases plasma oncotic pressure and pulls fluid into the intravascular space for up to 24–48 hours.
• Systemic antibiotic therapy is dictated by bacterial identification and sensitivity testing in patients with septic exudate ascites.

FOLLOW-UP

PATIENT MONITORING

• Varies with the underlying cause.
• Check sodium, potassium, BUN, creatinine, and weight fluctuations periodically if the patient is maintained on a diuretic.

POSSIBLE COMPLICATIONS

Aggressive diuretic administration may cause hypokalemia, which could predispose to metabolic alkalosis and exacerbation of hepatic encephalopathy in patients with underlying liver disease; alkalosis causes a shift from ammonium (NH_4) to ammonia (NH_3).

MISCELLANEOUS

AGE-RELATED FACTORS

N/A

PREGNANCY/FERTILITY/BREEDING

N/A

SYNONYMS

Abdominal effusion.

SEE ALSO

• Cirrhosis and Fibrosis of the Liver.
• Congestive Heart Failure, Right-Sided.
• Hypoalbuminemia.
• Nephrotic Syndrome.

ABBREVIATIONS

• BUN = blood urea nitrogen.
• CHF = congestive heart failure.

Suggested Reading

Gompf RE. The history and physical examination. In: Smith FWK, Tilley LP, Oyama MA, Sleeper MM, eds., Manual of Canine and Feline Cardiology, 5th ed. St. Louis, MO: Saunders Elsevier, 2016, pp. 3–24.

Kramer RE, Sokol RJ, Yerushalmi B, et al. Large-volume paracentesis in the management of ascites in children. J Ped Gastro Nutr 2001; 33:245–249.

Kumar KS, Srikala D. Ascites with right heart failure in a dog: diagnosis and management. J Adv Vet Anim Res 2014, 1(3):140–144.

Lewis LD, Morris ML Jr, Hand MS. Small Animal Clinical Nutrition, 3rd ed. Topeka, KS: Mark Morris Associates, 1987.

Li MK. Management of ascites. Hong Kong Med Di 2009; 14:27–29.

Pradham MS, Dakshinkar NP, Waghaye UG, Bodkhe AM. Successful treatment of ascites of hepatic origin in dog. Vet World 2008; 1(1):23.

Runyon BA. Management of adult patients with ascites due to cirrhosis. Hepatol 2004; 39:1–16.

Saravanan M, Sharma K, Kumar M, et al. Analysis of serum ascites albumin gradient test in ascitic dogs. Vet World 2012, 5(5):285–287.

Author Jerry A. Thornhill
Consulting Editor Michael Aherne

Client Education Handout available online

ASPERGILLOSIS, DISSEMINATED INVASIVE

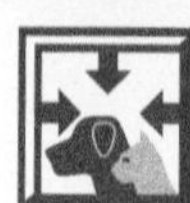

BASICS

OVERVIEW

- Opportunistic fungal infection caused by *Aspergillus* spp., common molds that are ubiquitous in the environment, forming spores in dust, straw, grass clippings, hay.
- Disseminated disease does not appear to be related to nasal form of disease.
- Disseminated disease—usually *A. terreus* or *A. deflectus*, but other *Aspergillus* species have also been described; *A. fumigatus* causes nasal or pulmonary disease; typically does not disseminate.
- Portal of entry not definitively established, possibly through respiratory tract or gastrointestinal tract, with subsequent hematogenous spread.
- Most commonly affects intervertebral discs, bones, thoracic lymph nodes, lung, renal pelvis; localized respiratory (bronchopulmonary aspergillosis) or, rarely, cornea or ear canal disease can occur, often with *Aspergillus* species other than *A. terreus* or *A. deflectus*.
- Sinoorbital aspergillosis has been described in cats; may be caused by variety of species including *Aspergillus felis*.

SIGNALMENT

Dogs

- Considerably more common in dogs than in cats.
- German shepherd dogs, and less so Rhodesian ridgebacks, overrepresented, but reported sporadically in many breeds; average age 3 years (range 2–8 years); females three times more likely to develop disease than males.

Cats

- Persians—overrepresented for sinoorbital aspergillosis.
- Disseminated cases mostly affect lungs and/or gastrointestinal tract.

SIGNS

Dogs

- May develop acutely or slowly over a period of several months.
- Lameness—fungal osteomyelitis, with focal pain and swelling.
- Neurologic—fungal discospondylitis causing paraparesis, paraplegia, spinal pain; central signs—vestibular signs, circling, seizures, hemiparesis, mental dullness, ataxia, vision impairment.
- Renal involvement—polyuria/polydipsia, vomiting, inappetence, weight loss.
- Respiratory—cough, increased respiratory effort, decreased lung sounds due to pleural effusion.
- Cardiac—arrhythmias.
- Gastrointestinal—abdominal distension, anorexia, vomiting, diarrhea.
- Ocular—uveitis, chorioretinitis, hyphema, panophthalmitis.
- Nonspecific—fever, weight loss, weakness, vomiting, lymphadenopathy.

Cats

- Usually nonspecific signs (e.g., lethargy, vomiting, and diarrhea).
- Ocular—exophthalmos.

CAUSES & RISK FACTORS

- Caused by *Aspergillus* species, most commonly *A. terreus or A. deflectus*, but other species have also been described (e.g., *A. niger*, *A. flavipes*, *A. versicolor*, *A. lentulus*, *A. alabamensis*).
- *A. felis* recently reported to cause fungal rhinosinusitis in cats, sinoorbital aspergillosis in cats, disseminated disease in dogs, pulmonary aspergillosis in humans.
- German shepherd dogs, purebred dogs, immunosuppressed animals at higher risk.
- Geographic/environmental conditions—may be factor, as some regions have higher incidence (e.g., California, Louisiana, Michigan, Georgia, Florida, Virginia in the United States; Western Australia; Barcelona; Milan).
- Cats—described in association with feline infectious peritonitis (FIP), feline panleukopenia virus, feline leukemia virus (FeLV), diabetes mellitus, chemotherapy.

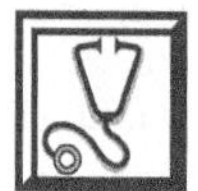

DIAGNOSIS

DIFFERENTIAL DIAGNOSIS

- Bacterial osteomyelitis/discospondylitis.
- Spinal neoplasia.
- Intervertebral disc disease.
- Skeletal neoplasia.
- Bacterial pyelonephritis.
- Bacterial pneumonia.
- Other causes of vestibular abnormalities or seizures.
- Other causes of uveitis (see Anterior Uveitis—Cats; Anterior Uveitis—Dogs).

CBC/BIOCHEMISTRY/URINALYSIS

- Nonspecific.
- CBC:
  - Dogs—mature neutrophilic leukocytosis, sometimes with eosinophilia and monocytosis; one-third have normocytic, normochromic, nonregenerative anemia.
  - Cats—may have nonregenerative anemia, leukopenia.
- Biochemistry—variable hyperglobulinemia, increases in activity of alkaline phosphatase (ALP), alanine aminotransferase (ALT), and amylase; increased concentrations of serum, creatinine, phosphate, blood urea nitrogen (BUN), and calcium.
- Urinalysis—possible isosthenuria, microscopic hematuria, pyuria, fungal hyphae in sediment.

OTHER LABORATORY TESTS

- Methods of detection include cytology, culture, histopathology.
- Definitive diagnosis by fungal culture from normally sterile body fluids and tissues (urine, bone, cerebrospinal fluid (CSF), blood, lymph node, pleural effusions, intervertebral disc aspirates, kidney, spleen); urine culture positive in 50% of dogs.
- Culture on Sabouraud's dextrose agar (requires 5–7 days).
- Antibody serology is highly insensitive for diagnosis of disseminated aspergillosis.
- Galactomannan antigen ELISA (urine or serum)—good sensitivity (89%) and specificity (89%); pulmonary and ocular infections have lower sensitivity; false positive in dogs treated with Plasmalyte or with other mycotic infections (*Penicillium*, *Paecilomyces*, *Cladosporidium*, *Geotrichum*, *Histoplasma*, *Cryptococcus*).
- Cats—test for FeLV and feline immunodeficiency virus (FIV).

IMAGING

Radiographic Findings

- Spinal views may show end-plate lysis, productive lesions with bridging spondylosis, lysis of vertebral bodies.
- Bony proliferation, lysis, periosteal reaction typical of osteomyelitis of diaphyseal region of long bones.
- Pulmonary involvement rare; mixed interstitial/alveolar pattern, enlarged sternal and/or tracheobronchial lymph nodes, pleural effusion; productive and destructive lesions of sternebrae; cavitary pulmonary lesions in dogs with chronic pulmonary localization.

Ultrasonographic Findings

- Kidneys—most common site to detect changes; renal pelvis dilation ± echogenic debris within pelvis, loss of corticomedullary distinction, renal distortion with mottled appearance of parenchyma, dilation of proximal ureter, renomegaly, nodules or masses, hydronephrosis.
- Spleen—hypoechoic, lacy, sharply demarcated areas with no Doppler signal (suggestive of infarct), nodules/masses, mottled parenchyma, splenic venous thrombosis.
- Other—abdominal lymphadenomegaly, diffuse hepatic hypoechogenicity, ascites, or evidence of venous thrombosis.

MRI Findings

Useful for further defining brain lesions in animals with CNS abnormalities; changes similar to other infectious and noninfectious inflammatory brain diseases; may identify subtle vertebral lesions in dogs with discospondylitis.

DIAGNOSTIC PROCEDURES

Area to collect sample relies on clinical presentation, but may include CSF tap, intervertebral disc space aspirates, abdominocentesis/thoracocentesis, aspirate of various organs (spleen, liver, kidney) or lymph nodes.

PATHOLOGIC FINDINGS

- Hyphae that branch at 45-degree angle; special stains assist organism detection.
- Focal osteomyelitis with multiple pale granulomas in kidneys, spleen, lymph node, myocardium, pancreas, liver.
- Pyogranulomatous inflammation can be found in lungs, eyes, thyroid, uterus, brain, prostate; contain numbers of septate, branching hyphae that may have characteristic lateral branching aleuriospores (*A. terreus*).
- Best visualized with periodic acid-Schiff, Gomori's methenamine silver, or Crocott's stain.

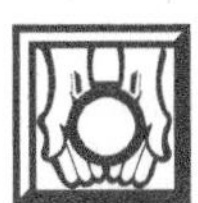

TREATMENT

DOGS

- Treatment rarely curative; may result in partial clinical remission or halt progression of clinical signs; severely ill dogs have poor prognosis.
- Fluid therapy—indicated by volume status, degree of renal compromise.
- Pulmonary lobectomy followed by systemic antifungals has been successful in dogs with cavitary lesions without evidence of dissemination.

CATS

Disseminated—likely difficult to treat; limited data.

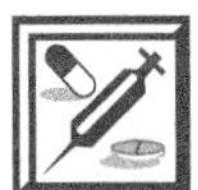

MEDICATIONS

DRUG(S) OF CHOICE

- Combination itraconazole (5–10 mg/kg PO q24h or divided q12h) and amphotericin B (dogs, 2–3 mg/kg IV 3 days/week for 9–12 treatments, to cumulative dose of 24–27 mg/kg)—treatment of choice.
- Itraconazole monotherapy has achieved remission for months to 1–2 years in small number of dogs.
- New triazoles—voriconazole and posaconazole both have activity against *Aspergillus*; some dogs treated with them have gone into remission for many months; *Aspergillus* spp. and other molds are intrinsically resistant to fluconazole, so it should not be used.
- Terbinifine (5–10 mg/kg PO q24h) alone or in combination with triazoles has been used to treat resistant infections, with unclear benefit.
- β-glucan synthase inhibitors caspofungin, micafungin, anidulafungin—limited clinical information in dogs, but efficacious in invasive aspergillosis in humans.

CONTRAINDICATIONS/POSSIBLE INTERACTIONS

- Amphotericin B—contraindicated in dogs with preexisting renal compromise or failure; amphotericin B lipid complex reduces likelihood of nephrotoxicity.
- Oral azoles—nausea, intermittent anorexia, liver enzyme elevation.
- Avoid midazolam and cisapride with azoles—fatal drug reactions noted in humans.
- Hepatotoxicity and ulcerative dermatitis more likely to occur at doses of itraconazole ≥10 mg/kg/day; discontinue itraconazole if adverse effects occur; may be able to reinstitute at lower dose once side effects have resolved.

FOLLOW-UP

- Disseminated—monitor serial radiographs every 1–2 months, renal function, and urine cultures.
- Prognosis poor, especially in purebred dogs that lack other reasons for immune compromise.

MISCELLANEOUS

ZOONOTIC POTENTIAL

None

ABBREVIATIONS

- ALP = alkaline phosphatase.
- ALT = alanine transaminase.
- BUN = blood urea nitrogen.
- CSF = cerebrospinal fluid.
- FeLV = feline leukemia virus.
- FIP = feline infectious peritonitis.
- FIV = feline immunodeficiency virus.

Suggested Reading

Maddison JE, Page SW, Church DB. Small Animal Clinical Pharmacology, 2nd ed. Edinburgh: Saunders, 2008, pp. 186–197.

Sykes, JE. Canine and Feline Infectious Diseases. Philadelphia, PA: Saunders, 2014, pp. 639–647.

Author Jane E. Sykes

Consulting Editor Amie Koenig

Acknowledgment The author and editors acknowledge the prior contributions of Hannah N. Pipe-Martin and Stephen C. Barr.

Client Education Handout available online

A

ASPERGILLOSIS, NASAL

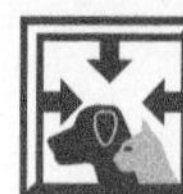

BASICS

DEFINITION

Nasal fungal disease caused by opportunistic ubiquitous saprophytic fungi that are members of the *Aspergillus fumigatus* species complex.

PATHOPHYSIOLOGY

- Inhalation of fungus leads to disease in the nasal cavity with destruction of turbinates, formation of plaque lesions, and overproduction of mucus, causing clinical signs of nasal disease; does not result in systemic mycosis.
- In dogs, confined to nasal cavity and frontal sinus—sinonasal form.
- In cats, can result in sinonasal or sino-orbital disease.

SYSTEMS AFFECTED

- Respiratory—sinonasal form in dogs and cats.
- Ophthalmic—sino-orbital form in cats.

GENETICS

Unknown

INCIDENCE/PREVALENCE

Unknown, but a common diagnosis in dogs with nasal discharge in many locations.

GEOGRAPHIC DISTRIBUTION

Worldwide

SIGNALMENT

Species

Dogs and cats (less common).

Breed Predilections

- Dogs—dolichocephalic and mesocephalic breeds.
- Cats—brachycephalic breeds may be overrepresented.

Mean Age and Range

Predominantly young to middle-aged.

Predominant Sex

None identified.

SIGNS

Historical Findings

- Unilateral or bilateral nasal discharge—typically mucoid, mucopurulent, or serosanguinous; may be primarily epistaxis.
- Sneezing.
- Typically chronic signs—several months.
- Many patients will have been treated with antibiotics for a possible bacterial infection, with variable response.

Physical Examination Findings

- Unilateral or bilateral nasal discharge.
- Typically increased nasal airflow on the affected side.
- Depigmentation with ulceration of the nasal planum.
- Facial pain.
- Ipsilateral mandibular lymphadenopathy.
- Sino-orbital disease in cats—stertor, exophthalmos, exposure keratitis, hard palate ulceration, facial asymmetry, loss of nasal airflow.

CAUSES

- No underlying cause identified, although preexisting foreign body or trauma is occasionally implicated.
- Likely due to inhalation of a large bolus of fungus from the environment, most commonly from the *Aspergillus fumigatus* species complex—*A. fumigatus* in sinonasal disease, *A. felis* in sino-orbital disease.

RISK FACTORS

Unknown

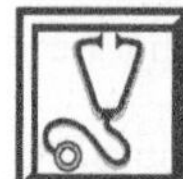

DIAGNOSIS

DIFFERENTIAL DIAGNOSIS

- Foreign body.
- Oronasal fistula.
- Lymphoplasmacytic rhinitis.
- Neoplasia.
- Nasopharyngeal polyp or cryptococcosis—cats.

CBC/BIOCHEMISTRY/URINALYSIS

- Often normal.
- Possible inflammatory leukogram.

OTHER LABORATORY TESTS

Serology

- Detects fungi-specific serum antibodies.
- Agar gel immunodiffusion (AGID)—commercially available; 98% specificity, 67% sensitivity in dogs; 43% sensitivity in cats. Serial serology does not appear to correlate with clinical status.
- ELISA—88% sensitivity, 97% specificity in dogs; 90% sensitivity in cats.
- Counter-immunoelectrophoresis—85% specificity in dogs.
- Serum galactomannan—unreliable.

Culture

- Tissue fungal culture—visualized biopsy sample taken from a region of suspected fungal growth showed 100% specificity, 81% sensitivity in dogs.
- Culture of nasal discharge is less sensitive and specific.

IMAGING

CT

- Imaging method of choice.
- Allows for evaluation of the cribriform plate.
- Cavitated turbinate lysis, thickening of the mucosa along the nasal turbinates.
- Frontal sinus proliferative mass effect.
- Cats—soft tissue mass in the choana or nasopharynx.

Skull Radiography

- Intraoral dorsoventral radiograph of the nasal cavity shows turbinate lysis.
- Rostrocaudal or skyline frontal sinus view may show increased soft tissue density in the frontal sinus.
- Cannot evaluate cribriform.

DIAGNOSTIC PROCEDURES

Rhinoscopy

- Allows for visualization of fungal plaques (white, yellow, black, or light green) on the mucosa of the nasal cavity and/or frontal sinus.
- Rigid rhinoscopy—examination of the nasal cavity alone; good visualization is possible due to large airspaces caused by turbinate lysis; excessive mucus and bleeding can make full examination difficult.
- Flexible rhinoscopy in dogs allows examination of the nasopharynx and frontal sinus if the opening of the nasofrontal duct is destroyed by fungal infection.
- Sinuscopy—may be required to confirm the diagnosis in dogs that lack nasal cavity plaques.

PATHOLOGIC FINDINGS

- Biopsies obtained of affected area under direct rhinoscopic visualization using cup biopsy instruments.
- Samples placed in formalin, routinely processed.
- Identification of septate, branching hyphae, and conidia on histopathology with surrounding inflammation.
- Blind biopsies in an unaffected area of the nasal cavity can result in a false diagnosis of inflammation.

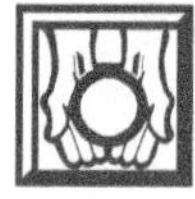

TREATMENT

APPROPRIATE HEALTH CARE

Overnight hospitalization advised after topical treatment or surgery.

NURSING CARE

Maintain the nares free of nasal discharge.

ACTIVITY

Restriction of activity is not required if no bleeding is documented.

DIET

N/A

CLIENT EDUCATION

- Dogs—inform client that multiple topical treatments may be necessary for cure.
- No established protocols for treatment in cats.

SURGICAL CONSIDERATIONS

Endoscopic Debridement

Extensive curettage and removal of fungal material from the nose and frontal sinus are essential for efficacy of topical medication.

Trephination of the Frontal Sinus

- May be required for dogs with frontal sinus involvement where access cannot be established via rhinoscopy.

• Performed using a Jacob's chuck and intramedullary pin.

Surgical Debridement and/or Exenteration

• Rhinotomy for debridement in some dogs.
• Exenteration in some cats with sino-orbital disease.

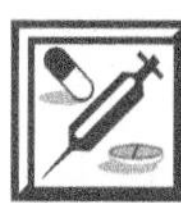

MEDICATIONS

DRUG(S) OF CHOICE

• Clotrimazole and enilconazole are the most widely used drugs topically in different formulations and protocols.
• Treatment is usually performed during the same anesthesia as diagnostics, after debridement.
• No consensus regarding the most effective therapy; three protocols are described here.

Clotrimazole Solution Infusion

• Clotrimazole solution 1% infused through catheters placed into the nasal cavity and frontal sinus via trephination, or in the nasal cavity only; reported efficacy of up to 87% in dogs with multiple treatments.
• Has been used in cats with sinonasal disease with varying success.

Combined Clotrimazole Irrigation and Depot Therapy

Frontal sinus trephination with flushing of 1% clotrimazole solution followed by 1% clotrimazole cream instilled as a depot agent; reported efficacy of 86% with multiple treatments needed in one dog.

Debridement and Clotrimazole Depot Therapy under Rhinoscopic Guidance

Debridement and sinus and nasal depot therapy with 1% clotrimazole cream under rhinoscopic guidance; reported efficacy of 100% with multiple treatments.

Systemic Therapy

• Antifungal triazole drugs should be considered if the cribriform is not intact; can also be combined with topical therapy.
• Used as primary therapy in some cats.
• May be cost-prohibitive.
• Itraconazole 5 mg/kg PO q12h in dogs; reported efficacy of 60–70%; 10 mg/kg PO q24h in cats.
• Posaconazole 5 mg/kg PO q12h with terbinafine 30 mg/kg PO q12h and doxycycline 5 mg/kg PO q12h for refractory disease; complete remission reported in 7/10 dogs, partial clinical remission in 3/10 dogs; 2/10 dogs relapsed after cessation of therapy.
• Voriconazole 5 mg/kg PO q12h in dogs; efficacy has not been established; neurotoxic in cats.
• Fluconazole is not recommended due to resistance.

CONTRAINDICATIONS

• A breach in the cribriform plate was thought to be a contraindication to topical treatment; two recent retrospective studies showed no adverse neurologic effects after topical treatment in dogs with lysis of the cribriform and/or frontal sinus floor.
• Sino-orbital disease in cats necessitates the use of systemic therapy.

PRECAUTIONS

Topical clotrimazole and enilconazole are caustic to mucosal surfaces; all staff in close contact should wear protective gear.

ALTERNATIVE DRUG(S)

Homeopathic remedy—aurum metallicum reported to have resulted in a resolution of clinical signs and clearance of organisms in a dog unresponsive to topical therapy.

FOLLOW-UP

PATIENT MONITORING

Dogs

• Reduction of clinical signs does not establish resolution of disease.
• Follow-up rhinoscopy with possible histopathology and culture is recommended to establish a response to treatment.
• Serial serology (AGID) appears not to correlate with disease status.
• Repeat CT should be considered for reassessment of the cribriform plate before repeat topical treatment if worsening clinical signs are seen.

Dogs and Cats

• Monitor liver enzymes on triazole therapy.
• Monitor renal parameters on amphotericin B.

PREVENTION/AVOIDANCE

N/A

POSSIBLE COMPLICATIONS

• Topical therapy—monitor for any complications such as swelling of oropharynx, neurologic signs, infection/swelling of trephine site.
• Triazoles can cause anorexia and can be hepatotoxic.
• Amphotericin B can be nephrotoxic.

EXPECTED COURSE AND PROGNOSIS

• The prognosis in dogs is good, though multiple topical treatments may be needed; recurrence or reinfection can occur years after supposedly successful therapy.
• The prognosis for cats with sinonasal disease is better than with the sino-orbital form.

MISCELLANEOUS

ASSOCIATED CONDITIONS

N/A

ZOONOTIC POTENTIAL

No documented cases of human infection from an affected dog or cat.

PREGNANCY/FERTILITY/BREEDING

N/A

ABBREVIATIONS

• AGID = agar gel immunodiffusion.

Suggested Reading

Barrs VR, Talbot JJ. Feline aspergillosis. Vet Clin North Am 2014, 44(1):51–73.
Friend E, Anderson DM, White RAS. Combined clotrimazole irrigation and depot therapy for canine nasal aspergillosis. J Small Anim Pract 2006, 47(6):312–315.
Mathews KG, Davidson AP, Koblik PD, et al. Comparison of topical administration of clotrimazole through surgically placed versus nonsurgically placed catheters for treatment of nasal aspergillosis in dogs: 60 cases (1990–1996). J Am Vet Med Assoc 1998, 213:501–506.
Sharman M, Mansfield CS. Sinonasal aspergillosis in dogs: a review. J Small Anim Pract 2012, 53:434–444.
Vedrine B, Fribourg-Blanc L-A. Treatment of sinonasal aspergillosis by debridement and sinonasal deposition therapy with clotrimazole under rhinoscopic guidance. J Am Anim Hosp Assoc 2018, 54:103–110.

Author Jill S. Pomrantz
Consulting Editor Elizabeth Rozanski

A

ASPIRIN TOXICOSIS

BASICS

OVERVIEW

- Given for its antipyretic, analgesic, anti-inflammatory, and antiplatelet effects.
- Aspirin inhibits cyclooxygenase, reducing the synthesis of prostaglandins and thromboxanes.
- Gastric irritation and hemorrhage can occur.
- Repeated doses can produce gastrointestinal ulceration and perforation and hepatic injury; renal injury is uncommon.
- Toxic hepatitis, marked metabolic acidosis, and anemia can occur, especially in cats (long half-life).
- Hepatic damage may not be dose related.

SIGNALMENT

Cats and less commonly dogs.

SIGNS

- Depression, lethargy.
- Anorexia.
- Vomiting ± blood.
- Diarrhea ± blood; melena.
- Tachypnea.
- Hyperthermia.
- Pallor.
- Polyuria/polydipsia (rare).
- Muscular weakness and ataxia.
- Ataxia, coma, seizures, and death in 1 or more days.

CAUSES & RISK FACTORS

- Owners employing human dosage guidelines to medicate cats and dogs.
- Dogs—single 25 mg/kg dose has resulted in gastric bleeding.
- Cats have a decreased ability to conjugate salicylate with glycine and glucuronic acid due to a deficiency in glucuronyl transferase.
- Half-life increases with dosage—cats, 22–27 hours for 5–12 mg/kg and approximately 44 hours for 25 mg/kg; responsible for higher risk in cats. Dogs, half-life = 7.5 hours.
- Elimination is slower in neonatal and geriatric patients.
- Patients with hypoalbuminemia may be at higher risk of toxicity because aspirin is highly protein bound to plasma albumin.

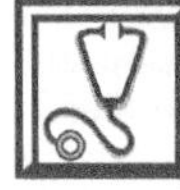

DIAGNOSIS

DIFFERENTIAL DIAGNOSIS

- Ethylene glycol or alcohol.
- Anticoagulant rodenticides.
- Other causes of liver failure, including acetaminophen, iron, metaldehyde, and blue-green algae.

CBC/BIOCHEMISTRY/URINALYSIS

- Cats—prone to Heinz body formation.
- Decreased packed cell volume (PCV); may be marked, especially in cats.
- Leukocytosis.
- Hypoproteinemia.
- Elevated liver enzymes.
- Elevated renal values (rare).

OTHER LABORATORY TESTS

- Initial respiratory alkalosis followed by marked metabolic acidosis.
- High ketones and pyruvic, lactic, and amino acid levels.
- Decreased sulfuric and phosphoric acid renal clearance.

IMAGING

- Abdominal imaging (perforation).

DIAGNOSTIC PROCEDURES

- Salicylic acid concentrations in serum.

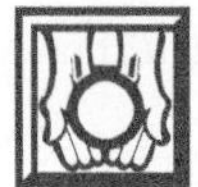

TREATMENT

- Inpatient—following general principles of poisoning management.
- Induced gastric emptying—gastric lavage or induced emesis.
- Correction of acid-base balance—continuous IV fluids; assisted ventilation and supplemental oxygen for severely affected animals.
- Whole blood transfusions for severe cases of hemorrhage and hypotension.
- Peritoneal dialysis and hemodialysis are advanced procedures that will increase salicylate clearance in severe cases.

MEDICATIONS

DRUG(S) OF CHOICE

- No specific antidote available.
- Activated charcoal—1–2 g/kg PO with a cathartic (sorbitol); monitor sodium concentration.
- 5% dextrose IV to correct dehydration.
- Gastrointestinal protectants—sucralfate and an H2 blocker or proton pump inhibitor; misoprostol for patients at higher risk for gastrointestinal hemorrhage.
- Sodium bicarbonate 1 mEq/kg IV in severe ingestions—alkalinizes urine; must closely monitor acid-base status.
- Diazepam 0.5–1 mg/kg IV or rectal as needed for seizures.

CONTRAINDICATIONS/POSSIBLE INTERACTIONS

N/A

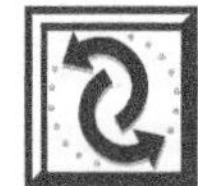

FOLLOW-UP

- Maintaining renal function and acid-base balance is vital.
- Severe acid-base disturbances, severe dehydration, toxic hepatitis, bone marrow depression, and coma are poor prognostic indicators.

MISCELLANEOUS

- Be sure that history of "aspirin" medication does not refer to other available pain medications.
- Question owner about any preexisting painful condition that may have prompted the aspirin administration.

ABBREVIATIONS

- PCV = packed cell volume.

Suggested Reading

Plumb DC. Aspirin. In: Plumb DC, ed., Plumb's Veterinary Drug Handbook, 9th ed. Ames, IA: Wiley-Blackwell, 2018, pp. 92–96.

Talcott PA, Gwaltney-Brant SM. Nonsteroidal anti-inflammatories. In: Peterson ME, Talcott PA, eds. Small Animal Toxicology, 3rd ed. St. Louis, MO: Elsevier, 2013, pp. 698–700.

Author Lisa A. Murphy

Consulting Editor Lynn R. Hovda

ASTHMA, BRONCHITIS—CATS

BASICS

DEFINITION

• Chronic bronchitis—neutrophilic inflammation of the lower airways (bronchi and bronchioles) lacking a specific etiology; chronic daily cough of greater than 2 months in duration. • Asthma—acute or chronic airway inflammation associated with increased airway responsiveness to various stimuli, airway narrowing due to smooth muscle hypertrophy or constriction, reversibility of airway constriction, and presence of eosinophils, lymphocytes, and mast cells within the airways. • Bronchitis is thought to result in airflow obstruction due to airway remodeling, while asthma is associated with airway constriction; however, clinically the two disease processes can appear similar. No physical examination findings or biomarkers can distinguish between the two syndromes, although reversal of airflow obstruction following administration of a beta-agonist is suggestive of the asthmatic form of disease.

PATHOPHYSIOLOGY

• Lower airway inflammation likely results from inhalation of irritant substances. • Bronchiolar smooth muscle constriction—can resolve spontaneously or with treatment. • Increase in mucosal goblet cells, mucus production, and edema of bronchial wall associated with inflammation. • Excessive mucus can cause bronchiolar obstruction, atelectasis, or bronchiectasis. • Smooth muscle hypertrophy implies chronicity—usually not reversible. • Chronic inflammation leads to airway remodeling and irreversible airflow obstruction.

SYSTEMS AFFECTED

• Respiratory. • Cardiac—pulmonary hypertension rarely.

GEOGRAPHIC DISTRIBUTION

Worldwide

SIGNALMENT

Species

Cat

Breed Predilections

Siamese overrepresented.

Mean Age and Range

Any age; more common between 2 and 8 years.

Predominant Sex

One study showed females overrepresented.

SIGNS

Historical Findings

• Coughing, tachypnea, labored breathing or wheezing. • Signs are typically episodic and can be acute or chronic.

Physical Examination Findings

• Severely affected cats present with open-mouth breathing, tachypnea, and cyanosis. • Increased tracheal sensitivity is common. • Chest auscultation may reveal crackles and/or expiratory wheezes, but can be normal. • Labored breathing with an abdominal push on expiration, increase in expiratory effort.

CAUSES

Triggers of airway inflammation unknown.

RISK FACTORS

• Cigarette smoke, poor environmental hygiene, dusty cat litter, hair sprays, and air fresheners can exacerbate disease. • Use of potassium bromide—implicated in causing signs of bronchitis/asthma in some cats.

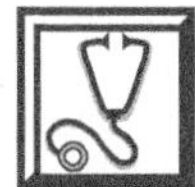

DIAGNOSIS

DIFFERENTIAL DIAGNOSIS

• Rule out infectious pneumonia (*Mycoplasma*, *Toxoplasma*, bacterial or fungal pneumonia). • Consider *Dirofilaria immitis* and primary lung parasites (*Aelurostrongylus abstrusus*, *Capillaria aerophilia*, *Paragonimus kellicotti*, *Troglostrongylus brevior*). More common in southern and midwest United States, and in outdoor and hunting cats in some geographic regions. • Primary or metastatic neoplasia can have similar clinical and radiographic appearance. • Clinical presentation of idiopathic pulmonary fibrosis may appear similar to feline bronchitis.

CBC/BIOCHEMISTRY/URINALYSIS

Frequently normal; ~40% of cats with bronchial disease have peripheral eosinophilia.

OTHER LABORATORY TESTS

• Fecal exams—flotation for *Capillaria*, sedimentation for *Paragonimus*, Baermann for *Aelurostrongylus*; false-negative results are common. • Heartworm antigen and antibody testing, particularly if coughing occurs in conjunction with vomiting. • Radioallergosorbent testing or intradermal skin testing—no correlation between skin allergies and respiratory disease currently documented.

IMAGING

Radiography

• Classically, diffuse bronchial wall thickening; interstitial or patchy alveolar patterns also possible. • Severity of radiographic changes does not necessarily correlate with clinical severity or duration, and normal radiographs can be found. • Hyperinflation of lung fields—flattened and caudally displaced diaphragm, increased distance between the heart and diaphragm, extension of lungs to the first lumbar vertebrae thought to reflect bronchoconstriction. • Collapse of right middle lung lobe due to mucus plugging and atelectasis reported in 11% of cases. • Pulmonary lobar arterial enlargement is suspicious for heartworm disease.

CT

Bronchial wall thickening, patchy alveolar patterns, and bronchiectasis.

Echocardiography

Useful to document heartworm disease or secondary pulmonary hypertension.

DIAGNOSTIC PROCEDURES

Transoral Tracheal Wash (TOTW)

Use a sterile endotracheal tube and polypropylene or red rubber catheter to collect airway fluids at the level of the carina.

Bronchoscopy

Allows visualization of trachea and bronchi. Excessive amounts of thick mucus are common with bronchitis. Mucosa of the airways is typically hyperemic and edematous.

Cytology of TOTW or Bronchoscopy/Bronchoalveolar Lavage (BAL)

• Eosinophils and neutrophils are most prominent cell types. • Up to 20% eosinophils on BAL cytology can be found in normal cats. • A mixed inflammatory cell population occurs in about 21% of cats.

Bacterial Cultures

• Quantitated cultures recommended; positive cultures frequently encountered, but bacterial colony counts >100–300 cfu/mL uncommon with bronchitis. • Specific *Mycoplasma* cultures and PCR for species detection.

Biopsy

Keyhole biopsy—can differentiate between idiopathic pulmonary fibrosis, neoplasia, and bronchitis if needed; rarely performed.

PATHOLOGIC FINDINGS

Hyperplasia/hypertrophy of goblet cells, hypertrophy of airway smooth muscle, epithelial erosion, and inflammatory infiltrates.

TREATMENT

APPROPRIATE HEALTH CARE

• Remove patient from environment that exacerbates disease. • Hospitalize for acute respiratory distress.

NURSING CARE

• Oxygen therapy, bronchodilators, and sedatives in an acute crisis. • Minimize manipulation in order to lessen stress and oxygen needs of the animal.

ACTIVITY

Usually self-limited by patient.

DIET

Calorie restriction for obese cats.

CLIENT EDUCATION

• Most causes are chronic and progressive. • Do not discontinue medical therapy when clinical signs have resolved—subclinical inflammation is common and can lead to progression of disease; lifelong medication and environmental changes usually necessary. • Some clients can be taught to give terbutaline subcutaneously and corticosteroid injections at home for a crisis situation.

MEDICATIONS

DRUG(S) OF CHOICE

Emergency Treatment

• Oxygen and a parenteral bronchodilator—injectable terbutaline (0.01 mg/kg IV/SC); repeat if no clinical improvement (decrease in respiratory rate or effort) in 20–30 minutes.
• A sedative can aid in decreasing anxiety (butorphanol tartrate at 0.2–0.4 mg/kg IV/IM, buprenorphine at 0.01 mg/kg IV/IM, or acepromazine at 0.01–0.05 mg/kg SC). • A short-acting parenteral corticosteroid may also be required—dexamethasone sodium phosphate (0.1–0.25 mg/kg IV/SC).

Long-Term Management

Corticosteroids

• Decrease inflammation. • Oral treatment is preferred over injectable for closer monitoring of dose and duration. • Prednisolone—0.5–1 mg/kg PO q12h; begin to taper dose (50% each week) after 1–2 weeks if clinical signs have improved; maintenance therapy 0.5–1 mg/kg PO q24–48h. • Longer-acting parenteral steroids (Vetalog® or Depo-Medrol®) should be reserved only for situations where owners are unable to administer oral or inhaled medication on a routine basis.

Inhaled Corticosteroids

• Requires a form-fitting facemask, spacer, and metered-dose inhaler (MDI); veterinary brand—Aerokat ® (Trudell Medical). • The most common corticosteroid used as an MDI is fluticasone propionate (Flovent®)—110 µg Flovent MDI is recommended (1–2 actuations, 7–10 breaths q12h); in one study, use of 44 µg Flovent decreased BAL eosinophil counts in cats with experimentally induced lower airway disease. • Flovent is used for long-term control of airway inflammation; takes 10–14 days to reach peak effect; use oral steroids concurrently during this time. • Results in some suppression of the hypothalamic–pituitary axis, but systemic side effects appear to be limited.

Bronchodilators

• Methylxanthines—sustained-release theophylline formulations recommended, and pharmacokinetics can vary greatly; only compounded generic currently available; dose at 15–20 mg/kg PO once daily in the evening.
• Beta-2 agonists (terbutaline, albuterol)—reverse smooth muscle constriction; oral terbutaline dose is 1/4 of a 2.5 mg tablet; initial albuterol dose is 1–2 puffs; avoid giving beta-2 agonists daily as tachyphylaxis may develop.

Anthelminthics

• Empirical therapy is indicated for cats with clinical signs of bronchial disease and eosinophilic airway cytology in an appropriate geographic location. • Consider fenbendazole, ivermectin, praziquantel, or milbemycin.

Antibiotics

Use based on a positive quantitative culture and susceptibility testing or *Mycoplasma* isolation.

CONTRAINDICATIONS

Beta-2 antagonists (e.g., propranolol) are contraindicated because of their ability to block sympathetically mediated bronchodilation.

PRECAUTIONS

• Long-term use of steroids increases risk of development of diabetes mellitus and predisposes to immunosuppression. • Use of corticosteroids in cats may precipitate congestive heart failure.
• Beta agonists could cause tachycardia and exacerbate underlying cardiac disease.

ALTERNATIVE DRUG(S)

• Leukotriene receptor blockers and inhibitors of generation—no evidence to support use.
• Tyrosine kinase inhibitors—masitinib is no longer on the market; side effects were dose limiting. • Antiserotonin and antihistamine drugs—no evidence to support use.
• Immunotherapy—allergen-specific rush immunotherapy (RIT) shows promise in treating asthma. • Omega 3 fatty acids/neutraceuticals—diminished hyperresponsiveness of airway, but did not resolve airway eosinophilia.

FOLLOW-UP

PATIENT MONITORING

• Owners should report any increase in coughing, sneezing, wheezing, or respiratory distress; medications should be increased appropriately, or additional therapy initiated if clinical signs worsen. • Follow-up radiographs may be helpful to detect onset of new disease.
• Owner should watch for signs of polyuria/polydipsia (PU/PD) that could indicate diabetes mellitus or renal disease; monitor blood glucose and urine cultures.

PREVENTION/AVOIDANCE

Eliminate any environmental factors that can trigger a crisis situation (see Risk Factors); change furnace and air-conditioner filters on a regular basis; consider dust-free litters.

POSSIBLE COMPLICATIONS

• Acute episodes can be life-threatening.
• Right-sided heart disease develops rarely as a result of long-term bronchitis.

EXPECTED COURSE AND PROGNOSIS

• Long-term therapy should be expected.
• Most cats do well if recurrence of clinical signs is carefully monitored and medical therapy appropriately adjusted. • A few cats will be refractory to treatment; these carry a much worse prognosis.

MISCELLANEOUS

ASSOCIATED CONDITIONS

Cor pulmonale can be a sequela to chronic lower airway disease.

PREGNANCY/FERTILITY/BREEDING

Glucocorticoids are contraindicated in the pregnant animal; bronchodilators should be used with caution.

SYNONYMS

• Allergic bronchitis. • Asthmatic bronchitis.
• Feline lower airway disease. • Extrinsic asthma. • Eosinophilic bronchitis.

SEE ALSO

• Heartworm Disease—Cats.
• Respiratory Parasites.

ABBREVIATIONS

• BAL = bronchoscopy/bronchoalveolar lavage.
• MDI = metered-dose inhaler. • PU/PD = polyuria/polydipsia. • RIT = rush immunotherapy. • TOTW = transoral tracheal wash.

INTERNET RESOURCES

• www.aerokat.com • www.fritzthebrave.com

Suggested Reading

Chang C, Cohn L, DeClue A, et al. Oral glucocorticoids diminish the efficacy of allergen-specific immunotherapy in experimental feline asthma. Vet J 2013, 197:268–272.
Chang DG, Dodam HR, Cohn LA, et al. An experimental janus kinase (JAK) inhibitor suppresses eosinophilic airway inflammation in feline asthma. ACVIM Forum Proceedings, 2013.
Cohn LA, DeClue AE, Cohen RL, Reinero CR. Effects of fluticasone propionate dosage in an experimental model of feline asthma. J Feline Med Surg 2010, 12(2):91–96.
Crisi P, DiCesare A, Boari A. Feline troglostrongylosis: current epizootiology, clinical features, and therapeutic pptions. Front Vet Sci 2018, 5:126.
Kirschvink J, Leemans J, Delvaux F, et al. Inhaled fluticasone reduces bronchial responsiveness and airway inflammation in cats with mild chronic bronchitis. J Feline Med Surg 2006, 8(1):45–54.
Schulz BS, Richter P, Weber K, et al. Detection of feline *Mycoplasma* species in cats with feline asthma and chronic bronchitis. J Feline Med Surg 2014, 16(12): 943–949.

Author Karah Burns DeMarle
Consulting Editor Elizabeth Rozanski
Acknowledgment The author and book editors acknowledge the prior contribution of Carrie J. Miller and Lynelle R. Johnson.

Client Education Handout available online

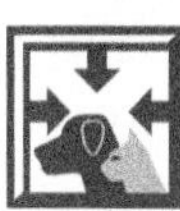

BASICS

OVERVIEW

• Glial cell neoplasm, most commonly affecting the brain and rarely the spinal cord. • Neoplastic cells are of astrocytic origin. • The most common intraaxial (situated inside of the brain parenchyma) intracranial neoplasm of dogs, but is rarely diagnosed in cats. • Tumors are often located in the pyriform area of the temporal lobe, the cerebral hemispheres, the thalamus, hypothalamus, or midbrain. • Biologic behavior of this tumor is dictated by the histopathologic grade (I–IV, from best to worst prognosis) and anatomic involvement. • Tumors typically do not penetrate the ventricular system or metastasize outside of the cranial vault.

SIGNALMENT

• Dog—often brachycephalic breeds >5 years of age; no sex predilection reported. • Cat—usually >9 years; no sex or breed predilection reported.

SIGNS

• Location and growth kinetic dependent. • Seizures. • Behavioral changes. • Apathy toward normal activities, including eating, playing, and societal interactions. • Disorientation. • Loss of conscious proprioception. • Cranial nerve abnormalities. • Head muscle atrophy. • Upper motor neuron tetraparesis.

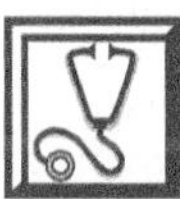

DIAGNOSIS

DIFFERENTIAL DIAGNOSIS

• Other primary tumors arising from tissues of the central nervous system. • Metastatic neoplasia with brain tropism such as hemangiosarcoma. • Granulomatous meningoencephalitis. • Trauma. Cerebrovascular infarction. • Meningitis.

CBC/BIOCHEMISTRY/URINALYSIS

Usually unremarkable.

OTHER LABORATORY TESTS

Cerebrospinal fluid (CSF) analysis may show albumin-cytologic dissociation (high protein with low number of nucleated cells). The CSF analysis is indicated to exclude infectious etiology, not to diagnose astrocytoma.

IMAGING

• MRI of brain is ideal for mass lesion confirmation, as it is superior to CT scanning for detecting lesions in the middle and caudal fossae. MRI is more sensitive than CT for detection infarcts, bleeding, and edema. • Brain MRI is useful in establishing a tentative differential diagnosis of a glial tumor, based on tumor characteristics highlighted in specific sequences.

DIAGNOSTIC PROCEDURES

• Neurologic exam. • Ophthalmic exam. • MRI. • CSF analysis. • Tumor biopsy for definitive diagnosis, when specific antineoplastic treatment is sought (surgery, curative-intent radiation therapy, experimental therapies).

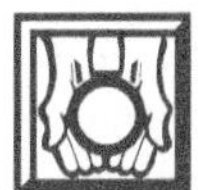

TREATMENT

• Surgery. • Radiation therapy can be very effective in improving neurologic signs. • Chemotherapy with lomustine, procarbazine, or temozolomide might exert cytoreductive activities. • Anti-inflammatory dosing with corticosteroids to reduce peritumoral edema. • Consultation with a neurosurgeon and a radiation oncologist is essential for appropriate patient management.

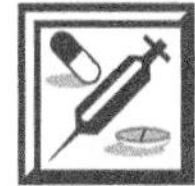

MEDICATIONS

DRUG(S) OF CHOICE

Seizure Control

• Status epilepticus—diazepam (0.5–1 mg/kg IV, up to three times to achieve effect); if no response to diazepam, use pentobarbital (5–15 mg/kg IV slowly to effect). • Long-term management—phenobarbital (1–4 mg/kg PO q12h) with or without adjuvant potassium bromide (20 mg/kg PO q24h).

Tumor Control

• Timely consultation with a neurosurgeon is of paramount importance for appropriate management of the patient. • Radiation therapy may be effective, and consultation with a radiation oncologist is recommended. Stereotactic radiosurgery or intensity-modulated radiation therapy may be considered as first-line treatment options. • Chemotherapy may be effective for treating dogs. Potential drugs that may exert measurable anticancer effects include CCNU (60–70 mg/m^2 PO every 3 weeks) or temozolomide (100–120 mg/m^2 PO q24h for 5 days every 3 weeks). • Prednisone (1 mg/kg q24h) may be effective in reducing peritumoral edema and improving neurologic signs. Patients may need to be on steroids long term, even after the definitive treatment of the tumor.

CONTRAINDICATIONS/POSSIBLE INTERACTIONS

• Prednisone and phenobarbital may cause polyphagia, polydipsia, and polyuria. • Phenobarbital may cause sedation for up to 2 weeks after initiation of treatment, and increase in hepatic enzymes on serum biochemical panel. • CBC and platelet count are recommended 7–10 days after chemotherapy and immediately before each dose of chemotherapy to monitor myelosuppression. • Chemotherapy has the potential to be synergistic with radiation therapy. Timely referral to a specialty center with neurosurgery, radiation therapy, and medical oncology capabilities is important for patients seeking more than palliative care.

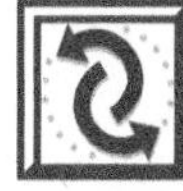

FOLLOW-UP

PATIENT MONITORING

• Blood phenobarbital concentration should be assessed after 7–10 days of treatment, with modifications to dosages for achieving target plasma concentrations. • Serial MRIs should be considered for documenting response if multimodality therapy is used. • Serial CBC and platelet counts should be performed to monitor myelotoxicity associated with chemotherapy.

EXPECTED COURSE AND PROGNOSIS

• Long-term prognosis is guarded. • Median survival after chemotherapy plus medical management may be up to 7 months. • Median survival after radiation therapy has been reported to be as high as 12 months.

MISCELLANEOUS

SEE ALSO

• Seizures (Convulsions, Status Epilepticus)—Cats
• Seizures (Convulsions, Status Epilepticus)—Dogs

ABBREVIATIONS

• CSF = cerebrospinal fluid.

Suggested Reading

Bentley RT, Ober CP, Anderson KL, et al. Canine intracranial gliomas: relationship between magnetic resonance imaging criteria and tumor type and grade. Vet J 2013, 198(2):463–471.

Stoica G, Levine J, Wolff J, Murphy K. Canine astrocytic tumors: a comparative review. Vet Pathol 2011, 48(1):266–275.

Troxel MT, Vite CH, Van Winkle TJ, et al. Feline intracranial neoplasia: retrospective review of 160 cases (1985–2001). J Vet Intern Med 2003, 17:850–859.

Author Nick Dervisis

Consulting Editor Timothy M. Fan

ATAXIA

BASICS

DEFINITION

- A sign of sensory dysfunction causing loss of coordination of the limbs, head, and/or trunk.
- Three clinical types—sensory (proprioceptive), vestibular, and cerebellar. All cause limb incoordination, but only vestibular and cerebellar ataxia cause head and neck incoordination.

PATHOPHYSIOLOGY

Sensory (Proprioceptive)

- Proprioceptive pathways in the spinal cord (i.e., fasciculus gracilis, fasciculus cuneatus, and spinocerebellar tracts) relay limb and trunk positions to the brain.
- When the spinal cord is slowly compressed, proprioceptive deficits are usually the first signs observed, because these tracts or pathways are located more superficially in the white matter and their larger axons are more susceptible to compression than are other tracts.
- Limb weakness (paresis) will occur if more centrally located motor tracts or pathways become involved; weakness is not always obvious early in the course of the disease.
- Ataxia can occur with spinal cord, brainstem, and cerebral lesions. Ataxia can be mild to absent with unilateral brainstem lesions, and subtle to absent with unilateral cerebral lesions.

Vestibular

- Changes in balance and head and neck positions are detected by vestibular receptors of the inner ear, relayed to the vestibulocochlear nerve, which is connected to vestibular nuclei in the brainstem.
- The inner ear's vestibular receptors and nerve are components of the peripheral nervous system, whereas brainstem vestibular nuclei are components of the central nervous system.
- Vestibular ataxia should be localized to either the peripheral or central vestibular nervous system, because prognosis and rule-outs differ for these two locations.
- Both locations of vestibular disease cause various degrees of vestibular ataxia, often manifested by head tilt and leaning, falling, or even rolling toward the side of the lesion.
- Central vestibular disease usually has vertical nystagmus or changing types of nystagmus; somnolence, stupor, or coma (due to involvement of the nearby ascending reticular activating system); multiple cranial nerve signs (e.g., trigeminal or facial nerve deficits); proprioceptive deficits and quadriparesis or hemiparesis.
- Peripheral vestibular disease does not typically show changes in mental status, vertical nystagmus, proprioceptive deficits, quadriparesis, or hemiparesis.
- Bilateral vestibular disease is uncommon and most often peripheral in origin. Typical vestibular signs are absent. Wide swinging back and forth head motions and poor to absent physiologic nystagmus are characteristic.

Cerebellar

- The cerebellum regulates, coordinates, and modulates motor activity.
- Proprioception is normal because the ascending proprioceptive pathways to the cortex are intact; weakness does not occur because the upper motor neurons are intact.
- While strength is preserved, affected animals have uncoordinated motor activity of limbs, head, and neck manifested by hypermetria; dysmetria; head tremors; intention tremors; and truncal sway. Menace responses may be absent without visual dysfunction.

SYSTEMS AFFECTED

Nervous—spinal cord (and brainstem and cortex), cerebellum, vestibular system.

SIGNALMENT

Any age, breed, or sex.

SIGNS

- Important to define the type of ataxia to localize the problem.
- Only one limb involved—rule out a musculoskeletal problem.
- Only hind limbs affected—likely a spinal cord disorder affecting the spinocerebellar tracts.
- All limbs or ipsilateral limbs affected—cervical spinal cord or cerebellar localization.
- Head tilt and/or nystagmus—vestibular localization.

CAUSES

Cerebellar

- Degenerative—abiotrophy (Kerry blue terrier, Gordon setter, rough-coated collie, Australian kelpie, Airedale, Bernese mountain dog, Finnish harrier, Brittany spaniel, border collie, beagle, Samoyed, wirehaired fox terrier, Labrador retriever, Great Dane, chow chow, Rhodesian ridgeback, domestic shorthair cats); storage diseases often have cerebellomedullary involvement.
- Anomalous—hypoplasia secondary to perinatal infection with panleukopenia virus (cats); malformed cerebellum due to herpesvirus infection (newborn puppies); arachnoid or epidermoid cyst located near fourth ventricle.
- Neoplastic—any CNS tumor (primary or secondary) localized to the cerebellum.
- Infectious—canine distemper virus; feline infectious peritonitis (FIP); and any other CNS infection affecting the cerebellum.
- Inflammatory, idiopathic, immune-mediated—meningoencephalomyelitis of undetermined etiology.
- Toxic—metronidazole.

Vestibular—CNS

- Infectious—FIP; canine distemper virus; rickettsial diseases.
- Inflammatory, idiopathic, immune-mediated—meningoencephalomyelitis of undetermined etiology.
- Nutritional—thiamine deficiency.
- Toxic—metronidazole.

Vestibular—Peripheral Nervous System

- Infectious—otitis media interna; *Cryptococcus* granuloma (cats).
- Inflammatory—nasopharyngeal (middle ear) polyps (cats).
- Idiopathic—geriatric vestibular disease (dogs); idiopathic vestibular syndrome (cats).
- Metabolic—hypothyroidism.
- Neoplastic—squamous cell carcinoma, bone tumors.
- Traumatic.

Spinal Cord

- Degenerative—degenerative myelopathy (old German shepherd, pug, boxer, Welsh corgi, others); degenerative disc disease.
- Vascular—fibrocartilaginous embolic myelopathy.
- Anomalous—hemivertebrae; dens hypoplasia with atlantoaxial subluxation-luxation; Chiari-like malformation; cervical spondylomyelopathy; spinal subarachnoid diverticulum; other spinal cord and vertebral malformation.
- Neoplastic—primary bone tumors; multiple myeloma and metastatic tumors that infiltrate the vertebral body; meningioma; others.
- Infectious—discospondylitis; myelitis.
- Traumatic—intervertebral disc herniation; fracture or luxation; atlantoaxial subluxation-luxation.

Metabolic

- Anemia.
- Polycythemia.
- Electrolyte disturbances—especially hypokalemia, hypocalcemia, and hypoglycemia.

Miscellaneous

- Drugs—acepromazine; antihistamines; antiepileptic drugs; flea and tick products.
- Respiratory compromise.
- Cardiac compromise—reverse patent ductus arteriosus, aortic thromboembolism.

RISK FACTORS

- Intervertebral disc disease—dachshund, poodle, cocker spaniel, beagle, and others.
- Cervical spondylomyelopathy—Doberman pinscher and Great Dane.
- Fibrocartilaginous embolism—young, large-breed dogs and miniature schnauzers.
- Dens hypoplasia and atlantoaxial luxation—small-breed dogs, poodles.
- Chiari-like malformation—cavalier King Charles spaniel, small-breed dogs.

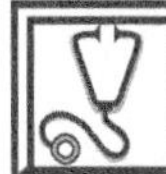

DIAGNOSIS

DIFFERENTIAL DIAGNOSIS

- Differentiate the types of ataxia.
- Differentiate from other disease processes that can affect gait—musculoskeletal, metabolic, cardiovascular, respiratory.
- Musculoskeletal disorders—typically produce lameness, pain, and a reluctance to move; degenerative joint disease signs often improve with increased movements.
- Systemic illness and endocrine, cardiovascular, and metabolic disorders—can cause intermittent ataxia, especially of the pelvic limbs; with fever, weight loss, murmurs, arrhythmias, hair loss, or collapse with exercise, suspect a non-neurologic cause; obtain minimum data from hemogram, biochemistry, and urinalysis.
- Head tilt or nystagmus—likely vestibular localization.
- Intention tremors of the head or hypermetria—likely cerebellar localization.
- All four limbs affected—lesion is in the cervical spinal cord, cerebellum, or is multifocal to diffuse.
- Only pelvic limbs affected—lesion is anywhere below the second thoracic vertebra.

CBC/BIOCHEMISTRY/URINALYSIS

Normal unless metabolic cause (e.g., hypoglycemia, electrolyte imbalance, anemia, polycythemia).

OTHER LABORATORY TESTS

- Hypoglycemia—determine serum insulin concentration on sample that has low glucose value; low glucose and higher than expected insulin value suggest insulin-secreting tumor.
- Anemia—differentiate as nonregenerative or regenerative on the basis of the reticulocyte count.
- Electrolyte imbalance—correct the problem; see if ataxia resolves.
- Antiepileptic drugs—if being administered, evaluate serum concentration for toxicity.

IMAGING

- Spinal radiography, myelography, CT, or MRI—if spinal cord dysfunction suspected.
- Bullae radiography—if peripheral vestibular disease suspected; CT or MRI superior; for inner ear disease, MRI superior to CT.
- Thoracic radiography—for older patients and patients suspected to have neoplasia or systemic fungal infection.
- CT or MRI—if cerebellar disease suspected; MRI superior to CT.
- Abdominal ultrasonography—if hepatic, renal, adrenal, or pancreatic dysfunction suspected.

DIAGNOSTIC PROCEDURES

- Cerebrospinal fluid analysis—helps confirm nervous system etiology.
- Cerebrospinal fluid culture, antibody titer, or polymerase chain reaction—helps confirm nervous system infectious etiology.

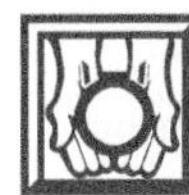

TREATMENT

- Usually outpatient, depending on severity and acuteness of clinical signs.
- Exercise—decrease or restrict if ataxia originates from spinal cord disease.
- Client should monitor gait for increasing dysfunction or weakness; if paresis worsens or paralysis develops, other testing is warranted.
- Avoid drugs that could contribute to the problem; may not be possible in patients on antiepileptic drugs for seizures.

MEDICATIONS

DRUG(S) OF CHOICE

Not recommended until the source or cause of the problem is identified.

FOLLOW-UP

PATIENT MONITORING

Periodic neurologic examinations to assess condition.

POSSIBLE COMPLICATIONS

- Spinal cord—progression to weakness and possibly paralysis.
- Hypoglycemia—seizures.
- Cerebellar disease—head tremors and bobbing.
- Brainstem disease—stupor, coma, death.

MISCELLANEOUS

SEE ALSO

- Cerebellar Degeneration.
- Head Tilt.
- Paralysis.

ABBREVIATIONS

- FIP = feline infectious peritonitis.

Suggested Reading

Cherubini GB, Lowrie M, Anderson J. Pelvic limb ataxia in the older dog. In Pract 2008, 30:386–391.

Davies C, Shell L. Neurological problems. In: Davies C, Lawrence T, Shell L, eds., Common Small Animal Medical Diagnoses: An Algorithmic Approach. Philadelphia, PA: Saunders, 2002, pp. 36–59.

Lowrie M. Vestibular disease: anatomy, physiology, and clinical signs. Compend Contin Educ Vet 2012, 34:E1–5.

Penderis J. The wobbly cat: diagnostic and therapeutic approach to generalised ataxia. J Fel Med Surg 2009, 11:349–359.

Rossmeisl JH Jr. Vestibular disease in dogs and cats. Vet Clin North Am Small Anim Pract 2010, 40:81–100.

Author Linda G. Shell

Client Education Handout available online

ATLANTOAXIAL INSTABILITY

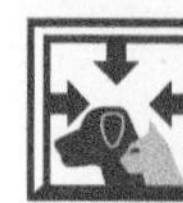

BASICS

OVERVIEW

- Results from malformation or disruption of the articulation between the first and second cervical vertebrae (atlas and axis, respectively); causes spinal cord compression.
- Can result in spinal cord trauma or compression at the junction between atlas and axis—may cause neck pain and/or varying degrees of general proprioceptive (GP) ataxia/upper motor neuron (UMN) tetraparesis, tetraplegia (with or without nociception), and death from respiratory arrest.

Etiology

- Congenital—anomaly of the dens (aplasia, hypoplasia, or malformation [dorsal angulation] of the dens) and its ligamentous attachments.
- Acquired—consequence of traumatic injury.

SIGNALMENT

- Congenital—toy-breed dogs (Yorkshire terrier, miniature or toy poodle, Chihuahua, Pekingese, and Pomeranian).
- Age at onset—usually before 12 months.
- Uncommon in larger-breed dogs, dogs >1 year old, and cats.
- No sex predilection.

SIGNS

- Intermittent or progressive ambulatory tetraparesis, usually with neck pain—most common.
- Neurologic signs vary from mild to moderate GP/UMN ambulatory tetraparesis to nonambulatory GP/UMN tetraparesis, or tetraplegia, depending on degree of spinal cord compression and secondary pathology (i.e., edema, hemorrhage, or gliosis).
- Animals may have only neck pain without concurrent neurologic deficits.
- Episodes of collapse secondary to weakness.
- Abnormal postural reactions with spinal reflexes that are normal to exaggerated, with normal to increased muscle tone in all four limbs.
- Acute death may occur when accompanied by trauma and respiratory arrest (uncommon).

CAUSES & RISK FACTORS

- Usually caused by abnormal development of the dens and/or ligamentous support structures, resulting in subluxation of the atlantoaxial joint.
- Fracture of the axis.
- Clinical signs often occur as a result of mild or insignificant trauma (e.g., jumping or playing).
- Clinical signs may be exacerbated by activity such as flexion of the neck.
- Toy-breed dogs—at risk for congenital malformation of the dens.

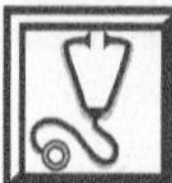

DIAGNOSIS

DIFFERENTIAL DIAGNOSIS

- Differential diagnoses are consistent with various causes of cervical myelopathies, including:
  - Other congenital malformation.
  - Trauma.
  - Meningitis or meningomyelitis, infectious or noninfectious (granulomatous meningoencephalomyelitis).
  - Fibrocartilaginous embolic myelopathy.
  - Disk herniation.
  - Neoplasia.

CBC/BIOCHEMISTRY/URINALYSIS

Normal

IMAGING

- Plain radiography of the cervical vertebral column:
  - Lateral view—caudal and dorsal displacement of the axis in relationship to the atlas, resulting in increased distance between vertebrae.
  - Ventral dorsal or oblique view—may reveal absence, hypoplasia, or malformation (dorsal angulation) of the dens.
- Cross-sectional imaging:
  - MRI.
  - Diagnosis based on observation of caudal and dorsal displacement of the axis in relationship to the atlas, as evidenced by the following features of the atlantoaxial articulation: (1) dorsal: displacement of the spinous process of the axis; (2) ventral: increased size of the occipito-atlas-axis joint cavity.
  - Allows identification of spinal cord compression.
  - Allows recognition of secondary spinal cord pathology such as edema, hemorrhage, or gliosis, which may impact prognosis.
- CT—may provide detailed visualization of bony structures, which allows for creation of three-dimensional reconstructed image to help surgical planning.
- Precautions:
  - Proper positioning will require sedation or general anesthesia.
  - Sedation or general anesthesia carries significant risk for iatrogenic trauma.
  - Care needs to be exercised when positioning animals.
  - *Avoid excessive flexion of the neck!*
  - Flexion may exacerbate compression, which may worsen clinical signs or cause death due to spinal cord trauma.
  - To protect against neck flexion during recovery, affected animals should be closely monitored until they are capable of maintaining normal head and neck carriage.

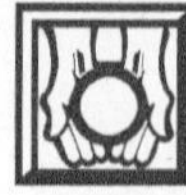

TREATMENT

- Prior to treatment, consultation with a board-certified neurologist or surgeon should be pursued.
- Improper treatment can lead to irreversible deterioration in neurologic function.

MEDICAL

- Neck brace (splint) to stabilize cervical vertebral column in extension.
  - Fiberglass cast material positioned ventrally from rostral aspect of mandible to xiphoid and incorporated into bandage material, which immobilizes head and neck.
  - Strict exercise restriction (cage confinement) for minimum of 8 weeks.
  - Frequent bandage/splint changes are needed.
- Adjunctive medication (see below).

Overall Prognosis

- Successful outcome observed in 62.5% of dogs.
- Improved prognosis associated with acute onset and short duration of clinical signs (<30 days).
- Surgery recommended to treat animals that fail to improve or experience recurrence of signs following medical treatment.

SURGERY

- Treatment of choice in majority of cases.
- Surgical approach; *ventral method is preferred.*
- Ventral approach—variety of methods:
  - Transarticular pinning or lag screw technique; ventral tips of pins incorporated in polymethylmethacrylate to prevent pin migration.
  - Transarticular pinning and ventral cortical screws or K-wires in bodies of atlas and axis ± K-wires applied longitudinally and wired to screws; screw heads and K-wires incorporated in polymethylmethacrylate to provide fixation.
- Dorsal approach—use wire or synthetic suture material to fix spinous process of axis to dorsal arch of atlas; provides less rigid fixation and may be associated with greater implant failure.
- Strict exercise restriction required for first month postoperatively, followed by gradual return to activity over additional month.
- Adjunctive medication (see below).
- Overall prognosis ranges from 63% to 91% success—improved prognosis associated with young (<24 months) dogs, duration of clinical signs <10 months, and mild neurologic deficits.

- Complications:
  - Failure to improve/worsening of neurologic deficits.
  - Implant failure/infection.
  - Respiratory—respiratory arrest, dyspnea, cough, and aspiration pneumonia.
  - Death.

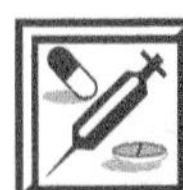

MEDICATIONS

DRUG(S) OF CHOICE

- Anti-inflammatory medication:
  - Corticosteroids—prednisone 0.5–1.0 mg/kg PO divided twice daily for 2 weeks, followed by tapering regime. Suggested protocol following initial dose: 0.5 mg/kg PO daily for 5 days, followed by 0.5 mg/kg PO every other day for 5 days.
  - Nonsteroidal anti-inflammatory drug (NSAID)—1- to 4-week course.
- Analgesia:
  - Tramadol 2.0–4.0 mg/kg PO q6–8h—questionable efficacy.
  - Gabapentin 10–20 mg/kg PO q6–8h.
  - Pregabalin 3–4 mg/kg (begin with 2 mg/kg) PO q8–12h.

CONTRAINDICATIONS/POSSIBLE INTERACTIONS

- Corticosteroid—use caution when given in conjunction with medical treatment; may reduce pain, resulting in increased activity and spinal cord trauma.
- Avoid NSAIDs in combination with corticosteroids in all patients—increases risk of life-threatening gastrointestinal hemorrhage.

FOLLOW-UP

- Dogs treated medically require frequent (weekly) bandage changes for associated soft tissue trauma.
- All dogs should be reevaluated at 1 and 3 months (postoperatively or after neck brace removal) and then monthly until neurologic deficits resolve or remain static over 2–3 months.
- More frequent rechecks may be needed for dogs experiencing complications or recurrence of signs.
- Untreated animals may experience deterioration in neurologic function, catastrophic acute spinal cord trauma, respiratory arrest, and death.

MISCELLANEOUS

- Rehabilitation may play a significant role in ultimate neurologic functional level of patient.
- Rehabilitation should only be considered in dogs >30 days postoperatively or after neck brace (splint) removal.

ABBREVIATIONS

- GP = general proprioceptive.
- NSAID = nonsteroidal anti-inflammatory drug.
- UMN = upper motor neuron.

INTERNET RESOURCES

www.acvs.org/small-animal/atlantoaxial-instability

Suggested Reading

Beaver DP, Ellison GW, Lewis DD. Risk factors affecting the outcome of surgery for atlantoaxial subluxation in dogs: 46 cases (1978–1998). J Am Vet Med Assoc 2000, 216(7):1104–1109.

Havig ME, Cornell KK, Hawthorne JC, et al. Evaluation of nonsurgical treatment of atlantoaxial subluxation in dogs: 19 cases (1992–2001). J Am Vet Med Assoc 2005, 227(2):257–262.

McCarthy RJ, Lewis DD, Hosgood G. Atlantoaxial subluxation in dogs. Compend Contin Educ Pract Vet 1995, 17:215–226.

Platt SR, Casimiro da Costa R. Cervical vertebral column. In: Johnston SA, Tobias KM, eds., Textbook of Small Animal Surgery, 2nd ed. St. Louis, MO: Elsevier, 2018, pp. 438–485.

Platt SR, Chambers JN, Cross A. A modified ventral fixation for surgical management of atlantoaxial subluxation in 19 dogs. Vet Surg 2004, 33(4):349–354.

Sanders SG, Bagley RS, Silver GM, et al. Outcomes and complications associated with ventral screws, pins, and polymethyl methacrylate for atlantoaxial instability in 12 dogs. J Am Anim Hosp Assoc 2004, 40:204–210.

Schulz KS, Waldron DR, Fahie M. Application of ventral pins and polymethylmethacrylate for the management of atlantoaxial instability: results in nine dogs. Vet Surg 1997, 26(4):317–325.

Author Mathieu M. Glassman

Consulting Editor Mathieu M. Glassman

ATOPIC DERMATITIS

BASICS

DEFINITION

• Genetically predisposed skin disease characterized by inflammation and pruritus. Clinical signs associated with immunoglobulin (Ig) E and most commonly directed against environmental allergens. • Differentiate from atopic-like dermatitis, in which clinical signs identical to atopic dermatitis but IgE response to environmental or other allergens cannot be demonstrated.

PATHOPHYSIOLOGY

• Allergen exposure in susceptible animals results in IgE production. Upon reexposure to allergen, mast cell degranulation and activation of T_H2 lymphocytes allow release of inflammatory cytokines, chemokines, histamine, proteolytic enzymes, and other chemical mediators. • Genetic defects—dogs: gene expression upregulated or downregulated; cats: not well documented. • Barrier function defects—dogs: impaired epidermal lipid barrier can lead to enhanced allergen penetration and increased transepidermal water loss (TEWL); filaggrin defect thought to be associated; cats: may not be as relevant as with dogs. • Immunologic defects—dogs: acute lesions characterized by increased T_H2 lymphocyte activity, while T_H1 cytokines predominate in chronic lesions; T_H2:T_H1 imbalance proposed; aberrant regulatory T-cell function reported; cats: T_H2-mediated dysfunction suspected, but cytokine pathways need further investigation. • Bacterial superantigens, auto-antigens released via keratinocyte damage, and *Malassezia* may play role in inflammation.

SYSTEMS AFFECTED

• Ophthalmic. • Respiratory. • Skin/exocrine.

GENETICS

• Dogs—inherited predisposition. • Cats—inherited predisposition less clear.

INCIDENCE/PREVALENCE

• Canine—3–27% of canine population estimated. • Feline—lower than for dogs.

GEOGRAPHIC DISTRIBUTION

Canine—worldwide; local factors influence seasonality, severity, and duration of signs.

SIGNALMENT

Species

Dogs and cats.

Breed Predilections

• United States—Boston terrier, boxer, Cairn terrier, Chinese Shar-Pei, cocker spaniel, Dalmatian, English bulldog, English and Irish setter, American Staffordshire terrier, Lhasa apso, miniature schnauzer, pug, Sealyham terrier, Scottish terrier, West Highland white terrier, wirehaired fox terrier, Labrador retriever. • Feline—Abyssinian, Devon Rex, domestic shorthaired cats.

Mean Age and Range

• Canine—6 months to 3 years. • Feline—6 months to 2 years, commonly under 3 years.

Predominant Sex

None reported.

SIGNS

General Comments

Cutaneous changes caused by self-induced trauma; primary lesions usually unrecognized.

Historical Findings

• Pruritus. • Early age of onset. •History in related individuals. • May be initially seasonal. • Recurring skin or ear infection.
• Temporary response to glucocorticosteroids.
• Signs worsen with time.

Physical Examination Findings

• Most common (dogs)—interdigital spaces, carpal/tarsal areas, muzzle, periocular, axillae, abdomen, pinnae; >40% can be generalized. • Most common (cats)—head and neck, mouth, abdomen, lateral thorax, hind limbs. • Lesions (dogs)—none to salivary staining, alopecia, erythema, papules, crusts, hyperpigmentation, lichenification, seborrhea sicca/oleosa, and/or hyperhidrosis.
• Lesions (cats)—miliary dermatitis (small crusted papules), alopecia, eosinophilic granuloma complex (indolent ulcers, eosinophilic granulomas, eosinophilic plaques). • Chronic relapsing bacterial and yeast skin/ear infections (common).
• Respiratory symptoms, conjunctivitis, and blepharitis possible.

CAUSES

• Pollens. • Mold spores. • *Malassezia.*
• House dust and storage mites. • Animal/human dander. • Insects.

RISK FACTORS

• Environments with long allergy seasons and high pollen and mold spore levels. • Concurrent hypersensitivities (summation effect). • Born during allergy season. • Breed predisposition.

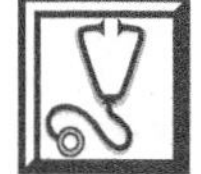

DIAGNOSIS

DIFFERENTIAL DIAGNOSIS

• Adverse food reaction. • Flea bite hypersensitivity. • Sarcoptic mange. • Bacterial folliculitis. • Yeast dermatitis. • Contact dermatitis (allergic or irritant).

CBC/BIOCHEMISTRY/URINALYSIS

Eosinophilia—rare in dogs without concurrent flea infestations; common in cats.

DIAGNOSTIC PROCEDURES

• Diagnosis made by history, physical examination, and ruling out differential diagnoses.
• Serology/intradermal test (IDT) *not* meant for diagnosis. • Greatest treatment success noted when immunotherapy based on results of both serum and intradermal testing.

Serologic Allergy Tests

• Measures allergen-specific IgE in serum.
• Advantages—readily available; clipping/sedation not required; concurrent/recent medications and infections less likely to affect results; similar hyposensitization success to IDT. • Disadvantages—fewer allergens tested; quality control/reliability varies with laboratory.

IDT

• Test allergens injected intradermally causing wheal formation. • Advantages—tests affected organ, results available immediately, many allergens tested; preferred where available. • Disadvantages—requires experience to interpret results, clipping and sedation needed, difficult to interpret in cats; drug withdrawal periods recommended, concurrent infection may affect results.

PATHOLOGIC FINDINGS

Skin biopsy—rule out other differential diagnoses; results not pathognomonic; superficial perivascular dermatitis with lymphocytic exocytosis ± eosinophils, mast cells; often with secondary bacterial folliculitis.

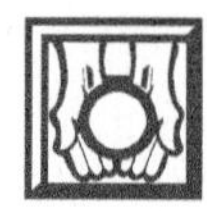

TREATMENT

APPROPRIATE HEALTH CARE

Outpatient

ACTIVITY

Avoid offending allergens when possible.

DIET

Diets rich in essential fatty acids may be beneficial.

CLIENT EDUCATION

Explain inheritable, progressive, and incurable nature of condition.

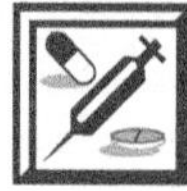

MEDICATIONS

DRUG(S) OF CHOICE

Immunotherapy (Hyposensitization)

• Subcutaneous or sublingual administration of causative allergens. • Allergen selection based on allergy test results, patient history, and knowledge of local exposure.
• Immunotherapy protocols not standardized and vary widely between clinicians.
• Preferred treatment in most cases.
• Successfully reduces pruritus in 50–90% of dogs and cats. • 3 months to 1 year for full effect. • May continue lifelong if effective.

Cyclosporine (Atopica® Preferred)

• Cyclosporine, modified (dogs, 5 mg/kg/day; cats, 7 mg/kg/day). • 1–4 weeks for effect—frequency of dosing may be reduced to maintain control of symptoms.
• Monitoring recommended. • Cats—drug blood level monitoring recommended; keep indoors, do *not* feed raw meat.

Corticosteroids

• For short-term relief or taper to lowest dosage/frequency. • Dogs—e.g., prednisolone (1 mg/kg PO q24h). • Cats—e.g., prednisolone (2 mg/kg q24h).

Antihistamines

• Less effective than corticosteroids. • 2 weeks for effect. • Dogs—cetirizine (1 mg/kg PO q12–24h), chlorpheniramine (0.4 mg/kg PO q8–12h), diphenhydramine (2.2 mg/kg PO q8–12h), amitriptyline (1–2 mg/kg q12h).
• Cats—cetirizine (5 mg/cat q24h), chlorpheniramine (2 mg/cat PO q12h), amitriptyline (5–10 mg/cat q24h); diphenhydramine may cause paradoxical excitation in cats.

Oclacitinib (Apoquel®)

• Dogs—onset time/response similar to glucocorticoids (0.4–0.6 mg/kg q12h for 14 days, then q24h for maintenance). • Cats—not licensed; limited short-term studies report effectiveness, but higher doses may be needed.

Lokivetmab (Cytopoint®)

Dogs only—anti-IL-31 monoclonal antibody injectable; repeated as needed up to frequency of every 4–6 weeks.

PRECAUTIONS

• Immunotherapy—anaphylaxis rare (accompanied by diarrhea, weakness, collapse), hives, facial swelling; monitor for 1 hour post injection; increased pruritus after injection may indicate change in schedule needed; pain or swelling at injection site uncommon. • Cyclosporine—may affect glucose homeostasis; increased incidence of urinary tract infection; vomiting and diarrhea most common side effects; gingival hyperplasia, papillomavirus, and hirsutism possible; risk of fatal toxoplasmosis in naïve cats. • Corticosteroids—avoid iatrogenic hyperglucocorticism/hyperadrenocorticism; possible aggravation of pyoderma and induction of demodicosis.
• Antihistamines—can produce drowsiness, rarely anorexia, vomiting, diarrhea, increased pruritus; use with caution in patients with cardiac arrhythmias. • Oclacitinib—not for use in dogs under 1 year of age; may cause existing parasitic skin infestations and/or prevent resolution of infections.

POSSIBLE INTERACTIONS

Concurrent use of cyclosporine and ketoconazole permits 50% dose reduction of each drug.

ALTERNATIVE DRUG(S)

• Frequent bathing (once to twice weekly) in cool water with antipruritic, antibacterial, antifungal, and/or moisturizing shampoos can be beneficial. • Fatty acids—diets rich in essential fatty acids typically provided higher amounts than with oral supplements.
• Pentoxifylline 25 mg/kg q12h. • Topical hydrocortisone or triamcinolone spray 0.015% (short-term use).

FOLLOW-UP

PATIENT MONITORING

• Examination every 2–8 weeks initially; once acceptable level of control achieved, examine every 3–6 months. • Monitor pruritus, self-trauma, development of secondary infection, possible adverse drug reactions. • CBC/blood chemistry/urinalysis with culture—recommended every 3–12 months for patients on chronic corticosteroid, cyclosporine, or oclacitinib therapy.

PREVENTION/AVOIDANCE

• Avoidance of allergens seldom possible.
• Minimize other sources of pruritus.

POSSIBLE COMPLICATIONS

• Secondary bacterial folliculitis or *Malassezia* dermatitis. • Concurrent hypersensitivities.

EXPECTED COURSE AND PROGNOSIS

• Pruritus and duration of signs usually worsen over time without intervention.
• Some cases spontaneously resolve.

MISCELLANEOUS

ASSOCIATED CONDITIONS

• Hypersensitivity (flea, food). • Bacterial folliculitis. • *Malassezia* dermatitis. • Otitis externa.

AGE-RELATED FACTORS

Severity worsens with age.

PREGNANCY/FERTILITY/BREEDING

• Corticosteroids—contraindicated during pregnancy. • Affected animals should not be used for breeding.

SYNONYMS

• Atopy. • Canine atopic disease.

SEE ALSO

• Eosinophilic Granuloma Complex.
• Flea Bite Hypersensitivity and Flea Control.
• Food Reactions, Dermatologic.
• Otitis Externa and Media.
• Pyoderma.

ABBREVIATIONS

• IDT = intradermal test.
• Ig = immunoglobulin.
• TEWL = transepidermal water loss.

Suggested Reading

Botoni LS, Torres SMF, Koch SN, et al. Comparison of demographic data, disease severity, and response to treatment, between dogs with atopic dermatitis and atopic-like dermatitis: a retrospective study. Vet Derm 2019, 30:10–e4.

Gedon NK, Mueller RS. Atopic dermatitis in cats and dogs: a difficult disease for animals and owners. Clin Transl Allergy 2018, 8:41.

Lappin MR, VanLare KA, Seewald W, et al. Effect of oral administration of cyclosporine on Toxoplasma gondii infection status of cats. Am J Vet Res 2015, 76(4):351–357.

Miller WH, Griffin CE, Campbell KL. Muller & Kirk's Small Animal Dermatology, 7th ed. St. Louis, MO: Elsevier Mosby, 2013.

Noli C, Matricoti I, Schievano C. A double blinded, randomized, methylprednisolone-controlled study on the efficacy of oclacitinib in the management of pruritus in cats with nonflea nonfood induced hypersensitivity dermatitis. Vet Derm 2019, 30(2):110–e30.

Author Heather D. Edginton
Consulting Editor Alexander H. Werner Resnick

Acknowledgment The author acknowledges the prior contribution of Alexander H. Werner Resnick.

Client Education Handout available online

ATRIAL FIBRILLATION AND ATRIAL FLUTTER

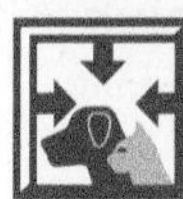

BASICS

DEFINITION

• Atrial fibrillation—rapid, irregularly irregular supraventricular rhythm. Two forms recognized: primary atrial fibrillation, an uncommon disease that occurs mostly in large dogs with no underlying cardiac disease; and secondary atrial fibrillation, which occurs in dogs and cats secondary to underlying cardiac disease. • Atrial flutter is similar to atrial fibrillation, but the atrial rate is generally slower and is characterized by saw-toothed flutter waves in the baseline of the ECG. The ventricular response is generally rapid, but may be regular or irregular.

ECG Features

Atrial Flutter

• Atrial rhythm usually regular; rate approximately 300–400 bpm. • P waves usually discerned as either discrete P waves or "saw-toothed" baseline. • Ventricular rhythm and rate generally depend on atrial rate and atrioventricular (AV) nodal conduction, but are generally regular or regularly irregular and rapid. • Conduction pattern to ventricles is variable—in some cases every other atrial depolarization produces a ventricular depolarization (2 : 1 conduction ratio), giving a regular ventricular rhythm (Figure 1); other times the conduction pattern appears random, giving an irregular ventricular rhythm that can mimic atrial fibrillation.

Secondary Atrial Fibrillation

• No P waves present—baseline may be flat or may have small irregular undulations ("f" waves); some undulations may look like P waves. • Ventricular rate often elevated—usually 180–240 bpm in dogs and >220 bpm in cats. • Interval between QRS complexes is irregularly irregular; QRS complexes usually appear normal (Figure 2).

Primary Atrial Fibrillation

Similar to secondary atrial fibrillation, except ventricular rate usually in normal range.

PATHOPHYSIOLOGY

• Atrial fibrillation—caused by numerous small reentrant pathways creating a rapid (>500 depolarizations/minute) and disorganized depolarization pattern in the atria that results in cessation of atrial contraction. Depolarizations continuously bombard the AV nodal tissue, which acts as a filter and does not allow all depolarizations to conduct to the ventricles. Many atrial depolarizations activate only a part of the atria, because the rapid rate renders portions of the atria refractory, and thus they cannot reach the AV junction. Other atrial impulses penetrate into the AV junctional tissue, but do not penetrate the entire length. Blocked impulses affect the conduction properties of the AV junctional tissue and alter conduction of subsequent electrical impulses; electrical impulses are conducted through the AV junction irregularly, producing an irregular ventricular rhythm. • Atrial flutter—probably originates from one site of reentry that moves continuously throughout the atrial myocardium and frequently and regularly stimulates the AV node. When the atrial rate becomes sufficiently fast, the refractory period of the AV node exceeds the cycle length (P to P interval) of the supraventricular tachycardia (SVT), and some atrial depolarizations are blocked from traversing the AV node (functional second-degree AV block).

SYSTEMS AFFECTED

Cardiovascular

Loss of atrial contraction may result in decreased stroke volume and cardiac output, depending on heart rate; high heart rate may result in deterioration in myocardial function (tachycardia-induced myocardial failure).

GENETICS

No breeding studies available.

SIGNALMENT

Species

Dog and cat.

Breed Predilections

Large- and giant-breed dogs more prone to primary atrial fibrillation.

Mean Age and Range

N/A

Predominant Sex

N/A

SIGNS

General Comments

• Generally relate to underlying disease process and/or congestive heart failure (CHF) rather than arrhythmia itself, but previously stable animals may decompensate. • Patients with primary atrial fibrillation are generally asymptomatic, but may demonstrate mild exercise intolerance.

Historical Findings

• Coughing/dyspnea/tachypnea. • Exercise intolerance. • Rarely, syncope. • Dogs with primary atrial fibrillation are typically asymptomatic.

Physical Examination Findings

• On auscultation, patients with atrial fibrillation have an erratic heart rhythm that sounds like "tennis shoes in a dryer." • First heart sound intensity in atrial fibrillation is variable; second heart sound only heard on beats with effective ejection, not on every beat. • Third heart sounds (gallop sounds) may be present. • Patients with atrial fibrillation have pulse deficits and variable pulse quality. • Signs of CHF often present (e.g., cough, dyspnea, cyanosis).

CAUSES

• Myxomatous valve disease. • Cardiomyopathy. • Congenital heart disease. • Digoxin toxicity. • Idiopathic. • Ventricular preexcitation (atrial flutter).

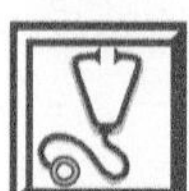

DIAGNOSIS

DIFFERENTIAL DIAGNOSIS

• Frequent atrial (supraventricular) premature depolarizations. • Supraventricular tachycardia with AV block. • Multifocal atrial tachycardia (irregular).

CBC/BIOCHEMISTRY/URINALYSIS

N/A

OTHER LABORATORY TESTS

N/A

IMAGING

• Echocardiography and radiography may characterize type and severity of underlying cardiac disease; moderate to severe heart enlargement common. • Typically normal in patients with primary atrial fibrillation, although mild left atrial enlargement may accompany hemodynamic alterations imposed by arrhythmia.

DIAGNOSTIC PROCEDURES

A baseline 24-hour Holter is recommended to determine if arrhythmia is chronic or paroxysmal. If it is chronic, drug therapy may be indicated.

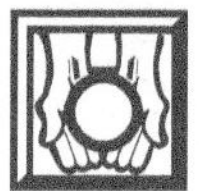

TREATMENT

APPROPRIATE HEALTH CARE

• Patients with fast (secondary) atrial fibrillation are treated medically to slow the ventricular rate. Converting the atrial fibrillation to sinus rhythm would be ideal, but such attempts in patients with severe underlying heart disease or left atrial enlargement are generally futile because of a low success rate and high rate of recurrence. Consider electrical cardioversion to sinus rhythm for a dog with primary atrial fibrillation and minimal structural heart disease. • Patients with primary atrial fibrillation may be converted back to normal sinus rhythm. The success rate depends on chronicity. Patients that have been in atrial fibrillation for >4 months generally have a lower success rate and a higher rate of recurrence. In these patients, rate control, if necessary, is the recommended treatment. • Electrical (DC) cardioversion—application of a transthoracic electrical shock at a specific time in the cardiac cycle; requires special equipment, trained personnel, and general anesthesia. Using a monophasic defibrillator: start with 4 J/kg; if no conversion occurs,

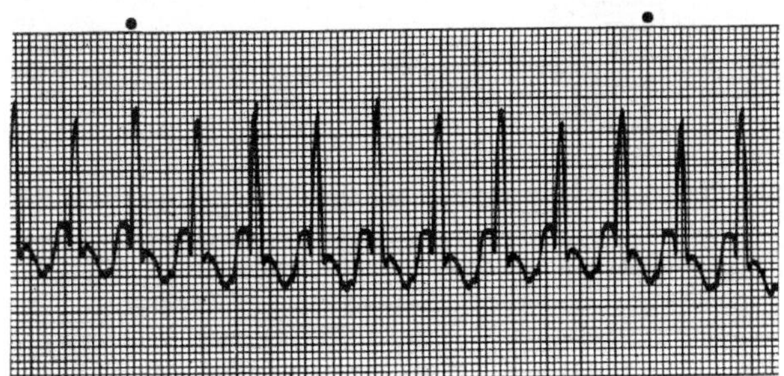

Figure 1.

Atrial flutter with 2 : 1 conduction at a ventricular rate of 330/minute in a dog with an atrial septal defect. This supraventricular tachycardia was associated with a Wolff-Parkinson-White pattern. (Source: From Tilley LP. Essentials of Canine and Feline Electrocardiography, 3rd ed. Baltimore, MD: Williams & Wilkins, 1992. Reprinted with permission of Wolters Kluwer.)

increase dose by 50 J and repeat until a max of 360 J. Using a biphasic defibrillator: start with 1–2 J/kg; if no cardioversion occurs, increase dose by 50 J and repeat until max of 360 J.
• For atrial flutter, conversion to sinus rhythm can be accomplished by drug therapy, electrical cardioversion, or rapid atrial pacing (transvenous pacing electrode).

NURSING CARE

As indicated for CHF.

ACTIVITY

Restrict activity until tachycardia is controlled.

DIET

Mild to moderate sodium restriction if CHF.

CLIENT EDUCATION

• Secondary atrial fibrillation and atrial flutter are usually associated with severe underlying heart disease; goal of therapy is to lower heart rate and control clinical signs. • Sustained conversion to sinus rhythm is unlikely with secondary atrial fibrillation.

SURGICAL CONSIDERATIONS

N/A

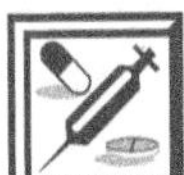

MEDICATIONS

DRUG(S) OF CHOICE

• Digoxin, β-adrenergic blockers, esmolol, and calcium channel blockers (diltiazem) are frequently used to slow conduction through the AV node; definition of an adequate heart rate response varies among clinicians, but in dogs is generally 130–150 bpm. • For atrial flutter, therapy is aimed at suppressing the atrial reentry circuit using sotalol, amiodarone, or procainamide.

Dogs

• Digoxin—maintenance oral dose 0.005–0.01 mg/kg PO q12h; to achieve therapeutic serum concentration more rapidly, maintenance dose can be doubled for the first day. If digoxin is administered alone and heart rate remains high, check digoxin level and adjust dose to bring level into therapeutic range. If heart rate remains high, consider adding calcium channel blocker or β-adrenergic blocker.
• Diltiazem—initially administered at dose of 0.5 mg/kg PO q8h, then titrated up to maximum of 1.5 mg/kg PO q8h or until adequate response is obtained. • Therapy for atrial flutter is aimed at suppressing atrial reentry circuit using sotalol, amiodarone, or procainamide. Conversion to normal sinus rhythm is usually unsuccessful.

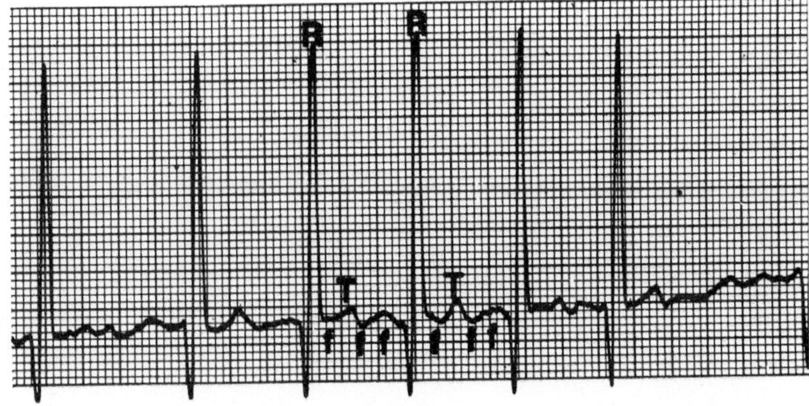

Figure 2.

"Coarse" atrial fibrillation in a dog with patent ductus arteriosus. The f waves are prominent. (Source: From Tilley LP. Essentials of Canine and Feline Electrocardiography, 3rd ed. Baltimore, MD: Williams & Wilkins, 1992. Reprinted with permission of Wolters Kluwer.)

ATRIAL FIBRILLATION AND ATRIAL FLUTTER (CONTINUED)

Cats

• Diltiazem (1–2.5 mg/kg PO q8h) or atenolol (6.25–12.5 mg/cat PO q12–24h) are drugs of choice in most cats. • If the heart rate is not sufficiently slowed with these drugs or myocardial failure is present, digoxin (5 µg/kg PO q24–48h) can be added.

CONTRAINDICATIONS

• Digoxin, diltiazem, propranolol, and atenolol should not be used in patients with preexisting AV block. • Use of calcium channel blockers in combination with beta blockers should be avoided because clinically significant bradyarrhythmias and/or AV block can develop.

PRECAUTIONS

• Calcium channel blockers and β-adrenergic blockers, both negative inotropes, should be used cautiously in animals with myocardial failure. • Using high-dose oral quinidine for conversion to sinus rhythm carries a risk of quinidine toxicity (e.g., hypotension, weakness, ataxia, and seizures)—administration of diazepam intravenously controls seizures; other signs abate within several hours of discontinuing quinidine administration.

POSSIBLE INTERACTIONS

Quinidine raises the digoxin level, generally necessitating a digoxin dose reduction.

FOLLOW-UP

PATIENT MONITORING

• Monitor heart rate and ECG closely. • As heart rates in the hospital and those measured on the surface ECG may be inaccurate (due to patient anxiety and other environmental factors), Holter monitoring provides a more accurate means for assessing the need for heart rate control and/or the efficacy of medical therapy for heart rate control.

POSSIBLE COMPLICATIONS

Worsening of cardiac function with onset of arrhythmia.

EXPECTED COURSE AND PROGNOSIS

• Secondary atrial fibrillation—often associated with severe structural heart disease, so a guarded to poor prognosis. • Primary atrial fibrillation with normal ultrasound findings—generally a good prognosis.

MISCELLANEOUS

ABBREVIATIONS

• AV = atrioventricular.
• CHF = congestive heart failure.
• SVT = supraventricular tachycardia.

Suggested Reading

Bright JM, Brunnen J. Chronicity of atrial fibrillation affects duration of sinus rhythm after transthoracic cardioversion of dogs with naturally occurring atrial fibrillation. J Vet Intern Med 2008, 22(1):114–119.

Gelzer RM, Kraus MS. Management of atrial fibrillation. Vet Clin North Am Small Anim Pract 2004, 34:1127–1144.

Gelzer ARM, Kraus MS, Moise NS, et al. Assessment of antiarrhythmic drug efficacy to control heart rate in dogs with atrial fibrillation using 24-hour ambulatory electrocardiographic (Holter) recordings. J Vet Intern Med 2004, 18(5):779.

Tilley LP, Smith FWK, Jr. Electrocardiography. In: Smith FWK, Tilley LP, Oyama M, Sleeper M., eds., Manual of Canine and Feline Cardiology, 5th ed. St. Louis, MO: Saunders Elsevier, 2016, pp. 49–76.

Santilli R, Moise NS, Pariaut R, Perego M. Electrocardiography of the Dog and Cat: Diagnosis of Arrhythmias, 2nd ed. Milan: Edra, 2018.

Tilley LP, Smith, F.W. Essentials of Electrocardiography: Interpretation and Treatment, 4th ed. Ames, IA: Wiley-Blackwell, 2016.

Willis R, Oliveira P, Mavropoulou A. Guide to Canine and Feline Electrocardiography. Ames, IA: Wiley-Blackwell, 2018.

Author Larry P. Tilley

Consulting Editor Michael Aherne

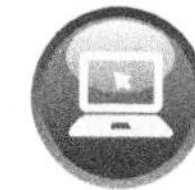

Client Education Handout available online

ATRIAL PREMATURE COMPLEXES

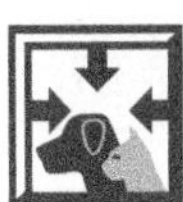

BASICS

DEFINITION

Premature atrial complexes or beats (APC) that originate outside the sinoatrial node and disrupt the normal sinus rhythm for 1 or more beats.

ECG Features

• Heart rate usually normal; rhythm irregular due to the premature P wave (called a P′ wave) that disrupts the normal P wave rhythm (Figure 1). • Ectopic P′ wave—premature; configuration differs from that of the sinus P waves and may be negative, positive, biphasic, or superimposed on the previous T wave. • QRS complex—premature; configuration usually normal (same as that of the sinus complexes). If the P′ wave occurs during the refractory period of the atrioventricular (AV) node, ventricular conduction does not occur (nonconducted APCs), so no QRS complex follows the P′ wave. If there is partial recovery in the AV node or intraventricular conduction systems, the P′ wave is conducted with a long P′–R interval or with an abnormal QRS configuration (aberrant conduction). The more premature the complex, the more marked the aberration. • In the P–QRS relationship, the P′–R interval is usually as long as, or longer than, the sinus P′–R interval. • A noncompensatory pause—when the R–R interval of the two normal sinus complexes enclosing an APC is less than the R–R intervals of three consecutive sinus complexes—usually follows an APC (Figure 2). The ectopic atrial impulse discharges the sinus node and resets the cycle.

PATHOPHYSIOLOGY

• Mechanisms—an increase in automaticity of atrial myocardial fibers or a single reentrant circuit. • May be normal finding in aged dogs; commonly seen in dogs with atrial enlargement secondary to chronic mitral valvular insufficiency; may also be observed in dogs or cats with any atrial disease. • May not cause hemodynamic problems; the clinical significance relates to their frequency, timing relative to other complexes, and the underlying clinical problems. • Can presage more serious rhythm disturbances (e.g., atrial fibrillation, atrial flutter, or atrial tachycardia).

SYSTEMS AFFECTED

Cardiovascular

GENETICS

N/A

INCIDENCE/PREVALENCE

Not documented.

SIGNALMENT

Species

Dog and cat.

Breed Predilections

Small-breed dogs.

Mean Age and Range

Geriatric animals, except those with congenital heart disease.

SIGNS

Historical Findings

• No signs. • Congestive heart failure (CHF). • Coughing and dyspnea. • Exercise intolerance. • Syncope.

Physical Examination Findings

• Myxomatous valve disease. • Cardiac murmur. • Gallop sound. • Signs of CHF.

CAUSES & RISK FACTORS

• Chronic valvular disease. • Congenital heart disease. • Cardiomyopathy. • Atrial myocarditis. • Electrolyte disorders. • Neoplasia. • Hyperthyroidism. • Toxemias. • Drug toxicity (e.g., digitalis). • Normal variation in aged animals.

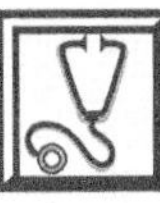

DIAGNOSIS

DIFFERENTIAL DIAGNOSIS

• Marked sinus arrhythmia. • Ventricular premature complexes when aberrant ventricular conduction follows an APC.

CBC/BIOCHEMISTRY/URINALYSIS

N/A

OTHER LABORATORY TESTS

N/A

IMAGING

Echocardiography and Doppler ultrasound may reveal the type and severity of the underlying heart disease.

DIAGNOSTIC PROCEDURES

• ECG. • Holter monitor to quantify APC frequency and event monitor/Holter ECG to correlate symptoms with rhythm.

PATHOLOGIC FINDINGS

Atrial enlargement; other features vary depending on underlying cause.

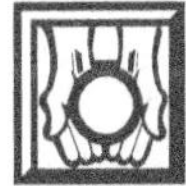

TREATMENT

APPROPRIATE HEALTH CARE

• Treat animal as inpatient or outpatient. • Treat the underlying CHF, cardiac disease, or other causes.

NURSING CARE

Usually not necessary; varies with underlying cause.

ACTIVITY

Restrict if symptomatic.

DIET

No modifications unless required for management of underlying condition (i.e., low-salt diet).

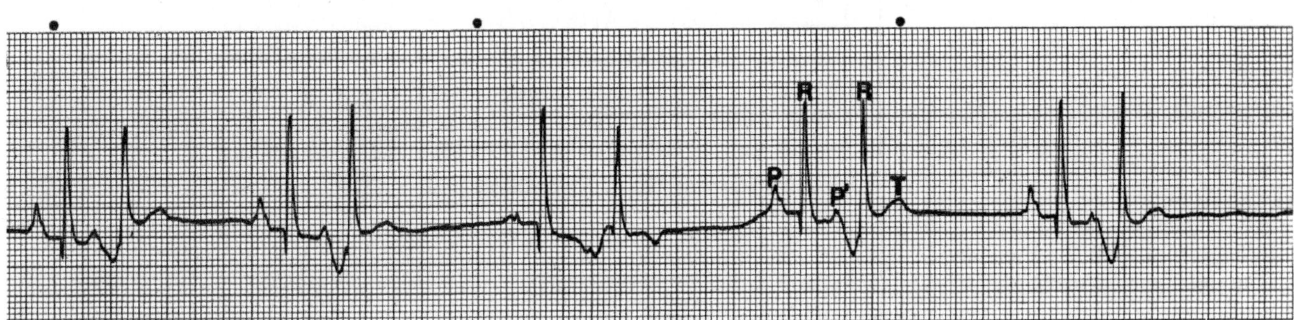

Figure 1.

APCs in a dog. P′ represents the premature P wave. The premature QRS resembles the normal (sinus) QRS. The upright P′ wave is superimposed on the T wave of the preceding complex. (Source: From Tilley LP. Essentials of Canine and Feline Electrocardiography, 3rd ed. Blackwell Publishing, 1992. Reprinted with permission of Wolters Kluwer.)

ATRIAL PREMATURE COMPLEXES (CONTINUED)

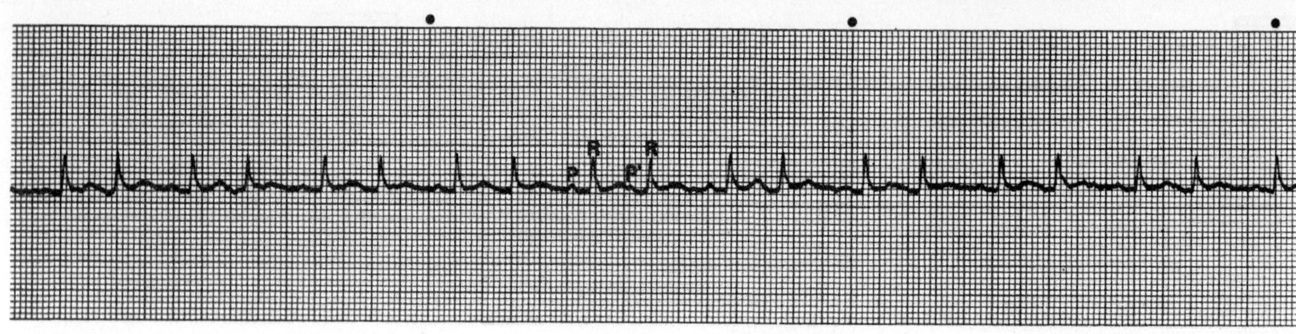

Figure 2.

APCs in bigeminy in a cat under general anesthesia. The second complex of each pair is an APC and the first is a sinus complex. The abnormality in rhythm disappeared after the anesthetic was stopped. (Source: From Tilley LP. Essentials of Canine and Feline Electrocardiography, 3rd ed. Baltimore: Williams & Wilkins, 1992. Reprinted with permission of Wolters Kluwer.)

CLIENT EDUCATION

APCs may not cause hemodynamic abnormalities; may be precursors of serious arrhythmias.

SURGICAL CONSIDERATIONS

N/A

MEDICATIONS

DRUG(S) OF CHOICE

Treat CHF and correct any electrolyte or acid/base imbalances.

Dogs

• Digoxin (0.005–0.01 mg/kg PO q12h, maintenance dosage), diltiazem (0.5–1.5 mg/kg PO q8h), or atenolol (0.25–1 mg/kg PO q12h) are used to treat clinically significant arrhythmias. • Digoxin—treatment of choice. • CHF is treated with appropriate dosage of diuretic, angiotensin-converting enzyme inhibitor, and pimobendan; appropriate management of CHF may reduce APC frequency.

Cats

• Cats with hypertrophic cardiomyopathy—diltiazem (1–2.5 mg/kg PO q8h) or atenolol (6.25–12.5 mg PO q12–24h). • Cats with dilated cardiomyopathy—digoxin (one-fourth of a 0.125 mg digoxin tablet q24h or q48h).

CONTRAINDICATIONS

Negative inotropic agents (e.g., propranolol) should be avoided in animals with CHF.

PRECAUTIONS

Use digoxin, diltiazem, atenolol, or propranolol cautiously in animals with underlying atrioventricular block or hypotension.

POSSIBLE INTERACTIONS

N/A

ALTERNATIVE DRUG(S)

N/A

FOLLOW-UP

PATIENT MONITORING

Monitor heart rate and rhythm with serial ECG.

PREVENTION/AVOIDANCE

N/A

POSSIBLE COMPLICATIONS

Frequent APCs may further diminish cardiac output in patients with underlying heart disease and worsen clinical symptoms.

EXPECTED COURSE AND PROGNOSIS

Even with optimal antiarrhythmic drug therapy, some animals have an increased frequency of APCs or deteriorate to more severe arrhythmia as the underlying disease progresses.

MISCELLANEOUS

ASSOCIATED CONDITIONS

None

AGE-RELATED FACTORS

Typically occurs in geriatric dogs.

PREGNANCY/FERTILITY/BREEDING

N/A

SYNONYMS

• Atrial extrasystoles. • Atrial premature contractions. • Atrial premature impulses. • Premature atrial complexes/contractions.

SEE ALSO

Supraventricular Tachycardia.

ABBREVIATIONS

• APC = atrial premature complex.
• AV = atrioventricular.
• CHF = congestive heart failure.

Suggested Reading

Jackson BL, Lehmkuhl LB, Adin DB. Heart rate and arrhythmia frequency of normal cats compared to cats with asymptomatic hypertrophic cardiomyopathy. J Vet Cardiol 2014, 16:215–225.

Santilli R, Moise NS, Pariaut R, Perego M. Electrocardiography of the Dog and Cat: Diagnosis of Arrhythmias, 2nd ed. Milan: Edra, 2018.

Tilley LP, Smith FWK Jr. Electrocardiography. In: Smith FWK, Tilley LP, Oyama M, Sleeper M, eds., Manual of Canine and Feline Cardiology, 5th ed. St. Louis, MO: Saunders Elsevier, 2016, pp. 49–76.

Willis R, Oliveira P, Mavropoulou A. Guide to Canine and Feline Electrocardiography. Ames, IA: Wiley-Blackwell, 2018.

Author Larry P. Tilley
Consulting Editor Michael Aherne

Client Education Handout available online

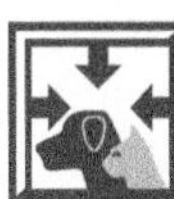

BASICS

OVERVIEW

• Congenital defect in which interatrial septum fails to develop normally, resulting in communication between atria. Unknown cause; genetic basis suspected. Acquired atrial septal defects (ASD) secondary to atrial rupture reported with canine degenerative mitral valve disease.
• Comprises 0.7–3.7% of congenital heart defects in dogs, <10% of congenital heart defects in cats. Significantly higher incidence (37.7%) noted in one study. • Three major types of ASD classified based on the location of the defect within the interatrial septum—ostium primum ASD (most apical portion of septum, adjacent to the atrioventricular [AV] valves), ostium secundum ASD (central portion of the septum, region of fossa ovalis), and sinus venosus ASD (adjacent to cranial or caudal vena cava). • Secundum ASD with left-to-right shunting is most common (98.7% in one study of dogs and cats). • Ostium primum ASD typically large; possible component of AV canal defect. • Sinus venosus ASD typically located at junction of cranial vena cava (less commonly caudal vena cava) and right atrium. Right pulmonary veins may be directed at right atrium through the defect. May be associated with anomalous pulmonary venous connections of some/all pulmonary veins.
• Isolated ASD typically shunts left to right. Magnitude of flow dependent on ASD size, relative systemic and pulmonary resistance, and relative ventricular compliance. Small restrictive defects allow atria to maintain normal differential pressure. Large defects may have significant left-to-right shunting, causing volume overload to right heart and pulmonary vessels. Secondary pulmonary hypertension can reverse shunting (i.e., right to left), termed Eisenmenger's physiology. ASD with concurrent defects causing increased right atrial pressure (i.e., pulmonic stenosis, tricuspid valve dysplasia, tricuspid valve stenosis) may have balanced or reversed shunting.

SIGNALMENT

• Dog and cat. • Various breeds affected; higher prevalence in boxer and standard poodle. • No sex predisposition.

SIGNS

General Comments

• Typically asymptomatic (73.7% in one study). • Severe cases may show signs of congestive heart failure (CHF). • Generalized cyanosis possible with reversed shunting.

Historical Findings

Clinical signs related to concurrent heart disease, CHF, or cyanosis; exercise intolerance, syncope, and dyspnea.

Physical Examination Findings

• Soft systolic murmur over left base due to increased blood flow across normal pulmonic valve. • Split S2 (fixed) due to delayed closure of pulmonic valve.
• Cyanosis with right-to-left shunting.
• Ascites and jugular vein distension with right CHF.

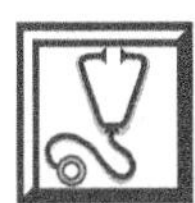

DIAGNOSIS

CBC/BIOCHEMISTRY/URINALYSIS

• Typically normal. • Polycythemia with right-to-left shunting.

IMAGING

Radiographic Findings

• None with small defects. • Right heart enlargement and vascular pattern (pulmonary overcirculation) with significant shunting.

Echocardiographic Findings

• Right atrial and/or right ventricular dilation. • Septal dropout (artifactual septal dropout is common and may lead to misdiagnosis). • Shunting across ASD by color-flow or spectral Doppler. • Increased pulmonic flow velocity. • Dilation of pulmonary trunk.

DIAGNOSTIC PROCEDURES

Electrocardiography

• Usually normal. • Right atrial and ventricular enlargement (tall P wave, deep S waves in lead II), right axis deviation.
• Arrhythmias and intraventricular conduction disturbances possible.

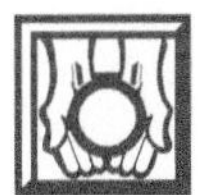

TREATMENT

GENERAL

• Long-term prognosis for small ASD is good; treatment typically unnecessary.
• Large ASD with hemodynamically significant shunting and right-sided enlargement warrants closure.

MEDICAL THERAPY

• Standard treatment of CHF—furosemide, pimobendan, angiotensin-converting enzyme (ACE) inhibitor). • Treatment of polycythemia (right-to-left shunting) if clinically indicated.

SURGICAL THERAPY

• Open heart surgery under cardiopulmonary bypass (surgical closure using patch graft). • Pulmonary artery banding as palliative measure to limit left-to-right shunting.

CATHETER-BASED THERAPY

• Amplatzer® atrial septal occluder (ASO) device delivered percutaneously through jugular vein possible for some secundum-type defects.
• Hybrid procedure involving surgical access and transatrial delivery of ASO device under inflow occlusion reported.

MEDICATIONS

See Congestive Heart Failure, Left-Sided; Congestive Heart Failure, Right-Sided; and Hypertension, Pulmonary.

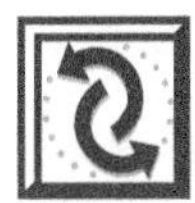

FOLLOW-UP

PATIENT MONITORING

• Periodic evaluation to assess cardiac structure and function. • Recheck when decompensation or other clinical signs develop.

EXPECTED COURSE AND PROGNOSIS

• Dependent on ASD size and coexisting defects.
• Small, isolated defects unlikely to cause clinical signs. • Defects >12 mm more likely to cause CHF.

MISCELLANEOUS

SEE ALSO

• Congestive Heart Failure, Left-Sided.
• Congestive Heart Failure, Right-Sided.
• Hypertension, Pulmonary.

ABBREVIATIONS

• ACE = angiotensin-converting enzyme.
• ASD = atrial septal defect.
• ASO = atrial septal occluder.
• AV = atrioventricular.
• CHF = congestive heart failure.

Suggested Reading

Bonagura JD, Lehmkuhl LB. Congenital heart disease. In: Fox PR, Sisson D, Moïse ND, eds., Textbook of Canine and Feline Cardiology, 2nd ed. Philadelphia, PA: Saunders 1999, pp. 471–535.

Chetboul V, Charles V, Nicolle A, et al. Retrospective study of 156 atrial septal defects in dogs and cats (2001–2005). J Vet Med Assoc 2006, 53(4):179–184.

Author Sandra P. Tou
Consulting Editor Michael Aherne

A

ATRIAL STANDSTILL

BASICS

DEFINITION

ECG rhythm characterized by absence of P waves; condition can be temporary (e.g., associated with hyperkalemia or drug induced), terminal (e.g., associated with severe hyperkalemia or dying heart), or persistent.

ECG Features

Persistent Atrial Standstill

- P waves absent.
- Heart rate usually slow (<60 bpm).
- Rhythm regular with supraventricular-type QRS complexes.
- Heart rate does not increase with atropine administration.

Hyperkalemic Atrial Standstill

- Heart rate normal or slow.
- Rhythm regular or irregular.
- QRS complexes tend to be wide and become wider as the potassium level rises; with severe hyperkalemia (potassium >10 mEq/L), the QRS complexes are replaced by a smooth biphasic curve.
- Heart rate may increase slightly with atropine.

PATHOPHYSIOLOGY

Persistent Atrial Standstill

Caused by an atrial muscular dystrophy/cardiomyopathy; skeletal muscle involvement common.

Hyperkalemic Atrial Standstill

Generally occurs with serum potassium levels >8.5 mEq/L; value influenced by serum sodium and calcium levels and acid-base status. Hyperkalemic patients with atrial standstill have sinus node function, but impulses do not activate atrial myocytes; thus, the associated rhythm is termed a sinoventricular rhythm. Since the sinus node is functional, an irregular rhythm may be due to sinus arrhythmia.

SYSTEMS AFFECTED

Cardiovascular

GENETICS

None

INCIDENCE/PREVALENCE

Rare rhythm disturbance.

GEOGRAPHIC DISTRIBUTION

None

SIGNALMENT

Species

Dog and cat.

Breed Predilections

Persistent atrial standstill—most common in English springer spaniels; other breeds occasionally affected.

Mean Age and Range

Most animals with persistent atrial standstill are young; animals with hypoadrenocorticism are usually young to middle-aged.

Predominant Sex

Hypoadrenocorticism more common in females (69%).

SIGNS

Historical Findings

- Vary with underlying cause.
- Lethargy common; syncope may occur.
- Patients with persistent atrial standstill may show signs of congestive heart failure (CHF).

Physical Examination Findings

- Vary with underlying cause.
- Bradycardia common.
- Patients with persistent atrial standstill may have skeletal muscle wasting of the antebrachium and scapula.

CAUSES

- Hyperkalemia.
- Atrial disease, often associated with atrial distension (e.g., cats with cardiomyopathy).
- Atrial myopathy (persistent atrial standstill).

RISK FACTORS

- Hyperkalemic atrial standstill.
- Hypoadrenocorticism.
- Conditions leading to obstruction or rupture of the urinary tract.
- Oliguric or anuric renal failure.

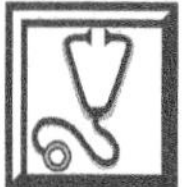

DIAGNOSIS

DIFFERENTIAL DIAGNOSIS

- Slow atrial fibrillation.
- Sinus bradycardia with small or hidden P waves.

CBC/BIOCHEMISTRY/URINALYSIS

Persistent Atrial Standstill

Normal

Hyperkalemic Atrial Standstill

- Hyperkalemia.
- Hyponatremia and sodium : potassium ratio <27 if atrial standstill secondary to hypoadrenocorticism.
- Azotemia and hyperphosphatemia with hypoadrenocorticism, renal failure, and rupture or obstruction of the urinary tract.

OTHER LABORATORY TESTS

Adrenocorticotropic hormone (ACTH) stimulation test if hypoadrenocorticism suspected.

IMAGING

Echocardiogram and electromyography if persistent atrial standstill suspected—cardiomegaly and depressed contractility may be seen.

DIAGNOSTIC PROCEDURES

Skeletal muscle biopsy in animals with persistent atrial standstill, particularly if skeletal muscle wasting noted.

PATHOLOGIC FINDINGS

Persistent Atrial Standstill

- Greatly enlarged and paper-thin atria; usually biatrial involvement, although one case of only left atrial involvement was reported.
- Severe scapular and brachial muscle wasting in some dogs.
- Marked fibrosis, fibroelastosis, chronic mononuclear cell inflammation, and steatosis throughout the atria and interatrial septum.

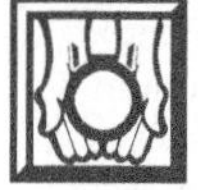

TREATMENT

APPROPRIATE HEALTH CARE

Persistent Atrial Standstill

Not life-threatening condition; animal can be treated as an outpatient.

Hyperkalemic Atrial Standstill

Potentially life-threatening; often requires aggressive treatment.

NURSING CARE

Aggressive fluid therapy with 0.9% saline often required to correct hypovolemia and lower serum potassium levels (see Hyperkalemia) in patients with hyperkalemic atrial standstill.

ACTIVITY

Restrict activity in patients with persistent atrial standstill and signs of CHF or syncope.

DIET

N/A

CLIENT EDUCATION

Persistent Atrial Standstill

Clinical signs generally improve after pacemaker implantation; signs of CHF may develop, and weakness and lethargy may persist even after heart rate and rhythm are corrected with the pacemaker.

SURGICAL CONSIDERATIONS

Persistent Atrial Standstill

Implant permanent ventricular pacemaker to regulate rate and rhythm.

Hyperkalemic Atrial Standstill

Hyperkalemia secondary to urinary tract obstruction or rupture may require surgery.

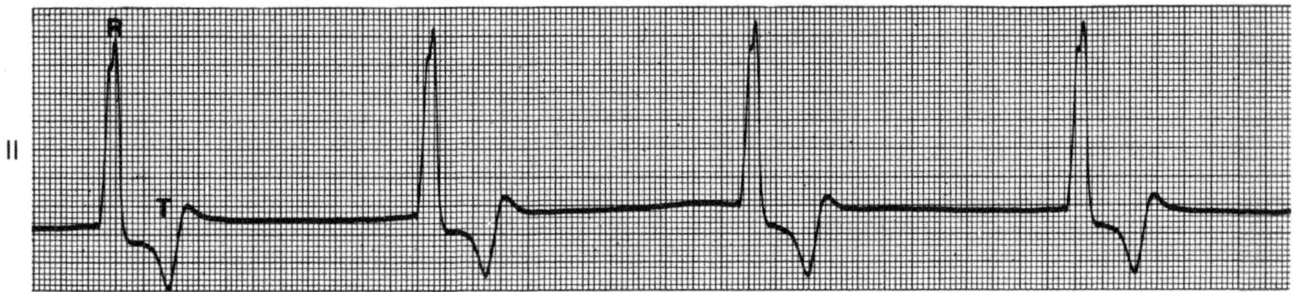

Figure 1.

Atrial standstill in a dog with a potassium of 9 mEq/L. Note the absence of P waves and wide QRS complexes.

MEDICATIONS

DRUG(S) OF CHOICE

Persistent Atrial Standstill

Treat with standard therapy (pimobendan, diuretics, and angiotensin-converting enzyme (ACE) inhibitor, e.g., enalapril or benazepril) if CHF develops.

Hyperkalemic Atrial Standstill

- Treat the underlying cause (e.g., oliguric renal failure, hypoadrenocorticism).
- Aggressive fluid therapy with 0.9% saline and possibly sodium bicarbonate or insulin with dextrose, as discussed under Hyperkalemia.
- Calcium gluconate—counters the cardiac effects of hyperkalemia; can be used in life-threatening situations while instituting treatment to lower potassium concentration.

CONTRAINDICATIONS

Avoid potassium-containing fluids or medications that increase potassium concentration in hyperkalemic patients.

PRECAUTIONS

Diuretics lower preload and may worsen weakness in dogs with persistent atrial standstill and CHF unless a pacemaker has been implanted.

POSSIBLE INTERACTIONS

N/A

ALTERNATIVE DRUG(S)

N/A

FOLLOW-UP

PATIENT MONITORING

- Monitor ECG during treatment of hyperkalemia and periodically in animals with a permanent ventricular pacemaker.
- Monitor electrolytes in patients with hyperkalemic atrial standstill.
- Monitor patients with persistent atrial standstill for signs of CHF.

PREVENTION/AVOIDANCE

N/A

POSSIBLE COMPLICATIONS

CHF in patients with persistent atrial standstill.

EXPECTED COURSE AND PROGNOSIS

Persistent Atrial Standstill

- Clinical signs generally improve after pacemaker implantation. Signs of CHF may develop, and weakness and lethargy may persist even after heart rate and rhythm are corrected with the pacemaker.
- Signs related to muscular dystrophy may persist.
- Median survival in 20 dogs with atrial standstill treated with a pacemaker was 866 days and was not influenced by breed or presence of heart failure at time of implantation.

Hyperkalemic Atrial Standstill

Long-term prognosis is excellent if underlying cause can be corrected and hyperkalemia reversed.

MISCELLANEOUS

ASSOCIATED CONDITIONS

Diseases causing hyperkalemia (e.g., hypoadrenocorticism, urethral obstruction or urinary tract tear, acidosis, and drugs).

AGE-RELATED FACTORS

Persistent atrial standstill—usually diagnosed in young animals; hypoadrenocorticism—usually diagnosed in young to middle-aged animals.

ZOONOTIC POTENTIAL

None

PREGNANCY/FERTILITY/BREEDING

N/A

SYNONYMS

Silent atrium.

SEE ALSO

- Digoxin Toxicity.
- Hyperkalemia.
- Hypoadrenocorticism (Addison's Disease).
- Urinary Tract Obstruction.

ABBREVIATIONS

- ACE = angiotensin-converting enzyme.
- ACTH = adrenocorticotropic hormone.
- CHF = congestive heart failure.

Suggested Reading

Cervenec RM, Stauthammer CD, Fine DM, et al. Survival time with pacemaker implantation for dogs diagnosed with persistent atrial standstill. J Vet Cardiol 2017, 19(3):240–246.

Kraus MS, Gelzer ARM, Moïse NS. Treatment of cardiac arrhythmias and conduction disturbances. In: Smith FWK, Tilley LP, Oyama MA, Sleeper MM, eds., Manual of Canine and Feline Cardiology, 5th ed. St. Louis, MO: Saunders Elsevier, 2016, pp. 313–329.

Tilley LP, Smith FWK Jr. Electrocardiography. In: Smith FWK, Tilley LP, Oyama MA, Sleeper MM, eds., Manual of Canine and Feline Cardiology, 5th ed. St. Louis, MO: Saunders Elsevier, 2016, pp. 49–76.

Author Francis W.K. Smith, Jr.

Consulting Editor Michael Aherne

Client Education Handout available online

ATRIAL WALL TEAR

BASICS

DEFINITION

- Endocardial splitting is a linear defect limited to the atrial endocardium (typically left atrium [LA]) resulting from distension of the atrial wall beyond its elastic limits.
- Atrial tear results if the split extends through the myocardium and epicardium, resulting in a full-thickness atrial wall defect and hemorrhage into the pericardial space.

PATHOPHYSIOLOGY

- Endocardial splitting typically results from increased LA pressure secondary to severe mitral regurgitation and mechanical trauma from the regurgitant jet; primary endocardial degeneration may also play a role.
- If split is incomplete, fibrin may seal the defect temporarily; either heals as a linear depression in endocardial surface or subsequently extends through myocardium, resulting in complete tear.
- LA tear results in peracute bleeding into pericardial sac and acute cardiac tamponade.
- If tear occurs in interatrial septum, an acquired atrial septal defect may form.
- Tearing of either atrium may also rarely occur secondary to blunt trauma, or iatrogenically during pericardiocentesis or cardiac catheterization.

SYSTEMS AFFECTED

- Cardiovascular.
- Respiratory.

GENETICS

Unknown

INCIDENCE/PREVALENCE

A rare cause of hemorrhagic pericardial effusion in the dog encompassing approximately 2% of pericardial effusion cases.

SIGNALMENT

Species

Dog; uncommon in cat.

Breed Predilections

- Any breed predisposed to degenerative valve disease.
- If traumatic, any breed may be represented.

Mean Age and Range

Middle-aged to older dogs.

Predominant Sex

Male dogs may be overrepresented.

SIGNS

Historical Findings

- Acute weakness and collapse; may progress quickly to respiratory or cardiopulmonary arrest.
- History of chronic cardiac disease; signs of congestive heart failure (CHF) in most patients.
- Acute worsening of cough or dyspnea is commonly observed.
- Possible history of blunt trauma.

Physical Examination Findings

- Collapse.
- Tachycardia.
- Weak pulses or pulsus paradoxus.
- Pale, muddy, or ashen mucous membranes; prolonged capillary refill time (CRT).
- Other signs of significant cardiac disease (e.g., murmur, gallop sound, arrhythmia, cough, dyspnea) typically present.
- May have signs of right CHF (e.g., ascites, jugular venous distension).
- Heart sounds may be muffled, or if murmur was heard before atrial wall tear occurred, it may be reduced in intensity.

CAUSES

- Myxomatous mitral valve disease.
- Chordae tendineae rupture.
- Chest trauma.
- Cardiac catheterization.

RISK FACTORS

- Severe mitral regurgitation; LA enlargement.
- May be precipitated by excitement, stress, or activity.

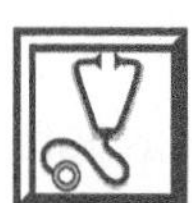

DIAGNOSIS

DIFFERENTIAL DIAGNOSIS

- Other causes of acute cardiovascular collapse or syncope.
- Pericardial effusion from other causes (e.g., neoplastic, idiopathic).
- CHF.
- Severe arrhythmias.

CBC/BIOCHEMISTRY/URINALYSIS

- Elevations in serum lactate; metabolic acidosis.
- Increased alanine aminotransferase/aspartate aminotransferase in some patients.
- Prerenal azotemia; hyponatremia or other electrolyte derangements may be seen.

OTHER LABORATORY TESTS

NT-proBNP and cardiac troponin I (cTnI) levels may be elevated.

IMAGING

Radiography

- Usually moderate to severe LA enlargement; cardiac silhouette may be rounded and further enlarged compared with previous radiographs.
- Interstitial to alveolar pulmonary infiltrates if left-sided CHF present.
- Pleural effusion, ascites, hepatomegaly, and large caudal vena cava if right-sided CHF.

ECG

- Pericardial effusion—volume may be relatively small as pericardium remains inelastic due to acute nature of bleed; characteristic linear, hyperechoic thrombus may be seen within pericardial sac.
- Actual tear often not identified, though associated thrombus occasionally visualized within LA.
- Evidence of cardiac tamponade.
- Signs of advanced myxomatous mitral valve disease with moderate to severe LA enlargement expected.

DIAGNOSTIC PROCEDURES

ECG

- Sinus tachycardia.
- Atrial or ventricular arrhythmias.
- Possible dampened QRS complexes.
- Electrical alternans.
- ST-segment abnormalities.
- Possible left ventricular or LA enlargement pattern.

PATHOLOGIC FINDINGS

- Endocardial splitting is noted grossly as pale linear depression in atrial endocardium.
- Atrial wall tears appear as full-thickness defects extending through atrial endocardium, myocardium, and epicardium; associated thrombus may or may not be present. Caudolateral aspect of LA most commonly affected, with many tears occurring at atrio-auricular junction.
- Hemorrhagic pericardial effusion or pericardial thrombus with acute tears.
- Myxomatous valve disease characterized by thickened leaflets with rolled edges; may have chordae tendineae rupture; possibly atrial jet lesions.
- Cardiomegaly with severe LA enlargement expected.

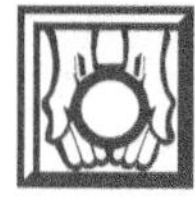

TREATMENT

APPROPRIATE HEALTH CARE

- If LA tear suspected, perform pericardiocentesis only if effusion causing symptomatic, life-threatening cardiac tamponade, since further hemorrhage into pericardial sac or exsanguination may occur once pericardial fluid removed; remove only enough fluid to improve clinical signs.
- Pericardiocentesis likely difficult given small volume of effusion typically present, severe cardiomegaly, and small size of most dogs with LA rupture; ultrasound guidance and continuous ECG monitoring highly recommended.
- Best practices for management of LA tear have not been clearly established; however, aggressive medical management to lower LA pressure using afterload and preload reducers recommended based on author's clinical experience.
- If fibrin clot forms over defect, patient may stabilize and recover.

NURSING CARE

- Administer oxygen to dyspneic or hemodynamically unstable dogs.

- Administer IV fluids only if evidence of hypovolemia present; most dogs volume overloaded and further intravascular volume expansion will increase LA pressure and potentially worsen tamponade.

ACTIVITY

Strict cage rest in acute period, followed by chronic exercise restriction.

DIET

Sodium restriction may be indicated for animals with advanced myxomatous valve disease with cardiomegaly.

CLIENT EDUCATION

LA tear typically accompanies advanced cardiac disease and chronic medical therapy is necessary; though prognosis is guarded for surviving acute event, some dogs have lived more than a year after the incident.

SURGICAL CONSIDERATIONS

Exploratory thoracotomy may be considered if hemorrhage persists or recurs, but should be undertaken cautiously given advanced state of cardiac disease typically present.

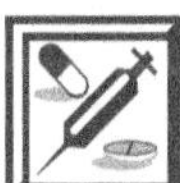

MEDICATIONS

DRUG(S) OF CHOICE

- Atrial tears occur secondary to elevated LA pressure; thus medical therapy should be focused on lowering LA pressures to reduce continued hemorrhage into pericardial space and permit fibrin clot formation at the tear; this may be accomplished with preload (e.g., diuretics, nitroglycerin paste) and/or afterload reducers (arterial vasodilators).
- Preload and afterload reduction must be undertaken cautiously to avoid worsening of hemodynamic compromise.
- If concurrent CHF present, afterload reduction may be achieved by conservative doses of sodium nitroprusside; low starting CRI dose of 0.5–1 µg/kg/min recommended to decrease LA pressure without precipitating significant hypotension; dose may be uptitrated as necessary every 15–30 min up to maximum of 10 µg/kg/min to improve clinical signs and/or reduce blood pressure by 10–15 mmHg.
- Alternatively, amlodipine may be started at 0.1–0.2 mg/kg PO q24h; chronic amlodipine therapy may be implemented in normotensive or hypertensive animals to reduce regurgitant fraction and lower LA pressure.
- Cautious diuretic use, if needed, to treat dyspnea associated with concomitant CHF (e.g., 1–2 mg/kg furosemide IV as needed); signs of left-sided CHF may worsen as cardiac tamponade resolves due to augmented preload—more aggressive diuretic therapy may then be required.
- Pimobendan (0.25–0.3 mg/kg PO q12h) may result in further LA pressure reduction, though studies have not specifically examined its use in setting of LA rupture.
- Once patient is stable, angiotensin-converting enzyme inhibitors (e.g., enalapril 0.5 mg/kg q12–24h) should be implemented for chronic management of accompanying CHF.

CONTRAINDICATIONS

- Antithrombotic medications.
- Arterial vasodilators, if significant hypotension present.

PRECAUTIONS

- Aggressive fluid therapy unwarranted; further volume expansion may increase LA pressure, worsen cardiac tamponade, and contribute to hemodynamic compromise.
- Best practices for management of LA tear not clearly established; choice of whether to perform pericardiocentesis, and whether to administer preload and/or afterload reducers, should be based on assessment of volume status, blood pressure, and clinical stability of patient.

POSSIBLE INTERACTIONS

Sodium nitroprusside should not be administered concurrently with phosphodiesterase-V inhibitors (e.g., sildenafil, tadalafil) due to potential for life-threatening systemic hypotension.

ALTERNATIVE DRUGS

N/A

FOLLOW-UP

PATIENT MONITORING

- Recommend close monitoring of respiratory rate and effort, mucous membrane color and CRT, pulse quality, and heart rate; blood pressure monitoring recommended if arterial vasodilators are implemented.
- Follow-up examination with echocardiography helps determine resolution of pericardial effusion and resorption of atrial or pericardial clot.
- Close follow-up every 2–3 months thereafter recommended for repeat pericardial fluid checks and medication adjustments as indicated.

PREVENTION/AVOIDANCE

Avoid strenuous physical activity and excitement.

POSSIBLE COMPLICATIONS

- Even if the tear seals, patient is prone to further tears because of underlying cardiac disease.
- Most dogs have or will develop concurrent CHF.

EXPECTED COURSE AND PROGNOSIS

Prognosis is guarded; however, some animals can do well for several months or more with exercise restriction and optimal medical management.

MISCELLANEOUS

ASSOCIATED CONDITIONS

- Myxomatous mitral valve disease.
- CHF.
- Mainstem bronchial compression.

AGE-RELATED FACTORS

Middle-aged to older dogs are predisposed.

ZOONOTIC POTENTIAL

N/A

PREGNANCY/FERTILITY/BREEDING

N/A

SYNONYMS

- Atrial rupture.
- Atrial splitting.

SEE ALSO

- Atrial Septal Defect.
- Congestive Heart Failure, Left-Sided.
- Congestive Heart Failure, Right-Sided.
- Myxomatous Mitral Valve Disease.
- Pericardial Disease.
- Syncope.

ABBREVIATIONS

- CHF = congestive heart failure.
- CRT = capillary refill time.
- cTnI = cardiac troponin I.
- LA = left atrium/atrial.

INTERNET RESOURCES

James Buchanan Cardiology Library: https://www.vin.com/apputil/content/defaultadv1.aspx?pId=84

Suggested Reading

Nakamura RK, Tompkins E, Russell NJ, et al. Left atrial rupture secondary to myxomatous mitral valve disease in 11 dogs. J Am Anim Hosp Assoc 2014, 50:405–408.

Peddle GD, Buchanan JW. Acquired atrial septal defects secondary to rupture of the atrial septum in dogs with degenerative mitral valve disease. J Vet Cardiol 2010, 12:129–134.

Reineke EL, Burkett DE, Drobatz KJ. Left atrial rupture in dogs: 14 cases (1990–2005). J Vet Emerg Crit Care 2008, 18:158–164.

Author Suzanne M. Cunningham
Consulting Editor Michael Aherne

A

ATRIOVENTRICULAR BLOCK, COMPLETE (THIRD DEGREE)

BASICS

DEFINITION

• All atrial impulses are blocked at the atrioventricular (AV) junction; atria and ventricles beat independently. A secondary "escape" pacemaker site (junctional or ventricular) stimulates the ventricles. • Atrial rate normal. • Idioventricular escape rhythm slow.

ECG Features

• Ventricular rate slower than atrial rate (more P waves than QRS complexes)—ventricular escape rhythm (idioventricular) usually <40 bpm; junctional escape rhythm (idiojunctional) 40–60 bpm in dogs and 60–100 bpm in cats. • P waves—usually normal configuration (Figures 1 and 2). • QRS complex—wide and bizarre when pacemaker located in the ventricle, or in the lower AV junction in a patient with bundle branch block; normal when escape pacemaker in the lower AV junction (above the bifurcation of the bundle of His) in a patient without bundle branch block. • No conduction between the atria and the ventricles; P waves have no constant relationship with QRS complexes; P–P and R–R intervals relatively constant (except for a sinus arrhythmia).

PATHOPHYSIOLOGY

Slow ventricular escape rhythms (<40 bpm) result in low cardiac output and eventual heart failure, often when animal is excited or exercised, since demand for greater cardiac output is not satisfied. As the heart fails, signs increase with mild activity.

SYSTEMS AFFECTED

Cardiovascular

GENETICS

Can be an isolated congenital defect.

INCIDENCE/PREVALENCE

Not documented.

GEOGRAPHIC DISTRIBUTION

N/A

SIGNALMENT

Species

Dog and cat.

Breed Predilections

• Cocker spaniel—can have idiopathic fibrosis. • Pug and Doberman pinscher—can have associated sudden death, AV conduction defects, and bundle of His lesions.

Mean Age and Range

Geriatric animals, except congenital heart disease patients. Median age for cats—14 years.

Predominant Sex

Intact female dogs.

SIGNS

Historical Findings

• Exercise intolerance. • Weakness or syncope. • Occasionally, congestive heart failure (CHF).

Physical Examination Findings

• Bradycardia. • Variable third and fourth heart sounds. • Variation in intensity of first heart sounds. • Signs of CHF possible. • Intermittent "cannon" A waves in jugular venous pulses. • Often bounding arterial pulses.

CAUSES & RISK FACTORS

• Isolated congenital defect. • Idiopathic fibrosis. • Infiltrative cardiomyopathy (amyloidosis or neoplasia). • Hypertrophic cardiomyopathy in cats. • Digitalis toxicity. • Hyperthyroidism in cats. • Myocarditis. • Endocarditis. • Electrolyte disorder. • Myocardial infarction. • Other congenital heart defects. • Lyme disease. • Chagas disease.

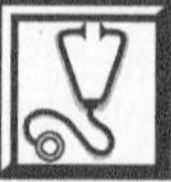

DIAGNOSIS

DIFFERENTIAL DIAGNOSIS

• Advanced second-degree AV block. • Atrial standstill. • Accelerated idioventricular rhythm.

CBC/BIOCHEMISTRY/URINALYSIS

• Abnormal serum electrolytes (e.g., hyperkalemia, hypokalemia) possible. • High white blood cell count with left shift in animals with bacterial endocarditis.

OTHER LABORATORY TESTS

• High serum digoxin concentration if AV block due to digoxin toxicity. • Lyme titer and accompanying clinical signs if AV block due to Lyme disease.

IMAGING

Echocardiography and Doppler ultrasound to assess cardiac structure and function.

DIAGNOSTIC PROCEDURES

• Electrocardiography. • His bundle electrogram to determine the site of the AV block is possible. • Long-term (Holter) ambulatory recording if AV block is intermittent.

PATHOLOGIC FINDINGS

Degeneration or fibrosis of the AV node and its bundle branches, associated with endocardial and myocardial fibrosis and organized endomyocarditis.

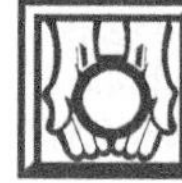

TREATMENT

APPROPRIATE HEALTH CARE

• Temporary or permanent cardiac pacemaker—only effective treatment in symptomatic patients. • Carefully monitor asymptomatic patients without a pacemaker for development of clinical signs.

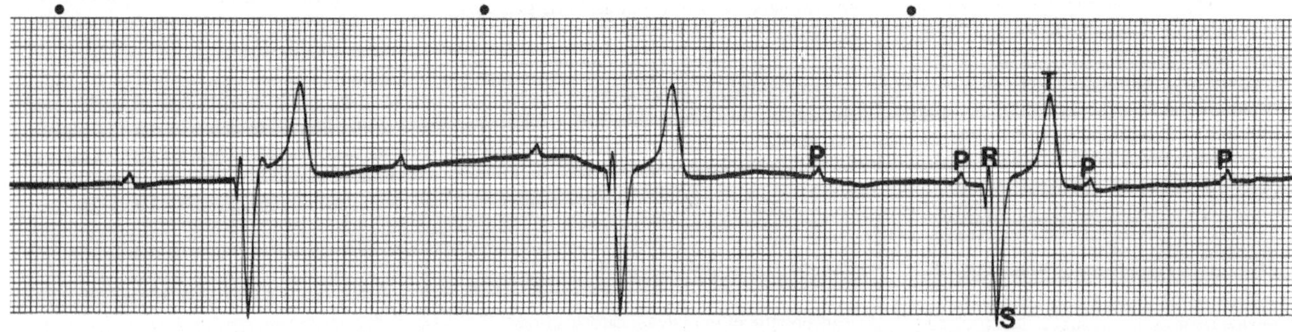

Figure 1.

Complete heart block in a dog. The P waves occur at a rate of 120, independent of the ventricular rate of 50. The QRS configuration is a right bundle branch block pattern. (Source: From Tilley LP. Essentials of Canine and Feline Electrocardiography, 3rd ed. Baltimore: Williams & Wilkins, 1992. Reprinted with permission of Wolters Kluwer.)

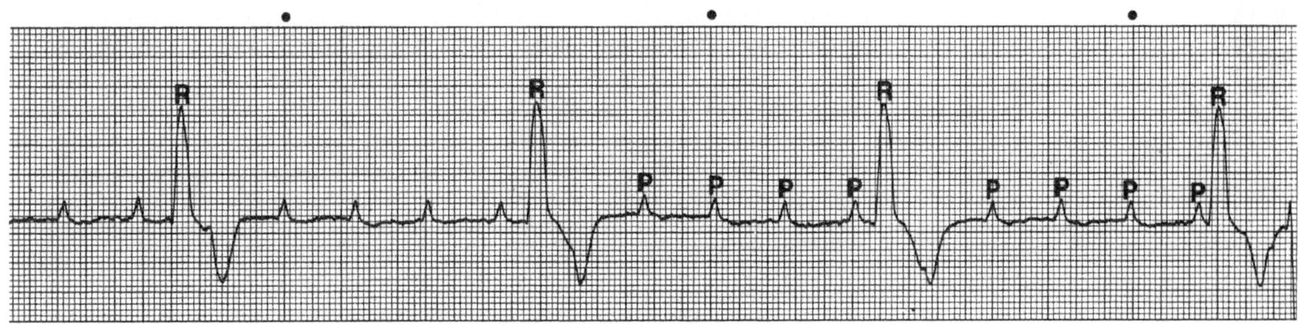

Figure 2.

Complete heart block in a cat. The P wave rate is 240/minute, independent of the ventricular rate of 48/minute. QRS configuration is a left bundle branch block pattern. (Source: From Tilley LP. Essentials of Canine and Feline Electrocardiography, 3rd ed. Baltimore: Williams & Wilkins, 1992. Reprinted with permission of Wolters Kluwer.)

NURSING CARE

Cage rest prior to pacemaker implantation; when the pulse generator is implanted into a subcutaneous pocket, a nonconstricting bandage is placed around the ventral neck or abdomen for 3–5 days to prevent seroma formation or pacemaker movement.

ACTIVITY

Restrict if symptomatic.

DIET

No modifications unless required to manage underlying condition (e.g., low-salt diet).

CLIENT EDUCATION

• Temporary or permanent cardiac pacemaker—only effective treatment in symptomatic patients. • Asymptomatic patients without a pacemaker—must be carefully monitored for development of clinical signs.

SURGICAL CONSIDERATIONS

• Most patients—at high anesthetic cardiopulmonary risk; usually paced preoperatively with a temporary external pacemaker system. • The small size of cats makes pacemaker implantation more difficult than in dogs.

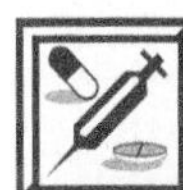

MEDICATIONS

DRUG(S) OF CHOICE

• Treatment with drugs—usually of no value. Traditionally used to treat complete AV block: atropine, isoproterenol, corticosteroids, and dobutamine. • Intravenous isoproterenol infusion may help increase the rate of the ventricular escape rhythm to stabilize hemodynamics. • If CHF—diuretic and vasodilator therapy may be needed before pacemaker implantation.

CONTRAINDICATIONS

Avoid digoxin, xylazine, acepromazine, beta blockers (e.g., propranolol and atenolol), and calcium channel blockers (e.g., verapamil and diltiazem); ventricular antiarrhythmic agents are dangerous because they suppress lower escape foci.

PRECAUTIONS

Vasodilators—may cause hypotension in animals with complete AV block; monitor closely if used, especially prior to pacemaker implantation.

FOLLOW-UP

PATIENT MONITORING

• Monitor—pacemaker function with serial electrocardiograms. • Radiographs—following pacemaker implantation, to confirm the position of the lead and generator.

PREVENTION/AVOIDANCE

N/A

POSSIBLE COMPLICATIONS

Pulse generators—pacemaker replacement necessary if battery becomes depleted, pulse generator malfunction occurs, or exit block develops; pacemaker leads can become dislodged and infected.

EXPECTED COURSE AND PROGNOSIS

Poor long-term prognosis if no cardiac pacemaker implanted, especially when the animal has clinical signs. Cats can sometimes survive >1 year without a permanent pacemaker.

MISCELLANEOUS

ASSOCIATED CONDITIONS

None

ABBREVIATIONS

• AV = atrioventricular.
• CHF = congestive heart failure.

Suggested Reading

Kellum HB, Stepien RL. Third-degree atrioventricular block in 21 cats (1997–2004). J Vet Intern Med 2006, 20:97–103.

Santilli R, Moise NS, Pariaut R, Perego M. Electrocardiography of the Dog and Cat: Diagnosis of Arrhythmias, 2nd ed. Milan: Edra, 2018.

Schrope DP, Kelch WJ. Signalment, clinical signs, and prognostic indicators associated with high-grade second or third-degree atrioventricular block in dogs: 124 cases (January 1, 1997–December 31, 1997). J Am Vet Med Assoc 2006, 228:1710–1717.

Tilley LP, Smith FWK Jr. Electrocardiography. In Smith FWK, Tilley LP, Oyama M, Sleeper M, eds., Manual of Canine and Feline Cardiology, 5th ed. St. Louis, MO: Saunders Elsevier, 2016, pp. 49–76.

Willis R, Oliveira P, Mavropoulou A. Guide to Canine and Feline Electrocardiography. Ames, IA: Wiley-Blackwell, 2018.

Author Larry P. Tilley
Consulting Editor Michael Aherne

Client Education Handout available online

ATRIOVENTRICULAR BLOCK, FIRST DEGREE

BASICS

DEFINITION

Refers to a delay in conduction that occurs between atrial and ventricular activation.

ECG Features

- Rate and rhythm—usually normal.
- Usually there are regularly occurring normal P waves and QRS complexes (Figures 1 and 2).
- Prolonged, consistent PR intervals—dogs, >0.13 sec; cats, >0.09 sec (Figures 1 and 2).

PATHOPHYSIOLOGY

- Virtually never causes clinical signs.
- May become a more severe atrioventricular (AV) conduction disturbance in some animals.
- Normally the PR interval tends to shorten with rapid heart rates.
- May be the result of intra-atrial conduction delay (prolongation of the PA interval on surface ECG and simultaneous His bundle electrogram) or delay of conduction within the AV node itself (prolongation of the AH interval on His bundle electrogram).

SYSTEMS AFFECTED

Cardiovascular

GENETICS

N/A

INCIDENCE/PREVALENCE

Common

GEOGRAPHIC DISTRIBUTION

None

SIGNALMENT

Species

Dog and cat.

Breed Predilections

American cocker spaniel, dachshund, brachycephalic dogs, Persian cats.

Mean Age and Range

- May occur in young, otherwise healthy dogs as a manifestation of high vagal tone.
- Intra-atrial conduction delay involving the right atrium may be seen with congenital heart disease, especially AV septal defects.
- May be noted in aged patients with degenerative conduction system disease, particularly cocker spaniels and dachshunds.
- Persian cats of any age with high vagal tone and in cats of any age with hypertrophic cardiomyopathy.

SIGNS

Historical Findings

- Most animals are asymptomatic.
- If drug induced, may have a history of clinical signs related to drug toxicity—anorexia, vomiting, and diarrhea with digoxin; weakness with calcium channel blockers or β-adrenergic antagonists.

Physical Examination Findings

Normal—unless also signs of more generalized myocardial disease, drug toxicity, or noncardiac disease.

CAUSES

- May occur in normal animals.
- Enhanced vagal stimulation resulting from noncardiac diseases—usually accompanied by sinus arrhythmia, sinus arrest, and/or Mobitz type I second-degree AV block.
- Pharmacologic agents—e.g., digoxin, β-adrenergic antagonists, calcium channel blocking agents, propafenone, amiodarone, α_2-adrenergic agonists, parasympathomimetic agents (bethanechol, physostigmine, pilocarpine), and severe procainamide or quinidine toxicity.
- Degenerative disease of the conduction system.
- Hypertrophic cardiomyopathy.
- Myocarditis (especially *Trypanosoma cruzi*, *Borrelia burgdorferi*, *Rickettsia rickettsii*).
- Infiltrative diseases (tumors, amyloid).
- Atropine administered intravenously may briefly prolong the PR interval.

RISK FACTORS

Any condition or intervention that raises vagal tone.

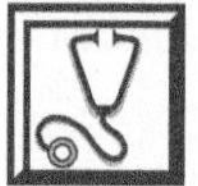

DIAGNOSIS

DIFFERENTIAL DIAGNOSIS

P waves superimposed upon preceding T waves because of first-degree AV block should be differentiated from bifid T waves.

CBC/BIOCHEMISTRY/URINALYSIS

- Serum electrolytes—hypokalemia and hyperkalemia may predispose to AV conduction disturbances.
- Leukocytosis—may be noted with bacterial endocarditis or myocarditis.

OTHER LABORATORY TESTS

- Serum digoxin concentration—may be high.
- *T. cruzi*, *B. burgdorferi*, *R. rickettsii* titers—may be high.
- Thyroxine (T_4)—may be high in cats if associated with thyrotoxic myocardial disease.

IMAGING

Echocardiographic examination—may reveal hypertrophic or infiltrative myocardial disorder.

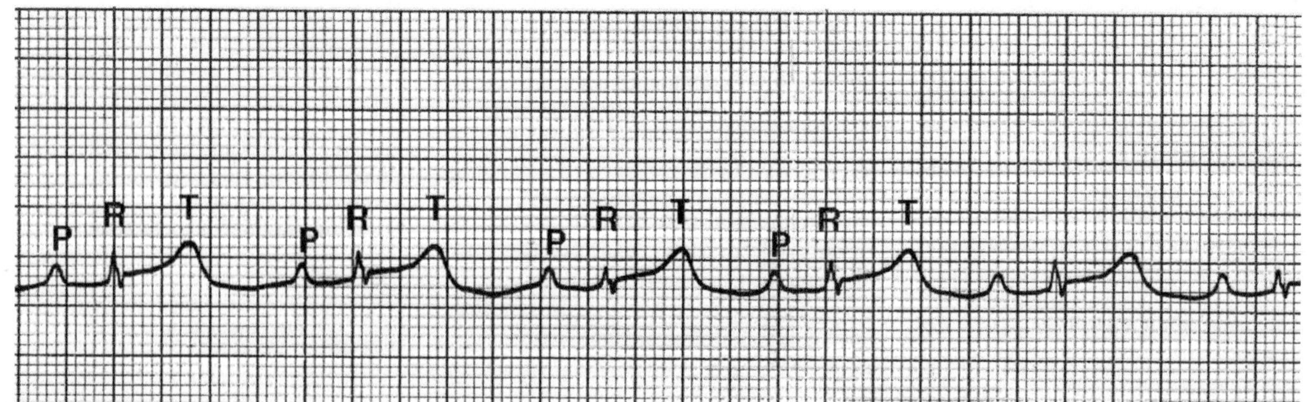

Figure 1.

Lead II ECG rhythm strip recorded from a cat with hypertrophic cardiomyopathy. There is sinus bradycardia (120 bpm) and first-degree AV conduction block. The PR interval is 0.12 second (paper speed = 50 mm/s).

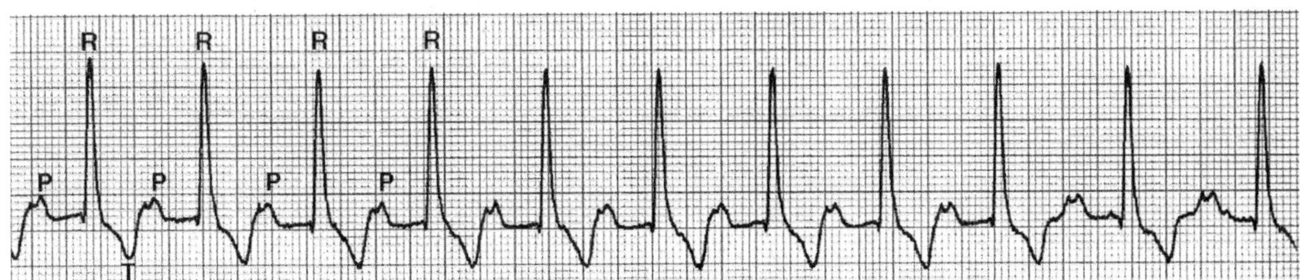

Figure 2.

Lead II ECG rhythm strip recorded from a dog showing sinus tachycardia (175 bpm) and first-degree AV conduction block. Because the heart rate is rapid, P waves are superimposed on the downslope of the preceding T waves. The PR interval exceeds 0.16 second (paper speed = 50 mm/s).

DIAGNOSTIC PROCEDURES

May be needed to identify causes of high vagal tone—upper airway disease, cervical and thoracic masses, gastrointestinal disorders, and high intraocular pressure.

PATHOLOGIC FINDINGS

Variable—depend on underlying cause.

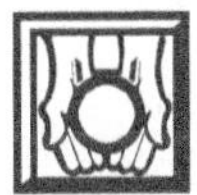

TREATMENT

APPROPRIATE HEALTH CARE

- Remove or treat underlying cause(s).
- Hospitalization may be necessary to manage the underlying cause (e.g., cardiomyopathy, gastrointestinal disease, airway disease).

NURSING CARE

N/A

ACTIVITY

Unrestricted; unless restriction required for an underlying condition.

DIET

No modifications or restrictions, unless required to manage an underlying condition.

CLIENT EDUCATION

Generally unnecessary.

SURGICAL CONSIDERATIONS

None, unless required to manage an underlying condition.

MEDICATIONS

DRUG(S) OF CHOICE

Medications used only if needed to manage an underlying condition.

CONTRAINDICATIONS

- Avoid hypokalemia—increases sensitivity to vagal tone; may potentiate AV conduction delay.
- Avoid drugs likely to impair impulse conduction further (calcium channel blocking agents, β-adrenergic antagonists, α_2-adrenergic agonists, amiodarone, propafenone).

PRECAUTIONS

Drugs with vagomimetic action (e.g., digoxin, bethanechol, physostigmine, pilocarpine) may potentiate first-degree block.

POSSIBLE INTERACTIONS

N/A

ALTERNATIVE DRUG(S)

N/A

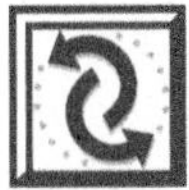

FOLLOW-UP

PATIENT MONITORING

Except in healthy young animals, monitor ECG to detect any progression in conduction disturbance.

PREVENTION/AVOIDANCE

N/A

POSSIBLE COMPLICATIONS

N/A

EXPECTED COURSE AND PROGNOSIS

- Depends on underlying cause.
- Prognosis usually excellent if no significant underlying disease is present.

MISCELLANEOUS

ASSOCIATED CONDITIONS

None

AGE-RELATED FACTORS

PR interval—tends to lengthen with advancing age.

ZOONOTIC POTENTIAL

None

PREGNANCY/FERTILITY/BREEDING

N/A

SEE ALSO

- Atrioventricular Block, Complete (Third Degree).
- Atrioventricular Block, Second Degree—Mobitz Type I.
- Atrioventricular Block, Second Degree—Mobitz Type II.

ABBREVIATIONS

- AV = atrioventricular
- T_4 = thyroxine

Suggested Reading

Berger MG, Rubenstein JC, Roth JA. Cardiac arrhythmias. In: Benjamin IJ, Griggs RC, Wing EJ, Fitz JG, eds., Andreoli and Carpenter's Cecil Essentials of Medicine, 9th ed. Philadelphia, PA: Saunders, 2016, pp. 110–135.

Miller MS, Tilley LP, Smith FWK, Fox PR. Electrocardiography. In: Fox PR, Sisson D, Moïse NS, eds., Textbook of Canine and Feline Cardiology. Philadelphia, PA: Saunders, 1999, pp. 67–106.

Santilli R, Moïse NS, Pariaut R, Perego M. Electrocardiography of the Dog and Cat: Diagnosis of Arrhythmias, 2nd ed. Milan: Edra, 2018.

Tilley LP, Smith FWK Jr. Electrocardiography. In: Smith FWK, Tilley LP, Oyama M, Sleeper M, eds., Manual of Canine and Feline Cardiology, 5th ed. St. Louis, MO: Saunders Elsevier, 2016, pp. 49–76.

Willis R, Oliveira P, Mavropoulou A. Guide to Canine and Feline Electrocardiography. Ames, IA: Wiley-Blackwell, 2018.

Authors Francis W.K. Smith, Jr. and Larry P. Tilley

Consulting Editor Michael Aherne

Client Education Handout available online

A

ATRIOVENTRICULAR BLOCK, SECOND DEGREE—MOBITZ TYPE I

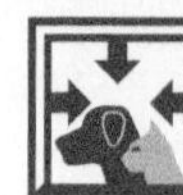

BASICS

DEFINITION

Second-degree atrioventricular (AV) block refers to failure of one or more P waves but not all P waves to be conducted. Mobitz type I second-degree AV block occurs when AV transmission is progressively delayed prior to a blocked P wave.

ECG Features

- PR interval—becomes progressively longer prior to the appearance of a P wave that is not followed by a QRS complex (Figure 1).
- Heart rate and QRS morphology—usually normal.
- Often cyclic.

PATHOPHYSIOLOGY

- Frequently associated with high resting vagal tone and sinus arrhythmia in dogs.
- Generally not pathologic or hemodynamically significant.
- This type of AV block usually results from conduction delay within the AV node itself (rather than delay in other segments of the AV conducting system) and is characterized by a progressive increase in AH interval, with eventual block between the A and H deflections on a His bundle recording.

SYSTEMS AFFECTED

Cardiovascular

GENETICS

N/A

INCIDENCE/PREVALENCE

Radiotelemetry studies have shown that this arrhythmia occurs in 64% of healthy adult dogs and 100% of healthy puppies 8–12 weeks of age.

GEOGRAPHIC DISTRIBUTION

N/A

SIGNALMENT

Species

Dog; uncommon in cat.

Breed Predilections

N/A

Mean Age and Range

- Usually occurs in young, otherwise healthy dogs as a manifestation of high vagal tone.
- Occasionally occurs in older dogs with abnormally strong vagal tone.
- Rarely noted in old dogs with degenerative conduction system disease.

SIGNS

Historical Findings

- Most animals are asymptomatic.
- If drug induced, owner may report signs of drug toxicity—anorexia, vomiting, and diarrhea with digoxin; weakness with calcium channel blockers or β-adrenergic antagonists.
- If heart rate is abnormally slow, syncope or weakness may occur.

Physical Examination Findings

- May be normal unless signs of more generalized myocardial disease or noncardiac disease are present.
- Intermittent pauses in the cardiac rhythm.
- First heart sound may become progressively softer, followed by a pause.
- An audible S4 may be heard unaccompanied by S1 and S2 when block occurs.

CAUSES

- Occasionally noted in normal animals.
- Enhanced vagal stimulation resulting from noncardiac diseases—usually accompanied by sinus arrhythmia, sinus arrest.
- Pharmacologic agents—digoxin, β-adrenergic antagonists, calcium channel blocking agents, propafenone, amiodarone, α_2-adrenergic agonists, opioids.

RISK FACTORS

Any condition or intervention that enhances vagal tone.

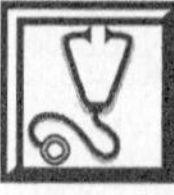

DIAGNOSIS

DIFFERENTIAL DIAGNOSIS

- Nonconducted P waves from supraventricular premature impulses or supraventricular tachycardias should be distinguished from second-degree AV block.
- Type II second-degree AV block (no variation in PR intervals).

CBC/BIOCHEMISTRY/URINALYSIS

Hypokalemia may predispose to AV conduction disturbances.

OTHER LABORATORY TESTS

Serum digoxin concentration—may be high.

IMAGING

N/A

DIAGNOSTIC PROCEDURES

- May be necessary to identify specific causes of enhanced vagal tone (e.g., upper airway disease, cervical and thoracic masses, gastrointestinal disorders, and high intraocular pressure).
- Atropine response test—administer 0.04 mg/kg atropine IM and repeat ECG in 20–30 minutes; may be used to determine whether AV block is due to vagal tone; resolution of AV block with atropine supports vagal cause.
- Electrophysiologic studies are generally unnecessary, but will confirm this type of second-degree AV block if surface ECG is equivocal.

PATHOLOGIC FINDINGS

Generally, no gross or histopathologic findings.

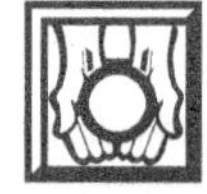

TREATMENT

APPROPRIATE HEALTH CARE

- Treatment usually unnecessary.
- Treat or remove underlying cause(s).

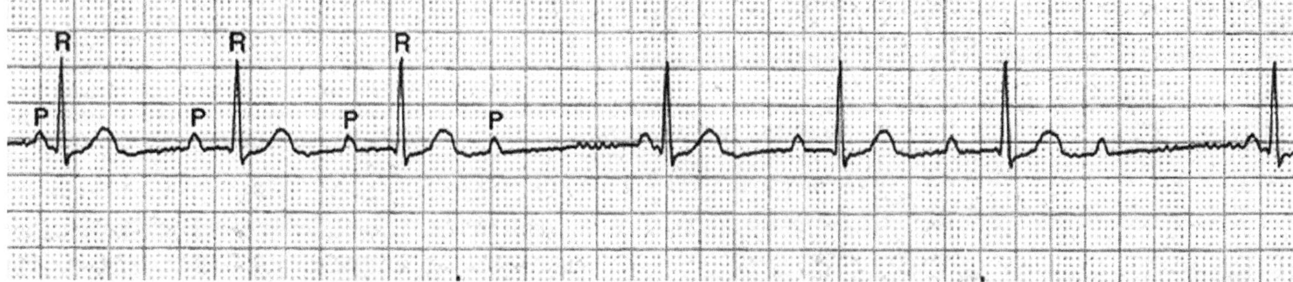

Figure 1.

Lead II ECG strip recorded from a dog with Mobitz type I, second-degree AV block. The PR intervals become progressively longer, with the longest PR intervals preceding nonconducted P waves (typical Wenckebach phenomenon) (paper speed = 50 mm/s).

NURSING CARE

Generally unnecessary.

ACTIVITY

Unrestricted

DIET

Modifications or restrictions only to manage an underlying condition.

CLIENT EDUCATION

Explain that any treatment is directed toward reversing or eliminating an underlying cause.

SURGICAL CONSIDERATIONS

N/A except to manage an underlying condition.

MEDICATIONS

DRUG(S) OF CHOICE

Only as needed to manage an underlying condition.

CONTRAINDICATIONS

Drugs with vagomimetic action (e.g., digoxin, bethanechol, physostigmine, pilocarpine) may potentiate block.

PRECAUTIONS

Hypokalemia increases the sensitivity to vagal tone and may potentiate AV conduction delay.

POSSIBLE INTERACTIONS

N/A

FOLLOW-UP

PATIENT MONITORING

Typically not necessary.

PREVENTION/AVOIDANCE

N/A

POSSIBLE COMPLICATIONS

N/A

MISCELLANEOUS

ASSOCIATED CONDITIONS

N/A

AGE-RELATED FACTORS

N/A

PREGNANCY/FERTILITY/BREEDING

N/A

SYNONYMS

- Wenckebach block.
- Wenckebach periodicity.
- Wenckebach phenomenon.

SEE ALSO

- Atrioventricular Block, Complete (Third Degree).
- Atrioventricular Block, First Degree.
- Atrioventricular Block, Second Degree—Mobitz Type II.

ABBREVIATIONS

- AV = atrioventricular.

Suggested Reading

Branch CE, Robertson BT, Williams JC. Frequency of second-degree atrioventricular heart block in dogs. Am J Vet Res 1975, 36:925–929.

Kittleson MD. Electrocardiography. In: Kittleson MD, Kienle RD, eds., Small Animal Cardiovascular Medicine. St. Louis, MO: Mosby, 1998, pp. 72–94.

Santilli R, Moïse NS, Pariaut R, Perego M. Electrocardiography of the Dog and Cat: Diagnosis of Arrhythmias, 2nd ed. Milan: Edra, 2018.

Tilley LP, Smith FWK Jr. Electrocardiography. In: Smith FWK, Tilley LP, Oyama M, Sleeper M, eds., Manual of Canine and Feline Cardiology, 5th ed. St. Louis, MO: Saunders Elsevier, 2016, pp. 49–76.

Willis R, Oliveira P, Mavropoulou A. Guide to Canine and Feline Electrocardiography. Ames, IA: Wiley-Blackwell, 2018.

Authors Francis W.K. Smith, Jr. and Larry P. Tilley

Consulting Editor Michael Aherne

Client Education Handout available online

A

ATRIOVENTRICULAR BLOCK, SECOND DEGREE—MOBITZ TYPE II

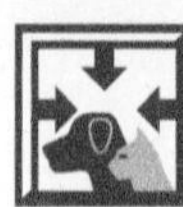

BASICS

DEFINITION

Second-degree atrioventricular (AV) block refers to failure of one or more P waves, but not all P waves, to be conducted. Mobitz type II second-degree AV block occurs when one or more P waves are blocked without a preceding progressive delay in AV transmission.

ECG Features

- One or more P waves not followed by a QRS complex; PR interval is constant, but may be either normal or consistently prolonged (Figure 1).
- Ventricular rate—usually slow.
- Fixed ratio of P waves to QRS complexes may occur (e.g., 2 : 1, 3 : 1, 4 : 1 AV block).
- High-grade (advanced) second-degree AV block is characterized by two or more consecutively blocked P waves.
- In second-degree AV block with a 2 : 1 conduction ratio or higher, it is impossible to observe prolongation of the PR interval before the block, so a designation of Mobitz type I vs. II is not appropriate.
- QRS complexes may appear normal, but may also be wide or have an abnormal morphology due to aberrant intraventricular conduction or ventricular enlargement.
- Abnormally wide QRS complexes may indicate serious, extensive cardiac disease.

PATHOPHYSIOLOGY

- Rare in healthy animals.
- May be hemodynamically important when ventricular rate is abnormally slow.
- May progress to complete AV block, particularly when accompanied by wide QRS complexes.
- Typically this type of AV block results from conduction delay within the AV node itself (rather than delay in another segment of the AV conducting system) that is characterized by normal or prolonged AH intervals, with intermittent block between A and H deflections on a His bundle electrogram.

SYSTEMS AFFECTED

- Cardiovascular.
- Central nervous or musculoskeletal systems if inadequate cardiac output.

GENETICS

May be heritable in pugs.

INCIDENCE/PREVALENCE

Unknown

GEOGRAPHIC DISTRIBUTION

N/A

SIGNALMENT

Species

Dog and cat.

Breed Predilections

American cocker spaniel, pug, dachshund, Airedale terrier, Doberman pinscher.

Mean Age and Range

Generally occurs in older animals.

Predominant Sex

N/A

SIGNS

Historical Findings

- Presenting complaint may be syncope, collapse, weakness, or lethargy.
- Some animals are asymptomatic.
- Animals may show signs of the underlying disease process if present.

Physical Examination Findings

- ± weakness.
- Bradycardia common.
- May be intermittent pauses in the cardiac rhythm.
- An S4 may be audible in lieu of the normally expected heart sounds (i.e., S1, S2) when the block occurs.
- If associated with digoxin intoxication, there may be vomiting, anorexia, and diarrhea.
- May be other abnormalities reflecting the underlying etiology.

CAUSES

- Heritable in pugs.
- Enhanced vagal stimulation from noncardiac diseases.
- Degenerative change within the cardiac conduction system—replacement of AV nodal cells and/or Purkinje fibers by fibrotic and adipose tissue in old cats and dogs.
- Pharmacologic agents (e.g., digoxin, β-adrenergic antagonists, calcium channel blocking agents, propafenone, α_2-adrenergic agonists, muscarinic cholinergic agonists, or severe procainamide or quinidine toxicity).
- Infiltrative myocardial disorders (neoplasia, amyloid).
- Endocarditis (particularly involving the aortic valve).
- Myocarditis (viral, bacterial, parasitic, idiopathic).
- Cardiomyopathy (especially in cats).
- Trauma.
- Atropine administered intravenously may cause a brief period of first- or second-degree heart block before increasing the heart rate.

RISK FACTORS

Any condition or intervention that enhances vagal tone.

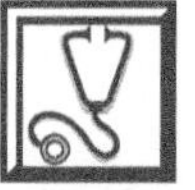

DIAGNOSIS

DIFFERENTIAL DIAGNOSIS

- High-grade (advanced) form must be distinguished from complete AV block.
- Nonconducted P waves arising from refractoriness of the conduction system during supraventricular tachycardias must be differentiated from pathologic conduction block.

CBC/BIOCHEMISTRY/URINALYSIS

- Serum electrolytes—hypokalemia and hyperkalemia may predispose to AV.
- Conduction disturbances.
- Leukocytosis—may be noted with bacterial endocarditis or myocarditis.
- Electrolyte abnormalities (e.g., severe hypokalemia, hyperkalemia, or hypercalcemia) may predispose to AV block.

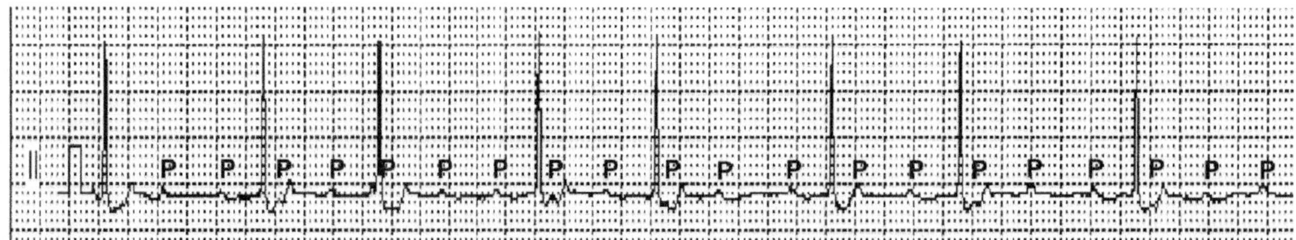

Figure 1.

Lead II ECG rhythm strip recorded from a dog with both first- and second-degree AV block. The second-degree AV block is high grade, with both 2 : 1 and 3 : 1 block resulting in variation in the RR intervals. The PR interval for the conducted beats is prolonged but constant (0.28 second) (paper speed = 25 mm/s).

OTHER LABORATORY TESTS

- Serum digoxin concentration—may be high.
- High thyroxine (T_4) in cats—if associated with hyperthyroidism.
- High arterial blood pressure—if associated with hypertensive heart disease.
- Positive *Borrelia*, *Rickettsia*, or *Trypanosoma cruzi* titers—if associated with one of these infectious agents.
- Blood cultures may be positive in patients with vegetative endocarditis.

IMAGING

Echocardiographic examination may reveal structural heart disease (e.g., endocarditis, neoplasia, or cardiomyopathy).

DIAGNOSTIC PROCEDURES

- Atropine response test—administer 0.04 mg/kg atropine IM and repeat ECG in 20–30 minutes; may be used to determine whether AV block is due to high vagal tone.
- Electrophysiologic testing is generally unnecessary, but can be done to confirm this type of AV block if surface ECG findings are equivocal.

PATHOLOGIC FINDINGS

- Variable—depend on underlying cause.
- Old animals with degenerative change of the conduction system may have focal mineralization of the interventricular septal crest visible grossly; chondroid metaplasia of the central fibrous body and increased fibrous connective tissue in the AV bundle is noted histopathologically.

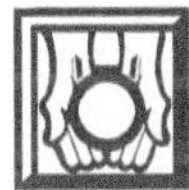

TREATMENT

APPROPRIATE HEALTH CARE

- Treatment—may be unnecessary if heart rate maintains adequate cardiac output.
- Positive dromotropic interventions are indicated for symptomatic patients.
- Treat or remove underlying cause(s).

NURSING CARE

Generally unnecessary.

ACTIVITY

Cage rest advised for symptomatic patients.

DIET

Modifications or restrictions only to manage an underlying condition.

CLIENT EDUCATION

- Need to seek and specifically treat underlying cause.
- Pharmacologic agents may not be effective long term.

SURGICAL CONSIDERATIONS

Permanent pacemaker may be required for long-term management of symptomatic patients.

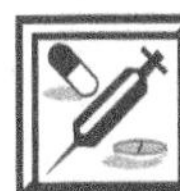

MEDICATIONS

DRUG(S) OF CHOICE

- Atropine (0.02–0.04 mg/kg IV/IM) or glycopyrrolate (5–10 µg/kg IV/IM) may be used short term if positive atropine response.
- Chronic anticholinergic therapy (propantheline 0.5–2 mg/kg PO q8–12h or hyoscyamine 3–6 µg/kg q8h)—indicated for symptomatic patients if improved AV conduction with atropine response test.
- Isoproterenol (0.04–0.09 µg/kg/min IV to effect) or dopamine (2–5 µg/kg/min IV to effect) may be administered in acute, life-threatening situations to enhance AV conduction and/or accelerate an escape focus.

CONTRAINDICATIONS

- Drugs with vagomimetic action (e.g., digoxin, bethanechol, physostigmine, pilocarpine) may potentiate block.
- Avoid drugs likely to impair impulse conduction further or depress a ventricular escape focus (e.g., procainamide, quinidine, lidocaine, calcium channel blocking agents, β-adrenergic blocking agents).

PRECAUTIONS

Hypokalemia—increases sensitivity to vagal tone and may potentiate AV conduction delay.

POSSIBLE INTERACTIONS

N/A

ALTERNATIVE DRUG(S)

N/A

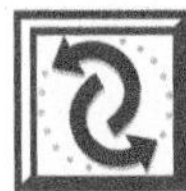

FOLLOW-UP

PATIENT MONITORING

Periodic ECG because risk of progression to complete (third-degree) AV block.

PREVENTION/AVOIDANCE

N/A

POSSIBLE COMPLICATIONS

Prolonged bradycardia may cause secondary congestive heart failure or inadequate renal perfusion.

EXPECTED COURSE AND PROGNOSIS

Variable—depends on cause. If degenerative disease of the cardiac conduction system, often progresses to complete (third-degree) AV block.

MISCELLANEOUS

ASSOCIATED CONDITIONS

May be noted in cats with primary or secondary myocardial disease.

AGE-RELATED FACTORS

N/A

ZOONOTIC POTENTIAL

N/A

PREGNANCY/FERTILITY/BREEDING

N/A

SEE ALSO

- Atrioventricular Block, Complete (Third Degree).
- Atrioventricular Block, Second Degree—Mobitz Type I.

ABBREVIATIONS

- AV = atrioventricular.
- T_4 = thyroxine.

Suggested Reading

Kittleson MD. Electrocardiography. In: Kittleson MD, Kienle RD, eds., Small Animal Cardiovascular Medicine. St. Louis, MO: Mosby, 1998, pp. 72–94.

Santilli R, Moise NS, Pariaut R, Perego M. Electrocardiography of the Dog and Cat: Diagnosis of Arrhythmias, 2nd ed. Milan: Edra, 2018.

Tilley LP, Smith FWK Jr. Electrocardiography. In: Smith FWK, Tilley LP, Oyama M, Sleeper M, eds., Manual of Canine and Feline Cardiology, 5th ed. St. Louis, MO: Saunders Elsevier, 2016, pp. 49–76.

Willis R, Oliveira P, Mavropoulou A. Guide to Canine and Feline Electrocardiography. Ames, IA: Wiley-Blackwell, 2018.

Authors Larry P. Tilley and Francis W.K. Smith, Jr.

Consulting Editors Michael Aherne

Client Education Handout available online

ATRIOVENTRICULAR VALVE DYSPLASIA

BASICS

DEFINITION

A congenital malformation of the mitral or tricuspid valve apparatus.

PATHOPHYSIOLOGY

• Atrioventricular valve dysplasia (AVVD) can result in valvular insufficiency, valvular stenosis, or dynamic outflow tract obstruction, depending on the anatomic abnormality. AVVD may occur alone or in association with abnormalities of the ipsilateral outflow tract (e.g., valvular or subvalvular aortic or pulmonic stenosis). It is not uncommon for mitral and tricuspid valve dysplasia to occur together in the same patient.
• Valvular insufficiency results in ipsilateral atrial dilation, eccentric hypertrophy of the associated ventricle, and, if severe, signs of congestive heart failure (CHF). Cardiomyopathy of chronic volume overload and elevated atrial pressures are the end result, culminating in pulmonary congestion (with mitral valve dysplasia [MVD]) or systemic congestion (with tricuspid valve dysplasia [TVD]).
• Valvular stenosis results in atrial dilation and hypertrophy and, if severe, hypoplasia of the receiving ventricle. The end result is atrial pressure elevation, also resulting in pulmonary congestion (mitral stenosis) or systemic congestion (tricuspid stenosis). Right-to-left shunting may occur in cases of tricuspid stenosis if there is an atrial septal defect or patent foramen ovale. Pulmonary hypertension is a common complication in animals with mitral valve stenosis.
• Dynamic outflow tract obstruction may occur in patients with MVD, with resultant concentric left ventricular (LV) hypertrophy that is proportional to the severity of the obstruction.
• Ebstein's anomaly is a rare form of TVD, characterized by apical displacement of the basal tricuspid leaflet attachments and resultant right atrial (RA) enlargement, with a small right ventricle ("atrialized" right ventricle). It can be accompanied by varying degrees of insufficiency or stenosis.

SYSTEMS AFFECTED

• Cardiovascular—chronic volume overload from valvular insufficiency and/or inflow obstruction due to valvular stenosis result in elevated pulmonary (MVD) or systemic (TVD) venous pressures.
• Respiratory—pulmonary edema may develop secondary to MVD; pulmonary hypertension is a common complication in animals with mitral stenosis.
• Neurologic—collapse and/or loss of consciousness, most often with exercise, may occur with severe disease due to low cardiac output/hypotension or ventricular arrhythmias in cases with severe dynamic outflow obstruction.

GENETICS

TVD appears to be inherited as an autosomal recessive trait in dogues de Bordeaux and an autosomal dominant with incomplete penetrance trait in Labrador retrievers.

INCIDENCE/PREVALENCE

These are common congenital cardiac anomalies in cats (17% of reported congenital cardiac defects in one study). Mitral valve malformations often are noted in cats with hypertrophic cardiomyopathy. Less frequently diagnosed in dogs.

SIGNALMENT

Species

Dog and cat.

Breed Predilections

• TVD—increased risk for Labrador retriever, German shepherd dog, great Pyrenees, possibly Old English sheepdog; also common in cats.
• MVD—increased risk in bull terrier, Newfoundland, Labrador retriever, Great Dane, golden retriever, Dalmatian, and Siamese cat.

Mean Age and Range

Variable; signs most often manifest within the first few years after birth.

Predominant Sex

Males are more likely to experience CHF.

SIGNS

Historical Findings

• Exercise intolerance.
• Abdominal distention, weight loss, and stunting may be observed with severe TVD.
• Labored respiration common with severe MVD.
• Syncope and collapse if critical atrioventricular (AV) valve stenosis, severe outflow tract obstruction, associated arrhythmias, or CHF.

Physical Examination Findings

• A holosystolic murmur is heard over the ipsilateral cardiac apex. In severe cases the murmur is accompanied by a thrill or gallop heart sounds. In animals with valvular stenosis, a soft diastolic murmur may be present in the same location, but many have no audible murmur. A labile systolic ejection murmur may be audible in animals with dynamic outflow tract obstruction. Silent tricuspid regurgitation is well documented in cats with a large regurgitant orifice and laminar regurgitant flow.
• Jugular venous distension/pulsation may be evident in patients with TVD.
• Evidence of left CHF (tachypnea, dyspnea, pulmonary crackles, cyanosis) in animals with severe MVD.
• Evidence of right CHF (ascites, peripheral edema) with severe TVD.

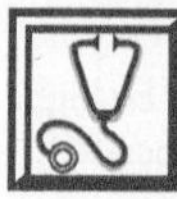

DIAGNOSIS

DIFFERENTIAL DIAGNOSIS

• Except for age of onset, congenital AV valve insufficiency resembles acquired degenerative AV valve insufficiency with regard to history, physical examination findings, and clinical sequelae.
• The right-sided murmur of tricuspid insufficiency may be confused with the right-sided murmur of a ventricular septal defect.
• Ascites caused by silent tricuspid regurgitation or tricuspid valve stenosis is often attributed to pericardial effusion, hepatic disease, or caudal vena caval obstruction.
• Dogs and cats with cor triatriatum share many of the clinical features of AV valve stenosis.
• There is no certain way to distinguish outflow tract obstruction due to MVD and obstructive hypertrophic cardiomyopathy. If the obstruction can be abolished with adrenergic beta blockers and LV hypertrophy resolves, it is likely that the primary abnormality was MVD.

IMAGING

Radiographic Findings

• Ipsilateral atrial and ventricular enlargement with valvular insufficiency. Isolated atrial enlargement with valvular stenosis. Mild left atrial (LA) enlargement with dynamic LV outflow obstruction. Cardiac silhouette may appear globoid with pronounced enlargement in cases of severe TVD.
• Evidence of left CHF—distended pulmonary veins, interstitial or alveolar edema in severe MVD.
• Evidence of right CHF—dilated caudal vena cava, hepatosplenomegaly, or ascites in severe TVD.

Echocardiography

• Valvular insufficiency results in ipsilateral atrial dilation and eccentric ventricular hypertrophy. Doppler echocardiography demonstrates a high velocity retrograde systolic jet and modestly increased transmitral or transtricuspid inflow velocities.
• Valvular stenosis results in ipsilateral atrial dilation, while the associated ventricular dimensions are normal or small. Valve leaflets are often thickened, relatively immobile, and fused. Doppler echocardiography demonstrates a high-velocity transmitral or transtricuspid diastolic jet with a reduced EF slope. There may also be evidence of concurrent AV valvular insufficiency, secondary pulmonary hypertension (in cases of mitral stenosis), or right-to-left shunting across a patent foramen ovale or associated atrial septal defect (in cases of tricuspid stenosis).

• With MVD, the LV papillary muscles are typically flattened and displaced dorsally. Chordae tendineae are often short and thickened. With TVD, papillary muscles and chordae tendineae may be fused, creating a curtain-like appearance of the tricuspid valve.
• Dynamic LV outflow obstruction in patients with MVD is characterized by systolic motion of the anterior mitral leaflet toward the interventricular septum, increased LV outflow tract velocities, eccentric mitral regurgitation, and concentric LV hypertrophy.

Cardiac Catheterization

• Indicated only for cases in which diagnosis cannot be confirmed by echocardiography or if surgical correction anticipated.
• Hemodynamic measurements should include ipsilateral atrial and ventricular pressures. Additional measurements in cases of MVD include pulmonary capillary wedge pressure (in lieu of direct LA pressure measurement), pulmonary artery pressures, and, in cases of dynamic obstruction, simultaneous aortic and LV pressure recording with medical provocation. Contrast studies are best performed with ventricular injection in cases of valvular insufficiency, and direct atrial injection in cases of valvular stenosis.

DIAGNOSTIC PROCEDURES

ECG

• Findings usually reflect pattern of chamber enlargement.
• Severe defects may be accompanied by arrhythmias, particularly atrial premature beats, supraventricular tachycardia, or atrial fibrillation.

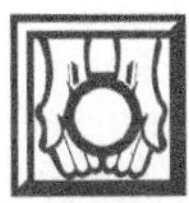

TREATMENT

APPROPRIATE HEALTH CARE

Inpatient treatment required for CHF.

DIET

Sodium restricted if overt or pending CHF.

CLIENT EDUCATION

Owners should be informed of heritability and advised against breeding.

SURGICAL CONSIDERATIONS

• Valve repair or replacement is available in a few centers.
• Balloon valvuloplasty is sometimes effective for valvular stenosis.

MEDICATIONS

DRUG(S) OF CHOICE

• For patients with CHF, furosemide (1–4 mg/kg q12–24h) and enalapril (0.5 mg/kg q12h) are used to control congestion, with the addition of pimobendan (0.3 mg/kg q12h) in cases of valvular insufficiency.
• Supraventricular tachyarrhythmias may be managed using digoxin (2–4 µg/kg q12h), a calcium channel blocker such as diltiazem (1–1.5 mg/kg q8h), or a beta blocker such as atenolol (0.5–1.5 mg/kg q12–24h). Heart rate should be maintained below 150 bpm.
• For dynamic outflow tract obstruction, beta blockers such as atenolol (0.5–1.5 mg/kg q12–24h) may be used to abolish or diminish severity of outflow obstruction; however, benefit has not been proven.

PRECAUTIONS

Standard patient monitoring for cardiac medication side effects (e.g., digitalis toxicity, azotemia).

FOLLOW-UP

PATIENT MONITORING

• Recheck yearly if no signs of CHF.
• Recheck every 3 months if signs of CHF (consider thoracic radiographs, ECG, and echocardiography).

PREVENTION/AVOIDANCE

Do not breed affected animals.

POSSIBLE COMPLICATIONS

• CHF—left-sided with MVD; right-sided with TVD.
• Collapse or syncope with exercise.
• Paroxysmal supraventricular tachycardia or atrial fibrillation with severe disease.

EXPECTED COURSE AND PROGNOSIS

• Depends on severity of underlying defect.
• Guarded to poor with serious defects.

MISCELLANEOUS

ASSOCIATED CONDITIONS

• MVD commonly accompanies valvular or subvalvular aortic stenosis as well as TVD.
• TVD commonly accompanies pulmonic stenosis as well as MVD.

PREGNANCY/FERTILITY/BREEDING

Breeding should be avoided—heritable defect and possibility of causing decompensated or worsening CHF.

SEE ALSO

• Congestive Heart Failure, Left-Sided.
• Congestive Heart Failure, Right-Sided.

ABBREVIATIONS

• AV = atrioventricular.
• AVVD = atrioventricular valve dysplasia.
• CHF = congestive heart failure.
• LA = left atrial.
• LV = left ventricular.
• MVD = mitral valve dysplasia.
• RA = right atrial.
• TVD = tricuspid valve dysplasia.

Suggested Reading

Bonagura JD, Lehmkuhl LB. Congenital heart disease. In: Fox PR, Sisson D, Moise NS. Textbook of Canine and Feline Cardiology: Principles and Clinical Practice, 2nd ed. Philadelphia, PA: Saunders, 1999, pp. 520–526.

Oyama MA, Sisson DD, Thomas WP, Bonagura JD. Congenital heart disease. In: Ettinger SJ, Feldman EC, eds., Textbook of Veterinary Internal Medicine, 7th ed. St. Louis, MO: Elsevier, 2010, pp. 1250–1298.

Strickland KN, Oyama MA. Congenital heart disease. In: Tilley LP, Smith FWK, Oyama MA, Sleeper MM, eds., Manual of Canine and Feline Cardiology, 5th ed. St. Louis, MO: Saunders Elsevier, 2016, pp. 218–238.

Author Michael Aherne

Consulting Editor Michael Aherne

Acknowledgment The author and book editors acknowledge the prior contribution of David D. Sisson.

Client Education Handout available online

A

ATRIOVENTRICULAR VALVULAR STENOSIS

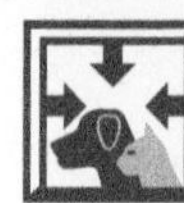

BASICS

DEFINITION

Atrioventricular (AV) valvular stenosis is a pathologic narrowing of the mitral or tricuspid valve orifice or the presence of an obstructive, supravalvular ring.

PATHOPHYSIOLOGY

- AV stenosis increases the resistance to ventricular filling.
- Ventricular filling in clinically significant disease requires a persistent diastolic pressure gradient between atrium and ventricle.
- Concomitant valvular regurgitation is common.
- The increased atrial pressure leads to atrial dilation, venous congestion, and often to congestive heart failure (CHF). Pulmonary edema occurs with mitral stenosis (MS); whereas ascites, pleural effusion, and chylothorax can develop in cases of severe tricuspid stenosis (TS).
- The foramen ovale can remain patent (PFO) in patients with TS, allowing right-to-left shunting with signs of cyanotic heart disease.
- Partial AV septal defect (primum atrial septal defect [ASD] and abnormal AV valve) is observed in some cats with supravalvular mitral (ring) stenosis.
- Cardiac output and therefore exercise capacity are limited.
- The atrial pressure increases disproportionally with faster heart rates, thereby creating the risk for "flash" pulmonary edema in dogs or cats with MS.
- Development of atrial tachyarrhythmias, especially atrial fibrillation (AF), is associated with cardiac decompensation.
- Pulmonary hypertension (PH) can develop consequent to MS, leading to exercise intolerance and right ventricular hypertrophy. This can be severe, especially in cats.

SYSTEMS AFFECTED

- Respiratory—with MS: bronchial compression from enlarged left atrium, pulmonary edema from left heart failure; potential for hemoptysis due to rupture of pulmonary venous–bronchial venous connections; pleural effusion with atelectasis in TS or in long-standing MS complicated by PH or AF.
- Hepatobiliary—with TS: hepatic congestion, ascites.

GENETICS

- Uncertain in most cases.
- Tricuspid valve dysplasia in Labrador retrievers has been localized to a defect in dog chromosome 9, inherited as an autosomal dominant trait with reduced penetrance. In dogue de Bordeaux, tricuspid valve dysplasia has been identified as an autosomal recessive trait.

INCIDENCE/PREVALENCE

Rare

GEOGRAPHIC DISTRIBUTION

Worldwide

SIGNALMENT

Species

Dog and cat.

Breed Predilections

- MS is overrepresented in bull terriers and Newfoundlands, and in Siamese cats.
- TS has been reported most often in Old English sheepdogs and Labrador retrievers.

Mean Age and Range

Most patients are presented at a young age, although exceptions occur, especially in cats.

Predominant Sex

N/A

SIGNS

Historical Findings

- Exercise intolerance.
- Syncope.
- Exertional dyspnea or tachypnea.
- Cough—MS.
- Cyanosis.
- Abdominal distention—TS.
- Acute posterior paresis—cats with MS and arterial thromboembolism.
- Stunted growth.
- Hemoptysis from rupture of intrapulmonary vessels—MS.

Physical Examination Findings

- Soft diastolic murmur with point of maximal intensity over left apex (MS) or right hemithorax (TS).
- Holosystolic murmur of mitral or tricuspid regurgitation is more often detected.
- Tachypnea, dyspnea from pulmonary edema or pleural effusion.
- Crackles from pulmonary edema.
- Jugular distention, jugular pulses, ascites, hepatomegaly with TS, or biventricular CHF associated with pulmonary hypertension and AF in chronic MS.
- Cyanosis from right-to-left shunting with TS and PFO or from pulmonary edema with MS.

CAUSES

- Usually due to congenital dysplasia of mitral or tricuspid valve.
- Supravalvular obstructing rings of tissue have been associated with AV stenosis; this is especially important in cats.
- Infective endocarditis, intracardiac neoplasia, and hypertrophic cardiomyopathy with scarring are rare causes of acquired AV valve stenosis.
- Acquired TS has been observed due to fibrous scarring of the tricuspid valve in dogs with transvenous pacing leads.

RISK FACTORS

Breed predispositions (see above); see Risk Factors for Endocarditis, Infective; permanent transvenous pacing.

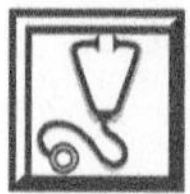

DIAGNOSIS

DIFFERENTIAL DIAGNOSIS

AV valvular stenosis must be differentiated from the more common causes of mitral and tricuspid regurgitation in the absence of stenosis. These include both congenital and acquired lesions of the AV valves and support apparatus. Cor triatriatum dexter, cor triatriatum sinister and double outlet right atrium can mimic some of the clinical findings of pure tricuspid and mitral valvular stenosis, respectively.

CBC/BIOCHEMISTRY/URINALYSIS

May be normal or reflect changes related to CHF or drug therapy for CHF.

IMAGING

Thoracic Radiography

- Atrial enlargement is the most common and outstanding feature; may see generalized cardiomegaly, especially with AV valve regurgitation.
- MS—may see pulmonary venous congestion and pulmonary edema; intrapulmonary hemorrhage can be misinterpreted as pneumonia or another parenchymal disease.
- TS—may see hepatomegaly; increased diameter of caudal vena cava.

Echocardiography

- Diagnostic test of choice.
- Two-dimensional echocardiography reveals a markedly dilated atrium and attenuated valve excursion during diastole, often with thickened, irregular AV valve leaflets; valve leaflets may appear to "dome" during diastole (see Web Video 1). A supravalvular obstructing ring also may be evident, as well as other lesions (see Causes).
- Color-flow imaging reveals a turbulent diastolic jet that originates proximal to the stenotic valve and projects toward the apex of the ventricle (see Web Video 2); AV valve regurgitation is often present (see Web Videos 3 and 4). Concurrent defects may also be noted, such as PFO, ASD, or bridging septal leaflet (see Web Video 5).
- M-mode studies show an enlarged atrium and concordant motion of the AV valve leaflets, indicating commissural fusion (see Web Figure 1); the E-to-F slope is decreased.
- Spectral Doppler studies show increased diastolic transvalvular flow velocities; prolonged calculated pressure half-time is a hallmark feature; E-wave/A-wave amplitude reversal is often evident in cases still in normal sinus rhythm (see Web Figures 2, 3, 4).

• Right-sided chamber enlargement in MS with pulmonary hypertension or with chronic AF (see Web Figure 4).

Angiography

• Right atrium—injection demonstrates markedly dilated atrium in TS; with concurrent PFO or ASD, opacification of the left atrium is also observed following right atrial injection.
• Might visualize thickened, irregular valve leaflets or a stenotic valve funnel.
• Ventricular injection often reveals valvular regurgitation.
• There can be delayed opacification of the ventricles and great vessels.

Cardiac Catheterization

• A diastolic pressure gradient is identified between atrium and ventricle. A large "A" wave is common if atrial function is preserved.
• High left atrial, pulmonary capillary wedge, and pulmonary artery pressures occur in MS.
• High right atrial and central venous pressures are present in TS.
• Ventricular pressure may be normal in the absence of concurrent defects.

DIAGNOSTIC PROCEDURES

ECG

• Variable enlargement and ventricular conduction patterns are observed. Widened or tall P-waves are commonly observed.
• Splintered R-waves are present in some dogs with tricuspid dysplasia.
• Axis deviation due to hypertrophy or ventricular conduction disturbances is relatively common in cats with mitral valve malformation.
• Ectopic rhythms, especially of atrial origin, are often observed. AF is the most important rhythm disturbance as atrial contribution to filling is lost and the R-to-R intervals vary with short cycles, increasing the mean diastolic gradient.

PATHOLOGIC FINDINGS

• The AV valve is abnormal, with thickened leaflets and fused commissures. Other lesions may be identified such as a supramitral ring (see Causes).
• Many cases also have abnormal chordae tendineae and papillary muscles.
• Atrial dilation and hypertrophy are common.
• PFO with TS or partial AV septal defect (primum ASD and bridging septal leaflet) with supravalvular mitral (ring) stenosis.

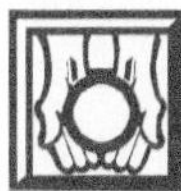

TREATMENT

APPROPRIATE HEALTH CARE

• Patients in overt CHF should be treated with inpatient medical management.
• Surgical or catheter-based interventions can be considered once heart failure has been stabilized.
• Control of heart rhythm disturbances, especially AF, is also important.
• These patients are typically complicated and consultation with a cardiologist is highly recommended.
• Electrocardioversion of AF should be considered, but advanced atrial disease can render the procedure less effective or limit the duration of sinus rhythm.

NURSING CARE

• Sedation with butorphanol is appropriate for dyspneic patients.
• Oxygen therapy should be administered to patients with dyspnea or hypoxemia from left-sided CHF.
• Fluid therapy is typically contraindicated in patients with overt CHF, except in cases of moderate to severe azotemia, renal compromise, or severe dehydration. Therapeutic paracentesis may be considered in patients with pleural effusion or tympanic ascites.

ACTIVITY

Exercise restriction is important to recommend for any animal with this condition, because tachycardia increases the mean gradient across the stenotic valve, predisposing to pulmonary edema or venous congestion (see Web Figures 3 and 4). Cage rest is ideal for patients with CHF.

DIET

Feed a sodium-restricted diet to patients in CHF.

CLIENT EDUCATION

Clients must be advised of symptoms associated with CHF and the urgency of treatment, particularly with left-sided CHF. Likelihood of recurrent bouts of CHF should also be discussed.

SURGICAL CONSIDERATIONS

• Surgical valve replacement or repair requires cardiopulmonary bypass or hypothermia; cost, availability, and high complication and mortality rates are greatly limiting factors.
• Balloon valvuloplasty is an alternative referral treatment and has been used successfully for managing some cases of AV stenosis.

MEDICATIONS

DRUG(S) OF CHOICE

CHF

• Diuretic—Furosemide: dogs, 2–4 mg/kg IV/IM/SC/PO q8–24h; cats, 1–4 mg/kg IV/IM/SC/PO q8–24h. Torsemide: dogs, 0.2–0.5 mg/kg PO q12–24h; cats, 1.25 mg PO q12–48h.
• Angiotensin-converting enzyme (ACE) inhibitor—enalapril or benazepril: dogs, 0.25–0.5 mg/kg PO q12h; cats, 0.25–0.5 mg/kg PO q12–24h; see Follow-Up for patient monitoring.
• Nitroglycerin paste (1/4 to 1 inch topically q12h) to reduce pulmonary venous pressures, but this has not been evaluated critically.

Atrial Tachyarrhythmias

• Digoxin—dogs, 3–5 µg/kg PO q12h; cats, one-fourth of a 0.125 mg tablet PO q24–48h; adjust dosage based on serum concentrations.
• Beta blockers such as atenolol or the calcium channel blocker diltiazem for suppression of frequent atrial premature complexes and for heart rate control in atrial tachyarrhythmias such as atrial tachycardia/flutter/fibrillation. Beware when using these drugs in uncontrolled CHF.
• Typical atenolol dosages—dogs, 0.25–1.0 mg/kg q12h; cats, 6.25–12.5 mg/cat q12–24h; start low and titrate to effect.
• Diltiazem dosages—dogs, 2–6 mg/kg daily in two (long-acting diltiazem) or three divided dosages; start low and titrate to effect; cats, 7.5 mg diltiazem HCl PO q8h. Higher dosages are sometimes needed.
• Sotalol for intractable/recurrent arrhythmias—dogs, 1–2.5 mg/kg PO q12h; cats, 10–20 mg/cat q12h.
• Dogs can be referred for electrocardioversion to convert AF to sinus rhythm (with follow-up therapy with sotalol or amiodarone); however, reversion to AF is common owing to marked atrial dilatation.

Pulmonary Hypertension

• Sildenafil—dogs, 0.5–3 mg/kg PO q8–12 hours.

CONTRAINDICATIONS

Primary afterload reducers such as hydralazine or amlodipine should be avoided in treatment of heart failure from pure MS due to risk of hypotension.

PRECAUTIONS

• As a general rule, pimobendan is relatively contraindicated in pure valvular stenosis; however, many dogs and cats with advanced CHF have been treated with this drug with apparent success, especially when there is combined stenosis/regurgitation of the valve.
• Use ACE inhibitors or other vasodilators judiciously in patients with CHF; cardiac output is limited and vasodilation may induce hypotension. Monitor arterial blood pressure and renal function.

POSSIBLE INTERACTIONS

• Furosemide and ACE inhibitors can affect kidney function, alter blood electrolytes, and reduce blood pressure; these parameters should be monitored.

A

ATRIOVENTRICULAR VALVULAR STENOSIS (CONTINUED)

• Sildenafil can also reduce systemic blood pressure and should not be used with nitroglycerin paste or other nitrates.

ALTERNATIVE DRUG(S)

Spironolactone (2 mg/kg PO q12–24h) should be considered as an ancillary diuretic and for its antifibrotic benefit (as an aldosterone antagonist).

FOLLOW-UP

PATIENT MONITORING

• Thoracic radiographs for pulmonary edema or pleural effusion.
• Echocardiography with Doppler studies—to estimate pulmonary pressures and subjectively assess right heart function if on sildenafil.
• Digoxin level—check 7–10 days following institution of therapy; 8- to 12-hour trough should be 0.8–1.5 ng/mL.
• Renal function, electrolyte status, and arterial blood pressure when on diuretic and/or ACE inhibitor.
• Standard rhythm ECG or Holter (ambulatory ECG) if arrhythmias are present.

POSSIBLE COMPLICATIONS

• CHF.
• Atrial fibrillation.
• Syncope.
• Arterial thromboembolism—cats with MS.
• Pulmonary hemorrhage with MS.

EXPECTED COURSE AND PROGNOSIS

• Morbidity is high; except for mild cases, prognosis is generally poor once an animal becomes symptomatic. However, some animals will live for many years even with relatively severe stenosis of the mitral or tricuspid valve.
• Surgical intervention or balloon valvuloplasty might alter course of disease, but data are limited.

MISCELLANEOUS

ASSOCIATED CONDITIONS

Concurrent congenital defects are common, e.g., subaortic stenosis in MS, PFO in TS, primum ASD in cats with supravalvular mitral (ring) stenosis.

PREGNANCY/FERTILITY/BREEDING

The possibility that this may be a heritable defect must be considered in assessing suitability of the animal for breeding, particularly in breeds with a predilection for this defect. The additional hemodynamic burden of gestation may be poorly tolerated by an already compromised heart. In general, breeding is strongly discouraged.

SYNONYMS

• AV dysplasia with stenosis.
• Supravalvular mitral ring.

SEE ALSO

• Atrioventricular Valve Dysplasia.
• Endocarditis, Infective.

ABBREVIATIONS

• ACE = angiotensin-converting enzyme.
• AF = atrial fibrillation.
• ASD = atrial septal defect.
• AV = atrioventricular.
• CHF = congestive heart failure.
• MS = mitral stenosis.
• PFO = patent foramen ovale.
• PH = pulmonary hypertension.
• TS = tricuspid stenosis.

Suggested Reading

Arndt JW, Oyama MA. Balloon valvuloplasty of congenital mitral stenosis. J Vet Cardiol 2013, 15:147–151.

Brown WA, Thomas WP. Balloon valvuloplasty of tricuspid stenosis in a Labrador retriever. J Vet Intern Med 1995, 9:419–424.

Campbell FE, Thomas WP. Congenital supravalvular mitral stenosis in 14 cats. J Vet Cardiol 2012, 14:281–292.

Lehmkuhl LB, Ware WA, Bonagura JD. Mitral stenosis in 15 dogs. J Vet Intern Med 1994, 8:2–17.

Stamoulis ME, Fox PR. Mitral valve stenosis in three cats. J Small Anim Pract 1993, 34:452–456.

Authors Lora S. Hitchcock and John D. Bonagura

Consulting Editor Michael Aherne

AZOTEMIA AND UREMIA

BASICS

DEFINITION

- Azotemia is an excess of urea, creatinine, or other nonprotein nitrogenous substances in blood, plasma, or serum.
- Uremia is the polysystemic toxic syndrome resulting from marked loss in kidney functions. Uremia occurs simultaneously in animals with increased quantities of urine constituents in blood (azotemia), but azotemia may occur in the absence of uremia.

PATHOPHYSIOLOGY

- Azotemia can be caused by (1) increased production of nonprotein nitrogenous substances, (2) decreased glomerular filtration rate (GFR), or (3) reabsorption of urine that has escaped from the urinary tract into the bloodstream. High production of nonprotein nitrogenous waste substances may result from high intake of protein (diet or gastrointestinal bleeding) or accelerated catabolism of endogenous proteins. GFR may decline because of reduced renal perfusion (prerenal azotemia), acute or chronic kidney disease (renal azotemia), or urinary obstruction (postrenal azotemia). Reabsorption of urine into the systemic circulation may also result from leakage of urine from the excretory pathways (also a form of postrenal azotemia).
- Pathophysiology of uremia—incompletely understood; may be related to (1) metabolic and toxic systemic effects of waste products retained because of renal excretory failure, (2) deranged renal regulation of fluid, electrolytes, and acid-base balance, and (3) impaired renal production and degradation of hormones and other substances (e.g., erythropoietin and 1,25-dihydroxycholecalciferol).

SYSTEMS AFFECTED

- Uremia affects all body systems.
- Cardiovascular—arterial hypertension, left ventricular hypertrophy, heart murmur, cardiomegaly, cardiac rhythm disturbances.
- Endocrine/metabolic—renal secondary hyperparathyroidism, inadequate production of calcitriol and erythropoietin, hypergastrinemia, weight loss.
- Gastrointestinal—anorexia, nausea, vomiting, diarrhea, uremic stomatitis, xerostomia, uremic breath, constipation.
- Hemic/lymph/immune—anemia and immunodeficiency.
- Neuromuscular—dullness, lethargy, fatigue, irritability, tremors, gait imbalance, flaccid muscle weakness, myoclonus, behavioral changes, dementia, isolated cranial nerve deficits, seizures, stupor, coma, impaired thermoregulation (hypothermia).
- Ophthalmic—scleral and conjunctival injection, retinopathy, acute-onset blindness.
- Respiratory—dyspnea.
- Skin/exocrine—pallor, bruising, increased shedding, unkempt appearance, loss of normal sheen to coat.

SIGNALMENT

Dog and cat.

SIGNS

General Comments

Azotemia may not be associated with historical or physical abnormalities. Unless patient has uremia, clinical findings are limited to disease responsible for azotemia.

Historical Findings

- Weight loss.
- Declining appetite or anorexia.
- Depression.
- Fatigue.
- Weakness.
- Vomiting.
- Diarrhea.
- Halitosis.
- Constipation.
- Polyuria.
- Changes in urine volume.
- Poor haircoat or unkempt appearance.

Physical Examination Findings

- Muscle wasting/sarcopenia/cachexia.
- Mental depression.
- Dehydration.
- Weakness.
- Pallor.
- Petechiae and ecchymoses.
- Dull and unkempt haircoat.
- Uremic breath.
- Uremic stomatitis (including oral ulcers, infarctions of the tongue).
- Scleral and conjunctival injection.
- Relative hypothermia.

CAUSES

Prerenal Azotemia

- Reduced renal perfusion due to low blood volume or low blood pressure.
- Accelerated production of nitrogenous waste products because of enhanced catabolism of tissues in association with infection, fever, trauma, corticosteroid excess, or burns.
- Increased gastrointestinal digestion and absorption of protein sources (diet or gastrointestinal hemorrhage).

Renal Azotemia

Acute or chronic kidney diseases (primary kidney disease affecting glomeruli, renal tubules, renal interstitium, and/or renal vasculature) that impair at least 75% of kidney function (GFR).

Postrenal Azotemia

Urinary obstruction; rupture of excretory pathway.

RISK FACTORS

- Medical conditions—kidney disease, hypoadrenocorticism, low cardiac output, hypotension, fever, sepsis, liver disease, pyometra, hypoalbuminemia, dehydration, acidosis, exposure to nephrotoxic chemicals, gastrointestinal hemorrhage, urolithiasis, urethral plugs in cats, urethral trauma, and neoplasia.
- Advanced age may be a risk factor.
- Drugs—potentially nephrotoxic drugs, nonsteroidal anti-inflammatory drugs, diuretics, antihypertensive medications; failure to adjust dosage of drugs primarily eliminated by the kidneys to correspond with decline in renal function.
- Toxins—ethylene glycol, grapes (dogs), lilies (cats).

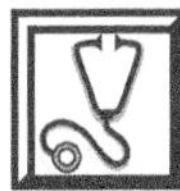

DIAGNOSIS

DIFFERENTIAL DIAGNOSIS

- Dehydration, poor peripheral perfusion, low cardiac output, history of recent fluid loss, high-protein diet—rule out prerenal azotemia.
- Recent onset of altered urine output (high or low), clinical signs consistent with uremia, exposure to possible nephrotoxicants or ischemic renal injury, or kidney size normal or enlarged—rule out acute kidney injury (AKI).
- Progressive weight loss, polyuria, polydipsia, small kidneys, disparate kidney size (cats—big kidney and little kidney), pallor, and signs of uremia that have developed over several weeks to months—rule out chronic kidney disease (CKD).
- Abrupt decline in urine output and onset of signs of uremia; disparate kidney size, dysuria, stranguria, and hematuria; large urinary bladder or fluid-filled abdomen—rule out postrenal azotemia.

CBC/BIOCHEMISTRY/URINALYSIS

CBC

- Nonregenerative anemia (normocytic, normochromic)—often present with CKD.
- Hemoconcentration—often present with prerenal azotemia; can also be seen with AKI and postrenal azotemia.

Biochemistry

- Serial determinations of serum urea nitrogen and creatinine concentrations may help differentiate the cause of azotemia. Appropriate therapy to restore renal perfusion typically yields a dramatic reduction in azotemia in patients with prerenal azotemia (typically within 24–48 hours). Correcting obstruction to urine flow or a rent in the excretory pathway typically is followed by a rapid reduction in the magnitude of azotemia.
- Hyperkalemia may be consistent with postrenal azotemia, primary renal azotemia due to oliguric renal failure, or prerenal azotemia associated with hypoadrenocorticism.
- Increased serum albumin and globulin concentration suggest prerenal component.

Urinalysis

- Urine specific gravity (USG) ≥1.030 (dog) and ≥1.035 (cat) supports a diagnosis of prerenal azotemia. Administration of fluid therapy before urine collection may interfere with interpretation of USG.
- Azotemic patients that have not been treated with fluids and have USG <1.030 (dog) and <1.035 (cat) typically have primary renal azotemia. A notable exception is glomerular

disease, which is sometimes characterized by glomerulotubular imbalance, where adequate urine-concentrating ability may persist despite sufficient renal glomerular damage to cause primary renal azotemia; these patients are recognized by moderate to marked proteinuria in the absence of hematuria and pyuria.
- USG is not useful in identifying postrenal azotemia.

OTHER LABORATORY TESTS

Endogenous or exogenous creatinine, iohexol, or inulin clearance tests or other specific tests of GFR may be used to confirm that azotemia is caused by reduced GFR.

IMAGING

- Abdominal radiographs—used to determine kidney size (small kidneys consistent with CKD; mild-to-moderate enlargement of kidneys may be consistent with AKI or urinary obstruction) and to rule out urinary obstruction (marked dilation of urinary bladder or mineral densities within excretory pathway).
- Ultrasonography—may detect changes in echogenicity of renal parenchyma and size and shape of kidneys; useful to rule out postrenal azotemia characterized by distension of excretory pathway and uroliths or masses within or impinging on excretory pathway and intra-abdominal fluid accumulation (with rupture of excretory pathway).
- Excretory urography, pyelography, or cystourethrography—may help establish diagnosis of postrenal azotemia due to urinary obstruction or rupture of excretory pathway.

DIAGNOSTIC PROCEDURES

Renal biopsy can confirm the diagnosis of primary kidney disease, to differentiate acute from chronic kidney disease, and to attempt to establish the underlying disease process responsible for kidney disease.

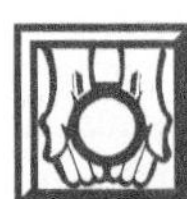

TREATMENT

- Prerenal azotemia caused by impaired renal perfusion—correct the underlying cause of renal hypoperfusion; aggressiveness of treatment depends on severity of underlying condition.
- Primary renal azotemia and associated uremia—(1) specific therapy directed at halting or reversing primary disease process affecting the kidneys, and (2) symptomatic, supportive, and palliative therapies that ameliorate clinical signs of uremia; minimize clinical impact of deficits and excesses in fluid, electrolyte, acid-base balances; minimize effects of inadequate renal biosynthesis of hormones and other substances; and maintain adequate nutrition.
- Postrenal azotemia—eliminate urinary obstruction or repair rents in excretory pathway; supplemental fluid administration often required to prevent dehydration that may develop during solute diuresis that follows correction of postrenal azotemia.
- Fluid therapy—indicated for most azotemic patients; isotonic balanced crystalloid is preferred replacement fluid, followed by hypotonic maintenance fluid administration. Determine fluid volume to administer on basis of severity of dehydration or volume depletion. If no clinical dehydration is evident, cautiously assume that patient is <5% dehydrated and administer corresponding volume of fluid. Provide 25% of calculated fluid deficit in first hour. Thereafter, serially monitor perfusion (capillary refill time, pulse pressure, heart rate, and temperature of feet), blood pressure, and urine output to assess adequacy of fluid therapy. If perfusion has not improved, additional fluid should be administered. Provide the remaining fluid deficit over the next 12–24 hours. Fluid therapy should be cautiously administered to patients with overt or suspected cardiac failure and patients that are oliguric or anuric.
- Consider feeding diets formulated for kidney disease to reduce magnitude of azotemia, hyperphosphatemia, and acidosis.

MEDICATIONS

DRUG(S) OF CHOICE

- Symptomatic therapy for myriad manifestations of uremia.
- Omeprazole (1 mg/kg q12h) may be used to reduce gastric hyperacidity.
- Antiemetics such as maropitant (1 mg/kg q24h) are indicated for vomiting.

CONTRAINDICATIONS

Administration of nephrotoxic drugs.

PRECAUTIONS

- Use caution when administering drugs requiring renal excretion. Consult appropriate references concerning dose-reduction schedules or adjustments of maintenance intervals.
- Cautiously administer fluids to oligoanuric patients. Monitor urine production rates and body weight during fluid therapy to minimize likelihood of inducing overhydration.
- Stop fluid therapy in overhydrated oliguric/anuric patients. Use caution in administering drugs that may promote hypovolemia or hypotension (e.g., diuretics); carefully monitor response to such drugs by assessing hydration status, peripheral perfusion, and blood pressure, with serial evaluation of renal function tests.
- Corticosteroids may worsen azotemia by increasing catabolism of endogenous proteins.

ALTERNATIVE DRUG(S)

N/A

FOLLOW-UP

PATIENT MONITORING

Serum urea nitrogen and creatinine concentrations 24 hours after initiating fluid administration; also urine production, blood pressure, body weight, and hydration status.

POSSIBLE COMPLICATIONS

- Failure to correct prerenal azotemia caused by renal hypoperfusion rapidly could result in ischemic primary kidney disease.
- Primary renal azotemia can progress to uremia.
- Failure to restore normal urine flow in patients with postrenal azotemia can result in progressive renal damage or death due to hyperkalemia and uremia.

MISCELLANEOUS

ASSOCIATED CONDITIONS

An association may exist between hypokalemia and azotemia in cats.

AGE-RELATED FACTORS

Primary renal failure may occur in animals of any age, but geriatric dogs and cats appear to be at substantially higher risk for both acute and chronic kidney disease; these patients are also at higher risk for prerenal and postrenal causes of azotemia.

ZOONOTIC POTENTIAL

Leptospirosis

PREGNANCY/FERTILITY/BREEDING

- Data on azotemia and pregnancy are very limited.
- Pregnant azotemic animals—pharmacologic agents excreted by nonrenal pathways are preferred.

SEE ALSO

- Acute Kidney Injury.
- Chronic Kidney Disease.
- Urinary Tract Obstruction.

ABBREVIATIONS

- AKI = acute kidney injury.
- CKD = chronic kidney disease.
- GFR = glomerular filtration rate.
- USG = urine specific gravity.

INTERNET RESOURCES

International Renal Interest Society (IRIS): www.iris-kidney.com.

Suggested Reading

Polzin D. Chronic kidney disease. In: Ettinger SJ, Feldman EC, eds., Textbook of Veterinary Internal Medicine, 7th ed. Philadelphia, PA: Saunders, 2010, pp. 2036–2067.

Ross L. Acute renal failure. In: Bonagura JD, Twedt DC, eds. Kirk's Veterinary Therapy XIV. Philadelphia, PA: Saunders, 2009, pp. 879–882.

Author David J. Polzin

Consulting Editor J.D. Foster

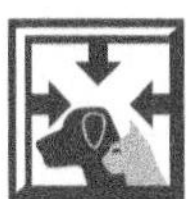

BASICS

OVERVIEW

• Caused by protozoal parasites of the genus *Babesia. Babesia* spp. infect mammalian red blood cells (RBCs). • Large *Babesia* spp. that infect dogs: ○ *Babesia vogeli* is transmitted by *Rhipicephalus sanguineus* and has a worldwide distribution. ○ *Babesia canis* is transmitted by *Dermacentor reticulatus* and is primarily found in Europe. ○ *Babesia rossi* is transmitted by *Haemaphysalis leachi* and is primarily found in Africa. ○ *Babesia* sp. (Coco)—tick vector is unknown; identified primarily in splenectomized and immune-suppressed dogs in the United States. • Small *Babesia* spp. (2–5 µm) that infect dogs: ○ *B. gibsoni*—worldwide distribution; most common *Babesia* sp. disease in the United States.
○ *B. conradae* (also *B. gibsoni* [United States/ California])— only reported in California.
○ *Babesia vulpes* (also *Theileria Vulpes*, Spanish dog piroplasm, and *B. microti*-like parasite)—reported in Europe and the United States. • Several case reports of novel *Babesia* sp. and other piroplasms (i.e., *T. equi)* infecting dogs. • Small piroplasms (2–5 µm) that infect cats: ○ *B. felis*—reported in Africa. ○ *Cytauxzoon felis*—reported in the United States. • Infection may occur either by tick transmission, direct transmission via blood transfer during dog bites, blood transfusions, or transplacentally.
• Incubation period averages approximately 2 weeks, but some cases are not clinically diagnosed for months to years. • Piroplasms infect and replicate in red blood cells (RBCs), resulting in both direct and immune-mediated hemolytic anemia. • Immune-mediated hemolytic anemia is more clinically important than parasite-induced RBC destruction, since severity of signs does not depend on degree of parasitemia.

Systems Affected

• Hemic/lymphatic/immune—anemia, thrombocytopenia (bleeding tendencies rare), fever, splenomegaly, lymphadenomegaly, vasculitis. • Hepatobiliary—mild to moderate increase in liver enzyme activities.
• Nervous—cerebral babesiosis, weakness, disorientation, collapse (most common with *B. canis rossi*). • Renal/urologic—renal failure (*B. rossi* and *B. vulpes*).

SIGNALMENT

• Any age or breed of dog can be infected.
• *B. vogeli* infections are more prevalent in greyhounds. • *B. gibsoni* infections are more prevalent in American pit bull terriers. • Any age or breed of cat can be infected, but to date, only *C. felis* has been reported in the United States.

SIGNS

• Similar in dogs and cats. • Peracute, acute, or chronic. • Some carrier animals have no detectable clinical signs. • Dogs—lethargy, anorexia, pale mucous membranes, fever, splenomegaly, lymphadenomegaly, pigmenturia, icterus, weight loss, discolored stool.
• Cats—lethargy, anorexia, pale mucous membranes, icterus.

CAUSES & RISK FACTORS

• History of tick attachment. • Splenectomized animals develop more severe clinical disease.
• History of splenectomy or chemotherapy is risk factor for *Babesia* sp. (Coco) infection. • Immune suppression may cause clinical signs and increased parasitemia in chronically infected dogs. • History of recent dog-bite wound is risk for *B. gibsoni* (Asia) infection. • Recent blood transfusion from subclinically infected donor.

DIAGNOSIS

DIFFERENTIAL DIAGNOSIS

• Any cause of immune-mediated hemolytic anemia or thrombocytopenia, including idiopathic immune-mediated hemolytic anemia or thrombocytopenia, ehrlichiosis, Rocky Mountain spotted fever, systemic lupus erythematosus, neoplasia, endocarditis, hemotropic mycoplasmosis (haemobartonellosis), and cytauxzoonosis. • A positive Coombs' test does not rule out babesiosis, since many animals with babesiosis are also Coombs' positive. • Non-immune-mediated hemolytic anemia, including microangiopathic anemia, caval syndrome, splenic torsion, disseminated intravascular coagulation (DIC), Heinz body anemia, pyruvate kinase deficiency, phosphofructokinase deficiency. • Hepatic and posthepatic jaundice.

CBC/BIOCHEMISTRY/URINALYSIS

• Anemia—absent to severe; usually regenerative (reticulocytosis) unless signs are very acute; in severe cases, packed cell volume (PCV) <10%. • Thrombocytopenia—usually moderate to severe; some animals have thrombocytopenia without anemia; most common hematologic abnormality. • Both leukocytosis and leukopenia reported. • Hyperbilirubinemia, depending on rate of hemolysis.
• Hyperglobulinemia is common in chronic infections and may be the only biochemical abnormality in some animals. • Mildly elevated liver enzyme activities from anemia/ hypoxia. • Proteinuria and hypoalbuminemia (protein-losing nephropathy) may occur.
• Azotemia and metabolic acidosis secondary to renal failure have been reported with *B. canis rossi*, *B. gibsoni*, and *B. vulpes*.
• Bilirubinuria is common.
• Hemoglobinuria is detected less commonly in United States than in Africa.

OTHER LABORATORY TESTS

• Microscopic examination of stained thin or thick blood smears—can provide definitive diagnosis (not to species level); sensitivity depends on microscopist experience and staining technique; most success using a quick modified Wright stain; capillary blood may enhance sensitivity. • Indirect fluorescent antibody (IFA)—serum antibody test; cross-reactive antibodies can prevent differentiation of species and subspecies; some infected animals, particularly young dogs, may have no detectable antibodies. • PCR—identifies presence of *Babesia* DNA in a biologic sample (usually ethylenediaminetetra-acetic acid [EDTA] anticoagulated whole blood); can differentiate subspecies and species.

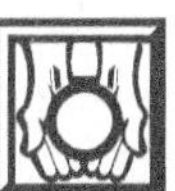

TREATMENT

• Inpatient or outpatient care depending on severity of disease. • Hypovolemic animals should receive aggressive fluid therapy.
• Severely anemic animals require blood transfusion.

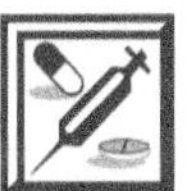

MEDICATIONS

DRUG(S) OF CHOICE

• Combination therapy of azithromycin (10 mg/kg PO q24h for 10 days) and atovaquone (13.5 mg/kg PO q8h for 10 days) is the treatment of choice and the only treatment that can potentially clear *B. gibsoni* (Asia) infections in dogs; in a controlled study, 85% of dogs cleared the infection after treatment. • Imidocarb dipropionate (FDA approved; 6.6 mg/kg SC/IM every 1–2 weeks) and diminazine aceturate (not FDA approved; 3.5–7 mg/kg SC/IM every 1–2 weeks) decrease morbidity and mortality in affected animals; they may completely clear *B. canis and B. vogeli* infections, but not *B. gibsoni.* • A combination of clindamycin (25 mg/kg PO q12h), metronidazole (15 mg/ kg PO q12h), and doxycycline (5 mg/kg PO q12h) had been associated with elimination or reduction of parasite below the limit of detection of PCR testing in dogs; unfortunately, a well-defined treatment course has not been established, with treatment times ranging from 24 to 92 days; minimum duration of therapy of 90 days recommended. • Combination of doxycycline (7–10 mg/kg PO q24h), enrofloxacin (2–2.5 mg/kg PO q12h), and

BABESIOSIS (CONTINUED)

metronidazole (5–15 mg/kg PO q12h) for 6 weeks was associated with clinical remission in 85% of dogs, but PCR was not performed to assess effect on parasitemia.
- Metronidazole (25–50 mg/kg PO q24h for 7 days), clindamycin (12.5–25 mg/kg PO q12h for 7–10 days), or doxycycline (10 mg/kg PO q12h for 7–10 days) as single-agent treatments may decrease clinical signs but not clear infections.
- Primaquine phosphate (1 mg/kg IM single injection) is the treatment of choice for *B. felis*.
- Since the anemia and thrombocytopenia are often immune mediated, immunosuppressive agents, such as prednisone (2.2 mg/kg/day PO), may be indicated in some cases that are not responding to antiprotozoal treatments alone; prolonged immune suppressive therapy *before* specific antiprotozoal therapy is contraindicated.
- Antibabesial drugs (imidocarb and diminazene) can cause cholinergic signs that can be minimized by administering atropine (0.02 mg/kg SC 30 min prior to administration).

CONTRAINDICATIONS/POSSIBLE INTERACTIONS

High doses of antibabesial drugs (imidocarb and diminazene) have resulted in liver and kidney failure.

FOLLOW-UP

- Recheck CBC and biochemistry as needed to monitor resolution of anemia, thrombocytopenia, icterus, etc.
- Most patients have clinical response within 1–2 weeks of treatment.
- 2–3 consecutive negative PCR tests beginning 2 months post treatment should be performed to rule out treatment failure and persistent parasitemia; IFA titers are not recommended for follow-up because titers may persist for years.
- Long-term follow-up of *B. conradae*, *B. vulpes*, or *B. felis* after treatment has not been reported.
- When a dog housed in a multidog kennel is diagnosed with babesiosis, all dogs in that kennel should be screened, since there is a high percentage of carrier animals in kennel situations.
- Coinfection with other vector-transmitted pathogens (e.g., *Ehrlichia*, hemotropic *Mycoplasma*, *Leishmania*) should be considered, especially in animals that fail to respond to treatment.

PREVENTION/AVOIDANCE

Recent studies suggest that using acaracides can reduce transmission with *Babesia* spp. All attached ticks should be removed as soon as possible. Vaccines for *B. canis* and *B. rossi* are available in Europe, but may not confer protection against other *Babesia* spp. Tick control is important for disease prevention.

MISCELLANEOUS

All potential blood donors should test negative for *Babesia* spp.

ZOONOTIC POTENTIAL

N/A

PREGNANCY/FERTILITY/BREEDING

Transplacental transmission.

ABBREVIATIONS

- DIC = disseminated intravascular coagulation.
- EDTA = ethylenediaminetetra-acetic acid.
- IFA = indirect fluorescent antibody.
- PCV = packed cell volume.
- RBC = red blood cell.

Suggested Reading

Birkenheuer AJ, Correa MT, Levy MG, Breitschwerdt EB. Geographic distribution of babesiosis among dogs in the United States and association with dog bites: 150 cases (2000–2003). J Am Vet Med Assoc 2005, 227(6):942–947.

Solano-Gallego L, Baneth G. Babesiosis in dogs and cats—expanding parasitological and clinical spectra. Vet Parasitol 2011, 181(1):48–60.

Author Adam J. Birkenheuer

Consulting Editor Amie Koenig

BASICS

OVERVIEW

• Baclofen is centrally acting skeletal muscle relaxant used to prevent spasticity in people with multiple sclerosis, cerebral palsy, and spinal disorders. • Binds to gamma-aminobutyric acid ($GABA_B$) receptors and prevents release of inhibitory neurotransmitters and substances.
• Has been used extra-label in dogs to reduce urethral resistance (1–2 mg/kg PO q8h), but is rarely recommended due to narrow margin of safety; use in cats not recommended. • Oral doses as low as 0.7 mg/kg in dogs have caused depression, dyspnea, and hypothermia. • Death has been documented in dogs at 2.3 mg/kg, but more likely at 8–16 mg/kg. • These organ systems are predominantly affected:
◦ Cardiovascular. ◦ Gastrointestinal.
◦ Musculoskeletal. ◦ Nervous. ◦ Respiratory.

SIGNALMENT

• Accidental exposure in dogs is more frequently reported than in cats, but any animal may be at risk for poisoning.
• Cats are extremely sensitive to baclofen.

SIGNS

• Signs begin within 15–90 minutes of ingestion but, rarely, may be delayed several hours. • Common signs—vocalization, vomiting, ataxia, disorientation, hypersalivation, depression, weakness, coma, flaccid paralysis, recumbency, seizures, and hypothermia.
• Life-threatening signs—dyspnea, respiratory depression, and arrest secondary to diaphragmatic/intercostal muscle paralysis.

CAUSES & RISK FACTORS

Pet owners with medical conditions such as multiple sclerosis, cerebral palsy, and spinal disorders are more likely to have baclofen in the home.

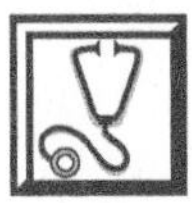

DIAGNOSIS

DIFFERENTIAL DIAGNOSIS

• Toxic—barbiturates, benzodiazepines, depressants, ethanol, ethylene glycol, cannabis/marijuana, illicit drugs (LSD, phencyclidine [PCP], hallucinogenic mushrooms), methanol, opioids, propylene glycol, tranquilizers, xylitol.
• Lower motor neuron disease (e.g., botulism, *Neospora*, tick paralysis, *Toxoplasma*). • Metabolic (e.g., hepatic encephalopathy, hypoglycemia, etc.).

CBC/BIOCHEMISTRY/URINALYSIS

No specific abnormalities expected, but should be used to rule out other causes.

OTHER LABORATORY TESTS

• Arterial blood gas analysis (hypoxemia, oxygenation, and ventilation).
• Pulse oximetry (hypoxemia). • End tidal CO_2 (hypercapnia or hypoventilation).
• Baclofen serum or urine concentrations to confirm exposure; not helpful for case management.

IMAGING

Thoracic radiographs (aspiration pneumonia secondary to severe sedation).

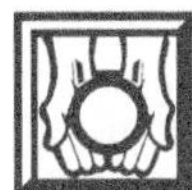

TREATMENT

• Many cases quickly become serious and referral to a 24-hour critical care center should be considered. • Treatment focused on decontamination and supportive care.
• Induce emesis following recent (<1 hour) ingestion in asymptomatic patients only if have not already vomited; consider gastric lavage for very large ingestions. • One dose of activated charcoal with sorbitol. • IV fluid crystalloids at 1.5–2.5 × maintenance to support organ perfusion and enhance elimination.
• Monitor for cardiac arrhythmias, hypoventilation, and aspiration pneumonia.
• Oxygen if respiratory depression; ventilator support if severe respiratory depression/failure.
• Monitor body temperature and provide warming/cooling measures as needed.
• Hemodialysis and hemoperfusion have successfully shortened elimination half-life and led to full recovery.

MEDICATIONS

DRUG(S) OF CHOICE

• Atropine for bradycardia (0.02–0.04 mg/kg IM/IV/SC PRN for dogs or cats). • Antiemetics as needed (e.g., maropitant 1 mg/kg SC q24h).
• Diazepam (0.25–1.0 mg/kg IV to effect) or midazolam (0.1–0.3 mg/kg IV/IM) for seizures; use lowest effective dose. • For seizures refractory to bolus diazepam or midazolam, use CRI of diazepam (0.1–0.5 mg/kg/h), midazolam (0.05–0.5 mg/kg/h), levetiracetam (dogs, 30–60 mg/kg IV; cats, 20 mg/kg IV), propofol (1–8 mg/kg IV to effect, followed by CRI dose of 0.1–0.6 mg/kg IV for dogs or cats), or inhalant anesthesia. • Agitation may be treated with diazepam or midazolam; acepromazine (0.05–0.2 mg/kg IV/IM/SC PRN for cats or dogs) should be used with caution.
• Cyproheptadine for vocalization/disorientation (dogs, 1.1 mg/kg PO or rectally q4–6h; cats, 2–4 mg total dose q4–6h). • IV lipid emulsion (ILE) has successfully treated dogs suffering from baclofen intoxication; should be reserved for critical cases; doses vary; using 20% emulsion, give 1.5 mL/kg IV bolus followed by CRI of 0.25 mL/kg/min for 30–60 min; if initial bolus fails to produce desired effect, consider *additional* doses of 1.5 mL/kg IV q4–6h for initial 24 hours; if after 3–5 boluses no clinical response is seen, discontinue use; do not exceed 8 mL/kg/day.

CONTRAINDICATIONS/POSSIBLE INTERACTIONS

• Use acepromazine cautiously due to risk of hypotension. • Use all sedatives cautiously as baclofen also causes sedation. • Avoid drugs that cause respiratory depression (e.g., phenobarbital).

FOLLOW-UP

PATIENT MONITORING

• Serious cases require intense, consistent patient monitoring including vital signs, blood pressure, blood gas analysis, pulse oximetry, and end tidal CO_2. • Nursing care should include turning/repositioning q6h, ocular lubrication, keeping patient dry/clean, passive range of motion of limbs, and soft bedding.

PREVENTION/AVOIDANCE

Educate pet owners about risks of leaving prescription drugs accessible to pets.

POSSIBLE COMPLICATIONS

Aspiration pneumonia due to combination of vomiting, sedation, seizures, and paralysis of diaphragm/intercostal muscles.

EXPECTED COURSE AND PROGNOSIS

• Patients suffering serious intoxications may take 5–7 days to fully recover. • Recovery often occurs with no residual effects.
• Prognosis good with early and appropriate care, but becomes poor if medical care delayed; seizures and aspiration pneumonia associated with guarded prognosis.

MISCELLANEOUS

ABBREVIATIONS

• GABA = gamma-aminobutyric acid.
• ILE = intravenous lipid emulsion.
• PCP = phencyclidine.

INTERNET RESOURCES

http://www.petpoisonhelpline.com/poison/baclofen

Suggested Reading

Khorzad R, Lee JA, Whelan M, et al. Baclofen toxicosis in dogs and cats: 145 cases (2004–2010). J Am Vet Med Assoc 2012, 241(8):1059–1064.

Author Ahna G. Brutlag
Consulting Editor Lynn R. Hovda

Client Education Handout available online

BARTONELLOSIS

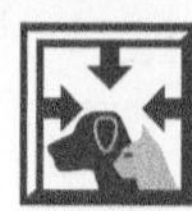

BASICS

OVERVIEW

• Small, facultative, fastidious intracellular argyrophilic, hemotrophic Gram-negative rod (bacilli) bacteria. • Emerging, vector-transmitted (fleas, ticks); adapted to reservoir hosts, establishes chronic, intraerythrocytic bacteremia. • Cats—usually asymptomatic, reservoir host. • Dogs—emerging clinical syndrome. • Seasonal—more cases reported between July and January. • Human syndrome—variable; cat scratch disease most common; worldwide, estimate >25,000 cases/year in United States; few fatalities.

SIGNALMENT

Dogs and cats.

SIGNS

Cats

• May have no clinical signs. • Lymphoid hyperplasia, uveitis, endocarditis (rare), self-limiting fever. • Between 5 and 60% seropositive, depending on geographic area.

Dogs

Nonspecific; include lethargy, fever, lymphadenomegaly, uveitis, or chorioretinitis, and may include signs consistent with endocarditis (e.g. weakness, cardiac arrhythmias), encephalitis (e.g. seizures, ataxia), myocarditis, vasculitis, rhinitis, angioproliferative lesions, or arthritis.

CAUSES & RISK FACTORS

• Dogs—flea and tick exposure, rural environment. • Bartonella associated with clinical illness in dogs and cats include *Bartonella henselae, B. clarridgeiae, B. koehlerae, B. quintana, B. vinsonii* ssp. *berkhoffii, B. rochalimae, B. elizabethae.*
• Human disease associated with contact with cats (>90%), particularly young cats with fleas.

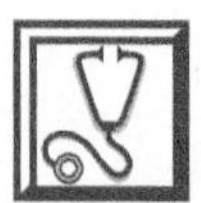

DIAGNOSIS

DIFFERENTIAL DIAGNOSIS

Other tick-borne infections (*Ehrlichia, Babesia*). Due to the broad spectrum of diseases associated with Bartonella, many differentials possible.

CBC/BIOCHEMISTRY/URINALYSIS

• Anemia, thrombocytopenia, eosinophilia.
• Hyperglobulinemia, signs of liver dysfunction, hypoglycemia possible.

OTHER LABORATORY TESTS

• Serology—indirect fluorescent antibody, ELISA, and western immunoblot.
∘ Fourfold rise in antibody titer over a 2–3-week period consistent with infection. ∘ Good specificity, poor sensitivity. ∘ Acutely ill bacteremic animals may not have detectable antibodies.
• PCR amplification of bacterial DNA—on blood, body fluids, fresh or fresh frozen tissue; for cases with negative culture and serology. • *Bartonella* alpha proteobacteria growth medium (BAPGM) culture—of blood, cerebrospinal fluid, joint fluid, effusions, or tissue biopsies; enriched media, requires 14–30 days; obtain culture before antibiotic therapy. • Combination BAPGM and PCR enhances diagnostic sensitivity.

PATHOLOGIC FINDINGS

• Histopathology of lymph nodes—nonspecific inflammatory reaction: granulomas, microabscesses, and necrosis. • Warthin–Starry silver stain—bacilli in lesions.
• Immunohistochemistry, alone or with PCR to identify bacteria.

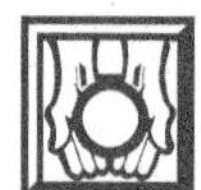

TREATMENT

Supportive care.

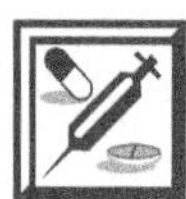

MEDICATIONS

DRUG(S) OF CHOICE

• Optimal protocols for treating *Bartonella* spp. have not been established; likely long-term (4–6 weeks) antibiotics required.
• Difficult to completely eliminate organism in cats; treatment reserved for symptomatic animals or those owned by immunocompromised people. • Single-agent antibiotic therapy not efficacious. • Antibiotic therapy: ∘ Cats—doxycycline, amoxicillin–clavulanate, fluoroquinolones, and azithromycin have been used. ∘ Dogs—fluoroquinolone + doxycycline good first choice; amoxicillin, gentamicin/amikacin, rifampin, erythromycin, azithromycin also options.
∘ Macrolides not recommended as first line due to rapid development of resistance.

FOLLOW-UP

PREVENTION/AVOIDANCE

• Immunocompromised people should avoid young cats. • Flea prevention.

POSSIBLE COMPLICATIONS

Caution with fluoroquinolones in cats and young dogs.

MISCELLANEOUS

• One episode appears to confer lifelong immunity. • Bacillary angiomatosis—vascular proliferative disease of skin; may be caused by *B. henselae*; responds to antimicrobial drugs.

ZOONOTIC POTENTIAL

• Risk of transfer of organisms from infected dogs and cats to people unknown. • Infected cats likely serve as source of organisms for fleas that transmit infection to humans (i.e., cat scratch disease). • Dogs may be chronically infected reservoirs for *Bartonella* species.
• Veterinarians are at occupational risk of infection from exposure. • Human disease manifested as erythema followed by unilateral regional lymphadenopathy (painful, often suppurative) in 3–10 days. Infection may be accompanied by fever, malaise, myalgia, nausea. Atypical infections may result in encephalopathy, meningitis, palpebral conjunctivitis, endocarditis, hepatitis, other systemic manifestations.

ABBREVIATIONS

• BAPGM = *Bartonella* alpha proteobacteria growth medium.

INTERNET RESOURCES

• www.cdc.gov/bartonella/index.html
• www.abcdcatsvets.org/feline-bartonellosis
• www.galaxydx.com

Suggested Reading

Álvarez-Fernández A, Breitschwerdt EB, Solano-Gallego L. Bartonella infections in cats and dogs including zoonotic aspects. Parasit Vectors 2018, 11(1):624.

Lappin MR. Update on flea and tick associated diseases of cats. Vet Parasitol 2018, 254:26–29.

Pultorak EL, Maggi RG, Breitschwerdt EB. Bartonellosis: a one health perspective. In: Yamada A, ed. Confronting Emerging Zoonoses. Tokyo: Springer, 2014, pp. 113–149.

Author J. Paul Woods
Consulting Editor Amie Koenig

BASICS

OVERVIEW

• Originates from the basal epithelial cells of both epidermal and adnexal origin.
• Majority of them are benign (e.g., basal cell epithelioma and basaloid tumor), with smaller occurrences of malignant (e.g., basal cell carcinoma) tumors.
• Metastasis is rare with the benign forms, and uncommon with malignant.

SIGNALMENT

• Most common skin tumor in cats (10–26%) and second to third most common skin tumor in dogs (4–12%).
• Median age—dogs, 6–9 years; cats, 10–11 years.
• Cocker spaniels, Kerry blue terriers, Siberian huskies, English springer spaniels, and poodles are predisposed for dogs. Persian, British Blue, Norwegian Forest Cat, Himalayan, and Siamese are predisposed for cats.

SIGNS

• Solitary, well-circumscribed, firm, often hairless, intradermal raised mass, typically located on the head, neck, limbs, or shoulders.
• Can vary greatly in size from a few millimeters to many centimeters in diameter.
• Feline basal cell tumors are frequently heavily pigmented, and occasionally cystic or ulcerated.

CAUSES & RISK FACTORS

• Breed (see Signalment).
• Contrary to human basal cell tumors, chronic ultraviolet exposure does not appear to play a role in pets.
• Possible association with papillomavirus in dogs and cats.

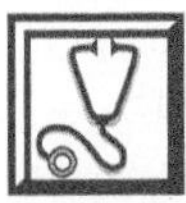

DIAGNOSIS

DIFFERENTIAL DIAGNOSIS

• Other skin tumors including mast cell tumor, extramedullary plasmacytoma, melanoma, hemangioma, hemangiosarcoma, histiocytoma.
• Melanoma is an especially important differential with the pigmented feline basal cell tumors.
• Intradermal cysts.

CBC/BIOCHEMISTRY/URINALYSIS

Normal

OTHER LABORATORY TESTS

N/A

IMAGING

N/A

DIAGNOSTIC PROCEDURES

• Cytologic evaluation of fine-needle aspiration sample reveals aggregates of round cells with basophilic cytoplasm; mitoses are not uncommon despite benign nature. In basal cell carcinomas, mitotic activity may be low to high with atypical mitotic figures.
• When clinically indicated, fine-needle aspiration of draining lymph nodes to confirm or deny the presence of regional metastases.
• Histopathologic examination required for definitive diagnosis; when highly pigmented, immunohistochemistry occasionally required to differentiate from melanoma.

PATHOLOGIC FINDINGS

• Histologic cellular patterns vary from solid to cystic to ribbon appearance.
• Tumor cells may contain melanin pigmentation; may have a fine eosinophilic stroma.
• Nuclear criteria might help predict risk of local recurrence in feline basal cell carcinomas.

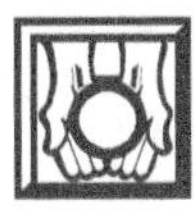

TREATMENT

• Surgical excision treatment of choice and generally curative for fully resectable tumors.
• Cryosurgery or plesiotherapy with strontium-90 can be used for smaller, superficial lesions (<1 cm).

MEDICATIONS

DRUG(S) OF CHOICE

N/A

CONTRAINDICATIONS/POSSIBLE INTERACTIONS

N/A

FOLLOW-UP

• Complete surgical excision is usually curative and associated with an excellent prognosis.
• Majority of tumors are locally confined and nonmetastatic. Long-term follow-up is generally unnecessary.

MISCELLANEOUS

Suggested Reading

Carpenter JL, Andrews LK, Holzworth J. Tumors and tumor-like lesions. In: Holzworth J, ed., Diseases of the Cat: Medicine and Surgery. Philadelphia, PA: Saunders, 1987, pp. 406–596.

Cowell RL, Tyler RD, Meinkoth JH. Diagnostic Cytology and Hematology of the Dog and Cat. St. Louis, MO: Mosby, 1999, pp. 40–42.

Ho NT, Smith KC, Dobromylskyj MJ. Retrospective study of more than 9000 feline cutaneous tumours in the UK: 2006–2013. J Feline Med Surg 2018, 20(2):128–134.

Pakhrin B, Kang MS, Bae IH, et al. Retrospective study of canine cutaneous tumors in Korea. J Vet Sci 2007, 8:229–236.

Ramos-Vara JA, Miller MA, Johnson GC, et al. Melan A and S100 protein immunohistochemistry in feline melanomas: 48 cases. Vet Pathol 2002, 39:127–132.

Simeonov R, Simeonova G. Nucleomorphometric analysis of feline basal cell carcinomas. Res Vet Sci 2008, 84:440–443.

Author Jason Pieper

Consulting Editor Timothy M. Fan

Acknowledgment The author and book editors acknowledge the prior contribution of Louis-Philippe de Lorimier.

BATTERY TOXICOSIS

BASICS

OVERVIEW

- Alkaline/acid-based batteries (generally referred to as dry cell batteries)—gastrointestinal tract (GIT) ulcers from leaking corrosive contents, oral injury from chewing on casing, rarely heavy metal toxicity from breakdown of casing in the GIT.
- Disc/button/lithium ion batteries—rapid necrosis to the esophagus and stomach due to electric current from the battery; significant necrosis can occur 15 minutes after contact.

SIGNALMENT

Dogs, cats, birds, and small mammals. Young animals are more commonly affected.

SIGNS

- Historical—finding chewed-up electronic equipment without the battery; chewed or mangled battery or battery packaging.
- Black debris in the oral cavity is evidence of leaked dry cell battery contents.
- Physical:
  - Oral ulcerations.
  - Oral injury from chewing on battery casing.
  - Anorexia, drooling, regurgitation, vomiting, diarrhea, melena, progressive weakness, dyspnea, coughing, stridor, pleuritis, pyothorax, and pneumo-mediastinum.

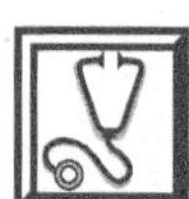

DIAGNOSIS

DIFFERENTIAL DIAGNOSIS

- Diagnosis based on history, complete oral exam, and full (esophagus and abdominal GIT) survey radiographs.
- Nonsteroidal anti-inflammatory drugs (NSAIDs), foreign body obstruction (FBO), pancreatitis, and other corrosive compounds (cleaning agents, drain cleaners, pool shocking agents, etc.).

CBC/BIOCHEMISTRY/URINALYSIS

- Anemia—secondary to bleeding GI ulceration.
- Leukocytosis—inflammation and secondary infection.
- Elevated total proteins/prerenal azotemia—secondary to dehydration.
- Elevated liver enzymes secondary to heavy metal toxicity from breakdown of casing.

IMAGING

- Full survey radiographs—determine if a battery was swallowed, assess location and condition of battery and casing; look for evidence of perforation and/or obstruction.
- Endoscopy—pending severity of signs, evaluate extent of damage to esophagus; may be able to remove battery or casing; use caution and do not damage esophagus.

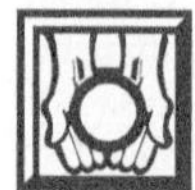

TREATMENT

- Lavage oral cavity for 10–15 minutes for alkaline batteries; for disc batteries give 10–20 mL of water every 15 minutes until battery is out of esophagus.
- Do *not* induce vomiting, as this may expose esophagus to further injury.
- NPO or slurry feeding for 24–48 hours if oral ulcerations are present.
- Ulceration may not be visible in the oral cavity until 48 hours post exposure.
- Wear gloves when cleaning up battery debris, as leaked acid could cause injury to hands.
- Small, intact dry cell batteries in stomach should pass within 48 hours; evaluate all stools and if battery has not passed the pylorus in 48 hours, surgical removal is recommended.
- Punctured dry cell batteries and disc/button/lithium ion batteries should be immediately removed by endoscopy or surgery.

MEDICATIONS

DRUG(S) OF CHOICE

- Analgesics:
  - Dogs—butorphanol 0.1–0.5 mg/kg IV/IM/SC; tramadol 4–10 mg/kg PO q6–8h.
  - Cats—buprenorphine 0.01–0.03 mg/kg buccal/IV/IM q6–8h.
- Antiemetics—maropitant 1 mg/kg PO/SC/IV q12h PRN.
- H2 blockers—pantoprazole 0.7–1 mg/kg IV over 15 min q24h; ranitidine 1–2 mg/kg PO/SC/IM/IV q8–12h; famotidine 0.5–1.1 mg/kg PO q12h.
- Sucralfate 0.25–1 g PO q8h on empty stomach.
- Antibiotics—as needed to prevent secondary infection when ulcers are present.

CONTRAINDICATIONS/ POSSIBLE INTERACTIONS

- Emetics—emesis should not be performed as it may worsen damage to the esophagus.
- Steroids—may reduce risk of esophageal stricture, but expected to slow healing time.
- NSAIDs—aid in pain management and swelling reduction, but may increase risk of gastric ulceration/perforation.

FOLLOW-UP

PATIENT MONITORING

Consider endoscopy 2 weeks post exposure to assess condition of esophagus.

POSSIBLE COMPLICATIONS

Esophageal perforation, esophageal stricture, gastrointestinal obstruction, heavy metal toxicity.

EXPECTED COURSE AND PROGNOSIS

- Nonruptured dry cell battery—excellent; most pets pass on own within 48 hours.
- Ruptured dry cell battery—guarded, pending location of corrosive exposure and amount of time before removal; esophageal injury worsens prognosis.
- Disc/button/lithium ion battery—guarded, rapid removal is needed; significant injury, including esophageal or gastric perforation, can occur within 15 minutes of ingestion.

MISCELLANEOUS

ASSOCIATED CONDITIONS

- Heavy metal toxicity.
- Esophagitis.
- Esophageal stricture.
- Esophageal perforation.
- Gastrointestinal obstruction.

ABBREVIATIONS

- FBO = foreign body obstruction.
- GIT = gastrointestinal tract.
- NSAID = nonsteroidal anti-inflammatory drug.

Suggested Reading

Angle CA. Batteries. In: Osweiler GD, Hovda LR, Brutlag AG, et al., eds. Blackwell's Five-Minute Clinical Companion, Small Animal Toxicology. Ames, IA: Wiley-Blackwell, 2016, pp. 617–623.

Yamashita M, Saito S, Koyama K, et al. Esophageal electrochemical burn by button-type alkaline batteries in dogs. Vet Hum Toxicol 1987, 29:226–230.

Author Tyne Hovda

Consulting Editor Lynn R. Hovda

Acknowledgment The author and book editors acknowledge the prior contribution of Catherine A. Angle.

Client Education Handout available online

BAYLISASCARIASIS

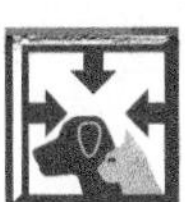

BASICS

OVERVIEW

• Disease caused by the raccoon roundworm, *Baylisascaris procyonis*.
• Two forms reported in dogs—intestinal infection occurring in adults; visceral disease caused by larval migration in puppies.
• Infection of raccoons occurs by ingestion of eggs or larvae in tissues of mammalian paratenic hosts.
• Dogs are infected by ingestion of infective eggs or paratenic hosts, from which they develop patent infections with adult worms in small intestine; puppies, probably infected by the ingestion of eggs, develop visceral disease.
• Dogs with intestinal infection are typically without signs; puppies with larval baylisascariasis show signs of neurologic disease.

SIGNALMENT

• Dogs.
• Intestinal form—adult animals.
• Larval form—puppies; suspect only severe cases have been reported; infection with only a few larvae probably does not cause severe disease in most puppies.

SIGNS

• Intestinal form—none.
• Larval form—weakness, ataxia, dysphagia, circling, recumbency.

CAUSES & RISK FACTORS

Sharing space with areas frequented by raccoons.

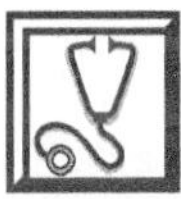

DIAGNOSIS

DIFFERENTIAL DIAGNOSIS

• Intestinal form—eggs in feces can be distinguished from those of either *Toxocara* or *Toxascaris*.
• Larval form—rabies, canine distemper, congenital neurologic defect, other infectious or inflammatory neurologic disease.

CBC/BIOCHEMISTRY/URINALYSIS

Usually normal; eosinophilia has been reported.

OTHER LABORATORY TESTS

N/A

IMAGING

• Larval form—based on lesions of toxocariasis or baylisascariasis in humans, lesions may appear on abdominal ultrasound or CT scans as small, single or multiple, ill-defined, oval or elongated, low-attenuating lesions in liver parenchyma.
• In neurologic lesions, MRI reveals diffuse periventricular white matter disease with atrophy.

DIAGNOSTIC PROCEDURES

• Intestinal form—direct fecal smear or fecal flotation (Web Figure 1).
• Larval form—ophthalmoscopic examination may show migratory tracks in retina, may use advanced imaging methods to visualize lesions in soft tissue or brain.

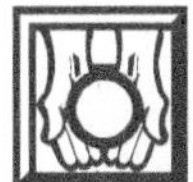

TREATMENT

• Intestinal form—may treat as inpatient to prevent environmental contamination with eggs and to ensure proper disposal (as biohazard) or destruction (incineration) of fecal material and worms after treatment.
• Larval form—no treatment to date.
• Client education—alert owner of potential risk to people who may frequent similar habitats to raccoons.

MEDICATIONS

DRUG(S) OF CHOICE

Intestinal Form

• Pyrantel pamoate—5–10 mg/kg PO.
• Fenbendazole (50 mg/kg q24h PO) for 3 days, repeat in 2 weeks.
• Febantel (25–35 mg/kg PO) with pyrantel pamoate (5–7 mg/kg PO) and praziquantel (5–7 mg/kg PO); Drontal Plus® label dose PO q24h for 5 days.
• Ivermectin (5 µg/kg PO) with pyrantel pamoate (5 mg/kg PO); Heartguard® approved label dosage, once monthly.
• Milbemycin (0.5–0.9 mg/kg PO), with lufenuron (10 mg/kg PO); Sentinel® approved label dosage, once monthly.

Larval Form

Corticosteroids and long-term albendazole (25–50 mg/kg/day PO for 10 days) may prove beneficial.

CONTRAINDICATIONS/POSSIBLE INTERACTIONS

N/A

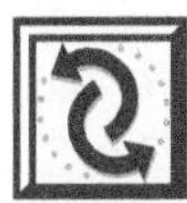

FOLLOW-UP

• Intestinal form—check feces 2 weeks after deworming and again 1 month later.
• Larval form—disease has proven fatal.

MISCELLANEOUS

ZOONOTIC POTENTIAL

• Intestinal form—eggs are not infectious when passed, but can develop in the environment in several days; ingestion of eggs containing infective larvae by humans can cause severe disease, i.e., larval baylisascariasis.
• Larval form—infected puppies pose no zoonotic threat.
• Alert owner of potential risk to people who may frequent similar habitats to raccoons.

Suggested Reading

Bauer C. Baylisascariosis—infections of animals and humans with "unusual" roundworms. Vet Parasitol 2013, 193:404–412.

Kazacos KR. *Baylisascaris* Larva Migrans. US Geological Survey, Circular 1412, 2016. doi: 10.3133/cir1412

Rowley HA, Uht RM, Kazacos KR, et al. Radiologic-pathologic findings in raccoon roundworm (*Baylisascaris procyonis*) encephalitis. Am J Neuroradiol 2000, 21:415–420.

Author Dwight D. Bowman
Consulting Editor Amie Koenig

BENIGN PROSTATIC HYPERPLASIA

BASICS

OVERVIEW

• Age-related pathologic change in prostate gland, making it nonpainfully large.
• Occurs in two phases, glandular and complex.
• Glandular phase characterized by high number of large prostatic cells and symmetrically large prostate gland.
• Complex phase characterized by glandular hyperplasia and atrophy, small cyst formation, chronic inflammation, and squamous metaplasia of epithelium.

SIGNALMENT

Prevalence increases with age; 60% of intact male dogs affected by 6 years and 95% of intact male dogs affected by 9 years of age.

SIGNS

Historical Findings

• None in most dogs.
• Serosanguinous urethral discharge.
• Hemospermia.
• Hematuria.
• Dysuria.
• Dyschezia.
• Ribbon-like stools.

Physical Examination Findings

• Symmetric, nonpainfully enlarged prostate gland.
• Prostatic pain in dogs with complication of bacterial infection or prostatic carcinoma.

CAUSES & RISK FACTORS

• Dihydrotestosterone (DHT; strongly) and testosterone (weakly).
• Estrogens.
• Aging as intact male.
• Risk eliminated by castration.

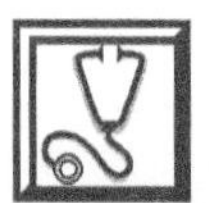

DIAGNOSIS

DIFFERENTIAL DIAGNOSIS

• Acute bacterial prostatitis—fever, depression, pain on rectal palpation, neutrophilia, pyuria, and bacteriuria; occurs concurrently with and secondary to benign prostatic hyperplasia (BPH).
• Chronic bacterial prostatitis—recurrent lower urinary tract infections and subfertility; occurs concurrently with and secondary to BPH.
• Prostatic adenocarcinoma—poor appetite, weight loss, hind limb weakness, dysuria, hematuria, and dyschezia; may see carcinoma cells in urine sediment.
• Prostatic and paraprostatic cysts—can cause palpable abdominal cystic mass filled with yellow to orange fluid.

CBC/BIOCHEMISTRY/URINALYSIS

• CBC and biochemistry—normal in BPH.
• Urinalysis—may be normal or reveal hematuria; pyuria and bacteriuria absent unless concurrent bacterial infection.

OTHER LABORATORY TESTS

Elevated serum concentration of canine prostate-specific arginine esterase correlates with histologic evidence of BPH.

IMAGING

• Radiography—abdominal radiographs reveal prostatomegaly.
• Ultrasonography—reveals enlarged prostate gland with uniform prostatic parenchymal echogenicity; small, fluid-filled cysts.

DIAGNOSTIC PROCEDURES

Prostatic fluid obtained by ejaculation or prostatic massage may be clear or hemorrhagic; red blood cell count high; white blood cell count normal; culture reveals <100,000 colony-forming units of bacteria/mL unless dog has concurrent bacterial infection.

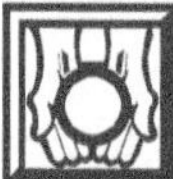

TREATMENT

• Not required if asymptomatic.
• Castration—most effective and prevents recurrence; if BPH complicated by acute bacterial prostatitis, delay surgery until infection resolved.
• Finasteride, if castration not desired, as long as dog is to remain intact.

MEDICATIONS

DRUG(S) OF CHOICE

• If castration not acceptable, the following are the most available and clinically useful:
  ○ Finasteride (0.1 mg/kg/day, not to exceed 5 mg/dog/day) for as long as dog remains intact—inhibits conversion of testosterone to DHT by enzyme 5-α-reductase.
  ○ Osaterone acetate (0.25 mg/kg PO once daily for 7 days)—competitively binds to androgen receptors, reduces 5-α-reductase, inhibits testosterone transport into prostate cells.
  ○ Delmadinone acetate (3 mg/kg SC once)—antiandrogenic activity due to competitive binding to androgen receptors.
  ○ Deslorelin acetate (subcutaneous implant administered every 6–12 months)—gonadotropin-releasing hormone (GnRH) agonist to inhibit hypothalamic–pituitary–gondal axis by negative feedback.

CONTRAINDICATIONS/POSSIBLE INTERACTIONS

• Potential for glucocorticoid insufficiency during stressful events for unspecified period after delmadinone acetate treatment.
• GnRH agonists contraindicated in breeding dogs as will inhibit fertility.

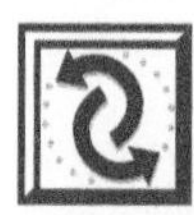

FOLLOW-UP

• Castration is treatment of choice for nonbreeding dogs, will result in 80% reduction in prostate volume within 12 weeks.
• Finasteride is treatment of choice for breeding males. Side effects in dogs reported. Prostate reduced 50–70% between 16 and 53 weeks of treatment. Testosterone preserved, thus finasteride not associated with decline in libido or semen quality. BPH will recur after withdrawal of finasteride; time until clinical signs recur is variable.

MISCELLANEOUS

ASSOCIATED CONDITIONS

• Bacterial prostatitis and prostatic carcinoma.
• Prostatomegaly in castrated dog strongly suggests prostatic carcinoma, as other prostatic diseases unlikely to occur in absence of androgenic influence.

SEE ALSO

• Prostatic Cysts.
• Prostatitis and Prostatic Abscess.
• Prostatomegaly.

ABBREVIATIONS

• BPH = benign prostatic hyperplasia.
• DHT = dihydrotestosterone.
• GnRH = gonadotropin-releasing hormone.

Suggested Reading

Christensen, BW. Canine prostate disease. Vet Clinics North Am Small Anim Pract 2018, 48(4):701–719.

Smith J. Canine prostatic disease: a review of anatomy, pathology, diagnosis, and treatment. Theriogenology 2008, 70:375–383.

Author Bruce Christensen

Consulting Editor J.D. Foster

Acknowledgments The author and book editors acknowledge the prior contributions of Carl A. Osborne and Jeffrey S. Klausner.

BENZODIAZEPINE AND OTHER SLEEP AIDS TOXICOSIS

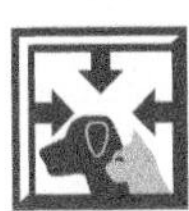

BASICS

DEFINITION

- Toxicosis due to ingestion of sleep aids or antianxiety medications commonly used in human and veterinary medicine.
- Benzodiazepine class—alprazolam (Xanax®), clonazepam (Klonopin®), diazepam (Valium®), lorazepam (Ativan®), midazolam (Versed®), temazepam (Restoril®), triazolam (Halcion®), and many more.
- Imidazopyridine class—eszopiclone (Lunesta®), zaleplon (Sonata®), and zolpidem (Ambien®, Ambien CR, Intermezzo®, Zolpimist®).

PATHOPHYSIOLOGY

- Benzodiazepines and imidazopyridines bind to receptors near the gamma-aminobutyric acid (GABA) receptor/chloride channel on neurons; they potentiate GABA's effect, which increases the opening of the chloride channel, leading to hyperpolarization of the nerve and decreased excitation.
- Imidazopyridines bind near the receptor subset that is responsible for sedation, while benzodiazepines bind to all receptor subsets and so not only mediate sedation, but are also anticonvulsant and anxiolytic.
- Paradoxical reactions can occur and are typically described as excitement, irritability, and aberrant demeanor in cats and excitement in dogs, when the expected effect is seizure control or sedation.
- Both classes are well absorbed orally and have rapid onset of actions, often less than 30 minutes.
- Duration of action depends on the drug and may last for hours to days.
- Both classes have wide margins of safety; lethal exposures are rare if a single agent is involved.
- Benzodiazepines—signs can be seen at therapeutic doses; however, the drugs have a wide margin of safety, with the minimal lethal dose being approximately 1,000 times the therapeutic dose. Cats may develop idiosyncratic hepatic failure with chronic oral dosing of diazepam and clonazepam.
- Zaleplon—based on a review of the American Society for the Prevention of Cruelty to Animals' Animal Poison Control Center (ASPCA APCC) Antox database: in dogs, doses >0.11 mg/kg have been associated with restlessness and hyperactivity; in cats, doses of >1.25 mg/kg caused paradoxical reactions.
- Zolpidem—based on a review of the ASPCA APCC Antox database: in dogs, dosages >0.2 mg/kg can cause mild sedation and ataxia; doses >0.6 mg/kg can cause paradoxical reactions. In cats, signs of paradoxical reactions were seen at 0.34 mg/kg or greater.

SYSTEMS AFFECTED

- Gastrointestinal—vomiting.
- Hepatic—acute necrosis and failure in cats with diazepam and clonazepam.
- Nervous—CNS depression and/or paradoxical reactions, ataxia, coma.
- Respiratory—depression.

GENETICS

N/A

INCIDENCE/PREVALENCE

Commonly prescribed drugs, so exposure is common.

GEOGRAPHIC DISTRIBUTION

None

SIGNALMENT

Species

Dogs and cats—acute toxicity; cats—idiosyncratic hepatic failure with chronic oral dosing of diazepam or clonazepam possible.

Breed Predilections

None

Mean Age and Range

None

Predominant Sex

None

SIGNS

General Comments

- Benzodiazepines can cause sedation with virtually any exposure (even at therapeutic doses).
- Imidazopyridines cause sedation at low doses, but likelihood of paradoxical reaction increases with increasing dose, especially in dogs.

Historical Findings

- Evidence of accidental ingestion of medication.
- Therapeutic use of drug.
- Lethargy.
- Ataxia.
- Sedation.
- Agitation.

Physical Examination Findings

- Depression.
- Ataxia.
- Sedation.
- Hypothermia.
- Agitation.
- Hyperthermia (secondary to agitation).
- Tachycardia.
- Icterus (in cats with idiopathic liver failure).

CAUSES

Accidental exposure, inappropriate administration, or therapeutic use.

RISK FACTORS

- Younger and older animals.
- Animals with preexisting conditions.

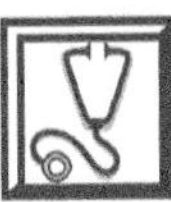

DIAGNOSIS

DIFFERENTIAL DIAGNOSIS

- CNS depression—barbiturates, ivermectin, ethylene glycol, alcohols (e.g., ethanol, methanol), marijuana, opioids, and antidepressants (low doses).
- Paradoxical reactions—amphetamines, pseudoephedrine, methylxanthines, cocaine, phenylpropanolamine, and serotonin syndrome (secondary to antidepressants).

CBC/BIOCHEMISTRY/URINALYSIS

- No abnormalities expected in acute overdoses.
- In cats with idiopathic liver failure, elevated liver enzymes and bilirubin.

OTHER LABORATORY TESTS

- Benzodiazepines can be detected in blood, urine, and liver; over-the-counter (OTC) drug-testing kits may be used to confirm exposure, but the label should be examined closely to be certain all benzodiazepines are included in the test kit.
- Imidazopyridines can be detected in blood and urine; OTC drug-testing kits are not yet readily available.

DIAGNOSTIC PROCEDURES

N/A

PATHOLOGIC FINDINGS

No gross or histologic changes are expected.

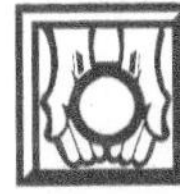

TREATMENT

APPROPRIATE HEALTH CARE

- Outpatient—most mildly affected animals can be managed at home with confinement (to avoid injury due to falls) and minimizing stimulation.
- Inpatient—animals who are comatose or showing paradoxical reactions.

NURSING CARE

- Intravenous fluids.
- Monitor and control body temperature.
- Good bedding and frequent turning for recumbent patients.
- Minimize sensory stimulation, especially with paradoxical reactions.

ACTIVITY

Restrict until recovered to avoid injury.

DIET

Cats with liver failure may require forced or tube feeding for support.

CLIENT EDUCATION

- Make all clients aware of proper storage of all medications.
- If prescribing diazepam or clonazepam to cats, have owner closely monitor the cat for the first week.

BENZODIAZEPINE AND OTHER SLEEP AIDS TOXICOSIS (CONTINUED)

SURGICAL CONSIDERATIONS

N/A

MEDICATIONS

DRUG(S) OF CHOICE

- Acepromazine 0.01–0.2 mg/kg IV/IM as needed to control paradoxical reactions.
- Cyproheptadine 1.1 mg/kg PO q4–6h or rectally for dogs; 2–4 mg/cat q4–6h for control of paradoxical reactions.
- Flumazenil—a benzodiazepine reversal agent: 0.01 mg/kg IV q1–2h as needed; it can be used to reverse both excessive sedation and paradoxical reaction; however, flumazenil can cause seizures, so its use is generally restricted to life-threatening situations.

CONTRAINDICATIONS

Do not give other benzodiazepines to control paradoxical reactions.

PRECAUTIONS

N/A

POSSIBLE INTERACTIONS

Care when using other depressant medications (e.g., barbiturates, phenothiazines), as these can potentiate the depressant effects of these drugs.

FOLLOW-UP

PATIENT MONITORING

TPR, blood pressure, respiratory effort.

PREVENTION/AVOIDANCE

Secure medications out of reach of dogs and cats.

POSSIBLE COMPLICATIONS

No long-term complications expected.

EXPECTED COURSE AND PROGNOSIS

- Prognosis for acute overdose is excellent with symptomatic care.
- Prognosis for acute hepatic failure in cats with diazepam is poor.

MISCELLANEOUS

ASSOCIATED CONDITIONS

N/A

AGE-RELATED FACTORS

- Young animals and those with preexisting liver disease may have prolonged signs due to reduced ability to clear the drugs.
- Younger animals may be more prone to paradoxical reactions.

ZOONOTIC POTENTIAL

None

PREGNANCY/FERTILITY/BREEDING

Benzodiazepines are considered teratogenic.

SEE ALSO

- Amphetamine and ADD/ADHD Medication Toxicosis.
- Antidepressant Toxicosis—SSRIs and SNRIs.
- Antidepressant Toxicosis—Tricyclic.
- Ethanol Toxicosis.
- Ethylene Glycol Toxicosis.
- Ivermectin and Other Macrocyclic Lactones Toxicosis.

ABBREVIATIONS

- ASPCA APCC = American Society for the Prevention of Cruelty to Animals' Animal Poison Control Center.
- GABA = gamma-aminobutyric acid.
- OTC = over-the-counter.

INTERNET RESOURCES

- http://www.aspca.org/pet-care/animal-poison-control
- http://www.petpoisonhelpline.com/poison/lunesta

Suggested Reading

Center SA, Elston TH, Rowland PH, et al. Fulminant hepatic failure associated with oral administration of diazepam in 11 cats. J Am Vet Med Assoc 1996, 209(3):618–625.

Czopowicz M, Szalus-Jordanow O, Frymus T. Zolpidem poisoning in a cat. Aust Vet J 2010, 88(8):326–327.

Lancaster AR, Lee JA, Hovda LR, et al. Sleep aid toxicosis in dogs: 317 cases (2004–2010). J Vet Emerg Crit Care 2011, 21(6):658–665.

Author Eric K. Dunayer

Consulting Editor Lynn R. Hovda

BETA RECEPTOR ANTAGONIST (BETA BLOCKERS) TOXICOSIS

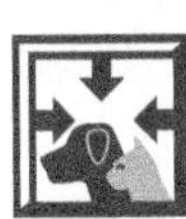

BASICS

OVERVIEW

- Beta receptor antagonists—class II anti-dysrhythmics used to treat hypertrophic or hypertrophic obstructive cardiomyopathy in cats and hypertension and tachydysrhythmias in dogs and cats.
- β_1 receptors—primarily located in heart, eye, and kidney.
- β_2 receptors—primarily located in bronchial smooth muscle, gastrointestinal tract, pancreas, liver, skeletal muscle, vascular smooth muscle, and endothelium.
- Systems affected include:
  - Cardiovascular—bradycardia, hypotension.
  - Respiratory—bronchospasm.
  - Nervous—decreased mentation, seizures.
  - Endocrine/metabolic—hypoglycemia, metabolic acidosis secondary to hypoperfusion.
  - Renal/urologic—acute kidney injury secondary to prolonged hypoperfusion.

SIGNALMENT

Dogs and cats equally affected with no breed, age, or sex predilection.

SIGNS

- Bradycardia, atrioventricular (AV) block.
- Hypotension.
- Decreased mentation.
- Respiratory distress/bronchospasm.
- Seizures.
- Coma.
- Death.

CAUSES & RISK FACTORS

Therapeutic overdose or ingestion of medication.

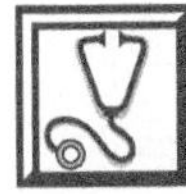

DIAGNOSIS

DIFFERENTIAL DIAGNOSIS

- Calcium channel blocker overdose.
- Cardiac disease with bradyarrhythmias.
- Cardiovascular drug overdose (e.g., clonidine, digoxin toxicosis).
- Sedative overdose (e.g., opioid or baclofen toxicosis).
- Sick sinus syndrome.
- Hyperkalemia.
- Decompensated shock.

CBC/CHEMISTRY/URINALYSIS

- Hypoglycemia.
- Hyperkalemia (mild).
- Azotemia and elevated liver enzymes with prolonged hypoperfusion.

OTHER LABORATORY TESTS

Blood gas—metabolic acidosis.

DIAGNOSTIC PROCEDURES

- ECG—first, second, and third degree AV block; prolonged PR, QRS, and QT intervals.
- Echocardiogram—negative inotropy, decreased cardiac output.

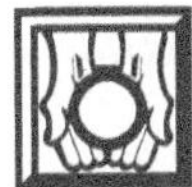

TREATMENT

- Emesis if asymptomatic and recent ingestion (<2 hours).
- Consider gastric lavage if decreased mental status and large number of pills ingested.
- Volume resuscitation with IV fluid bolus over 15–20 minutes for hypotension—cats, 10–20 mL/kg for cats; dogs, 20–30 mL/kg.
- Consider temporary cardiac pacing and hemodialysis (drug removal) in severe intoxications.

MEDICATIONS

DRUG(S) OF CHOICE

- Activated charcoal (1–2 g/kg) within 2 hours post exposure; repeat activated charcoal for ER formulations.
- Atropine (0.02–0.04 mg/kg IV) for sinus bradycardia.
- Intravenous fat emulsion (IFE)—may bind lipid-soluble drugs, increase Ca available for muscle contraction, and provide energy source for heart muscle. IFE 20% dose—1.5 mL/kg IV bolus over 1 min followed by CRI of 0.25 mL/kg/min for 30–60 min. Additional IV doses—1.5 ml/kg every 4–6 hours or CRI of 0.5 mL/kg/h; monitor serum for lipemia every 2–4 hours to determine if additional dosing needed.
- High-dose insulin euglycemia (HIE) treatment—may provide energy for heart muscle and increase Ca available for muscle contraction. Recommended treatment:
  - Check blood glucose (BG) concentration and administer dextrose if BG <100 mg/dL.
  - Administer regular insulin at 1 unit/kg IV followed by CRI at 0.5–2 units/kg/h. Increase every 10 min as needed up to maximum dose of 10 units/kg/h. When clinical signs resolve, decrease insulin by 1–2 units/kg/h.
  - Monitor BG every 10 min while titrating insulin dosing. Once insulin dosing is stabilized, check BG every 30–60 min. Dextrose supplementation IV will be needed to maintain normal BG concentrations. Central line placement recommended for frequent glucose monitoring and dextrose administration during HIE treatment. May need to continue dextrose supplementation up to 24 hours after discontinuation of insulin.
  - Monitor potassium concentration every hour during titration, then every 6 hours. Administer potassium chloride to keep potassium concentrations within normal range.
- Calcium gluconate 10% 0.5–1.5 ml/kg IV over 10–20 min, followed by CRI 0.1–0.15 ml/kg/h. May increase calcium available for heart muscle contraction.
- Glucagon—0.05–0.2 mg/kg slow IV bolus followed by CRI of 0.1–0.15 mg/kg/h. May not be as effective as IFE or HIE therapy.
- Sympathomimetics or vasopressin should only be used in cases refractory to other treatments.

CONTRAINDICATION/POSSIBLE INTERACTIONS

Vasopressors/sympathomimetics may not be as effective as other therapy and may make patients less responsive to treatment.

FOLLOW-UP

PATIENT MONITORING

- Monitor for 8 hours with immediate release preparations and 12–24 hours for extended release (ER) preparations.
- Heart rate/ECG.
- Blood pressure.
- Potassium levels.
- Blood glucose.

POSSIBLE COMPLICATIONS

Renal failure can occur secondary to prolonged hypoperfusion.

EXPECTED COURSE AND PROGNOSIS

- Ingestion of immediate release preparations typically result in clinical signs in 6 hours.
- Sustained release (SR) or ER preparations may take 12–24 hours for clinical signs to develop.
- Prognosis depends on dose ingested and response to therapy, but generally good.

MISCELLANEOUS

ABBREVIATIONS

- AV = atrioventricular.
- BG = blood glucose.
- ER = extended release.
- HIE = high-dose insulin euglycemia.
- IFE = intravenous fat emulsion.
- SR = sustained release.

Suggested Reading

Engebretsen KM, Kaczarek KM, Morgan J, Holger JS. High dose insulin therapy in beta-blocker and calcium channel-blocker poisoning. Clin Toxicol 2011, 49(4):277–283.

Author Katherine L. Peterson

Consulting Editor Lynn R. Hovda

Client Education Handout available online

BETA-2 AGONIST INHALER TOXICOSIS

B

BASICS

OVERVIEW

- Beta-2 agonist inhaler toxicosis occurs when dogs chew and puncture pressurized inhalers containing albuterol (salbutamol), levalbuterol, or salmeterol.
- Loss of beta-2 adrenergic selectivity with overdose results in beta-1 stimulation (sinus tachycardia). Failure of the myocardium to effectively oxygenate during extreme periods of tachycardia can result in other tachyarrhythmias such as ventricular premature contractions (VPCs) and ventricular tachycardia.
- Generalized adrenergic stimulation releases catecholamines that exacerbate cardiovascular (CV) stimulation, stimulate the CNS and respiratory systems, and can result in significant intracellular translocation of potassium and phosphorus.
- Propellants are now hydrofluoroalkanes (HFAs) and are expected to sensitize the myocardium less to catecholamines than older chlorofluorocarbon propellants.

Systems Affected

- Behavioral—hyperactivity, apprehension, nervousness, restlessness.
- Cardiovascular—sinus tachycardia, other tachyarrhythmias.
- Endocrine/metabolic—hypokalemia, hypophosphatemia.
- Gastrointestinal—mild vomiting.
- Musculoskeletal—tremors, weakness with catecholamine depletion.
- Nervous—anxiety, apprehension initially, depression with catecholamine depletion.
- Neuromuscular—tremors.
- Respiratory—tachypnea.

SIGNALMENT

Young dogs are overrepresented due to their predilection for dietary indiscretion.

SIGNS

- Tachycardia, other tachyarrhythmias.
- Lethargy, weakness, depression.
- Hyperactivity, apprehension, nervousness, restlessness.
- Tachypnea.
- Vomiting.
- Tremors.

CAUSES & RISK FACTORS

- Puncture of inhalers containing beta-2 agonists.
- Pets prone to dietary indiscretion with access to inhalers.

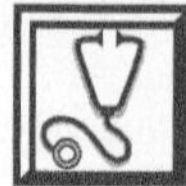

DIAGNOSIS

DIFFERENTIAL DIAGNOSIS

- Amphetamines and related drugs such as those used for attention deficit hyperactivity disorder (ADHD).
- Sympathomimetics (e.g., phenylpropanolamine, pseudoephedrine, phenylephrine, ephedrine).
- Methylxanthines (e.g., caffeine, theobromine).
- Metaldehyde.
- Illicit drugs including methamphetamine.
- Thyroxine.
- Tremorgenic mycotoxins.
- Hops (*Humulus lupulus*).
- Nicotine.

CBC/BIOCHEMISTRY/URINALYSIS

- Hypokalemia.
- Hypophosphatemia.

DIAGNOSTIC PROCEDURES

ECG to confirm, monitor for arrhythmias.

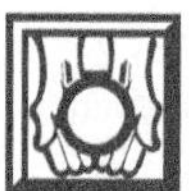

TREATMENT

- Inpatient treatment—initiate medical management and emergency care as soon as possible following exposure.
- Nursing care required—fluid support.
- Altered activity—cage rest, quiet environment.
- NPO if vomiting.
- Discuss with owner timing of presentation relative to exposure; patients that have delayed presentation and prolonged, untreated CNS and CV stimulation may be at greater risk for more serious arrhythmias and slower recovery.
- No surgical or anesthetic considerations.

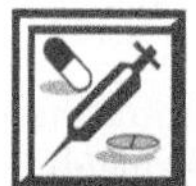

MEDICATIONS

DRUG(S) OF CHOICE

- Benzodiazepines PRN for anxiety, nervousness, tremors—diazepam: 0.5–1 mg/kg IV or 1 mg/kg rectally, repeat PRN; midazolam: 0.1–0.3 mg/kg IV, IM, repeat PRN.
- Beta blockers for severe tachycardia (HR >160 in large dogs; >200 in miniature breeds), hypokalemia—propranolol (preferred, nonspecific blocker): dogs, 0.02–0.06 mg/kg IV to effect; esmolol (blocks beta-1 only; ultra-short acting): dogs, 0.25–0.5 mg/kg IV as slow bolus then CRI of 0.01–0.2 mg/kg/min.
- Potassium chloride supplementation—up to 0.5 mEq potassium/kg/h IV maximum, based on degree of hypokalemia.
- Potassium phosphate if phosphorus <1 mg/dL—0.01–0.03 mM/kg/h IV.
- Lidocaine for ventricular arrhythmias—dogs, 2–4 mg/kg IV (max 8 mg/kg over 1–2 mins) followed by CRI of 25–100 µg/kg/min; cats, 0.25–0.5 mg/kg IV slowly (special caution for use in cats due to predilection for CNS and CV toxicity).

CONTRAINDICATIONS/POSSIBLE INTERACTIONS

N/A

FOLLOW-UP

PATIENT MONITORING

- Electrolytes (potassium, phosphorus) q12h or PRN if ECG changes, weakness (potassium), hemolysis (phosphorus). *Note*: Monitor for rebound hyperkalemia.
- ECG.
- Mentation.

POSSIBLE COMPLICATIONS

- Rarely fatal. Persistent, severe tachycardia can result in myocardial hypoxia and more serious arrhythmias or other cardiac sequelae.
- Catecholamine depletion can result in weakness and depression once the stimulatory effects wane.

EXPECTED COURSE AND PROGNOSIS

Excellent prognosis with prompt and appropriate treatment in an otherwise healthy patient.

MISCELLANEOUS

PREGNANCY/FERTILITY/BREEDING

- Albuterol crosses the placenta. Overdose effects are expected to be similar for the fetus. Hypoxia with cardiac compromise in the bitch may harm the fetus.
- No adverse effects expected with regard to fertility.

ABBREVIATIONS

- ADHD = attention deficit hyperactivity disorder.
- CV = cardiovascular.
- HFA = hydrofluoroalkane.
- VPC = ventricular premature contraction.

Suggested Reading

Mensching D, Volmer PA. Breathe with ease when managing beta-2 agonist inhaler toxicoses in dogs. Vet Med, 2007, June:369–373.

Author Lynn R. Hovda

Consulting Editor Lynn R. Hovda

Acknowledgments The author and book editors acknowledge the prior contribution of Donna Mensching.

BILE DUCT CARCINOMA

BASICS

OVERVIEW

• Epithelial neoplasia that arises from the cells lining the biliary ducts or gallbladder. • Second most common malignant hepatic tumor in dogs, representing 22–41% of all malignant canine liver tumors. • Most common malignant hepatobiliary tumor in cats, but less common than benign biliary cystadenoma. • Benign biliary cystadenomas may undergo malignant transformation into cystadenocarcinomas, although time period over which this occurs is unknown. • Common metastatic sites include lungs, regional lymph nodes, and peritoneum (carcinomatosis); other metastatic sites include intestine, pancreas, heart, spleen, kidney, spinal cord, urinary bladder, bone, and rarely bone marrow.

SIGNALMENT

• Dogs and cats. • Possible predilection for Labrador retrievers. • Affected animals typically >10 years of age. • Possible predisposition for female dogs.

SIGNS

Historical Findings

• Anorexia. • Lethargy. • Weight loss.
• Vomiting. • Polyuria/polydipsia. • Icterus.
• Abdominal distension.

Physical Examination Findings

• Hepatomegaly/cranial abdominal mass effect. • Ascites. • Icterus. • Paraneoplastic alopecia (ventral abdomen) associated with feline biliary carcinoma.

CAUSES & RISK FACTORS

• Potential association between canine cholangiocarcinoma and trematode (hookworms, whipworms) infection. • Canine biliary carcinoma has been experimentally induced by N-ethyl-N′-nitro-N-nitrosoguanidine.

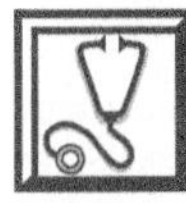

DIAGNOSIS

DIFFERENTIAL DIAGNOSIS

• Hepatocellular adenoma (hepatoma).
• Hepatocellular carcinoma. • Biliary adenoma/cystadenoma. • Nodular hyperplasia.
• Cirrhosis. • Chronic active hepatitis.
• Hepatic myelolipoma. • Carcinoids.
• Hepatic abscess.

CBC/BIOCHEMISTRY/URINALYSIS

• Anemia. • Leukocytosis. • Elevated serum enzyme (alkaline phosphatase [ALP], gamma-glutamyl transferase [GGT], alanine aminotransferase [ALT], aspartate aminotransferase [AST]) activity.
• Hyperbilirubinemia.

OTHER LABORATORY TESTS

• α-fetoprotein (an oncofetal glycoprotein) is elevated in 55% of dogs with bile duct carcinoma; may differentiate neoplastic from non-neoplastic lesions in dogs. • Coagulation profile (prothrombin time [PT], partial thromboplastin time [PTT]) recommended before biopsy or surgical procedures.
• Pre- and postprandial bile acids can help assess hepatobiliary function.

IMAGING

• Abdominal radiography—may localize a mass to the liver, show displacement of the stomach, or demonstrate loss of detail in patients with peritoneal effusion. • Abdominal ultrasonography—can be used to assess location and character of lesion, detect and sample peritoneal effusion, and guide tumor biopsy. • Thoracic radiography—should be used to screen for pulmonary metastasis.
• CT and MRI—more sensitive techniques that are more likely to detect smaller lesions not visible on ultrasound and radiography.

DIAGNOSTIC PROCEDURES

• Abdominocentesis and cytologic evaluation of peritoneal fluid. • Cytology or needle core (Tru-Cut®) biopsy samples via ultrasound guidance. • Laparoscopy or laparotomy may be needed to obtain larger samples for definitive diagnosis.

PATHOLOGIC FINDINGS

• Gross findings—morphologic types include massive (37–46%), nodular (0–21%), or diffuse (17–54%). Can be intrahepatic (most common in dogs), extrahepatic, or within the gall bladder (rare). • Histopathology findings—histologic subtypes include solid (cholangiocarcinoma) and cystic (biliary cystadenocarcinoma); subtype does not influence prognosis; immunohistochemistry (hepatocyte paraffin-1 and Claudin-7) can distinguish poorly differentiated hepatocellular carcinoma from biliary carcinoma.

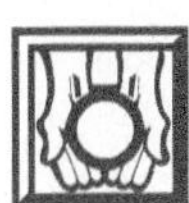

TREATMENT

• Complete surgical excision is treatment of choice; surgery not applicable for nodular/diffuse forms. • Up to 80% of liver can be resected if remaining liver tissue is functional.
• Interventional techniques (chemoembolization) may be utilized as palliative procedures for nonresectable solitary tumors.

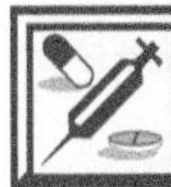

MEDICATIONS

DRUG(S) OF CHOICE

• Chemotherapy—no effective protocol identified. Tyrosine kinase inhibitors have been used anecdotally.

CONTRAINDICATIONS/POSSIBLE INTERACTIONS

Medications requiring metabolism by hepatobiliary system should be used with caution if evidence of dysfunction is present.

FOLLOW-UP

PATIENT MONITORING

Periodic physical examination, lab work, abdominal ultrasonography, and thoracic radiography after tumor resection.

PREVENTION/AVOIDANCE

Anthelmintic therapy is warranted due to potential association between canine bile duct carcinoma and infection with hookworms or whipworms.

POSSIBLE COMPLICATIONS

• Tumor rupture/hemorrhage, esp. if the massive form. • Biliary obstruction.

EXPECTED COURSE AND PROGNOSIS

• Aggressive tumor with a guarded to poor prognosis, especially if nonresectable. • High rate of metastasis (up to 88%) in both dogs and cats; widespread intraperitoneal carcinomatosis common in cats. • Most patients die within 6 months of surgery due to local recurrence or metastasis.

MISCELLANEOUS

PREGNANCY/FERTILITY/BREEDING

Chemotherapy drugs may be carcinogenic and mutagenic.

ABBREVIATIONS

• PT = Prothrombin time.
• PTT = Partial thromboplastin time.

Suggested Reading

Kinsey JR, Gilson SD, Hauptman J, et al. Factors associated with long-term survival in dogs undergoing liver lobectomy for liver tumors. Can Vet J 2015, 56:598–604.

Liptak JM. Hepatobiliary tumors. In: Withrow SJ, Vail DM, eds., Small Animal Clinical Oncology, 5th ed. St. Louis, MO: Saunders Elsevier, 2013, pp. 405–410.

Selmic LE. Hepatobiliary neoplasia. Vet Clin Small Anim Pract 2017, 47:725–735.

Authors Christine Mullin and Craig A. Clifford

Consulting Editor Timothy M. Fan

BILE DUCT OBSTRUCTION (EXTRAHEPATIC)

BASICS

DEFINITION

Extrahepatic bile duct obstruction (EHBDO) is biliary tree obstruction at the level of either the common bile duct (CBD) or the hepatic ducts, where it may involve one, several, or all hepatic ducts. Obstruction may be partial or complete.

PATHOPHYSIOLOGY

- EHBDO caused by abnormalities within biliary system or secondary to diseases affecting organs surrounding biliary tree; see Causes.
- Serious hepatobiliary injury follows within weeks of complete duct obstruction.
- Gallbladder (GB) bile may become colorless (white bile) if canalicular green pigmented hepatic bile not diverted into GB.
- Increased risk of bacterial infection of bile with stasis of bile flow.
- EHBDO progresses to biliary cirrhosis within 6 weeks; exception is pancreatitis causing EHBDO that may self-resolve within 2–3 weeks.

SYSTEMS AFFECTED

Hepatobiliary

SIGNALMENT

Species

Dog and cat.

Breed Predilection

- Some breeds predisposed to pancreatitis, choleliths, GB mucocele (GBM), dyslipidemias.
- Animals with large duct ductal plate malformation (DPM) phenotypes—predisposed to infection and cholelithiasis.
- Choleliths appear more common in small-breed dogs and cats.
- Neoplasia involving CBD more common in older animals and cats with chronic inflammation of biliary tree.

Mean Age and Range

Middle-aged to old animals with acquired disease; younger animals with DPM.

Predominant Sex

None

SIGNS

Historical Findings

- Depend on underlying disorder and "completeness" of EHBDO.
- Progressive lethargy and vague illness associated with progressive jaundice.
- Pale (acholic) stools—complete EHBDO in absence of enteric bleeding.
- Polyphagia—complete EHBDO causes nutrient malassimilation (fat).
- Bleeding tendencies—within 10 days of complete EHBDO, more severe/overt in cats.

Physical Examination Findings

- Depend on underlying cause.
- Weight loss.
- Severe jaundice.
- Hepatomegaly unless biliary cirrhosis.
- Cranial mass effect—extrahepatic biliary structures (small dogs and cats) or pancreatic involvement.
- Vague cranial abdominal discomfort.
- Acholic feces—unless enteric bleeding (hemoglobin pigment evolves pigmented feces).
- Bleeding tendencies and bruising—chronic EHBDO.
- Orange urine—severe bilirubinuria.

CAUSES & RISK FACTORS

- Diverse primary disorders.
- Cholelithiasis.
- Choledochitis.
- Neoplasia.
- Bile duct malformations—DPM phenotypes: choledochal cysts (cats), Caroli's malformation (dogs, cats), rare cystadenoma encroaching on porta hepatis (cats).
- Parasitic infestation—flukes (cats).
- Extrinsic compression—lymph nodes, neoplasia, pancreatitis, CBD entrapment in diaphragmatic hernia; foreign body obstruction of sphincter of Oddi in duodenum.
- Duct fibrosis—trauma, peritonitis, pancreatitis; major duct involvement in feline cholangitis/cholangiohepatitis syndrome (CCHS).
- Duct stricture—blunt trauma, iatrogenic surgical manipulations, e.g., after cholecystectomy.

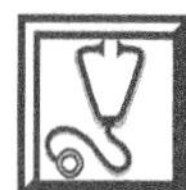

DIAGNOSIS

DIFFERENTIAL DIAGNOSIS

- Mass lesions—primary or metastatic hepatobiliary neoplasia; adjacent viscera.
- Diffuse infiltrative liver disease—neoplastic, inflammatory, hepatic lipidosis (HL), amyloid (rare).
- Infectious hepatitis—bacterial, viral, trematodes, protozoal.
- Severe hepatic fibrosis/cirrhosis.
- Decompensated chronic hepatitis.
- Copper-associated hepatopathy.
- Fulminant hepatic failure.
- Biliary cysts—DPM phenotypes: choledochal (cats), cystadenoma compressing CBD at porta hepatis.
- Pancreatitis—CBD stenosis/stricture, choleliths in cats: fused bile and pancreatic ducts.
- HL—cats: canalicular collapse causes jaundice.
- CCHS—cats, lymphocytic sclerosing or destructive cholangitis.

CBC/BIOCHEMISTRY/URINALYSIS

CBC

- Anemia—mild nonregenerative (chronic disease) or regenerative (enteric bleeding, Heinz body hemolysis).
- Microcytosis—uncommon.
- Leukogram—variable, neutrophilic leukocytosis, left-shifted leukogram with sepsis.
- Plasma—markedly jaundiced.

Biochemistry

- Liver enzymes—variable; marked increases in alkaline phosphatase (ALP) and gamma glutamyltransferase (GGT) reflect ductal injury; high alanine aminotransferase (ALT) and aspartate transaminase (AST) reflect periportal hepatocyte injury or multifocal injury associated with sepsis.
- Total bilirubin—moderate to markedly high; less than observed with hemolysis or HL; hyperbilirubinemia markedly escalated subsequent to blood transfusion.
- Albumin—variable, usually normal except when EHBDO >6 weeks (biliary cirrhosis); low albumin reflects synthetic failure or loss into abdominal effusion if syndrome complicated by GB rupture, suppurative hepatitis, or hepatic fibrosis leading to ascites.
- Globulins—normal or increased.
- Glucose—normal or low if biliary cirrhosis or sepsis; high if diabetes with pancreatitis.
- Hypercholesterolemia—common.

Urinalysis

- Bilirubinuria and bilirubin crystal formation.
- Absence of urobilinogen—unless enteric bleeding; unreliable test for EHBDO.

OTHER LABORATORY TESTS

- Serum bile acids—always markedly increased; superfluous test if hepatobiliary jaundice already suspected.
- Coagulation abnormalities—within 10 days of EHBDO develop vitamin K deficiency; may develop disseminated intravascular coagulation (DIC).
- Fecal examination—acholic stools consistent with EHBDO, but may be masked by small-volume melena; trematode eggs may be verified in fluke infestation (cats).

IMAGING

- Abdominal radiography—inconsistent hepatomegaly; variable mass effect in area of gallbladder or CBD, pattern consistent with pancreatitis, mineralized cholelith(s).
- Cholecystography—rarely provides additional practical information.
- Abdominal ultrasonography—evidence of obstruction in 72–96 hours (distended, tortuous CBD, cystic duct, intrahepatic bile ducts); may disclose underlying or primary disorder (e.g., pancreatitis, cystic lesions, mass

lesions, choleliths). *Caution*: GB bile "sludge" and full GB common in anorectic or fasted patients—do not mistake for EHBDO.

- *Caution*: Feline CBD serpiginous compared to canine—always inspect liver image for distended intrahepatic bile ducts and confirm that "tubes" are ducts rather than vasculature with color flow Doppler.

DIAGNOSTIC PROCEDURES

- Hepatic aspiration cytology—used to rule in HL (cats) or sample mass lesions; most clinicians avoid aspiration of obstructed biliary structures to avoid iatrogenic bile leakage and peritonitis.
- Ultrasound-guided needle biopsy—strongly contraindicated; may cause iatrogenic bile peritonitis.
- Laparotomy—best approach; allows tissue biopsy; biliary decompression; mass excision: cholelith or inspissated bile removal; cholecystectomy or creation of biliary-enteric anastomosis; CBD stent insertion.
- Laparoscopic procedures *not prioritized* because of need to completely evaluate biliary structures, ensure bile duct patency, and provide biliary decompressive surgeries.

PATHOLOGIC FINDINGS

- Gross—distended, tortuous bile duct, distended GB: cause often grossly apparent; obstruction >2 weeks: large, dark green to dark mahogany-colored liver; chronic complete obstruction often associates with white or clear GB bile.

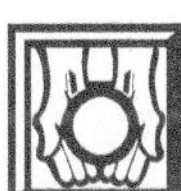

TREATMENT

APPROPRIATE HEALTH CARE

Inpatient—surgical intervention for EHBDO unless the cause is pancreatitis with prospect for resolution with supportive care.

NURSING CARE

- Fluid therapy—depends on underlying conditions; rehydrate and provide maintenance fluids before general anesthesia and surgical interventions.
- Water-soluble vitamins—in IV fluids; B complex (2 mL/L polyionic fluids).
- Initiate antibiotic therapy before surgery—see Drug(s) of Choice.
- Vitamin K_1—parenteral administration if EHBDO >5–7 days (see Drug(s) of Choice) before surgical interventions, abdominal or visceral aspiration cytology, placement of central lines or urinary catheters.

ACTIVITY

Depends on patient status and coagulopathy.

DIET

- Maintain nitrogen balance—avoid protein restriction.
- Restrict fat *if* overt fat malassimilation caused by lack of enteric bile acids in chronic EHBDO—rare.
- Supplement fat-soluble vitamins—vitamins E and K most urgent; supplements of vitamins D and A can lead to toxicity, thus careful use only in chronic unresolvable EHBDO.
- Water-soluble vitamin E—necessary in chronic EHBDO (see Drug(s) of Choice).
- Vitamin K—parenteral only, use SC or IM routes only.

CLIENT EDUCATION

- Inform client that surgical biliary decompression essential (unless resolvable pancreatitis or cholelith obstruction).
- Warn client that surgical success contingent on underlying cause, results of liver biopsy, infection, and individual variables.

SURGICAL CONSIDERATIONS

- Surgical exploration—imperative for determining underlying cause and for implementing definitive treatment unless obvious pancreatitis with hope for resolution.
- Excise masses, remove choleliths and inspissated bile; ensure common duct patency.
- Resect GB—if necrotizing cholecystitis, GBM, or GB cholelithiasis.
- Biliary-enteric anastomosis—if irresolvable occlusion of CBD: e.g., fibrosing pancreatitis, or neoplasia; anastomotic stoma at least 2.5 cm wide; chronic recurrent infection likely after biliary-enteric anastomosis; warn clients that temporary stenting instead of biliary-enteric anastomosis may be complicated by infection and stent obstruction, esp. in cats.
- Hypotension and bradycardia (vasovagal reflex)—may develop during biliary tree manipulation; ensure availability of emergency drugs (anticholinergics) and ventilatory support for rescue endeavors.
- Cholangiovenous reflux—bacteria and endotoxins during surgery from biliary tree manipulations in septic conditions; contributes to perioperative hypotension; all suspected EHBDO patients should be given broad-spectrum IV antimicrobials pre-, intra-, and postoperatively (during surgery after tissue and bile collection for bacterial culture).
- Ensure IV catheter access and volume expansion before surgery—use colloids only when plasma unavailable; be prepared for hemorrhage (have whole blood or packed red blood cells [RBCs] available).
- Surgical biopsies—submit tissue and particulate bile for aerobic and anaerobic bacterial culture; submit tissue for histology. Culture biliary debris; if GB removed, scrape wall to collect mucoid wall adherent material. Also collect GB wall, liquid bile, and liver tissue for culture. Combine all samples into a single culture for best bacterial recovery.
- Cytology—tissue and bile; cytology may detect bacterial infection and fluke eggs not recognized in biopsy sections; bile, biliary debris, and GB wall: more likely to harbor bacteria.
- Sclerosing or destructive feline cholangitis (intrahepatic ductopenia associated with lymphocytic or nonsuppurative or suppurative CCHS) may clinically emulate EHBDO; does not respond to biliary tree decompression; liver biopsy necessary for definitive diagnosis.

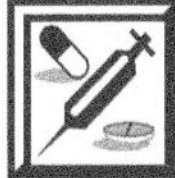

MEDICATIONS

DRUG(S) OF CHOICE

Vitamin K_1

- Provide 12–36h before surgery—0.5–1.5 mg/kg IM/SC, 3 doses at 12h intervals. *Caution*: avoid IV, may cause anaphylaxis.
- If chronic EHBDO not resolvable, parenteral vitamin K_1 given chronically with frequency titrated using prothrombin time (PT); too much vitamin K_1 causes hemolytic (Heinz body) anemia in cats.
- Oral vitamin K ineffectual owing to low bioavailability in EHBDO.

Vitamin E

- If chronic EHBDO nonresolvable, use water-soluble vitamin E (d-α-tocopheryl polyethylene glycol succinate [TPGS]-vitamin E)—10 U/kg/day PO.
- Treat early to allow response before invasive catheterizations, sampling, or surgical procedures.

Antibiotics

Before surgery—broad-spectrum antimicrobials for potential biliary infection because surgical manipulations may disseminate bacteremia; initially use antibiotics with wide spectrum, e.g., triad of ticarcillin 25 mg/kg IV q8h, metronidazole 7.5 mg/kg IV/PO q12h, enrofloxacin 5 mg/kg PO q12–24h (24h dose in cats no greater than 5 mg/kg/24h to avoid retinopathy).

Antioxidants

- Vitamin E (α-tocopherol acetate)—10–100 IU/kg; a larger than normal (normal = 10 IU/kg/day) oral dose needed in chronic EHBDO if fat-soluble vitamin used; lower dose used with water-soluble vitamin E (preferred, see previous).
- *S*-adenosylmethionine (SAMe)—20-40 mg/kg/day PO enteric-coated tablet 1–2h before feeding; choleretic with high-dose administration via glutathione (GSH) provoked bile flow.

Ursodeoxycholic Acid

- 10–15 mg/kg PO per day—*after biliary decompression* as a choleretic; ensure adequate hydration to achieve choleresis; *inappropriate before* biliary decompression: can accelerate liver injury in EHBDO.

BILE DUCT OBSTRUCTION (EXTRAHEPATIC) (CONTINUED)

- Beneficial effects: antifibrotic, anti-endotoxic, hepatoprotectant, anti-apoptotic, immunomodulator.

Bowel Preparation before Surgery

- Mechanical cleansing of colon with water or crystalloid fluids—may reduce endotoxemia potentiating perioperative hypotension.
- Acutely alter enteric flora to reduce enteric translocation of opportunistic pathogen with medications given either PO or by high enema instillation—neomycin 22 mg/kg q8h; lactulose 1–2 mL/kg q8h; metronidazole 7.5 mg/kg q12h; enrofloxacin 2.5 mg/kg q12h PO; rifaximin 5–10 mg/kg q12h, at present limited experience with rifaximin in dogs and cats; probiotic bacteria, empirical product dose but has unproven efficacy.

Gastrointestinal Protectants

- Agents reducing gastric acidity—omeprazole or pantoprazole (pump inhibitors) or famotidine (H2 blocker) combined with sucralfate for local cytoprotection if PO medications tolerated and enteric bleeding recognized (stagger sucralfate administration from other oral medications to avoid drug interactions).
- Antiemetics—maropitant (Cerenia®) or ondansetron.

CONTRAINDICATIONS

- Provide biliary decompression before institution of ursodeoxycholic acid.
- Take care to reduce drug dosages for medications eliminated in bile if EHBDO.
- Avoid invasive procedures—sampling, biopsy, surgical interventions before vitamin K_1.

PRECAUTIONS

See Surgical Considerations.

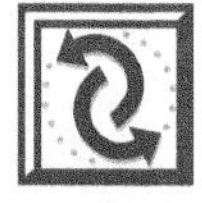

FOLLOW-UP

PATIENT MONITORING

- Depends on underlying condition.
- Total bilirubin values acutely reflect biliary decompression; values normalize within days.
- Liver enzyme activities—decline slowly.
- CBC—repeat q2–3 days initially if septic.
- Bile peritonitis—evaluate abdominal girth, body weight, and fluid accumulation.
- Determine necessity for pancreatic enzyme supplementation based on site of biliary-enteric anastomosis; patients with cholecystojejunostomy may benefit from enzyme supplementation; cannot rely on trypsin-like immunoreactive (TLI) substance to estimate pancreatic exocrine adequacy in this circumstance; sequentially evaluate body weight and condition, check feces for steatorrhea; only relevant if animal is fed a normal fat-containing diet; if steatorrheic after biliary-enteric anastomosis and patient is anicteric, reduce dietary fat intake and supplement pancreatic enzymes. *Warning*: pancreatic enzymes can induce oral or esophageal injury, especially in cats—must be mixed in food or administered in capsule or tablet form, followed by liquid or food to prevent mucosal adherence and injury.

POSSIBLE COMPLICATIONS

- Bile peritonitis.
- Restenosis of bile duct—if not bypassed and only stented to achieve biliary decompression.
- Stenosis of biliary-enteric anastomosis.
- Severe enteric hemorrhage with EHBDO—hypertensive enteric vasculopathy with coagulopathy (vitamin K deficiency).
- Hemorrhage during surgery.
- Septic bacteremia or systemic inflammatory response syndrome (SIRS) during or after surgery.
- Perioperative unresponsive hypotension—persistent vasovagal reflex or sepsis related.
- Vasovagal reflex.
- Cholangiovenous reflux.

EXPECTED COURSE AND PROGNOSIS

- Depends on underlying disease.
- Prognosis good if fibrosing pancreatitis and pancreatic inflammation resolve; bile duct patency may return without surgery.
- *Beware*: biliary tree distention often persists (ultrasound imaging) after EHBDO resolution.
- Permanent peribiliary fibrosis from EHBDO.
- Cats with sclerosing cholangitis or ductopenia mimic EHBDO but show no response to biliary decompression; liver biopsy is essential for diagnosis.

Considerations/Precautions

- Anticipate bleeding tendencies, vasovagal reflex, and cholangiovenous reflux during surgical procedures.
- Always submit liver and biliary tree biopsies for histology; all tissues, crushed choleliths, and biliary debris for bacterial culture (aerobic, anaerobic).

MISCELLANEOUS

ASSOCIATED CONDITIONS

- See Causes.
- Sclerosing or destructive lymphocytic cholangitis (cats) and destructive suppurative cholangitis causing ductopenia and idiopathic or toxic ductopenia are confused with EHBDO.

SEE ALSO

- Cholangitis/Cholangiohepatitis Syndrome.
- Gallbladder Mucocele.

ABBREVIATIONS

- ALP = alkaline phosphatase.
- ALT = alanine aminotransferase.
- AST = aspartate transaminase.
- CBD = common bile duct.
- CCHS = cholangitis/cholangiohepatitis syndrome.
- DIC = disseminated intravascular coagulation.
- DPM = ductal plate malformation.
- EHBDO = extrahepatic bile duct obstruction.
- GB = gallbladder.
- GBM = gallbladder mucocele.
- GGT = gamma glutamyltransferase.
- GSH = glutathione.
- HL = hepatic lipidosis.
- PT = prothrombin time.
- RBC = red blood cell.
- SAMe = *S*-adenosylmethionine.
- SIRS = systemic inflammatory response syndrome.
- TLI = trypsin-like immunoreactive.
- TPGS-Vitamin E = d-α-tocopheryl polyethylene glycol succinate.

Suggested Reading

Center SA. Diseases of the gallbladder and biliary tree. Vet Clin North Am Small Anim Pract 2009, 39(3):543–598.

Mehler SJ, Mayhew PD, Drobatz KJ, et al. Variables associated with outcome in dogs undergoing extrahepatic biliary surgery: 60 cases (1988–2002). Vet Surg 2004, 33:644–649.

Author Sharon A. Center

Consulting Editor Kate Holan

Client Education Handout available online

BILE PERITONITIS

BASICS

OVERVIEW

- Chemical peritonitis due to release of free bile into the abdominal cavity.
- Can involve focal or diffuse peritoneal inflammation, depending on chronicity and causal factors, and omental adhesions.

SIGNALMENT

- More common in dog than in cat.
- No age, breed, or sex predilection.

SIGNS

Historical Findings

- Acute presentation if septic peritonitis.
- May have chronic illness if nonseptic.
- Rare asymptomatic biliary rupture associated with omental encapsulation of leakage.
- Abdominal discomfort—vague.
- Lethargy.
- Gastrointestinal signs—anorexia, vomiting, diarrhea.
- Weight loss.
- ± Abdominal distention.
- Variable jaundice.
- Collapse, if septic.

Physical Examination Findings

- Lethargy.
- Variable (cranial) abdominal pain.
- Jaundice.
- Abdominal effusion.
- ± Fever.
- ± Endotoxic shock, if septic.

CAUSES & RISK FACTORS

- Limited arterial perfusion (cystic artery) to gallbladder (GB) fundus predisposes to ischemic necrosis and GB rupture.
- Trauma to biliary structures—automobile injuries, surgical, animal bites, gunshot wounds, cystic artery laceration during cholecystocentesis.
- Common bile duct (CBD)—frequent site of rupture with blunt trauma.
- Cholecystitis/choledochitis—may derive from GB mucocele (GBM); sepsis more common with necrotizing cholecystitis.
- Extrahepatic bile duct obstruction (EHBDO)—may derive from neoplasia, cholelithiasis, pancreatitis, duct stricture.
- Focal, small-volume, bile peritonitis—associated with cholecystitis; may reflect omental entrapment of bile or transmural bile leakage without rupture.
- Chemical peritonitis due to bile—predisposes to septic peritonitis.

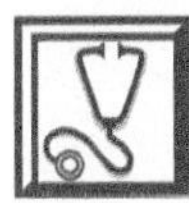

DIAGNOSIS

DIFFERENTIAL DIAGNOSIS

- Conditions promoting inflammation/devitalization of biliary structures—e.g., cholecystitis, choledochitis, neoplasia, GBM, neoplasia, blunt trauma.
- Conditions causing EHBDO—e.g., neoplasia, choleliths, pancreatitis, duct stricture/fibrosis.
- Sepsis or endotoxemia.
- Ascites—in jaundiced cirrhotic patient.
- Nonhepatic conditions causing abdominal effusion and jaundice.

CBC/BIOCHEMISTRY/URINALYSIS

CBC

Inflammatory leukogram—left shift and toxic neutrophils if necrotizing cholecystitis or sepsis; nonregenerative anemia if chronic inflammation.

Biochemistry

- High liver enzymes, especially alkaline phosphatase (ALP); hyperbilirubinemia; ± hypoalbuminemia; ± prerenal azotemia.
- Electrolyte, fluid, and acid-base disturbances; hyponatremia common.

Urinalysis

Bilirubinuria

OTHER LABORATORY TESTS

Coagulation tests—abnormal if sepsis syndrome, disseminated intravascular coagulation (DIC), or chronic EHBDO.

IMAGING

- Abdominal radiography—reduced abdominal detail, generalized or focal in GB area; cranial abdominal mass effect; rare mineralized cholelith or biliary gas (emphysematous cholecystitis).
- Thoracic radiography—rare bicavity effusion (pleural effusion), signs of trauma (e.g., fractured rib, hernia).
- Abdominal ultrasonography—effusion; EHBDO—distended GB or CBD; cholecystitis/choledochitis— thick GB or duct wall; necrotizing cholecystitis—segmental GB wall hyperechogenicity, laminated wall (represents necrosis); pericholecystic fluid; hepatic/pancreatic mass effect: common with bile peritonitis; choleliths or GBM ("kiwifruit sign"); gas in GB or bile ducts (emphysematous inflammation, implicates gas-forming organisms) casting acoustic shadow; ruptured GB may be difficult to image; liver size usually normal; variable parenchymal echogenicity reflects hepatic pathology (e.g., ascending cholangitis/cholangiohepatitis [CCHS]).

DIAGNOSTIC PROCEDURES

- Abdominocentesis—physicochemical, cytologic, and culture evaluations; ultrasound guidance optimizes sampling; sample close to biliary structures but avoid structure penetration.
- Cytology—impression smears of GB, liver, and bile (with particulate material) used for immediate detection of infection and neoplasia; modified transudate or exudate, phagocytized/free bile, and bilirubin.
- Acellular mucinous material reflects biliary mucin production; GBM material may be free within abdominal cavity.
- Ratio of bilirubin in effusion : serum usually ≥2–3 : 1.
- Bacterial aerobic/anaerobic culture and sensitivity—effusion, GB wall, liver, GB contents; Gram-negative enteric opportunists and anaerobes most common; polymicrobial infection possible.
- Exploratory laparotomy—appropriate for definitive diagnosis and treatment; permits cholecystectomy, cholecysto-enterostomy, duct or GB repair.
- Liver biopsy—important, evaluates for antecedent or coexistent disease, sample distant to the GB to avoid artifacts.

PATHOLOGIC FINDINGS

Depend on cause and site of rupture.

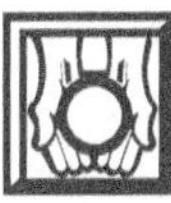

TREATMENT

- Inpatient—expediency of surgery depends on patient condition: achieve euhydration, correct electrolyte and acid-base status, provide preoperative antimicrobial treatment for best survival.
- Abdominal lavage to reduce peritoneal contamination if surgery delayed; use warm polyionic fluids and aseptic technique.
- Surgical experience important for best outcome—complicated resections and anastomoses may be required.
- Need for cholecystectomy decided at surgery; discolored GB wall indicates ischemic devitalized wall.

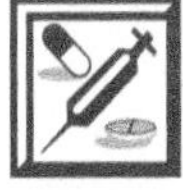

MEDICATIONS

DRUG(S) OF CHOICE

- Antimicrobials—in all patients, initiate broad-spectrum antimicrobials *before* surgical intervention; enteric Gram-negative and anaerobic organisms most common opportunists (good initial choices: ticarcillin, piperacillin, or third-generation cephalosporins, with enro-floxacin and metronidazole); customized antimicrobial treatment, thereafter based on cultures; continue antimicrobials ≥4–8 weeks if signs of infection confirmed by culture or on cytology.
- Vitamin K_1 (0.5–1.5 mg/kg IM/SC q12h for up to 3 doses)—all jaundiced patients *before* surgery.
- Prepare for blood component ± synthetic colloid therapy.
- Antiemetics if patient is vomiting—metoclopramide (0.2–0.5 mg/kg PO/SC q6–8h or 1–2 mg/kg/24h IV by CRI); ondansetron (0.5–1.0 mg/kg q12h IV/PO

BILE PERITONITIS (CONTINUED)

30 min before feeding); maropitant (1.0 mg/kg/day IV/SC/PO max 5 days).
- Proton pump inhibitor if gastric bleeding—pantoprazole (0.7–1.0 mg/kg IV q12–24h); omeprazole (0.5–1.0 mg/kg PO q12–24h); H2-receptor antagonists if proton pump inhibitor is not available: famotidine (0.5–2.0 mg/kg PO/IV/SC q12–24h); sucralfate (0.25–1.0 g PO q8–12h).
- Ursodeoxycholic acid as choleretic and hepatoprotectant if GBM, choleliths, CCHS, or chronic hepatitis—may administer chronically if GBM or cholelithiasis: 10–15 mg/kg PO daily, divided, with food for best bioavailability.
- Antioxidants—vitamin E (10 IU/kg/24h); *S*-adenosylmethionine (SAMe, with proven bioavailability and efficacy) 20 mg/kg PO daily 2h before feeding until enzymes normalize, indefinitely if chronic hepatitis or CCHS, GBM, inspissated bile syndrome; choleretic influence requires higher dose (40 mg/kg/day).

FOLLOW-UP

PATIENT MONITORING

- Sequential hematologic, biochemical, and imaging tests.
- Repeat abdominocentesis to assess continued infection and/or bile leakage as indicated.

POSSIBLE COMPLICATIONS

- Cholangitis/cholangiohepatitis.
- Pancreatitis.
- Recurrent bacterial cholangitis if biliary-enteric anastomosis required.

EXPECTED COURSE AND PROGNOSIS

- High survival rate for dogs with sterile bile peritonitis, if successful surgery, depending on underlying cause.
- Higher mortality in septic bile peritonitis (up to 73%).
- Anticipate slow clinical recovery and normalization of liver enzymes, but rapid resolution of hyperbilirubinemia with successful surgery.

MISCELLANEOUS

SEE ALSO

- Cholecystitis and Choledochitis.
- Cholelithiasis.
- Gallbladder Mucocele.
- Hepatitis, Chronic.

ABBREVIATIONS

- ALP = alkaline phosphatase.
- CBD = common bile duct.
- CCHS = cholangitis/cholangiohepatitis.
- DIC = disseminated intravascular coagulation.
- EHBDO = extrahepatic bile duct obstruction.
- GB = gallbladder.
- GBM = GB mucocele.
- SAMe = *S*-adenosylmethionine.

Suggested Reading

Mayhew PD, Holt DE, McLear RC, et al. Pathogenesis and outcome of extrahepatic biliary obstruction in cats. J Small Anim Pract 2002, 43:247–253.

Mehler SJ. Complications of the extrahepatic biliary surgery in companion animals. Vet Clin North Am Small Anim Pract 2011, 41:949–967.

Mehler SJ, Mayhew PD, Drobatz KJ, et al. Variables associated with outcome in dogs undergoing extrahepatic biliary surgery: 60 cases (1988–2002). Vet Surg 2004, 33:644–649.

Author Sharon A. Center

Consulting Editor Kate Holan

BILIOUS VOMITING SYNDROME

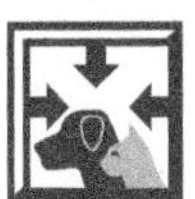

BASICS

OVERVIEW

• Bilious vomiting syndrome (BVS) is suspected to be secondary to alterations in normal gastrointestinal (GI) motility. BVS is associated with chronic intermittent vomiting of bile, thought to be the result of reflux of intestinal contents (bile) into the stomach. The normal aboral gastric and intestinal motility and functional pylorus prevent the reflux of bile back into the stomach. When bile is refluxed into the stomach it is normally rapidly removed by subsequent peristaltic contractions. Bile remaining in the gastric lumen along with gastric acid and pepsin can subsequently cause gastric mucosal damage. • Clinical signs often occur early in the morning, suggesting that prolonged fasting or gastric inactivity may modify normal motility patterns, resulting in bile reflux. • System affected—GI.

SIGNALMENT

• Commonly observed in dogs, rarely in cats.
• Most animals are young or middle-aged.
• No breed or sex predisposition.

SIGNS

• Chronic intermittent vomiting of bile associated with empty stomach. Signs generally occur late at night or early in morning. Signs may occur daily, but usually intermittent. Between episodes, animal appears normal and most dogs appear healthy immediately after vomiting episodes. • Results of physical examination usually unremarkable.

CAUSES & RISK FACTORS

• Cause unknown (idiopathic). • Primary gastric hypomotility or abnormal intestinal peristaltic motility are suspected as probable underlying causes. • Conditions causing gastritis, duodenitis, or intestinal obstructive disease may be responsible for altered proximal GI motility and can cause bile reflux; investigate for parasitism (e.g., *Giardia*), inflammatory bowel disease (IBD), intestinal neoplasia, or obstructions as possible etiologies.
• Previous pyloric opening or resection surgery can increase risk of enterogastric reflux.

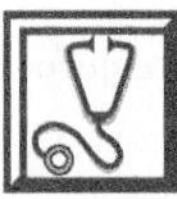

DIAGNOSIS

DIFFERENTIAL DIAGNOSIS

• Any number of GI and non-GI disorders can cause chronic vomiting. *Giardia* should be excluded since signs of this disease may mimic those of BVS. • IBD can result in bile reflux. • Intestinal obstruction or partial obstructions should be ruled out.

CBC/BIOCHEMISTRY/URINALYSIS

Results usually unremarkable.

OTHER LABORATORY TESTS

• Fecal examination to detect *Giardia* or other parasites. • Baseline cortisol to rule out hypoadrenocorticism. • GI panel—pancreatic lipase immunoreactivity (PLI), trypsin-like-immunoreactivity (TLI), cobalamin, folate.

IMAGING

• Barium contrast study may reveal delayed gastric emptying, although finding must be interpreted with caution. • Barium given with meals, radiopaque markers, or using special motility capsule (Smartpill®) may also demonstrate delayed gastric motility.

DIAGNOSTIC PROCEDURES

• Endoscopic findings frequently unremarkable and help rule out underlying GI disease. • May be evidence of bile in stomach or gastritis in antral region of stomach. • Endoscopy useful to rule out structural or inflammatory disease, since BVS is diagnosis of exclusion.

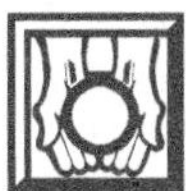

TREATMENT

• Generally not serious debilitating disorder if truly BVS, but important to rule out major conditions such as gastritis, IBD, or GI neoplasia. • Idiopathic bilious vomiting cases generally treated symptomatically on an outpatient basis and treatment response supports suspected diagnosis. • Feeding the animal small frequent meals, including late evening meal, often resolves clinical signs; food possibly could act as buffer to refluxed bile or may in some way enhance GI motility.
• Trial with hypoallergenic diet (novel protein or hydrolyzed protein) can also improve clinical signs, which may actually suggest underlying food-responsive enteropathy. • If diet modification fails, medical treatment should be considered.

MEDICATIONS

DRUG(S) OF CHOICE

• Choices include agents for gastric mucosal protection against refluxed bile or use of gastric prokinetic agents to improve motility.
• Often single evening dose of medication may be all that is required to prevent clinical signs if signs occur at night. • Drugs for gastric mucosal protection include various antacids or sucralfate (1 g/25 kg q8h).
• Drugs that block gastric acid production, including famotidine (0.5–1.0 mg/kg q12h–24h), ranitidine (1–2 mg/kg q8–12h), and omeprazole (0.7–1.5 mg/kg q12–24h) may be beneficial; ranitidine has mild gastric prokinetic effects in vitro and may be beneficial, but is less effective acid reducer.
• Specific gastric prokinetic agents include metoclopramide (0.2–0.4 mg/kg PO q6–8h) and cisapride (0.5 mg/kg PO q8–12h); cisapride only available through compounding pharmacies. • Erythromycin (0.5–1 mg/kg q8h) stimulates gastric motility by activation of motilin receptors and may also resolve signs.

CONTRAINDICATIONS/POSSIBLE INTERACTIONS

• Gastric prokinetic agents should not be administered in patients with GI obstruction.
• Metoclopramide can cause nervousness, anxiety, or depression. • Cisapride at higher doses can cause vomiting, diarrhea, or abdominal cramping. • Erythromycin can cause vomiting.

FOLLOW-UP

• Most patients respond to one of these treatments and clinical response supports the diagnosis. • Failure to respond suggests another underlying or causative factor.

MISCELLANEOUS

ASSOCIATED CONDITIONS

Gastroesophageal reflux.

SEE ALSO

• Gastric Motility Disorders.
• Gastroesophageal Reflux.

ABBREVIATIONS

• BVS = bilious vomiting syndrome.
• GI = gastrointestinal.
• IBD = inflammatory bowel disease.
• PLI = pancreatic lipase immunoreactivity.
• TLI = trypsin-like-immunoreactivity.

Suggested Reading

Ferguson LE, Wennogle SA, Webb CB. Bilious vomiting in dogs: retrospective study of 20 cases (2002–2012). J Am Anim Hosp Assoc 2016, 52:157–161.

Washabau RJ. Gastrointestinal motility disorders and gastrointestinal prokinetic therapy. Vet Clin North Am Small Anim Pract 2003, 33(5):1007–1028.

Webb C, Twedt DC. Canine gastritis. Vet Clin North Am Small Anim Pract 2003, 33(5):969–985.

Author Leah Ferguson

Consulting Editor Mark P. Rondeau

Acknowledgment The author and book editors acknowledge the prior contribution of David C. Twedt.

BLASTOMYCOSIS

BASICS

DEFINITION

A systemic, mycotic infection caused by the dimorphic soil organism *Blastomyces dermatitidis.*

PATHOPHYSIOLOGY

- A small spore (conidia) shed from the mycelial phase (*Ajellomyces dermatitidis*) of the organism growing in soil is inhaled, entering the terminal airway.
- At body temperature, spore transforms to its yeast form, which may initiate infection in lungs.
- From a focus of mycotic pneumonia, yeast may disseminate hematogenously throughout the body.
- Immune response produces pyogranulomatous inflammation.

SYSTEMS AFFECTED

- Respiratory—85% of affected dogs.
- Eyes, skin, subcutaneous tissues, lymphatic, and musculoskeletal—commonly affected.
- Reproductive, nasal cavity, and heart—less commonly affected.
- Subclinical infection is uncommon.

INCIDENCE/PREVALENCE

Depends on environmental and soil conditions that favor growth of *Blastomyces.* Growth of organism requires sandy, acidic soil and proximity to water.

GEOGRAPHIC DISTRIBUTION

Most common along the Mississippi, Ohio, and Tennessee river basins. Also reported in Great Lakes and St. Lawrence River areas, southern Canada, mid-Atlantic states; has been found outside endemic area in Colorado.

SIGNALMENT

Species

- Predominantly dog.
- Occasionally cat.

Breed Predilections

Large-breed dogs weighing ≥25 kg, especially sporting breeds; may reflect increased exposure rather than susceptibility.

Mean Age and Range

- Dogs—most common in those 1–5 years of age; uncommon after 7 years of age.
- Cats—no age predilection noted.

Predominant Sex

- Dogs—males in most studies.
- Cats—none noted.

SIGNS

Historical Findings

- Weight loss, hyporexia.
- Cough, dyspnea.
- Ocular inflammation/discharge.
- Draining skin lesions.
- Lymphadenitis.
- Lameness.
- Seizures or neurologic deficits with CNS involvement.
- Syncope if cardiac involvement.

Physical Examination Findings

Dogs

- Fever up to 104 °F (40 °C) in ~50% of patients.
- Harsh, dry lung sounds, increased respiratory effort.
- Generalized or regional lymphadenopathy with or without skin lesions or subcutaneous swellings.
- Uveitis with or without secondary glaucoma and conjunctivitis, ocular exudates, and corneal edema.
- Lameness—bone involvement in up to 30%.
- Testicular enlargement and prostatomegaly—occasional.
- Murmur and atrioventricular (AV) block—with endocarditis and myocarditis.

Cats

- Increased respiratory effort.
- Granulomatous skin lesions.
- Visual impairment.

RISK FACTORS

- Wet environment—banks of rivers, streams, lakes or swamps; most affected dogs live within 400 meters of water.
- Exposure to recently excavated areas.
- Reported in indoor-only cats.

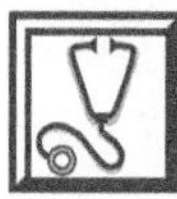

DIAGNOSIS

DIFFERENTIAL DIAGNOSIS

- Respiratory signs—bacterial pneumonia, metastatic neoplasia, heart failure, pleural effusion, or other fungal infection.
- Lymphadenopathy—similar to lymphoma.
- Combination of respiratory disease with ocular, bony, or skin/subcutaneous involvement in a young dog supports the diagnosis.

CBC/BIOCHEMISTRY/URINALYSIS

- CBC reflects inflammation; mild anemia in chronic cases.
- High serum globulins, borderline hypoalbuminemia with chronic infection.
- Hypercalcemia (generally mild) in some dogs.
- *Blastomyces* yeasts may be found in urine of dogs with prostatic involvement; mild proteinuria can be present.

OTHER LABORATORY TESTS

- Urine or serum antigen testing—sensitivity >90%; sensitivity greater with urine test; cross-reacts with other fungal infections (e.g., histoplasmosis).
- Agar gel immunodiffusion (AGID)—not sensitive early in disease, but very specific for infection.

IMAGING

Radiographs

- Lungs—generalized interstitial to nodular infiltrate, may be nonuniform distribution.
- Tracheobronchial lymphadenopathy.
- Changes may resemble metastatic neoplasia.
- Pleural effusion has been reported in dogs.
- Focal bone lesions—lytic and proliferative; can be mistaken for osteosarcoma.

DIAGNOSTIC PROCEDURES

- Cytology of lymph node aspirates, lung, or lytic bone aspirates, tracheal wash fluid, or impression smears of skin lesions—best method for diagnosis.
- Histopathology of bone biopsies or enucleated eyes.
- Organisms—usually plentiful in tissues; may be scarce in tracheal washes if there is no productive cough.

PATHOLOGIC FINDINGS

- Lesions—pyogranulomatous with budding 5–20 μm diameter yeast; thick, refractile, double-contoured cell wall; occasionally very fibrous with few organisms found.
- Special fungal stains—facilitate organism detection.

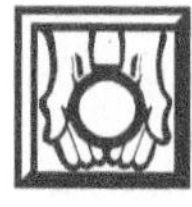

TREATMENT

NURSING CARE

Severely dyspneic dogs—require prolonged oxygen support; about 25% of dogs have worsening of respiratory disease during first days of treatment, attributed to an inflammatory response.

ACTIVITY

Patients with respiratory compromise must be restricted.

DIET

N/A

CLIENT EDUCATION

- Treatment is costly and long term.
- Infected dogs are not contagious to other animals or people.

SURGICAL CONSIDERATIONS

- Removal of abscessed lung lobe may be required if medical treatment ineffective.
- Blind eyes should be enucleated to remove potential sites of residual infection.

MEDICATIONS

DRUG(S) OF CHOICE

Itraconazole

- Dogs—5 mg/kg PO q12h with a fat-rich meal (e.g., canned dog food) for the first 3 days, then reduce to 5 mg/kg PO q24h.

- Cats—5 mg/kg PO q12h; open the 100 mg capsules containing pellets and mix with palatable food.
- Avoid antacid drugs as absorption best in acidic environment.
- Treat for minimum 90 days, or for 1 month after all signs of disease have resolved (whichever is longer).
- Absorption of compounded itraconazole is unreliable and use is not recommended.

Fluconazole

- Dogs—5 mg/kg PO q12h.
- Cats—5–10 mg/kg PO q12–24h; 50 mg/cat.
- Inexpensive, but may require longer treatment duration.

Amphotericin B

- For dogs with neurologic signs or life-threatening disease.
- 0.5–1.0 mg/kg IV q48h; use lipid complex for dogs with renal dysfunction.

CONTRAINDICATIONS

Corticosteroids—may allow continued proliferation of organisms; patients with previous steroid therapy require longer treatment duration; for dogs with life-threatening dyspnea, dexamethasone (0.1–0.2 mg/kg/day IV) for 2–3 days may be given with itraconazole treatment; taper and discontinue corticosteroids as soon as possible.

PRECAUTIONS

Itraconazole and Fluconazole Toxicity

- Anorexia—most common sign; attributed to liver toxicity; monitor serum alanine aminotransferase (ALT) activity monthly or when anorexia occurs; temporarily discontinue drug for patients with anorexia and moderate ALT activity elevation; after appetite improves, restart at half the previous dose.
- Ulcerative dermatitis—in some dogs due to vasculitis; dose related; temporarily discontinue drug until ulcers resolve, then restart at half the previous dose.

Amphotericin B Toxicity

- Only absolute contraindication to therapy is anaphylaxis, but major limiting factor is cumulative nephrotoxicity.
- Monitor serum creatinine concentration throughout therapy—elevation above normal or 20% greater than baseline considered significant.

FOLLOW-UP

PATIENT MONITORING

Serum chemistry—monthly to monitor for hepatic toxicity, or if anorexia develops.

Thoracic Radiographs

- Considerable permanent pulmonary changes (fibrosis/scarring) may occur after the infection resolves, making determination of persistent active disease difficult.
- At 90 days of treatment—if active pulmonary disease, continue treatment for additional 30 days.
- If lungs appear normal, stop treatment and repeat radiographs again in 30 days.
- At 120 days of treatment—if the lungs appear the same as day 90, changes are residual (fibrosis); if clearer than day 90, continue treatment for 30 more days. If lesions are significantly worse than at 90 days, consider a change in therapeutic agent.
- Continue treatment as long as improvement is noted in the lungs; if there is no further improvement and no indication of active disease, the lesions are likely the result of scarring.

Urine Antigen Testing

- Positive test is generally related to active disease.
- If other signs have resolved, a negative test supports treatment discontinuation.

PREVENTION/AVOIDANCE

- Location of environmental growth of *Blastomyces* organisms unknown, thus difficult to avoid exposure; exposure to lakes and streams may be restricted (but limited practicality).
- Dogs that recover from the infection may be immune to reinfection.

EXPECTED COURSE AND PROGNOSIS

- Death—25% of dogs die during first week of treatment; early diagnosis improves chance of survival.
- Severe pulmonary disease and CNS involvement decrease prognosis.
- Recurrence—approximately 20% of dogs; usually within 3–6 months after completion of treatment; may occur >1 year after treatment; a second course of azole treatment cures most patients; drug resistance has not been observed.
- With early detection of blastomycosis, the prognosis in cats appears similar to dogs.

MISCELLANEOUS

ZOONOTIC POTENTIAL

- Yeast form is not spread from animals to humans, except through bite wounds; inoculation of organisms from dog bites has occurred.
- Avoid cuts during necropsy of infected dogs and avoid needle sticks when aspirating lesions.
- Warn clients that blastomycosis is acquired from an environmental source and that they may have been exposed to the source; the incidence in dogs is 10 times that in humans.
- Encourage clients with respiratory and skin lesions to inform their physicians that they may have been exposed to blastomycosis.

PREGNANCY/FERTILITY/BREEDING

Azole drugs can have teratogenic effects (embryotoxicity found at high doses) and should ideally be avoided during pregnancy (but the risk of not treating the mother must be balanced with the theoretical risk of azole therapy to the fetuses).

ABBREVIATIONS

- AGID = agar gel immunodiffusion.
- ALT = alanine transaminase.
- AV = atrioventricular.

INTERNET RESOURCES

Information on antigen testing: www.miravistalabs.com

Suggested Reading

Crews LJ, Feeney DA, Jessen CR, et al. Radiographic findings in dogs with pulmonary blastomycosis: 125 cases (1989–2006). J Am Vet Med Assoc 2008, 232:215–221.

Foy DS, Trepanier LA, Kirsch EJ, et al. Serum and urine Blastomyces antigen concentrations as markers of clinical remission in dogs treated for systemic blastomycosis. J Vet Intern Med 2014, 28:305–310.

Legendre AM, Rohrbach BW, Toal RL, et al. Treatment of blastomycosis with itraconazole in 112 dogs. J Vet Intern Med 1996, 10:365–371.

Mazepa AS, Trepanir LA, Foy DS. Retrospective comparison of the efficacy of fluconazole or itraconazole for the treatment of systemic blastomycosis in dogs. J Vet Intern Med 2011, 25:440–445.

Spector D, Legendre AM, Wheat J, et al. Antigen and antibody testing for the diagnosis of blastomycosis in dogs. J Vet Intern Med 2008, 22:839–843.

Author Daniel S. Foy
Consulting Editor Amie Koenig

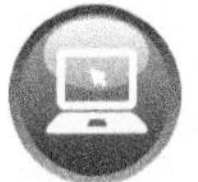

Client Education Handout available online

BLEPHARITIS

BASICS

DEFINITION

Inflammation of outer (skin) and middle (muscle, connective tissue, and glands) portions of eyelid, usually with secondary inflammation of palpebral conjunctiva.

PATHOPHYSIOLOGY

• Inflammation—immune mediated, infectious, endocrine mediated, self- and external trauma, parasitic, radiation, nutritional. Inflammatory response often exaggerated because conjunctiva is rich in mast cells and densely vascularized.
• Meibomian gland dysfunction—bacterial lipases alter meibomian lipids and plug gland; produce irritating fatty acids, enhance bacterial growth, and destabilize tear film.

SYSTEMS AFFECTED

Ophthalmic

SIGNALMENT

See Causes.

SIGNS

• Serous, mucoid, or mucopurulent ocular discharge. • Blepharospasm. • Eyelid hyperemia, edema, and thickening.
• Pruritus. • Excoriation. • Depigmentation—skin, hair (in Siamese-type cats with color points, lightening of hair on affected lids due to increased skin temperature). • Alopecia.
• Swollen, cream-colored meibomian glands.
• Elevated, pinpoint meibomian gland orifices. • Abscesses. • Scales, crusts, papules, or pustules. • Single or multiple nodular hyperemic swellings. • Concurrent conjunctivitis and/or keratitis.

CAUSES

Congenital

• Eyelid abnormalities—may promote self-trauma or moist dermatitis. • Prominent nasal folds, medial trichiasis, and lower lid entropion—shih tzu, Pekingese, English bulldog, Lhasa apso, pug; Persian and Himalayan cat. • Distichia—shih tzu, pug, golden retriever, Labrador retriever, poodle, English bulldog. • Ectopic cilia. • Lateral lid entropion—Chinese Shar-Pei, chow chow, Labrador retriever, Rottweiler.
• Lagophthalmos—brachycephalic dogs; Persian, Himalayan, and Burmese cats. • Deep medial canthal pocket—dolichocephalic dogs.
• Dermoids—Rottweiler, dachshund, and others; Burmese cat.

Allergic

• Type I (immediate)—atopy, food, insect bite, inhalant, *Staphylococcus* hypersensitivity (SH). • Type II (cytotoxic)—pemphigus, pemphigoid, drug eruption • Type III (immune complex)—systemic lupus erythematosus (SLE), SH, drug eruption.
• Type IV (cell mediated)—contact and flea bite hypersensitivity; drug eruption.

Bacterial

• Hordeolum—localized abscess of eyelid glands, usually staphylococcal; may be external (sty in young dogs, glands of Zeis) or internal (in old dogs, meibomian glands). • Generalized bacterial blepharitis and meibomianitis—usually *Staphylococcus* or *Streptococcus*. • *Bartonella henselae*—chronic blepharoconjunctivitis in cats.
• Pyogranulomas. • SH—young and old dogs.

Neoplastic

• Sebaceous adenomas and adenocarcinomas—from meibomian gland.
• Squamous cell carcinoma—white cats.
• Mast cell—may appear as swollen, hyperemic lesion.

Other

• External trauma—eyelid lacerations, thermal or chemical burns. • Mycotic—dermatophytosis; systemic fungal granulomas.
• Parasitic—demodicosis; sarcoptic mange; *Cuterebra* and *Notoedres cati. Note: Demodex injai* has a propensity for sebaceous glands and can be associated with meibomian gland dysfunction in dogs, including chalazia and granulomatous blepharitis. • Chalazia—sterile, yellow-white, painless meibomian gland swellings caused by granulomatous inflammatory response to meibum in surrounding eyelid tissue. • Nutritional—zinc-responsive dermatosis (Siberian husky, Alaskan Malamute, puppies), fatty acid deficiency.
• Endocrine—hypothyroidism (dogs); hyperadrenocorticism (dogs); diabetic dermatosis. • Viral—chronic blepharitis in cats (feline herpesvirus type 1 [FHV-1]).
• Irritant—drug reaction (e.g., neomycin); smoke in environment; post-parotid duct transposition. • Familial canine dermatomyositis—collie and Shetland sheepdog.
• Nodular granulomatous episclerokeratitis—fibrous histiocytoma and collie granuloma; may affect eyelids, cornea, or conjunctiva.
• Eosinophilic granuloma—cats; may affect eyelids, cornea, or conjunctiva. • Eyelid contact with tear overflow and purulent exudate (tear burn). • Keratitis, conjunctivitis, dacryocystitis. • Dry eye.
• Orbital disease. • Radiotherapy. • Idiopathic—especially Persians and Himalayans.

RISK FACTORS

• Breed predisposition to eyelid abnormalities (e.g., entropion, ectropion).
• Hypothyroidism—may promote chronic bacterial disease in dogs. • Canine seborrhea—may promote chronic generalized meibomianitis, with predisposition for *Demodex injai* infection.

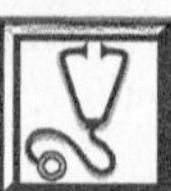

DIAGNOSIS

DIFFERENTIAL DIAGNOSIS

Clinical signs are diagnostic.

CBC/BIOCHEMISTRY/URINALYSIS

Usually normal unless metabolic cause (e.g., diabetic dermatosis).

OTHER LABORATORY TESTS

Indicated for systemic disorders, including hypothyroidism.

DIAGNOSTIC PROCEDURES

• Eye examination—inciting cause, corneal ulcer, foreign body, distichia, ectopic cilia, keratoconjunctivitis sicca (KCS). • Ancillary ocular tests— fluorescein, Schirmer tear test.
• Thorough history and dermatologic exam: ○ Cytology—deep skin scrape, conjunctival scrape, or exudate from glands and pustules. ○ Wood's light evaluation, dermatophyte culture. ○ KOH preparation. ○ Intradermal skin testing, other testing for hypersensitivity-induced disease. ○ Consider referral to a dermatologist for refractory cases. • Aerobic bacterial culture and sensitivity—of exudate from skin, conjunctiva, expressed meibomian glands, or pustules; often will not recover *Staphylococcus* from patients with chronic meibomianitis and suspected SH. • Immunofluorescent antibody assay or PCR for FHV-1 and *Chlamydia*—in conjunctival scrapings from cats with primary conjunctivitis or keratitis.
• Full-thickness wedge biopsy of eyelid.

PATHOLOGIC FINDINGS

Routine histopathology often nondiagnostic in chronic disease.

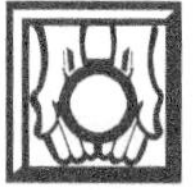

TREATMENT

APPROPRIATE HEALTH CARE

See Nursing Care.

NURSING CARE

• Prevent self-trauma—Elizabethan collar.
• Cleanse eyelids—to remove crusts; warm compresses applied for 5–15 minutes 3–4 times daily, avoiding ocular surfaces. Use saline, lactated Ringer's solution, or a commercial ocular cleansing agent (e.g., I-Lid 'n Lash®); clip periocular hair short.
• Common underlying cause in cats is FHV-1 infection; minimize stress.

DIET

Only if food allergy.

CLIENT EDUCATION

In cats with FHV-1-related blepharitis, inform client that there is no cure and that clinical signs often recur when animal is stressed.

SURGICAL CONSIDERATIONS

• Temporary everting eyelid sutures—spastic entropion; or in puppies before permanent surgical correction. • Repair eyelid lacerations. • Lancing—large abscesses only; lance and curette hordeola that resist medical treatment and chalazia that have hardened and cause keratitis; manually express infected meibomian secretions.

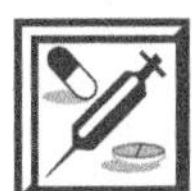

MEDICATIONS

DRUG(S) OF CHOICE

Antibiotics

• Systemic—for bacterial eyelid infections (e.g., cephalexin 20 mg/kg IV q8h). For *Bartonella henselae* infection in cats, therapy may include doxycycline (10 mg/kg PO q12h for 3 weeks), pradofloxacin (5–10 mg/kg PO q12–24h for 28–42 days), or azithromycin (10 mg/kg PO q24h for 3 weeks). • Topical—neomycin, polymyxin B, and bacitracin combination or chloramphenicol.

Congenital

• Topical antibiotic ointment—q6–12h to prevent frictional rubbing of eyelid hairs or cilia on ocular surface. • Regularly flush debris from deep medial canthal pocket using saline, lactated Ringer's solution, or ocular irrigant.

External Trauma

• Topical antibiotic ointment—q6–12h; in patients with spastic entropion and blepharospasm until surgical correction. • Systemic antibiotics.

Allergic

• SH blepharitis—systemic broad-spectrum antibiotics and systemic corticosteroids (prednisolone 0.5 mg/kg PO q12h for 3–5 days, then taper); many patients respond to systemic corticosteroids alone; systemic cyclosporine (5 mg/kg PO q24h until remission, then q48–72h) if refractory to corticosteroids; failure of treatment—consider injections of *Staphylococcus aureus* bacterin (Staphage Lysate®). • Infected meibomian glands—oral tetracycline (15–20 mg/kg PO q8h), doxycycline (3–5 mg/kg PO q12h), or cephalexin (22 mg/kg PO q8h) for 3 weeks (the former two are lipophilic and cause decreased production of bacterial lipases and irritating fatty acids); topical polymyxin B and neomycin with 0.1% dexamethasone (q6–8h) or topical 0.02% tacrolimus compounded ointment (q8–12h). *Some affected dogs might also require treatment for demodecosis.* • Eyelid lesions associated with puppy strangles—treat generalized condition. • Atopy—see Atopic Dermatitis.

Bacterial

• Based on culture and sensitivity or serologic testing. • Pending results—topical polymyxin B and neomycin with 0.1% dexamethasone ointment (q4–6h) and systemic broad-spectrum antibiotic.

Mycotic

Microsporium canis infection—see Dermatophytosis.

Parasitic

Demodicosis, *Notoedres* infection, sarcoptic mange—see relevant chapters.

Idiopathic

Clinical signs often controlled with topical polymyxin B and neomycin with 0.1% dexamethasone (q8–24h or as needed); occasionally may need prednisolone (0.5 mg/kg PO q12h for 3–5 days, then taper) and/or systemic antibiotic.

CONTRAINDICATIONS

• Topical corticosteroids—do not use with corneal ulceration. • Many cats with presumed idiopathic blepharoconjunctivitis have FHV-1 infection; topical and systemic corticosteroids may exacerbate infection. • Oral tetracycline and doxycycline—do not use in puppies and kittens. • Neomycin—avoid topical use if possible cause of blepharitis. • Neomycin, bacitracin, and polymyxin—avoid topical ophthalmic use in cats due to rare but potentially fatal anaphylactic reaction.

PRECAUTIONS

• Ectoparasitism—wear gloves; do not contact ocular surfaces with a drug topically applied to skin; apply artificial tear ointment to eyes for protection. • Topical gentamicin, neomycin, terramycin, and most ointments—may cause irritant blepharoconjunctivitis (rare); withdrawal may resolve condition.

POSSIBLE INTERACTIONS

Staphylococcal bacterin may cause anaphylactic reaction (rare).

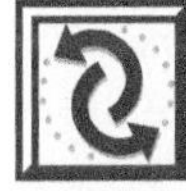

FOLLOW-UP

PATIENT MONITORING

• Depends on cause, therapy. • Bacterial—systemic and topical treatment for at least 3 weeks; should notice improvement within 10 days. • Most common causes of treatment failure—use of subinhibitory antibiotic dosages, failure to correct one or more predisposing factors, early discontinuation of medications.

PREVENTION/AVOIDANCE

Depends on cause.

POSSIBLE COMPLICATIONS

• Cicatricial lid contracture—results in trichiasis, ectropion, or lagophthalmos. • Spastic entropion—because of blepharospasm and pain. • Qualitative tear film deficiency—loss of proper meibum secretion. • Recurrence of bacterial infection or FHV-1 blepharoconjunctivitis.

EXPECTED COURSE AND PROGNOSIS

Depend on cause.

MISCELLANEOUS

ZOONOTIC POTENTIAL

• Dermatophytosis.
• Sarcoptic mange.

SEE ALSO

• Atopic Dermatitis.
• Conjunctivitis—Cats.
• Conjunctivitis—Dogs.
• Dermatophytosis.
• Epiphora.
• Keratitis—Nonulcerative.
• Keratitis—Ulcerative.
• Red Eye.

ABBREVIATIONS

• FHV-1 = feline herpesvirus type 1.
• KCS = keratoconjunctivitis sicca.
• SH = *Staphylococcus* hypersensitivity.
• SLE = systemic lupus erythematosus.

Suggested Reading

Bettany S, Mueller R, Maggs D. Diseases of the eyelids. In: Maggs DJ, Miller PE, Ofri R, eds., Slatter's Fundamentals of Veterinary Ophthalmology, 6th ed. St. Louis, MO: Saunders, 2018, pp. 127–157.

Author Terri L. McCalla
Consulting Editor Kathern E. Myrna

Client Education Handout available online

BLIND QUIET EYE

BASICS

DEFINITION

Loss of vision in one or both eyes without ocular vascular injection or other externally apparent signs of ocular inflammation.

PATHOPHYSIOLOGY

Results from abnormalities in focusing images on the retina, the retina detecting an image, optic nerve transmission, or the brain not interpreting images correctly.

SYSTEMS AFFECTED

• Nervous. • Ophthalmic.

SIGNALMENT

• Dog and cat. • Any age, breed, or sex.
• Many causes (e.g., cataracts and progressive retinal atrophy) have a genetic basis and are often highly breed and age specific.
• Sudden acquired retinal degeneration syndrome (SARDS)—tends to occur in older dogs. • Optic nerve hypoplasia—congenital.

SIGNS

Historical Findings

• Vary with underlying cause. • Bumping into objects. • Clumsy behavior. • Reluctance to move. • Impaired vision in dim light.

Physical Examination Findings

• Vary with underlying cause. • Decreased or absent menace or dazzle response. • Impaired visual placing responses.

CAUSES

• Cataracts—entire lens must become opaque to produce complete blindness; incomplete opacification may reduce performance of visually demanding tasks. • Loss of focusing power of the lens—rarely completely blinding; substantial hyperopia (far-sightedness) occurs when the optical power of the lens is not replaced after lens extraction or if the lens luxates posteriorly out of the pupillary plane and into the vitreous. • Retina—SARDS, progressive retinal atrophy (PRA), retinal detachment, taurine deficiency (cats), enrofloxacin toxicity (cats), ivermectin toxicity (dogs, cats). • Optic nerve—optic neuritis, neoplasia of the optic nerve or adjacent tissues, trauma, optic nerve hypoplasia, lead toxicity, excessive traction on the optic nerve during enucleation resulting in trauma to the contralateral optic nerve or optic chiasm (especially cats and brachycephalic dogs). • CNS (amaurosis)—lesions of the optic chiasm or tract, optic radiation, or visual cortex. CNS-associated vision loss that occurs at a level higher than the optic chiasm often has vague visual disturbances in which the patient has some vision, but clearly does not have normal vision.

RISK FACTORS

• Poorly regulated diabetes mellitus—cataracts.
• Related animals with genetic cataracts or PRA.
• Systemic hypertension—retinal detachment.
• CNS hypoxia—blindness may become apparent after excessively deep anesthesia or revival from cardiac arrest.

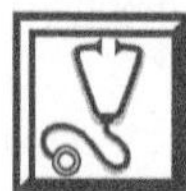

DIAGNOSIS

DIFFERENTIAL DIAGNOSIS

Signs

• Anterior segment inflammation and glaucoma—conjunctiva typically injected.
• Young patients—may lack menace responses, but will successfully navigate a maze or visually track hand movements or cotton balls.
• Postictal period—transient vision loss.
• Abnormal mentation—may be difficult to determine whether an animal is visual; other neurologic abnormalities help localize the lesion.

Causes

• Optic neuritis, retinal detachment, SARDS, or visual cortex hypoxia—sudden vision loss (over hours to weeks). • SARDS—often preceded by polyuria, polydipsia, polyphagia, and weight gain. • PRA—gradual vision loss, especially in dim light; apparently acute vision loss with sudden change in environment. • Cataract—either gradual or rapidly increasing opacification and vision loss in a quiet eye. • Optic nerve hypoplasia—congenital; may be unilateral or bilateral.
• Optic neuropathy or CNS disease—other signs of neurologic abnormalities. • Pupillary light responses—usually normal with cataracts or visual cortex lesions; sluggish to absent with retinal or optic nerve diseases.
• Ophthalmoscopy—normal with early SARDS, retrobulbar optic neuritis, and higher visual pathway lesions; abnormal with retinal detachment and disorders of optic nerve head.

CBC/BIOCHEMISTRY/URINALYSIS

• Usually normal, unless underlying systemic disease. • Hyperglycemia or glucosuria—may note with diabetic cataracts. • Elevated alkaline phosphatase (ALP) enzyme activity and changes consistent with hyperadrenocorticism (Cushing's syndrome)—suggest SARDS.
• Retinal detachment secondary to systemic hypertension (cats)—azotemia or changes consistent with hyperthyroidism.

OTHER LABORATORY TESTS

• Blood lead and serology for deep fungal or viral infections—consider for suspected optic neuritis (see Optic Neuritis and Papilledema).
• Low-dose dexamethasone suppression test—may help rule out Cushing's syndrome with SARDS. • Sex hormone abnormalities are common in patients with SARDS.

IMAGING

• Ocular ultrasound—may demonstrate retinal detachment (especially if the ocular media are opaque) or optic nerve mass lesion.
• Plain skull radiographs—seldom informative. • CT or MRI—often helpful with orbital or CNS lesions.

DIAGNOSTIC PROCEDURES

See Figure 1.
• Ophthalmic examination with a penlight—usually permits diagnosis of cataracts or retinal detachments severe enough to cause blindness.
• Ophthalmoscopy—may show PRA, late SARDS, or optic nerve disease; normal exam suggests early SARDS, retrobulbar optic neuritis, or a CNS lesion. • Systemic arterial blood pressure—determine in patients with retinal detachment. • Electroretinography—differentiates retinal from optic nerve or CNS disease. • Cerebrospinal fluid (CSF) tap—may be of value with a neurogenic cause of vision loss.

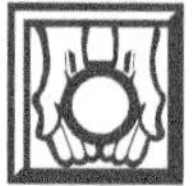

TREATMENT

• Try to obtain a definitive diagnosis on an outpatient basis before initiating treatment.
• Consider referral before attempting empirical therapy. • Most causes are not fatal, but must perform a workup to rule out potentially fatal diseases. • Reassure client that most causes of a blind quiet eye are not painful and that blind animals can lead relatively normal and functional lives.
• Warn client that the environment should be examined for potential hazards to a blind animal. • Advise client that patients with PRA or genetic cataracts should not be bred and related animals should be examined.
• Retinal detachment—restrict exercise until the retina is firmly reattached. • Calorie-restricted diet—to prevent obesity owing to reduced activity level. • Cats with nutritionally induced retinopathy—ensure diet has adequate levels of taurine. • SARDS, PRA, optic nerve atrophy, and optic nerve hypoplasia—no effective treatment.
• Cataracts, luxated lenses, and some forms of retinal detachment—best treated surgically.

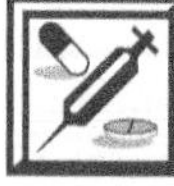

MEDICATIONS

DRUG(S) OF CHOICE

• Depend on cause. • If workup is declined, infectious disease is unlikely, and the likely diagnosis is either SARDS or retrobulbar optic neuritis—consider systemic prednisolone (1–2 mg/kg/day PO for 7–14 days, then taper); may concurrently administer oral broad-spectrum antibiotic.

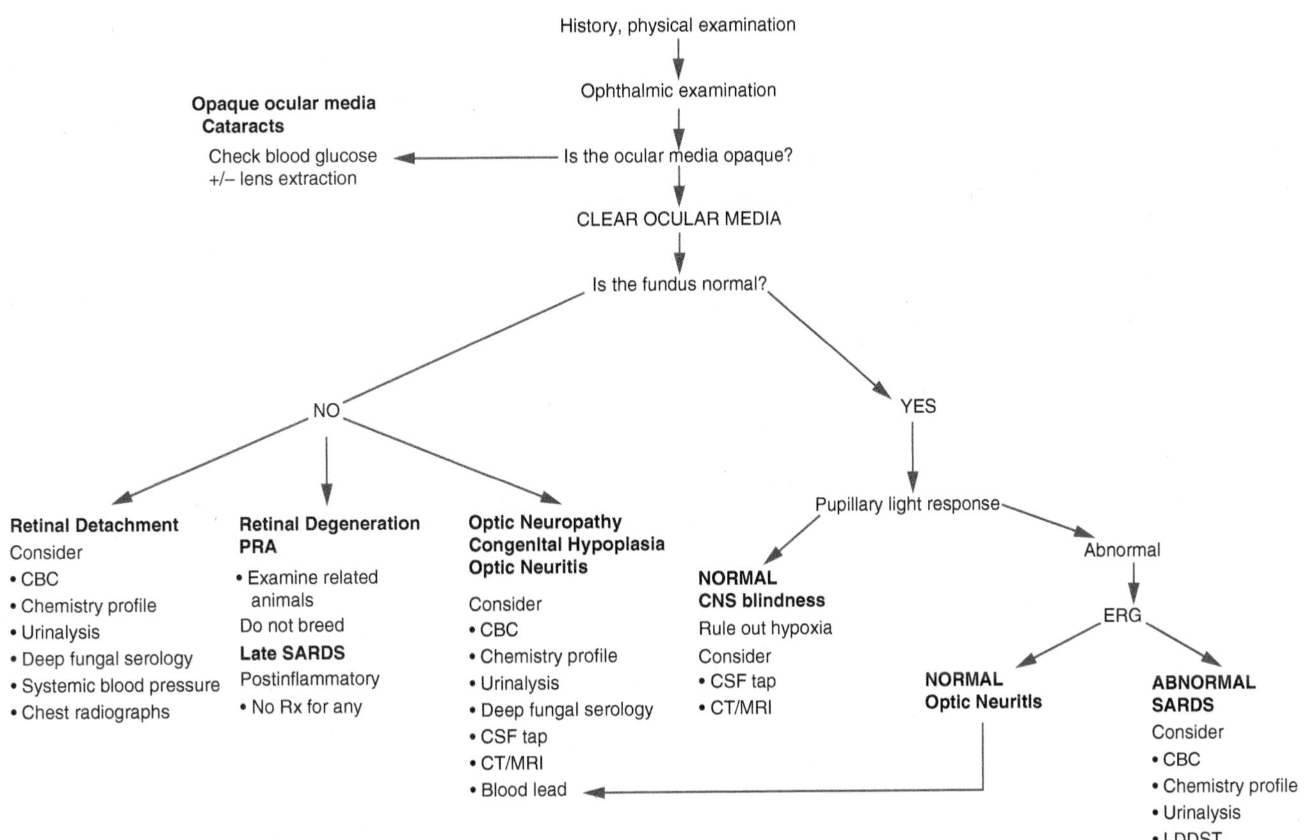

Figure 1.

CONTRAINDICATIONS

Do not use systemic corticosteroids or other immunosuppressive drugs with optic neuritis and retinal detachments that are infectious in origin.

PRECAUTIONS

Pretreatment with corticosteroids may mimic or mask liver enzyme changes in SARDS.

POSSIBLE INTERACTIONS

N/A

ALTERNATIVE DRUG(S)

Oral azathioprine 1–2 mg/kg/day PO for 3–7 days, then taper; may be used to treat immune-mediated retinal detachments if systemic corticosteroids are not effective; perform a CBC, platelet count, and liver enzyme every 1–2 weeks for the first 8 weeks, then periodically.

FOLLOW-UP

PATIENT MONITORING

• Repeat ophthalmic examinations—as required to ensure that ocular inflammation is controlled and, if possible, vision is maintained. • Recurrence of vision loss—common in optic neuritis; may occur weeks, months, or years after initial presentation.

POSSIBLE COMPLICATIONS

• Death. • Permanent vision loss. • Loss of the eye. • Chronic ocular inflammation and pain. • Obesity from inactivity or as a sequela of SARDS.

MISCELLANEOUS

ASSOCIATED CONDITIONS

• SARDS (dogs)—signs similar to those of hyperadrenocorticism. • Neurologic disease—may note seizures, behavior or personality changes, circling or other CNS signs.
• Cardiomyopathy (cats)—taurine deficiency.

AGE-RELATED FACTORS

• PRA and many cataracts—breed-specific ages of onset. • SARDS—tends to occur in older dogs. • Optic nerve hypoplasia—congenital.

ZOONOTIC POTENTIAL

N/A

PREGNANCY/FERTILITY/BREEDING

Corticosteroids and immunosuppressive drugs may complicate pregnancy.

SEE ALSO

Optic Neuritis and Papilledema.

ABBREVIATIONS

• ALP = alkaline phosphatase. • CSF = cerebrospinal fluid. • PRA = progressive retinal atrophy. • SARDS = sudden acquired retinal degeneration syndrome.

INTERNET RESOURCES

• https://muffinshalo.com •http://www.pepedog.com •https://www.akc.org/expert-advice/health/seven-ways-to-keep-the-light-in-your-blind-dogs-life

Suggested Reading

Maggs DJ, Miller PE, Ofri R. Fundamentals of Veterinary Ophthalmology, 6th ed. St Louis, MO: Elsevier, 2018.

Rubin LF. Inherited Eye Disease in Purebred Dogs. Baltimore, MD: Williams & Wilkins, 1989.

Author Paul E. Miller

Consulting Editor Kathern E. Myrna

Client Education Handout available online

BLOOD TRANSFUSION REACTIONS

BASICS

OVERVIEW

• Reaction to donor blood cells can result in minor (fever, urticaria) or major (hemolysis, anaphylactic shock) reactions, usually acute but can be delayed. • Can occur with administration of any blood-derived product.

SIGNALMENT

• Dogs and cats. • No sex predilection. • All ages affected.

SIGNS

Acute Nonhemolytic Reaction

• Fever, urticaria, erythema, pruritus (in 10–25% of transfusions). • Septic shock from bacterial contamination of blood products.
• Transfusion-associated circulatory overload (TACO)—dyspnea, cough, cyanosis (congestive heart failure). • Transfusion-associated acute lung injury (TRALI)—dyspnea, cyanosis.
• Citrate toxicity—facial pruritis, weakness.
• Hyperammonemia—encephalopathy.

Acute Hemolytic Reaction

• Occurs in 1–5% of transfusions.
• Tachycardia, shock, anaphylaxis, death.
• Collapse, lethargy, weakness. • Vomiting, diarrhea. • Pigmenturia, potential for pigmentary nephropathy. • Restlessness, hypersalivation, urticaria, facial swelling.
• Hemolysis of transfused red blood cells (RBCs).

Delayed Hemolytic Reaction

Clinical signs of anemia may recur.

Delayed Nonhemolytic Reaction

Signs of blood-borne disease (e.g., *Babesia, Mycoplasma haemofelis, Ehrlichia*).

CAUSES & RISK FACTORS

Cats and previously transfused dogs have higher risk of transfusion reactions.

Acute Nonhemolytic Reaction

• Anaphylaxis/immune reaction to donor cells, major histocompatibility complex (MHC) or plasma antigens, release of inflammatory mediators and pyrogens. • RBC membrane fragility (from depleted adenosine triphosphate [ATP]) can result in mechanical destruction during transfusion; degradation of ATP causes hyperammonemia in stored blood.
• Contamination of blood can result from lack of aseptic collection or poor storage conditions. • TACO results from rapid transfusion or excessive transfusion volume.
• Citrate toxicity causes hypocalcemia.

Acute Hemolysis

• Type II hypersensitivity reaction caused by naturally occurring or acquired antibodies against donor RBCs (cats have existing alloantibodies against other blood type, dogs require prior sensitization). • Transfusion of damaged RBCs.

Delayed Hemolysis

Immune reaction to RBC antigens (5–14 days after transfusion).

Delayed Nonhemolytic Reaction

Transmission of blood-borne disease.

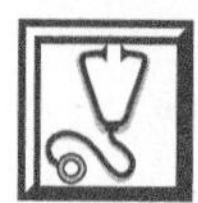

DIAGNOSIS

DIFFERENTIAL DIAGNOSIS

• Hemolysis—other hemolytic disease (e.g., immune-mediated hemolytic anemia, *Babesia*, zinc toxicity). • Fever, hypotension—infectious/inflammatory disease, contamination of IV catheter sites. • Urticaria/pruritis—allergic reaction; avoid coadministration of medications during transfusion to distinguish drug vs. transfusion reaction. • Pigmenturia—hematuria or myoglobinuria vs. hemoglobinuria.

CBC/BIOCHEMISTRY/URINALYSIS

Hemoglobinemia, leukocytosis, thrombocytopenia possible, bilirubinemia, pigmenturia (hemoglobin/bilirubinuria).

OTHER LABORATORY TESTS

• Cross-match to confirm incompatibility.
• Bacterial culture or microscopic examination of blood may reveal contamination.
• Centrifugation of donor blood may show hemolysis.

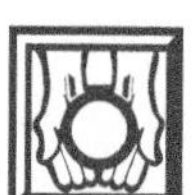

TREATMENT

• *Acute, nonhemolytic reaction*—stop transfusion: if signs resolve, restart at slower rate, if signs recur, discontinue transfusion; if dyspnea, supplemental oxygen; if volume overload/congestive heart failure, furosemide; animals with TRALI may require mechanical ventilation. • *Acute, hemolytic reaction*—stop transfusion and administer IV fluids to maintain blood pressure and treat shock; in hypotensive patients, administer isotonic crystalloids (20–30 mL/kg, repeat as necessary); epinephrine and vasopressor therapy for severe anaphylaxis.

MEDICATIONS

DRUG(S) OF CHOICE

• For anaphylaxis—IV crystalloid as above, epinephrine 0.01 mg/kg IV. • For urticaria, fever—diphenhydramine (1–2 mg/kg IM); dexamethasone sodium phosphate (0.1 mg/kg IV once). • If septic shock suspected—broad-spectrum IV antibiotics, IV fluid therapy.
• Volume overload—furosemide 2–4 mg/kg IV, oxygen. • Hypocalcemia—calcium gluconate 50–150 mg/kg IV slowly (monitor ECG).

FOLLOW-UP

PATIENT MONITORING

• Check attitude, rectal temperature, and vital signs before, during, and after transfusion. • For acute hemolytic reactions or septicemia—intensive monitoring and supportive care required. • Measure PCV or hematocrit 2 hours post transfusion, sooner if clinical signs warrant.

PREVENTION/AVOIDANCE

• Record any transfusion reaction in the medical file. • Pretransfusion testing: ◦ Screen donors for infectious disease. ◦ Blood type donors and recipients (imperative in cats).
◦ Cross-match patients receiving repeated transfusions. • Have standard transfusion protocols, dedicated storage for blood products.
• Transfusion administration should start slowly but be completed within 4 hours.
• Leukoreduction of RBC-containing products may decrease incidence of reactions. • Older stored blood more likely to result in reaction.

POSSIBLE COMPLICATIONS

Fulminant hemolysis may cause acute renal failure, multiorgan dysfunction, coagulopathies, and cardiac arrhythmias.

EXPECTED COURSE AND PROGNOSIS

• Acute course in most animals; nonhemolytic reactions have good prognosis.
• Prognosis guarded in animals with severe reactions or hemolysis.

MISCELLANEOUS

SEE ALSO

Sepsis and Bacteremia.

ABBREVIATIONS

• ATP = adenosine triphosphate. • MHC = major histocompatibility complex. • RBC = red blood cells. • TACO = transfusion-associated circulatory overload. • TRALI = transfusion-associated acute lung injury.

Suggested Reading

Hann L, Brown DC, King LG, Callan MB. Effect of duration of packed red blood cell storage on morbidity and mortality in dogs after transfusion: 3,095 cases (2001–2010). J Vet Intern Med 2014, 28(6):1830–1837.

Maglaras CH, Koenig A, Bedard DL, Brainard BM. Retrospective evaluation of the effect of red blood cell product age on occurrence of acute transfusion-related complications in dogs: 210 cases (2010–2012). JVECC 2017, 27(1):108–120.

Wardrop KJ. Update on canine and feline blood donor screening for blood-borne pathogens. J Vet Intern Med 2016, 30(1):15–35.

Author Jörg Bucheler

Consulting Editor Melinda S. Camus

BLUE-GREEN ALGAE TOXICOSIS

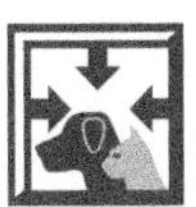

BASICS

OVERVIEW

• Cyanobacterial blooms can occur in fresh and brackish waters, and in backyard ponds where algal material is concentrated. • Nutrient-rich runoff, increased water temperatures, and stagnant water conditions favor toxic bloom formation. • Blue-green algae exposure can lead to acute hepato- or neurotoxicosis in animals and humans. • Skin irritation following exposure to cyanobacteria-contaminated water may occur. • Hepatotoxic blue-green algae poisonings are more frequently reported than neurotoxic algal intoxication. • Toxin-producing cyanobacteria include *Microcystis*, *Anabena*, *Aphanizomenon*, *Oscillatoria*, *Lyngbya*, and *Planktothrix* spp. • Microcystins are hepatotoxic blue-green algae toxins that have been found worldwide. • Anatoxins, which include anatoxin-a and anatoxin-as, are neurotoxic blue-green algae toxins.

SIGNALMENT

• Dogs—no breed, sex, or age predilection.
• Cats—no cases reported.

SIGNS

Hepatotoxic

• Diarrhea, weakness, shock. • Rapid progression to depression, coma, and death.

Neurotoxic

• Onset of rigidity and muscle tremors within minutes to a few hours after exposure.
• Rapid progression to paralysis, cyanosis, and death.

Dermatotoxic

• Pruritus, erythema, urticaria. • Secondary skin infection.

CAUSES & RISK FACTORS

• Access to and ingestion of toxin-contaminated water and/or algal material.
• Exposure to dietary supplements containing the blue-green algae *Spirulina platensis* and *Aphanizomenon flos aquae* that are contaminated with microcystins. • Blooms more common in nutrient-rich water in warmer months. • Blooms concentrated through wind or by removal into containers. • Certain algae reside in the benthic zone, e.g., in sediment; dogs mouthing material such as rocks from sediment can be at risk.

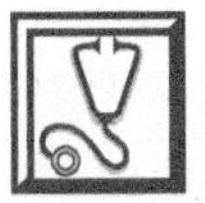

DIAGNOSIS

DIFFERENTIAL DIAGNOSIS

Hepatotoxic

• Amanitins, xylitol, cycad palms, acetaminophen, manganese, pennyroyal oil, cocklebur. • Other causes of acute liver failure—infectious, metabolic, dietary.

Neurotoxic

• Strychnine, metaldehyde, avitrol, pyrethrins/pyrethroids, zinc phosphide, bromethalin.
• Organophosphorus, carbamate, and organochlorine insecticides. • Penitrem A, methylxanthines. • Poisonous plants (*Brunfelsia* spp., cyanide, oleander, poison hemlock).
• Illicit substances (amphetamine and derivatives), ephedra-containing compounds.
• Neurotoxic mushrooms.

Dermatotoxic

Other causes of pruritus—allergies, infectious, parasitic, dietary, endocrine.

CBC/BIOCHEMISTRY/URINALYSIS

Hepatotoxic

• Elevated serum liver enzymes—alanine transaminase (ALT), aspartate transaminase (AST), alkaline phosphatase (ALP), bilirubin.
• Hypoalbuminemia. • Hypoglycemia.

Neurotoxic and Dermatotoxic

No specific changes.

DIAGNOSTIC PROCEDURES

Morphologic algal ID in suspect water, algal material, or stomach content. Positive ID confirms hazard but is not confirmatory for the toxin because toxicity is strain specific.

Hepatotoxic

• Detection of algal material on fur or in stomach contents. • Analysis of stomach contents and water/algal source for microcystins.

Neurotoxic

• Detection of anatoxin-a in gastric contents, urine, bile, and suspect source material.
• Depressed blood cholinesterase activity with anatoxin-as poisoning.

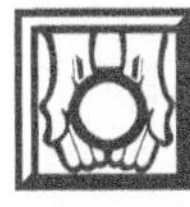

TREATMENT

• No antidote available. • Rapid onset typically prevents timely therapeutic intervention.
• Gastrointestinal decontamination with activated charcoal can be attempted, but efficacy not known. • Hepatotoxic—supportive care, close monitoring, and case-specific IV fluids to correct electrolytes and hypoglycemia, vitamin K_1, and plasma transfusions. • Neurotoxic—supportive care and seizure control.
• Dermatotoxic—supportive care and treatment for secondary skin infections.

MEDICATIONS

DRUG(S) OF CHOICE

• Activated charcoal—1 g/kg PO q6-8h until 2–3 days post ingestion; mix activated charcoal in water at 1 g/5 mL of water. • IV fluids—maintain hydration, induce diuresis, correct hypoglycemia. • Dextrose—50% dextrose 1 mL/kg IV slow bolus (1–3 min). • Vitamin K_1—0.5–1.5 mg/kg SC/IM q12h; 1–5 mg/kg PO q24h. • Blood products—dependent on hemostatic test results. • Diazepam (2–5 mg/kg IV, repeat in 30 min if necessary) for seizure control. • Phenobarbital (2–5 mg/kg IV q6–12h) for seizure control. • Methocarbamol (55–220 mg/kg IV) for muscle relaxation.

Alternative Drugs

• S-adenosylmethionine (SAMe)—antioxidant and hepatoprotectant; no data on efficacy in hepatotoxic cyanotoxin toxicosis available; dose 20 mg/kg PO q24h. • Ascorbic acid and cimetidine—hepatocyte protectors; no data on efficacy in hepatotoxic cyanotoxin poisoning available. • N-acetylcysteine (NAC)—antioxidant; no data on efficacy in hepatotoxic cyanotoxin toxicosis available; glutathione precursor that can be included in treatment regimen for acute hepatic failure at 140 mg/kg IV load, followed by 70 mg/kg IV q6h for 7 treatments.

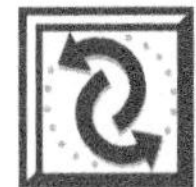

FOLLOW-UP

PATIENT MONITORING

• Hepatotoxic—liver enzymes/function, coagulation status. • Neurotoxic—thermoregulation, respiratory function, blood gases.

PREVENTION/AVOIDANCE

• Deny access to water with visible algal blooms. • Remove algal blooms from ponds immediately and discard material safely.

EXPECTED COURSE AND PROGNOSIS

• Prognosis poor to guarded for hepatotoxic and neurotoxic; good for dermatotoxic.
• Rapid onset and progression; often lethal.

MISCELLANEOUS

ABBREVIATIONS

• ALP = alkaline phosphatase. • ALT = alanine transaminase. • AST = aspartate transaminase. • NAC = N-acetylcysteine.
• SAMe = S-adenosylmethionine.

INTERNET RESOURCES

http://www.cdc.gov/habs

Suggested Reading

Bautista AC, Moore CE, Lin Y, et al. Hepatopathy following consumption of a commercially available blue-green algae dietary supplement in a dog. BMC Vet Res 2015, 11:136.

Puschner B, Bautista AC, Wong C. Debromoaplysiatoxin as the causative agent of dermatitis in a dog after exposure to freshwater in California. Front Vet Sci 2017, 4:50.

Authors Birgit Puschner and Adrienne C. Bautista

Consulting Editor Lynn R. Hovda

Client Education Handout available online

BOTULISM

BASICS

OVERVIEW

• Paralytic illness caused by preformed neurotoxin produced by bacterium *Clostridium botulinum* (Gram +, anaerobe) contained in uncooked food, carrion, and contaminated or improperly stored silage.
• Most cases in dogs caused by *Clostridium botulinum* neurotoxin serotype C; neurotoxin interferes with release of acetylcholine at neuromuscular junction, resulting in diffuse lower motor neuron signs. • Heavy molecular weight of the toxin seems to preclude its transfer to placenta.

SIGNALMENT

Dogs (naturally infected) and cats (experimentally infected except for one case report of natural *Clostridium botulinum* type C toxicosis).

SIGNS

Historical Findings

• Signs appear a few hours to 6 days after toxin ingestion. • Other dogs living in the same environment may be affected. • Acute, symmetric, progressive weakness develops, starting in the pelvic limbs and ascending to the trunk, thoracic limbs, neck, and muscles innervated by the cranial nerves; severe tetraparesis or tetraplegia ensues.

Physical Examination

• Possible increased or decreased heart rate.
• In severe cases—diaphragmatic respiration.

Neurologic Examination Findings

• Mental status—normal. • Cranial nerves—may reveal sluggish pupillary light reflexes (PLR), diminished palpebral reflexes, decreased jaw tone, decreased gag reflex, salivation, and dysphonia. • Gait and posture—a stiff, short-stride gait (no ataxia) is initially observed until recumbence develops (usually within 12–24 hours). • Spinal reflexes—decreased to absent with decreased muscle tone (to atonia) and muscle atrophy.
• Autonomic signs—mydriasis with decreased PLR, decreased lacrimation, ileus, and urine retention or frequent voiding of small volumes. • No hyperesthesia.

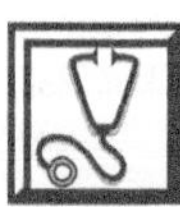

DIAGNOSIS

DIFFERENTIAL DIAGNOSIS

• Acute canine polyradiculoneuritis (coonhound paralysis). • Myasthenia gravis.
• Tick bite paralysis. • Coral snake venom toxicity. • Dumb form of rabies. • Lasalocid (growth promoter in ruminants) toxicosis.

CBC/BIOCHEMISTRY/URINALYSIS

Usually normal.

OTHER LABORATORY TESTS

• Definitive diagnosis is based on detection of botulinum toxin in serum, feces, vomitus, or ingested food sample; by neutralization test in small rodents; or by in vitro test that measures toxin antigenicity rather than toxicity. • Detection of anti-C botulinum neurotoxin antibodies may help support clinical diagnosis.

IMAGING

Thoracic radiographs—possible megaesophagus and/or signs of aspiration pneumonia.

DIAGNOSTIC PROCEDURES

• Electromyography may reveal fibrillation potentials and positive sharp waves in affected muscles. • Motor nerve conduction velocity may be normal or decreased, with reduced amplitude of evoked muscle action potentials; compound muscle action potentials can be decreased after low-frequency repetitive nerve stimulations.

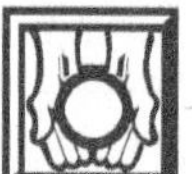

TREATMENT

• If recent ingestion—gastric lavage, cathartics (avoid agents containing magnesium), or enemas may be useful.
• Mildly affected dogs recover over a period of several days with supportive treatment including physical therapy, frequent turning, good bedding (to prevent decubital sores), bladder care (catheterization), artificial tears (to prevent corneal ulceration), and feeding from an elevated position (when megaesophagus present). • Dogs with respiratory difficulties require intensive care monitoring with arterial blood gas, intermittent esophageal suction, alimentation by nasogastric or gastrotomy tube, and eventually ventilatory support.

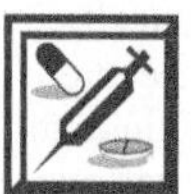

MEDICATIONS

DRUG(S) OF CHOICE

• Type C antitoxin may cause anaphylaxis; not effective when the toxin is already fixed at the nerve ending. • Antibiotics are not recommended since they might increase the release of toxins through bacterial lysis or by promoting intestinal infection; to be used only if secondary infections occur.

CONTRAINDICATIONS/POSSIBLE INTERACTIONS

Aminoglycosides, procaine penicillin, tetracyclines, phenothiazines, antiarrhythmic agents, and magnesium should be avoided (neuromuscular transmission blockade).

FOLLOW-UP

PATIENT MONITORING

Monitor patients for respiratory failure, aspiration pneumonia, progressive lower motor neuron signs, urinary tract infection, and ocular complications.

PREVENTION/AVOIDANCE

• Prevent access to carrion and feed dogs cooked food. • Avoid contact with spoiled raw meat. • Samples should be refrigerated (not frozen) and manipulated with caution, since humans are also sensitive to the toxin.

POSSIBLE COMPLICATIONS

• Respiratory failure and death in severe cases.
• Aspiration pneumonia from megaesophagus and regurgitations. • Keratoconjunctivitis sicca and corneal ulceration. • Prolonged recumbence—pulmonary atelectasia and infection; decubital sores; urine scalding.

EXPECTED COURSE AND PROGNOSIS

• Maximum severity of signs usually reached within 12–24 hours. • Neurologic signs disappear in reverse order of appearance; complete recovery usually occurs within 1–3 weeks, and requires the formation of new nerve terminals and functional neuromuscular junctions.

MISCELLANEOUS

SEE ALSO

• Coonhound Paralysis (Acute Polyradiculoneuritis). • Myasthenia Gravis.
• Snake Venom Toxicosis—Coral Snakes.
• Tick Bite Paralysis.

ABBREVIATIONS

• PLR = pupillary light reflex.

Suggested Reading

Añor S. Acute lower motor neuron tetraparesis. Vet Clin North Am Small Anim Pract 2014, 44(6):1201–1222,

Barsanti J, Greene C, eds. Infectious Diseases of the Dog and Cat, 4th ed. St. Louis, MO: Saunders Elsevier, 2012, pp. 416–422.

Elad D, Yas-Natan E, Aroch I, et al. Natural Clostridium type C toxicosis in a group of cats. J Clin Microbiol 2004, 42(11):5406–5408.

Lamoureux A, Pouzot-Nevoret C, Escriou C. A case of type B botulism in a pregnant bitch. J Small Anim Pract 2015, 56(5):348–350.

Silva R, Martins R, Assis R, et al. Type C botulism in domestic chickens, dogs and black-pencilled marmoset (*Callithrix penicillata*) in Minas Gerais, Brazil. Anaerobe 2018, 51:47–49.

Uriarte A, Thibaud J, Blot S. Botulism in 2 urban dogs. Can Vet J 2010, 51:1139–1142.

Author Hélène L.M. Ruel

Acknowledgment The author and book editors acknowledge the prior contribution of Roberto Poma (deceased).

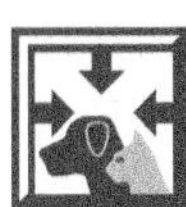

BASICS

OVERVIEW

• Trauma with traction and/or severe abduction of a forelimb causes avulsion of nerve rootlets from their spinal cord attachment. • Ventral (motor) nerve roots are more susceptible than dorsal (sensory) roots. • It is important to rule out nerve root avulsions in traumatized animals that are not able to bear weight on a forelimb, especially before surgical repair of orthopedic injuries.

SIGNALMENT

• Dogs and cats. • No age, sex, or breed predilection.

SIGNS

• Depend on the extent and distribution of rootlet damage. • Motor signs—paresis/ weakness (partial damage) to paralysis (complete ventral root avulsion). • Sensory signs—decreased to absent pain perception (dorsal root damage). • Muscle atrophy—begins within a week of injury. • Complete avulsion—spinal nerves C5 to T2; most common; combines cranial and caudal avulsion deficits. • Cranial avulsion—C5 to C7 nerves: supraspinatus and infraspinatus muscle atrophy, loss of shoulder and elbow movement flexion (dropped elbow), analgesia of craniodorsal scapula and medial forearm, possible diaphragm hemiplegia detected by fluoroscopy (phrenic nerve roots C5 to C7); if roots C8 to T2 are preserved, weight bearing remains almost normal. • Caudal avulsion—spinal nerves C7 to T2: inability to bear weight with knuckling over dorsum of paw; if C5 to C7 are spared, the limb is held in a flexed position and there is analgesia distal to the elbow (except for a small area on the medial aspect of the forearm); T1 to T2 involvement causes an ipsilateral partial Horner's syndrome (anisocoria only) and lack of ipsilateral cutaneous trunci reflex (reflex present contralaterally). • Bilateral avulsion—rarely encountered, caused by a significant fall with sternal landing and splaying of limbs. • Over time, complications of self-trauma may occur as a result of paresthesia in the most severe cases.

CAUSES & RISK FACTORS

Trauma—road accident; hung by foot; dragged; fall.

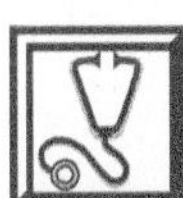

DIAGNOSIS

DIFFERENTIAL DIAGNOSIS

• Brachial plexus trauma without avulsion—rare; temporary deficit owing to root contusion (neurapraxia). • Brachial plexus tumor—usually chronic, progressive onset. • Brachial plexus neuritis or neuropathy—rare, bilateral deficits, unknown etiology; acute onset; no trauma. • Fibrocartilaginous embolic myelopathy—deficits of ipsilateral hind limb and mild deficits of contralateral forelimb and hind limb are usually present. • Migrating foreign body – slow onset and no history of trauma. • Pure radial nerve paralysis caused by fracture of humerus or first rib—no nerve root sign. • Lateralized intervertebral disc protrusion.

IMAGING

CT or MRI—visualize lesion; rarely needed for diagnosis.

DIAGNOSTIC PROCEDURES

• Clinical—history of trauma with sudden onset of typical neurologic deficits. • Define involved spinal nerve roots—map motor and sensory deficits; note signs of Horner's syndrome; determine if cutaneous trunci reflex is present. • Electromyography (EMG) and nerve conduction studies (NCS) may help further define deficits and detect signs of recovery—from 5–7 days post injury, EMG shows denervation in affected muscles.

PATHOLOGIC FINDINGS

• Ventral and dorsal root avulsions—intradurally at level of root–spinal cord junction (most fragile area because it lacks protective perineurium). • Neuroma formation may develop over time on pial surface of spinal cord.

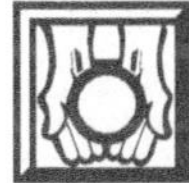

TREATMENT

Appropriate Health Care

• No specific treatment. • Outcome depends on initial damage. • Amputation of limb—may be necessary for patients showing complications (infections/self-mutilation, likely as a result of paresthesia) and no improvement. • Carpal fusion (arthrodesis) and transposition of biceps muscle tendon—consider only with adequate function of triceps and musculocutaneous muscles.

Nursing Care

• Protective wrap or boot to protect distal paw if patient walks a lot/walks on rough surfaces—increased skin fragility and lack of protective reflexes due to sensory deficits can result in severe excoriations when animal walks on affected limb. • Early and sustained physical therapy—crucial to prevent severe muscle atrophy and tendon contraction to keep joints and muscles mobile during recovery of reversible injuries; passive range of motion, massage therapy. • Monitor noncomplicated cases for 4–6 months before considering amputation.

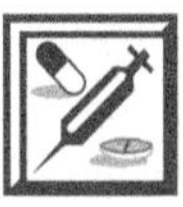

MEDICATIONS

DRUG(S) OF CHOICE

Prednisolone (prednisone)—1-week anti-inflammatory course may decrease early edema and favor healing of reversible injuries.

FOLLOW-UP

POSSIBLE COMPLICATIONS

• Skin excoriation and secondary infection—from trauma to unprotected paw. • Trophic ulcers—thin, traumatized skin, especially over arthrodesis sites. • Paresthesia may lead to self-mutilation.

EXPECTED COURSE AND PROGNOSIS

• Preserved pain sensation (dorsal roots intact)—suggests less severe injury to ventral nerve roots. • Cranial avulsion—better prognosis with preserved sensation to distal limb and ability to bear weight. • Complete avulsion—poor prognosis for recovery, amputation likely. • Rarely, mild cases may resolve after 2–3 months.

MISCELLANEOUS

SEE ALSO

Polyneuropathies (Peripheral Neuropathies).

ABBREVIATIONS

• EMG = electromyography. • NCS = nerve conduction studies.

Suggested Reading

Bailey CS. Patterns of cutaneous anesthesia associated with brachial plexus avulsions in the dog. JAVMA 1984, 185:889–899.

Braund KG. Neuropathic disorders. In: Braund KG, ed., Clinical Neurology in Small Animals: Localization, Diagnosis and Treatment. Ithaca, NY: IVIS, 2003. http://www.ivis.org/advances/Vite/braund20b/chapter_frm.asp.

Walmsley G, Scurrell E, Summers B, et al. Foreign body induced neuritis masquerading as a canine brachial plexus nerve sheath tumour. Vet Comp Orthop Traumatol 2009, 22(5):427–429.

Author Christine F. Berthelin-Baker

BRACHYCEPHALIC AIRWAY SYNDROME

BASICS

DEFINITION

Partial upper airway obstruction in brachycephalic dogs and cats caused by any of the following: stenotic nares, overlong soft palate, everted laryngeal saccules, and laryngeal collapse. Hypoplastic trachea can also be present and worsen respiratory distress.

PATHOPHYSIOLOGY

• In normal dogs, the upper airway accounts for 50–70% of total airway resistance. Brachycephalic breeds have increased upper airway resistance due to stenosis of nares, aberrant formation of nasal conchae, and presence of nasopharyngeal turbinates. Skull bones are shortened in length but normal in width, and soft tissues are not proportionately reduced, resulting in redundant tissue and narrowed air passages. • Increased airway resistance leads to more negative intra-airway pressures—may result in secondary eversion of laryngeal saccules, further elongation of palate, and laryngeal collapse. • Recruitment of pharyngeal dilator muscles (sternohyoid) becomes necessary to maintain airway patency; sleep apnea may occur secondary to relaxation of these muscles.

SYSTEMS AFFECTED

• Respiratory—respiratory distress, hypoxemia, hypercarbia, hyperthermia, aspiration pneumonia, noncardiogenic pulmonary edema from airway obstruction.
• Cardiovascular—cardiovascular collapse if complete airway obstruction or severe hyperthermia occurs. • Gastrointestinal—may be reluctant to eat or drink; increased airway resistance can exacerbate hiatal hernia, gastroesophageal reflux, and esophagitis.

GENETICS

Brachycephalic head shape—inherited defect in development of skull bones perpetuated by selective breeding.

INCIDENCE/PREVALENCE

• Dogs—common in brachycephalic breeds.
• Cats—less commonly severe enough to require treatment.

GEOGRAPHIC DISTRIBUTION

Worldwide

SIGNALMENT

Species

Dog and cat.

Breed Predilections

• Dogs—brachycephalic breeds (English bulldogs most common—up to 55% of breed, French bulldog, pug, Boston terrier); Norwich terriers and Cavalier King Charles spaniels affected by a variant of the syndrome.
• Cats—Persians and Himalayans.

Mean Age and Range

• Young adults, most diagnosed by 2–3 years.
• If diagnosed later than 4 years, look for concurrent disease or exacerbating circumstances.
• Laryngeal collapse reported in brachycephalic breed puppies as young as 6–7 months.

Predominant Sex

No sex predilection.

SIGNS

Historical Findings

• Snoring, stridor, stertorous breathing.
• Tachypnea, frequent panting. • Coughing and gagging. • Difficulty eating and swallowing. • Ptyalism, regurgitation, and vomiting. • Syncope or collapse.

Physical Examination Findings

• Stridor and stertorous breathing.
• Stenotic nares—medial collapse of lateral nasal cartilage. • Increased respiratory effort—retraction of the commissures of lips, open-mouth breathing or constant panting, increased respiratory rate, abduction of forelimbs, increased abdominal component of respiration, recruitment of secondary muscles of respiration. • In severe distress, may see paradoxical abdominal movement, inward collapse of intercostal muscles during inspiration, orthopnea, and cyanosis. Hyperthermia may be present.

CAUSES

• Inherited or congenital defects in conformation. • Elongated soft palate—over 90% of surgical cases in dogs. • Stenotic nares—about 50% of dogs; most common defect in cats. • Aberrant formation of rostral and caudal nasal conchae. • Presence of nasopharyngeal turbinates (20% of dogs) and 100% of English bulldogs. • Laryngeal disease—everted laryngeal saccules (>50% of dogs) and/or laryngeal collapse (~10% of dogs).

RISK FACTORS

• Breed. • Obesity—worsens airway obstruction, associated with poorer outcome postoperatively, and may contribute to gastroesophageal reflux and aspiration pneumonia.
• Excitement and/or warm, humid weather—increased panting can lead to airway edema, further compromise of the lumen, and hyperthermia. • Exercise—dogs are often exercise intolerant due to airway compromise and hypoxia. • Sedation—relaxation of muscles of pharynx and palate can cause complete airway obstruction. • Respiratory infection or concurrent pulmonary disease—will cause further respiratory compromise.
• Endocrine disease (hypothyroidism and hyperadrenocorticism)—could worsen weight gain and panting.

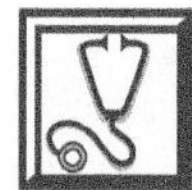

DIAGNOSIS

DIFFERENTIAL DIAGNOSIS

• Foreign bodies of nasopharynx, larynx, or trachea. • Infection—upper respiratory infection, nasopharyngeal abscess.
• Neoplasia obstructing the nasopharynx, glottis, larynx, or trachea. • Laryngeal paralysis. • Pharyngeal mucocoele.
• Nasopharyngeal polyp or cyst.

CBC/BIOCHEMISTRY/URINALYSIS

CBC—usually normal, but polycythemia can occur with chronic hypoxia, and leukocytosis if concurrent infection or severe stress.

OTHER LABORATORY TESTS

• Arterial blood gas—to diagnose respiratory acidosis and hypoxemia, and response to oxygen supplementation. • Pulse oximetry—to diagnose hypoxemia.

IMAGING

Radiographic Findings

• If stable, cervical and thoracic radiographs recommended. • Cervical radiographs may show thickened, elongated soft palate and suggest tracheal hypoplasia. • Thoracic radiographs can reveal aspiration pneumonia, pulmonary edema, air in esophagus, and hypoplastic trachea (TD/TI = tracheal diameter at the level of thoracic inlet/thoracic inlet distance, which is the distance from the sternum to the ventral surface of TI. A ratio <0.13 in bulldogs and <0.16 in other brachycephalic breeds suggests hypoplastic trachea).

Fluoroscopy

Gives information about degree of dynamic pharyngeal obstruction by palate and concurrent disease such as collapsing trachea (uncommon in brachycephalic dogs).

DIAGNOSTIC PROCEDURES

Laryngoscopy/Pharyngoscopy

• Performed under general anesthesia. • Due to risk of airway obstruction, owner should be prepared for surgical intervention if deemed necessary. • Overlong soft palate extends more than just a few millimeters beyond tip of epiglottis and hangs down into glottis. • Soft palate is often thickened and inflamed. • May have inflammation and edema of arytenoid cartilages. • Everted laryngeal saccules are diagnosed by visualizing two smooth, round, glistening masses in ventral half of laryngeal opening—they often obscure visualization of vocal folds.
• Laryngeal collapse can also be seen.
• Flexible endoscopy with retroflexed view of nasopharynx can detect nasopharyngeal turbinates.

Tracheoscopy

• Can reveal hypoplastic trachea with overlap of dorsal tracheal rings and dorsal tracheal membrane. • Collapsing trachea can also be diagnosed.

CT Scan

Can identify and grade aberrant nasopharyngeal turbinates.

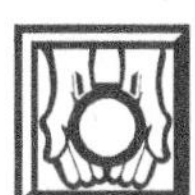

TREATMENT

APPROPRIATE HEALTH CARE

• Surgery recommended for patients with significant clinical signs or to prevent progressive respiratory dysfunction. • Severe respiratory distress requires rapid intervention including O_2 supplementation, cautious use of antianxiety medication. • If hyperthermic, cool via convective losses by wetting patient with cool water and placing fan to blow over them; administer IV fluids, up to a shock rate if extremely hyperthermic (T° >106 °F [41 °C]).
• If complete airway obstruction, immediate orotracheal intubation and/or temporary tracheostomy is indicated. • Dexamethasone sodium phosphate can be administered (0.1 mg/kg IV) to reduce inflammation.

NURSING CARE

• Patients require 24-hour monitoring because of risk of acute airway obstruction and death. • Monitor respiratory rate, effort, heart rate, pulse quality, mucous membrane color, capillary refill time, temperature, and other physical parameters before and after surgery. • Pulse oximetry and arterial blood gases, depending on severity of condition.
• Administer IV fluids at maintenance rate and minimize handling and stress. • O_2 therapy and cooling as necessary.

ACTIVITY

Usually self-limited.

DIET

• Weight loss is recommended if overweight.
• For obese, stable patients, weight loss is recommended prior to surgery.

CLIENT EDUCATION

• Avoidance of risk factors is critical. • Inform owners that dogs with brachycephalic airway syndrome are at increased anesthetic risk, especially if obese, or have cardiac disease or aspiration pneumonia. • Inform owners that surgery often improves but does not normalize airway.

SURGICAL CONSIDERATIONS

• Evaluation for elongated soft palate performed under general anesthesia when patient is stable. • Temporary tracheostomy can be placed to facilitate exposure or to treat airway obstruction. • Stenotic nares are corrected by resection of a wedge of the dorsolateral nasal cartilage and planum; hemorrhage is controlled with pressure followed by closure of the surgical wound with 3 or 4 sutures of 3-0 or 4-0 absorbable suture material. • Elongated soft palate is resected using scissors, carbon dioxide laser, or bipolar sealing device; remove only enough to allow contact of center of soft palate with tip of epiglottis. • Sacculectomy performed by grasping tissue with Allis tissue forceps and trimming all mucosal tissue with curved scissors. • Severe laryngeal collapse might require cricoarytenoid and thyroarytenoid caudolateralization or permanent tracheostomy.

MEDICATIONS

DRUG(S) OF CHOICE

• Dexamethasone sodium phosphate for 12–24h pre- or postoperatively at 0.1 mg/kg IV q12–24h to reduce edema and inflammation.
• Broad-spectrum antibiotics indicated if aspiration pneumonia present until culture and sensitivity results obtained. • Omeprazole 0.7 mg/kg q24h or pantoprazole 1 mg/kg q24h, cisapride 0.2 mg/kg q8h, and sucralfate 0.5–1 g q12h for dogs with concurrent esophagitis, gastritis, and/or duodenitis.

CONTRAINDICATIONS

Overuse of steroids can lead to panting, weight gain, and gastrointestinal ulceration, which can exacerbate signs of brachycephalic airway syndrome.

PRECAUTIONS

Sedation should be used with caution because of risk of upper airway obstruction with muscle relaxation.

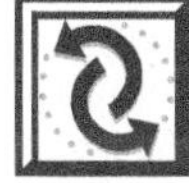

FOLLOW-UP

PATIENT MONITORING

Postoperatively, 24-hour monitoring to observe for airway swelling and obstruction that may require temporary tracheostomy.

PREVENTION/AVOIDANCE

• Selection by breeders for dogs without severe conformational changes—difficult because breed standards encourage these.
• Avoid risk factors, particularly weight gain.

POSSIBLE COMPLICATIONS

• Hyperthermia and heat stroke. • Aspiration pneumonia. • Death in about 10% of patients from airway disease. • Most common postoperative complication is airway swelling and obstruction within first 24 hours, may necessitate temporary tracheostomy.
• Continued respiratory difficulty after corrective surgery. • Excessive resection of palate resulting in nasal aspiration of food contents due to inability to close pharynx during swallowing. • Progressive laryngeal collapse resulting in need for permanent tracheostomy.

EXPECTED COURSE AND PROGNOSIS

• Prognosis good for improvement in breathing (80% or more have good to excellent results), but airway still abnormal. • Prognosis better for dogs other than English bulldogs and for dogs that have correction of both stenotic nares and elongated soft palate. • Without surgery, prognosis poor due to continued progression of acquired components of brachycephalic airway syndrome. • Lifelong avoidance of risk factors recommended.

MISCELLANEOUS

ASSOCIATED CONDITIONS

• Aspiration pneumonia. • Heat stroke.
• Hiatal hernia. • Hypoplastic trachea.

AGE-RELATED FACTORS

Older dogs may have a worse outcome postoperatively, but most have some improvement.

PREGNANCY/FERTILITY/BREEDING

Enlarged abdomen and pressure on the diaphragm in the pregnant bitch can further compromise respiratory function by decreasing tidal volume.

INTERNET RESOURCES

https://www.acvs.org/small-animal/brachycephalic-syndrome

Suggested Reading

Ginn JA, Kumar MSA, McKiernan BC, Powers BE. Nasopharyngeal turbinates in brachycephalic dogs and cats. J Am Anim Hosp Assoc 2008, 44(5):243–249.
Monnet E. Brachycephalic airway syndrome. In: Slatter D, ed., Textbook of Small Animal Surgery, 3rd ed. Philadelphia, PA: Saunders, 2003, pp. 808–813.
Poncet CM, Dupre GP, Freiche VG, Bouvy BM. Long-term results of upper respiratory syndrome surgery and gastrointestinal tract medical treatment in 51 brachycephalic dogs. J Small Anim Pract 2006, 47(3):137–142.
Poncet CM, Dupre GP, Freiche VG, et al. Prevalence of gastrointestinal tract lesions in brachycephalic dogs with upper respiratory syndrome: clinical study in 73 cases (2000–2003). J Small Anim Pract 2005, 46:273–279.
Riecks TW, Birchard SJ, Stephens JA. Surgical correction of brachycephalic syndrome in dogs: 62 cases (1991–2004). J Am Vet Med Assoc 2007, 230(9):1324–1328.
White RN. Surgical management of laryngeal collapse associated with brachycephalic airway obstruction syndrome in dogs. J Small Anim Pract 2012, 53:44–50.

Authors David A. Puerto and Lori S. Waddell
Consulting Editor Elizabeth Rozanski

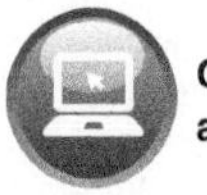

Client Education Handout available online

BRAIN INJURY

BASICS

DEFINITION

• Traumatic—external forces. • Nontraumatic—hypoxia, metabolic disorders, vascular disruption, infection, toxicity, neoplasia. • Primary—direct initial insult when tissue and vessels are stretched, compressed, or torn. • Secondary—alterations of brain vasculature and tissue following primary injury.

PATHOPHYSIOLOGY

• Acceleration, deceleration, and rotational forces traumatize brain tissue. • The brain has high oxygen and glucose requirements; reduced blood flow puts it at great risk for hypoxia. • Oxygen delivery dependent on cerebral blood flow (CBF) and cerebral perfusion pressure (CPP) (= mean arterial pressure [MAP] – intracranial pressure [ICP]). • Intracranial bleeding, edema (vasogenic and cytotoxic), vasodilation, and/or vasospasms increase ICP, causing low CBF, ischemia, brain swelling, and herniation; slow, progressive increase in ICP better tolerated than small, acute rise. • Hypotension, hypoxia—major contributors to secondary injury.

SYSTEMS AFFECTED

• Nervous—altered mentation, cranial nerve deficit, seizures, twitching, postural changes. • Cardiovascular—arrhythmia. • Endocrine/metabolic—alteration in antidiuretic hormone (ADH) release and sodium concentration; central temperature dysregulation; insulin resistance; depletion of cortisol. • Ophthalmic—changes in eye position, eye movements, pupillary light reflex, papilledema. • Respiratory—hyper- or hypocapnea; abnormal breathing patterns; neurogenic pulmonary edema.

INCIDENCE/PREVALENCE

• Head and neck injuries found in up to 34% of dogs and cats suffering blunt force trauma. • Head trauma reported in up to 25% of dogs with severe blunt force trauma and in 50% of dogs and cats injured by motor vehicles and crush injuries. • Additional causes—penetrating injuries, fall from heights, human-inflicted trauma. • Parenchymal and extradural hematomas found in 10% of dogs and cats with signs of mild head injury and in up to 80% with severe head injury.

SIGNALMENT

Species

Dog and cat.

SIGNS

Historical Findings

• Determine cause—trauma, cardiac arrest, heart failure, hypertension, toxins, vascular event, coagulopathy, severe respiratory compromise, prolonged seizures, hypoglycemia, jaundice. • Decline in neurologic condition—implies progression from intracranial bleeding, cerebral edema, ischemia. • Seizure activity—cerebral or diencephalon involvement.

Physical Examination Findings

• Evidence of head trauma—open wounds, epistaxis, blood in ear canal. • Cardiac or respiratory insufficiency—hypoxia, cyanosis, hypoventilation. • Poor perfusion—weak pulse, pale mucous membranes. • Skull palpation—fracture, open fontanelle. • Sustained bradycardia—midbrain, pontine, or medullary lesion. • Cushing reflex—bradycardia and hypertension. • Ecchymosis, petechiae, retinal hemorrhages, or distended vessels—hypertension, coagulopathy. • Papilledema—cerebral edema. • Retinal detachment—infectious, neoplastic, or hypertensive cause.

Neurologic Examination Findings

Mental Status

• Level of consciousness and cranial nerve deficits—cerebral cortex (better prognosis), midbrain/brainstem, or multifocal. • Postural changes—decerebrate rigidity with midbrain lesion; decerebellate rigidity with cerebellar lesion. • Peracute focal deficits—vascular or neoplastic causes.

Pupillary Light Reflexes

• Miotic responsive pupils—cerebral or diencephalic lesion (rule out traumatic uveitis, Horner's syndrome). • Pinpointed unresponsive pupils—diencephalic, pontine, or medullary lesion. • Dilated unresponsive pupil(s) or midpoint fixed unresponsive pupils—midbrain lesion.

Cranial Nerves

• Normal with altered mentation—cerebrum/diencephalic lesion. • CN II—loss of menace and dazzle response with dilated unresponsive pupils; cranial forebrain. • Loss of physiologic nystagmus—brainstem lesion. • CN III—midbrain lesion. • CN V–XII—pontine or medullary lesion.

Respiratory Patterns

• Cheyne-Stokes—severe diffuse cerebral or diencephalon lesion. • Hyperventilation—midbrain lesion. • Ataxic or apneustic—pontine or medullary lesion.

CAUSES

• Trauma. • Prolonged hypoxia or ischemia. • Prolonged shock. • Severe hypoglycemia. • Prolonged seizures. • Severe hyper- or hypothermia. • Alterations in serum osmolality. • Toxins. • Neoplasia. • Hypertension. • Hemorrhage. • Inflammatory, infectious, immune-mediated diseases. • Thiamin deficiency. • Hydrocephalus. • Parasitic migration.

RISK FACTORS

• Free-roaming—trauma, toxins. • Coexisting cardiac, respiratory, hematologic, hepatic disease. • Diabetes mellitus—insulin therapy.

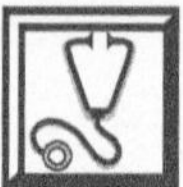

DIAGNOSIS

DIFFERENTIAL DIAGNOSIS

Systemic causes of altered states of consciousness or central vestibular signs—metabolic disease; toxins; drugs; infection.

CBC/BIOCHEMISTRY/URINALYSIS

• Reflect systemic effects of neurologic signs. • Alterations in serum sodium suggest central ADH abnormalities.

OTHER LABORATORY TESTS

• Arterial blood gas. • Coagulation profile. • Infectious disease titers.

IMAGING

• Skull radiographs—detect fractures, lytic lesion. • CT—detect acute hemorrhage, infarcts, fractures, lytic lesion, penetrating foreign bodies, hydrocephalus, herniation. • MRI—detect cerebral edema, hemorrhage, mass, hydrocephalus, infiltrative diseases, inflammation, herniation, fractures. • Ultrasound optic disk—more than 3 mm diameter may be associated with brain edema.

DIAGNOSTIC PROCEDURES

• ECG—detects arrhythmias. • BP—assess perfusion. • Cerebrospinal fluid (CSF) analysis—if cause unknown and no contra-indications.

PATHOLOGIC FINDINGS

• Brain edema, inflammation. • Herniation. • Hemorrhage. • Hydrocephalus. • Infarct. • Laceration, contusion. • Hematoma. • Skull fracture, lytic lesion. • Necrosis. • Apoptosis.

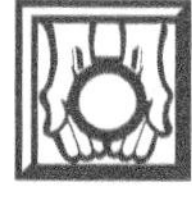

TREATMENT

APPROPRIATE HEALTH CARE

• Goals of therapy—support oxygenation and ventilation; maintain BP and CPP; decrease ICP; decrease cerebral metabolic rate. • Maintain systolic BP >90 mmHg and partial pressure of carbon dioxide (PCO_2) at 35–40 mmHg; with suspected elevated ICP, hyperventilation to 32–35 mmHg. • Maintain partial pressure of oxygen (PaO_2) >60 mmHg, arterial oxygen saturation (SaO_2) >90%, peripheral oxygen saturation (SpO_2) >94%. • Avoid cough or sneeze reflex during intubation or nasal oxygen supplementation; lidocaine (dogs: topical and 1–2 mg/kg IV) before. • Do not compress jugular veins. • Orotracheal intubation if gag reflex lost.

NURSING CARE

• Aggressive therapy for midbrain/brainstem lesion or declining neurologic signs. • Overzealous fluid resuscitation can contribute to brain edema. • Small-volume fluid resuscitation techniques to maintain systolic BP >90 mmHg with normal heart rate. • Combination of

isotonic crystalloids (10–20 mL/kg increments) with hydroxyethyl starch (5 mL/kg increments) over 5–8 minutes. • Avoid hypertension.
• Level head with body or elevate head and neck to 20° angle. • Keep airway unobstructed; use suction and humidify if intubated; hyperoxygenate, consider IV lidocaine prior to suctioning. • Lubricate eyes. • Reposition every 2–4 hours to avoid hypostatic pulmonary congestion, pressure sores. • Prevent fecal/urine soiling. • Maintain normal body temperature.
• Maintain hydration with balanced crystalloid solution. • Rehabilitation exercises.

ACTIVITY

• Restricted. • Consult rehabilitation specialist for appropriate exercises to maintain muscle tone.

CLIENT EDUCATION

• Neurologic signs may worsen before improving.
• Neurologic recovery may not be evident for several days; possibly >6 months for residual neurologic deficits. • Serious systemic abnormalities contribute to CNS instability.

SURGICAL CONSIDERATIONS

Depressed skull fracture, penetrating foreign body, uncontrollable ICP elevation (insufficient CSF drainage, hematoma/mass evacuation, herniation).

MEDICATIONS

DRUG(S) OF CHOICE

Elevated ICP

• Ensure systolic BP >90 mmHg; lower ICP by hyperventilation, drug therapy, drainage of CSF from ventricles, or surgical decompression.
• 7% hypertonic saline—2–4 mL/kg IV.
• Furosemide—0.75 mg/kg IV; may decrease CSF production. • Mannitol—0.5–1 g/kg IV bolus repeated at 2h intervals 3–4 times in dogs, and 2–3 three times in cats; repeated doses must be given on time; improves CBF and lowers ICP; may exacerbate hemorrhage.
• Glucocorticosteroids—no benefit in acute management and long-term outcome in human traumatic brain injury (TBI); anti-inflammatory doses (prednisone 1 mg/kg/day) may be of benefit with brain edema related to intracranial neoplasia and infectious meningoencephalomyelitis (MEM); immunosuppressive doses (2 mg/kg/day) in combination with additional immunosuppressive drugs in immune-mediated MEM. • Provide analgesia/sedatives (e.g., fentanyl 3–5 µg/kg IV, then 3–5 µg/kg/h CRI ± lidocaine 3–5 mg/kg/h) as indicated; avoid agents that can reduce CPP. Avoid ketamine with obstructive intracranial lesions. • Thrashing, seizures, or uncontrolled motor activity—diazepam CRI (0.5–1 mg/kg/h), midazolam CRI (0.2–0.4 mg/kg IV), or propofol (3–6 mg/kg IV titrated to effect; 0.1–0.6 mg/kg/min CRI); monitor for hypotension; intubate if unable to protect airway.
• Levetiracetam—20–30 mg/kg IV/IM/PO/rectal q8h if seizure activity.

Other

• Reducing cerebral metabolic rate with heavy sedation using dexmedetomidine (3 µg/kg slow bolus followed by 3–7 µg/kg/h CRI IV) with ketamine (1 µg/kg slow bolus followed by 1 µg/kg/h CRI IV) with uncontrolled seizures or propofol (2–4 mg/kg IV then 0.1–0.4 mg/kg/min); must intubate and support blood pressure, oxygenation, and ventilation. • Cooling patient to 32–33 °C (89–91 °F) for 48h may provide cerebral protection when administered within 6 hours of global ischemia or severe brain injury.
• Glucose regulation. • Careful nasogastric tube feeding for early trickle flow feeding; cisapride (0.5 mg/kg PO q8–12h) and metoclopramide (1–2 mg/kg/day) may promote gastrointestinal motility. • Desmopressin for refractory hypernatremia; emergency dosage not established for animals (dogs: 4 µg topical conjunctival q12h; cats: 5 µg SC q12h).

CONTRAINDICATIONS

Drugs that cause hypertension, hypotension, hyperexcitability, or increase in metabolic rate.

PRECAUTIONS

• Avoid hypotension, hypoxemia, hypertension, hyperglycemia, hypoglycemia, hypernatremia, hypo- or hypervolemia.
• Keep head and neck above plane of body.
• Do not compress jugular veins.
• Furosemide, mannitol, and hypertonic saline—can cause hypovolemia and hypotension. • Maintain PCO_2 >32 mmHg; avoid hyperventilation in the first 24–8h and do not perform therapeutic hyperventilation (32–35 mmHg) for extended periods (>48h).

FOLLOW-UP

PATIENT MONITORING

• Repeated neurologic examinations—deterioration warrants aggressive therapeutic intervention. • BP—maintain systolic BP >90 mmHg. • Blood gases, pulse oximetry, end-tidal CO_2—to assess need for oxygen supplementation or ventilation. • Blood glucose—avoid severe persistent hyperglycemia and hypoglycemia. • ECG—arrhythmias may affect perfusion, oxygenation, and CBF.
• ICP—to detect elevations and monitor response to therapy.

PREVENTION/AVOIDANCE

Keep pets in a confined area or leashed.

POSSIBLE COMPLICATIONS

• Seizures. • Brain herniation. • Intracranial hemorrhage. • Progression from cerebral cortical to midbrain signs. • Malnutrition. • Aspiration pneumonia. • Hypostatic pulmonary congestion. • Corneal desiccation. • Urine scalding. • Airway obstruction from mucus.
• Arrhythmias. • Hypotension. • Hypernatremia.
• Hypokalemia. • Respiratory failure. • Residual neurologic deficits. • Death.

EXPECTED COURSE AND PROGNOSIS

• Young animals, minimal primary brain injury, secondary injury consisting of cerebral edema—best prognosis. • No deterioration for 48 hours—better prognosis. • Rapid resuscitation of systolic BP to >90 mmHg and avoiding hypoxemia—better neurologic outcome. • Modified Glasgow Coma Score may offer prognostic insight.

MISCELLANEOUS

SYNONYMS

• Head trauma. • TBI.

SEE ALSO

Stupor and Coma.

ABBREVIATIONS

• ADH = antidiuretic hormone. • CBF = cerebral blood flow. • CPP = cerebral perfusion pressure. • CRI = continuous rate infusion
• CSF = cerebrospinal fluid. • ICP = intracranial pressure. • MAP = mean arterial pressure.
• MEM = meningoencephalomyelitis. • PaO_2 = partial pressure of oxygen. • PCO_2 = partial pressure of carbon dioxide. • SaO_2 = arterial oxygen saturation. • SpO_2 = peripheral oxygen saturation. • TBI = traumatic brain injury.

INTERNET RESOURCES

http://www.traumaticbraininjury.com

Suggested Reading

Dewey CW, Downs MO, Aron DN, et al. Acute traumatic intracranial haemorrhage in dogs and cats. Vet Comp Orthop Traumatol 1993, 6:29–35.
Dewey CW, Fletcher DJ. Head trauma management. In: Dewey CW, ed., A Practical Guide to Canine and Feline Neurology, 2nd ed. Ames, IA: Wiley, 2008, pp. 221–235.
Fletcher D, Syring R. Traumatic brain injury. In: Silverstein D, Hopper K, eds., Small Animal Critical Care Medicine. St. Louis, MO: W.B. Saunders, 2014, pp. 723–727.
Freeman C, Platt SR. Head trauma, In: Platt SR, Garosi LS, eds., Small Animal Neurological Emergencies. London: Manson, 2012, pp. 363–382.
Sande A, West C. Traumatic brain injury: a review of pathophysiology and management. J Vet Emerg Crit Care 2010, 20:177–190.

Author Elke Rudloff

Acknowledgment The author and book editors acknowledge the prior contribution of Rebecca Kirby.

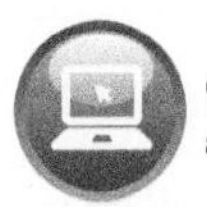

Client Education Handout available online

BRAIN TUMORS

BASICS

DEFINITION

• Brain tumors of cats and dogs may be classified as either primary or secondary, depending on the cell type of origin. • Primary brain tumors originate from cells normally found within the brain and meninges, including the neuroepithelium, lymphoid tissues, germ cells, endothelial cells, and malformed tissues. • Secondary tumors are either neoplasms that have reached the brain by hematogenous metastasis from a primary tumor outside the nervous system, or neoplasms that affect the brain by local invasion, or extension, from adjacent non-neural tissues such as bone. • Pituitary gland neoplasms (adenomas or carcinomas) and tumors arising from cranial nerves (e.g., nerve sheath tumor of trigeminal, oculomotor, or vestibulocochlear nerves) are considered secondary brain tumors.

PATHOPHYSIOLOGY

• Brain tumors result in cerebral dysfunction by causing both primary effects, such as infiltration of nervous tissue or compression of adjacent anatomic structures, and secondary effects, such as hydrocephalus. • Additional primary effects include disruption of cerebral circulation and local necrosis, which may result in further damage to neural tissue. • The most important secondary effects of a primary brain tumor include disturbance of cerebrospinal fluid (CSF) flow dynamics, elevated intracranial pressure (ICP), cerebral edema, or brain herniation. • Secondary effects usually are more diffuse or generalized in their clinical manifestations and may mask the precise location of a focal intracranial lesion.

SYSTEMS AFFECTED

Nervous (brain).

GENETICS

• An unusually high incidence of meningiomas has been reported in cats with mucopolysaccharidosis type I. • Specific genetic factors associated with breed predisposition have not been identified. • Brachycephaly provisionally has been associated with the *SMOC*-2 and *thrombospondin-2* genes on canine chromosome 1, and a component of glioma susceptibility provisionally has been mapped to a region on canine chromosome 2. • Molecular and genetic classification of brain tumors may permit targeted therapies in the future.

INCIDENCE/PREVALENCE

• Brain tumors appear to be more common in dogs than in other domestic species. • Reported incidence in dogs is 10–20 per 100,000 animals, or 1–3% of all deaths where necropsy was done. • Primary nervous system tumors in dogs account for 60–80% of all such tumors reported in domestic animals (10–20% in cats; 10–20% in other species). • The most common sites for neoplasia to occur in immature dogs (<6 months), in decreasing order, are the hematopoietic system, brain, and skin. • Reported incidence in cats is 3.5/100000.

SIGNALMENT

Breed Predilections

• Meningiomas occur most frequently in dolichocephalic breeds of dog. • Glial cell tumors and pituitary tumors occur commonly in brachycephalic breeds of dog. • Canine breeds overrepresented include boxer, golden retriever, Doberman pinscher, Scottish terrier, and Old English sheepdog. • There does not appear to be a breed predisposition for development of brain tumors in cats.

Mean Age and Range

• Brain tumors occur in dogs and cats of any age. • Most frequent in older dogs, with greatest incidence in dogs >5 years of age. • Median age for diagnosis of meningiomas, gliomas, and choroid plexus tumors in dogs has been reported as 10–11 years, 8 years, and 5–6 years, respectively.

Predominant Sex

Older male cats appear to be most susceptible to meningiomas.

SIGNS

• Vary with tumor location. • The most frequently recognized clinical sign associated with a brain tumor of a dog or cat is seizures, particularly should first seizure occur after 5 years of age. • Other clinical signs frequently associated with brain tumor are abnormal behavior and mentation, visual deficits, circling, ataxia, head tilt, and cervical spinal hyperesthesia. • Signs that result from disease in given location in nervous system are similar, regardless of precise cause. • On basis of signalment, history, and results of complete physical and neurologic examinations, it is possible to localize a problem to the brain and, in some cases, to determine the approximate location.

CAUSES

• Uncertain. • Dietary, environmental, genetic, chemical, viral, traumatic, and immunologic factors may be considered.

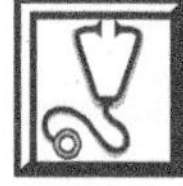

DIAGNOSIS

DIFFERENTIAL DIAGNOSIS

Categories of disease that may result in clinical signs similar to those of a brain tumor include congenital disorders, infections, immunologic and metabolic disorders, toxicities, nutritional disorders, trauma, vascular disorders, degeneration, and idiopathic disorders.

CBC/BIOCHEMISTRY/URINALYSIS

The major objective in the completion of these tests is to eliminate extracranial causes for signs of cerebral dysfunction.

OTHER LABORATORY TESTS

N/A

IMAGING

• Survey radiographs of the thorax and abdominal ultrasound—to rule out primary malignancy elsewhere in body. • Skull radiographs—of limited value; may detect neoplasms of skull or nasal cavity that involve brain by local extension. • Occasionally, lysis or hyperostosis of skull may accompany primary brain tumor (e.g., meningioma of cats), or there may be radiographically visible mineralization within a neoplasm. • CT—provides accurate determination of presence, location, size, and anatomic relationships of many intracranial neoplasms. • MRI—considered superior to CT in localization and characterization of most brain tumors.

DIAGNOSTIC PROCEDURES

CSF Analysis

• CSF—may help to rule out inflammatory causes of cerebral dysfunction: in some cases may support diagnosis of brain tumor. • Care should be used in collection of CSF, because increased ICP may be present in association with brain tumor, and pressure alterations associated with CSF collection may lead to brain herniation. • CSF collection usually delayed until advanced imaging has been completed to evaluate factors such as presence of cerebral edema or hemorrhage. • In general, increased CSF protein content and normal to increased CSF white blood cell count have been considered "typical" of a brain neoplasm.

Biopsy

• Cytologic evaluation of smear preparations from biopsy tissue, rapidly fixed in 95% alcohol and stained with hematoxylin and eosin, may be done within minutes of biopsy collection. • Tissue biopsy remains sole method available for definitive diagnosis of brain tumor type in cats or dogs, and is essential consideration prior to any type of therapy. • Biopsy not always attempted because of practical considerations, such as cost and morbidity. • CT-guided stereotactic biopsy systems provide relatively rapid and extremely accurate means of tumor biopsy, with low rate of complications.

PATHOLOGIC FINDINGS

• Classification of CNS tumors in dogs and cats primarily is based on the characteristics of their constituent cell type, pathologic

behavior, topographic pattern, and secondary changes present within and surrounding the tumor. • Meningioma is most common intracranial neoplasm of dogs and cats.
• Classification of glial subset of neuroepithelial tumors is based on predominant cell type (e.g., astrocyte or oligodendrocyte).

Dogs

• Embryonal tumors have been consolidated under single term "primitive neuroectodermal tumors" (or PNETs) to accommodate their anaplastic nature. • Brain tumors arising from lymphoreticular cells traditionally have been grouped under a heading of reticulosis or histiocytic lymphoma.
• Skull tumors that affect the brain by local extension include osteosarcoma, chondrosarcoma, and multilobular osteochondrosarcoma. • The most frequently seen secondary tumors of dogs include local extension of nasal adenocarcinoma; metastases from mammary, prostatic, or pulmonary adenocarcinoma; metastases from hemangiosarcoma; and extension of pituitary adenoma or carcinoma. • Nerve sheath tumors arising from cranial nerves (particularly oculomotor nerve and trigeminal nerve) may occur in dogs.

Cats

• Meningiomas involving multiple intracranial sites (including third ventricle) relatively common in cats. • Primary brain tumors other than meningiomas occur infrequently in cats. • Tumors that have been reported include astrocytoma, ependymoma, oligodendroglioma, choroid plexus papilloma, medulloblastoma, lymphoma, olfactory neuroblastoma, and gangliocytoma.
• Lymphoma of the brain may be primary or secondary, or may be an aspect of multicentric lymphoma of cats. • Secondary tumors that have been reported to occur in the brain of cats include pituitary macroadenomas and macrocarcinomas, and metastatic carcinoma.
• Local extension may occur either from tumors of middle ear cavity (e.g., squamous cell carcinoma), nasal cavity (e.g., nasal adenocarcinoma), or skull (e.g., osteosarcoma).

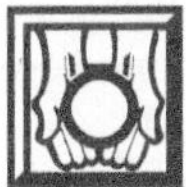

TREATMENT

APPROPRIATE HEALTH CARE

• Beyond general efforts to maintain homeostasis, major goals of therapy for brain tumor are to control secondary effects, such as increased ICP or cerebral edema, and to eradicate the tumor or reduce its size.
• Beyond palliative care, three methods of therapy for a brain tumor currently are available for use in dogs and cats: surgery, irradiation, and chemotherapy.

Surgery

• Neurosurgical intervention is an essential consideration in management of brain tumors in cats or dogs, whether for complete excision, partial removal, or biopsy. • Meningiomas, particularly those located over cerebral convexities or in frontal lobes of cerebrum, may be completely (or almost completely) removed by surgery, especially in cats.
• Primary calvarial tumors also may be removed surgically prior to other types of therapy.

Radiation Therapy

• Irradiation may be used either alone or in combination with other treatments for either primary or secondary brain tumors. • Careful treatment planning by qualified and experienced radiation therapist is essential to success of radiation therapy. • A major development in radiation therapy is emergence of more precise protocols that spare tissues surrounding the brain tumor (e.g., stereotactic radiotherapy).

Chemotherapy

Alkylating agents (e.g., carmustine [BCNU], lomustine [CCNU], and temozolomide), antimetabolic agents (e.g., cytosine arabinoside), and ribonucleotide reductase inhibitors (e.g., hydroxuurea) may result in reduction of tumor size and improvement of clinical signs in dogs with glial cell tumors; however, evidence of efficacy in animals is lacking.

MEDICATIONS

DRUG(S) OF CHOICE

• Glucocorticoids may be used for edema reduction and, in some cases (e.g., lymphoma), for retardation of tumor growth. • Some animals with brain tumor demonstrate dramatic improvement in clinical signs for weeks or months with sustained glucocorticoid therapy. • Antiepileptic drugs (e.g., phenobarbital, bromide, levetiracetam) may be utilized for control of generalized seizures.
• Mannitol and hypertonic saline are agents best suited for effective reduction of increased ICP.

FOLLOW-UP

PATIENT MONITORING

• Serial neurologic examinations. • Serial CT or MRI examinations.

POSSIBLE COMPLICATIONS

• Aspiration pneumonia due to depressed swallowing reflexes associated with increased ICP. • Seizures.

EXPECTED COURSE AND PROGNOSIS

• Little information available concerning survival times of dogs or cats with brain tumor that have received only palliative therapy (i.e., therapy to control secondary effects of a tumor without an attempt to eradicate the tumor). • Results of one study indicate mean and median survival of 81 days and 56 days, respectively, following CT diagnosis of primary brain tumor in each of 8 dogs. • Results from several studies confirm that prognosis for a dog or cat with a primary brain tumor may be significantly improved by surgical removal and irradiation, either alone or in combination.

MISCELLANEOUS

ASSOCIATED CONDITIONS

Dogs that have been treated for a brain tumor may develop a second type of tumor elsewhere in the body.

ABBREVIATIONS

• CSF = cerebrospinal fluid.
• ICP = intracranial pressure.
• PNET = primitive neuroectodermal tumor.

Suggested Reading

Dickinson PJ. Advances in diagnostic and treatment modalities for intracranial tumors. J Vet Intern Med 2014, 28:1165–1185.
Dickinson PJ. Intracranial tumors in dogs. Vet Focus 2014, 24(2):2–10.
Hicks J, Platt S, Kent M, Haley A. Canine brain tumors: a model for human disease? Vet Comp Oncol 2017, 15(1):252–272.
Kohler RJ, Arnold SA, Eck DJ, et al. Incidence of and risk factors for major complications or death in dogs undergoing cytoreductive surgery for treatment of suspected primary intracranial masses. J Am Vet Med Assoc 2018, 253(12):1594–1603.
Rossmeisl JH. New treatment modalities for brain tumors in dogs and cats. Vet Clin Small Anim 2014, 44:1013–1038.

Author Richard A. LeCouteur

Client Education Handout available online

BREEDING, TIMING

BASICS

DEFINITION

Timing of insemination(s) to maximize pregnancy risk and litter size.

PATHOPHYSIOLOGY

Dogs

• Must determine ovulation day so that breeding(s) occur(s) at proper time. • Fresh, chilled, or frozen semen—usually limited to one or two inseminations; insemination must be timed relative to ovulation for maximum fertility. • Ovulation may vary relative to onset of heat (proestrus), standing heat (estrus), vaginal cytology. • Luteinizing hormone (LH)—controls ovulation; peaks on same day or after full cornification is observed; ovulation occurs approximately 2 days after peak; 2–3 days (54–72 hours) more required for oocyte maturation; mature oocytes viable for minimum 2–3 days; thus fertile period is 4–8 days after LH peak, and maximum fertility is 5–6 days after LH peak. • Serum progesterone concentration—increase closely associated with LH peak.

Cats

• Ovulation—usually induced; timing of breeding is not as critical as with dogs; depends on adequate gonadotropin-releasing hormone (GnRH) and then LH release triggered by vaginal stimulation. • Adequate stimulation—characterized by copulatory cry and postcoital reaction; frequency of coital stimuli important in determining adequacy of coital contact. • LH—peak concentration and duration of elevation determine number of follicles ovulating; higher concentration with multiple copulations; response to copulation depends on day of estrus (greater release on estrus day 3 than on estrus day 1); release partially depends on duration of exposure to estrogen.

SYSTEMS AFFECTED

Reproductive

GENETICS

N/A

INCIDENCE/PREVALENCE

N/A

GEOGRAPHIC DISTRIBUTION

N/A

SIGNALMENT

Dog and cat.

SIGNS

General Comments

Dogs

• Onset of estrus—usually associated with a change in the vaginal discharge from sanguineous to barely red and decreased vulvar edema; sanguineous discharge may continue during estrus and cease only at the onset of diestrus. • Physical signs alone—unreliable for precise determination of fertile period. • Receptivity—may be detected by touching the perineum near the vulva; if receptive, female will "flag" by elevating the tail to one side and lifting the vulva dorsally.

Cats

LH response to a single mating—may vary substantially.

Historical Findings

Dogs

Sanguineous vulvar discharge during estrus.

Cats

Return to estrus in <30 days may indicate failure to ovulate; interestrus usually 8–10 days, but highly variable even within queen; some queens will breed while pregnant.

Physical Examination Findings

Dogs

• Interest shown by male. • Vulva less turgid. • Vaginal discharge—less color and amount. • Flagging. • Females show mounting behavior. • Fully cornified and crenulated pale vaginal epithelium. • Digital palpation of vagina may be resented by bitch in proestrus, improving throughout proestrus until estrus. May feel edematous mass on floor of caudal vagina, just cranial to urethral os, that should shrink as optimal breeding period approaches.

Cats

• Fully cornified vaginal epithelium. • Interest shown by male. • No changes in external genitalia. • Vocalizes, rubs objects. • Lordosis.

CAUSES

Dogs

• Limited number of breedings. • Female unreceptive to male. • Artificial insemination (fresh, chilled, or frozen semen).

Cats

• Coitus—too early or too late in estrus; too few times. • Artificial insemination.

RISK FACTORS

N/A

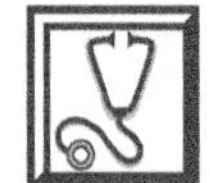

DIAGNOSIS

DIFFERENTIAL DIAGNOSIS

• Vaginal discharge—proestrus or estrus; vaginitis; neoplasia, pyometra, urinary tract infection. • Refusal to allow intromission—anatomic abnormalities of Mullerian duct development, vulvovestibular or vestibulo-vaginal junction, acquired abnormality from dystocia or breeding trauma, vaginal hyperplasia, behavioral.

CBC/BIOCHEMISTRY/URINALYSIS

N/A

OTHER LABORATORY TESTS

Dogs

• Semi-quantitative progesterone ELISA—adjunct to vaginal cytologic examination. • Quantitative serum progesterone testing—preferred when breeding with frozen semen; especially useful in animals with reduced fertility. Commercial labs or in-house machines available. ○ Progesterone concentration <1 ng/mL (3.18 nmol/L) before LH peak, 1.5–4 ng/mL (4.8–12.7 nmol/L) at LH peak, 4–10 ng/mL (12.7–31.8 nmol/L) at ovulation; continues to rise during diestrus/pregnancy. ○ Commercial laboratories use various methods of progesterone concentration measurement, so values indicative of LH and ovulation vary among labs. ○ Documenting rapid rise in progesterone concentration subsequent to initial rise is more reliable indicator of ovulation than single measurement of LH peak or initial rise in progesterone. • LH testing—must sample daily to observe LH peak; can use serum progesterone to signal when to start testing or use the initial rise in progesterone concentration as surrogate for LH peak.

Cats

Serum progesterone testing to verify ovulation.

IMAGING

Ultrasonographic imaging of ovaries—may help determine ovulation; perform daily, best if using color flow Doppler.

DIAGNOSTIC PROCEDURES

Dogs

• Vaginal cytologic examination—imprecise indicator of fertile period; cornification of vaginal epithelium with clear background usually coincides with sexual receptivity. ○ Proestrus (in breeder terms, "day 1," first sign of hemorrhagic vaginal discharge)—most epithelial cells are noncornified. ○ Percentage of cornified cells (cells with angular cytoplasm and pyknotic nuclei or nuclei that fail to take up stain) increases during proestrus. ○ Estrus—90% or more cornified cells, background of slide free of debris. ○ Breeders refer to estrus by day, usually occurs day 10–18 in breeder terms. ○ Diestrus—abrupt decline in percentage of cornified cells (20–50%) in a single day: day 1 of diestrus (D1); normal to see neutrophils on days 1–4 of diestrus. • Vaginoscopy—edematous vaginal folds until LH peak, then vagina pale with slight wrinkling (crenulation) as edema decreases with estradiol decline; by optimum breeding period crenulation is obvious, until diestrus when folds are flat and edema disappears.

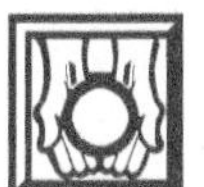

TREATMENT

APPROPRIATE HEALTH CARE

Dogs

• Fresh semen, multiple breedings—inseminate q48h, starting 48–96h after initial rise in serum progesterone concentration is observed until D1. • Fresh semen, two breedings—inseminate either on days 3 and 5 or on days 4 and 6 after LH peak or initial rise in serum progesterone concentration; use standard artificial insemination (AI) pipettes or modified Foley catheters (several sizes available); vaginal insemination on or after day 5 may be associated with reduced pregnancy rates and litter sizes due to beginning of cervical closure. • Frozen or chilled semen—frozen semen is less viable than chilled, thus timing is more critical; one or two intrauterine inseminations most common: inseminate on day 5 or 6 after LH peak or initial rise in serum progesterone concentration (day 0) or 3 days after serum progesterone concentration ≥5 ng/mL (16 nmol/L); for intrauterine insemination via transcervical endoscopy (TCI) or surgical insemination, serum progesterone concentration on day of insemination should be ≥12 ng/mL (38 nmol/L; value is laboratory dependent). • Timing insemination based on serum progesterone concentration improves chance of conception and increased litter size.
• Blood collection and vaginal examination q48h are adequate in most cases.

Cats

• Increase likelihood of ovulation and litter size by maximizing number of matings; breed on successive days. • Breed at least 4 times daily at least 2–3 hours apart on days 2 and 3 of estrus to maximize LH release. • May induce ovulation by administration of exogenous hormones—GnRH or human chorionic gonadotropin (hCG) after mating.

ACTIVITY

• No alteration in activity necessary except confinement—bitch will search for male.
• Keep strictly away from unintended sexually intact males.

CLIENT EDUCATION

Client education on physical, behavioral, and endocrinologic changes that occur during estrous cycle, and how variable timing of these changes can be from animal to animal, can improve owner compliance and satisfaction.

SURGICAL CONSIDERATIONS

Surgical AI requires standard postoperative care.

MEDICATIONS

DRUG(S) OF CHOICE

Cats—hCG (100–500 IU/cat IM); GnRH (25–50 μg/cat IM).

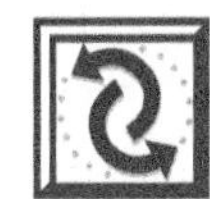

FOLLOW-UP

PATIENT MONITORING

• Dogs—serial vaginal cytology to determine D1; ovulation is ~6 days before D1. • Dogs—whelping is 65 ± 1 days from LH peak, 63 ± 1 days from ovulation, or 57 ± 1 days from D1; for fresh, chilled, or frozen semen: repeat quantitative serum progesterone measurement after initial progesterone rise or LH peak to verify >10 ng/mL (32 nmol/L). • Cats—use serum progesterone assay 1 week post insemination to verify ovulation. • Cats—queening is 62–71 days from first breeding.

PREVENTION/AVOIDANCE

N/A

POSSIBLE COMPLICATIONS

Dogs

• Vaginal cytologic examinations—compare D1 with prospective estimation based on progesterone; if estimates differ, pregnancy rates are reduced. • Semi-quantitative progesterone kits—must come to room temperature before use; concentrations falsely elevated when using a cold kit. • Serum progesterone concentration—allow blood to clot at room temperature; separate cells from serum 20 minutes after collection; falsely low concentrations occur when using serum mixed with red blood cells (progesterone binds to erythrocytes). • Hemolyzed or lipemic specimen—may give falsely low progesterone concentration. • Quantitative (chemiluminescence assay, fluorescence, ELISA) progesterone assay—more accurate than semi-quantitative kits; several in-house analyzers available; turnaround times should be less than 24 hours. • Serum separator tubes cause false elevations in chemiluminescence progesterone assay; anticoagulant may affect reported concentration (serum > heparin plasma > EDTA plasma).

MISCELLANEOUS

AGE-RELATED FACTORS

Split heats in young bitches—period of proestrus (may be prolonged to 6 weeks or more), followed by cessation of signs, and subsequent resumption of estrus cycle (1–3 weeks later); no initial rise in progesterone or LH concentration occurs with first proestrus/estrus; subsequent estrus usually normal.

PREGNANCY/FERTILITY/BREEDING

Ultrasound—conceptuses can first be detected 18–20 days after LH peak (requires high-resolution, high-frequency probe, easier in toy breeds) or 2–3 days earlier in cats; commonly done 4 weeks post breeding; recommend earlier exam in bitches with history of pregnancy loss or infertility.

SEE ALSO

• Infertility, Female—Dogs.
• Ovulatory Failure.
• Vaginal Discharge.
• Vaginal Malformations and Acquired Lesions.

ABBREVIATIONS

• AI = artificial insemination.
• D1 = first day of diestrus.
• GnRH = gonadotropin-releasing hormone.
• hCG = human chorionic gonadotropin.
• LH = luteinizing hormone.
• TCI = endoscopic transcervical insemination.

Suggested Reading

Johnston SD, Root Kustritz MV, Olson PN. Breeding management, artificial insemination, in vitro fertilization, and embryo transfer in the queen. In: Johnston SD, Root Kustritz MV, Olson-Schultz P, eds., Canine and Feline Theriogenology. Philadelphia, PA: Saunders, 2001, pp. 406–413.

Author Cathy J. Gartley
Consulting Editor Erin E. Runcan

BRONCHIECTASIS

BASICS

OVERVIEW

- Clinical condition seen primarily in dogs; irreversible dilatation of the bronchi; caused by chronic infectious or inflammatory airway disease, foreign body pneumonia, or associated with primary ciliary dyskinesia.
- Occurs in cats as a sequela to longstanding inflammatory lung disease or neoplasia.
- Airways are pulled open by surrounding lung tissue; pooling of secretions can occur, which perpetuates lung damage and allows colonization by bacteria.
- Can be cylindrical or saccular, focal or diffuse.

SIGNALMENT

- Primarily dogs but radiographically detected in many cats.
- Cocker spaniels and perhaps West Highland white terriers predisposed.
- Young animals (<1 year) with primary ciliary dyskinesia.
- Middle-aged to old dogs with chronic pulmonary disease.

SIGNS

- Chronic cough—usually moist and productive; hemoptysis.
- Recurrent fever.
- Exercise intolerance.
- Tachypnea or respiratory distress.
- Chronic nasal discharge or sinusitis, particularly with primary ciliary dyskinesia.
- Moist, harsh inspiratory crackles; loud expiratory lung sounds or wheezes on physical exam.
- Tracheal hypersensitivity.

CAUSES & RISK FACTORS

- Primary ciliary dyskinesia.
- Inadequately treated infectious or inflammatory lung conditions (pneumonia, bronchitis, or eosinophilic lung disease).
- Smoke inhalation, chronic aspiration pneumonia, radiation injury, and inhalation of environmental toxins—predispose animal to airway injury and colonization by bacteria.
- Chronic bronchial obstruction or foreign body pneumonia—development of bronchiectasis distal to the obstructed region common.
- Signs related to bronchiectasis may not be recognized until long after the primary injury.

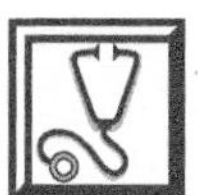

DIAGNOSIS

DIFFERENTIAL DIAGNOSIS

- Recurrent bacterial bronchopneumonia.
- Fungal pneumonia.
- Chronic bronchitis.
- Infectious or parasitic bronchitis.
- Foreign body pneumonia.
- Neoplasia.

CBC/BIOCHEMISTRY/URINALYSIS

- Neutrophilia and monocytosis.
- Hyperglobulinemia.
- Proteinuria—can be seen with secondary amyloidosis, glomerulonephritis, or sepsis.

OTHER LABORATORY TESTS

Arterial blood gas analysis—hypoxemia; widened alveolar–arterial oxygen gradient.

IMAGING

- Radiography—insensitive for the diagnosis. Abnormalities visible late in the course of disease include dilatation of the lobar bronchi with lack of normal tapering in the periphery; diffuse thickening of bronchial walls; mixed bronchial, interstitial, and alveolar pattern.
- Changes can be focal or diffuse.
- CT—bronchus >2 times the width of the adjacent pulmonary artery in dogs, abnormally dilated bronchi near the lung periphery; thickened airways; cystic dilatations of the bronchi with or without pulmonaray consolidation.

DIAGNOSTIC PROCEDURES

- Bronchoscopy—saccular or tubular dilatation of the airways.
- Airway sampling—cytologic examination of bronchoalveolar lavage fluid or tracheal wash specimens; culture for aerobic and anaerobic bacteria and *Mycoplasma*; typically find suppurative inflammation with high numbers of neutrophils, or increased eosinophils indicating eosinophilic bronchopneumopathy; may culture a mixed population of bacteria; some cases appear to have sterile inflammation.

PATHOLOGIC FINDINGS

- Dilated bronchi.
- Diffuse peribronchial and alveolar inflammation and fibrosis.
- Squamous metaplasia of bronchial epithelium.

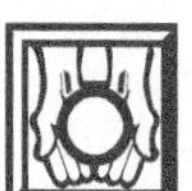

TREATMENT

- Inpatient—severe condition: intravenous fluids and antibiotics; oxygen administration.
- Airway nebulization and coupage to facilitate removal of viscid pulmonary secretions, often lifelong.
- Gentle activity enhances clearance of secretions.
- Long-term antibiotic administration.
- Stress to owner the importance of appropriate follow-up care.
- Single affected lung lobe or bronchial obstruction—lung lobectomy can be curative.

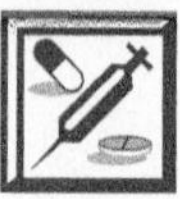

MEDICATIONS

DRUG(S) OF CHOICE

- Intravenous antibiotics—may be required initially; good choices: ampicillin (10–20 mg/kg IV q6–8h) and enrofloxacin (5–10 mg/kg q24h).
- Broad-spectrum agents with efficacy against both aerobes and anaerobes and that offer good penetration of pulmonary tissue—preferred; combination of enrofloxacin (5–20 mg/kg PO q24h) and clindamycin (5–11 mg/kg PO q12h) or amoxicillin–clavulanate often effective.
- Azithromycin can be a good alternative antibiotic for outpatient care.
- Long-term use of antibiotics (2 months to lifelong)—based on bacterial culture and sensitivity testing; may be required even if culture of airway specimens yields no growth.
- Bronchodilators—may be beneficial, although animals usually have irreversible airflow limitation; extended release theophylline advised.
- Eosinophilic lung disease requires treatment with glucocorticoids.
- Saline nebulization and coupage highly beneficial in removing secretions.

CONTRAINDICATIONS/POSSIBLE INTERACTIONS

- Theophylline derivatives and fluoroquinolones—concurrent use causes high and possibly toxic plasma theophylline concentration.
- Furosemide—avoid; dries airway secretions.
- Cough suppressants—avoid; will trap secretions and bacteria in lower airway and perpetuate damage.

FOLLOW-UP

PATIENT MONITORING

- Clinical response—outpatient.
- Serial CBC, blood gas analysis, and thoracic radiographs.

PREVENTION/AVOIDANCE

- Antibiotics—complete a full course of therapy in patients that appear to have parenchymal involvement.
- Early recognition and resolution of foreign body pneumonia.
- Appropriate treatment of eosinophilic pneumonia.

POSSIBLE COMPLICATIONS

Chronic recurrent pulmonary infection likely.

EXPECTED COURSE AND PROGNOSIS

- Chronic and recurrent clinical signs expected; some degree of coughing will always be present.

- Animals can live for years with bronchiectasis if managed properly.
- Some patients succumb to respiratory failure.
- Other organs may fail if bacteremia or glomerulonephritis develops.

MISCELLANEOUS

ASSOCIATED CONDITIONS

- Primary ciliary dyskinesia.
- Chronic sinusitis.
- Chronic bronchitis.
- Pneumonia—bacterial, eosinophilic aspiration, foreign body.
- Smoke inhalation.

Suggested Reading

Cannon MS, Johnson LR, Pesavento PA, et al. Quantitative and qualitative computed tomographic imaging features of bronchiectasis in dogs. Vet Rad US 2013, 54(4):351–357.

Hawkins EC, Basseches J, Berry CR, et al. Demographic, clinical, and radiographic features of bronchiectasis in dogs: 316 cases (1988–2000). J Am Vet Med Assoc 2003, 223(11):1628–1635.

Johnson LR, Johnson EG, Vernau W, et al. Bronchoscopy, imaging, and concurrent diseases in dogs with bronchiectasis (2003–2014). J Vet Int Med 2016, 30(1):247–254.

Author Lynelle R. Johnson

Consulting Editor Elizabeth Rozanski

BRONCHITIS, CHRONIC

BASICS

DEFINITION

• Chronic coughing for longer than 2 months that is not attributable to another cause (e.g., neoplasia, congestive heart failure, eosinophilic pneumonia, or infectious bronchitis). • Partly nonreversible and often slowly progressive condition owing to accompanying pathologic airway changes.

PATHOPHYSIOLOGY

• Recurrent airway inflammation suspected, but a specific cause is rarely determined. • Persistent tracheobronchial irritation—causes chronic coughing; leads to changes in tracheobronchial epithelium and submucosa. • Airway inflammation, epithelial edema, and thickening—prominent. • Excess production of thickened mucus is a hallmark. • In severe, very chronic cases—probable increased lung resistance; decreased expiratory airflow, especially in cats; in dogs, possible sequelae such as broncholamacia and bronchiectasis.

SYSTEMS AFFECTED

• Respiratory • Cardiovascular—pulmonary hypertension, cor pulmonale. • Nervous—syncope (infrequent).

INCIDENCE/PREVALENCE

Common in dogs and cats.

GEOGRAPHIC DISTRIBUTION

Worldwide

SIGNALMENT

Species

Dogs and cats.

Breed Predilections

• Dogs—small and toy breeds common; also observed in large breeds. • Siamese cats and domestic shorthairs affected.

Mean Age and Range

Most often affects middle-aged and old animals.

Predominant Sex

N/A, although spayed females are often overrepresented (might be due to weight gain).

SIGNS

Historical Findings

• Coughing—hallmark of tracheobronchial irritation; usually harsh and dry; post-tussive gagging common (owners often misinterpret this as vomiting, especially in dogs). • Exercise intolerance, difficult breathing, wheezing (in cats). • Cyanosis and even syncope may be noted in severe cases.

Physical Examination Findings

• Patients usually bright, alert, and afebrile. • Tracheal palpation—typically results in coughing because of increased tracheal sensitivity. • Small airway disease—assumed when expiratory abdominal push (during quiet breathing) or end-expiratory wheezing is detected. • Bronchovesicular lung sounds, end-inspiratory crackles, and wheezing (result of airflow into obstructed airways) may be heard. • Loud end-expiratory snap is suggestive of concurrent airway collapse. • Cardiac auscultation—murmurs secondary to valvular insufficiency common in dogs, but not always associated with congestive heart failure; chronic bronchitis usually results in normal or slower than normal resting heart rate and pronounced sinus arrhythmia; in cats, tachycardia is possible. • Obesity— common; important complicating factor. • Severe dental disease may predispose to lower airway colonization and possible infection (dogs).

CAUSES

Chronic airway inflammation initiated by multiple causes, although specific cause rarely identified.

RISK FACTORS

• Long-term exposure to inhaled irritants. • Obesity. • Recurrent bacterial infection. • Dental disease and laryngeal disease—result in bacterial showering of lower airways.

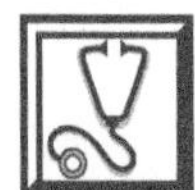

DIAGNOSIS

DIFFERENTIAL DIAGNOSIS

• Bronchiectasis. • Eosinophilic bronchopneumopathy. • Foreign bodies. • Heartworm disease. • Bacterial, pneumonia. • Neoplasia—metastatic more than primary. • Pulmonary parasites or parasitic larval migration. • Pulmonary fibrosis—cats and dogs. • Pulmonary granulomatosis. • Congestive heart failure—typically associated with high resting heart rate and left atrial enlargement, which may lead to collapse of left principal bronchus.

CBC/BIOCHEMISTRY/URINALYSIS

• Rarely diagnostic. • Neutrophilic leukocytosis common. • Absolute eosinophilia—suggests but not diagnostic for allergic bronchitis. • Polycythemia secondary to chronic hypoxia—may be seen. • Liver enzymes and bile acids may be elevated due to passive congestion.

OTHER LABORATORY TESTS

• Fecal and heartworm tests—rule out pulmonary parasites. • Pulse oximetry—useful for detecting hemoglobin desaturation. • Arterial blood gas analysis—collect, ice, and have analyzed at a local hospital; mild to moderately low partial pressure of oxygen (PaO_2) seen with severe condition; aids in prognosis and monitoring treatment. • As hyperadrenocorticism could be responsible for obesity and/or enlarged liver/abdomen, testing should be considered if clinically indicated.

IMAGING

Thoracic Radiography (High Resolution Computed Topography)

Common features (in descending order of frequency)—bronchial thickening; interstitial pattern; middle lung lobe consolidation (cats); atelectasis; hyperinflation and diaphragmatic flattening (primarily cats).

Echocardiography

• May reveal right heart enlargement with pulmonary hypertension. • Helps rule out cardiac disease as a cause of coughing. • Check for pulmonary hypertension via Doppler echocardiography.

DIAGNOSTIC PROCEDURES

Bronchoscopy

Preferred test for assessing the lower airways. • Allows direct visualization of structural as well as functional (dynamic) changes; allows selected airway sampling (e.g., biopsy and lavage). • Gross changes—excess mucoid to mucopurulent secretions; epithelial edema or thickening with blunting of bronchial bifurcations; irregular or granular mucosa; mucosal polypoid proliferations can indicate chronic bronchitis or chronic eosinophilic pneumonia. • Large airway caliber changes (e.g., static or dynamic airway collapse and bronchiectasis)—may be detected as complicating problems.

Evaluation of Airway Secretions

• Must collect from lower airways—helps to establish underlying cause if present or to determine the severity of inflammation. • Throat swab cultures are not representative of lower airway flora • Tracheal aspiration or bronchoalveolar lavage—collect specimens for cytologic examination and bacterial/mycoplasmal culture or qPRC assessment. • Quantitated aerobic bronchoalveolar lavage (BAL) cultures help differentiate infection versus airway colonization; reported cutoff is >1.7 × 10^3 colony-forming units (CFU) for infection in dogs. Anaerobic and *Mycoplasma* cultures recommended as well. • Cytology—inflammation primary finding; most cells are neutrophils, eosinophils, or macrophages; evaluate for bacteria, parasites, neoplastic cells, and contamination with foreign material. • Recurrent infections—implicated in pathogenesis of bronchitis; however, positive cultures are not frequently reported; *Mycoplasma* infection discussed but rarely confirmed as a cause.

PATHOLOGIC FINDINGS

See Bronchoscopy under Diagnostic Procedures.

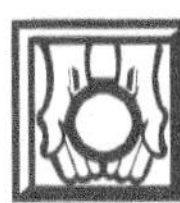

TREATMENT

APPROPRIATE HEALTH CARE

• Usually outpatient—oxygen can be given at home in chronic cases. • Inpatient—if requires oxygen therapy, parenteral medication, or aerosol therapy; patients that owners cannot keep calm at home during initial stages of therapy.

NURSING CARE

Consider saline nebulization followed by coupage and/or gentle exercise to encourage removal of airway secretions.

ACTIVITY

• Exercise—moderate (not forced) useful in clearing secretions; assists with weight loss.
• Limit if exertion causes excessive coughing.
• Use a harness instead of a collar.

DIET

Weight loss critical—improves PaO_2, attitude, and exercise tolerance in obese patients; reduces cough frequency.

CLIENT EDUCATION

• Warn client that chronic bronchitis is an incurable disease and complete suppression of all coughing is an unattainable goal. • Stress that aggressive treatment (including weight control, avoiding risk factors, and medical treatment) minimizes the severity of the coughing and slows disease progression in most patients.

SURGICAL CONSIDERATIONS

Treat severe dental disease to minimize secondary bacterial complications.

MEDICATIONS

DRUG(S) OF CHOICE

Corticosteroids

• Diminish airway inflammation and coughing regardless of the underlying cause.
• Indicated for noninfectious conditions.
• With allergic or hypersensitivity reactions—require long-term administration; attempt to wean off steroids or determine lowest effective dosage. • Prednisolone preferred in cats.
• Prednisone or prednisolone usually initiated at 0.5–1 mg/kg PO q12h for a variable time, with tapering of the dosage based on clinical signs. • Inhaled agents (e.g., budenoside or fluticasone 1–3 puffs using metered dose inhalers [variable concentrations exist] a day) are often effective and can be used to reduce systemic side effects of corticosteroids; they are delivered via a spacer chamber and face mask (e.g., AeroDawg); however, the most adequate dose is not clearly established.

Bronchodilators

Commonly prescribed, although limited evidence of efficacy.

Antibiotics

• Select on basis of quantitated culture and sensitivity test results.

Antitussives

• Indicated for nonproductive, paroxysmal, continuous, or debilitating cough. • Dogs—butorphanol (0.55 mg/kg PO q6–12h; 0.055–0.11 mg/kg SC); hydrocodone (0.1–0.3 mg/kg q6–8h PO). Over-the-counter cough suppressants are rarely effective; gabapentin 2–5mg.kg by mouth every eight hours (but unestablished efficacy).

CONTRAINDICATIONS

Lasix and atropine—do not use because of drying effects on tracheobronchial secretions.

PRECAUTIONS

• Beta agonists (e.g., terbutaline and albuterol)—may cause tachycardia, nervousness, and muscle tremors; typically transient. • Theophylline—may cause tachycardia, restlessness, excitability, vomiting, and diarrhea; evaluate ethylene diamine tetra-acetate (EDTA) plasma sample for peak plasma concentration (ideally 5–20 μg/mL); toxicity may be more common with generic formulations.

POSSIBLE INTERACTIONS

Fluoroquinolones decrease theophylline clearance in dogs and can result in theophylline toxicity.

ALTERNATIVE DRUG(S)

Maropitant (some antitussive properties suggested, but not advised yet).

FOLLOW-UP

PATIENT MONITORING

• Follow abnormalities revealed by physical examination and selected diagnostic tests—determine response to treatment. • Monitor weight; arterial blood gases usually improve after significant weight loss.

PREVENTION/AVOIDANCE

Avoid and address risk factors (see Risk Factors).

POSSIBLE COMPLICATIONS

• Syncope—possible complication of chronic coughing, particularly in toy-breed dogs. • Pulmonary hypertension and cor pulmonale—most serious complications. • Bronchectasis and airway remodeling.

EXPECTED COURSE AND PROGNOSIS

• Progressive airway changes—syncopal episodes, chronic hypoxia, right ventricular hypertrophy, and pulmonary hypertension.
• Acute exacerbations—common with seasonal changes, air quality changes, worsened inflammation, and potentially development of secondary infection.

MISCELLANEOUS

ASSOCIATED CONDITIONS

• Syncope—secondary to chronic coughing or development of pulmonary hypertension.
• Increased susceptibility to airway infection, chronic hypoxia, pulmonary hypertension, and cor pulmonale.

PREGNANCY/FERTILITY/BREEDING

Safety in pregnant animals not established for most of the recommended drugs.

SYNONYMS

Chronic bronchitis.

SEE ALSO

• Asthma, Bronchitis—Cats. • Bronchiectasis.
• Cough. • Hypoxemia. • Tracheal Collapse.

ABBREVIATIONS

• BAL = bronchoalveolar lavage. • CFU = colony-forming unit. • EDTA = ethylene diamine tetra-acetate. • PaO_2 = partial pressure of oxygen.

Suggested Reading

Grotheer M, Hirschberger J, Hartmann K, et al., Comparison of signalment, clinical, laboratory and radiographic parameters in cats with feline asthma and chronic bronchitis. J Feline Med Surg. 2020, 22(7):649–655.

Reinero CR, Masseau I, Grobman M, et al., Perspectives in veterinary medicine: Description and classification of bronchiolar disorders in cats. J Vet Intern Med. 2019, 33(3):1201–1221.

Rozanski E. Canine chronic bronchitis. An update . Vet Clin N Am Small Anim Pract 2020, 50:393–404.

Author Cécile Clercx
Consulting Editor Elizabeth Rozanski

Client Education Handout available online

BRUCELLOSIS

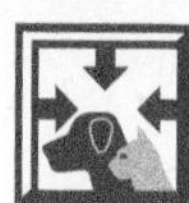

BASICS

DEFINITION

• Contagious disease of dogs caused by *Brucella canis*. • Rarely caused by *B. suis, B. abortus, or B. mellitensis*. • Characterized by abortion and infertility in females, epididymitis and testicular atrophy in males.

PATHOPHYSIOLOGY

B. canis—a small, intracellular Gram-negative bacterium; has propensity for growth in lymphatic, placental, and male genital (epididymis and prostate) tissues.

SYSTEMS AFFECTED

• Hemic/lymph/immune—lymph nodes, spleen, bone marrow, mononuclear leukocytes.
• Reproductive—target tissues of gonadal steroids (gravid uterus, fetus, testes epididymides, prostate gland). • Other tissues—intervertebral discs, anterior uvea, meninges (uncommon).

GENETICS

No known genetic predisposition.

INCIDENCE/PREVALENCE

• Incidence unknown. • Seroprevalence—not well defined; false-positive results common with agglutination tests. • Prevalence—1–18% in United States, Japan; higher in rural United States; 25–30% in stray dogs in Mexico, Peru.

GEOGRAPHIC DISTRIBUTION

United States, Mexico, Japan, South America; Spain, Tunisia, China, Bulgaria; individual outbreaks in Germany, Czech Republic.

SIGNALMENT

Species

Dogs

Breed Predilections

• No evidence of breed susceptibility, reportedly high prevalence in beagles. • Pure breeds in commercial kennels ("puppy mills").

Mean Age and Range

• Any age. • Most common in sexually mature dogs.

Predominant Sex

Most common in females.

SIGNS

General Comments

Suspect with abortions, reproductive failures, or genital disease.

Historical Findings

• Animals may appear healthy or have vague signs of illness. • Lethargy. • Loss of libido.
• Swollen lymph nodes. • Back or neck pain.
• Abortion—commonly 6–8 weeks after conception, although pregnancy may terminate at any stage.

Physical Examination Findings

• Peripheral lymphadenopathy. • Males—swollen scrotum with scrotal dermatitis, enlarged firm epididymides, orchitis, prostatitis. • Chronic infection—unilateral or bilateral testicular atrophy, spinal pain, discospondylitis, posterior weakness, ataxia.
• Chronic recurrent anterior uveitis without signs of systemic disease; also iris hyperpigmentation, vitreal infiltrates, multifocal chorioretinitis. • Vaginal discharge—may last several weeks after abortion. • Fever (rare).

CAUSES

B. canis—Gram-negative coccobacillus; morphologically indistinguishable from other members of genus.

RISK FACTORS

• Breeding kennels, pack hounds. • Contact with strays in endemic areas.

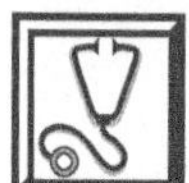

DIAGNOSIS

DIFFERENTIAL DIAGNOSIS

• Abortions—maternal, fetal, or placental abnormalities. • Systemic infections—canine distemper, canine herpesvirus, *B. abortus*, hemolytic streptococci, *E. coli*, leptospirosis, toxoplasmosis. • Inguinal hernia.
• Discospondylitis—fungal infections, actinomycosis, staphylococcal infections, nocardiosis, streptococci, or *Corynebacterium* diphtheroids.

CBC/BIOCHEMISTRY/URINALYSIS

• Normal in uncomplicated cases. • Chronic infection—hyperglobulinemia and hypoalbuminemia. • Cerebrospinal fluid—neutrophilic pleocytosis, elevated protein (meningoencephalitis); normal in discospondylitis. • Urinalysis usually normal.

OTHER LABORATORY TESTS

Serologic testing—most common diagnostic method; subject to error due to false-positive reactions to several species of bacteria common with tube agglutination tests; chronically infected dogs may test negative.

Rapid 2-Mercaptoethanol Slide Agglutination Test (RSAT)

• Simple, inexpensive, rapid. • Detects infected dogs 3–4 weeks after infection; accurate in identifying noninfected dogs.
• Screening test—sensitive, not specific; high rate (50%) of false-positive tests. • Confirm results with other tests.

Mercaptoethanol Tube Agglutination Test (2ME)

• Semi-quantitative—similar information to RSAT, but inactivates immunoglobulin (Ig) M.
• Good screening test (lacks specificity). • If positive RSAT and negative 2ME, retest in 2–4 weeks.

Agar Gel Immunodiffusion (AGID) Test

• Soluble antigen test—recommended; employs antigens highly specific for antibodies against *Brucella* spp. (including *B. canis, B. abortus*, and *B. suis*); reactive antibodies appear 4–12 weeks after infection and persist; may be positive after other tests become equivocal or negative.
• ELISA—using purified cytoplasmic antigens; not yet commercially available.
• PCR—available at some diagnostic laboratories; high sensitivity and specificity.
• Cell wall antigen test—not recommended; highly sensitive but not standardized; frequent false positives.

IMAGING

Discospondylitis—radiographic changes slow to develop, may not be seen even when spinal pain is present.

DIAGNOSTIC PROCEDURES

Isolation of Organism

• Blood cultures—when clinical and serologic findings suggest diagnosis, can be isolated from blood of infected dogs if they have not received antibiotics; onset of bacteremia 2–4 weeks after oral-nasal exposure, persists for 8 months to 5.5 years. Culture is preferred method for diagnosis in endemic situations or with known exposure (1–8 weeks ago); must specifically request *Brucella* culture. • Culture or PCR of vaginal fluids or vaginal swab after abortion. • Semen or urine—PCR more practical than culture. • Tissue samples—culture or PCR of prostate, testicle, epididymis, lochia, or placenta. • Contaminated samples—media that contain antibiotics (e.g., Thayer–Martin medium) have proven useful.

Semen Quality

• Sperm motility, immature sperm, inflammatory cells (neutrophils) with epididymitis.
• Abnormalities usually evident by 5–8 weeks post infection; conspicuous by 20 weeks.
• Azoospermia without inflammatory cells common with bilateral testicular atrophy.

Lymph Node Biopsy

• Tissues (lymph node, uterus, testes) should be sterilely obtained, cultured on appropriate media, and submitted for histopathology.
• Lymphoid hyperplasia—large numbers of plasma cells. • Intracellular bacteria—may be observed in macrophages with special stains (e.g., Brown–Brenn stain). • Histopathologic examination of testes—necrotizing vasculitis, inflammatory cells, granulomatous lesions.

PATHOLOGIC FINDINGS

• Gross findings—lymph node enlargement, splenomegaly, enlarged and firm epididymides, scrotal edema, or atrophy of one or both testes; chronic infection: anterior uveitis and discospondylitis. • Microscopic changes—

diffuse lymphoreticular hyperplasia; chronic infection: lymph node sinusoids with plasma cells and macrophages that contain bacteria, diffuse lymphocytic infiltration and granulomatous lesions in all genitourinary organs (especially prostate, epididymis, uterus, and scrotum); inflammatory cell infiltration and necrosis of prostate parenchyma, seminiferous tubules. • Ocular changes—granulomatous iridocyclitis; exudative retinitis; leukocytic exudates in anterior chamber.

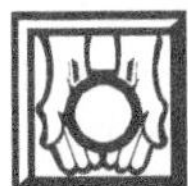

TREATMENT

APPROPRIATE HEALTH CARE

Outpatient

ACTIVITY

Restricted

CLIENT EDUCATION

• Goal is eradication of *B. canis* from animal (seronegative, no bacteremia for at least 3 months); sometimes result is persistent low antibody titers with no systemic infection.
• Antibiotic treatment is expensive, time consuming, and controversial (because outcomes are uncertain, and organism has potential to recrudesce). • Euthanasia is strongly recommended for breeding or commercial kennels; treatment is only recommended for spayed or castrated dogs if the owner is willing to accept the ongoing zoonotic risk. • Before treatment is attempted for an intact household pet or breeding dog, client must clearly agree that animal will be neutered and potentially euthanized if treatment fails. • Zoonotic infection is a possibility; discuss proper sanitation and prevention of exposure.

SURGICAL CONSIDERATIONS

Neuter/spay plus treatment—when euthanasia is unacceptable to owner.

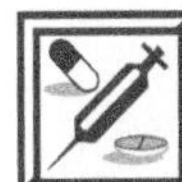

MEDICATIONS

DRUG(S) OF CHOICE

• Several therapeutic regimens have been evaluated, results have been equivocal; treatment duration longer than 30 days may be required. • Most successful—combination of a tetracycline (tetracycline hydrochloride, chlortetracycline, or minocycline: 25 mg/kg PO q8h for 4 weeks) or doxycycline (10 mg/kg PO q12h for 4 weeks) and dihydrostreptomycin (10 mg/kg IM q8h during weeks 1 and 4). • Enrofloxacin (10–20 mg/kg PO q24h for 30 days)—not recommended: variable results.

CONTRAINDICATIONS

Tetracyclines—do not use in immature animals.

ALTERNATIVE DRUG(S)

Gentamicin—6–15 mg/kg IM/SC q12h; limited success; insufficient data on efficacy combined with tetracycline.

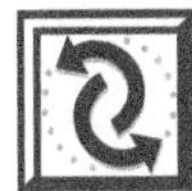

FOLLOW-UP

PATIENT MONITORING

• Serologic tests—monthly at least 3 months after completion of treatment; continuous, persistent decline in antibodies to negative status indicates successful treatment.
• Recrudescent infections (rise in antibody levels, recurrence of bacteremia after therapy)—retreat, neuter and retreat, or euthanize.
• Blood cultures—negative for at least 3 months after completion of treatment.

PREVENTION/AVOIDANCE

• Vaccine—none. • Testing—all females before estrus if breeding is planned; breeding males at frequent intervals. • Quarantine and test all new dogs twice at monthly intervals before entering breeding kennel; test all breeding animals yearly.

POSSIBLE COMPLICATIONS

• Owner reluctance to neuter or euthanize valuable dogs, regardless of treatment failure.
• Remind owners of ethical considerations, obligation not to sell or distribute infected dogs.

EXPECTED COURSE AND PROGNOSIS

• Prognosis guarded. • Infected for <3–4 months—likely to respond to treatment.
• Chronic infections—may not respond to therapy. • Discospondylitis—may need repeated or long-term drug treatment, rarely surgical intervention. • Combination therapy with gentamicin or streptomycin, doxycycline, enrofloxacin, and rifampin has successfully treated ocular disease in dogs. • Successfully treated (seronegative) dogs are susceptible to reinfection.

MISCELLANEOUS

ZOONOTIC POTENTIAL

• Human infections possible; usually mild flu-like symptoms. • Severe infections, including hepatomegaly, splenomegaly, meningitis, endocarditis reported in immunocompromised children and adults.

PREGNANCY/FERTILITY/BREEDING

• Abortions at 45–60 days of gestation typical. • Pups from infected bitches may be infected or normal.

SYNONYMS

Contagious canine abortion.

ABBREVIATIONS

• 2-ME = mercaptoethanol tube agglutination test.
• AGID = agar gel immunodiffusion.
• Ig = immunoglobulin.
• RSAT = rapid 2-mercaptoethanol slide agglutination test.

Suggested Reading

Greene CE, Carmichael LE. Canine brucellosis. In: Greene CE, ed., Infectious Diseases of the Dog and Cat, 3rd ed. St. Louis, MO: Saunders Elsevier, 2012, pp. 398–411.

Johnson CA, Carter TD, Dunn JR, et al. Investigation and characterization of Brucella canis infections in pet-quality dogs and associated human exposures during a 2007–2016 outbreak in Michigan. JAVMA 2018, 253:322–336.

Kauffman LK, Petersen CA. Canine brucellosis old foe and reemerging scourge. Vet Clin Small Anim 2019, 49:763–779.

Keid LB, Soares RM, Vasconcellos SA, et al. Comparison of agar gel immunodiffusion test, rapid slide agglutination test, microbiological culture, and PCR for the diagnosis of canine brucellosis. Res Vet Sci 2009, 86:22–26.

Author Robyn Ellerbrock

Consulting Editor Amie Koenig

Acknowledgment The author and book editors acknowledge the prior contribution of Stephen C. Barr.

Client Education Handout available online

CALCIPOTRIENE/CALCIPOTRIOL TOXICOSIS

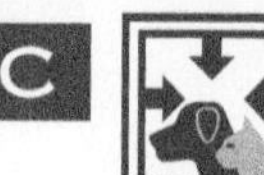

BASICS

OVERVIEW

• Calcipotriene, also known as calcipotriol, is a synthetic analogue of calcitriol, an active metabolite of Vitamin D3. • Calcitriol activity: • Anti-psoriatic—increases epithelial cell differentiation and decreases keratinocyte proliferation. • Promotes calcium retention—triggers intestinal absorption, renal reabsorption, and mobilization of bone resorption of calcium. • Toxic exposure leads to hypercalcemia with soft tissue mineralization (hypercalcemic nephropathy), cardiac conduction disturbance, and gastrointestinal ulceration. • Cream, ointment, foam, and solution formulation for treatment of human psoriasis; common tradenames—Calcitrene®, Dovonex®, Sorilux®, Taclonex®. • Very low margin of safety—consider *all* exposures toxic. • Organ systems affected—cardiovascular, endocrine/metabolic, gastrointestinal, musculoskeletal, nervous, renal/urologic.

SIGNALMENT

Dogs and cats, with small or young animals at increased risk for toxicity.

SIGNS

• Early (0–24 hours)—vomiting, anorexia, diarrhea, depression, polyuria, polydipsia. • Late (18–72 hours)—hypercalcemia, hyperphosphatemia, azotemia/acute renal injury. • Other—bradycardia, arrhythmias, hematemesis, melena, abdominal pain, oliguria. • End stage—anuria, acute renal failure/dystrophic calcification of soft tissue, coma, death.

CAUSES & RISK FACTORS

Toxic exposure occurs when pets chew product tube/bottle or lick skin of human where product has been applied.

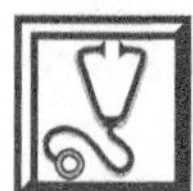

DIAGNOSIS

DIFFERENTIAL DIAGNOSIS

• Vitamin D toxicity—vitamin D supplements, cholecalciferol rodenticide. • Ethylene glycol toxicity. • Grape/raisin toxicity. • Renal failure—acute or chronic. • Infectious disease—blastomycosis, heterobilharziasis, histomoniasis, bacterial osteomyelitis. • Hypoadrenocorticism. • Hypercalcemia of malignancy. • Hyperparathyroidism, primary. • Idiopathic hypercalcemia of cats. • Large-volume ingestion of calcinogenic plants—*Cestrum diurnum, Solanum malacoxylon.* • Severe dehydration.

CBC/CHEMISTRY/URINALYSIS

• Hyperphosphatemia. • Hypercalcemia. • Azotemia. • Hyposthenuria, isosthenuria. • Neutrophilia.

OTHER LABORATORY TESTS

Ionized calcium preferred over serum calcium.

IMAGING

Thoracic and abdominal radiographs—mineralization of soft tissue structure including kidneys, blood vessels, lungs, and intestine.

PATHOLOGIC FINDINGS

Coronary artery mineralization, gastrointestinal hemorrhage and mineralization, renal tubular necrosis and renal cortical mineralization, pulmonary mineralization.

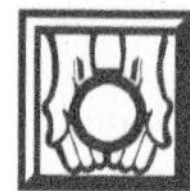

TREATMENT

• Therapy immediately post ingestion focuses on decontamination and serial monitoring; if hypercalcemia occurs, weeks-long therapy is necessary due to slow release of stored product from fat/muscle tissue. • Oral irrigation with water if patient has recently licked product. • Early emesis or gastric lavage. • Activated charcoal (1–2 gm/kg) with a cathartic × 1, followed by activated charcoal only q6–8h × 2 doses; monitor sodium concentration. • Fluid therapy—if hypercalcemic: IV 0.9%NaCl rehydrate prn then 2× maintenance to encourage calciuresis; *if* normocalcemic: IV or SC fluids PRN to maintain hydration. • Diet—*if* hypercalcemic: calcium-restricted prescription diet or veterinary nutritionist-guided homemade diet.

MEDICATIONS

• Antiemetics PRN (e.g. maropitant 1mg/kg SC/IV, 2mg/kg PO q24h). • Proton pump inhibitor (e.g., omeprazole 1 mg/kg PO q24h) or H2 blocker (e.g., famotidine 1mg/kg IM/IV/PO/SC q 12-24h; slow IV administration advised for cats). • Sucralfate (0.25–1g PO q8h on empty stomach). • Cholestyramine (0.3–1 g/kg PO q8h × 4 days post ingestion); may reduce enterohepatic recirculation of vitamin D by reducing reabsorption of vitamin D–bound bile acids. • *If* hypercalcemic: ○ Treatment goals—serum calcium <12.5 mg/dL or ionized calcium <1.33 mmol/L. ○ Bisphosphonate tx (e.g., pamidronate sodium 1.3–2.0mg/kg diluted in 150cc saline IV CRI × 2–4 h or zoledronate 0.25 mg/kg in 50cc saline IV CRI x 15 min); bisphosphonates block dissolution of calcium hydroxyapatite and inhibit osteoclastic bone resorption; reduction in calcium level seen in 1–3 days; rebound hypercalcemia may occur and repeat dosing necessary in 3–7 days. ○ Prednisone 1 mg/kg PO BID or dexamethasone 0.2 mg/kg IV BID; initially or at a later time; wean slowly. • Furosemide 1 mg/kg PO BID or 0.1–0.66mg/kg/h IV CRI- only in well-hydrated patients. • If hyperphosphatemic - aluminum hydroxide: 30–90 mg/kg/day divided; with meals.

CONTRAINDICATIONS/POSSIBLE INTERACTIONS

• Bisphosphonate use may result in hypocalcemia. • Long-term adverse effects from use of bisphosphonates in juvenile/growing dog or cat unknown.

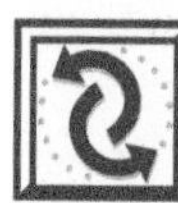

FOLLOW-UP

PATIENT MONITORING

• Baseline CBC, serum chemistry, urinalysis; monitor renal values, hydration parameters, and calcium/phosphorous levels q12–24h × 4 days minimum; *if* hypercalcemia/hyperphosphatemia occurs continued monitoring of calcium/phosphorous, renal values, and hydration parameters advised until normalized—up to 3–4 weeks. • Urine output. • Appetite. • Heart rate/blood pressure.

PREVENTION/AVOIDANCE

• Do not allow pets to lick humans where calcipotriene was applied. • Keep medication inaccessible to pets.

POSSIBLE COMPLICATIONS

Dystrophic mineralization of soft tissue, acute kidney failure, death.

EXPECTED COURSE AND PROGNOSIS

Good prognosis if rapid, aggressive, and continuing therapy is provided and hypercalcemia/hypophosphatemia minimized. Guarded to poor prognosis if soft tissue mineralization occurs.

MISCELLANEOUS

Suggested Reading

Gwaltney-Brant S, Calcipotriene/calcipotriol. In: Hovda LR, Brutlag A, Poppenga R, Peterson K, eds., Blackwell's Five-Minute Veterinary Consult Clinical Companion: Small Animal Toxicology, 2nd ed. Ames, IA: Wiley-Blackwell, 2016, pp. 172–177.

Author Susan Holland
Consulting Editor Lynn R. Hovda

CALCIUM CHANNEL BLOCKER TOXICOSIS

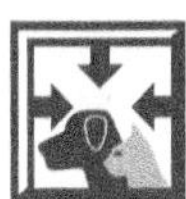

BASICS

OVERVIEW

• Calcium channel blockers (CCBs): class IV antidysrhythmics used to treat systemic hypertension, cardiac disease, tachydysrhythmias, and oliguric/anuric renal failure in dogs and cats. • CCBs inhibit movement of Ca through L-type voltage-gated slow Ca channels located on cardiac muscle, atrioventricular (AV) and sinoatrial (SA) nodes, vasculature smooth muscle, and pancreatic beta cells. • Three classes of CCBs—phenylalkylamine, benzothiazepine, dihydropyridine; CCB class determines the effect on the body.

SIGNS

Systems affected include: • Cardiovascular—bradycardia, AV dissociation and AV block (first, second, or third degree), hypotension. • Gastrointestinal—vomiting, diarrhea, ileus. • Respiratory—pulmonary edema. • Nervous—decreased mentation, weakness, collapse, seizures. • Endocrine/metabolic—hyperglycemia, metabolic acidosis secondary to hypoperfusion.

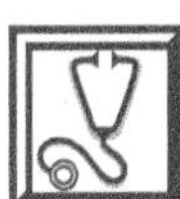

DIAGNOSIS

DIFFERENTIAL DIAGNOSIS

• Beta blocker antagonist toxicosis. • Cardiac disease with bradyarrhythmias. • Cardiovascular drug overdose (e.g., clonidine, digoxin toxicosis). • Sedative overdose (e.g., opioid or baclofen toxicosis). • Sick sinus syndrome. • Hyperkalemia. • Decompensated shock.

CBC/CHEMISTRY/URINALYSIS

• Hyperglycemia. • Azotemia and elevated liver enzymes with prolonged hypoperfusion.

OTHER LABORATORY TESTS

Blood gas—metabolic acidosis.

IMAGING

Chest radiographs to evaluate for pulmonary edema with respiratory signs.

DIAGNOSTIC PROCEDURES

• ECG—first-, second-, and third-degree AV block; prolonged PR, QRS, and QT intervals. • Echocardiogram—negative inotropy, decreased cardiac output.

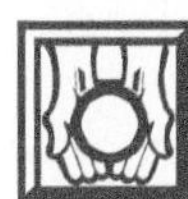

TREATMENT

• Emesis if asymptomatic and <2 hours after exposure. • Gastric lavage if decreased mental status and large number of pills ingested. • Temporary cardiac pacing when medical therapy fails. • IV fluid bolus over 15–20 min for hypotension—cats, 10–20 mL/kg; dogs, 20–30 mL/kg.

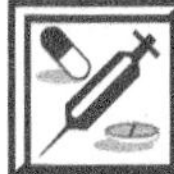

MEDICATIONS

DRUG(S) OF CHOICE

• Activated charcoal (1–2 g/kg) PO, repeat activated charcoal for extended-release (ER) formulations. • Atropine (0.02–0.04 mg/kg IV) for sinus bradycardia. • Calcium infusion—first-line therapy despite normocalcemia to increase Ca availability for muscle function and improve contractility. ◦ Ca gluconate 10% bolus 0.5–1.5 mL/kg IV over 5–10 min followed by CRI of 0.5–1.5 mL/kg/h, titrated to effect; monitor continuous ECG and infusion should be slowed or stopped if bradycardia or conduction blockade worsens. ◦ Ca chloride 10% bolus 0.15–0.5 mL/kg IV; central line recommended due to risk of tissue injury secondary to drug extravasation. • Intravenous fat emulsion (IFE)—may bind lipid-soluble drugs, increase Ca available for muscle contraction, and provide an energy source for heart muscle. ◦ IFE 20% solution dose—1.5 mL/kg IV bolus over 1 min; follow with CRI of 0.25 mL/kg/min for 30–60 min; additional IV doses: 1.5 ml/kg every 4–6h or CRI of 0.5 mL/kg/h; monitor serum for lipemia every 2–4h to determine if additional dosing is needed. • High-dose insulin euglycemia (HIE) treatment—may provide energy for heart muscle and increase Ca available for muscle contraction. Recommended treatment: ◦ Check blood glucose (BG) concentration and administer dextrose if BG <100 mg/dL. ◦ Administer regular insulin at 1 unit/kg IV, followed by CRI at 0.5–2 units/kg/h; may increase every 10 min up to maximum dose of 10 units/kg/h; when signs resolve, decrease insulin by 1–2 units/kg/h. ◦ Monitor BG every 10 min while titrating insulin dose; once stabilized, check BG every 30–60 min; central line placement recommended for frequent glucose monitoring and dextrose administration during HIE treatment; dextrose supplementation will be needed to maintain normal BG concentrations and continued up to 24h after discontinuation of insulin therapy. ◦ Monitor potassium concentration every hour during titration, then every 6h; administer potassium chloride to keep potassium concentrations within normal range. • Glucagon—may not be as effective as HIE or IFE; dose is 0.05–0.2 mg/kg slowly IV bolus, followed by CRI of 0.05–0.1 mg/kg/h.

CONTRAINDICATION/POSSIBLE INTERACTIONS

Vasopressors/sympathomimetics may not be as effective as other therapy and may make patients less response to other therapy.

FOLLOW-UP

PATIENT MONITORING

Monitor heart rate/ECG, BP, and BG for 6–12h with immediate-release preparations and 12–24h for ER/sustained-release (SR) preparations, depending on peak drug levels.

EXPECTED COURSE AND PROGNOSIS

• Ingestion of immediate-release preparations typically result in clinical signs in 8–12h. • SR or ER preparations may take 12–24h for clinical signs to develop. • Prognosis depends on dose ingested and response to therapy. • Toxicosis normally results in bradycardia, hypotension, and in severe cases decreased mental status, coma, and apnea.

MISCELLANEOUS

ABBREVIATIONS

- AV = atrioventricular.
- BG = blood glucose.
- CCB = calcium channel blocker.
- ER = extended release.
- HIE = high-dose insulin euglycemia.
- IFE = Intravenous fat emulsion.
- SA = sinoatrial.
- SR = sustained release.

Suggested Reading

Hayes CL, Knight M. Calcium channel blocker toxicity in dogs and cats. Vet Clin North Am Small Anim Pract 2012: 42:263–277.

Author Katherine L. Peterson
Consulting Editor Lynn R. Hovda

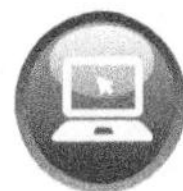

Client Education Handout available online

CAMPYLOBACTERIOSIS

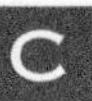

BASICS

OVERVIEW

• *Campylobacter jejuni*—fastidious, microaerophilic, Gram-negative curved bacteria; often isolated from healthy dogs and cats; may cause superficial erosive enterocolitis. • Infection—fecal–oral route from contaminated food, water, raw meat (especially chicken), environment; localized in crypts of intestine; motile; produces multiple enterotoxins. • Invasion of gut mucosa—hematochezia, inflammation, ulceration, edema; bacteria shed in feces for weeks to months. • Up to 49% of dogs without diarrhea and 45% of normal cats carry *C. jejuni* and shed it in feces.

SIGNALMENT

• Dogs; less commonly cats. • Prevalence—higher in puppies and kittens up to 6 months. • Can cause chronic disease.

SIGNS

• Diarrhea—varies; mucoid and watery, hemorrhagic; may be chronic. • Tenesmus. • Fever, anorexia, intermittent vomiting possible. • Adults—may be asymptomatic carriers. • Abortion and perinatal death.

CAUSES & RISK FACTORS

• *C. jejuni*, *C. coli*, *C. upsaliensis*, *C. helviticus*, *C. lari*, and more uncommon species. • Kennels/intensive housing, poor sanitation/hygiene, fecal contamination in environment. • Young animals—debilitated, immunosuppressed, parasitized. • Nosocomial infection in hospitalized patients. • Adults—concurrent intestinal infections (e.g., *Salmonella*, parvovirus, hookworms). • Feeding homemade or commercially available raw meat–based diets.

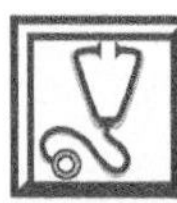

DIAGNOSIS

DIFFERENTIAL DIAGNOSIS

• Bacterial enterocolitis—*Salmonella*, *Yersinia enterocolitica*, *Clostridium difficile*, *Clostridium perfringens*. • Parasitic—helminths (whipworms); protozoa (*Giardia*, *Isospora*). • Viral—parvovirus; signs often more severe. • Dietary indiscretion, intolerance. • Drugs, toxins. • Pancreatitis. • Intussusception, other causes of abdominal pain. • Distinguish from other causes of chronic diarrhea. • Primary intestinal disease.

CBC/BIOCHEMISTRY/URINALYSIS

• Leukocytosis—possible. • Biochemistry abnormalities—effects of diarrhea, dehydration (e.g., azotemia, electrolyte disturbances).

DIAGNOSTIC PROCEDURES

• Fecal leukocytes—in gastrointestinal tract and stool. • Fecal culture—submit feces in Amies transport medium with charcoal or Cary-Blair medium kept refrigerated at 4 °C in transit. • Species-specific quantitative PCR—current methodology may be biased to detect *C. jejuni* and *C. coli*.

Direct Examination of Feces

• Gram stain—make smear; leave Gram safranin on for longer period. • Wet mount—large numbers of highly motile bacteria (characteristic darting motility).

PATHOLOGIC FINDINGS

• Gross—diffuse colon thickening, congestion/edema; hyperemia of small intestine; enlarged mesenteric lymph nodes. • Thickening of intestinal smooth muscle in cats.

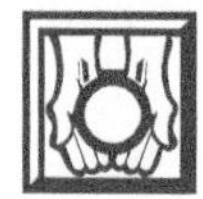

TREATMENT

Mild Enterocolitis

• Outpatient. • Usually self-limiting.

Severe Enterocolitis

• Inpatient, especially if very young, fever, hematochezia, melena. • Severe neonatal disease—isolate; aggressive therapy. • NPO for 24 hours; then bland diet. • Mild dehydration—oral fluid therapy with enteric fluid replacement solution. • Severe dehydration—intravenous fluid therapy with balanced isotonic replacement solution. • Plasma transfusion may be required. • Locally acting intestinal adsorbents/protectants.

MEDICATIONS

DRUG(S) OF CHOICE

• Antibiotics—for systemic illness (e.g., high fever, dehydration), when diarrhea or abnormal clinical signs persist >7 days, in immune-suppressed patients. • Erythromycin 10–20 mg/kg PO q8h for 5 days; drug of choice. • Enrofloxacin—dog, 10 mg/kg PO/IV/IM q24h; cat, 5 mg/kg PO/IM/IV q24h. • Tylosin 11 mg/kg PO q8h for 7 days. • Septicemia—parenteral broad-spectrum antibiotics indicated. • Multidrug resistance (vs. macrolides, quinolones) becoming more common.

CONTRAINDICATIONS/POSSIBLE INTERACTIONS

• Antidiarrheal drugs that reduce intestinal motility are contraindicated. • Enrofloxacin—may induce arthropathy in dogs <28 weeks of age; caution with use in cats.

FOLLOW-UP

PATIENT MONITORING

Repeat fecal culture after treatment.

PREVENTION/AVOIDANCE

• Good hygiene (hand washing). • Routinely clean and disinfect runs, food and water bowls. • Do not feed raw-meat diets to companion animals.

EXPECTED COURSE AND PROGNOSIS

• Adults—usually self-limiting. • Juveniles with severe or persistent enterocolitis—prognosis good with appropriate intervention.

MISCELLANEOUS

ASSOCIATED CONDITIONS

Concurrent infection with other pathogenic bacteria, enteric parasites, viruses.

ZOONOTIC POTENTIAL

High (*C. jejuni*, *C. coli*, *C. upsaliensis*).

PREGNANCY/FERTILITY/BREEDING

Erythromycin—safe in early pregnancy.

INTERNET RESOURCES

http://www.cfsph.iastate.edu/DiseaseInfo/disease.php?name=campylobacteriosis&lang=en

Suggested Reading

Acke E. Campylobacteriosis in dogs and cats: a review. N Z Vet J 2018, 66:221–228.

Marks SL, Rankin SC, Byrne BA, et al. Enteropathogenic bacteria in dogs and cats: diagnosis, epidemiology, treatment, and control. J Vet Intern Med 2011, 25:1195–1208.

Montgomery MP, Robertson S, Koski L, et al. MDR Campylobacter jejuni outbreak linked to puppy exposure. MMWR Morb Mortal Wkly Rep. 2018, 67:1032–1035.

Author Patrick L. McDonough

Consulting Editor Amie Koenig

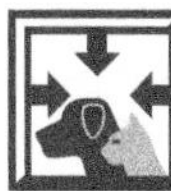

BASICS

OVERVIEW

- *Candida*—dimorphic fungus with the yeast phase (*Candida* spp.) being part of the normal flora of the mouth, nose, ears, and gastrointestinal (GI) and urogenital tracts of dogs and cats.
- *C. albicans* and *C. parapsilosis* most commonly cultured from clinically healthy dogs.
- Recovery from mucosal surfaces does not imply disease; organisms may cause opportunistic infection, colonize damaged tissues, or invade normal tissues of immunosuppressed animals.
- Pathogenic role determined by infiltration of organisms into tissues, or detection of organisms in presumed sterile sites (e.g., urinary bladder, peritoneal cavity).
- Organ systems most affected include GI, renal/urologic, skin, and respiratory.
- Conditions that suppress the immune system (e.g., feline immunodeficiency virus [FIV] infection) increase the likelihood of isolation in asymptomatic animals.

SIGNALMENT

Cats and dogs—any age and breed.

SIGNS

- Nonhealing ulcers in the oral, upper respiratory, GI, or urogenital mucosa—signs reflect location/extent of disease:
    - Cystitis—hematuria, stranguria, and pollakiuria.
    - Otitis—head shaking, scratching.
    - Oral cavity—drooling.
- Inflammation around IV catheters or gastrotomy tubes.
- Ulcerative, red skin lesions.
- Systemic disease with fever, cardiac and/or neurologic abnormalities can be seen.

CAUSES & RISK FACTORS

- Infection—rare; associated with neutropenia, parvovirus or FIV infection, endocrinopathies, glucocorticoid therapy, gastrotomy tubes, indwelling urinary catheters/urethrostomy, IV catheters, and incomplete bladder emptying.
- Lower urinary tract disease may predispose to candiduria.
- Administration of antibiotics in prior 30 days.
- Occasionally local or systemic infection is seen in animals without predisposing conditions.
- Skin damaged by burns, trauma, or necrotizing dermatitis.

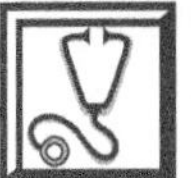

DIAGNOSIS

DIFFERENTIAL DIAGNOSIS

Considered whenever the primary condition does not respond as expected.

CBC/BIOCHEMISTRY/URINALYSIS

- Reflect underlying inflammation and organ involvement (unless neutropenic).
- Urinalysis—may show yeast or clumps of mycelial elements (pseudohyphae) with inflammatory cells; concurrent bacterial urinary tract infection common.

OTHER LABORATORY TESTS

- Cytology—spherical to oval yeast cells 5–7 µm in diameter; pseudohyphae and septate hyphae 3–5 µm wide.
- Culture—grows well on blood agar and often is isolated from specimens submitted for bacterial culture; more easily isolated from urine than blood.
- PCR and antigen tests available.

DIAGNOSTIC PROCEDURES

- Lesions—to determine if *Candida* is truly a pathogen, requires demonstration of organisms penetrating the tissues.
- Urine sample—cystocentesis; culture of multiple colonies of *Candida* supports diagnosis.
- Otitis (dogs)—culture of *Candida* spp. or identification of yeast or mycelial elements on ear cytology suggests diagnosis.
- In febrile patients, culture catheter tips.

PATHOLOGIC FINDINGS

- White caseous foci in the infected tissue.
- Large numbers of both yeast and pseudohyphae in tissues surrounded by necrosis and suppurative inflammatory reaction.
- May be pyogranulomatous in more chronic infections.

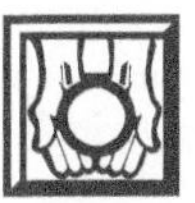

TREATMENT

- Treat underlying causes of immunosuppression.
- Remove indwelling catheters, if possible.

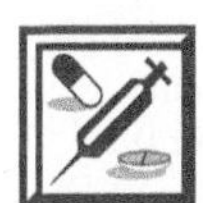

MEDICATIONS

DRUG(S) OF CHOICE

- Topical therapy (mucosal lesions)—nystatin or amphotericin B.
- Fluconazole—5 mg/kg PO q12h; very effective and excreted unchanged in urine (high concentration in commonly infected sites).
- Itraconazole—5–10 mg/kg PO q12h; effective, can use if organism resistant to fluconazole; not recommended for urinary tract infection (poor urinary excretion).
- In lower urinary tract *Candida* infections resistant to fluconazole—infuse 10–30 mL of 1% clotrimazole into the bladder every other day for three treatments.
- *Candida* may develop drug resistance—consider drug sensitivity testing if suspected.
- Caspofungin—may be option for resistant isolates.

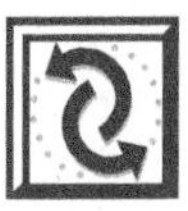

FOLLOW-UP

PATIENT MONITORING

- Fluconazole and itraconazole—hepatic toxicity; monitor serum alanine aminotransferase (ALT) activity monthly initially and check if patient becomes anorexic.
- After signs have resolved—reculture sites of infection; continue treatment for 2 weeks beyond negative culture; repeat cultures 2 weeks after completion of treatment and again if signs recur.

EXPECTED COURSE AND PROGNOSIS

- Should resolve within 2–4 weeks of treatment with correction of immunosuppression.
- Control of the underlying disease is necessary to prevent recurrence.
- May resolve spontaneously if the underlying condition is corrected.

MISCELLANEOUS

ZOONOTIC POTENTIAL

Genetic similarities between human and animal isolates suggest a potential for transfer of *C. albicans* between species.

ABBREVIATIONS

- ALT = alanine aminotransferase.
- FIV = feline immunodeficiency virus.
- GI = gastrointestinal.

Suggested Reading

Reagan KL, Dear JD, Kass PH, et al. Risk factors for Candida urinary tract infections in dogs and cats. J Vet Intern Med 2019, 33:648–653.

Author Daniel S. Foy
Consulting Editor Amie Koenig

CANINE CORONAVIRUS INFECTIONS

C

BASICS

OVERVIEW

- Canine enteric coronavirus (CCoV)—sporadic outbreaks of enteritis in dogs; worldwide distribution.
- Canine pantropic coronavirus (CPCoV)—variant of CCoV, fatal disease in dogs <6 months, described principally in Europe.
- CCoV, CPCoV—closely related to feline infectious peritonitis (FIP) virus, feline enteric coronavirus.
- Canine respiratory coronavirus (CRCoV)—associated with canine infectious respiratory disease complex (kennel cough); worldwide distribution; genetically and serologically distinct from CCoV.
- Incubation period 1–3 days.
- CCoV infection—usually inapparent; mild to severe enteritis possible; death reported in young pups; infects upper two-thirds of small intestine and associated lymph nodes; crypt cells spared.
- Simultaneous infection with canine parvovirus (CPV)-2 possible; severe, often fatal.
- CPCoV—infects intestinal tract, after short viremia distributes to organs like spleen, lungs, brain.
- Coronaviruses undergo rapid evolution, are highly variable; differences in virulence likely between isolates.

SIGNALMENT

- Dogs of all ages, breeds; disease more severe in young.
- CRCoV infections more common in winter, in shelters.

SIGNS

- Vary greatly—CPCoV virulent isolates cause systemic disease.
- Adults—most infections inapparent.
- Puppies—mild to severe, occasionally fatal, enteritis.
- Diarrhea—may be explosive; yellow-green or orange; loose or liquid; typically malodorous (characteristic); may persist for days to >3 weeks; may recur; young dogs may suffer severe, protracted diarrhea, dehydration.
- Vomiting.
- Coughing, dyspnea—CRCoV associated with kennel cough complex.
- Anorexia, lethargy.
- For CPCoV—pyrexia, anorexia, depression, vomiting, hemorrhagic enteritis, respiratory distress, and leukopenia that persists >1 week; ataxia, seizures, and death also possible.

CAUSES & RISK FACTORS

- Stress—greatest risk; sporadic outbreaks have occurred in dogs attending shows, in kennels where new dogs frequently introduced; crowding and unsanitary conditions promote illness.
- For CCoV, CPCoV—feces primary source of infection; virus shed for 2 weeks.
- For CRCoV—respiratory secretions, fomites likely sources of infection.

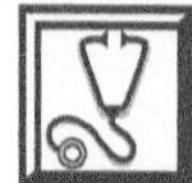

DIAGNOSIS

DIFFERENTIAL DIAGNOSIS

- Infections caused by enteric bacteria, protozoa, other viruses; canine kennel cough complex pathogens.
- Other mild to moderate upper respiratory disease.
- Food intoxication or intolerance.

CBC/BIOCHEMISTRY/URINALYSIS

Normal; lymphopenia with more virulent CCoV isolates.

OTHER LABORATORY TESTS

Serologic tests—available; not standardized, difficult to interpret due to frequent asymptomatic infection.

DIAGNOSTIC PROCEDURES

- Viral isolation for CCoV, CRCoV—possible but not recommended.
- Specific reverse transcriptase polymerase chain reaction (RT-PCR)—using feces for CCoV, respiratory swabs for CRCoV; CPCoV defined by presence of virus in extraintestinal organs.
- Immunofluorescence of small intestine—fatal cases; may show viral antigen in cells lining villous epithelium.

PATHOLOGIC FINDINGS

- Gross—dilated small intestine filled with gas, watery green-yellow material.
- Bowel loops congested, hemorrhagic; mesenteric lymph nodes enlarged, edematous.
- Histopathology—atrophy and fusion of intestinal villi, deepening of crypts, increased cellularity of lamina propria, epithelial cell flattening, increased goblet cells.
- CPCoV—hemorrhagic lesions in various organs (lungs, small intestines, spleen, lymph nodes).

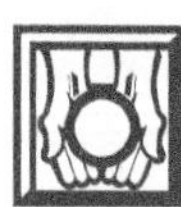

TREATMENT

- Most dogs recover without treatment.
- CCoV—fluid, electrolyte treatment if dehydration severe.
- CRCoV—as for canine kennel cough complex.

MEDICATIONS

DRUG(S) OF CHOICE

Antibiotics—not usually indicated, except with enteritis, sepsis, severe respiratory illness.

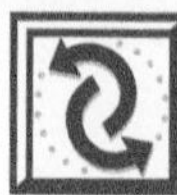

FOLLOW-UP

PREVENTION/AVOIDANCE

- CCoV vaccines—controversial; inactivated and live viral vaccines; appear safe; moderate efficacy may be due to variability of CCoV strains; not recommended; do not cross-protect against CPCoV, CRCoV.
- Strict quarantine, sanitation essential in kennels: susceptible to common disinfectants.
- CCoV, CRCoV—highly contagious; spread rapidly.

POSSIBLE COMPLICATIONS

Diarrhea with CCoV—may persist 10–12 days, may recur.

EXPECTED COURSE AND PROGNOSIS

- Prognosis—good, except severe infections of young pups.
- Majority recover after short illness.

MISCELLANEOUS

ASSOCIATED CONDITIONS

- Concurrent infection with CPV or other agent.
- Infections with other respiratory pathogens with CRCoV.

ABBREVIATIONS

- CCoV = canine enteric coronavirus.
- CPCoV= canine pantropic coronavirus.
- CPV = canine parvovirus.
- CRCoV = canine respiratory coronavirus.
- FIP = feline infectious peritonitis.
- RT-PCR = reverse transcriptase polymerase chain reaction.

Suggested Reading

Decaro N, Cordonnier N, Demeter Z, et al. European surveillance for pantropic canine coronavirus. J Clin Microbiol 2013, 51:83–88.

Mitchell JA, Cardwell JM, Leach H. European surveillance of emerging pathogens associated with canine infectious respiratory disease. Vet Microbiol 2017, 212:31–38.

Author Sophie Le Poder

Consulting Editor Amie Koenig

Acknowledgment The author and book editors acknowledge the prior contribution of John S. Parker.

CANINE DEGENERATIVE MYELOPATHY

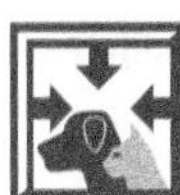

BASICS

DEFINITION

Canine progressive adult-onset fatal neurodegenerative disease that has recently been shown in many breeds to be a result of a mutation in the superoxide dismutase 1 gene (*SOD1*). Mutations in *SOD1* are known to cause some forms of amyotrophic lateral sclerosis (ALS), also known as Lou Gehrig's disease. Initial signs of progressive upper motor neuron spastic paresis and general proprioceptive ataxia in the pelvic limbs occur in older dogs. If euthanasia is delayed, clinical signs progress to flaccid tetraparesis/plegia and other lower motor neuron signs.

PATHOPHYSIOLOGY

- A *c.118 G>A* transition in Exon 2 of *SOD1* that predicts an E40K missense mutation underlies most degenerative myelopathy (DM); a second *SOD1* missense mutation (*c.52 A>T*) has been seen only in Bernese mountain dogs.
- Lesions may represent a multisystem central-peripheral axonopathy.
- Predilection for lesion severity in mid-thoracic spinal cord may be a result of lower percentages of radicular artery contributions and small-diameter vessels when compared to other spinal cord regions.
- Paucity of vascular supply in thoracic spinal cord may predispose it to damage from oxidative and metabolic disturbances.

SYSTEMS AFFECTED

- Central and peripheral nervous systems.
- Thoracolumbar spinal cord in early stage.
- Progresses to involve the cervical and lumbar spinal cord and peripheral nervous system later in the course of the disease.
- Neurons in the brainstem also may be affected.
- Disease also involves the sensory nerve roots and dorsal root ganglia.

GENETICS

- Most commonly autosomal recessive inheritance.
- Due to preponderance of purebred dogs affected, a familial inheritance is currently suspected.
- Mutations in *SOD1* are causative for DM but are incompletely penetrant.
- Dogs that are homozygous for the mutant allele are *at highest risk* for developing DM; not all dogs that test homozygous for the mutation will develop DM, but dogs that test normal (clear) are highly unlikely to develop DM; dogs that test carrier are less likely to develop DM, but this has been documented in some breeds.

INCIDENCE/PREVALENCE

Prevalence rate of DM reported for all dogs collected from the Veterinary Medical Database (1990–1999) was 0.19%.

GEOGRAPHIC DISTRIBUTION

Worldwide

SIGNALMENT

Breed Predilections

So far the DM-associated *SOD1:c.118A* allele is in >150 breeds or varieties; a second *SOD1* mutation (*c.52 A>T*) was found only in Bernese mountain dogs. DM has been histopathologically confirmed in many purebred and mixed-breed dogs.

Mean Age and Range

- Mean—9 years of age in large dogs; mean age at onset is 11 years in Pembroke Welsh corgi.
- Range—between 8 and 14 years.

Predominant Sex

No known sex predilection.

SIGNS

- Early:
  - Upper motor neuron paraparesis.
  - Insidious, progressive, asymmetric general proprioceptive ataxia; gait shows long-strided spastic paraparesis.
  - Paw replacement deficits.
  - Spinal reflexes usually present or exaggerated (patellar reflex may be reduced).
  - Presence of crossed-extensor reflex is variable.
  - Lack of paraspinal hyperesthesia is key clinical feature.
- Later:
  - Pelvic limb paresis leading to plegia, eventually progressing to tetraparesis/plegia.
  - Mild to moderate loss of muscle mass in pelvic limbs due to neurogenic atrophy.
  - Reduced spinal reflexes in pelvic limbs.
  - ± Urinary and fecal incontinence.
- End stage:
  - Flaccid tetraplegia.
  - Difficulty with swallowing and tongue movements.
  - Absence of spinal reflexes in all limbs.
  - Reduced to absent cutaneous trunci reflex.
  - Profound generalized muscle wasting.
  - Urinary and fecal incontinence.

CAUSES

- Hereditary disease and genetic predisposition.
- Other hypothesized causes include immune-mediated, metabolic deficiencies, toxic, and oxidative stress.

RISK FACTORS

- Dogs homozygous for the mutant allele(s) are at highest risk.
- There may be other environmental factors and modifying genes; studies underway.

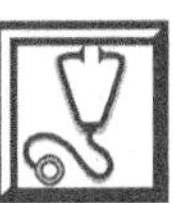

DIAGNOSIS

DIFFERENTIAL DIAGNOSIS

- Type II intervertebral disc herniation.
- Intramedullary spinal cord neoplasia.
- Degenerative lumbosacral stenosis.
- Hip dysplasia.
- Other coexisting orthopedic disease.

CBC/BIOCHEMISTRY/URINALYSIS

- Usually normal.
- Performed to rule out other underlying metabolic disease.
- Urinalysis may identify secondary urinary tract infection.

OTHER LABORATORY TESTS

- Urine culture and sensitivity testing.
- Thyroid function testing.
- Electrodiagnostic testing results are normal in early diagnosis of DM.
- Genetic testing—test result of at-risk can support a presumptive diagnosis of DM in light of typical clinical signs and normal findings on neuroimaging and cerebrospinal fluid analysis.

IMAGING

- Survey spinal radiography.
- Myelography evaluates for compressive spinal cord disease.
- Myelography combined with CT—more sensitive technique to evaluate suspicious lesions.
- MRI—preferred technique to evaluate for extramedullary compressive and intramedullary lesions.

DIAGNOSTIC PROCEDURES

- CSF analysis evaluates for inflammatory disease.
- Definitive diagnosis is determined by post-mortem histopathology of spinal cord.

PATHOLOGIC FINDINGS

- Spinal cord axons and myelin affected most severely in dorsal and dorsal portion of lateral funiculi.
- Vacuolated axon cylinders/myelin sheaths most extensive in mid-thoracic spinal cord.
- Astroglial proliferation is prominent in severely affected areas of lesion distribution.
- Usually, lesion distribution is described as asymmetric and discontinuous; however, more recent evidence describes lesion distribution as symmetric and continuous in dogs that survive for long periods with DM.
- Neuronal cell body loss in ventral horn is evident at terminal or end-stage disease.
- Nerve specimens show fiber loss resulting from axonal degeneration and secondary demyelination.
- Muscle specimens show large and small groups of atrophic fibers typical of denervation.

CANINE DEGENERATIVE MYELOPATHY (CONTINUED)

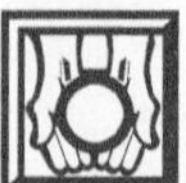

TREATMENT

APPROPRIATE HEALTH CARE

- Supportive care.
- Breeds of small size may survive longer with DM because the pet owner is able to more easily give the appropriate care.

NURSING CARE

- When dog becomes nonambulatory, keep on a well-padded surface to prevent decubitus ulceration over bony prominences.
- Keep hair trimmed, and skin clean and dry to prevent urine scald secondary to incontinence.
- Urine should be monitored for odor and color change, which may indicate urinary tract infection.
- Physical therapy using range-of-motion and active exercises may help maintain limb mobility and muscle strength.

ACTIVITY

- Exercise is encouraged to slow disuse atrophy of pelvic limbs, but fatigue should be monitored and exercise intensity adjusted.
- Hydrotherapy can involve use of an underwater treadmill setup.
- A wheel cart may assist with patient mobility.

DIET

- Maintain balanced diet.
- Prevent weight gain.

CLIENT EDUCATION

- Long-term prognosis is poor.
- Meticulous nursing care is crucial to preventing secondary complications in a recumbent patient.

SURGICAL CONSIDERATIONS

None

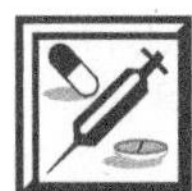

MEDICATIONS

DRUG(S) OF CHOICE

Clinical trials are underway to determine effectiveness in slowing or halting disease progression.

FOLLOW-UP

PATIENT MONITORING

- Repeat neurologic examinations.
- Urine retention.
- Urinalysis and urine culture to monitor for urinary tract infection.

PREVENTION/AVOIDANCE

- Decubitus ulceration.
- Urine retention.
- Dermatitis from urine scald.
- Weight gain.

POSSIBLE COMPLICATIONS

- Urine retention may predispose to urinary tract infections.
- Local skin infections from decubitus ulceration.

EXPECTED COURSE AND PROGNOSIS

- Nonambulatory paraparesis occurs within 9–12 months from time of onset of signs.
- Tetraparesis may be evident within 3 years from time of onset of signs.
- Long-term prognosis is poor.

MISCELLANEOUS

ASSOCIATED CONDITIONS

- Other neurologic diseases associated with old-age onset.
- Spinal cord neoplasia.
- Intervertebral disc disease.
- Orthopedic disease.

AGE-RELATED FACTORS

Older dogs commonly affected.

ZOONOTIC POTENTIAL

None

PREGNANCY/FERTILITY/BREEDING

N/A

SYNONYMS

- Canine ALS.
- DM.
- Degenerative radiculomyelopathy.
- German Shepherd dog myelopathy.

SEE ALSO

- Intervertebral Disc Disease, Cervical.
- Intervertebral Disc Disease, Thoracolumbar.
- Lumbosacral Stenosis and Cauda Equina Syndrome.

ABBREVIATIONS

- ALS = amyotrophic lateral sclerosis.
- DM = degenerative myelopathy.
- *SOD1* = superoxide dismutase 1.

INTERNET RESOURCES

- www.caninegeneticdiseases.net/dm/maindm.htm
- www.ofa.org/diseases/dna-tested-diseases/dm

Suggested Reading

Awano T, Johnson GS, Wade C, et al. Genome-wide association analysis reveals a *SOD1* missense mutation canine degenerative myelopathy that resembles amyotrophic lateral sclerosis. Proc Natl Acad Sci USA 2009, 106:2794–2799.

Coates JR, March PA, Ogelsbee M, et al. Clinical characterization of a familial degenerative myelopathy in Pembroke Welsh Corgi dogs. J Vet Intern Med 2007, 21:1323–1331.

Coates JR, Wininger FA. Canine degenerative myelopathy. Vet Clin North Am Small Anim Pract 2010, 40:929–950.

March PA, Coates JR, Abyad R, et al. Degenerative myelopathy in 18 Pembroke Welsh Corgi dogs. Vet Pathol 2009, 46:241–250.

Ogawa M, Uchida K, Yamato O, et al. Neuronal loss and decreased GLT-1 expression observed in the spinal cord of Pembroke Welsh Corgi Dogs with canine degenerative myelopathy. Vet Pathol 2014, 51:591–602.

Wininger FA, Zeng R, Johnson GS, et al. Degenerative myelopathy in a Bernese Mountain Dog with a novel *SOD1* missense mutation. J Vet Intern Med 2011, 25:1166–1170.

Zeng R, Coates JR, Johnson GC, et al. Breed distribution of *SOD1* alleles previously associated with canine degenerative myelopathy. J Vet Intern Med 2014, 28:515–521.

Author Joan R. Coates

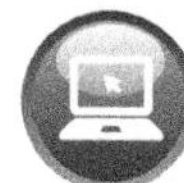

Client Education Handout available online

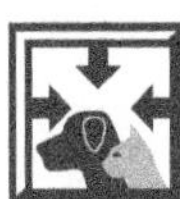

BASICS

DEFINITION

• Acute to subacute, contagious, febrile, often fatal disease with respiratory, urogenital, gastrointestinal, ocular, and CNS manifestations.
• Caused by canine distemper virus (CDV), a *Morbillivirus* in the *Paramyxoviridae* family.
• Affects many Carnivora species; mortality rate varies greatly.

PATHOPHYSIOLOGY

• Natural route of infection—airborne and droplet exposure; from nasal cavity, pharynx, and lungs, virus replication occurs in local lymph nodes; within 1 week, viral shedding occurs (mainly in respiratory exudates but also urine) and virtually all lymphatic tissues become infected; spreads via viremia to surface epithelium of respiratory, gastrointestinal, and urogenital tracts and to CNS.
• Disease progression depends on virus strain and host immune response:
  ◦ Strong cellular and humoral immune response—subclinical infection.
  ◦ Weak immune response—subacute infection; longer survival.
  ◦ Failed immune response—death within 2–4 weeks after infection; frequently due to CNS manifestations.
  ◦ Gray matter disease—affects cerebral cortex, brainstem, and spinal cord and may cause a nonsuppurative meningitis, seizures, mentation change, and ataxia; dogs may die in 2–3 weeks; some dogs recover (associated with prompt humoral and cell-mediated immunity), others develop white matter disease.
  ◦ White matter disease—multifocal disease, commonly cerebellovestibular signs, paresis, ataxia, occasionally myoclonus; some dogs die 4–5 weeks after initial infection with noninflammatory, demyelinating disease; some dogs may recover with minimal CNS injury.
• Optic neuritis and retinal lesions may occur; anterior uveitis, keratoconjunctivitis sicca possible.
• Hardening of footpads (hyperkeratosis) and nose—some virus strains; uncommon.
• Enamel hypoplasia of teeth after neonatal infection.
• Viral excretion can occur for up to 2–3 months.

SYSTEMS AFFECTED

• Multisystemic—all lymphatic tissues, surface epithelium in respiratory, alimentary, and urogenital tracts, skin, endocrine and exocrine glands.
• CNS—brain and/or spinal cord.

INCIDENCE/PREVALENCE

• Dogs—sporadic outbreaks.
• Wildlife (raccoons, skunks, fox, tigers)—fairly common.

GEOGRAPHIC DISTRIBUTION

Worldwide

SIGNALMENT

Species

Most species of the order Carnivora; has been reported in large exotic cats.

Mean Age and Range

Young, especially unvaccinated animals are most susceptible.

SIGNS

• Fever—intermittent peaks starting 3–6 days after infection.
• Gastrointestinal and/or respiratory signs—nasal and ocular discharge, depression, anorexia, vomiting, diarrhea; often exacerbated by secondary bacterial infection.
• CNS—common; generally after systemic disease (depends on virus strain).

CAUSES

• CDV exposure.
• Incompletely attenuated vaccines (rare).

RISK FACTORS

Contact of nonimmunized animals with CDV-infected animals (dogs, wild carnivores).

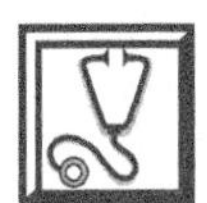

DIAGNOSIS

DIFFERENTIAL DIAGNOSIS

• Diagnosis based on clinical suspicion; combination of respiratory and gastrointestinal, ± CNS disease, in unvaccinated dog.
• Respiratory signs—can mimic kennel cough.
• Enteric signs—differentiate from canine parvovirus, coronavirus, parasitism (giardiasis), bacterial infections, gastroenteritis from toxin ingestion, inflammatory bowel disease.
• CNS form—differentiate from autoimmune meningoencephalitis (granulomatous meningoencephalomyelitis, necrotizing encephalitis, meningoencephalitis of unknown etiology), protozoal (e.g., toxoplasmosis, neosporosis), fungal (e.g., cryptococcosis), and rickettsial (e.g., ehrlichiosis, Rocky Mountain spotted fever) meningoencephalitis, rabies.

CBC/BIOCHEMISTRY/URINALYSIS

Lymphopenia in early infection; rare thrombocytopenia; intracytoplasmic inclusions in white and red blood cells.

OTHER LABORATORY TESTS

• Serology—positive antibody tests do *not* differentiate between vaccination and exposure to virulent virus; patient may die from acute disease before neutralizing antibody is produced. Immunoglobulin (Ig) M responses may occur up to 3 months after exposure to virulent virus, up to 3 weeks after vaccination; rising IgG titers in unvaccinated dog are suggestive of infection; may be useful for risk assessment of clinically healthy dogs in shelter environment.
• CDV antibody in cerebrospinal fluid (CSF)—indicative of distemper encephalitis, false negatives possible.

IMAGING

• Radiographs—evaluate pulmonary disease.
• CT and MRI—may or may not show lesions; MRI sensitive for demyelination.

DIAGNOSTIC PROCEDURES

• Immunohistochemical detection in haired skin, nasal mucosa, and footpad epithelium.
• Viral antigen or viral inclusions—in buffy coat cells, urine sediment, conjunctival or vaginal imprints, trans-tracheal wash (negative results do not rule out CDV).
• Reverse transcriptase polymerase chain reaction (RT-PCR)—on buffy coat, urine sediment cells, respiratory secretions, conjunctival swabs, CSF; false negatives possible, false positives with recent vaccination (uncommon).
• CSF—moderate mononuclear pleocytosis, elevated concentrations of CDV-specific antibody, interferon, and viral antigen early in disease course.

PATHOLOGIC FINDINGS

Gross

• Thymus—greatly reduced in size (young animals); sometimes gelatinous.
• Lungs—patchy consolidation.
• Footpads, nose—hyperkeratosis.
• Mucopurulent discharges—from eyes and nose, bronchopneumonia, catarrhal enteritis, skin pustules (secondary bacterial infection).

Histologic

• Intracytoplasmic eosinophilic inclusion bodies—in epithelium of bronchi, stomach, urinary bladder; also in reticulum cells and leukocytes in lymphatic tissues.
• Inclusion bodies in glial cells and neurons—frequently intranuclear; also in cytoplasm.
• Immunofluorescence and/or immunocytochemistry, virus isolation, and/or RT-PCR performed on tissues from lungs, stomach, urinary bladder, lymph nodes, brain.

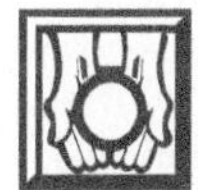

TREATMENT

APPROPRIATE HEALTH CARE

Inpatient medical management to intensive care as indicated; isolate patient to prevent spread to other dogs.

NURSING CARE

• Symptomatic.
• IV fluids—for hypovolemia, support.
• Oxygen therapy, nebulization, and coupage—for pneumonia.
• Clean ocular, nasal discharges.

ACTIVITY

Limited, to reduce spread.

DIET

Depends on extent of gastrointestinal involvement.

CLIENT EDUCATION

- Inform client that mortality rate is about 50%.
- Inform client that dogs appearing to recover from early catarrhal signs may develop fatal CNS disease.
- Presenting neurologic abnormalities usually not reversible.

MEDICATIONS

DRUG(S) OF CHOICE

- Antiviral drugs—none known to be effective.
- Broad-spectrum antibiotics—for secondary bacterial infection (CDV is immunosuppressive), beta-lactams or cephalosporins are good initial choices.
- Anticonvulsant therapy—phenobarbital, potassium bromide, levetiracetam.
- Myoclonus—no proven treatment; single case report describes use of botulinum toxin type A.

CONTRAINDICATIONS

Corticosteroids—use anti-inflammatory dosages with caution; may provide short-term control. Immunosuppressive dosages may enhance viral dissemination.

PRECAUTIONS

Tetracycline, fluoroquinolones—avoid in growing animals.

FOLLOW-UP

PATIENT MONITORING

- Monitor for CNS abnormalities, particularly seizures.
- Monitor for respiratory distress or dehydration in acute phase.

PREVENTION/AVOIDANCE

- Vaccination.
- Isolate puppies to prevent infection from wildlife (e.g., raccoons, foxes, skunks), CDV-infected dogs, ferrets.
- Recovered dogs may shed virus for up to 4 months; isolate for this time period or until multiple negative RT-PCR tests.

Vaccines

- Duration of immunity from most vaccines is >3 years.
- Modified live vaccine for CDV (MLV-CD)—prevents infection and disease; two types available:
  - Canine tissue culture-adapted vaccines (e.g., Rockborn strain)—induce complete immunity in virtually 100% of susceptible dogs; rarely, a postvaccinal fatal encephalitis develops 7–14 days after vaccination, especially in immunosuppressed animals.
  - Chick embryo-adapted vaccines (e.g., Lederle strain)—safer; postvaccinal encephalitis does not occur; only about 80% of susceptible dogs seroconvert.
  - Other species—chick embryo can safely be used in variety of wildlife species (e.g., gray fox); Rockborn type fatal in these animals.
- Killed vaccines—useful for species in which either type of MLV-CD is fatal (e.g., red panda, blackfooted ferret).
- Canarypox recombinant CDV vaccine.

Maternal Antibody

- Important.
- Most puppies lose protection from maternal antibody at 6–12 weeks of age; 2–3 vaccinations should be given during this period.
- Heterotypic (measles virus) vaccination—recommended for puppies that have maternal antibody; induces protection from disease but not from infection.

POSSIBLE COMPLICATIONS

Possibility of CNS signs developing for 2–3 months after catarrhal signs have subsided.

EXPECTED COURSE AND PROGNOSIS

- Depends on strain and individual host response—subclinical, acute, subacute, fatal, or nonfatal infection.
- Mild CNS signs—patient may recover; myoclonus may continue for several months or indefinitely.
- Death—2 weeks to 3 months after infection; mortality rate ~50%.
- Euthanasia—owner may elect if or when neurologic signs develop; indicated if uncontrollable seizures occur.

MISCELLANEOUS

ASSOCIATED CONDITIONS

- Persistent or latent *Toxoplasma gondii* infections—may be reactivated due to immunosuppressive state.
- Respiratory infections with *Bordetella bronchiseptica* (kennel cough).

AGE-RELATED FACTORS

- Young puppies—more susceptible; mortality rate is higher.
- Nonimmunized old dogs—highly susceptible to infection and disease.

ZOONOTIC POTENTIAL

Possible that humans may become subclinically infected with CDV; immunization against measles virus also protects against CDV infection.

PREGNANCY/FERTILITY/BREEDING

In utero infection—occurs in antibody-negative bitches; rare; may lead to abortion or to persistent infection; infected neonates may develop fatal disease by 4–6 weeks of age.

SYNONYMS

- Canine distemper.
- Hard pad disease.

SEE ALSO

Myoclonus

ABBREVIATIONS

- CDV = canine distemper virus.
- CSF = cerebrospinal fluid.
- Ig = immunoglobulin.
- MLV-CD = modified live virus of canine distemper.
- RT-PCR = reverse transcriptase polymerase chain reaction.

INTERNET RESOURCES

https://www.uwsheltermedicine.com/library/resources/canine-distemper-cdv

Suggested Reading

Greene CE, Vendevelde M. Canine distemper. In: Greene CE, ed., Infectious Diseases of the Dog and Cat, 4th ed. St. Louis, MO: Saunders Elsevier, 2012, pp. 25–42.

Lempp C, Spitzbarth I, Puff C, et al. New aspects of pathogenesis of canine distemper leukoencephalitis. Viruses 2014, 6:2571–2601.

Loots AK, Mitchell E, Dalton DL, et al. Advances in canine distemper virus pathogenesis research: a wildlife perspective. J Gen Virol 2017, 98:311–321.

Pesavento PA, Murphy BG. Common and emerging infectious disease in the animal shelter. Vet Pathol 2014, 51:478–491.

Author Michelle C. Tensley

Consulting Editor Amie Koenig

Acknowledgment The author and book editors acknowledge the prior contribution of Stephen C. Barr.

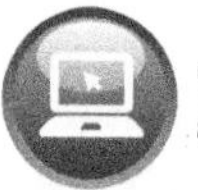

Client Education Handout available online

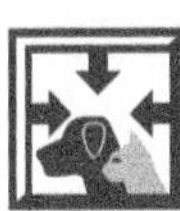

BASICS

DEFINITION

- Viral, enteropathogenic bacterial, protozoal, or parasitic etiologies; small, large, or mixed-bowel diarrhea.
- Secondary systemic signs with canine parvovirus (CPV)-2 and salmonellosis.
- Presence of organisms on diagnostic screening does not indicate causation; patient factors (clinical signs, age, environmental exposure) should be considered before treatment.
- Some dogs will have self-resolution; diagnostic testing appropriate for more severely affected animals or if clinical signs are persistent having ruled out other causes of acute or chronic diarrhea.
- Puppies with acute diarrhea should be screened for CPV-2.

PATHOPHYSIOLOGY

- Typically, fecal–oral route of infection.
- Diarrhea from enterotoxins, osmotic diarrhea, or invasion of epithelium resulting in inflammation.
- Up to 50% of dogs may have coinfections.

SYSTEMS AFFECTED

- Gastrointestinal (GI)—vomiting, diarrhea.
- Cardiovascular—fluid balance.

INCIDENCE/PREVALENCE

- Prevalence of most pathogens similar in dogs with or without diarrhea.
  - Coronavirus more common in dogs with diarrhea.
  - Dogs with diarrhea more likely to have >1 enteropathogen.
- Specific prevalence in dogs in United States:
  - 0–6%—CPV-2, Salmonella spp., Cystoisospora spp., Dipylidum caninum, Campylobacter spp., C. difficile toxin A and B, ascarids.
  - 7–20%—whipworms, *Giardia* spp., *Cryptosporidium*, circovirus.
  - 35–60%—*C. perfringens* enterotoxin A or alpha toxin gene, hookworm.

GEOGRAPHIC DISTRIBUTION

- Widespread.
- Prevalence of etiologies varies by location.

SIGNALMENT

- Species—dog.
- Breed predilections—none.
- Mean age and range—largely pediatric and young adult dogs; older animals if in high-risk environments.

SIGNS

- General comments—range from mild to severely affected.
- Historical findings—acute or chronic, small or large bowel diarrhea; possibly vomiting, weight loss, hyporexia; no history of dietary indiscretion.
- Physical examination findings—depends on etiology and severity; may include dehydration, poor body condition, borborygmus, flatulence, hematochezia, melena, visualization of worms on rectal exam or peri-anal, signs of sepsis or systemic inflammatory response syndrome (SIRS).

CAUSES

- Viral—coronavirus, CPV-2, circovirus.
- Bacterial—*Campylobacter spp., Clostridium perfringens* enterotoxin, *Clostridium difficile* toxins, *Salmonella* spp.
- Parasitic—*Toxocara* spp., *Ancylostoma* spp., *Toxascaris leonine, Dipyldium caninum, Trichuris vulpis.*
- Protozoal—*Giardia* spp.
- Coccidial—*Cryptosporidium* spp., *Cystoisospora* spp.

RISK FACTORS

- Pediatric and young adult dogs more commonly affected, particularly for viral enteritis, *Cryptosporidium* spp., roundworm (*Toxocara* and *Toxascaris*), *Cystoisospora* spp., and *Campylobacter* spp.
- Administration of antimicrobials and immunosuppressive drugs increase risk for hospital-associated colonization of *C. difficile.*
- Crowding and poor sanitation.
- Lack of regular parasiticide administration.
- Dogs with environmental exposure to livestock or wildlife for *Cryptosporidium* spp., *Campylobacter* spp., *Giardia* spp.

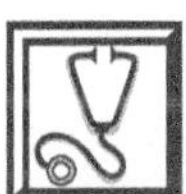

DIAGNOSIS

DIFFERENTIAL DIAGNOSIS

- Acute diarrhea—dietary indiscretion, foreign body, pancreatitis, GI neoplasia; non-GI diseases: hepatotoxicity, renal disease, other systemic diseases (commonly other clinical signs such as hyporexia, vomiting, icterus).
- Chronic diarrhea—chronic enteropathy (dietary responsive, antibiotic responsive, or inflammatory bowel disease), chronic pancreatitis, primary GI neoplasia, and non-GI diseases of other organs.

CBC/BIOCHEMISTRY/URINALYSIS

- Eosinophilia—possible with intestinal parasitism.
- Anemia and/or microcytosis—GI hemorrhage or iron deficiency, particularly with high worm burden (e.g., *T. vulpis*) or GI mucosal shedding (e.g., CPV).
- Leukopenia—parvoviral enteritis (bacterial translocation or bone marrow suppression) or systemic salmonellosis.
- Hyponatremia and hyperkalemia with large bowel diarrhea—*T. vulpis.*
- Azotemia and electrolyte derangements with dehydration.
- Hypoglycemia—parvoviral enteritis and systemic salmonellosis.
- Panhypoproteinemia and hypocholesterolemia if secondary protein-losing enteropathy or GI blood loss.

IMAGING

- Abdominal radiographs if no response to symptomatic care to rule out other causes of diarrhea.
- Abdominal ultrasound recommended in nonpediatric patients with diarrhea that is nonresponsive to symptomatic care.

DIAGNOSTIC PROCEDURES

- Fecal flotation—for intestinal parasitism; false negatives possible (ova are intermittently shed); dogs suspected to have intestinal parasitism should have multiple fecal flotations performed or be treated with anthelmintics.
- Fecal cytology—bacterial morphology (frequent spirochetes, spores) or presence of fungal or protozoal organisms.
- *Giardia* ELISA.
- Infectious diarrhea PCR panels detect a range of possible causes of diarrhea; however, caution should be used in interpretation of these assays, as a positive result does not necessarily indicate causation and false-negative results are possible.

PATHOLOGIC FINDINGS

- Gross examination of intestinal mucosa may demonstrate parasites attached to intestinal mucosa with multifocal hemorrhagic ulcerations, submucosal congestion or hemorrhage, intestinal wall thickening.
- Histopathology of intestine may show eosinophilic, neutrophilic, or lymphoplasmacytic enteritis with varying degrees of hemorrhage and necrosis, depending on etiology.

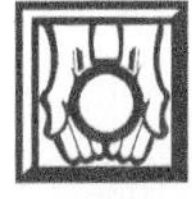

TREATMENT

APPROPRIATE HEALTH CARE

- Mildly affected dogs—outpatient basis.
- Moderate to severely affected dogs may require IV administration of isotonic balanced electrolyte solution for dehydration.
- Electrolyte and acid-base imbalances should be corrected with fluid therapy and monitored closely.
- Dextrose should be supplemented parenterally in dogs with hypoglycemia.
- Packed red blood cell or plasma transfusions should be given as needed for severe anemia or coagulopathies from sepsis (rare).

DIET

- Easily digestible diets until clinical signs have resolved, followed by slow transition (3–4 days) to maintenance diet.
- In anorexic pediatric patients, nasogastric tube feeding of liquid diet recommended if anorexia persists ≥48 hours.

CANINE INFECTIOUS DIARRHEA (CONTINUED)

C

CLIENT EDUCATION

- For most infectious organisms, environmental decontamination prevents transmission to other pets/people and reinfection; isolation during hospitalization may be warranted depending on underlying cause.
- Appropriate vaccination and deworming schedules should be followed.
- Dogs with identified infectious causes of diarrhea should be isolated from other dogs if possible until clinical signs resolve.

SURGICAL CONSIDERATIONS

Viral and parasitic enterocolitis can result in intussusceptions, especially in puppies.

MEDICATIONS

DRUG(S) OF CHOICE

- Many cases will self-resolve with supportive care and time.
- Empiric therapy pending diagnostics, if clinical signs persist—probiotics, or metronidazole (10 mg/kg PO q12h) and fenbendazole (50 mg/kg PO q24h for 5 days).
- Anthelmintics—fenbendazole (50 mg/kg PO q24h for 5 days), pyrantel pamoate (5–10 mg/kg PO for 3 days).
- Coccidiostatic—sulfadimethoxine (50–60 mg/kg PO q24h for 5–10 days), ponazuril (50 mg/kg PO once).
- Antiprotozoal drugs—fenbendazole (50 mg/kg PO q24h for 5 days).
- Campylobacteriosis with persistent clinical signs—erythromycin (10–15 mg/kg PO q8h) or azithromycin (5–10 mg/kg PO q24h).
- Probiotics may be of benefit for dogs with bacterial enteritis with acute or chronic signs; probiotics should be selected with evidence of efficacy (e.g., Visbiome®).
- Patients with systemic illness, leukopenia, or suspected GI mucosal barrier breakdown (evidenced by blood in the feces) should be treated with broad-spectrum antimicrobial agents and as indicated by specific etiology.
- Dogs with confirmed salmonella should *not* be treated with antibiotics unless systemically ill.

PRECAUTIONS

Metronidazole dose should be reduced in animals with hepatic insufficiency.

POSSIBLE INTERACTIONS

- Metronidazole given at higher doses for giardiasis or long-term use can lead to vestibular signs.
- Some dogs may be sensitive to sulfa-containing medications used for treatment of coccidiosis.

FOLLOW-UP

PATIENT MONITORING

- Case-based, may include reassessment of anemia, leukopenia, or electrolyte derangements as appropriate.
- Persistent clinical signs after appropriate treatment is suggestive for alternative cause of diarrhea.
- Patients with recurrent clinical signs should be retested, particularly if environmental reinfection is possible (e.g., giardiasis, campylobacteriosis).

PREVENTION/AVOIDANCE

- Routine vaccination.
- Monthly flea/tick or heartworm preventative with combination anthelmintic therapy.
- Avoid subjecting poorly vaccinated or immunocompromised animals to high-traffic areas, including but not limited to pet supply stores, dog parks, or newly introduced poorly vaccinated pets.

POSSIBLE COMPLICATIONS

- Sepsis.
- Anemia.
- Electrolyte disturbances.
- Aspiration pneumonia if concurrent vomiting (uncommon).

EXPECTED COURSE AND PROGNOSIS

- Usually good to excellent; underlying immunosuppressive conditions may increase susceptibility to infection and worsen prognosis.
- Parvoviral enteritis carries guarded to poor prognosis without treatment; appropriate supportive care provides full recovery rates of 90% or more.

MISCELLANEOUS

AGE-RELATED FACTORS

Puppies and young dogs affected.

ZOONOTIC POTENTIAL

- Giardiasis—low risk of transmission.
- Cryptosporidiosis.
- Salmonellosis.
- *Campylobacter jejuni.*
- *Toxocara* spp. (ascarids)—visceral larval migrans in humans, most common in children.
- *Ancylostoma* (hookworms)—cutaneous larval migrans in humans, most common in children.

PREGNANCY/FERTILITY/BREEDING

If heavy endoparasite load, fenbendazole can be administered to pregnant bitches from 14th day of gestation through to 14th day of lactation. If risk of infection is high, all puppies (and mothers) should be treated with appropriate anthelmintics at 2, 4, 6, and 8 weeks of age.

SEE ALSO

- Acute Diarrhea.
- Campylobacteriosis.
- Canine Coronavirus Infections.
- Canine Parvovirus.
- Clostridial Enterotoxicosis.
- Coccidiosis.
- Diarrhea, Chronic—Dogs.
- Giardiasis.
- Hookworms (Ancylostomiasis).
- Roundworms (Ascariasis).
- Salmonellosis.
- Whipworms (Trichuriasis).

ABBREVIATIONS

- CPV-2 = canine parvovirus.
- GI = gastrointestinal.
- SIRS = systemic inflammatory response syndrome.

Suggested Reading

Gookin JL. Infection, large intestine. In: Washabau RJ, Day MJ, eds., Canine & Feline Gastroenterology. St. Louis, MO: Saunders Elsevier, 2013, pp. 745–757.

Lappin MR. Infection, small intestine. In: Washabau RJ, Day MJ, eds., Canine & Feline Gastroenterology. St. Louis, MO: Saunders Elsevier, 2013, pp. 683–695.

Authors Kasey E. Mabry and Tracy Hill

Consulting Editor Amie Koenig

CANINE INFECTIOUS RESPIRATORY DISEASE

BASICS

DEFINITION
A multifaceted disease whereby infectious disease and environment contribute to the genesis of cough and other respiratory signs in dogs.

PATHOPHYSIOLOGY
Initiated by injury to the respiratory epithelium by viral infection followed by invasion of damaged tissue by bacterial, mycoplasmal, or other virulent organisms, resulting in further damage and clinical signs.

SYSTEMS AFFECTED
Respiratory—upper and lower airways can be involved. Multisystemic—cases that develop sepsis.

GENETICS
None

INCIDENCE/PREVALENCE
Most common in areas of high density with immunologically naïve or immunosuppressed patients (i.e., training kennels, shelters, veterinary hospitals).

GEOGRAPHIC DISTRIBUTION
Worldwide

SIGNALMENT

Species
Dog

Breed Predilections
None

Mean Age and Range
• Most severe in puppies 6 weeks–6 months old. • Can develop in dogs of all ages, particularly with preexisting airway disease.

Predominant Sex
None

SIGNS

General Comments
• Related to the degree of respiratory tract damage and age of the affected dog and virulence of infectious organism. • Can be subclinical, mild, or severe with pneumonia. • Most viral, bacterial, and mycoplasmal agents spread rapidly from seemingly healthy dogs to others in the same environment; signs usually begin about 3–7 days after exposure to the infecting agent(s).

Historical Findings
• Uncomplicated—acute-onset cough in an otherwise healthy animal; dry and hacking, soft and dry, moist and hacking, or paroxysmal, followed by gagging, retching, and expectoration of mucus; excitement, exercise, and pressure on the trachea induce coughing spells.
• Complicated (severe)—inappetence to anorexia; cough is moist and productive; lethargy, difficulty breathing, hemoptysis, and exercise intolerance can occur.

Physical Examination Findings
• Uncomplicated—cough readily induced with minimal tracheal pressure; lung sounds often normal; systemically healthy. • Complicated—low-grade or intermittent fever (39.4–40.0 °C; 103–104 °F); increased intensity of normal lung sounds, crackles or wheezes possible.

CAUSES
• Viral—canine distemper virus (CDV); canine adenovirus (CAV-2); canine parainfluenza (CPIV); canine respiratory coronavirus (CRCoV), canine reovirus; canine herpesvirus-1 (CHV-1); canine influenza virus (CIV; H3N8 or H3N2); canine bocavirus, canine hepacivirus; canine pneumovirus (CnPnV). • Most viral pathogens (except CHV and CDV) primarily infect epithelial and lymphoid tissue of the upper and lower respiratory tract; in severe cases, causing desquamation of the epithelium and aggregation of inflammatory cells in the lungs, leading to secondary bacterial colonization and infection; CRCoV infection leads to loss of cilia associated with the respiratory epithelium, increasing the severity and duration of secondary infections. • Bacterial—*Bordetella bronchiseptica*, with no other respiratory pathogens, produces clinical signs indistinguishable from those of other bacterial causes; *Streptococcus equi* subsp. *zooepidemicus* is associated with a particularly virulent course that can progress to death; *Pseudomonas, Escherichia coli, Klebsiella, Pasteurella, Streptococcus, Mycoplasma*, and other species equally likely.

RISK FACTORS
• Substandard hygienic conditions and overcrowding—encountered in some pet shops, shelters, research facilities, and boarding and training kennels. • Coexisting subclinical airway disease—congenital anomalies; chronic bronchitis; bronchiectasis.

DIAGNOSIS

DIFFERENTIAL DIAGNOSIS
• In systemically well dogs—parasitic bronchitis, irritant tracheobronchitis, airway foreign body, airway collapse. • In a dog with systemic signs—fungal or bacterial (aspiration) pneumonia, primary or metastatic neoplasia, congestive heart failure, migrating foreign body. • Provisional diagnosis of infectious tracheobronchitis is made in a dog with compelling clinical signs and a history of exposure to the implicated organisms. • See Cough.

CBC/BIOCHEMISTRY/URINALYSIS
• Early, mild leukopenia (5,000–6,000 cells/dL)—can be detected; suggests viral cause.
• Neutrophilic leukocytosis with a toxic left shift—frequently found with severe pneumonia.

OTHER LABORATORY TESTS
Pulse oximetry and arterial blood gas analysis—can reveal hypoxemia in pneumonia.

IMAGING
• Uncomplicated disease—radiographs: unremarkable; most useful for ruling out other differential diagnoses. • Complicated disease—radiographs: interstitial and alveolar lung pattern with a cranioventral distribution typical of bacterial pneumonia; can see diffuse interstitial lung pattern typical of viral pneumonia; mixed lung pattern can be present.

DIAGNOSTIC PROCEDURES
• In cases with severe disease—ideally perform bronchoalveolar lavage via bronchoscopy for cytology and microbial culture; tracheal wash sample acceptable, but increased likelihood for upper airway contamination. • Antimicrobial sensitivity pattern of cultured bacteria—identification aids markedly in providing an effective treatment plan. • PCR from bronchoalveolar lavage, nasal, ocular, or pharyngeal secretions can be used to detect virus, though there is difficulty in interpreting results as many healthy animals shed virus in the absence of clinical signs.

PATHOLOGIC FINDINGS
• CPIV—causes few to no clinical signs; lungs of infected dogs 6–10 days after exposure may contain petechial hemorrhages that are evenly distributed over the surfaces; detected by immunofluorescence in columnar epithelial cells of the bronchi and bronchioles 6–10 days after aerosol exposure. • CAV-2—lesions confined to the respiratory system; large intranuclear inclusion bodies found in bronchial epithelial cells and alveolar septal cells; clinical signs tend to be mild and short-lasting; lesions persist for at least a month after infection. • CIV (H3N8, H3N2)—fulminant disease characterized by secondary *Mycoplasma* or bacterial infection and pulmonary hemorrhage. • CRCoV—characterized by marked inflammation of the trachea and nares with cilia loss in the former; detected by immunohistochemistry of the trachea or bronchioles. • *Streptococcus equi* subsp. *zooepidemicus* infection—acute, fibrinosuppurative pneumonia with large numbers of cocci found within the pulmonary parenchyma and, often, septic thomboemboli.
• Bordetellosis and severe bacterial infection—evidence of purulent bronchitis, tracheitis, and rhinitis with hyperemia and enlargement of the bronchial, mediastinal, and retropharyngeal lymph nodes; may see large numbers of Gram-positive or Gram-negative organisms in the mucus of the tracheal and bronchial epithelium.

CANINE INFECTIOUS RESPIRATORY DISEASE (CONTINUED)

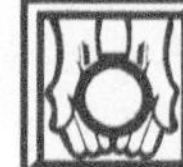

TREATMENT

APPROPRIATE HEALTH CARE

• Outpatient—strongly recommended for uncomplicated disease. • Inpatient—strongly recommended for complicated disease and/or pneumonia.

NURSING CARE

Fluid administration—indicated for complicated disease and/or pneumonia.

ACTIVITY

Enforced rest—14–21 days with uncomplicated disease; for at least the duration of radiographic evidence of pneumonia in severely affected dogs.

DIET

Good-quality commercial food.

CLIENT EDUCATION

• Isolate patient from other animals; infected dogs can transmit the agent(s) before onset of clinical signs and afterward until immunity develops. • Dogs with uncomplicated disease should respond to treatment in 10–14 days. • Once infection spreads in a kennel, it can be controlled by evacuation for 1–2 weeks and disinfection with commonly used chemicals, such as sodium hypochlorite (1 : 30 dilution), chlorhexidine, and benzalkonium.

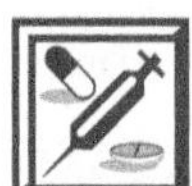

MEDICATIONS

DRUG(S) OF CHOICE

• Amoxicillin/clavulanic acid (12.5–25 mg/kg PO q12h) or doxycycline (5 mg/kg PO q12h or 10 mg/kg PO q24h)—initial treatment of uncomplicated disease. • Penicillin (ampicillin 10–20 mg/kg IV q6–8h or ticarcillin 40–50 mg/kg IV q6–8h) with aminoglycoside (gentamicin 2–4 mg/kg IV/IM/SC q6–8h or amikacin 6.5 mg/kg IV/IM/SC q8h) or fluoroquinolone (enrofloxacin 5–10 mg/kg PO/IM/IV q24h)—usually effective for severe disease.
• Antimicrobial therapy—continue for at least 10 days beyond radiographic resolution. • *B. bronchiseptica* and other resistant species—some antimicrobials may not reach adequate therapeutic concentrations in the lumen of the lower respiratory tract, so oral or parenteral administration may have limited effectiveness; nebulization with gentamicin (3–5 mg/kg) can decrease bacterial numbers when administered daily for 3–5 days; use in conjunction with systemic antibiotics in dogs with parenchymal disease. • Butorphanol (0.55 mg/kg PO q8–12h) or hydrocodone bitartrate (0.22 mg/kg PO q6–8h)—effective suppression of dry, nonproductive cough not associated with bacterial infection. • Bronchodilators (e.g., terbutaline 0.625–5 mg/dog q8–12h)—may be used to control bronchospasm and wheeze.

CONTRAINDICATIONS

• Do not use cough suppressants in patients with pneumonia. • Employ glucocorticoids only in cases with significant inflammatory disease refractory to conventional supportive care.

PRECAUTIONS

None

POSSIBLE INTERACTIONS

Fluoroquinolones and theophylline derivatives—concurrent use causes high and possibly toxic plasma theophylline concentration. Dose reduce theophylline while concurrently administering fluoroquinolones.

ALTERNATIVE DRUG(S)

None

FOLLOW-UP

PATIENT MONITORING

• Uncomplicated disease—should resolve spontaneously or respond to treatment in 10–14 days; if patient continues to cough 14 days or more after establishment of an adequate treatment plan, question the diagnosis of uncomplicated disease. • Complicated disease—repeat thoracic radiography until at least 7 days beyond resolution of all clinical signs.

PREVENTION/AVOIDANCE

Shedding of the causative agent(s) of infectious respiratory disease in airway secretions of dogs undoubtedly accounts for the persistence of this problem in kennels, animal shelters, boarding facilities, and veterinary hospitals.

Viral and Bacterial Vaccines

• Modified live CDV and CAV-2 vaccines provide reliable protection and are considered core vaccines for all puppies; can be administered at 6 weeks of age, every 2–4 weeks. • *B. bronchiseptica* and CPIV vaccine—can vaccinate puppies mucosally or intranasally as early as 2–4 weeks of age without interference from maternal antibody and follow with annual revaccination; can vaccinate mature dogs with a one-dose intranasal vaccination (at the same time as their puppies or when they receive their annual vaccinations). • Inactivated *B. bronchiseptica* parenteral vaccine—administered as two doses, 2–4 weeks apart; initial vaccination of puppies is recommended at or about 6–8 weeks of age; revaccinate at 4 months of age. • Inactivated CIV vaccines (H3N2 and H3N8) available to reduce severity and duration of clinical signs but considered noncore; can be administered starting at 6 weeks as two doses, 2–4 weeks apart; results in seroconversion.

POSSIBLE COMPLICATIONS

N/A

EXPECTED COURSE AND PROGNOSIS

• Natural course of uncomplicated disease, if untreated—10–14 days; simple restriction of exercise and prevention of excitement shortens the course. • Typical course of severe disease—2–6 weeks; patients that die often develop severe pneumonia that affects multiple lung lobes and multiple organ dysfunction due to sepsis.

MISCELLANEOUS

ASSOCIATED CONDITIONS

May accompany other respiratory tract anomalies.

AGE-RELATED FACTORS

Most severe in puppies 6 weeks–6 months old and in puppies from commercial pet shops and humane society shelters.

ZOONOTIC POTENTIAL

Potential zoonotic risk of *Streptococcus equi* subsp. *zooepidemicus* and *B. bronchispetica* reported in single case reports.

PREGNANCY/FERTILITY/BREEDING

High risk in dogs on extensive medical treatment; especially risky for dogs in overcrowded breeding facilities.

SYNONYMS

• Kennel cough. • Infectious tracheobronchitis—uncomplicated disease.

ABBREVIATIONS

• CAV-2 = canine adenovírus. • CDV = canine distemper vírus. • CHV-1 = canine herpesvirus-1. • CIV = canine influenza virus. • CnPnV = canine pneumovirus. • CPIV = canine parainfluenza. • CRCoV = canine respiratory coronavirus.

INTERNET RESOURCES

https://www.cdc.gov/flu/other/canine-flu

Suggested Reading

Bemis DA. Bordetella and Mycoplasma respiratory infection in dogs. Vet Clin North Am Small Anim Pract 1992, 22:1173–1186.

Buonavoglia C, Martella V. Canine respiratory viruses. Vet Res 2007, 38(2):355–373.

Chalker VJ, Owen WM, Paterson C, et al. Mycoplasmas associated with canine infectious respiratory disease. Microbiology 2004, 150(Pt 10):3491–3497.

Erles K, Dubovi E, Brooks HW, Brownlie J. Longitudinal study of viruses associated with canine infectious respiratory disease. J Clin Micro 2004, 42:4524–4529.

Priestnall SL, Mitchell JA, Walker CA, et al. New and emerging pathogens in canine infectious respiratory disease. Vet Path 2014, 51(2):492–504.

Author Jonathan D. Dear
Consulting Editor Elizabeth Rozanski

Client Education Handout available online

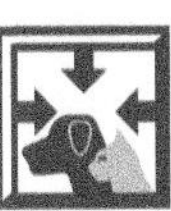

BASICS

DEFINITION

- An acute systemic illness characterized by vomiting, hemorrhagic enteritis, and leukopenia.
- Myocardial form was observed in puppies in late 1970s, now rare.
- Most puppies protected against neonatal infection by maternal antibodies.
- Monoclonal antibodies have revealed antigenic changes in canine parvovirus (CPV)-2; CPV2a, b, and c strains have been identified.
- Original virus now virtually extinct in domestic dogs.
- CPV2c viruses are more virulent, and mortality rates higher.
- CPV-2 is closely related to feline panleukopenia virus (FPV).

PATHOPHYSIOLOGY

- Parvoviruses require actively dividing cells for growth.
- After ingestion of virus there is a 2–4-day period of viremia.
- Early lymphatic infection is accompanied by lymphopenia and precedes intestinal infection and clinical signs.
- By postinfection (PI) day 3, rapidly dividing crypt cells of small intestine are infected.
- Viral shedding in feces starts ~3–4 days PI, peaks with clinical signs.
- Virus ceases to be shed in detectable amounts by PI days 8–12.
- Absorption of bacterial endotoxins from damaged intestinal mucosa plays a role in CPV-2 disease.
- Intensity of illness related to viral dose and antigenic type.

SYSTEMS AFFECTED

- Cardiovascular—myocarditis (uncommon), hypovolemia.
- Gastrointestinal.
- Hemic/lymphatic/immune.

GENETICS

Unknown

INCIDENCE/PREVALENCE

Common in breeding kennels, animal shelters, pet stores.

GEOGRAPHIC DISTRIBUTION

Worldwide

SIGNALMENT

Species

Dog

Breed Predilections

- Certain breeds are at increased risk, including Rottweiler, Doberman pinscher, American pit bull terrier, Labrador retriever, German shepherd dog, and Yorkshire terrier.
- Higher fatality rates are seen in hounds, gundogs, and nonsporting pedigree groups.

Mean Age and Range

- Illness occurs at any age.
- Most severe in dogs 6–24 weeks of age.

Predominant Sex

None

SIGNS

General Comments

Suspect CPV-2 infection whenever puppies have an enteric illness.

Historical Findings

- Sudden onset of bloody diarrhea, anorexia, and vomiting.
- Some dogs may collapse in a shock-like state and die without enteric signs.
- In breeding kennels, several littermates may become ill simultaneously or within a short period.
- Occasionally, one or two puppies in a litter have minimal signs, followed by death of littermates, which may reflect degree of virus exposure.

Physical Examination Findings

- Hypovolemic shock—weak pulse, tachycardia, dull mentation.
- Severe hemorrhagic diarrhea.
- Fluid-filled intestinal loops may be palpated.
- Dehydration, weight loss, abdominal discomfort.
- May have fever or hypothermia.

CAUSES

CPV-2.

RISK FACTORS

- Unvaccinated dogs.
- Dogs <4 months of age.
- Co-pathogens such as parasites, viruses, and certain bacterial species (e.g., *Campylobacter* spp., *Clostridium* spp.) may exacerbate illness.
- Severe, often fatal parvoviral infections have been demonstrated in puppies exposed simultaneously to CPV-2 and canine coronavirus.
- Crowding and poor sanitation.

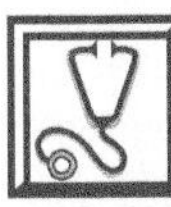

DIAGNOSIS

DIFFERENTIAL DIAGNOSIS

- Canine coronavirus infection.
- Salmonellosis; colibacillosis; other enteric bacterial infections.
- Gastrointestinal foreign bodies.
- Gastrointestinal parasites.
- Acute hemorrhagic diarrhea syndrome (previously hemorrhagic gastroenteritis).
- Intussusception (may be concurrent).
- Toxin ingestion.

CBC/BIOCHEMISTRY/URINALYSIS

- Lymphopenia—characteristic; commonly occurs PI days 4–6.
- Severely affected dogs exhibit severe neutropenia with onset of intestinal damage.
- Leukocytosis during recovery.
- Serum chemistry profiles help assess electrolyte disturbances (especially hypokalemia), presence of azotemia, panhypoproteinemia, hypoglycemia.

OTHER LABORATORY TESTS

- Virus antigen detection in stool at onset of disease and for 2–4 days afterward; many commercial point-of-care ELISA assays available, also PCR and quantitative PCR methodologies.
- Serologic tests are not diagnostic because dogs often have high titers from vaccination and/or maternal antibodies.

IMAGING

- Abdominal radiographs—generalized small intestinal ileus; exercise caution to prevent misdiagnosis of intestinal obstruction, but intussusception may cause obstructive pattern.
- Abdominal ultrasound—fluid-filled, atonic small and large intestines, duodenal and jejunal mucosal layer thinning with or without indistinct wall layers and irregular luminal-mucosal surfaces, extensive duodenal and/or jejunal hyperechoic mucosal speckling, and duodenal and/or jejunal corrugations; intussusceptions can be identified.

DIAGNOSTIC PROCEDURES

- Electron microscopy detects fecal virus during early stages of infection.
- Samples for virus detection should be submitted during acute phase of infection; ship specimens refrigerated, not frozen.

PATHOLOGIC FINDINGS

- Gross changes include subserosal congestion and hemorrhage or frank hemorrhage into small intestinal lumen, or intestines that are empty or contain yellow or blood-tinged fluid.
- Mesenteric lymph nodes often enlarged and edematous, with hemorrhages in cortex.
- Thymic atrophy in young dogs.
- Pulmonary edema and hydropericardium may be only gross change in dogs with myocarditis and heart failure.
- Histopathology reveals intestinal inflammation and necrosis, with severe villus atrophy.

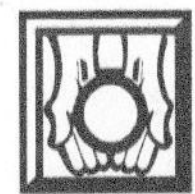

TREATMENT

APPROPRIATE HEALTH CARE

- Symptomatic and supportive (see Acute Vomiting; Acute Diarrhea; Gastroenteritis, Acute Hemorrhagic Diarrhea Syndrome), including IV fluids, antibiotics, antiemetics, and analgesics.
- Intensity depends on severity of signs; both in- and outpatient treatment protocols exist.

CANINE PARVOVIRUS (CONTINUED)

C

• Goals are to provide intestinal nutrients, restore and maintain fluid and electrolyte balance, and resolve shock, sepsis, and endotoxemia.
• Fecal microbiota transplant may speed resolution of diarrhea.
• Prompt, intensive inpatient care leads to treatment success.
• Proper, strict isolation procedures are essential.
• Exercise care to prevent spread of CPV-2, a very stable virus.
• Antiviral drugs have not yet been shown to be a critical part of treatment.

NURSING CARE

• Hospitalize patients and monitor for dehydration and electrolyte imbalance.
• Fluids are usually supplemented with potassium chloride, 5% dextrose, and possibly sodium bicarbonate (if severe metabolic acidosis due to bicarbonate loss).

ACTIVITY

Restrict until symptoms abate.

DIET

Puppies receiving early enteral nutrition via a nasoesophageal tube (compared to puppies that received nothing enterally until cessation of vomiting) showed earlier clinical improvement, significant weight gain, and improved gut barrier function, which could limit bacterial or endotoxin translocation.

CLIENT EDUCATION

• Inform about need for thorough disinfection, especially if other dogs are on premises; strict sanitation is essential; a 1 : 30 dilution of bleach (5% sodium hypochlorite) destroys CPV-2 in a few minutes.
• If possible, isolate puppies until they reach 3 months of age and vaccinate repeatedly; typical protocols involve vaccination at 6, 9, and 12 weeks of age.
• Puppies can be infected with virulent virus before any vaccine will confer immunity.
• CPV-2 is shed for less than 2 weeks after infection; no carrier state has been substantiated.

SURGICAL CONSIDERATIONS

• Exercise caution to prevent misdiagnosis of intestinal obstruction, especially if vomiting is only clinical sign.
• Intussusceptions can occur.

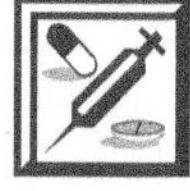

MEDICATIONS

See Acute Vomiting; Acute Diarrhea; Gastroenteritis, Acute Hemorrhagic Diarrhea Syndrome.

DRUG(S) OF CHOICE

Additional recommended drugs include parenteral antibiotics (ampicillin and gentamicin) and antiemetics (e.g., ondansetron, maropitant).

PRECAUTIONS

Gentamicin may cause renal toxicity in dehydrated puppies.

FOLLOW-UP

PATIENT MONITORING

There is an increased incidence of discospondylitis in puppies that had parvovirus infection.

PREVENTION/AVOIDANCE

• Inactivated and live vaccines are available for prophylaxis, and vaccines differ in their capacity to immunize puppies with maternal antibodies.
• Vaccination with a modified live vaccine at 4 weeks of age in puppies with high maternally derived antibody concentrations resulted in seroconversion rates of up to 80%; this may lead to a decreased window of susceptibility to CPV infection and might be an adjunct control method in contaminated environments.
• Control of CPV-2 requires efficacious vaccines, isolation of puppies, and stringent hygiene.

POSSIBLE COMPLICATIONS

• Septicemia/endotoxemia.
• Bacterial pneumonia.
• Intussusception.
• Discospondylitis.

EXPECTED COURSE AND PROGNOSIS

• Prognosis is guarded in severely affected puppies.
• Prognosis is good for dogs that receive prompt initial treatment and survive initial crisis—approximately 80% survival rate.
• Poor prognosis if a patient is purebred, has a low bodyweight, and if the following biomarker levels are present after 24 hours of intensive therapy: severe persistent leuko- and lymphopenia, persistently elevated or rising serum cortisol concentration (>8.1 μg/dL), severe hypothyroxinemia (<0.2 μg/dL), hypocholesterolemia (<100 mg/dL), and persistently elevated serum C-reactive protein (>97.3 mg/L).
• Conversely, puppies with a good prognosis are of mixed breed, >6 months old, and show the following biomarker values: total leukocyte count >4.5 × 10^3/μL, lymphocyte count >1 × 10^3/μL, and mature neutrophil count >3 × 10^3/μL. Additionally, a serum cortisol concentration <8.1 μg/dL at 48 hours after admission is associated with 96% survival, and a serum thyroxine concentration >0.2 μg/dL at 24 hours after admission is associated with 100% survival. An HDL-cholesterol concentration >50.2 mg/dL at admission is associated with 100% survival.

MISCELLANEOUS

ASSOCIATED CONDITIONS

Coinfection with intestinal helminths and *Giardia* are indicative of unhygienic housing conditions and can worsen clinical signs and contribute to morbidity.

AGE-RELATED FACTORS

Infection less likely in dogs >1 year of age, but can still occur, especially if unvaccinated.

ZOONOTIC POTENTIAL

Parvovirus per se is not zoonotic, but these puppies may harbor coinfections with *Giardia,* which can be zoonotic.

PREGNANCY/FERTILITY/BREEDING

Pregnant animals are likely to abort.

SEE ALSO

• Acute Diarrhea.
• Acute Vomiting.
• Canine Coronavirus Infections.
• Gastroenteritis, Acute Hemorrhagic Diarrhea Syndrome.
• Sepsis and Bacteremia.
• Shock, Septic.

ABBREVIATIONS

• CPV = canine parvovirus.
• FPV = feline panleukopenia virus.
• PI = postinfection.

Suggested Reading

Mohr AJ, Leisewitz AL, Jacobson LS, et al. Effect of early enteral nutrition on intestinal permeability, intestinal protein loss, and outcome in dogs with severe parvoviral enteritis. J Vet Intern Med 2003, 17:791–798.

Schoeman JP, Goddard A, Herrtage ME. Serum cortisol and thyroxine concentrations as predictors of death in critically ill puppies with parvoviral diarrhea. J Am Vet Med Assoc 2007, 231:1534–1539.

Venn EC, Preisner K, Boscan PL, et al. Evaluation of an outpatient protocol in the treatment of canine parvoviral enteritis. J Vet Emerg Crit Care 2017, 27:52–65.

Author Johan P. Schoeman
Consulting Editor Amie Koenig

Client Education Handout available online

CANINE SCHISTOSOMIASIS (HETEROBILHARZIASIS)

BASICS

OVERVIEW

- *Heterobilharzia americanum* is a trematode of the genus Schistosoma that has fresh water lymnaeid snails as intermediate hosts and raccoons as the natural definitive host.
- Eggs passed in the feces of raccoons hatch to release miracidia that penetrate freshwater snail hosts. After a period of development and asexual multiplication, the snails release cercariae that infect the next host by skin penetration. After penetrating skin, larvae undergo a migration to the lung and then make their way to mesenteric veins, where separate males and females form pairs. Eggs laid by female worms are carried to the intestinal wall, where they erode their way through to the lumen to be passed in the feces. Other eggs are carried to the liver or other organs by the bloodstream, where they lodge and cause granulomatous disease.
- Dogs become infected in contact with freshwater containing cercariae.
- Endemic in raccoons in southeastern United States; canine cases reported from Arkansas, Indiana, Florida, Georgia, Kansas, Louisiana, North Carolina, Oklahoma, and Texas.

SIGNALMENT

Dogs, typically adult, that have access to swampy areas or bayous.

SIGNS

- Lethargy (most common sign), weight loss, and decreased appetite.
- Other signs include vomiting, diarrhea, anorexia, polyuria/polydipsia; more rarely melena, borborygmus, ascites.

CAUSES & RISK FACTORS

Swimming in freshwater in areas contaminated with cercariae from miracidia.

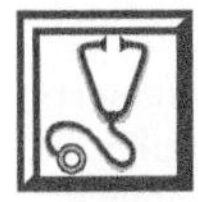

DIAGNOSIS

DIFFERENTIAL DIAGNOSIS

- Coccidiosis.
- Bacterial diarrhea.
- Viral enteritis.
- Hepatopathies.

CBC/BIOCHEMISTRY/URINALYSIS

- CBC—anemia, lymphopenia, eosinopenia or eosinophilia, thrombocytopenia.
- Biochemistry—elevated liver enzyme activities, azotemia, hypercalcemia, hypernatremia, hyperglobulinemia, hypoalbuminemia.
- Urinalysis—proteinuria.

OTHER LABORATORY TESTS

- Elevated parathyroid hormone-related protein (PTH-rp) reported in dogs with hypercalcemia.
- PCR on feces (Texas A&M Gastrointestinal Laboratory).

IMAGING

Contrast radiographs and ultrasound may reveal thickened bowel walls; calcified eggs disseminated into tissues may give the false impression of soft tissue mineralization.

DIAGNOSTIC PROCEDURES

- Eggs with miracidia can be identified in feces, but feces must be kept in saline (not water) or miracidia will spontaneously hatch, making diagnosis impossible.
- Fecal direct or sedimentation methods are preferred to fecal flotation; routine fecal flotation will not detect these heavy eggs; if used, requires flotation with sugar solution with specific gravity of 1.3.
- Histopathology—trematode eggs in multiple organs (especially liver, intestine, pancreas, lymph nodes); lymphoplasmacytic, histiocytic, and eosinophilic to granulomatous enteritis, hepatitis with possible peri-portal fibrosis, dystrophic mineralization of multiple tissues.

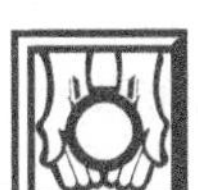

TREATMENT

Inpatient care for the first few days of treatment may be warranted, as the response to worm kill may require supportive care.

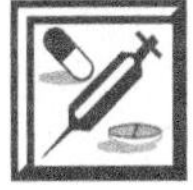

MEDICATIONS

DRUG(S) OF CHOICE

- Praziquantel—25 mg/kg PO q8h for 2–3 days.
- Fenbendazole—50 mg/kg PO q24h for 10 days; clinical improvement without parasite elimination has been reported with fenbendazole.

FOLLOW-UP

- Check feces after treatment to ensure that it does not contain eggs.
- Reinfection from environment is possible.

MISCELLANEOUS

In Japan and other countries with endemic *Schistosoma japonicum*, dogs can be infected with this human and zoonotic species.

ZOONOTIC POTENTIAL

Stages in the dog pose no threat to people; with shared waterway exposure, cercariae can cause skin lesions in people.

SYNONYMS

- Schistosomiasis.
- Swimmer's itch (human, skin penetration of cercariae).

ABBREVIATIONS

- PTH-rp = parathyroid hormone-related protein.

Suggested Reading

Fabrick C, Bugbee A, Fosgate G. Clinical features and outcome of *Heterobilharzia americana* infection in dogs. J Vet Intern Med 2010, 24:140–144.

Flowers JR, Hammerberg B, Wood SL, et al. *Heterobilharzia americana* infection in a dog. J Am Vet Med Assoc 2002, 220:193–196.

Stone RH, Frontera-Acevedo K, Saba CF, et al. Lymphosarcoma associated with *Heterobilharzia americana* infection in a dog. J Vet Diag Invest 2011, 23:1065–1070.

Author Dwight D. Bowman

Consulting Editor Amie Koenig

CAR RIDE ANXIETY—DOGS AND CATS

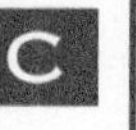

BASICS

DEFINITION

Excessive or disruptive distress, fear, or panic associated with vehicle travel. Anxiety exhibited during travel can be mistaken for excitement.

PATHOPHYSIOLOGY

Unknown or not definitively determined. Lack of car ride experience, generalized anxiety disorder, nausea, previous negative experience with car rides; fear, anxiety, or arousal related to visual or auditory stimuli.

SYSTEMS AFFECTED

- Behavioral.
- Gastrointestinal.
- Neuromuscular.

GENETICS

May be genetic component, but experiential learning may be more significant.

INCIDENCE/PREVALENCE

Reported in over 50% of cats and over 20% of dogs.

SIGNALMENT

Dog and cat.

Breed Predilections

None

Mean Age and Range

Any. Young or ill animals may be predisposed to motion sickness.

Predominant Sex

None

SIGNS

Historical Findings

- May include pacing, restlessness, inappetence, vigilance, excitability, and vocalization including whining or high-pitched barking in dogs and growling, hissing, meowing, or yowling in cats.
- Locomotion varies between individuals—some may pace while others remain immobile; fear that manifests as freezing or hiding may be underrecognized and underreported.
- Pet-related panic, vocalization, and pacing may impair owner's ability to drive safely.
- Travel-related anxiety may prevent owners from taking pets to destinations (e.g., veterinary visits, grooming, social events, training).

Physiologic and Physical Signs

May include panting, rapid heart rate, drooling, urination, vomiting, defecation.

Physical Examination

Normal unless underlying medical problems.

CAUSES & RISK FACTORS

- Behavioral causes include unruliness, inadequate or poor prior experience traveling; insufficient adaptation to carriers, leashes, or restraint devices; fear and reactivity to visual stimuli such as people, animals, bikes, or cars; and generalized anxiety.
- Prior stressful or uncomfortable experiences following car rides such as veterinary visits, boarding, or shelter relinquishment.
- Traumatic events such as sudden stops or car accidents.
- Medical conditions may exacerbate or manifest as anxiety—motion sickness, musculoskeletal pain or discomfort, dental disease or pain, gastrointestinal upset, sensory hypersensitivity.

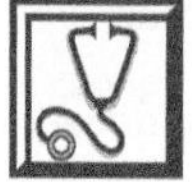

DIAGNOSIS

DIFFERENTIAL DIAGNOSIS

- Fear and anxiety-related behavior.
- Manifestation of pain, nausea, or physical discomfort.
- Acute onset or abrupt change in car ride anxiety warrants ruling out contributory medical conditions.

CBC/BIOCHEMISTRY/URINALYSIS

If indicated by clinical signs and prior to drug therapy.

OTHER LABORATORY TESTS

If indicated by clinical signs.

IMAGING

If indicated by clinical signs.

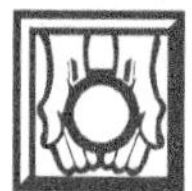

TREATMENT

ACTIVITY

Normal. Recommend adequate exercise and play before car ride.

DIET

- Normal.
- Providing highly palatable food during car travel may distract, reduce stress, and promote a positive association with car travel.
- If the pet has experienced nausea or vomiting in association with car travel, fasting is recommended.

CLIENT EDUCATION

A complete behavior program includes empathy, environmental management, and behavior modification together with supplements or medication where indicated.

Compassion

- Give thoughtful preparation and consideration for the pet's perspective before traveling; allow time for travel and be patient.
- Anticipate and avoid evoking the pet's fears to prevent exacerbating established fears; for example, when carrying a pet in a carrier, consider their viewpoint and the unsettling motion that may be experienced.
- Avoid reprimands or scolding.
- Avoid forcing pets that are unfamiliar or do not get along to be in close proximity.

Management and Safety

- Provide stable footing and secure resting locations.
- Consider crating if pet acclimated to crate confinement; pet seat belts, barriers, and seat slings can also be beneficial.
- A nondriver should accompany highly distressed pets.

Anxiety Reduction

- Multimodal comforting and anxiolytic support provides the best outcome.
- Window shades, covered crates, solid wall carriers, or products for dogs such as Doggles® or Thundercap® may alleviate anxiety related to visual stimuli.
- Classical music or psychoacoustically designed music for dogs or cats may help to calm; music or white noise may mute perception of fear-evoking sounds.
- Comforting pressure wraps may alleviate anxiety.
- Synthetic pheromone analogues (Adaptil®, Feliway®) sprayed into carriers, onto bedding, or on a bandana (for dogs) may reduce anxiety.
- Anxiety-reducing supplements or medications should be considered.

Behavior Modification

- Rehearse settle and relax positions when not traveling.
- Teach the dog to get in and out of the car by positive reinforcement (e.g., food or toy reward).
- Teach cats and small dogs to go in and out of carriers willingly; they should be acclimated to the motion of being in a carrier that is being carried.
- Practice training when travel is not imminent; use positive reinforcement training and avoid reprimand or intimidation training; animals should never receive corrections from shock, prong, or choke collars.
- During travel, provide comforting activities such as toys, food chews, or feeding puzzles that may distract the pet, reduce anxiety, or counter-condition the pet to car rides.

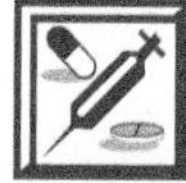

MEDICATIONS

DRUG(S) OF CHOICE

General Comments

- Psychotropic medication, supplements, or pheromones may be beneficial or necessary

Table 1

Benzodiazepine doses		
	Canine	*Feline*
Alprazolam	0.02–0.1 mg/kg PO q6–12h	0.025–0.1 mg/kg PO q8–24h
Clonazepam	0.1–1.0 mg/kg PO q8–12h	0.02–0.2 mg/kg PO q12–24h
Diazepam	0.5–2 mg/kg PO PRN (e.g., q6h)	
Lorazepam	0.025–0.2 mg/kg PO q24h to PRN	0.025–0.05 mg/kg PO 12–24h
Oxazepam	0.2–1 mg/kg PO q12–24h	0.2–0.5 mg/kg PO 12–24h

as an adjunct to the behavior program; short-acting anxiolytics are appropriate for pets traveling occasionally; administer anxiolytics so that optimal effect precedes onset of anxiety; the effect of anxiolytics may be overcome by severe anxiety or distress; high or repeated doses, extreme anxiety, and other medical conditions increase the risk for profound sedation and drug reactions.

- Drugs should be trial dosed in advance to determine effects, side effects, optimal dose, and duration.
- Address concurrent behavioral conditions (e.g., separation anxiety, fears, phobias, anxiety, reactivity) that may warrant ongoing anxiolytics (e.g., tricyclic antidepressants [TCAs] or selective serotonin reuptake inhibitors [SSRIs]) in conjunction with the treatment of travel-related anxiety.

Benzodiazepines

- Anxiolytic; see Table 1 for drug options and dosing information.
- Give 30–60 minutes prior to travel.
- Side effects—incoordination, hyperphagia, paradoxical excitability, muscle relaxation, possible amnesic effect that might interfere with learning.
- Hyperphagia may be advantageous for pets with stress anorexia.
- Oxazepam and lorazepam have no active intermediate metabolites and may be safer if hepatic function compromised; injectable midazolam may be useful if administered in the veterinary hospital before home travel.

Maropitant

- May be indicated for nausea related to travel and prior to opioid sedation.
- Dog—1–2 mg/kg PO 2h before travel; for motion sickness 8 mg/kg given with a small amount of food 1–2h before travel.
- Cat—1 mg/kg SC daily.

Trazodone

- Dog—2–5 mg/kg; titrate up to 5–10 mg/kg based on effect; higher doses may be utilized by experienced clinicians; may be started twice daily 12–48h in advance.
- Cat—25–50 mg/cat for car travel.
- Side effects—sedation, lethargy, incoordination, cardiac conduction disturbances, agitation.

Gabapentin

- Cat—20 mg/kg (50–150 mg/cat) 2–3h before travel.
- Dog—10–30 mg/kg PRN to BID; may be started twice daily 12–48h in advance.
- Side effects—sedation, ataxia.

Clonidine

- Dog—0.01–0.05 mg/kg PO; begin at low dose and titrate to most effective dose; maximum effect may take up to 2h with faster absorption on an empty stomach; may be started twice daily 12–48h in advance.
- Side effects—transient hyperglycemia, anticholinergic, hypotension, collapse, bradycardia, agitation; use with caution in cardiac disease or compromised renal or liver function.

Dexmedetomidine Oromucosal Gel

- Dogs—125 μg/m^2 onto oral mucosa 30–60 min prior to travel; can be repeated in 2h.
- Licensed for use in dogs with noise aversion.
- Side effects—sedation, paradoxical excitement, pale mucous membranes, emesis.

Acepromazine

- Dog and cat—0.5–2.2 mg/kg PO.
- Not for sole use; may be combined with anxiolytic medication for added sedation.
- Side effects—ataxia, inhibits thermoregulation, peripheral vasodilation, muscle tremor or spasm, altered noise reactivity.

Pheromone

F3 cheek gland pheromone or dog-appeasing pheromone given 30–60 min before travel.

Natural Supplements

- For mild to moderate anxiety or adjunctive therapy—alpha-casosopene alone or in a diet in combination with l-tryptophan; l-theanine alone or in combination products containing whey protein, *Phellodendron amurense*, and *Magnolia officinalis*; melatonin; *Souroubea* and *Plantanus*; or a calming probiotic supplement.
- Lavender essential oils may have a calming effect in dogs, but avoid in cats since floral scents may be aversive.

CONTRAINDICATIONS

Avoid use or use with caution in combination with any drug that enhances serotonin transmission (e.g., trazodone, SSRIs, TCAs) and that may pose an increased risk for serotonin syndrome.

PRECAUTIONS

All listed medications are extra-label or off-label (except maropitant). Use with informed consent.

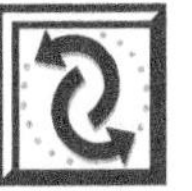

FOLLOW-UP

PATIENT MONITORING

Ask about travel-related distress as part of wellness assessment, and recommend early intervention and prevention. Travel-related difficulties pose a barrier for bringing pets to the veterinary hospital.

PREVENTION/AVOIDANCE

- Provide preventive guidance on making travel positive and carrier training at first puppy or kitten visit.
- Avoid travel for severely affected pets.
- Use appropriate medication when travel required.

EXPECTED COURSE AND PROGNOSIS

Likely to worsen if untreated.

MISCELLANEOUS

ASSOCIATED CONDITIONS

- Generalized anxiety disorder, noise-related fears and phobias, separation anxiety; hyperattachment.
- Dental disease or pain.

AGE-RELATED FACTORS

Cognitive decline may exacerbate anxiety.

ZOONOTIC POTENTIAL

A distressed pet may cause distraction and put drivers at risk for accidents.

PREGNANCY/FERTILITY/BREEDING

Drug use in breeding, pregnant, or lactating animals should be avoided.

SEE ALSO

- Fear and Aggression in Veterinary Visits—Cats.
- Fear and Aggression in Veterinary Visits—Dogs.
- Fears, Phobias, and Anxieties—Cats.
- Fears, Phobias, and Anxieties—Dogs.

ABBREVIATIONS

- SSRI = selective serotonin reuptake inhibitor.
- TCA = tricyclic antidepressant.

INTERNET RESOURCES

www.catalystcouncil.org/resources/video

Suggested Reading

Crowell-Davis SL, Murray T, Dantas L. Veterinary Psychopharmacology, 2nd ed. Hoboken, NJ: Wiley, 2019.

Horwitz D, ed. Blackwell's 5 Minute Consult Clinical Companion: Canine and Feline Behavior, 2nd ed. Hoboken, NJ: Wiley, 2018, pp. 873–884.

Author Theresa L. DePorter
Consulting Editor Gary M. Landsberg

CARBON MONOXIDE TOXICOSIS

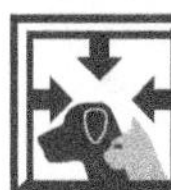

BASICS

OVERVIEW

- Carbon monoxide (CO)—odorless, colorless, nonirritating gas produced by inefficient combustion of carbon fuels.
- Common sources are fires, automotive exhaust, leaking coal, oil, or natural gas/propane furnaces, gas appliances or fireplaces, and some paint strippers and sprays.
- CO is absorbed into the blood, forming carboxyhemoglobin (COHb).
- Affinity of CO for hemoglobin is approximately 240 times that of oxygen.
- COHb cannot bind oxygen and impairs oxyhemoglobin from releasing oxygen to the tissues.
- Major effect is acute cellular hypoxia, leading to death.
- Survivors may have cardiac damage, acute and delayed neurotoxicity.
- Lethal concentration is approximately 1,000 ppm (0.1%) for 1 hour.

SIGNALMENT

Dogs and cats equally affected.

SIGNS

Acute Exposure

- Acute signs progress within minutes to hours.
- Neurologic signs—lethargy or agitation, weakness, ataxia, depressed mentation, deafness, coma, seizures.
- Respiratory—tachypnea and dyspnea.
- Cardiovascular—tachycardia, dysrhythmias, hypotension.
- Hyperemic skin and mucous membranes are rarely apparent in animals.

Chronic Exposure

- Nausea, vomiting, decreased activity, and cough; may mimic other diseases.
- Disturbance of postural and position reflexes and gait.

CAUSES & RISK FACTORS

- Housed in areas with blocked exhaust vents, furnaces, appliances, or chimneys; exposure to automobile exhaust or kerosene heaters in closed spaces with poor ventilation.
- Trapped in house or kennel fires.
- Animals with impaired cardiac or pulmonary function.

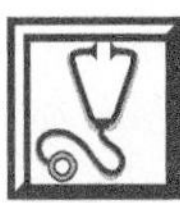

DIAGNOSIS

DIFFERENTIAL DIAGNOSIS

- Sedatives, ethanol, ethylene glycol, petroleum hydrocarbons, lead poisoning; cyanide or hydrogen sulfide gas toxicosis.
- Smoke inhalation, primary neurologic disease, and severe metabolic disease.

CBC/BIOCHEMISTRY/URINALYSIS

Biochemistry—may see liver and kidney value elevations secondary to hypoxia.

OTHER LABORATORY TESTS

- Carboxyhemoglobin can be measured via co-oximetry; may return to normal within hours after removal from CO source. Available at human hospital or veterinary specialty/diagnostic lab.
- Blood gas—metabolic acidosis due to lactic acidosis; arterial blood gas may have normal partial pressure of oxygen (PaO_2).

IMAGING

Thoracic radiographs—evaluate for pulmonary injury and rule out other causes of respiratory signs.

DIAGNOSTIC PROCEDURES

- Pulse oximetry may overestimate hemoglobin saturation (SpO_2); COHb and oxyhemoglobin absorb light at the same wavelength.
- ECG—sinus tachycardia or cardiac dysrhythmia, ST-T depression with myocardial hypoxia/anoxia.
- Blood pressure—hypotension common in shock.

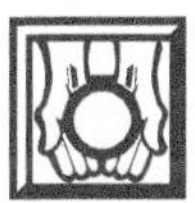

TREATMENT

- Supplemental oxygen (flow-by, mask, nasal, oxygen cage, or intubation ± mechanical ventilation)—improves oxygen delivery to vital organs, especially brain and heart; decreases half-life of COHb.
- Hyperbaric oxygen therapy use is controversial and not readily available in veterinary medicine, but will further reduce half-life of COHb.
- IV fluid therapy for hydration and perfusion and to correct metabolic acidosis.

MEDICATIONS

DRUG(S) OF CHOICE

- Sedatives and anxiolytics may be needed to allow oxygen supplementation—diazepam 0.1–0.5 mg/kg IV q6–8h.
- Short-acting opioids such as fentanyl (2–5 µg/kg IV followed by CRI 2–5 µg/kg/h) can be used for pain and sedation.

CONTRAINDICATIONS/POSSIBLE INTERACTIONS

Limit 100% oxygen to <24 hours to avoid oxygen toxicosis.

FOLLOW-UP

- Patient monitoring—neurologic status, BP and ECG during hospitalization; frequency depends on stability of patient.
- Possible complications—delayed neurologic signs within days to weeks of initial improvement; deafness may occur/persist in survivors.
- Expected course and prognosis—respond and improve rapidly to oxygen therapy (within 30–60 minutes); prognosis guarded to poor with persistent or worsening respiratory and neurologic signs.
- Prevention—use adequate ventilation with use of kerosene heaters in kennels and use CO detectors.

MISCELLANEOUS

ASSOCIATED CONDITIONS

Animals in house fires may have dermal burns, thermal and smoke inhalation injury to the airways, corneal ulcerations, or other injuries.

ZOONOTIC POTENTIAL

People and other pets in the same CO-contaminated environment are at risk.

PREGNANCY/FERTILITY/BREEDING

CO reduces oxygen-carrying ability of maternal blood, producing fetal hypoxia, abortion, or neurologic impairment of the fetus, often with minimal effects on the dam.

ABBREVIATIONS

- COHb = carboxyhemoglobin.
- PaO_2 = partial pressure of oxygen.
- SpO_2 = oxygen saturation.

Suggested Reading

Berent AC, Todd J, Sergeeff J, et al. Carbon monoxide toxicity: a case series. J Vet Emerg Crit Care 2005, 15(2):128–135.

Fitzgerald KT. Carbon monoxide. In: Peterson ME, Talcott PA, eds. Small Animal Toxicology, 3rd ed. St. Louis, MO: Elsevier Saunders, 2013, pp. 479–487.

Vaughn L, Beckel N. Severe burn injury, burn shock, and smoke inhalation injury in small animals. Part 1: Burn classification and pathophysiology. J Vet Emerg Crit Care 2012, 22(2):179–186.

Vaughn L, Beckel N, Walters P. Severe burn injury, burn shock, and smoke inhalation injury in small animals. Part 2: Diagnosis, therapy, complications, and prognosis. J Vet Emerg Crit Care 2012, 22(2):187–200.

Author Katherine L. Peterson

Consulting Editor Lynn R. Hovda

Acknowledgment The author and book editors acknowledge the prior contribution of Gary D. Osweiler.

CARCINOID AND CARCINOID SYNDROME

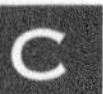

BASICS

OVERVIEW

- Carcinoid tumors are neuroendocrine tumors arising from amine precursor uptake and decarboxylation (APUD) cells.
- Carcinoids originate from enterochromaffin and enterochromaffin-like cells of the gastrointestinal tract, but can be found in the liver, gall bladder, pancreas, tracheobronchial tree and genitourinary system due to embryologic origins.
- Carcinoids may secrete amines such as histamine, serotonin, prostaglandin, and peptides such as bradykinins and tachykinins.
- In humans, secretion causes "carcinoid syndrome." This occurs in approximately 5–10% of patients with metastatic carcinoid tumors. Hepatic degradation of excess amines, notably seratonin, is bypassed, causing clinical signs. Human carcinoid syndrome is characterized by flushing, abdominal pain, diarrhea, bronchospasm, and cyanosis. This syndrome has not been reported in small animals, although a recent report describes a dog with episodic collapse and melena and an ileocecal carcinoid.
- Morbidity and mortality are more often a function of tumor size and gastrointestinal blockage.
- Primary carcinoid tumors in dogs have been reported in the stomach, small intestine, colon, lung, gallbladder, and liver. In cats, carcinoids have been found in the stomach, small intestine, liver, and heart.

SIGNALMENT

- Dog—rare, generally >8–9 years of age.
- Cat—rare, generally >7–8 years of age.

SIGNS

Clinical signs depend on the location of the primary tumor or metastases and may include anorexia, vomiting, dyschezia, melena, collapse, ascites, weight loss, and signs of hepatic failure or gall bladder obstruction.

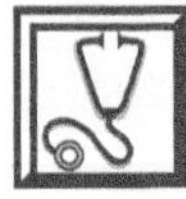

DIAGNOSIS

DIFFERENTIAL DIAGNOSIS

Differentials include primary gastrointestinal diseases—neoplasia, infection, inflammation, parasites, foreign body, dietary indiscretion, or hepatic/biliary disease.

CBC/BIOCHEMISTRY/URINALYSIS

- Normal, possible mild nonregenerative anemia.
- Electrolyte abnormalities, elevated liver enzyme activities, and hyperbilirubinemia can be present.

OTHER LABORATORY TESTS

- Serum serotonin, serum chromogranin A, and urinary 5-hydroxyindoleacetic acid are measured in humans suspected of carcinoid tumors; these tests are more diagnostic than direct measurement of serum amine and peptides.
- Serum serotonin levels were found to be increased tenfold in a dog with an intestinal carcinoid; other testing has not been documented in animals with carcinoid tumors.

IMAGING

- Radiography and ultrasound can identify primary tumors and metastases.
- CT scan and MRI may also be useful.
- In humans, more sensitive molecular imaging includes radiolabeled somatostatin receptor scintigraphy (OctreoScan); radioiodinated metaiodobenzylguanidine (MIBG) imaging; and PET scans.

DIAGNOSTIC PROCEDURES

- Biopsy often confirms diagnosis.
- If histopathologic results are equivocal, electron microscopy and/or immunohistochemistry (looking for chromogranin A and/or synaptophysin expression) may be used to confirm a carcinoid tumor.

PATHOLOGIC FINDINGS

Tumors have a fine fibrovascular stroma with minimal to moderate cellular pleomorphism. Cytoplasm is eosinophilic and usually contains secretory granules that stain argyrophilic and/or argentaffin-positive (silver stains).

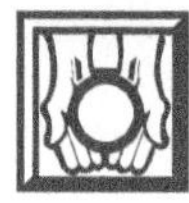

TREATMENT

In some cases, surgical excision can be curative, especially if no metastasis. Debulking can decrease hormone secretion in humans, and it may relieve tumor-related gastrointestinal obstruction.

MEDICATIONS

DRUG(S) OF CHOICE

- Octreotide, a somatostatin analogue that inhibits hormone secretion from the tumor cells, is used in humans for palliative therapy; as carcinoid syndrome has not been reliably reported in animals with carcinoid tumors, octreotide may be of little benefit.
- High-dose radioiodinated MIBG is used in humans with nonresectable or metastatic carcinoid.
- Interferons have demonstrated limited success in humans with carcinoid tumors.
- Chemotherapy and radiotherapy have minimal efficacy in humans with carcinoid tumors.
- Adjuvant carboplatin therapy has been reported in a dog with a completely excised nonmetastatic jejunal carcinoid.

FOLLOW-UP

Abdominal ultrasound and thoracic radiographs should be performed regularly to identify metastasis.

EXPECTED COURSE AND PROGNOSIS

- Limited survival data exists (few reported cases).
- Survival of 18 months seen in dog with intestinal carcinoid treated with surgery and carboplatin.
- Survival of 12 months reported in cats with extrahepatic carcinoids.

MISCELLANEOUS

ABBREVIATIONS

- APUD = amine precursor uptake and decarboxylation.
- MIBG = metaiodobenzylguanidine.

INTERNET RESOURCES

https://www.carcinoid.com

Suggested Reading

Corrigan A, Bechtel S. APUDomas: diagnosis, supportive care, and definitive treatment. Proceedings of the American College of Veterinary Internal Medicine Forum, Indianapolis, Indiana, 2015.

Rossmeisl JH Jr., Forrester SD, Robertson JL, Cook WT. Chronic vomiting associated with a gastric carcinoid in a cat. J Am Anim Hosp Assoc 2002, 38(1):61–66.

Author Virginia L. Gill

Consulting Editor Patty A. Lathan

CARDIAC GLYCOSIDE PLANT TOXICOSIS

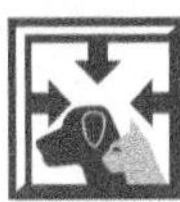

BASICS

OVERVIEW

- Same toxic profile as digoxin, in particular cardiovascular (CV) and gastrointestinal (GI) signs.
- All plant parts, fresh or dry, are considered toxic, but the concentration varies depending on specific plant and plant part.
- Plants are best identified by scientific name.
- Common plants include *Adenium obesum* (desert rose); *Apocynum cannabinum* (dogbane); *Asclepias* spp. (milkweed); *Calatropis* spp. (giant milkweed); *Convallaria majalis* (lily of the valley); *Digitalis lanata* (wooly foxglove); *Digitalis purpurea* (common or purple foxglove); *Kalanchoe* spp. (mother of millions); *Nerium oleander* (oleander); *Ornithogalum umbellatum* (star of Bethlehem); *Thevetia peruviana* (yellow oleander).

SIGNALMENT

- Cats are more sensitive to some of the plant toxins than dogs.
- Dogs with the ABCB1-1Δ gene mutation *may* be more sensitive to toxins.

SIGNS

- CV—bradycardia (rarely tachycardia), atrioventricular (AV) block, all forms of arrhythmias, death from asystole.
- GI (most frequent)—hypersalivation, vomiting ± blood, diarrhea ± blood.
- Neuromuscular—coma, tremors, seizures (rarely); may be related to decreased cardiac output.

CAUSES & RISK FACTORS

- Cardiac glycoside–containing plants inhibit the ATPase sodium/potassium pump, resulting in an increase in intracellular sodium and a decrease in intracellular potassium; increased intracellular (myocyte) calcium results in increased cardiac contractions.
- Animals with a prior history of cardiac or renal disease and receiving digoxin or other cardiac glycoside drugs are at risk.

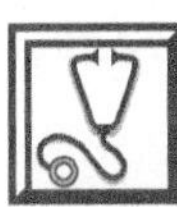

DIAGNOSIS

DIFFERENTIAL DIAGNOSIS

- Beta blocker or calcium channel blocker toxicosis.
- Cardiac disease in general.
- Digoxin/digitoxin toxicosis.
- Ingestion of medications with known cardiac effects.
- Ingestion of other plants with known cardiac effects such as *Taxus* spp. (yew), *Rhododendron* spp. (azalea, rhododendron), *Kalmia* spp. (mountain laurel, lambkill), and *Pieris japonica* (Japanese pieris).

CBC/BIOCHEMISTRY/URINALYSIS

Serum chemistry—hyperkalemia early and severe, may switch to hypokalemia.

OTHER LABORATORY TESTS

Serum digoxin levels may be useful in some ingestions.

DIAGNOSTIC PROCEDURES

- Presence of plant pieces in vomit or stool.
- ECG monitoring for cardiac arrhythmias.

PATHOLOGIC FINDINGS

Sudden death is common. Plant pieces are often found in the stomach and small intestine. Clotted blood may be present in the ventricles with a mottled appearance to the epicardium. Histopathology findings are similar to digoxin toxicosis.

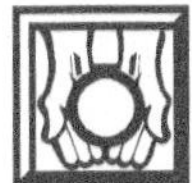

TREATMENT

- Emesis *quickly after ingestion*.
- Activated charcoal (1–2 g/kg) with a cathartic × 1, followed by activated charcoal without a cathartic every 6–8 hours × 2 doses.
- Asymptomatic animals—hospitalize and monitor for 12 hours.
- Symptomatic animals—hospitalize and monitor with an ECG for 24 hours; administer appropriate IV fluids (dependent on serum potassium) to maintain blood pressure but not overload the CV system; monitor blood pressure closely, as hypotension may be persistent.

MEDICATIONS

DRUG(S) OF CHOICE

- Digoxin-specific fragment antigen binding (Fab; Digibind®) may be useful in some cases, especially oleander toxicosis.
- Antiemetics if vomiting is severe or persistent—maropitant 1 mg/kg SC/IV/PO q24h in dogs and cats; ondansetron 0.5–1 mg/kg IV, SC, PO q8–12h in dogs and cats.
- Bradycardia—atropine 0.02–0.04 mg/kg IV/IM/SC in dogs and cats; repeat q4–6h as needed.
- Antiarrhythmics may be necessary in patients with ventricular dysrhythmias, evidence of poor perfusion, or who remain tachycardic despite IV fluid therapy—lidocaine: dogs, 2–4 mg/kg IV to effect.
- GI protectants as needed—H2 blockers such as famotidine (0.5–1 mg/kg PO/SC/IM/IV q12h); omeprazole (0.5 mg/kg PO daily); or sucralfate (0.25–1 g PO q8h).

CONTRAINDICATIONS/POSSIBLE INTERACTIONS

Beta blockers and calcium channel blockers may have an additive effect on AV conduction and cause complete heart block.

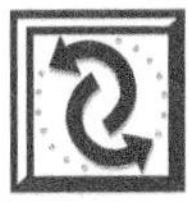

FOLLOW-UP

PATIENT MONITORING

- ECG and blood pressure monitoring for first 24 hours, then PRN.
- Strict attention to serum electrolytes.

PREVENTION/AVOIDANCE

- Identify and recognize plants.
- Oleander grows seemingly everywhere in parts of the SW United States and off-leash dogs and cats should be monitored closely.

POSSIBLE COMPLICATIONS

Sudden death.

EXPECTED COURSE AND PROGNOSIS

- Good nursing care for 5–7 days.
- Prognosis is good with early and appropriate care.
- Cardiac arrhythmias prolong treatment and hospitalization.

MISCELLANEOUS

ABBREVIATIONS

- AV = atrioventricular.
- CV = cardiovascular.
- Fab = fragment antigen binding.
- GI = gastrointestinal.

INTERNET RESOURCES

- http://www.petpoisonhelpline.com/poisons
- http://www.aspca.org/pet-care/animal-poison-control/toxic-and-non-toxic-plants

Suggested Reading

Eucher J. Cardiac glycosides. In: Hovda LR, Brutlag A, Poppenga RH, Peterson K, eds. Blackwell's Five-Minute Veterinary Consult Clinical Companion: Small Animal Toxicology. Ames, IA: Wiley-Blackwell, 2016, pp. 760–769.

Author Lynn R. Hovda
Consulting Editor Lynn R. Hovda

Client Education Handout available online

CARDIOMYOPATHY, ARRHYTHMOGENIC RIGHT VENTRICULAR—CATS

BASICS

OVERVIEW

Arrhythmogenic right ventricular cardiomyopathy (ARVC) is a rare primary cardiomyopathy characterized by progressive atrophy of the right ventricular (RV) and/or right atrial (RA) myocardium, with replacement by fatty or fibrofatty tissue that may act as an arrhythmogenic substrate. The condition in cats typically manifests as signs of right-sided congestive heart failure (CHF) due to progressive RV dysfunction. A variety of arrhythmias have been observed in cats with ARVC; however, sudden death does not appear to be well recognized in this species.

SIGNALMENT

- Cats.
- One study reported mean age at presentation of 7.3 years (range: 1–20 years).
- Breed or sex predilections unknown.

SIGNS

General Comments

Compared to dogs and humans, sudden death does not appear to be as well recognized in cats with ARVC, despite the wide variety of arrhythmias documented with this condition.

Historical Findings

- Lethargy.
- Anorexia.
- Dyspnea.
- Tachypnea.
- Abdominal distention may be noted.

Physical Examination Findings

- Signs consistent with right-sided CHF.
- Dyspnea.
- Tachypnea.
- Jugular venous distention.
- Ascites.
- Heart and/or lung sounds may be muffled.
- Weak femoral pulses.
- Hepatosplenomegaly.
- Thoracic percussion may reveal presence of pleural effusion.
- May auscult arrhythmia.

CAUSES & RISK FACTORS

- Unknown.
- A genetic mutation in the striatin (desmosomal protein) gene is associated with ARVC in some dogs. Genetic mutations are identified in approximately 60% of humans with ARVC, with mutations identified in at least 13 genes. Genetic studies in feline ARVC are lacking.

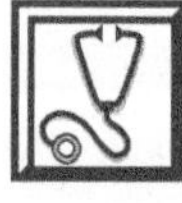

DIAGNOSIS

DIFFERENTIAL DIAGNOSIS

Uhl's anomaly—a congenital abnormality characterized by partial or complete absence of myocardium in the RV free wall. Histopathology is required to distinguish this from ARVC and demonstrates apposing endocardial and epicardial surfaces, without any interposed adipose tissue or any evidence of inflammation or necrosis.

CBC/BIOCHEMISTRY/URINALYSIS

Alanine aminotransferase may be elevated secondary to hepatic congestion.

IMAGING

Radiographic Findings

- Cardiomegaly, typically in regions of right atrium and right ventricle; left atrial enlargement may also be noted.
- Pleural effusion.
- Ascites.
- Pericardial effusion.
- Caudal vena caval dilation.

Echocardiographic Findings

- Severe RA and RV dilation.
- RV systolic dysfunction/hypokinesis.
- Tricuspid regurgitation.
- Paradoxical septal motion.
- Focal aneurysms may be observed in the RV wall, often toward the apex.
- Left atrial enlargement sometimes seen.

DIAGNOSTIC PROCEDURES

ECG

- A variety of various arrhythmias have been observed in cats with ARVC.
- Ventricular premature complexes (right-sided or left-sided in origin).
- Ventricular tachycardia.
- Atrial fibrillation.
- Supraventricular tachycardia.
- Ventricular premature complexes.
- Right bundle branch block.
- First-degree atrioventricular block.
- Third-degree atrioventricular block.
- RA and RV enlargement (tall P wave, deep S waves in lead II), right axis deviation.

Paracentesis and Fluid Analysis

Fluid analysis of pleural or abdominal effusions typically reveals modified transudate consistent with right-sided CHF.

PATHOLOGIC FINDINGS

Gross Pathology

- Moderate-to-severe RA and RV dilation.
- Severe thinning of RA and RV walls, which are easily trans-illuminated.
- Left atrial dilation and rarely left ventricular dilation may be seen in some cats.
- Thrombi sometimes identified.

Histopathology

- RV myocardial atrophy with replacement by fatty or fibrofatty tissue.
- Fibrosis may also be observed in right atrium, left ventricular free wall, and interventricular septum.
- Focal or multifocal myocarditis.
- Apoptotic cardiomyocytes.

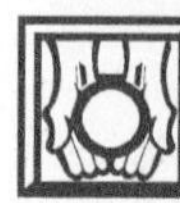

TREATMENT

- Medical management of right-sided CHF is the mainstay of treatment for clinically affected cats with ARVC.
- Anti-arrhythmic therapy is not routinely required, but in cases with hemodynamically significant arrhythmias, anti-arrhythmic drugs should be selected based on the suspected underlying mechanism of the arrhythmia.

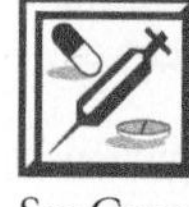

MEDICATIONS

See Congestive Heart Failure, Right-Sided.

FOLLOW-UP

PATIENT MONITORING

Recheck when decompensation or other clinical signs develop.

EXPECTED COURSE AND PROGNOSIS

Prognosis appears to be very poor in cats identified with ARVC. Reported median survival time after development of clinical signs of approximately 1 month (range: 2 days to 4 months). Most cats die or are euthanized due to signs of right-sided CHF or thromboembolic complications.

MISCELLANEOUS

SEE ALSO

- Cardiomyopathy, Arrhythmogenic Right Ventricular—Dogs.
- Congestive Heart Failure, Right-Sided.

ABBREVIATIONS

- ARVC = arrhythmogenic right ventricular cardiomyopathy.
- CHF = congestive heart failure.
- RA = right atrial.
- RV = right ventricular.

Suggested Reading

Fox P, Maron B, Basso C, et al. Spontaneously occurring arrhythmogenic right ventricular cardiomyopathy in the domestic cat: a new animal model similar to the human disease. Circulation 2000, 102(15):1863–1870.

Author Michael Aherne
Consulting Editor Michael Aherne

CARDIOMYOPATHY, ARRHYTHMOGENIC RIGHT VENTRICULAR—DOGS

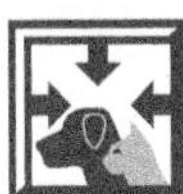

BASICS

OVERVIEW

A myocardial disease commonly characterized by ventricular tachyarrhythmias that can be accompanied by syncope or sudden death. A small percentage (<5%) develop congestive heart failure with systolic dysfunction, comparable to the dilated cardiomyopathy observed in other breeds.

SIGNALMENT

- Dog.
- Specific to the boxer, although a similar presentation is infrequently observed in the English bulldog.
- Usually observed in mature dogs between 5 and 8 years of age. Dogs as young as 6 months have been reported and some affected dogs may not develop clinical signs until >10 years of age.

SIGNS

- Usually one of three presentations:
  - Asymptomatic dog with ventricular premature complexes (VPCs) detected on routine examination.
  - Syncope with VPCs detected on ECG or Holter monitor.
  - Signs of left heart failure (e.g., tachypnea, coughing) or biventricular failure (e.g., ascites, tachypnea, coughing) with VPCs; this presentation is least common.
- Sudden death may occur before development of obvious clinical signs.

CAUSES & RISK FACTORS

- Adult onset, inherited (autosomal dominant).
- A genetic mutation (deletion) in a cardiac desmosomal gene (striatin) is associated with the development of the disease. Dogs that are homozygous for the striatin deletion appear to be more likely to be more severely affected with a higher number of VPCs, and are more likely to have cardiac dilation and myocardial dysfunction. Sudden death is more common. It is not yet known if this is the only genetic cause or if additional genetic mutations will be identified.
- At least one family of boxers with VPCs, ventricular dilation, and systolic dysfunction was found to have decreased myocardial l-carnitine levels and demonstrated some clinical improvement when supplemented with l-carnitine. The cause and effect of this relationship is unclear, and response to this supplementation does not occur in all dogs with myocardial dysfunction.

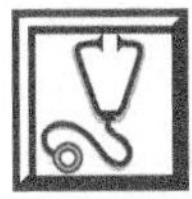

DIAGNOSIS

DIFFERENTIAL DIAGNOSIS

- Aortic stenosis—moderate and severe forms can be associated with VPCs.
- Uncommon forms of acquired cardiac disease (neoplasia, endocarditis).
- Abdominal disease (especially splenic disease) can be associated with VPCs.
- Echocardiography and abdominal ultrasonography can be used to differentiate other causes of cardiac and abdominal disease.

OTHER LABORATORY TESTS

- Genetic testing can now be performed to screen for the genetic mutation (https://cvm.ncsu.edu/genetics) associated with arrhythmogenic right ventricular cardiomyopathy. Submission samples can be either a blood sample in an EDTA tube or a buccal swab of the oral mucosal surface.
- Plasma l-carnitine levels may be evaluated in boxers with ventricular dilation and systolic dysfunction. However, plasma levels are not always reflective of myocardial levels. If plasma levels are not low, it is still possible to have low myocardial levels, and supplementation with l-carnitine might be considered.

IMAGING

Thoracic Radiography

- Normal in most affected dogs.
- Dogs with ventricular dilation and systolic dysfunction may have cardiac enlargement and evidence of heart failure (e.g., pulmonary edema).

Echocardiography

- Normal in most affected dogs.
- A small percentage of dogs have ventricular dilation and systolic dysfunction, particularly if they are homozygous for the deletion mutation.

DIAGNOSTIC PROCEDURES

ECG

- Many dogs will not have VPCs on an ECG of brief duration since the arrhythmia can be intermittent. However, some dogs will have one or more upright VPCs on a brief lead II ECG.
- In either case, if suspicion of disease is present, Holter monitoring is recommended to determine the severity and complexity of the arrhythmia and to have a baseline for comparison once treatment is started. If Holter monitoring is not available and the dog is symptomatic with upright VPCs on an ECG, therapy should be considered.

PATHOLOGIC FINDINGS

- Gross pathology is nonspecific in most cases. In a small percentage of cases, left and right ventricular dilation may be observed.
- Histopathologic abnormalities include a fatty and fibrous infiltrate into the right ventricular (and sometimes interventricular and left ventricular) free wall.

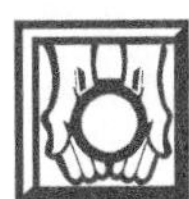

TREATMENT

- The goals of therapy include reduction of the number of VPCs, reduction of clinical signs, and reduction of the risk of sudden cardiac death. Unfortunately, there is no evidence that therapy can reduce the risk of sudden death. The decision to start therapy in the asymptomatic boxer with VPCs is controversial, since all antiarrhythmics have the potential to make the arrhythmia worse. However, dogs with as few as 300 VPCs/24 hours have been observed to die suddenly. In general, initiate antiarrhythmic drugs if there are >1,000 VPCs/24 hours and/or significant runs of ventricular tachycardia or other signs of arrhythmia complexity (e.g., bigeminy, couplets), or clinical signs (syncope, exercise intolerance) related to the VPCs.
- Syncope and sudden cardiac death may be more frequently associated with stress and excitement. Reduce stress and effort when possible. There is no direct relationship between exercise restriction and survivability. Some dogs die while asleep. Thus, strict exercise restriction is not recommended.

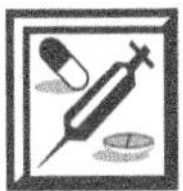

MEDICATIONS

DRUG(S) OF CHOICE

- The two best choices for treating the ventricular arrhythmia are sotalol (1.5–2.0 mg/kg PO q12h) or mexiletine (5–6 mg/kg PO q8h). Some cases continue to have significant ventricular ectopy after treatment with one of these; such cases seem to respond well to the combination of sotalol and mexiletine. These drugs have different mechanisms and appear to work in a safe and complementary fashion.
- In dogs with systolic dysfunction and heart failure, consider treatment with furosemide, enalapril, pimobendan, spironolactone, and l-carnitine.

CONTRAINDICATIONS/POSSIBLE INTERACTIONS

Any antiarrhythmic drug has the potential to make an arrhythmia worse.

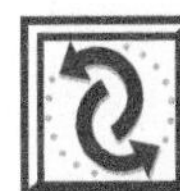

FOLLOW-UP

- If possible, repeat the Holter monitor 2–3 weeks after starting therapy to evaluate for a response. Affected dogs can have an 85% day-to-day variability in VPC number before medications; therefore, a good response to therapy would be an 85% reduction in VPC number. It is also anticipated that the complexity of the arrhythmia (bigeminy,

trigeminy, couplets, triplets, runs of ventricular tachycardia) will be reduced once on therapy. It may not always be possible to achieve an 85% reduction in VPC number; in those cases an improvement in arrhythmia complexity and clinical signs would be reasonable goals.
- Annual Holter monitoring and echocardiography are suggested, since in some cases the disease can be progressive.
- Advise owners that dogs are always at risk of sudden death. However, the majority of affected dogs can be maintained on antiarrhythmics for years with good quality of life. Dogs with systolic dysfunction and dilation have the worst prognosis, although some of these dogs do show improvement and a decreased rate of progression on l-carnitine supplementation.

MISCELLANEOUS

SYNONYMS

Boxer cardiomyopathy.

SEE ALSO

- Ventricular Premature Complexes.
- Ventricular Tachycardia.

ABBREVIATIONS

- VPC = ventricular premature complex.

Author Kathryn M. Meurs
Consulting Editor Michael Aherne

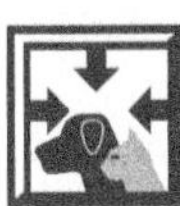

BASICS

DEFINITION

• Dilated cardiomyopathy (DCM) is a disease of the heart muscle characterized by systolic myocardial failure and a dilated, volume-overloaded heart that leads to signs of congestive heart failure (CHF) or low cardiac output.
• Before 1987, DCM was the second most commonly diagnosed heart disease in cats. Most cats had a secondary DCM as a result of taurine deficiency. Primary idiopathic DCM is now an uncommon cause of heart disease in cats.

PATHOPHYSIOLOGY

• Histopathologically, the myocardium of cats with idiopathic DCM has evidence of myocytolysis, fibrosis, myofibril fragmentation, and vacuolization. Gross examination reveals global eccentric enlargement of all four cardiac chambers.
• These anatomic changes are associated with progressive myocardial systolic failure, decreased contractility, decreased compliance, and secondary mitral valve regurgitation due to mitral valve annular dilation. These changes are typically identified by echocardiography.
• Eventually, the chronic myocardial dysfunction leads to CHF and clinical signs.

SYSTEMS AFFECTED

• Cardiovascular—DCM is a primary myocardial disease and primarily affects the heart and its ability to maintain an adequate cardiac output to maintain the body's needs.
• Musculoskeletal—cats with DCM can present with aortic thromboembolism (ATE), which causes acute paraparesis or monoparesis.
• Renal/urologic—cats with DCM and CHF often have poor renal perfusion and commonly have prerenal azotemia.
• Respiratory—cats usually present with tachypnea or dyspnea due to CHF with DCM. These cats can develop both pulmonary edema and pleural effusion.

GENETICS

Because of the human experience with DCM, it is likely that feline DCM also has a genetic basis, either inherited or de novo, as the cause of the disease. No definitive mutation has been identified in the cat to date; however, a quantitative genetic evaluation of a large cattery suggested an inherited factor in the development of DCM.

INCIDENCE/PREVALENCE

Idiopathic feline DCM is relatively uncommon now that taurine is adequately supplemented in cat foods. A retrospective survey of 106 cats with feline myocardial disease from 1994 to 2001 from Europe revealed that DCM was diagnosed in approximately 10% of the cases in this series. In the author's experience, the prevalence of feline idiopathic DCM may be less than 10%.

SIGNALMENT

Species

Cat

Breed Predilections

Because the prevalence is low, breed predilections are not clearly defined. That said, the Burmese cat may have an increased incidence.

Mean Age and Range

9 years (5–13 years).

Predominant Sex

None. (One study cites a male predisposition, while another states a female overrepresentation.)

SIGNS

General Comments

• Cats with idiopathic DCM usually present for signs of CHF.
• They are rarely diagnosed prior to onset of clinical signs.

Historical Findings

• Signs related to low cardiac output—anorexia, weakness, depression.
• Signs related to CHF—dyspnea, tachypnea.
• Signs related to ATE—sudden-onset pain and paraparesis.

Physical Examination Findings

• Heart rate can be fast, normal, or slow.
• Soft systolic heart murmur.
• Weak left cardiac impulse.
• Gallop sound.
• Possible arrhythmia.
• Hypothermia.
• Prolonged capillary refill time.
• Tachypnea.
• Quiet lung sounds (pleural effusion).
• Crackles (pulmonary edema).
• Ascites.
• Hypokinetic femoral pulses.
• Possibly, posterior paresis and pain as a result of ATE.

CAUSES

The underlying etiology of idiopathic DCM remains unknown, although a genetic predisposition has been identified in some families of cats. Taurine deficiency was a common cause of secondary myocardial failure before 1987.

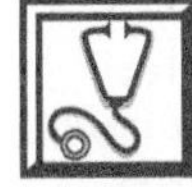

DIAGNOSIS

DIFFERENTIAL DIAGNOSIS

• Taurine deficiency DCM; because primary idiopathic DCM and taurine deficiency have similar clinical presentations, cats with myocardial failure should be assumed to have taurine deficiency until shown to be unresponsive to taurine.
• Myocardial failure secondary to long-standing congenital or acquired left ventricular volume overload diseases.
• End-staged remodeled hypertrophic cardiomyopathy may manifest with a dilated hypocontractile heart.
• Arrhythmogenic right ventricular cardiomyopathy.

CBC/BIOCHEMISTRY/URINALYSIS

Many cats will have prerenal azotemia related to low cardiac output.

OTHER LABORATORY TESTS

• Ensure that thyroid concentrations are normal.
• Plasma taurine concentrations less than 40 nmol/L or whole blood taurine concentrations less than 250 nmol/L, are subnormal and suggestive of taurine deficiency DCM. Taurine assays are performed at a limited number of institutions and require special handling.
• Cardiac biomarkers such as plasma amine terminal B-type natriuretic peptide (NT-proBNP) and cardiac troponin I (cTnI) concentrations would be elevated in a cat with CHF due to idiopathic DCM.

IMAGING

Radiography

• Radiography often shows pleural effusion or pulmonary edema.
• Generalized cardiomegaly.

Echocardiography

• Diagnostic modality of choice.
• Characteristic findings include thin ventricular walls, enlarged left ventricular end-systolic and end-diastolic dimensions, left atrial enlargement, and low fractional shortening.
• Pleural and pericardial effusion may be visualized.
• Spontaneous echocardiographic contrast or a thrombus may be visualized.

DIAGNOSTIC PROCEDURES

ECG

• ECG may be normal or may show left atrial or ventricular enlargement patterns.
• Both ventricular and supraventricular arrhythmias can be seen.

Pleural Effusion Analysis

• Pleural effusion typically is a modified transudate with total protein <4 g/dL and nucleated cell counts of less than 2,500/mL; chylous effusion may also be present.
• Analysis of the pleural effusion is important to rule out other causes of pleural effusion such as pyothorax, infectious peritonitis, or lymphosarcoma.

PATHOLOGIC FINDINGS

• Heart : body ratio is increased.
• All four cardiac chambers are dilated;

ventricular walls are thin and left ventricular lumen is enlarged.

- Valve anatomy is normal.
- Histopathology shows myocytolysis and myocardial fibrosis.

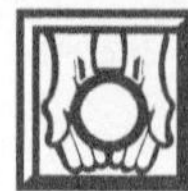

TREATMENT

APPROPRIATE HEALTH CARE

These cats usually present in CHF and should be treated as inpatients, typically in an intensive care setting until more stable.

NURSING CARE

- Thoracocentesis is often utilized for both therapeutic and diagnostic purposes.
- Supplemental oxygen therapy is beneficial for cats in CHF to decrease the work of breathing.
- If hypothermic, cautious external heat (incubator or heating water pad) is recommended.

ACTIVITY

Indoors only after hospital discharge to reduce stress. Let cat dictate its own activity.

DIET

These cats typically are anorexic, thus tempting their appetite with many types of food may be necessary. Eventually, a low-sodium diet is recommended.

CLIENT EDUCATION

Some cats will need chronic intermittent thoracocentesis to manage significant accumulations of pleural effusion despite medical therapy.

MEDICATIONS

DRUG(S) OF CHOICE

- Furosemide is recommended to manage pulmonary edema and pleural effusion. Recommended dose range is 1–4 mg/kg q8–12h. Initially, administer parenterally then switch to oral. Chronically the lowest effective dose of furosemide is recommended.
- Pimobendan, an inodilator, is also recommended to strengthen contractility and provide some vasodilation. Recommended dose range is 0.1–0.3 mg/kg PO q12h. Although pimobendan is not currently licensed for use in cats, several recent publications have demonstrated its safety in cats and possibly a beneficial effect, albeit in retrospective studies. One study in cats with non-taurine-responsive DCM that were treated with pimobendan had a median survival time that was four times longer than the cats not treated with pimobendan (49 vs. 12 days).
- Taurine supplementation is recommended initially in all cats with DCM at 250 mg PO q12h, until it is demonstrated that the patient is unresponsive to taurine or is not taurine deficient based on diagnostic testing.
- Nitroglycerin (2% ointment) one-fourth to one-half inch applied topically can be used in conjunction with diuretics in the acute management of severe CHF to further reduce preload. Nitroglycerin will lower the dose of furosemide and is particularly useful in patients with hypothermia or dehydration.
- Enalapril or benazepril, at a dose of 0.25–0.5 mg/kg PO q24h, is recommended to reduce afterload and preload as soon as the cat is able to take oral medications and is clinically stable. Use with caution and possibly avoid if creatinine >2.5 mg/dL.
- Digoxin is optionally recommended to strengthen contractility and for its positive neurohumoral effects at a dose of 0.03 mg/cat (one-fourth of a 0.125 mg tablet) or 0.01 mg/kg PO q48h. Digoxin can be given concurrently with pimobendan. However, digoxin is often omitted when pimobendan is given because of the difficulties in giving a cat several pills and digoxin's side-effect profile.
- Dobutamine at extremely low dosages can be given to a patient with severe signs of CHF and low cardiac output that cannot take oral medications. Dose varies 0.25–5 µg/kg/minute IV CRI. ECG monitoring is recommended.
- Because ATE is a concern, an antithrombotic agent is also recommended. Clopidogrel given at a dose of 18.75 mg (one-fourth of a 75 mg tablet) PO q24h is generally the author's preferred antithrombotic agent. Other options include aspirin 81 mg PO q72h (with food) or low molecular weight heparin (e.g., dalteparin 100–150 units/kg SC q8–24h or enoxaparin 1 mg/kg SC q12–24h).
- Antiarrhythmic drugs may also be needed to control supraventricular or ventricular arrhythmias. If hemodynamically significant supraventricular tachycardia or rapid atrial fibrillation is present, diltiazem is recommended. Usually, diltiazem is given orally in either a non-sustained-release formulation (7.5 mg/cat PO q8h) or a sustained-release oral formulation (Cardizem CD® at 10 mg/kg PO q24h or Dilacor XR® 30 mg/cat [or 1/2 of an inner 60 mg tablet] PO q12h). Diltiazem is also available in an injectable formulation for urgent control of a supraventricular arrhythmia in a cat that cannot take oral medications (0.05–0.1 mg/kg slow IV, repeated PRN up to 0.25 mg/kg). If rapid and sustained ventricular tachycardia, lidocaine slow IV 0.2–0.5 mg/kg (repeat once or twice max) or sotalol PO 2 mg/kg q12h is recommended.
- Beta blockers, such as atenolol, may be useful in the chronic management of both supraventricular and ventricular arrhythmias. Beta blockers are used in the long-term management of DCM in humans because of their positive myocardial effects and survival benefit. Clinical experience is limited in feline DCM and they must be used cautiously, as they acutely decrease contractility and could worsen CHF. Recommended dose ranges from 3.125 to 6.25 mg PO q12–24h. Start low and titrate up based on heart rate and clinical signs.

PRECAUTIONS

- Unless needed for acute cardiac rhythm control, drugs such as calcium channel blockers (diltiazem) or beta-adrenergic blockers may reduce contractility and lower cardiac output. Use cautiously.
- Overzealous diuretic and vasodilation therapy may cause azotemia and electrolyte disturbances.
- Digoxin should not be used if renal insufficiency is documented or suspected.
- Enalapril or benazepril should be used with caution and possibly withheld if serum creatinine is >2.5 mg/dL.
- Dobutamine may cause seizures and cardiac tachyarrhythmias.

FOLLOW-UP

PATIENT MONITORING

- Repeat examination with ideally blood pressure, diagnostic imaging (either a thoracic radiograph or focused thoracic ultrasound for fluid assessment), and chemistry panel within 1 week to determine response of therapy.
- Home resting respiratory rate monitoring is helpful to determine need for diuretic dose adjustment or thoracocentesis.
- Periodically monitor electrolyte and renal parameters. Periodically monitor for CHF fluid accumulation with diagnostic imaging.
- If using digoxin, serum blood concentrations should be measured approximately 10–14 days after initiating therapy. Therapeutic range is 0.5–1.5 ng/dL 8–12 hours post-pill.
- Repeat diagnostic echocardiogram in 2–3 months after initiating taurine supplementation to determine echocardiographic response to therapy. Although echocardiographic response may take 2–3 months to assess, one should see dramatic clinical response within 2 weeks of initiating taurine therapy if cat has taurine-responsive DCM.

PREVENTION/AVOIDANCE

Ensure that cats eat a high-protein diet with sufficient dietary taurine. No vegetarian diets.

POSSIBLE COMPLICATIONS

ATE is the most feared complication of any feline myocardial disease.

EXPECTED COURSE AND PROGNOSIS

- These cats have a poor prognosis despite intensive therapy. If cat is not taurine responsive, survival is usually weeks to months.
- CHF can be medically refractory and recurrent despite appropriate medical therapy.
- Repeated thoracocentesis may be necessary.

MISCELLANEOUS

ASSOCIATED CONDITIONS

- CHF.
- ATE.
- Pleural effusion.
- Cardiac arrhythmias.

SYNONYMS

Cardiomyopathy

SEE ALSO

- Aortic Thromboembolism.
- Congestive Heart Failure, Left-Sided.
- Congestive Heart Failure, Right-Sided.

ABBREVIATIONS

- ATE = aortic thromboembolism.
- CHF = congestive heart failure.
- cTnI = cardiac troponin I.
- DCM = dilated cardiomyopathy.

Suggested Reading

Ferasin L, Sturgess CP, Cannon MJ, et al. Feline idiopathic cardiomyopathy: a retrospective study of 106 cats (1994–2001). J Feline Med Surg 2003; 5:151–159.

Hambrook LE, Bennett PF. Effect of pimobendan on the clinical outcome and survival of cats with non-taurine responsive dilated cardiomyopathy. J Feline Med Surg 2012; 14:233–239.

Kittleson MD. Feline myocardial disease. In: Ettinger SJ, Feldman EC, eds. Textbook of Veterinary Internal Medicine, 6th ed. St. Louis, MO: Elsevier, 2005, pp. 1082–1103.

Lawler DF, Templeton AJ, Monti KL. Evidence of genetic involvement in feline dilated cardiomyopathy. J Vet Intern Med 1993; 7:383–387.

Pion PD, Kittleson MD, Rogers QR, et al. Myocardial failure in cats associated with low plasma taurine: a reversible cardiomyopathy. Science 1987; 237:764–768.

Author Teresa C. DeFrancesco

Consulting Editor Michael Aherne

CARDIOMYOPATHY, DILATED—DOGS

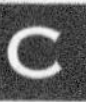

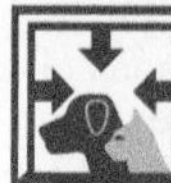

BASICS

DEFINITION

Dilated cardiomyopathy (DCM) characterized by left- and right-sided dilation, normal coronary arteries, anatomically normal although commonly insufficient atrioventricular valves, significantly decreased inotropic state, and myocardial dysfunction occurring primarily during systole; however, progressive diastolic dysfunction with restrictive physiology may also be present and is a negative predictor of survival.

PATHOPHYSIOLOGY

- Myocardial failure leads to reduced cardiac output and congestive heart failure (CHF).
- Atrioventricular (AV) annulus dilation and altered papillary muscle function promote valvular insufficiency.
- Although left-sided signs commonly predominate, evidence of severe right-sided disease can occur and infrequently is the dominant clinical scenario.

SYSTEMS AFFECTED

- Cardiovascular.
- Renal/urologic—prerenal azotemia.
- Respiratory—pulmonary edema, infrequently pulmonary hypertension.
- All organ systems are affected by reductions in cardiac output.

GENETICS

- Genetic cause or heritable susceptibility strongly suspected in most breeds and documented in some (Portuguese water dog, boxer, and Doberman pinscher) with variable forms of inheritance.
- A genetic test is commercially available for causative mutations in boxer dogs (striatin) and Doberman pinscher (NCSU DCM 1—pyruvate dehydrogenase kinase; NCSU DCM 2—titin).
- These mutations are not causative in other predisposed breeds in which they have been evaluated.
- Correlations between genotype and phenotype have shown that Doberman pinschers with both mutations have, on average, an earlier onset of clinical disease with a predisposition to sudden death; boxers homozygous for the mutation are more likely to develop the DCM phenotype.

INCIDENCE/PREVALENCE

Estimated at 0.5–1.1% in predisposed breeds and perhaps higher in specific geographic regions.

GEOGRAPHIC DISTRIBUTION

None with the exception of Chagas' cardiomyopathy, which is limited to the southern United States (Gulf Coast) and both Central and South America.

SIGNALMENT

Species

Dog

Breed Predilections

- Doberman pinscher, boxer.
- Giant breeds—Scottish deerhound, Irish wolfhound, Great Dane, St. Bernard, Newfoundland.
- Cocker spaniel, Portuguese water dog (juvenile).

Mean Age and Range

4–10 years.

Predominant Sex

Males > females in most but not all breeds (minor predisposition).

SIGNS

Historical Findings

- Respiratory—tachypnea, dyspnea, coughing.
- Weight loss, typically of lean muscle mass.
- Weakness, lethargy, anorexia.
- Abdominal distention.
- Syncope, usually associated with arrhythmias (atrial fibrillation; ventricular tachycardia).
- Some dogs are asymptomatic, having what is termed preclinical DCM, the diagnosis of which in specific breeds is well described.
- Breed-specific echocardiographic parameters coupled with cardiac biomarkers (NT-proBNP; cardiac troponin I [cTnI]) may help identify dogs with preclinical DCM.

Physical Examination Findings

- May be completely normal with preclinical DCM.
- Weakness, possibly cardiogenic shock.
- Hypokinetic femoral pulse from low cardiac output.
- Pulse deficits with atrial fibrillation, ventricular or supraventricular premature contractions, and paroxysmal ventricular tachycardia.
- Jugular pulses from tricuspid regurgitation, arrhythmias, or right-sided CHF.
- Breath sounds—muffled with pleural effusion; crackles with pulmonary edema.
- S3 or summation gallop sounds.
- Mitral and/or tricuspid regurgitation murmurs are common but usually focal and soft.
- Auscultatory evidence of cardiac arrhythmia is common.
- Slow capillary refill time, infrequent cyanosis.
- Hepatomegaly with or without ascites.

CAUSES

- Majority of cases represent familial abnormalities of structural, energetic, or contractile cardiac proteins, some of which have been identified.
- Nutritional deficiencies (taurine and/or carnitine) have been documented in several breeds including golden retriever, boxer, Newfoundland, and cocker spaniel; diet-associated DCM, which may be associated with taurine deficiency, commonly secondary to boutique, exotic-ingredient, or grain free (BEG) diets, is increasing recognized and potentially reversible.
- Viral, protozoal, and immune-mediated mechanisms have been proposed but not proven.
- Doxorubicin toxicity.
- Hypothyroidism and persistent tachyarrhythmias (sometimes associated with congenital tricuspid valve malformation) may cause reversible myocardial failure.

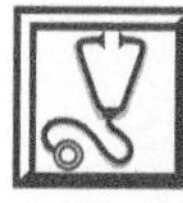

DIAGNOSIS

DIFFERENTIAL DIAGNOSIS

- Myxomatous valvular degeneration.
- Congenital heart disease.
- Heartworm disease.
- Bacterial endocarditis.
- Cardiac tumors and pericardial effusion.
- Airway obstruction—foreign body, neoplasm, laryngeal paralysis.
- Primary pulmonary disease—bronchial disease, pneumonia, neoplasia, aspiration, vascular disease (e.g., heartworms).
- Noncardiogenic pleural effusions (e.g., pyothorax, hemothorax, chylothorax).
- Trauma resulting in diaphragmatic hernia, pulmonary hemorrhage, hemothorax, pneumothorax.

CBC/BIOCHEMISTRY/URINALYSIS

Routine hematologic tests and urinalysis are usually normal unless altered by severe reductions in cardiac output or severe elevations in venous pressures (e.g., prerenal azotemia, high alanine aminotransferase, hyponatremia), therapy for heart failure (e.g., hyponatremia, hypokalemia, hypochloremia, azotemia, and metabolic alkalosis from diuresis), or concurrent disease.

OTHER LABORATORY TESTS

Cardiac biomarkers including NT-proBNP and cTnI are elevated in both the preclinical and clinical stages of the disease. Clinical studies investigating use of these markers for diagnosis, prognosis, and optimization of therapy are ongoing.

IMAGING

Radiography

- Typically normal in the preclinical phase.
- Generalized cardiomegaly and signs of CHF are common.
- Left ventricular (LV) enlargement and left atrial enlargement may be most evident in early cases.
- In some cases, the degree of cardiomegaly may be less than expected for the severity of clinical signs; it is also often substantially less than would be expected in a dog with

primary valvular heart disease and comparable clinical signs.
- Pleural effusion, hepatomegaly, ascites.

Echocardiography

- Gold standard for diagnosis.
- LV dilation often precedes overt reductions in indices of systolic function.
- Ventricular and atrial dilation.
- Indices of myocardial systolic function (fractional shortening [FS%]), ejection fraction, area shortening, and mitral annular motion by tissue Doppler imaging may be reduced.
- Spectral Doppler studies may confirm decreased velocity and/or acceleration of trans-aortic flow as well as mitral regurgitation and/or tricuspid regurgitation.
- Doppler evidence of restrictive LV filling is associated with decreased survival.

DIAGNOSTIC TESTS

ECG

- Sinus rhythm or sinus tachycardia with isolated atrial or ventricular premature complexes.
- Atrial fibrillation and ventricular tachycardia (paroxysmal or sustained) are very common in Doberman pinschers.
- Boxers commonly have isolated ventricular arrhythmias without evidence of functional or anatomic heart disease.
- Prolonged QRS (>0.06 second), possible increased voltages (R >3 mV lead II), suggesting LV enlargement.
- May have "sloppy" R wave descent with ST-T coving, suggesting myocardial disease or LV ischemia.
- May have low voltages (pleural or pericardial effusion, concurrent hypothyroidism).

PATHOLOGIC FINDINGS

- Dilation of all chambers with or without thinning of chamber walls.
- Slightly thickened endocardium with pale areas within myocardium (necrosis, fibrosis).
- Two histologically distinct forms—fatty infiltration: degenerative type seen in boxers and Doberman pinschers; and attenuated wavy fiber type: seen in many giant-, large-, and medium-sized breeds, including some boxers and Doberman pinschers.

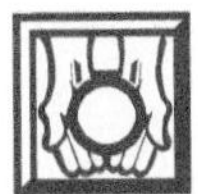

TREATMENT

APPROPRIATE HEALTH CARE

With the exception of severely affected dogs (life-threatening arrhythmias, severe pulmonary edema, cardiogenic shock), most therapy can be administered on an outpatient basis.

ACTIVITY

Allow the dog to choose its own level of activity.

DIET

- During initial therapy for clinical signs, simply maintaining adequate caloric intake is paramount.
- Goal—reduce dietary sodium intake to <12–15 mg/kg/day.
- Severe sodium restriction is typically not necessary when using potent cardioactive therapy and may adversely affect appetite.
- Best to use commercially prepared diets.

CLIENT EDUCATION

- Emphasize potential signs associated with progression of disease and adverse side effects of medication.
- Monitoring sleeping respiratory rate often gives insight into impending decompensation.

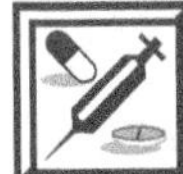

MEDICATIONS

DRUG(S) OF CHOICE

First identify patient problems—CHF (left or right-sided), arrhythmia, hypothermia, renal failure, shock.

Preclinical Disease

- There is clinical evidence (PROTECT Trial) that early intervention with pimobendan monotherapy substantially changes the course of preclinical disease in Doberman pinschers.
- These results are routinely extrapolated to other breeds, but have not been proven.
- Critical evaluation suggests that early intervention with monotherapy using an angiotensin-converting enzyme (ACE) inhibitor is of minimal or no survival benefit in preclinical disease.

Initial Stabilization

- Treat hypoxemia with oxygen administration; prevent heat loss if hypothermic (warm environment).
- If pulmonary edema—furosemide (1–4 mg/kg IM/IV, then 1–2 mg/kg q6–12h for first 1–3 days), or CRI 1–2 mg/kg/h (author's preference).
- 2% topical nitroglycerin for first 24–48h for severe pulmonary edema—apply 1 inch–2 inches q8h (beware of hypotension in both patients and staff).
- If significant pleural effusion—drain each hemithorax.
- If severe heart failure and cardiogenic shock—dobutamine may be indicated; this drug may exacerbate arrhythmias, particularly in hypoxic dogs; oral pimobendan (see dosing below) may have important acute (2–4h) hemodynamic benefit as well; IV pimobendan (0.15 mg/kg) is available in select countries.
- Dobutamine 5–15 µg/kg/min infused for 24–72h with care (start low and gradually up-titrate based on response).
- If paroxysmal ventricular tachycardia is present—administer lidocaine slowly in 2 mg/kg boluses (up to 8 mg/kg total over 30 min) to convert to sinus rhythm; follow with lidocaine infusion (50–100 µg/kg/min).
- If lidocaine is ineffective—administer procainamide slowly at dose of 2–5 mg/kg (up to 15 mg/kg) IV to convert to sinus rhythm; follow with 25–50 µg/kg/min CRI (beware of proarrhythmia and infrequently hypotension).

Maintenance Therapy

- ACE inhibitors (enalapril, benazepril, lisinopril) are considered cornerstone of therapy for DCM.
- Enalapril (0.25–0.5 mg/kg PO q12h), benazepril (0.5 mg/kg PO q12–24h), or lisinopril (0.5 mg/kg PO q 12–24h) should be initiated early in the therapeutic regimen.
- Furosemide (1–4 mg/kg PO q8–12h) is used to control signs of congestion.
- Torsemide (0.1–0.4 mg/kg PO q8–12h) is commonly employed as an alternative to furosemide, particularly in later-stage disease.
- Spironolactone (1–2 mg/kg PO q12h) may impart an independent survival benefit by blocking aldosterone; higher doses can be used for refractory heart failure (2–4 mg/kg PO q12h).
- Hydrochlorthiazide (1–2 mg/kg PO q12h) may be beneficial as a third diuretic.
- Beta blockers can be used cautiously once heart failure is controlled with other drugs (see Precautions); if tolerated, they may improve myocardial function with chronic use; carvedilol (0.25–1.25 mg/kg PO q12h) is an alpha and beta blocker with antioxidant activity: start at the low end of the dose range and gradually up-titrate over a 6-week period if tolerated; consult with a cardiologist before using beta blockers in clinical DCM patients as can result in rapid and profound clinical deterioration.
- Pimobendan (0.25–0.3 mg/kg PO q12h) is a calcium-sensitizing drug and a vasodilating, positive inotrope (inodilator) that, when added to furosemide, ACE inhibitors, and spironolactone improves functional heart failure class and in Doberman pinschers increases survival time; the author has administered pimobendan 0.5 mg/kg PO q8h in refractory cases with perceived clinical benefit.
- The role of carnitine and taurine in therapy of DCM remains controversial; however, American cocker spaniels with DCM generally respond favorably to taurine and l-carnitine supplementation, but still require additional cardiac medications.

Arrhythmias

- In atrial fibrillation, slowing of ventricular rate response typically achieved with chronic administration of extended-release diltiazem

(Dilacor®) 2–7 mg/kg PO q12h, or atenolol 0.75–1.5 mg/kg PO q12h (never start in patient with active CHF), occasionally combined with digitalis at dose of 0.005 mg/kg PO q12h; therapeutic drug monitoring recommended when administering digoxin.
• Therapeutic goal is obtaining resting ventricular rate of 100–140 bpm.
• At-home monitoring with AliveCor Kardia device.
• This therapy merely controls ventricular rate, by depressing atrioventricular nodal conduction; generally does not convert rhythm from atrial fibrillation to sinus rhythm.
• Amiodarone (10–15 mg/kg PO q24h for 7–10 days followed by 5–10 mg/kg PO q24h) may either control ventricular response rate or in some cases result in conversion to normal sinus rhythm.
• Chronic oral therapy for ventricular tachycardia includes sotalol (1–2 mg/kg PO q12h), mexiletine (5–10 mg/kg PO q8h), or amiodarone (5–10 mg/kg PO q24h).
• Mexiletine can be combined with sotalol if necessary.

CONTRAINDICATIONS

Digoxin should be avoided in severe uncontrolled paroxysmal ventricular tachycardia, in animals with compromised renal function, and in animals with important hypokalemia.

PRECAUTIONS

• Calcium channel blockers and notably beta blockers are negative inotropes and may have acute adverse effect on myocardial function; numerous human studies, however, have suggested that chronic administration of beta blockers may be of benefit in DCM.
• Combination of diuretics and ACE inhibitors may result in azotemia, especially in patients with severe heart failure or preexisting renal dysfunction, and must be closely monitored.

POSSIBLE INTERACTIONS

• Quinidine, amiodarone, and diltiazem may increase serum digoxin levels and predispose to digitalis intoxication.
• Renal dysfunction, hypothyroidism, and hypokalemia predispose to digitalis intoxication.

ALTERNATIVE DRUG(S)

• Other vasodilators, including hydralazine and amlodipine, may be used instead of or in addition to ACE inhibitors (beware of hypotension).
• Role of co-enzyme Q10, fish oil, and arginine remains to be determined.

FOLLOW-UP

PATIENT MONITORING

• Serial clinical examinations, thoracic radiographs, blood pressure measurements, routine serum biochemical evaluations (including electrolytes), and electrocardiography are most helpful.
• Repeat echocardiography is rarely informative or indicated.
• Serial evaluation of serum digoxin levels (therapeutic range: 0.5–1 ng/mL) taken 6–8 hours post-pill and serum biochemistries may help prevent iatrogenic problems.

POSSIBLE COMPLICATIONS

• Sudden death due most commonly to arrhythmias.
• Iatrogenic problems associated with medical management (see above).

EXPECTED COURSE AND PROGNOSIS

• Always fatal unless associated with nutritional deficiencies.
• Death usually occurs 6–24 months following diagnosis.
• Dobermans typically have worst prognosis; however, with addition of pimobendan, survival following identification in *preclinical* phase averages over 700 days.
• Atrial fibrillation, paroxysmal ventricular tachycardia, Doppler evidence of restrictive LV filling, markedly decreased FS%, homozygosity for known mutations (boxer), or presence of multiple mutations (Doberman pinschers) are believed to be markers for shortened survival and increased risk for sudden arrhythmogenic death.

MISCELLANEOUS

ASSOCIATED CONDITIONS

Prevalence increases with age.

SYNONYMS

• Congestive cardiomyopathy.
• Giant-breed cardiomyopathy.

SEE ALSO

• Atrial Fibrillation and Atrial Flutter.
• Ventricular Tachycardia.

ABBREVIATIONS

• ACE = angiotensin-converting enzyme.
• AV = atrioventricular.
• BEG = boutique, exotic-ingredient, or grain free.
• CHF = congestive heart failure.
• cTnI = cardiac troponin I.
• DCM = dilated cardiomyopathy.
• FS% = percent fractional shortening.
• LV = left ventricular.

INTERNET RESOURCES

https://cardiaceducationgroup.org

Author Matthew W. Miller
Consulting Editor Michael Aherne

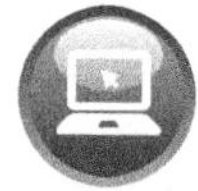

Client Education Handout available online

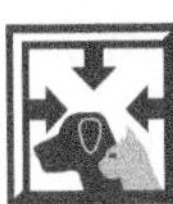

BASICS

DEFINITION

Inappropriate concentric hypertrophy of the ventricular free wall and/or the interventricular septum of the nondilated left ventricle. The disease occurs independently of other cardiac or systemic disorders.

PATHOPHYSIOLOGY

- Diastolic dysfunction results from a thickened, less compliant left ventricle.
- High left ventricular filling pressure develops, causing left atrial (LA) enlargement.
- Pulmonary venous hypertension causes pulmonary edema. Some cats develop biventricular failure (i.e., pulmonary edema, pleural effusion, small volume pericardial effusion without tamponade, and infrequently ascites).
- Stasis of blood in the large left atrium predisposes the patient to aortic thromboembolism (ATE).
- Dynamic aortic outflow obstruction and systolic anterior mitral motion (SAM) with secondary mitral insufficiency may occur, but unlike in humans, appears not to affect prognosis.
- Recent evidence suggests that some cats with apparent hypertrophic cardiomyopathy (HCM) and congestive heart failure (CHF) actually have transient myocardial thickening, often associated with high serum troponin I concentrations. These cats are younger than average for HCM, with on average less severe left ventricular (LV) hypertrophy, and they can experience resolution of both CHF and LV hypertrophy.

SYSTEMS AFFECTED

- Cardiovascular—CHF, ATE, and arrhythmias.
- Pulmonary—dyspnea if CHF develops.
- Renal/urologic—prerenal azotemia.

GENETICS

Some families of cats have been identified with a high prevalence of the disease, and the disease appears to be an autosomal dominant trait in Maine coon cats and ragdoll cats, due to a mutation in the myosin-binding protein C (MyBPC) gene. The genetics have not been definitively determined in other breeds; however, the Maine coon and ragdoll mutations have not been identified in affected Sphynx, Norwegian forest cats, Bengals, Siberians, or British shorthair cats.

INCIDENCE/PREVALENCE

Unknown, but relatively common. May be as high as 15% of the population.

SIGNALMENT

Species

Cat

Breed Predilections

Maine coon cats, ragdolls, Sphynx, British and American shorthairs, and Persians.

Mean Age and Range

- 5–7 years, with reported ages of 3 months–17 years. Some breeds of cats including ragdolls and Sphynx may develop the disease at a younger age (average of 2 years).
- HCM is most often a disease of young to middle-aged cats; unexplained murmurs in geriatric cats are more likely associated with hyperthyroidism or hypertension.

Predominant Sex

Male

SIGNS

Historical Findings

- Dyspnea, tachypnea.
- Anorexia.
- Exercise intolerance.
- Vomiting.
- Collapse.
- Sudden death.
- Coughing is uncommon in cats with HCM and suggests primary pulmonary disease.

Physical Examination Findings

- Gallop rhythm (S3 or S4).
- Systolic murmur in approximately half of affected cats.
- Apex heartbeat may be exaggerated.
- Muffled heart sounds, lack of chest compliance, and dyspnea characterized by rapid shallow respirations may be associated with pleural effusion.
- Dyspnea and crackles if pulmonary edema is present.
- Weak femoral pulse.
- Acute pelvic limb paralysis with cyanotic pads and nailbeds, cold limbs, and absence of femoral pulse in animals with ATE; emboli rarely affect thoracic limbs.
- Arrhythmia in some animals.
- May have no clinical signs.

CAUSES

- Usually unknown—multiple causes exist.
- MyBPC mutations in some cats with HCM.

Possible Causes

- Abnormalities of contractile protein myosin or other sarcomeric proteins (e.g., troponin, myosin-binding proteins, tropomyosin).
- Abnormality affecting catecholamine-influenced excitation contraction coupling.
- Abnormal myocardial calcium metabolism.
- Collagen or other intercellular matrix abnormality.
- Growth hormone excess.
- Dynamic LV outflow obstruction may contribute to secondary LV hypertrophy.

RISK FACTORS

Offspring of animals with familial mutations of MyBPC.

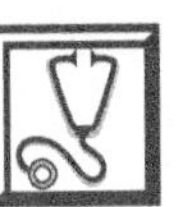

DIAGNOSIS

DIFFERENTIAL DIAGNOSIS

- Other forms of cardiomyopathy.
- Hyperthyroidism.
- Aortic stenosis.
- Systemic hypertension.
- Acromegaly.
- Noncardiac causes of pleural effusion.

CBC/BIOCHEMISTRY/URINALYSIS

- Results usually normal.
- Prerenal azotemia in some animals.

OTHER LABORATORY TESTS

- MyBPC assay; mutation differs for Maine coon cats and ragdoll cats.
- In cats >6 years old, check thyroid hormone concentration; hyperthyroidism causes myocardial hypertrophy that might be confused with HCM.
- Serum NT-proBNP concentrations higher in cats with HCM than in normal cats, and higher still in cats with symptomatic HCM. SNAP NT-proBNP point-of-care testing is also available to help differentiate symptomatic cats with HCM from those that are symptomatic from other causes. Send-out serum NT-proBNP testing is useful in identifying cats with suspicion of HCM from asymptomatic cats with abnormal physical exam findings (e.g., murmur). Follow-up echocardiography indicated in cats with serum NT-proBNP concentrations in "equivocal" or "high" range, or positive SNAP results.

IMAGING

Radiography

- Dorsoventral radiographs often reveal a valentine-appearing heart because of atrial enlargement and a left ventricle that comes to a point.
- Pulmonary edema, pleural effusion, or both in some animals.
- Radiographs may be normal in asymptomatic cats.
- Different forms of cardiomyopathy cannot be reliably differentiated by radiography.

Echocardiography

- Hypertrophy of interventricular septum (IVS) or LV posterior wall (diastolic wall thickness >6 mm).
- Hypertrophy may be symmetric (affecting IVS and posterior wall) or asymmetric (affecting IVS or posterior wall, but not both).
- Hypertrophy of papillary muscles.
- Normal or high fractional shortening.
- Normal or reduced LV lumen.
- LA enlargement.
- Systolic anterior motion of mitral valve (some animals).
- LV outflow obstruction (some animals); specialized Doppler studies performed by

CARDIOMYOPATHY, HYPERTROPHIC—CATS (CONTINUED)

C

experienced sonographers often reveal LV relaxation abnormalities (e.g., mitral inflow E : A wave reversal).
• Thrombus in left atrium (rare).
• *Note:* there is some overlap between normal cats (especially ketaminized or dehydrated) and cats with mild HCM. Correlate echo findings with physical findings. Presence of LA enlargement favors HCM.

DIAGNOSTIC PROCEDURES

ECG

• Sinus tachycardia (heart rate >240) common with heart failure; however, some cats with severe heart failure and hypothermia are bradycardic.
• Atrial and ventricular premature complexes seen more often in cats with cardiomyopathy, but also occasionally seen in normal cats.
• Atrial fibrillation seen in some advanced cases.
• Left axis deviation often seen.
• Prolongation of QT interval and QTc (QT interval corrected for heart rate) often seen with LV hypertrophy.
• Cannot differentiate different forms of cardiomyopathy; may be normal.

Systemic Blood Pressure

• Normotensive or hypotensive.
• Evaluate blood pressure in all patients with myocardial hypertrophy to rule out systemic hypertension as cause of hypertrophy.

PATHOLOGIC FINDINGS

• Nondilated left ventricle with hypertrophy of IVS or LV free wall.
• Hypertrophy of papillary muscles.
• LA enlargement.
• Mitral valve thickening.
• Myocardial hypertrophy with disorganized alignment of myocytes (myofiber disarray).
• Interstitial fibrosis.
• Myocardial scarring.
• Hypertrophy and luminal narrowing of intramural coronary arteries.

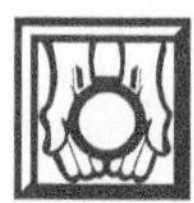

TREATMENT

APPROPRIATE HEALTH CARE

Cats with CHF should be hospitalized.

NURSING CARE

• Minimize stress.
• Oxygen if dyspneic.
• Warm environment if hypothermic.

ACTIVITY

Restricted with CHF.

DIET

Modest to moderate sodium restriction in animals with CHF.

CLIENT EDUCATION

• Many cats diagnosed while asymptomatic eventually develop CHF and may develop ATE and die suddenly.
• If cat is receiving warfarin, dalteparin, enoxaparin (Lovenox®), or combination of clopidogrel and any of those medications, minimize potential for trauma and subsequent hemorrhage.

MEDICATIONS

DRUG(S) OF CHOICE

Furosemide

• Dosage—1–2 mg/kg PO/IM/IV q8–24h.
• Critically dyspneic animals often require high dosage (4 mg/kg IV); this dose can be repeated in 1 hour if cat still severely dyspneic; indicated to treat pulmonary edema, pleural effusion, and ascites.
• Cats are sensitive to furosemide and prone to dehydration, prerenal azotemia, and hypokalemia.
• Once pulmonary edema resolves, taper to lowest effective dose.

Pimobendan

• Dosage—0.25–0.3 mg/kg PO q12h.
• Appears to be useful in management of CHF (e.g., pulmonary edema or pleural effusion) in cats with HCM, possibly by enhancing diastolic function and LA fractional shortening; not used in management of asymptomatic HCM at this time.
• Not currently licensed for use in cats.

Angiotensin-Converting Enzyme (ACE) Inhibitors

• Dosage—enalapril or benazepril 0.25–0.5 mg/kg PO q24h.
• Indications in cats with HCM not well defined—authors currently use for CHF.

Beta Blockers

• Dosage—atenolol (6.25–12.5 mg/cat PO q12h).
• Beneficial effects may include slowing of sinus rate, correcting atrial and ventricular arrhythmias, platelet inhibition.
• More effective than diltiazem in controlling dynamic outflow tract obstruction.
• Role in asymptomatic patients unresolved, but many clinicians use if dynamic outflow obstruction and hypertrophy present.
• Contraindicated in presence of CHF.

Diltiazem

• Dosage—7.5–15 mg/cat PO q8h or 10 mg/kg PO q24h (Cardizem® CD) or 30 mg/cat q12h (Dilacor XR®).
• Beneficial effects may include slower sinus rate, resolution of supraventricular arrhythmias, improved diastolic relaxation, coronary and peripheral vasodilation, platelet inhibition.
• May reduce hypertrophy and LA dimensions in some cats.
• Role in asymptomatic patients unresolved.

Aspirin

• Dosage—81 mg/cat q2–3 days if severe atrial enlargement.
• Depresses platelet aggregation, hopefully minimizing risk of thromboembolism.
• Warn owners that thrombi can still develop despite aspirin administration; aspirin appears to be not as effective as clopidogrel (1/4 of 75 mg tablet PO q24h) in prevention of ATE, at least in cats with previous embolic episode.

Nitroglycerin Ointment

• Dosage—one-fourth inch/cat topically applied q6–8h or 2.5 mg/24h patch.
• Often used in acute stabilization of cats with severe pulmonary edema or pleural effusion.
• When used intermittently, may be useful for long-term management of refractory cases.

CONTRAINDICATIONS

Avoid beta blockers in cats with emboli; these agents cause peripheral vasoconstriction. If beta blockers must be used in this setting for arrhythmia control, choose beta-1 selective blocker such as atenolol.

PRECAUTIONS

Use ACE inhibitors cautiously in azotemic animals.

ALTERNATIVE DRUG(S)

Torsemide

• Dosage—0.1–0.5 mg/kg q24h, sometimes with dose escalation to q12h.
• Used as substitute for furosemide in refractory pulmonary edema or pleural effusion in cats with apparently normal (or at least stable) renal function.
• Monitor renal function closely in first days after switching to torsemide.

Spironolactone

• Dosage—1 mg/kg q12–24h.
• Used in conjunction with furosemide in cats with CHF, especially refractory effusions.
• May cause facial pruritis.

Warfarin and Low Molecular Weight Heparin

• Used sometimes in cats at high risk for thromboembolism.
• See Aortic Thromboembolism.

Clopidogrel

• Dosage—18.75 mg/cat/day.
• Platelet function inhibitor, superior to aspirin in cats with previous ATE.

Beta Blocker plus Diltiazem

• Cats that remain tachycardic on a single agent can be treated cautiously with a combination of a beta blocker and diltiazem.
• Monitor for bradycardia and hypotension.

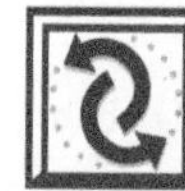

FOLLOW-UP

PATIENT MONITORING

• Observe closely for dyspnea, lethargy, weakness, anorexia, and painful posterior paralysis or paresis.

- If treating with warfarin, monitor prothrombin time.
- If treating with ACE inhibitor or spironolactone, monitor renal function and electrolytes.
- Repeat echocardiogram in 6 months to assess efficacy of treatment for hypertrophy. If beta blocker or diltiazem was prescribed in asymptomatic animal and there is evidence of progressive hypertrophy/LA enlargement, consider switching to another class of medications (or adding an ACE inhibitor) and recheck 4–6 months later.
- Echocardiographic evaluations that reveal LA diameters >2 cm or loss of LV systolic function should prompt more aggressive prophylaxis against ATE (e.g., clopidogrel with low molecular weight heparin).

PREVENTION/AVOIDANCE

Avoid stressful situations that might precipitate CHF.

POSSIBLE COMPLICATIONS

- Heart failure.
- ATE and paralysis.
- Cardiac arrhythmias/sudden death.

EXPECTED COURSE AND PROGNOSIS

- Animals homozygous for MyBPC mutations more likely to develop severe HCM and at earlier age than heterozygous animals.
- Prognosis varies considerably, probably because there are multiple causes. In one study of cats with HCM living at least 24 hours following presentation:
    - Asymptomatic cats—median survival 563 days (range: 2–3,778 days).
    - Cats with syncope—median survival 654 days (range: 28–1,505 days).
    - Cats with CHF—median survival 563 days (range: 2–4,418 days).
    - Cats with ATE—median survival 184 days (range: 2–2,278 days).
    - Older age and larger left atria predicted shorter survival.

MISCELLANEOUS

ASSOCIATED CONDITIONS

Aortic thromboembolism.

PREGNANCY/FERTILITY/BREEDING

- High risk of complications.
- Avoid aspirin.

SEE ALSO

- Aortic Thromboembolism.
- Congestive Heart Failure, Left-Sided.
- Hypersomatotropism/Acromegaly in Cats.
- Hypertension, Systemic Arterial.
- Hyperthyroidism.
- Murmurs, Heart.

ABBREVIATIONS

- ACE = angiotensin-converting enzyme.
- ATE = aortic thromboembolism.
- CHF = congestive heart failure.
- HCM = hypertrophic cardiomyopathy.
- IVS = interventricular septum.
- LA = left atrial.
- LV = left ventricular.
- MyBPC = myosin-binding protein C.
- QTc = QT interval corrected for heart rate.
- SAM = systolic anterior mitral motion.

Suggested Reading

Fox PR, Keene BW, Lamb K, et al. International collaborative study to assess cardiovascular risk and evaluate long-term health in cats with preclinical hypertrophic cardiomyopathy and apparently healthy cats: the REVEAL study. J Vet Intern Med 2018, 32(3):930–943.

McDonald K. Feline cardiomyopathy. In: Smith FWK, Tilley LP, Oyama MA, Sleeper MM, eds. Manual of Canine and Feline Cardiology, 5th ed. St. Louis, MO: Saunders Elsevier, 2016, pp. 153–180.

Novo Matos J, Pereira N, Glaus T, et al. Transient myocardial thickening in cats associated with heart failure. J Vet Intern Med 2018, 32(1):48–56.

Romito G, Guglielmini C, Mazzarella MO, et al. Diagnostic and prognostic utility of surface electrocardiography in cats with left ventricular hypertrophy. J Vet Cardiol 2018, 20(5):364–375.

Authors Francis W.K. Smith, Jr., Bruce W. Keene, and Kathryn M. Meurs

Consulting Editor Michael Aherne

Client Education Handout available online

CARDIOMYOPATHY, HYPERTROPHIC—DOGS

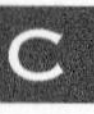

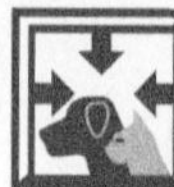

BASICS

OVERVIEW

Hypertrophic cardiomyopathy (HCM) is defined as inappropriate myocardial hypertrophy of a nondilated left ventricle, occurring in the absence of an identifiable stimulus. HCM is rare in dogs, and is characterized by left ventricular (LV) concentric hypertrophy (increased wall thickness). The primary disease process is confined to the heart and only affects other organ systems when congestive heart failure (CHF) is present. Increased LV wall thickness leads to impaired ventricular filling (due to lack of compliance and abnormal relaxation), with resultant increases in LV end-diastolic pressure and left atrial (LA) pressure. LA enlargement is usually in response to increased LV end-diastolic pressure. Mitral insufficiency and/or dynamic LV outflow tract obstruction commonly occur secondary to structural and/or functional changes of the mitral valve apparatus caused by papillary muscle malalignment due to hypertrophy.

SIGNALMENT

- The incidence of HCM in dogs is very low, thus accurate accounts of signalment are lacking.
- Young (<3 years) male dogs.
- Rottweiler, Dalmatian, German shepherd, pointer breeds and Boston terriers have been reported.

SIGNS

Historical Findings

- Most are asymptomatic.
- Signs of left CHF predominate in symptomatic dogs.
- Syncope, generally during activity or exercise.
- Sudden death is the most commonly reported clinical sign.

Physical Examination Findings

- ± Systolic heart murmur.
- ± Gallop heart sound.
- ± Signs of left CHF (e.g., dyspnea, cyanosis, exercise intolerance, cough).

CAUSES & RISK FACTORS

The cause of canine HCM is unknown. Genetic abnormalities in genes coding for myocardial contractile proteins have been documented in humans and cats.

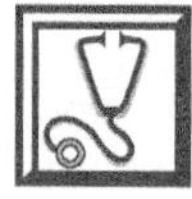

DIAGNOSIS

DIFFERENTIAL DIAGNOSIS

- Systemic hypertension.
- Infiltrative cardiac disorders.
- Thyrotoxicosis.
- Mitral dysplasia.

IMAGING

Radiography

- May be normal or may show LA or LV enlargement.
- Pulmonary edema present with left CHF.

Echocardiography

- Severe cases usually have marked LV and papillary muscle hypertrophy, and LA enlargement. Hypertrophy is usually global, but can be more regional or segmental (asymmetric). Milder forms may have subtle LV hypertrophy.
- Systolic anterior motion of the mitral valve, suggesting dynamic LV outflow tract obstruction (LVOTO), is common in dogs with HCM.

DIAGNOSTIC PROCEDURES

ECG

- May be normal.
- ST segment and T wave abnormalities have been reported.
- Atrial or ventricular ectopic arrhythmias may rarely occur.

Blood Pressure

Usually normal. Should be evaluated to rule out systemic hypertension as the cause of LV hypertrophy.

PATHOLOGIC FINDINGS

- Abnormal heart : body weight ratio.
- LV concentric hypertrophy.
- The interventricular septum may have an impact lesion, varying from a small opaque lesion to a thickened plaque.
- The mitral valve is often thickened and elongated.
- Varying degrees of LA enlargement may be present.

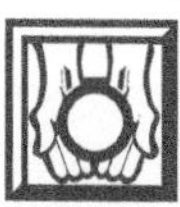

TREATMENT

Treatment is generally only pursued if there is evidence of CHF, severe arrhythmias, or frequent syncope. Exercise restriction and sodium restriction are beneficial.

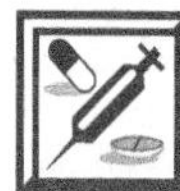

MEDICATIONS

DRUG(S) OF CHOICE

- In patients with left CHF, diuretics and angiotensin-converting enzyme (ACE) inhibitor therapy are advocated.
- In dogs with severe dynamic LVOTO, administration of beta blockers or calcium channel blockers has been advocated; however, benefit has not been proven.
- Beta blockers or calcium channel blockers may also improve myocardial oxygenation, reduce heart rate, improve LV diastolic function, and control arrhythmias, and therefore may be useful in dogs with left CHF; however, benefit has also not been proven.

CONTRAINDICATIONS/POSSIBLE INTERACTIONS

- Positive inotropes may worsen dynamic LVOTO.
- Avoid calcium channel blockers in combination with beta blockers, as clinically significant bradyarrhythmias can develop.
- Avoid potent arteriolar dilators in cases with dynamic LVOTO. The use of milder vasodilators such as ACE inhibitors in dogs with CHF is generally well tolerated.

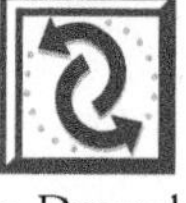

FOLLOW-UP

- Depends on clinical severity. Serial radiography and/or echocardiography may help characterize disease progression and guide medication adjustments.
- Due to the rarity of canine HCM, prognostic information is lacking. In dogs with severe CHF or other complications, prognosis is generally guarded.

MISCELLANEOUS

ABBREVIATIONS

- ACE = angiotensin-converting enzyme.
- CHF = congestive heart failure.
- HCM = hypertrophic cardiomyopathy.
- LA = left atrial.
- LV = left ventricular.
- LVOTO = left ventricular outflow tract obstruction.

Suggested Reading

Oyama MA. Canine cardiomyopathy. In: Smith FWK, Tilley LP, Oyama MA, Sleeper MM, eds., Manual of Canine and Feline Cardiology, 5th ed. St. Louis, MO: Saunders Elsevier, 2016, pp. 141–152.

Ware WA. Myocardial diseases of the dog. In: Ware WA, Cardiovascular Disease in Small Animal Medicine. London: Manson/Veterinary Press, 2011, pp. 280–299.

Author Michael Aherne

Consulting Editors Michael Aherne

Acknowledgment The author and book editors acknowledge the prior contribution of Larry P. Tilley.

BASICS

OVERVIEW

• Nutritional imbalances, such as taurine and L-carnitine deficiency, can lead to the development of dilated cardiomyopathy (DCM) in some dogs and cats. Deficiencies of other nutrients (e.g., selenium, zinc, vitamin E, thiamine, copper, iron) or nutrient toxicities (e.g., iron, cobalt) also have the potential to alter myocardial function, resulting in clinical manifestations of heart disease. Additionally, relative nutritional deficiencies or toxicities may interact with other toxic, infectious, or genetic insults in certain individuals to produce DCM.
• Taurine is the most abundant free amino acid found in cardiac muscle, playing an important role in myocardial calcium regulation. Taurine deficiency was first reported as a cause of reversible DCM in cats in 1987, prompting an increase in the dietary taurine requirement for commercial cat foods, and since then DCM in cats is uncommon. Unlike cats, dogs should be able to endogenously synthesize taurine; however, several breeds (e.g., American cocker spaniel, Newfoundland, Irish wolfhound, golden retriever) have reported predispositions to taurine deficiency and resultant DCM. Additionally, some commercial dog foods such as grain-free, high-legume, lamb and rice formulations and high-fiber foods, have been associated with taurine deficiency. Oral taurine supplementation can effect disease reversal in deficient cats and significant improvement in dogs.
• L-carnitine, a quaternary amine, is an important part of enzyme systems that transport fatty acids into mitochondria for oxidization to make energy. It also has other important cellular metabolic and scavenging functions. Carnitine deficiency complicates some cases of DCM in dogs. Plasma L-carnitine deficiency in association with cardiomyopathy does not mean that the deficiency is the sole cause of the myopathy, although correcting the deficiency, if possible, makes medical and physiologic sense. In the dog, dietary carnitine intake influences plasma concentrations significantly, and oral carnitine supplementation is usually an effective means of raising plasma and subsequently muscle carnitine levels.
• A perceived increase in recognition of DCM in dogs eating boutique, exotic-ingredient, or grain-free (BEG) dog foods in 2018 prompted an FDA investigation into a possible relationship between BEG diets and canine DCM. The majority of affected dogs eating BEG diets do not appear to be taurine or L-carnitine deficient; however, golden retrievers appear to be more susceptible to taurine deficiency when eating these foods. The underlying cause has not yet (as of writing) been identified, and causation has not been proven. Nutritional management, involving diet change and in some cases taurine supplementation, has resulted in improvement or resolution of cardiomyopathy over a period of 3–12 months. Investigations are ongoing.

SIGNALMENT

Dogs

• Golden retrievers, American cocker spaniels, Newfoundlands, English setters, St. Bernards, and Irish wolfhounds are reported to be predisposed to taurine-deficient DCM.
• L-carnitine deficiency has been reported in a family of boxers.
• Dogs eating BEG diets that are affected with suspected nutritional DCM have been of varied ages and breeds.

Cats

Taurine deficiency is rare in cats fed commercial, nutritionally balanced diets. Taurine-deficient DCM can occur in cats fed vegetarian or home-prepared diets.

SIGNS

• Clinical signs of taurine-deficient DCM are related to poor myocardial contractility, which can lead to congestive heart failure in some cases; these signs include lethargy, weakness, syncope, dyspnea and tachypnea.
• Cats may also present for reproductive failure, poor growth, or blindness due to central retinal degeneration.
• Clinical signs of carnitine deficiency can be diverse, ranging from clinical manifestations of DCM to skeletal muscle pain and exercise intolerance.
• See Cardiomyopathy, Dilated—Dogs.

CAUSES & RISK FACTORS

• Vegetarian and home-prepared diets increase the risk of taurine-deficient DCM in cats if taurine is not exogenously supplemented adequately.
• Factors predisposing to taurine deficiency in dogs include breed (possible genetic causes) and dietary components; high-fiber diets, low-protein diets, lamb and rice diets, and beet pulp ingredients have been associated with taurine deficiency; dietary predisposition to taurine deficiency with these factors could be a result of inadequate taurine precursors (methionine and cysteine), low bioavailability of taurine and/or precursors, reduced entero-hepatic bile acid recycling due to high dietary fiber, excessive urinary taurine wasting, or gastrointestinal microbial interaction with taurine.
• Some dogs with DCM have been documented to have carnitine transport defects, in which muscle carnitine is low despite adequate plasma concentrations. In cases in which a mitochondrial enzyme defect causes the accumulation of a metabolite to toxic levels within the mitochondria (e.g., multiple Co-A dehydrogenase defects), free L-carnitine is used to "scavenge" potentially toxic excess metabolites, which appear harmlessly in the plasma and eventually the urine as carnitine esters; in these cases, the total amount of carnitine (free carnitine plus that esterified to other molecules) in the plasma or muscle may be normal or even high, but the ratio of free to esterified carnitine is decreased; this situation is known as carnitine insufficiency (since although the concentration of free carnitine may be within the normal range, it is insufficient to meet the body's pathologically increased need for free carnitine).
• Certain families of boxers appear to be at especially high risk of developing symptomatic DCM in association with, and probably caused by, carnitine deficiency; a known first-degree relative with cardiomyopathy should increase the index of suspicion.
• The cause of the apparent, although unproven, link between BEG diets and canine DCM is unknown; however, the commonality of ingredients in these diets has drawn the attention of veterinary nutritionists; the high legume content of these foods (e.g., lentils and peas), less studied protein sources (e.g., kangaroo, alligator, bison), and other unusual ingredients (e.g., flaxseed) raise the possibility of a nutrient deficiency, toxicity, or nutrient–nutrient interaction that may predispose to the development of DCM in some dogs.

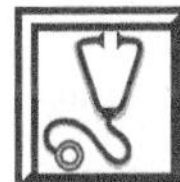

DIAGNOSIS

CBC/BIOCHEMISTRY/URINALYSIS

Normal

OTHER LABORATORY TESTS

• Ideally, both whole blood and plasma taurine concentrations should be evaluated to assess for taurine deficiency in any dog with DCM; if only one blood sample can be analyzed, whole blood is considered a better indicator of long-term taurine status. Blood for taurine concentrations should be drawn into lithium heparin tubes and frozen immediately. The normal whole blood taurine concentration range for dogs (200–350 nmol/mL) has been questioned recently, especially in golden retrievers, where normal has been proposed to be 213–377 nmol/mL. Historically, taurine-deficient DCM is diagnosed when whole blood concentrations are <150 nmol/mL in dogs and <200 nmol/mL in cats, or when plasma taurine concentrations are <40 nmol/mL in both species; values ≤213 nmol/mL (whole blood) and ≤63 nmol/mL (plasma) have been proposed for DCM diagnosis in golden retrievers.
• Plasma carnitine concentrations appear to be a specific but insensitive indicator of

myocardial or skeletal muscle carnitine deficiency. Plasma free carnitine concentrations of less than 8 μmol/L are considered diagnostic of systemic carnitine deficiency; plasma concentrations in the normal or supernormal range do not rule out myocardial carnitine deficiency or insufficiency.

• There is no confirmatory laboratory test currently available to diagnose nutritional DCM associated with BEG diets; dogs should be assessed for taurine and carnitine deficiency, and the diagnosis is solidified by response to nutritional management.

IMAGING

Echocardiography is used to diagnose DCM.

DIAGNOSTIC PROCEDURES

• Endomyocardial biopsy is the gold standard to assess myocardial carnitine levels, since plasma carnitine concentrations are an insensitive indicator of muscle carnitine deficiency.
• Myocardial free carnitine concentrations <3.5 nmol/mg of noncollagenous protein are considered diagnostic of myocardial carnitine deficiency.
• Ratio of esterified to free carnitine >0.4 is considered diagnostic of carnitine insufficiency.

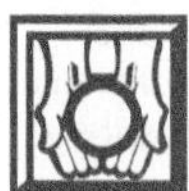

TREATMENT

• Response to nutritional manipulation and supplementation can take months, so patients will require medications to support myocardial function (e.g., pimobendan), antagonize neurohormonal activation (e.g., angiotensin-converting enzyme inhibitors and spironolactone), and diuretic therapy if congestive heart failure is present (e.g., furosemide).
• Taurine supplementation if taurine deficiency is diagnosed; if blood concentrations are not measured, it is reasonable to trial with supplementation and assess response to treatment; taurine deficiency associated with DCM in American cocker spaniels is reported to respond to both taurine and L-carnitine supplementation.
• Treatment with L-carnitine is indicated in addition to conventional treatment for DCM; however, some dogs, including some families of carnitine-deficient boxers, fail to respond clinically to supplementation. While supplementation dramatically improves a small percentage of dogs with DCM, the overall efficacy of L-carnitine supplementation for treatment of DCM is untested. If a trial of metabolic supplementation is desired in the absence of known L-carnitine deficiency, the combination of L-carnitine with taurine and CoQ10 (100 mg as ubiquinol q8–12h) seems prudent.
• Transition to a high-quality, scientifically backed, grain-based food with a well-studied protein source is critical to the recovery of nutritional DCM associated with BEG diets. The role of taurine supplementation in the absence of deficiency is uncertain; however, there is no known detriment to empiric supplementation, and taurine may have therapeutic benefits apart from correction of deficiency.

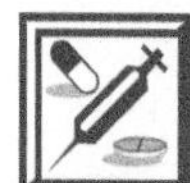

MEDICATIONS

DRUG(S) OF CHOICE

Taurine

• Dogs—250 mg PO q12h if <10 kg; 500 mg PO q12h if 10–25 kg; 1000 mg PO q12h if >25 kg.
• Cats—250 mg PO q12h.

L-Carnitine

• Large-breed dogs—2 g (approximately 1 tsp L-carnitine powder) q8–12h.
• American cocker spaniels—(in combination with taurine) 1 g (approximately 0.5 tsp L-carnitine powder) q8–12h.

FOLLOW-UP

Repeat echocardiogram 3–6 months after nutritional manipulation, including amino acid supplementation and/or diet change. Improvement in myocardial function may take up to a year for dogs with nutritional cardiomyopathy.

MISCELLANEOUS

ASSOCIATED CONDITIONS

N/A

AGE-RELATED FACTORS

N/A

ZOONOTIC POTENTIAL

None

PREGNANCY/FERTILITY/BREEDING

Taurine deficiency may cause reproductive failure in cats.

SEE ALSO

• Cardiomyopathy, Dilated—Cats.
• Cardiomyopathy, Dilated—Dogs.

ABBREVIATIONS

• BEG = boutique, exotic-ingredient, grain-free.
• DCM = dilated cardiomyopathy.

Suggested Reading

Adin D, DeFrancesco T, Keene B, et al. Echocardiographic phenotype of DCM differs based on diet type. J Vet Cardiol 2019, 21:1–9.

Authors Darcy B. Adin and Bruce W. Keene
Consulting Editor Michael Aherne

CARDIOMYOPATHY, RESTRICTIVE—CATS

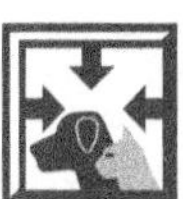

BASICS

DEFINITION

A rare, primary heart muscle disease characterized *functionally* by severe diastolic dysfunction with restrictive left ventricular (LV) filling and normal to near normal systolic function, *morphologically* by a nondilated, nonhypertrophied left ventricle with increased endocardial and/or myocardial fibrosis and severe atrial enlargement, and *clinically* by congestive heart failure (CHF), thromboembolic disease, and cardiac death.

PATHOPHYSIOLOGY

• Increased cardiomyofilament Ca^{2+} sensitivity leading to severely impaired myocardial relaxation, high myocardial stiffness due to endomyocardial fibrosis (endomyocardial type) and/or interstitial fibrosis (myocardial type), and disorganized myofiber architecture (disarray) are main characteristics of primary restricted cardiomyopathy (RCM); RCM-like myocardial changes and clinical syndromes can result from myocardial remodeling and dysfunction secondary to other causes (e.g., endomyocarditis, immune-mediated disease, or end-stage hypertrophic cardiomyopathy). • Diastolic heart failure and cardiogenic arterial thromboembolism (ATE) lead to high mortality.

SYSTEMS AFFECTED

• Cardiovascular. • Respiratory.

GENETICS

Primary RCM can be a spontaneous or familial disease, but is generally considered of genetic cause in humans with an autosomal dominant pattern of inheritance; several genes encoding sarcomeric and nonsarcomeric proteins can be affected; RCM-causing mutations have not been identified in cats.

INCIDENCE/PREVALENCE

Primary feline RCM is rare—prevalence ranging from 1% to 5% of all myocardial diseases in cats.

SIGNALMENT

• Cats. • Higher prevalence in Siamese and oriental cats. • Middle-aged to older cats. • Male predisposition.

SIGNS

Historical Findings

• Lethargy. • Weight loss. • Paresis or paralysis (i.e., signs of ATE). • Labored breathing. • Tachypnea. • Ascites. • Jugular venous distension. • Cyanosis.

Physical Examination Findings

• If not in CHF—arrhythmias. ○ Prominent gallop sounds are a hallmark. ○ Heart murmur uncommon. • If in CHF—above signs plus the following: ○ Tachypnea. ○ Labored breathing. ○ Cyanosis. ○ Hepatomegaly or ascites with jugular venous distention. ○ Pulmonary crackles. ○ Muffled cardiac or respiratory sounds if pleural effusion. ○ Paralysis or paresis with loss of femoral pulses; one or more extremities cold and painful (ATE).

CAUSES

• Primary RCM—currently unknown; genetic cause documented in humans. • Secondary RCM—late or end stage of underlying disease (e.g., hypertrophic cardiomyopathy); link between prior interstitial pneumonia and feline endomyocarditis leading to RCM suspected in one study.

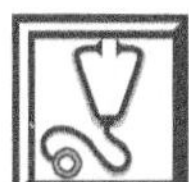

DIAGNOSIS

DIFFERENTIAL DIAGNOSIS

• Advanced stages of other feline cardiomyopathies: ○ Hypertrophic, dilated, arrhythmogenic right ventricular, non-specific phenotype, and tachycardia-induced cardiomyopathy. ○ Myocardial infarct. ○ CHF secondary to thyrotoxicosis or hypertensive heart disease.

CBC/BIOCHEMISTRY/URINALYSIS

Routine chemistry panel and urinalysis helpful to document concurrent or complicating conditions (e.g., renal failure and potassium depletion).

OTHER LABORATORY TESTS

• Plasma T_4 concentration in cats ≥6 years old. • Plasma cardiac troponin I concentration (more specific if ischemic heart disease or myocarditis suspected).

IMAGING

Thoracic Radiography

• Cardiomegaly with severe biatrial enlargement ("valentine" heart on v/d projections). • Interstitial or alveolar infiltrates or pleural effusion with pulmonary venous distention if in CHF.

Echocardiography

• *Note:* definitive diagnostic criteria are *poorly* defined and remain controversial. Early (noncongestive) RCM has rarely been documented in cats. • Anatomic findings characterizing the RCM phenotype include: ○ Severe biatrial enlargement. ○ Nonhypertrophied, nondilated left ventricle (normal chamber dimension, normal wall thickness). ○ Severe enlargement of the left atrium with spontaneous echocardiographic contrast or thrombi frequently seen. ○ Prominent, often diffuse echogenic scar ("moderator bands," false tendons) leading to a small LV lumen and narrowing at the midventricle (endomyocardial fibrosis or "bridging" fibrosis). ○ Focal areas of highly echogenic and often thin myocardium indicative of ischemia or scarring. ○ Myocardium can appear normal with pure myocardial form of RCM. ○ Pleural effusion and pericardial effusion may be present.
• Functional findings (echocardiographic): ○ Severe LV diastolic dysfunction on Doppler echocardiography—restrictive LV filling with a peak velocity of early : late transmitral flow (E : A) ratio >2.0, short isovolumic relaxation time (<37 msec), shortened deceleration time of E (<45 msec), low peak velocity of mitral annular motion (E′), and E : E′ ≫15. ○ Normal to low normal LV systolic function (in some cases LV systolic dysfunction is present). ○ Regional wall motion abnormalities possible. ○ Left atrial dysfunction. ○ Severe left atrial appendage enlargement with evidence of blood stasis. ○ Midventricular obstruction with flow turbulence in cats with bridging endomyocardial fibrosis. ○ In cats with other causes of restrictive physiology, characteristics of the underlying disease can predominate; however, severe atrial enlargement and restrictive LV filling will be present in nearly all cats.

DIAGNOSTIC PROCEDURES

ECG

• *Note*: ECG findings are neither sensitive nor specific. • Sinus tachycardia is common, but cats with severe CHF and hypothermia may be bradycardic. • Ventricular or supraventricular ectopic beats, paroxysmal or sustained supraventricular or ventricular tachycardia, or atrial fibrillation. • Atrial or ventricular enlargement patterns. • ST segment changes.

Pathology

• *Note*: histopathologic confirmation is needed to diagnose RCM. • Increased heart weight (>19 g). • Severe biatrial dilatation. • Locally or diffusely thickened opaque endocardium. • False tendons ("moderator bands") present in some cats. • Normal luminal size of the left and right ventricles. • Diffuse or focal cardiomyocyte disarray. • Increased interstitial and replacement fibrosis. • Abnormal intramural coronary arterioles with medial hypertrophy and narrowed lumen. • Increased number of inflammatory cells seen only in cats with acute endomyocarditis—this finding is commonly absent in cats with endocardial fibrosis.

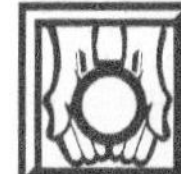

TREATMENT

APPROPRIATE HEALTH CARE

• Patients with severe CHF are hospitalized for emergency care. • Mildly symptomatic animals can be treated with outpatient medical management.

NURSING CARE

• Cats with respiratory distress should receive oxygen. • Sedation is usually beneficial. • Thoracocentesis if relevant pleural effusion. • Maintain a low-stress environment (e.g., cage rest, minimize handling). • Heating pad for hypothermic patients. • Respiratory rate should be used to monitor immediate treatment success.

CARDIOMYOPATHY, RESTRICTIVE—CATS (CONTINUED)

C

ACTIVITY

Cage rest for CHF patients.

DIET

In acute heart failure, maintain intake with hand feeding if necessary.

CLIENT EDUCATION

Owner should be counseled regarding technique of pill administration in cats, possible adverse effects of medications, importance of maintaining stable food and water intake, and monitoring their cat's resting respiratory rate at home.

MEDICATIONS

DRUG(S) OF CHOICE

Acute CHF

• Parenteral administration of furosemide (1–2 mg/kg IV/IM/SC q2–6h); CRI may be considered. • Dermal application of nitroglycerin ointment (2%, one-fourth inch q12h). • Oxygen delivered by cage, mask, nasal prongs, or flow-by. • Thoracocentesis if relevant pleural effusion. • Dobutamine only if cats are hypotensive (systolic blood pressure <90 mmHg); 1–5 µg/kg/minute as CRI, start a lower dose and increase over 0.5–1h. • Severe supraventricular tachyarrhythmias can be treated with diltiazem CRI (2–6 µg/kg/min IV). • Ventricular tachycardia may resolve with resolution of CHF. • Acute therapy of ventricular tachycardia may include lidocaine (0.25–0.5 mg/kg IV *slowly*); monitor closely for neurologic signs of toxicity. • Pimobendan (0.25 mg/kg PO q12h) may be helpful to increase cardiac performance in acute heart failure, but is only used in animals that cannot be stabilized and systemic hypotension cannot be corrected. *Note*: pimobendan is not approved for clinical use in cats and clinical safety and efficacy data are limited. • Antiplatelet medication (clopidogrel bisulfate 18.75 mg PO q24h) or anticoagulants (e.g., unfractionated heparin 150–250 IU/kg SC q6h) may be administered, in particular in cats with severe left atrial enlargement and spontaneous echocardiographic contrast.

Chronic Therapy

• Furosemide is gradually decreased to lowest effective dose. • Angiotensin-converting enzyme (ACE) inhibitors may reduce fluid retention, decrease the need for diuretics, and counterbalance adverse effects of diuretics (e.g., enalapril 0.25–0.5 mg/kg PO q12–24h). • Diltiazem (1.5–2.5 mg/kg regular diltiazem or 10 mg/kg q24h extended-release diltiazem) decreases heart rate and improves supraventricular arrhythmias in affected cats; the addition of digoxin (0.007 mg/kg PO q48h) may allow better control of ventricular response rate in cats with atrial fibrillation; cats with hemodynamically important ventricular and supraventricular ectopy can also benefit from sotalol (1.0–2.0 mg/kg PO q12h). • Pimobendan (0.25 mg/cat PO q12h) may be helpful in the management of chronic heart failure; *note*: pimobendan is not approved for clinical use in cats. • Treat associated conditions (e.g., dehydration, hypothermia, hypokalemia). • Clopidogrel (one-fourth of a 75 mg tablet PO q24h) to inhibit platelets chronically; aspirin (25 mg/kg PO q72h) may also be considered, but efficacy is questionable; in cases of echogenic smoke or prior ATE, dual platelet inhibition (clopidogrel and aspirin) may be used. • Addition of low molecular weight heparin (enoxaparin [Lovenox®] at 1–2 mg/kg q12h SC) may be considered in cats at high risk for thromboembolic disease; apixaban (Eliquis®) at 0.625 mg/cat q12h in cats <5 kg bodyweight and 1.25 mg/cat q12h in cats ≥5 kg has been recommended, but published evidence is not available. • Treatment of cats with preclinical RCM has rarely been reported, but includes ACE inhibitors and antiplatelet drugs; there is currently no specific drug for LV diastolic dysfunction.

CONTRAINDICATIONS

• Beta blockers should never be administered in cats with RCM. • For diltiazem—bradycardia, atrioventricular block, myocardial failure, and hypotension. • For furosemide—severe dehydration, severe hypokalemia, and moderate to severe azotemia. • For ACE inhibitors—moderate to severe azotemia, hypotension, and hyperkalemia.

POSSIBLE INTERACTIONS

• Combination of ACE inhibitors and furosemide—hypotension and renal failure. • Chronic aspirin therapy may increase risk of renal side effects of ACE inhibitors and may lead to inappetence and gastrointestinal upset. • Combining antiplatelets and anticoagulants may increase risk of bleeding.

FOLLOW-UP

PATIENT MONITORING

• Frequent physical reexaminations to assess response to treatment. • Frequent reevaluation of hydration status and renal function, particularly in first few days of therapy to avoid dehydration, hypokalemia, and azotemia. • Repeated thoracocentesis if necessary. • "Hands-off" hourly assessment of respiratory rate in first 12–24 hours can be used to monitor efficacy of CHF therapy. • Radiographs may be repeated in 12–24 hours to monitor pulmonary infiltrate resolution. • Repeat physical examination and analysis of blood biochemistries after 3–7 days' treatment of acute CHF. • Stable patients reevaluated every 2–4 months or more frequently if problems occur.

PREVENTION/AVOIDANCE

No known preventative measures for RCM.

POSSIBLE COMPLICATIONS

Tissue necrosis or loss of function in limbs affected by thromboembolic complications, adverse effects of medications, sudden death, and euthanasia due to refractory heart failure.

EXPECTED COURSE AND PROGNOSIS

Variable, but most cats have a grave prognosis.

MISCELLANEOUS

ASSOCIATED CONDITIONS

Aortic thromboembolism and CHF.

AGE-RELATED FACTORS

Hyperthyroidism should be ruled out with appropriate testing in feline patients with heart disease ≥6 years of age.

SYNONYMS

• Intermediate cardiomyopathy. • Unclassified cardiomyopathy.

SEE ALSO

• Aortic Thromboembolism. • Congestive Heart Failure, Left-Sided. • Congestive Heart Failure, Right-Sided.

ABBREVIATIONS

• A = peak velocity of late transmitral flow. • ACE = angiotensin-converting enzyme. • ATE = arterial thromboembolism. • CHF = congestive heart failure. • E = peak velocity of early transmitral flow. • E′ = peak velocity of mitral annular motion. • LV = left ventricular. • RCM = restrictive cardiomyopathy.

Suggested Reading

Charles PY, Li YJ, Nan CL, Huang XP. Insights into restrictive cardiomyopathy from clinical and animal studies. J Geriatr Cardiol 2011, 8:168–183.

Fox PR. Endomyocardial fibrosis and restrictive cardiomyopathy: pathologic and clinical features. J Vet Cardiol 2004, 6:25–31.

Author Karsten E. Schober

Consulting Editor Michael Aherne

Client Education Handout available online

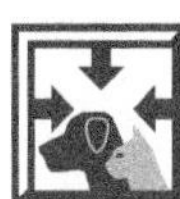

BASICS

DEFINITION

• Cessation of effective perfusion and ventilation because of loss of coordinated cardiac and respiratory function.
• Cardiac arrest invariably follows respiratory arrest if not recognized and corrected.

PATHOPHYSIOLOGY

• Generalized or cellular hypoxia may be cause or effect of sudden death.
• After 1–4 minutes of airway obstruction, breathing efforts stop while circulation remains intact.
• If obstruction continues for 6–9 minutes, severe hypotension and bradycardia lead to dilated pupils, absence of heart sounds, and lack of palpable peripheral pulse.
• After 6–9 minutes, myocardial contractions cease even though ECG may look normal—pulseless electrical activity (formerly electrical mechanical dissociation).
• Ventricular fibrillation, ventricular asystole, and pulseless electrical activity are rhythms indicating cessation of myocardial contractility.

SYSTEMS AFFECTED

• All systems are affected, but those requiring greatest supply of oxygen and nutrients affected first.
• Cardiovascular.
• Renal/urologic.
• Neurologic.

SIGNALMENT

• Dog and cat.
• Any age, breed, or sex.

SIGNS

• Lack of response to stimulation.
• Loss of consciousness.
• Dilated pupils.
• Cyanosis.
• Agonal gasping or absence of ventilation.
• Absence of peripheral pulses.
• Hypothermia.
• Absence of audible heart sounds.

CAUSES

• Hypoxemia caused by ventilation–perfusion mismatch, diffusion barrier impairment, hypoventilation, or shunting.
• Poor oxygen delivery due to anemia or vasoconstriction.
• Myocardial disease—infectious, inflammatory, infiltrative, traumatic, neoplastic, or embolic.
• Acid-base abnormalities.
• Electrolyte derangements—hyperkalemia, hypocalcemia, and hypomagnesemia.
• Hypovolemia.
• Shock.
• Anesthetic agents.
• Sepsis/septic shock.
• CNS trauma.
• Electrical shock.

RISK FACTORS

• Cardiovascular disease.
• Respiratory disease.
• Trauma.
• Anesthesia.
• Septicemia.
• Endotoxemia.
• Ventricular arrhythmias—ventricular tachycardia, R on T phenomenon, multiform ventricular complexes.
• Increased parasympathetic tone—gastrointestinal disease, respiratory disease, manipulation of eyes, larynx, or abdominal viscera.
• Prolonged seizing.
• Invasive cardiovascular manipulation—pericardiocentesis, surgery, angiography.

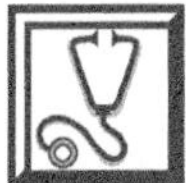

DIAGNOSIS

• Sudden cardiovascular collapse associated with inadequate cardiac output leading to severe consequences.
• Quick assessment and diagnosis are critical.
• Assess the ABCs—airway, breathing, circulation.

DIFFERENTIAL DIAGNOSIS

• Severe hypovolemia and absence of palpable pulses.
• Pericardial effusion with cardiac tamponade, decreased cardiac output, and muffled heart sounds.
• Pleural effusion with respiratory arrest.
• Respiratory arrest can be confused with cardiopulmonary arrest (CPA).
• Upper airway obstruction can rapidly progress to CPA.

CBC/BIOCHEMISTRY/URINALYSIS

May help identify underlying cause for CPA, but should not be part of initial triage.

OTHER LABORATORY TESTS

• Arterial blood gas evaluation may be useful during or after resuscitative procedures, but is not part of initial emergency management.
• Venous blood gas evaluation may be more useful during cardiopulmonary resuscitation (CPR) than arterial blood gas and provides electrolyte and lactate concentrations.

IMAGING

• Thoracic/abdominal focused assessment with sonography for trauma (TFAST®/AFAST®) may be useful in identifying underlying disease; additional terminology being introduced, such as POCUS (point of care ultrasound) and eFAST (extended FAST).
• Thoracic or abdominal radiographs or abdominal ultrasound may help identify underlying disease processes, but only consider after patient has been stabilized.
• Echocardiography may confirm pericardial effusion or underlying myocardial disease, but should not interfere with resuscitative procedures.

DIAGNOSTIC PROCEDURES

Once CPA has developed, continuous ECG monitoring, blood pressure monitoring, pulse oximetry, and capnography are useful in monitoring effectiveness of resuscitative procedures.

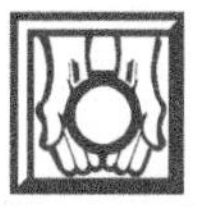

TREATMENT

Institute CPR immediately upon diagnosing CPA; CPR in veterinary patients should follow Reassessment Campaign on Veterinary Resuscitation (RECOVER) evidence-based guidelines, published in 2012 and divided into five domains. It is recommended the reader read the original publication.

Basic Life Support (Domain 2)

Immediate Recognition of CPA

If patient is identified as being nonresponsive and apneic, start CPR immediately, do not take time to confirm via palpation of pulse or ECG.

Chest Compressions

• Perform CPR in continuous, uninterrupted, 2-minute cycles when possible.
• Use the cardiac pump in patients weighing <10 kg bodyweight; with the patient in right lateral recumbency, perform compressions directly over the heart (intercostal spaces 3–5); this can be performed using one or two hands.
• Use the thoracic pump for patients weighing >10 kg bodyweight; with the patient in right lateral recumbency, apply thoracic compressions at the widest portion of the thorax.
• Different compression and ventilation regimes have been reported.
• Providing appropriate compressions (100–120 per minute) and appropriate ventilations (10 per minute) without stopping compressions for ventilations and without trying to synchronize ventilations with compressions is the goal; the chest should be displaced ~30–50%.
• Try to minimize discontinuing compressions to interpret ECG.
• Avoid leaning on the patient during chest compressions and allow full chest wall recoil.
• Interposing abdominal compressions between chest compressions enhances cerebral and coronary blood flow by increasing aortic diastolic pressure; this technique has not been shown to improve survival, but should be considered if adequate personnel are available.

Airway and Ventilation

• Visualize the airway by extending the patient's head and neck and pulling the tongue forward; clear any debris (e.g., secretions,

blood, or vomitus) manually or with suction; use of a laryngoscope is advised.
- Establish an airway by either oral endotracheal intubation or, if complete obstruction, emergency tracheostomy.
- Correct endotracheal tube placement should be confirmed visually, by auscultation and/or capnography.
- 10 breaths per minute with a tidal volume of 10 mL/kg and an inspiratory time of 1 second; peak airway pressures should not exceed 20 cm H_2O.
- Techniques for ventilation include mouth to mouth, mouth to nose, or mouth to endotracheal tube; these techniques provide ~16% oxygen; use of a mechanical resuscitator (Ambu® bag) and room air provides 21% oxygen.
- The preferred technique is endotracheal intubation and ventilation with 100% oxygen using an Ambu bag or an anesthesia machine.
- The suggested rate of oxygen administration is 150 mL/kg/minute.

Circulation
- Assessment—palpate peripheral pulses and auscultate heart to confirm CPA.
- External thoracic compression provides at best ~30% of normal cardiac output; internal cardiac compression is two to three times more effective in improving cerebral and coronary perfusion.

Open-Chest CPR
- Indicated if closed-chest CPR is ineffective or preexisting conditions such as flail chest, obesity, diaphragmatic hernia, pericardial effusion, or other significant intrathoracic disease preclude closed-chest techniques.
- Perform through a left thoracotomy at the fifth or sixth intercostal space.
- Perform a pericardectomy.
- The palmar surface of the fingers and thumb is used to push the ventricular blood toward the great vessel; digital compression of the descending aorta may help improve coronary and cerebral perfusion.

Advanced Life Support (Domain 4)

This includes drug therapy and additional resuscitation techniques. Drugs should be administered every other CPR cycle (~q4 minutes).

Epinephrine
- Epinephrine low dose—0.01 mg/kg IV (1 : 10,000) 1 mL/10 kg patient.
- Epinephrine high dose—0.1 mg/kg IV (1 : 1000) can be used in protracted CPR.

Vasopressin

May be used as alternative to epinephrine 0.8 U/kg IV (20 U/ml; ~0.5 ml/10 kg patient); may be used in combination with epinephrine, especially if protracted CPR.

Atropine
- Atropine—0.04 mg/kg IV (0.4 mg/mL) 1 mL/10 kg patient.
- Limited data to suggest benefit unless arrest is due to increased vagal tone.

Fluids

Administer fluids cautiously unless known hypovolemia has led to CPA. Crystalloids, colloids, or blood products may be considered, including Oxyglobin®.

MEDICATIONS

DRUG(S) OF CHOICE
- See Advanced Life Support.
- Administer drugs via intravenous, intraosseous, or intratracheal routes in descending order of preference; volumes should be doubled if administering via the intratracheal route and diluted in saline.
- Intracardiac administration should not be used unless open-chest CPR is being performed; administration of epinephrine into the left ventricle with concurrent digital or mechanical compression of descending aorta is optimal.

PRECAUTIONS
Fluid administration should be used cautiously and only if there is a known history of hypovolemia; excessive fluid administration may lead to decreased coronary perfusion.

FOLLOW-UP

PATIENT MONITORING
- Maintain normal heart rate and blood pressure with fluids and inotropic agents.
- Arterial blood pressure.
- Central venous pressure.
- Blood gas analysis.
- Support respiration with artificial ventilation and supplemental oxygen.
- Neurologic status—if signs of increased intracranial pressure develop, consider mannitol, corticosteroids, and furosemide.
- ECG—continuously.
- Urine output.
- Body temperature.
- Radiograph thorax to assess resuscitative injury.
- Diagnose and correct factors that led to initial CPA.

PREVENTION/AVOIDANCE
Careful monitoring of all critically ill patients.

POSSIBLE COMPLICATIONS
- Vomiting.
- Aspiration pneumonia.
- Fractured ribs or sternebrae.
- Pulmonary contusions and edema.
- Pneumothorax.
- Acute renal failure.
- Neurologic deficits.
- Cardiac arrhythmias.

EXPECTED COURSE AND PROGNOSIS
- Prognosis depends on underlying disease process.
- Rapid return to spontaneous cardiac and respiratory function improves the prognosis.
- Overall prognosis is poor; <10% of patients are discharged.

MISCELLANEOUS

ZOONOTIC POTENTIAL
None

SYNONYMS
- For CPA—cardiac arrest, heart attack.
- For CPR—cardiopulmonary cerebral resuscitation (CPCR).

SEE ALSO
- Ventricular Fibrillation.
- Ventricular Standstill (Asystole).

ABBREVIATIONS
- CPA = cardiopulmonary arrest.
- CPCR = cardiopulmonary cerebral resuscitation.
- CPR = cardiopulmonary resuscitation.
- FAST = focused assessment with sonography for trauma.
- POCUS = point of care ultrasound.
- RECOVER = Reassessment Campaign on Veterinary Resuscitation.

Suggested Reading

Fletcher DJ, Boller M, Brainard BM, et al. RECOVER evidence and knowledge gap analysis on veterinary CPR. Part 7: Clinical guidelines. J Vet Emerg Crit Care 2012, 22(S1):102–131.

McIntyre RL, Hopper K, Epstein SE, et al. Assessment of cardiopulmonary resuscitation in 121 dogs and 30 cats at a university teaching hospital (2009–2012). J Vet Emerg Crit Care 2014, 24(6):693–704.

Author Steven L. Marks

Consulting Editor Michael Aherne

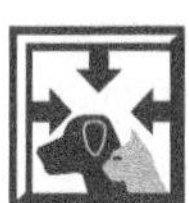

BASICS

DEFINITION

Opacification of the lens (focal or diffuse).

PATHOPHYSIOLOGY

- The normal lens is composed of perfectly aligned lens fibers that create a transparent structure. A clear capsule surrounds the cortex and nucleus. New lens fibers are continually produced at the equator of the lens cortex throughout life. The aqueous humor provides nutrition to the lens.
- A cataract occurs when there is derangement of lens fibers due to changes in lens nutrition, energy metabolism, protein synthesis or metabolism, or osmotic balance.
- Anterior uveitis is a common cause of altered lens nutrition.
- Genetics can result in altered protein and energy metabolism, or protein synthesis, in the lens.
- Diabetes mellitus affects the osmotic balance in the lens. Hyperglycemia increases glucose in the aqueous and lens overwhelming the glycolysis pathway; glucose is shunted to the sorbitol pathway; sorbitol creates an osmotic gradient that draws water into the lens and rapid cataract formation. The sorbitol pathway requires aldose reductase enzyme and dogs have more aldose reductase than cats, making cats more resistant to developing diabetic cataracts. The enzyme levels vary between individuals, which may explain dogs that are resistant to cataract development.

SYSTEMS AFFECTED

Ophthalmic

GENETICS

- Inheritance has been established for many dog breeds; the most common mode of inheritance is autosomal recessive.
- Inheritance has been established in the Himalayan cat (autosomal recessive).

INCIDENCE/PREVALENCE

- One of the leading causes of blindness in dogs.
- The prevalence of genetic cataracts varies significantly; up to 10% in some breeds.
- Most diabetic dogs will develop cataracts regardless of their diabetic control.
- Cataracts are rare in cats.

SIGNALMENT

Species

Dogs and cats.

Breed Predilections

Over 135 dog breeds are suspected as being predisposed to hereditary cataracts.

Mean Age and Range

Cataracts can develop at any age; genetic cataracts can develop as early as 6 months of age.

SIGNS

Historical Findings

- Cloudy/white appearance of the lens.
- Vision loss when the cataracts are bilateral and diabetic cataracts with a rapid, bilateral onset.
- Polyuria/polydipsia is noticed prior to cataract development in diabetic dogs.

Physical Examination Findings

- General physical examination findings—unremarkable unless the dog is an undiagnosed diabetic.
- Ophthalmic examination findings—opacification in one or both lenses.
  - Incipient stage—small, focal opacity/opacities in the lens that does not interfere with the view of the fundus; no vision deficits.
  - Immature stage—diffusely cloudy appearance to the lens with the tapetal reflection still visible and some portions of the fundus visible through a dilated pupil; the menace reflex is positive.
  - Mature stage—completely opaque lens with no tapetal reflection visible; blind.
  - Hypermature stage—wrinkled lens capsule, areas of dense white mineralization, may have portions of liquefied cortex (white, sparkly to clear); deep anterior chamber; blind unless there is a large area of clear liquefied cortex.
  - Intumescent mature cataract—opaque, swollen lens usually due to the hyperosmotic effect of diabetes; shallow anterior chamber.

CAUSES

- Hereditary—most common cause in dogs.
- Diabetes mellitus.
- Anterior uveitis—either by altered nutrition of the lens from the abnormal aqueous, or by posterior synechia and inflammatory debris causing opacification of the anterior lens capsule.
- Trauma—perforating injury that disrupts the anterior lens capsule, most commonly a cat claw injury, especially in puppies and kittens.
- Senile—slowly progressive cataract in geriatric animals, usually beginning as dense nuclear sclerosis followed by gradual spoke-like opacities extending into the cortex.
- Congenital—due to heredity, in utero insult, or associated with other congenital ocular anomalies such as persistent pupillary membranes, persistent hyperplastic primary vitreous/persistent tunica vasculosa lentis, or a hyaloid artery attachment.
- Surgery—transpupillary laser energy, intraocular instrument trauma.
- Toxic—long-term ketoconazole therapy; suspected secondary to toxic by-products of degenerating photoreceptors in dogs with progressive retinal atrophy.
- Radiation—when the eye is in the radiation treatment field for neoplasia of the mouth or head.
- Hypocalcemia—can cause bilateral, diffuse punctate or incipient cataracts.
- Nutritional—use of unbalanced milk replacers in bottle-fed puppies and kittens.
- Electrical shock—chewing electrical cords or lightning strike.

RISK FACTORS

- Diabetes mellitus (dogs).
- Chronic anterior uveitis.
- Progressive retinal atrophy.

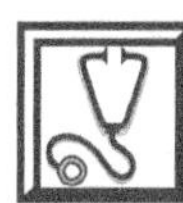

DIAGNOSIS

DIFFERENTIAL DIAGNOSIS

Lenticular nuclear sclerosis—normal aging change in the lens of dogs and cats starting at 6 years of age due to compression of older lens fibers in the center of the lens; gradually becomes more visible with age and can be mistaken for a cataract in geriatric patients; definitive diagnosis can be made using mydriasis (1% tropicamide) and the observation of a perfectly round, bilaterally symmetric, homogeneous nucleus in the center of each lens, and the ability to view the fundus through the lens; vision is rarely affected and treatment is not indicated.

CBC/BIOCHEMISTRY/URINALYSIS

Dogs with diabetic cataracts may have hyperglycemia and glucosuria.

IMAGING

Ocular ultrasound can be used to evaluate the posterior lens capsule for any sign of rupture and can evaluate for retinal detachment prior to cataract surgery.

DIAGNOSTIC PROCEDURES

ERG is performed prior to cataract surgery to evaluate for retinal degeneration when the fundus is not visible due to the cataract.

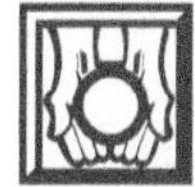

TREATMENT

ACTIVITY

For safety, blind animals should not be allowed access to an in-ground swimming pool or elevated decks with open railings; use caution near stairs; restrict outside activity to fenced yards or leash walks.

CLIENT EDUCATION

- Cataract surgery is routinely performed, with an overall 80–90% success rate.
- Once the cataracts are removed they cannot return.
- Artificial lens implants will restore essentially normal vision.
- Evaluation for surgery should be done early in the course of cataract development to avoid complications that may result in the cataract becoming inoperable, to allow time to plan

CATARACTS (CONTINUED)

C

for the surgery, and in some cases to eliminate the need and extra cost for an ocular ultrasound and ERG.

SURGICAL CONSIDERATIONS

- Phacoemulsification (removal of the cataract through a corneal incision using ultrasonic waves to emulsify and aspirate the lens) is the most common technique for cataract removal.
- The ideal time for cataract surgery is the immature/early mature stage.
- Inherited, diabetic, and senile cataracts are potentially good candidates for surgery; cataracts secondary to anterior uveitis are normally poor surgical candidates.
- Artificial intraocular lenses are routinely placed inside the patient's lens capsule; lens implants restore normal focus and help minimize posterior capsular fibrosis; if a lens cannot be implanted (e.g., due to an unstable lens capsule or luxated lens), the dog or cat will still have functional vision.
- Traumatic lens perforation with release of lens cortex into the anterior chamber may require surgery to remove the lens, depending on the size of the capsular tear.

MEDICATIONS

DRUG(S) OF CHOICE

- Topical anti-inflammatory medication is recommended q6–24h to help prevent or treat lens-induced uveitis with immature, mature, and hypermature cataracts; this can be a topical nonsteroidal anti-inflammatory drug (NSAID) such as flurbiprofen, diclofenac, or ketorolac, or a topical steroid such as prednisolone acetate 1% or dexamethasone 0.1%; topical NSAIDs may be preferable in diabetic patients.
- Topical atropine q8–24h is indicated for lens-induced uveitis; *contraindicated with glaucoma.*
- Oral NSAIDs (carprofen, meloxicam, deracoxib) are also used to treat lens-induced uveitis.
- Topical antioxidants are advertised as able to reverse cataract changes; to date there have been no published data conclusively showing a significant reversal, or delay in progression; time spent trying medical therapy will delay evaluation for surgery, resulting in surgery being performed at a suboptimal stage, or complications from the cataract making it inoperable.
- A topical aldose reductase inhibitor, Kinostat®, is in the final stage of FDA approval. When made available, it may prove helpful in delaying the onset of diabetic cataracts in dogs.

FOLLOW-UP

PATIENT MONITORING

- Incipient or early immature cataracts should be monitored regularly for progression in order to select the ideal time for surgery and to avoid complications associated with cataracts.
- Postoperative monitoring by the surgeon is critical for the success of surgery and should be clearly discussed with the owner prior to surgery.

PREVENTION/AVOIDANCE

Do not breed animals with cataracts.

POSSIBLE COMPLICATIONS

- Lens-induced uveitis—associated with hypermature cataracts and cataracts that progress rapidly; caused by antigenic lens proteins leaking through the lens capsule. Clinical signs can be subtle (e.g., low intraocular pressure) to extreme (granulomatous uveitis with aqueous flare, miosis, synechia, keratic precipitates); preoperative uveitis increases postoperative complications.
- Secondary glaucoma—impaired aqueous outflow from intraocular changes associated with lens-induced uveitis, or from an intumescent cataract causing a forward displacement of the iris, narrowing the iridocorneal angle.
- Retinal detachment—associated with hypermature cataracts and cataracts in young dogs with a rapid onset and cortical liquefaction.
- Lens luxation—associated with hypermature cataracts in which the lens and capsule shrink, causing the zonules to stretch and break, resulting in a lens subluxation or luxation.

EXPECTED COURSE AND PROGNOSIS

- Most cataracts are progressive, although the rate of progression can vary widely depending on age, breed, and location of the cataract.
- Long-term prognosis following cataract surgery is very good; however, some patients have increased risk for postoperative complications.
- Those that do not pursue surgery should be monitored for uveitis and glaucoma.

MISCELLANEOUS

ASSOCIATED CONDITIONS

- Retinal detachment.
- Lens-induced uveitis.
- Congenital ocular anomalies.

AGE-RELATED FACTORS

- Immediate referral for cataracts in young dogs (<2 years of age) is recommended because the cataract can progress very rapidly, with partial cortical liquefaction followed by retinal detachment.
- Nuclear sclerosis is prominent in geriatric animals; a dilated exam may be necessary to definitively distinguish nuclear sclerosis from cataract.

SEE ALSO

- Anterior Uveitis—Cats.
- Anterior Uveitis—Dogs.
- Diabetes Mellitus Without Complication—Cats.
- Diabetes Mellitus Without Complication—Dogs

ABBREVIATION

- NSAID = nonsteroidal anti-inflammatory drug.

Author Margi A. Gilmour
Consulting Editor Kathern E. Myrna

Client Education Handout available online

CEREBELLAR DEGENERATION

BASICS

OVERVIEW

• Progressive and non-progressive etiologies. Progressive - premature aging and neuronal death; may be due to failure of neuronal energy supply, ion regulation, excitotoxicity, autoimmunity/inflammation, or inappropriate apoptosis; neonatal, postnatal, and adult onset (rare). • Nonprogressive - due to abnormal cerebellar development following in utero or neonatal viral infection in cats (feline panleukopenia) and dogs (canine herpesvirus, canine parvovirus).

SIGNALMENT

Progressive

• Dog and cat. • Described in over 40 dog breeds, often affecting a single family or individual. • Eight causal mutations, all with autosomal recessive mode of inheritance, have been identified. Beagle (onset of clinical signs before 1 month); Finnish hound (2 months), Parson Russell terrier (2 months), Jack Russell terrier (2–12 months) Hungarian Vizsla (3 months); Kerry blue terrier and Chinese crested (3–4 months); Old English sheepdog and Gordon setter (6 months – 3 years).
• Immune-mediated disorder described in Coton de Tulear (2 months). • Sporadic reports in miniature poodle (neonatal), papillon (5 months); Scottish terrier, Border Collie, Lagotto Romagnolo, Australian Kelpie, Labrador Retriever, Bavarian mountain dogs, Italian hound (2 months – 1 year); English bulldog (5–8 months); American Staffordshire terrier (2–9 years).
• Late onset disorder described in Labrador Retriever, Bern running dog, Irish setter, and Brittany spaniel (signs at 5–13 years).
• Cerebellar degeneration and coat color dilution reported in one family of Rhodesian ridgebacks. • X-linked mode of inheritance suspected in English pointer (only males affected). • Both early- (days to weeks) and late- (years) onset in domestic shorthair cat.
• Described in two Havana brown kittens from the same litter. Signs observed at one month. Heritable nature suspected.

Nonprogressive

• Two causal mutations identified in two dog breeds. • Non-inflammatory disorder with autosomal recessive mode of inheritance reported in six litters of Coton de Tulear (signs by 2 weeks). • Eurasier dog (2 months).

SIGNS

• Cerebellar ataxia- hypermetria; broad-based stance; swaying of body, intention tremors.
• Lack of menace responses with normal vision and pupillary light reflexes. • Head tilt and episodes of vestibular ataxia with resting or positional nystagmus. • Diffuse tapetal hyperreflectivity on funduscopic exam.
• Decerebellate posture—opisthotonos with extensor rigidity of the forelimbs and flexed hind limbs. • Cerebellar degeneration is not characterized by altered mentation, proprioceptive deficits, or paresis. • Progression of signs varies. • Use caution in interpreting progression of clinical signs—cerebellar ataxia in a puppy or kitten with cerebellar degeneration caused by in utero or neonatal infection may appear to worsen as the animal grows and becomes more active; the underlying disease process itself is nonprogressive.

CAUSES & RISK FACTORS

• Causal mutations associated with progressive cerebellar degeneration have been identified in several breeds. • In utero or neonatal exposure to feline panleukopenia or canine herpesvirus infection. • Poor vaccination history or exposure to modified live virus during gestation. • A syndrome of hepatocerebellar degeneration has been described in a litter of Bernese mountain dogs.
• Paraneoplastic cerebellar degeneration has been reported in humans.

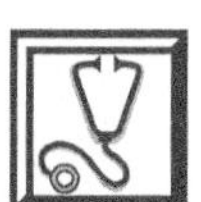

DIAGNOSIS

DIFFERENTIAL DIAGNOSIS

• Lysosomal storage diseases—diffuse diseases of the CNS; differentiate by presence of signs of involvement of parts of the CNS outside of the cerebellum. • Toxicity (e.g., hexachlorophene)—differentiate by history of exposure. • Inflammatory diseases—infectious (e.g., canine distemper and feline infectious peritonitis [FIP]) and immune-mediated (dogs). Differentiate from cerebellar degeneration by MRI and cerebrospinal fluid (CSF) analysis. Infectious diseases are frequently accompanied or preceded by systemic signs of illness. • Cerebellar cyst—differentiate by advanced imaging (MRI).
• Medulloblastoma (cerebellar tumor)—reported in dogs and cats <1 year old; differentiate by advanced imaging (MRI) and CSF analysis. • Other primary and metastatic tumors in adult dogs.

IMAGING

• MRI is preferred imaging modality—cerebellum may be smaller than normal.
• CT can aid in diagnosis of other conditions (e.g., cyst); if MRI is not accessible, CT may have some value.

DIAGNOSTIC PROCEDURES

• CSF analysis—normal with nonprogressive disease; normal-to-high protein concentration and normal cell counts with progressive disease.
• Cerebellar biopsy—may be only definitive means of antemortem diagnosis.

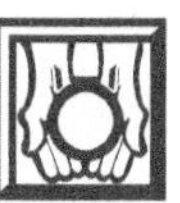

TREATMENT

• Restrict to supervised activity in safe areas; leash-walks only; avoid stairs, furniture, proximity to swimming pools, etc.
• Amantadine has potentiating effects on dopaminergic neurotransmission in CNS and anticholinergic activity; buspirone is serotonin agonist; research models demonstrate some potential benefit for progressive cerebellar degeneration; guidelines and clinical evidence are lacking. • Neuroprotective agents (such as coenzyme Q10 and acetyl-L-carnitine) may have promising effects.

MEDICATIONS

DRUG(S) OF CHOICE

N/A

FOLLOW-UP

• Neurologic status—examine at weekly-to-monthly intervals if progression of signs is uncertain; consider videotaping patient to determine progression objectively.
• Progression of signs—rate varies depending on etiology; ranges from days to years.
• Nonprogressive disease—patient may show improvements as they learn to compensate for deficits. • Do not vaccinate pregnant animals with modified live virus. • Do not breed animals with familial history of cerebellar disease.

MISCELLANEOUS

ABBREVIATIONS

• CSF = cerebrospinal fluid.
• FIP = feline infectious peritonitis.

Suggested Reading

de Lahunta A, Glass E, Kent M. Cerebellum. In: de Lahunta A, Glass E, eds., Veterinary Neuroanatomy and Clinical Neurology, 4th ed. St. Louis, MO: W.B. Saunders, 2015, pp. 368–408.

Dewey CW, da Costa RC. A Practical Guide to Canine and Feline Neurology, 3rd ed. Ames, IA: Wiley-Blackwell, 2016, pp. 183–191.

Urkasemsin, G, Nielsen DM, Singleton A, et al. Genetics of hereditary ataxia in Scottish Terriers. J Vet Intern Med, 2017, 31(4):1132–1139.

Authors Richard J. Joseph and Anne E. Buglione

CEREBELLAR HYPOPLASIA

C

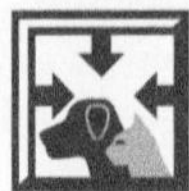

BASICS

OVERVIEW

Caused by incomplete development of parts of the cerebellum owing to intrinsic (inherited) or extrinsic (infectious, toxic, or nutritional) factors.

SIGNALMENT

- Symptoms may not be visible until puppies and kittens begin to stand/walk (usually by 6 weeks old).
- Hereditary in Airedale, chow chow, Boston terrier, Labrador retriever, Weimaraner, shih tzu, miniature schnauzer, and bull terrier.

SIGNS

- Symmetric, nonprogressive cerebellar disorder—head bobbing; limb tremors; aggravated by movement or eating and disappear during sleep (intention tremors).
- Cerebellar ataxia, wide-base stance.
- Dysmetria and disequilibrium—falling, flipping over.

CAUSES & RISK FACTORS

- Cats—usually transplacental or perinatal infection with panleukopenia virus (wild or from modified live virus used in some vaccines), which selectively attacks rapidly dividing cells, e.g., external germinal layer of the cerebellum at birth and for 2 weeks postnatal.
- Dogs—hereditary in some breeds (autosomal recessive).

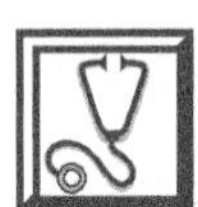

DIAGNOSIS

DIFFERENTIAL DIAGNOSIS

- Age, breed, history, typical symmetric and nonprogressive symptoms—usually sufficient for tentative diagnosis.
- Early cerebellar abiotrophy—postnatal degeneration after normal development; slow progression of signs over weeks to months; neonatal onset (beagle, Samoyed, Rhodesian ridgeback, Irish setter, Jack Russell terrier, miniature poodle) or postnatal onset (Australian kelpie at 5–6 weeks; Kerry blue terrier at 8–16 weeks; rough-coated collie at 4–8 weeks; bullmastiff at 4–9 weeks).
- Neuroaxonal dystrophy—slowly progressive cerebellar signs starting around 5 weeks of age in cats and 7 weeks in Chihuahuas.
- Cerebellar sequels of systemic canine herpesvirus infection—follow systemic illness.
- Concomitant seizures or other cerebral signs—suggest other malformations, such as lissencephaly (wirehaired fox terrier and Irish setter) or hydrocephalus.
- Final diagnosis possible only at necropsy.

CBC/BIOCHEMISTRY/URINALYSIS

Usually normal.

IMAGING

MRI—cerebellar atrophy or malformation (incomplete or asymmetric filling of the caudal cranial fossa by the cerebellum); rule out other malformations.

PATHOLOGIC FINDINGS

- Cerebellum—normally very small in newborn kitten or puppy (cerebellar development continues for up to 10 weeks postnatal); subtle to marked atrophy; as necropsy is performed weeks to months after birth, there is no sign of active inflammation.
- Transverse fibers of the pons—decreased size associated with marked cortical cerebellar atrophy.
- Hydrocephalus—may be concomitant, resulting from multifocal inflammation or multiple malformations (e.g., Dandy–Walker syndrome).
- Microscopic—depletion of cerebellar cortex cellular layers.

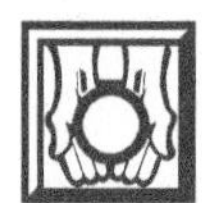

TREATMENT

None

Care

- Restrict environment to prevent injuries and road accidents—no climbing, falling, or escaping.
- Nutritional support as needed.
- Euthanasia—severely affected animals that are unable to feed, groom, or be housetrained.

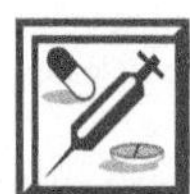

MEDICATIONS

DRUG(S) OF CHOICE

N/A

CONTRAINDICATIONS/POSSIBLE INTERACTIONS

N/A

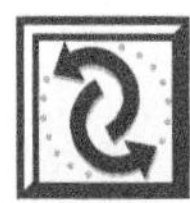

FOLLOW-UP

PATIENT MONITORING

Helps confirm the diagnosis (as necessary).

PREVENTION/AVOIDANCE

Avoid using modified live panleukopenia vaccines in reproducing female cats and keep cats vaccinated against panleukopenia.

POSSIBLE COMPLICATIONS

N/A

EXPECTED COURSE AND PROGNOSIS

- Slight improvement may occur as patient compensates for deficits.
- Deficits—permanent; do not progress; compatible with a normal lifespan.
- Some patients may be acceptable indoor pets.

MISCELLANEOUS

Suggested Reading

de Lahunta A, Glass E, Kent M. Veterinary Neuroanatomy and Clinical Neurology, 4th ed. St. Louis, MO: W.B. Saunders, 2015, pp. 389–390.

Author Christine F. Berthelin-Baker

CEREBROVASCULAR ACCIDENTS

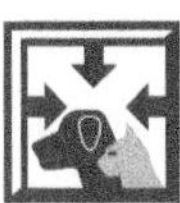

BASICS

DEFINITION

• Sudden onset of nonprogressive focal brain signs. • Signs must remain for >24 hours for a diagnosis of cerebrovascular accident (CVA). • Permanent brain damage usually ensues. • Called transient ischemic attack or TIA if clinical signs resolve within 24 hours.

PATHOPHYSIOLOGY

• Cerebrovascular diseases are the underlying cause of CVA. • Brain abnormality resulting from a pathologic process that compromises the blood supply to the brain. • Lesions affecting the cerebral blood vessels are divided into two broad categories: ◦ Hemorrhagic stroke—ruptured blood vessel with hemorrhage into or around the brain. ◦ Ischemic stroke—abrupt disruption of blood flow from blockage of an artery depriving the brain tissue of oxygen and glucose.

SYSTEMS AFFECTED

• Nervous. • Multisystemic—if underlying cause present.

INCIDENCE/PREVALENCE

Unknown; supposed low compared to human.

SIGNALMENT

Species

Dog and cat.

Breed Predilections

• Ischemic stroke—cavalier King Charles spaniel and greyhound seem predisposed; small breed (≤15 kg) more likely to have cerebellar infarct; large breed (>15 kg) more likely to have midbrain or thalamic infarct. • Hemorrhagic stroke—unknown.

SIGNS

Historical Findings

• Ischemic stroke—peracute to acute nonprogressive focal brain signs. • Hemorrhagic stroke—acute to subacute focal or multifocal brain signs that can progress over a short period of time.

Physical Examination Findings

• Fundus examination—may reveal tortuous vessels (systemic hypertension), hemorrhage (coagulopathy or systemic hypertension), or papilledema (elevated intracranial pressure [ICP]). • Coagulation defects—may underlie hemorrhagic stroke and cause hemorrhage in any tissue or organ and anemia.

Neurologic Examination Findings

• Ischemic stroke—signs depend on the localization of the vascular insult (prosencephalon, midbrain, pons, medulla, cerebellum). • Hemorrhagic stroke—signs relate to increased ICP with nonspecific forebrain and/or brainstem disturbance.

CAUSES

Ischemic Stroke

Dogs

• Unknown in 50% of cases. • Endocrine diseases—hyperadrenocorticism, hypothyroidism, diabetes. • Embolism, thromboembolism—neoplastic (hemangiosarcoma, lymphoma), infectious (associated with bacterial endocarditis or other sources of infection), and aortic or cardiac. • Systemic hypertension—chronic kidney disease, protein losing enteropathy. • Fibrocartilaginous embolism. • Intravascular lymphoma. • Parasite migration (*Cuterebra*) or embolism (*Dirofilaria immitis*).

Cats

• High likelihood of concurrent disease. • Parasite migration (*Cuterebra* or heartworms). • Systemic hypertension—hyperthyroidism, chronic kidney disease, heart disease. • Neoplastic embolism. • Intracranial telangiectasia. • Hypertropic cardiomyopathy. • Hyperthyroidism. • Pulmonary disease. • Liver disease. • Neoplasia elsewhere in the body.

Hemorrhagic Stroke

Dogs

• Ruptured congenital vascular anomalies. • Primary and secondary brain tumors. • Inflammatory disease of arteries and veins (vasculitis). • Intravascular lymphoma. • Brain hemorrhagic infarction. • Impaired coagulation.

Cats

• Primary and secondary brain tumors. • Inflammatory disease of arteries and veins (vasculitis). • Brain hemorrhagic infarction. • Impaired coagulation—cerebral amyloid angiopathy. • Systemic hypertension.

RISK FACTORS

• Ischemic stroke—systemic hypertension, systemic conditions associated with hypercoagulability syndrome. • Hemorrhagic stroke—systemic hypertension, coagulopathy.

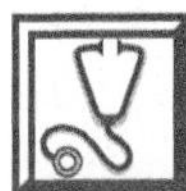

DIAGNOSIS

DIFFERENTIAL DIAGNOSIS

• Head trauma—history and physical findings suggestive of trauma. • Decompensation from primary or metastatic brain tumor—signs are progressive. • Infectious and noninfectious encephalitis—acute to subacute clinical signs that gradually worsen. • Neurotoxicity—bilateral, symmetric neurologic deficits.

CBC/BIOCHEMISTRY/URINALYSIS

Most often normal; may show changes reflecting underlying cause.

OTHER LABORATORY TESTS

• Cerebrospinal fluid—unlikely to confirm CVA, may help rule out inflammatory CNS disease. Variable findings; either normal, or mild mononuclear or neutrophilic pleocytosis; protein concentration occasionally elevated. • Prothrombin time—screening test for extrinsic mechanism defects. • Activated partial thromboplastin time—screening test for intrinsic mechanism defects. • Bleeding time—prolonged in patients with von Willebrand's disease; normal with most other coagulation defects, except disseminated intravascular coagulation. • Thromboelastography, D-dimer assay, and antithrombin III—screening tests for hypercoagulability syndrome as possible cause of ischemic stroke. • Endocrine testing—hyperadrenocorticism, thyroid disease, and pheochromocytoma. • Renal disease—urine protein/creatinine ratio.

IMAGING

Ischemic Stroke

• CT—often normal during acute phase. • MRI—within 12–24 hours of onset to distinguish hemorrhage from infarction; T2-weighted and fluid-attenuated inversion recovery (FLAIR) images particularly useful; T2*-weighted (gradient echo) images to show presence of or exclude intracranial hemorrhage; diffusion-weighted imaging (DWI) sequence: ideal for identification of hyperacute stroke, excluding stroke mimics; perfusion-weighted MRI can be used to depict brain regions of hypoperfusion and derive the tissue at risk by comparing the results with the findings on DWI. • Time of flight magnetic resonance angiography (MRA) and contrast-enhanced MRA can be used to assess intracranial vascular status of stroke patients.

Hemorrhagic Stroke

• CT—very sensitive for detection of acute hemorrhage; hyperdensity due to hyperattenuation of X-ray beam by the globin portion of blood; attenuation decreases until the hematoma is isodense at about 1 month from onset; periphery of hematoma contrast-enhances from 6 days to 6 weeks after onset due to revascularization. • MRI—signal intensity of intracranial hemorrhage is influenced by several intrinsic (time from ictus, source, size and location of hemorrhage) and extrinsic (pulse sequence and field strength) factors; as hematoma ages, oxyhemoglobin in blood breaks down sequentially into several paramagnetic products (deoxyhemoglobin, methemoglobin, hemosiderin), each with different MRI signal intensities; compared to other conventional sequences, T2*-weighted (gradient echo) images demonstrate readily detectable hypointensity regardless of time from ictus, source and location of hemorrhage, or field strength. • Multiple hemorrhagic lesions <5 mm—most often associated with hyperadrenocorticism, hypertension, chronic kidney disease, or hypothyroidism. • Single hemorrhagic lesion—most often associated with *Angiostrongylus vasorum*. • Multiple hemorrhagic lesions ≥5 mm—most often associated with *Angiostrongylus vasorum*, primary extracranial neoplasia with metastases (haemangiosarcoma).

DIAGNOSTIC PROCEDURES

Diagnosis of potential underlying causes.

Ischemic Stroke

Evaluate for hypertension (and potential underlying causes), endocrine disease (hyperadrenocorticism, hypothyroidism, hyperthyroidism, diabetes mellitus), chronic kidney disease (especially protein-losing nephropathy), protein-losing enteropathy, heart disease, and metastatic diseases (particularly hemangiosarcoma).

Hemorrhagic Stroke

Evaluate for coagulopathy (and potential underlying causes), hypertension (and potential underlying causes), and metastatic diseases (particularly hemangiosarcoma).

PATHOLOGIC FINDINGS

Ischemic Stroke

• Ischemic necrosis centered on gray matter due to selective vulnerability. • Lesions limited to brain area vascularized by the affected vessel with sharply demarcated borders; normal surrounding brain tissue; minimal to no mass effect. • Global brain ischemia usually affects a dense area of selectively vulnerable neurons; specific anatomic areas including cerebral cortex, hippocampus, certain basal nuclei (e.g., caudate nuclei), thalamus, and cerebellar Purkinje cell layers are more susceptible to hypoxic injury. • Early ischemic cell changes occur rapidly and are a result of energy deprivation with swelling of the mitochondria and endoplasmic reticulum, which causes cytoplasmic microvacuolation; more chronic lesions are characterized by postnecrotic atrophy of the brain parenchyma, endothelial proliferation in viable capillaries, and accumulation of Gitter cells.

Hemorrhagic Stroke

• Parenchymal bleeding results from rupture of the small penetrating brain arteries; most acute cases reveal fresh hemorrhage and acute neuronal necrosis that is slowly removed by macrophages, leaving over time a cystic cavity lined by fibrillary astrocytes. • Histology is characterized by presence of edema, neuronal damage, macrophages, and neutrophils in the region surrounding the hematoma. • While some cerebral hemorrhages stop quickly as a result of clotting and tamponade by the surrounding regions, others tend to expand over time; the latter is a result of continued bleeding from the primary source and to the mechanical disruption of surrounding vessels; the hemorrhage spreads between planes of white matter cleavage with minimal destruction, leaving nests of intact neural tissue within and surrounding the hematoma.

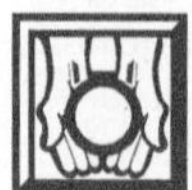

TREATMENT

NURSING CARE

Ischemic Stroke

• Monitoring and correction of basic physiologic variables (e.g., oxygen level, fluid balance, blood pressure, body temperature). • Maintenance of systemic arterial blood pressure within physiologic range; aggressive lowering of blood pressure should be avoided during acute stages unless the patient is at high risk of end-stage organ damage (systolic blood pressures >180 mmHg); hypertension can develop as a physiologic response to a stroke to ensure adequate cerebral perfusion pressure; elevated blood pressure can persist for up to 72 hours after the onset of injury. • No evidence that glucocorticoid provides beneficial neuroprotection; most neuroprotective agents tested have either failed to prove their efficacy in clinical trials or are awaiting further investigation.

Hemorrhagic Stroke

• Patient stabilization (airway protection, monitoring and correction of vital signs). • Assessment and monitoring of neurologic status. • Determination and treatment of potential underlying causes of hemorrhage. • Assessment for the need of specific treatment measures including management of raised ICP, which revolves around reducing cerebral edema, optimizing cerebral blood volume, and eliminating space-occupying mass. • Risk of neurologic deterioration and cardiovascular instability highest during the first 24 hours after onset of intracranial hemorrhage, as the space-occupying lesion slowly expands and cerebral vasogenic edema develops.

MEDICATIONS

DRUG(S) OF CHOICE

Ischemic Stroke

• Antihypertensive—consider if systemic BP >180 mmHg on serial evaluation and/or severe ocular manifestations of hypertension. • Angiotensin-converting enzyme (ACE) inhibitor—enalapril (0.25–0.5 mg/kg q12h) or benazepril (0.25–0.5 mg/kg q12h) and/or calcium channel blockers such as amlodipine (0.1–0.25 mg/kg q24h); amlodipine is more effective in severe hypertension. • Prevention of clot formation—consider in proven cardiac sources of embolism; antiplatelet therapy with low-dose aspirin (0.5 mg/kg PO q24h) or clopidogrel (2–4 mg/kg PO q24h) and low molecular weight heparin can be used prophylactically; low molecular weight heparin 80–150 IU/kg SC can be used in suspected or confirmed case of hypercoagulable state; anti-factor Xa activity should be monitored, although this may not be practical.

Hemorrhagic Stroke

Mannitol—if suspected elevated ICP unresponsive to extracranial stabilization measures (0.25–2 g/kg IV over 10–20 min up to q4-8h).

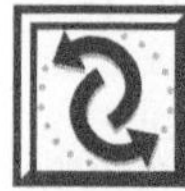

FOLLOW-UP

PATIENT MONITORING

Frequent neurologic evaluations in the first 48–72 hours to monitor progress.

EXPECTED COURSE AND PROGNOSIS

• Maximum severity of signs usually reached within 24h for ischemic stroke. • Resolution of signs—gradual within 2–10 weeks; some dogs/cats may be left with permanent neurologic signs due to irreversible brain damage. • Dogs with causal medical condition significantly more likely to relapse and have significant shorter survival time than dogs with no identifiable medical condition. • Despite having a high likelihood of concurrent disease, cat with ischemic stroke have been reported to have a favorable short-term outcome, if neither clinical presentation nor concurrent disease was severe. • Prognosis for global brain ischemia difficult to predict as there are no controlled studies.

MISCELLANEOUS

SYNONYMS

Stroke

ABBREVIATIONS

• ACE = angiotensin-converting enzyme. • CVA = cerebrovascular accident. • DWI = diffusion-weighted imaging. • FLAIR = fluid-attenuated inversion recovery. • ICP = intracranial pressure. • MRA = magnetic resonance angiography. • TIA = transient ischemic attack.

Suggested Reading

Lowrie M., De Risio L, Dennis R, et al. Concurrent medical conditions and long-term outcome in dogs with nontraumatic intracranial hemorrhage. Vet Radiol Ultrasound, 2012, 53:381–388.

Whittaker DE, Drees R, Beltran E. MRI and clinical characteristics of suspected cerebrovascular accident in nine cats. J Feline Med Surg, 2017, 20:674–684.

Author Laurent Garosi

CERUMINOUS GLAND ADENOCARCINOMA, EAR

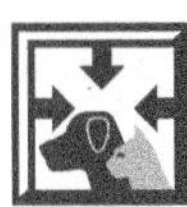

BASICS

OVERVIEW

- Most common primary malignant tumor of the external ear canal, arising from modified apocrine sweat glands (ceruminous glands).
- Often locally invasive, but associated with a low metastatic rate.

SIGNALMENT

- Uncommon overall, but the most common malignant tumor of the ear canal in both dogs and cats, followed by carcinoma of undetermined origin and squamous cell carcinoma.
- Cocker spaniels and German shepherd dogs are overrepresented.
- Mean age—dogs, 10 years; cats, 11 years.
- No known sex predisposition.

SIGNS

- Progressive hearing loss.
- Similar to chronic, recurrent otitis externa—discharge, odor, pruritus, inflammation.
- Early appearance—pale pink, friable, ulcerative, bleeding nodular mass(es) within the external ear canal.
- Late appearance—large mass(es) filling the canal and invading through canal wall into surrounding structures.
- Regional lymph node enlargement.
- Neurologic signs (vestibular signs, Horner's syndrome) may be present secondary to middle ear involvement.
- Signs of pain and discomfort; pain upon opening the mouth.

CAUSES & RISK FACTORS

Chronic inflammation and ceruminous gland hyperplasia/dysplasia appear to play a role in tumor development.

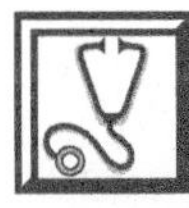

DIAGNOSIS

DIFFERENTIAL DIAGNOSIS

- Proliferative chronic otitis externa with ceruminous gland hyperplasia.
- Inflammatory polyps.
- Other tumors including squamous cell carcinoma, basal cell tumor, mast cell tumor, papilloma, sebaceous gland tumor, ceruminous gland adenoma.

CBC/BIOCHEMISTRY/URINALYSIS

Usually normal.

OTHER LABORATORY TESTS

- Ear swab cytology for bacteria and yeast.
- Bacterial culture and sensitivity as needed.

IMAGING

- Skull radiography to assess potential involvement of the tympanic bulla, but this is difficult to interpret due to superimposition of bones in the skull.
- Thoracic radiography to evaluate for pulmonary metastasis.
- CT or MRI is most useful for loco-regional staging and before surgery and radiation therapy, providing greater detail than with radiographs.

DIAGNOSTIC PROCEDURES

- Cytologic examination of aspirate from regional lymph nodes.
- Cytologic examination of fine-needle aspirate from mass.
- Biopsy and histopathology.

PATHOLOGIC FINDINGS

- Cytology from fine-needle aspirate—round to polygonal epithelial cells arranged both singly and in large clusters with deep blue to lavender-gray cytoplasm and a variable quantity of black, intracytoplasmic granular material; unable to differentiate adenocarcinoma from adenoma consistently with cytology.
- Histopathologic characteristics—apocrine type differentiation from ceruminous glands and local invasion into stroma; neoplastic cells show moderate to marked nuclear atypia with frequent mitotic figures.

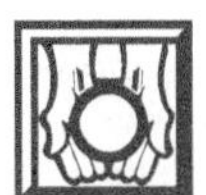

TREATMENT

- Total ear canal ablation and lateral bulla osteotomy (TECABO) is the preferred surgical approach over lateral ear resection.
- Radiation therapy may be considered for either large (palliative intent) or incompletely excised masses (curative intent).

MEDICATIONS

DRUG(S) OF CHOICE

- Chemotherapy not evaluated, but occasionally considered based on histologic information and clinical staging results.
- Multimodal therapy incorporating corticosteroids or nonsteroidal anti-inflammatory drugs (NSAIDs) and other analgesics.

CONTRAINDICATIONS/POSSIBLE INTERACTIONS

N/A

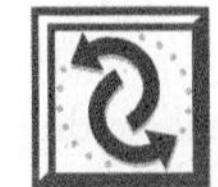

FOLLOW-UP

PATIENT MONITORING

- Physical examination and thoracic radiography at regular intervals following therapy (every 3–4 months) is recommended for the first year postoperatively.
- Serial CT or MRI to monitor for local tumor regrowth may be recommended.

POSSIBLE COMPLICATIONS

- Permanent or transient Horner's syndrome secondary to surgery.
- Permanent or transient facial paralysis following surgery (more frequent in cats).

EXPECTED COURSE AND PROGNOSIS

- Median survival after lateral ear resection is around 10 months for both dogs and cats.
- Median survival after TECABO is >3 years in both dogs and cats.
- Median survival after radiation therapy is >3 years, but published information is on small numbers only.
- Poor prognosis associated with extensive tumor involvement (advanced stage), preoperative neurologic signs, and conservative therapy (e.g., lateral ear canal ablation alone).

MISCELLANEOUS

ASSOCIATED CONDITIONS

- Otitis externa.
- Peripheral vestibular disease, Horner's syndrome.
- Chronic pain.

ABBREVIATIONS

- NSAID = nonsteroidal anti-inflammatory drug.
- TECABO = total ear canal ablation and bulla osteotomy.

Suggested Reading

Bacon NJ, Gilbert RL, Bostock DE, White RA. Total ear canal ablation in the cat: indications, morbidity and long-term survival. J Small Anim Pract 2003, 44:430–434.

De Lorenzi D, Bonfanti U, Masserdotti C, Tranquillo M. Fine-needle biopsy of external ear canal masses in the cat: cytologic results and histologic correlations in 27 cases. Vet Clin Pathol 2005, 34:100–105.

Moisan PG, Watson GL. Ceruminous gland tumors in dogs and cats: a review of 124 cases. J Am Anim Hosp Assoc 1996, 32:448–452.

Théon AP, Barthez PY, Madewell BR, Griffey SM. Radiation therapy of ceruminous gland carcinomas in dogs and cats. J Am Vet Med Assoc 1994, 205:566–569.

Author Jason Pieper

Consulting Editor Timothy M. Fan

Acknowledgment The author and book editors acknowledge the prior contribution of Louis-Philippe de Lorimier.

CERVICAL SPONDYLOMYELOPATHY (WOBBLER SYNDROME)

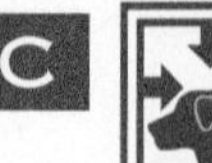

BASICS

DEFINITION

- Cervical spondylomyelopathy (CSM) or wobbler syndrome is a disease of the cervical spine of large- and giant-breed dogs.
- CSM is characterized by compression of the spinal cord and/or nerve roots associated with neurologic deficits and/or cervical pain.

PATHOPHYSIOLOGY

- Compressive lesion caused by intervertebral disc herniation, osseous malformation, thickened ligaments, or a combination, in a stenotic vertebral canal.
- Disc-associated compression—dogs >3 years; intervertebral disc degeneration and subsequent protrusion might be secondary to abnormal articular facet articulation in Doberman pinschers, which predisposes to increased rotational strain in the intervertebral discs.
- Vertebral malformation (bony-associated compression)—most commonly seen in giant breeds of dogs, usually in young adult dogs (<4 years); the osseous malformation can compress the spinal cord dorsoventrally (vertebral arch malformation), dorsolaterally (articular process malformation/osteoarthritic lesions), or laterally (pedicular malformation/osteoarthritic lesions).
- Dynamic spinal cord compression (one that changes with movements of the cervical spine) is always a component of the pathophysiology with any type of compression.
- Current evidence does not suggest that instability has a primary role in the pathogenesis of CSM.

SYSTEMS AFFECTED

Nervous

GENETICS

- Heritable basis proposed for borzoi and basset hound.
- Recent evidence suggests that the disease is inherited as an autosomal dominant trait (with incomplete penetrance) in Doberman pinscher.

INCIDENCE/PREVALENCE

CSM is probably the most common neurologic disorder of the cervical spine of large- and giant-breed dogs.

GEOGRAPHIC DISTRIBUTION

N/A

SIGNALMENT

Breed Predilections

- Doberman pinscher and Great Dane are the most commonly affected breeds, with approximately 60–70% of cases seen in these breeds.
- Other breeds with a high incidence include Rottweiler, German shepherd, Weimaraner, Labrador, and Dalmatian.
- CSM can be seen in any breed, including small-breed dogs.

Mean Age and Range

- Doberman pinschers and other large-breed dogs are usually presented >3 years of age, with a mean age of 6 years.
- Giant-breed dogs are usually presented <3 years of age, although late presentations can be seen.

Predominant Sex

Males overrepresented, primarily in giant-breed dogs.

SIGNS

General Comments

The classic clinical presentation is a slowly progressive pelvic limb ataxia with less severe thoracic limb involvement.

Historical Findings

- Chronic, slowly progressive gait dysfunction is characteristic; acute presentations are usually associated with neck pain; occasionally, acute worsening of a dog with chronic history is observed.
- Neck pain or cervical hyperesthesia is a common historical finding; it occurs in approximately 65–70% of Dobermans, and 40–50% of other breeds.

Neurologic Examination Findings

- Cervical pain is the primary complaint in only approximately 5% of patients.
- Gait changes are characterized by proprioceptive ataxia and paresis (weakness); the ataxia and paresis are more obvious in the pelvic limbs, with lesions in the caudal cervical spine (C5–6, C6–7); compressive lesions in the mid-cervical spine tend to cause ataxia in all four limbs.
- The thoracic limb gait can appear short-strided, spastic with a floating appearance, or very weak.
- Proprioceptive positioning deficits are usually present, but dogs with chronic ataxia may not display them; the gait exam (presence of ataxia) provides a more sensitive indication of myelopathy than proprioceptive positioning deficits.
- Dogs can present nonambulatory.
- Supraspinatus muscle atrophy and worn toenails can be seen in some cases.
- Extensor muscle tone is commonly increased in all four limbs.
- Patellar reflexes are normal or increased; flexor reflex may be difficult to elicit in the thoracic limbs due to increased extensor tone.

CAUSES

- Nutrition—excess protein, calcium, and caloric intake were proposed in Great Danes; nutrition does not appear to play a role in the development of CSM in large-breed dogs.
- The cause of CSM is likely multifactorial.

RISK FACTORS

- Body conformation—large head and long neck have been proposed, but later studies found no correlation between body dimensions and incidence of CSM.
- Fast growth rate has been proposed, but not confirmed by other studies.

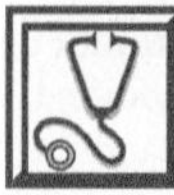

DIAGNOSIS

DIFFERENTIAL DIAGNOSIS

- Orthopedic conditions such as hip dysplasia and cruciate ligament rupture; differentiated by neurologic examination (absence of ataxia).
- Spinal neoplasia, spinal subarachnoid diverticulum, spinal synovial cysts, discospondylitis, osteomyelitis, meningomyelitis, trauma; differentiated by results of survey radiographs, cerebrospinal fluid (CSF), myelography, CT, CT myelography, or MRI findings.

CBC/BIOCHEMISTRY/URINALYSIS

N/A

IMAGING

Survey Cervical Radiographs

- Survey radiographs serve as a screening tool to rule out bony disorders; although intervertebral disc narrowing or vertebral tipping can be seen, these findings are not specific for CSM since they can be observed in clinically normal large-breed dogs.
- Osteoarthritic changes of the articular processes can be seen in giant breeds.

Myelography

- Myelography can define the location(s) and direction (ventral, dorsal, lateral) of the spinal cord compression.
- Stressed views (flexion or extension) may cause significant risk of neurologic deterioration.
- Linear traction myelography is a safer procedure and can distinguish a static from a dynamic lesion.

Advanced Imaging

- CT myelography—cross-sectional visualization of the spinal cord compression and determination of sites with spinal cord atrophy.
- MRI—visualization of the spinal cord parenchyma, intervertebral disc, soft tissues, and nerve roots; images can be obtained in sagittal, transverse, and dorsal planes; spinal cord signal changes allow more precise identification of the main site of compression than CT and myelography; kinematic MRI is a novel procedure that allows more precise identification of dorsal and ventral lesions, primarily when the vertebral column is placed in extension.

DIAGNOSTIC PROCEDURES

CSF analysis—usually normal; mild mixed or neutrophilic pleocytosis can be seen in dogs with acute presentations; elevated protein concentrations can be observed with chronic presentations.

PATHOLOGIC FINDINGS

- Spinal cord white matter tract demyelination at the site of spinal cord compression; axonal damage can lead to Wallerian degeneration in the ascending and descending white matter tracts.
- Neuronal loss, gliosis, and necrosis can be observed in the gray matter.
- Chronic severe focal spinal cord compression can lead to focal myelomalacia.

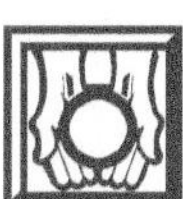

TREATMENT

APPROPRIATE HEALTH CARE

- Inpatient if surgical treatment is elected.
- Outpatient if medical management is chosen.

NURSING CARE

- Nonambulatory dogs—keep patients on soft bedding and alternate recumbence side every 4 hours to avoid bed sores.
- Bladder catheterization.
- Physical therapy is essential to avoid muscle atrophy and ankylosis, and to hasten recovery.

ACTIVITY

- Medically treated dogs should have restricted activity for at least 2 months.
- Restriction of activity is also important for the first 2 or 3 months postoperatively to allow bone fusion and prevent implant displacement.

DIET

Avoid excess of protein, calcium, or caloric intake in giant-breed dogs with osseous compression.

CLIENT EDUCATION

Inform that surgery offers the best chance of improvement (approximately 80%), but there is a 1–5% risk of significant complications associated with cervical surgical procedures.

SURGICAL CONSIDERATIONS

- Ventral slot—commonly used and recommended for single ventral compressions; could also be used for two ventral compressions.
- Dorsal laminectomy—primary indication for dorsal or dorsolateral compressions; can also be used for multiple ventral compressions; hemilaminectomy is an alternative for lateralized osseous compressions.
- Distraction/stabilization/fusion techniques are recommended primarily for single dynamic ventral compressions, but could be used for multiple compressions.
- Cervical disc arthroplasty—novel technique that appears safe and as effective as the traditional procedures; it can be used for multiple compressions.
- Recurrence rate is approximately 20% with any surgical technique.
- Fenestration provides a very low success rate and is not recommended.

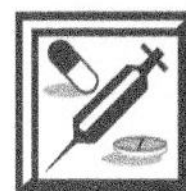

MEDICATIONS

DRUG(S) OF CHOICE

- Corticosteroids—prednisone 1 mg/kg q24h or 0.5 mg/kg q12h, progressively decreasing dosage and frequency; most dogs can have prednisone discontinued after 4–8 weeks of treatment; dexamethasone 0.1–0.25 mg/kg q24h can be used as an alternative to prednisone in dogs severely affected; corticosteroids act by reducing the vasogenic edema often present in chronic compressive spinal cord lesions.
- Gabapentin—10 mg/kg q8–12h can be used for analgesia in cases of more severe cervical pain.

CONTRAINDICATIONS

N/A

PRECAUTIONS

Monitor for signs of gastroenteritis, gastric hemorrhage, and cystitis. A proton pump inhibitor may be used to minimize the risk of gastrointestinal bleeding.

POSSIBLE INTERACTIONS

Do not use corticosteroids in combination with nonsteroidal anti-inflammatory drugs (NSAIDs).

ALTERNATIVE DRUG(S)

NSAIDs (all kinds) can be used in dogs with only cervical hyperesthesia or mild ataxia.

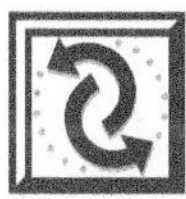

FOLLOW-UP

PATIENT MONITORING

Repeat neurologic evaluation as often as needed to monitor response to treatment.

PREVENTION/AVOIDANCE

- Excessive activity, jumping, and running should be avoided.
- Avoid use of neck collars; use a body harness instead.

POSSIBLE COMPLICATIONS

Recurrence of clinical signs can occur in dogs treated medically or surgically.

EXPECTED COURSE AND PROGNOSIS

- About 80% of patients improve with surgery.
- Approximately 50% of patients improve with medical treatment (restricted activity ± corticosteroids) and 25% remain stable.

MISCELLANEOUS

ASSOCIATED CONDITIONS

Dilated cardiomyopathy, hypothyroidism, and von Willebrand's disease are common in Doberman pinscher dogs; these diseases can affect diagnostic and treatment options. Doberman pinschers suspected of having CSM should be routinely evaluated for these conditions.

AGE-RELATED FACTORS

- Young giant- or large-breed dogs—vertebral malformation and compression.
- Older dogs—disc-associated compression.

ZOONOTIC POTENTIAL

N/A

PREGNANCY/FERTILITY/BREEDING

N/A

SYNONYMS

- Cervical malformation-malarticulation.
- Cervical spondylopathy.
- Cervical vertebral instability.

SEE ALSO

Intervertebral Disc Disease—Cats.

ABBREVIATIONS

- CSF = cerebrospinal fluid.
- CSM = cervical spondylomyelopathy.
- NSAID = nonsteroidal anti-inflammatory drug.

Suggested Reading

da Costa RC. Cervical spondylomyelopathy (wobbler syndrome). Vet Clin North Am Small Anim Pract 2010, 40:881–913.

da Costa RC, Parent JM. Outcome of medical and surgical treatment in dogs with cervical spondylomyelopathy: 104 cases. J Am Vet Med Assoc 2008, 233:1284–1290.

De Decker SD, da Costa RC, Volk HA, et al. Current insights and controversies in the pathogenesis and diagnosis of disc-associated cervical spondylomyelopathy in dogs. Vet Rec 2012, 171:531–537.

Jeffery ND, McKee WM. Surgery for disc-associated wobbler syndrome in the dog—an examination of the controversy. J Small Anim Pract 2001, 42:574–581.

Martin-Vaquero P, da Costa RC, Drost WT. Comparison of noncontrast computed tomography and high field magnetic resonance imaging in the evaluation of Great Danes with cervical spondylomyelopathy. Vet Radiol Ultrasound 2014, 55:4.

Provencher M, Habing A, Moore SA, et al. Evaluation of osseous-associated cervical spondylomyelopathy in dogs using kinematic magnetic resonance imaging. Vet Radiol Ultrasound 2017, 58:4.

Provencher M, Habing A, Moore SA, et al. Kinematic magnetic resonance imaging for evaluation of disc-associated cervical spondylomyelopathy in Doberman Pinschers. J Vet Intern Med, 2016 30:4.

Author Ronaldo Casimiro da Costa

Client Education Handout available online

CHAGAS DISEASE (AMERICAN TRYPANOSOMIASIS)

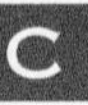

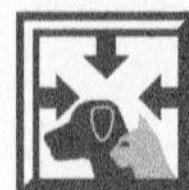

BASICS

OVERVIEW

- Caused by hemoflagellate protozoan *Trypanosoma cruzi.*
- Transmission through contact with infected feces of the Reduviid ("kissing") bug, ingestion of bug vector, through blood transfusion, or vertical transmission to offspring.
- After multiplication at entry site (5 days postinfection [PI]), hematogenous spread to heart, brain, and other organs.
- Maximal parasitemia at 14 days PI; associated with acute myocarditis and (less commonly) encephalitis.
- Infection becomes subpatent 30 days PI.
- Dogs then enter long asymptomatic period (months to years); subset develop cardiomyopathy.
- South and Central America—endemic in humans and pets; infected animals are sentinels for human risk.
- United States—in southern states with infected vectors and reservoir hosts (raccoons, opossums, armadillos, mice, rats, squirrels).

SIGNALMENT

- Dogs of any age, breed:
    - Acute infection—more severe in dogs <2 years old.
    - Chronic infection—adults.
    - Sporting breeds and outdoor-housed dogs more likely to be in contact with vectors or reservoir host.
- Cats—more recent evidence of infection and organ pathology.

SIGNS

General Comments

Two syndromes can be difficult to distinguish—acute myocarditis/encephalitis and chronic arrhythmias and myocardial dysfunction.

Historical Findings

- Lethargy, weakness.
- Anorexia.
- Abdominal distension (ascites).
- Cough, dyspnea.
- Syncope, sudden death.
- Ataxia, seizures.

Physical Examination Findings

- Tachy- or bradyarrhythmia.
- Heart murmur.
- Congestive heart failure (tachypnea, dyspnea, ascites).
- Hepatomegaly.
- Generalized lymphadenopathy (acute).
- Neurologic—weakness, ataxia, seizures (acute).

CAUSES & RISK FACTORS

Lives in or travels to endemic area.

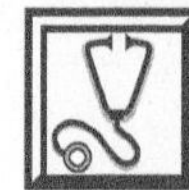

DIAGNOSIS

DIFFERENTIAL DIAGNOSIS

- Cardiomyopathy.
- Congenital heart defect (tricuspid valve dysplasia).
- Myocarditis.
- Distemper, other causes of meningoencephalitis.

CBC/BIOCHEMISTRY/URINALYSIS

Generally normal.

OTHER LABORATORY TESTS

- Cardiac troponin I—elevation indicates myocardial damage.
- Serology—presence of *T. cruzi* serum antibodies (present by 16 days PI) confirms infection, but not necessarily clinical disease.
- Tests can cross-react with *Leishmania.*
- Cytology—trypomastigote (blood form) occasionally on blood smear, lymph node aspirate, abdominal effusion, or buffy coat during period of high parasitemia.
- Cytology—amastigote (intracellular form) identified on lymph node aspirate or impression.
- PCR—detect parasite DNA in blood or tissue with high specificity; low sensitivity in chronic stage if parasite levels low.

IMAGING

- Thoracic radiography—cardiomegaly, pulmonary edema, pleural effusion.
- Echocardiography—dilation of heart chambers, systolic dysfunction.

DIAGNOSTIC PROCEDURES

ECG

- Supraventricular and ventricular arrhythmias, atrioventricular block (any degree), bundle branch block.
- Ambulatory ECG (Holter) to document abnormalities.

PATHOLOGIC FINDINGS

- Acute—diffuse granulomatous myocarditis, myocardial necrosis, parasitic pseudocysts with intracellular amastigotes.
- Chronic—lymphoplasmacytic inflammation, loss of myocardial fibers, severe interstitial fibrosis.
- *T. cruzi* amastigotes in heart, lymph nodes, liver, spleen, brain.

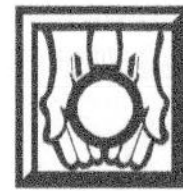

TREATMENT

- No currently approved treatment for *T. cruzi.*
- Manage heart failure (see Congestive Heart Failure, Left-Sided; Congestive Heart Failure, Right-Sided).
- Tachyarrhythmias—anti-arrhythmic drugs.
- Bradyarrhythmias—pacemaker implantation.

Client Education

- Test housemates/littermates of infected dogs.
- Take measures to eliminate the insect vector—remove brush, pyrethroid insecticide.
- Alert owner to possible zoonotic risk and potential for sudden death.
- Infected female can transfer infection to offspring.
- Cardiology tests (ECG, echocardiography) can identify dogs at risk of developing clinical signs or sudden death.

MEDICATIONS

DRUG(S) OF CHOICE

Limited therapeutic options for treating infection. Variable clinical response to Benznidazole; treated dogs still develop myocardial damage. Other drug protocols under investigation.

FOLLOW-UP

- Monitor positive dogs for clinical disease.
- Prognosis unknown for asymptomatic, positive dogs.
- Dogs with clinical signs or arrhythmias have guarded prognosis.

MISCELLANEOUS

ZOONOTIC POTENTIAL

- Public health concern with limited treatment options.
- Risk of human acquiring infection directly from infected dog is low, but infected animal indicates presence of infected vectors or reservoir hosts.

ABBREVIATIONS

- PI = postinfection.

Internet Resources

https://www.cdc.gov/parasites/chagas

Suggested Reading

Barr SC, Saunders AB, Sykes J. Trypanosomiasis. In: Sykes J, ed., Canine and Feline Infectious Diseases. Philadelphia, PA: Saunders Elsevier, 2013, p. 760.

Meyers AC, Hamer SA, Matthews D, et al. Risk factors and select cardiac characteristics in dogs naturally infected with *Trypanosoma cruzi.* J Vet Int Med 2019, 33:1695–1706.

Author Ashley B. Saunders

Consulting Editor Amie Koenig

Acknowledgment The author and book editors acknowledges the prior contribution of Stephen C. Barr.

CHEDIAK-HIGASHI SYNDROME

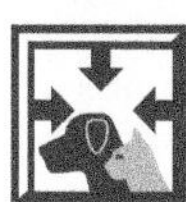

BASICS

OVERVIEW

- Autosomal recessive inherited disorder of Persian cats characterized by abnormalities in cellular morphology and pigment formation.
- Large intracytoplasmic granules in circulating leukocytes and melanocytes formed by fusion of preexisting granules.
- Storage pool deficiency of adenosine diphosphate (ADP), adenosine triphosphate (ATP), magnesium, and serotonin results from lack of platelet-dense granules.
- Prolonged bleeding from trauma, venipuncture, or minor surgery occurs because of impaired platelet aggregation and release reaction.
- Normal coagulation times.
- Depressed chemotaxis.
- No change in rates of infection.
- Mildly depressed neutrophil count, but within reference interval.
- In humans, it is associated with one of eight mutations in the LYST gene.

SIGNALMENT

- Persian cats with dilute smoke-blue coat color and yellow-green irises (and white tigers).
- Not reported in dogs.

SIGNS

Historical Findings

Prolonged bleeding from trauma, venipuncture, or minor surgery.

Physical Examination Findings

- Red fundic reflex (lack of choroidal pigment).
- Dilute smoke-blue coat color and yellow-green irises.
- Photophobia (blepharospasm and epiphora) in bright light.

CAUSES & RISK FACTORS

Genetic disease.

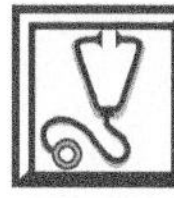

DIAGNOSIS

DIFFERENTIAL DIAGNOSIS

Lysosomal storage diseases (e.g., mucopolysaccharoidoses), therapy with antiplatelet agents (e.g., aspirin, clopidogrel), other inherited platelet function defect.

CBC/BIOCHEMISTRY/URINALYSIS

Romanowsky-stained blood smear—leukocytes, especially neutrophils, contain pink to magenta cytoplasmic inclusions approximately 2 μm in diameter.

OTHER LABORATORY TESTS

None

IMAGING

N/A

DIAGNOSTIC PROCEDURES

Advanced platelet function testing or electron microscopy of platelets may provide additional evidence for diagnosis.

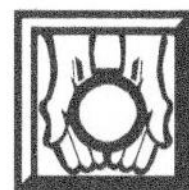

TREATMENT

- Provide ascorbic acid (vitamin C) to increase cyclic guanosine monophosphate (cGMP) concentration and to improve cell and platelet function (no controlled studies in cats).
- Transfusion of platelet-rich plasma or fresh whole blood from healthy cats will temporarily normalize bleeding time in affected individuals.
- Experimentally, bone marrow transplantation has restored neutrophil and platelet function in cats, but is impractical for general clinical use.

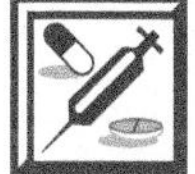

MEDICATIONS

DRUG(S) OF CHOICE

Ascorbic acid (100 mg PO q8h).

CONTRAINDICATIONS/POSSIBLE INTERACTIONS

None

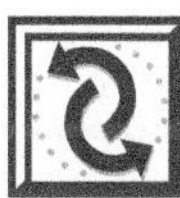

FOLLOW-UP

PATIENT MONITORING

None

PREVENTION/AVOIDANCE

Advise owner of potential for prolonged bleeding after trauma, venipuncture, or minor surgery.

POSSIBLE COMPLICATIONS

Prolonged bleeding time.

EXPECTED COURSE AND PROGNOSIS

Normal lifespan, with avoidance of trauma or other situations that may predispose to bleeding.

MISCELLANEOUS

PREGNANCY/FERTILITY/BREEDING

- Provide genetic counseling to eliminate Chediak-Higashi syndrome from animals used for breeding.
- Neuter affected and carrier animals or advise owner not to breed.

ABBREVIATIONS

- ADP = adenosine diphosphate.
- ATP = adenosine triphosphate.
- cGMP = cyclic guanosine monophosphate.

Suggested Reading

August JR. Consultations in Feline Internal Medicine, 2nd ed. Philadelphia, PA: Saunders, 1994.

Colgan SP, Hull-Thrall MA, Gasper PW, et al. Restoration of neutrophil and platelet function in feline Chediak-Higashi syndrome by bone marrow transplantation. Bone Marrow Transplant 1991, 7:365–374.

Cowles BE, Meyers KM, Wardrop KJ, et al. Prolonged bleeding time of Chediak-Higashi cats corrected by platelet transfusion. Throm Haemost 1992, 67:708–712.

Author Kenneth S. Latimer

Consulting Editor Melinda S. Camus

CHEMODECTOMA

BASICS

OVERVIEW

- Chemodectomas are tumors arising from the chemoreceptor cells (such as in the aortic body and the carotid body).
- Other names—aortic body tumors, cardiac paraganglioma, APUDoma (amine precursor uptake decarboxylase), and glomus body tumor.
- Aortic body tumors more common (80–90%) in dogs than carotid body tumors (10–20%).

SIGNALMENT

- Rare in cats.
- Dogs—age 6–15 years.
- Any breeds—but brachycephalic breeds predisposed, especially boxers, Boston terriers, English bulldogs, and German shepherd dogs.
- Males predisposed for aortic body tumors; no sex predilection for carotid body tumors.

SIGNS

- Nonspecific and dependent upon tumor size and anatomic localization, and can include lethargy, anorexia, weakness, collapse, coughing, respiratory distress, exercise intolerance, distended abdomen, vomiting, sudden death.
- Carotid body tumor—may notice neck mass, regurgitation, dyspnea, Horner's syndrome, head tilt, facial nerve paralysis, or laryngeal paralysis.
- May be associated with pericardial effusion and cardiac tamponade—muffled heart sounds, poor pulses, tachycardia, tachypnea, weak pulses, slow capillary refill time, ascites.
- May be associated with cranial vena cava syndrome (edema of head, neck, and forelimbs).
- May be associated with ascites secondary to right heart failure.
- May be associated with pleural effusion—decreased lung sounds ventrally, cyanosis.
- Cardiac arrhythmias with pulse deficits.

CAUSES & RISK FACTORS

Chronic hypoxia may play a role in the development of this disease in brachycephalic breeds.

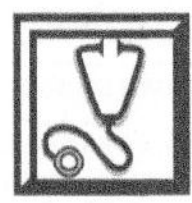

DIAGNOSIS

DIFFERENTIAL DIAGNOSIS

- Other masses located at the heart base (i.e., hemangiosarcoma, thymoma, ectopic thyroid carcinoma, mesothelioma, abscess, and granuloma).
- Idiopathic pericardial effusion.
- Pericarditis.
- Cardiomyopathy.
- Valvular insufficiency.

CBC/BIOCHEMISTRY/URINALYSIS

Typically normal, but 36% of patients can have nucleated red blood cells without anemia.

OTHER LABORATORY TESTS

N/A

IMAGING

- Thoracic radiography—to evaluate for mass in the region of the heart base, pericardial effusion, metastatic lesions in the lungs.
- Cervical ultrasound, CT, or MRI—to evaluate for masses arising in the neck.
- Echocardiography—to image mass and aorta/pulmonary arteries/veins.

DIAGNOSTIC PROCEDURES

- Biopsy of mass.
- ECG—if evidence of arrhythmia, may see low-amplitude QRS complexes with pericardial or pleural effusion, or electrical alternans with pericardial effusion.

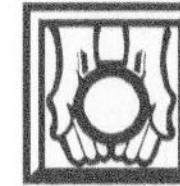

TREATMENT

Aortic Body Tumors

- Surgical removal of mass—if possible.
- Subphrenic pericardectomy has been shown to prolong survival.
- Symptomatic pericardiocentesis or thoracocentesis.
- Conformal radiation therapy or stereotactic body radiation therapy—discuss with owners possible complications including cough, tachyarrhythmias, and congestive heart failure.
- Palliative thoracoscopic-guided pericardial window.

Carotid Body Tumors

Surgical removal if possible—discuss with owners possibility of postoperative Horner's syndrome and laryngeal paralysis.

Both

Possible role of chemotherapy (doxorubicin)—however, definitive studies are lacking.

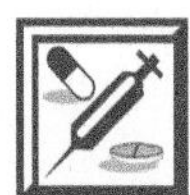

MEDICATIONS

DRUG(S) OF CHOICE

- The role of chemotherapy in this disease has not been published.
- Pharmacologic intervention for cardiac insufficiency.

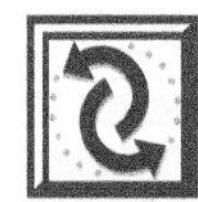

FOLLOW-UP

PATIENT MONITORING

Serial thoracic radiography or advanced imaging for monitoring tumor progression and metastasis.

EXPECTED COURSE AND PROGNOSIS

- Carotid body tumors treated with surgery—median survival time (MST) 25.5 months.
- Aortic body tumors—animals treated with pericardectomy MST 730 days vs. animals that did not have pericardectomy MST 42 days. Larger tumors (as determined by tumor weight to body weight ratio) more likely associated with metastasis.
- Conformal radiation therapy in 1 dog—survival >42 months.
- Stereotactic body radiation therapy in 6 dogs—tumor reduction by 30–76% in 4 dogs, 3 dogs alive 408–751 days post radiation therapy, 2 dogs died suddenly at 150 days and 294 days post radiation therapy, and 1 dog died of unrelated causes 1228 days post radiation.

MISCELLANEOUS

PREGNANCY/FERTILITY/BREEDING

It is not recommended to breed animals with cancer. Chemotherapy is teratogenic—do not give to pregnant animals.

SEE ALSO

Pericardial Disease.

ABBREVIATIONS

- APUD = amine precursor uptake decarboxylase.
- MST = median survival time.

Suggested Reading

Kisseberth WC. Neoplasia of the heart. In: Withrow SJ, Vail DE, Page RL, eds., Small Animal Clinical Oncology, 5th ed. Philadelphia, PA: Saunders, 2013, pp. 700–706.

Author Rebecca G. Newman

Consulting Editor Timothy M. Fan

Cheyletiellosis

BASICS

OVERVIEW

- Contagious parasitic skin disease caused by surface-living mites.
- Signs of mild pruritus and scaling resemble other more common dermatoses.
- Potential zoonosis.
- System affected—skin/exocrine.

SIGNALMENT

- Dogs and cats.
- More severe in young animals.
- Cocker spaniels, poodles, and longhaired cats may be inapparent carriers.

SIGNS

Historical Findings

- Referred to as "walking dandruff," because of the large mite size and excessive scaling.
- Prevalence varies by geographic region owing to mite susceptibility to common flea-control insecticides and differences in climate.
- Pruritus—usually absent to mild, but can be severe: hypersensitivity to mite allergens may develop, producing clinical signs similar to infestations with *Sarcoptes* or *Notoedres* mites.
- Infestation often suspected only after lesions in human beings develop (pseudo-scabies).

Physical Examination Findings

- Scaling— diffuse or plaque like; more severe in chronically infested or debilitated animals.
- Lesions—dorsal orientation commonly noted; head can be affected in cats.
- Underlying skin irritation may be minimal.
- Cats may exhibit bilaterally symmetric alopecia, bizarre behavior, head shaking, or excessive grooming.

CAUSES & RISK FACTORS

- Partial host specificity—dogs: *C. yasguri*. Cats: *C. blakei*. Rabbits: *C. parasitovorax*.
- Cheyletiellosis should be considered in every animal that shows scaling, with or without pruritus.
- Contagion by direct contact or by fomites.
- Common sources of infestation—animal shelters, breeders, and grooming facilities.
- Adult female mites may survive in the environment up to 10 days.
- Eggs can be found on shed hair.

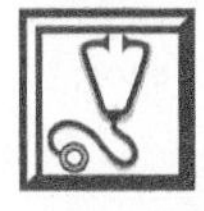

DIAGNOSIS

DIFFERENTIAL DIAGNOSIS

- Keratinization disorders.
- Cutaneous hypersensitivity.
- *Sarcoptes* and *Notoedres* spp. mite infestation; other fur mites.
- Endocrinopathy.
- Dermatophytosis.
- Pediculosis.

CBC/BIOCHEMISTRY/URINALYSIS

Usually normal.

DIAGNOSTIC PROCEDURES

- Examination of epidermal debris—*Cheyletiella* mites are large and can be visualized with a hand lens or microscope (10× objective); scales and hair may be examined under low magnification; finding mite eggs is diagnostic.
- Mite numbers may be low—concentration of debris for examination increases the likelihood of diagnosis; collection of debris: flea combing (most effective), skin scraping, hair plucking, acetate tape preparation, scale collection, and fecal flotation.
- Response to insecticide treatment may be required to definitively diagnose suspicious cases in which mites cannot be identified.

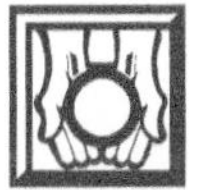

TREATMENT

- All animals in the same household must be treated.
- Clip long coats to facilitate treatment.
- Weekly baths to remove scale, followed by rinses with an insecticide.
- Lime-sulfur rinses—cats, kittens, dogs, and puppies.
- Routine flea sprays—not always effective: treat all animals in the home before introducing a new pet.
- Environmental treatment with frequent cleanings and insecticide sprays—reduces possibility of reinfestation.
- Continue treatment for at least 6–8 weeks to prevent reinfestation from shed eggs.
- Combs, brushes, and grooming tools—discard or thoroughly disinfect before reuse.

MEDICATIONS

DRUG(S) OF CHOICE

- Amitraz rinses—dogs only; 2-week intervals for 4 applications.
- Fipronil—2-week intervals for 1–4 applications.
- Ivermectin—300 µg/kg PO/SC 3 times at 2-week intervals; dogs and cats >3 months old; pour-on forms have shown efficacy in cats (500 µg/kg 2 times at 2-week intervals; non-FDA-approved usage; see Contraindications/Possible Interactions).
- Selamectin—apply every 2–4 weeks for 3 applications (non-FDA-approved usage).
- Imidacloprid/moxidectin—apply every 2 weeks for 3 applications (non-FDA-approved usage); imidacloprid alone: not effective.
- Milbemycin oxime—2 mg/kg PO once weekly for 4 weeks.
- Moxidectin—subcutaneous injection every 2 weeks for 3 treatments (non-FDA-approved usage: dogs).
- Doramectin—subcutaneous injection every week for three treatments (non-FDA-approved usage: dogs).

CONTRAINDICATIONS/POSSIBLE INTERACTIONS

Prevent ingestion/avoid use of avermectins in sensitive dogs (*MDR1*/*ABCB1* gene mutation, collie, sheltie, Australian shepherd, Old English sheepdog)—selamectin may be used in these dog breeds.

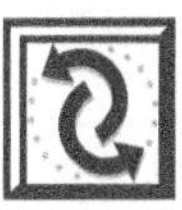

FOLLOW-UP

- Treatment failure requires a thorough reevaluation for other causes of pruritus and scaling.
- Reinfestation may indicate contact with an asymptomatic carrier or the presence of an unidentified source of mites

MISCELLANEOUS

ZOONOTIC POTENTIAL

Pruritic papular rash may develop in human beings.

Suggested Reading

Hnilica KA, Paterson A. Small Animal Dermatology: A Color Atlas and Therapeutic Guide, 4th ed. St. Louis, MO: Elsevier, 2017.

Saari S, Näreaho A, Nikander S. Canine Parasites and Parasitic Diseases. London: Academic Press, 2019.

Taylor MA, Coop RL, Wall RL. Veterinary Parasitology. Ames, IA: Wiley-Blackwell, 2016.

Author Guillermina Manigot

Consulting Editor Alexander H. Werner Resnick

CHLAMYDIOSIS—CATS

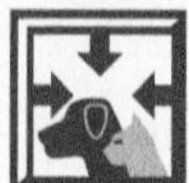

BASICS

DEFINITION

A chronic respiratory infection of cats caused by an intracellular bacterium, characterized by mild to severe conjunctivitis, mild upper respiratory signs, and mild pneumonitis.

PATHOPHYSIOLOGY

- *Chlamydophila felis* (previously *Chlamydia psittaci var. felis*)—a Gram-negative, obligate intracellular bacterium spread through close contact, aerosolization, or genital contact during parturition.
- Replicates on the mucosa of the upper and lower respiratory epithelium; produces a persistent commensal flora that causes local irritation, resulting in mild upper and lower respiratory signs and conjunctivitis; can also colonize the mucosa of the gastrointestinal and reproductive tracts.
- Incubation period—7–10 days (longer than that of other common feline respiratory pathogens).

SYSTEMS AFFECTED

- Gastrointestinal—cat: infection without clinical disease; other species: may have clinical gastroenteritis.
- Ophthalmic—acute or chronic conjunctivitis, unilateral often progresses to bilateral.
- Reproductive—infection without clinical disease.
- Respiratory—mild rhinitis, bronchitis, and bronchiolitis.

GENETICS

None

INCIDENCE/PREVALENCE

- Incidence of clinical disease—sporadic; outbreaks of respiratory disease may occur, especially in multicat facilities.
- Prevalence of *C. felis* in the feline population: ~5–10% chronically infected.

GEOGRAPHIC DISTRIBUTION

Worldwide

SIGNALMENT

Species

- Cat
- Human

Breed Predilections

None

Mean Age and Range

Usually cats >8 weeks and <1 year of age; any age of cat possible.

Predominant Sex

None

SIGNS

General Comments

- Commonly associated with feline conjunctivitis.
- Infection often subclinical.
- Clinical disease—commonly coinfection with other organisms, such as feline herpesvirus (FHV) and feline coronavirus (FCV).

Historical Findings

- Primarily signs of ocular discharge, blepharospasm.
- Mild upper respiratory infection, with possible sneezing and oculonasal discharge.
- Varying degrees of anorexia, lethargy.
- Lameness possible (uncommon).

Physical Examination Findings

- Conjunctivitis—unilateral or bilateral chemosis, blepharospasm, conjunctival and third eyelid hyperemia; serous to mucopurulent discharge without keratitis.
- Mild nasal discharge.
- Fever.
- Dyspnea and cough extremely unlikely; rales with pneumonitis.

CAUSES & RISK FACTORS

- Concurrent infections with other respiratory pathogens (FHV, FCV, *Bordetella bronchiseptica*, *Mycoplasma felis*).
- Lack of vaccination.
- Multicat facilities, especially adoption shelters and breeding catteries.
- Stress.
- Presence of asymptomatic shedders.

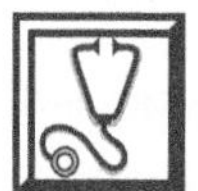

DIAGNOSIS

DIFFERENTIAL DIAGNOSIS

- Feline herpesvirus infection—short incubation period (4–5 days), rapid bilateral conjunctivitis, severe sneezing, and ulcerative keratitis.
- Feline calicivirus infection—short incubation period (3–5 days), ulcerative stomatitis, and potentially pneumonia.
- *Mycoplasma felis.*

CBC/BIOCHEMISTRY/URINALYSIS

Leukocytosis possible.

IMAGING

Thoracic radiographs—consolidation of lung tissue with pneumonia.

DIAGNOSTIC PROCEDURES

- PCR—preferred; best sensitivity; submit conjunctival swab in a sterile red top tube with a small amount of sterile saline.
- Culture—obtain conjunctival swab with vigorous exfoliation and submit on ice within 24 hours in special transport media such as 2-sucrose-phosphate (2-SP).
- Conjunctival cytology—characteristic intracytoplasmic basophilic inclusions may be seen with Giemsa staining early in disease.
- Serum antibody titers—limited diagnostic value.
- ELISA kits—variable sensitivity and specificity.

PATHOLOGIC FINDINGS

- Gross—chronic conjunctivitis with mucopurulent ocular discharge; minor rhinitis with nasal discharge; sometimes lung changes indicative of pneumonitis.
- Histopathologic (conjunctiva)—an early intense infiltration of neutrophils; inflammatory response changes to lymphocytes and plasma cells; inclusions detected with special stains (inclusions invisible with routine H&E stains).

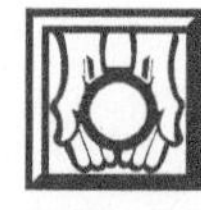

TREATMENT

APPROPRIATE HEALTH CARE

Generally outpatient.

NURSING CARE

- Clean eyes and nose as necessary with warm water or saline.
- Provide access to steam, such as in a bathroom, to clear secretions.
- Provide palatable, soft foods; warming food can improve cat's olfaction.
- Generally does not require other supportive therapy (e.g., fluids), unless complicated by concurrent infections.

ACTIVITY

- Quarantine affected cats from contact with other cats.
- Do not allow affected cats to go outside.

DIET

- No restrictions.
- Special diets—to entice anorectic cats to resume eating.

CLIENT EDUCATION

Inform clients of the causative organism, the anticipated chronic course of disease, and the opportunity to vaccinate other cats before exposure.

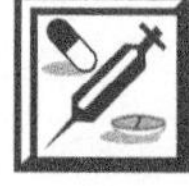

MEDICATIONS

DRUG(S) OF CHOICE

- Ophthalmic ointments—usually beneficial; oxytetracycline 3-4 times daily for 3 weeks; preparations with polymyxin may be irritating for cats; alternatively erythromycin or fluoroquinolone ointment; resistant to bacitracin, neomycin, gentamicin.
- Systemic antibiotics—tetracyclines are antibiotic of choice; doxycycline (10 mg/kg PO q24h or 5 mg/kg PO q12h for 4 weeks to prevent recrudescence); amoxicillin-clavulanate (20–25 mg/kg PO q12h) as alternative for young kittens.

CONTRAINDICATIONS

Tetracyclines—risk for esophagitis; may affect growing teeth of young kittens.

PRECAUTIONS

Colonies/shelters/breeding catteries—all cats may have to be treated; treatment should be continued for 4 weeks.

POSSIBLE INTERACTIONS

None

ALTERNATIVE DRUG(S)

None

FOLLOW-UP

PATIENT MONITORING

Monitor for improved health as treatment proceeds.

PREVENTION/AVOIDANCE

Vaccines

- Both inactivated and modified live vaccines available.
- Vaccines do not prevent infection; rather, they reduce severity and duration of clinical disease.
- American Association of Feline Practitioners—noncore vaccine; for at-risk cats, give a single vaccination at initial visit as early as 9 weeks of age, repeat in 3–4 weeks; revaccinate annually where *C. felis* is endemic.
- Adverse vaccine reactions—mild clinical disease with modified live vaccines in small percentage of vaccinated cats.

Environmental Management

- Quarantine affected cats by >4 ft perimeter.
- Practice appropriate hygiene and beware of fomites.
- *C. felis* readily inactivated with common disinfectants.

POSSIBLE COMPLICATIONS

- If kittens are affected <2 weeks of age, eyelids may need to be surgically opened to allow for drainage of purulent material (ophthalmia neonatorum).
- If entire course of antibiotics are not completed, persistently infected cats can become asymptomatic shedders.
- Coinfections increase morbidity.

EXPECTED COURSE AND PROGNOSIS

- Without treatment, tends to be chronic, lasting for several weeks or months.
- Prognosis good with appropriate antibiotic therapy.
- Improvement in 1–2 days with therapy; 28 days of treatment needed to clear organism.
- Look for coinfections if not improving as expected.

MISCELLANEOUS

ASSOCIATED CONDITIONS

Affected cats may be concurrently infected with FHV or FCV, especially in multicat and breeding facilities.

AGE-RELATED FACTORS

Primarily a disease of young cats.

ZOONOTIC POTENTIAL

C. felis can infect humans, especially immuno-compromised individuals; limited number of reports of mild conjunctivitis in humans transmitted from infected cats.

PREGNANCY/FERTILITY/BREEDING

- Endemic breeding catteries—treat all cats with doxycycline for at least 4 weeks; then vaccinate.
- Role of *C. felis* as a pathogen during pregnancy—unclear; can colonize the reproductive mucosa; severe ophthalmia neonatorum can occur in neonatal kittens infected at or shortly after birth.

SYNONYMS

Feline pneumonitis.

SEE ALSO

- Conjunctivitis—Cats.
- Feline Calicivirus Infection.
- Feline Herpesvirus Infection.
- Feline (Upper) Respiratory Infections.
- Mycoplasmosis.
- Ophthalmia Neonatorum.

ABBREVIATIONS

- 2-SP = 2-sucrose-phosphate.
- FCV = feline calicivirus.
- FHV = feline herpesvirus.

INTERNET RESOURCES

http://www.abcdcatsvets.org/chlamydia-chlamydophila-felis

Suggested Reading

Hartmann AD, Hawley J, Werckenthin C, et al. Detection of bacterial and viral organisms from the conjunctiva of cats with conjunctivitis and upper respiratory tract disease. J Feline Med Surg 2010; 12:775–782.

Scherk MA, Ford RB, Gaskell RM, et al. 2013 AAFP Feline Vaccination Advisory Panel Report. J Feline Med Surg 2013; 15:785–808.

Sykes JE. Pediatric feline upper respiratory disease. Vet Clin North Am Small Anim Pract 2014; 44:331–342.

Sykes JE, Greene CE. Chlamydial infections. In: Greene CE, ed., Infectious Diseases of the Dog and Cat, 4th ed. St. Louis, MO: Saunders Elsevier, 2012, pp. 270–276.

Author Sara E. Gonzalez

Consulting Editor Amie Koenig

Acknowledgment The author and book editors acknowledge the prior contribution of Fred W. Scott.

Client Education Handout available online

CHOCOLATE TOXICOSIS

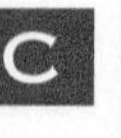

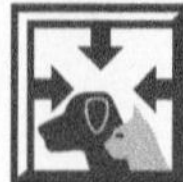

BASICS

DEFINITION

• Chocolate, derived from the seed of the *Theobroma cacao* plant, contains the naturally occurring methylxanthine alkaloids theobromine and caffeine. • Excessive intake can lead to dose-dependent gastroenteric, cardiac, and neurologic toxicosis. • Theobromine is the largest fraction of methylxanthines in chocolate products; lower concentration of caffeine is present (Table 1). Other sources of methylxanthines include coffee, tea, diet pills, over-the-counter (OTC) stimulants, and herbal medications.

PATHOPHYSIOLOGY

• Variably absorbed orally (caffeine <1 hour; theobromine 10 hours), metabolized by liver, undergo enterohepatic recirculation; metabolites primarily excreted via urine and may be reabsorbed from urinary bladder. • Estimated theobromine and caffeine half-lives in dogs 17.5 hours and 4.5 hours, respectively.
• Methylxanthines inhibit phosphodiesterase to increase intracellular cyclic adenosine monophosphate (cAMP), stimulate catecholamine release, and increase intracellular calcium, which results in vasoconstriction, increased myocardial and skeletal muscle contractility, and CNS stimulation. • Toxic dosages:
∘ Theobromine—LD_{50} (dog) 250–500 mg/kg; LD_{50} (cat) 200 mg/kg. Mild signs (agitation, vomiting, diarrhea): 20 mg theobromine/kg. Moderate signs (tachycardia): 40–50 mg theobromine/kg. Severe signs (seizures): 60 mg theobromine/kg. ∘ Caffeine—LD_{50} (dog) 140 mg/kg; LD_{50} (cat) 80–150 mg/kg. Clinical signs: >15 mg caffeine/kg. Moderate signs: >25 mg caffeine/kg. Cardiotoxic signs: >50 mg caffeine/kg. • Several aids to assess canine risk from chocolate can be found online—see Internet Resources.

SYSTEMS AFFECTED

• Cardiovascular—tachycardia, hypertension, ventricular premature contractions (VPCs), other tachyarrhythmias, bradycardia (rare).
• Gastrointestinal (GI)—vomiting, diarrhea, regurgitation. • Metabolic—hypokalemia, hyperthermia, dehydration. • Nervous—agitation, tremors, seizures, ataxia, muscle rigidity, hyperreflexia. • Renal/urologic—polyuria, polydipsia. • Respiratory—panting, tachypnea, cyanosis, respiratory failure.

INCIDENCE/PREVALENCE

• Dogs—among 10 most common poisonings reported by small animal practices and animal poison control centers. • More common at holidays when chocolate products readily available.

GEOGRAPHIC DISTRIBUTION

Indoor dogs at risk owing to closer proximity to chocolate products.

SIGNALMENT

Species

• Dogs most frequently poisoned based on proximity to methylxanthine products and propensity for dietary indiscretion leading to excessive ingestion. • Cats rarely affected.

Breed Predilections

• Small dogs may be at higher risk due to smaller body weight relative to amount of chocolate consumed. • Breeds prone to dietary indiscretion, such as Labrador retrievers.

SIGNS

Historical Findings

• History of ingestion. • Evidence of chewed packaging. • Vomiting and diarrhea—vomit often contains evidence of chocolate and may be first sign noted. • Early restlessness and hyperactivity. • Polydipsia.

Physical Examination Findings

• Physical exam may be normal after recent ingestion (<1–2 hours). • Vomiting. • Diarrhea.
• Restlessness and hyperactivity. • Panting.
• Polyuria/polydipsia. • Dehydration.
• Tachycardia. • Cardiac arrhythmias such as VPCs. • Hypertension. • Hyperthermia.
• Tremors. • Hyperreflexia and muscle rigidity. • Seizures. • Advanced signs with severe toxicosis—cardiac failure, weakness, cyanosis, coma, and death. • Death—12–48 hours after ingestion.

CAUSES

Excessive ingestion of chocolate and other methylxanthine products.

RISK FACTORS

• Access to chocolate, which is palatable and attractive to dogs, often readily available, and unprotected in homes and kitchens. • Dogs with preexisting heart disease may be more sensitive to cardiac effects.

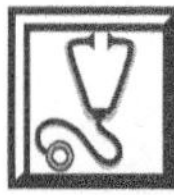

DIAGNOSIS

DIFFERENTIAL DIAGNOSIS

• Convulsant or excitatory alkaloids—strychnine, amphetamine, nicotine, 4-aminopyridine. • Convulsant pesticides such as pyrethroids, organochlorines, bromethalin, zinc phosphide, metaldehyde.
• Tremorgenic mycotoxins. • Acute psychogenic drugs—LSD, cocaine. • Medications such as phenylpropanolamine, pseudoephedrine, tricyclic and selective serotonin reuptake inhibitor antidepressants. • Cardioactive glycosides—*Digitalis* spp., *Nerium oleander*.
• Primary GI, cardiac, or neurologic disease.

CBC/BIOCHEMISTRY/URINALYSIS

• Hyperglycemia or hypoglycemia.
• Hypokalemia, especially with caffeine overdose. • Urine may be dilute due to polydipsia.

OTHER LABORATORY TESTS

• Methylxanthine assay—rarely necessary as history and clinical signs usually sufficient for diagnosis; can be performed on stomach contents, plasma, serum, urine, or liver.

DIAGNOSTIC PROCEDURES

• ECG monitoring—sinus tachycardia, VPCs, and ventricular tachyarrhythmias.
• Blood pressure monitoring.

PATHOLOGIC FINDINGS

• Presence of chocolate in GI tract. • Nonspecific gastroenteritis. • No distinctive microscopic lesions.

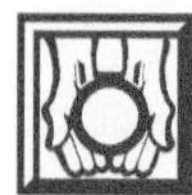

TREATMENT

APPROPRIATE HEALTH CARE

• Emesis in stable patients considered low risk for aspiration; chocolate is slowly absorbed from a dog's stomach, so emesis may be rewarding up to 6–8 hours after ingestion. • Gastric lavage with cuffed tube in symptomatic patients with large-volume ingestions once stabilized.
• Activated charcoal may not be necessary with lower-dose exposures or in cases where most of the chocolate was recovered by induction of vomiting or gastric lavage; monitor electrolytes for hypernatremia if giving multiple doses of activated charcoal. • IV fluid therapy to correct dehydration, promote urinary excretion of methylxanthines, and avoid hypernatremia; SC fluids may suffice with lower-dose exposures; potassium may be supplemented in fluids, if needed. • Control hyperthermia. • Urine voiding every 4 hours or urinary catheterization may reduce urinary bladder resorption. • GI support as needed (see Medications). • Control hyperactivity and agitation, tremors, seizures (see Medications).
• Treat tachycardia with beta blockers, if sedation not effective; treat arrhythmias with anti-arrhythmic drugs as appropriate (see Medications).

NURSING CARE

Fluid therapy used to correct electrolyte disturbances and dehydration and to enhance excretion of methylxanthines.

ACTIVITY

Avoid stress and limit activity until recovered.

DIET

• No food until vomiting is controlled.
• Convalescence—bland, low-fat diet to aid recovery from gastroenteritis and/or pancreatitis.

CLIENT EDUCATION

Warn owners about toxicologic hazards of chocolate, and advise keeping chocolate out of reach of dogs.

MEDICATIONS

DRUG(S) OF CHOICE

• Induce emesis—*only if patient is stable with low risk of aspiration*; apomorphine

Table 1

Comparative concentrations of caffeine and theobromine

Caffeine Source	*Amount (mg/g)*	*Amount (mg/oz)**
Coffee beans	10–20	284–570
Drip coffee	90–100 mg/6 oz cup	15–20
Cola drinks	30–71 mg/12 oz can	2.5–6
Baking chocolate (unsweetened)	0.8	23
Dark chocolate	0.43–0.8	12–23
Milk chocolate	0.2	6
Cocoa powder (unsweetened)	2.3	70
Guarana	30–50	850–1,400
Caffeine stimulant tablets	50–200 mg/tablet	————
OTC migraine pain control	65 mg/tablet	————
Theobromine Source	*Amount (mg/g)*	*Amount (mg/oz)*
Cacao beans	10–50	300–1500
Baking chocolate (unsweetened)	13–16	370–454
Milk chocolate	1.5–2	42–57
Cacao bean hulls	5–9	142–256
Cacao bean mulch	2–30	57–852
Cocoa powder (unsweetened)	14–29	398–832

* To convert mg/g to mg/oz, multiply by 28.4.

(0.02–0.04 mg/kg IV); hydrogen peroxide 3% (1–2 mL/kg PO); do not exceed 50 mL in dogs. • Activated charcoal 1–2 g/kg PO with cathartic × 1 dose. With large ingestions, repeat activated charcoal (no cathartic) q8 up to 24h to prevent enterohepatic recirculation. • Hyperactivity—acepromazine (0.02–0.04 mg/kg IV/IM/SC) or butorphanol (0.2–0.5 mg/kg IM/IV), with doses repeated/titrated to effect. • Seizures—diazepam (0.5–1 mg/kg IV) or phenobarbital (2–6 mg/kg IV) as needed to effect. • Tremors—diazepam (0.5–1 mg/kg IV) or methocarbamol (50–220 mg/kg IV slowly, up to daily dose of 330 mg/kg). • Vomiting—maropitant (1 mg/kg SC or IV) q24h as needed. • Persistent ventricular tachycardia—metoprolol (0.04–0.06 mg/kg IV), esmolol (initial loading dose 0.25–0.5 mg/kg IV slowly over 1–2 min, followed by CRI at 10–200 μg/kg/min) or propranolol (0.02–0.06 mg/kg IV); metoprolol or esmolol preferred but may be difficult to obtain. • Ventricular arrhythmias (dogs)—lidocaine (2–4 mg/kg IV followed by 25–100 μg/kg/min IV CRI); lidocaine not recommended in cats. • In rare instance of bradycardia—atropine 0.02–0.04 mg/kg IV/IM/SC; rule out reflex bradycardia from hypertension before use.

CONTRAINDICATIONS

• Do not use epinephrine concurrent with lidocaine. • Avoid erythromycin and corticosteroids, which may reduce excretion of methylxanthines. • Do not use lidocaine in cats due to risk of seizures.

PRECAUTIONS

Keep patient under observation until recovered and treatment no longer needed.

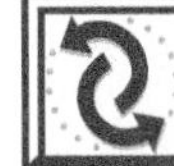

FOLLOW-UP

PATIENT MONITORING

Monitor heart rate, blood pressure, ECG, mentation, and temperature closely while hospitalized.

PREVENTION/AVOIDANCE

Warn owners about toxicologic hazards of chocolate and advise keeping chocolate out of reach of dogs.

POSSIBLE COMPLICATIONS

• Aspiration can occur rarely secondary to vomiting. • Pancreatitis can occur in some patients that consume chocolate.

EXPECTED COURSE AND PROGNOSIS

• Expected course—12–36 hours, up to 72 hours in severe cases, depending on dosage and effectiveness of decontamination and treatment. • Successfully treated patients—usually recover completely. • Prognosis—good if prompt oral decontamination occurs, but guarded with advanced signs of seizures and arrhythmias.

MISCELLANEOUS

PREGNANCY/FERTILITY/BREEDING

Methylxanthines cross the placenta and are excreted in milk.

SEE ALSO

- Antidepressant Toxicosis—SSRIs and SNRIs.
- Metaldehyde Toxicosis.
- Poisoning (Intoxication) Therapy.

ABBREVIATIONS

- cAMP = cyclic adenosine monophosphate.
- GI = gastrointestinal.
- OTC = over the counter.
- VPC = ventricular premature contraction.

INTERNET RESOURCES

- https://www.aspca.org/pet-care/animal-poison-control/apcc-mobile-app
- https://www.merckvetmanual.com/en-ca/toxicology/food-hazards/chocolate

Suggested Reading

Dolder LK. Methylxanthines. In: Peterson M, Talcott P, eds., Small Animal Toxicology, 3rd ed. St. Louis, MO: Elsevier Saunders, 2013, pp. 647–652.

Hoffberg JE. Chocolate and caffeine. In: Hovda LR, Brutlag AG, Osweiler G, Peterson K. The 5 Minute Veterinary Clinical Companion Consult: Small Animal Toxicology, 2nd ed. Ames, IA: Wiley-Blackwell, 2016, pp. 479–484.

Luiz JA, Heseltine J. Five common toxins ingested by dogs and cats. Compend Contin Educ Pract Vet 2008, 30:578–587.

Author Charlotte Flint

Consulting Editor Lynn R. Hovda

Acknowledgment The author and book editors acknowledge the prior contribution of Gary D. Osweiler.

Client Education Handout available online

CHOLANGITIS/CHOLANGIOHEPATITIS SYNDROME

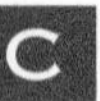

BASICS

DEFINITION

- Cholangitis—bile duct inflammation.
- Cholangiohepatitis—inflammation of bile ducts and adjacent liver parenchyma.
- Cholangitis/cholangiohepatitis syndrome (CCHS)—more common in cats; histologically classified as suppurative (predominant neutrophilic inflammation, S-CCHS); nonsuppurative (lymphocytic, plasmacytic, NS-CCHS); lymphoproliferative (may transition to lymphosarcoma); or granulomatous.

PATHOPHYSIOLOGY

- Antecedent or coexisting conditions—inflammation or obstruction involving extrahepatic bile duct (EHBDO) or pancreatic duct (cat), pancreatitis or inflammatory bowel disease (IBD; dog, cat); chronic interstitial nephritis (CIN; cat).
- Bacterial infection may be primary or secondary.
- Acute or chronic cholangitis—associates with biliary epithelial hyperplasia and ductular reaction.
- Chronic inflammation—may cause bile duct dystrophic mineralization or cholelithiasis.
- S-CCHS—usually positive bacterial culture or bacteria observed cytologically (tissue or bile); rarely observed in liver tissue, may observe in gallbladder (GB).
- NS-CCHS—immune-mediated and self-perpetuating, may evolve from S-CCHS.
- Sclerosing or destructive cholangitis—bile duct involution/destruction, may be immune mediated or infectious; leads to loss of small and medium-sized bile ducts (ductopenia) with "sclerosing" circumferential fibrosis; ductopenia is severe lesion.
- Pyogranulomatous CCHS—infectious or immune mechanisms (dog or cat).
- Lymphoproliferative disease—speculated transition stage of inflammation to neoplasia.

SYSTEMS AFFECTED

- Hepatobiliary—liver and biliary system.
- Gastrointestinal (GI)—pancreas and intestines.

INCIDENCE/PREVALENCE

NS-CCHS—most common chronic liver disorder in cats.

SIGNALMENT

Species

Cat (common), dog (uncommon).

Breed Predilections

Possibly Himalayan, Persian, Siamese cats.

Mean Age and Range

- S-CCHS—range: 0.4–16 years; mostly young to middle-aged cats.
- NS-CCHS—range: 2–17 years; mostly middle-aged cats.

Predominant Sex

- S-CCHS—male cats may be predisposed.
- NS-CCHS—no sex prevalence.

SIGNS

General Comments

- S-CCHS—most severe clinical illness, acute onset (often <5 days); abdominal pain, pyrexia; associated with EHBDO and cholelithiasis.
- NS-CCHS—ill >3 weeks (months to years).

Historical Findings

Feline CCHS—cyclic illness with chronic vague signs: lethargy, vomiting, anorexia, weight loss; ductopenic cats demonstrate polyphagia, acholic stools, variable steatorrhea, reduced uptake of fat-soluble substances.

Physical Examination Findings

- S-CCHS—fever; painful abdomen; ± jaundice; dehydration; shock.
- NS-CCHS—few physical abnormalities other than variable hepatomegaly; thickened intestines with IBD; variable jaundice; rare abdominal effusion.
- Ductopenia (cats)—unkempt coat, cyclic lateral thoracoabdominal alopecia; jaundiced; acholic feces (may be cyclic).

CAUSES

Suppurative CCHS

- Infections acquired as result of ductal plate malformations (DPM), all phenotypes but most commonly choledochal cyst and caroli phenotypes.
- Bacterial infection—more common in cats: *E coli and Enterococcus* most common, but numerous bacteria (e.g., *Enterobacter*, β-hemolytic *Streptococcus*, *Klebsiella*, *Actinomyces*, *Clostridia*, *Bacteroides*); rare toxoplasmosis; dogs: usually enteric opportunists; rare *Campylobacter*, *Salmonella*, *Leptospirosis*, others.
- Aerobic infections commonest, polymicrobial infections in ~30%.
- May represent sequela to intermittent mechanical bile flow stasis or EHBDO; DPM with cholelithiasis most common associated disorder.

Nonsuppurative CCHS

Concurrent disorders—cholecystitis, cholelithiasis, pancreatitis, EHBDO, IBD (dogs, cats); CIN (cats).

RISK FACTORS

- S-CCHS—EHBDO; cholelithiasis; DPM; other causes of cholestasis; infections elsewhere (dental, splenic abscess, pyelonephritis).
- Feline NS-CCHS—IBD, pancreatitis, EHBDO, cholelithiasis, CIN; may evolve from chronic intermittent S-CCHS.

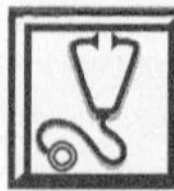

DIAGNOSIS

DIFFERENTIAL DIAGNOSES

- Feline hepatic lipidosis (FHL)—may coexist; similar enzyme patterns with jaundice but low γ-glutamyl transferase (GGT) unless concurrent biliary or pancreatic inflammation.
- EHBDO and obstructive cholelithiasis; variable jaundice, increased alkaline phosphatase (ALP), GGT, transaminase activities; increased cholesterol.
- Pancreatitis—may reflect cholelithiasis-initiated CCHS in cats; lipemia, high cholesterol, hyperbilirubinemia; inconsistent high feline pancreatic lipase activity (fPLI); high fPLI implicates pancreatic inflammation but also may reflect IBD, pancreatic duct inflammation/obstruction from cholelithiasis; ultrasound may differentiate.
- Lymphoproliferative disease and lymphoma—may involve any enteric segment, mesenteric/thoracic lymphadenopathy; shares clinical features with CCHS; hepatic infiltrates may require immunohistochemical characterization and clone evaluation to differentiate lymphoproliferative or lymphoma from NS-CCHS.
- Jaundice of septicemia—hyperbilirubinemia dominates clinical biochemical features, usually disproportionate to magnitude of liver enzyme activity unless concurrent CCHS.
- DPM occur in dogs, cats, esp. longhaired cats (Persian and Himalayan)—normal or modestly increased liver enzymes (see Ductal Plate Malformations); variable mild to moderate suppurative or nonsuppurative portal aggregates, cholangitis, or CCHS.

CBC/BIOCHEMISTRY/URINALYSIS

CBC

- Poikilocytes; nonregenerative anemia; anemia of chronic disease; Heinz body hemolysis.
- S-CCHS—variable neutrophilic leukocytosis, left shift, toxic neutrophils; NS-CCHS—may be normal; lymphoproliferative disorder or lymphoma may have lymphocytosis ± abnormal cell morphology.

Serum Biochemistry

- Consistent findings—high alanine aminotransferase (ALT), aspartate aminotransferase (AST), ALP, variable GGT.
- Variable findings—high total serum bile acids, bilirubin, cholesterol: depends on severity and extent of cholestasis, coexistent illness, liver dysfunction, cholelithiasis, DPM-associated hepatic fibrosis.

OTHER LABORATORY TESTS

- Species-specific PLI—may be high with pancreatitis, enteritis, or cholelith occlusion of bile duct ampulla in cats.
- Vitamin B_{12}—low values indicate small bowel malabsorption, exocrine pancreatic disease, chronic oral antimicrobials (dysbiosis).
- Coagulation tests—variable results; prothrombin time most sensitive for vitamin K_1–induced coagulopathy.
- T_4—rules out hyperthyroidism as cause of increased liver enzyme activity in cats.

IMAGING

- Thoracic radiography—sternal lymphadenopathy may reflect abdominal inflammation or lymphoma, general lymphadenopathy suggests lymphoma.
- Abdominal radiography—normal to large liver in NS-CCHS; mineralized choleliths or biliary structures in S-CCHS or NS-CCHS.
- Abdominal US—normal to large liver; thick extrahepatic bile duct or GB wall if choledochitis or cholecystitis; echogenic intraluminal debris; choleliths; focal parenchymal lesions (abscess, infiltrates: inflammation, neoplasia); lymphadenopathy suggests pancreatic, liver, intestinal inflammation or neoplasia; hepatic parenchymal hyperechogenicity (concurrent FHL, fibrosis); hypoechogenicity (inflammation); cysts (DPM, cystadenoma). *Note*: no US lesions apparent in some animals with CCHS.

DIAGNOSTIC PROCEDURES

Fine-Needle Aspiration Cytology

- Hepatic aspiration—for culture and diagnosis of FHL; cytology may reveal bacteria not visualized by light microscopy of biopsy sections. *Note*: cytology is diagnostic for FHL but unreliable for diagnosis of NS-CCHS; hepatocyte vacuolation common in ill cats, may implicate FHL as primary process when consequence of primary hepatic disease.
- Cholecystocentesis—may disclose suppuration, bacteria, trematode eggs, or neoplasia.

Percutaneous Biopsy

- US-guided core-needle biopsy—small sample size may misdiagnose CCHS; need min 15 portal triads for accuracy; if 18-G core needle used, collect min 4 samples.
- Inaccuracy with needle biopsy in feline CCHS reflects biopsy of single liver lobe in syndrome with differential lobe involvement or small sample size.
- Postbiopsy complications—esp. cats: collapse due to vasovagal response; biliary trauma; cats and tiny dogs: unintentional sampling of nonhepatic tissues.

Laparoscopy

- Permits direct visualization of GB, common bile duct (CBD), porta hepatis, pancreas, perihepatic and peripancreatic lymph nodes; allows biopsy of multiple liver lobes, pancreas, aspiration collection of bile.
- In EHBDO—not recommended, see Laparotomy.

Laparotomy

- Esp. if suspected EHBDO or choleliths in CBD or GB.
- Permits inspection and flushing of extrahepatic biliary conduits; biliary decompression and biliary enteric anastomosis.
- May be preferable approach in cats with CCHS as allows biopsy of liver, biliary structures, pancreas, intestines, lymph nodes, bile collection.

Tissue Sampling

If NS-CCHS suspected, also biopsy bowel, pancreas, and suspicious lymph nodes.

Bile and Tissue Cultures

- Aerobic and anaerobic bacterial cultures—of liver, bile, any choleliths (crushed); bile sample should include particulate debris (empty GB to collect mucin-laden bile: site of bacterial biofilm).
- If cholecystectomy done—scrape portion of GB wall and cut section of GB wall for culture.
- Put bile, GB wall, crushed cholelith, liver in same culture transport medium.

Molecular Genetics

Genetic test for feline polycystic disease may be appropriate if DPM diagnosis, especially if breeding animal.

PATHOLOGIC FINDINGS

- S-CCHS—normal or swollen liver, sharp or blunt edges, focal discolorations; may note erythematous, necrotic, or thick-walled GB; peripancreatic steatonecrosis or fat saponification (pancreatitis); perihepatic and peripancreatic lymphadenopathy; EHBDO: may observe choleliths or cystic lesions (DPM) or neoplastic mass lesions.
- NS-CCHS—variable liver size, normal to firm texture; sharp or blunt margins; variable surface irregularity; choleliths or cystic lesions (DPM phenotypes).
- If concurrent FHL—pale yellow friable parenchyma, liver floats in formalin.

TREATMENT

APPROPRIATE HEALTH CARE

Inpatient Management

- *S-CCHS with acute febrile illness, painful abdomen, left-shifted leukogram*—hydration support, "best guess" bactericidal antimicrobials: initially based on cytology and Gram stain or start trimodal antibiotics, esp. if EHBDO or cholecystitis suspected. Antibiotics essential *before* surgery; continue antibiotics ≥4 weeks with choleretic therapy until enzymes normalize or signs resolve (see Medications).
- *NS-symptomatic cats*—fluid therapy as necessary; if jaundiced: vitamin K_1 (0.5–1.5 mg/kg SC/IM q12h for 3 doses) before invasive diagnostics; cats with CCHS may need blood transfusion consequent to surgery or biopsy.
- Polyionic fluids—with B-soluble vitamins (2 mL/L), KCl, and K phosphate if refeeding syndrome possible; avoid dextrose supplements unless hypoglycemia (see Hepatic Lipidosis).

Outpatient Management

- S-CCHS—after acute crisis managed.
- NS-CCHS—after resolution of acute crisis, provide lifelong immunomodulation (if no bacteria observed or cultured), antioxidants, hepatoprotectants.

ACTIVITY

Restricted while symptomatic.

DIET

Nutritional support—avoid FHL in cats by feeding balanced high-protein, high-calorie feline diet; supplement water-soluble vitamins; antigen-restricted diet if concurrent IBD; fat-restricted diet if steatorrhea due to chronic EHBDO or severe ductopenia or chronic pancreatitis causing maldigestion; may require feeding tube; rarely require parenteral nutrition (may provoke FHL).

CLIENT EDUCATION

Emphasize chronic nature of NS-CCHS and requirement for lifelong therapy.

SURGICAL CONSIDERATIONS

- Cholecystectomy—if cholecystitis.
- Cholecystoenterostomy—may be necessary for some causes of EHBDO; if choleliths in GB: perform cholecystectomy.

MEDICATIONS

DRUG(S) OF CHOICE

Antibiotics: S-CCHS

- Bactericidal—against enteric opportunists; initial combination of ticarcillin or clavamox with enrofloxacin and metronidazole (7.5–15 mg/kg PO q12h; low dose if jaundiced).
- Modify initial empiric antimicrobials based on culture and sensitivity reports; resistant enterococcus may require vancomycin (10 mg/kg q12h IV slow infusion for 7–10 days).

Immunomodulation: NS-CCHS

- Glucocorticoids—prednisolone (dogs: 2 mg/kg/day prednisone or prednisolone; cats: 2–4 mg/kg/day prednisolone only) for 14–21 days, taper to lowest effective alternate-day dose based on ALT and clinical signs.

- Metronidazole—used for cell-mediated immunomodulation, antiendotoxin and antibacterial effects, esp. for IBD; as chronic bacterial involvement possible in feline NS-CCHS, chronic antibiotic treatment may be beneficial.
- Cats with confirmed ductopenia—aggressive immunomodulation; *do not use azathioprine*; clinical experience suggests combination of prednisolone, metronidazole with pulsed methotrexate (see below) *or* chlorambucil 1–2 mg per cat, load q24h for 3 days then every 3 days.
- *Methotrexate protocol feline destructive or sclerosing NS-CCHS:* 0.4 mg *total dose* given in 3 divided doses *on 1 day* (0.13 mg total at 0, 12, and 24h), repeated at 7–10-day intervals), PO/IV/IM (parenteral routes require 50% dose reduction); concurrently provide folate (folinic acid) 0.25 mg/kg daily. If lymphoproliferative or neoplastic infiltrates, use chemotherapy protocols developed for enteric lymphoma.

Antioxidants

- Vitamin E (α-tocopherol acetate)—10 IU/kg), using oral water-soluble form in chronic EHBDO or ductopenia (fat malabsorption).
- S-adenosylmethionine (SAMe)—20 mg/kg/day enteric-coated tablet PO 2h before feeding; benefits include anti-inflammatory influence; high dose for glutathione choleresis: 40 mg/kg/day.

Other

- Ursodeoxycholic acid (UDCA)—10–15 mg/kg/day PO divided, given with food for best bioavailability; provides immunomodulatory, hepatoprotectant, choleretic, antifibrotic, antioxidant effects; in immune-mediated NS-CCHS with developing ductopenia, use is controversial based on work in humans and animal models of immune-mediated destructive cholangitis: findings indicate may hasten small duct injury; liver biopsy recommended before prescribing UDCA for cats with "suspected" chronic CCHS; taurine supplementation (250 mg/day) should be considered in cats with poor appetite given chronic UDCA because of obligatory bile acid taurine conjugation.
- B vitamin supplementation—thiamine (B_1) and B_{12}: thiamine 50–100 mg PO q24h for 3 days, then in water-soluble vitamin supplements while hospitalized; B_{12} 0.25–1.0 mg SC if suspect gut malabsorption, using initial and sequential plasma B_{12} concentrations to guide need for chronic supplementation.

CONTRAINDICATIONS

Adjust drug dosages with regard to liver function and cholestasis. Caution with metronidazole to avoid neurotoxicity—if jaundiced use 7.5 mg/kg PO BID.

FOLLOW-UP

PATIENT MONITORING

- S-CCHS—follow body temperature, CBC, biochemical profile initially q7–14 days; continue antibiotics until clinical features normalize; if DPM may require lifelong antimicrobials.
- Animals with intrahepatic cholelithiasis and S-CCHS require long-term antibiotics, UDCA, high-dose SAMe, and monitoring for recurrent sepsis, stone migration (e.g., CBD, EHBDO).
- NS-CCHS—initially monitor enzymes and bilirubin q7–14 days, then monthly for 3 months to judiciously adjust immunomodulatory protocol, then quarterly.
- Serum bile acid measurements complicated by ursodeoxycholic acid administration and superfluous in circumstance of hepatobiliary jaundice

PREVENTION/AVOIDANCE

- Control IBD.
- If S-CCHS in animals with DPM—manage long term with appropriate antibiotics (see Ductal Plate Malformation).
- If choleliths in CBD or GB—surgically intervene: cholecystectomy if GB choleliths; flushing CBD free of lithic material essential if EHBDO.

POSSIBLE COMPLICATIONS

- S-CCHS may transform to NS-CCHS or sclerosing CCHS.
- Diabetes mellitus develops in ~30% of cats with sclerosing CCHS treated with prednisolone.
- FHL may develop due to inadequate nutritional intake or as side effect of glucocorticoids.

EXPECTED COURSE AND PROGNOSIS

- S-CCHS—may be cured.
- NS-CCHS—chronic, long-term, vacillating illness or remission possible (survival >8 years documented in some cats).

MISCELLANEOUS

ASSOCIATED CONDITIONS

- Pancreatitis.
- Hepatic lipidosis.
- DPM.
- Lymphosarcoma.
- Lymphoproliferative disease.
- Cholangiocarcinoma—may develop in some cats with chronic NS-CCHS or DPM.

SEE ALSO

- Bile Duct Obstruction (Extrahepatic).
- Cholecystitis and Choledochitis.
- Cholelithiasis.
- Ductal Plate Malformation (Congenital Hepatic Fibrosis).
- Hepatic Lipidosis.
- Inflammatory Bowel Disease.
- Pancreatitis—Cats.
- Pancreatitis—Dogs.

ABBREVIATIONS

- ALP = alkaline phosphatase.
- ALT = alanine aminotransferase.
- AST = aspartate amino transferase.
- CBD = common bile duct.
- CCHS = cholangitis/cholangiohepatitis syndrome.
- CIN = chronic interstitial nephritis.
- DPM = ductal plate malformation.
- EHBDO = extrahepatic bile duct obstruction.
- FHL = hepatic lipidosis.
- fPLI = feline pancreatic lipase activity.
- GB = gallbladder.
- GGT = γ-glutamyltransferase.
- GI = gastrointestinal.
- IBD = inflammatory bowel disease.
- NS-CCHS = nonsuppurative CCHS.
- SAMe = S-adenosylmethionine.
- S-CCHS = suppurative CCHS.
- UDCA = ursodeoxycholic acid.

Suggested Reading

Center SA. Diseases of the gallbladder and biliary tree. Vet Clin North Am Small Anim Pract 2009, 39:543–598.

Warren AE, Center SA, McDonough SE, et al. Histopathologic features, immunophenotyping, clonality and eubacterial FISH in cats with nonsuppurative cholangitis/cholangiohepatitis. Vet Pathol 2011, 48:627–634.

Author Sharon A. Center

Consulting Editor Kate Holan

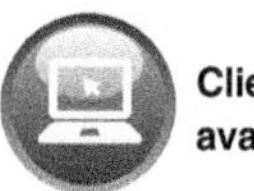

Client Education Handout available online

CHOLECYSTITIS AND CHOLEDOCHITIS

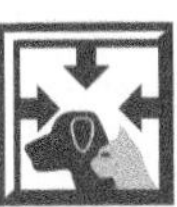

BASICS

OVERVIEW

• Cholecystitis = gallbladder (GB) inflammation. • Choledochitis = large bile duct inflammation. • Associated with cholelithiasis; secondary to GB mucocele (GBM); extrahepatic bile duct obstruction (EHBDO); inflammation of intrahepatic biliary structures (common in ductal plate malformation [DPM]). • Severe GB inflammation can lead to rupture and subsequent bile peritonitis, necessitating combined surgical and medical interventions. • Bile duct obstruction increases risk for biliary infection: enteric bacteria transmigrate bowel wall, pass into portal circulation, disseminate within liver, bile, and then GB, dispersing endotoxins and bacteria that may cause systemic sepsis or septic peritonitis.

SIGNALMENT

• Dog and cat. • No breed or sex predilection. • Necrotizing cholecystitis (dogs)—usually middle-aged or older animals. • GBM—predisposition for elderly dogs, dogs with hyperlipidemia or hypercholesterolemia (e.g., endocrinopathies [hyperadrenocorticism, hypothyroidism, diabetes mellitus]), pancreatitis, glucocorticoid administration, nephrotic syndrome, idiopathic hyperlipidemia (e.g., Shetland sheepdogs, miniature schnauzers, beagles, others); leads to cholestasis and possible cholecystitis (see Gallbladder Mucocele).

SIGNS

• Choledochitis—vague signs, variable icterus. • Sudden onset—inappetence, lethargy, vomiting, vague abdominal pain (may be postprandial with cholecystitis or GBM, reflecting post-meal GB contraction).
• Chronic postprandial discomfort/distress—position of comfort, stretching, pacing, panting. • Mild to moderate jaundice and fever common. • Severe disease—shock due to endotoxemia, bacteremia, hypovolemia.
• Soft tissue mass in right cranial abdomen palpable in small dogs and cats, reflecting inflammation or adhesions between GB and pericholecystic tissues.

CAUSES & RISK FACTORS

• Impaired bile flow at cystic duct or GB (cholelithiasis, mass lesions), GB dysmotility, or ischemic insult to GB wall (from GB distention)—may precede cholecystitis ± necrotizing lesions. • Irritants in sludged bile (e.g., lysolecithin, prostaglandins, choleliths, flukes) or retrograde flow of pancreatic enzyme into bile duct in cats may initiate/augment GB or duct inflammation.
• Previous enteric disorders, trauma, abdominal surgery—may be contributing factors. • Anomalous GB or duct development—DPM lesions including choledochal cysts (cats > dogs). • Bacterial infection—common; retrograde duct bacterial invasion from intestines or hematogenous dispersal from splanchnic circulation. • Toxoplasmosis and biliary coccidiosis—rare causes. • Necrotizing cholecystitis (dogs)—ruptured GB (common, often secondary to cholelithiasis or hypermature GBM); *E. coli* and *Enterococcus* spp.: common isolates.
• Emphysematous cholecystitis/choledochitis—rare, associated with diabetes mellitus, traumatic GB ischemia, acute cholecystitis (with or without cholelithiasis); common gas-forming organisms: *Clostridia* spp. and *E. coli*.

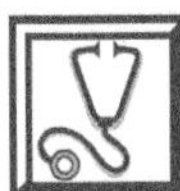

DIAGNOSIS

DIFFERENTIAL DIAGNOSIS

• EHBDO. • GBM. • Cholelithiasis.
• Cholangitis/cholangiohepatitis. • Pancreatitis.
• Focal or diffuse peritonitis. • Bile peritonitis.
• Gastroenteritis with biliary involvement.
• Hepatic necrosis or abscessation. • Septicemia.

CBC/BIOCHEMISTRY/URINALYSIS

• Variable leukocytosis with toxic neutrophils and inconsistent left shift if necrosis or sepsis.
• High bilirubin and bilirubinuria common.
• High alanine aminotransferase (ALT), aspartate aminotransferase (AST), alkaline phosphatase (ALP), and γ-glutamyl transferase (GGT) activity. • Low albumin with peritonitis. • High cholesterol and bilirubin if EHBDO. • Hypercholesterolemia and/or hypertriglyceridemia—breed related, endocrine related, pancreatitis, nephrotic syndrome, EHBDO, GBM.

OTHER LABORATORY TESTS

• Abdominocentesis—inflammatory effusion (see Bile Peritonitis). • Bile culture (dogs and cats)—*E. coli*, *Enterococcus* spp., *Klebsiella* spp., *Pseudomonas* spp., *Clostridium* spp., many others. • Coagulation tests—abnormal if chronic EHBDO (vitamin K deficiency) or disseminated intravascular coagulation (DIC) in severe conditions with sepsis; cats display coagulopathy with EHBDO early.

IMAGING

• Abdominal radiography—may reveal loss of cranial abdominal detail with focal or diffuse peritonitis or effusion; ileus; radiodense choleliths; gas in biliary structures; radiodense GB (dystrophic mineralization due to chronic inflammation; porcelain GB is rare).
• Ultrasonography—diffusely thick GB wall, segmental hyperechogenicity and/or laminated wall or double-rimmed GB wall observed with necrotizing cholecystitis; double-rimmed GB wall also observed with acute cholecystitis, hepatitis, cholangiohepatitis; GB lumen filled with amorphous echogenic stellate or finely striated pattern, resembling sliced kiwi fruit ("kiwi sign") in mature GBM; GB rupture implicated by discontinuous GB wall, pericholecystic fluid, or generalized effusion, and hyperechogenicity of pericholicystic tissue; failure to image GB: may implicate rupture or agenesis; mineralized GB wall may indicate dystrophic mineralization (limey or porcelain GB) due to chronic cholecystis often associated with sacculated GB or bile ducts in DPM: Caroli's phenotype; intrahepatic bile ducts may be difficult to visualize or be thick and prominent: ascending cholangitis or EHBDO (dilated ducts, "too many tubes signs" defined with color-flow Doppler); pericholecystic fluid: necrotizing cholecystitis and surgical emergency. • Choledochitis involving common bile duct (CBD)—thick wall, intraluminal debris, extends into hepatic ducts.

PATHOLOGIC FINDINGS

• Gross appearance—erythematous GB; may appear green-black if necrotizing lesion; tenacious "inspissated" biliary material common with GBM; pigmented choleliths if infection; dark black or frank blood if hemobilia; CBD with thick wall, variable intraductal debris (e.g., biliary particulates, cholelithiasis, suppurative inflammation).
• Microscopic features of GBM without cholecystitis are benign, with wall thinning, mucosal cystic hyperplasia, elongated mucosal fronds extending from flattened mucosa, without granulation response in GB wall; if chronic GBM may involve arterial thrombi and/or transformation to chronic cholecystitis. • Microscopic features of cholecystitis include inflammatory infiltrates in lamina propria (lymphoplasmacytic or suppurative with macrophages, rarely eosinophilic, occasional lymphoid follicular hyperplasia), intraluminal suppurative/necrotic debris; if chronic cholecystitis—submucosal granulation tissue with variable ulcerative/necrotic mucosa, occasional hemobilia, occasional arterial thrombi; if cholelithiasis—hyperplastic mucosa with dense elongated mucosal fronds and glands contrasting with flattened appearance of GBM.

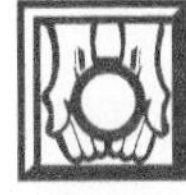

TREATMENT

• Inpatient—provision of critical care during diagnostic/presurgical evaluations or if septic. • Place IV catheter in peripheral vein for polyionic fluids and blood component therapy as needed. • Restore fluid and electrolyte balance; monitor electrolytes frequently. • Vitamin K—if jaundiced; give parenterally (see Medications) before surgical interventions, cystocentesis, jugular venipuncture, other iatrogenic trauma. • Plasma—preferred colloid; indicated if hypoalbuminemia *and* coagulopathy or if anticipated surgical

CHOLECYSTITIS AND CHOLEDOCHITIS (CONTINUED)

interventions and complicating coagulopathy uncorrected. • Whole blood or fresh frozen plasma—for surgical cases with bleeding tendencies; if septic, artificial colloids may delay recovery; if bleeding, some artificial colloids impair platelet aggregation. • Monitor urine output. • Remain vigilant for vasovagal reflex (abrupt bradycardia, hypotension, cardiac arrest) during biliary tree manipulation or cholecystocentesis; be prepared with anticholinergics (atropine) and pressor drugs. • Remain vigilant for cholangiovenous reflux—systemic dispersal of endotoxin or bacteria while handling septic biliary tree: give IV antibiotics promptly (but after culture collection). • GB resection advised for cholecystis, best based on surgical evaluations, ultrasound images, bedside cytology of bile—bacterial infection mandates cholecystectomy.

MEDICATIONS

DRUG(S) OF CHOICE

• Antibiotics—*before surgery*; broad spectrum; surgical manipulations may cause bacteremia; select antibiotics for *Enterococcus* spp., enteric Gram-negative and anaerobic flora; refine treatment using culture and sensitivity results; good initial choice is triad combination of metronidazole, ticarcillin (or clavamox), and a fluorinated quinolone; reduce standard dose for metronidazole by 50% if cholestatic jaundice. • Ursodeoxycholic acid—10–15 mg/kg PO daily divided BID with food; requires decompression of EHBDO *prior to treatment*. • Antioxidants—vitamin E (α-tocopherol acetate): 10 IU/kg (see Bile Duct Obstruction (Extrahepatic); use water-soluble form if EHBDO); S-adenosylmethionine (SAMe): use enteric-coated bioavailable product; on empty stomach: used as glutathione (GSH) donor (20 mg/kg PO q24h), 2h before feeding; nonbile acid-dependent (GSH) choleresis (40 mg/kg PO q24h); n-acetylcysteine (NAC) IV if oral administration of antioxidants not possible; loading dose 140 mg/kg IV over 20 min, follow by 70 mg/kg over 20 min q6–8h. • Vitamin K_1—0.5–1.5 mg/kg SC/IM q12h for 3 doses; *caution*: never administer IV (anaphylactoid reaction); treat early to allow response before surgical manipulations.

CONTRAINDICATIONS/POSSIBLE INTERACTIONS

Ursodeoxycholic acid—contraindicated in uncorrected EHBDO or bile peritonitis.

FOLLOW-UP

PATIENT MONITORING

• After critical crisis resolution and surgery—physical examination and pertinent diagnostic testing: repeat every 1–2 weeks until abnormalities resolve. • If septic—continue antibiotics until enzymes, hyperbilirubinemia, leukocytosis, left shift, and fever resolve.

POSSIBLE COMPLICATIONS

Anticipate protracted clinical course with ruptured biliary tract or peritonitis; postoperative pancreatitis.

MISCELLANEOUS

ASSOCIATED CONDITIONS

• Cholelithiasis. • DPM. • EHBDO. • GBM. • Bile peritonitis.

AGE-RELATED FACTORS

Congenital malformations of biliary structures do not predispose patients to cholecystitis, but do predispose to choledochitis and cholelithiasis that lead to GB disease and infection.

ZOONOTIC POTENTIAL

Campylobacter and *Salmonella* may cause cholecystitis in dogs; advise owner if diagnosed.

SEE ALSO

- Bile Peritonitis.
- Gallbladder Mucocele.

ABBREVIATIONS

- ALP = alkaline phosphatase.
- ALT = alanine aminotransferase.
- AST = aspartate aminotransferase.
- CBD = common bile duct.
- DIC = disseminated intravascular coagulation.
- DPM = ductal plate malformation.
- EHBDO = extrahepatic bile duct obstruction.
- GB = gallbladder.
- GBM = gallbladder mucocele.
- GGT = γ-glutamyltransferase.
- GSH = glutathione.
- NAC = n-acetylcysteine.
- SAMe = S-adenosylmethionine.

Suggested Reading

Center SA. Diseases of the gallbladder and biliary tree. Vet Clin North Am Small Anim Pract 2009, 39(3):543–598.

Lawrence YA, Ruaux CG, Nemanic S, et al. Characterization, treatment, and outcome of bacterial cholecystitis and bactibilia in dogs. J Am Vet Med Assoc 2015, 246:982–989.

Tamborini A, Jahns H, McAllister H, et al. Bacterial cholangitis, cholecystitis, or both in dogs. J Vet Intern Med 2016, 30:1046–1055.

Author Sharon A. Center

Consulting Editor Kate Holan

BASICS

OVERVIEW

- Radiopaque or radiolucent calculi in common bile ducts (CBD), gallbladder (GB), or less commonly in intrahepatic bile ducts (hepatolithiasis); gallbladder mucocele (GBM) qualifies as a form of cholelithiasis (see Gallbladder Mucocele).
- May be asymptomatic.
- Symptomatic—signs reflect sludging of bile, extrahepatic bile duct obstruction (EHBDO), cholecystitis, cholangiohepatitis, or bile peritonitis.
- Primary constituents of choleliths—mucin, glycoprotein, calcium carbonate, and bilirubin pigments; while dog bile is less lithogenic than human bile (lower cholesterol saturation), dog bile forms calcium bilirubinate sludge upon fasting.
- 50% feline choleliths are mineralized; may be radiographically visible (calcium carbonate).
- Surgical treatment—not recommended without clinical signs or clinicopathologic abnormalities (current or historical), with the exception of preemptive GBM removal.

SIGNALMENT

- Cat and dog.
- Small-breed dogs may be predisposed; animals with ductal plate malformations (DPM) predisposed: particularly Caroli DPM phenotypes (i.e., malformative dilated large ducts causing bile stasis in sacculated ducts); microhepatolithiasis encountered more often in DPM.
- Hyperlipidemic and hypercholesterolemic dogs—predisposed to GBM; may relate to endocrine disorders, idiopathic condition, or other disorders (see Gallbladder Mucocele).

SIGNS

- May be asymptomatic.
- When accompanied by infection or causing intermittent or complete EHBDO (with or without peritonitis)—vomiting; meal-related discomfort, vague abdominal pain; fever; ± jaundice.
- Episodic vague peri- or postprandial abdominal pain or behavior seeking position of relief.

CAUSES & RISK FACTORS

- Predisposing factors—stasis of bile flow: GB dysmotility, choledochal cysts (cat especially, form of DPM); lith nidus may evolve from inflammatory debris, infection, epithelial irregularity/exfoliation, neoplasia, residual suture material; bile supersaturation: heme-bilirubin pigments, hemobilia, calcium-bilirubinate, enhanced mucin production (inflammation, prostaglandins), cholesterol.
- Fused feline pancreatic and bile duct predisposes to concurrent biliary/pancreatic cholelithiasis, choledochitis, and bile stasis progressing to EHBDO as well as cholelith-initiated pancreatitis or signs mistaken for pancreatitis.
- Bile sludge associated with GB distention—may enhance mucin production and coalescence of bile particulates increasing risk for choleliths; but EHBDO does not cause choleliths.
- Inflammatory mediators and bacterial enzymes associated with cholecystitis—increase risk for stone precipitation.
- Hemobilia—bleeding into GB or bile ducts or chronic hemolysis can lead to heme-initiated cholelith formation.
- Low-methionine and high-cholesterol experimental diet in dogs is proven lithogenic.

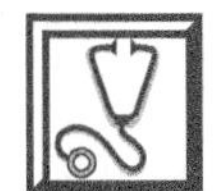

DIAGNOSIS

DIFFERENTIAL DIAGNOSIS

- EHBDO—inflammatory, infectious, or neoplastic conditions involving liver, CBD, or extrahepatic tissues adjacent to porta hepatis; suggested by marked increases in alkaline phosphatase (ALP), γ-glutamyltransferase (GGT), bilirubin, and gradual increase in cholesterol.
- Cholangiohepatitis.
- Cholecystitis/choledochitis.
- Bile peritonitis.
- GBM.
- Consequence of DPM.
- Chronic hypercalcemia may increase risk.

CBC/BIOCHEMISTRY/URINALYSIS

- May have no clinicopathologic abnormalities—asymptomatic cholelithiasis.
- CBC—may be normal; may reflect bacterial infection, endotoxemia, biliary obstruction, or other underlying causal factors; inflammatory leukogram in some cases.
- Biochemistry—if symptomatic: variable hyperbilirubinemia, increase ALP, GGT, alanine aminotransferase (ALT), and aspartate aminotransferase (AST) activities; also see Bile Duct Obstruction (Extrahepatic).

OTHER LABORATORY TESTS

- Bacterial culture—bile: aerobic and anaerobic bacteria often confirmed in symptomatic patients if crushed cholelith, sludged bile, ± GB wall (if cholecystectomy) submitted for cultures.
- Cholelith nidus—may house associated bacterial infection.
- Coagulation profile—bleeding associated with prolonged clotting times may develop with EHBDO of ≥7–10 days; see Bile Duct Obstruction (Extrahepatic); responsive to parenteral vitamin K_1 administration.
- Cholelith analysis—infrequently done; submit to laboratory equipped for cholelith analyses.

IMAGING

- Abdominal radiography—limited value in delineating GB structure/content; choleliths often small, may be radiolucent; rarely mistaken for dystrophic biliary mineralization in animals with chronic cholangitis or Caroli DPM phenotype.
- Ultrasonography—can detect: choleliths ≥2 mm diameter, thickened GB wall, distended biliary tract, increased hepatic parenchymal echogenicity and extrahepatic ductal involvement; may facilitate specimen collection for culture, cytology, and histopathology; may detect evidence of EHBDO within 72h; *caution*: distended GB with bile "sludge" is common in anorectic or fasted patients; do not mistake for GB obstruction. Hepatolithiasis usually casts acoustic shadows. Imaging of choleliths within extrahepatic ducts may be difficult owing to enteric gas obstructing imaging "window"; confirmation of distended intrahepatic bile duct done with color-flow Doppler.

DIAGNOSTIC PROCEDURES

Histopathologic evaluation of liver necessary in patients undergoing surgical cholelith removal to detect comorbid conditions influencing treatment and prognosis, i.e., suppurative cholangitis, nonsuppurative cholangitis, DPM, neoplasia.

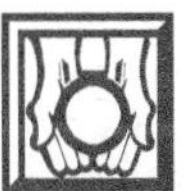

TREATMENT

- Controversial whether choleresis with ursodeoxycholate (UDCA) is beneficial in animals lacking clinical or clinicopathologic signs; can resolve cholesterol choleliths in humans, but these are rare in dogs or cats; choleresis with UDCA may help move sludged biliary debris.
- Supportive fluids—if hospitalized, according to hydration, electrolyte, and acid-base status.
- If hyperlipidemia coexistent—prescribe fat-restricted diet, identify and manage endocrinopathies; if failure to control hyperlipidemia, may require additional medical management.
- Control predisposing conditions, especially biliary tree infection (with antimicrobials) and GB dysmotility (by GB removal).
- Exploratory surgery, choledochotomy, cholecystotomy, and possibly cholecystectomy or biliary-enteric anastomosis—indicated in symptomatic cases according to circumstances.
- Warn client that cholelithiasis is chronic problem and that stones may reform even after surgical removal despite chronic medical treatment; choleliths in GB is strong

CHOLELITHIASIS (CONTINUED)

indication for cholecystectomy unless GB needed for biliary enteric anastomosis in certain conditions.

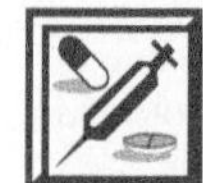

MEDICATIONS

DRUG(S) OF CHOICE

- Antibiotics—based on culture of bile, tissue, and cholelith nidus, cytology and Gram staining of biliary debris or crushed lith if cultures negative; if culture negative then directed against enteric microbial opportunists; initial treatment with Timentin or Clavamox® with metronidazole, combined with a fluoroquinolone, usually successful.
- Ursodeoxycholic acid—10–15 mg/kg/day PO, divided BID, given with food to increase bioavailability; provides choleretic, hepatoprotectant, anti-endotoxic, antifibrotic effects, and may facilitate cholesterol stone dissolution; therapy often continued lifelong if no cause for cholelithiasis identified to augment choleresis thwarting bile stasis.
- Vitamin K_1—parenterally; 0.5–1.5 mg/kg to max 3 doses in 24–36h in jaundiced patients; do not administer IV (anaphylaxis).

Antioxidants

- Vitamin E (α-tocopherol acetate)—10 IU/kg per day for patients with high liver enzymes or confirmed hepatobiliary inflammation; use water-soluble form if EHBDO.
- S-adenosylmethionine (SAMe; use form with proven bioavailability and efficacy)—glutathione (GSH) donor (important hepatic antioxidant, GSH also provides driving force for non-bile acid–dependent choleresis) and thus is potential choleretic for patients with high liver enzymes or confirmed hepatobiliary inflammation; 20–40 mg/kg using enteric-coated tablet PO q24h, administer 2h before feeding; higher dose recommended for choleresis; also provides antifibrotic and antiinflammatory benefits.

CONTRAINDICATIONS/POSSIBLE INTERACTIONS

Ursodeoxycholic acid—contraindicated with EHBDO before biliary decompression.

FOLLOW-UP

PATIENT MONITORING

- Physical examination and pertinent diagnostic testing q2–4 weeks postoperatively until clinical signs and clinicopathologic abnormalities resolve.
- Periodic ultrasonography—assess cholelith status, integrity/distention of biliary tract, hepatic parenchymal changes.

POSSIBLE COMPLICATIONS

Sudden onset of fever, abdominal pain, and malaise—may signify bile peritonitis and/or sepsis from breakdown in bile containment, or recurrent cholelith lodged in sphincter of Oddi (duodenal papilla) or obstructing pancreatic duct (cats only).

EXPECTED COURSE AND PROGNOSIS

- May be asymptomatic.
- Symptomatic disease—reflects existing infection, EHBDO, cholecystitis, DPM, or bile peritonitis.

MISCELLANEOUS

SEE ALSO

- Bile Duct Obstruction (Extrahepatic).
- Cholecystitis and Choledochitis.
- Ductal Plate Malformation (Congenital Hepatic Fibrosis).
- Gallbladder Mucocele.

ABBREVIATIONS

- ALP = alkaline phosphatase.
- ALT = alanine aminotransferase.
- AST = aspartate aminotransferase.
- CBD = common bile duct.
- DPM = ductal plate malformation.
- EHBDO = extrahepatic bile duct obstruction.
- GB = gallbladder.
- GBM = gallbladder mucocele.
- GGT = γ-glutamyltransferase.
- GSH = glutathione.
- SAMe = S-adenosylmethionine.
- UDCA = ursodeoxycholate.

Suggested Reading

Center SA. Diseases of the gallbladder and biliary tree. Vet Clin North Am Small Anim Pract 2009, 39:543–598.

van Geffen C, Savary-Bataille K, Chiers K, et al. Bilirubin cholelithiasis and haemosiderosis in an anaemic pyruvate kinase-deficient Somali cat. J Small Anim Pract 2008, 49:479–482.

Author Sharon A. Center

Consulting Editor Kate Holan

BASICS

OVERVIEW

• Chondrosarcoma (CSA) is a malignant mesenchymal tumor arising from cartilage and characterized by production of chondroid and fibrillar matrix. • CSA is the second most common primary bone tumor in dogs and accounts for 5–10% of all primary bone tumors; primary bone tumors are uncommon in cats, and CSA is third in incidence behind osteosarcoma and fibrosarcoma. • Dogs—majority of CSAs arise from flat bones (axial skeleton); approximately 30% occur in nasal cavity and 20% of CSAs arise from ribs; 20% of CSAs in dogs arise from appendicular skeleton; sites are generally similar to where osteosarcoma typically occurs. • Cats: 66% of CSAs arise in appendicular skeleton, with 33% occurring in the axial skeleton. • Rarely, CSA can arise in soft tissue (extraskeletal) sites.

SIGNALMENT

• Dogs—medium- to large-breed dogs, with mixed-breed dogs, golden retrievers, boxers, and German shepherd dogs overrepresented; median age is 8 years (range: 1–15 years). • Cats—median age is 9 years (range: 2–18 years), with males twice as likely to be affected.

SIGNS

Historical Findings

• Patients often present with a visible mass at the affected site. • History of lameness if involvement of weight-bearing bone. • Rarely, CSA of the rib may be associated with respiratory signs. • Additional clinical signs vary with site of involvement.

Physical Examination Findings

• Findings depend on anatomic location. • A firm to hard mass often is palpable, with variable degrees of pain elicited on palpation. • CSA of the rib occurs most commonly at the costochondral junction; dyspnea is rare and associated with space-occupying effect.

CAUSES & RISK FACTORS

• Etiology largely unknown. • Osteochondromatosis (multiple cartilaginous exostosis) lesions can transform into CSA.

DIAGNOSIS

DIFFERENTIAL DIAGNOSIS

• Other primary bone tumors (osteosarcoma, fibrosarcoma, hemangiosarcoma). • Metastatic bone tumors (transitional cell, prostatic, mammary, thyroid, apocrine gland, anal sac carcinomas). • Tumors that locally invade adjacent bone (especially oral, nasal, digital, and joint tumors). • Fungal osteomyelitis.

CBC/BIOCHEMISTRY/URINALYSIS

Usually normal.

IMAGING

• Radiographs of affected area show features of aggressive bone lesion (cortical lysis, nonhomogenous reactive bone formation, ill-defined zone of transition). • Thoracic radiographs recommended to screen for pulmonary metastasis. • CT recommended for axial tumors to more accurately stage local disease and plan for surgery and/or radiation therapy; concurrent CT imaging of thorax recommended as more sensitive way to screen for pulmonary metastasis. • MRI, alone or in combination with CT, may be recommended for treatment planning for vertebral CSA.

DIAGNOSTIC PROCEDURES

• Histopathology needed for definitive diagnosis. • Fine-needle aspirate bone cytology may provide supportive diagnosis; differentiation of CSA from other sarcomas may be challenging if sample contains sparse amounts of matrix.

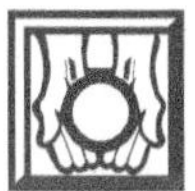

TREATMENT

• Amputation recommended for appendicular tumors. • For axial tumors, wide surgical excision recommended whenever possible. • Stereotactic radiation therapy provides effective local control for canine osteosarcoma and might be alternative to surgery for patients with CSA. • Palliative therapy recommended for patients with nonresectable local disease or gross metastasis, or when definitive therapy is declined; palliative care focuses on pain control.

MEDICATIONS

DRUG(S) OF CHOICE

Pain Management

• Nonsteroidal anti-inflammatory drugs (NSAIDs). • Tramadol. • Gabapentin. • IV aminobisphosphonates (e.g., pamidronate, zoledronate) might alleviate bone pain and slow pathologic bone resorption.

Chemotherapy

Role of chemotherapy has not been defined in veterinary oncology, but does not improve outcome in humans.

CONTRAINDICATIONS/POSSIBLE INTERACTIONS

• Use NSAIDs cautiously in all cats and in dogs with renal insufficiency. • Do not combine NSAIDs with corticosteroids.

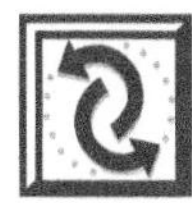

FOLLOW-UP

PATIENT MONITORING

Physical examination every 2–3 months and thoracic radiographs every 3–4 months to monitor for local tumor control and distant metastases, respectively.

EXPECTED COURSE AND PROGNOSIS

• Overall, 15–30% of dogs will develop metastatic disease, with lungs being most commonly affected site; metastatic rates approach 50% for high-grade canine tumors; development of metastasis rare for cats with CSA. • With curative-intent surgery, median survival >3 years; depending on tumor location and completeness of excision, up to 40% will develop local recurrence. • With palliative care alone, survival times of >1 year still possible.

MISCELLANEOUS

SEE ALSO

- Chondrosarcoma, Nasal and Paranasal Sinus.
- Chondrosarcoma, Oral.
- Fibrosarcoma, Bone.
- Osteosarcoma.

ABBREVIATIONS

- CSA = chondrosarcoma.
- NSAID = nonsteroidal anti-inflammatory drug.

Suggested Reading

Durham AC, Popovitch CA, Goldschmidt MH. Feline chondrosarcoma: a retrospective study of 67 cats (1987–2005). J Am Anim Hosp Assoc 2008, 44(3):124–130.

Farese JP, Kirpensteijn J, Kik M, et al. Biologic behavior and clinical outcome of 25 dogs with canine appendicular chondrosarcoma treated by amputation: a Veterinary Society of Surgical Oncology retrospective study. Vet Surg 2009, 38:914–919.

Author Jenna H. Burton

Consulting Editor Timothy M. Fan

Acknowledgment The author and book editors acknowledge the prior contribution of Dennis B. Bailey.

CHONDROSARCOMA, NASAL AND PARANASAL SINUS

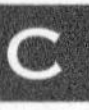

BASICS

OVERVIEW

• Chondrosarcoma (CSA) is a malignant mesenchymal tumor arising from cartilage and characterized by production of chondroid and fibrillar matrix. • Nasal CSA arises most commonly from the nasal turbinates. • In dogs, CSA accounts for 15% of all nasal tumors.

SIGNALMENT

• Mixed-breed dogs, Labrador retrievers, golden retrievers, boxers, and German shepherd dogs are overrepresented. • Median age is 7 years (range: 2–13 years). • CSA tends to develop at a younger age than other nasal tumors. • Rare in cats, with no obvious breed or sex predilections.

SIGNS

Historical Findings

• Intermittent unilateral epistaxis and/or mucopurulent discharge, may progress to bilateral involvement. • Sneezing, stertorous breathing, and/or facial deformity. • Decreased appetite and/or halitosis secondary to oral cavity invasion. • Seizures, behavior changes, and/or obtundation secondary to cranial invasion.

Physical Examination Findings

• Epistaxis and/or nasal discharge, initially unilateral but can progress to bilateral.
• Decreased nasal air flow (unilateral or bilateral). • Pain on nasal or paranasal sinus palpation or percussion. • Facial deformity, decreased ocular retropulsion, exophthalmia, or epiphora. • Visible mass effect protruding through the palate into the oral cavity.

CAUSES & RISK FACTORS

Unknown

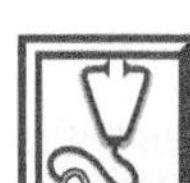

DIAGNOSIS

DIFFERENTIAL DIAGNOSIS

• Other nasal tumors—adenocarcinoma, squamous cell carcinoma, osteosarcoma, fibrosarcoma, lymphoma, transmissible venereal tumor (dogs), nasopharyngeal polyp (cats). • Fungal rhinitis—aspergillosis and penicilliosis (dogs), cryptococcus (cats), sporotrichosis (both). • Rhinosporidiosis (dogs). • Foreign body. • Thrombocytopenia or other coagulopathy. • Tooth root abscess.
• Oronasal fistula.

CBC/BIOCHEMISTRY/URINALYSIS

Usually normal—evaluate for thrombocytopenia if signs of epistaxis.

OTHER LABORATORY TESTS

• Nasal flush for cytology and culture—rarely helpful. • Coagulation profile. • Buccal mucosal bleeding time.

IMAGING

• Thoracic radiographs to screen for pulmonary metastasis (uncommon). • CT for detecting soft tissue opacity within nasal cavity and surrounding sinuses, bony destruction, and extension through cribriform plate into brain. • If CT scan is not accessible, skull radiographs can be performed to assess for soft tissue opacity in nasal cavity and/or frontal sinuses.

DIAGNOSTIC PROCEDURES

• Blood pressure, to rule out systemic hypertension as cause for epistaxis. • Mandibular lymph node cytology to screen for possible metastasis. • Rhinoscopy is helpful for visualization of mass or fungal plaque and guiding subsequent tissue biopsy. • Tissue biopsy and histopathology needed for definitive diagnosis; biopsy instrument should not pass caudal to level of medial canthus of eye to avoid penetrating cribriform plate.
• Intranasal approach to obtaining tissue biopsy preferable if treatment radiation therapy planned.

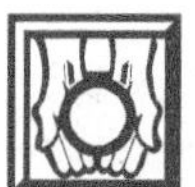

TREATMENT

• Radiation therapy is treatment of choice.
• Conventional linear accelerator used most commonly; however, if available, stereotactic radiation therapy can reduce number of radiation treatments and reduce adverse effects. • Palliative radiation protocols (fewer treatments and lower total radiation dose) might be preferable for dogs with very advanced disease.

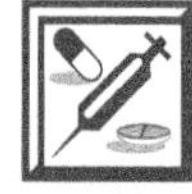

MEDICATIONS

DRUG(S) OF CHOICE

• Nonsteroidal anti-inflammatory drugs (NSAIDs) for pain control. • Prednisone (0.5–1 mg/kg PO q24h) to help relieve nasal congestion. • Phenylephrine nasal spray can be used intermittently to help with epistaxis.
• Empiric antibiotic therapy can be considered for secondary bacterial infections.

CONTRAINDICATIONS/POSSIBLE INTERACTIONS

• Use NSAIDs cautiously in all cats and in dogs with renal insufficiency. • Do not combine NSAIDs with corticosteroids.

FOLLOW-UP

PATIENT MONITORING

• Physical examinations every 2–3 months and thoracic radiographs every 3–4 months.
• CT of skull can be considered when clinical signs recur or progress.

EXPECTED COURSE AND PROGNOSIS

• <10% develop metastasis (lungs affected most commonly). • Median survival with palliative care alone is 3 months. • With definitive daily radiation therapy, median survival is around 17 months, and 2-year survival rate is around 30%; median survival with palliative radiation protocols is about 9 months. • Recurrence/progression of tumor and recurrence of clinical signs generally life-limiting event for nasal CSA. • Brain involvement is poor prognostic sign.
• Unilateral versus bilateral involvement is not significant prognostic factor.

MISCELLANEOUS

SEE ALSO

• Adenocarcinoma, Nasal.
• Chondrosarcoma, Bone.
• Chondrosarcoma, Oral.
• Epistaxis.

ABBREVIATIONS

• CSA = chondrosarcoma.
• NSAID = nonsteroidal anti-inflammatory drug.

Suggested Reading

Patnaik AK, Lieberman PH, Erlandson RA, et al. Canine sinonasal skeletal neoplasms: chondrosarcomas and osteosarcomas. Vet Pathol 1984, 21(5):475–482.

Sones E, Smith A, Schleis S, et al. Survival times for canine intranasal sarcomas treated with radiation therapy: 86 cases (1996–2011). Vet Radiol Ultrasound 2013, 54(2):194–201.

Author Jenna H. Burton

Consulting Editor Timothy M. Fan

Acknowledgment The author and book editors acknowledge the prior contribution of Dennis B. Bailey.

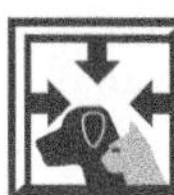

BASICS

OVERVIEW

- Chondrosarcoma (CSA) is a malignant mesenchymal tumor arising from cartilage and characterized by production of chondroid and fibrillar matrix.
- CSA accounts for 5–10% of all primary bone tumors; mandibular and maxillary CSAs have been reported in dogs, but these are not common locations for this tumor (see Chondrosarcoma, Bone, and Chondrosarcoma, Nasal and Paranasal Sinus).

SIGNALMENT

- Dogs—medium- to large-breed dogs, with mixed-breed dogs, golden retrievers, boxers, and German shepherd dogs overrepresented; median age is 8 years (range: 1–15 years).
- Cats—rarely affected.

SIGNS

Historical Findings

- Visible mass involving the mandible or maxilla.
- Halitosis, dysphagia, and/or hypersalivation.
- Bloody oral discharge and oral pain.
- Weight loss secondary to a prolonged decrease in food intake.

Physical Examination Findings

- A firm to hard mass centered on the maxilla or mandible is seen most commonly.
- The overlying gingival mucosa usually is intact, although trauma and ulceration from the occlusal teeth are common with larger tumors.
- Loose or missing teeth.
- Difficulty or pain when opening the mouth (especially caudal tumors).
- Facial deformity.
- Mandibular lymphadenopathy.
- Nasal discharge, epistaxis, or decreased air flow through the nares (maxillary tumors).

CAUSES & RISK FACTORS

None identified.

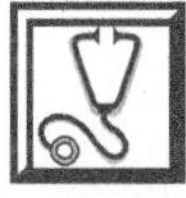

DIAGNOSIS

DIFFERENTIAL DIAGNOSIS

- Other primary oral tumors, including melanoma, fibrosarcoma, squamous cell carcinoma, osteosarcoma, and acanthomatous ameloblastoma.
- Maxillary invasion of primary nasal CSA.
- Craniomandibular osteopathy.
- Dentigerous cyst, tooth root abscess, or osteomyelitis.

CBC/BIOCHEMISTRY/URINALYSIS

Usually normal.

IMAGING

- Thoracic radiographs are recommended to screen for pulmonary metastasis.
- Skull radiographs often will show features of an aggressive bone lesion (bone lysis, cortical destruction, nonhomogenous bone formation, ill-defined zone of transition); however, normal radiographs do not exclude bone involvement.
- High-detail dental radiographs may be appropriate for imaging smaller lesions.
- CT imaging can more accurately determine extent of local disease and is useful for surgical planning, particularly caudal lesions; CT is generally required for radiation therapy planning.

DIAGNOSTIC PROCEDURES

- Fine-needle aspiration (FNA) and cytology of the mass may provide provisional diagnosis. FNA and cytology are recommended for mandibular lymph nodes, especially if they are enlarged.
- Histopathology is required to reach a definitive diagnosis; preoperative incisional biopsy is recommended.
- If curative-intent surgery is performed, all excised tissue should be submitted to the pathologist *en bloc* for evaluation of surgical margin.

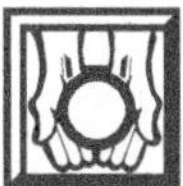

TREATMENT

- Surgical excision—removal of the affected segment of bone (maxillectomy or mandibulectomy) with a margin of at least 2 cm is recommended whenever possible.
- If excision is incomplete, adjuvant radiation therapy might help improve local control, although there is little information regarding efficacy.
- Radiation therapy can be considered as a sole local treatment modality but, because of the chondroid matrix produced by CSAs, radiation therapy likely will stabilize tumor size and not necessarily cause substantial shrinkage.
- Chemotherapy has not been evaluated, but is not thought to be effective.
- Palliative care focuses on pain control.

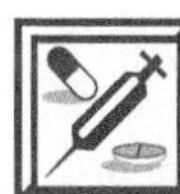

MEDICATIONS

DRUG(S) OF CHOICE

- Nonsteroidal anti-inflammatory drugs.
- Tramadol.
- Gabapentin.
- Intravenous aminobisphosphonates (pamidronate or zoledronate) might alleviate bone pain and attenuate bone resorption.
- Empiric antibiotic therapy can be considered for secondary bacterial infections.

FOLLOW-UP

PATIENT MONITORING

Physical examination with thorough oral examination every 2–3 months and thoracic radiographs every 3–4 months to monitor for local tumor control and distant metastases, respectively.

EXPECTED COURSE AND PROGNOSIS

- Prognosis depends on tumor size and location, and surgical resectability; with complete excision, long-term control may be possible.
- Most patients die or are euthanized due to local disease progression.
- Overall CSA metastatic rate is 15–30%, with the lungs being affected most commonly; metastatic rates approach 50% for high-grade tumors.

MISCELLANEOUS

SEE ALSO

- Chondrosarcoma, Bone.
- Chondrosarcoma, Nasal and Paranasal Sinus.

ABBREVIATIONS

- CSA = chondrosarcoma.
- FNA = fine-needle aspiration.

Suggested Reading

Verstraete FJ. Mandibulectomy and maxillectomy. Vet Clin North Am Small Anim Pract 2005, 35(4):1009–1039.

Waltman SS, Seguin B, Cooper BJ, Kent M. Clinical outcome of nonnasal chondrosarcoma in dogs: thirty-one cases (1986–2003). Vet Surg 2007, 36:266–271.

Author Jenna H. Burton

Consulting Editor Timothy M. Fan

Acknowledgment The author and book editors acknowledge the prior contribution of Dennis B. Bailey.

CHORIORETINITIS

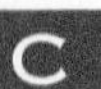

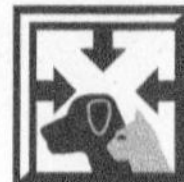

BASICS

DEFINITION

- Inflammation of the choroid and retina.
- Choroid is also called posterior uvea.
- Diffuse inflammation may result in retinal detachment.

PATHOPHYSIOLOGY

- Caused by infectious agents, neoplastic cells, or immune complexes (immune-mediated diseases); hematogenous pathogenic factors inducing choroidal inflammation is most common.
- Choroid and retina—closely apposed; physiologically interdependent; inflammation of one usually results in inflammation of the other.
- May also occur as a retinochoroiditis—retinal inflammation preceding and inducing choroidal inflammation.

SYSTEMS AFFECTED

- Nervous.
- Ophthalmic.
- Other systems if underlying disease is systemic.

INCIDENCE/PREVALENCE

- Fairly common.
- Exact incidence unknown.

GEOGRAPHIC DISTRIBUTION

Varies with endemic infectious diseases (e.g., systemic mycoses, rickettsial disease).

SIGNALMENT

Species

Dog and cat.

Breed Predilections

- Systemic mycoses—more common in hunting dogs.
- Uveodermatologic syndrome—Akita, chow chow, and Siberian husky predisposed.
- Chorioretinopathy—borzoi, border collie, beagle, German shepherd dog.
- Systemic histiocytosis—Bernese mountain dog, golden retriever.

Mean Age and Range

Depends on underlying cause.

Predominant Sex

Uveodermatologic syndrome—more common in young male dogs.

SIGNS

- Not usually painful, except with concurrent anterior uveitis, secondary glaucoma, or inflammatory retrobulbar disease.
- Vitreous abnormalities—may note exudate, hemorrhage, or syneresis (liquefaction).
- Interruption or alteration of the course of retinal blood vessels—due to retinal elevation.
- Ophthalmomyiasis (cats)—curvilinear tracts from migrating larvae.
- Others—related to underlying systemic disease, retrobulbar disease.

Lesions

- Active—indistinct margins, tapetal hyporeflectivity, white-gray color, altered course of retinal blood vessels.
- Few or small lesions—no apparent visual deficits.
- Extensive lesions involving larger areas of the retina—blindness or reduced vision.
- Inactive (scars)—discrete margins, tapetal hyperreflectivity with hyperpigmented central areas, depigmented in the nontapetum and some surrounding or central hyperpigmentation.

CAUSES

Infectious

Dogs

- Viral—canine distemper, herpesvirus (rare, usually neonates), rabies.
- Bacterial—leptospirosis, brucellosis, pyometra (toxic uveitis), borreliosis, ehrlichiosis, Rocky Mountain spotted fever, bartonellosis; discospondylitis, endocarditis may be present with bacteremia.
- Fungal—aspergillosis, blastomycosis, coccidioidomycosis, histoplasmosis, cryptococcosis, acremoniosis, pseudallescheriasis, candidiasis, geotrichosis.
- Algal—protothecosis.
- Protozoal—toxoplasmosis, leishmaniasis (rare), neosporosis, and sarcocystosis (dogs).
- Parasitic—ocular larval migrans (*Strongyles, Ascarids, Baylisascaris*), *Sarcocystis neurona*, and ophthalmomyiasis interna (Diptera larval migrans).
- Retrobulbar abscess/cellulitis—uncommon.

Cats

- Viral—feline leukemia virus (FeLV), feline immunodeficiency virus (FIV), feline infectious peritonitis (FIP).
- Bacterial—septicemia or bacteremia, bartonellosis.
- Fungal—cryptococcosis, histoplasmosis, blastomycosis.
- Parasitic—toxoplasmosis, ophthalmomyiasis interna (Diptera, Cuterebra), ocular larval migrans, leishmaniasis (rare).
- Protozoal—toxoplasmosis.

Idiopathic

- Common.
- Multifocal chorioretinitis or chorioretinopathy—acquired syndrome; affected dogs have multifocal retinal edema or chorioretinal atrophy.
- German shepherd dog—choroidal scars in police dogs: possibly due to physical exertion or circulatory disorders; affected dogs had lower amplitude ERG.

Immune

- Any immune-mediated disease may cause vasculitis or inflammation, resulting in exudative retinal detachment or chorioretinitis. Thrombocytopenia may result in small multifocal or large retinal or vitreal hemorrhages with inflammation.
- Dogs—Vogt-Koyanagi-Harada-like (uveodermatologic) syndrome: target is melanin pigment granule (abundant in uveal tissue), leading to severe anterior and posterior inflammation (affected dogs may also exhibit depigmentation of the skin, especially at mucocutaneous junctions); systemic lupus erythematosus (SLE).
- Cats—periarteritis nodosa, SLE.

Metabolic

Early hypertensive retinopathy may result in multifocal localized lesions.

Neoplastic

Neoplasia (multiple myeloma, lymphoma, malignant histiocytosis) can metastasize to the eye.

Toxic

- Ethylene glycol, idiosyncratic drug reactions (e.g., trimethoprim-sulfa), ivermectin.
- Photic injury—exposure to bright light can burn the retina.

Trauma

Perforating wound or migrating foreign body.

RISK FACTORS

- FeLV or FIV infection—may predispose cat to ocular toxoplasmosis or other infectious disease.
- Immunosuppressive therapy.

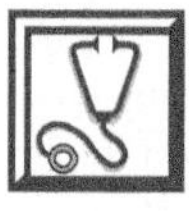

DIAGNOSIS

DIFFERENTIAL DIAGNOSIS

- Blindness or impaired vision—optic neuritis, CNS disease, diffuse retinal inflammation.
- Retinal dysplasia—bilateral, symmetric folds or geographic clumps of pigment or altered fundus reflectivity; no associated signs of inflammation in the eye.

CBC/BIOCHEMISTRY/URINALYSIS

Normal if problem confined to the eye, otherwise may have signs of systemic disease.

OTHER LABORATORY TESTS

- Anti-nuclear antibody (ANA)—for suspected SLE.
- Bence-Jones proteinuria—for multiple myeloma.
- Skin biopsy—SLE, uveodermatologic syndrome.
- Coagulation profile.
- Bacterial culture of ocular or body fluids.
- Serologic or PCR testing—infectious disease (see Causes).
- Cytology of lymph node, mass, or organ aspirates.
- Histopathology of enucleated eyes.
- Bartonella—PCR, culture on special media (BAPGM).

IMAGING

- Thoracic radiography—may show infectious or neoplastic disease.
- Spinal radiography— may show discospondylitis or multiple myeloma.
- Ocular ultrasound—retinal detachment, intraocular masses; especially helpful if the ocular media are not clear; can identify retrobulbar disease.
- Abdominal ultrasound—screen for neoplasia, systemic disease.
- CT/MRI—if signs of retrobulbar or CNS disease.

DIAGNOSTIC PROCEDURES

- Indirect ophthalmoscopy—screens a large area of the retina.
- Direct ophthalmoscopy—facilitates examination of suspicious areas.
- Cerebrospinal fluid (CSF) tap—indicated for diagnosis of some CNS disease or optic neuritis.
- Vitreocentesis or subretinal aspirate—if other diagnostic tests fail or to identify infectious agent or neoplasia; vitreocentesis may worsen inflammation or induce hemorrhage or retinal detachment, reducing chances for restoration of vision.
- Choroidal aspirate—of thickened areas, ideally ultrasound guided; procedure may aggravate inflammation, induce hemorrhage or retinal detachment.
- Measurement of blood pressure.

PATHOLOGIC FINDINGS

- Masses or retinal or choroidal exudates.
- Fungal organisms in exudates and inflammatory cells.
- Perivascular inflammation with vasculitis, FIP.
- Inactive lesions—retinal and choroidal atrophy (thinning); may note retinal pigment epithelium hyperpigmentation and tapetal destruction.

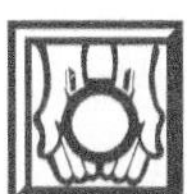

TREATMENT

APPROPRIATE HEALTH CARE

Depends on physical condition of patient, usually outpatient.

NURSING CARE

Therapy for systemic disease, depending on patient status.

CLIENT EDUCATION

- Chorioretinitis may be a sign of systemic disease, so diagnostic testing is important.
- Immune-mediated disease requires lifelong therapy.
- Dogs with uveodermatologic syndrome may have anterior uveitis and secondary glaucoma, which necessitate treatment or eye removal; dermatitis may also require management.

MEDICATIONS

DRUG(S) OF CHOICE

- Identify and treat underlying systemic disease (see specific chapters).
- Topical medications—not effective in dogs with intact lenses; systemic therapy required.
  - 1% prednisolone acetate or 0.1% dexamethasone q6–8h to treat anterior uveitis.
  - Parasympatholytics (e.g., 1% atropine) can be given at a frequency that dilates the pupil and reduces pain.
  - 0.5% timolol maleate or 2% dorzolamide may be used to treat secondary glaucoma.
- Corticosteroids at anti-inflammatory doses—prednisone 0.5–1 mg/kg PO q24h (dog), prednisolone 1–2 mg/kg q24h (cat), then taper; avoid use unless large areas of the retina are affected and vision is severely threatened.
- Prednisone for immunosuppression—2–4 mg/kg PO divided q12 for 3–10 days (dog, cat), then taper slowly over months (do not exceed 80 mg per day).

CONTRAINDICATIONS

Systemically administered corticosteroids—do not use if systemic infectious disease is present. Exception: sometimes steroids are used when infectious cause has been identified and is being treated.

ALTERNATIVE DRUG(S)

Uveodermatologic syndrome or known autoimmune etiology—may require corticosteroids and concurrent use of or transition to other immunosuppressive medications (e.g., azathioprine, cyclosporine, leflunomide, or mycophenolate mofetil; see Retinal Detachment).

FOLLOW-UP

PATIENT MONITORING

- As appropriate for underlying cause and type of medical treatment.
- For bartonella treatment in cats, consider follow-up testing to help assess response.
- CBC, platelet count, and liver enzymes—monitor for side effects of systemic immunosuppressive drugs.
- Intraocular pressure monitoring—for anterior uveitis.

PREVENTION/AVOIDANCE

Tick and flea control measures.

POSSIBLE COMPLICATIONS

- Permanent blindness.
- Cataracts.
- Glaucoma.
- Chronic ocular pain.
- Death—secondary to systemic disease.

EXPECTED COURSE AND PROGNOSIS

- Prognosis for vision—guarded to good, depending on amount of retina affected; visual deficits or blindness if large areas of the retina were destroyed; focal and multifocal disease do not markedly impair vision but do leave scars.
- Prognosis for life—guarded to good, depending on underlying cause.
- Prognosis for globe—secondary glaucoma may necessitate removal of blind painful eye.

MISCELLANEOUS

ASSOCIATED CONDITIONS

Several systemic diseases.

ZOONOTIC POTENTIAL

- Toxoplasmosis—may be transmitted to humans if patient is shedding oocysts in feces.
- Vector-borne diseases—infected animals may act as reservoirs, i.e., bartonella (cat scratch disease), rickettsia, others.

SYNONYMS

Retinochoroiditis

SEE ALSO

- Retinal Degeneration.
- Retinal Detachment.
- Uveodermatologic Syndrome (VKH).

ABBREVIATIONS

- ANA = antinuclear antibody.
- CSF = cerebrospinal fluid.
- FeLV = feline leukemia virus.
- FIP = feline infectious peritonitis.
- FIV = feline immunodeficiency virus.
- SLE = systemic lupus erythematosus.

Suggested Reading

Narfström K, Petersen-Jones S. Diseases of the canine ocular fundus. In: Gelatt KN, ed., Veterinary Ophthalmology, 5th ed. Ames, IA: Blackwell, 2013, pp. 2087–2235.

Stiles J. Infectious diseases and the eye. Vet Clin North Am Small Anim Pract 2000, 30:971–1167.

Author Patricia J. Smith

Consulting Editor Kathern E. Myrna

Client Education Handout available online

CHRONIC KIDNEY DISEASE

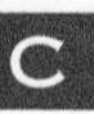

BASICS

DEFINITION

Chronic kidney disease (CKD) encompasses functional or structural lesions (in one or both kidneys as detected by blood or urine tests, imaging studies, or kidney biopsy) that have been present for >3 months. This definition includes all cases previously described by the terms renal insufficiency or renal failure, as well as less advanced forms of kidney disease. Patients are categorized into stages along a continuum of progressive CKD (IRIS CKD stages 1–4; www.iris-kidney.com) based on >2 serum creatinine values obtained over several weeks when the patient is fasted and well hydrated. The IRIS system uses the term "kidney" rather than "renal" because it is more universally recognized by pet owners.

PATHOPHYSIOLOGY

More than ~67–75% reduction in renal function results in impaired urine-concentrating ability (leading to polyuria/polydipsia [PU/PD]) and retention of nitrogenous waste products of protein catabolism (azotemia). CKD is progressive; more advanced CKD results in uremia. Decreased renal erythropoietin and calcitriol production results in hypoproliferative anemia and renal secondary hyperparathyroidism, respectively.

SYSTEMS AFFECTED

- Cardiovascular—hypertension; uremic pericarditis.
- Endocrine/metabolic—renal secondary hyperparathyroidism, activation of renin-angiotensin-aldosterone system, erythropoietin deficiency.
- Gastrointestinal—uremic stomatitis and halitosis, nausea, vomiting, anorexia, gastrointestinal bleeding, diarrhea.
- Hemic/lymphatic/immune—anemia; hemorrhagic diathesis.
- Musculoskeletal—renal osteodystrophy; sarcopenia.
- Neuromuscular—seizures and other neurologic signs, muscle tremors, muscle wasting.
- Ophthalmic—retinal detachment, hemorrhage, or edema due to hypertension.
- Reproductive—impaired reproductive capacity.
- Respiratory—uremic pneumonitis.

GENETICS

- Inherited in these breeds (mode of inheritance indicated in parentheses)—Abyssinian cat (dominant with incomplete penetrance); Persian cat (dominant); bull terrier (dominant); Cairn terrier (recessive); German shepherd (dominant); Samoyed (X-linked dominant); English cocker spaniel (recessive).
- Renal dysplasia—shih tzu, Lhasa apso, golden retriever, Norwegian elkhound, chow chow, standard poodle, soft-coated wheaten terrier, Alaskan Malamute, miniature schnauzer, Dutch kooiker, and many other breeds.

INCIDENCE/PREVALENCE

- 9 cases per 1,000 dogs and 16 cases per 1,000 cats examined.
- Prevalence increases with age—age >15 years, reportedly 57 cases per 1,000 dogs and 153 cases per 1,000 cats examined.

GEOGRAPHIC DISTRIBUTION

Worldwide

SIGNALMENT

Species

Dog and cat.

Breed Predilections

See Genetics.

Mean Age and Range

Mean age at diagnosis is 7 years in dogs and 9 years in cats. Animals of any age can be affected; prevalence increases with age.

Predominant Sex

None

SIGNS

General Comments

- Clinical signs related to stage of CKD and complications such as proteinuria and hypertension.
- CKD stages 1 and 2 may be asymptomatic; overt clinical signs typically become apparent in stages 3 and 4.
- Animals with stable CKD (particularly stages 3 and 4) may decompensate, resulting in uremic crisis.

Historical Findings

- PU/PD.
- Anorexia.
- Lethargy.
- Vomiting.
- Weight loss.
- Nocturia.
- Constipation.
- Diarrhea.
- Acute blindness.
- Seizures or coma.
- Cats may have ptyalism and muscle weakness with cervical ventroflexion.

Physical Examination Findings

- Kidneys may be small, irregular, enlarged (secondary to polycystic kidney disease or lymphoma), or normal.
- Dehydration.
- Cachexia.
- Weakness.
- Mucous membrane pallor.
- Oral ulceration.
- Uremic halitosis.
- Hypertensive retinopathy.
- Renal osteodystrophy may manifest as bone pain, particularly in skull.
- Reduced body temperature with uremia.

CAUSES

- Unknown in most cases due to late diagnosis.
- Familial and congenital renal disease, nephrotoxins, hypercalcemia, hypokalemic nephropathy, glomerulopathies, amyloidosis, pyelonephritis, polycystic kidney disease, nephroliths, chronic urinary obstruction, drugs, lymphoma, leptospirosis (following acute kidney injury [AKI]), feline infectious peritonitis.

RISK FACTORS

Age, proteinuria, hypercalcemia, hypokalemia, hypertension, urinary tract infection (UTI).

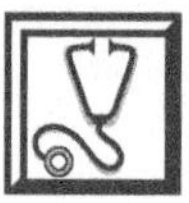

DIAGNOSIS

DIFFERENTIAL DIAGNOSIS

- See Polyuria and Polydipsia for differential diagnosis.
- Azotemia—includes causes of prerenal and postrenal azotemia, AKI, and hypoadrenocorticism.
- Prerenal azotemia—azotemia with urine specific gravity (USG) >1.030 in dogs and >1.035 in cats; rapid reduction in azotemia after correcting hypoperfusion indicates prerenal azotemia; prerenal azotemia commonly occurs concurrent with primary renal azotemia when gastrointestinal signs of uremia are present.
- Postrenal azotemia—obstruction or rupture of excretory system; rapid correction of azotemia following elimination of obstruction or resolution of leakage from urinary tract supports postrenal azotemia.
- AKI—differentiated by normal to large renal size, cylindruria, lack of indications of chronicity, and history of recent nephrotoxin exposure or hypotensive episode; AKI can also occur in patients with CKD where rapid developing increase in serum creatinine concentration and uremic signs suggests acute-onset CKD.
- Hypoadrenocorticism—characterized by hyponatremia and hyperkalemia with hypocortisolemia.

CBC/BIOCHEMISTRY/URINALYSIS

- Hypoproliferative anemia.
- High blood urea nitrogen (BUN), creatinine, and symmetric dimethylarginine (SDMA).
- Hyperphosphatemia.
- Metabolic acidosis (normal or high anion gap).
- Hypokalemia or hyperkalemia.
- Hypercalcemia or hypocalcemia.

- USG <1.030 in dogs and <1.035 in cats.
- Proteinuria.

OTHER LABORATORY TESTS

Urinary protein : creatinine ratio to assess proteinuria.

IMAGING

- Abdominal radiographs may demonstrate small kidneys, or large kidneys secondary to polycystic kidney disease or lymphoma.
- Ultrasound demonstrates small kidneys and hyperechoic renal parenchyma with less apparent distinction between cortex and medulla in some animals. Animals with lymphoma often have renomegaly with hypoechoic renal parenchyma.

DIAGNOSTIC PROCEDURES

- Blood pressure measurement to detect hypertension.
- Measurement of glomerular filtration rate may be useful for detection of loss of kidney function before onset of azotemia.
- Renal biopsy may be indicated in proteinuric patients with normal to large kidneys.

PATHOLOGIC FINDINGS

- Gross—small kidneys with irregular surface; fewer glomeruli found on visualizing cut across renal cortex.
- Histopathologic—variable; complete evaluation of biopsy material requires light, immunofluorescent, and electron microscopy; advanced CKD has nonspecific changes including interstitial fibrosis and foci of interstitial mononuclear cells, chronic generalized nephropathy.
- Findings may be specific for diseases causing CKD in some patients with less advanced disease.

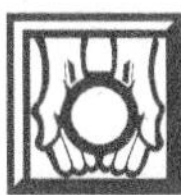

TREATMENT

APPROPRIATE HEALTH CARE

Patients with compensated CKD may be managed as outpatients; patients in uremic crisis should be managed as inpatients.

NURSING CARE

- Uremic crisis—correct fluid and electrolyte deficits with IV fluids, providing 25% of calculated fluid deficit in first hour; thereafter, serially monitor perfusion, blood pressure, and urine output to assess adequacy of fluid therapy; if perfusion not improved, additional fluid should cautiously be administered. Provide remaining fluid deficit over next 12–24 hours. Overhydration can result in anuria; once patient has been hydrated, only sufficient fluid to sustain hydration should be administered.
- Subcutaneous fluid therapy may benefit patients with moderate to severe CKD. Continue therapy only if clinical improvement noted.

ACTIVITY

Unrestricted

DIET

- Diets designed for CKD delay onset of uremic crisis and extend survival in dogs and cats with CKD stages 2–4; they are standard of care for these patients.
- Important components of renal foods—reduced protein, phosphorus, sodium, and net acid content, supplementation of n-3 fatty acids and antioxidants.
- Free access to fresh water.

CLIENT EDUCATION

- CKD typically progresses to terminal kidney failure over months to years, but may not be progressive in some cats, which may live for years
- Higher levels of proteinuria associated with shorter survival; may be mitigated by anti-proteinuria therapy.
- Heritability of familial renal diseases.

SURGICAL CONSIDERATIONS

- Avoid hypotension during anesthesia.
- Renal transplantation has been successfully performed in cats with CKD.

MEDICATIONS

DRUG(S) OF CHOICE

Uremic Crisis

- Antiemetics (maropitant 1 mg/kg q24h; or ondansetron 0.2–1 mg/kg IV q12h) to minimize vomiting and hyporexia due to nausea.
- Potassium chloride in IV fluids or potassium gluconate PO (2–6 mEq/cat/day) as needed to correct hypokalemia.
- Sodium bicarbonate to correct metabolic acidosis (IV to raise blood pH >7.1).

Compensated CKD

- Antiemetic (maropitant) and potassium gluconate as above.
- Mirtazapine (cats, 1.88 mg PO q 24–47h) to promote appetite.
- Intestinal phosphate binders as needed to correct hyperphosphatemia (see Hyperparathyroidism, Renal Secondary).
- Darbepoetin (see Anemia of Chronic Kidney Disease).
- Amlodipine (dogs, 0.1–0.6 mg/kg PO q24h; cats, 0.625–1.25 mg/cat PO q24h) or angiotensin-converting enzyme (ACE) inhibitors (0.5 mg/kg PO q24h) or angiotensin receptor blockers (ARB; e.g., telmisartan 1–3 mg/kg PO q24h) as needed for hypertension; amlodipine and telmisartan are more effective than ACE inhibitors for CKD-induced hypertension; if refractory to monotherapy, consider combination of amlodipine and ACE inhibitor or ARB, with frequent monitoring of blood pressure and electrolytes.
- ACE inhibitor (start at 0.5 mg/kg PO q24h; increase to 1 mg/kg PO q12h) or ARB (telmisartan 1–3 mg/kg PO q24h) for proteinuria.

CONTRAINDICATIONS

Avoid nephrotoxic drugs (aminoglycosides, cisplatin, amphotericin B) and corticosteroids.

PRECAUTIONS

- Drug dosage or dosing interval may need to be modified for some drugs eliminated by the kidneys.
- Use ACE inhibitors and ARB cautiously; monitor for worsening of azotemia,
- Generally avoid nonsteroidal anti-inflammatory drugs.

POSSIBLE INTERACTIONS

Cimetidine or trimethoprim may cause artifactual increases in serum creatinine concentration by reducing tubular secretion in dogs with CKD.

ALTERNATIVE DRUG(S)

- Metoclopramide (0.2–0.4 mg PO/SC q6–8h) can be used to treat uremic vomiting.
- Hemodialysis and renal transplantation are available at selected referral hospitals.

FOLLOW-UP

PATIENT MONITORING

- Monitor at regular intervals; initially weekly for patients receiving erythropoietin; every 1–3 months for stable patients with CKD stages 3 and 4.
- Proteinuric patients—monitor at least every 3–4 months (minimum: serum creatinine and urine protein : creatine ratio).

PREVENTION/AVOIDANCE

- Do not breed animals with familial renal disease.
- Include urinalysis and serum creatinine in yearly examination for older pets; if serum creatinine increases, increase frequency to every 4–6 months.

POSSIBLE COMPLICATIONS

- Systemic hypertension.
- Uremia.
- Anemia.
- UTI.
- Nephrouretrolithiasis.

EXPECTED COURSE AND PROGNOSIS

- Short term—depends on severity.
- Long term—guarded to poor in dogs (CKD tends to be progressive over months to years); poor to good in cats (CKD does not progress in some cats).

MISCELLANEOUS

ASSOCIATED CONDITIONS

- Renal secondary hyperparathyroidism.
- Systemic hypertension.
- Nephroureterolithiasis.

CHRONIC KIDNEY DISEASE (CONTINUED)

AGE-RELATED FACTORS

Renal function may decrease with aging.

ZOONOTIC POTENTIAL

None

PREGNANCY/FERTILITY/BREEDING

Patients with mild CKD may maintain pregnancy; those with moderate to severe disease may be infertile or have spontaneous abortions; breeding of females not recommended.

SYNONYMS

- Chronic kidney failure.
- Chronic renal disease or failure.

SEE ALSO

- Acute Kidney Injury.
- Anemia of Chronic Kidney Disease.
- Azotemia and Uremia.
- Congenital and Developmental Renal Diseases.
- Hydronephrosis.
- Hyperparathyroidism, Renal Secondary.
- Hypertension, Systemic Arterial.
- Nephrolithiasis.
- Polycystic Kidney Disease.
- Polyuria and Polydipsia.
- Proteinuria.
- Pyelonephritis.
- Urinary Tract Obstruction.

ABBREVIATIONS

- ACE = angiotensin-converting enzyme.
- AKI = acute kidney injury.
- ARB = angiotensin receptor blocker.
- BUN = blood urea nitrogen.
- CKD = chronic kidney disease.
- PU/PD = polyuria/polydipsia.
- SDMA = symmetric dimethylarginine.
- USG = urine specific gravity.
- UTI = urinary tract infection.

INTERNET RESOURCES

www.iris-kidney.com

Suggested Reading

Polzin DJ. Chronic kidney disease. In: Ettinger SJ, Feldman EC, eds., Textbook of Veterinary Internal Medicine, 7th ed. St. Louis, MO: Elsevier, 2010, pp. 1990–2021.

Ross SJ, Polzin DJ, Osborne CA. Clinical progression of early chronic renal failure and implications for management. In: August JR, ed., Consultations in Feline Internal Medicine. St. Louis, MO: Elsevier, 2006, pp. 389–398.

Author David J. Polzin
Consulting Editor J.D. Foster

Client Education Handout available online

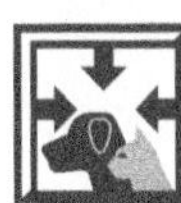

BASICS

DEFINITION

• Accumulation of chyle in the pleural space. • Chyle—triglyceride-rich fluid from the intestinal lymphatics that empties into the venous system (usually cranial cava/jugular vein) in the thorax. • Pseudochylous effusion—effusion that contains less triglycerides and more cholesterol compared to serum, but appears fatty grossly. • Thoracic lymphangiectasia—tortuous, dilated lymphatics found in many animals with chylothorax. • Fibrosing pleuritis—condition in which pleural thickening leads to constriction of lung lobes; when severe, results in marked restriction of ventilation; can be caused by any chronic pleural exudate, but is most commonly associated with chylothorax and pyothorax.

PATHOPHYSIOLOGY

• Alteration of flow through thoracic duct (TD) leading to leakage of chyle—can be related to increased pressure or permeability in TD or venous obstruction downstream. • Can be caused by any disease or process that increases systemic venous pressure at the entrance of the TD to the venous system. • Cardiac causes—pericardial disease, cardiomyopathy, heartworm disease, other causes of right-sided heart failure; thrombosis around pacing lead wire. • Noncardiac causes—neoplasia (especially mediastinal lymphoma in cats), lung lobe torsion, diaphragmatic hernia, venous granuloma, venous thrombus. • Rare TD rupture/trauma—surgical (thoracotomy), nonsurgical (e.g., hit by car). • Idiopathic considered most common.

SYSTEMS AFFECTED

• Respiratory—due to reduced lung expansion. • Systemic signs can be present secondary to the respiratory distress (e.g., decreased appetite, weight loss).

GENETICS

Unknown

INCIDENCE/PREVALENCE

Unknown

GEOGRAPHIC DISTRIBUTION

Worldwide

SIGNALMENT

Species

Dog and cat.

Breed Predilections

• Dogs—Afghan hound and Shiba Inu. • Cats—oriental breeds (e.g., Siamese and Himalayan).

Mean Age and Range

• Any age affected. • Cats—more common in older cats; could indicate an association with neoplasia. • Afghan hound—develop when middle-aged. • Shiba Inu—develop when young (<1–2 years of age).

Predominant Sex

None identified.

SIGNS

General Comments

• Signs will depend on the rate of fluid accumulation and volume of pleural effusion. • Usually not exhibited until there is marked impairment of ventilation. • Many patients appear to have the condition for prolonged periods before diagnosis.

Historical Findings

• Tachypnea and respiratory difficulty. • Coughing—can be present for months before examination, likely due to lung compression associated with pleural effusion. • Lethargy. • Anorexia and weight loss. • Exercise intolerance.

Physical Examination Findings

• Vary with cause of effusion. • Muffled heart and lung sounds ventrally. • Increased bronchovesicular sounds, particularly in dorsal lung fields. • Pale mucous membranes or cyanosis. • Arrhythmia. • Heart murmur. • Signs of right-sided heart failure (e.g., jugular pulses, ascites, hepatomegaly). • Decreased compressibility of anterior chest—common in cats with a cranial mediastinal mass.

CAUSES

• Cranial mediastinal masses—lymphoma, thymoma. • Cardiac disease—heartworm, cardiomyopathy, pericardial disease, congenital diseases. • Lung lobe torsion. • Venous obstruction—granuloma, thrombi. • Congenital abnormality of TD. • Cardiac or thoracic surgery. • Idiopathic—most common cause.

RISK FACTORS

Unknown

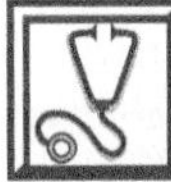

DIAGNOSIS

DIFFERENTIAL DIAGNOSIS

Other causes of pleural effusion—neoplasia, pyothorax, heart failure, feline infectious peritonitis (FIP).

CBC/BIOCHEMISTRY/URINALYSIS

• Often normal. • Lymphopenia and hypoalbuminemia—can be found; hyponatremia and hyperkalemia sometimes noted due to fluid shifts with repeat thoracocentesis.

OTHER LABORATORY TESTS

Heartworm testing.

Fluid Analysis

• Classified as an exudate. • Color will depend on fat content from diet and presence of concurrent hemorrhage—usually milky white and opaque, but can appear serosanguinous and range from yellow to pink. • Protein content varies, and high lipid content will make refractive index inaccurate. • Total nucleated cell count—usually <10,000 cells/µL. • Fluid triglycerides—higher compared to serum. • Fluid cholesterol—lower compared to serum.

Cytology

• Place sample in an EDTA tube to allow cell count to be performed. • Initially, cytology comprises primarily small lymphocytes, neutrophils, and macrophages containing lipid. • Chronic effusions contain fewer lymphocytes due to continued loss and more nondegenerate neutrophils due to inflammation from multiple thoracocenteses or irritation of pleural lining by chyle. • Atypical lymphocytes—suggestive of underlying neoplasia.

IMAGING

Thoracic Radiography

• Two to four views if patient is stable—pleural effusion. • Dorsoventral view associated with less stress than ventrodorsal view in animal with respiratory difficulty. • Repeat radiographs after thoracocentesis to assess for underlying causes of effusion or evidence of fibrosing pleuritis; if collapsed lung lobes do not appear to reexpand after pleural fluid is removed or if respiratory distress persists with only minimal fluid present, suspect underlying pulmonary parenchymal or pleural disease (e.g., fibrosing pleuritis).

Ultrasonography/Echocardiography

• Should be performed before thoracocentesis if patient is stable—fluid acts as an acoustic window, enhancing visualization of thoracic structures. • Assess for underlying causes—detect abnormal cardiac structure and function, pericardial disease, and mediastinal masses.

CT Lymphangiography

• Can quantify TD branches more accurately than standard radiographic lymphangiography. • In dogs, percutaneously inject 1–2 mL of nonionic contrast material into mesenteric lymph nodes using ultrasound or CT guidance. • Acquire helical thoracic CT images before and after injection of contrast media. • Can document location and character of TD and its tributary lymphatics; likely useful for surgical planning.

PATHOLOGIC FINDINGS

• Lymphatics (including TD)—difficult to identify at necropsy. • Fibrosing pleuritis—lungs appear shrunken; pleural layers (visceral and parietal) are diffusely thickened. • Fibrosing pleuritis—characterized histologically by diffuse, moderate to marked thickening of the pleura by fibrous connective tissue with moderate infiltrates of lymphocytes, macrophages, and plasma cells.

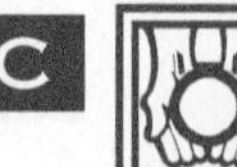

TREATMENT

APPROPRIATE HEALTH CARE

• Dyspneic animal—immediate thoracocentesis; removal of even small amounts of pleural effusion can markedly improve ventilation. • Identify and treat the underlying cause, if possible. • Medical management—usually treated on outpatient basis with intermittent thoracocentesis as needed based on clinical signs (see Medications). • Chest tubes—place *only* in patients with suspected chylothorax secondary to trauma (very rare), in cases with rapid fluid accumulation, or after surgery. • Surgery if medical management does not resolve the problem in 2–3 months (see Surgical Considerations); some clinicians believe earlier intervention is better to avoid potential for development of restrictive pleuritis.

NURSING CARE

• Patients undergoing multiple thoracocenteses can rarely develop electrolyte abnormalities (hyponatremia, hyperkalemia) that may need to be corrected with fluid therapy. • Thoracocentesis—perform under aseptic conditions to reduce risk of iatrogenic infection; antibiotic prophylaxis generally unnecessary if proper technique is used.

ACTIVITY

Patients will usually restrict their own exercise as pleural fluid volume increases or if they develop fibrosing pleuritis.

DIET

• Low fat—potentially decreases the amount of fat in the effusion, which would improve the patient's ability to resorb fluid from the thoracic cavity; not a cure; may help in management by facilitating reabsorption. • Medium-chain triglycerides are transported via the TD in dogs and are no longer recommended.

CLIENT EDUCATION

• Inform client that no specific treatment will stop the effusion in all patients with the idiopathic form of the disease. • Inform client that the condition can spontaneously resolve in some patients after several weeks or months.

SURGICAL CONSIDERATIONS

TD Ligation and Pericardiectomy

• Recommended in patients that do not respond to medical management. • The duct usually has multiple branches in the caudal thorax where ligation is performed; failure to occlude all branches results in continued pleural effusion. • Always perform in conjunction with lymphangiography; methylene blue injected in the mesenteric lymph node greatly facilitates visualization and complete occlusion of all branches. • Thickening of the pericardium can prevent formation of lymphaticovenous communications—perform pericardiectomy simultaneously with TD ligation; reports of up to 100% success rate when both techniques are performed; second surgery can be necessary if all branches are not occluded. • Video-assisted thorascopic surgery for thoracic duct ligation and pericardiectomy is reported to have similar success rates to thoracotomy (86%).

Other

• Success rates of 83–88% reported for cysterna chyli ablation in combination with TD ligation. • Salvage procedures for recurrence after TD ligation include cisterna chyli and TD glue embolization, pleuroperitoneal or pleurovenous shunts, or placement of a PleuralPort®.

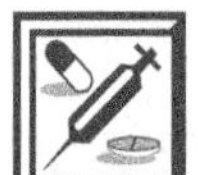

MEDICATIONS

DRUG(S) OF CHOICE

• Rutin 50–100 mg/kg PO q8h; believed to increase macrophage removal of proteins, which promotes absorption of fluid; complete resolution of effusion appears to occur in some patients; further study is required to determine whether resolution occurs spontaneously or in response to this therapy. • Somatostatin analog (octreotide)—a naturally occurring substance that inhibits gastric, pancreatic, and biliary secretions and prolongs gastrointestinal transit time, decreases jejunal secretion, and stimulates gastrointestinal water absorption; in traumatic chylothorax, reduction of gastrointestinal secretions may aid healing of the TD by decreasing TD lymphatic flows; resolution of pleural fluid has occurred in dogs and cats with idiopathic chylothorax in which octreotide has been administered, but the mechanism is unknown; octreotide (Sandostatin®; 10 µg/kg SC q8h for 2–3 weeks) is a synthetic analog of somatostatin that has a prolonged half-life and minimal side effects.

CONTRAINDICATIONS

Cardiac disease or neoplasia—treat the underlying disease rather than the effusion (other than heartworm disease in cats where TD ligation may be beneficial while the heartworm infection clears).

FOLLOW-UP

PATIENT MONITORING

• Monitor for signs of recurrence of pleural effusion (tachypnea, labored breathing, respiratory distress)—perform thoracentesis as needed. • Periodically reevaluate for several years to detect recurrence.

POSSIBLE COMPLICATIONS

• Fibrosing pleuritis. • Iatrogenic infection with repeated thoracocentesis—important to use aseptic technique.

EXPECTED COURSE AND PROGNOSIS

• Can resolve spontaneously or after surgery. • Untreated or chronic disease—can result in severe fibrosing pleuritis and persistent dyspnea. • Euthanasia—frequently performed in patients that do not respond to surgery or medical management.

MISCELLANEOUS

ASSOCIATED CONDITIONS

Diffuse lymphatic abnormalities (e.g., intestinal lymphangiectasia, hepatic lymphangiectasia, pulmonary lymphangiectasia, and chylous ascites)—may be noted; may worsen the prognosis.

AGE-RELATED FACTORS

Young patients may have a better prognosis than old animals because of the association of neoplasia with advanced age.

ABBREVIATIONS

• FIP = feline infectious peritonitis.
• TD = thoracic duct.

Suggested Reading

Allman DA, Radlinsky MG, Ralph AG, Rawlings CA. Thoracoscopic thoracic duct ligation and thoracoscopic pericardiectomy for treatment of chylothorax in dogs. Vet Surg 2010, 39(1):21–27.

Fossum TW, Mertens MM, Miller MW, et al. Thoracic duct ligation and pericardectomy for treatment of idiopathic chylothorax. J Vet Intern Med 2004, 18:307–310.

Johnson EG, Wisner ER, Kyles A, et al. Computed tomographic lymphography of the thoracic duct by mesenteric lymph node injection. Vet Surg 2009, 38(3):361–367.

Author Elizabeth Rozanski

Consulting Editor Elizabeth Rozanski

Acknowledgment The author and book editors acknowledge the prior contribution of Jill S. Pomrantz.

Client Education Handout available online

CIRRHOSIS AND FIBROSIS OF THE LIVER

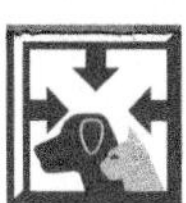

BASICS

DEFINITION

- Hepatic fibrosis—replacement/effacement of hepatic parenchyma, intrasinusoidal, variable zonal, deposition of extracellular matrix (ECM).
- Cirrhosis—regenerative nodules with dissecting fibrotic partitions and regions of parenchymal extinction, deranging hepatic architecture; usually reflects chronic necro-inflammatory liver injury.

PATHOPHYSIOLOGY

- Fibrosis—usually reflects injury-associated release of cytokines/mediators stimulating production and accumulation of ECM; exception: ductal plate malformation (DPM), with congenital hepatic fibrosis (CHF) phenotype (severe portal-to-portal bridging fibrosis without chronic inflammation).
- Cirrhosis—consequence of chronic hepatic injury, fibrogenesis, and hepatic regeneration; typified by regenerative nodules, reduced functional hepatic mass, collagen deposition in sinusoids (space of Disse) or portal tracts, compromising parenchymal perfusion.
- Cirrhosis/fibrosis—leads to hepatic dysfunction, capillarization of hepatic sinusoids, collagenization of sinusoids, development of sinusoidal hypertension, intrahepatic shunting through collagenized sinusoids, recanalized vascular pathways in fibrotic partitions between regenerative nodules; these microcirculatory disturbances impair exchanges between blood and hepatocytes.
- Sinusoidal hypertension—leads to hepatofugal portal flow (away from liver); splanchnic hypertension; acquired portosystemic shunt (APSS) formation; episodic hepatic encephalopathy (HE); splanchnic pooling of blood, decreased effective systemic blood volume, stimulation of renal sodium and water retention, with ascites formation; hypertensive splanchnic vasculopathy predisposing to enteric bleeding.

SYSTEMS AFFECTED

- Gastrointestinal (GI)—splanchnic portal hypertension leads to ascites and propensity for enteric bleeding.
- Neurologic—HE.
- Hemic—red blood cell (RBC) microcytosis reflects APSS; bleeding tendencies: failed factor synthesis or activation, thrombocytopenia; reduced anticoagulants increases risk for thrombosis.
- Renal/urologic—ammonium biurate crystalluria; isosthenuria: polyuria/polydipsia (PU/PD); hepatorenal syndrome (rare) may follow therapeutic paracentesis of large-volume ascites (postcentesis hypotension syndrome [PHS]).
- Endocrine/metabolic—hypoglycemia if end-stage liver failure.
- Respiratory—tachypnea if tense ascites or pleural effusion.
- Skin—superficial necrolytic dermatitis, unkempt coat.

GENETICS

Familial predisposition for chronic hepatitis—Doberman pinscher, cocker spaniel, Labrador retriever, Maltese, Bedlington terrier (copper related), West Highland white terrier, others.

INCIDENCE/PREVALENCE

High in dogs with chronic necroinflammatory liver disease, animals with chronic extrahepatic bile duct occlusion (EHBDO), dogs with severe hepatic copper accumulation.

SIGNALMENT

Species

- Cirrhosis—dogs with chronic hepatitis; cats with chronic cholangitis/cholangiohepatitis; dogs and cats with chronic EHBDO.
- Severe fibrosis—dogs and cats with severe DPM-CHF phenotype.

Breed Predilection

- Many breeds and mixed-breed dogs.
- Copper associated hepatopathy (CuAH)—genetics proven only in Bedlington terriers and partially in Labrador retrievers; Doberman pinschers, West Highland white terriers, and Dalmatians appear predisposed; but all breeds at risk for CuAH due to dietary Cu intake.
- DPM-CHF phenotype—boxers may be predisposed, many breeds of dogs and cats; cats with polycystic malformations at risk.

Mean Age and Range

- Cirrhosis (dogs)—any age; more common in middle-aged to older; CuAH any age.
- Biliary cirrhosis (cats)—with chronic cholangiohepatitis often >7 years old.
- Fibrosis—DPM-CHF phenotype (dogs, cats)—ECM accumulates with aging (suspected), genetic cause (see Ductal Plate Malformation).

Predominant Gender

- Cocker spaniels—may be higher in males.
- Doberman pinschers and Labrador retrievers—no sex predilection.
- DPM—no gender predilection.

SIGNS

General Comments

- Initially—vague and nonspecific.
- Later—relate to complications of portal hypertension (e.g., HE, ascites, gastroduodenal bleeding) and impaired hepatic function.

Historical Findings

- Chronic intermittent lethargy, anorexia, reduced body condition.
- GI signs—vomiting, diarrhea or constipation. Melena—late stage or as APSS develop.
- PU/PD.
- Late onset—ascites, bleeding, HE.
- Jaundice—with necroinflammatory disease; DPM usually anicteric.
- Cats—ascites uncommon with acquired necroinflammatory disease, more common with DPM; ptyalism, aggression, seizures with HE.

Physical Examination Findings

- Lethargy.
- Poor body condition/coat.
- ± Variable jaundice.
- ± Ascites.
- ± HE.
- Obstructive uropathy—ammonium biurates.
- Anasarca—rare; may develop with over-zealous fluid therapy.
- Liver size—dogs: microhepatia; cats: variable.
- Coagulopathy—variable, uncommon in DPM.
- Cutaneous lesions—superficial necrolytic dermatitis.

CAUSES

- Chronic necroinflammatory, oxidant, or immune-mediated liver injury has many causes; may develop subsequent to chronic inflammatory bowel disease (IBD) or pancreatitis.
- CuAH.
- Drug- or toxin-induced liver injury—anticonvulsants; azole antifungals; nonsteroidal anti-inflammatory drug (NSAID) oxibendazole; trimethoprimsulfamethoxazole; chronic food-borne toxins (aflatoxins), others.
- Infections—leptospirosis, canine adenovirus I, leishmanial, histoplasmosis, protozoal (toxoplasmosis).
- Chronic cholangiohepatitis (cats).
- Chronic EHBDO (>6 weeks, dogs and cats).
- Single episode of massive hepatic necrosis; sago palm (cycad toxicity), xylitol, NSAIDs in dogs with substantial Cu accumulation.

RISK FACTORS

- Breed predisposition.
- Dietary Cu intake >patient tolerance.
- Hepatic iron accumulation—supplementation.
- Chronic hepatobiliary inflammation.
- Chronic EHBDO.
- Chronic phenobarbital administration (dogs).
- NSAIDS—dogs, especially carprofen.

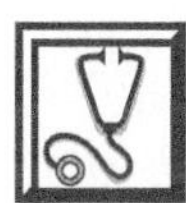

DIAGNOSIS

DIFFERENTIAL DIAGNOSIS

- Chronic hepatitis—common in dogs.
- Cholangiohepatitis—common in cats.
- Noncirrhotic portal hypertension—dogs.
- Chronic EHBDO.
- Chronic IBD or pancreatitis.
- Hepatic neoplasia.
- Metastatic neoplasia or carcinomatosis.
- Congenital portosystemic vascular anomaly (shunt).
- Congenital portal atresia—intrahepatic or extrahepatic.
- Right-sided heart failure, pericardial disease.

CIRRHOSIS AND FIBROSIS OF THE LIVER (CONTINUED)

C

- Cats—hepatic lipidosis, feline infectious peritonitis, toxoplasmosis.
- Hemolytic anemia (jaundice differential).

CBC/BIOCHEMISTRY/URINALYSIS

CBC

- Microcytic RBCs: APSS; mild anemia: small RBCs with normal cell count; anemia of chronic disease; microangiopathic shearing: sinusoidal fibrosis, APSS.
- Mild thrombocytopenia variable.
- Leukogram variable.

Biochemistry

- Bilirubin variable.
- Liver enzyme activities—high (alanine transaminase [ALT] > alkaline phosphatase [ALP]) noted before clinical signs or liver dysfunction; at end-stage enzymes may decline.
- Normal to hypoalbuminemia.
- Normal to hyperglobulinemia.
- Hypocholesterolemia—reflects APSS.
- Low blood urea nitrogen (BUN)—reduced urea cycle activity, APSS, protein-restricted diet, PU/PD.
- Hypoglycemia—rare.
- Hypokalemia—may predispose to HE.
- Hyponatremia—fluid imbalance with ascites.

Urinalysis

- Isosthenuria—with PU/PD.
- Ammonium biurate crystalluria.
- Bilirubinuria, bilirubin crystalluria.

OTHER LABORATORY TESTS

- Ascitic fluid—pure or modified transudate.
- Coagulation tests—inconsistently prolonged prothrombin time (PT), activated partial thromboplastin time, buccal mucosal bleeding time (BMBT).
- Low protein C and antithrombin activity—reflects APSS, synthetic failure, or disseminated intravascular coagulation (DIC).
- Serum bile acids—high; reflects APSS or cholestasis in cirrhosis.
- Hyperammonemia—inferred from ammonium biurate crystalluria.

IMAGING

Radiography

Abdominal—small to normal-sized liver; ascites may obscure details; urate calculi radiolucent unless calcium complexed.

Ultrasonography

- Abdominal—hyperechoic or mixed echogenic liver parenchyma; ± nodularity; often small with cirrhosis; abdominal effusion (ascites); APSS (color-flow Doppler); enlarged portal lymph nodes; no parenchymal change in some cases.
- Doppler interrogation of portal vasculature—may confirm hepatofugal flow or nests of APSS, esp. near left kidney or splenic vessels.

DIAGNOSTIC PROCEDURES

- Fine-needle aspiration cytology—helps rule out neoplasia; rule in bacterial infection; *cannot define fibrosis* or *nonsuppurative inflammation.*
- Liver biopsy—for definitive diagnosis; accuracy increased by multiple biopsy samples.
- Ultrasound guided—14–16G.
- Laparoscopy/laparotomy—best methods, permits gross visualization, documents APSS, biopsy access to multiple liver lobes and focal lesions.

PATHOLOGIC FINDINGS

Gross

- Fibrosis—small, firm irregular to finely nodular liver; DPM-CHF may not be small; fibrotic liver may display APSS, ± ascites.
- Cirrhosis—firm irregular liver; prominent micro- or macronodules, APSS, ± ascites.

Histopathology

- Immune-mediated hepatitis—periportal, lobular, or centrilobular lymphoplasmacytic infiltrates, hepatic cord disorganization, sinusoidal fibrosis, biliary hyperplasia.
- CuAH—initially centrilobular, may evolve immune-mediated hepatitis; single necrotic hepatocytes; significant fibrotic tissue may falsely decrease quantitative Cu concentration measurements in biopsy samples.
- DPM—bridging partitions with proliferative nonfunctional embryonic bile ducts embedded in ECM interconnecting portal regions.
- Postnecrotic fibrosis—fibrosis marks regenerative repair, disorganized wide hepatic cords; engorged lymphatics reflect sinusoidal hypertension.
- Cirrhosis—diffuse lesion; fibrosis, nodular regeneration distorting lobular architecture, periportal or sinusoidal fibrosis depending on zone of chronic injury, engorged lymphatics; single hepatocyte necrosis if active disease.

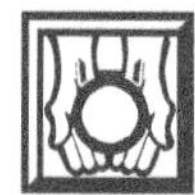

TREATMENT

APPROPRIATE HEALTH CARE

- Outpatient—minimally symptomatic patients.
- Inpatient—diagnostic tests; treatment for dehydration, severe HE, enteric bleeding, tense ascites.

NURSING CARE

- Fluids—avoid lactate if hepatic failure; avoid sodium loading if ascites.
- B complex vitamins (esp. cats)—2 mL/L fluid advised.
- Vitamin K_1—0.5–1.5 mg/kg SC q12h for 3 doses initially; titrate with proteins invoked by vitamin K absence or antagonism (PIVKA; if available) or PT.
- Glucose—if hypoglycemia; 2.5–5% dextrose in polyionic solution; titrate to response.
- Potassium chloride—in fluids, as needed.
- Avoid alkalosis—worsens HE.
- Therapeutic large-volume abdominocentesis if tense ascites nonresponsive to medical treatment; *caution*: PHS—hypotensive crisis and acute renal failure.

ACTIVITY

Limit

DIET

- Withhold oral food in acute severe HE if stupor, coma, or vomiting associated with enteric bleeding or pancreatitis.
- Consider partial parenteral nutrition or total parenteral nutrition.
- If HE—restrict protein intake, use soy or dairy protein sources (dogs) with medical interventions to increase nitrogen tolerance (see Hepatic Encephalopathy).
- Supplement water-soluble vitamins.

CLIENT EDUCATION

- Treatment palliative and symptomatic.
- Fibrosis diminished by control of inflammation and provocative diseases.
- Attenuate factors provoking HE—azotemia, dehydration; infection; catabolism; high-protein meals, hypokalemia; alkalemia; constipation, endoparasitism; enteric bleeding; certain drugs.

SURGICAL CONSIDERATIONS

- Cirrhosis—high anesthetic risk; gas anesthesia preferred: isoflurane or sevoflurane.
- Coagulopathy—predisposes to bleeding; BMBT may better assess risk for bleeding.
- Postoperative intensive care—avoid HE, maintain hydration, euglycemia, electrolytes, acid-base balance (avoid alkalemia).
- Predisposed to enteric bacterial translocation—judiciously administer antibiotics, esp. if surgical procedures involve alimentary canal or biliary structures.

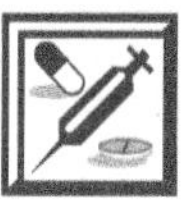

MEDICATIONS

DRUG(S) OF CHOICE

- Treatments for specific etiologies—chelate Cu if CuAH; withdraw potentially hepatotoxic drugs, herbal or natural remedies.
- No clinical trials prove efficacy of specific regimens in animals.

Immune Modulation

- Prednisolone/prednisone—1–2 mg/kg q24h PO; taper to 0.5 mg/kg q48h; do not exceed 40 mg/day/dog.
- Azathioprine—2 mg/kg (or 50 mg/m^2) q24h for 14 days, then q48h; contraindicated in cats (toxic); dogs: with prednisone, antioxidants, antifibrotics, and polyenylphosphatidylcholine (PPC).
- Cyclosporine—5 mg/kg BID tapered to q24h; has been successful as single agent or with corticosteroids.
- Mycophenolate—10–15 mg/kg BID; has been successful as first- or second-line treatment with corticosteroids.

Antifibrotics

- Immunomodulation, S-adenosylmethionine (SAMe), silybin, vitamin E—considered antifibrotics as well as hepatoprotectants.

- Ursodiol—7.5 mg/kg/day PO q12h with food; use indefinitely.
- Polyunsaturated phosphatidylcholine with dilinolylphosphatidylcholine (PhosChol®)—25 mg/kg/q24h, mix with food.
- Colchicine—0.025–0.03 mg/kg q24–48h; no evidence of chronic benefit; side effects complicate use; no longer recommended.
- Losartan and telmisartan—losartan: 0.5 mg/kg/q24h; telmisartan: 0.5–1 mg/kg q24h initial dose; closely monitor blood pressure, renal function, and potassium, reducing dose if hypotension or hyperkalemia; angiotensin receptor blockers used in humans as antihypertensives and have been shown to be nephroprotective, to protect against some forms of drug-induced hepatotoxicity, and to inconsistently limit hepatic fibrosis.

Antioxidants

- Necroinflammatory disorders.
- SAMe—20 mg/kg q24h PO, *empty stomach.*
- Vitamin E mixed tocopherols—10 U/kg q24h PO with food.

Hepatoprotectants

- Necroinflammatory disorders.
- Ursodeoxycholate, vitamin E, SAMe.
- Silibinin—efficacy unclear, use PPC complexed form (bioavailable), 2–5 mg/kg q24h PO.
- Elemental zinc—1.5–3 mg PO q24h (if low liver zinc confirmed); adjust dose with plasma zinc measurements; avoid ≥800 µg/dL; contraindicated with concurrent d-penicillamine administration.

Gastroprotectants

- Gastric acid inhibitors—if enteric bleeding (see Hepatitis, Chronic).
- Eliminate endoparasitism.

Ascites

- Restrict activity and sodium intake combined with diuretic therapy.
- Dietary sodium restriction (0.2% dry matter basis or <0.05 g/100 kcal).
- Diuretics (see Hypertension, Portal; Hepatitis, Chronic); slowly mobilize effusion: furosemide (0.5–1 mg/kg IV/SC/PO q12h) with spironolactone (0.5–2 mg/kg PO q12h); adjust dose to response (7–10 day recheck; if no response titrate up q3–5d to max dose 4 mg/kg/day).
- Therapeutic large-volume abdominocentesis if nonresponsive ascites mobilization after 7–14 days of diuretics and sodium restriction.
- Consider vasopressin V_2 antagonists with low-dose diuretics for treatment-resistant ascites (no published data for dogs or cats).

CONTRAINDICATIONS

NSAIDs—avoid; potentiate enteric bleeding; may worsen ascites; potentiate centrilobular hepatic necrosis-hepatotoxic metabolites and CuAH.

PRECAUTIONS

- Diuretics—dehydration, hypokalemia, alkalemia worsen HE.
- Glucocorticoids—increase susceptibility to infection, enteric bleeding, sodium and water retention, ascites, protein catabolism, HE.
- Avoid drugs or reduce dose if first-pass hepatic extraction, if require hepatic conjugation or biotransformation (e.g., metronidazole—reduce conventional dose to 7.5 mg/kg PO q12h, as used for HE).

ALTERNATIVE DRUG(S)

- Dexamethasone—if ascites, replace prednisone/prednisolone to avoid mineralocorticoid effect); divide dose by 7–10, administer q3–4 days; taper dose to efficacy.

FOLLOW-UP

PATIENT MONITORING

- Liver enzymes, albumin, BUN, cholesterol, bilirubin—monthly to quarterly.
- Serial monitoring of total serum bile acids—adds no prognostic or diagnostic information.
- Body condition score, weight, muscle mass—reflects nutritional adequacy/nitrogen balance.
- Abdominal girth—reflects ascites volume.
- Azathioprine, mycophenolate, colchicine—monitor for bone marrow toxicity (serial CBCs) and other side effects.

POSSIBLE COMPLICATIONS

HE, septicemia, bleeding—may be life-threatening; DIC—may be terminal event.

EXPECTED COURSE AND PROGNOSIS

- Flare-ups of HE and ascites may require hospitalization to adjust nutritional and medical interventions.
- Sodium restriction and diuretics may require titration to achieve optimal control of ascites.
- Presence of ascites indicates severe disease.
- DPM—survival up to 12 years after diagnosis.
- Cirrhosis—variable: poor long-term prognosis in limited studies, <6 months; however, some can survive years (>5) with careful interventional management depending on whether histologic changes truly "end-stage" or not.

MISCELLANEOUS

ZOONOTIC POTENTIAL

Dogs with leptospirosis-associated chronic liver disease (rare) may shed organisms.

SEE ALSO

- Coagulopathy of Liver Disease.
- Copper Associated Hepatopathy.
- Ductal Plate Malformation (Congenital Hepatic Fibrosis).
- Hepatic Encephalopathy.
- Hepatitis, Chronic.
- Hypertension, Portal.

ABBREVIATIONS

- ALP = alkaline phosphatase.
- ALR = alanine transaminase.
- APSS = acquired portosystemic shunt.
- BMBT = buccal mucosal bleeding time.
- BUN = blood urea nitrogen.
- CHF = congenital hepatic fibrosis.
- CuAH = copper associated hepatopathy.
- DIC = disseminated intravascular coagulation.
- DPM = ductal plate malformation.
- ECM = extracellular matrix.
- EHBDO = extrahepatic bile duct occlusion.
- GI = gastrointestinal.
- HE = hepatic encephalopathy.
- IBD = inflammatory bowel disease.
- NSAID = nonsteroidal anti-inflammatory drug.
- PHS = postcentesis hypotension syndrome.
- PIVKA = proteins invoked by vitamin K absence or antagonism.
- PPC = polyenylphosphatidylcholine.
- PT = prothrombin time.
- PU/PD = polyuria/polydipsia.
- RBC = red blood cell.
- SAMe = S-adenosylmethionine.

Suggested Reading

Center SA. Metabolic, antioxidant, nutraceutical, probiotic, and herbal therapies relating to the management of hepatobiliary disorders. Vet Clin North Am Small Anim Pract 2004, 34:67–172.

Eulenberg VM, Lidbury JA. Hepatic fibrosis in dogs. J Vet Intern Med. 2018, 32:26–41.

Strickland JM, Buchweitz JP, Smedley RC, et al. Hepatic copper concentrations in 546 dogs (1982–2015). J Vet Intern Med 2018, 32:1943–1950.

Webster CRL, Center SA, Cullen JM, et al. ACVIM consensus statement on the diagnosis and treatment of chronic hepatitis in dogs. J Vet Intern Med 2019, 33(3):1173–1200.

Authors Alysha Vincent and Kate Holan
Consulting Editor Kate Holan

Acknowledgment The author and book editors acknowledge the prior contribution of Sharon A. Center.

Client Education Handout available online

CLAW AND CLAWFOLD DISORDERS

BASICS

DEFINITION

- Ungual fold—crescent-shaped tissue surrounding the proximal claw.
- Coronary band and dorsal ridge (dorsal ridge of the ungual crest)—produces most of the claw; contributes to the curvature of the claw.
- Paronychia—inflammation of soft tissue around the claw.
- Onychomycosis—fungal infection of the claw.
- Onychorrhexis—brittle claws that tend to split or break.
- Onychomadesis—sloughing of the claw.
- Onychodystrophy—deformity caused by abnormal growth; often a sequela of a disorder.
- Onychomalacia—softening of the claw.

PATHOPHYSIOLOGY

- Claws and ungual folds—subject to trauma, infection, vascular insufficiency, immune-mediated disease, parasites, neoplasia, defects in keratinization, and congenital abnormalities.
- A particular claw deformity may be caused by a variety of diseases—claw disease is most often associated with other dermatoses: rarely the only epithelial structure affected.
- A single disease can present with various claw lesions.
- One foot affected—top differentials include foreign body, neoplasia, trauma, fungal infection, bacterial infection.
- Multiple feet affected—allergy, endocrine, secondary infections, demodicosis, immune-mediated disorders, epidermolysis bullosa, symmetric lupoid onychodystrophy (SLO), plasma cell pododermatitis, superficial necrolytic dermatitis, nutritional deficiencies, psychogenic dermatoses, idiopathic.

SIGNALMENT

- Dog and cat.
- Claw and clawfold diseases—1.3% of dogs and 2.2% of cats.
- Mean age range—SLO 3–8 years.
- No predominant sex reported.
- Dachshunds—onychorrhexis.
- German shepherd dogs, Rottweilers, possibly giant schnauzers and Doberman pinschers—SLO.
- Siberian huskies, dachshunds, Rhodesian ridgebacks, Rottweilers, cocker spaniels—idiopathic onychodystrophy.
- German shepherd dogs, whippets, English springer spaniels—idiopathic onychomadesis
- Shorthair dog breeds—paronychia in multiple digits.
- Devon Rex cats—*Malassezia* paronychia.

SIGNS

- Licking at the feet and/or ungual folds.
- Lameness.
- Pain.
- Swelling, erythema, and exudate of ungual fold.
- Deformity or band formation of claw.
- Sloughing of claw.
- Discoloration of claw.
- Hemorrhage from claw or at loss of a claw.

CAUSES

Paronychia

- Infection—bacteria, dermatophyte, yeast (*Candida, Malassezia*).
- Demodicosis.
- Immune-mediated—pemphigus, bullous pemphigoid, systemic lupus erythematosus (SLE), drug eruption, SLO.
- Neoplasia—subungual squamous cell carcinoma, melanoma, eccrine carcinoma, osteosarcoma, subungual keratoacanthoma, inverted squamous papilloma.
- Arteriovenous fistula.

Onychomycosis

- Dogs—*Trichophyton mentagrophytes*—usually generalized.
- Cats—*Microsporum canis.*

Onychorrhexis

- Idiopathic—especially in dachshunds; multiple claws.
- Trauma.
- Infection—dermatophytosis, leishmaniasis.

Onychomadesis

- Trauma.
- Infection.
- Immune-mediated—pemphigus, bullous pemphigoid, SLE, drug eruption, SLO.
- Vascular insufficiency—vasculitis, cold agglutinin disease.
- Neoplasia—see above.
- Idiopathic.

Claw Dystrophy

- Acromegaly.
- Feline hyperthyroidism.
- Zinc-responsive dermatosis.
- Congenital malformations.
- Leishmaniasis.

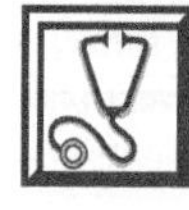

DIAGNOSIS

DIFFERENTIAL DIAGNOSIS

- Trauma or neoplasia often affects a single claw.
- Involvement of multiple claws suggests a systemic disease.
- Immune-mediated diseases (except SLO) usually have other skin lesions in addition to claw or ungual fold lesions.

CBC/BIOCHEMISTRY/URINALYSIS

May show evidence of SLE, diabetes mellitus, hyperthyroidism, or other systemic illness.

OTHER LABORATORY TESTS

- Feline leukemia virus (FeLV).
- Serum thyroxine.
- Antinuclear antibody (ANA) titer.

IMAGING

Radiographs—osteomyelitis of third phalanx, neoplastic change.

DIAGNOSTIC PROCEDURES

- Biopsy—often involves a third phalanx amputation; inclusion of the coronary band required for diagnosis of most diseases; punch biopsy of the claw (onychobiopsy).
- Cytology of exudate from the claw and/or fold.
- Skin scraping.
- Bacterial and fungal culture.

TREATMENT

PARONYCHIA

- Surgical removal of claw plate (shell).
- Antimicrobial soaks.
- Systemic antibiotics as per culture results.
- Identify underlying condition and treat specifically.

Onychomycosis

- Antifungal soaks—chlorhexidine, povidone iodine, lime sulfur.
- Surgical removal of claw plate—may improve response to systemic medication.
- Amputation of third phalanx.

Onychorrhexis

- Repair with fingernail glue (type used to attach false nails in humans).
- Remove splintered pieces and maintain with rotary sander (Dremel).
- Treat underlying cause.
- Amputate third phalanx, last resort.

Onychomadesis

- Antimicrobial soaks.
- Treat underlying cause.

Neoplasia

- Determined by biologic behavior of specific tumor.
- Surgical excision.
- Amputation of digit or leg.
- Chemotherapy and/or radiation therapy.

Claw Dystrophy

Treat underlying cause.

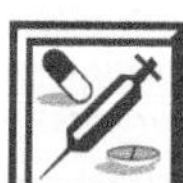

MEDICATIONS

DRUG(S) OF CHOICE

- Bacterial paronychia—systemic antibiotics based on culture and sensitivity.
- Yeast paronychia—*Candida* or *Malassezia* paronychia: ketoconazole (5–10 mg/kg PO q12–24h); topical nystatin or miconazole.

- Onychomycosis—griseofulvin (50–150 mg/kg PO/day) or ketoconazole (5–10 mg/kg PO q12h) for 6–12 months until negative cultures; itraconazole (10 mg/kg PO q24h) for 3 weeks and then pulse therapy until resolved.
- Onychomadesis—determined by cause; immunomodulation therapy for immune-mediated diseases (e.g., SLO); options include essential fatty acid supplementation; cycline antibiotics: tetracycline 250 mg PO TID for dogs <10 kg; 500 mg PO TID dogs >10 kg); doxycycline 10 mg/kg PO q24h; minocycline 5 mg/kg PO BID, often administered with niacinamide 250 mg PO for dogs <10 kg and 500 mg PO for dogs >10 kg; pentoxifylline 10–15 mg/kg PO BID to TID; corticosteroids and cyclosporine 5 mg/kg PO q24h; vitamin E; appropriate chemotherapeutic agents (e.g., azathioprine, chlorambucil).
- Nonsteroidal anti-inflammatory drugs (NSAIDs) or tramadol if pain is present.

PRECAUTIONS

- Griseofulvin—teratogenic; may cause bone marrow suppression, anorexia, vomiting, and diarrhea; absorption enhanced if given with a high-fat meal.
- Ketoconazole—avoid use in cats; may cause anorexia, gastric irritation, hepatic toxicity, and lightening of the hair coat.

FOLLOW-UP

EXPECTED COURSE AND PROGNOSIS

- Slow claw growth cycle may require 6–8 months of therapy to fully correct an abnormality; improvement may be noted after 6–8 weeks of appropriate treatment.
- Bacterial or yeast paronychia and onychomycosis—treatment may be prolonged and response may be influenced by underlying factors; weight reduction in obese patients.
- Onychorrhexis—may require amputation of the third phalanx for resolution.
- Onychomadesis—prognosis determined by underlying cause; immune-mediated diseases and vascular problems carry a more guarded prognosis than do trauma or infectious causes.
- Neoplasia—excised by amputation of the digit; malignant tumors metastasize by the time of diagnosis.

MISCELLANEOUS

ABBREVIATIONS

- ANA = antinuclear antibody.
- FeLV = feline leukemia virus.
- NSAID = nonsteroidal anti-inflammatory drug.
- SLE = systemic lupus erythematosus.
- SLO = symmetric lupoid onychodystrophy.

Suggested Reading

Helton Rhodes KA, Werner A. Blackwell's Five-Minute Veterinary Consult: Clinical Companion: Small Animal Dermatology, 3rd ed. Hoboken, NJ: Wiley-Blackwell, 2018.

Miller WH, Griffin CE, Campbell KL. Muller & Kirk's Small Animal Dermatology, 7th ed. St. Louis, MO: Elsevier Mosby, 2013.

Author Guillermina Manigot

Consulting Editor Alexander H. Werner Resnick

Acknowledgment The author and book editors acknowledge the prior contribution of Karen Helton Rhodes.

Client Education Handout available online

CLOSTRIDIAL ENTEROTOXICOSIS

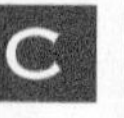

BASICS

DEFINITION

A complex disorder characterized by diarrhea in dogs and cats associated with *Clostridium perfringens* enterotoxins (CPEs).

PATHOPHYSIOLOGY

• *Clostridium perfringens* (CP) is a Gram-positive, spore-forming, strictly anaerobic bacterium. • CP is a normal commensal organism found in the intestinal tract of humans and animals. • A strong link between canine acute hemorrhagic diarrhea syndrome (AHDS; formerly hemorrhagic gastroenteritis [HGE]) and the presence of CP has been identified. • Certain strains of CP (primarily Type A) produce a potent enterotoxin (CPE) as well as pore-forming toxins (NetE and NetF). • CPE is a cytotoxic enterotoxin that causes tissue destruction; it has been identified in the feces of up to 14% of dogs without diarrhea, thus its role in causing diarrhea is unclear. • NetF-producing CP isolates have not been found in healthy dogs. • Not all strains of CP produce CPE or NetF and not all dogs that have CPE in feces are clinical, therefore it is undetermined why some develop diarrhea. • CPE production is coregulated with sporulation of the organism; conditions that precipitate sporulation in animals include a sudden change in diet, dietary indiscretion, injudicious use of antibiotics causing a severe dysbiosis, and underlying intestinal disease.

SYSTEMS AFFECTED

Gastrointestinal (GI).

INCIDENCE/PREVALENCE

Incidence is unknown; up to 34% of canine diarrhea cases are suspected to be CP related. The infection is far less common in cats.

SIGNALMENT

Species

Dog and cat.

Mean Age and Range

Any age.

SIGNS

General Comments

Can include both large and small bowel diarrhea.

Historical Findings

• Large bowel diarrhea—tenesmus, mucous, frank blood, and increased frequency of defecation. • Small bowel diarrhea—large volumes of soft to liquid diarrhea. • Vomiting and abdominal discomfort. • Severity varies from mild, self-limiting diarrhea to fatal, acute, hemorrhagic diarrhea.

Physical Examination Findings

• Abdominal discomfort. • Hematochezia.
• Mucoid feces. • Dehydration if there has been voluminous diarrhea or vomiting.
• Fever is uncommon. • Evidence of systemic illness or debilitation is rare.

CAUSES

• In humans, CP-associated diarrhea is usually due to ingestion of enterotoxigenic isolates. In dogs, it is thought to be secondary to disruption of the intestinal microenvironment. • Anything that disrupts normal enteric microbiota can lead to CP overgrowth and diarrhea. • CP toxins have been implicated in dogs with AHDS.

RISK FACTORS

• Dietary changes. • Antibiotic use. • Stress.
• Primary small intestinal bacterial overgrowth.

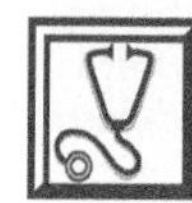

DIAGNOSIS

• Diagnostic testing should occur during the acute phase. • In the absence of sepsis, antibiotic therapy has not been shown to alter resolution of clinical signs, therefore response to antibiotics cannot be used as diagnostic criterion.

DIFFERENTIAL DIAGNOSIS

Any cause of diarrhea can be considered, including, but not limited to, viral, bacterial, or parasitic infection, dietary indiscretion, chronic enteropathy, metabolic disease, neoplasia.

CBC/BIOCHEMISTRY/URINALYSIS

• If dehydration is present—increased packed cell volume (PCV) from hemoconcentration, increased total plasma protein, increased amylase, and increased blood urea nitrogen (BUN) from prerenal azotemia.
• Dogs with AHDS will often have increased PCV with discordantly low total plasma protein. • Leukocytosis with neutrophilia and monocytosis. • Decreased albumin secondary to loss and decreased production. • Increased alanine aminotransferase (ALT) and aspartate aminotransferase (AST) activities from organ hypoxia secondary to hypovolemia.

OTHER LABORATORY TESTS

There is no gold standard diagnostic test for confirming CP-associated diarrhea.

Microbiology

• Fecal culture alone should not be used to diagnose CP-associated illness because the organism is a normal commensal; CP can be isolated from feces of >80% of healthy dogs and 43–63% of normal cats. • Fecal endospore cultures are not useful, as sporulation of enterotoxigenic strains of CP occurs in dogs with and without diarrhea.

Enterotoxin Assay

• Fecal ELISA for identification of CPE in patients with diarrhea suspected to be due to CP is the current recommendation; since CPE is present in the feces of 5–14% of clinically normal dogs, this may or may not be clinically useful. • Fecal ELISA should be run in conjunction with PCR to detect enterotoxigenic strains. • Real-time polymerase chain reaction (RT-PCR) for detection of the CPE gene and the alpha toxin gene is available; the CPE gene has been found in up to 33.7% of healthy dogs, therefore its presence in a dog with GI disease does not confirm that CP is the cause.

Fecal Cytology

• CP endospores, characterized by "safety-pin" appearance with oval form and dense body at one end of spore wall, can be seen on microscopic evaluation of heat-fixed thin fecal smear stained with Romanowsky-type stain (e.g., Diff-Quik®), Wright's stain, or new methylene blue. • High numbers of CP endospores on fecal cytology correlates poorly with clinical disease or fecal CPE activity.
• High numbers of fecal endospores can be found in feces of healthy dogs.

DIAGNOSTIC PROCEDURES

• Abdominal ultrasound can help rule out other causes of GI disease. • Colonoscopy and endoscopy with biopsy can be used to confirm presence of acute mucosal necrosis and neutrophilic infiltration, as well as adherence of rod-shaped bacteria to these necrotic areas, and can rule out other causes of GI disease.

PATHOLOGIC FINDINGS

• Grossly hyperemic or ulcerated mucosa. • Acute intestinal mucosal destruction and neutrophilic infiltration. • Immunohistochemical staining of bacterial plaques on necrotic areas may be clostridial antigen positive.

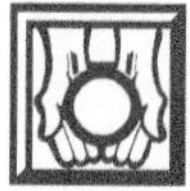

TREATMENT

APPROPRIATE HEALTH CARE

• There are no research-based recommendations for optimal treatment of patients with CP-associated illness. • If vomiting or diarrhea is not severe, animals may be treated as outpatients with antiemetics and subcutaneous fluids. • If more severe diarrhea, vomiting, dehydration, or evidence of hypovolemia, hospitalization with IV replacement crystalloids and antiemetics is recommended.

DIET

• Diet change plays a role in treatment and management of cases with chronic recurring disease; diets high in either soluble (fermentable) or insoluble fiber often result in clinical improvement by reducing enteric CP

number, possibly through acidification of the distal intestine, which limits CP sporulation and enterotoxin production.
• Commercial diets can be supplemented with psyllium (1/2–2 tsp/day) as a source of soluble fiber.
• Diets low in fiber should be supplemented with fiber (coarse bran 1–3 tbs/day) as a source of insoluble fiber or psyllium added as a source of soluble fiber. • Probiotics might help restore the normal intestinal microbiota, thereby reducing risk of recurrent CP-associated diarrhea.

CLIENT EDUCATION

• Acute disease is often self-limiting. • There have been no documented reports of transmission of CP from animals to humans; however, if there are immunosuppressed members in the household, strict hygiene protocols should be followed.

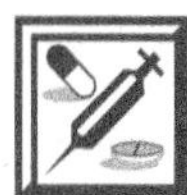

MEDICATIONS

DRUG(S) OF CHOICE

Antiemetics

• Maropitant—1 mg/kg IV/SC q 24h.
• Ondansetron—0.5–1 mg/kg IV/PO q24h.

Antibiotics

• Antibiotics are unnecessary in animals with mild disease as the infection is typically self-limiting. • If signs of systemic disease or sepsis are present, antibiotics should be administered. • Antibiotics that are recommended are ampicillin: 22 mg/kg IV q8h; amoxicillin: 22 mg/kg PO q8h; metronidazole: 10–25 mg/kg IV/PO q12h for 5–7 days; tylosin: 5–10 mg/kg PO q24h.
• Tetracyclines are no longer recommended due to resistance of CP isolates.

ALTERNATIVE DRUGS(S)

• Probiotics (e.g., lactobacillus) may alter the intestinal microbiota, reducing likelihood of recurrences. • One study reported faster resolution of clinical signs with use of probiotics than with no treatment. • Diet change can be instituted following resolution of clinical signs.

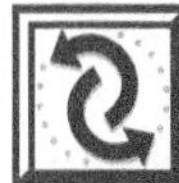

FOLLOW-UP

PATIENT MONITORING

• Ensure adequate hydration and intravascular volume, with replacement fluid administration as needed. • Monitor PCV, total plasma protein, acid-base balance, and electrolyte concentrations.

PREVENTION/AVOIDANCE

• Regular use of high-fiber diets or probiotics. • Avoiding or anticipating stressful events (e.g., kenneling) and using anxiolytics.

EXPECTED COURSE AND PROGNOSIS

• Overall excellent prognosis; many animals will have resolution of clinical signs without in-hospital treatment. • Acute hemorrhagic diarrheal events should be addressed with aggressive resuscitation and hospitalization; if the animal responds to therapy, the prognosis is good.

MISCELLANEOUS

ASSOCIATED CONDITIONS

• CP enterotoxicosis can be associated with AHDS. • The connection to chronic enteropathies is less well understood.

ZOONOTIC POTENTIAL

Unknown

PREGNANCY/FERTILITY/BREEDING

Antibiotic therapy may be contraindicated.

SEE ALSO

• Colitis and Proctitis.
• Small Intestinal Dysbiosis.

ABBREVIATIONS

• AHDS = acute hemorrhagic diarrhea syndrome.
• ALT = alanine aminotransferase.
• AST = aspartate aminotransferase.
• BUN = blood urea nitrogen.
• CP = *Clostridium perfringens.*
• CPE = *Clostridium perfringens* enterotoxin.
• GI = gastrointestinal.
• HGE = hemorrhagic gastroenteritis.
• PCV = packed cell volume.
• RT-PCR = real-time polymerase chain reaction.

Suggested Reading

Albini S, Brodard I, Jaussi A. Real-time multiplex PCR assays for reliable detection of Clostridium perfringens toxin genes in animal isolates. Vet Microbiol 2008, 127:179–185.

Marks SL, Rankin SC, Byrne BA, et al. ACVIM Consensus Statement: enteropathogenic bacteria in dogs and cats: diagnosis, epidemiology, treatment, and control. J Vet Intern Med 2011, 25:1195–1208.

Minamoto Y, Dhanani N, Markel ME, et al. Prevalence of Clostridium perfringens, Clostridium perfringens enterotoxin and dysbiosis in fecal samples of dogs with diarrhea. Vet Microbiol 2014, 174:463–473.

Weese SJ, Staempfli HR, Prescott JF, et al. The roles of Clostridium difficile and enterotoxigenic Clostridium perfringens in diarrhea in dogs. JVIM 2001, 15:374–378.

Ziese AL, Suchodolski JS, Hartmann K, et al. Effect of probiotic treatment on the clinical course, intestinal microbiome, and toxigenic Clostridium perfringens in dogs with acute hemorrhagic diarrhea. Plos One 2018, 13(9):e0204691.

Author Jennifer Good

Consulting Editor Amie Koenig

Acknowledgment The author and book editors acknowledge the prior contribution of Stanley L. Marks.

Client Education Handout available online

COAGULATION FACTOR DEFICIENCY

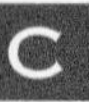

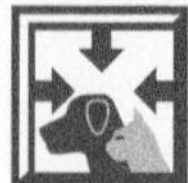

BASICS

DEFINITION

Hemostatic defects characterized by a lack of one or more procoagulant proteins (coagulation factors).

PATHOPHYSIOLOGY

- Coagulation involves a complex series of enzymatic reactions that generate a burst of thrombin (factor IIa) at sites of blood vessel injury; thrombin then cleaves plasma fibrinogen into fibrin monomers that subsequently polymerize and cross-link to form an insoluble fibrin clot.
- Functional and/or quantitative coagulation factor deficiencies cause a failure of fibrin clot formation.
- The liver is the sole or primary site of synthesis of most coagulation factors; after synthesis, factors II, VII, IX, and X require a vitamin K–dependent modification to become fully active.

SYSTEMS AFFECTED

- Coagulation factor deficiency can cause spontaneous hemorrhage, prolonged post-traumatic hemorrhage, and ultimately blood loss anemia.
- Spontaneous hemorrhage—often develops in body cavities or potential spaces (i.e., hemothorax, hemoperitoneum, hemarthrosis, subcutaneous, or intramuscular hematoma).

GENETICS

- Hemophilia A and B (factor VIII and IX deficiencies)—X-linked recessive traits.
- All other factor deficiencies are autosomal traits.
- Specific defects are more likely to be propagated within a single breed, but all breeds are at risk for developing new mutations.

SIGNALMENT

- Dog and cat.
- Hereditary factor deficiencies—severe defects manifest by 3–6 months of age, milder hemostatic defects manifest after surgery or trauma.
- For X-linked recessive traits, males express the bleeding tendency, female carriers are clinically normal.
- For autosomal traits, males and females express signs with equal frequency.
- Hemophilia A is a common hereditary factor deficiency and may be seen in all breeds and mixed-breed dogs and cats.
- Factor XII deficiency is common in cats, but does not cause a clinical bleeding tendency.
- Acquired factor deficiencies—depends on underlying disease process.

SIGNS

- Hematoma formation.
- Intracavitary hemorrhage.
- Prolonged hemorrhage after surgery or trauma.
- Blood loss anemia.

CAUSES

- Acquired—synthetic failure (liver disease); vitamin K deficiency (cholestasis, anticoagulant rodenticide toxicity, malabsorption, long-term antibiotics, coumadin); factor inhibition (anticoagulant overdose, envenomation, auto- or alloantibodies); factor consumption and depletion (disseminated intravascular coagulopathy [DIC]); factor dilution (high-volume transfusion, crystalloid, or colloid fluid therapy); hyperfibrinolysis (secondary fibrinogen depletion).
- Hereditary—distinct mutations in coagulation factor genes.

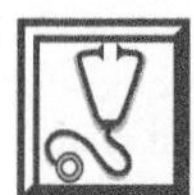

DIAGNOSIS

DIFFERENTIAL DIAGNOSIS

- Thrombocytopenia should be the first rule-out for any patient with abnormal hemorrhage; thrombocytopathies may also cause bleeding (see Thrombocytopenia, Thrombocytopathies).
- Hereditary coagulation factor deficiencies cause prolongation of coagulation screening tests, whereas vonWillebrand disease (vWD) does not.
- Hyperfibrinolysis may cause hemorrhage in patients with hypovolemic shock, acute blood loss, or trauma, but generally does not cause prolongation of activated partial thromboplastin time (APTT) or prothrombin time (PT) tests; a breed predisposition for hyperfibrinolysis may exist in sighthounds.
- Acquired coagulopathies often develop because of liver disease, anticoagulant rodenticide ingestion, or DIC.
- Liver disease is accompanied by changes in the chemistry profile (see Coagulopathy of Liver Disease).
- Anticoagulant rodenticide toxicity prolongs the PT and/or APTT, but does not affect thrombin clotting time (TCT) or fibrinogen concentration.
- DIC always develops secondary to systemic disease (especially sepsis, neoplasia, other inflammatory conditions) and is often accompanied by low or falling platelet count.
- Massive transfusion (>1 blood volume) with stored blood products may dilute functional factors, fibrinogen, and platelets below hemostatic levels; hypocalcemia may also result.
- Contamination of blood samples (e.g., with heparin flush) or delayed processing can generate spurious PT and APTT abnormalities.

CBC/BIOCHEMISTRY/URINALYSIS

- Regenerative anemia develops over the course of days after blood loss.
- Platelet count is normal unless the patient has DIC or massive bleeding.
- Resorption of blood from a large hematoma may cause hyperbilirubinemia.

OTHER LABORATORY TESTS

- Coagulation screening tests (activated clotting time [ACT], APTT, PT, TCT) are functional tests that measure the time for in vitro clot formation; coagulation factor and fibrinogen deficiencies prolong clotting time (see Figure 1).
- ACT is a point-of-care screening test that detects severe deficiencies of all factors (except factor VII); ACT may be influenced by anemia, thrombocytopenia, and changes in blood viscosity.
- APTT is a screening test of the contact pathway (prekallikrein, high molecular weight kininogen, factor XII), intrinsic system (factors XI, IX, VIII), common system (factors X, V, II), and severe fibrinogen deficiency.
- PT is a screening test of factor VII, common system, and severe fibrinogen deficiency.
- The TCT is a screening test of functional fibrinogen and is sensitive to the presence of fibrinogen inhibitors.
- Acquired coagulation factor deficiencies generally cause prolongation of more than one screening test; the most common hereditary factor deficiencies (hemophilia and factor XII deficiency) specifically prolong APTT.
- Individual factor assays can be performed for definitive diagnosis of hereditary or complex coagulopathies.

Drugs That May Alter Laboratory Results

Therapeutic dosages of unfractionated heparin, coumadin, and plasma expanders (dextran, hetastarch) prolong coagulation screening tests.

Disorders That May Alter Laboratory Results

- Improper sample collection (poor venipuncture technique, partially or overfilled citrate collection tubes, use of heparin or clot activator tubes) will invalidate coagulation test results.
- Extreme lipemia, hemoglobinemia, or icterus may interfere with clot detection by photo-optical coagulation analyzers.
- Because of factor lability, samples should be assayed on site or plasma separated and sent on ice to the laboratory.

Valid if Run in Human Laboratory?

- Interpretation of coagulation assay results requires same-species reference intervals and controls; for example, human APTT values are generally twice those of dogs and cats.
- The laboratory should confirm cross-reactivity of antigenic assays and optimization of functional tests for animal species.

DIAGNOSTIC PROCEDURES

Buccal mucosal bleeding time (BMBT) is prolonged in patients with severe thrombocytopenia, platelet dysfunction, vWD, and fibrinogen deficiency, but BMBT is insensitive to coagulation factor deficiencies.

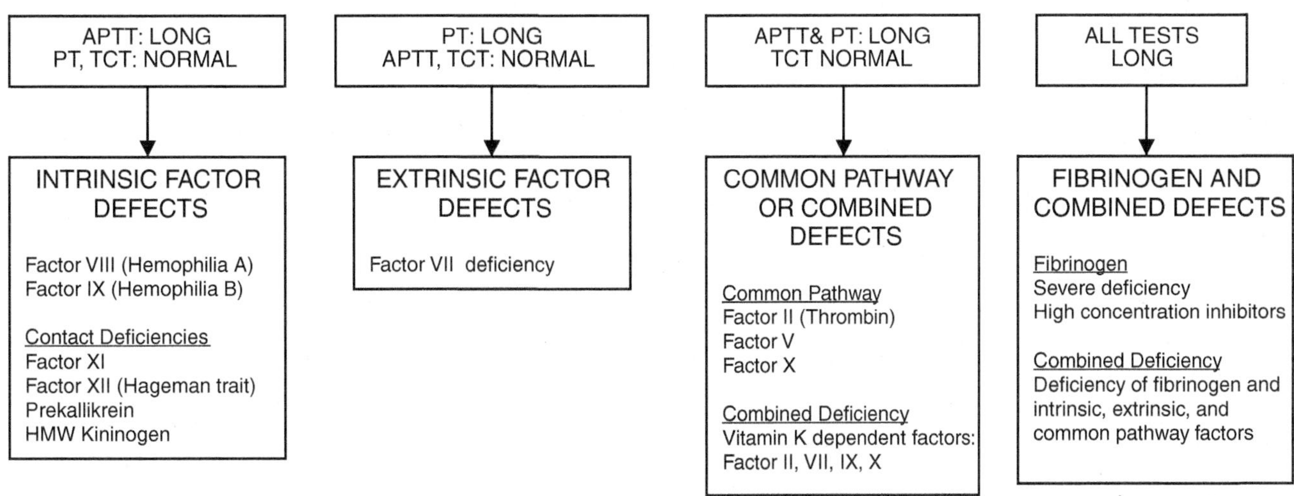

Figure 1.

Diagnostic algorithm for coagulation factor deficiencies

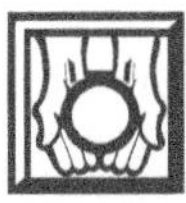

TREATMENT

- Transfusion of fresh whole blood, fresh plasma, and fresh frozen plasma will supply all coagulation factors.
- Cryoprecipitate is a specific source of factor VIII, fibrinogen, and von Willebrand factor; cryo-supernatant plasma supplies all other factors.
- Component therapy is preferred for surgical prophylaxis and nonanemic patients to prevent red cell sensitization and volume overload.
- Patients with severe acquired or hereditary factor deficiencies may require repeated transfusion (q8–12h) to control or prevent hemorrhage.

MEDICATIONS

DRUG(S) OF CHOICE

Vitamin K_1 (1.0 to 2.0 mg/kg SQ using a small needle, or preferably PO q24h) is an effective treatment for patients with anticoagulant rodenticide poisoning and other causes of vitamin K deficiency.

CONTRAINDICATIONS

Nonsteroidal anti-inflammatory drugs (NSAIDs), anticoagulants, and plasma expanders should be avoided to prevent further compromise of hemostasis.

PRECAUTIONS

- IM injections and jugular venipuncture should be avoided, when possible, because of the risk of inducing additional bleeding.
- Intravenous administration of vitamin K is not recommended because of the risk of anaphylaxis.

ALTERNATIVE DRUG(S)

Antifibrinolytic drugs (aminocaproic acid and tranexamic acid) help correct coagulopathy due to acute trauma and reduce transfusion requirements for orthopedic procedures in humans, and have shown benefit to prevent postoperative bleeding in greyhounds. These drugs may also be used topically (e.g., bleeding from tooth extraction).

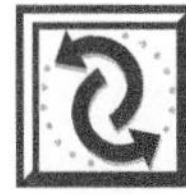

FOLLOW-UP

PATIENT MONITORING

- PT or factor VII assays can be used to monitor effectiveness of vitamin K administration in animals with anticoagulant toxicity; test results should normalize after 24–48 hours of initiating therapy.
- ACT is a less specific but reasonable substitute for monitoring response to vitamin K.
- Hereditary defects can be monitored by cessation of bleeding, stabilization of hematocrit, resolution of hematoma, and, if needed, specific factor analyses.

POSSIBLE COMPLICATIONS

Transfusion poses a risk of immune and nonimmune reactions (see Blood Transfusion Reactions).

MISCELLANEOUS

PREGNANCY/FERTILITY/BREEDING

Patients with hereditary factor deficiencies should not be bred.

SYNONYMS

- Coagulation defects.
- Coagulopathies.

SEE ALSO

- Coagulopathy of Liver Disease.
- Disseminated Intravascular Coagulation.
- Thrombocytopathies.
- Thrombocytopenia.
- Von Willebrand Disease.

ABBREVIATIONS

- ACT = activated clotting time.
- APTT = activated partial thromboplastin time.
- BMBT = buccal mucosal bleeding time.
- DIC = disseminated intravascular coagulation.
- NSAID = nonsteroidal anti-inflammatory drug.
- PT = prothrombin time.
- TCT = thrombin clotting time.
- vWD = von Willebrand disease.

INTERNET RESOURCES

http://eclinpath.com/hemostasis

Suggested Reading

Brooks MB and DeLaforcade A. Acquired coagulopathies. In: Weiss DJ, Wardrop KJ, eds., Schalm's Veterinary Hematology, 6th ed. Ames, IA: Wiley-Blackwell, 2010, pp. 654–660.

Author Marjory B. Brooks
Consulting Editor Melinda S. Camus

COAGULOPATHY OF LIVER DISEASE

C

BASICS

OVERVIEW

- The liver is the sole/primary site of synthesis of procoagulant, anticoagulant, and fibrinolytic proteins, except factors V, VIII, von Willebrand factor (vWF), tissue plasminogen activator (TPA).
- Some patients develop prolonged in vitro clotting times, but few exhibit spontaneous bleeding.
- Causes of hemostatic imbalance:
  - reduced synthesis or activation of procoagulant proteins;
  - vitamin K deficiency;
  - dysfibrinogenemia due to abnormal fibrin polymerization;
  - reduced clearance of fibrin/fibrinogen degradation products (FDP);
  - thrombocytopenia or thrombocytopathy;
  - enhanced fibrinolysis.
- Vitamin K deficiency—linked to severe intra- or extrahepatic cholestasis, steatorrhea, or prolonged oral antibiotic administration.

SIGNALMENT

Dog and cat of any age, breed, or sex.

SIGNS

- Often minor or absent.
- Melena, hematemesis, hematochezia, hematuria.
- Prolonged bleeding if provoked—venipuncture, cystocentesis, biopsy, surgical wounds.
- Spontaneous bruising/hematomas—rare unless severe vitamin K deficiency or fulminant disseminated intravascular coagulation (DIC).

CAUSES & RISK FACTORS

- Severe hepatic failure of any etiology.
- Acute viral liver disease.
- Extrahepatic bile duct obstruction (EHBDO).
- Chronic liver disease—especially cirrhosis.
- Concurrent small bowel disease (e.g., cats with cholangiohepatitis or hepatic lipidosis) predisposing to vitamin K deficiency.
- High central venous pressure (CVP) and portal hypertension.
- Portosystemic vascular anomaly (PSVA)—asymptomatic factor deficiency common; overt bleeding uncommon.

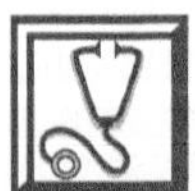

DIAGNOSIS

DIFFERENTIAL DIAGNOSIS

- Toxicities—see Hepatotoxins.
- Hereditary hemostatic defects.
- Thrombocytopenia.
- DIC—any cause.
- Hepatic amyloidosis.
- Abdominal trauma, gastrointestinal infiltrative disorders.

CBC/BIOCHEMISTRY/URINALYSIS

- CBC—normal or regenerative anemia; microcytosis; thrombocytopenia.
- Biochemistry—high liver enzymes; bilirubinemia; low albumin; hypoglobulinemia; low cholesterol.
- Urinalysis—hematuria; bilirubinuria.

OTHER LABORATORY TESTS

Hemostatic tests—thrombocytopenia; prolonged APTT (activated clotting time [ACT]), prothrombin time (PT), thrombin clotting time (TCT), and proteins induced by vitamin K absence (PIVKA); low fibrinogen and coagulation factors; low anticoagulant factors (antithrombin [AT], protein C); high FDP and D-dimer.

IMAGING

Abdominal Ultrasonography

- Effusion (ascites, hemorrhage).
- Liver changes—variable.
- Abnormal enteric motility, thickening in area of bleeding.

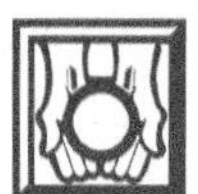

TREATMENT

- Not necessary unless invasive procedures planned or spontaneous hemorrhage noted.
- Fresh whole blood—provides replacement of red cells, coagulation factors, functional platelets.
- Fresh frozen plasma—provides coagulation factors, other hemostatic proteins, and reduces risk of red cell sensitization or volume overload.
- Cryoprecipitate—for severe hypofibrinogenemia or bleeding with coexistent von Willebrand's disease (vWD).
- Platelet-rich plasma—rarely indicated.
- Avoid synthetic colloids if bleeding tendencies observed.

Biopsy

- High risk for bleeding—PIVKA, PT, APTT, or ACT prolonged by >50%; thrombocytopenia <50,000/μL; prolonged mucosal bleeding time.
- Iatrogenic hemorrhage—grave prognosis if spontaneous bleeding with undetermined cause.
- Hemostasis support—postprocedure bleeding.
- Ultrasound-guided needle core—highest risk; observe biopsy site for 15 minutes, then sequentially over several hours postprocedure.
- Laparoscopy—affords visibility and allows hemostasis (cautery, Gelfoam pack biopsy site).
- Laparotomy—wedge biopsy; ill-advised in patients with overt bleeding.

MEDICATIONS

DRUG(S) OF CHOICE

- Based on cause of hepatic abnormality.
- Vitamin K deficiency—parenteral vitamin K_1 (0.5–1.5 mg/kg q12h SC up to 3 doses in 24h interval initially); vitamin K_1 PO (Mephyton®, 1 mg/kg q24h) if normal enteric bile acid uptake.
- DIC—correct primary disease; consider heparin for overt thrombosis (unfractionated heparin [UFH]: 200 U/kg q6–12h; or low molecular weight heparin [enoxaparin]: 1 mg/kg q12–24h), dose titration based on clinical status and laboratory monitoring (ACT, APTT [UFH], heparin anti-Xa activity [all heparins]).
- Blood products—fresh whole blood: 12–20 mL/kg q24h; fresh frozen plasma: 10–20 mL/kg q12h; plasma cryosupernatant (albumin, vitamin K–dependent factors): 10–20 mL/kg q12h; cryoprecipitate (fibrinogen, vWF, factor VIII): 1 U/10 kg or dose to effect.
- Desmopressin acetate (DDAVP)—0.5–1 μg/kg IV in saline; may increase coagulation factors, shortens bleeding times, reduces bleeding tendencies; empirically used for biopsy-induced bleeding.
- Antifibrinolytics—epsilon aminocaproic acid (EACA): 100 mg/kg loading, 30 mg/kg/h up to 8h; tranexamic acid: 25 mg/kg q8h; if evidence of hyperfibrinolysis.

CONTRAINDICATIONS/POSSIBLE INTERACTIONS

- Stored whole blood—may provoke hepatic encephalopathy (HE).
- Vitamin K_1 (cats)—high dose causes Heinz body hemolysis and oxidant liver injury.
- Aspirin or other nonsteroidal anti-inflammatory drugs (NSAIDs)—may predispose to renal failure, worsen ascites, provoke emesis and spontaneous bleeding,
- High-volume transfusion in citrate-based anticoagulants (especially in animals <5 kg) may induce symptomatic hypocalcemia.
- Avoid provocative procedures—e.g., jugular venipuncture or catheter placement, cystocentesis, if recognized bleeding tendencies.

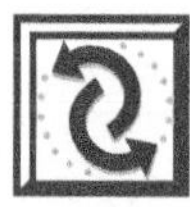

FOLLOW-UP

PATIENT MONITORING

- PT, PIVKA (limited availability), factor VII—most sensitive coagulation tests to detect vitamin K deficiency; if no improvement after 48h of vitamin K_1 injection, unlikely correction by further dosing.

- Heart rate, blood pressure, mucous membrane color and refill, packed cell volume (PCV), and total solids to monitor response if active bleeding.
- Biopsy site—observe immediately and sequentially (ultrasonography) for hemorrhage.
- Sample abdominal effusion to differentiate hemorrhage from ascites.

PREVENTION/AVOIDANCE

- Well-balanced diet replete with vitamins.
- Consider impaired vitamin K availability or synthesis from chronic oral antimicrobials.
- Invasive procedures—anticipate bleeding; pretreat with vitamin K_1; give DDAVP within 20 min of anticipated biopsy or if bleeding tendencies persist despite vitamin K_1 therapy (repeated DDAVP of no use); fresh frozen plasma for factor/fibrinogen replacement and active bleeding; avoid volume overload and increased CVP.
- Eliminate enteric parasitism.

POSSIBLE COMPLICATIONS

Hemorrhage, anemia, hypovolemia, HE.

EXPECTED COURSE AND PROGNOSIS

Spontaneous hemorrhage, refractory coagulopathy, and DIC—poor prognosis.

MISCELLANEOUS

SEE ALSO

- Hepatotoxins.

ABBREVIATIONS

- ACT = activated clotting time.
- APTT = activated partial thromboplastin time.
- AT = antithrombin.
- CVP = central venous pressure.
- DDAVP = desmopressin acetate.
- DIC = disseminated intravascular coagulation.
- EACA = epsilon aminocaproic acid.
- EHBDO = extrahepatic bile duct obstruction.
- FDP = fibrin/fibrinogen degradation product.
- HE = hepatic encephalopathy.
- NSAID = nonsteroidal anti-inflammatory drug.
- PCV = packed cell volume.
- PIVKA = proteins induced by vitamin K absence.
- PSVA = portosystemic vascular anomaly.
- PT = prothrombin time.
- TCT = thrombin clotting time.
- TPA = tissue plasminogen activator.
- UFH = unfractionated heparin.
- vWD = von Willebrand's disease.
- vWF = von Willebrand factor.

Author Marjory B. Brooks

Consulting Editor Kate Holan

COBALAMIN DEFICIENCY

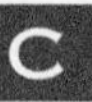

BASICS

OVERVIEW

• Cobalamin deficiency occurs in patients with cobalamin malabsorption when all body stores of cobalamin have been utilized and cobalamin is deficient on a cellular level.
• Cobalamin is required by virtually all cells in the body and plays a major role in beta-oxidation, conversion of certain amino acids, and the formation of tetrahydrofolate, and is thus crucial for energy production, amino acid metabolism, and DNA and RNA synthesis.
• Cobalamin deficiency is associated with gastrointestinal (GI) signs and systemic complications, such as immunodeficiencies, central neuropathies, and peripheral neuropathies.
• Cobalamin is absorbed exclusively in the ileum of dogs and cats via a receptor-mediated mechanism.
• The main causes of cobalamin deficiency in dogs and cats include chronic GI disease involving the ileum (e.g., inflammatory bowel disease, small intestinal dysbiosis, intestinal lymphoma), exocrine pancreatic insufficiency (EPI), short bowel syndrome, and, in rare cases, inherited cobalamin malabsorption or dietary deficiencies.

SIGNALMENT

• In the United States, Chinese Shar-Pei have a high prevalence of cobalamin deficiency. Isolated families of other breeds, such as the giant schnauzer, beagle, border collie, and Australian shepherd dog, have also been described as having cobalamin deficiency.
• No other breed, sex, or age predilections are known for canine or feline patients with cobalamin deficiency.

SIGNS

• Clinical signs attributable to the underlying disease process:
  ◦ Chronic enteropathy—diarrhea, weight loss, vomiting, poor appetite, or others.
  ◦ EPI—weight loss, failure to thrive, loose stools, steatorrhea, polyphagia or pica, borborygmus, flatulence.
• Clinical signs attributable to cobalamin deficiency—weight loss, failure to thrive, poor hair coat, lethargy, anorexia; less commonly signs of peripheral and central neuropathy such as a plantigrade stance or encephalopathy.

CAUSES & RISK FACTORS

• Intestinal disease involving the distal small intestine (i.e., the ileum)—inflammatory bowel disease, food-responsive enteropathy, lymphoma, others.
• EPI.
• Short bowel syndrome.
• Hereditary (Chinese Shar-Pei, giant schnauzer, beagle, border collie, Australian shepherd dog).
• Dietary—being fed exclusively vegan or vegetarian diet without concurrent supplementation.

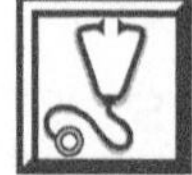

DIAGNOSIS

DIFFERENTIAL DIAGNOSIS

Other diseases causing chronic GI disease, immunosuppression, central neuropathies, or peripheral neuropathies.

CBC/BIOCHEMISTRY/URINALYSIS

• May be within normal limits.
• May show changes associated with underlying disease process (e.g., hypoalbuminemia in patients with severe inflammatory bowel disease).
• May show anemia, neutrophilia with left shift, or neutropenia. Rubricytes have been documented in cobalamin-deficient dogs and have been interpreted as evidence of ineffective erythropoiesis. Hypersegmented neutrophils can also be observed.

OTHER LABORATORY TESTS

• Serum and urine methylmalonic acid concentrations are increased in patients with cobalamin deficiency.
• Decreased or low normal serum cobalamin concentrations. Studies measuring methylmalonic acid in serum from dogs and cats have shown that patients with low normal serum cobalamin concentrations may be cobalamin deficient on a cellular level. Note that all assays used for the measurement of serum cobalamin concentration in dogs and cats have been developed for use in humans and thus must be analytically validated for dogs and cats before routine clinical use. In addition, each laboratory should develop specific reference intervals.

IMAGING

Not useful, other than for evaluation of underlying intestinal disease.

DIAGNOSTIC PROCEDURES

None for the diagnosis of cobalamin deficiency. However, intestinal biopsies may be useful to confirm and characterize chronic enteropathies.

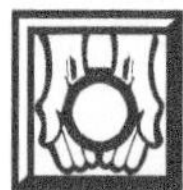

TREATMENT

Treatment of the underlying disease process, if identified (e.g., inflammatory bowel disease, EPI, lymphoma, small intestinal dysbiosis).

MEDICATIONS

DRUG(S) OF CHOICE

• Cobalamin supplements:
  ◦ Cyanocobalamin—usually at 1,000 µg/mL for parenteral use; or 1,000 µg tablets or 250 µg and 1000 µg chewable tablets for oral use.
  ◦ Hydroxocobalamin—usually at 1,000 µg/mL; for parenteral use.
  ◦ Methylcobalamin—usually 1 mg capsule; for oral use.
• Traditionally, cobalamin supplementation in cobalamin-deficient patients has been administered parenterally (usually SC) using cyanocobalamin or rarely hydroxocobalamin.
  ◦ Cats receive 250 µg/injection; dogs receive between 250 µg (small dog) and 1,500 µg (giant dog) per injection; doses should approximate 50 µg/kg per injection within this dose range.
  ◦ In either species there are 6 weekly injections, one more injection a month later, and reevaluation of serum cobalamin concentration a month later.
• Recent studies have shown that oral cobalamin supplementation with cyanocobalamin is equally efficacious regardless of the underlying cause of cobalamin deficiency.
  ◦ Cats receive 250 µg/day; dogs receive between 250 µg (small dog) and 1,000 µg (giant dog) per day.
  ◦ Reevaluation of serum cobalamin concentration 2–4 weeks after the last dose.
• Continue therapy at the original dosing scheme if serum cobalamin is still low; continue at a decreased interval if cobalamin is in the mid-normal range; discontinue if serum cobalamin is in the high end of the reference interval.

CONTRAINDICATIONS/POSSIBLE INTERACTIONS

None known.

FOLLOW-UP

Depending on the severity of the underlying disease process, the complications from cobalamin deficiency, and treatment response.

PATIENT MONITORING

• See above; reevaluation of serum cobalamin concentration either 1 month after the last cobalamin injection or 2–4 weeks after the last oral dose of cobalamin.
• Additional monitoring as required for the underlying disease process.

MISCELLANEOUS

SEE ALSO

- Diarrhea, Chronic—Cats.
- Diarrhea, Chronic—Dogs.
- Exocrine Pancreatic Insufficiency.
- Inflammatory Bowel Disease.
- Protein-Losing Enteropathy.

ABBREVIATIONS

- EPI = exocrine pancreatic insufficiency.
- GI = gastrointestinal.

INTERNET RESOURCES

http://vetmed.tamu.edu/gilab

Suggested Reading

Batchelor DJ, Noble P-JM, Taylor RH, et al. Prognostic factors in canine exocrine pancreatic insufficiency: prolonged survival is likely if clinical remission is achieved. J Vet Intern Med 2007, 21:54–60.

Berghoff N, Parnell NK, Hill SL, et al. Serum cobalamin and methylmalonic acid concentrations in dogs with chronic gastrointestinal disease. American J Vet Res 2013, 74:84–89.

Bishop MA, Xenoulis PG, Berghoff N, et al. Partial characterization of cobalamin deficiency in Chinese Shar-Peis. Vet J 2011, 191:41–45.

Maunder CL, Day MJ, Hibbert A, et al. Serum cobalamin concentrations in cats with gastrointestinal signs: correlation with histopathological findings and duration of clinical sigs. J Feline Med Surg 2012, 14:686–693.

Toresson L, Steiner JM, Suchodolski JS, et al. Oral cobalamin supplementation in dogs with chronic enteropathies and hypocobalaminemia. J Vet Intern Med 2016, 30:101–107.

Author Jörg M. Steiner
Consulting Editor Mark P. Rondeau

COCCIDIOIDOMYCOSIS

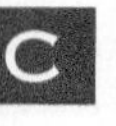

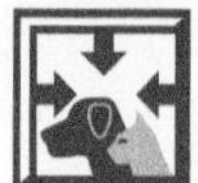

BASICS

DEFINITION

A systemic mycosis caused by the inhalation of infective arthroconidia of the soil-borne fungus *Coccidioides immitis*.

PATHOPHYSIOLOGY

• Grows in soil in the mycelial state.
• Inhalation of infective arthroconidia is the primary route of infection; at body temperature, all but one nucleus is shed and an immature spherule is produced within 2–3 days. • Spherule matures and ruptures, releasing 200–300 endospores that can produce new spherules. • Neutrophils cannot penetrate the spherule wall but can phagocytize the endospores. • Fewer than 10 inhaled arthrospores are sufficient to cause disease in susceptible animals. • Respiratory signs are often noted 1–3 weeks after exposure; signs of dissemination may not be evident for several months. • Most infections are mild or subclinical, although dogs appear more susceptible than cats to development of disseminated disease. • Fever, lethargy, inappetence, coughing, and joint pain or stiffness may be noticed. • Dissemination may occur within 10 days, resulting in signs related to the organ system involved; skin lesions are usually associated with dissemination.

SYSTEMS AFFECTED

• Respiratory—site of initial infection.
• Extrapulmonary—musculoskeletal, ophthalmic, cardiovascular, skin, neuromuscular, reproductive, and visceral organs.

INCIDENCE/PREVALENCE

Not an uncommon disease in endemic areas, rare in nonendemic areas. It occurs more commonly in dogs and rarely in cats.

GEOGRAPHIC DISTRIBUTION

• *C. immitis* is found in the southwestern United States in the geographic Lower Sonoran life zone. • More common in southern California, Arizona, and southwest Texas. • Less prevalent in New Mexico, Nevada, and Utah.

SIGNALMENT

Species

Dog and cat.

Breed Predilections

None

Mean Age and Range

Though most commonly diagnosed in young animals (<4 years of age), it is seen in animals of all ages.

Predominant Sex

None

SIGNS

Historical Findings

• Coughing (ranges from dry/harsh to wet/productive). • Fever unresponsive to antibiotics. • Anorexia, weight loss. • Weakness, lameness (bone or joint involvement).
• Seizures, paraparesis, back and neck pain (CNS involvement). • Visual changes (ophthalmic involvement).

Physical Examination Findings

Dogs

• Signs with pulmonary involvement—coughing and dyspnea. • Fever. • Bone swelling, joint enlargement, and lameness.
• Lymphadenomegaly, skin lesions, and draining tracts. • Neurologic dysfunction including ataxia, spinal or cranial nerve deficits, and behavioral changes. • Blindness, uveitis, keratitis, and iritis.

Cats

Like dogs, although skin lesions are most common type of infection in cats.

CAUSES

C. immitis grows several inches deep in the soil, where it survives high ambient temperatures and low moisture. After a period of rainfall, the organism returns to the soil surface where it sporulates, releasing many arthroconidia that disseminate by wind and dust storms.

RISK FACTORS

• Aggressive nosing in contaminated soil and underbrush may expose susceptible animals to large numbers of arthroconidia. • Dust storms after the rainy season; increased incidence noted after earthquakes. • Land development with earth disruption may lead to increased exposure.

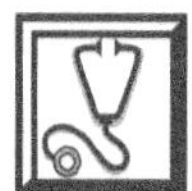

DIAGNOSIS

DIFFERENTIAL DIAGNOSIS

• Pulmonary lesions may resemble those of other systemic mycoses (e.g., histoplasmosis, blastomycosis) or neoplasia (single mass or multiple nodules). • Lymphadenomegaly may be seen in lymphoma, other systemic mycoses, and localized bacterial infections. • Bone lesions may resemble those caused by primary or metastatic bone tumors or bacterial osteomyelitis. • Skin lesions must be differentiated from routine abscesses or other infective processes. • For seizures and ataxia, consider inflammatory and neoplastic etiologies.

CBC/BIOCHEMISTRY/URINALYSIS

• Hemogram—mild nonregenerative anemia, neutrophilic leukocytosis, monocytosis.
• Serum chemistry profile—hyperglobulinemia, hypoalbuminemia, other changes may be consistent with organ of involvement.
• Urinalysis—proteinuria with inflammatory glomerulonephritis.

OTHER LABORATORY TESTS

• Serologic tests (generally by agar gel immunodiffusion [AGID] or ELISA) for antibody to *C. immitis* may provide a presumptive diagnosis; may aid in monitoring response to therapy. • Antigen testing has not proven to be sensitive.

IMAGING

• Radiography of lung (interstitial infiltrates, granulomas, tracheobronchial lymphadenopathy) and bone lesions (osteolysis) may aid in diagnosis. • MRI may help in diagnosing granulomas in the CNS.

DIAGNOSTIC PROCEDURES

• Serologic testing; repeat serology titers in 4–6 weeks when low titers are accompanied by clinical signs. • Microscopic identification of the large spherule form of *C. immitis* in lesion or biopsy material is the definitive method of diagnosis (large 10–80 μm round, double-walled structure containing endospores).
• Lymph node aspirates and impression smears of skin lesions or draining exudate may yield organisms. • Cultures should be performed by trained laboratory personnel using protective hoods. • Biopsy of infected tissue often is preferred to avoid false-negative results; tissues involved, however, may not be readily accessible and finding the organism can be challenging; therefore, serologic testing is often a more logical approach.

PATHOLOGIC FINDINGS

• Granulomatous, suppurative, or pyogranulomatous inflammation present in many tissues. • Presence of the characteristic spherule forms in affected tissues.

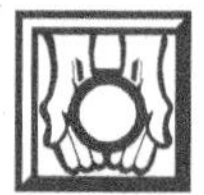

TREATMENT

APPROPRIATE HEALTH CARE

• Generally treated as outpatient.
• Concurrent clinical symptoms (e.g., seizures, pain, coughing) should be treated appropriately.

ACTIVITY

Restrict activity until clinical signs begin to subside.

DIET

Feed a high-quality palatable diet to maintain body weight.

CLIENT EDUCATION

• Treatment is potentially long (>6–9 months) and expensive. • Relapse (especially with disseminated disease) is common.
• Reassure client that infection is not zoonotic.

SURGICAL CONSIDERATIONS

In cases of focal granulomatous organ involvement (e.g., consolidated pulmonary lung lobe, eye, kidney), surgical removal of the affected organ may be indicated.

C

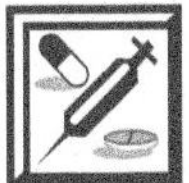

MEDICATIONS

DRUG(S) OF CHOICE

Coccidioidomycosis is considered one of the most severe and life-threatening of the systemic mycoses. Treatment of disseminated disease often requires at least 1 year of aggressive antifungal therapy.

Dogs

- Ketoconazole (KTZ)—5–10 mg/kg PO q12h; ideally given with food; treatment typically requires at least 1 year of therapy; if titers rise or clinical signs deteriorate over first 4–6 weeks of treatment, alternative therapy should be considered. • Fluconazole (FCZ)—10 mg/kg PO q12h; noted to greatly increase success of treatment; cost of the drug has significantly decreased with availability of medical-grade generic compound; treatment failures have been noted with use of chemical-grade compounded formulations.
- Itraconazole (ITZ)—5 mg/kg PO q12h; administered similarly to KTZ, it has been reported to have higher penetration rate than KTZ; some suggest greater efficacy of ITZ over FCZ. • Amphotericin B (AMB) is rarely recommended because most patients do not require this aggressive therapy and effective oral medications are readily available; AMB can be administered at a dosage of 0.5 mg/kg IV 3 times per week, for a total cumulative dosage of 8–10 mg/kg; given IV either as a slow infusion (in dogs that are gravely ill) or as a rapid bolus (in fairly healthy dogs); for slow infusion, add AMB to 250–500 mL of 5% dextrose solution and administer as a drip over 4–6 hours; to lessen adverse renal effects of AMB, consider 0.9% NaCl (2 mL/kg/h) for several hours before initiating AMB therapy.

Cats

Any of the following azoles may be used in cats: KTZ 50 mg total dose PO q12h; FCZ 25–50 mg total dose PO q12h; ITZ 25–50 mg total dose PO q12h.

CONTRAINDICATIONS

- Drugs metabolized primarily by the liver should be used with caution alongside azole drugs.
- Drugs metabolized primarily by the kidneys should be used with caution alongside AMB.

PRECAUTIONS

- Side effects of azoles include inappetence, vomiting, and hepatotoxicity (typically alanine transaminase [ALT] > alkaline phosphatase [ALP]); liver values should be monitored monthly initially; drugs may be stopped until signs abate and restarted at a lower dose, which may be slowly increased to the recommended dose if the animal is able to tolerate the drug; newer azoles (ITZ and FCZ) have fewer side effects. • Side effects of AMB therapy can be severe, especially renal dysfunction, fever; use with caution if patient is azotemic, but not an absolute contraindication if the infection is life-threatening.

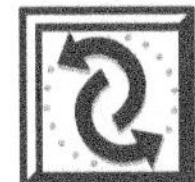

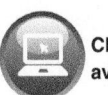

FOLLOW-UP

PATIENT MONITORING

- Serologic titers should be monitored every 3–4 months; animals should be treated until clinical and radiographic signs resolve/stabilize and their titers ideally fall to less than 1 : 4; titers frequently do not become negative throughout treatment. • Consider ITZ levels (2–4h post pill) in patients showing poor response to ITZ therapy, especially if using generic or compounded formulation.
- Creatinine and urinalysis should be monitored in all animals treated with AMB; treatment should be temporarily discontinued if creatinine rises above reference range or greater than 20% above baseline, or if granular casts are noted in urine.

PREVENTION/AVOIDANCE

- No vaccine is available for dogs or cats.
- Contaminated soil in endemic areas should be avoided, particularly during dust storms after the rainy season.

POSSIBLE COMPLICATIONS

Pulmonary disease resulting in severe coughing may temporarily worsen after therapy is begun owing to inflammation in the lungs. Anti-inflammatory short-term (2 weeks to 2 months) oral prednisone and cough suppressants may be required to alleviate the respiratory signs.

EXPECTED COURSE AND PROGNOSIS

- Prognosis for localized respiratory disease is good. • Prognosis for disseminated disease is guarded; many dogs will improve following oral therapy with resolution of signs reported in up to 90% cases; however, relapses may be common, especially if therapy is shortened; overall recovery rate has been estimated at 60%. • Prognosis with CNS involvement may be guarded to poor. • Prognosis for cats is not well documented, but long-term therapy should be anticipated and relapses are common. • Serologic testing every 3–4 months after completion of therapy is recommended to monitor possibility of rising titer and potential relapse. • Spontaneous recovery from disseminated coccidioidomycosis without treatment is extremely rare.

MISCELLANEOUS

ZOONOTIC POTENTIAL

- The spherule form of the fungus, as found in animal tissues, is not directly transmissible to humans or to other animals. • Under certain rare circumstances, however, there could be reversion to growth of the infective mold form of the fungus on or within bandages placed over a draining lesion or in contaminated bedding; draining lesions can lead to contamination of the environment with arthrospores; care should be exercised whenever handling an infected draining lesion. • Special precautions should be recommended to households in which the owners may be immunosuppressed.

PREGNANCY/FERTILITY/BREEDING

Azole drugs can be teratogenic and should be used in pregnant animals only if the potential benefit justifies the potential risk to offspring.

SYNONYMS

- Desert rheumatism (in humans).
- San Joaquin Valley fever. • Valley fever.

ABBREVIATIONS

- AGID = agar gel immunodiffusion.
- ALP = alkaline phosphatase.
- ALT = alanine transaminase.
- AMB = amphotericin B.
- FCZ = fluconazole.
- ITZ = itraconazole.
- KTZ = ketoconazole.

Suggested Reading

Arbona N, Butkiewicz CD, Keyes M, et al. Clinical features of cats diagnosed with coccidioidomycosis in Arizona, 2004–2018. J Feline Med Surg 2020, 22(2):129–137.

Graupmann-Kuzma A, Valentine BA, Shubitz LF, et al. Coccidioidomycosis in dogs and cats: a review. J Am Anim Hosp Assoc 2008, 44:226–235.

Johnson LR, Herrgesell EJ, Davidson AP, et al. Clinical, clinicopathologic, and radiographic findings in dogs with coccidioidomycosis: 24 cases (1995–2000). J Am Vet Med Assoc 2003, 222:461–466.

Shubitz LE, Butkiewicz CD, Dial SM, et al. Incidence of coccidioides infection among dogs residing in a region in which the organism is endemic. J Am Vet Med Assoc 2005, 226:1846–1850.

Author Daniel S. Foy

Consulting Editor Amie Koenig

Client Education Handout available online

COCCIDIOSIS

BASICS

OVERVIEW

- An enteric infection, traditionally associated with *Cystoisospora canis* (dogs) and *Cystoisospora felis* (cats) as potential pathogens; other species of *Cystoisospora* may be present.
- Strictly host specific (i.e., no cross-transmission).
- *Eimeria* spp. are not parasitic for dogs or cats.
- *Cryptosporidium* can cause an acute, life-threatening coccidiosis (cryptosporidiosis) in neonatal pups and kittens; can also cause non-life-threatening small bowel diarrhea in dogs and cats (see Cryptosporidiosis)
- Voluminous watery diarrhea is characteristic; auto-infection and recycling within the intestinal tract result in a rapid loss of mucosal lining with cryptosporidiosis.

SIGNALMENT

Dog and cat (especially puppies and kittens).

SIGNS

- Watery to mucoid, sometimes blood-tinged, diarrhea; vomiting; abdominal discomfort; inappetence.
- Weak puppies and kittens.
- Immunocompromised animals.

CAUSES & RISK FACTORS

- Infected dogs or cats contaminating environment with oocysts of *Cystoisospora* spp. or *Cryptosporidium* spp.
- Stress.
- Immunocompromise.

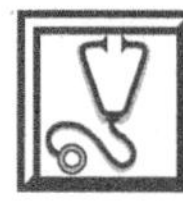

DIAGNOSIS

DIFFERENTIAL DIAGNOSIS

Enteric viral infections and other intestinal parasites.

CBC/BIOCHEMISTRY/URINALYSIS

Usually unremarkable; may be hemoconcentrated if dehydrated.

OTHER LABORATORY TESTS

N/A

IMAGING

N/A

DIAGNOSTIC PROCEDURES

- Fecal flotation (preferably centrifugation flotation technique) for oocysts (distinguish from pseudoparasitic *Eimeria* sp.); use sucrose solution or zinc sulfate; acid-fast stains should be considered for detection of *Cryptosporidium* spp.
- Direct fluorescent antibody (DFA) assay is a sensitive dual assay (can detect *Giardia* cysts and *Cryptosporidium* oocysts very well) and can be performed at reference laboratories or university parasitology laboratories.
- *Cystoisospora* oocysts should be 40 µm long; cysts of *Cryptosporidium* are approximately 5 µm diameter.

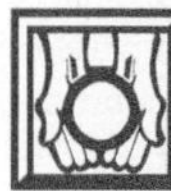

TREATMENT

- Usually treated as an outpatient.
- Inpatient if debilitated.
- Fluid therapy if dehydrated.

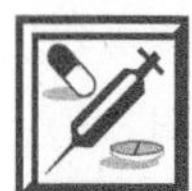

MEDICATIONS

DRUG(S) OF CHOICE

- Sulfadimethoxine—55 mg/kg PO on the first day, then 25–50 mg/kg PO q24h for up to 10–14 days, or until dog is asymptomatic for *Cystoisospora* and fecal examination is negative for oocysts.
- Sulfadiazine/trimethoprim—15–30 mg/kg sulfadiazine PO q24h up to 10 days.
- Amprolium (extra-label)—dogs: 100–400 mg (total dose) PO q24h for 7 days; cats with *Cystoisospora*: 60–100 mg (total dose) PO q24h for 7 days.
- No effective or approved treatment for *Cryptosporidium*—paromomycin 165 mg/kg PO q12h for 5 days has been suggested (extra-label); however, the drug is potentially nephrotoxic and ototoxic in cats and should not be used; azithromycin has been used at a dosage of 7–10 mg/kg PO q12h for 7 days for eradication of *Cryptosporidium* spp. in dogs and cats; however, efficacy is unknown.
- Ponazuril at 30–50 mg/kg PO q24h for 1–7 consecutive days in dogs, or 15 mg/kg PO q24h for 7 consecutive days in cats; treatment can be repeated after 3- to 5-day break to increase efficacy; single doses of the drug are generally ineffective.
- Toltrazuril—10–30 mg/kg PO q24h for 1–6 consecutive days in dogs.

Precautions

- Mild gastrointestinal upset with antibiotics.
- Amprolium—not recommended to be used for more than 12 consecutive days in puppies, exogenous thiamine in high doses may decrease efficacy; neurologic abnormalities have been reported in some dogs: if observed, discontinue medication and begin thiamine supplementation.
- Sulfadimethoxine—caution with diminished hepatic or renal function.
- Sulfadiazine/trimethoprim—potentially teratogenic; dog: associated with irreversible keratoconjunctivitis sicca, type 1 or type 3 hypersensitivity (especially in larger-breed dogs), thrombocytopenia; cat: anorexia, leukopenia, anemia, hematuria.

CONTRAINDICATIONS/POSSIBLE INTERACTIONS

Sulfa medications—caution in patients with preexisting renal or hepatic disease.

FOLLOW-UP

Fecal flotation (for *Cystoisospora* spp. oocysts) or DFA (for *Cryptosporidium* spp. oocysts) 1–2 weeks following treatment.

MISCELLANEOUS

AGE-RELATED FACTORS

More severe disease in young or immunocompromised patients.

SEE ALSO

- Cryptosporidiosis.
- Toxoplasmosis.

ABBREVIATIONS

- DFA = direct fluorescent antibody.

Suggested Reading

Bowman DD, Lynn RC, Eberhard ML. Georgis' Parasitology for Veterinarians, 8th ed. St. Louis, MO: Saunders (Elsevier Science), 2003, pp. 92–100.

Dubey JP, Greene CE. Enteric coccidiosis. In: Greene CE, ed., Infectious Diseases of the Dog and Cat, 4th ed. St. Louis, MO: Elsevier Saunders, 2012, pp. 828–839.

Lappin, MR. Update on the diagnosis and management of *Isospora* spp. infections in dogs and cats. Top Companion Anim Med 2010, 25(3):133–135.

Author Gavin L. Olsen
Consulting Editor Amie Koenig

COGNITIVE DYSFUNCTION SYNDROME

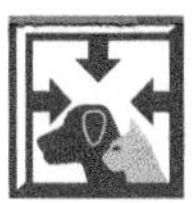

BASICS

DEFINITION

Syndrome associated with brain aging. Leads to alterations in awareness, decreased responsiveness to stimuli, deficits in learning and memory, agitation, and anxiety. Subtle signs seen in early stages of cognitive decline may include alterations in activity, social interactions and increasing anxiety.

PATHOPHYSIOLOGY

• Neuronal loss, decreased frontal lobe volume, increased ventricular volume, and neurotoxic deposits including lipofuscin and beta-amyloid. • Toxic free radicals (reactive oxygen species) increase with age because of illness and stressors, age-related decline in mitochondrial efficiency, and decreased clearance mechanisms. • Unclear which changes are associated with the clinical signs; possible correlation between cognitive decline, amount of beta-amyloid in the cerebral cortex, and increases in toxic free radicals. • Compromised cerebral vascular blood flow and infarcts may be contributory. • Neurotransmission is compromised; may be a decline in catecholamine and cholinergic transmission.

SYSTEMS AFFECTED

• Behavioral. • Nervous.

GENETICS

Unknown; may be genetic factors contributing to beta-amyloid deposition and the age at which it begins to accumulate.

INCIDENCE/PREVALENCE

• Clinical signs of cognitive dysfunction syndrome (CDS) have been reported to arise in 41–68% (or higher) of dogs over 14. • Overall prevalence in dogs over 10 estimated as at least 14.2%. • Clinical signs reported to arise in 50% of cats over 15. • Prevalence in cats over 10 estimated at 35%. • Progressive—over 6 months, 24% of dogs with mild signs progressed to moderate and 42% with no impairment progressed to mild.

SIGNALMENT

Species

Dogs and cats.

Mean Age and Range

• Increased prevalence with increasing age. • Neuropsychological testing in dogs and cats has identified a decline in memory and learning as early as 6–8 years of age. • Initial signs may not be noticed by pet owners, except perhaps in dogs trained to perform more specialized tasks (e.g., guide and hearing dogs, drug detection, agility).

SIGNS

Historical Findings

• Clinical signs have been categorized using the acronym DISHAA. • **D**isorientation, including getting lost in familiar environments, confusion, inability to navigate through familiar routes (e.g., goes to hinge side of door), dropping food and not retrieving. • **I**nteractions with humans or other animals may be altered (irritability, decreased interest in play/affection, or increased attention seeking). • **S**leep–wake cycle alterations including night waking, vocalization, and/or increased sleep during the day. • **H**ousetraining and other previously learned behaviors might deteriorate. • **A**ctivity may be altered—including a decline in activity level, exploration, and self-care; however, as the condition progresses, activity may increase with signs of restlessness, pacing, aimless wandering, vocalization, or excessive licking. • **A**nxiety and agitation.

Physical Examination

• No specific abnormalities associated with cognitive dysfunction. • Other age-related medical disorders might be noted.

CAUSES

• Exact cause is unknown and animals are variably affected. • Environmental factors may contribute to age-related degeneration. • May be predisposing genetic factors. • Diet, enrichment, and stress management may be in part preventive. • See Pathophysiology.

RISK FACTORS

• Chronic oxidative stress and chronic low-grade inflammation. • Conditions that affect cerebral vascular blood supply (e.g., systemic hypertension, anemia). • Deficiency in docosahexaenoic acid (DHA), B6, B12, and folic acid, high homocysteine, low-quality diets.

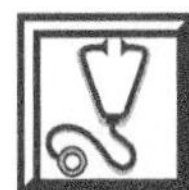

DIAGNOSIS

DIFFERENTIAL DIAGNOSIS

• Any medical condition that affects the pet's mental attitude or behavior must be ruled out. • Pain (e.g., arthritis, dental disease) can lead to increased irritability, anxiety, and altered response to stimuli. • If mobility is affected, the pet may be less able to avoid fearful stimuli and less able to access its elimination area. • Impaired sight or hearing might lead to decreased responsiveness or increased reactivity to stimuli. • Diseases of the urinary or gastrointestinal tract can cause house-soiling. • Organ failure, tumors, immune diseases, and endocrinopathies can also affect behavior. • Diseases that affect the CNS or its circulation can affect behavior.

CBC/BIOCHEMICAL/URINALYSIS

Normal with CDS, but concurrent disease processes common in aged dogs.

OTHER LABORATORY TESTS

Normal with CDS.

IMAGING

• Used to rule out primary organic/structural cause. • Most important when there are abnormalities on the neurologic examination or when the onset is sudden; less likely to be of diagnostic value if signs are slowly progressive in the absence of other neurologic findings.

DIAGNOSTIC PROCEDURES

• Diagnosis is based on identifying clinical signs on screening questionnaire, e.g., DISHAA (Pan et al.), CADEs (Madari et al.), and CCDR (Salvin et al.), ruling out possible medical causes. • Early and mild signs not likely to be reported; therefore veterinarians must ask (e.g., with screening questionnaire). • Endoscopy, radiography, ultrasound, and other specialized diagnostic procedures may be necessary to rule out other causes of the clinical signs. • Further ophthalmic and neurologic assessment if indicated to rule out visual or auditory deficits and neurologic disease. • Therapeutic trial might be considered to rule out and treat other potential causes of the signs, e.g., pain.

PATHOLOGIC FINDINGS

Loss of frontal and temporal lobe volume, neuronal loss, meningeal calcification, microhemorrhage and infarcts, beta-amyloid deposition and hyperphosphorylated tau.

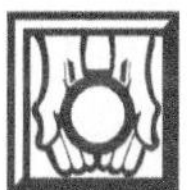

TREATMENT

NURSING CARE

Support and home care by pet owners.

ACTIVITY

• Maintain exercise, play, reward-based training, work, feeding enrichment (e.g., food-filled toys), and daily routines that are appropriate for the pet's age and health. • Maintaining mental stimulation and physical activity have been shown to reduce or slow progression of cognitive decline.

DIET

• Diet should be fed that meets and prioritizes medical and cognitive health care needs. • For dogs, diet supplemented with antioxidants including vitamins E and C, selenium, beta carotene, and flavonoids and carotenoids, omega-3 fatty acids, and carnitine and alpha lipoic acid (for mitochondrial health) has been shown to improve memory, learning ability, and clinical signs of cognitive dysfunction (Hills Prescription Diet b/d). • As cerebral glucose metabolism declines with increasing age in dogs, a diet supplemented with 5.5% medium-chain triglyceride (MCT) oil to provide ketone bodies as an alternative source of energy for aging neurons has been demonstrated to improve cognitive function in middle-aged and senior dogs (e.g., Purina ProPlan Bright Mind 7+®). • A brain support blend containing arginine (to enhance nitrous oxide synthesis), antioxidants including vitamins C, E, and selenium; B vitamins; and omega-3 fatty acids has been demonstrated to improve cognitive function in laboratory studies in senior dogs and middle-aged cats. • A combination of the brain support blend and 6.5% MCT supplementation has been demonstrated to improve clinical signs of cognitive dysfunction in dogs (Purina Pro Plan Veterinary Diets NC NeuroCare®). • For dogs—supplements containing phosphatidylserine (Senilife, CEVA Animal Health and Activait, VetPlus), S-adenosyl-L-methionine-tosylate disulfate (SAMe; Novifit, Virbac Animal Health), and apoaequorin have demonstrated some evidence of efficacy. • For cats—SAMe and diets containing fish oil, arginine, B vitamins, and antioxidants have demonstrated beneficial effects.

CLIENT EDUCATION

• Lifelong therapy is required, and concurrent medications may be necessary if the pet has multiple problems. • Any changes in the pet's health or behavior should be reported immediately, as this may be due to cognitive dysfunction or new health problems. • Considering the pet's health and cognitive status, the owner must be advised on any limitations on what might be achieved. • Signs are generally progressive; treatment is aimed at slowing the progression of the disease, not cure.

MEDICATIONS

DRUG(S) OF CHOICE

Dogs

• Selegiline—monoamine oxidase (MAO) B inhibitor, may contribute to improved catecholamine transmission, decrease in free radicals, and neuroprotective effect; 0.5–1 mg/kg PO q24h in the morning and maintained if effective; reevaluate clinical signs for improvement after 1–2 months; side effects might include occasional gastrointestinal upset and restlessness, and repetitive behavior at higher doses.
• Propentofylline—not licensed in North America but is licensed in other countries; xanthine derivative; purported to inhibit platelet aggregation and thrombus formation, make the red cells more pliable, and increase blood flow; may increase oxygen supply to CNS without increasing glucose demand; 3–5 mg/kg PO q12h.
• Nicergoline—alpha-adrenergic antagonist that may improve cognitive function through vasodilatory effects on cerebral circulation; 0.25–0.5 mg/kg PO q24h.

Cats

• No therapeutic agents licensed for treatment of CDS. • Selegiline (0.5–1 mg/kg PO q24h), propentofylline (1/4 of 50 mg tablet PO q24h), and nicergoline (0.25–0.5 mg/kg PO q24h) have been used off-label in cats, with anecdotal evidence of effect.

CONTRAINDICATIONS

• Selegiline should not be used concurrently with MAO inhibitors such as amitraz, narcotics, alpha-adrenergic agents such as phenylpropanolamine or ephedrine, or selective serotonin reuptake inhibitors (e.g., fluoxetine) or tricyclic antidepressants (e.g., clomipramine). • A 2-week washout is suggested following most tricyclic antidepressants and up to 5 weeks following fluoxetine before starting selegiline.

PRECAUTIONS

• Choose medications that are least sedating and least anticholinergic. • Potential drug interactions must be considered with concurrent use of drugs and over-the-counter medications.

POSSIBLE INTERACTIONS

See Contraindications.

ALTERNATIVE DRUG(S)

• Consider potential benefits vs. risks including contraindications, side effects, off-label use, and evidence of effect. • Anti-inflammatory medications and natural supplements such as gingko biloba and curcumin might be considered based on preliminary work in other species.
• Medication used in humans for Alzheimer's disease to enhance cholinergic transmission might be useful, but doses and pharmacokinetics in dogs have not been determined; side effects might include nausea, vomiting, diarrhea, and sleep-wake disturbances. • For anxiety, agitation, apathy, and night waking consider adjunctive therapeutics including buspirone or fluoxetine for ongoing use, or trazodone, benzodiazepines, and alpha-2 agonists for as needed use. • Natural supplements including pheromones, melatonin, valerian, l-theanine, alpha-casozepine, γ-aminobutyric acid (GABA), magnolia and phellodendron (Solliquin®), or Souroubea (Zentrol®) might help to reduce signs related to anxiety and night-time waking.

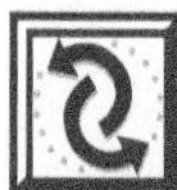

FOLLOW-UP

PATIENT MONITORING

• If a drug or diet for CDS is dispensed, therapeutic response should be evaluated after 30–60 days and the dose adjusted or treatment changed if there is insufficient improvement. • If the pet is stable, twice-yearly checkups are recommended unless new problems arise before reassessment is due.

PREVENTION/AVOIDANCE

• Providing an enriched environment, ongoing training, and physical activity that is appropriate and practical for the pet's age and health may help to prevent or delay the onset of cognitive decline. • Early CDS dietary intervention may address risk factors and slow the progression of disease.

EXPECTED COURSE AND PROGNOSIS

Diet and medication may improve signs and slow progression in most cases; however, with increasing age, CDS may progress and other concurrent health problems will ultimately arise.

MISCELLANEOUS

SYNONYMS

• Age-related cognitive and affective disorders, involutional depression, dysthymia.
• Dementia. • Senility.

ABBREVIATIONS

• CDS = cognitive dysfunction syndrome.
• DHA = docosahexaenoic acid. • GABA = γ-aminobutyric acid. • MAO = monoamine oxidase. • MCT = medium-chain triglyceride.
• SAMe = S-adenosyl-L-methionine-tosylate disulfate.

Suggested Reading

Landsberg GM, Madari A, Zilka N., eds. Canine and Feline Dementia: Molecular Basis, Diagnostics, and Therapy. Cham: Springer, 2017.

Madari A, Farbakova J, Katina S, et al. Assessment of severity and progression of canine cognitive dysfunction syndrome using the Canine Dementia Scale (CADES). Appl Anim Behav Sci 2015, 17:138–145.

Pan Y, Landsberg G, Mougeot I, et al. Efficacy of a therapeutic diet on dogs with signs of cognitive dysfunction syndrome (CDS): a prospective double blinded placebo controlled clinical trial. Front Nutr, 2018, doi: 10.3389/fnut.2018.00127.

Salvin HE, McGreevy PD, Sachdev PS, et al. The canine cognitive dysfunction rating scale (CCDR): a data-driven and ecologically relevant assessment tool. Vet J 2011, 188:331–336.

Authors Gary M. Landsberg and Sagi Denenberg

Consulting Editor Gary M. Landsberg

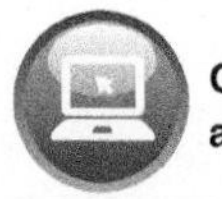

Client Education Handout available online

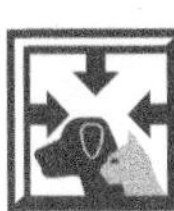

BASICS

OVERVIEW

- Rare type II autoimmune disorder in which anti-erythrocyte antibodies have enhanced activity at temperatures <99 °F (37.2 °C).
- Cold agglutinins are typically immunoglobulin (Ig) M, although IgG alone and in combination with IgM may result in disease.
- Cold agglutinins cause direct erythrocyte agglutination at low body temperatures (primarily peripheral microvasculature), leading to vaso-occlusive disease, initiated or intensified by cold exposure.
- Fixation of complement and hemolysis is a warm reactive process occurring at higher body temperatures; at those temperatures cold agglutinins have eluted off the red blood cells (RBCs), lowering the rate of complement binding; therefore, acute hemolytic anemias are uncommon with this condition.
- Most cold agglutinins cause little or no shortening of erythrocyte lifespan.
- High thermal amplitude cold agglutinins (rare)—may cause mild chronic hemolysis, but exposure to cold may greatly augment binding of cold agglutinins and cause intravascular hemolysis.

SIGNALMENT

- Rare; genetics, age, breed, and sex predilections unknown.
- Low titer of cold agglutinins (1 : 32 or less) may be found in healthy pets without clinical significance.
- More likely to occur following exposure to cold temperatures.

SIGNS

- Cyanosis of the extremities associated with sludging of erythrocyte agglutinates in microvasculature.
- Erythema, skin ulceration with secondary crusting.
- Dry, gangrenous necrosis of ear tips, tail tip, nose, and feet.
- Anemia may cause signs of pallor, tachycardia, tachypnea, icterus, and pigmenturia.

CAUSES & RISK FACTORS

- Idiopathic; cold exposure is a risk factor.
- Secondary disease—associated with upper respiratory infection (cats), neonatal isoerythrolysis, lead intoxication (dogs), *Mycoplasma* pneumonia, and neoplasia.

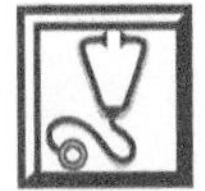

DIAGNOSIS

DIFFERENTIAL DIAGNOSIS

- Skin lesions—vasculitis, hepatocutaneous syndrome, toxic epidermal necrolysis, dermatomyositis, systemic lupus erythematosus (SLE), lymphoma, frostbite, lead poisoning, and pemphigus.
- Other causes of anemia (including hemolytic anemias).

CBC/BIOCHEMISTRY/URINALYSIS

- Laboratory abnormalities secondary to hemolysis, if present.
- Autoagglutination of RBCs may be observed at room temperature.

OTHER LABORATORY TESTS

- Cold agglutinins should be suspected when blood in heparin or EDTA on a glass slide agglutinates spontaneously at room temperature with enhancement at 39 °F (3.9 °C), and the erythrocytes disperse again upon warming to 99 °F (37.2 °C).
- If no agglutination can be induced in vitro, it will not occur in vivo in extremities.
- Coombs' test at 99 °F—cold agglutinins usually not detected because they may be eluted off the erythrocytes during washing; thus test requires the use of anti-complement factor serum.
- Coombs' test at 39 °F—incidence of a positive result in healthy dogs has been reported to be >50%, which may be caused by unspecific binding of the reagent itself or by binding of naturally occurring nonpathogenic low-titer cold agglutinins.
- The globulin class can be established by immunoelectrophoresis of the patient's erythrocytes, which may be important for prognosis and treatment.

PATHOLOGIC FINDINGS

- Dermal necrosis and ulceration with possible opportunistic infections.
- Vascular thrombosis, ischemic necrosis.

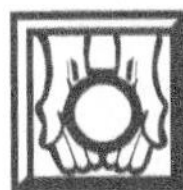

TREATMENT

- Hospitalization in a warm environment until the disease is nonprogressive.
- Supportive care and wound management.
- Splenectomy is of little benefit in patients with IgM-mediated hemolysis, but may be helpful in those with IgG-mediated hemolysis.
- Inform the client to keep the patient in a warm environment at all times to prevent relapse.
- Exercise restriction.
- In humans, plasmapheresis, IV gamma globulins, and rituximab with or without fludarabine have been tried.

MEDICATIONS

DRUG(S) OF CHOICE

- IgM cold agglutinins—immunosuppressive therapy not very effective against IgM-mediated disorders, but can be tried (i.e., corticosteroids, leflunomide, cyclosporine).
- IgG cold agglutinins—immunosuppressive therapy.

CONTRAINDICATIONS/POSSIBLE INTERACTIONS

Use warmed IV fluids if indicated.

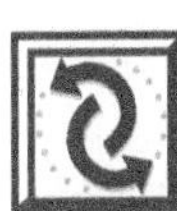

FOLLOW-UP

- Keep patient in warm environments.
- Cold agglutinin disease usually characterized by acute onset and rapid progression.
- Prognosis is guarded to fair; recovery may take weeks.

MISCELLANEOUS

SEE ALSO

Anemia, Immune-Mediated.

ABBREVIATIONS

- Ig = immunoglobulin.
- RBC = red blood cell.
- SLE = systemic lupus erythematosus.

Suggested Reading

Dickson NJ. Cold agglutinin disease in a puppy associated with lead intoxication. J Small Anim Pract 1990, 31:105–108.

Author Jörg Bucheler

Consulting Editor Melinda S. Camus

COLIBACILLOSIS

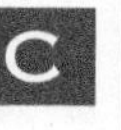

BASICS

DEFINITION

- *Escherichia coli* (EC)—Gram-negative member of the *Enterobacteriaceae*; normal inhabitant of intestine of most mammals.
- Acute infection of puppies and kittens in first week of life characterized by septicemia and multiple organ involvement.
- Isolation from stool of young animals—inconclusive evidence of pathogenic potential because it is normal flora; molecular methods can assess virulence potential.
- Isolation from blood cultures or internal organs—better evidence of causality.
- Infection of older dogs and cats—documented; virulence of individual strains poorly characterized.

PATHOPHYSIOLOGY

- Virulence factors—not well defined; likely EC as a cause of septicemia in neonatal dogs and cats reflects balance between immunologic immaturity and intestinal barrier function of host and resident enteric EC rather than a single virulent strain.
- Enterotoxigenic EC (ETEC), attaching and effacing EC (AEEC), uropathogenic EC (UPEC), cytotoxic necrotizing factor (CNF) + EC strains—recovered from dogs, similar in cats.
- Intestinal strains colonize and multiply in small intestine; ETEC then elaborates uncharacterized adhesins and enterotoxins (STa); attaching and effacing factor of AEEC (intimin [eae]+).
- Many strains of EC from dogs and cats are hemolytic.
- An EC reported in boxer dogs with granulomatous colitis characterized by ability to adhere, invade, and replicate in macrophages, resulting in massive inflammatory response within intestinal wall.

SYSTEMS AFFECTED

- Neonates—small intestine (enteritis); multiple body systems (septicemia).
- Puppies/kittens and adults—small intestine (enteritis); urogenital (cystitis, endometritis, pyelonephritis, prostatitis); mammary gland (mastitis); large intestine (colitis).

GENETICS

Boxer dogs may be predisposed.

INCIDENCE/PREVALENCE

- Few statistics available.
- More common in neonatal puppies and kittens <1 week old that have not received any or adequate amounts of colostrum.
- Problem in overpopulated kennels and catteries.
- Sporadic accounts in older dogs and cats (mainly diarrhea and urogenital problems).
- Purulent skin disease, otitis, meningoencephalomyelitis.

Dogs

- ETEC—2.7–29.5% of diarrheic dogs; strains: STa/STb+/–, and CNF+ isolated from diarrheic dogs along with hemolysin.
- β-hemolytic EC—major cause of septicemia in newborn puppies exposed in utero, during birth, or from mastitic milk.

Cats

- AEEC/enteropathic EC (EPEC)—diarrheic cats; strains: eae+, hemolysin.
- Extraintestinal pathogenic EC (ExPEC)—acute necrotizing and hemorrhagic pneumonia and pleuritis; strains: CNF-1 plus other adhesions.
- UPEC—cystitis; strains: CNF-1+, P-fimbria, hemolysin.

GEOGRAPHIC DISTRIBUTION

Worldwide

SIGNALMENT

Species

Dog and cat.

Breed Predilections

Boxer dogs may be predisposed to colitis.

Mean Age and Range

- Neonatal infections common (diarrhea, septicemia) up to 2 weeks of age.
- Puppies/kittens and adult animals—sporadic disease often associated with other infectious agents.

Predominant Sex

None

SIGNS

General Comments

One of the most common causes of septicemia and death in puppies and kittens.

Historical Findings

- Neonates—sudden-onset vomiting, weakness/lethargy, diarrhea, cold skin; one or more animals affected in a litter.
- Puppies/kittens and adults—vomiting and diarrhea.

Physical Examination Findings

- Neonates—acute depression, anorexia, vomiting, tachycardia, weakness, hypothermia, cyanosis, watery diarrhea.
- Puppies/kittens and adults—ETEC associated with acute vomiting, diarrhea, anorexia, rapid dehydration, fever.

CAUSES

- EC—endogenous microbial flora of adult gastrointestinal tract, prepuce, and vagina.
- Many strains; poorly characterized regarding virulence factors; need molecular methods to assess virulence.
- Often found in older dogs and cats concurrently with other infectious agents.

RISK FACTORS

Neonates

- Bitch/queen in poor health and nutritional status—unable to provide good care and colostrum.
- Lack of colostrum or insufficient colostrum.
- Dirty birthing environment.
- Difficult or prolonged labor and birth.
- Crowded facilities—feces in environment, chance for fecal–oral spread.

Puppies/Kittens and Adults

- Concurrent disease—parvovirus, heavy parasitism.
- Antimicrobial drugs—upset gastrointestinal microbial flora.
- Immunosuppression.
- Postparturient mastitis.

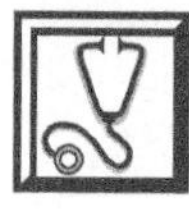

DIAGNOSIS

DIFFERENTIAL DIAGNOSIS

- Infectious enteritis—viral: feline panleukopenia, feline leukemia virus, feline immunodeficiency virus, enteric coronavirus, canine parvovirus, rotavirus, canine distemper; bacterial: *Salmonella*, *E. coli*, *Campylobacter jejuni*, *Yersinia enterocolitica*, bacterial overgrowth syndrome, *Clostridium difficile*, *Clostridium perfringens*; parasitic: hookworms, ascarids, whipworms, *Strongyloides*, *Giardia*, coccidia, cryptosporidia, rickettsiae (salmon poisoning).
- Dietary-induced enteritis—overeating, abrupt changes, starvation, thirst, food intolerance or allergy, indiscretions (e.g., foreign material, garbage).
- Drug- or toxin-induced enteritis—antimicrobial agents, antineoplastic agents, anthelmintics, heavy metals, organophosphates.
- Extraintestinal disorders or metabolic diseases—acute pancreatitis; hypoadrenocorticism; liver or kidney disease; pyometra; peritonitis.
- Functional or mechanical ileus— gastrointestinal obstruction, intussusception, electrolyte disorder, gastrointestinal foreign body.
- Neurologic disorders—vestibular disease, psychogenic (e.g., fear, excitement, pain).
- Fading neonates.

CBC/BIOCHEMISTRY/URINALYSIS

- Few abnormalities noted, owing to rapidity of death in puppies.
- Adults with enteritis may show nonspecific abnormalities, depending on condition.

DIAGNOSTIC PROCEDURES

- Routine bacterial culture and identification of EC from blood (antemortem) or necropsy tissue (bone marrow, heart blood, liver, spleen, brain, mesenteric lymph node) required.

- False-negative results can occur if antimicrobials are used before obtaining bacterial cultures.
- Appropriate testing of strains—identify adhesins and toxins (by DNA colony hybridization, PCR) in ETEC and verotoxigenic EC (VTEC) strains.

PATHOLOGIC FINDINGS

- Acute enteritis.
- Inflammation of small intestinal mucosa.
- Petechiae and hemorrhagic lesions on serosal surface of gastrointestinal mucosae and all body cavities.
- Fibrin on abdominal wall.
- Necrosis of liver/spleen.

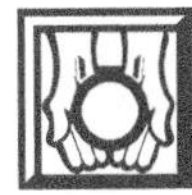

TREATMENT

APPROPRIATE HEALTH CARE

Acutely ill puppies/kittens—inpatient care.

NURSING CARE

- Balanced parenteral polyionic isotonic solution (e.g., lactated Ringer's)—restore fluid balance.
- Oral hypertonic glucose solution—for secretory diarrhea, as indicated.

ACTIVITY

Acutely ill immature puppies/kittens (bacteremic/septicemic)—restricted activity, cage rest, monitoring, and warmth.

DIET

Puppies—likely to still be nursing when affected; good nursing care needed with bottle-feeding and/or IV nutrients.

CLIENT EDUCATION

Neonates—life-threatening with poor prognosis.

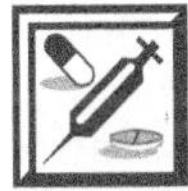

MEDICATIONS

DRUG(S) OF CHOICE

- Antimicrobial therapy—septicemia.
- Guided by culture and susceptibility (and minimal inhibitory concentration) testing of EC; empiric therapy until results available. Extended-spectrum β-lactamase (ESBL) and/or plasmid mediated AmpC (pAmpC) strains becoming more common.
- Amikacin—dog and cat: 15–20 mg/kg IV q24h.
- Cefazolin—dog and cat: 15–35 mg/kg IV q6–8h.
- Cefoxitin—dog and cat: 30 mg/kg IV once, then 15 mg/kg IV q6–8h.
- Enrofloxacin—dog: 10–15 mg/kg IM/IV q24h; cat: 5 mg/kg IV q24h.
- Ticarcillin–clavulanate—dogs and cats: 50 mg/kg IV q6h.

CONTRAINDICATIONS

Fluoroquinolones—avoid use in pregnant, neonatal, or growing animals (medium-sized dogs <8 months of age; large or giant breeds <12–18 months of age) because of potential cartilage lesions.

PRECAUTIONS

Ensure adequate hydration and perfusion when using aminoglycosides.

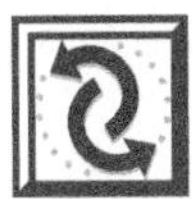

FOLLOW-UP

PATIENT MONITORING

- Physical exam—mentation, rectal temperature, pulse quality.
- Behavior—puppies should be eating, drinking, and/or nursing; adequate weight gain.

PREVENTION/AVOIDANCE

- Bitch/queen—good health; vaccinated; good nutritional status.
- Clean and disinfect parturition environment (1 : 32 dilution of bleach); clean bedding frequently after birth.
- Ensure adequate colostrum intake of all littermates.
- Separate mother with nursing litter from other cats or dogs.
- Keep density low in kennel or cattery rooms.
- Wash hands and change clothes and shoes after handling other cats/dogs and before dealing with neonates.

EXPECTED COURSE AND PROGNOSIS

- Neonates—life-threatening; prognosis often poor; neonate may rapidly succumb; quick treatment with supportive care essential for survival.
- Adults—self-limiting with supportive care, depending on degree of dehydration and existence of other diseases.

MISCELLANEOUS

AGE-RELATED FACTORS

Neonates—greatest risk of infection and subsequent septicemia.

ZOONOTIC POTENTIAL

- Little information of virulence potential of EC strains from dogs or cats for humans, although recently similarities have been found between canine fecal and UPEC and human EC associated with urinary tract infections, sepsis, and meningitis.
- Growing concern for presence of multidrug resistance determinants in EC strains from companion animals.
- Children and immunosuppressed persons should be kept away from pets with diarrhea.
- Whole genome sequencing has linked commercially available raw meat diets to pathogens found in dogs and cats, including EC, *Salmonella*, and *Listeria*.

SYNONYMS

- *E. coli* septicemia.
- Neonatal enteritis.

ABBREVIATIONS

- AEEC = attaching and effacing *E. coli*.
- CNF = cytotoxic necrotizing factor.
- EC = *Escherichia coli*.
- EPEC = enteropathogenic *E. coli*.
- ESBL = extended spectrum beta-lactamase.
- ETEC = enterotoxigenic *E. coli*.
- ExPEC = extraintestinal pathogenic *E. coli*.
- UPEC = uropathogenic *E. coli*.
- VTEC = verotoxigenic *E. coli*.

Suggested Reading

Craven M, Mansfield CS, Simpson KW. Granulomatous colitis of boxer dogs. Vet Clin North Am Small Anim Pract, 2011 41:433–445.

Marks SL, Rankin SC, Byrne BA, et al. Enteropathogenic bacteria in dogs and cats: diagnosis, epidemiology, treatment, and control. J Vet Intern Med 2011, 25:1195–208.

Sabshin SJ, Levy JK, Tupler T, et al. Enteropathogens identified in cats entering a Florida animal shelter with normal feces or diarrhea. J Am Vet Med Assoc 2012, 241:331–337.

Tupler T, Levy JK, Sabshin SJ, et al. Enteropathogens identified in dogs entering a Florida animal shelter with normal feces or diarrhea. J Am Vet Med Assoc 2012, 241:338–343.

Weese JS. Bacterial enteritis in dogs and cats: diagnosis, therapy, and zoonotic potential. Vet Clin North Am Small Anim Pract 2011, 41:287–309.

Author Patrick L. McDonough
Consulting Editor Amie Koenig

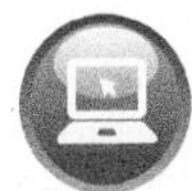

Client Education Handout available online

COLITIS AND PROCTITIS

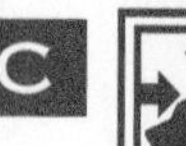

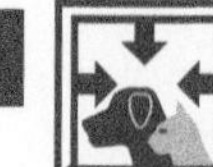

BASICS

DEFINITION

• Colitis—inflammation of the colon (large intestine); colitis may be acute and self-limiting or chronic. • Colitis does not infer causality, and an underlying cause of the colitis should be investigated, particularly in chronic cases. • Proctitis—inflammation of the rectum.

PATHOPHYSIOLOGY

• Inflammation of the colon causes accumulation of inflammatory cytokines, disrupts tight junctions between epithelial cells, stimulates colonic secretion, stimulates goblet cell secretion of mucus, and disrupts motility. • These mechanisms reduce the ability of the colon to absorb water and electrolytes, and store feces, which causes frequent diarrhea, often with mucus and/or frank blood.

SYSTEMS AFFECTED

Gastrointestinal

GENETICS

• Breeds predisposed to histiocytic ulcerative colitis (granulomatous colitis [GC]) include boxers, French bulldogs, and, less commonly, border collies. • German shepherd dogs are predisposed to perianal fistulae (anal furunculosis) that can be associated with colitis.

INCIDENCE/PREVALENCE

• Approximately 30% of dogs with chronic diarrhea examined at one university hospital. • 71% of dogs with a food-responsive enteropathy had clinical signs of colitis (either alone or in association with enteritis (enterocolitis). • Prevalence of colitis probably higher than perceived, because many diarrheic dogs and cats manifesting small bowel diarrhea have evidence of colitis histopathologically when biopsied.

GEOGRAPHIC DISTRIBUTION

• N/A except for certain infectious diseases. • Pythiosis—predominantly Gulf Coast and southeast United States, although becoming more widespread, including California. • Histoplasmosis—Midwest, eastern United States. • *Prototheca* spp.—ubiquitous in nature, especially prevalent in warm, humid climates (e.g., southern and southeastern United States, northeastern Australia, southern continental Europe, Japan) in aqueous environments where decaying organic matter present. • *Entamoeba histolytica*—prevalent in tropical and subtropical regions worldwide; in United States, much higher rate of amebiasis-related mortality in California and Texas, which might be caused by their proximity to *E. histolytica*-endemic areas, such as Mexico, other parts of Latin America, and Asia. • *Tritrichomonas blagburni*—widespread distribution in North America, Australasia, Europe, and Asia.

SIGNALMENT

Species

Dog and cat.

Breed Predilections

• Boxers, French bulldogs, border collies (GC). • German shepherd dogs—perianal fistulas and concurrent colitis.

Mean Age and Range

• Any age; boxers and French bulldogs are typically younger (<2 years). • Cats infected with *Tritrichomonas blagburni* are typically younger (<2 years), but can also be infected when older.

SIGNS

Historical Findings

• Fecal consistency can be variable from semi-formed to liquid. • Marked increase in frequency of defecation (6–15 times per day) with small fecal volume. • Tenesmus. • Increased fecal mucus. • Hematochezia; cats may have formed feces with hematochezia. • Occasional dyschezia (painful defecation). • Increased urgency to defecate. • Vomiting in approximately 30% of dogs and cats with colitis.

Physical Examination Findings

• Usually unremarkable. • Rectal examination may reveal thickened and irregular colorectal mucosa. • Dogs with GC may show systemic signs of weight loss and anorexia.

CAUSES

• Dietary—food-responsive enteropathy is common and important cause of colitis; dietary indiscretion; food intolerance. • Drug administration (antibiotics, nonsteroidal anti-inflammatory drugs [NSAIDs]). • Infectious—*Trichuris vulpis, Entamoeba histolytica, Balantidium coli, Tritrichomonas blagburni, Clostridium perfringens and Clostridium difficile, Campylobacter jejuni and Campylobacter coli, Yersinia enterocolitica, Prototheca, Histoplasma capsulatum*, pythiosis/phycomycosis. • Traumatic—foreign body, abrasive material. • Inflammatory—secondary to pancreatitis (transverse colitis). • Inflammatory/immune—inflammatory bowel disease (lymphoplasmacytic, eosinophilic, granulomatous) colitis.

DIAGNOSIS

DIFFERENTIAL DIAGNOSIS

• Neoplasia—colonic lymphoma, adenocarcinoma, sarcomas. • Irritable bowel syndrome. • Colorectal polyps do not typically cause signs of colitis, but instead cause hematochezia in association with formed stool defecated at normal frequency. • Cecal inversion. • Ileocecocolic intussusception.

CBC/BIOCHEMISTRY/URINALYSIS

• Results usually unremarkable; neutrophilia with left shift can be seen with severe inflammatory causes; eosinophilia secondary to eosinophilic colitis, parasitism, histoplasmosis, pythiosis/phycomycosis. • Mild microcytic, hypochromic anemia may occur secondary to chronic intestinal bleeding and iron deficiency. • Hyperglobulinemia in some patients (especially cats) with chronic disease.

OTHER LABORATORY TESTS

• Examination of fecal centrifugation flotation, direct fecal smear (only on fresh diarrheic feces), detection of netE and netF toxin genes of *C. perfringens* and *C. difficile* toxins A and B genes via PCR, serum ELISA test for *Pythium* when indicated. • Rectal scraping for cytology for *Histoplasma* organisms and *Prototheca* spp. • Biopsy of colon or regional lymph nodes for detection of *Prototheca* spp., or biopsy of gastrointestinal tract and regional lymph nodes for detection of *Histoplasma* organisms. • Microscopic examination of urine sediment or cerebrospinal fluid (CSF) in dogs with disseminated protothecosis and associated clinical signs can be excellent means of detecting organisms. • Culture and sensitivity testing for diagnosis of *Prototheca* spp. • MVista® Histoplasma quantitative antigen test performed on serum, plasma, urine, or CSF can aid diagnosis and management of histoplasmosis. • Fecal PCR or In Pouch TF medium for culture of *Tritrichomonas foetus*.

IMAGING

• Abdominal radiographs—usually unremarkable. • Abdominal ultrasonography—may reveal masses, diffuse thickening or altered architecture of the colon, or enlarged associated lymph nodes. • Contrast studies—barium may be administered transcolonically to evaluate colorectal mucosa for irregularities or filling defects and colorectal strictures; however, procedure rarely indicated in dogs and cats with colitis and of low sensitivity in general.

DIAGNOSTIC PROCEDURES

• Colonoscopy with biopsy—procedure of choice for diagnosis of chronic or refractory cases; animals must be adequately prepared for colonoscopy by being fasted and administered osmotic cathartics such as OsmoPrep® or GoLYTELY®; mucosal changes visible grossly in animals with colitis include disappearance of submucosal blood vessels, granular appearance of mucosa, hyperemia, excessive mucus, ulceration, pinpoint hemorrhage (small ulcerations), or mass(es). • Always obtain multiple biopsy specimens from multiple locations (ascending colon, transverse colon, descending colon, rectum) because extent of mucosal change assessed histologically does not necessarily reflect severity of colitis or proctitis.

PATHOLOGIC FINDINGS

Histopathologic findings depend on histologic type of colitis—lymphoplasmacytic, eosinophilic, or histiocytic represent most common subtypes; hyperplastic mucosa may be seen with irritable bowel syndrome; various infectious agents may be seen with special stains.

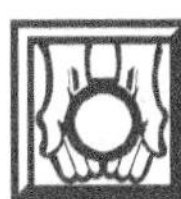

TREATMENT

DIET

• No inherent benefit to fasting patients with diarrhea, unless cause of diarrhea has osmotic component. • Animals that do not have severe clinical signs can be managed with elimination diet or hypoallergenic diet for 2 weeks; response to dietary therapy typically seen within first 5–7 days following dietary implementation; obtain comprehensive dietary history to optimize selection of novel, single protein source diet; strict dietary compliance pivotal during this trial period to optimize interpretation of response. • Fiber supplementation with poorly fermented fiber (e.g., bran and alphacellulose) recommended to increase fecal bulk, improve colonic muscle contractility, and bind fecal water to produce formed feces. • Some fermentable fiber sources (e.g., psyllium or diet containing beet pulp or fructooligosaccharides) may be beneficial—short-chain fatty acids produced by fermentation may be beneficial for colonocyte function.

SURGICAL CONSIDERATIONS

Segments of colon severely affected by fibrosis from chronic inflammation and subsequent stricture formation may need surgical excision, especially in patients with granulomatous form of disease; cecal inversion and ileocecocolic intussusception require surgical intervention; pythiosis/phycomycosis often requires surgical excision or debulking.

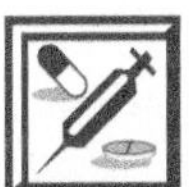

MEDICATIONS

DRUG(S) OF CHOICE

Antimicrobial Drugs

• *Trichuris*—fenbendazole (50 mg/kg PO q24h for 5 consecutive days, repeat in 3 months). • *Entamoeba, Balantidium*—metronidazole (25 mg/kg PO q12h for 5–7 days). • *Tritrichomonas blagburni*—ronidazole (30 mg/kg q24h for 14 days). • *Clostridium perfringens*—metronidazole (10 mg/kg PO q12h for 5 days), tylosin (5–10 mg/kg PO q24h for 5 days), ampicillin or amoxicillin (20 mg/kg PO q8h for 5 days); diarrhea, including acute hemorrhagic diarrheal syndrome, can be self-limiting and avoidance of antimicrobials recommended whenever feasible. • *Clostridium difficile*—metronidazole (10 mg/kg PO q12h for 5 days). • *Campylobacter jejuni*—erythromycin (10–15 mg/kg PO q8h) or azithromycin (5–10 mg/kg PO q24h) can be given for 7–10 days; azithromycin better tolerated than erythromycin. • *Yersinia* spp.—select drug on basis of bacterial culture and sensitivity testing. • *Prototheca*—combination therapy with amphotericin B and itraconazole, although disseminated cases typically fatal. • *Histoplasma*—itraconazole (dogs: 10 mg/kg PO q24h; cats: 5 mg/kg PO q12h; several months of therapy necessary); amphotericin B (0.25–0.5mg/kg slow IV q48h up to cumulative dose of 4–8 mg/kg) in advanced cases. • Pythiosis—itraconazole (10 mg/kg PO q24h) and terbinafine (10 mg/kg PO q24h) are drugs of choice following surgical debridement of affected portions of bowel; however, combination of itraconazole, terbinafine, and prednisone (without surgical resection) was shown to be highly effective in small cohort of dogs with focal involvement of colon; antifungal therapy often administered for 3–4 months or longer in affected animals.

Anti-inflammatory and Immunosuppressive Drugs for Inflammatory/Immune Colitis

• Sulfasalazine (dogs: 25–40 mg/kg PO q8h for 3–6 weeks with progressive tapering of dose throughout course of drug therapy; cats: 20 mg/kg PO q12h for 3 weeks); use with caution, particularly in cats, in which adverse effects on gastrointestinal tract and kidneys can be observed; sulfasalazine has been associated with irreversible keratoconjunctivitis sicca (KCS). • Corticosteroids—prednisone for dogs and prednisolone for cats: 1–2 mg/kg PO q12h for 5–7 weeks with gradual, progressive tapering of dose; most cats can be started on 5 mg (per cat) q12h with gradual taper; never use more than 50 mg total of prednisone (per day) for any animal, regardless of size. • Azathioprine (dogs) 1–2 mg/kg PO q24h for 10–14 days, followed by taper to 1–2 mg/kg q48h for 4–6 weeks; drug is markedly myelosuppressive in cats and should be avoided even though lower dose (0.3 mg/kg PO q48h) for this species has been published. • Chlorambucil—effective immunomodulator in both dogs and cats and usually administered in conjunction with prednisone or prednisolone; several dosing regimens have been published—cats: 2 mg per cat q3–4 days for 2–3 months (or longer if managing lymphoma) or 15 mg/m^2 given for 4 consecutive days every 3 weeks for 2–3 months; dogs: 0.1–0.2 mg/kg PO q24h for 8–12 weeks for immune disease, with gradual tapering of dose over course of therapy. • Cyclosporine (5 mg/kg PO q12–24h for 6 weeks for immune disease). • GC (histiocytic ulcerative colitis) usually managed with fluoroquinolones such as enrofloxacin at 10 mg/kg q24h for 6–8 weeks; however, evidence of marked increase in antimicrobial resistance to this class of drugs underscores importance of culture and sensitivity testing to optimize antimicrobial therapy. • Reconsider diagnosis of food-responsive colitis or nonspecific colitis carefully in dogs that do not respond to dietary therapy, fenbendazole administration, and tylosin therapy.

Motility Modifiers

• Indicated for symptomatic relief only in animals with intractable diarrhea; must be avoided in all animals with suspected infectious enteropathy. • Loperamide—0.1 mg/kg PO q8–12h. • Diphenoxylate—0.1–0.2 mg/kg PO q8h. • Propantheline bromide—0.25–0.5 mg/kg PO q8h, if colonic spasm contributing to clinical signs.

Anthelminthics

• Broad-spectrum anthelminthics such as fenbendazole (50 mg/kg q24h for 5 consecutive days) or Drontal® Plus in conjunction with dietary therapy (elimination diet) for first 2 weeks is mainstay of therapy for most patients with chronic colitis, unless a boxer breed that should have endoscopy and biopsy to confirm presence of GC, which has different therapy and prognosis. • Tylosin is highly effective antimicrobial that can be administered following assessment of response to dietary and anthelminthic therapy.

PRECAUTIONS

• Monitor patients on sulfasalazine for signs of KCS; measure tear production (Schirmer tear test) at baseline and every 2 weeks throughout course of therapy; discontinue drug if tear production decreases; use of sulfasalazine therapy has decreased markedly over past decade in light of excellent response to dietary and tylosin therapy in most dogs. • Monitor patients on azathioprine for bone marrow suppression—CBC every 2–3 weeks; stop treatment or go to alternate day if white blood cell count falls below 3,000 cells/μL. • Azathioprine can also increase risk of pancreatitis and should be used extremely cautiously in any dog at increased risk for pancreatitis; azathioprine can also cause hepatopathy. • Chlorambucil can cause progressive neutropenia and CBC should be repeated q2–3 weeks in all animals receiving this drug. • Cyclosporine can cause hepatotoxicity and chemistry panel should be performed as baseline before starting the drug and repeated q2–3 months.
• Amphotericin B is nephrotoxic and requires close assessment of renal function

COLITIS AND PROCTITIS (CONTINUED)

via urinalyses and serum biochemistry panels. • Enrofloxacin-resistant cases of GC are increasing in prevalence due to antimicrobial resistance, necessitating alternative antimicrobial therapy in select cases.

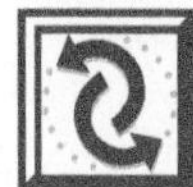

FOLLOW-UP

PATIENT MONITORING

• Infrequent recheck examinations or client communication by phone. • Recheck of CBC is important for animals on immunomodulatory therapy.

EXPECTED COURSE AND PROGNOSIS

• Most bacterial and parasitic infectious causes have excellent prognosis, with high likelihood of cure following therapy.
• *Prototheca*—grave; no known treatment except excision and itraconazole and amphotericin B following early diagnosis and before dissemination. • *Histoplasma* spp.—poor in advanced or disseminated disease; mild to moderate cases generally respond to therapy. • Pythiosis/phycomycosis—poor long-term prognosis in most animals, despite surgical intervention, given advanced stage of disease at diagnosis; addition of anti-inflammatory dose of prednisone with antifungal therapy appears to enhance effectiveness and benefit of therapy. • Cecal inversion, ileocecocolic intussusception—good with surgical resection if diagnosed in timely fashion. • Inflammatory—fair to good with treatment in patients with lymphoplasmacytic or eosinophilic colitis or GC. • Most dogs with mild to moderate nonspecific colitis respond favorable to combination of fenbendazole, feeding of elimination or hypoallergenic diet, and tylosin therapy.

MISCELLANEOUS

ZOONOTIC POTENTIAL

Entamoeba, *Balantidium*, *Campylobacter jejuni*, *Yersinia* in immunosuppressed individuals.

SYNONYMS

• Inflammatory bowel disease. • Large bowel diarrhea.

ABBREVIATIONS

• CSF = cerebrospinal fluid.
• GC = granulomatous colitis.
• KCS = keratoconjunctivitis sicca.
• NSAID = nonsteroidal anti-inflammatory drug.

Suggested Reading

Marks SL, Kather EJ, Kass PH, et al. Genotypic and phenotypic characterization of *Clostridium perfringens* and *Clostridium difficile* in diarrheic and healthy dogs. J Vet Intern Med 2002, 16:533–540.

Reagan KL, Marks SL, Pesavento PA, et al. Successful management of 3 dogs with colonic pythiosis using itraconzaole, terbinafine, and prednisone. J Vet Intern Med 2019, 33(3):1434–1439.

Author Stanley L. Marks
Consulting Editor Mark P. Rondeau

Client Education Handout available online

COLITIS, HISTIOCYTIC ULCERATIVE

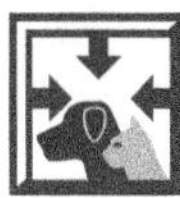

BASICS

OVERVIEW

• Relatively common cause of colitis in Boxer breeds and infrequently seen in French bulldogs and border collies. • Boxer colitis is also referred to as granulomatous colitis (GC) in light of the granulomatous inflammation (macrophages) in the colon. • Etiology of GC is an adherent-invasive *E. coli* (AIEC) strain.

SIGNALMENT

• Dogs—primarily affects young Boxers, usually <3 years of age. • Reported in French bulldogs and border collies less frequently.

SIGNS

• Bloody, mucoid diarrhea with marked increase in frequency of defecation. • Tenesmus. • Weight loss and anorexia can occur and debilitation may develop.

CAUSES & RISK FACTORS

GC appears to be a genetic disorder in boxer breeds associated with reduced macrophage phagocytic function and inability to kill AIEC.

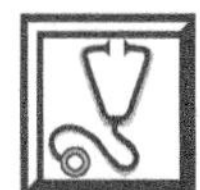

DIAGNOSIS

DIFFERENTIAL DIAGNOSIS

• Other causes of colitis—nonhistiocytic inflammatory bowel disease (IBD), lymphocytic, plasmacytic, eosinophilic colitis, other infectious causes of colitis (pythiosis, protothecosis, entamoeba), parasitic colitis (whipworms), food-responsive diarrhea. • Cecal inversion. • Ileocolic intussusception. • Neoplasia—lymphoma, adenocarcinoma. • Foreign body. • Colorectal polyps—dogs with colorectal polyps do not have diarrhea or increased mucus in stools, and instead have normal defecation frequency with formed stools (can have altered shape) coated with frank blood. • Irritable bowel syndrome. • Differentiate by clarifying history (colitis vs. colorectal neoplaia), fecal flotations, abdominal imaging, and colonoscopy or proctoscopy and biopsy.

CBC/BIOCHEMISTRY/URINALYSIS

• Usually unremarkable; microcytic anemia may be present in Boxer dogs with GC secondary to intestinal bleeding. • Chemistry panel may reveal hypoalbuminemia, electrolyte abnormalities, and prerenal azotemia in dogs with severe diarrhea and anorexia.

IMAGING

Abdominal ultrasound in Boxer dogs with GC often reveals mild or moderate mesenteric or sublumbar lymphadenomegaly, and colonic wall can appear thickened.

DIAGNOSTIC PROCEDURES

• Proctoscopy or colonoscopy to obtain colonic biopsies. • Most Boxer dogs with GC have involvement of descending colon, underscoring diagnostic utility of proctoscopy. • Common changes in appearance to colonic wall include erythema, irregularity, and ulceration of colonic and rectal wall.

Microbiologic Testing

E. coli commonly isolated on routine bacteriologic media from feces of both healthy dogs and dogs with diarrhea; however, attempts to isolate *E. coli* from colonic biopsies is recommended for sensitivity testing and optimization of antimicrobial therapy.

PATHOLOGIC FINDINGS

• Histopathologic lesions include neutrophilic inflammation, epithelial ulceration, crypt hyperplasia and distortion, decreased numbers of goblet cells, and large numbers of macrophages that stain positive with periodic acid–Schiff (PAS) stain. • Presence of *E. coli* within macrophages can be confirmed using fluorescent in-situ hybridization (FISH).

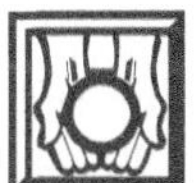

TREATMENT

• Outpatient medical management following confirmation of diagnosis. • Antimicrobial therapy utilizing fluoroquinolones (unless resistance is observed) is mainstay of therapy. • Diet change to include moderately fermentable fiber source can be used in cases that do not show complete resolution of diarrhea.

MEDICATIONS

DRUG(S) OF CHOICE

Antimicrobials—First-Line Therapy

• Enrofloxacin (10 mg/kg q24h) for minimum duration of 6–8 weeks is typically associated with rapid resolution of clinical signs and resolution of histopathologic abnormalities. • Because enrofloxacin resistance has been documented in up to 70% of isolates from dogs with GC, attempts to isolate *E. coli* from colonic biopsies before treatment recommended such that antimicrobial susceptibility testing can be performed. • Antimicrobials that penetrate intracellularly, such as fluoroquinolones, chloramphenicol, rifampin, or trimethoprim-sulfonamides, should be preferentially chosen for treatment based on results of antimicrobial susceptibility testing. • Chloramphenicol, trimethoprim-sulfa, clarithromycin, imipenem, and meropenem should be considered for cases resistant to fluoroquinolones.

Anti-inflammatory/Immunosuppressive Drugs

• Rarely indicated in dogs with GC, and used at anti-inflammatory dose in conjunction with appropriate antimicrobial therapy. • Diagnosis must be reconsidered if no dramatic improvement in clinical signs following administration of fluoroquinolone therapy, because not all boxers with signs of colitis have GC.

CONTRAINDICATIONS/POSSIBLE INTERACTIONS

Avoid anticholinergics or other motility modifiers such as Imodium® in dogs with infectious cause of diarrhea.

FOLLOW-UP

PATIENT MONITORING

• Monitor clinical signs, stool consistency and frequency, and body weight. • Dogs showing favorable response should improve within 5 days of starting effective antimicrobial therapy.

EXPECTED COURSE AND PROGNOSIS

• Generally good prognosis following appropriate antimicrobial therapy. • Increasing injudicious administration of fluoroquinolones to dogs is increasing resistance of *E. coli* to this class of antimicrobials, necessitating use of alternative antimicrobials in a subset of dogs.

MISCELLANEOUS

PREGNANCY/FERTILITY/BREEDING

Boxers, French bulldogs, and border collies with GC should not be bred.

SEE ALSO

Colitis and Proctitis.

ABBREVIATIONS

• AIEC = adherent-invasive *E. coli*. • FISH = fluorescent in-situ hybridization. • GC = granulomatous colitis. • IBD = inflammatory bowel disease. • PAS = periodic acid–Schiff.

Suggested Reading

Craven M, Dogan B, Schukken A, et al. Antimicrobial resistance impacts clinical outcome of granulomatous colitis in boxer dogs. J Vet Intern Med 2010, 24(4):819–824.

Manchester AC, Hill S, Sabation B, et al. Association between granulomatous colitis in French Bulldogs and invasive *Escherichia coli* and response to fluoroquinolone antimicrobials. J Vet Int Med 2013, 27(1):56–61.

Author Stanley L. Marks
Consulting Editor Mark P. Rondeau

COMPULSIVE DISORDERS—CATS

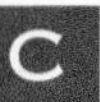

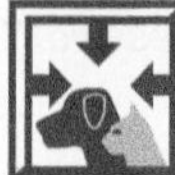

BASICS

DEFINITION

• Compulsive disorders are relatively invariant exaggerated behavior patterns, often derived from normal behaviors but out of context and repetitive, without apparent function; may be performed to the exclusion of other normal behaviors or to the detriment of the animal. • May be a heterogeneous group of conditions with differing pathologies including compulsive, stereotypic, and neurologic; therefore abnormal repetitive behaviors might be used to describe the clinical presentation. • Considered here are psychogenic dermatitis/alopecia, compulsive fabric chewing/sucking, and hyperesthesia syndrome.

PATHOPHYSIOLOGY

• Diagnosis of exclusion; must rule out pathophysiologic causes, including psychomotor seizures, before a presumptive diagnosis is made. • Can be a behavioral response to confinement, specific anxiety-producing event, or undefined environmental conditions (e.g., conflict, stress, anxiety, frustration); over time, can become fixed and independent of the environment; affected cats may lack control of onset or termination. • Behaviors may be self-reinforcing—allowing some animals to cope with conditions that do not meet their species-specific needs.

SYSTEMS AFFECTED

• Behavioral. • Gastrointestinal—fabric chewing/sucking. • Musculoskeletal—feline hyperesthesia (involves cutaneous trunci muscle), tail attack/mutilation. • Skin/exocrine—psychogenic dermatitis/alopecia. • Nervous—feline hyperesthesia syndrome.

GENETICS

None identified, although the association of compulsive fabric chewing/sucking with Asian breeds suggests a heritable component.

INCIDENCE/PREVALENCE

Unknown, uncommon.

SIGNALMENT

Species

Cat

Breed Predispositions

Siamese, Burmese, Birman, and crosses may be overrepresented for fabric chewing and sucking.

Mean Age and Range

• Compulsive disorders can develop at any time, generally not seen in kittens. • Psychogenic dermatitis/alopecia—6 months to 12 years. • Fabric chewing/sucking—12–49 months; generally around 24 months. • Hyperesthesia syndrome—1–5 years.

Predominant Sex

None

SIGNS

General Comments

• Behaviors may quickly increase in frequency if reinforced with attention by owner. • Scolding or punishment may increase cat anxiety and stress and worsen expression of behavior.

Historical Findings

• Onset may be coincident with environmental change (e.g., move or new household member) suggesting stress effect; cat may hide to avoid punishment. • Psychogenic dermatitis/alopecia—may be associated with excessive grooming to exclusion of other activities; may be history of flea exposure or diet change. • Compulsive fabric chewing/sucking—some patients show preference for specific fabric type such as wool or may have general texture preference; grind fabric with molars; may ingest fabric leading to foreign body obstruction. • Hyperesthesia syndrome—may be triggered by tactile contact (petting along dorsum and rump); may be episodic; flea exposure.

Physical Examination Findings

• Psychogenic dermatitis/alopecia—focal, partial, and bilateral dermatitis or alopecia; most common locations: groin, ventrum, and medial or caudal thigh regions; appearance of skin variable (normal or abnormal; erythematous to abraded). • Fabric chewing/sucking—often normal; secondary gastrointestinal inflammation or obstruction may occur if cat ingests material. • Hyperesthesia syndrome—episode may be prompted by petting or scratching dorsum; signs may include dilated pupils, salivation, alarming vocalization, "rippling skin" (hyperresponsive cutaneous trunci muscle), inappropriate urination or defecation, tail twitching, frantic grooming, self-directed (especially to tail) or owner-directed aggression, escape behavior.

CAUSES

Unidentified

RISK FACTORS

• Changes in environment might predispose cat to compulsive disorder. • More commonly reported in indoor cats. • Cats fed ad libitum may have lower prevalence of fabric chewing/sucking; must be balanced with nutritional needs.

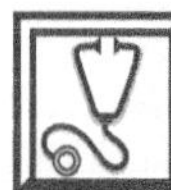

DIAGNOSIS

DIFFERENTIAL DIAGNOSIS

Rule out medical, including psychomotor seizures, before behavioral diagnosis is made.

Psychogenic Dermatitis/Alopecia

• Skin conditions—especially if associated with pruritus including external parasites; hypersensitivity to parasites, fleas, or food; atopy; neoplasia; fungal or bacterial dermatitis. • Nervous system disorders. • Disk rupture and associated neuritis. • Feline hyperesthesia syndrome. • Pain/neuropathy.

Fabric Chewing/Sucking

• Lead intoxication. • Hyperthyroidism. • Thiamin deficiency. • Gastrointestinal upset.

Hyperesthesia Syndrome

• Seizure disorder. • Skin disorders including external parasites, hypersensitivity to food, flea bites, and parasites; atopy. • Spinal disorder/neuropathy. • Myositis, myopathy.

CBC/BIOCHEMISTRY/URINALYSIS

Minimum database to rule out metabolic abnormalities. No consistent clinicopathologies associated with compulsive disorders.

OTHER LABORATORY TESTS

Psychogenic Alopecia

Microscopic examination of hairs (trichogram), skin scraping, skin biopsy, fungal culture, bacterial culture, examination for external parasites, exclusion diet to rule out dermatologic condition.

Fabric Chewing

• Serum lead level—if indicated for pica. • Serum T_4.

Hyperesthesia Syndrome

Rule out dermatologic conditions as above.

IMAGING

• CT or MRI—if indicated by abnormalities on examination, i.e., to diagnose neurologic, pain. • Fabric chewing/sucking—imaging gastrointestinal tract if obstruction or foreign body suspected.

DIAGNOSTIC PROCEDURES

Psychogenic Alopecia

Complete dermatologic evaluation.

Hyperesthesia Syndrome

Skin and/or muscle biopsy (as necessary).

PATHOLOGIC FINDINGS

Psychogenic Alopecia

• Microscopic examination of hairs—typically shafts are cleanly broken off at variable length as a result of trauma from the tongue. • If primarily behavioral, results of other dermatologic testing will be generally normal.

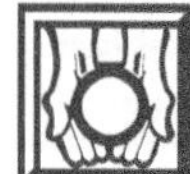

TREATMENT

APPROPRIATE HEALTH CARE

Supportive care.

NURSING CARE

Fabric chewing/sucking—create a "safe place" for when the cat is left alone, devoid of fabric of the sort favored for chewing.

ACTIVITY

Increase opportunities for play and social interactions by providing outlets favored by the affected cat. Insure environmental needs are fully addressed.

Table 1

Drugs and dosages used to manage feline compulsive disorder.

Drug	*Drug Class*	*Oral Dosage in Cats*	*Frequency*	*Side Effects—Usually Transient*
Fluoxetine	SSRI	0.5–1.0 mg/kg	q24h	Decreased appetite, sleepiness
Paroxetine	SSRI	0.25–0.50 mg/kg	q24h	Constipation
Clomipramine	TCA	0.25–1.0 mg/kg	q24h	Sleepiness, urine retention
Amitriptyline	TCA	0.25–1.0 mg/kg	q24h	Sleepiness, urine retention
Gabapentin	Anticonvulsant	3–5 mg/kg	q12h	Sleepiness, sedation

DIET

• Fabric chewing—increasing fiber in the diet has been suggested. • Presumptive psychogenic alopecia—exclusion diet.

CLIENT EDUCATION

• Identify and remove triggers for the behavior, if applicable. • Do not reward the behavior. • Ignore the behavior as much as possible; distract the cat and initiate an acceptable behavior. • Note details of the time, place, and social milieu so that an alternative behavior (play or feeding or food-dispensing toy) may be scheduled prior to initiation of the compulsive behavior. • Punishment is contraindicated and can increase the unpredictability of the patient's environment, increase patient fear or aggressive behavior, and disrupt the human–animal bond. • Reduce environmental stress—increase the predictability of household events (feeding, play, exercise, and social time with the client); eliminate unpredictable events as much as possible.

SURGICAL CONSIDERATIONS

N/A unless obstructed.

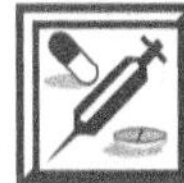

MEDICATIONS

DRUG(S) OF CHOICE

• If a specific etiology cannot be identified, anti-compulsive or anti-anxiety drugs may be helpful; relatively high doses may be required (Table 1). • Goal—use the drugs until control is achieved for 2 months; attempt gradual withdrawal by decreasing dosage at 2-week intervals; treatment should be resumed at the last effective dose at the first sign of relapse; may be life-long. • Drugs are listed with dosage used to manage behavior and common side effects. • Hyperesthesia syndrome—gabapentin has been reported anecdotally to reduce the frequency and intensity of bouts.

CONTRAINDICATIONS

• Selective serotonin reuptake inhibitors (SSRIs)—depending on agent: poor appetite, constipation, sedation. • Tricyclic antidepressants (TCAs)—cats with history of cardiac conduction disturbances, urinary or fecal retention, megacolon, lower urinary tract blockages, seizures, and glaucoma. • Transdermal route does not appear to consistently produce satisfactory drug levels.

PRECAUTIONS

• Start behavioral drugs at low dose to avoid side effects; may give at bedtime to reduce complaints of sedation; may be given with food. • No drugs approved by FDA for treatment of these disorders in cats; inform client of extra-label use and risks involved; document the discussion in the medical record or with a release form.

POSSIBLE INTERACTIONS

Do not use TCAs or SSRIs with monoamine oxidase inhibitors, including selegiline.

ALTERNATIVE DRUG(S)

• Phenobarbital if seizure disorder suspected. • Selegiline if cognitive dysfunction. • Presumptive psychogenic alopecia—exclusion diet, parasite treatment/preventative, trial course of steroids.

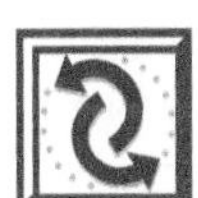

FOLLOW-UP

PATIENT MONITORING

• Before initiating treatment, record frequency of compulsive behavior so that progress can be monitored. • Successful treatment requires a schedule of follow-up examinations; a recommended schedule is a phone check 1 week after the initial consultation and an office recheck 4–6 weeks later; if improvement is evident, the treatment regime should be continued; if there is no improvement, differential diagnoses should be considered or an alternative drug should be considered. • If a medication is not effective after dosage adjustment, select an agent from another drug class.

PREVENTION/AVOIDANCE

Create an enriched environment with distributed resources, safe and accessible elevated resting sites, exercise and play opportunities, and predictable social interactions with people.

POSSIBLE COMPLICATIONS

• Treatment failure. • Realistic expectations must be created; immediate control of a longstanding problem is unlikely.

EXPECTED COURSE AND PROGNOSIS

With treatment, prognosis for improvement is good; treatment can be lifelong.

MISCELLANEOUS

ASSOCIATED CONDITIONS

Avoidance behavior or aggression toward the owner—if the owner punishes the patient when it exhibits a compulsive behavior.

AGE-RELATED FACTORS

None

ZOONOTIC POTENTIAL

None

PREGNANCY/FERTILITY/BREEDING

• Do not breed animals that display compulsive behavior. • TCAs—contraindicated in pregnant animals.

SYNONYMS

• Psychogenic alopecia—barbering, overgrooming. • Hyperesthesia syndrome—rippling skin disease, neurodermatitis.

SEE ALSO

Compulsive Disorders—Dogs.

ABBREVIATIONS

• SSRI = selective serotonin reuptake inhibitor. • TCA = tricyclic antidepressant.

INTERNET RESOURCES

https://www.vet.cornell.edu/departments-centers-and-institutes/cornell-feline-health-center/health-information/feline-health-topics

Suggested Reading

Horwitz D, ed. Blackwell's 5 Minute Consult Clinical Companion: Canine and Feline Behavior, 2nd ed. Ames, IA: Wiley-Blackwell, 2018, pp. 391–403, 425–455, 481–492.

Landsberg G. Stereotypic and compulsive disorders. In: Landsberg G, Hunthausen W, Ackerman L. Behavior Problems of the Dog and Cat, 3rd ed. New York: Saunders/Elsevier, 2013, pp. 163–179.

Tynes VV, Sinn L. Abnormal repetitive behaviors in dogs and cats: a guide for practitioners. Vet Clin Small Anim Pract 2014, 44:543–564.

Authors Margaret E. Gruen and Barbara L. Sherman

Consulting Editor Gary M. Landsberg

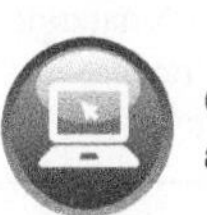

Client Education Handout available

COMPULSIVE DISORDERS—DOGS

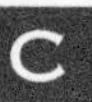

BASICS

DEFINITION

• Heterogeneous group of abnormal repetitive behaviors with differing pathologies (compulsive, stereotypic, neurologic). • Categorized as locomotor (spinning, tail chasing, circling, fence running, pacing, light/shadow chasing); oral (licking, sucking/mouthing an object/body part, e.g., flank, tail, limb; pica, excessive drinking, "fly biting"); or hallucinatory ("fly biting," hind end checking, freezing, staring), with/without vocal and affective responses.
• Compulsive disorders (CDs) are abnormal, repetitive, exaggerated, and/or sustained, variable in form and fixated on a goal; they are derived from normal maintenance behaviors (e.g., grooming, predation, ingestion); motivational conflict or frustration appears to trigger the behaviors in specific contexts often associated with high arousal; with repeated/sustained conflict, the behavior becomes emancipated from the original trigger(s) and displayed in diverse contexts; the animal may lack control of onset or termination.
• Stereotypies are repetitive behaviors that are unvaried in sequence and have no obvious function or purpose; they may arise in situations of conflict/frustration related to confinement or husbandry practices, when the environment lacks sufficient outlets for the normal behavior repertoire, and with maternal deprivation.

PATHOPHYSIOLOGY

• Alterations in brain neurotransmitter functions likely—primarily serotonin; also dopamine, glutamate, endorphins; different CDs may preferentially involve different brain regions. • Abnormal serotonin transmission has been identified as a primary mechanism by which compulsive disorders are induced; stereotypies might be induced by dopaminergic stimulation.

SYSTEMS AFFECTED

• Behavioral—fear, anxiety, aggression.
• Cardiovascular—tachycardia. • Endocrine/metabolic— hypothalamic–pituitary–adrenal (HPA) axis upregulation. • Gastrointestinal—inappetence, gastroenteritis, foreign body obstruction. • Hemic/lymphatic/immune—stress leukogram. • Musculoskeletal—weight loss, self-injury. • Respiratory—tachypnea.
• Skin/exocrine—abrasions/wounds/infections secondary to self-trauma.

GENETICS

• Higher than expected occurrence among first-generation relatives (manifestations may differ). • Certain breeds overrepresented for specific CDs. • Genetic studies implicate N-methyl-D-aspartate (NMDA) glutamatergic neurotransmission, particularly via neural cadherin (*CDH2*); also serotonergic transmission via the 5-HT3 receptor, as well as other aspects of synaptic transmission.

INCIDENCE/PREVALENCE

Generally uncommon, although recent studies report in up to 16%; more common in certain breeds/families.

SIGNALMENT

Species

Dog

Breed Predispositions

Bull terrier—spinning, freezing/"trancing"; German shepherd—spinning, tail chasing; Great Dane, German shorthaired pointer—self-directed oral behaviors, fence running, hallucinations; Doberman—flank/blanket sucking; miniature schnauzer—hind end checking; border collie—light/shadow chasing; cavalier King Charles spaniel—fly catching.

Mean Age and Range

May be presented at any age; usually develops from onset of sexual (6 months) to social (12–24 months) maturity; earlier onset (3–6 months) reported for some CDs.

Predominant Sex

Some CDs may be more common in males.

SIGNS

General Comments

• Wide variety of manifestations—behaviors may be repetitive or static (e.g., freezing).
• Signs may not be observed during examination; descriptions may be unclear; video aids diagnosis and treatment planning.

Historical Findings

• May be other signs of anxiety/concurrent behavioral diagnoses (e.g., separation anxiety, fears, aggression) and/or a history of stress (e.g., inadequate stimulation, punishment, change in routine/household). • Behavior may first be displayed as play or in situations of high arousal/stress; eventually may occur in multiple contexts independent of identifiable triggers. • Certain repetitive behaviors are expressed in situations with little to no external stimulation or evidence of arousal (e.g., blanket sucking). • May occur whether or not the owner is present; if punished, pet may avoid detection. • Hallmarks—behavior is ritualized, often exaggerated in form, and with time increases in frequency, intensity, and duration. • Behavior may be difficult/impossible to interrupt. • Behavior may interfere with normal functioning (e.g., eating, sleeping, social interactions).

Physical Examination Findings

• May be unremarkable. • May see skin lesions/injuries related to self-trauma (especially tail, forelimbs, distal extremities); excessive tooth wear/damage; lameness or poor body condition.

CAUSES

No direct cause.

RISK FACTORS

• Environmental stress (e.g., kenneling—spinning), management. • Owner/environmental reinforcement of the behavior. • Punishment of the behavior further contributing to stress and conflict. • Medical disease, pain, neuropathy—may increase anxiety or may be primary cause.
• Sensory abnormalities (e.g., visual deficits) may contribute.

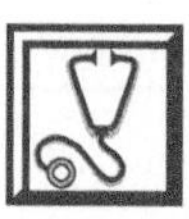

DIAGNOSIS

DIFFERENTIAL DIAGNOSIS

• Dermatologic (e.g., atopy). • Gastrointestinal (e.g., inflammatory bowel disease [IBD], neoplasia, gastroesophageal reflux).
• Metabolic/endocrine (e.g., Cushing's).
• Neurologic (e.g., seizure focus, forebrain neoplasia, neurodegenerative disorder).
• Orthopedic (e.g., degenerative joint disease [DJD]). • Any disorder causing abnormalities of sensation such as dysesthesia, paresthesia (e.g., sensory neuropathy). • Other problem behaviors—displacement/conflict behaviors, play and attention seeking, behaviors occurring secondary to lack of stimulation or due to resource restriction (e.g., water restriction—excessive drinking). • Rule out physical/medical causes.

CBC/BIOCHEMISTRY/URINALYSIS

• Usually within reference range—use for general health screening; prior to drug use.
• Hematocrit, cholesterol, triglyceride increases have been reported.

OTHER LABORATORY TESTS

Specific to differential diagnoses (e.g., endoscopy, biopsy, echocardiography).

IMAGING

• For neurologic differentials, CT or MRI to rule out structural brain/spinal disease; altered brain/gray matter volume/density reported in CD. • Radiography, ultrasound if needed to rule out underlying physical causes.

DIAGNOSTIC PROCEDURES

History, video clips.

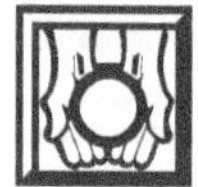

TREATMENT

Repetitive behaviors may represent a normal coping mechanism. If not harmful nor interfering with normal functioning, health, or human–animal bond, intervention may be unnecessary or contraindicated.

APPROPRIATE HEALTH CARE

• Generally outpatient. • Sedation—stop-gap measure; if needed to stop serious self-mutilation. • Treat associated physical conditions (primary or secondary).
• Combination of environmental modification, behavior modification, and

pharmacologic treatment. • Pharmacologic intervention—implement early; reduction of anxiety facilitates behavioral therapy.
• Environmental modification—reduce stress and anxiety; identify and remove sources (e.g., triggers) and/or begin desensitization and counter-conditioning exercises.
• Punishment—contraindicated; increases anxiety, may worsen behavior and increase patient secrecy. • Provide structured, consistent interactions, routine, and sufficient exercise, enrichment/mental stimulation appropriate to species and individual; includes interactive play, food puzzles, and reward-based training. • Behavior modification—teach the patient to relax in a variety of settings; also teach a calm, desirable behavior incompatible with the stereotypic one, coupled to a verbal cue (e.g., for circling, teach to lie down with head and neck outstretched in response to "Head down"). In some cases, a head collar (e.g., Gentle Leader, Halti) left on the dog (when the owner is home) in the problem contexts may allow the owner to use gentle physical guidance along with verbal encouragement/cues to interrupt the behavior and redirect it more effectively; monitor for situation in which behavior occurs and preempt it by engaging the pet in an incompatible activity; if behavior occurs, disrupt immediately, redirect the animal to alternative incompatible activity and reward (with food/play/other reinforcer); dogs with CD may be more perseverant and thus not respond well to extinction procedures. • Have clients monitor behaviors via videos and written logs (e.g., rate severity) for objective assessment of response to therapy; improvement may be seen in frequency and/or intensity. • Bandages, collars, braces, and crates increase distress, do not address the behavioral condition, and may worsen it; if needed to ensure healing, use as briefly as possible.

ACTIVITY

Environmental enrichment.

CLIENT EDUCATION

• Cure unlikely; usually requires lifelong management. • Teach client to recognize all body language/behaviors reflecting anxiety.

SURGICAL CONSIDERATIONS

Tail/limb mutilation—avoid amputation unless medically indicated; will not resolve the CD.

MEDICATIONS

DRUG(S) OF CHOICE

• Selective serotonin reuptake inhibitors (SSRIs) and tricyclic antidepressants (TCAs)—CNS serotonin effects. • Generally treat at low end of dose range for 4–6 weeks; gradually increase dosage if ineffective and no adverse events. • SSRIs—fluoxetine 1–2 mg/kg q24h; sertraline 1–3 mg/kg q24h; paroxetine 1–2 mg/kg q24h. • TCAs—clomipramine is most serotonergic (most effective, fewest side effects): 2–3 mg/kg q12h. • If symptoms resolve, continue medication for >1 month; taper dose no faster than 25% every two weeks; recurrence common.

CONTRAINDICATIONS

• Hepatic or renal compromise—medications metabolized by these organs. • Cardiac conduction anomalies—TCAs. • Use extreme care combining serotonergic drugs (e.g., SSRI with tramadol); risk of serotonin syndrome.
• Do not use SSRIs or TCAs within 2 weeks of monoamine oxidase (MAO) inhibitors (e.g., selegiline, amitraz).

PRECAUTIONS

• Use of listed medications for CD is extra- or off-label. • TCA overdose—cardiac conduction disturbances. • TCA/SSRI overdose—serotonin syndrome. • Side effects of SSRIs and TCAs—most common: lethargy, appetite change; less common: increased anxiety/reactivity, vomiting/diarrhea; severe side effects may necessitate discontinuation.

POSSIBLE INTERACTIONS

SSRIs competitively inhibit cytochrome P450 enzymes: may increase warfarin, many TCAs, some benzodiazepines and anticonvulsants, other medications; check compatibility and adjust dosage if necessary.

ALTERNATIVE DRUG(S)

• Synthetic pheromones (Adaptil), l-theanine, or alpha-casozepine—may reduce anxiety.
• Adjunctive use of memantine (NMDA receptor antagonist) 0.3–1 mg/kg q12h; second-line TCAs, e.g., amitriptyline 1–6 mg/kg q12h. • Selegiline (MAO inhibitor) 0.5–1 mg/kg q24h—may be effective in some cases. • Narcotic antagonists (e.g., naltrexone, naloxone)—may be effective but not a practical therapeutic option. • Antipsychotics (e.g., thioridazine, haloperidol)—not recommended: risk of adverse effects, efficacy undocumented.

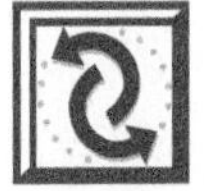

FOLLOW-UP

PATIENT MONITORING

• CBC, biochemistry, T_4 (TCAs may artificially lower), and urinalysis—semi-annually to yearly if chronic treatment; adjust dosages accordingly. • Medications may take 8–12 weeks or longer to affect CDs; first sign of efficacy may be reduced duration/frequency. • Relapses common during stressful situations; manage with increased intensity of behavior modification, addition of short-term, shorter-acting anxiolytics (e.g., benzodiazepines).

PREVENTION/AVOIDANCE

Monitor for affected relatives; early recognition and intervention.

POSSIBLE COMPLICATIONS

Dermatologic/musculoskeletal injury; gastrointestinal disorders.

EXPECTED COURSE AND PROGNOSIS

• Untreated CDs almost always progress.
• >50% reduction in CD in approximately two-thirds of cases with appropriate medication and behavioral and environmental modification.

MISCELLANEOUS

ASSOCIATED CONDITIONS

Various; specific to type of CD.

PREGNANCY/FERTILITY/BREEDING

• Listed medications not evaluated/contraindicated in pregnant animals; avoid use. • Do not breed affected animals.

SYNONYMS

Obsessive-compulsive disorder.

SEE ALSO

Acral Lick Dermatitis.

ABBREVIATIONS

• CD = compulsive disorder. • DJD = degenerative joint disease. • HPA = hypothalamic–pituitary–adrenal. • IBD = inflammatory bowel disease. • MAO = monoamine oxidase. • NMDA = N-methyl-D-aspartate. • SSRI = selective serotonin reuptake inhibitor. • TCA = tricyclic antidepressant.

Suggested Reading

Crowell-Davis SL, Murray T, Dantas L. Veterinary Psychopharmacology, 2nd ed. Hoboken, NJ: Wiley, 2019.

Overall KL, Dunham AE. Clinical features and outcome in dogs and cats with obsessive-compulsive disorder; 126 cases (1989–2000). J Am Vet Med Assoc 2002, 221:1445–1452.

Tynes VV, Sinn L. Abnormal repetitive behaviors in dogs and cats: a guide for practitioners. Vet Clin Small Anim Pract 2014, 44:543–564.

Author Mary P. Klinck

Consulting Editor Gary M. Landsberg

Acknowledgment The author and book editors acknowledge the prior contribution of Karen L. Overall

Client Education Handout available online

CONGENITAL AND DEVELOPMENTAL RENAL DISEASES

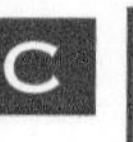

BASICS

DEFINITION

• Functional or morphologic abnormalities resulting from heritable (genetic) or acquired disease processes affecting differentiation and growth of the developing kidney. • Renal agenesis—complete absence of one or both kidneys. • Renal dysplasia—disorganized renal parenchymal development. • Renal ectopia—congenital malposition of one or both kidneys. • Glomerulopathy—glomerular disease of any type. • Polycystic renal disease—formation of multiple, variable-sized cysts throughout the renal medulla and cortex. • Renal telangiectasia—multifocal vascular malformations involving the kidneys and other organs. • Renal amyloidosis—extracellular deposition of amyloid in glomerular capillaries, glomeruli, and interstitium. • Nephroblastoma—congenital renal neoplasm arising from the pluripotent metanephric blastema. • Multifocal renal cystadenocarcinoma—hereditary renal neoplasm in dogs. • Fanconi syndrome—generalized renal tubular functional anomaly characterized by impaired reabsorption of glucose, phosphate, electrolytes, amino acids, and uric acid. • Primary renal glucosuria—defect in renal tubular reabsorption of glucose. • Cystinuria—excessive urinary excretion of cystine due to defect in renal tubular reabsorption of cystine and other amino acids. • Xanthinuria—excessive urinary excretion of xanthine caused by a deficiency in xanthine oxidase. • Hyperuricuria—excessive urinary excretion of uric acid, sodium urate, or ammonium urate. • Primary hyperoxaluria—intermittent hyperoxaluria, l-glyceric aciduria, and oxalate nephropathy. • Congenital nephrogenic diabetes insipidus—polyuria caused by diminished renal responsiveness to antidiuretic hormone.

PATHOPHYSIOLOGY

Many congenital and developmental renal disorders are caused by genetic abnormalities that disrupt the normal development and interaction of multiple embryonic tissues involved in formation of the mature kidney. Nongenetic factors are also possible.

SYSTEMS AFFECTED

Renal/urologic.

GENETICS

• Familial renal disorders have been reported in the following breeds: ◦ Renal agenesis—beagle, Doberman pinscher, Shetland sheepdog. ◦ Renal dysplasia—Alaskan Malamute, border terrier, boxer, bullmastiff, bulldog, Cairn terrier, cavalier King Charles spaniel, chow chow, cocker spaniel, Dutch kookier, golden retriever, Finnish harrier, keeshond, Lhasa apso, miniature schnauzer, Norwegian elkhound, Rhodesian ridgeback, shih tzu, soft-coated wheaten terrier, standard poodle. ◦ Glomerulopathy—Airedale terrier, beagle, Belgian shepherd, Bernese mountain dog, Brittany spaniel, bull terrier, bullmastiff, Dalmatian, Doberman pinscher, English cocker spaniel, Newfoundland, Pembroke Welsh corgi, Rottweiler, Samoyed, soft-coated wheaten terrier. ◦ Polycystic renal disease—beagle, bull terrier, Cairn terrier, West Highland white terrier; Persian, exotic shorthair, Himalayan, British blue cats. ◦ Renal telangiectasia—Pembroke Welsh corgi. ◦ Renal amyloidosis—Abyssinian, oriental shorthair, Siamese cats; beagle, English foxhound, shar-pei. ◦ Renal cystadenocarcinoma—German shepherd. ◦ Fanconi syndrome—basenji and border terrier. ◦ Primary renal glucosuria—Norwegian elkhound, Scottish terrier, basenji. ◦ Cystinuria—American pit bull terrier, basset hound, English bulldog, dachshund, mastiff, Newfoundland, Rottweiler, among others. ◦ Xanthinuria—cavalier King Charles spaniel, wirehaired dachshund; domestic shorthair cats. ◦ Hyperuricuria—Dalmatian, black Russian terrier, English bulldog. ◦ Primary hyperoxaluria—domestic shorthair cats; Tibetan spaniel.

INCIDENCE/PREVALENCE

Uncommonly recognized, but occur more frequently in related animals from more than one generation than in the general population.

SIGNALMENT

Species

Dog and cat.

Breed Predilections

Sporadic cases can occur without apparent familial predisposition in any breed of dog or cat.

Mean Age and Range

Most are <5 years old at time of diagnosis.

Predominant Sex

• Familial cystinuria occurs primarily in male dogs. • Samoyed hereditary glomerulopathy more common in males. • Familial glomerulonephropathy of Bernese mountain dogs is more common in females.

SIGNS

General Comments

Most congenital and developmental disorders cannot be distinguished from acquired renal disease without kidney biopsy.

Historical Findings

• Indicate chronic kidney disease. • Some glomerulopathies associated with abdominal distension, edema, or other signs of nephrotic syndrome. • Abdominal distension in some patients with polycystic kidneys or renal neoplasms. • Hematuria or abdominal pain in some patients with renal telangiectasia or renal neoplasms. • Patients with unilateral renal agenesis, ectopic kidneys, and isolated renal tubular transport defects are frequently asymptomatic.

Physical Examination Findings

• Signs associated with advanced chronic kidney disease. • Ascites or pitting edema in some patients with protein-losing glomerulopathies or amyloidosis. • Renomegaly or abdominal mass lesions in some patients with polycystic kidneys, renal neoplasms, or fused ectopic kidneys.

CAUSES

Nonhereditary

• Infectious agents—feline panleukopenia virus and canine herpesvirus infection associated with renal dysplasia. • Drugs—corticosteroids, diphenylamine, and biphenyls associated with polycystic kidneys; chlorambucil and sodium arsenate associated with renal agenesis. • Dietary factors—hypo- or hypervitaminosis A associated with renal ectopia.

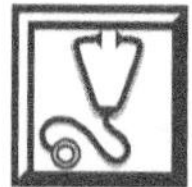

DIAGNOSIS

DIFFERENTIAL DIAGNOSIS

• Rule out acquired and nondevelopmental causes of primary renal disease. • Rule out nonrenal causes of hematuria, proteinuria, glucosuria, abdominal distention, or ascites.

CBC/BIOCHEMISTRY/URINALYSIS

• Nonregenerative anemia. • Azotemia and urine specific gravity <1.030 in dogs and <1.035 in cats. • Proteinuria, hypoalbuminemia, and hypercholesterolemia with nephrotic syndrome. • Normoglycemic glucosuria in Fanconi syndrome or primary renal glucosuria. • Hematuria with congenital renal neoplasia or renal telangiectasia. • Cystine crystalluria with cystinuria. • Xanthine crystalluria with xanthinuria. • Urate crystalluria with hyperuricuria.

OTHER LABORATORY TESTS

Genetic tests are available for some specific genetic mutations associated with hereditary renal disorders.

IMAGING

Survey abdominal radiography, renal ultrasonography, and excretory urography may identify and characterize congenital and developmental renal disorders and their associated sequelae.

DIAGNOSTIC PROCEDURES

Consider light microscopic evaluation of kidney biopsy specimens from patients with morphologic or functional abnormalities of the kidney for which a definitive diagnosis has not been established.

PATHOLOGIC FINDINGS

• Renal dysplasia—primary lesions include immature glomeruli, persistent mesenchyme, persistent metanephric ducts, atypical tubular epithelium, and dysontogenic metaplasia; primary lesions usually associated with, and may be obscured by, secondary degenerative, inflammatory, and compensatory lesions. • Glomerulopathies—usually normal-to-small kidneys; most are characterized by a primary membranoproliferative glomerulonephritis with variable degrees of tubulointerstitial disease, others have cystic atrophic membranous glomerulopathy. • Polycystic renal disease—see Polycystic Kidney Disease. • Renal amyloidosis—see Amyloidosis. • Renal telangiectasia—multiple, variable-sized, red-black, blood-filled nodules and clots in the renal cortex and medulla, interstitial fibrosis, interstitial mononuclear cell infiltrate, and hydronephrosis. • Nephroblastoma—unilateral renal mass; contains both embryonic mesenchymal and epithelial tissue components. • Multifocal renal cystadenocarcinoma—bilaterally enlarged kidneys with irregular protruding cystic structures or multifocal neoplastic renal tubular epithelial cell proliferations. • Renal ectopia—kidneys abnormally located in the retroperitoneal space or abdomen; horseshoe kidneys are symmetrically fused along the medial border of either pole. • Fanconi syndrome—inconsistent findings of tubular atrophy, interstitial fibrosis, and acute papillary necrosis. • Primary hyperoxaluria—large, irregularly shaped kidneys; renal tubular deposition of calcium oxalate crystals and variable interstitial and periglomerular fibrosis.

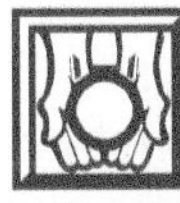

TREATMENT

• Congenital and developmental renal disorders often have no specific treatment. • Supportive strategies are similar to those for acquired chronic kidney disease and may improve quality of life and minimize progression in patients with renal dysfunction. • Refer to chapters describing specific renal diseases or clinical syndromes.

MEDICATIONS

DRUG(S) OF CHOICE

Refer to chapters describing specific renal diseases or clinical syndromes.

CONTRAINDICATIONS

Avoid potentially nephrotoxic drugs or anesthetic agents that decrease renal function.

PRECAUTIONS

Avoid drugs requiring renal excretion in patients with renal failure; if necessary, modify dosage regimens to compensate for decreased renal clearance of drugs and other metabolites.

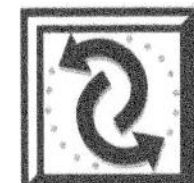

FOLLOW-UP

PATIENT MONITORING

Refer to chapters describing specific renal diseases or clinical syndromes.

PREVENTION/AVOIDANCE

Congenital and developmental renal disorders are irreversible, so control lies in preventing breeding of affected animals.

POSSIBLE COMPLICATIONS

• Acute or chronic renal failure. • Nephrotic syndrome. • Urolithiasis. • Hydronephrosis. • Urinary tract infection.

EXPECTED COURSE AND PROGNOSIS

• Highly variable; depends on the specific disorder, the extent of primary lesions, and the severity of renal dysfunction. • Congenital and developmental disorders are irreversible and may result in advanced chronic kidney disease; some patients with mild to moderate renal dysfunction may remain stable for long periods. • Patients with some disorders may remain asymptomatic unless the disorder is complicated by urolithiasis, infection, or other disease processes that promote progressive renal dysfunction.

MISCELLANEOUS

ASSOCIATED CONDITIONS

• Polycystic renal disease associated with hepatic biliary cysts. • Cystinuria, xanthinuria, and hyperuricuria associated with formation of uroliths. • Amyloidosis in Chinese Shar-Pei dogs associated with intermittent pyrexia or swelling of the hocks. • Renal neoplasms associated with hypertrophic osteoarthropathy, polycythemia, or other paraneoplastic syndromes.

SYNONYMS

• Familial renal disease. • Juvenile renal disease.

SEE ALSO

- Acute Kidney Injury.
- Amyloidosis.
- Anemia of Chronic Kidney Disease.
- Chronic Kidney Disease.
- Fanconi Syndrome.
- Hematuria.
- Hyperparathyroidism, Renal Secondary.
- Nephrotic Syndrome.
- Oliguria and Anuria.
- Polycystic Kidney Disease.
- Polyuria and Polydipsia.
- Renal Tubular Acidosis.
- Renomegaly.
- Urolithiasis, Cystine.

Suggested Reading

Segev G. Familial and congenital renal diseases of cats and dogs. In: Ettinger SJ, Feldman EC, Cote E, eds., Textbook of Veterinary Internal Medicine, 8th ed. St. Louis, MO: Elsevier, 2017, pp. 1981–1984.

Author John M. Kruger

Consulting Editor J.D. Foster

Acknowledgment The author and book editors acknowledge the prior contributions of Carl A. Osborne, and Scott D. Fitzgerald.

Client Education Handout available online

CONGENITAL OCULAR ANOMALIES

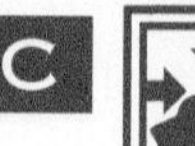

BASICS

DEFINITION

Solitary or multiple abnormalities that affect the globe or its adnexa; observed in dogs and cats at birth or within the first 6–8 weeks of life.

PATHOPHYSIOLOGY

- Breed-related inherited defects.
- Spontaneous malformations.
- In utero systemic infections and inflammations, exposure to toxic compounds, and lack of specific nutrients in pregnant dams or bitches.

SYSTEMS AFFECTED

Ophthalmic—entire eye or any part; unilateral or bilateral.

GENETICS

- * Indicates availability of genetic testing for all or most affected breeds.
- Congenital keratoconjunctivitis sicca (KCS) and KCS ichthyosiform dermatosis (KCSID)*—cavalier King Charles spaniel (dry eye and curly coat syndrome): recessive trait.
- Persistent pupillary membranes (PPM)—Basenji and other breeds: unknown mode of inheritance.
- Persistent hyperplastic tunica vasculosa lentis (PHTVL) and persistent hyperplastic primary vitreous (PHPV)—Doberman pinscher and Staffordshire bull terrier: dominant allele with variable expression.
- Retinal dysplasia—English springer spaniel: recessive trait.
- Collie eye abnormality (CEA)*—collie and other dog breeds: recessive trait.
- Merle ocular dysgenesis (MOD)—Australian shepherd: autosomal recessive trait with incomplete penetrance.
- Oculo-skeletal dysplasia (OSD)*—Labrador retriever and Samoyed: autosomal dominant trait with incomplete penetrance.
- Retinal dystrophy*—Briard: recessive trait.
- Rod cone dysplasia*—collies, Irish setter, Cardigan Welsh corgi, sloughi: recessive traits; nonallelic disease.
- Early retinal degeneration*—Norwegian elkhound: recessive trait.
- Photoreceptor dysplasia—Belgian shepherd.
- Cone rod dystrophy*—American pit bull terrier, American Staffordshire terrier, springer spaniel, long-, short- and wirehaired dachshunds: recessive traits; nonallelic disease.
- Cone degeneration, achromatopsia, or day blindness*—Alaskan Malamute, Australian shepherd, German shepherd dog, miniature American shepherd, German shorthaired pointer, Australian cobberdog, Labrador retriever and Labrador crosses (incl. Labradoodles): recessive traits.
- Optic nerve hypoplasia—miniature and toy poodle, sporadically in other breeds: unknown mode of inheritance.
- Photoreceptor dysplasia*—Abyssinian, Somali, and Ocicat cat breeds: dominant trait.

INCIDENCE/PREVALENCE

- Incidence—low; dogs > cats.
- CEA—>50% in collies, lower in other breeds.

SIGNALMENT

Species

Dog and cat.

Breed Predilections

See Genetics.

SIGNS

General Comments

- Depends on defect.
- May cause no signs of disease; often incidental finding.
- May be congenitally blinding disease.

Historical Findings

Ranges from none to severe visual impairment to blindness.

Physical Examination Findings

- Anophthalmos—congenital lack of globe; rare.
- Microphthalmos—congenitally small eye; often associated with other hereditary defects, including MOD.
- Eyelid agenesis or colobomas of eyelids in cats—result in congenitally open eyelids; affects temporal portion of upper eyelid; may cause blepharospasm, epiphora, and corneal changes as result of trichiasis.
- Dermoids—islands of aberrant skin tissue involving either eyelids, conjunctiva, or cornea; may cause blepharospasm and epiphora (see Web Figure 1).
- Atresia and imperforate puncta of lacrimal system, common in dogs—results in tear streak at nasal canthus.
- Congenital KCS—usually unilateral; affected eye appears smaller; thick mucous discharge from red and irritated eye.
- KCSID—therapy-resistant KCS, curly coat and progressive dermatologic signs, including footpad hyperkeratosis that can cause lameness.
- PPMs—remnants of pupillary membrane spanning from iris collarette to another portion of iris, lens, or cornea; may coexist with other defects (see Web Figures 2 and 3).
- Iris cysts—pigmented or nonpigmented spherical structures may float freely in anterior chamber or be attached to posterior iris, ciliary body, or corneal endothelium (see Web Figure 4).
- Congenital glaucoma—rare; buphthalmic eye, often associated with multiple anterior segment changes.
- Pupillary abnormalities—polycoria, acorea, aniridia, or dyscoria.
- Congenital cataracts—primary, inherited, or developmental defect; associated with anomalies of lens, including microphakia, lenticonus or lentiglobus, and coloboma (see Web Figures 5 and 6).
- PHTVL and PHPV—persistence of parts of hyaloid vasculature; developmental aberrations of vitreous, lens, and lens capsule; may show leukocoria as result of retrolental fibrovascular plaques and/or cataracts, or reddish sheen from pupillary area with intralenticular bleeding.
- Retinal dysplasia—effect on retinal structure depends on severity; ranges from focal neuroretinal folds (multifocal defects often along major blood vessels in central tapetal fundus) to geographic dysplasia (abnormal central tapetal fundus area with elevated retina and surrounding hyperpigmentation and scarring) to complete retinal detachment.
- CEA—bilateral area of choroidal hypoplasia temporal to optic nerve head: focal increased visibility of white sclera and scarce, irregularly shaped choroidal blood vessels; visual impairment or blindness can be caused by optic nerve coloboma and retinal detachment.
- MOD—microphthalmia, microcornea, heterochromia irides, pupillary abnormalities, cataract, fundus coloboma, retinal detachment, intraocular hemorrhage.
- Coloboma of posterior segment—primary or in conjunction with CEA or MOD; focal, well-defined tissue depression, typically at 6 o'clock position in optic nerve head in CEA, or in fundus periphery in MOD; may be in other locations of fundus near optic nerve head.
- OSD—heterozygous carriers typically display signs of focal/multifocal retinal dysplasia, whereas homozygous animals display complete phenotype, including skeletal (short-limbed dwarfism) and ocular defects (ranging from retinal dysplasia to retinal detachments; corneal and lens opacities also possible).
- Retinal dystrophy—congenital night blindness, variable severity and progression of day blindness.
- Rod cone dysplasia, early retinal degeneration, photoreceptor dysplasia, and cone rod dystrophy—pupillary abnormalities and visual impairment in first few months of life; disease progression depends on specific disease and breed affected.
- Cone degeneration—apparent day blindness from 8–10 weeks of age; vision in dim light never affected.
- Retinal detachment—often in conjunction with other hereditary ocular diseases; signs depend on extent of detachment and include widely dilated pupils, weak to absent

pupillary light reflexes; presence of fundus areas that appear out of focus, vascularized membranous structure (retina) visible within pupillary aperture behind lens, blindness with complete bilateral detachment.
• Optic nerve hypoplasia—avascular, dark, abnormally small, circular optic nerve head, may result in blindness.

CAUSES

• Genetic.
• Spontaneous malformations.
• Infections or inflammation during pregnancy.
• Toxicity during pregnancy.
• Nutritional deficiencies.

RISK FACTORS

Breeding dogs or cats that are homozygous or heterozygous for hereditary disease with recessive inheritance, or affected animals where disease has dominant inheritance.

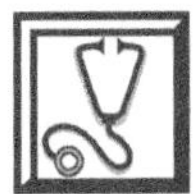

DIAGNOSIS

DIFFERENTIAL DIAGNOSIS

• Infectious and inflammatory processes in adnexa—may mimic and mask congenital abnormalities.
• Cataracts induced at early age may be interpreted as congenital.
• Postinflammatory ophthalmic lesions with anterior or posterior synechia—easily confused with iris to cornea or iris to lens PPMs.
• Tumors of anterior segment may be confused with iris cysts.
• Focal, multifocal, or generalized retinopathy of inflammatory origin—resulting retinal atrophy may appear to be retinal dysplasia or photoreceptor dysplasia.
• Retinal detachment as result of trauma or uveitis in young dogs.
• Optic nerve atrophy due to inflammatory process may be difficult to differentiate from congenital optic nerve hypoplasia.

IMAGING

• Routine ophthalmic ultrasound—use of 10–20 MHz probes for evaluation of intraocular changes in case of opacities that prevent proper ophthalmic examination.
• High-resolution ultrasound—use of 20–50 MHz probes for evaluation and measurement of corneal and anterior chamber structures, e.g., anterior chamber cysts or iridocorneal angle.

DIAGNOSTIC PROCEDURES

• Examination with diffuse and focal illumination, including slit-lamp biomicroscopy—evaluation of adnexal and anterior segment anomalies, including lens and anterior vitreous (following pharmacologic pupil dilation).
• Schirmer tear test—evaluate tear production.
• Tonometry—when glaucoma or uveitis suspected.
• Direct and/or indirect ophthalmoscopy—evaluation of posterior segment anomalies; pharmacologic pupil dilation necessary; difficult to perform in patients with opacities in cornea, anterior chamber, lens, or anterior vitreous.
• Gonioscopy—evaluation of width of and presence of signs of dysgenesis in iridocorneal angle when glaucoma suspected; critical to include examination of unaffected eye.
• Electroretinography (ERG).
• Optical coherence tomography (OCT).
• Referral to ophthalmologist necessary for gonioscopic, ERG, and OCT examinations.

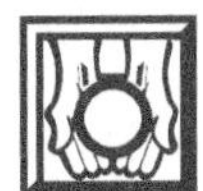

TREATMENT

APPROPRIATE HEALTH CARE

• Patients usually referred to ophthalmologist.
• No treatment for most congenital abnormalities, except symptomatic treatment or surgery.

NURSING CARE

• In KCS—removing discharge and flushing with saline.
• Accommodate handicap of blind animals—leash walking, supervision.

ACTIVITY

Visually impaired or blind animals need adequate exercise.

DIET

Provide diet adequate in vitamins, antioxidants, and omega-3 fatty acids, especially in photoreceptor degenerations.

CLIENT EDUCATION

Discuss visual capacity, possible progression, and sequelae.

SURGICAL CONSIDERATIONS

• Adnexal abnormalities—surgery as soon as possible.
• Congenital KCS—parotid duct transposition.
• Cataract extraction—congenital cataract may be associated with other anomalies, decreasing chances for visual rehabilitation or causing surgical complications; presurgical evaluation should include imaging and ERG.
• Congenital glaucoma—surgical options depend on presence of vision, size of patient/eye, and level of motivation of owners; enucleation or intrascleral prosthesis typical treatments of choice; consider euthanasia if bilateral.
• Barrier retinopexy to prevent occurrence of retinal detachments with large colobomatous or dysplastic lesions of fundus—carries risk of inducing retinal detachment.

MEDICATIONS

DRUG(S) OF CHOICE

• Congenital KCS—frequent application of tear substitutes; antibiotics may be added; cyclosporine ophthalmic ointment q12h.
• Congenital cataracts—if only in nuclear region of lens, mydriatics used to increase visual capability.

FOLLOW-UP

PATIENT MONITORING

• Congenital KCS—repeated monitoring of tear production and status of external eye.
• Congenital cataracts and severe PHTVL and PHPV—regular checkups, usually on 6-month basis; monitor progression.
• Large colobomatous defects of the fundus and geographic retinal dysplasia—regular checkups to monitor possible retinal detachment.

PREVENTION/AVOIDANCE

Restrict breeding of affected animals and of known carriers of hereditary defects; DNA-based tests available for various diseases (see Internet Resources).

POSSIBLE COMPLICATIONS

• In congenital KCS with parotid duct transposition, keratitis and dermatitis may occur due to excessive deposition of minerals from saliva.
• Cataract surgery can result in glaucoma, retinal detachment, and corneal scarring in puppies and kittens; surgery seldom recommended before age 8–12 weeks.

EXPECTED COURSE AND PROGNOSIS

• Most abnormalities affecting adnexa can be corrected in young dogs and cats.
• Prognosis for most anterior segment abnormalities good to fair.
• Prognosis for glaucoma poor.
• For photoreceptor abnormalities prognosis for vision poor, but eyes should remain comfortable.
• For most other abnormalities prognosis depends on severity of condition.

MISCELLANEOUS

PREGNANCY/FERTILITY/BREEDING

• Dogs and cats affected with congenital ocular anomalies resulting in blindness and/or pain should not be used for breeding.
• Many congenital ocular anomalies are hereditary and use of affected animals in breeding should be prohibited or severely

restricted. Breeding advice should be sought from kennel club and breed associations.

ABBREVIATIONS

- CEA = collie eye anomaly.
- ERG = electroretinography.
- KCS = keratoconjunctivitis sicca.
- KCSID = KCS ichthyosiform dermatosis.
- MOD = merle ocular dysgenesis.
- OSD = oculo-skeletal dysplasia.
- PHPV = persistent hyperplastic primary vitreous.
- PHTVL = persistent hyperplastic tunica vasculosa lentis.
- PPM = persistent pupillary membrane.

INTERNET RESOURCES

- These laboratories offer DNA-based tests:
  - www.antagene.com
  - www.CatDNAtest.org
  - www.aht.org.uk
  - www.laboklin.co.uk
  - https://breeder.wisdompanel.com/
  - https://vgl.ucdavis.edu/services
  - www.vetgen.com
  - www.caninegeneticdiseases.net
  - www.optimal-selection.com
  - www.mydogdna.com
  - www.pawprintgenetics.com
  - https://www.vet.upenn.edu/research/academic-departments/clinical-sciences-advanced-medicine/research-labs-centers/penngen/penngen-tests
- Good summaries of genetic basis and clinical signs of diseases, relevance of test results, and relevant references are listed on most of these websites.

Suggested Reading

Gelatt KN, Gilger BC, Kern TJ, ed. Veterinary Ophthalmology, 5th ed. Ames, IA: Wiley-Blackwell, 2013.

Maggs DJ, Miller PE, Ofri R, ed. Slatter's Fundamentals of Veterinary Ophthalmology, 6th ed. St. Louis, MO: Saunders, 2017.

Author Simon A. Pot

Consulting Editor Kathern E. Myrna

Client Education Handout available online

CONGENITAL SPINAL AND VERTEBRAL MALFORMATIONS

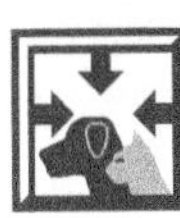

BASICS

DEFINITION

Anomalous development of spinal structures, which are apparent at birth or within the first weeks of life.

PATHOPHYSIOLOGY

- Malformation of the occipital bones, atlas, and axis; malformation of the odontoid process; occipitoatlantoaxial malformation; and occipital dysplasia—may cause atlanto-axial subluxation with secondary compression and trauma to the first segments of the cervical spinal cord.
- Other embryonic or developmental anomalies of the vertebrae such as hemivertebra, transitional vertebra, block vertebra, and butterfly vertebra—these defects cause deformity and instability of the vertebral canal and, on rare occasions, compression of the associated spinal cord or nerve roots.
- Sacrococcygeal dysgenesis—characterized by absence or partial development of the sacrocaudal spinal cord segments; often associated with additional malformations (e.g., spina bifida).
- Spina bifida—caused by failure of fusion of the vertebral arches; may be associated with protrusion of the spinal cord and meninges; other malformations often linked to this syndrome include spinal dysplasia, dysraphism, syringomyelia/hydromyelia, and myelodysplasia.
- Congenital spinal stenosis—can occur when vertebral malformations cause segmental or diffuse narrowing of the spinal cord; inborn errors in skeletal growth, hypertrophy of ligamentum flavum, and bony proliferation may also contribute to the stenosis.

SYSTEMS AFFECTED

Nervous—spinal cord; spinal nerve roots; and vertebral column.

GENETICS

- A genetic background, with unknown mode of inheritance, is suspected in most congenital spinal diseases.
- Sacrococcygeal dysgenesis—autosomal dominant.
- Thoracic hemivertebra of German shorthaired pointers—autosomal recessive.

GEOGRAPHIC DISTRIBUTION

N/A

SIGNALMENT

Species and Breed Predilections

- Malformation of the occipital bones, atlas, and axis—most common in small-breed dogs.
- Hemivertebra, transitional vertebra, block vertebra, and butterfly vertebra—most common in brachycephalic, "screw-tailed" breeds (e.g., French and English bulldog, pug, Boston terrier).
- Sacrococcygeal dysgenesis—Manx cat.
- Spina bifida—bulldog, Manx cat, and other screw-tailed breeds.
- Spinal dysraphism—Weimaraner.
- Congenital spinal stenosis—Doberman pinscher; chondrodystrophic breeds.

Mean Age and Range

- Often silent, vertebral malformation may cause clinical disease during the rapid growth of the animal (e.g., 5–9 months of age).
- Spinal cord anomalies cause clinical disease from birth on.

SIGNS

- Distortion of the spinal column—lordosis; kyphosis; and scoliosis in cases of vertebral malformations.
- Ataxia and paresis associated with spinal cord compression and trauma.
- Signs vary with spinal cord segment(s) involved.

CAUSES

Breed-related inherited defects are suspected for most congenital spinal abnormalities, although interactions between several genes and environmental factors (e.g., teratogenic compounds, nutritional deficiencies) are likely involved and would explain some of these complex pathologic changes.

RISK FACTORS

- Teratogenic compounds.
- Toxins.
- Nutritional deficiencies.
- Stress.

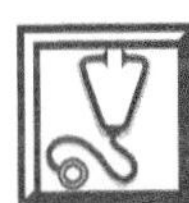

DIAGNOSIS

DIFFERENTIAL DIAGNOSIS

- Metabolic disease (e.g., storage diseases).
- Nutritional disease (e.g., hypovitaminosis and hypervitaminosis A, thiamine deficiency).
- Early-onset inflammatory or infectious processes (e.g., viral, protozoal, and rarely bacterial).
- Toxin exposure (e.g., lead, organophosphates, hexachlorophene, organochlorine).
- Trauma.

CBC/BIOCHEMISTRY/URINALYSIS

Usually within normal limits.

OTHER LABORATORY TESTS

N/A

IMAGING

- Survey radiography—to reveal vertebral malformation(s) and deviation of the spinal column.
- Myelography—to determine the level(s) of spinal cord compression; flexed and extended views may cause neurologic deterioration if instability present.
- CT myelography and 3D reconstructed imaging—to characterize bony abnormalities and associated spinal cord compression.
- MRI—sensitive modality to visualize abnormalities of spinal cord parenchyma, cauda equina, nerve roots, and surrounding soft tissues.

DIAGNOSTIC PROCEDURES

Cerebrospinal fluid analysis to rule out infectious/inflammatory conditions.

PATHOLOGIC FINDINGS

- Multiple congenital malformations—often present concomitantly; pathologic changes reflect several disease processes.
- Acute compression of the spinal cord secondary to congenital malformation(s)—may result in spinal cord ischemia, hemorrhage, ballooning of the myelin sheath at the point of compression or trauma, and axonal swelling or loss; in chronic spinal cord compression, myelin degeneration, astrocytosis, and fibrosis are more prominent; at spinal sites, cranial and caudal to the primary injury, Wallerian degeneration can be observed in ascending or descending pathways, respectively.
- Chronic changes—may result from vertebral malformations secondary to bony proliferation, thickening of the joint capsule, hypertrophy of articular processes, and thickening of the ligaments surrounding the spinal cord.
- Atlantoaxial subluxation—congenital aplasia or hypoplasia of the odontoid process and surrounding ligaments.
- Occipitoatlantoaxial malformations—fusion of the atlas to the occipital bone (cats) and dorsal angulation of the dens (dogs).
- Occipital dysplasia—anomaly of the foramen magnum in which the occipital bone is incompletely formed and fibrous tissue membrane covers the caudal cerebellum.
- Sacrococcygeal dysgenesis—caudal vertebral aplasia or hypoplasia.
- Spina bifida—incomplete fusion of the dorsal vertebral arches where the meninges or spinal cord can protrude; most commonly seen in the caudal lumbar or sacral area; a dimple can be observed in a few cases secondary to the lack of separation between the neuroectoderm and other ectodermal structures, leaving a small attachment between the spinal cord or meninges and the skin; often seen with myelodysplasia, central canal defects, syringomyelia or hydromyelia, and abnormal gray-matter differentiation.
- Spinal stenosis—pathologic changes observed within the spinal cord are most commonly chronic and are caused by focal or diffuse narrowing of the spinal canal.

CONGENITAL SPINAL AND VERTEBRAL MALFORMATIONS (CONTINUED)

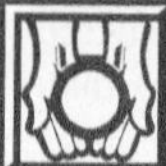

TREATMENT

APPROPRIATE HEALTH CARE

- Depends on severity of neurologic deficits.
- Outpatient—if animal is ambulatory.
- Inpatient—if animal is nonambulatory or requires emergency surgical treatment (e.g., for atlantoaxial subluxation).

NURSING CARE

- Restricted activity combined with physical therapy—may help neurologically disabled patients in the postoperative period; a cart may be necessary for severely affected patients.
- Management of urination—essential for cases in which disorders of micturition accompany the spinal injury.

ACTIVITY

Restricted, especially if vertebral subluxation is present.

DIET

Maintaining a lean bodyweight limits stress on the spinal column.

CLIENT EDUCATION

- Many congenital vertebral malformations are clinically silent.
- Perform a thorough workup when a congenial malformation results in neurologic abnormalities.
- Heritability is suspected; avoid breeding.
- Many neurologically affected dogs and cats left untreated are euthanized.
- Early surgical intervention often necessary to alleviate compression of the spinal cord and prevent further damage.

SURGICAL CONSIDERATIONS

- In general, surgical decompression is required when congenital malformation(s) cause narrowing of the spinal canal and compression of the spinal cord. In cases of chronic or diffuse spinal cord compression, improvement following surgery is minimal.
- Atlantoaxial subluxation—surgical ventral decompression combined with stabilization of the atlantoaxial joint with pins or screws is the treatment of choice.
- Spina bifida—meningoceles can be closed surgically to prevent leakage of cerebrospinal fluid and infections; surgery usually not attempted when the spinal cord parenchyma is involved.

MEDICATIONS

DRUG(S) OF CHOICE

Corticosteroids may be used in some cases, with variable results.

CONTRAINDICATIONS

Avoid steroids with concomitant infections.

PRECAUTIONS

Steroids may cause ulcerations of the gastrointestinal tract and inhibit bone growth.

POSSIBLE INTERACTIONS

Steroids reduce immune response following vaccination.

ALTERNATIVE DRUG(S)

N/A

FOLLOW-UP

PATIENT MONITORING

- Frequent neurologic examinations—to monitor the progression of clinical signs in developing animals (e.g., every 4–6 weeks).
- Neuroimaging—repeat as needed.

PREVENTION/AVOIDANCE

Avoid breeding affected animals.

POSSIBLE COMPLICATIONS

- Depend on the type and severity of neurologic signs. In cases of subluxation of the atlantoaxial joint, acute death may occur.
- Acute paralysis can also be seen with vertebral subluxation, with further trauma and spinal cord compression.
- Implant failure may be observed after surgical decompression/stabilization.

EXPECTED COURSE AND PROGNOSIS

- Prognosis varies depending on the type of malformation, degree of spinal cord compression or injury, and surgical decompression or stabilization techniques.
- Vertebral malformation without compression of the spinal cord—prognosis is good.
- Atlantoaxial subluxation following surgical decompression or stabilization—prognosis is fair to good.
- Spinal cord compression treated surgically—prognosis is fair.
- Spina bifida associated with spinal cord malformation, chronic neurologic disease despite surgical treatment, and lower motor neuron incontinence—prognosis is poor.
- Medical treatment usually is insufficient to alleviate moderate to severe neurologic signs caused by spinal cord compression secondary to congenital vertebral malformation(s).

MISCELLANEOUS

ASSOCIATED CONDITIONS

N/A

AGE-RELATED FACTORS

N/A

ZOONOTIC POTENTIAL

N/A

PREGNANCY/FERTILITY/BREEDING

N/A

SEE ALSO

- Ataxia.
- Atlantoaxial Instability.
- Cervical Spondylomyelopathy (Wobbler Syndrome).
- Paralysis.
- Spinal Dysraphism.

Suggested Reading

de Lahunta A, Glass E, Kent M. Veterinary Neuroanatomy and Clinical Neurology, 4th ed. St Louis, MO: W.B. Saunders, 2015, pp. 45–77.

Dewey CW, Da Costa RC. Myelopathies: disorders of the spinal cord. In: Dewey CW & Da Costa RC, ed., Practical Guide to Canine and Feline Neurology, 3rd ed. Ames, IA: John Wiley & Sons, Inc. 2016, pp. 361–371, 412–415.

Summer BA, Cummings JF, de Lahunta A. Veterinary Pathology. Philadelphia, PA: Mosby-Year Book, 1995, pp. 86–90.

Wyatt S, Gonçalves R, Gutierrez-Quintana & al. Outcomes of nonsurgical treatment for congenital thoracic vertebral body malformations in dogs: 13 cases (2009–2016). J Am Vet Med Assoc 2016;253:768–773.

Author Joane M. Parent.

Client Education Handout available online

CONGESTIVE HEART FAILURE, LEFT-SIDED

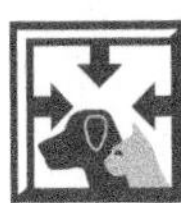

BASICS

DEFINITION

Failure of the left side of the heart to advance blood at a sufficient rate to meet the metabolic needs of the patient or to prevent blood from pooling within the pulmonary venous circulation.

PATHOPHYSIOLOGY

- Low cardiac output causes lethargy, exercise intolerance, syncope, and prerenal azotemia.
- High hydrostatic pulmonary venous pressure causes leakage of fluid from pulmonary venous circulation into pulmonary interstitium and alveoli; when fluid leakage exceeds ability of lymphatics to drain affected areas, pulmonary edema develops.

SYSTEMS AFFECTED

- All systems can be affected by poor perfusion. • Respiratory—increased rate and effort because of elevated pulmonary venous pressures/edema. • Cardiovascular.

GENETICS

Some congenital heart defects, cardiomyopathies, and valvular heart disease have genetic basis in some breeds.

INCIDENCE/PREVALENCE

Common

GEOGRAPHIC DISTRIBUTION

Seen everywhere; prevalence of causes varies with location.

SIGNALMENT

Species

Dog and cat.

Breed Predilections

Varies with cause.

Mean Age and Range

Varies with cause.

Predominant Sex

Varies with cause.

SIGNS

General Comments

Signs vary with underlying cause and species.

Historical Findings

- Weakness, lethargy, exercise intolerance.
- Coughing (dogs with large left atria, concurrent tracheobronchial disease, or such severe edema that large airways affected) and dyspnea (increased respiratory rate and effort); respiratory signs often worsen at night and may require assuming standing, sternal, or "elbows abducted" position (orthopnea). • Cats rarely cough from heart failure; coughing should prompt search for primary airway disease.

Physical Examination Findings

- Tachypnea and dyspnea. • Coughing, often soft in conjunction with tachypnea (dogs).
- Pulmonary crackles and wheezes. • Pale/gray/cyanotic mucous membranes.
- Prolonged capillary refill time. • Possible murmur or gallop. • Weak femoral pulses.

CAUSES

Pump (Muscle) Failure of Left Ventricle

- Dilated cardiomyopathy (DCM)/diet-induced DCM. • Trypanosomiasis (rare). • Doxorubicin cardiotoxicity (dogs). • Hypothyroidism (rare).
- Hyperthyroidism (rarely causes pump failure; more commonly causes high output failure).
- Tachycardia-induced cardiomyopathy (caused by persistent pathologic supraventricular or ventricular tachyarrhythmia).

Pressure Overload of Left Heart

- Systemic hypertension (uncommon cause of heart failure in animals). • Subaortic stenosis. • Aortic coarctation (rare; Airedale predisposed). • Left ventricular tumors (rare).

Volume Overload of Left Heart

- Degenerative mitral valve disease (dogs).
- Mitral valve dysplasia (cats and dogs).
- Patent ductus arteriosus (dogs). • Ventricular septal defect, especially if complicated by aortic valve insufficiency. • Aortic valve insufficiency secondary to endocarditis (dogs). • Chronic, severe anemia. • Inadvertent high-volume fluid administration. • Steroid administration (cats, often with previously asymptomatic underlying hypertrophic cardiomyopathy [HCM]).

Impediment to Filling of Left Ventricle

- Restrictive cardiomyopathy (rare in dogs, more common in cats). • Pulmonary vein stenosis (rare). • HCM. • Left atrial masses (e.g., tumor or thrombus). • Mitral stenosis (rare). • Cor triatriatum sinister (cats, rare).

Rhythm Disturbances

- Bradyarrhythmia (high-grade atrioventricular block). • Tachyarrhythmia (e.g., atrial fibrillation, sustained supraventricular tachycardia, ventricular tachycardia).

RISK FACTORS

Conditions causing chronic high cardiac output (e.g., hyperthyroidism and anemia).

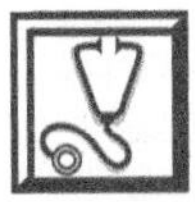

DIAGNOSIS

DIFFERENTIAL DIAGNOSIS

Must differentiate from other causes of coughing, dyspnea, and weakness.

CBC/BIOCHEMISTRY/URINALYSIS

- CBC usually normal; maybe stress leukogram. • Mild to moderate liver enzyme elevation; bilirubin generally normal.
- Prerenal azotemia in some animals.

OTHER LABORATORY TESTS

- Thyroid disorders may be detected.
- Serum NT-proBNP and cardiac troponin I concentrations higher in animals with left-sided congestive heart failure (L-CHF) than in normal animals.

IMAGING

Radiography

- Left heart and pulmonary veins enlarged.
- Pulmonary edema, often hilar, especially involving right caudal lung lobe in acute edema of dog, but may be patchy, especially in cats; acute pulmonary edema may begin in right caudal lung lobe.

Echocardiography

- Findings vary markedly with cause, but left atrial enlargement relatively consistent finding in cardiogenic pulmonary edema. • Diagnostic test of choice for documenting congenital defects, cardiac masses, and pericardial effusion.

DIAGNOSTIC PROCEDURES

ECG

- Atrial or ventricular arrhythmias.
- Evidence of left cardiomegaly (e.g., wide P waves, tall and wide QRS complexes, and left axis orientation). • May be normal.

PATHOLOGIC FINDINGS

Cardiac findings vary with disease.

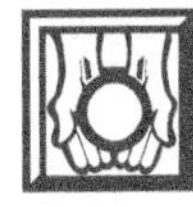

TREATMENT

APPROPRIATE HEALTH CARE

- Usually treat as outpatient unless dyspneic or severely hypotensive. • Identify and correct underlying cause whenever possible.
- Minimize handling of critically dyspneic animals—stress can kill!

NURSING CARE

Oxygen supplementation and postural support in dyspneic patients.

ACTIVITY

Restrict activity when dyspneic or tachypneic.

DIET

Initiate moderately sodium-restricted diet with adequate protein and calories. Severe sodium restriction indicated with advanced disease.

CLIENT EDUCATION

With few exceptions (e.g., animals with thyroid disorders, anemia, arrhythmias, nutritionally responsive heart disease, congenital heart disease), L-CHF is not curable.

SURGICAL CONSIDERATIONS

- Surgical intervention, coil embolization, Amplatz occluder placement, or balloon valvuloplasty may benefit selected patients with some forms of congenital and acquired valvular heart disease; response to these interventions varies. • Pericardiocentesis in animals with pericardial effusion.

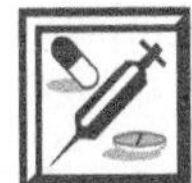

MEDICATIONS

DRUG(S) OF CHOICE

Diuretics

- Furosemide (1–2 mg/kg q8–24h) or other loop diuretic is initial diuretic of choice; diuretics indicated to reduce preload and remove pulmonary edema; critically dyspneic animals often require high doses (2–4 mg/kg) IV to

CONGESTIVE HEART FAILURE, LEFT-SIDED (CONTINUED)

stabilize; dose can be repeated in 1h if animal still severely dyspneic; IV bolus of 0.66 mg/kg followed by CRI of 0.66–1 mg/kg/h for 1–4h causes greater diuresis than equal dose divided into two IV boluses given 4h apart; once edema resolves, taper to lowest effective dose.
• Spironolactone (0.5–2 mg/kg PO q12–24h) increases survival in humans with CHF and is in clinical trials in dogs; use in combination with furosemide. • Thiazide diuretics can be added to furosemide and spironolactone in refractory heart failure cases. • Torsemide (0.2–0.8 mg/kg q24h) may be useful as substitute for furosemide in animals requiring daily furosemide dosing in excess of 12 mg/kg, and it may be more effective than furosemide at delaying death due to cardiac disease in dogs with CHF secondary to degenerative valve disease.

Angiotensin-Converting Enzyme ACE) Inhibitors

• ACE inhibitors such as enalapril (0.5 mg/kg q12–24h) or benazepril (0.25–0.5 mg/kg q12–24h) indicated in most animals with L-CHF. • ACE inhibitors improve survival and quality of life in dogs with L-CHF secondary to degenerative valve disease and DCM.

Positive Inotropes

• Pimobendan (0.25–0.3 mg/kg PO q12h) is a calcium channel sensitizer that dilates arteries and increases myocardial contractility; first-line agent in treating DCM or CHF due to degenerative valve disease efficacy in cats with CHF is not known, but possibly beneficial. • Dobutamine (dogs: 2.5–10 μg/kg/min; cats: 0.5–5 μg/kg/min) is a potent positive inotropic agent that may provide valuable short-term support of a heart failure patient with poor cardiac contractility. • Positive inotropes in general are potentially arrhythmogenic—monitor carefully.

Venodilators

• Nitroglycerin ointment (one-fourth inch/5 kg q6–8h) causes venodilation, lowering left atrial filling pressures. • Used for acute stabilization of patients with severe pulmonary edema and dyspnea, but uncertain benefit.

Antiarrhythmic Agents

Treat arrhythmias if clinically indicated.

CONTRAINDICATIONS

Avoid vasodilators in patients with pericardial effusion or fixed outflow obstruction.

PRECAUTIONS

• ACE inhibitors and arterial dilators must be used with caution in patients with possible outflow obstruction. • Pulmonary hypertension, hypothyroidism, and hypoxia increase risk for digoxin toxicity; hyperthyroidism diminishes effects of digoxin. • ACE inhibitors and digoxin—use cautiously in patients with renal disease. • Dobutamine—use cautiously in cats.
• Spironolactone—may cause facial pruritis in cats.

POSSIBLE INTERACTIONS

• Combination of high-dose diuretics and ACE inhibitors may cause azotemia, especially in animals with severe sodium restriction. • Combination diuretic therapy adds to risk of dehydration and electrolyte disturbances. • Combination vasodilator therapy predisposes animal to hypotension.

ALTERNATIVE DRUG(S)

Arterial Dilators

• Hydralazine (0.5–2 mg/kg PO q12h; 0.5 mg/kg PO to start when added to ACE inhibitor) or amlodipine (0.05–0.2 mg/kg PO q24h) can be substituted for ACE inhibitor in patients that do not tolerate the drug or have advanced renal failure; monitor for hypotension and tachycardia; can be cautiously added to ACE inhibitor in animals with refractory L-CHF. • Nitroprusside (1–10 μg/kg/min) is potent arterial dilator usually reserved for short-term support of patients with life-threatening edema.

Digoxin

• Digoxin (dogs: 0.22 mg/m^2 q12h; cats: 0.01 mg/kg q48h) is used in animals with atrial fibrillation and myocardial failure (e.g., DCM); commonly used in combination with diltiazem to control rate of atrial fibrillation.
• Digoxin is also indicated to treat dogs with refractory heart failure from either myocardial failure or volume loads; however, its use as a primary agent in myocardial failure has been replaced by pimobendan.

Calcium Channel Blockers

Diltiazem (0.5–1.5 mg/kg PO q8h) is frequently used in L-CHF patients for rate control in animals with supraventricular arrhythmias.

Beta Blockers

• Atenolol and metoprolol are sometimes used for rate control in animals with supraventricular tachycardia, hypertrophic cardiomyopathy, and hyperthyroidism. • Used alone or with a class 1 antiarrhythmic drug for control of ventricular arrhythmias; these drugs depress contractility (negative inotropes), so use cautiously in patients with myocardial failure or active signs of CHF.
• On basis of human studies, may enhance survival in animals with idiopathic DCM; treatment is best initiated under guidance of a cardiologist, starting with very low dosage and gradually increasing; carvedilol is sometimes used for this purpose, starting at 0.1 mg/kg q24h and titrating to 0.5 mg/kg q12h.

Nutritional Supplements

• Potassium and magnesium supplementation if deficiency is documented; use potassium supplements cautiously in animals receiving ACE inhibitor or spironolactone. • Taurine supplementation in cats with DCM and dogs with DCM and taurine deficiency (e.g., American cocker spaniels) • L-carnitine supplementation may help some dogs with DCM. • Coenzyme Q_{10} is of potential value based on results in humans with DCM.
• Ensure animal receiving a nutritionally balanced diet (see Cardiomyopathy, Nutritional).

FOLLOW-UP

PATIENT MONITORING

• Monitor resting respiratory rate and effort, appetite, renal status, electrolytes, hydration, heart rate, bodyweight. • If azotemia develops, reduce diuretic dose; if azotemia persists and animal is also on ACE inhibitor, reduce or discontinue ACE inhibitor; use digoxin with caution if azotemic. • Monitor ECG if arrhythmias suspected. • Check digoxin concentration (0.5–1.5 ng/mL, 8–10 hours post dose).

PREVENTION/AVOIDANCE

• Minimize stress, exercise, and sodium intake in patients with heart disease.
• Pimobendan delays onset of CHF in Doberman pinschers, and in dogs with hemodynamically significant myxomatous mitral valve regurgitation; prescribing an ACE inhibitor with pimobendan early in course of heart disease in patients with DCM may slow progression of heart disease and delay onset of CHF; role of ACE inhibitors in asymptomatic animals with mitral valve disease remains controversial.

POSSIBLE COMPLICATIONS

• Syncope. • Aortic thromboembolism (cats).
• Arrhythmias. • Electrolyte imbalances.
• Digoxin toxicity. • Azotemia and renal failure.

EXPECTED COURSE AND PROGNOSIS

Prognosis varies with underlying cause; cats and dogs that survive initial episode of pulmonary edema and can be reliably medicated often survive months to more than a year with good quality of life. Animals with reversible causes of L-CHF may recover to normal lives.

MISCELLANEOUS

AGE-RELATED FACTORS

• Congenital causes seen in young animals.
• Degenerative heart conditions and neoplasia generally seen in old animals.

SEE ALSO

Pulmonary Edema, Noncardiogenic.

ABBREVIATIONS

• ACE = angiotensin-converting enzyme.
• DCM = dilated cardiomyopathy.
• HCM = hypertrophic cardiomyopathy.
• L-CHF = left-sided congestive heart failure.

Authors Francis W.K. Smith, Jr. and Bruce W. Keene

Consulting Editor Michael Aherne

Client Education Handout available online

CONGESTIVE HEART FAILURE, RIGHT-SIDED

BASICS

DEFINITION

Failure of the right side of the heart to advance blood at a sufficient rate to meet the metabolic needs of the patient or to prevent blood from pooling within the systemic venous circulation.

PATHOPHYSIOLOGY

• High hydrostatic pressure leads to leakage of fluid from venous circulation into the pleural and peritoneal space and potentially into the pericardium and interstitium of peripheral tissue. • When fluid leakage exceeds ability of lymphatics to drain the affected areas, pleural effusion, ascites, pericardial effusion, and peripheral edema develop.

SYSTEMS AFFECTED

All systems can be affected by either poor delivery of blood or the effects of passive congestion from backup of venous blood.

GENETICS

• Some congenital cardiac defects have a genetic basis in certain breeds. • Arrhythmogenic right ventricular cardiomyopathy (ARVC) appears to have a genetic basis in boxers and possibly some cats.

INCIDENCE/PREVALENCE

Common

GEOGRAPHIC DISTRIBUTION

Syndrome seen everywhere; prevalence of various causes varies with location.

SIGNALMENT

Species

Dog and cat.

Breed Predilections

Vary with cause.

Mean Age and Range

Vary with cause.

Predominant Sex

Varies with cause.

SIGNS

General Comments

• Signs vary with underlying cause and between species. • Pleural effusion without ascites and hepatomegaly is rare in dogs with right-sided congestive heart failure (R-CHF). • Ascites without pleural effusion is rare in cats with R-CHF. • Small-volume pericardial effusion without tamponade is relatively common in cats with R-CHF. • Interstitial peripheral edema is a rare manifestation of R-CHF in both species.

Historical Findings

• Weakness. • Lethargy. • Exercise intolerance. • Abdominal distension. • Dyspnea, tachypnea.

Physical Examination Findings

• Jugular venous distention. • Hepatojugular reflux. • Jugular pulse in some animals. • Hepatomegaly. • Ascites common in dogs and rare in cats with R-CHF. • Possible regurgitant murmur in tricuspid valve region or ejection murmur at left heart base (pulmonic stenosis). • Muffled heart sounds if animal has pleural or pericardial effusion. • Weak femoral pulses. • Rapid, shallow respiration if animal has pleural effusion or severe ascites.• Peripheral edema (infrequent).

CAUSES

Pump (Myocardial) Failure of Right Ventricle

• Idiopathic dilated cardiomyopathy (DCM). • ARVC. • Hypertrophic cardiomyopathy (cats). • Restrictive cardiomyopathy (cats). • Trypanosomiasis. • Doxorubicin cardiotoxicity. • Chronic hyperthyroidism.

Volume Overload of Right Ventricle

• Chronic atrioventricular (AV) valve (mitral ± tricuspid) insufficiency due to myxomatous valvular degeneration. • Tricuspid valve dysplasia. • Large atrial septal defect.

Pressure Overload of Right Ventricle

• Heartworm disease. • Chronic obstructive pulmonary disease with pulmonary hypertension. • Pulmonary thromboembolism. • Pulmonic stenosis. • Tetralogy of Fallot. • Right ventricular tumors. • Heart base tumors (occasionally, compression of the pulmonary artery). • Primary pulmonary hypertension.

Impediment to Right Ventricular Filling

• Pericardial effusion (tamponade). • Constrictive/restrictive pericarditis. • Right atrial or caval masses. • Tricuspid stenosis. • Cor triatriatum dexter.

Rhythm Disturbances

• Bradycardia, generally complete AV block. • Tachyarrhythmias, generally sustained supraventricular tachycardia.

RISK FACTORS

• No heartworm prophylaxis. • Offspring of animal with right-sided congenital cardiac defect. • Conditions that augment demand for cardiac output (e.g., hyperthyroidism, anemia, pregnancy).

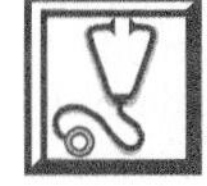

DIAGNOSIS

DIFFERENTIAL DIAGNOSIS

• Must differentiate from other causes of pleural effusion and ascites; generally requires complete diagnostic workup including CBC, biochemistry profile, heartworm test, thoraco- or abdominocentesis with fluid analysis and cytology, and sometimes thoracic and abdominal ultrasound. • Animals with ascites or pleural effusion due to heart failure should have jugular venous distension.

CBC/BIOCHEMISTRY/URINALYSIS

• CBC usually normal; animals with heartworm disease may have eosinophilia. • Mild to moderately high alanine aminotransferase, aspartate aminotransferase, and alkaline phosphatase due to passive liver congestion; bilirubin generally normal. • Prerenal azotemia in some animals.

OTHER LABORATORY TESTS

• Heartworm test may be positive. • NT-proBNP concentrations higher in animals with cardiac causes of fluid accumulation.

IMAGING

Thoracic Radiography

• Right cardiomegaly in some animals. • Dilated caudal vena cava (diameter greater than the length of the vertebra directly above the heart). • Pleural effusion (especially cats). • Hepatosplenomegaly and possible ascites (especially dogs).

Echocardiography

• Findings vary with underlying cause; especially useful for documenting congenital defect, cardiac mass, and pericardial effusion. • Abdominal ultrasound reveals hepatomegaly with hepatic vein dilation, flow reversal in the hepatic veins (Doppler), and possibly ascites.

DIAGNOSTIC PROCEDURES

ECG Findings

• Small (<1 mV) QRS complexes in all frontal axis leads if pericardial or pleural effusion. • Electrical alternans or elevated ST segment with pericardial effusion. • Evidence of right cardiomegaly (e.g., tall [>0.4 mV] P waves in lead II, deep S waves in leads I, II, aVF, and right axis deviation). • Atrial or ventricular arrhythmias. • ECG may be normal.

Abdominocentesis

Analysis of ascitic fluid in patients with R-CHF generally reveals modified transudate with total protein >2.5 mg/dL.

Thoracentesis

• Cats with pleural effusion associated with R-CHF may have transudate, modified transudate, or chylous effusion. • Dogs with pleural effusion and R-CHF may have transudate or modified transudate.

Central Venous Pressure

Central venous pressure is high (>9 cmH_2O) or rises dramatically to that level and remains elevated for more than 1h following a fluid bolus (e.g., 5–10 mL/kg IV).

PATHOLOGIC FINDINGS

• Cardiac findings vary with disease. • Hepatomegaly in animals with centrolobular necrosis (chronic condition).

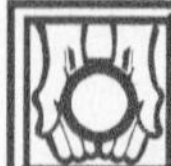

TREATMENT

APPROPRIATE HEALTH CARE

Most animals treated as outpatients unless dyspneic or collapsed (e.g., significant pleural or pericardial effusion).

NURSING CARE

Thoracentesis and abdominocentesis may be required periodically for patients no longer responsive to medical management or those with severe dyspnea due to pleural effusion or ascites.

ACTIVITY

Restrict activity.

DIET

Restrict sodium moderately; severe sodium restriction indicated for animals with advanced disease.

CLIENT EDUCATION

• With few exceptions (e.g., in heartworm disease, arrhythmias, hyperthyroidism, and idiopathic pericardial effusion), R-CHF is not curable. • Most patients improve with initial treatment but often have recurrent failure.

SURGICAL CONSIDERATIONS

• Surgical intervention or balloon valvuloplasty is indicated to treat certain congenital defects such as pulmonic stenosis or cor triatriatum dexter, and Amplatz occluder placement for morphologically appropriate atrial septal defects. • Pericardiocentesis or pericardectomy for pericardial effusion. • Removal of heartworms from the heart via the jugular vein in dogs with caval syndrome.

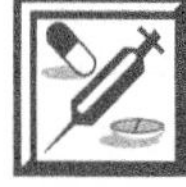

MEDICATIONS

DRUG(S) OF CHOICE

Drugs should be administered only after a definitive diagnosis is made.

Diuretics

• Furosemide (1–2 mg/kg q8–24h) or another loop diuretic is the initial diuretic of choice; diuretics are indicated to remove excess fluid accumulation. • Torsemide (0.2–0.8 mg/kg q24h) may be a useful substitute for furosemide in animals requiring a daily furosemide dose in excess of 12 mg/kg. • Spironolactone (2 mg/kg PO q12–24h) increases survival in humans with heart failure; use in combination with furosemide.

Vasodilators

• Angiotensin-converting enzyme (ACE) inhibitors such as enalapril (0.5 mg/kg q12–24h) or benazepril (0.25–0.5 mg/kg q24h) are helpful when CHF is secondary to DCM or chronic AV valve insufficiency.
• Sildenafil (0.5–1 mg/kg PO q12h up to 2–3 mg/kg q8h) may be beneficial for pulmonary hypertension.

Pimobendan

• Calcium sensitizer that acts as an inodilator, causing arterial vasodilation and increasing myocardial contractility. • Especially useful in myocardial failure. • Dose—0.25–0.3 mg/kg PO q12h.

Digoxin

• Digoxin (dogs: 0.22 mg/m^2 q12h; cats: 0.01 mg/kg q48 h) is used in animals with myocardial failure (e.g., DCM) and atrial fibrillation. • Digoxin indicated in animals with refractory CHF that have supraventricular arrhythmias.

CONTRAINDICATIONS

• Avoid diuretics in patients with pericardial effusion/tamponade. • Avoid vasodilators in patients with pericardial effusion or fixed outflow obstructions.

PRECAUTIONS

• ACE inhibitors and arterial dilators must be used with caution in patients with possible outflow obstructions. • Pulmonary hypertension, hypothyroidism, and hypoxia increase risk for digoxin toxicity; hyperthyroidism diminishes effects of digoxin. • ACE inhibitors and digoxin—use cautiously with renal disease. • Dobutamine—use cautiously in cats. • Spironolactone—may cause facial pruritis in cats.

POSSIBLE INTERACTIONS

• Combination of high-dose diuretics and ACE inhibitors may alter renal perfusion and cause azotemia. • Combination diuretic therapy promotes risk of dehydration and electrolyte disturbances.

ALTERNATIVE DRUG(S)

• Patients unresponsive to furosemide, spironolactone, vasodilator, pimobendan, and digoxin (if indicated) may benefit from triple diuretic therapy by adding a thiazide diuretic, or substitution of torsemide for furosemide, generally at 0.1–0.2 mg of torsemide for each 1 mg of furosemide previously administered.
• Potassium and magnesium supplementation if deficiency documented; use potassium supplements cautiously in animals receiving ACE inhibitors or spironolactone. • Treat arrhythmias if clinically indicated. • Taurine supplementation in cats with DCM and dogs with DCM and taurine deficiency. • Carnitine supplementation may help some dogs with DCM (e.g., cocker spaniels and boxers).

FOLLOW-UP

PATIENT MONITORING

• Monitor renal status, electrolytes, hydration, respiratory rate and effort, bodyweight, and abdominal girth (dogs). • If azotemia develops, reduce diuretic dosage; if azotemia persists and the animal is also on an ACE inhibitor, reduce or discontinue this drug; if azotemia develops, reduce digoxin dosage to avoid toxicity.
• Monitor ECG periodically to detect arrhythmias. • Monitor digoxin concentrations—normal value 0.5–1.5 ng/mL for serum sample obtained 8–10h after dose is administered.

POSSIBLE COMPLICATIONS

• Pulmonary thromboembolism. • Arrhythmias.
• Electrolyte imbalances. • Digoxin toxicity.
• Azotemia and renal failure.

EXPECTED COURSE AND PROGNOSIS

Prognosis varies with underlying cause.

MISCELLANEOUS

AGE-RELATED FACTORS

• Congenital causes seen in young animals.
• Degenerative heart conditions and neoplasia generally seen in old animals.

SEE ALSO

• Ascites.
• Chylothorax.
• Pleural Effusion.

ABBREVIATIONS

• ACE = angiotensin-converting enzyme.
• ARVC = arrhythmogenic right ventricular cardiomyopathy.
• AV = atrioventricular.
• DCM = dilated cardiomyopathy.
• R-CHF = right-sided congestive heart failure.

Authors Francis W.K. Smith, Jr. and Bruce W. Keene

Consulting Editor Michael Aherne

Client Education Handout available online

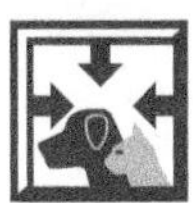

BASICS

DEFINITION

Inflammation of the conjunctiva, the vascularized mucous membrane that covers the anterior sclera (bulbar conjunctiva), lines the eyelids (palpebral conjunctiva), and lines the third eyelid.

PATHOPHYSIOLOGY

May be primary or secondary to adnexal or ocular disease.

SYSTEMS AFFECTED

Ophthalmic

GENETICS

N/A

INCIDENCE/PREVALENCE

Common

GEOGRAPHIC DISTRIBUTION

N/A

SIGNALMENT

Species

Cat

Breed Predilections

Infectious—purebred cats may be predisposed.

Mean Age and Range

Infectious—commonly affects young animals.

Predominant Sex

N/A

SIGNS

• Blepharospasm. • Conjunctival hyperemia. • Ocular discharge—serous, mucoid, or mucopurulent. • Chemosis. • Conjunctival follicles. • Upper respiratory infection—possible with infectious etiologies.

CAUSES

Viral

• Feline herpesvirus (FHV)—most common infectious cause; only one that leads to corneal changes (e.g., dendritic or geographic ulcers). • Calicivirus—may cause conjunctival ulcerations.

Bacterial

• *Chlamydophila felis*—chemosis is common clinical sign. • *Mycoplasma* spp.—may be overgrowth of normal flora. • Conjunctivitis neonatorum—accumulation of exudates under closed eyelids prior to natural opening; bacterial or viral component.

Immune-Mediated

• Eosinophilic. • Lipogranulomatous. • Allergic. • Related to systemic immune-mediated disease.

Trauma or Environmental Causes

• Conjunctival foreign body. • Irritation from dust, smoke, chemicals, or ophthalmic medications.

Secondary to Adnexal Disease

• May develop keratoconjunctivitis sicca (KCS) as a result of scarring. • Eyelid diseases (e.g., entropion, trichiasis, distichia, or eyelid agenesis)—cause frictional irritation or exposure. • Dacryocystitis or nasolacrimal system outflow obstruction.

Referred Inflammation from Other Ocular or Periocular Diseases

• Ulcerative keratitis. • Corneal sequestrum. • Anterior uveitis. • Glaucoma. • Orbital disease. • Pyoderma.

RISK FACTORS

Stress or immune system compromise (FHV).

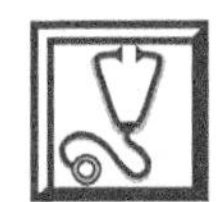

DIAGNOSIS

DIFFERENTIAL DIAGNOSIS

• Must distinguish primary conjunctivitis from secondary conjunctival hyperemia. • Thorough ophthalmic exam rules out other diseases (e.g., ulcers, uveitis, glaucoma, orbital disease); assess pupil size and symmetry, look for aqueous flare, perform intraocular pressure testing and fluorescein staining. • Deeper, darker, more linear and immobile blood vessel injection indicates episcleral vasculature congested due to intraocular disease. • Conjunctival mass biopsy will identify neoplasia (lymphoma and squamous cell carcinoma most common).

CBC/BIOCHEMISTRY/URINALYSIS

Normal, except with systemic disease.

OTHER LABORATORY TESTS

Infectious—serologic testing for feline leukemia virus (FeLV) and feline immunodeficiency virus (FIV).

IMAGING

N/A

DIAGNOSTIC PROCEDURES

• Thorough adnexal examination—rule out eyelid abnormalities and foreign bodies under eyelids or third eyelid. • Complete ophthalmic examination—rule out other ocular disease (e.g., uveitis, glaucoma). • Fluorescein stain—assess for corneal ulceration or dendritic lesions (FHV) and observe nares for stain passage to indicate nasolacrimal system patency. • Nasolacrimal flush—considered to rule out dacryocystitis or nasolacrimal system obstruction. • Schirmer tear test—measures aqueous tears to diagnose or rule out KCS; performed before anything is placed in the eye. • Conjunctival cytology—rarely reveals cause; eosinophils with eosinophilic conjunctivitis; degenerate neutrophils and intracytoplasmic bacteria indicate bacterial infection; intracytoplasmic inclusion bodies indicate chlamydial or mycoplasmal infection; rarely see intranuclear FHV inclusions.
• Conjunctival biopsy—"snip biopsy" may be useful with mass lesions and immune-mediated disease or chronic disease. • PCR testing for chlamydia or FHV. • Virus isolation or immunofluorescence antibody (IFA) testing for FHV; false-positive result if fluorescein staining is done before IFA testing.
• Serologic test for FHV antibodies—not useful (widespread exposure, vaccination).

PATHOLOGIC FINDINGS

• Biopsy—signs of inflammation, possible infectious agents. • Histopathology of mass lesions may reveal neoplasia (e.g., squamous cell carcinoma and lymphoma).

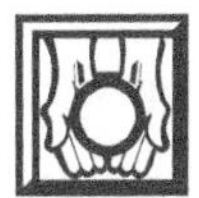

TREATMENT

APPROPRIATE HEALTH CARE

• Primary—often outpatient. • Secondary to other diseases (ulcerative keratitis, uveitis, glaucoma)—may need hospitalization to address severe underlying ophthalmic issue.

NURSING CARE

• Irritant-induced conjunctivitis—flush ocular surfaces and remove foreign body if observed.
• Topical hyaluronate-based artificial tear, q8h to benefit tear film. • Frequent cleaning of eyelid margins and periocular skin to remove ocular discharge.

ACTIVITY

• Generally, no restrictions. • Suspected contact irritant or acute allergic disease—prevent contact with the offending agent. • Suspected FHV—minimize stress. • Do not expose patients with infectious disease to susceptible animals.

DIET

• No change for most patients. • Suspected underlying skin disease and/or food allergy—food elimination diet.

CLIENT EDUCATION

• When solutions and ointments are prescribed, instruct the client to use solution(s) before ointment(s) and wait at least 5 minutes between treatments. • If copious discharge is noted, instruct client to clean eyes before giving medication. • Instruct client to call for instructions if condition fails to improve or worsens.

SURGICAL CONSIDERATIONS

• Lipogranulomatous conjunctivitis—surgical incision and curettage of glandular material and inflammatory infiltrates. • Entropion, distichia, or other eyelid disease—perform temporary or permanent surgery depending on the findings, signalment, and history.
• Nasolacrimal duct obstruction—difficult; treatment often not recommended (see Epiphora). • Conjunctival neoplasia—depending on tumor type and extent of involvement, may involve local excision and adjunctive therapy (β-irradiation, cryotherapy), enucleation, or exenteration. • Symblepharon

CONJUNCTIVITIS—CATS (CONTINUED)

C

(adhesions between the conjunctiva and cornea)—adhesions may require surgical resection (poor prognosis). • Corneal sequestration—keratectomy often recommended (see Corneal Sequestrum—Cats).

MEDICATIONS

DRUG(S) OF CHOICE

Herpetic

• Condition usually mild and self-limiting.
• Antiviral treatment—indicated for severe intractable conjunctivitis, herpetic keratitis, and before keratectomy for corneal sequestra suspected to be related to FHV; for all antivirals treat 2 weeks past resolution of clinical signs. • 0.5% cidofovir solution (available from compounding pharmacies)—topical, q12h. • 0.1% idoxuridine solution or 0.5% ointment (compounding pharmacies)—topical, q4h. • Vidarabine 3% ointment—topical, q4h. • Trifluridine 1% solution—topical, q4h; potentially irritating.
• Oral famciclovir is effective and safe; recommended dosage 90 mg/kg PO q12h.
• Lysine 500 mg PO q12h for adult cat (250 mg PO q12h for kitten). • FortiFlora® probiotic PO q24h may decrease incidence of conjunctivitis associated with FHV.

Chlamydial or Mycoplasmal

• Tetracycline, erythromycin, or chloramphenicol ophthalmic ointment—topically q6–8h; continue for several days past resolution of all clinical signs; recurrence or reinfection common. • Topical ciprofloxacin ophthalmic solution q6–8h as alternative to ophthalmic ointment. • Doxycycline 10 mg/kg PO q24h for 3–4 weeks may be superior to or used along with topical treatment. • Based on bacterial culture and sensitivity results.

Neonatal

Carefully open the eyelid margins (medial to temporal), establish drainage, and treat with topical antibiotic ointment q6–8h and an antiviral for suspected FHV.

Eosinophilic

• Topical corticosteroid—0.1% dexamethasone sodium phosphate q6–8h generally effective; taper gradually to lowest effective dose or transition to cyclosporine. • Cyclosporine 0.2% ointment 1–2% compounded solution, or tacrolimus 0.03% compounded solution—topical therapy q8–24h. • Topical 0.5% megestrol acetate solution (available from compounding pharmacies)—q8–12h; safe with concurrent corneal ulceration and/or concurrent FHV ocular disease. • Oral megestrol acetate—may help resistant condition, but rarely used given possible systemic side effects.

CONTRAINDICATIONS

• Topical corticosteroids—avoid with known or suspected infectious conjunctivitis; may result in FHV recrudescence and predispose to corneal sequestrum formation; never use if corneal ulceration is noted. • Valacyclovir should never be used in cats.

PRECAUTIONS

• Topical medications may be irritating.
• Monitor all patients treated with topical corticosteroids for signs of corneal ulceration; discontinue agent immediately if corneal ulceration occurs.

POSSIBLE INTERACTIONS

N/A

ALTERNATIVE DRUG(S)

Other corticosteroids—1% prednisolone acetate.

FOLLOW-UP

PATIENT MONITORING

Recheck shortly after beginning treatment (at 5 days), then in 2 weeks or as needed.

PREVENTION/AVOIDANCE

• Treat any underlying disease that may be exacerbating the conjunctivitis. • Minimize stress for patients with herpetic disease. • Isolate patients with infectious conjunctivitis to prevent spread. • Prevent reexposure to infectious sources. • Vaccination recommended; infection is still possible if the cat was exposed to an infectious agent before being vaccinated (e.g., FHV infection from an infected queen).

POSSIBLE COMPLICATIONS

• Corneal sequestration (see Corneal Sequestrum—Cats)—usually requires surgical keratectomy. • Symblepharon—may require surgery. • KCS—most likely from chronic FHV.

EXPECTED COURSE AND PROGNOSIS

• FHV—most patients become chronic carriers; may see repeated exacerbations, but episodes less common as patient matures; more severe clinical signs at times of stress or immunocompromise. • Bacterial conjunctivitis—usually resolves with appropriate administration of antibiotic. • Immune-mediated diseases (e.g., eosinophilic)—control not cure; may require chronic treatment at lowest level possible. • If underlying disease is found (e.g., KCS, entropion), resolution may depend on appropriate treatment of the disease.

MISCELLANEOUS

ASSOCIATED CONDITIONS

FeLV and FIV—may predispose patient to chronic carrier state of FHV conjunctivitis.

AGE-RELATED FACTORS

FHV—tends to be more severe in kittens and in old cats with waning immunity.

ZOONOTIC POTENTIAL

Chlamydophila felis—low.

PREGNANCY/FERTILITY/BREEDING

Use topical and systemic medications with caution, if at all, in pregnant animals.

SEE ALSO

- Corneal Sequestrum—Cats.
- Keratoconjunctivitis Sicca.
- Ophthalmia Neonatorum.
- Red Eye.

ABBREVIATIONS

- FeLV = feline leukemia virus.
- FHV = feline herpesvirus.
- FIV = feline immunodeficiency virus.
- IFA = immunofluorescent antibody.
- KCS = keratoconjunctivitis sicca.

Suggested Reading

Maggs DJ, Miller PE, Ofri R. Slatter's Fundamentals of Veterinary Ophthalmology, 6th ed. St. Louis, MO: Elsevier, 2018, pp. 158–177.

Author Rachel A. Allbaugh
Consulting Editor Kathern E. Myrna

Client Education Handout available online

BASICS

DEFINITION

Inflammation of the conjunctiva, the vascularized mucous membrane that covers the anterior sclera (bulbar conjunctiva), lines the eyelids (palpebral conjunctiva), and lines the third eyelid.

PATHOPHYSIOLOGY

- Primary—allergic, infectious, environmental.
- Secondary to other ocular disease—keratoconjunctivitis sicca (KCS), entropion, distichiasis.

SYSTEMS AFFECTED

Ophthalmic

GENETICS

N/A

INCIDENCE/PREVALENCE

Common

GEOGRAPHIC DISTRIBUTION

N/A

SIGNALMENT

Species

Dog

Breed Predilection

Breeds predisposed to allergic or immune-mediated skin diseases (e.g., atopy) tend to have more problems with allergic conjunctivitis or KCS.

Mean Age and Range

N/A

Predominant Sex

None

SIGNS

- Blepharospasm. • Conjunctival hyperemia. • Ocular discharge—serous, mucoid, or mucopurulent. • Chemosis. • Follicle formation on posterior third eyelid surface.
- Enophthalmos and third eyelid elevation.

CAUSES

Infectious

- Bacterial—rare as primary condition, usually secondary to KCS; conjunctivitis neonatorum involves accumulation of exudates under closed eyelids prior to natural opening. • Viral—canine herpes virus-1, canine distemper virus, or canine adenovirus-2. • Parasitic—*Leishmania*, *Onchocerca*, or *Thelazia*. • Conjunctival manifestation of systemic infectious disease

Immune-Mediated

- Allergic—especially in atopic patients.
- Follicular conjunctivitis—common in dogs <18 months, secondary to chronic antigenic stimulation. • Lymphocytic/plasmacytic conjunctivitis—especially in German shepherd dogs with or without chronic superficial keratitis (pannus).
- Systemic immune-mediated disease (e.g., pemphigus).

Trauma or Environmental Causes

- Conjunctival foreign body. • Irritation (dust, smoke, ophthalmic medications). • Toxin or chemical contact.

Other

Ligneous conjunctivitis—rare, young female Dobermans may be predisposed.

Secondary to Adnexal Disease

- Aqueous tear film deficiency (KCS) or qualitative tear deficiency. • Eyelid diseases—entropion, ectropion, medial canthal pocket syndrome, eyelid mass. • Hair or eyelash disorders—trichiasis, distichiasis, ectopic cilia.
- Exposure—facial nerve paralysis, lagophthalmos. • Dacryocystitis or nasolacrimal system outflow obstruction (e.g., obstructed duct or imperforate punctum).

Referred Inflammation from Other Ocular or Periocular Diseases

- Ulcerative keratitis. • Nodular episcleritis.
- Anterior uveitis. • Glaucoma. • Orbital disease. • Pyoderma.

RISK FACTORS

Atopy, KCS.

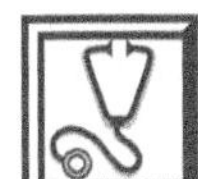

DIAGNOSIS

DIFFERENTIAL DIAGNOSIS

- Distinguish primary conjunctivitis from secondary conjunctival hyperemia. • Thorough systematic ophthalmic exam identifies other potential diseases (e.g., KCS, ulcers, uveitis, glaucoma, orbital disease); assess pupil size and symmetry, look for aqueous flare, attempt globe retropulsion, perform Schirmer tear test, intraocular pressure measurement, and fluorescein staining. • Deeper, darker, more linear and immobile blood vessel injection indicates congested episcleral vasculature due to episcleritis or intraocular disease. • Mass biopsy will differentiate conjunctival neoplasia (rare: squamous cell carcinoma, melanoma, hemangioma/sarcoma, lymphoma, papilloma, mast cell tumor) or episcleritis.

CBC/BIOCHEMISTRY/URINALYSIS

Normal unless systemic disease.

OTHER LABORATORY TESTS

N/A

IMAGING

N/A

DIAGNOSTIC PROCEDURES

- Adnexal examination—rule out facial nerve paralysis, lagophthalmos, eyelid abnormalities, hair or eyelash disorders, and foreign bodies in cul-de-sacs or under third eyelid. • Schirmer tear test—rule out KCS; perform before anything else is placed in eye. • Fluorescein stain—no corneal retention rules out ulcerative keratitis; stain flow to nares rules out nasolacrimal disease.
- Tear film breakup time—assesses tear film stability to rule out qualitative tear deficiency.
- Intraocular pressures—rule out glaucoma.
- Globe retropulsion—rule out orbital disease.
- Examine for signs of anterior uveitis (e.g., hypotony, aqueous flare, miosis) or other intraocular disease (e.g., cataracts, lens luxation).
- Consider nasolacrimal duct flush if fluorescein stain did not pass to nares. • Conjunctival cytology—lymphocytes and plasma cells diagnostic for lymphocytic/plasmacytic conjunctivitis; eosinophils in allergic conjunctivitis; degenerate neutrophils and intracellular bacteria with bacterial infection; rarely distemper virus intracytoplasmic inclusions. • Conjunctival biopsy—may be useful with mass lesions and nodular episcleritis or chronic undiagnosed disease. • PCR or viral isolation testing for canine herpesvirus-1.
- Intradermal skin testing—if suspect allergic conjunctivitis.

PATHOLOGIC FINDINGS

- Biopsy—inflammation, may note infectious agents, neoplasia, or nodular episcleritis.
- Ligneous conjunctivitis—thick, amorphous eosinophilic hyaline-like material.

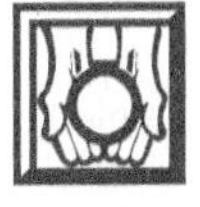

TREATMENT

APPROPRIATE HEALTH CARE

- Primary—outpatient. • Secondary to other disease (e.g., ulcerative keratitis, uveitis, glaucoma, lens luxation)—may require hospitalization to address underlying ophthalmic issue.

NURSING CARE

- Irritant-induced conjunctivitis—flush ocular surfaces and remove foreign body if observed.
- Allergic or follicular conjunctivitis—apply viscous artificial tear gel to both eyes before patient is active outdoors (q8–12h), then flush ocular surface with eye wash when returning indoors to remove "trapped" allergens.
- Secondary to ectropion or medial canthal pocket syndrome—flush ocular surface with eye wash daily to remove dust, dirt, or other matter that collects ventrally. • Warm pack eyelids and periocular skin to soften crusted secretions and improve comfort.

ACTIVITY

- No restriction for most. • Suspected contact irritant or allergic disease—prevent contact with offending agent. • Do not expose patients with infectious viral disease to susceptible animals.

DIET

- No change for most. • Suspected underlying skin disease and/or food allergy—food elimination diet trial.

CONJUNCTIVITIS—DOGS (CONTINUED)

C

CLIENT EDUCATION

• When solutions and ointments are prescribed, the client should use solution(s) before ointment(s) and wait 5 minutes between treatments. • If copious discharge is noted, clean eyes before giving medication. • Call for instructions if condition fails to improve or worsens. • An Elizabethan collar should be placed on the patient to prevent self-trauma.

SURGICAL CONSIDERATIONS

• Follicular conjunctivitis—if follicles are unresponsive to medication, consider debridement. • Entropion, distichia, ectopic cilia, or other eyelid disease—perform temporary or permanent surgery depending on findings, signalment, and history. • Nasolacrimal duct obstruction—if repeated flushing attempts at weekly intervals along with medical therapy are unsuccessful, consider contrast study and surgery (see Epiphora). • Conjunctival neoplasia—depending on tumor type and extent of involvement, may involve local excision and adjunctive therapy (β-irradiation, cryotherapy), enucleation, or exenteration.

MEDICATIONS

DRUG(S) OF CHOICE

Bacterial

• Initial treatment—broad-spectrum topical triple antibiotic q6–8h continuing several days past resolution of clinical signs; revise based on bacterial culture and sensitivity results. • Systemic antibiotic (e.g., cephalosporin)—occasionally indicated, especially for more generalized disease (e.g., pyoderma).

Neonatal

Carefully open eyelid margins (medial to lateral), establish drainage, and treat with topical antibiotic ointment q6–8h.

Herpetic

• Condition usually mild and self-limiting. • Antiviral treatment—indicated for severe intractable canine herpesvirus-1 conjunctivitis or herpetic keratitis. • 0.15% ganciclovir gel—topical q4h for 7 days, then q8h. • 1% trifluridine solution—topical q4h for 2 days, then q6h. • 0.1% idoxuridine solution (compounding pharmacies)—topical q4h for 2 days, then q6h. • 0.5% cidofovir solution (compounding pharmacies)—topical q12h; generally avoided: reduces duration of shedding but may worsen clinical disease due to local ocular toxic effects.

Immune-Mediated

• Depends on severity. • Allergic and follicular conjunctivitis—attempt nursing care first with viscous artificial tear gel lubricants and ocular flushing q8–12h; if nonresponsive consider antihistamine eye drops (e.g., ketotifen) q8–12h, or topical corticosteroid (e.g., dexamethasone) q8–12h. • Lymphocytic/plasmacytic conjunctivitis—0.1% dexamethasone q8h, then taper gradually to lowest effective dose; could attempt transition to cyclosporine 0.2% ointment, cyclosporine 1–2% compounded solution q12–24h, or tacrolimus 0.03% compounded solution q12–24h. • Treatment of any underlying disease (e.g., atopy) often improves clinical signs of allergic conjunctivitis.

Tear Deficiencies

• Aqueous tear film deficiency (see Keratoconjunctivitis Sicca). • Qualitative tear deficiency—cyclosporine 0.2% ointment, cyclosporine 1–2% compounded solution q12h, or tacrolimus 0.03% compounded solution q12–24h, and viscous artificial tear lubricants q6–12h.

CONTRAINDICATIONS

Topical corticosteroids—avoid if corneal ulceration is present, patient is at high risk for ulceration (e.g., entropion, lagophthalmos, severe KCS), or with known or suspected infectious conjunctivitis.

PRECAUTIONS

• Topical medications may be irritating. • Topical corticosteroids—monitor all patients carefully for signs of corneal ulceration; discontinue agent immediately if corneal ulceration occurs.

POSSIBLE INTERACTIONS

N/A

ALTERNATIVE DRUG(S)

Other corticosteroids—1% prednisolone acetate, betamethasone, hydrocortisone.

FOLLOW-UP

PATIENT MONITORING

Recheck shortly after beginning treatment (at 5 days), then recheck in 2 weeks or as needed.

PREVENTION/AVOIDANCE

Treat any underlying disease that may be exacerbating the conjunctivitis (e.g., KCS, allergic or immune-mediated skin disease).

POSSIBLE COMPLICATIONS

N/A

EXPECTED COURSE AND PROGNOSIS

• Good prognosis when underlying cause identified and treated (e.g., KCS, adnexal disease, eyelash disorder). • Bacterial—usually resolves with appropriate antibiotics; may depend on control of underlying disease (e.g., KCS). • Allergic or follicular—nursing care or medical treatment may be needed during peak allergy times. • Lymphocytic/plasmacytic—tend to be controlled and not cured; may require chronic treatment at lowest level possible.

MISCELLANEOUS

ASSOCIATED CONDITIONS

• Atopy. • Pyoderma.

AGE-RELATED FACTORS

N/A

ZOONOTIC POTENTIAL

N/A

PREGNANCY/FERTILITY/BREEDING

Use topical and systemic medications with caution, if at all, in pregnant animals.

SEE ALSO

• Epiphora.
• Keratoconjunctivitis Sicca.
• Red Eye.

ABBREVIATIONS

• KCS = keratoconjunctivitis sicca.

Suggested Reading

Hendrix DVH. Diseases and surgery of the canine conjunctiva and nictitating membrane. In: Gelatt KN, Gilger BC, Kern T, eds., Veterinary Ophthalmology, 5th ed. Ames, IA: Wiley-Blackwell, 2013, pp. 945–975.

Maggs DJ, Miller PE, Ofri R. Slatter's Fundamentals of Veterinary Ophthalmology, 6th ed. St. Louis, MO: Elsevier, 2018, pp. 158–177.

Author Rachel A. Allbaugh
Consulting Editor Kathern E. Myrna

Client Education Handout available online

CONSTIPATION AND OBSTIPATION

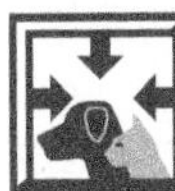

BASICS

DEFINITION

• *Constipation* is defined as infrequent, incomplete, or difficult defecation with passage of hard or dry feces. This does not imply abnormal motility or loss of function. • *Obstipation* denotes intractable constipation that has failed several consecutive treatments; defecation is impossible in the obstipated patient.

PATHOPHYSIOLOGY

• Constipation can develop with any disease that impairs the passage of feces through the colon. Potential causes include congenital vertebral malformation, spinal cord disease, pelvic canal narrowing (trauma), rectal mass lesions causing obstruction, and perianal disease causing painful defecation. Often in cats no underlying etiology can be identified. • Delayed fecal transit allows removal of additional salt and water, producing drier feces. Clinical signs are attributable to dehydration and potential toxemia resulting from fecal retention. • Peristaltic contractions may increase during constipation, but eventually motility diminishes because of smooth muscle degeneration secondary to chronic overdistension.

SYSTEMS AFFECTED

Gastrointestinal.

GENETICS

N/A

INCIDENCE/PREVALENCE

Common clinical problem in older cats; less common in dogs.

GEOGRAPHIC DISTRIBUTION

N/A

SIGNALMENT

Species

• Dog and cat. • More common in cat.

Breed Predilections

N/A

Mean Age and Range

Any age; most common in older cats.

Predominant Sex

N/A

SIGNS

Historical Findings

• Reduced, absent, or painful defecation. • Hard, dry feces. • Small amount of liquid, mucoid stool, sometimes with blood present produced after prolonged tenesmus. • Occasional vomiting, inappetence, and/or lethargy.

Physical Examination Findings

• Colon filled with hard feces. Severe impaction may cause abdominal distention. • Other findings depend on underlying cause. • Rectal examination may reveal mass, stricture, perineal hernia, anal sac disease, foreign body or material, prostatic enlargement, or narrowed pelvic canal.

CAUSES

Dietary

• Bones. • Hair. • Foreign material. • Excessive fiber. • Inadequate water intake.

Environmental

• Lack of exercise. • Change of environment—hospitalization, dirty litter box. • Inability to ambulate.

Drugs

• Anticholinergics. • Antihistamines. • Opioids. • Barium sulfate. • Sucralfate. • Antacids. • Kaopectolin. • Iron supplements. • Diuretics.

Painful Defecation (Dyschezia)

• Anorectal disease—anal sacculitis, anal sac abscess, perianal fistula, anal stricture, anal spasm, rectal foreign body, rectal prolapse, proctitis. • Trauma—fractured pelvis, fractured limb, dislocated hip, perianal bite wound or laceration, perineal abscess.

Mechanical Obstruction

• Extraluminal—healed pelvic fracture with narrowed pelvic canal, prostatic hypertrophy, prostatitis, prostatic neoplasia, intrapelvic neoplasia, sublumbar lymphadenopathy. • Intraluminal and intramural—colonic or rectal neoplasia or polyp, rectal stricture, rectal foreign body, rectal diverticulum, perineal hernia, rectal prolapse, congenital defect (atresia ani).

Neuromuscular Disease

• Central nervous system—paraplegia, spinal cord disease, intervertebral disc disease, cerebral disease (lead toxicity, rabies). • Peripheral nervous system—dysautonomia, sacral nerve disease, sacral nerve trauma (e.g., tail fracture/pull injury). • Colonic smooth muscle dysfunction—idiopathic megacolon in cats.

Metabolic and Endocrine Disease

• Impaired colonic smooth muscle function—hyperparathyroidism, hypothyroidism, hypokalemia (chronic renal failure), hypercalcemia. • Debility—general muscle weakness, dehydration, neoplasia.

RISK FACTORS

• Manx cats may be predisposed due to vertebral (sacral) abnormalities. • Drug therapy—anticholinergics, narcotics, barium sulfate. • Metabolic disease causing dehydration. • Feline dysautonomia. • Intact male—perineal hernia, benign or infectious prostatic disease. • Castrated male—prostatic neoplasia. • Perianal fistula.

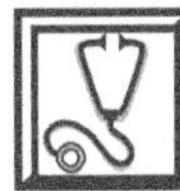

DIAGNOSIS

DIFFERENTIAL DIAGNOSIS

• Dyschezia and tenesmus (e.g., caused by colitis or proctitis)—unlike constipation, associated with increased frequency of attempts to defecate and frequent production of small amounts of liquid feces containing blood and/or mucus; rectal examination reveals diarrhea and lack of hard stool. • Stranguria (e.g., caused by cystitis/urethritis)—unlike constipation, can be associated with hematuria and abnormal findings on urinalysis (pyuria, crystalluria, bacteruria).

CBC/BIOCHEMISTRY/URINALYSIS

• Usually unremarkable. • May detect hypokalemia, hypercalcemia. • High packed cell volume (PCV) and total protein in dehydrated patients. • High white blood cell (WBC) count in patients with severe obstipation secondary to bacterial or endotoxin translocation, abscess, perianal fistula, prostatic disease. • Pyuria and hematuria with prostatitis.

OTHER LABORATORY TESTS

• If patient is hypercholesterolemic, consider thyroid panel to rule out hypothyroidism. • If patient is hypercalcemic, consider parathyroid hormone assay.

IMAGING

• Abdominal radiography documents severity of colonic impaction. Other findings may include colonic or rectal foreign body, colonic or rectal mass, prostatic enlargement, fractured pelvis, dislocated hip, or perineal hernias. • Pneumocolon (after enemas to clean colon) may better define intraluminal mass or stricture. • Ultrasonography may help define extraluminal mass and prostatic disease.

DIAGNOSTIC PROCEDURES

Colonoscopy may be needed to identify a mass, stricture, or other colonic or rectal lesion; rectal/colonic mucosal biopsy specimens should always be obtained.

PATHOLOGIC FINDINGS

Dependent on underlying disease process.

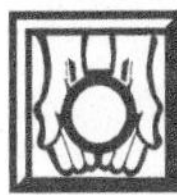

TREATMENT

APPROPRIATE HEALTH CARE

• Remove or ameliorate any underlying cause if possible. • Discontinue any medications that may cause constipation. • May need to treat as inpatient if obstipation and/or dehydration present.

CONSTIPATION AND OBSTIPATION (CONTINUED)

C

NURSING CARE

Dehydrated patients should receive IV (preferably) or SC balanced electrolyte solutions (with potassium supplementation if indicated).

ACTIVITY

Encourage activity.

DIET

Dietary supplementation with a bulk-forming agent (bran, methylcellulose, canned pumpkin, psyllium) is often helpful, though they can sometimes worsen colonic fecal distension; in this instance, feed a low-residue diet.

CLIENT EDUCATION

• Feed appropriate diet and encourage activity. • Survey cat boxes daily to ensure level of defecation activity.

SURGICAL CONSIDERATIONS

• Manual removal of feces through the anus with the animal under general anesthesia (after rehydration) may be required if enemas and medications are unsuccessful. • Subtotal colectomy may be required with recurring obstipation that responds poorly to assertive medical therapy.

MEDICATIONS

DRUG(S) OF CHOICE

• Emollient laxatives—docusate sodium or docusate calcium (dogs: 50–100 mg PO q12–24h; cats: 50 mg PO q12–24h).
• Stimulant laxatives—bisacodyl (5 mg/animal PO q8–24h). Ensure that animal is not obstructed prior to use of stimulant laxatives. • Saline laxatives—isosmotic mixture of polyethylene glycol and poorly absorbed salts; usually administered as a trickle amount via nasoesophageal tube over 6–12h. • Disaccharide laxative—lactulose (1 mL/4.5 kg PO q8–12h to effect). • Warm water enemas may be needed; a small amount of mild soap or docusate sodium can be added but is usually not needed; sodium phosphate retention enemas (e.g., Fleet®) are contraindicated because of their association with severe hypocalcemia.
• Suppositories can be used as a replacement for enemas; use glycerol, bisocodyl, or docusate sodium products. • Motility modifiers can be administered—cisapride (dogs: 0.3–0.5 mg/kg PO q8–12h; cats: 2.5–10 mg/cat PO q8–12h) may stimulate colonic motility; indicated with early megacolon.

CONTRAINDICATIONS

• Lubricants such as mineral oil and white petrolatum are *not* recommended because of the danger of fatal lipid aspiration pneumonia due to their lack of taste. • Fleet (sodium phosphate) enemas. • Anticholinergics.
• Diuretics.

PRECAUTIONS

Cisapride and cholinergics—can be used with caution; contraindicated in obstructive processes. Avoid the use of metoclopramide because it does not affect the colon.

POSSIBLE INTERACTIONS

N/A

ALTERNATIVE DRUG(S)

• Ranitidine causes contraction of colonic smooth muscle in vitro. • Misoprostol causes contraction of colonic smooth muscle in vitro. • Newer-generation cisapride-like drugs may be available soon. • One recent pilot study using multistrain probiotic SLAB51® showed clinical improvement in a feline cohort having chronic constipation and idiopathic megacolon.

FOLLOW-UP

PATIENT MONITORING

Monitor frequency of defecation and stool consistency at least twice a week initially, then weekly or biweekly in response to dietary and/or drug therapy.

PREVENTION/AVOIDANCE

Keep pet active and feed appropriate diet. Subcutaneous fluids to ensure hydration can help reduce frequency of constipation, particularly in cats.

POSSIBLE COMPLICATIONS

• Chronic constipation or recurrent obstipation can lead to acquired megacolon.
• Overuse of laxatives and enemas can cause diarrhea. • Colonic mucosa can be damaged by improper enema technique, repeated rough mechanical breakdown of feces, or ischemic necrosis secondary to pressure of hard feces. • Perineal irritation and ulceration can lead to fecal incontinence.

EXPECTED COURSE AND PROGNOSIS

• Fair to good prognosis with early diagnosis and intervention. • Recurring bouts of constipation/obstipation may occur dependent on underlying cause.

MISCELLANEOUS

ASSOCIATED CONDITIONS

Vomiting—with severe/prolonged obstipation.

AGE-RELATED FACTORS

N/A

ZOONOTIC POTENTIAL

N/A

PREGNANCY/FERTILITY/BREEDING

N/A

SYNONYMS

• Colonic impaction. • Fecal impaction.

SEE ALSO

Megacolon

ABBREVIATIONS

• PCV = packed cell volume.
• WBC = white blood cell.

Suggested Reading

Chandler M. Focus on nutrition: dietary management of gastrointestinal disease. Compend Contin Educ Vet 2013, 35(6):E1–E3.

Rossi G, Jergens A, Cerquetella M, et al. Effects of a probiotic (SLAB51™) on clinical and histologic variables and microbiota of cats with chronic constipation/megacolon: a pilot study. Benef Microbes 2018, 9:101–110.

Tam FM, Carr AP, Myers SL. Safety and palatability of polyethylene glycol 3350 as an oral laxative in cats. J Feline Med Surg 2011, 13(10):694–697.

Author Albert E. Jergens
Consulting Editor Mark P. Rondeau

Client Education Handout available online

CONTACT DERMATITIS

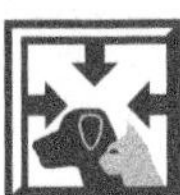

BASICS

OVERVIEW

• Irritant and allergic contact dermatitis—rare syndromes with similar clinical signs but different pathophysiology; differentiation may be more conceptual. • Irritant contact dermatitis (ICD)—direct damage to keratinocytes by exposure to particular irritant or sensitizer induces inflammatory response directed at skin without prior sensitization. • Allergic contact dermatitis (ACD)—type IV (delayed) hypersensitivity: immunologic event requiring sensitization and elicitation; Langerhans cells and keratinocytes interact with environmental haptens to create antigens, leading to sensitization of T-lymphocytes and activation following reexposure with release of cytokines (mainly tumor necrosis factor alpha • [TNF-α], IL1βGM-CSF). • Recent reports blur distinction between ICD, ACD, and atopic dermatitis.

SIGNALMENT

• ICD—Any age as direct result of irritation from offending chemical. • ACD—older dogs; chronic exposure to antigen (months to years); extremely rare in cats, (except exposure to d-limonene-containing insecticides). • ACD—German shepherd dog, poodle, wirehaired fox terrier, Scottish terrier, West Highland white terrier, Labrador and golden retriever.

SIGNS

Lesions

• Location determined by antigen contact; commonly limited to glabrous skin and regions frequently in direct contact with the environment. • Extreme erythroderma stops abruptly at hairline. • Initial erythema, edema, and papules leading to crusts and excoriations; lichenification and hyperpigmentation with chronicity; vesicles uncommon.

Others

• Localized reactions to topical medications.
• Generalized reactions to shampoos or insecticide sprays. • Pruritus—moderate to severe (most common). • Seasonal incidence may indicate plant or outdoor antigen.

CAUSES & RISK FACTORS

• Reported offending substances—plants, mulch, cedar chips, fabrics, rugs, carpets, plastics, rubber, leather, nickel, cobalt, concrete, soaps, detergents, floor waxes, epoxy resin, carpet and litter deodorizers, herbicides, fertilizers, insecticides (including topical flea treatments), flea collars, topical preparations (neomycin). • Increased incidence with atopic disease.

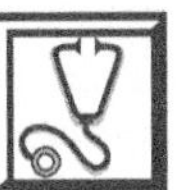

DIAGNOSIS

DIFFERENTIAL DIAGNOSIS

• Hypersensitivity dermatitis. • Drug reaction.
• Pelodera dermatitis. • Hookworm dermatitis.
• Pyoderma. • *Malassezia* dermatitis.
• Demodicosis. • Solar dermatitis. • Thermal injuries. • Trauma from rough surfaces.

DIAGNOSTIC PROCEDURES

• ACD—closed-patch test (corticosteroids and nonsteroidal anti-inflammatory drugs [NSAIDs] must be discontinued for 3–6 weeks); materials taken from environment or home applied to upper thorax skin under bandage; examine for erythema, edema, pruritus at 48, 72 hours, and 7 days.
• ICD—eliminate exposure to contact irritant or antigen, followed by provocation. • Open patch test—apply substance to inside pinnae; monitor for mild erythema, edema, pruritus; examine daily for 5–15 days. • Human patch test kits (TRUE Test®). • Skin biopsy.

PATHOLOGIC FINDINGS

• Intraepidermal vesiculation and spongiosis; superficial dermal edema with perivascular mononuclear cell infiltrate in ICD and ACD; polymorphonuclear cell infiltrate in ICD; leukocyte exocytosis common. • Lymphocytic spongiotic or eosinophilic and lymphocytic spongiotic infiltrate with intraepidermal eosinophilic pustules in canine ACD.

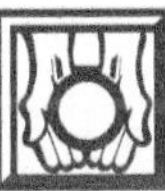

TREATMENT

• Eliminate offending substance(s). • Bathe with hypoallergenic shampoos to remove antigen from skin. • Create mechanical barriers, if possible—socks, shirts, restriction from environment.

MEDICATIONS

DRUG(S) OF CHOICE

• Prednisolone (1 mg/kg PO q24h for 5–7 days, then q48h for 2 weeks). • Topical corticosteroids for focal lesions. • Topical tacrolimus. • Pentoxifylline (10–25 mg/kg PO q8–12h initially). • Cyclosporine (modified, 5 mg/kg q24h).

CONTRAINDICATIONS/POSSIBLE INTERACTIONS

Pentoxifylline—do not administer with alkylating agents, cisplatin, or amphotericin B; cimetidine may increase serum levels of pentoxifylline.

FOLLOW-UP

PREVENTION/AVOIDANCE

Remove offending substances from the environment.

EXPECTED COURSE AND PROGNOSIS

ICD

• Acute condition—may occur after only one exposure; can be manifested within 24 hours of exposure. • Corticosteroids rarely helpful.
• Lesions resolve 1–2 days after irritant removal.

ACD

• Requires chronic exposure for hypersensitivity to develop. • Reexposure results in development of clinical signs within 1–5 days; signs may persist for several weeks. • Responds well to corticosteroids; pruritus returns after discontinuation if antigenic stimulus persists.
• Hyposensitization not effective. • Prognosis—good if allergen is identified and removed, otherwise poor: may require lifelong treatment.

MISCELLANEOUS

ABBREVIATIONS

• ACD = allergic contact dermatitis.
• ICD = irritant contact dermatitis.
• NSAID = nonsteroidal anti-inflammatory drug.
• TNF-α = tumor necrosis factor alpha.

Suggested Reading

Ho KK, Campbell KL, Lavergne SN. Contact dermatitis: a comparative and translational review of the literature. Vet Dermatol 2015; 26:314–327.

Author Liora Waldman
Consulting Editor Alexander H. Werner Resnick

COONHOUND PARALYSIS (ACUTE POLYRADICULONEURITIS)

C

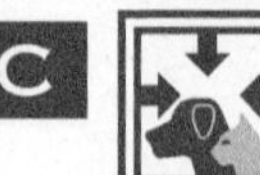

BASICS

DEFINITION

• Acute inflammatory disorder involving the axons and myelin of nerve roots, spinal nerves, and peripheral nerves in dogs, with or without a previous history of contact with raccoon saliva, vaccination, or a gastrointestinal or respiratory infection. • Proposed animal model for Guillain-Barré syndrome in humans.

PATHOPHYSIOLOGY

• Etiology uncertain, appears to be immune mediated. • Immune-mediated inflammation develops 7–14 days after antecedent event (delayed hypersensitivity reaction?).
• Thought to be the dog's immune system reaction to a cross-reacting antigen (suspect molecular mimicry phenomenon between external antigen and gangliosides from dog's neural tissue, with the development of antiganglioside autoantibodies). • Coonhound paralysis (CHP)—antecedent event is recent contact with raccoon saliva. • Acute canine idiopathic polyradiculoneuritis (ACIP)—affected dogs with identical clinical signs to those with CHP but without a history of raccoon exposure; may have history of recent respiratory or gastrointestinal infection.
• Postvaccinal polyradiculoneuritis—antecedent event is recent vaccination (rare).
• *Toxoplasma gondii* infection—dogs with ACIP more likely to have positive titers than control dogs (possible triggering factor?).

SYSTEMS AFFECTED

• Peripheral nervous system—most severe involvement in the ventral (motor) nerve roots and ventral root components of the spinal nerves; lumbosacral nerve roots affected more severely than cervical and thoracic nerve roots. • Cranial nerves—nerve VII often affected; nerves IX, X occasionally affected. • Respiratory failure—secondary to intercostal and/or phrenic nerve involvement in some patients.

GENETICS

No proven basis.

INCIDENCE/PREVALENCE

• Most commonly recognized acute polyneuropathy in dogs. • Low incidence.

GEOGRAPHIC DISTRIBUTION

• CHP—relative to distribution of raccoons (e.g., North and Central America; parts of South America). • ACIP—worldwide.

SIGNALMENT

Species

Dog, very occasionally cat.

Breed Predilections

• CHP—Coonhounds; any breed in contact with raccoons susceptible. • ACIP, postvaccinal polyradiculoneuritis—none.

Mean Age and Range

N/A

Predominant Sex

N/A

SIGNS

Historical Findings

• Appear 7–14 days after contact with raccoon saliva (bite or scratch), receipt of vaccination, or development of respiratory or gastrointestinal infection. • Initial signs—stiff, stilted gait in all limbs, typically starting in the pelvic limbs and eventually progressing to the thoracic limbs. • Rapid progression (2–4 days) to a flaccid, lower motor neuron tetraparesis to tetraplegia. • Owners may notice loss or change of voice. • Appetite and water consumption—usually normal.
• Urination and defecation—normal.
• Progressive phase of the disease—clinical signs can continue to worsen up to 5–10 days after onset.

Neurologic Examination Findings

• Usually symmetric. • Stiff, stilted gait that usually progresses rapidly to lower motor neuron tetraparesis or tetraplegia; some dogs may remain ambulatory tetraparetic.
• Generalized hyporeflexia to areflexia, with the exception of a normal perineal reflex.
• Generalized hypotonia to atonia, severe neurogenic muscle atrophy. • Affected dogs often show inability to hold the head up.
• Aphonia or dysphonia common; no megaesophagus. • Facial paresis—bilateral incomplete palpebral closure in some patients. • Respiration—labored in severely affected dogs; occasional progression to respiratory paralysis. • Pain sensation intact; hyperesthesia common—may reflect variable dorsal nerve root inflammation. • Motor dysfunction—always predominates; even tetraplegic patient can usually wag its tail.
• Mental status, urination, and defecation—unaffected.

CAUSES

• CHP—contact with a raccoon; perhaps more important, contact with raccoon saliva.
• ACIP—none proven; possibly previous respiratory or gastrointestinal viral or bacterial infection. • Postvaccinal polyradiculoneuritis—recent vaccination (rare).

RISK FACTORS

• CHP—coonhounds tend to be predisposed primarily because of the nature of their activities; previous disease does not confer immunity and may increase risk of redevelopment; multiple bouts not uncommon. • ACIP—unknown.

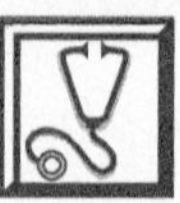

DIAGNOSIS

DIFFERENTIAL DIAGNOSIS

• Other acute polyneuropathy (i.e., paraneoplastic neuropathy). • Distal denervating disease. • Botulism. • Tick bite paralysis.
• Fulminant myasthenia gravis. • Black widow spider bite envenomation, coral snake envenomation. • Intoxications (lasalocid, blue-green algae). • Generalized (diffuse) or multifocal myelopathy (involving both cervical and lumbosacral intumescences).

CBC/BIOCHEMISTRY/URINALYSIS

Usually normal.

OTHER LABORATORY TESTS

• Serum immunoglobulins (Ig)—high serum IgG but not IgM in some patients.
• Immunologic—serum reaction to raccoon saliva on ELISA; dogs with CHP have a strong positive reaction that decreases in intensity over time; dogs without disease but with raccoon contact have a strong positive reaction; dogs with ACIP but with no raccoon contact have a negative reaction. • Immunologic—for dogs with ACIP, identification of anti-GM2 ganglioside antibodies reached a diagnostic sensitivity of 60% and a specificity of 97%.

IMAGING

Thoracic radiographs and abdominal ultrasound—normal.

DIAGNOSTIC PROCEDURES

Cerebrospinal Fluid Analysis

• Lumbar—high protein without an increase in leukocytes at all stages of disease. • Albumin leakage across the disrupted blood–nerve barrier of the affected ventral nerve roots is the primary cause of the protein increase.

Electrodiagnostics

• Electromyography (EMG)—generalized spontaneous activity (fibrillation potentials and positive sharp waves) consistent with denervation; EMG normal in first 4–5 days. • Markedly low compound muscle action potential amplitudes after motor nerve stimulation. • F waves (late waves that indicate proximal motor nerve and ventral nerve root function)—prolonged minimum latencies, increased F ratio, decreased amplitudes. • Motor nerve conduction velocities—usually normal; severely affected patients may have mildly decreased values. • Sensory nerve function—usually normal. • Abnormalities provide evidence of severe peripheral motor axonopathy (more severe in proximal portions of nerves and ventral nerve roots), along with demyelination in the proximal motor nerves and ventral nerve roots.

PATHOLOGIC FINDINGS

• Ventral nerve roots and the ventral root components of the spinal nerves—most severe lesions, various degrees of axonal degeneration, paranodal and segmental demyelination, and leukocyte infiltration (predominantly monocytes and macrophages). • Peripheral nerves—affected to a lesser degree; might be normal. • Dorsal nerve roots—much less severely affected.

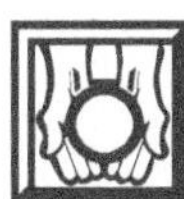

TREATMENT

APPROPRIATE HEALTH CARE

• Inpatient—closely monitor patients in the progressive phase of the disease (especially during first 5 days) for respiratory problems. • Severe respiratory compromise—mechanical ventilation as required. • IV fluid therapy—administer if patient is dehydrated. • Outpatient—once patient is stable and the progressive phase of the disease is over.

NURSING CARE

• Patients are usually able to eat and drink; hand feed in sternal position until able to reach food and water. • Intensive physical therapy—important to decrease muscle atrophy; severe neurogenic muscle atrophy is inevitable. • Frequent turning and excellent padding—essential to prevent pressure sores.

ACTIVITY

Encourage as much movement as possible.

DIET

• No restrictions. • Make sure patient is able to reach food and water. • Cervical weakness—may need to hand feed patient in sternal position.

CLIENT EDUCATION

• Inform client that good nursing care is essential. • Discuss importance of preventing pressure sores and urine scalding and of limiting the degree of muscle atrophy by frequent daily physical therapy (passive limb movement, swimming as the patient's strength begins to improve). • Patient needs soft bedding that must be kept free of urine and feces, frequent turning (every 3–4 hours), frequent bathing, and adequate nutrition.

SURGICAL CONSIDERATIONS

N/A

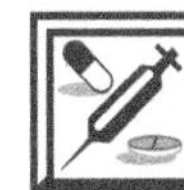

MEDICATIONS

DRUG(S) OF CHOICE

• None proven effective. • Immunoglobulin—1 g/kg IV daily for 2 consecutive days, 0.5 g/kg IV daily for 3 consecutive days, or 0.4 g/kg IV daily for 5 consecutive days; given early may shorten recovery time in ACIP.

CONTRAINDICATIONS

Corticosteroids—do not improve clinical signs or shorten course of disease; may reduce survival in humans with Guillain-Barré syndrome.

PRECAUTIONS

Monitor for possible adverse reactions (anaphylaxis, hematuria) after IV immunoglobulin administration.

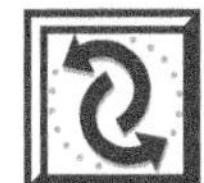

FOLLOW-UP

PATIENT MONITORING

• Outpatient—keep in close contact with client regarding complications or changes in the patient's condition. • Urinalysis—perform periodically to check for cystitis in tetraplegic or severely tetraparetic patients. • Ideally, reevaluate at least every 2 weeks.

PREVENTION/AVOIDANCE

• CHP—if possible, avoid contact with raccoons. • Postvaccinal polyradiculoneuritis—if strong association with a specific vaccination, avoid that particular vaccine in the future.

POSSIBLE COMPLICATIONS

• Respiratory paralysis—in progressive phase of disease. • Pressure sores, urine scalding, cystitis—common in chronically recumbent dogs.

EXPECTED COURSE AND PROGNOSIS

• Signs stabilize once progressive phase of disease is over. • Most affected dogs recover fully over 3–6 weeks; severely affected cases may take up to 3–4 months to recover; incomplete recoveries can happen.

MISCELLANEOUS

ASSOCIATED CONDITIONS

N/A

AGE-RELATED FACTORS

N/A

ZOONOTIC POTENTIAL

N/A

PREGNANCY/FERTILITY/BREEDING

Unknown effect on the fetuses of an affected bitch.

SYNONYMS

Coondog paralysis.

SEE ALSO

- Botulism.
- Myasthenia Gravis.
- Polyneuropathies (Peripheral Neuropathies).
- Tick Bite Paralysis.

ABBREVIATIONS

- ACIP = acute canine idiopathic polyradiculoneuritis.
- CHP = coonhound paralysis.
- EMG = electromyography.
- Ig = immunoglobulin.

Suggested Reading

Añor S. Acute lower motor neuron tetraparesis. Vet Clin North Am Small Anim 2014, 44:1201–1222.

Cuddon PA. Electrophysiologic assessment of acute polyradiculoneuropathy in dogs: comparison with Guillain-Barré syndrome in people. J Vet Intern Med 1998, 12:294–303.

Cummings JF, de Lahunta A, Holmes DF, Schultz RD. Coonhound paralysis: further clinical studies and electron microscopic observations. Acta Neuropathol 1982, 56:167–178.

Hirschvogel K, Jurina K, Steinberg TA, et al. Clinical course of acute canine polyradiculoneuritis following treatment with human IV immunoglobulin. J Am Anim Hosp Assoc 2012, 48:299–309.

Northington JW, Brown MJ. Acute canine idiopathic polyneuropathy: a Guillain-Barré-like syndrome in dogs. J Neurol Sci 1982, 56:259–273.

Author Paula Martín Vaquera

COPPER ASSOCIATED HEPATOPATHY

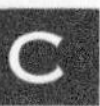

BASICS

DEFINITION

- Severe hepatic accumulation of copper (Cu) causes acute or chronic hepatitis leading to cirrhosis or death from liver failure.
- Mild to moderate hepatic Cu accumulation augments oxidative injury and increases risk for liver disease caused by other hepatobiliary insults, notably hepatotoxicity from nonsteroidal anti-inflammatory drugs (NSAIDs).
- *Primary copper associated hepatopathy* (CuAH) depicts copper accumulation in the absence of other liver disorders or *as the major cause of liver injury.*
- *Secondary CuAH* depicts Cu accumulation caused by severe chronic cholestasis in cats (not dogs) or fulminant hepatic failure (rare).
- *Genetic primary CuAH*—only proven in Bedlington terriers.
- *Acquired primary CuAH*—most common canine cause of CuAH, reflects dietary Cu availability in commercial dog food that exceeds individual's tolerance limit.
- *Congenital primary CuAH* (no gene mutation characterized)—comparatively rare in cats.
- Some animals with primary CuAH accumulate Cu without histologic evidence of liver damage despite vacillating liver enzyme activity (alanine aminotransferase [ALT] most common); in absence of inflammation or hepatocyte necrosis, the term *hepatopathy* is most correct.

PATHOPHYSIOLOGY

- Hepatic Cu homeostasis involves complex regulatory system including protein transporters, chaperones, membrane receptors, intracellular binding proteins, canalicular egress pumps; Cu absorbed from small intestine, stored in liver, with excess excreted in bile.
- A single gene mutation (*COMMD1*) causes genetic primary CuAH in Bedlington terriers.
- More commonly, canine hepatic Cu accumulation reflects Cu intake exceeding capacity to maintain neutral Cu balance; suspected pharmacogenetic basis.
- Secondary CuAH reflects reduced canalicular Cu egress associated with severe cholestasis (cats only) or severe panlobular liver injury (fulminant hepatic failure, rare).
- Primary CuAH—hepatocyte cytosolic Cu first accumulates in zone 3 (centrilobular region).
- Secondary CuAH (cats)—hepatocyte cytosolic Cu accumulates in zone 1 (periportal) or adjacent to injured regions.
- Hepatic Cu concentrations widely variable—primary CuAH: range 500 to >10,000 μg/g dry weight liver (DWL); secondary CuAH in cats rarely exceeds 1,000 μg/g DWL.
- Cu accumulation causes oxidative membrane injury—cell and organelles; high hepatic Cu concentration not always associated with histologic evidence of liver injury.
- Focal hepatitis initiated by Cu may progress to chronic hepatitis, eventually cirrhosis.
- Rarely, acute severe hepatic necrosis releases Cu into systemic circulation causing hemolysis and/or acute-onset acquired Fanconi syndrome (proximal renal tubular injury causing euglycemic glucosuria).

SYSTEMS AFFECTED

- Hepatobiliary—centrilobular hepatitis, chronic hepatitis, eventual cirrhosis.
- Hemic/lymphatic—hemolytic anemia rare sequel to acute hepatic necrosis in dogs.
- Renal—rare reversible Fanconi syndrome causes euglycemic glycosuria, granular casts, ± clinicopathologic evidence of compromised renal function.

GENETICS

- Autosomal recessive *COMMD1* mutation in Bedlington terriers reduces biliary Cu excretion.
- Gene mutations remain unproven in other breeds and in cats; gene associations may modify susceptibility in Labrador retrievers, but no genetic test and liver biopsy remains gold standard for diagnosis of CuAH.
- Predisposition to CuAH recognized in Labrador retriever, West Highland white terrier, Doberman pinscher, Dalmatian, keeshond, corgi, Staffordshire terrier, and other breeds.

INCIDENCE/PREVALENCE

- Bedlington terrier—at one time up to 2/3 of dogs carried *COMMD1* mutation; incidence significantly declined with genetic testing.
- Prevalence of excess hepatic Cu remains high in West Highland white terrier, Labrador retriever, Doberman pinscher, and other breeds.
- CuAH currently most common cause of chronically increased ALT activity in dogs (since mid-1990s) likely caused by increased Cu availability in manufactured dog foods.
- CuAH comprises ≥20% of liver biopsy submissions for abnormal enzyme activity in dogs.
- Primary congenital CuAH occurs in cats but comparatively rare.

GEOGRAPHIC DISTRIBUTION

Reported worldwide.

SIGNALMENT

Species

Dog and cat; more common in dog.

Breed Predilections

Bedlington terrier, West Highland white terrier, Labrador retriever, Doberman pinscher, Dalmatian, Welsh corgi, keeshond, Staffordshire terrier with observed increased incidence of high hepatic Cu concentrations; no canine breed exempt.

Mean Age and Range

- Bedlington terrier—Cu slowly accumulates to max at ~6 years of age; dogs can be clinically affected at any age; most present as middle-aged to older dogs with chronic hepatitis.
- West Highland white terrier—maximum Cu accumulation observed by 12 months of age and may vacillate or decline with clinical disease at any time; *however*, some dogs with high hepatic Cu survive to old age (15 years) without evidence of liver injury.
- Labrador retriever, Doberman pinscher, Dalmatian, other breeds—young adult to middle-aged at diagnosis for chronic hepatitis.
- Doberman pinscher—often develop hepatitis with ALT increases and Cu accumulation at 1–3 years of age; clinical signs of liver disease often recognized by 5–7 years of age.

Predominant Sex

None

SIGNS

Historical Findings

- Primary CuAH—4 categories:
  - no clinical signs;
  - subclinical disease: increased ALT activity with no clinical illness;
  - acute disease associated with severe acute hepatic necrosis;
  - chronic progressive hepatitis eventually evolving cirrhosis.
- Secondary CuAH accompanies feline cholestatic necroinflammatory liver disease (cholangiohepatitis) or rarely in dogs with fulminant liver necrosis.
- Acute signs—with extreme hepatic Cu accumulation, sudden-onset lethargy, anorexia, vomiting; may have rapid course, dogs succumb despite intensive supportive care.
- Chronic signs—variable, intermittent lethargy, hyporexia, weight loss, vomiting, diarrhea, with later polydipsia and polyuria; eventual liver injury leads to ascites, jaundice, bleeding tendencies, hepatic encephalopathy (HE).

Physical Examination Findings

- Acute signs—lethargy, weakness, jaundice, pallor (anemia), vomiting, diarrhea, dark urine (bilirubinuria); rare hemoglobinemia and hemoglobinuria if intravascular Cu-mediated hemolysis.
- Chronic signs—weight loss, ascites, jaundice, nodular microhepatia; melena and petechial hemorrhage in animals with significant panlobular injury.

CAUSES

- Genetic primary CuAH—single gene mutation in Bedlington terriers.
- Acquired primary CuAH—either Bedlington mutation or suspected pharmacogenetic differences involving regulatory pathways influencing Cu homeostasis, making them intolerant to current levels of dietary Cu supplementation.
- Secondary acquired CuAH—necroinflammatory chronic cholestatic liver disease in cats or diffuse severe panlobular injury in dogs or cats (rare).

RISK FACTORS

- Primary—feeding diets or providing water with Cu concentrations exceeding individual's tolerance to maintain neutral Cu balance.
- Stress or concurrent illnesses may precipitate acute illness in dogs with hepatocyte Cu accumulation.
- Asymptomatic dogs with primary CuAH may become symptomatic when additional disease processes or toxicities (e.g., NSAID administration; CCNU chemotherapy) impose oxidative challenge, expose hepatocytes to inflammatory cytokines, or another primary liver disease develops.

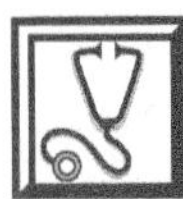

DIAGNOSIS

DIFFERENTIAL DIAGNOSIS

- Acute diseases—infectious (e.g., infectious canine hepatitis, leptospirosis, septicemia, suppurative bacterial cholangiohepatitis), acute hepatic necrosis, hepatic abscess, drug- or toxin-induced hepatic injury, acute pancreatitis, hepatic lymphoma, immune-mediated hemolytic anemia, zinc toxicity.
- Chronic diseases—chronic hepatitis or cholangiohepatitis of any other cause, drug- or toxin-induced liver injury, severe diffuse glycogen-type vacuolar hepatopathy (dogs), infectious hepatitis, chronic obstructive biliary disease, chronic fibrosing pancreatitis, congenital portosystemic shunt, primary or metastatic hepatic neoplasia.

CBC/BIOCHEMISTRY/URINALYSIS

- *CBC*—may be normal; regenerative anemia, leukocytosis, neutrophilia if acute Cu-associated hemolysis; microcytic or normocytic, normochromic nonregenerative anemia in chronic progressive liver injury; microcytosis usually reflects acquired portosystemic shunting.
- *Biochemistry*—increased liver enzymes (ALT, aspartate transaminase [AST], γ-glutamyl transferase [GGT], and alkaline phosphatase [ALP] with increase in ALT > ALP); hyperbilirubinemia in dogs with severe liver injury; increased ALT without clinical signs increases suspicion for early or cyclic CuAH necrosis.
- As hepatic function deteriorates—onset of hypoalbuminemia, ± hyperglobulinemia, low blood urea nitrogen (BUN), hypoglycemia, hypocholesterolemia.
- *Urinalysis*—usually normal, bilirubinuria escalates with hyperbilirubinemia; hepatic insufficiency: dilute urine, ammonium biurate crystalluria reflects acquired portosystemic shunts (APSS); glucosuria, granular casts if acquired Fanconi syndrome.

OTHER LABORATORY TESTS

- High fasting or postprandial total serum bile acid (TSBA) values—dogs with severe liver injury, remodeling, or portal hypertension associated with APSS.
- Prolonged prothrombin time (PT), activated partial thromboplastin time (APTT), activated clotting time (ACT), mucosal bleeding time in severe liver injury.
- Rare increased serum Cu concentration—dogs with acute severe CuAH liver necrosis; otherwise serum Cu does not reflect liver Cu concentrations; low-yield screening test.
- Hepatic Cu measurements *must* be reconciled with histopathologic findings.
- Genetic marker testing in Bedlington terrier—microsatellite markers or specific *COMMD1* mutation; however, kindreds of Bedlington terriers with CuAH have had negative PCR-based gene tests.

IMAGING

- Radiography—unremarkable in most dogs; small liver in chronic hepatic injury, poor abdominal detail if ascites.
- Ultrasonography—early: normal hepatic imaging; later: hyperechoic to heterogeneous nodular echogenicity; ascites in some cases.

DIAGNOSTIC PROCEDURES

- *Liver biopsy*—gold standard diagnostic test; confirms and characterizes liver injury; needle samples may not provide adequate liver lobe assessment as Cu is differentially distributed across lobes and liver sections; biopsy at least 3 lobes.
- Routine H&E staining—can overlook pathologic Cu accumulation.
- Cu-specific staining—rhodanine (preferred); confirms Cu-protein aggregates, details zonal distribution.
- Semi-quantitative scoring system—estimates severity of Cu accumulation; variation among interpreters confounds comparisons between biopsy reports.
- Cu measurements—can be completed on fresh, frozen, formalin fixed liver, liver tissue extracted from paraffin blocks, or liver sections.
- Distribution of hepatocytes with cytosolic Cu granules and quantification of Cu should be reconciled—areas of dense fibrosis, parenchymal extinction, regenerative nodules contain lower Cu concentrations than unremodeled liver tissue; this phenomenon causes discordance between measured and assessed Cu accumulations.
- In dogs with severe illness with high risk for general anesthesia and liver biopsy, hepatic aspiration cytology with samples stained with rhodanine may identify Cu accumulation; qualitative with variable accuracy; *not* recommended method for definitive diagnosis.

Cu Measurement

- *Atomic absorption spectroscopy*—gold standard method of Cu determination; requires at least full needle biopsy (≥16 g) sample; larger samples improve accuracy.
- Cu must be expressed per DWL.
- *Digital scanning of rhodanine-stained biopsy sections*—validated against atomic absorption spectroscopy, accurately quantifies liver Cu (Cornell University) on biopsy sections; allows rhodanine staining of all sections to determine accurate hepatic Cu distribution and quantification.

Hepatic Cu Concentrations (DWL)

- Normal hepatic Cu ≤400 μg/g.
- Hepatic Cu concentration in dogs with primary diet-induced or genetic CuAH (μg/g DWL)—Bedlington terrier (*COMMD1* mutation): 850–12,000; West Highland white terrier: up to 3,500; Labrador retriever: 400–9,000; Doberman pinscher: 1,000–10,000; Dalmatian: 750–22,000; cat: 700–8,000.
- *Avoid* analytic methods "estimating" sample hydration or reporting Cu on wet weight basis.

PATHOLOGIC FINDINGS

- Cu accumulates in lysosomes and mitochondria in zone 3 (centrilobular) hepatocytes in dogs.
- Oxidative injury—mechanism of hepatocellular injury.
- In some cases, apparent immune-mediated hepatitis accompanies CuAH injury.
- Rhodanine Cu staining confirms affiliation of Cu with histologic injury.
- Histologic features commonly include formation of "copper granulomas" in areas of hepatocyte necrosis—reflects response to oxidatively mediated hepatocyte necrosis; adjacent copper-laden hepatocytes.
- Chronic untreated necroinflammatory injury progresses to chronic hepatitis, parenchymal extinction, liver fibrosis, eventually to cirrhosis and formation of APSS.
- CuAH causing necroinflammatory liver injury leads to development of microhepatia, regenerative nodules, fibrotic "firm" liver texture.

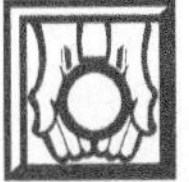

TREATMENT

APPROPRIATE HEALTH CARE

- Outpatient for most dogs.
- Inpatient evaluation and treatment for dogs with hepatic failure or severe acute hepatitis.
- See Hepatitis, Chronic; Cirrhosis and Fibrosis of the Liver for detailed management of liver disease.

NURSING CARE

- Animals in liver failure require fluid and electrolyte correction; may require treatment for HE and coagulopathies and should be treated with IV N-acetylcysteine (NAC) for oxidative injury, d-penicillamine chelation protocol started as soon as oral treatment possible.
- Dogs with hemolytic anemia may require whole or packed red blood cell (RBC) transfusion, IV NAC.

COPPER ASSOCIATED HEPATOPATHY (CONTINUED)

C

- Dogs with acquired Fanconi syndrome require IV fluid therapy and IV NAC to protect against acute renal failure.

ACTIVITY

Normal; rest if severe acute hepatic necrosis.

DIET

- Feed Cu-restricted diets to all affected dogs *for their lifetime.*
- Merely feeding Cu-restricted diet is unreliable intervention for dogs with pathologic hepatic Cu accumulation (see Suggested Reading).
- Avoid Cu in water if copper pipes—run water for 5 min to remove eluted Cu; restrict access to water with Cu >0.2 ppm.
- Prescription-type liver diets contain lowest Cu content, only provide 2.2–2.5 g protein/kg body weight when fed for maintenance energy requirements; *however*, dietary protein content should *only be reduced* for dogs exhibiting signs of HE or developing ammonium biurate crystalluria.
- Supplemental protein added to base prescription "liver" diets to increase protein intake by 0.5 g up to 1.5 g protein/kg body weight using low Cu-containing foods; select supplemental low Cu-containing protein sources using USDA food tables (freely available on internet).
- Alternative dietary management—balanced homemade Cu-restricted diets (*avoid* organ meats, nuts, certain grains) formulated by veterinary clinical nutritionist.
- Supplement water-soluble vitamins but avoid ascorbate (vitamin C supplements) during Cu hepatotoxicity as may augment oxidative injury.
- Avoid mineral supplements containing Cu if homemade diet; use specifically formulated supplements (e.g., Balance-It®).
- Chelation protocol must be adjunctively used with commercial diets for initial Cu removal.

CLIENT EDUCATION

- Educate all Bedlington terrier owners about genetic basis of CuAH in this breed and appropriate genetic testing, but inform that some dogs require liver biopsy for diagnosis.
- Other breeds—monitor for increased ALT activity with liver biopsy.
- Dogs receiving NSAIDs with circumstantial increase in ALT activity should be investigated for potential asymptomatic or "silent" hepatic Cu accumulation.
- Dietary management and chronic intermittent chelation or zinc administration needed for life in most dogs rescued from CuAH.

SURGICAL CONSIDERATIONS

- Animals with hepatic failure are surgical and anesthetic risks.
- Hypoxia encountered during anesthesia or surgery can provoke Cu-driven oxidative injury.

MEDICATIONS

DRUG(S) OF CHOICE

See other liver topics for specific treatments of chronic hepatitis and cirrhosis.

Chelation

d-Penicillamine

- 10–15 mg/kg PO q12h on empty stomach (1h before feeding); bioavailability reduced 50% if given with food.
- Mechanism—chelates Cu, promotes urinary excretion of Cu, other Cu-protective effects.
- Supplement vitamin B6 (pyridoxine)—25 mg PO q24h for duration of d-penicillamine treatment.
- Initiate treatment in dogs with increased ALT activity associated with biopsy-confirmed centrilobular Cu accumulation in >25% centrilobular hepatocytes or that reconciles with lobular injury/remodeling and Cu affiliation.
- Hepatic Cu as low as 600 µg/g DWL may require chelation and chronic management.
- Dogs with hepatic Cu <1,500 µg/g DWL usually cleared with 6 months of d-penicillamine chelation based on cases with biopsy-proven response.
- Dogs with hepatic Cu >3,000 µg/g may require ≥9–12 months chelation or longer.
- Drug-associated vomiting or hyporexia—abated with starting ½ dose d-penicillamine and titrating upward or concurrent low-dose prednisone; giving with morsel of meat anecdotally reported to solve nausea but may compromise drug bioavailability.
- Monitoring—most clinicians use ALT as surrogate marker because of cost and risks associated with follow-up liver biopsy; post-treatment biopsy optimal.
- Expect substantial decline in ALT by 8 weeks of chelation; do not discontinue daily chelation until ALT within normal range for several months, coordinating with anticipated chelation duration based on hepatic biopsy Cu quantification.
- Successful chelation achieves remarkable histologic improvement and resolution of ALT activity.

Trientine hydrochloride

- Alternative Cu chelator—as effective as d-penicillamine with similar guidelines; dose: 5–7 mg/kg PO q12h given 1h before meals; higher dosing associated with acute renal injury.
- Trientine currently restrictively expensive and difficult to acquire.
- Ammonium tetrathiomolybdate—alternative method for chelating Cu in circulation, from liver, and blocking enteric uptake in humans with Wilson's disease; limited use in dogs.

Zinc—Blocking Enteric Cu Uptake

- Zinc oral administration may assist in chronic control of CuAH; zinc use predicated on study of only 6 dogs.
- Reduces intestinal Cu absorption—study demonstrated reduced hepatic Cu concentrations after 2 years.
- 100 mg elemental zinc PO q12h 1h before feeding as loading dose for 2 months, then 25–50 mg PO q12h for Bedlington terrier-sized dog; zinc acetate best tolerated as zinc source.
- In humans, zinc therapy *less effective* than chelation for chronic management.
- May be useful in early CuAH with lower hepatic Cu concentrations: <1,000 µg/g DWL.
- Effects too slow to achieve therapeutic utility in dogs with high Cu concentrations and hepatitis where chelation therapy required for acute Cu mobilization and elimination.
- Coadministration of zinc and Cu *strongly contraindicated* as will negate efficacy of each treatment.
- Vomiting and inappetence commonly associated with zinc-induced gastritis.
- Evidence suggests low zinc utility in CuAH in dogs—low concentrations of oral zinc concurrent with Cu-restricted diet in previously chelated Labrador retrievers provided no additional benefit (see Suggested Reading).

Antioxidants

- d-α-tocopherol (vitamin E)—10 U/kg q24h PO; may be mixed in food.
- S-adenosylmethionine (SAMe)—20 mg/kg q24h, given on empty stomach.

Hepatoprotectants

- Silibinin (milk thistle extract, form bound to phosphatidylcholine [PPC] improves bioavailability)—5 mg/kg PO q24h; no proven benefit aside from high-dose IV silibinin for Amanita toxicity.
- Ursodeoxycholic acid—10–15 mg/kg PO divided BID given with food for best bioavailability (see Hepatitis, Chronic).
- Polyunsaturated PPC (dilinolylphosphatidylcholine [DLPC])—20–50 mg/kg PO q24h (soy bean extract; PhosChol® form providing 52% DLPC) mixed with food, advised for membrane-protectant and antifibrotic effects; apparent benefit with described chelation protocol based on post-treatment biopsy evaluations.

CONTRAINDICATIONS

- Ascorbic acid (vitamin C) may augment Cu hepatotoxicity.
- Avoid treatment with NSAIDs in affected dogs.

PRECAUTIONS

- Remain aware of altered drug metabolism related to reduced first-pass extraction if APSS develop or altered hepatic metabolism/biotransformation in dogs with severe centrilobular necrosis and remodeling.
- Avoid NSAID administration.

POSSIBLE INTERACTIONS

Penicillamine or trientine may not be effective if giving concurrent zinc therapy.

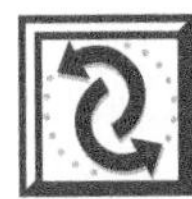

FOLLOW-UP

PATIENT MONITORING

- Liver enzymes initially q2–4 weeks for 8 weeks, then q2-4 months.
- Evaluate body weight and condition.
- Optimal reassessment—hepatic biopsy with determination of hepatic Cu concentration within 1 year of initiated treatment.
- If using zinc therapy—assess serum zinc concentrations initially, then during first 2–3 weeks until stable to insure values increase but remain within nontoxic range (200–500 µg/dL), then q6 months; plasma zinc does not reflect liver zinc concentrations.

PREVENTION/AVOIDANCE

- Breed only Bedlington terriers without *COMMD1* mutation; liver registry available for Bedlington terriers proven unaffected on basis of hepatic Cu concentration <400 µg/g DWL at 1 year of age or by gene testing.
- Other breeds noted previously may have recognized kindred predispositions.

POSSIBLE COMPLICATIONS

- d-Penicillamine can cause anorexia and vomiting; start at low end of dose range for first week; give 1h before meals; small amount of food may reduce nausea but reduces treatment efficacy.
- d-Penicillamine can induce glycogen-type vacuolar hepatopathy and ALP activity.
- d-Penicillamine side effects—glomerulonephritis, polyarthritis, drug-associated hepatopathy, or autoimmune-like vesicular disease of mucocutaneous junctions that resolves on drug withdrawal; *note*: assess urine for proteinuria before initiating therapy; rare hepatotoxicity: indicated by escalation of ALT activity; drug known to induce ALP.
- Excess zinc (oral dose >200 mg/day or blood concentration >800 µg/dL) can cause hemolytic anemia.

EXPECTED COURSE AND PROGNOSIS

- Prognosis poor in acutely affected young dogs with fulminant hepatic failure or older dogs with cirrhosis; however, some respond to acute care and chelation.
- Dogs with mild to moderate acute hepatic injury usually have good prognosis.
- Even dogs with nodular hepatopathy and microhepatia and ascites can respond well to described protocol with resolution of many histologic changes, including fibrosis.
- Good prognosis warranted if CuAH detected before liver remodeling or development of hepatitis.

MISCELLANEOUS

AGE-RELATED FACTORS

- Health evaluations that include ALT measurement help identify at-risk dogs.
- Important to evaluate ALT in any dog placed on chronic NSAIDs where Cu retention appears to augment centrilobular hepatotoxicity; measure ALT before and 2–4 weeks after NSAID initiation (sooner if patient demonstrates inappetence, vomiting, lethargy).

PREGNANCY/FERTILITY/BREEDING

- Do not breed affected Bedlington terriers or carriers.
- Genetics of other at-risk breeds unknown—some kindred predispositions recognized.

SYNONYMS

- Bedlington hepatitis.
- Chronic active hepatitis.
- Chronic Cu toxicity.
- Cu toxicosis.

SEE ALSO

- Cirrhosis and Fibrosis of the Liver.
- Hepatitis, Chronic.

ABBREVIATIONS

- ACT = activated clotting time.
- ALT = alanine aminotransferase.
- APSS = acquired portosystemic shunt.
- APTT= activated partial thromboplastin time.
- AST = aspartate transaminase.
- BUN = blood urea nitrogen.
- CuAH = copper associated hepatopathy.
- DLPC = dilinolylphosphatidylcholin.
- DWL = dry weight liver.
- GGT = γ-glutamyl transferase.
- HE = hepatic encephalopathy.
- NAC = N-acetylcysteine.
- NSAID = nonsteroidal anti-inflammatory drug.
- PPC = phosphatidylcholine.
- PT = prothrombin time.
- RBC = red blood cell.
- SAMe = S-adenosylmethionine.
- TSBA = total serum bile acid.

INTERNET RESOURCES

www.vetgen.com for genetic screening in Bedlington terriers

Suggested Reading

Fieten H, Biourge VC, Watson AL, et al. Dietary management of Labrador retrievers with subclinical hepatic copper accumulation. J Vet Intern Med. 2015, 29:822–827.

Fieten H, Hooijer-Nouwens BD, Biourge VC, et al. Association of dietary copper and zinc levels with hepatic copper and zinc concentration in Labrador Retrievers. J Vet Intern Med 2012, 26:1274–1280.

Hoffmann G, van den Ingh TS, Bode, P, et al. Cu-associated chronic hepatitis in Labrador Retrievers. J Vet Intern Med 2006, 20(4):856–861.

Johnston AN, Center SA, McDonough SP, et al. Hepatic copper concentrations in Labrador Retrievers with and without chronic hepatitis: 72 cases (1980–2010). J Am Vet Med Assoc 2013, 242(3):372–380.

Strickland JM, Buchweitz JP, Smedley RC, et al. Hepatic copper concentrations in 546 dogs (1982-2015). J Vet Intern Med 2018, 32:1943–1950.

Author Sharon A. Center

Consulting Editor Kate Holan

Acknowledgment The author and book editors acknowledge the prior contribution of Sean P. McDonough.

Client Education Handout available online

COPROPHAGIA AND PICA

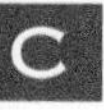

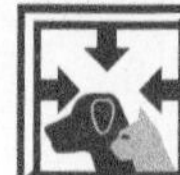

BASICS

DEFINITION

Pica is an abnormal ingestive behavior in which nonfood items are consumed. Coprophagia is a form of pica in which feces is consumed.

PATHOPHYSIOLOGY

• The pathophysiology of pica is unclear. • Coprophagia is not usually a pathologic condition. • Pica is a sign that may be associated with a variety of different conditions—any medical condition leading to nutritional deficiencies, electrolyte imbalances, gastrointestinal (GI) disturbances, polyphagia, or CNS disturbances may lead to pica and/or coprophagia. • Severely calorie-restricted diets or imbalanced diets leading to insufficiencies may also lead to pica and/or coprophagia.

SYSTEMS AFFECTED

GI—foreign body obstruction, GI upset leading to vomiting and diarrhea; increased chance of GI parasitism with coprophagia.

GENETICS

None known.

INCIDENCE/PREVALENCE

• Pica—unknown. • Coprophagia—occurrence has been estimated at 16–23% in dogs.

SIGNALMENT

Species

Coprophagia is common in dogs but rare in cats. Pica is seen in both dogs and cats.

Breed Predilections

Oriental cat breeds such as Siamese may be at greater risk of pica.

Mean Age and Range

Pica occurs more often in puppies than in adult dogs. Pica in cats is most likely to begin prior to 18 months of age.

SIGNS

Historical Findings

• In dogs, ingestion of inappropriate items such as rocks, clothing, and/or feces. • In cats, ingestion of fabrics, plastic, shoelaces, string, thread, or other inappropriate items.

Physical Examination Findings

• Halitosis if coprophagia is the presenting problem. • Dental trauma if the dog targets hard objects. • Pallor or weakness if anemia is a contributing condition. • Poor body condition if malabsorption or maldigestion is a contributing condition. • Neurologic signs if caused by neurologic disease. • May be abnormalities on abdominal palpation if gastroenteritis or foreign body.

CAUSES

Behavioral Causes

• Coprophagia is considered normal maternal behavior; the dam or queen licks the anogenital region of the neonate to stimulate elimination and then consumes the excreta. • Coprophagia may be considered a normal exploratory behavior in puppies; it has been postulated that high levels of deoxycholic acid in feces may contribute to neurologic development. • It is normal for dogs to seek out cat feces because it is high in protein—odor and taste may also be appealing. • Ungulate feces is also appealing to dogs, apparently due to partially digested vegetable matter. • Dogs described as "greedy eaters" have higher incidence of coprophagy; therefore a voracious appetite may predispose to coprophagia. • Feces may be appetizing to some dogs, so the behavior might be self-rewarding. • Dogs that have been punished for eliminating in the house could learn to eat their own feces in an apparent attempt to avoid punishment. • Dogs may also eat their own feces as a form of "nest cleaning." • Coprophagia may be attention-seeking behavior if a dog learns that it reliably leads to immediate owner attention. • Coprophagia may also develop in response to anxiety or frustration. • Pica may occur secondary to stealing behavior when the dog is highly motivated to prevent the owner from retrieving the stolen object or when the object has ingestive appeal. • Pica may develop as a result of anxiety or frustration that leads to destruction and subsequent consumption of an item.

Medical Causes

• Anemia. • Malnutrition leading to polyphagia. • Endocrinopathies—hyperthyroidism, diabetes mellitus, hyperadrenocorticism. • Maldigestion/malabsorption (e.g., exocrine pancreatic insufficiency). • Inflammatory bowel disease. • Small intestinal bacterial overgrowth. • CNS disease. • Portosystemic shunt. • Intestinal parasitism.

Drug-Induced Causes

Administration of drugs such as corticosteroids, progestins, phenobarbital, or benzodiazepines can lead to polyphagia.

RISK FACTORS

• Early weaning of kittens has been postulated to lead to sucking and ingestion of fabrics. • Cats fed low-roughage diets and/or not allowed access to roughage sources such as grass. • Dogs lacking appropriately stimulating environment, adequate activity, or social interactions may be at risk for pica and/or coprophagia. • Long periods of confinement, especially in a barren environment, may predispose to coprophagia. • Dogs in multidog households may be at higher risk of demonstrating coprophagia.

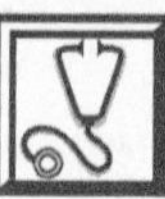

DIAGNOSIS

DIFFERENTIAL DIAGNOSIS

• Diagnosis is based on history and description of the behavior. • History should include: ○ Description of the problem—when and where it happens. ○ Age of onset. ○ Owner's usual response, any corrections attempted so far, and their results. ○ Changes in household, schedule, diet, or health associated with onset of problem. ○ Feeding routine of pets—when, where fed, by whom. ○ Any other unusual oral behaviors. ○ Other behavioral problems. ○ House training status—when and where the pet eliminates. ○ How the pet was house trained. ○ Relationships with other pets. • Environment, including daily schedule for play, exercise, attention, or training. • Medical health should be evaluated, including appetite and weight, any signs of nausea or GI upset such as excessive lip licking or surface licking, and color, consistency, and frequency of feces. • Pica must be differentiated from destructive chewing, where items may be torn apart but not consumed. • Pica must also be differentiated from instances where an animal consumes a nonfood item because the item smells and/or tastes appealing.

CBC/BIOCHEMISTRY/URINALYSIS

• Results suggesting diabetes mellitus, hyperadrenocorticism, hyperthyroidism, or drug-induced causes of polyphagia. • Anemia or hypoproteinemia. • Results suggesting presence of a portosystemic shunt—microcytosis, target cells, hypoalbuminemia, low blood urea nitrogen (BUN), ammonium biurate crystalluria. • Peripheral eosinophilia may occur due to gastrointestinal parasitism or eosinophilic inflammatory bowel disease.

OTHER LABORATORY TESTS

• Trypsin-like immunoreactivity (TLI)—may be low if exocrine pancreatic insufficiency exists. • Serum folate and cobalamin to evaluate for small intestinal bacterial overgrowth and small intestinal mucosal disease. • Fecal fat and fecal trypsin may help to evaluate for exocrine pancreatic insufficiency and other malabsorption/maldigestion-related conditions. • Thyroid panel to determine if hyperthyroid. • Fecal examinations to screen for intestinal parasites; *note*: coprophagia can result in false-positive tests for helminths in dogs. • Bile acids to evaluate for presence of a portosystemic shunt. • Adrenocorticotropic hormone (ACTH) stimulation if hyperadrenocorticism a consideration.

IMAGING

Survey abdominal radiographs and/or abdominal ultrasonography if indicated to rule out foreign body obstruction. May also demonstrate microhepatica if a portosystemic shunt is present.

DIAGNOSTIC PROCEDURES

• GI scoping and biopsy may be needed to evaluate for gastric and small bowel disease. • Cultures if indicated to evaluate for small intestinal bacterial overgrowth.

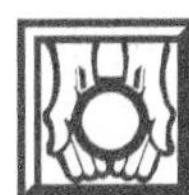

TREATMENT

APPROPRIATE HEALTH CARE

Treatment of Pica

• Prevent access to nonfood items that are likely targets—physical barriers to prevent access or confine animal away from targeted nonfood items; teach dog to wear basket muzzle. • Change to diet higher in fiber. • Provide feeding toys and acceptable foraging opportunities (e.g., green plants such as grass or catnip for cats). • Teach dogs a "Drop it" or "Leave it" command so the owner can prevent consumption of inappropriate items. • If diagnosis consistent with compulsive disorder, see appropriate section in text for treatment.

Treatment of Coprophagia

• Prevent access to feces. • Walk dog on leash and pick up feces immediately. • Teach dog to wear basket muzzle. • Head collar for increased ability to guide pet away from feces and reward "turning away" after defecation; dogs should then be rewarded with a tasty treat for returning to the owner on command. • There is no evidence that changing the taste or texture of the stool helps to decrease coprophagia or that any product marketed for the treatment of coprophagia reliably stops the behavior. • Taste aversion might be taught by treating the feces with a strongly distasteful substance (e.g., hot sauce, cayenne pepper, etc.); all feces that the dog can come in contact with must be treated in order for this to be effective; however, even if effective, dogs can learn to recognize which feces are treated, and ingest untreated feces.

ACTIVITY

• Increased mental and physical enrichment may help in treatment and prevention of pica and coprophagia and keep the pet engaged in alternative desirable activities. • Regular, predictable schedules of interaction and exercise can decrease anxiety and may aid in treatment of pica and coprophagia.

DIET

Dietary changes may be helpful in some cases of coprophagia. A more highly digestible diet or the addition of plant-based enzyme supplements or meat tenderizers is rarely successful in decreasing coprophagia.

CLIENT EDUCATION

• Owners should be counseled that coprophagia is, in most cases, normal canine behavior and not harmful unless the dog consumes feces containing pathogens or infective parasites. • Owners should avoid the use of any form of direct or confrontational punishment for pica or coprophagia due to the risk of increasing anxiety, possibly worsening the behavior, and/or leading to other problem behaviors. Close supervision and prevention of access are the best approach.

MEDICATIONS

DRUG(S) OF CHOICE

If the behavior is determined to be a compulsive disorder or secondary to anxiety, psychoactive drugs or anxiolytic drug therapy may be indicated.

CONTRAINDICATIONS

The use of any drugs that might contribute to polyphagia should be avoided when possible.

PRECAUTIONS

If drugs are indicated, precautions should be considered for the specific drug.

POSSIBLE INTERACTIONS

If drugs are prescribed, interactions should be considered for the specific drug.

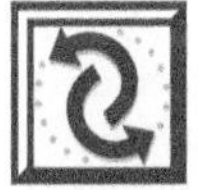

FOLLOW-UP

PATIENT MONITORING

• Client should be contacted in 1–2 weeks to verify compliance and determine if there is improvement. • If no or minimal improvement, further diagnostics should be recommended.

PREVENTION/AVOIDANCE

• Prevent access to the items likely to be consumed. • Careful supervision during house training may help to prevent puppy exploration of feces and reinforcement of coprophagia. • Administration of monthly parasiticide to control GI parasites.

POSSIBLE COMPLICATIONS

Foreign body obstruction is most common sequela to pica in both dogs and cats.

EXPECTED COURSE AND PROGNOSIS

◦ Prognosis is guarded if the condition has been present for a long period of time; or the owner is not willing to closely supervise the dog when it eliminates or prevent access to inappropriate items that the pet attempts to consume. • If owner is willing to supervise the dog and comply with treatment recommendations, prognosis improves.

C

MISCELLANEOUS

AGE-RELATED FACTORS

In adult or geriatric onset of pica or coprophagia, primary underlying medical conditions should be strongly suspected.

PREGNANCY/FERTILITY/BREEDING

• Owners of wool-sucking cats should be cautioned that the behavior appears to have a breed disposition, so avoiding breeding of this individual may be prudent and responsible action. • If this behavior is believed to be associated with a compulsive disorder, the animal should not be bred, as compulsive disorders appear to have a hereditary basis.

SYNONYMS

• Depraved appetite. • Wool sucking or wool chewing in cats.

SEE ALSO

• Compulsive Disorders—Cats.
• Compulsive Disorders—Dogs.
• Fear, Phobias and Anxieties—Cats.
• Fear, Phobias, and Anxieties—Dogs.

ABBREVIATIONS

• ACTH = adrenocorticotropic hormone.
• BUN = blood urea nitrogen.
• GI = gastrointestinal.
• TLI = trypsin-like immunoreactivity.

Suggested Reading

Horwitz D, ed. Blackwell's 5 Minute Consult Clinical Companion: Canine and Feline Behavior, 2nd ed. Ames, IA: Wiley-Blackwell, 2018, pp. 436–446, 754–760.

Houpt KA. Domestic Animal Behavior, 4th ed. Ames, IA: Blackwell, 2005, pp. 321–334.

Landsberg G, Hunthausen W, Ackerman L. Behavior Problems of the Dog and Cat, 3rd ed. St. Louis, MO: Saunders Elsevier, 2013, pp. 78–79, 157–158.

Author Valarie V. Tynes

Consulting Editor Gary M. Landsberg

Client Education Handout available online

CORNEAL AND SCLERAL LACERATIONS

BASICS

DEFINITION

• Penetrating—a wound or foreign body enters but does not pass through the cornea or sclera. • Perforating—a wound or foreign body completely passes through the cornea or sclera; greater risk of vision loss than penetrating. • Simple—only the cornea or sclera, penetrating or perforating, other eye structures intact. • Complicated—perforating, involves other ocular structures, uveal, vitreal, or retinal incarceration or prolapse through the wound, traumatic cataract, hyphema, lid lacerations.

PATHOPHYSIOLOGY

• Sharp trauma—wounds by an outside-in mechanism. • Blunt trauma—wounds by an inside-out mechanism; eye undergoes sudden changes in its equatorial and axial dimensions and intraocular pressure (IOP); actual wound may be distant from point of impact; often more damaging than sharp trauma. • All or a portion of foreign object initiating injury may be retained in wound or eye.

SYSTEMS AFFECTED

• Musculoskeletal—surrounding skull or orbital tissue. • Nervous—brain injury. • Ophthalmic.

INCIDENCE/PREVALENCE

Common

SIGNALMENT

Species

Dog and cat.

SIGNS

Historical Findings

• Usually acute onset. • History of running through vegetation, hit by projectiles (gunshot etc.), scratched by a cat. • Trauma may not be observed.

Physical Examination Findings

• Varies with tissues affected. • Corneal, scleral, or eyelid deformity, edema, or hemorrhage. • May see retained foreign body. • Often rapidly seals; may appear only as subconjunctival hematoma. • May also see iris defects, pupil distortion, hyphema, cataract, vitreal hemorrhage, retinal detachment, and exophthalmia.

CAUSES

Blunt or sharp trauma.

RISK FACTORS

• Preexisting visual impairment. • Young, naïve, or highly excitable animals. • Hunting or running through heavy vegetation. • Fighting.

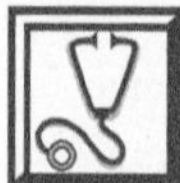

DIAGNOSIS

DIFFERENTIAL DIAGNOSIS

• Traumatic event not observed and no foreign body found—consider nontraumatic causes of ocular injury. • Traumatic hyphema—generally accompanied by corneal or scleral lesions and subconjunctival or periocular hemorrhage. • Traumatic cataracts—disrupted lens capsule. • Traumatic retinal detachment—accompanied by intraocular hemorrhage.

CBC/BIOCHEMISTRY/URINALYSIS

Normal, or related to other injuries.

OTHER LABORATORY TESTS

• Cytologic examination and aerobic culture and sensitivity of the wound and foreign body—recommended even if infection is not apparent; specimen may be collected under general anesthesia at time of surgery. • Consider other tests (platelet count, coagulation profile, etc.) if nontraumatic causes possible.

IMAGING

• Ocular ultrasonography—if ocular media are opaque; may clarify extent and nature of intraocular disease, may detect foreign body. • Orbital radiographs, CT, or MRI (if nonmetallic)—may help determine projectile's course; may detect foreign body.

DIAGNOSTIC PROCEDURES

• Determine nature, force, and direction of impact of object—to identify which tissues may be involved. • Do not put pressure on eye until rupture or laceration of globe has been ruled out. • Assess vision—menace response; aversion to bright light. • Periocular skin and orbit—examine for lacerations or deformities; suspect globe involvement if lid laceration crosses eyelid margin or penetrates orbital septum; entry sites often small and quickly seal. • Abnormal ocular motility—suggests extraocular muscle trauma, orbital hemorrhage or edema, retained foreign bodies, or peripheral nerve or CNS damage. • Scleral rupture—consider if subconjunctival hemorrhage, especially if anterior chamber is deep or shallow, there is vitreal hemorrhage, or eye is abnormally soft. • Pupils—assess size, shape, symmetry, direct and consensual light reflexes. • Detailed ophthalmoscopy—assess clarity of ocular media and fundus integrity, rule out intraocular foreign body. • Seidel test—if any question of corneal or scleral leaking; use a dry to slightly moist fluorescein strip to paint a thin coat of fluorescein over the surface of the defect; leaking aqueous combines with the orange fluorescein, forming a bright green rivulet (seen best with cobalt illumination).

PATHOLOGIC FINDINGS

• Depends on wound and affected tissues. • Usually correlates with clinical examination findings. • Vitreal hemorrhage—may organize into a fibrous band that causes traction retinal detachment. • Post-traumatic sarcoma (cats)—may occur months to years after severe ocular trauma.

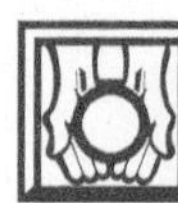

TREATMENT

APPROPRIATE HEALTH CARE

• Depends on severity. • Outpatient—if integrity of globe is ensured.

NURSING CARE

• Sedation—consider for excited or fractious patients. • When walking—apply an Elizabethan collar (E-collar) and use a harness or put ipsilateral foreleg through the leash to avoid increasing IOP in affected eye.

Injuries Considered for Medical Treatment

• Complicated wounds, those with retained plant material, and those caused by blunt trauma with tissue devitalization—infection common. • Bacterial endophthalmitis—5–7% of perforations; very rare in wounds that only penetrate but do not perforate the cornea. • Nonperforating wounds with no wound edge override or gape—apply an E-collar; give topical antibiotic or atropine ophthalmic solutions. • Nonperforating wounds with mild wound gape or shelved edges—apply a therapeutic soft contact lens and an E-collar; give topical antibiotic or atropine ophthalmic solutions. • Simple full-thickness, pinpoint corneal perforation with a negative Seidel test that has a formed anterior chamber and no uveal prolapse—sedentary patients; use a therapeutic soft contact lens and an E-collar; give topical antibiotic or atropine ophthalmic solutions; reexamine a few hours after applying the lens and at 24 and 48 hours.

ACTIVITY

• Usually confined indoors (cats) or limited to leash walks until healing is complete. • A harness is preferred to a collar to reduce pressure on the neck and the risk of increased IOP and wound leaks.

CLIENT EDUCATION

Warn client that the full extent of the injury (cataracts, retinal detachment, infection) may not be apparent until days or weeks after the injury and that long-term follow-up is necessary.

SURGICAL CONSIDERATIONS

Injuries Requiring Surgical Exploration or Repair

• Full-thickness corneal lacerations with a positive Seidel test. • Full-thickness wounds with iris incarceration or prolapse. • Full-thickness scleral or corneoscleral lacerations. • Suspected retained foreign body or posterior scleral rupture. • Simple nonperforating wound with edges that are moderately or overtly gaping and that are long or more than two-thirds the corneal thickness.

Injuries Considered for Surgical Exploration or Repair

• Small full-thickness corneal lacerations with a negative Seidel test and no uveal prolapse. • Large conjunctival lacerations. • Partial-thickness corneal or scleral lacerations in an active patient.

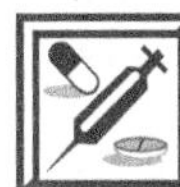

MEDICATIONS

DRUG(S) OF CHOICE

Antibiotics

• Penetrating—topical antibiotics alone (e.g., neomycin, polymyxin B, and bacitracin) or gentamicin solution q6–8h; usually sufficient. • Perforating wounds with negative Seidel test—systemic ciprofloxacin (dogs: 10–20 mg/kg PO q24h); topical cefazolin (add injectable cefazolin to artificial tears to concentration of 33 mg/mL) and either topical ophthalmic ciprofloxacin or ofloxacin; both drugs q4–6h. • Perforating wounds with positive Seidel test—systemic ciprofloxacin (dogs: 10–20 mg/kg PO q24h); topical antibiotics as noted above, only after defect has been made watertight.

Anti-Inflammatories

• Topical 1% prednisolone acetate or 0.1% dexamethasone solution q6–12h; as soon as wound is sutured or has epithelialized (becomes fluorescein stain negative), as long as infection is not present. • Systemic prednisone 0.5–1 mg/kg PO q12–24h; for sutured or epithelialized wounds when inflammation is severe, when lens or posterior structures are involved, or when wound is infected or not epithelialized and control of inflammation is mandatory to preserve the eye. • Topical nonsteroidal anti-inflammtory drugs (NSAIDs)—flurbiprofen or others; if topical corticosteroids are contraindicated and control of inflammation is mandatory to preserve the eye.

Mydriatics

1% atropine ophthalmic solution q6–12h—when there is significant miosis.

Analgesics

• Topical atropine may provide sufficient pain relief. • Carprofen 2.2 mg/kg PO q12h or 4.4 mg/kg PO q24h. • Tramadol—2–5 mg/kg PO q12h.

CONTRAINDICATIONS

• Topical ophthalmic ointments—avoid in Seidel-positive perforations until wound closed. • Systemic ciprofloxacin—avoid in young dogs.

PRECAUTIONS

• Aminoglycosides—topical application may be irritating and may impede reepithelization if used frequently or at high concentrations; possibility for renal toxicity. • Topical solutions may be preferable to ointments if corneal integrity is questionable. • Atropine—may exacerbate keratoconjunctivitis sicca and glaucoma. • Topical or systemic NSAIDs—use cautiously with hyphema; unknown safety in cats.

POSSIBLE INTERACTIONS

Systemic NSAIDs—may potentiate nephrotoxicity of aminoglycosides; ensure good hydration and adequate renal function.

ALTERNATIVE DRUG(S)

Topical ciprofloxacin ophthalmic solution—may be used instead of combination of topical cefazolin and fortified aminoglycoside; some streptococcus are resistant.

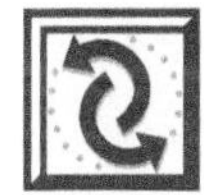

FOLLOW-UP

PATIENT MONITORING

• Deep or long penetrating wounds that have not been sutured and perforating wounds—recheck q24–48h for first several days to ensure integrity of globe, to monitor for infection, and to check control of ocular inflammation. • Superficial penetrating wounds—usually recheck at 3–5-day intervals until healed. • Antibiotic therapy—alter according to culture and sensitivity.

PREVENTION/AVOIDANCE

• Take care when introducing new puppies to households with cats. • Minimize running through dense vegetation; owner should consider having bottle of saline eyewash to irrigate foreign debris from eye. • Minimize visually impaired dog's exposure to dense vegetation.

POSSIBLE COMPLICATIONS

• Loss of eye or vision. • Chronic ocular inflammation or pain. • Post-traumatic sarcoma—may develop in cat eyes following trauma.

EXPECTED COURSE AND PROGNOSIS

• Most eyes with corneal lacerations or a retained corneal foreign body are salvageable. • The more posterior the injury, the poorer the prognosis for retention of vision. • Poor prognosis—scleral or uveal involvement, no light perception, perforating injuries involving the lens or with significant vitreal hemorrhage or retinal detachment. • Penetrating injuries usually better prognosis than perforating injuries. • Blunt trauma carries poorer prognosis than sharp trauma.

MISCELLANEOUS

ASSOCIATED CONDITIONS

Depends on nature and extent of injury.

PREGNANCY/FERTILITY/BREEDING

• Systemic corticosteroids—may complicate pregnancy. • Systemic ciprofloxacin—should be avoided during pregnancy.

SEE ALSO

- Cataracts.
- Hyphema.
- Keratitis—Ulcerative.
- Proptosis.
- Retinal Detachment.

ABBREVIATIONS

- E-collar = Elizabethan collar.
- IOP = intraocular pressure.
- NSAID = nonsteroidal anti-inflammatory drug.

Suggested Reading

Ledbetter EC, Gilger BC. Diseases and surgery of the canine cornea and sclera. In: Gelatt KN, Gilger BC, Kern TJ, eds., Veterinary Ophthalmology, 5th ed. Ames, IA: Wiley-Blackwell, 2013, pp. 976–1049.

Maggs DJ. Diseases of the Cornea and Sclera. In: Maggs DJ, Miller PE, Ofri R, eds., Slatter's Fundamentals of Veterinary Ophthalmology, 6th ed. St. Louis, MO: Elsevier, 2018, pp. 213–253.

Author Paul E. Miller

Consulting Editor Kathern E. Myrna

Client Education Handout available online

CORNEAL OPACITIES—DEGENERATIONS AND INFILTRATES

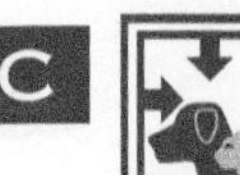

BASICS

OVERVIEW

Acquired corneal disorder characterized by lipid or calcium deposition. May be unilateral or bilateral, have distinct margins, and occur secondary to other ocular or systemic disorders.

SIGNALMENT

Primarily in dogs, uncommon in cats. Lipid deposition most common in geriatric dogs. May be associated with systemic hyperlipoproteinemia.

SIGNS

- Lipid deposits—gray-white or crystalline; band-shaped, irregular, or circular.
- Calcium deposits—dense white to crystalline; irregular, punctate to band-shaped lesions in the superficial stroma.
- Frequently associated with inflammatory disorders such as keratitis or uveitis.
- Corneal vascularization, edema, and pigmentation often present.
- With progression the cornea may develop a roughened appearance; disruption of epithelium can lead to ulceration.
- Associated ocular conditions that may lead to corneal degeneration—corneal scars, keratoconjunctivitis sicca (KCS), exposure keratitis, chronic uveitis, episcleritis, phthisis bulbi, chronic topical steroid therapy, limbal neoplasia.
- When lipid deposition occurs secondary to hyperlipoproteinemia, perilimbal annular ring may form with clear zone between affected cornea and limbus; often bilateral but may be asymmetric; vascularization is variable.

CAUSES & RISK FACTORS

- Lipid—hyperlipoproteinemia may increase risk or worsen existing deposits; can be secondary to hypothyroidism, diabetes mellitus, hyperadrenocorticism, diet, pancreatitis, nephrotic syndrome, liver disease, hyperlipidemia of miniature schnauzers.
- Calcium—hypercalcemia, hyperphosphatemia, hypervitaminosis D, hyperadrenocorticism, uremia.
- Lipid and calcium deposits are frequently seen together.

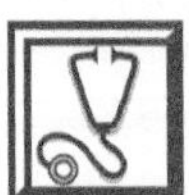

DIAGNOSIS

DIFFERENTIAL DIAGNOSIS

- Corneal scar—nonpainful lesion, gray to white; fluorescein negative; relatively smooth corneal surface; distinct margins.
- Corneal stromal dystrophies—bilateral, often symmetric foci of gray to white deposition, distinct margins; heritable, not associated with ocular inflammation; do not retain fluorescein stain; often occur away from the limbus.
- Edema—bluish to gray; usually homogeneous; varies in size depending on severity; indistinct margins; can retain fluorescein stain if corneal erosion/ulceration present.
- Corneal ulcer—ocular pain, retains fluorescein stain, varying degrees of edema around the lesion.
- Inflammatory cell infiltrates—ocular pain, gray to tan to yellow with indistinct margins; cytologic examination of cornea reveals white blood cells, microorganisms.

CBC/BIOCHEMISTRY/URINALYSIS

- *Systemic tests only necessary if hyperlipidemia is suspected; no systemic tests necessary for most cases.*
- Lipid—evaluate fasting cholesterol, triglyceride, blood glucose concentrations.
- Calcium—evaluate ionized calcium concentration.

OTHER LABORATORY TESTS

Endocrinopathy testing—thyroid function, adrenocorticotropic hormone (ACTH) stimulation test.

DIAGNOSTIC PROCEDURES

Fluorescein staining—may retain dye around margins of deposit if raised.

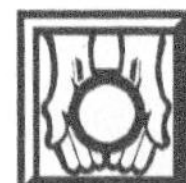

TREATMENT

- Treat primary ocular disease if present.
- Corneal deposits causing patient discomfort or impaired vision may benefit from corneal debridement or superficial keratectomy followed by medical treatment; deposits likely to recur if underlying cause not corrected.
- Hyperlipoproteinemia may resolve with low-fat diet and treatment of systemic disease if present; both may slow or stop progression of ocular disease.

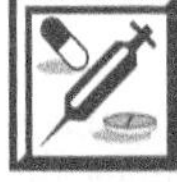

MEDICATIONS

DRUG(S) OF CHOICE

- Topical broad-spectrum antibiotics (i.e., triple antibiotic) for ulcerated cornea; frequency depends on severity; usually uncomplicated ulcers treated q8–12h.
- Topical nonsteroidal anti-inflammatory drug q8–12h—indicated if uveitis noted.
- Topical 0.2% cyclosporine—to improve tear film quality, reduce inflammation.
- Topical 1% atropine q8–24h—indicated to reduce pain if uveitis or ulceration is present.
- Topical ethylene diamine tetra-acetate (EDTA) solution 0.5–3% q6h; may help minimize calcium deposits; usually used following debulking procedure to improve efficacy.
- Artificial tear ointment q6–12h; may prevent or reduce frequency of secondary corneal ulceration; provides lubrication and improves comfort when corneal surface is irregular.

CONTRAINDICATIONS/POSSIBLE COMPLICATIONS

- Topical corticosteroids—not recommended, may worsen severity; contraindicated with corneal ulceration.
- Topical atropine—contraindicated with KCS, glaucoma, lens luxations.

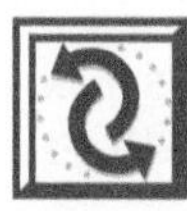

FOLLOW-UP

PATIENT MONITORING

Monitor serum cholesterol and triglycerides to assess efficacy of dietary management in hyperlipidemic patients; monitor treatment of primary disease if present.

EXPECTED COURSE AND PROGNOSIS

- Corneal ulceration—associated with worsening of disease.
- Vision—may be affected in advanced disease; may be severe if primary ocular disease (e.g., uveitis) present.
- Deposits may recur following superficial keratectomy.

MISCELLANEOUS

SEE ALSO

- Corneal Opacities—Dystrophies.
- Keratitis—Ulcerative.

ABBREVIATIONS

- ACTH = adrenocorticotropic hormone.
- EDTA = ethylene diamine tetra-acetate.
- KCS = keratoconjunctivitis sicca.

INTERNET RESOURCES

https://www.columbiaeye.org/education/digital-reference-of-ophthalmology/cornea-external-diseases/degenerations

Suggested Reading

Crispin SM, Barnett KC. Dystrophy, degeneration and infiltration of the canine cornea. J Small Anim Pract 1983, 24:63–83.

Author Kathern E. Myrna

Consulting Editor Kathern E. Myrna

Acknowledgment The author and book editors acknowledge the prior contribution of Amber L. Labelle

CORNEAL OPACITIES—DYSTROPHIES

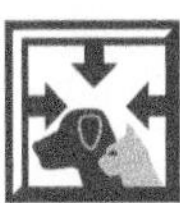

BASICS

OVERVIEW

• Primary, inherited (or familial), bilateral, and often symmetric condition of the cornea that is not associated with other ocular or systemic diseases. • Three types based on anatomic location—epithelial: characterized by dyskeratotic and necrotic epithelial cells, focal absence of epithelial basement membrane, and cell infiltrate in anterior corneal stroma; stromal: lipid deposition within corneal stroma; endothelial: characterized by abnormal, dystrophic endothelial cells.

SIGNALMENT

Usually dogs; rare in cats.

Epithelial

Shetland Sheepdogs—age of onset 6 months–6 years; slow progression.

Stromal

• Usually young adult dogs at age of onset. • Affected breeds—Afghan hound, Airedale terrier, Alaskan Malamute, American cocker spaniel, beagle, bearded collie, bichon frisé, cavalier King Charles spaniel, German shepherd, Lhasa apso, mastiff, miniature pinscher, rough collie, Samoyed, Siberian husky, Weimaraner, whippet, and others; inheritance pattern identified in few breeds.

Endothelial

• Dogs—primarily Boston terriers, Chihuahuas, and dachshunds; may affect other breeds; typically middle-aged or older at onset of clinical signs; female predilection suggested. • Cats—affects young animals; described most often in domestic shorthairs; a similar condition without endothelial disease is inherited as an autosomal recessive disorder in Manx.

SIGNS

All cause some degree of opacity in cornea.

Epithelial

• Can be asymptomatic or have blepharospasm; multifocal white or gray circular to irregular opacities or rings; sometimes associated with multifocal corneal erosions. • Vision usually not affected.

Stromal

• Usually asymptomatic without inflammation. • Central—most common; gray, white, or silver oval to circular opacity of central or paracentral cornea; with magnification may note multiple fibrillar to coalescing opacities that have crystalline or ground-glass appearance (crystalline corneal dystrophy). • Diffuse—affects Airedales; more diffuse, dense opacity than with central dystrophy. • Annular—commonly affects Siberian huskies; doughnut-shaped opacity of paracentral or peripheral cornea. • Vision—usually not affected; visual deficit possible with advanced or diffuse disease.

Endothelial

• Asymptomatic in early stages. • Edema of temporal or inferio-temporal cornea that usually progresses to entire cornea after months to years. • Corneal epithelial bullae (bullous keratopathy) and subsequent corneal erosion ulceration may develop; erosions or ulceration may cause blepharospasm due to pain. • Vision—may be impaired with advanced disease.

CAUSES & RISK FACTORS

• Epithelial—result of degenerative or innate abnormalities of corneal epithelium and/or basement membrane. • Stromal—innate abnormality or localized error in corneal lipid metabolism; may be affected by hyperlipoproteinemia (may increase opacity). • Endothelium—degeneration of endothelial cell layer; subsequent loss of endothelial cell pump function results in corneal edema.

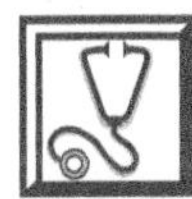

DIAGNOSIS

DIFFERENTIAL DIAGNOSIS

• Epithelial, stromal—other causes of corneal opacity: corneal degenerations, ulcers, scars, inflammatory cell infiltrates. • Endothelial—other causes of diffuse corneal edema: uveitis and glaucoma.

CBC/BIOCHEMISTRY/URINALYSIS

Epithelial, stromal—high concentrations of cholesterol and triglyceride levels may modify course of disease, but are not the cause.

DIAGNOSTIC PROCEDURES

• Stromal—usually does not retain fluorescein stain. • Epithelial or endothelial—may retain fluorescein stain, often in multifocal punctate areas, particularly with advanced disease. • Tonometry—to eliminate glaucoma as cause of corneal edema.

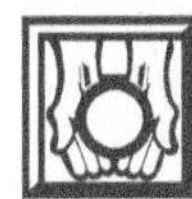

TREATMENT

• Advanced epithelial or endothelial disease with ulceration—may require treatment for ulcerative keratitis. • Stromal—usually none required; may perform superficial keratectomy to remove lipid deposits if severe, but usually unnecessary and deposits may recur. • Inform client that some corneal dystrophies are inherited. • Advanced endothelial dystrophy—may use therapeutic soft contact lens with or without debridement of redundant corneal epithelial tags, conjunctival flap surgery, or thermal cautery of cornea.

MEDICATIONS

DRUG(S) OF CHOICE

• Corneal ulceration—topical antibiotics and possibly atropine (see Keratitis—Ulcerative). • Epithelial—1–2% cyclosporine in oil or 0.2% ointment q8–24h to relieve clinical signs. • Endothelial—topical 5% sodium chloride ointment; palliative treatment; does not markedly clear cornea, but may prevent progression and rupture of corneal epithelial bullae.

CONTRAINDICATIONS/POSSIBLE INTERACTIONS

Topical corticosteroids—no benefit to lipid (stromal) dystrophy, of questionable benefit to other forms of dystrophy.

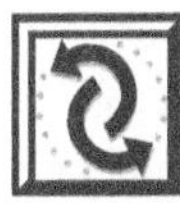

FOLLOW-UP

• Reexamination—necessary only if ocular pain or corneal ulceration develops. • Corneal opacity—may wax and wane with lipid dystrophy; unlikely to resolve. • Corneal ulceration—may accompany progression of epithelial or endothelial dystrophy. • Vision—not substantially affected except in advanced cases.

MISCELLANEOUS

SEE ALSO

• Corneal Opacities—Degenerations and Infiltrates.
• Keratitis—Ulcerative.

Suggested Reading

Crispin SM, Barnett KC. Dystrophy, degeneration and infiltration of the canine cornea. J Small Anim Pract 1983, 24:63–83.

Author Ellison Bentley
Consulting Editor Kathern E. Myrna

CORNEAL SEQUESTRUM—CATS

BASICS

OVERVIEW

- A focal, light brown to black, plaque-like area of stromal coagulation necrosis usually located axially.
- Usually caused by chronic corneal ulceration, trauma, or exposure.
- Synonym—keratitis nigrum.

SIGNALMENT

- Cats—any breed, age.
- Brachycephalic breeds, Siamese predisposed.
- Colorpoints may be genetically predisposed.

SIGNS

- Unilateral or bilateral, focal round to oval, variably sized areas of corneal discoloration ranging from translucent golden-brown (early) to opaque black (chronic).
- Often with chronic nonhealing corneal ulcer.
- Corneal vascularization and edema.
- History of feline herpesvirus-1 (FHV-1) keratoconjunctivitis.
- Blepharospasm or ocular discharge.
- Conjunctival hyperemia and chemosis.
- Miotic pupil.
- May be static for long periods or may rapidly progress.
- With chronicity, corneal vascularization may extrude plaque.

CAUSES & RISK FACTORS

- Thought to involve chronic mechanical corneal irritation or ulceration with corneal necrosis and desiccation.
- Risk factors include chronic corneal ulceration, chronic trichiasis or entropion, brachycephalic conformation, lagophthalmia, keratoconjunctivitis sicca (KCS), qualitative tear film disorders (lipid or mucin deficiency), FHV-1 infection, topical corticosteroids, and iatrogenic trauma (grid keratotomy).

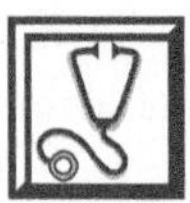

DIAGNOSIS

DIFFERENTIAL DIAGNOSIS

- Corneal perforation/iris prolapse—protruding iris is fleshy and yellow to light brown.
- Corneal foreign body.
- Corneal pigmentation—rare in cats.
- Corneal neoplasia—melanocytoma occurs at limbus and is typically nonpainful.

CBC/BIOCHEMISTRY/URINALYSIS

No specific abnormalities.

OTHER LABORATORY TESTS

- Schirmer tear test—very low values suggest KCS, but some normal cats have low values.
- Corneal culture and cytology to rule out corneal infection.
- Fluorescein stain.
- Tear film breakup time (TBUT)—normal time to breakup of fluorescein-stained tear film is 21 seconds; TBUT may be decreased in cats with sequestra or FHV-1 due to mucin tear film deficiency or secondary to corneal disease.
- Corneal histopathology—confirm diagnosis and evaluate completeness of excision.
- PCR for FHV-1— limited value.
- Conjunctival biopsy—goblet cell numbers may decrease with conjunctival inflammation or FHV-1.

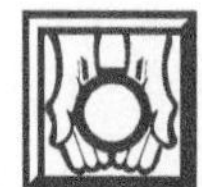

TREATMENT

- Lesion depth, degree of ocular pain, and cost are important factors.
- Medical—supportive care, wait for sequestrum to spontaneously slough; ocular pain may persist for months and sloughing of sequestrum may lead to deep corneal ulceration or perforation.

Surgical Considerations

- Lamellar keratectomy—if performed early, can relieve ocular pain, promote corneal healing, and may prevent lesion from involving deeper corneal stroma.
- Corneal grafting should be performed if ≥50% of corneal stroma has been excised; options include conjunctival pedicle grafting, grafting with synthetic, autogenous, or heterologous biomaterials, and corneoscleral transposition.
- Diamond burr debridement may be used to remove superficial sequestra.
- Postoperative management—broad-spectrum topical antibiotic, atropine ointment, and tear supplement.

MEDICATIONS

DRUG(S) OF CHOICE

- Topical oxytetracycline with polymyxin B or bacitracin-neomycin-polymyxin B q6–8h (prophylactic).
- Topical 1% atropine sulfate ointment q12–24h (improve ocular comfort).
- Topical lubricants (e.g., carboxymethylcellulose gel) q6–8h (reduce mechanical irritation and corneal desiccation); may prevent progression of nonulcerated sequestra.
- Topical or systemic antiviral therapy in cats with history or clinical signs of FHV-1 infection.

CONTRAINDICATIONS/POSSIBLE INTERACTIONS

Topical antibiotics (neomycin) may be irritating and cause chemical conjunctivitis.

FOLLOW-UP

PATIENT MONITORING

- If managing medically, examine as needed to monitor progression and for complications associated with sloughing of sequestrum.
- If managed by keratectomy, examine q5–7 days until corneal defect has reepithelialized (usually 7–14 days).
- Sequestra may recur or occur in contralateral eye; recurrence more likely in cats with low Schirmer tear tests, full-thickness lesions, or in cases in which keratectomy did not result in complete excision of pigmented corneal tissue or predisposing cause was not addressed.

POSSIBLE COMPLICATIONS

Corneal perforation may occur if sequestrum sloughs, leaving full-thickness defect, or if sloughing results in deep stromal corneal ulcer that becomes malacic or infected.

MISCELLANEOUS

ASSOCIATED CONDITIONS

- Corneal ulceration—cats.
- Eyelid conformational abnormalities (trichiasis, entropion, etc.).

ABBREVIATIONS

- FHV-1 = feline herpesvirus-1.
- KCS = keratoconjunctivitis sicca.
- TBUT = tear film breakup time.

Suggested Reading

Featherstone HJ, Sansom J. Feline corneal sequestra: a review of 64 cases (80 eyes) from 1993 to 2000. Vet Ophthalmol 2004, 7(4):213–227.

Stiles J. Feline ophthalmology. In: Gelatt KN, Gilger BC, Kern TJ, eds., Veterinary Ophthalmology, 5th ed. Ames, IA: Wiley, 2013, pp. 1495–1496.

Author Anne J. Gemensky Metzler

Consulting Editor Kathern E. Myrna

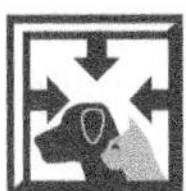

BASICS

DEFINITION

• A sudden and often repetitively occurring defense reflex that helps clear large airways of excess secretions, irritants, foreign particles, and microbes, or clear foreign material from upper airways. • The cough reflex consists of three phases: inhalation, forced exhalation against a closed glottis, and violent expulsion of air from the lungs following opening of the glottis, usually accompanied by a sudden noise. Coughing can happen voluntarily as well as involuntarily, although in dogs and cats it is presumed to be essentially involuntary. Coughing should not be confused with other airway sounds (cf differential diagnosis).

PATHOPHYSIOLOGY

• A physiologic reflex in healthy animals that protects the lower airways from inhalation of foreign particles and helps clear particles that have been entrapped in the mucus; acts in conjunction with the mucociliary clearance mechanism. • The cough pathway includes cough receptors, which are made up of sensory nerves in the airways, the vagus nerve, the central cough center, and effector muscles. • The cough pathway can be stimulated by mechanical or chemical factors; endogenous triggers include airway secretions and inflammation; exogenous triggers include smoke and aspirated foreign material. • Cough receptors include rapidly adapting stretch receptors (sensitive to mechanical stimuli) that are located within the mucosa of the tracheobronchial tree (especially larynx and trachea), and pulmonary/bronchial C-fibers, which are more sensitive to chemical stimulation; coughing mechanisms and pathways are very complex and are not fully understood, even in humans.

SYSTEMS AFFECTED

• Respiratory—cough of any origin can be an inciting factor for aggravation or precipitation of signs associated with tracheal collapse in susceptible breeds. • Cardiovascular—enlargement or impaired function of the right ventricle can result from a respiratory disorder causing tissue damage, hypoxic injury, and/or chronic hypoxic pulmonary vasoconstriction (cor pulmonale).

SIGNALMENT

• Dogs and cats of all ages and breeds. • Much more common clinical sign in dogs than in cats. • Cough of tracheal origin is less common in cats than in dogs. • Age, breed, and sex predispositions vary with inciting cause.

SIGNS

• Cough must be differentiated from similar signs such as reverse sneezing, gagging, retching. • Description of the cough and/or smartphone recording of suspect sounds are helpful in identification of the anatomic structures involved in dogs (i.e., honking cough is typical of tracheal collapse, harsh sonorous cough followed by terminal retch characterizes cough of tracheal or bronchial origin, faint moist cough is heard in moderate to severe pneumonia). • Cough can be described as dry or moist, productive, honking, short or harsh, faint or sonorous, followed by gagging or retching. • Cough can be elicited by traction on the collar (laryngeal or tracheal origin), aggravated by exercise or excitation (tracheal collapse), or can occur after a period of rest (cough due to heart failure). • Can be accompanied by stertor or stridor (laryngeal, tracheal origin) or dyspnea (many areas).

CAUSES

Upper Respiratory Tract Diseases

• A variety of sinonasal conditions cause extension of inflammation and/or secretions into the pharynx and/or larynx and can lead to the upper airway cough syndrome (UACS), previously referred to as postnasal drip syndrome. • Laryngeal and/or pharyngeal disease (inflammation, paralysis, tumor, granuloma, collapse). • Tracheal disease (inflammation, infection, foreign body, collapse, stenosis, tumor).

Lower Respiratory Tract Diseases (Tracheobronchial or Bronchopulmonary Disease)

• Inflammatory (feline bronchitis syndrome; dogs: chronic bronchitis, eosinophilic broncho-pneumopathy). • Infectious—bacterial, viral (dog: distemper, kennel cough; cat: feline leukemia virus [FeLV], feline immuno-deficiency virus [FIV], feline infectious peritonitis [FIP], calicivirus, herpesvirus), parasitic (dog: *Filaroides* spp., *Angiostrongylus vasorum*, *Capillaria aerophilia*, *Crenosoma vulpis*; cat: *Aerulostrongylus abstrusus*; dog, cat: *Paragonimus kellicotti*, *Dirofilaria immitis*), protozoal (cat: toxoplasmosis; dog: pneumo-cystosis), fungal (blastomycosis, histoplasmosis, coccidiomycosis, cryptococcosis, aspergillosis). • Neoplastic (primary, metastatic, compression due to enlarged lymph nodes). • Chemical or traumatic (aspiration, near drowning, noxious fumes, foreign body, trauma, hemorrhage). • Chronic disorders of unknown origin (interstitial pulmonary fibrosis).

Other Diseases

• Cardiovascular diseases (pulmonary edema, left atrial enlargement, heart-base tumor, embolism). • Gastroesophageal reflux. • Compression of respiratory structures by adjacent organs (cardiomegaly, megaesophagus, hilar lymph node enlargement). • Noncardiogenic pulmonary edema (multiple causes). • Passive smoking inhalation. • Adverse drug reaction—potassium bromide in cats.

RISK FACTORS

Breed

• Toy and miniature breeds at risk for tracheal collapse. • Terrier breeds at risk for pulmonary fibrosis. • Husky, Rottweiler, Labrador, and Jack Russell terrier at risk for eosinophilic bronchopneumopathy. • Giant breeds at risk for dilated cardiomyopathy. • Labrador retriever, large breeds at risk for laryngeal paralysis. • Siamese cats at risk for feline bronchitis syndrome.

Environmental Factors

Longhaired cats that are infrequently groomed will periodically retch, cough, and vomit up mats of hair.

Drugs

Potassium bromide in cats.

Geographic Area (or Travel History)

Certain diseases are common in specific areas (e.g., dirofilariasis, angiostrongylosis).

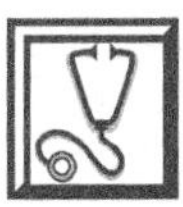

DIAGNOSIS

DIFFERENTIAL DIAGNOSIS

• Similar signs. • Coughing may be confused with other signs such as sneezing, reverse sneezing, gagging, panting, retching, and vomiting; presence of terminal retch is often misinterpreted as vomiting. • Honking noise coughing in case of severe tracheal collapse can be descried by owners as severe stertor.

CBC/BIOCHEMISTRY/URINALYSIS

Minimum database may suggest acute bacterial infection (leukocytosis with left shift) or eosinophilic airway disease (periph-eral eosinophilia).

OTHER LABORATORY TESTS

• Filter test for microfilaria and/or heartworm antigen serology—for heartworm disease. • Serum antibody titer—toxoplasmosis, FIV, FIP, distemper, *Angiostrongylus vasorum*. • Coagulation profile—for any patient that presents with cough associated with either epistaxis or hemoptysis. • Feces examination (Baermann test: identification of *Angistrongylus* (dogs), *Aerulostrongylus* (cat), or other parasites (*Filarial*, *Crenosoma*). • PCR diagnosis available for several microorganisms. • Tests for evaluation of possible hyperadrenocorticism (potentially causing pulmonary thromboembolism).

IMAGING

• Thoracic radiographs are first step prior to any additional test—provide essential information about intrathoracic airways, lung parenchyma, pleural space, mediastinum, and cardiovascular system. • Thoracic computed tomography is being more and more often used for identification of respiratory intrathoracic problems. • Fluoroscopy—helpful to investigate diseases in which dynamic obstruction is suspected (tracheal collapse, bronchial collapse, bronchomalacia). • Echocardiography—helpful when heart failure or dysfunction is suspected. • Thoracic ultrasonography—in case of pleural effusion or when a pulmonary or mediastinal mass is suspected.

DIAGNOSTIC PROCEDURES

• Endoscopy allows visualization of both static (tumor, granuloma, abnormal mucosa, excessive secretions) and dynamic (laryngeal paralysis, dynamic airway collapse) airway abnormalities. • When bronchial and/or alveolar infiltrates are present—samples from lower airways can be obtained for diagnostic purpose (cytology, bacterial/mycologic cultures) by bronchoalveolar lavage or tracheal wash. • Transthoracic (fine-needle aspiration) biopsy or thoracoscopy—allows biopsy sample when interstitial infiltration is prominent. • Thoracocentesis—allows sampling of pleural fluid, can be performed under ultrasonographic guidance. • Pulse oximetry and blood gas determination. • Pulmonary function tests—require sophisticated material and/or experienced technicians, not readily available in private practice.

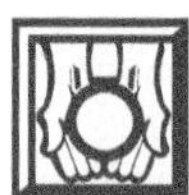

TREATMENT

• Usually treated as outpatient. • Most successful management of cough involves treatment and resolution of underlying cause rather than use of medications that suppress signs. • If chronic cough is related to acute or chronic inflammation, anti-inflammatory therapy preferred to cough suppressant therapy. • Use of cough suppressant therapy must be limited to cases in which the cause of the cough can neither be treated medically nor resolved, and in which excessive coughing leads to exhaustion of the patient or insomnia of the owners, as well as aggravation of the disease.

MEDICATIONS

DRUG(S) OF CHOICE

Antimicrobial Therapy

Indicated for tracheo-broncho-pulmonary disease of bacterial origin. Better selected based in culture and antimicrobial susceptibility testing.

Anti-inflammatory Therapy

• Indicated in feline bronchitis syndrome, canine chronic bronchitis, or canine eosinophilic bronchopneumopathy. • Oral prednisolone 0.5 mg/kg q12h in dogs and cats, then taper the dose progressively to q48h. • Nebulized fluticasone or budesonide 100–200 µg q12h with metered dose inhaler including spacer with face mask and inspiratory valve.

Antitussives

• Hydrocodone (dog only)—0.2–0.3 mg/kg PO q 6–12h. • Butorphanol (dog only)—0.25–1.1 mg/kg every 8–12h. • No antitussive available for cats. • In humans, gabapentin (neuromodulator) recently described to treat refractory chronic cough. • Gabapentin in dogs, 2–5 mg/kg by mouth every 8h, but unestablished efficacy.

Bronchodilators

Theophylline (for Dogs and Cats)

• Pharmacokinetics are form and species dependent; slow-release formulations exist. • Beneficial effects of theophylline include relaxation of bronchial smooth muscle, improved diaphragmatic contraction, and probably some anti-inflammatory effects but primary antitussive action not demonstrated. • Side effects are related to inotropic and chronotropic effects, as well as to an increase in blood pressure; can also cause nausea, diarrhea, arrhythmias, and CNS excitation.

Beta-2 Agonists (Cats Only)

• Delivered mostly via a meter dose inhaler (MDI); administered IV in emergency situations. Short-acting (salbutamol, terbutaline, fenoterol) or long-acting (salmeterol, formoterol) drugs. • May be administered temporarily to cause immediate and temporary relief, but not as long-term management; have limited effect. • Side effects include dry mouth, tachycardia, nausea; regular inhalation of racemic and S-albuterol (but not R-albuterol) induces airway inflammation in both healthy and asthmatic cats.

Expectorants

Guafenesin—included in some preparations but benefit not extensively studied or proven.

CONTRAINDICATIONS

Antitussive agents are strictly contraindicated when cough is needed to clean the airways, i.e., in infectious or inflammatory airway disease.

PRECAUTIONS

See side effects of respective drugs.

POSSIBLE INTERACTIONS

Theophylline—clearance may be inhibited by other drugs such as fluoroquinolones, increasing risk of theophylline toxicity.

FOLLOW-UP

PATIENT MONITORING

• Acute cough must be adequately treated in order to avoid chronic cough, leading to possibly irreversible lesions. • Conditions leading to chronic cough sometimes can only be alleviated but not cured; communicate with client to ensure successful management of cough.

POSSIBLE COMPLICATIONS

• Aggravation of tracheal collapse. • Progression toward chronic bronchitis, chronic obstructive pulmonary disease, lung emphysema, irreversible bronchial and parenchymal remodeling, bronchiectasis. • Acute severe cough might lead to syncope, rib fracture, or pneumothorax. • Right heart dysfunction.

MISCELLANEOUS

AGE-RELATED FACTORS

• In dogs with anatomic disorders of inherited (e.g., primary ciliary dyskinesia) or congenital origin, signs might start early in life. • Puppies and kittens more likely to suffer from infectious disease. • Inflammatory disorders affect middle-aged adults. • Heart failure and tumors more frequent in older animals.

PREGNANCY/FERTILITY/BREEDING

• Dogs affected with primary ciliary dyskinesia. • Possible decreased fertility (in male and female dogs) as cilia from urogenital tract and flagellated cells can be affected. • Proven hereditary in some breeds (Old English sheepdog; carrier test detection exists).

SEE ALSO

• Asthma, Bronchitis—Cats.
• Bronchitis, Chronic.
• Congestive Heart Failure, Left-Sided.
• Hypoxemia.
• Nasal Discharge.
• Pneumonia, Bacterial.
• Pneumonia, Eosinophilic.
• Respiratory Parasites.
• Sneezing, Reverse Sneezing, Gagging.
• Tracheal Collapse.

ABBREVIATIONS

• FeLV = feline leukemia virus.
• FIP = feline infectious peritonitis.
• FIV = feline immunodeficiency virus.
• UACS = upper airway cough syndrome.

Suggested Reading

Ferasin L. Coughing. In Ettinger SJ, Feldman EC, Côté E. Textbook of Veterinary Internal Medicine, 8th ed. St. Louis, MO: Elsevier, 2016, 107–111.

Rozanski AE, Rush JE. Acute and chronic cough. In: Ettinger SJ, Feldman EC, eds., Textbook of Veterinary Internal Medicine, 6th ed. St. Louis, MO: Elsevier, 2005, pp. 189–195.

Author Cécile Clercx

Consulting Editor Elizabeth Rozanski

Acknowledgment The author and book editors acknowledge the prior contribution of Dominique Peeters.

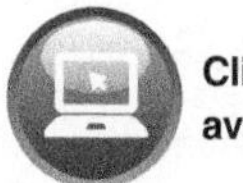

Client Education Handout available online

CRANIOMANDIBULAR OSTEOPATHY

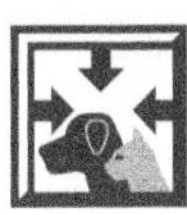

BASICS

OVERVIEW

• A non-neoplastic, noninflammatory proliferative disease of the bones of the head. • Primary bones affected—mandibular rami; occipital and parietal; tympanic bullae; zygomatic portion of the temporal. • Bilateral symmetric involvement most common. • Affects musculoskeletal system.

SIGNALMENT

• Scottish, Cairn, and West Highland white terrier breeds—most common. • Labrador retrievers, Great Danes, Boston terriers, Doberman pinschers, Irish setters, English bulldogs, bullmastiffs, Shetland sheepdogs, and boxers—may be affected. • Usually growing puppies 4–8 months of age. • No gender predilection. • Neutering may increase incidence.

SIGNS

Historical Findings

• Usually relate to pain around the mouth and difficulty opening the mouth progressively worsening. • Difficulty in prehension and mastication—may lead to starvation.

Physical Examination Findings

• Temporal and masseter muscle atrophy—common. • Palpable irregular thickening of mandibular rami and/or temporomandibular joint (TMJ) region. • Inability to fully open jaw, even under general anesthesia. • Intermittent pyrexia. • Bilateral exophthalmos.

CAUSES & RISK FACTORS

• Believed to be hereditary—occurs in certain breeds and families. • West Highland white terriers—autosomal recessive trait. • Scottish terriers—possible predisposition. • Young terrier with periosteal long bone disease—monitor for disease.

DIAGNOSIS

DIFFERENTIAL DIAGNOSIS

• Osteomyelitis—bones not symmetrically affected; generally not as extensive; lysis; lack of breed predilection; history of penetrating wound. • Traumatic periostitis—bones not symmetrically affected; generally not as extensive; history of trauma. • Neoplasia—mature patient; not symmetrically affected; more lytic bone reaction; metastatic disease. • Calvarial hyperostosis—young patient: frontal, parietal, and occipital bones; does not involve mandible; may have long bone involvement.

CBC/BIOCHEMISTRY/URINALYSIS

• Serum alkaline phosphatase (ALP) and inorganic phosphate—may be high. • May note hypogammaglobulinemia or α_2-hyperglobulinemia.

OTHER LABORATORY TESTS

Serology—rule out fungal agents; indicated in atypical cases.

IMAGING

• Skull radiography—reveals uneven, bead-like osseous proliferation of the mandible or tympanic bullae (bilateral); extensive, periosteal new bone formation (exostoses) affecting one or more bones around the TMJ; may show fusion of the tympanic bullae and angular process of the mandible. • CT—may help evaluate osseous involvement of TMJ.

DIAGNOSTIC PROCEDURES

Bone biopsy and culture (bacterial and fungal)—necessary only in atypical cases; rule out neoplasia and osteomyelitis.

PATHOLOGIC FINDINGS

• Bone biopsy—reveals normal lamellar bone being replaced by enlarged coarse-fiber bone and osteoclastic osteolysis of periosteal or subperiosteal region. • Bone marrow—replaced by vascular fibrous-type stroma. • Inflammatory cells—occasionally seen at periphery of bony lesion.

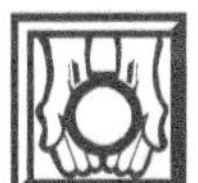

TREATMENT

• Palliative only. • Surgical excision of exostoses—results in regrowth within weeks. • High-calorie, protein-rich gruel diet—helps maintain nutritional balance. • Surgical placement of pharyngostomy, esophagostomy, or gastrostomy tube—considered to help maintain nutritional balance.

MEDICATIONS

DRUG(S) OF CHOICE

• Analgesics and anti-inflammatory drugs—palliative use warranted.
• Nonsteroidal anti-inflammatory drugs (NSAIDs)—inhibit cyclooxygenase enzymes. • Deracoxib (1–2 mg/kg PO q24h, chewable). • Carprofen (2.2 mg/kg PO q12h or 4.4 mg/kg q24h). • Meloxicam (load 0.2 mg/kg PO, then 0.1 mg/kg PO q24h, liquid). • Grapiprant (2 mg/kg PO q24h). • Firocoxib (5 mg/kg PO q24h).

FOLLOW-UP

PATIENT MONITORING

Frequent reexaminations—mandatory to ensure adequate nutritional balance and pain control.

PREVENTION/AVOIDANCE

• Do not repeat dam–sire breedings that resulted in affected offspring. • Discourage breeding of affected animals.

EXPECTED COURSE AND PROGNOSIS

• Pain and discomfort may diminish at skeletal maturity (10–12 months of age); exostoses may regress. • Prognosis—depends on involvement of bones surrounding TMJ.
• Elective euthanasia may be necessary.

MISCELLANEOUS

SYNONYMS

• Lion jaw. • Craniomandibular osteoarthropathy.
• Craniomandibular osteodystrophy. • Mandibular periostitis. • Westie jaw. • Scotty jaw.

ABBREVIATIONS

• ALP = alkaline phosphatase.
• NSAID = nonsteroidal anti-inflammatory drug.
• TMJ = temporomandibular joint.

Suggested Reading

Franch J, Cesari JR, Font J. Craniomandibular osteopathy in two Pyrenean mountain dogs. Vet Record 1998, 142(17):455–459.
Huchkowsky SL. Craniomandibular osteopathy in a bullmastiff. Can Vet J 2002, 43(11):883–885.
LaFond E, Breur GJ, Austin CC. Breed susceptibility for developmental orthopedic diseases in dogs. J Am Anim Hosp Assoc 2002, 38(5):467–477.
McConnell JF, Hayes A, Platt SR, Smith KC. Calvarial hyperostosis syndrome in two bullmastiffs. Vet Radiol Ultrasound 2006, 47(1):72–77.
Padgett GA, Mostosky UV. The mode of inheritance of craniomandibular osteopathy in West Highland White terrier dogs. Am J Med Genet 1986, 25(1):9–13.
Pastor KF, Boulay JP, Schelling SH, Carpenter JL. Idiopathic hyperostosis of the calvaria in five young bullmastiffs. J Am Anim Hosp Assoc 2000, 36(5):439–445.
Taylor SM, Remedios A, Myers S. Craniomandibular osteopathy in a Shetland sheepdog. Can Vet J 1995, 36(7):437–439.
Watson ADJ, Adams WM, Thomas CB. Craniomandibular osteopathy in dogs. Compend Contin Educ Pract Vet 1995, 17:911–921.

Author Steven M. Cogar
Consulting Editor Mathieu M. Glassman

CRUCIATE LIGAMENT DISEASE, CRANIAL

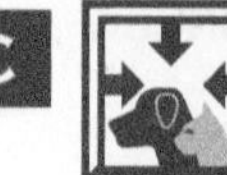

BASICS

DEFINITION

The acute or progressive failure of the cranial cruciate ligament (CrCL), which results in partial to complete instability of the stifle joint.

PATHOPHYSIOLOGY

• Function of the CrCL includes passive constraint of the stifle joint by limiting internal rotation of the tibia, hyperextension of the stifle, and cranial displacement of the tibia relative to the femur. • Two distinct bands—craniomedial band is taut on both flexion and extension of the joint (primary check) and caudolateral band is taut in extension and lax in flexion (secondary check).
• Types of injury:
o Avulsion—skeletally immature animals in which acute load results in avulsion of the origin or insertion of the ligament.
o Acute (traumatic) rupture—result of hyperextension, limb overloading, or internal rotation; mid-substance tear of the CrCL; most common cause in cats.
o Progressive (chronic) degeneration pathogenesis remains elusive; decreases in elasticity, stress/strain energy, failure to maintain collagen fiber organization, and chondroid metaplasia—most common cause in dogs.
• Repetitive subclinical injury may be due to neuromuscular incoordination, aging, conformational abnormalities (excessive tibial plateau angle (TPA), medial luxating patella, narrow intercondylar notch), breed variations, poor muscle tone related to sedentary habits or limb immobilization, and possibly immune-mediated damage. • Complete and partial tears exist in varying degrees. • Untreated instability leads to degenerative osteoarthritic changes within a few weeks; severe within a few months. • Medial meniscal (caudal horn) damage occurs in 33.2–77% of cases—due to shearing force during drawer.

SYSTEMS AFFECTED

Musculoskeletal, ± neurologic.

GENETICS

Suspected

INCIDENCE/PREVALENCE

Most common cause of hind limb lameness in dogs; major cause of degenerative joint disease (DJD) in the stifle joint.

SIGNALMENT

SPECIES

Dog and cat.

Breed Predilections

• All susceptible. • Rottweiler and Labrador retriever—increased incidence when <4 years of age. • West Highland white terrier—over-represented affected small breed.

Mean Age and Range

• Incidence increases with age >5 years.
• Large- to giant-breed dogs may present earlier in life; approx. 2 years of age.

Predominant Sex

Female—neutered.

SIGNS

General Comments

Severity of lameness—related to degree of rupture (partial vs. complete), mode of rupture (acute vs. chronic), occurrence of meniscal injury, and severity of inflammation and DJD. Condition and therefore lameness may be bilateral.

Historical Findings

• Athletic or traumatic events—generally precede acute injuries. • Normal activity resulting in acute lameness—suggests degenerative rupture. • Subtle to marked intermittent lameness (for weeks to months)—consistent with partial tears that are progressing to complete rupture.

Physical Examination Findings

• Varying degrees of lameness and joint effusion, pain, and/or crepitus; affected limb generally held in partial flexion while standing. • Cranial drawer test—diagnostic for rupture; test in flexion, normal standing angle, and extension. • Tibial compression test—cranial movement of tibia relative to femur when tightening gastrocnemius by flexing hock. • Medial periarticular thickening (medial buttress). • Presence of click or pop—63% accurate in detecting meniscal injury. • Hind limb muscle atrophy—especially quadriceps muscle group. • False-negative drawer or compression tests with chronic or partial tears and in painful or anxious patients that are not sedated or anesthetized. • Earliest sign of partial rupture is pain on hyperextension of stifle.

CAUSES

• Trauma. • Repetitive microinjury; excessive stifle loading. • Progressive degeneration.

RISK FACTORS

• Obesity. • Patella luxation. • Conformational abnormalities. • Excessive caudal slope of tibial plateau. • Narrowed intercondylar notch.

DIAGNOSIS

DIFFERENTIAL DIAGNOSIS

• Puppy laxity—positive drawer motion that stops abruptly as CrCL is stretched taut.
• Patella luxation (medial or lateral). • Collateral ligament injury, long digital extensor tendon injury. • Osteochondritis dissecans of femoral condyle. • Neoplasia (e.g., synovial sarcoma, osteosarcoma, chondrosarcoma). • Traumatic fractures or avulsions. • Caudal cruciate ligament rupture—uncommon and generally only seen with significant trauma.

CBC/BIOCHEMISTRY/URINALYSIS

N/A

OTHER LABORATORY TESTS

N/A

IMAGING

Radiography

• Verify secondary intra-articular changes such as DJD and rule out other differentials.
• Common findings—joint effusion with capsular distention and effacement of infrapatellar fat pad; periarticular osteophytes; enthesiophytes; CrCL avulsion fractures; calcification of CrCL and/or menisci. • Cats commonly have mineralized menisci present (incidental finding). • Necessary for preoperative planning with osteotomy procedures.

Alternative Diagnostic Imaging

Ultrasound and MRI—facility and operator dependent.

DIAGNOSTIC PROCEDURES

• Arthrocentesis—rule out sepsis or immune-mediated disease. • Arthroscopy—gold standard; direct visualization and magnification of cruciate ligaments, menisci, and other intra-articular structures.

PATHOLOGIC FINDINGS

• Varying degrees of synovitis, cartilage fibrillation, and erosion. • Periarticular osteophyte formation. • Meniscal damage.
• Ruptured fibers of CrCL—hyalinization; fibrous tissue invasion; necrosis; loss of parallel orientation of ligament bundles.

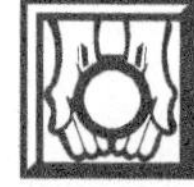

TREATMENT

APPROPRIATE HEALTH CARE

• Stabilization surgery—recommended; speeds rate of recovery; reduces degenerative changes; enhances function. • Conservative management—diet, nonsteroidal anti-inflammatory drugs (NSAIDs), physical rehabilitation, weight loss; approx. 66% of patients have improved function over course of >1 year; DJD is progressive; not generally recommended.

NURSING CARE

Postsurgery—restricted activity with physical rehabilitation (e.g., ice packing, range-of-motion exercises, massage, and muscle electrical stimulation); important for improving mobility and strength.

ACTIVITY

Restricted—duration depends on method of treatment and progress of patient.

DIET

• Weight control—important for decreasing load and thus stress on stifle joint. • Joint-health diets rich in omega-3 fatty acids and chondroprotectants may support overall joint health.

CLIENT EDUCATION

• Regardless of treatment, DJD is common and progressive. • Return to full athletic function is possible, but requires early surgical intervention and rehabilitation. • Rupture of contralateral CrCL can occur in 37–48% of patients.

SURGICAL CONSIDERATIONS

• No one technique has proven consistently superior, clinically or radiographically. • Recent force plate studies show slight differences between common techniques; dogs with tibial plateau leveling osteotomy (TPLO) procedure achieve normal limb loading faster than with extracapsular procedure.

Extra-articular Methods

• Wide variety of techniques that use an implant to mimic CrCL and restore stability; these techniques rely on periarticular fibrosis for long-term stability. • Alternative method includes fibular head transposition to realign and tension lateral collateral ligament in order to restrict internal rotation and cranial drawer.

Intra-articular Methods

Designed to replace CrCL anatomically with autografts (patellar ligament, fascia), allografts, xenografts, and synthetic materials.

Osteotomy Procedures

Cranial Tibial Closing Wedge Osteotomy

• Levels TPA by removing cranially based wedge of bone from proximal tibia and eliminates cranial thrust. • Held in place with bone plate and screws. • Can potentially shorten tibia and alter stifle biomechanics.

TPLO

• Rotational osteotomy of proximal tibia to level TPA and neutralize cranial tibial thrust. • Held in place with bone plate and screws. • Can accomplish correction for angular and torsional deformities.

Tibial Tuberosity Advancement

• Tibial crest osteotomy; crest is held in advanced position with cage and plate; bone graft fills defect. • Active control of cranial tibial displacement improved, which helps stabilize stifle. • Can combine technique with lateral transposition of tibial tuberosity to correct concurrent medial luxating patella.

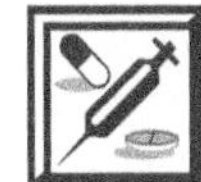

MEDICATIONS

DRUG(S) OF CHOICE

NSAIDs—minimize pain; decrease inflammation.

CONTRAINDICATIONS

Avoid concurrent use of corticosteroids with NSAIDs.

PRECAUTIONS

NSAIDs—gastrointestinal irritation or renal/hepatic toxicity may preclude use in some patients.

POSSIBLE INTERACTIONS

N/A

ALTERNATIVE DRUG(S)

• Chondroprotective drugs (polysulfated glycosaminoglycans, glucosamine, and chondroitin sulfate) may help reduce cartilage damage and improve regeneration.
• Omega-3 fatty acid supplementation to reduce inflammation is recommended.

FOLLOW-UP

PATIENT MONITORING

Most techniques require 2–4 months of rehabilitation.

PREVENTION/AVOIDANCE

Avoid breeding animals with conformational abnormalities.

POSSIBLE COMPLICATIONS

• Subsequent meniscal injury can occur in 6–22% of patients. • Incisional and/or implant-related infection. • Tibial tuberosity avulsion and/or fractures. • Patellar luxation.
• Delayed bone healing (osteotomy procedures). • Pivot shift—unknown clinical significance <2% (self-limiting).

EXPECTED COURSE AND PROGNOSIS

Regardless of surgical technique, success rate better than 85%.

MISCELLANEOUS

ASSOCIATED CONDITIONS

Meniscal damage.

AGE-RELATED FACTORS

See Pathophysiology.

ZOONOTIC POTENTIAL

N/A

PREGNANCY/FERTILITY/BREEDING

N/A

SEE ALSO

• Arthritis (Osteoarthritis).
• Patellar Luxation.

ABBREVIATIONS

• CrCL = cranial cruciate ligament.
• DJD = degenerative joint disease.
• NSAID = nonsteroidal anti-inflammatory drug.
• TPA = tibial plateau angle.
• TPLO = tibial plateau leveling osteotomy.

Suggested Reading

Aragon CL, Budsberg SC. Applications of evidence-based medicine: cranial cruciate ligament injury repair in the dog. Vet Surg 2005, 34:93–98.

Balzter WI, Smith-Ostrin S, Warnock JJ, Ruaux CG. Evaluation of the clinical effects of diet and physical rehabilitation in dogs following tibial plateau leveling osteotomy. J Am Vet Med Assoc 2018, 252:686–700.

Christopher SA, Beetem J, Cook JL. Comparison of long-term outcomes associated with three surgical techniques for treatment of cranial cruciate ligament disease in dogs. Vet Surg 2013, 42(3):329–334.

Comerford EJ, Smith K, Hayashi K. Update on the aetiopathogenesis of canine cranial cruciate ligament disease. Vet Comp Orthop Traumatol 2011, 24:91–98.

Krotscheck U, Nelson SA, Todhunter RJ, et al. Long-term functional outcome of Tibial Tuberosity Advancement vs. Tibial Plateau Leveling Osteotomy and extracapsular repair in a heterogenous population of dogs. Vet Surg 2016, 45(2):261–268.

Wucherer KL, Conzemius MG, Evans R, Wilke VL. Short-term and long-term outcomes for overweight dogs with cranial cruciate ligament rupture treated surgically or nonsurgically. J Am Vet Med Assoc 2013, 242:1364–1372.

Author Marian E. Benitez
Consulting Editor Mathieu M. Glassman

Client Education Handout available online

CRYPTOCOCCOSIS

BASICS

DEFINITION

A localized or systemic fungal infection caused by the environmental yeast *Cryptococcus* spp., most commonly *C. neoformans* and *C. gattii.*

PATHOPHYSIOLOGY

• *C. neoformans*—grows in bird droppings and decaying vegetation; soil disturbance increases risk of infection. • Dogs and cats inhale the yeast and a focus of infection is established, usually in nasal passages; smaller dried, shrunken organisms may reach the terminal airways (uncommon). • There may be colonization or subclinical infection of nasal passages that spontaneously resolves. • Stomach and intestinal infections suggest that primary gastrointestinal entry can occur. • Dissemination—hematogenously spread via macrophages from nasal passages to brain, eyes, lungs, and other tissues; by extension to skin of nose, eyes, retro-orbital tissues, and draining lymph nodes.

SYSTEMS AFFECTED

• Cats—mainly respiratory (nose, nasopharynx, and sinuses), skin (nasal planum), nervous, ophthalmic, and lymphatic.
• Dogs—mainly skin (over nose and sinuses), respiratory (nasal passages, occasionally lungs), nervous (brain), lymphatic, and ophthalmic.

INCIDENCE/PREVALENCE

• Dogs—rare in United States; prevalence 0.00013%. • Cats—7–10 times more common than in dogs; most common systemic mycoses of cats.

GEOGRAPHIC DISTRIBUTION

• Worldwide. • Some areas of southern California and Australia have an increased incidence and an outbreak has occurred on Vancouver Island in British Columbia, Canada. • *C. gattii* grows well around eucalyptus trees.

SIGNALMENT

Species

Dog and cat.

Breed Predilections

• Dogs—American cocker spaniels (United States), Doberman pinschers and German shepherd dogs (Australia) may be overrepresented. • Cats—Siamese may be at increased risk.

Mean Age and Range

• Most commonly cats and dogs <6 years of age. • Can occur at any age.

Predominant Sex

• Dogs—none. • Cats—males may be overrepresented.

SIGNS

Historical Findings

• Lethargy. • Varies depending on organ systems involved. • May have signs/problems for weeks to months.

Dogs

• Neurologic—seizures, ataxia, paresis.
• Ocular signs—periorbital swelling, blindness, uveitis, hyphema. • Skin ulceration.
• Lymphadenopathy. • Respiratory—upper respiratory signs, labored breathing, coughing.
• Vomiting, diarrhea, and anorexia.

Cats

• Nasal discharge and ocular signs.
• Neurologic signs—seizures, disorientation, vestibular signs. • Granulomatous tissue seen at the nares. • Firm swellings over the bridge of the nose. • Lymphadenopathy. • Respiratory abnormalities less commonly noted.

Physical Examination Findings

• Mild fever—<50% of patients. • Dogs—nasal discharge, multifocal CNS abnormalities, ataxia, anterior uveitis.
• Cats—respiratory noise (stertor), nasofacial swelling, ulcerated crusting skin lesions on the head, lymphadenopathy, neurologic abnormalities (behavior change, circling, vestibular signs, ataxia), ocular abnormalities (blindness, optic neuritis, retinal detachment).

CAUSES

Exposure to cryptococcal organisms and inability of immune system to prevent colonization and tissue invasion.

RISK FACTORS

• Exposure to disrupted soil. • Infection with feline leukemia virus (FeLV) or feline immunodeficiency virus (FIV).

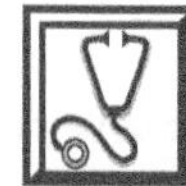

DIAGNOSIS

DIFFERENTIAL DIAGNOSIS

Dogs

• Other causes of focal or diffuse neurologic disease—distemper, inflammatory meningoencephalomyelitis, infectious meningoencephalitis (bacterial, rickettsial, protozoal), neoplasia, fungal diseases (depending on geography). • Nasal lesions, especially at mucocutaneous junction—immune-mediated, neoplasia (squamous cell carcinoma).
• Lymphadenopathy—lymphoma, fungal disease. • Chorioretinitis and optic neuritis—fungal infections, distemper, neoplasia.

Cats

• Nasal disease—nasal tumors, chronic rhinitis, chronic sinusitis. • Ulcerative skin changes—bacterial infection, trauma, neoplasia (squamous cell carcinoma). • Ocular and neurologic abnormalities—lymphoma, feline infectious peritonitis (FIP), other infections (fungal, *Toxoplasma*).

CBC/BIOCHEMISTRY/URINALYSIS

• Mild anemia in some cats. • Eosinophilia occasionally seen. • Chemistry usually normal.

OTHER LABORATORY TESTS

• Latex agglutination or ELISA—detect cryptococcal capsular antigen in serum or cerebrospinal fluid (CSF); highly sensitive assay; most infected animals have measurable capsular antigen titers; magnitude of titer correlates with extent of infection. • May be less sensitive in dogs. • May be positive with colonization alone; antigen titers 1 : 32 or greater seen with fungal invasion.

IMAGING

• Nasal radiographs (cats)—soft tissue density material in nasal passage; bone destruction of nasal dorsum. • Contrast-enhanced CT or MRI best for identifying brain and nasal lesions. • Thoracic radiographs—can identify lower respiratory tract disease.

DIAGNOSTIC PROCEDURES

Dogs

Neurologic disease—additional procedures: cytologic examination and culture of CSF, other CSF infectious disease testing, measurement of CSF capsular antigen.

Cats

• Cytology of impression smears or aspirates of mucoid material from nasal passages, or biopsy of granulomatous tissue protruding from nares—characteristic yeast with large negatively- staining (clear) capsule. • Aspirates of lymph nodes or subcutaneous swellings often high yield. • Sedated oropharyngeal exam—in patients with upper respiratory obstruction/noise: may identify granuloma in nasopharynx (spay hook or endoscope to expose the mass).
• Biopsy—skin lesions. • Cultures—confirm diagnosis; determine drug susceptibility.

PATHOLOGIC FINDINGS

• Gross lesions—gray, gelatinous mass produced by polysaccharide capsule; in nose, sinuses, and nasopharynx of cats; skin lesions usually ulcerative. • Neurologic lesions—more common in dogs; diffuse or focal CNS granulomas.
• Chorioretinitis with or without retinal detachment or optic neuritis. • Histologic response—usually pyogranulomatous; inflammatory cell infiltrate may be mild as polysaccharide capsule interferes with neutrophil migration; organism characterized by capsulate yeast with narrow-neck budding.

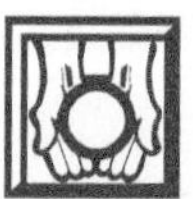

TREATMENT

APPROPRIATE HEALTH CARE

• Outpatient if stable. • Neurologic signs—may initially require inpatient supportive care.

NURSING CARE

Cats—nasal obstruction influences appetite; encourage to eat by offering warmed, palatable food.

ACTIVITY

N/A

DIET

Patients treated with itraconazole—give medication in fatty food (e.g., canned food) to improve absorption.

CLIENT EDUCATION

• Inform client that this is a chronic disease that requires months of treatment. • Reassure client that infection is not zoonotic.

SURGICAL CONSIDERATIONS

Remove granulomatous masses in nasopharynx to reduce respiratory difficulties.

MEDICATIONS

DRUG(S) OF CHOICE

• Fluconazole—preferred for ocular or CNS disease (water soluble and better penetrates CNS); cats: 50 mg/cat PO q12–24h; dogs: 5 mg/kg PO q12h; most economical drug choice. • Itraconazole—cats: 10 mg/kg PO q24h; dogs: 5 mg/kg PO q12h; pellets in capsule can be mixed with fatty food; itraconazole liquid has better absorption on empty stomach and compounded itraconazole is not recommended. • Amphotericin B may have some advantage in severe disease at a dosage of 0.25 mg/kg IV q48h, given slowly over 3–4h, up to a total cumulative dose of 4–16 mg/kg; monitor renal function closely. • Terbinafine (5 mg/kg PO q12h, 10 mg/kg PO q24h) effective for treatment of cats with resistant infections. • Flucytosine—25–50 mg/kg PO q6h; synergistic with amphotericin B, may allow lower doses and decrease renal toxicity. Do not use as single agent.

CONTRAINDICATIONS

Caution with concurrent steroid use (immunosuppression).

PRECAUTIONS

• Triazoles—hepatotoxicity; anorexia signals problems; monitor liver enzyme activities monthly initially. • Itraconazole—ulcerative dermatitis (differentiate from skin lesions of cryptococcosis); new skin lesions after disease is much improved should be considered a drug reaction. • Amphotericin B—nephrotoxicity; caution if patient is azotemic, but not absolute contraindication if life-threatening infection. • Terbinafine—monitor for hepatic toxicity and anorexia.

ALTERNATIVE DRUG(S)

Cryptococcal organisms are prone to becoming resistant to antifungal treatment.

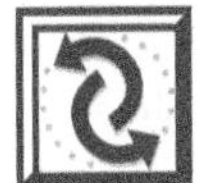

FOLLOW-UP

PATIENT MONITORING

• Monitor liver enzyme activities monthly (especially early in treatment) in patients receiving triazole antifungal agent. • Improvement in clinical signs, resolution of lesions, improvement in wellbeing, and return of appetite measure response to treatment. • Capsular antigen titers—after 2–3 months of treatment, titers should decrease if treatment is effective; if ineffective, try terbinafine, because organism may become resistant. • Continue monitoring antigen titers every 1–2 months during treatment and after discontinuing treatment. • Ideally treat until cryptococcal antigen titers reach zero (may take >2 years).

PREVENTION/AVOIDANCE

The organism is ubiquitous and cannot be avoided.

POSSIBLE COMPLICATIONS

Patients with neurologic disease may have seizures and permanent neurologic deficits.

EXPECTED COURSE AND PROGNOSIS

Treatment—anticipated duration 4 months to ≥1 year; patients with CNS disease may require lifelong maintenance; median time of successful treatment with fluconazole 4 months; median time for itraconazole treatment 8 months.

MISCELLANEOUS

ASSOCIATED CONDITIONS

N/A

AGE-RELATED FACTORS

N/A

ZOONOTIC POTENTIAL

• Not considered zoonotic, but possibility of transmission through bite wounds. • Inform client that organism was acquired from the environment and that he or she could be at increased risk, especially if immunosuppressed.

PREGNANCY/FERTILITY/BREEDING

Azole drugs can be teratogenic and should be used in pregnant animals only if the potential benefit justifies the potential risk to offspring.

ABBREVIATIONS

- CSF = cerebrospinal fluid.
- FeLV = feline leukemia virus.
- FIP = feline infectious peritonitis.
- FIV = feline immunodeficiency virus.

Suggested Reading

O'Brien CR, Krockenberger MB, Martin P, et al. Long-term outcome of therapy for 59 cats and 11 dogs with cryptococcosis. Aust Vet J 2006, 84:384–392.

O'Brien CR, Krockenberger MB, Wigney DI, et al. Retrospective study of feline and canine cryptococcosis in Australia from 1981 to 2001: 195 cases. Med Mycol 2004, 42:449–460.

Pennisi MG, Hartmann K, Lloret A, et al. Cryptococcosis in cats: ABCD guidelines on prevention and management. J Feline Med Surg 2013, 15:611–618.

Sykes JE, Hodge G, Singapuri A, et al. In vivo development of fluconazole resistance in serial Cryptococcus gattii isolates from a cat. Med Mycol 2017, 55:396–401.

Trivedi SR, Sykes JE, Cannon MS, et al. Clinical features and epidemiology of cryptococcosis in cats and dogs in California: 93 cases (1988–2010). J Am Vet Med Assoc 2011, 239:357–369.

Author Daniel S. Foy

Consulting Editor Amie Koenig

Client Education Handout available online

CRYPTORCHIDISM

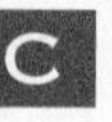

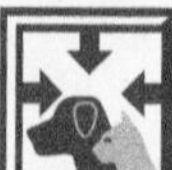

BASICS

OVERVIEW

- Incomplete scrotal descent of one or both testes; most common testicular congenital anomaly.
- Abdominal or inguinal location for undescended testis or testes.
- Diagnosis usually made at 2 months of age (i.e., descent to scrotal position should occur before this time), with some exceptions of full descent occurring between 2 and 6 months of age.
- Abdominally retained testicles typically lack spermatozoa and have only Sertoli cells in the seminiferous tubules; estradiol (E2) and testosterone (T) can be present in normal systemic concentrations in affected animals.
- Unilaterally cryptorchid animals are typically fertile.

SIGNALMENT

- Cats—purebred cats have higher incidence.
- Dogs—toy and miniature breeds at 2.7 times greater risk than large breeds of being affected; high rates in miniature schnauzers with persistent Müllerian duct syndrome (PMDS).
- Incidence—rates up to 24.1% in some purebred dogs (compared to 2.1% in overall population) with 50% incidence in dogs with PMDS; in cats observed rates range from 1.3 to 6.2%.
- Unilateral more common than bilateral; right testis retained twice as often in dogs, but with equal frequency in cats.
- Genetics—estimated medium level of heritability with multifactorial genetic basis; females act as genetic carriers for the trait.

SIGNS

- Absence of one, or both, testicles from the scrotum in a patient without history of castration.
- Cats—strong urine odor, tom cat marking behavior, presence of penile spines.
- Abdominal pain, lameness, vomiting—increased risk exists for spermatic cord torsion of neoplastic, retained testes.
- Feminizing paraneoplastic syndrome—estrogen-secreting Sertoli cell tumors produce feminizing signs including gynecomastia, symmetric alopecia of trunk and flanks, hyperpigmentation of inguinal skin, pendulous preputial sheath, prostatic squamous metaplasia.

CAUSES & RISK FACTORS

- Affected males or carriers (i.e., females or nonaffected males of cryptorchid littermates) present in breeding lines.
- Carriers produce increased number of males per litter and increased litter size; efforts to eliminate cryptorchidism difficult in these circumstances.

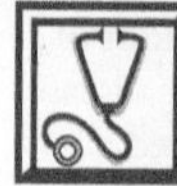

DIAGNOSIS

DIFFERENTIAL DIAGNOSIS

- Bilateral—previously castrated patient.
- Unilateral—remaining abdominal or inguinal testis after removal of single scrotal testis.

DIAGNOSTIC PROCEDURES

Transrectal prostate exam—intact males have pronounced prostate; prostate of larger breeds may be beyond reach.

OTHER LABORATORY TESTS

- Human chorionic gonadotropin (hCG) or gonadotropin-releasing hormone (GnRH) stimulation test (differentiate cryptorchidism from castrated)—collect blood sample for baseline T analysis; administer 750 IU hCG IV or 50 µg GnRH IM; repeat sample collection for T analysis in 2–3 hours; twofold increase in T from baseline indicates presence of testicular tissue.
- Canine anti-Müllerian hormone concentration—increased level indicates testicular Sertoli cells present.

IMAGING

Ultrasonography—highly sensitive for identification of inguinal or abdominal testes.

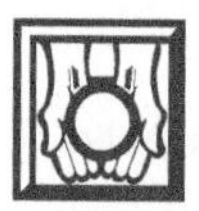

TREATMENT

- Identification and removal of undescended testis or testes.
- Orchiopexy—surgical tacking of retained testis into scrotum; results in misrepresentation of individual's true phenotype and genotype.
- hCG or GnRH—little controlled evidence establishing efficacy or protocol; ethical concerns same as with orchiopexy.
- Failure to remove retained testis—increased risk of testicular neoplasia (13.6 times greater), spermatic cord torsion; 53% of Sertoli cell tumors and 36% of seminomas occur in retained testes.

MEDICATIONS

DRUG(S) OF CHOICE

To possibly induce descent of retained testicle:

- hCG (dogs)—100–1,000 IU IM 4 times in 2-week period before 16 weeks of age.
- GnRH (dogs)—50–750 µg IM 1–6 times between 2 and 4 months of age.
- Buserelin (GnRH analogue; dogs)—10 µg, once weekly, for 3 doses.

FOLLOW-UP

Migration of testes into the scrotum after 4 months is unlikely; rare after 6 months.

MISCELLANEOUS

ASSOCIATED CONDITIONS

- Inguinal or umbilical hernia.
- Hip dysplasia.
- Patellar luxation.
- Penile and preputial defects (e.g., hypospadias).

SEE ALSO

- Seminoma.
- Sertoli Cell Tumor.
- Sexual Development Disorders.

ABBREVIATIONS

- E2 = estradiol.
- hCG = human chorionic gonadotropin.
- GnRH = gonadotropin-releasing hormone.
- PMDS = persistent Mullerian duct syndrome.
- T = testosterone.

Suggested Reading

Feldman EC, Nelson RW. Canine and Feline Endocrinology and Reproduction. Philadelphia, PA: Saunders, 1987, pp. 697–699.

Felumlee AE, Reichle JK, Hecht S, et al. Use of ultrasound to locate retained testes in dogs and cats. Vet Radiol Ultrasound 2012, 53(5):581–585.

Khan FA, Gartley CJ, Khanam A. Canine cryptorchidism: an update. Reprod Dom Anim 2018, 53(6):1263–1270.

Little S. Feline reproduction: problems and clinical challenges. J Feline Med Surg 2011, 13:508–515.

Author Candace C. Lyman

Consulting Editor Erin E. Runcan

Acknowledgment The author and book editors acknowledge the prior contribution of Carlos R.F. Pinto.

CRYPTOSPORIDIOSIS

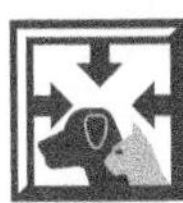

BASICS

OVERVIEW

- *Cryptosporidium* spp.—apicomplexan protozoan causing gastrointestinal disease; ubiquitous in nature with worldwide distribution.
- Infection—sporulated oocysts are ingested, sporozoites are released and penetrate intestinal epithelial cells; after asexual reproduction, merozoites released to infect other cells, sexual reproduction follows, then oocyst shedding.
- Prepatent period—5–10 days (cats).
- Immunocompetent animals—intestinal disease.
- Immunocompromised animals—intestinal, liver, gallbladder, pancreatic, respiratory infection.
- Dogs—prevalence 0.5% worldwide; 2–17% in the United States.
- Cats—prevalence 0–29% worldwide; 2–15% in the United States.

SIGNALMENT

- No sex or breed predilection.
- Dogs—virtually all clinical cases in immunocompromised animals or animals <6 months of age; older dogs can excrete oocysts without clinical signs.
- Cats—more common in immunocompromised cats or kittens <6 months of age.

SIGNS

- Most infections subclinical.
- Principally small bowel diarrhea; large bowel diarrhea reported.

CAUSES & RISK FACTORS

- *C. canis* (dogs), *C. felis* (cats)—ingestion of contaminated water or feces.
- Morphologically, intestinal *Cryptosporidium* species very similar.
- Some species are host specific (*C. canis*, *C. felis*); others (*C. parvum*, *C. muris*) infect multiple species.
- Immunosuppression—major risk factor; common causes feline leukemia virus, canine distemper virus, canine parvovirus, intestinal lymphoma.
- Immunocompetent animals—usually asymptomatic infection with fecal oocyst shedding.

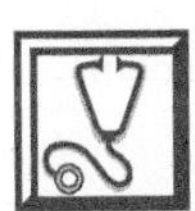

DIAGNOSIS

DIFFERENTIAL DIAGNOSIS

- Parasites—giardiasis, trichuriasis.
- Infectious agents—parvovirus, coronavirus, feline infectious peritonitis, *Salmonella*, *Campylobacter*, *Rickettsia*, *Histoplasma*.
- Metabolic—hypoadrenocorticism, hyperthyroidism (cats).
- Infiltrative diseases—e.g., inflammatory bowel disease, intestinal lymphoma.
- Dietary indiscretion or intolerance.
- Toxicities—medications, lead, etc.

CBC/BIOCHEMISTRY/URINALYSIS

Usually normal, can reflect underlying disease.

DIAGNOSTIC PROCEDURES

- Sugar and zinc sulfate centrifugal flotation—specific gravity = 1.18–1.3; concentrates fecal oocysts (oocysts are 5 µm, routine salt flotation often fails); oocysts best seen with modified acid-fast stain, may have slight pink color.
- Fecal antigen detection test (ProSpecT *Cryptosporidium* Microtiter Assay, Color-Vue *Cryptosporidium*) available for humans.
- Fluorescent antibody assay—veterinary diagnostic laboratories.
- PCR—commercial laboratories; more sensitive for diagnosis than other techniques.
- Submitting feces to laboratory—laboratory-specific protocols; can mix 1 part 100% formalin with 9 parts feces to inactivate oocysts and decrease health risk to laboratory personnel.

PATHOLOGIC FINDINGS

- Gross lesions—enlarged mesenteric lymph nodes, hyperemic intestinal (especially ileal) mucosa; fix specimens in Bouin's or formalin solution within hours of death; autolysis causes rapid loss of intestinal surface with organisms.
- Microscopic lesions—villous atrophy, reactive lymphoid tissue, inflammatory infiltrates in lamina propria; parasites throughout intestines, most numerous in distal small intestine.

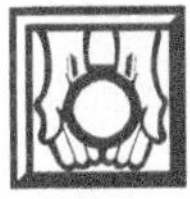

TREATMENT

- Outpatient.
- In immunocompetent animals—diarrhea usually mild and self-limiting; withhold food for 24–48h to control diarrhea; oral glucose-electrolyte solution if mild diarrhea; parenteral fluids (isotonic with potassium added) if severe diarrhea.

MEDICATIONS

DRUG(S) OF CHOICE

- No drugs currently labeled for animal use in United States.
- Paromomycin (Humatin®)—125–165 mg/kg PO q12h for 5 days; aminoglycoside effective in humans with acute intestinal symptoms; may cause nephropathy in young animals with damaged gastrointestinal barrier; monitor urine for casts during therapy.
- Tylosin—11 mg/kg PO q12h for 28 days; reported effective in cat with concurrent lymphocytic duodenitis.
- Nitazoxanide (Alinia®)—25 mg/kg PO q24h for 7–28 days; reduces oocyst shedding in cats; associated with vomiting (responsive to antiemetics); used in limited number of cats.

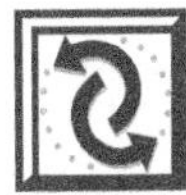

FOLLOW-UP

- Treatment efficacy based on clinical improvement.
- Monitor oocyst shedding in feces 2 weeks after treatment completion or if signs persist.
- Prognosis excellent if underlying disease treated.

MISCELLANEOUS

ZOONOTIC POTENTIAL

Possible—transmission of infection from dogs and cats to humans possible; in general, transmission from pets to people rare.

Disinfection

- 10% formaldehyde solution or 5% ammonia solution will kill oocysts, but requires 18 hours of exposure; 50% ammonia solution kills oocysts in 30 minutes.
- Resistant to commercial bleach (5.25% sodium hypochlorite) and chlorination of drinking water.
- Moist heat (steam or pasteurization, >55 °C), freezing and thawing or thorough drying also effective.

Suggested Reading

Lucio-Forster A, Griffiths JK, Cama VA, et al. Minimal zoonotic risk of cryptosporidiosis from pet dogs and cats. Trends Parasitol 2010, 26:174–179.

Authors Matt Brewer and Jeba R.J. Jesudoss Chelladurai

Consulting Editor Amie Koenig

CRYSTALLURIA

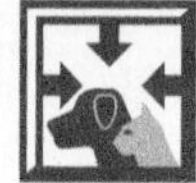

BASICS

DEFINITION

Appearance of crystals in urine. This finding may be normal, clinically significant or artifactual.

PATHOPHYSIOLOGY

- Identification of crystals formed in vitro does not justify therapy.
- Crystals form only in urine that is, or recently has been, supersaturated with crystallogenic substances; thus in vivo crystalluria represents risk factor for urolithiasis.
- Certain crystal types such as cystine, urate, or 2,8-dihydroxyadenine may indicate underlying disease; proper identification and interpretation of urine crystals important in formulation of medical protocols to dissolve uroliths.
- Crystalluria in individuals with anatomically and functionally normal urinary tracts usually harmless because crystals eliminated before they grow large enough to interfere with normal urinary function; however, they represent a risk factor for urolithiasis.
- Crystals that form following elimination or removal of urine from the patient often are of little clinical importance; in recent studies following time and temperature changes, crystals formed in 28% of dog and cat samples that were initially free of crystals.
- Detection of some types of crystals (e.g., cystine and ammonium urate) in clinically asymptomatic patients or detection of any form of crystals in fresh urine collected from patients with confirmed urolithiasis may have diagnostic, prognostic, or therapeutic importance.
- Drug crystals detected in patients administered high doses of medications such as allopurinol, sulfadiazines, or fluoroquinolones should prompt therapy changes due to risk for formation of drug-containing uroliths.

SYSTEMS AFFECTED

Renal/urologic/hepatic.

SIGNALMENT

- Calcium oxalate in miniature schnauzer, bichon frisé, Yorkshire terrier, Lhasa apso, miniature poodle dogs; Burmese, Himalayan, Persian cats.
- Cystine in dachshunds, English bulldogs, Newfoundlands, and others.
- Ammonium urate in Dalmatians and English bulldogs.
- Struvite in any dog with concomitant urinary tract infection (UTI).
- Struvite in cats not typically associated with UTIs.
- Xanthine in cavalier King Charles spaniels.
- 2,8-dihydroxyadenine in North American indigenous dogs and wolves.

SIGNS

None, or those caused by concomitant urolithiasis.

CAUSES

In Vivo Variables

- Concentration of crystallogenic substances in urine (in turn influenced by rate of excretion and urine concentration).
- Urine pH (struvite and calcium phosphate most common in neutral-to-alkaline urine; ammonium urate, sodium urate, calcium oxalate, cystine, and xanthine crystals most common in acid-to-neutral urine).
- Solubility of crystallogenic substances in urine.
- Excretion of diagnostic agents (e.g., radiopaque contrast agents) and medications (e.g., sulfonamides).
- Dietary influence—hospital diet may differ from home diet; timing of sample collection (fasting vs. postprandial) may influence evidence of crystalluria.

In Vitro Variables

- Temperature.
- Evaporation.
- pH changes following sample collection.
- Technique of specimen preparation—centrifugation versus noncentrifugation, volume of urine examined.
- Important in vitro changes that occur following urine collection may enhance formation or dissolution of crystals; when knowledge of in vivo urine crystal type and quantity especially important, examine fresh specimens, ideally at body temperature; if not possible, they should be at room temperature, not refrigeration temperature.
- Collection container—spurious crystals may be contaminants from unclean collection containers.

RISK FACTORS

See preceding discussion.

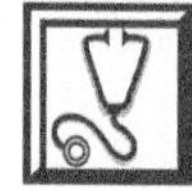

DIAGNOSIS

DIFFERENTIAL DIAGNOSIS

Ammonium Urate, Sodium Urate, and Amorphous Urate Crystalluria

- Uncommonly seen in apparently healthy dogs and cats.
- Frequently seen in dogs and occasionally in cats with portal vascular anomalies, with or without concomitant ammonium urate uroliths.
- Observed in some dogs and cats with urate uroliths caused by disorders other than portal vascular anomalies, such as canine breeds identified as carriers of hyperuricosuria gene.

Bilirubin Crystalluria

- Observed in highly concentrated urine from some healthy dogs.
- Large numbers in serial samples raises suspicion of abnormality in bilirubin metabolism.
- Usually associated with underlying diseases in cats.

Calcium Oxalate Monohydrate and Calcium Oxalate Dihydrate Crystalluria

- May be observed in apparently healthy dogs and cats and in dogs and cats with uroliths primarily composed of calcium oxalate.
- Calcium oxalate monohydrate crystals most commonly associated with ethylene glycol toxicity, but calcium oxalate dihydrate may be observed, or ethylene glycol toxicity may occur without crystalluria.

Calcium Phosphate Crystalluria

- Large numbers of crystals presumed to be composed of calcium phosphate have been observed in apparently healthy dogs, dogs with persistently alkaline urine, dogs with calcium phosphate uroliths, and dogs with uroliths composed of mixture of calcium phosphate and calcium oxalate.
- Small numbers of calcium phosphate crystals may occur in association with infection-induced struvite crystalluria.
- May be observed in dogs and cats with primary hyperparathyroidism, and renal tubular acidosis.

Struvite Crystalluria

- Observed in many dogs and cats that are healthy and as an artifact.
- Observed in dogs and cats with urinary tract disease without uroliths.
- Observed in dogs and cats with infection-induced struvite uroliths, sterile struvite uroliths, nonstruvite uroliths, and uroliths of mixed composition (e.g., nucleus composed of calcium oxalate and shell composed of struvite).

Cystine Crystalluria

Observed in dogs and cats with inborn errors of metabolism characterized by abnormal transport of cystine and other dibasic amino acids; this metabolism defect can also lead to dilated cardiomyopathy in cats.

Uric Acid Crystalluria

- Uncommon in dogs and cats.
- Importance as described for ammonium and amorphous urates.

Xanthine Crystalluria

- Suggests administration of excessive dosages of allopurinol in conjunction with consumption of relatively high amounts of dietary purine precursors.
- Primary xanthinuria has been observed in cavalier King Charles spaniels.
- Primary xanthinuria and xanthine uroliths occur in cats.

Miscellaneous Crystalluria

- Uric acid monohydrate crystals from melamine/cyanuric acid toxicosis.
- Cholesterol crystals—observed in humans with excessive tissue destruction, nephrotic syndrome, and chyluria; observed in apparently healthy dogs.
- Hippuric acid crystals—apparently rare in dogs and cats; importance unknown.
- Leucine crystals in dogs—importance not determined; may occur in association with cystinuria.
- Tyrosine crystals—occur in association with severe liver disease in humans; uncommonly observed in dogs and cats with liver disorders; sodium urate needle-like appearance commonly misinterpreted as tyrosine needles.
- 2,8-dihydroxyadenine—a genetic disorder, the result of metabolic abnormality due to deficiency of enzyme adenine phosphoribosyl transferase (APRT).

Drug-Induced Crystalluria

- May be observed following administration of radiopaque contrast agents.
- May be observed following treatment with sulfadiazine, fluoroquinolones, xanthine oxidase inhibitors, and tetracycline.

LABORATORY FINDINGS

Drugs That May Alter Laboratory Results

- Urinary acidifiers (e.g., d-, l-methionine and ammonium chloride).
- Urinary alkalinizers (e.g., sodium bicarbonate and potassium citrate).

CBC/BIOCHEMISTRY/URINALYSIS

- Bilirubin crystals may be associated with bilirubinemia and other laboratory abnormalities of hepatic disorders.
- Most dogs and cats with calcium oxalate and calcium phosphate crystalluria are normocalcemic; some are hypercalcemic; calciuria may be used as a future index for calcium oxalate stone formation and treatment evaluation.
- Some dogs and cats with calcium oxalate crystalluria may be acidemic.
- Serially examine fresh specimens for knowledge of in vivo urine crystals.
- Definitive identification of crystal composition depends on one or more of optical crystallography, infrared spectroscopy, X-ray diffraction, and electron microprobe analysis.

OTHER LABORATORY TESTS

- Struvite crystalluria is not synonymous with infection and may be the result of normal in vivo or in vitro factors; when accompanied by elevated pH, bacteriuria, or pyuria on cystocentesis, UTI should be considered; imaging must be performed to assess for stones.
- Dogs and cats with ammonium urate crystalluria and portosystemic shunts often have high serum bile acid levels and hyperammonemia.
- Ammonium urate and amorphous urate crystals are insoluble in acetic acid; addition of 10% acetic acid to urine sediment containing these crystals often yields uric acid and sometimes sodium urate crystals.
- Dogs and cats with calcium oxalate monohydrate crystalluria secondary to ethylene glycol poisoning have detectable levels of ethylene glycol in serum and urine up to 48 hours after ingestion.
- Cystine crystals are insoluble in acetic acid while struvite crystals are soluble; a urine nitroprusside test is positive for cystine.
- Sulfonamide crystalluria may be associated with a positive lignin test.

IMAGING

- Crystalluria may be associated with radiographically or ultrasonographically detectable uroliths.
- Abdominal radiographs should include the entire urethra.
- 25% of radiopaque stones are not seen on ultrasound.

DIAGNOSTIC PROCEDURES

- Empirical therapy for struvite urolithiasis if stone identified on radiographs and concurrent UTI caused by urease-producing bacteria.
- Basket retrieval, voiding urohydropropulsion, or aspiration through a transurethral catheter to retrieve small urocystoliths.

TREATMENT

- Manage clinically important in vivo crystalluria by managing underlying cause(s) or associated risk factors.
- Minimize clinically important crystalluria by increasing urine volume, encouraging complete and frequent voiding, modifying diet, appropriate drug therapy, neutering where appropriate, and in some instances modifying pH.

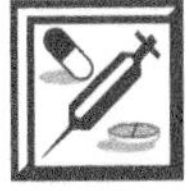

MEDICATIONS

DRUG(S) OF CHOICE

See comments on urate crystalluria and cystinuria.

FOLLOW-UP

PATIENT MONITORING

- Recheck urinalysis to determine if crystalluria is persistent.
- Re-radiograph or ultrasound, depending on crystal type, to determine if crystalluria has clinical significance or not.
- See specific urolith types for monitoring urolithiasis.

POSSIBLE COMPLICATIONS

- Persistent crystalluria may contribute to formation of uroliths.
- Crystalluria may solidify crystalline-matrix plugs as in male pugs and cats, resulting in urethral obstruction.

MISCELLANEOUS

SEE ALSO

- Nephrolithiasis.
- Urolithiasis, Calcium Oxalate.
- Urolithiasis, Calcium Phosphate.
- Urolithiasis, Cystine.
- Urolithiasis, Pseudo (Dried Blood, Ossified Material).
- Urolithiasis, Struvite—Cats.
- Urolithiasis, Struvite—Dogs.
- Urolithiasis, Urate.
- Urolithiasis, Xanthine.

ABBREVIATIONS

- APRT = adenine phosphoribosyl transferase.
- UTI= urinary tract infection.

Author Ewan D.S. Wolff

Consulting Editor J.D. Foster

Acknowledgment The author and book editors acknowledge the prior contributions of Carl A. Osborne and Lisa K. Ulrich.

CUTANEOUS DRUG ERUPTIONS

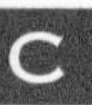

BASICS

OVERVIEW

- A wide spectrum of diseases and clinical signs that vary markedly in clinical appearance.
- Mild eruptions may go unnoticed or unreported; incidence rates for specific drugs are unknown.

SIGNALMENT

- Dogs and cats.
- May have a familial basis (e.g., rabies vaccine reactions in canine littermates).

SIGNS

- Pruritus.
- Macular and papular rashes—commonly accompany pruritus as nonspecific sign of inflammation.
- Exfoliative erythroderma—diffuse erythematous response caused by vasodilation; often leads to exfoliation (diffuse scaling).
- Urticaria/angioedema—immediate (type I) hypersensitivity; requires prior sensitization; increased vascular permeability leads to fluid leakage.
- Hypersensitivity vasculitis—type III response; inflammation of cutaneous vasculature; results in poor blood flow and anoxic injury to recipient tissue.
- Eosinophilic dermatitis with edema (Wells-like syndrome) of dogs—deeply erythematous plaques or macules (may be targetoid) accompanied by marked edema; localized, regional, or generalized distribution; clinical appearance of lesions may be indistinguishable from vasculitis and erythema multiforme (EM).
- EM—erythematous macules or plaques expand peripherally and may clear in center (targetoid); multiple shapes/forms noted.
- Stevens-Johnson syndrome (SJS)—similar to toxic epidermal necrolysis (TEN) with less extensive epidermal detachment (<30%) and often involvement of oral mucosa.
- TEN—extensive (>30%) necrosis and sloughing of epidermis in sheets; results in moist and intensely inflamed skin surface.
- Drug-induced pemphigus/pemphigoid—least common drug reaction in animals; can closely mimic autoimmune (spontaneous) disease; symptoms may persist after drug withdrawal.

CAUSES & RISK FACTORS

- Any drug.
- Can occur after first dose or after weeks to months of administration.
- Exfoliative erythroderma—most often associated with shampoos and dips; also reaction to topical ear medications (in ear canals and on concave pinnae).
- Eosinophilic dermatitis with edema—strong association with concurrent acute gastrointestinal disease.
- Pemphigus foliaceus—may be triggered by specific topical flea and tick control products; lesions may include "splash zone" where product was applied.

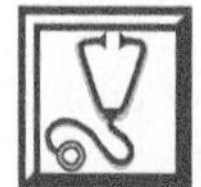

DIAGNOSIS

DIFFERENTIAL DIAGNOSIS

- Pruritus, macular/papular rashes, and urticaria/angioedema—allergic and parasitic diseases (atopic diseases, contact hypersensitivity, flea-bite hypersensitivity, scabies, stinging insects).
- Exfoliative erythroderma—epitheliotropic lymphoma in old dogs and cats.
- Vasculitis—infectious, neoplastic, autoimmune disease and idiopathic.
- EM/SJS/TEN—respiratory infections, herpes virus, parvovirus, bacterial infection (noncutaneous), and internal neoplasia; idiopathic/chronic form of EM occurs in older adult dogs.
- Pemphigus/pemphigoid—consider drug reaction whenever these diseases diagnosed; however, spontaneously occurring disease more common.

CBC/BIOCHEMISTRY/URINALYSIS

Potential for concurrent hepatic, renal, and gastrointestinal disease with cases of vasculitis.

OTHER LABORATORY TESTS

- Dogs with vasculitis—rickettsial serology.
- Cats with vasculitis—feline immunodeficiency virus (FIV) and feline leukemia virus (FeLV) serology, rule out feline infectious peritonitis (FIP).
- Bacterial and fungal cultures with vasculitis or pyogranulomatous inflammation.

DIAGNOSTIC PROCEDURES

Skin biopsy—mandatory for diagnosis of most drug-induced diseases.

PATHOLOGIC FINDINGS

Determined by specific disease process.

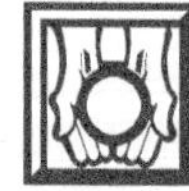

TREATMENT

- Discontinue use of offending or suspect drug.
- SJS/TEN—intensive supportive care and fluid/nutritional support because of fluid and protein exudation and risk of sepsis.
- Pain relief when indicated—minimal drug use recommended when drug eruption suspected.

MEDICATIONS

DRUG(S) OF CHOICE

Most conditions respond to immunosuppressive therapy if withdrawal of offending drug alone is insufficient (controversial in case of SJS/TEN).

CONTRAINDICATIONS/POSSIBLE INTERACTIONS

Avoid offending drug or any other drug in same class or family.

FOLLOW-UP

PATIENT MONITORING

Inpatient—if debilitated.

POSSIBLE COMPLICATIONS

- Secondary infection.
- Electrolyte and plasma protein depletion (SJS/TEN).

EXPECTED COURSE AND PROGNOSIS

- Some reactions appear to activate self-perpetuating immune responses.
- Some drug metabolites may persist for days to weeks and provoke continued response.
- TEN—prognosis poor.
- Vasculitis—prognosis guarded when systemic complications.

MISCELLANEOUS

ABBREVIATIONS

- EM = erythema multiforme.
- FeLV = feline leukemia virus.
- FIP = feline infectious peritonitis.
- FIV = feline immunodeficiency virus.
- SJS = Stevens-Johnson syndrome.
- TEN = toxic epidermal necrolysis.

Suggested Reading

Helton Rhodes KA, Werner A. Blackwell's Five-Minute Veterinary Consult: Clinical Companion: Small Animal Dermatology, 3rd ed. Hoboken, NJ: Wiley-Blackwell, 2018.

Author Daniel O. Morris

Consulting Editor Alexander H. Werner Resnick

CUTEREBRIASIS

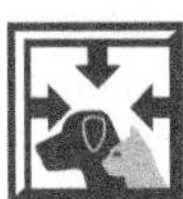

BASICS

OVERVIEW

- Flies of the genus *Cuterebra* are found in the Americas, where they are obligatory parasites of rodents and lagomorphs. Adult flies lay eggs on blades of grass or in nests; they hatch and crawl onto the skin of passing host. The small maggots enter a body orifice, migrate through various internal tissues, and ultimately over several weeks to months make their way to the skin, where they establish a warble. The mature maggots, which may be an inch long, then drop out of the rodent or rabbit host and pupate in the soil.
- Dogs and cats become infected when they contact a blade of grass upon which an egg containing an infective maggot is stimulated to hatch and attach onto the passing animal. The maggots then crawl around on the cat or dog until they find an orifice in which to enter.
- Dogs and cats can develop maggots in warbles or can develop signs associated with larvae migrating within their tissues.
- Dogs and cats can present with respiratory signs, neurologic signs, ophthalmic lesions, or maggots in their skin.

SIGNALMENT

- Dogs and cats—all ages.
- In northern United States, most cases occur in late summer and early autumn, based on time of emergence of adult egg-laying females in spring and early summer.

SIGNS

- Dermatologic—warble containing bot with protruding spiracles.
- Neurologic—ataxia, circling, paralysis, blindness, recumbency.
- Ophthalmic lesions—larva in conjunctiva.
- Respiratory—eosinophilic respiratory disease.

CAUSES & RISK FACTORS

- Dogs and cats with access to outdoors, where they contact eggs and larvae.
- Neonatal cats have been infected, presumably with larvae carried on queen's fur.

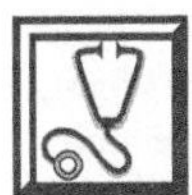

DIAGNOSIS

DIFFERENTIAL DIAGNOSIS

- Respiratory—allergies, lungworms, migrating ascarids or hookworms.
- Neurologic—rabies, distemper, angiostrongylosis.
- Ophthalmic lesions—larval *Hypoderma* or *Oestrus*.
- Dermatologic—mature warble unmistakable, young warble may present as pustule or papule.

CBC/BIOCHEMISTRY/URINALYSIS

Eosinophilia may be present, otherwise no specific findings.

OTHER LABORATORY TESTS

N/A

IMAGING

CT, MRI—may show intracranial lesions in cats.

DIAGNOSTIC PROCEDURES

N/A

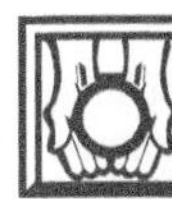

TREATMENT

- Can remove maggots from subcutaneous lesions, eyes, or nares (see Web Video 1).
- Manifestations of lung migration may be alleviated by corticosteroids.
- Neurologic disease has poor prognosis.

MEDICATIONS

DRUG(S) OF CHOICE

- Ivermectin 0.2 mg/kg SC should kill migrating maggots; can be administered either to alleviate signs caused by maggots suspected of migrating in lungs, or to kill larvae in other tissues, including CNS; pretreatment with corticosteroids may mitigate inflammatory reaction to dying worms.
- Products containing isoxazolines (i.e., afoxolaner, fluralaner, lotilaner, andsarolaner), when routinely given to cats and and dogs, may prevent migration and warble formation by *Cuterebra* spp. Efficacy and potential side effects in patients with migrating maggots has not been reported.

FOLLOW-UP

Good return of function following ivermectin treatment is possible.

MISCELLANEOUS

- In northern United States disease is seasonal, with most cases occurring in late summer and early fall when adult flies are active; seasonality is less demarcated in areas where warmer temperatures and active flies occur through longer periods of the year.
- Does not appear to result in prolonged immunity; the same animal can develop skin lesions several years in a row.
- Application of monthly heartworm preventatives (avermectin-containing products), flea development control products (lufenuron-containing products), or topical flea and tick treatments may either prevent the maggots from developing, or may kill them before they access an orifice for entry. However, based on anecdotal information, some cats and dogs on these products still develop warbles with maggots.

ZOONOTIC POTENTIAL

The maggots in the dog or cat pose no zoonotic threat.

Suggested Reading

Bordelon JT, Newcomb BT, Rochat MC. Surgical removal of a *Cuterebra* larva from the cervical trachea of a cat. J Am Anim Hosp Assoc 2009, 45:52–54.

Edelmann ML, Lucio-Forster A, Kern TJ, et al. Ophthalmomyiasis interna anterior in a dog: keratotomy and extraction of a Cuterebra sp. larva. Vet Ophthalmol 2014, 17:448–453.

Thawley VJ, Suran, JN, Boller EM. 2013 Presumptive central nervous system cuterebriasis and concurrent protein-losing nephropathy in a dog. J Vet Emerg Crit Care 2013, 23:335–339.

Author Dwight D. Bowman

Consulting Editor Amie Koenig

CYANOSIS

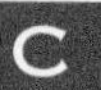

BASICS

DEFINITION

A bluish discoloration of the skin and mucous membranes owing to an increase in the amount of reduced, or deoxygenated, hemoglobin within the blood.

PATHOPHYSIOLOGY

• Concentration of deoxygenated hemoglobin—must be >5 g/dL to detect condition; thus anemia may obscure recognition of cyanosis. • Central—associated with systemic arterial hypoxemia or hemoglobin abnormalities. • Peripheral—limited to one or more extremities of the body; associated with diminished peripheral blood flow; arterial oxygen tension and saturation typically normal.

Arterial Hypoxemia

• Low partial pressure of inspired oxygen (e.g., high altitude). • Hypoventilation due to primary neurologic disorders affecting brain, cervical spinal cord, or lower motor neuron; centrally acting respiratory depressant drugs; chest wall injuries; pleural space diseases; upper airway obstructions. • Ventilation–perfusion mismatching resulting in impaired gas exchange (e.g., pulmonary parenchymal or thromboembolic diseases). • Diffusion impairment fromthickening of alveolar barrier through which oxygen must pass to reach red blood cells (RBCs); interstitial lung disease may cause this. • Addition of deoxygenated venous blood to arterial circulation—congenital right-to-left shunting cardiac defects (e.g., tetralogy of Fallot, transposition of great vessels); reversed shunting cardiac defects caused by high pulmonary vascular resistance (e.g., right-to-left shunting patent ductus arteriosus [PDA], atrial septal defect [ASD], ventricular septal defect [VSD]).

Abnormal Hemoglobin

• Methemoglobin—most common abnormal heme pigment; unable to bind oxygen; normally formed at low rate in erythrocytes; cats with significant exposure to acetaminophen will appear cyanotic. • Nicotinamide adenine dinucleotide dependent methemoglobin reductase (NADH-MR)—intracellular reductive enzyme; maintains methemoglobin : hemoglobin ratio at <2%; deficiency and/or exposure to oxidizing agents causes methemoglobinemia. • Hypoxia—when >20–40% of hemoglobin has been oxidized to methemoglobin.

Other

• Peripheral cyanosis—results from increased oxygen extraction from arterial supply to an area (e.g., a limb); caused by severe vasoconstriction, poor peripheral blood flow, obstruction to flow associated with arterial thromboembolism, or stagnation or obstruction of venous blood flow; difficult to see, with exception of discolored paw pads in cats with arterial thromboembolism. • Differential cyanosis—with reverse shunting PDA, head and neck receive oxygenated blood via brachiocephalic trunk and left subclavian artery, which arise from aortic arch; rest of the body receives desaturated blood through ductus located in descending aorta.

SYSTEMS AFFECTED

• Central—all systems affected.
• Peripheral—may diminish or abolish neuromuscular function of affected limb(s).

SIGNALMENT

• Right-to-left cardiac shunts in association with high pulmonary vascular resistance and pulmonary hypertension (Eisenmenger physiology)—dogs: Keeshond, English bulldog, klee kai, and beagle; some cats; generally young animals. • Tracheal collapse—usually young or middle-aged small-breed dogs (e.g., Pomeranian, Yorkshire terrier, poodles). • Acquired laryngeal paralysis—most common in old large-breed dogs (e.g., retrievers). • Hypoplastic trachea—identified in young English bulldogs; occasionally other breeds. • Brachycephalic airway syndrome—dogs: English and French bulldogs, Pekinese, pugs, Boston terrier, and other brachycephalic breeds. • Asthma—cats: higher incidence reported in Siamese.

SIGNS

Historical Findings

• Central—stridor; respiratory distress; cough; voice change; episodic weakness; syncope; exposure to oxidizing substances or drugs causing methemoglobinemia.
• Peripheral—limb paresis or paralysis.

Physical Examination Findings

• Heart murmur or splitting of second heart sound—with cardiac disease or pulmonary hypertension. • Pulmonary crackles or wheezes—with pulmonary edema or respiratory disease. • Muffled heart sounds—owing to pleural space or pericardial disease.
• Upper airway stridor with laryngeal paralysis.
• Honking cough—typical of tracheal collapse; often induced by tracheal palpation.
• Dyspnea—may be inspiratory, expiratory, or a combination (see Differential Diagnosis).
• Limbs—may be cyanotic, cool, pale, painful, and edematous; can lack a pulse in conditions causing peripheral cyanosis. • Weakness—can be generalized and persistent with severe cardiac diseases; can be episodic and especially noticeable with exercise or excitement.
• Posterior paresis or paralysis—can be seen with distal aorta arterial thromboembolism; differentiated from primary neuromuscular disease by absence (or near absence) of pulses.

CAUSES

Respiratory System

• Larynx—paralysis (acquired or congenital); collapse; spasm; edema; trauma; neoplasia; granulomatous disease. • Trachea—collapse; neoplasia; foreign body; trauma; hypoplasia.
• Lower airway and parenchyma—pneumonia (viral, bacterial, fungal, eosinophilic, mycobacteria, aspiration); chronic bronchitis; hypersensitivity bronchial disease or asthma; bronchiectasis; neoplasia; foreign body; parasites (*Filaroides*, *Paragonimus*, *Pneumocystis jiroveci*, toxoplasmosis, *Aelurostrongylus* spp.); pulmonary contusion or hemorrhage; noncardiogenic edema (smoke inhalation, snake bite, electric shock); near drowning.
• Pleural space—pneumothorax; infectious (bacterial, fungal, feline infectious peritonitis [FIP]); chylothorax; hemothorax; pyothorax; neoplasia; trauma. • Thoracic wall or diaphragm—congenital (pericardial, diaphragmatic hernia); trauma (diaphragmatic hernia, fractured ribs, flail chest); neuromuscular disease (tick bite paralysis, coonhound paralysis).

Cardiovascular System

• Congenital defects—Eisenmenger physiology (right-to-left shunting PDA, VSD, ASD); tetralogy of Fallot; truncus arteriosus; double outlet right ventricle; anomalous pulmonary venous return; atresia of aortic or tricuspid or pulmonary valves. • Acquired disease—mitral valve disease; cardiomyopathy.
• Pericardial effusion—idiopathic disease; neoplasia. • Pulmonary thromboembolic disease—hyperadrenocorticism; immune-mediated hemolytic anemia; protein-losing nephropathy; dirofilariasis; severe, acute pancreatitis. • Pulmonary hypertension—idiopathic; right-to-left cardiac shunts.
• Peripheral vascular disease—arterial thromboembolism (feline cardiomyopathies); venous obstruction; reduced cardiac output; shock, arteriolar constriction.

Neuromusculoskeletal System

• Brainstem dysfunction—encephalitis; trauma; hemorrhage; neoplasia; drug-induced depression of respiratory center (morphine, barbiturates). • Cervical spinal cord dysfunction—edema; trauma; vertebral fractures; disk prolapse. • Neuromuscular dysfunction—overdose of paralytic agents (succinylcholine, pancuronium); tick bite paralysis; botulism; tetanus; acute polyradiculoneuritis (coonhound paralysis); dysautonomia; myasthenia gravis.

Methemoglobinemia

• Congenital—NADH-MR deficiency (dogs).
• Ingestion of oxidant chemicals—acetaminophen; nitrates; nitrites; phenacetin; sulfonamides; benzocaine; aniline dyes; dapsone.

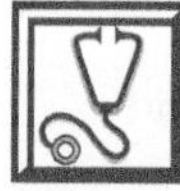

DIAGNOSIS

DIFFERENTIAL DIAGNOSIS

• Generalized—systemic hypoxemia or heme abnormality. • Peripheral only—reduced blood flow to extremities. • Caudal body—right-to-left shunting PDA. • Cardiac versus respiratory causes—differentiation can be difficult; cardiac murmur may suggest cardiac disease, but murmurs are often heard in older patients with primary respiratory disease; higher hematocrit may make murmurs harder to hear; thoracic radiography and echocardiography useful for differentiation. • Central or peripheral neurologic signs—should prompt concern for arterial hypoxemia owing to primary neuromuscular disease.

Breathing Pattern

• May help define cause. • Inspiratory effort—often associated with obstructive upper airway or pleural space disease; stridor frequently localizes problem to larynx or cervical trachea. • Expiratory effort—generally seen with obstructive lower airway disease. • Rapid shallow (restrictive)—may be associated with pleural space disease or neuromuscular abnormalities of thoracic wall.

CBC/BIOCHEMISTRY/URINALYSIS

• Color of blood—may be darkened; chocolate brown with methemoglobinemia. • Polycythemia—often accompanies congenital heart disease; may occur with chronic hypoxemia owing to severe respiratory disease. • Proteinuria—accompanies protein-losing nephropathies, which may result in secondary pulmonary thromboembolism. • Panhypoproteinemia—accompanies protein-losing enteropathies, which may lead to pulmonary thromboembolism.

OTHER LABORATORY TESTS

• Co-oximetry to estimate percent of methemoglobin or carboxyhemoglobin. • Arterial blood gas analysis. • Urine protein : creatinine ratio—with suspected pulmonary thromboembolism secondary to protein-losing nephropathy.

IMAGING

• Radiography—essential for determining cause. • Echocardiography—aids in diagnosis of congenital or acquired cardiac disease, pulmonary hypertension, and pulmonary thromboembolism. • CT/angiography—can further define obstructive nasal, pulmonary, or pleural space disease; gold standard for diagnosing pulmonary embolism in humans.

DIAGNOSTIC PROCEDURES

• Pulse oximetry to estimate oxygen saturation; inaccurate when carboxyhemoglobin or methemoglobin present. • Laryngoscopic examination—evaluate laryngeal structure and arytenoid function. • Bronchoscopy—often useful in diagnosis of airway and pulmonary diseases. • Transtracheal wash, bronchoalveolar lavage, or fine-needle lung aspirate—often required to characterize bronchopulmonary diseases. • Thoracocentesis—required for diagnosis and treatment of pleural space disorders. • Electrocardiography—may reveal heart enlargement changes; unreliable; echocardiography better. • Lung biopsy—can be necessary for diagnosis of interstitial lung disease.

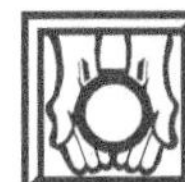

TREATMENT

• Inpatient—immediate diagnostic testing and treatment. • Stabilization therapy (e.g., oxygen, thoracocentesis, tracheostomy)—usually instituted before aggressive diagnostics. • Specific therapy—depends on ultimate diagnosis; usually exercise restriction and dietary modification required. • Surgical treatment—depends on primary disease process and extent of cardiac or respiratory involvement. • Warn the client when admitting the patient that diseases associated with cyanosis can have dire outcomes.

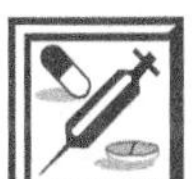

MEDICATIONS

DRUG(S) OF CHOICE

• Oxygen therapy—provide as soon as possible. • Additional drug therapy depends on final diagnosis. • Furosemide—aggressive use indicated with suspected cardiogenic pulmonary edema. • Methemoglobinemia as result of ingestion of oxidizing substances (acetaminophen)—give acetylcysteine as soon as possible (140 mg/kg PO/IV; then 70 mg/kg q4h for five treatments); cimetidine (10 mg/kg PO; then 5 mg/kg PO q6h for 48h) is useful adjunct to acetylcysteine; ascorbic acid (30 mg/kg PO q6h for seven treatments) may be of some value, but do not use as sole agent; methylene blue given IV followed by oral supplementation reported as successful treatment modality in dogs. • Sildenafil citrate—phosphodiesterase type 5 inhibitor used to treat pulmonary arterial hypertension at 1–3 mg/kg PO q8–12h.

CONTRAINDICATIONS

Avoid using paralytic agents (succinylcholine, pancuronium) and agents that cause profound depression of respiratory center (morphine, barbiturates).

FOLLOW-UP

PATIENT MONITORING

• Patients in an oxygen cage should be disturbed as infrequently as possible for monitoring. • Assess efficacy of therapy—changes in depth and rate of respiration; color of mucous membranes (should return to normal pink color if cause is not anatomic shunt and patient has adequate reserves); pulse oximetry or arterial blood analysis. • Instruct client to monitor mucous membrane color and respiratory effort, and advise immediate veterinary care if cyanotic condition returns.

POSSIBLE COMPLICATIONS

Advanced pulmonary or airway disease and severe cardiac disease—poor long-term prognosis.

MISCELLANEOUS

ASSOCIATED CONDITIONS

• Obesity—can complicate or exacerbate underlying respiratory or cardiac diseases. • Ascites—can complicate or exacerbate respiratory effort and reduce lung capacity due to cranial displacement of diaphragm.

AGE-RELATED FACTORS

Congenital cardiac abnormalities—usually the cause in young patients.

PREGNANCY/FERTILITY/BREEDING

• Advanced pregnancy may exacerbate signs because of pressure on diaphragm and reduced lung expansion. • Fetuses likely to be harmed or aborted by hypoxemia associated with cyanosis.

SEE ALSO

• Dyspnea and Respiratory Distress.
• Panting and Tachypnea.
• Stertor and Stridor.

ABBREVIATIONS

• ASD = atrial septal defect.
• FIP = feline infectious peritonitis.
• NADH-MR = nicotinamide adenine dinucleotide dependent methemoglobin reductase.
• PDA = patent ductus arteriosus.
• RBC = red blood cell.
• VSD = ventricular septal defect.

Author Sean B. Majoy
Consulting Editor Elizabeth Rozanski
Acknowledgment The author and book editors acknowledge the prior contribution of Ned F. Kuehn.

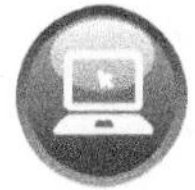

Client Education Handout available online

CYCLIC HEMATOPOIESIS

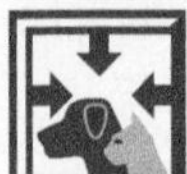

BASICS

OVERVIEW

- Cyclic hematopoiesis in color-dilute gray collie pups, also known as gray collie syndrome, is characterized by frequent episodes of infection with failure to thrive and early death. Systems affected are hematopoietic, ocular, respiratory, gastrointestinal, and skin. Pups may appear normal for the first 4–6 weeks and then develop diarrhea, conjunctivitis, gingivitis, pneumonia, skin infections, joint pain, and fever.
- Episodes of illness, varying from inactivity accompanied by fever to life-threatening infection, repeat at 11–14-day intervals.
- Affected pups are usually smaller than their littermates at birth, weak, and often pushed aside by their mothers.

SIGNALMENT

- Cyclic hematopoiesis in the collie breed is present only in the color-dilute pups. The color dilution and bone marrow disorder are inherited as an autosomal recessive trait. This condition has also been reported in crossbred collie/beagle pups.
- Clinical signs occur as early as 1–2 weeks of age and are always apparent by 4–6 weeks of age. Affected dogs rarely live beyond 2–3 years of age.
- An apparently similar disease was reported in normal-colored pups in two border collie litters in the UK. Cyclic hematopoiesis has also been reported in Pomeranians, Cocker Spaniels, and a Basset Hound, but the disease is not well characterized in these breeds.
- Cyclic hematopoiesis has been observed in two cats with feline leukemia virus (FeLV) infection.

SIGNS

Historical Findings

- Weakness.
- Failure to thrive.
- Conjunctivitis.
- Gingivitis.
- Diarrhea.
- Pneumonia.
- Skin infections.
- Joint pain.
- Coagulopathies.

Physical Examination Findings

- Dilute coat color with color dilution of nasal epithelium.
- Smaller and weaker than normal-colored littermates.
- Fever.
- Watery eyes, reddened gums, tonsillitis, and diarrhea nearly always present during phase of hematopoietic cycle when clinical signs are evident; other signs vary depending on presence of infection in various body systems.
- Signs and symptoms of FeLV in cats.

CAUSES & RISK FACTORS

- Inherited disease in purebred or crossbred collie dogs.
- FeLV infection in cats.

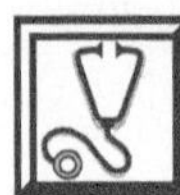

DIAGNOSIS

DIFFERENTIAL DIAGNOSIS

- Coat color dilution and nasal epithelial color dilution are always present in collies or collie mixed breeds with cyclic hematopoiesis.
- Coat color dilution as a result of dilute gene expression is also observed in collies. These dogs have blue or lilac coat color with normal color intensity on nose and do not develop cyclic hematopoiesis.
- Trapped neutrophil syndrome is another autosomal recessive inherited neutropenia in border collie pups who present with recurrent infections and musculoskeletal disease, usually between 6 and 12 weeks of age. Unlike cyclic neutropenia, affected pups have persistent neutropenia. A DNA test for this disease is available.
- Cats will present with signs and symptoms consistent with FeLV infection.

CBC/BIOCHEMISTRY/URINALYSIS

- CBC—severe neutropenia, lasting 2–5 days, followed by neutrophilia, and occurring at 11–14-day intervals with mild normocytic to microcytic anemia in dogs; slight to moderate normocytic or macrocytic anemia in cats.
- Local swelling, redness, and systemic signs of infection usually occur during first days of neutrophilic phase of disease cycle; therefore, on initial CBC examination, neutrophilia with moderate monocytosis is usually observed.

OTHER LABORATORY TESTS

A DNA mutation test is available for canine cyclic hematopoiesis from Animal Genetics.

TREATMENT

- Recombinant G-CSF or lentivirus-mediated G-CSF can be administered to shorten period of neutropenia and reduce infections.
- Antibiotics and supportive therapy to treat or relieve symptoms.
- Bone marrow transplantation eliminates cyclic hematopoiesis and can be curative.

MEDICATIONS

DRUG(S) OF CHOICE

Antibiotics and intravenous fluids as indicated for infections.

FOLLOW-UP

PATIENT MONITORING

Owner advised to watch for signs of infection.

PREVENTION/AVOIDANCE

Dogs should not be boarded with other animals.

POSSIBLE COMPLICATIONS

Infections can be life threatening if untreated.

EXPECTED COURSE AND PROGNOSIS

Intermittent infections are expected. Prognosis is guarded.

MISCELLANEOUS

PREGNANCY/FERTILITY/BREEDING

Carriers or affected collies should not be bred.

SEE ALSO

- Neutropenia.
- Thrombocytopathies.

ABBREVIATIONS

- FeLV = feline leukemia virus.
- G-CSF = granulocyte colony-stimulating factor.

Suggested Reading

Harvey JW. Veterinary Hematology: A Diagnostic Guide and Color Atlas. St. Louis, MO: Elsevier Health Sciences, 2012, p.148.

Author June C. Huang

Consulting Editor Melinda S. Camus

Acknowledgment The author and book editors acknowledge the prior contribution of Alan H. Rebar.

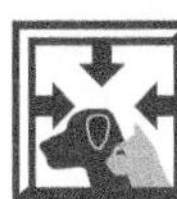

BASICS

OVERVIEW

• Increased number of casts in urine sediment. • Occasional hyaline and granular casts can be found in clinically normal animals. • High numbers of casts indicate tubular pathology, but do not correlate with degree of damage. • Can develop with primary renal disease or systemic disorders that secondarily affect kidneys. • Absence of casts does not exclude possibility of renal tubular disease. • Systems affected—renal/ urologic.

SIGNALMENT

Dog and cat.

CAUSES & RISK FACTORS

Nephrotoxicosis

• Toxins—ethylene glycol, grape/raisin ingestion (dogs), lily ingestion (cats), hypercalcemia. • Nephrotoxic drugs—e.g., aminoglycosides, amphotericin B, cisplatin, nonsteroidal anti-inflammatory drugs, angiotensin-converting enzyme inhibitors, radiocontrast agents.

Renal Ischemia

• Dehydration. • Low cardiac output. • Renal vessel thrombosis. • Hemoglobinuria.
• Myoglobulinuria.

Renal Inflammation

Infectious diseases (e.g., pyelonephritis, leptospirosis, feline infectious peritonitis, tick/vector-borne disease).

Glomerular Disease

• Glomerulonephritis. • Amyloidosis.

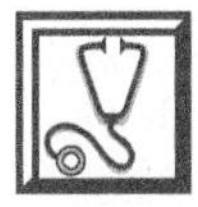

DIAGNOSIS

DIFFERENTIAL DIAGNOSIS

• Cylindruria with azotemia and adequately concentrated urine (specific gravity >1.030 in dogs and >1.040 in cats)—consider prerenal disorders such as dehydration. • Cylindruria with azotemia and inadequately concentrated urine—consider renal failure. • Cylindruria with leukocytosis—consider pyelonephritis or other infectious and inflammatory disorders.
• Cylindruria with glucosuria and proteinuria—consider renal tubular necrosis. • Transient hyaline and/or granular casts can be seen after strenuous exercise.

CBC/BIOCHEMISTRY/URINALYSIS

• Casts classified by appearance and quantified per low power field. • Granular casts (fine or coarse) associated with tubular degeneration, inflammation, or necrosis.
• Hyaline casts can be seen with proteinuria, dehydration, and after diuresis. • Waxy casts usually seen with chronic kidney disease.
• Epithelial casts formed from degeneration of renal tubular epithelial cells; most commonly seen with acute tubular injury.
• White blood cell (WBC) casts indicate renal inflammation (e.g., pyelonephritis).
• Red blood cell (RBC) casts indicate renal hemorrhage. • Fatty casts suggest renal tubular injury. • Chemistry profile may show azotemia and hyperphosphatemia. • CBC may show anemia, erythrocytosis, leukocytosis, and/or thrombocytopenia depending on underlying pathology.

OTHER LABORATORY TESTS

• Determine urine protein : creatinine ratio to evaluate magnitude of proteinuria.
• Perform urine culture to rule out urinary tract infection in patients with pyuria or WBC casts. Also consider ultrasound ± radiography to assess for pyelonephritis, nephroliths, etc. • Test for systemic infections as indicated. • If thrombocytopenic or RBC casts are present, perform coagulation studies to rule out consumptive coagulopathy such as disseminated intravascular coagulation.

Disorders That May Alter Laboratory Results

• Delayed processing of urinalysis and examination of urine sediment may result in disappearance of casts; ideally should be examined within 30 minutes of collection.
• Alkaline urine can cause dissolution of casts. • Low speed centrifugation necessary to prevent cast destruction.

Valid If Run in Human Laboratory?

Yes

DIAGNOSTIC PROCEDURES

Consider renal biopsy if kidney disease persists or progresses and cause cannot be determined from routine diagnostic tests.

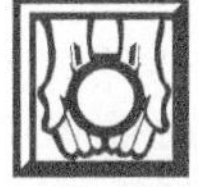

TREATMENT

• Manage as outpatient unless patient is dehydrated or has decompensated kidney failure.
• Acute kidney injury and chronic kidney disease should be managed according to standard recommendations. • If patient cannot maintain hydration, administer parenteral fluid therapy. • Consider dialysis if toxin exposure or leptospirosis infection.

MEDICATIONS

CONTRAINDICATIONS/POSSIBLE INTERACTIONS

Avoid nephrotoxic drugs.

FOLLOW-UP

PATIENT MONITORING

• Physical examination including patient's weight to assess hydration status. • Blood pressure monitoring. • CBC/chemistry/ urinalysis monitoring.

PREVENTION/AVOIDANCE

Avoid or correct risk factors (e.g., exposure to toxins, infectious disease prevention, etc.).

POSSIBLE COMPLICATIONS

Irreversible renal disease, depending on underlying cause of cylindruria.

MISCELLANEOUS

ZOONOTIC POTENTIAL

Possible in patients with leptospirosis. Use safety precautions when handing urine.

SEE ALSO

Nephrotoxicity, Drug-Induced.

ABBREVIATIONS

• RBC = red blood cell.
• WBC = white blood cell.

Suggested Reading

Latimer K. Duncan and Prasse's Veterinary Laboratory Medicine Clinical Pathology, 5th ed. Ames, IA: Wiley-Blackwell, 2011, pp. 264–272.

Sink C, Weinstein N. Practical Veterinary Urinalysis. Ames, IA: Wiley-Blackwell, 2012, pp. 69–84.

Stockham S, Scott M. Fundamentals of Veterinary Clinical Pathology, 2nd ed. Ames, IA: Wiley-Blackwell, 2008, pp. 472–473.

Author Tracie D. Romsland

Consulting Editor J.D. Foster

Acknowledgment The authors and book editors acknowledge the prior contributions of Allyson C. Berent and Cathy E. Langston.

CYTAUXZOONOSIS

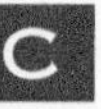

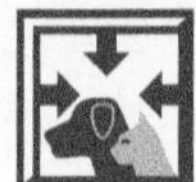

BASICS

OVERVIEW

- Infection with the protozoan *Cytauxzoon felis*.
- Affects vascular system of lungs, liver, spleen, kidneys, and brain; bone marrow and developmental stages of red blood cells (RBCs) affected as well.
- Uncommon in most regions, but common during the spring and summer in endemic regions.
- Affects feral and domestic cats in south-central, southeastern, and mid-Atlantic United States; range appears to be expanding towards eastern and northeastern United States.
- Related *Cytauxzoon* spp. have been identified in Europe and Asia, but have not been associated with classic Cytauxzoonosis (see Signs) as seen in North America.

SIGNALMENT

- Domestic cats of all ages.
- Wild felids are also at risk.
- No breed or sex predilection, although most cases are diagnosed in young cats that have access to outdoors.

SIGNS

- Most cats have severe illness at presentation.
- Pale mucous membranes.
- Depression.
- Anorexia.
- Dehydration.
- High fever.
- Icterus.
- Splenomegaly.
- Hepatomegaly.
- Some cats may be infected but asymptomatic.

CAUSES & RISK FACTORS

- Bite of infected tick (primarily *Amblyomma americanum* or *Dermacentor variabilis*).
- Roaming in areas shared by reservoir hosts (bobcats).
- Living in same household/region as cat diagnosed with cytauxzoonosis.

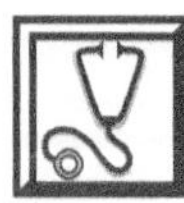

DIAGNOSIS

DIFFERENTIAL DIAGNOSIS

- Other causes of pancytopenia such as sepsis and panleukopenia.
- Other causes of fever and jaundice such as pancreatitis, hepatitis, and cholangitis.

CBC/BIOCHEMISTRY/URINALYSIS

- Bicytopenia or pancytopenia are the most common findings; thrombocytopenia is almost always present.
- Moderate hyperbilirubinemia and bilirubinuria.
- Mild hyperglycemia.
- If present, anemia is believed to be secondary to hemolysis.

OTHER LABORATORY TESTS

- Fresh blood smear—*Cytauxzoon* erythrocytic form; 1–3 µm in diameter; shape of signet ring or safety pin.
- Schizont-infected monocyte/macrophages may be observed on feathered edge of thin blood smears.
- Splenic, lymph node, liver, or bone marrow aspirate—best suited to demonstrate extra-erythrocytic schizont forms.
- PCR assay is commercially available.
- Blood type in all cats prior to transfusion.

IMAGING

Radiographs or ultrasound may assist in identifying pleural effusion or pulmonary edema.

DIAGNOSTIC PROCEDURES

N/A

PATHOLOGIC FINDINGS

Organisms inside myeloid cells in bone marrow aspirate and in dramatically enlarged myeloid cells in vessels of multiple organs including lung, liver, spleen, kidney, and brain.

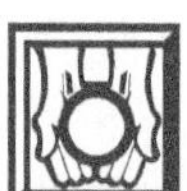

TREATMENT

- Inpatient with aggressive supportive therapy including supplemental oxygen.
- Blood transfusion.
- Feeding tube for medication and nutritional support.

MEDICATIONS

DRUG(S) OF CHOICE

- Combination of atovaquone (15 mg/kg PO q8h with a fatty meal) and azithromycin (10 mg/kg PO q24h) and supportive care is associated with survival rates of 60%.
- Imidocarb dipropionate—5 mg IM two injections 14 days apart has been recommended, but is associated with survival rates of approximately 27%.
- Heparin (100–300 U/kg SC q8h or 300–900 U/kg/day as IV CRI) until time of discharge (longer if significant thrombosis such as pulmonary thromoboembolism is present).

CONTRAINDICATIONS/POSSIBLE INTERACTIONS

N/A

FOLLOW-UP

EXPECTED COURSE AND PROGNOSIS

- With aggressive supportive care and treatment, expect 3–7 days of hospitalization with severe illness.
- Some cats develop pleural effusion and require thoracocentesis.
- Cats that survive will return to normal within 2–4 weeks of discharge and appear immune to reinfection.
- Some cats remain persistently infected with the intraerythrocytic form without overt signs.
- Without treatment, most cats with acute cytauxzoonosis have died within 5 days of presentation.

MISCELLANEOUS

ZOONOTIC POTENTIAL

- No known risk to humans.
- Cannot be directly transmitted to another cat except by blood or tissue inoculation.

ABBREVIATIONS

- RBC = red blood cell.

Suggested Reading

Cohn LA, Birkenheuer AJ, Brunker JD, et al. Efficacy of atovaquone and azithromycin or imidocarb dipropionate in cats with acute cytauxzoonosis. J Vet Intern Med 2011, 25(1):55–60.

Reichard MV, Thomas JE, Arther RG, et al. Efficacy of an imidacloprid 10%/flumethrin 4.5% collar (Seresto®, Bayer) for preventing the transmission of *Cytauxzoon felis* to domestic cats by *Amblyomma americanum*. Parasitol Res 2013, 112(Suppl. 1):11–20.

Author Adam J. Birkenheuer
Consulting Editor Amie Koenig

DEAFNESS

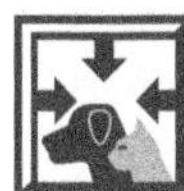

BASICS

DEFINITION

- Partial or complete hearing loss.
- Two forms:
  - Sensorineural deafness—caused by damage to receptors in cochlea, cochlear nerve, or auditory pathways in CNS.
  - Conduction deafness—caused by inability to conduct sound vibration through external to inner-ear structures.

PATHOPHYSIOLOGY

Sensorineural Deafness

- Hereditary—breed-related cochlear degeneration closely associated with the recessive alleles of the piebald locus and the dominant allele of the merle locus in dogs and with the dominant allele of the white locus in cats. These genes alter the ability of neural crest melanocytes to populate regions of the body including skin, hair, iris, ocular tapetum, and portions of the cochlea. The absence of melanocytes in the stria vascularis of the cochlea is associated with early postnatal degeneration of this structure. Can also be non-pigment-associated and in some cases also affect the vestibular system, such as in Doberman pinschers (associated with a mutation in the PTPRQ gene).
- Acquired—cochlear degeneration due to chronic infection, ototoxicity, neoplasia, chronic exposure to loud noises, anesthesia-associated, or age-related loss of hair cells and spiral ganglion cells (presbycusis).

Conduction Deafness

- Congenital defects in external ear canal, tympanic membrane, or ossicles that transmit vibration in middle ear are rare. Hereditary predisposition in primary secretory otitis media in the cavalier King Charles spaniel.
- Acquired defects resulting in stenosis/ obstruction of external ear canal, rupture of tympanic membrane, or fusion of bony ossicles; most commonly associated with chronic otitis or middle ear polyps.

SYSTEMS AFFECTED

Nervous—inner ear.

GENETICS

Genetics of congenital deafness not fully understood, although strong association with the piebald and the merle locus in dogs and dominant white locus in cats (pigment-associated genes related to coat color).

INCIDENCE/PREVALENCE

Prevalence of congenital deafness in one or both ears available for the following breeds—Dalmatian: 30% in United States, 18% in UK, 17% in Switzerland, 20% in Germany; Jack Russell terrier: 4% in United States; Australian cattle dog: 15% in United States, 10% in Australia; English bull terrier: 11% (20% if white) in UK; English setter: 8% in United States; English cocker spaniel: 7% in United States; border collie: 2–3% in UK; purebred white cats: 20% in United States and Germany; non-purebred white cats: 50% in UK and United States.

GEOGRAPHIC DISTRIBUTION

Prevalence for different breeds varies between countries.

SIGNALMENT

- Breed-related congenital cochlear degeneration described in >90 breeds of dogs. Most breeds have a large amount of white pigmentation associated with merle or piebald genes, except for Doberman pinscher, puli, Shropshire terrier. Congenital sensorineural deafness present by 6 weeks of age, although has late onset in border collie (5 years) and Rhodesian ridgeback (4–12 months).
- No association with gender. Dogs with blue iris color have a higher incidence of congenital deafness.
- Mixed-breed cats with white hair coat and blue irises—high incidence of deafness. Purebred white cats that carry the Siamese gene for blue eyes have a lower incidence of congenital deafness.
- Acquired deafness may occur in any breed or age of dog and cat.

SIGNS

- Unilateral deafness often goes unnoticed. Rarely, dogs have difficulty localizing sound.
- With bilateral disease, animals do not respond to auditory cues such as calling their name or rattling food dish. Often they are easily startled. Commonly have heightened response to vibration and visual cues.

CAUSES

Sensorineural Deafness

- Genetic etiology likely in neonates.
- Acquired cochlea and cochlear nerve damage—infectious (otitis interna), neoplasia of bony labyrinth or nerve, trauma (physical or noise), systemic or topically applied drugs or toxins (antibiotics: aminoglycosides, polymyxin, erythromycin, vancomycin, chloramphenicol; antiseptics: ethanol, chlorhexidine, cetrimide; antineoplastics: cisplatin, carboplatin; diuretics: furosemide; heavy metals: arsenic, lead, mercury; miscellaneous: ceruminolytic agents, propylene glycol, salicylates), presbycusis, anesthesia-induced.

Conduction Deafness

- Otitis externa and other external ear canal disease (e.g., stenosis of canal, foreign bodies, neoplasia, or ruptured tympanum).
- Otitis media, middle-ear polyps, primary secretory otitis media.

RISK FACTORS

- Merle, piebald gene, or white coat color; blue eye color.
- Chronic otitis externa, media, or interna.
- Use of ototoxic drugs.
- General anesthesia.

D

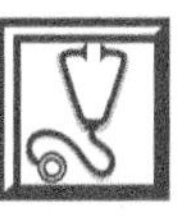

DIAGNOSIS

DIFFERENTIAL DIAGNOSIS

- Early age of onset—suggests congenital causes in predisposed breeds.
- Use of ototoxic drugs, recent anesthesia, or chronic ear disease—suggests acquired causes.
- Evaluate for brain disease.

CBC/BIOCHEMISTRY/URINALYSIS

Usually normal.

OTHER LABORATORY TESTS

- Bacterial culture and sensitivity of ear canal if otitis externa.
- Myringotomy with culture of aspirates if otitis media.

IMAGING

- Tympanic bullae and skull radiographs—may show soft tissue opacity and bone remodeling of tympanic bulla; often unremarkable in cases with otitis media/interna.
- Ultrasound of tympanic bullae—may show anechoic content in cases with otitis media/ interna, but low sensitivity.
- CT/MRI—higher sensitivity for middle–inner ear disease and intracranial pathology.

DIAGNOSTIC PROCEDURES

- Brainstem auditory evoked response (BAER)—gold standard test for evaluation of hearing. Measures electrical response of cochlea and auditory pathways in the brain to an auditory stimulus; reliable to identify dogs with unilateral disease or partial hearing loss. Bone conduction stimulation can be useful to distinguish sensorineural from conduction deafness. Can be used to determine the hearing threshold.
- Otoacoustic emissions (OAEs)—low-level sounds produced by inner ear as part of the normal hearing process that can be measured by placing a probe containing a microphone in the external ear canal. Two forms have been used in dogs for assessment of sensorineural deafness—transient evoked OAEs (TEOAEs) and distortion product OAEs (DPOAEs). OAE is best suited for cases with congenital deafness, as it tests outer hair cell function and is not affected by inner hair cell, synapse, or cochlear nerve deficiencies. DPOAEs may show benefits in assessing age-related and noise-induced hearing loss and may reduce cost and testing times in congenital sensorineural deafness compared to BAER.

PATHOLOGIC FINDINGS

- Congenital deafness—degeneration of the stria vascularis with subsequent collapse of membranous labyrinth structures. Bony labyrinth remains intact.

DEAFNESS (CONTINUED)

- Acquired deafness—related to primary disease such as otitis or neoplasia.
- Ototoxicity—degeneration of otic hair cells, cochlear nerve degeneration, and loss of stria vascularis.

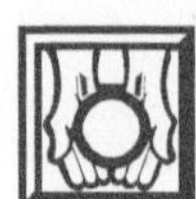

TREATMENT

CLIENT EDUCATION

Deaf animals may be functional pets, but require patience, specialized training, and extra protection from traffic.

SURGICAL CONSIDERATIONS

- Directed toward acquired causes; congenital deafness irreversible.
- Otitis externa, media, or interna—medical or surgical approaches depend on culture and sensitivity test results, response to antibiotics, and imaging findings. Conduction may improve as otitis externa or media resolves.
- Cochlear implants can be used in dogs with moderate to profound deafness, but only preliminary data available and very expensive.

MEDICATIONS

DRUG(S) OF CHOICE

- None for congenital deafness.
- Treat otitis based on culture and sensitivity results.

PRECAUTIONS

- Aminoglycosides or other ototoxic drugs—use with caution.
- Topical treatment of external ear canal—avoid if tympanic membrane is ruptured.

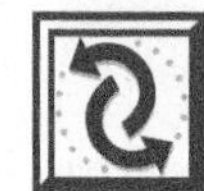

FOLLOW-UP

PATIENT MONITORING

As needed for management of otitis.

POSSIBLE COMPLICATIONS

Deaf dogs need protected environments and training to be functional pets.

MISCELLANEOUS

PREGNANCY/FERTILITY/BREEDING

Dogs homozygous for recessive merle gene can be blind and sterile.

ABBREVIATIONS

- BAER = brainstem auditory evoked response.
- DPOAE = distortion product OAE.
- OAE = otoacoustic emission.
- TEOAE = transient evoked OAE.

Author Rita Gonçalves

Client Education Handout available online

DECIDUOUS TEETH, PERSISTENT (RETAINED)

BASICS

OVERVIEW

• A persistent (retained) deciduous tooth is one that is still present when the permanent tooth begins to erupt or has fully erupted. • Numerous factors influence the exfoliation of deciduous teeth—lack of a permanent successor; ankylosis of the deciduous crown or root to the alveolus; failure of the developing permanent crown to contact the deciduous root, preventing resorption of the deciduous root during eruption.

SIGNALMENT

• More common in dogs than cats. • More common in small-breed dogs (e.g., Maltese, poodle, Yorkshire terrier, Pomeranian, etc.). • Occurs during permanent tooth eruption phase, which begins at 3 months of age for incisors and 5–7 months of age for canine teeth and molars. • Persistent deciduous teeth may not be detected or diagnosed until later in life. • No sex predilection.

SIGNS

General Comments

• Persistent deciduous teeth can cause the permanent teeth to erupt in an abnormal position resulting in a malocclusion; early recognition and intervention are essential. • Maxillary canine teeth erupt mesial (rostral) to the persistent deciduous canine teeth; this can result in a diastema (space) between the maxillary canine tooth and the third incisor that is too narrow to accommodate the crown zcanine position is referred to as mesioversion. • Mandibular canine teeth erupt lingual to the persistent deciduous teeth; this can result in a narrow space between the lower canines resulting in impingement on the soft tissue of the hard palate. The mandibular canine position is referred to as linguoversion. • All permanent incisors erupt lingual to the persistent deciduous incisors; this can result in a rostral crossbite.

Physical Examination Findings

• Presence of a deciduous tooth with the permanent tooth erupting or fully erupted. • Abnormal position of the permanent tooth due to persistence of the deciduous tooth. • Oral malodor from accumulation of debris and plaque due to crowding of the permanent tooth and the persistent deciduous tooth. • Local gingivitis and periodontal disease due to plaque accumulation from crowding. • Oronasal fistula from linguoversion of the permanent mandibular canine teeth. • Deciduous tooth crown is usually smaller than the permanent tooth. • Deciduous tooth might not have an underlying permanent tooth, and will often remain intact and vital.

CAUSES & RISK FACTORS

• Cause is unknown, but is suspected to have a genetic basis. • Small-breed dogs are predisposed.

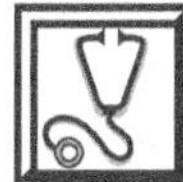

DIAGNOSIS

DIFFERENTIAL DIAGNOSIS

• Supernumerary teeth. • Gemination of the crown.

CBC/BIOCHEMISTRY/URINALYSIS

N/A

IMAGING

Intraoral Radiography

• Distinguish between permanent tooth and deciduous tooth. • Provide evidence or extent of root resorption of the deciduous tooth. • Identify dental abnormalities prior to extraction, including persistent deciduous tooth with no permanent successor, retained root with crown missing, and unerupted permanent tooth. • Identify relationship of deciduous root and permanent crown prior to extraction.

DIAGNOSTIC PROCEDURES

• Complete oral examination—chart oral cavity to indicate presence of persistent deciduous teeth, malpositioned teeth, missing teeth, soft tissue trauma, and other oral abnormalities. • Appropriate preoperative diagnostics prior to procedure to include intraoral radiography.

PATHOLOGIC FINDINGS

N/A

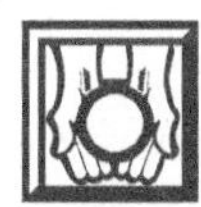

TREATMENT

Client Education

• Persistent deciduous teeth may be prevalent in certain breeds. • Start looking at teeth from the first puppy or kitten visit. • Inform owners that you will be evaluating for exfoliation of deciduous teeth as well as for proper eruption of permanent teeth.

Surgical Considerations

• Extract the deciduous tooth as soon as the permanent tooth has erupted through the gingiva. • Pain management - local/regional and systemic. • Intraoral radiographs. • General anesthesia with endotracheal tube in place and cuff inflated. • Elevation of deciduous tooth. • Careful, gentle elevation is critical; excessive force or pressure can damage the developing permanent tooth (and other underlying structures). • A fractured or retained root may need to be removed with a gingival flap. • If a permanent tooth has erupted in an abnormal position, full root extraction of the deciduous tooth is necessary. • If the deciduous root has undergone resorption, it may not need to be extracted.

MEDICATIONS

DRUG(S) OF CHOICE

• Topical oral antimicrobial rinse prior to extraction. • Pain management prior to, during, and following extraction.

CONTRAINDICATIONS/POSSIBLE INTERACTIONS

N/A

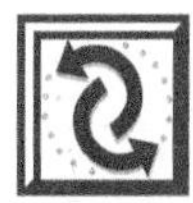

FOLLOW-UP

PATIENT MONITORING

• After surgery, restrict activity for the rest of the day. • Analgesia (nonsteroidal anti-inflammatory drug [NSAID]) for 24–36 hours postop. • Soft diet for 3 days—canned food or moistened dry kibble. • No chew toys for 3 days; no "tug of war" for 1 week. • Oral chlorhexidine rinse for 3–5 days. • Continue daily tooth brushing after 24 hours.

PREVENTION/AVOIDANCE

May be prevalent in certain breeds and lines—avoid similar breeding.

POSSIBLE COMPLICATIONS

• Malocclusion that results after full eruption of permanent teeth may require treatment. • Linguoversion of one or both mandibular canine teeth. • Mesioversion of one or both maxillary canine teeth.

EXPECTED COURSE AND PROGNOSIS

• Once extracted, there should be no further problems. • Resulting malocclusion needs further evaluation. • Gingiva generally heals uneventfully.

MISCELLANEOUS

SEE ALSO

Malocclusions—Skeletal and Dental.

ABBREVIATIONS

• NSAID = nonsteroidal anti-inflammatory drug.

INTERNET RESOURCES

http://www.avdc.org/avdc-nomenclature

Suggested Reading

Lobprise HB, Dodd JR eds. Wiggs's Veterinary Dentistry: Principles and Practice, 2nd. Hoboken, NJ, Wiley-Blackwell; 2019.

Author Randi Brannan

Consulting Editor Heidi B. Lobprise

DEEP CUTANEOUS MYCOSES

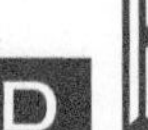

BASICS

DEFINITION

• Fungal infections that may secondarily disseminate by hematogenous route to the skin.
• Most often caused by cryptococcosis, blastomycosis, and coccidioidomycosis.

PATHOPHYSIOLOGY

Cryptococcosis

Main route of infection is inhalation and colonization of nasal mucosa, followed by hematogenous spread to lymph nodes, skin, bones, and CNS.

Blastomycosis

• Infection by inhalation of spores produced from mycelial growth in the environment.
• Spores settle in airways, transform into yeast forms, and establish a primary infection of the lungs, followed by dissemination via blood and lymphatic vessels.
• Colonize lymph nodes, skin, eyes, bones, CNS, and testes.

Coccidioidomycosis

• Infection by inhalation of arthroconidia.
• In the lungs, arthroconidia transform into spherules filled with endospores, which disseminate by hematogenous routes to bones, skin, eyes, heart, testes, CNS, liver, and kidneys, among others.

SYSTEMS AFFECTED

Systemic infections via inhalation with hematogenous dissemination to multiple organs—skin, lymph nodes, eyes, bones, CNS, testes.

GENETICS

N/A

INCIDENCE/PREVALENCE

• Uncommon diseases,
• Incidence depends on geographic location; can be very high (e.g., coccidioidomycosis in areas of Arizona).

GEOGRAPHIC DISTRIBUTION

Cryptococcosis

• *C. neoformans* worldwide distribution.
• *C. gattii* associated with tropical and subtropical climates.
• Recognized also in North America and British Columbia (Vancouver Island).

Blastomycosis

Areas of the United States and Canada surrounding the Ohio and Mississippi River valleys, the Great Lakes, and the Saint Lawrence River.

Coccidioidomycosis

Southwestern United States, Mexico, and areas of Central and South America.

SIGNALMENT

Cryptococcosis

• Young dogs and cats; more common in cats.
• Siamese, Birman, and ragdoll cats
• Doberman pinscher, German shepherd dogs, and cocker spaniels.

Blastomycosis

• Young dogs (1–3 years); rare in cats.
• Doberman pinscher.
• Increased incidence in male dogs

Coccidioidomycosis

• Young dogs; rare in cats.
• Boxer and Doberman pinscher predisposed.
• Increased incidence in males.

SIGNS

Historical Findings

• Nonspecific clinical signs (asthenia, weakness, anorexia, weight loss), respiratory signs, or the appearance of skin lesions in the animal.
• Upper respiratory signs—cryptococcosis and blastomycosis.
• Lameness—coccidioidomycosis.

Physical Examination Findings (Skin)

Cryptococcosis

• Cat—multiple papules, nodules, abscesses, and ulcers; bridge of nose/dorsal muzzle (primary site) or any skin ara; lesions may drain a serous exudate.
• Dog—papules, dermal-subcutaneous nodules or ulcers; located on any portion of the integument, lips, tongue, or claw beds.

Blastomycosis

Dog—draining tracts and abscesses in one-third of cases; *Planum nasale*, face, and claw bed most frequent locations.

Coccidioidomycosis

Dog—dermal nodules that progress to abscesses and ulcers, or draining tracts over sites of infected bone; *Coccidioides* infection may also be asymptomatic.

CAUSES

Cryptococcosis

• Dimorphic fungi.
• Filamentous form in the environment.
• Yeast phase in mammalian tissues.
• Genus *Cryptococcus* includes 40 species—most infections in dogs and cats caused by *C. neoformans* and *C. gattii.*
• *C. neoformans* often found in soils associated with bird excrement.
• *C. gattii* found in soils, especially in those covered with leaves of some tree species (eucalyptus), and in the bark of some trees (oak, maple, cedar).

Blastomycosis

• Dimorphic fungus.
• Mycelial form lives in moist soil and in decomposing organic matter such as wood and leaves.
• Yeast form in the mammal host causes disseminated infection.

Coccidioidomycosis

• Dimorphic saprophytic fungi.
• Found in sandy, alkaline soils with high environmental temperature.
• Main infectious species *Coccidioides immitis* and *C. posadasi.*

RISK FACTORS

• Immunosuppressed hosts are more predisposed to develop cryptococcosis caused by *C. neoformans.*
• Living in or visiting endemic areas increases risk of cryptococcosis (*C. gattii*), blastomycosis, and coccidioidomycosis.

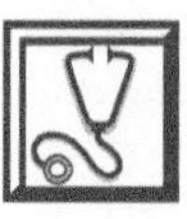

DIAGNOSIS

DIFFERENTIAL DIAGNOSIS

• Deep staphylococcal pyoderma.
• Nocardiosis.
• Actinomycosis.
• Mycobacterial infections.
• Pseudomycetoma (cat).
• Chromoblastomycosis.
• Pheohyphomycosis.
• Hyalohyphomycosis.
• Leishmaniasis.
• Sterile nodular panniculitis.
• Sterile pyogranuloma syndrome.
• Eosinophilic granuloma.

CBC/BIOCHEMISTRY/URINALYSIS

• Generally nonspecific—nonregenerative anemia, leukocytosis, monocytosis, eosinophilia.
• Serum biochemical profile may reflect specific organ involvement; hypoalbuminemia and hyperglobulinemia common.

OTHER LABORATORY TESTS

Cryptococcosis

• Detection of cryptococcal polysaccharide capsular antigen in serum using a latex agglutination technique.
• Organism can be cultured in Sabouraud agar from skin lesions.

Blastomycosis

Measuring antibodies in serum (agar gel immunodiffusion [AGID], ELISA) assists in diagnosis of blastomycosis when organisms cannot be specifically identified in cytologic or histologic specimens.

Coccidioidomycosis

• Conclusively diagnosed by cytologic or histologic visualization of the organism.
• Detection of antibodies (AGID, ELISA) commonly used when the organism cannot be demonstrated in cytology or biopsy samples.
• *Coccidioides* grows in common culture media.

- Exposure to mycelial growth in cultures a potential hazard to humans—organism should not be cultured outside of qualified laboratories with proper warning of the differential diagnosis.

IMAGING

- Radiographs-- evaluate for the presence of lesions in the upper airways, lungs, and bones.
- Ultrasound imaging—to evaluate for the presence of lesions in the abdominal cavity.

DIAGNOSTIC PROCEDURES

- Cytologic evaluation of all cutaneous lesions (papules, nodules, abscesses) by fine-needle aspirate of solid lesions or impression smears of exudates.
- Cytologic preparations usually reveal a pyogranulomatous exudate with the presence of the causal organism.
- Cryptococcosis—number of organisms is very high and they are easily detected.
- Blastomycosis and coccidioidomycosis—detection of the fungal elements more difficult. If cytologic preparations are inconclusive, a skin biopsy for histopathologic examination should be obtained.
- Histologically, these diseases are characterized by a nodular to diffuse pyogranulomatous dermatitis and panniculitis, with the presence of the causal organisms.

PATHOLOGIC FINDINGS

Chronic pyogranulomatous reaction with the presence of organisms in tissues.

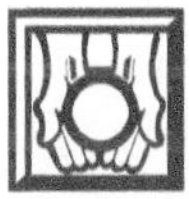

TREATMENT

APPROPRIATE HEALTH CARE

Outpatient medical management, unless severe internal lesions (meningoencephalitis, severe kidney disease).

NURSING CARE

N/A

ACTIVITY

Normal activity.

DIET

N/A

CLIENT EDUCATION

Owners should be informed of the risk involved in visiting areas where these infections are endemic.

SURGICAL CONSIDERATIONS

Surgical excision of large tissue masses infected with *Cryptococcus* (skin nodules, lymph nodes, nasopharyngeal masses) when possible.

MEDICATIONS

DRUG(S) OF CHOICE

Cryptococcosis

- Itraconazole (5 mg/kg PO q12–24h).
- Fluconazole (10 mg/kg PO q12–24h).
- Treatment maintained for 6–18 months—until resolution of clinical disease.
- Some authors recommend continued antifungal therapy until the cryptococcal antigen is zero.

Blastomycosis

- Itraconazole (5 mg/kg PO q12–24h).
- Fluconazole (10 mg/kg PO q12–24h).
- Treatment continued for at least 60 days and at least 1 month after all signs of disease have resolved.

Coccidioidomycosis

- Fluconazole (10 mg/kg PO q12–24h).
- Itraconazole (5 mg/kg PO q12–24h).
- Treatment is prolonged—treat for at least 1 year and/or until resolution of clinical disease.

PRECAUTIONS

N/A

POSSIBLE INTERACTIONS

Azole antifungals, especially ketoconazole, are inhibitors of cytochrome P450 (CYP) and can increase serum levels of other drugs that are metabolized by this route (e.g., cyclosporine).

ALTERNATIVE DRUG(S)

Cryptococcosis

Amphotericin B and flucytosine for CNS and/or resistant infection.

Blastomycosis

Amphotericin B for resistant infection.

Coccidioidomycosis

- Ketoconazole (5–10 mg/kg PO q12–24h)—if fluconazole or itraconazole is not available.
- Side effects more common and more severe with ketoconazole than with the other two azoles in cats.

CONTRAINDICATIONS

- Ketoconazole is hepatotoxic and should not be prescribed to patients with liver damage.
- Amphotericin B is nephrotoxic and is contraindicated in patients with kidney damage.

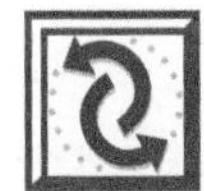

FOLLOW-UP

PATIENT MONITORING

The frequency of monitoring depends on the severity and location of the lesions.

PREVENTION/AVOIDANCE

Avoid visiting areas where these infections are endemic.

POSSIBLE COMPLICATIONS

N/A

EXPECTED COURSE AND PROGNOSIS

- Prognosis is guarded; depends on the affected organs.
- Poor prognosis with CNS involvement in cryptococcosis.

MISCELLANEOUS

ASSOCIATED CONDITIONS

N/A

ZOONOTIC POTENTIAL

- Cryptococcosis, blastomycosis, and coccidioidomycosis are not considered zoonoses.
- Infected dogs and cats pose no public health threat because infective forms are not produced in tissues.
- Handling mycelial cultures of the organism in the laboratory is dangerous.

PREGNANCY/FERTILITY/BREEDING

- Vertical transmission of cryptococcosis and blastomycosis has been reported in humans—considered extremely rare and not reported in dogs and cats.
- Intrauterine transmission of coccidioidomycosis not likely to occur because of the large size of the spherules.

SYNONYMS

- Cryptococcosis—torulosis, European blastomycosis.
- Blastomycosis—Gilchrist disease, Chicago disease.
- Coccidioidomycosis—valley fever, San Joaquín Valley fever.

ABBREVIATIONS

- AGID = agar gel immunodiffusion.

INTERNET RESOURCES

https://www.cdc.gov/fungal

Suggested Reading

Greene CG. Infectious Diseases of the Dog and Cat, 4th ed. St. Louis, MO: Elsevier, 2012.

Helton Rhodes KA, Werner A. Blackwell's Five-Minute Veterinary Consult Clinical Companion: Small Animal Dermatology, 3rd ed. Hoboken, NJ: Wiley-Blackwell, 2018.

Author Lluís Ferrer

Consulting Editor Alexander H. Werner Resnick

D

DEMODICOSIS

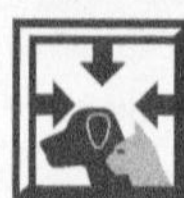

BASICS

DEFINITION

An inflammatory parasitic disease of dogs and cats characterized by an increased number of demodectic mites in the hair follicles and on the epidermis.

PATHOPHYSIOLOGY

Dogs

• Three species of mites identified in the dog: ○ *Demodex canis*—follicular mite; part of the normal fauna of the skin; typically present in small numbers; resides in the hair follicles and sebaceous glands of the skin, transmitted from the mother to the neonate during the first 2–3 days of nursing. ○ *Demodex injai*—large, long-bodied mite found in the pilosebaceous unit, mode of transmission unknown; only associated with adult-onset disease, with highest incidence noted in the terrier breeds often along the dorsal midline (West Highland white terrier and wirehaired fox terrier).○ *Demodex cornei*—lives in the stratum corneum of the epidermis; mode of transmission unknown; most likely a morphologic variant of *D. canis*. • Proliferation of mites may be the result of immunologic disorder, either genetic or iatrogenic. • Pruritus occurs when a secondary bacterial infection is present.

Cats

• Two species of mites identified in the cat: ○ *Demodex gatoi*—contagious; can be asymptomatic, but most commonly is associated with pruritic dermatitis leading to self-trauma, alopecia, and barbering. ○ *Demodex cati*— often associated with immunosuppressive and metabolic disease; these mites cause folliculitis and alopecia, but are rarely pruritic.

SYSTEMS AFFECTED

Skin/exocrine.

GENETICS

Initial proliferation of mites may be the result of a genetic disorder.

INCIDENCE/PREVALENCE

• Dogs—*D. canis* is very common. • Cats—depending on geographic location, *D. gatoi* may be common or rare; *D. cati* is rare.

SIGNALMENT

Species

Dogs and cats.

Breed Predilections

• *D. canis*—American Staffordshire terrier, shar-pei, Boston terrier, English bulldog, and West Highland white terrier. • *D. injai*—West Highland white and wirehaired fox terriers, shih tzu. • Potential increased incidence in Siamese and Burmese cats.

Mean Age and Range

• Juvenile onset, localized—usually in dogs <1 year of age; median 3–6 months, typically <5 lesions. • Generalized—both young and old animals. • *D. cati* may be more common in middle-aged or older cats; *D. gatoi* seems to be more common in younger cats and kittens, but any age can be affected.

SIGNS

Dogs

• Patchy alopecia—most common site is the face, especially around the perioral and periocular areas and forelegs; may also be seen on the trunk and feet. • Pododemodicosis—lesions localized to the feet. • Disease can progress to become or begin with a generalized distribution. • Usually not pruritic unless secondarily infected. • Hair follicles distended with large numbers of mites, lose hair and develop secondary bacterial folliculitis, followed by rupturing of the follicles (furunculosis). • With progression, the skin becomes severely inflamed, exudative, and granulomatous. • *D. injai* may be associated with greasy seborrheic dermatitis of the dorsal trunk, comedones, erythema, alopecia, and hyperpigmentation.

Cats

• *D. cati*—partial to complete alopecia of the eyelids, periocular region, head, neck, flank, and ventrum. • *D. gatoi*—pruritus with dramatic scaling, erythema, and/or crusting due to inflammation and self-trauma. • Ceruminous otitis externa has been reported. • *D. cati* often associated with immunosuppressive disease.

CAUSES

• Dog—*D. canis*, *D. injai*, and *D. cornei*. • Cat—*D. cati* and *D. gatoi*.

RISK FACTORS

Dogs

• Exact immunopathologic mechanism unknown. • Dogs with generalized demodicosis may have abnormal or depressed T-cell function. • Development associated with oclacitinib treatment. • Genetic factors (especially juvenile onset), immunosuppression, and/or metabolic diseases may predispose animal.

Cats

• *D. cati*—often associated with metabolic diseases that affect the immune system (e.g., feline immunodeficiency virus [FIV], hyperadrenocorticism, diabetes mellitus). • *D. gatoi*—considered contagious; cats in contact with other cats are at risk.

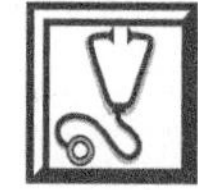

DIAGNOSIS

DIFFERENTIAL DIAGNOSIS

Dogs

• Bacterial folliculitis/ furunculosis. • Dermatophytosis. • Any cause of inflammatory alopecia.

Cats

• Allergic dermatitis. • Dermatophytosis. • Any cause of alopecia or pruritus.

CBC/BIOCHEMISTRY/URINALYSIS

Normal unless there is an underlying process.

OTHER LABORATORY TESTS

• Feline leukemia virus (FeLV) and FIV serology. • Fecal samples—rare finding of mites in feces; more common with cats.

DIAGNOSTIC PROCEDURES

• Skin scrapings diagnostic for finding mites in most cases—*D. gatoi* may be difficult to find. • Hair plucking can be used in areas such as eyelids. • Skin biopsy—may be needed when lesions are chronic, granulomatous, and fibrotic (especially on the foot); may be needed to diagnose demodicosis in the shar pei breed.

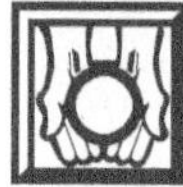

TREATMENT

APPROPRIATE HEALTH CARE

• Localized *D. canis* lesions often (90%) resolve spontaneously. • Evaluate the health status of patients presenting with generalized lesions of demodicosis.

CLIENT EDUCATION

• Localized—most cases resolve spontaneously. • Generalized—frequent management problem due to chronicity. Juvenile onset considered to have an inheritable predisposition—breeding of affected animals is not recommended.

MEDICATIONS

DRUG(S) OF CHOICE

Dogs

Isoxazolines antiparasitics

• Treatment of choice—excellent efficacy against demodicosis at label doses for fleas; safe for avermectin-sensitive dogs. • Side effects uncommon—vomiting, diarrhea, inappetence, or neurologic signs including seizures.

Ivermectin

• 0.3–0.6 mg/kg q24h PO very effective; initiate therapy with a test dose of 0.12 mg/kg q24h for first week to observe for any signs of sensitivity. • Treat for 30–60 days beyond negative skin scrapings (average 3–8 months). • Non-FDA-approved usage—do not use in avermectin-sensitive (ABCB-1 mutation) breeds.

Milbemycin Oxime

• 1–2 mg/kg PO q24h cures 50% of cases; 2 mg/kg PO q24h cures 85% of cases.

• ABCB-1 mutation individuals may have neurologic signs with higher doses; tolerate milbemycin better than other drugs in this class. • Non-FDA-approved usage.

Moxidectin

• 0.3 mg/kg PO q24h or topical application once weekly. • Non-FDA-approved usage—do not use in avermectin-sensitive (ABCB-1 mutation) breeds.

Amitraz

• Applied in the United States as a 250 ppm (0.025%) dip every 14 days and in Europe as a 500 ppm (0.05%) dip every 7 days. See adverse effects below. • Clipping the hair coat and bathing with a benzoyl peroxide shampoo before application of the rinse assist response. • Amitraz-containing collars and spot-ons are not effective. • Efficacy is proportional to the frequency of administration and the concentration of the rinse. • Poor compliance limits efficacy. • 11% and 30% of cases will not be cured; may need to try an alternative therapy or control with maintenance rinse every 2–8 weeks.

DRUG(S) OF CHOICE

Cats

Isoxazoline antiparasitics

• Treatment of choice at label doses for fleas. • Side effects uncommon but include drooling, vomiting, diarrhea, inappetence, or neurologic signs including seizures.

2% lime sulfur

• Can be diluted, sponged over the cat, and allowed to dry without rinsing once weekly for 6 treatments. • Malodorous, staining, and difficult to apply to the face. • Patient should be restricted from grooming after application.

Alternatives

Alternative but less effective options for the treatment of *D. gatoi*:

• Milbemycin oxime—1 mg/kg PO q24h.
• Doramectin—0.6 mg/kg SC weekly
• Ivermectin—0.2–0.3 mg/kg PO q24–48h. Neurologic side effects such as ataxia are possible with ivermectin.

CONTRAINDICATIONS

Do not use ivermectin in avermectin-sensitive breeds—collies, Shetland sheepdogs, Old English sheepdogs, Australian shepherds, other herding breeds, and crosses with these breeds. Screening for the ABCB-1 mutation is recommended.

PRECAUTIONS

Amitraz

• Side effects—somnolence, lethargy, depression, anorexia seen in 30% of patients for 12–36 hours after treatment. • Rare side effects—vomiting, diarrhea, pruritus, polyuria, mydriasis, bradycardia, hypoventilation, hypotension, hypothermia, ataxia, ileus, bloat, hyperglycemia, convulsions, death. • Yohimbine at 0.11 mg/kg IV is an antidote, as is atipamezole. • Incidence and severity of side effects do not appear to be proportional to dose or frequency of use. • Apply in a well-ventilated area; owners should wear aprons and gloves so they do not come in contact with the dip. • Human beings can develop dermatitis, headaches, and respiratory difficulty after exposure. Amitraz should not be used by people taking monoamine oxidase (MAO) inhibitors (e.g., some antihistamines, antidepressants, and antihypertensives). • Can dysregulate blood sugar in diabetics.

Ivermectin and Milbemycin

Signs of toxicity—salivation, vomiting, mydriasis, confusion, ataxia, hypersensitivity to sound, weakness, recumbency, coma, and death.

POSSIBLE INTERACTIONS

• Amitraz—may interact with heterocyclic antidepressants, xylazine, benzodiazepines, and macrocyclic lactones. • Ivermectin and milbemycin—cause elevated levels of monoamine neurotransmitter metabolites, which could result in adverse drug interactions with amitraz and benzodiazepines. • Spinosad and other drugs in that class are contraindicated with ivermectin therapy.

FOLLOW-UP

PATIENT MONITORING

Repeat skin scrapings and evidence of clinical resolution are used to monitor progress, generally repeated every 2–4 weeks until resolution, and then treatments are continued 1–2 months beyond negative scrapings.

PREVENTION/AVOIDANCE

Do not breed animals with generalized disease.

POSSIBLE COMPLICATIONS

Secondary bacterial folliculitis and furunculosis.

EXPECTED COURSE AND PROGNOSIS

Prognosis is very good for elimination of the demodicosis with isoxazoline treatment. Prognosis depends heavily on compliance, and genetic, immunologic, and underlying diseases. Severe, generalized cases with underlying disease may be refractory to treatments other than isoxazoline.

MISCELLANEOUS

D

ASSOCIATED CONDITIONS

• Adult-onset demodicosis—sudden occurrence is associated with internal disease, malignant neoplasia, and/or immunosuppressive disease; approximately 25% of cases are idiopathic over a follow-up period of 1–2 years. • *D. cati* associated with FeLV, FIV, toxoplasmosis, iatrogenic immune suppressants, papillomaviral plaques, and systemic lupus erythematosus (SLE).

AGE-RELATED FACTORS

Young dogs are often predisposed to a localized form.

ZOONOTIC POTENTIAL

None

PREGNANCY/FERTILITY/BREEDING

Do not breed animals with the generalized form.

SYNONYMS

• Mange. • Red mange.

SEE ALSO

Ivermectin and Other Macrocyclic Lactones Toxicosis.

ABBREVIATIONS

• FeLV = feline leukemia virus.
• FIV = feline immunodeficiency virus.
• MAO = monoamine oxidase.
• SLE = systemic lupus erythematosus.

Suggested Reading

Sastre N, Ravera I, Villanueva S, et al. Phylogenetic relationships in three species of canine *Demodex* mite based on partial sequences of mitochondrial 16S rDNA. Vet Derm 2012, 23(6):509–e101.

Author Melissa N.C. Eisenschenk

Consulting Editor Alexander H. Werner Resnick

Acknowledgment The author and book editors acknowledge the prior contribution of Karen Helton Rhodes.

Client Education Handout available online

DENTAL CARIES

BASICS

OVERVIEW

- Caries is the decay of the dental hard tissues (enamel, cementum, and dentin) due to the effects of oral bacteria on fermentable carbohydrates on the tooth surface.
- The word "caries" is Latin for rottenness and is both the singular and plural form.
- Oral bacteria ferment carbohydrates on the tooth surface, resulting in the production of acids leading to demineralization of the hard tissues, thus allowing bacterial and leukocytic digestion of the organic matrix of the tooth.
- Caries has been very common in humans in "westernized" society, where diets rich in highly refined carbohydrates are the norm. Aggressive public education and preventive measures have resulted in a decline in incidence over the past several decades.
- In humans, *Streptococcus mutans* is particularly implicated in the development of caries.
- For various reasons (e.g., diet lower in refined carbohydrates, higher salivary pH, lower salivary amylase, conical crown shape, wider interdental spacing, different indigenous oral flora), caries is not common in the domestic dog, but it does occur and should be looked for.
- A study published in the *Journal of Veterinary Dentistry* in 1998 (see Suggested Reading) reported that 5.3% of dogs 1 year of age or older had one or more caries lesions, with 52% having bilaterally symmetric lesions.
- Caries can affect the crown or roots of the teeth and is classified as pit-and-fissure, smooth-surface, or root caries.

SIGNALMENT

- Caries occurs in dogs.
- Reported in cats; tooth resorption (feline odontoclastic resorptive lesions [FORL]) has sometimes been misnamed feline caries. To the author's knowledge, there are no published reports of true dental caries occurring in the domestic cat, though it is theoretically possible.
- There is no reported breed, age, or gender predilection.
- Anecdotally, the author has observed a higher incidence of pit-and-fissure lesions in the occlusal tables of the maxillary first molar teeth in large-breed dogs such as Labrador retrievers and German shepherds.

SIGNS

- Incipient smooth-surface caries—appears as an area of dull, frosty-white enamel.
- Clinical caries—appears as a structural defect on the surface of the crown or root.
- The defect is frequently filled with or lined by dark, soft necrotic dentin. The defect may also trap and hold food debris.
- Affected dentin will yield to a dental explorer and can be removed with a dental excavator or curette.

CAUSES & RISK FACTORS

- Caries is caused by oral bacteria fermenting carbohydrates on the tooth surface, leading to the production of acids (acetic, lactic, propionic) that demineralize the enamel, cementum, and dentin, followed by digestion of the organic matrix of the tooth by oral bacteria and/or leukocytes.
- There is a constant exchange of minerals between the tooth surfaces (enamel, any exposed dentin or root cementum) and the oral fluids; if there is a net loss of mineral, caries develops.
- Early (incipient) caries may be reversible through remineralization.
- Once the protein matrix collapses, the lesion is irreversible.
- Any factors that allow prolonged retention of fermentable carbohydrates and bacterial plaque on the tooth surface predispose to the development of caries.
- A deep occlusal pit on the maxillary first molar is the most common place for caries to develop.
- Dental surfaces in close contact with an established caries are at risk of developing a lesion by extension.
- Deep occlusal pits and developmental grooves on the crown surface predispose to pit-and-fissure caries.
- Tight interdental contacts predispose to smooth-surface caries.
- Deep periodontal pockets predispose to root caries.
- Animals with poorly mineralized enamel, lower salivary pH, diets high in fermentable carbohydrates, and poor oral hygiene are at risk of developing caries.
- Loss of enamel through any means (hypocalcification at the developmental stage, abrasive wear or attrition, traumatic fracture) that exposes the softer, underlying dentin may increase the risk for the development of caries.

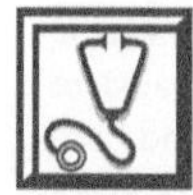

DIAGNOSIS

DIFFERENTIAL DIAGNOSIS

- Crown fracture, abrasive wear or attrition with exposed tertiary dentin, or extrinsic staining.
- Enamel hypocalcification with exposed and stained dentin.
- Tooth resorption (FORL) has been misnamed feline caries in the past.
- Tooth resorption can also occur in dogs and may be mistaken for caries.
- Sound dentin is hard and will not yield to a dental explorer, whereas carious dentin is soft and will yield to a sharp instrument.
- Root caries may be confused with external root resorption, though the distinction would often be academic, as either usually indicates the need for extraction.
- The lesion should be staged as to the depth of the pathology.
- Table 1 is adapted from the American Veterinary Dental College approved nomenclature for tooth resorption as published on its website.

CBC/BIOCHEMISTRY/URINALYSIS

N/A

IMAGING

Intraoral Dental Radiography

- Areas of demineralization and tissue loss will appear as lucent areas contrasted against radiodense normal dental tissues.
- If the lesion has penetrated into the pulp chamber, there will be endodontic disease, and periapical disease may be evident if the lesion is sufficiently longstanding.

Table 1

Stage 1	Defect involves enamel or cementum only.
Stage 2	Defect extends into dentin but not into pulp chamber.
Stage 3	Deep dental hard tissue loss (cementum and/or enamel with loss of dentin that extends to the pulp cavity); most of the tooth retains its integrity.
Stage 4	Extensive dental hard tissue loss (cementum and/or enamel with loss of dentin that extends to the pulp cavity); most of the tooth has lost its integrity.
Stage 5	Majority of crown lost; root remnants remaining.

• Small lesions may be difficult to demonstrate due to superimposition of normal, radiodense tissues (dental and skeletal).

DIAGNOSTIC PROCEDURES

• Visual examination of the clean, dry tooth surface under good light and with the aid of magnification.
• Exploration with a sharp dental explorer—the explorer will sink into carious dentin and stick, providing the sensation of "tug-back" upon withdrawal.
• Subgingival exploration—reveals irregularities in the root surface.
• Caries detection dyes have been used by human and veterinary dentists to aid in the differentiation between sound and carious dentinal tissue. However, their use may lead to false-positive results and overtreatment through the removal of excess tissue. Reliance on visual, tactile, and radiographic findings is preferable.

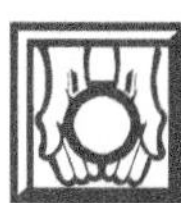

TREATMENT

• Focus on prevention—examine the adult dentition of adolescent dogs (6–8 months of age) to identify anatomically compromised areas at risk for the development of caries. Deep pits in the occlusal surface of the maxillary first molar (for example) can be filled with a pit-and-fissure sealant or fluoride-releasing dental bonding agent to prevent caries development if identified prior to the development of any decay.
• Incipient caries—can be arrested and possibly reversed by application of a fluoride varnish or fluoride-releasing dental bonding agent and modification of the risk factors.
• Lesions that result in mild to moderate coronal tissue loss (stage 1 or 2)—remove carious dentin and unsupported enamel using hand instruments and power rotary dental instruments, then restore the coronal anatomy with a bonded, composite restoration or prosthetic restoration.
• Lesions that extend into pulp tissue (stage 3)—endodontic treatment must precede restorative treatment. Alternatively, extraction may be indicated. As the pulp tissue in the roots will be contaminated, complete removal of all root remnants is essential if extraction is performed.
• Lesions that result in extensive coronal tissue loss (stage 4 or 5)—extraction is typically the only treatment option. As the pulp tissue in the roots will be contaminated, complete removal of all root remnants is essential.
• Root caries—if the periodontal disease can be managed and the restoration placed supragingivally, restoration may be possible; however, for most teeth with root caries, extraction will be the treatment of choice.
• If only one root of a multirooted tooth is carious—extraction of the affected root with endodontic treatment of the remaining root(s) is also an option.
• For high-risk patients—application of a pit-and-fissure sealant and/or fluoride-releasing dental bonding agent on remaining teeth with occlusal surfaces may be considered.

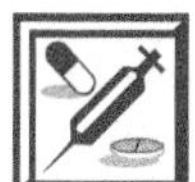

MEDICATIONS

DRUG(S) OF CHOICE

• Postoperative broad-spectrum antibiotics—may be indicated if there is pulp involvement necessitating endodontic treatment or extraction.
• Postoperative analgesia with nonsteroidal anti-inflammatory drugs and/or narcotics is indicated following endodontic or exodontic treatment or extensive restorative work of vital teeth.

CONTRAINDICATIONS/POSSIBLE INTERACTIONS

N/A

FOLLOW-UP

PATIENT MONITORING

• Examine and radiograph treated teeth 6 months postoperatively, then annually or as the opportunity presents.
• Evaluate the integrity of the restorations, assess for further decay at the margins or under the restorations, assess for the development of endodontic disease.
• As affected individuals frequently have more than one caries, examine all teeth carefully (clinically and radiographically) at any opportunity to monitor for the development of new lesions.

PREVENTION/AVOIDANCE

Avoidance of diet and treats high in refined carbohydrates may reduce the risk of the development of further caries.

EXPECTED COURSE AND PROGNOSIS

If a lesion has been properly debrided and restored it should have an excellent prognosis. Appropriate staging and case selection, thorough removal of all carious tissues, and adherence to restorative principles are essential.

MISCELLANEOUS

SYNONYMS

• Cavities.
• Dental decay.

ABBREVIATIONS

• FORL = feline odontoclastic resorptive lesions.

INTERNET RESOURCES

• http://www.toothvet.ca/PDFfiles/DentalCaries.pdf
• https://avdc.org/avdc-nomenclature
• http://www.toothvet.ca/PDFfiles/Tooth_resorption_in_cats.pdf
• http://www.toothvet.ca/PDFfiles/RLs_in_Dogs.pdf

Suggested Reading

Hale FA. Dental caries (cavities). In: Lobprise HB, ed., Blackwell's Five-Minute Veterinary Consult Clinical Companion: Small Animal Dentistry. Ames, IA: Blackwell, 2007, pp. 212–224.
Hale FA. Dental caries in the dog. J Vet Dent 1998, 15:79–83.
Hale FA. Veterinary dentistry. Dental caries in the dog. CVJ 2009, 50:1301–1304.
McComb D. Caries-detector dyes—how accurate and useful are they? J Can Dent Assoc 2000, 66:195–198. http://www.cda-adc.ca/jcda/vol-66/issue-4/195.html

Author Fraser A. Hale
Consulting Editor Heidi B. Lobprise

DENTIGEROUS CYST

D

BASICS

OVERVIEW

Cyst formation originating from tissue surrounding the crown of an unerupted tooth.

SIGNALMENT

- Any breed that is at an increased risk for impaired eruption.
- Boxers, bulldogs—mandibular first premolars, often bilateral.
- Unerupted teeth at 6–7 months of age, but cystic development may not occur until much later, if at all.

SIGNS

- Cystic changes may be initially unapparent without diagnostic imaging.
- "Missing" tooth.
- Formation of a soft swelling at the site of a missing tooth, often fluctuant with fluid.
- Patient may present, with no previous indication of a problem, for a pathologic fracture of the mandible due to cystic destruction of the surrounding bone.

CAUSES & RISK FACTORS

Unerupted teeth.

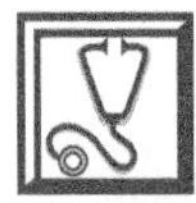

DIAGNOSIS

DIFFERENTIAL DIAGNOSIS

- Odontogenic keratocyst—cyst of the jaw demonstrating aggressive expansion that may, or may not, be associated with unerupted teeth.
- Primordial cyst—cystic degeneration of a tooth bud before enamel/dentin formation (cyst without a tooth).
- Oral mass—odontoma (complex or compound): tooth structures (enamel, dentin, cementum, and pulp) sometimes contained within cystic structure, but with different levels of organization.
- Transformation to ameloblastomas have been reported in humans; histologic evaluation of the cyst lining is highly recommended.

CBC/BIOCHEMISTRY/URINALYSIS

- No abnormalities typically found.
- Preoperative diagnostics where appropriate for safe administration of general anesthesia.

IMAGING

- Definitive diagnosis from radiography.
- Radiographs are essential in any instance of missing or unerupted teeth.
- Radiographically—radiolucent cyst originating from the remnant enamel organ at the neck of the tooth and encompassing the crown (a halo).
- CT studies of the head should evaluate for presence of unerupted teeth.

DIAGNOSTIC PROCEDURES

Histopathologic assessment if atypical radiographic findings (any unerupted teeth demonstrating radiolucency surrounding the unerupted crown should be submitted for histologic evaluation).

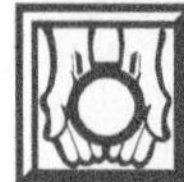

TREATMENT

- Appropriate preoperative antimicrobial and pain management therapy when indicated.
- Appropriate patient monitoring and support during anesthetic procedure.
- If cystic formation is present—surgical extraction, complete debridement of cyst lining, and histologic evaluation.
- If an embedded tooth has been present in a mature animal—assess for any cystic structure or other pathologic changes involving the tooth; continued monitoring (minimally yearly) may be reasonable if surgical extraction would damage large amounts of bone.
- If a nonstrategic tooth can be easily extracted, it would be best to do so, even if cystic changes are not present.

MEDICATIONS

DRUG(S) OF CHOICE

Postoperative analgesics, as necessary.

CONTRAINDICATIONS/POSSIBLE INTERACTIONS

N/A

FOLLOW-UP

POSSIBLE COMPLICATIONS

- Pathologic fracture may occur if dentigerous cyst is not diagnosed and treated.
- Fracture of mandible at time of extraction, due to compromised supporting bone.
- Cyst development and expansion result in weakening of the bone at that location and may risk causing root resorption or devitalization of neighboring teeth.

EXPECTED COURSE AND PROGNOSIS

- Extraction should be performed to avoid risk for future cyst development.
- Good with early detection and extraction.
- Fair to guarded with extensive bone destruction or pathologic fracture.

MISCELLANEOUS

INTERNET RESOURCES

https://avdc.org/avdc-nomenclature

Suggested Reading

Babbitt SG, Krakowski Volker M, Luskin IR. Incidence of radiographic cystic lesions associated with unerupted teeth in dogs. J Vet Dent 2016, 33(4):226–233.

Lobprise HB. Blackwell's Five-Minute Veterinary Consult Clinical Companion: Small Animal Dentistry. Ames, IA: Blackwell, 2007.

Lobprise HB, Dodd JR. Wigg's Veterinary Dentistry: Principles and Practice, 2nd ed. Ames, IA: Wiley-Blackwell, 2019.

Verstraete FJM, Zin BP, Kass PH, et al. Clinical signs and histologic findings in dogs with odontogenic cysts: 41 cases (1995–2010). J Am Vet Med Assoc 2011, 239(11):1470–1476.

White SC, Pharoah MJ. Oral Radiology Principles and Interpretation, 5th ed. St. Louis, MO: Mosby, 2004, pp. 388–392.

Author Christopher J. Snyder

Consulting Editor Heidi B. Lobprise

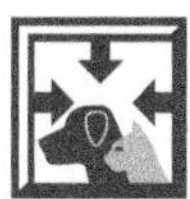

BASICS

DEFINITION

An inheritable inflammatory disease of the skin, muscles, and vasculature that develops in young collies, Shetland sheepdogs, and their crossbreeds.

PATHOPHYSIOLOGY

- The exact pathogenesis of dermatomyositis is unknown.
- A familial predisposition has been reported in collies and Shetland sheepdogs; however, possible triggers for the disease include infectious agents (especially viral), vaccines, drugs, malignancy, toxins, infection—as seen with ischemic dermatopathy in other breeds.
- Based on the clinical and histopathologic evidence, an immune-mediated or autoimmune process may be involved.

SYSTEMS AFFECTED

- Skin/exocrine.
- Musculoskeletal.

GENETICS

Autosomal dominant inheritance, with variable expression in collies and Shetland sheepdogs.

INCIDENCE/PREVALENCE

Exact prevalence is unknown.

SIGNALMENT

Species

Dogs

Breed Predilections

- Inheritable disease in collie, Shetland sheepdog and their crossbreeds, Beauceron shepherd, Belgian Tervuren, Rottweiler, kelpie, and Portuguese water dog.
- Similar symptoms reported in the mongrel, Welsh corgi, Lakeland terrier, chow chow, German shepherd dog, schipperke, and kuvasz.
- Dogs of other breeds with similar signs are classified as ischemic dermatopathy (dermatomyositis-like), and not dermatomyositis as previously reported.

Mean Age and Range

- Cutaneous lesions typically develop before 6 months, and may develop as early as 7 weeks of age.
- Full extent of lesions usually present by 1 year of age, and may lessen thereafter.
- Adult-onset dermatomyositis can occur, but is rare, and is usually less severe.

Predominant Sex

None reported.

SIGNS

General Comments

- Clinical signs vary from subtle skin lesions and subclinical myositis to severe skin lesions with generalized muscle atrophy, abnormal gait, and megaesophagus.
- Several littermates may be affected, but the severity of the disease often varies significantly among affected dogs.

Physical Examination Findings

- Waxing and waning lesions.
- Usually seen in affected dogs before 6 months of age.
- Begins around the eyes and lips, face, inner ear pinnae, tip of the tail, and bony prominences—the entire face may be involved.
- Pressure points over bony prominences, especially the carpal and tarsal regions.
- Characterized by variable degrees of crusted erosions, ulcers, and alopecia, with erythema, scaling, and scarring.
- Foot pad and oral ulcers, as well as nail abnormality or loss may occur.
- Scarring—often a sequela to the initial skin lesions.
- Atrophy of the masseter and temporal muscles—severe cases may have difficulty eating, drinking, and swallowing.
- Stiff or high-stepping gait.
- Myositis—signs may be absent or vary from subtle decrease in the mass of the temporalis muscles to generalized symmetric muscle atrophy and stiff high-stepping gait.
- Dogs with megaesophagus may present with aspiration pneumonia.

CAUSES

- Hereditary in collies, Shetland sheepdogs, and their crosses.
- Infectious agents, toxins, malignancy, vaccines, or drugs may be a triggering event.
- Immune-mediated disease in other breeds.

RISK FACTORS

Mechanical pressure and trauma, and ultraviolet light exposure may worsen cutaneous lesions.

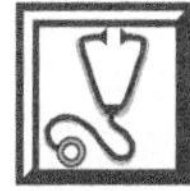

DIAGNOSIS

DIFFERENTIAL DIAGNOSIS

- Demodicosis.
- Dermatophytosis.
- Bacterial folliculitis.
- Juvenile cellulitis.
- Discoid lupus erythematosus.
- Systemic lupus erythematosus.
- Polymyositis.
- Ischemic dermatopathy.
- Epidermolysis bullosa simplex.

CBC/BIOCHEMISTRY/URINALYSIS

Serum creatine kinase may be elevated due to muscle damage.

OTHER LABORATORY TESTS

- Antinuclear antibody titers—rule out systemic lupus erythematosus.
- Elevated levels of immunoglobulin G and circulating immune complex correlated with disease severity.

DIAGNOSTIC PROCEDURES

- Skin biopsy—may be diagnostic for dermatomyositis, although this disease can be difficult to definitively diagnose; avoid infected and scarred lesions.
- Muscle biopsy—proper muscle selection can be difficult because pathologic changes may be mild consisting of muscle necrosis and atrophy.
- Electromyography (EMG)—ideally, used to select affected muscles for biopsy; if EMG is not available, atrophied muscles should be biopsied.

PATHOLOGIC FINDINGS

Skin Biopsy

- Scattered apoptosis or vacuolation of individual and follicular basal cells; may lead to intrabasal or subepidermal clefting.
- Mild pigmentary incontinence.
- Superficial, mild, diffuse dermal and perivascular cellular infiltrates—composed of lymphocytes, plasma cells, and histiocytes.
- Follicular atrophy and perifollicular fibrosis in chronic cases.
- Secondary epidermal ulceration and dermal scarring—may be present.
- Histopathologic features may be subtle and consist mostly of atrophic changes; however, the combination of epidermal and follicular basal cell degeneration, perivascular inflammation, and follicular atrophy with fibrosis is highly suggestive of dermatomyositis.

Muscle Biopsy

- Variable multifocal accumulations of inflammatory cells, including lymphocytes, plasma cells, macrophages, and neutrophils.
- Myofibril degeneration—characterized by fragmentation, vacuolation, atrophy, fibrosis, and regeneration.

EMG

EMG abnormalities are present especially in the muscles of the head and distal limbs; findings include fibrillation potentials (rapid, irregular, and unsynchronized contraction of muscle fibers) and positive sharp waves.

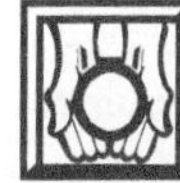

TREATMENT

APPROPRIATE HEALTH CARE

- Most dogs treated as outpatients.
- Dogs with severe myositis and megaesophagus may need hospitalization for supportive care.
- Severe cases may warrant euthanasia.
- Assist to eat if muscles of mastication are affected; feed at an elevated position if megaesophagus develops.
- Nonspecific supportive therapy includes gentle bathing and soaking to remove crusts, and treatment of secondary bacterial folliculitis (if present).

DERMATOMYOSITIS (CONTINUED)

D

ACTIVITY

- Avoid activities that may traumatize the skin.
- Keep indoors during the day to avoid solar radiation.

DIET

N/A

CLIENT EDUCATION

- Discuss the hereditary nature of the disease.
- Note that affected dogs should not be bred.
- Inform the owner that the disease is not curable, although spontaneous resolution or waxing and waning of symptoms may occur.
- Discuss prognosis and possible complications, especially in severely affected dogs.
- Therapeutic efficacy of medical treatment can be difficult to assess because the disease tends to be cyclic in nature and is often self-limiting.

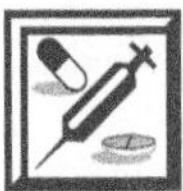

MEDICATIONS

DRUG(S) OF CHOICE

- Vitamin E 200–800 IU PO q12–24h.
- Essential fatty acid supplement.
- Prednisolone 1–2 mg/kg PO q12–24h until remission, then alternate-day to twice-weekly administration using the lowest dosage possible for long-term control.
- Nonsteroidal anti-inflammatory medication (if steroids contraindicated).
- Pentoxifylline 10–20 mg/kg PO q12h.
- Tetracycline (250 mg >10 kg, 500 mg <10 kg PO q8–12h), doxycycline (10 mg/kg q24h), minocycline (5 mg/kg q12h), with niacinamide (250 mg >10kg, 500 mg <10 kg PO q8–12h).
- Tacrolimus 0.1% applied q12h.
- Oclacitinib 0.4-0.6mg/kg BID.

PRECAUTIONS

- Pentoxifylline—rarely causes gastric irritation; can affect clotting times (prothrombin time [PT]/partial thromboplastin time [PTT] prolongation and thrombocytopenia) and dogs receiving anticoagulant therapy should be monitored carefully when treated with this drug; possible rare seizure or reduction of seizure threshold in epileptics.
- Glucocorticoids—discuss possible side effects with the owner.
- Tacrolimus can cause local irritation.

POSSIBLE INTERACTIONS

Glucocorticoids and nonsteroidal anti-inflammatory medications can cause gastrointestinal bleeding if used concurrently.

ALTERNATIVE DRUG(S)

N/A

FOLLOW-UP

PREVENTION/AVOIDANCE

- Do not breed affected animals.
- Neuter intact animals to reduce hormonal influence on symptoms.
- Minimize trauma and exposure to sunlight.

POSSIBLE COMPLICATIONS

- Secondary bacterial folliculitis.
- Mildly to moderately affected dogs may have residual scarring.
- Severely affected dogs may have trouble chewing, drinking, and swallowing due to scarring of the masticatory and esophageal muscles.
- Megaesophagus may develop, predisposing the dog to aspiration pneumonia.
- Dogs may be lame due to damage of the muscles of the extremities.

EXPECTED COURSE AND PROGNOSIS

- Long-term prognosis—variable, depending on severity of disease.
- Minimal disease—prognosis good; tends to spontaneously resolve with no evidence of scarring.
- Mild to moderate disease—tends to resolve spontaneously, but residual scarring is common.
- Severe disease—prognosis for long-term survival is poor as damage to the skin and muscle may be lifelong.

MISCELLANEOUS

ASSOCIATED CONDITIONS

None

AGE-RELATED FACTORS

- Initial clinical signs usually occur in dogs younger than 6 months.
- Adult onset—rare; more commonly seen in dogs that had subtle lesions as puppies.

ZOONOTIC POTENTIAL

None

PREGNANCY/FERTILITY/BREEDING

- Do not breed affected dogs.
- Pregnancy may exacerbate clinical symptoms.
- Estrus may exacerbate clinical symptoms.

SYNONYMS

- Familial canine dermatomyositis.
- Canine familial dermatomyositis.
- Ischemic dermatopathy in collies and Shetland sheepdogs.

SEE ALSO

- Lupus Erythematosus, Cutaneous (Discoid).
- Lupus Erythematosus, Systemic (SLE).

ABBREVIATIONS

- EMG = electromyography, electromyographic.
- PT = prothrombin time.
- PTT = partial thromboplastin time.

Suggested Reading

Bresciani F, Zagnoli L, Fracassi F, et al. Dermatomyositis-like disease in Rottweiler. Vet Dermatol 2014, 25(3):229–e62.

Carlotti DN, Grucker S, Germain PA. Dermatomyositis in a four month old schipperke. Pratique Medicale et Chirurgicale de l'Animal de Compagnie 2005, 40(3):141–144.

Gross TL, Ihrike PJ, Walder EJ, Affolter VK. Skin Diseases of the Dog and Cat, 2nd ed. Oxford: Blackwell Science, 2005, pp. 49–52, 503–505.

Hargis AM, Mundell AC. Familial canine dermatomyositis. Compend Contin Educ Pract Vet 1992, 14:855–864.

Helton Rhodes KA, Werner A. Blackwell's Five-Minute Veterinary Consult Clinical Companion: Small Animal Dermatology, 3rd ed. Hoboken, NJ: Wiley-Blackwell, 2018.

Levy BJ, Linder KE, Olivry T. The role of oclacitinib in the management of ischemic dermatopathy in four dogs. Vet Dermatol 2019, 30(3): 201–208.

Rothing A, Rufenacht S, Welle MM. Dermatomyositis in family of working Kelpies. Tierarztl Prax Ausg K Kleintiere Heimtiere 2015, 43(5):331–336.

Wahl JM, Clark LA, Skalli O, et al. Analysis of gene transcript profiling and immunobiology in Shetland sheepdog with dermatomyositis. Vet Dermatol 2008, 19(2):52–58.

Author Liora Waldman

Consulting Editor Alexander H. Werner Resnick

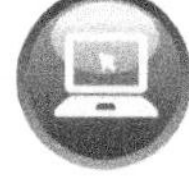

Client Education Handout available online

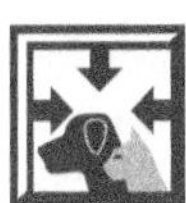

BASICS

OVERVIEW

• "Mud rash" or "mud fever." • Caused by *Dermatophilus congolensis*. • Rare crusting dermatitis (dogs). • Rare nodular subcutaneous and oral disease (cats). • Systems affected—skin/exocrine.

SIGNALMENT

• Dogs and cats. • No age, breed, or sex predilection.

SIGNS

Historical Findings

• Association with cattle, sheep, or horses.
• Occasionally free-roaming dogs. • Cats with subcutaneous disease—episode of trauma; existence of a foreign body; lesions generally chronic; no systemic clinical signs, except when internal organs or large oral lesions develop.

Physical Examination Findings

• Dogs—lesions: circular to coalescent, papular, crusted skin lesions on the head and/or trunk, lesions resemble superficial bacterial pyoderma caused by *Staphylococcus pseudintermedius*; lesions may resemble dermatophilosis in horses (adherent thick, gray-yellow crusts that incorporate hair and leave a circular, glistening, shallow erosion when removed); pruritus is variable. • Cats—subcutaneous, oral, or internal ulcerated and fistulated nodules or abscesses similar to lesions caused by other actinomycetes in this species; superficial pyogenic crusting disease of the face has been reported.

CAUSES & RISK FACTORS

• *D. congolensis*—causative agent; Gram-positive, branching filamentous bacterium classified as an actinomycete; very common cause of crusting dermatoses in hoofed animals; persists in the environment within crusts. • Dogs, cats, and humans can be exposed directly from lesions on large animals or from environmental exposure. • Infectious stage—requires wetting for activation; cannot penetrate intact epithelium; minor trauma or mechanical transmission by biting ectoparasites (*Amblyomma variegatum*) may help in establishing infection.
• Deeper infections—require traumatic inoculation of infectious material.

DIAGNOSIS

DIFFERENTIAL DIAGNOSIS

Dogs

• Staphylococcal folliculitis. • Acute moist dermatitis. • Dermatophytosis. • Pemphigus foliaceus. • Keratinization disorder.

Cats

• Infections—actinomycosis, nocardiosis, sporotrichosis, cryptococcosis, opportunistic mycobacterial granuloma, *Rhodococcus equi*.• Foreign body. • Bite wound abscess.
• Cutaneous or mucosal neoplasia.

CBC/BIOCHEMISTRY/URINALYSIS

Usually normal.

DIAGNOSTIC PROCEDURES

Dogs

• Cytologic examination of exudate from under crusts or of macerated crusts.
• Biopsy—crusts contain organisms; submit with tissue samples. • Distinctive morphology of organism in cytologic and histopathologic preparations; bacterium forms branching chains of small diplococci resembling "railroad tracks." • Real-time quantitative polymerase chain reaction (RT-qPCR)—crust samples and hair.

Cats

• Histopathologic examination—biopsy of nodules; procedure of choice. • Culture from crusts or tissues—alert laboratory of differential; requires use of special selective medium; isolation is possible but usually very difficult.
• RT-qPCR—crust samples and hair.

PATHOLOGIC FINDINGS

• Dogs—crusting and superficial pustular dermatitis; palisading of the crusts with orthokeratotic and parakeratotic hyperkeratosis; organism visualized within the crusts. • Cats—pyogranulomatous inflammation; central necrosis; fistulous tract formation; organism visualized near the necrotic center of granulomas, especially with Gram stain.

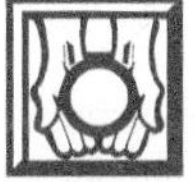

TREATMENT

• Dogs—antibacterial shampoo with gentle removal of crusts: iodine or lime-sulfur may also be used. • Cats—for pyogranulomas and abscesses: surgical debridement; exploration for foreign body; establishment of drainage for exudate.

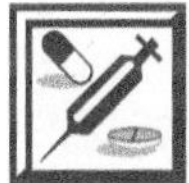

MEDICATIONS

DRUG(S) OF CHOICE

• Treatment should be continued for 10–20 days. • Penicillin V (10 mg/kg PO q12h) for 10–20 days; drug of choice. • Tetracycline (22–30 mg/kg PO q8h); doxycycline (5–10 mg/kg PO q12h); minocycline (5–12 mg/kg PO q12h. • Ampicillin 10–20 mg/kg PO q12h. • Amoxicillin 10–20 mg/kg PO q12h.

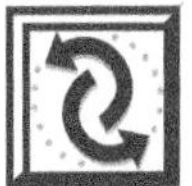

FOLLOW-UP

PATIENT MONITORING

• Dogs—reexamine after 2 weeks of treatment to ensure complete resolution; give an additional 7 days of systemic therapy if indicated. • Cats—monitor biweekly for 1 month after apparent resolution of lesions, depending on location.

EXPECTED COURSE AND PROGNOSIS

• Dogs—excellent. • Cats—varies with the location of lesions and extent of surgical debridement; complete resolution can be achieved with early diagnosis and medical/surgical therapy.

MISCELLANEOUS

ZOONOTIC POTENTIAL

• Veterinarians and animal care workers—infection uncommon even with exposure to infected farm animals.
• Dogs and cats—very unlikely to serve as a source for human infection; caution is warranted for exposure of immunocompromised individuals.

ABBREVIATIONS

• RT-qPCR = real-time quantitative polymerase chain reaction.

Suggested Reading

Frank LA, Kania SA, Weyant E. RT-qPCR for the diagnosis of dermatophilosis in horses. Vet Dermatol 2016, 27(5):431–e112.

Hirazumi M, Tagawa Y. Isolation and characterization of flagellar filament from zoospores of Dermatophilus congolensis. Vet Microbiol 2014, 173(1–2):141–146.

Author Mitchell D. Song

Consulting Editor Alexander H. Werner Resnick

DERMATOPHYTOSIS

BASICS

DEFINITION

- Cutaneous fungal infection affecting the cornified regions of hair, claws, and occasionally the superficial layers of the skin.
- *Microsporum* and *Trichophyton* dermatophytes are most commonly isolated.

PATHOPHYSIOLOGY

- Dermatophytes—grow in the keratinized layers of hair, claw, and skin; do not thrive in living tissue.
- Exposure to or contact with a dermatophyte does not necessarily result in an infection. Infection may not result in clinical signs.
- 2–4-week incubation period.
- Infective spores must contact the skin surface and defeat host-protective mechanisms (innate immunity, normal flora, sebum, grooming) in order for infection to occur.
- Factors that favor the development of disease—stress, trauma, ectoparasite infestations, and immunosuppression.
- Infected animals may remain as asymptomatic (inapparent) carriers for a prolonged period of time; some animals never become symptomatic.

SYSTEMS AFFECTED

Skin/exocrine.

INCIDENCE/PREVALENCE

- Lesions may mimic many dermatologic conditions; overdiagnosis is likely common.
- Infection rates (inapparent and clinical) vary widely, depending on the population studied.

GEOGRAPHIC DISTRIBUTION

- More common in hot, humid climates.
- Incidence of dermatophyte species may vary seasonally and geographically.
- *M. canis*—cats: UK, southern United States, Italy, and Brazil; source most often infected cat.
- *M. gypseum*—dogs: southern United States; less than 1% in UK; source most often soil.
- *M. persicolor*—India, Brazil, and North America; source most often associated with rodents.
- *T. mentagrophytes*—India and UK; less common in southern United States, Italy, and Brazil; source most often associated with rodents.

SIGNALMENT

Species

Dog, cat, and many others.

Breed Predilections

- Cat—longhaired breeds (Persian and Himalayan).
- Dog—Yorkshire terrier and Manchester terrier. Increased exposure in working and hunting dogs.

Mean Age and Range

- *M. canis* is more common in younger animals.
- Generalized dermatophytosis in older dogs associated with immunosuppression.

SIGNS

Physical Examination Findings

- Inapparent carrier state—cats.
- Extreme variability of clinical signs.
- Classic lesion—slowly expanding circular patch of alopecia with scale.
- Seborrheic or greasy hair coat.
- Papular or pustular eruptions.

CAUSES

Multiple species identified; majority of cases caused by *M. canis*, *M. gypseum*, *T. mentagrophytes*, and *M. persicolor* (nonfollicular).

RISK FACTORS

- Immunocompromise caused by medications or disease.
- High population density.
- Poor management practices.

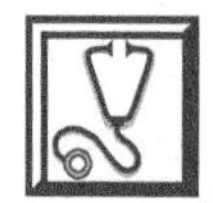

DIAGNOSIS

DIFFERENTIAL DIAGNOSIS

- Staphylococcal folliculitis.
- Demodicosis.
- Allergic dermatitis.
- Pemphigus foliaceus.
- Keratinization defect.

DIAGNOSTIC PROCEDURES

Wood's Lamp Examination

- Can be misleading—not all *M. canis* isolates fluoresce; most other pathogenic dermatophytes do not fluoresce.
- True positive reaction—apple-green fluorescence of the hair shaft. False-positive and false-negative results commonly due to debris on the hair and skin, inadequate equipment, and/or poor technique.

Microscopic Examination of Hair

- Choose hairs that fluoresce under Wood's lamp illumination to increase success.
- Hyphae and arthrospores seen invading hair shafts.

Fungal Culture with Identification

- Choose hairs that fluoresce under Wood's lamp if possible.
- Pluck hairs from the periphery of an alopecic area or brush haircoat with a sterile toothbrush or carpet square (especially inapparent or treated patients).
- Dermatophyte test media—dermatophytes change media color to red during the early growing phase of the culture; saprophytes cause color change after significant colony growth; examine inoculated media daily.
- Fungal colonies are nonpigmented/white to slightly yellow. Contaminants are often darker.
- Microscopic examination of the growth for microconidia and macroconidia—necessary to confirm pathogenic dermatophyte and to identify genus and species; helps identify source of infection.
- Positive culture—indicates presence of a dermatophyte; however, organisms may be transient (i.e., geophilic dermatophytes on the feet).

Skin Biopsy

- Not usually required for diagnosis.
- Can be helpful in confirming true invasion and infection, or to diagnose suspicious cases with negative fungal culture.

PCR

PCR of the dermatophyte DNA on the hair samples may be helpful. Positive PCR does not necessarily indicate active infection—dead fungal organisms from a successfully treated infection may be detected on PCR, as will inapparent carriers.

PATHOLOGIC FINDINGS

- Folliculitis, perifolliculitis, or furunculosis.
- Fungal hyphae seen in H&E-stained sections; special stains allow easier visualization of the organism.

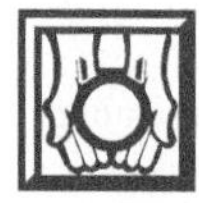

TREATMENT

APPROPRIATE HEALTH CARE

Quarantine owing to the infective and zoonotic nature of the disease.

CLIENT EDUCATION

- Many shorthaired cats and many dogs will undergo spontaneous remission within 3 months.
- Longhaired animals should be clipped to reduce environmental contamination.
- Decontamination of the environment reduces the risk of false positive fungal cultures, which can lead to prolonged treatment and confinement.
- Infective spores are shed into the environment, but do not multiply in the environment; transmission of the disease strictly from a contaminated environment (i.e., no direct contact with an infected animal) is extremely rare.
- Effective disinfectants.
- Diluted sodium hypochlorite (0.5%)—concentrations ranging from 1 : 10 to 1 : 100 effective with short contact times.
- Enilconazole (0.2%)—available as a concentrated spray or fogger; 10-minute contact time recommended. Not available in the United States.
- Accelerated hydrogen peroxide—should not be mixed with concentrated sodium hypochlorite products; 10-minute contact time recommended.
- Washable textiles—decontaminate via mechanical washing; two washings on the

longest wash cycle in a washing machine found to be effective.
• Treatment can be both frustrating and expensive, especially in multianimal households or with recurrent cases; consider referral to a veterinary dermatologist.

MEDICATIONS

DRUG(S) OF CHOICE

• Topical therapy and clipping— recommended concurrently with systemic therapy; may help prevent environmental contamination.
• Lime-sulfur (1 : 16 dilution or 8 oz per gallon of water), miconazole/chlorhexidine (0.2%), or enilconazole (0.2%) applied once to twice weekly; lime sulfur is odoriferous and can stain; enilconazole is not currently approved for use in companion animals in the United States. Shampoos containing 1–2% ketoconazole, miconazole, or 0.5% climbazole; a minimum of a 3-minute contact time is recommended; little to no residual effect.
• Use of an Elizabethan collar, particularly in cats, is recommended to prevent ingestion of these products.
• Itraconazole—dogs and cats: 5–10 mg/kg PO q24h in one-week-on, one-week-off schedule for minimum of 3 cycles; manufactured drug preferred over compounded formulations due to absorption/concentration variability. Compounded formulations have been shown to be of extremely variable efficacy.
• Ketoconazole—resistance reported (10 mg/kg q24h PO); not recommended in cats.
• Griseofulvin—effective, but use declining due to cost and requirement for monitoring.
• Terbinafine—effective, may be helpful in cases resistant to azole drugs; dogs: 20–30 mg/kg q12–24h for 4–8 weeks; cats: 20–40 mg/kg q24–48h for 4–8 weeks; dermatophyte carriers: 8.25 mg/kg q24h for 4–8 weeks; side effects may include gastrointestinal upset, hepatotoxicity, neutropenia, and pancytopenia.
• Antifungal vaccines have not been shown to protect against challenge exposure.

CONTRAINDICATIONS

• Corticosteroids—can modulate inflammation and prolong the infection.
• Griseofulvin—do not administer to cats with feline leukemia virus (FeLV) or feline immunodeficiency virus (FIV); teratogen.

PRECAUTIONS

Ketoconazole

• Hepatopathy has been reported and can be severe in cats.
• Inhibits endogenous production of steroid hormones in dogs.

Itraconazole

• Rare vasculitis and ulcerative skin lesions at doses of 5 mg/kg q12h; not noted in patients receiving 5 mg/kg q24h.
• Hepatotoxicity reported infrequently in dogs.

Terbinafine

• Gastrointestinal upset, hepatotoxicity, and bone marrow suppression (pancytopenia, neutropenia).
• Decrease dosage with renal and/or hepatic insufficiency.
• Concurrent administration with Cimetidine increases blood concentration; rifampin decreases blood concentration.

Lime-Sulfur Solution

Ingestion of lime-sulfur may lead to oral erosions.

ALTERNATIVE DRUG(S)

• Lufenuron—a chitin synthesis inhibitor used in flea control; not effective in controlled studies.
• Fluconazole—less effective option, but less expensive than itraconazole.

FOLLOW-UP

PATIENT MONITORING

• Dermatophyte culture required to monitor response to therapy; many animals clinically improve but remain culture-positive.
• Continue treatment until at least two subsequent cultures are negative.
• In resistant cases, cultures should be repeated weekly using the toothbrush technique.
• Weekly or biweekly CBC if treating with griseofulvin; periodic evaluation of liver enzymes if treating with ketoconazole, itraconazole, or terbinafine.
• Depending on which systemic medications used, appropriate follow-up should be performed due to potential side effects.

PREVENTION/AVOIDANCE

• Initiate a quarantine period and obtain dermatophyte cultures of all animals entering the household to prevent reinfection from inapparent carriers.
• Consider exposure based on species isolated.
• Decontaminate the environment.
• Consider prophylactic treatment of exposed animals.

POSSIBLE COMPLICATIONS

False-negative dermatophyte culture.

EXPECTED COURSE AND PROGNOSIS

• Many animals will "self-clear" infection over a period of a few months.
• Treatment hastens clinical cure and helps reduce environmental contamination.
• Some infections, particularly in longhaired cats or multianimal situations, can be persistent.

MISCELLANEOUS

ZOONOTIC POTENTIAL

• Dermatophytosis is zoonotic.
• Considered a low-level pathogen; disease is not life-threatening, can be easily treated, but may cause scarring.

PREGNANCY/FERTILITY/BREEDING

• Griseofulvin is teratogenic.
• Ketoconazole can affect steroidal hormone synthesis, especially testosterone.

SYNONYMS

Ringworm

ABBREVIATIONS

• FeLV = feline leukemia virus.
• FIV = feline immunodeficiency virus.

Suggested Reading

Bond R. Superficial veterinary mycoses. Clin Dermatol 2010, 28(2):226–236. doi: 10.1016/j.clindermatol.2009.12.012

Miller WH, Griffin CE, Campbell KL. Muller & Kirk's Small Animal Dermatology, 7th ed. Philadelphia, PA: Saunders, 2013, pp. 5226–5241.

Moriello KA, Coyner K, Paterson S, Mignon B. Diagnosis and treatment of dermatophytosis in dogs and cats. Vet Dermatol 2017, 28(3). doi: 10.1111/vde.12440

Authors W. Dunbar Gram and Andhika Putra

Consulting Editor Alexander H. Werner Resnick

Acknowledgment The authors and book editors acknowledge the previous contribution of Sheena Narine-Reece

Client Education Handout available online

DERMATOSES, DEPIGMENTING DISORDERS

D

BASICS

DEFINITION

• Pathologic or cosmetic condition involving loss of pigmentation of the skin and/or hair coat, either by lack of pigmentation or by melanocyte damage. • Leukotrichia—whitening of the hair (nonspecific location). • Poliosis—whitening of hair on the head/face. • Leukoderma—whitening of the skin.

PATHOPHYSIOLOGY

• Melanocytes may be damaged or destroyed by toxins (including toxic melanin precursors), inflammatory mediators, auto-antibodies, and/or inhibitors of melanogenesis. • Diseases may be distinguished clinically by depigmentation as the initial symptom versus depigmentation occurring secondary to inflammation.

SYSTEMS AFFECTED

• Skin/exocrine. • Ophthalmic.

SIGNALMENT

• Mucocutaneous pyoderma—German shepherd dog. • Systemic lupus erythematosus (SLE)—German shepherd dog. • Discoid lupus erythematosus (DLE)—collie, Shetland sheepdog, German shepherd dog, Siberian husky; may occur more often in females. • Pemphigus foliaceus (PF)—chow chow, Akita, cocker spaniel, dachshund, Labrador retriever. • Uveodermatologic syndrome—Akita, Samoyed, Siberian husky. • Vitiligo—dogs: Belgian Tervuren, German shepherd dog, Doberman pinscher, Rottweiler, German shorthaired pointer, Old English sheepdog, dachshund; usually less than 3 years of age; cats: Siamese. • Seasonal nasal hypopigmentation—Siberian husky, Alaskan Malamute, Labrador retriever, golden retriever. • Epitheliotropic lymphoma (mycosis fungoides)—typically dogs >10 years old. • Proliferative arteritis of the nasal philtrum—Saint Bernard, giant schnauzer. • Periocular leukotrichia—Siamese cat. • Chediak-Higashi syndrome—Persian cat.

SIGNS

• Leukotrichia. • Leukoderma. • Lightening of the pigmentation in the skin (seen as a "graying" or "browning" of previously pigmented areas). • Erythema. • Erosion and ulcerations.

CAUSES

• Mucocutaneous pyoderma. • DLE. • SLE. • PF. • Pemphigus erythematosus (PE). • Uveodermatologic syndrome. • Contact hypersensitivity. • Vitiligo. • Seasonal nasal depigmentation. • Albinism. • Schnauzer gilding syndrome. • Endocrinopathy. • Drug reaction. • Erythema multiforme (EM). • Proliferative arteritis of the nasal philtrum. • Postinflammatory depigmentation. • Immune-mediated pigmentary incontinence. • Oculocutaneous albinism.

RISK FACTORS

• Sun exposure—DLE, SLE, and PE. • Drug triggered—PF, EM.

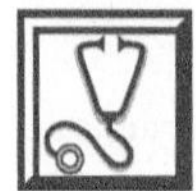

DIAGNOSIS

DIFFERENTIAL DIAGNOSIS

Mucocutaneous Pyoderma

• Biopsy—epidermal hyperplasia with superficial pustulation. • Depigmentation is secondary and develops with chronicity. • Skin lesions—affects the lips, perioral area, and nasal/alar folds. • Clinically similar to intertrigo (skinfold bacterial folliculitis). • Swelling and fissuring lead to erosions and crusts. • ++Biopsy—epidermal hyperplasia with superficial pustulation. • Antibiotic responsive. • Frequent recurrence if due to an underlying cause.

Nasal Solar Dermatitis

• Depigmentation is secondary and develops with chronicity. • Lesions confined primarily to dorsal muzzle and precipitated by sun exposure. • Begins in poorly pigmented skin at the junction of the nasal planum and dorsal muzzle. • Negative for direct immunofluorescence. • Solar vasculopathy may appear similar.

DLE

• Depigmentation is a primary symptom. • Primarily affects nasal area, eyelid margins, and lip margins. • Exacerbated by sun exposure. • Positive direct immunofluorescence at basement membrane zone. • Biopsy—interface dermatitis.

SLE

• Depigmentation is a primary symptom. • Multisystemic disease. • Skin lesions—often involve nose, face, and mucocutaneous junctions; multifocal or generalized. • Antinuclear antibody (ANA)—may be positive. • Positive direct immunofluorescence at basement membrane zone.

PF

• Depigmentation develops with chronicity. • Initial lesions on face and ears; commonly involve footpads; eventually generalized. • Biopsy—subcorneal pustules with acantholysis. • Positive direct immunofluorescence in intercellular spaces of epidermis.

PE

• Depigmentation is a primary symptom. • Lesions—primarily confined to face and ears, nasal planum, and lip margins. • Depigmentation often precedes significant lesions. • Exacerbated by sun exposure. • Biopsy—intraepidermal pustules with acantholysis and interface dermatitis. • Positive direct immunofluorescence at basement membrane zone and intercellular spaces. • ANA—occasionally positive.

Uveodermatologic Syndrome

• Depigmentation is a primary symptom. • Uveitis—usually precedes dermatologic disease. • Cutaneous macular depigmentation with inflammation on nose, lips, and eyelids. • Striking poliosis and leukotrichia. • Biopsy of early lesions—interface dermatitis, pigmentary incontinence.

Others

• Contact dermatitis (uncommon)—depigmentation secondary due to chronicity; erythema of rostral nasal planum and lips; no ulceration and minimal crusting; history of exposure. • Vitiligo—depigmentation often without inflammation; cutaneous macular depigmentation on nose, lips, eyelids, footpads, and nails; concurrent leukotrichia. • Seasonal nasal hypopigmentation—depigmentation is a primary symptom; normal black coloration of nasal planum fades to light tan or pink; usually seasonal or slowly progressive with age. • Albinism—hereditary lack of pigment of the skin, hair coat, and irises (not a depigmenting process). • Aurotrichia—young miniature gray schnauzers may develop idiopathic golden hair coat coloration, primarily of the trunk. • Endocrinopathy may cause coat color change, mainly from black to reddish-brown. • Drug reaction—depigmentation is often secondary; resembles many cutaneous disorders such as DLE, SLE, PF, and PE; pruritus is variable; onset of symptoms is usually within 2 weeks of administration. • Proliferative arteritis of the nasal philtrum—depigmentation is secondary and develops with chronicity; marked focal ulceration of the nasal planum often resulting in acute, severe hemorrhage; no additional skin lesions noted; this may be an idiopathic syndrome associated with allergy. • Dermatophytosis— depigmentation is secondary and develops with chronicity; especially develops on the dorsal muzzle and face; hyperpigmentation may also occur, especially with *Tricophyton mentagrophytes* infection. • Epitheliotropic lymphoma—depigmentation is secondary and develops with chronicity; occurs in mucocutaneous areas, nose, and skin. • EM in dogs—classic annular lesions with a clear center; depigmentation is secondary and develops with chronicity. • Zinc deficiency—depigmentation may be a primary or secondary symptom; zinc is required for normal melanin synthesis. • Chediak-Higashi syndrome—depigmentation is a primary symptom; young Persian cats (blue smoke color); ophthalmologic signs, prolonged bleeding. • Cyclic neutropenia in young silver-gray collie dogs with light-colored nose.

CBC/BIOCHEMISTRY/URINALYSIS

• Usually normal. • SLE—may see hemolytic anemia, thrombocytopenia, or evidence of glomerulonephritis. • Hematologic abnormalities in Persian cats with Chediak-Higashi syndrome. • Cyclic neutropenia in collie dogs (cyclic hematopoiesis anomalies).

OTHER LABORATORY TESTS

• Fungal culture—dermatophytosis.
• ANA—positive in SLE.

DIAGNOSTIC PROCEDURES

• Cytology—acantholytic cells (pemphigus), neoplastic lymphocytes (epitheliotropic lymphoma). • Joint tap—evidence of polyarthritis in SLE. • Ocular examination—uveitis in uveodermatologic syndrome. • Direct immunofluorescence—deposition of immunoglobulin at the basement membrane zone with DLE, SLE, and PE, and in the intercellular spaces of the epidermis with PF and PE. • Skin biopsy. • Genetic testing for oculocutaneous albinism.

PATHOLOGIC FINDINGS

Histopathologic Examination of the Skin

• Interface dermatitis—DLE, SLE, uveodermatologic syndrome. • Pigmentary incontinence—DLE, PE. • Intraepidermal pustules with acantholysis—PF and PE.
• Hypomelanosis—vitiligo, uveodermatologic syndrome, seasonal nasal hypopigmentation, and Auriotrichosis. • Apoptosis (individual cell necrosis of keratinocytes)—drug reaction and EM. • Proliferation of spindle cells of dermal arteries and arterioles—proliferative arteritis. • Infiltration of neoplastic lymphocytes— epitheliotropic lymphoma.

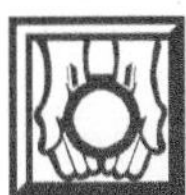

TREATMENT

• Outpatient, except for SLE, EM, and cutaneous lymphoma with systemic involvement. • Reduce exposure to sunlight—DLE, SLE, and PE. • Immunosuppressive therapy—SLE, PF, and PE. • Avoid contact with topical drugs. • Contact dermatitis—avoid irritant; replace plastic or rubber dishes: particularly if roughened edges cause abrasions.
• Application of water-resistant sunblock ointments or gels with an SPF/UVA and UVB >30 to depigmented and sun-exposed areas of skin. • Uveodermatologic syndrome—management by veterinary ophthalmologist recommended. • Appropriate antibiotics—pyoderma. • Appropriate antifungals— dermatophytosis.

MEDICATIONS

DRUG(S) OF CHOICE

• Auto-immune dermatoses—immunosuppressive therapy with prednisolone or dexamethasone and azathioprine (dogs) or chlorambucil (cats); see specific diseases.
• Topical corticosteroids—PE, DLE.
• Vitiligo and nasal depigmentation—no treatment. • Epitheliotropic lymphoma—multiple treatment protocols.

CONTRAINDICATIONS

Azathioprine therapy—not recommended in cats; may cause fatal leukopenia or thrombocytopenia.

ADVERSE REACTIONS

Ketoconazole may cause lightening of the hair coat, elevated alkaline phosphatase, and gastrointestinal distress.

ALTERNATIVE DRUG(S)

• Cyclosporine, modified—5 mg/kg/day for auto-immune disorders. • Tacrolimus—0.1% gel applied daily to lesions in combination with or to replace corticosteroids; may sting; avoid licking; wear latex gloves to apply.
• Pimecrolimus—1% cream applied daily to lesions in combination with or to replace corticosteroids; may sting; avoid licking; wear latex gloves to apply.

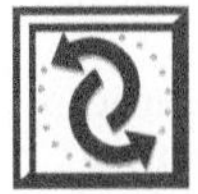

FOLLOW-UP

PATIENT MONITORING

• Varies with specific disease and treatment prescribed. • Postinflammatory depigmentation should resolve when the cause of inflammation is treated.

POSSIBLE COMPLICATIONS

• Sunburn in areas of depigmentation.
• Squamous cell carcinoma—in cases of solar damage and actinic keratosis of depigmented areas. • SLE—associated scarring with ulcerative dermatitis.

MISCELLANEOUS

ZOONOTIC POTENTIAL

Dermatophytosis—can cause infection in humans.

SEE ALSO

• Cutaneous Drug Eruptions.
• Lupus Erythematosus, Cutaneous (Discoid).
• Lupus Erythematosus, Systemic (SLE).
• Lymphoma, Cutaneous Epitheliotropic.
• Pemphigus.
• Uveodermatologic Syndrome (VKH).

ABBREVIATIONS

• ANA = antinuclear antibody.
• DLE = discoid lupus erythematosus.
• EM = erythema multiforme.
• PE = pemphigus erythematosus.
• PF = pemphigus foliaceus.
• SLE = systemic lupus erythematosus.

Suggested Reading

Mealey KL. Pharmacotherapeutics for Veterinary Dispensing. Ames, IA: Wiley-Blackwell, 2019.
Miller W, Griffin C, Campbell, K. Muller and Kirk's Small Animal Dermatology, 7th ed. St. Louis, MO: Elsevier, 2013.
Morris DO, Kennis RA. Clinical dermatology, special issue. Vet Clin Small Anim Pract 2013, 43(1).
Torres SMF, Roudebush P, eds., Advances in Veterinary Dermatology, Vol. 8. Hoboken, NJ: Wiley, 2017.

Author Guillermina Manigot
Consulting Editor Alexander H. Werner Resnick

Client Education Handout available online

DERMATOSES, EROSIVE OR ULCERATIVE

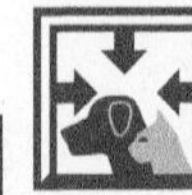

BASICS

DEFINITION

A heterogenous group of skin disorders characterized by disruption of the epidermis (erosions) or, if the basement membrane is compromised, the epidermis and dermis (ulcers).

PATHOPHYSIOLOGY

Varies widely, depending on the cause; may include congenital or developmental disorders that compromise tissue cohesion; cell-mediated (inflammatory or neoplastic) injury; anoxic injury; antigen-specific auto-immune disorders; and necrosis due to trauma, toxins, contactants (irritants), microbial organisms, or parasitic migration.

SYSTEMS AFFECTED

Skin/exocrine.

GENETICS

Some diseases are likely heritable due to breed predilections; however, there are no genetic screening tests available for any of the diseases listed.

INCIDENCE/PREVALENCE

Rare to common, depending on the cause.

SIGNALMENT

Species

Dogs and cats.

Breed Predilections

Some specific causes (see below) have strong breed predilections, e.g., lupoid disorders, familial dermatomyositis, and zinc-responsive dermatosis.

Mean Age and Range

- Highly variable according to etiology.
- Canine juvenile cellulitis and several congenital diseases (see below) are diagnosed in very young animals.

Predominant Sex

Sex predispositions may vary according to the disease in question.

SIGNS

Historical Findings

- Pruritus may result in ulcers or erosions due to self-trauma; especially ectoparasitism, superficial pyoderma, and *Malassezia* dermatitis.
- Exposure to caustic chemicals, burns, cold stress, venomous reptiles and insects, etc.
- Some infectious diseases (e.g., pythiosis, coccidioidomycosis, feline cow pox) have very restricted ranges.
- Previous or concurrent systemic signs or illness.

Physical Examination Findings

- Lesions may be heterogenous in gross appearance; some diseases result in erythematous erosions with minimal crust or scale, while others cause scale or crusting that (when removed) results in erosion.
- Ulcers may be shallow/superficial or deep; deep ulceration can present as sinuses with draining tracts, cavitated lesions with well-demarcated borders, or exudative crusted lesions.
- Some specific diseases are typically accompanied by fever and malaise, especially auto-immune disorders and infectious etiologies.
- May be associated with extracutaneous disease (e.g., superficial necrolytic dermatitis and hyper-eosinophilic syndrome of cats).

CAUSES

Autoimmune

- Pemphigus foliaceus—crusting with erosion.
- Pemphigus vulgaris—superficial ulcerative.
- Bullous pemphigoid and epidermolysis bullosa acquisita—superficial ulcerative.
- Discoid lupus erythematosus and muco-cutaneous lupus erythematosus—erosive or superficial ulcerative.
- Exfoliative lupus (German shorthaired pointers)—scaling with erosion.
- Vesicular lupus (rough collies and Shetland sheepdogs)—superficial ulcerative.
- Cold agglutinin disease—deep ulcerative.

Immune-Mediated

- Erythema multiforme, Stevens–Johnson syndrome, and toxic epidermal necrolysis (may be drug induced)—erosive to superficial ulcerative.
- Vasculitis—superficial to deep ulcerative (may be cavitated).
- Idiopathic panniculitis—deep ulcerative (usually exudative with crusting).
- Canine eosinophilic furunculosis of the face (may be insect related)—ulcerative and crusting.
- Canine juvenile cellulitis (puppy strangles)—erosive to superficial or deep ulcerative.
- Feline indolent ulcer (rodent ulcer)—erosive to superficial or deep ulcerative.

Infectious

- Surface pyoderma—acute moist pyotraumatic dermatitis: erosive.
- Superficial staphylococcal folliculitis—erosive to superficial ulcerative.
- Bacterial folliculitis/furunculosis—deep ulcerative.
- Superficial fungal (*Malassezia* dermatitis, dermatophytosis)—erosive to superficial ulcerative.
- Deep fungal (sporotrichosis, cryptococcosis, histoplasmosis, blastomycosis, coccidioidomycosis)—deep ulcerative with or without sinuses and draining tracts.
- Opportunistic mycobacteriosis—deep ulcerative nodules with sinuses and draining tracts.
- Actinomycetic bacteria (*Nocardia* spp., *Actinomyces* spp., *Streptomyces* spp.)—deep ulcerative nodules with sinuses and draining tracts.
- Pythiosis/lagenidiosis and protothecosis— ulcerative, proliferative with or without draining tracts.
- Leishmaniasis—erosive to superficial or deep ulcerative.
- Feline cow pox—deep ulcerative.
- Feline immunodeficiency virus (FIV)/feline leukemia virus (FeLV) related—erosive to superficial ulcerative.
- Feline herpesvirus-associated dermatosis—ulcerative with crusting.

Parasitic

- Demodicosis—ulcerative with crusting (especially with secondary bacterial folliculitis).
- Sarcoptic/notoedric mange—erosive with crusting.
- Flea bite allergy—erosive to ulcerative.
- Feline mosquito bite hypersensitivity—erosive to superficial or deep ulcerative.
- *Pelodera* and hookworm migration—deep ulcerative.

Congenital/Hereditary

- Canine familial dermatomyositis (predominantly in collies and Shetland sheepdogs)—erosive.
- Epidermolysis bullosa—superficial ulcerative.
- Cutaneous asthenia (Ehlers–Danlos syndrome)—skin tears easily.

Metabolic

- Superficial necrolytic dermatitis (usually associated with advanced hepatic disease or pancreatic glucagonoma)—crusting with erosion.
- Hyperadrenocorticism—erosive to ulcerative when complicated by secondary infections or calcinosis cutis.
- Uremia (mucous membranes)—superficial ulcerative.

Neoplastic

- Squamous cell carcinoma—erosive to ulcerative with scale or crust.
- Feline squamous cell carcinoma in situ (Bowenoid in situ carcinoma)—erosive with scale or crust.
- Mast cell tumors—superficial to deep ulcerative.
- Epitheliotropic lymphoma (mycosis fungoides)—erosive to superficial ulcerative.
- Feline thymoma-associated exfoliative dermatosis—scaling with erosion.
- Feline paraneoplastic alopecia—erosive.

Nutritional

Zinc-responsive dermatosis—crusting with erosion.

Physical/Conformational Dermatoses

- Pressure point ulcers—deep ulcerative.
- Intertrigo (skinfold pyoderma)—erosive.

Idiopathic

- Feline dorsal neck ulcer—deep ulcerative with crusting.
- Canine and feline acne—erosive to ulcerative.
- Feline plasma cell pododermatitis—superficial to deep ulcerative.

Miscellaneous

Thermal (heat/cold), electrical, solar, or chemical irritant/burns—depth of lesions depends on severity of insult.

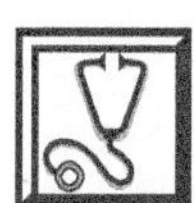

DIAGNOSIS

DIFFERENTIAL DIAGNOSIS

Depends upon presentation.

CBC/BIOCHEMISTRY/URINALYSIS

May be abnormal with metabolic or systemic disease.

IMAGING

• Rarely indicated. • Thoracic radiographs—deep/systemic fungal diseases, feline thymoma-associated exfoliative dermatitis, or systemic neoplasia. • Abdominal ultrasound—superficial necrolytic dermatitis (dogs) or paraneoplastic alopecia (cats).

DIAGNOSTIC PROCEDURES

• Skin scraping—ectoparasitism. • Direct impression cytology—bacteria, yeast, or acantholytic keratinocytes in pemphigus. • Fine-needle aspirate with cytology— indurated or nodular lesions. • Culture: bacterial (aerobic and anaerobic), mycobacterial, and/or fungal—suspected infectious disease. • Fungal serology and serology for pythiosis and lagenidiosis may be indicated on a case-by-case basis and depending upon geographic location. • PCR and immunohistochemistry are adjuncts to the histologic diagnosis of feline herpesvirus-associated dermatitis.

PATHOLOGIC FINDINGS

Skin Biopsy

• For cavitated lesions, the leading edge (elliptical full-thickness biopsy) should be harvested with a scalpel blade if the defect is too large to be excised in total. • Punch biopsy sufficient for diffuse erosive lesions; should take normal skin near a lesion and lesions that are both early and late in development.

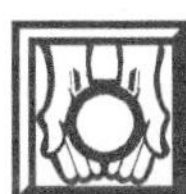

TREATMENT

APPROPRIATE HEALTH CARE

• Outpatient for most diseases. • Varies widely according to the cause.

DIET

• Nutritional support may be necessary in debilitated animals, especially those with superficial necrolytic dermatitis. • Correcting dietary deficiencies is the only treatment for generic dog-food dermatosis. • Supplementation of zinc is necessary for zinc-responsive dermatosis.

CLIENT EDUCATION

Variable by diagnosis; most important with suspected or confirmed zoonotic disease.

SURGICAL CONSIDERATIONS

• Indicated as curative treatment for feline thymoma-associated exfoliative dermatitis. • May be curative for nonmetastatic pancreatic or hepatobiliary tumors causing paraneoplastic alopecia. • Radical surgical excision of nodules and draining tracts may be an adjunct to antimicrobial therapy of infections caused by rapid-growing *Mycobacteria* spp. and *Nocardia* spp. in cats and pythiosis or lagenidiosis in dogs.

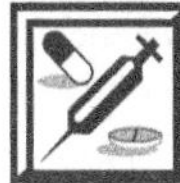

MEDICATIONS

DRUG(S) OF CHOICE

Variable by cause.

PRECAUTIONS

Side effects—associated with many antimicrobial, immunosuppressive, and antineoplastic drugs.

POSSIBLE INTERACTIONS

Dependent on medications administered.

FOLLOW-UP

PATIENT MONITORING

Dependent on disease process, concurrent systemic disease(s), drugs used, and potential side effects expected.

PREVENTION/AVOIDANCE

• Incidence of many feline infectious diseases can be minimized by restricting outdoor activity. • Some autoimmune diseases (lupus and pemphigus) are aggravated by ultraviolet light exposure; patients should be restricted from sun exposure during peak hours of the day.

POSSIBLE COMPLICATIONS

• Determined by cause. • Some diseases are potentially life-threatening. • Some diseases have zoonotic potential. • Infections and drug side effects are possible in cases requiring immunosuppression.

EXPECTED COURSE AND PROGNOSIS

• Some infectious diseases (nocardiosis, atypical mycobacteriosis) may be controlled with chronic antimicrobial therapy, but are generally not curable if lesion progression is extensive by the time of diagnosis. • Pythiosis/lagenidiosis—prognosis is extremely poor for response to therapy and survival when lesions are extensive.

MISCELLANEOUS

ZOONOTIC POTENTIAL

• Sarcoptic acariasis. • Dermatophytosis. • Sporotrichosis. • Mycelial phase of some fungi (e.g., *Coccidioides immitis, Blastomyces dermatitidis*), when grown on culture media, can be infectious to humans through inhalation. In-clinic fungal culturing (other than for dermatophytes) is not advised.

PREGNANCY/FERTILITY/BREEDING

• Due to the potential severity of clinical signs and syndromes, any patient diagnosed with an erosive/ulcerative disease that occurs with moderate to strong breed predilections should not be used for breeding. • Many drugs used to treat the auto-immune, immune-mediated, and infectious diseases listed may be teratogens.

SYNONYMS

Superficial necrolytic dermatitis = necrolytic migratory erythema, metabolic epidermal necrosis, hepatocutaneous syndrome.

SEE ALSO

- Acne—Cats.
- Acne—Dogs.
- Actinomycosis & Nocardia.
- Azotemia and Uremia.
- Blastomycosis.
- Coccidioidomycosis.
- Cold Agglutinin Disease.
- Cryptococcosis.
- Demodicosis.
- Dermatophytosis.
- Feline Herpesvirus Infection.
- Feline Immunodeficiency Virus (FIV) Infection.
- Feline Leukemia Virus (FeLV) Infection.
- Feline Paraneoplastic Alopecia.
- Flea Bite Hypersensitivity and Flea Control.
- Histoplasmosis.
- Hookworms (Ancylostomiasis).
- Hyperadrenocorticism (Cushing's Syndrome—Dogs.
- Hyperadrenocorticism (Cushing's Syndrome—Cats.
- Leishmaniosis, Cutaneous.
- Lupus Erythematosus, Cutaneous (Discoid).
- Lymphoma, Cutaneous Epitheliotropic.
- Malassezia Dermatitis.
- Mast Cell Tumors.
- Mycobacterial Infections.
- Notoedric Mange.
- Panniculitis/Steatitis.
- Pemphigus.
- Pododermatitis.
- Protothecosis.
- Puppy Strangles (Juvenile Cellulitis).
- Pyoderma.
- Pythiosis.
- Sarcoptic Mange.
- Sporotrichosis.
- Squamous Cell Carcinoma, Skin.
- Superficial Necrolytic Dermatitis.
- Vasculitis, Cutaneous.

ABBREVIATIONS

- FeLV = feline leukemia virus.
- FIV = feline immunodeficiency virus.

Suggested Reading

Mason IS. Erosions and ulcerations. In: Ettinger SH, Feldman EC, eds., Textbook of Veterinary Internal Medicine, 7th ed. St. Louis, MO: Saunders Elsevier, 2010, pp. 79–83.

Author Daniel O. Morris

Consulting Editor Alexander H. Werner Resnick

Client Education Handout available online

D

DERMATOSES, EXFOLIATIVE

D

BASICS

DEFINITION

Excessive or abnormal shedding of epidermal cells resulting in the clinical presentation of cutaneous scaling.

PATHOPHYSIOLOGY

- An increase in the production, an increase in the desquamation, or a decrease in the cohesion of keratinocytes results in abnormal shedding of epidermal cells individually (fine scale) or in sheets (coarse scale).
- Primary exfoliative disorders—keratinization defects: genetic control of epidermal cell proliferation and maturation is abnormal.
- Secondary exfoliative disorders—disease alters the normal maturation and proliferation of epidermal cells.
- Anomalies in sebaceous or apocrine gland function may be present or causative.

SYSTEMS AFFECTED

Skin/exocrine.

SIGNALMENT

- Dog and cat.
- Primary—apparent by 2 years of age; characteristic in affected breeds.
- Secondary—any age; any breed of dog or cat.

SIGNS

Physical Examination Findings

- Dry or greasy collections of fine or coarse scale located diffusely throughout the hair coat or focally in keratinaceous plaques.
- Oily skin and hair.
- Malodor.
- Comedones.
- Follicular casts.
- Candle wax–like deposits on hair.
- Silver scales, mostly affecting nose, face, and ears.
- Alopecia.
- Pruritus.
- Secondary bacterial folliculitis and/or *Malassezia* dermatitis.

CAUSES

Primary

- Primary idiopathic seborrhea (primary keratinization disorder)—primary cellular defect; accelerated epidermopoiesis and hyperproliferation of the epidermis, follicular infundibulum, and sebaceous gland; cocker and springer spaniel, West Highland white terrier, basset hound, Doberman pinscher, Irish setter, and Labrador retriever.
- Vitamin A–responsive dermatosis—young cocker spaniels; clinically similar to severe idiopathic seborrhea; identified by response to oral vitamin A supplementation.
- Zinc-responsive dermatosis—alopecia, dry scaling, crusting, and erythema around the eyes, ears, feet, lips, and external orifices; two syndromes: young adult dogs (mainly Siberian husky and Alaskan Malamute) and rapidly growing large-breed puppies; nutritionally responsive.
- Ectodermal defects—follicular dysplasias; color mutant or dilution alopecia; represent anomalies in melanization of the hair shaft and structural hair growth; keratinization defects theorized as causative for several syndromes; Doberman pinscher, Irish setter, dachshund, chow chow, Yorkshire terrier, poodle, Great Dane, whippet, saluki, and Italian greyhound; failure to regrow blue or fawn hair with normal "point" hair growth, excessive scaliness, comedone formation, secondary pyoderma.
- Idiopathic nasodigital hyperkeratosis—excessive build-up of scale and crusts on the nasal planum and footpad margins; possibly a senile change; generally asymptomatic; spaniels and retrievers; cracking and secondary bacterial infection can cause pain.
- Sebaceous adenitis—inflammatory disease targeting sebaceous glands and ducts causing patchy or diffuse hair loss and excessive scaling; tightly adherent follicular casts; standard poodle, Akita, Samoyed, German shepherd, Havanese, Bernese Mountain dog, and vizsla.
- Ichthyosis—rare and severe congenital disorder of keratinization; West Highland white terrier, golden retriever, cavalier King Charles spaniel, and Norfolk terrier; generalized accumulations of scale and crusts at an early age; secondary infections (bacterial and yeast) common.
- Primary seborrhea in Persian kittens.

Secondary

- Cutaneous hypersensitivity—with pruritus, secondary skin trauma, and irritation.
- Ectoparasitism—scabies, demodicosis, and cheyletiellosis; with inflammation and exfoliation.
- Bacterial folliculitis—bacterial enzymatic disadhesion with increased exfoliation of keratinocytes.
- Dermatophytosis—increased exfoliation as a skin mechanism in resolving infection.
- Cutaneous Leishmaniasis in endemic regions of the world; systemic signs might be present.
- Endocrinopathy—hypothyroidism: abnormalities in keratinization, failure to regrow hair, and excessive sebum production; hyperadrenocorticism: abnormal keratinization and decreased follicular activity; excessive scaling and secondary pyoderma common in both syndromes; other hormonal abnormalities may also be associated with excessive scaling.
- Age—dull, brittle, and scaly hair coat due to alterations caused by natural changes in epidermal metabolism associated with age; no specific defect identified.
- Nutritional disorders—malnutrition and generic dog food dermatosis; auto-immune dermatoses—pemphigus complex: may appear exfoliative; vesicles become scaly and crusty; cutaneous and systemic lupus erythematosus: cutaneous signs often appear as areas of alopecia and scaling.
- Neoplasia—primary epidermal neoplasia (epitheliotropic lymphoma): with alopecia and scaling as epidermal structures are damaged by infiltrating lymphocytes; preneoplastic conditions (actinic keratosis): initially appear exfoliative.
- Miscellaneous—any disease process may result in excessive scale formation due to a metabolic disorder or to cutaneous inflammation.
- Exfoliative disorders—rare in cats: tail gland hyperplasia, feline thymoma-associated exfoliative dermatitis.

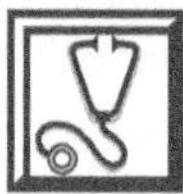

DIAGNOSIS

DIFFERENTIAL DIAGNOSIS

Based on signalment and history (breed-associated vs. age of onset), presence/absence of pruritus (hypersensitivity vs. secondary infection), and concurrent signs (endocrinopathy).

CBC/BIOCHEMISTRY/URINALYSIS

- Normal with primary keratinization disorders.
- Mild, nonregenerative anemia and hypercholesteremia are consistent with hypothyroidism.
- Neutrophilia, monocytosis, eosinopenia, lymphopenia, elevated serum alkaline phosphatase, hypercholesterolemia, and hyposthenuria suggest hyperadrenocorticism.

OTHER LABORATORY TESTS

Thyroid hormone levels and adrenal function tests if an endocrinopathy is suspected; see specific chapters for test recommendations. Serology, PCR, cytology, and histopathology for Leishmaniasis; see specific chapter.

IMAGING

Thoracic radiographs—feline thymoma-associated exfoliative dermatitis.

DIAGNOSTIC PROCEDURES

- Skin scraping.
- Skin biopsy—rule out particular differential diagnoses; strongly recommended for most cases.
- Intradermal allergy test.
- Restricted ingredient food trial.
- Cytology of skin surface.
- Microscopic examination of plucked hairs—macromelanosomes and structural anomalies in follicular dysplasia and color dilution alopecia.

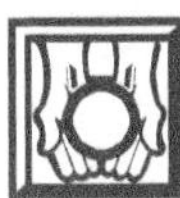

TREATMENT

- Frequent and adequate topical therapy.
- Diagnose and control treatable primary and secondary diseases.
- Recurrence of secondary infections may require repeated therapy and further diagnostics.
- Maintaining control is often lifelong.
- Prioritize restoration of epidermal barrier integrity and function.

MEDICATIONS

DRUG(S) OF CHOICE

Shampoos

- Contact time—5–15 minutes required; >15 minutes discouraged, may result in epidermal maceration, loss of barrier function, and excessive epidermal drying and irritation.
- Relative keratolytic activity—hypoallergenic < sulfur/salicylic acid < benzoyl peroxide.
- Ethyl lactate—less keratolytic/less drying; useful for moderate bacterial folliculitis and dry scale.
- Chlorhexidine—antimicrobial; mildly drying; useful for moderate bacterial folliculitis and *Malassezia* dermatitis.
- Tar—keratolytic, keratoplastic, and antipruritic; useful for moderate scale associated with pruritus.

Moisturizers/Barrier Restoration

- Restore skin hydration and increases effectiveness of subsequent shampoos.
- Humectants—enhance hydration of the stratum corneum by attracting water from the dermis; at high concentrations may be keratolytic.
- Propylene glycol spray (50–75% dilution with water) applied frequently.
- Microencapsulation—may improve residual activity of moisturizers by allowing sustained release after bathing.
- Emollients—coat the skin; smooth the roughened surfaces produced by excessive scaling; usually combined with occlusives to promote hydration of the epidermis.
- Barrier restoration—phytosphingosines, ceramides.

Systemic Therapy

- Specific disease (e.g., thyroxine replacement for hypothyroidism).
- Systemic antibiotics—secondary pyoderma.
- Retinoids—varied success for idiopathic or primary seborrhea; reports of individual response in refractory cases; isotretinoin (1 mg/kg PO q12–24h); if response is seen, taper dosage (1 mg/kg q48h or 0.5 mg/kg q24h); difficult to dispense due to strict prescription procedures.
- Cyclosporine (modified) 5 mg/kg/day until controlled, then decreased to minimal effective maintenance dosage for individual cases of keratinization disorder associated with hypersensitivity, sebaceous adenitis, epidermal dysplasia, ichthyosis, and/or *Malassezia* dermatitis.

PRECAUTIONS

- Corticosteroids—use judiciously to control the inflammation resulting from exfoliative disorders; may mask signs of pyoderma and prevent accurate diagnosis of primary disease.
- Vitamin A and D analogues—side effects can be severe; patients should be referred to a dermatologist before being treated with these drugs; teratogenic.

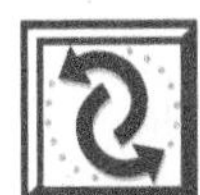

FOLLOW-UP

PATIENT MONITORING

- Antibiotics and topical therapy—monitor response every 3 weeks; patients may respond differently to the various topical therapies.
- Development of additional diseases and recurrence of pyoderma—reevaluation critical to determine if new factors are involved and if changes in therapy are necessary.
- Endocrinopathy—specific laboratory testing for disease management.
- Selective autoimmune disorders—clinical evaluation and laboratory monitoring frequent initially; based on diagnosis and treatment protocols.
- Retinoid drugs—serum chemistries, including triglycerides, and Schirmer tear tests.

MISCELLANEOUS

AGE-RELATED FACTORS

Skin aging might be related to increase in exfoliative disorders or relapses.

ZOONOTIC POTENTIAL

- Dermatophytosis and several ectoparasites have zoonotic potential.
- Leishmaniasis is a reportable disease.

PREGNANCY/FERTILITY/BREEDING

Systemic retinoids and vitamin A in therapeutic dosages—extreme teratogen; do not use in intact females because of severe and predictable teratogenicity and extremely long withdrawal period; women of childbearing age should not handle these medications.

SYNONYMS

- Keratinization disorder, seborrhea, idiopathic seborrhea, keratinization defect, dyskeratinization.
- Eczema, psoriasis, dandruff—incorrect human terms.
- Sebopsoriasis—correct term to describe similarities between some human and canine keratinization defects.

SEE ALSO

- Atopic Dermatitis.
- Demodicosis.
- Hyperadrenocorticism (Cushing's Syndrome)—Cats.
- Hyperadrenocorticism (Cushing's Syndrome)—Dogs.
- Hypothyroidism.
- Leishmaniosis
- Malassezia Dermatitis.
- Pyoderma.
- Sarcoptic Mange.

Suggested Reading

Gross TL, Ihrke PJ, Walder EJ, Affolter V. Skin Diseases of the Dog and Cat: Clinical and Histopathologic Diagnosis, 2nd ed. Oxford: Blackwell Science, 2005.

Miller W, Griffin C, Campbell, K. Muller and Kirk's Small Animal Dermatology, 7th ed. St. Louis, MO: Elsevier, 2013.

Torres SMF, Roudebush P, eds., Advances in Veterinary Dermatology, Vol. 8. Hoboken, NJ: Wiley, 2017.

Author Guillermina Manigot

Consulting Editor Alexander H. Werner Resnick

Client Education Handout available online

DERMATOSES, NEOPLASTIC

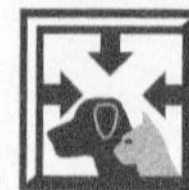

BASICS

DEFINITION

• Neoplastic proliferation of cells derived from the skin or migrating to the skin. • Epidermal tumors include those arising from keratinocytes, melanocytes, Merkel cells, and Langerhans cells, and epitheliotropic lymphoma. • Adnexal tumors include those arising from hair follicles, sebaceous glands, and sweat glands. • Dermal and subcutaneous skin tumors include those of mesenchymal origin and tumors of round cell origin. • Secondary or metastatic skin tumors result from the proliferation of cells from primary neoplasms of other organs in the skin.

PATHOPHYSIOLOGY

• Neoplasia develops as a result of changes in genes controlling cell proliferation and homeostasis. • More than 100 cancer-related genes have been identified. • Oncogenes encode proteins that promote cell growth; tumor-suppressor genes encode proteins that restrict cell proliferation and differentiation. • Mutations in *p53*, a tumor-suppressor gene, are found in approximately 50% of cancers in humans and have also been found in many tumors affecting dogs and cats. • Ultraviolet light promotes tumor development by damaging DNA and suppressing the immune system. • Many viruses promote tumor growth through stimulating cell proliferation and/or suppressing the immune system. • Reports of specific cutaneous neoplasia associated with medications and/or vaccinations.

SYSTEMS AFFECTED

Skin/exocrine.

GENETICS

• Breed predispositions have been reported for specific tumors, but the mode of inheritance in these breeds has not been determined. Mutations in oncogenes and/or tumor-suppressor genes (e.g., *p53*) are present in many types of skin tumors.

INCIDENCE/PREVALENCE

• The combined incidence rate for skin tumors has been reported as 728/100,000 (0.728%) for dogs and 84/100,000 (0.084%) for cats. • The skin is the most common site of occurrence of neoplasia in the dog (30% of total tumors) and the second most common site in the cat (20% of total tumors). • Canine skin tumors are approximately 55% mesenchymal, 40% epithelial, and 5% melanocytic. • The most frequently reported cutaneous or subcutaneous tumors in descending order for dogs are lipoma, sebaceous gland adenoma, mast cell tumor, papilloma, and histiocytoma. • Feline skin tumors are approximately 50% epithelial, 48% mesenchymal, and 2% melanocytic. • The most frequently reported cutaneous or subcutaneous tumors in cats are basal cell tumor, squamous cell carcinoma, mast cell tumor, and fibrosarcoma. • Skin tumors in cats are more frequently malignant; skin tumors in dogs are more frequently benign.

GEOGRAPHIC DISTRIBUTION

Geographic regions near the equator, with high altitude, or with sand or other reflective surfaces, have a higher incidence of solar-induced neoplastic dermatoses.

SIGNALMENT

Species

Dogs and cats.

Breed Predilections

• Canine breeds with the highest overall incidence of skin tumors include boxer, Scottish terrier, bullmastiff, basset hound, Weimaraner, Kerry blue terrier, and Norwegian elkhound. • Feline breeds with the highest overall incidence of skin tumors include Siamese and Persian. • Certain breeds are predisposed to specific types of tumors (see Suggested Reading). • Dog—breeds associated with the most common cutaneous neoplasms: ◦ Lipoma—cocker spaniel, dachshund, Doberman pinscher, Labrador retriever, miniature schnauzer, Weimaraner. ◦ Sebaceous gland tumor—beagle, cocker spaniel, dachshund, Irish setter, Lhasa apso, Malamute, miniature schnauzer, poodle, shih tzu, Siberian husky. ◦ Mast cell tumor—American Staffordshire terrier, beagle, Boston terrier, boxer, bull terrier, dachshund, English bulldog, fox terrier, golden retriever, Labrador retriever, pug, shar-pei, Weimaraner. ◦ Histiocytoma—American Staffordshire terrier, Boston terrier, boxer, cocker spaniel, dachshund, Doberman pinscher, English springer spaniel, Great Dane, Labrador retriever, miniature schnauzer, Rottweiler, Scottish terrier, shar-pei, Shetland sheepdog, West Highland white terrier. ◦ Papilloma—cocker spaniel, Kerry blue terrier. • Cat—breeds associated with the most common cutaneous neoplasms: ◦ Basal cell tumor—Persian, Himalayan (basal cell carcinoma—Siamese). ◦ Squamous cell carcinoma—no predisposed breed reported. ◦ Mast cell tumor—Siamese. ◦ Fibrosarcoma—no predisposed breed reported.

Mean Age and Range

• The median age for cutaneous neoplasia is 10.5 years in dogs and 12 years in cats. • The peak age period for cutaneous neoplasia in dogs and cats is 6–14 years.

Predominant Sex

• Females have a higher incidence of tumors in dogs (56%). • Males have a higher incidence of tumors in cats (56%).

SIGNS

General Comments

Most common clinical sign is a cutaneous or subcutaneous nodule; some tumors have an ulcerated surface; others may result in excessive scaling or in the formation of cutaneous plaques.

Historical Findings

• Tumors are most often slow growing; the owner may find them during petting, bathing, or grooming of the pet. • Tumors may be rapidly growing and appear (or increase in size) quickly (e.g., histiocytoma).

Physical Examination Findings

• Nodules—cutaneous or subcutaneous. • Cutaneous ulcers. • Excessive scaling. • Cutaneous papillomas. • Cutaneous plaques.

CAUSES

• Genetic (gene mutations). • Environmental (e.g., ultraviolet light, radiation exposure). • Viruses (e.g., papillomaviruses, feline leukemia virus, feline immunodeficiency virus). • Toxins (e.g., tars). • Drugs (e.g., immunosuppressive agents, chemotherapeutic agents). ◦ Epidermal neoplasms: ◦ Keratinocytes—papillomas, squamous cell carcinoma, basal cell carcinoma, basosquamous carcinoma. ◦ Melanocytes—melanoma. ◦ Merkel cells—Merkel cell carcinoma. ◦ Langerhans cells—histiocytoma and malignant histiocytosis. ◦ Epitheliotropic lymphoma—T lymphocytes. • Adnexal neoplasms: ◦ Hair follicles—trichofolliculoma, trichoepithelioma, infundibular keratinizing acanthoma, tricholemmoma, pilomatrixoma, trichoblastoma. ◦ Sebaceous glands—sebaceous adenoma, sebaceous epithelioma, sebaceous adenocarcinoma, perianal gland epithelioma, perianal gland carcinoma. ◦ Sweat glands—apocrine cystadenoma, apocrine secretory adenoma/adenocarcinoma, apocrine ductal adenoma/carcinoma, eccrine carcinoma. • Dermal and subcutaneous neoplasms: ◦ Mesenchymal origin—soft tissue sarcoma: fibroma/fibrosarcoma, myxoma/myxosarcoma, hemangiopericytoma, lymphangioma/lymphangiosarcoma, hemangioma/hemangiosarcoma, lipoma/liposarcoma, neurofibrosarcoma, leiomyoma/leiomyosarcoma, synovioma/synovial sarcoma, rhabdomyoma/rhabdomyosarcoma. ◦ Round cell origin—transmissible venereal tumor, mast cell tumor, plasmacytoma, lymphoma, histocytoma, and histocytic tumors. • Secondary or metastatic skin tumors result from the metastasis or primary neoplasms in other organs to the skin.

RISK FACTORS

• Hair coat color and length (e.g., hairless breeds, white hair coat, lightly pigmented skin—increased risk for squamous cell carcinoma). • Age (e.g., young animals highest risk for viral infections, older animals at highest risk for environment-associated neoplasia). • Sunlight exposure (e.g., dogs and cats that sunbathe or spend time outdoors on reflective surfaces have higher risk of ultraviolet light–induced skin tumors). • Genetics—certain breeds have higher risk of developing specific types of tumors (see above and Suggested Reading).

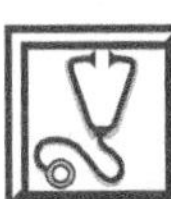

DIAGNOSIS

DIFFERENTIAL DIAGNOSIS

• Cyst. • Abscess. • Inflammatory nodule/granuloma/plaque—sterile granulomatous and pyogranulomatous disease, sterile panniculitis, fungal infection, mycobacterial infection, foreign body. • Trauma/self-induced skin ulceration. • Hamartoma/nevus.

CBC/BIOCHEMISTRY/URINALYSIS

N/A

OTHER LABORATORY TESTS

• Cytology (fine-needle aspirate or impression smear). • Regional lymph node aspirate (for staging).

IMAGING

Thoracic radiographs and abdominal ultrasonography useful for staging (evaluate for metastatic disease or underlying primary neoplasia).

DIAGNOSTIC PROCEDURES

• Cytology. • Biopsy with histopathologic examination. • Immunohistochemistry (useful in confirming certain types of tumors).

PATHOLOGIC FINDINGS

Varies with tumor type; see specific tumors for additional information.

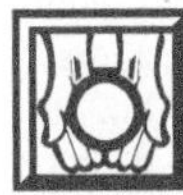

TREATMENT

APPROPRIATE HEALTH CARE

• Varies with tumor type. • Observation is appropriate for some benign tumors.
• Surgical excision, cryosurgery, radiation therapy, and/or tumor-specific chemotherapy or immunotherapy may be curative or palliative.

NURSING CARE

• Varies with tumor type and location. • Traumatized tumors may become secondarily infected.

ACTIVITY

Varies with tumor type and location.

DIET

Diets high in omega-3 fatty acids, arginine, and protein may be beneficial in boosting the immune response and preventing cancer-associated cachexia.

CLIENT EDUCATION

Varies with tumor type and location.

SURGICAL CONSIDERATIONS

• Vary with tumor type and location—wide margins may be needed to prevent reoccurrence of infiltrative tumors.
• Pretreatment with antihistamines appropriate when excising mast cell tumors.

MEDICATIONS

DRUG(S) OF CHOICE

Vary with tumor type—chemotherapy protocols are useful in some cases.

CONTRAINDICATIONS

Vary with tumor type and presence of concurrent disease.

PRECAUTIONS

Vary with tumor type and location.

POSSIBLE INTERACTIONS

Vary with tumor type and location.

ALTERNATIVE DRUG(S)

Vary with tumor type and location.

FOLLOW-UP

PATIENT MONITORING

Varies with tumor type and location.

PREVENTION/AVOIDANCE

• Varies with tumor type and location.
• Minimize exposure to ultraviolet light to help prevent some types of tumors.

POSSIBLE COMPLICATIONS

Vary with tumor type and location.

EXPECTED COURSE AND PROGNOSIS

Vary with tumor type and location.

MISCELLANEOUS

ASSOCIATED CONDITIONS

Vary with tumor type and location.

AGE-RELATED FACTORS

Vary with tumor type and location.

ZOONOTIC POTENTIAL

None

PREGNANCY/FERTILITY/BREEDING

Varies with tumor type; some may have a genetic predisposition.

SYNONYMS

N/A

SEE ALSO

• Adenocarcinoma, Skin (Sweat Gland, Sebaceous).
• Basal Cell Tumor.
• Fibrosarcoma, Bone.
• Lipoma, Infiltrative.
• Malignant Fibrous Histiocytoma.
• Mast Cell Tumors.
• Papillomatosis.
• Squamous Cell Carcinoma, Skin.

INTERNET RESOURCES

• http://www.oncolink.org/types/section.cfm?c=22&s=69
• http://www.vetcancersociety.org

Suggested Reading

Campbell KL, ed. Small Animal Dermatology Secrets. Philadelphia, PA: Hanley & Belfus, 2004, pp. 385–458.

Goldschmidt MH, Shofer FS. Skin Tumors of the Dog and Cat. Oxford: Butterworth Heinemann, 1992.

Gross TL, Ihrke PJ, Walder EJ, et al. Skin Diseases of the Dog and Cat: Clinical and Histopathologic Diagnosis, 2nd ed. Oxford: Blackwell, 2005, pp. 561–893.

Martin PD, Argyle DJ. Advances in the management of skin cancer. Vet Dermatol 2013, 24:173–180.

Miller WH, Griffin CE, Campbell KL, eds. Muller & Kirk's Small Animal Dermatology, 7th ed. Philadelphia, PA: Elsevier, 2013, pp. 774–843.

Shearer D, Dobson J. An approach to nodules and draining sinuses. In: Foster A, Foil C, BSAVA Manual of Small Animal Dermatology, 2nd ed. Gloucester: BSAVA, pp. 55–65.

Author Karen L. Campbell
Consulting Editor Alexander H. Werner Resnick

D

DERMATOSES, PAPULONODULAR

BASICS

DEFINITION

- Diseases whose primary lesions manifest as papules and nodules.
- Papule—solid, elevated lesion of the skin less than 1 cm in diameter.
- Nodule—solid, elevated lesion of the skin more than 1 cm in diameter that extends into deeper layers of the skin.

PATHOPHYSIOLOGY

- Papules—usually the result of tissue infiltration by inflammatory cells; accompanying intraepidermal edema or epidermal hyperplasia and dermal edema.
- Nodules—usually the result of a massive infiltration of inflammatory or neoplastic cells into the dermis or subcutis.

SYSTEMS AFFECTED

Skin/exocrine.

GENETICS

Determined by cause; specific diseases may be more commonly seen in certain breeds.

INCIDENCE/PREVALENCE

Determined by cause.

GEOGRAPHIC DISTRIBUTION

Determined by cause.

SIGNALMENT

Species

Dogs and cats.

Breed Predilection

Determined by cause.

Mean Age and Range

Determined by cause.

Predominant Sex

Determined by cause.

SIGNS

- Papules and/or nodules with distribution characteristic of the cause.
- Accompanying crusting, inflammation, pigmentation changes, and hair coat changes often noted; also characteristic of the cause.

CAUSES

- Superficial and deep bacterial folliculitis (e.g., *Staphylococcus*).
- Other bacterial—mycobacterial, actinomycosis, nocardiosis, abscess.
- Fungal—dermatophytosis (including pseudomycetoma/kerion), histoplasmosis, cryptococcosis, coccidiomycosis, sporotrichosis, blastomycosis, phaeohyphomycosis.
- Sebaceous adenitis, granulomatous.
- Canine and feline acne.
- Parasitic—demodicosis, Leishmaniasis, flea bite hypersensitivity, sarcoptic mange, pelodera dermatitis.
- Sterile nodular—sterile pyogranulomatous dermatitis and panniculitis, reactive histiocytosis.
- Metabolic—cutaneous xanthomatosis, calcinosis circumscripta.
- Hypersensitivity—feline eosinophilic dermatitis.
- Neoplasia.

RISK FACTORS

- Bacterial folliculitis, dermatophytosis, and demodicosis—any disease or medication that causes immune compromise or interferes with the barrier function of the skin.
- Pelodera dermatitis—may be associated with contact with decaying organic debris (straw or hay) containing *Pelodera strongyloides*.

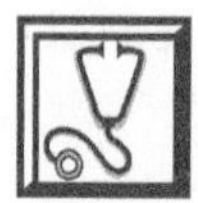

DIAGNOSIS

DIFFERENTIAL DIAGNOSIS

Determined by cause.

CBC/BIOCHEMISTRY/URINALYSIS

Usually normal—determined by cause.

OTHER LABORATORY TESTS

Determined by cause.

IMAGING

N/A

DIAGNOSTIC PROCEDURES

- Skin scraping—parasites.
- Dermatophyte cultures—dermatophytes.
- Pustule (if present) impression smear cytology—bacteria and degenerative neutrophils compatible with bacterial folliculitis; eosinophils can be compatible with hypersensitivity and/or with rupturing folliculitis or furunculosis; acantholytic keratinocytes consistent with an inflammatory folliculitis or pemphigus disease.
- Culture from tissue (fungal, bacterial, mycobacterial)—identify deep/systemic infection; possible susceptibility report for treatment.
- Aspirate and cytology from nodule—identify cellular infiltrate; presence of organisms.
- Skin biopsy— determine definitive diagnosis; especially if baseline diagnostic procedures are normal and/or initial empiric treatment is ineffective.

PATHOLOGIC FINDINGS

Depends upon underlying disease process.

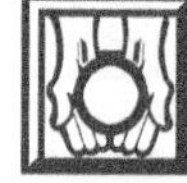

TREATMENT

APPROPRIATE HEALTH CARE

- Outpatient for nearly all causes (except some cases of neoplasia).
- Generalized demodicosis with secondary sepsis requires hospitalization.

NURSING CARE

Depends upon underlying issue.

ACTIVITY

No specific alteration of activity recommended.

DIET

No specific alteration of diet recommended.

CLIENT EDUCATION

- For fungal infections, treatment may be expensive and prognosis can be guarded for deep/systemic fungal infections.
- For immune-mediated processes, treatment may be for the duration of the patient's life.

SURGICAL CONSIDERATIONS

Rarely necessary unless neoplasia is diagnosed.

MEDICATIONS

DRUG(S) OF CHOICE

Bacterial Folliculitis

- Superficial pyoderma—appropriate antibiotics based on bacterial culture and susceptibility testing for at least 3–4 weeks, or 1 week beyond resolution of clinical signs.
- Deep pyoderma—appropriate antibiotics based on bacterial culture and susceptibility testing for at least 6–8 weeks, or 2 weeks beyond resolution of clinical signs.
- Identify and control underlying cause to prevent recurrence.
- See Pyoderma for additional recommendations.

Sebaceous Adenitis

- Appropriate antibiotics if secondary bacterial infection present.
- Propylene glycol and water (50–75% dilution) once daily as a spray to affected areas helpful in mild cases.
- Essential fatty acid dietary supplements (omega-3 and omega-6 PO).
- Topical therapy—antiseborrheic shampoos, emollient rinses (baby oil), and humectants.
- Cyclosporine, modified (5 mg/kg PO q24h).
- Vitamin A (10,000–30,000 IU PO daily or 1000 IU/kg PO daily).
- Refractory cases—isotretinoin (1 mg/kg PO q12–24h); if response is seen, taper dosage (1 mg/kg q48h or 0.5 mg/kg q24h); the synthetic retinoids have become difficult to dispense due to strict prescription procedures.
- Most cases are refractory to corticosteroids.
- See Sebaceous Adenitis, Granulomatous for additional recommendations.

Canine and Feline Acne

- May resolve without therapy in mild cases.
- Warm water soaks or Epsom salt solution (2 T/quart or 30 m/L of water) for 5–10 min.
- Chlorhexidine-based pads, or acetic acid/boric acid pads/wipes, or benzoyl peroxide gels used daily or alternated daily; topical ceramide/EFA preparations may be helpful.

• Topical creams/ointments—mupirocin 2% ointment: topical antibiotic; apply q24h; should not be used in cats with deep lesions; metronidazole, 0.05% Vitamin A acid cream, clindamycin are alternative options.
• Secondary bacterial infection—systemic antibiotics.
• Underlying cause(s) should be determined and treated accordingly.
• Refractory cases—isotretinoin (1–2 mg/kg PO q24h); oral synthetic retinoids have become difficult to dispense due to strict prescription procedures; prednisolone PO (1–2 mg/kg/day for 10–14 days and taper) may reduce scar tissue formation.
• See Acne—Cats and Acne—Dogs for additional recommendations.

Pelodera Dermatitis

• Remove and destroy bedding.
• Wash kennels, beds, and cages and treat with a premise insecticide or flea spray.
• Bathe affected animal and remove crusts.
• Parasiticidal dip or ivermectin as recommended for sarcoptic mange.
• Corticosteroids as needed for inflammation.
• Severe infection—may require use of antibiotics.

Sterile Nodular Dermatoses

• Attempt to identify underlying cause.
• Cyclosporine, modified 5 mg/kg PO q24h.
• Tetracycline (250 mg <10 kg, 500 mg >10 kg q8–12h), doxycycline (10 mg/kg q24h), or minocycline (5 mg/kg q12h) with niacinamide (250 mg <10 kg, 500 mg >10 kg q8–12h).
• Corticosteroids at immunosuppressive doses and taper according to response.
• Chemotherapeutic drugs (chlorambucil or azathioprine or mycophenolate mofetil).

Other

• Dermatophytosis—itraconazole, ketoconazole, or terbinafine; see Dermatophytosis.
• Kerion—see Dermatophytosis.
• Demodicosis/sarcoptic mange—see Demodicosis, Sarcoptic Mange.
• Other bacterial infection—antibiotics dependent upon culture and sensitivity results.
• Deep/systemic fungal infection.
• Feline eosinophilic dermatitis—look for underlying cause.
• Neoplasia—see Dermatoses, Neoplastic.

CONTRAINDICATIONS

Corticosteroids and immunosuppressive medications should be avoided with folliculitis, dermatophytosis, kerion, and demodicosis.

PRECAUTIONS

• Side effects more common and more severe with ketoconazole than with other azoles in cats.
• Cats can be sensitive to the irritant effects of benzoyl peroxide.
• Fatty acids—use with caution in dogs with inflammatory bowel disease or recurrent pancreatitis.
• Isotretinoin—may cause keratoconjunctivitis sicca, hyperactivity, pinnal pruritus, erythematous mucocutaneous junctions, swollen tongue, lethargy with anorexia or vomiting, abdominal distension, or collapse; CBC and chemistry screen abnormalities include high platelet count, hypertriglyceridemia, hypercholesterolemia, and high alanine transaminase; teratogen.
• Cyclosporine—may cause vomiting and diarrhea, gingival hyperplasia, B lymphocyte hyperplasia, hirsutism, papillomatous skin eruptions, and increased incidence of infection; decreased glucose homeostasis; potential toxic reactions rare and include nephrotoxicity and hepatotoxicity.
• Azathioprine, mycophenolate mofetil, and chlorambucil—potential for bone marrow suppression, gastrointestinal upset; azathioprine can cause hepatotoxicity and possibly pancreatitis.

POSSIBLE INTERACTIONS

• Cyclosporine and corticosteroids interact with several medications; an appropriate drug formulary should be consulted prior to usage.
• Referral to a veterinary dermatologist should be considered if the etiology remains undetermined and/or prior to prescribing unfamiliar medications.

ALTERNATIVE DRUG(S)

N/A

FOLLOW-UP

PATIENT MONITORING

• CBC, chemistry screen, urinalysis, and urine cultures—monitor periodically in patients receiving immunosuppressive medications; monitoring will depend upon medication and dosage.
• CBC, chemistry screen, and urinalysis—monitor monthly for 4–6 months in patients receiving synthetic retinoid therapy.
• Tear production—monitor monthly for 4–6 months, then every 6 months in patients receiving synthetic retinoid therapy or sulfonamide-containing antibiotics.
• Skin scraping—monitor therapy in patients with Demodicosis (see Demodicosis).
• Repeat fungal culture—monitor therapy in patients with dermatophytosis (see Dermatophytosis).
• Resolution of lesions—monitor progress of sebaceous adenitis, actinic conditions, and all other diseases.

POSSIBLE COMPLICATIONS

Dependent upon specific disease.

MISCELLANEOUS

ASSOCIATED CONDITIONS

N/A

AGE-RELATED FACTORS

N/A

ZOONOTIC POTENTIAL

• Dermatophytosis—incidence in humans reported in 30–50% of cases of *Microsporum canis*, but possible with all dermatophytosis cases.
• Fungal infections—potential depends upon organism.
• Sarcoptic mange.

PREGNANCY/FERTILITY/BREEDING

• Synthetic retinoids—teratogens; do not use in pregnant animals, animals intended for reproduction, or intact female animals; should not be handled by women of childbearing age.
• Corticosteroids—avoid use in pregnant animals.
• Cyclosporine—avoid during pregnancy unless necessary; dosages two to five times normal have been fetotoxic and embryotoxic in rats and rabbits.
• Antifungal agents should be avoided in pregnant animals.
• All drugs should be used with caution in pregnant and breeding animals.

SEE ALSO

• Acne—Cats.
• Acne—Dogs.
• Demodicosis.
• Dermatophytosis.
• Pyoderma.
• Sebaceous Adenitis, Granulomatous.

Suggested Reading

Helton Rhodes KA, Werner A. Blackwell's Five-Minute Veterinary Consult Clinical Companion: Small Animal Dermatology, 3rd ed. Hoboken, NJ: Wiley-Blackwell, 2018.

Author Karen A. Kuhl
Consulting Editor Alexander H. Werner Resnick

Client Education Handout available online

DERMATOSES, STERILE NODULAR/GRANULOMATOUS

BASICS

DEFINITION

Sterile diseases with primary lesions of nodules and/or plaques.

PATHOPHYSIOLOGY

- Nodules/plaques—usually result from an infiltration of inflammatory cells into the dermis and subcutis; may be secondary to endogenous or exogenous stimuli.
- Inflammation is typically, but not always, granulomatous to pyogranulomatous.

SYSTEMS AFFECTED

Skin/exocrine.

GENETICS

Oligogenic transmission is proposed for histiocytic sarcoma for Bernese mountain dogs.

SIGNALMENT

- Collagenous nevi—German shepherd dogs 3–5 years old.
- Calcinosis circumscripta—German shepherd dogs <2 years old.
- Systemic histiocytosis and malignant histiocytosis—Bernese mountain dogs (primarily), Rottweilers, and retrievers (golden and Labrador).
- Eosinophilic granuloma—Siberian huskies <3 years, males.

SIGNS

- Characterized by single to multiple dermal to subcutaneous nodules and/or plaques.
- Firm to fluctuant.
- Occasionally painful.
- Overlying epidermis may be normal to ulcerated.

CAUSES

- Amyloidosis.
- Foreign body reaction.
- Spherulocytosis.
- Idiopathic sterile granuloma and pyogranuloma.
- Canine eosinophilic granuloma.
- Calcinosis cutis.
- Calcinosis circumscripta.
- Reactive (cutaneous, systemic) or malignant histiocytosis (disseminated histiocytic sarcoma).
- Sterile nodular panniculitis.
- Collagenous nevi (nodular dermatofibrosis).
- Cutaneous xanthoma.

RISK FACTORS

- Foreign body reaction—induced by exposure to any irritating material.
- Calcinosis cutis—increased risk with exposure to high doses of exogenous or endogenous glucocorticosteroids.
- Panniculitis—increased risk with vitamin E–deficient diet.
- Cutaneous xanthoma—high-fat treats or diet, diabetes mellitus, hyperlipidemia.

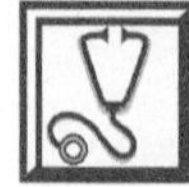

DIAGNOSIS

DIFFERENTIAL DIAGNOSIS

- Sterile nodular dermatoses must be differentiated from deep bacterial and fungal infections and dermal neoplasia.
- Diagnosis by histopathology and deep tissue cultures.
- Immunohistochemistry—differentiating histiocytic conditions.
- Immunohistochemical staining and PCR testing—diagnose Leishmaniasis and mycobacterial infections.

CBC/BIOCHEMISTRY/URINALYSIS

- Amyloidosis—possible changes in biochemistry and/or urinalysis if internal organs are affected.
- Malignant histiocytosis—pancytopenia.
- Calcinosis cutis—changes characteristic of hyperglucocorticoidism.
- Cutaneous xanthomas—may have glucosuria, hyperglycemia, and/or lipid profile abnormalities.
- Sterile panniculitis—possible biochemistry changes associated with pancreatitis, hepatic disease, or systemic lupus erythematosus.

IMAGING

Radiology and ultrasonography—involvement of internal organs in amyloidosis and histiocytosis; areas of dystrophic calcification and/or adrenal enlargement or tumor in dogs with calcinosis cutis; renal or uterine tumors in German shepherd dogs with collagenous nevi.

DIAGNOSTIC PROCEDURES

- Skin biopsy for histopathology and cultures (fungal, aerobic, anaerobic, and mycobacterial).
- Biopsies should be excisional and taken from an intact or early (nondraining) nodule if possible.
- Culture samples should be taken from nodular tissue, not exudates.
- Special histopathologic stains for bacteria, mycobacteria, and fungi.

PATHOLOGIC FINDINGS

- Amyloidosis—accumulation of amorphous eosinophilic deposits that may extend into the subcutis; deposits stain apple green with Congo red in polarized light.
- Foreign body reaction—suppurative to pyogranulomatous inflammation that affects the dermis, subcutis, and occasionally the underlying muscle.
- Spherulocytosis—histiocytes surrounding thin-walled parent bodies filled with homogeneous eosinophilic spherules.
- Idiopathic sterile granuloma and pyogranuloma—granulomatous to pyogranulomatous inflammation that can extend from the dermis to the panniculus; differentiated from infectious diseases by obtaining negative cultures.
- Canine eosinophilic granuloma—accumulation of eosinophils with edema, possible mucin, and collagen degeneration.
- Calcinosis cutis—diffuse calcium deposition of the dermal collagen and adnexa that may extend into the deeper tissue.
- Calcinosis circumscripta—focal to multifocal deposits of mineral that efface the soft tissue.
- Reactive histiocytosis (cutaneous and systemic)—markedly angiocentric infiltrate of histiocytes that do not form granulomas or pyogranulomas.
- Malignant histiocytosis (disseminated histiocytic sarcoma)—dense pleomorphic cell proliferation of spindle or round cells that efface normal tissue architecture; tumors from other spindle and round cell tumors differentiated by immunohistochemistry; see specific chapters.
- Sterile nodular panniculitis—neutrophilic to pyogranulomatous inflammation that affects the deep dermis and panniculus predominantly; adipocytes may be necrotic or may be infiltrated by foamy macrophages; differentiated from infectious diseases by obtaining negative cultures.
- Collagenous nevi—focal but often subtle dermal thickening of normal collagen bundles.
- Cutaneous xanthoma—diffuse granulomatous inflammation composed of large foamy macrophages; lakes of extracellular amorphous lipid deposits and cholesterol clefts.

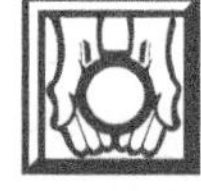

TREATMENT

APPROPRIATE HEALTH CARE

- Most of these disorders can be treated on an outpatient basis.
- Neoplastic or metabolic disorders may require hospitalization and supportive care.

NURSING CARE

Gentle bathing and soaking to clean the skin and remove debris.

DIET

Animals with xanthoma should be on a low-fat diet.

CLIENT EDUCATION

- Malignant histiocytosis, amyloidosis, collagenous nevi of German shepherd dogs, and systemic reactive histiocytosis are almost always fatal.
- Prognoses for cutaneous reactive histiocytic disease, sterile panniculitis, and sterile pyogranuloma are guarded since they may

require long-term immunosuppressive therapy; a few of these cases will not respond to therapy at all.

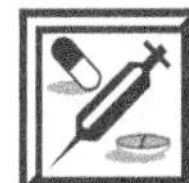

MEDICATIONS

DRUG(S) OF CHOICE

- Amyloidosis—no known therapy, unless the lesion is solitary and can be surgically removed.
- Spherulocytosis—only effective treatment is surgical removal.
- Idiopathic sterile granuloma and pyogranuloma:
  - Prednisolone (2.2–4.4 mg/kg divided PO q12h) is the first line of therapy; continue steroids for 7–14 days after complete remission, then taper dose.
  - Azathioprine (2.2 mg/kg q48h) or cyclosporine (modified, 5–10 mg/kg q24h) added as a steroid-sparing drug.
- Foreign body reactions—removal of the offending substance; secondary deep bacterial infections require treatment with both topical and systemic antibiotics.
- Canine eosinophilic granuloma—prednisolone (1.1–2.2 mg/kg PO q24h) usually effective.
- Cutaneous/systemic or malignant histiocytosis—no effective long-term therapy; see Histiocytosis, Cutaneous.
- Calcinosis cutis—underlying disease must be controlled if possible; most cases require antibiotics to control secondary bacterial infections; hydrotherapy and frequent bathing in antibacterial shampoos minimize secondary infection; topical dimethyl sulfoxide (DMSO) is useful (applied to no more than one-third of the body once daily until lesions resolve); if lesions are extensive, serum calcium levels should be monitored closely while using DMSO.
- Calcinosis circumscripta—surgical excision.
- Sterile nodular panniculitis:
  - Single lesions can be removed surgically.
  - Prednisolone (2.2–4.4 mg/kg PO q24h or divided PO q12h) treatment of choice; administer until lesions regress, then taper; some dogs remain in long-term remission, others require prolonged alternate-day therapy.
  - Azathioprine (2.2 mg/kg q48h) can be used together with prednisolone as a corticosteroid-sparing agent.
  - Cyclosporine, modified (5–10 mg/kg 24h) can be used together with prednisolone or as an alternative to glucocorticosteroid therapy if the patient is steroid intolerant or steroids are not sufficiently effective.
  - Tetracycline (250 mg <10 kg, 500 mg >10 kg q8–12h), doxycycline (10 mg/kg q24h), or minocycline (5 mg/kg q12h) with niacinamide (250 mg <10 kg, 500 mg >10 kg q8–12h) can also be used as an alternative to glucocorticoid therapy; this is effective only in mild cases.
- Collagenous nevi—no therapy for most cases since cystadenocarcinomas are usually bilateral; for rare unilateral case of cystadenocarcinoma or cystadenoma, removal of single affected kidney may be helpful; ovariohysterectomy should be performed in intact females to remove leiomyomas.
- Cutaneous xanthoma—correction of underlying diabetes mellitus or hyperlipoproteinemia usually curative.

CONTRAINDICATIONS

Corticosteroids and other immunosuppressive drugs should be avoided, if possible, in any animal with secondary bacterial folliculitis.

PRECAUTIONS

DMSO—handle with care; monitor serum calcium levels if used to treat calcinosis cutis.

FOLLOW-UP

PATIENT MONITORING

- Patients on long-term immunosuppressive therapy should have CBC, chemistry screen, urinalysis, and urine culture performed at least every 6 months.
- Dogs treated with DMSO for calcinosis cutis should have calcium levels checked every 7–14 days for first month of therapy if large areas are affected.

POSSIBLE COMPLICATIONS

Long-term use of immunosuppressive therapy (especially glucocorticosteroids) may make patients more susceptible to other dermatoses such as bacterial folliculitis, demodicosis, and dermatophytosis, as well as systemic side effects.

EXPECTED COURSE AND PROGNOSIS

- Systemic amyloidosis, malignant histiocytosis, systemic reactive histiocytosis, and nodular dermatofibrosis—invariably fatal.
- Many of the other conditions have a guarded prognosis; many require lifelong immunosuppressive therapy to remain in remission.

D

MISCELLANEOUS

ASSOCIATED CONDITIONS

- Calcinosis cutis—hyperglucocorticoidism, chronic renal failure, and diabetes mellitus.
- Calcinosis circumscripta—(occasionally) hypertrophic osteodystrophy and idiopathic polyarthritis.
- Collagenous nevi—renal cystadenoma/cystadenocarcinoma and uterine, leiomyoma/leiomyosarcoma.
- Cutaneous xanthoma—diabetes mellitus and hyperlipoproteinemia.

SEE ALSO

- Adenocarcinoma, Renal.
- Amyloidosis.
- Hyperadrenocorticism (Cushing's Syndrome)—Dogs.

ABBREVIATIONS

- DMSO = dimethyl sulfoxide

INTERNET RESOURCES

http://www.histiocytosis.ucdavis.edu

Suggested Reading

Helton Rhodes KA, Werner A. Blackwell's Five-Minute Veterinary Consult Clinical Companion: Small Animal Dermatology, 3rd ed. Hoboken, NJ: Wiley-Blackwell, 2018.

O'Kell AL, Inteeworn N, Diaz SF, et al. Canine sterile nodular panniculitis: retrospective study of 14 cases. J Vet Intern Med 2010, 24:278–284.

Santoro D, Prisco M, Ciaramella P. Cutaneous sterile granulomas/pyogranulomas, leishmaniasis and mycobacterial infections. J Small Anim Pract 2008, 49:552–561.

Schissler J. Sterile pyogranulomatous dermatitis and panniculitis. Vet Clin Small Anim 2019, 49:27–36.

Author Dawn E. Logas

Consulting Editor Alexander H. Werner Resnick

Client Education Handout available online

DERMATOSES, SUN-INDUCED

D

BASICS

OVERVIEW

The hair coat and epidermal pigmentation protect the skin from damage caused by UV light radiation. Excessive UV exposure damages keratinocytes (producing mutation), causes inflammation, and decreases cutaneous immune system surveillance. UVA (320–400 nm) penetrates more deeply than UVB (290–320 nm). Prolonged and repeated damage leads to preneoplastic changes and eventual neoplasia. Prolonged sun exposure in darkly pigmented individuals may cause thermal burn. UV exposure may exacerbate symptoms of pemphigus erythematosus (PE), discoid lupus erythematosus (DLE), systemic lupus erythematosus (SLE), and dermatomyositis.

SIGNALMENT

- Dogs—Dalmatian, bull terrier, boxer, bulldog, basset hound, beagle, whippet, American Staffordshire terrier, Australian shepherd (nasal solar dermatitis).
- Cats—white cats.

SIGNS

- Dogs—glabrous areas especially axillae, flanks, ventral abdomen, lateral extremities.
- Cats—pinnae, nasal planum, dorsal muzzle, eyelids.
- Solar dermatitis—photodermatitis.
  - Nasal—erythema and scaling at junction of haired and hairless skin of nose; expands caudally followed by scarring.
  - Truncal—erythema, scaling, and lichenification; gradual palpable thickening of white areas (adjacent dark areas are normal), comedones; secondary deep pyoderma.
- Actinic keratosis— premalignant epithelial dysplasia capable of becoming invasive squamous cell carcinomas (SCC); indurated, crusted, hyperkeratotic plaques.
- Hemangioma—well-circumscribed plaques or nodules, firm to fluctuant, bluish to purplish.
- Hemangiosarcoma—poorly circumscribed dermal dark red to purple, fluctuant nodules; may become large; commonly ulcerate and bleed; subcutaneous hemangiosarcomas usually not solar induced.
- SCC—proliferative and ulcerated plaques; easily traumatized; secondary pyoderma common; locally invasive and slow to metastasize.
- Solar-induced thermal burn (dorsal thermal necrosis)—alopecia, erythema, ulceration, eschars/necrosis, and crusts on the dorsal parts of the body; dogs with dark shorthair coats at increased risk.
- Cutaneous horns—firm hornlike projections, may originate from actinic keratoses, SCC, or other neoplasia; the base of a horn must be inspected for underlying cause.

CAUSES & RISK FACTORS

- White-haired and lightly haired individuals with poorly pigmented skin.
- History of sunbathing.
- Outdoor housing.
- Regions with greater sun exposure, high altitudes; usually occurs in summer, but also in winter as result of reflection from snow.

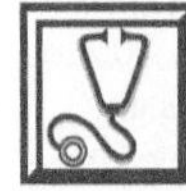

DIAGNOSIS

DIFFERENTIAL DIAGNOSIS

- Dermatophytosis.
- Demodicosis.
- DLE.
- PE.
- Pemphigus foliaceus.
- Drug eruption.
- Contact dermatitis.
- Chemical burn.

DIAGNOSTIC PROCEDURES

- Biopsy/histopathology—definitive diagnosis.
- Solar dermatitis—epidermal hyperplasia, apoptotic keratinocytes, perivascular inflammation, vascular dilatation, dermal fibrosis and elastosis.
- Actinic keratosis—parakeratotic hyperkeratosis with epidermal atypia and solar elastosis.
- Hemangioma—proliferative blood-filled vascular channels with minimal atypia or mitosis.
- Hemangiosarcoma—invasive proliferation of atypical endothelial cells with areas of vascular space formation.
- SCC—invasion of dermis by keratinocytes; keratin "pearls," mitoses, atypia.
- Solar-induced thermal burn—partial/full thickness necrosis of the epidermis, adnexa, dermis; coagulation necrosis.

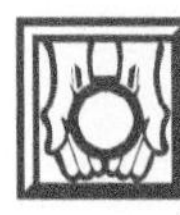

TREATMENT

- Sun avoidance—keep indoors during day; avoid reflected sunlight; apply waterproof (>30 SPF) sunscreen (without zinc oxide and PABA); sun-protective clothing.
- Surgical excision of neoplastic lesions.

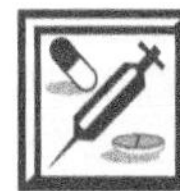

MEDICATIONS

DRUG(S) OF CHOICE

- Cyclooxygenase-2 (COX2) inhibitors—overexpression by sun-damaged cells; inhibition of COX2 demonstrated improvement: firocoxib 5 mg/kg/day PO.
- Glucocorticoids—reduced inflammation noted in acute cases; prednisolone 0.5–1 mg/kg PO tapering dosage; discontinue when possible.
- Imiquimod 5% cream—induces local immune response; for individual lesions, esp. actinic keratosis; apply q48h until resolution.
- Cryosurgery—actinic keratosis, SCC.
- Antibiotics—control secondary pyoderma (see Pyoderma).

CONTRAINDICATIONS/POSSIBLE INTERACTIONS

Firocoxib—gastrointestinal upset; elevated liver enzymes.

FOLLOW-UP

- Patients should be regularly screened for development and removal of new lesions.
- Sun-induced dermatoses rarely metastasize.
- Long-term therapy necessary following extended periods of sun damage.

ABBREVIATIONS

- COX2 = cyclooxygenase-2.
- DLE = discoid lupus erythematosus.
- PE = pemphigus erythematosus.
- SCC = squamous cell carcinoma.
- SLE = systemic lupus erythematosus.

Suggested Reading

Albanese F, Abramo F, Caporali C, et al. Clinical outcome and cyclo-oxygenase-2 expression in 5 dogs with solar dermatitis/actinic keratosis treated with firocoxib. Vet Dermatol 2013, 24(6):606–e147.

Burrows AK. Actinic dermatoses and sun protection. In: Kirk's Current Veterinary Therapy XV. St. Louis, MO: Elsevier, 2014, pp. 480–482.

Author Clarissa P. Souza

Consulting Editor Alexander H. Werner Resnick

Acknowledgment The author acknowledges the prior contribution of Alexander H. Werner Resnick.

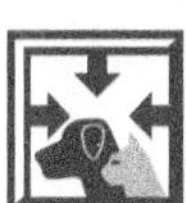

BASICS

DEFINITION

- Pustule—small (<1 cm), circumscribed elevation of the epidermis filled with pus.
- Vesicle—small (<1 cm), circumscribed elevation of the epidermis filled with clear fluid.

PATHOPHYSIOLOGY

Pustules and vesicles—produced by edema, acantholysis (pemphigus), ballooning degeneration (viral infections), proteolytic enzymes from neutrophils (pyoderma), degeneration of basal cells (lupus), or dermoepidermal separation (bullous pemphigoid).

SYSTEMS AFFECTED

Skin/exocrine.

SIGNALMENT

- Lupus—collies, Shetland sheepdogs, and German shepherd dogs may be predisposed.
- Pemphigus erythematosus—collies and German shepherd dogs may be predisposed.
- Pemphigus foliaceus—Akitas, chow chows, dachshunds, bearded collies, Labrador retrievers, Newfoundlands, Doberman pinschers, and schipperkes may be predisposed.
- Bullous pemphigoid—collies and Doberman pinschers may be predisposed.
- Dermatomyositis—young collies and Shetland sheepdogs.
- Subcorneal pustular dermatosis—schnauzers affected most frequently.
- Linear immunoglobulin (Ig) A dermatosis—dachshunds exclusively; very rare.
- Dermatophytosis—young animals.

SIGNS

N/A

CAUSES

Pustules/Vesicles

- Superficial pyoderma—impetigo, superficial spreading pyoderma, superficial bacterial folliculitis, canine or feline acne.
- Pemphigus complex—pemphigus foliaceus, pemphigus erythematosus, panepidermal pemphigus; pemphigus vulgaris produces deep clefts that rapidly erode into ulcers.
- Subcorneal pustular dermatosis.
- Dermatophytosis.
- Demodicosis.
- Sterile eosinophilic pustulosis.
- Linear IgA dermatosis.
- Systemic lupus erythematosus (SLE).
- Discoid lupus erythematosus (DLE).
- Bullous pemphigoid
- Dermatomyositis.
- Cutaneous drug eruption.
- Epidermolysis bullosa.

RISK FACTORS

- Drug exposure—SLE and bullous pemphigoid.
- Bacterial folliculitis usually secondary to a predisposing factor (e.g., demodicosis, hypothyroidism, allergy, or corticosteroid administration).
- UV light—pemphigus erythematosus, bullous pemphigoid, SLE, DLE, and dermatomyositis.

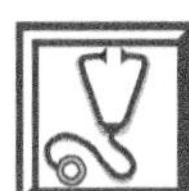

DIAGNOSIS

DIFFERENTIAL DIAGNOSIS

Superficial Pyoderma

- Most common cause.
- Readily responds to appropriate antibiotic therapy if underlying cause is effectively managed.
- Intact pustule—direct smear reveals neutrophils engulfing bacteria; most often *Staphylococcus pseudintermedius*; biopsy demonstrates intraepidermal neutrophilic pustules or folliculitis with bacteria.

Pemphigus Complex

- Group of immune-mediated diseases characterized histologically by disadhesion of keratinocytes within the epidermis (acantholytic keratinocytes).
- Direct smears—many acantholytic keratinocytes, nondegenerate neutrophils, eosinophils, and few to no bacteria.
- Culture of an intact pustule negative.
- Direct immunofluorescence—deposits in the intercellular spaces of the epidermis in approximately 50% of cases.
- Tends to wax and wane irrespective of antibiotic therapy; responds to immunosuppressive therapy.
- Pemphigus foliaceus and erythematosus—superficial acantholysis leading to erosions; face, pinnae, and footpads (foliaceus) commonly affected; mucous membranes not affected; biopsy: subcorneal acantholysis; interface and lichenoid inflammation with pemphigus erythematosus.
- Pemphigus vulgaris—severe and deep form of pemphigus; characterized by erosions rapidly leading to ulcerations of oral cavity, mucocutaneous junctions, and skin; biopsy: suprabasal acantholysis and cleft formation.
- Direct immunofluorescence positive at the intercellular spaces of the deeper epidermis.

Subcorneal Pustular Dermatosis

- Rare idiopathic pustular dermatosis of dogs.
- Tends to wax and wane.
- Intact pustules—direct smears reveal numerous neutrophils, no bacteria, and occasional acantholytic keratinocytes; cultures negative.
- Direct immunofluorescence negative.
- Poor response to glucocorticosteroids and antibiotics.

Dermatophytosis

- Common disease of both dogs and cats.
- Dermatophyte culture positive.
- Secondary bacterial folliculitis common.
- Skin biopsy—folliculitis with fungal elements.

Sterile Eosinophilic Pustulosis

- Rare idiopathic dermatosis of dogs.
- Direct smears—numerous eosinophils, nondegenerate neutrophils, occasional acantholytic keratinocytes, and no bacteria.
- Biopsy—eosinophilic intraepidermal pustules, folliculitis, and furunculosis.
- Direct immunofluorescence negative.
- Rapid response to glucocorticosteroids.

Linear IgA Dermatosis

- Rare idiopathic dermatosis of dachshunds.
- Tends to wax and wane.
- Pustules—sterile and subcorneal.
- Direct immunofluorescence positive for IgA at basement membrane zone.

SLE

- Multisystemic disease with variable clinical signs and cutaneous manifestations, including mucocutaneous ulceration.
- Direct immunofluorescence positive at the basement membrane zone.
- Antinuclear antibody (ANA) positive.

DLE

- Affects only the skin; lesions usually confined to the head.
- Depigmentation, erythema, and ulceration of the nasal planum common.
- Skin biopsy—interface and lichenoid dermatitis.
- Direct immunofluorescence positive at the basement membrane zone.
- ANA negative.

Bullous Pemphigoid

- Ulcerative disorder of the skin and/or mucous membranes.
- Skin biopsy—subepidermal cleft formation.
- Direct immunofluorescence positive at the basement membrane zone.
- No acantholysis.

Dermatomyositis

- Idiopathic inflammatory disease of the skin and muscle of young collies and Shetland sheepdogs; seen rarely in adult animals.
- Lesions affect the face, ear tips, tail tip, and pressure points of the extremities.
- Characterized by alopecia, crusting, pigmentation disturbances, erosions/ulceration, and scarring.
- Skin biopsy—follicular atrophy, perifolliculitis, and hydropic degeneration of the basal cells.
- Direct immunofluorescence negative.
- Muscle biopsy and electromyography (EMG)—evidence of inflammation.

CBC/BIOCHEMISTRY/URINALYSIS

- Usually unremarkable.
- SLE—possible anemia, thrombocytopenia, or glomerulonephritis.

- Eosinophilic pustular dermatosis—most affected dogs have peripheral eosinophilia.

OTHER LABORATORY TESTS

ANA titer—may be positive with SLE.

DIAGNOSTIC PROCEDURES

- Direct smear from intact pustule/vesicle.
- Culture of intact pustule/vesicle.
- Skin biopsy for histopathology.
- Direct immunofluorescence, including IgA.
- EMG—fibrillation potentials (rapid, irregular, and unsynchronized contraction of muscle fibers) and positive sharp waves in dermatomyositis.
- Muscle biopsy—myofibril degeneration, characterized by fragmentation, vacuolation, atrophy, fibrosis, and regeneration in dermatomyositis.

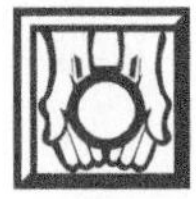

TREATMENT

APPROPRIATE HEALTH CARE

- Periodic bathing with an antimicrobial shampoo—helps remove surface debris and control secondary bacterial folliculitis.
- Usually treated as outpatient.
- SLE, pemphigus vulgaris, and bullous pemphigoid may be life-threatening and require inpatient intensive care.

MEDICATIONS

DRUG(S) OF CHOICE

See specific disease chapters for more information.

Bacterial Folliculitis

- Empiric choices—cephalexin (22 mg/kg PO q12h); clindamycin (11 mg/kg PO q24h); amoxicillin–clavulanic acid (12.5–15 mg/kg PO q12h).
- Appropriate antibiotic choice based on cultures from intact pustules.

Pemphigus Complex/Bullous Pemphigoid

Immunosuppressive/combination therapy:

- Corticosteroids—prednisolone 2.2–4.4 mg/kg PO tapering dosage; see Pemphigus.
- Azathioprine—2 mg/kg PO q48h to twice weekly.
- Chlorambucil—2 mg/m^2 PO q48h.
- Tetracycline—250 mg <10 kg, 500 mg >10 kg PO q8–12h.
- Doxycycline—10 mg/kg PO q24h.
- Minocycline—5 mg/kg PO q12h with niacinamide: 250 mg <10 kg, 500 mg >10 kg PO q8–12h.
- Cyclosporine, modified—5 mg/kg PO q24h.

Subcorneal Pustular Dermatosis

- Dapsone—1 mg/kg PO q8h until remission; tapered to 1 mg/kg q24h or twice weekly.
- Sulfasalazine—10–20 mg/kg PO q8h until remission; then as needed.

Linear IgA Dermatosis

- Prednisolone—2.2–4.4 mg/kg PO q24h until remission; taper to alternate-day therapy.
- Dapsone—1 mg/kg PO q8h until remission; taper and give as needed.

Sterile Eosinophilic Pustulosis

Prednisolone—2.2–4.4 mg/kg PO q24h until remission; then as needed to prevent relapses (usually long-term, alternate-day therapy required).

PRECAUTIONS

Prednisolone

- Secondary infection.
- Iatrogenic Cushing's syndrome.
- Muscle wasting.
- Steroid hepatopathy.
- Behavioral changes.
- Polydipsia, polyuria.
- Polyphagia.

Dapsone

- Dogs—mild anemia, mild leukopenia, and mild elevation of alanine aminotransferase (ALT), not associated with clinical signs; usually return to normal when dosage is reduced for maintenance.
- Rare fatal thrombocytopenia or severe leukopenia.
- Occasional vomiting, diarrhea, or pruritic skin eruption.
- Cats—more susceptible to dapsone toxicity; hemolytic anemia and neurotoxicity reported.

Sulfasalazine

Keratoconjunctivitis sicca.

Azathioprine and Chlorambucil

Potential for bone marrow suppression, gastrointestinal upset; azathioprine can cause hepatotoxicity and possibly pancreatitis.

Cyclosporine

May cause vomiting and diarrhea, gingival hyperplasia, B-lymphocyte hyperplasia, hirsutism, papillomatous skin eruptions, and increased incidence of infection; decreased glucose homeostasis; potential toxic reactions rare and include nephrotoxicity and hepatotoxicity.

POSSIBLE INTERACTIONS

N/A

ALTERNATIVE DRUG(S)

N/A

FOLLOW-UP

PATIENT MONITORING

- Dapsone—monitor hemogram, platelet count, and ALT every 2 weeks initially and if any clinical side effects develop.
- Long-term sulfasalazine therapy—monitor tear production.
- Immunosuppressive therapy—monitor every 1–2 weeks initially; then every 3–4 months during maintenance therapy.

MISCELLANEOUS

AGE-RELATED FACTORS

N/A

ZOONOTIC POTENTIAL

Dermatophytosis: may infect human beings in the household.

PREGNANCY/FERTILITY/BREEDING

N/A

SEE ALSO

- Acne—Cats.
- Acne—Dogs.
- Dermatomyositis.
- Dermatophytosis.
- Lupus Erythematosus, Cutaneous (Discoid).
- Lupus Erythematosus, Systemic (SLE).
- Pemphigus.
- Pyoderma.

ABBREVIATIONS

- ALT = alanine aminotransferase.
- ANA = antinuclear antibody.
- DLE = discoid lupus erythematosus.
- EMG = electromyography.
- Ig = immunoglobulin.
- SLE = systemic lupus erythematosus.

Suggested Reading

Helton Rhodes KA, Werner A. Blackwell's Five-Minute Veterinary Consult Clinical Companion: Small Animal Dermatology, number="3">3rd ed. Hoboken, NJ: Wiley-Blackwell, 2018.

Nuttall T, Eisenschenk M, Heinrich NA, Harvey RG. Skin Diseases of the Dog and Cat, 3rd ed. London: CRC Press, 2018.

Author Guillermina Manigot

Consulting Editor Alexander H. Werner Resnick

Acknowledgment The author and book editors acknowledge the prior contribution of Karen Helton Rhodes.

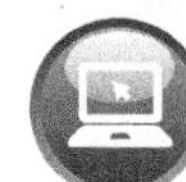

Client Education Handout available online

Dermatoses, Viral (Non-Papillomatosis)

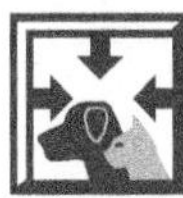

BASICS

OVERVIEW

• Dermatoses caused by viral infection within keratinized structures. • Viral replication may cause cytosuppressive effects or upregulate keratinization, resulting in hyperplastic or crusted conditions.

SIGNALMENT

• Young to young adult dogs. • Cats of any age.

SIGNS

• Facial involvement or involvement of head is common. • Lesions often asymmetric in distribution. • Paws and/or foot pads may be affected as well as mucocutaneous junctions. • Acute or gradual onset; lesions may be associated with bite wound or fight.
• Variable pruritus; can progress to self-mutilation. • Crusts. • Abscess.
• Paronychia. • Poor wound healing.
• Seborrhea. • Exfoliative dermatitis.
• Cutaneous horns. • Gingivitis/stomatitis.
• Cutaneous or oral ulceration. • Nasodigital hyperkeratosis. • Pigmented macules or plaques. • Progression to bowenoid in situ carcinoma (feline immunodeficiency virus [FIV], papillomavirus). • Multiple mast cell tumors (FIV). • Systemic signs of illness may be present. • Signs consistent with upper respiratory infection may or may not be present prior to development of skin lesions.

CAUSES & RISK FACTORS

• Feline leukemia virus (FeLV). • FIV.
• Feline cowpox virus infection. • Feline infectious peritonitis. • Feline papillomavirus.
• Canine papillomavirus. • Canine distemper. • Contagious viral pustular dermatitis (orf [parapoxvirus]). • Pseudorabies (α-herpesvirus). • Feline rhinotracheitis infection (α-herpesvirus-1). • Feline calicivirus infection. • Fighting or hunting behavior, multiple animal households, exposure to infected animals, and/or ingestion of infected material increases risk of exposure.

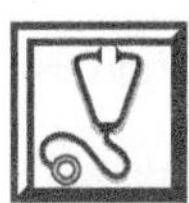

DIAGNOSIS

DIFFERENTIAL DIAGNOSIS

• Crusting diseases—drug eruption, actinic keratoses, pemphigus foliaceus, systemic lupus erythematosus, other causes for exfoliative dermatitis. • Allergic disorders—usually pruritic: atopy, fleas, food. • Feline herpesvirus dermatitis lesions can mimic lesions of eosinophilic granuloma complex.
• Parasitic diseases—canine and/or feline scabies, demodicosis, cheyletiellosis.
• Infectious diseases—superficial and deep bacterial and fungal infections, leishmaniasis.
• Dogs—zinc deficiency syndromes, hepatocutaneous syndrome, nasal hyperkeratosis. • Neoplasia—with extensive crusting and ulceration; squamous cell carcinoma, mast cell tumor, epitheliotropic lymphoma.

CBC/BIOCHEMISTRY/URINALYSIS

Nonspecific

OTHER LABORATORY TESTS

• Skin biopsy—necessary to prove viral origin of skin lesions; not always conclusive; if considering herpesvirus dermatitis, inform pathologist of suspicion. • Virus isolation.
• Serology—confirms FeLV, FIV, or other viral infection.

DIAGNOSTIC PROCEDURES

• Skin scrapings, trichograms—parasitic infestations. • Dermatophyte culture—fungal infections. • Epidermal cytology—bacterial folliculitis. • Skin biopsy is definitive diagnostic test. • Immunohistochemical staining for viral particles. • Viral serology and/or PCR.

PATHOLOGIC FINDINGS

• Irregular hyperplasia. • Ballooning degeneration. • Hydropic interface dermatitis. • Syncytial-type giant cell formation within epidermis and/or outer root sheath of hair follicle with associated apoptotic keratinocytes. • Keratinocyte inclusion bodies. • Epidermal ulceration with dermal necrosis, necrosis of epitrichial sweat glands, neutrophilic and/or eosinophilic inflammation.

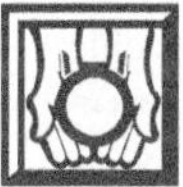

TREATMENT

• Usually outpatient, except for systemically ill patients. • Prevent exposure to other animals that could become infected.

MEDICATIONS

DRUG(S) OF CHOICE

• Supportive care and treatment of secondary infections. • Cats—herpesvirus: L-lysine 200–500 mg/cat q12h (questionable efficacy); interferon-α 30 units/cat/day PO; famcyclovir 125 mg q12h or 40–90mg/kg q12h, use of topical acyclovir reported.
• Cats—bowenoid in situ carcinoma: imiquimod. • Dogs—individual papillomas: surgical excision; imiquimod.

CONTRAINDICATIONS/POSSIBLE INTERACTIONS

Immunosuppressive therapies.

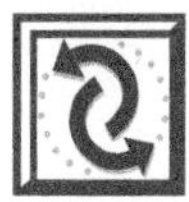

FOLLOW-UP

PATIENT MONITORING

Varies based on viral infection and presence or absence of systemic involvement.

PREVENTION/AVOIDANCE

Prevent hunting behavior and exposure to potentially infectious materials and infected animals.

EXPECTED COURSE AND PROGNOSIS

• Skin lesions may not respond to therapy.
• Systemic signs may eventually develop as result of viral infection. • Dependent on causal virus, animals may self-cure. • In cats, papillomavirus infection may progress to bowenoid in situ carcinoma.

MISCELLANEOUS

AGE-RELATED FACTORS

Dependent on viral cause.

ZOONOTIC POTENTIAL

Feline cowpox virus and contagious viral pustular dermatitis (parapoxvirus) can be transmitted to other dogs, humans, and cats.

SEE ALSO

• Canine Distemper.
• Feline Herpesvirus Infection.
• Feline Immunodeficiency Virus (FIV) Infection.
• Feline Leukemia Virus (FeLV) Infection.

ABBREVIATIONS

• FeLV = feline leukemia virus.
• FIV = feline immunodeficiency virus.

Suggested Reading

Helton Rhodes KA, Werner A. Blackwell's Five-Minute Veterinary Consult Clinical Companion: Small Animal Dermatology, 3rd ed. Hoboken, NJ: Wiley-Blackwell, 2018.

Author Elizabeth R. Drake
Consulting Editor Alexander H. Werner Resnick

DESTRUCTIVE AND SCRATCHING BEHAVIOR—CATS

BASICS

OVERVIEW

• Behavior that causes damage to an owner's home or belongings. • Primary destructive behaviors are normal feline behaviors that occur during exploration and play; scratching may be part of normal nail maintenance and communication with visual and scent marks. • Secondary destructive behavior may be a sign of other behavioral conditions and disease states.

Systems Affected

• Gastrointestinal—damage to teeth; vomiting, diarrhea, obstruction if items ingested.
• Ingestion of toxic material could affect any organ system.

SIGNALMENT

• Any breed or gender; may be genetic basis for sucking or chewing fabric in Siamese, Burmese, and Birman. • Primary destructive behavior is more common in young cats.

SIGNS

Primary Destructive Behavior

• No specific environmental trigger.
• Common targets for scratching are furniture, door frames, carpet, speakers.
• Curtains and furniture may be damaged when cats climb to explore or play. • May chew houseplants. • Items resembling string, including thread, shoelaces, and rubber bands, are often chewed and ingested; small items that are batted about may be accidentally swallowed.

Secondary Destructive Behavior

• Attention-seeking—destructive behavior in presence of owner. • Separation-related distress—destructive behavior in absence of the owner. • Compulsive behavior—licking, chewing, sucking, or ingesting nonfood items.
• Scratching may occur secondary to household conflict.

CAUSES & RISK FACTORS

• Lack of suitable outlets for scratching, climbing, perching, play, and resting. • Inadequate supervision, particularly in young cats.

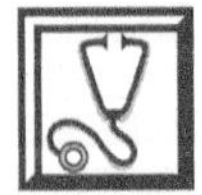

DIAGNOSIS

DIFFERENTIAL DIAGNOSIS

• Rule out medical conditions, especially if onset in mature cat. • Conditions affecting digestion, absorption, and appetite, including recent diet change. • Gastrointestinal disease and medical conditions associated with pain or anxiety.

CBC/BIOCHEMISTRY/URINALYSIS

Usually normal.

OTHER LABORATORY TESTS

As indicated to rule out medical conditions (T_4).

IMAGING

As indicated to rule out medical conditions.

DIAGNOSTIC PROCEDURES

For chewing/ingestive behavior, attention to oral cavity and scoping if indicated to rule out gastrointestinal causes.

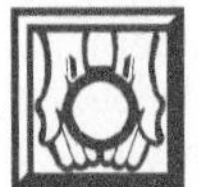

TREATMENT

Treat underlying disease.

Primary Destructive Behavior

• Keep claws trimmed. • Supervise/confine until appropriate behavior patterns have been established; provide food, litter, toys, and scratching posts in confinement area. • Prevent access to potential targets. • Provide acceptable scratching substrate such as sisal, cardboard, and loosely woven carpet in locations and orientation (horizontal or vertical) based on cat's preference.
• Apply feline interdigital pheromone to scratching posts. • Provide climbing towers, interactive play, feeding stations at different levels, food-dispensing toys, and multiple small meals.
• Reward appropriate behavior. • Reduce appeal of target areas and objects—e.g., double-sided sticky tape. • Provide indoor grass gardens.
• Declawing is banned in a number of countries and jurisdictions for ethical and humane reasons; where still legally permissible it should be a last resort after owners have been counseled on all alternative options. • While behavior modification is being implemented, plastic claw covers may be applied to prevent further damage.

Secondary Destructive Behavior

• Attention-seeking behavior—provide owner-initiated interactions. • Separation-related distress—provide opportunities for independent play and exploration.
• Compulsive disorder—identify and reduce sources of anxiety; offer appropriate outlets for play, chewing, and food-filled toys; some cats will chew rawhide; prevent access to target items. • Reduce household conflict.

MEDICATIONS

DRUG(S) OF CHOICE

• Medication is not indicated for primary destructive or attention-seeking behaviors.
• Medication may be indicated in combination with behavior management and modification for anxiety-based conditions and compulsive disorders. • See Fear, Phobias, and Anxieties—Cats; Compulsive Disorders—Cats.

Pheromones and Nutraceuticals

• Feline interdigital pheromone applied to scratching posts to encourage scratching. • F3 facial pheromone, cat-appeasing pheromone, alpha-casozepine, and l-theanine may reduce anxiety.

FOLLOW-UP

PATIENT MONITORING

Weekly follow-up to support owners.

PREVENTION/AVOIDANCE

• Destructive behavior is normal and self-rewarding. • Frequency may be reduced through client education during the first well-care visit, regardless of the age of the patient. • Provide information on suitable outlets for scratching, chewing, exploration, play, and enrichment.

POSSIBLE COMPLICATIONS

• Owners become frustrated, resulting in declawing or relinquishment. • Punishment can trigger fear or aggression. • Obstruction due to foreign body, including string foreign body.

EXPECTED COURSE AND PROGNOSIS

• Resolution of normal exploratory behavior usually within weeks. • Anxiety-based conditions and compulsive disorders often require long-term management, including psychotropic medication.

MISCELLANEOUS

AGE-RELATED FACTORS

Rule out medical conditions in adult onset.

PREGNANCY/FERTILITY/BREEDING

Preparturient destructive behavior (nesting).

SEE ALSO

• Compulsive Disorders—Cats.
• Fears, Phobias, and Anxieties—Cats.
• Kitten Behavior Problems.

INTERNET RESOURCES

• https://fearfreehappyhomes.com/category/explore/exercise-enrichment • https://catvets.com/guidelines/practice-guidelines/environmental- needs-guidelines • https://indoorpet.osu.edu/cats

Suggested Reading

Heath S. Canine and feline enrichment in the home and kennel: a guide for practitioners. Vet Clin North Am Small Anim Pract 2014, 44:427–449.
Landsberg G, Hunthausen W, Ackerman L. Behavior Problems of the Dog and Cat, 3rd ed. Philadelphia, PA: Elsevier Saunders, 2013.

Author Ellen M. Lindell
Consulting Editor Gary M. Landsberg

DESTRUCTIVE BEHAVIOR—DOGS

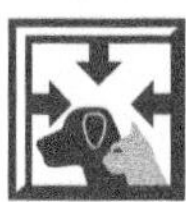

BASICS

DEFINITION

- Behavior that causes damage to an owner's home, property, or belongings.
- Primary destructive behavior is normal behavior that includes exploratory and play-based behavior.
- Secondary destructive behavior is a clinical sign of another behavior condition.

PATHOPHYSIOLOGY

- Dogs normally explore and engage with their environment. When access to appropriate outlets and enrichment is not readily available and in the absence of supervision and guidance, owner's property may be targeted.
- Insufficient opportunities for social interactions can contribute to destructive behavior.
- Dogs may dig for comfort or cooling, and to escape confinement. Digging can be triggered by sounds of burrowed animals and scents of food sources.
- Though manipulating the environment results in property damage, it may be self-rewarding and self-soothing.
- Conditions causing distress, including pain, fear, anxiety, and frustration, can contribute to destructive behavior.

SYSTEMS AFFECTED

- Behavioral—frustration or anxiety.
- Gastrointestinal (GI)—damage to teeth or oral mucosa; pharyngitis or esophagitis; vomiting, diarrhea, or obstruction if ingested.
- Musculoskeletal—trauma caused by scratching, chewing, or digging.
- Skin—excoriation, nail damage secondary to trauma.
- Ingestion of toxic material could affect any organ system.

GENETICS

None

INCIDENCE/PREVALENCE

Normal canine behavior—problem reported by approximately 12% of owners.

GEOGRAPHIC DISTRIBUTION

None

SIGNALMENT

- Species—dog.
- Breed predilections—certain breeds are by nature more active and, if insufficient outlets for exploratory and/or social engagement, may engage in destructive behavior. Northern breeds may dig for resting and thermoregulation. Some terrier and hound breeds may dig when burrowing for prey.
- Mean age and range—primary destructive behavior most often seen in puppies and young dogs; secondary destructive behavior seen at any age.
- Predominant sex—N/A.

SIGNS

- Destructive behavior is a clinical sign rather than a diagnosis.
- Dogs may use their teeth or claws to damage floors, furniture, walls, or frames of doors and windows or dig at fencing. Some dogs chew or even ingest small personal items.
- Clients may ascribe the underlying motivation to spite or suggest a diagnosis such as separation anxiety. Though barriers are often targeted in association with separation-related distress or territorial behavior, no focus of damage is pathognomonic.
- Knowledge of the contexts in which destructive behavior occurs is critical for diagnosis.
- Physical examination findings—fractured teeth; excoriations on nose; broken front claws; digital pain.

CAUSES

- Primary destructive behavior:
  - Inadequate supervision provides access to self-rewarding behavior.
  - Lack of access to preferred chewable and/or interactive toys.
  - Insufficient cognitive enrichment.
  - Inadequate social enrichment.
- Secondary destructive behavior:
  - Confinement in presence of an inciting trigger.
  - Confinement frustration.
  - Separation-related distress—inadequate habituation to absence of owner.
  - Noise phobia.
  - Territorial behavior.
  - Unintentional reinforcement by owner.
  - Medical conditions associated with pain.

RISK FACTORS

Early environmental experiences including prior emotional trauma are risk factors for development of fear and anxiety-related conditions.

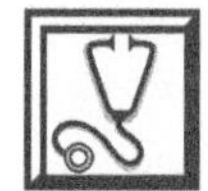

DIAGNOSIS

DIFFERENTIAL DIAGNOSIS

- Pathologic conditions—index of suspicion for underlying medical condition should be high in adult patients with sudden onset of destructive behavior in absence of notable environmental changes.
- GI disease—if pica accompanies destructive chewing: rule out conditions affecting digestion, absorption, and polyphagia, including recent diet changes that can affect satiety; licking of surfaces such as floors, carpet, and nonfood items may be associated with upper GI disease.
- Separation-related distress.
- Noise phobia, storm phobia—distress in response to stimulus.
- Territorial behavior—destructive behavior related to presence of triggers; window frames and doorways are damaged.
- Cognitive dysfunction syndrome—destructive behavior related to agitation, anxiety, and abnormal repetitive behaviors with onset or progression in patients 7 years or older; other signs of cognitive dysfunction are typically present.

CBC/BIOCHEMISTRY/URINALYSIS

No pathology expected.

OTHER LABORATORY TESTS

As indicated to rule out medical conditions.

DIAGNOSTIC PROCEDURES

As indicated to rule out medical conditions.

PATHOLOGIC FINDINGS

N/A except lesions secondary to self-trauma.

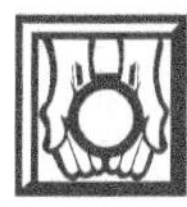

TREATMENT

APPROPRIATE HEALTH CARE

- Traumatic injuries are typically minor and can be managed with outpatient care. Traumatic dental injuries and GI foreign bodies may require surgical intervention.
- Behavioral treatment protocols include behavior modification to address frustration or anxiety; determination of safe methods for supervision, confinement; and customized enrichment protocol based on patient preferences and owner lifestyle.
- All toys carry a potential risk of injury to the patient, including inadvertent ingestion and dental injury.
- Environmental management:
  - Prevent or supervise access to potential targets of destruction.
  - Provide thermoregulation options (kiddie pool, dog house) to reduce digging.
- Behavior modification may include:
  - Providing for and reinforcing alternative desirable activities and outlets.
  - Relaxation exercises to reduce inadvertent reinforcement of undesirable behavior.
  - Habituation to crate or gate confinement.
- Environmental enrichment:
  - Preference testing of appropriate toys and chew items.
  - Provide acceptable substrate and location for digging—treats and toys can be buried to encourage digging in area.
- Design a schedule for provision of exercise, cognitive enrichment, social enrichment, and reward-based training.
- Design a behavioral log to record progress and preferences.

NURSING CARE

Behavioral appointments can be scheduled with veterinarian or trained nursing staff.

ACTIVITY

- Aerobic exercise schedule should consider the patient's physical health. Healthy dogs may benefit from two half-hour exercise sessions each day.

- Cognitive stimulation may be provided with reward-based training and food puzzles.
- Provide opportunities for dogs to engage in breed-typical normal behaviors, including sniffing and "hunting" (tracking, nosework).

DIET

- Some patients benefit from feeding via puzzles and food-stuffed toys.
- Food toys may not be appropriate for pets that exhibit possessive or food-related aggression.

CLIENT EDUCATION

- Clients should take an active role in managing destructive behavior.
- Preadoption counseling provides an opportunity to educate clients regarding providing for pets' needs, including social and exploratory play and safe toys.
- Provide a plan for supervision and enrichment.
- Teach clients to communicate expectations by reinforcing desired behaviors and preventing access to undesirable behaviors, including dog proofing and confinement training.
- Provide references for local trainers who support positive reinforcement rather than confrontation.

Aversive Products and Punishment

- Application of nontoxic bitter-tasting products to targeted objects is sometimes used to manage primary destructive behavior in conjunction with supervision.
- It is essential that, upon discovering an unpleasant taste, the dog has immediate access to an appropriate item; it is more effective and appropriate to supervise and quietly guide dogs toward appropriate items.
- Punishment is not an accepted tool for managing destructive behavior; it does not address the underlying motivation and can lead to fear, anxiety, or aggression.

SURGICAL CONSIDERATIONS

N/A

MEDICATIONS

DRUG(S) OF CHOICE

- Medication is not indicated for treating primary destructive behaviors or attention-seeking behavior.
- Medication complements behavior modification and may provide more rapid resolution when treating anxiety-based conditions.

Selective Serotonin Reuptake Inhibitors (SSRIs)

Fluoxetine—0.5–2 mg/kg PO q24h.

Tricyclic Antidepressants (TCAs)

Clomipramine—1–3 mg/kg PO q12h.

For Situational Anxiety (Alone or Together with SSRI or TCA)

- Alprazolam—0.01–0.1 mg/kg PO prior to event.
- Trazodone—3–10 mg/kg PO prior to event.
- Clonidine—0.01–0.05 mg/kg PO prior to event.

CONTRAINDICATIONS

TCAs—contraindicated in animals with cardiac conduction disturbances or glaucoma.

PRECAUTIONS

Benzodiazepines may disinhibit aggression—use with caution in dogs with a history of aggressive behavior.

POSSIBLE INTERACTIONS

- SSRIs, TCAs, and trazodone should not be used with monoamine oxidase inhibitors, including amitraz and selegiline.
- Combining drugs that increase serotonin (e.g., SSRI or TCA with trazodone) should be done with caution to avoid serotonin syndrome.

ALTERNATIVE DRUGS

Dog-appeasing pheromone, nutraceuticals containing L-theanine or alpha-casozepine, or a calming probiotic may be used to reduce mild anxiety. The safety margin is wide.

FOLLOW-UP

PATIENT MONITORING

Weekly calls to confirm compliance and adjust enrichment based on patient preferences. Most patients benefit from one-on-one behavior modification sessions every 2 weeks.

PREVENTION/AVOIDANCE

Client education during the first visit, regardless of the age of the patient. Provide information on suitable outlets for chewing, digging, exercise, reward training, and the importance of both cognitive and social enrichment.

POSSIBLE COMPLICATIONS

Without adequate support, owners may become frustrated, resulting in relinquishment of the dog. Owners may seek advice from individuals offering "quick fixes" that could ultimately jeopardize the patient.

EXPECTED COURSE AND PROGNOSIS

Prognosis is excellent. Resolution of normal exploratory behavior is usually rapid.

MISCELLANEOUS

ASSOCIATED CONDITIONS

Destructive behavior is often associated with attention-seeking behavior.

AGE-RELATED FACTORS

Young dogs are at increased risk for normal destructive behavior.

ZOONOTIC POTENTIAL

None

PREGNANCY/FERTILITY/BREEDING

Preparturient destructive behavior (nesting).

SEE ALSO

- Cognitive Dysfunction Syndrome.
- Marking, Roaming, and Mounting Behavior—Dogs.
- Puppy Behavior Problems.
- Separation Anxiety Syndrome.
- Thunderstorm and Noise Phobias.
- Unruly Behaviors: Jumping, Pulling, Chasing, Stealing—Dogs.

ABBREVIATIONS

- GI = gastrointestinal.
- SSRI = selective serotonin reuptake inhibitor.
- TCA = tricyclic antidepressant.

INTERNET RESOURCES

- fearfreehappyhomes.com
- https://indoorpet.osu.edu/dogs/environmental_enrichment_dogs

Suggested Reading

Heath S. Canine and feline enrichment in the home and kennel: a guide for practitioners. Vet Clin North Am Small Anim Pract 2014, 44:427–449.

Horwitz D, ed. Blackwell's 5 Minute Consult Clinical Companion: Canine and Feline Behavior, 2nd ed. Hoboken, NJ: Wiley, 2018, pp. 745–753, 767–773.

Author Ellen M. Lindell

Consulting Editor Gary M. Landsberg

BASICS

DEFINITION

Diabetes insipidus (DI) is a disorder of water metabolism characterized by polyuria (PU), urine of low specific gravity or osmolality (so-called insipid, or tasteless, urine), and polydipsia (PD).

PATHOPHYSIOLOGY

- Central DI (CDI)—deficiency in the secretion of antidiuretic hormone (ADH).
- Nephrogenic DI (NDI)—renal insensitivity to ADH.

SYSTEMS AFFECTED

- Endocrine/metabolic.
- Renal/urologic.

INCIDENCE/PREVALENCE

- Primary CDI—rare.
- Primary NDI—rare.

SIGNALMENT

Species

Dog and cat.

Breed Predilections

None

Mean Age and Range

- Congenital forms <1 year.
- Acquired forms, any age.

SIGNS

- PU.
- PD.
- Incontinence—occasional.
- Signs of intracranial mass if due to pituitary tumor.
- Dehydration and weakness in animals with uncompensated free water loss.

CAUSES

Inadequate Secretion of ADH

- Congenital defect.
- Idiopathic.
- Trauma.
- Neoplasia.

Renal Insensitivity to ADH

- Congenital—defect in aquaporin (renal tubular channel that allows free water reabsorption).
- Secondary to drugs (e.g., lithium, demeclocycline).
- Secondary to endocrine and metabolic disorders (e.g., hyperadrenocorticism, hyponatremia, hypercalcemia).
- Secondary to renal disease or infection (e.g., pyelonephritis, chronic kidney disease, pyometra).

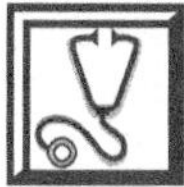

DIAGNOSIS

DIFFERENTIAL DIAGNOSIS

Polyuric Disorders

- Hyperadrenocorticism.
- Diabetes mellitus.
- Renal disease.
- Hyperthyroidism—cats.
- Hyperadrenocorticism.
- Liver disease—portosystemic shunt.
- Pyometra.
- Pyelonephritis.
- Hypercalcemia.
- Primary PD.

CBC/BIOCHEMISTRY/URINALYSIS

- Usually normal; hypernatremia in patients with excessive free water loss.
- Urinary specific gravity low (<1.006, hyposthenuria).

OTHER LABORATORY TESTS

Plasma ADH (not commercially available).

IMAGING

- MRI or CT scan if pituitary tumor is suspected.
- Abdominal radiographs or ultrasound may help rule out other polyuric disorders.

DIAGNOSTIC PROCEDURES

- ADH supplementation trial—preferred to water deprivation test; therapeutic trial with synthetic ADH (desmopressin [DDAVP]); positive response (water intake decreases by 50% in 5–7 days).
- Modified water deprivation test (see Appendix II for protocol)—not routinely recommended due to risk of complications.
- Rule out all other causes of PU/PD before considering primary CDI.

PATHOLOGIC FINDINGS

Degeneration and death of neurosecretory neurons in neurohypophysis (primary CDI).

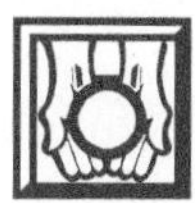

TREATMENT

APPROPRIATE HEALTH CARE

- Patients should be hospitalized for modified water deprivation test; the ADH trial is often performed as an outpatient procedure.
- Animals with NDI should have underlying disease diagnosed and treated.

ACTIVITY

Not restricted.

DIET

Normal, with free access to water.

CLIENT EDUCATION

- Review dosage of DDAVP and administration technique.
- Importance of having water available at all times.

SURGICAL CONSIDERATIONS

Pyometra is a surgical emergency and should be removed as soon as the patient is stabilized.

MEDICATIONS

DRUG(S) OF CHOICE

- CDI—DDAVP (1–2 drops of intranasal preparation in conjunctival sac q12–24h to control PU/PD); alternatively, intranasal preparation may be given SC (2–5 μg, q12–24h). Oral preparation of DDAVP is available in 0.1–0.2 mg tablets, with each 0.1 mg comparable to 1 large drop of intranasal preparation.
- NDI—hydrochlorothiazide (2–4 mg/kg PO q12h), in addition to treatment of any underlying cause.

CONTRAINDICATIONS

None

PRECAUTIONS

Overdose of DDAVP can cause water intoxication.

FOLLOW-UP

PATIENT MONITORING

- Adjust treatment according to patient's signs; ideal dosage and frequency of DDAVP administration based on water intake.
- Laboratory tests such as PCV, total solids, and serum sodium concentration, and patient weight to detect dehydration (inadequate DDAVP replacement).

PREVENTION/AVOIDANCE

Circumstances that might increase water loss.

POSSIBLE COMPLICATIONS

Anticipate complications of primary disease (e.g., pituitary tumor).

EXPECTED COURSE AND PROGNOSIS

- CDI usually permanent, except in patients in which condition was trauma induced.
- NDI usually resolves with treatment of underlying disorder.
- Prognosis generally good, depending on underlying disorder.
- Without treatment, dehydration can lead to stupor, coma, and death.

MISCELLANEOUS

AGE-RELATED FACTORS

- Congenital CDI and NDI usually manifest before 6 months of age.
- CDI related to pituitary tumors usually seen in dogs >5 years old.

DIABETES INSIPIDUS (CONTINUED)

D

SYNONYMS
- Cranial diabetes insipidus.
- ADH-responsive diabetes insipidus.

SEE ALSO
Hyposthenuria

ABBREVIATIONS
- ADH = antidiuretic hormone.
- CDI = central diabetes insipidus.
- DI = diabetes insipidus.
- NDI = nephrogenic diabetes insipidus.
- PD = polydipsia.
- PU = polyuria.

Suggested Reading

Feldman EC, Nelson RW, Reusch CE, Scott-Moncrieff JCR. Canine and Feline Endocrinology, 4th ed. Philadelphia, PA: Saunders, 2015.

Author Patty A. Lathan
Consulting Editor Patty A. Lathan
Acknowledgment The author and book editors acknowledge the prior contribution of Rhett Nichols.

Client Education Handout available online

Diabetes Mellitus With Hyperosmolar Hyperglycemic State

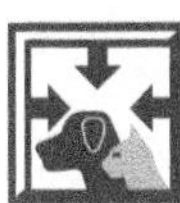

BASICS

DEFINITION

• The hyperosmolar hyperglycemic state (HHS) is a complicated form of diabetes mellitus (DM) characterized by severe hyperglycemia and dehydration that produces a marked elevation in serum osmolarity. Unlike diabetic ketoacidosis (DKA), ketone production and metabolic acidosis are not major features of HHS. • Specific guidelines for HHS diagnosis are lacking in dogs and cats, but serum effective osmolarity >320 mOsm/L, glucose concentration >600 mg/dL, and bicarbonate concentration >18 mEq/L, along with minimal ketonuria, are criteria in humans.

PATHOPHYSIOLOGY

• Hyperglycemia is due to insulin deficiency from DM; insulinopenia reduces tissue glucose utilization and increases hepatic glucose production, leading to increased extracellular glucose concentrations; the magnitude of hyperglycemia in HHS is usually greater than in DKA. • Hyperosmolarity develops secondary to hyperglycemia and is exacerbated by dehydration and reduced extracellular fluid volume; the contribution of glucose to total plasma osmolarity is significant in HHS.
• Dehydration and volume deficit are typically severe and are caused by several factors, including reduced water intake and volume losses via gastrointestinal and renal systems.
• Reduced plasma volume decreases glomerular filtration rate and urine production, leading to azotemia; in HHS, severe volume contraction with reduced urinary glucose excretion results in severe hyperglycemia and plasma hyperosmolarity.
• Hyperketonemia and ketonuria are not major features of HHS; lactic acidosis secondary to volume depletion, tissue hypoperfusion, and impaired glucose metabolism is the major cause of acidosis in patients with HHS.

SYSTEMS AFFECTED

• Endocrine. • Renal/urologic—prerenal azotemia due to decreased extracellular fluid volume; urine production usually maintained by glucose-induced diuresis unless volume deficit is severe or acute kidney injury is present. • Cardiovascular—hypovolemia; metabolic acidosis and electrolyte abnormalities may contribute to hypotension and poor myocardial contractility. • Nervous—hyperosmolarity promotes intracellular dehydration and neuronal dysfunction.

GENETICS

N/A

INCIDENCE/PREVALENCE

Uncommon

GEOGRAPHIC DISTRIBUTION

N/A

SIGNALMENT

Species

Dog and cat (more frequent).

Breed Predilections

N/A

Mean Age and Range

Most common in middle-aged dogs (mean 9 years) and cats (mean 12 years).

Predominant Sex

N/A

SIGNS

Historical Findings

• All patients have DM; in some, diagnosis of DM occurs prior to HHS. • Some patients have concurrent chronic illness. • Signs caused by DM—may not be appreciated after HHS onset: ◦ Polydipsia. ◦ Polyuria. ◦ Polyphagia. ◦ Weight loss. • Signs caused by HHS: ◦ Weakness/lethargy. ◦ Vomiting. ◦ Reduced appetite. ◦ Neurologic complaints—abnormal responsiveness, coma.

Physical Examination Findings

• Findings associated with dehydration and hypovolemia: ◦ Decreased skin turgor. ◦ Prolonged capillary refill time. ◦ Reduced pulse pressure. ◦ Tachycardia. ◦ Hypothermia.
• Findings associated with hyperosmolarity: ◦ Lethargy, depressed mentation, stupor, or coma. ◦ Seizure. • Findings associated with DM: ◦ Low body condition score. ◦ Cataracts (dogs).

CAUSES

• Develops in patients with DM and severe dehydration/volume loss. • Reduced water intake may precede onset of HHS.
• Comorbid conditions common.

RISK FACTORS

Risk for HHS may be higher in diabetic animals with concurrent disorders, including heart disease, renal insufficiency, hyperadrenocorticism, acute pancreatitis, and neoplasia.

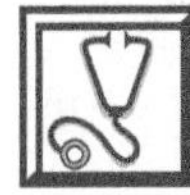

DIAGNOSIS

DIFFERENTIAL DIAGNOSIS

• DM—may be uncomplicated to complicated, including DKA and HHS; all have similar clinical signs and laboratory findings, but can be subcategorized based on magnitude of hyperglycemia and hyperketonemia.
• Hypernatremia—severe hypernatremia produces CNS signs similar to HHS, but with sodium as major osmole; polyuria and polydipsia may be present, particularly if hypernatremia develops secondary to diabetes insipidus. • Hyperosmolarity of any cause—may produce similar CNS abnormalities; toxins (e.g., ethylene glycol or alcohol) or CNS lesions (e.g., causing adipsia) may cause hyperosmolarity. • CNS disease—primary CNS disorders may produce clinical signs of HHS; marked fluid deficits are not expected.
• Myxedema coma—manifestation of severe hypothyroidism with similar clinical signs without hyperosmolarity or hyperglycemia; low total thyroxine and elevated thyroid-stimulating hormone present.

CBC/BIOCHEMISTRY/URINALYSIS

• Hyperglycemia—blood glucose concentration frequently exceeds 600 mg/dL and severe hyperglycemia (1500–2000+ mg/dL) exists in some patients. • Azotemia—elevated blood urea nitrogen (BUN) and serum creatinine concentrations are common, usually prerenal, but renal azotemia occurs in some patients. • Sodium—hypo- or hypernatremia may be observed; hyperosmolarity is most severe with concurrent hyperglycemia and hypernatremia. • Potassium—hypokalemia is common; hyperkalemia is associated with acute kidney injury or reduced urine output.
• Acidosis—metabolic acidosis is less severe than DKA; hypobicarbonemia and hyperlactatemia occur secondary to hypovolemia or renal failure. • Glucosuria—present; mild ketonuria possible. • Urine specific gravity (USG) variable; may be misleading due to glucosuria, which increases USG.

OTHER LABORATORY TESTS

• Blood and urine osmolarity—serum osmolarity >320 mosm/L consistent with HHS; urine osmolality elevated due to glucosuria. • Serum osmolarity can be estimated from routine serum chemistry results: $2\,([Na^+]+[K^+]) + [BUN]/2.8 + [Glucose]/18$; if results are in IU, equation is modified: $2\,([Na^+]+[K^+]) + [BUN] + [Glucose]$.

IMAGING

N/A

DIAGNOSTIC PROCEDURES

N/A

PATHOLOGIC FINDINGS

• Pancreas—consistent with DM: islet atrophy and loss (dogs and cats) and islet amyloid (cats). • Brain—changes not specific for HHS; evidence of CNS edema.

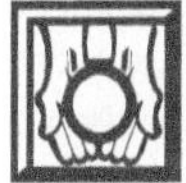

TREATMENT

APPROPRIATE HEALTH CARE

Life-threatening medical emergency requiring inpatient treatment. After HHS resolution, patients require treatment and follow-up for DM.

NURSING CARE

• Correction of fluid deficits—major treatment goal, begin prior to insulin replacement; IV fluid replacement indicated for ill patients; enteral water can assist with free water replacement in patients that tolerate oral intake. • Fluid type and rate depend on patient's hydration and volume status and magnitude of metabolic derangements; fluid deficit is estimated using the equation: %volume depletion * body weight(kg) = fluid deficit (L). • Hypo- and normonatremic patients—isotonic crystalloid solution is appropriate for initial volume replacement; replacement of volume deficit should occur over 12–24h; patients with hypotension or shock due to hypovolemia should receive fluid bolus of 20–25% of estimated blood volume (dog: 80 mL/kg; cat: 50 ml/kg), which can be repeated until blood pressure is adequate; once blood pressure is restored, the remaining deficit is replaced over 12–24h. • Hypernatremic patients—hypernatremia implies a free water deficit and its occurrence with hyperglycemia in HHS may result in life-threatening hyperosmolarity; isotonic (0.9%) saline solution appropriate for initial volume replacement in hypernatremic patients with hypovolemic hypotension; if hypernatremia persists after blood pressure and urine output are restored, use of hypotonic (0.45%) saline solution indicated to replace free water and reduce sodium, unless oral water intake possible; recommended that serum sodium concentration reduction should not exceed 12 mEq/day (see Hypernatremia). • Electrolyte replacement—potassium deficiency is expected, and should be replaced unless hyperkalemia is present; dosage based on magnitude of hypokalemia; potassium replacement by IV infusion should not exceed 0.5 mEq K^+/kg/h and fluids with supplemented K^+ should be avoided during rapid volume infusion; supplementation of other electrolytes (e.g., magnesium, phosphorous) may also be necessary. • Glucose supplementation—some protocols recommend using dextrose infusion to prevent hypoglycemia during insulin therapy; 2.5–5% dextrose CRI used as needed to maintain blood glucose concentrations between 150 and 250 mg/dL.

ACTIVITY

N/A

DIET

N/A

CLIENT EDUCATION

• Patients frequently have a serious concurrent disorder(s) that affects prognosis. • Permanent DM is expected and survivors will require lifelong treatment for DM.

SURGICAL CONSIDERATIONS

N/A

MEDICATIONS

DRUG(S) OF CHOICE

• CRI of regular insulin is recommended for initial glucose control; insulin therapy should be started 2–6h after starting fluid therapy so initial decrease in serum glucose is not extreme. • CRI preparation—regular insulin at 2.2 U/kg/24h (some protocols recommend 1.1 U/kg/24h dose in cats) added to 250 mL of 0.9% NaCl; prior to beginning CRI, 50 mL of solution should pass through plastic administration tubing and be discarded (insulin binds to some plastics); CRI started at 5 mL/h (cat) or 10 mL/h (dog) and infusion rate adjusted as needed to reduce hyperglycemia at desired rate and maintain target glucose concentration. • Once HHS is resolved and patient stable, discontinue insulin CRI and transition to longer-acting insulin to be used for chronic DM management.

CONTRAINDICATIONS

N/A

PRECAUTIONS

• Brain edema may occur when hyperosmolarity is corrected too rapidly; patients with edema develop worsening neurologic status during treatment; minimizing rapid decreases in glucose and sodium during treatment lowers edema risk. • Insulin administration can result in hypokalemia; electrolytes should be monitored frequently (q4–6h) until stable.

POSSIBLE INTERACTIONS

N/A

ALTERNATIVE DRUG(S)

• Ultrashort-acting insulins (insulin aspart or insulin lispro) may be substituted for regular insulin in CRI protocols. • Protocol for intermittent IM use of regular insulin (when CRI not available)—0.2 U/kg IM initially, followed by 0.1 U/kg IM q1h until glucose <250 mg/dL; subsequent doses 0.5–1.0 U/kg IM q4–6h to maintain glucose concentration between 150 and 250 mg/dL.

FOLLOW-UP

PATIENT MONITORING

• Volume and hydration status—monitor heart rate, pulse quality, capillary refill time, blood pressure, bodyweight, and urine output. • Blood glucose—monitor q1–2h to guide insulin therapy; aim for gradual reduction of serum glucose (50–100 mg/dL/h) to 150–250 mg/dL without hypoglycemia. • Monitor serum Na^+ and K^+ concentrations, especially during correction of hypernatremia or K^+ supplementation; magnesium and phosphorous should be monitored, especially after start of insulin therapy. • After stabilization, long-term monitoring appropriate for DM is indicated.

PREVENTION/AVOIDANCE

• Adequate insulin therapy and monitoring of glycemia in patients with DM may reduce risk of HHS. • Early recognition and effective treatment of new-onset DM may reduce risk of DKA or HHS.

POSSIBLE COMPLICATIONS

• Hypoglycemia or electrolyte disturbances may develop during treatment. • Severe neurologic signs, including coma and death, may occur. • Dehydration and shock can precipitate acute kidney injury. • Death due to shock or coma may occur in untreated animals.

EXPECTED COURSE AND PROGNOSIS

• Hydration and blood pressure should improve within a few hours of initiating fluid therapy and resolve over 12–24h; hyperglycemia is corrected over 6–12h once insulin therapy started.
• Electrolyte derangements must be managed to avoid osmotic complications secondary to sodium fluctuations, and to avoid hypo-/hyperkalemia, hypophosphatemia, or hypomagnesemia. • Depending on patient response, prognosis is guarded; worse if severe neurologic compromise or renal failure is present.

MISCELLANEOUS

ASSOCIATED CONDITIONS

• DKA and HHS have significant overlap in clinical signs and laboratory abnormalities.
• Patients with HHS should be evaluated for concurrent conditions (cardiac or renal failure, pancreatitis, neoplasia, etc.).

SYNONYMS

• Diabetic coma. • Hyperosmolar nonketotic syndrome.

SEE ALSO

• Diabetes Mellitus With Ketoacidosis.
• Diabetes Mellitus Without Complication—Cats. • Diabetes Mellitus Without Complication—Dogs. • Hyperglycemia.
• Hyperosmolarity.

ABBREVIATIONS

• BUN = blood urea nitrogen. • DKA = diabetic ketoacidosis. • DM = diabetes mellitus.
• HHS = hyperosmolar hyperglycemic state.
• USG = urine specific gravity.

Suggested Reading

Koenig A, Drobatz KJ, Beale AB, King LG. Hyperglycemic, hyperosmolar syndrome in feline diabetics: 17 cases (1995–2001). J Vet Emerg Crit Care 2004, 14:30–40.
O'Brien MA. Diabetic emergencies in small animals. Vet Clin North Am Small Anim Pract 2010, 40:317–333.
Rand JS. Diabetic ketoacidosis and hyperosmola hyperglycemia in cats. Vet Clin North Am Small Anim Pract 2013, 43:367–379.
Trotman, TK, Drobatz KJ, Hess RS. Retrospective evaluation of hyperosmolar hyperglycemia in 66 dogs (1993–2008). J Vet Emerg Crit Care 2013, 23:557–564.

Author Thomas Schermerhorn
Consulting Editor Patty A. Lathan
Acknowledgment The author and book editors acknowledge the prior contribution of Deborah S. Greco.

DIABETES MELLITUS WITH KETOACIDOSIS

BASICS

DEFINITION

A medical emergency secondary to absolute or relative insulin deficiency, characterized by hyperglycemia, ketonemia, metabolic acidosis, dehydration, and electrolyte depletion.

PATHOPHYSIOLOGY

- Insulin deficiency causes an increase in lipolysis, resulting in excessive ketone body production and metabolic acidosis; an inability to maintain fluid and electrolyte homeostasis causes dehydration, prerenal azotemia, electrolyte disorders, obtundation, and death.
- Many patients with diabetic ketoacidosis (DKA) have underlying conditions such as infection, inflammation, or heart disease that cause stress hormone (e.g., glucagon, cortisol, growth hormone, epinephrine) secretion; this probably contributes to development of insulin resistance and DKA by promoting lipolysis, ketogenesis, gluconeogenesis, and glycogenolysis.
- Dehydration and electrolyte abnormalities result from osmotic diuresis, promoting the loss of total body water and electrolytes.

SYSTEMS AFFECTED

- Endocrine/metabolic.
- Gastrointestinal.
- Hematologic (cats).

GENETICS

None

INCIDENCE/PREVALENCE

Unknown

GEOGRAPHIC DISTRIBUTION

None

SIGNALMENT

Species

Dog and cat.

Breed Predilections

- Dog—miniature poodle and dachshund.
- Cat—none.

Mean Age and Range

- Dog—mean age 8.4 years.
- Cat—median age 11 years (range: 1–19 years).

Predominant Sex

- Dogs—females 1.5 times more prevalent than males.
- Cats—males 2 times more prevalent than females.

SIGNS

- Shock.
- Dehydration.
- Hypothermia.
- Polyuria.
- Polydipsia or adipsia.
- Anorexia.
- Weakness.
- Vomiting.
- Lethargy.
- Tachypnea.
- Muscle wasting and weight loss.
- Unkempt haircoat.
- Thin body condition.
- Ketone odor on breath.
- Icterus.
- Dandruff.

CAUSES

- Diabetes mellitus.
- Infection (e.g., pyoderma, pneumonia, urinary tract infection, prostatis, pyelonephritis, pyometra).
- Concurrent disease (e.g., heart failure, pancreatitis, renal insufficiency or failure, asthma, neoplasia, acromegaly).
- Estrus.
- Idiopathic.
- Medication noncompliance.
- Stress.
- Surgery.

RISK FACTORS

- Any condition that leads to absolute or relative insulin deficiency.
- History of corticosteroid or beta blocker administration.

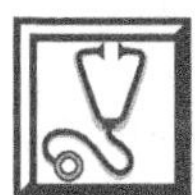

DIAGNOSIS

DIFFERENTIAL DIAGNOSIS

- Hyperosmolar hyperglycemic state.
- Acute hypoglycemic coma/insulin overdose.
- Uremia/azotemia due to renal disease or postrenal obstruction.
- Other cause of metabolic acidosis (e.g., lactic acidosis, ethylene glycol intoxication, renal tubular acidosis).

CBC/BIOCHEMISTRY/URINALYSIS

- Leukocytosis with mature neutrophilia.
- Hyperglycemia—blood glucose concentration usually >250 mg/dL.
- High liver enzyme activity.
- Hypercholesterolemia and lipemia.
- Azotemia.
- Hypochloremia.
- Hypokalemia.
- Hyponatremia.
- Hypophosphatemia.
- Hypomagnesemia.
- High anion gap—anion gap = (sodium + potassium) – (chloride + bicarbonate); normal is 16 ± 4.
- Glucosuria and ketonuria.
- Variable urinary specific gravity with active or inactive sediment.
- Hyperproteinemia.
- Heinz body anemia (cats).

OTHER LABORATORY TESTS

- Metabolic acidosis—HCO_3^- <15 mEq/L (total CO_2 estimates HCO_3^-).
- Hyperosmolarity (>330 mOsm/kg).
- Bacterial culture of urine and blood.

DIAGNOSTIC PROCEDURES

- Abdominal and thoracic radiography and ultrasound may be necessary to identify comorbid diseases.
- ECG and blood pressure monitoring indicated for patients with shock or electrolyte abnormalities.

PATHOLOGIC FINDINGS

Pancreatic islet cell atrophy.

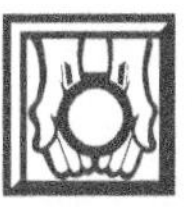

TREATMENT

APPROPRIATE HEALTH CARE

- If the animal is bright, alert, and well hydrated, intensive care and IV fluid administration are not required; start SC administration of insulin (short- or intermediate-acting insulin), offer food, and supply constant access to water; monitor closely for signs of illness (e.g., anorexia, lethargy, vomiting).
- Treatment of animals with DKA that are systemically ill requires intensive inpatient care; goals are to correct depletion of water and electrolytes, reverse ketonemia and acidosis, and increase rate of glucose use by insulin-dependent tissues.

NURSING CARE

- Fluids—necessary to ensure adequate cardiac output and tissue perfusion and to maintain vascular volume; also reduce blood glucose concentration.
- IV administration of isotonic crystalloid supplemented with potassium is initial fluid of choice; volume and rate determined by fluid replacement needs plus maintenance requirements; replace over 24–48h.

ACTIVITY

N/A

DIET

Following stabilization, diet should be adjusted to account for patient's diabetes, concurrent disease, and body condition. High-fiber diets are not recommended in underweight pets.

CLIENT EDUCATION

Serious medical condition requiring lifelong insulin administration in most patients. Confirm that client is prepared to inject twice daily insulin prior to treatment of DKA.

SURGICAL CONSIDERATIONS

N/A

MEDICATIONS

DRUG(S) OF CHOICE

Insulin

- Regular insulin is the insulin of choice until eating; lispro insulin may also be considered.
- Initial dosage—0.2 U/kg IM (or SC if hydration normal).
- Subsequent dosage 0.1–0.2 U/kg IM given 3–6h later—may be given hourly if patient is closely monitored; response to previous insulin dosage should be considered when calculating

DIABETES MELLITUS WITH KETOACIDOSIS (CONTINUED)

subsequent dosages; ideally, glucose concentration should drop by 50–100 mg/dL/h.
• Regular insulin can also be administered as CRI via designated catheter. Dogs: 2.2 units/kg in 250 mL of 0.9% NaCl; Cats: 1.1 units/kg in 250 mL 0.9% NaCl. Then, allow 50 mL of dilute insulin to flow through IV tubing and discard. If blood glucose >250 mg/dL, administer at 10 mL/h; if blood glucose 200–250 mg/dL, administer at 7 mL/h; if blood glucose 150–200 mg/dL, administer at 5 mL/h; if blood glucose 100–150 mg/dL, administer at 5 mL/h and add 2.5% dextrose to IV crystalloid fluids; if blood glucose <100 mg/dL, discontinue IV insulin infusion and continue 2.5–5% dextrose in IV crystalloid infusion.
• Check blood glucose q1–3h using automated test strip analyzer (Accu-Chek® III, Alpha Trak® II glucometer), corrected for patient's PCV as indicated.
• Monitor urine or serum ketones daily.
• Administer longer-acting insulin once patient is eating, drinking, and ketosis is resolved; the dosage is based on that of short-acting insulin given in hospital.

Potassium Supplementation

• Total body potassium is depleted and treatment (e.g., fluids and insulin) will further lower serum potassium.
• If possible, check potassium concentration before initiating insulin therapy to guide supplementation; if extremely low, insulin therapy may need to be delayed (hours) until serum potassium concentration increases.
• Refractory hypokalemia may indicate hypomagnesemia, requiring magnesium replacement at 0.75–1 mEq/kg/24h IV as magnesium chloride or magnesium sulfate.
• Supplementation of potassium should start at 0.2 mEq/kg/h, which can be adjusted to max 0.5 mEq/kg/h. Potassium concentration should be measured q6-8h until stabilized.

Dextrose Supplementation

• Because insulin is required to correct the ketoacidotic state, the supplementation of dextrose allows continuous insulin administration without hypoglycemia.
• Whenever blood glucose <200 mg/dL, 50% dextrose should be added to fluids to produce 2.5% dextrose solution (increase to 5% dextrose if glucose <100 mg/dL). Discontinue dextrose once glucose is maintained above 250 mg/dL.
• Insulin therapy is continued as long as blood glucose >100 mg/dL

Bicarbonate Supplementation

• Controversial; consider if patient's venous blood pH <7.0 or HCO_3^- <11 mEq/L; of little benefit if pH >7.0.
• Dosage—bodyweight (kg) × 0.3 × base deficit (base deficit = normal serum bicarbonate – patient's serum bicarbonate); *slowly* administer ¼ to ½ of dose IV and give remainder in fluids over 3–6h.
• Recheck blood gas or serum total carbon dioxide (TCO_2) before further supplementation.

Phosphorus Supplementation

• Pretreatment serum phosphorus is usually normal; however, treatment of ketoacidosis reduces phosphorus, and serum concentrations should be checked q12–24h once supplementation is initiated.
• Dosage—0.01–0.03 mmol/kg/h for 6–12h in IV fluids (may need to increase dose to 0.06 mmol/kg/h). Remember to account for additional potassium in potassium phosphate if supplemented.

CONTRAINDICATIONS

If the patient anuric or oliguric or if blood potassium concentration >5 mEq/L, do not supplement potassium until urine flow is established or potassium concentration decreases.

PRECAUTIONS

• Use bicarbonate with caution in patients without normal ventilation (cannot excrete carbon dioxide created during treatment).
• Acidosis results in falsely elevated blood ionized calcium concentrations; calcium should be rechecked as acidosis resolves and supplemented as necessary.

POSSIBLE INTERACTIONS

None

ALTERNATIVE DRUG(S)

None

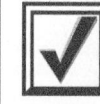

FOLLOW-UP

PATIENT MONITORING

• Attitude, hydration, cardiopulmonary status, urine output, and bodyweight.
• Blood glucose q1–3h initially; q6h once stable.
• Electrolytes q4–8h initially; q24h once stable.
• Acid-base status q8–12h initially; q24h once stable.

PREVENTION/AVOIDANCE

Appropriate insulin administration.

POSSIBLE COMPLICATIONS

• Hypokalemia.
• Hypoglycemia.
• Hypophosphatemia.
• Cerebral edema.
• Pulmonary edema/heart failure.
• Renal failure.

EXPECTED COURSE AND PROGNOSIS

Guarded

MISCELLANEOUS

ASSOCIATED CONDITIONS

• Pancreatitis.
• Hyperadrenocorticism.
• Diestrus.
• Bacterial infection.
• Electrolyte depletion.

AGE-RELATED FACTORS

N/A

ZOONOTIC POTENTIAL

N/A

PREGNANCY/FERTILITY/BREEDING

• Risk of fetal death may be relatively high.
• Glucose regulation is often difficult in pregnant animals.

SYNONYMS

N/A

SEE ALSO

• Diabetes Mellitus Without Complication—Cats.
• Diabetes Mellitus Without Complication—Dogs.

ABBREVIATIONS

• DKA = diabetic ketoacidosis.
• TCO_2 = total carbon dioxide.

Suggested Reading

Behrend E, Holford A, Lathan P, et al. 2018 AAHA diabetes management guidelines for dogs and cats. J Am Anim Hosp Assoc 2018, 54:1–21.
Difazio J, Fletcher DJ. Retrospective comparison of early- versus late-insulin therapy regarding effect on time to resolution of diabetic ketosis and ketoacidosis in dogs and cats: 60 cases (2003–2013). J Vet Emerg Crit Care 2016, 26:108–115.
Hume DZ, Drobatz KJ, Hess RS. Outcome of dogs with diabetic ketoacidosis: 127 dogs (1993–2003). J Vet Intern Med 2006, 20(3):547–555.
Kerl ME. Diabetic ketoacidosis: pathophysiology and clinical and laboratory presentation. Comp Cont Educ Pract Vet 2001, 23:220–228.
Kerl ME. Diabetic ketoacidosis: treatment recommendations. Comp Cont Educ Pract Vet 2001, 23:330–339.
Malerba E, Mazzarino M, Del Baldo F, et al. Use of lispro insulin for treatment of diabetic ketoacidosis in cats. J Fel Med Surg 2019, 21:115–123.
Sieber-Ruckstuhl NS, Klev S, Tschuor F, et al. Remission of diabetes mellitus in cats with diabetic ketoacidosis. J Vet Intern Med 2008, 22:1326–1332.

Author Katherine Gerken
Consulting Editor Patty A. Lathan
Acknowledgment The author and book editors acknowledge the prior contribution of Deborah S. Greco.

Client Education Handout available online

DIABETES MELLITUS WITHOUT COMPLICATION—CATS

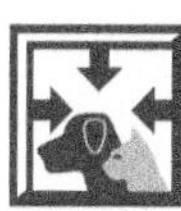

BASICS

DEFINITION

• Disorder of carbohydrate, fat, and protein metabolism caused by an absolute or relative insulin deficiency, resulting in the hallmark abnormality of persistent hyperglycemia.
• The most common form in cats resembles Type II or non-insulin-dependent diabetes mellitus (DM) of humans.

PATHOPHYSIOLOGY

• Insulin resistance impairs the ability of tissues (especially muscle, adipose tissue, and liver) to use carbohydrates, fats, and proteins.
• Impaired systemic glucose utilization coupled with ongoing hepatic gluconeogenesis causes persistent hyperglycemia, which directly impairs insulin secretion by reducing functional beta cell mass ("glucose toxicity").
• Initial beta cell dysfunction progresses to irreversible failure of insulin production as reactive oxidative species, inflammatory cytokines, and amyloid deposition perpetuate beta cell injury and loss.

SYSTEMS AFFECTED

• Endocrine/metabolic—electrolyte depletion, metabolic acidosis.
• Hepatobiliary—chronic pancreatitis, hepatic lipidosis.
• Neuromuscular—muscle wasting, peripheral neuropathy.
• Renal/urologic—osmotic diuresis with compensatory polydipsia (PD); urinary tract infection.

GENETICS

Genetic susceptibility suspected in certain breeds (e.g., European Burmese cats).

INCIDENCE/PREVALENCE

Reported at between ~1 : 250 (0.4%) to ~1 : 100 (1.2%) cats.

GEOGRAPHIC DISTRIBUTION

N/A

SIGNALMENT

Species

Cat

Breed Predilections

Breeds with possible increased susceptibility include Burmese (Europe, Australia, and New Zealand), Maine Coon, Russian Blue, Siamese, and Norwegian Forest cats.

Mean Age and Range

Over 80% of cases are 7 years or older at diagnosis; range: 1–19 years.

Predominant Sex

Males are overrepresented, but common in both sexes.

SIGNS

Historical Findings

• Obesity often present prior to diagnosis.
• Polyuria (PU)/PD, polyphagia, weight loss, generalized muscle wasting, poor coat quality.
• Signs suggesting a complication—anorexia, lethargy, depression, vomiting, jaundice.

Physical Exam Findings

Hepatomegaly, dehydration, plantigrade stance (diabetic neuropathy).

CAUSES

• Genetic susceptibility.
• Islet amyloid deposition.
• Pancreatitis.
• Diseases causing insulin resistance (e.g., hyperadrenocorticism and acromegaly).
• Drugs (e.g., glucocorticoids and progestogens).

RISK FACTORS

• Obesity.
• Advanced age.

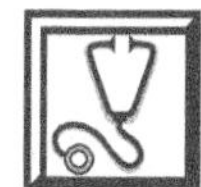

DIAGNOSIS

DIFFERENTIAL DIAGNOSIS

• Stress hyperglycemia—no PU/PD or weight loss; blood glucose concentration normal if sample taken when cat is not stressed; normal fructosamine concentration.
• Renal glucosuria—absence of hyperglycemia; usually does not cause PU/PD or weight loss.

CBC/BIOCHEMISTRY/URINALYSIS

• Mild normocytic, normochromic anemia possible.
• Glucose >150 mg/dL.
• High alkaline phosphatase (ALP), alanine aminotransferase (ALT), and aspartate aminotransferase (AST) activities.
• Hypercholesterolemia, hyperbilirubinemia, and hypertriglyceridemia.
• Total CO_2 or HCO_3 low with ketoacidosis or severe dehydration.
• Glucosuria, ketonuria uncommon in uncomplicated DM.
• Isosthenuria, proteinuria.

OTHER LABORATORY TESTS

• Fructosamine >350 μmol/L—confirms persistence of hyperglycemia.
• Feline pancreas-specific lipase >3.50 μg/L—identifies presence of pancreatitis.
• Urine culture—positive in 10–15% of newly diagnosed DM.

IMAGING

• Thoracic and abdominal radiography— to evaluate for concurrent or underlying disease (e.g., neoplasia, cystic or renal calculi, emphysematous cystitis, or cholecystitis).
• Abdominal ultrasonography—in selected patients, particularly those with jaundice, to evaluate for hepatic lipidosis, cholangiohepatitis, and pancreatitis.

DIAGNOSTIC PROCEDURES

Liver fine-needle aspiration—if concern for hepatic lipidosis.

PATHOLOGIC FINDINGS

• Usually no gross necropsy changes; pancreatic weight may be increased.
• Histopathology—normal, more likely to reveal islet amyloidosis, vacuolar or hydropic degeneration of the islets of Langerhans; lymphoplasmacytic pancreatic infiltration rare in cats.

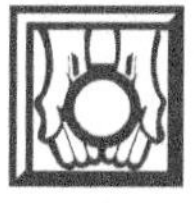

TREATMENT

APPROPRIATE HEALTH CARE

• Compensated cats can be managed as outpatients if they are alert, hydrated, and eating and drinking without vomiting.
• For decompensated patients, see Diabetes Mellitus With Ketoacidosis.

NURSING CARE

Fluid therapy—in decompensated patients.

ACTIVITY

Strenuous activity may lower insulin requirements; consistent daily activity level is helpful.

DIET

Ultra-low-carbohydrate (<12% metabolizable energy) and high protein (>40% metabolizable energy) canned diets may improve glycemic control, and increase the likelihood of diabetic remission in newly diagnosed diabetic cats.

CLIENT EDUCATION

• Discuss maintaining a consistent daily feeding and medication schedule, home glucose monitoring, signs of hypoglycemia and what to do, and when to seek veterinary assistance.
• Clients are encouraged to chart pertinent daily information about the pet, such as any home-obtained glucose readings or patterns of exhibited clinical signs (e.g., PU/PD or appetite).

SURGICAL CONSIDERATIONS

Intact females should have ovariohysterectomy when stable; progesterone secreted during diestrus makes management of DM difficult.

MEDICATIONS

DRUG(S) OF CHOICE

• Insulin is treatment of choice and should be initiated at 1–2 units per cat SC q12h; based on routine monitoring, some cats may eventually be reduced to once-daily dosing.
• Two U-40 insulin formulations are FDA-approved for use in cats—protamine zinc (PZI) and porcine zinc lente insulin suspension.

DIABETES MELLITUS WITHOUT COMPLICATION—CATS (CONTINUED)

D

• Most consensus recommendations support the use of PZI or glargine (U-100) as first-choice insulin therapy for cats.

PRECAUTIONS

Glucocorticoids, megestrol acetate, and progesterone cause insulin resistance. If steroid therapy is necessary, use oral methylprednisolone. Avoid injectable steroids.

POSSIBLE INTERACTIONS

• Drugs that may increase insulin sensitivity—angiotensin-converting enzyme inhibitors, sulfonamides, tetracycline, beta blockers, monoamine oxidase inhibitors, salicylates.
• Drugs that increase insulin resistance—glucocorticoids, estrogen supplements, furosemide, thiazide diuretics, and calcium channel blockers.
• Always consult a new medication's product insert.

ALTERNATIVE DRUG(S)

• Oral sulfonylureas (e.g., glipizide)—only considered when insulin therapy is not possible (e.g., owner considering euthanasia instead of injections). Initial does of 2.5 mg PO q12h can be used and monitored similar to insulin. If DM is not controlled after 2 weeks, dose of 5 mg PO q12h may be tried; however, response is seen in <40% of cats and often not sustained long term. Potential side effects are hypoglycemia, hepatic enzyme alterations, icterus, and vomiting.
• Acarbose—an alpha-glucosidase inhibitor used to limit intestinal glucose absorption. Often used in combination with diet and insulin at a starting dose of 12.5 mg PO q12h; diarrhea is most common side effect.
• Drugs warranting further study for utility in managing feline DM include once-weekly injected glucagon-like peptide 1 analogues and oral renal tubular transporter inhibitors.

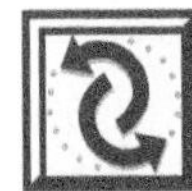

FOLLOW-UP

PATIENT MONITORING

• Owner-assessed clinical signs (PU/PD, appetite, attitude) and bodyweight—if signs are normal and weight stable to increasing, disease is likely to be regulated.
• Glucose curves—ideally generated by the owner at home. Perform 5–14 days after starting insulin or after any dose adjustments until controlled, then again at 1 month, and every 3–6 months thereafter.
• Fructosamine—maintain <400 µmol/L. Recheck monthly during initial regulation, then every 3–6 months as part of routine monitoring visits.
• Urinary monitoring—useful for identifying ketones in chronically unregulated patients or persistently negative glucose in cats likely entering remission.
• Flash glucose monitoring system (FreeStyle Libre®)—24-hour glucose monitoring system that measures blood glucose BG every 5 minutes for up to 14 days; use reported in dogs, but not cats. Anecdotal evidence suggests the device is not 100% accurate, but helpful in assessing BG trends in cats in which a BG curve is not possible.

PREVENTION/AVOIDANCE

Prevent or correct obesity; avoid unnecessary use of glucocorticoids or megestrol acetate.

POSSIBLE COMPLICATIONS

• Seizure, blindness, or coma with insulin overdose.
• Diabetic ketoacidosis or hyperglycemic hyperosmolar syndrome.

EXPECTED COURSE AND PROGNOSIS

• Prognosis with treatment and monitoring is good; most animals have a normal lifespan.
• Some cats may recover insulin-secreting ability ("diabetic remission"), typically if glycemic control is achieved within 6 months of diagnosis; however, relapse is common (~30%).
• Reported remission rates vary greatly (0–100%); however, studies surveying general practitioners have suggested ~25–30% is reasonable expectation.

MISCELLANEOUS

ASSOCIATED CONDITIONS

Urinary tract infection, chronic pancreatitis.

AGE-RELATED FACTORS

Congenital and juvenile forms of DM are rare (<3% of cases are under 2 years of age) and may be more difficult to manage.

ZOONOTIC POTENTIAL

None

PREGNANCY/FERTILITY/BREEDING

• Insulin requirements should be monitored closely during pregnancy as they are expected to fluctuate.
• Severe maternal hypoglycemia can negatively impact fetal viability and neonatal neurologic function, therefore should be avoided during gestation.

SYNONYMS

N/A

SEE ALSO

• Diabetes Mellitus With Ketoacidosis.
• Diabetes Mellitus With Hyperosmolar Hyperglycemic State.

ABBREVIATIONS

• ALP = alkaline phosphatase.
• ALT = alanine aminotransferase.
• AST = aspartate aminotransferase.
• BG = blood glucose.
• DM = diabetes mellitus.
• PU/PD = polyuria and polydipsia.
• PZI = protamine zinc insulin.

INTERNET RESOURCES

https://www.aaha.org/guidelines/diabetes_guidelines/default.aspx

Suggested Reading

Behrend E, Holford A, Lathan P, et al. 2018 AAHA diabetes management guidelines for dogs and cats. J Am Anim Hosp Assoc 2018, 54:1–21.

Sparkes A, Cannon M, Church D, et al. ISFM consensus guidelines on the practical management of diabetes mellitus in cats. J Feline Med Surg 2015, 17:235–250.

Author Andrew C. Bugbee

Consulting Editor Patty A. Lathan

Acknowledgment The author and book editors acknowledge the prior contribution of Deborah S. Greco.

Client Education Handout available online

DIABETES MELLITUS WITHOUT COMPLICATION—DOGS

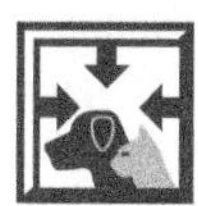

BASICS

DEFINITION

• Fasting hyperglycemia of sufficient magnitude to result in characteristic clinical signs including weight loss with normal or increased appetite, polydipsia (PD), and polyuria (PU) caused by glucosuria.
• Disorder of carbohydrate, fat, and protein metabolism caused by absolute or relative insulin deficiency. • Generally canine diabetes mellitus (DM) is characterized by loss of insulin-secreting ability through presumed immune-mediated destruction of pancreatic beta cells. • Far less frequently, canine DM may develop as result of combination of relative insulin-deficient state with concurrent peripheral insulin resistance.

PATHOPHYSIOLOGY

• Absolute or relative insulin deficiency results in accelerated tissue catabolism, impaired ability to maintain carbohydrate, lipid, and protein homeostasis, as well as insulin resistance. • Reduced insulin-secreting ability, peripheral insulin resistance, and continued hepatic gluconeogenesis result in persistent hyperglycemia of sufficient severity to overload renal tubular glucose resorption; leading to glucosuria, osmotic diuresis, PU accompanied by compensatory PD. • Loss of insulin-dependent glucose-mediated hypothalamic satiation signaling results in polyphagia. • Decreased insulin-dependent utilization of glucose results in catabolic protein breakdown with weight loss and increased lipid mobilization (hyperlipidemia, hepatic lipidosis, production of ketoacids). • Accumulation of large amounts of ketone bodies leads to metabolic acidosis (see Diabetes Mellitus With Ketoacidosis).

SYSTEMS AFFECTED

• Endocrine/metabolic—electrolyte depletion and metabolic acidosis. • Hepatobiliary—hepatic lipidosis. • Ophthalmic—cataracts.
• Renal/urologic—glucosuria resulting in osmotic diuresis and increased likelihood of bacterial urinary tract infections, particularly of upper urinary tract.

GENETICS

Certain breeds dramatically over- and underrepresented, suggesting inherited susceptibility to immune-mediated "isletitis."

INCIDENCE/PREVALENCE

• Prevalence varies between 1 : 400 and 1 : 500. • Onset has seasonal incidence; more animals diagnosed in autumn and winter.

SIGNALMENT

Species

Dog

Breed Predilections

• Samoyed, Tibetan terrier, Cairn terrier, golden retriever (United States only) overrepresented. • Keeshond, poodle, dachshund, miniature schnauzer, beagle may have increased predisposition. • Boxer, German shepherd, golden retriever (UK only) underrepresented.

Mean Age and Range

Mean ~8 years; range: 4–14 years (excluding rare juvenile form).

Predominant Sex

Female

SIGNS

• PU/PD, polyphagia with weight loss.
• Hepatomegaly. • Cataracts common finding—approximately 80% of dogs with DM for >12 months will have cataracts regardless of level of control. • Lethargy, depression, inappetence, anorexia, and vomiting may occur in animals with ketoacidosis.

CAUSES

• Immune-mediated isletitis. • Disorders that predispose to secondary immune-mediated isletitis—pancreatitis, viral illness.

RISK FACTORS

• Diestrus. • Genetic susceptibility. • Use of glucocorticoids or progestins.

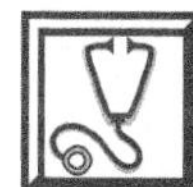

DIAGNOSIS

DIFFERENTIAL DIAGNOSIS

Renal glucosuria—not associated with hyperglycemia, usually no weight loss or polyphagia.

CBC/BIOCHEMISTRY/URINALYSIS

• Hemogram usually normal. • Glucose >200 mg/dL, possible ketonemia. • High serum alkaline phosphatase (ALP) and alanine aminotransferase (ALT) enzyme activities, generally with greater proportionate increase in ALP. • Hypercholesterolemia, lipemia. • Electrolyte alterations vary; hypokalemia and hypophosphatemia may be present. • Total CO_2 or HCO_3 will be low with ketoacidosis or severe dehydration.
• Glucosuria, ketonuria in some dogs.
• Urinary specific gravity variable depending on degree of glucosuria.

OTHER LABORATORY TESTS

• Anion gap—high in patients with ketoacidosis. • Glycated proteins—fructosamine or glycosylated hemoglobin: extent of glycosylation directly related to blood glucose concentration over lifespan of protein in circulation (10–20 days for fructosamine, 4–8 weeks for hemoglobin).
∘ Glycated protein concentration modified by changes in albumin or hemoglobin concentrations; accelerated albumin turnover (e.g., glomerulonephropathy, liver dysfunction, gastrointestinal disease) will lower fructosamine level for given average blood glucose. ∘ Best used for ongoing management of relatively stable diabetic patients; fructosamine concentration in upper third of reference range reflects excellent diabetic control; concentration in lower third is more suggestive of overzealous diabetic control and possible increased risk of hypoglycemia. • Plasma insulin concentrations not particularly helpful—while low insulin concentration suggests insulin deficiency, may be reflection of reversible islet exhaustion (persistent hyperglycemia can impair insulin secretory activity, even if functional beta cells present).

IMAGING

• Radiography—useful to look for comorbidities (e.g., cystic or renal calculi, emphysematous cystitis, cholecystitis, pancreatitis). • Ultrasonography—indicated in selected patients, particularly those with jaundice, to evaluate for presence of obstructive hepatopathy or pancreatitis.

DIAGNOSTIC PROCEDURES

Liver biopsy (percutaneous)—indicated in some jaundiced patients to evaluate other causes for hepatopathy.

PATHOLOGIC FINDINGS

• Necropsy findings—hepatomegaly with significant hepatic lipid accumulation.
• Histopathologic findings generally reveal dramatic reduction in size and number of pancreatic islets with relatively normal exocrine tissue architecture.

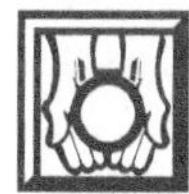

TREATMENT

APPROPRIATE HEALTH CARE

• Compensated dogs generally alert, well hydrated, eating and drinking without vomiting, and can be managed as outpatients.
• For management of decompensated patients, see Diabetes Mellitus With Ketoacidosis.

DIET

• Diet should be calorically and constitutively consistent. • Ideally glucose-lowering effects of insulin should match glucose-raising effects of the meal. ∘ Most insulins act maximally 2–4h after SC administration, and most food absorbed within 1h of consumption, so glycemic control almost always improved if dog fed 60–90 min *after* q12h insulin dosing.
∘ Animals that "graze" throughout day can be fed dry food ad libitum and given 2 small meals of canned food as above. ∘ If insulin can only be administered once daily, feed total daily caloric intake in 2 or 3 meals within first 6–8h after insulin dosing. • Feed caloric quantity appropriate for animal's ideal

bodyweight (~60 kcal/kg); food should be something dog will eat reliably and within short period. • Obese diabetic dogs—feed restricted caloric intake to ensure ideal bodyweight achieved within 2–4 months using high-fiber, low-calorie food; while high-fiber diet may improve patient satiety and possibly owner satisfaction, has no role in improving diabetic control. • While snacks should generally be avoided, small treats given at time of injection to positively reinforce owner–patient interaction should be encouraged.

CLIENT EDUCATION

• Most important that insulin and feeding regime are discussed and agreed with owner and they feel comfortable with plan; effective management requires significant owner–patient interaction; flexibility in establishing best management regime is thus paramount and rigid "one size fits all protocols" should be avoided. • Discuss daily feeding and medication schedule, home monitoring, signs of hypoglycemia and what to do, and when to call or visit veterinarian. • Clients encouraged to keep chart of pertinent information about pet, such as daily water consumption, weekly bodyweight, current insulin dose, and amount of food consumed; use of standardized clinical scoring tool should be encouraged to maintain consistency across veterinary and tech teams involved in managing both dog and owner.

SURGICAL CONSIDERATIONS

Intact females should have ovariohysterectomy when stable; progesterone secreted during diestrus makes management of DM more unpredictable.

MEDICATIONS

DRUG(S) OF CHOICE

• Insulin—almost always required • Vetsulin® (porcine-origin lente) 0.75 units/kg SC q12h initial dose; *note*: U-40 insulin—must use with U-40 insulin syringe; availability may be limited. • Humulin N—intermediate-acting, human insulin; 0.75 units/kg SC q12h initial dose. • Novolin N—intermediate-acting, human insulin; 0.75 units/kg SC q12h initial dose. • PZI Vet® (intermediate- to longer-acting protamine zinc human insulin) rarely used in dogs; *note*: U-40 insulin—must use with U-40 syringe. • Detemir insulin—longer-acting, synthetic insulin; part of reason for its delayed release is because bound to albumin; unlike insulins mentioned above, starting dose should be considerably lower: 0.1 unit/kg SC q12h initial dose. • Glargine insulin—longer-acting, synthetic insulin; 0.75 units/kg SC q12h initial dose. • Species of origin of insulin may affect pharmacokinetics; canine and porcine insulin have identical amino acid sequence, hence Vetsulin does not produce significant insulin antibody response, whereas most other commercially available insulins do; however, no evidence the development of insulin antibodies has any clinical significance.

PRECAUTIONS

• Glucocorticoids, megestrol acetate, and progesterone cause insulin resistance.
• Hyperosmotic agents (e.g., mannitol and radiographic contrast agents) should be avoided if patient is already hyperosmolar from hyperglycemia.

ALTERNATIVE DRUG(S)

Oral hypoglycemic agents are generally not recommended.

FOLLOW-UP

PATIENT MONITORING

• Diabetic dogs require regular contact between owner and veterinary team; visits should occur every 3–4 months if animal is stable and clinical signs are controlled, or more frequently if control is poor or variable. Criteria to assess control include: ○ Clinical signs—degree of PU/PD, appetite, and bodyweight; if within acceptable limits, disease likely well regulated; consider using standardized clinical scoring system to consistently evaluate clinical phenotype.
○ Glycated proteins—fructosamine or glycosylated hemoglobin; see above.
○ Glucose curve—provides information on insulin effectiveness, duration of action, nadir (lowest blood glucose level achieved during dosing interval), and potential for rebound hyperglycemia; results subject to influence of stress (hospitalization, multiple blood draws) and "normal" conditions should be mimicked as much as possible; used most effectively when establishing initial control, changing insulin type, dose, or frequency, or problem solving for difficult diabetic; duration of curve ideally matches dosing interval (12 or 24 hours)—identification of nadir (to avoid iatrogenic hypoglycemia) and glucose level at time of dosing are most important aspects of curve; goal is to establish effective insulin dose (decline in blood glucose to 100–200 mg/dL) for appropriate duration (majority of 12- or 24-hour dosing interval) with nadir >80 mg/dL and <150 mg/dL; in dogs average glucose levels for 12-hour period overnight are lower than during daylight period. • Home glucose monitoring using serial blood glucose estimations or real-time measures using SC glucose monitoring devices—requires owner commitment, compliance, and competence; most useful as early indicator of need for reduction in dose in patients with well-controlled clinical signs; should never be used by owner to make independent adjustment of insulin dose; owner-measured urine glucose levels not particularly useful.

PREVENTION/AVOIDANCE

• Neuter females; avoid unnecessary use of megestrol acetate. • No evidence exists to suggest obesity increases risk of DM in neutered dogs.

POSSIBLE COMPLICATIONS

• Cataracts can occur even with good glycemic control. • Weakness, especially with exercise; seizures or coma may occur with insulin overdose.

EXPECTED COURSE AND PROGNOSIS

• Dogs generally have permanent disease unless affected during estrus cycle, where neutering may resolve diabetes for a period.
• Prognosis with twice-daily insulin treatment and feeding aligned with insulin's maximum effects is good.

MISCELLANEOUS

ASSOCIATED CONDITIONS

• Urinary tract infection. • Cataracts.

AGE-RELATED FACTORS

Juvenile DM is rare and may be more difficult to manage.

PREGNANCY/FERTILITY/BREEDING

• DM can develop during pregnancy, in which case pregnancy is difficult to maintain.
• Exogenous insulin administration may cause fetal oversize and dystocia. • Insulin resistance develops, making hyperglycemia difficult to control. • Pregnant bitch is prone to ketoacidosis; emergency ovariohysterectomy may be necessary. • Do not breed dogs with DM.

ABBREVIATIONS

• ALP = alkaline phosphatase.
• ALT = alanine aminotransferase.
• DM = diabetes mellitus.
• PD = polydipsia.
• PU = polyuria.

Author David B. Church
Consulting Editor Patty A. Lathan

Client Education Handout available online

BASICS

OVERVIEW

• Protrusion of an abdominal organ through an abnormal opening in the diaphragm, either as an acquired injury or as a congenital defect. • Congenital—pleuroperitoneal (PIPDH) or peritoneopericardial diaphragmatic hernia (PPDH). • Traumatic—most often the result of a motor vehicle accident. • Impaired lung expansion. • Myocardial trauma. • Evidence of shock. • Systems affected—respiratory, cardiovascular, gastrointestinal.

SIGNALMENT

• Dogs and cats. • Acquired—no breed predilection. • Congenital (PPDH)—Weimaraner, Maine coon cat, and Persian cats. • Congenital PIPDH—golden retriever, cavalier King Charles spaniel. • Young animals at higher risk for both congenital and traumatic causes (median age 1.2 and 3.1 years, respectively). • No sex predilection.

SIGNS

Traumatic

• Can be acute, subacute, or chronic. • Possible known history of blunt trauma. • Difficulty breathing. • Evidence of shock (tachycardia, pale mucous membranes, weak pulses). • Gastrointestinal sounds ausculted in thorax. • Empty abdomen on abdominal palpation. • Signs may be progressive.

Congenital

• May not have clinical signs or may develop clinical signs later in life. • Difficulty breathing. • Gastrointestinal signs. • Signs may be progressive. • Evidence of shock (tachycardia, pale mucous membranes, weak pulses). • Evidence of cardiac tamponade. • Arrhythmias. • Muffled heart sounds.

CAUSES & RISK FACTORS

Traumatic

• Motor vehicle accident. • Other blunt trauma. • Penetrating trauma (e.g., bite wounds).

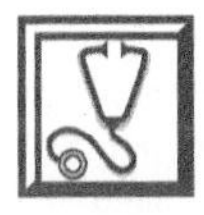

DIAGNOSIS

DIFFERENTIAL DIAGNOSIS

• Pneumothorax. • Pulmonary contusion. • Hemothorax.

CBC/BIOCHEMISTRY/URINALYSIS

Nonspecific changes due to trauma may be noted.

OTHER LABORATORY TESTS

Serum lactate—may be significantly elevated following trauma.

IMAGING

Point-of-Care Ultrasound (POCUS)

• Thoracic-focused assessment with sonography for trauma (TFAST®). • Abdominal focused assessment with sonography for trauma (AFAST®).

Standard Imaging

• Three-view thoracic and abdominal radiography. • Horizontal beam radiography. • Ultrasonography.

Additional Imaging

• Contrast radiography—upper gastrointestinal positive contrast series; peritoneography. • CT.

Imaging Findings

• Identification of gastrointestinal viscera within pleural space and/or absence from abdominal cavity makes diagnosis of diaphragmatic herniation often uncomplicated. • Other radiographic signs include loss of diaphragmatic outline and cardiac silhouette, displacement of lung fields, presence of gas-filled viscera, and pleural effusion.• For congenital PPDH cardiac silhouette is markedly enlarged and may have evidence of gas-filled structures within it. • Contrast or advanced imaging is often unnecessary.

DIAGNOSTIC PROCEDURES

• Thoracocentesis for pleural effusion. • Pericardiocentesis for pericardial effusion.

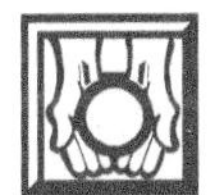

TREATMENT

Emergency Inpatient Intensive Care Management

• Address shock. • Improve ventilation and cardiac output. • Manage concurrent injury. • Gastric decompression if indicated.

Surgical Management

• Exploratory laparotomy. • Reduction and assessment of herniated abdominal viscera. • Surgical repair of diaphragmatic rent. • Additional surgical procedures (e.g., splenectomy, intestinal resection and anastomosis, liver lobectomy). • Pleural space evacuation (thoracostomy tube placement, thoracocentesis).

Nursing Care

• IV fluid therapy. • Oxygen supplementation. • Pain management.

Surgical Considerations

• Anesthesia and surgery should be delayed until animal is hemodynamically stable. • Emergency surgery indicated with evidence of gastrothorax, gastrointestinal entrapment, or persistent respiratory distress. • Long lasting absorbable monofilament suture (e.g., Maxon® or PDS®) should be used to close the diaphragm in a full-thickness simple continuous pattern. • Care should be taken around caval foramen, esophageal hiatus, and aortic hiatus.

MEDICATIONS

DRUG(S) OF CHOICE

• Appropriate postoperative pain medications; consider local analgesia. • Antiarrhythmic agents as indicated.

CONTRAINDICATIONS

Avoid nonsteroidal anti-inflammatories for at least 24–48 hours following trauma.

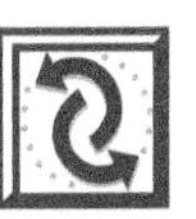

FOLLOW-UP

PATIENT MONITORING

• Frequent or continuous ECG monitoring. • Observation of ventilation. • Pulse oximetry. • Serial arterial blood gas evaluation.

POSSIBLE COMPLICATIONS

• Respiratory distress—due to concurrent injury or pneumothorax. • Reexpansion pulmonary edema (RPE) is uncommon but often fatal complication; to minimize risk of RPE, avoid aggressive positive-pressure ventilation following reduction of herniated organs, and avoid aggressive evacuation of pleural space in postoperative period. • Recurrence uncommon, but most often associated with inadequate surgical repair.

EXPECTED COURSE AND PROGNOSIS

If animal survives for first 12–24 hours after surgery, prognosis is excellent. Reported survival rates range from 80 to 90%. Death most often due to concurrent injury.

MISCELLANEOUS

ASSOCIATED CONDITIONS

• Congenital PPDH may be associated with other congenital midline defects. • Animals suffering trauma may have significant concurrent injuries.

ABBREVIATIONS

• AFAST® = abdominal focused assessment with sonography for trauma.
• PIPDH = pleuroperitoneal diaphragmatic hernia.
• POCUS = point-of-care ultrasound.
• PPDH = peritoneopericardial diaphragmatic hernia.
• RPE = reexpansion pulmonary edema.
• TFAST® = thoracic-focused assessment with sonography for trauma.

Suggested Reading

Burns CG, Bergh MS, McLoughlin MA. Surgical and nonsurgical treatment of peritoneopericardial diaphragmatic hernia in dogs and cats: 58 cases (1999–2008). J Am Vet Med Assoc 2013, 242:643–650.

Legallet C, Thieman Mankin K, Selmic LE. Prognostic indicators for perioperative survival after diaphragmatic herniorrhaphy in cats and dogs: 96 cases (2001–2013). BMC Vet Res 2017, 13:16.

Author Catriona M. MacPhail

Consulting Editor Elizabeth Rozanski

DIARRHEA, ANTIBIOTIC RESPONSIVE

BASICS

OVERVIEW

• Defined as chronic diarrhea with no identifiable underlying etiology that responds to antibiotic therapy. • Antibiotic-responsive diarrhea (ARD) was previously termed idiopathic (primary) small intestinal bacterial overgrowth (SIBO); this term is no longer used as it was based on quantitative culture of bacteria in the upper gastrointestinal tract that could not be confirmed by newer PCR-based methods; secondary SIBO is a result of concurrent gastrointestinal diseases (e.g., exocrine pancreatic insufficiency [EPI]). • Current theories center on the possibility of immune dysregulation, possibly associated with abnormal CD4+ T-cells, immunoglobulin (Ig) A plasma cells, cytokine expression, and, in German shepherd dogs, mutations in pattern recognition receptors.

SIGNALMENT

Species

Dog

Breed Predilections

Increased incidence in German shepherd, boxer, and Chinese Shar-Pei.

Mean Age and Range

More common in young dogs, with median age of 2 years.

Predominant Sex

N/A

SIGNS

Historical Findings

• Small bowel signs—inappetence or anorexia, vomiting, weight loss, large-volume diarrhea.
• Large bowel signs—tenesmus, hematochezia, increased frequency of defecation.

Physical Examination Findings

Weight loss, poor body condition, borborygmus, and flatulence may be detected; hematochezia may be present if there is large bowel involvement.

CAUSES & RISK FACTORS

• Genetic mutations in pattern recognition genes (*TLR4* and *TLR5*) have been associated with the disease. • Certain enteropathogenic bacteria (*Clostridium perfringens*, *Escherichia coli*, and *Lawsonia intracellularis*) have been suspected but not proven to be etiologic agents.

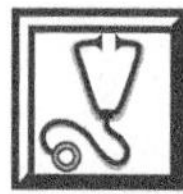

DIAGNOSIS

DIFFERENTIAL DIAGNOSIS

• Secondary SIBO. • EPI. • Parasitic infection. • Inflammatory bowel disease.
• Food-responsive diarrhea. • Neoplasia.

CBC/BIOCHEMISTRY/URINALYSIS

• Typically normal. • Hypoalbuminemia is uncommon finding.

OTHER LABORATORY TESTS

• Fecal examination for parasites should be performed. • Serum cobalamin levels may be low and folate levels may be increased or decreased. • Serum trypsin-like immunoreactivity (measured to rule out EPI) is normal.

IMAGING

Routine abdominal imaging (radiographs and ultrasound) should be performed to rule out other causes for diarrhea. These tests are unremarkable in cases of ARD.

DIAGNOSTIC PROCEDURES

Diagnosis depends upon ruling out all other causes for chronic diarrhea (especially food-responsive diarrhea) and a clinical response to an appropriate course of antibiotic therapy.

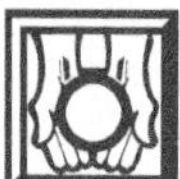

TREATMENT

• Hospitalization generally not indicated; treated on outpatient basis. • Role of diet in ARD is unknown; current recommendations are to feed low-fat, highly digestible food or elimination or hydrolyzed diet.

MEDICATIONS

DRUG(S) OF CHOICE

• Several options for antibiotics available—tylosin (5–10 mg/kg PO q24h); metronidazole (10–15 mg/kg PO q12h); oxytetracycline (10–20 mg/kg PO q8h). • In some cases, combination therapy may be necessary.
• Antibiotic therapy administered for 4–6 weeks and then discontinued. • If serum cobalamin levels decreased, cobalamin supplementation should be pursued; dogs: 50 µg/kg up to max dose of 1,500 µg parenteral cobalamin; doses given as SC injections once weekly for 6 weeks, then once every other week for 6 weeks; serum cobalamin levels should be reassessed at end of therapy; oral cobalamin supplementation is effective at dosage of 0.25–1.0 mg PO daily.

CONTRAINDICATIONS/POSSIBLE INTERACTIONS

• Oxytetracycline may cause staining of tooth enamel; doses should be decreased in animals with hepatic or renal insufficiency; oxytetracycline has been associated with high incidence of bacterial transfer of resistance genes. • Metronidazole undergoes extensive hepatic metabolism; dosages should be reduced in animals with hepatic insufficiency.
• Long-term administration of both tylosin and metronidazole has been found to induce long-term dysbiosis in ARD dogs, which is very difficult to correct; this dysbiosis is associated with changes in bile acid metabolism and serum metabolome, and persists for over 6 months after discontinuing treatment.

FOLLOW-UP

• Clinical resolution of diarrhea is most important criterion. • Weight gain may also be seen; hypoalbuminemia (if present) should resolve. • Relapses usually occur when antibiotics are discontinued; some dogs can be maintained on very low doses of antibiotics long term, however the development of antimicrobial resistance in these dogs is a concern. • Recent studies suggest ARD dogs have poor long-term prognosis, possibly due to induction of dysbiosis; many dogs eventually will become steroid resistant or will be euthanized because of treatment resistance.

MISCELLANEOUS

SEE ALSO

Small Intestinal Dysbiosis.

ABBREVIATIONS

• ARD = antibiotic-responsive diarrhea.
• EPI = exocrine pancreatic insufficiency.
• Ig = immunoglobulin.
• SIBO = small intestinal bacterial overgrowth.

Suggested Reading

Allenspach K, Culverwell C, Chan D. Long-term outcome in dogs with chronic enteropathies: 203 cases. Vet Rec 2016, 178(15):368. doi: 10.1136/vr.103557

German AJ, Day MJ, Ruaux CG, et al. Comparison of direct and indirect tests for small intestinal bacterial overgrowth and antibiotic-responsive diarrhea in dogs. J Vet Intern Med 2003, 17:33–43.

Toresson L, Steiner JM, Spodsberg E, et al. Effects of oral versus parenteral cobalamin supplementation on methylmalonic acid and homocysteine concentrations in dogs with chronic enteropathies and low cobalamin concentrations. Vet J 2019, 243:8–14. doi: 10.1016/j.tvjl.2018.11.004

Westermarck E, Skrzypczak T, Harmoinen J, et al. Tylosin-responsive chronic diarrhea in dogs. J Vet Intern Med 2005, 19:177–186.

Author Karin Allenspach
Consulting Editor Mark P. Rondeau

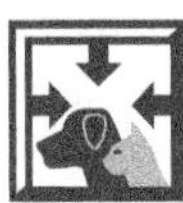

BASICS

DEFINITION

• A change in the frequency, consistency, and volume of feces for more than 3 weeks or with a pattern of episodic recurrence. • Can be either small bowel, large bowel, or mixed in origin.

PATHOPHYSIOLOGY

• High solute and fluid secretion—secretory diarrhea. • Low solute and fluid absorption—osmotic diarrhea. • High intestinal permeability. • Abnormal gastrointestinal (GI) motility. • Many cases involve various combinations of these four basic pathophysiologic mechanisms.

SYSTEMS AFFECTED

• Endocrine/metabolic—fluid, electrolyte, and acid-base. • Exocrine. • GI. • Lymphatic.

GENETICS

N/A

INCIDENCE/PREVALENCE

Unknown

GEOGRAPHIC DISTRIBUTION

Worldwide

SIGNALMENT

Species

Cat

Breed Predilections

None

Mean Age and Range

Any age.

Predominant Sex

None

SIGNS

General Comments

• Underlying disease process determines extent of clinical signs. • 2–3% increase of water content of stool results in gross description of diarrhea. • Classification of small, large, and mixed bowel types of diarrhea may have overlap of descriptive findings.

Historical Findings

• Small bowel diarrhea can include—normal to increased volume; normal to moderately increased (2–4 times/day) defecation frequency; weight loss; polyphagia; melena; flatulence and borborygmus; vomiting: variable. • Large bowel diarrhea can include—smaller volume; frequency of defecation is increased (>4 times/day); often hematochezia and mucus; tenesmus, urgency, dyschezia; flatulence and borborygmus: variable; vomiting: variable.

Physical Examination Findings

Small Bowel

• Poor body condition associated with malabsorption, maldigestion, and protein-losing enteropathy (PLE). • Variable dehydration. • Abdominal palpation may reveal segmental or diffusely thickened small bowel loops associated with infiltrative disease, abdominal effusion, foreign body, neoplastic mass, intussusception, or enlarged mesenteric lymph nodes. • Rectal palpation typically unremarkable.

Large Bowel

• Body condition typically unremarkable. • Dehydration—uncommon. • Abdominal palpation may reveal thickened large bowel, foreign body, neoplastic mass, intussusception, or enlarged mesocolic lymph nodes. • Rectal palpation may reveal irregularity of rectal mucosa, intraluminal or extraluminal rectal masses, rectal stricture, or sublumbar lymphadenopathy.

CAUSES

Small and Large Intestinal Diseases

Primary Disease

• Inflammatory bowel disease (IBD)—e.g., lymphoplasmacytic enteritis, eosinophilic enteritis, granulomatous enteritis. • Neoplasia—e.g., lymphoma, including large cell (B-cell lymphoma) and small cell alimentary lymphoma (T-cell), adenocarcinoma, mast cell neoplasia. • Bacterial—e.g., *Salmonella* spp., enterotoxic *Escherichia coli*, other enterobacteriaceae species, *Clostridia* spp.: usually acute diarrhea. • Viral—e.g., enteric coronavirus (usually acute diarrhea unless combined with other viral infections or co-factors), feline infectious peritonitis, feline leukemia virus (FeLV) associated, feline immunodeficiency virus (FIV) associated. • Mycotic—e.g., histoplasmosis. • Algal—e.g., protothecosis, pythiosis. • Parasites—e.g., *Giardia*, *Toxocara* spp., *Ancylostoma*, *Toxascaris leonina*, *Cryptosporidium* spp., *Cystoisospora* spp., *Tritrichomonas foetus*. • Partial obstruction—e.g., foreign body, intussusception, neoplasia. • Secondary lymphangiectasia—very rare in cats. • Intestinal microbial dysbiosis—cause vs. effect. • Short bowel syndrome. • GI ulceration—rare in cats.

Maldigestion

• Hepatobiliary disease—lack of bile salts needed for intraluminal digestion. • Exocrine pancreatic insufficiency (EPI).

Dietary

• Dietary intolerance (food-responsive diarrhea). • Food allergy.

Metabolic Disorders

• Hyperthyroidism. • Cobalamin deficiency—typically secondary to underlying IBD or lymphoma. • Renal disease. • Hepatobiliary disease. • Adverse drug reactions.

Congenital Anomalies

• Short colon. • Portosystemic shunt. • Persistent pancreaticomesojejunal ligament.

RISK FACTORS

Dietary changes, feeding poorly digestible or high-fat diets.

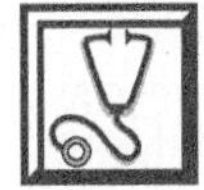

DIAGNOSIS

DIFFERENTIAL DIAGNOSIS

First localize the origin of the diarrhea to the small or large bowel (or both) on the basis of historical signs.

CBC/BIOCHEMISTRY/URINALYSIS

• Eosinophilia in some cats with parasitism, eosinophilic enterocolitis, hypereosinophilic syndrome, or neoplasia. • Macrocytosis in some cats with hyperthyroidism or FeLV infection. • Anemia that is variably regenerative and may show microcytosis suggests chronic GI bleeding and iron deficiency. • Leukopenia in some cats with FeLV or FIV infection. • Panhypoproteinemia caused by PLE is uncommon in cats with intestinal disease, but can occur; hypoalbuminemia can be seen. • Biochemical profiles and urinalysis abnormalities may suggest renal disease, hypoproteinemia, hepatobiliary disease, or endocrinopathy.

OTHER LABORATORY TESTS

Fecal and/or Rectal Scraping Exam

• Direct wet prep, routine centrifugation fecal flotation, fecal ELISA testing may indicate GI parasites. • Cytologic examination of rectal scrapings may reveal specific organisms, such as *Histoplasma*, *Prototheca*, or *Tritrichomas*. • PCR fecal testing should be interpreted with caution, because positive results for toxin genes or infectious agents may or may not correlate with clinical disease; interpret PCR results in light of patient signalment, history, clinical presentation, vaccination history, and other laboratory data. • PCR for *Tritrichomonas*—most sensitive test; be certain to send fresh fecal sample, colonic lavage fluid, or loop scraping for testing. • Culture feces if *Salmonella* is suspected—special media required.

Thyroid Function Tests

• High total T_4 or free T_4 concentration indicates hyperthyroidism. • If hyperthyroidism is suspected but T_4 is normal, perform a T_3 suppression test, repeat the T_4 a few months later, or perform a technetium scan of the thyroid glands.

Serologic Testing

Test for FeLV and FIV—especially if hematologic abnormalities are present.

Test for Exocrine Pancreatic Function

Feline-specific trypsin-like immunoreactivity—test of choice for diagnosis of EPI.

IMAGING

• Survey abdominal radiography may indicate abnormal intestinal pattern, organomegaly, mass, foreign body, pancreatic disease, hepatobiliary disease, urinary disease, or abdominal effusion; low yield in most cats with chronic diarrhea. • Contrast radiography (upper GI series or barium enema) may indicate bowel wall thickening, intestinal ulcers, mucosal irregularities, mass, radiolucent foreign body, or stricture; procedure performed infrequently in cats in light of advantages of abdominal ultrasonography. • Abdominal ultrasonography may demonstrate bowel wall thickening, abnormal bowel wall layering, GI or extra-GI masses, intussusception, foreign body, ileus, abdominal effusion, hepatobiliary disease, pancreatitis, renal disease, or mesenteric or mesocolic lymphadenopathy.

DIAGNOSTIC PROCEDURES

If maldigestive (EPI), metabolic, parasitic, dietary, and infectious causes have been excluded, consider empiric dietary therapy, utilizing an elimination diet for 2 weeks before performing endoscopy and biopsy or a laparotomy for definitive diagnosis.

Endoscopy/Laparoscopy

• Upper GI flexible endoscopy allows examination and biopsy of gastric and duodenal mucosa; always obtain multiple (8–10) mucosal specimens from each segment/area. • Flexible colonoscopy allows examination of entire rectum, colon, cecum, and ileum; always obtain multiple mucosal specimens (8–10) from each segment. • Visual impressions of GI mucosal detail may not reflect histopathologic changes; always take biopsies. • Endoscopic biopsies rely upon infiltrative and inflammatory diseases being represented in first two layers of the intestinal wall, and segments biopsied being representative of disease process. • Full-thickness biopsies can be obtained via laparoscopy from one or more segments of small intestine (not large intestine) via exteriorization of the segment(s), but are not typically necessary as most diseases can be diagnosed endoscopically.

Surgical Biopsy

Surgical approach beneficial if biopsies of multiple organs (small intestine, lymph nodes, stomach, pancreas, liver) are desired.

Ultrasound-Guided GI Aspiration or Biopsy

• Can perform ultrasound-guided fine-needle aspiration on some GI mass lesions, but cytologic interpretation accuracy is subject to sample quality, expertise, and limitations of technique; small cell alimentary lymphoma cannot be diagnosed by cytology, as cells will be small lymphocytes. • Paracentesis of peritoneal fluid for fluid analysis, culture, and cytology is recommended. • Concern has been expressed for risk of translocation of cancer cells or infective organisms with these procedures.

PATHOLOGIC FINDINGS

Vary with underlying disease.

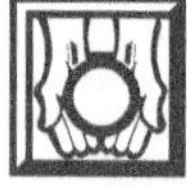

TREATMENT

APPROPRIATE HEALTH CARE

• Outpatient medical management most common. • Treat underlying cause.

NURSING CARE

• Give fluid therapy with balanced electrolyte solution as needed. • Correct electrolyte and acid-base imbalances.

ACTIVITY

No restriction.

DIET

• Feeding elimination diet (intact novel protein source or hydrolyzed protein) will resolve diarrhea in 40–60% of cats with chronic enteropathy; response should be detected within 2–3 weeks following dietary implementation. • Repeated changes of diet made in order to maintain a symptom-free situation suggest that further testing needed.

CLIENT EDUCATION

Complete resolution of signs is not always possible in cats with IBD, neoplasia, or fungal disease despite proper treatment.

SURGICAL CONSIDERATIONS

Pursue exploratory laparotomy and surgical biopsy if evidence of obstruction, intestinal mass, or mid-small bowel disease unreachable via endoscopic procedure.

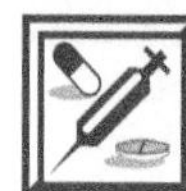

MEDICATIONS

DRUG(S) OF CHOICE

• Disease specific. • Prednisolone (1–2 mg/kg BID) for management of IBD; chlorambucil (2 mg/cat q48–72h) should be considered together with prednisolone in severe IBD cases that are refractory to steroids alone or for management of small cell intestinal lymphoma. • Supplementation with cyanocobalamin at 250 ug SC per cat on a weekly basis for 6 consecutive weeks, followed by every 3 weeks for the indefinite future. • Probiotics can be beneficial in some patients with chronic nonspecific diarrhea.

CONTRAINDICATIONS

Anticholinergics exacerbate most types of chronic diarrhea and should not be used for empirical treatment.

PRECAUTIONS

Opiate antidiarrheals such as diphenoxylate and loperamide can cause hyperactivity and respiratory depression in cats and should not be used for more than 3 days.

POSSIBLE INTERACTIONS

N/A

ALTERNATIVE DRUG(S)

N/A

FOLLOW-UP

PATIENT MONITORING

• Assess changes in frequency and severity of diarrhea and bodyweight. • Resolution usually occurs within 2–3 weeks following successful implementation of dietary therapy; consider reevaluating diagnosis if diarrhea does not resolve.

PREVENTION/AVOIDANCE

N/A

POSSIBLE COMPLICATIONS

• Dehydration. • Lowered body condition. • Abdominal effusions as related to specific cause of chronic diarrhea.

EXPECTED COURSE AND PROGNOSIS

Vary with underlying disease.

MISCELLANEOUS

ASSOCIATED CONDITIONS

N/A

AGE-RELATED FACTORS

N/A

ZOONOTIC POTENTIAL

• Toxoplasmosis. • Giardiasis (low zoonotic potential). • Cryptosporidiosis. • Salmonellosis. • *Campylobacter jejuni.*

PREGNANCY/FERTILITY/BREEDING

N/A

SYNONYMS

None

SEE ALSO

• Cobalamin Deficiency. • Diarrhea, Antibiotic Responsive. • Exocrine Pancreatic Insufficiency. • Food Reactions (Gastrointestinal), Adverse. • Inflammatory Bowel Disease. • Small Intestinal Dysbiosis.

ABBREVIATIONS

• EPI = exocrine pancreatic insufficiency. • FeLV = feline leukemia virus. • FIV = feline immunodeficiency virus. • GI = gastrointestinal. • IBD = inflammatory bowel disease. • PLE = protein-losing enteropathy.

Suggested Reading

Evans SE, Bonczynski JJ, Broussard JD, et al. Comparison of endoscopic and full-thickness biopsy specimens for diagnosis of inflammatory bowel disease and alimentary tract lymphoma in cats. J Am Vet Med Assoc 2006, 229(9):1447–1450.

Sabattini S, Bottero E, Turba ME, et al. Differentiating feline inflammatory bowel disease from alimentary lymphoma in duodenal endoscopic biopsies. J Small Anim Pract 2016, 57(8):396–401. doi: 10.1111/jsap.12494

Tolbert MK, Gookin JL. Tritrichomonas foetus: a new agent of feline diarrhea. Compend Contin Educ Pract Vet 2009, 31(8):374–381.

Willard MD, Mansell J, Fosgate GT, et al. Effect of sample quality on the sensitivity of endoscopic biopsy for detecting gastric and duodenal lesions in dogs and cats. J Vet Intern Med 2008, 22(5):1084–1089.

Author Karin Allenspach

Consulting Editor Mark P. Rondeau

Acknowledgment The author and book editors acknowledge the prior contribution of Mark E. Hitt.

Client Education Handout available online

DIARRHEA, CHRONIC—DOGS

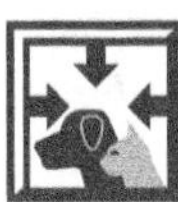

BASICS

DEFINITION

• A change in the frequency, consistency, and volume of feces for more than 3 weeks. • Can be small bowel, large bowel, or mixed.

PATHOPHYSIOLOGY

• Secretory diarrhea. • Osmotic diarrhea. • Increased permeability. • Abnormal gastrointestinal (GI) motility. • Many cases involve combinations of these pathophysiologic mechanisms.

SYSTEMS AFFECTED

• Endocrine/metabolic. • Exocrine. • Cardiovascular (fluid balance). • GI. • Lymphatic.

GENETICS

N/A

INCIDENCE/PREVALENCE

Unknown

GEOGRAPHIC DISTRIBUTION

Pythiosis occurs often in young, large-breed dogs living in rural areas, with a higher incidence in states bordering the Gulf of Mexico.

SIGNALMENT

Species

Dog

Breed Predilections

• Yorkshire terrier, West Highland white terrier, Rottweiler, soft-coated wheaten terrier—lymphangiectasia secondary to inflammatory bowel disease (IBD). • Boxer and French bulldog—granulomatous colitis.

Mean Age and Range

Any age.

Predominant Sex

None

SIGNS

General Comments

• Disease processes determine extent of clinical signs. • 2–3% increase of water content of stool results in gross description of diarrhea. • Classification of small, large, and mixed bowel types of diarrhea may have overlap of descriptive findings.

Historical Findings

• Small bowel diarrhea can include—normal to increased volume; normal to moderately increased (2–4 times/day) defecation frequency; weight loss; polyphagia; melena; flatulence and borborygmus; vomiting—variable. • Large bowel diarrhea can include—smaller volume; frequency of defecation increased (>4 times/day); often hematochezia and mucus; tenesmus, urgency, dyschezia; flatulence and borborygmus—variable; vomiting—variable.

Physical Examination Findings

Small Bowel

• Poor body condition associated with malabsorption, maldigestion, and protein-losing enteropathy (PLE). • Variable dehydration. • Abdominal palpation may reveal thickened small bowel loops (diffuse or segmental) associated with infiltrative disease, abdominal effusion, foreign body, neoplastic mass, intussusception, or enlarged mesenteric lymph nodes. • Rectal palpation typically unremarkable.

Large Bowel

• Body condition more typically normal. • Dehydration—uncommon. • Abdominal palpation may reveal thickened large bowel, foreign body, neoplastic mass, intussusception, or enlarged mesocolic lymph nodes. • Rectal palpation may reveal irregularity of colorectal mucosa, intraluminal or extraluminal rectal masses, rectal stricture, or sublumbar lymphadenopathy.

CAUSES

Small Bowel

Primary Small Intestinal Disease

• Inflammatory bowel disease (e.g., lymphoplasmacytic enteritis, eosinophilic enteritis, granulomatous enteritis, immunoproliferative enteropathy of Basenjis). • Primary or secondary lymphangiectasia. • Neoplasia. • Bacterial (*Campylobacter jejuni*, *Salmonella* spp., invasive adherent or enterotoxic *Escherichia coli*, other enterobacteriaceae species). • Mycotic (e.g., histoplasmosis). • Algal (e.g., protothecosis, pythiosis). • Parasites (e.g., *Giardia*, *Toxocara* spp., *Ancylostoma*, *Toxascaris leonina*, *Cryptosporidium* spp., *Cystoisospora* spp.). • Partial obstruction (e.g., foreign body, intussusception, neoplasia). • Antibiotic-responsive diarrhea (ARD; intestinal microbial dysbiosis). • Short bowel syndrome.

Maldigestion

• Exocrine pancreatic insufficiency (EPI). • Hepatobiliary disease—lack of intraluminal bile.

Dietary

• Food-responsive enteropathy. • Food allergy.

Metabolic Disorders

• Hepatobiliary disease. • Hypoadrenocorticism. • Uremic gastroenteritis. • Toxins—enterotoxins, aflatoxins, exotoxins, food poisoning. • Adverse drug reactions.

Large Bowel

Primary Large Intestinal Disease

• Inflammatory bowel disease (e.g., lymphoplasmacytic colitis, eosinophilic colitis, granulomatous colitis). • Neoplasia. • Infection (e.g., histoplasmosis, adherent invasive *E. coli* [granulomatous colitis], *Prototheca*, pythiosis). • Parasites (e.g., *Trichuris vulpis*, *Giardia intestinalis*, *Entamoeba histolytica*, *Balantidium coli*). • Ileocolic intussusception and cecal inversion.

Dietary

• Diet—dietary indiscretion, diet changes, food-responsive enteropathy, foreign material (e.g., bones, plastic, wood, hair). • Fiber-responsive large bowel diarrhea.

Miscellaneous

Irritable bowel syndrome.

RISK FACTORS

Small Bowel

• Large-breed, younger, and less severely affected dogs have higher risk of food-responsive diarrhea. • Yorkshire terrier, West Highland white terrier, Rottweiler, soft-coated wheaten terrier predisposed to lymphangiectasia secondary to IBD.

Large Bowel

• Dietary changes or indiscretion, stress, and psychological factors may play a role. • Granulomatous colitis (invasive adherent *E. coli*–associated)—boxer, French bulldog <3 years old. • Pythiosis more common in large-breed dogs that spend more time outside (roaming, hunting).

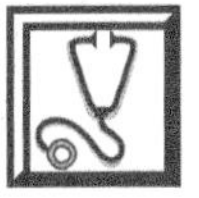

DIAGNOSIS

DIFFERENTIAL DIAGNOSIS

First localize the origin to the small or large bowel (or both).

CBC/BIOCHEMISTRY/URINALYSIS

• Eosinophilia may be associated with parasitism, eosinophilic enterocolitis, hypoadrenocorticism, paraneoplastic causes, or pythiosis. • Lymphopenia and hypocholesterolemia may be associated with lymphangiectasia. • Anemia and microcytosis suggest chronic GI bleeding and iron deficiency. • Panhypoproteinemia resulting from PLE associated with infiltrative small bowel disorders and lymphangiectasia. • Biochemical profiles and urinalysis abnormalities may suggest renal disease, hepatobiliary disease, or endocrinopathy.

OTHER LABORATORY TESTS

Fecal and/or Rectal Scraping Exam

• Direct wet-prep examination, fecal ELISA testing, and zinc sulfate centrifugation (for *Giardia*) may indicate GI parasites; multiple samples may be required for whipworm infestations. • Cytologic examination of rectal scrapings may reveal specific organisms, such as *Histoplasma* or *Prototheca*. • PCR fecal testing can be helpful when screening for uncommon or difficult to diagnose infections; interpret with caution as many of the microorganisms can be found in healthy, nondiarrheic animals (e.g., viral enteritis, cryptosporidiosis, *Giardia*, *Salmonella*, *C. perfringens* enterotoxin gene, *C. difficile*, *Campylobacter jejuni*); PCR testing should be interpreted in light of patient signalment, history, clinical presentation, vaccination history, and other laboratory data. • Culture feces if *Campylobacter* or *Salmonella* suspected—special media required; check with laboratory prior to submission.

Tests of Exocrine Pancreatic Function

Canine-specific trypsin-like immunoreactivity (TLI)—test of choice for confirming EPI.

Tests for Malabsorption

• Serum folate—low serum folate may be associated with proximal small intestinal malabsorption. • Cobalamin—low serum cobalamin may be associated with EPI or ileal malabsorption; primary cobalamin deficiency syndromes are rare (border collie, giant schnauzer).

Tests for Metabolic Disease

• Resting cortisol—value <2.0 µg/dL should be followed up with adrenocorticotrophic hormone stimulation test to evaluate for hypoadrenocorticism. • Fasting and 2-hour postprandial serum bile acids—test if hepatobiliary disease suspected; significantly increased values suggest hepatic dysfunction or portosystemic shunting.

IMAGING

• Survey abdominal radiography may indicate abnormal intestinal pattern, organomegaly, mass, foreign body, pancreatic disease, hepatobiliary disease, urinary disease, or abdominal effusion.
• Contrast radiography (upper GI series or barium enema) may indicate bowel wall thickening, intestinal ulcers, mucosal irregularities, mass, radiolucent foreign body, or stricture; utility of contrast radiography has been replaced with ultrasound in most patients.
• Abdominal ultrasonography may demonstrate bowel wall thickening, abnormal bowel wall layering, GI or extra-GI masses, intussusception, foreign body, ileus, abdominal effusion, hepatobiliary disease, or mesenteric or mesocolic lymphadenopathy.

DIAGNOSTIC PROCEDURES

If maldigestive (EPI), metabolic, parasitic, dietary, and infectious causes have been excluded, then consider dietary trial using elimination diet (novel, single protein source) or hydrolyzed diet for 2 weeks in stable dogs prior to performing advanced diagnostics (endoscopy or laparotomy and biopsy). Up to 75% of dogs in referral practices have been shown to be diet responsive.

Endoscopy/Laparoscopy

• Upper GI flexible endoscopy allows examination and biopsy of gastric and duodenal mucosa; always obtain multiple (8–10) mucosal specimens from each segment. • Flexible colonoscopy allows examination of rectum, colon, cecum, and ileum; always obtain multiple mucosal specimens (8–10) from each segment. • Gross appearance of mucosa does not always correlate with histopathology; always take biopsies. • Endoscopic biopsies rely upon diseases being represented in first two layers of intestinal wall and segments biopsied being representative of others not reached. • Full-thickness biopsies not indicated as most diseases can be diagnosed endoscopically. • Surgical approach can be advantageous if biopsies of multiple organs (e.g., small intestine, lymph nodes, stomach, pancreas, liver) are desired

Ultrasound-Guided GI Aspirates

• Ultrasound-guided fine-needle aspiration of GI mass lesions can be helpful for diagnosing mast cell tumors, carcinomas, and large-cell lymphoma.
• Seeding of neoplastic cells is a concern.

Capsule Endoscopy

Capsule endoscopy procedures can help identify location of bleeding ulcers in the jejunum.

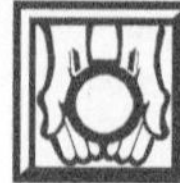

TREATMENT

APPROPRIATE HEALTH CARE

• Outpatient medical management most common. • Treat underlying cause.

NURSING CARE

• Fluid therapy with balanced electrolyte solutions as needed. • Correct electrolyte and acid-base imbalances.

ACTIVITY

No restrictions.

DIET

• Therapy with elimination diets or hydrolyzed diets can be beneficial in up to 75% of dogs with uncomplicated chronic enteropathies.
• Feeding lower-fat, novel (for the patient) protein source, highly digestible, or fiber-supplemented diets for 3–4 weeks may resolve diarrhea due to dietary intolerance or allergy; repeated changes of diet to maintain symptom-free situation suggests further testing needed.

CLIENT EDUCATION

Complete resolution of signs is not always possible in dogs with severe IBD, lymphangiectasia, intestinal neoplasia, and pythiosis.

SURGICAL CONSIDERATIONS

Pursue laparotomy and biopsy if evidence of obstruction, intestinal mass, or mid-small bowel disease unreachable via ultrasound-guided procedure, or if diagnosis based on endoscopic biopsy or ultrasound-guided procedure is questioned because of poor response to therapy.

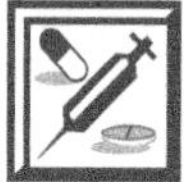

MEDICATIONS

DRUG(S) OF CHOICE

• Disease-specific. • Prednisone (2 mg/kg BID for 2 weeks, with slow tapering over 6 weeks) for IBD.
• Cyclosporine has shown to rescue dogs with steroid-refractory IBD. • Need for cyanocobalamin supplementation must be assessed in all dogs with chronic enteropathy. • Probiotics beneficial in some dogs with chronic enteropathy.

CONTRAINDICATIONS

Anticholinergics can exacerbate the situation with many causes of chronic diarrhea; they are sometimes used to relieve cramping associated with irritable bowel syndrome.

PRECAUTIONS

N/A

POSSIBLE INTERACTIONS

N/A

ALTERNATIVE DRUGS

N/A

FOLLOW-UP

PATIENT MONITORING

• Frequency and consistency of stool, appetite, and bodyweight. • In dogs with PLE—serum proteins, cholesterol, and clinical signs (ascites, subcutaneous edema, pleural effusion). • Resolution of diarrhea usually gradual with treatment; if does not resolve, reevaluate diagnosis.

PREVENTION/AVOIDANCE

N/A

POSSIBLE COMPLICATIONS

• Dehydration. • Lowered body condition.
• Abdominal effusions as related to specific cause of chronic diarrhea. • Ascites, subcutaneous edema, and/or pleural effusion with hypoalbuminemia from PLE.

EXPECTED COURSE AND PROGNOSIS

Vary with underlying disease.

MISCELLANEOUS

ASSOCIATED CONDITIONS

N/A

AGE-RELATED FACTORS

N/A

ZOONOTIC POTENTIAL

• Giardiasis (low risk of transmission).
• Salmonellosis. • *Campylobacter jejuni.*
• Ascaridiasis.

PREGNANCY/FERTILITY/BREEDING

N/A

SYNONYMS

N/A

SEE ALSO

• Colitis, Histiocytic Ulcerative. • Diarrhea, Antibiotic Responsive. • Fiber-Responsive Large Bowel Diarrhea. • Food Reactions (Gastrointestinal), Adverse. • Inflammatory Bowel Disease. • Lymphangiectasia. • Protein-Losing Enteropathy. • Small Intestinal Dysbiosis.

ABBREVIATIONS

• ARD = antibiotic-responsive diarrhea.
• EPI = exocrine pancreatic insufficiency.
• GI = gastrointestinal. • IBD = inflammatory bowel disease. • PLE = protein-losing enteropathy. • TLI = trypsin-like immunoreactivity.

Suggested Reading

Allenspach K, Culverwell C, Chan D. Long-term outcome in dogs with chronic enteropathies: 203 cases. Vet Rec 2016, 178(15):368. doi: 10.1136/vr.103557

Willard MD, Mansell J, Fosgate GT, et al. Effect of sample quality on the sensitivity of endoscopic biopsy for detecting gastric and duodenal lesions in dogs and cats. J Vet Intern Med 2008, 22(5):1084–1089.

Author Karin Allenspach
Consulting Editor Mark P. Rondeau
Acknowledgment The author and book editors acknowledge the prior contribution of Mark E. Hitt.

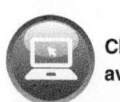

Client Education Handout available online

DIGOXIN TOXICITY

BASICS

OVERVIEW

Not uncommon in patients treated with digoxin due to digoxin's narrow therapeutic index and prevalence of renal impairment in elderly patients with cardiac disease. Becoming less common in clinical practice as use of digoxin has decreased in management of heart failure.

SIGNALMENT

- Dog and cat.
- More common in geriatric patients.

SIGNS

Historical Findings

- Anorexia.
- Vomiting.
- Diarrhea.
- Lethargy.
- Depression.

Physical Examination Findings

Heart rate may range from severe bradycardia to severe tachycardia.

CAUSES & RISK FACTORS

- Renal disease—impairs digoxin elimination.
- Chronic pulmonary disease—results in hypoxia and acid-base disturbances.
- Obesity—if dosage not calculated on lean bodyweight.
- Drugs and conditions that alter digoxin metabolism or elimination (e.g., quinidine and hypothyroidism).
- Rapid IV digitalization.
- Overdosage or accidental ingestion of owner's medication.
- Administration of diuretic leading to hypokalemia.

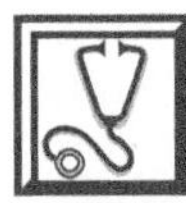

DIAGNOSIS

DIFFERENTIAL DIAGNOSIS

- Arrhythmias and conduction disturbances—may reflect structural heart disease, not digoxin toxicity.
- Anorexia—common in animals with heart failure.

CBC/BIOCHEMISTRY/URINALYSIS

Animals with hypokalemia, hypercalcemia, hypomagnesemia, and renal failure are predisposed to toxicity.

OTHER LABORATORY TESTS

- Consider checking thyroid status.
- Obtain digoxin serum concentration 8–10 hours after an oral dose—therapeutic range is 0.5–1.5 ng/mL. A recent study in humans found digoxin levels greater than 1 mg/ml were associated with increased mortality; not all patients with concentrations >1.5 ng/mL have signs of toxicity; some with values in the normal range have signs of toxicity, especially if hypokalemic. To minimize the risk of toxicity, the author aims to achieve a digoxin level between 0.5 and 1 ng/mL.

IMAGING

N/A

DIAGNOSTIC PROCEDURES

ECG

- Conduction disturbances—atrioventricular (AV) block, arrhythmias, and ST segment depression in some patients.
- Digoxin can cause any arrhythmia.

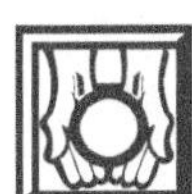

TREATMENT

- Discontinue digoxin until signs of toxicity resolve (24–72 hours); reevaluate need for the medication; if necessary, resume treatment at a dosage based on the serum digoxin concentration.
- Maintain hydration and correct any electrolyte disturbance (especially hypokalemia) with parenteral fluid administration.
- Discontinue drugs that slow digoxin metabolism or elimination (e.g., quinidine, verapamil, amiodarone).
- Severe arrhythmias (ventricular tachycardia) and conduction disturbances—can be life-threatening; require hospitalization for treatment and monitoring.

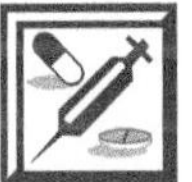

MEDICATIONS

DRUG(S) OF CHOICE

- Treat clinically important bradyarrhythmias with atropine or a temporary transvenous pacemaker.
- Treat clinically important ventricular arrhythmias with lidocaine or phenytoin; phenytoin also reverses high-degree AV block.
- Digoxin-binding antibodies (e.g., Digibind®) rapidly drop digoxin concentration in critically ill animals; the use of these products is limited in veterinary practice by their exorbitant cost.
- Thyroxin supplementation if hypothyroidism confirmed.

CONTRAINDICATIONS/POSSIBLE INTERACTIONS

- Avoid or discontinue drugs that slow digoxin elimination or metabolism (e.g., quinidine, verapamil, and diltiazem).
- Avoid drugs that could worsen conduction disturbances (e.g., beta blockers and calcium channel blockers).
- Class 1A antiarrhythmic drugs (e.g., quinidine and procainamide) may worsen AV block.

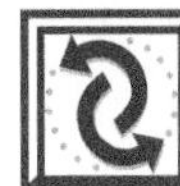

FOLLOW-UP

- Inform owner that reduction in appetite is an early indication of digoxin toxicity.
- Monitor renal function and electrolytes frequently in patients receiving digoxin; lower digoxin dose if renal disease develops.
- Monitor serum digoxin concentration periodically.
- Monitor ECG periodically to assess for arrhythmias or conduction disturbances that may suggest digoxin toxicity.
- Monitor bodyweight frequently; alter digoxin dosage accordingly; patients with congestive heart failure often lose weight.

MISCELLANEOUS

SEE ALSO

- Atrioventricular Block, Complete (Third Degree).
- Atrioventricular Block, First Degree.
- Atrioventricular Block, Second Degree—Mobitz Type I.
- Atrioventricular Block, Second Degree—Mobitz Type II.
- Ventricular Tachycardia.

ABBREVIATIONS

- AV = atrioventricular.

Suggested Reading

Teerlink JR, Gersh BJ, Opie LH. Heart failure. In: Opie LH, Gersh BJ, eds., Drugs for the Heart, 8th ed. Philadelphia, PA: Elsevier Saunders, 2013, pp. 169–223.

Author Francis W.K. Smith, Jr.
Consulting Editor Michael Aherne

DIISOCYANATE GLUES

D

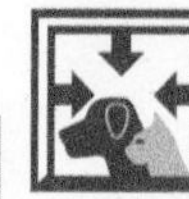

BASICS

OVERVIEW

• Diisocyanate glues include wood glue, construction glue, and some "high-strength or extra strength" glues.
• Gorilla Glue is one popular brand name. There are non-Gorilla brand glue types that contain diisocyanate as the active ingredient and not all types of Gorilla Glue contain diisocyanates. Confirm the actual product with the owner, using the packaging if necessary.
• Typically, the owner finds a chewed bottle of glue or glue stuck on the animal.
• Diisocyanate glue rapidly expands in the moist environment of the stomach, causing bloat and foreign body obstruction (FBO). The glue is not absorbed and does not cause systemic toxicity. Ingestions as small as 2 oz (56 g) can require surgical intervention to resolve obstruction.
• Glue is also adhesive and an irritant to the paws, oral cavity, and stomach lining.
• Inhalation may cause irritation to the lungs.

SIGNALMENT

Dogs and less commonly cats, birds, and small mammals. Young animals are more often affected.

SIGNS

• Occur within 15 minutes to 24 hours after ingestion.
• Ingestion—consistent with FBO and may include gagging, retching, vomiting, anorexia, abdominal distension, abdominal pain; hematemesis in prolonged or severe cases.
• Inhalation—coughing, sneezing, increased secretions within 4–8 hours.
• Dermal—irritation, redness, rash.

CAUSES & RISK FACTORS

Pets with access to diisocyanate glue products.

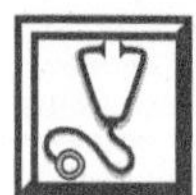

DIAGNOSIS

DIFFERENTIAL DIAGNOSIS

• History of exposure and clinical signs generally facilitate diagnosis.
• Presenting signs are consistent with gastric dilatation-volvulus (GDV), bloat, pancreatitis, inflammatory bowel disease, and other causes of FBO.
• Radiographs are highly suggestive of FBO (see Web Figure 1).

CBC/BIOCHEMISTRY/URINALYSIS

• CBC—generally no significant changes.
• Electrolyte disturbances—consistent with gastrointestinal (GI) obstruction and anorexia.
• Elevated total proteins/prerenal azotemia—may occur secondary to dehydration from vomiting.

IMAGING

Survey radiographs (4–24 hours post exposure)—glue appears as a mottled gas and soft tissue opacity distending the stomach. The appearance can resemble recent food ingestion (see Web Figure 1).

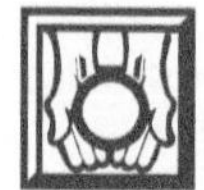

TREATMENT

• Generally, not recommended due to risk of esophageal or GI obstruction. Potential use immediately after a large ingestion.
• Gastric lavage is rarely of benefit as glue expands too rapidly.
• Dilution with water or other fluids should be avoided as excess moisture allows further expansion of the glue.
• IV fluids as needed for dehydration.
• Wash exposed skin with warm soapy water, rub vegetable oil into the hair, or clip hair to remove as much glue as possible. Glue can be left adhered to the skin if nonirritating and will fall off over time.
• Oxygen as needed for signs related to inhalation.
• Surgical removal of the expanded glue foreign body is almost always indicated in ingestions greater than 2 oz or with lesser amounts in smaller animals.

MEDICATIONS

DRUG(S) OF CHOICE

• Antiemetic—maropitant citrate 1 mg/kg SC/IV q24h.
• H2 blocker (for gastric inflammation or ulceration)—ranitidine 1–2 mg/kg PO/IM/SC/IV q6–12h; famotidine 0.5–1.1 mg/kg PO q12h; pantoprazole 0.7–1 mg/kg IV over 15 minutes q24h.
• Sucralfate (for a gastric ulcer if present)—0.5–1 g PO TID on an empty stomach.

CONTRAINDICATIONS

• Emetics—emesis should not be performed unless done immediately after a witnessed ingestion. Expansion of the glue is rapid: late emesis stresses the stomach wall and could damage the esophagus.
• Do *not* dilute with water as exposure to moisture leads to rapid expansion of the glue.

FOLLOW-UP

PATIENT MONITORING

Monitor in hospital until eating and drinking normally. Recheck 10–14 days post surgery.

PREVENTION/AVOIDANCE

Prevent exposure.

EXPECTED COURSE AND PROGNOSIS

• With removal of FBO, prognosis is excellent.
• Without surgical removal, the FBO is not expected to resolve on its own.

MISCELLANEOUS

ASSOCIATED CONDITIONS

• Gastritis.
• Dermatitis.

ABBREVIATIONS

• FBO = foreign body obstruction.
• GDV = gastric dilatation-volvulus.
• GI = gastrointestinal.

Suggested Reading

Horstman CL, Eubig PA, Cornell KK, et al. Gastric outflow obstruction after ingestion of wood glue in a dog. J Am Anim Hosp Assoc 2003, 39:47–51.
Peterson KL. Glues and adhesives. In: Hovda LR, Brutlag A, Poppenga R, Peterson K, eds., Blackwell's Five Minute Veterinary Consult: Small Animal Toxicology, 2nd ed. Ames, IA: Wiley-Blackwell, 2016, pp. 95–100.

Author Tyne Hovda
Consulting Editor Lynn R. Hovda
Acknowledgment: The author and book editors acknowledge the prior contribution of Catherine A. Angle.

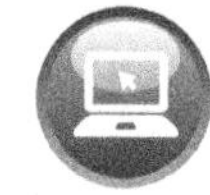

Client Education Handout available online

DISCOLORED TOOTH/TEETH

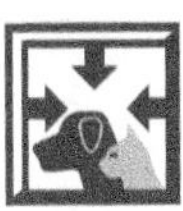

BASICS

DEFINITION

- Normal tooth color varies and depends on the shade, translucency, and thickness of enamel. Translucent enamel is bluish-white, opaque enamel is gray-white.
- Extrinsic—from surface accumulation of exogenous pigment.
- Intrinsic—secondary to endogenous factors discoloring the underlying dentin.

PATHOPHYSIOLOGY

Extrinsic Discoloration

- Bacterial stains—chromogenic bacteria: green to black-brown to orange color, usually 1 mm above the gingival margin on the tooth.
- Plaque related—a black-brown stain; usually secondary to the formation of ferric sulfide from the interaction of bacterial ferric sulfide and iron in the saliva. Plaque is usually white.
- Foods—charcoal biscuits and similar products penetrate the pits and fissures of the enamel; food with abundant chlorophyll can produce a green discoloration.
- Gingival hemorrhage—green or black staining from the breakdown of hemoglobin into green biliverdin.
- Dental restorative materials—amalgam: black-gray discoloration.
- Medications—products containing iron or iodine give a black discoloration; sulfides, silver nitrate, or manganese: gray-to-yellow to brown-to-black discoloration; copper or nickel: green discoloration; cadmium, yellow to golden brown discoloration (e.g., 8% stannous fluoride combines with bacterial sulfides, giving a black stain; chlorhexidine gives a yellowish-brown discoloration).
- Metals—wear from chewing on cages or food dishes.
- From removed orthodontic brackets or bands.
- Crown fragments—less translucency due to dehydration of fragment.
- Discolored restorations.
- Tooth wear with dentin exposure—tertiary dentin, reparative dentin, secondary dentin.
- A calculus-covered crown ranges in color from dark yellow to dark brown.

Intrinsic Discoloration

- Hyperbilirubinemia—affects all teeth; during dentin formation bilirubin accumulates in the dentin from excess red blood cell breakdown; extent of discoloration depends on the length of hyperbilirubinemia (lines of resolution occur once the condition has been resolved); green discoloration.
- Localized red blood cell destruction, one tooth or focal area—usually follows a traumatic injury to the tooth; discoloration from hemoglobin breakdown within the pulp with release into adjacent dentinal tubules; discoloration goes from pink to purple (pulpitis) to gray (pulpal necrosis) to black (liquefactive necrosis).
- Amelogenesis imperfecta—developmental alteration in the structure of enamel affecting all teeth; chalky appearance with a pinkish hue; problem in the formation of the organic matrix, mineralization of the matrix, or the maturation of the matrix.
- Dentinogenesis imperfecta—developmental alteration in dentin formation; enamel separates easily from the dentin, resulting in grayish discoloration.
- Infectious agents (systemic)—parvovirus, distemper virus, or any agent that causes a sustained body temperature rise; affects the formation of enamel; a distinct line of resolution is visible on the teeth; affects all teeth developing at the time of the insult; results in enamel hypoplasia or hypocalcification where the abnormal enamel can have black edges and the dentin is brownish.
- Dental fluorosis—affects all teeth; excess fluoride consumption affects the maturation of enamel, resulting in pits (enamel hypoplasia) with black edges; the enamel is a lusterless, opaque white, with yellow-brown zones of discoloration.
- Tooth erosion from constant vomiting results in enamel pitting and darkened staining.
- Attrition—tooth-to-tooth wear results in crown loss and reparative dentin formation (yellow-brown color).
- Abrasion—tooth wear against another surface; chewing on tennis balls or from a dermatologic condition. Reparative dentin (yellow-brown color) forms.
- Aging—older animals' dentition is more yellow and less translucent.
- Malnutrition (generalized, vitamin D deficiency, and vitamin A deficiency)—if severe can result in demarcated opacities on the enamel.

Internal/External Resorption

- Internal—follows pulpal injury (trauma) causing vascular changes with increased oxygen tension and decreased pH, resulting in destruction (resorption) of the tooth from within the pulp from odontoclasts; tooth has pinkish hue.
- External—many factors possible: trauma, orthodontic treatment, excessive occlusal forces, periodontal disease (and treatment), tumors, periapical inflammation, and unknown factors; resorption can start anywhere along the periodontal ligament and can extend to the pulp and into the crown causing a pinkish discoloration; osteoclasts and odontoclasts resorb the tooth structure.

Medications and Discoloration

- Tetracycline—during enamel formation, it binds to calcium, forming a calcium orthophosphate complex in the collagen matrix of enamel; occurs on multiple teeth; results in a yellow-brown discoloration. Long-term use of tetracyclines in mature animals can involve secondary dentin formation.
- Amalgam (as with extrinsic stains).
- Iodine/essential oils.
- In endodontically treated teeth from the medicants penetrating the dentinal tubules.
- Macrolide antibiotic (reported in humans)—results in vacuolar degeneration of the ameloblast and cystic change at maturation and hypocalcification, giving a white discolored lesion with horizontal stripes on the enamel.
- Bacterial "creeping" (leakage)—occurs around the margins of a restoration and usually is blackish in color.

SYSTEMS AFFECTED

Gastrointestinal—oral cavity.

GENETICS

- Amelogenesis imperfecta and dentinogenesis imperfecta in humans are inherited conditions that have many modes of inheritance. The mode of inheritance in animals has not been studied.
- Congenital hypothyroidism.
- Metabolic diseases.

INCIDENCE/PREVALENCE

- Discoloration of the teeth or a tooth is extremely common in all animals.
- Extrinsic staining is very common, especially bacterial stains; others are less common.
- Intrinsic staining is likewise very common, especially internal and external resorption, followed by localized red blood cell destruction; the other causes are rare.

GEOGRAPHIC DISTRIBUTION

- Heavy metals from mining operations.
- Fluoridation forms areas of excessive fluoride in the drinking water.
- Otherwise none.

SIGNALMENT

Species

Dogs and cats.

Mean Age and Range

The reported age range varies—when the condition affects the developing enamel or dentin it can be first noted after tooth eruption (6 months of age).

Predominant Sex

None

SIGNS

Historical Findings

Owner reports a variation in color of a tooth or teeth.

Physical Examination Findings

- Abnormal coloration of tooth or teeth.
- Pitted enamel with staining.

DISCOLORED TOOTH/TEETH (CONTINUED)

- Fractured tooth.
- Rings or lines of discoloration around tooth or teeth.
- Wear on crowns of the dentition or in selected areas as in behavioral causes (cage biters—distal aspect of the canines is affected).
- Erosion of enamel.

CAUSES & RISK FACTORS

- Extrinsic discoloration—bacterial stains from plaque and calculus; foods; gingival hemorrhage; dental restorative materials, medications (chlorhexidine, 8% stannous fluoride), metal.
- Intrinsic discoloration—internal (trauma); external tooth resorption; localized red blood cell destruction in the tooth (trauma); systemic infections; medications (tetracycline); fluorosis; hyperbilirubinemia; amelogenesis imperfecta; dentinogenesis imperfecta.

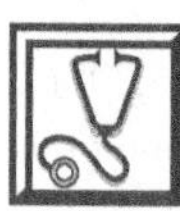

DIAGNOSIS

DIFFERENTIAL DIAGNOSIS

- Calculus on the teeth.
- Normal tooth aging—increased translucence.
- Food debris lodged in the spaces between the teeth (diastema).

CBC/BIOCHEMISTRY/URINALYSIS

- Anemia—blood-related disorders.
- Bilirubin—increased with liver diseases.

OTHER LABORATORY TESTS

- T_3/T_4—low in congenital hypothyroidism.
- Specific metabolic enzyme decrease or absence—tyrosinemia.

IMAGING

Dental radiography is extremely useful in identifying internal or external resorption, restorative materials, or bacterial stain from coronal percolation.

DIAGNOSTIC PROCEDURES

- If many teeth are affected, one tooth can be extracted and sent for histologic evaluation (see below).
- Transillumination with a strong fiberoptic light may help distinguish between vital and necrotic pulp.
- Appropriate preoperative diagnostics when indicated prior to procedure.

PATHOLOGIC FINDINGS

See Pathophysiology.

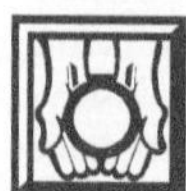

TREATMENT

APPROPRIATE HEALTH CARE

- Extrinsic stain removal—mainly cosmetic.
- Intrinsic stain treatment—functional and pain relieving.

NURSING CARE

- Extrinsic stain—remove inciting cause.
- Intrinsic stain—soft food; remove chew toys.

ACTIVITY

Curtail or treat specific behavioral abnormalities (cage biting).

DIET

N/A

CLIENT EDUCATION

- To prevent it in future animals or litters if preventable (medication use).
- Intrinsic causes—irregular enamel surfaces are more likely to accumulate plaque and calculus, leading to subsequent periodontal disease. Abnormally formed teeth or teeth that have localized red blood cell destruction are more prone to fracture or development of tooth abscessation.
- Some causes are painful (tooth resorption).

SURGICAL CONSIDERATIONS

- Extrinsic stain (cosmetic)—internal and/or external bleaching; veneers or crowns. Polishing the affected teeth with 3% hydrogen peroxide in pumice will help remove external stain. Also good home care with plaque control will minimize redevelopment of some stains (plaque/calculus/bacteria stain).
- Intrinsic stain (functional and pain relief)—possible endodontic treatment (internal resorption and localized red blood cell destruction).
- Restorative procedures such as crowns or veneers to protect both tooth and pulp.
- Extraction of affected teeth may be required, especially with external resorption.

MEDICATIONS

DRUG(S) OF CHOICE

N/A

FOLLOW-UP

PREVENTION/AVOIDANCE

- See Pathophysiology.
- Good oral care at home will help prevent the reoccurrence of certain specific stains.

POSSIBLE COMPLICATIONS

See Client Education.

EXPECTED COURSE AND PROGNOSIS

Vary dependent upon the etiology, but can range from mere aesthetics to significant pain.

MISCELLANEOUS

ASSOCIATED CONDITIONS

- Enamel hypoplasia/hypocalcification
- Juvenile purpura.

AGE-RELATED FACTORS

All ages affected, depends on the cause.

ZOONOTIC POTENTIAL

None.

PREGNANCY/FERTILITY/BREEDING

- Tetracycline administration during pregnancy may result in permanent tooth discoloration in offspring.
- See Genetics.

SYNONYMS

- Chlorhexidine staining.
- Extrinsic staining.
- Intrinsic staining.
- Tetracycline staining.

Suggested Reading

Hale FA. Localized intrinsic staining of teeth due to pulpitis and pulp necrosis in dogs. J Vet Dent, 2001, 18(1):14–20.

Lobprise HB, Dodd JR. Wiggs' Veterinary Dentistry Principles and Practice. Hoboken, NJ: Wiley-Blackwell, 2019.

Author Kristin M. Bannon

Consulting Editor Heidi B. Lobprise

DISCOSPONDYLITIS

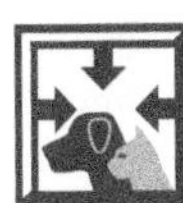

BASICS

DEFINITION

A bacterial, fungal, and rarely algal infection of the intervertebral end plates, discs, and adjacent vertebral bodies.

PATHOPHYSIOLOGY

- Hematogenous spread of bacterial or fungal organisms—most common cause.
- Seeding secondary to migrating foreign body (grass awn) is also reported.
- Neurologic dysfunction—may occur; usually the result of spinal cord compression caused by proliferation of bone and fibrous tissue; less commonly owing to luxation or pathologic fracture of the spine, epidural abscess, or extension of infection to the meninges and spinal cord.

SYSTEMS AFFECTED

- Musculoskeletal—infection and inflammation of the spine.
- Nervous—compression and/or infection of the spinal cord.

GENETICS

- No definite predisposition identified.
- An inherited immunodeficiency has been detected in a few cases.

INCIDENCE/PREVALENCE

Approximately 0.1–0.8% of dog hospital admissions.

GEOGRAPHIC DISTRIBUTION

- More common in the southeastern United States.
- Grass awn migration and coccidiomycosis—more common in certain regions.

SIGNALMENT

Species

Dog; rare in cat.

Breed Predilections

Large and giant breeds, especially German shepherd and Great Dane.

Mean Age and Range

- Mean age—4–5 years.
- Range—5 months–12 years.

Predominant Sex

Males outnumber females by ~2 : 1.

SIGNS

Historical Findings

- Onset usually relatively acute; however, some patients may have mild signs for several months before presenting for examination.
- Pain—difficulty rising, reluctance to jump, and stilted gait are most common signs.
- Ataxia or paresis.
- Weight loss and anorexia.
- Lameness.

Physical Examination Findings

- Focal or multifocal areas of spinal pain in >80% of patients.
- Any disc space may be affected; lumbosacral space is most commonly involved.
- Paresis or paralysis, especially in chronic, untreated cases.
- Fever in ~30% of patients.
- Lameness.

CAUSES

- Bacterial—*Staphylococcus pseudintermedius* is most common. Others include *Streptococcus, Brucella canis*, and *Escherichia coli*, but virtually any bacteria can be causative.
- Fungal—*Aspergillus, Paecilomyces, Scedosporium apiospermum*, and *Coccidioides immitis*.
- Grass awn migration is often associated with mixed infections, especially *Actinomyces*; tends to affect the L2–L4 disc spaces and vertebrae.
- Other causes—surgery, bite wounds.

RISK FACTORS

- Urinary tract infection; reproductive tract infection.
- Periodontal disease.
- Bacterial endocarditis.
- Pyoderma.
- Immunodeficiency.
- Recent steroid administration.
- Intact male status.

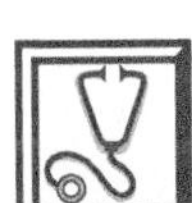

DIAGNOSIS

DIFFERENTIAL DIAGNOSIS

- Intervertebral disc protrusion—may cause similar clinical signs; differentiated on the basis of radiography and myelography.
- Vertebral fracture or luxation—detected on radiographs.
- Vertebral neoplasia—usually does not affect adjacent vertebral end plates.
- Spondylosis deformans—rarely causes clinical signs; has similar radiographic features, including sclerosis, ventral spur formation, and collapse of the disc space; rarely causes lysis of the vertebral end plates.
- Focal meningomyelitis—often identified by cerebrospinal fluid (CSF) analysis.

CBC/BIOCHEMISTRY/URINALYSIS

- Hemogram—often normal; may see leukocytosis.
- Urinalysis—may reveal pyuria and/or bacteriuria with concurrent urinary tract infections.

OTHER LABORATORY TESTS

- Aerobic, anaerobic, and fungal blood cultures identify the causative organism in about 35% of cases; obtain if available.
- Sensitivity testing—indicated if cultures are positive.
- Urine cultures—indicated; positive in about 30% of patients.
- Organisms other than *Staphylococcus* spp.—may not be the cause.
- Serologic testing for *Brucella canis*—indicated as this presents zoonotic potential.

IMAGING

- Spinal radiography—usually reveals lysis of vertebral end plates adjacent to the affected disc, collapse of the disc space, and varying degrees of sclerosis of the end plates and ventral spur formation; may not see lesions until 3–4 weeks after infection (therefore normal radiographs do not rule out).
- Myelography—indicated with substantial neurologic deficits; determine location and degree of spinal cord compression, especially if considering decompressive surgery; spinal cord compression caused by discospondylitis typically displays an extradural pattern.
- CT or MRI—more sensitive than radiography; indicated when radiographs are normal or inconclusive.

DIAGNOSTIC PROCEDURES

- CSF analysis—occasionally indicated to rule out meningomyelitis; usually normal or reveals mildly high protein.
- Bone scintigraphy—occasionally useful for detecting early lesions; helps clarify if radiographic changes are infectious or degenerative (spondylosis deformans).
- Fluoroscopically guided fine-needle aspiration of the disc—valuable for obtaining tissue for culture when blood and urine cultures are negative and there is no improvement with empiric antibiotic therapy.

PATHOLOGIC FINDINGS

- Gross—loss of normal disc space; bony proliferation of adjacent vertebrae.
- Microscopic—fibrosing pyogranulomatous destruction of the disc and vertebral bodies.

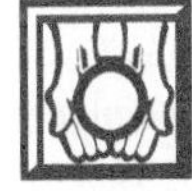

TREATMENT

APPROPRIATE HEALTH CARE

- Outpatient—mild pain managed with medication.
- Inpatient—severe pain or progressive neurologic deficits require intensive care and monitoring.

NURSING CARE

Nonambulatory patients—keep on clean, dry, well-padded surface to prevent decubital ulceration.

ACTIVITY

Restricted

CLIENT EDUCATION

- Explain that observation of response to treatment is very important in determining the need for further diagnostic or therapeutic procedures.

DISCOSPONDYLITIS

- Instruct the client to immediately contact the veterinarian if clinical signs progress or recur or if neurologic deficits develop.

SURGICAL CONSIDERATIONS

- Curettage of a single affected disc space—occasionally necessary for patients that are refractory to antibiotic therapy.
- Goals—remove infected tissue; obtain tissue for culture and histologic evaluation.
- Decompression of the spinal cord by hemilaminectomy or dorsal laminectomy—indicated for substantial neurologic deficits and spinal cord compression evident on MRI or myelography when there is no improvement with antibiotic therapy; also perform curettage of the infected disc space; it may be necessary to perform surgical stabilization if more than one articular facet is removed from a disc site.

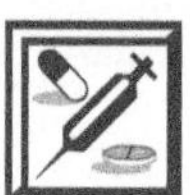

MEDICATIONS

DRUG(S) OF CHOICE

Antibiotics

- Selection based on results of blood cultures and serology or end plate aspirate culture and sensitivity.
- Negative culture and serology—assume causative organism is *Staphylococcus* spp.; treat with a cephalosporin (e.g., cephalexin 22 mg/kg PO q8h) for 8–12 weeks.
- Acutely progressive signs or substantial neurologic deficits—initially treated with parenteral antibiotics (e.g., cefazolin; dogs and cats: 22 mg/kg IV q8h).
- Brucellosis—treated with tetracycline (dogs: 15 mg/kg PO q8h) and streptomycin (dogs: 3.4 mg/kg IM q24h) or enrofloxacin (dogs: 10 mg/kg PO q24h).
- One study suggested that antibiosis be continued until radiographic signs were resolved (range of 40–80 weeks). The roll of imaging in definitively determining length of treatment has not been proven, however.

Analgesics

- Signs of severe pain—treated with an analgesic (e.g., oxymorphone; dogs: 0.05–0.2 mg/kg IV/IM/SC q4–6h).
- Taper dosage after 3–5 days to gauge effectiveness of antibiotic therapy.

CONTRAINDICATIONS

Glucocorticoids

PRECAUTIONS

Use nonsteroidal anti-inflammatory drugs (NSAIDs) and other analgesics cautiously—may cause temporary resolution of clinical signs even when infection is progressing; when used, discontinue after 3–5 days to assess efficacy of antibiotic therapy.

POSSIBLE INTERACTIONS

None

ALTERNATIVE DRUG(S)

- Initial therapy—cephradine (dogs: 20 mg/kg PO q8h); amoxicillin trihydrate/clavulanate potassium (dogs: 13.75–22 mg/kg PO q12h).
- Refractory patients—clindamycin (dogs and cats: 10 mg/kg PO q12h), enrofloxacin (dogs: 10 mg/kg PO q24h; cats: 5 mg/kg PO q24h), orbifloxacin (dogs and cats: 2.5–7.5 mg/kg PO q24h).

FOLLOW-UP

PATIENT MONITORING

- Reevaluate after 5 days of therapy.
- No improvement in pain, fever, or appetite—reassess therapy; consider a different antibiotic, percutaneous aspiration of the affected disc space, or surgery.
- Improvement—evaluate clinically and radiographically every 4 weeks.

PREVENTION/AVOIDANCE

Early identification of predisposing causes and prompt diagnosis and treatment—help reduce progression of clinical symptoms and neurologic deterioration.

POSSIBLE COMPLICATIONS

- Spinal cord compression owing to proliferative bony and fibrous tissue.
- Vertebral fracture or luxation.
- Meningitis or meningomyelitis.
- Epidural abscess.

EXPECTED COURSE AND PROGNOSIS

- Recurrence is common if antibiotic therapy is stopped prematurely (before 8–12 weeks of treatment).
- Some patients require prolonged therapy (1 year or more).
- Prognosis—depends on causative organism and degree of spinal cord damage.
- Mild or no neurologic dysfunction (dogs)—usually respond within 5 days of starting antibiotic therapy.
- Substantial paresis or paralysis (dogs)—prognosis guarded; may note gradual resolution of neurologic dysfunction after several weeks of therapy; treatment warranted.
- *Brucella canis*—signs usually resolve with therapy; infection may not be eradicated; recurrence common.

MISCELLANEOUS

ASSOCIATED CONDITIONS

See Risk Factors.

AGE-RELATED FACTORS

N/A

ZOONOTIC POTENTIAL

Brucella canis—human infection uncommon but may occur.

PREGNANCY/FERTILITY/BREEDING

N/A

SYNONYMS

- Diskitis.
- Intervertebral disc infection.
- Intradiskal osteomyelitis.
- Vertebral osteomyelitis.

SEE ALSO

Brucellosis

ABBREVIATIONS

- CSF = cerebrospinal fluid.
- NSAID = nonsteroidal anti-inflammatory drug.

Suggested Reading

Ameel L, Martlè V, Gielen I, et al. Discospondylitis in the dog: a retrospective study of 18 cases. Vlaams Diergeneeskundig Tijdschrift 2009, 78(5):347–353.

Bagley RS. Diskospondylitis. Fundam Clin Neuro 2005, 172–173(283–285):346.

Braund KG, Sharp NJH. Discospondylitis. In: Vite C, ed., Braund's Clinical Neurology in Small Animals: Localisation, Diagnosis and Treatment. Ithaca, NY: IVIS, 2003. https://www.ivis.org/library/braunds-clinical-neurology-small-animals-localization-diagnosis-and-treatment/degenerative

Burkert BA, Kerwin SC, Hosgood GL, et al. Signalment and clinical features of diskospondylitis in dogs: 513 cases (1980–2001). J Am Vet Med Assoc 2005, 227(2):268–275.

Fischer A, Mahaffey MB, Oliver JE. Fluoroscopically guided percutaneous disk aspiration in 10 dogs with diskospondylitis. J Vet Intern Med 1997, 11:284–287.

Johnson RG, Prata RG. Intradiskal osteomyelitis: a conservative approach. JAAHA 1983, 19:743–750.

Kerwin SC, Lewis DD, Hribernik TN, et al. Diskospondylitis associated with Brucella canis infection in dogs: 14 cases (1989–1991). J Am Vet Med Assoc 1992, 201:1253–1257.

Kornegay JN. Diskospondylitis. In: Kirk RW, ed., Current Veterinary Therapy IX. Philadelphia, PA: Saunders, 1986, pp. 810–814.

Ruoff CM, Kerwin SC, Taylor AR. Diagnostic imaging of discospondylitis. Vet Clin North Am Small Anim Pract 2018, 48:85–94.

Thomas WB. Diskospondylitis and other vertebral infections. Vet Clin North Am Small Anim Pract 2000, 30:169–182.

Author Mathieu M. Glassman
Consulting Editor Mathieu M. Glassman

Client Education Handout available online

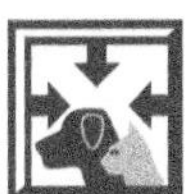

BASICS

DEFINITION

An acquired complex hemostatic defect arising from a variety of inciting causes that leads to intravascular activation of coagulation and consumption of clotting factors. It results in widespread formation of microthrombi with clinical manifestations of thrombosis and/or hemorrhage. Non-overt disseminated intravascular coagulation (DIC) is the early, compensated form of DIC that features consumption of coagulation factors and generation of microthrombi without clear clinical signs. Overt (decompensated) DIC refers to the classic phenotype associated with hemorrhage, thrombosis, and organ failure.

PATHOPHYSIOLOGY

- DIC represents a complication of a variety of primary conditions. It begins with a hypercoagulable state that leads to production or embolization of microthrombi in small vessels.
- The primary conditions act through increased exposure/production of tissue factor (TF) that activates the extrinsic coagulation pathway.
- TF is normally restricted from intravascular exposure. Increased TF exposure occurs through widespread endothelial injury and/or inflammation.
- Inflammation activates endothelial cells, platelets, and monocytes leading to membrane expression of TF. Inflammatory cytokines also induce vesiculation of these membranes, releasing large quantities of microparticles into circulation that are enriched with both TF and phosphatidylserine (PS) and facilitate initiation of coagulation. Some neoplastic cells constitutively produce membrane TF and also release microparticles.
- Microparticles provide a suitable membrane surface for amplifying intrinsic and common pathway coagulation, potentially leading to uncontrolled production of thrombin that overwhelms endogenous coagulation inhibitors. Fibrin clots generated by thrombin can cause vascular occlusion and lead to organ dysfunction.
- Widespread microthrombus formation consumes coagulation factors and platelets while initiating fibrinolysis. By-products of fibrinolysis (fibrin degradation products [FDPs]) have anticoagulant properties and inhibit platelet function. Hemorrhage at a variety of sites can follow.
- Uncontrolled progression leads to widespread tissue hypoxia, multiorgan dysfunction, and death.

SYSTEMS AFFECTED

Multisystemic syndrome.

INCIDENCE/PREVALENCE

Associated with severe systemic inflammatory disease.

SIGNALMENT

Species

Dogs and cats; diagnosed more in dogs.

Breed Predilections

None

Mean Age and Range

Depends on the primary disease.

Predominant Sex

None

SIGNS

- Vary with the primary disease and with DIC-associated organ dysfunction.
- Petechiae.
- Bleeding from venipuncture sites, mucosa, or into body cavities.
- Bleeding is infrequent in cats, possibly leading to underdiagnosis.

CAUSES

- Gastric dilatation-volvulus.
- Heart failure.
- Heartworm disease.
- Heat stroke.
- Hemolysis, especially immune mediated.
- Hemorrhagic gastroenteritis.
- Infectious diseases, systemic (especially endotoxemia).
- Inflammation, severe—regardless of underlying cause.
- Liver disease, severe.
- Malignancies, especially hemangiosarcoma, mammary carcinoma, and pulmonary adenocarcinoma in dogs and lymphoma in cats.
- Pancreatitis.
- Protein-losing nephropathy.
- Shock, hypoxia, acidosis.
- Thrombocytopenia, especially immune-mediated.
- Transfusion incompatibility.
- Trauma.
- Envenomation.

RISK FACTORS

Vary with cause.

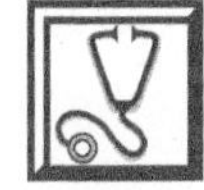

DIAGNOSIS

DIFFERENTIAL DIAGNOSIS

- Key differentials—immune-mediated thrombocytopenia, anticoagulant toxicity, coagulation factor deficiency, paraproteinemia.
- Highly variable diagnostic pattern includes thrombocytopenia, prolonged clotting times (prothrombin time [PT], activated partial thromboplastin time [APTT]), decreased fibrinogen, decreased antithrombin (AT), and increased products of fibrinolysis (FDPs, D-dimers).
- Suspect DIC any time thrombocytopenia and prolonged clotting tests are seen together.
- Patients showing predisposing conditions should have laboratory monitoring every 24–48 hours. A sudden drop in platelet count and a 20–30% prolongation in APTT is suspicious for non-overt DIC. This is a critical stage for intervention to prevent progression to overt DIC.
- Hepatic insufficiency may mimic DIC. Decreased production of clotting factors is common. Decreased clearance of normal fibrin(ogen)olytic by-products may increase FDP values. Mild idiopathic thrombocytopenia may also be seen. Spontaneous bleeding is uncommon unless DIC is present.

CBC/BIOCHEMISTRY/URINALYSIS

- Inflammatory leukogram, often with a stress component.
- Mild to moderate thrombocytopenia ($40–100 \times 10^3/\mu L$); less reliable in cats.
- Anemia is possible. Red blood cell (RBC) fragmentation is a supportive finding.
- Biochemical changes reflect affected organs; acute kidney injury may result in isosthenuria, oligo-anuria, or the identification of casts in urine sediment.

OTHER LABORATORY TESTS

- Prolonged clotting tests (PT, APTT); APTT is prolonged first, PT becomes prolonged with transition to overt DIC.
- Hypofibrinogenemia, although inflammatory increase may mask consumption.
- Increased FDPs and D-dimers. D-dimers are very sensitive and specific. DIC is unlikely if D-dimers are low/negative. Neither test is specific enough alone to diagnose DIC.
- Decreased AT; may be a positive acute phase reactant in cats, masking consumption.
- Thromboelastography may provide evidence of hypocoagulability or fibrinolysis.

DIAGNOSTIC PROCEDURES

Diagnostic procedures should be focused on identifying the inciting cause of inflammation, and may include imaging, tissue biopsy, or surgery as dictated by clinical signs.

PATHOLOGIC FINDINGS

- Usually related to the primary disease or DIC-affected organs.
- Petechiae common.

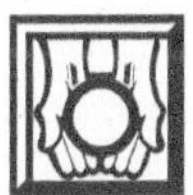

TREATMENT

APPROPRIATE HEALTH CARE

- Requires intensive inpatient treatment.
- Aggressive treatment of the primary disease is essential (e.g., antimicrobials for sepsis).

DISSEMINATED INTRAVASCULAR COAGULATION (CONTINUED)

D

NURSING CARE

- Maintain tissue perfusion and oxygenation using fluids, transfusions, and oxygen therapy.
- Restore depleted factors by blood/plasma transfusions. Use fresh frozen plasma (10–20 mL/kg) to correct bleeding due to factor deficiency.

ACTIVITY

Limited by disease severity.

DIET

Maintain nutritional support as appropriate for the clinical condition of the patient.

CLIENT EDUCATION

Inform the owner that the condition is life-threatening with a guarded to poor prognosis.

SURGICAL CONSIDERATIONS

Related to primary disease. Plasma or whole blood transfusion to restore clotting factors is a presurgical consideration. Surgery may be contraindicated with uncontrolled bleeding.

MEDICATIONS

DRUG(S) OF CHOICE

- There is no specific pharmacologic therapy for DIC per se.
- Heparin may be used in patients that have overt thrombosis or in those at high risk of thrombosis with normal coagulation times. Unfractionated heparin is preferred to low molecular weight heparin in human patients with DIC.
- Heparin binds to and potentiates the action of AT. Plasma or blood transfusions may be needed to replenish AT for heparin to be an effective anticoagulant.
- Starting doses for unfractionated heparin are 150–200 U/kg SC q8h. It may also be given as a CRI starting at 20–30 U/kg/h IV (i.e., same total daily dosage). Therapy should be monitored using serial measurements of APTT or anti-Xa activity.

CONTRAINDICATIONS

- Heparin therapy should be avoided in patients with coagulopathy.
- Inhibitors of fibrinolysis should not be used.
- The use of antiplatelet medications in thrombocytopenic patients is not indicated.
- Corticosteroids impair function of mononuclear phagocytes and do not have a clear indication for DIC unless important for therapy of the underlying disease (e.g., lymphoma).

PRECAUTIONS

- Heparin may cause hemorrhage, and therapy should be monitored.
- Volume overload may occur in cases with renal or pulmonary compromise.

POSSIBLE INTERACTIONS

None

FOLLOW-UP

PATIENT MONITORING

- Clinical improvement and the arrest of bleeding are key positive findings.
- Daily lab testing (e.g., coagulation tests, fibrinogen, platelet counts) is warranted in severe cases to identify positive or negative trends. Less frequent testing may suffice in milder cases.
- Coagulation times and fibrinogen often normalize more rapidly than FDPs and platelet counts.

PREVENTION/AVOIDANCE

Early detection of non-overt DIC can allow therapy before disease progresses to overt DIC.

POSSIBLE COMPLICATIONS

Aside from the primary disease, affected organs may have permanent dysfunction or marginal reserve capacity.

EXPECTED COURSE AND PROGNOSIS

For overt DIC, mortality rates for dogs range from 50% to 77%. For cats, rates may be >90%.

MISCELLANEOUS

PREGNANCY/FERTILITY/BREEDING

Unlike in humans, obstetric complications are not a common cause in dogs and cats.

SYNONYMS

- Consumptive coagulopathy.
- Disseminated intravascular coagulopathy.

SEE ALSO

- Coagulation Factor Deficiency.
- Thrombocytopenia.

ABBREVIATIONS

- APTT = activated partial thromboplastin time.
- AT = antithrombin.
- DIC = disseminated intravascular coagulation.
- FDP = fibrin degradation product.
- PS = phosphatidylserine.
- PT = prothrombin time.
- RBC = red blood cell.
- TF = tissue factor.

Suggested Reading

Dunn ME. Acquired coagulopathies. In: Ettinger SJ, Feldman EC, eds. Textbook of Veterinary Internal Medicine: Diseases of the Dog and Cat, 7th ed. St. Louis, MO: Saunders, 2010, pp. 797–801.

O'Brien M. The reciprocal relationship between inflammation and coagulation. Top Companion Anim Med 2012, 27:46–52.

Ralph AG, Brainard MB. Update on disseminated intravascular coagulation: when to consider it, when to expect it, when to treat it. Top Companion Anim Med 2012, 27:65–72.

Stokol T. Laboratory diagnosis of disseminated intravascular coagulation in dogs and cats: the past, the present, and the future. Vet Clin North Am Small Anim Pract 2012, 42:189–202.

Author John A. Christian

Consulting Editor Melinda S. Camus

Client Education Handout available online

DROWNING (NEAR DROWNING)

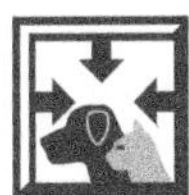

BASICS

OVERVIEW

• Defined as process of experiencing respiratory impairment from submersion or immersion in liquid; near drowning defined as water submersion followed by survival for at least 24 hours; recent changes in terminology prefer the use of "death, morbidity or no morbidity following a drowning episode." • Following submersion, elevations in CO_2 levels in the bloodstream stimulate respiration, and subsequent aspiration of water occurs. • Fresh water aspiration dilutes pulmonary surfactant, leading to alveolar collapse ± infectious pneumonia; hypertonic seawater aspiration leads to diffusion of interstitial water into alveoli; large volumes of water are not typically aspirated, but any amount results in ventilation–perfusion mismatch, hypoxemia, and metabolic acidosis. • Submersion time, temperature of water, and type of water (fresh vs. salt vs. chemical water) significantly affect development of organ damage.

SIGNALMENT

Dogs and cats. Approximately half of animals involved in immersion accidents are <4 months of age.

SIGNS

- Noted acutely after exposure to water.
- Cyanosis, apnea, respiratory distress.
- Coughing ± clear to frothy red sputum.
- Vomiting. • Obtunded to comatose.
- Crackles or wheezes auscultated over chest.
- Tachycardia or bradycardia, asystole.

CAUSES & RISK FACTORS

• Greater risk near bodies of water (including pools, buckets, bathtubs) or ice. • Owner negligence or inadequate safety precautions vs. purposeful harm. • Animals in or near water at time of seizure, head trauma, hypoglycemic event, cardiac arrhythmia, or syncopal episode are at risk of drowning.

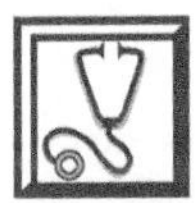

DIAGNOSIS

DIFFERENTIAL DIAGNOSIS

- Hypothermia, neck trauma, and meningitis.
- With drowning secondary to seizure, head trauma, hypoglycemic event, cardiac arrhythmia, or syncopal episode, history at time of presentation may be informative.

CBC/BIOCHEMISTRY/URINALYSIS

- Fresh water inhalation/ingestion—hemodilution, hemolysis, and decreases in sodium, chloride, and urine specific gravity.
- Hypertonic salt water ingestion/inhalation—hemoconcentration and increases in sodium, chloride, and urine specific gravity.

OTHER LABORATORY TESTS

Arterial blood gas reveals hypoxemia (partial pressure of oxygen [PaO_2] <80 mmHg), hypoventilation (partial pressure of carbon dioxide [$PaCO_2$] >50 mmHg), and acid-base derangements.

IMAGING

• Radiographic changes may not be detectable for 24–48 hours. • Focal or diffuse alveolar pattern due to aspiration pneumonia or noncardiogenic pulmonary edema. • Mixed patterns may be present, ± radiopaque material filling the airways ("sand bronchogram"). • Foreign body inhalation may produce segmental atelectasis. • Progression of pulmonary injury to acute respiratory distress syndrome (ARDS) is possible and may appear as bilateral, diffuse, symmetric alveolar infiltrates.

DIAGNOSTIC PROCEDURES

• Endotracheal or transtracheal wash with cytologic evaluation and culture with sensitivity indicated if animal is stable. • ECG monitoring. • Cervical radiographs, CT or MRI of brain, and brainstem auditory evoked response (BAER) assessment in select cases.

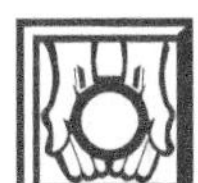

TREATMENT

• Initiate mouth-to-muzzle resuscitation on-site. • Emergency inpatient care is required. • Airway clearance, if obstructed, is first priority. • Cardiopulmonary resuscitation (CPR), if necessary. • Oxygen supplementation. • Intubation and mechanical ventilation with positive end-expiratory pressure may be required in animals with severe hypoxemia, hypercapnia, or imminent respiratory fatigue. • Fluid therapy and acid-base/electrolyte management are crucial. • Gradually rewarm (over 2–3 hours) hypothermic animals. • Gravitational drainage or abdominal thrusts (Heimlich maneuver) are not recommended in absence of airway obstruction owing to high risk of regurgitation and subsequent aspiration of stomach contents. • Continuous venovenous filtration may decrease mortality following salt water drowning.

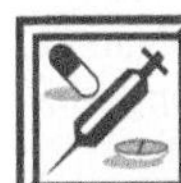

MEDICATIONS

DRUG(S) OF CHOICE

• Mannitol 0.5 g/kg IV over 30 min may be beneficial in animals with suspected cerebral edema. • Broad-spectrum antibiotics (e.g., ampicillin 22 mg/kg IV q8h; enrofloxacin 10–20 mg/kg IV q24h in the dog, 5 mg/kg IV q24h in the cat) for aspiration pneumonia. • Beta-2 agonists may help animals with suspected bronchospasm. • Pentoxifylline decreased incidence of lung injury in dogs with experimental freshwater aspiration.

CONTRAINDICATIONS/POSSIBLE INTERACTIONS

• Corticosteroid therapy not indicated; use could be detrimental in animals with aspiration pneumonia. • Use of enrofloxacin in young animals may result in cartilage erosion.

FOLLOW-UP

PATIENT MONITORING

• Continuous monitoring of heart rate and rhythm, respiratory rate, mucous membrane color and capillary refill time, urine output, arterial blood pressure, rectal temperature, and neurologic status. • Arterial blood gas, CBC, biochemical profile, coagulation profile, and acid-base status checked as needed.

PREVENTION/AVOIDANCE

Close monitoring of animals (especially young and old/debilitated animals) near bodies of water. Place barriers around bodies of water, life jackets on animals, train owners to perform CPR.

POSSIBLE COMPLICATIONS

Aspiration pneumonia, noncardiogenic pulmonary edema, ARDS, gastrointestinal bleeding, diarrhea, vomiting, acute kidney injury, permanent neurologic derangements, disseminated intravascular coagulation, central diabetes insipidus.

EXPECTED COURSE AND PROGNOSIS

Directly related to animal's status at time of admission—animals that present comatose, severely acidotic (pH <7.0), or requiring cardiopulmonary resuscitation or mechanical ventilation have poor prognosis. Animals that present conscious have good prognosis if no complications ensue; 37.5% mortality rate in 15 dogs and 1 cat with freshwater aspiration.

MISCELLANEOUS

ABBREVIATIONS

• ARDS = acute respiratory distress syndrome. • BAER = brainstem auditory evoked response. • CPR = cardiopulmonary resuscitation. • $PaCO_2$ = partial pressure of carbon dioxide. • PaO_2 partial pressure of oxygen.

Author Deborah C. Silverstein
Consulting Editor Elizabeth Rozanski

DUCTAL PLATE MALFORMATION (CONGENITAL HEPATIC FIBROSIS)

D

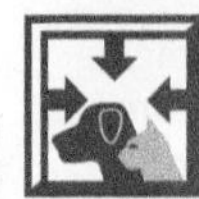

BASICS

DEFINITION

• Ductal plate malformations (DPMs) are congenital noninflammatory hepatopathies subject to complicating bacterial cholangitis; recognized most often in juvenile and young adult dogs or cats and reflect malformation of biliary structures. • DPMs reflect aberrant development, differentiation, proliferation, or intussusceptive resorption of embryonic anlage of bile ducts during development of ductal plate, embryologic precursor of portal tract structures (predominantly bile ducts).
• Pathomechanisms leading to DPM interfere with tubulogenesis—may affect kidneys, liver, or pancreatic ductal structures.
• Four DPM phenotypes defined based on involved structures and severity of coexistent portal tract fibrosis, severity of fibroductal bridging trabeculae, development of presinusoidal portal hypertension (PH) causing splanchnic hypertension, and development of acquired portosystemic shunts (APSS). • Animals with DPM have propensity for septic suppurative cholangitis, choledochitis, cholelithiasis, or extrahepatic bile duct obstruction (EHBDO).

MAJOR DPM PHENOTYPES

• *Choledochal cyst*—diverticulum protruding from common bile duct (CBD) or cystic duct; propensity for infection similar to appendicitis in humans; may cause systemic sepsis, EHBDO, and cranial abdominal mass effect; complex confusing US appearance. • *Caroli's malformation*—irregular duct silhouettes (sacculation, invagination, or "budding" protrusions) with occasional periductal satellite ductal elements surrounding large ducts; malformations variably involve hepatic, interlobular, or large intralobular bile ducts; biliary epithelium may appear normal, hyperplastic, attenuated, or vacuolated; intraluminal debris in large ducts; develop choleliths, dystrophic mineralization, septic cholangitis. • *Small proliferative-like phenotype*—diffuse intralobular bile duct malformation without *or* with bridging portal-to-portal fibroductular trabeculae: if fibrosis severe may evolve presinusoidal PH and consequent splanchnic hypertension = *congenital hepatic fibrosis (CHF) phenotype*—involves small intralobular bile duct malformation with densely packed proliferative-like ductule structures (± luminal apertures) within excessive extracellular matrix (ECM); ECM accrual varies in severity, but appears progressive with aging; histologic features characterized by amalgamation of proliferative bile ductules with numerous stout (muscular) entangling arterials and inconspicuous portal veins within exuberant ECM that dimensionally expands portal tracts; variable fibroductal bridging partitions may interconnect portal regions; because ECM accrues with aging, transformation to CHF may occur over time. • *von Meyenburg's complexes (VMCs)*—isolated single microscopic DPM composed of clustered proliferative intralobular bile duct profiles embedded in expanded ECM; also termed bile duct hamartomas; usually located adjacent to liver capsule; inconsequential malformation.
• Progression of portal tract fibrosis with aging can lead to gradual onset of presinusoidal PH, formation of APSS, ascites, and hepatic encephalopathy (HE). • Gallbladder (GB) agenesis and severe hypoplasia or agenesis of entire liver lobes may occur. • Liver lobes may be variably affected with DPM; unaffected liver lobes possible.

PATHOPHYSIOLOGY

• DPMs not associated with increased liver enzymes or jaundice unless complicated by infection, choleliths, EHBDO, or choledochitis.
• Different phenotypes acquire different disease manifestations. • *Choledochal cysts*—not recognized until cystic luminal contents contaminated by bacteria with ensuing infection and cyst expansion, development of choledochitis or EHBDO; until compromised CBD patency patient remains anicteric, usually asymptomatic.
• *Caroli's malformation*—serendipitously recognized on abdominal radiography (limy gallbladder, mineralized sacculated intrahepatic large bile ducts), or on abdominal US as distended intra- or extrahepatic bile ducts, mineralized ducts, association with cholelithiasis, or thickened duct walls (infection, choledochitis).
• *Diffuse DPM without extensive bridging fibrosis or presinusoidal PH*—not associated with increased liver enzymes or jaundice, usually normal total serum bile acid (TSBA) concentrations; diagnosed when infection increases liver enzyme activity leading to liver biopsy. • *Diffuse DPM with bridging fibrosis (CHF) causes presinusoidal PH*—these patients may present for ascites, increased TSBA concentrations, ± increased liver enzymes reflecting secondary cholangitis, or for HE; not jaundiced unless infected or have concurrent EHBDO.

SYSTEMS AFFECTED

• Liver—variable size (small, normal, large); may have GB agenesis or maldevelopment of entire liver lobe(s); rare concurrent congenital intrahepatic or extrahepatic congenital portosystemic vascular anomaly (shunt, PSVA); jaundice due to EHBDO from choledochal cyst, cholelithiasis, rare cholangiocarcinoma, or due to sepsis (Caroli's malformation, choledochal cyst); increased liver enzymes may reflect suppurative cholangitis or unrelated copper associated hepatopathy (CuAH) in dogs.
• Gastrointestinal (GI)—anorexia; intermittent vomiting or diarrhea reflects concurrent inflammatory bowel disease (IBD) or enteric hypertensive vasculopathy (splanchnic hypertension from presinusoidal PH).
• Nervous—episodic HE if APSS associated with CHF or if concurrent PSVA.
• Musculoskeletal—stunted growth and poor body condition if CHF and APSS or if concurrent PSVA; also may reflect chronic disease, inappetence, or enteric malassimilation.
• Urogenital—polyuria and polydipsia (PU/PD); possible polycystic renal phenotype; ammonium biurate urolithiasis reflects APSS or rare concurrent PSVA. • Hemic/lymphatic/immune—red blood cell (RBC) microcytosis reflects APSS or PSVA; neutrophilic leukocytosis with toxic neutrophils and left-shifted leukon reflects sepsis due to suppurative bacterial cholangitis/choledochitis or infected choledochal cyst.

SIGNALMENT

• Dog and cat, no sex predilection. • Juvenile and young adults predominate; dogs: mean age 1.5–2.5 years (0.2–12) years. • May affect multiple littermates. • Boxer dogs may be predisposed. • Persian cats and descendent breeds with or without polycystic renal disease appear predisposed.

SIGNS

• May be asymptomatic. • Stunted growth, poor body condition if CHF with APSS or concurrent PSVA. • GI signs—inappetence, emesis, diarrhea, enteric hemorrhage; especially if concurrent IBD. • PU/PD if APSS or rare concurrent PSVA, or polycystic renal disease. • ± Increased liver enzymes.
• ± Fever, leukocytosis, hyperbilirubinemia—due to sepsis evolved from bacterial cholangitis, choledochitis, or choledochal cyst infection or infection-related cholelithiasis. • ± Abdominal distention—ascites with APSS in CHF; CHF with PSVA no ascites unless PSVA attenuated.
• ± Episodic CNS signs due to HE if APSS in CHF or rare concurrent PSVA. • ± Urolithiasis (ammonium urates) if APSS in CHF or rare concurrent PSVA.

CAUSES & RISK FACTORS

• In humans (and knockout mouse models) DPM reflects gene mutations influencing structure or function of primary cilia; polycystic kidney disease in Persian cats involves polycystin-1 precursor gene, one gene influencing primary ciliary function; ~15% develop hepatic DPM. • Clinical signs usually reflect acquired complications.

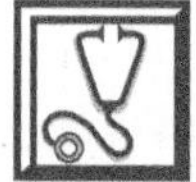

DIAGNOSIS

DIFFERENTIAL DIAGNOSIS

• Stunted growth, increased TSBA concentrations—PSVA, severe portal vein atresia, splanchnic portal vein thromboembolism (TE). • Increased liver enzymes ± hyperbilirubinemia—chronic hepatitis, CuAH, hepatotoxicity, liver abscess, primary hepatic neoplasia, cholangiohepatitis, choledochitis, or cholecystitis. • Jaundice—acute liver injury, hepatotoxicosis, chronic hepatitis, CuAH, cholelithiasis, ruptured GB, EHBDO, hemolysis. • CNS signs—infectious disorders (distemper); toxicities (lead); hydrocephalus; epilepsy; metabolic disorders (severe hypoglycemia, hypokalemia, hyperkalemia, hypophosphatemia); thiamine deficiency. • Ascites—pure transudate, many causes (see Hypertension, Portal). • HE—APSS, PSVA, portal TE, other causes.

CBC/BIOCHEMISTRY/URINALYSIS

• CBC—RBC microcytosis: reflects APSS; target cells associated in dogs.
• Biochemistry—if APSS with CHF: ± low albumin, cholesterol, blood urea nitrogen, variable globulin; all DPM phenotypes: ± increased alkaline phosphatase and alanine aminotransferase activity with cholangitis; hyperbilirubinemia: if EHBDO due to choledochal cyst or cholelithiasis or if septic.
• Urinalysis—ammonium biurate crystalluria if APSS in CHF phenotype.

OTHER LABORATORY TESTS

• Routine coagulation tests—variable abnormalities (see Coagulopathy of Liver Disease); low protein C and antithrombin activity may reflect APSS in CHF phenotype.
• TSBA—increased concentrations in anicteric patients reflect APSS or rare concurrent PSVA. • Peritoneal fluid analysis—pure transudate (protein <2.5 g/dL); modified transudate if chronic: only in CHF phenotype.

IMAGING

Radiography

• Abdominal radiography—variable liver size.
• Abdominal effusion—APSS in CHF phenotype. • Ammonium biurate calculi—radiolucent unless radiodense mineral shell.
• Thoracic radiography—normal.

Abdominal US

• Variable liver size—small to large. • GB may not be discovered if atretic or may be tiny. • May disclose intra- or extrahepatic biliary malformations (sacculated or cystic ductal structures); variable liver texture; unremarkable vasculature to portal hypoperfusion. • Choledochal cyst—may be difficult to decipher owing to overlying enteric gas and confusion with CBD and cystic duct. • Abdominal effusion—if APSS in CHF. • APSS—confirm using color-flow Doppler; rule out portal TE and intrahepatic arteriovenous malformations as causes of APSS. • Uroliths—renal pelvis or urinary bladder.

Additional Imaging

• Colorectal or splenoportal scintigraphy with Technetium-^{99m} pertechnetate (see Portosystemic Vascular Anomaly, Congenital)—sensitive noninvasive test confirming macroscopic shunting, but cannot differentiate PSVA from APSS. • Multisector CT—gold standard imaging modality: confirms APSS or PSVA; dual-phase angiogram can reveal asymmetric liver development (liver lobe absence or atresia), GB atresia, choledochal cyst, sacculated interlobular and cystic ducts, cholelithiasis, and APSS.

DIAGNOSTIC PROCEDURES

• Fine-needle aspiration cytology—cannot diagnose DPM, sometimes identifies complicating bacterial infection especially if bile collected. • Liver biopsy—mandatory for definitive diagnosis; open surgical wedge, laparoscopic cup samples; needle core sample may be adequate; collect biopsies from several liver lobes. • Echocardiography—if ascites present.

PATHOLOGIC FINDINGS

• Gross—depends on phenotype.
○ *Choledochal cyst*—predominantly occurs in cats, variable size (as large as 10 cm) with thick or thin wall; contents acholic or mucinous white bile; may be purulent or bile laden; may envelop CBD. ○ *Caroli's malformation*—grossly distended hepatic, interlobular, or segmental bile ducts, thick walls if choledochitis, wall may be mineralized, may have pigmented-calcium carbonate choleliths. ○ *Small-proliferative-type DPM*—firm fibrotic hepatic parenchyma, fine nodular to smooth capsular surface, may have splanchnic APSS if CHF phenotype. ○ *von Meyenburg complexes*—inapparent or tiny pale foci on liver margin. • Possible GB atresia, PSVA, other vascular malformations, liver lobe agenesis. • Microscopic—variable severity as described (see Major DPM Phenotypes); stereotypic histologic features of portal venous hypoperfusion are common; direct intersection of proliferative-like bile ductules and hepatocytes is signature histologic feature of DPM in absence of inflammatory infiltrates; islands of hepatocytes may be encircled or isolated by portal-to-portal fibroductal partitions.

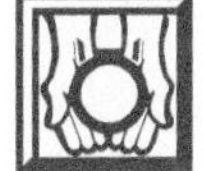

TREATMENT

APPROPRIATE HEALTH CARE

• Inpatient—for septic complications or severe HE. • Surgical intervention—choledochal cyst: best managed by resection but depends on anatomic malformation and location; may be marsupialized or anastomosed to intestine. • Outpatient—stable patients.
• Avoid endoparasitism. • Treat infections promptly—DPM patients (except VMC) predisposed to bacterial cholangitis, choledochitis, and associated cholelithiasis because of blind-ended noncontiguous ductal structures; in CHF with APSS reduced Kupffer cell surveillance increases risk for infection and systemic sepsis. • In CHF—remain vigilant for ammonium biurate obstructive uropathy. • If APSS—avoid nonsteroidal anti-inflammatories that may augment ascites and GI bleeding provoking HE; adjust dosage of drugs with high first-pass hepatic extraction. • CuAH diagnosed by liver biopsy should be treated.

NURSING CARE

• HE—eliminate causal factors; individualize diet, supplement water-soluble vitamins, vitamin E, and K depending on prothrombin/activated partial thromboplastin time tests or presence of EHBDO; provide multiple small feedings daily.
• Ascites—see Hypertension, Portal.

MEDICATIONS

DRUG(S) OF CHOICE

Strategy for DPM is to treat syndrome complications.

HE

• Lactulose (0.5–1.0 mL/kg PO q8–12h)—achieve several soft stools daily; may withdraw with optimal diet modification. • Oral antibiotics—modify encephalogenic enteric toxin production: first choices metronidazole (7.5 mg/kg PO q12h) or amoxicillin (22 mg/kg PO q12h); avoid neomycin (20 mg/kg PO q8–12h): potential for enteric absorption (esp. if concurrent IBD) causing ototoxicity (deafness) and nephrotoxicity.

Ascites

• Dietary sodium restriction. • Diuretics—furosemide (1–4 mg/kg PO/IM/IV q12–24h): potassium wasting effect modulated by combination with spironolactone (1–4 mg/kg PO q12h, loading dose then maintenance dose 2–4 mg/kg PO q24h); potassium sparing; less potent than furosemide.
• Diuretic-resistant ascites—consider therapeutic abdominocentesis (see Hypertension, Portal for other medical options). • Antifibrotic—not proven effective in humans with DPM; liver transplant common, unknown in veterinary medicine; colchicine not effective.
• Telmisartan—angiotensin receptor blocker safe for use in dogs and cats; attenuated progressive ECM accrual in DPM rodent model; adverse effects if coadministered with spironolactone or angiotensin-converting enzyme (ACE) inhibitor: leads to serious hypotension (collapse, acute renal failure); initial dose 0.5 mg/kg/day titrated to max of 1 mg/kg/day.

Antioxidant Medications

Indicated if chronic cholangitis, CuAH, chronic increased liver enzymes, or CHF.

Bleeding Tendencies

Rare in CHF; may encounter if chronic EHBDO caused by choledochal cyst or cholelithiasis.

GI Hemorrhage

Hypertensive enteric vasculopathy may be encountered with CHF because of APSS.

CONTRAINDICATIONS/POSSIBLE INTERACTIONS

- Avoid or reduce dosage of drugs relying on first-pass hepatic metabolism if APSS; avoid drugs reacting with GABA-benzodiazepine receptors if intermittent HE in patients with APSS-CHF phenotype; avoid drugs inhibiting biotransformation and metabolism of other drugs (e.g., cimetidine, chloramphenicol, quinidine, some calcium channel blockers); if jaundiced avoid drugs undergoing biliary elimination. • Avoid metoclopramide if spironolactone used as diuretic (augments aldosterone). • Avoid combination of spironolactone with telmisartan or ACE inhibitor.

FOLLOW-UP

PATIENT MONITORING

- Instruct owners to monitor body temperature, appetite, activity, for jaundice or other signs of infection or complications.
- Biochemistry—initially monitor q2–4 weeks until stabile in animals presenting with sepsis or EHBDO, then q4–6 months or if cyclically ill or febrile; monitor for recurrent septic cholangitis/choledochitis, development of septic effusion; HE decompensation.

POSSIBLE COMPLICATIONS

CHF associated with HE—requires indefinite nutritional and medical management. If concurrent PSVA—likely cannot be attenuated without causing APSS.

EXPECTED COURSE AND PROGNOSIS

- Long-term survival (years) possible.
- Guarded prognosis if CHF phenotype with APSS. • Short-term or lifelong treatments may be required. • Flare-ups of HE and ascites may require hospitalizations for adjustment of nutritional and medical interventions.

MISCELLANEOUS

ASSOCIATED CONDITIONS

- HE. • Ascites. • GI bleeding. • APSS.

AGE-RELATED FACTORS

- Prognosis depends on degree of fibrosis and APSS in CHF; severity of relapsing septic cholangitis or choledochal cyst infection; intrahepatic infected cholelithiasis; evidence of hepatic insufficiency and APSS at initial diagnosis. • Fibrosis progressive with aging in some patients.

SEE ALSO

- Ascites.
- Hepatic Encephalopathy.
- Hypertension, Portal.
- Portosystemic Shunting, Acquired.

ABBREVIATIONS

- ACE = angiotensin-converting enzyme.
- APSS = acquired portosystemic shunts.
- CBD = common bile duct.
- CHF = congenital hepatic fibrosis.
- CuAH = copper associated hepatopathy.
- DPM = ductal plate malformation.
- ECM = extracellular matrix.
- EHBDO = extrahepatic bile duct occlusion.
- GB = gallbladder.
- GI = gastrointestinal.
- HE = hepatic encephalopathy.
- IBD = inflammatory bowel disease.
- PH = portal hypertension.
- PSVA = portosystemic vascular anomaly.
- PU/PD = polyuria/polydipsia.
- RBC = red blood cell.
- TE = thromboembolism.
- TSBA = total serum bile acid.
- VMC = von Meyenburg's complex.

Suggested Reading

Brown DL, Van Winkle T, Cecere T, et al. Congenital hepatic fibrosis in 5 dogs. Vet Pathol 2010, 47:102–107.

Pillai S, Center SA, McDonough SP, et al. Ductal plate malformation in the liver of boxer dogs: clinical and histological features. Vet Pathol 2016, 53:602–613.

Author Sharon A. Center

Consulting Editor Kate Holan

DYSAUTONOMIA (KEY-GASKELL SYNDROME)

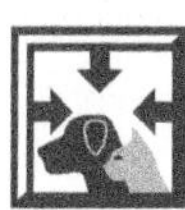

BASICS

OVERVIEW

• Failure of autonomic function in multiple organs with minimal motor or sensory involvement. • Young adult, rural dogs in specific states at greatest risk. • Treatment is symptomatic and prognosis guarded.

SIGNALMENT

• Dog and less commonly cat. • No breed or sex predilection. • Median age is 18 months but any age animal may be affected.

SIGNS

• Acute to subacute onset (5–14 days).
• Various combinations of signs may be present, but both sympathetic and parasympathetic signs in various organs are necessary to be confident of diagnosis.
• Sensory or motor deficits are minimal.

Presenting Complaints

• Most commonly gastrointestinal (GI) signs of vomiting or regurgitation, diarrhea, or occasionally constipation. • Straining to urinate and dribbling urine. • Photophobia and third-eyelid elevation. • Dyspnea, coughing, and purulent nasal discharge.
• Depression, anorexia, and weight loss.

Examination Findings

• Variable combinations of autonomic dysfunction. • Loss of anal sphincter tone.
• Dry nose and mucous membranes; lack of tear production. • Distended, easily expressed bladder. • Pupils midrange to maximally dilated with no pupillary light reflex but intact vision. • Third-eyelid elevation, ptosis, and enophthalmos. • Lack of gut sounds and occasional abdominal pain. • Heart rate and blood pressure typically in low end of normal range but do not rise in response to stress.
• Secondary aspiration pneumonia or rhinitis. • Cachexia. • Occasionally mild proprioceptive deficits or weakness.

CAUSES & RISK FACTORS

• Cause unknown. • Highest incidence in Missouri, Oklahoma, and Kansas as well as Wyoming and northern Colorado, but occasional cases reported throughout United States.
• Free-roaming, rural dogs at greatest risk.

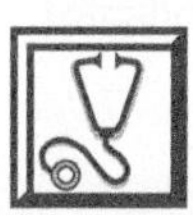

DIAGNOSIS

DIFFERENTIAL DIAGNOSIS

• Anticholinergic toxicity. • Other differential diagnoses depend upon specific clinical signs: e.g., urinary tract infection for dysuria, corneal ulcer for photophobia, dehydration for dry mucous membranes.

CBC/BIOCHEMISTRY/URINALYSIS

Unremarkable

IMAGING

• Megaesophagus ± aspiration pneumonia.
• Distended bowel loops with no peristalsis.
• Distended urinary bladder.
• Echocardiography may show systolic dysfunction as reduced fractional shortening.

DIAGNOSTIC PROCEDURES

• If pupils affected, 0.05% pilocarpine drops in one eye will produce miosis within 60 minutes; rules out anticholinergic toxicity.
• Atropine (0.03 mg/kg IV) may not produce expected rise in heart rate; suggests loss of vagal tone. • Intradermal histamine may produce no response or wheal but no flare; demonstrates loss of sympathetic innervation of arterioles.

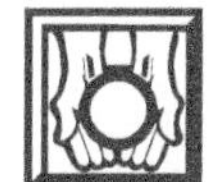

TREATMENT

• IV fluids to prevent dehydration. • High-calorie food; feeding tube to ensure adequate nutrition if megaesophagus present; if GI motility absent, parenteral nutrition may be necessary. • Lubricating eye drops if tear production insufficient. • Humidification of air may help with dry mucous membranes.
• Manual bladder expression.

MEDICATIONS

DRUG(S) OF CHOICE

• Antibiotics as needed to treat secondary infections. • Prokinetic drug such as metoclopramide if GI motility affected.
• Bethanechol to stimulate lacrimation and urination (start at 0.05 mg/kg q8–12h and adjust dose based on response); manual expression of bladder more reliable.
• Ocular pilocarpine to relieve photophobia.
• Pimobendan if poor cardiac contractility.

CONTRAINDICATIONS/POSSIBLE INTERACTIONS

• Animals with dysautonomia develop denervation supersensitivity to direct acting cholinergic or adrenergic drugs. • Great care must be exercised in using such drugs, particularly adrenergic drugs that could precipitate fatal tachyarrhythmias; best to start at <10% of low end of dose range when using direct-acting drugs and escalate dose as needed to produce desired effect.

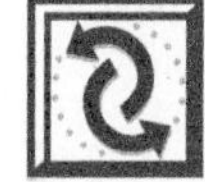

FOLLOW-UP

• Prognosis guarded; most animals die of aspiration pneumonia or euthanasia due to poor quality of life. • Animals who survive often have some degree of permanent autonomic dysfunction that may require constant care.

MISCELLANEOUS

• Necropsy identification of neuronal loss in ganglia confirms diagnosis. • Clinical diagnosis based on autonomic failure in multiple organs without underlying cause or significant motor or sensory involvement and appropriate response to pharmacologic testing.

ABBREVIATIONS

• GI = gastrointestinal.

Suggested Reading

Berghaus RD, O'Brien DP, Johnson GC, Thorne JG. Risk factors for development of dysautonomia in dogs. J Am Vet Med Assoc 2001, 218:1285–1292.

Harkin KR, Andrews GA, Nietfeld JC. Dysautonomia in dogs: 65 cases (1993–2000). J Am Vet Med Assoc 2002, 220:633–644.

Harkin KR, Bulmer BJ, Biller DS. Echocardiographic evaluation of dogs with dysautonomia. J Am Vet Med Assoc 2009, 235:1431–1436.

Kidder AC, Johannes C, O'Brien DP, et al. Feline dysautonomia in the Midwestern United States: a retrospective study of nine cases. J Fel Med Surg 2008, 10:130–136.

Longshore RC, O'Brien DP, Johnson GC, et al. Dysautonomia in dogs—a retrospective study. J Vet Intern Med 1996, 10(3):103–109.

O'Brien DP, Johnson GC. Dysautonomia and autonomic neuropathies. Vet Clin North Am Small Anim Pract 2002, 32:251–265.

Author Dennis P. O'Brien

DYSCHEZIA AND HEMATOCHEZIA

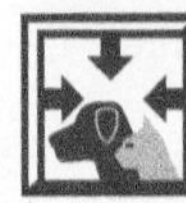

BASICS

DEFINITION

- Dyschezia—painful or difficult defecation.
- Hematochezia—bright red blood in or on the feces.

PATHOPHYSIOLOGY

Results from inflammatory, infectious, or neoplastic conditions affecting the colon, rectum, or anus.

SYSTEMS AFFECTED

Gastrointestinal

SIGNALMENT

- Dog and cat.
- No breed or sex predilection.

SIGNS

Historical Findings

- Vocalizing and whimpering during defecation.
- Tenesmus.
- Decreased frequency of defecation in association with severe dyschezia (animal resists defecating due to pain), resulting in constipation or obstipation.
- Mucoid, bloody diarrhea with a marked increase in frequency and scant fecal volume in patients with colitis.
- Scooting behavior in association with anal gland infection or impaction.
- It is pivotal to differentiate hematochezia secondary to colitis from hematochezia secondary to a colorectal mass—the histories are profoundly different and a rectal examination should always be performed to further differentiate these two disorders (see below).

Physical Examination Findings

- Rectal examination may reveal hard feces (constipation or obstipation), diarrhea (colorectal disease), colorectal masses, anorectal thickening, rectal or colonic strictures, anal sac enlargement/pain, prostatomegaly, or perineal hernias.
- Fistulous tracts around anus occur with perianal fistulae.
- Anal occlusion with matted hair and feces occurs with pseudocoprostasis.

CAUSES

Rectal/Anal Disease

- Stricture or spasm.
- Anal sacculitis or abscess.
- Perianal fistulae.
- Rectal or anal foreign body.
- Pseudocoprostasis.
- Rectal prolapse.
- Trauma—bite wounds, etc.
- Neoplasia—adenocarcinoma, lymphoma, and anal sac tumors.
- Rectal polyps.
- Mucocutaneous lupus erythematosus.

Colonic Disease

- Neoplasia—adenocarcinoma, lymphoma, other tumors.
- Idiopathic megacolon—cats.
- Inflammation—inflammatory bowel disease, infectious parasitic agents, colitis secondary to dietary-responsive enteropathy (see Colitis and Proctitis).
- Constipation (see Constipation and Obstipation).

Extraintestinal Disease

- Fractured pelvis or pelvic limb.
- Prostatic disease.
- Perineal hernia.
- Intrapelvic neoplasia.

RISK FACTORS

- Ingestion of hair, bone, or foreign material may contribute to constipation and subsequent dyschezia.
- Environmental factors such as a dirty litter pan or infrequent outside walks may contribute to constipation and subsequent dyschezia.

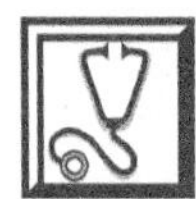

DIAGNOSIS

It is pivotal to recognize that hematochezia in animals can be seen with both diffuse colitis as well as with focal or discrete colorectal neoplasms. The fundamental differences in the clinical presentation between the two disorders can usually be recognized during the history and following a thorough physical examination, including a rectal examination. Dogs with colorectal neoplasms do not have diarrhea, and the most important and frequent clinical sign is hematochezia in the absence of an increase in defecation frequency or change in stool consistency. Pencil-thin or ribbon-like stools can be seen when the colorectal neoplasm is advanced, causing a change in the shape of the stool. *A rectal examination must be performed on every patient with a history of hematochezia or dyschezia.*

DIFFERENTIAL DIAGNOSIS

- Dysuria, stranguria, or hematuria—abnormal findings on urinalysis, such as pyuria, crystalluria, or bacteriuria. The history and physical examination should differentiate whether the animal is having difficulty urinating or defecating.
- Dystocia—differentiate with history and imaging.

CBC/BIOCHEMISTRY/URINALYSIS

- Usually unremarkable, unless there is a history of chronic blood loss with secondary iron deficiency causing a microcytic and hypochromic nonregenerative anemia.
- Mild neutrophilia (with or without a left shift) with infection or inflammation.

OTHER LABORATORY TESTS

Centrifugation fecal flotation to help rule out parasitic causes of colitis.

IMAGING

- Pelvic radiographs may reveal intrapelvic disease, foreign body, or fracture.
- Ultrasonography may demonstrate prostatic disease or caudal abdominal masses; however, a portion of the descending colon cannot be visualized because of the pelvis.

DIAGNOSTIC PROCEDURES

Colonoscopy/proctoscopy to evaluate for inflammatory or neoplastic disease.

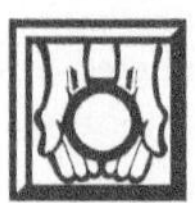

TREATMENT

- Depends on the underlying cause.
- Colonic strictures secondary to neoplasms can be managed via surgical excision or balloon catheter dilation.
- Consider laxatives (lactulose) to ease defecation and discomfort in animals with colorectal strictures or masses.
- Colorectal masses are best removed surgically or via endoscopy (snare and cauterization for polyps).

MEDICATIONS

DRUG(S) OF CHOICE

- Antibiotics—if bacterial infection (e.g., anal sac abscess); amoxicillin/clavulanic acid 15 mg/kg PO q12h for 7–10 days.
- Anti-inflammatory drugs—sulfasalazine or prednisone (dogs) and prednisolone (cats) if colitis is present (see Colitis and Proctitis; Colitis, Histiocytic Ulcerative).
- Cyclosporine (5 mg/kg q12h for 3–4 months with gradual taper thereafter) for dogs with perianal fistulae.
- Laxatives—lactulose 1 mL/4.5 kg PO q8–12h to effect; docusate sodium or docusate calcium: dogs: 50–100 mg PO q12–24h; cats: 50 mg PO q12–24h.
- Cisapride—prokinetic indicated for cats with moderate to severe megacolon (and no evidence of obstruction) in conjunction with lactulose and dietary therapy at a dose of 5 mg/cat q12h.

CONTRAINDICATIONS

Avoid agents that cause increased fecal bulk (insoluble fiber), unless specifically indicated (colitis).

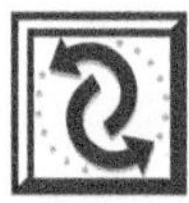

FOLLOW-UP

- The need for follow-up depends on the underlying cause. Dogs and cats that are undergoing balloon dilation of colorectal strictures usually require multiple procedures to manage the stricture properly. Animals should always be rechecked at suture removal or 10–14 days following surgical resection of colorectal masses.

- Animals with hematochezia secondary to colitis should have a marked improvement or resolution of their clinical signs within 5–7 days following implementation of elimination dietary therapy.

PATIENT MONITORING

Daily monitoring by the owner with periodic phone calls to the clinician every 2–3 weeks during the beginning of treatment.

POSSIBLE COMPLICATIONS

- May see fecal incontinence following surgical resection of anal sacs or colorectal tumors if anal sphincter is compromised.
- Secondary megacolon may occur if obstipation is severe and long term.

MISCELLANEOUS

ASSOCIATED CONDITIONS

N/A

PREGNANCY/FERTILITY/BREEDING

Caution with corticosteroids, antibiotics.

SEE ALSO

- Colitis and Proctitis.
- Constipation and Obstipation.

Suggested Reading

Adamovich-Rippe KN, Mayhew PD, Marks SL, et al. Colonoscopic and histologic features of rectal masses in dogs: 82 cases (1995–2012). J Am Vet Med Assoc 2017, 250(4):424–430.

Webb CB. Anal-rectal disease. In: Bonagura JD, Twedt DC, eds., Current Veterinary Therapy XIV. St. Louis, MO: Elsevier, 2009, pp. 527–531.

Zoran DL. Rectoanal disease. In: Ettinger SJ, Feldman EC, eds., Textbook of Veterinary Internal Medicine, 6th ed. St. Louis, MO: Elsevier, 2005, pp. 1408–1420.

Author Stanley L. Marks

Consulting Editor Mark P. Rondeau

DYSPHAGIA

BASICS

DEFINITION

- Dysphagia refers to difficulty in swallowing and is far more commonly seen in dogs than cats.
- Dysphagia is divided into three main categories—oropharyngeal, esophageal, and gastroesophageal causes.
- Oropharyngeal causes of dysphagia can be further subcategorized into oral, pharyngeal, or cricopharyngeal.
- Any disorder causing difficulty with prehension or mastication can cause dysphagia.
- Odynophagia refers to painful swallowing and is most commonly seen in association with pharyngitis, pharyngeal foreign bodies, esophageal foreign bodies, or severe esophagitis.
- Esophageal dysphagia is discussed in Megaesophagus and in Regurgitation.

PATHOPHYSIOLOGY

- The *oral preparatory phase* is voluntary and begins as food or liquid enters the mouth. Mastication and lubrication of food are the hallmarks of this phase. Abnormalities of the oral preparatory phase usually are associated with dental disease, xerostomia, weakness of the lips (cranial nerves [CN] V and VII), tongue (CN XII), and cheeks (CN V and VII).
- The *oral phase* of swallowing consists of the muscular events responsible for movement of the bolus from the tongue to the pharynx and is facilitated by tongue, jaw, and hyoid muscle movements.
- The *pharyngeal phase* begins as the bolus reaches the tonsils and is characterized by elevation of the soft palate to prevent the bolus from entering the nasopharynx, elevation and forward movement of the larynx and hyoid, retroflexion of the epiglottis and closure of the vocal folds to close the entrance into the larynx, contraction of the muscles of the pharynx, and relaxation of the cricopharyngeus muscle that makes up much of the proximal esophageal sphincter (PES) to allow passage of the bolus into the esophagus. Respiration is briefly halted (apneic moment) during the pharyngeal phase.
- Abnormalities of the pharyngeal phase of swallowing are associated with pharyngeal weakness secondary to neuropathies or myopathies, pharyngeal tumors or foreign bodies, or cricopharyngeus muscle disorders.
- The *esophageal phase* is involuntary and begins with relaxation of the PES and movement of the bolus into the esophagus.

SYSTEMS AFFECTED

- Gastrointestinal.
- Nervous.
- Neuromuscular.
- Respiratory.

GENETICS

Breeds that have a hereditary predisposition or high incidence of dysphagia include golden retriever (pharyngeal weakness, cricopharyngeal muscle dysfunction), cocker and springer spaniels (cricopharyngeal muscle dysfunction), Bouvier des Flandres and cavalier King Charles spaniel (muscular dystrophy), and boxer (inflammatory myopathy). In addition, large and giant-breed dogs are predisposed to acquired megaesophagus.

INCIDENCE/PREVALENCE

Variable depending on underlying etiology. Megaesophagus one of the most common causes of dysphagia in dogs.

GEOGRAPHIC DISTRIBUTION

None

SIGNALMENT

- Dog and cat.
- Congenital disorders that cause dysphagia (e.g., cricopharyngeal muscle achalasia, cleft palate, hiatal hernia) usually diagnosed in animals <1 year old.
- Acquired esophageal dysmotility and pharyngeal weakness more common in older patients.

SIGNS

Historical Findings

- Drooling (due to pain or inability to swallow saliva), gagging, ravenous appetite, repeated or exaggerated attempts at swallowing, swallowing with head in abnormal position, nasal discharge (due to nasal reflux of food and liquids into nasopharynx), coughing (due to aspiration), regurgitation, painful swallowing, and occasionally anorexia and weight loss. If tongue is not functioning normally, problems with prehension and mastication may be seen.
- Ascertain onset and progression. Foreign bodies cause acute dysphagia; pharyngeal dysphagia may be chronic and insidious in onset.

Physical Examination Findings

- Physical examination must include careful examination of oropharynx using sedation or anesthesia if necessary to help rule out morphologic abnormalities such as dental disease, foreign bodies, cleft palate, glossal abnormalities, and oropharyngeal tumors.
- Evaluation of cranial nerves should be performed, including assessment of tongue and jaw tone, and of laryngeal function.
- Complete physical and neurologic examination may identify clinical signs supporting generalized neuromuscular disorder, including muscle atrophy, stiffness, or decreased or absent spinal reflexes.
- Evaluate gag reflex by placing a finger in the pharynx; however, presence or absence of gag reflex does not correlate with efficacy of pharyngeal swallow nor adequacy of deglutitive airway protection.
- The importance of the clinician's carefully observing the dysphagic animal while eating (kibble and canned food) and drinking in hospital (or at home via video) is pivotal, and such observation helps localize the problem to oral cavity, pharynx, or esophagus.

Oral Dysphagia

- Modified eating behavior (e.g., eating with head tilted to one side or having difficulty prehending the bolus or opening the mouth).
- Tongue paralysis or dystrophy, dental disease, masticatory muscle myositis, temporal muscle atrophy, or pain, and food packed in buccal folds suggest oral dysphagia.

Pharyngeal Dysphagia

- Prehension of food is normal.
- Repeated attempts at swallowing with food falling out of mouth and excessive gagging suggest pharyngeal dysphagia.
- Saliva-coated food retained in buccal folds, diminished gag reflex, and nasal discharge may also exist.

Cricopharyngeal Muscle Dysfunction

- Patients make repeated, nonproductive efforts to swallow, gag, and cough, then forcibly regurgitate immediately after swallowing.
- Gag reflex and prehension are normal.
- Nasal reflux commonly observed when food hits closed PES.
- Coughing commonly observed secondary to aspiration pneumonia.

Esophageal Dysphagia

- Most common causes include megaesophagus, esophagitis, esophageal stricture, esophageal foreign bodies, and esophageal dysmotility.
- Diagnosis made with survey radiographs of thorax and neck followed by videofluoroscopic swallow assessment.

Gastroesophageal Dysphagia

Most common cause is sliding hiatal hernia in brachycephalic breeds, often associated with gastroesophageal reflux and subsequent esophagitis.

CAUSES

- Anatomic or mechanical lesions include pharyngeal inflammation (e.g., abscess, inflammatory polyps, oral eosinophilic granuloma), neoplasia, pharyngeal and retropharyngeal foreign body, sialocele, temporomandibular joint disorders (e.g., luxation, fracture, craniomandibular osteopathy), mandibular fracture, cleft or congenitally short palate, cricopharyngeal muscle achalasia, lingual frenulum disorder, pharyngeal trauma.
- Pain as result of dental disease (e.g., tooth fractures and abscess), mandibular trauma, stomatitis, glossitis, and pharyngeal inflammation may disrupt normal prehension,

bolus formation, and swallowing. Stomatitis, glossitis, and pharyngitis may be secondary to feline viral rhinotracheitis, feline leukemia virus (FeLV)/feline immunodeficiency virus (FIV), pemphigus, systemic lupus erythematosus (SLE), uremia, and ingestion of caustic agents or foreign bodies.

- Neuromuscular disorders that impair prehension and bolus formation include CN deficits (e.g., idiopathic trigeminal neuropathy CN V, lingual paralysis CN XII) and masticatory muscle myositis.
- Pharyngeal weakness, paresis, or paralysis can be caused by infectious polymyositis (e.g., toxoplasmosis and neosporosis), immune-mediated polymyositis, muscular dystrophy, polyneuropathies, and myoneural junction disorders (e.g., myasthenia gravis, tick bite paralysis, botulism).
- Other CNS disorders, especially those involving the brainstem.
- Rabies can cause dysphagia by affecting both brainstem and peripheral nerves.

RISK FACTORS

Many causative neuromuscular conditions have breed predispositions.

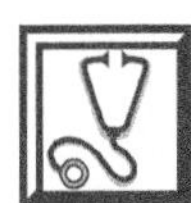

DIAGNOSIS

DIFFERENTIAL DIAGNOSIS

- Differentiate vomiting from regurgitation.
- Vomiting is typically associated with abdominal contractions; dysphagia is not.

CBC/BIOCHEMISTRY/URINALYSIS

- Inflammatory conditions often cause a leukocytosis, sometimes with a left shift.
- High serum creatine kinase activity is usually suggestive of a myopathy.
- May find evidence of renal disease (e.g., azotemia and low urine concentration) in patients with oral and lingual ulcers secondary to uremia.

OTHER LABORATORY TESTS

- Type 2M muscle antibody serology (masticatory muscle myositis).
- Acetylcholine receptor antibody serology (acquired myasthenia gravis).
- Antinuclear antibody serology (immune-mediated diseases).
- T_4, free T_4, thyroid-stimulating hormone (TSH), anti-thyroglobulin antibodies to rule out hypothyroidism.
- Resting cortisol and/or adrenocorticotropic hormone (ACTH) stimulation test to rule out Addison's disease.

IMAGING

- Obtain survey radiographs of thorax (3-views) and neck in all dysphagic animals for which oral cause of dysphagia has been ruled out.
- Ultrasonography of pharynx may be useful in patients with mass lesions and for obtaining ultrasound-guided biopsy specimens.
- Fluoroscopy with barium is useful in evaluating pharyngeal and esophageal motility as well as proper coordination of upper and lower esophageal sphincters.
- CT and/or MRI for suspected intracranial mass.
- Esophagram (liquid barium administered orally followed by immediate survey radiographs of the thorax) is helpful for diagnosing radiolucent esophageal foreign bodies and esophageal strictures, but is insensitive for diagnosing esophageal functional disorders.

DIAGNOSTIC PROCEDURES

- Endoscopy of nasopharynx—retroflexion of endoscope over soft palate to look for foreign bodies and evaluate esophagus and lower esophageal sphincter.
- Electromyography of skeletal musculature to confirm presence of myopathy.
- Repetitive nerve stimulation and edrophonium chloride (0.1–0.2 mg/kg IV) test for suspected myasthenia gravis.
- Cerebrospinal fluid analysis in patients with a CNS disorder.

PATHOLOGIC FINDINGS

Variable depending on underlying etiology. Myopathies can be inflammatory or dystrophic.

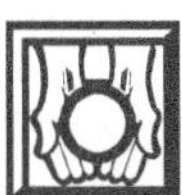

TREATMENT

APPROPRIATE HEALTH CARE

- Determine underlying cause to optimize therapy and outcome.
- Most patients can be managed on outpatient basis unless there are other complicating factors such as aspiration pneumonia, dehydration, or weakness.

NURSING CARE

- Supportive care may be necessary if patient is dehydrated (IV fluids).
- Other supportive modalities may be necessary in case of aspiration pneumonia (oxygen, coupage, etc.).
- For patients with generalized weakness due to myopathies, good nursing care is required, such as rotating position, good padding, and physical therapy.

ACTIVITY

Alterations in activity should be based on underlying etiology.

DIET

- Nutritional support is important for all dysphagic patients, and consistency of diet should be altered to optimize swallowing in affected animals.
- Elevating head and neck during feeding and for 10–15 minutes after feeding may help patients with esophageal disease. Consider altering consistency of diet. Dogs with cricopharyngeal muscle dysfunction are able to handle kibble better than canned food or water.
- If nutritional requirements cannot be met orally, gastrostomy tube may be necessary.

CLIENT EDUCATION

- Variable dependent on underlying cause.
- Educate the client that not all diseases can be cured, but managed.
- Changes in feeding (see above) may be long term.
- Clients should be taught to monitor for signs of possible aspiration pneumonia (mucopurulent nasal discharge, increased respiratory rate at rest, coughing, dyspnea, tachypnea).

SURGICAL CONSIDERATIONS

- Cricopharyngeal myectomy (bilateral removal) may benefit patients with cricopharyngeal muscle dysfunction; correct diagnosis is essential using videofluoroscopy before surgery, and to rule out other myopathic or neuropathic causes of dysphagia.
- Hiatal hernia surgery generally involves left-sided gastropexy with esophageal hiatal plication and esophagopexy.

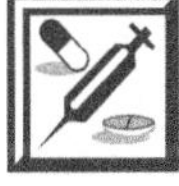

MEDICATIONS

DRUG(S) OF CHOICE

Dysphagia is not immediately life-threatening; direct drug therapy at the underlying cause.

PRECAUTIONS

- Use barium sulfate with caution in patients with evidence of aspiration.
- Use corticosteroids with caution or not at all in patients with evidence of, or at risk for, aspiration.

FOLLOW-UP

PATIENT MONITORING

- Daily for signs of aspiration pneumonia (e.g., lethargy, fever, mucopurulent nasal discharge, coughing, dyspnea).
- Body condition and hydration status daily; if oral nutrition does not meet requirements, use gastrostomy tube feeding.

POSSIBLE COMPLICATIONS

Aspiration pneumonia and malnutrition.

MISCELLANEOUS

ASSOCIATED CONDITIONS

- Aspiration pneumonia.
- Megaesophagus.
- Malnutrition.

AGE-RELATED FACTORS

- Puppies are more likely to have congenital abnormalities such as cricopharyngeal muscle achalasia, congenital megaesophagus, vascular ring anomalies, and cleft palates.
- Puppies with vascular ring anomalies will typically present with signs of regurgitation shortly after being weaned onto solid food at 6–8 weeks of age.
- Puppies with cleft palates usually have milk or food refluxing from the nasal passage during mastication and swallowing.
- Puppies with cricopharyngeal muscle achalasia typically present with repeated bouts of swallowing, gagging, and retching during swallowing with nasal reflux of water or food.
- Puppies are more likely to ingest foreign objects that can lodge in the esophagus and cause esophagitis and stricture formation.
- Older dogs, in particular Labrador retrievers, are more likely to have esophageal dysmotility secondary to a polyneuropathy (geriatric onset laryngeal paralysis polyneuropathy or GOLPP).

ZOONOTIC POTENTIAL

- Consider rabies in any patient with oropharyngeal dysphagia, especially if animal's rabies vaccination status is unknown or questionable or it has been exposed to a potentially rabid animal.
- If a dysphagic animal dies of rapidly progressive neurologic disease, submit the head to a qualified laboratory designated by the local or state health department for rabies examination.

SEE ALSO

- Megaesophagus.
- Pneumonia, Bacterial.
- Regurgitation.

ABBREVIATIONS

- ACTH = adrenocorticotropic hormone.
- CN = cranial nerve.
- FeLV = feline leukemia virus.
- FIV = feline immunodeficiency virus.
- GOLPP = geriatric onset laryngeal paralysis polyneuropathy.
- PES = proximal esophageal sphincter.
- SLE = systemic lupus erythematosus.
- TSH = thyroid-stimulating hormone.

Suggested Reading

Kook PH. Gastroesophageal reflux. In: Bonagura JD, Twedt DC, eds., Kirk's Current Veterinary Therapy XV. St Louis, MO: Elsevier Saunders, 2014, pp. 501–504.

Marks SL. Oropharyngeal dysphagia. In: Bonagura JD, Twedt DC, eds., Kirk's Current Veterinary Therapy XV. St Louis, MO: Elsevier Saunders, 2014, pp. 495–500.

Pollard RE, Marks SL, Cheney DM. Diagnostic outcome of contrast videofluoroscopic swallowing studies in 216 dysphagic dogs. Vet Radiol Ultrasound 2017, 58(4):373–380.

Warnock JJ, Marks SL, Pollard R, et al. Surgical management of cricopharyngeal dysphagia in dogs: 14 cases (1989–2001). J Am Vet Med Assoc 2003, 223(10):1462–1468.

Author Stanley L. Marks

Consulting Editor Mark P. Rondeau

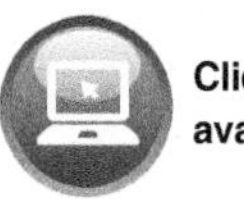

Client Education Handout available online

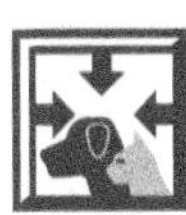

BASICS

DEFINITION

Dyspnea—a subjective term that in human medicine means "an uncomfortable sensation in breathing" or a sensation of air hunger; in veterinary medicine, it is used to indicate difficulty breathing or respiratory distress.

PATHOPHYSIOLOGY

Dyspnea and respiratory distress are believed to occur when the CNS notes a difference between the afferent feedback from a given efferent motor drive signal (ventilation demanded) and what the brain had anticipated would be the appropriate afferent response (ventilation achieved).

SYSTEMS AFFECTED

Respiratory

SIGNALMENT

Dogs and cats; age, breed, and sex predisposition vary with inciting cause.

SIGNS

Historical Findings

• Acute or chronic onset.
• Often associated with tachypnea, coughing, exercise intolerance, lethargy, inappetence.

Physical Examination Findings

• General signs of respiratory distress—tachypnea, increased abdominal effort, nasal flaring, open-mouth breathing, cyanosis, orthopnea (neck extension, elbow abduction), altered mentation; other signs depend on underlying cause.
• Nasal disease—stertor, nasal discharge, lack of airflow through nostrils; dyspnea improves with open-mouth breathing.
• Upper airway/laryngeal disease—stridor, panting, cough, hyperthermia, dysphonia, respiratory effort and noise on inspiration, fixed obstruction such as a mass or foreign body in a large airway: dyspnea on inspiration and expiration.
• Tracheal collapse—honking cough, tracheal sensitivity, respiratory effort and noise: inspiratory effort if cervical tracheal collapse, expiratory effort if intrathoracic tracheal collapse.
• Lower airway disease—cough, expiratory wheezes on auscultation, abdominal effort.
• Pulmonary parenchymal disease—may have crackles, harsh or moist lung sounds on auscultation.
• Pneumonia—fever, may have tracheal sensitivity.
• Cardiogenic pulmonary edema—heart murmur, arrhythmia, hypothermia, pale mucous membranes, prolonged capillary refill time.
• Pleural space disease—diminished breath sounds: ventrally—fluid; dorsally—air; unilaterally—space-occupying lesions or pyothorax/chylothorax. Paradoxical respiratory pattern (inward movement of the abdominal wall during inspiration).
• Thoracic wall disease—can have paradoxical respiratory pattern, visible or palpable trauma (open pneumothorax, flail chest).
• Pulmonary thromboembolism (PTE)—may have clinical signs of underlying disease predisposing to thrombosis, e.g., hyperadrenocorticism, immune-mediated hemolytic anemia (IMHA), systemic inflammatory response syndrome (SIRS)/sepsis, protein-losing nephropathy (PLN), protein-losing enteropathy (PLE), neoplasia.
• Other signs will pertain to the underlying disease, e.g., shock, trauma.

CAUSES & RISK FACTORS

Upper Airway Disease

• Nasal obstruction—stenotic nares, nasopharyngeal polyp or stenosis, infection, inflammation, neoplasia, trauma, foreign body, coagulopathy.
• Pharynx—elongated soft palate, foreign body, neoplasia, granuloma, stenosis.
• Larynx—laryngeal paralysis, everted laryngeal saccules, edema, collapse, foreign body, neoplasia, inflammation, trauma, webbing.
• Trachea—collapse, stenosis, trauma, foreign body, neoplasia, parasites, extraluminal compression (lymphadenopathy, enlarged left atrium, heart-base tumors).

Lower Airway Disease

Allergic disease, inflammatory, infectious (*Mycoplasma*), parasitic, neoplastic (bronchogenic carcinoma).

Pulmonary Parenchymal Disease

• Edema—cardiogenic or noncardiogenic.
• Pneumonia—infectious; parasitic; aspiration; eosinophilic; interstitial.
• Neoplasia (primary or metastatic).
• Inflammatory— acute respiratory distress syndrome (ARDS); uremic pneumonitis; smoke inhalation.
• Hemorrhage—trauma; coagulopathy.
• PTE—IMHA; PLN, PLE; heartworm disease; hyperadrenocorticism; neoplasia.
• Others—lung lobe torsion, atelectasis.

Pleural Space Disease

• Pneumothorax—traumatic; iatrogenic; secondary to pulmonary parenchymal disease; ruptured bulla; migrating foreign body; primary spontaneous (no underlying cause).
• Pleural effusion—transudates, exudates; hemothorax; chylothorax.
• Soft tissue—neoplasia; diaphragmatic hernia.
• Fibrosing pleuritis.

Thoracic Wall Disease

• Open pneumothorax—trauma.
• Flail segment—trauma.
• Neoplasia.
• Paralysis due to cervical spinal disease, botulism, polyradiculoneuritis, tick bite paralysis, myasthenia gravis, elapid snake envenomation, hypokalemia.

Diaphragmatic Disease

• Trauma—rupture; hernia.
• Phrenic nerve disease.
• Neoplasia.
• Fibrosis.

Abdominal Distention

Organomegaly—hyperplasia; neoplasia, pregnancy; obesity; ascites; gastric dilatation, torsion.

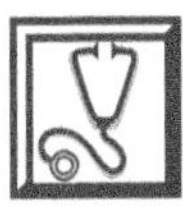

DIAGNOSIS

DIFFERENTIAL DIAGNOSIS

• Inspiratory dyspnea—suggests extrathoracic upper airway disease.
• Expiratory dyspnea—suggests intrathoracic airway disease.
• Dyspnea on inspiration and expiration can occur with fixed upper airway obstructions and severe intrathoracic disease.
• Congestive heart failure—murmur, arrhythmia, tachycardia, poor pulse quality, jugular pulses, hypothermia, crackles on auscultation, fluid dripping from nose.

CBC/BIOCHEMISTRY/URINALYSIS

• Anemia—can cause nonrespiratory dyspnea.
• Polycythemia—chronic hypoxia.
• Inflammatory leukogram—pneumonia, pneumonitis, pyothorax.
• Eosinophilia—hypersensitivity or parasitic airway disease.
• Thrombocytosis—hyperadrenocorticism predisposes to PTE.
• Sodium : potassium ratio <27—can be seen with pleural or abdominal effusions.
• Azotemia—if severe may lead to uremic pneumonitis.
• Proteinuria—can predispose to PTE.
• Multiple organ dysfunction—ARDS.
• Hypoproteinemia—may suggest protein-losing disease that can predispose to PTE or pleural effusion.

OTHER LABORATORY TESTS

• Pleural fluid analysis.
• Fecal examination for parasites if indicated
• Serum antigen or antibody titers—heartworm, toxoplasmosis, distemper, feline leukemia virus (FeLV), feline immunodeficiency virus (FIV).
• Increased urine protein : creatinine ratio with PLN could indicate loss of antithrombin and hypercoagulability resulting in PTE.
• PaO_2—partial pressure of oxygen dissolved in arterial blood; normoxemia: PaO_2 80–120 mmHg (room air, sea level); hypoxemia: PaO_2 <80 mmHg; FIO_2—fraction of inspired oxygen ranges from 0.21 (room air) to 1.0; PaO_2/FIO_2 ratio—measure

of lung efficiency during oxygen therapy; PaO_2/FIO_2 ≥400—normal lung efficiency; 300–400—mild insufficiency; 200–300—moderate insufficiency; <200—severe insufficiency. Reduction in lung efficiency can be due to venous admixture, hypoventilation, low inspired oxygen.

- $PaCO_2$ or $PvCO_2$—partial pressure of CO_2 dissolved in arterial or venous blood; measure of ventilation; normal 30 mmHg $< PCO_2 <$ 40 mmHg. $PCO_2 >$ 45 mmHg = hypercapnia = hypoventilation = decreased alveolar minute ventilation (MV).
- Coagulation testing—if suspect hemothorax and/or pulmonary hemorrhage.
- Plasma NT-proBNP and cardiac troponin-I (cTNI) concentrations may aid in differentiation of cardiac and noncardiac causes of dyspnea.

IMAGING

- Cervical and thoracic radiography—upper airway disease: soft palate elongation, large airway narrowing, lymphadenopathy, intraluminal abnormalities. Lower airway disease: bronchial thickening, middle lung lobe consolidation (cats), atelectasis, hyperinflation, and diaphragmatic flattening (primarily cats). Pneumonia: alveolar infiltrates; aspiration pneumonia usually cranioventral distribution or middle lobe affected. Cardiogenic pulmonary edema: enlarged cardiac silhouette, pulmonary venous distention, enlarged left atrium with perihilar pulmonary infiltrates in dogs; infiltrates can be of any distribution in cats. Noncardiogenic pulmonary edema: usually caudodorsal distribution. ARDS: diffuse, symmetric alveolar infiltrates. Pulmonary vascular abnormalities: PTE, heartworm disease. Pleural space disease: pneumothorax, pleural effusion, mass lesions, diaphragmatic hernias. Thoracic wall disease: rib fractures, neoplasia.
- Thoracic ultrasonography—evaluation of distribution of pleural effusion, pneumothorax (absence of "glide sign"), and parenchymal disease (presence of "comet tail" artifact). Pulmonary mass identification: guide fine-needle aspiration; mediastinal evaluation.
- Echocardiography—evaluate cardiac function and chamber size if cardiogenic pulmonary edema or pleural effusion suspected; elevated pulmonary artery pressure, right ventricular overload with ventricular septal flattening can support diagnosis of PTE; visualize heart-based masses.
- Abdominal radiography or ultrasound—evaluation of abdominal distention.
- Fluoroscopy—evaluate tracheal and bronchial collapse; evaluate diaphragmatic function.
- CT—airway, pulmonary parenchymal, and pleural space disease can be evaluated; can detect lesions not clearly defined on radiographs.
- Pulmonary vascular angiography—gold standard for diagnosis of PTE.
- Ventilation perfusion scintigraphy—abnormal perfusion scan is considered supportive of PTE.

DIAGNOSTIC PROCEDURES

- Pulse oximetry—SpO_2; peripheral capillary hemoglobin oxygen saturation. The relationship between PaO_2 and SpO_2 is defined by the oxygen hemoglobin dissociation curve: PaO_2 of 60 mmHg = SpO_2 of 90%; PaO_2 of 80 mmHg = SpO_2 of 95%; PaO_2 of >100 mmHg = SpO_2 of 100%. Below 95%, small changes in SpO_2 signify large changes in PaO_2. SpO_2 measurements in animals on high inspired oxygen lack sensitivity.
- Thoracentesis—fluid analysis and culture.
- Laryngoscopy/nasopharyngoscopy/tracheoscopy—evaluate upper airway; laryngeal paralysis, tracheal collapse, foreign bodies, masses.
- Bronchoscopy—evaluate upper and lower airways; perform bronchoalveolar lavage for cytology and culture. Requires anesthesia, perform only when stabilized.

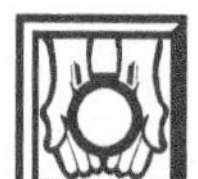

TREATMENT

APPROPRIATE HEALTH CARE

- Inpatient care until the cause is identified and treated or determined not to be life-threatening; therapy dependent on underlying cause.
- *Always* administer oxygen and keep patient in sternal recumbency until ability to oxygenate is determined.
- May require intubation and positive-pressure ventilation in patients with severe respiratory distress refractory to oxygen therapy.
- Upper airway disease—use sedation to reduce respiratory effort. Check body temperature and actively cool patients as needed.
- Lower airway disease—bronchodilators; systemic corticosteroids may be required to stabilize cats with acute bronchoconstriction.
- Pulmonary parenchymal disease—antibiotics if pneumonia; treat coagulation disorders; cardiogenic edema requires furosemide ± vasodilators. Noncardiogenic edema requires oxygen therapy, may require positive-pressure ventilation.
- Pleural space disease—thoracocentesis for air and fluid. Place a chest tube if repeated thoracocentesis is necessary to keep patient stable.
- Thoracic wall disease—surgery as indicated, particularly if open chest wound is present; flail chest may require surgery if medical management fails or there is a severe displacement of fractures. Thoracic wall paralysis/muscle fatigue: positive-pressure ventilation if severely hypercapnic.
- Abdominal distention—drain ascites as needed; relieve gastric distention.

NURSING CARE

- Oxygen therapy via cage, nasal cannula, Elizabethan collar covered in plastic wrap, mask, or flow-by. Humidify oxygen source if giving oxygen therapy for more than a few hours.
- Maintain in sternal recumbency and turn hips every 3–4 hours if patient cannot tolerate lateral recumbency.
- Monitor temperature regularly, as excess work of breathing results in hyperthermia, which augments respiratory distress.

DIET

Weight-reducing diet if obesity is a contributing cause.

SURGICAL CONSIDERATIONS

- Anesthesia must be carefully tailored to the patient. Securing an airway is essential and rapid intravenous induction is important. The ability to positive-pressure ventilate patients is often required.
- Animals with upper airway obstruction are fragile and can rapidly decompensate. Have multiple-sized endotracheal tubes available.
- Dyspnea associated with a laryngeal mass can respond to debulking surgery, but edema and hemorrhage can lead to worsened obstruction. Warn owners of increased likelihood of aspiration pneumonia complications in animals with laryngeal disease.
- Avoid positive-pressure ventilation in patients with a closed pneumothorax. Must monitor oxygenation status of anesthetized patients with pulse oximetry and when possible arterial blood gases.

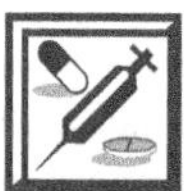

MEDICATIONS

DRUG(S) OF CHOICE

Varies with underlying cause (see Appropriate Health Care).

FOLLOW-UP

PATIENT MONITORING

- Patients receiving oxygen therapy can be monitored by assessing the degree of respiratory effort. As the animal stabilizes, perform a room air trial and reevaluate the level of respiratory difficulty. Arterial and venous blood gases can be a useful assessment.
- Pulse oximetry is an effective and noninvasive tool for monitoring patients on room air.
- Repeat radiographs are often indicated in assessing pulmonary parenchymal disease and pleural space disease.

MISCELLANEOUS

SEE ALSO

- Acute Respiratory Distress Syndrome.
- Asthma, Bronchitis—Cats.
- Brachycephalic Airway Syndrome.
- Congestive Heart Failure, Left-Sided.
- Congestive Heart Failure, Right-Sided.
- Laryngeal Diseases.
- Panting and Tachypnea.
- Pneumonia, Aspiration.
- Pneumothorax.
- Pulmonary Edema, Noncardiogenic.

ABBREVIATIONS

- ARDS = acute respiratory distress syndrome.
- cTNI = cardiac troponin-I.
- FeLV = feline leukemia virus.
- FIO_2 = fraction of inspired oxygen.
- FIV = feline immunodeficiency virus.
- IMHA = immune-mediated hemolytic anemia.
- MV = minute ventilation.
- $PaCO_2$ = partial pressure of carbon dioxide.
- PaO_2 = partial pressure of oxygen.
- PLE = protein-losing enteropathy.
- PLN = protein-losing nephropathy.
- PTE = pulmonary thromboembolism.
- SIRS = systemic inflammatory response syndrome.
- SpO_2 = oxygen saturation.

Suggested Reading

Herndon WE, Rishniw M, Schrope D, et al. Assessment of plasma cardiac troponin I concentration as a means to differentiate cardiac and noncardiac causes of dyspnea in cats. JAVMA 2008, 233:1261–1264.

Mellema MS. The neurophysiology of dyspnea. J Vet Emerg Crit Care 2008, 18:561–571.

Rozanski E. Respiratory distress. In: Drobatz KJ, Hopper K, Rozanski EA, et al. Textbook of Small Animal Emergency Medicine. Hoboken, NJ: Wiley, 2018, pp. 18–21.

Smith KF, Quinn RL, Rahilly LJ. Biomarkers for differentiation of causes of respiratory distress in dogs and cats: Part 1 – Cardiac disease and pulmonary hypertension. J Vet Emerg Crit Care 2015, 25(3):311–329.

Author Yu Ueda

Consulting Editor Elizabeth Rozanski

Acknowledgement The author and book editors acknowledge the prior contribution of Kate Hopper.

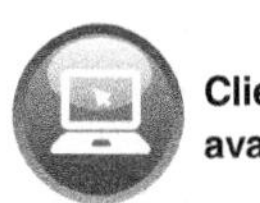

Client Education Handout available online

D

DYSTOCIA

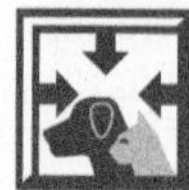

BASICS

DEFINITION

Difficult birth.

PATHOPHYSIOLOGY

- Dystocia may occur due to maternal or fetal factors and may occur during any stage of labor.
- May be caused by abnormal fetal presentation, posture, or position.
- Normal stages of labor:

Stage 1

- Onset of uterine contractions and relaxation of cervix; ends with rupture of first chorioallantoic sac—averages 6–12h (up to 36h in primiparous bitch).
- Bitch—may be restless, nervous, shiver, pant, pace, and nest.
- Queen—tend to vocalize initially; purr and socialize as Stage 1 progresses.

Stage 2

- Delivery of fetuses.
- Bitch—obvious abdominal contractions; beginning of stage 2 to delivery of first offspring usually <4h; average time to delivery of subsequent fetus 20–60 min (may be as long as 2–3h).
- Queen—average length of parturition 16h, with range of 4–42h (up to 3 days in some cases); important to consider this variability when intervening.
- Number of fetuses present may significantly affect length of stages 2 and 3.

Stage 3

- Delivery of fetal membranes.
- May alternate between stage 2 and 3 with multiple fetuses.

INCIDENCE/PREVALENCE

- Dog—incidence unknown due to breed variability and breeder intervention.
- Cat—3.3–5.8% of parturitions; mixed-breed cats 0.4%, higher in pedigree cats, to 18.2% in Devon Rex.

SIGNALMENT

Breed Predilections

Dogs

- Higher incidence with miniature and small breeds (small litter size, concurrent large fetal size); may occur in large breeds with large or singleton litters.
- Brachycephalic breeds—broad head and narrow pelvis.
- Large fetal head : maternal pelvis ratio—Sealyham terrier, Scottish terrier.
- Uterine inertia—Scottish terrier, dachshund, border terrier, Aberdeen terrier, Labrador retriever.
- Other breeds with increased incidence of dystocia—chihuahua, dachshund, Pekingese, Yorkshire terrier, miniature poodle, Pomeranian.

Cats

Brachycephalic (Persian, Himalayan) or dolichocephalic (Devon Rex) breeds.

SIGNS

Historical Findings

- More than 30 min of persistent, strong, abdominal contractions without fetal delivery.
- More than 4h from onset of stage 2 to delivery of first fetus (bitch).
- More than 2h between delivery of fetuses (bitch).
- Failure to commence stage 1 labor within 24h of rectal temperature drop below 37.2 °C (99 °F) or within 36h of serum progesterone concentration <2 ng/mL (bitch).
- Female cries, displays signs of pain, and constantly licks vulvar area when contracting.
- Prolonged gestation—more than 72 days from day of first mating (bitch); more than 59 days from first day of cytologic diestrus (bitch); more than 66 days from luteinizing hormone (LH) peak (bitch); more than 68 days from last day of mating (queen).

Physical Examination Findings

- Presence of greenish-black discharge (uteroverdin) preceding birth of first fetus by more than 2h or increasing amounts before delivery of first fetus.
- Bloody discharge prior to delivery of first fetus.
- Diminished or absent Ferguson's reflex (stimulation or pressure to dorsal vaginal wall to elicit abdominal straining: "feathering") indicates uterine inertia.

CAUSES

Fetal

- Oversize; fetal monsters, fetal anasarca, fetal hydrocephalus, prolonged gestation due to inability of singleton fetus to initiate labor.
- Abnormal presentation, position, or posture of fetus in birth canal.
- Fetal death.

Maternal

- Inadequate uterine contractions (primary or secondary uterine inertia)—myometrial defect, hypocalcemia electrolyte imbalance, psychogenic disturbance, exhaustion.
- Ineffective abdominal press—pain, fear, debility (exhaustion), diaphragmatic hernia, age.
- Placentitis, metritis, endometritis.
- Pregnancy toxemia, gestational diabetes.
- Abnormal pelvic canal—previous pelvic injury, abnormal conformation, pelvic immaturity.
- Congenitally small pelvis—Welsh corgis, brachycephalic breeds.
- Inguinal hernia.
- Abnormality of vaginal vault—stricture, septae, vaginal hyperplasia, hypoplastic vagina, intra- or extraluminal cysts, neoplasia.
- Abnormal vulvar opening—stricture, fibrosis from trauma, neoplasia.
- Insufficient cervical dilation.
- Lack of adequate lubrication.
- Uterine torsion.
- Uterine rupture.
- Uterine neoplasia, cysts, or adhesions.

RISK FACTORS

- Age.
- Brachycephalic and toy breeds.
- Persian, Himalayan, and Devon Rex breeds.
- Obesity.
- Abrupt changes in peripartum environment.
- Previous history of dystocia.

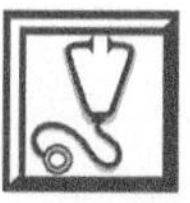

DIAGNOSIS

DIFFERENTIAL DIAGNOSIS

Uterine inertia—hypocalcemia versus hypoglycemia.

Physical Examination

- Complete physical examination—careful abdominal palpation to confirm presence of fetuses.
- Digital vaginal examination—fetus or fetal membranes in vaginal canal, assess maternal pelvic canal, Ferguson's reflex.
- Bitch unresponsive to oxytocin or lacking Ferguson's reflex—uterine inertia more likely than obstructive dystocia unless obstructed for several hours.

CBC/BIOCHEMISTRY/URINALYSIS

Minimum database—packed cell volume (PCV), total protein, serum glucose, urea nitrogen, and calcium (ionized preferable to total concentration corrected for albumin) concentrations. Pregnant females have mild anemia.

OTHER LABORATORY TESTS

Serum progesterone concentration.

IMAGING

- Radiography—determine pelvic conformation, number and position of fetuses, evidence of fetal obstruction, oversize, or death.
- Fetal death—collapse of fetal skeletons, abnormal association of fetal bones to axial skeleton, presence of air/gas surrounding fetus, fetal balling.
- Ultrasonography—recommended for monitoring fetal viability, heart rate (fetal heart rate <180 bpm indicates fetal stress, >260 bpm indicates need for close monitoring), placental separation, and character of fetal fluids (presence of meconium or blood in amniotic fluid).

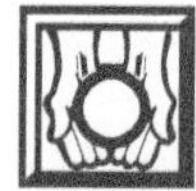

TREATMENT

APPROPRIATE HEALTH CARE

- Inpatient—until delivery of all fetuses and dam is stable.
- Treat hypoglycemia and hypocalcemia.
- Uterine inertia—medical treatment if no evidence of fetal stress.

• Ecbolic agents contraindicated with possible obstructive dystocia—may accelerate placental separation and fetal death or cause uterine rupture.
• WhelpWise® tocodynamometer monitors fetal heart rates and uterine contraction patterns; useful for bitches with large litters or history of uterine inertia to determine need for intervention.

Manual Delivery

Fetus lodged in vaginal vault:
• Lubricate liberally.
• Digital manipulation—least amount of damage to fetus and dam. Apply traction in postero-ventral direction.
• Instrument delivery not recommended due to inadequate space—may mutilate fetus or lacerate dam.
• Never apply traction to distal extremities or tail of a live fetus.
• Failure to deliver fetus located in vaginal canal within 30 min—Cesarean section (C-section) indicated.

SURGICAL CONSIDERATIONS

• Indications for C-section—uterine inertia unresponsive to oxytocin or uterine inertia with more than four fetuses remaining in utero (maximizes fetal survivability), pelvic or vaginal obstruction, inability to correct fetal malposition, fetal oversize, fetal stress, in utero fetal death.
• Elective C-section—breeds prone to dystocia, bitches with a history of dystocia, bitches with singleton or large litter size, performed to maximize fetal survivability.

General Comments

• Provide fluid therapy with balanced electrolyte solution before, during, and after surgery.
• Gravid uterus can compress great vessels and place pressure on diaphragm, compromising venous return and tidal volume.
• Preoxygenation of patient before anesthesia is indicated.
• Anesthetic protocol for C-section:
  ○ Premedication can include glycopyrrolate (bitches, queens: 0.01 mg/kg IV/IM) if fetal heart rates are normal; or atropine (bitches, queens: 0.04 mg/kg IM) if fetal bradycardia present.
  ○ Alpha-2 agonist agents (xylazine, dexmedetomidine) are contraindicated.
  ○ Rapidly acting induction agents include propofol or alfaxalone; ketamine may cause dose-dependent neonatal respiratory and neurologic depression; severely depressed or exhausted patients may be induced with combination of opioid and benzodiazepine with supplemental propofol or alfaxalone for intubation, if needed.
  ○ Maintenance may include inhalant anesthetics or propofol IV CRI.
  ○ Use of a midline lidocaine line block (1–2 mg/kg SC) can decrease inhalant anesthetic requirement.
• Epidural—0.5% bupivacaine (0.2 mg/kg) and preservative-free morphine (0.1 mg/kg) or 2% lidocaine (2–4 mg/kg).
• Postoperative analgesia may be provided with opioids, although they are excreted in the milk to varying degrees.
• Reversal agents—repeated dosing may be necessary until neonate has processed all anesthetic drugs:
  ○ Opioids used during anesthesia can be reversed in neonate with naloxone (0.04 mg/kg IV/IM/SC/sublingual/intranasal).
  ○ Benzodiazepines used during anesthesia can be reversed in neonate with flumazenil (0.01 mg/kg IV/IM/SC/sublingual/intranasal).

MEDICATIONS

DRUG(S) OF CHOICE

• Hypoglycemia—treat prior to hypocalcemia:
  ○ Bolus 0.5 g/kg IV (diluted 1 : 3).
  ○ Add 5% dextrose to balanced electrolyte solution and infuse IV at 60–80 mL/kg/day.
• Hypocalcemia:
  ○ Bitch—10% calcium gluconate 0.2 mL/kg IV over 10 min; monitor for bradycardia. Repeat q4–6h as needed.
  ○ May also be given SC at a dose of 0.5 mL/4.5 kg diluted 1:1 with sterile saline. If using 23% solution, dilute at least 1:3 prior to administration.
  ○ Queen—10% calcium gluconate 0.5–1.0 mL/cat IV over 10 min—use with caution; risk of uterine rupture increased due to strong uterine contractions following calcium.
• Oxytocin—once calcium and glucose deficits are treated: microdose at 0.5–3.0 IU IM/SC depending on size of bitch and response to treatment. May repeat q30 min as long as delivery progresses. Consider C-section if more than three doses of oxytocin per fetus are required or more than four fetuses remain.

CONTRAINDICATIONS

Oxytocin—contraindicated with obstructive dystocia, fetal stress, longstanding in utero fetal death, uterine rupture, uterine torsion.

FOLLOW-UP

PREVENTION/AVOIDANCE

• Schedule elective C-section for bitches with abnormal pelvic canal, anatomic abnormalities, predisposition to dystocia, previous history of uterine inertia.
• Scheduling surgery—extremely important that D1 diestrus, LH peak, or ovulation is identified during breeding to ensure acceptable fetal survivability. If ovulation timing is not available, ultrasonographic gestational aging and maturation assessment is necessary.

EXPECTED COURSE AND PROGNOSIS

• If dystocia is identified promptly and intervention is successful—good to fair for survival of dam; fair for fetuses.
• If dystocia unrecognized or untreated for 24–48h—poor to guarded for life of dam; fetal survival unlikely.

MISCELLANEOUS

PREGNANCY/FERTILITY/BREEDING

Dystocia may or may not impact future fertility, but may recur depending on cause. Resolution of dystocia by C-section does not preclude natural whelping for future deliveries.

SEE ALSO

• Breeding, Timing.
• Uterine Inertia.
• Vaginal Malformations and Acquired Lesions.

ABBREVIATIONS

• C-section = Cesarean section.
• LH = luteinizing hormone.
• PCV = packed cell volume.

Suggested Reading

Johnston SD, Root Kustritz MV, Olson PNS. Canine parturition; Feline parturition. In: Canine and Feline Theriogenology. Philadelphia, PA: Saunders, 2001, pp. 105–128, 431–437.

Author Cheryl Lopate
Consulting Editor Erin E. Runcan

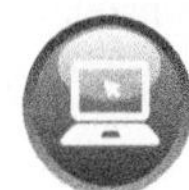

Client Education Handout available online

DYSURIA, POLLAKIURIA, AND STRANGURIA

D

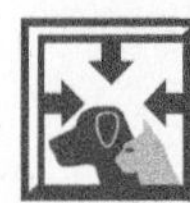

BASICS

DEFINITION

- Dysuria—difficult or painful urination.
- Pollakiuria—voiding small quantities of urine with increased frequency.
- Stranguria—straining to urinate.

PATHOPHYSIOLOGY

The urinary bladder and urethra normally serve as a reservoir for urine. Inflammatory and noninflammatory disorders of the lower urinary tract including the urethral orifice may decrease bladder compliance and storage capacity by damaging structural components of the bladder wall or by stimulating sensory nerve endings located in the bladder or urethra. Sensations of bladder fullness, urgency, and pain stimulate premature micturition and reduce functional bladder capacity. Dysuria and pollakiuria are caused by lesions of the urinary bladder and/or urethra and provide unequivocal evidence of lower urinary tract disease; these clinical signs do not exclude concurrent involvement of the upper urinary tract or disorders of other body systems. Stranguria may be caused by bladder, intraluminal, and extraluminal urethral disease.

SYSTEMS AFFECTED

Renal/urologic/pelvic structures—bladder, urethra, prostate gland, colon, others.

SIGNALMENT

Dog and cat.

CAUSES

Urinary Bladder

- Urinary tract infection (UTI)—bacterial, fungal, mycoplasmal, parasitic, or viral.
- Cystolithiasis.
- Neoplasia—e.g., transitional cell carcinoma.
- Trauma.
- Anatomic abnormalities—e.g., ureterocele/urethrocele, ectopic ureter, persistent uterus masculinus, perineal hernias containing the urinary bladder, and spay granulomas.
- Detrusor atony—e.g., chronic partial obstruction, neurologic damage, and dysautonomia.
- Chemicals/drugs—e.g., cyclophosphamide.
- Iatrogenic—e.g., catheterization, palpation, reverse flushing, overdistension of the bladder during contrast radiography, urohydropropulsion, urethrocystoscopy, and surgery/interventional hardware (e.g., ureteral stent, subcutaneous ureteral bypass, stent, hydraulic occluder).
- Idiopathic—e.g., feline idiopathic cystitis.

Urethra

- UTI—see above.
- Urethrolithiasis—see above.
- Urethral plugs—e.g., matrix and matrix-crystalline.
- Neoplasia—see above; local invasion by malignant neoplasms of adjacent structures.
- Trauma.
- Anatomic anomalies—e.g., congenital or acquired strictures, urethrorectal fistulas, pseudohermaphrodites.
- Urethral sphincter hypertonicity—e.g., upper motor neuron spinal cord lesions, reflex dyssynergia, urethral spasm/urethritis.
- Proliferative urethritis—secondary to chronic UTI.

Prostate Gland

- Prostatitis, prostatic, or paraprostatic cyst or prostatic abscess.
- Neoplasia—adenocarcinoma, transitional cell carcinoma.

RISK FACTORS

- Diseases, diagnostic procedures, or treatments that alter normal host urinary tract defenses and predispose to infection, predispose to formation of uroliths, or damage urothelium or other tissues of lower urinary tract.
- Mural or extramural diseases that compress bladder or urethral lumen.
- Diseases that encourage repeated urination despite full void such as juvenile vaginitis may present as stranguria.

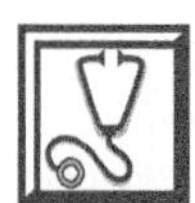

DIAGNOSIS

DIFFERENTIAL DIAGNOSIS

Differentiating from Other Abnormal Patterns of Micturition

- Polyuria—increased frequency and volume of urine >2 mL/kg/h and urine specific gravity <1.025.
- Rule out urethral obstruction—anuria, overdistended urinary bladder, signs of postrenal uremia.
- Urinary incontinence—involuntary urination, urine dribbling, enuresis, incomplete bladder emptying.
- Behavioral causes.

Differentiate Causes of Dysuria, Pollakiuria, Stranguria

- Rule out UTI—hematuria; malodorous or cloudy urine; small, painful, thickened bladder (also evaluate for mineralization or gas in wall).
- Rule out urolithiasis—hematuria; palpable uroliths in urethra or bladder.
- Rule out neoplasia—hematuria; palpable masses in urethra or bladder.
- Rule out neurogenic disorders—flaccid bladder wall; residual urine in bladder lumen after micturition; other neurologic deficits to hind legs, tail, perineum, and anal sphincter.
- Rule out prostatic diseases—urethral discharge, prostatomegaly, pyrexia, depression, tenesmus, caudal abdominal pain, stiff gait.
- Rule out colorectal disease for stranguria.
- Rule out cyclophosphamide cystitis—history.
- Rule out iatrogenic disorders—history of catheterization, reverse flushing, contrast radiography, urohydropropulsion, urethrocystoscopy, or surgery/complications from interventional devices.

CBC/BIOCHEMISTRY/URINALYSIS

- Results of bloodwork often normal. Lower urinary tract disease complicated by urethral obstruction may be associated with azotemia, hyperphosphatemia, acidosis, and hyperkalemia. Patients with concurrent pyelonephritis may have impaired urine-concentrating capacity, leukocytosis, azotemia, and thrombocytopenia if ureteral obstruction occurs concurrently. Patients with acute prostatitis or prostatic abscesses may have leukocytosis, discospondylitis, and/or heart murmur. Dehydrated patients may have elevated total plasma protein.
- Disorders of urinary bladder are best evaluated with urine specimen collected by cystocentesis. Urethral disorders best evaluated with mid-catch voided urine sample or by comparison of results of analysis of voided and cystocentesis samples. (Caution: cystocentesis may induce hematuria.)
- Pyuria, hematuria, and proteinuria indicate urinary tract inflammation, but are nonspecific findings that may result from infectious and noninfectious causes of lower urinary tract disease.
- Identification of bacteria, fungi, or parasite ova in urine sediment suggests, but does not prove, that UTI causing or complicating lower urinary tract disease. Consider contamination of urine during collection and storage when interpreting urinalyses.
- Identification of neoplastic cells in urine sediment indicates urinary tract neoplasia. Use caution in establishing diagnosis of neoplasia based on urine sediment examination. Urinary tract inflammation or extremes in urine pH or osmolality can cause epithelial cell atypia that is difficult to differentiate from neoplasia. Follow up with traumatic catheterization, cystoscopic biopsies, or urine BRAF assay.
- Crystalluria occurs in normal patients, patients with urolithiasis, or patients with lower urinary tract disease unassociated with uroliths. Interpret significance of crystalluria cautiously.
- Hematuria, proteinuria, and variable crystalluria occur in cats with nonobstructive idiopathic cystitis. Significant pyuria is rare.

OTHER LABORATORY TESTS

- Quantitative urine culture—most definitive means of identifying and characterizing bacterial UTI. If not affordable then rapid culture can still be performed for species identification at limited cost.

• Cytologic evaluation of urine sediment, prostatic fluid, urethral or vaginal discharges, or biopsy specimens obtained by catheter or needle aspiration—may help in evaluating patients with localized urinary tract disease; may establish definitive diagnosis of urinary tract neoplasia, but cannot rule it out.

IMAGING

Survey abdominal radiography, urinary tract ultrasonography, cystoscopy, and fluoroscopic urography are important means of identifying and localizing causes of dysuria, pollakiuria, and stranguria.

DIAGNOSTIC PROCEDURES

• Use cystoscopy in patients with persistent lesions of lower urinary tract for which no definitive diagnosis has been established by other, less invasive means.
• Use light microscopic evaluation of tissue biopsy specimens from patients with persistent lesions of urinary tract. Tissue specimens may be obtained by traumatic catheterization, cystoscopy and biopsy, or surgery.

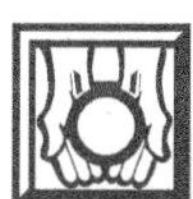

TREATMENT

• Patients with nonobstructive lower urinary tract diseases typically managed as outpatients; diagnostic evaluation may require brief hospitalization.
• Dysuria, pollakiuria, and stranguria associated with systemic signs of illness (e.g., pyrexia, depression, anorexia, vomiting, and dehydration) or laboratory findings of azotemia or leukocytosis warrant aggressive diagnostic evaluation and initiation of supportive and symptomatic treatment.
• Treatment depends on underlying cause and specific sites involved.
• Clinical signs of dysuria, pollakiuria often resolve rapidly following specific treatment of underlying cause(s). If not related to infection, stranguria may be more challenging to resolve.

MEDICATIONS

DRUG(S) OF CHOICE

• Patients with urge incontinence, severe or persistent signs, or untreatable lower urinary tract disease may benefit from symptomatic therapy with propantheline or oxybutynin that may reduce the force and frequency of uncontrolled detrusor contractions.
• Propantheline—dogs: 0.2 mg/kg PO q6–8h; cats: 0.25–0.5 mg/kg PO q12–24h. Oxybutynin—dogs: 0.2 mg/kg PO q8–12h; cats: 0.5–1.25 mg/cat PO q8–12h.
• Stranguria due to physiologic causes may be treated with prazosin in female dogs or cats, or in male dogs or cats with tamsulosin. If secondary to inflammation, meloxicam or carprofen can be utilized (caution with elevated liver values and azotemia), although short-term catheterization may also be warranted.
• Patients with transitional cell carcinoma of the urinary bladder or urethra may be treated with piroxicam (0.3 mg/kg PO q24h), which reduces the severity of clinical signs, improves quality of life, and in some cases induces tumor remission. Chemotherapeutic and radiation oncology treatment options are also available, as is urethral stenting.

CONTRAINDICATIONS

• Glucocorticoids or other immunosuppressive agents in patients suspected of having urinary or genital tract infection.
• Potentially nephrotoxic drugs (e.g., gentamicin) in patients that are febrile, dehydrated, or azotemic or that are suspected of having pyelonephritis, septicemia, or preexisting renal disease.

PRECAUTIONS

N/A

POSSIBLE INTERACTIONS

N/A

ALTERNATIVE DRUG(S)

N/A

FOLLOW-UP

PATIENT MONITORING

Monitor response to treatment by status of clinical signs, serial physical examination, laboratory testing, and imaging evaluations appropriate for each specific case.

POSSIBLE COMPLICATIONS

• Dysuria and pollakiuria may be associated with formation of macroscopic vesicourachal diverticula.
• Refer to specific chapters describing diseases listed under Causes.

MISCELLANEOUS

ASSOCIATED CONDITIONS

• Hematuria, pyuria, and proteinuria.
• Disorders predisposing to UTI.
• Disorders predisposing to formation of uroliths.
• Macroscopic vesicourachal diverticula.

SYNONYMS

• Feline urological syndrome.
• Lower urinary tract disease.

SEE ALSO

• Feline Idiopathic Lower Urinary Tract Disease.
• Lower Urinary Tract Infection, Bacterial.
• Lower Urinary Tract Infection, Fungal.
• Urinary Retention, Functional.
• Urinary Tract Obstruction.
• Urolithiasis, Calcium Oxalate.
• Urolithiasis, Calcium Phosphate.
• Urolithiasis, Cystine.
• Urolithiasis, Pseudo (Dried Blood, Ossified Material).
• Urolithiasis, Struvite—Cats.
• Urolithiasis, Struvite—Dogs.
• Urolithiasis, Urate.
• Urolithiasis, Xanthine.
• Vesicourachal Diverticula.

ABBREVIATIONS

• UTI = urinary tract infection.

Author Ewan D.S. Wolff
Consulting Editor J.D. Foster
Acknowledgment The author and book editors acknowledge the prior contributions of John M. Kruger and Carl A. Osborne

EAR MITES

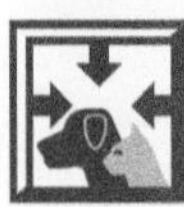

BASICS

E

OVERVIEW

Otodectes cynotis mites infest primarily the external ear canal and cause variable degrees of otic discharge and pruritus.

SIGNALMENT

- Common in young dogs and cats, although it may occur at any age.
- No breed or sex predilection.

SIGNS

- Pruritus is usually present, but can be minimal.
- Pruritus primarily located around the ears, head, and neck; occasionally generalized.
- Thick, red-brown, or black otic exudate ("coffee grounds" appearance)—usually seen in the outer ear.
- Otic exudate and pruritus demonstrate individual variability.
- Crusting and scales may occur on the neck, rump, and tail (dogs).
- Excoriations on the convex surface of the pinnae often occur, owing to the intense pruritus.

CAUSES & RISK FACTORS

Otodectes cynotis.

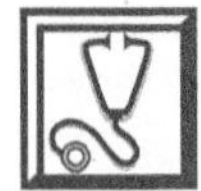

DIAGNOSIS

DIFFERENTIAL DIAGNOSIS

- Pediculosis.
- *Pelodera* dermatitis.
- Sarcoptic mange.
- Notoedric mange.
- Chiggers.
- Otitis externa secondary to allergy/hypersensitivity.
- Flea bite hypersensitivity.

CBC/BIOCHEMISTRY/URINALYSIS

Normal

OTHER LABORATORY TESTS

N/A

DIAGNOSTIC PROCEDURES

- Ear swabs placed in mineral oil—usually effective means of identification.
- Skin scrapings—may identify mites if signs are generalized.
- Mites may be visualized in external ear canal.
- Diagnosis may be made by response to treatment.

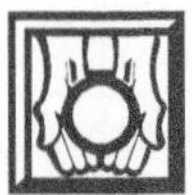

TREATMENT

- Outpatient.
- Diet and activity—no alteration necessary.
- Very contagious—all animals in contact with the affected animal must be treated.
- Thoroughly clean and treat the environment.

MEDICATIONS

DRUG(S) OF CHOICE

- Ears should be thoroughly cleaned with a commercial ear cleaner.
- Otic parasiticides should be used for 7–10 days to eradicate mites and eggs; effective topical commercial products contain pyrethrins, thiabendazole, ivermectin, and milbemycin; treat during alternative weeks for two to three treatment cycles recommended to prevent reinfestation from eggs.
- Selamectin—per label instructions or repeated at 2 weeks.
- Imidacloprid/moxidectin (Advantage Multi/Advocate)—per label instructions.
- Ivermectin—200–300 μg/kg PO (three treatments) or SC (two treatments) at 14-day intervals; non-FDA-approved usage.
- Isoxazolines—per label instructions; non-FDA-approved usage.
- Flea treatments should be applied to animal for elimination of ectopic mites.
- Mites may persist in the environment; environmental treatment may be helpful.

CONTRAINDICATIONS/POSSIBLE INTERACTIONS

- Ivermectin and moxidectin—sensitivity in ABCB-1 mutant dogs; do not use orally or by injection in collies, shelties, their crosses, or other herding breeds; use only if absolutely necessary in animals <6 months of age; an increasing number of toxic reactions have been reported in kittens.
- Ivermectin and milbemycin—cause elevated levels of monoamine neurotransmitter metabolites, which could result in adverse drug interactions with amitraz and benzodiazepines.
- Isoxazolines—use with caution in pets with previous history of seizures.

FOLLOW-UP

- Ear swab and physical examination should be done 1 month after therapy commences.
- Prognosis is good.
- If signs persist after treatment, an additional, underlying cause may be present.
- Repeat infestation indicates an uncontrolled source of mites.

MISCELLANEOUS

ZOONOTIC POTENTIAL

Transient papular dermatitis in human beings.

Suggested Reading

Helton Rhodes KA, Werner A. Blackwell's Five-Minute Veterinary Consult Clinical Companion: Small Animal Dermatology, 3rd ed. Hoboken, NJ: Wiley-Blackwell, 2018.

Thomas RC. Treatment of ectoparasites. In: Bonagura JD, Twedt DC, eds. Current Veterinary Therapy XV. St. Louis, MO: Elsevier Saunders, 2014, pp. 428–432.

Author Karen A. Kuhl
Consulting Editor Alexander H. Werner Resnick

BASICS

OVERVIEW

- Postparturient hypocalcemia.
- Usually develops 1–4 weeks postpartum; may occur at term, prepartum, or during late lactation.
- Hypocalcemia alters cell membrane potentials, causing spontaneous discharge of nerve fibers and tonic–clonic contraction of skeletal muscles.
- Life-threatening tetany and convulsions, leading to hyperthermia.
- Cerebral edema possible.

SIGNALMENT

- Dog—postpartum bitch; most common in toy breeds; higher incidence with first litter.
- Most common prior to day 40 postpartum; occasionally occurs prepartum.
- Breeds at increased risk—chihuahua, miniature pinscher, shih tzu, miniature poodle, Xoloitzcuintli, Pomeranian.
- Cat—rare.

SIGNS

Historical Findings

- Poor mothering.
- Restlessness, nervousness.
- Panting, whining.
- Vomiting, diarrhea.
- Ataxia, stiff gait, limb pain.
- Facial pruritis.
- Muscle tremors, tetany, convulsions.
- Recumbency, extensor rigidity—usually seen 8–12 hours after onset of signs.

Physical Examination Findings

- Hyperthermia.
- Rapid respiratory rate.
- Dilated pupils, sluggish pupillary light responses.
- Muscle tremors, muscular rigidity, convulsions.

CAUSES & RISK FACTORS

- Calcium supplementation during gestation, including dairy products.
- Inappropriate Ca : P ratio in gestational diet.
- Low bodyweight : litter size ratio.
- Poor prenatal nutrition.
- First litter.
- Large litter size.

DIAGNOSIS

DIFFERENTIAL DIAGNOSIS

- Hypoglycemia—may be concurrent; hypoglycemia alone does not cause muscular rigidity.
- Toxicosis—distinguished by signalment and history.
- Epilepsy or other neurologic disorder—differentiated by signalment; calcium concentration diagnostic.

CBC/BIOCHEMISTRY/URINALYSIS

- Total serum calcium <9 mg/dL in bitches; <8 mg/dL in queens.
- Although ionized calcium (<2.4–3.2 mg/dL) is the form important for normal neuromuscular function, measurement of total serum calcium is usually sufficient for diagnosis.
- Hypoglycemia—may be concurrent.
- Hypomagnesemia has been reported in 44% of affected bitches; may promote tetany.
- Serum potassium elevated in 56% of cases, due to metabolic acidosis or respiratory alkalosis.

OTHER LABORATORY TESTS

N/A

IMAGING

N/A

DIAGNOSTIC PROCEDURES

ECG may show prolonged QT interval, bradycardia, tachycardia, or ventricular premature complexes.

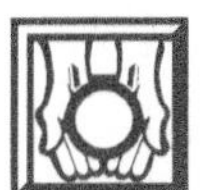

TREATMENT

- Emergency inpatient.
- Hyperthermia—cool by wetting haircoat and exposing to breeze from fan.
- Puppies—remove from dam onto a foster dam or hand-raise; if not possible or undesirable due to behavioral need for contact with dam, remove pups from dam for 24 hours, or until serum calcium is stabilized, and provide supplemental calcium for remainder of lactation; continue to monitor serum calcium level.

MEDICATIONS

DRUG(S) OF CHOICE

- Calcium gluconate—10% solution 0.22–0.44 mL/kg IV given slowly to effect over 5 min; monitor heart rate or ECG during administration; corresponds to dosage of 50–150 mg/kg.
- Correct hypoglycemia—50% dextrose: 0.5 g/kg diluted 1 : 3 with saline IV; can supplement maintenance IV fluids to 2.5% or 5% dextrose for longer-term treatment.
- Diazepam—0.5 mg/kg IV; for unresponsive seizures.
- Cerebral edema—if present, can treat with mannitol: 0.25–0.5 g/kg IV over 20 min, or 7.2% hypertonic saline 1–3 mL/kg IV over 15–20 min.
- Long-term therapy—calcium carbonate or calcium gluconate 10–30 mg/kg PO q8h until lactation ends (calcium carbonate 500 mg tablets supply 200 mg calcium).
- Magnesium supplementation may be helpful in hypomagnesemic bitches.
- Start puppies/kittens on solid food at 3–4 weeks of age.

E

CONTRAINDICATIONS/POSSIBLE INTERACTIONS

Corticosteroids—avoid; cause decreased intestinal absorption and increased renal excretion of calcium.

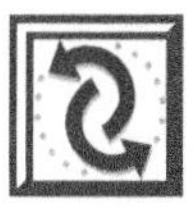

FOLLOW-UP

PATIENT MONITORING

- Serum calcium concentration—monitor until stabilized in the normal range.
- Avoid calcium supplementation during gestation.
- Diet—maternal: ensure calcium : phosphorus ratio of 1.1 : 1 or 1.2 : 1; avoid high-phytate foods (e.g., soybeans); puppies: supplement feeding for large litters.

POSSIBLE COMPLICATIONS

- Cerebral edema.
- Death.
- Hand-raising of puppies.

EXPECTED COURSE AND PROGNOSIS

- Probably will recur with subsequent litters; calcium supplementation can be started after parturition for bitches with history of eclampsia in prior litters.
- Prognosis—good with immediate treatment; poor with delayed treatment.

MISCELLANEOUS

Suggested Reading

Davidson AP. Reproductive causes of hypocalcemia. Topics Compan Anim Med 2012, 27:165–166.

Drobatz KJ, Casey KK. Eclampsia in dogs: 31 cases (1995–1998). J Am Vet Med Assoc 2000, 217(2):216–219.

Gonzalez, K. Peripariturient diseases in the dam. Vet Clin North Am Small Anim Pract 2018, 48(4):663–681.

Author Joni L. Freshman

Consulting Editor Erin E. Runcan

ECTOPIC URETER

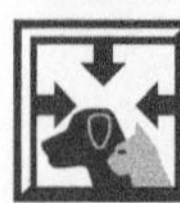

BASICS

OVERVIEW

- Congenital ureteral orifice(s) is inappropriately positioned caudal to the bladder trigone (i.e., trigone, urethra, vagina, vestibule, uterus, or prostate), resulting in incontinence.
- A common cause of urinary incontinence in juvenile female dogs. Also seen in adult dogs.
- Dogs—>95% tunnel intramurally, traversing the urethra in the submucosa.
- Male dogs—commonly associated with severe hydronephrosis and hydroureter due to ureteral opening stenosis.
- Commonly associated with multiple anomalies of the urinary tract—including concurrent urethral sphincter mechanism incompetence (USMI), hydroureter, hydronephrosis, short urethra/intrapelvic bladder.

SIGNALMENT

- Dog and cat.
- Juvenile incontinent dogs.
- Infrequently reported in cats and male dogs; 20 : 1 ratio of female : male dogs.
- Dog breeds may be predisposed—retrievers, Siberian huskies, Newfoundlands, poodles, terriers.

SIGNS

- Constant or intermittent incontinence since birth.
- Normal voiding in some.
- Chronic urinary tract infection(s) (UTIs).
- May be asymptomatic (male dogs) and can have moderate to severe hydroureter/hydronephrosis.

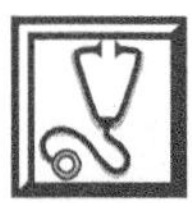

DIAGNOSIS

DIFFERENTIAL DIAGNOSIS

- USMI.
- Inappropriate urination—urge incontinence, "overactive bladder," behavioral (conscious urination).
- UTI—pollakiuria and urge incontinence.
- Vaginal pooling.
- Congenital hydroureter/hydronephrosis—male dogs with ectopic ureter(s) (EUs) often continent.
- Short urethra/intrapelvic bladder syndrome.

CBC/BIOCHEMISTRY/URINALYSIS

Labwork is typically normal, except when patients have concurrent anomalies (e.g., renal dysplasia, pyelonephritis).

OTHER LABORATORY TESTS

Urine bacterial culture and sensitivity—via cystocentesis.

IMAGING

- Cystoscopy (96% sensitivity).
- CT (91% sensitivity).
- Urinary tract ultrasonography (60–91% sensitivity) can provide accurate diagnosis and anatomic information of the upper urinary tract. Color-flow Doppler ultrasonography can provide location of ureteral jets, but does not guarantee the absence of a multifenestrated ureter.
- Excretory urography (50–75% sensitivity) with positive contrast cystogram or a pneumocystogram.
- Retrograde urethrography (47% sensitivity).

DIAGNOSTIC PROCEDURES

Cystoscopy—definitive diagnosis and characterization of EU, short urethra syndrome, location of ectopic orifice in the genitourinary tract. Also allows for simultaneous treatment.

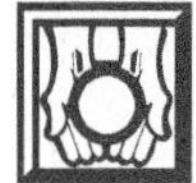

TREATMENT

- Cystoscopic-guided laser ablation (CLA)—performed for intramural EU only. Opens ureteral tract in a minimally invasive manner; addresses concurrent vaginal defects, which may lead to considerable deviation of the urethra. Patients treated with CLA typically discharged the same day.
- Surgical—treatment of choice for extramural EU: neoureterostomy, reimplantation, or rarely ureteronephrectomy; complication rates range between 14% and 25% including ureteral strictures, leakage, and infection.

MEDICATIONS

DRUG(S) OF CHOICE

- Use if incontinence persists after surgery.
- Phenylpropanolamine (1–1.5 mg/kg PO q8h) will improve continence after surgery/laser therapy in 10–20% of dogs, improving continence levels to 50–60%.
- Testosterone propionate (2.2 mg/kg IM q2–3 days) or methyltestosterone (0.5 mg/kg/day) is administered to male dogs. For longer action, testosterone cypionate (2.2 mg/kg IM q30 days) can be used; this approach is not advised in immature or intact males.
- Estriol (2 mg once daily per dog for 14 days, followed by the lowest effective daily dose tapered every 7 days).

Other

Treatment for persistent incontinence after surgery/laser ablation—transurethral submucosal bulking agent injections: can improve continence to ~60–65%; placement of an artificial urethral sphincter (called a hydraulic occluder) can improve continence to ~80–90%.

FOLLOW-UP

EXPECTED COURSE AND PROGNOSIS

- Warn owners that incontinence may continue in some patients after surgery. Many patients become continent with the addition of medications, collagen bulking, and/or placement of a hydraulic occlude.
- Dogs—continence with surgery (25–50%) or laser ablation (40–55%) alone, which improves to 60% with medications, 65% with bulking agent injection, and ~80–90% with placement of a hydraulic occlude.

MISCELLANEOUS

ASSOCIATED CONDITIONS

- Hydronephrosis.
- Hydroureter.
- Ureterocele.
- Pelvic bladder.
- Persistent paramesonephric remnant.
- Vaginal septum.
- Renal dysplasia.
- Renal agenesis.
- USMI.
- Short urethra/intrapelvic bladder.

SEE ALSO

- Incontinence, Urinary.
- Pelvic Bladder.

ABBREVIATIONS

- CLA = cystoscopic-guided laser ablation.
- EU = ectopic ureter.
- USMI = urethral sphincter mechanism incompetence.
- UTI = urinary tract infection.

Author Ewan D.S. Wolff

Consulting Editor J.D. Foster

Acknowledgment The author and book editors acknowledge the prior contribution of Allyson C. Berent.

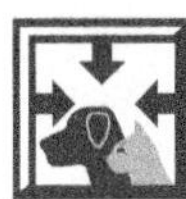

BASICS

OVERVIEW

- Eversion or rolling out of the eyelid margin, resulting in exposure of the palpebral conjunctiva.
- Can be conformational/congenital (primary) or acquired (secondary).
- Exposure and poor tear retention/ distribution may predispose patient to irritation, recurrent infections, and sight-threatening corneal disease.

SIGNALMENT

- Dogs, seldom cats.
- Breeds with higher than average prevalence—sporting breeds (e.g., spaniels, hounds, and retrievers); giant breeds (e.g., Saint Bernard, mastiff); any breed with loose facial skin (especially bloodhounds).
- Primary—genetic predisposition in listed breeds; may occur in dogs <1 year old.
- Acquired—noted in other breeds; occurs late in life secondary to age-related loss of facial muscle tone and skin laxity.
- Intermittent—caused by fatigue; may be observed after strenuous exercise or when drowsy.

SIGNS

- Eversion of the lower eyelid with lack of contact of the lower lid to the globe and exposure of the palpebral conjunctiva and third eyelid.
  - Often excessively long palpebral fissure (macroblepharon).
  - Conjunctivitis and history of mucoid to mucopurulent discharge caused by chronic exposure to air and debris. Debris generally located between lid and globe in inferior conjunctival cul-de-sac.
  - Tear staining of periocular skin caused by poor tear drainage.
- History of bacterial conjunctivitis.

CAUSES & RISK FACTORS

- Primary disease—most common due to breed-associated facial conformation and alterations in eyelid support.
- Acquired disease—from marked weight loss or muscle mass loss about the head and orbits, tragic facial expression in hypothyroid dogs, and cicatricial ectropion from scarring of the eyelids secondary to injury or from surgical overcorrection of entropion.

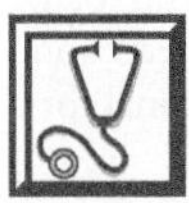

DIAGNOSIS

DIFFERENTIAL DIAGNOSIS

- Usually clinically obvious.
- Look for any underlying disorder in nonpredisposed breeds and dogs with late-age onset.
- Loss of orbital or periorbital mass—may occur in patients with masticatory myositis.
- Facial nerve paralysis—associated with lack of muscle tone of orbicularis oculi muscles.

CBC/BIOCHEMISTRY/URINALYSIS

N/A

OTHER LABORATORY TESTS

- Possible masticatory myositis—test for auto-antibodies against type 2M muscle fibers.
- Palpebral nerve paralysis or tragic facial expression—consider testing for hypothyroidism.

IMAGING

N/A

DIAGNOSTIC PROCEDURES

- Palpebral nerve paralysis—full neurologic evaluation; potential for hypothyroidism.
- Secondary conjunctivitis—flush fornix and examine for follicles.
- Fluorescein or rose Bengal staining of cornea and conjunctiva—to identify corneal ulcerations; may reveal severity of exposure problem.

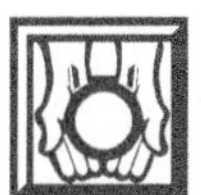

TREATMENT

- Supportive care (topical lubricant, rinsing eyes with eyewash after being outside to remove debris) and good ocular and facial hygiene—sufficient for most mild disease.
- Surgical treatment—eyelid shortening or radical facelift; necessary for severely affected patients that have chronic ocular irritation.
- Intermittent, fatigue-induced condition—do not treat surgically.

MEDICATIONS

DRUG(S) OF CHOICE

- Topical broad-spectrum ophthalmic antibiotics—bacterial conjunctivitis or corneal ulceration. Neomycin/polymyxin B/ bacitracin (or based on culture and sensitivity) q6–8h.
- Lubricant ointments (e.g., Puralube®)—reduce conjunctival and corneal desiccation secondary to exposure.
- Hypothyroid and masticatory myositis-induced conditions—may respond well to appropriate medical treatment of underlying disease.

CONTRAINDICATIONS/POSSIBLE INTERACTIONS

N/A

FOLLOW-UP

- May become more severe as patient ages.
- Nonsurgically treated patient—monitor for signs of infectious conjunctivitis, exposure keratopathy, corneal ulceration, and facial dermatitis.

MISCELLANEOUS

ASSOCIATED CONDITIONS

- Hypothyroidism.
- Masticatory myositis, extraocular myositis.

AGE-RELATED FACTORS

Old animals more likely to have ectropion secondary to loss of facial muscle tone.

SEE ALSO

- Hypothyroidism.
- Myopathy – Masticatory and Extraocular Myositis.

Suggested Reading

Stades FC, van der Woerdt A. Diseases and surgery of the canine eyelid. In: Gelatt KN, Gilger BC, Kern TJ, eds., Veterinary Ophthalmology, 5th ed. Ames, IA: Wiley-Blackwell, 2013, pp. 853–864.

Author Sarah L. Czerwinski
Consulting Editor Kathern E. Myrna

Acknowledgment The author and book editor acknowledge the prior contribution of J. Phillip Pickett.

EHRLICHIOSIS AND ANAPLASMOSIS

BASICS

E

DEFINITION

Caused by *Ehrlichia* and *Anaplasma*—tick-borne rickettsial disease.

Dogs

• Obligate intracellular pathogens in three genera: *Ehrlichia*, *Anaplasma*, and *Neorickettsia*. • *Ehrlichia*—predominant species: *E. canis*: canine monocytic ehrlichiosis (CME); *E. ewingii*: granulocytic ehrlichiosis; *E. chaffeensis*: primarily human pathogen, may cause canine disease. • *Anaplasma*—*A. phagocytophilum*: granulocytic anaplasmosis; *A. platys*: thrombocytic anaplasmosis. • *Neorickettsia*—infect mononuclear cells (monocytes and macrophages): *N. risticii*: Potomac horse fever; rarely infects dogs; acquired by ingesting infected vectors; serum from infected dogs does not cross-react with *Ehrlichia*; *N. helminthoeca*: salmon poisoning, primarily northwestern United States.

Cats

Feline ehrlichiosis (rare)—serologic, PCR, and cytologic evidence for *Ehrlichia* (*E. canis*, *E. canis*-like, *E. chaffeensis*, *E. ewingii*) and *Anaplasma* (*A. phagocytophilum*); clinical signs may include fever, lethargy, joint pain, anemia, hyperglobulinemia, and thrombocytopenia; may also be asymptomatic.

PATHOPHYSIOLOGY

• *Anaplasma* and *Ehrlichia* transmitted via tick bite; transmission time between 3h (*E. canis*) and 18h; can occur via blood transfusion. • *E. canis*—*Rhipicephalus sanguineus* tick vector; infects mononuclear cells; 1–3-week incubation period; three stages of canine disease: ○ Acute (2–4 weeks)—spread to spleen, liver, lymph nodes; causes endothelial cell and perivascular inflammation, thrombocytopenia (possible antiplatelet antibodies), mild anemia; infections may be subclinical. ○ Subclinical (months–years)—organism persists; hyperglobulinemia; mild thrombocytopenia; dogs may eliminate infection, others remain persistently infected or develop chronic disease. ○ Chronic—myelosuppression; pancytopenia. • *E. ewingii*—*Amblyomma americanum* tick vector; infects granulocytes; dogs can be persistently infected and asymptomatic; acute clinical signs include fever, neutrophilic polyarthritis, neutrophilia, reactive lymphocytes, and proteinuria; bleeding disorders uncommon.
• *A. phagocytophilum*—*Ixodes* spp. tick vector; infects granulocytes; infections can be asymptomatic and self-limiting; acute clinical signs include fever, lameness, thrombocytopenia, and lymphopenia. • *A. platys*—tick vector likely *R. sanguineus*; infects platelets; persistent or cyclic thrombocytopenia.

SYSTEMS AFFECTED

• Multisystemic disease. • Vasculature—bleeding tendencies (thrombocytopenia and vascular inflammation). • Hemic/lymphatic/immune—bone marrow, spleen, lymph nodes. • Nervous (meningitis, cerebral hemorrhage). • Ophthalmic (anterior uveitis). • Joint (neutrophilic arthritis).

PREVALENCE/GEOGRAPHIC DISTRIBUTION

• *E. canis*—year round, worldwide; higher prevalence in warm climates. • *E. ewingii*—warmer months; seroprevalence eastern and midwest United States.
• *A. phagocytophilum*—warmer months; eastern, upper midwest, and Pacific coast United States.

SIGNALMENT

Species

Dogs and cats (infrequent).

Breed Predilections

Chronic CME—German shepherd dogs, Belgian Malinois.

Mean Age and Range

• Average age 5.2 years. • Range 2 months–14 years.

SIGNS

General Comments

Vary in severity and duration, dependent on host, coinfections, and strain variations.

Historical Findings

• Fever, lethargy, anorexia, weight loss.
• Spontaneous bleeding—sneezing, epistaxis, petechia, ecchymosis. • Ocular discharge/pain. • Lameness. • Ataxia, head tilt

Physical Examination Findings

Acute

• Bleeding diathesis. • Fever. • Generalized lymphadenopathy. • Organomegaly (spleen, liver). • Ocular discharge. • Lameness. • Ticks.

Chronic E. canis

• Pale mucous membranes (anemia).
• Ulcerative stomatitis. • Hind limb or scrotal edema. • Uveitis, hyphema, retinal hemorrhages. • Ataxia, vestibular dysfunction, cervical pain.

RISK FACTORS

Coinfection with other vector-borne diseases (VBDs).

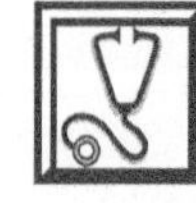

DIAGNOSIS

DIFFERENTIAL DIAGNOSIS

• Rocky Mountain spotted fever (*Rickettsia rickettsii*)—seasonal (Mar–Oct); diagnose with serology; same treatment. • Immune-mediated thrombocytopenia—no fever or lymphadenopathy; rule out VBD. • Systemic lupus erythematosus—positive antinuclear antibody (ANA) test. • Multiple myeloma—monoclonal gammopathy, bony lesions.
• Chronic lymphocytic leukemia—bone marrow cytology; PCR for antigen receptor rearrangements (PARR; *E. canis* infrequently PARR negative). • Brucellosis.

CBC/BIOCHEMISTRY/URINALYSIS

Acute

• Thrombocytopenia, anemia, leukopenia (lymphopenia, neutropenia, and eosinopenia), or leukocytosis (granular lymphocytosis, monocytosis). • Morulae—intracytoplasmic inclusions in leukocytes, rare. • Hyperglobulinemia—progressive increase 1–3 weeks postinfection. • Hypoalbuminemia. • Mild increases in liver enzyme activities, azotemia, hyperbilirubinemia.
• Proteinuria.

Chronic

• Pancytopenia—anemia, thrombocytopenia, neutropenia, but monocytosis and lymphocytosis possible. • Hyperglobulinemia—magnitude correlates with duration of infection; usually polyclonal gammopathy, occasionally monoclonal. • Hypoalbuminemia.

OTHER LABORATORY TESTS

Serologic Testing

• Antibodies present ~3 weeks postinfection.
• Immunofluorescent antibody test (IFAT)—sensitive; cross-reactivity between *Ehrlichia* species; use same laboratory to compare acute and convalescent titers; fourfold increase paired in convalescent titer indicates active infection; detection at one time-point may represent past exposure or active infection.
• Rapid point-of-care (POC) screening test—sensitivity and specificity vary depending on test; overtly healthy dogs with positive POC tests should have CBC, Biochemistry, UA, PCR or paired IFAT to identify evidence of infection before treatment; animals can remain seropositive by POC for years, even after infection cleared.

PCR Testing

• Detects pathogen DNA; sensitive indicator of active or recent infection. • Whole blood or tissue (spleen, lymph node, liver, bone marrow); identifies species; detect as early as 7 days postinfection. • Negative PCR result cannot rule out VBD infections; false negative can occur due to low organism load; genetic variations can prevent PCR detection.
• Combining serology and PCR optimal for accurate diagnosis.

Additional Tests

• Coombs' positive anemia; indicates concurrent immune-mediated erythrocyte destruction; may be positive in dogs with babesiosis, other VBD. • Test for VBD coinfections. • Culture and sensitivity testing (blood, urine) indicated in febrile patients.

DIAGNOSTIC PROCEDURES

Bone Marrow Aspirate

• Acute—hypercellularity of megakaryocytic and myeloid series. • Chronic—erythroid hypoplasia with increased M : E ratio, plasmacytosis. • Increased number of mast cells.

PATHOLOGIC FINDINGS

• Acute—serosal and mucosal petechiae; lymphadenopathy, splenomegaly, hepatomegaly, and red bone marrow; perivascular infiltrates of macrophages and lymphocytes (lung); periportal infiltrates of lymphocytes and macrophages (liver); lymphoid hyperplasia (spleen). • Chronic—pale marrow, subcutaneous edema; histologically, perivascular plasma cell infiltrates in organs; multifocal nonsuppurative meningoencephalitis with lymphoplasmacytic infiltrate.

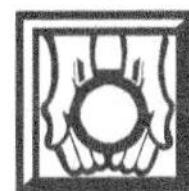

TREATMENT

APPROPRIATE HEALTH CARE

• Inpatient—medical stabilization for acute signs. • Outpatient—stable patients; frequent monitoring for therapeutic response.

NURSING CARE

• Balanced electrolyte solution IV. • Blood or platelet-rich plasma transfusion for severe anemia or thrombocytopenia.

CLIENT EDUCATION

• Acute—prognosis excellent with appropriate therapy. • Chronic—prognosis guarded; cytopenia resolution may take ≥6 months; prognosis poor if hypoplastic bone marrow.
• Progression to chronic prevented by early effective treatment; serological tests may stay positive (IFAT ≤1 year and POC for years); reinfection can occur if animals reexposed.
• Breed risks for chronic CME.

MEDICATIONS

DRUG(S) OF CHOICE

• Doxycycline—5 mg/kg PO q12h or 10 mg/kg PO q24h for 3–4 weeks; clinical response usually in 1–2 days; slower response in chronic ehrlichiosis or neurologic disease.
• Prednisolone or prednisone, use with antibiotics; anti-inflammatory (0.5–1 mg/kg PO q12–24h for 3–5 days) for polyarthritis; immunosuppressive (1–2 mg/kg PO q12h for 5 days; rarely exceed 60 mg/dog/day) when immune-mediated disease suspected. • For CME, prophylactic antibiotics if neutrophils <1000 cells/μl for >1 week.

CONTRAINDICATIONS

• Glucocorticoids in myelosuppressive CME.
• Glucocorticoids in animals with diabetes mellitus, gastrointestinal ulceration, concurrent or recent nonsteroidal anti-inflammatory drug (NSAID) use.

PRECAUTIONS

• Prolonged immunosuppressive corticosteroid use may interfere with elimination of *E. canis*. • Doxycycline in dogs with liver disease or abnormal liver enzyme values.

ALTERNATIVE DRUG(S)

• Minocycline—10 mg/kg PO q12h for 3–4 weeks. • Rifampicin: 10 mg/kg PO q24h for 3 weeks (do not exceed 10 mg/kg/day in dogs); less effective.

FOLLOW-UP

PATIENT MONITORING

• CBC, blood smear examination—2, 4, 8 weeks after starting antibiotics; recurrence of clinical signs post treatment suggests treatment failure, reinfection, or concurrent infection with pathogen partially sensitive to therapy (*Babesia*, *Bartonella*). • IFAT—9 months post treatment; most dogs become seronegative; extended seropositivity may indicate reinfection or ineffective treatment. • PCR—1–2 months post treatment for evidence of pathogen clearance; if PCR positive, repeat antibiotics for 4–6 weeks, ensure use of acaricides; if persistently negative, change drug. • POC assay—not used to monitor treatment response.

PREVENTION/AVOIDANCE

• Control tick infestation—acaricides: topical (spot treatments and collars)—imidacloprid/flumethrin, fipronil, permethrin, deltamethrin, and amitraz (do not use permethrin, deltamethrin, or amitraz on cats); systemic—isoxazolines. • Manually remove ticks; use gloves; ensure removal of mouth parts.

EXPECTED COURSE AND PROGNOSIS

• Acute—excellent prognosis with appropriate treatment; most immunocompetent dogs recover, enter subclinical phase, or clear infection; treatment accelerates recovery, may prevent chronic phase.
• Chronic—may take 4 weeks for clinical response, 6 months for cytopenia rebound; prognosis poor and expensive medical management with hypoplastic marrow.
• *Ehrlichia* and *Anaplasma* antibodies do not protect against reinfection.

MISCELLANEOUS

ASSOCIATED CONDITIONS

• *Babesia*. • *Bartonella*. • Hemotropic *Mycoplasma*. • *Leishmania*.

ZOONOTIC POTENTIAL

E. canis, *E. ewingii*, *E. chaffeensis*, *A. phagocytophilum*, and *A. platys* can infect humans via tick bite; *R. sanguineus* prefers dogs, will bite humans in living conditions with high vector population; *A. americanum* bites humans; *Ixodes* bite humans and transmit *Borrelia burgdorferi*, *Babesia microti*, likely *E. muris*.

SYNONYMS

• Canine hemorrhagic fever. • Canine rickettsiosis. • Canine typhus. • Tracker dog disease. • Tropical canine pancytopenia.

ABBREVIATIONS

• ANA = antinuclear antibody. • CME = canine monocytic ehrlichiosis. • IFAT = indirect fluorescent antibody test. • NSAID = nonsteroidal anti-inflammatory drug.
• PARR = PCR for antigen receptor rearrangements. • POC = point of care.
• VBD = vector-borne disease.

Suggested Reading

Mylonakis ME, Harrus S, Breitschwerdt EB. An update on the treatment of canine monocytic ehrlichiosis (Ehrlichia canis). Vet J 2019, 246:45–53.

Author Barbara Qurollo

Consulting Editor Amie Koenig

Acknowledgment The author and book editors acknowledge the prior contribution of Stephen C. Barr.

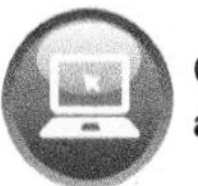

Client Education Handout available online

ELBOW DYSPLASIA

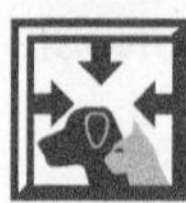

BASICS

E

DEFINITION

A group of developmental abnormalities that lead to malformation, degeneration, and secondary osteoarthritis of the elbow joint.

PATHOPHYSIOLOGY

- Four abnormalities—un-united anconeal process (UAP), osteochondritis dissecans (OCD), fragmented medial coronoid process (FMCP), and incongruity; alone or in combination; may be seen in one or both elbows; bilateral disease common (50% of cases).
- Terminology— medial compartment disease (MCompD) involves any pathology within the medial compartment, while medial coronoid process disease (MCD) is used to describe all pathologies of the medial coronoid process such as fissuring, fragmenting, sclerosis, microfracture, and cartilage damage.
- FMCP and incongruity are the most common documented MCompD pathologies.
- UAP—delayed closure of growth plate between anconeal process and proximal ulnar metaphysis (olecranon) by 5 months of age; may be result of abnormal mechanical stress on anconeal process.
- OCD—affects medial aspect of humeral condyle; disturbance in endochondral ossification causes retention of articular cartilage and subsequent mechanical stress leads to cartilage flap lesion.
- FMCP—chondral or osteochondral fragmentation or fissure of medial coronoid process of ulna; possibly manifestation of osteochondrosis of coronoid process; coronoid does not have separate ossification center; may be result of abnormal mechanical stress on medial coronoid process considered to be due to incongruity.
- Incongruity—asynchronous growth between radius and ulna may lead to abnormal loading, wearing, and erosion of cartilage in humeroulnar compartment. Malformation of trochlear notch of ulna; elliptical trochlear notch with decreased arc of curvature is too small to articulate with humeral trochlea—resulting in major points of contact at anconeal process, coronoid process, and medial humeral condyle.

SYSTEMS AFFECTED

Musculoskeletal

GENETICS

High heritability

INCIDENCE/PREVALENCE

- Most common cause for elbow pain and lameness.
- One of the most common causes for thoracic lameness in large-breed dogs.

GEOGRAPHIC DISTRIBUTION

N/A

SIGNALMENT

Species

Dog

Breed Predilections

Large and giant breeds—Labrador retrievers; Rottweilers; golden retrievers; German shepherds; Bernese mountain dogs; chow chows; bearded collies; Newfoundlands.

Mean Age and Range

- Age at onset of clinical signs—typically 4–10 months.
- Age at diagnosis—generally 4–18 months.
- Onset of symptoms related to degenerative joint disease (DJD)—any age.

Predominant Sex

- FMCP—males predisposed.
- UAP, OCD, incongruity—none established.

SIGNS

General Comments

- Lameness—if no distinct abnormalities noted on physical examination or radiographs, early intervention may demand advanced imaging.
- Any resistance at all in flexion in immature dog should raise suspicion of elbow dysplasia.
- Not all patients are symptomatic when young.
- Intermittent episodes of elbow lameness due to advanced DJD changes in mature patient—common.

Historical Findings

Intermittent or persistent thoracic limb lameness—exacerbated by exercise; progressed from stiffness seen only after rest.

Physical Examination Findings

- Pain—elicited on elbow hyperflexion or extension; elicited when holding elbow and carpus at 90° while pronating and supinating carpus and applying pressure to medial compartment.
- Affected limb—tendency to be held in abduction and supination.
- Joint effusion and capsular distension—especially noted between lateral epicondyle and olecranon.
- Crepitus—may be palpated with advanced DJD.
- Diminished range of motion.

CAUSES

- Genetic.
- Developmental.
- Nutritional.

RISK FACTORS

- Rapid growth and weight gain.
- High-calorie diet.

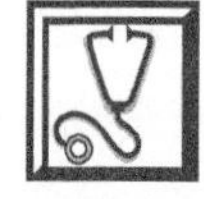

DIAGNOSIS

DIFFERENTIAL DIAGNOSIS

- Trauma.
- Septic arthritis.
- Panosteitis.
- Avulsion or calcification of flexor muscles.
- Synovial sarcoma.

CBC/BIOCHEMISTRY/URINALYSIS

N/A

IMAGING

Radiography

- Image both elbows—high incidence of bilateral disease.
- UAP, OCD, FMCP, and incongruity—elbow DJD recognized by osteophytes on cranial margin of radial head (37%), anconeal process (70%), and epicondyles (medial and lateral), and medial coronoid process; sclerosis of ulna caudal to coronoid process and trochlear notch; stairstep between joint surface of radius and lateral coronoid.
- UAP—best diagnosed from mediolateral hyperflexed view; may see lack of bony union. Comparison to contralateral elbow may be helpful, although high incidence of bilateral disease should be kept in mind.
- OCD—best diagnosed from craniocaudal and craniocaudal-lateromedial oblique views; reveals radiolucent defect or flattening of medial aspect of humeral condyle.
- FMCP—may not be visualized in some cases; diagnosis then presumptive based on DJD and lack of UAP or OCD lesions; commonly see trochlear sclerosis and/or early osteophyte formation on proximal caudal surface of anconeal process with FMCP.

Other

CT, MRI, and linear tomography—can provide more definitive evidence for fissures and nondisplaced fragments. CT is necessary in many cases of MCD as survey radiographs have low sensitivity.

DIAGNOSTIC PROCEDURES

- Joint tap and analysis of synovial fluid—confirm involvement of joint.
- Synovial fluid—should be straw colored with normal to decreased viscosity; cytology reveals <5,000 nucleated cells/μL (>90% are mononuclear cells); normal results do not necessarily rule out the diagnosis.
- Arthroscopy—may help diagnose UAP, MCD, OCD, and incongruity.

PATHOLOGIC FINDINGS

- UAP—fibrous union between anconeal process and proximal ulnar metaphysis; fibrous tissue invasion and degeneration of anconeal process; DJD.
- OCD—chondral flap on medial humeral condyle; sclerosis of underlying subchondral bone with fibrous tissue invasion; erosive lesion on apposing coronoid cartilage; DJD.
- FMCP—chondral or osteochondral fragmentation of cranial tip or lateral margin of medial coronoid; erosive lesion on cartilage of apposing medial aspect of humeral condyle; DJD.

- Incongruity—a step greater than 2 mm noted between medial border of radial head and lateral border of medial coronoid process.
- MCompD—erosive lesions involving part or all of medial coronoid process and apposing articular cartilage of medial aspect of humeral condyle; DJD; linear striations in articular cartilage.

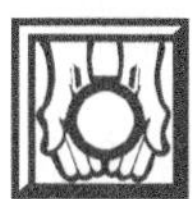

TREATMENT

APPROPRIATE HEALTH CARE

Surgery—controversial but recommended for most patients.

NURSING CARE

- Cold packing elbow joint—perform immediately post surgery to help decrease swelling and control pain; perform at least 20 minutes q8h for 3–5 days.
- Passive range-of-motion exercises—beneficial until patient can bear weight on limb(s), then progress into static and dynamic therapeutic exercises.
- If osteoarthritis is present, then multimodal management is necessary as for arthritic management of any joint.

ACTIVITY

- Restricted for all patients postoperatively.
- Consideration for avoidance of high concussive activities for life.

DIET

- Weight control—important for decreasing load and stress on affected joint(s).
- Restricted weight gain and growth in young dogs—may decrease incidence and severity.

CLIENT EDUCATION

- Discuss heritability of disease.
- Discuss likelihood of DJD progression regardless of intervention.
- Discuss influence of excessive intake of nutrients that promote rapid growth.

SURGICAL CONSIDERATIONS

- Severity of DJD and advanced age of patient—negatively influence outcome. Generally DJD progresses faster without treatment.
- UAP—four options: removal, lag screw fixation, dynamic proximal ulnar osteotomy, and lag screw fixation plus dynamic proximal osteotomy; base decision on degree of DJD, patient's age, and surgical expertise.
- OCD and FMCP—medial approach to elbow (diagnostic differentiation not necessary); removal of loose fragment(s).
- Incongruity—controversial; four options: no surgery, subtotal coronoidectomy, dynamic proximal ulnar osteotomy, intra-articular osteotomy; base decision on type of incongruity, degree of DJD, patient's age, and surgical expertise.
- Arthroscopic diagnosis and treatment—excellent option for FMCP, OCD, and incongruity; benefits: superior visualization, minimally invasive, superior to arthrotomy in outcome.

MEDICATIONS

DRUG(S) OF CHOICE

- None that promotes healing of osteochondral or chondral fragments.
- Nonsteroidal anti-inflammatory drugs (NSAIDs)—minimize pain, decrease inflammation, symptomatically treat associated DJD.
- Deracoxib (3–4 mg/kg PO q24h, chewable).
- Carprofen (2.2 mg/kg PO q12h or q24h).
- Meloxicam (load 0.2 mg/kg PO, then 0.1 mg/kg PO q24h—liquid).
- Tepoxalin (load 20 mg/kg, then 10 mg/kg PO q24h).

CONTRAINDICATIONS

Avoid corticosteroids—potential side effects; articular cartilage damage associated with long-term use.

PRECAUTIONS

NSAIDs—gastrointestinal irritation may preclude use in some patients.

POSSIBLE INTERACTIONS

N/A

ALTERNATIVE DRUG(S)

Chondroprotective drugs (e.g., polysulfated glycosaminoglycans, glucosamine, and chondroitin sulfate)—may help limit cartilage damage and degeneration; may help alleviate pain and inflammation.

FOLLOW-UP

PATIENT MONITORING

- Post surgery—limit activity for minimum of 12 weeks; encourage early, active, controlled movement of affected joint(s); consider formal rehabilitation therapy.
- Yearly to twice-yearly examinations—recommended to evaluate progression of DJD.

PREVENTION/AVOIDANCE

- Discourage breeding of affected animals.
- Do not repeat dam–sire breeding that resulted in affected offspring.

POSSIBLE COMPLICATIONS

N/A

EXPECTED COURSE AND PROGNOSIS

- Progression of DJD—expected.
- Prognosis—fair to good for all forms.

MISCELLANEOUS

ASSOCIATED CONDITIONS

N/A

AGE-RELATED FACTORS

N/A

ZOONOTIC POTENTIAL

N/A

PREGNANCY/FERTILITY/BREEDING

N/A

SYNONYMS

Elbow osteochondrosis.

SEE ALSO

Osteochondrosis

ABBREVIATIONS

- DJD = degenerative joint disease.
- FMCP = fragmented medial coronoid process.
- MCD = medial coronoid process disease.
- MCompD = medial compartment disease.
- NSAID = nonsteroidal anti-inflammatory drugs.
- OCD = osteochondritis dissecans.
- UAP = un-united anconeal process.

INTERNET RESOURCES

https://www.ofa.org/diseases/elbow-dysplasia

Suggested Reading

Cook CR, Cook JL. Diagnostic imaging of canine elbow dysplasia: a review. Vet Surg 2009, 38(2):144–153.

Fitzpatrick N, Yeadon R. Working algorithm for treatment decision making for developmental disease of the medial compartment of the elbow in dogs. Vet Surg 2009, 38(2):285–300.

Sallander MH, Hedhammar A, Trogen ME. Diet, exercise, and weight as risk factors in hip dysplasia and elbow arthrosis in Labrador retrievers. J Nutr 2006, 136(7 Suppl):2050S–2052S.

Samoy Y, Van Ryssen B, Gielen I, et al. Review of the literature: elbow incongruity in the dog. Vet Comp Orthop Traumatol 2006, 19(1):1–8.

Author David Dycus

Consulting Editor Mathieu M. Glassman

Acknowledgment The author and book editors acknowledge the prior contribution of Walter C. Renberg.

Client Education Handout available online

ELECTRIC CORD INJURY

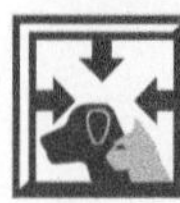

BASICS

OVERVIEW

• Electric cord injury is an uncommon event that occurs when an animal bites an electric cord. • Other causes of electrocution are uncommon in dogs and cats but can occur. • Household electrical currents are alternating (50–60 Hz), 110–120 or 220–240 volts depending on geographic location, and are dangerous. • Injury can be caused due to thermal injury or due to disruption of normal electrophysiologic activity of excitable tissue. • Pulmonary edema can be a sequela to electrocution and the pathophysiology is thought to be neurogenic and centrally mediated, leading to pulmonary hypertension. • Cataract formation is reported following electrocution.

SIGNALMENT

• Most commonly dogs; also cats. • Most commonly young animals; in published report age ranged from 5 months to 1.5 years. • No breed or sex predilections. • No genetic basis.

SIGNS

• Burns associated with gingiva, tongue, palate. • Singed hair or whiskers. • Most common clinical signs are related to acute dyspnea. • Coughing. • Tachypnea. • Orthopnea. • Increased respiratory effort. • Cyanosis. • Crackles during pulmonary auscultation. • Tachycardia. • Muscle tremors. • Tonic–clonic activity. • Collapse.

CAUSES & RISK FACTORS

• Chewing electric cord. • Young animals.

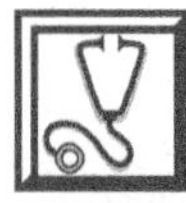

DIAGNOSIS

DIFFERENTIAL DIAGNOSIS

• Left-sided congestive heart failure due to congenital or acquired heart disease; the presence of cardiac murmur or dysrhythmia may help differentiate; however, dysrhythmias may be seen with electric cord injury. • Vitamin K antagonist, rodenticide intoxication history (pulmonary hemorrhage). • Thoracic trauma (pulmonary contusions)—history, thoracic radiographs. • Other causes of noncardiogenic pulmonary edema. • Pleural space disease—muffled lung sounds during auscultation, thoracic radiographs. • Thermal or chemical injuries—history, physical examination, thoracic radiographs. • Exposure to fire and smoke inhalation—history, physical examination. • Atypical pneumonia—history, physical examination, thoracic radiographs.

CBC/BIOCHEMISTRY/URINALYSIS

May help rule out other systemic causes of noncardiogenic pulmonary edema.

OTHER LABORATORY TESTS

Arterial blood gas analysis may be useful to document hypoxemia; this may be difficult to perform in unstable patients.

IMAGING

• Thoracic radiographs may help distinguish between cardiogenic and noncardiogenic causes of pulmonary edema. • Radiographic pattern is usually a generalized, mixed alveolar bronchial pattern; edema is often most notable in caudal dorsal lung fields. • Pulmonary venous congestion is absent with noncardiogenic pulmonary edema. • Echocardiography may help identify or rule out underlying cardiac disease.

DIAGNOSTIC PROCEDURES

• ECG—may help distinguish cardiogenic disease from noncardiogenic disease; however, dysrhythmias may be seen with electrocution and other causes of noncardiogenic pulmonary edema.

PATHOLOGIC FINDINGS

• Pink, frothy fluid in airways. • Fluid-filled, congested lungs. • Subendocardial and subepicardial petechiae. • Circumscribed, pale gray or tan oral lesions.

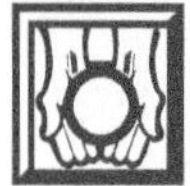

TREATMENT

• If patient is close to live wire, turn off electricity and/or remove patient to safe area. • Establish patent airway if patient is unconscious. • Oxygen supplementation. • Mechanical ventilation may be required. • Establish venous access.

MEDICATIONS

DRUG(S) OF CHOICE

• If in shock—treat with intravenous crystalloids (90 mL/kg/h in dog, 45–60 mL/kg/h in cat) or colloids (20 mL/kg in dogs, 5–10 mL/kg in cats). • If pulmonary edema is present—furosemide 2–4 mg/kg IV; this is controversial as this is a form of noncardiogenic pulmonary edema. • Anxiolytic therapy if dyspneic—butorphanol 0.1–0.2 mg/kg IV. • Corticosteroids have been employed, but are controversial and of unknown value. • Inotropic support if required. • Antiarrhythmic therapy if required. • Oral and cutaneous burns—treated symptomatically.

FOLLOW-UP

PATIENT MONITORING

• Patient should be monitored until stable. • Physical examination. • Monitor oral lesion; may prevent patient from eating. • ECG. • Central venous pressure. • Blood pressure. • Arterial blood gas. • Thoracic radiographs.

PREVENTION/AVOIDANCE

• Damaged electric cords should be discarded. • Avoid animal exposure to electric cords. • Follow child safety rules for a safe home.

POSSIBLE COMPLICATIONS

• Infected burn wounds can occur but are uncommon. • Oronasal fistula due to severe burns.

EXPECTED COURSE AND PROGNOSIS

• Prognosis based on response to therapy. • Pulmonary edema can develop as soon as 1 hour and as late as 36 hours after incident. • Pulmonary edema associated with electrocution is associated with high mortality (38.5%). • If patient survives first 24 hours, prognosis improves. • Resolution of pulmonary edema may take 3–5 days. • Most oral lesions resolve. • Inappetence related to oral lesions resolves.

MISCELLANEOUS

ASSOCIATED CONDITIONS

Cataracts have been reported in one dog 18 months after electrocution.

Suggested Reading

Brightman AH, Brogdon JD, Helper LC, Everds N. Electrical cataracts in the canine: a case report. J Am Anim Hosp Assoc 1984, 20:895–898.

Drobatz KJ, Saunders HM, Pugh CR, Hendricks JC. Noncardiogenic pulmonary edema in dogs and cats: 26 cases (1987–1995). J Am Vet Med Assoc 1995, 206:1732–1736.

Kolata RJ, Burrows CF. The clinical features of injury by chewing electrical cords in dogs and cats. J Am Anim Hosp Assoc 1981, 17:219–222.

Author Steven L. Marks

Consulting Editor Michael Aherne

ENAMEL HYPOPLASIA/HYPOCALCIFICATION

BASICS

OVERVIEW

- Enamel hypoplasia is the inadequate deposition of normal enamel matrix, affecting one or several teeth.
- The crowns can have areas of normal enamel next to hypoplastic or missing enamel.
- Apparent defect in enamel surfaces, often pitted and discolored; focal or generalized, due to disruption of normal enamel formation.
- Most cases are primarily aesthetic; some have extensive structural damage, even root involvement. The dentin is rarely exposed with hypoplasia.
- Enamel hypoplasia is less common than hypocalcification.
- Enamel hypocalcification refers to inadequate mineralization (calcification) of enamel, affecting several or all teeth. The crowns are covered by poorly formed, rough enamel that may easily be worn or flaked away and have light brown discoloration. There can be areas of normal enamel next to areas of abnormal enamel.
- Systemic influences during enamel formation (e.g., distemper, fever) over an extended time may cause generalized changes; local or focal influences (e.g., trauma, even from deciduous tooth extraction) over a short time may cause specific patterns or bands.
- Teeth may be more sensitive with exposed dentin, and occasionally fractures of severely compromised teeth occur; usually they remain fully functional.

SIGNALMENT

- Dogs and less commonly cats.
- Often apparent at time of tooth eruption (after 6 months of age) or shortly thereafter (with signs of wear).

SIGNS

Historical Findings

Discolored teeth.

Physical Examination Findings

- Irregular, pitted, or flaky enamel surface with discoloration of diseased enamel and potential exposure and staining of underlying dentin (light brown).
- Early or rapid accumulation of plaque and calculus on roughened tooth surface; possible gingivitis and/or accelerated periodontal disease.
- Teeth may fracture easily.
- Animals may show cold sensitivity (avoiding outdoor water or refrigerated food).

CAUSES & RISK FACTORS

- Insult during enamel formation.
- Canine distemper virus, fever, trauma (e.g., accidents, fractured deciduous tooth, excessive force during deciduous tooth extraction).

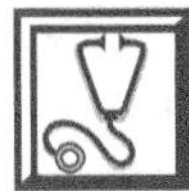

DIAGNOSIS

DIFFERENTIAL DIAGNOSIS

- Enamel staining—discolored but smooth surface (tetracycline).
- Carious lesions—cavities with decay.
- Amelogenesis imperfecta—genetic and/or developmental formation and maturation abnormalities other than hypomineralization.
- Tooth resorption—similar to that found in cats, also found in dogs.

CBC/BIOCHEMISTRY/URINALYSIS

- Usually normal.
- Appropriate preanesthetic diagnostic when indicated.

OTHER LABORATORY TESTS

N/A

IMAGING

- Intraoral radiographs are necessary to determine the structure and viability of roots.
- Cases reported of abnormal root formation, no root formation, or separated crown and root.

DIAGNOSTIC PROCEDURES

None

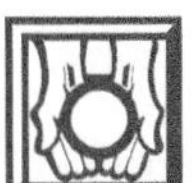

TREATMENT

- Treatment depends upon extent of lesions and equipment and materials available.
- Goal is to provide the smoothest surface possible.
- Enamel hypoplasia typically does not require treatment as the enamel is normal, just decreased in thickness. Enamel hypocalcification typically benefits from treatment.

Optimal Treatment

- Gently remove diseased enamel (enamel scrub) with white stone burs or finishing disks on high-speed handpiece (adequate water coolant).
- Take care not to damage the tooth—excess enamel/dentin removal; hyperthermic damage to pulp.
- Focal defects may be amenable to composite restoration; many restorative materials (bonding agents, composites) require use of light-curing units and appropriate skill levels.
- Bonding agent recommended to seal exposed dentinal tubules and protect surfaces.
- Extraction is recommended if the root is significantly malformed; extraction or root canal therapy if tooth is radiographically nonvital.

Alternative Treatment

- Soft, diseased enamel can sometimes be removed with ultrasonic scalers or hand instruments, but avoid excessive removal and hyperthermia.
- Fluoride treatment can be used to decrease sensitivity and enhance enamel strength.

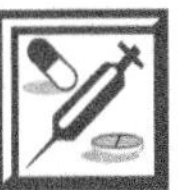

MEDICATIONS

DRUG(S) OF CHOICE

N/A

FOLLOW-UP

PATIENT MONITORING

Inform the owner that further degeneration of remaining enamel may occur, necessitating additional therapy in the future, or that affected teeth may become nonvital over time, requiring root canal therapy or extraction.

PREVENTION/AVOIDANCE

- Regular professional dental cleaning and a routine homecare program (brushing); may include weekly application of stannous fluoride at home (minimize ingestion because of toxicity).
- Avoid chewing on hard objects.

MISCELLANEOUS

INTERNET RESOURCES

https://avdc.org/avdc-nomenclature

Suggested Reading

Bittegeko SB, Arnbjerg J, Nkya R, Tevik A. Multiple dental developmental abnormalities following canine distemper infection. J Am Anim Hosp Assoc 1995, 31(1):42–45.

Lobprise HB, Dodd JR. Wiggs' Veterinary Dentistry Principles and Practice. Hoboken, NJ: Wiley-Blackwell, 2019.

Author Kristin M. Bannon

Consulting Editor Heidi B. Lobprise

ENCEPHALITIS

BASICS

DEFINITION

Inflammation of the brain with or without concurrent inflammation of the meninges and spinal cord.

PATHOPHYSIOLOGY

• Immune-mediated mechanism, usually of unknown triggering factor. • Infection of the brain.

SYSTEMS AFFECTED

• Nervous. • Multisystemic signs—usually seen if infectious cause.

INCIDENCE/PREVALENCE

Unknown

GEOGRAPHIC DISTRIBUTION

• Immune-mediated—worldwide.
• Infectious—varies depending on infectious agent distribution.

SIGNALMENT

Species

Dog and cat.

Breed Predilections

Immune Mediated

• Meningoencephalitis of unknown origin (MUO) can happen in any breed.
• Granulomatous meningoencephalitis (GME)—toy poodle and terrier. • Necrotizing meningoencephalitis (NME)—pug and chihuahua. • Necrotizing leukoencephalitis (NLE)—Yorkshire terrier and French bulldog.
• Eosinophilic meningoencephalitis (EME)—golden retriever and Rottweiler. • Idiopathic tremor syndrome—West Highland white terrier, Maltese. • Greyhound nonsuppurative meningoencephalitis—greyhound.

Infectious

• Pyogranulomatous meningoencephalomyelitis—pointer dogs. • Aspergillosis—German shepherd. • Protothecosis—boxer, collie.
• Cryptococcosis—American cocker spaniel.

Feline Infectious Peritonitis (FIP)

Burmese

Mean Age and Range

Immune Mediated

• Peak 3–7 years old; can happen at any age in dogs older than 4 months old. • GME—peak 4–8 years old. • NME and NLE—mean 2.5 years old (6 months–7 years). • Cats—mean 9 years old.

Infectious

Two peaks: <2 years and >8 years.

Predominant Sex

MUO—females slightly predisposed.

SIGNS

Historical Findings

• Immune mediated—acute to chronic onset and progression (days to months).
• Infectious—acute onset with rapid progression (days).

Physical Examination Findings

• Immune mediated—none. • Infectious—fever, lethargy, diffuse pain, ocular lesions, coughing, diarrhea.

Neurologic Examination Findings

• Rostral fossa—seizures, blindness, abnormal mentation, absent menace and nasal septum stimulation responses, delayed postural reactions. • Caudal fossa—lethargy, cranial nerve deficits, ataxia (proprioceptive, vestibular, and/or cerebellar), paresis. • Progression (e.g., anisocoria, pinpoint pupils, decreasing level of consciousness, poor physiologic nystagmus)—suggests increased intracranial pressure with potential brain herniation.

CAUSES

Dogs

• Idiopathic—MUO, GME, NME, NLE, EME, pyogranulomatous meningoencephalomyelitis, greyhound nonsuppurative meningoencephalitis, idiopathic tremor syndrome.
• Postvaccinal—distemper, rabies. • Viral—distemper, rabies, pseudorabies, herpesvirus, parvovirus, coronarivus, parainfluenza, West Nile virus, eastern, western and Venezuelan equine encephalomyelitis virus, *Bunyaviridae*, *Flaviviridae*. • Rickettsial—*Ehrlichia canis*, *Neorickettsia helminthoeca*, *Anaplasma phagocytophilum*, Rocky mountain spotted fever.
• Bacterial—aerobic, anaerobic, mycoplasma, mycobacterium. • Fungal—*Blastomyces*, *Histoplasma*, *Cryptococcus*, *Coccidioidomyces*, *Aspergillus*, *Phaeohyphomyces*. • Protozoal—*Toxoplasma*, *Neospora*. • Algal—*Prototheca*.
• Parasitic—sarcocystis, encephalitozoon, larva migrans (*Dirofilaria*, *Toxocara*, *Ancylostoma*, *Cuterebra*, *Baylisascaris*, *Cysticercus*), trypanosoma.

Cats

• Viral—FIP, rabies, feline immunodeficiency virus (FIV), pseudorabies, paramyxovirus, Borna disease virus, West Nile virus, *Bunyaviridae*. • Bacterial—aerobic, anaerobic, mycoplasma, mycobacterium. • Fungal—*Cryptococcus*, *Blastomyces*, *Histoplasma*, *Coccidioidomyces*. • Protozoal—*Toxoplasma*.
• Algal—*Prototheca*. • Parasitic—larva migrans (*Dirofilaria*, *Toxocara*, *Ancylostoma*, *Cuterebra*, *Baylisascaris*, *Cysticercus*). • Idiopathic—lymphohistiocytic meningoencephalomyelitis.

RISK FACTORS

• Immunosuppressive drugs and FIV or feline leukemia virus (FeLV) infection—infectious encephalitides. • FIP: recent stress, multicat environment. • Tick-infected areas—tick-borne rickettsial and viral infections. • Travel history—geographically localized infectious agents.

DIAGNOSIS

DIFFERENTIAL DIAGNOSIS

• Cerebrovascular accident—should not progress after 24 hours. • Congenital anomaly—primarily young animals.
• Trauma—usually reported in history.
• Metabolic encephalopathy—usually symmetric deficits, CBC/biochemistry abnormalities common. • Toxic—usually acute. • Neoplasia—signs may be similar; usually in older patients. • Degenerative—usually slow, progressive signs.

CBC/BIOCHEMISTRY/URINALYSIS

• Immune mediated—usually normal.
• Infectious—CBC: leukocytosis if systemic signs; distemper: lymphopenia; FIP: lymphopenia, anemia; rickettsial disease: anemia, thrombocytopenia; fungal/parasitic: occasionally eosinophilia; biochemistry: FIP: hyperglobulinemia; distemper: hyper/hypoglobulinemia; rickettsial disease: hyperglobulinemia; some fungal diseases: hypoalbuminemia, hyperglobulinemia, hypercalcemia; urinalysis: fungus rarely seen.

OTHER LABORATORY TESTS

• Serology—in serum or cerebrospinal fluid (CSF); available for fungal, protozoal, rickettsial, and viral diseases; may not differentiate exposed/vaccinated animals from active disease; antibodies appear 2–3 weeks after infection; immunoglobulin (Ig) M higher predictive positive value than IgG for *Toxoplasma*, preferred test for *Neospora*, low sensitivity/specificity for FIP. • Histology—postmortem; lacks specificity; may reveal specific inclusion bodies for viral infections (e.g., distemper, rabies). • Immunohistochemistry—postmortem; usually high sensitivity and specificity; best test to confirm FIP. • PCR—available for viral, fungal, rickettsial, protozoal diseases in blood and CSF; highly sensitive for distemper; low sensitivity but high specificity for FIP. • Culture—bacterial culture of CSF commonly unrewarding despite bacterial infection; fungal and viral culture unrewarding and potential zoonoses. • Urine galactomannan assay (ELISA)—high sensitivity and specificity for *Blastomyces*, *Aspergillus*, and *Histoplasma*.
• Blood/urine cultures—low sensitivity and specificity; may help discriminate agent in bacterial encephalitis and help in antibiotics choice. • Rabies—no premortem diagnostic test.

IMAGING

• Thoracic radiographs—may reveal fungal/toxoplasma infection or concurrent bacterial pneumonia. • Spine radiographs—may reveal concurrent fungal/bacterial discospondylitis.
• Brain MRI—shows focal/multifocal lesions.
• Brain CT—may show focal/multifocal brain lesions; less sensitive and specific than MRI

DIAGNOSTIC PROCEDURES

• CSF cytology—used to confirm inflammation; may be normal if meninges not affected. ○ Immune mediated—increased protein and cellular content (lymphocytes and/or macrophages), increased eosinophils in EME; predominantly neutrophilic in some cases. ○ Viral—predominantly lymphocytic. ○ Bacterial—predominantly degenerated neutrophils. ○ Fungal—mixed inflammation.

• Infectious agent rarely seen (except *Cryptococcus*).

PATHOLOGIC FINDINGS

Findings depend on specific type of immune-mediated inflammation (e.g., granulomatous, necrotic) and infectious agent.

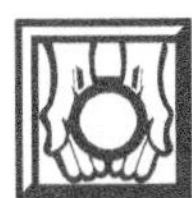

TREATMENT

APPROPRIATE HEALTH CARE

Inpatient medical management—may require initial intensive care management if elevated intracranial pressure.

NURSING CARE

• Increased intracranial pressure—hypertonic saline, mannitol, dexamethasone. • Anti-seizure treatment—diazepam, phenobarbital, levetiracetam in boluses or CRI. • Analgesic medication—necessary if painful from associated meningitis: opioids, gabapentin. • Nursing care for nonambulatory patients—bedding, switching sides, physiotherapy.

ACTIVITY

As tolerated.

DIET

No oral intake if unable to swallow, e.g., depressed, dysphagia, vomiting.

CLIENT EDUCATION

Relapse possible with both immune-mediated and infectious encephalitis.

SURGICAL CONSIDERATIONS

Brain biopsy—may be needed in specific cases.

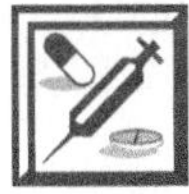

MEDICATIONS

DRUG(S) OF CHOICE

• Apply specific therapy once diagnosis is reached or highly suspected. • Immune mediated—prednisone/prednisolone 2 mg/kg/day until most of recovery achieved (usually 1–2 weeks), then tapered progressively each month over 6 months; initially, dexamethasone 0.25 mg/kg q24h can be given IV. • Viral—no specific: treat symptomatically. • Bacterial—broad-spectrum IV antibiotics initially (e.g., fluoroquinolones + amoxicillin/clavulanate); continue PO depending on sensitivity or with broad-spectrum if agent unknown. • Fungal—itraconazole (*Aspergillus*), fluconazole (may be preferred if intra-axial), amphotericin B, voriconazole. • Protozoal—clindamycin, trimethoprim/sulfamides. • Rickettsial—doxycycline. • Parasitic—ivermectin, albendazole.

CONTRAINDICATIONS

• Prednisone not to be used more than a few days if infectious. • Puppies <6 months of age—doxycycline contraindicated. • Puppies <8 months of age—enrofloxacin contra-indicated. • Cats - ocular toxicity with enrofloxacin > 5mg/kg/day.

POSSIBLE INTERACTIONS

Prior corticosteroid treatment may alter MRI and CSF results and decrease chance of diagnosis.

ALTERNATIVE DRUG(S)

• Some patients may have better response if treated with prednisone plus another immunosuppressive drug compared to prednisone alone; no increased benefits of using 3 or more drugs; second immunosuppressive drug progressively tapered once prednisone dose is 0.5 mg/kg/day. • Cytosine arabinoside—first administration IV CRI 100 mg/m^2/24h for 24–48h, then 100 mg/m^2 IV CRI over 8–24h every 3 weeks for 6 months; time between administration progressively lengthened thereafter; SC injection protocol exists but likely less efficient. • Azathioprine—2 mg/kg PO q24h. • Cyclosporine—5–10 mg/kg PO q12h. • Mycophenolate—10–20 mg/kg PO q12h. • Leflunomide—2–4 mg/kg PO q24h. • Radiation therapy—reported.

FOLLOW-UP

PATIENT MONITORING

• Frequent neurologic evaluations in first 48–72 hours to monitor progress. • Recheck CBC/biochemistry every month initially and then every 3–6 months while on immunosuppressive therapy. • Relapse as medication is withdrawn—chance of relapse increased if abnormal recheck MRI and CSF before stopping treatment. • Stop treatment for fungal diseases when antigen titers negative.

PREVENTION/AVOIDANCE

• Avoid outdoor roaming and use effective tick control in endemic areas. • No definitive association between immune-mediated encephalitis and vaccination.

POSSIBLE COMPLICATIONS

• General anesthesia and CSF collection—contraindicated in unstable patients with increased intracranial pressure.
• Immunosuppressive drugs—predispose to infections. • Long-term corticosteroid therapy—signs of iatrogenic hyperadrenocorticism and related side effects. • Increased intracranial pressure—poor prognosis factor, increased chance of death early in course of disease.

EXPECTED COURSE AND PROGNOSIS

• Resolution progressive—2–8 weeks.
• Rickettsial, bacterial, protozoal—fair chance of survival if treated early. • Fungal, algal, viral—almost always fatal. • Immune mediated—necrotic encephalitis has worse prognosis. • Idiopathic tremor syndrome—excellent prognosis with complete resolution.

MISCELLANEOUS

ZOONOTIC POTENTIAL

• Rabies—consider in endemic areas if patient is outdoor animal that has rapidly progressive encephalitis. • Humans may be infected by the same vector tick that affected the patient.
• Exudates and diagnostic samples from animals with mycosis can be contagious.

SYNONYMS

• Meningoencephalitis of unknown etiology (MUE). • Idiopathic tremor syndrome—white shaker syndrome.

SEE ALSO

• Seizures (Convulsions, Status Epilepticus)—Cats.
• Seizures (Convulsions, Status Epilepticus)—Dogs.
• Stupor and Coma.
• Vestibular Disease, Geriatric—Dogs.
• Vestibular Disease, Idiopathic—Cats.

ABBREVIATIONS

• CSF = cerebrospinal fluid. • EME = eosinophilic meningoencephalitis. • FeLV = feline leukemia virus. • FIP = feline infectious peritonitis. • FIV = feline immunodeficiency virus. • GME = granulomatous meningoencephalitis. • Ig = immunoglobulin. • MUE = meningoencephalitis of unknown etiology.
• MUO = meningoencephalitis of unknown origin. • NLE = necrotizing leukoencephalitis.
• NME = necrotizing meningoencephalitis.

Suggested Reading

Bentley RT, Taylor AR, Thomovsky SA. Fungal infections of the central nervous system in small animals. Vet Clin North Am Small Anim Pract 2018, 48:63–83.
Coates JR, Jeffery ND. Perspectives on meningoencephalomyelitis of unknown origin. Vet Clin North Am Small Anim Pract 2014, 44:1157–1185.
Cornelis I, Van Ham L, Gielen I, et al. Clinical presentation, diagnostic findings, prognostic factors, treatment and outcome in dogs with meningoencephalomyelitis of unknown origin: a review. Vet J 2019, 244:37–44.
Sykes JE, Greene CE. Infectious Diseases of the Dog and Cat, 4th ed. St. Louis, MO: Elsevier Health Sciences, 2011.

Author Thomas Parmentier

Acknowledgment The author and book editors acknowledge the prior contribution of Allen Franklin Sisson.

Client Education Handout available online

ENCEPHALITIS SECONDARY TO PARASITIC MIGRATION

BASICS

E

OVERVIEW

- Aberrant parasitic migration into the CNS.
- Parasites usually affect another organ system of the same host (e.g., *Dirofilaria immitis*, *Taenia*, *Ancylostoma caninum*, *Angiostrongylus*, or *Toxocara canis*) or a different host species (e.g., raccoon roundworm, *Baylisascaris procyonis*; skunk roundworm, *B. columnaris*; *Coenurus* spp.; or *Cysticercus cellulosae*).
- Access to CNS—hematogenously (dirofilariasis) or through adjacent tissues, including the middle ear, skull foramina, cribriform plate through nasal cavities, or open fontanelles (cuterebraiasis).

SIGNALMENT

- Dirofilariasis—adult animals only.
- Other parasites—young dogs and cats with access to outdoors: rare and sporadic occurrence.

SIGNS

- Vary with the portion of CNS affected.
- Likely asymmetric.
- May suggest a focal mass lesion or a multifocal disease process.
- Cuterebriasis—seasonal (July–October) acute or peracute onset of behavior changes, seizures, visual deficits, etc.; previous history of respiratory disease is common.
- Rat parasite, *Angiostrongylus cantonensis* (Australia)—lumbosacral syndrome (hind limbs, tail, and bladder paralysis/paresis) in puppies that may ascend to thoracic limbs and cranial nerves.

CAUSES & RISK FACTORS

Housing in a cage previously occupied by wildlife (raccoons, skunks).

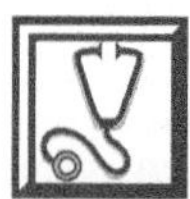

DIAGNOSIS

DIFFERENTIAL DIAGNOSIS

- Rule out other causes of focal encephalopathy—infectious diseases (viral, bacterial, protozoan, or fungal); granulomatous meningoencephalomyelitis; brain tumor.
- Diagnosis often made on necropsy.

CBC/BIOCHEMISTRY/URINALYSIS

Normal unless the parasite also affects non-neural tissues.

OTHER LABORATORY TESTS

Cerebrospinal fluid (CSF)—may show eosinophilic, neutrophilic, or mononuclear pleocytosis (also found in protozoal, fungal, and prototheca encephalitides); may be normal (strictly parenchymal lesions).

IMAGING

CT or MRI—brain; focal lesion and/or cerebral infarction from occlusion of cerebral vessels. Nonspecific and often inconclusive, but could lead to surgical exploration and removal of migrating parasite.

PATHOLOGIC FINDINGS

- The parasite or its tracts may or may not be identified.
- Infarction, vascular rupture, and hemorrhage or vascular emboli may cause local to extensive necrosis and malacia; there may be granulomatous proliferation or/and obstructive hydrocephalus.
- *Dirofilaria immitis*—intravascular or extravascular.
- Worms produce focal inflammation.
- Cuterebriasis is the suspected cause of feline ischemic encephalopathy.

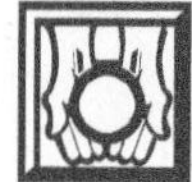

TREATMENT

- Surgical removal of intracranial cuterebra.
- Parasiticides (see below) could potentiate illness.
- Supportive and nursing care.

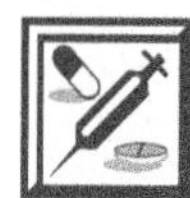

MEDICATIONS

DRUG(S) OF CHOICE

- Dirofilariasis and neural angiostrongylosis—anthelmintic treatment may cause worsening of signs and sometimes death.
- Mild neural angiostrongylosis—puppies may recover with supportive care and corticosteroid therapy.
- A single dose of ivermectin (400 mg/kg SC) may kill cuterebra larvae in cats with suspected cuterebriasis; pretreatment with diphenhydramine (4 mg/kg) and intravenous dexamethasone (0.1 mg/kg) may mitigate allergic/anaphylactic reactions to dead or dying larvae.
- Treat inflammation and secondary infections—corticosteroids/nonsteroidal anti-inflammatory drugs (NSAIDs), antibiotics.

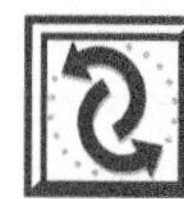

FOLLOW-UP

PATIENT MONITORING

As necessary.

PREVENTION/AVOIDANCE

- Keep pets indoors or/and segregated from wildlife.
- Use preventive anthelmintics and dirofilaricides.

EXPECTED COURSE AND PROGNOSIS

Acute or insidious onset, then usually progressive.

MISCELLANEOUS

SEE ALSO

- Encephalitis.
- Feline Ischemic Encephalopathy.
- Heartworm Disease—Cats.
- Heartworm Disease—Dogs.

ABBREVIATIONS

- CSF = cerebrospinal fluid.
- NSAID = nonsteroidal anti-inflammatory drug.

Suggested Reading

Braund KG. Neurovascular disorders. In: Vite CH, ed., Clinical Neurology in Small Animals—Localization, Diagnosis and Treatment. Ithaca, NY: IVIS, 2003. https://www.ivis.org/library/braunds-clinical-neurology-small-animals-localization-diagnosis-and-treatment/neurovascular

Dewey CW. Verminous encephalitis. In: Dewey CW, ed., A Practical Guide to Canine and Feline Neurology, 2nd ed. Ames, IA: Wiley-Blackwell, 2008, pp. 184–185.

Glass EN, Cornetta AM, deLahunta A, et al. Clinical and clinicopathologic features in 11 cats with Cuterebra Larvae myiasis of the central nervous system. J Vet Intern Med 1998, 12:365–368.

James FMK, Poma R. Neurological manifestations of feline cuterebriasis. Can Vet J 2010, 51:213–215.

Vite CH. Inflammatory diseases of the central nervous system. In: Vite CH, ed., Clinical Neurology in Small Animals—Localization, Diagnosis and Treatment. Ithaca, NY: IVIS, 2005.

Williams KJ, Summers BA, de Lahunta A. Cerebrospinal cuterebriasis in cats and its association with feline ischemic encephalopathy. Vet Pathol 1998, 35:330–343.

Author Christine F. Berthelin-Baker

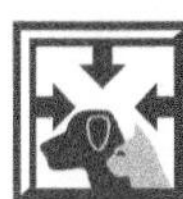

BASICS

DEFINITION

The invasion of the cardiac endocardium, usually the valves, by infectious agents. Usually Gram-positive bacteria, especially staphylococci or streptococci. Occasionally *Rickettsia* or *Bartonella* in dogs. Rarely fungi in dogs. Culture-negative cases may be due to *Bartonella* or fungi (e.g., *Aspergillus*). Less likely due to *Brucella, Coxiella, Corynebacterium*, and *Chlamydia*.

PATHOPHYSIOLOGY

• Bacteremia from various portals of entry; bacteria invade and colonize the heart valves—usually the aortic, occasionally the mitral, and rarely the tricuspid and pulmonic valves. • Endocardial ulceration exposes collagen causing platelet aggregation, activation of the coagulation cascade, and formation of vegetations. • Vegetations on heart valves are composed of an inner layer of platelets, fibrin, red blood cells, and bacteria; a middle layer of bacteria; and an outer layer of fibrin. • Valvular insufficiency develops in virtually all patients; aortic insufficiency almost invariably leads to intractable left-sided congestive heart failure (CHF) within weeks to several months. • CHF is less frequent and latent when only the mitral valve is affected. • Vegetative lesions may dislodge causing infarction or metastatic infection to any organ; organs commonly infected include the spleen, kidneys, brain, and skeletal muscles.

SYSTEMS AFFECTED

• Cardiovascular—valvular insufficiency; arrhythmias, myocarditis. • Nervous—para/tetraparesis; cranial nerve deficits; abnormal mentation. • Hemic/lymphatic/immune—hypercoagulation; disseminated intravascular coagulation. • Musculoskeletal—septic or immune-mediated polyarthropathy; hypertrophic osteopathy; discospondylitis. • Renal/urologic—renal infarction; immune-mediated glomerulonephritis; urinary tract infections.
• Respiratory—pulmonary edema and/or emboli.

SIGNALMENT

Species

Dog; rarely cat.

Breed Predilections

• Medium to large breeds. • Breeds predisposed to subaortic stenosis (SAS).

Mean Age and Range

Most affected dogs are 4–8 years of age; infection can occur at any age.

Predominant Sex

Most studies report male predominance—may be as great as 2 : 1.

SIGNS

General Comments

• Gram-negative bacteremia results in peracute or acute signs; Gram-positive bacteremia results in subacute or chronic clinical signs. • Systemic signs secondary to infarction, infection (inflammation), toxemia, or immune-mediated damage; usually override cardiac signs.

Historical Findings

• Infectious disease involving skin, oral, gastrointestinal (GI), or genital tracts (e.g., prostatitis). • Predisposing factors—immunosuppressive drug therapy, SAS, recent surgery, infected wound, abscess, pyoderma, or recent implantation of cardiovascular device (i.e., pacemaker, Amplatz® canine ductal occluder). • Presenting complaints include lethargy, paresis, fever, anorexia, GI disturbance, and lameness; in cats, cardiac decompensation and/or locomotor abnormalities are common presenting complaints.

Physical Examination Findings

• Usually diverse and misleading—the "great imitator." • Pyrexia and general malaise.
• Dyspnea due to CHF. • Arrhythmias (ventricular, supraventricular, or heart block).
• Single or shifting leg lameness. • Systolic heart murmur. • "To-and-fro" murmur—associated with aortic valve vegetation causing systolic turbulence and diastolic regurgitation.
• Diastolic murmur with hyperdynamic femoral pulses are a strong indication of advanced aortic endocarditis.

CAUSES

• Bacterial infection associated with oral cavity, bone, prostate, skin, and other sites.
• Invasive diagnostic or surgical procedures causing bacteremia.

RISK FACTORS

• SAS. • Immunosuppression from long-term or high-dose corticosteroids, neoplasia, or cytotoxic drug administration.

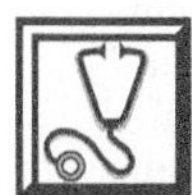

DIAGNOSIS

DIFFERENTIAL DIAGNOSIS

• Bacteremia of any cause. • Polysystemic, immune-mediated disorders. • Left-sided CHF caused by dilated cardiomyopathy or SAS.

CBC/BIOCHEMISTRY/URINALYSIS

• Inflammatory leukogram (i.e., neutrophilia, left shift, and monocytosis)—patients with chronic, relatively inactive, or walled-off infection may have normal or nearly normal leukogram; those with chronic infection may have mature neutrophilia with monocytosis.
• Nonregenerative anemia.
• Thrombocytopenia—variable severity.
• Low-normal or low albumin, low-normal or low glucose, and high serum alkaline phosphatase/bilirubin activity are inconsistently associated with sepsis (septic triad). • Renal azotemia—secondary to renal emboli, pyelonephritis, and/or hypovolemia-induced renal failure.
• Proteinuria caused by septic emboli, immune-mediated glomerulonephritis, or renal infarction; hematuria, pyuria, and granular casts associated with pyelonephritis.

OTHER LABORATORY TESTS

• Blood culture—three samples taken at least 1 hour apart over 24 hours; at least two should yield the same microbe; both aerobic and anaerobic cultures recommended; antibiotic removal systems available for diagnosis of patients given antibiotics. • PCR with bacterial 16s primers, in combination with blood culture, increases likelihood of identification of bacteremia. • Culture-negative bacteremia often due to prior antibiotic administration or fastidious microbes, especially *Bartonella*.
• Catheter tips—culture. • Urine culture (not a substitute for blood culture)—easy; often positive; does not necessarily incriminate the urinary tract as the source of infection. • Tests for prostate, kidney, and bone infection may be warranted. • Positive antinuclear antibody, lupus erythematosus, rheumatoid factor, and Coombs' test results occasionally found—nonspecific; tend to confound the diagnosis.
• Bartonella alpha-Proteobacteria growth medium (BAPGM) and PCR—for *Bartonella*.

IMAGING

Radiography

Left cardiomegaly; rarely, calcification of one or more heart valves.

Echocardiography

Best test—vegetative aortic endocarditis easily discerned; mitral valve infection may be difficult to differentiate from degenerative valve disease; hyperechoic with chronicity.

DIAGNOSTIC PROCEDURES

Arthrocentesis

Joint taps for cytology and culture—cytology usually does not differentiate septic from immune-mediated arthritis; either, though usually not septic, can exist with infective endocarditis; usually nondegenerate neutrophils regardless of cause.

ECG

• May be normal; occasionally reflects left cardiomegaly; often detects ventricular tachyarrhythmias; occasionally heart block of variable severity or supraventricular tachyarrhythmias. • Heart block suggests aortic valve involvement with infection or infarction of the adjacent septum.

PATHOLOGIC FINDINGS

• Cardiomegaly, almost always left sided when present. • Vegetations and thrombi on one or more valves. • Infection, hemorrhage, and infarction of adjacent myocardium.
• Renal infarcts usually present. • Primary or secondary sites of infection, especially

ENDOCARDITIS, INFECTIVE (CONTINUED)

kidneys and spleen. • Pulmonary hemorrhage or edema.

E

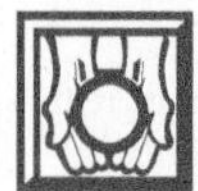

TREATMENT

Early index of suspicion with aggressive, rapid diagnostic testing, followed by appropriate treatment are imperative for cure. Cure is a reasonable expectation when mitral valve (alone) endocarditis is identified early in its course and treatment is aggressive.

NURSING CARE

• Aggressive fluid therapy—overt or impending CHF limits fluid volumes that can be administered; this problem is virtually insurmountable in patients with concomitant renal failure. • Imminent CHF—provide no more than maintenance volumes of fluid; alternate 5% dextrose in water (D5W) with lactated Ringer's solution (LRS; or 2.5% dextrose in half-strength LRS); potassium supplementation usually required.

CLIENT EDUCATION

Guarded prognosis if only mitral valve involved. Grave prognosis if aortic valve is involved.

MEDICATIONS

DRUG(S) OF CHOICE

Treatment variable—depends on severity of sepsis and presence or absence of CHF.

Antibiotics

• Backbone of treatment but usually do not eradicate infection before irreversible aortic valve damage occurs; more than minimal damage to the aortic valve is life-threatening because aortic insufficiency tends to be a lethal complication. • High-dose IV administration of bactericidal antibiotics is imperative and recommended for as long as feasible (at least 1 week), followed by SC administration for 1 or more weeks. • Oral administration—recommended only after at least 4 weeks of injectable therapy and at least 1 week after hematologic and clinical signs of infection and inflammation have disappeared; long-term (>4 months) treatment may be required to eradicate the infection from vegetations. • Selection determined by both urgency of septic complications and results of bacterial culture; coagulase-positive staphylococci and streptococci are most often incriminated, so choices can be logically made before culture results are obtained.
• Coagulase-positive staphylococci—usually resistant to penicillin, hetacillin, amoxicillin, and ampicillin. • Streptococci—often resistant to aminoglycosides and fluoroquinolones. • Gram-negative bacteria—often sensitive to third-generation cephalosporins, fluoroquinolones, and aminoglycosides. • *Bartonella*—only aminoglycosides appear bactericidal; can try doxycycline, fluoroquinolone, rifampin, or azithromycin. • First-generation cephalosporins—reasonable choice for stable patients until culture results are obtained. • Treat life-threatening sepsis immediately with drug combinations; pending culture results, one of three regimens is recommended: ○ Penicillin, ampicillin, ticarcillin, or a first-generation cephalosporin is combined with an aminoglycoside; aminoglycosides are not good choices for animals with overt or impending CHF or those with renal azotemia; gentamicin (2 mg/kg q8h) is recommended for only 5–10 days because of renal toxicity; a fluoroquinolone may be substituted for an aminoglycoside.
○ Clindamycin (2–10 mg/kg IV q8h) plus enrofloxacin (10 mg/kg q24h given diluted 1 : 1 in sterile water and injected slowly over 15–20 min). ○ Advanced-generation cephalosporins or ticarcillin–clavulanic acid (Timentin®)—high dosages, but only normal dosages if patient has renal failure.

Treatment of CHF

• Pimobendan, angiotensin-converting enzyme inhibitor, spironolactone, and furosemide (± amlodipine) indicated for patients with overt or impending CHF.
• Oxygen, high-dose furosemide—2–8 mg/kg IV (± nitroglycerin and/or hydralazine 1–2 mg/kg q12h) for patients with acute, severe pulmonary edema.

CONTRAINDICATIONS

• Avoid antibiotics that cannot penetrate fibrin (e.g., sulfonamides). • Corticosteroids.

ALTERNATIVE DRUG(S)

• Anticoagulant therapy—controversial in the prevention of embolization; heparin not recommended in human medicine as it increases risk of hemorrhage. • Aspirin (5–7 mg/kg PO q24h) and/or dalteparin (100 U/kg SC q8h) and/or clopidogrel (2–4 mg/kg PO q24h)—may reduce bacterial dissemination and embolization.

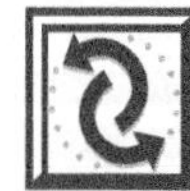

FOLLOW-UP

PATIENT MONITORING

• Emergence of antibiotic resistance—relapsing fever and inflammatory leukogram; imperative to adjust treatment based on culture results. • Frequent examination and CBC after discharge. • Repeat blood cultures 1 week after antibiotics are discontinued or if fever recurs.

PREVENTION/AVOIDANCE

• Indwelling catheters—restrict to appropriate indications; aseptic placement; replace within 3–5 days. • Administer antibiotics to dogs with moderate to severe SAS during dentistry or "dirty" procedures.
• Avoid careless use of corticosteroids.

POSSIBLE COMPLICATIONS

• CHF. • Renal failure. • Septic embolization of many tissues and organs. • Persistent or latent immune-mediated polyarthropathy.

EXPECTED COURSE AND PROGNOSIS

• Best prognosis associated with short history of bacteremia, rapid diagnosis, and aggressive treatment; given that diagnosis is often delayed in cats, prognosis is often grave.
• Mortality relatively higher in animals recently given corticosteroids. • Grave prognosis for patients with aortic valve endocarditis. • Patients with mitral valve endocarditis can be saved with appropriate treatment. • Latent CHF can occur with advanced, late diagnosis, or inadequate treatment for mitral valve endocarditis.

MISCELLANEOUS

ASSOCIATED CONDITIONS

Congenital heart defects (usually SAS) in some animals.

SYNONYMS

• Bacterial endocarditis. • Vegetative endocarditis.

SEE ALSO

• Bartonellosis. • Congestive Heart Failure, Left-Sided. • Discospondylitis. • Prostatitis and Prostatic Abscess. • Sepsis and Bacteremia.

ABBREVIATIONS

• BAPGM = Bartonella alpha-Proteobacteria growth medium. • CHF = congestive heart failure. • D5W = 5% dextrose in water.
• GI = gastrointestinal. • LRS = lactated Ringer's solution. • SAS = subaortic stenosis.

Suggested Reading

Calvert C, Thomason J. Cardiovascular infections. In: Greene CE, ed., Infectious Diseases of the Dog and Cat. St. Louis, MO: Saunders Elsevier, 2012: 912–936.

Palerme JS, Jones AE, Ward JL, et al. Infective endocarditis in 13 Cats. J Vet Cardiol 2016, 18:213–225.

Author Justin D. Thomason

Consulting Editor Michael Aherne

Acknowledgment The author and book editors acknowledge the prior contribution of Clay A. Calvert

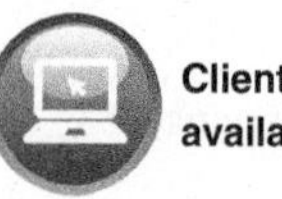

Client Education Handout available online

ENDOMYOCARDIAL DISEASES—CATS

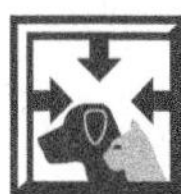

BASICS

OVERVIEW

- Endomyocarditis—acute cardiopulmonary disease that typically develops following a stressful event; characterized by interstitial pneumonia and endomyocardial inflammation; pneumonia is usually severe and commonly causes death; one report recorded the incidence of endomyocarditis at postmortem to be equivalent to that of hypertrophic cardiomyopathy.
- Endocardial fibroelastosis—congenital heart disease in which severe fibrous endocardial thickening leads to heart failure secondary to diastolic and systolic failure.
- Excessive moderator bands (EMBs)—a rare and unique pathologic disease; moderator bands are normal muscular bands in the right ventricle, but they can sometimes occur in the left ventricle.

SIGNALMENT

- Cats.
- Endomyocarditis—predominantly males (62%) age 1–4 years.
- Endocardial fibroelastosis—early development of biventricular or left heart failure, usually prior to 6 months of age.
- EMBs—can be seen in any age of cat.

SIGNS

Historical Findings

Endomyocarditis

- Dyspnea following a stressful event in a young, healthy cat.
- Respiratory signs usually occur 5–21 days after the stressor.
- In one report, 73% of cases presented between August and September.

Endocardial Fibroelastosis and EMBs

- Lethargy, weakness, collapse, syncope.
- Poor appetite and weight loss.
- Dyspnea.
- Tachypnea.
- Cyanosis.
- Abdominal distention.
- Paresis or paralysis; signs of thromboembolic disease.

Physical Examination Findings

Endomyocarditis

- Severe dyspnea.
- Occasional crackles.
- May have murmur or gallop; murmur may vary in intensity.
- May have evidence of thromboembolic disease.
- Typically no significant abnormalities prior to the stressful event.

Endocardial Fibroelastosis and EMBs

- Gallop.
- Systolic murmur, possible mitral regurgitation.
- Dyspnea and increased lung sounds or crackles.
- Paresis or paralysis with weak or absent femoral pulses.
- Arrhythmias possible.

CAUSES & RISK FACTORS

- Cause unknown for all three diseases.
- Risk factors for endomyocarditis include stressful incidents such as anesthesia (commonly associated with neutering or declawing), vaccination, relocation, or bathing.
- Endocardial fibroelastosis may be familial in Burmese and Siamese cats.
- Appearance of EMBs in a young cat would suggest a congenital malformation.

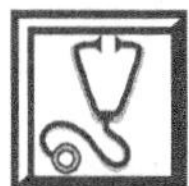

DIAGNOSIS

DIFFERENTIAL DIAGNOSIS

Other Causes of Cardiac Disease

- Hypertrophic cardiomyopathy.
- Unclassified cardiomyopathy.
- Restrictive cardiomyopathy.
- Dilated cardiomyopathy.
- Congenital heart malformations.

Other Causes of Dyspnea

- Other forms of cardiac disease as above.
- Primary respiratory disease.
- Pleural space disease.
- Mediastinal disorders, infection, trauma, neoplasia.
- Hemoglobin disorders, anemia, methemoglobinemia, causes of central cyanosis.

Other Causes of Collapse, Weakness, or Syncope

- Arrhythmias.
- Neurologic or musculoskeletal disease.
- Metabolic disease or electrolyte disorders.
- Other forms of paresis or paralysis.
- Arterial thromboembolism secondary to any form of cardiac disease or neoplasia.
- Neurologic or musculoskeletal disease.
- Neoplasia.

CBC/BIOCHEMISTRY/URINALYSIS

Not diagnostic.

OTHER LABORATORY TESTS

N/A

IMAGING

Thoracic Radiographic Findings for All Three Diseases

- Cardiomegaly.
- Interstitial or alveolar infiltrates or pleural effusion if congestion has developed.

Echocardiographic Findings

Endomyocarditis

- Normal to mildly large left atrium.
- Left ventricular wall thickness can be normal to mildly thick (0.6–0.7 cm).
- Hyperechoic endomyocardium reported—incidence seems to vary and is subjective; in one report it was as high as 86%.

Endocardial Fibroelastosis

- Limited data available.
- Reduced left ventricular function and enlarged left atrium.

EMBs

Many findings can overlap with restrictive cardiomyopathy. A network of false tendons can sometimes be imaged with 2D echocardiography.

DIAGNOSTIC PROCEDURES

ECG Findings

- Endomyocarditis—sinus tachycardia common; ventricular premature complexes, atrial premature complexes, bundle branch block, and complete atrioventricular (AV) block reported.
- Endocardial fibroelastosis—evidence for left-sided enlargement; sinus rhythm typically present, but various arrhythmias possible.
- EMBs—various electrocardiographic findings have been reported: AV block, sinus bradycardia, right bundle branch block, and left axis deviation.

PATHOLOGIC FINDINGS

Endomyocarditis

- Interstitial pneumonia.
- Left heart enlargement and opacity of the left ventricular endomyocardium with foci of hemorrhage; fibroplasia of the endocardium is striking.
- Varying degrees of endomyocardial inflammation with infiltrates of neutrophils, lymphocytes, plasma cells, histiocytes, and macrophages seen histologically.

Endocardial Fibroelastosis

- Left ventricular and atrial dilation with severe diffuse white opaque thickening of the endocardium.
- Diffuse hypocellular, fibroelastic thickening of the endomyocardium; prominent endomyocardial edema with dilation of lymphatics.

EMBs

Changes typically include an irregular left ventricular endocardial contour with a rounded apex and numerous irregular left ventricular false tendons; heart weight can be greater than normal; the moderator bands are composed of central Purkinje fibers and collagen.

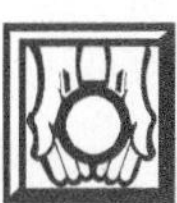

TREATMENT

Endomyocarditis

- No single therapy protocol to date.
- Small percentage of cats have survived; these cats do not require long-term therapy.

ENDOMYOCARDIAL DISEASES—CATS (CONTINUED)

E

- Supportive care with oxygen and possibly ventilation.

Endocardial Fibroelastosis and EMBs

- Oxygen therapy via cage delivery is least stressful.
- Thoracocentesis if pleural effusion.

MEDICATIONS

DRUG(S) OF CHOICE

Endomyocarditis

Steroids, furosemide, and vasodilators have been tried, but efficacy is unknown.

Endocardial Fibroelastosis and EMBs with Acute Congestive Heart Failure (CHF)

- Parenteral administration of furosemide 0.5–1 mg/kg IV/IM q1–6h.
- Dermal application of 2% nitroglycerin ointment one-eighth to one-fourth inch q4–6h has been suggested but is of unknown efficacy.
- Arrhythmias may resolve with stabilization. If there is rapid atrial fibrillation (heart rate >200), a calcium channel blocker or beta blocker can be considered to control the ventricular response. If there is dilated cardiomyopathy, digoxin may be a better choice for controlling the atrial fibrillation rate. For other supraventricular (SV) arrhythmias and ventricular arrhythmias, waiting for a response to heart failure therapy may be wise before starting antiarrhythmic therapy.
- Intractable edema—nitroprusside 1–5 μg/kg/min may be helpful.

Chronic CHF

- Treat as other CHF, with furosemide and angiotensin-converting enzyme inhibitors (e.g., enalapril, benazepril).
- Digoxin can be added for SV arrhythmia control when patient is stable and eating.

CONTRAINDICATIONS

N/A

FOLLOW-UP

EXPECTED COURSE AND P ROGNOSIS

- Endomyocarditis—poor, although some animals survive; animals that survive respiratory phase may progress to left ventricular endocardial fibrosis.
- Endocardial fibroelastosis and EMBs—medical treatment of CHF may prolong life, but recovery is unlikely.

MISCELLANEOUS

ASSOCIATED CONDITIONS

- Aortic thromboembolism.
- Relationship possible between endomyocarditis and left ventricular endocardial fibrosis.

SEE ALSO

- Aortic Thromboembolism.
- Congestive Heart Failure, Left-Sided.
- Congestive Heart Failure, Right-Sided.
- Myocarditis.

ABBREVIATIONS

- AV = atrioventricular.
- CHF = congestive heart failure.
- EMB = excessive moderator band.
- SV= supraventricular.

Suggested Reading

Bossbaly MB, Stalis I, Knight D, Van Winkle T. Feline endomyocarditis: a clinical/pathological study of 44 cases. Proceedings of the 12th ACVIM Forum, 1994, p. 975.

Liu S, Tilley LP. Excessive moderator bands in the left ventricle of 21 cats. JAVMA 1982, 180:1215–1219.

Stalis IH, Bossbaly MJ, Van Winkle TJ. Feline endomyocarditis and left ventricular endocardial fibrosis. Vet Pathol 1995, 32(2):122–126.

Wray JD, Gajanayake I, Smith SH. Congestive heart failure associated with a large transverse left ventricular moderator band in a cat. J Feline Med Surg 2007, 9:56–60.

Author Carl D. Sammarco

Consulting Editors Michael Aherne

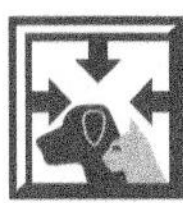

BASICS

OVERVIEW

- Inversion or rolling in of eyelid margin, resulting in frictional irritation of cornea and/or conjunctiva from contact with outer surface of eyelid.
- May result in keratitis, corneal ulceration, or corneal perforation.
- Can be conformational/congenital (primary) or acquired (secondary).
- Severe corneal disease may threaten vision.

SIGNALMENT

- Common in dogs—seen in chow chow, Chinese Shar-Pei, Norwegian elkhound, sporting breeds (e.g., spaniel, retriever), brachycephalic breeds, toy breeds, and giant breeds; age—puppies as early as 2–6 weeks old; usually identified in dogs <1 year old.
- Cats—usually in brachycephalic breeds, in young cats due to chronic ocular surface disease, and older animals due to retrobulbar fat loss.

SIGNS

- Mild, medial—chronic epiphora and medial pigmentary keratitis (toy dogs and brachycephalic dogs and cats).
- Mild, lateral—chronic mucoid to mucopurulent ocular discharge (giant-breed dogs).
- Upper lid, lower lid, or lateral canthal—severe blepharospasm, purulent discharge, pigmentary or ulcerative keratitis, potential cornea rupture (chow chow, shar-pei, bloodhound, sporting breeds).
- Cats—often have associated keratoconjunctivitis, corneal ulceration, or corneal sequestrum (brown-black corneal opacity).

CAUSES & RISK FACTORS

- Genetic predisposition—based on facial conformation and eyelid support.
- Brachycephalic breeds (dogs and cats)—excessive tension on ligamentous structures of medial canthus plus nasal folds and facial conformation results in rolling inward of medial aspects of upper and lower eyelids at the medial canthus.
- Giant breeds and breeds with excessive eyelid length (macroblepharon), heavy/loose facial skin, or excessive facial folds—laxity of lateral canthus allows entropion of upper and lower eyelids and lateral canthus.
- Spastic entropion—from ocular irritation (e.g., distichia, ectopic cilia, trichiasis, foreign body, irritant conjunctivitis); leads to excessive blepharospasm.
- Non-predisposed breeds—may be primary irritant causing secondary spastic entropion.
- Loss of orbital fat or periorbital musculature may lead to enophthalmos and entropion.
- Secondary cicatricial entropion—from scarring due to eyelid wounds or eyelid surgery.
- Cats—chronic infectious conjunctivitis or keratitis: may lead to functional entropion caused by chronic blepharospasm (spastic entropion); also in older cats due to enophthalmos from retrobulbar fat loss.

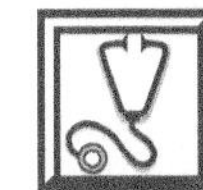

DIAGNOSIS

DIFFERENTIAL DIAGNOSIS

- Underlying causes of spastic entropion (eyelid hair anomalies, foreign bodies, infectious keratitis/conjunctivitis) should be ruled out and corrected, if possible, before an attempt at surgical correction is made.
- Puppies—common for first-time breeders of chow chows and Chinese Shar-Peis to mistakenly think that eyelids have not opened at 4–5 weeks of age, when puppies actually have severe blepharospasm and spastic entropion.

CBC/BIOCHEMISTRY/URINALYSIS

N/A

OTHER LABORATORY TESTS

N/A

IMAGING

N/A

DIAGNOSTIC PROCEDURES

- Observe patient with minimal restraint to assess degree of entropion without distortion from tension on eyelids or periocular area.
- Apply a topical anesthetic to reduce spastic component to differentiate spastic versus physiologic entropion.

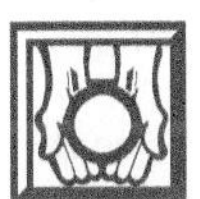

TREATMENT

Puppies

- Do *not* initially perform skin resection surgery.
- If cornea ulcerated—topical antibiotic (e.g., neomycin/polymyxin B/bacitracin) ointment q6–8h.
- If mildly entropic and cornea not ulcerated, lubricate with artificial tear ointment q8–12h.
- If moderate to severe entropion with or without corneal ulceration, temporarily evert eyelid margins with sutures to break the irritation–spasm cycle; if successful, permanent procedure is unnecessary; may need to be repeated every 2–4 weeks until adult facial conformation is achieved.
- Semi-permanent eyelid eversion with hyaluronic acid filler injection—lasts up to several months, often until adult facial conformation is achieved.
- Permanent skin resection technique—postponed until patient's facial conformation matures (usually 1.5–2 years).

Medial Entropion

- Temporary eversion of medial canthus with sutures may aid in determining contribution of medial entropion to epiphora.
- Medial canthoplasty should be considered if entropion results in pigmentary keratitis, chronic epiphora, or corneal scarring.

Mature Dogs and Cats

- Chronic entropion—requires eyelid margin–everting surgery; ranges from simple Hotz-Celsus procedure to more radical lateral canthoplasty procedures; often combined with lid-shortening procedures.
- No history of previous entropion and clinical signs of acute condition—identify cause of spastic condition and correct; may attempt temporary eversion sutures before permanent skin resection.

E

MEDICATIONS

DRUG(S) OF CHOICE

- Topical ophthalmic ointment—triple antibiotic (in dogs only, q6–12h) or antibiotic based on culture and sensitivity testing; may be used if cornea is ulcerated, postoperatively, or as presurgical lubricant.
- Topical petrolatum-based artificial tear ointments (e.g., Puralube® q8–12h) may be used temporarily in mild cases without corneal ulceration.

CONTRAINDICATIONS/POSSIBLE INTERACTIONS

N/A

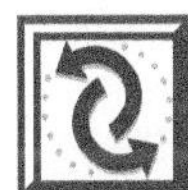

FOLLOW-UP

Temporary eversion suture technique—entropion may revert when sutures are removed or spontaneously pull through the skin; repeat as necessary until patient is mature enough to undergo more permanent repair. Consider hyaluronic acid filler injection as alternative.

MISCELLANEOUS

Suggested Reading

Stades FC, van der Woerdt A. Diseases and surgery of the canine eyelid. In: Gelatt KN, Gilger BC, Kern TJ, eds., Veterinary Ophthalmology, 5th ed. Ames, IA: Wiley-Blackwell, 2013, pp. 843–864.

Williams DL, Kim JY. Feline entropion: a case series of 50 affected animals (2003–2008). Vet Ophthalmol 2009, 12(4):221–226.

Author Sarah L. Czerwinski

Consulting Editor Kathern E. Myrna

Acknowledgment The author and book editors acknowledge the prior contribution of J. Phillip Pickett.

EOSINOPHILIA

E

BASICS

OVERVIEW

• Eosinophilia refers to an increased number of circulating eosinophils.
• Reference intervals may be difficult to accurately determine, as numbers do not tend to have normal (Gaussian) distribution. Absolute counts >1.5 x $10^3/\mu l$ often indicate clinically significant eosinophilia.
• Diseases associated with eosinophilia are highly variable. However, they often involve those causing release of cytokines including IL-5, IL-2, IL-3, and/or GM-CSF.
• Prevalence varies; 4.8% of cats and 10% of dogs have been identified with eosinophilia in large retrospective studies.

SIGNALMENT

• Breed and sex predilections are directly correlated to the characteristics of specific diseases.
• Rottweilers and German shepherd dogs show the highest overall prevalence of eosinophilia.

SIGNS

• Clinical signs directly associated with eosinophilia per se are lacking.
• Specific clinical signs are dependent on the disease causing the eosinophilia.

CAUSES & RISK FACTORS

• Diseases associated with eosinophilia are widely variable and can be categorized in many ways.
• Infectious diseases typically involve tissues rather than peripheral blood, and are more likely to be parasitic than bacterial.
• Tissues involved are frequently those that contain abundant mast cells, such as skin, lungs, and intestine, and often involve hypersensitivity.
• Metabolic—hypoadrenocortisim.
• Neoplastic—mast cell tumor; eosinophilic leukemia; lymphoma (both T-cell and B-cell); thymoma; mammary carcinoma; oral fibrosarcoma; transitional cell carcinoma.
• Immune mediated—hypereosinophilic syndrome (HES); idiopathic HES in Rottweilers; feline asthma; eosinophilic bronchopneumopathy; feline gastro-intestinal eosinophilic sclerosing fibroplasia; flea bite allergy; eosinophilic granuloma complex.
• Infectious—*Angiostrongylus vasorum*; heartworm disease (*Dirofilaria immitis*); *Ehrlichia* spp. infections; *Anaplasma* spp. infections; histoplasmosis; sarcocytosis; *Aelurostrongylus* spp.; larval migration of various parasites.
• Toxic methimazole therapy.

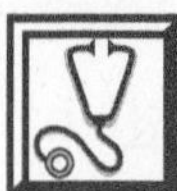

DIAGNOSIS

DIFFERENTIAL DIAGNOSIS

• HES represents an idiopathic response that may be due to an occult immunologic stimulus.
• Eosinophilic leukemia is a myeloproliferative disease that often has immature forms in circulation and in the bone marrow.
• Differentiation between HES and eosinophilic leukemia can be extremely difficult and is somewhat controversial.

CBC/BIOCHEMISTRY/URINALYSIS

• Caution should be taken in interpreting the results of some in-house hematology analyzers, as they only show good correlation with gold standard instruments. A blood smear should *always* be evaluated as part of the CBC.
• Eosinophils tend to be larger and hypolobulated compared to neutrophils.
• Feline eosinophils have small, rod-shaped granules.
• Sight hounds and sporadic other individuals have "gray eosinophils," which have poorly staining granules and occasionally empty vacuoles in their cytoplasm.
• Eosinophils are grouped into one large category; bands, metamyelocytes, etc. are typically not divided out, as they are with neutrophils.

OTHER LABORATORY TESTS

Additional testing (e.g., adrenocorticotropic hormone (ACTH) stimulation test, fecal flotation, cytology, etc.) are dependent on the differential diagnosis/disease in question.

IMAGING

Diagnostic imaging utilized (e.g., radio-graphs, ultrasound, CT, etc.) is dependent on the differential diagnosis/disease in question.

DIAGNOSTIC PROCEDURES

Diagnostic procedures utilized (e.g., transtracheal wash, endoscopy, serologic testing, biopsy, etc.) are dependent on the differential diagnosis/disease in question.

PATHOLOGIC FINDINGS

• No specific lesions are ascribed solely to eosinophilia other than peripheral blood findings.
• Lesions are dependent on the disease(s) present.

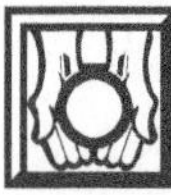

TREATMENT

• No specific treatment is described exclusively for eosinophilia.
• The treatment employed is dependent on the cause of the eosinophilia.

MEDICATIONS

Dependent on cause.

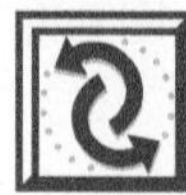

FOLLOW-UP

Dependent on cause.

MISCELLANEOUS

SEE ALSO

Hypereosinophilic Syndrome (HES).

ABBREVIATIONS

• ACTH = adrenocorticotropic hormone.
• HES = hypereosinophilic syndrome.

Suggested Reading

Center SA, Randolph JR, Erb HN, Reiter S. Eosinophilia in the cat: a retrospective study of 312 cases. J Am Anim Hosp Assoc 1990, 26(4):349–358.

Lillieöök I, Gunnardsson L, Zakrisson G, Tvedten H. Diseases associated with pronounced eosinophilia: a study of 105 dogs in Sweden. J Small Anim Pract 2000, 41(6):248–253.

Lillieöök I, Tvedten H. Investigation of hypereosinophilia and potential treatments. Vet Clin North Am Small Anim Pract 2003, 33(6):1359–1378.

Author Craig A. Thompson
Consulting Editor Melinda S. Camus

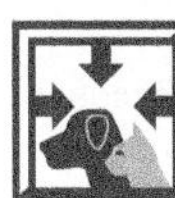

BASICS

DEFINITION

• Cats—also called feline eosinophilic skin disease; term used for three distinct syndromes: eosinophilic plaque, eosinophilic granuloma, and indolent ulcer; grouped primarily according to their clinical similarities, their frequent concurrent (and recurrent) development, and their positive response to corticosteroids; reaction pattern and not a final diagnosis unless idiopathic. • Dogs—eosinophilic granuloma in dogs (EGD) rare; specific differences from cats listed separately.

PATHOPHYSIOLOGY

• Eosinophil—major infiltrative cell for eosinophilic granuloma and eosinophilic plaque, but not typically with indolent ulcer; most often associated with allergic or parasitic conditions but has a more general role in inflammatory reactions. • Eosinophilic granuloma complex (EGC)—most often in cats with hypersensitivities to inhaled allergens, food, or insects, but can also be idiopathic with possible genetic causes. • EGD—may have both a genetic predisposition and a hypersensitivity cause (especially in non-genetically susceptible breeds).

SYSTEMS AFFECTED

Skin/exocrine.

GENETICS

• Related individuals with disease development in a colony of specific pathogen-free cats indicate that genetic predisposition (possible inheritable dysfunction of eosinophilic regulation) may be significant component for development. • Genetically predisposed development of hypersensitivity.

GEOGRAPHIC DISTRIBUTION

Seasonal incidence in some geographic locations—insect or environmental allergen exposure.

SIGNALMENT

Species

• Cats—eosinophilic granuloma, eosinophilic plaque, indolent ulcer. • Dogs—eosinophilic granuloma.

Breed Predilections

• Cats—none. • Dogs—EGD: Siberian husky (76% of cases), cavalier King Charles spaniel.

Mean Age and Range

• Eosinophilic granuloma and plaque—younger cats. • Spontaneously regressing eosinophilic granuloma—<1 year. • Indolent ulcer—any age. • EGD— usually <3 years of age (80%).

Predominant Sex

• Cats (eosinophilic granuloma, indolent ulcer)—predilection for females reported; eosinophilic plaque: no sex predilection. • EGD—males (72% of cases).

SIGNS

General Comments—Cats

• Distinguishing among the syndromes depends on clinical signs. • Lesions of more than one syndrome may occur simultaneously or may change over time.

Historical Findings—Cats

• Lesions may develop spontaneously and acutely. • Eosinophilic granuloma—variable but typically nonpruritic. • Eosinophilic plaque—severe pruritus. • Indolent ulcer—pain and pruritus rare. • Seasonal incidence possible (related to insects and allergy). • Waxing and waning of clinical signs common in all syndromes.

Physical Examination Findings

• *Eosinophilic plaque*—single or multiple, alopecic, erythematous, eroded/ulcerated well-demarcated and flat-topped ± white necrotic foci; most commonly seen on the abdomen and medial thighs, but may also see in mucocutaneous junctions and other areas of the skin; frequently moist or glistening; may appear oval or linear due to pattern of licking. • *Eosinophilic granuloma*—caudal thigh (linear granuloma)—distinctly linear orientation on the caudal thigh; chin ("pouting cats")—lip margin and chin swelling; paw pads—footpad swelling, pain, and lameness; oral cavity—ulceration common (especially on the tongue, palate): cats with oral lesions may be dysphagic, have halitosis, and may drool; can be located anywhere on the body; spontaneous regression—especially in young cats with the inheritable form. • *Indolent ulcer*—classically concave and indurated ulcerations with a granular, orange-yellow color, confined to the upper lips near philtrum or upper canine teeth. • Peripheral lymphadenopathy possible for EGC lesions. • *EGD*—ulcerated plaques and nodules; green/orange color; most often affects the tongue and palatine arches; uncommon cutaneous lesions on the abdomen, cheek, digits, prepuce, and flanks. • Cavalier King Charles spaniels—lesions on the soft palate or near the tonsils.

CAUSES

• Hypersensitivity—flea or insect (mosquito bite), food hypersensitivity, and atopy; a heritable dysfunction has been proposed. • Idiopathic. • EGD—unknown; genetics in susceptible breeds; a hypersensitivity reaction often suspected (insect bite) in non-genetically susceptible breeds.

DIAGNOSIS

DIFFERENTIAL DIAGNOSIS

• Herpes virus dermatitis. • Feline leukemia virus (FeLV) or feline immunodeficiency virus (FIV). • Unresponsive lesions—pemphigus foliaceus, dermatophytosis and deep fungal infection, demodicosis, pyoderma, and neoplasia (metastatic adenocarcinoma, squamous cell carcinoma, and lymphoma). • EGD—neoplasia, infectious and noninfectious granuloma.

CBC/BIOCHEMISTRY/URINALYSIS

CBC—mild to moderate eosinophilia.

OTHER LABORATORY TESTS

FeLV and FIV.

DIAGNOSTIC PROCEDURES

• Impression smears (cytology) from lesions—large numbers of eosinophils (indolent ulcer may be more neutrophilic). • Comprehensive flea and insect control—assist in excluding flea or mosquito bite hypersensitivity. • Food elimination trial and provocation—appropriate in all cases. • Atopy—intradermal skin testing (preferred) or serum allergy testing followed by immunotherapy. • Biopsy.

PATHOLOGIC FINDINGS

• Histopathologic diagnosis—mainly to rule out other differentials. • Eosinophilic granuloma—nodular to diffuse granulomatous dermatitis with flame figures, eosinophils, multinucleated histiocytic giant cells; mucinosis of epidermis/hair follicle outer root sheath, mural eosinophilic folliculitis/furunculosis, eosinophilic panniculitis possible. • Eosinophilic plaque—superficial to deep perivascular dermatitis with eosinophilia to interstitial to diffuse eosinophilia; mucinosis of epidermis/hair follicle outer root sheath, diffuse spongiosis of outer root sheath, eosinophilic microvesicles/microabscesses possible. • Indolent ulcer—variable; may be predominantly neutrophilic or eosinophilic. • EGD—foci of palisading granulomas and flame figures; infiltrate with eosinophils mixed with macrophages.

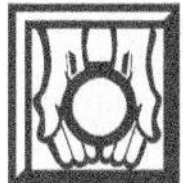

TREATMENT

APPROPRIATE HEALTH CARE

• Most patients treated as outpatients unless severe oral disease prevents adequate fluid intake. • Identify and eliminate offending allergen(s) before providing medical intervention. • Atopy—immunotherapy: successful in a majority of cases; preferable to long-term corticosteroid administration.

NURSING CARE

Discourage patient from damaging lesions by excessive grooming.

DIET

No restrictions unless a food allergy is suspected. Elimination diet for suspected food allergy.

EOSINOPHILIC GRANULOMA COMPLEX (CONTINUED)

CLIENT EDUCATION

• Inform clients about the possible allergic or heritable causes. • Discuss the waxing and waning nature of these diseases.

SURGICAL CONSIDERATIONS

EGD—individual lesions may be excised/removed by carbon dioxide laser if being mechanically traumatized and medically unresponsive.

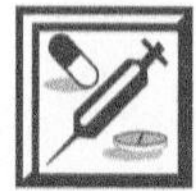

MEDICATIONS

DRUG(S) OF CHOICE

• Cases may improve with antibiotics—amoxicillin trihydrate–clavulanate 10–20 mg/kg q12h; cefovecin 8 mg/kg every 14 days; or clindamycin 11–22 mg/kg q24h. • Oral corticosteroids—ongoing treatment necessary unless the primary cause is controlled; prednisolone 2–4 mg/kg q24h, then as required to control lesions; steroid tachyphylaxis may occur and may be specific to the drug administered; may be useful to change the form; other drugs: methylprednisolone 2–3 mg/kg q24h, dexamethasone 0.1–0.2 mg/kg q24–72h, and triamcinolone 0.2–0.3 mg/kg q24–72h; higher induction dosages may be required but should be tapered as quickly as possible. • Cyclosporine modified, 7 mg/kg q24–48h. • Topical—fluocinolone/dimethyl sulfoxide (DMSO; Synotic® lotion) to individual lesions; not practical and/or may cause systemic effects in patients with large numbers of lesions.

Alternate Therapies

• Chlorambucil 0.1–0.2 mg/kg q24–72h.
• α-interferon 300–1000 IU/day; limited success. • Megestrol acetate—significant side effects (e.g., diabetes, mammary cancer, pyometra); use not recommended except in severe, recalcitrant cases.

EGD

• Oral prednisolone 0.5–2.2 mg/kg/day initially; then taper gradually. • Some may undergo spontaneous remission.

FOLLOW-UP

PATIENT MONITORING

• Corticosteroids—baseline and frequent hemograms, serum chemistry profiles, and urinalyses with culture; excessive or too-frequent use of corticosteroids increases risk for development of diabetes mellitus and acquired skin fragility. • Cyclosporine—baseline and frequent hemograms, serum chemistry profiles, and urinalyses with culture; measurement of plasma cyclosporine levels as needed to establish dosage within therapeutic levels (especially cats); avoid raw meat and keep cats indoors. • Selective immunosuppressant drugs—frequent hemograms (biweekly at first, then monthly or bimonthly as therapy continues) to monitor for bone marrow suppression; routine serum chemistry profiles and urinalyses with culture (monthly at first, then every 3 months) to monitor for complications (renal disease, diabetes mellitus, and urinary tract infection).

EXPECTED COURSE AND PROGNOSIS

• Lesions should resolve permanently if a primary cause can be identified and controlled. • Most lesions wax and wane, with or without therapy; an unpredictable schedule of recurrence should be anticipated.
• Drug dosages should be tapered to the lowest possible level (or discontinued, if possible) once the lesions have resolved.
• Lesions in cats with the inheritable disease may resolve spontaneously after several years.
• EGD—lesions may be recalcitrant to medical intervention.

MISCELLANEOUS

PREGNANCY/FERTILITY/BREEDING

Systemic glucocorticoids and immunosuppressive drugs should not be used during pregnancy.

SYNONYMS

• Eosinophilic granuloma—feline collagenolytic granuloma; feline linear granuloma. • Indolent ulcer—eosinophilic ulcer; rodent ulcer; feline upper lip ulcerative dermatitis.

SEE ALSO

• Atopic Dermatitis.
• Food Reactions, Dermatologic.

ABBREVIATIONS

• DMSO = dimethyl sulfoxide.
• EGC = eosinophilic granuloma complex.
• EGD = eosinophilic granulomas in dogs.
• FeLV = feline leukemia virus.
• FIV = feline immunodeficiency virus.

Suggested Reading

Buckley L, Nuttall, T. Feline eosinophilic granuloma complex(ities): some clinical clarification. J Feline Med Surg 2012, 14:471–481.

King S, Favrot C, Messinger L, et al. A randomized double-blinded placebo-controlled study to evaluate an effective ciclosporin dose for the treatment of feline hypersensitivity dermatitis. Vet Derm 2012, 23:440–e84.

Knight EC, Shipstone MA. Canine eosinophilic granuloma of the digits treated with prednisolone and chlorambucil. Vet Derm 2016, 27:446–e119.

Miller WH, Griffin CE, Campbell KL. Muller & Kirk's Small Animal Dermatology, 7th ed. St. Louis, MO: Elsevier Mosby, 2013.

Rosenkrantz WS. Feline eosinophilic granuloma complex. In: Griffin CE, Kwochka KW, MacDonald JM, eds., Current Veterinary Dermatology: The Science and Art of Therapy. St. Louis, MO: Mosby, 1993, p. 319.

Author Heather D. Edgington

Consulting Editor Alexander H. Werner Resnick

Acknowledgment The author acknowledges the prior contribution of Alexander H. Werner Resnick.

Client Education Handout available online

EPIDIDYMITIS/ORCHITIS

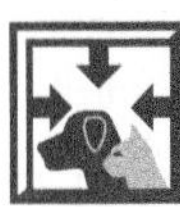

BASICS

OVERVIEW

• Epididymitis—inflammation of an epididymis; a prominent clinical sign of brucellosis. • Orchitis—inflammation of testis; may be concurrent with epididymitis (orchiepididymitis). • May be acute or chronic.

SIGNALMENT

• Often unilateral. • Infrequent in dogs; rare in cats. • No genetic basis or breed predilections. • Mean age 3.7 years; range: 11 months–10 years.

SIGNS

• Swollen testis. • Pain (if acute). • Pyrexia. • Infertility. • Anorexia. • Listlessness. • Reluctance to walk. • Reluctance to breed. • Scrotal wound or abscess. • Scrotal dermatitis (from licking behavior).

CAUSES & RISK FACTORS

• Infectious—*Brucella canis* (brucellosis), canine distemper virus, *Rickettsia rickettsii* (Rocky Mountain spotted fever). • Urethritis, prostatitis, cystitis. • Blunt abdominal or scrotal trauma, including scrotal bite or puncture wounds. • Auto-immune response to spermatozoa antigens—secondary to trauma or inflammation. • Lymphoplasmacytic auto-immune orchitis with, or without, thyroiditis.

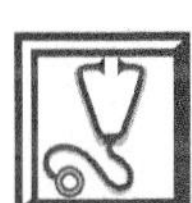

DIAGNOSIS

DIFFERENTIAL DIAGNOSIS

• Inguinoscrotal hernia. • Scrotal dermatitis. • Torsion of the spermatic cord. • Hydrocele. • Sperm granuloma. • Testicular neoplasia. • Prostatitis. • Cystitis.

CBC/BIOCHEMISTRY/URINALYSIS

• Leukocytosis—may be found with acute or infectious orchitis. • Pyuria, hematuria, proteinuria—may be found if epididymitis/orchitis is secondary to prostatitis or cystitis.

OTHER LABORATORY TESTS

• Serology—tests identifying *B. canis* antibodies or antigens may take up to 12 weeks to become detectable: perform immediate testing in any dog with scrotal enlargement (see Brucellosis). • Rapid slide agglutination test (RSAT)—screening test; sensitive but not specific. • Due to occurrence of false positives with RSAT, retest all positives for *B. canis* with a more specific test method: modified rapid slide agglutination test (ME-RSAT), agar gel immunodiffusion test (AGID), tube agglutination test (TAT), PCR, or bacterial culture of whole blood or lymph node aspirate.

IMAGING

• Ultrasonographic evaluation of testes and epididymides—inflamed testes have patchy hypoechoic areas; inflamed epididymides have irregular contours and hypoechoic or hyperechoic areas; obtain measurements for future comparisons. • Ultrasonographic evaluation of prostate to identify underlying causes (i.e., prostatitis).

DIAGNOSTIC PROCEDURES

• Bacterial culture of semen (differentiate results from normal flora). • Semen cytologic evaluation—leukocytes; bacteria; spermatozoa with morphologic abnormalities; head-to-head agglutination (*B. canis*). • Prostate fluid cytologic examination and bacterial culture; sample collected aseptically by performing prostatic massage (per rectum) after urethral catheter placed where tip can be palpated (per rectum), followed with 5 mL saline infusion and aspiration. • Open wounds—bacterial culture. • Fine-needle aspirate—sample enlarged testes/epididymides for cytology and culture; leukocytes vary from numerous neutrophils (suppurative) to minimal inflammatory cells (granulomatous).

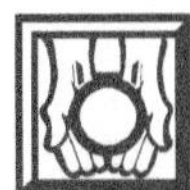

TREATMENT

• Castration—if fertility is not a priority; before castration, culture appropriate specimen; administer antibiotics perioperatively to avoid scirrhous cord. • Unilateral castration—for unilateral orchitis when patient's fertility must be maintained; administer appropriate perioperative antibiotics.

MEDICATIONS

DRUG(S) OF CHOICE

• If *B. canis* is diagnosed, removal of affected testicle(s) is strongly recommended due to zoonotic potential. • If infection present, antibiotic choice should be based on culture and sensitivity if available; broad-spectrum antibiotics (e.g., ampicillin sulbactam 22–30 mg/kg IV q8h) may be administered until cultures are available. • If attempting to treat *B. canis*, combined antibiotic regimes generally more successful; treatments may fail to completely clear infection. • Reported success with doxycycline (10 mg/kg PO q12h), gentamicin (5 mg/kg SC q24h for 7 days and repeated every 3 weeks), rifampin (5 mg/kg PO q24h), or enrofloxacin (5 mg/kg PO q12h) for 1–3 months.

CONTRAINDICATIONS/POSSIBLE INTERACTIONS

N/A

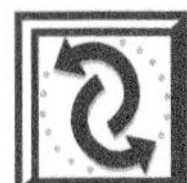

FOLLOW-UP

• Prognosis for fertility—guarded to poor, especially with bilateral orchitis. • Testicular degeneration of remaining contralateral testis may occur due to elevated intrascrotal temperature (inflammation), even following unilateral castration. • Trauma or inflammation can cause obstruction of efferent tubules or epididymal duct, leading to spermatocele or sperm granuloma. • Semen—evaluate characteristics 3 months after treatment for orchitis is completed (dogs).

MISCELLANEOUS

SEE ALSO

• Brucellosis
• Torsion of thr Spermatic Cord

ABBREVIATIONS

• AGID = agar gel immunodiffusion.
• ME-RSAT = modified rapid slide agglutination test.
• RSAT = rapid slide agglutination test.
• TAT = tube agglutination test.

Suggested Reading

Hollett RB. Canine brucellosis: outbreaks and compliance. Theriogenology 2006, 66(3):575–587.

Johnston SD, Root Kustritz MV, Olson PNS. Disorders of the canine testes and epididymides. In: Johnston SD, Kustritz MVR, Olson PN, eds., Canine and Feline Theriogenology. Philadelphia, OA: Saunders, 2001, pp. 313–317.

Kauffman LK, Petersen CA. Canine brucellosis: old foe and reemerging scourge. Vet Clin North Am Small Anim Pract 2019, 49(4):763–779.

Author Candace C. Lyman

Consulting Editor Erin E. Runcan

Acknowledgment The author and book editors acknowledge the prior contribution of Carlos R.F. Pinto.

E

EPILEPSY, GENETIC (IDIOPATHIC)—DOGS

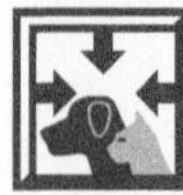

BASICS

DEFINITION

Syndrome that is only epilepsy, with no demonstrable underlying brain lesion or other neurologic signs or symptoms; age-related; assumed genetic. The term "idiopathic" replaced by "genetic" according to the International League Against Epilepsy (ILAE) classification (see Appendix IX).

PATHOPHYSIOLOGY

• Exact mechanism unknown. • Likely different mechanisms between breeds.

SYSTEMS AFFECTED

Nervous

GENETICS

Genetic basis suspected in Australian shepherd, beagle, Belgian shepherd (Groenendael and Tervuren), Bernese mountain dog, border collie, dachshund, English springer spaniel, Finnish spitz, German shepherd, golden retriever, keeshond, Irish wolfhound, Italian spinone, Labrador retriever, Shetland sheepdog, standard poodle, vizsla.

INCIDENCE/PREVALENCE

0.5–2.3% of all dogs.

GEOGRAPHIC DISTRIBUTION

Widespread

SIGNALMENT

Species

Dog

Breed Predilections

Beagles; all shepherds (German, Australian, Belgian); Bernese mountain dogs; boxers; cocker spaniels; border collies; dachshunds; golden retrievers; Irish setters; Labrador retrievers; poodles (all sizes); Saint Bernards; Shetland sheepdogs; Siberian huskies; springer spaniels; Welsh corgis; wirehaired fox terriers. Can occur in any breed.

Mean Age and Range

• Mean age 10 months–3 years. • Range 6 months–5 years.

Predominant Sex

Male predisposition in Bernese mountain dog.

SIGNS

General Comments

• Seizures may be generalized (convulsive) from onset, or have a short aura (focal onset) with rapid secondary generalization. • An aura (animal appears frightened, dazed, seeks attention, or hides, etc.) frequently precedes the generalized seizure. • Focal seizures reported in the border collie, Finnish spitz, English springer spaniel, Labrador retriever, viszla, Belgian shepherd, standard poodle.

Historical Findings

• First seizure—between 6 months and 5 years. • Seizures—often when patient is resting or asleep; often at night or early morning; frequency tends to increase if left untreated; affected animal falls on its side, becomes stiff, chomps its jaw, salivates profusely, urinates, defecates, vocalizes, and paddles with all limbs in varying combinations; short duration (30–90 seconds). • Postictal behavior—confusion, disorientation; aimless, compulsive, blind, pacing; frequent polydipsia and polyphagia; recovery immediate or may take up to 24 hours. • Dogs with established epilepsy might have clustered generalized seizures at intervals of 1–4 weeks. • No asymmetry should be observed during seizure, e.g., twitching more pronounced on one side, limb contractions on one side, compulsive circling just prior to or after the seizure.
• Stimulus-induced seizures—seizures only upon specific stimulus (sound, event).

Physical Examination Findings

• Patients often have recovered at time of presentation. • Patients may have postictal behavior.

CAUSES

Genetic in some breeds; of unknown cause in others.

RISK FACTORS

Known epilepsy in the family line.

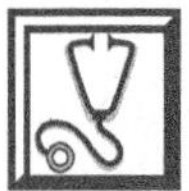

DIAGNOSIS

DIFFERENTIAL DIAGNOSIS

• Seizure pattern (breed, age at onset, type and frequency of seizures)—most important factor toward diagnosis. • Acute onset of cluster seizures or status epilepticus—rule out toxicity or structural brain disease. • >2 seizures within the first week of onset—consider diagnosis other than genetic epilepsy. • Seizures at <6 months or >5 years of age—consider metabolic or intracranial structural disease; rule out hypoglycemia in older dogs. • Focal seizures or presence of neurologic deficits—rule out intracranial structural disease.

CBC/BIOCHEMISTRY/URINALYSIS

• Usually normal. • Perform before initiating drug therapy as baseline data.

OTHER LABORATORY TESTS

Bile acids to rule out hepatic encephalopathy unnecessary in dogs with seizures without accompanying episodic abnormal behavior.

IMAGING

MRI—if seizure pattern does not fit genetic (idiopathic) epilepsy, neurologic deficits are present, or intracranial structural disease is suspected.

DIAGNOSTIC PROCEDURES

• Cerebrospinal fluid (CSF)—for suspected structural intracranial diseases.
• Electroencephalography—may see interictal spikes, polyspikes, and spike slow wave complexes.

PATHOLOGIC FINDINGS

• No primary lesion. • Secondary neuronal loss and gliosis from prolonged seizures.

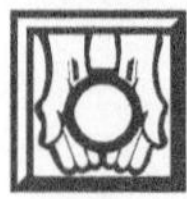

TREATMENT

APPROPRIATE HEALTH CARE

• Outpatient—recurrence of isolated seizures.
• Inpatient—for cluster seizures (>1 seizure q24h) or status epilepticus.

NURSING CARE

Inpatients with seizure disorders require constant monitoring.

DIET

• Dogs on chronic phenobarbital (PB) and potassium bromide (KBr) treatment often become overweight; weight-reducing program as necessary. • KBr treatment—insure steady levels of salt in diet; increase in salt causes increase in bromide excretion preferentially over chloride, with subsequent decreased serum KBr levels; alternatively, decreased salt content increases KBr serum level. • Trial with high-fat, low-carbohydrate diet—no improvement in seizure control.

CLIENT EDUCATION

• Severe cluster seizures and status epilepticus are life-threatening emergencies requiring immediate medical attention. • Keep seizure calendar noting date, time, length, and severity of seizures to assess response to treatment. • Once treatment instituted, medication is lifelong in most cases. • Abrupt drug withdrawal may cause seizures.

MEDICATIONS

DRUG(S) OF CHOICE

• Initiate treatment at second generalized seizure if dog <2 years; when interictal period gradually shortens in others. • Antiepileptic treatment—decreases frequency, severity, and length of seizures; perfect control rarely achieved. • Tolerance and refractoriness to treatment may develop.

Phenobarbital

• Most efficacious antiepileptic drug (AED) in the dog. • Traditional first-line drug; initial dosage 3–5 mg/kg PO q12h; steady state reached at 12–15 days, but levels decrease significantly in first 6 months owing to activation of lysosomal enzymes. • Optimal therapeutic serum levels—100–120 μmol/L or 23–28 μg/mL. • Oral loading dose (if needed)—6–10 mg/kg PO q12h for 2–3 days to reach therapeutic range rapidly.

Zonisamide

First-line drug when seizure frequency allows (<1/week); 5 mg/kg PO q12h; 10 mg/kg PO q12h as add-on to PB; half-life 15 hours;

steady state 4 days; therapeutic range in human 10–45 µg/mL.

Levetiracetam

First-line drug when seizures have focal onset; <1 seizure/week; 20–70 mg/kg (smaller breeds require higher dosage) PO q8h; must be given q8h to reach adequate levels; no hepatic metabolism; safe; steady state 3 days; therapeutic range in human 10–40 µg/mL.

Potassium Bromide

- Traditional first-line drug; initial dosage 30 mg/kg PO q24h or divided q12h; half-life 24–46 days; steady state 3–4 months; varies with salt concentration in diet; bioavailability differs between dogs. • Optimal therapeutic serum levels—20–25 mmol/L or 1.6–2 mg/mL; if sole antiepileptic drug, 25–32 mmol/L or 2–2.25 mg/mL can be safely used. • Add on to PB if seizures uncontrolled with optimal PB level—beneficial and synergistic effect. • Loading dose—may cause vomiting, diarrhea, profound longstanding sedation; if needed, double daily PO doses for 2 weeks.
- Renal insufficiency decreases bromide elimination; half initial dosage.

Diazepam (At-Home Use)

- To abort ongoing seizures—dogs with cluster seizures or status epilepticus. • Insert 0.5–1 mg/kg injectable drug in rectum (or intranasal) via 1 inch teat cannula as soon as a seizure occurs; repeat 20 and 40 minutes later for a total of 3 insertions within 40 minutes; can be safely repeated once more in 24h period. • Given early in course of ongoing seizures, helps abort subsequent seizures. • Intransal midazolam can also be used 0.5 mg/kg. Can be repeated once after 20 minutes.

CONTRAINDICATIONS

Aminophylline, theophylline.

PRECAUTIONS

α-adrenergic agonists (e.g., phenylpropanolamine)—CNS excitation.

POSSIBLE INTERACTIONS

- Cimetidine and chloramphenicol—interfere with PB metabolism; may cause toxic PB levels.
- PB lowers serum levels of zonisamide and levetiracetam. • PB may lower T_4 and cause upward trend in thyroid-stimulating hormore (TSH) without signs of hypothyroidism. • PB does not interfere with low-dose dexamethasone suppression tests regardless of dose and treatment. • Zonisamide decreases total T_4. • Whenever animals on lifetime medication, refer to manufacturer's drug profile or to pharmacist for interaction information.

ALTERNATIVE DRUG(S)

- With polypharmacy, initiate add-on gradually to avoid sedation. • Gabapentin 10–20 mg/kg PO q8h; low efficacy as add-on; newer analog pregabalin may be more efficacious, 2–4 mg/kg q8h PO.
- Clorazepate 0.5–1 mg/kg PO q8h.
- Felbamate 30–70 mg/kg q12h–8h.
- Topiramate 2–10 mg/kg PO q12h.
- Phenytoin, valproic acid, carbamazepine, and ethosuximide—unsuitable pharmacokinetics in dogs. • Others—acupuncture, vagal nerve stimulation, transcranial magnetic motor stimulation. • CBD-infused oil 2.5 mg/kg (1.1 mg/lb) q12h.

FOLLOW-UP

PATIENT MONITORING

- Serum drug levels—preferentially at trough, at same time for each sampling; use same laboratory. • Phenobarbital—measure PB level 4 weeks after initiating therapy; adjust dose as needed; then repeat level every 2 weeks until optimal levels reached; with chronic use perform CBC, biochemistry, and PB level every 6–12 months; tabulate albumin, liver enzymes, and serum drug levels to monitor trend; drug essentially hepatotoxic; most dogs eventually develop hepatotoxicity if serum levels >140 µmol/L (>33 µg/mL) for long time (>6–8 months); if hepatotoxicity suspected, perform bile acids. • KBr—serum level (along with PB level) 4–6 weeks after initiating (should be 8–12 mmol/L or 0.5–1 mg/mL) and at 3–4 months; if diet change required, consider diet salt content; monitor level accordingly; monitor KBr level closely if renal insufficiency (isosthenuria or azotemia). • Zonisamide—measure level at 1 week; monitor electrolytes and acid-base status to check for renal tubular acidosis.
- Levetiracetam—measure level at 4 days.

PREVENTION/AVOIDANCE

- Abrupt discontinuation of medication may precipitate seizures. • Avoid salty treats in dogs treated with KBr.

POSSIBLE COMPLICATIONS

- Recurrent episodes of cluster seizures and status epilepticus. • PB and KBr—polyuria, polydipsia, polyphagia, weight gain.
- Phenobarbital-induced corticosteroid alkaline phosphatase (C-AP) elevation occurs frequently; may be early sign of hepatotoxicity, but of less concern if alanine aminotransferase (ALT) is within reference range. • PB-induced hepatotoxicity—after chronic treatment at high serum levels (>140 µmol/L or >33 µg/mL); often insidious in onset; only biochemical abnormality may be decreased albumin.
- Higher incidence of pancreatitis in patients treated with PB and/or KBr; once pancreatitis develops, recurrence is frequent.
- Phenobarbital—rare bone marrow suppression with severe neutropenia (± sepsis) early in course of treatment; discontinue drug.
- Paradoxical hyperexcitability; discontinue drug; risk factor for superficial necrolytic dermatitis. • KBr—when levels are >22 mmol/L or >1.8 mg/mL, owners may complain of patient's unsteadiness while managing stairs.
- Zonisamide—mild sedation, decreased appetite, gastrointestinal signs. • One case of renal tubular acidosis and one case of acute idiosyncratic hepatic necrosis reported.
- Levetiracetam—transient sedation.

EXPECTED COURSE AND PROGNOSIS

- Treatment for life. • Some dogs are well controlled with same drug and dosage for years; others remain poorly controlled despite polypharmacy. • Patient may develop status epilepticus and die. • Early treatment does not decrease occurrence of status epilepticus.
- Normal expected lifespan, but survival time shorter if episodes of status epilepticus.
- Treatment with 2 AEDs not linked to poor prognosis. • Increased risk of premature death. • Marked breed differences in incidence and mortality rates. • Prognosis depends on combined veterinary expertise, therapeutic success, and owner's motivation.

MISCELLANEOUS

ASSOCIATED CONDITIONS

Idiopathic epilepsy can be a reason for euthyroid sick syndrome in dogs.

AGE-RELATED FACTORS

If onset <2 years of age, epilepsy more likely to be difficult to control; condition may become intractable.

PREGNANCY/FERTILITY/BREEDING

- Avoid breeding affected animals. • Reported association between estrus and onset of seizures in intact bitches with presumptive "idiopathic" epilepsy; two hormonally based patterns recognized: during heat; and during a specific time point at the end of diestrus.

SEE ALSO

- Seizures (Convulsions, Status Epilepticus)—Cats. • Seizures (Convulsions, Status epilepticus)—Dogs.

ABBREVIATIONS

- AED = antiepileptic drug.
- ALT = alanine aminotransferase. • C-AP = corticosteroid alkaline phosphatase. • CSF = cerebrospinal fluid. • ILAE = International League Against Epilepsy. • KBr = potassium bromide. • PB = phenobarbital. • TSH = thyroid-stimulating hormone.

INTERNET RESOURCES

http://www.canine-epilepsy.net

Suggested Reading

Muñana KR. Management of refractory epilepsy. Top Companion Anim Med 2013, 28:67–71.

Podell M. Antiepileptic drug therapy and monitoring. Top Companion Anim Med 2013, 28:59–66.

Author Joane M. Parent.

Client Education Handout available online

EPIPHORA

BASICS

DEFINITION

Abnormal overflow of the aqueous portion of the precorneal tear film.

PATHOPHYSIOLOGY

Caused by one of three common problems: overproduction of the aqueous portion of tears (usually in response to ocular irritation); poor eyelid function secondary to eyelid malformation, breed conformation, or deformity; or blockage of the nasolacrimal drainage system.

SYSTEMS AFFECTED

Eye and periocular skin.

SIGNALMENT

Dogs and (less frequently) cats. See Causes.

SIGNS

N/A

CAUSES

Overproduction of Tears Secondary to Ocular Irritants

Congenital

- Distichiasis or trichiasis—common in young Shetland sheepdogs, shih tzus, Lhasa apsos, cocker spaniels, miniature poodles.
- Entropion—Chinese Shar-Peis, chow chows, Labrador retrievers.
- Eyelid agenesis—domestic shorthair cats.

Acquired

- Corneal or conjunctival foreign bodies—usually young, large-breed, active, outdoor dogs.
- Eyelid neoplasms—old dogs (all breeds).
- Blepharitis—infectious or immune mediated.
- Conjunctivitis—infectious or immune mediated.
- Ulcerative keratitis (traumatic or viral).
- Anterior uveitis.
- Glaucoma.

Eyelid Abnormalities or Poor Eyelid Function

- Abnormal eyelid function does not direct tears toward the medial canthus and nasolacrimal puncta.
- Tears never reach the nasolacrimal puncta and subsequently spill over the eyelid margin.

Congenital

- Macropalpebral fissures—brachycephalic breeds.
- Ectropion—Great Danes; bloodhounds; spaniels.
- Entropion—brachycephalic dogs: medial lower eyelid; Labrador retrievers: lateral lower eyelid.

Acquired

- Post-traumatic eyelid scarring.
- Facial nerve paralysis.

Obstruction of the Nasolacrimal Drainage System

Congenital

- Imperforate nasolacrimal puncta—Bedlington terriers, cocker spaniels, bulldogs, poodles.
- Ectopic nasolacrimal openings—extra openings along the side of the face ventral to the medial canthus.
- Nasolacrimal atresia—lack of distal openings into the nose.
- Punctal displacement.
- Lack of ventral canaliculus, nasolacrimal sac, or nasolacrimal duct.

Acquired

- Rhinitis or sinusitis—causes swelling adjacent to the nasolacrimal duct.
- Trauma—resulting in fractures of the lacrimal or maxillary bones or laceration of the nasolacrimal duct.
- Foreign bodies—grass awns, seeds, sand, parasites.
- Neoplasia—of third eyelid, conjunctiva, medial eyelids, nasal cavity, maxillary bone, or periocular sinuses causing invasion or compression of the nasolacrimal system.
- Dacryocystitis—inflammation of canaliculi, lacrimal sac, or nasolacrimal ducts.

RISK FACTORS

- Breeds prone to congenital eyelid abnormalities (see Causes).
- Active outdoor dogs—at risk for foreign bodies.

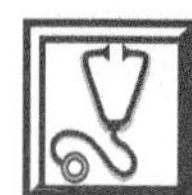

DIAGNOSIS

DIFFERENTIAL DIAGNOSIS

- Other ocular discharges (e.g., mucous or purulent)—epiphora is a watery, serous discharge.
- Primary ocular abnormalities—usually the eye is red when the epiphora is caused by overproduction and quiet when secondary to impaired outflow.
- Irritative causes and some congenital causes of obstruction—thorough ocular examination.
- Acute onset, unilateral condition with ocular pain (blepharospasm)—usually indicates a foreign body or corneal injury.
- Chronic, bilateral condition—usually indicates a congenital problem.
- Facial pain, swelling, nasal discharge, or sneezing—may indicate nasal or sinus infection; may indicate obstruction from neoplasm.
- With mucous or purulent discharge at the medial canthus—may indicate dacryocystitis.

CBC/BIOCHEMISTRY/URINALYSIS

N/A

OTHER LABORATORY TESTS

N/A

IMAGING

- Skull radiographs—may show a nasal, sinus, or maxillary bone lesion.
- Dacryocystorhinography—radiopaque contrast material to help localize obstruction.
- MRI or CT—may help localize obstruction (usually with contrast media) and characterize associated lesions.

DIAGNOSTIC PROCEDURES

- Bacterial culture and sensitivity testing and cytologic examination of purulent material from the puncta (e.g., dacryocystitis); performed before instilling any substance into the eye.
- Jones test—topical fluorescein dye application to the eye; most physiologic test for nasolacrimal function; should be performed first (after culture); dye flows through the nasolacrimal system and reaches the external nares in approximately 10 seconds (or longer) in normal dogs, 15 seconds to 1 minute in cats.
- Nasolacrimal irrigation—see below.
- Rhinoscopy—with or without biopsy or bacterial culture; may be indicated if previous tests suggest a nasal or sinus lesion.
- Exploratory surgery—may be the only way to obtain a definitive diagnosis.
- Temporary tacking out of the lower medial eyelid with suture—may help determine whether repair of medial lower entropion or repositioning of the eyelid would reduce epiphora secondary to eyelid conformational abnormalities.

Nasolacrimal Irrigation

- Confirms obstruction.
- May dislodge foreign material.
- A nasolacrimal cannula or 22- or 24-gauge IV catheter without stylet is inserted into the upper nasolacrimal punctum.
- Eyewash in a 6 ml syringe is attached and irrigated through the cannula or catheter—if fluid does not exit the lower nasolacrimal punctum, the obstruction is in the upper or lower canaliculi, the nasolacrimal sac, or the lower punctum (imperforate).
- Lower punctum is manually obstructed—if flushed fluid does not exit the external nares, the obstruction is in the nasolacrimal duct or at its distal opening (atresia or blockage from a nasal sinus lesion).

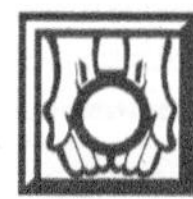

TREATMENT

- Remove cause of ocular irritation—removal of a conjunctival or corneal foreign body, treatment of the primary ocular disease (e.g., conjunctivitis, ulcerative keratitis, and uveitis), cryosurgery or electroepilation for distichiasis, entropion correction, medial or lateral canthoplasty (for medial trichiasis and macropalpebral fissures), correction of cicatricial eyelid abnormalities.

- Treat primary obstruction (e.g., third eyelid mass, nasal or sinus mass, and infection)—successful management may allow normal nasolacrimal flow to resume.
- In patients predisposed to nasolacrimal obstruction, recurrence is common.
- Inform client that early detection and intervention provide better long-term prognosis.

SURGICAL CONSIDERATIONS

Imperforate Puncta

- Surgical opening of the puncta is indicated.
- If one of the puncta is patent (usually the upper punctum), flushing eyewash through the upper opening will cause "tenting" of the conjunctiva at the site of the lower punctum. Place patient under topical or general anesthesia. Grasp conjunctiva overlying the lower canaliculi with forceps and cut with scissors to leave a patent punctum.
- Puncta closed by conjunctival scarring (symblepharon) caused by severe conjunctivitis (e.g., herpesvirus conjunctivitis in cats)—use same procedure.
- Recurrent disease—may be necessary to suture Silastic® tubing in place to prevent stricture formation.

Obstructed or Obliterated Distal Nasolacrimal Duct

- Dacryocystorhinotomy, conjunctivorhinostomy, conjunctival maxiallary sinusostomy, conjunctival buccostomy—create an opening to drain the tears into the nasal cavity or oral cavity.
- See Suggested Reading for surgical technique.

MEDICATIONS

DRUG(S) OF CHOICE

- Topical broad-spectrum antibiotic ophthalmic solutions—while awaiting results of bacterial culture; q4–6h; may try neomycin, gramicidin, polymyxin B triple ophthalmic antibiotic solution, or ophthalmic ciprofloxacin solution.
- Dacryocystitis—based on bacterial culture and sensitivity test results; continue antibiotic therapy for at least 21 days.

CONTRAINDICATIONS

- Topical corticosteroids or antibiotic–corticosteroid combinations—avoid unless a definitive diagnosis has been made.
- Topical corticosteroids—never use if the cornea retains fluorescein stain (corneal ulcer present).

PRECAUTIONS

N/A

POSSIBLE INTERACTIONS

N/A

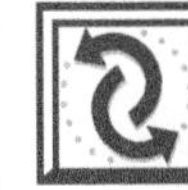

FOLLOW-UP

PATIENT MONITORING

Dacryocystitis

- Reevaluate every 7 days until the condition is resolved.
- Continue treatment for at least 7 days after resolution of clinical signs.
- If problem persists more than 7–10 days with treatment or recurs soon after cessation of treatment—indicates a foreign body or nidus of persistent infection; requires further diagnostics (e.g., dacryocystorhinography).
- Nasolacrimal catheter; commonly required for persistent dacryocystitis, maintains patency of the duct and prevents stricturing.
- Procedure—pass 2-0 nylon via the upper punctum and thread it through the nasolacrimal duct to exit the external nares; pass Silastic or polyethylene (PE90) tubing retrograde over the suture; suture the upper and lower portions of the tubing to the face. Most dogs tolerate the tubing well; however, an Elizabethan collar may be needed to prevent self-trauma. Continue topical antibiotics as before. Leave in place 2–4 weeks.

Dacryocystorhinotomy/ Conjunctivorhinostomy

- Tubing—reevaluate every 7 days to ensure it remains intact; may need to resuture if it becomes loosened or dislodged.
- After tubing has been removed—reevaluate in 14 days; for this and future examinations, place fluorescein on the eye and check nasolacrimal patency by examining the external nares for fluorescein; may evaluate further by cannulating and flushing with eyewash.
- Dacryocystorhinography contrast study—repeated 3–4 months after surgery to evaluate size of nasal opening; repeated for recurrence or with no nasolacrimal fluorescein drainage.

POSSIBLE COMPLICATIONS

Recurrence—most common complication; caused by recurrence of ocular irritation (e.g., corneal ulceration, distichiasis, entropion), recurrence of dacryocystitis, or closure of the dacryocystorhinotomy or conjunctivorhinostomy openings into the nasal cavity.

MISCELLANEOUS

ASSOCIATED CONDITIONS

- Chronic conjunctivitis.
- Recurrent eye "infections."
- Moist dermatitis (hot spots) ventral to the medial canthus.
- Nasal discharge.

AGE-RELATED FACTORS

N/A

ZOONOTIC POTENTIAL

N/A

PREGNANCY/FERTILITY/BREEDING

N/A

SEE ALSO

- Conjunctivitis—Cats.
- Conjunctivitis—Dogs.
- Eyelash Disorders (Trichiasis/Distichiasis/ Ectopic Cilia).
- Keratitis—Ulcerative.
- Third Eyelid Protrusion.

Suggested Reading

Binder DR, Herring IP. Evaluation of nasolacrimal fluorescein transit time in ophthalmically normal dogs and nonbracycephalic cats. Am J Vet Res 2010, 71:570–574.

Giuliano EA. Diseases and surgery of the canine nasolacrimal system. In: Gelatt KN, Gilger BC, Kern T, eds., Veterinary Ophthalmology, 5th ed. Ames, IA: Wiley-Blackwell, 2013, pp. 912–944.

Miller PE. Lacrimal system. In: Maggs DJ, Miller PE, Ofri R, Slatter's Fundamentals of Veterinary Ophthalmology, 6th ed. St. Louis, MO: Elsevier, 2018, pp. 186—203.

Author Silvia G. Pryor

Consulting Editor Kathern E. Myrna

Acknowledgment The author and book editors acknowledge the prior contribution of Brian C. Gilger.

Client Education Handout available online

EPISCLERITIS

BASICS

OVERVIEW

- Focal or diffuse infiltration of episclera and/or scleral stroma by inflammatory cells and fibroblasts.
- Primary—affects only the eye; probably immune mediated; appears either as a perilimbal episcleral/scleral nodule (nodular episcleritis) or as a diffuse thickening of the episclera (diffuse episcleritis); nodular form may affect cornea and third eyelid with nodules.
- Secondary—usually diffuse; from spillover of inflammatory cells into the episclera from other ocular disorders (e.g., endophthalmitis and panophthalmitis); may affect virtually any other organ system.

SIGNALMENT

- Dog.
- Young to middle-aged collie, Shetland sheepdog.

SIGNS

- Nodular—typically appears as a smooth, painless, localized, raised, pink-tan, firm episcleral/scleral mass.
- Diffuse—less common; appears as a diffuse reddening and thickening of the entire episclera/sclera; accompanied by variable amounts of ocular pain.
- Secondary—uveitis often pronounced.
- Conjunctiva—usually moves freely over the surface of the lesion.
- Nodules—tend to be slowly progressive, bilateral, and prone to recurrence.

CAUSES & RISK FACTORS

- Nodular and diffuse primary—idiopathic; believed to be immune mediated.
- Secondary—may result from deep fungal or bacterial ocular infection, lymphoma, systemic histiocytosis in Bernese mountain dogs, chronic glaucoma, and ocular trauma.

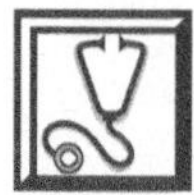

DIAGNOSIS

DIFFERENTIAL DIAGNOSIS

- Other causes of a red eye—differentiated by complete ophthalmic examination.
- Other mass-like lesions—differentiated by biopsy or cytologic examination.
- Neoplasia—lymphoma, squamous cell carcinoma, extension of intraocular mass, other tumors.
- Granuloma—deep fungal infection, retained foreign body.
- Granulation tissue—trauma, healing corneal ulcer, globe perforation with uveal prolapse.

CBC/BIOCHEMISTRY/URINALYSIS

- Usually normal if lesion is confined to eye or adnexa.
- Secondary—may see abnormalities consistent with systemic disease.

OTHER LABORATORY TESTS

Serologic testing—may help diagnose fungal infection.

IMAGING

- Abdominal ultrasound, thoracic and abdominal radiographs—may help rule out fungal infection or disseminated neoplasia.
- Ocular ultrasound—may reveal other abnormalities if ocular media opacities prevent thorough ocular examination.

DIAGNOSTIC PROCEDURES

- Incisional biopsy and histopathologic examination of affected tissue.
- Nodular—varying numbers of histiocytes, lymphocytes, plasma cells, and fibroblasts.
- If uveitis prominent—see Anterior Uveitis—Dogs.

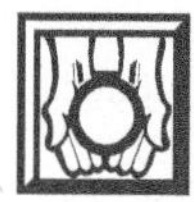

TREATMENT

- Verify the diagnosis histologically or cytologically before treatment.
- Primary nodular—benign course; observation alone may be appropriate with mild disease.
- Outpatient treatment if ocular pain, diffuse scleral involvement, eyelid function is disrupted, cornea is affected, or vision is threatened.

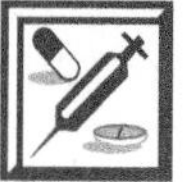

MEDICATIONS

DRUG(S) OF CHOICE

- Progress down the list only if the previous modality was ineffective.
- Topical 1% prednisolone acetate q4h for 1 week, then q6h for 2 weeks, then tapered.
- Systemic prednisolone 1–2 mg/kg/day PO; taper with improvement.
- Systemic azathioprine 1–2 mg/kg/day PO for 3–7 days; then tapered to as low as possible.
- Cryosurgery or attempted excision.
- Alternative to listed drugs or surgery—may try a combination of tetracycline and niacinamide (q8h PO); 250 mg each for dogs <10 kg; 500 mg each for dogs >10 kg; may not observe good clinical response for at least 8 weeks; side effects uncommon and primarily the result of gastrointestinal upset by niacinamide.

CONTRAINDICATIONS/POSSIBLE INTERACTIONS

- Avoid systemic immunosuppressive drugs with fungal infections.
- Systemically administered prednisolone—may precipitate pancreatitis, iatrogenic hyperadrenocorticism.
- Azathioprine—may induce potentially fatal myelosuppression, hepatotoxicosis.
- Niacin—do not substitute for niacinamide.

FOLLOW-UP

PATIENT MONITORING

- Primary—monitor for nodule regression or reduction in episcleral thickening or reddening every 2–3 weeks for 6–9 weeks and then as needed; prognosis usually good; may require therapy for months to rest of life.
- Secondary—follow-up, prognosis, and complications depend on primary disease.
- Azathioprine—repeat CBC, platelet count, and measurement of liver enzymes every 1–2 weeks for first 8 weeks, then periodically.

POSSIBLE COMPLICATIONS

- Vision loss.
- Chronic ocular pain.
- Uveitis.
- Secondary glaucoma.

MISCELLANEOUS

SYNONYMS

- Collie granuloma.
- Fibrous histiocytoma.
- Limbal granuloma.
- Necrogranulomatous sclerouveitis.
- Nodular fasciitis.
- Nodular granulomatous episcleritis.
- Proliferative keratoconjunctivitis.

Suggested Reading

Maggs DJ. Diseases of the cornea and sclera. In: Maggs DJ, Miller PE, Ofri R, Slatter's Fundamentals of Veterinary Ophthalmology, 6th ed. St. Louis, MO: Elsevier 2018, pp. 213–253.

Rothstein E, Scott DW, Riis RC. Tetracycline and niacinamide for the treatment of sterile pyogranuloma/granuloma syndrome in a dog. J Am Anim Hosp Assoc 1997, 33:540–543.

Author Paul E. Miller

Consulting Editor Kathern E. Myrna

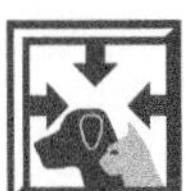

BASICS

DEFINITION

Bleeding from the nose.

PATHOPHYSIOLOGY

Results from one of three abnormalities—coagulopathy; local disease or space-occupying lesion; vascular or systemic disease.

SYSTEMS AFFECTED

- Respiratory—hemorrhage; sneezing
- Gastrointestinal (GI)—melena.
- Hemic/lymphatic/immune—anemia.

GENETICS

Varies depending on underlying cause.

INCIDENCE/PREVALENCE

Varies depending on underlying cause.

SIGNALMENT

Species

Dog and cat.

Age, Breed, and Sex Predilections

Vary depending on underlying cause.

SIGNS

Historical Findings

- Nasal hemorrhage—unilateral or bilateral possible.
- Sneezing and/or stertorous respiration.
- Melena.
- With coagulopathy—hematochezia, melena, hematuria, or hemorrhage from other areas of the body.
- With hypertension—possibly blindness, intraocular hemorrhage, neurologic signs, cardiac or renal signs.

Physical Examination Findings

- Nasal hemorrhage.
- Melena—from swallowing blood or concurrent upper GI hemorrhage.
- Nasal stridor—may be present with neoplasia, foreign body, or advanced inflammatory disease.
- With coagulopathy—possibly petechiae, ecchymosis, hematomas, intracavitary bleeds, hematochezia, melena, and hematuria.
- With coagulopathy or hypertension—possibly retinal or intraocular hemorrhages or retinal detachment; with hypertension—possibly heart murmur or arrhythmia.

CAUSES

Coagulopathy

Thrombocytopenia

- Immune-mediated disease—idiopathic disease; drug reaction; modified live virus (MLV) vaccine reaction.
- Infectious disease—ehrlichiosis; anaplasmosis; Rocky Mountain spotted fever, babesiosis, feline leukemia virus (FeLV) or feline immunodeficiency virus (FIV)-related illness.
- Bone marrow disease—neoplasia; aplastic anemia; infectious (fungal, rickettsial, or viral).
- Paraneoplastic disorder.
- Disseminated intravascular coagulation (DIC).

Thrombopathia

- Congenital—von Willebrand disease; thrombasthenia; thrombopathia.
- Acquired—nonsteroidal anti-inflammatory drugs (NSAIDs); clopidogrel; hyperglobulinemia (*Ehrlichia*, multiple myeloma); uremia; DIC.

Coagulation Factor Defects

- Congenital—hemophilia A (factor VIIIc deficiency) and hemophilia B (factor IX deficiency).
- Acquired—anticoagulant rodenticide (warfarin) intoxication, hepatobiliary disease, DIC.

Local Lesion

- Foreign body.
- Trauma.
- Infection—fungal (*Aspergillus*, *Cryptococcus*, *Rhinosporidium*); viral or bacterial. Usually blood-tinged mucopurulent exudate rather than frank hemorrhage.
- Neoplasia—adenocarcinoma; carcinoma; chondrosarcoma; squamous cell carcinoma; fibrosarcoma; lymphoma; transmissible venereal tumor.
- Dental disease—oronasal fistula, tooth root abscess.
- Lymphoplasmacytic rhinitis.

Vascular or Systemic Disease

- Hypertension—renal disease; hyperthyroidism; hyperadrenocorticism; pheochromocytoma; idiopathic disease.
- Hyperviscosity—hyperglobulinemia (multiple myeloma, *Ehrlichia*); polycythemia.
- Vasculitis—immune-mediated and rickettsial diseases.

RISK FACTORS

Coagulopathy

- Immune-mediated disease—young to middle-aged, small-to medium-sized female dogs.
- Infectious disease—dogs living in or traveling to endemic areas; tick exposure.
- Thrombasthenia—otter hounds.
- Thrombopathia—basset hounds, spitz.
- von Willebrand disease—Doberman pinschers, Airedales, German shepherds, Scottish terriers, Chesapeake Bay retrievers, and many other breeds; cats.
- Hemophilia A—German shepherds and many other breeds; cats.
- Hemophilia B—Cairn terriers, coonhounds, Saint Bernards, and other breeds; cats.

Space-Occupying Lesions

- Aspergillosis—German shepherds, Rottweilers, mesocephalic and dolichocephalic breeds.
- Neoplasia—dolichocephalic breeds.

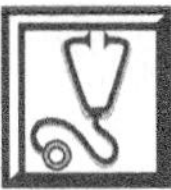

DIAGNOSIS

DIFFERENTIAL DIAGNOSIS

See Causes.

CBC/BIOCHEMISTRY/URINALYSIS

- Anemia—if enough hemorrhage has occurred.
- Thrombocytopenia—possible.
- Neutrophilia—infection; neoplasia.
- Pancytopenia—if bone marrow disease.
- Hypoproteinemia—if enough hemorrhage has occurred.
- High blood urea nitrogen (BUN) with normal creatinine—possible, owing to blood ingestion.
- Hyperglobulinemia—possible with ehrlichiosis, multiple myeloma.
- Azotemia—with renal failure-induced hypertension.
- High alanine transaminase (ALT), aspartate aminotransferase (AST), and total bilirubin—with coagulopathy from severe hepatic disease.
- Urinalysis—usually normal; possible to see hematuria (if coagulopathy), isosthenuria (if renal failure–induced hypertension), and proteinuria (if glomerulotubular disease and hypertension).

OTHER LABORATORY TESTS

- Coagulation profile—prolonged times with coagulation factor defects; normal with thrombocytopenia and thrombopathia.
- Platelet function testing (e.g., buccal mucosal bleeding time, von Willebrand factor analysis)—may be abnormal with platelet dysfunction (platelet count and coagulation profile may be normal).
- *Ehrlichia*, *Anaplasma*, Rocky Mountain spotted fever, or *Babesia* testing—may be positive in thrombocytopenia or thrombopathia-induced epistaxis.
- *Aspergillus* serology—may help establish a diagnosis of fungal rhinitis; false-negative results are common, so results must be interpreted in light of other clinical and diagnostic findings.
- Thyroid hormone assay—elevated in cats with epistaxis due to hyperthyroid-induced hypertension.

IMAGING

- Thoracic radiograph—screen for metastasis.
- Nasal series—under anesthesia, including open-mouth ventrodorsal and skyline sinus views when space-occupying or local lesion is suspected; osteolysis with neoplasia and fungal sinusitis; foreign bodies usually not seen; dental disease may be identified.
- CT or MRI—more sensitive than radiographs.

DIAGNOSTIC PROCEDURES

- Blood pressure evaluation—indicated when coagulopathies and space-occupying lesions have been ruled out and particularly when azotemia or proteinuria is noted.

EPISTAXIS (CONTINUED)

E

• Rhinoscopy, nasal lavage, nasal biopsy (blind or guided via rhinoscopy or CT)—indicated for space-occupying disease; aimed at removing foreign bodies and evaluating and sampling nasal tissue for causal diagnosis (e.g., evaluate nasal tissue samples for neoplasia, inflammation, and infection via cytology and/or histopathology and bacterial/fungal culture and sensitivity testing).
• Bone marrow aspiration biopsy—indicated if pancytopenia identified.

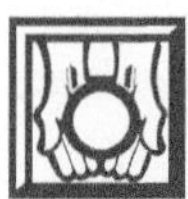

TREATMENT

APPROPRIATE HEALTH CARE

• Coagulopathy—usually inpatient management.
• Space-occupying lesion or vascular or systemic disease—outpatient or inpatient management, depending on disease and its severity.
• Nasal tumors—radiotherapy; various response rates.

NURSING CARE

Provide basic supportive care if needed (fluids, nutrition).

ACTIVITY

Minimize activity or stimuli that precipitate hemorrhage episodes.

CLIENT EDUCATION

• Inform client about the disease process.
• Teach client how to recognize a serious hemorrhage (e.g., weakness, collapse, pallor, and blood loss >30 mL/kg bodyweight).

SURGICAL CONSIDERATIONS

• Surgery indicated if a foreign body is unable to be removed by rhinoscopy or blind attempt.
• Fungal rhinitis (e.g., *Aspergillus* and *Rhinosporidium*) require debulking (also see Medications).

MEDICATIONS

DRUG(S) OF CHOICE

General

• Whole blood, packed red blood cell (RBC), or hemoglobin solution transfusion—can be needed with severe anemia.
• Acepromazine (0.05–0.1 mg/kg SC/IV if normothermic and no platelet disorder present) to lower blood pressure and promote clotting; may help control serious hemorrhage.
• Discontinue all NSAIDs.

Coagulopathy

• Immune-mediated thrombocytopenia—prednisone (1.1 mg/kg q12h; taper over 4–6 months); other drugs can be used in addition to prednisone for refractive cases (see Thrombocytopenia, Primary Immune Mediated).
• Infectious disease—rickettsial disease (doxycycline 5 mg/kg PO q12h for 3–6 weeks); *Babesia* (imidocarb 6.6 mg/kg SC 2 doses 2 weeks apart, diminazene aceturate 5 mg/kg IM once, or 10 days of atovaquone 13.3 mg/kg PO q8h with azithromycin 10 mg/kg PO q24h).
• Bone marrow neoplasia—see Myeloproliferative Disorders.
• Thrombopathia and thrombasthenia—no treatment unless lymphoproliferative disease.
• von Willebrand disease—plasma or cryoprecipitate for acute bleeding; 1-desamino-8-d-arginine vasopressin (DDAVP) 1 µg/kg SC/IV diluted in 20 mL 0.9% NaCl given over 10 min may help control or prevent hemorrhage prior to invasive procedures; intranasal formulation (less expensive) may be used after passing through a bacteriostatic filter.
• Hemophilia A—plasma or cryoprecipitate for acute bleeding; no long-term treatment.
• Hemophilia B—plasma for acute bleeding; no long-term treatment.
• Anticoagulant rodenticide intoxication—plasma for acute bleeding; vitamin K at 5 mg/kg loading dose followed by 1.25 mg/kg q12h for 1 week (if warfarin formulation) to 4 weeks (longer-acting formulation).
• Hyperglobulinemia—plasmapheresis.
• Polycythemia—phlebotomy; hydroxyurea.
• Liver disease and DIC—treat and support underlying cause; plasma may be beneficial.

Space-Occupying Lesion

• Secondary bacterial infection—antibiotics based on culture and sensitivity testing.
• Fungal infection—for aspergillosis, topical treatment of nasal cavity and frontal sinuses with 1% clotrimazole in polyethylene glycol (see Precautions) or 1–5% enilconazole (see Aspergillosis, Nasal for protocol); for cryptococcosis—oral and injectable antifungal agents (see Cryptococcosis); for rhinosporidiosis—surgery followed by dapsone (1 mg/kg PO q8h for 2 weeks, then 1 mg/kg PO q12h for 4 months).

Vascular or Systemic Disease

• Hyperviscosity—treat underlying disease (e.g., ehrlichiosis, multiple myeloma, or polycythemia); plasmapheresis.
• Vasculitis— doxycycline for rickettsial disease (5 mg/kg q12h for 3–6 weeks); prednisone for immune-mediated disease (1.1 mg/kg q12h; taper over 4–6 months).

Hypertension

• Treat underlying disease—renal disease, hyperthyroidism, hyperadrenocorticism.
• Reduce weight if overconditioned.
• Restrict sodium.
• Calcium channel blockers—amlodipine (dogs: 0.1 mg/kg PO q12–24h; cats: 0.625–1.25 mg/cat PO q12–24h); treatment of choice.
• ACE inhibitors—benazepril (0.5 mg/kg q24h); enalapril (0.25–0.5 mg/kg q12–24h).
• Beta blockers—propranolol (0.5–1 mg/kg q8h); atenolol (0.25–1.0 mg/kg q12–24h).
• Diuretics—hydrochlorothiazide (2–4 mg/kg q12h); furosemide (0.5–2 mg/kg q8–12h).
• Phenoxybenzamine (0.2–1.5 mg/kg q12h) for pheochromocytoma.

CONTRAINDICATIONS

• Avoid drugs that may predispose patient to hemorrhage—NSAIDs; heparin; clopidogrel; phenothiazine tranquilizers.
• Topical antifungals—do not use in patients with disruption of the cribriform plate.

PRECAUTIONS

• Chemotherapeutic drugs (immune-mediated thrombocytopenia therapy, e.g., azathioprine)—monitor neutrophil counts and liver enzymes weekly until a pattern has been established that shows that the patient is tolerating the drug.
• Enalapril and/or diuretics—closely monitor patients with renal failure; avoid severe salt restriction when using angiotensin-converting enzyme (ACE) inhibitors.
• Avoid topical clotrimazole preparations with propylene glycol, as life-threatening mucosal irritation, ulceration, and nasopharyngeal swelling can occur.

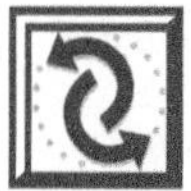

FOLLOW-UP

PATIENT MONITORING

• Platelet count with thrombocytopenia.
• Coagulation profile with coagulation factor defects.
• Blood pressure with hypertension.
• Clinical signs.

PREVENTION/AVOIDANCE

• Restrict access to areas that might contain anticoagulant rodenticides.
• Practice dental preventative care.

POSSIBLE COMPLICATIONS

Anemia and collapse (rare).

EXPECTED COURSE AND PROGNOSIS

Varies depending on underlying cause.

MISCELLANEOUS

PREGNANCY/FERTILITY/BREEDING

Avoid teratogenic drugs (e.g., itraconazole).

ABBREVIATIONS

• ACE = angiotensin-converting enzyme.
• ALT = alanine transaminase.
• AST = aspartate aminotransferase.
• BUN = blood urea nitrogen.
• DDAVP = 1-desamino-8-d-arginine vasopressin.
• DIC = disseminated intravascular coagulation.
• FeLV = feline leukemia virus.
• FIV = feline immunodeficiency virus.

- GI = gastrointestinal.
- MLV = modified live virus.
- NSAID = nonsteroidal anti-inflammatory drug.
- RBC = red blood cell.

Suggested Reading

Bissett SA, Drobatz KJ, McKnight A, Degernes LA. Prevalence, clinical features, and causes of epistaxis in dogs: 176 cases (1996–2001). J Am Vet Med Assoc 2007, 231:1843–1850.

Brooks MB, Catalfamo JL. Immune-mediated thrombocytopenia, von Willebrand disease, and platelet disorders. In: Ettinger SJ, Feldman EC, eds., Textbook of Veterinary Internal Medicine, 7th ed. St. Louis, MO: Saunders Elsevier, 2010, pp. 772–783.

Dunn ME. Acquired coagulopathies. In: Ettinger SJ, Feldman EC, eds., Textbook of Veterinary Internal Medicine, 7th ed. St. Louis, MO: Saunders Elsevier, 2010, pp. 797–801.

Venker-van Haagen AJ, Herrtage ME. Diseases of the nose and nasal sinuses. In: Ettinger SJ, Feldman EC, eds., Textbook of Veterinary Internal Medicine, 7th ed. St. Louis, MO: Saunders Elsevier, 2010, pp. 1030–1040.

Author Meghan Vaught
Consulting Editor Elizabeth Rozanski
Acknowledgment The author and book editors acknowledge the prior contribution of Mitchell A. Crystal.

Client Education Handout available online

ERYTHROCYTOSIS

BASICS

DEFINITION

An increase in packed cell volume (PCV), hemoglobin concentration, or red blood cell (RBC) count above the reference interval due to a relative or absolute increase in the number of circulating RBCs.

PATHOPHYSIOLOGY

- Circulating RBC numbers are affected by changes in plasma volume, rate of RBC destruction or loss, splenic contraction, erythropoietin (EPO) secretion, and bone marrow production.
- Erythropoiesis is also affected by hormones from the adrenal cortex, thyroid gland, ovary, testis, and anterior pituitary gland; normal PCV is maintained by an endocrine loop.
- Erythrocytosis is either relative or absolute.
- Relative—develops when hemoconcentration or splenic contraction produces an increase in circulating RBCs.
- Absolute—increase in circulating RBC mass due to an increase in bone marrow production; either primary or secondary to an increase in the production of EPO.
- Primary absolute (polycythemia vera)—myeloproliferative disorder characterized by neoplastic proliferation of all marrow cell precursors independent of EPO.
- Secondary absolute—caused by physiologically appropriate release of EPO due to chronic hypoxemia, excessive production of EPO or an EPO-like substance in an animal with normal partial pressure of oxygen (PaO_2), or by excessive exogenous administration of EPO or darbepoetin.

SYSTEMS AFFECTED

Cardiovascular, respiratory, nervous, renal/urologic—blood hyperviscosity causes poor perfusion and oxygen delivery to tissues.

GENETICS

Mutations of the JAK2 gene have been associated with polycythemia vera in humans.

INCIDENCE/PREVALENCE

Relative erythrocytosis due to hemoconcentration or splenic contraction is the most common cause of erythrocytosis.

GEOGRAPHIC DISTRIBUTION

- Reference intervals for PCV, hemoglobin, and RBC count vary with geographic location and breed.
- Animals living at high altitudes have higher PCV than those at sea level.

SIGNALMENT

Species

Dog and cat.

Breed Predilections

- Excitable breeds and cats are prone to splenic contraction.
- Greyhounds have higher PCV values (reference interval is 50–65%).

Mean Age and Range

Primary absolute polycythemia vera—cats 6–7 years; dogs 7 years or older.

Predominant Sex

Male cats, female dogs.

SIGNS

Historical Findings

- Relative—excitement or dehydration.
- Absolute—lethargy, seizures, altered mentation, anorexia, epistaxis, mucous membrane hyperemia.

Physical Examination Findings

- Relative—dehydration and clinical evidence of fluid loss.
- Absolute—lethargy, low exercise tolerance, behavioral change, brick red or cyanotic mucous membranes, sneezing, epistaxis, large size and tortuosity of retinal and sublingual vessels, cardiopulmonary impairment.
- Primary absolute—variable degrees of splenomegaly, hepatomegaly, thrombosis, and hemorrhage; seizures.
- Secondary appropriate absolute—clinical signs of hypoxemia caused by chronic pulmonary disease, cardiac disease with right-to-left shunting, or hemoglobinopathy.
- Secondary absolute (inappropriate EPO secretion)—signs associated with neoplasia, space-occupying renal lesion, or endocrine disorder.

CAUSES

- Relative—hemoconcentration/dehydration or splenic contraction due to excitement.
- Primary absolute—rare myeloproliferative disorder.
- Secondary appropriate absolute—chronic pulmonary disease, cardiac disease or anomaly with right-to-left shunting, high altitude, methemoglobinemia, and impairment of renal blood supply.
- Secondary absolute caused by inappropriate EPO secretion (rare)—neoplasia (e.g., T-cell lymphoma, nasal fibrosarcoma, renal carcinoma, pheochromocytoma, cecal leiomyosarcoma), hyperadrenocorticism, hyperthyroidism, hyperandrogenism.
- Secondary absolute caused by inappropriate EPO or darbepoetin administration in animals undergoing therapy for anemia.

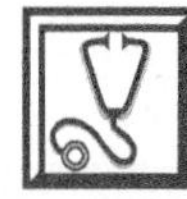

DIAGNOSIS

DIFFERENTIAL DIAGNOSIS

- Moderately high PCV and total plasma protein with concurrent dehydration—suggest relative polycythemia.
- Secondary absolute—caused by diseases that produce chronic hypoxemia or by space-occupying lesions of the kidney, endocrine disorders, neoplasms that produce EPO or an EPO-like substance independent of hypoxia, history of EPO administration.
- Polycythemia vera—diagnosed by elimination of other causes.

CBC/BIOCHEMISTRY/URINALYSIS

- Increased PCV or hematocrit.
- Physiologic leukocytosis (neutrophilia and lymphocytosis) may occur with splenic contraction.

OTHER LABORATORY TESTS

- Serial monitoring of PCV—diagnosis of polycythemia vera requires an unexplained high PCV documented on multiple occasions (several weeks) with no underlying cause.
- Arterial blood gas analysis may demonstrate a low PaO_2 in cases of secondary appropriate absolute erythrocytosis; pulse oximetry may also be used to assess oxygen saturation (SpO_2).
- EPO measurement—not currently recommended due to lack of veterinary-specific assays and extensive overlap in EPO concentration between normal and affected animals.
- Thyroid testing (cats).

IMAGING

Radiography and abdominal ultrasonography to detect cardiopulmonary disease and neoplasia.

DIAGNOSTIC PROCEDURES

- Biopsy of any masses.
- Bone marrow aspirate.

PATHOLOGIC FINDINGS

Polycythemia vera—gross findings: generalized vascular congestion, arterial thrombosis, splenomegaly, diffusely red bone marrow with reduced fat; microscopic findings: hyperplastic bone marrow with normal or reduced myeloid/erythroid ratio and reduced iron content.

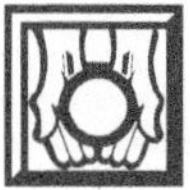

TREATMENT

APPROPRIATE HEALTH CARE

- Relative—rehydration with IV fluids appropriate for primary cause; assessment of renal function, gastrointestinal system, acid-base status, and electrolyte balance; if not hemoconcentrated, allow patient to calm down.
- Absolute—phlebotomy recommended (20 mL/kg over 1 to several days) to reduce RBC mass to PCV of 55%; blood volume should be replaced concurrently with isotonic fluids.
- Secondary inappropriate absolute—phlebotomy combined with identification and removal of EPO source.
- Secondary appropriate absolute—phlebotomy and hydroxyurea. The high PCV

is an appropriate compensatory response; thus, phlebotomy may be dangerous; if indicated, remove blood at a lower volume (5 mL/kg). A higher PCV (60–65%) may be necessary to sustain life until the cause of hypoxemia can be corrected.
- Polycythemia vera—phlebotomy (20 mL/kg) and hydroxyurea; frequency of bleeding and dosage adjusted to maintain a PCV of 55% in dogs and 45% in cats.

NURSING CARE

Oxygen therapy may be indicated for patients with cyanosis, hypoxemia, cardiopulmonary disease, or weakness following phlebotomy.

ACTIVITY

Excessive exercise should be avoided.

DIET

Normal diet, free-choice water.

CLIENT EDUCATION

- Patients need to be observed at home for changes in activity, difficulty breathing, or bleeding.
- Patients treated with EPO for anemia must have PCV rechecked and dose adjusted at regular intervals.

SURGICAL CONSIDERATIONS

If surgery is necessary, preoperative phlebotomy and close monitoring of oxygenation and vital parameters may be necessary. Postoperatively, monitor for bleeding or thrombosis.

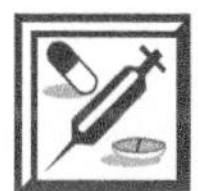

MEDICATIONS

DRUG(S) OF CHOICE

- Polycythemia vera—hydroxyurea (dogs: 40–50 mg/kg PO divided twice daily; cats: 30 mg/kg PO q24h).
- Erythrocytosis secondary to hypoxemia—hydroxyurea (40–50 mg/kg PO q48h).

CONTRAINDICATIONS

Phlebotomy may be contraindicated in hypoxemic patients.

PRECAUTIONS

- Rapid removal of blood can cause hypotension and cardiovascular collapse.
- Adverse effects of hydroxyurea include bone marrow hypoplasia with thrombocytopenia, anemia, and neutropenia, alopecia, changes in skin pigmentation, and sloughing of toenails.
- Methemoglobinemia and hemolytic anemia reported in cats treated with hydroxyurea.

ALTERNATIVE DRUG(S)

Polycythemia vera—chlorambucil (dogs and cats: 0.2 mg/kg PO q24h) or busulfan (dogs: 2–4 mg/m^2 PO q24h).

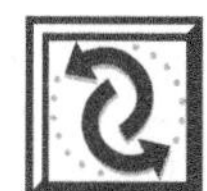

FOLLOW-UP

PATIENT MONITORING

- PCV, total protein, urine output, and bodyweight daily in severely dehydrated animals.
- Patients treated for polycythemia vera by chemotherapy—monitor weekly for changes in PCV, leukocytes, and platelets during initial treatment; then monthly for adjustment of chemotherapy and periodic phlebotomy.
- Periodic assessment of bone marrow iron stores or serum iron levels is indicated to detect iron deficiency.

POSSIBLE COMPLICATIONS

- Hyperviscosity in patients with absolute polycythemia, especially polycythemia vera, may lead to thrombosis, infarction, or hemorrhage.
- Chemotherapy may cause bone marrow suppression.
- Patients undergoing repeated phlebotomies can develop iron deficiency, hypoproteinemia, and peripheral edema.

EXPECTED COURSE AND PROGNOSIS

- Relative erythrocytosis—fair to good prognosis depending on primary cause.
- Secondary absolute appropriate erythrocytosis—clinical course and prognosis are determined by the severity of the lesion causing hypoxemia.
- Secondary inappropriate absolute erythrocytosis—if the tissue source of excessive EPO secretion can be identified and removed or corrected, prognosis is good to fair depending on cause.
- Primary absolute erythrocytosis (polycythemia vera)—prognosis is guarded, although cats have had survival times up to 5 years.

E

MISCELLANEOUS

PREGNANCY/FERTILITY/BREEDING

Hydroxyurea may arrest or inhibit spermatogenesis.

SYNONYMS

Polycythemia—although use of this term should be avoided, due to its similarity with polycythemia vera.

SEE ALSO

- Hyperviscosity Syndrome.
- Polycythemia Vera.

ABBREVIATIONS

- EPO = erythropoietin.
- PaO_2 = partial pressure of oxygen.
- PCV = packed cell volume.
- RBC = red blood cell.
- SpO_2 = oxygen saturation.

Suggested Reading

Cook SM, Lothrop CD. Serum erythropoietin concentrations measured by radioimmunoassay in normal, polycythemic, and anemic dogs and cats. J Vet Intern Med 1994, 8:18–25.

Darcy H, Simpson K, Gajanayake I, et al. Feline primary erythrocytosis: a multicenter case series of 18 cats. J Fel Med Surg 2018, 1:1–7.

Randolph JF, Peterson ME, Stokol T. 2010. Erythrocytosis and polycythemia. In: Weiss DJ, Wardrop KJ, eds., Schalm's Veterinary Hematology, 6th ed. Ames, IA: Wiley-Blackwell, 2010, pp. 162–166.

Author Bridget C. Garner

Consulting Editor Melinda S. Camus

Acknowledgment The author and book editors acknowledge the prior contribution of Alan H. Rebar.

Client Education Handout available online

ESOPHAGEAL DIVERTICULA

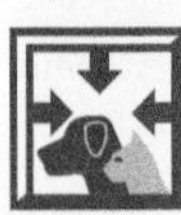

BASICS

OVERVIEW

- Pouch-like sacculations of the esophageal wall that accumulate fluids and ingesta.
- Diverticula may be congenital or acquired and are rare.
- Pulsion diverticula occur secondary to increased intraluminal pressure. Seen with esophageal obstructive disorders such as foreign body or mass lesions.
- Traction diverticula occur secondary to periesophageal inflammation where fibrosis contracts and pulls out the wall of the esophagus into a pouch.
- Localized inflammation around (esophagitis) and lining the diverticulum may be present.
- Potential complications include ingesta impaction, mechanical obstruction (large diverticulum), and/or esophageal hypomotility.
- Organ systems affected include gastrointestinal (regurgitation), musculoskeletal (weight loss), and respiratory (aspiration pneumonia).

SIGNALMENT

- Rare; more common in dog than cat.
- Congenital or acquired (no genetic basis proven).
- No important breed or sex predisposition.

SIGNS

- Postprandial regurgitation, dysphagia, anorexia, coughing.
- Weight loss, respiratory distress.

CAUSES & RISK FACTORS

Pulsion Diverticulum

- Embryonic developmental disorders of the esophageal wall.
- Esophageal foreign body, mass or focal motility disturbances (uncommon).

Traction Diverticulum

Inflammatory processes associated with the trachea, lungs, hilar lymph nodes, or pericardium; resultant fibrous connective tissue adheres to the esophageal wall.

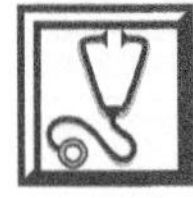

DIAGNOSIS

DIFFERENTIAL DIAGNOSIS

- Esophageal redundancy—barium contrast accumulation in the region of the thoracic inlet can occur normally in young dogs (especially brachycephalic breeds and Chinese Shar-Pei).
- Periesophageal mass—esophagram or esophagoscopy should differentiate the presence of a mass causing luminal narrowing.
- Esophagitis.
- Esophageal foreign body.
- Hiatal hernia.
- Gastroesophageal intussusception.

CBC/BIOCHEMISTRY/URINALYSIS

Usually within normal limits.

OTHER LABORATORY TESTS

N/A

IMAGING

- Thoracic radiography—may show air or soft tissue opacity cranial to the diaphragm or cranial to the thoracic inlet.
- Contrast esophagram—shows contrast accumulation within the diverticulum.
- Videofluoroscopy—useful to evaluate for disturbances in esophageal motility.

DIAGNOSTIC PROCEDURES

Esophagoscopy confirms ingesta/debris within outpouchings of the esophagus.

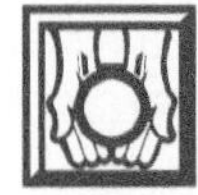

TREATMENT

- If the diverticulum is small and not causing significant clinical signs, treat conservatively with elevated feedings of a soft, bland diet followed by copious liquids or a semi-liquid diet.
- If the diverticulum is large or is associated with significant clinical signs, surgical resection is recommended.
- Client education should include the importance of dietary management and the potential for aspiration pneumonia.
- Fluid therapy, antibiotics, and aggressive nursing, if concurrent aspiration pneumonia is present; alternative enteral nutrition via gastrostomy tube may be necessary in patients with aspiration pneumonia.
- Treat for esophagitis if present.

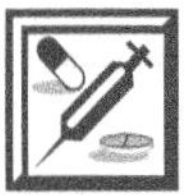

MEDICATIONS

DRUG(S) OF CHOICE

- Drug therapy for esophagitis, if present.
- Proton pump inhibitors, such as omeprazole or pantoprazole, are potent and effective anti-secretory agents (omeprazole: 0.7–1.5 mg/kg PO q12h; pantoprazole: 0.7–1.5 mg/kg IV once daily) for treatment of severe esophagitis.
- Use broad-spectrum antibiotics if patient has concurrent aspiration pneumonia; if recurrent or severe pneumonia is present, base antibiotic selection on culture and sensitivity of samples obtained by transtracheal wash or bronchoalveolar lavage.

CONTRAINDICATIONS/POSSIBLE INTERACTIONS

N/A

FOLLOW-UP

PATIENT MONITORING

- Evaluate for evidence of infection or aspiration pneumonia.
- Maintain positive nutritional balance throughout disease process.

POSSIBLE COMPLICATIONS

Patients with diverticula and impaction are predisposed to perforation, fistula, stricture, and postoperative incisional dehiscence.

EXPECTED COURSE AND PROGNOSIS

- Prognosis is guarded in patients with large diverticula and overt clinical signs.
- Motility disturbances may persist post-surgery.

MISCELLANEOUS

INTERNET RESOURCES

https://www.vin.com/vin/default.aspx

Suggested Reading

Marks SL. Diseases of the pharynx and esophagus. In: Ettinger SJ, Feldman EC, eds., Textbook of Veterinary Internal Medicine, 8th ed. Philadelphia, PA: Saunders, 2017.

Sherding RG, Johnson SE. Esophagoscopy. In: Tams TR, Rawlings CA, eds., Small Animal Endoscopy, 3rd ed. Philadelphia, PA: Mosby, 2011, pp. 41–95.

Author Albert E. Jergens

Consulting Editor Mark P. Rondeau

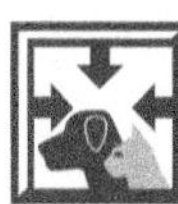

BASICS

DEFINITION

Ingestion of foreign material or foodstuffs too large to pass through the esophagus, causing partial or complete luminal obstruction.

PATHOPHYSIOLOGY

Esophageal foreign bodies cause mechanical obstruction, mucosal inflammation with edema, and possibly ischemic necrosis and esophageal perforation.

SYSTEMS AFFECTED

- Gastrointestinal.
- Respiratory—if aspiration pneumonia.

GENETICS

N/A

INCIDENCE/PREVALENCE

Unknown

GEOGRAPHIC DISTRIBUTION

N/A

SIGNALMENT

Species

Due to the indiscriminate eating habits of many dogs, they have a higher incidence than cats.

Breed Predilections

More common in small-breed dogs; terrier breeds often overrepresented.

Mean Age and Range

More common in young to middle-aged animals.

Predominant Sex

N/A

SIGNS

General Comments

The pet may have been observed ingesting a foreign body.

Historical Findings

Most common include retching, gagging, lethargy, anorexia, ptyalism, regurgitation, restlessness, dysphagia, odynophagia, and persistent gulping.

Physical Examination Findings

- Ptyalism.
- Can be unremarkable.
- Occasional discomfort when palpating the neck or cranial abdomen.

CAUSES

Occurs most often with an object whose size, shape, or texture does not allow free movement through the esophagus, causing it to become lodged before it can pass.

RISK FACTORS

- Indiscriminate eating habits.
- Access to foreign materials.

DIAGNOSIS

DIFFERENTIAL DIAGNOSIS

- Esophagitis.
- Esophageal stricture.
- Esophageal neoplasia.
- Megaesophagus.
- Other esophageal disorders.

CBC/BIOCHEMISTRY/URINALYSIS

- Usually unremarkable.
- Occasionally, electrolyte abnormalities, an inflammatory leukogram, and/or hemoconcentration, depending upon the severity of signs and degree of dehydration.

OTHER LABORATORY TESTS

N/A

IMAGING

Thoracic Radiography

- Most esophageal foreign bodies are radiodense and are readily visualized. These objects most commonly lodge at points of minimal esophageal distension, including the thoracic inlet, base of the heart, and esophageal hiatus.
- Esophageal distension with air may be visualized cranial to the foreign body. Retained air in the esophagus is not always associated with esophageal foreign bodies.
- A contrast esophagram or videofluoroscopy is required to identify radiolucent objects. If perforation is suspected, use an aqueous organic iodide contrast agent for imaging studies.
- Air and/or fluid in the mediastinum or pleural space suggests esophageal perforation; depending on severity, this can be an indication for surgery versus esophagoscopy.
- Pulmonary infiltrates suggest aspiration pneumonia.

DIAGNOSTIC PROCEDURES

Esophagoscopy allows removal of most (80%) foreign bodies using retrieval forceps. It also allows for visual inspection of the mucosa for trauma after foreign body removal. Use of an endoscope with an accessory channel diameter of >2.8 mm will allow use of the largest types of retrieval forceps.

PATHOLOGIC FINDINGS

N/A

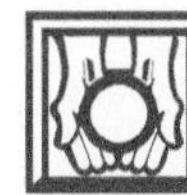

TREATMENT

APPROPRIATE HEALTH CARE

- Emergencies—treat as inpatient and perform endoscopy as soon as possible after diagnosis.
- If endoscopic retrieval of the foreign body succeeds *and* esophageal damage is minimal, the patient may be discharged the same day.
- Foreign bodies which cannot be removed through the mouth may be pushed aborally into the stomach.

NURSING CARE

- If the procedure to remove the foreign body is atraumatic and the esophagus has sustained minimal damage, no special aftercare is needed.
- Severe mucosal trauma may require placing a gastrostomy tube for enteral nutritional support during esophageal healing. Fluid therapy may also be required to maintain normal hydration status during periods of prolonged esophageal rest.

ACTIVITY

The patient may resume normal activity after a foreign body has been routinely removed.

DIET

- No change needed other than, perhaps, altering the food to a more liquid consistency.
- Feeding should be withheld 12–24 hours following foreign body removal.

CLIENT EDUCATION

Discuss the possibility of complications and repeat offenders.

SURGICAL CONSIDERATIONS

- Surgery is indicated when endoscopy fails to retrieve the foreign body; when endoscopy enables advancement of the object into the gastric lumen but it is too large to pass through the gastrointestinal tract; or when a large esophageal perforation or area of necrosis requires resection.
- The short-term prognosis for esophageal surgery is dogs and cats is favorable (~90%).
- It is often less traumatic to advance a bone foreign body into the stomach than to attempt retrieval transorally via endoscopy. Gastrostomy, if required, may then be performed.
- Most bone foreign bodies can be safely left to dissolve in the stomach without need for surgical removal. Nondigestible foreign objects (wood, metal, plastic) passed into the stomach may need to be removed surgically.

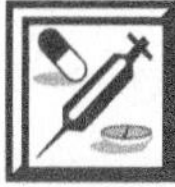

MEDICATIONS

DRUG(S) OF CHOICE

If there is significant mucosal injury (i.e., esophagitis), recommendations include:

- Sucralfate slurry (0.5–1 g/dog PO q8h) for mucosal cytoprotection and healing.
- Proton pump inhibitor (omeprazole or pantoprazole at 1 mg/kg q12h) for robust suppression of gastric acid secretions that may contribute to reflux esophagitis.
- Broad-spectrum antibiotics (amoxicillin or Clavamox®) are only administered to animals with mucosal perforation.

ESOPHAGEAL FOREIGN BODIES (CONTINUED)

- Metoclopramide (0.2–0.5 mg/kg IV/SC/PO q8h) or cisapride (0.5 mg/kg q8–12h PO) to stimulate gastric motility and minimize reflux esophagitis.
- Gastrostomy tube placement for enteral nutrition in animals with severe mucosal trauma.

CONTRAINDICATIONS

N/A

PRECAUTIONS

N/A

POSSIBLE INTERACTIONS

N/A

ALTERNATIVE DRUG(S)

N/A

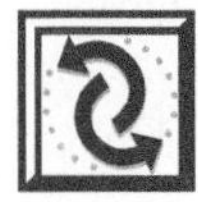

FOLLOW-UP

PATIENT MONITORING

- Examine the esophagus closely via endoscopy for mucosal damage after foreign body removal.
- Mild erythema/erosions are not uncommon and tend to heal uneventfully.
- If an esophageal laceration/perforation is detected—gastrostomy tube feedings allow esophageal rest and healing.
- Advise post-procedural survey thoracic radiographs to assess for pneumomediastinum/pneumothorax.
- Monitor at least 2–3 weeks for evidence of stricture formation.
- Esophageal stricture—most common clinical sign is regurgitation with evidence of odynophagia in many animals; esophagram or videofluoroscopy and/or esophagoscopy may be indicated to confirm a stricture.

PREVENTION/AVOIDANCE

Carefully monitor the environment and what is fed to the pet.

POSSIBLE COMPLICATIONS

- Approximately 25% of patients with foreign bodies develop complications.
- Complications most frequently encountered include esophageal perforation, esophageal strictures, esophageal fistulas, and severe esophagitis. Focal, transient esophageal motility disturbances can occur secondary to esophageal trauma.
- Pneumomediastinum, pneumothorax, pneumonia, pleuritis, mediastinitis, and bronchoesophageal fistulas can all occur secondary to perforation.

EXPECTED COURSE AND PROGNOSIS

- Most patients do well and recover uneventfully.
- With complications, the prognosis is guarded.

MISCELLANEOUS

ASSOCIATED CONDITIONS

None

AGE-RELATED FACTORS

N/A

ZOONOTIC POTENTIAL

None

PREGNANCY/FERTILITY/BREEDING

N/A

SEE ALSO

- Esophageal Diverticula.
- Esophageal Stricture.
- Regurgitation.

INTERNET RESOURCES

https://www.vin.com

Suggested Reading

Deroy C, Corcuff JB, Billen F, et al. Removal of oesophageal foreign bodies: comparison between oesophagoscopy and oesophagotomy in 39 dogs. J Small Anim Pract 2015, 56:613–617.

Pratt CL, Reineke EL, Drobatz KJ. Sewing needle foreign body ingestion in dogs and cats: 65 cases (2000–2012). J Am Vet Med Assoc 2014, 245(3):302–308.

Sutton JS, Culp WTN, Scotti K, et al. Perioperative morbidity and outcome of esophageal surgery in dogs and cats: 72 cases (1993-2013). J Am Vet Med Assoc 2016, 249(7):787–793.

Tams TR. Endoscopic removal of gastrointestinal foreign bodies. In: Tams TR, Rawlings CA, eds., Small Animal Endoscopy, 3rd ed. Philadelphia, PA: Mosby, 2011, pp. 247–295.

Author Albert E. Jergens

Consulting Editor Mark P. Rondeau

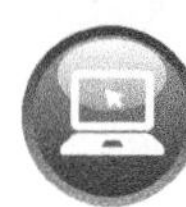

Client Education Handout available online

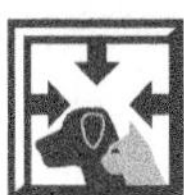

BASICS

DEFINITION

A fixed narrowing of the esophagus resulting in partial or complete obstruction.

PATHOPHYSIOLOGY

• Benign strictures occur when there is circumferential erosion and ulceration of the esophageal mucosa; regardless of the initiating event, once esophagitis develops there is a decrease in the lower esophageal sphincter (LES) tone; this results in more acid reflux and subsequent worsening of esophagitis; once severe esophagitis is present, damage can extend to the lamina propria and muscularis layers of the esophagus; this incites fibroblastic proliferation and contraction, leading to stricture formation. • Malignant strictures occur rarely in dogs and cats, and result from direct tumor invasion.

SYSTEMS AFFECTED

• Gastrointestinal—a single site of stricture is most common, although multiple strictures can occur anywhere through the esophagus.
• Respiratory—regurgitation is common with strictures, increasing risk for aspiration pneumonia.

GENETICS

N/A

INCIDENCE/PREVALENCE

Infrequent

GEOGRAPHIC DISTRIBUTION

Spirocerca lupi granuloma occurs in the southern United States, parts of Europe, South Africa, and Israel.

SIGNALMENT

Species

Dog and cat.

Breed Predilections

None

Mean Age and Range

Any. Puppies and kittens with extraluminal compression of the esophagus from a vascular ring anomaly typically become symptomatic at weaning.

Predominant Sex

None

SIGNS

Historical Findings

• Odynophagia, dysphagia, increased salivation, regurgitation, anorexia, and weight loss; signs tend to be progressive as the stricture progressively narrows. • If regurgitation leads to aspiration pneumonia, cough and dyspnea can develop.

Physical Examination Findings

May have poor body condition secondary to malnutrition.

CAUSES

• Reflux during anesthesia is the most common cause of benign esophageal stricture, accounting for about 65% of cases; decreased LES tone during anesthesia may promote gastroesophageal reflux, resulting in subsequent acid injury to the esophageal mucosa. • Esophageal foreign bodies (if >270° mucosal damage occurs). • Esophagitis from certain tablets and capsules; commonly incriminated drugs are doxycycline, clindamycin, alendronate, and aspirin.
• Gastroesophageal reflux. • Prolonged vomiting of gastric contents. • Swallowing of caustic substances. • Esophageal neoplasia (squamous cell carcinoma and lymphoma most common). • *Spirocerca lupi* granuloma.
• Iatrogenic trauma during endoscopy.
• Vascular ring anomaly as an extraluminal cause for focal esophageal narrowing.

RISK FACTORS

• General anesthesia, especially with drugs that decrease LES tone, when the patient is in Trendelenburg position, and in large-breed, deep-chested dogs positioned in sternal recumbency. • Oral medications given with a dry swallow. • Foreign body ingestion.

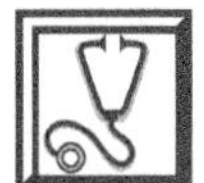

DIAGNOSIS

DIFFERENTIAL DIAGNOSIS

• Megaesophagus. • Esophageal foreign body.
• Esophageal neoplasia. • Extrinsic esophageal compression (mass, abscess). • Gastroesophageal reflux. • Vomiting (any cause). • Oropharyngeal dysphagia. • Vascular ring anomaly.

CBC/BIOCHEMISTRY/URINALYSIS

Usually unremarkable.

OTHER LABORATORY TESTS

Usually unremarkable.

IMAGING

• Thoracic radiographs—usually unremarkable unless aspiration pneumonia develops.
• Videofluoroscopic barium swallow should identify most strictures; if videofluoroscopy is not available, barium swallow of liquid, paste, or food followed immediately by radiography is performed; peristalsis proximal to the stricture site can be abnormal with concurrent esophagitis; may demonstrate more than one stricture.

DIAGNOSTIC PROCEDURES

• Endoscopy—diagnostic test of choice.
• A focal narrowing (single or multiple) is easily identified; there is an abrupt decrease in luminal diameter at the stricture site.
• Usually the mucosa is normal (smooth and pink), but can appear hyperemic and ulcerated if esophagitis is present.

PATHOLOGIC FINDINGS

• If an esophageal mass is present, biopsy with histopathology is warranted; otherwise, benign strictures are not typically biopsied. • Strictures can be focal, multifocal, or coalescing.

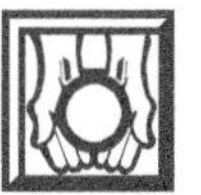

TREATMENT

APPROPRIATE HEALTH CARE

• Outpatient medical management is only successful for mild strictures; most strictures require intervention. • If there are complications (esophageal perforation, aspiration pneumonia), then inpatient care is required.

NURSING CARE

IV fluids may be necessary if the animal is dehydrated.

ACTIVITY

• Exercise restriction is not necessary after dilation. • If pneumonia is present, the degree of hypoxia will determine appropriate activity level.

DIET

• Recommend feeding a fat-restricted diet to enhance gastric emptying. • Canned food can be fed in small frequent amounts following dilation. • If a balloon esophagostomy (BE) tube is placed, supplemental nutrition can be provided as needed through the tube; for refractory cases, placement of a percutaneous endoscopic gastrostomy tube could be considered.

CLIENT EDUCATION

• Owners should be aware that dilation procedures are not always successful, and that multiple attempts are required in many patients; it is important that medical management for esophagitis be diligently employed following dilation procedures to reduce the risk of restricture. • Placement of a BE tube could be discussed if multiple dilation procedures are not feasible or desired, or in the case of severe stricture.

SURGICAL CONSIDERATIONS

• First-line treatment of benign esophageal strictures is mechanical dilatation of the stricture; techniques have evolved from rigid bougienage, to flexible bougies, to balloon dilation; the theoretical advantage of balloon dilatation is that the forces applied to the stricture are a radial stretch, whereas some of the forces applied with bougienage are longitudinal, resulting in possibly greater potential for esophageal perforation.
• Esophageal dilatation balloons are made of special plastic that makes the balloon extremely rigid when maximally inflated at high pressures; balloons are positioned within the stricture under direct endoscopic visualization; the balloon is slowly inflated with saline using a commercially available

E

inflation device until it reaches the manufacturer's rated pressure for that balloon; to ensure adequate dilation of the stricture has occurred, inflation of the balloon with ioxhexol and fluoroscopic monitoring during inflation is recommended; inadequate stricture effacement is commonly seen if this procedure is only performed with endoscopy.
• Initial balloon diameter is ideally selected following measured diameters of normal esophagus obtained via a contrast study during the procedure; if fluoroscopy is not available, a balloon diameter 50–100% larger than the estimated stricture diameter can be selected; it is important to avoid assuming size based on weight of the animal as this can result in under- or overestimation; the sequence of subsequent larger dilations is then determined by the degree of mucosal tearing, ideally visualized fluoroscopically; the final dilation diameter is usually chosen by the degree of mucosal tearing and the size of the normal esophagus for the patient. • BE tube placement is a newer treatment option; this device allows for balloon dilation twice daily for 4–6 weeks at home to prevent stricture recurrence; the small number of reported patients have had improved short- and long-term outcomes compared to other treatments; the BE tube is placed similarly to a standard esophagostomy tube after balloon dilation is performed; placement of the balloon is confirmed with fluoroscopy to ensure the balloon spans the length of the stricture and does not interfere with the upper or lower esophageal sphincter. • For persistent strictures, despite multiple balloon dilations, a salvage procedure with placement of a self-expanding or bioabsorbable stent can be employed; it is important that the stent be secured with sutures to prevent migration; esophageal stenting has been associated with adverse effects including ptyalism, regurgitation, megaesophagus requiring removal, and incision infection/drainage; given the unpredictability for which patients will tolerate stent placement, this procedure should be considered only for highly refractory cases that fail BE tube placement.
• Surgical management (resection and anastomosis) is typically only performed as a last resort.

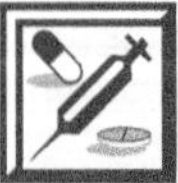

MEDICATIONS

DRUG(S) OF CHOICE

• Following dilation, give sucralfate suspension (0.5–1 g/patient PO q6h) to reduce esophagitis and pain. • Medications for esophagitis are used, including cisapride (0.5–0.75 mg/kg PO q8h) to increase LES tone and enhance gastric emptying, and omeprazole (1 mg/kg PO q12h) to decrease gastric acidity.

CONTRAINDICATIONS

Caustic substances and emetic medications.

PRECAUTIONS

• Esophageal perforation can occur with overzealous balloon dilation of the stricture, therefore incremental increase in balloon diameter is recommended. • Ineffective balloon dilation can occur with incomplete tearing of the stricture; monitoring with videofluoroscopy could be considered to monitor for this. • Using a balloon over a guidewire is the safest way to perform this procedure; perforation is most common when a guidewire is not used through the lumen of the balloon and the balloon tip is advanced accidentally into the esophageal wall—use caution.

POSSIBLE INTERACTIONS

Sucralfate may inhibit the absorption of other drugs.

ALTERNATIVE DRUG(S)

• Metoclopramide can be used to increase LES tone. • Histamine H2-receptor blockers can be used to decrease gastric acid.

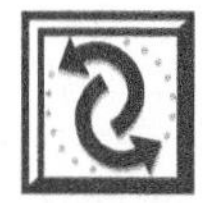

FOLLOW-UP

PATIENT MONITORING

Patients are monitored for signs of recurrent stricture, including regurgitation and gagging.

PREVENTION/AVOIDANCE

• Preanesthetic administration of cisapride decreases the number of reflux events in anesthetized dogs. • Preanesthetic administration of omeprazole will minimize the likelihood of acid reflux. • Medications with ulcerogenic potential should be given with at least 6 mL of water or food.

POSSIBLE COMPLICATIONS

• Complications of balloon dilatation include perforation, severe mucosal tearing and esophagitis, and stricture recurrence; with BE tube placement additional complications include infection at the tube site and migration of the tube beyond the stricture; this is typically well tolerated.
• Complications with stent placement include hyperplastic tissue ingrowth or overgrowth, dysphagia, gagging, perceived discomfort, and stricture recurrence.
• Aspiration pneumonia secondary to regurgitation.

EXPECTED COURSE AND PROGNOSIS

• With standard balloon dilation, reported successful outcomes defined as ability to swallow at least semi-solid food range from 71.4% to 88.0%, with 12–23.1% able to eat a normal diet. • With BE tube placement, the majority (66.7%; 8/12) of patients were able to eat a normal diet with no dysphagia. • The prognosis for esophageal neoplasia is poor, but these cases tolerate esophageal stents well.

MISCELLANEOUS

ASSOCIATED CONDITIONS

• Aspiration pneumonia. • Esophagitis.

AGE-RELATED FACTORS

None.

ZOONOTIC POTENTIAL

None.

PREGNANCY/FERTILITY/BREEDING

N/A

SYNONYMS

• Esophageal narrowing. • Esophageal blockage or obstruction.

SEE ALSO

- Dysphagia.
- Esophageal Foreign Bodies.
- Esophagitis.
- Regurgitation.

ABBREVIATIONS

- BE = balloon esophagostomy.
- LES = lower esophageal sphincter.

Suggested Reading

Lam N, Weisse C, Berent A, et al. Esophageal stenting for treatment of refractory benign esophageal strictures in dogs. J Vet Intern Med 2013, 27(5):1064–1070.

Leib MS, Dinnel H, Ward DL, et al. Endoscopic balloon dilation of benign esophageal strictures in dogs and cats. J Vet Intern Med 2001, 15:547–552.

Tan DK, Weisse CW, Berent AB, Lamb KE. Prospective evaluation of an indwelling esophageal balloon dilation feeding tube for treatment of benign esophageal strictures in cats and dogs. J Vet Intern Med 2018, 32:693–700.

Authors Melissa L. Milligan and Allyson Berent

Consulting Editor Mark P. Rondeau

Acknowledgment The author and book editors acknowledge the prior contribution of Keith Richter

Client Education Handout available online

ESOPHAGITIS

BASICS

DEFINITION

Inflammation of the esophagus typically affecting the esophageal body and lower esophageal sphincter (LES).

PATHOPHYSIOLOGY

- Disruption of esophageal defense mechanisms can result in esophageal inflammation, most commonly due to the effects of gastric acid from gastroesophageal reflux (GER) or vomiting.
- Esophagitis can result in impaired esophageal motility and LES incompetence, which may result in further GER perpetuating esophageal damage.

SYSTEMS AFFECTED

- Gastrointestinal (GI)—esophagus and in the vomiting patient primary or secondary GI disease.
- Respiratory—regurgitation and GER may lead to aspiration pneumonia, reflux laryngitis, pharyngitis and/or rhinitis; respiratory signs may be covert presentation for GER.

INCIDENCE/PREVALENCE

Unknown—relatively common; probably underestimated, as most cases are not definitively diagnosed.

GEOGRAPHIC DISTRIBUTION

Worldwide, except when caused by *Pythium* spp. (US Gulf Coast) and *Spirocerca lupi* (southern states).

SIGNALMENT

Species

Dog and cat.

Breed Predilections

Reflux esophagitis in brachycephalic breeds due to negative intrathoracic pressure upon inspiration increasing the tendency for GER and hiatal hernia (HH).

Mean Age and Range

- Any age.
- Young animals with congenital esophageal HH and older animals that are anesthetized are at greater risk of developing reflux esophagitis.

Predominant Sex

None

SIGNS

Historical Findings

- Regurgitation.
- Ptyalism.
- Dysphagia (difficulty swallowing, gagging, retching).
- Odynophagia (pain when swallowing, repeated swallowing efforts, and extension of head and neck during swallowing).
- Hyporexia or anorexia.
- Weight loss.
- Coughing and/or nasal discharge with aspiration pneumonia, reflux laryngitis, pharyngitis, and/or rhinitis.

Physical Examination Findings

- Often normal.
- Oral and pharyngeal inflammation and/or ulceration with ingestion of caustic substances or oropharyngeal reflux of gastric acid.
- Fever and pain with ulcerative esophagitis or aspiration pneumonia.
- Halitosis, ptyalism, possibly pain on palpation of neck.
- Cachexia and weight loss, with chronicity.
- Nasal discharge and congestion with reflux rhinitis.
- Cough, increased bronchovesicular sound, pulmonary crackles, and dyspnea with aspiration pneumonia.

CAUSES

- Most commonly GER secondary to general anesthesia (Web Figure 1), hiatal hernia (Web Figure 2), persistent or chronic vomiting, and GI disease resulting in delayed gastric emptying.
- Gastroesophageal reflux disease (GERD) secondary to primary LES abnormality is poorly understood in veterinary patients.
- Esophageal retention of tablets or capsules (doxycycline, clindamycin, nonsteroidal anti-inflammatory drugs [NSAIDs], alendronate).
- Esophageal foreign body (Web Figure 3).
- Infectious agents—*Pythium* spp., *Spirocerca lupi*, *Candida* infection secondary to immune suppression.
- Uncommonly esophageal tumors, radiation injury, megaesophagus, vascular ring anomalies, gastrinoma, eosinophilic esophagitis and esophageal tubes.
- Idiopathic.

RISK FACTORS

- General anesthesia.
- HH.
- GI or metabolic/endocrine disease resulting in vomiting or gastric hyperacidity.
- Preanesthetic fasting for prolonged periods (≥24h) increases risk for GER and gastric hyperacidity.

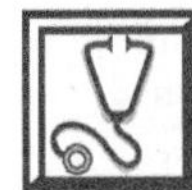

DIAGNOSIS

DIFFERENTIAL DIAGNOSIS

- Esophageal foreign body—usually detected by survey radiography or esophagoscopy.
- Esophageal stricture—revealed by barium contrast radiography or esophagoscopy.
- Oropharyngeal dysphagia—diagnosed with videofluoroscopic swallow study.
- HH—may be diagnosed by thoracic radiographs or esophagoscopy; contrast esophagram with fluoroscopy may be required to document (Web Figure 2).
- Megaesophagus—survey radiography revealing diffuse dilation of esophageal body.
- Esophageal diverticula—detected by survey or contrast radiography or esophagoscopy.
- Vascular ring anomaly—usually revealed by leftward deviation of trachea at heart base on survey thoracic radiographs, or barium contrast radiography as focal dilation of proximal esophageal body.
- Esophageal neoplasia—mass effect with possible esophageal dilation diagnosed with survey or contrast radiography, thoracic CT, or esophagoscopy.

CBC/BIOCHEMISTRY/URINALYSIS

Usually unremarkable; patients with ulcerative esophagitis or aspiration pneumonia may have leukocytosis and neutrophilia.

IMAGING

- Survey thoracic radiography—often unremarkable, but may reveal mild esophageal dilation or fluid accumulation in distal esophagus; aspiration pneumonia may be evident; dilation of esophagus cranial to a stricture; esophageal foreign body, HH, or esophageal mass may be detected.
- Barium contrast esophagram (static images and/or fluoroscopic)—may reveal esophageal dilation with retention of barium, strictures, foreign bodies, or masses; fluoroscopic studies allow for evaluation of swallowing, esophageal motility, strictures that may not be apparent on a static esophagram, sliding HH (Web Figure 2), and GER (the latter two conditions may require abdominal compressions to demonstrate).
- Thoracic CT can be helpful for esophageal masses, foreign bodies, and HHs.

DIAGNOSTIC PROCEDURES

- Endoscopy and biopsy—most reliable means of diagnosis (Web Figures 1 and 3). Mild cases of esophagitis may appear normal. Visual findings of mucosal hyperemia and edema are common and in more severe cases ulceration. With GER, changes usually most apparent in distal third of esophagus. Gastroduodenoscopy may also be performed to evaluate for GI causes of vomiting that caused esophagitis.
- Histopathology provides most definitive evidence of esophagitis, although endoscopy and biopsies usually reserved for cases unresponsive to therapy. Diagnostic quality esophageal biopsies difficult to obtain endoscopically due to tough stratified squamous epithelium.
- Endotracheal or transtracheal aspiration and/or bronchoalveolar lavage for cytology, and culture and sensitivity testing, may be considered in patients with aspiration pneumonia.

PATHOLOGIC FINDINGS

Mucosal squamous hyperplasia or dysplasia with erosions and ulcers; lymphocytic plasmacytic and neutrophilic inflammation.

ESOPHAGITIS (CONTINUED)

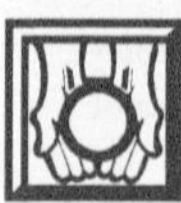

TREATMENT

APPROPRIATE HEALTH CARE

- Mildly affected animals can be managed as outpatients; those with more severe esophagitis (persistent regurgitation, dehydration) and complications (aspiration pneumonia) require hospitalization.
- Successful treatment of esophagitis involves addressing underlying risk factors and predisposing conditions when possible; gastric acid suppression to reduce esophageal mucosal injury; increasing LES pressure and promoting gastric emptying to reduce GER; and protecting esophageal mucosa from further injury.

NURSING CARE

- Upright or elevated feeding will be of benefit with regurgitation associated with abnormal esophageal motility secondary to esophagitis.
- Coupage and nebulization are provided for patients with aspiration pneumonia.
- IV fluids to maintain hydration in severe cases.
- Oxygen therapy may be necessary in patients with aspiration pneumonia.

DIET

- Fat-restricted diets recommended to minimize gastric acid production.
- With severe esophagitis oral food and water may need to be withheld until regurgitation resolved; gastrostomy tube feedings may be required.

CLIENT EDUCATION

- Advise upright or elevated feeding when there is esophageal dysmotility.
- Discuss potential complications, including aspiration pneumonia, esophageal stricture, esophageal perforation, and/or esophageal motility abnormalities.

SURGICAL CONSIDERATIONS

- Percutaneous endoscopic gastrostomy or surgical gastrostomy tube placement in severe cases.
- Surgical correction for HH when medical management not effective.
- Esophageal surgery may be necessary for large perforations, difficult esophageal foreign bodies, or esophageal neoplasia, but should be avoided if possible.

MEDICATIONS

DRUG(S) OF CHOICE

Acid Suppression

- Most important therapy for treatment of GERD and associated esophagitis. H2-receptor antagonists (H2RAs) and proton pump inhibitors (PPIs) are two main classes of acid suppressors. PPIs provide superior gastric acid suppression compared to H2RAs.
- PPIs should be administered at dose of 1 mg/kg PO or IV q12h. Most common PPIs prescribed are omeprazole and pantoprazole. Other choices include lansoprazole and esomeprazole.
- Fractionated enteric-coated omeprazole tablets remain effective despite disruption of the enteric coating. Tablets need to be cleanly split and cannot be crushed.
- In humans widespread media attention has concerned potential adverse effects of PPIs. Current evidence is inadequate to establish cause and effect for most associations. Caution should be exercised when prescribing PPIs as they are among the most overprescribed drugs in humans and veterinary medicine.
- Famotidine is most effective and commonly recommended H2RA given at dose of 0.5–1.0 mg/kg PO/SC/IV q12h. Has diminished effect over time with repeated administration. Is appropriate for short-term gastric acid suppression, but long-term administration not advised.
- When prescribing a PPI, overlap with an H2RA during initial dosing is unnecessary.
- When discontinuing a PPI after >3–4 weeks of therapy, PPI should be gradually tapered by 50% increments over 2–3 weeks to avoid rebound gastric hyperacidity.
- Dosing for metabolic disease (renal failure and liver failure) not established; lower dose or longer dose interval may be appropriate for these conditions.

GI Prokinetics

- Second most common class of drugs used to treat GER and esophagitis. Increase LES pressure and promote gastric emptying, therefore reducing GER.
- Most effective is cisapride at 0.5–1.0 mg/kg PO q8h. Readily available from compounding pharmacies.
- Metoclopramide is GI prokinetic with antiemetic effects in dogs dosed at 0.2–1.0 mg/kg PO/SC q8h or 1.0–3.0 mg/kg/day as CRI.

Mucosal Protectants

- Sucralfate 0.25–1.0 g PO q6–8h is given as suspension mixed into slurry with water and administered on empty stomach. Forms insoluble complex that binds to inflamed tissue, creating protective barrier and preventing further damage caused by pepsin, acid, and bile. Additionally increases mucosal defense and repair mechanisms through stimulation of bicarbonate and prostaglandin E production and binding of epidermal growth factor, at neutral pH. Reported to relieve symptoms in humans.
- Antibiotics indicated with aspiration pneumonia, severe esophageal ulceration, and esophageal perforation.
- Analgesics, especially in severe cases—lidocaine solution (2.0 mg/kg PO q4–6h) for local analgesia; tramadol 2–4 mg/kg PO q8–12h.
- Anti-inflammatory dosage of corticosteroids (e.g., prednisone 0.5–1 mg/kg PO per day or divided q12h) may decrease fibrosis and esophageal stricture formation in severe cases; controversial and efficacy not been supported by literature. Avoid when evidence of aspiration pneumonia.

CONTRAINDICATIONS

None

PRECAUTIONS

None

POSSIBLE INTERACTIONS

Sucralfate may interfere with GI absorption of other drugs and it is best to separate dosing by 2 hours from other drugs; may not be clinically important.

ALTERNATIVE DRUG(S)

- Narcotic analgesics including buprenorphine, methadone, and fentanyl may be necessary in severe cases of painful esophagitis.
- Ranitidine 2.0 mg/kg PO q12h, nizatidine 2.5–5.0 mg/kg PO q24h, and erythromycin 0.5–1.0 mg/kg PO/IV have GI prokinetic effects and may be alternate or additive drugs.

FOLLOW-UP

PATIENT MONITORING

- For patients with mild esophagitis, monitoring of clinical signs is sufficient.
- Consider follow-up endoscopy in patients with ulcerative esophagitis and those at risk for esophageal stricture.

PREVENTION/AVOIDANCE

- Consider two doses of omeprazole 1 mg/kg PO or famotidine 1 mg/kg PO given 12–24h and 1–4h prior to anesthesia to reduce gastric acidity.
- Prokinetic drug (cisapride 1 mg/kg PO; metoclopramide 0.2–1.0 mg/kg PO/SC) with acid suppressor may also help reduce GER during anesthesia and surgery.
- Maropitant useful to prevent vomiting and regurgitation associated with opioid premedications and anesthesia.
- If GER is cause of esophagitis, owners should avoid late-night feedings that tend to diminish LES pressure during sleep.
- Proper patient preanesthesia fasting decreases risk of GER. Withholding water for 4–8h and food for 8–12h prior to anesthesia is recommended.
- Follow oral administration of capsules and tablets with 5–10 mL bolus of water (especially for doxycycline) amd a meal, or give with a treat such as a pill pocket to hasten

transit time of pills to stomach. Coating pills with butter or applying Nutri-Cal® to the nose to stimulate licking after administration of tablets may also be effective.

POSSIBLE COMPLICATIONS

- Esophageal stricture formation.
- Aspiration pneumonia.
- Chronic reflux esophagitis.
- Permanent esophageal dysmotility.
- Chronic cough due to laryngopharyngeal aspiration or tracheal microaspiration.
- Esophageal perforation (rare).
- Barrett's esophagus (rare complication of chronic reflux esophagitis reported in cats).

EXPECTED COURSE AND PROGNOSIS

- Best results when treated with gastric acid suppressant, GI prokinetic, and possibly mucosal protectant.
- Mild esophagitis—good to excellent prognosis.
- Severe or ulcerative esophagitis—greater potential for complications, which warrants guarded prognosis.
- Complete recovery can be expected especially when treated before serious complications develop.

MISCELLANEOUS

ZOONOTIC POTENTIAL

None

PREGNANCY/FERTILITY/BREEDING

H2RAs, PPIs, and glucocorticoids should all be used with caution during pregnancy.

SYNONYMS

Esophageal inflammation.

SEE ALSO

- Dysphagia.
- Esophageal Diverticula.
- Esophageal Foreign Bodies.
- Esophageal Stricture.
- Gastroesophageal Reflux.
- Hiatal Hernia.
- Megaesophagus.
- Regurgitation.

ABBREVIATIONS

- GER = gastroesophageal reflux.
- GERD = gastroesophageal reflux disease.
- GI = gastrointestinal.
- H2RA = H2 receptor antagonist.
- HH = hiatal hernia.
- LES = lower esophageal sphincter.
- NSAID = nonsteroidal anti-inflammatory drug.
- PPI = proton pump inhibitor.

Suggested Reading

Garcia RS, Belafsky PC, DellaMaggiore A, et al. Prevalence of gastroesophageal reflux in cats during anesthesia and effect of omeprazole on gastric pH. J Vet Intern Med 2017, 31(3):734–742.

Golly E, Odunayo A, Daves M, et al. The frequency of oral famotidine administration influences its effect on gastric pH in cats over time. J Vet Intern Med 2019, 33(2);544–550.

Marks SL, Kook PH, Papich MG, et al. ACVIM consensus statement: Support for rational administration of gastrointestinal protectants in dogs and cats. J Vet Intern Med 2018, 32:1823–1840.

Tolbert K, Odunayo A, Howell RS, et al. Efficacy of intravenous administration of combined acid suppressants in healthy dogs. J Vet Intern Med 2015, 29:556–560.

Author Steve Hill

Consulting Editor Mark P. Rondeau

Client Education Handout available online

ESSENTIAL OILS TOXICOSIS

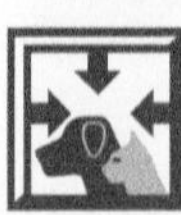

BASICS

E

OVERVIEW

• Essential oils—volatile, organic constituents extracted from plants; contribute to fragrance/taste. Often used as natural remedies by owners for their own medical issues. Essential oil insecticides (low %) manufactured for use on animals.
• Known toxicants to *cats*—D-Limonene (citrus oil), pine oil, ylang ylang oil, peppermint oil, cinnamon oil.
• Known toxicants to *cats and dogs*—wintergreen oil, sweet birch oil, eucalyptus oil, clove oil, tea tree (aka melaleuca) oil.
• Known toxicants to *dogs*—pennyroyal oil.

Systems Affected

• Cardiovascular—bradycardia, peripheral vasodilation.
• Endocrine/metabolic—hypothermia.
• Gastrointestinal (GI)—hypersalivation, vomiting.
• Hepatobiliary—elevated liver enzymes (LEs), hepatic failure.
• Nervous—ataxia, tremors, CNS depression.
• Respiratory—respiratory irritation/distress.
• Skin—irritation, possible ulceration.

SIGNALMENT

Cats are more sensitive than dogs. Cats lack glucuronyl transferase; cannot metabolize/eliminate toxins via hepatic glucuronidation.

SIGNS

• Signs vary based on type/concentration of oil. Higher the concentration the greater the risk. Only 7–8 drops of 100% oil may be needed to cause toxicosis.
• Onset—1–8 hours post exposure.
• Animal may smell of oil (hair coat, skin, breath) or feel greasy.
• Nausea, hypersalivation, vomiting, abdominal pain.
• Hypothermia.
• Ataxia, tremors, CNS depression.
• Coughing, wheezing, panting, tachypnea, and dyspnea.
• Bradycardia, hypotension.
• Elevated LEs (cats, sometimes dogs—pennyroyal oil).

CAUSES & RISK FACTORS

• Passive oil diffusers—animals inhale odor, develop mild to severe respiratory irritation/distress.
• Active diffusers—release micro-droplets of oil. Respiratory difficulties, but droplets can land on animal's coat causing direct absorption or ingestion via grooming.
• History of preexisting respiratory issues (e.g., asthmatic cats) places animals at greater risk.
• Indirect ingestion—essential oils used on human skin, animal licks skin.
• Direct dermal or oral use as owners try natural remedies (e.g., flea control) on their animals.

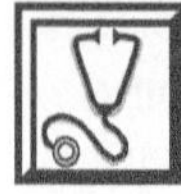

DIAGNOSIS

DIFFERENTIAL DIAGNOSIS

• Aspirin toxicity—wintergreen and sweet birch oil contain methyl salicylate; anemia/GI hemorrhage may develop.
• Hepatotoxins xylitol, acetaminophen, cycads (sago palm), others.
• Toxins or conditions that affect CNS—ethylene glycol, hypoglycemia, hypotension, drug overdoses.

CBC/BIOCHEMISTRY/URINALYSIS

• Most often no specific diagnostic features.
• CBC and chemistry—possible increase in LEs.

IMAGING

• Thoracic radiographs with respiratory irritation/distress.
• Abdominal radiographs if abdominal pain.

PATHOLOGIC FINDINGS

Limited data—lesions of severe hepatic necrosis with pennyroyal oil.

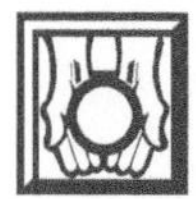

TREATMENT

Appropriate Health Care

Fresh air, emergency examination, bathing, inpatient care until signs resolve.

Nursing Care

• Intravenous crystalloids.
• Prevent aspiration of vomitus.
• Oxygen therapy.
• Monitor BP, heart rate, thermoregulation.

Diet

Do not feed patients that are vomiting, having CNS signs, or are in respiratory distress.

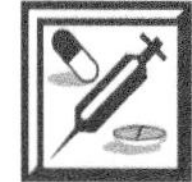

MEDICATIONS

DRUG(S) OF CHOICE

• No specific antidote.
• Bathe with warm water and liquid hand dishwashing detergent.
• Activated charcoal (AC) with a cathartic × 1 in large or concentrated oral ingestions. Repeat AC only q8h × 2 doses if tea tree oil (enterohepatic recirculation).
• Fluid boluses or vasopressors as needed for hypotension.
• Anticholinergics if bradycardic, as long as normotensive.
• Bronchodilators with respiratory distress.
• Anti-emetics.
• Hepatoprotectants with elevated LEs.

CONTRAINDICATIONS/POSSIBLE INTERACTIONS

Do not induce vomiting. Do not give AC to a patient with CNS signs.

Precautions

Use hepatically metabolized medications with caution in the presence of LE elevation.

FOLLOW-UP

PATIENT MONITORING

Recheck LEs 48–72 hours post discharge, then as needed based on values and clinical signs.

PREVENTION/AVOIDANCE

• Do not apply essential oils directly to animals.
• Use essential oil products manufactured for use on animals with caution.
• Avoid using essential oil diffusers.

POSSIBLE COMPLICATIONS

• Aspiration pneumonia—if neurologic patient with concurrent GI signs.
• Pennyroyal oil—disseminated intravascular coagulation, chronic hepatic insufficiency.

EXPECTED COURSE AND PROGNOSIS

• Prognosis—good if treated early and aggressively. May take several days for complete resolution.
• More guarded prognosis with use of 100% oil (i.e., tea tree oil, pennyroyal oil), especially if treatment is delayed or inadequate. Fatalities can occur.

MISCELLANEOUS

ABBREVIATIONS

• AC = activated charcoal.
• GI = gastrointestinal.
• LEs = liver enzymes.

Suggested Reading

Hovda L, Brutlag A, Poppenga R, et al. Essential oils/liquid potpourri; Tea tree oil/melaleuca oil. In: Hovda LR, Brutlag AG, Poppenga RH, Peterson KL, eds., Five-Minute Veterinary Consult Clinical Companion: Small Animal Toxicology, 2nd ed. Ames, IA: Wiley-Blackwell, 2016, pp. 585–591, 592–597.

Author Kia J. Benson
Consulting Editor Lynn R. Hovda

ETHANOL TOXICOSIS

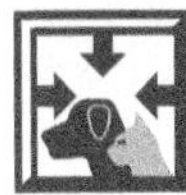

BASICS

OVERVIEW

- Ethanol (CH3CH2OH)—short-chain alcohol; highly miscible with water; less volatile than comparable hydrocarbons (e.g., ethane); solvent for medications; component of alcoholic beverages; metabolized to acetaldehyde.
- Used intravenously to treat ethylene glycol poisoning.
- Denatured forms may contain other toxic fractions (e.g., acetone, benzene, camphor, castor oil, phthalates, kerosene, sulfuric acid, terpinols); may complicate effects.
- Ethanol concentration—expressed as proof (twice the % concentration).
- Acute oral lowest toxic dosage—5–8 mL/kg as pure alcohol; consider % alcohol in specific product consumed.
- Other alcohols—toxicity of methanol is similar to that of ethanol; the LD_{50} of 70% isopropanol is 2 mL/kg.
- Cell membrane damage; impaired sodium and potassium nerve conduction.
- May inhibit glutamate receptors in brain with reduction of cyclic guanosine monophosphate (GMP).

SIGNALMENT

- Most common in dogs.
- No breed or sex predilections.
- Young, curious animals more susceptible.

SIGNS

- CNS—develop within 15–30 minutes after ingestion on an empty stomach or 1–2 hours on a full stomach; ataxia, reduced reflexes, behavioral changes, excitement, depression.
- Cardiovascular—cardiac arrest.
- Gastrointestinal—flatulence (bread dough).
- Respiratory—respiratory depression, narcosis.
- Urologic—polyuria, incontinence.
- Hypothermia.

CAUSES & RISK FACTORS

- Alcoholic beverages, either accidental or intentional, are most common source.
- Exposure to deicers, sanitizers, mouthwash, dyes, inks, some fuels, paint, varnishes, perfume, pharmaceuticals.
- Exposure to rising bread doughs containing active yeast.
- Fermented products—rotten apples, garbage.
- Dermal exposure—alcohol-containing products.

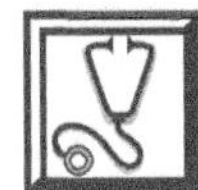

DIAGNOSIS

DIFFERENTIAL DIAGNOSIS

- Other alcohols—methanol, isopropanol, butanol.
- Human drugs of abuse—marijuana, barbiturates, benzodiazepines.
- Early stages of ethylene glycol (antifreeze) toxicosis.
- Early stages of xylitol toxicosis.
- Halogenated or aliphatic hydrocarbon solvents.
- Hypoglycemia inducing metabolic and neurologic disorders.
- Pesticides—amitraz, macrolide antiparasiticides.

CBC/BIOCHEMISTRY/URINALYSIS

- PCV and total solids.
- Monitor for hypoglycemia; blood glucose <60 mg/dL considered serious.
- Metabolic acidosis likely from ethanol-induced lactic acidemia.

OTHER LABORATORY TESTS

- Blood ethanol levels routinely available at reference labs—clinical signs in puppies at >0.6 mg/mL and in adults at >1–4 mg/mL.
- Blood methanol and isopropanol levels available at some reference labs.
- Blood gases and increased anion gap—evaluate potential acidosis.

DIAGNOSTIC PROCEDURES

N/A

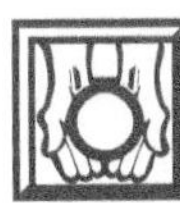

TREATMENT

- Activated charcoal—not effective.
- Emesis or gastric lavage—only in very recent exposures (less than 15 minutes) due to rapid absorption and rapid onset of clinical signs.
- Respiratory depression—provide artificial ventilation.
- IV isotonic crystalloid fluids—correct dehydration.
- Acidosis—sodium bicarbonate if pH <7.0, BE <15 mmHg, HCO_3 <11 mmHg.
- Cardiac arrest—cardiac therapy (see Cardiopulmonary Arrest).
- Hemodialysis—may aid in elimination of ethanol after life-threatening exposure.
- Yohimbine may be effective for CNS depression.

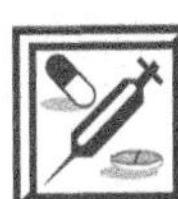

MEDICATIONS

DRUG(S) OF CHOICE

- Dextrose—0.5–1.5 ml/kg 50% dextrose diluted 1 : 4 in 0.9% NaCl as a bolus for immediate correction of severe hypoglycemia; 2.5–5% dextrose supplementation in fluids for hypoglycemia.
- Fomepizole (4-methylpyrazole)—not specifically cleared for use in ethanol intoxication
- Sodium bicarbonate (if needed)—mEq of bicarbonate required = 0.5 × bodyweight in kg × (desired total CO_2 mEq/L − measured CO_2 mEq/L); give half the total calculated dose slowly over 3–4 hours IV; recheck blood gases and clinical status of the animal.

CONTRAINDICATIONS/POSSIBLE INTERACTIONS

Avoid other CNS depressants.

FOLLOW-UP

- Monitor for metabolic acidosis—blood pH, blood gases, urine pH, anion gap.
- Recovery from clinical signs—usually within 8–12 hours.

MISCELLANEOUS

ABBREVIATIONS

- GMP = guanosine monophosphate.

Suggested Reading

Dorman DC. Alcohols (ethanol, methanol, isopropanol). In: Hovda LR, Brutlag AG, Poppenga RH, Peterson KL, eds., Blackwell's Five-Minute Veterinary Consult: Small Animal Toxicology, 2nd ed. Ames, IA: Wiley-Blackwell, 2016, pp. 71–77.

Kammerer M, Sachot E, Blanchot D. Ethanol toxicosis from ingestion of rotten apples by a dog. Vet Hum Toxicol 2001, 43(6):349–350.

Means C. Bread dough toxicosis in dogs. J Vet Emerg Crit Care 2003, 13(1):39–41.

Author Tabatha J. Regehr

Consulting Editor Lynn R. Hovda

Acknowledgment The author and book editors acknowledge the prior contribution of Gary D. Osweiler

ETHYLENE GLYCOL TOXICOSIS

BASICS

DEFINITION

Results primarily from ingesting substances containing ethylene glycol (EG; e.g., antifreeze). Rarely from other products.

PATHOPHYSIOLOGY

• EG—rapidly absorbed from the gastrointestinal tract; food in the stomach delays absorption. • Toxicity—initially causes CNS depression, ataxia, gastrointestinal irritation, and polyuria or polydipsia; rapidly metabolized in the liver by alcohol dehydrogenase to glycoaldehyde, glycolic acid, glyoxalic acid, and oxalic acid; leads to severe metabolic acidosis and renal epithelial damage. • Minimum lethal dosage—cats: 1.4 mL/kg; dogs: 6.6 mL/kg.

SYSTEMS AFFECTED

• Gastrointestinal—irritated mucosa. • Nervous—inebriation from EG and glycoaldehyde owing to inhibition of respiration, glucose metabolism, and serotonin metabolism, and alteration of amine concentrations. • Renal/urologic—initially, osmotic diuresis; later, metabolites, especially calcium oxalate monohydrate crystals, are directly cytotoxic to renal tubular epithelium, resulting in renal failure; mechanism of toxicity is now thought to involve attachment of oxalate to cell plasma membrane, activation of enzyme activity, and production of free radicals and lipid peroxidation, leading to cell necrosis.

INCIDENCE/PREVALENCE

• Common in small animals. • Highest fatality rate of all poisons; fatality rates higher for cats than dogs. • Incidence similar in cats and dogs.

GEOGRAPHIC DISTRIBUTION

Higher incidence in colder areas where antifreeze is more commonly used.

SIGNALMENT

Species

Dogs, cats, and many other species, including birds.

Mean Age and Range

• Any age susceptible (3 months–13 years). • Mean: 3 years.

SIGNS

General Comments

• Dose dependent. • Almost always acute. • Caused by unmetabolized EG and its toxic metabolites (frequently fatal).

Physical Examination Findings

• Early—from 30 minutes to 12 hours post ingestion in dogs: nausea and vomiting; mild to severe depression; ataxia and knuckling; muscle fasciculations; nystagmus; head tremors; decreased withdrawal reflexes and righting ability; polyuria and polydipsia. • Dogs—with increasing depression, patient drinks less but polyuria continues, resulting in dehydration; CNS signs abate transiently after approximately 12 hours, but recur later. • Cats—usually remain markedly depressed; do not exhibit polydipsia. • Oliguria (dogs: 36–72 hours; cats: 12–24 hours) and anuria (72–96 hours post ingestion)—often develop if untreated. • May note severe hypothermia. • Severe lethargy or coma. • Seizures. • Anorexia. • Vomiting. • Oral ulcers. • Salivation. • Kidneys—often swollen and painful, particularly in cats.

CAUSES

Ingestion of EG, the principal component (95%) of most antifreeze solutions.

RISK FACTORS

Access to EG—widespread availability; somewhat pleasant taste; small minimum lethal dose; lack of public awareness of toxicity.

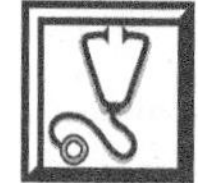

DIAGNOSIS

DIFFERENTIAL DIAGNOSIS

• Acute (30 minutes–12 hours post ingestion)—ethanol, methanol, and marijuana toxicosis; ketoacidotic diabetes mellitus; pancreatitis; gastroenteritis. • Renal stage—acute renal failure by nephrotoxins, e.g., aminoglycoside antibiotics, amphotericin B, cancer chemotherapeutic drugs, ibuprofen, oxalate-containing plants such as philodendrons, plants of the lily family (cats), cyclosporin, grape and raisin toxicosis (causes hypercalcemia, unlike EG toxicosis), and heavy metals; leptospirosis, tubulointerstitial nephritis; glomerular and vascular disease; renal ischemia (hypoperfusion).

CBC/BIOCHEMISTRY/URINALYSIS

• Packed cell volume (PCV) and total protein—often high owing to dehydration. • Stress leukogram— common. • High blood urea nitrogen (BUN) and creatinine—dog: 36–48 hours post ingestion; cat: 12 hours post ingestion. • Hyperphosphatemia may occur transiently 3–6 hours post ingestion, owing to phosphate rust inhibitors in antifreeze; hyperphosphatemia is also seen with azotemia owing to decreased glomerular filtration. • Hyperkalemia if oliguric or anuric. • Hypocalcemia—occurs in approximately half of patients, owing to chelation of calcium by oxalic acid; clinical signs infrequently observed because of acidosis. • Hyperglycemia—occurs in approximately half of patients, owing to inhibition of glucose metabolism by aldehydes, increased epinephrine and endogenous corticosteroids, and uremia. • Isosthenuria—by 3 hours post ingestion, owing to osmotic diuresis and serum hyperosmolality-induced polydipsia; continues in later stages of toxicosis because of renal dysfunction. • Calcium oxalate crystalluria—consistent finding; as early as 3 hours post ingestion in cats and 6 hours in dogs; monohydrate form more common. • Urine—pH consistently decreases; inconsistent findings—hematuria; proteinuria; glucosuria; may note granular and cellular casts, white blood cells (WBCs), red blood cells (RBCs), and renal epithelial cells.

OTHER LABORATORY TESTS

Blood Gases

• Metabolites cause severe metabolic acidosis. • Total CO_2, plasma bicarbonate concentration, and blood pH—low by 3 hours post ingestion; markedly low by 12 hours. • Partial pressure of CO_2 (PCO_2) decreases, owing to partial respiratory compensation. • Anion gap—increased by 3 hours post ingestion; peaks at 6 hours post ingestion; remains increased for approximately 48 hours (EG metabolites are unmeasured anions. Glycolate, a metabolite of EG, can result in a false increase in plasma lactate, which could lead to the assumption that acidosis is due to increased lactate, rather than EG toxicosis.

Other

• Serum osmolality and osmole gap—high by 1 hour post ingestion, in parallel with serum EG concentrations; dose related; usually remain high for approximately 18 hours post ingestion; EG toxicosis most common cause of high osmolal gap. • EG serum concentration— peaks 1–6 hours post ingestion; usually not detectable in serum or urine by 72 hours. • Commercial kits—PRN Pharmacal REACT EG measures concentrations at >50 mg/dL; estimate by multiplying osmole gap by 6.2. ◦ Test does not detect metabolites, so must be used within the first few hours post ingestion. ◦ Results available in 6 minutes but should not be read over 10 minutes. ◦ Labeled for dogs and cats; some cats may have toxicosis at levels below 50 mg/dL. ◦ False-positive test results can be seen with propylene glycol, glycerol, mannitol, and sorbitol. Ethanol may combine with propylene glycol or glycerol to give a false positive. • Wood's lamp examination of urine, face, paws, or vomitus may detect fluorescein that is sometimes added to antifreeze to detect radiator leaks. This method is nonspecific and may be unreliable; fluorescein has a half-life of approximately 4 hours.

IMAGING

Ultrasonography—renal cortices may be hyperechoic as a result of crystals.

DIAGNOSTIC PROCEDURES

• Kidney biopsy—with anuria; confirm diagnosis. • Cytologic examination of kidney imprints—often diagnostic; numerous calcium oxalate crystals.

PATHOLOGIC FINDINGS

- Kidneys often swollen.
- Postmortem examination of kidney reveals the presence of calcium oxalate crystals in the tubules.

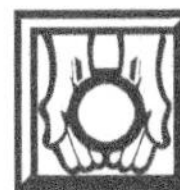

TREATMENT

APPROPRIATE HEALTH CARE

- Cats—usually inpatient.
- Dogs—usually outpatient if <5 hours post ingestion and treated with fomepizole; inpatient if >5 hours for IV fluids to correct dehydration, increase tissue perfusion, and promote diuresis.

NURSING CARE

- Goals—prevent absorption; increase excretion; prevent metabolism. • Induction of vomiting and gastric lavage with activated charcoal not recommended unless can be performed in first 30 minutes following ingestion due to rapid absorption of EG. • IV fluids—correct dehydration, increase tissue perfusion, and promote diuresis; accompanied by bicarbonate given slowly IV to correct metabolic acidosis. • Monitor serial plasma bicarbonate concentrations—0.5 × body weight (kg) × (24 – plasma bicarbonate) = sodium bicarbonate needed (mEq).
- Monitor urine pH in response to therapy.
- Azotemia and oliguric renal failure (dogs)—most of the EG has been metabolized; little benefit from inhibition of alcohol dehydrogenase (ADH); correct fluid, electrolyte, and acid-base disorders; establish diuresis; diuretics (particularly mannitol) may help; hemodialysis or peritoneal dialysis may be useful; may need extended treatment (several weeks) before renal function reestablished.

SURGICAL CONSIDERATIONS

Kidney transplantation—successfully employed in cats with EG-induced renal failure.

MEDICATIONS

DRUG(S) OF CHOICE

Dogs

Fomepizole (4-methyl pyrazole, available from Kacey Diagnostics)—effective and nontoxic liver ADH inhibitor; much more expensive than ethanol but less intensive care required; 5% (50 mg/mL) at 20 mg/kg IV initially; then 15 mg/kg IV at 12 and 24 hours; then 5 mg/kg IV at 36 hours.

Cats

- Fomepizole—cats must be given a higher dose of fomepizole than dogs; 125 mg/kg IV initially, then 31.25 mg/kg at 12, 24, and 36 hours.
- Ethanol—use if fomepizole not available; 20% at 5mL/kg diluted in fluids and given in an IV drip over 6 hours for 5 treatments; then over 8 hours for 4 more treatments.

CONTRAINDICATIONS

Avoid drugs that cause CNS depression, including ethanol.

PRECAUTIONS

- Competitive substrates (alcohols, such as ethanol) contribute to CNS depression; monitor respiration. • Cats may become hypothermic; require heat. • Other pyrazoles—may be toxic to the marrow and liver; do not substitute for fomepizole.

POSSIBLE INTERACTIONS

- Fomepizole—contributes slightly to CNS depression in cats; none in dogs. • Ethanol—contributes to CNS depression; further increases serum osmolality.

ALTERNATIVE DRUG(S)

- Ethanol, propylene glycol, and 1,3-butanediol—have higher affinity for ADH than does EG; effectively inhibit EG metabolism; may cause CNS depression and increase serum osmolality; constant serum ethanol concentrations of 100 mg/dL will inhibit most EG metabolism.
- Ethanol treatment requires hospitalization, constant IV infusion (ethanol and fluids); continuous monitoring for respiratory and acid-base status.

FOLLOW-UP

PATIENT MONITORING

BUN, creatinine, acid-base status, and urine output—monitored daily.

PREVENTION/AVOIDANCE

- Increasing client awareness of toxicity—helps prevent exposure; earlier treatment of patients. • Use of antifreeze products (e.g., Sierra®, Prestone LowTox®) that contain propylene glycol, which is much less toxic.

POSSIBLE COMPLICATIONS

- Without azotemia—usually no complications. • Urine concentrating ability—may be impaired with azotemia; may recover.

EXPECTED COURSE AND PROGNOSIS

- Untreated—oliguric renal failure (dogs: 36–72 hours; cats: 12–24 hours); anuria by 72–96 hours post ingestion. • Dogs treated <5 hours post ingestion—prognosis excellent with fomepizole treatment. • Dogs treated up to 8 hours post ingestion—most recover.
- Dogs treated up to 36 hours post ingestion—may be of benefit to prevent metabolism of any remaining EG. • Cats treated within 3 hours post ingestion—prognosis good. • If a large quantity of EG is ingested, prognosis is poor, unless treated within 4 hours of ingestion.
- Patients with azotemia and oliguric renal failure—prognosis poor; almost all of the EG will have been metabolized.

MISCELLANEOUS

AGE-RELATED FACTORS

Patients <6 months of age with oliguric renal failure sometimes fully recover.

SYNONYMS

Antifreeze poisoning.

SEE ALSO

Hyperosmolarity

ABBREVIATIONS

- ADH = alcohol dehydrogenase. • BUN = blood urea nitrogen. • EG = ethylene glycol.
- PCO_2 = partial pressure of carbon dioxide.
- PCV = packed cell volume. • RBC = red blood cell. • WBC = white blood cell.

Suggested Reading

Connally HE, Thrall MA, Forney SD, et al. Safety and efficacy of 4-methylpyrazole as treatment for suspected or confirmed ethylene glycol intoxication in dogs: 107 cases (1983–1995). J Am Vet Med Assoc 1996, 209:1880–1883.

Connally HE, Thrall MA, Hamar DW. Safety and efficacy of high-dose fomepizole compared with ethanol as therapy for ethylene glycol intoxication in cats. J Vet Emerg Crit Care 2010, 20(2):191–206.

Tart KM, Powell LL. 4-Methylpyrazole as a treatment in naturally occurring ethylene glycol intoxication in cats. J Vet Emerg Crit Care 2011, 21(3):268–272.

Authors Mary Anna Thrall, Gregory F. Grauer, Heather E. Connally, and Sharon M. Dial

Consulting Editor Lynn R. Hovda

Acknowledgment The author and book editors acknowledge the prior contribution of Gary D. Osweiler.

Client Education Handout available online

EXCESSIVE VOCALIZATION AND WAKING AT NIGHT—DOGS AND CATS

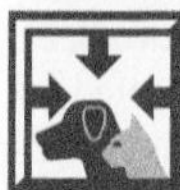

BASICS

DEFINITION

- Vocalization that is uncontrollable, excessive, at inappropriate times of day or night, or that disrupts owners, neighbors, or other animals.
- In night-time waking, the pet wakes during the night, does not fall asleep at bedtime, or awakens early, leading to disruption of owner's sleep.

PATHOPHYSIOLOGY

- Varies with cause.
- Barking may be normal canine communication (social, threat, warning, care-soliciting) but unacceptable to owners.
- Owner responses may reinforce or increase anxiety (punishment).
- Cats are crepuscular, so early morning waking may be normal.
- May be due to medical conditions that cause anxiety, discomfort, irritability, or altered sleep–wake cycles.
- Hearing decline may be associated with increased vocalization.
- Cognitive dysfunction syndrome (CDS) can lead to sleep disturbances, anxiety, and excessive vocalization.
- Night waking may be due to a change in schedule, environment, or activity, especially in senior pets that are more sensitive to change.

SYSTEMS AFFECTED

- Behavioral.
- Diseases of other systems may cause or contribute to signs.

GENETICS

N/A

INCIDENCE/PREVALENCE

Unknown

SIGNALMENT

Species

Dog and cat.

Breed Predilections

- Asian breeds of cats may be prone to excess vocalization.
- Working and hunting breeds may be more prone to barking.

Mean Age and Range

- Puppies may not be able to sleep through the night without waking to eliminate.
- Senior pets may be more prone to vocalization and night waking due to underlying medical conditions.

Predominant Sex

Intact females during estrus and mating.

SIGNS

Historical Findings

- Vocalization at times or in intensity that disturbs owners or neighbors.
- Sleeping pattern altered—does not fall asleep at bedtime, awakens during the night, or sleeps more during the day.
- Signs reported vary with how disruptive they are to the family, neighbors, and the pet's quality of life.
- Pets with CDS may pace, wander aimlessly, have decreased interest in social interactions, be less responsive to stimuli and increasingly anxious.
- Additional signs related to medical causes.

Physical Examination Findings

Signs associated with underlying medical issues.

CAUSES

- Vocalization and night waking—medical: gastrointestinal, metabolic (renal, hepatic), urogenital, CNS disorders, CDS, hypertension, hyperadrenocorticism or hypothyroidism (dog), hyperthyroidism (cat), pain, sensory decline.
- Vocalization:
    - Anxiety or conflict.
    - Normal for individual or breed.
    - Alarm barking—response to novel stimuli.
    - Territorial—warning or guarding.
    - Owner inadvertently reinforces.
    - Also reinforced each time stimulus retreats.
    - Distress vocalization, e.g., howl or whine may be related to separation from social group.
    - Growl—associated with agonistic displays.
    - Stereotypic behaviors—dog.
    - Mating/sexual—cat.
- Night waking:
    - Normal crepuscular rhythm—cat.
    - Changes in routine and/or environment—insufficient enrichment/scheduling.
    - Owner inadvertently reinforces.
    - Hyperactivity/hyperkinesis—dog.
    - Mating/sexual—cat.

RISK FACTORS

- Increasing age.
- Changes in schedule or environment.

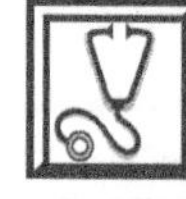

DIAGNOSIS

DIFFERENTIAL DIAGNOSIS

Sleep disorders.

CBC/BIOCHEMISTRY/URINALYSIS

To determine if underlying medical cause.

OTHER LABORATORY TESTS

- T_4 and blood pressure—senior cats.
- Rule out hypothyroidism and hyperadrenocorticism in dogs.

IMAGING

To rule out medical/neurologic if indicated.

DIAGNOSTIC PROCEDURES

- Behavioral diagnosis based on history; observation of pet, owner, and their interactions; video if available.
- Intraocular pressure.
- Brainstem auditory evoked response (BAER) if indicated to rule out auditory decline.
- Endoscopy and biopsy if gastrointestinal cause suspected.

PATHOLOGIC FINDINGS

N/A

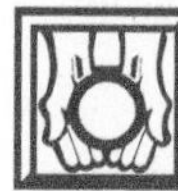

TREATMENT

APPROPRIATE HEALTH CARE

If any medical issues.

NURSING CARE

If any medical issues.

ACTIVITY

Insure behavioral needs (e.g., social interactions, exercise, elimination, routine, and mental stimulation) are adequately met each day.

DIET

- Feed from toys to encourage normal hunting and scavenging behaviors.
- Timed feeders and multiple small meals.

CLIENT EDUCATION

Individualize for the pet, home, and problem.

Behavior Modification

- Identify and minimize or avoid exposure to inciting stimuli.
- Provide a quiet and calm environment for security, rest, and sleep.
- Structure all interactions (i.e., calm sit or down and quiet behavior for all rewards).
- Reward-based training to teach calm/settle on cue ("Sit," "Down," "Mat").
- Response substitution—use settle commands to train alternative acceptable behavior.
- Head halter may provide more immediate control to quiet and calm.
- Eliminate any owner reinforcement.
- Owner anxiety, verbal reprimands, and punishment may increase anxiety and potentiate barking.
- Desensitize and countercondition—expose the pet to the inciting stimulus at a low level (under the response threshold) and pair a favored reward (e.g., food treat) with each exposure to change the emotional response. Gradually progress to more intense stimulus.
- Interrupting vocalization by directing into an alternative behavior may help to achieve

quiet, which can then be reinforced; however, aversive techniques may increase anxiety.

Environmental Modification

Modify environment to avoid or minimize exposure to stimuli that incite vocalization or wake the pet, e.g., covered crate, quiet room, thunder cap, classical music, white noise or fan.

SURGICAL CONSIDERATIONS

N/A

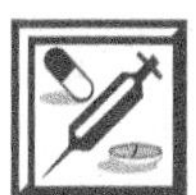

MEDICATIONS

DRUG(S) OF CHOICE

• Short term or as needed for situations of anxiety or for inducing sleep.
• Benzodiazepines—dog: clonazepam 0.05–0.25 mg/kg, diazepam 0.5–2.2 mg/kg; cat: oxazepam 0.2–0.5 mg/kg, alprazolam 0.125–0.25 mg/cat, clonazepam 0.02–0.2 mg/kg.
• Trazodone—dog: 5–10 mg/kg; cat: 25–50 mg/cat.
• Gabapentin—dog: 20–30 mg/kg; cat: 50–100 mg/cat.
• Melatonin—dog and cat: 3–6 mg (1.5–12 mg).
• For ongoing therapy for chronic anxiety or compulsive disorders—clomipramine (tricyclic antidepressant [TCA]): dog: 1–3 mg/kg PO q12h, cat: 0.5–1 mg/kg PO q24h; fluoxetine or paroxetine (selective serotonin reuptake inhibitors [SSRIs]): dog: 1–2 mg/kg PO q24h, cat: 0.5–1.5 mg/kg PO q24h.
• Natural products that might be used adjunctively for anxiety—Adaptil®, Feliway®, l-theanine, alpha-casozepine, Harmonease®, S-adenosyl-L-methionine-tosylate disulfate (SAMe), or aromatherapy (lavender).
• For CDS—selegiline and cognitive supplements (see Cognitive Dysfunction Syndrome).

CONTRAINDICATIONS

Review contraindications and side effects for each drug used.

PRECAUTIONS

• Caution with drugs that might sedate in elderly pets.
• Monitor for undesirable behavioral effects.
• Avoid anticholinergic drugs in pets with CDS.

POSSIBLE INTERACTIONS

Do not use SSRIs and TCAs together with monoamine oxide (MAO) inhibitors such as selegiline and amitraz, and use cautiously or avoid with buspirone and tramadol.

ALTERNATIVE DRUG(S)

• Concurrent sedation with acepromazine 0.5–2.2 mg/kg might be considered, but it is not anxiolytic and may increase noise sensitivity and vocalization.
• For a less sedating anxiolytic consider buspirone at 0.5–1 mg/kg (dogs: q8–12h; cats: q12h).
• Analgesics for pain control.

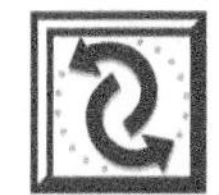

FOLLOW-UP

PATIENT MONITORING

Modify the program based on response to therapy.

PREVENTION/AVOIDANCE

• Train calm and settle on cue (sit, down, go to mat).
• Predictable interactions, e.g., insure calm sit or down and quiet before any reward given.
• Reward desirable, do not punish undesirable behavior.
• Socialize and habituate pet when young to a wide range of people, pets, stimuli, and environments.
• Provide enrichment to meet needs including food puzzles and multiple small meals for cats.

POSSIBLE COMPLICATIONS

• Night-time waking can lead to fatigue, increased irritability, and possibly aggression.
• Both night waking and vocalization can be particularly distressing to the pet owner's health and wellbeing and greatly weaken the bond.

EXPECTED COURSE AND PROGNOSIS

• Variable—based on diagnosis, environment, pet, and owner expectations.
• Most can be improved over time, but might not be eliminated.

MISCELLANEOUS

ASSOCIATED CONDITIONS

CDS

AGE-RELATED FACTORS

Increased anxiety and night waking more common in senior pets.

ZOONOTIC POTENTIAL

None, but sleep disruption and anxiety in pets can contribute to sleep disruption and anxiety in owners.

PREGNANCY/FERTILITY/BREEDING

N/A

SYNONYMS

Sleep disturbances.

SEE ALSO

• Cognitive Dysfunction Syndrome.
• Compulsive Disorders—Cats.
• Compulsive Disorders—Dogs.
• Separation Anxiety Syndrome.

ABBREVIATIONS

• BAER = brainstem auditory evoked response.
• CDS = cognitive dysfunction syndrome.
• MAO = monoamine oxide.
• SAMe = S-adenosyl-L-methionine-tosylate disulfate.
• SSRI = selective serotonin reuptake inhibitor.
• TCA = tricyclic antidepressant.

Suggested Reading

Landsberg GM, DePorter T, Araujo JA. Management of anxiety, sleeplessness and cognitive dysfunction in the senior pet. Vet Clin North Am Small Anim Pract 2011, 41(3):565–590.

Horwitz DF (ed.). Blackwell's Five-Minute Veterinary Consult Clinical Companion: Canine and Feline Behavior, 2nd ed. Hoboken: NJ: Wiley, 2018, pp. 885–894.

Authors Sagi Denenberg and Gary M. Landsberg

Consulting Editor Gary M. Landsberg

EXERCISE-INDUCED WEAKNESS/COLLAPSE IN LABRADOR RETRIEVERS

BASICS

DEFINITION

Inherited nervous system disorder causing weakness and collapse during intensive exercise in otherwise normal Labrador retrievers and a few other breeds.

SIGNALMENT

- Labrador retrievers—approximately 6% of all pet, show, and field Labrador retrievers are affected.
- Also occurs in Chesapeake Bay retrievers, curly-coated retrievers, and Boykin spaniels, and rarely in Old English sheepdogs, German wirehaired pointers, Bouvier des Flandres, Pembroke Welsh corgis, and cocker spaniels.
- No sex or color predilection.

SIGNS

General Comments

- No systemic signs.
- Episodes of collapse first occur between 5 months and 3 years of age.
- Collapse episodes occur only with extremes of exciting exercise.
- Dogs can engage normally in hiking, swimming, jogging, and other activities.

Physical Examination Findings

Between weakness/collapse episodes, physical and neurologic examinations are normal.

Features of Weakness/Collapse Episodes

- Weakness occurs after 5–20 minutes of intense exercise with excitement or stress.
- Rear limbs become weak and unable to support weight.
- Rear limb muscles are flaccid during collapse and there is a loss of patellar reflexes.
- Dogs may continue to run, dragging their rear limbs in a crouched posture.
- During a severe episode, all four limbs can be affected; rarely the dog may become recumbent and unable to move its limbs or raise its head.
- Dogs remain conscious and fully alert during episodes.
- There is no apparent pain or discomfort on palpation or manipulation of the muscles, joints, or spine during or after collapse.
- Complete recovery occurs within 5–30 minutes.
- Rectal temperature is elevated (mean >107 °F; >41.6 °C), but not different from Labradors without exercise-induced collapse doing similar exercise.
- A few dogs with exercise-induced collapse (EIC) have died during collapse—death is usually preceded by a short generalized seizure. The cause of death is uncertain, but weakness of the respiratory muscles and extreme hyperthermia are suspected.

CAUSES

- Genetic disorder—inherited as an autosomal recessive trait.
- Symptomatic dogs are homozygous for a mutation in the dynamin 1 gene. Dynamin 1 (*DNM1*) is a protein important in neurotransmission in the brain and spinal cord during high-level neuronal activity. There is evidence that the *DNM1* mutation associated with EIC has its most profound effect on *DNM1* function when body temperature is elevated, as normally occurs with exercise.

RISK FACTORS

- Genetically affected dogs are at risk for collapse when participating in high-intensity exercise with concurrent excitement or stress.
- Trigger activities most likely to induce collapse include repetitive fun or training retrieves, upland bird hunting, intense play with other dogs, and running alongside an all-terrain vehicle.
- Increased ambient temperature and humidity increase the risk of collapse in affected dogs.
- Most genetically affected dogs (>80%) will have at least one episode of collapse before they reach 3 years of age, but affected dogs with a sedentary lifestyle or calm temperament may never exhibit weakness or collapse.

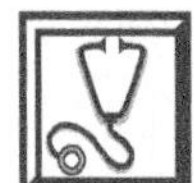

DIAGNOSIS

DIFFERENTIAL DIAGNOSIS

- The episodic nature of the collapse, association with exercise and excitement, typical features of collapse including rear limb weakness and normal mentation, progression of weakness during an episode, and rapid complete recovery should lead to a presumptive diagnosis of EIC in an otherwise healthy Labrador retriever. Physical and neurologic examinations are normal; further evaluation should be performed to eliminate other causes of weakness and collapse. Genetic testing is required to confirm the diagnosis of EIC.
- The disorder most often confused with EIC is a focal seizure/movement disorder characterized by brief episodes of abnormal crouched gait, disequilibrium, head-bobbing, or incoordination. Episodes are often induced by exercise/excitement, leading to confusion with EIC. The onset of signs is peracute, the episodes are short (usually less than 5 minutes), all limbs are involved, and recovery is immediate, helping to distinguish this disorder from the more progressive gait disturbance caused by EIC. Diagnosis can only be made by ruling out other disorders (including EIC) with testing.
- Dogs with metabolic myopathies, polymyositis, and myasthenia gravis are typically much more exercise intolerant than dogs with EIC and they collapse with mild exercise of short duration.
- Centronuclear myopathy—inherited muscle disorder in Labrador retrievers that causes generalized muscle atrophy, constant weakness that worsens with exercise, and absent patellar reflexes at rest. Diagnosis of this disorder is by muscle biopsy or DNA testing (http://labradorcnm.vet-alfort.fr/pages/site/Overview_history.html).
- Cardiac arrhythmia—as a cause of exercise intolerance can be ruled out by cardiac auscultation, palpation of femoral pulses, and performing an ECG at rest and during collapse. Holter monitor or an ECG event recorder may be required to rule out intermittent cardiac arrhythmia.
- Pulmonary hypertension—can cause exercise intolerance and syncopal episodes as exercise and excitement increase systolic pressure in an already overloaded right ventricle and pulmonary arteries, resulting in reflex bradycardia, vasodilation, and hypotension.
- Hypoglycemia—ruled out by measuring blood glucose during an episode.
- Hypo- or hyperkalemia—ruled out by measuring potassium during collapse.
- Hypoadrenocorticism (Addison's disease)—can cause exercise-induced hypoglycemic collapse or seizures; should be ruled out with adrenocorticotropin hormone (ACTH) stimulation test.
- Cataplexy—peracute, nonprogressive, brief episodes of flaccid paralysis.
- Heat stroke—collapse due to heat stroke is usually associated with bleeding, shock, and abnormal mentation. Acute renal failure, disseminated intravascular coagulation (DIC), and death are common. Recovery, if it does occur, is prolonged.
- Malignant hyperthermia—hypermetabolic state triggered by certain anesthetics, extreme heat, intense activity, or psychologic stress in genetically susceptible dogs. Hyperthermia, generalized skeletal muscle contraction, rhabdomyolysis, and DIC occur and many dogs die. Recovery, if it does occur, is prolonged. In vitro contracture tests on muscle biopsies or identification of the causative genetic mutation of the ryanodine receptor (*RYR1*) is required for diagnosis.

CBC/BIOCHEMISTRY/URINALYSIS

Normal at rest and during collapse.

OTHER LABORATORY TESTS

- Arterial blood gas—normal at rest, respiratory alkalosis and metabolic acidosis during collapse identical to intensively exercising Labradors without EIC.
- Lactate and pyruvate—normal at rest, not different during collapse from exercising Labradors without EIC.
- Thyroid evaluation—normal.
- ACTH stimulation test—normal.

- Analysis for mutation in *RYR1* causing malignant hyperthermia—negative.
- Testing for acetylcholine receptor antibodies causing acquired myasthenia gravis— negative.

IMAGING

Thoracic and abdominal radiographs, abdominal ultrasound, echocardiography—normal.

DIAGNOSTIC PROCEDURES

ECG findings at rest and during collapse—normal.

DNA Testing

- Definitive diagnosis requires demonstration that a dog has two copies of the causative *DNM1* mutation.
- Testing can be performed on blood, cheek swabs, puppy dewclaws, or semen.
- Approximately 6% of all tested Labrador retrievers have two copies of the *DNM1* mutation (affected); >35% of all tested Labrador retrievers have one copy of the *DNM1* mutation (carrier).
- Finding two copies of the *DNM1* mutation confirms that a dog is EIC affected and susceptible to collapse, but does not rule out other causes of exercise intolerance or collapse. It is important to do the necessary tests to rule out other causes of collapse that may be potentially more treatable.

PATHOLOGIC FINDINGS

- Muscle histology—normal.
- Complete postmortem examinations of dogs dying during collapse due to EIC—normal.

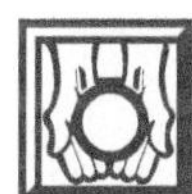

TREATMENT

ACTIVITY

Most affected dogs can live normal active lives if specific trigger activities are avoided or done in moderation.

CLIENT EDUCATION

- Signs commonly worsen in the 3–5 minutes after exercise is terminated; some (<5%) affected dogs die during collapse.
- All activity should be halted at the first sign of weakness or incoordination.
- Consider offering cool water orally, spraying with water, or immersing in water to lower body temperature.

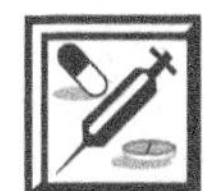

MEDICATIONS

DRUG(S) OF CHOICE

There is no recommended drug therapy for this disorder.

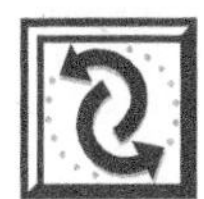

FOLLOW-UP

Most affected dogs can be managed effectively by avoiding trigger activities and carefully observing for the first signs of weakness.

MISCELLANEOUS

ASSOCIATED CONDITIONS

Dogs with EIC do not develop other associated medical conditions as they age.

AGE-RELATED FACTORS

Episodes of collapse may become less frequent as dogs age, perhaps because of less excitement associated with trigger activities.

PREGNANCY/FERTILITY/BREEDING

- Animals should be tested to establish their EIC status prior to breeding.
- Affected dogs (with two copies of the *DNM1* mutation) should not be bred or should be bred only to known noncarriers to avoid producing affected offspring.
- Carrier dogs (with one copy of the *DNM1* mutation) should only be bred to known noncarriers to avoid producing affected offspring.

ABBREVIATIONS

- ACTH = adrenocorticotropin hormone.
- DIC = disseminated intravascular coagulation.
- EIC = exercise-induced collapse.

INTERNET RESOURCES

https://www.vetmed.umn.edu/research/labs/canine-genetics-lab/genetic-testing/exercise-induced-collapse

Suggested Reading

Furrow E, Minor KM, Taylor SM, et al. Relationship between Dynamin-1 mutation status and phenotype in 109 Labrador retrievers with recurrent collapse during exercise. J Am Vet Med Assoc 2013, 242:786–791.

Patterson EE, Minor KM, Tchernatynskaia AV, et al. A canine DNM1 mutation is highly associated with the syndrome of exercise-induced collapse. Nat Genet 2008, 40(10):1235–1239.

Taylor SM, Shmon CL, Adams VJ, et al. Evaluations of Labrador retrievers with exercise-induced collapse, including response to a standardized strenuous exercise protocol. J Am Anim Hosp Assoc 2009, 45:3–13.

Taylor SM, Shmon CL, Shelton GD, et al. Exercise induced collapse of Labrador retrievers: survey results and preliminary investigation of heritability. J Am Animal Hosp Assoc 2008, 44:295–301.

Author Susan M. Taylor

EXOCRINE PANCREATIC INSUFFICIENCY

BASICS

E

DEFINITION

Syndrome that is caused by inadequate amounts of pancreatic digestive enzymes in the small intestinal lumen.

PATHOPHYSIOLOGY

• Most commonly caused by insufficient synthesis and secretion of pancreatic enzymes by the exocrine pancreas. • In rare cases can be caused by an obstruction of the pancreatic duct or isolated lipase deficiency.
• Insufficient synthesis of pancreatic digestive enzymes can be due to destruction of acinar cells resulting from chronic pancreatitis (approximately 50% of cases in dogs and almost all cases in cats) or can be due to idiopathic pancreatic acinar atrophy (PAA; most common cause of exocrine pancreatic insufficiency in German shepherd dogs).
• Deficient exocrine pancreatic secretion results in maldigestion and nutrient malabsorption, leading to weight loss and loose stools with steatorrhea. • Malabsorption contributes to small intestinal dysbiosis.

SYSTEMS AFFECTED

Nutritional—protein-calorie malnourishment.

GENETICS

Assumed to be hereditary in the German shepherd dog and probably transmitted by a complex trait (early studies have suggested an autosomal recessive trait, but this is no longer believed to be the case).

INCIDENCE/PREVALENCE

• PAA is very commonly seen in the German shepherd dog; it is less commonly seen in rough-coated collies and Eurasians. • Other causes of exocrine pancreatic insufficiency (EPI) may be seen in all dog and cat breeds.
• Less common in cats than in dogs.

GEOGRAPHIC DISTRIBUTION

None

SIGNALMENT

Species

Dog and cat.

Breed Predilections

German shepherd dogs, rough-coated collies, and Eurasians.

Mean Age and Range

• PAA in young adult dogs. • Chronic pancreatitis in dogs and cats of any age.

Predominant Sex

No sex predilection.

SIGNS

General Comments

• Consider in young adult (age range approximately 1–4 years) German shepherd dogs with weight loss and loose stools.
• Severity—varies depending on time until diagnosis and therapy.

Historical Findings

• Weight loss with normal to increased appetite. • Chronically loose stools or diarrhea. • Fecal volumes are larger than normal and may be associated with steatorrhea. • Flatulence and borborygmus are commonly reported, especially in dogs.
• May show coprophagia and/or pica. • May be accompanied by polyuria/polydipsia with diabetes mellitus as a sequel to chronic pancreatitis.

Physical Examination Findings

• Thin body condition. • Decreased muscle mass. • Poor-quality hair coat. • Cats with steatorrhea may have greasy "soiling" of the hair coat in the perineal area, but this is seen in the minority of cases.

CAUSES

• PAA. • Chronic pancreatitis. • Pancreatic adenocarcinoma or other abdominal tumor leading to pancreatic duct obstruction

RISK FACTORS

• Breed—German shepherd dogs, rough-coated collies, and Eurasians. • Any condition predisposing dogs or cats to chronic pancreatitis.

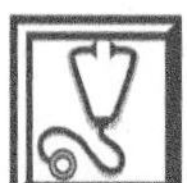

DIAGNOSIS

DIFFERENTIAL DIAGNOSIS

• Secondary causes of chronic diarrhea and weight loss (e.g., hepatic failure, renal failure, hypoadrenocorticism, and hyperthyroidism in cats). • Primary gastrointestinal disease (e.g., infectious, inflammatory, neoplastic, mechanical, or toxic).

CBC/BIOCHEMISTRY/URINALYSIS

Usually normal.

OTHER LABORATORY TESTS

Direct/Indirect Fecal Examinations

Negative for parasites.

Exocrine Pancreatic Function Tests—Trypsin-Like Immunoreactivity (TLI)

• Diagnostic test of choice in both dogs and cats. • Principle of test—serum TLI can be measured by an assay that detects trypsinogen and trypsin that is directly released into the blood from pancreatic acinar cells; serum TLI is detected in the serum of all normal dogs and cats with a functional exocrine pancreatic mass.
• Serum TLI concentrations are dramatically reduced with EPI—dogs: cTLI ≤2.5 μg/L; cats: fTLI ≤8.0 μg/L. • The TLI tests are species specific. • Advantages—simple; quick; single serum specimen (fasted); highly sensitive and specific for EPI in both species.

Other Exocrine Pancreatic Function Tests

• Assays of fecal proteolytic activity using casein-based substrates have been used to diagnose EPI in both dogs and cats; however, fecal proteolytic activity is associated with false-positive and false-negative test results and should only be used in exotic species for which a serum TLI test is not available. • An assay for the measurement of fecal elastase has been validated for the dog; however, this test is associated with a high rate of false-positive test results; therefore a positive test result, suggesting EPI, must be verified by measurement of a serum cTLI concentration.

Screening Tests for Malassimilation

Microscopic examination of feces for undigested food, assessment of fecal proteolytic activity, and the plasma turbidity test are unreliable and *not* recommended.

Cobalamin and Folate

• Often run as a panel with TLI. • Used to assess for concurrent small intestinal dysbiosis or concurrent small intestinal disease (such as inflammatory bowel disease [IBD]). • Cobalamin (vitamin B_{12}) is frequently deficient in both dogs and cats with EPI and can lead to treatment failure or complications if not addressed.

IMAGING

Abdominal radiography and ultrasonography are unremarkable unless the patient has concurrent conditions.

DIAGNOSTIC PROCEDURES

N/A

PATHOLOGIC FINDINGS

• Chronic pancreatitis—microscopically, acini and possibly islets are depleted and replaced by fibrous tissue; there may also be an active inflammatory infiltration. • PAA—marked atrophy/absence of pancreatic acinar tissue on gross and histopathologic inspection in dogs with PAA.

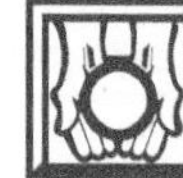

TREATMENT

APPROPRIATE HEALTH CARE

• Outpatient medical management.
• Patients with concurrent diabetes mellitus may initially require hospitalization if ill (e.g., diabetic ketoacidosis).

NURSING CARE

N/A

ACTIVITY

No restriction.

DIET

• Type of diet does not play a role in the management of EPI in dogs and cats.
• However, low-fat and high-fiber diets should be avoided.

CLIENT EDUCATION

• Discuss hereditary nature in German shepherd dogs. • Discuss expense of pancreatic enzyme supplementation and need for lifelong therapy. • Discuss the possibility of diabetes mellitus in patients with chronic pancreatitis.

SURGICAL CONSIDERATIONS

Mesenteric torsion has been reported in German shepherd dogs with EPI in Finland, but not North America.

MEDICATIONS

DRUG(S) OF CHOICE

• Powdered pancreatic enzymes are the treatment of choice (as a reference these products should contain at least 70,000 USP of lipase per teaspoon). • In Europe, microencapsulated products are available; because the lipase is protected from gastric inactivation a much smaller amount is needed for treatment. • Initially—mix enzyme powder in food at a dosage of 1 teaspoon/10 kg body weight with each meal; feed at least two meals daily to promote weight gain. • Preincubation of enzymes with food does *not* improve the effectiveness of oral enzyme therapy, but may negatively impact owner compliance. • Approximately 85% of all dogs with EPI and virtually all cats with EPI are cobalamin deficient and require parenteral or oral cobalamin supplementation (see Cobalamin Deficiency for dosing). • Administration of a proton pump inhibitor (e.g., omeprazole at 0.7–1.0 mg/kg q12h) may improve the condition in nonresponsive patients. • Most dogs and cats respond to therapy within 5–7 days; after a complete response has been achieved, the amount of pancreatic enzyme supplement may be gradually reduced to a dose that prevents return of clinical signs. • Oral antibiotic therapy (tylosin: 25 mg/kg PO q12h) may be required for 4–6 weeks in patients with concurrent dysbiosis, but in most patients dysbiosis resolves spontaneously upon commencement of enzyme replacement therapy. • Severely malnourished dogs may also require supplementation with tocopherol; body stores of other fat-soluble vitamins are probably also decreased in dogs and cats with EPI, but supplementation does not appear to be crucial.

CONTRAINDICATIONS

Avoid tablets and capsules, as mixing of enzymes and chyme is unpredictable.

PRECAUTIONS

N/A

POSSIBLE INTERACTIONS

N/A

ALTERNATIVE DRUG(S)

• The cost of pancreatic enzyme replacement is very high; also, some cats refuse to consume the pancreatic enzyme supplement; these patients can often be successfully managed by addition of fish oil to the enzyme supplement or administration of raw beef, pork, or game pancreas. • Each teaspoon of pancreatic enzyme supplement needs to be replaced with 1–3 ounces (approximately 30–90 g) of raw chopped pancreas. • Raw pancreas can be kept frozen for months without losing enzymatic activity.

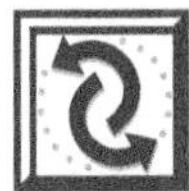

FOLLOW-UP

PATIENT MONITORING

• Weekly for first month of therapy. • Diarrhea improves markedly—fecal consistency typically normalizes within 1 week. • Gain in bodyweight. • Patients that fail to respond after 2 weeks of enzyme therapy and cobalamin supplemenation should be treated for secondary intestinal dysbiosis. • Once bodyweight and condition normalize, gradually reduce daily dosage of enzyme supplements to a level that maintains normal fecal quality and bodyweight.

PREVENTION/AVOIDANCE

Do not breed patients that belong to a breed predisposed to PAA.

POSSIBLE COMPLICATIONS

• Approximately 20% of dogs fail to respond to pancreatic enzymes and need further evaluation and therapy. • Most patients with EPI have cobalamin deficiency and need to be managed accordingly. • Some dogs and cats treated with pancreatic enzyme supplements develop oral ulcerations; in most of these patients the dose of pancreatic enzyme supplements can be decreased, while maintaining therapeutic response; in a few patients, the dose of the pancreatic enzyme supplement needs to be adjusted frequently to avoid treatment failure and oral ulceration. • Two cats with EPI and vitamin K–responsive coagulopathy have been reported; thus, patients that present with a bleeding diathesis should be further evaluated and possibly treated with parenteral vitamin K supplementation.

EXPECTED COURSE AND PROGNOSIS

• Most causes are irreversible, and lifelong therapy is required. • Patients with EPI alone have a good prognosis with appropriate enzyme supplementation and supportive management. • Prognosis is more guarded in patients with EPI and concurrent diabetes mellitus.

MISCELLANEOUS

ASSOCIATED CONDITIONS

• Dysbiosis. • Cobalamin deficiency. • IBD. • Diabetes mellitus. • Associated vitamin K–responsive coagulopathy.

AGE-RELATED FACTORS

Consider EPI in young adult German shepherd dogs with weight loss and loose stools.

ZOONOTIC POTENTIAL

None

PREGNANCY/FERTILITY/BREEDING

Do not breed animals with EPI suspected to be due to PAA.

SYNONYMS

None

SEE ALSO

- Cobalamin Deficiency.
- Diarrhea, Chronic—Cats.
- Diarrhea, Chronic—Dogs.
- Pancreatitis—Cats.
- Small Intestinal Dysbiosis.

ABBREVIATIONS

- cTLI = canine trypsin-like immunoreactivity.
- EPI = exocrine pancreatic insufficiency.
- fTLI = feline trypsin-like immunoreactivity.
- IBD = inflammatory bowel disease.
- PAA = pancreatic acinar atrophy.
- TLI = trypsin-like immunoreactivity.

INTERNET RESOURCES

http://www.vetmed.tamu.edu/gilab

Suggested Reading

Batchelor DJ, Noble PJ, Taylor RH, et al. Prognostic factors in canine exocrine pancreatic insufficiency: prolonged survival is likely if clinical remission is achieved. J Vet Intern Med 2007, 21:54–60.

German AJ. Exocrine pancreatic insufficiency in the dog: breed associations, nutritional considerations, and long-term outcome. Top Companion Anim Med 2012, 27:104–108.

Steiner JM. Exocrine pancreas. In: Steiner JM, ed., Small Animal Gastroenterology. Hanover: Schlütersche-Verlagsgesellschaft, 2008, pp. 283–306.

Thompson KA, Parnell NK, Hohenhaus AE, et al. Feline exocrine pancreatic insufficiency: 16 cases (1992–2007). J Feline Med Surg 2009, 11:935–940.

Westermarck E, Wiberg M. Exocrine pancreatic insufficiency in the dog: historical background, diagnosis, and treatment. Top Companion Anim Med 2012, 27:96–103.

Xenoulis PG, Zoran DL, Fosgate GT, et al. Feline exocrine pancreatic insufficiency: a retrospective study of 150 cases. J Vet Intern Med 2016, 30:1790–1797.

Author Jörg M. Steiner

Consulting Editor Mark P. Rondeau

Client Education Handout available online

E

EYELASH DISORDERS (TRICHIASIS/DISTICHIASIS/ECTOPIC CILIA)

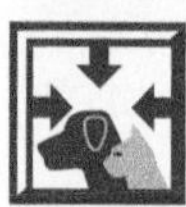

BASICS

OVERVIEW

• Trichiasis—normal hair from the skin contacting corneal or conjunctival surface. • Distichiasis—abnormal hairs that emerge from the meibomian glands along the eyelid margin; may contact corneal or conjunctival surface. • Ectopic cilia—abnormal hairs that emerge through the palpebral conjunctiva several millimeters from the lid margin; contact the corneal surface.

SIGNALMENT

• *Trichiasis*: ○ Facial fold trichiasis—brachycephalic dogs with prominent facial folds or a shallow orbit and prominent globe (e.g., Pekingese, pug, English bulldog). ○ Entropion—rolling in of eyelid margin; conformational (primary) entropion common in young dogs in predisposed breeds (shar pei, retrievers, chow chow, English bulldog, among others); secondary (acquired) entropion may occur in dogs and cats of any breed or age. ○ Eyelid agenesis (eyelid coloboma)—congenital in cats; sporadic occurrence. • *Distichiasis*— common in young dogs; rare in cats; some predisposed breeds include spaniels, English bulldog, flat-coated retriever, and dachshund. • *Ectopic cilia*—common in young dogs, rare in cats; predisposed breeds include Pekingese, shih tzu, and English bulldog.

SIGNS

Facial-Fold Trichiasis

• Commonly bilateral. • Epiphora. • Pigmentary keratitis (especially nasally). • Often associated with lagophthalmos (incomplete blink). • Blepharospasm if ulcerative keratitis present.

Trichiasis Associated with Entropion

• Bilateral if primary. • Blepharospasm. • Epiphora. • Conjunctivitis. • Keratitis (vascularization, pigmentation, possibly ulcerative).

Eyelid Agenesis

• Typically bilateral. • Absent portion of dorsal-lateral eyelid margin. • Other intraocular congenital abnormalities are common. • Conjunctivitis. • Keratitis (vascularization, pigmentation; possibly ulcerative). • Lagophthalmos. • Blepharospasm.

Distichiasis

• Involves upper and/or lower eyelid margin; unilateral or bilateral. • Soft hairs and those directed away from the cornea: asymptomatic. • Stiff, stout cilia contacting the cornea: blepharospasm, epiphora, conjunctivitis, and keratitis (vascularization, pigmentation; possibly ulcerative).

Ectopic Cilia

• Unilateral or bilateral; typically central/upper eyelid. • Hair may be pigmented or nonpigmented. • Severe blepharospasm. • Epiphora. • Conjunctivitis. • Recurrent superficial corneal ulcers.

CAUSES & RISK FACTORS

• Trichiasis—often related to conformation. • Secondary (acquired) entropion may be associated with pain (spastic entropion), scarring (cicatricial entropion), or enophthalmos; occasionally seen in cats. • Distichiasis—considered to be inherited; many predisposed breeds. • Eyelid agenesis (eyelid coloboma)—may be hereditable or due to in utero viral infection. • Ectopic cilia—multiple breeds predisposed.

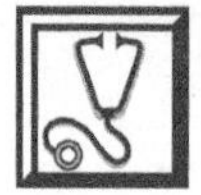

DIAGNOSIS

DIFFERENTIAL DIAGNOSIS

• Other adnexal abnormalities. • Keratoconjunctivitis sicca. • Conjunctival foreign body. • Infectious or inflammatory conjunctivitis. • Diagnosis based on observation of abnormal cilia and lid/facial conformation.

CBC/BIOCHEMISTRY/URINALYSIS

N/A

OTHER LABORATORY TESTS

N/A

IMAGING

N/A

DIAGNOSTIC PROCEDURES

Ocular examination with magnification.

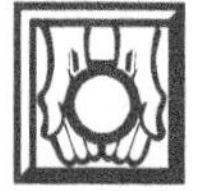

TREATMENT

Trichiasis

• Conservative management—topical lubricating ointments. • Clipping hair on facial folds may cause hairs to become stiffer and more irritating. • Surgical correction of adnexal abnormalities (primary entropion, eyelid agenesis). • Reduce/remove facial folds in contact with ocular surface. • Medial canthoplasty—for nasal trichiasis; reduces lagophthalmos and medial entropion. • Treat underlying cause (e.g., spastic entropion, enophthalmia); temporary eyelid tacking may be indicated.

Distichiasis

• If asymptomatic, no treatment is required. • Symptomatic—mechanical removal (periodic manual epilation) or surgical destruction of hair follicles by cryoepilation, electroepilation, or transconjunctival electrocautery. • Avoid lid-splitting and partial tarsal plate excision techniques; may predispose to cicatricial entropion and impaired lid function.

Ectopic Cilia

• Surgical treatment—en bloc resection of the cilia and associated meibomian gland. • Cryotherapy—may be used as sole treatment or adjunct after resection. • May develop ectopic cilia at other locations. • Recheck if clinical signs recur.

MEDICATIONS

DRUG(S) OF CHOICE

• Rarely indicated. • Lubricant ointments—lessen irritation before surgical correction. • Soft contact lens—temporary relief of clinical signs before surgical correction. • Topical antibiotics—for ulcerative keratitis, prophylactic following surgical eyelid procedures.

CONTRAINDICATIONS/POSSIBLE INTERACTIONS

N/A

FOLLOW-UP

• Trichiasis—good prognosis; some corneal changes may be permanent. • Distichiasis—regrowth may occur; destructive procedures must be done conservatively to minimize lid damage. • Ectopic cilia—good prognosis; regrowth may occur.

MISCELLANEOUS

Suggested Reading

Bettenay S, Mueller RS, Maggs DJ. Diseases of the eyelids. In: Maggs DJ, Miller PE, Ofri R, Slatter's Fundamentals of Veterinary Ophthalmology, 6th ed. St. Louis, MO: Saunders, 2018, pp. 127–157.

Gelatt KN, Plummer CE. Canine eyelids. In: Gelatt KN, Plummer CE, eds., Color Atlas of Veterinary Ophthalmology, 2nd ed. Wiley-Blackwell, 2017, pp. 67–85.

Author Renee T. Carter

Consulting Editor Kathern E. Myrna

Acknowledgment The author and book editors acknowledge the prior contribution of Filipe Espinheira.

FACIAL NERVE PARESIS AND PARALYSIS

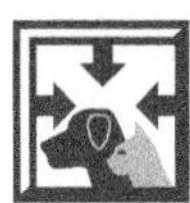

BASICS

DEFINITION

Dysfunction of the facial nerve (cranial nerve [CN] VII) causing paresis (weakness) or paralysis of the muscles of facial expression, which include the ears, eyelids, lips, and nostrils.

PATHOPHYSIOLOGY

- Central—impairment of the facial nucleus within the rostral medulla (brainstem).
- Peripheral—impairment of the facial nerve anywhere along its length or at the neuromuscular junction.

SYSTEMS AFFECTED

- Nervous—facial nerve peripherally or its nucleus centrally.
- Ophthalmic—if parasympathetic preganglionic neurons that supply the lacrimal gland and gland of the third eyelid that course with the facial nerve proximally are affected, keratoconjunctivitis sicca (KCS) develops due to lack of tear secretion.

GENETICS

N/A

INCIDENCE/PREVALENCE

More common in dogs than cats.

SIGNALMENT

Species

Dog and cat.

Breed Predilections

Idiopathic paralysis—cocker spaniel, beagle, Pembroke Welsh corgi, boxer, English setter, golden retriever, and domestic longhair cats.

Mean Age and Range

Adults

Predominant Sex

N/A

SIGNS

General Comments

- Assess strength of palpebral closure—there should be full eyelid closure when a finger is gently passed over the eyelids.
- Idiopathic—unaffected side may become affected within a few weeks to months; may rarely occur bilaterally at first presentation; can have concurrent idiopathic vestibular neuropathy.
- Most patients with bilateral nerve involvement have polyneuropathy-associated systemic disease—look for other nerve deficits.
- May accompany other clinical signs and/or neurologic deficits—always perform a full neurologic examination.
- Ear droop is not always evident in cats and dogs with erect ears.

Historical Findings

- Messy eating; food left around mouth.
- Excessive drooling on affected side.
- Facial asymmetry.
- Eye—inability to close eyelids, rubbing, ocular discharge, ulceration.

Physical Examination Findings

- Facial asymmetry—lip and ear droop, wide palpebral fissure, collapse of nostril.
- Decreased or absent palpebral reflex.
- Decreased or absent menace response (may see eye retraction rather than lid closure).
- Inability to close eyelids.
- Excessive drooling or food falling from mouth on affected side.
- Chronically, patients may have facial muscle contraction toward the affected side due to muscle fibrosis subsequent to paralysis and denervation.
- Decreased Schirmer tear test, mucopurulent discharge from affected eye, and exposure conjunctivitis or keratitis with concurrent KCS.
- Altered mentation (e.g., somnolence or stupor) and/or other cranial nerve abnormalities and gait disturbances may be noted when secondary to intracranial (brainstem) disease.
- Hemifacial spasms (facial nerve tetanus) may be infrequently observed in lesions affecting the facial nerve such as neuritis or otitis media. These patients have sustained contraction of the facial muscles, giving a "grinning" appearance to the affected side of the face. This is a dynamic process and at times the face will appear normal, only to begin the "grinning" appearance once again. If one notices this clinical presentation, middle ear disease should be investigated thoroughly.
- Intermittent facial paresis can be observed in patients with a contralateral thalamocortical lesion when patient is relaxed—due to "release" of upper motor neuron influence on lower motor neuron (CN VII).
- Concurrent heat tilt on ipsilateral side with concurrent otitis interna.
- Concurrent head tilt on ipsilateral side with concurrent idiopathic vestibular neuropathy.
- Abnormal tympanum (bulging, opaque, rupture) on otoscopic examination. Obvious external ear disease may not be present with otitis media.

CAUSES

Unilateral Peripheral

- Idiopathic.
- Metabolic—hypothyroidism.
- Infectious—otitis media–interna (dogs and cats).
- Inflammatory—nasopharyngeal polyps (cats), neuritis.
- Iatrogenic—secondary to surgical ablation of external ear canal or bulla osteotomy; secondary to exuberant ear cleaning; idiosyncratic reaction to potentiated sulfonamides (dogs).
- Neoplastic—aural cholesteatoma, squamous cell carcinoma.
- Trauma—fracture of petrous temporal bone, direct injury to facial nerve by laceration, or compression by hematoma or other mass.
- Toxic—tick bite paralysis (*Dermacentor* spp. (humans), *Ixodes holocyclus*).

Bilateral Peripheral

- Idiopathic.
- Immune-mediated—polyradiculoneuritis (coonhound paralysis), polyneuropathy, myasthenia gravis.
- Metabolic—paraneoplastic polyneuropathy (e.g., insulinoma), hypothyroidism.
- Toxic—botulism.

CNS

- Most unilateral.
- Infectious—viral, bacterial, fungal, rickettsial, protozoal encephalitis.
- Inflammatory—meningoencephalitis of unknown etiology (MUE).
- Neoplastic—primary such as meningioma, choroid plexus tumor, lymphoma; metastatic tumor such as hemangiosarcoma, carcinoma.

RISK FACTORS

Chronic otitis externa and otitis media.

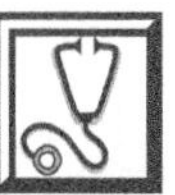

DIAGNOSIS

DIFFERENTIAL DIAGNOSIS

- Differentiate unilateral from bilateral involvement.
- Look for other neurologic deficits—behavior change, gait disturbance, other CN deficits.
- Idiopathic—diagnosis of exclusion; no historical or physical signs of ear disease and no other neurologic deficits.
- Hypothyroidism—with clinical evidence (e.g., lethargy, poor hair coat, weight gain, anemia, hypercholesterolemia, ↓FT4, ↑canine thyroid-stimulating hormone [cTSH]).
- Otitis media–interna—Horner's syndrome, head tilt, and KCS may be simultaneously present.
- CNS disease—if there is somnolence, gait disturbances, or other CN deficits.

CBC/BIOCHEMISTRY/URINALYSIS

- Usually normal in idiopathic facial paralysis.
- Fasting hypercholesterolemia, normocytic/normochromic nonregenerative anemia may be observed with hypothyroidism-associated facial paralysis.
- Hypoglycemia with insulinoma.

OTHER LABORATORY TESTS

- Indicated for patients with suspected underlying disease
- Insulin : glucose ratio to detect insulinoma.
- Acetylcholine receptor antibodies to diagnose myasthenia gravis.

FACIAL NERVE PARESIS AND PARALYSIS (CONTINUED)

- Free T_4 (ideally by equilibrium dialysis) and cTSH to diagnose hypothyroidism.

IMAGING

- CT—sensitive to evaluate middle–inner ear diseases, preferred modality to evaluate bony structures in middle ear.
- MRI—superior to CT for intracranial imaging, preferable for CNS disease; contrast enhancement of facial nerve in dogs with idiopathic facial nerve paralysis; the greater the extent of enhancement, the poorer the prognosis for return to function.
- Bullae radiographs—four views; two obliques, 30° open mouth, dorso-ventral; not sensitive for middle–inner ear diseases.

DIAGNOSTIC PROCEDURES

- Schirmer test—evaluate tear production (normal >15 mm in 60 seconds), should always be performed when evaluating a patient with facial paresis/paralysis.
- Fluorescein test—evaluate for presence of corneal ulceration secondary to KCS.
- Otoscopic examination—evaluate integrity of tympanic membrane and for evidence of otitis media.
- Cerebrospinal fluid (CSF)—evaluate for evidence of intracranial disease; not sensitive if used alone, should be combined with diagnostic imaging (e.g., MRI).
- Facial muscle electromyography—evaluate for denervation and neuromuscular disease.
- Facial and trigeminal nerve reflex electrodiagnostic testing—evaluate peripheral nerve integrity, distinguish between peripheral and central lesions.

PATHOLOGIC FINDINGS

Idiopathic—may see degeneration of large and small myelinated fibers without evidence of inflammation.

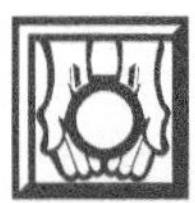

TREATMENT

APPROPRIATE HEALTH CARE

- Outpatient—idiopathic facial paralysis.
- Inpatient—initial medical workup and management of systemic or CNS disease if present.

DIET

No change required.

CLIENT EDUCATION

- Clinical signs may be permanent; however, as muscle fibrosis develops, there is a natural "tuck up" of the affected side that reduces asymmetry; drooling usually stops within 2–4 weeks.
- Inform client that other side can become affected.
- Discuss eye care—cornea on affected side may need lubrication; extra care may be needed if animal is a breed with natural exophthalmia; client must regularly check eyes for redness, discharge, or pain that may indicate corneal ulcer.
- Inform client that most animals tolerate this nerve deficit well; there is no significant impact on quality of life.

SURGICAL CONSIDERATIONS

Bulla osteotomy may be indicated for patients with disorders of middle ear.

MEDICATIONS

DRUG(S) OF CHOICE

- Treat specific disease if possible (e.g., thyroxine for hypothyroidism).
- Idiopathic disease—no treatment required; efficacy of corticosteroids unknown and used commonly in humans to treat Bell's palsy, however are not recommended in veterinary medicine at this time.
- Tear replacement if Schirmer test value low (<15 mm), in patients with KCS or with exophthalmic globes.

CONTRAINDICATIONS

If middle ear disease is suspected, and tympanic membrane may be ruptured, do not use topical ear cleaning solutions due to risk of ototoxicity.

PRECAUTIONS

N/A

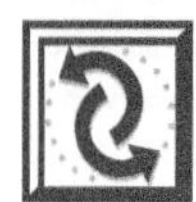

FOLLOW-UP

PATIENT MONITORING

- Reevaluate early for evidence of corneal ulcers.
- Reassess monthly (for 2–3 months) for menace responses, palpebral reflexes, and lip and ear movements to evaluate return of function, condition of affected eye, and development of other neurologic deficits that would indicate progressive disease.

PREVENTION/AVOIDANCE

N/A

POSSIBLE COMPLICATIONS

- KCS.
- Corneal ulcers.
- Permanent facial asymmetry (aesthetic only).

EXPECTED COURSE AND PROGNOSIS

- Depends on underlying cause if one is present.
- Idiopathic disease—prognosis guarded for full recovery.
- Improvement may take weeks or months or may never occur.
- Lip contracture sometimes develops.
- Corneal ulcers may perforate and require enucleation.

MISCELLANEOUS

ASSOCIATED CONDITIONS

Otitis

AGE-RELATED FACTORS

N/A

PREGNANCY/FERTILITY/BREEDING

N/A

SYNONYMS

- Facial neuritis.
- Facial palsy.
- Idiopathic facial neuropathy.

SEE ALSO

- Hypothyroidism.
- Keratitis—Ulcerative.
- Keratoconjunctivitis Sicca.
- Otitis Media and Interna.

ABBREVIATIONS

- CN = cranial nerve.
- CSF = cerebrospinal fluid.
- cTSH = canine thyroid-stimulating hormone.
- KCS = keratoconjunctivitis sicca.
- MUE = meningoencephalitis of unknown etiology.

Suggested Reading

Cook LB. Neurologic evaluation of the ear. Vet Clin North Am Small Anim Pract 2004, 34:425–435.

de Lahunta A, Glass EN, Kent M. Veterinary Neuroanatomy and Clinical Neurology, 4th ed. St. Louis, MO: Elsevier Saunders, 2015, pp. 172–180.

Jeandel A, Thibaud JL, Blot S. Facial and vestibular neuropathy of unknown origin in 16 dogs. J Small Anim Pract 2016, 57:74–78.

Kern TJ, Erb HN. Facial neuropathy in dogs and cats: 95 cases (1975–1985). J Am Vet Med Assoc 1987, 191(12):1604–1609.

Varejao AS, Munoz A, Lorenzo V. Magnetic resonance imaging of the intratemporal facial nerve in idiopathic facial paralysis in the dog. Vet Radiol Ultrasound 2006, 47(4):328–333.

Author Andrea M. Finnen

Client Education Handout available online

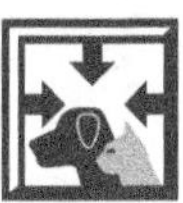

BASICS

DEFINITION

- Physical and behavioral changes resulting from normal hormonal changes during diestrus and early anestrus in the nonpregnant bitch. The term false pregnancy is a misnomer, since the pattern of hormonal changes is normal.
- Physical, hormonal, and behavioral changes following a nonfertile mating or spontaneous ovulation in the queen.

PATHOPHYSIOLOGY

- Hormone profile of pregnant and nonpregnant bitch very similar following ovulation.
- All cycling bitches undergo a lengthy (2+ months) diestrus following ovulation.
- Mammary development and behavioral changes occur under the influence of progesterone and prolactin in late diestrus.
- Galactorrhea (excessive production and inappropriate excretion of milk) is seen following a rise in serum prolactin at the end of diestrus, and also in dogs with severe hypothyroidism due to resulting hyperprolactinemia.
- False pregnancies in the bitch are thought to occur as a holdover from a period in evolution when females of a pack would cycle at the same time, but only dominant individuals would become pregnant. Nonpregnant pack members were available to nurse puppies of the more dominant females.
- Any event that results in an abrupt drop in serum progesterone and rise in prolactin can lead to a clinically overt false pregnancy. Signs are frequently created iatrogenically when ovariectomy (OVE) or ovariohysterectomy (OHE) is performed during mid to late diestrus.
- Queens that ovulate spontaneously or ovulate following mating but do not become pregnant experience a 6–7-week period of diestrus due to elevated progesterone concentrations; some queens develop a clinically overt false pregnancy during this time.

SYSTEMS AFFECTED

- Reproductive.
- Behavioral.
- Endocrine.

GENETICS

N/A

INCIDENCE/PREVALENCE

- False pregnancies occur in 100% of bitches following ovulation.
- >60% of cycling bitches exhibit signs of false pregnancy.
- Spontaneous ovulation occurs frequently in the queen (35–85%) depending on presence of other queens and tom. False pregnancy occurs after every nonpregnant ovulation in the queen, but overt symptoms are uncommon.

SIGNALMENT

Species

Dog and cat.

Breed Predilections

None

Mean Age and Range

Any age.

Predominant Sex

Female only.

SIGNS

General Comments

- Although all cycling bitches have similar progesterone and prolactin hormone profiles during late diestrus and early anestrus, they vary in the magnitude of clinical symptoms associated with the false pregnancy. This may be due in part to individual sensitivities to prolactin.
- Some bitches experience repeated overt false pregnancies, while others have covert false pregnancies.
- The magnitude of symptoms can vary during individual false pregnancies for the same bitch.
- Overt symptoms are uncommon in queens.

Historical Findings

- Estrus—bitch: ~6–12 weeks previously; queen: ~40 days previously.
- OVE or OHE during diestrus, 3–14 days prior to presentation.
- Mammary gland development.
- Galactorrhea.
- Weight gain.
- Behavior change including nesting, maternal behavior, aggression, lethargy.
- Inappetence.
- Abdominal distension (rare).

Physical Examination Findings

- Mammary gland hypertrophy.
- Galactorrhea—fluid can be clear to milky to brown in color.

CAUSES

- Decline in serum progesterone concentration and rise in serum prolactin concentration.
- Decline in serum progesterone concentrations due to OVE or OHE during diestrus.
- Hyperprolactinemia—can be due to severe hypothyroidism.

RISK FACTORS

- OHE or OVE during diestrus.
- Does not impact future fertility.

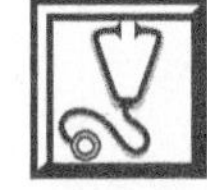

DIAGNOSIS

DIFFERENTIAL DIAGNOSIS

- Pregnancy.
- Mastitis.
- Mammary neoplasia.
- Mammary hyperplasia (queens).
- Pyometra.
- Other causes of abdominal distension (organomegaly, ascites).
- Hypothyroidism.
- Pituitary tumor causing hyperprolactinemia (rare).

CBC/BIOCHEMISTRY/URINALYSIS

- Normocytic, normochromic anemia—17–21% decrease in hematocrit during late diestrus.
- Hypercholesterolemia—75–94% increase during diestrus.

OTHER LABORATORY TESTS

Serum progesterone concentrations elevated if tested during diestrus.

IMAGING

- Ultrasonography—uterine enlargement; performed after 25 days from mating; can be used to evaluate for pregnancy and uterine fluid accumulation.
- Radiography—normal; performed after 54 days from mating; can be used to detect presence of fetal skeletons and uterine fluid accumulation.

DIAGNOSTIC PROCEDURES

N/A

PATHOLOGIC FINDINGS

N/A

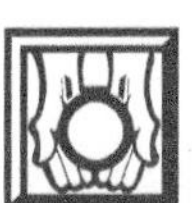

TREATMENT

APPROPRIATE HEALTH CARE

- Usually no treatment needed.
- Outpatient treatment for medical management of severe clinical signs of false pregnancy.

NURSING CARE

- Prevent mammary gland stimulation from self-nursing with Elizabethan collar or body suit.
- Owners can cold pack mammary glands to reduce mammary gland activity.

ACTIVITY

Increase activity in sedentary dogs and cats to increase caloric expenditure and decrease calories available for lactation.

DIET

Decrease caloric intake for several days to reduce energy available for lactation.

CLIENT EDUCATION

- False pregnancies are normal in bitches and do not impact future fertility.
- Advise cat owners that pyometra can develop following spontaneous ovulations.

SURGICAL CONSIDERATIONS

- OVE or OHE if bitch or queen is not intended for use in a breeding program.
- Perform OVE or OHE during anestrus or early diestrus when possible.

FALSE PREGNANCY (CONTINUED)

MEDICATIONS

DRUG(S) OF CHOICE

- Dopamine agonists—reduce milk production and some maternal behaviors by inhibiting prolactin release.
- Cabergoline 5 µg/kg PO q24h for 5–7 days.
- Bromocriptine 10 µg/kg PO q8h for 5–7 days.

CONTRAINDICATIONS

Dopamine agonists can cause abortion if given to a pregnant bitch or queen, as prolactin is luteotrophic. Drugs that suppress prolactin will terminate pregnancy by reducing progesterone and can cause premature parturition (abortion).

PRECAUTIONS

- Incidence of vomiting with bromocriptine administration reduced if given with food; cabergoline has fewer side effects and higher efficacy, but is more costly.
- Coat color changes in dogs possible with prolonged dopamine agonist treatment (uncommon).

POSSIBLE INTERACTIONS

Avoid acepromazine and metoclopramide; both can promote lactation and reduce efficacy of dopamine agonists.

ALTERNATIVE DRUG(S)

- Short-term therapy with diazepam can be useful for bitches with extreme behavioral signs.
- Mibolerone 16 µg/kg PO q24h for 5–7 days to reduce symptoms of false pregnancy. Can also be used at 2.6 µg/kg/day PO starting at least 1 month prior to the next heat cycle to suppress estrus in bitches, which will prevent recurrence. Side effect and risks of treatment should be explained and owners should give informed consent prior to treatment. Do not give to cats.

FOLLOW-UP

PATIENT MONITORING

Have owners monitor mammary glands for inflammation and discoloration that could indicate mastitis.

PREVENTION/AVOIDANCE

- Perform OVE or OHE during anestrus or early diestrus when possible.
- Estrus suppression.

POSSIBLE COMPLICATIONS

Mastitis with significant mammary gland hypertrophy, galactostasis, and ascending infection.

EXPECTED COURSE AND PROGNOSIS

- Typically resolves in 4–6 weeks without treatment.
- Resolution in 10–14 days with dopamine agonist or mibolerone.
- May recur after any ovulation.

MISCELLANEOUS

ASSOCIATED CONDITIONS

N/A

AGE-RELATED FACTORS

N/A

ZOONOTIC POTENTIAL

N/A

PREGNANCY/FERTILITY/BREEDING

- The tendency to display overt false pregnancies has no impact on fertility.
- Bitches and queens should be evaluated for possible pregnancy before treating for false pregnancy.

SYNONYMS

- Pseudopregnancy.
- Pseudocyesis.
- Pseudogestation.
- Phantom pregnancy.
- False whelping.

ABBREVIATIONS

- OHE = ovariohysterectomy.
- OVE = ovariectomy.

Suggested Reading

Gobello C, De La Sota RL, Goya RG. A review of canine pseudocyesis. Reprod Dom Anim. 2001, 36:283–288.

Kowalewski MP. Endocrine and molecular control of luteal and placental function in dogs: a review. Reprod Domest Anim 2012, 47(Suppl 6):19–24.

Lee WM, Kooistra HS, Mol JA, et al. Ovariectomy during the luteal phase influences secretion of prolactin, growth hormone, and insulin-like growth factor-I in the bitch. Theriogenology 2006, 66(2):484–490.

Root AL, Parkin TD, Hutchison P, et al. Canine pseudopregnancy: an evaluation of prevalence and current treatment protocols in the UK. BMC Vet Res 2018, 14(1):170.

Verstegen-Onclin K, Verstegen J. Endocrinology of pregnancy in the dog: a review. Theriogenology 2008, 70:291–299.

Author Milan Hess

Consulting Editor Erin E. Runcan

Client Education Handout available online

FAMILIAL SHAR-PEI FEVER

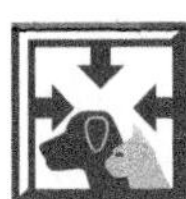

BASICS

DEFINITION

A hereditary autoinflammatory disease in the Chinese Shar-Pei dog characterized by episodic fever and progressive systemic amyloidosis.

PATHOPHYSIOLOGY

- Multifactorial disorder caused by genetic defects that induce chronic inflammation and reactive amyloidosis. Environmental factors and gene modifiers play a role.
- Associated with the thick skin phenotype, resulting from an excessive dermal deposition of hyaluronic acid (HA) by increased expression of hyaluronic acid synthase 2 (HAS2).
- Overabundant HA is degraded into low molecular weight HA, triggering release of inflammatory interleukins.
- Elevated inflammatory cytokines increase serum amyloid A (SAA) concentration. SAA is deposited extracellularly throughout the tissues.
- Amyloid deposition may cause organ failure, particularly in kidneys and liver.

SYSTEMS AFFECTED

- Musculoskeletal—nonerosive polyarthropathy, frequently affecting the tibiotarsal joints.
- Skin—periarticular edema, especially around the tibiotarsal region, swollen muzzle, icterus, skin sloughing.
- Renal/urologic—amyloid deposition in renal medulla, glomerular amyloidosis, renal failure, proteinuria.
- Hepatobiliary—impaired hepatic function; hepatomegaly; friable liver, hepatic rupture and hemoabdomen (rare).
- Hemic/lymphatic/immune—inflammatory response; anemia; coagulation defects; hypercoagulability; hyperglobulinemia; occasionally decreased immunoglobulin (Ig) A or IgG levels.
- Gastrointestinal (GI)—submucosal amyloid deposition; GI ulceration due to renal or hepatic failure.
- Cardiovascular—venous thrombosis; systemic hypertension.
- Nervous—vascular accident; hepatic encephalopathy.
- Ophthalmic—retinal detachment.
- Respiratory—pleural effusion; pulmonary thromboembolism.

GENETICS

- Autosomal recessive inherited disorder. Different modes of inheritance proposed.
- A greater number of mutations in the “meatmouth” (or heavily wrinkled) shar-pei phenotype increases risk.

INCIDENCE/PREVALENCE

- Estimated 23–28% of shar-pei dogs.
- Estimated 53% of shar-pei dogs with fever.

SIGNALMENT

- Mean age—4 years.
- Range—19 weeks–9 years.
- Sex predisposition—female (female : male, 2.5 : 1).

SIGNS

General Comments

Findings vary depending on distribution and severity of amyloidosis.

Historical Findings

- Episodic anorexia, lethargy, stiffness, swollen hocks and/or muzzle—self-limiting (12–36 hours) or responsive to nonsteroidal anti-inflammatory drugs (NSAIDs).
- Intermittent abdominal pain, vomiting, and/or diarrhea.
- Polyuria and polydipsia.
- Weight loss.

Physical Examination Findings

- Marked fever 39.4–41.7 °C (103–107 °F) of 12–36-hour duration.
- Lethargy and dehydration.
- Edematous periarticular soft tissue swellings.
- Joint effusion.
- Swollen muzzle.
- Abdominal pain.
- Reluctance to move/hunched posture.
- Tachypnea or dyspnea.
- Hepatomegaly, ascites, and icterus.
- Pale mucous membranes secondary to chronic anemia or rarely hemoperitoneum.

CAUSES

Dysregulation of inflammatory processes in the shar-pei dog induces reactive amyloidosis.

RISK FACTORS

Stress may trigger a fever episode.

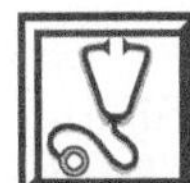

DIAGNOSIS

DIFFERENTIAL DIAGNOSIS

- Infectious or immune-mediated causes of polyarthritis (see Polyarthritis, Nonerosive, Immune-Mediated, Dogs).
- Infectious or immune-mediated causes of fever (see Fever).

CBC/BIOCHEMISTRY/URINALYSIS

- Nonregenerative anemia.
- Neutrophilia with or without left shift.
- Acute kidney injury (e.g., azotemia, hyperphosphatemia, metabolic acidosis, isosthenuria).
- Hypoalbuminemia—secondary to proteinuria or liver failure.
- Hypercholesterolemia—consistent with nephrotic syndrome.
- Elevations in serum alkaline phosphatase (ALP) and alanine aminotransferase (ALT) activities and bilirubin concentration.
- Proteinuria—in cases of glomerular amyloidosis.
- Bilirubinuria—secondary to cholestasis or hepatic failure.

OTHER LABORATORY TESTS

- Genetic tests are available for HAS2 and MDM2 binding protein (MTBP) defects.
- Coombs' test, antinuclear antibody test, and rheumatoid factor identify concurrent underlying immune-mediated disease.
- Prothrombin time (PT) and partial thromboplastin time (PTT)—can be prolonged with liver failure and disseminated intravascular coagulation (DIC); DIC may result in increased D-dimer concentration.
- Antithrombin activity—may be low (urinary loss).
- Thromboelastography/elastometry—hypercoagulability.
- IgA or IgG levels—may be low.
- Urine protein : creatinine ratio (UPC)—severely elevated with glomerular deposition of amyloid.

IMAGING

- Abdominal radiography—hepatomegaly or decreased detail due to peritoneal effusion.
- Thoracic radiography—pleural effusion.
- Joint radiography—periarticular swelling of the soft tissues without bony involvement.
- Abdominal ultrasonography—diffusely hypoechoic liver with rounded edges; kidneys may appear hyperechoic with loss of corticomedullary distinction.

DIAGNOSTIC PROCEDURES

- Synovial fluid analysis—may reveal acute synovitis.
- Kidney and/or liver fine-needle aspiration or biopsy (pending coagulation testing, biopsy preferred)—amyloid deposition, confirmed by Congo red staining and polarized light.

PATHOLOGIC FINDINGS

Deposition of amyloid in multiple organs, associated primarily with vessels or within the parenchyma.

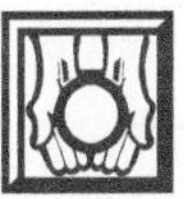

TREATMENT

APPROPRIATE HEALTH CARE

- Minor episodes of pain and fever—outpatient care.
- Inpatient care required for severe fever, anorexia, dehydration, lameness or nonspecific pain, vomiting and/or diarrhea.
- Intensive care may be required to treat organ failure or sequelae of thromboembolism.

FAMILIAL SHAR-PEI FEVER (CONTINUED)

F

NURSING CARE

- IV isotonic crystalloid fluids—for dehydration, anorexia, vomiting and/or diarrhea.
- Oxygen—to treat hypoxemia.
- Abdominocentesis/thoracocentesis—if effusion causes respiratory compromise or elevated intra-abdominal pressure.
- Blood transfusions—to treat anemia.
- Fresh frozen plasma—consider for coagulopathies, DIC.

DIET

- Protein and phosphorus restriction in accordance with IRIS renal staging.
- Dogs with hepatic encephalopathy should be fed protein-restricted diet.
- Omega-3 fatty acids may be beneficial for glomerular disease.

CLIENT EDUCATION

- There is no cure; therapy is palliative and lifelong.
- Early therapy may decrease further deposition of amyloid.
- Diagnostics should be performed to ensure there is no underlying or concurrent disorder.
- Affected dogs should not be bred; genetic testing available.

MEDICATIONS

DRUG(S) OF CHOICE

- Colchicine 0.03 mg/kg PO q24h; advised early in course of disease to delay amyloid deposition; unknown if beneficial once amyloid has been deposited.
- Corticosteroids—if concurrent immune-mediated disease is present.
- Clopidogrel (1–2 mg/kg PO q24h) if concerned about hypercoagulability.
- Angiotensin-converting enzyme (ACE) inhibitor (e.g., enalapril or benazepril 0.25–0.5 mg/kg PO q12–24h) or angiotensin receptor blocker (ARB; e.g., telmisartan 1 mg/kg PO q24h) for proteinuria (may cause transient worsening of azotemia).
- Anti-hypertensive therapy if indicated.
- Antibiotics—for concurrent infection or sepsis.
- NSAIDs/analgesics for fever and pain, unless corticosteroids have been given.
- Gastroprotectants—if gastric ulcer suspected.

CONTRAINDICATIONS

- NSAIDs contraindicated in patients with renal disease, GI upset, and in combination with corticosteroid therapy.
- ACE inhibitors/ARBs contraindicated in dehydrated or hypovolemic patients.

PRECAUTIONS

Colchicine can cause GI upset; chronic use can be associated with bone marrow suppression.

POSSIBLE INTERACTIONS

Concurrent use of colchicine and cyclosporine increases risk of colchicine toxicity.

FOLLOW-UP

PATIENT MONITORING

- Body temperature.
- Blood pressure measurement and fundic examination—monitor for hypertension.
- Urinalysis and UPC.
- Biochemistry panel—renal and hepatic parameters, including albumin.
- CBC—to assess anemia and inflammation.

PREVENTION/AVOIDANCE

Avoid puppies from lines that have a history of shar-pei fever.

POSSIBLE COMPLICATIONS

- Death—due to hepatic rupture or pulmonary thromboembolism (PTE).
- Neutrophilic vasculitis causing severe skin sloughing; streptococcal toxic shock syndrome causing localized necrotizing fasciitis and/or concurrent shock and multiorgan failure.

EXPECTED COURSE AND PROGNOSIS

- Waxing and waning, progressive disorder with a fair to poor prognosis, depending on timing of diagnosis.
- Inevitably fatal due to chronic kidney disease or hepatic failure.
- Time course may be weeks to more than 10 years.

MISCELLANEOUS

AGE-RELATED FACTORS

Most severe in cases diagnosed at an early age.

PREGNANCY/FERTILITY/BREEDING

Do not breed affected dogs.

SYNONYMS

- Swollen hock syndrome.
- Shar-pei autoinflammatory disorder.

SEE ALSO

- Hepatic Encephalopathy.
- Icterus.
- Nephrotic Syndrome.
- Proteinuria.

ABBREVIATIONS

- ACE = angiotensin-converting enzyme.
- ALP = alkaline phosphatase.
- ALT = alanine aminotransferase.
- ARB = angiotensin receptor blocker.
- DIC = disseminated intravascular coagulation.
- GI = gastrointestinal.
- HA = hyaluronic acid.
- HAS2 =hyaluronic acid synthase 2.
- Ig = immunoglobulin.
- MTBP = MDM2 binding protein.
- NSAID = nonsteroidal anti-inflammatory drug.
- PT = prothrombin time.
- PTE = pulmonary thromboembolism.
- PTT = partial thromboplastin time.
- SAA = serum amyloid A.
- UPC = urine protein : creatinine ratio.

INTERNET RESOURCES

- www.drjwv.com
- www.iris-kidney.com
- www.wvc.vetsuite.com

Suggested Reading

DiBartola SP, Tarr MJ, Webb DM, et al. Familial renal amyloidosis in Chinese Shar Pei dogs. J Am Vet Med Assoc 1990, 197:483–487.

May C, Hammill J, Bennett D. Chinese shar pei fever: A preliminary report. Vet Rec 1992, 26:586–587.

Metzger J, Nolte A, Uhde AK, et al. Whole genome sequencing identifies missense mutation in MTBP in Shar-Pei affected with Autoinflammatory Disease (SPAID). BMC Genomics 2017, 18(1):348.

Olsson M, Tintle L, Kierczak M, et al. Thorough investigation of a canine autoinflammatory disease (AID) confirms one main risk locus and suggests a modifier locus for amyloidosis. PLoS One 2013, 8(10):e75242.

Author Bianca N. Lourenço

Consulting Editor Melinda S. Camus

Acknowledgment The author and book editors acknowledge the prior contribution of Julie Armstrong.

FANCONI SYNDROME

BASICS

OVERVIEW

Defective proximal renal tubular reabsorption of glucose, electrolytes, and amino acids.

SIGNALMENT

Species

Dogs and rarely cats.

Breed Predilections

Sporadically reported in several breeds, idiopathic Fanconi syndrome primarily affects the basenji breed (approximately 75% of cases). In America, 10–30% of basenjis are affected. It is presumed to be inherited in this breed, but the mode of inheritance is unknown.

Mean Age and Range

Age at diagnosis: 10 weeks–11 years. Affected basenjis usually are >2 years of age; most develop clinical signs from 4 to 7 years.

Predominant Sex

None

SIGNS

- Depends on the severity of specific solute losses and residual renal function.
- Loss of amino acids and glucose—usually not associated with clinical signs other than polyuria and polydipsia.
- Weight loss.
- Uremia, lethargy, decreased appetite.
- Abnormal growth (rickets) may occur in young animals.

CAUSES & RISK FACTORS

- Inherited in basenjis and possibly Irish wolfhounds.
- Acquired Fanconi syndrome has been reported in dogs given gentamicin, streptozotocin, maleic acid, amoxicillin, chlorambucil (cats), and chicken or duck jerky treats, many of which have originated from China; also reported secondary to primary hypoparathyroidism, copper associated hepatopathy, and lead toxicity.

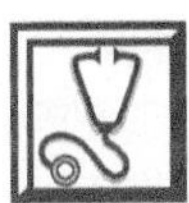

DIAGNOSIS

DIFFERENTIAL DIAGNOSIS

Primary renal glucosuria causes glucosuria despite normoglycemia; documentation of aminoaciduria, mild proteinuria, or a hyperchloremic normal anion gap metabolic acidosis suggests Fanconi syndrome.

CBC/BIOCHEMISTRY/URINALYSIS

- CBC usually normal.
- Hypokalemia.
- Hyperchloremic metabolic acidosis.
- Azotemia if renal failure develops.
- Hypophosphatemia and hypocalcemia may occur in affected young, growing animals.
- Urine specific gravity usually low (1.005–1.018); mild proteinuria common; ketonuria may be present.
- Granular or lipid casts and bacteria were seen in 27–40% of dogs.

OTHER LABORATORY TESTS

Hyperchloremic normal anion gap metabolic acidosis due to bicarbonaturia with urine pH <5.5. Urine pH >6.0 in distal renal tubular acidosis, which is key diagnostic difference to proximal renal tubular acidosis (Fanconi syndrome).

IMAGING

Radiography—young growing dogs may have rickets and angular limb deformities; adults may have decreased bone density.

DIAGNOSTIC PROCEDURES

Urinary clearance studies to document excessive excretion of glucose, amino acids, and electrolytes needed for confirmation. Do not test animals <8 weeks of age because false-positive results may occur. Urine can be evaluated at PennGen for aminoaciduria. Fractional reabsorption of amino acids in affected dogs ranges from 50% to 96% (normal 97–100%).

PATHOLOGIC FINDINGS

Renal papillary necrosis may occur in late disease.

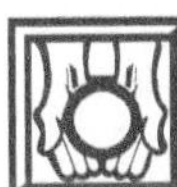

TREATMENT

- Discontinue any drug or treats that may cause Fanconi syndrome or treat for specific intoxication.
- No treatment reverses transport defects in dogs with inherited or idiopathic disease.
- Because magnitude of transport defects varies among affected animals, treatment must be individualized.
- Treat for metabolic acidosis if blood bicarbonate concentration <12 mEq/L. Large doses of alkalinizing agents may be required because decreased proximal tubular resorptive capacity results in marked bicarbonaturia. Goal of alkali therapy to maintain blood bicarbonate concentration 12–18 mEq/L.
- Young, growing dogs may require vitamin D, calcium, and phosphorus supplementation.

MEDICATIONS

DRUG(S) OF CHOICE

Use potassium citrate or sodium bicarbonate (start with low dosage) as dictated by blood gas and electrolyte data.

CONTRAINDICATIONS/POSSIBLE INTERACTIONS

- Avoid drugs that are nephrotoxic or have potential to cause Fanconi syndrome (see Causes & Risk Factors).
- Avoid potassium chloride if hyperchloremic.

FOLLOW-UP

- Monitor serum biochemistry at 14-day intervals to assess treatment response; monitor serum potassium concentration regularly as bicarbonate therapy may aggravate renal potassium loss; once stable, monitor biochemistry at 3-month intervals.
- Clinical course varies; some dogs remain stable for years, others develop rapidly progressive renal failure over a few months; cause of death usually acute kidney injury with severe metabolic acidosis.
- Some dogs (18% in one study) developed seizures or other neurologic signs several years after diagnosis.

MISCELLANEOUS

SEE ALSO

- Acute Kidney Injury.
- Chronic Kidney Disease.

INTERNET RESOURCES

- https://www.vet.upenn.edu/research/academic-departments/clinical-sciences-advanced-medicine/research-labs-centers/penngen
- http://www.basenji.org/ClubDocs/fanconiprotocol2003.pdf

Suggested Reading

Thompson M, Fleeman L, et al. Acquired proximal renal tubulopathy in dogs exposed to a common dried chicken treat: retrospective study of 108 cases (2007–2009). Aust Vet J 2013, 91(9):368–373.

Authors Joao Felipe de Brito Galvao and Stephen P. DiBartola

Consulting Editor J.D. Foster

FEAR AND AGGRESSION IN VETERINARY VISITS—CATS

BASICS

DEFINITION

• Fear—involuntary, negative emotional state caused by anticipation/awareness of danger. • Aggression—warning/intent to cause harm/increase distance to perceived threat.

PATHOPHYSIOLOGY

See Causes and Risk Factors.

SYSTEMS AFFECTED

• Behavioral—neurochemical input between limbic system and forebrain. • Sympathetic nervous system arousal.

GENETICS

Fearful/fractious temperaments are heritable.

INCIDENCE/PREVALENCE

Up to 85% of cats stressed at physical exam.

GEOGRAPHIC DISTRIBUTION

None

SIGNALMENT

Species

Cat

Breed Predilections

Any

Mean Age and Range

Any

Predominant Sex

Any

SIGNS

Fearful body language—dilated pupils, ears back, crouching, hissing, growling, tail thrashing, swatting.

CAUSES

• Previous frightening/painful experience.
• Fearful temperament.

RISK FACTORS

History of fearful/fractious behavior to handling, unfamiliar people, travel, or at previous visits.

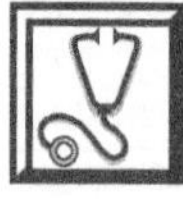

DIAGNOSIS

DIFFERENTIAL DIAGNOSIS

• Pain. • Irritability from illness. • Forebrain lesion. • Cognitive dysfunction syndrome.

CBC/BIOCHEMISTRY/URINALYSIS

Stress leukogram; hyperglycemia; glucosuria.

IMAGING

If indicated to rule out medical conditions, e.g., pain.

DIAGNOSTIC PROCEDURES

If indicated to rule out medical conditions.

PATHOLOGIC FINDINGS

Stress related increase in blood pressure, heart rate, temperature, respiratory rate.

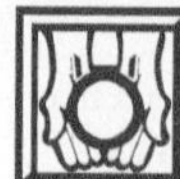

TREATMENT

APPROPRIATE HEALTH CARE

Prior to Handling

Assess environment, patient, and veterinary personnel. What cats see, smell, feel, taste, and hear affects emotional state and can lower aggression threshold.

Assess Environment: Make Cat Comfortable

• Reduce carrier/transport stress. • Eliminate/avoid triggers. • Modify environmental stimuli—light, noises, sound level (stress at ≥80 DB), movement, touch, temperature (30–36 °C).
• Comfortable exam site (no slippery, shiny, cold surfaces). • Allow cats to hide, feel secure.

Assess Animal: Anxiety/Fear/Arousal Fuel Aggression

• Body language interpretation is critical.
• Track willingness to approach, interact with environment and people. • Intervene early.
• Change in location (examination vs. treatment area), interaction, procedure, personnel can affect patient.

Assess Yourself: Avoid Perceived Threats, Track Body Postures and Behavior

• Avoid direct eye contact or putting face near fearful cat. • Avoid petting top of head, grabbing body, or reaching into carrier.
• Remove carrier tops—do not pull or dump cat. • Allow time to sniff your hand; gently scratch under chin and side of head if postures indicate safety; avoid petting beyond shoulder—often overarousing. • Start exam at head or middle and move back; save socially invasive (head, feet, rear, belly) or painful areas for last.
• Talk softly; work quietly; avoid sudden movements. • Often narrow window of opportunity before fear/arousal escalates. • Not approaching indicates use of social distance to cope; anticipate approach may lead to aggressive response—make a plan. • Fear or frustration by handler increases cat fear. • Use language that is scientifically accurate and promotes patient empathy—fearful, painful, confused; avoid labels that result in poor handling and offend clients—evil, spiteful, mean, bad, stupid.
• Strictly avoid punishment (verbal or physical).

Make Handling Plan

• Handling plans unique to individual cats, environment, and procedures and require adjustments based on patient response. • Make plan for safety, decreased handling time, patient welfare, client satisfaction. • Maintain record of likes and dislikes to plan future visits.

Patient Handling Plan Guidelines

• Determine cat's preferred food/treat for distraction and counter-conditioning (CC).
• Select restraint for individual cat/procedures.
• Select handling tools that increase safety and decrease patient fear/arousal. • Critically consider procedures—must it be done today? Consider rescheduling to add oral sedative/anxiolytics and/or divide treatment into shorter visits with fewer procedures. • Place required procedures in order of most important to least in case not all are tolerated. • Place procedures in order of least to most aversive so early procedures do not inhibit completion of later ones. • Consider pain, invasiveness, number of procedures, how patient is coping. • Use chemical restraint immediately, prior to any necessary procedures in which fear may escalate above mild. • Have chemical restraint prepared for at-risk patients—use before arousal to promote efficacy, safety, reduce future fear.

CC

• Learning where cat's negative emotional response (fear) to stimulus (veterinary setting) is changed to positive one (pleasure). • Food is easiest/most powerful way to create this shift.
• Palatability must be high (e.g., meat baby food, squeeze cheese, canned food) to maximize cat's interest/increase positive emotional response.
• Offer food while cat relaxed/feels safe, then just before/during/after any (aversive) procedure.
• Stressed cats may need food for duration of handling to prevent escalation of fear/arousal.
• Barometer—stressed cats often reject food.

Guidelines for Restraint

• Create safe handling plan for each procedure; use least restraint required. • Avoid over-restraint—causes more stress than procedure itself. • If greater restraint needed, use balanced pressure with global support. • Prevent flailing—control head/rear. • Avoid scruffing—use only for cats comfortable with technique.
• Avoid stretching—use lateral recumbency only if procedure requires. • Avoid multiple bouts of restraint; adjust position by sliding hands along body instead of release/regrab. • Struggling 2 seconds—stop, reposition, try again; wait for cat to relax to resume. • Second attempt—if not relaxed and/or starts to get fractious, stop; is procedure essential? • If essential—use chemical restraint. • If nonessential—send home with handling plan and medication if indicated for return visit. • Owner presence—can provide secure base and reduce stress.

Handling Tools

Expedite procedures by reducing patient fear, minimizing manual restraint, and increasing safety.

Pheromones: F3 Cheek Gland (Feliway® Classic)

• Diffusers—reception, exam rooms, wards.
• Spray/wipes—travel, examination, cages.

Muzzles

Toweling preferred.

Towels

• Towel/thick bedding for immobilization—protects cat from flailing, handler from bites/scratches. • Provides head/body control, avoids visual stimuli, firm global pressure—can modify to gain head/jugular or front/back leg access.
• Allows auscultation, abdominal palpation.
• Safe restraint of fleeing/fearful cats, removal from carrier/cage, chemical restraint injection.

Music

Classical music and cat-specific music may mask stressful external sounds, relax patients, have potential calming effects on clients and staff.

Cat Carrier

• Positively condition/train cats to carrier prior to travel. • Select carrier that allows cat to easily exit or remain in lower portion for exam (removable top). • Provides familiar area, prevents fleeing, promotes hiding. • Soft-sided/mesh panels—can press mesh against cat's body for safe IM injection. • Place carrier in cage of hospitalized cat—offers familiarity, encourages faster return to eating.

Restraint Nets (EZ Nabber)

• Provides safe option for catch/restraint for prompt administration of IM injections. • Very effective for cats housed in wall unit cages. • Cover with towel once cat inside—reduces visual stimulation, protects handler.

NURSING CARE

N/A

ACTIVITY

N/A

DIET

N/A

CLIENT EDUCATION

• Preventive counseling (start at first visit)—positive carrier training, travel, handling, feline communication, reward training, avoid use of punishment. • Provide kitten classes in veterinary clinic. See Internet Resources.

SURGICAL CONSIDERATIONS

N/A

MEDICATIONS

DRUG(S) OF CHOICE

Chemical Restraint

• Allows safe handling, effective completion of procedures. • Blocks/prevents fear, discomfort, pain, further distress, and fear escalation. • Minimal or no physical restraint. • Injectable sedation (IM) most effective for safe handling of fractious/highly fearful patients. • Base protocol on age, temperament, health. • Pre-travel oral anxiolytics/sedatives reduce fear, facilitate gentle handling, promote safety for injection, reduce injectable doses.

Oral Sedative/Anxiolytics

• Administer 60–90 min prior to travel for mild/moderate fear, or to facilitate administering chemical restraint. • May give first dose 12h in advance. • Also may be required for inpatients. • Gabapentin—10–20 mg/kg PO (50–150 mg/cat). • Trazodone—25–50 mg/cat PO. • Lorazepam—0.05–0.25 mg/kg PO (0.125–0.25 mg/cat). • Buprenorphine—0.01–0.03 mg/kg oral transmucosal (OTM). • For additional sedation can add acepromazine—0.5–2.2 mg/kg PO.

Injectable Sedation/Chemical Restraint

• *Young/healthy*—dexmedetomidine 10–20 µg/kg *or* acepromazine 0.1 mg/kg + opioid; for additional sedation can add ketamine 3–5 mg/kg IM. • *Alternative*—tiletamine/zolazepam 5–10 mg/kg IM. • *Geriatric/ill*—acepromazine 0.01–0.05 mg/kg *or* dexmedetomidine 5–10 µg/kg + opioid: for greater sedation add ketamine 3–5 mg/kg IM; hydromorphone 0.05 mg/kg + midazolam 0.1–0.2 mg/kg ± ketamine 3–5 mg/kg ± acepromazine 0.01–0.05 mg/kg; alfaxalone 1–2 mg/kg + midazolam 0.2 mg/kg ± opioid ± acepromazine 0.01–0.05 mg/kg. • Can reverse dexmedetomidine—½ volume atipamezole to volume of dexmedetomidine administered IM. • Dexmedetomidine/ketamine protocols—to avoid dysphoria wait 45–60 min to reverse. • Opioid choices (full Mu agonist superior for pain control)—butorphanol 0.2 mg/kg; buprenorphine 0.01–0.03 mg/kg; morphine 0.2 mg/kg; hydromorphone 0.05–0.1 mg/kg; oxymorphone 0.1 mg/kg.

CONTRAINDICATIONS

Reports of acute hepatic necrosis with oral diazepam.

PRECAUTIONS

• Have client perform drug trial at home to determine response/ideal dose. • Agitation, gastrointestinal upset, sedation, appetite changes possible with above oral medications. • Benzodiazepines—disinhibition of aggression uncommon but possible. • Gabapentin—caution with chronic renal disease.

POSSIBLE INTERACTIONS

N/A

ALTERNATIVE DRUG(S)

Natural products including pheromones and supplements containing l-theanine or alpha-casozepine.

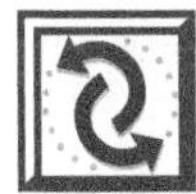

FOLLOW-UP

PATIENT MONITORING

• Evaluate physiologic/behavioral parameters. • Evaluate and record response to handling, location, personnel, products, drugs.

PREVENTION/AVOIDANCE

• Prevention—more effective, safer, less expense, improves healthcare compliance, avoids fear sensitization. • Low Stress handling and CC during all kitten and adult visits recommended.

POSSIBLE COMPLICATIONS

Fearful and/or aggressive behavior negatively impacts frequency and level of veterinary care.

EXPECTED COURSE AND PROGNOSIS

Effective implementation of Fear Free, Low Stress, and Cat Friendly visits reduces fear, anxiety, and stress and improves frequency and quality of veterinary care.

MISCELLANEOUS

ASSOCIATED CONDITIONS

Fearful/fractious cats in veterinary setting often have comorbid behavioral problems at home, such as aggression to owners or strangers, undesirable elimination, and anxiety disorders.

AGE-RELATED FACTORS

• Socialization period (2–7 weeks)—time where positive early exposure minimizes fear. • Regular, gentle, brief exposure to handling paired with positive experience (food) leads to less fear/improved future handling.

F

ZOONOTIC POTENTIAL

Bite wounds and associated infections.

PREGNANCY/FERTILITY/BREEDING

Fearful/aggressive temperaments are heritable.

SYNONYMS

• Fear aggression. • Defensive aggression. • Phobic behavior.

SEE ALSO

• Car Ride Anxiety—Dogs and Cats. • Fears, Phobias, and Anxieties—Cats. • Kitten Socialization and Kitten Classes.

ABBREVIATIONS

• CC = counter-conditioning. • OTM = oral transmucosal.

INTERNET RESOURCES

Travel

• https://catfriendly.com/be-a-cat-friendly-caregiver/getting-cat-veterinarian • www.catalystcouncil.org/resources/health_welfare/cat_carrier_video/index.aspx

Veterinary Visits

• https://https://fearfreehappyhomes.com/courses/how-to-prepare-your-pet-for-vet-visit/ • https://fearfreehappyhomes.com/courses/how-to-make-trip-to-vet-fear-free/

Body Language

• https://www.dacvb.org/page/cats • https://fearfreehappyhomes.com/courses/cat-body-language-101

General

• http://www.fearfreepets.com • http://www.catalystcouncil.org • https://www.partnersforhealthypets.org/practice_feline.aspx • https://lowstresshandling.com • https://www.catvets.com/guidelines/practice-guidelines/handling-guidelines • https://www.aaha.org/aaha-guidelines/behavior-management/behavior-management-home/ • http://www.catalystcouncil.org/resources/health_welfare/cat_friendly_practices • https://icatcare.org/advice/cat-handling-videos

Suggested Reading

Herron M, Shreyer T. The pet friendly veterinary practice: a guide for practitioners. Vet Clin North Am Small Anim Pract 2014, 44:451–481.

Yin S. Low Stress Handling, Restraint, and Behavior Modification of Dogs and Cats. Davis, CA: Cattle Dog Publishing, 2009.

Authors Meghan E. Herron and Traci A. Shreyer

Consulting Editor Gary M. Landsberg

FEAR AND AGGRESSION IN VETERINARY VISITS—DOGS

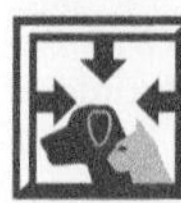

BASICS

DEFINITION

• Fear—involuntary, negative emotional state caused by anticipation/awareness of danger.
• Aggression—warning/intent to cause harm/ increase distance in response to perceived threat.

PATHOPHYSIOLOGY

See Causes and Risk Factors.

SYSTEMS AFFECTED

• Behavioral—neurochemical input between limbic system and forebrain. • Activation of hypothalamic pituitary axis (HPA) and sympathetic nervous system.

GENETICS

Fearful temperament may be heritable.

INCIDENCE/PREVALENCE

Over 75% fearful when examined.

SIGNALMENT

Species

Dog

Breed Predilections

Any

Mean Age and Range

Any

Predominant Sex

Any

SIGNS

Fearful body language—ears back, gaze avoidance, crouching, tail tucked, yawning, panting, lip licking, scanning.

CAUSES

• Previous frightening/painful experiences.
• Fearful temperament (genetics, peri/ postnatal experience, socialization).

RISK FACTORS

History of fearful behavior to handling, unfamiliar people, noises, environments, or previous visits.

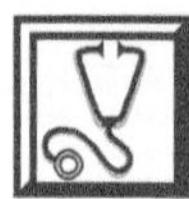

DIAGNOSIS

DIFFERENTIAL DIAGNOSIS

• Pain. • Irritability from illness.
• Forebrain lesion. • Cognitive dysfunction syndrome.

CBC/BIOCHEMISTRY/URINALYSIS

Stress leukogram; glucosuria.

OTHER LABORATORY TESTS

As indicated to rule out medical conditions.

DIAGNOSTIC PROCEDURES

As indicated to rule out medical conditions.

PATHOLOGIC FINDINGS

Stress-induced increase in blood pressure, heart rate, temperature, panting.

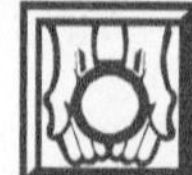

TREATMENT

APPROPRIATE HEALTH CARE

Prior to Handling

Assess environment, dog, and veterinary personnel. What dogs see, smell, feel, taste, and hear affects emotional state and lowers aggression threshold.

Assess Environment: Make Dog Comfortable

• Eliminate known triggers. • Modify environmental stimuli including light, noises, sound level (stress at ≥80 DB), movement, touch, temperature (15–30 °C). • Owner presence—can provide secure base, reduce stress.
• Comfortable exam site (no slippery, shiny, cold surfaces). • Allow fearful dogs to hide, feel secure.

Assess Dog

• Anxiety/fear/arousal leading to aggression.
• Body language interpretation critical.
• Track willingness to approach, interact with environment/people. • Intervene early.
• Change in location (examination vs. treatment area), interaction, procedure, personnel can affect patients.

Assess Yourself: Avoid Perceived Threats, Track Body Postures and Behavior

• Avoid direct eye contact, bending over, putting face near fearful dog, loud talking, sudden movements. • Bend at knee, turn to side, squat (when safe). • Avoid reaching out, petting top of head, grabbing collar. • Encourage patients to approach or have handler they trust move them to you. ○ Hand at your side, pat your leg gently, soft verbal encouragement. ○ Palm open with valued treats. ○ Allow dog to sniff/investigate. ○ Gently pet under chin/neck. ○ Test acceptance—stop petting, does dog reengage. ○ If no: stop, make a plan. ○ If yes: pet again, slowly move to desired exam position. ○ Start exam in middle, slowly work to rear, back to center, to head. ○ Monitor/be prepared for any fear- or pain-evoking handling. • Not approaching indicates use of social distance to cope; approach may lead to aggressive response—make a plan. • Avoid front-facing interactions or cover dog's head; work at side, just behind point of shoulder, facing same direction as dog. • Often narrow window of opportunity before fear/arousal escalates. • Fear or frustration by handler or veterinary personnel increases pet fear; use scientifically accurate language that promotes patient empathy—fearful, painful, confused; avoid labels that result in poor handling/offend clients—mean, bad, spiteful, dominant. • Strictly avoid punishment (verbal or physical).

Make Handling Plan

• Handling plans unique to individual dogs, environment, and procedure and require adjustments based on dog's response. • Make plan for safety, decreased handling time, patient welfare, and client satisfaction. • Maintain record of likes and dislikes to plan further visits.

Patient Handling Plan Guidelines

• Determine most motivating food/treats for distraction and counter-conditioning (CC).
• Select restraint for individual dog/procedures.
• Select handling tools that increase safety and decrease patient fear/arousal. • Critically consider procedures—must it be done today? Consider rescheduling to add oral sedative/ anxiolytics and/or divide treatment into shorter visits with fewer procedures. • Place required procedures in order of most important to least in case not all are tolerated. • Place procedures in order of least to most aversive, so early procedures do not inhibit completion of later ones. • Consider pain, invasiveness, number of procedures, how dog is coping. • Use chemical restraint immediately for any necessary procedures in which fear escalates beyond mild; use before arousal to promote efficacy, safety, escalation, learning.

CC

• Learning where dog's negative emotional response (fear) to stimulus (veterinary setting) is changed to positive one (pleasure). • Food easiest/most powerful way to create shift.
• Palatability must be high (meat baby food, squeeze cheese, canned food) to maximize dog's interest/increase positive emotional response. • Offer food while dog relaxed/feels safe, then just before/during/after any (aversive) procedure. • Stressed dogs may need food for duration of handling to distract and prevent escalation of fear/arousal.
• Barometer—stressed dogs often reject food.

Restraint

• Create safe handling plan for each procedure.
• Use least restraint required—increased restraint increases stress. • If greater restraint needed, use gentle, balanced pressure with global support.
• Prevent flailing by controlling head/rear.
• Avoid lateral recumbency—only if procedure requires. • Avoid multiple bouts of restraint—adjust positioning by sliding hands along body.
• Struggling 3 seconds—stop, reposition, try again; wait for dog to relax to begin. • Second attempt—if fear increases or starts to get fractious, stop; is procedure essential?
• Essential—use chemical restraint.
• Nonessential:—send home with handling plan and pre-visit meds if indicated for return visit.

Handling Tools

Expedite procedures by reducing dog fear, minimizing manual restraint, and increasing safety.

Music

Music and sources of white noise may mask stressful external sounds. Classical music may relax dogs and have calming effects on clients and staff.

Dog-Appeasing Pheromone (Adaptil®)

• Diffusers—reception, exam rooms, wards.
• Spray/wipes—travel, examination, cages.

Muzzles

• For safety, assessment/evaluation, avoid human fear response, injectable sedation. • Home desensitization (DS)/CC—enters wearing comfortably. • Basket muzzle preferred—allows panting: safer for longer procedures/kenneling; allows CC: inserted food or smeared along inside. • Nylon sleeve—short procedures or facilitate essential injection.

Elizabethan Collar

Muzzle alternative for avoiding/reducing visual stimuli.

Towels

• Towels/thick bedding can help immobilize—especially small dogs: head/body control, reduced visual stimuli, global pressure. • Roll towels (cervical collar)—head control.

Eye Covers (e.g., ThunderCap®)

Reduce visual stimuli/triggers for fear and anxiety during travel, exam, injections.

Compression Garments (e.g., ThunderShirt®)

Swaddles—may relax patients with balanced body pressure.

NURSING CARE

N/A

ACTIVITY

N/A

DIET

N/A

CLIENT EDUCATION

Preventive counseling at first puppy visit ± puppy classes in clinic to review positive travel, handling, communication, reward training, and avoiding punishment. See Internet Resources.

SURGICAL CONSIDERATIONS

N/A

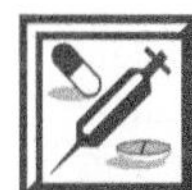

MEDICATIONS

DRUG(S) OF CHOICE

Chemical Restraint

• Allows safe, effective, minimal handling and successful completion of procedures. • Blocks or prevents distress, discomfort, pain, escalation, and fear sensitization. • Injectable sedation (IM)—most effective for safe handling fractious/fearful dogs. • Base protocol on age, temperament, health. • Pre-travel oral sedative/anxiolytics reduce fear, facilitate gentle handling, safety for injection, reduce injectable doses.

Oral Sedative/Anxiolytics

• Administer 1.5–2 hours pre-travel for mild/moderate fear or to facilitate restraint injection; may give first dose 12 hours in advance; repeat dosing as needed if patient is hospitalized.
• Trazodone—4.0–10 mg/kg (up to 18 mg/kg); maximum 300 mg per dose. • Clonidine—0.01–0.05 mg/kg. • Dexmedetomidine oromucosal gel—125 μg/m². • Gabapentin—20–50 mg/kg. • Lorazepam—0.05–0.5 mg/kg.
• Diazepam—0.5–2.2 mg/kg. • Alprazolam—0.01–0.1 mg/kg. • For additional sedation can add acepromazine—0.55–2.2 mg/kg. • Can combine trazodone, clonidine, gabapentin, benzodiazepines. • Avoid acepromazine as sole agent—ineffective anxiolysis

Injectable Restraint

• *Young/healthy*—dexmedetomidine 10–20 μg/kg + opioid: for additional sedation can add ketamine 3–5 mg/kg IM. • *Alternative*—tiletamine/zolazepam 5–10 mg/kg IM (not practical for dogs >20 kg due to volume).
• *Geriatric/ill*—acepromazine 0.01–0.05 mg/kg *or* dexmedetomidine 5–10 μg/kg + opioid: for additional sedation add ketamine 2–5 mg/kg IM; alfaxalone 1–2 mg/kg (not practical for dogs >10 kg due to volume) + midazolam 0.2 mg/kg ± opioid ± acepromazine 0.01–0.05 mg/kg.
• Can reverse dexmedetomidine—equivolume atipamezole to volume of dexmedetomidine IM.
• Dexmedetomidine/ketamine protocols—to avoid dysphoria wait 45–60 min to reverse; opioid choices (full Mu agonist superior for pain control): butorphanol 0.2–0.4 mg/kg; morphine 0.2–0.4 mg/kg; hydromorphone 0.05–0.2 mg/kg; methadone 0.3–0.5 mg/kg.

Oral Transmucosal (OTM)

• *Young/healthy*—dexmedetomidine 10–40 μg/kg ± opioid (e.g., morphine 10 mg/kg or butorphanol 0.2 mg/kg) OTM; can reverse dexmedetomidine with atipamezole (½ volume of dexmedetomidine). • DS/CC to syringe in buccal pouch. • Up to 1h to effect. • Mucosal contact time improves absorption—mix with syrup.

CONTRAINDICATIONS

Avoid clonidine with cardiovascular output issues.

PRECAUTIONS

• Have client perform oral medication trial at home to determine dose/response. • Agitation, gastrointestinal upset, sedation, appetite changes possible. • Benzodiazepines—disinhibition of aggression possible. • Gabapentin—caution with chronic renal disease.

POSSIBLE INTERACTIONS

Avoid combining oral acepromazine with clonidine—potential blood pressure fluctuation.

ALTERNATIVE DRUG(S)

Natural products including pheromones, supplements containing l-theanine or alpha-casozepine and calming probiotic.

FOLLOW-UP

PATIENT MONITORING

• Evaluate and monitor physiologic/behavioral parameters. • Maintain record of response to handling, location, personnel, products, and drugs.

PREVENTION/AVOIDANCE

• Prevention—more effective, safer, less expense, improved healthcare compliance, and avoids fear sensitization. • Also see Client Education.

POSSIBLE COMPLICATIONS

Dogs with fearful and/or aggressive behavior may not receive adequate veterinary care including wellness care, diagnostics, and treatment.

EXPECTED COURSE AND PROGNOSIS

Effective implementation of Fear Free, Low Stress care prevents and reduces fear, anxiety, and stress and improves frequency and quality of veterinary care.

MISCELLANEOUS

ASSOCIATED CONDITIONS

Dogs with fearful/fractious behavior in veterinary setting often have comorbid behavioral problems, including aggression to owners or strangers, leash reactivity, resource guarding, anxiety disorders.

AGE-RELATED FACTORS

• Socialization period (3–12 weeks)—sensitive period where positive exposure minimizes fear; gentle, brief handling paired with positive experience (food) leads to less fear and improved handling. • Fear period (8–10 weeks of age and between 4 and 11 months)—susceptible to single-event learning, highly sensitive to negative experiences. • Social maturity (1–3 years)—fearful puppies/adolescents may begin to show fear and aggression at this time; prompt recognition and intervention essential at first signs of fear to establish handling plan.

ZOONOTIC POTENTIAL

Bite wounds and associated infections.

PREGNANCY/FERTILITY/BREEDING

Fearful/aggressive temperaments heritable.

SYNONYMS

• Fear aggression. • Defensive aggression.
• Phobic behavior.

SEE ALSO

• Car Ride Anxiety—Dogs and Cats.
• Fears, Phobias, and Anxieties—Dogs.
• Puppy Socialization and Puppy Classes.

ABBREVIATIONS

• CC = counter-conditioning.
• DS = desensitization.
• HPA = hypothalamic pituitary axis.
• OTM = oral transmucosal.

INTERNET RESOURCES

• https://fearfreehappyhomes.com/courses/how-to-prepare-your-pet-for-vet-visit/
• https://fearfreehappyhomes.com/courses/how-to-make-trip-to-vet-fear-free/ • https://fearfreehappyhomes.com/courses/dog-body-language-101 • http://www.fearfreepets.com
• https://lowstresshandling.com/

Suggested Reading

Herron M, Shreyer T. The pet friendly veterinary practice: a guide for practitioners. Vet Clin Small Anim 2014, 44:451–481.

Yin S. Low Stress Handling, Restraint, and Behavior Modification of Dogs and Cats. Davis, CA: Cattle Dog Publishing, 2009.

Authors Meghan E. Herron and Traci A. Shreyer

Consulting Editor Gary M. Landsberg

FEARS, PHOBIAS, AND ANXIETIES—CATS

BASICS

DEFINITION

• Fear is the feeling of apprehension resulting from the nearness of some situation or object presenting an external threat. The response of the autonomic nervous system prepares the body for "freeze, fight, or flight." As such, it is a normal behavior, essential for adaptation and survival.
• Anxiety is the anticipation of dangers from unknown or imagined origins that results in physiologic reactions associated with fear. Anxiety may occur in the aftermath of a fear-producing event or as a result of unrelated environmental changes that are unpredictable.
• A phobia is a persistent and excessive fear of a specific stimulus, such as a thunderstorm or separation from an attachment figure.

PATHOPHYSIOLOGY

• Stress responses become problematic when the individual is not able to control the stressful situation by their actions or escape from it through appropriate behavioral responses.
• Chronic anxiety or fear can lead to secondary behavior problems, such as overgrooming, spraying, or intercat aggression, or predispose the cat to health problems owing to a compromised immune system.

SYSTEMS AFFECTED

• Behavioral—hypervigilance, avoidance behaviors, possible aggression.
• Cardiovascular—increased heart rate and blood flow to internal organs during fear-evoking incidents.
• Endocrine/metabolic—glucose release into bloodstream, release of glucocorticoids.
• Gastrointestinal (GI)—decreased appetite.
• Hemic/lymphatic/immune—chronic stress effects on immune function.
• Musculoskeletal—weight loss in response to chronic stress effects on appetite, decreased food intake due to hiding behavior.
• Neuromuscular—decrease in activity due to avoidance and hiding; fearful/anxious reaction may also include pacing, trembling, repetitive activity.
• Ophthalmic—dilated pupils in response to autonomic nervous system stimulation.
• Respiratory—increased respiratory rate when anxious or frightened.
• Skin/exocrine—overgrooming in response to stressors.

GENETICS

• Genetic component possible.
• Breed/coat color and paternal personality have been linked to individual personality traits in cats.

SIGNALMENT

Any age, sex, or breed.

SIGNS

General Comments

• Signs of fear or anxiety can vary between individuals and with different stimuli that may be specific (a particular individual, sound, etc.) or more generalized.
• In mild cases of anxiety or fear the cat may become tense and more reactive to environmental stimuli. Some individuals may retreat to perceived safe hiding places or show little movement.
• Cats in panic can become very aggressive or destructive in an attempt to retreat from the fearful stimulus.

Historical Findings

• Clear description of the cat's body language, behavior, and events or situations that consistently trigger anxiety or fear is helpful in setting up behavioral modification and environmental management program.
• Body postures associated with fearful behavior include ears flattened to back or side of head, crouched body posture when resting or moving, lowered head, tail tucked alongside body or held low, piloerection, dilated pupils, shaking, panting, drooling, "Halloween cat" silhouette.
• If fear is intense, cat may lose bladder and bowel control and express its anal sacs.
• Vocalizations are usually minimal, unless cat is showing defensive behavior in response to perceived threat.
• Cat may pace, vocalize, and solicit attention from owner.
• Urine spraying and destructive scratching may be seen in anxious cats.

Physical Examination Findings

Usually unremarkable unless cat has injured itself trying to escape or while seeking shelter.

CAUSES & RISK FACTORS

Fearful behavior in cats can be related to genetic influences on temperament; lack of positive early experience and socialization, observational learning from fearful mother, other adult cats; learning from negative experiences; social stress, population pressure.

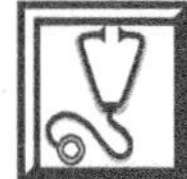

DIAGNOSIS

DIFFERENTIAL DIAGNOSIS

Thorough medical history and physical examination will help differentiate fearful behavior from withdrawal due to illness.

CBC/BIOCHEMISTRY/URINALYSIS

As indicated to rule out medical conditions and as baseline prior to medication use and as premedication screen.

OTHER LABORATORY TESTS

As indicated, including T4 in middle age and older.

IMAGING

As indicated.

TREATMENT

ACTIVITY

Normal social interactions and play should be encouraged, but contact should not be forced.

DIET

Placement of food, water, and litter box may need to be altered if anxious or fearful behavior is limiting access.

CLIENT EDUCATION

General Comments

• Educate owners to read and understand cat communication language for early recognition of signs.
• Discuss behavioral expectations. Owner expectations in regard to social interactions with humans or other cats may be contributing to the problem and could affect prognosis.
• Treatment plan involving case-tailored behavioral modification, environmental adjustments, and support material will help owner better understand situation and implement treatment.

Behavioral Therapy

• Identify and avoid exposure to fear-evoking stimuli and situations. Provide ways for cat to manage situation by creating "safe places" for cat to go to avoid the stimulus.
• If cat must be handled while fearful, caution and gentle physical restraint aids (cat muzzles, head covers, towel wraps, etc.) should be used to prevent injury and decrease stress.
• Desensitization and counter-conditioning to help decrease reactivity to fear-producing stimulus. Systematic desensitization is program of slowly increasing exposure to fearful stimulus or situation. Counter-conditioning consists of enhancing internal and external environment with food rewards or other pleasurable stimuli such as playing with toys.
• Address secondary problems such as strained social interactions subsequent to defensive aggression directed toward humans or other cats, or elimination problems that may be result of fears or anxieties.

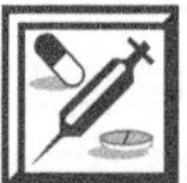

MEDICATIONS

DRUG(S) OF CHOICE

• Medication can be helpful adjunct to behavioral modification, if animal's fearful or anxious behavior is so intense that it interferes with quality of life.

- No drug is approved by FDA for use in cats for fearful behavior; therefore, clients must be advised that information concerning efficacy, contraindications, and side effects is limited.
- If there are questions or concerns about a specific patient or medication, consultation with a veterinary behaviorist may be helpful.
- Selective serotonin reuptake inhibitors (SSRIs)—fluoxetine or paroxetine 0.5–1 mg/kg PO q24h. Side effects—decreased appetite and irritability; paroxetine has anticholinergic effects.
- Tricyclic antidepressants (TCAs)—clomipramine 0.5 mg/kg PO q24h (2.5–5 mg/cat). Side effects—sedation, anticholinergic effects, possible cardiac conduction disturbances in predisposed animals.
- Buspirone—0.5–1.0 mg/kg q8–24h. Side effects—GI upset, mild sedation.
- Benzodiazepines—oxazepam 0.2–0.5 mg/kg q12–24h; alprazolam 0.125–0.25 mg/cat q12h or as needed prior to event; lorazepam 0.025–0.05 mg/kg (or 0.125–0.5 mg/cat) q12h or as needed prior to event. Side effects—sedation, increased appetite, agitation.
- Buspirone and benzodiazepines might reduce fear and build confidence in fearful cat that does not retaliate or fight back.

CONTRAINDICATIONS

- Cats with renal or hepatic disease.
- Caution with TCAs and SSRIs in diabetics.
- TCAs in patients with cardiac abnormalities.

PRECAUTIONS

- Laboratory screening tests suggested before placing animal on psychotropic medication for health assessment and baseline for comparison.
- Compounding medications in more palatable form can ease administration and improve compliance.
- Assess all medications and natural supplements being administered for potential contraindications.

POSSIBLE INTERACTIONS

- TCAs and SSRIs should not be used together.
- Mirtazapine should be used cautiously in combination with TCA or SSRI.
- Practitioner should verify safety when combining psychoactive drugs with other medications.

ALTERNATIVE DRUG(S)

- Natural products that might aid in reducing anxiety alone or in conjunction with drugs—S-adenosylmethionine (SAMe) 100 mg PO q24h; alpha-casozepine 75 mg (15 mg/kg or greater) PO q24h; l-theanine 25 mg PO daily.
- Cat-appeasing pheromone (Feliway® Multicat or Friends); F3 cheek gland pheromone (Feliway).
- Calming and stress diets containing alpha-casozepine and l-tryptophan.

FOLLOW-UP

PATIENT MONITORING

Frequent follow-up either in person or by telephone is necessary, especially during first few months of treatment, to motivate client and monitor effectiveness of any adjunct drug treatment.

PREVENTION/AVOIDANCE

- Early socialization to people, places, and things up to 7 weeks of age, and ongoing positive exposure during first year, may help prevent some later problems with fearful behavior.
- Calm interactions and positive associations with fear-producing stimuli may help keep fear-based reactions to minimum.

POSSIBLE COMPLICATIONS

Secondary behavior problems may arise or persist after fearful or anxious behavior has diminished and will need specific treatment.

EXPECTED COURSE AND PROGNOSIS

- Realistic "end point" depends on animal's background (socialization history, genetic and individual differences in personality), home situation, and other confounding factors such as frequency of natural exposure to fear-producing stimuli.
- Medication may improve but not totally ameliorate signs.

MISCELLANEOUS

ASSOCIATED CONDITIONS

- Stereotypic or compulsive disorders.
- Urine marking, inappropriate elimination.
- Defensive aggression directed toward humans, other animals; may also make cat target for aggression from other cats.

ZOONOTIC POTENTIAL

N/A except for bite and scratch wounds.

PREGNANCY/FERTILITY/BREEDING

Drug use in pregnant animals should be avoided.

SEE ALSO

- Aggression, Overview—Cats.
- Compulsive Disorders—Cats.
- Fear and Aggression in Veterinary Visits—Cats.
- Housesoiling—Cats.
- Marking, Roaming, and Mounting Behavior—Cats.

ABBREVIATIONS

- GI = gastrointestinal.
- SAMe = S-adenosylmethionine.
- SSRI = selective serotonin reuptake inhibitor.
- TCA = tricyclic antidepressant.

INTERNET RESOURCES

- https://www.catvets.com
- https://fearfreehappyhomes.com/courses/cat-body-language-101

Suggested Reading

Herron, M. E., Horwitz, D., Siracusa, C., & Dale, S. (2020). Decoding your cat: The ultimate experts explain common cat behaviors and reveal how to prevent or change unwanted ones. Boston: Houghton Mifflin Harcourt.

Landsberg G, Hunthausen W, Ackerman L. Behavior Problems of the Dog and Cat, 3rd ed. Edinburgh: Saunders Elsevier, 2013.

Levine ED. Feline fear and anxiety. Vet Clin North Am Small Anim Pract 2008, 38(5):1065–1079.

Overall KL. Manual of Clinical Behavioral Medicine for Dogs and Cats. St. Louis, MO: Elsevier Mosby, 2013.

Author Leslie Larson Cooper
Consulting Editor Gary M. Landsberg

FEARS, PHOBIAS, AND ANXIETIES—DOGS

BASICS

DEFINITION

• *Fear*—an emotion consisting of a physiologic stress response (PSR) and a psychologic response to the presence of a stimulus perceived as dangerous (e.g., person, animal, situation, sound, object, scent) inducing an adaptive, avoidance reaction. • *Phobia*—marked, irrational, and excessive fear of a stimulus (e.g., animal, situation, person, sound, object, scent) consisting of a PSR and psychologic response resulting in a maladaptive reaction. • *Anxiety*—reaction consisting of a PSR and psychologic response triggered by anticipation of future or memory of past dangers.

PATHOPHYSIOLOGY

• Information about a fear-inducing stimulus is perceived by sensory organs and transmitted to the central nucleus of the amygdala; the central nucleus sends output to the central grey matter (musculoskeletal response), lateral hypothalamus (autonomic nervous system [ANS] response), and stria terminalis (hormonal response) causing a PSR. • The PSR is graded based on the animal's perceived level of control, coping strategy, and level of difficulty. • Any neutral stimulus in the environment can be paired with the PSR through classical conditioning triggering a PSR to the conditioned stimulus. • Hormones and neurotransmitters released during the PSR enhance learning, memory consolidation, and retrieval. • There is evidence that while frightening memories can be significantly reduced, they cannot be "erased."

SYSTEMS AFFECTED

• Psychologic—immobility, restlessness, pacing, circling, hyperattachment, escape, avoidance, approach/retreat, destructiveness, vocalization, aggression. • Cardiovascular—tachycardia, hypertension. • Endocrine/metabolic—alterations in hypothalamic pituitary–adrenal axis, increased blood glucose. • Gastrointestinal—inappetence, hypersalivation, vomiting, diarrhea, defecation. • Hemic/lymphatic/immune—stress leukogram. • Musculoskeletal—self-injury. • Neurologic—increased motor activity, trembling, decreased pain perception, catatonia, partial seizure. • Ophthalmic—episcleral injection, mydriasis. • Renal/urologic—urination. • Respiratory—tachypnea. • Skin/exocrine—traumatic injury, acral lick dermatitis (ALD).

GENETICS

Heredity influences development of fears and phobias, although unclear at this time to what extent specific fears (e.g., noise) are heritable.

INCIDENCE/PREVALENCE

• Separation anxiety—13–40%. • Sound aversion, fear, and phobia—up to 50%. • General fearfulness—26%. • Reactivity to people—7%. • Fear of veterinarian—up to 78.5%.

SIGNALMENT

No age, breed, or sex overrepresented.

SIGNS

General Comments

Hypervigilance, ANS arousal, catatonia, increased motor activity, elimination, destruction, vocalization, hypersalivation, panting, hiding, trembling, escape behaviors, fearful body language.

Historical Findings

Traumatic experience, inadequate socialization, fearful/anxious dam or sire, history of inability to escape stimulus (e.g., locked in crate).

Physical Examination Findings

May be unremarkable; self-induced injuries possible.

CAUSES

• Inadequate socialization, traumatic event, hereditary, cognitive dysfunction syndrome (CDS), previous learning. • Illness or pain may contribute to development of fears, phobias, and anxieties.

RISK FACTORS

General—existing fears, anxieties, and phobias; inadequate socialization, rehoming, anxious/fearful/physically ill dam, traumatic event.

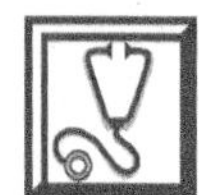

DIAGNOSIS

DIFFERENTIAL DIAGNOSIS

• Psychologic—CDS; incomplete housetraining; urine/fecal marking; territorial aggression; separation-related disorders; attention-seeking; storm, noise, or environmental phobias; generalized anxiety; neophobia; fear-induced aggression. • Medical—neoplasia (e.g., intracranial), endocrinopathy (e.g., Cushing's, hypothyroidism), cystitis, pyelonephritis, diabetes, gastrointestinal disease (e.g., inflammatory bowel disease), neurologic disease (e.g., seizures), dermatologic (e.g., ALD, atopy, food allergies), toxicity (e.g., lead, recreational drugs).

CBC/BIOCHEMISTRY/URINALYSIS

Perform before initiating drug treatment.

OTHER LABORATORY TESTS

• Thyroid status. • Adrenal tests if indicated by history, signalment, physical examination, and laboratory tests.

IMAGING

CT or MRI if indicated to rule out CNS disorder. Other imaging if indicated (e.g., pain).

DIAGNOSTIC PROCEDURES

• Thorough behavioral history and observation of patient (video of behavior is helpful). • Exposure to stimulus if safe.

TREATMENT

APPROPRIATE HEALTH CARE

• Typically outpatient. • Inpatient (dayboarding/daycare)—if fear-/anxiety-/phobia-inducing stimulus unavoidable, patient causing self-injury, medication not yet effective, hospitalization to stabilize patient on medication. • Treatment includes owner education, safety, behavior modification to change emotional state of patient, environmental modification to avoid triggers and distract patient during episodes, reduction of anxiety. • Diagnose and treat any conditions that may cause pain, discomfort, or changes in mood as well as any injuries.

Safety

• Owner—should not push, pull, grab, or reach for dog showing clinical signs, as this can result in owner-directed aggression; instead, use food or toy to move patient. • Patient—if intense escape attempts or self-injury are present, avoid crating and limit dog's access to windows, doors, electrical wiring, and water lines; consider dayboarding. • Public—avoid situations where stimulus is present until treatment is complete.

Behavior Modification

• Avoid stimulus for 2–8 weeks depending on severity of reaction while teaching coping skills to patient (e.g., sit, watch, look at that, leave it, relaxation) and setting up safe spot. • Structured interactions with owner (e.g., sit for all interactions). • Independence exercises—down/stay with food toy. • Punishment (e.g., shock/choke collar correction, yelling, hitting) contraindicated. • Client should distract dog and redirect to play or food toy when frightened or anxious. • Desensitization and counter-conditioning (DS/CC)—can begin after coping tools have been taught; can be attempted with supervision of highly qualified positive reinforcement trainer or veterinary behavior technician; DS/CC can sensitize animal to stimulus, causing behavior disorder to worsen.

Environmental Modification

• Create safe spot/safe haven where exposure to fear-producing stimulus can be limited. • Consider dayboarding/daycare. • Limit use of crate until dog uses readily and does not panic when confined. • Environmental enrichment (e.g., rotate toys, food toys, exercise).

NURSING CARE

Behavior treatment appointments can be scheduled with veterinary technicians. Consider short-term or day boarding for regulation of medications or avoidance of stimulus.

ACTIVITY

• Increased exercise will act as environmental enrichment for patient but will not significantly lower anxiety/fear disorders. • Exercise should avoid any exposure to fear-inducing stimulus.

CLIENT EDUCATION

• Advise owners that patient is not spiteful or guilty; may be long course of treatment; will most likely be managed, not cured. • Help client understand subtlety of signs involved and learn to recognize signs associated with fear, anxiety, and stress.

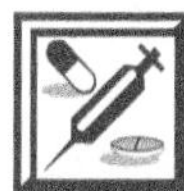

MEDICATIONS

DRUG(S) OF CHOICE

• Should always be prescribed with complete treatment plan in order to be compliant with standard of care. • Most treatment will be long term, possibly years; minimum treatment generally 6 months with concurrent behavior modification; if dog has significantly improved in 6 months, try slow weaning by reducing dose by 25–50% every 14 days. • Situational, mild PRN drug indicated, e.g., benzodiazepine, serotonin reuptake inhibitor/antagonist (SARI) either alone if stimulus is occasional and predictable, or more commonly concurrent with selective serotonin reuptake inhibitor (SSRI) or tricyclic antidepressant (TCA) prior to event.
○ Best administered before any signs of anxiety, fear, or panic; minimally 60–90 min before anticipated provocative stimulus.
○ Benzodiazepines—diazepam 0.50–2 mg/kg PO up to q8h; clorazepate 0.50–2 mg/kg PO up to q6h; alprazolam 0.01–0.1 mg/kg PO up to q4h. ○ SARI: trazodone 3.0–10 mg/kg PO up to q8h (up to 15 mg/kg). ○ Alpha-2 agonist—clonidine 0.01–0.05 mg/kg PO up to q8h.
• Dexmedetomidine oromucosal gel—125 μg/m^2 onto oral mucosa 30–60 min prior to fear-evoking event. • Generalized, stimulus unavoidable or severe—daily administered drug indicated. ○ Both TCAs and SSRIs can take up to 6 weeks to take effect; start at low end of dosing range and then slowly increase in 2–4-week increments based on response to avoid side effects. ○ TCA—clomipramine 1.0–3.0 mg/kg PO q12h. ○ SSRI—sertraline 1.0–3.0 mg/kg PO q24h; fluoxetine or paroxetine 0.5–2.0 mg/kg PO q24h.

PRECAUTIONS

• All listed medications are extra-label except clomipramine and fluoxetine for treatment of separation anxiety and dexmedetomidine oro-mucosal gel for noise aversion in dogs in the United States—follow Health and Human Services recommendations. • Cardiac conduction anomalies—use caution and monitoring when giving TCAs. • Use caution when prescribing drugs to geriatric patients or patients with hepatic or renal compromise—review metabolism and elimination of medication before prescribing.
• Clients should receive drug information handouts with potential side effects listed.
• Mood-altering medications have potential to increase agitation, fear, and aggression.

POSSIBLE INTERACTIONS

• Use caution when prescribing multiple medications concurrently that have same mode of action; review drug monographs for each drug before prescribing. • Do not use SARIs, SSRIs, or TCAs with monoamine oxidase inhibitor (MAOIs), including but not limited to selegiline and amitraz.
• Do not use SSRIs and TCAs together—possible risk of serotonin syndrome, which can be fatal.

ALTERNATIVE DRUG(S)

Buspirone (daily)—0.5–1.0 mg/kg BID–TID.

Supplements

Natural products that may aid in reducing anxiety—dog-appeasing pheromone (Adaptil®); alpha-casosopene (Zykene®) alone or in diet together with l-tryptophan (Royal Canin Calm® diet); l-theanine alone (Anxitane®) or in combination product containing whey protein, *Phellodendron amurense*, and *Magnolia officinalis* (Solliquin®); melatonin; S-adenosylmethionine (SAMe); Souroubea and Plantanus (Zentrol®), or a probiotic supplement (Calming Care®).

FOLLOW-UP

PATIENT MONITORING

• Clients should contact veterinary healthcare team with updates at 2-week intervals for first 6–8 weeks of treatment; typically, treatment plan will have to be altered. • CBC, biochemistry, urinalysis, T_4, fT_4, q12 months for animals <8 years on daily administered medications; senior dogs may require more frequent reassessment based on age and health.

PREVENTION/AVOIDANCE

• Proper socialization—8–12 weeks, including puppy classes starting at 8 weeks.
• Structured relationship with owner (e.g., sit for all interactions). • Basic obedience.
• Treat traumatic experiences immediately.

POSSIBLE COMPLICATIONS

If left untreated or treated with medication only, worsening clinical signs likely.

EXPECTED COURSE AND PROGNOSIS

• Depends on response to medication, suitability of environment, and client's ability to perform behavior modification.
• Treatment duration varies from 2 to 12 months depending on severity and number of problems; only dogs who respond well to behavior modification and environmental management can be expected to be weaned off medication.
• Typically, treatment will continue to some extent throughout dog's life.

F

MISCELLANEOUS

AGE-RELATED FACTORS

CDS can present as nonspecific fear.

PREGNANCY/FERTILITY/BREEDING

Most listed medications are not evaluated in or contraindicated in pregnant animals.

SYNONYMS

• Generalized anxiety. • Neophobia.

SEE ALSO

• Aggression – Overview Dogs.
• Fear and Aggression – Veterinary Visits Dogs.
• Separation Anxiety Syndrome.
• Thunderstorm and Noise Phobias – Dogs.

ABBREVIATIONS

• ALD = acral lick dermatitis.
• ANS = autonomic nervous system.
• CDS = cognitive dysfunction syndrome.
• DS/CC = desensitization and counter-conditioning.
• MAOI = monoamine oxidase inhibitor.
• PSR = physiologic stress response.
• SAMe = S-adenosylmethionine.
• SARI = serotonin reuptake inhibitor/antagonist.
• SSRI = selective serotonin reuptake inhibitor.
• TCA = tricyclic antidepressant.

INTERNET RESOURCES

• https://www.dacvb.org • https://avsab.org
• https://fearfreehappyhomes.com/courses/dog-body-language-101

Suggested Reading

Becker M, Radosta L, Sung W, et al. From Fearful to Fear Free. Irvine, CA: Lumina Media, 2017.

Horwitz D, ed. Blackwell's 5 Minute Consult Clinical Companion: Canine and Feline Behavior, 2nd ed. Chichester: Wiley, 2018, pp. 253–388.

Horwitz D, Mills D, eds. BSAVA Manual of Canine and Feline Behavioural Medicine, 2nd ed. Gloucester: BSAVA, 2009.

Landsberg G, Hunthausen W, Ackerman L. Behavior Problems of the Dog and Cat, 3rd ed. Philadelphia, PA: Elsevier Saunders, 2013.

Author Lisa Radosta
Consulting Editor Gary M. Landsberg

Client Education Handout available online

FELINE ALVEOLAR OSTEITIS

OVERVIEW

Thickening of bone over the jugum of tooth roots due to inflammation. Alveolar osteitis most commonly occurs over the maxillary canine tooth roots of middle-aged and older cats (sometimes also called buttressing). This process appears to be secondary to periodontal inflammation. Tooth resorption and extrusion (supereruption) may also be seen in affected teeth. Feline alveolar osteitis should be distinguished from benign alveolar bone expansion (also called buccal bone expansion), which is devoid of inflammation.

SIGNALMENT

Although alveolar osteitis can occur in dogs, it is far more common in cats. There are no established breed or sex predilections, and no established genetic basis. Middle-aged and older cats are most commonly affected.

SIGNS

History

- Owner may report thickening or bulging over the maxillary canine teeth roots, usually bilateral, but can be unilateral.
- Evidence of oral pain is not often noted by pet owners.
  - Discomfort may occur with mobile teeth.
  - Discomfort may occur when extruded maxillary canine teeth contact the lower lip or the opposing canine, resulting in an acquired malocclusion.

Clinical Findings

- Bulging of alveolar bone on the buccal surface of the root; variable degree of gingival inflammation.
- Patient may have abnormal periodontal pocket depths on probing (normal sulcus depth for cats is 0–1 mm); patients often exhibit vertical bone loss with infrabony pockets.
- Patients may exhibit extrusion (supereruption) of one or more teeth; extended tooth length may cause trauma to lower lip or malocclusion with opposing mandibular canine tooth.
- May progress to tooth mobility and acquired dental malocclusion due to contact between maxillary and mandibular canine teeth.

CAUSES & RISK FACTORS

Cause is unknown, but buttressing in humans is considered to be an attempt by the body to stabilize a diseased tooth. Cats that are prone to periodontal disease may be at a higher risk for developing alveolar osteitis.

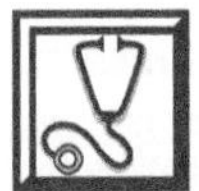

DIAGNOSIS

DIFFERENTIAL DIAGNOSIS

Alveolar bone expansion, also known as buccal bone expansion, is an enlargement of alveolar bone that looks similar to alveolar osteitis. However, when biopsied, alveolar bone expansion may show no signs of inflammation.

CBC/BIOCHEMISTRY/URINALYSIS

No specific abnormalities seen related to alveolar osteitis.

IMAGING

Intraoral dental radiographs typically show evidence of vertical periodontal bone loss along the long axis of the root on the palatal and buccal surface of the root. The expanded bone may be less dense than normal adjacent alveolar bone.

DIAGNOSTIC PROCEDURES

- Appropriate preanesthetic diagnostics when indicated prior to procedure.
- Complete oral examination with periodontal probing—assess for periodontal pockets, gingival bleeding or tooth mobility; pay particular attention to probing depth of palatal surface of maxillary canine teeth.
- Intraoral radiographs under anesthesia—assess extent of osseous changes; assess root stability, attachment loss, and evidence of tooth resorption.
- Consider biopsy if bone changes are unilateral or if aggressive osseous changes are seen on dental radiographs.

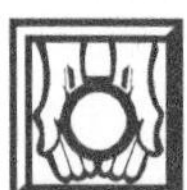

TREATMENT

- If mild periodontal changes are present (moderate pocket depth, no tooth mobility, minimal extrusion, no oronasal fistulation), a professional ultrasonic dental cleaning with root planing and subgingival curettage ± placement of periodontal pocket antimicrobial treatment ± osseous surgery.
- If extensive periodontal disease is present (deep periodontal pocket, tooth mobility, extensive extrusion, patient discomfort, oronasal fistula), consider extraction. Buccal attached gingiva may be very thin, making it difficult to elevate a gingival flap. Ostectomy/osteoplasty of buccal alveolar bulge is necessary after raising the gingival flap and prior to closure. Biopsy of buccal alveolar bone can be accomplished with rongeurs once a mucogingival flap has been elevated. Gently elevate palatal mucosal edge to facilitate closure.

MEDICATIONS

DRUG(S) OF CHOICE

Appropriate antimicrobials and pain medications when indicated.

CONTRAINDICATIONS/POSSIBLE INTERACTIONS

N/A

FOLLOW-UP

PATIENT MONITORING

Recheck patient at 2 weeks postoperatively, with regular reevaluations depending on what treatment was chosen.

PREVENTION/AVOIDANCE

No known methods of prevention.

POSSIBLE COMPLICATIONS

Complications include those that may occur when extracting teeth (perforation of mucogingival flap, dehiscence, iatrogenic oronasal fistula, etc.).

EXPECTED COURSE AND PROGNOSIS

Good with appropriate treatment, unless neoplasia is diagnosed with biopsy.

Suggested Reading

Beebe DE, Gengler WR. Osseous surgery to augment treatment of chronic periodontitis of canine teeth in a cat. J Vet Dent 2007, 24(1):30–38.

Author John R. Lewis

Consulting Editor Heidi B. Lobprise

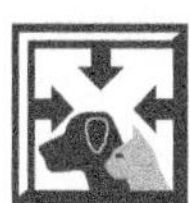

BASICS

DEFINITION

A common viral respiratory disease of domestic and exotic cats characterized by upper respiratory disease and oral ulceration, occasionally pneumonia or arthritis, and rarely a highly fatal systemic hemorrhagic disease (FCV–VSD).

PATHOPHYSIOLOGY

- Spread through ocular, nasal, and oral secretions.
- Transmission typically occurs through direct contact or fomite exposure; droplet transmission possible within 4–5 feet; replication takes place primarily in respiratory and oral tissues.
- Rapid cytolysis of infected cells results in tissue pathology and clinical disease.

SYSTEMS AFFECTED

- Gastrointestinal—ulceration of the tongue common; occasional ulceration of the hard palate and lips.
- Hemic/lymphatic/immune—hemorrhage; splenic necrosis (FCV–VSD).
- Hepatobiliary—hepatic necrosis (FCV–VSD).
- Musculoskeletal—acute arthritis.
- Ophthalmic—acute serous conjunctivitis without keratitis or corneal ulcers.
- Respiratory—rhinitis; interstitial pneumonia; ulceration of nose tip.
- Skin/exocrine—subcutaneous edema; ulcerations of pinnae or pawpads; pancreatic necrosis (FCV–VSD).

GENETICS

None

INCIDENCE/PREVALENCE

- Persistent infection common, resulting in virus-shedding carriers.
- Clinical disease—common in multicat facilities, shelters, breeding catteries.
- Routine vaccination—reduces incidence and severity of clinical disease; has not decreased prevalence of the virus.

GEOGRAPHIC DISTRIBUTION

Worldwide

SIGNALMENT

Species

Cat

Breed Predilections

None

Mean Age and Range

- Young kittens >6 weeks old—most common.
- Cats of any age may show clinical disease.

Predominant Sex

None

SIGNS

General Comments

Severity of disease is dependent on host immune status, virulence of infecting strain, and presence of co-infections. Most common manifestation involves self-limiting upper respiratory tract disease and oral ulceration.

Historical Findings

- Sudden onset.
- Anorexia.
- Serous ocular or nasal discharge, usually with little or no sneezing.
- Ulcers on tongue, hard palate, lips, tip of nose, or around claws.
- Dyspnea from pneumonia.
- Acute, painful lameness.

Physical Examination Findings

- Ranging from generally alert and in good condition to lethargy and decreased mentation.
- Fever.
- Ulcers of tongue/mouth may occur without other signs.
- Hypersalivation.
- Upper to lower respiratory tract disease—nasal discharge, or stertor; wheezes, crackles, or increased bronchovesicular sounds on pulmonary auscultation,
- Epistaxis or hematochezia with systemic hemorrhage (FCV–VSD).
- Facial and limb edema with crusting/ ulcerations of face, pinnae, and feet due to vasculitis (FCV–VSD).
- Icterus (FCV–VSD).

CAUSES

- A small, nonenveloped single-stranded RNA virus, feline calicivirus (FCV).
- Numerous strains exist in nature, with varying degrees of antigenic cross-reactivity.
- More than one serotype.
- Relatively stable and resistant to many disinfectants.

RISK FACTORS

- Lack of vaccination or improper vaccination.
- Multicat facilities.
- Concurrent infections with other pathogens, e.g., feline herpesvirus (FHV), feline panleukopenia virus (FPV), feline immunodeficiency virus (FIV), feline leukemia virus (FeLV).
- Poor ventilation.
- Stress.

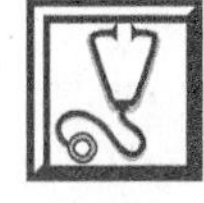

DIAGNOSIS

DIFFERENTIAL DIAGNOSIS

- FHV.
- Chlamydiosis.
- *Bordetella bronchiseptica*.

CBC/BIOCHEMISTRY/URINALYSIS

No characteristic or consistent findings.

OTHER LABORATORY TESTS

Often diagnosed on clinical signs.

IMAGING

Radiographs of lungs—consolidated lung tissue in cats with pneumonia.

DIAGNOSTIC PROCEDURES

- PCR—oropharyngeal swabs most likely to detect virus; positive result does not prove that FCV is causative agent for disease due to persistently shedding cats.
- Cell cultures to isolate virus—oral pharynx; lung tissue; feces; blood; secretions from nose and conjunctiva.
- Immunofluorescent assays of lung tissue—viral antigen.
- Serologic testing on paired serum samples—detect rise in neutralizing antibody titers against virus; vaccination interferes with results from serum neutralization testing.

PATHOLOGIC FINDINGS

- Gross—upper respiratory infection; ocular and nasal discharge; pneumonia with consolidation of large portions of individual lung lobes; possible ulcerations on tongue, lips, and hard palate; systemic hemorrhages.
- Histopathologic—interstitial pneumonia of large portions of individual lung lobes; ulcerations on epithelium of tongue, lips, and hard palate; mild inflammatory reactions in nose and conjunctiva; systemic hemorrhages, vasculitis, or necrosis.

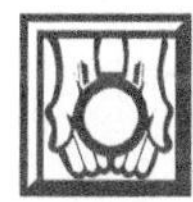

TREATMENT

APPROPRIATE HEALTH CARE

Outpatient, unless severe pneumonia, hemorrhage, or severe systemic disease.

NURSING CARE

- Clean eyes and nose as indicated with warm water or saline.
- Provide access to steam, such as in a bathroom, to clear secretions.
- Provide palatable, soft foods.
- Oxygen—with severe pneumonia.

ACTIVITY

Patients should be restricted from contact with other cats to prevent transmission of causative virus.

DIET

- No restrictions.
- Special diets—to entice anorectic cats to resume eating.
- Soft foods—if ulcerations restrict eating.

CLIENT EDUCATION

Discuss need for proper vaccination and to modify vaccination protocol in breeding catteries to include kittens before they

FELINE CALICIVIRUS INFECTION (CONTINUED)

become infected (often at 6–8 weeks of age) from a carrier queen.

SURGICAL CONSIDERATIONS

None

MEDICATIONS

DRUG(S) OF CHOICE

- No specific antiviral drugs are clearly indicated.
- Broad-spectrum antibiotics—indicated for treatment of secondary bacterial infections (e.g., amoxicillin or amoxicillin–clavulanate at 22 mg/kg PO q12h; doxycycline at 5 mg/kg PO q12h).
- Secondary bacterial infections of affected cats not nearly as important as with FHV-1 infections.
- Antibiotic eye ointments—to reduce secondary bacterial infections of conjunctiva.
- Pain medication—as indicated for arthritis pain or significant ulceration.

CONTRAINDICATIONS

None

PRECAUTIONS

None

POSSIBLE INTERACTIONS

None

ALTERNATIVE DRUG(S)

None

FOLLOW-UP

PATIENT MONITORING

- Monitor for sudden development of dyspnea associated with pneumonia.
- No specific laboratory tests.

PREVENTION/AVOIDANCE

- American Association of Feline Practitioners—classifies FHV, FPV, and FCV as core vaccines; vaccinate all cats with either a modified live virus (MLV) or inactivated core vaccine on initial visit (as early as 6 weeks of age), repeat every 3–4 weeks until 16 weeks of age, and booster 1 year after last kitten vaccine; revaccinate every 3 years.
- Breeding catteries—respiratory disease is a problem; vaccinate kittens at earlier age, either with additional vaccination at 4–5 weeks or with intranasal vaccine at 10–14 days; follow-up vaccinations every 3–4 weeks until 16 weeks of age.
- Vaccination will not prevent virus infection in subsequent exposure, but can prevent serious clinical disease caused by most strains; FCV–VSD can occur in vaccinated cats.
- Environmental management—decrease housing density; isolate affected cats by >4 ft; beware of hygiene and fomites; disinfect with dilute (1 : 30) bleach.

POSSIBLE COMPLICATIONS

- Interstitial pneumonia—most serious complication; can be life-threatening.
- Secondary bacterial infections of lungs or upper airways.

EXPECTED COURSE AND PROGNOSIS

- Clinical disease—usually appears 3–4 days after exposure.
- With supportive care, infection usually self-limiting and cats with upper respiratory signs respond favorably within 7–10 days.
- Oral ulcerations typically improve in 2–3 weeks.
- Lameness usually resolves in 1–2 days.
- Prognosis excellent, unless severe pneumonia or systemic hemorrhagic disease develops.
- FCV–VSD may be severe and fatal.
- Recovered cats—persistently infected for long periods; will shed small quantities of virus in oral secretions continuously.

MISCELLANEOUS

ASSOCIATED CONDITIONS

Affected cats may also be concurrently infected with FHV-1, especially in multicat and breeding facilities. FCV has been implicated in development of feline chronic gingivostomatitis.

AGE-RELATED FACTORS

Usually occurs in young kittens whose maternally derived immunity has waned.

ZOONOTIC POTENTIAL

None

PREGNANCY/FERTILITY/BREEDING

Generally no problem, because most cats have been exposed or vaccinated before becoming pregnant.

SYNONYMS

- Feline picornavirus infection—FCV originally classified as a picornavirus; older literature refers to the infection by this name; no known picornavirus infects cats.
- Limping kitten syndrome.
- Hemorrhagic calicivirus.

SEE ALSO

- Chlamydiosis—Cats.
- Feline Herpesvirus Infection.
- Feline (Upper) Respiratory Infections.
- Rhinitis and Sinusitis.
- Stomatitis and Oral Ulceration.

ABBREVIATIONS

- FCV = feline calicivirus.
- FCV–VSD = feline calicivirus–virulent systemic disease.
- FeLV = feline leukemia virus.
- FHV = feline herpesvirus.
- FIV = feline immunodeficiency virus.
- FPV = feline panleukopenia virus.
- MLV = modified live virus.

INTERNET RESOURCES

http://www.abcdcatsvets.org/feline-calicivirus-infection-2012-edition

Suggested Reading

Afonso MM, Gaskell RM, Radford A. Feline upper respiratory infections. In: Ettinger SJ, Feldman EC, Côté, E, eds. Textbook of Veterinary Internal Medicine: Diseases of the Dog and Cat, 8th ed. St. Louis, MO: Elsevier, 2017, pp. 1013–1016.

Gaskell RM, Dawson S, Radford AD. Feline respiratory disease. In: Greene CE, ed., Infectious Diseases of the Dog and Cat, 4th ed. St. Louis, MO: Saunders Elsevier, 2012, pp. 151–162.

Pedersen NC, Elliot JB, Glasgow A, et al. An isolated epizootic of hemorrhagic-like fever in cats caused by a novel and highly virulent strain of feline calicivirus. Vet Microbiol 2000, 73:281–300.

Scherk MA, Ford RB, Gaskell RM, et al. 2013 AAFP Feline Vaccination Advisory Panel Report. J Feline Med Surg 2013; 15:785–808.

Author Sara E. Gonzalez

Consulting Editor Amie Koenig

Acknowledgment The author and book editors acknowledge the prior contribution of Fred W. Scott.

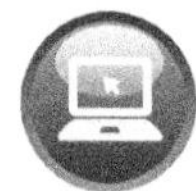

Client Education Handout available online

FELINE HERPESVIRUS INFECTION

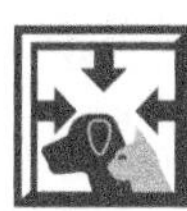

BASICS

DEFINITION

An acute disease in cats characterized by sneezing, fever, rhinitis, conjunctivitis, and ulcerative keratitis.

PATHOPHYSIOLOGY

Feline herpesvirus-1 (FHV-1) causes acute cytolytic infection of respiratory or ocular epithelium after oral, intranasal, or conjunctival exposure. The intracellular virus travels from cell to cell and does not stimulate a strong immune response from the host.

SYSTEMS AFFECTED

- Integumentary—herpes dermatitis near the nares.
- Ophthalmic—conjunctivitis with serous or purulent ocular discharge; ulcerative keratitis or panophthalmitis.
- Reproductive—in utero infection (infected pregnant queen) may result in severe neonatal herpetic infection.
- Respiratory—rhinitis with sneezing and serous to purulent nasal discharge; chronic sinusitis may result; tracheitis possible.
- Neurologic—latent virus found in optic nerve, ciliary ganglion, brainstem, cerebellum, and olfactory bulb.

GENETICS

N/A

INCIDENCE/PREVALENCE

- Common, especially in multicat households or facilities housing large numbers of cats; catteries and shelters are source of most infections.
- Perpetuated by latent carriers that harbor virus in nerve (especially trigeminal) ganglia.

GEOGRAPHIC DISTRIBUTION

Worldwide

SIGNALMENT

Species

All domestic and many exotic cats.

Breed Predilections

- None.
- Brachycephalic breeds have more severe corneal disease and are more likely to have corneal sequestra.

Mean Age and Range

- All ages.
- Kittens most susceptible.

Predominant Sex

N/A

SIGNS

Historical Findings

- Acute onset of paroxysmal sneezing.
- Blepharospasm and ocular discharge.
- Anorexia (from high fever, general malaise, or inability to smell).
- Recurrent signs—carriers.
- Abortion.

Physical Examination Findings

- Fever—up to 106 °F (41 °C).
- Rhinitis—serous, mucopurulent, or purulent discharge.
- Conjunctivitis—serous, mucopurulent, or purulent discharge.
- Chronic rhinitis/sinusitis—chronic purulent nasal discharge.
- Keratitis—ulceration, descemetocele, panophthalmitis.

CAUSES

FHV-1

RISK FACTORS

- Lack of vaccination for FHV-1, although vaccines do not bestow sterilizing immunity.
- Multicat facilities with overcrowding, poor ventilation, poor sanitation, poor nutrition, or physical or psychologic stress.
- Pregnancy and lactation.
- Concomitant disease, especially owing to immunosuppressive organisms or other respiratory organisms.
- Kittens born to carrier queens—infected ~5 weeks of age.

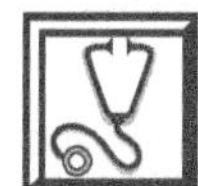

DIAGNOSIS

DIFFERENTIAL DIAGNOSIS

- Feline calicivirus infection—less sneezing than FHV-1, conjunctivitis, ulcerative keratitis; may cause ulcerative stomatitis, pneumonia.
- Feline *Chlamydophila* infection—more chronic conjunctivitis, which may be unilateral; pneumonitis; intracytoplasmic inclusions in conjunctival scrapings; responds to tetracyclines or chloramphenicol.
- Bacterial infection (*Bordetella*, *Haemophilus*, or *Pasteurella*)—less nasal and ocular involvement; often respond to antibiotics.

CBC/BIOCHEMISTRY/URINALYSIS

- Nonspecific.
- Transient leukopenia followed by leukocytosis may occur.

OTHER LABORATORY TESTS

- PCR testing from pharyngeal and conjunctival swabs will identify presence of virus; more sensitive than other diagnostic modalities; may be transiently positive following vaccination with modified live virus (MLV) vaccine for FHV-1.
- Immunofluorescent assay—nasal or conjunctival scrapings; viral detection.
- Viral isolation—pharyngeal swab sample.
- Stained conjunctival smears—detect intranuclear inclusion bodies.

IMAGING

- Radiography—open-mouth ventrodorsal and rostrocaudal (skyline) views of skull reveal presence of chronic disease in nasal cavity and frontal sinuses; infection cannot be reliably distinguished from neoplasia and inflammatory polyps; no abnormal radiographic findings with acute disease.
- CT provides more accurate assessment of disease in nasal cavity and frontal sinus compared to radiographs; CT may differentiate neoplasia from inflammation based on amount of bony destruction.

DIAGNOSTIC PROCEDURES

N/A

PATHOLOGIC FINDINGS

- Gross—ocular and nasal discharge, mucosal edema of upper airway epithelium, tracheitis, sinusitis, ulcerative keratitis, panophthalmitis.
- Microscopic—submucosal edema, inflammatory cell infiltrates of upper respiratory and conjunctival tissues, chronic sinusitis, intranuclear inclusion bodies in epithelial cells.

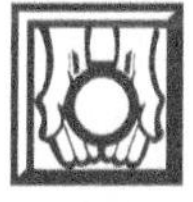

TREATMENT

APPROPRIATE HEALTH CARE

- Inpatient—nutritional and fluid support to anorectic cats.
- Outpatient—if eating and afebrile.

NURSING CARE

- Outpatient—keep patient indoors to prevent environmentally induced stress, which may lengthen disease course.
- Fluids—IV or SC; to correct and prevent dehydration; to keep nasal secretions thin.
- Appetite stimulant as needed (mirtazapine—1.8 mg/cat PO q24–48h).

ACTIVITY

Isolate affected cats during acute phase because they are contagious.

DIET

- Outpatient—encourage food consumption to avoid anorexia; offer foods with appealing tastes and smells; warming food may enhance smell.
- Inpatient—forced enteral feeding for anorectic cats; remove nasal secretions (so nasal breathing can occur) before starting orogastric or esophagostomy tube feeding; avoid nasoesophageal tubes because of rhinitis.

CLIENT EDUCATION

- Inform client of contagious nature of disease.
- Discuss proper vaccination protocols and early vaccination of cats in multicat facilities and households.

FELINE HERPESVIRUS INFECTION (CONTINUED)

• Inform client that early weaning and isolation from all other cats except littermates may prevent infections.

SURGICAL CONSIDERATIONS

Surgically implanted feeding tubes (esophagostomy tube, gastrostomy tube) may be needed to manage prolonged anorexia.

MEDICATIONS

DRUG(S) OF CHOICE

• Antibiotics not recommended if nasal discharge is serous and lacks purulent or mucopurulent component; antibiotics recommended only if fever, lethargy, or anorexia present concurrently with mucopurulent nasal discharge.
• Doxycycline (10 mg/kg PO q24h) recommended; amoxicillin (22 mg/kg PO/IM/SC q8–12h) or ampicillin (10–20 mg/kg IV/IM/SC q6–8h) for secondary bacterial infections.
• Famciclovir (40–90 mg/kg PO 12h) may shorten course and severity of disease.
• Ophthalmic antibiotics—for keratitis.
• Ophthalmic antivirals for herpetic ulcers in order of efficacy—trifluridine, cidofovir, idoxuridine, ganciclovir, aciclovir; must be instilled q2h for significant effect, except for cidofovir which can be given q12h, making it ophthalmic drug of choice, although it must be compounded.
• Some evidence that administration of intranasal vaccine 2–6 days prior to exposure will result in lessening of clinical signs; may be helpful in outbreak in multicat setting.

CONTRAINDICATIONS

• Idoxuridine ophthalmic—may be painful; discontinue medication.
• Cidofovir ophthalmic—scarring of nasolacrimal duct reported in humans, rabbits.
• Trifluridine, idoxuridine, acyclovir—toxic if given systemically.
• Systemic corticosteroids—may induce relapse in chronically infected cats.
• Ophthalmic corticosteroids—may predispose to ulcerative keratitis
• Nasal decongestant drops—0.25% oxymetazoline HCl; decrease nasal discharge; contraindicated because some cats object and some experience rebound rhinorrhea.

PRECAUTIONS

• Oral doxycycline tablets can cause esophageal ulceration.
• Death usually result of inadequate nutritional and fluid support or immunosuppression due to feline leukemia virus (FeLV) or feline immunodeficiency virus (FIV).

ALTERNATIVE DRUG(S)

• Lysine (500 mg PO q12h) might reduce viral shedding, clinical signs.
• Lysine-lactoferrin (500 mg PO q12h) more effective than lysine alone for treatment.
• Penciclovir—effectively inhibits FHV-1, doses unknown at this time.

FOLLOW-UP

PATIENT MONITORING

Monitor appetite closely; hospitalize for fluids and tube feeding if anorexia develops.

PREVENTION/AVOIDANCE

Can survive in environment for several hours; drying and most disinfectants effectively kill the virus.

Vaccines

• Routine vaccination with MLV or inactivated virus vaccine—prevents development of severe disease; does not prevent infection and local viral replication with mild clinical disease and virus shedding.
• Vaccinate at 8–10 weeks, 12–14 weeks, and 16–18 weeks of age and with annual boosters for reasonable protection, especially in high-risk populations.
• Endemic multicat facilities or households—vaccinate kittens with dose of intranasal vaccine at 10–14 days of age, then parenterally at 6, 10, and 14 weeks of age; isolate litter from *all* other cats at 3–5 weeks of age; then use kitten vaccination protocol to prevent early infections.

POSSIBLE COMPLICATIONS

• Chronic rhinitis or rhinosinusitis with long-term sneezing and nasal discharge.
• Herpetic ulcerative keratitis.
• Corneal sequestrum that must be removed surgically.
• Permanent closure of nasolacrimal duct with chronic ocular discharge.

EXPECTED COURSE AND PROGNOSIS

• 7–10 days followed by spontaneous remission, if secondary bacterial infections do not occur.
• Prognosis generally good, if fluid and nutritional therapy are adequate.
• Correlation between severity of acute signs and degree of latent infection.
• May become chronically affected and exhibit respiratory signs long term.

MISCELLANEOUS

ASSOCIATED CONDITIONS

Simultaneous viral or bacterial respiratory diseases.

AGE-RELATED FACTORS

More severe in young kittens.

ZOONOTIC POTENTIAL

None

PREGNANCY/FERTILITY/BREEDING

Pregnant cats with FHV infection may transmit FHV-1 to kittens in utero, resulting in abortion or neonatal disease.

SYNONYMS

• Coryza.
• Feline rhinotracheitis.
• Rhino.

SEE ALSO

Feline Calicivirus Infection.

ABBREVIATIONS

• FeLV = feline leukemia virus.
• FHV-1 = feline herpesvirus type 1.
• FIV = feline immunodeficiency virus.
• MLV = modified live virus.

Suggested Reading

Bol S, Bunnik EM. Lysine supplementation is not effective for the prevention or treatment of feline herpesvirus 1 infection in cats: a systematic review. BMC Vet Res 2015, 11:284.

Horzinek MC, Addie D, Sándor B, et al. ABCD: update of the 2009 guidelines on prevention and management of feline infectious diseases. J Feline Med Surg 2013, 15:530–539.

Lappin MR, Blondeau J, Boothe D, et al. Antimicrobial use guidelines for treatment of respiratory tract disease in dogs and cats. J Vet Intern Med 2017, 31:279–294.

Malik R, Lessels NS, Webb S, et al. Treatment of feline herpesvirus-1 associated disease. J Feline Med Surg 2009, 11(1):40–48.

Thiry E, Addie D, Belak S, et al. Feline herpesvirus infection: ABCD guidelines on prevention and management. J Feline Med Surg 2009, 11(7):547–555.

Thomasy SM, Maggs DJ. A review of antiviral drugs and other compounds with activity against feline herpesvirus-1. Vet Ophthalmol 2016, 19(Suppl 1):119–130.

Author Lisa Restine

Consulting Editor Amie Koenig

Acknowledgment The author and book editors acknowledge the prior contribution of Gary D. Norsworthy.

Client Education Handout available online

FELINE HYPERESTHESIA SYNDROME

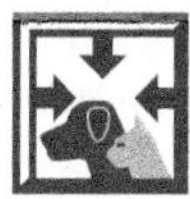

BASICS

OVERVIEW

• Idiopathic disorder of cats characterized by paroxysmal agitation, focal epaxial muscle spasms, vocalization, and intense biting or licking of the back, tail, and pelvic limbs. • Also known as atypical neurodermatitis, rolling skin disease, apparent neuritis, and twitchy cat disease. • Pathophysiology unknown. • Organ systems affected—behavioral, nervous, neuromuscular, skin/exocrine.

SIGNALMENT

Species

Cat

Breed Predilections

Can be seen in any breed; Siamese, Abyssinian, Burmese, and Himalayan may be predisposed.

Mean Age and Range

Most common at 1–7 years of age.

SIGNS

• Episodes of twitching of skin over lumbar area, violent swishing of tail, vocalizing, and biting or licking of flank, pelvic region, or tail. • Pupils often dilate, and cats can become aggressive or appear agitated and run wildly about the environment. • Episodes are several seconds to several minutes in length; cats are typically normal between episodes, but may be intolerant of being stroked along the back. • General physical examination often reveals no abnormalities aside from possible alopecia and broken hair over lumbar area from self-mutilation; many cats resent palpation of thoracolumbar musculature, and manipulation of area may elicit an episode; no neurologic deficits present.

CAUSES & RISK FACTORS

• Not known whether this syndrome is manifestation of underlying behavioral problem, dermatopathy, focal seizure disorder, or abnormal sensory state causing neuropathic pain or itch; speculated that cause is multifactorial, or that syndrome is not distinct entity with single cause, but rather can develop from variety of different factors. • Cats that tend to be nervous or hyperexcitable may be at increased risk; environmental stressors can serve as trigger.

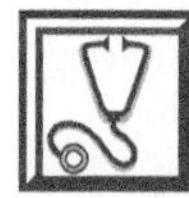

DIAGNOSIS

DIFFERENTIAL DIAGNOSIS

• Dermatologic conditions causing pruritus—parasitic (e.g., flea, *Notoedres*, *Cheyletiella*), fungal (e.g., dermatophytosis), or allergic (e.g., parasitic, inhalant, dietary); evaluate for underlying dermatitis; skin scrapings and fungal cultures can help confirm diagnosis. • Diseases of spinal cord, nerve roots, epaxial muscles, or vertebral column causing pain—degenerative (intervertebral disc disease), inflammatory (discospondylitis, meningitis, myositis), neoplastic, or traumatic; spinal radiographs helpful in evaluating for abnormalities; further diagnostics (e.g., advanced imaging, serology for infectious agents, cerebrospinal fluid [CSF] analysis) may be necessary. • Forebrain disease causing behavioral changes and/or seizures—metabolic (hepatic encephalopathy), infectious/inflammatory (feline leukemia virus, feline immunodeficiency virus, feline infectious peritonitis, cryptococcosis, toxoplasmosis), neoplastic, vascular; complete diagnostic evaluation including bile acid tolerance, testing for infectious causes, CSF analysis, and brain imaging may be indicated. • Behavioral condition—compulsive disorder; exclusion diagnosis.

CBC/BIOCHEMISTRY/URINALYSIS

Frequently normal.

IMAGING

None required aside from that necessary to exclude differential diagnoses.

DIAGNOSTIC PROCEDURES

• Diagnosis based on characteristic history and clinical findings, and by excluding other diseases that can cause similar signs. • No test or group of tests support definitive diagnosis. • Electromyography (EMG)—evidence of abnormal spontaneous activity in thoracolumbar epaxial muscles in one study of affected cats. • Muscle biopsy—if EMG changes; isolated report of vacuoles within epaxial muscles, with antibody labeling characteristics similar to those described with inclusion body myositis/myopathy in humans.

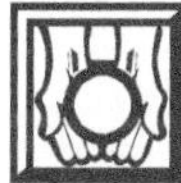

TREATMENT

• Outpatient. • Eliminate environmental changes that can precipitate episodes. • Behavioral modification has been successful in reducing clinical manifestations in some cats. • In severe cases of self-mutilation, Elizabethan collar or tail bandaging may be necessary.

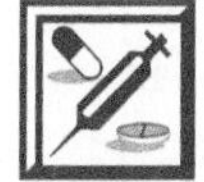

MEDICATIONS

DRUG(S) OF CHOICE

• Several pharmacologic agents recommended, based on suspected underlying cause. • Prednisolone indicated if pruritic dermatitis suspected. • Antiepileptic drugs often utilized; phenobarbital (1–2 mg/kg PO q12h) effective in some cats; gabapentin (5–10 mg/kg PO q12h) can be used for both antiepileptic and analgesic properties; topiramate (5 mg/kg PO q12h) is antiepileptic that has also been used to treat self-mutilation in cats. • Selective serotonin reuptake inhibitors (fluoxetine 0.5–2.0 mg/kg PO q24h), tricyclic antidepressants (clomipramine 0.5–1.0 mg/kg PO q24h), or benzodiazepines (lorazepam 0.125–0.50 mg per cat PO q8–24h) recommended when primary behavioral disorder suspected. • Combination therapy often required. • Treatment response variable; in cats that respond, therapy often lifelong as episodes tend to resume after medication discontinued.

CONTRAINDICATIONS/POSSIBLE INTERACTIONS

Fluoxetine inhibits the cytochrome P450 system and should be used cautiously with other drugs that undergo extensive hepatic metabolism, including phenobarbital, benzodiazepines, and tricyclic antidepressants.

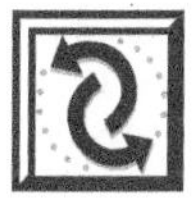

FOLLOW-UP

PATIENT MONITORING

Cats administered phenobarbital—check serum drug concentrations in 2–3 weeks and adjust dosage as needed to maintain levels of 20–30 μg/mL (85–130 μmol/L); CBC and biochemistry profile at 6–12-month intervals to monitor for adverse effects.

EXPECTED COURSE AND PROGNOSIS

Prognosis depends on whether underlying cause is identified, response to medication, and frequency and severity of episodes.

MISCELLANEOUS

ABBREVIATIONS

• CSF = cerebrospinal fluid.
• EMG = electromyography.

Suggested Reading

Amengual Batle P, Rusbridge C, Nuttall T, et al. Feline hyperaesthesia syndrome with self-trauma to the tail: retrospective study of seven cases and proposal for integrated multidisciplinary diagnostic approach. J Feline Med Surg 2019, 21(2):178–185. doi: 10.1177/1098612X18764246

Author Karen R. Muñana

F

FELINE IDIOPATHIC LOWER URINARY TRACT DISEASE

BASICS

DEFINITION

Idiopathic lower urinary tract disease, commonly referred to as feline idiopathic cystitis (FIC), is a nonmalignant, sterile, inflammatory disease of the urinary bladder and urethra. It is the most common urinary disorder of young to middle-aged cats and is characterized by dysuria, pollakiuria, hematuria, periuria, and in some cases urinary obstruction. Clinical observations suggest that FIC is associated with different clinical phenotypes (acute self-limiting, chronic, nonobstructive, and obstructive forms) and pathologic phenotypes (ulcerative, inflammatory, hyperplastic, nonulcerative, and noninflammatory forms). Regardless of form, the terms idiopathic lower urinary tract disease and FIC represent an exclusionary diagnosis established only after known causes have been eliminated.

PATHOPHYSIOLOGY

- Etiopathogenesis is uncertain.
- Urinary bladder abnormalities include alterations in urothelial barrier structure and function, differentiation and repair, signaling, eicosanoid biosynthesis, and innate immune and inflammatory responses.
- Association of FIC with stress (environmental, psychologic, physiologic, or comorbid pathologic stressors) and identification of multiple abnormalities of nervous and endocrine systems have led to hypothesis that systemic psychoneuroendocrine factors may have a role in the pathogenesis.
- Clinical and morphologic features of chronic forms of FIC are similar to those of an idiopathic cystopathy of humans called interstitial cystitis/painful bladder syndrome (IC/PBS). However, the extent to which the feline and human forms share pathogenic mechanisms has not yet been fully defined.

SYSTEMS AFFECTED

- Renal/urologic—lower urinary tract.
- Persistent urethral outflow obstruction results in postrenal azotemia.

INCIDENCE/PREVALENCE

- Incidence of hematuria, dysuria, and/or urethral obstruction (UO) in domestic cats has been previously reported to be ~0.5–1% per year.
- Hospital morbidity rate for FIC in cats with lower urinary tract signs is ~65%; it is the single most common cause of lower urinary tract signs in cats.

SIGNALMENT

Species

Cat

Mean Age and Range

- May occur at any age, but most commonly recognized in young to middle-aged adults (mean 3.5 years, range: 2–7 years).
- Uncommon in cats <1 and >10 years old.

SIGNS

Historical Findings

- Dysuria.
- Hematuria.
- Pollakiuria.
- Periuria.
- Urge incontinence.
- Outflow obstruction.

Physical Examination Findings

Thickened, firm, contracted bladder wall.

CAUSES

See Pathophysiology.

RISK FACTORS

- Male, middle-aged, and overweight cats, as well as cats housed indoors or living in a home with other cats, are at increased risk.
- Feeding dry food has not been consistently recognized as a risk factor.
- Stress may play a role in precipitating or exacerbating signs.

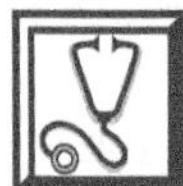

DIAGNOSIS

DIFFERENTIAL DIAGNOSIS

- Metabolic disorders including various types of uroliths/urethral plugs.
- Urinary tract infection (UTI) from bacteria, mycoplasma/ureaplasma, fungal agents, and parasites.
- Trauma.
- Neurogenic disorders including reflex dyssynergia, urethral spasm, and hypotonic or atonic bladder.
- Iatrogenic disease including reverse flushing solutions, indwelling and postsurgical urethral catheters, and urethrostomy complications.
- Anatomic abnormalities including urachal anomalies and acquired urethral strictures.
- Neoplasia.
- Clinical signs may be confused with constipation.

CBC/BIOCHEMISTRY/URINALYSIS

- Hematuria and proteinuria without significant pyuria or bacteriuria—usually present.
- If UO persists, serum chemistry profiles reveal azotemia, hyperphosphatemia, hyperkalemia, and acidosis.

OTHER LABORATORY TESTS

- Absence of bacteriuria—verify by quantitative urine culture; collect urine specimens by cystocentesis to avoid contamination.
- Transmission electron microscopy has revealed calicivirus-like particles in some urethral plugs.

IMAGING

- Survey radiography may exclude radiopaque uroliths or urethral plugs.
- Ultrasonography may exclude uroliths and thickening of bladder wall due to inflammation or neoplasia.
- Contrast cystography may exclude small or radiolucent uroliths, blood clots, urethral stricture, vesicourachal diverticula, and thickening of bladder wall due to inflammation or neoplasia.

DIAGNOSTIC PROCEDURES

- Cystoscopy may exclude uroliths and diverticula.
- Biopsies of urinary bladder wall may permit morphologic characterization of inflammatory or neoplastic lesions.

PATHOLOGIC FINDINGS

- Cystoscopy may reveal petechial hemorrhages (glomerulations) of urinary bladder mucosa.
- Mucosal ulceration or hyperplasia, submucosal edema, hemorrhage, neovascularization, fibrosis, and mononuclear inflammatory cell infiltrates are prominent features of chronic FIC.

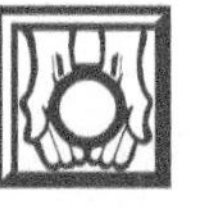

TREATMENT

APPROPRIATE HEALTH CARE

- Patients with nonobstructive lower urinary tract diseases—typically managed as outpatients; diagnostic evaluation may require brief hospitalization.
- Patients with obstructive lower urinary tract diseases—usually hospitalized for diagnosis and management.

DIET

- Results of prospective, randomized, double-masked, controlled clinical trial provided evidence that feeding specific multipurpose therapeutic urinary food (Hill's c/d Multicare) enriched with omega-3 fatty acids (EPA and DHA) and antioxidants significantly reduced rate of recurrent episodes of FIC signs.
- Low-grade evidence that recurrence of signs may be minimized by feeding moist foods.
- Appropriate dietary management for persistent crystalluria associated with matrix-crystalline urethral plugs.

CLIENT EDUCATION

- Hematuria, dysuria, and pollakiuria—often self-limiting within 4–7 days in most cats. Signs may recur unpredictably; up to 65% of cats experience ≥1 episodes within 1–2 years.
- A lack of controlled studies demonstrating efficacy of most drugs used to treat this disorder symptomatically.
- Reduce environmental stress by minimizing impact of changes in the home and maintaining a constant diet. Environmental enrichment for indoor-housed cats consists of provision of necessary resources (food, water, litter boxes, space, play), providing a safe place to hide, refinement of cat–owner interactions, and management of conflict.

- Provide proper litter box hygiene.
- Males should be monitored for signs of UO.

SURGICAL CONSIDERATIONS

Do not perform perineal urethrostomy to minimize recurrent UO without localizing obstructive disease to penile urethra by contrast urethrography.

MEDICATIONS

DRUG(S) OF CHOICE

- Amitriptyline—empirically advocated to treat cats with severe recurrent or persistent signs; suggested dosage is 5–10 mg/cat q24h given at night; not recommended for treatment of acute, self-limiting episodes of FIC.
- Butorphanol, buprenorphine, and fentanyl—have been empirically recommended for short-term analgesia in cats with FIC; there have been no reports of controlled studies to evaluate their safety or efficacy.
- Prazosin—may be used to minimize reflex dyssynergia and functional urethral outflow obstruction; suggested dosage is 0.25–0.5 mg/cat PO q12–24h.
- Tolteridine may be considered as an anticholinergic and antispasmodic to minimize hyperactivity of bladder detrusor muscle and urge incontinence; suggested dose is 0.05 mg/kg PO q12h; there have been no controlled studies to evaluate its safety or efficacy.
- Glycosaminoglycans—empirically recommended to help repair glycosaminoglycan coating of urothelium; results of controlled clinical studies have not demonstrated any beneficial effects on reducing severity or frequency of clinical signs in cats with FIC.
- Feline facial pheromone—empirically recommended to decrease signs of stress in cats with FIC; results of controlled clinical studies have not demonstrated any beneficial effects in management of FIC.
- Corticosteroids—no detectable effect on remission of acute clinical signs demonstrated; predispose to bacterial UTIs, especially in cats with indwelling transurethral catheters.
- Nonsteroidal anti-inflammatory drugs (NSAIDs)—empirically recommended by some because of their anti-inflammatory and analgesic properties; the safety of NSAIDs in the treatment of FIC has not been evaluated by controlled clinical trials.
- Antibiotics—no detectable effect on remission of clinical signs in cats demonstrated.

CONTRAINDICATIONS

- Phenazopyridine—may result in methemoglobinemia and irreversible oxidative changes in hemoglobin resulting in formation of Heinz bodies and anemia.
- Methylene blue—may cause Heinz bodies and severe anemia.
- Bethanechol—do not use in patients with UO.

PRECAUTIONS

- Cats with UO and postrenal azotemia are at increased risk for adverse drug events, especially with drugs and anesthetics that depend on renal elimination or metabolism.
- Indwelling transurethral catheters, especially when associated with fluid-induced diuresis, predispose patients to bacterial UTIs.

FOLLOW-UP

PATIENT MONITORING

Monitor hematuria by urinalysis; cystocentesis may cause iatrogenic hematuria, so naturally voided samples are preferred.

PREVENTION/AVOIDANCE

Best evidence suggests that multimodal approach to managing cats with acute nonobstructive FIC is advised, including multipurpose therapeutic urinary food proven to reduce rate of recurrent episodes of FIC signs (Hill's c/d Multicare); environmental enrichment; feeding moist food; and short-term administration of analgesics to control signs of pain.

POSSIBLE COMPLICATIONS

- Indwelling transurethral catheters—cause trauma; predispose to ascending bacterial UTIs.
- Perineal urethrostomies—predispose to bacterial UTIs and urethral strictures.

EXPECTED COURSE AND PROGNOSIS

Hematuria, dysuria, and pollakiuria often self-limiting within 4–7 days in most patients. These signs often recur unpredictably.

F

MISCELLANEOUS

AGE-RELATED FACTORS

Frequency of recurrence appears to decline with advancing age.

SYNONYMS

- Feline idiopathic cystitis.
- Feline interstitial cystitis.

SEE ALSO

- Dysuria, Pollakiuria, and Stranguria.
- Hematuria.
- Lower Urinary Tract Infection, Bacterial.
- Lower Urinary Tract Infection, Fungal.
- Urolithiasis, Struvite—Cats.

ABBREVIATIONS

- FIC = feline idiopathic cystitis.
- IC/PBS = interstitial cystitis/painful bladder syndrome.
- NSAID = nonsteroidal anti-inflammatory drug.
- UO = urethral obstruction.
- UTI = urinary tract infection.

Suggested Reading

Forrester SD, Towell TL. Feline idiopathic cystitis. Vet Clin Small Anim 2015, 45:783–806.

Kruger JM, Lulich JP, MacLeay J, et al. A randomized, double-masked, multicenter, clinical trial of two foods for long-term management of acute nonobstructive feline idiopathic cystitis (FIC). J Am Vet Med Assoc 2015; 247:508–517.

Author John M. Kruger

Consulting Editor J.D. Foster

Acknowledgment The author and book editors acknowledge the prior contributions of Carl A. Osborne and Jody P. Lulich

Client Education Handout available online

FELINE IMMUNODEFICIENCY VIRUS (FIV) INFECTION

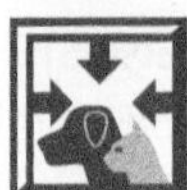

BASICS

DEFINITION

A complex retrovirus that causes immunodeficiency in domestic cats; same genus (*Lentivirus*) as human immunodeficiency virus (HIV).

PATHOPHYSIOLOGY

- Infection causes immune dysfunction due to cytokine alterations, nonspecific hyperactivation of B and T lymphocytes, and apoptosis of T cells.
- Strain or subtype influences pathogenicity; subtypes A and B are most common in the United States.
- Acute infection—virus spreads from site of entry to lymph tissues and thymus via dendritic cells, first infecting T lymphocytes, then macrophages.
- Primary receptor is feline CD134; uses chemokine receptor CXCR4 as co-receptor.
- CD4+ and CD8+ T cells can be infected; virus selectively and progressively decreases CD4+ (T-helper) cells; inversion of the CD4+ : CD8+ ratio (from ~2 : 1 to <1 : 1) develops slowly, with absolute decrease of CD4+ T cells after several months of infection.
- Early infection and activation of CD4+ CD25+ regulatory T cells may limit effective immune response to FIV infection.
- Cats clinically asymptomatic until cell-mediated immunity is disrupted; humoral immune function declines in advanced stages of infection.
- T cells and macrophages—main cellular reservoirs of virus in affected cats; lymphoid tissues are reservoirs throughout the body.
- Astrocyte and microglial cells in brain and megakaryocytes and mononuclear bone marrow cells may be infected; neuronal loss may occur.
- Co-infection with feline leukemia virus (FeLV) may increase expression of FIV in many tissues, including kidney, brain, and liver.

SYSTEMS AFFECTED

- Hemic/lymphatic/immune—loss of CD4+ T cells; lymphocytic/plasmocytic infiltrates in tissues (especially gingiva, lymphoid tissues); lymphomas, mast cell tumors.
- Gastrointestinal—panleukopenia-like syndrome.
- Nervous—alterations in astrocyte function and neurotransmitter expression.
- Ophthalmic—anterior uveitis.
- Renal/urologic—nephropathy.
- Reproductive—fetal death or perinatal infections.
- Cardiovascular—possible myocarditis.
- Other body systems—secondary infections.

GENETICS

No predisposition for infection, but may play role in progression and severity.

INCIDENCE/PREVALENCE

United States and Canada—1–3% prevalence in healthy cat populations; 9–15% in sick cats.

GEOGRAPHIC DISTRIBUTION

Worldwide; variable seroprevalence.

SIGNALMENT

Species

Cat

Mean Age and Range

- Prevalence of infection increases with age.
- Mean age—6 years at time of diagnosis.

Predominant Sex

Male—more aggressive; roaming.

SIGNS

General Comments

- Diverse due to immunosuppressive nature.
- Cannot be clinically distinguished from FeLV-associated immunodeficiency.

Historical Findings

Recurrent minor illnesses, especially upper respiratory and gastrointestinal.

Physical Examination Findings

- Opportunistic infections.
- Lymphadenomegaly—mild to moderate.
- Gingivitis, stomatitis, periodontitis (25–50% of cases).
- Rhinitis, conjunctivitis, keratitis (30% of cases); often associated with feline herpesvirus and calicivirus infections.
- Persistent diarrhea (10–20% of cases); bacterial or fungal overgrowth, parasite-induced inflammation; direct effect of FIV on gastrointestinal epithelium.
- Chronic, nonresponsive, or recurrent infections of external ear and skin—bacterial infections or dermatophytosis.
- Fever and wasting—especially in later stage.
- Ocular disease—anterior uveitis; pars planitis; glaucoma.
- Neurologic abnormalities—disruption of normal sleep patterns; behavioral changes (pacing and aggression); motor and neurocognitive deficits; peripheral neuropathies.

CAUSES

- Cat-to-cat transmission—usually by bite wounds.
- Occasional perinatal transmission.
- Sexual transmission uncommon, although FIV has been detected in semen.

RISK FACTORS

- Male.
- Free-roaming or feral.

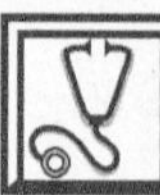

DIAGNOSIS

DIFFERENTIAL DIAGNOSIS

- Primary bacterial, parasitic, fungal, or viral infections, especially FeLV.
- Toxoplasmosis—neurologic and ocular manifestations may be the result of *Toxoplasma* infection, FIV infection, or both.
- Nonviral neoplastic diseases.
- Chronic kidney disease.

CBC/BIOCHEMISTRY/URINALYSIS

- Anemia, lymphopenia, or neutropenia—common; but neutrophilia may occur in response to secondary infections; may also be normal.
- Urinalysis and serum chemistry profile—hypergammaglobulinemia, azotemia with isosthenuria, proteinuria (immune-mediated glomerulonephritis).

OTHER LABORATORY TESTS

Serologic Testing

- Detects antibodies to FIV.
- ELISA—routine screening; point-of-care and diagnostic laboratory kits; confirm positive results with additional testing, especially in healthy, low-risk cats.
- Western blot (immunoblot)—confirmatory testing of ELISA-positive samples.
- Kittens—when <6 months old may test positive owing to passive transfer of antibodies from FIV-positive queen; positive test does not indicate infection; retest at 8–12 months to determine infection.
- Vaccinated cats may test positive for FIV antibodies.

Others

- Virus isolation and subtyping.
- Reverse transcriptase polymerase chain reaction (RT-PCR)—useful in vaccinated cats or kittens with maternal antibody.
- CD4+ : CD8+ evaluation—helps determine extent of immunosuppression.

IMAGING

N/A

DIAGNOSTIC PROCEDURES

N/A

PATHOLOGIC FINDINGS

- Lymphadenopathy—initially, follicular hyperplasia and paracortical infiltration of plasmacytes; later, follicular hyperplasia with follicular depletion or involution; in terminal stages, lymphoid depletion.
- Lymphocytic and plasmacytic infiltrates—gingiva, lymph nodes and other lymphoid tissues, spleen, kidney, liver, and brain.
- Perivascular cuffing, gliosis, neuronal loss, white matter vacuolization, and occasional giant cells in the brain.

- Intestinal lesions similar to those seen with feline parvovirus infection.

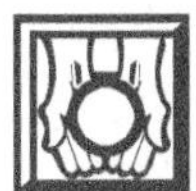

TREATMENT

APPROPRIATE HEALTH CARE

- Outpatient sufficient for most patients.
- Inpatient—with severe secondary infections until stable.

NURSING CARE

- Primary consideration—manage secondary and opportunistic infections.
- Supportive therapy—parenteral fluids and nutrition, as required.

ACTIVITY

Normal

DIET

Normal, may alter as necessary for cats with diarrhea, kidney disease.

CLIENT EDUCATION

- Inform client that infection is slowly progressive and healthy antibody-positive cats may remain healthy for years.
- Advise client that cats with clinical signs will have recurrent or chronic health problems that require medical attention.
- Discuss importance of keeping cats indoors to protect them from exposure to secondary pathogens and to prevent spread of FIV.

SURGICAL CONSIDERATIONS

- Oral treatment or surgery—dental cleaning, tooth extraction, gingival biopsy as needed; gingivitis and stomatitis may be refractory to treatment.
- Biopsy or removal of neoplastic lesions.

MEDICATIONS

DRUG(S) OF CHOICE

- Zidovudine (Retrovir®) 5–10 mg/kg PO q12h—antiviral agent; most effective against acute infection; monitor for bone marrow toxicity.
- Immunomodulatory drugs—may alleviate some clinical signs:
  - α-interferon (Roferon®-A)—diluted in saline at 30 units/day PO for 7 days, every other week; may increase survival rates and improve clinical status.
  - Feline omega-interferon (Virbagen® Omega)—1 million units/kg/day SC q24h for 5 days at 3 intervals (d0–4, d14–18, d60–64); lower-dose oral protocols may be effective.
- Antibacterial or antimycotic drugs—as indicated; prolonged therapy or high dosages may be required.
- Corticosteroids or gold salts—judicious but aggressive use may help control immune-mediated inflammation.
- Topical corticosteroids—for anterior uveitis; long-term response may be incomplete or poor; pars planitis often regresses spontaneously and may recur.
- Glaucoma—standard treatment.
- Vaccinate for respiratory and enteric pathogens based on individual risk assessment. Rabies vaccination according to regulatory guidelines.

CONTRAINDICATIONS

- Griseofulvin—avoid or use with extreme caution in FIV-positive cats; may induce severe neutropenia; neutropenia is reversible if drug is withdrawn early enough, but secondary infections can be life-threatening.

PRECAUTIONS

Systemic corticosteroids—use with caution; may lead to further immunosuppression.

ALTERNATIVE DRUG(S)

- *Propionibacterium acnes* (ImmunoRegulin®)—0.5 mL/cat IV once or twice weekly.
- Acemannan (Carrisyn®)—100 mg/cat PO q24h.

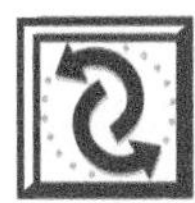

FOLLOW-UP

PATIENT MONITORING

Varies according to secondary infections and other manifestations of disease.

PREVENTION/AVOIDANCE

- Prevent contact with FIV-positive cats.
- Quarantine and test incoming cats before introducing into multicat households.
- Vaccine no longer available in the U.S.

EXPECTED COURSE AND PROGNOSIS

- Approx. 20% of cats die within 2 years of diagnosis or 4.5–6 years after estimated time of infection, but >50% remain asymptomatic.
- In late stages of disease (wasting and frequent or severe opportunistic infections), life expectancy ≤1 year.
- Overall survival time and quality of life for many FIV-positive cats will be similar to uninfected cats.

MISCELLANEOUS

ASSOCIATED CONDITIONS

- Secondary bacterial, viral, fungal, and parasitic disease.
- Lymphoid tumors.
- Immune-mediated disease.

AGE-RELATED FACTORS

Kittens (up to 4–6 months old) may test positive because of passive antibody transfer.

ZOONOTIC POTENTIAL

- None known.
- Potential transmission of secondary pathogens (e.g., *Toxoplasma gondii*) to immunocompromised humans.

PREGNANCY/FERTILITY/BREEDING

FIV-positive queens—reported abortions and stillbirths; transmission to kittens infrequent if queen is antibody-positive before conception; rate of transmission may be subtype or strain-dependent (>90% for experimental infections with some strains).

SYNONYMS

Feline immunodeficiency syndrome.

SEE ALSO

- Feline Calicivirus Infection.
- Feline Herpesvirus Infection.
- Feline Leukemia Virus (FeLV) Infection.
- Feline Stomatitis—Feline Chronic Gingivostomatitis (FCGS).
- Gingival Enlargement/Hyperplasia.

INTERNET RESOURCES

https://catvets.com/public/PDFs/PracticeGuidelines/RetrovirusGLS-Summary.pdf

ABBREVIATIONS

- FeLV = feline leukemia virus.
- FIV = feline immunodeficiency virus.
- HIV = human immunodeficiency virus.
- RT-PCR = reverse transcriptase polymerase chain reaction.

Suggested Reading

Hartmann K, Wooding A, Bergmann M. Efficacy of antiviral drugs against feline immunodeficiency virus. Vet Sci 2015, 2:456–476.

Levy JK, Crawford CP, Tucker SJ. Performance of 4 point-of-care screening tests for feline leukemia and feline immunodeficiency virus. J Vet Intern Med 2017, 31:521–526.

Little S, Levy J, Hartmann K, et al. 2020 AAFP feline retrovirus testing and management guidelines. J Feline Med Surg 2020, 22:5–30.

Sykes JE. Feline immunodeficiency virus infection. In: Sykes JE, ed., Canine and Feline Infectious Diseases. St. Louis, MO: Elsevier Saunders, 2014, pp. 209–223.

Author Margaret C. Barr
Consulting Editor Amie Koenig

Client Education Handout available online

FELINE INFECTIOUS DIARRHEA

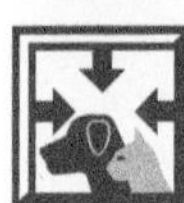

BASICS

DEFINITION

- Diarrhea is defined as excess fecal water, increased quantity of fecal material, or increased frequency of bowel movements.
- Etiologies include viral, enteropathogenic bacterial, protozoal, fungal, or helminths; small bowel, large bowel, or mixed bowel diarrhea.
- Secondary systemic signs likely with infection by feline immunodeficiency virus (FIV), feline leukemia virus (FeLV), feline enteric coronavirus (FECV), feline parvovirus (FPV), histoplasmosis.
- Presence of organisms on diagnostic screening does not indicate causation; patient factors (clinical signs, age, environmental exposure) should be considered before treatment.
- Some cats will have self-resolution; diagnostic testing may be appropriate for more severely affected animals or if clinical signs are persistent despite supportive care and having ruled out other causes of acute or chronic diarrhea; kittens with acute diarrhea should be screened for FPV.

PATHOPHYSIOLOGY

- Typically, fecal–oral route of infection.
- Diarrhea may result from decreased intestinal absorption or increased intestinal secretion caused by enterotoxins, osmotic forces, or epithelial damage.
- Immune response to infectious organisms can contribute to development of diarrhea; activated white blood cells release inflammatory mediators that stimulate secretion and damage intestinal epithelium.

SYSTEMS AFFECTED

- Cardiovascular—fluid balance.
- Gastrointestinal (GI).

GENETICS

Feline infectious peritonitis (FIP) more likely in purebred cats.

INCIDENCE/PREVALENCE

- 84% of cats from shelters had entero-pathogens—no difference with or without diarrhea.
- FECV more common in cats with diarrhea.

GEOGRAPHIC DISTRIBUTION

- Widespread.
- Prevalence of etiologies varies by region.
- Histoplasma more common in eastern United States, Latin America.

SIGNALMENT

Species

Cat

Breed Predilections

Purebred cats have higher prevalence of FIP.

Mean Age/Range

Young cats more likely to develop diarrhea from FECV, FPV, *Cryptosporidium*, helminths; FIP has bimodal distribution (young and old).

Predominant Sex

FIP more frequent in males.

SIGNS

General Comments

Range from mild to severe.

Historical Findings

- Acute or chronic, small or large bowel diarrhea.
- Possibly lethargy, vomiting, weakness, weight loss, hyporexia.
- Crowded environment.

Physical Examination Findings

- Dehydration.
- Poor body condition.
- Fluid/gas-filled intestinal loops.
- Signs of sepsis or systemic inflammatory response syndrome (SIRS) possible—tachycardia, hypotension, hyper/hypothermia, tachypnea, pale mucous membranes.
- Abdominal masses or enlarged lymph nodes may be palpable (histoplasmosis, FIP).
- With systemic infections may note chorioretinitis, icterus, neurologic deficits.

CAUSES

- Viral—FECV, FPV, astrovirus, calicivirus, FIV, FeLV, torovirus-like agent.
- Bacterial—*Campylobacter* spp., *Clostridium perfringens* enterotoxin A, *Clostridium difficile* toxins, *Salmonella* spp., *Escherichia coli, Yersinia spp.*
- Helminth—*Toxocara* spp., *Ancylostoma* spp., *Strongyloides* spp., *Toxascaris leonine, Spirometra* spp., *Trichuris vulpis.*
- Protozoal—*Giardia* spp., *Tritrichomonas foetus, Toxoplasma gondii.*
- Coccidial—*Cryptosporidium* spp., *Cystoisospora* spp.
- Fungal—*Histoplasma capsulatum.*

RISK FACTORS

- Pediatric, young adult cats more commonly affected, particularly with helminths, viral, and coccidial disease.
- Crowding, poor sanitation increase risk of transmission.

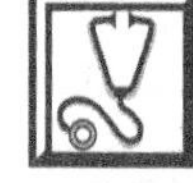

DIAGNOSIS

DIFFERENTIAL DIAGNOSIS

- Acute diarrhea—dietary indiscretion, foreign body, GI neoplasia; non-GI diseases: hyperthyroidism, iatrogenic, hepatotoxicity, renal disease, and other systemic diseases (frequently have hyporexia, vomiting, icterus).
- Chronic diarrhea—chronic enteropathy (dietary responsive, antibiotic responsive, dysbiosis, or inflammatory bowel disease), primary GI neoplasia, pancreatic insufficiency, and hepatic or renal disease.

CBC/BIOCHEMISTRY/URINALYSIS

- Eosinophilia with intestinal parasitism or histoplasmosis.
- Leukopenia with FPV, sepsis from salmonellosis or translocation, bone marrow involvement with histoplasmosis or FeLV.
- Anemia and microcytosis suggest GI hemorrhage or iron deficiency, particularly with high worm burden.
- Elevated liver enzyme activities or creatine kinase with toxoplasmosis.
- Hyperglobulinemia, elevated total bilirubin with FIP.
- Hemoconcentration, prerenal azotemia, electrolyte derangements with dehydration.
- Panhypoproteinemia if protein-losing enteropathy or GI blood loss.

IMAGING

- Abdominal radiographs if no response to symptomatic care to rule out other causes of diarrhea.
- Abdominal ultrasound recommended in nonpediatric patients with diarrhea nonresponsive to symptomatic care.
- Thoracic radiographs may show pulmonary disease or enlarged lymph nodes with histoplasmosis or toxoplasmosis.

DIAGNOSTIC PROCEDURES

- Fecal flotation—for intestinal parasitism; false negatives are possible as ova are intermittently shed; cats suspected to have intestinal parasitism should have multiple fecal flotations or be treated with anthelmintics.
- Fecal cytology—bacterial morphology (frequent spirochetes, spores) or presence of fungal or protozoal organisms.
- *Giardia* ELISA.
- Tritrichomonas PCR using "colonic flush" technique.
- Histoplasma enzyme immunoassay (EIA)—urine.
- Toxoplasmosis immunofluorescence antibody test (IFA) for immunoglobulin (Ig) G and IgM, rising titer between acute and convalescent samples.
- FIV antibody, FeLV antigen ELISA.
- Infectious diarrhea PCR panels assess for range of infectious causes of diarrhea; caution should be used in interpretation; positive results do not necessarily indicate causation and false-negative results possible.

PATHOLOGIC FINDINGS

- Gross examination of intestinal mucosa may demonstrate parasites attached to intestinal mucosa with multifocal hemorrhagic ulcerations, submucosal congestion or hemorrhage, intestinal wall thickening, lymphadenopathy.
- Histopathology of intestine may show eosinophilic, neutrophilic, pyogranulomatous, or lymphoplasmacytic enteritis with varying

degrees of hemorrhage and necrosis, depending on etiology; may visualize causative agent.

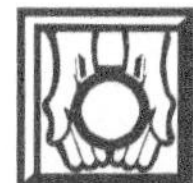

TREATMENT

APPROPRIATE HEALTH CARE

- Mildly affected cats treated as outpatients.
- Moderate to severely affected cats may require IV fluids for dehydration/electrolyte management.
- Dextrose should be supplemented parenterally for hypoglycemia,

ACTIVITY

N/A

DIET

- Diets high in easily digestible protein, including adequate taurine.
- In anorexic pediatric patients, nasogastric tube feeding of liquid diet recommended if anorexia >48 hours.

CLIENT EDUCATION

- For most infectious organisms, environmental decontamination prevents reinfection and transmission to other pets/humans; isolation during hospitalization may be warranted depending on cause.
- Appropriate vaccination and deworming schedules should be followed.
- Cats with identified infectious causes of diarrhea should be isolated from other cats until clinical signs resolve; *Histoplasma* not directly transmitted from cat to other hosts.

SURGICAL CONSIDERATIONS

Viral and parasitic enterocolitis can result in intussusceptions.

MEDICATIONS

DRUG(S) OF CHOICE

- Many cases self-resolve with supportive care and time.
- Empiric therapy, pending diagnostics if clinical signs persist—probiotics (Visbiome® 112.5 billion bacteria/cat/day), or metronidazole 10 mg/kg PO q12h, with fenbendazole 50 mg/kg PO q24h for 5 days.
- Anthelmintics—fenbendazole 50 mg/kg PO q24h for 5 days; pyrantel pamoate 10 g/kg PO q24h for 3 days.
- Coccidiostatic—sulfadimethoxine 50–60 mg/kg PO q24h for 5–10 days; ponazuril 50 mg/kg PO once.
- Campylobacteriosis with persistent clinical signs—erythromycin 10–15 mg/kg PO q8h; azithromycin 5–10 mg/kg PO q24h.
- Histoplasmosis—itraconazole 5–10 mg/kg PO q12–24h: do not use compounded formulations.
- Toxoplasmosis—clindamycin 10–17 mg/kg PO/IM/IV q8–12h for 4 weeks.
- Trichomoniasis—ronidazole 30 mg/kg PO q24h for 14 days.
- Patients with sepsis or leukopenia should be treated with broad-spectrum antibiotics.
- Cats with confirmed salmonella should *not* be treated with antibiotics unless systemically ill.

CONTRAINDICATIONS

N/A

PRECAUTIONS

- Metronidazole dose should be reduced in animals with hepatic insufficiency.
- Clindamycin should be given with food or water to prevent development of esophageal strictures.
- Ronidazole can cause neurotoxicity and should be discontinued if clinical signs including anorexia develop.

POSSIBLE INTERACTIONS

Dependent on drug used; itraconazole has many interactions.

FOLLOW-UP

PATIENT MONITORING

- Case-based, may include reassessment of anemia, leukopenia, or electrolyte derangements as appropriate.
- Persistent clinical signs after appropriate treatment suggest alternative cause of diarrhea.
- Patients with recurrent clinical signs should be retested, particularly if environmental reinfection possible (e.g., giardiasis, campylobacteriosis).

PREVENTION/AVOIDANCE

- Routine vaccination.
- Monthly flea and heartworm preventative with combination anthelmintic therapy.
- Maintain clean facilities and quarantine ill patients.
- Do not allow nonimmunocompetent patients to contact other animals until determined to be low risk.

POSSIBLE COMPLICATIONS

- Sepsis.
- Anemia.
- Dehydration, electrolyte, acid-base disturbances.

EXPECTED COURSE AND PROGNOSIS

- Usually good to excellent; underlying immunosuppressive conditions may increase susceptibility to infection and worsen prognosis.
- Infectious agents that cause systemic illness likely have worse prognosis.

MISCELLANEOUS

ASSOCIATED CONDITIONS

N/A

AGE-RELATED FACTORS

Young animals more susceptible.

ZOONOTIC POTENTIAL

- Toxoplasmosis—human abortion.
- Giardiasis—low risk of transmission.
- Cryptosporidiosis.
- Salmonellosis.
- *Campylobacter jejuni*.
- *Toxocara* spp. (ascarids)—visceral larval migrans, most common in children.
- *Ancylostoma* (hookworms)—cutaneous larval migrans, most common in children.

PREGNANCY/FERTILITY/BREEDING

Patients exhibiting clinical signs of illness should not be bred. If illness develops while pregnant, take caution regarding drug choice.

SEE ALSO

- Acute Diarrhea.
- Campylobacteriosis.
- Clostridial Enterotoxicosis.
- Coccidiosis.
- Diarrhea, Chronic—Cats.
- Feline Infectious Peritonitis (FIP).
- Feline Panleukopenia.
- Giardiasis.
- Histoplasmosis.
- Hookworms (Ancylostomiasis).
- Roundworms (Ascariasis).
- Salmonellosis.
- Toxoplasmosis.
- Whipworms (Tricuriasis).

ABBREVIATIONS

- EIA = enzyme immunoassay.
- FECV = feline enteric coronavirus.
- FeLV = feline leukemia virus.
- FIP = feline infectious peritonitis.
- FIV = feline immunodeficiency virus.
- FPV = feline parvovirus.
- GI = gastrointestinal.
- IFA = immunofluorescence antibody test.
- Ig = immunoglobulin.
- SIRS = systemic inflammatory response syndrome.

Suggested Reading

Green CE. Infectious Diseases of the Dog and Cat, 4th ed. St. Louis, MO: Elsevier Saunders, 2012.

Little SE. The Cat: Clinical Medicine and Management. St. Louis, MO: Elsevier Saunders, 2012.

Author Genna Atiee

Consulting Editor Amie Koenig

F

FELINE INFECTIOUS PERITONITIS (FIP)

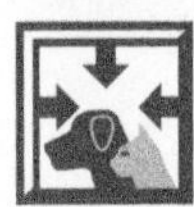

BASICS

DEFINITION

A systemic, immune-mediated, viral disease of cats characterized by insidious onset, persistent fever, pyogranulomatous tissue reaction, exudative effusions in body cavities, and high mortality.

PATHOPHYSIOLOGY

- The term feline coronavirus (FCoV) encompasses feline enteric coronavirus (FECV) and feline infectious peritonitis virus (FIPV).
- FECV is common and highly infectious; replicates locally in intestinal tract.
- FIPV infects monocytes/macrophages, which disseminate virus throughout body; localizes at vein wall and perivascular sites.
- FIP is an immune-mediated disease—perivascular accumulation of virus-infected macrophages and inflammatory cells produces pyogranulomatous inflammation in various organs.

SYSTEMS AFFECTED

- Multisystemic—pyogranulomatous or granulomatous lesions on omentum, serosal surface of abdominal organs, within abdominal lymph nodes, and submucosa of intestinal tract.
- Nervous—vascular lesions throughout CNS, especially in meninges.
- Ophthalmic—uveitis, chorioretinitis, and iritis.
- Respiratory—lesions on lung surfaces, pleural effusion.

INCIDENCE/PREVALENCE

- Prevalence of antibodies against FCoV—high, due to widespread presence of FECV, especially in multicat facilities.
- Incidence of FIP—low in most populations, especially in single-cat households.
- Because of difficulty in diagnosis, control, and prevention, outbreaks within breeding catteries may be catastrophic; in endemic catteries, risk of FCoV antibody–positive cat eventually developing FIP is usually <10%.

GEOGRAPHIC DISTRIBUTION

Worldwide

SIGNALMENT

Species

Cats—domestic and exotic.

Breed Predilections

Some bloodlines or breeds of cats may be more susceptible.

Mean Age and Range

Highest incidence in kittens 3 months–2 years of age.

SIGNS

General Comments

- Variable, depending on effectiveness of cell-mediated immune response, and organ system(s) affected.
- Two classic forms—wet (effusive) and dry (noneffusive); depends on presence of effusion in body cavities; dry form may become wet form with disease progression.

Historical Findings

- Insidious onset.
- Gradual weight loss and inappetence.
- Stunted growth in kittens.
- Gradual increase in size of abdomen due to effusion.
- Persistent fever—fluctuating, antibiotic unresponsive.

Physical Examination Findings

- Depression.
- Fever.
- Poor condition.
- Stunted growth.
- Dull, rough hair coat.
- Icterus.
- Abdominal and/or pleural effusion.
- Palpable abdominal masses (granulomas or pyogranulomas).
- Ocular—anterior uveitis, keratic precipitates, iris color change, irregularly shaped pupil.
- Neurologic—seizure, ataxia, paresis/paralysis, abnormal behavior, cranial nerve deficits.

CAUSES

- Prevailing theory is that FECV mutates to FIPV during FECV infection in individual cats; weak cell-mediated immunity plays a role in development of FIP.
- FCoV has two genomic types (FCoV type 1 and 2) and two biotypes (FECV and FIPV).
- FCoV type 1 is predominant (>85%); both types 1 and 2 can cause FIP.
- FECV—enteritis; highly transmissible among cats.
- FIPV—systemic, fatal disease (FIP); cat-to-cat transmission unlikely.

RISK FACTORS

- Contact with FECV-shedding cat; >30% of cats are chronic shedders.
- Breeding catteries or multicat facilities.
- Less than 2 years of age.
- Feline leukemia virus (FeLV) or feline immunodeficiency virus (FIV) infection.
- Certain cat breeds have higher incidence of FIP, especially dry form; some breeding pairs are prone to producing litters that develop FIP.

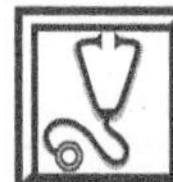

DIAGNOSIS

- Wet form—straightforward clinical diagnosis.
- Dry form—difficult to diagnose.
- Reverse-transcription polymerase chain reaction (RT-PCR) or immunohistochemistry on effusion or affected tissue confirmatory.
- No single diagnostic laboratory test.

DIFFERENTIAL DIAGNOSIS

- Fever of unknown origin—infection, inflammation.
- Pleural effusion—cardiac disease; cardiac effusion has low specific gravity and cell count.
- Neoplasia—lymphoma, other causing abdominal organ enlargement/effusion.
- CNS signs—neoplasia, toxoplasmosis.
- Anemia and icterus—blood parasites causing hemolysis.
- Pansteatitis (yellow fat disease)—classic feel and appearance of fat within abdominal cavity; pain on abdominal palpation; often a fish-only diet.
- Leukopenia, enteritis—panleukopenia (see Feline Panleukopenia).

CBC/BIOCHEMISTRY/URINALYSIS

- Leukocytosis with neutrophilia and lymphopenia.
- Mild to severe anemia.
- High total plasma protein, specifically globulin fraction (serum albumin : globulin typically <0.8).
- Hyperbilirubinemia and hyperbilirubinuria.

OTHER LABORATORY TESTS

- Serum antibody tests—detect antibodies against FCoV; positive tests not diagnostic of FIP (indicate only previous FECV infection); likelihood of FIP increases with titers ≥1 : 3200, but low titers do not exclude FIP.
- RT-PCR—detect viral genome; positive tests on blood or stool not diagnostic of FIP; positive tests on effusion or tissues confirm FIP.
- Immunohistochemistry—detect virus in biopsy or tissue samples; excellent for confirming cause of specific lesions, especially abdominal disease, which often is not diagnosed as FIP.

IMAGING

- May confirm abdominal and pleural effusions.
- May detect granulomatous lesions.

DIAGNOSTIC PROCEDURES

- Thoracocentesis and/or abdominocentesis—fluid pale to straw colored, viscous with flecks of fibrin, specific gravity 1.017–1.047; fluid may be used for RT-PCR or immunohistochemistry.
- Laparoscopy—to observe specific lesions of peritoneal cavity and obtain biopsy samples.
- Exploratory laparotomy—may be indicated for difficult-to-diagnose patients.

PATHOLOGIC FINDINGS

Gross

- Variable, patient generally emaciated, with rough hair coat.

- Abdomen and/or thoracic cavity—may contain thick, viscous exudates.
- White, rough, pyogranulomatous plaques or granulomas—may be on serosal surface of abdominal organs and omentum; fibrous strands may extend between organs.
- Discolored iris with anterior uveitis—may see keratic precipitates.
- Lesions in brain and/or spinal cord possible

Histopathologic

- Granulomas or pyogranulomas in any affected tissue.
- Lesions—perivascular; increase in size, involving large portions of tissue; microscopic appearance suggests diagnosis.

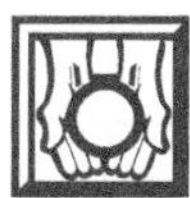

TREATMENT

APPROPRIATE HEALTH CARE

Inpatient or outpatient, depending on severity of disease and owner's willingness and ability to provide good supportive care.

NURSING CARE

- Therapeutic paracentesis—to relieve pressure/ dyspnea from ascites or pleural effusions.
- Encourage cat to eat.

ACTIVITY

FIP transmission to other cats unlikely; no or low levels of FIPV shedding.

DIET

Any food that will entice patient to eat.

CLIENT EDUCATION

- Discuss various aspects of disease, including grave prognosis; once clinical FIP is confirmed, nearly 100% of cats will die of disease.
- Inform client of high prevalence of FECV infection but low incidence of FIP; <10% of FCoV antibody–positive cats <2 years of age eventually develop clinical disease.

SURGICAL CONSIDERATIONS

- Generally none.
- Rarely, inflammatory abdominal disease from FIP may cause intestinal obstruction.

MEDICATIONS

DRUG(S) OF CHOICE

- No cure; only symptomatic treatment is available.
- Immunosuppressive drugs (e.g., oral prednisolone)—may alleviate some symptoms.
- Feline omega interferon—unclear effectiveness in symptomatic management.
- Antibiotics—generally not necessary.

ALTERNATIVE DRUG(S)

Direct-acting antiviral drugs for FIP have shown effectiveness in treatment and are under development.

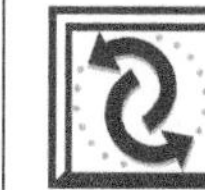

FOLLOW-UP

PATIENT MONITORING

Monitor for development of pleural effusion or neurologic disease.

PREVENTION/AVOIDANCE

- Modified live intranasal vaccine—against FIPV; low efficacy; cannot rely on vaccination alone for control; will produce antibody-positive cats, complicating monitoring in catteries or colonies; not generally recommended.
- Mother/offspring—main method of transmission appears to be from asymptomatic carrier queens to their kittens at 4–7 weeks of age, after maternal immunity wanes; break cycle of transmission by early weaning at 4–5 weeks of age and isolating litter from direct contact with other cats, including queen.
- Routine disinfection to reduce FECV transmission—premises, cages, and water/ food dishes; common disinfectants readily inactivate virus.
- Introduce only FCoV antibody–negative cats to catteries or colonies that are free of virus.
- Avoid breeding pairs that are prone to producing litters that develop FIP.

POSSIBLE COMPLICATIONS

Pleural effusion may require thoracocentesis; supportive care for other clinical signs.

EXPECTED COURSE AND PROGNOSIS

- Clinical course—a few days to several months until euthanasia is warranted.
- Prognosis grave once clinical signs occur; mortality nearly 100%.

MISCELLANEOUS

ASSOCIATED CONDITIONS

FeLV or FIV-positive cats—more prone to developing FIP.

PREGNANCY/FERTILITY/BREEDING

FIPV transmission from mother to offspring during pregnancy is presumed rare.

SYNONYMS

- Feline coronaviral polyserositis.
- Feline coronaviral vasculitis.
- Systemic feline coronavirus infection.

ABBREVIATIONS

- FCoV = feline coronavirus.
- FECV = feline enteric coronavirus.
- FeLV = feline leukemia virus.
- FIP = feline infectious peritonitis.
- FIPV = feline infectious peritonitis virus.
- FIV = feline immunodeficiency virus.
- RT-PCR = reverse-transcription polymerase chain reaction.

F

INTERNET RESOURCES

https://www.vet.cornell.edu/departments-centers-and-institutes/cornell-feline-health-center/health-information/feline-health-topics/feline-infectious-peritonitis

Suggested Reading

Addie D, Belák S, Boucraut-Baralon C, et al. Feline infectious peritonitis: ABCD guidelines on prevention and management. J Feline Med Surg 2009, 11:594–604.

Addie D, Jarrett O. Feline coronaviral infections. In: Sykes JE, Greene CE, ed., Infectious Diseases of the Dog and Cat, 4th ed. St. Louis, MO: Saunders Elsevier, 2011, pp. 54–67.

Brown MA, Troyer JL, Pecon-Slattery J, et al. Genetics and pathogenesis of feline infectious peritonitis virus. Emerg Infect Dis 2009; 15:1445–1452.

Drechsler V, Alcaraz A, Bossong FJ, et al. Feline coronavirus in multicat environments. Vet Clin North Am Small Anim Pract 2011, 1133–1169.

Hartmann K, Binder C, Hirschberger J, et al. Comparison of different tests to diagnose feline infectious peritonitis. J Vet Intern Med 2003, 17:781–790.

Pederson NC. An update on feline infectious peritonitis: diagnostics and therapeutics. Vet J 2014b, 201:133–141.

Pederson NC. An update on feline infectious peritonitis: virology and immunopathogenesis. Vet J 2014a, 201:123–132.

Richards JR, Elston TH, Ford RB, et al. The 2006 American Association of Feline Practitioners Feline Vaccine Advisory Panel Report. J Am Vet Med Assoc 2006, 229: 1405–1441.

Scherk MA, Ford RB, Gaskell RM, et al. 2013 AAFP Feline Vaccination Advisory Panel Report. J Feline Med Surg 2013, 15:785–808.

Author Yunjeong Kim

Consulting Editor Amie Koenig

Acknowledgment The author and book editors acknowledge the prior contribution of Fred W. Scott.

Client Education Handout available online

FELINE ISCHEMIC ENCEPHALOPATHY

BASICS

DEFINITION

- Seasonal neurologic disease that occurs in outdoor cats or those with access to outdoors in North America during late spring, summer, and early fall; usually results in sudden onset of seizures, circling, altered mentation, and/or blindness; however, any neurologic abnormalities can be found in these cats.
- Aberrant migration of *Cuterebra* larva in the brain of a cat that often causes thrombosis or vasospasm of middle cerebral artery with ensuing ischemic necrosis; degeneration of superficial layers of cerebral cortex and parenchymal destruction associated with physical migration of larva in brain parenchyma.
- Must be differentiated from other causes of vascular diseases affecting brains of cats as well as other neurologic diseases of cats.

PATHOPHYSIOLOGY

- In feline ischemic encephalopathy (FIE), *Cuterebra* larva enters nasal passage of cat, migrates through cribriform plate into olfactory bulb of the brain, then along olfactory peduncle and sometimes continues in parenchyma of brain, or alternatively in subarachnoid space; parasite then, if still alive, migrates caudally, where it may compromise the middle cerebral artery (MCA) physically through spines on the larvae's body, or possibly via chemical agent secreted by parasite causing vasospasm to vessel; or vasospasm may be secondary to hemorrhage caused by parasite; parasite may then die in subarachnoid space (SAS) or within parenchyma.
- Adult botfly lays eggs by entrance of rodent's den; eggs hatch into L1 stage of larva, which attaches to hair of mouse or rabbit and enters body through a normal orifice (mouth, nose, eye, or anus) and migrates into associated tissues (nasopharynx, trachea, thoracic cavity, diaphragm, abdominal cavity); then larva continues its migration to reach subcutaneous site in inguinal or thoracic region where it matures first to L2 stage and then within warble to L3 larval stage, emerges through skin, drops off host, pupates in soil over winter, and then emerges in spring as an adult botfly. Adult lays eggs near entrance of rodent's den; eggs hatch to form L1 larvae… When cat hunts near rodent's den, L1 larva attaches to cat's hair and gains access to nasal passage of cat and begins catastrophic pathway of FIE.
- Occasionally larva does not migrate through cribriform plate but embeds in nasal passage or respiratory tract of cat, causing focal respiratory signs; larva has also been found in the eye and oropharyngeal region.

SYSTEMS AFFECTED

- Brain and less commonly spinal cord.
- Larvae can also be found in skin, nasal passage, pharynx, larynx, eye, trachea, and thorax of cats.

GENETICS

None

INCIDENCE/PREVALENCE

Not known.

GEOGRAPHIC DISTRIBUTION

- North America only.
- Same distribution as *Cuterebra* botfly.
- Disease not recognized in locations that do not have *Cuterebra* botfly, such as Australia and Japan.

SIGNALMENT

Breed Predilections

None

Mean Age and Range

- Median age—2 years old.
- Range—1–7 years old.

Predominant Sex

None

SIGNS

- Sudden onset of neurologic signs.
- Often preceded by upper respiratory signs 1–3 weeks prior to neurologic signs (due to migration of the parasite in the nasal passage).
- Often prosencephalic signs.
- Most commonly—seizures, circling, altered mentation, blindness.
- Sometimes multifocal neurologic signs.
- Rarely spinal cord signs.
- May stop meowing/develop aphasia.

CAUSES

Cuterebra larvae.

RISK FACTORS

- Outdoor cats; access to outdoors.
- Not reported in indoor only cats.
- July, August, and September in northeast United States and southeast Canada; can be found in May and June in southeast United States.
- Hunting cats.

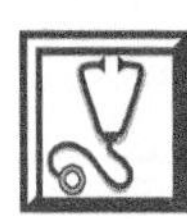

DIAGNOSIS

DIFFERENTIAL DIAGNOSIS

- Other causes of vascular accidents in brain such as renal disease and hyperthyroidism with hypertension.
- External trauma.
- Tumors—usually progressive rather than sudden in onset.
- Infectious/inflammatory diseases—such as those caused by *Cryptococcus* sp., *Toxoplasma gondii*, feline infectious peritonitis (FIP) virus, and feline immunodeficiency virus (FIV).

CBC/BIOCHEMISTRY/URINALYSIS

- Usually normal.
- CBC—occasionally neutrophilia, leukocytosis, or eosinophilia.
- Chemistry—occasionally elevated globulins or hyperglycemia.

OTHER LABORATORY TESTS

- Serology for feline leukemia virus (FeLV), FIV, FIP—negative.
- Cryptococcal antigen titers—negative.
- Toxoplasma immunoglobulin (Ig) G and IgM—negative.

IMAGING

- MRI—diagnostic modality of choice; detect track lesion extending from cribriform plate into olfactory bulb and frontal, parietal, and temporal lobes best recognized on dorsal sequences; may see abnormalities in ipsilateral nasal passage; may also see area of ischemic infarction in brain; if performed soon after onset of signs, increased signal intensity on T2 weighted, proton density weighted, and fluid attenuated inversion recovery (FLAIR) images associated with ischemia of superficial layers of cerebral cortex, or the area supplied by MCA; scant parenchymal enhancement in area of infarction after administration of contrast. If MRI is done more then 2–3 weeks after onset of signs, may find loss of overlying gray matter in region supplied by MCA and associated hydrocephalus ex vacuo. Magnetic resonance angiography (MRA; time of flight or postcontrast) may be of some utility in some cases.
- CT—limited value.

DIAGNOSTIC PROCEDURES

Cerebrospinal fluid—normal or nonsuppurative inflammation with macrophages, lymphocytes, or eosinophils.

PATHOLOGIC FINDINGS

- Local areas of malacia and hemorrhage involving olfactory bulbs and peduncles on brain transverse sections. Thorough examination of nasal passage, cribriform plate, olfactory bulbs, and peduncles, as well as remaining parenchyma, meninges, and overlying calvaria, may reveal the larva, which is approximately 5–10 mm in length (stage 2 larva), tan, and with concentric rings of spines along length of body.
- Histopathologic features may include necrosis and hemorrhage of parasitic track, or less specific findings such as superficial laminar cerebrocortical necrosis, cerebral infarction, subependymal rarefaction, and astrogliosis and subpial astrogliosis.

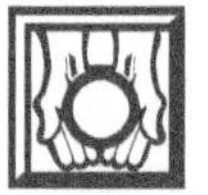

TREATMENT

NURSING CARE

- Padded cage may be necessary if cat is having seizures.
- Swivel IV line can be used if patient exhibits propulsive/compulsive circling or loss of balance.

CLIENT EDUCATION

- Only occurs in outdoor cats and those with access to outdoors; strictly indoor cats do not develop FIE.
- Only occurs in summer months, with majority of patients seen during July, August, and September in the northeast United States and southeast Canada.
- May not occur in major metropolitan areas that do not have normal appropriate hosts such as cottontail rabbit.

SURGICAL CONSIDERATIONS

Successful removal of parasite from the brain/spinal cord has not been reported in cats, but may be possible if neuroimaging is available early after onset of clinical signs.

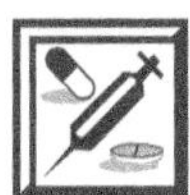

MEDICATIONS

DRUG(S) OF CHOICE

- Supportive care including antiepileptic drugs and appropriate fluid supplementation, which may include thiamine administration and additional potassium IV depending on nutritional status of patient; typically phenobarbital is used at maintenance dose of 7.5–15 mg PO/IM/IV q12h/cat; in addition phenobarbital can be loaded at a total loading dose of 16 mg/kg IV/PO/IM; this dose is usually divided over 24–48h (e.g., 4 mg/kg q12h for 2 days); then maintenance dose is started; diazepam can be used at 2.5–5 mg IV to stop cluster seizures or status epilepticus; other anticonvulsants, such as levetiracetam, may also be utilized.
- Cocktail treatment has been proposed for recently affected cats—diphenhydramine IM at 4 mg/kg 1–2h before giving ivermectin SC at 200–500 µg/kg and prednisolone sodium succinate at 30 mg/kg IV; treatment is repeated at 24h and 48h after first injection of ivermectin; in addition patients receive prednisone at 5 mg/cat q12h PO for 14 days and enrofloxacin at 22.7 mg PO q12h for 14 days. Because of concerns of blindness in some cats with administration of enrofloxacin, pradofloxacin or other antibiotics with broad-spectrum utility can be considered; ivermectin is not approved for use against *Cuterebra* larva so appropriate client permission must be obtained prior to administration; this cocktail treatment is not for patients with clinical signs >1 week as parasite is likely already dead.

CONTRAINDICATIONS

Do not use ivermectin in cats with known sensitivity.

PRECAUTIONS

No adverse effects from ivermectin have been noted; however, anaphylactic or allergic reaction could occur if *Cuterebra* larva suddenly dies and releases possible foreign antigens.

ALTERNATIVE DRUG(S)

Can use dexamethasone instead of prednisone.

FOLLOW-UP

PATIENT MONITORING

Sequential neurologic evaluations.

PREVENTION/AVOIDANCE

- Keep cat indoors.
- Use of monthly fipronil, imidacloprid, selamectin, or ivermectin has been suggested to prevent infections with *Cuterebra* parasite in outdoor cats.

POSSIBLE COMPLICATIONS

- May continue to have uncontrolled seizures.
- May continue to circle compulsively/propulsively.
- May have behavioral changes such as aggression, especially in cats with damage to piriform lobe.
- May stop meowing/develop aphasia in some cats.

EXPECTED COURSE AND PROGNOSIS

After initial onset, many patients improve and become acceptable pets; there may be persistent deficits, seizures, circling, and undesirable behavior such as aggression; may develop aphasia; persistent clinical signs depend on damage caused by infarction and parasitic migration.

MISCELLANEOUS

ASSOCIATED CONDITIONS

None

AGE-RELATED FACTORS

N/A

ZOONOTIC POTENTIAL

None; however, aberrant *Cuterebra* larva migration has been reported in humans, most commonly as ocular form in children.

SYNONYMS

CNS cuterebriasis.

ABBREVIATIONS

- FeLV = feline leukemia virus.
- FIE = feline ischemic encephalopathy.
- FIP = feline infectious peritonitis.
- FIV = feline immunodeficiency virus.
- FLAIR = fluid attenuated inversion recovery.
- Ig = immunoglobulin.
- MCA = middle cerebral artery.
- MRA = magnetic resonance angiography.
- SAS = subarachnoid space.

INTERNET RESOURCES

http://www.neurovideos.vet.cornell.edu
Videos 14-8, 14-9, 12-20

Suggested Reading

Bowman DD, Hendrix CM, Lindsay DS, et al. Feline Clinical Parasitology. Ames, IA: Iowa State University Press, 2002, pp. 430–439.

de Lahunta A, Glass EN, Kent M. Veterinary Neuroanatomy and Clinical Neurology, 4th ed. St. Louis, MO: Elsevier-Saunders, 2015, pp. 433–436, 549–550.

Glass EN, Cornetta AM, de Lahunta A, et al. Clinical and clinicopathologic features in 11 cats with *Cuterebra* larvae myiasis of the central nervous system. J Vet Intern Med 1998, 12:365–368.

Williams KJ, Summers BA, de Lahunta A. Cerebrospinal cuterebriasis in cats and its association with feline ischemic encephalopathy. Vet Pathol 1998, 35:330–343.

Authors Eric N. Glass and Alexander de Lahunta

Client Education Handout available online

F

FELINE LEUKEMIA VIRUS (FELV) INFECTION

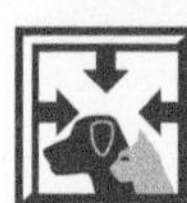

BASICS

DEFINITION

A simple retrovirus (*Gammaretrovirus* genus) that causes immunodeficiency and neoplastic disease in domestic cats.

F

PATHOPHYSIOLOGY

- Four subgroups of feline leukemia virus (FeLV)—A, B, C, and T; FeLV-A most transmissible and present in all isolates; FeLV-B arises from recombination of FeLV-A *env* gene with endogenous retroviral sequences (50% of isolates); FeLV-C (1% of isolates) arises from mutation in *env* gene sequences; FeLV-T infects only T cells.
- Early infection (five stages)—(1) viral replication in tonsils and pharyngeal lymph nodes; (2) infection of circulating B lymphocytes and macrophages that disseminate virus; (3) replication in lymphoid tissues, intestinal crypt epithelial cells, bone marrow precursor cells; (4) release of infected neutrophils and platelets from bone marrow; and (5) infection of epithelial and glandular tissues, subsequent shedding of virus into saliva, urine.
- *Abortive infection*—if virus replication terminated at stage 1; no viremia.
- *Regressive or nonproductive infection*—immune response stops progression at stage 2 or 3 (4–8 weeks after exposure) and forces virus into latency after transient viremia; may be reactivated with immune suppression or other viral infections.
- *Progressive or productive infection*—immune response not effective, persistent viremia (stages 4 and 5) from 4–12 weeks after infection.
- Tumor induction—DNA provirus integrates into cat chromosomal DNA in critical regions near oncogenes (e.g., *c-myc* or genes influencing *c-myc* expression); thymic lymphosarcoma results.
- Feline sarcoma viruses—FeLV mutants; arise by recombination between FeLV and host genes; virus–host fusion proteins responsible for induction of fibrosarcomas.
- Pathogenesis influenced by presence of other viruses (e.g., feline foamy virus, feline coronavirus, feline immunodeficiency virus [FIV]) or endogenous retroviruses.

SYSTEMS AFFECTED

- Hemic/lymphatic/immune—bone marrow dyscrasia, neoplasia, immunosuppression.
- Nervous—degenerative myelopathy, neoplasia.
- Other body systems—immunosuppression with secondary infections or neoplasia.

GENETICS

N/A

INCIDENCE/PREVALENCE

- In United States, 2–3% in healthy cat population; worldwide infection rate 1–8% in healthy cats; 3–4 times greater in clinically ill cats.
- Decline in US prevalence since 1980s.

GEOGRAPHIC DISTRIBUTION

Worldwide

SIGNALMENT

Species

Cat

Mean Age and Range

- Prevalence highest between 1 and 6 years of age.
- Mean—3 years.

Predominant Sex

Male : female ratio—1.7 : 1.

SIGNS

General Comments

- Onset of FeLV-associated disease—months to years after infection.
- Associated diseases—non-neoplastic or neoplastic; most non-neoplastic or degenerative diseases result from immunosuppression.
- Regressive infections may be associated with cardiomyopathies, lymphomas, leukemias, anemia, other infections.
- Clinical signs of FeLV-induced immunodeficiency cannot be distinguished from FIV-induced immunodeficiency.

Historical Findings

- Outdoor cat.
- Multicat household.

Physical Examination Findings

- Depend on type of disease (neoplastic or non-neoplastic) and secondary infections.
- Lymphadenomegaly—mild to severe.
- Fever, wasting.
- Upper respiratory tract—rhinitis, conjunctivitis, keratitis.
- Persistent diarrhea—bacterial or fungal overgrowth, parasite-induced inflammation, direct effect on crypt cells.
- Gingivitis, stomatitis, periodontitis.
- Nonresponsive or recurrent infections of external ear and skin.
- Lymphoma—risk increased 62-fold in FeLV-infected cats; thymic and multicentric; extranodal lymphoma can affect eye, nervous system.
- Erythroid and myelomonocytic leukemias.
- Fibrosarcomas—coinfection with mutated sarcoma virus; frequently young cats.
- Peripheral neuropathies; progressive ataxia.

CAUSES

- Cat-to-cat transmission—close casual contact (grooming), shared dishes or litter pans, bites.
- Perinatal transmission—transplacental and transmammary transmission in $\geq$20% of surviving kittens from infected queens.

RISK FACTORS

- Age—kittens more susceptible than adults.
- Male—result of behavior.
- Free-roaming.
- Multicat household.

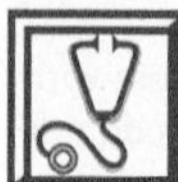

DIAGNOSIS

DIFFERENTIAL DIAGNOSIS

- FIV.
- Other infections—bacterial, parasitic, viral, or fungal.
- Nonviral neoplastic diseases.

CBC/BIOCHEMISTRY/URINALYSIS

- Anemia—often severe, often nonregenerative; regenerative anemias usually associated with *Mycoplasma haemofelis* or *M. haemominutum* coinfections.
- Lymphopenia or lymphocytosis.
- Neutropenia—sometimes cyclic; may be response to secondary infections or immune-mediated disease.
- Thrombocytopenia and immune-mediated hemolytic anemia.
- Biochemistry/urinalysis abnormalities depend on affected organs.

OTHER LABORATORY TESTS

- Immunochromatography (lateral flow) and ELISA—point-of-care screening, detect antigen in plasma, serum, saliva, tears; more sensitive than immunofluorescent antibody (IFA) for early or transient infection; single positive test does not predict persistent viremia (retest in 12 weeks); confirm positive tests with another method.
- IFA—identify FeLV antigen in leukocytes and platelets in fixed smears of whole blood or buffy coat; positive result indicates productive bone marrow infection; 97% of IFA-positive cats persistently infected and viremic for life; antigen usually detected by 4 weeks after infection, but may be up to 12 weeks; for leukopenic cats, use buffy coat smears rather than whole blood smears; confirm positive tests.
- FeLV vaccination does not interfere with antigen testing.
- PCR for proviral DNA in blood or tissue—denotes exposure, confirm with antigen test; proviral DNA detectable 1–2 weeks after infection; proviral loads can differentiate cats with regressive versus progressive infections.
- Reverse transcription PCR (RT-PCR) for viral RNA (virus circulating or replicating within cells) in saliva or blood—denotes viremia and FeLV shedding; first test to become positive as early as 1 week after infection.
- Multiple tests over several months may be needed to clarify FeLV status and whether infection progressive or regressive; a few cats have persistently discordant ELISA-positive and IFA-negative tests or test positive only sporadically.

IMAGING

Thymic atrophy (fading kittens); mediastinal mass and pleural effusion with thymic lymphoma.

DIAGNOSTIC PROCEDURES

Bone marrow aspiration or biopsy—arrest in erythroid differentiation; true aplastic anemia with hypocellular bone marrow may be seen; some cases of anemia result from myelopthesis.

PATHOLOGIC FINDINGS

- Bone marrow hypercellularity with neoplastic disease.
- Lymphocytic and plasmacytic infiltrates of gingiva, lymph nodes, other lymphoid tissues, spleen, kidney, liver.
- Intestinal lesions—feline panleukopenia-like syndrome.

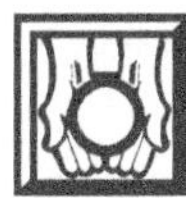

TREATMENT

APPROPRIATE HEALTH CARE

- Outpatient for most cats.
- Inpatient—may be required with severe secondary infections, anemia, cachexia.
- Blood transfusions—emergency support; may need multiple transfusions; passive antibody transfer (if vaccinated donor) reduces level of FeLV antigenemia in some.
- Management of secondary and opportunistic infections.

NURSING CARE

Supportive therapy (e.g., parenteral fluids, nutritional supplements) as indicated.

ACTIVITY

Normal

DIET

Normal, may alter as necessary for cats with diarrhea, kidney disease.

CLIENT EDUCATION

- Keep cats indoors and separated from FeLV-negative cats to protect from secondary pathogens and prevent spread of FeLV.
- Discuss good nutrition, routine husbandry to control secondary infections.

SURGICAL CONSIDERATIONS

- Biopsy or removal of tumors.
- Oral treatment or surgery—dental cleaning, tooth extraction, gingival biopsy.

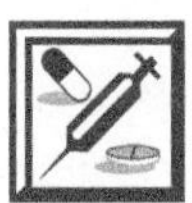

MEDICATIONS

DRUG(S) OF CHOICE

- Antiretroviral therapy not routinely indicated due to inconsistent evidence of efficacy and potential adverse effects; immune modulator therapy also unproven.
  - Zidovudine (Retrovir® 5–10 mg/kg PO q12h)—clinical improvement, does not clear virus.
  - α-interferon (Roferon®-A in saline 30 U/day PO for 7 days every other week).
  - Feline recombinant interferon omega (Virbagen® Omega 1 million U/kg SC for 5 days starting days 0, 14, 60)—may increase survival rates and improve clinical status.
- *Mycoplasma haemofelis* infection—see Mycoplasmosis for recommended treatment.
- Lymphoma—management with standard chemotherapy protocols; remission periods average 3–4 months.
- Myeloproliferative disease, leukemias—more refractory to treatment.
- Vaccinate for respiratory and enteric pathogens based on individual risk assessment. Rabies vaccination according to regulatory guidelines.

CONTRAINDICATIONS

Modified live vaccines—potential for disease in severely immunosuppressed cats.

PRECAUTIONS

Systemic corticosteroids—potential for further immunosuppression.

POSSIBLE INTERACTIONS

N/A

ALTERNATIVE DRUG(S)

Immunomodulatory drugs—*Propionibacterium acnes* (ImmunoRegulin® 0.5 mL/cat IV once or twice weekly); acemannan (Carrisyn® 100 mg/cat/day PO).

FOLLOW-UP

PATIENT MONITORING

Varies according to clinical manifestations.

PREVENTION/AVOIDANCE

- Prevent contact with FeLV-positive cats.
- Quarantine and test incoming cats before introduction to multicat households.
- Screen blood donor cats for FeLV-regressive infections using PCR for proviral DNA.

Vaccines

- Most commercial vaccines induce virus-neutralizing antibodies, reported efficacy ranges from <20% to almost 100%, depending on methodology; canarypox–FeLV recombinant vaccine does not contain adjuvant.
- Test cats for FeLV before initial vaccination.
- Vaccinate kittens at 8–9 and 12 weeks of age; boost at 1 year of age; revaccinate every 2–3 years if cat is in low risk environment; annually if high risk..

EXPECTED COURSE AND PROGNOSIS

Persistently viremic cats: >50% succumb to related diseases within 2–3 years after infection.

MISCELLANEOUS

ASSOCIATED CONDITIONS

- Secondary infections.
- Neoplasia (lymphoid, fibrosarcoma).
- Immune-mediated disease.

AGE-RELATED FACTORS

- Neonatal kittens—most (70–100%) susceptible to infection.
- Older kittens—<30% susceptible to infection by 16 weeks of age; may develop regressive infections.

ZOONOTIC POTENTIAL

Probably low, but controversial.

PREGNANCY/FERTILITY/BREEDING

- Abortions, stillbirths, and fetal resorptions occur in about 80% of FeLV-positive queens.
- Transmission from queen to kittens—in at least 20% of live births.

SEE ALSO

- Anemia, Nonregenerative.
- Feline Immunodeficiency Virus (FIV) Infection.
- Feline Stomatitis—Feline Chronic Gingivostomatitis (FCGS).
- Lymphoma—Cats.
- Myeloproliferative Disorders.

ABBREVIATIONS

- FeLV = feline leukemia virus.
- FIV = feline immunodeficiency virus.
- IFA = immunofluorescent antibody.
- RT-PCR = reverse transcription polymerase chain reaction.

INTERNET RESOURCES

http://www.abcdcatsvets.org/feline-leukaemia-virus-infection

Suggested Reading

Little S, Levy J, Hartmann K, et al. 2020 AAFP feline retrovirus testing and management guidelines. J Feline Med Surg 2020, 22:5–30.

Sykes JE. Feline leukemia virus infection. In: Sykes JE, ed., Canine and Feline Infectious Diseases. St. Louis, MO: Elsevier Saunders, 2014, pp. 224–238.

Willett BJ, Hosie MJ. Feline leukaemia virus: half a century since its discovery. Vet J 2013, 195:16–23.

Author Margaret C. Barr

Consulting Editor Amie Koenig

Client Education Handout available online

F

FELINE PANLEUKOPENIA

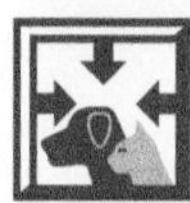

BASICS

DEFINITION

A viral infection of cats characterized by sudden onset, vomiting and diarrhea, severe dehydration, and high mortality.

PATHOPHYSIOLOGY

Feline parvovirus (FPV) infects and causes acute death of rapidly dividing cells.

SYSTEMS AFFECTED

- Gastrointestinal—crypt cells of jejunum and ileum are destroyed causing blunted villi; malabsorption of nutrients; acute vomiting and diarrhea; dehydration; and secondary bacteremia.
- Hemic/lymphatic/immune—severe panleukopenia; atrophy of thymus.
- Nervous and ophthalmic—in neonates, rapidly dividing granular cells of cerebellum and retinal cells of eye destroyed; cerebellar hypoplasia with ataxia and retinal dysplasia result.
- Reproductive—in utero infection in nonimmune queens leads to fetal death or neurologic abnormalities.

GENETICS

N/A

INCIDENCE/PREVALENCE

- Unvaccinated populations—most severe and important feline infectious disease.
- Routine vaccination—almost total control of disease.
- Extremely contagious.
- Extremely stable virus, survives for years on contaminated premises.

GEOGRAPHIC DISTRIBUTION

Worldwide in unvaccinated populations.

SIGNALMENT

Species

- Felidae—all, domestic and exotic.
- Canidae—susceptible to canine parvovirus; some exotic canids may be susceptible to FPV.
- Mustelidae—especially mink; may be susceptible.
- Procyonidae—raccoon and coatimundi; susceptible.

Breed Predilections

None

Mean Age and Range

- Unvaccinated and previously unexposed cats of any age can become infected once maternal immunity has been lost.
- Kittens 2–6 months of age—most susceptible to develop severe disease.
- Adults—often mild or subclinical infection.

Predominant Sex

N/A

SIGNS

Historical Findings

- History of recent exposure (e.g., from shelter population).
- Newly acquired kitten.
- Kitten 2–4 months old from premises with history of feline panleukopenia (FP).
- No vaccination history or last vaccinated when <16 weeks of age.
- Sudden onset, with vomiting, diarrhea, depression, complete anorexia.

Physical Examination Findings

- Mental dullness/lethargy.
- Typical "panleukopenia posture"—sternum and chin resting on floor, feet tucked under body, top of scapulae elevated above the back.
- Dehydration—appears rapidly; may be severe.
- Vomiting, diarrhea.
- Body temperature—usually mild to moderately increased or decreased in early stages; becomes severely low as patients become moribund.
- Abdominal pain.
- Small intestine—either turgid or flaccid.
- Subclinical or mild infections common, especially in adults.
- Ataxia from cerebellar hypoplasia—kittens infected in utero or neonatally; evident at 10–14 days of age and persist for life: hypermetria; dysmetria; base-wide stance; alert, afebrile, and otherwise normal; retinal dysplasia sometimes seen.

CAUSES

FPV

- Small, single-stranded DNA virus.
- Single antigenic serotype.
- Antigenic cross-reactivity with canine parvovirus (CPV) type 2 and mink enteritis virus.
- Extremely stable against environmental factors, temperature, and most disinfectants.
- Requires a mitotic cell for replication.

CPV Types 2a, 2b, and 2c

- CPV-2a, CPV-2b, and CPV-2c can produce FP in domestic and/or exotic cats.
- Properties of CPV similar to FPV.

RISK FACTORS

- Factors that increase mitotic activity of small intestinal crypt cells such as intestinal parasites or pathogenic bacteria.
- Secondary or coinfections—viral upper respiratory infections.

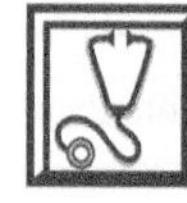

DIAGNOSIS

DIFFERENTIAL DIAGNOSIS

- Panleukopenia-like syndrome of feline leukemia virus (FeLV) infection—chronic enteritis and panleukopenia, frequently anemia; patient positive for FeLV antigen.
- Salmonellosis—can cause severe gastroenteritis; white blood cell (WBC) count usually high.
- Acute poisoning—similar to acute disease; depression; subnormal temperature; WBC count normal.
- Many diseases cause mild clinical signs hard to differentiate from mild FP; total WBC count always low during acute infection with FPV, even in subclinical infections.

CBC/BIOCHEMISTRY/URINALYSIS

- Panleukopenia—most consistent finding; WBC counts usually between 500 and 3,000 cells/μL during acute disease.
- Biochemical findings usually nonspecific—hypoproteinemia, hypoalbuminemia, hypocholesterolemia possible.

OTHER LABORATORY TESTS

- CPV antigen fecal immunoassay (Cite Canine Parvovirus Test Kit, IDEXX Labs)—not licensed for FP; detects FPV antigen in feces.
- Chromatographic test strip—feces for FPV and CPV.
- Serologic testing—paired serum samples detect rising antibody titer.
- PCR testing–confirms FPV in blood, feces, or tissue; positive result with recent modified live virus (MLV) vaccination.

DIAGNOSTIC PROCEDURES

- Viral isolation from feces or affected tissues (e.g., thymus, small intestine, spleen).
- Electron microscopy of feces—detects parvovirus, presumably FPV.

PATHOLOGIC FINDINGS

Gross

- Rough hair coat, weight loss.
- Severe dehydration.
- Evidence of vomiting and diarrhea.
- Edematous, turgid small intestine.
- Petechial or ecchymotic hemorrhages in jejunum and ileum.
- Thymic atrophy.
- Gelatinous or liquid bone marrow.
- In utero or neonatal infection—gross hypoplasia of cerebellum.

Microscopic

- Dilated small intestinal crypts with sloughing of epithelial cells.
- Shortened and blunt intestinal villi.
- Lymphocytic depletion of follicles of lymph nodes, Peyer's patches, spleen.
- Neonatal and fetal infection—disorientation and depletion of granular and Purkinje cells of cerebellum.
- Eosinophilic intranuclear inclusions in affected tissues during early infection.

TREATMENT

APPROPRIATE HEALTH CARE

- Main principles of treatment—rehydration; antibiotic therapy; supportive care (antiemetics and analgesics as needed).
- Inpatient—severe cases.
- Outpatient—mild cases.

NURSING CARE

- IV fluid therapy—essential in severe cases: correct dehydration and provide electrolytes; add dextrose if patient is hypoglycemic.
- SC fluids—mild cases without dehydration or shock.
- Antiemetic therapy should be considered in vomiting patients.
- Whole blood, packed red blood cells, or fresh frozen plasma transfusions—if clinical signs of anemia are present or serum albumin <2 g/dL.

ACTIVITY

Keep patient indoors during acute disease.

DIET

Temporarily withhold food until vomiting is controlled.

CLIENT EDUCATION

- Inform client that current and future cats in household must be vaccinated for FPV before exposure.
- Inform client that virus will remain infectious for years unless environment can be adequately disinfected with dilute bleach.

SURGICAL CONSIDERATIONS

None

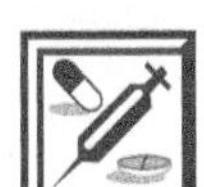

MEDICATIONS

DRUG(S) OF CHOICE

Broad-spectrum antibiotics (e.g., ampicillin or ampicillin–sulbactam IV, amoxicillin or amoxicillin–clavulanate PO)—counter secondary bacteremia from intestinal bacterial translocation.

CONTRAINDICATIONS

Oral medications until vomiting/gastroenteritis has been controlled.

ALTERNATIVE DRUG(S)

None

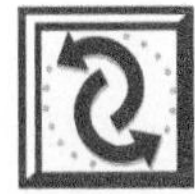

FOLLOW-UP

PATIENT MONITORING

- Monitor hydration and electrolyte balance closely.
- Monitor CBC every 24–48h until recovery.

PREVENTION/AVOIDANCE

- Contaminated environments (e.g., cages, floors, food and water dishes) should be disinfected with 1 : 32 dilution of bleach.
- FPV resistant to most commercial disinfectants.

Vaccines

- FP vaccines are core vaccines—to be given to all cats.
- FP is preventable by routine vaccination of kittens.
- MLV vaccines are available for parenteral injection or intranasal administration; MLV vaccine is preferred, with exceptions, as it may provide better protection.
- Inactivated vaccine is available for parenteral injection.
- Do not use MLV vaccines in pregnant cats or kittens younger than 4 weeks old.
- Immunity—long duration, perhaps even for life.
- Kittens—vaccinate as early as 6 weeks of age, then every 3–4 weeks until 16–20 weeks of age; American Association of Feline Practitioners vaccination guidelines now recommend the last vaccine to be given when kitten is at least 16 weeks old, instead of 12 weeks, because maternal antibodies may not have waned until 16 weeks of age.
- Boosters—1 year after last kitten vaccine; then repeat every 3 years.

POSSIBLE COMPLICATIONS

- Shock, sepsis—severe dehydration, hypoglycemia, hypoproteinemia bacterial translocation, electrolyte imbalance.
- Chronic enteritis—fungal or other cause.
- Teratogenic effects (cerebellar hypoplasia resulting in ataxia for life)—virus infection of fetus.
- Concurrent infection with intestinal parasites.

EXPECTED COURSE AND PROGNOSIS

- Most cases acute, lasting only 5–7 days.
- Guarded prognosis during acute disease, especially if WBC count <2,000 cells/μL.
- Approximately 50% mortality has been reported.
- If patient survives acute disease, recovery usually rapid and uncomplicated.

MISCELLANEOUS

ASSOCIATED CONDITIONS

Viral upper respiratory diseases—feline viral rhinotracheitis and feline calicivirus infection.

AGE-RELATED FACTORS

- Clinical—typically in kittens.
- Subclinical—usually adults.

ZOONOTIC POTENTIAL

None

PREGNANCY/FERTILITY/BREEDING

- Unvaccinated pregnant cats at great risk of infection.
- Fetuses almost always become infected with fatal or teratogenic effects, even when dam has subclinical infection.
- Fetal resorption, abortion, fetal mummification, stillbirth, or birth of weak, fading kittens.
- Kittens may have cerebellar hypoplasia.

SYNONYMS

- Feline distemper.
- Feline parvovirus infection.
- Feline viral enteritis.

ABBREVIATIONS

- CPV = canine parvovirus.
- FeLV = feline leukemia virus.
- FP = feline panleukopenia.
- FPV = feline parvovirus.
- MLV = modified live virus.
- WBC = white blood cell.

Suggested Reading

Greene CE. Feline enteric viral infections. In: Greene CE, ed., Infectious Diseases of the Dog and Cat, 4th ed. St. Louis, MO: Saunders Elsevier, 2012, pp. 80–91.

Kruse BD, Unterer S, Horlacher K, et al. Prognostic factors in cats with feline panleukopenia. J Vet Intern Med 2010, 24:1271–1276.

Lappin MR, Veir J, Hawley J. Feline panleukopenia virus, feline herpesvirus-1, and feline calicivirus antibody responses in seronegative specific pathogen-free cats after a single administration of two different modified live FVRCP vaccines. J Feline Med Surg 2009, 11:159–162.

Porporato F, Horzinek MC, Hoffman-Lehmann R, et al. Survival estimates and outcome predictors for shelter cats with feline panleukopenia virus infection. J Am Vet Med Assoc 2018, 253:188–195.

Scherk MA, Ford RB, Gaskell RM, et al. 2013 AAFP Feline Vaccination Advisory Panel Report. J Feline Med Surg 2013, 15:785–808.

Truyen U, Addie D, Belák S, et al. Feline panleukopenia: ABCD guidelines on prevention and management. J Feline Med Surg 2009, 11:538–546.

Author Julie M. Walker

Consulting Editor Amie Koenig

Acknowledgment The author and book editors acknowledge the prior contribution of Fred W. Scott.

Client Education Handout available online

FELINE PARANEOPLASTIC ALOPECIA

BASICS

OVERVIEW

- Rare condition characterized by cutaneous lesions that serve as markers of internal neoplasia.
- Most affected cats have pancreatic adenocarcinoma with metastases to liver, lungs, pleura, and/or peritoneum; reports of other neoplasias.
- Link between internal malignancies and cutaneous lesions is unknown; may involve cytokines producing atrophy of hair follicles.

SIGNALMENT

- Domestic shorthair cats only reported cases. Median age—13 years; range: 7–16 years.

SIGNS

- Decrease in appetite followed by rapid weight loss and excessive shedding.
- Pruritus—variable; sometimes with excessive grooming.
- Hairs epilate easily leading to severe alopecia on ventral neck, abdomen, medial thighs; rapidly progressive.
- Stratum corneum may "peel," leading to glistening appearance to skin.
- Alopecic skin is shiny, inelastic, and thin, but not fragile.
- Gray lentigines may develop in alopecic areas.
- Footpads may be fissured and/or scaly; often painful.

CAUSES & RISK FACTORS

- Majority of cases are associated with underlying pancreatic adenocarcinoma.
- Other associated tumor types include cholangiocarcinoma, hepatocellular carcinoma, intestinal carcinoma, neuroendocrine pancreatic neoplasia, and hepatosplenic plasma cell tumor.

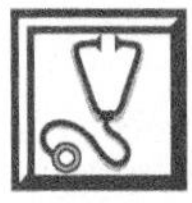

DIAGNOSIS

DIFFERENTIAL DIAGNOSIS

- Hyperadrenocorticism—polyuria, polydipsia, and skin fragility.
- Hyperthyroidism—polyphagia.
- Feline symmetrical alopecia—hair loss self-induced; not associated with easy epilation.
- Thymoma—skin is thick, scaly, and fissured; lymphocytic interface dermatitis; radiographs reveal thoracic mass.
- Demodicosis—mites not associated with paraneoplastic alopecia.
- Dermatophytosis—hair loss often associated with breakage, not spontaneous shedding; inappetence and weight loss rare.
- Alopecia areata—rarely involves entire ventral surface; inappetence and weight loss rare.
- Telogen effluvium—not associated with miniaturization of hair follicles.
- Skin fragility syndrome—markedly thin skin with lacerations; not always associated with exfoliation.
- Superficial necrolytic dermatitis—not associated with marked exfoliation and miniaturization of hair follicles.

CBC/BIOCHEMISTRY/URINALYSIS

No consistent abnormalities; may be helpful in ruling out other differentials.

OTHER LABORATORY TESTS

- Endocrine (thyroid profiles and dexamethasone suppression test)—endocrine disease.
- Skin scrapings—demodicosis.
- KOH examination of hairs and/or fungal culture—dermatophytosis.
- Skin cytology—possible secondary *Malassezia* infection (causing pruritus).

IMAGING

- Ultrasonography—pancreatic mass and/or nodular lesions in liver, intestines, or peritoneal cavity; failure to demonstrate nodules does not exclude the diagnosis, neoplasia may be too small for detection.
- Thoracic radiographs—metastatic lesions in lungs or pleural cavity.

DIAGNOSTIC PROCEDURES

- Skin biopsy.
- Laparoscopy or exploratory laparotomy—identify primary and metastatic tumors.

PATHOLOGIC FINDINGS

- Skin—nonscarring alopecia; severe atrophy of hair follicles and adnexa; miniaturization of hair bulbs; mild to severe acanthosis; variable absence of stratum corneum; variable mixed superficial perivascular infiltrates of neutrophils, eosinophils, and mononuclear cells; some have secondary *Malassezia* infections.
- Primary tumor—usually pancreatic adenocarcinoma, rarely primary bile duct cholangiocarcinoma, hepatocellular or intestinal carcinomas, other pancreatic tumors (neuroendocrine), and hepatosplenic plasma cell tumor. • Metastatic nodules—common in liver, lungs, pleura, and peritoneum.

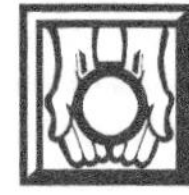

TREATMENT

- Removal of tumor via surgery may be curative; prognosis guarded, as majority of cases have metastatic disease.
- Chemotherapy or other medications—no reported response.
- Affected animals rapidly deteriorate; euthanasia should be suggested.
- Supportive care—only if owners refuse to consider euthanasia; feed highly palatable, nutrient-dense foods and/or tube feed.

MEDICATIONS

DRUG(S) OF CHOICE

N/A

FOLLOW-UP

EXPECTED COURSE AND PROGNOSIS

- Progressive deterioration.
- Supportive care—ultrasonography and thoracic radiographs may demonstrate progression of metastatic disease.
- Death most often occurs within 2–20 weeks after onset of skin lesions.

MISCELLANEOUS

SEE ALSO

Adenocarcinoma, Pancreas.

Suggested Reading

Caporali C, Albanese F, Binanti D, Abramos F. Two cases of feline paraneoplastic alopecia associated with a neuroendocrine pancreatic neoplasia and a hepatosplenic plasma cell tumour. Vet Dermatol 2016, 27:508–513.

Grandt LM, Roethig A, Schroeder S, et al. Feline paraneoplastic alopecia associated with metastasising intestinal carcinoma. J Fel Med Surg 2015, 1(2):2055116915621582. doi: 10.1177/2055116915621582

Outerbridge CA. Cutaneous manifestations of internal diseases. Vet Clin North Am Small Anim Pract 2013, 43:135–152.

Author Karen L. Campbell

Consulting Editor Alexander H. Werner Resnick

FELINE STOMATITIS—FELINE CHRONIC GINGIVOSTOMATITIS (FCGS)

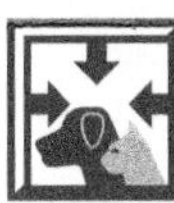

BASICS

OVERVIEW

- Inflammatory response affecting the oral cavity in cats.
- FCGS oropharyngeal inflammation is classified by location as:
  - Alveolar mucositis (alveolar stomatitis)—inflammation of alveolar mucosa (i.e., mucosa overlying the alveolar process and extending from the mucogingival junction without obvious demarcation to the vestibular sulcus and to the floor of the mouth).
  - Caudal mucositis—inflammation of mucosa of the caudal oral cavity, bordered medially by the palatoglossal folds and fauces, dorsally by the hard and soft palate, and rostrally by alveolar and buccal mucosa.
  - Glossitis—inflammation of mucosa of the dorsal and/or ventral surface of the tongue.
  - Stomatitis—inflammation of the mucous lining of any of the structures in the mouth; in clinical use the term should be reserved to describe widespread oral inflammation (beyond gingivitis and periodontitis) that may also extend into submucosal tissues.

SIGNALMENT

- Cats.
- Purebred breeds predisposed—Abyssinian, Persian, Himalayan, Burmese, Siamese, and Somali.

SIGNS

- Ptyalism.
- Halitosis.
- Dysphagia.
- Anorexia—and/or prefers soft food.
- Weight loss.
- Scruffy hair coat from lack of grooming.
- Erythematous, ulcerative, proliferative lesions affecting gingiva, glossopalatine arches, tongue, lips, buccal mucosa, and/or hard palate.
- Gingival inflammation commonly completely surrounds the tooth, compared with gingivitis, which usually occurs on buccal and labial surfaces.
- May extend to glossopharyngeal arches as well as palate.

CAUSES & RISK FACTORS

- Cause unknown; bacterial, viral, and immunologic etiologies suspected.
- Significant findings of feline calicivirus; however, calicivirus load does not correlate with degree of inflammation or prognosis of positive therapy.
- Immunosuppression from feline leukemia virus (FeLV) or feline immunodeficiency virus (FIV) can also lead to poorly responsive infections; most affected cats are negative for FeLV. Concomitant FIV infection is not uncommon.

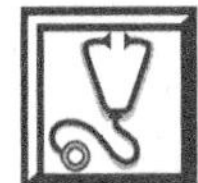

DIAGNOSIS

DIFFERENTIAL DIAGNOSIS

- Periodontal disease.
- Oral malignancy.
- Eosinophilic granuloma complex.

CBC/BIOCHEMISTRY/URINALYSIS

- Elevated globulin—polyclonal gammopathy secondary to antibody production following bacterial invasion into periodontal tissues.
- Leukocytosis and eosinophilia may be present.

IMAGING

Intraoral radiographs to evaluate periodontal disease and tooth resorption.

DIAGNOSTIC PROCEDURES

- Biopsy (especially unilateral lesions) to rule out neoplasia—primarily squamous cell carcinoma.
- Calicivirus, *Bartonella*, and oral bacterial culture and sensitivity testing not recommended.

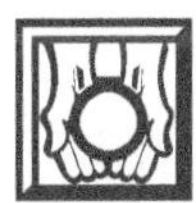

TREATMENT

- Prognosis for cats whose lesions do not include caudal oral mucosa is better than those affected by caudal stomatitis.
- Initial therapy for early cases of alveolar mucositis involves dental scaling above and below gingiva and treatment (extraction) for teeth affected with grades 3 and 4 periodontal disease and/or tooth resorption.
- For cases of focal vestibular and alveolar mucositis, extraction of locally affected teeth in proximity to lesions usually results in resolution.
- For cases of moderate to marked caudal stomatitis, extraction of all maxillary and mandibular teeth (including root fragments) or those distal to canines (if no clinical evidence of disease affecting canines and incisors) resulted in resolution of inflammation in ~60% of cases without further need for medication, with ~20% of cases requiring control with medication, and ~20% refractory.
- To aid extractions—create a gingival flap in all quadrants for exposure; after completely elevating all roots, use high-speed drill with water spray to create trough of bone where roots were, removing most of keratinized gingiva, periodontal ligament, and periradicular alveolar bone; before suturing, "smooth down" alveolar margin to remove sharp edges with round or football-shaped diamond bur.
- CO_2 laser has been effective as treatment adjunct during initial care, especially in cases of moderate to marked caudal stomatitis; laser helps to remove some of inflamed tissue and bacterial load; laser is set to 4 W of continuous energy; after shielding airway from laser energy with moistened gauze, inflamed areas can be rastered; relasering recommended monthly for 3 months if inflammation persists.
- If patients do not respond to extraction of teeth distal to canines, consider trial of prednisolone 2 mg/kg every other day to control the inflammation, or remove all teeth; when extracting teeth, pay meticulous attention to removing all dental hard tissue; take intraoral radiographs before and after surgery; postoperative application of fluocinonide 0.05% (Lidex Gel) to gingival margin may help healing.
- Refractory cases with extensive proliferative lesion in caudal oral cavity and pharynx warrant more guarded prognosis.

F

MEDICATIONS

DRUG(S) OF CHOICE

- Medication and other therapies have been used with limited long-term success; lack of permanent response to conventional oral hygiene, antibiotics, anti-inflammatory drugs, and immunosuppressive drugs is typical; medications should not be regarded as primary method to control oropharyngeal inflammation.
- Antibiotics—clindamycin 5 mg/kg q12h, metronidazole, amoxicillin, ampicillin, enrofloxacin, tetracycline.
- Corticosteroids—prednisone 2 mg/kg initially daily, followed by every other day; methylprednisolone acetate 2 mg/kg q7–30 days may also help control inflammation.
- Gold salts—Solganal 1 mg/kg IM weekly until improvement (up to 4 months), then every 14–35 days.
- Chlorambucil—2 mg/m^2 PO every other day or 20 mg/m^2 every other week.
- Bovine lactoferrin—40 mg/kg applied to oral mucous membranes.
- Interferon—alpha or omega 30 IU/day 7 days on, 7 days off, indefinitely.
- CO_2 laser to decrease inflamed tissue.
- Cyclosporine—2 mg/kg BID.

FOLLOW-UP

PATIENT MONITORING

- Recommend 2- and 4-week postoperative examinations to determine success of surgical procedure.
- Soft diet should be encouraged for 2 weeks postoperatively, though some cats may not accept any dietary changes well.

PREVENTION/AVOIDANCE

N/A

POSSIBLE COMPLICATIONS

Wound dehiscence; inappetence, refractory caudal inflammation.

EXPECTED COURSE AND PROGNOSIS

- Caudal mouth extractions have been shown to greatly improve large percentage of patients; full-mouth extractions sometimes warranted.
- Refractory cases with extensive proliferative lesion in caudal oral cavity and pharynx warrant more guarded prognosis.

MISCELLANEOUS

ASSOCIATED CONDITIONS

- Lymphocytic plasmacytic stomatitis.
- Stomatitis.

ABBREVIATIONS

- FeLV = feline leukemia virus.
- FIV = feline immunodeficiency virus.

INTERNET RESOURCES

https://avdc.org/avdc-nomenclature

Suggested Reading

Bellows, JE. Feline Dentistry. Oxford: Wiley-Blackwell, 2010.

Druet I, Hennet P, Relationship between *Feline calicivirus* load, oral lesions, and outcome in feline chronic gingivostomatitis (caudal stomatitis): retrospective study in 104 cats. Front Vet Sci 2017, 4:209. doi: 10.3389/fvets.2017.00209

Wiggs RB, Lobrise HB. Veterinary Dentistry: Principles and Practice. Philadelphia, PA: Lippincott-Raven, 1997.

Author Jan Bellows

Consulting Editor Heidi B. Lobprise

Client Education Handout available online

FELINE SYMMETRICAL ALOPECIA

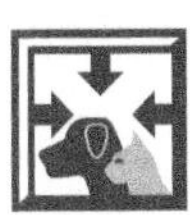

BASICS

OVERVIEW

- Alopecia in a symmetrical pattern with no gross changes in the skin.
- Common clinical presentation in cats.
- Similar manifestation for many different underlying disorders.

SIGNALMENT

No age, breed, or sex predilection reported.

SIGNS

- Total to partial hair loss; most often symmetrical but can occur in a patchy distribution.
- Areas of the body commonly affected—ventrum, caudal dorsum, and lateral and caudal thighs.
- Affected areas are often those accessible for grooming.
- Patchy areas of hair loss (unsymmetrical) on distal extremities or body.

CAUSES & RISK FACTORS

- Cutaneous hypersensitivity—flea allergic dermatitis, food, atopy.
- Ectoparasites—flea bite dermatitis, Cheyletiellosis, *Otodectes cynotis*.
- Infection—dermatophytosis.
- Neurologic or behavioral—"psychogenic alopecia" (uncommon as primary cause of symptoms).
- Stress or metabolic—telogen effluvium.
- Neoplasia—pancreatic neoplasia (paraneoplastic alopecia).
- Hyperadrenocorticism.
- Alopecia areata.
- Hyperthyroidism (early sign).

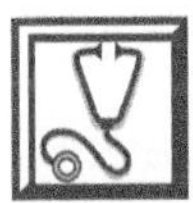

DIAGNOSIS

DIFFERENTIAL DIAGNOSIS

See Causes & Risk Factors.

CBC/BIOCHEMISTRY/URINALYSIS

Eosinophilia may occur with hypersensitivities.

OTHER LABORATORY TESTS

Serum thyroxine—hyperthyroidism.

IMAGING

N/A

DIAGNOSTIC PROCEDURES

- Flea combing—identify fleas, flea excrement, or both.
- Microscopic examination of hair—self-induced hair loss results in broken blunt shafts; endogenous hair loss results in tapered ends (telogen hairs).
- Fecal examination—excess hair, mites, and ova (*Cheyletiella*), tapeworm, or fleas.
- Food elimination diet trial—adverse reactions to food.
- Intradermal allergy testing—atopy.
- Skin biopsy—confirm/exclude presence of underlying cause (e.g., hypersensitivity dermatitis vs. psychogenic, or rarely systemic disease).
- Cytology of papules or crusts, if present, may have large numbers of eosinophils.
- Microscopic examination of skin scrapings—ectoparasites.
- Hair plucks (trichogram)—dermatophyte arthrospores or *Demodex* mites adjacent to hair shafts.

PATHOLOGIC FINDINGS

- Histopathologic findings—vary depending on cause.
- Feline psychogenic alopecia—hair follicles and skin normal.
- High numbers of mast cells, eosinophils, lymphocytes, or macrophages suggest allergic dermatitis.
- Alopecia areata—lymphocytic inflammation that encircles bulb portions of hair follicles; rare.

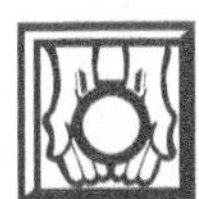

TREATMENT

- Management of underlying cause.
- Inform the owner of the diagnostic plan and the time it could take to see a response (hair coat regrowth).
- Environmental enrichment in cases of true psychogenic cause.

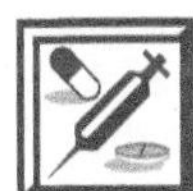

MEDICATIONS

DRUG(S) OF CHOICE

- Antihistamines—e.g., chlorpheniramine 0.5 mg/kg PO q8h; cetirizine 5 mg/cat q12–24h.
- Glucocorticosteroid—prednisolone 0.5 mg/kg PO, tapering/alternate-day therapy.
- Amitriptyline—1–2 mg/kg PO daily.
- Clomipramine hydrochloride—0.5 mg/kg q24h.
- Cyclosporine, modified—5–7 mg/kg PO daily; tapering therapy.

CONTRAINDICATIONS/POSSIBLE INTERACTIONS

- Glucocorticosteroids—can cause alopecia, diabetes mellitus, polydipsia, polyuria, polyphagia, and weight gain; can suppress pruritus, making it difficult to determine underlying cause.
- Withdraw antipruritic medications (including glucocorticosteroids) as diagnostic tests near completion (e.g., restricted-ingredient food trials).

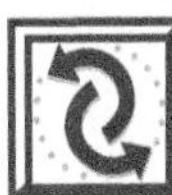

FOLLOW-UP

- Frequent examinations are essential in confirming differential diagnoses.
- Successful identification of underlying cause offers best prognosis, if cause can be controlled (e.g., flea bites or food hypersensitivity).

MISCELLANEOUS

INTERNET RESOURCES

https://indoorpet.osu.edu/cats

Suggested Reading

Helton Rhodes KA, Werner A. Blackwell's Five-Minute Veterinary Consult Clinical Companion: Small Animal Dermatology, 3rd ed. Hoboken, NJ: Wiley-Blackwell, 2018.

Mertens PA, Torres S, Jessen C. The effects of clomipramine hydrochloride in cats with psychogenic alopecia: a prospective study. J Am Anim Hosp Assoc 2006, 42(5):336–343.

Sawyer LS, Moon-Fanelli AA, Dodman NH. Psychogenic alopecia in cats: 11 cases (1993–1996). J Am Vet Med Assoc 1999, 214(1):71–74.

Waisglass SE, Landsberg GM, Yager JA, Hall JA. Underlying medical conditions in cats with presumptive psychogenic alopecia. J Am Vet Med Assoc 2006, 228(11):1705–1709.

Author David D. Duclos

Consulting Editor Alexander H. Werner Resnick

FELINE TOOTH RESORPTION (ODONTOCLASTIC RESORPTION)

BASICS

DEFINITION

Tooth resorption (TR) is resorption of dental hard tissues (cementum, dentin, and in late stages also enamel).

PATHOPHYSIOLOGY

- Odontoclasts deriving from hematopoietic stem cells migrate to the external root surface, where they start resorption of cementum and dentin.
- TR is often preceded by dentoalveolar ankylosis (fusion between alveolar bone and the root with disappearance of the periodontal ligament space). The alveolar bone (already in a state of constant resorption and apposition) will then include the tooth in its normal remodeling process, which results in noninflammatory replacement resorption. If TR progresses coronally and emerges at the gingival margin, an inflammatory component through contact with oral bacteria joins the initially noninflammatory process, and inflamed granulation tissue may form to cover defects in the crown of the tooth (inflammatory resorption).
- TR in cats most commonly starts anywhere on the external root (not crown) surface and not just close to the cementoenamel junction.

SYSTEMS AFFECTED

Gastrointestinal—oral cavity.

INCIDENCE/PREVALENCE

At least one-third of cats may develop TR during life, with the risk of developing TR increasing with age. Reported prevalence (25–75%) greatly depends on the population of animals investigated (general practice versus dental specialist practice) and the diagnostic methods applied (observation only, tactile exploration with an instrument, and/or use of dental radiography).

SIGNALMENT

Species

Cats

Breed Predilections

Persian longhaired cats reported to have TR at a younger age compared with other breeds.

Mean Age and Range

Rarely seen in cats less than 2 years of age; first teeth usually affected at 4–6 years of age.

SIGNS

Historical Findings

Most affected cats do not show clinical signs, in particular when teeth are affected by replacement resorption only (which is asymptomatic) and the TR is located apical to the gingival attachment (not yet exposed to oral bacteria); some show dropping of food while eating, reluctance to eat hard food, and repetitive lower jaw motions ("chattering").

Physical Examination Findings

- Dental deposits, hyperplastic gingiva, and granulation tissue often cover a clinically evident TR emerging at the gingival margin. A dental explorer can be used under general anesthesia to detect irregularities at the tooth surface near the gingival margin.
- TR occurs more often on the labial and buccal aspects of premolar and molar teeth, and less commonly on canine and incisor teeth. The mandibular third premolar teeth are usually the first teeth affected by TR.
- Canine teeth (in particular maxillary) often appear to extrude excessively (abnormal tooth extrusion), leading to exposure of the root surface. Thickening of alveolar bone with local osteomyelitis (alveolar bone expansion) is often associated with this phenomenon.

Classification of Tooth Resorption

- American Veterinary Dental College (AVDC) currently suggests classification based on the severity (stages 1–5) and radiographic appearance of the resorption (types 1–3):
    - Stage 1 (TR1)—mild dental hard tissue loss (cementum or cementum and enamel).
    - Stage 2 (TR2)—moderate dental hard tissue loss (cementum or cementum and enamel with loss of dentin that does not extend to the pulp cavity).
    - Stage 3 (TR3)—deep dental hard tissue loss (cementum or cementum and enamel with loss of dentin that extends to the pulp cavity) with most of the tooth still retaining its integrity.
    - Stage 4 (TR4)—extensive dental hard tissue loss (cementum or cementum and enamel with loss of dentin that extends to the pulp cavity) with most of the tooth having lost its integrity; there are substages TR4a (crown and root equally affected), TR4b (crown more severely affected than root, and TR4c (root more severely affected than crown).
    - Stage 5 (TR5)—remnants of dental hard tissue are visible only as irregular radiopacities with complete gingival covering.
- See Imaging for additional classification scheme (types 1–3).

CAUSES

- Etiology is unknown; possibly multifactorial (e.g., nutritional, inflammatory, and hereditary).
- One hypothesis is that chronic dietary intake of excess vitamin D would lead to periodontal ligament degeneration, hypercementosis, hyperosteoidosis, narrowing of the periodontal ligament space, dentoalveolar ankylosis, and replacement resorption. If such a process occurred close to the gingival attachment, an inflammatory component would join the initially noninflammatory disease.

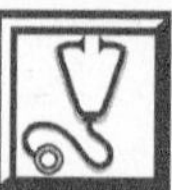

DIAGNOSIS

DIFFERENTIAL DIAGNOSIS

Periodontal disease, stomatitis.

IMAGING

- Without dental radiography, TR below the gingival attachment (and thus the vast majority of TR) will not be detectable.
- On a radiograph of a tooth with type 1 resorption, a focal or multifocal radiolucency is present in the tooth with otherwise normal radiopacity and normal-appearing periodontal ligament space. On a radiograph of a tooth with type 2 resorption, there is narrowing or disappearance of the periodontal ligament space in at least some areas and decreased radiopacity of part of the tooth. On a radiograph of a tooth with type 3 resorption, features of both type 1 and type 2 resorptions are present in the same tooth; the affected tooth shows areas of normal and narrow or lost periodontal ligament space, and there is focal or multifocal radiolucency in the tooth and decreased radiopacity in other areas of the tooth.
- For example, a clinically evident TR emerging at the gingival margin (inflammatory resorption) will generally be visible as a notched radiolucency in the tooth with sharp or scalloped margins (type 1 resorption). The periodontal ligament space may be of normal width apical to the TR, but there will be horizontal or vertical loss of alveolar bone adjacent to the TR. Lesions on mesial and distal tooth surfaces or in the furcation area usually are more obvious on radiographs than those on labial/buccal and lingual/palatal tooth surfaces.
- Fusion of the root and alveolar bone (dentoalveolar ankylosis) results in focalized or generalized disappearance of the periodontal ligament space and lamina dura on radiographs. Resorbed dental tissue will gradually be replaced by bone (replacement resorption). The root will take on a striated or moth-eaten appearance ("ghost roots"), and the periodontal ligament space and lamina dura will disappear on radiographs (type 2 resorption). Unlike inflammatory resorption, adjacent bone usually is not resorbed.

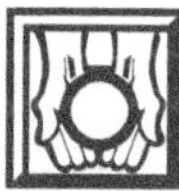

TREATMENT

DIET

Add water to hard kibble to soften it.

CLIENT EDUCATION

Daily tooth brushing or other means of home oral hygiene may help control plaque and allow for earlier detection of teeth affected by TR.

SURGICAL CONSIDERATIONS

- The treatment of choice for teeth with TR is complete extraction. Multirooted teeth are sectioned after creation of a flap and removal of alveolar bone on labial and buccal aspects of the roots so that each single-rooted crown–root segment can be elevated and removed. Resorbing root remnants under noninflamed and intact gingiva (often appearing as a small gingival bulge) and without periapical pathology on dental radiographs may be left where they are. However, root remnants underneath inflamed gingiva with sinus tracts must be extracted.
- Teeth with dentoalveolar ankylosis and replacement resorption can be treated by means of crown amputation and intentional retention of resorbing root tissue. A flap is made, the crown is removed with a water-cooled round bur to, or slightly below, the level of the alveolar margin, and the wound is rinsed and closed by suturing. Contraindications include periodontitis, endodontic and periapical disease, and stomatitis.
- Canine teeth exhibiting moderate to severe abnormal extrusion and alveolar bone expansion should be treated with an open extraction so that a flap can be used to close the wound.

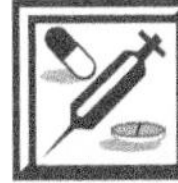

MEDICATIONS

Topical chlorhexidine or zinc ascorbate gel applied to the mouth once a day.

FOLLOW-UP

PATIENT MONITORING

- Recommend 2-week postoperative examination to determine success of surgical procedure.
- Soft diet should be encouraged for 2 weeks postoperatively, though some cats may not accept any dietary changes well.

PREVENTION/AVOIDANCE

N/A

POSSIBLE COMPLICATIONS

Wound dehiscence.

EXPECTED COURSE AND PROGNOSIS

Additional teeth may develop TR in the future, so monitoring with dental radiographs is warranted.

MISCELLANEOUS

SYNONYMS

Feline odontoclastic resorptive lesion (FORL).

ABBREVIATIONS

- TR = Tooth resorption.

Author Alexander M. Reiter

Consulting Editor Heidi B. Lobprise

Acknowledgment The author and book editors acknowledge the prior contribution of Jan Bellows.

Client Education Handout available online

F

FELINE (UPPER) RESPIRATORY INFECTIONS

BASICS

DEFINITION

- Viral, bacterial, fungal etiologies.
- Most cats harbor viral causes and become clinical with stress.
- Viral upper respiratory infection (URI) very common, secondary bacterial infections common; primary bacterial rhinitis uncommon.
- Most organisms spread through direct contact, air (droplets from coughing, sneezing, or discharge), and contaminated surfaces (e.g., shared bowls, cages).
- Illness typified by rhinosinusitis, conjunctivitis, lacrimation, salivation, oral ulcerations.

PATHOPHYSIOLOGY

- Feline herpesvirus (FHV) induces marked rhinitis, sneezing, and conjunctivitis, and may lead to chronic signs; cats are infected for life, with latent virus sequestered in trigeminal nerve ganglion.
- FHV infects epithelial cells of respiratory tract, conjunctiva, and/or cornea; during primary infection or recrudescence, direct effect is cytolysis of infected cells and necrosis of affected tissues; inflammatory disease can occur via immune-mediated response to infection; turbinate lysis can occur.
- Feline calicivirus (FCV) has predilection for epithelial cells of oral cavity and upper respiratory tract; causes rhinitis, stomatitis, oral ulceration: ulcers start as vesicles; some strains infect lungs and can cause focal alveolitis and interstitial pneumonia; other strains cause "limping syndrome."
- FCV–virulent systemic disease (VSD) caused by hypervirulent strains that can infect endothelium of liver, lungs, and pancreas, leading to severe systemic illness characterized by vasculitis; results in edema, alopecia, ulcers, and can cause multiple organ dysfunction syndrome (MODS), systemic inflammatory response syndrome (SIRS), disseminated intravascular coagulation, death.
- *Chlamydophila felis* predominantly infects conjunctiva and causes conjunctivitis; has also been associated with URI.
- Bacterial infection—often secondary to viral disease, trauma, allergic rhinitis.
- *Cryptococcus* affects rostral nasal cavity resulting in rhinitis and turbinate lysis; granulomatous protuberances can occur; destruction of adjacent facial bones facilitates spread of infection to contiguous regions, such as bridge and side of nose, nasal planum, or hard palate, resulting in facial distortion; infection can spread through cribriform plate, resulting in meningoencephalitis, cryptococcal optic neuritis, secondary retinitis.

SYSTEMS AFFECTED

- Respiratory—nasal and upper airway, including sinuses, lower airway.
- Ophthalmologic—conjunctiva.
- Musculoskeletal—FCV.
- Integument/mucous membranes—FHV, *Cryptococcus*.
- Neurologic—*Cryptococcus*, lymph.
- VSD can affect many organ systems.

GENETICS

N/A

INCIDENCE/PREVALENCE

- FHV and FCV most common causes of URI.
- Over 90% of cats are seropositive for FHV.
- Conjunctivitis is most common disease caused by FHV, most common feline ophthalmic disease.
- Carrier states exist for FHV, FCV (10–75%).
- *C. felis*—1–5% for cats without signs of respiratory tract disease, 10–30% for cats with conjunctivitis or URI.
- *Bordetella bronchiseptica*—seroprevalence of 24–79%, isolation rates up to 47% reported.

GEOGRAPHIC DISTRIBUTION

- Ubiquitous.
- *Cryptococcus*—worldwide, associated with pigeon guano.

SIGNALMENT

- Species—cat.
- Breed predilection—N/A.
- Mean age/range—more common in younger cats, though viral flare-ups can occur through life.
- Predominant sex—N/A.

SIGNS

Historical Findings

- Exposure to other cats common; stress, steroids, immunosuppression may precipitate clinical signs for viral causes.
- Caretakers may report upper respiratory signs, weight loss, anorexia, gagging, halitosis, depression.

Physical Examination Findings

- Depend on organism.
- Frequently—sneezing, nasal discharge, stertor, halitosis, ocular discharge, inappetence.
- FHV—fever, sneezing, nasal discharge, conjunctivitis, ulcerative stomatitis, ulcerative keratitis, blepharospasm, salivation, depression, anorexia.
- FCV—fever, salivation and ulceration of tongue, hard palate, or nostrils, stomatitis, gingivitis, rhinitis, conjunctivitis, coughing, dyspnea, lameness.
- With VSD—peripheral edema, dermal ulcers, icterus possible.
- *B. bronchiseptica*—fever, sneezing, ocular discharge, nasal discharge, lymphadenopathy, coughing, dyspnea, cyanosis.
- *Cryptococcus*—sneezing, nasal discharge, ocular discharge, gagging, dysphagia, stertor, upper airway obstruction, facial deformity, lymphadenopathy, neurologic abnormalities, optic neuritis, chorioretinitis.
- *C. felis*—conjunctivitis, occasional sneeze, fever.
- *Mycoplasma* spp.—conjunctivitis, ocular and nasal discharge, dyspnea.

CAUSES

- Viral—FHV, FCV, influenza.
- Primary bacterial—*B. bronchiseptica, C. felis, Streptococcus canis, Mycoplasma* spp.
- Secondary bacterial invaders—*Corynebacterium* spp., *Escherichia coli, Pasturella multocida, Pseudomonas aeruginosa, Streptococcus* spp., *Staphylococcus* spp.
- Fungal—*Cryptococcus neoformans, Sporothrix schenckii, Aspergillus* spp., *Penicillium* spp.

RISK FACTORS

- Stress/steroids.
- Decreased immune function, feline immunodeficiency virus (FIV)/feline leukemia virus (FeLV) infection.
- Multicat households, shelters, young cats.

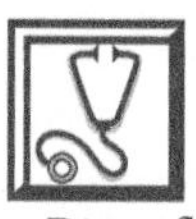

DIAGNOSIS

- Direct fluorescent staining of conjunctival scraping—FHV.
- PCR for *B. bronchiseptica* (controversial if positive), *Chlamydophila felis*, FCV, FHV, H7N2 influenza virus, influenza A virus (including H7N2, H3N2, H1N1, H3N8), *Mycoplasma felis*.
- Viral isolation.
- Mycoplasma culture.
- *Cryptococcus*—direct microscopic visualization of organisms in nasal discharge or tissue: cytology or histopathology, culture, serology; latex agglutination to identify antigen.

DIFFERENTIAL DIAGNOSIS

- Nasopharyngeal polyps.
- Nasopharyngeal stenosis.
- Foreign body.
- Neoplasia.
- Dental disease—tooth root abscess.
- Anatomic defects.
- Trauma.
- Burn—caustic agent or electrical.

CBC/BIOCHEMISTRY/URINALYSIS

Generally normal with most etiologies—with virulent systemic FCV may see inflammatory leukogram, thrombocytopenia, elevated liver enzymes/total bilirubin.

OTHER LABORATORY TESTS

- Culture of upper airways.
- Lymph node cytology.
- Nasal biopsies.

IMAGING

- Skull radiographs generally not helpful.
- Thoracic radiography—generally normal, may see pulmonary involvement if fungal disease or pneumonia.

• CT of head—may show mass, turbinate lysis, increased soft tissue within nasal passages, lymphadenopathy.

DIAGNOSTIC PROCEDURES

• Conjunctival scraping may identify FHV.
• Rhinoscopy—in cats with *Cryptococcus.*
• Upper airway exam.
• Bronchoalveolar lavage if pneumonia suspected.
• FIV antibody, FeLV antigen testing.

PATHOLOGIC FINDINGS

Histopathology—lymphoplasmacytic stomatitis: FCV; vasculitis: FCV–VSD; bacterial rhinitis, suppurative inflammation; *Cryptococcus* organisms on nasal or lymph node biopsy.

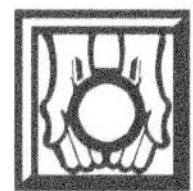

TREATMENT

APPROPRIATE HEALTH CARE

• Most cats managed as outpatient; isolate if hospitalized, as many organisms highly contagious and airborne.
• Moderate to severely affected cats may require IV fluids for hydration.
• May require supplemental oxygen.

ACTIVITY

N/A

DIET

• Enteral feeding recommended if anorexia persists >48 hours.
• Nasogastric feeding may not be appropriate if there is severe nasal discharge.
• Cats with severe oral ulceration may need enteric feeding while ulcers heal.

CLIENT EDUCATION

Most agents are contagious.

SURGICAL CONSIDERATIONS

Corneal ulcers can be deep, may require surgical intervention.

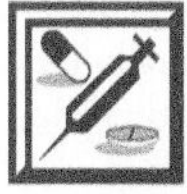

MEDICATIONS

DRUG(S) OF CHOICE

• Many cases will self-resolve.
• Antibiotics not recommended for cats with only serous discharge; observation without antibiotics recommended for up to 10 days for acute-onset mucopurulent/purulent discharge without systemic signs (fever, lethargy, anorexia) or specific etiology identified by exam or history; susceptibility profiles of organism may be helpful for chronic cases.
  ◦ First choices—doxycycline 10 mg/kg PO q24h, usually effective for *B. bronchiseptica, C. felis, Mycoplasma* spp.; amoxicillin 22 mg/kg, PO, q12h.
  ◦ Other options—amoxicillin–clavulanate 15–20 mg/kg PO q12h, azithromycin 5–15 mg/kg PO q24h, marbofloxacin 2.5–5 mg/kg PO q24h, pradofloxacin 5–10 mg/kg PO q24h.
• Antifungals—fluconazole 50 mg/cat PO q12–24h, itraconazole 10 mg/kg PO q24h; compounded formulations not recommended.
• Antivirals—famciclovir 62.5 mg/cat PO q12h, cidofovir topical 0.5% 1 drop OU q12h.

CONTRAINDICATIONS

Use azole drugs with caution in patients with liver disease.

PRECAUTIONS

Doxycycline can cause esophagitis and esophageal strictures—follow with food and/or water.

POSSIBLE INTERACTIONS

Azole antifungals have many drug interactions.

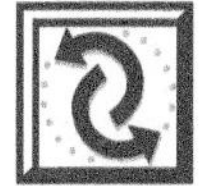

FOLLOW-UP

PATIENT MONITORING

• Viral—most cases improve within 1 week; could take up to 6 weeks to resolve.
• Persistent clinical signs after appropriate treatment suggest alternative cause.

PREVENTION/AVOIDANCE

• Vaccination.
• FCV, FHV—core vaccines; modified live and inactivated virus vaccines give reasonable protection, mild clinical signs may be seen; vaccines do not prevent infection or viral latency, although shedding post challenge may be reduced.
• Vaccination against *C. felis* and *B. bronchiseptica* is noncore.
• Do not allow non-immunocompetent patients to contact other animals until determined to be low risk.
• Bleach diluted 1 : 30 with water mixed with detergent is effective at eliminating most respiratory pathogens from environment.

POSSIBLE COMPLICATIONS

• Pneumonia.
• Septicemia (rare).

EXPECTED COURSE AND PROGNOSIS

• Good to excellent; underlying immunosuppression may increase susceptibility to infection, worsen prognosis.
• FHV—generally, mortality low and prognosis good, except for young kittens and aged cats.
• FCV–VSD—poor, mortality >50%.

MISCELLANEOUS

AGE-RELATED FACTORS

Young animals more susceptible.

ZOONOTIC POTENTIAL

• *B. bronchiseptica* rare cause of zoonotic infections.
• Human conjunctivitis caused by feline chlamydia has been reported.

PREGNANCY/FERTILITY/BREEDING

Animals who are actively ill should not be bred. FHV can cause abortions.

SEE ALSO

• Chlamydiosis—Cats.
• Cryptococcosis.
• Feline Calicivirus Infection.
• Feline Herpesvirus Infection.
• Mycoplasmosis.
• Rhinitis and Sinusitis.

ABBREVIATIONS

• FCV = feline calicivirus.
• FeLV = feline leukemia virus.
• FHV = feline herpesvirus-1.
• FIV = feline immunodeficiency virus.
• MODS = multiple organ dysfunction syndrome.
• SIRS = systemic inflammatory response syndrome.
• VSD = virulent systemic disease.
• URI = upper respiratory infection.

INTERNET RESOURCES

https://catvets.com/guidelines/practice-guidelines/feline-vaccination-guidelines

Suggested Reading

Green CE. Infectious Diseases of the Dog and Cat, 4th ed. St. Louis, MO: Elsevier Saunders, 2012.
Lappin MR, Blondeau J, Boothe D, et al. Antimicrobial use guidelines for treatment of respiratory tract disease in dogs and cats. J Vet Intern Med 2017, 31:279–294.
Little SE. The Cat: Clinical Medicine and Management. St. Louis, MO: Elsevier Saunders, 2012.

Author Genna Atiee
Consulting Editor Amie Koenig

F

FEVER

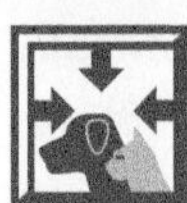

BASICS

DEFINITION

Higher than normal body temperature because of changed thermoregulatory set point in hypothalamus; normal body temperature in dogs and cats 100.2–102.8 °F (37.8–39.3 °C). Fever of unknown origin (FUO)—at least 103.5 °F (39.7 °C) on at least four occasions over 14-day period and illness of 14 days' duration without obvious cause.

PATHOPHYSIOLOGY

Exogenous or endogenous pyrogens reset thermoregulatory center to higher temperature, activating physiologic responses to raise body temperature. Physiologic consequences include increased metabolic demands, muscle catabolism, bone marrow suppression, heightened fluid and caloric requirements, and possibly disseminated intravascular coagulation (DIC) and shock.

SYSTEMS AFFECTED

- Cardiovascular—tachycardia.
- Hemic/lymphatic/immune—bone marrow depression, DIC.
- Nervous—cerebral edema, depression.

SIGNALMENT

Species

Dog and cat.

Breed Predilections

Some breed-associated conditions may result in FUO (e.g., shar-pei fever).

SIGNS

General Comments

- Fever lowers bacterial division and increases immune competence.
- Prolonged fever >105 °F (>40.5 °C) leads to dehydration and anorexia.
- Fevers >106 °F (>41.1 °C) may lead to cerebral edema, bone marrow depression, arrhythmia, electrolyte disorders, multiorgan damage, DIC.

Historical Findings

- Clinical history (e.g., contact with infectious agents, lifestyle, travel, recent vaccination, drug administration, insect bites, previous illness, allergies) and physical examination (including retinal examination) may help identify underlying disease condition.
- Fever patterns (e.g., sustained, intermittent) rarely helpful.

Physical Examination Findings

- Hyperthermia.
- Lethargy.
- Inappetence.
- Tachycardia.
- Tachypnea.
- Hyperemic mucous membranes.
- Dehydration.
- Shock.

CAUSES

Infectious Agents

- Viruses—feline leukemia virus (FeLV), feline immunodeficiency virus (FIV), parvo, distemper, herpes, calici.
- Bacteria—endotoxins, *Mycoplasma*, *Bartonella*, *Leptospira*, *Borrelia burgdorferi*, others.
- Systemic fungi—*Histoplasma*, *Blastomyces*, *Coccidioidomyces*, *Cryptococcus*.
- Vector borne—*Rickettsia*, *Borrelia*, *Ehrlichia*, *Anaplasma*, *Neorickettsia*.
- Parasites and protozoa—*Babesia*, *Toxoplasma*, aberrant larva migrans, *Dirofilaria* thromboemboli, *Leishmania*, *Cytauxzoon*, *Hepatozoon*, *Neospora*.

Immune-Mediated Processes

Systemic lupus erythematosus, immune-mediated hemolytic anemia, immune-mediated thrombocytopenia, pemphigus, polyarthritis, polymyositis, rheumatoid arthritis, vasculitis, hypersensitivity reaction, transfusion reaction, infection secondary to inherited or acquired immune defects.

Endocrine and Metabolic

Hyperthyroidism, hypoadrenocorticism (rare), pheochromocytoma, hyperlipidemia, hypernatremia.

Neoplasia

Lymphoma, myeloproliferative disease, plasma cell neoplasm, mast cell tumor, malignant histiocytosis, metastatic disease, necrotic tumor, and solid tumor, particularly in liver, kidney, bone, lung, lymph nodes.

Other Inflammatory Conditions

Cholangiohepatitis, hepatic lipidosis, toxic hepatopathy, cirrhosis, inflammatory bowel disease, pancreatitis, peritonitis, pleuritis, granulomatous diseases, portosystemic shunting, thrombophlebitis, infarctions, pansteatitis, panosteitis panniculitis, hypertrophic osteodystrophy, blunt trauma, cyclic neutropenia, intracranial lesions, pulmonary thromboembolism.

Drugs and Toxins

Tetracycline, sulfonamide, penicillins, nitrofurantoin, amphotericin B, barbiturates, iodine, atropine, cimetidine, salicylates, antihistamines, procainamide, heavy metals.

FUO—Dogs

- Infection (28%)—discospondylitis, fungal infections, endocarditis, abscesses, bacteremia, septic arthritis, septic meningitis, pyothorax, pulmonary foreign body/abscess, stump pyometra, pneumonia, osteomyelitis, peritonitis, prostatitis, pancreatitis, pyelonephritis, sepsis secondary to immunodeficiency, leptospirosis, leishmaniasis, toxoplasmosis, Lyme disease, infection with *Ehrlichia*, *Anaplasma*, *Bartonella*, others.
- Immune-mediated disease (27%)—polyarthritis, meningitis, vasculitis, others.
- Bone marrow disease, including neoplasia (16%).
- Neoplasia (7%).
- Miscellaneous (10%)—hypertrophic osteodystrophy, lymphadenitis, panosteitis, portosystemic shunting, shar-pei fever.
- Undiagnosed (12%).

FUO—Cats

- Most virally mediated (e.g., FeLV, FIV, feline infectious peritonitis [FIP], less commonly parvo, herpes, calici).
- Occult bacterial infection with atypical bacteria, sometimes secondary to bite wounds (e.g., *Yersinia*, *Mycobacteria*, *Nocardia*, *Actinomyces*, *Brucella*).
- Pyothorax.
- Additional causes—pyelonephritis, blunt trauma, penetrating intestinal lesion, dental abscess, systemic fungal disease, lymphoma, solid tumors.
- Immune disorders, endometritis, discospondylitis, pneumonia, endocarditis rare.

RISK FACTORS

- Recent travel.
- Exposure to biologic agents.
- Immunosuppression.
- Very young or old animals.

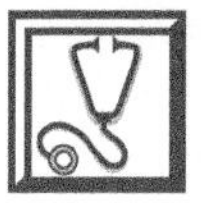

DIAGNOSIS

DIFFERENTIAL DIAGNOSIS

Differentiate fever from hyperthermia. Temperatures up to 103 °F (39.4 °C) may be caused by stress or illness. Temperatures >104 °F (>40 °C) almost always important. Temperatures >107 °F (>41.7 °C) usually not fever, more likely to be primary hyperthermia.

CBC/BIOCHEMISTRY/URINALYSIS

- CBC and blood smear—leukopenia or leukocytosis, left shift, monocytosis, lymphocytosis, thrombocytopenia or thrombocytosis, spherocytes, organisms.
- Biochemistry profile and urinalysis vary with organ system involved.

OTHER LABORATORY TESTS

- If infectious disease suspected, attempt to culture an organism—urine culture, blood cultures (i.e., three anaerobic/aerobic cultures, taken 20 min apart; try to use as much volume as possible to increase diagnostic yield; use special blood culture bottles), fungal and cerebrospinal fluid cultures, synovial and prostatic fluid, biopsy specimens.

• FeLV and FIV test, Snap 4DX test, serologic tests or PCR for *Toxoplasma*, *Borrelia*, *Mycoplasma*, *Bartonella*, *Anaplasma*, *Ehrlichia*, *Rickettsia*, FIP, systemic mycoses.
• Fecal examination.
• Tracheal wash or bronchoalveolar lavage.
• If immune disorders suspected—cytologic examination of synovial fluid; Coombs' test, rheumatoid factor, antinuclear antibodies.
• Pancreatic lipase immunoreactivity.
• T_4 in cats.

IMAGING

Radiography

• Abdominal radiographs—tumors and effusion.
• Thoracic radiographs—pneumonia, neoplasia, pyothorax.
• Survey skeletal radiographs—bone tumors, multiple myeloma, osteomyelitis, discospondylitis, panosteitis, hypertrophic osteopathy, hypertrophic osteodystrophy.
• Dental/skull radiographs—tooth root abscess, sinus infections, foreign bodies, neoplasia.
• Contrast radiography (e.g., gastrointestinal and excretory urography).

Ultrasonography

• Abdominal (plus directed aspirate or biopsy)—abdominal neoplasia, abscess or other site of infection (e.g., pyelonephritis, pancreatitis, pyometra).
• Echocardiography if endocarditis suspected.

Nuclear Imaging

• Radionuclide scanning procedures to evaluate for bone tumors, osteomyelitis, pulmonary embolism.
• CT, MRI, or positron emission tomography scan if indicated.

DIAGNOSTIC PROCEDURES

• Arthrocentesis (culture and cytology).
• Bone marrow aspirate and biopsy if malignancy or myelodysplasia suspected.
• Lymph node, skin, or muscle biopsy if clinically indicated.
• Fine-needle aspirate or biopsy of any mass or abnormal organ.
• Central spinal fluid tap if neurologic signs.
• Endoscopy and biopsy if gastrointestinal signs.
• Exploratory laparotomy—last resort if all other diagnostic tests fail to determine cause and patient not improving.

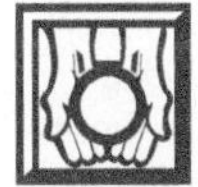

TREATMENT

APPROPRIATE HEALTH CARE

Goals of treatment—reset thermoregulatory set point to lower level; remove underlying cause.

NURSING CARE

• Fluid administration (IV) often lowers body temperature.
• Topical cooling if fever is severe (convection cooling with fans, evaporative cooling with alcohol on foot pads, axilla, and groin).
• Only use antipyretic treatment when fever is prolonged and life-threatening (>106 °F, >41.1 °C) and topical cooling is unsuccessful. Impaired patients (e.g., with heart failure, seizures, or respiratory disease) require antipyretic treatment earlier. Antipyretic treatment may preclude elucidation of cause, delay correct treatment, and complicate patient monitoring (e.g., reduction of fever is important indication of response to treatment).

DIET

Febrile patients in hypercatabolic state require high caloric intake.

CLIENT EDUCATION

Work-up of patients with FUO often extensive, expensive, and invasive, and may not result in definitive diagnosis.

SURGICAL CONSIDERATIONS

Surgery may be necessary in some animals (e.g., pyometra, peritonitis, pyothorax, liver abscess, neoplasms).

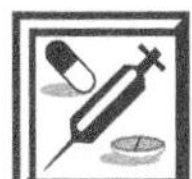

MEDICATIONS

DRUG(S) OF CHOICE

Do not use broad-spectrum (i.e., "shotgun") treatment in place of thorough diagnostic workup unless patient's status is critical and deteriorating rapidly.

Antibiotics

• Based on results of bacterial culture or serology.
• In emergency situations, combination antibiotic therapy can be started after culture specimens obtained (e.g., cephalothin 20 mg/kg IV q6–8h; combined with enrofloxacin 10 mg/kg IV q24h). Additional antimicrobials depend on main clinical suspicion based on preliminary laboratory and clinical evidence.
• Do not give antibiotics longer than 1–2 weeks if ineffective.

Antipyretics

• Aspirin—dogs: 10 mg/kg PO q12h; cats: 6 mg/kg PO q48h.
• Deracoxib—dogs: 1–2 mg/kg/day.
• Carprofen—dogs: 2 mg/kg q12h.
• Meloxicam—0.1 mg/kg/day.
• Dipyrone—dogs: 25 mg/kg IV.
• Flunixin meglumine—dogs: 0.25 mg/kg SC once (give IV fluids).

Glucocorticoids

• Do not use unless infectious causes have been ruled out.
• May mask clinical signs, may lead to immunosuppression, and not recommended for use as antipyretics; administration of corticosteroids to cats with intractable FUO after ruling out infectious diseases may promote favorable response.
• Primarily indicated for fever associated with immune-mediated disease and certain steroid-responsive tumors (e.g., lymphoma).

PRECAUTIONS

Side effects of antipyretics include emesis, diarrhea, gastrointestinal ulceration, renal damage, hemolysis, hepatotoxicity.

POSSIBLE INTERACTIONS

Combination of nonsteroidal anti-inflammatory drugs and steroids raises risk of gastrointestinal hemorrhage.

FOLLOW-UP

PATIENT MONITORING

• Body temperature at least q12h.
• If cause of fever not found, repeat history and physical exam along with screening laboratory tests.
• If fever develops or worsens during hospitalization, consider nosocomial infection or superinfection.

EXPECTED COURSE AND PROGNOSIS

Vary with cause; in some patients (more commonly cats), underlying cause cannot be determined.

MISCELLANEOUS

ASSOCIATED CONDITIONS

• Young animals—infectious disease more common; prognosis better.
• Old animals—neoplasia and intra-abdominal infection more common; signs tend to be more nonspecific; prognosis often guarded.

SYNONYMS

Pyrexia

SEE ALSO

Heat Stroke and Hyperthermia.

ABBREVIATIONS

• DIC = disseminated intravascular coagulation.
• FeLV = feline leukemia virus.
• FIP = feline infectious peritonitis.
• FIV = feline immunodeficiency virus.
• FUO = fever of unknown origin.

Authors Maria Vianna and Jörg Bucheler
Consulting Editor Michael Aherne

F

FIBER-RESPONSIVE LARGE BOWEL DIARRHEA

BASICS

OVERVIEW

- A form of chronic idiopathic large bowel diarrhea that occurs in dogs and usually responds favorably to dietary soluble fiber supplementation.
- At the author's institution, chronic idiopathic large bowel diarrhea is diagnosed in approximately 25% of dogs referred for evaluation of chronic large bowel diarrhea.
- Exclusion diagnosis that requires eliminating known causes of chronic large bowel diarrhea and clinical response to dietary fiber supplementation.
- No pathophysiologic studies have been performed.
- Only 3 reports in dogs comprising 83 cases.
- May overlap with a stress-associated poorly defined syndrome that has been called irritable bowel syndrome, also referred to as nervous colitis, spastic colon, or mucus colitis. Some dogs with irritable bowel syndrome respond to dietary fiber supplementation, while others require stress alleviation, antispasmodic medications, and/or anti-anxiety drugs.

SIGNALMENT

- Dogs of all ages (0.5–14 years); median 6 years.
- Many breeds, including mixed breeds; common breeds include German shepherd dog, miniature schnauzer, cocker spaniel, and miniature or toy poodle.

SIGNS

- Chronic diarrhea (soft to liquid) with classic large bowel characteristics; tenesmus, excess fecal mucus, hematochezia, increased frequency (median 3.5 times/day), and urgency.
- Diarrhea usually episodic alternating with periods of normal stool; diarrhea may be continuous in approximately 25% of dogs.
- Less common signs include occasional vomiting, decreased appetite during episodes of diarrhea, abdominal pain, and anal pruritus.
- Weight loss rare.
- Stress factors or abnormal personality traits in approximately 35% of dogs; household visitation, travel, moving, construction, instillation of an invisible fence; recent adoption or considered nervous, high-strung, sensitive, or aggressive; or possess noise phobia, anxiety, or depressive disorders.
- Physical examination reveals no significant findings related to gastrointestinal tract.
- Digital rectal examination is usually normal. Feces may be normal due to episodic nature of the disease. Loose stool may be present and it may contain hematochezia (red blood) or excess mucus.

CAUSES & RISK FACTORS

- Unknown; stress or abnormal personality traits may play a role in some.
- Clinical response to dietary soluble fiber supplementation suggests abnormal colonic motility and/or dysbiosis. Dysbiosis is defined as a microbial imbalance within the gastrointestinal tract. Soluble dietary fiber is a prebiotic, fermented by colonic bacteria resulting in altered composition or activity of bacteria. Prebiotics are not digested by mammalian digestive enzymes and "feed" colonic bacteria, potentially correcting dysbiosis. Soluble fibers also adsorb water, improving stool quality. Fermentation of soluble fiber by colonic bacteria produces volatile fatty acids, which are energy source for colonic epithelial cells.

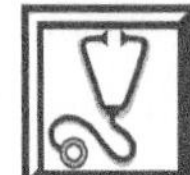

DIAGNOSIS

DIFFERENTIAL DIAGNOSIS

- Dietary indiscretion.
- Highly digestible diet-responsive diarrhea.
- Hypoallergenic diet-responsive diarrhea.
- Whipworms.
- *Clostridium perfringens*–associated diarrhea.
- Lymphocytic plasmacytic colitis.
- Eosinophilic colitis.
- Miscellaneous types of colitis.
- Irritable bowel syndrome.
- Colonic neoplasia (adenocarcinoma, lymphoma, and adenoma are most common).
- Cecal inversion.

CBC/BIOCHEMISTRY/URINALYSIS

No consistent or specific abnormalities, although can recognize peripheral eosinophilia occasionally in dogs with colonic whipworms, eosinophilic colitis, and food allergy.

OTHER LABORATORY TESTS

Multiple fecal flotations by zinc sulfate; negative for whipworms and other parasites.

IMAGING

- Abdominal radiographs within normal limits.
- Abdominal ultrasound within normal limits.

DIAGNOSTIC PROCEDURES

- *Clostridium perfringens* enterotoxin fecal ELISA; negative.
- Therapeutic deworming for whipworms (fenbendazole 50 mg/kg PO q24h for 5 days); no improvement.
- Highly digestible diet trial for 2–3 weeks; no improvement in stool quality. During the food trial the dog must not receive any other nutrients. These diets are highly digestible, low in fiber, and restricted in fat. If the dog's stool becomes normal during this diet trial, no further diagnostic tests are indicated. The highly digestible diet can be fed for another 2–4 weeks and then the original diet can be slowly introduced. Some dogs develop diarrhea again, others can be maintained on their original diet.
- Hypoallergenic diet trial for 2–3 weeks; no improvement in stool quality. During the food trial the dog must not receive any other nutrients, including flavored heartworm preventatives, vitamins, or any other supplements. For this diet trial the author recommends using a hydrolyzed diet. The hydrolyzed protein in these diets is hypoallergenic. If the dog's stool becomes normal during this diet trial a diagnosis of dietary hypersensitivity or inflammatory bowel disease can be made. These hydrolyzed diets are also highly digestible, low in fiber, and restricted in fat. Some clinicians skip the highly digestible diet trial and go directly to the hydrolyzed diet trial. Without performing a highly digestible diet trial first, response to the hydrolyzed diet trial could also be due to digestibility, fat, and fiber content and not due to dietary hypersensitivity. Many dogs that respond to a hypoallergenic food trial can be slowly switched back to their original diet after 12–14 weeks.
- Colonoscopy; usually within normal limits or only mild nonspecific findings such as slight increases in mucosal granularity or friability.

PATHOLOGIC FINDINGS

- Histopathologic evaluation of colonic biopsy samples; within normal limits.
- Multiple biopsy samples should be evaluated from throughout the colon from the cecum to the rectum. Usually at least 5–6 locations are sampled.

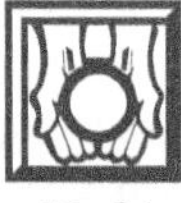

TREATMENT

- Health care can be provided on an outpatient basis and consists of dietary fiber supplementation.
- Activity level does not have to be modified.
- A highly digestible "GI" diet should initially be supplemented with 1–3 tbsp daily of psyllium hydrophobic mucilloid (Metamucil 10.2 g psyllium/tbsp).
- Psyllium is a soluble fiber that adsorbs water, improving fecal consistency, and acts as a prebiotic promoting bacterial fermentation and production of volatile fatty acids, which are an energy source for colonic epithelial cells. Psyllium comes from the seeds or husks of the plant ispaghul and consists of approximately 90% soluble fiber. Psyllium has been shown to be an effective treatment in some children with chronic nonspecific diarrhea and in other people with several diarrheal disorders.
- Median dose is 2 tbsp/day, or 0.13 tbsp/kg/day, or 1.3 g psyllium/kg/day.

- Initial response to lower amounts of fiber supplementation or use of other types of fiber is not as successful.
- After 2–3 months without diarrhea, the amount of fiber can be slowly reduced successfully in approximately 50% of dogs.
- After resolution of diarrhea with psyllium supplementation, owners may attempt to switch to a commercial high-fiber (insoluble fiber) diet that may be more convenient to feed; however diarrhea may return in 50% of dogs. Insoluble dietary fiber helps to distend the colonic lumen; distention is necessary for normal fecal storage and colonic motility.
- After resolution of diarrhea with psyllium supplementation, owners may be able to switch from the highly digestible "GI" diet to a high-quality maintenance dog food.
- Lack of initial response to fiber supplementation suggests that chronic idiopathic large bowel diarrhea may be due to irritable bowel syndrome, and pharmacologic management of that disorder should be instituted.

MEDICATIONS

None indicated.

CONTRAINDICATIONS/POSSIBLE INTERACTIONS

No known interactions of fiber supplementation with commonly used drugs.

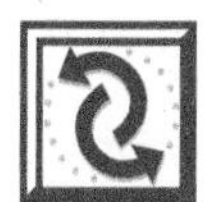

FOLLOW-UP

- Patient monitoring requires periodic assessment of stool quality, performed during recheck office examinations or via telephone interviews.
- If stresses were initially identified, stress reduction should be attempted.
- If abnormal personality traits were initially identified, they should be modified.
- Dietary soluble fiber supplementation can occasionally produce excessive flatulence, which can be managed by reduction in fiber dosage.
- Prognosis is very favorable, as approximately 85% of dogs have excellent or very good long-term response to fiber supplementation.

MISCELLANEOUS

- There are no known associated conditions.
- Age does not play a role in diagnosis or treatment.
- There is no known zoonotic potential.
- There are no special considerations regarding pregnancy, fertility, or breeding.

Suggested Reading

Lecoindre P, Gaschen FP. Chronic idiopathic large bowel diarrhea in the dog. Vet Clin North Am 2011, 41:447–456.

Leib M. Treatment of chronic idiopathic large bowel diarrhea in dogs with a highly digestible diet and soluble fiber: a retrospective review of 37 cases. J Vet Int Med 2000, 14:27–32.

Author Michael S. Leib

Consulting Editor Mark P. Rondeau

FIBROCARTILAGINOUS EMBOLIC MYELOPATHY

F

BASICS

DEFINITION

Acute ischemic necrosis of the spinal cord caused when fibrocartilaginous emboli become lodged in the spinal vasculature.

PATHOPHYSIOLOGY

• Emboli—found in spinal cord vasculature; histologically and histochemically identical to nucleus pulposus of the intervertebral disc.
• Exact mechanism of entry into the spinal vasculature unknown.

SYSTEMS AFFECTED

Nervous

GENETICS

N/A

INCIDENCE/PREVALENCE

• Common cause of spinal cord disease in nonchondrodystrophic breeds of dogs.
• Rarely reported in chondrodystrophic breeds.
• Uncommon in cats.

SIGNALMENT

Species

Dog and cat.

Breed Predilections

• Giant- and large-breed dogs most common, but seen in small breeds as well.
• Miniature schnauzers overrepresented.

Mean Age and Range

• Median age 5 years.
• Range: 8 weeks–14.5 years.

Predominant Sex

Males overrepresented.

SIGNS

Historical Findings

• May be associated with trauma or physical activity at or immediately before onset of signs.
• Sudden onset, generally nonprogressive and nonpainful.
• Discomfort occasionally noted at onset but resolves rapidly (minutes to hours).
• Signs of paresis or paralysis develop over a matter of seconds, minutes, or hours.
• Condition typically stabilizes within 24 hours.

Physical Examination Findings

N/A

Neurologic Examination Findings

• Localization—any spinal cord segment can be affected; T3–L3 and L4–S3 most common; multifocal lesions may rarely be seen; may see spinal shock with T3–L3 lesions, which can give the appearance of a multifocal spinal cord lesion.
• Deficits—commonly lateralized (due to spinal vascular anatomy) but can be symmetric; contralateral side may be mildly affected or normal.
• Severity of deficits—related to severity of infarction. Most display nonambulatory paresis, or plegia with intact nociception; fewer patients display ambulatory paresis, or plegia with absent nociception.
• Spinal pain—may be present briefly at onset of signs (owner report) and generally resolves by the time patient is examined.

CAUSES

Unknown

RISK FACTORS

• Trauma/physical activity may precede the incident.
• Hyperlipoproteinemia may be a comorbidity in miniature schnauzers and Shetland sheepdogs.

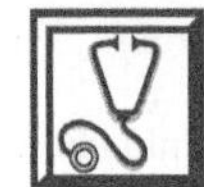

DIAGNOSIS

DIFFERENTIAL DIAGNOSIS

• Acute noncompressive nucleus pulposus extrusion (ANNPE)—most important clinical difference may be persistent spinal pain beyond 24 hours; differentiate with cross-sectional imaging; may be indistinguishable but treated the same.
• Thrombi/emboli from other sources can cause similar ischemic injury to the spinal cord—consider underlying predisposing conditions (cardiomyopathy, hypothyroidism, hyperthyroidism, hyperadrenocorticism, chronic kidney disease, hypertension, hyperlipidemia; especially in cats).
• Intervertebral disc disease; discospondylitis; neoplasia; fracture and luxation—typically painful with symmetric deficits; survey radiography, MRI, CT, and/or myelography help confirm the diagnosis.
• Intra- and extramedullary hemorrhage secondary to coagulopathy (e.g., anticoagulant rodenticide ingestion, thrombocytopenia, or disseminated intravascular coagulation)—rule out by examining for underlying causes of hemorrhage, performing platelet count, and determining blood clotting times.
• Infectious/immune-mediated focal myelitis—differentiate on progressive history and cerebrospinal fluid (CSF) analysis.
• Acute, nonprogressive, asymmetric, and nonpainful spinal cord disease—presence of these characteristics greatly helps in diagnosis of fibrocartilaginous embolic myelopathy (FCE).

CBC/BIOCHEMISTRY/URINALYSIS

Usually normal.

IMAGING

• Survey spinal radiograph—usually normal, used to rule out other causes of myelopathy such as fracture, neoplasia, or discospondylitis.
• Myelography and CT myelography—in acute stage often demonstrates focal intramedullary swelling at embolic site; later, often normal or shows area of cord atrophy.
• MRI—preferred imaging modality for antemortem diagnosis: may see increased T2 signal intensity within spinal cord at site of lesion; may see mild contrast enhancement.

DIAGNOSTIC PROCEDURES

CSF Analysis

• Normal or nonspecific changes (mild pleocytosis/elevated protein concentration). Profound elevations in cell count can occasionally be observed with severe necrosis.
• Results depend on location (lumbar vs. cerebellomedullary cistern) and time of collection in relation to onset of clinical signs.

PATHOLOGIC FINDINGS

• Gross—focal spinal cord swelling ± hemorrhage.
• Microscopic—emboli of fibrocartilage in arteries and/or veins of spinal cord within or near area of focal spinal cord swelling; gray matter generally more affected than white matter.
• Histologic examination required for definitive diagnosis. Presumptive antemortem diagnosis is based on typical presentation and exclusion of other causes of acute myelopathy.

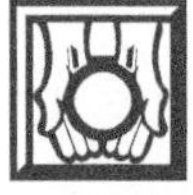

TREATMENT

APPROPRIATE HEALTH CARE

Inpatient—for immediate medical treatment and diagnostic procedures.

NURSING CARE

• Keep recumbent patients on padded surface; turn frequently to prevent pressure sores.
• Assist and encourage patients to ambulate as soon as possible.
• Assist bladder emptying (catheterize or express) several times daily if needed.
• Physical rehabilitation therapy may improve recovery and reduce residual neurologic deficits.
• Sling or harness support for assisted walking at home.

ACTIVITY

• Restrict until diagnosis is made in case of vertebral column instability from other causes such as intervertebral disc herniation or fracture/luxation.
• Once FCE is confirmed, activity should be encouraged, not restricted.

DIET

Normal unless other general health comorbidities are present.

CLIENT EDUCATION

• Gradual recovery from paresis or paralysis; most will recover ambulation, but residual neurologic deficits are common. Patients who

are paraplegic with absent nociception have a more guarded prognosis for return of function.
• Most patients need considerable home care during recovery, including bladder management.

SURGICAL CONSIDERATIONS

N/A

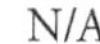

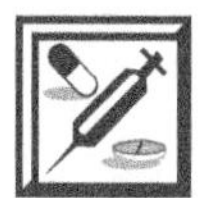

MEDICATIONS

DRUG(S) OF CHOICE

No specific medications are indicated for the treatment of FCE. Use of steroids such as methylprednisolone sodium succinate is controversial and unlikely to be of benefit.

CONTRAINDICATIONS

Nonsteroidal analgesics should not be administered with methylprednisolone sodium succinate.

PRECAUTIONS

N/A

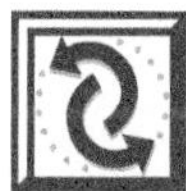

FOLLOW-UP

PATIENT MONITORING

• Sequential neurologic evaluations—during first 12–24 hours after initial examination.
• Neurologic status—at 2, 3, and 4 weeks after onset of clinical signs.
• Urinary incontinence—manually express bladder in patients who are not voluntarily urinating. Urinalysis and culture/sensitivity to detect urinary tract infection.

PREVENTION/AVOIDANCE

• Recurrence highly unlikely but possible.
• No known method of prevention in most cases.

POSSIBLE COMPLICATIONS

• Fecal and urinary incontinence.
• Urinary tract infection.
• Urine scalding and pressure sores.

EXPECTED COURSE AND PROGNOSIS

• Generally good prognosis for recovery of ambulation.
• Most patients (85%) recover ambulation within 3 weeks (range: 3 days–12 weeks).
• Most patients retain some permanent neurologic deficits despite recovering ambulation.
• Paraplegia with loss of pain perception at presentation implies more guarded prognosis.

MISCELLANEOUS

ASSOCIATED CONDITIONS

Disorders that lead to compromise in circulatory function may predispose or mimic FCE—hyperadrenocorticism; hypothyroidism; high systemic blood pressure; hyperviscosity syndrome; hyperlipidemia; bleeding diathesis; bacterial endocarditis.

AGE-RELATED FACTORS

N/A

ZOONOTIC POTENTIAL

N/A

PREGNANCY/FERTILITY/BREEDING

High-dose corticosteroid administration—may cause premature delivery.

ABBREVIATIONS

• ANNPE = acute noncompressive nucleus pulposus extrusion.
• FCE = fibrocartilaginous embolic myelopathy.
• CSF = cerebrospinal fluid.

Suggested Reading

Bartholomew KA, Stover KE, Olby NJ, Moore SA. Clinical characteristics of canine fibrocartilaginous embolic myelopathy (FCE): a systematic review of 393 cases (1973–2013). Vet Rec 2016, 179:650.

De Risio L, Adams V, Dennis R, et al. Magnetic resonance imaging findings and clinical associations in 52 dogs with suspected ischemic myelopathy. J Vet Int Med 2007, 21:1290–1298.

De Risio L, Platt SR. Fibrocartilaginous embolic myelopathy in small animals. Vet Clin North Am Small Anim Pract 2010, 233:129–135.

Gandini G, Cizinauska S, Lang J, et al. Fibrocartilaginous embolism in 75 dogs: clinical findings and factors influencing the recovery rate. J Small Anim Pract 2003, 44:76–80.

Hawthorne JC, Wallace LJ, Fenner WR, et al. Fibrocartilaginous embolic myelopathy in miniature schnauzers. J Am Anim Hosp Assoc 2001, 37:374–383.

Mikszewski JS, Van Winkle TJ, Troxel MT. Fibrocartilaginous embolic myelopathy in five cats. J Am Anim Hosp Assoc 2006, 42:226–233.

Summers BA, Cummings JF, de Lahunta A. Veterinary Neuropathology. St Louis, MO: Mosby, 1995, pp. 246–249.

Authors Kristen Bartholomew and Sarah A. Moore

Acknowledgment The authors and book editors acknowledge the prior contribution of Allen Franklin Sisson

FIBROSARCOMA, BONE

BASICS

OVERVIEW

- Primary bone fibrosarcoma (FSA) arises from stromal elements within the marrow cavity and is characterized by malignant spindle cells that produce varying amounts of collagen but not any osteoid or cartilage.
- In dogs, FSA accounts for <8% of all primary bone tumors, with 60% occurring in the axial skeleton and 40% arising in the appendicular skeleton.
- Bone tumors are rare in cats. FSA is the second most common bone tumor in cats and can involve the maxilla, mandible, humerus, scapula, carpus, digits, ribs, and sacrum.

SIGNALMENT

- Dog and cat; no obvious breed or gender predilections in either species.
- Mean age of dogs 9.7 years (range: 2–15 years).
- Affected cats tended to be older, but have been reported as young as 1.5 years old.

SIGNS

Historical Findings

Appendicular FSA

- Lameness, usually progressive, but occasionally acute if there is a pathologic fracture.
- A palpable swelling may be present.

Axial FSA

- Localized swelling with or without pain is common; however, anatomic site dependent.
- Tumors arising from the mandible or maxilla can be associated with halitosis, dysphagia, pain on opening the mouth, or nasal discharge.
- Vertebral tumors may induce neurologic deficits secondary to spinal cord compression.
- Rib tumors are rarely associated with respiratory signs unless large and causing space-occupying effects. Rib tumors can grow asymmetrically, with majority of growth occurring within the intrathoracic space.

Physical Examination Findings

- For appendicular FSA, lameness and a palpable swelling may be present.
- Physical examination findings may be variable for FSA for the axial skeleton depending on the size and location of the tumor; a mass may be visible or palpable.

CAUSES & RISK FACTORS

Unknown

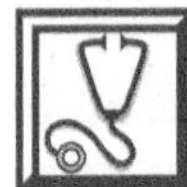

DIAGNOSIS

DIFFERENTIAL DIAGNOSIS

- Other primary bone tumors (osteosarcoma, chondrosarcoma, hemangiosarcoma, histiocytic sarcoma, etc.).
- Metastatic bone tumors (transitional cell, prostatic, mammary, thyroid, apocrine gland anal sac carcinomas).
- Tumors that locally invade adjacent bone (nasal carcinoma; oral squamous cell carcinoma, melanoma, fibrosarcoma, ameloblastoma; synovial sarcoma; histiocytic sarcoma; digital squamous cell carcinoma, melanoma).
- Hematopoietic tumors (myeloma, lymphoma).
- Bacterial or fungal osteomyelitis.

CBC/BIOCHEMISTRY/URINALYSIS

Usually normal.

IMAGING

- Radiographs of the primary lesion show features of an aggressive bone lesion (bone lysis, cortical destruction, nonhomogenous bone formation, ill-defined zone of transition).
- Thoracic radiographs are recommended to screen for pulmonary metastasis (uncommon).
- CT is recommended for axial tumors to plan for surgery and/or radiation therapy.

DIAGNOSTIC PROCEDURES

- Histopathology is needed for a definitive diagnosis.
- Primary bone FSA has been reported to metastasize to a variety of locations—lungs, regional lymph nodes, other bones, skin, kidneys, pericardium, and myocardium. Consider additional diagnostic evaluation as indicated to rule out metastasis to these or other locations.

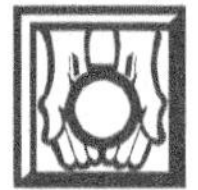

TREATMENT

- Amputation is recommended for appendicular tumors.
- For axial tumors, wide surgical excision is recommended whenever possible. If surgical excision is incomplete, adjuvant radiation therapy might help improve local control.
- Palliative analgesic therapy is recommended for patients with nonresectable local disease or gross metastasis, or when definitive therapy is declined.

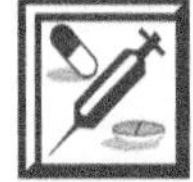

MEDICATIONS

DRUG(S) OF CHOICE

- Nonsteroidal anti-inflammatory drugs (NSAIDs).
- Tramadol (2–5 mg/kg PO q6–12h).
- Gabapentin (3–10 mg/kg PO q8–24h).
- Intravenous aminobisphosphonates (pamidronate, zoledronate) might alleviate bone pain and attenuate bone resorption.
- The benefit of adjuvant chemotherapy is unknown, but it may be considered for high-grade tumors; consult a veterinary oncologist for current recommendations.

CONTRAINDICATIONS/POSSIBLE INTERACTIONS

- Use NSAIDs cautiously in all cats and in dogs with renal insufficiency.
- Do not combine NSAIDs with corticosteroids.

FOLLOW-UP

PATIENT MONITORING

Physical examination and thoracic radiographs every 2–3 months.

EXPECTED COURSE AND PROGNOSIS

- There is limited information regarding long-term prognosis.
- Complete excision of the primary tumor can potentially provide long-term control.
- Patients with high-grade primary bone FSA may be more likely to develop metastasis.

MISCELLANEOUS

SEE ALSO

- Chondrosarcoma, Bone.
- Osteosarcoma.

ABBREVIATIONS

- FSA = fibrosarcoma.
- NSAID = nonsteroidal anti-inflammatory drug.

Suggested Reading

Albin LW, Berg J, Schelling SH. Fibrosarcoma of the canine appendicular skeleton. JAAHA 1991, 27:303–309.

Author Jenna H. Burton

Consulting Editor Timothy M. Fan

Acknowledgment The author and book editors acknowledge the prior contribution of Dennis B. Bailey

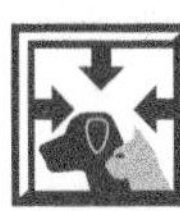

BASICS

OVERVIEW

- Fibrosarcoma (FSA) is a malignant tumor of spindle cells that produce varying amounts of collagenous (fibrous) extracellular matrix and associated stroma.
- Oral FSA arises most commonly in the gingiva; occasionally involves lips and rarely tongue; invasion into bone is common.
- In dogs, FSA is third most common oral malignancy (20% of all oral tumors).
- In cats, FSA is second most common oral malignancy (5–15% of all oral tumors).

SIGNALMENT

- Dogs—overall, large-breed dogs are predisposed; median age 9 years (range: 1–13 years).
- Golden retrievers are overrepresented specifically for histologically low-grade but biologically high-grade FSA variant (see Pathologic Findings).
- Cats—no breed predilections; median age 8–10 years (range: 1–21 years).

SIGNS

Historical Findings

- Visible mass arising within oral cavity or causing facial deformity.
- Halitosis, hypersalivation, dysphagia, and/or bloody oral discharge.
- Oral pain—head-shy behavior and/or decreased food intake despite showing interest in food; change in food preference (favor soft vs. hard foods).

Physical Examination Findings

- Firm, smooth oral mass with intact overlying mucosa is commonly observed.
- Halitosis, hypersalivation, and/or oral bleeding.
- Difficulty or pain when opening mouth and/or facial deformity.
- Ipsilateral mandibular lymphadenopathy.
- Nasal discharge, epistaxis, or decreased nasal air flow (maxillary tumors) can be identified.

CAUSES & RISK FACTORS

None identified.

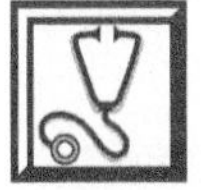

DIAGNOSIS

DIFFERENTIAL DIAGNOSIS

- Other malignant oral tumors, including melanoma, squamous cell carcinoma, or osteosarcoma.
- Benign tumors such as acanthomatous ameloblastoma, peripheral odontogenic fibroma (epulis), or osteoma.
- Tooth root abscess or osteomyelitis.
- Dentigerous cyst.
- Craniomandibular osteopathy (lion's jaw).

IMAGING

- Skull radiographs recommended to evaluate for bone involvement (present in 60–70%).
- Thoracic radiographs to screen for pulmonary metastasis (uncommon).
- CT imaging can more accurately determine extent of local disease and useful for planning surgery and/or radiation therapy.

DIAGNOSTIC PROCEDURES

- Histopathology required for definitive diagnosis.
- Cytology or histopathology of ipsilateral mandibular lymph node recommended to screen for metastasis.

PATHOLOGIC FINDINGS

Histologically low-grade yet biologically high-grade tumors are a distinct subset of oral FSA that tend to occur in large pure-breed dogs, particularly golden retrievers. These tumors classified as benign lesions (nodular fasciitis, chronic inflammatory nodules, granulation tissue) or low-grade FSA on histopathology. However, aggressive biologic behavior, including rapid tumor growth, bone destruction (75%), lymph node metastasis (20%), and pulmonary metastasis (12%), observed in affected dogs.

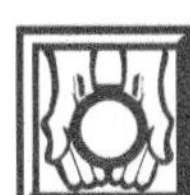

TREATMENT

- Surgical excision—removal of mass and adjacent bone (maxillectomy or mandibulectomy) with margin of at least 2–3 cm recommended whenever anatomically possible.
- If tumor margins observed to be incomplete or narrow on histopathology, adjuvant radiation therapy recommended to improve local control.
- Radiation therapy can be considered as sole local treatment modality when surgery not possible or declined; however, treatment intent might not be curative in nature.
- Palliative care focuses on pain control.

MEDICATIONS

DRUG(S) OF CHOICE

- Nonsteroidal anti-inflammatory drugs (NSAIDs).
- Tramadol (2–5 mg/kg PO q6–12h).
- Gabapentin (3–10 mg/kg PO q8–24h).
- Empiric antibiotic therapy can be considered for secondary bacterial infections.
- IV aminobisphosphonates might alleviate bone pain for dogs treated palliatively.

CONTRAINDICATIONS/POSSIBLE INTERACTIONS

Use NSAIDs cautiously in all cats and in dogs with renal insufficiency.

FOLLOW-UP

PATIENT MONITORING

Physical examination every 2–3 months and thoracic radiographs every 3–4 months.

EXPECTED COURSE AND PROGNOSIS

- Most patients die or are euthanized due to progression or recurrence of local disease.
- Overall metastatic rate is 25% (regional lymph nodes and lungs).
- Prognosis with surgery alone depends on tumor size and location, with reported median survival times 9–24 months; long-term control is possible with complete excision.
- Combining surgery with radiation therapy, median survival is 18 months.
- With radiation therapy alone, median progression-free survival is 45 months for tumors <2 cm, 31 months for tumors 2–4 cm, and 7 months for tumors >4 cm.

MISCELLANEOUS

ABBREVIATIONS

- FSA = fibrosarcoma.
- NSAID = nonsteroidal anti-inflammatory drug.

Suggested Reading

Ciekot PA, Powers BE, Withrow SJ, et al. Histologically low-grade, yet biologically high-grade, fibrosarcomas of the mandible and maxilla in dogs: 25 cases (1982–1991). J Am Vet Med Assoc 1994, 204(4):610–615.

Gardner H, Fidel J, Haldorson G, et al. Canine oral fibrosarcomas: a retrospective analysis of 65 cases (1998–2010). Vet Comp Oncol 2015, 13(1):40–47.

Author Jenna H. Burton

Consulting Editor Timothy M. Fan

Acknowledgment The author and book editors acknowledge the prior contribution of Dennis B. Bailey

F

FIBROSARCOMA, NASAL AND PARANASAL SINUS

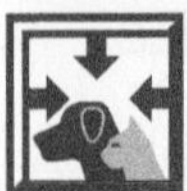

BASICS

OVERVIEW

- Fibrosarcoma (FSA) is a malignant tumor of spindle cells that produce varying amounts of collagenous (fibrous) extracellular matrix and associated stroma.
- In dogs, FSA accounts for up to 5% of all canine sinonasal tumors.
- Nasal FSA uncommon in cats.

SIGNALMENT

- In dogs, no breed or gender predilections identified. Median age 9 years (range: 1–16 years).
- Uncommon in cats—no identified predilections.

SIGNS

Historical Findings

- Intermittent unilateral epistaxis and/or mucopurulent discharge, may progress to bilateral involvement.
- Sneezing, stertorous breathing, and/or facial deformity.
- Decreased appetite and/or halitosis secondary to oral cavity invasion.
- Seizures, behavior changes, and/or obtundation secondary to cranial invasion (uncommon).

Physical Examination Findings

- Epistaxis and/or nasal discharge, initially unilateral but can progress to bilateral.
- Decreased nasal air flow (unilateral or bilateral).
- Pain on nasal or paranasal sinus palpation or percussion.
- Facial deformity decreased ocular retropulsion, exophthalmia, or epiphora.
- Visible mass effect protruding through palate into oral cavity.

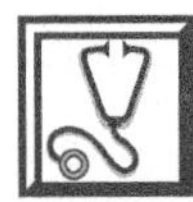

DIAGNOSIS

DIFFERENTIAL DIAGNOSIS

- Other nasal tumors—adenocarcinoma, squamous cell carcinoma, chondrosarcoma, osteosarcoma, lymphoma, transmissible venereal tumor (dogs), nasopharyngeal polyp (cats).
- Fungal rhinitis—aspergillosis and penicilliosis (dogs), *Cryptococcus* (cats), sporotrichosis (both).
- Rhinosporidiosis (dogs).
- Foreign body.
- Thrombocytopenia or other coagulopathy.
- Tooth root abscess or oronasal fistula.

CBC/BIOCHEMISTRY/URINALYSIS

Usually normal—evaluate for thrombocytopenia if signs of epistaxis.

OTHER LABORATORY TESTS

- Nasal flush for cytology and culture—rarely helpful.
- Coagulation profile.
- Buccal mucosal bleeding time.

IMAGING

- Thoracic radiographs to screen for pulmonary metastasis (distant metastases uncommon).
- CT for detecting soft tissue opacity within nasal cavity and surrounding sinuses, bony destruction, extension through cribriform plate into brain.
- If CT scan not accessible, skull radiographs can be performed to assess for soft tissue opacity in nasal cavity and/or frontal sinuses.

DIAGNOSTIC PROCEDURES

- Blood pressure measurement to rule out systemic hypertension as cause for epistaxis.
- Mandibular lymph node cytology to screen for possible regional metastasis (uncommon).
- Rhinoscopy helpful for visualization of mass or fungal plaque and guiding subsequent tissue biopsy.
- Tissue biopsy and histopathology needed for definitive diagnosis; biopsy instrument should not pass the level of the medial canthus of the eye to avoid penetrating the cribriform plate.
- Intranasal approach to obtaining tissue biopsy preferable if treatment with radiation therapy planned.

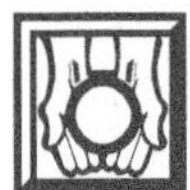

TREATMENT

- Radiation therapy is treatment of choice.
- Conventional linear accelerator is used most commonly; however, if available, stereotactic radiation therapy can reduce number of radiation treatments and reduce adverse effects while maintaining treatment efficacy.
- Palliative radiation protocols (fewer treatments and lower total radiation dose) might be preferable for dogs with very advanced disease or if intent of treatment is primarily symptomatic.
- Surgery alone is ineffective.

MEDICATIONS

DRUG(S) OF CHOICE

- Nonsteroidal anti-inflammatory drugs (NSAIDs) for pain control.
- Prednisone (0.5–1 mg/kg PO q24h) to help relieve nasal congestion.
- Phenylephrine nasal spray can be used intermittently to help with epistaxis.
- Empiric antibiotic therapy can be considered for secondary bacterial infections.

CONTRAINDICATIONS/POSSIBLE INTERACTIONS

- Use NSAIDs cautiously in all cats and in dogs with renal insufficiency.
- Do not combine NSAIDs with corticosteroids.

FOLLOW-UP

PATIENT MONITORING

- Physical examinations every 2–3 months and thoracic radiographs every 3–4 months.
- CT of nasal cavity can be considered to monitor disease regression or if clinical signs recur or worsen.

EXPECTED COURSE AND PROGNOSIS

- Overall metastatic rate <20% (usually involve regional lymph nodes and/or lungs).
- Median survival with palliative care alone 3 months.
- With definitive radiation therapy, 1-year relapse-free survival rate around 50% and 2-year relapse-free survival rate around 30%.
- Recurrence/progression of tumor and recurrence of clinical signs is generally life-limiting event for nasal/paranasal FSA.
- Brain involvement is poor prognostic factor.
- Unilateral versus bilateral involvement is not a significant prognostic factor.

MISCELLANEOUS

SEE ALSO

- Adenocarcinoma, Nasal.
- Chondrosarcoma, Nasal and Paranasal Sinus.
- Epistaxis.

ABBREVIATIONS

- FSA = fibrosarcoma.
- NSAID = nonsteroidal anti-inflammatory drug.

Suggested Reading

Sones E, Smith A, Schleis S, et al. Survival times for canine intranasal sarcomas treated with radiation therapy: 86 cases (1996–2011). Vet Radiol Ultrasound 2013, 54(2):194–201.

Author Jenna H. Burton

Consulting Editor Timothy M. Fan

Acknowledgment The author and book editors acknowledge the prior contribution of Dennis B. Bailey

FIPRONIL TOXICOSIS

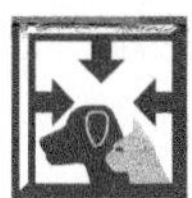

BASICS

OVERVIEW

- Phenylpyrazole compound with selective toxicity against insects.
- Discovered in 1987, registered as a pesticide in the United States in 1996; used worldwide today.
- Blocks chloride passage through γ-aminobutyric acid (GABA) and glutamate gated chloride channels.
- Except for rabbits, low mammalian toxicity—GABA receptors less sensitive and lack mammals lack glutamate gated chloride channels.
- Uses:
    - Topical flea and tick spot-on products ("plus" versions include S-methoprene).
    - Roach and ant-bait stations. Flea and tick sprays for pets.
    - Granular turf products.
    - Soil treatment.
    - Crop pest control.

SIGNALMENT

Dogs

- Accidental ingestion and/or licking of topical spot-on products.
- Chewing ant and roach-bait stations or licking gel products.
- Ingesting liquid from bottles or granules from bags containing product.

Cats

Accidental ingestion of topical spot-on product from grooming.

Rabbits

- Inappropriate application of spot on products to rabbits.

SIGNS

- Dermal—skin irritation, alopecia, or dermal hypersensitivity reaction.
- Oral—hypersalivation, nausea, vomiting, diarrhea.
- Ingestion of large doses—CNS: hyperexcitability, tremors, convulsions, seizures, death.

Rabbits

Dermal and oral exposure (any amount) can cause anorexia, hypersalivation, ataxia, tremors, seizures and death.

CAUSES & RISK FACTORS

- Ingestion by dogs, especially young dogs, occurs more frequently due to behavioral factors.
- With chronic studies in dogs, severe neurotoxic signs were observed at a dose of 20 mg/kg.
- Wide availability and frequent access to products.
- Biggest concern is exposure to concentrated products frequently found on farms and ranches or used by pesticide control applicators.

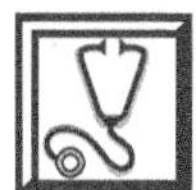

DIAGNOSIS

- History of exposure.
- Detected in blood, tissue, hair with gas chromatography/mass spectrometry (GC/MS).
- Differential diagnosis—dogs and cats: exposure to agents that can cause dermal hypersensitivity or CNS signs.

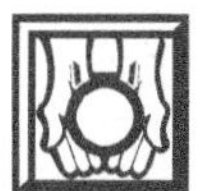

TREATMENT

- Baseline CBC, chemistry profile, and urinalysis should be performed to rule out preexisting organ dysfunction, which could increase the risk for toxicosis.
- For dermal reaction, bathe with liquid dishwashing detergent and rinse thoroughly.
- Antihistamine or steroids for dermal hypersensitivity reaction.
- With ingestion of a large dose, one dose of activated charcoal with sorbitol may be beneficial.
- Methocarbamol for tremors.
- Anticonvulsants for seizures.
- IV fluids (balanced crystalloid) at twice maintenance if CNS signs occur.

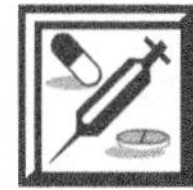

MEDICATIONS

- Activated charcoal 1–2 g/kg PO and an osmotic cathartic (sorbitol) × 1 dose for large ingestions.
- Methocarbamol for tremors—55–220 mg/kg IV; titrate as needed; max daily dose 330 mg/kg/day (cats and dogs).
- Anticonvulsants for seizures—diazepam 0.5–1 mg/kg IV (dogs and cats); phenobarbital 2–6 mg/kg IV (dogs and cats).
- Diphenhydramine 2–4 mg/kg q8–12h PO; 0.5–2 mg/kg q8–12h IM/SC/IV.
- Dexamethasone 0.5–1 mg/kg IV/IM (dogs); 0.125–0.5 mg/kg IV/IM (cats).

FOLLOW-UP

Patients usually recover well with symptomatic and supportive care; no long-term organ damage is expected to occur.

MISCELLANEOUS

- Puppies/young dogs are less discriminating and more likely to chew up product containers.
- Young and geriatric animals may have lower detoxification capabilities.

PREGNANCY/FERTILITY/BREEDING

Fipronil was administered to rats (route of exposure not included) to determine reproductive effects. No reproductive effects were noted at 30 ppm (2.54 mg/kg/day in males and 2.74 mg/kg/day in females). The lowest dosage at which reproductive effects were observed was 300 ppm (26.0 mg/kg/day in males and 28.4 mg/kg/day in females) based on unspecified clinical signs in the offspring, reduced litter size, decreased bodyweights, decreased mating, reduced fertility, reduced postimplantation and offspring survival, and delay in physical development.

F

ABBREVIATIONS

- GABA = γ-aminobutyric acid.
- GC/MS = gas chromatography/mass spectrometry.

INTERNET RESOURCES

http://npic.orst.edu/factsheets/fipronil.html

Suggested Reading

Anadon A, Gupta RC. Fipronil. In: Gupta RC, ed., Veterinary Toxicology Basic and Clinical Principles, 2nd ed. Waltham, MA: Elsevier, 2012, pp. 604–608.

Gupta RC. Fipronil. In: Veterinary toxicology: basic and clinical principles. 2nd ed. Amsterdam: Elsevier, 2012;604–608.

Hovda LR, Hooser SB. Toxicology of newer pesticides for use in dogs and cats. Vet Clin North Am Small Anim Pract 2002, 32:455–467.

Stern L, Fipronil toxicosis in rabbits, DVM360, 10/13/2015.

Wismer T. Novel insecticides: fipronil. In: Plumlee KH, ed. Clinical veterinary toxicology. St. Louis: Mosby, 2004;183–184.

Author Sharon L. Rippel

Consulting Editor Lynn R. Hovda

FLATULENCE

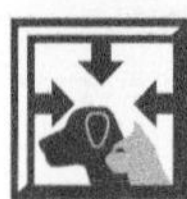

BASICS

DEFINITION

The act of expelling gases formed in the gastrointestinal (GI) tract through the anus. "Flatus" refers to gas formed in the GI tract.

PATHOPHYSIOLOGY

- Passing flatus is a normal physiologic function in the dog and cat. Variations in the volume, odor, and frequency of the pet's flatus may cause the owner to perceive the act of flatulence as a problem.
- Swallowed air (aerophagia), bacterial fermentation of nutrients, the interaction of gastric acid and pancreatic/salivary bicarbonate, and diffusion of gases from blood are the main sources of GI gas.
- Odorless gases comprise more than 99% of GI gases; these include nitrogen, oxygen, hydrogen, carbon dioxide, and methane.
- Malodorous gases containing volatile sulfur compounds comprise less than 1% of GI gases; these include ammonia, hydrogen sulfide, methanethiol, dimethylsulfide, indole, skatole, volatile amines, and short-chain fatty acids.
- Dogs and cats lack digestive enzymes to cleave oligosaccharides (commonly of vegetable source) into absorbable monosaccharides. Diets high in oligosaccharides provide substrate for colonic microbiota fermentation and lead to excessive gas formation.
- Foods containing fermentable fibers (including pectins, gums, and carrageenan) contribute to flatus directly by fermentation of the fiber by colonic microbiota.
- Dogs and cats are lactose intolerant; a dietary concentration of 1.5 g/kg/day (there is 11 g lactose in 1 cup of milk) may produce flatulence and diarrhea.
- Hypersensitivity or intolerance to certain proteins or carbohydrates is often responsible for increased volume or odor of flatus.
- Disease states causing malassimilation of nutrients (such as protein-losing enteropathies [PLEs] and exocrine pancreatic insufficiency), making them available for colonic fermentation, can cause increased flatulence.
- Infection with certain enteropathogenic organisms, such as *Giardia* sp., can cause increased flatulence.
- Antibiotics that alter the colonic microbiota may cause increased flatulence.

SYSTEMS AFFECTED

GI

GENETICS

No known genetic basis, although brachycephalic breeds are overrepresented.

INCIDENCE/PREVALENCE

Excessive flatulence was reported in 10% of dogs in the United States, with 1 out of 4 experiencing daily episodes.

GEOGRAPHIC DISTRIBUTION

N/A

SIGNALMENT

Species

Dog (common); cat (rare).

Breed Predilections

Excessive aerophagia is seen in brachycephalic breeds, sporting dogs, and those with gluttonous/competitive eating behavior.

Mean Age and Range

Any age.

Predominant Sex

None

SIGNS

Historical Findings

- "He who smelt it dealt it"—a pet who turns around frequently to sniff or look at its rear end.
- Increased frequency, volume, or objectionable odor of flatus reported by the pet owner.
- When excessive flatulence is due to pancreatic or GI disease, concurrent GI signs such as diarrhea, vomiting, borborygmus, changes in appetite, and weight loss may be present.

Physical Examination Findings

- May be normal.
- Abdominal discomfort due to GI gas distention.
- Increased borborygmus on abdominal auscultation or decreased gut sounds suggesting ileus.
- Low body condition score may indicate underlying pancreatic insufficiency or GI disease.
- Obesity may suggest a sedentary lifestyle or gluttonous eating habits.
- When excessive flatulence is due to aerophagia, concurrent respiratory signs such as excessive panting, increased upper- or lower-airway sounds, dyspnea, and tachypnea may be present.

CAUSES

Aerophagia

- Gluttony or competitive eating.
- Respiratory disease or any cause of increased respiratory rate or effort.
- Brachycephalic breeds.

Diet-Related

- Diets high in nonabsorbable oligosaccharides—soybeans, peas, beans.
- Diets high in fermentable fiber—pectin, gums, carrageenan, inulin, psyllium, oat bran.
- Spoiled foods.
- Dairy products.
- Abrupt changes in diet.

Disease Conditions

- Acute and chronic intestinal disease—including protein-losing enteropathies; intestinal dysbiosis; neoplasia; irritable bowel syndrome; parasitism; bacterial, protozoal, or viral enteritis; and food allergy or intolerance.
- Exocrine pancreatic insufficiency.

RISK FACTORS

- Nervous, gluttonous, or competitive eating.
- Eating soon after exercise.
- Brachycephalic breeds.
- Large-breed dogs.
- Abrupt dietary changes.
- Inappropriate (table food that is likely to be fermented) or spoiled foods.
- Lack of regular exercise.

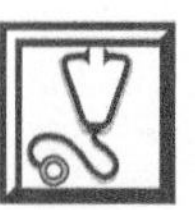

DIAGNOSIS

DIFFERENTIAL DIAGNOSIS

- Differential diagnoses include excessive aerophagia, dietary factors, motility disorders, malabsorption, and changes in the colonic microbiota.
- Distinguish dietary and behavioral causes of flatus from GI disease by thorough evaluation of the patient history; this allows the clinician to ascertain the type of diet, amount fed, frequency of feeding, frequency of dietary changes or additions, the environment in which the patient is fed, and frequency of exercise.

CBC/BIOCHEMISTRY/URINALYSIS

Usually normal unless significant pancreatic or GI disease is present (e.g., hypoalbuminemia in PLE).

OTHER LABORATORY TESTS

- Rectal cytology to evaluate presence of neoplasia, parasites, protozoa, or fungal organisms.
- Zinc sulfate flotation tests and fecal PCR, ELISA, or culture to detect *Giardia* sp., *Tritrichomonas* (cats), and other parasitic, bacterial, viral, and protozoal infections.
- Serum trypsin-like immunoreactivity to diagnose exocrine pancreatic insufficiency.
- Serum cobalamin and folate concentrations to investigate small intestinal malabsorptive disease.

IMAGING

- Thoracic and abdominal radiographs can show the distribution of gas in the alimentary tract, as well as reveal specific reasons such as gastric dilatation volvulus, pulmonary infiltrates, and megaesophagus.
- Abdominal ultrasonography to evaluate GI thickness and rule out masses.
- Contrast studies may be needed in some cases to detect an obstructive pattern and provide insight into GI transit time.
- Assessment of gut motility using motility capsules and scintigraphic markers may be available in certain referral hospitals.

DIAGNOSTIC PROCEDURES

GI biopsy specimens obtained at surgery or via endoscopy to detect infiltrative GI disease.

PATHOLOGIC FINDINGS

N/A

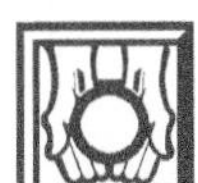

TREATMENT

APPROPRIATE HEALTH CARE

Outpatient—treat any underlying pancreatic or GI disease.

NURSING CARE

None

ACTIVITY

Encourage an active lifestyle—exercise increases GI motility, which will help decrease gas retention and increase regularity of defecation.

DIET

- Feed smaller meals more frequently in an isolated, quiet environment.
- Provide interactive/modified feeding containers to slow the rate of food intake.
- Change diet to one that is highly digestible, with low fermentable fiber and fat content. If food intolerance is suspected, consider a trial of hydrolyzed protein diet or novel protein diet.
- Limit vegetables, which are generally high in fermentable fibers, in pet's diet.

CLIENT EDUCATION

- Encourage a consistent diet.
- Encourage routine exercise.
- Prevent coprophagia by leash-walking and cleaning up fecal waste daily.

SURGICAL CONSIDERATIONS

None

MEDICATIONS

DRUG(S) OF CHOICE

- Carminatives are medications or remedies that relieve flatulence; there are few studies to show safety or benefit of these drugs in dogs or cats.
- Zinc acetate and bismuth are divalent cations that bind sulfhydryl compounds (e.g., hydrogen sulfide) and can decrease odor of flatulence.
- *Yucca schidigera* decreases odor by binding ammonia and by decreasing the production and release of hydrogen sulfide in the intestinal tract.
- Dry activated charcoal adsorbs virtually all odiferous gases due to its large surface area.
- Inclusion of activated charcoal (0.32 g/5 kg), *Y. schidigera* (2.45 mg/5 kg), and zinc acetate (17 mg/5 kg) in a treat reduced the frequency of highly odiferous episodes in dogs.
- Bismuth subsalicylate (dogs: 1 mL/kg/day PO, in divided doses) adsorbs hydrogen sulfide and has antibacterial properties. Do not use in cats due to potential for salicylate toxicity.
- Simethicone (25–200 mg PO q6h) is an antifoaming agent that reduces the surface tension of gas bubbles, allowing easier coalescence and release of intestinal gas; its effectiveness in controlling flatulence in animals is unknown.
- Pancreatic enzyme supplements reduce flatulence in patients with exocrine pancreatic insufficiency.
- Probiotics, specifically *Enterococcus faecium* SF 68, the probiotic in Purina Veterinary Diets® FortiFlora® Canine Nutritional Supplement, has been shown to help nutritionally manage dogs with flatulence by promoting greater beneficial intestinal microflora.
- Nonabsorbed antibacterials such as neomycin and rifaximin may have a role in normalizing gut microbiota and decreasing flatulence.

CONTRAINDICATIONS

Avoid bismuth subsalicylate in cats and in dogs with gastroduodenal ulceration and bleeding disorders.

PRECAUTIONS

N/A

POSSIBLE INTERACTIONS

N/A

ALTERNATIVE DRUG(S)

More than 30 herbal and botanical carminatives are available; however, the dosage, safety, and efficacy are unknown.

FOLLOW-UP

PATIENT MONITORING

Response to therapy.

PREVENTION/AVOIDANCE

- Avoid diets high in nonabsorbable oligosaccharides and high in fermentable or nonfermentable fibers.
- Avoid milk products, spoiled diets, and abrupt changes in diet.
- Do not feed shortly after exercise.

POSSIBLE COMPLICATIONS

None

EXPECTED COURSE AND PROGNOSIS

N/A

MISCELLANEOUS

ASSOCIATED CONDITIONS

GI disease.

AGE-RELATED FACTORS

N/A

ZOONOTIC POTENTIAL

N/A PREGNANCY/FERTILITY/ BREEDING

N/A

SYNONYMS

N/A

SEE ALSO

- Exocrine Pancreatic Insufficiency.
- Inflammatory Bowel Disease.
- Small Intestinal Dysbiosis.

ABBREVIATIONS

- GI = gastrointestinal.
- PLE = protein-losing enteropathy.

Suggested Reading

German AJ. Flatulence. In: Ettinger SJ, Feldman EC, Côté E, eds., Textbook of Veterinary Internal Medicine, 8th ed. St. Louis, MO: Elsevier Saunders, 2017, pp. 175–178.

Giffard CJ, Collins SB, Stoodley NC. Administration of charcoal, Yucca schidigera, and zinc acetate to reduce malodorous flatulence in dogs. J Am Vet Med Assoc. 2001 (281)6:892–896.

Roudebush P. Flatulence. In: Bonagura JD, Twedt DC, eds., Kirk's Current Veterinary Therapy XV. St. Louis, MO: Elsevier Saunders, 2014, pp. e247–e251.

Waldron, M. GI exchange: a nutritional approach to managing dogs with flatulence. https://www.purinaproplanvets.com/media/1155/50174-5_gi_tradecolumn_nov.pdf

Author Andrea Wang Munk

Consulting Editor Mark P. Rondeau

Acknowledgment The author and book editors acknowledge the prior contributions of Debra L. Zoran

Client Education Handout available online

FLEA BITE HYPERSENSITIVITY AND FLEA CONTROL

BASICS

DEFINITION

Flea bite hypersensitivity (FBH)—allergic reaction to antigens in flea saliva.

Flea Life Cycle

• *Ctenocephalides felis* (cat flea)—not host specific: parasitizes cats, dogs, wildlife. • Adult fleas mate on host and within 24 hours females lay up to 50 eggs per day. • Eggs fall off pets into the environment and hatch. • Larvae have negative phototropism and infest carpets, upholstery, and under furniture. • Eggs from wildlife and feral cats survive in moist, protected areas. • Larvae undergo molts until they pupate; the cocoon enhances survival. • Adults emerge when environmental conditions and host availability are favorable. • Less than 5% of the total flea burden is found as adults on the pet. • The majority of the biomass is found as immature stages in the home and in peridomestic areas.

PATHOPHYSIOLOGY

• Antigens in flea saliva cause FBH. • Major allergen—*Ctef1*, an 18-kD protein. • Flea saliva—contains histamine-like compounds that irritate skin. • Both immunoglobulin (Ig) E and IgG anti-flea antibodies reported. • Immediate and delayed hypersensitivity reactions reported. • Mast cell degranulation follows antigen exposure. • FBH is associated with a T_H2 response.

SYSTEMS AFFECTED

Skin

GENETICS

No known inheritance pattern.

INCIDENCE/PREVALENCE

• Varies with climatic conditions and flea population.
• In areas where fleas are prevalent, FBH is considered the most common skin disease.

GEOGRAPHIC DISTRIBUTION

May occur anywhere; nonseasonal in climates that are warm and humid.

SIGNALMENT

Species

Dogs and cats.

Breed Predilections

None

Mean Age and Range

Typically signs by 5 years of age, but may be seen at any age.

SIGNS

Historical Findings

• Pruritus. • Lack of consistent or effective flea control.

Physical Examination Findings

• Determined by the severity of the reaction. • Finding fleas and flea dirt is supportive but not essential for diagnosis. • Sensitive animals require a low exposure and tend to overgroom, removing evidence of infestation. • Dogs—lesions concentrated in the caudal-dorsal lumbosacral region; caudal-lateral aspect of the thighs, lower abdomen, and inguinal region; primary lesions are papules; secondary lesions (hyperpigmentation, lichenification, alopecia, and scaling) and pyotraumatic dermatitis ("hotspots") are common. Erythema and papules around the umbilicus are highly suggestive ("peri-umbilical rush") • Cats—head and neck pruritic papular dermatitis and/or a generalized distribution including dorsal lumbosacral area, caudomedial thighs, and abdomen. Also common clinical signs are self-induced symmetrical alopecia and lesions of the eosinophilic granuloma complex.

CAUSES

See Pathophysiology.

RISK FACTORS

Exposure to fleas; atopy may predispose dogs to FBH.

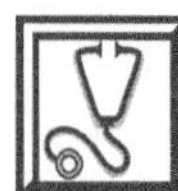

DIAGNOSIS

DIFFERENTIAL DIAGNOSIS

• Food allergy. • Atopy. • Ectoparasitism. • Dermatophytosis. • Pyoderma. • Any pruritic skin disease.

CBC/BIOCHEMISTRY/URINALYSIS

• Usually normal. • Cats—occasional eosinophilia.

OTHER LABORATORY TESTS

• Skin scrapings—negative. • Flea combings—may find fleas or flea dirt. • Intradermal allergen testing (IDT), radioallergosorbent test (RAST), and ELISA—variable accuracy; both false-positive and false-negative results reported.

DIAGNOSTIC PROCEDURES

• Diagnosis based on historical information, clinical signs, and response to anti-flea treatment. • Fleas or flea dirt is supportive but not mandatory. • Identification of *Dipylidium caninum* segments in stool is supportive. • The only way to confirm FBH is by response to treatment.

PATHOLOGIC FINDINGS

• Superficial perivascular to interstitial dermatitis. • Eosinophils often the predominant cell type.• Eosinophilic intra-epidermal microabscesses may be visible. • In cats—superficial or deep perivascular to interstitial dermatitis with numerous eosinophils and mast calls. • Histopathologic evaluation—does not differentiate FBH from other hypersensitivities.

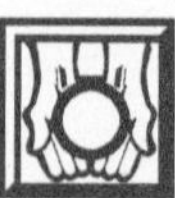

TREATMENT

APPROPRIATE HEALTH CARE

Outpatient therapy.

NURSING CARE

N/A

DIET

N/A

CLIENT EDUCATION

• Inform owners that there is no cure for FBH; flea-allergic animals often become more sensitive to flea bites as they age. • Hyposensitization is not effective. • Medications that stop itching are meant to bring relief while flea control is instituted.

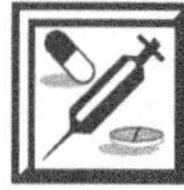

MEDICATIONS

DRUG(S) OF CHOICE

Itch Relief

Corticosteroids

• Anti-inflammatory dosages for symptomatic relief while instituting adequate flea control. Use only as much as is needed and for the shortest duration to achieve the desired effect. • Oral—prednisolone: cats, 1–2 mg/kg PO q24h for 5–7 days then taper; dogs, 0.5–1 mg/kg PO q24h for 7 days then taper, or for 4 days without tapering.

Oclacitinib

• Anti-itch, mild to moderate anti-inflammatory properties approved for allergic itch relief in dogs only. Usually a 7–10-day period is enough to control the itch while the anti-flea treatment is enhanced. • Oral: 0.4–0.6 mg/kg q12h for 14 days, then reduce frequency to q24h.

Antihistamines

Little to no effect.

Flea Control

The most important therapy is the immediate reduction or elimination of adult fleas on the host. In a highly infested environment, it is recommended to treat the surroundings as well.

Pet-Targeted Flea Control

• Oral: ○ Nitenpyram—adulticide; has the fastest onset, but short acting; for dogs q24h, for cats q48h. ○ Spinosad—monthly oral treatment for dogs and cats. ○ Isoxazolines—very effective antiparasitic drugs, lotilaner, and sarolaner monthly and fluralaner trimonthly. • Topical/spot-on: ○ Dinotefuran/pyriproxyfen—rapid-acting spot-on product for dogs and cats; a second canine product

contains high-dose permethrin and should not be used on cats. o Fipronil plus insect growth regulator (IGR)—spot-on treatment for cats and dogs (spray treatment for dogs).
o Imidacloprid plus IGR—monthly spot-on treatment for cats and dogs; a second canine product contains permethrin and should not be used on cats; also available as a collar.
o Indoxycarb—monthly spot-on, dogs only, activated by flea digestive enzymes, contains permethrin, should not be used on cats.
o Selamectin—for dogs and cats, monthly spot-on; also has insect development inhibitor (IDI) action. o Selamectin plus sarolaner spot-on for cats—monthly spot-on.
o Fluralaner spot-on for dogs and cats—tri-monthly treatment. • Sprays—usually contain pyrethrins and pyrethroids with IGR.

IGRs

S-methoprene and pyriproxyfen are analogues of insect juvenile hormone that bind to immature stages and prevent maturation.

IDIs

Lufenuron and selamectin inhibit chitin synthesis in egg shell, immature stages, and adults.

Premises-Targeted Flea Control

• Indoor treatment: o Vacuuming significantly reduces the flea burden: removing eggs, larvae, and adult fleas; particularly carpets, furniture and the floor under furniture. o "Foggers/bombs" and premises sprays—contain organophosphates, pyrethrins, and/or IGRs. Etofenprox plus IGR and permethrin/pyrethrin plus IGR, available in inverted aerosol sprays; apply according to manufacturer's directions; treat all areas of the house; can be applied by the owner. o Foggers/bombs do not effectively penetrate all areas commonly inhabited by fleas such as under furniture; handheld sprays are highly effective against biomass, may be directed where flea populations reside, and have long residual activity. • Professional exterminator—discuss products with representative.

Environment-Targeted Flea Control

• Outdoor treatment—concentrate in shaded areas; sprays usually contain pyrethroids or organophosphates and an IGR; owners should be educated on areas of application based on likelihood of reinfestation from feral cats and wildlife.
• Nematode (*Steinerma carpocapsae*)—may kill *C. felis* larvae and pupae, but efficacy is unknown; no knowledge of the effects these worms might have on beneficial insects, mammals, or humans.

CONTRAINDICATIONS

N/A

PRECAUTIONS

• Label instructions—must be strictly followed.
• Spinosad can potentiate neurologic side effects of high-dose ivermectin—but is safe when combined with heartworm preventive dose. • Isoxazolines should be used with caution in animals with preexisting epilepsy.
• Pyrethrin/pyrethroid-type flea products—adverse reactions include depression, hypersalivation, muscle tremors, vomiting, ataxia, dyspnea, and anorexia: do not use in cats.
• Organophosphates—inappropriate given the current alternatives.

ALTERNATIVE DRUG(S)

• Powders and dips—adverse reactions and toxicity make their use inappropriate given the current alternatives. Shampoos containing D-limonene on cats can cause acute necrotizing dermatitis and septicemia.
• Over-the-counter products often contain the same ingredient(s), but the absence of proper education frequently leads to failure in flea control.

FOLLOW-UP

PATIENT MONITORING

• Pruritus—a decrease means the FBH is being controlled. • Fleas and flea dirt—absence is not always a reliable indicator of successful treatment.

PREVENTION/AVOIDANCE

• Warm climates and infested premises require year-round flea control. • Seasonally warm climates—begin flea control when temperatures consistently remain above freezing.

POSSIBLE COMPLICATIONS

• Secondary bacterial folliculitis. • Acute moist dermatitis. • Acral lick dermatitis.

EXPECTED COURSE AND PROGNOSIS

Prognosis is excellent if strict flea control is instituted.

MISCELLANEOUS

ASSOCIATED CONDITIONS

• Anemia—could result from heavy flea burden, especially in puppies or kittens. • *Dipylidium caninum* due to ingestion of the flea.

AGE-RELATED FACTORS

Package should be consulted for the minimum approved age for application.

ZOONOTIC POTENTIAL

• Humans can be bitten by fleas; the resulting papular rash can be mild to extensive, depending on numbers of fleas and individual hypersensitivity reactions. • *C. felis* can transmit zoonotic agents, including *B. henselae* (cat scratch disease), *R. felis* (murine typhus, flea-borne typhus), and *D. caninum* (tapeworms).

PREGNANCY/FERTILITY/BREEDING

• Corticosteroids and organophosphates—do not use in pregnant bitches and queens.
• The safe use of sarolaner and afoxolaner has not been evaluated in breeding, pregnant, or lactating dogs.

SYNONYMS

• Flea bite allergy. • Flea allergy dermatitis.

ABBREVIATIONS

• ELISA = enzyme-linked immunosorbent assay.
• FBH = flea bite hypersensitivity.
• IDI = insect development inhibitor.
• IDT = intradermal allergen testing.
• Ig = immunoglobulin.
• IGR = insect growth regulator.
• RAST = radioallergosorbent test.

INTERNET RESOURCES

http://capcvet.org

Suggested Reading

Rust MK. The biology and ecology of cat fleas and advancements in their pest management: a review. Insects 2017, 8:118.

Author Ronnie Kaufmann
Consulting Editor Alexander H. Werner Resnick
Acknowledgment The author and book editors acknowledge the prior contribution of Steven A. Levy.

Client Education Handout available online

F

FOOD REACTIONS, DERMATOLOGIC

BASICS

DEFINITION

• Adverse reactions to food affecting the skin. • Associated with ingestion of one or more substances. • Reaction may be immunologic or idiosyncratic.

PATHOPHYSIOLOGY

• Pathogenesis not completely understood. • Food hypersensitivity—immediate and delayed reactions to specific ingredients documented; immediate reactions presumed to be type I hypersensitivity reactions; delayed presumed to be type III or IV. • Failure or prevention of the development of oral tolerance to food allergens may encourage sensitization. • Food intolerance—nonimmunologic, idiosyncratic reaction; involves metabolic, toxic, or pharmacologic effects of offending ingredients. • Adverse food reaction is the most common term used, and does not distinguish between immunologic and idiosyncratic reactions. • Adverse food reactions patients associated with an increased predisposition to atopy. • Cutaneous adverse food reactions can trigger flares of atopic dermatitis.

SYSTEMS AFFECTED

• Skin/exocrine. • Gastrointestinal. • Nervous.

GENETICS

N/A

INCIDENCE/PREVALENCE

• Approximately 5% of all dermatitis and 10–15% of allergic dermatitis in dogs and cats are caused by adverse reactions to food. • 13–30% of food allergic dogs have concurrent atopy or flea bite hypersensitivity. • Third most common pruritic skin disease in the dog; second most common in the cat. • Percentages vary greatly with clinicians and geographic location.

SIGNALMENT

Species

Dogs and cats.

Breed Predilections

• Dogs—none reported; breeds associated with atopic dermatitis overrepresented. • Cats—Siamese.

Mean Age and Range

• Any age—dogs: possibly increased development (over other allergic dermatoses) in patients <12 months or >7 years of age; 40% of cases develop at <12 months of age in one study; cats: patients <2 years or >5 years of age. • Most adult patients have been fed the offending allergen for over 2 years prior to becoming symptomatic.

Predominant Sex

None reported.

SIGNS

General Comments

• Symptoms similar to other hypersensitivity reactions. • Pruritus is the main dermatologic sign.

Historical Findings

• Pruritus of any bodily location. • Usually nonseasonal. • Poor response to anti-inflammatory doses of glucocorticosteroids, or oclacitinib or lokivetmab. • Recurrent bacterial folliculitis with or without pruritus. • Persistent otitis externa. • Concurrent gastrointestinal symptoms in a minority of cases—vomiting and/or diarrhea, excessive borborygmus, flatulence, and frequent bowel movements. • Very rare association of neurologic signs (seizures) with food hypersensitivity. • Respiratory signs have been reported in dogs.

Physical Examination Findings

• Dogs—rump, perineum, axillae, groin, face, and interdigital areas frequently affected. • Cats—face, neck, and ears frequently affected. • Cats—lesions of the eosinophilic granuloma complex. • Otitis externa. • Malassezia dermatitis.
• Secondary bacterial folliculitis.
• Plaques. • Pustules. • Erythema.
• Crusts. • Scale. • Self-induced alopecia.
• Excoriation. • Lichenification.
• Hyperpigmentation. • Urticaria.
• Angioedema. • Pyotraumatic dermatitis.
• Acral lick dermatitis.

CAUSES

• Immune-mediated reactions (food hypersensitivity)—result from the ingestion and subsequent presentation to the immune system of one or more glycoproteins (allergens) either before or after digestion; sensitization may occur at the gastrointestinal mucosa, after the substance is absorbed, or both; cross-reactivity between various food allergens, and between food and pollen allergens, has been demonstrated. • Non-immune-mediated reactions (food intolerance)—result of ingestion of foods with high levels of histamine or substances that induce histamine either directly or through histamine-releasing factors.

RISK FACTORS

• Unknown. • Intestinal parasites, infection, or inflammation may damage the intestinal mucosa, resulting in the abnormal absorption of allergens and subsequent sensitization.

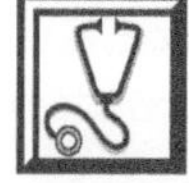

DIAGNOSIS

DIFFERENTIAL DIAGNOSIS

• Flea bite hypersensitivity—usually confined to the caudal half of the body; often seasonal. • Atopy—similar clinical symptoms, but typically develop between 1 and 3 years of age; 20–30% of dogs with adverse reactions to food also have atopic dermatitis. • Drug reactions—history of drug administration before the development of signs and improvement after withdrawal of the suspected drug. • Scabies mites—pruritus usually specific to the ears, elbows, and hocks (dogs) and head, ears, and neck (cats); mites in skin scrapings and/or response to specific therapy.

CBC/BIOCHEMISTRY/URINALYSIS

N/A

OTHER LABORATORY TESTS

In vitro (serum, hair, saliva) allergy tests; poor correlation between test results and food exposure; poor correlation between diet trial and test results; neither sensitive or specific; significant discrepancy between labs; currently no standard to enable comparisons between techniques; not recommended either as a diagnostic test for food allergy or for choosing appropriate ingredients for food trials.

DIAGNOSTIC PROCEDURES

Diagnosis requires response to dietary exclusion in the form of restricted-ingredient food trials followed by challenge and redevelopment of symptoms.

Food Elimination Diet

• Definitive test for adverse food reactions. • Tailored to the individual patient. • Diet must be restricted to one novel protein and one novel carbohydrate—veterinary prescription novel protein or hydrolyzed diets strongly recommended over over-the-counter novel protein diets; multiple studies report contamination of over-the-counter diets with proteins not listed on the label. • Most patients will improve within 6–8 weeks. • Food trials should be continued up to 10 weeks unless improvement occurs earlier. • Home-cooked food trials remove possible sources of antigen due to processing, storage, and cross-contamination from other ingredients.

Challenge and Provocation Diet Trials

• Used if the patient improves on the elimination diet.
• Challenge—feed the patient the original diet; a return of the signs confirms that the original diet contains an inciting ingredient; the challenge period should last until the signs return, but no longer than 10 days.
• Provoke (provocation diet trial)—if the challenge confirmed the presence of an adverse food reaction, add single ingredients to the elimination diet; test ingredients include a full range of meats (beef, chicken, fish, pork, lamb), a full range of carbohydrates (corn, wheat, soybean, rice), eggs, and dairy products; the provocation period for each ingredient should last up to 10 days or less if signs develop sooner; results

guide the selection of commercial foods that do not contain the offending substance(s).

PATHOLOGIC FINDINGS

• Skin biopsy—not diagnostic; may be helpful to confirm or eliminate other differential diagnoses. • Histopathologic findings—variable; common findings suggest hypersensitivity; secondary bacterial folliculitis or Malassezia dermatitis may be present.

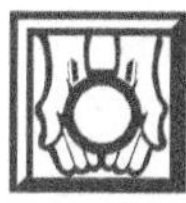

TREATMENT

Avoidance of the offending food substance(s).

APPROPRIATE HEALTH CARE

Outpatient management.

DIET

Avoid any food substances that caused the clinical signs to return during the provocation phase of the diagnosis.

CLIENT EDUCATION

• Explain the principles involved in each phase of the diagnostic test diets. • Instruct client to eliminate treats, chewable toys, vitamins, medication wraps, and flavored medications (e.g., parasiticides), as these may contain previously fed ingredients. • If a home-cooked diet is needed, the website www.balanceit.com is useful to create a diet with adequate supplementation. • Outdoor pets must be confined to prevent foraging and hunting. • Advise all family members to adhere to the restricted-ingredient diet trial protocol.

MEDICATIONS

DRUG(S) OF CHOICE

• Systemic antipruritic drugs—may be useful during the first 2–3 weeks of diet trial to control self-mutilation. • Antibiotics or antifungal medications—useful for secondary bacterial folliculitis or Malassezia dermatitis.

CONTRAINDICATIONS

• Antibiotics that are known to have anti-inflammatory effects (e.g., tetracycline, doxycycline, erythromycin, and trimethoprim-potentiated sulfas) may confuse response to dietary trials. • Chewable medications may contain a food protein such as chicken or beef to which the animal is allergic. • Glucocorticosteroids and antihistamines should be discontinued for at least 10–14 days while on the diet trial to allow correct assessment of the animal's response.

PRECAUTIONS

N/A

POSSIBLE INTERACTIONS

None

ALTERNATIVE DRUG(S)

None

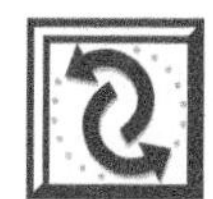

FOLLOW-UP

PATIENT MONITORING

Examine patient and evaluate and document the pruritus and clinical signs every 3–4 weeks.

PREVENTION/AVOIDANCE

Avoid intake of any of the ingredients included in the previous diet, including treats and chewable vitamins and toys.

POSSIBLE COMPLICATIONS

Other causes of pruritus, such as bacterial or yeast infections, as well as parasites such as fleas or mites, must be eliminated or controlled to permit accurate assessment of the effect of dietary antigens on clinical signs.

EXPECTED COURSE AND PROGNOSIS

• Prognosis is good if food ingredients are the only cause of pruritus and offending ingredients are avoided. • Rarely a dog or cat may develop hypersensitivity to new substances, requiring a new elimination diet trial. • A partial response to a food elimination diet trial suggests a combined food reaction with atopy or with another cause of pruritus.

MISCELLANEOUS

ASSOCIATED CONDITIONS

• Superficial bacterial folliculitis. • Malassezia dermatitis. • Otitis externa. • Atopic dermatitis.

AGE-RELATED FACTORS

None, except age ranges during which symptoms of food allergy most often develop.

ZOONOTIC POTENTIAL

None

PREGNANCY/FERTILITY/BREEDING

N/A

SYNONYMS

• Adverse reactions to food. • Food allergy. • Food hypersensitivity. • Food intolerance.

SEE ALSO

• Atopic Dermatitis. • Contact Dermatitis. • Flea Bite Hypersensitivity and Flea Control. • Malassezia Dermatitis. • Otitis Externa and Media. • Pyoderma.

Suggested Reading

Foster AP, Knowles TG, Moore AH, et al. Serum IgE and IgG responses to food antigens in normal and atopic dogs, and dogs with gastrointestinal disease. Vet Immunol Immunopathol 2003, 92(3–4):113–124.

Hillier A, Griffin CE. The ACVD task force on canine atopic dermatitis (X): Is there a relationship between canine atopic dermatitis and cutaneous adverse food reactions? Vet Immunol Immunopathol 2001, 81(3–4):227–231.

Olivry T, DeBoer DJ, Prélaud P, et al. International Task Force on Canine Atopic Dermatitis. Vet Dermatol 2006, 17:223–235.

Olivry T, Mueller RS. Critically appraised topic on adverse food reactions of companion animals (3): prevalence of cutaneous adverse food reactions in dogs and cats. BMC Vet Res 2017, 13(1):51.

Verlinden A, Hesta M, Millet S, Janssens GP. Food allergy in dogs and cats: a review. Crit Rev Food Sci Nutr 2006, 46(3):259–273.

Author David D. Duclos

Consulting Editor Alexander H. Werner Resnick

Client Education Handout available online

FOOD REACTIONS (GASTROINTESTINAL), ADVERSE

BASICS

DEFINITION

• Adverse food reactions encompass disorders with an immunologic (food allergy), non-immunologic (food intolerance), and toxic basis (food intoxication). • Food allergy, food intolerance, and food intoxication may have similar signs, diagnostics, and treatments and may not be easily distinguishable.

PATHOPHYSIOLOGY

• The pathogenesis of food allergy involves complex immunologic events—a leaky intestinal mucosal barrier, dysregulated immune responses, and loss of oral tolerance. Most food allergies are due to type 1 hypersensitivity reactions. Major food allergens include milk, eggs, beef, chicken, and plant proteins from corn, wheat, and soybeans. • Food intolerance may be due to idiosyncratic reactions to dietary ingredients or additives, pharmacologic reactions to compounds in the diet, defects or deficiencies in the metabolic pathways needed to use the food, or a toxicity reaction to food ingredients or spoiled foodstuffs. Unlike food allergy, food intolerance requires no previous exposure to the food product. • Toxic reactions to food may occur when a foodstuff is ingested in large amounts (e.g., onion poisoning). • Toxicity reactions occur when food contains toxins (e.g., aflatoxin, a hepatotoxin produced by *Aspergillus* spp.) or has spoiled or been contaminated by bacterial growth.

SYSTEMS AFFECTED

• Gastrointestinal (GI)—small intestine, colon, and/or stomach can be affected by adverse food reactions. • Skin/exocrine—food allergy can manifest with concurrent dermatologic signs or exclusive dermatologic signs.

GENETICS

Gluten sensitivity in Irish setters has a genetic basis.

INCIDENCE/PREVALENCE

Up to 50% of dogs and cats with chronic GI signs respond to an elimination diet.

GEOGRAPHIC DISTRIBUTION

N/A

SIGNALMENT

Species

Dog and cat.

Breed Predilections

• Soft-coated wheaten terriers affected with the syndrome of protein-losing enteropathy (PLE) and/or protein-losing nephropathy (PLN) have been shown to be affected by food allergies, which may play a role in the development of PLE/PLN. • Gluten-sensitive enteropathy is an autosomal recessive trait seen in some Irish setters.

Mean Age and Range

• Dogs affected with diet-responsive chronic enteropathy tend to be young (median age 3.4 years in one study). • Cats of all ages have been reported to be affected (median age 5 years).

Predominant Sex

None

SIGNS

General Comments

• Food intolerance commonly produces diarrhea (small or large bowel), vomiting, flatulence, anorexia, and abdominal discomfort. • Food allergy may cause cutaneous signs, such as pruritus and hair loss, which may be associated with GI signs.

Historical Findings

• Acute food intolerance may accompany feeding a novel foodstuff, a new food source, or dietary change. • Clients may report cessation of clinical signs in the fasted state or within days of an elimination diet trial.

Physical Examination Findings

The physical examination is generally nonspecific, but may show abdominal discomfort, flatulence, bloating, or patchy areas of alopecia along the pinnae of the ears and periorbital regions, especially in cats.

CAUSES

• Idiosyncratic reactions to food additives—colorings, preservatives (butylated hydroxyanisole, monosodium glutamate, sodium nitrate, sulfur dioxide, etc.), spices, propylene glycol, etc. • Pharmacologic reactions—vasoactive substances (i.e., histamine), psychoactive agents, stimulants (i.e., theobromine, caffeine), etc. • Metabolic defects or deficiencies—brush border enzyme defects (i.e., lactase deficiency), inborn errors of metabolism, aminopeptidase N (in gluten-sensitive enteropathy). • Toxic reactions to foods or spoiled foods—spices, oxalate toxicity, lectin toxicity, *N*-propyl disulfide aflatoxicosis, ergotism, botulism, dietary indiscretion, etc. • Genetic mutations in innate immunity genes regulating host responses to dietary constituents.

RISK FACTORS

• Young Irish setters susceptible to gluten-sensitive enteropathy may be at greater risk of developing the disease if exposed to gluten at an early age. • Host genetic susceptibility is suspected in wheaten terriers and German shepherd dogs.

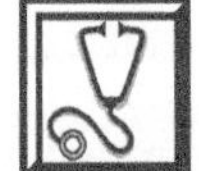

DIAGNOSIS

DIFFERENTIAL DIAGNOSIS

• Infectious diseases—intestinal nematodes, *Giardia*, histoplasmosis, salmonellosis, toxoplasmosis (cats), feline infectious peritonitis. • Infiltrative GI diseases—inflammatory bowel disease, histiocytic ulcerative colitis (boxers, French bulldogs). • Endocrine diseases—hypoadrenocorticism, hyperthyroidism (cats). • Exocrine pancreatic insufficiency. • Lymphangiectasia. • GI motility disorders. • Pancreatitis. • Metabolic diseases (renal disease, liver disease).

CBC/BIOCHEMISTRY/URINALYSIS

Usually normal; animals with food allergy may occasionally have eosinophilia.

OTHER LABORATORY TESTS

• Few diagnostic tests are specific to adverse food reactions, but the following are helpful to rule out differential diagnoses and to identify complicating factors. • Serum cobalamin and folate—can help determine involvement of proximal and distal small intestine as well as identify possible need for supplementation. • Trypsin-like immunoreactivity—for exocrine pancreatic insufficiency. • Baseline cortisol or adrenocorticotropic hormone stimulation test—to rule out hypoadrenocorticism if clinically suspected. • Total T_4 (cats)—to evaluate for hyperthyroidism if clinically suspected. • Fecal alpha-1 proteinase inhibitor—this test can be performed if there is a suspicion of PLE, but other lab results are equivocal, or there is complicating proteinuria. • Perinuclear antineutrophilic cytoplasmic autoantibodies—this test is currently limited to use in a research setting, but has shown promise in early detection of PLE and PLN, believed to be due to underlying food allergy, in soft-coated wheaten terriers. Additionally, it may help to differentiate between dogs with diet-responsive enteropathies and enteropathies requiring treatment with glucocorticoids. • Fecal flotation and fecal smear—perform 2–3 tests over several days to increase sensitivity. • Empiric deworming with a broad-spectrum anthelminthic may be considered to address possible undetected parasitism.

IMAGING

• Abdominal radiographs or ultrasound may be useful in eliminating differential diagnoses. • Doppler evaluation (ultrasound) may detect alterations in blood flow through the celiac and cranial mesenteric arteries of dogs.

DIAGNOSTIC PROCEDURES

• Perform an elimination diet trial of 2 weeks in cats and 3 weeks in dogs with GI signs. • Following improvement on an elimination diet, use challenge exposure to sequential single ingredients to specifically identify the incriminating dietary ingredient. While technically the gold standard, this is generally impractical in a clinical setting.

• Exclusive feeding with a hydrolyzed or novel protein source indefinitely is generally required to prevent clinical relapse. • Perform urinalysis and urine protein : creatinine ratio (if indicated) in diet-responsive wheaten terriers to screen for concurrent glomerular injury with urinary protein loss.

PATHOLOGIC FINDINGS

Villous atrophy and mild lymphoplasmacytic enteritis may be seen with food allergy.

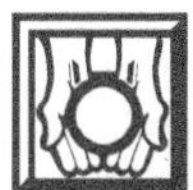

TREATMENT

APPROPRIATE HEALTH CARE

Generally treat on an outpatient basis.

NURSING CARE

If an adverse food reaction is severe, IV fluid therapy, administration of antiemetics, and nutritional support via enteral-assisted feeding may be temporarily required.

ACTIVITY

No restrictions.

DIET

• Lifelong dietary management is essential for animals with food intolerance and food allergy. • Diets that can be chosen for an elimination diet trial include veterinary prescription hydrolyzed protein diets, commercial novel protein diets (available as veterinary prescription diets or over-the-counter products), or a home-cooked novel protein diet. • Novel protein diets are foods containing only protein sources to which the animal has not been previously exposed and are selected based on a careful dietary history. • Over-the-counter novel protein diets have been found to contain proteins other than those listed on the label, which may be due to contamination during processing; veterinary prescription products are prepared specifically for animals with food allergy and should be chosen when possible. • Home-prepared novel protein diets can uncommonly result in a beneficial response in animals who did not respond to a commercial diet containing the same protein. Considerations for home-prepared novel protein diets are that many are not suitable for long-term feeding (unless the diet is complete and balanced with the help of a veterinary nutritionist) and create inconvenience for the owner, which may limit compliance. • Hydrolyzed protein diets are created by enzymatic hydrolysis of the intact protein into peptides small enough to reduce the potential of the protein to induce an allergic response. • Hydrolyzed diets are ideal when an animal has been exposed to many different protein sources or when a reliable dietary history cannot be obtained. • Hydrolyzed protein diets can retain some antigenicity and, if possible, the parent protein of the hydrolyzed diet should be a protein to which the animal does not have a known sensitivity. • Hydrolyzed protein diets may also benefit animals without true food allergy due to the improved digestibility of the diet.

CLIENT EDUCATION

• Owners should be aware of possible sources of food antigen during an elimination trial that may make the animal's response difficult to interpret, including table scraps, flavored medications and toothpastes, and coprophagy. • Counsel clients on the necessity of lifelong avoidance of ingredients to which their animal is sensitive.

SURGICAL CONSIDERATIONS

N/A

MEDICATIONS

N/A

FOLLOW-UP

PATIENT MONITORING

• Assess efficacy of elimination diet trial by observing improvement in GI signs. • Failure to improve in 2–3 weeks may warrant a subsequent trial with another diet if adverse food reaction is strongly suspected, or continued work-up for other causes of GI signs, including endoscopy with biopsies.

PREVENTION AND AVOIDANCE

Avoid foods, treats, and flavored medications outside of the elimination diet.

POSSIBLE COMPLICATIONS

N/A

EXPECTED COURSE AND PROGNOSIS

The prognosis is excellent as long as the offending dietary components are successfully identified and avoided.

MISCELLANEOUS

ASSOCIATED CONDITIONS

N/A

AGE-RELATED FACTORS

N/A

ZOONOTIC POTENTIAL

None

PREGNANCY/FERTILITY/BREEDING

N/A

SYNONYMS

• Food intolerance. • Food allergy. • Dietary sensitivity. • Food-responsive enteropathy.

SEE ALSO

- Acute Diarrhea.
- Diarrhea, Chronic—Cats.
- Diarrhea, Chronic—Dogs.
- Gluten Enteropathy in Irish Setters.

ABBREVIATIONS

- GI = gastrointestinal.
- PLE = protein-losing enteropathy.
- PLN = protein-losing nephropathy.

INTERNET RESOURCES

https://www.vin.com/VIN.plx

Suggested Reading

Gaschen FP, Merchant SR. Adverse food reactions in dogs and cats. Vet Clin North Am Small Anim Pract 2011, 41(2):361–379.

Guilford WG. Food sensitivity in cats with chronic idiopathic gastrointestinal problems. J Vet Intern Med 2001, 15:7–13.

Roudebush P. Ingredients and foods associated with adverse reactions in dogs and cats. Vet Dermatol 2013, 24(2):293–294.

Author Albert E. Jergens

Consulting Editor Mark P. Rondeau

Client Education Handout available online

GALLBLADDER MUCOCELE

G

BASICS

OVERVIEW

• Gallbladder (GB) accumulation of tenacious, thick, mucin-rich, inspissated bile conglomerate (sludge) impairing GB reservoir capacity and GB contraction, thereby thwarting periprandial bile expulsion; often associated with episodic abdominal pain.
• Organized sludge expands GB lumen, flattens/thins GB wall; when severe, provokes necrotizing cholecystitis and occasional GB rupture. • Canine syndrome, rare in cats.
• Initiated by GB dysmotility.

SIGNALMENT

• Dog. • Shetland sheepdogs, miniature schnauzers, cocker spaniels, bichon frisé, shih tzu overrepresented in one study of 219 dogs. • Middle-aged to older adults.
• No sex predilection. • Associated with endocrinopathies—adrenal hyperplasia (typical or sex hormone atypical form), hypothyroidism, diabetes mellitus, and administration of glucocorticoids; these likely associated with GB dysmotility, hypertriglyceridemia, or hypercholesterolemia that may impart negative influence on GB contraction. • Notably associated with hypertriglyceridemic syndromes.

SIGNS

General Comments

• Symptomatic or asymptomatic—depending on stage at diagnosis: mature vs. immature gall bladder mucocele (GBM). • Asymptomatic GBM—often serendipitously discovered on abdominal US.

Historical Findings: Symptomatic

• Episodic periprandial abdominal discomfort. • Anorexia. • Vomiting.
• Lethargy. • ± Polyuria/polydipsia—reflects underlying endocrinopathy. • Collapse—vasovagal episode or bile peritonitis.

Physical Examination Findings

• May demonstrate no physical signs if immature GBM. • ± Lethargy. • ± Cranial abdominal discomfort—GB dysmotility and maturing GBM. • Jaundice late in syndrome.
• ± Dehydration. • ± Fever—secondary infection.

CAUSES & RISK FACTORS

• Inborn errors of lipid metabolism (hypertriglyceridemia)—miniature schnauzer, Shetland sheepdogs, beagles, others.
• Medical/dietary conditions provoking hypercholesterolemia or dyslipidemia—endocrinopathies, recurrent pancreatitis, feeding high-fat diet to dog with predisposing disorder or dyslipidemia. • GB dysmotility.
• Cystic mucosal hyperplasia—common in older dogs; may be aggravated by sex hormones (e.g., progestins).

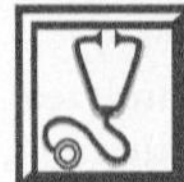

DIAGNOSIS

DIFFERENTIAL DIAGNOSIS

Conditions causing GB bile stasis—GB dysmotility; or other causes of incomplete GB emptying such as cystic duct or GB wall neoplasia, pedunculated adenomatous mucosal lesions, ball-valve cholelith obstructions.

CBC/BIOCHEMISTRY/URINALYSIS

CBC

• Inflammatory leukogram—variable, depends on GB wall viability and hepatic impact of GBM. • Stress leukogram—if underlying hyperadrenocorticism.
• Nonregenerative anemia—if chronic inflammation or hypothyroidism.

Biochemistry

• High liver enzymes—may be noted on acute presentation for GBM or serendipitously discovered on routine health assessments; alkaline phosphatase (ALP), γ-glutamyltransferase (GGT), alanine aminotransferase (ALT), ± aspartate aminotransferase (AST) variably affected; ALP activity predominant.
• High ALP—often associates with glycogen-type vacuolar hepatopathy (VH), may reflect adrenal endocrinopathy or glucocorticoid therapy. • Variable hyperbilirubinemia; depends on GBM maturation and common bile duct patency. • Low albumin—if ruptured biliary tree and bile peritonitis.
• Prerenal azotemia—if ruptured GB, sepsis, or dehydration from vomiting. • Electrolyte abnormalities with fluid and acid-base disturbances—due to bile peritonitis or persistent vomiting.

Urinalysis

No specific features.

OTHER LABORATORY TESTS

• Triglyceride concentrations.
• Coagulation tests—normal unless chronic extrahepatic bile duct obstruction (EHBDO), GB rupture, bile peritonitis, sepsis, or disseminated intravascular coagulation (DIC).

IMAGING

• Abdominal radiography—normal or large liver; loss of detail in cranial abdomen if focal peritonitis with GB rupture or concurrent pancreatitis; rarely intrahepatic gas. • Abdominal US—liver may be large, with rounded margins, or normal sized; diffuse to multifocal hyperechoic hepatic parenchyma (associated with glycogen-type VH); may have hypoechoic nodular appearance if severe VH; typical GBM US image: lumen filled with amorphous echogenic "organizing" nongravitational debris with stellate or finely striated pattern resembling sliced kiwi fruit ("kiwi sign"); distended GB (>1.2 mL/kg bodyweight) and sometimes distended common bile duct ± cystic duct if EHBDO; pericholecystic edema may enhance GB wall imaging; pericholecystic or generalized effusion with hyperechogenicity of surrounding tissues may indicate focal peritonitis and bile leakage (even if GB wall not ruptured); diffusely thick GB wall with segmental hyperechogenicity and double-rimmed or laminated appearance associates with necrotizing cholecystitis; GB rupture associated with discontinuous GB wall or difficult-to-image GB; ruptured GBM may have inspissated congealed biliary material released into abdominal cavity where discrete free-floating "mass" may be discovered; intrahepatic bile ducts may be difficult to visualize or appear prominent or distended.
• GB motility study—indicated if suspected developing GBM serendipitously recognized if GB volume ≥1.2 mL/kg bodyweight; sequential GB volume measurements determined after meal ingestion (100 g food; may include 0.5 mg/kg erythromycin as motilin agonist provoking GB contraction if no response with food alone). Normal GB contraction results in ≥25% decline of initial or baseline GB volume on one or more recorded postprandial images. Procedure: image GB at 0, 15, 30, 45, 60, 90, 120 min relative to feeding. • GB volume in mL = [length (cm) × width (cm) × height (cm)] × 0.52.

DIAGNOSTIC PROCEDURES

• Aspiration sampling—fluid adjacent to biliary structures or free in abdominal cavity; clarifies GB rupture and/or infection; *caution*: do *not* perform cholecystocentesis on suspected GBM as this may cause bile peritonitis.
• Laparotomy—for diagnosis, cholecystectomy, perhaps cholecystenterostomy.
• Laparoscopy—*not* advised as CBD should be flushed to patency. • Liver biopsy—collect biopsy distant to GB; biopsy from GB area often interpreted as severely fibrotic or as cholangitis. • Bacterial culture/sensitivity—any effusion; GB wall, mucinous debris clinging to GB wall (scrape GB wall for best sample), liver (single inoculum); request aerobic and anaerobic bacterial culture. Positive ranging from 17% to 33% in different studies; histologic identification of bacteria unreliable.
• Cytology—impression smears of GB wall mucinous debris and liver assist prompt recognition of suppurative septic inflammation or rarely neoplasia.

PATHOLOGIC FINDINGS

• Gross—mature GBM: GB distended, wall may appear normal, erythematous, or hemorrhagic ± focal areas of necrosis; may be evidence of focal peritonitis with adhesions; liver and extrahepatic biliary structures usually appear normal but EHBDO possible; GB contents: dark green-black, tenacious, firm, or organized as solid light green-yellow rubbery conglomerate. Slender long proliferative mucosal projections or cystic mucosal hyperplasia on GB mucosa are common. Immature GBM: normal to distended GB with thick dark black green bile with black particulate calcium bilirubinate debris.

• Microscopic—mature GBM demonstrates mural thinning with elongate mucosal fronds ± cystic mucosal hyperplasia and laminated dehydrated mucin; occasional particulate bilirubinate conglomerates in GB sections; mixed inflammatory infiltrates and fibrosis in chronic GBM; focal areas of necrosis usually caused by arterial thrombosis; Gram stain and modified Steiner's stains should be used to detect intraluminal bacteria as not all cultures recover infectious organisms. If GB not sectioned before fixation, mucosa may not fix and will appear necrotic. Liver biopsy collected distant to GB often discloses glycogen-type VH with no evidence of mechanical bile stasis if immature GBM and underling endocrinopathy; ascending suppurative cholangitis and cholangiohepatitis may be secondary complications.

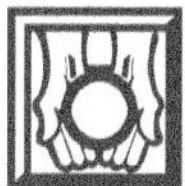

TREATMENT

• Outpatient management—ursodeoxycholic acid and *S*-adenosylmethionine (SAMe) induce bile acid and non-bile acid mediated choleresis and provide hepatoprotection—*but* medical therapy is *not* advised to resolve GBM. While medical management has occasionally resolved immature GBM in some dogs, these patients remain at risk for GBM recurrence. Naïve unmonitored treatment with choleretics may eventuate in ruptured GB. • Inpatient—depends on whether patient presents with severe acute necrotizing cholecystitis, suppurative cholecystitis, intact nonurgent mature GBM, or incidentally discovered immature GBM. • If patient hyperlipidemic, investigate cause, restrict dietary fat, avoid glucocorticoids. • Symptomatic patients require exploratory surgery for cholecystectomy and evaluation/treatment for potential bile peritonitis. • Cholecystotomy and mucocele removal with GB retention *not* advised; high risk for recurrent GBM and potential bile peritonitis. • Fluid therapy—balanced polyionic solutions to correct hydration and electrolyte status. • Be prepared for blood component therapy.
• Abdominal lavage—at surgery if bile peritonitis encountered.

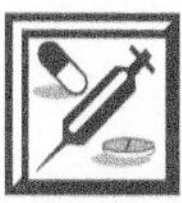

MEDICATIONS

DRUG(S) OF CHOICE

Antimicrobials

Initiate combined broad-spectrum antimicrobials *before* surgery; continue treatment 4–8 weeks if septic complications; adjust drugs based on culture and sensitivity test reports and biochemical appraisals. If no histologic or culture evidence of infection and postoperative recovery unremarkable, discontinue antimicrobials 7–10 days after surgery.

Vitamin K1

0.5–1.5 mg/kg IM/SC q12h for three doses—*if jaundiced*; oral route ineffective if EHBDO.

Antiemetics/Antacids/Gastroprotectants

• Antiemetics—may be needed during preoperative interval. Maropitant citrate (Cerenia®), NK-1 antagonist—2 mg/kg PO or 1 mg SC q24h up to 5 days. Ondansetron—0.1–0.3 mg/kg PO 30 min before feeding, maximum q8h, or 0.1–0.2 mg/kg slow IV push q6–12h if vomiting. • Antacids—preoperative interval, proton pump inhibitors preferred: omeprazole 0.7–1.0 mg/kg PO/IV q24h or pantoprazole 0.7–1.0 mg/kg IV q24h. • Gastric prokinetics—if postoperative gastric atony: metoclopramide 0.2–0.5 mg/kg PO/IV/SC q6–8h or 1–2 mg/kg/day CRI.
• Gastroprotectant—if suspected gastritis, esophagitis, or upper gastrointestinal bleeding: sucralfate—0.5–1.0 g PO q8–12h.

Choleretics

• Maintain hydration status to optimize choleresis. • Ursodeoxycholic acid—choleretic, hepatoprotectant, anti-inflammatory, anti-endotoxic effects: 10–15 mg/kg PO divided BID daily with food for best bioavailability; treat until complete biochemical recovery or chronically if suspect persistent cholangitis. • SAMe—choleretic, antioxidant, and metabolic benefits; choleretic dose (40 mg/kg PO q24h on empty stomach) higher than antioxidant dose.

Antioxidants

• Vitamin E—α-tocopherol 10 IU/kg/day PO with food: antioxidant, anti-inflammatory, antifibrotic influence.
• SAMe—20 mg/kg PO daily 2h before feeding: give until liver enzymes normalize or indefinitely if chronic hepatitis or cholangitis.

CONTRAINDICATIONS/POSSIBLE INTERACTIONS

N/A

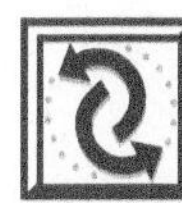

FOLLOW-UP

PATIENT MONITORING

• Repeat sequential hematology, biochemistry, and imaging to monitor surgical recovery; if GBM caused clinicopathologic abnormalities, all changes should resolve within weeks. • Persistent clinicopathologic abnormalities implicate underlying endocrinopathy, intrahepatic cholangiopathy, or other liver disease.
• At-risk dogs should have US assessment of GB as part of routine health appraisal when middle-aged to geriatric.

POSSIBLE COMPLICATIONS

• Suppurative cholangitis or cholangiohepatitis. • Bile peritonitis. • EHBDO.

EXPECTED COURSE AND PROGNOSIS

• Good with successful surgery, chronic choleretic therapy, correction/management of comorbid conditions, dietary and/or medical management of hypertriglyceridemia.
• Anticipate protracted clinical course if ruptured biliary tract or peritonitis—dogs with ruptured GBM 2–3 times more likely to succumb to GBM-related illness.
• Recrudescence may occur if mucocele contents removed and GB retained, with or without chronic medical therapy. • Chronic postoperative jaundice may reflect iatrogenic stricture at site of cholecystectomy.

MISCELLANEOUS

SEE ALSO

- Bile Peritonitis.
- Cholecystitis and Choledochitis.
- Cholelithiasis.
- Glycogen-Type Vacuolar Hepatopathy.
- Hepatitis, Chronic.

ABBREVIATIONS

- ALP = alkaline phosphatase.
- ALT = alanine aminotransferase.
- AST = aspartate aminotransferase.
- DIC = disseminated intravascular coagulation.
- EHBDO = extrahepatic bile duct obstruction.
- GB = gallbladder.
- GBM = gallbladder mucocele.
- GGT = γ-glutamyltransferase.
- SAMe = *S*-adenosylmethionine.
- VH = vacuolar hepatopathy.

Suggested Reading

Aguirre AL, Center SA, Randolph JF. Gallbladder disease in Shetland Sheepdogs: 38 cases (1995–2005). J Am Vet Med Assoc 2007, 231:79–88.

Jaffey JA, Graham A, VanEerde E, et al. Gallbladder mucocele: variables associated with outcome and the utility of ultrasonography to identify gallbladder rupture in 219 dogs (2007–2016). J Vet Intern Med 2018, 32:195–200.

Author Sharon A. Center
Consulting Editor Kate Holan

GASTRIC DILATION AND VOLVULUS SYNDROME

DEFINITION

Gastric dilation and volvulus syndrome (GDV) is a disease in which the stomach rotates around its short axis, with or without distention of the stomach.

PATHOPHYSIOLOGY

The mechanism and etiology are poorly understood. Many risk factors have been evaluated. Rotation of the stomach can occur in any direction, but the majority occur in clockwise rotation. The pylorus, pyloric antrum, and proximal duodenum move from dorsal to ventral, from right to left of the patient, continuing from the ventral abdomen to the left, and eventually are located in the left dorsal quadrant of the peritoneal cavity. With distention of the stomach, intra-abdominal pressure increases. Collapse of the compliant abdominal venous network leads to decreased venous return to the heart and portal hypertension. As the disease progresses, hypovolemic shock and decreased organ perfusion lead to local and systemic inflammatory response, visceral and myocardial ischemia, disseminated intravascular coagulation (DIC), and eventually cardiovascular collapse and death.

SYSTEMS AFFECTED

• Gastrointestinal (GI)—rotation of the stomach causes venous congestion of the stomach, spleen, pancreas, and proximal small intestine and arterial compromise of the stomach. • Hemic/lymphatic/immune—splenic engorgement, vascular compromise, ischemia, and thrombosis are common.
• Cardiovascular—both distributive and obstructive hypovolemic shock may be seen; cardiac arrhythmias are common. • Renal/urologic—acute kidney injury (AKI) may occur secondary to shock and renal vascular compression. • Endocrine/metabolic—nephrogenic diabetes insipidus has been reported, likely secondary to AKI, endotoxemia, and systemic inflammatory responses.

GENETICS

• Having a first-order relative with a history of GDV markedly increases the risk of developing GDV. • While the genetic basis is unknown, it is likely to be a complex, multifactorial (or polygenic) disorder.

INCIDENCE/PREVALENCE

One study indicated that likelihood of a purebred large- or giant-breed dog developing GDV during its lifetime is approximately 24% and 21.6%, respectively.

GEOGRAPHIC DISTRIBUTION

N/A

SIGNALMENT

Species

Dog (common) and cat (rare).

Breed Predilections

• German shepherd dog. • Great Dane.
• Standard poodle. • Labrador retriever.
• Akita. • Golden retriever. • Saint Bernard.
• Doberman pinscher. • Chow chow. • Collie.
• Rottweiler. • Mastiff. • Weimaraner.
• Bloodhound. • Basset hound. • Belgian shepherd. • Great Pyrenees. • Boxer. • Husky.
• German shorthaired pointer. • Samoyed.
• Newfoundland. • Bernese mountain dog.
• Smaller breeds are reported, including dachshund, corgi, and Pekingese.

Mean Age and Range

Any age. Risk increases with age in large- and giant-breed dogs.

Predominant Sex

Male > female.

SIGNS

Historical Findings

• Restlessness. • Anxiety. • Vomiting progressing to nonproductive retching or nonproductive retching alone. • Abdominal distension and/or pain. • Ptyalism.
• Lethargy. • Collapse.

Physical Examination Findings

• Distended abdomen; may not be noted in deep-chested dogs. • Tachycardia.
• Tachypnea or dyspnea. • Weak pulses.
• Pale or hyperemic mucus membranes and prolonged or rapid capillary refill time.

CAUSES

• Multifactorial. • Genetic. • Conformational.
• Environmental. • Secondary to gastric, hepatic, or splenic neoplasia. • Any cause of aerophagia. • Massive food consumption or other cause of gas or liquid gastric distention.
• Pyloric outflow obstruction.

RISK FACTORS

• Direct relative with a history of GDV.
• Large- or giant-breed dog. • Deep-chested body conformation. • History of splenic torsion, colonic torsion, or mesenteric volvulus. • Gastric motility disorder. • Rapid consumption of large amounts of food and water with or without excessive postprandial activity. • Altered microbiome. • Trauma. • Anxious temperament.

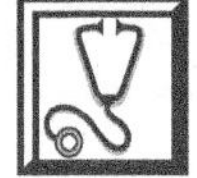

DIAGNOSIS

DIFFERENTIAL DIAGNOSIS

• Gastric dilation without volvulus.
• Abdominal effusion. • Any cause of abdominal pain. • Gastric or intestinal obstruction. • Urinary tract obstruction.
• Pyometra. • Splenic torsion. • Mesenteric volvulus. • Colonic torsion. • Hepatic, gastric, or splenic mass.

CBC/BIOCHEMISTRY/URINALYSIS

• Stress leukogram; hemoconcentration; thrombocytopenia from consumption if DIC is present or if significant intra-abdominal hemorrhage has occurred. • Electrolyte abnormalities; increased liver enzymes; azotemia, either prerenal or due to AKI.
• Increased specific gravity with dehydration; isosthenuria with AKI.

OTHER LABORATORY TESTS

• Plasma lactate—initial lactate and trends are useful in predicting gastric necrosis and prognosis. ○ Dogs with initial lactate >9 mmol/L had reduced survival (13/24 = 54%) compared to those with initial lactate ≤9 mmol/L (36/40 = 90%). ○ Dogs with initial lactate >9 mmol/L that did not decrease by ≥4 mmol/L had 10% survival rate, while those whose lactate decreased by ≥4 mmol/L with presurgical stabilization had 90% survival rate. ○ Decrease in plasma lactate by ≥50% within 12 hours is associated with a good outcome. • Coagulation testing—may show evidence for DIC.

IMAGING

• Abdominal radiography—right lateral abdominal radiograph is imaging modality of choice. ○ In a normal patient, the pylorus would be filled with fluid. ○ In a patient with GDV, the pylorus, which is now on the left side of the peritoneal cavity, is filled with gas and visualized as such, showing the classic compartmentalization of the stomach, which is considered to be pathognomonic. ○ Gas bubbles within the gastric wall indicate gastric necrosis. ○ Pneumoperitoneum may be evident. • Thoracic radiographs—three views to screen for aspiration pneumonia and metastatic disease; may also see evidence of hypovolemia (microcardia, small-caliber vessels). • Abdominal ultrasound—may show fluid due to small volume hemoabdomen, serosanguinous effusion, or gastric perforation.

DIAGNOSTIC PROCEDURES

ECG to detect presence of cardiac arrhythmias.

PATHOLOGIC FINDINGS

• Splenic engorgement, ischemia, malposition, and/or venous thrombosis.
• Gastric wall may appear edematous and thickened, or areas may be extremely thinned.

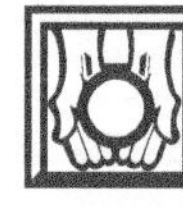

TREATMENT

APPROPRIATE HEALTH CARE

• GDV is a medical and surgical emergency.
• Aggressive emergency medical stabilization is initiated. • Subsequent to cardiovascular stabilization, gastric decompression should be performed, ideally via orogastric intubation; the patient should be intubated with a cuffed endotracheal tube prior to performing orogastric intubation and decompression to minimize the risk of aspiration pneumonia.
• If orogastric intubation is unsuccessful,

percutaneous gastrocentesis may be performed for decompression by locating the point of maximal tympany, which typically corresponds to an area of the stomach that is gas filled. ○ The largest-diameter needle or catheter that the clinician is comfortable using is passed into the stomach at this area. ○ Considerable time is necessary to achieve gastric decompression using this technique. • Recent studies suggest that when comparing orogastric decompression and percutaneous decompression, there is no difference in complication rates or outcome. Therefore, clinicians should select the technique that they are most familiar and comfortable with. • Surgical management occurs once the patient is stable.

NURSING CARE

• IV fluid therapy is initiated and type, rate, and duration are based on individual patient needs and personal preference. ○ Avoid use of saphenous veins for emergency resuscitation, as venous return from the caudal half of the body is compromised. ○ Crystalloids, colloids, or a combination can be used; initial fluid resuscitation efforts may require crystalloid boluses at 15–30 mL/kg increments, up to 90 mL/kg total; colloid boluses up to 5–10 mL/kg total may be required. • Physical therapy may be necessary, as many patients will be recumbent for several days in the postoperative period.

ACTIVITY

Restriction of activity for 2 weeks postoperatively is recommended.

DIET

• Enteral nutrition is recommended as soon as adequate recovery from anesthesia has been achieved to stimulate GI mucosal healing and motility. • Optimal diet is unknown; consider fat-restricted diets to improve gastric emptying.

CLIENT EDUCATION

• Clients should be aware of the critical nature of GDV. • Patients can still experience gastric dilation after gastropexy, as many have gastric motility disorders.

SURGICAL CONSIDERATIONS

• Surgery is required after medical stabilization. • Goals of surgery are: ○ Continue decompression. ○ Assess stomach and spleen for evidence of devitalization and necrosis that necessitates partial gastrectomy or splenectomy. ○ Reposition stomach and spleen. ○ Perform systematic and thorough exploratory laparotomy. ○ Perform gastropexy to prevent recurrence of GDV—should always be performed; decreases risk of recurrent GDV from 80% to <5%; incorporating gastropexy and gastrocolopexy are associated with higher rates of recurrence of GDV and should not be performed.

MEDICATIONS

DRUG(S) OF CHOICE

• Lidocaine beginning with a 2 mg/kg IV bolus, followed by a CRI (0.05 mg/kg/min for 24h) in perioperative period improves morbidity but not mortality. ○ Fewer cardiac arrhythmias. ○ Lower incidence of AKI. ○ Shorter hospitalization. • Perioperative antibiotics are indicated. ○ For patients with moderate to severe disease in which there is a risk of visceral perforation or hematogenous bacterial translocation from the GI tract, cefoxitin sodium (30 mg/kg IV q6–8h) may be an appropriate choice. ○ For patients in which no entry into the GI tract has occurred, cefazolin sodium (22 mg/kg IVq2h intra-operatively) is sufficient. • Treatment for esophagitis and gastritis or gastric ulceration is indicated. ○ Pantoprazole (1 mg/kg IV q12h) or omeprazole (1 mg/kg PO q12h) for acid suppression. ○ Metoclopramide (2 mg/kg/day IV as CRI) or cisapride (0.5–1 mg/kg PO q8–12h) as a prokinetic. ○ Sucralfate 0.25–1 g PO as a slurry q6–8h if gastric ulceration is present. • Pain management based on patient needs postoperatively.

CONTRAINDICATIONS

Synthetic colloids should be used cautiously in patients with DIC or AKI.

PRECAUTIONS

Patients may decompensate at any time, particularly under anesthetic intervention. Emergency drug dosages should be calculated for the patient before anesthesia and be readily available.

POSSIBLE INTERACTIONS

N/A

ALTERNATIVE DRUG(S)

There is conflicting evidence to support the use of physiologic corticosteroids in patients with GDV. Use is not currently recommended.

FOLLOW-UP

PATIENT MONITORING

• Intermittent or continuous ECG postoperatively to monitor for arrhythmias. • Monitor urine production and renal function postoperatively.

PREVENTION/AVOIDANCE

While not proven, the following have been suggested to decrease risk of GDV: elevation of food bowl; avoiding exercise after eating or drinking; slowing rate of consumption of meals; feeding multiple smaller meals.

POSSIBLE COMPLICATIONS

• Gastric dilation without volvulus may recur, even after a gastropexy is performed, because of a possible underlying motility disorder. • Failure to resect all necrotic or devitalized gastric tissue may result in eventual stomach perforation and septic peritonitis. • Cardiac arrhythmias, DIC, esophagitis, AKI, and gastric ulceration may also occur.

EXPECTED COURSE AND PROGNOSIS

• Prognosis in dogs treated appropriately that do not have gastric necrosis is excellent, with a reported survival rate of 98%. • Dogs with gastric necrosis have a more guarded prognosis, with a reported survival rate of 66%. • Potential negative prognostic indicators include hypotension, DIC, peritonitis, and the need to perform both a splenectomy and a partial gastrectomy.

MISCELLANEOUS

ASSOCIATED CONDITIONS

N/A

AGE-RELATED FACTORS

More common in middle-aged to older dogs.

ZOONOTIC POTENTIAL

None

PREGNANCY/FERTILITY/BREEDING

Affected dogs should not be bred due to potential genetic predisposition.

SYNONYMS

• Bloat. • Gastric torsion. • Gastric volvulus.

ABBREVIATIONS

• AKI = acute kidney injury. • DIC = disseminated intravascular coagulation. • GDV = gastric dilation and volvulus syndrome. • GI = gastrointestinal.

Suggested Reading

Allen P, Paul A. Gastropexy for prevention of gastric dilation-volvulus in dogs: history and techniques. Top Companion Anim Med. 2014, 29:77–80.

Beck JJ, Staatz AJ, Pelsue DH, et al. Risk factors associated with short-term outcome and development of perioperative complications in dogs undergoing surgery because of gastric dilatation-volvulus: 166 cases (1992–2003). J Am Vet Med Assoc 2006, 229:1934–1939.

Zacher LA, Berg J, Shaw SP, Kudej RK. Association between outcome and changes in plasma lactate concentration during pre-surgical treatment in dogs with gastric dilation-volvulus: 64 cases (2004–2009). J Am Vet Med Assoc 2010, 236:892–897.

Author Stephen Mehler

Consulting Editor Mark P. Rondeau

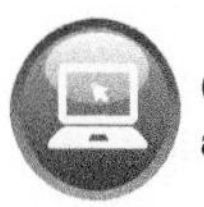

Client Education Handout available online

G

GASTRIC MOTILITY DISORDERS

BASICS

DEFINITION

Gastric motility disorders result from conditions that disrupt normal peristalsis and, consequently, gastric emptying. This abnormal gastric retention may, in turn, cause gastric distention, and subsequent signs of anorexia, nausea, bloating, and vomiting.

PATHOPHYSIOLOGY

The stomach has two distinct motor regions. The proximal stomach (fundus and body) relaxes to accommodate ingested food and regulates the expulsion of liquids. Intrinsic slow contractions of this region push liquids toward the pylorus. The distal stomach (antrum) mechanically breaks down solids through strong peristaltic contractions and ultimately expels them. The gastric pacemaker, an area of intrinsic electrical activity located in the greater curvature of the stomach, regulates distal gastric motility and emptying. Gastric electrical activity, dietary composition, and extrinsic factors (e.g., vagal and sympathetic innervation) all influence emptying. During fasting, indigestible solids are expelled from the stomach by migrating myoelectric complexes (MMCs). These produce strong "digestive housekeeper" contractions that, in the fasted state, sweep through the stomach and small intestine to mid-jejunum every 2 hours, preparing the gastrointestinal (GI) tract for the next meal. MMCs are regulated by the hormone motilin. Dysrhythmias in normal gastric electrical activity may be fundamental in the pathophysiology of disorders affecting gastric motility, but may also be secondary to gastric inflammation, neoplasia, and overdistension.

SYSTEMS AFFECTED

GI

GENETICS

N/A

INCIDENCE/PREVALENCE

Unknown. Many factors can alter gastric emptying, although they may not result in clinical disease or may only partially contribute to signs.

GEOGRAPHIC DISTRIBUTION

N/A

SIGNALMENT

Species

Dog and cat.

Breed Predilections

Unknown

Mean Age and Range

Signs occur at any age, though it is uncommon to observe primary motility disorders in young animals.

Predominant Sex

N/A

SIGNS

General Comments

Clinical signs are often secondary to the primary etiology causing the gastric motility disorder.

Historical Findings

• Major clinical sign is chronic postprandial vomiting of food; stomach should normally be empty after average-sized meal in approx 6–8 hours in dogs and 4–6 hours in cats (note: normal emptying times vary greatly from animal to animal and are influenced by meal volume, caloric density, fiber content, and environmental factors, e.g., stress); vomiting of undigested food >12 hours following meal suggests abnormal gastric motility or outflow obstruction; vomiting can occur, however, any time after eating. • Gastric distention, nausea, anorexia, belching, bloating, pica, and weight loss may occur. • Distal esophageal sphincter may be incompetent with gastric hypomotility and signs associated with reflux esophagitis may occur.

Physical Examination Findings

• Normal or findings associated with underlying cause. • Palpation of large, distended stomach. • Decreased gastric sounds on abdominal auscultation.

CAUSES

• Rarely, idiopathic gastric motility disorders arise from primary defects in normal myoelectric activity, e.g., myenteric ganglionitis, intestinal leiomyositis; most motility disorders occur secondary to other conditions. • Metabolic disorders include hypokalemia, uremia, hepatic encephalopathy, and hypothyroidism. • Nervous inhibition as result of stress, fear, pain, or trauma. • Drugs such as anticholinergics, beta-adrenergic agonists, narcotics, and chemotherapeutics. • Primary gastric disease such as outflow obstructions, gastritis, gastric ulcers, parvovirus, and gastric surgery. • Gastric dilatation and volvulus syndrome (GDV) is suspected to be, in part, result of abnormal gastric motility associated with changes in myoelectric and mechanical activity, although whether primary or secondary to overstretching of gastric wall is unknown; some dogs with GDV may continue to have signs of gastric hypomotility following surgical gastropexy. • Gastroesophageal reflux and enterogastric reflux (see Bilious Vomiting Syndrome) may result from primary gastric hypomotility. • Dysautonomia may affect GI tract and result in abnormal esophageal, gastric, and intestinal motility.

RISK FACTORS

Any gastric disease may result in secondary hypomotility.

DIAGNOSIS

DIFFERENTIAL DIAGNOSIS

Differential diagnosis is extensive and should consider any gastric condition causing vomiting, including gastritis, gastric ulcers, neoplasia, gastric surgery, and GDV. Gastric outflow obstruction as cause of delayed gastric emptying must always be ruled out.

CBC/BIOCHEMISTRY/URINALYSIS

Abnormalities may result from underlying cause of gastric hypomotility. Continued vomiting may result in changes indicative of dehydration, electrolyte abnormalities, or acid-base imbalance.

OTHER LABORATORY TESTS

Specialized testing may be required to determine specific cause of gastric hypomotility, and is individualized for each patient.

IMAGING

Survey Radiographs

Abdominal radiographs may reveal gas-, fluid-, or ingesta-distended stomach. (Note: important to determine when patient was last fed in relationship to when radiographs were taken.)

Barium Contrast Study

May be evidence of delayed gastric emptying and decreased gastric contractions if evaluated using fluoroscopy. Some cases may have normal emptying of liquids but abnormal emptying of solids. Normal dogs should empty stomachs by approx. 6–8 hours. (Note: stress of radiographs may decrease gastric emptying even in normal animal.)

Ultrasonography

Ultrasound can evaluate antral and pyloric motility.

Tests Available in Specialized Practices

Radionuclide Emission Scintigraphy

Radionuclide markers mixed with a meal give most clinically accurate measurement of emptying. Gastric emptying times (time for standard meal to leave stomach) range from 4 to 8 hours.

Stable Isotope Breath Tests

C-14-labeled foods are fed and time to onset of $^{14}CO_2$ emission in breath is marker of gastric emptying.

Smartpill

This is noninvasive wireless sensor capsule that is given orally and transmits data on pressures, transit time, luminal pH, and temperature as it passes through stomach and small and large bowel. Has been validated for use in healthy dog but, as yet, limited reports evaluating clinical conditions.

DIAGNOSTIC PROCEDURES

Endoscopy

Endoscopic findings frequently normal in primary gastric motility disorders. Food may be found in stomach when it should be empty following 12-hour pre-endoscopic fast. Endoscopy will detect obstructive or inflammatory/ulcerative diseases of stomach.

PATHOLOGIC FINDINGS

• Idiopathic conditions have normal gastric mucosa; special staining may reveal disruption of enteric nervous system. • Gastric histology may identify inflammatory or neoplastic causes of gastric hypomotility.

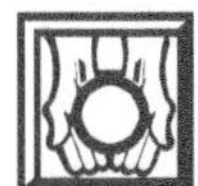

TREATMENT

APPROPRIATE HEALTH CARE

• Most treated as outpatients. • With severe vomiting or dehydration and electrolyte imbalance, hospitalization, fluid support, and specific therapy required.

NURSING CARE

Dehydration with fluid and electrolyte imbalance requires appropriate fluid replacement. Drugs that inhibit gastric motility (e.g., opioids) should be withdrawn.

ACTIVITY

Dependent on underlying disease.

DIET

• Dietary manipulation important in management of primary gastric motility disorders in order to speed gastric emptying. • Optimal diets liquid or semi-liquid consistency and low in fat and fiber content. • Small-volume meals with frequent feeding should be given. • Occasionally dietary manipulation alone is successful.

CLIENT EDUCATION

Discuss possible underlying etiologies and that response to therapy varies with individual cases.

SURGICAL CONSIDERATIONS

• Large-breed dogs with chronic GDV syndrome and gastric retention should have surgical gastropexy. • Following gastric surgery generally takes several days but up to 14 days for return of normal motility. • Mechanical gastric outflow obstructions require surgical correction.

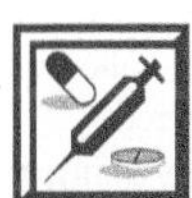

MEDICATIONS

DRUG(S) OF CHOICE

Gastric Prokinetic Agents

• Metoclopramide increases amplitude of antral contractions, inhibits fundic receptive relaxation, and coordinates duodenal and gastric motility; dopamine receptor antagonism in proximal GI tract results in increased release of acetylcholine from enteric neurons; at higher concentrations it has serotonin ($5HT_4$) agonist effects; also has antiemetic effects, blocking chemoreceptor trigger zone in dogs, but not in cats. ০ Oral dosage 0.2–0.5 mg/kg q8h given 30 min before meals (use lower dose in cats) or as CRI at 1–2 mg/kg q24h. ০ Metoclopramide generally considered to be weak prokinetic agent in dogs and recent studies suggest it has little effect at increasing lower esophageal sphincter pressure. • Cisapride works directly by cholinergic neurotransmission ($5HT_4$ agonist) of GI smooth muscle, stimulating motility; proposed mechanism of action is enhancement of release of acetylcholine at myenteric plexus; increases lower esophageal sphincter pressure, improves gastric emptying, and promotes motility of small and large intestine. ০ Oral dosage 0.2–0.5 mg/kg PO q8–12h given before meals. ০ Cisapride currently available through compounding pharmacies—human product has been removed from market because of associated cardiac arrhythmias not yet noted to occur in dogs or cats. ০ Mosapride (0.5–2 mg/kg PO q12–24h) and prucalopride (0.02–0.6 mg/kg PO q12–24h) are also $5HT_4$ agonist prokinetic agents. • Macrolide antibiotics, such as erythromycin, are motilin receptor agonists and increase GI motility; motilin is hormone that promotes MMC-associated motility. ০ Erythromycin given at low (submicrobiologic) doses binds motilin receptors promoting acetylcholine release, which speeds gastric emptying; dose of erythromycin for specific motility effects is 0.5–1 mg/kg PO q8–12h, given 30 min before meals. ০ Chronic use of submicrobiologic doses of antibiotics not recommended. • H_2 receptor antagonists ranitidine (1–2 mg/kg q8h) and nizatidine (2.5–5 mg/kg q24h) have reported prokinetic effects on gastric motility due to acetylcholinesterase inhibition; are considered poor prokinetic drugs and recent studies question ranitidine's prokinetic activity in dogs; neither cimetidine nor famotidine affects gastric emptying.

CONTRAINDICATIONS

Gastric prokinetic agents are contraindicated in patients with gastric outflow obstruction.

PRECAUTIONS

• Metoclopramide may cause nervousness, anxiety, or depression. • Cisapride may cause depression, vomiting, diarrhea, or abdominal cramping. • Erythromycin may cause vomiting.

POSSIBLE INTERACTIONS

Metoclopramide contraindicated with concurrent phenothiazine and narcotic administration or in animals with epilepsy.

ALTERNATIVE DRUG(S)

• Domperidone is peripheral dopamine receptor antagonist that regulates motility of gastric and small intestinal smooth muscle similar to metoclopramide. • Mirtazapine is noradrenergic and specific serotonergic antidepressant and has reported gastric prokinetic effects in dogs. • Acotiamide is acetylcholine esterase inhibitor that facilitates muscarinic activity and has been shown to stimulate postprandial gastroduodenal activity in dogs at dose of 30 mg/kg, but only available in Asia.

FOLLOW-UP

PATIENT MONITORING

• Response to therapy varies with underlying cause. • Clinical signs are primary indicator of response.

PREVENTION/AVOIDANCE

N/A

POSSIBLE COMPLICATIONS

GDV

EXPECTED COURSE AND PROGNOSIS

Length of treatment depends on ability to resolve underlying cause.

MISCELLANEOUS

ASSOCIATED CONDITIONS

Gastric hypomotility may be associated with reflux esophagitis and reflux gastritis (see Bilious Vomiting Syndrome).

AGE-RELATED FACTORS

N/A

ZOONOTIC POTENTIAL

N/A

PREGNANCY/FERTILITY/BREEDING

Avoid gastric prokinetic agents in pregnant animals.

SYNONYMS

• Delayed gastric emptying. • Gastric atony. • Gastric hypomotility.

SEE ALSO

• Bilious Vomiting Syndrome.
• Gastric Dilation and Volvulus Syndrome.
• Gastritis, Chronic.
• Gastroesophageal Reflux.

ABBREVIATIONS

• GDV = gastric dilation and volvulus syndrome.
• GI = gastrointestinal.
• MMC = migrating myoelectric complex.

Suggested Reading

Gaschen FP. Gastric and intestinal motility disorders. In: Bonagura JB, Twedt DC, eds., Current Veterinary Therapy XV. St. Louis, MO: Elsevier, 2014, pp. 513–518.

Washabau RJ. Prokinetic agents. In: Washabau RJ, Day MJ, eds. Canine and Feline Gastroenterology. St. Louis, MO: Elsevier, 2013, pp. 530–536.

Wyse CA, McLellan AM, Dickie DGM, et al. A review of methods for the assessment of the rate of gastric emptying in the dog and cat: 1898–2002. J Vet Intern Med 2003, 17:609–621.

Author Edward J. Hall

Consulting Editor Mark P. Rondeau

Acknowledgment The author and book editors acknowledge the prior contribution of David Twedt

Client Education Handout available online

G

GASTRITIS, CHRONIC

BASICS

DEFINITION

Inflammation of the stomach leading to clinical signs of >3 weeks' duration.

PATHOPHYSIOLOGY

• Inflammation may be secondary to drugs, infection, neoplasia, toxins/irritants, foreign material, food antigens or bacterial antigens; may be primary as a form of inflammatory bowel disease (IBD). • Visceral receptors stimulated by inflammation, distension, etc. send signals via vagal and sympathetic nerves to vomiting center (medulla oblangata).

SYSTEMS AFFECTED

• Gastrointestinal (GI). • Musculoskeletal—weight loss, muscle wasting, weakness.
• Integument—hair coat changes. • Respiratory—aspiration pneumonia.

GENETICS

N/A

INCIDENCE/PREVALENCE

Common

GEOGRAPHIC DISTRIBUTION

N/A

SIGNALMENT

Species

Dog and cat.

Breed Predilections

• Norwegian lundehund—chronic atrophic gastritis with IBD (lymphoplasmacytic); can progress to adenocarcinoma. • Basenji and Drentse patrijshond—chronic hypertrophic gastritis.

Mean Age and Range

Any age.

Predominant Sex

None

SIGNS

Historical Findings

• Vomiting is most common—digested or undigested food, bile, frank blood, digested blood ("coffee grounds"); variable frequency.
• Hyporexia to anorexia. • Melena. • Polydipsia.
• Diarrhea with concurrent intestinal disease.
• Retching. • Burping. • Weight loss.

Physical Examination Findings

• Abdominal distension ± pain. • Ptyalism.
• Muscle wasting, weight loss, coat changes.
• Pallor if bleeding ulcer. • Dehydration or hypovolemia.

CAUSES

• Food sensitivity. • IBD. • Toxins, e.g., heavy metals, environmental irritants (cleaners, herbicides). • Metabolic/endocrine disease—renal disease, liver disease, hypoadrenocorticism, pancreatitis, hyperthyroidism. • Neoplasia—large or small cell lymphoma, adenocarcinoma, polyp, gastrinoma, leiomyosarcoma, plasma cell tumor, mast cell tumor. • Foreign material.
• Drugs—nonsteroidal anti-inflammatory drugs (NSAIDs), antibiotics, chemotherapeutics.
• Parasitism—*Toxocara* spp., *Physaloptera* spp. (dogs and cats), *Ollulanus tricuspis* (cats).
• *Helicobacter* spp. • Pythiosis. • Canine distemper virus. • Hypergastrinemia—gastrinoma, achlorhydria, Basenji gastroenteropathy, hepatic or renal disease. • Miscellaneous—stress, emphysematous gastritis (gas-forming organisms/severe signs), benign gastric emphysema (milder disease/air trapping), eosinophilic sclerosing fibroplasia.

RISK FACTORS

• Drugs (e.g., NSAIDs). • Unsupervised/free-roaming pets—exposure to toxin.

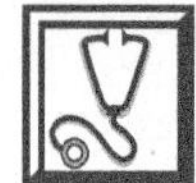

DIAGNOSIS

DIFFERENTIAL DIAGNOSIS

• Any cause of GI signs. • Esophageal disease—differentiate vomiting from regurgitation. • Hypertrophic pyloric gastropathy. • Bilious vomiting syndrome.

CBC/BIOCHEMISTRY/URINALYSIS

• Hemoconcentration if dehydrated.
• Anemia—if blood loss (regenerative anemia if acute blood loss such as ulceration; microcytic, hypochromic with chronic blood loss. • Thrombocytosis with chronic blood loss leading to iron deficiency. • Eosinophilia with parasitism, neoplasia, or eosinophilic gastritis.
• Biochemistry—prerenal or renal azotemia; increased blood urea nitrogen (BUN) : creatinine ratio with GI bleeding; hyperkalemia and hyponatremia with hypoadrenocorticism; hypochloremic metabolic alkalosis with gastric outflow obstruction. • Urinalysis—unremarkable.

OTHER LABORATORY TESTS

• Gastrin levels—elevated with gastrinoma; may be elevated with azotemia or use of antacids. • T_4. • Fecal float. • Baseline cortisol ± adrenocorticotropic hormone (ACTH) stimulation test. • Pythium ELISA.
• Iron panel (iron deficiency with bleeding).

IMAGING

• Abdominal radiographs—radiopaque foreign material, thickened gastric wall, gastric distension. • Contrast radiography—radiolucent foreign material, outflow obstruction, delayed emptying, wall defects or thickening.
• Ultrasonography—wall thickening, layering loss, ulcer, foreign object, mass.

DIAGNOSTIC PROCEDURES

• Upper GI endoscopy—visualize gastric mucosa, identify ulcer or mass, retrieve foreign object, biopsy (even when grossly normal), removal of small mass lesions (cautery), evaluate duodenum. • Exploratory laparotomy—perforated ulcer, full-thickness biopsy, partial gastrectomy, mass removal.
• Wireless capsule endoscopy—identify mass or ulcer.

PATHOLOGIC FINDINGS

• IBD—variable inflammatory infiltrate: lymphoplasmacytic, eosinophilic, neutrophilic, granulomatous/histiocytic gastritis (investigate for infectious cause).
• *Helicobacter* spp. do not always convey pathology—significant populations deep in gastric glands may warrant treatment.
• Special stains—further evaluation of potential neoplasia and infectious organisms.

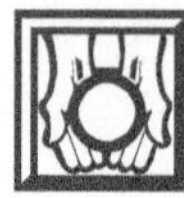

TREATMENT

APPROPRIATE HEALTH CARE

• Many treated as outpatients pending diagnostic testing or treatment trials (i.e., diet, drugs). • Inpatient management warranted if significant dehydration or hypovolemia present.

NURSING CARE

• IV fluids based on patient status; *caution* for fluid overload with hypoproteinemia.
• Enteral nutrition (nasoesophageal, nasogastric, or esophageal tubes) with persistent anorexia. • Severe hypoalbuminemia—consider albumin, plasma, or colloids.

ACTIVITY

Restrict postoperatively if surgery performed.

DIET

• Novel protein or hydrolyzed diet when allergy or IBD suspected; initial response expected within 2 weeks; worsening warrants diet change or other intervention; if improvement noted, continue beneficial diet for several months before reintroducing other foods to assess tolerance.
• Challenge with original diet can prove food hypersensitivity; rarely pursued. • Low-fat diet if hyperacidity or gastric ulcer. • Frequent, small meals (q4–6h) may provide benefit. • Small late-night meal may decrease bilious vomiting.
• Calorie requirement/diet guideline increases compliance. • Unflavored or topical flea, tick, and heartworm preventatives. • Treats limited to prescription diet. • If commercial diet declined, consider home-cooked diet formulated by veterinary nutritionist.

CLIENT EDUCATION

• Review multiple etiologies. • Least invasive testing first when patient status allows; biopsy for definitive diagnosis if extra-intestinal causes ruled out and patient fails diet and drug trial (i.e.. anthelminthic).

SURGICAL CONSIDERATIONS

• Obstructive lesion or material. • Perforated ulcer. • Removal of foreign objects if endoscopy unsuccessful or not available. • Full-thickness biopsy. • Mass resection and biopsy.

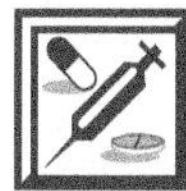

MEDICATIONS

DRUG(S) OF CHOICE

• Anthelminthic—fenbendazole (50 mg/kg PO q24h for 5 days), pyrantel pamoate + febantel. • Gastroprotectants—proton pump inhibitor (PPI), i.e., omeprazole (1 mg/kg PO q12h 30–60 min before meal); also consider sucralfate, H2 receptor antagonist, and others per ACVIM consensus (see Suggested Reading). • Antiemetics—maropitant (1 mg/kg SC or IV q24h; 2 mg/kg PO q24h), ondansetron, metoclopramide, mirtazapine. • Prokinetics—metoclopramide (0.2–0.4 mg/kg PO q8h; CRI 1–2 mg/kg/day), cisapride, ranitidine, low-dose erythromycin. • IBD suspected/confirmed—glucocorticoid (i.e., prednisone 2 mg/kg PO q24h or divided q12h; prednisolone for cat) when no clinical response to other therapeutic trials or in advanced disease; taper by 20–25% increments over time to lowest effective dose; discontinue when possible; total dose not >60 mg per day (dog); use with diet. • If glucocorticoid not tolerated and/or relapse, consider second drug; see Alternative Drug(s). • *Helicobacter* gastritis—several protocols have been described (e.g., metronidazole, amoxicillin, clarithromycin); see Suggested Reading.

CONTRAINDICATIONS

• Do not use prokinetics if GI obstruction possible. • Do not use antacids or PPIs with atrophic gastritis and achlorhydria.

PRECAUTIONS

• Immune modulation predisposes to secondary infections. • Steroids can cause GI ulceration, diabetes mellitus. or fluid overload (especially cat: congestive heart failure); patient monitoring and client education are vital to success. • Prolonged use of antacids or PPIs can lead to overgrowth of bacteria.

POSSIBLE INTERACTIONS

• Sucralfate will decrease absorption of other medications; separate by 2 hours from other medications. • Omeprazole affects clearance of many drugs. • Never use NSAIDs with glucocorticoids; high risk for GI erosion or ulcer.

ALTERNATIVE DRUG(S)

• IBD—if steroid and diet alone do not achieve disease remission, if patient relapses, and/or if steroid side effects are undesirable, second agent may be considered; options: cyclosporine, mycophenolate, chlorambucil, azathioprine (never in cats); find lowest effective dose. • Monitoring—exam, labwork (CBC, chemistry) for myelosuppression and other concerns (i.e., hepatic toxicity with cyclosporine, chlorambucil, and azathioprine). • Budesonide (steroid; 1–3 mg/patient depending on size) may have fewer systemic side effects; adrenal pituitary axis is affected.

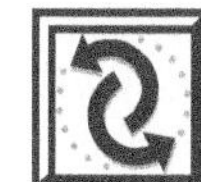

FOLLOW-UP

PATIENT MONITORING

• Depends on patient severity and medication chosen; minimum—physical exam within 2 weeks of starting treatment. • Recheck abnormal labwork (i.e., electrolytes, proteins) and monitor for medication side effects (i.e., hyperglycemia, anemia, myelosuppression, heptaopathy, etc. based on specific drugs selected). • Recurrence warrants repeat diagnostics; repeat biopsy may be indicated (i.e., patients previously in remission of IBD can progress to lymphoma). • Lack of response—change in medical management (i.e., alternative diet or drug); repeat biopsy (primary disease may have been missed) and labwork (CBC, chemistry, fecal, T_4) for emerging comorbidity.

PREVENTION/AVOIDANCE

• Avoid drugs with high incidence of GI upset (i.e., doxycycline, NSAIDs). • Avoid rapid diet change. • Prevent free-roaming and potential for dietary indiscretion—may need basket muzzle in dogs.

POSSIBLE COMPLICATIONS

• Gastroesophageal reflux. • Delayed gastric emptying/motility disorders. • Erosions/ulcers. • Aspiration pneumonia. • Electrolyte or acid-base imbalances. • Progression from superficial to atrophic gastritis. • Debilitation/death in refractory cases. • Steroids—diabetes mellitus, heart failure, calcinosis cutis, muscle weakness, ulcers. • Other immune-modulating drugs—bone marrow suppression, pancreatitis, hepatitis, GI upset.

EXPECTED COURSE AND PROGNOSIS

• Varies with cause. • Medication tapered to lowest effective dose ± stopped with diet.

MISCELLANEOUS

ASSOCIATED CONDITIONS

N/A

AGE-RELATED FACTORS

• Foreign objects—more common in young animals. • Food-responsive enteropathy—often younger animals. • IBD—often middle-aged to older. • Neoplasia—middle-aged to older animals more common.

ZOONOTIC POTENTIAL

Potential/uncommon concern secondary to parasites (i.e., *Toxocara spp.*—larval migrans).

PREGNANCY/FERTILITY/BREEDING

• Prednisone—abortion, teratogenic, can induce parturition. • Azathioprine—fetal harm; decrease sperm production. • Cyclosporine—fetal toxicity.

SEE ALSO

- Bilious Vomiting Syndrome.
- Gastroduodenal Ulceration/Erosion.
- Gastroenteritis, Eosinophilic.
- *Helicobacter* spp.
- Hypertrophic Pyloric Gastropathy, Chronic.

ABBREVIATIONS

- ACTH = adrenocorticotropic hormone.
- GI = gastrointestinal.
- IBD = inflammatory bowel disease.
- NSAID = nonsteroidal anti-inflammatory drug.
- PPI = proton pump inhibitor.

INTERNET RESOURCES

• https://veterinarypartner.vin.com/default.aspx?pid=19239&id=4951472 • https://veterinarypartner.vin.com/default.aspx?pid=19239&id=4951476

Suggested Reading

Leib MS. Gastric Helicobacter Species and Chronic Vomiting in Dogs. In: Bonagura J., Twedt D, eds., Kirk's Current Veterinary Therapy XVI. St. Louis, MO: Elsevier, pp. 508–513.

Marks SL, Kook PH, Papich MG, et al. ACVIM consensus for rational administration of gastrointestinal protectants to dogs and cats. J Vet Intern Med 2018; 32:1823–1840.

Simpson KW. Diseases of the stomach. In: Ettinger SJ, Feldman EC, eds., Textbook of Veterinary Internal Medicine, 8th ed. St. Louis, MO: Elsevier, 2017, pp. 1495–1515.

Author Kathryn M. McGonigle

Consulting Editor Mark P. Rondeau

Acknowledgment The author and book editors acknowledge the prior contribution of Michelle Pressel

Client Education Handout available online

G

GASTRODUODENAL ULCERATION/EROSION

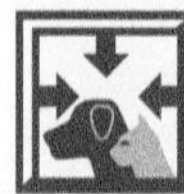

BASICS

DEFINITION

Ulcers are defects that extend completely through the mucosa; erosions extend part way through the mucosa.

G

PATHOPHYSIOLOGY

• Gastroduodenal ulceration/erosion (GUE) results from factors that damage or overwhelm normal gastric mucosal defense and repair mechanisms. • Factors protecting the stomach from GUE include the mucus/bicarbonate layer, gastric epithelial cell turnover, gastric mucosal blood flow, and local prostaglandins.

SYSTEMS AFFECTED

• Gastrointestinal (GI)—ulcers and erosion are most common in stomach, followed by proximal duodenum; however, neoplasia and some drugs (e.g., flunixin meglumine) can cause ulceration anywhere in GI tract. • Cardiovascular—hemorrhage may cause anemia, tachycardia, systolic heart murmur, and/or hypotension. • Peritoneal cavity—perforation may cause peritonitis/sepsis/systemic inflammatory response syndrome (SIRS).

INCIDENCE/PREVALENCE

• 40–60% in racing Alaskan sled dogs.
• Fairly common in dogs receiving nonsteroidal anti-inflammatory drugs (NSAIDs) or dexamethasone.

SIGNALMENT

Species

Dogs; rare in cats.

Breed Predilections

Chow chows, rough-coated collies, Staffordshire bull terriers, and Belgian shepherd dogs have increased incidence of gastric carcinoma.

Mean Age and Range

Any age.

Predominant Sex

Male dogs are predisposed to gastric carcinoma.

SIGNS

General Comments

Severity of clinical signs is not necessarily proportional to size/number of GUEs.

Historical Findings

• Some animals are asymptomatic (e.g., patients taking NSAIDs or dexamethasone, dogs working in extreme environments).
• Hyporexia is the most common clinical sign. • Vomiting, hematemesis, and/or melena may be seen (in decreasing order of frequency). • Cranial abdominal pain ("praying position") is rarely seen.
• Weakness, pallor, lethargy, and/or collapse if severe anemia or SIRS develops.

Physical Examination Findings

• Often normal. • Melena is rare. • Pale mucous membranes and weakness if severely anemic. • Tachycardia, hypotension, and prolonged capillary refill time if hypovolemic shock or perforation/SIRS.

CAUSES

Drugs

• NSAIDs—cyclooxygenase (COX)-2 selective NSAIDs are usually safer than nonselective NSAIDs; however, GUE and perforation can occur with all NSAIDs. Coadministration of glucocorticoids (either systemic or local) enhances ulcerogenic potential of NSAIDs. Some NSAIDs are renowned for being extremely ulcerogenic (flunixin meglumine, naproxen, indomethacin). • Glucocorticoids—dexamethasone is most ulcerogenic. Prednisolone less likely to cause clinically significant GUE unless there are additional stress factors (e.g., hypoxemia, hypoperfusion).

GI Diseases

• GI neoplasia—carcinomas are most common cause of neoplastic ulceration, but leiomyomas/leiomyosarcomas may cause severe hemorrhage. • Foreign bodies can be associated with GUE, but not a common cause. Intestinal foreign bodies (especially linear foreign bodies) commonly cause intestinal ulceration/perforation. • Gastric hyperacidity.

Infectious Diseases

Pythiosis can cause severe GUE. It is regionally important and is becoming increasingly widespread in North America.

Metabolic Diseases

• Hepatic disease. • Hypoadrenocorticism.

Toxicity

Heavy metal poisoning (arsenic, zinc, thallium, iron, and lead are rare causes).

Neoplasia

• GI neoplasia (carcinoma, lymphoma, leiomyoma, GI stromal tumor). • Paraneoplastic hyperacidity (mastocytosis, gastrinoma).

Stress/Major Medical Illness

• Shock/severe hypotension (e.g., secondary to trauma or surgery). • SIRS (heat stroke, sepsis). • Burns. • Sustained strenuous exercise (especially in extreme environments, either cold or hot).

RISK FACTORS

• Ulcerogenic drugs (NSAIDs, dexamethasone). • Hypovolemic shock/SIRS. • Extreme exercise.

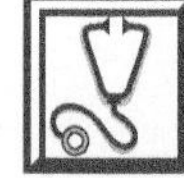

DIAGNOSIS

DIFFERENTIAL DIAGNOSIS

• Esophageal disease (neoplasia, esophagitis, foreign body)—diagnose with radiography and/or esophagoscopy. • Coagulopathies (thrombocytopenia, anticoagulant poisoning)—diagnose with platelet count, coagulation testing. • Bronchopulmonary disease causing hemoptysis—diagnose with radiography and/or bronchoscopy. • Regurgitation or vomiting blood (hematemesis) swallowed from respiratory tract or swallowed with food.
• Pepto-Bismol and activated charcoal cause stool to resemble melena.

CBC/BIOCHEMISTRY/URINALYSIS

• Acute blood loss (≤3–5 days)—nonregenerative anemia/hypoproteinemia. • Blood loss >7 days—regenerative anemia/hypoproteinemia. • Chronic blood loss—iron deficiency anemia (i.e., low mean corpuscular volume [MCV], high red cell distribution width [RDW], hypochromic, variable reticulocytosis) and hypoproteinemia. • Blood urea nitrogen (BUN) : creatinine ratio may be elevated with acute, severe GI hemorrhage, but this is hard to evaluate without recent pre-bleed laboratory values.

OTHER LABORATORY TESTS

• Fecal flotation (parasitism). • Bile acids (hepatic insufficiency). • Resting serum cortisol (screen for hypoadrenocorticism). • Serum gastrin concentrations (gastrinoma is rare).

IMAGING

• Abdominal radiography (GI foreign body, abdominal mass, pneumoperitoneum, effusion, hepatic disease). • Barium contrast radiography very insensitive for GUE.
• Ultrasonography specific but poorly sensitive for GI lesions (e.g., infiltrates, altered layering, ulcer); cannot detect erosions.

DIAGNOSTIC PROCEDURES

• Endoscopy most sensitive test for GUE. Allows biopsy of the lesion; best to biopsy normal-appearing tissue around GUE plus periphery of ulcer. Be careful biopsying center of ulcers as this rarely causes perforation. • Capsule endoscopy less expensive and does not require anesthesia, but not as sensitive as regular gastroscopy and does not allow for biopsy.
• Fine-needle aspirates or biopsies of infiltrative lesions in GI tract. • Abdominocentesis may reveal septic peritonitis if ulcer perforates.
• Exploratory surgery can be done to look for GUE, but easy to miss mucosal lesions from serosal surface. Can easily look into stomach through gastrostomy incision and miss lesions.

PATHOLOGIC FINDINGS

• GUEs are grossly visible. • Gastric body and antrum most common sites of GUE (especially from NSAIDs and steroids), but GUE can occur anywhere in stomach.
• Proximal duodenal ulceration classic but not diagnostic for excessive gastric acid secretion (mast cell tumor, gastrinoma).
• Microscopically can see inflammation, neoplasia, or fungal organisms.

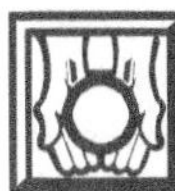

TREATMENT

APPROPRIATE HEALTH CARE

Very important: remove underlying cause if possible (e.g., drugs, toxins, poor perfusion). Many GUEs resolve spontaneously if cause is removed.

NURSING CARE

• IV fluids if needed to maintain hydration, gastric mucosal perfusion, and/or treat shock. • Transfusions if patient is severely anemic or has vigorous GI hemorrhage.

ACTIVITY

Based upon patient's condition.

DIET

• Discontinue oral intake if vomiting. • When feeding resumed, feed small amounts of low-fat/low-fiber diet.

CLIENT EDUCATION

• Dogs are especially prone to NSAID-induced GUE because these drugs have a longer half-life in dogs than in humans. • Never administer NSAID (especially if sold for human use) unless specifically prescribed by veterinarian (e.g., low dose of aspirin [0.5 mg/kg q24h] is safe when used to prevent thromboembolic disease in dogs being treated with steroids). • NSAID-associated GUE reduced by giving drug with food. • Proton pump inhibitors (PPIs) as effective as misoprostol in preventing NSAID-induced GUE. • No drug shown to be effective in preventing steroid-induced GUE.

SURGICAL CONSIDERATIONS

• If GI blood loss potentially life threatening, perform gastroduodenoscopy to identify sites of hemorrhage; then either surgically resect lesions or cauterize sites endoscopically (electrically or chemically). • Surgical excision of ulcers indicated if medical treatment shows no evidence of benefit after 5–7 days. • May need intraoperative endoscopy to locate lesions that cannot be found at surgery. • Rarely need surgeon to telescope intestines over tip of endoscope to thoroughly examine entire duodenal and jejunal mucosa.

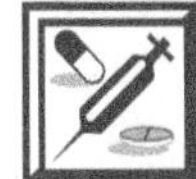

MEDICATIONS

DRUG(S) OF CHOICE

• PPIs most potent inhibitors of gastric acid secretion. Require 3–5 days to achieve maximum efficacy. Used as prophylactic drugs and as first-line therapy for existing GUE; primary therapy for gastrinomas. Omeprazole (1–2 mg/kg PO q12h) administered orally; pantoprazole (1 mg/kg IV q12h) can be administered parenterally. • Histamine (H2) receptor antagonists also inhibit gastric acid secretion. Famotidine (0.5–1 mg/kg PO/IV q12–24h) most potent, but all of these drugs inferior to PPIs. • Sucralfate (0.5–1 g PO q6–8h) protects ulcerated tissue by binding to it and stimulating prostaglandin synthesis (use suspension instead of tablets). No benefit in combining with PPIs. • Misoprostol (2–5 µg/kg PO q12h) effective, but has many side effects. • Antiemetics if vomiting frequent or nausea severe. Maropitant (1 mg/kg SC q24h; 2 mg/kg PO q24h); ondansetron (0.2–0.5 mg/kg PO/IV q8–12h). • Oral antacids (e.g., calcium carbonate) poorly effective and not recommended.

POSSIBLE INTERACTIONS

• Sucralfate may slow absorption of other drugs. • Antacids may slow absorption of other drugs. • H2 receptor antagonists decrease effectiveness of PPIs. • Do not use misoprostol in pregnant patients.

FOLLOW-UP

PATIENT MONITORING

Effective medical therapy should result in clinical improvement within 5–7 days.

PREVENTION/AVOIDANCE

• Administer NSAIDs with food. • PPIs generally as effective as misoprostol at preventing NSAID-induced GUE. • COX-2 selective or dual lipoxygenase (LOX)/COX inhibitors less likely to cause GUE than nonselective NSAIDs, but can still cause GUE and perforation/peritonitis.

POSSIBLE COMPLICATIONS

Hemorrhage, perforation, septic peritonitis.

EXPECTED COURSE AND PROGNOSIS

• Varies with underlying causes. • GUE not due to local malignancy can usually be treated successfully medically (especially if one can remove cause). However, if perforation has occurred, surgery is necessary.

MISCELLANEOUS

ASSOCIATED CONDITIONS

Anemia

AGE-RELATED FACTORS

Neoplasia more common in older animals.

SEE ALSO

- Hematemesis.
- Melena.

ABBREVIATIONS

- ACTH = adrenocorticotropic hormone.
- BUN = blood urea nitrogen.
- COX = cyclooxygenase.
- DIC = disseminated intravascular coagulation.
- GI = gastrointestinal.
- GUE = gastric ulceration/erosion.
- LOX = lipoxygenase.
- MCV = mean corpuscular volume.
- NSAID = nonsteroidal anti-inflammatory drug.
- PPI = proton pump inhibitor.
- RDW = red cell distribution width.
- SIRS = systemic inflammatory response syndrome.

Suggested Reading

Mansfield CS, Abraham LA. Ulcer. In: Washabau RJ, Day MJ, eds., Canine and Feline Gastroenterology. St. Louis, MO: Elsevier Saunders, 2013, pp. 637–642.

Neiger R. Gastric ulceration. In: Bonagura JD, Twedt DC, eds., Kirk's Current Veterinary Therapy XIV. St. Louis, MO: Elsevier Saunders, 2009, pp. 497–501.

Simpson KW. Diseases of the stomach. In: Ettinger SJ, Feldman EC, Cote E, eds., Textbook of Veterinary Internal Medicine, 8th ed. St. Louis, MO: Elsevier, 2017, pp. 1495–1516.

Author Michael D. Willard
Consulting Editor Mark P. Rondeau

Client Education Handout available online

G

GASTROENTERITIS, ACUTE HEMORRHAGIC DIARRHEA SYNDROME

BASICS

DEFINITION

A peracute hemorrhagic enteritis of dogs characterized by a sudden onset of severe bloody diarrhea that is often explosive, with vomiting (typically the first clinical sign observed by the owner), hypovolemia, and usually marked hemoconcentration due to a dramatic loss of fluid into the intestinal lumen.

PATHOPHYSIOLOGY

• Many conditions result in hemorrhagic diarrhea, but the acute hemorrhagic diarrhea syndrome (AHDS) of dogs appears to have unique clinical features that distinguish it from other conditions. • AHDS results in a peracute loss of intestinal mucosal integrity with the rapid movement of fluid and electrolytes into the gut lumen. Dehydration and hypovolemic shock occur quickly. In proportion to fluid loss, blood loss is usually minor. This has to be differentiated from true gastrointestinal (GI) bleeding, in which anemia is usually observed. Protein loss can be substantial in some cases, resulting in severe hypoalbuminemia. Translocation of bacteria or toxins through the damaged intestinal mucosa can usually be compensated. In a few cases the immune defense mechanisms can be overwhelmed, resulting in septicemia/septic shock.

SYSTEMS AFFECTED

• GI. • Cardiovascular.

GENETICS

Unknown; small or toy breeds appear to be overrepresented.

INCIDENCE/PREVALENCE

Unknown; appears to be common.

GEOGRAPHIC DISTRIBUTION

N/A

SIGNALMENT

Species

Dog

Breed Predilections

• Any breed can be affected; incidence is greater in small and toy breeds. • Breeds most represented include Yorkshire terrier, miniature pinscher, miniature schnauzer, miniature poodle, and Maltese.

Mean Age and Range

Usually in adult dogs with a mean age of 5 years.

Predominant Sex

N/A

SIGNS

General Comments

• Mucosal lesions are restricted to the intestines and cannot be detected in the stomach histologically; therefore, it is suggested to replace the term hemorrhagic gastroenteritis (HGE), implicating gastric inflammation, with AHDS. • Most animals affected are previously healthy with no historical environmental changes; some dogs have a history of chronic intermittent GI disease. • Clinical findings are variable in both the course and severity of the disease; the disease is usually acute to peracute; with adequate fluid and symptomatic treatment, rapid clinical improvement is typically observed in the first 48 hours.

Historical Findings

• Acute vomiting, anorexia, and lethargy, followed by watery diarrhea quickly changing to bloody diarrhea. • Signs progress rapidly and become severe within a period of <12 hours as a result of hypovolemic shock and hemoconcentration.

Physical Examination Findings

• Evidence of hypovolemia; lethargy, weakness, tachycardia, prolonged capillary refill time, and weak pulse pressure. • Skin turgor as a reflection of dehydration may appear normal owing to the peracute nature of the disease and the lag time in compartmental fluid shifts. • Abdominal pain and fluid-filled bowel can be detected. • Rectal examination identifies bloody diarrhea, and later in the course of disease a "raspberry jam" characteristic stool develops. • Often normo- or hypothermia; fever is unusual and represents an important feature differentiating uncomplicated AHDS cases from dogs with infection and systemic reaction to an enteropathogen or septicemia following bacterial translocation.

CAUSES

• There is increasing evidence to suggest that *Clostridium perfringens* type A is involved, as these bacteria have been identified on necrotic mucosal surfaces closely associated with epithelial lesions. • A novel pore-forming toxin designated NetF was detected in *C. perfringens* type A strains, which were involved in AHDS; compared to healthy control dogs (prevalence: 0–10%), the prevalence of *C. perfringens* encoding the *netF* gene is significantly higher in dogs with AHDS (50–55%). • Other undetected clostridial toxins might be involved in the disease process; it is also possible that different etiologies are responsible for this syndrome in different patients.

RISK FACTORS

• Unknown. • Some dogs have a history of chronic intermittent diarrhea.

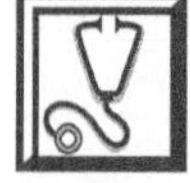

DIAGNOSIS

DIFFERENTIAL DIAGNOSIS

• Drugs/toxins causing mucosal irritation (e.g., nonsteroidal anti-inflammatory drugs, high-dose corticosteroids, doxycycline). • Parvovirus. • Circovirus. • Acute GI ulceration. • Bacterial enteritis such as salmonellosis or campylobacteriosis. • Conditions resulting in endotoxic or hypovolemic shock. • Intestinal obstruction or intussusception. • Hypoadrenocorticism. • Heat stroke. • Pancreatitis. • Coagulopathy.

CBC/BIOCHEMISTRY/URINALYSIS

• Marked hemoconcentration with packed cell volume (PCV) usually >60%, with discordant plasma proteins that are normal to decreased due to protein loss into the GI tract; some dogs show significant hypoalbuminemia after rehydration; usually a stress leukogram. • Biochemistry profile may reveal secondary hepatic enzyme elevations and high blood urea nitrogen (BUN) due to prerenal causes.

OTHER LABORATORY TESTS

Fecal Tests

• Stool is negative for parasites. • ELISA and PCR for parvovirus are negative. • Fecal cytology shows many red blood cells (RBCs) and occasional white blood cells (WBCs). • *Clostridium* spp. may be cultured from healthy dogs and should not be used as a diagnostic test for AHDS. Fecal ELISA test for detection of *C. perfringens* enterotoxin is often positive. A culture for other enteric pathogens is not diagnostic, since many enteropathogens can be found in feces of healthy dogs. Fecal PCR for detection of *C. perfringens* alpha toxin gene alone is not sufficient to diagnose this disorder. A positive PCR for *netF* encoding *C. perfringens* strains is suggestive for AHDS.

Coagulogram

Usually normal, but rarely secondary disseminated intravascular coagulation (DIC) is a complication.

IMAGING

Abdominal radiographs or ultrasound show fluid- and gas-filled small and large intestine. Ultrasonography often reveals fluid-filled intestinal loops without peristaltic movements due to the presence of a paralytic ileus.

DIAGNOSTIC PROCEDURES

Endoscopy

• Rarely indicated. • Stomach may appear normal, but small and large intestine will show diffuse mucosal hemorrhage, and hyperemia.

PATHOLOGIC FINDINGS

• Gross findings include intestinal congestion. • Histological examination of the intestinal tract shows superficial mucosal hemorrhagic necrosis without significant inflammation. • Frequently, layers of rod-shaped bacteria (e.g., *C. perfringens*) can be detected on the surface of the intestinal mucosa. • Gastric mucosa is spared.

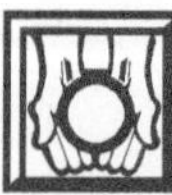

TREATMENT

APPROPRIATE HEALTH CARE

Patients suspected of having AHDS should be hospitalized and treated aggressively, because clinical deterioration is often rapid and can be fatal.

NURSING CARE

• Rapid volume replacement through a large-bore IV catheter is required in all cases.
• Balanced electrolyte solutions are given up to the rate of 40–60 mL/kg/hour IV until PCV <50%. • Shock fluids can also be given as fast as 30 mL/kg in 10 min; this bolus can be repeated up to three times if needed. • A moderate rate of maintenance fluids is given to maintain circulatory function and correct any potassium or other electrolyte deficits during the recovery period. • Continued GI fluid losses should be estimated and that volume added to the fluid requirements. • Hypoproteinemic animals may require colloids, plasma, or albumin solutions (canine preferred over human, if available).

ACTIVITY

Restricted

DIET

• NPO during acute phase as long as dogs are vomiting. • Trickle feeding with oral glutamine solution or low-fat (liquid) diet as long as the dog is not eating. • During recovery period a bland, low-fat, low-fiber GI diet should be fed for several days before returning to normal diet. • Consider increased dietary fiber to alter the intestinal microbiota to reduce the likelihood of recurrence of *C. perfringens*–associated diarrhea.

CLIENT EDUCATION

• Discuss the need for immediate and aggressive medical management; with appropriate therapy, mortality is usually low.
• Recurrence is reported in about 10% of cases.

SURGICAL CONSIDERATIONS

N/A

MEDICATIONS

DRUG(S) OF CHOICE

• Antibiotics should be restricted to dogs with signs of systemic infection, immunosuppression, and reduced liver function, as well as to dogs inadequately responding to symptomatic therapy; amoxicillin/sulbactam (50 mg/kg q8h IV) is suggested prophylactically in dogs that cannot be monitored closely. • An antiemetic such as maropitant (1 mg/kg q24h IV) is suggested to control nausea and vomiting.
• Analgesics (e.g., buprenorphine 0.01 mg/kg q6–8h IV) should be administered at the clinician's discretion. • Excessive blood loss may require blood transfusion (very rare).

CONTRAINDICATIONS

N/A

PRECAUTIONS

Septic and or hypovolemic shock can occur quickly and consequently the animal should be monitored closely.

POSSIBLE INTERACTIONS

N/A

ALTERNATIVE DRUG(S)

• Oral antibiotics and intestinal protectants are of little benefit and generally not administered.
• Administration of mucosal protectants such as sucralfate is of questionable value.
• Antidiarrheal drugs are contraindicated.
• High-dose, multistrain probiotic therapy might help to displace *C. perfringens* strains from the GI tract, though clinical efficacy has not been evaluated. • Long-term administration of probiotics could theoretically alter the intestinal microbiota to reduce the likelihood of recurrence of *C. perfringens*–associated diarrhea, though clinical efficacy has not been evaluated.

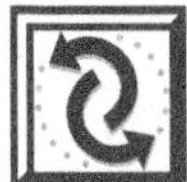

FOLLOW-UP

PATIENT MONITORING

• Check response to fluid therapy by assessing heart rate, capillary refill time, pulse pressure, as well as mental status and urine production every hour until considering the dog stable.
• Monitor PCV and total solids frequently (at least every 4–6 hours). • Modify fluid replacement based on patient status. • If there is failure of clinical improvement in 24–48 hours, reevaluate the patient, as other causes of hemorrhagic diarrhea are probable.

PREVENTION/AVOIDANCE

N/A

POSSIBLE COMPLICATIONS

• Occasionally DIC may develop. • Neurologic signs or seizures secondary to hemoconcentration may occur. • Cardiac arrhythmias occur from suspected myocardial reperfusion injury.

EXPECTED COURSE AND PROGNOSIS

• Most dogs recover; mortality rate can be high in untreated dogs; fewer than 10% of treated dogs die, and 10–15% have repeated occurrences. • The course of the disease is generally short, lasting from 24 to 72 hours.
• About 50% of dogs still have soft feces on day 5. • Time to complete normalization of stool consistency can be up to 7–10 days.

MISCELLANEOUS

ASSOCIATED CONDITIONS

N/A

AGE-RELATED FACTORS

N/A

ZOONOTIC POTENTIAL

Unknown

PREGNANCY/FERTILITY/BREEDING

N/A

SYNONYMS

(Acute) HGE.

SEE ALSO

• Acute Diarrhea. • Acute Vomiting.

ABBREVIATIONS

• AHDS = acute hemorrhagic diarrhea syndrome. • BUN = blood urea nitrogen.
• DIC = disseminated intravascular coagulation. • GI = gastrointestinal. • HGE = hemorrhagic gastroenteritis. • PCV = packed cell volume. • RBC = red blood cell.
• WBC = white blood cell.

Suggested Reading

Busch K, Suchodolski JS, Kuhner KA, et al. Clostridium perfringens enterotoxin and Clostridium difficile toxin A/B do not play a role in acute haemorrhagic diarrhoea syndrome in dogs. Vet Rec 2015, 176:253.

Hall JH. Small intestine. In: Washabau RJ, Day MJ, eds., Canine and Feline Gastroenterology. St. Louis, MO: Elsevier, 2013, pp. 651–728.

Marks SL, Rankin SC, Byrne BA, et al. Enteropathogenic bacteria in dogs and cats: diagnosis, epidemiology, treatment, and control. J Vet Intern Med 2011, 25:1195–1208.

Mehdizadeh Gohari I, Parreira VR, Nowell VJ, et al. A novel pore-forming toxin in type A Clostridium perfringens is associated with both fatal canine hemorrhagic gastroenteritis and fatal foal necrotizing enterocolitis. PLoS One 2015, 10:e0122684.

Mortier F, Strohmeyer K, Hartmann K, et al. Acute haemorrhagic diarrhoea syndrome in dogs: 108 cases. Vet Rec 2015, 176:627.

Sasaki J, Goryo M, Asahina M, et al. Hemorrhagic enteritis associated with *Clostridium perfringens* type A in a dog. J Vet Med Sci 1999, 61:175–177.

Spielman BL, Garvey MS. Hemorrhagic gastroenteritis in dogs. J Am Anim Hosp Assoc 1993, 29:341–344.

Unterer S, Busch K, Leipig M, et al. Endoscopically visualized lesions, histologic findings, and bacterial invasion in the gastrointestinal mucosa of dogs with acute hemorrhagic diarrhea syndrome. J Vet Intern Med 2014, 28:52–58.

Unterer S, Lechner E, Mueller RS, et al. Prospective study of bacteraemia in acute haemorrhagic diarrhoea syndrome in dogs. Vet Rec 2015, 176:309.

Unterer S, Strohmeyer K, Kruse BD, et al. Treatment of aseptic dogs with hemorrhagic gastroenteritis with amoxicillin/clavulanic acid: a prospective blinded study. J Vet Intern Med 2011, 25:973–979.

Author Stefan Unterer

Consulting Editor Mark P. Rondeau

Acknowledgment The author and book editors acknowledge the prior contribution of David C. Twedt.

Client Education Handout available online

GASTROENTERITIS, EOSINOPHILIC

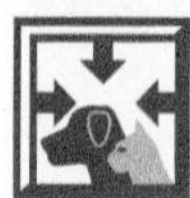

BASICS

DEFINITION

• Disease of gastrointestinal (GI) tract caused by primary infiltrate of eosinophils. • When other causes of eosinophilic infiltrates are ruled out, this is considered a form of inflammatory bowel disease (IBD).

PATHOPHYSIOLOGY

• Eosinophils involved in innate, acquired, and adaptive immunity; antigenic stimulation causes eosinophilic recruitment to GI tract.
• Stimulation from food hypersensitivity, parasitic infection, neoplasia (i.e., mast cell, lymphoma), fungi, viruses, bacteria, disease affecting mast cells, or idiopathic. • Small and large eosinophil granules release substances cytoxic to microorganisms and recruit other immune defenses; also damaging to self tissues. • Eosinophils activate mast cells directly causing continued tissue destruction.

SYSTEMS AFFECTED

• GI—primarily stomach and small intestine; large intestine less commonly affected; esophagus rarely affected. • Hemic/lymphatic/immune—hypereosinophilic syndrome (HES) and certain neoplasms affect spleen and lymph nodes.
• Hepatobiliary—HES may affect liver.
• Respiratory—aspiration pneumonia secondary to vomiting. • Musculoskeletal—weight loss, muscle wasting, weakness. • Integument—hair coat changes with nutritional deficiencies.

GENETICS

Unknown

INCIDENCE/PREVALENCE

• Unknown. • Second most common form of IBD.

GEOGRAPHIC DISTRIBUTION

N/A

SIGNALMENT

Species

Dog and cat.

Breed Predilections

German shepherd, boxer, Rottweiler, Doberman pinscher, and shar-pei.

Mean Age and Range

• Any age. • Dogs—commonly young (<5 years). • Cats—commonly middle-aged.

Predominant Sex

None

SIGNS

General Comments

Signs vary with severity of illness and sites affected.

Historical Findings

• Vomiting, small bowel diarrhea > large bowel diarrhea. • Abdominal pain.
• Anorexia/hyporexia. • Weight loss.
• Occasional melena.

Physical Examination Findings

• Cats > dogs—thickened bowel loops on abdominal palpation. • HES—skin lesions, enlarged peripheral lymph nodes, hepatosplenomegaly. • Abdominal pain. • Muscle wasting, weight loss, ± coat changes. • Pale mucous membranes with bleeding ulcer.
• Dehydration, hypovolemia. • Palpable abdominal mass lesion.

CAUSES

• IBD. • Parasites—e.g., *Physaloptera* spp., *Ollulanus tricuspis*, *Spirocerca* spp. • Fungal, viral, bacterial infection. • Loss of tolerance to normal intestinal flora. • Systemic mastocytosis. • HES.
• Neoplasia—mast cell tumor, lymphoma.

RISK FACTORS

N/A

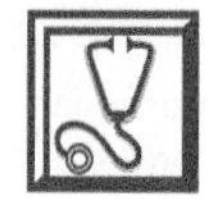

DIAGNOSIS

DIFFERENTIAL DIAGNOSIS

• Any cause of GI signs. • Feline GI eosinophilic sclerosing fibroplasia (ulcerated intramural mass at pyloric sphincter or ileocecocolic junction most common).

CBC/BIOCHEMISTRY/URINALYSIS

• Hemogram—unremarkable, mild to marked peripheral eosinophilia (cats > dogs).
• Biochemistry—blood urea nitrogen (BUN) elevation alone or disproportionally higher than creatinine suggests GI bleeding; hypoproteinemia and hypocholesterolemia common with significant disease; increased liver enzyme activity and/or azotemia may be seen with HES; prerenal azotemia with dehydration.
• Urinalysis—usually unremarkable.

OTHER LABORATORY TESTS

• Buffy-coat smear—evaluate for systemic mastocytosis. • Serum cobalamin and folate—screen for evidence of intestinal malabsorption. • Fecal float, multiple.
• Baseline cortisol ± adrenocorticotropic hormone (ACTH) stimulation test. • Based on location or travel history, testing for fungal organisms (i.e., histoplasmosis). • Expanded infectious disease testing depending on patient risk and exposure.

IMAGING

• Abdominal radiography—rules out other disease causing clinical signs; does not diagnose this condition; hepatosplenomegaly may be seen with HES. • Barium contrast radiography may demonstrate thick intestinal walls and mucosal irregularities, but does not provide etiology.
• Ultrasonography—assess stomach and intestinal wall thickness; assess for mass lesions, ulcer, and obstruction; rule out other diseases; examine liver, spleen, and mesenteric lymph nodes with suspected HES or metastatic disease.

DIAGNOSTIC PROCEDURES

• Upper and lower GI endoscopy—visualize mucosa; identify ulcer or mass; biopsy (even when grossly normal); thickened rugal folds, increased mucosal friability, villous blunting, edema, and erythema are commonly visualized; intestinal parasites may be seen.
• Fine-needle aspirate and cytology of enlarged liver, spleen, and/or lymph nodes.
• Bone marrow aspirate cytology—when systemic mastocytosis or severe peripheral eosinophilia is present. • Exploratory laparotomy—perforated ulcer; full-thickness biopsy; removal of obstructive lesion and/or biopsy of other affected organs (lymph node, spleen, liver).

PATHOLOGIC FINDINGS

• Eosinophilic infiltrates can be patchy in intestine; multiple biopsies always recommended. • Histopathology reveals diffuse mucosal infiltrate of eosinophils; submucosa and muscularis are less commonly involved in the dog (more common in the cat); infiltrate of muscularis layer associated with obstructive eosinophilic lesions; eosinophilic inflammation within fibroplasia seen in feline GI eosinophilic sclerosing fibroplasia; WSAVA guidelines from international GI Standardization Group should be followed for interpretation of normal vs. pathologic numbers of eosinophils.

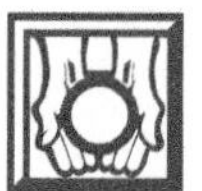

TREATMENT

APPROPRIATE HEALTH CARE

• Many treated as outpatients (minimal dehydration) after obstruction excluded, pending diagnostic testing or treatment trials (i.e., diet trial, drugs). • Inpatient medical management if significant dehydration or intractable vomiting.

NURSING CARE

• IV fluids to restore volume and correct dehydration when indicated; *caution* for fluid overload with hypoproteinemia. • Enteral nutrition (nasoesophageal, nasogastric, or esophageal tubes) with persistent anorexia.
• Severe hypoalbuminemia—consider albumin, plasma, or colloids.

ACTIVITY

Restrict postoperatively if surgery performed.

DIET

• Novel protein or hydrolyzed diet when allergy or IBD suspected; initial response expected within 2 weeks; worsening warrants diet change or other intervention; if improvement noted, continue diet for several months before reintroducing other foods to assess tolerance. • Challenge with original diet can prove food hypersensitivity; rarely pursued. • Calorie requirement/diet guideline increases compliance. • Unflavored or topical flea, tick, and heartworm preventatives.
• Treats limited to prescription diet. • If commercial diet declined, consider home-cooked diet formulated by veterinary nutritionist.

CLIENT EDUCATION

• Review multiple etiologies. • Least invasive testing first when patient status allows; biopsy for definitive diagnosis if extra-intestinal causes ruled out and patient fails diet and drug trial (i.e., anthelminthic, antimicrobial). • Potential for waxing and waning nature; necessity for lifelong vigilance regarding inciting factors; potential for long-term therapy.

SURGICAL CONSIDERATIONS

• Obstructive lesion. • Perforated ulcer.
• Full-thickness biopsy.

MEDICATIONS

DRUG(S) OF CHOICE

• Gastroprotectants and antiemetics often needed to control clinical symptoms initially.
• Gastroprotectants—proton pump inhibitor (PPI), i.e., omeprazole 1 mg/kg PO q12h 30–60 min before meal; also consider sucralfate, H2 receptor antagonist, and others per ACVIM consensus (see Suggested Reading). • Antiemetics—maropitant (1 mg/kg SC/IV q24h; 2 mg/kg PO q24h); ondansetron, metoclopramide, mirtazapine.
• Prokinetics—metoclopramide (0.2–0.4 mg/kg PO q8h; CRI 1–2 mg/kg/day), cisapride, ranitidine, low-dose erythromycin.
•Anthelminthic—fenbendazole (50 mg/kg PO q24h for 5 days), pyrantel pamoate + febantel. • Antimicrobial—metronidazole (10 mg/kg PO q12h for 2–4 weeks), tylosin (11–20 mg/kg PO q12h for 2–4 weeks).
• IBD suspected/confirmed—glucocorticoid (i.e., prednisone 2 mg/kg PO q24h or divided q12h; prednisolone for cat) when no clinical response to other therapeutic trials or in advanced disease; taper by 20–25% increments over time to lowest effective dose; discontinue when possible; total dose not >60 mg per day (dog); use with diet. • If glucocorticoid not tolerated and/or relapse, consider second drug; see Alternative Drug(s).

CONTRAINDICATIONS

Do not use prokinetics if GI obstruction possible.

PRECAUTIONS

• Immune modulation predisposes to secondary infections. • Steroids can cause GI ulceration, diabetes mellitus, or fluid overload (especially cat: congestive heart failure); patient monitoring and client education are vital to success. • Prolonged use of antacids or PPIs can lead to overgrowth of bacteria.

POSSIBLE INTERACTIONS

• Sucralfate will decrease absorption of other medications; separate by 2 hours from other medications. • Omeprazole affects clearance of many drugs. • Never use nonsteroidal anti-inflammatory drugs (NSAIDs) with glucocorticoid; high risk of GI erosion/ulcer.

ALTERNATIVE DRUG(S)

• IBD—if steroid and diet alone do not achieve disease remission, if patient relapses, and/or if steroid side effects undesirable, second agent may be considered; options: cyclosporine, mycophenolate, chlorambucil, and azathioprine (never in cats); find lowest effective dose. • Monitoring—exam, labwork (CBC, chemistry) for myelosuppression and other concerns (i.e., hepatic toxicity with cyclosporine, chlorambucil, and azathioprine).
• Leukotriene receptor blockers (i.e., montelukast) have been successful in humans.
• Budesonide (steroid; 1–3 mg/patient depending on size) may have fewer systemic side effects; adrenal pituitary axis affected.

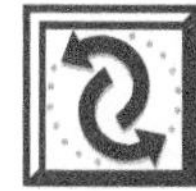

FOLLOW-UP

PATIENT MONITORING

• Depends on patient severity and medication chosen; minimum: physical exam within 2 weeks of starting treatment.
• Monitoring peripheral eosinophil count if initially elevated. • Recheck abnormal labwork (i.e., electrolytes, proteins) and monitor for medication side effects (i.e., hyperglycemia, anemia, myelosuppression, heptaopathy, etc. based on specific drugs selected). • Recurrence warrants repeat diagnostics; repeat biopsy may be indicated (i.e., patients previously in remission of IBD can progress to lymphoma). • Lack of response—change in medical management (i.e., alternative diet or drug); repeat biopsy (primary disease may have been missed) and labwork (CBC, chemistry, fecal, T_4) for emerging comorbidity.

PREVENTION/AVOIDANCE

• Avoid rapid diet change. • Prevent free-roaming and potential for dietary indiscretion—may need basket muzzle in dogs.

POSSIBLE COMPLICATIONS

• Gastroesophageal reflux disease (GERD).
• Delayed gastric emptying/motility disorders.
• Erosions/ulcers. • Aspiration pneumonia.
• Electrolyte, acid-base imbalances.
• Debilitation/death in refractory cases.
• Steroid—diabetes mellitus, heart failure, calcinosis cutis, muscle weakness, ulcers. • Other immune-modulating drugs—bone marrow suppression, pancreatitis, hepatitis, GI upset.

EXPECTED COURSE AND PROGNOSIS

• Vary with cause. • Medication tapered to lowest effective dose ± stopped with diet.

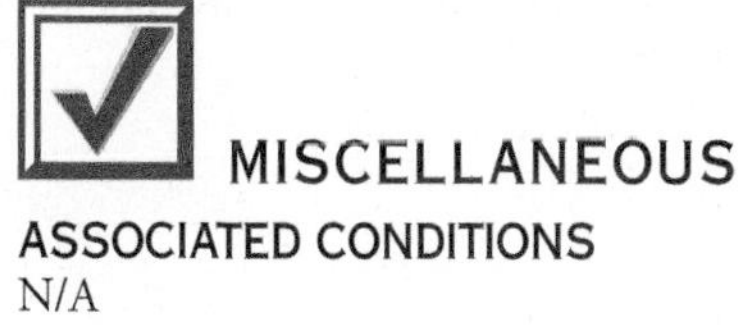

MISCELLANEOUS

ASSOCIATED CONDITIONS

N/A

AGE-RELATED FACTORS

• Food-responsive enteropathy—often younger. • IBD—often middle-aged to older.
• Neoplasia—middle-aged to older animals more common.

ZOONOTIC POTENTIAL

Potential/uncommon concern secondary to parasites (i.e., *Toxocara* spp.—larval migrans).

G

PREGNANCY/FERTILITY/BREEDING

• Prednisone—abortion, teratogenic, can induce parturition. • Azathioprine—fetal harm; decreases sperm production.
• Cyclosporine—fetal toxicity.

SEE ALSO

• Gastroduodenal Ulceration/Erosion.
• Inflammatory Bowel Disease.

ABBREVIATIONS

• ACTH = adrenocorticotropic hormone.
• BUN = blood urea nitrogen. • GERD = gastroesophageal reflux disease. • GI = gastrointestinal. • HES = hypereosinophilic syndrome. • IBD = inflammatory bowel disease.
• NSAID = nonsteroidal anti-inflammatory drug. • PPI = proton pump inhibitor.

INTERNET RESOURCES

• https://veterinarypartner.vin.com/default.aspx?pid=19239&id=7393377 • https://veterinarypartner.vin.com/default.aspx?pid=19239&id=4951476

Suggested Reading

Hall EJ, Day MK. Diseases of the small intestine. In: Ettinger SJ, Feldman EC, eds., Textbook of Veterinary Internal Medicine, 8th ed. St. Louis, MO: Elsevier, 2017, pp. 1516–1564.

Linton M, Nimmo JS, Norris JM, et al. Feline gastrointestinal eosinophilic sclerosing fibroplasia: 13 cases and review of an emerging clinical entity. J Feline Med Surg 2015, 17:392–404.

Marks SL, Kook PH, Papich MG, et al. ACVIM consensus statement: support for rational administration of gastrointestinal protectants to dogs and cats. J Vet Intern Med 2018, 32:1823–1840.

Sattasathuchana O, Steiner JM. Canine eosinophilic gastrointestinal disorders. Anim Health Res Rev 2014, 15(1):76–86.

Author Kathryn M. McGonigle

Consulting Editor Mark P. Rondeau

Acknowledgment The author and book editors acknowledge the prior contribution of Michelle Pressel

Client Education Handout available online

GASTROESOPHAGEAL REFLUX

G

BASICS

OVERVIEW

- Reflux of gastric or intestinal fluid into the esophageal lumen.
- Incidence unknown; probably more common than clinically recognized.
- Transient relaxation of the lower esophageal sphincter (LES) or chronic vomiting may permit reflux of gastrointestinal juices into the esophageal lumen. Reflux is common in dogs with sliding hiatal hernias. A small amount of gastroesophageal reflux (GER) is a normal phenomenon in dogs and cats.
- Gastric acid, pepsin, trypsin, bicarbonate, and bile salts are all injurious to the esophageal mucosa with prolonged or repetitive contact.
- Sequelae of GER may vary from mild inflammation of the superficial mucosa to severe ulceration involving the submucosa and muscularis.
- Systems affected include gastrointestinal (regurgitation) and respiratory (aspiration pneumonia).

SIGNALMENT

- Dog and cats; male or female.
- No breed predilections reported.
- May be associated with congenital hiatal hernia seen in Chinese Shar-Pei dogs and brachycephalic breeds.
- Occurs at any age; younger animals may be at increased risk because of developmental immaturity of the gastroesophageal sphincter.

SIGNS

- Regurgitation.
- Hypersalivation.
- Painful swallowing (odynophagia).
- Anorexia.

CAUSES & RISK FACTORS

- General anesthesia.
- Retained gastric contents.
- Acquired or congenital hiatal hernia.
- Chronic vomiting with secondary esophagitis.
- Brachycephalic airway syndrome.

DIAGNOSIS

DIFFERENTIAL DIAGNOSIS

- Oral or pharyngeal disease.
- Ingestion of caustic agent.
- Esophageal foreign body.
- Esophageal tumor.
- Megaesophagus.
- Hiatal hernia.
- Gastroesophageal intussusception.

CBC/BIOCHEMISTRY/URINALYSIS

Usually normal.

OTHER LABORATORY TESTS

N/A

IMAGING

- Survey thoracic radiography—usually unremarkable; may be air or fluid in the distal esophagus (nonspecific finding).
- Barium contrast radiography—reveals GER in some, but not all, animals; videofluoroscopy is superior to esophagram; aspiration pneumonia may be evident in the dependent portions of the lung.

DIAGNOSTIC PROCEDURES

Esophagoscopy—the best means of confirming esophagitis: irregular mucosal surface with hyperemia or active bleeding often present in the distal esophagus. Refluxed gastroduodenal secretions may be seen pooling in the distal esophagus near the LES, which may or may not be open.

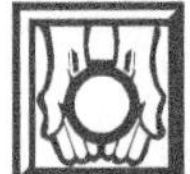

TREATMENT

- Generally managed as outpatient.
- Not necessary to restrict activity.
- Moderate to severe cases—may withhold food for 24 hours to promote esophageal rest and to minimize further GER; thereafter, feed low-fat, low-protein meals in small, frequent feedings; dietary fat decreases gastroesophageal sphincter pressure and delays gastric emptying; protein stimulates gastric acid secretion and may precipitate GER.

MEDICATIONS

DRUG(S) OF CHOICE

- Drug therapy is recommended if significant mucosal injury is present.
- Oral sucralfate slurry (0.5–1 g PO q8h).
- Proton pump inhibitors (omeprazole: 0.7–1.5 mg/kg PO q12h or pantoprazole: 1 mg/kg IV q12–24h) for robust suppression of gastric acid production.
- Prokinetic agents—cisapride (0.5 mg/kg PO q8–12h) or metoclopramide (0.5 mg/kg PO q6–8h or 1–2 mg/kg q24h as CRI).
- Gastrostomy tube placement for enteral nutrition in animals with severe mucosal trauma.

CONTRAINDICATIONS/POSSIBLE INTERACTIONS

Sucralfate may interfere with the absorption of other drugs.

FOLLOW-UP

PATIENT MONITORING

- It is appropriate in most patients to monitor clinical signs.
- Consider endoscopy for patients that do not respond to empirical medical therapies. Severe mucosal damage (esophagitis) may progress to stricture.

PREVENTION/AVOIDANCE

Clients should avoid feeding high-fat foods; they promote gastric retention and might exacerbate GER.

POSSIBLE COMPLICATIONS

Esophagitis and stricture formation.

EXPECTED COURSE AND PROGNOSIS

Most animals respond well to medical management and have a good prognosis.

MISCELLANEOUS

ASSOCIATED CONDITIONS

Hiatal hernia.

AGE-RELATED FACTORS

May be worse in younger animals because of developmental immaturity of the gastroesophageal sphincter mechanism.

ZOONOTIC POTENTIAL

N/A

PREGNANCY/FERTILITY/BREEDING

N/A

SEE ALSO

- Esophageal stricture.
- Esophagitis.

ABBREVIATIONS

- GER = gastroesophageal reflux.
- LES = lower esophageal sphincter.

Suggested Reading

Kook PH, Kempf J, Ruetten M, Reusch CE. Wireless ambulatory esophageal pH monitoring in dogs with clinical signs interpreted as gastroesophageal reflux. J Vet Intern Med 2014, 28(6):1716–1723.

Zacuto AC, Marks SL, Osborn J, et al. The influence of esomeprazole and cisapride on gastroesophageal reflux during anesthesia in dogs. J Vet Intern Med 2012, 26(3):518–525.

Author Albert E. Jergens

Consulting Editor Mark P. Rondeau

Client Education Handout available online

BASICS

DEFINITION

The partial or complete physical impedance to the flow of ingesta and/or secretions aborally through the pylorus into the duodenum (gastric outflow tract obstruction [GOTO]) or through the small intestine. Obstructions in the pharynx, esophagus, large intestine, and rectum, and motility disorders, are addressed in separate chapters.

PATHOPHYSIOLOGY

• Mechanical obstruction commonly results from indiscriminate ingestion of foreign material, the presence of a gastrointestinal (GI) mass, or intussusception. • The accumulation of ingesta and GI secretions orad to the obstruction causes local vascular compromise, resulting in intestinal wall edema, necrosis, and possible sepsis.
• Decreased oral intake, vomiting, and sequestration of GI secretions result in acid-base and electrolyte imbalances.

SYSTEMS AFFECTED

• Cardiovascular—hypovolemic or septic shock can result from fluid loss or GI translocation of bacteria. • GI—GI obstructions cause pathology by distension and compression of the GI tract orad to the obstruction; this results in decreased blood flow to the area with subsequent edema, ulceration, and necrosis of the mucosa; direct physical damage to the GI mucosa by foreign bodies (especially linear foreign bodies) can result in ulceration and possible perforation of the intestinal wall. • Hemic/lymphatic/immune—sepsis secondary to necrosis and/or bacterial translocation.

GENETICS

Unknown

INCIDENCE/PREVALENCE

Common

SIGNALMENT

Species

Dog and cat.

Breed Predilections

Gastric dilation and volvulus (GDV) is common in large- and giant-breed dogs (Great Dane, German shepherd).

Mean Age and Range

• Foreign bodies—more common in young animals, but can occur at any age. • Pyloric stenosis—occurs most often in young animals. • Chronic hypertrophic gastropathy (CHG)—more common in middle-aged and older animals. • Intussusceptions—most common in young animals.

Predominant Sex

None

SIGNS

Historical Findings

• Severity of clinical signs is influenced by location and completeness of obstruction.
• Patients with GOTO tend to have acute onset of severe vomiting; some patients can present as acute abdomen (acute and severe abdominal pain, vomiting); partial obstructions can have more chronic and intermittent clinical signs. • Duration of clinical signs varies, but usually 2–3 days.
• Patients may have vomiting, anorexia, and/or lethargy.

Physical Examination Findings

• Moderate to severe dehydration is common.
• Careful oral examination is recommended as linear foreign bodies can often be lodged at the base of the tongue. • Abdominal palpation will often elicit a painful response; sometimes patients will vomit in response to palpation. • Abdominal mass may be palpated. • Cranial abdominal distension and tympany often seen with GDV.

CAUSES

• Benign pyloric outflow tract obstruction.
• Foreign body. • Gastroenteritis (infectious, granulomatous). • GDV. • GI neoplasia.
• Intussusception. • Mesenteric torsion/volvulus. • Pyloric stenosis. • Stricture.

RISK FACTORS

• Foreign bodies more commonly found in young dogs and cats (mean age 2–4 years) due to indiscriminate eating behavior.
• Linear foreign bodies found more commonly in cats. • GI tumors more common in older cats and dogs.

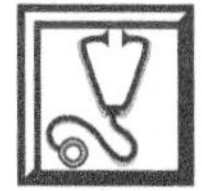

DIAGNOSIS

DIFFERENTIAL DIAGNOSIS

• Metabolic disease (e.g., renal failure, hepatic disease, diabetic ketoacidosis, hypoadrenocorticism). • Infectious gastroenteritis (e.g., viral, bacterial, parasitic).
• Nonspecific gastroenteritis. • Pancreatitis.
• Peritonitis. • Gastroduodenal ulcer and erosion. • CNS disease.

CBC/BIOCHEMISTRY/URINALYSIS

• CBC—will often reflect systemic consequences of obstruction; variable degrees of neutrophilia with left shift and possible toxic changes seen with cases of sepsis.
• Biochemistry—often reveals changes secondary to dehydration (increased blood urea nitrogen [BUN] and creatinine) as well as electrolyte and acid-base disturbances; animals with GOTO classically have hypokalemic and hypochloremic metabolic alkalosis.
• Urinalysis—urine specific gravity may be increased secondary to dehydration.

OTHER LABORATORY TESTS

Lactate—hypoperfusion results in hyperlactatemia (>2.5 mmol/L).

IMAGING

• Survey abdominal radiographs—radiopaque foreign material may be seen in GI lumen; presence of soft tissue opacity in the stomach in a patient with recent history of vomiting and anorexia is highly suspicious for GOTO; indirect signs of GI obstruction can include gastric or intestinal distension with fluid or gas; linear foreign bodies characteristically cause grouping of intestinal loops on right of midline with small luminal gas bubbles (apostrophe shaped); presence of free gas in abdomen is consistent with GI perforation and septic peritonitis. • Contrast abdominal radiographs—positive contrast agents (liquid barium) can be used to identify radiolucent material in GI lumen; retained contrast material in stomach 4–6 hours after administration is consistent with GOTO; use of barium contrast agents contraindicated if GI perforation is suspected; in these instances, use of iodinated contrast agents is recommended. • Abdominal ultrasound—ultrasound can be very effective at identifying GI foreign bodies and intraluminal masses as well as assessing for integrity of GI tract and presence of abdominal fluid/air; luminal foreign bodies will cause distal acoustic shadowing, while linear foreign bodies often appear as hyperechoic linear objects within intestinal lumen.

DIAGNOSTIC PROCEDURES

• In cases where intestinal neoplasia is suspected, advanced imaging techniques such as CT may provide additional information such as the nature of the mass and its degree of invasion. • GI endoscopy may be used for removal of gastric foreign bodies causing GOTO.

PATHOLOGIC FINDINGS

Histopathology of GI masses causing obstruction can reveal granulomatous inflammation, fungal infection (e.g., pythiosis), and neoplasia.

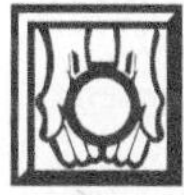

TREATMENT

APPROPRIATE HEALTH CARE

• *Emergency intervention is required to relieve the obstruction.*
• Prior to definitive treatment of the obstruction, stabilization of the patient and correction of dehydration as well as electrolyte and acid-base abnormalities are imperative.
• Dogs with GDV should have gastric decompression first using orogastric intubation or percutaneous gastrocentesis in order to relieve gastric pressure.

G

GASTROINTESTINAL OBSTRUCTION (CONTINUED)

NURSING CARE

• Aggressive IV administration of isotonic crystalloids is recommended to correct dehydration and hypovolemia, if present; recommendation is to administer ¼ shock bolus of 20 mL/kg (dog) or 10 mL/kg (cat) over 15 min and reevaluate patient's status (heart rate, blood pressure, blood lactate); repeat 1–2 times if vital parameters fail to normalize; if crystalloid therapy not successful in stabilizing patient, colloid solutions such as hetastarch can be administered at 5 mL/kg (dog) and 2.5 mL/kg (cat), to max 20 mL/kg (dog) and 10 mL/kg (cat). • Colloids should be used with caution, especially in cases where sepsis is suspected, due to their association with acute kidney injury.

ACTIVITY

Restricted for first 10–14 days post surgery.

DIET

• Nothing by mouth until relief of obstruction and resolution of vomiting; then feed bland fat-restricted diet for 1–2 days, with gradual return to normal diet. • Enteral tube feeding or parenteral feeding may be required postoperatively.

CLIENT EDUCATION

Animals with a history of GI foreign bodies have a tendency to repeat this behavior; owners should be counseled on ways to minimize ingestion of these objects.

SURGICAL CONSIDERATIONS

• Surgical exploration of the abdomen allows for removal of the foreign body as well as resection of any nonviable tissue; if the obstruction is neoplastic, infectious, or inflammatory in nature, surgical intervention can be therapeutic as well as diagnostic as long as excised tissue is submitted for histopathology and culture. • When GI obstruction is caused by a gastric foreign body, endoscopic removal can be attempted; if unsuccessful, foreign material can be removed from the stomach by gastrotomy.
• GOTO—GDV should be corrected and future volvulus prevented with a gastropexy.
• Intestinal obstruction—the full length of the intestinal tract should be examined and palpated; enterotomy should be performed to remove any luminal foreign material; if nonviable or perforated sections are present, resection and anastomosis should be performed. • Although intussusceptions can be percutaneously reduced, recurrence is very common; surgical reduction and/or resection with or without enteropexy is recommended.

MEDICATIONS

DRUG(S) OF CHOICE

• Parenteral broad-spectrum IV antibiotic therapy (ampicillin–sulbactam 30 mg/kg IV q8h with enrofloxacin 10 mg/kg IV q24h) should be initiated as soon as possible in patients with suspected GI obstruction. • In cases where GI ulceration is suspected or confirmed, use of a proton pump inhibitor is recommended (omeprazole or pantoprazole 1 mg/kg q12h PO or IV, respectively).
• Appropriate analgesia should be provided before, during, and after surgery; mu-agonist opioids (fentanyl 2–5 μg/kg/h IV as CRI or hydromorphone 0.1 mg/kg IV q4–6h) are recommended given their strong analgesic effect.

CONTRAINDICATIONS

Prokinetic agents (e.g., metoclopramide, cisapride) must be avoided until obstruction is resolved.

PRECAUTIONS

• Use of antiemetic medications is contraindicated in patients with suspected GI obstruction. • Nonsteroidal anti-inflammatory drugs should not be used in patients with GI obstructions due to their adverse effects on the GI mucosa and renal function in patients that are not hemodynamically stable.

POSSIBLE INTERACTIONS

N/A

ALTERNATIVE DRUG(S)

N/A

FOLLOW-UP

PATIENT MONITORING

• Dehiscence of gastrotomy and enterotomy sites can occur 3–5 days postoperatively; patients should be watched closely during this period for signs of lethargy, recurrence of vomiting, and fever. • Ventricular arrhythmias are documented in approximately 40% of GDV patients; in these cases, electrolyte and acid-base disturbances should be identified and treated, if present.

PREVENTION/AVOIDANCE

Efforts to prevent repeat ingestion of foreign bodies.

POSSIBLE COMPLICATIONS

• Aspiration pneumonia. • Septic peritonitis.
• Functional ileus.

EXPECTED COURSE AND PROGNOSIS

• With rapid surgical intervention of uncomplicated cases of GI foreign bodies, prognosis is good (>95%); however, prognosis associated with septic peritonitis is significantly lower (50%); negative prognostic factors that have been identified include longer duration of clinical signs, presence of linear foreign body, and multiple surgical procedures. • With intestinal neoplasia, prognosis remains guarded to poor, with the exception of small cell lymphoma in cats; with gastric carcinoma, complete surgical excision is rarely attainable and intestinal carcinoma has high rate of metastasis at time of diagnosis; large cell GI lymphoma has relatively poor response rate to commonly used chemotherapy protocols, and median survival times in cats and dogs are 4–6 months and 110 days, respectively.

MISCELLANEOUS

ASSOCIATED CONDITIONS

N/A

AGE-RELATED FACTORS

See Signalment.

ZOONOTIC POTENTIAL

N/A

PREGNANCY/FERTILITY/BREEDING

N/A

SYNONYMS

N/A

SEE ALSO

- Acute Abdomen.
- Acute Vomiting.
- Gastric Dilation and Volvulus Syndrome.
- Gastric Motility Disorders.
- Hypertrophic Pyloric Gastropathy, Chronic.
- Intussusception.
- Peritonitis.
- Pythiosis.
- Vomiting, Chronic.

ABBREVIATIONS

- BUN = blood urea nitrogen.
- CHG = chronic hypertrophic gastropathy.
- GDV = gastric dilation and volvulus.
- GI = gastrointestinal.
- GOTO = gastric outflow tract obstruction.

Suggested Reading

Boag AK, Coe RJ, Martinez TA, Hughes D. Acid-base and electrolyte abnormalities in dogs with gastrointestinal foreign bodies. J Vet Intern Med 2005, 19:816–821.

Hayes G. Gastrointestinal foreign bodies in dogs and cats: a retrospective study of 208 cases. J Small Anim Pract 2009, 50:576–583.

Hobday MM, Pachtinger GE, Drobatz KJ, Syring RS. Linear versus non-linear gastrointestinal foreign bodies in 499 dogs: clinical presentation, management and short-term outcome. J Small Anim Pract 2014, 55:560–565.

Author Albert E. Jergens

Consulting Editor Mark P. Rondeau

Acknowledgment The author and book editors acknowledge the prior contribution of Steven L. Marks.

Client Education Handout available online

GESTATIONAL DIABETES MELLITUS

OVERVIEW

Diabetes mellitus (DM), which occurs during mid to late gestation, most likely due to insulin resistance from increased progesterone and growth hormone production by the mammary glands.

SIGNALMENT

- Middle-aged intact female dogs.
- Mean age—6 years.
- Nordic spitz breeds are overrepresented.
- Not reported in cats.

SIGNS

- Polyuria.
- Polydipsia.
- Polyphagia.
- Weight loss.
- Lethargy.
- Vomiting.
- Ketosis.

CAUSES & RISK FACTORS

- Late-term pregnancy.
- Diestrus.
- Exogenous progesterone supplementation.
- Acromegaly.

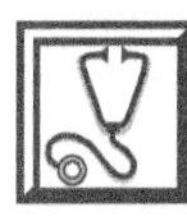

DIAGNOSIS

DIFFERENTIAL DIAGNOSIS

Acromegaly—affected bitches are listless and have increased abdominal size, increased interdental spaces, polyuria/polydipsia, weight gain, and excessive skin folds in the facial/neck areas.

CBC/Biochemistry/Urinalysis

- Hyperglycemia.
- Glucosuria.
- Metabolic acidosis if ketonemic or ketonuric.

Other Laboratory Tests

Urine culture—urinary tract infections can contribute to insulin resistance.

Imaging

- Ultrasonography—assess fetal viability; deceased puppies may affect treatment decisions.
- Radiographs—determine fetal size and relative risk for dystocia.

Diagnostic Procedures

N/A

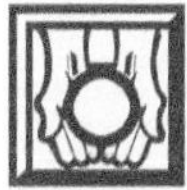

TREATMENT

- Nonpharmacologic considerations—management of gestational DM requires intensive fluid and insulin therapy. Continued glucose toxicity can destroy the pancreatic beta cells' capacity to produce insulin, leading to permanent DM.
- Ovariohysterectomy is recommended. While the diabetes may resolve at the end of diestrus or after parturition, it will return on subsequent cycles and then has a greater potential to become permanent.

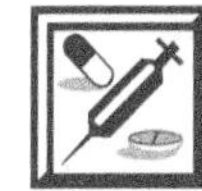

MEDICATIONS

DRUG(S) OF CHOICE

- Insulin—if ketosis not present, start at an insulin dose of 0.25 U/kg SC q12h of intermediate or long-acting insulin; will likely need to increase the dose to achieve glycemic control. If ketoacidosis is present, regular insulin (0.1–0.2 U/kg IM q4–6h) may be necessary to achieve initial glycemic control before switching to longer-acting insulin.
- Aglepristone—10 mg/kg SC days 1, 2, 9, and 17 from diagnosis. This medication is a progesterone receptor blocker, but does not affect progesterone levels. Treatment reserved for cases in which ovariohysterectomy is not possible or authorized by the owners.

CONTRAINDICATIONS/POSSIBLE INTERACTIONS

N/A

FOLLOW-UP

PATIENT MONITORING

Care must be taken to avoid insulin overdose causing hypoglycemia during the immediate postpartum period (or the end of diestrus), because the speed at which insulin resistance resolves and exogenous insulin requirements decrease is unpredictable.

PREVENTION/AVOIDANCE

Ovariohysterectomy to remove source of progesterone.

POSSIBLE COMPLICATIONS

Lack of prompt resolution of hyperglycemia may result in diabetes mellitus becoming permanent.

EXPECTED COURSE AND PROGNOSIS

- Diabetes usually resolves at parturition or at the end of diestrus. More likely to be transient DM if pregnancy terminated, whereas insulin-treated bitches more likely to develop permanent DM.
- May abort the litter or have dystocia as a result of the effects of chronic hyperglycemia.
- Small, unthrifty puppies may result from an abnormal placental blood supply. Conversely, some fetuses in a hyperglycemic environment experience an abnormally increased growth rate (macrosomia). These puppies tend to be large, leading to dystocia.

MISCELLANEOUS

ASSOCIATED CONDITIONS

Pregnancy

AGE-RELATED FACTORS

Older bitches are more likely to develop permanent DM.

ZOONOTIC POTENTIAL

N/A

PREGNANCY/FERTILITY/BREEDING

May abort the litter or have dystocia as a result of the effects of chronic hyperglycemia. There is thought to be a genetic component, due to a breed predisposition. It is not advised to continue to breed affected individuals.

SEE ALSO

Diabetes Mellitus without Complication—Dogs.

ABBREVIATIONS

- DM = diabetes mellitus.

Suggested Reading

Johnson CA. Glucose homeostasis during canine pregnancy: insulin resistance, ketosis, and hypoglycemia. Theriogenology 2008, 70(9):1418–1423.

Author Carla Barstow
Consulting Editor Erin E. Runcan

G

GIARDIASIS

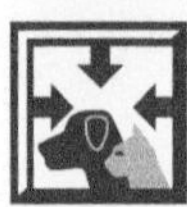

BASICS

OVERVIEW

- Enteric infection of dogs and cats with protozoan parasite, *Giardia duodenalis.*
- Direct transmission by ingestion of cysts that are immediately infective when shed in feces.
- Trophozoites, motile (flagellated) organisms released from ingested cysts, attach to surface of enterocytes in small intestine with ventral sucking disc; move from site to site.
- Can cause small bowel diarrhea, but infection often asymptomatic.

SIGNALMENT

More common in dogs than cats.

SIGNS

- Clinical signs more common in young hosts; adults usually asymptomatic.
- Signs can be acute, transient, intermittent, or chronic.
- Malabsorption syndrome with soft, frothy, greasy, voluminous feces (diarrhea), usually with rancid odor.

CAUSES & RISK FACTORS

- Transmitted by ingestion of cysts from feces in/on food, water, environment, or fur.
- Indirect water-borne transmission most common; cool, moist conditions favor cyst survival.
- Higher risk of infection in puppies and kittens, in high-density populations, and in animals with compromised immunity.

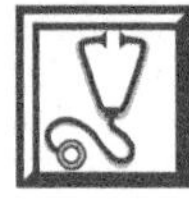

DIAGNOSIS

DIFFERENTIAL DIAGNOSIS

- Infectious and noninfectious causes of small bowel diarrhea, maldigestion, and malabsorption syndromes, especially pancreatic exocrine insufficiency or inflammatory bowel disease.
- In cats, differentiate from infection with *Tritrichomonas foetus.*

CBC/BIOCHEMISTRY/URINALYSIS

Generally within normal limits.

OTHER LABORATORY TESTS

N/A

IMAGING

N/A

DIAGNOSTIC PROCEDURES

- Detection of *Giardia* trophozoites, cysts, or antigen in feces.
- Trophozoites (15 × 8 μm) detectable in fresh feces (especially diarrheic feces) and in duodenal aspirates obtained by endoscopy; trophozoites identified on Diff-Quik® or Lugol's iodine-stained fecal smear by teardrop shape with two prominent nuclei. Trophozoites identified in wet mount diluted in saline by "falling leaf" motility; flotation media may lyse trophozoites, interfering with accurate identification.
- Cysts, ~12 μm long, oval with 2–4 nuclei, shed intermittently; centrifugal flotation of fresh feces in zinc sulfate (specific gravity 1.18) preferred method for identification of cysts. Three samples collected at 2–3-day intervals should be examined to detect >70% of infections; cysts become distorted (crescent-shaped) in sugar or other flotation solution with specific gravity >1.25; formalin–ethyl acetate sedimentation is useful in cases of steatorrhea.
- ELISA-based kits available for in-house detection of *Giardia* antigen in feces have high sensitivity; kits should be used to confirm suspicious cases rather than for screening healthy animals; if clinical signs resolve, continued antigen testing not recommended.
- PCR testing—commercial laboratories; studies have shown variable (usually poorer) sensitivity compared to other methods.

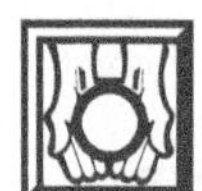

TREATMENT

- Outpatient, unless debilitated or dehydrated.
- Drug therapy should be combined with environmental cleaning and disinfection plus bathing of patient.
- *Giardia* vaccines commercially available; efficacy is poor and vaccine not widely used.

MEDICATIONS

DRUG(S) OF CHOICE

- All extra-label.
- Fenbendazole—50 mg/kg PO q24h for 3 days (dogs) or 5 days (cats); second course of treatment may be necessary.
- Metronidazole—20–22 mg/kg PO q12h for 5–8 days in dogs.
- Metronidazole benzoate—22–25 mg/kg PO q12h for 5–7 days in cats.
- Fenbendazole (50 mg/kg PO q24h) plus metronidazole (25 mg/kg PO q12h) for 5 days—may provide better resolution and reduction in cyst shedding.
- Combination febantel, pyrantel pamoate, and praziquantel product—use for 3 days at label dose for *Giardia.*

CONTRAINDICATIONS/POSSIBLE INTERACTIONS

- Metronidazole—efficacy reportedly 50–67% in dogs; bitter taste; can cause anorexia, vomiting, vestibular signs.
- Albendazole (25 mg/kg PO q12h for 2 days in dogs or 5 days in cats) is effective but not recommended because it can be teratogenic and cause anorexia, depression, vomiting, ataxia, diarrhea, abortion, and myelosuppression.

FOLLOW-UP

- Repeat fecal examinations to confirm efficacy of treatment and detect reinfection.
- Chronic infection can lead to debilitation.

MISCELLANEOUS

ZOONOTIC POTENTIAL

- In North America, *Giardia* is the most common intestinal parasite in humans. Dog and cat isolates are host specific, with little data to demonstrate transmission from pets to humans.
- Most *Giardia* infections in humans are anthroponotic or originate from livestock.
- Zoonotic transmission from pets to immunosuppressed humans may occur.

PREGNANCY/FERTILITY/BREEDING

Do not use albendazole in pregnant animals.

INTERNET RESOURCES

- https://capcvet.org
- https://www.cdc.gov/parasites/giardia

Suggested Reading

Bowman DD. Georgis' Parasitology for Veterinarians, 9th ed. St. Louis, MO: Elsevier Science, 2009, pp. 89–91.

Uehlinger FD, Naqvi SA, Greenwood SJ, et al. Comparison of five diagnostic tests for Giardia duodenalis in fecal samples from young dogs. Vet Parasitol. 2017, 244:91–96.

Authors Matt Brewer and Katy A. Martin
Consulting Editor Amie Koenig

Gingival Enlargement/Hyperplasia

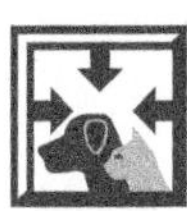

BASICS

OVERVIEW

- Enlargement of gingival tissue due to proliferation of its elements (abnormal multiplication or increase in the normal number of cells in normal arrangement).
- Probable familial tendency—boxers.

SIGNALMENT

- Dogs and rarely cats.
- Breed predilections—boxers, Great Danes, collies, Doberman pinschers, Dalmatians.

SIGNS

- Thickening and increase in height of attached gingiva and gingival margin—sometimes completely covers tooth surface.
- Resultant formation of "pseudopockets"—increase in pocket depth due to increased gingival height; not due to loss of attachment, unless untreated and progresses to concurrent periodontal disease.
- Gingival margin may be thickened in a labial to lingual direction, especially at incisors.
- Locally affected areas possible (shelties), but typically more generalized pattern found.
- Focally affected areas, other than the marginal gingiva, may develop hyperplastic areas due to chronic irritation, such as the "gum chewer's lesion." These areas should be evaluated for therapeutic need (excision).
- May form as protuberant masses (grape cluster) at gingival margins—biopsy necessary to rule out neoplasia.

CAUSES

Chronic inflammatory response to presence of bacteria in plaque associated with periodontal disease.

RISK FACTORS

- Breed predilection (see Signalment).
- Chronic drug administration—diphenylhydantoin, cyclosporine, nitrendipine, nifedipine, amlodipine.

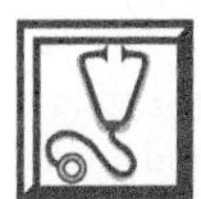

DIAGNOSIS

DIFFERENTIAL DIAGNOSIS

- Presumptive diagnosis based on clinical appearance, especially if generalized and found in breed with high predilection.
- Oral neoplasia—e.g., peripheral odontogenic fibromas; usually not generalized; sometimes osseous changes present.
- Oral papillomatosis—papilloma usually on mucosal surfaces.
- Operculum—seen in young animals during eruption phase of teeth; incomplete loss and/or persistence of gingival tissue covering erupting tooth.
- Chronic sublingual or buccal trauma with proliferation—"gum chewer's lesion."

IMAGING

Intraoral radiography—to rule out any underlying osseous changes (more common with epulides or tumors).

DIAGNOSTIC PROCEDURES

- Biopsy—focal area or areas that do not respond to standard therapy.
- Histopathology—to rule out neoplasia and other causes; histologic evaluation is only way to confirm.

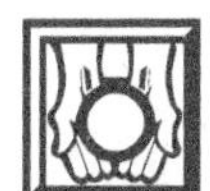

TREATMENT

Appropriate Health Care

Regular dental cleanings and homecare—to minimize effects of plaque and bacterial accumulation.

Client Education

- Chronic, recurring problem that often needs repeated therapy.
- Encourage the highest level of home care and regular professional cleaning.

Surgical Considerations

Gingivectomy (Excising Excess Tissue) and Gingivoplasty (Recontouring)

- To remove excess gingival tissue and return pocket depths to normal.
- Provide appropriate patient monitoring and support during anesthetic procedures.
- Regional and local anesthetic injections or topical gels.
- Periodontal probe—to determine depth of pseudopocket; can mark pocket depth on outside of pocket with end of probe to mark with a bleeding "dot."
- Excise excess tissue and reshape gingival margin.
- Cold steel—sharp, stout scissors (crown and collar scissors) or scalpel blade.
- Connect dots made by probe with blade to approximate normal gingival margin or use scissors, following pocket depth to remove bulk tissue.
- Twelve-fluted bur on high-speed handpiece—contour margin to feather angle; assists in hemostasis.
- Electrocautery or radiosurgery—use fully or partially rectified current; avoid damage to underlying bone or tissue.
- Laser—use appropriately and avoid damage to tooth and bone.
- Excessive thickness (incisor and canine region)—modified Widman technique; envelope flap to lift gingiva off tooth surfaces; excise tissue wedge to remove gingiva at inside of pocket to provide narrower width of attached gingiva; suture interdentally to secure gingiva; use digital pressure to reposition.
- Tincture of myrrh and benzoin—use dropper; coat cut margins and dry; 4–5 layers.
- Hemostatic solutions—to aid in hemorrhage control as needed.

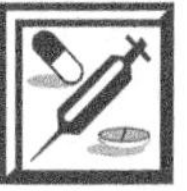

MEDICATIONS

DRUG(S) OF CHOICE

- Oral antimicrobials—chlorhexidine; zinc ascorbate gel.
- Postoperative pain management.

CONTRAINDICATIONS/POSSIBLE INTERACTIONS

Patients on chronic administration of amlodipine, diphenylhydantoin or cyclosporine may be predisposed to hyperplastic changes. Dose reduction may decrease extent of gingival enlargement.

FOLLOW-UP

PATIENT MONITORING

- Postoperative comfort—give pain medication as needed.
- Regular examinations and professional cleaning and treatment—to avoid recurrence, which is common.

PREVENTION/AVOIDANCE

Regular professional cleaning, meticulous home care.

POSSIBLE COMPLICATIONS

- Possible exacerbation of periodontal disease in pseudopockets if left untreated; deeper pockets are more susceptible to anaerobic bacterial infections.
- Excessive heat with electrosurgical treatment may result in damaged teeth (pulpitis, pulpal death) and alveolar bone.

EXPECTED COURSE AND PROGNOSIS

- Good prognosis with regular care.
- Recurrence common.

MISCELLANEOUS

INTERNET RESOURCES

https://avdc.org/avdc-nomenclature

Suggested Reading

Lobprise HB. Blackwell's Five-Minute Veterinary Consult Clinical Companion: Small Animal Dentistry, 2nd ed. Ames, IA: Blackwell, 2012 (for additional topics, including diagnostics and techniques).

Lobprise HB, Dodd JR. Wiggs' Veterinary Dentistry Principles and Practice. Hoboken, NJ, Wiley-Blackwell, 2019.

Author Heidi B. Lobprise

Consulting Editor Heidi B. Lobprise

G

GLAUCOMA

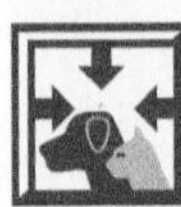

BASICS

DEFINITION

- A group of diseases where elevated intraocular pressure (IOP) causes optic nerve and retinal degeneration with subsequent loss of vision.
- Diagnosis—IOP >20 mmHg (dogs) or >25 mmHg (cats) as determined by tonometry, with changes in vision or the appearance of the globe, optic nerve, and/or retina.

PATHOPHYSIOLOGY

- Multifactorial disease where obstruction of aqueous humor outflow leads to increased IOP and optic nerve degeneration.
- Elevated IOP induces mechanical changes (stretching of sclera in lamina cribosa damages optic nerve axons) and vascular changes (decreased ocular perfusion causes ischemic damage to retina), resulting in ganglion cell death and optic nerve atrophy.

SYSTEMS AFFECTED

- Ophthalmic.
- Nervous.

GENETICS

- Primary angle-closure glaucoma (PACG; dogs)—complex trait with multiple genetic risk factors and uncertain mode of inheritance.
- Primary open-angle glaucoma (POAG; dogs)—monogenic (*ADAMTS10*) and autosomal recessive.
- Primary congenital glaucoma (PCG; cats)—monogenic (*LTBP2*) and autosomal recessive.

INCIDENCE/PREVALENCE

- Dogs—prevalence depends on breed; primary and secondary glaucoma are each listed as approximately 0.8% of all hospital admissions in the North American Veterinary Medical Database (NAVMDB).
- Cats—relatively uncommon; less than 0.3% of diagnoses in NAVMDB.

SIGNALMENT

Species

- Dog—primary and secondary common.
- Cat—primary rare; secondary more common (due to intraocular neoplasia or chronic uveitis).

Breed Predilections

- PACG—Alaskan Malamute, American cocker spaniel, Australian cattle dog, basset hound, Boston terrier, bouvier des Flandres, bullmastiff, Chinese Shar-Pei, chow chow, Dalmatian, Dandie Dinmont terrier, English cocker spaniel, English springer spaniel, flat-coated retriever, golden retriever, Great Dane, Labrador retriever, Newfoundland, poodle, Samoyed, Shiba Inu, shih tzu, Siberian husky, Welsh springer spaniel.
- POAG—beagle, Norwegian elkhound, petit basset griffon Vendéen.
- PCG—Siamese cats.
- Other forms of primary glaucoma—Burmese, Persian, Siamese cats.

Mean Age and Range

- Primary (dogs)—any age; predominantly affects middle-aged (4–9 years).
- Secondary (cats)—usually affects older cats (>6 years).

Predominant Sex

Females suffer PACG compared to males at a ratio of 2 : 1.

SIGNS

General Comments

All well-equipped small animal hospitals should have a tonometer.

Historical Findings

- Dogs—owners may note pain (blepharospasm, tenderness about the head), serous to seromucoid ocular discharge, red or cloudy eye, dilated pupil, or altered vision; in chronic cases, globe enlargement may be apparent.
- Cats—signs are more subtle; eye may not appear painful, red, or cloudy; owners may note dilated pupil, vision changes, or enlarged globe.

Physical Examination Findings

Acute Primary

- High IOP (often >30 mmHg).
- Blepharospasm.
- Enophthalmos with elevated third eyelid.
- Episcleral injection.
- Diffuse corneal edema.
- Mydriasis.
- Vision loss—may be detected by lack of menace response, dazzle reflex, and/or direct or consensual pupillary light reflex.
- Optic nerve may be normal or swollen and hyperemic.

Chronic (End Stage)

- High or normal IOP.
- Buphthalmos.
- Descemet's streaks (Haab's striae).
- Subluxated lens with an aphakic crescent.
- Optic nerve head atrophy will appear dark and cupped.
- Retinal atrophy detected by peripapillary or generalized tapetal hyper-reflectivity.

Secondary

- High IOP.
- Episcleral injection.
- Corneal edema.
- Aqueous flare.
- Iris changes (miosis or mydriasis, posterior synechia, iris bombé).
- Hyphema.
- Anterior lens luxation.
- Intumescent cataracts.
- Intraocular mass.

CAUSES

- Congenital—severe dysgenesis/lack of formation of the iridocorneal angle.
- Primary—developmental iridocorneal angle anomalies that impede aqueous humor outflow.
- Secondary—obstruction of aqueous humor outflow by various mechanisms, e.g., uveitis (inflammatory cells or debris), anterior lens luxation (lens or attached vitreous), red blood cells, or neoplastic cells.

RISK FACTORS

- Age.
- Breed.
- Chronic uveitis.
- Goniodysgenesis—developmental defect of iridocorneal angle.
- Lens luxation.
- Hypermature or intumescent cataracts.
- Hyphema.
- Intraocular neoplasia.
- Topically applied mydriatics—may precipitate acute glaucoma in predisposed animals.
- Primary glaucoma is bilateral and often asymmetric; the unaffected fellow eye is at risk for developing glaucoma.

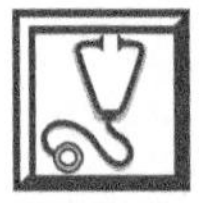

DIAGNOSIS

DIFFERENTIAL DIAGNOSIS

- See Red Eye.
- Conjunctivitis—normal IOP and pupil size with conjunctival hyperemia (diffuse, red discoloration) instead of episcleral vessel engorgement.
- Uveitis—initially low IOP with miotic pupil.

IMAGING

Ocular ultrasound—facilitates evaluation of eye with opaque ocular media; may identify cause of secondary glaucoma (lens luxation, intraocular tumor).

DIAGNOSTIC PROCEDURES

- Rebound or applanation tonometry—essential for diagnosis of glaucoma.
- Gonioscopy—referral procedure that allows for evaluation of iridocorneal angle and assists with diagnosis of primary vs. secondary glaucoma.
- Systemic workup may be indicated in cases of secondary glaucoma due to chronic uveitis, hyphema, or intraocular neoplasia.

PATHOLOGIC FINDINGS

- Histopathologic evaluation is required for all eyes enucleated due to intractable glaucoma.
- Iridocorneal angle morphology assists diagnosis of primary vs. secondary glaucoma.
- Loss of retinal ganglion cells.
- Gliosis and "cupping" of optic nerve head.

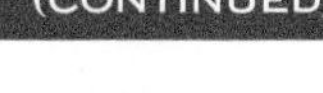

TREATMENT

APPROPRIATE HEALTH CARE

- Acute—outpatient medical management vs. referral.
- Chronic—outpatient medical management vs. salvage surgical management.

CLIENT EDUCATION

- Warn client that primary glaucoma is a bilateral disease; more than 50% of dogs develop glaucoma in the other eye within 8 months without prophylactic therapy.
- Warn client that up to 50% of dogs will be blind in the affected eye within the first year regardless of therapy.

SURGICAL CONSIDERATIONS

- Acute, visual eyes (dogs)—referral surgical procedures aim to control IOP by decreasing aqueous humor production (transscleral or endoscopic cyclophotocoagulation), increasing outflow (gonioimplants), or both; medical treatment is still required long term to control IOP and inflammation.
- Blind, painful eyes (dogs and cats)—salvage procedures include enucleation, evisceration with intrascleral prosthesis (if no intraocular infection or neoplasia), and intravitreal gentamicin or cidofovir injection to minimize long-term medical therapy.

MEDICATIONS

DRUG(S) OF CHOICE

Use multiple agents to lower IOP into the normal range as quickly as possible in an attempt to salvage vision and maintain comfort. Topical hypotensive drugs have largely replaced systemic therapy due to higher efficacy and fewer side effects.

Acute Primary (Dogs)

- Prostaglandin analog—latanoprost 0.005% q12h. In emergency, apply one drop to affected eye, followed by another drop in 30 min. Recheck IOP in 1–2 hours.
- Carbonic anhydrase inhibitor—dorzolamide 2% q8h. Use in combination with latanoprost for long-term therapy.
- Topical corticosteroids—0.1% dexamethasone or 1% prednisolone acetate q12h. Use to control intraocular inflammation from initial hypertensive episode.
- ± Topical beta blocker—timolol maleate 0.5% q12h. Minimal effect on lowering IOP in companion animals. Use as auxiliary or prophylactic medication.
- ± Hyperosmotic agent—mannitol 1–2 g/kg IV over 20 min. In emergency, use to dehydrate vitreous humor and lower IOP if topical medications ineffective.

Secondary (Dogs and Cats)

- Identify and treat primary disease.
- Topical corticosteroids—to reduce inflammation if no ulcerative keratitis.
- Topical carbonic anhydrase inhibitors.
- ± Topical beta blockers.

CONTRAINDICATIONS

- Topical atropine—do not use with glaucoma.
- Prostaglandin analogs/miotic agents—do not use with primary anterior lens luxation or uveitis; mostly ineffective in cats.

PRECAUTIONS

- Systemic absorption of topical beta blockers may cause bronchoconstriction and bradycardia in small dogs and cats.
- Hyperosmotic agents may initiate acute pulmonary edema in patients with cardiovascular disease or hypervolemia.

POSSIBLE INTERACTIONS

Concurrent administration of latanoprost with a topical nonsteroidal anti-inflammatory drug such as flurbiprofen 0.03% may decrease its hypotensive effect.

ALTERNATIVE DRUG(S)

- Prostaglandin analogs—travoprost 0.004% q12h, bimatoprost 0.03% q12h.
- Carbonic anhydrase inhibitor—brinzolamide 1% q8h.
- Beta blockers—levobunalol 0.5% q12h, betaxolol 0.5% q12h.
- Osmotic agents—hypertonic hydroxyethyl starch 6–7.5% (4 mL/kg IV over 15–20 min).

FOLLOW-UP

PATIENT MONITORING

- IOP—monitored often (weekly to monthly) after starting initial therapy, then q3-4 months long term. Client's daily observation of comfort and vision is most important.
- Monitor for drug reactions.

PREVENTION/AVOIDANCE

- Primary—bilateral disease; recommend that a veterinary ophthalmologist examine the unaffected eye to determine its risk of developing glaucoma.
- Prophylactic therapy for the predisposed, unaffected eye delays onset of glaucoma—0.25% demecarium bromide (miotic) q12h, or 0.5% timolol maleate q12h, or 2% dorzolamide q8–12h.

POSSIBLE COMPLICATIONS

- Blindness.
- Chronic ocular pain.

EXPECTED COURSE AND PROGNOSIS

- Chronic disease that requires constant medical treatment (even with surgical intervention).
- With medical treatment only—most patients ultimately become blind.
- Referral surgical treatment—better chance of retaining vision longer; most patients do not remain visual for more than 2 years after initial diagnosis.
- Secondary to lens luxation—may carry fair prognosis with referral for successful removal of luxated lens and postoperative medical therapy.
- Secondary to anterior uveitis—may carry fair prognosis with control of uveitis.

MISCELLANEOUS

PREGNANCY/FERTILITY/BREEDING

- All listed drugs may affect pregnancy.
- Primary and lens luxation cases—inherited; do not breed affected animals.

SEE ALSO

- Anterior Uveitis—Cats.
- Anterior Uveitis—Dogs.
- Lens Luxation.
- Red Eye.

ABBREVIATIONS

- IOP = intraocular pressure.
- PACG = Primary angle-closure glaucoma.
- POAG = Primary open-angle glaucoma.
- PCG = Primary congenital glaucoma.
- NAVMDB = North American Veterinary Medical Database.

Suggested Reading

Miller PE. The glaucomas. In: Maggs DJ, Miller PE, Ofri R, eds. Slatter's Fundamentals of Veterinary Ophthalmology, 6th ed. St. Louis, MO: Elsevier, 2018, pp. 279–305.

Pizzirani S, ed. Glaucoma. Vet Clin Small Anim 2015, 45(6): 1102–1378.

Author Erin M. Scott

Consulting Editor Kathern E. Myrna

Acknowledgment The author and book editors acknowledge the prior contribution of J. Phillip Pickett.

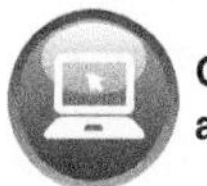

Client Education Handout available online

GLOMERULONEPHRITIS

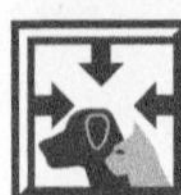

BASICS

DEFINITION

Glomerulonephritis (GN) is a term often used to describe proteinuria of glomerular origin; however, GN is immune-mediated inflammation within the glomerulus (immune complex glomerulonephritis [ICGN]). Because this can only be diagnosed from a renal biopsy, many noninflammatory conditions (glomerulosclerosis, amyloidosis, etc.) may be incorrectly labeled GN in patients who have not undergone evaluation via renal histology.

PATHOPHYSIOLOGY

- Circulating antigen–antibody complexes become entrapped or antibodies can attach in situ to glomerular antigens or soluble antigens entrapped within the glomerular basement membrane; complement component C3 and/or immunoglobulins (Ig) G, M, or A may be involved in complexes, which alter glomerular permeability and induce inflammation, causing proteinuria, nephron injury, fibrosis, and progressive loss of renal function.
- ICGN has several different morphologies depending on the location of immune-complex deposition as well as the glomerular response to injury; membranoproliferative, membranous nephropathy, proliferative, IgA nephropathy, and minimal change disease are recognized ICGN in small animals.
- Inflammation and altered glomerular permeability result in proteinuria; subsequent oxidative damage and tubular obstruction cause renal injury, progressive nephron loss, and decreased glomerular filtration; azotemia and uremia may ensue.
- Hypercoagulability, hypoalbuminemia, and hypertension (HTN) are common complications.

SYSTEMS AFFECTED

- Renal/urologic—proteinuria is the initial symptom; both acute kidney injury (AKI) and chronic kidney disease (CKD) may occur secondarily.
- Cardiovascular—HTN is common; ascites and edema occur in nephrotic syndrome (NS); hypercoagulability and thromboembolism (TE).
- Endocrine/metabolic—hypercholesterolemia in NS.

GENETICS

Many breeds have inheritable glomerular disease leading to protein-losing nephropathy (PLN). Most are non-ICGN; however, several breeds are more frequently affected by GN (see below).

INCIDENCE/PREVALENCE

Glomerular disease is present in most patients with kidney disease; however, not all are ICGN. Approximately 50% of dogs and cats that have undergone renal biopsy have ICGN. GN may be clinically silent and undiagnosed in many patients.

GEOGRAPHIC DISTRIBUTION

Worldwide

SIGNALMENT

- Species—dog and cat.
- Breed predilections—American foxhound, Bernese mountain dog, Doberman pinscher, German shepherd, golden retriever, greyhound, Labrador retriever, Shetland sheepdog, and soft-coated wheaten terrier.
- Mean age and range—middle age (4–8 years), although may occur at any time; cats often younger—mean 4 years.
- Predominant sex—dogs: none; cats: majority are male.

SIGNS

- Proteinuria caused by albuminuria is hallmark.
- Historical findings—nonspecific and include weight loss, muscle wasting, decreased appetite, lethargy, vomiting, and polyuria/polydipsia.
- Physical examination findings—may be normal; subcutaneous edema, peritoneal and/or pleural effusion seen in NS; acute dyspnea and hypoxia may be present in pulmonary TE.

CAUSES

- Most patients have ICGN secondary to systemic infection or inflammation; many patients will not have an obvious trigger identified. * Infectious causes include rickettsial infection (*Borrelia*, *Ehrlichia*, *Anaplasma*, Rocky Mountain spotted fever), babesiosis, bartonellosis, leishmaniasis, brucellosis, dirofilariasis, leptospirosis, systemic fungal infections, and hepatozoonosis.
- Inflammatory conditions include pancreatitis, polyarthritis, pyometra, and systemic lupus erythematosus; reactions to sulfonamides and vaccines is possible; paraneoplastic GN is uncommon.

RISK FACTORS

Lyme-associated GN is a severe and progressive form of ICGN found in dogs with positive *Borrelia* serology, but causation unknown. Labrador retrievers, golden retrievers, and several other breeds are more at risk.

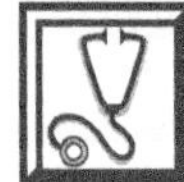

DIAGNOSIS

DIFFERENTIAL DIAGNOSIS

- Proteinuria—commonly occurs for reasons other than GN (see Proteinuria).
- Hypoalbuminemia—may result from decreased hepatic synthesis or protein-losing enteropathy.
- Azotemia—can also be due to AKI or CKD, which may not be caused by ICGN.

CBC/BIOCHEMISTRY/URINALYSIS

- CBC may reveal thrombocytopenia, uncommonly leukocytosis; usually unremarkable.
- Hypoalbuminemia with normal or increased serum globulins; hypercholesterolemia seen in NS; azotemia may be present.
- Persistent proteinuria; some patients may be azotemic with preservation of urine concentration.

OTHER LABORATORY TESTS

- Urine protein : creatinine ratio (UPC) is gold standard test for diagnosing, quantifying, and monitoring proteinuria.
- Testing for underlying systemic infectious/inflammatory causes should be performed as indicated.
- Urine electrophoresis can be performed to fraction proteins by molecular weight to discriminate glomerular and tubular causes of proteinuria.
- Blood pressure measurement should be performed.

IMAGING

Thoracic radiographs and abdominal ultrasound to evaluate for systemic disease.

DIAGNOSTIC PROCEDURES

- Renal biopsy is the only way to diagnose GN and determine the subtype; it characterizes fibrosis and chronicity, which may help predict recovery of renal function following treatment; percutaneous ultrasound-guided needle biopsy is commonly performed; small patients or those with congenital disease may benefit from a surgical wedge/punch biopsy; biopsy contraindications include uncontrolled hypertension, severe thrombocytopenia, and anticoagulant therapy.
- Histology using multiple stains, immunofluorescence, and electron microscopy is required for definitive diagnosis of ICGN; biopsies should be submitted to a veterinary nephropathologist.
- Some patients are too unstable to have renal biopsy performed (thrombocytopenic, rapidly progressing azotemia, etc.); empiric immunosuppression should be given when ICGN is suspected in the absence of biopsy.

PATHOLOGIC FINDINGS

- Definitive diagnosis of ICGN depends on ultrastructural findings of electron-dense immune within glomeruli; positive immunofluorescence.
- Secondary changes to glomerular basement membrane, hypercellularity, and sclerosis.

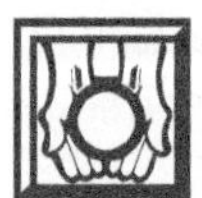

TREATMENT

APPROPRIATE HEALTH CARE

- Many require inpatient therapy to correct hypovolemia, nausea, and anorexia; once

stabilized, patients can be managed as outpatient.
• Patients with AKI may require dialysis to treat severe uremia.
• Therapeutic plasma exchange may be considered.

NURSING CARE

IV crystalloids should be used judiciously. Hypervolemia is a common complication of aggressive fluid therapy.

ACTIVITY

No specific need for activity restriction; patients often have limited endurance.

DIET

• Ideal diets are protein and sodium restricted; prescription "renal" diets are most appropriate; home-prepared diets may be used after consultation with a nutritionist.
• Feeding tubes allow for delivery of supplemental nutrition and medication.

CLIENT EDUCATION

• Prognosis is guarded for azotemic patients; however, complete recovery may occur.
• Dialysis and plasma exchange may allow for more rapid control of disease and promote renal recovery.

SURGICAL CONSIDERATIONS

• Avoid hypotension and renal hypoperfusion.
• Discontinue anticoagulant 1 week before biopsy.

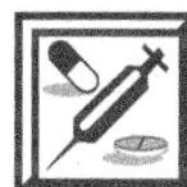

MEDICATIONS

DRUG(S) OF CHOICE

• ICGN requires immunosuppression; mycophenolate (5–10 mg/kg q12h) is most commonly used; GI upset is most frequently observed side effect; peripheral edema is rare; short course of corticosteroids (prednisone 2 mg/kg/day) can be used as mycophenolate may require 2 weeks to take effect.
• Cyclophosphamide (50 mg/m^2 4 days/week); sterile hemorrhagic cystitis and bone marrow suppression are side effects.
• Anti-proteinuric therapy includes angiotensin-converting enzyme (ACE) inhibitors (enalapril/benazepril 0.5–1 mg/kg q12h) or angiotensin receptor blockers (ARB; telmisartan 1–3 mg/kg q24h); these have modest antihypertensive effects; begin at low doses and increase if response is inadequate; cautious use in severely azotemic patients.
• HTN treated with amlodipine (0.25–0.8 mg/kg q24h) or telmisartan (1–3 mg/kg q24h).
• Systemic anticoagulation to prevent TE—clopidogrel (1–4 mg/kg q24h) or aspirin (2–5 mg/kg q24h); newer direct factor X inhibitors may also be considered.

CONTRAINDICATIONS

• ACE inhibitors and ARBs should not be used if patient is dehydrated or hypovolemic.
• Anticoagulation should be avoided in thrombocytopenic patients until platelet count is normal.

PRECAUTIONS

• ACE inhibitors and ARBs should be used cautiously in patients with serum creatinine >3.5, as they may exacerbate uremia; 30% increase in serum creatinine is generally tolerated, if uremic symptoms do not occur; hyperkalemia may occur at higher doses.
• Hypoalbuminemic patients poorly tolerate parenteral fluids; enteral hydration via feeding tube may be better tolerated.
• Immunosuppression increases risk of opportunistic infections.

POSSIBLE INTERACTIONS

Dual therapy of ACE inhibitor and ARB increases risk of hyperkalemia.

ALTERNATIVE DRUG(S)

• Corticosteroids not used for long-term management, but may be considered if other therapies cannot be afforded.
• Patients who fail initial immunosuppressive therapy may benefit from alternative immunosuppression.

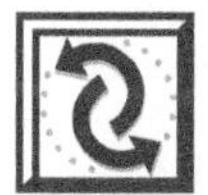

FOLLOW-UP

PATIENT MONITORING

• Renal values, electrolytes, blood pressure, and urinalysis with UPC should be checked 1–2 weeks after starting therapy; reduction in proteinuria may take 4–6 weeks; subsequent rechecks should occur every 1–4 months.
• Complete remission is obtaining UPC <0.5; partial remission is >50% reduction and therapeutic failure is <50% reduction in UPC.
• Normalization of serum creatinine expected with complete response to therapy; many patients will have partial remission with improved but not normal serum creatinine.
• Goal to obtain serum albumin >2.0 mg/dL.
• Repeat renal biopsy can document resolution of immune complexes and guide duration of immunosuppression.

PREVENTION/AVOIDANCE

Avoiding exposure to fleas and ticks may reduce risk of vector-borne infections causing ICGN; preventative therapies should be used.

POSSIBLE COMPLICATIONS

• AKI or CKD.
• HTN.
• NS.
• TE.

EXPECTED COURSE AND PROGNOSIS

Guarded prognosis. Short survival has been reported for azotemic proteinuric dogs. Disease may progress despite therapy. Complete resolution of disease may occur with immunosuppression.

MISCELLANEOUS

ASSOCIATED CONDITIONS

• HTN.
• Hypoalbuminemia.
• Hypercoagulability.

AGE-RELATED FACTORS

None

ZOONOTIC POTENTIAL

N/A

PREGNANCY/FERTILITY/BREEDING

Patients with suspected genetic disease should not be bred.

SYNONYMS

• Glomerulonephropathy.
• Protein-losing nephropathy.

SEE ALSO

• Amyloidosis.
• Nephrotic syndrome.
• Proteinuria.

ABBREVIATIONS

• ACE = angiotensin-converting enzyme.
• AKI = acute kidney injury.
• ARB = angiotensin receptor blocker.
• CKD = chronic kidney disease.
• GN = glomerulonephritis.
• HTN = hypertension.
• ICGN = immune complex glomerulonephritis.
• Ig = immunoglobulin.
• NS = nephrotic syndrome.
• PLN = protein-losing nephropathy.
• TE = thromboembolism.
• UPC = urine protein : creatinine ratio.

INTERNET RESOURCES

www.iris-kidney.com

Suggested Reading

Brown S, ed. Special issue: International Renal Interest Society consensus clinical practice guidelines for glomerular disease in dogs. J Vet Intern Med 2013, 27:S1–S75.
Littman MP. Protein-losing nephropathy in small animals. Vet Clin North Am Small Anim Pract 2011, 41(1):31–62.

Author J.D. Foster
Consulting Editor J.D. Foster

GLUCAGONOMA

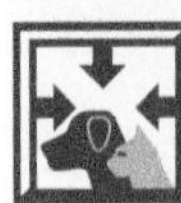

BASICS

OVERVIEW

- Glucagonoma is an uncommon pancreatic islet cell tumor originating from alpha cells, which secrete glucagon. They occasionally arise in extra-pancreatic locations (i.e., liver). Glucagonomas may secrete other hormones, such as gastrin, pancreatic polypeptide, and (rarely) insulin.
- Excess circulating glucagon activates glycogenolysis and gluconeogenesis and inhibits glycogenesis. This increases protein catabolism and lipolysis. Glucagon excess can inhibit erythropoiesis. The culmination of these biochemical changes results in hyperglycemia and occasionally diabetes mellitus (DM), hypoaminoacidemia, anemia, and weight loss. Glucagon can exert a secretory effect on the small intestine, leading to diarrhea.
- Glucagonomas may cause an overall decrease in plasma amino acid concentrations, with epidermal protein depletion in the skin, leading to the classic dermatopathy associated with glucagonoma (necrolytic migratory erythema [NME]).
- Glucagonomas can affect numerous organ systems, including musculoskeletal, integumentary, endocrine, gastrointestinal, nervous/behavioral, and hepatobiliary.

SIGNALMENT

- Dog—rare; older animals.
- Cat—rare.

SIGNS

- The hallmark sign is NME, although this may be caused by glucagonoma or hepatocutaneous syndrome. NME has also been described in veterinary medicine as metabolic epidermal necrosis and superficial necrolytic dermatitis.
- Skin lesions include erythema, erosions, and crusting, generally located around mucocutaneous junctions (perineum, face, and genitalia), distal extremities, and footpads. Lesions are often pruritic with hyperkeratotic and painful footpads. In many cases, footpads are the only affected area.
- Other systemic signs include lethargy, polyuria, polydipsia, diarrhea, secondary pyoderma or yeast infection, anorexia, and weight loss.

CAUSES & RISK FACTORS

Component of the multiple endocrine neoplasia syndrome.

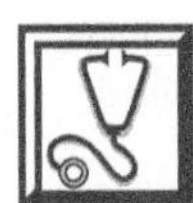

DIAGNOSIS

DIFFERENTIAL DIAGNOSIS

- Other diseases that produce skin lesions consistent with NME are nonspecific liver disease, hypoaminoacidemia, DM, and pancreatic tumors.
- Other similar dermatopathies include pemphigus foliaceus, systemic lupus erythematosus, vasculitis, food dermatoses, vitamin A responsive dermatosis, and zinc deficiency dermatopathy.
- Mild–moderate hyperglucagonemia can result from nonglucagonoma diseases such as liver disease, pancreatic disease, chronic kidney disease, starvation, bacteremia, diabetic ketoacidosis, and hyperadrenocorticism.

CBC/BIOCHEMISTRY/URINALYSIS

- CBC—may be normal or show a normocytic, normochromic anemia or mature neutrophilia.
- Biochemistry—may be normal or show mild elevations in liver enzyme activity or total bilirubin concentration, with mild hyperglycemia and hypoalbuminemia.
- Liver function tests (e.g., bile acid concentrations) are generally normal.
- Urinalysis—decreased urine specific gravity, glucosuria with DM.

OTHER LABORATORY TESTS

- Plasma glucagon levels are generally extremely elevated (>1,000 pg/mL); however, normal to mild elevation does not rule out glucagonoma.
- Plasma amino acid concentrations are generally severely reduced and are thought to be associated with the development of NME.
- Plasma zinc concentration is generally reduced and also thought to be associated with the development of NME.
- Serum fructosamine may be elevated in patients with DM.

IMAGING

- Ultrasonography—to detect pancreatic glucagonomas, peripancreatic metastases, and hepatic metastases; however, ultrasound was normal in 4/9 dogs with glucagonoma. A honeycomb pattern has been described in the liver of patients with NME.
- CT, MRI, PET scans, selective visceral angiography, and somatostatin receptor scintigraphy (octreoscan and radioiodinated MIBG) are used to detect glucagonoma in humans.

DIAGNOSTIC PROCEDURES

- Increased serum glucagon and clinical signs consistent with NME are indicative of glucagonoma, but the definitive diagnosis can only be made by biopsy, histopathologic examination, and immunohistochemical documentation of glucagon expression.
- Immunohistochemical assays for other pancreatic and gastrointestinal hormones may also be performed.

PATHOLOGIC FINDINGS

- Skin biopsies taken from glucagon-associated NME lesions typically exhibit severe superficial to mid-epidermal edema, diffuse parakeratotic hyperkeratosis, and irregular epidermal hyperplasia.
- Biopsies taken from the primary glucagonoma (and/or metastases) typically exhibit pleomorphic islet cells with fine cytoplasmic granules and occasional mitoses with immunohistochemical glucagon (and often other secretory hormone) expression.

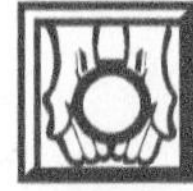

TREATMENT

- Surgical excision of nonmetastatic primary pancreatic glucagonoma is the best chance for cure. There is a high rate of postoperative morbidity and mortality in dogs, often secondary to pancreatitis. Glucagonoma syndrome reported in people is associated with thromboembolic disease.
- Combined debulking (primary tumor and/or metastases) and octreotide therapy can temporarily resolve skin lesions and provide relief of clinical signs.
- If surgery and/or octreotide therapy are not possible, symptomatic palliative therapies may be beneficial and include high-protein diet with egg whites (approximately two to four egg whites/day for a 25 kg dog), zinc supplementation (beneficial even in the face of normal serum zinc concentration), and fatty acid supplementation.
- IV amino acid therapy may be beneficial in patients with NME.
- Secondary bacterial and/or yeast skin infections are common and should be appropriately treated.
- Concurrent DM should be treated.

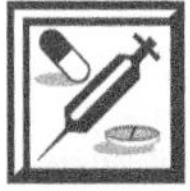

MEDICATIONS

DRUG(S) OF CHOICE

- Octreotide—somatostatin analogue that inhibits conversion of preproglucagon to glucagon; may be beneficial in patients with unresectable or metastatic glucagonoma. Side effects reported in humans include injection site pain, vomiting, diarrhea, and cholestasis. A safe and effective dosage has not been reported in dogs; however, 10–20 μg/dog SC q8–12h has been used, and a one-time dose of 50 μg/dog SC is reported to be safe in healthy dogs. Octreotide can be difficult to obtain.
- Chemotherapeutics in humans with glucagonoma include doxorubicin and streptozotocin, although efficacy may be limited. The use of streptozotocin as an islet-cell lytic agent has been reported in a small number of dogs with insulinoma, but not in dogs with glucagonoma.

• Glucocorticoids may improve the pruritis of NME skin lesions, but are not recommended for use in glucagonomas as they are likely to exacerbate hyperglycemia associated with secondary DM.
• IV amino acids (500 mL of essential amino acids added to saline or lactated Ringer's solution over 12h, or 10% amino acid solution 24 mL/kg over 8–12h) have resulted in variable improvement in NME skin lesions in dogs. Treatments may be repeated every 1–2 weeks if effective until clinical signs abate or resolve.
• Sulfur/salicylic acid–based shampoos or very mild shampoos may help remove crusts, soften skin, and improve pain and pruritus associated with footpad or skin lesions.
• Oral zinc sulfate (10 mg/kg/day PO), zinc methionine (2 mg/kg/day PO), or zinc gluconate (3 mg/kg/day PO) may be considered.
• Supplementation with oral fatty acids (80 mg/kg PO) may also be of benefit.

CONTRAINDICATIONS/POSSIBLE INTERACTIONS

Glucocorticoids may exacerbate hyperglycemia if DM is present.

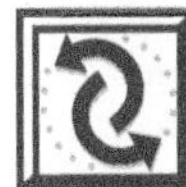

FOLLOW-UP

PATIENT MONITORING

• Serial blood work should be performed postoperatively to confirm that hyperglucagonemia (and any other abnormalities) is resolving.
• Strong considerations should be given to serial ultrasounds and chest radiographs to monitor for regrowth or metastasis.

POSSIBLE COMPLICATIONS

• Pancreatitis.
• Thromboembolic disease.
• DM.

EXPECTED COURSE AND PROGNOSIS

• Prognosis is considered poor in dogs.
• Transient improvement in skin lesions and clinical signs may be noted in patients treated with octreotride and amino acids.
• One cat had a survival time of 11 months following surgery.

MISCELLANEOUS

SEE ALSO

• Glycogen-Type Vacuolar Hepatopathy.
• Superficial Necrolytic Dermatitis.

ABBREVIATIONS

• DM = diabetes mellitus.
• NME = necrolytic migratory erythema.

Suggested Reading

Allenspach K, Arnold P, Glaus T, et al. Glucagon-producing neuroendocrine tumour associated with hypoaminoacidemia and skin lesions. J Small Anim Pract 2000, 41:402–406.

Asawaka MG, Cullen JM, Linder KE. Necrolytic migratory erythema associated with a glucagon-producing primary hepatic neuroendocrine tumor in a cat. Vet Dermal 2013, 24:466–469.

Chastain MA. The glucagonoma syndrome: a review of its features and discussion of new perspectives. Am J Med Sci 2001, 321(5):306–320.

Feldman EC, Nelson RW. Gastrinoma, glucagonoma and other APUDomas. In: Canine and Feline Endocrinology and Reproduction, 3rd ed. St. Louis, MO: Saunders, 2004, pp. 654–655.

Langer NB, Jergens AE, Miles KG. Canine glucagonoma. Compend Contin Educ Pract Vet 2003, 25(1):56–63.

Author Virginia L. Gill

Consulting Editor Patty A. Lathan

GLUCOSURIA

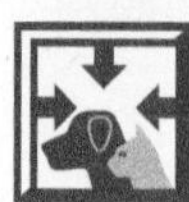

BASICS

DEFINITION

Glucosuria is detected via routine laboratory testing, most commonly with reagent test strips. Persistent glucosuria is an abnormal finding.

G

PATHOPHYSIOLOGY

• Glucose is a small molecule that is freely filtered through the glomerulus into the ultrafiltrate. • Glucose is actively reabsorbed in the proximal renal tubule by a sodium–glucose co-transport system. Physiologic levels of filtered glucose are mostly reabsorbed, leaving excreted levels too low to detect using screening tests.

Hyperglycemic Glucosuria

• Glucosuria will be present when blood glucose concentration exceeds renal tubular epithelial transport maximum. This varies by species, with dogs typically above 180 mg/dL and cats typically above 280 mg/dL. • If hyperglycemia is present, determine whether glucosuria transient or persistent.

Transient

• Physiologic—usually transient and associated with release of endogenous "stress" hormones (catecholamines, glucagon, corticosteroids); especially common in cats. Serum may be normoglycemic or hyperglycemic at urine collection because different concentrations of glucose excreted in urine over time equilibrate in bladder.
• Pharmacologic—may occur following administration of glucose-containing solutions (e.g., dextrose); administration of drugs (glucocorticoids, growth hormone, thiazide diuretics, morphine, epinephrine) may also result in hyperglycemia and glucosuria. • Toxic—ethylene glycol.
• Pathologic—possible with acute pancreatitis.

Persistent

Pathologic conditions that can result in persistent glucosuria (due to hyperglycemia) include diabetes mellitus, hyperadrenocorticism, acromegaly, extreme stress, hyperthyroidism in cats.

Normoglycemic Glucosuria

Impaired renal proximal tubular epithelial cell reabsorptive capacity.

Congenital

Primary glucosuria—Scottish terriers; Fanconi syndrome: basenji dogs; also sporadic in Norwegian elkhounds, Shetland sheepdogs, miniature schnauzers, Labrador retrievers, border terriers, whippets, Yorkshire terriers, and mixed-breed dogs; decreased reabsorption of glucose, amino acids, and phosphorus plus decreased secretion of hydrogen ions.

Acquired

• Fanconi syndrome due to toxicity such as heavy metal poisoning (e.g., lead, mercury, copper, copper associated hepatitis) or dried chicken treats made in China, drugs (e.g., gentamicin, cephalosporins, outdated tetracycline, cisplatin, streptozotocin), chemicals (Lysol, maleic acid), other miscellaneous causes. • Acute renal failure with significant tubular lesions.

SYSTEMS AFFECTED

• Renal—normoglycemic patients have abnormal renal tubular epithelial cell function; dogs with Fanconi syndrome may develop metabolic acidosis and chronic kidney disease (CKD) with secondary multisystem involvement; glucosuria predisposes to bacterial urinary tract infection. • Endocrine—hyperglycemic patients may have diabetes mellitus and/or hyperadrenocorticism. • Liver—copper associated hepatitis; centrilobular hepatitis with copper accumulation.

SIGNALMENT

• Adult dogs and cats develop persistent hyperglycemic glucosuria due to adult-onset diabetes mellitus. • Dogs with congenital Fanconi syndrome typically develop clinical disease due to defective reabsorption of glucose and amino acids at 4–5 years of age; no sex predilection. • Familial renal tubular disorders have been reported (see Pathophysiology). • Primary renal glucosuria (Scottish terriers) may be recognized at early age as incidental finding. • Copper associated hepatitis with acquired Fanconi syndrome (Labrador retrievers). • Dogs (any breed or age) fed dried chicken treats made in China.

SIGNS

Clinical signs variable depending upon primary cause.

Historical Findings

• Persistent glucosuria results in polyuria (osmotic diuresis), leading to compensatory polydipsia. • Glucosuria predisposes to urinary tract infections; clinical signs associated with upper and/or lower urinary tract infection. • Breed and therapeutic history (see Pathophysiology) are important.

Physical Examination Findings

• Patients with hyperglycemic glucosuria may exhibit systemic signs; see diabetes mellitus chapters. • Patients with normoglycemic glucosuria may have normal body functions.
• Dogs with Fanconi syndrome may develop signs of metabolic acidosis, electrolyte abnormalities, and CKD.

CAUSES

Hyperglycemic Glucosuria Transient

• Physiologic—stress; common in cats.
• Pharmacologic—see Pathophysiology.

Persistent

• Diabetes mellitus; insulin deficiency or resistance. • Hyperadrenocorticism; insulin resistance. • Acute pancreatitis; insulin deficiency or resistance. • Less common causes include pheochromocytoma, acromegaly, hyperglucagonemia, hyperpituitarism, hyperthyroidism, and chronic liver failure (due to failure to metabolize glucagon).

Normoglycemic Glucosuria

Congenital

• Primary renal glucosuria (Scottish terrier).
• Fanconi syndrome. • Congenital diseases may be associated with renal dysfunction (Norwegian elkhound).

Acquired

• Acute kidney injury associated with proximal tubular dysfunction. • Fanconi syndrome. • CKD (rare).

RISK FACTORS

Vary with underlying causes.

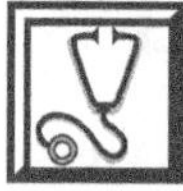

DIAGNOSIS

DIFFERENTIAL DIAGNOSIS

• Persistent hyperglycemic glucosuria in fasted patients is frequently associated with endocrinopathies (diabetes mellitus, hyperadrenocorticism). • Acute pancreatitis.
• Renal tubular reabsorptive dysfunctions cause normoglycemic glucosuria. • Stressed patients exhibit mild transient hyperglycemia and glucosuria.

LABORATORY FINDINGS

Screening Tests

Normally negative (urine glucose concentration below detection).

Glucose Oxidase Tests

• Reagent strips use glucose oxidase method that is specific for glucose; positive values occur with urine glucose concentrations greater than 100 mg/dL. • Methodology is a two-step enzymatic process—glucose oxidase catalyzes glucose and produces gluconic acid and hydrogen peroxide; peroxidase catalyzes reaction of hydrogen with chromagen to produce color change on reagent pad; the test is time dependent, which varies with manufacturer; pigmenturia can complicate color interpretation. • False negatives can be seen with ascorbic acid, exposure to formalin, ketonuria, marked bilirubinuria, highly concentrated urine, and refrigerated urine samples that have not been warmed to room temperature prior to performing the test.
• False positives can be seen with exposure to oxidizing agents such as hydrogen peroxide or chlorine bleach (most commonly with samples obtained from table top or floor).
• Specific for glucose; more sensitive

(~40–100 mg/dL) than copper reduction methods.

$$\text{Glucose} + O_2\,(\text{air}) + H_2O \xrightarrow{\text{oxidase}} \text{glucuronic acid} + H_2O$$

$$H_2O_2 \xrightarrow[\text{peroxidase}]{\text{horseradish}} H_2O + O(\text{nascent oxygen})$$

$$O + \text{color indicator} \longrightarrow \text{oxidized color change complex}$$

Copper Reduction Tests

• Not specific for glucose; less sensitive (250 mg/dL) and higher detection limit than glucose oxidase methods; more often used in human medicine, but can be used in veterinary medicine to verify questionable reagent strip result. • Testing method uses copper, which reacts with reducing substance (e.g., glucose, fructose, lactose, etc.) to produce cuprous oxide and cuprous hydroxide, which results in color change.
• Results are semiquantitative and reported as negative, approximately 250 mg/dl, approximately 500 mg/dL, approximately 750 mg/dl, approximately 1000 mg/dL, or approximately 2000 mg/dL. • Less affected by pigmenturia; false positives can be seen with cephalosporins, formaldehyde, reactions with other sugars, and high concentrations of ascorbic acid.

$$\underset{(\text{blue})}{\text{Cupric ions}} + \text{glucose} \xrightarrow[\text{alkali}]{} \underset{(\text{orange-red})}{\text{cuprous ions}} + \text{oxidized glucose}$$

Confirmatory Tests

Hexokinase or glucokinase dehydrogenase tests using automated chemistry analyzer may be used to confirm presence or absence of glucose when unexpected results or pigmented urine encountered.

Drugs That May Alter Laboratory Results

See Screening Tests.

Disorders That May Alter Laboratory Results

See Screening Tests.

Valid if Run in Human Laboratory?

Yes

CBC/BIOCHEMISTRY/URINALYSIS

Hyperglycemic Glucosuria

• Hyperglycemia with glucosuria and ketonuria indicates diabetic ketoacidosis; persistent hyperglycemia and glucosuria with appropriate clinical signs support diabetes mellitus. • Dogs with pancreatitis may have leukocytosis, fever, abdominal pain and effusion, elevations in pancreatic specific enzymes, and characteristic ultrasonographic abnormalities. • Dogs with markedly increased serum alkaline phosphatase activity, hyperglycemia, glucosuria (also hypercholesterolemia, hypertriglyceridemia) should be evaluated for hyperadrenocorticism. • Mild glucosuria with transient hyperglycemia is likely physiologic in stressed patients.

OTHER LABORATORY TESTS

• Hyperglycemic glucosuria—conduct appropriate screening test if hyperadrenocorticism suspected. • Normoglycemic glucosuria—measurement of phosphorus, glucose, and amino acid concentrations in timed urine samples may help differentiate Fanconi syndrome and primary renal glucosuria; also evaluation of hepatic function for acquired Fanconi syndrome due to copper associated hepatitis.

IMAGING

Ultrasonography aids in diagnosis of hyperadrenocorticism and pancreatitis.

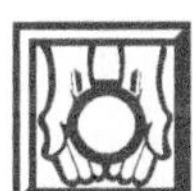

TREATMENT

• Discontinue any drugs associated with acquired renal tubular transport defects.
• Treatment varies with cause; see chapters related to specific causes.

MEDICATIONS

DRUG(S) OF CHOICE

• Hyperglycemic glucosuria—treat diabetes mellitus with insulin. • Normoglycemic glucosuria—no treatment required for tubular transport disorders unless metabolic acidosis, electrolyte abnormalities, or hepatic abnormalities present (e.g., Fanconi syndrome).

CONTRAINDICATIONS

Patients with diabetes mellitus should not be given diabetogenic drugs such as corticosteroids or dextrose-containing fluids.

FOLLOW-UP

PATIENT MONITORING

Variable, depending upon underlying condition.

POSSIBLE COMPLICATIONS

• Persistent glucosuria predisposes to development of bacterial urinary tract infections (cystitis, ascending pyelonephritis).
• Osmotic diuresis with obligatory polyuria results in polydipsia, necessitating access to water to prevent dehydration.

MISCELLANEOUS

Growth hormone–secreting pituitary tumors in older cats (especially male) may induce diabetes mellitus (insulin resistant).

ASSOCIATED CONDITIONS

• Urinary tract infections. • CKD.
• Diabetic retinopathy or cataracts. • Copper associated hepatitis.

PREGNANCY/FERTILITY/BREEDING

Excess progesterone secretion in intact female dogs may induce diabetes mellitus (insulin resistant).

SEE ALSO

• Congenital and Developmental Renal Diseases.
• Diabetes Mellitus without Complication—Cats.
• Diabetes Mellitus without Complication—Dogs.
• Fanconi Syndrome.
• Hyperadrenocorticism (Cushing's Syndrome)—Cats.
• Hyperadrenocorticism (Cushing's Syndrome)—Dogs.
• Pancreatitis—Cats.
• Pancreatitis—Dogs.

ABBREVIATIONS

• CKD = chronic kidney disease.

Suggested Reading

Latimer K. Duncan and Prasse's Veterinary Laboratory Medicine Clinical Pathology, 5th ed. Ames, IA: Wiley-Blackwell, 2011, pp 257–264.
Sink C, Weinstein N. Practical Veterinary Urinalysis. Ames, IA: Wiley-Blackwell, 2012, pp. 38–40.
Stockham S and Scott M. Fundamentals of Veterinary Clinical Pathology, 2nd ed. Ames, IA: Wiley-Blackwell, 2008, pp. 462–464.

Author Tracie D. Romsland
Consulting Editor J.D. Foster
Acknowledgment The author and book editors acknowledge the prior contributions of Cheryl L. Swenson and Carl A. Osborne.

GLUTEN ENTEROPATHY IN IRISH SETTERS

BASICS

OVERVIEW

A rarely confirmed, inherited, intestinal disease in which sensitivity develops to dietary gluten (present in wheat) and similar proteins present in related grains (i.e., rye and barley). In affected dogs, the enteropathy is characterized by partial villous atrophy, reduced brush border enzyme expression, lymphocytic infiltration of the intestinal mucosa, and goblet cell hyperplasia; changes that are reversed by feeding a gluten-free diet.

G

SIGNALMENT

- Irish setter breed—the line of affected setters originally described in the UK has been bred out.
- Signs develop in young dogs, but are modulated by the age of first exposure to gluten.
- Genetic transmission of gluten sensitive enteropathy is likely under the control of a single major autosomal recessive locus.
- Gluten enteropathy has been suspected but not proven in other dog breeds and cats.

SIGNS

- Poor weight gain (or weight loss).
- Poor body condition.
- Mild small intestinal diarrhea that can be intermittent.

CAUSES & RISK FACTORS

The enteropathy and clinical signs are triggered by gluten-containing diets. Abnormal mucosal permeability precedes the development of signs, implying there is abnormal entry of gluten across the mucosal barrier. Gluten is then either directly toxic to the intestinal mucosa or induces an immune-mediated reaction. An analogous condition in humans (celiac disease) is characterized by the presence of antibodies cross-reacting to gluten and tissue transglutaminase, but they have not been tested for in affected setters. These antibodies have been demonstrated in Border terriers with gluten-sensitive dyskinesia.

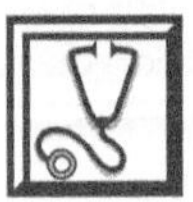

DIAGNOSIS

DIFFERENTIAL DIAGNOSIS

- Canine chronic enteropathy—food-responsive enteropathy, inflammatory bowel disease.
- Infectious diseases such as *Giardia*, hookworms, and roundworms.
- Metabolic abnormalities.
- Exocrine pancreatic insufficiency.

CBC/BIOCHEMISTRY/URINALYSIS

- Biochemistry can be unremarkable or may show panhypoproteinemia.
- CBC may show eosinophilia.

OTHER LABORATORY TESTS

- Serum folate concentrations are subnormal in some patients, reflecting malabsorption.
- Other tests are recommended to rule out other differentials, such as fecal flotation to rule out enteric parasites and serum trypsin-like immunoreactivity (TLI) to rule out exocrine pancreatic insufficiency.
- Serum TLI and cobalamin concentrations are usually unremarkable.

IMAGING

Only useful to rule out other conditions.

DIAGNOSTIC PROCEDURES

Intestinal biopsy specimens obtained via endoscopy or laparotomy may be helpful, but proof of gluten sensitivity requires histologic resolution in biopsies repeated following a clinically successful gluten-free diet trial.

PATHOLOGIC FINDINGS

- Histologic examination of jejunal biopsy specimens from affected dogs reared on a wheat-containing diet reveals partial villus atrophy and accumulation of intraepithelial lymphocytes.
- Jejunal abnormalities improve following gluten withdrawal, but recur with gluten challenge.

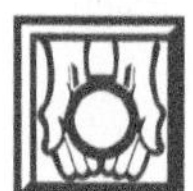

TREATMENT

Treatment is on an outpatient basis. Avoid diets containing gluten (wheat, rye, barley, triticale, brewer's yeast, and wheat starch) for the life of the animal.

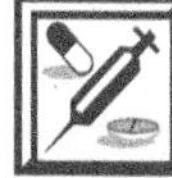

MEDICATIONS

DRUG(S) OF CHOICE

Folate (0.5–2 mg PO q24h for 2–4 weeks) if serum folate concentration is markedly subnormal (<4 μg/L).

CONTRAINDICATIONS/POSSIBLE INTERACTIONS

N/A

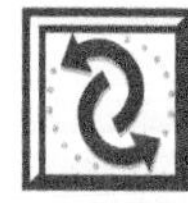

FOLLOW-UP

Consider periodic assay of serum folate (q6–12 months) if initially decreased.

MISCELLANEOUS

ABBREVIATIONS

- TLI = trypsin-like immunoreactivity

Suggested Reading

Cave N. Adverse food reactions. In: Washabau RJ, Day MJ, eds., Canine and Feline Gastroenterology. St. Louis, MO: Elsevier, 2013, p. 403.

Hall EJ, Day MJ. Diseases of the small intestine. In: Ettinger SJ, Feldman EC, Côté E, eds., Textbook of Veterinary Internal Medicine, 8th ed. St. Louis, MO: Elsevier, 2017, p. 1547.

Lowrie M, Garden OA, Hadjivassiliou M, et al. Characterization of paroxysmal gluten-sensitive dyskinesia in Border terriers using serological markers. J Vet Intern Med 2018, 32(2):775.

Author Edward J. Hall

Consulting Editor Mark P. Rondeau

Acknowledgment The author and book editors acknowledge the prior contribution of Krysta Deitz

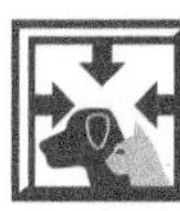

BASICS

OVERVIEW

• Also known as glycogenosis—rare inherited disorders of defective or deficient enzyme activity governing glycogen metabolism. • Tissue glycogen accumulation—leads to organ enlargement and dysfunction; may affect liver, heart, skeletal muscle, kidney, and CNS. • Impaired hepatic glycogenolysis—leads to symptomatic hypoglycemia (neuroglycopenia). • Classification—based on enzymatic defect and primary organ(s) involvement: more than 12 types in humans, 4 types in dogs (Ia, II, III, and VII), 1 type in cats (IV).

SIGNALMENT

• Clinical signs manifest in juveniles—may be days to months after birth. • Type Ia (von Gierke's disease)—Maltese puppies; autosomal recessive mutation of glucose-6-phosphatase gene (gene symbol: *G6PC*). • Type II (Pompe's disease)—Swedish Lapland, Finnish and Swedish Lapphund dogs; onset by 6 months of age; autosomal recessive, single mutation in acid α-glucosidase (gene symbol: *GAA*). • Type III (Cori's disease)—young female German shepherds, curly-coated retrievers; autosomal recessive mutation in glycogen debranching enzyme (gene symbol: *AGL*). • Type IV (Andersen disease)—Norwegian forest cats; may be stillborn or fade shortly after birth; may manifest signs at 5–7 months with progressive neurologic decline; autosomal recessive mutation in glycogen branching enzyme (complex rearrangement mutation; gene symbol *GBE1*). • Type VII (Tarui disease)—English springer, American cocker, whippets, mixed breeds; PFK (M-PFK) muscle isoform single missense mutation; different missense mutation in wachtelhunds; adult dogs, no sex predilection. • Autosomal recessive inheritance—Maltese, Lapland, Lapphund, English springer spaniels, Norwegian forest cats, other M-PFK affected breeds; also suspected in German shepherds.

SIGNS

• Depend on enzymatic defect. • Type Ia (Maltese puppies)—failure to thrive; mental depression; hypoglycemia; abdominal distention; hepatomegaly; death or euthanasia by 60 days of age. • Type II (Lapland dogs)—vomiting and regurgitation related to megaesophagus; progressive muscle weakness; cardiac changes; death before 2 years of age. • Type III (German shepherds, curly-coated retrievers)—depression; weakness; stunted; abdominal distention from hepatomegaly; mild hypoglycemia, high liver enzymes and creatine kinase. • Type IV (Norwegian forest cats)—perinatal death common; intermittent fever; generalized muscle tremors; muscle atrophy, weakness progressing to tetraplegia; sudden death from myocardial degeneration and terminal dysrhythmia; glucose administration can enable cats to survive to adulthood. • Type VII (English springer spaniels)—compensated hemolytic anemia; episodic weakness, exercise-induced with intravascular hemolysis; hemoglobinuria; one patient with a progressive myopathy at 11 years of age: no liver effect.

CAUSES & RISK FACTORS

Deficiencies

• Type Ia—glucose-6-phosphatase. • Type II—acid-α–glucosidase. • Type III—amylo-1,6-glucosidase. • Type IV—glycogen branching enzyme (α-1,4-d-glucan).
• Type VII—phosphofructokinase.

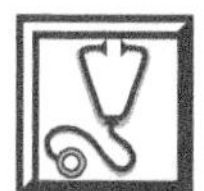

DIAGNOSIS

DIFFERENTIAL DIAGNOSIS

• High index of suspicion for diagnosis.
• Breed affiliation—familial history.
• Differentiate other causes of juvenile hypoglycemia—malnutrition; endoparasitism; transient fasting hypoglycemia; portosystemic vascular anomaly. • Other causes of muscular weakness—infectious diseases; endocrinopathy; immune-mediated causes; hypokalemia; other neuromyopathies.

CBC/BIOCHEMISTRY/URINALYSIS

• Types I and III—hypoglycemia. • Type I—lactic acidemia, increased: cholesterol, triglycerides, uric acid. • Type VII—anemia; reticulocytosis; pigmenturia, no hepatic effects.

OTHER LABORATORY TESTS

Genetic testing—type I: in Maltese dogs, type II: in Lapland and Lapphund dogs, type III: in curly-coated retrievers, type IV: in Norwegian forest cats, type VII: in breeds listed previously and in vitro erythrocyte testing.

IMAGING

• Type II—thoracic radiography; cardiomegaly and megaesophagus. • Types Ia and III—abdominal radiography; hepatomegaly.
• Abdominal ultrasonography—hepatomegaly, hyperechoic parenchyma consistent with hepatic glycogen accumulation. • Types II and IV—echocardiography may reveal cardiac changes.

DIAGNOSTIC PROCEDURES

• Tissue enzyme analysis and glycogen determination. • Electromyography—depends on disorder. • ECG—depends on disorder.
• Genetic testing.

PATHOLOGIC FINDINGS

• Type Ia—emaciation; massive hepatomegaly due to hepatocyte glycogen and lipid vacuolation and similar change in renal tubular epithelium. • Type II—glycogen accumulation in skeletal, smooth, and cardiac muscle. • Type III—hepatomegaly due to hepatic glycogen accumulation; also in skeletal muscle. • Type IV—generalized muscle atrophy; glycogen accumulation: skeletal muscle, CNS, and peripheral nervous system. • Type VII—polysaccharide deposits in skeletal muscle.

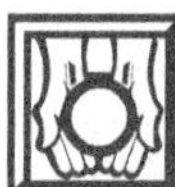

TREATMENT

Nursing Care

• Supportive care. • Types I and III—may require IV/SC dextrose for management of hypoglycemic crisis; long-term management usually futile. • Gene therapy with adeno-associated virus vector experimentally for type 1a dogs resulted in survival.

Diet

Control hypoglycemia (types I and III) with frequent feedings of a high-carbohydrate diet until diagnosis is confirmed; glucose solutions usually used.

Client Education

• Advise that specimens be submitted for genetic/enzyme characterizations. • Discuss known mechanisms of inheritance to modify breeding programs.

MEDICATIONS

DRUG(S) OF CHOICE

N/A

FOLLOW-UP

• Monitor for hypoglycemia. • Cull parents from breeding programs. • Prognosis—poor; most patients with glycogen storage disorders causing hypoglycemia and hepatomegaly and stunted growth die or are euthanized owing to progressive deterioration.

MISCELLANEOUS

SEE ALSO

• Lysosomal Storage Diseases.
• Mucopolysaccharidosis. • Portosystemic Vascular Anomaly, Congenital.

Suggested Reading

Walvoort HC. Glycogen storage disease type II in the Lapland dog. Vet Q 1985, 7:187–190.

Author Sharon A. Center
Consulting Editor Kate Holan

G

GLYCOGEN-TYPE VACUOLAR HEPATOPATHY

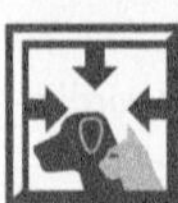

BASICS

DEFINITION

• Glycogen-type vacuolar hepatopathy (VH)—reversible hepatocellular cytosolic vacuolation.
• Reflects many primary disorders including glucocorticoid treatment, hyperadrenocorticism, atypical adrenal hyperplasia (sex hormone hyperplasia), chronic systemic illnesses (inflammatory, neoplastic), and rarely congenital glycogen storage disorders.
• Typified by high alkaline phosphatase (ALP) activity—usually without hyperbilirubinemia or hepatic insufficiency.
• Similar but remarkably severe VH in hepatocutaneous disease; may reflect chronic phenobarbital administration.
• Glycogen VH may coexist with cytosolic lipid vacuolation—comparatively rare in dogs, but may associate with idiopathic hyperlipidemia, diabetes mellitus, hypothyroidism, and rare inborn errors of glycogen/lipid metabolism.

PATHOPHYSIOLOGY

• Glucocorticoids—induce reversible increase in hepatocyte glycogen within 2–3 days; injectable or reposital drug induces most severe VH compared to PO or topical (ocular, cutaneous, aural) routes.
• Cell expansion—causes hepatomegaly, ballooning degeneration leads to parenchymal collapse; when severe, nodularity grossly mistaken for cirrhosis.
• Variable response to glucocorticoids among dogs relates to drug type; route; dose; treatment duration; individual sensitivity—VH may follow low-dose, short-term oral treatment.
• VH may reflect stress response, cytokines, or acute-phase response initiated by nonhepatic systemic disorders or neoplasia (especially lymphoma), without exogenous glucocorticoid exposure or adrenal disease.
• VH common in dogs with gallbladder mucocele.

SYSTEMS AFFECTED

• Hepatobiliary—normal hepatic function usually; severe degenerative VH can lead to hepatic dysfunction, jaundice, ascites, liver failure.
• All systems affected by steroid hormones or primary systemic disease.

INCIDENCE/PREVALENCE

• Dogs—common, often accompanies primary necroinflammatory liver disorders.
• Cats—rare; liver vacuolation with triglyceride accumulation more common (see Hepatic Lipidosis).

SIGNALMENT

Species

Dog; rarely cat.

Breed Predilections

Breeds predisposed to hyperadrenocorticism develop glycogen VH (e.g., miniature poodles, dachshunds, boxers, Boston terriers), Scottish terriers (sex hormone adrenal hyperplasia, hyperlipidemia), and others with hyperlipidemia (miniature schnauzers, Shetland sheepdogs) may develop mixed glycogen/lipid VH.

Mean Age and Range

• Middle-aged to old dogs—spontaneous hyperadrenocorticism (>75% older than 9 years); chronic systemic inflammation or neoplasia.
• Dogs of any age—iatrogenic VH subsequent to glucocorticoid administration.
• Young dogs or cats—genetic glycogen storage disease.

SIGNS

General Comments

• Reflect glucocorticoids or underlying systemic illness.
• Rarely, signs of hepatic disease or failure; hepatic failure can develop with severe chronic VH.
• Hepatic encephalopathy observed in some dogs with hepatocutaneous syndrome.

Historical Findings

• Glucocorticoid excess—polyuria and polydipsia; polyphagia; endocrine alopecia; abdominal distention: weak muscles, loss of elasticity; skeletal muscle weakness; excessive panting; lethargy; friable skin; bruising tendencies; urinary tract infections, may be asymptomatic; corneal ulcer.
• Adrenal sex hormone hyperplasia—may display some signs of glucocorticoid excess but often fewer and less severe; endocrine alopecia may be only sign; some dogs remain asymptomatic except for chronic progressive marked ALP activity and degenerative VH.
• Other causes—depend on system affected; chronic phenobarbital may cause severe VH.
• Sex hormone hyperplasia causing VH may increase risk for dysplastic hepatic foci and hepatocellular carcinoma (e.g., Scottish terriers).

Physical Examination Findings

• Hepatomegaly.
• Relate to steroid hormone excess or underlying disease; depend on severity and duration.

CAUSES

• Glucocorticoid administration.
• Typical hyperadrenocorticism (spontaneous).
• Atypical adrenal hyperplasia—overproduction of cortisol precursor sex hormones (spontaneous).
• Systemic disease provoking acute-phase response or stress—e.g., severe dental disease, inflammatory bowel disease, chronic pancreatitis, systemic neoplasia (especially lymphoma), chronic infections (urinary tract, skin), hypothyroidism, many others.

RISK FACTORS

• Pharmacologic doses of glucocorticoids.
• Breeds at risk for hyperadrenocorticism.
• Breeds at risk for hyperlipidemia—often also demonstrate combined glycogen VH: miniature schnauzers, Shetland sheepdogs, beagles.
• Dogs receiving chronic phenobarbital.

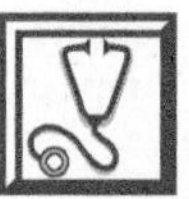

DIAGNOSIS

DIFFERENTIAL DIAGNOSES

• Other diffuse hepatopathies (especially those causing hepatomegaly and increased ALP activity)—passive congestion; neoplasia (primary or metastatic to liver); necroinflammatory liver disease; anticonvulsant hepatopathy; hepatomegaly due to amyloid (rare).
• VH distinguishing features—most dogs have increase in ALP > alanine aminotransferase (ALT) or aspartate aminotransferase (AST); increased cholesterol, normal serum bilirubin; normal/mild increase in total serum bile acids (TSBA); heterogeneous or homogeneous hyperechoic hepatic parenchyma on ultrasonography (nodules or "Swiss cheese" pattern); characteristic cytology: hepatocytes engorged due to expanded "rarified" cytoplasm.

CBC/BIOCHEMISTRY/URINALYSIS

CBC

• Depends on underlying disease.
• Nonregenerative anemia—anemia of chronic disease or hypothyroidism.
• Relative polycythemia—steroid excess.
• Stress leukogram—hyperadrenocorticism; glucocorticoid exposure; stress of illness.
• Thrombocytosis—neoplasia; hyperadrenocorticism; splenic disease.

Biochemistry

• ALP markedly increased; ALP glucocorticoid isoenzyme cannot differentiate cause of VH as other liver disorders also induce this isoenzyme; variable γ-glutamyltransferase (GGT), ALT, AST activity.
• Serum albumin and total bilirubin—usually normal; high bilirubin typically implicates another hepatobiliary or hemolytic process.
• Hypercholesterolemia—hyperadrenocorticism, sex hormone adrenal hyperplasia; breed-related hyperlipidemias; hypothyroidism; pancreatitis; nephrotic syndrome.

OTHER LABORATORY TESTS

- ALP glucocorticoid isoenzyme—see above, lacks specificity and thus clinical utility.
- TSBA—may be modestly increased; ammonia tolerance test: usually normal.
- Pituitary adrenal axis—adrenocorticotropic hormone (ACTH) response test or low-dose ± high-dose dexamethasone suppression test (LDDST ± HDDST) and endogenous ACTH may help differentiate nonadrenal illness, adrenal or pituitary disorders.
- Urine cortisol : creatinine ratio—at-home urine collection helps rule out hyperadrenocorticism; high ratio may reflect stress or nonadrenal illness.
- Adrenal ultrasound imaging—nodules, adrenomegaly; consider dog size and age.
- If VH confirmed (liver biopsy) and underlying cause not evident, patient asymptomatic or symptomatic for adrenal disease—assess cortisol and sex hormone panel with ACTH response test.
- Thyroid testing—rules out hypothyroidism.
- Triglycerides (fasting)—hyperlipidemia.
- Canine pancreatic lipase immunoreactivity (cPLI)—may indicate "subclinical" pancreatic inflammation or inflammatory bowel disease.

IMAGING

- Abdominal radiography—reveals hepatomegaly or other underlying conditions.
- Thoracic radiography—may reveal lymphadenopathy, metastatic disease, cardiac or pulmonary disorders.
- Abdominal ultrasonography—discloses hepatomegaly, diffuse hyperechoic hepatic parenchyma or multifocal nodular "mottling"; multifocal lesions suggest nodules ("Swiss cheese pattern") formed by progressive hepatocellular ballooning degeneration; may disclose underlying primary visceral abnormalities (e.g., mesenteric lymphadenopathy, neoplasia) or adrenal disorders (size/shape): adrenals may be large with hyperadrenocorticism, sex hormone adrenal hyperplasia, chronic stress, or neoplasia.

DIAGNOSTIC PROCEDURES

- Hepatic fine-needle aspiration cytology—22 gauge, 2.5–3.75 cm (1–1.5 in) US-guided needle aspiration; target nodules and normal parenchyma.
- Cytology—glycogen vacuolation common in many primary liver disorders; used to rule out vacuolar change; cannot definitively confirm illness caused only by VH.
- Hepatic biopsy—verifies VH; excludes other primary hepatic disease; pursue if systemic disorder not discovered explaining high ALP and VH; use US-guided Tru-Cut® needle biopsy to confirm VH, but may miss primary hepatic disease, laparoscopy (recommended), or laparotomy (if visceral inspections and biopsies indicated).
- Cytologic features—hepatocellular cytosolic distention: "rarefication" or granular appearance with increased cell fragility; canalicular bile casts may be observed; primary VH not associated with inflammatory infiltrates; common association with extramedullary hematopoiesis (EMH) may be misinterpreted as suppurative inflammation.
- Tissue culture and sensitivity—if suppurative inflammation suspected, submit aerobic and anaerobic bacterial cultures.
- Coagulation assessments—prothrombin time (PT), activated partial thromboplastin time (APTT), fibrinogen, and mucosal bleeding time: usually normal; bench assessments have low predictive value in predicting iatrogenic hemorrhage; buccal mucosal bleeding time may be more relevant.

PATHOLOGIC FINDINGS

- Gross—variable; normal to moderate hepatomegaly; inconsistent surface irregularity; tan or pale color; confusion with cirrhosis if nodular severe degenerative VH.
- Microscopic—marked vacuolization and ballooning of hepatocytes; no consistent zonal distribution, foci of hepatic degeneration; focal aggregates of neutrophils due to EMH; severe degenerative VH leads to parenchymal collapse, forming nodules surrounded by a thin partition with minimal collagen deposition.

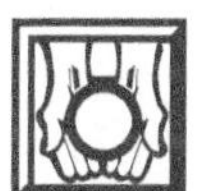

TREATMENT

DIET

- Hyperlipidemia or pancreatitis—restrict dietary fat and fatty supplements.
- Obesity—gradual energy restriction; treat predisposing disorders.

SURGICAL CONSIDERATIONS

- Depend on underlying conditions.
- Adrenal masses may be resected.
- Hypophyseal masses—resection only by experienced surgeons; pituitary mass lesions may respond to radiation therapy.

MEDICATIONS

DRUG(S) OF CHOICE

- Depend on underlying disease.
- Pituitary-dependent hyperadrenocorticism or adrenal hyperplasia syndrome (sex hormone)—usually treated medically: op'-DDD (mitotane or Lysodren®), trilostane, or ketoconazole; op'-DDD preferred for sex hormone adrenal hyperplasia, as trilostane augments sex hormone accumulation; l-deprenyl and melatonin ineffective.
- Manage primary inflammatory disorders necessitating immunosuppressive or anti-inflammatory medications—use polypharmacy to minimize glucocorticoid exposure if symptomatic or progressive VH; see Alternative Drug(s).
- Neoplasia—tumor resection, chemotherapy, or radiation, as appropriate.
- Dental disease—antibiotics and dentistry.
- Inflammatory bowel disease—hypoallergenic/hydrolyzed protein diets and immunomodulation (avoid glucocorticoids).
- Pyelonephritis, chronic dermatitis, or other infectious disorders—long-term antimicrobial treatment based on microbial culture and sensitivity tests; other appropriate medications.
- Hypothyroidism—supplemental thyroxine.

CONTRAINDICATIONS

- Avoid hepatotoxic drugs if severe VH.
- Beware of drug interactions if using ketoconazole for adrenal disease.
- Avoid drugs with hepatic ALP induction effects.

PRECAUTIONS

Glucocorticoids—caution in VH patients; use lowest effective dose regimen (e.g., alternate-day protocol if prednisone or prednisolone); special caution in hyperlipidemia: may worsen clinical signs of abdominal pain, vomiting, pancreatitis; increase insulin requirements in diabetes mellitus; may augment gallbladder mucocele formation; may provoke hepatic lipidosis in cats.

ALTERNATIVE DRUG(S)

Polypharmacy protocol—may reduce glucocorticoid usage in management of immune-mediated or inflammatory disorders; e.g., metronidazole, azathioprine, chlorambucil, cyclophosphamide, mycophenolate, or cyclosporine.

FOLLOW-UP

PATIENT MONITORING

- Hepatomegaly—abdominal palpation; imaging.
- Normalizing enzymes—biochemistry.
- Adrenal function—ACTH stimulation tests.
- Neoplasia—physical exams and imaging.
- Control of infection—repeat cultures.
- Hyperlipidemia—assess gross plasma lipemia; measure triglycerides and cholesterol.

PREVENTION/AVOIDANCE

- Limit glucocorticoid exposure.
- Use alternate-day therapy with prednisone/prednisolone; titrate to lowest effective dose; use alternative medications to control primary illness.

GLYCOGEN-TYPE VACUOLAR HEPATOPATHY (CONTINUED)

G

POSSIBLE COMPLICATIONS

Numerous—related to multisystemic effects of glucocorticoids and associated conditions.

EXPECTED COURSE AND PROGNOSIS

- Most patients are asymptomatic for VH despite high ALP; however, progressive degenerative hepatopathy leading to diffuse nodule formation and hepatic insufficiency may develop in chronic VH in dogs with high ALP activity.
- Laboratory and pathologic features reversible before degenerative parenchymal collapse.
- Dogs with sex hormone hyperplasia, VH, and dysplastic hepatocellular foci appear at risk for development of hepatocellular carcinoma.

MISCELLANEOUS

ASSOCIATED CONDITIONS

- Pulmonary thromboembolism and myopathy due to hyperadrenocorticism.
- Pancreatitis associated with hyperlipidemia.
- Gallbladder mucocele.

PREGNANCY/FERTILITY/BREEDING

Reproductive failure with glucocorticoid excess—testicular atrophy; abnormal estrus.

SYNONYMS

- Glucocorticoid hepatopathy.
- Steroid hepatopathy.
- Corticosteroid hepatopathy.
- Vacuolar change.

SEE ALSO

- Gallbladder Mucocele.
- Hyperadrenocorticism (Cushing's Disease)—Cats.
- Hyperadrenocorticism (Cushing's Disease)—Dogs.
- Hyperlipidemia.

ABBREVIATIONS

- ACTH = adrenocorticotropic hormone.
- ALP = alkaline phosphatase.
- ALT = alanine aminotransferase.
- APTT = activated partial thromboplastin time.
- AST = aspartate aminotransferase.
- cPLI = canine pancreatic lipase immunoreactivity.
- EMH = extramedullary hematopoiesis.
- GGT = γ-glutamyltransferase.
- HDDST = high-dose dexamethasone suppression test.
- LDDST = low-dose dexamethasone suppression test.
- PT = prothrombin time.
- TSBA = total serum bile acids.
- VH = vacuolar hepatopathy.

Suggested Reading

Cortright CC, Center SA, Randolph JF, et al. Clinical features of progressive vacuolar hepatopathy in Scottish Terriers with and without hepatocellular carcinoma: 114 cases (1980–2013). J Am Vet Med Assoc 2014, 245:797–808.

Sepesy LM, Center SA, Randolph JF, et al. Vacuolar hepatopathy in dogs: 336 cases (1993–2005). J Am Vet Med Assoc 2006: 229:246–252.

Author Sharon A. Center

Consulting Editor Kate Holan

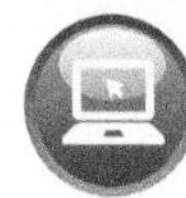

Client Education Handout available online

GRAPE AND RAISIN TOXICOSIS

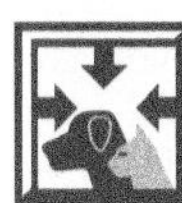

BASICS

OVERVIEW

Syndrome resulting from ingestion of grapes, raisins, sultanas, or Zante currants (*Vitis vinifera*).

SIGNALMENT

- Dogs are the only species in which toxicosis has been well described.
- No breed, sex, or age predisposition noted.
- Anecdotal reports of toxicosis in cats and ferrets exist, but data are lacking to confirm.

SIGNS

- Vomiting within 24 hours of ingestion; vomitus frequently contains ingested fruit.
- Diarrhea, anorexia, lethargy, and abdominal pain may occur; stools may contain ingested fruit.
- Within 24 hours to several days, dehydration with oliguria or anuria occurs.
- Death due to anuric renal failure or euthanasia.

CAUSES & RISK FACTORS

- Although amounts of raisins and grapes reported to cause toxicosis lie in the range 2.8–9.6 g/kg and 11–31 g/kg, respectively, a minimum toxic dose has not been established. Additionally, not all exposures of dogs to *Vitis vinifera* have resulted in clinical evidence of renal injury.
- Ingestion of sultanas, Zante currants, and other varieties of *Vitis vinifera* has also been associated with renal injury in dogs, but amounts associated with toxicosis have not been reported.
- Mechanism of toxicity and toxic principle are unknown. Inconsistent development of clinical signs resulting from ingestion of *Vitis vinifera* may reflect idiosyncratic reactions of individual dogs or a toxic principle that is of variable presence in the fruit due to variances in growing conditions.
- Until further toxicity data are available, all exposures of dogs to *Vitis vinifera* should merit veterinary attention.

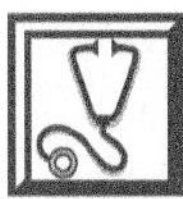

DIAGNOSIS

DIFFERENTIAL DIAGNOSIS

Other causes of acute renal failure—ethylene glycol, heavy metal toxicosis, nephrotoxic antibiotics (e.g., aminoglycosides), nonsteroidal anti-inflammatory drug toxicosis, hemoglobinuria, myoglobinuria, leptospirosis, borreliosis, and vitamin D toxicosis.

CBC/BIOCHEMISTRY/URINALYSIS

- Hypercalcemia, hyperphosphatemia, high creatinine and blood urea nitrogen (BUN) may develop within 24–48 hours of ingestion. Elevated creatinine and hyperphosphatemia tend to develop first, followed by elevation of BUN, with calcium elevation tending to increase 48–72 hours after exposure. Differentiate from vitamin D3 toxicosis, where calcium and phosphorus elevate first followed by elevations in BUN and creatinine as kidney injury develops. Not all cases develop hypercalcemia or hyperphosphatemia.
- Hyperkalemia, hyperamylasemia, hyperlipasemia, and elevated alanine aminotransferase (ALT) also occasionally occur.
- Isosthenuria, hyposthenuria, proteinuria, hematuria, and glucosuria have been reported.
- Granular casts may occur in the urine.

OTHER LABORATORY TESTS

Histopathology of kidneys reveals acute diffuse renal tubular degeneration and necrosis.

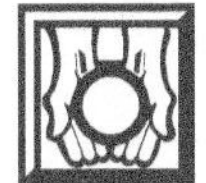

TREATMENT

- Gastrointestinal decontamination (induction of emesis, administration of activated charcoal) should follow ingestion of grapes or raisins by dogs.
- Fluid diuresis (2–3 times maintenance) for minimum of 48 hours is recommended, longer if renal failure develops. Fluid choice may vary with circumstance, but 0.9% NaCl is most commonly recommended.
- Monitor serum chemistry values, particularly renal values, for minimum of 72 hours, longer if renal failure develops.
- Correct fluid imbalances (e.g., dehydration).
- Monitor fluid in/out.
- Diuretics (e.g., furosemide, mannitol, dopamine) if oliguria or anuria develops.
- Hemodialysis or peritoneal dialysis may be required in anuric patients.

MEDICATIONS

DRUG(S) OF CHOICE

- Emetics—3% hydrogen peroxide 2.2 mL/kg up to a maximum of 45 mL/dog PO; may repeat once if first dose unsuccessful; *or* apomorphine crushed and diluted with sterile saline and instilled in conjunctival sac, rinse eye after emesis, or 0.03 mg/kg IV.
- Activated charcoal—1–3 g/kg PO.

Management of Oliguric or Anuric Renal Failure

- Mannitol 0.25–0.5 g/kg of 20–25% solution IV over 15–20 min, repeat q4–6h or administer as CRI of 8–10% solution for 12–24h.
- Furosemide 2 mg/kg IV, repeat at 4 mg/kg if no diuresis within 1h; use with dopamine for best results.
- Dopamine 0.5–3 µg/kg/min.

CONTRAINDICATIONS/POSSIBLE INTERACTIONS

N/A

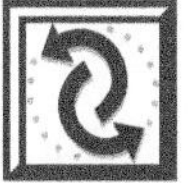

FOLLOW-UP

- In dogs developing renal insufficiency, monitor renal values until they return to normal.
- Some dogs may develop irreversible renal injury requiring lifelong management.
- Evidence of pancreatitis developed in 3 of 43 dogs with acute renal injury following *Vitis vinifera* ingestion.

MISCELLANEOUS

ABBREVIATIONS

- ALT = alanine aminotransferase.
- BUN = blood urea nitrogen.

INTERNET RESOURCES

https://www.aspcapro.org/animal-health-toxicology-poison-control/people-pet-food-dangers

Suggested Reading

Eubig PA, Brady MS, Gwaltney-Brant S, et al. Acute renal failure in dogs after ingestion of grapes or raisins: a retrospective evaluation of 43 dogs (1992–2002). J Vet Intern Med 2005;19:663–674.

Mostrom MS. Grapes and raisins. In: Peterson M, Talcott PA, eds., Small Animal Toxicology, 3rd ed. St. Louis, MO: Saunders, 2006, pp. 569–572.

Author Sharon Gwaltney-Brant

Consulting Editor Lynn R. Hovda

G

HAIR FOLLICLE TUMORS

H

BASICS

OVERVIEW

• Five types—trichoepithelioma and trichoblastoma are most common types, but uncommon types include infundibular keratinizing acanthoma, tricholemmoma, and pilomatricoma; these are differentiated based on their origin: trichoepithelioma, trichoblastoma, infundibular keratinizing acanthoma, and tricholemmoma, which arise from keratinocytes in the outer root sheath of the hair follicle (± hair matrix); and pilomatricoma, which arises from the hair matrix. • All types—generally benign; a few published reports of malignant trichoepitheliomas, trichoblastomas, and pilomatricomas.
• Approximately 5% of all skin tumors in dogs and 1% of all skin tumors in cats.

SIGNALMENT

• Dog and cat. • Age—usually >5 years. • No sex predisposition. • Trichoepithelioma—common in dogs; rare in cats; golden retrievers, basset hounds, German shepherds, cocker spaniels, Irish setters, English springer spaniels, miniature schnauzers, and standard poodles may be predisposed; Persian and Siamese cats. • Trichoblastoma—common in dogs; common in cats; poodles and cocker spaniels may be predisposed; no known breed predisposition in cats. • Infundibular keratinizing acanthoma—uncommon in dogs and cats; Norwegian elkhound, keeshond, and German shepherd dog may be predisposed; no known breed predisposition in cats.
• Tricholemmoma—uncommon in dogs and cats; Afghan hounds may be predisposed; no known breed predisposition in cats.
• Pilomatricoma—uncommon in dogs and cats; Kerry blue terriers, Old English sheepdogs, and miniature poodles may be predisposed; no known breed predisposition in cats.

SIGNS

• Usually a solitary mass. • Trichoepithelioma—common on the lateral thorax and dorsal lumbar area (dogs) and head (cats).
• Trichoblastoma—common on the head and neck, especially the base of the ear (dogs) and cranial half of the trunk (cats). • Infundibular keratinizing acanthoma—common on the back, neck, and limbs (dogs). • Tricholemmoma—common on the head and neck (dogs).
• Pilomatricoma—common on the back, limbs, shoulders, flanks, and tail. • Firm, round, elevated, well-circumscribed, often hairless, or ulcerated dermoepithelial masses or nodules.

CAUSES & RISK FACTORS

Unknown, some genetic predisposition.

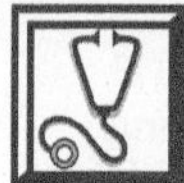

DIAGNOSIS

DIFFERENTIAL DIAGNOSIS

Distinguish from other tumors, including basal cell tumor and squamous cell carcinoma, and from epidermal inclusion cysts.

CBC/BIOCHEMISTRY/URINALYSIS

Usually normal.

DIAGNOSTIC PROCEDURES

• Fine-needle aspiration and cytopathology.
• Tissue biopsy and histopathology.

PATHOLOGIC FINDINGS

• Fine-needle aspiration cytology is very similar among all hair follicle tumors with basaloid and ghost cells; the exception to this rule is trichoblastomas, which have abundant pink matrix and scattered spindle cells.
• Trichoepithelioma—varies in degree of differentiation and site of origin (root sheath or hair matrix); horn cysts, lack of desmosomes, and differentiation toward hair follicle-like structures and formation of hair common.
• Trichoblastoma—four basic subtypes including ribbon, trabecular, granular, and clear cell; ribbon have basaloid cells in branding, winding, and radiating columns; trabecular have basaloid cells with prominent peripheral palisading; granular is identical to ribbon type but many of the cells are larger cells with granular or vacuolated cytoplasm; clear cell have basaloid cells in ribbon pattern with some cells having sebaceous differentiation. • Infundibular keratinizing acanthoma—characterized by keratin-filled crypt in the dermis that opens to the skin surface.
• Tricholemmoma—characterized by nodular proliferation of keratinocytes, of which many are clear and surrounded by thickened basement membrane. • Pilomatricoma—characterized by a variable proliferation of basophilic cells resembling hair matrix cells and fully keratinized, faintly eosinophilic cells with a central unstained nucleus (shadow cells); calcification common; features of malignancy are present with the occasional malignant pilomatricoma.

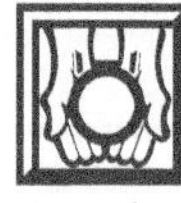

TREATMENT

Complete excision, cryotherapy, or electrosurgery—curative with most cases.

MEDICATIONS

DRUG(S) OF CHOICE

• Isotretinoin (1 mg/kg q24h PO) was used to successfully control multiple pilomatricomas in one dog and multiple infundibular keratinizing acanthomas in some dogs. • Multimodal analgesia recommended for painful lesions.

CONTRAINDICATIONS/POSSIBLE INTERACTIONS

N/A

FOLLOW-UP

• Monitor for local recurrence. • Prognosis usually excellent; multiple reports of metastatic disease with the less common canine malignant pilomatricomas.

MISCELLANEOUS

Suggested Reading

Abramo F, Pratesi F, Cantile C, et al. Survey of canine and feline follicular tumours and tumour-like lesions in central Italy. J Small Anim Pract 1999, 40:479–481.
Adedeji AO, Affolter VK, Christopher MM. Cytologic features of cutaneous follicular tumors and cysts in dogs. Vet Clin Pathol 2017; 46(1):143–150.
Beck A, Huber D, Šćuric V, et al. A four year retrospective study of the prevalence of canine follicular tumours in Croatia. Veterinarski Arhiv 2016, 86(3):453–466.
Toma S, Noli C. Isotretinoin in the treatment of multiple benign pilomatrixomas in a mixed-breed dog. Vet Dermatol 2005, 16(5):346–350.

Author Jason Pieper
Consulting Editor Timothy M. Fan
Acknowledgment The author and book editors acknowledge the prior contribution of Louis-Philippe de Lorimier.

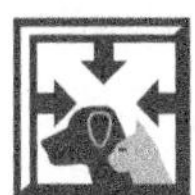

BASICS

DEFINITION

An offensive odor emanating from the oral cavity.

PATHOPHYSIOLOGY

- The sour milk odor accompanying periodontal disease may result from bacterial populations associated with plaque, calculus, unhealthy oral cavity tissues, decomposing food particles retained within the oral cavity, and tissue necrosis.
- Contrary to common belief, neither normal lung air nor stomach aroma contributes.
- The most common cause is periodontal diseases caused by plaque bacteria.
- A bacterial biofilm forms over a freshly cleaned and polished tooth as soon as the patient starts to salivate; bacteria attach to the pellicle within 6–8 hours; within days, the plaque becomes mineralized, producing calculus; as plaque ages gingival inflammation (gingivitis) may occur and progress into periodontitis (tooth support loss). Eventually the bacterial flora changes from a predominantly nonmotile Gram-positive aerobic coccoid flora to a more motile, Gram-negative anaerobic population including *Prophyromonas*, *Bacteroides*, *Fusobacterium*, and *Actinomyces* spp.
- The rough surface of calculus attracts more bacteria-laden biofilm, irritating the free gingiva; as the inflammation continues, the gingival sulcus is transformed into a periodontal pocket, which accumulates food debris and bacterial breakdown products, generating oral malodor (halitosis).
- The primary cause of malodor is Gram-negative anaerobic bacteria that generate volatile sulfur compounds (VSCs), such as hydrogen sulfide, methyl mercaptan, dimethyl sulfide, and volatile fatty acids.
- VSCs may also play a role in periodontal disease, affecting the integrity of the tissue barrier, allowing endotoxins to produce periodontal destruction, endotoxemia, and bacteremia.

SYSTEMS AFFECTED

Gastrointestinal—oral cavity.

SIGNALMENT

Species

Dogs and cats.

Breed Predilections

Small breeds and brachycephalic breeds are more prone to oral disease because the teeth are closer together, smaller animals live longer, and their owners tend to feed softer food.

Mean Age and Range

Older animals are predisposed.

SIGNS

- When oral malodor is secondary to oral disease, ptyalism (with or without blood), pawing at mouth, and anorexia may occur.
- In most cases, no clinical signs are present other than the odor.

CAUSES

- Eating malodorous food.
- Metabolic—diabetes, uremia.
- Respiratory—rhinitis, sinusitis, neoplasia.
- Gastrointestinal—megaesophagus, neoplasia, foreign body.
- Dermatologic—lip-fold pyoderma.
- Dietary—fetid foodstuffs, coprophagy.
- Oral disease—periodontal disease and ulceration, orthodontic, pharyngitis, tonsillitis, neoplasia, foreign bodies.
- Trauma—electric cord injury, open fractures, caustic agents damaging oral cavity.
- Infectious—bacterial, fungal, viral infections of oral cavity.
- Autoimmune diseases of oral cavity.
- Eosinophilic granuloma complex.

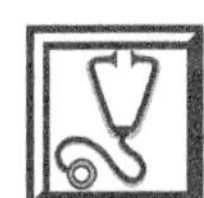

DIAGNOSIS

CBC/BIOCHEMISTRY/URINALYSIS

Usually normal. Might see changes consistent with diabetes mellitus or renal disease.

IMAGING

Intraoral radiographs are appropriate to help diagnose causes of halitosis.

DIAGNOSTIC PROCEDURES

- Hydrogen sulfide, mercaptans, and volatile fatty acids are the primary components of halitosis; an industrial sulfide monitor can be used to measure sulfide concentration in peak parts per billion.
- Additional diagnostic procedures to evaluate periodontal disease include intraoral radiography, probing pocket depths, attachment levels, and tooth mobility.

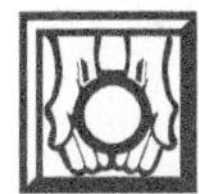

TREATMENT

APPROPRIATE HEALTH CARE

- Following appropriate tooth-by-tooth diagnostics (periodontal probing, intraoral imaging, mobility evaluation), under anesthesia all teeth should be ultrasonically scaled, and polished; a curette should be used to remove remaining plaque and calculus accessible subgingivally.
- Once the specific cause of halitosis is known, direct therapy at correcting existing pathology; often multiple teeth need to be extracted when advanced periodontal disease is the cause of halitosis.

CLIENT EDUCATION

- Halitosis is generally a sign of an unhealthy oral cavity and should prompt oral assessment under general anesthesia, treatment, and prevention.
- Initiate preventive measures to ensure good oral health (e.g., twice-daily brushing or wiping teeth, recommend accepted Veterinary Oral Heath Council products).

SURGICAL CONSIDERATIONS

Oral assessment performed under general anesthesia with intraoral radiographs and probing treatment including extraction of teeth with greater than 50% support loss.

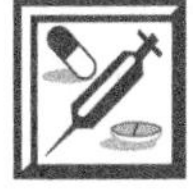

MEDICATIONS

DRUG(S) OF CHOICE

- Antibiotics are not indicated to treat halitosis.
- Controlling periodontal pathogens helps control dental infections and accompanying malodor; when accompanied by follow-up home care, has been shown to decrease pocket depth.
- Weekly application of a plaque-retardant gel has been shown to decrease plaque in dogs and cats.
- The use of oral care products that contain metal ions, especially zinc, inhibits odor due to the affinity of the metal ion to sulfur; zinc complexes with hydrogen sulfide to form insoluble zinc sulfide; zinc interferes with microbial proliferation and calcification of microbial deposits (by interfering with the crystal development of calculus). Topical treatment with zinc ascorbate cysteine gel usually reduces halitosis within 30 minutes.

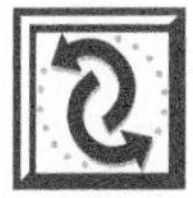

FOLLOW-UP

PATIENT MONITORING

Evaluate for recurrence of signs.

PREVENTION/AVOIDANCE

- Daily brushing or friction wipes to remove plaque and control dental disease and odor; periodic veterinary examinations to monitor care.
- Veterinary Oral Health Council (VOHC.org) was created to accept products that decrease the accumulation of plaque and/or tartar; additionally those products accepted are considered safe to use.

EXPECTED COURSE AND PROGNOSIS

Varies with underlying cause.

MISCELLANEOUS

SYNONYMS

- Bad breath.
- Fetor ex ore.
- Fetor oris.
- Foul breath.
- Malodor.

SEE ALSO

Periodontal Disease.

ABBREVIATIONS

- VSC = volatile sulfur compounds.

Suggested Reading

Di Cerbo A, Pezzuto F, Canello S, et al. Therapeutic effectiveness of a dietary supplement for management of halitosis in dogs. J Vis Exp 2015, 101:e52717. doi: 10.3791/52717

Eubanks DL. Canine oral malodor. J Am Anim Hosp Assoc 2006, 42(1):77–79.

Eubanks DL. "Doggy breath": what causes it, how do I evaluate it, and what can I do about it? J Vet Dent 2009, 26(3):192–193.

Jeusette IC, Román AM, Torre C, et al. 24-hour evaluation of dental plaque bacteria and halitosis after consumption of a single placebo or dental treat by dogs. Am J Vet Res 2016, 77(6):613–619. doi: 10.2460/ajvr.77.6.613

Wiggs RB, Lobprise HB. Veterinary Dentistry: Principles and Practice. Philadelphia, PA: Lippincott-Raven, 1997.

Author Jan Bellows

Consulting Editor Heidi B. Lobprise

Client Education Handout available online

HEAD PRESSING

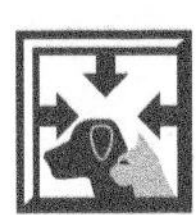

BASICS

DEFINITION

Compulsive pressing of the head against a wall or other object for no apparent reason.

PATHOPHYSIOLOGY

- Alterations in behavior—caused by lesions in the prosencephalon (i.e., cerebrum, limbic system, thalamus, and hypothalamus), particularly those affecting the limbic system and frontal and temporal cortices.
- Lesions may result in compulsive pacing; when an obstacle (e.g., a wall) is reached, the animal may press its head against it for long periods of time, apparently unable to turn and move away.
- Apparent inability to voluntarily move away—may reflect impaired integration of sensory information, leading to inappropriate behavior.

SYSTEMS AFFECTED

Nervous

GENETICS

N/A

INCIDENCE/PREVALENCE

N/A

SIGNALMENT

Dogs and cats of any age, breed, and sex.

SIGNS

- Head pressing—just one sign of prosencephalon disease.
- Compulsive pacing and circling toward the side of the lesion; circling can be toward either side if lesion is centrally located.
- Change in learned behavior, including loss of sleep cycles.
- Seizures.
- Contralateral postural reaction deficits.
- Contralateral visual deficits with normal pupillary light reflexes.
- Contralateral facial hypalgesia.

CAUSES & RISK FACTORS

- Anatomic—hydrocephalus, most commonly in young toy-breed dogs; lissencephaly (Lhasa apsos).
- Metabolic—hepatic encephalopathy as a result of a portosystemic shunt or severe hepatic disease; severe hyper- or hyponatremia.
- Nutritional—very unusual since most pets are fed compounded diets; thiamine deficiency can occur in cats fed a diet of raw fish, if thiamine supplementation in canned food is insufficient or in cats with severe malabsorptive syndromes; however, vestibular signs predominate.
- Neoplastic—primary (e.g., glioma, meningioma) or metastatic (e.g., hemangiosarcoma) tumors affecting the brain; more common in older animals (>6 years).
- Immune-mediated/inflammatory—granulomatous meningoencephalitis; necrotizing encephalitides (Maltese encephalitis, pug encephalitis); meningoencephalitis of unknown etiology.
- Infectious (dogs)—viral (rabies virus, canine distemper virus), rickettsial (*Ehrlichia canis*, Rocky Mountain spotted fever), protozoal (*Toxoplasma gondii, Neospora caninum*), or fungal (*Blastomyces, Cryptococcus*); rabies is of particular importance because neurons in the limbic system are frequently infected in carnivores.
- Infectious (cats)—viral (rabies, feline infectious peritonitis, feline leukemia virus: associated immunosuppression predisposes to other encephalitides and neoplasia; feline immunodeficiency virus: can cause encephalopathy primarily and can predispose to other encephalitides and neoplasia due to immunosuppression); *Bartonella henselae*; *Cuterebra* migration; toxoplasmosis; *Cryptococcus* and other fungal infections.
- Toxic—e.g., lead poisoning.
- Trauma.
- Vascular—intracranial hemorrhage as a result of hypertension (consider in older cats with hyperthyroidism, diabetes, or chronic renal insufficiency); bleeding disorder (either primary or secondary to rodenticide toxicity); ischemia (feline ischemic encephalopathy or secondary to systemic metabolic, inflammatory, or neoplastic disease).

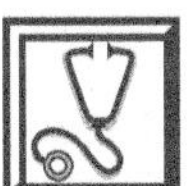

DIAGNOSIS

DIFFERENTIAL DIAGNOSIS

A newly blind animal might bump into objects, but rapidly recognizes its environment and acts visual; an animal with a prosencephalic lesion continues bumping into objects despite normal ocular exam.

CBC/BIOCHEMISTRY/URINALYSIS

- May reflect a metabolic or toxic cause.
- Hepatic encephalopathy—decreased serum albumin, blood urea nitrogen, cholesterol, and glucose concentrations, with or without elevated alanine phosphatase (ALP), alanine aminotransferase (ALT), and bilirubin concentrations; microcytic anemia may be present; ammonium biurate crystals may be present in the urine.
- Lead toxicity—basophilic stippling of erythrocytes; presence of reticulocytes and nucleated red blood cells (RBCs) in the absence of anemia.
- Encephalitis—findings often unremarkable, but may reflect an inflammatory process (e.g., with fungal infection).
- CNS lymphoma—may see evidence of bone marrow involvement.

OTHER LABORATORY TESTS

- Bile acid tolerance—to diagnose hepatic encephalopathy; blood ammonia concentrations may also be elevated.
- Acute and convalescent serologic titers—to diagnose rickettsial, protozoal, fungal, and viral diseases; for some infections (e.g., canine distemper virus, *Toxoplasma, Cryptococcus*) also measure cerebrospinal fluid (CSF) antibody or antigen (*Cryptococcus*) titers.
- PCR on CSF and serum—to diagnose rickettsial, bacterial, protozoal, fungal, and viral diseases; sensitive and specific if the infectious agent is present in CSF or serum.
- Blood lead concentration—to diagnose lead toxicity.

IMAGING

- Thoracic radiography—recommended for older patients to identify metastatic disease.
- Abdominal ultrasonography— recommended for older patients if intra-abdominal neoplasia is suspected; indicated if a portosystemic shunt or other hepatic disease is suspected.
- Rectal scintigraphy—may be used to definitively diagnose a portosystemic shunt.
- Brain CT or MRI—to identify intracranial masses, malformations, skull fractures, inflammation, and hemorrhage.
- Ultrasonography of the brain via persistent fontanels—may be used to diagnose hydrocephalus in young dogs.

DIAGNOSTIC PROCEDURES

- Fundic examination—to identify chorioretinitis (evidence of infectious/inflammatory disease) and vascular lesions.
- Blood pressure measurement to identify hypertension.
- CSF analysis—to diagnose encephalitis.

PATHOLOGIC FINDINGS

Findings at necropsy will reflect the etiology.

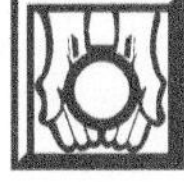

TREATMENT

APPROPRIATE HEALTH CARE

- Severe clinical signs—hospitalization for diagnostic workup and treatment.
- Suspected rabies—quarantine outdoor animal with no vaccination or unknown vaccination history when rapidly progressive neurologic signs are present and animal lives in a rabies-endemic area; minimize the number of people in contact with the animal, and maintain a contact log; if neurologic signs deteriorate rapidly, euthanize the animal and send it to a public health laboratory to be tested for rabies.

HEAD PRESSING

(CONTINUED)

H

NURSING CARE

- When hospitalized, patients should be monitored closely for deterioration in mental status and for seizures.
- Maintenance IV fluids may be necessary for patients with severe prosencephalic syndrome.
- The cage may need to be padded to avoid self-trauma if constantly head pressing and pacing.
- Eyes should be monitored regularly for development of corneal ulcers due to self-induced trauma.
- Central IV catheters should be placed in the saphenous vein rather than the jugular vein if possible, to avoid increasing intracranial pressure by occlusion of the jugular veins.

ACTIVITY

N/A

DIET

- Suspected hepatic encephalopathy—appropriate low-protein diet.
- Hand-feeding may be necessary in severely encephalopathic patients; risk of aspiration if the patient fails to prehend and swallow correctly.

CLIENT EDUCATION

- Specific to the underlying condition.
- Clients should be warned about the possibility of seizures, be provided with a description of a seizure, and given instructions on what to do if a seizure occurs.
- Clients should be provided with a description of signs of acute decompensation due to brain herniation.

SURGICAL CONSIDERATIONS

- If signs are due to intracranial disease, elevated intracranial pressure is likely and therefore there is a risk of herniation during anesthesia, with induction and recovery from anesthesia posing the highest risk; patients should be ventilated carefully to ensure that their partial pressure of carbon dioxide (pCO_2) remains within normal limits (35–45 mmHg).
- Hydrocephalus can be treated by placement of a ventriculo-peritoneal shunt.
- Brain neoplasia, in particular extra-axial tumors such as meningiomas, can be treated surgically if tumor location accessible.

MEDICATIONS

DRUG(S) OF CHOICE

- Different causes require different treatment; do not initiate therapy until a diagnosis has been established.
- If patient's mental status deteriorates suggesting impending brain herniation, mannitol (0.25–1 g/kg IV over 10–30 min) or hypertonic saline (4 mL/kg of 7.5% or 5.3 mL/kg of 3%) can be used to transiently reduce intracranial pressure; treatment can be repeated, but recurrent use will simply result in dehydration.
- Furosemide (0.7 mg/kg IV) given prior to administration of mannitol can complement the use of mannitol and prolong its effect.

CONTRAINDICATIONS

N/A

PRECAUTIONS

Sedatives should be used with caution in patients exhibiting head pressing, because they prevent assessment of mental status changes and might suppress respiratory drive, causing an increase in pCO_2 and thus causing an increase in intracranial pressure.

ALTERNATIVE DRUG(S)

N/A

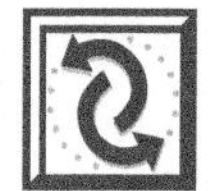

FOLLOW-UP

PATIENT MONITORING

- Periodic repeat neurologic examinations to monitor progress.
- See specific diseases.

POSSIBLE COMPLICATIONS

N/A

EXPECTED COURSE AND PROGNOSIS

N/A

MISCELLANEOUS

ASSOCIATED CONDITIONS

N/A

AGE-RELATED FACTORS

N/A

ZOONOTIC POTENTIAL

- Rabies should be considered in endemic areas.
- Fungal infections may be zoonotic if spores are released; most likely to occur if exudative skin lesions are present.

SEE ALSO

- Brain Injury.
- Encephalitis.
- Hepatic Encephalopathy.
- Hydrocephalus.

ABBREVIATIONS

- ALP = alanine phosphatase.
- ALT = alanine aminotransferase.
- CSF = cerebrospinal fluid.
- pCO_2 = partial pressure of carbon dioxide.
- RBC = red blood cell.

INTERNET RESOURCES

http://www.ivis.org/advances/Vite/braund1/chapter_frm.asp?LA=1#Cerebral_Syndrome

Suggested Reading

Bagley RS, Platt SR. Coma, stupor and mentation changes. In: Platt SR, Olby NJ, eds. BSAVA Manual of Canine and Feline Neurology, 4th ed. Gloucester: BSAVA, 2013, pp. 136–166.

Dewey CW. Encephalopathies: disorders of the brain. In: Dewey CW. ed. A Practical Guide to Canine and Feline Neurology, 2nd ed. Ames, IA: Wiley-Blackwell, 2008, pp. 115–220.

Author Natasha J. Olby

BASICS

DEFINITION

Tilting of the head away from its normal orientation with the trunk and limbs; usually associated with disorders of the vestibular system.

PATHOPHYSIOLOGY

- Vestibular system—coordinates position and movement of the head with that of the eyes, trunk, and limbs by detecting linear acceleration and rotational movements of the head; includes vestibular nuclei in the rostral medulla of the brainstem, vestibular portion of the vestibulocochlear nerve (cranial nerve [CN] VIII), and receptors in the semicircular canals of the inner ear.
- Head tilt—most consistent sign of diseases affecting the vestibular system and its projections to the cerebellum, spinal cord, cerebral cortex, reticular formation, and extraocular muscles (via medial longitudinal fasciculus); usually ipsilateral to the lesion.

SYSTEMS AFFECTED

Nervous—peripheral or CNS.

SIGNS

- Ensure that abnormal head posture is true head tilt and not a head turn; i.e., turning of the head and neck to the side as if to turn in a circle.
- Head tilt may not be present if disease is bilateral.

CAUSES

Peripheral Disease

- Anatomic—congenital head tilt.
- Metabolic—hypothyroidism; pituitary chromophobe adenoma; paraneoplastic disease.
- Neoplastic—nerve sheath tumor of CN VIII; neoplasia of the bone and surrounding tissue (e.g., osteosarcoma, fibrosarcoma, chondrosarcoma, and squamous cell carcinoma).
- Inflammatory—otitis media and interna; primarily bacterial but also parasitic (e.g., *Otodectes*), and fungal; foreign body; nasopharyngeal polyp(s).
- Idiopathic—canine geriatric vestibular disease; feline idiopathic vestibular disease.
- Immune-mediated—cranial nerve neuropathy.
- Toxic—aminoglycosides, lead, hexachlorophene.
- Traumatic—fracture of tympanic bulla or petrosal bone; ear flush.

Central Disease

- Degenerative—storage disease; demyelinating disease; vascular event.
- Anatomic—hydrocephalus.
- Neoplastic—glioma, choroid plexus papilloma, meningioma, lymphoma, nerve sheath tumor, medulloblastoma, skull tumor (e.g., osteosarcoma); metastasis (e.g., hemangiosarcoma, melanoma).
- Nutritional—thiamin deficiency.
- Inflammatory, infectious—viral (e.g., feline infectious peritonitis [FIP], canine distemper); protozoal (e.g., toxoplasmosis, neosporosis); fungal (e.g., cryptococcosis, blastomycosis, histoplasmosis, coccidioidomycosis, nocardiosis); bacterial (e.g., extension from otitis media and interna); parasitic (e.g., *Cuterebra* larvae); rickettsial (e.g., ehrlichiosis); algae (protothecosis).
- Inflammatory, noninfectious—granulomatous meningoencephalomyelitis (GME), meningoencephalitis of unknown etiology/origin (MUE/MUO), breed-specific meningoencephalitis (e.g., necrotizing encephalitis).
- Trauma—fracture petrosal bone with brainstem injury.
- Toxic—metronidazole.

RISK FACTORS

- Hypothyroidism.
- Administration of ototoxic drugs.
- Metronidazole treatment.
- Thiamin-deficient diet.
- Otitis externa, media, and interna.

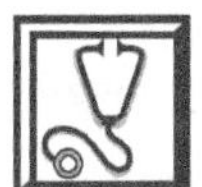

DIAGNOSIS

DIFFERENTIAL DIAGNOSIS

Vestibular Disease

- Unilateral disease—head tilt usually toward side of lesion; usually accompanied by other vestibular signs, e.g., abnormal nystagmus (resting, positional) with fast phase usually in the direction opposite the tilt; ventral deviation of the eye (vestibular strabismus) ipsilateral to the tilt observed with elevation of the head; ataxia and disequilibrium with tendency to fall, lean, and/or circle toward the side of the tilt.
- Bilateral disease—head tilt may be absent or mild on the more severely affected side; abnormal nystagmus may be present; physiologic nystagmus (i.e., normal vestibular nystagmus) may be depressed or absent; may have wide side-to-side swaying movements of the head (especially evident in cats); may have wide-based stance or crouched posture with reluctance to move.
- Head tilt—localizes either to *peripheral* (e.g., vestibular portion of CN VIII or receptors in the inner ear) or *central* (e.g., vestibular nuclei and their neuronal pathways) nervous system.
- Peripheral deficits—horizontal or rotatory nystagmus with fast phase opposite the head tilt; possible concomitant ipsilateral facial nerve paresis or paralysis and/or Horner's syndrome, and/or decreased tear production because of the close association of CN VIII with CN VII and the sympathetic nervous system in the petrosal bone and tympanic bulla.
- Central deficits—vertical, horizontal, or rotatory nystagmus that can change direction with position of the head; altered mentation; ipsilateral paresis and/or proprioceptive deficits; central signs related to cerebellum, rostral medulla, and pons; in some patients, multiple CN involvement.
- Paradoxical vestibular syndrome—with lesions in the caudal cerebellar peduncles, or flocculonodular lobes of cerebellum; vestibular signs (e.g., head tilt, nystagmus) contralateral to the lesion, whereas the cerebellar signs and proprioceptive deficits are ipsilateral to the lesion.

Nonvestibular Head Tilt and Head Posture

- Uncommon.
- Unilateral midbrain lesions can cause severe rotation of the head (>90°) toward the side opposite the lesion; no other vestibular signs; tilt corrects when patient is blindfolded.
- Adversive syndrome—observed with rostral thalamic or frontoparietal lobe lesions; head turn, neck curvature, and/or compulsive circling can be misinterpreted as vestibular deficits; may have postural reaction, menace, and/or sensory deficits that are contralateral to the lesion; compulsive turning is usually in large circles and is without the disequilibrium and true head tilt of vestibular disease.

CBC/BIOCHEMISTRY/URINALYSIS

- Usually normal.
- Mild anemia—hypothyroidism.
- Leukocytosis with neutrophilia—otitis media and interna.
- Thrombocytopenia—ehrlichiosis.
- Hypercholesterolemia—hypothyroidism.
- High serum globulin concentration—FIP.

OTHER LABORATORY TESTS

- T_4, free T_4, free T_4 by equilibrium dialysis ($FT_4 E_QD$), and endogenous thyroid-stimulating hormone (TSH) levels—if hypothyroidism is suspected based on physical examination and associated unilateral or bilateral involvement of CN VIII and possibly VII.
- Bacterial culture and sensitivity—sample from myringotomy or surgical drainage of tympanic bulla if otitis media/interna is suspected.
- Microscopic examination of ear swab—parasites (e.g., *Otodectes*).
- Serologic testing—infectious causes (e.g., canine distemper; FIP; protozoal, fungal, rickettsial diseases).

IMAGING

- Radiographs of tympanic bullae and skull—normal radiographs do not rule out bulla disease.
- CT and MRI—valuable to confirm bulla lesions, CNS extension from peripheral

H

HEAD TILT (CONTINUED)

disease, localize tumor, granuloma, and document extent of inflammation.

DIAGNOSTIC PROCEDURES

- Cerebrospinal fluid (CSF)—from cerebellomedullary cistern; for evaluating central vestibular disease; detects inflammatory process; protein electrophoresis and titers to match with serologic testing if indicated; collection may put the patient at risk for herniation if elevated intracranial pressure.
- Brainstem auditory-evoked response (BAER)—assess cochlear portion of CN VIII and brainstem auditory pathways; particularly valuable for evaluating peripheral vestibular disease, because some diseases may cause ipsilateral deafness (e.g., otitis media/interna), whereas other diseases (e.g., canine geriatric and feline idiopathic vestibular diseases) affect only the vestibular portion of CN VIII.
- Biopsy—bone, tissue in tympanic bulla when a tumor, polyp, or osteomyelitis is suspected; brainstem mass (e.g., cerebellomedullary angle) difficult to approach and remove surgically.

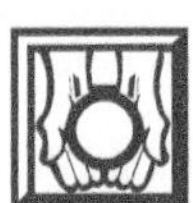

TREATMENT

- Inpatient versus outpatient—depends on severity of signs (especially vestibular ataxia), size and age of patient, and need for supportive care.
- Supportive fluids—replacement or maintenance IV fluids may be required in acute phase when disorientation, nausea, and vomiting preclude oral intake; especially important in geriatric patients; maropitant—dog: 1 mg/kg SC q24h for up to 5 days or 2 mg/kg PO q24h for up to 5 days; cat: 1 mg/kg SC/PO for up to 5 days to help manage nausea (questionable benefit).
- Diet—as usual unless there is thiamin deficiency (e.g., exclusively fish diet without vitamin supplementation); restrict oral intake if nausea and vomiting; caution: aspiration secondary to abnormal body posture in patients with severe head tilt and disequilibrium or brainstem dysfunction.
- Discontinue drug if toxicity suspected.
- Sedative for severe disorientation and ataxia—e.g., dog: acepromazine 0.02–0.05 mg/kg IV/IM/SC to max 2 mg; dexmedetomidine 1–2 µg/kg IV; diazepam 2–10 mg/dog PO/IV q8h.
- Surgical treatment—to drain bulla with otitis media, remove nasopharyngeal polyp in cats, and resect tumor, if accessible.

MEDICATIONS

DRUG(S) OF CHOICE

- Otitis media and interna—broad-spectrum antibiotic (parenteral or oral) that penetrates bone while awaiting culture results; trimethoprim-sulfa (15 mg/kg PO q12h or 30 mg/kg PO q12–24h); first-generation cephalosporins, such as cephalexin (10–30 mg/kg PO q6–8h) or amoxicillin-clavulanic acid (Clavamox®—dogs: 12.5 mg/kg PO q12h; cats: 62.5 mg/cat PO q12h; Clavaseptin® 12.5 mg/kg PO q12h); treatment for 4–6 weeks.
- Hypothyroidism—T_4 replacement (dogs: levothyroxine 22 µg/kg PO q12h) should be introduced gradually in geriatric patients, especially with cardiac disease; response varies, partly depending on duration of signs (i.e., in some patients neuropathy is not reversible).
- Infectious CNS—specific treatment, if indicated; for bacterial diseases, antibiotic that penetrates the blood–brain barrier (e.g., trimethoprim-sulfa 15 mg/kg PO q12h; metronidazole 15 mg/kg q12h or 10 mg/kg q8h PO or slowly IV; third-generation cephalosporin, e.g., cefotaxime 25–50 mg/kg IV q8h); for protozoal diseases, clindamycin (12.5–25 mg/kg PO q12h); for fungal diseases, itraconazole (dogs: 2.5 mg/kg PO q12h or 5 mg/kg PO q24h; cats: 5 mg/kg PO q12h), fluconazole (dogs: 5–8 mg/kg PO q12h, 10–12 mg/kg PO q24h; cats: 50 mg/cat PO q12–24h); prognosis usually poor for protozoal, fungal, and viral diseases (e.g., FIP).
- GME/MUE/MUO—usually initially treated with steroids: dexamethasone (0.25 mg/kg PO, IM q12h for 3 days; followed by or starting with prednisone 2 mg/kg PO q24h for a minimum of 2 weeks; then decrease slowly); depending on progress, may need stronger immunosuppression, e.g., cytosine arabinoside 50 mg/m^2 q12h for four treatments repeated every 3 weeks (need to monitor CBC) or preferably starting with CRI of cytosine arabinoside at 200 mg/m^2 administered IV over 4h, then follow every 3 weeks with SC injections; also consider cyclosporine and/or leflunomide or radiation therapy.
- Trauma—supportive care (e.g., anti-inflammatory drugs, antibiotics, IV fluid administration); specific fracture repair or hematoma removal is potentially difficult considering the location.
- Canine geriatric and feline idiopathic vestibular disease—supportive care; maropitant—dog: 1 mg/kg SC q24h for up to 5 days or 2 mg/kg PO q24h for up to 5 days; cat: 1 mg/kg SC/PO for up to 5 days to help manage nausea (questionable benefit).
- Cranial nerve polyneuropathy—response to prednisone good if the patient has a primary immune disorder.
- Thiamin deficiency—diet modification and thiamin supplementation.

PRECAUTIONS

- Trimethoprim-sulfa administration—keratoconjunctivitis sicca (dry eye).
- Avoid administering drugs into external ear canal (especially oil-based) if tympanic membrane is ruptured.

FOLLOW-UP

PATIENT MONITORING

- Repeat the neurologic examination as dictated by underlying cause.
- Head tilt may persist.
- Hypothyroidism—measure T_4 concentration 4–6 hours after treatment 3–4 weeks after initiation of thyroid therapy or dosing change.
- Repeat CSF and brain imaging—with some central vestibular disorders.
- Monitor tear production (Schirmer tear test) with trimethoprim-sulfa administration.

EXPECTED COURSE AND PROGNOSIS

- Prognosis for central vestibular disorders usually poorer than peripheral vestibular disorders.
- Prognosis for canine geriatric and feline idiopathic vestibular syndromes is excellent.

MISCELLANEOUS

ASSOCIATED CONDITIONS

- Facial nerve paresis or paralysis.
- Horner's syndrome.

SEE ALSO

- Encephalitis.
- Otitis Media and Interna.
- Vestibular Disease, Geriatric—Dogs.
- Vestibular Disease, Idiopathic—Cats.

ABBREVIATIONS

- BAER = brainstem auditory-evoked response.
- CN = cranial nerve.
- CSF = cerebrospinal fluid.
- FIP = feline infectious peritonitis.
- FT_4 E_QD = free T_4 by equilibrium dialysis.
- GME = granulomatous meningoencephalomyelitis.
- MUE/MUO = meningoencephalitis of unknown etiology/origin.
- TSH = thyroid-stimulating hormone.

Suggested Reading

Garosi L. Head tilt and nystagmus. In: Platt S, Garosi L, eds. Small Animal Neurological Emergencies. London: Manson, 2012, pp. 253–263.

Rossmeisl JH. Vestibular disease in dogs and cats. Vet Clin North Am Small Anim Pract 2010, 40:81–100.

Author Susan M. Cochrane

Client Education Handout available online

HEAD TREMORS (BOBBING), IDIOPATHIC—DOGS

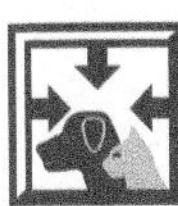

BASICS

OVERVIEW

- Common, very specific, benign, often self-limiting, head and neck tremors in dogs.
- Synonyms—head bobbing, wobbling, nodding, shaking, tremors; episodic head tremor syndrome; bobble head doll syndrome.
- A movement disorder (paroxysmal dyskinesia) was suspected, but the pathophysiology remains unknown and a recent electroencephalographic (EEG) study may support an epileptic syndrome.

SIGNALMENT

- All dog breeds can be affected.
- Not reported in cats.
- English bulldog (EB), French bulldog, boxer, Doberman pinscher (DP), and Labrador retriever are predisposed.
- Reported prevalence of 19–38% in EB.
- Reports that males are overrepresented in DP and EB.
- Generally starts early in life (<3 years old), but can start at any age.

SIGNS

Historical Findings

- Acute onset of head tremor episodes.
- Possible recent stressful event (heat, whelping with lactation, vaccination, illness, etc.).
- Littermates may be affected (familial form identified in DP ≤1 year old).

Physical Examination Findings

- None if not currently experiencing an episode.
- Typical vertical or horizontal rapid (4–8 Hertz or movements per second) head tremors—episodes last from a few seconds to a few hours.
- Variable tremor episode frequency, duration, and interepisode interval.
- Occasional reports of abnormal dystonic posture (subtle head tilt, stiffness, floppiness) during episodes, but not between episodes.
- Occasional reports of abnormal behavior (disorientation, sleepiness, agitation) immediately prior to episode.
- All dogs are reported to be responsive to their surroundings during the episode.
- Rare reports of associated generalized seizure.
- Episodes can often be interrupted by distraction or treats.
- Other neurologic abnormalities (ataxia, proprioceptive deficits, paresis) consistent with concurrent, unrelated neurologic disease (cervical spondylomyelopathy in DP, hemivertebrae in bulldogs) are often noted.

CAUSES & RISK FACTORS

- Unknown pathophysiology.
- Anatomic, neoplastic, and traumatic causes have been ruled out by different studies.
- Genetic basis suspected but unproven.
- May be triggered by a recent stressful event.

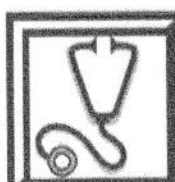

DIAGNOSIS

DIFFERENTIAL DIAGNOSIS

- Tremorgenic toxin (mycotoxin, permethrins, etc.).
- Corticosteroid responsive shaker/tremor syndrome.
- Hypomyelinating/dysmyelinating congenital or degenerative disease.
- Cerebellar disease (intention tremor).
- Hypocalcemia.
- Hypoglycemia.
- Hypoadrenocorticism (electrolyte imbalance).
- Epilepsy (focal or generalized seizures) or reactive seizures.
- Stress.
- Muscle fatigue following exercise or associated with generalized weakness from myopathy, neuropathy, or neuromuscular disease.
- History, signalment, and viewing of a video helps greatly in identifying this typical head movement and differentiating it from other types of tremor.
- Variation from the above-described typical pattern should be video-filmed and reviewed.

CBC/BIOCHEMISTRY/URINALYSIS

Usually normal.

IMAGING

MRI might be considered if abnormalities other than typical head tremor noted.

DIAGNOSTIC PROCEDURES

Cerebrospinal fluid analysis and electrodiagnostic testing might be considered if abnormalities other than typical head bobbing episodes noted. Video-EEG may show seizure activity during an episode, but has been normal between episodes in one multicentric case series study.

PATHOLOGIC FINDINGS

Have not been studied.

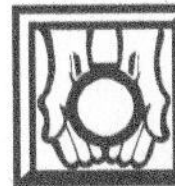

TREATMENT

- No known effective treatment.
- Interrupting the episodes by distracting the dog should be tried by the client.
- If head bobbing episodes significantly impair crucial life functions such as eating or sleeping, consult a veterinary neurologist for further recommendations.

MEDICATIONS

DRUG(S) OF CHOICE

No known effective medication.

CONTRAINDICATIONS/POSSIBLE INTERACTIONS

Commonly used antiepileptic drugs (phenobarbital, potassium bromide) have multiple significant side effects and have not been proven successful at treating head bobbing. Their use is not warranted with this condition.

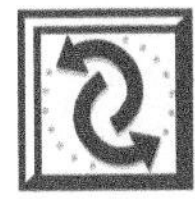

FOLLOW-UP

PREVENTION/AVOIDANCE

N/A

EXPECTED COURSE AND PROGNOSIS

- Self-limiting in 49% of EB in one study.
- Benign head tremor episodes may continue lifelong at a variable frequency, usually decreasing over time.
- Prognosis is excellent as head bobbing is not associated with a life-threatening condition.

MISCELLANEOUS

ASSOCIATED CONDITIONS

Concurrent epilepsy may be present.

PREGNANCY/FERTILITY/BREEDING

There is potential genetic transmission.

ABBREVIATIONS

- DP = Doberman pinschers.
- EB = English bulldog.
- EEG = Electroencephalography.

Suggested Reading

Guevar J, De Decker S, Van Ham LML, Fisher A, Volk HA. Idiopathic head tremor in English Bulldogs. Mov Disord 2014, 29(2):191–194.

Wolf M, Bruehschwein A, Sauter-Louis C, Sewell AC, Fisher A. An inherited Episodic Head tremor Syndrome in Doberman Pinscher Dogs. Mov Disord 2011, 26(13):2381–2386.

Author Stéphanie Dugas

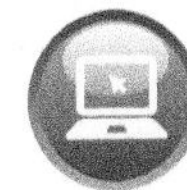

Client Education Handout available online

H

HEARTWORM DISEASE—CATS

BASICS

OVERVIEW

• Disease caused by infection with *Dirofilaria immitis*. • Microfilaremia uncommon (<20%) and usually transient if present. • Prevalence one-tenth that of unprotected dogs. • Low average worm burden. • Worms are physically smaller but recent evidence suggests lifespan is similar to that in the dog.

SIGNALMENT

• No age or breed predisposition. • Males more commonly infected naturally and easier to infect experimentally.

SIGNS

Historical Findings

• Coughing (this sign is relatively uncommon with heart failure). • Cough will commonly occur early in disease prior to established adult infection. • Heartworm-associated respiratory disease (HARD)—clinical signs and pulmonary pathology that occur 2–4 months post infection even when adult infection is never established. • Dyspnea.
• Vomiting (undetermined cause).
• Pulmonary thromboembolism (PTE) frequently results in acute respiratory failure and death. • Vomiting and respiratory signs predominate in chronic disease.

Physical Examination Findings

• Usually normal. • Increased bronchovesicular sounds. • Arrhythmia, murmur, or gallop rhythm should increase suspicion of primary cardiac disease.

CAUSES & RISK FACTORS

• Outdoor cats at increased risk (2 : 1).
• Feline leukemia virus (FeLV) infection not predisposing factor.

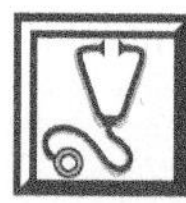

DIAGNOSIS

DIFFERENTIAL DIAGNOSIS

• Asthma. • Cardiomyopathy. • Chylothorax.
• *Aelurostrongylus abstrusus* infection.
• *Paragonimus kellicotti* infection.

CBC/BIOCHEMISTRY/URINALYSIS

• Varies with stage of disease. • Mild nonregenerative anemia. • Eosinophilia inconsistent. • Concurrent basophilia should increase suspicion. • Hyperglobulinemia.

OTHER LABORATORY TESTS

Microfilaria Concentration Tests

Very low sensitivity, high specificity.

Heartworm Antigen Tests

• ELISA or immunochromatographic tests.
• Tests that detect circulating adult heartworm antigen (HWAg) more specific than antibody tests. • Positive antigen test result is strong evidence of adult heartworm infection. • Low worm burdens (fewer than five worms) and single-sex infections commonly result in false-negative antigen tests. • Data suggest heat treatment of samples prior to testing may significantly increase test sensitivity; negative result does not rule out heartworm disease: more than 40% of cats with adult infection are antigen-negative; many cats are symptomatic (HARD) well before antigen test would become positive.

Heartworm Antibody Tests

• ELISA or immunochromatographic tests.
• Tests that detect circulating antibodies to immature and adult heartworm antigen are most sensitive tests for feline heartworm disease.
• Positive result does not confirm *adult* infection; usually becomes positive within 4 months of infection. • The more intense the antibody response, the more likely adult infection. • May become negative in adult infections perhaps associated with Ag:Ab complexing.

IMAGING

Radiography

• Enlarged (pulmonary artery, >1.6 times width of ninth rib). • Blunted, tortuous pulmonary arteries. • Patchy perivascular pulmonary infiltrates. • Pleural effusion may be present.
• Chylothorax has been documented with spontaneously occurring and experimentally induced heartworm infections in cats.

Echocardiography

• Dilated main pulmonary artery.
• Identification of worms in heart or main pulmonary artery; most commonly seen in right pulmonary artery but also in right ventricle and atrium (hyperechoic "=" sign). • Sensitive test in hands of experienced echocardiographer.
• Excludes or confirms other primary cardiac diseases (cardiomyopathy).

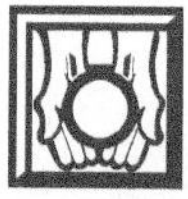

TREATMENT

• Currently no approved or recommended medical adulticide therapy. • Surgical or catheter-based extraction may be most reasonable option. • Symptomatic cats should be stabilized (see below) prior to consideration of worm extraction. • Spontaneous "cure" probably more common in cats than dogs.

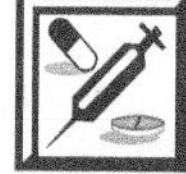

MEDICATIONS

DRUG(S) OF CHOICE

Initial Stabilization

• Supplemental oxygen. • Theophylline (sustained-release formulation) 15–25 mg/kg PO q24h in evening. • Prednisolone 1–2 mg/kg PO q12–24h for 10–14 days; then gradually taper and discontinue. • Doxycycline therapy 10 mg/kg PO q24h for 30 days (to eliminate endosymbiont *Wolbachia*) may hasten worm death and reduce severity of pulmonary inflammation secondary to worm embolization.
• Cautious balanced fluid therapy if indicated.
• Medical adulticide therapy not currently recommended. • Supportive care for PTE the same as initial stabilization (see above).

CONTRAINDICATIONS/POSSIBLE INTERACTIONS

• Aspirin therapy—no documented benefit.
• Current information does not support use of melarsomine (Immiticide®) in cats.

FOLLOW-UP

PATIENT MONITORING

Serial evaluation of clinical response, thoracic radiographs, and heartworm antigen and antibody tests is most informative.

PREVENTION/AVOIDANCE

• Ivermectin 24 µg/kg PO q30 days.
• Milbemycin oxime 0.5 mg/kg PO q30 days. • Selamectin 6.6–12 mg/kg cutaneously q30 days. • Moxidectin 1–2 mg/kg cutaneously q30 days. • Administration of these drugs in cats is not precluded by antibody or antigen seropositivity.

MISCELLANEOUS

ABBREVIATIONS

• FeLV = feline leukemia virus.
• HARD = heartworm-associated respiratory disease.
• HWAg = adult heartworm antigen.
• PTE = pulmonary thromboembolism.

INTERNET RESOURCES

https://www.heartwormsociety.org/veterinary-resources/american-heartworm-society-guidelines

Suggested Reading

Little SE, Raymond MR, Thomas JE, et al. Heat treatment prior to testing allows detection of antigen of *Dirofilaria immitis* in feline serum. Parasit Vectors 2014, 7:1.

Thomason JD, Calvert CA. Heartworm disease. In: Smith FWK, Tilley LP, Oyama MA, Sleeper MM, eds., Manual of Canine and Feline Cardiology, 5th ed. St. Louis, MO: Saunders Elsevier, 2016.

Author Michael Aherne

Consulting Editor Michael Aherne

Acknowledgment The author and book editors acknowledge the prior contribution of Matthew W. Miller

Client Education Handout available online

BASICS

DEFINITION

Disease caused by infestation with *Dirofilaria immitis*.

PATHOPHYSIOLOGY

• Severity directly related to worm number, duration of infestation, host response, and host activity level. • Endothelial damage leads to myointimal proliferation and inflammation predisposing to periarterial edema. • Lobar arterial enlargement, tortuosity, and obstruction cause impaired compliance, loss of collateral recruitment, pulmonary hypertension (PH), right-sided congestive heart failure (rCHF), thrombosis.
• Pulmonary damage exacerbated after death of adult worms and with exercise.

SYSTEMS AFFECTED

• Respiratory—PH, thromboembolism, allergic pneumonitis (some occult infections), eosinophilic granulomatosis (uncommon).
• Cardiovascular—severe PH causes right ventricular hypertrophy and, in some dogs, rCHF (ascites). • Hemic/lymphatic/immune—venous inflow to the heart can become obstructed by worms causing traumatic hemolytic anemia and cardiogenic shock (caval syndrome). • Renal/urologic—immune-complex glomerulonephritis.

INCIDENCE/PREVALENCE

Virtually 100% in unprotected dogs living in highly endemic regions.

GEOGRAPHIC DISTRIBUTION

• Most common in tropical and subtropical zones; endemic in North, Central, and South America, southern Europe, and Australia.
• Diagnosed in all 50 states of United States; common along Atlantic/Gulf coasts and Ohio/Mississippi river basins. • Ubiquitous mosquito vector in endemic areas.

SIGNALMENT

Breed Predilections

• Medium-to-large breed dogs > small dogs.
• Outdoor dogs > indoor dogs.

Mean Age and Range

Infestation can occur at any age; most affected dogs 3–8 years old.

Predominant Sex

Males > females.

SIGNS

Historical Findings

• Dogs often asymptomatic or exhibit minimal signs such as occasional coughing (mild infestation). • Coughing and exercise intolerance associated with moderate pulmonary damage (moderate infestation).
• Cachexia, exercise intolerance, syncope, and/or abdominal distention (rCHF) in severely affected dogs. • Cardiogenic shock, pigmenturia, abdominal distention (rCHF) in dogs with caval syndrome.

Physical Examination Findings

• No abnormalities—dogs with mild and some with moderate infestation. • Labored breathing and/or crackles—dogs with severe PH or pulmonary thromboembolism (PTE).
• Tachycardia, weight loss, exercise intolerance, syncope, coughing, pale or light pink mucous membranes, dyspnea. • Ascites, jugular vein distention/pulsation, hepatomegaly (rCHF).
• Hemoptysis—occasionally. • Pale mucous membranes, dyspnea, weak pulses.

RISK FACTORS

• Residence in endemic areas. • Outside habitat. • Lack of prophylaxis.
• Environmental temperature >57 °F (14 °C).

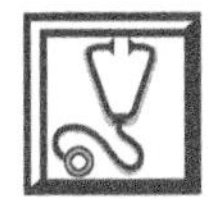

DIAGNOSIS

DIFFERENTIAL DIAGNOSIS

• Other causes of PH and thrombosis (e.g., hyperadrenocorticism, protein-losing nephropathy or enteropathy). • Chronic obstructive lung disease. • Pneumonia.
• Allergic lung disease. • Other causes of ascites (e.g., dilated cardiomyopathy).
• Other causes of hemolytic anemia (e.g., immune-mediated).

CBC/BIOCHEMISTRY/URINALYSIS

• Anemia—absent, mild, or moderate depending on chronicity, severity, thromboembolic complications. • Eosinophilia and basophilia—vary. • Inflammatory leukogram and thrombocytopenia associated with thromboembolism. • Hyperglobulinemia—inconsistent finding. • Hemoglobinemia—evident with caval syndrome and less often thromboembolism. • Proteinuria—common with severe and chronic infestation; due to immune-complex glomerulonephritis or amyloidosis. • Hemoglobinuria—caval syndrome or severe lysis with thromboembolism.

OTHER LABORATORY TESTS

• Highly specific, sensitive serologic tests identify adult female *D. immitis* antigen; test 7 months after end of previous transmission season; false positives possible with *Spirocerca* infestation; in author's experience, false negatives occur more commonly in shelter animals due to antigen-antibody complexes (antigen blocking); if infestation suspected with negative antigen test, consider heartworm heat treatment antigen ELISA testing.
• Antigenemia absent in absence of adult female worms. • Weak positive test verified by repeat testing using different test and/or microfilaria testing. • Strong reaction indicates relative high worm burden or recent worm death and highly predictive of thromboembolic complications post adulticide therapy.
• Microfilaria testing—mainly to confirm weak positive antigen tests, determine microfilarial status prior to using milbemycin preventatives, and identify microfilaria that may contribute to development of resistance when treated chronically with macrolide preventative.

IMAGING

Radiography

• Use DV projection. • Main pulmonary artery segment enlargement, lobar arterial enlargement, tortuosity/pruning vary from absent to severe; right caudal artery > left caudal artery > cranial arteries. • Parenchymal lung infiltrates of variable severity—surround lobar arteries; may extend into most or all of one or multiple lung lobes with thromboembolism and/or PH. • Diffuse, symmetric, alveolar, interstitial infiltrates occur secondary to allergic reaction to microfilaria (allergic pneumonitis) in about 10% of occult infestations.

Echocardiography

• Often unremarkable; may reflect right ventricular dilation and wall hypertrophy, tricuspid regurgitation, PH, small left heart due to underloading (pulmonary obstruction/hypertension). • Parallel, linear echodensities produced by heartworms may be detected in right ventricle, right atrium, pulmonary arteries.

DIAGNOSTIC PROCEDURES

ECG

• Usually normal. • May reflect right ventricular hypertrophy in dogs with severe infestation. • Heart rhythm disturbances—occasionally seen (atrial premature contractions and atrial fibrillation most common) in severe infestation.

PATHOLOGIC FINDINGS

• Large right heart. • Pulmonary arterial myointimal proliferation. • PTE.
• Pulmonary hemorrhage. • Hepatomegaly and congestion in dogs with rCHF.

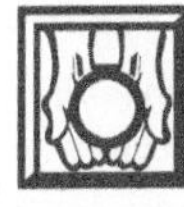

TREATMENT

APPROPRIATE HEALTH CARE

• Most dogs hospitalized during adulticide administration. • Eliminate microfilaria with monthly prophylaxis and doxycycline/minocycline; milbemycin may cause rapid decrease in microfilaria numbers and should be used with caution in that scenario; dogs should be rendered microfilaria free 3-4 months post diagnosis. • Hospitalization recommended for dogs experiencing thromboembolic complications.

ACTIVITY

Severely restrict activity for 4–6 weeks after adulticide administration.

HEARTWORM DISEASE—DOGS (CONTINUED)

CLIENT EDUCATION

• Good prognosis for animals with mild to moderate disease. • Post-adulticide pulmonary complications likely in patients with moderate to severe pulmonary artery pathology and those with high worm burden. • Reinfestation can occur without appropriate prophylaxis.

SURGICAL CONSIDERATIONS

• Treatment of choice for caval syndrome. • Worm removal from right heart and pulmonary artery via jugular vein, by use of fluoroscopy and long, flexible alligator forceps or horsehair brush, highly effective for treating high worm burden when employed by experienced operator.

MEDICATIONS

DRUG(S) OF CHOICE

• Stabilize animals in rCHF with diuretics, angiotensin-converting enzyme (ACE) inhibitor, pimobendan, sildenafil, cage rest, and moderate sodium restriction before adulticide treatment. • Stabilize pulmonary failure with oxygen supplementation, antithrombotics (e.g., clopidogrel and heparin), and/or anti-inflammatory dosages of corticosteroid depending on clinical and radiographic findings. • Doxycycline/minocycline (5–10 mg/kg PO q12h) for 4 weeks followed by 1 month wait period is used prior to adulticide therapy to kill *Wolbachia*, a Gram-negative, endo-symbiotic, intrafilarial bacterium associated with inflammation of the lungs and kidneys; the author practices adulticide therapy after 4 weeks of treatment. • Adulticide—melarsomine dihydrochloride (2.5 mg/kg IM/dose): injections given into epaxial muscles using 22-gauge needles; apply pressure over injection site during and after needle withdrawal. • Graded-kill protocol recommended in most cases—administer one injection followed in 1 month by two injections (first injection on left or right epaxial muscles, followed by injection on opposite side 24h later). • For severe heartworm infestation with high worm burdens, administer one injection every 4–6 weeks for a total of three injections; maintain strictest patient confinement practical for 4–6 weeks; perform antigen test 6 months after third injection. • Allergic pneumonitis—administer prednisone or prednisolone (2 mg/kg PO q12–24h for several days) and then immediately administer melarsomine. • Rapid microfilaricidal therapy (e.g., milbemycin or high-dose ivermectin) not recommended—eliminate microfilaria with monthly prophylaxis and doxycycline/minocycline; confirm elimination of microfilaria by testing 3–4 months after initiating therapy.

PRECAUTIONS

• Adulticide treatment—not indicated in patients with renal failure, hepatic failure (icterus), or nephrotic syndrome. • Caval syndrome—remove worms surgically and stabilize patient with conservative management for at least 1 month prior to adulticide therapy.

ALTERNATIVE DRUG(S)

• Sodium heparin (75–100 units/kg SC q8h), clopidogrel (2–4 mg/kg PO q24h), or low molecular weight heparin (dalteparin: 100 units/kg SC q12–24h) for 1–3 weeks before, during, and for 3 weeks after adulticide administration are controversial recommendations for most severe cases; therapy is combined with strict, extended cage confinement. • Sodium heparin (200–500 units/kg SC q8h) recommended for dogs with PTE or hemoglobinuria with goal of prolonging activated partial thromboplastin time (APTT) 1.5–2 times baseline. • Soft or slow kill methods using any macrocyclic lactone alone are not recommended.

FOLLOW-UP

PATIENT MONITORING

• Perform antigen test 6 months after adulticide treatment; some dogs with persistent, low-grade antigenemia may not require retreatment. • Weak antigenemia indicates most worms killed, pulmonary pathology will improve, and ivermectin prophylaxis will likely eventually kill remaining worms.

PREVENTION/AVOIDANCE

• Heartworm prophylaxis should be provided for all dogs at risk—author recommends year-round prophylaxis; otherwise begin with mosquito season and continue for 1 month following first frost. • In highly endemic areas, consider combination of heartworm prophylaxis, insect repellents, and ectoparasiticides. • Antigen test 7 months after end of previous season. • Ivermectin (Heartgard®, Iverhart®, Tri-Heart®)—highly effective, monthly preventative; safe for microfilaremic dogs. • Milbemycin oxime (Interceptor®, Sentinel®, Trifexis®)—highly effective, monthly prophylaxis; acute reactions may occur when given to microfilaremic dogs. • Moxidectin (Advantage® Multi, ProHeart® 6)—topical solution administered monthly; slow-release injectable formulation (ProHeart® SR12) available in some countries. • Selamectin (Revolution®)—highly effective monthly topical preparation. • Administer to puppies as soon after 8 weeks of age as dictated by seasonal risk. • All prophylactic drugs can be administered safely to collies at labeled dosages. • For dogs infected with adult worms not already on prophylaxis, any of above drugs can be started immediately and should be started within 1 month of diagnosis; author recommends against using milbemycin in microfilaremic dogs. • All macrocyclic lactones combined with 1 month doxycycline/minocycline therapy should eliminate microfilaria in 1–3 months. • Due to recent increase in number of lack of efficacy reports and concern of possible heartworm resistance to current heartworm preventatives, dogs should be rendered microfilaria free 3–4 months post diagnosis.

POSSIBLE COMPLICATIONS

• Post-adulticide PTE—may occur up to 4–6 weeks after treatment; more likely in dogs with severe disease and those not properly confined. • Thrombocytopenia and disseminated intravascular coagulation. • Melarsomine adverse effects—PTE (usually 7–30 days post therapy); anorexia; injection site reaction: myositis; lethargy or depression; elevation of hepatic enzymes; paresis/paralysis/altered mentation; lack of efficacy.

EXPECTED COURSE AND PROGNOSIS

• Mild—usually uneventful with excellent prognosis. • Severe or caval syndrome—guarded prognosis with higher risk of complications.

MISCELLANEOUS

When anesthesia/surgery required, delay heartworm treatment until after procedure.

ASSOCIATED CONDITIONS

Wolbachia

PREGNANCY/FERTILITY/BREEDING

• Delay adulticide treatment.
• Transplacental infestation by microfilaria can occur.

SEE ALSO

• Congestive Heart Failure, Right-Sided.
• Disseminated Intravascular Coagulation.
• Hypertension, Pulmonary.
• Nephrotic Syndrome.
• Pulmonary Thromboembolism.

ABBREVIATIONS

• ACE = angiotensin-converting enzyme.
• APTT = activated partial thromboplastin time.
• PH = pulmonary hypertension.
• PTE = pulmonary thromboembolism.
• rCHF = right-sided congestive heart failure.

INTERNET RESOURCES

www.heartwormsociety.org

Author Justin D. Thomason
Consulting Editor Michael Aherne
Acknowledgment The author and book editors acknowledge the prior contribution of Clay A. Calvert

Client Education Handout available online

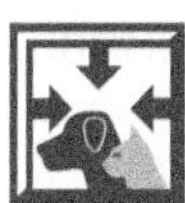

BASICS

DEFINITION

• Hyperthermia is defined as an elevation in body temperature above the normal range; although published normal values for dogs and cats vary slightly, it is generally accepted that body temperatures >103 °F (39.4 °C) are abnormal. • Hyperthermia can be categorized into pyrogenic hyperthermia (pyrexia or fever) and nonpyrogenic hyperthermia. • Heat stroke is a form of nonpyrogenic hyperthermia that occurs when heat-dissipating mechanisms of the body cannot accommodate excessive heat; this can lead to multisystem organ dysfunction; temperatures of ≥106 °F (41.1 °C) without signs of inflammation are suggestive of nonpyrogenic hyperthermia. • Malignant hyperthermia is an uncommon familial form of nonpyrogenic hyperthermia that can occur secondary to some anesthetic agents. • Other causes of nonpyrogenic hyperthermia include excessive exercise, thyrotoxicosis, and hypothalamic lesions.

PATHOPHYSIOLOGY

• The hypothalamic set point is changed with true fever; this is most likely mediated via the endogenous pyrogen interleukin-1.
• Nonpyrogenic hyperthermia does not change the hypothalamic set point. • The critical temperature leading to multiple organ dysfunction is 109 °F (42.7 °C). • The primary pathophysiologic processes of heat stroke are related to thermal damage, which can lead to cellular necrosis, hypoxemia, and protein denaturalization. • Heat stroke and its sequelae can lead to systemic inflammatory response syndrome (SIRS).

SYSTEMS AFFECTED

• Cardiovascular—hypovolemia, cardiac arrhythmias, myocardial ischemia, necrosis.
• Gastrointestinal—mucosal ischemia and ulceration, bacterial translocation and endotoxemia. • Hemic/lymphatic/immune—hemoconcentration, thrombocytopenia, disseminated intravascular coagulation (DIC).
• Hepatobiliary—hepatocellular necrosis.
• Musculoskeletal—rhabdomyolysis.
• Nervous—neuronal damage, parenchymal hemorrhage, cerebral edema. • Renal/urologic—acute renal failure.

GEOGRAPHIC DISTRIBUTION

May occur in any climate but more common in warm and/or humid environments.

SIGNALMENT

Species

Dog and, uncommonly, cat.

Breed Predilections

• May occur in any breed. • Longhaired animals. • Brachycephalic breeds.

Mean Age and Range

• All ages but often age extremes. • Young dogs may tend to overexert. • Old dogs with preexisting disease.

SIGNS

Historical Findings

• Identifiable underlying cause—warm environmental conditions, locked in car or other confined area without adequate ventilation, grooming accident associated with drying cages, excessive exercise, restricted access to water. • Predisposing underlying disease—laryngeal paralysis, brachycephalic obstructive disease, cardiovascular disease, neuromuscular disease, previous history of heat-related disease.

Physical Examination Findings

• Panting. • Hypersalivation. • Hyperthermia.
• Hyperemic mucous membranes. • Pale mucous membranes. • Cyanosis.
• Tachycardia. • Cardiac dysrhythmias.
• Shock. • Respiratory distress.
• Hematemesis. • Hematochezia. • Melena.
• Petechiation. • Changes in mentation.
• Seizures. • Muscle tremors. • Ataxia.
• Coma. • Oliguria/anuria. • Respiratory arrest. • Cardiopulmonary arrest.

CAUSES

• Excessive environmental heat and humidity (may be due to weather conditions or accidents such as enclosed in unventilated room, car, or grooming dryer cage). • Upper airway disease. • Exercise. • Toxicosis (some compounds that lead to seizures, i.e., strychnine and metaldehyde). • Anesthesia (malignant hyperthermia).

RISK FACTORS

• Previous history of heat-related disease.
• Age extremes. • Heat intolerance due to poor acclimatization. • Obesity. • Poor cardiopulmonary conditioning.
• Hyperthyroidism. • Underlying cardiopulmonary disease. • Brachycephalic breeds.
• Thick hair coat. • Dehydration.

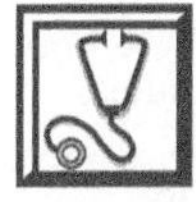

DIAGNOSIS

DIFFERENTIAL DIAGNOSIS

• If temperature exceeds 106 °F (41.1 °C) without evidence of inflammation should consider heat stroke. • Panting and hypersalivation may not be seen with true fever as hypothalamic set point has been raised.

CBC/BIOCHEMISTRY/URINALYSIS

• May help identify underlying disease process and/or sequelae to hyperthermia. • CBC abnormalities may include stress leukogram, leukopenia, anemia, nucleated red blood cells, thrombocytopenia, or hemoconcentration.
• Biochemistry profile may show azotemia, hyperalbuminemia, elevations in serum enzymes (alanine aminotransferase, aspartate aminotransferase, creatine kinase), hypernatremia, hyperchloremia, hyperglycemia, hypoglycemia, hyperphosphatemia, hyperkalemia, hypokalemia, hyperbilirubinemia. • Urinalysis may show hypersthenuria, proteinuria, cylindruria, hemoglobinuria, myoglobinuria.

OTHER LABORATORY TESTS

• Blood gas analysis may show mixed acid-base disorder, respiratory alkalosis, or metabolic acidosis. • Lactate concentrations may be elevated due to impaired perfusion.
• Coagulation profile may indicate prolonged activated clotting time (ACT), prothrombin time (PT), or partial thromboplastin time (PTT); fibrin degradation products (FDP) or D-dimers may be positive; DIC may be present if PT and PTT are prolonged along with positive FDPs or D-dimers and thrombocytopenia; if available measurement of antithrombin may be valuable.
• Thromboelastography may document hyper- or hypocoagulability.

IMAGING

• Thoracic/abdominal radiographs and/or ultrasound may help identify underlying cardiopulmonary disease or predisposing factors. • CT or MRI may help identify hypothalamic lesion.

DIAGNOSTIC PROCEDURES

Continuous temperature monitoring.

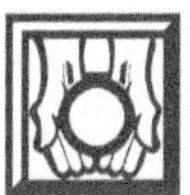

TREATMENT

• Early recognition is key. • Immediate correction of hyperthermia—spray with water or immerse in water prior to transport to veterinary facility; convection cooling with fans; evaporative cooling such as alcohol on foot pads, axilla, and groin.
• Stop cooling procedures when temperature reaches 103 °F (39.4 °C) to avoid hypothermia. • Oxygen supplementation via oxygen cage, mask, or nasal catheter. • Airway management in cases of laryngeal paralysis or edema. • Ventilatory support if required.
• Fluid support with shock doses of crystalloids or colloids. • Treat complications, seizures, DIC, renal injury, cerebral edema. • Treat underlying disease or correct predisposing factors.

APPROPRIATE HEALTH CARE

• Patients should be hospitalized until temperature is stabilized. • Most patients need intensive care for several days.

NURSING CARE

• External cooling—try to avoid ice as this may cause peripheral vasoconstriction and impede heat elimination; shivering response is also undesirable as this creates heat. • Fluid therapy—isotonic crystalloids can be administered at shock rates (dogs: 90 ml/kg/h; cats: 45–60 mL/kg/h) based on clinical assessment; synthetic colloids may also be

HEAT STROKE AND HYPERTHERMIA (CONTINUED)

used to treat shock (dogs: 20 mL/kg, 5 mL/kg IV boluses; cats: 5–10 mL/kg, 1–2 mL/kg boluses). • Oxygen supplementation—can be administered via mask, cage, or nasal cannula.

ACTIVITY

Restricted

DIET

Nil PO until animal is stable.

H

CLIENT EDUCATION

• Be aware of clinical signs. • Know how to cool off animals. • Seek veterinary care immediately. • An episode of heat stroke may predispose pets to additional episodes.

SURGICAL CONSIDERATIONS

Tracheostomy may be required if upper airway obstruction is underlying cause or contributing factor.

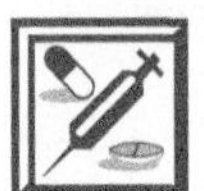

MEDICATIONS

DRUG(S) OF CHOICE

• No specific drugs for hyperthermia or heat stroke; therapy dependent on clinical presentation. • Prophylactic broad-spectrum antimicrobials may decrease incidence of bacterial translocation; first-generation cephalosporins or potentiated penicillins (clavulanate/amoxicillin, sulbactam/ampicillin) in combination with fluoroquinolones provide excellent four-quadrant coverage. • Acute renal failure—dopamine CRI (2–5 µg/kg/min), furosemide (2–4 mg/kg IV PRN), mannitol 0.5–1 g/kg as slow IV/CRI. • Cerebral edema—mannitol (1 g/kg IV over 15–30 min), furosemide (1 mg/kg IV) 30 min following mannitol infusion, corticosteroids: dexamethasone sodium phosphate (1–2 mg/kg IV), prednisone sodium succinate (10–20 mg/kg IV), methyl prednisolone (15 mg/kg IV); see Contraindications. • Ventricular arrhythmia—lidocaine bolus (2 mg/kg IV) followed by CRI (25–75 µg/kg/min); procainamide (6–8 mg/kg IV). • Metabolic acidosis—sodium bicarbonate (0.3 × BW [kg] × base excess) give ⅓ to ½ as IV bolus. • DIC—fresh frozen plasma (20 mL/kg); heparin doses vary widely (300–500 U/kg SC q 6–8h). • Thrombocytopenia—severe thrombocytopenia with active bleeding can be treated with fresh whole blood, platelet-rich plasma, lyophilized platelets, or frozen platelet concentrate. • Hematochezia or melena—broad-spectrum antibiotics, H2-antagonists, or proton pump inhibitors in combination with sucralfate. • Seizures—diazepam (0.5–1 mg/kg IV) or midazolam; phenobarbital (6 mg/kg IV PRN).

CONTRAINDICATIONS

• Nonsteroidal anti-inflammatory agents are not indicated in nonpyrogenic hyperthermia because the hypothalamic set point is not altered. • Corticosteroid use considered controversial in heat stroke due to possible adverse effects.

PRECAUTIONS

N/A

POSSIBLE INTERACTIONS

N/A

FOLLOW-UP

PATIENT MONITORING

• Patients should be closely monitored during cooling-down period and for a minimum of 24 hours post episode; most animals must be monitored for several days depending on clinical presentation and clinical complications. • Thorough physical examination should be performed daily; in addition the following parameters should be given consideration: ○ Body temperature. ○ Body weight. ○ Blood pressure. ○ Central venous pressure. ○ ACT. ○ PT/PTT. ○ D-dimers. ○ ECG. ○ Thoracic auscultation. ○ Urinalysis and urine output. ○ Packed cell volume, total protein. ○ CBC, biochemical profile. ○ Venous blood gas analysis (electrolytes, lactate).

POSSIBLE COMPLICATIONS

• Cardiac dysrhythmias. • Organ failure. • Coma. • Seizures. • Acute renal failure. • DIC. • SIRS. • Sepsis/septic shock. • Pulmonary edema—acute respiratory distress syndrome (ARDS). • Rhabdomyolysis. • Hepatocellular necrosis. • Respiratory arrest. • Cardiopulmonary arrest.

EXPECTED COURSE AND PROGNOSIS

• Depends on underlying cause or disease process. • Prognosis may depend on time lag between event and hospital admission. • Prognosis is guarded—dependent on complications (renal failure and DIC) and duration of episode. • May predispose animal to further episodes due to damage to thermoregulatory center.

MISCELLANEOUS

SYNONYMS

• Heat exhaustion. • Heat prostration. • Heat-related disease. • Heat stroke.

SEE ALSO

Fever

ABBREVIATIONS

• ACT = activated clotting time.
• ARDS = acute respiratory distress syndrome.
• DIC = disseminated intravascular coagulation.
• FDP = fibrin degradation products.
• PT = prothrombin time.
• PTT = partial thromboplastin time.
• SIRS = systemic inflammatory response syndrome.

Suggested Reading

Bruchim Y, Klement E, Saragusty J, et al. Heat stroke in dogs: a retrospective study of 54 cases (1999–2004) and analysis of risk factors for death. J Vet Intern Med 2006; 20:38–46.

Gfeller R. Heat stroke. In: Ettinger SJ, Feldman EC, eds. Textbook of Veterinary Internal Medicine, 6th ed. St. Louis, MO: Elsevier, 2005, pp. 437–440.

Johnson SI, McMichael M, White G. Heatstroke in small animal medicine: a clinical practice review. J Vet Emerg Crit Care 2006; 16(2):112–119.

Author Steven L. Marks
Consulting Editor Michael Aherne

Client Education Handout available online

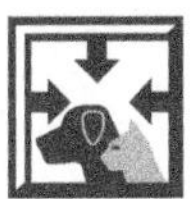

BASICS

DEFINITION

Helicobacter spp. are microaerophilic, Gram-negative, urease-positive bacteria ranging in shape from coccoid to curved to spiral.

PATHOPHYSIOLOGY

Helicobacter spp. in the Stomach

• The association of *Helicobacter pylori* with gastritis, peptic ulceration, and gastric neoplasia fundamentally changed understanding of gastric disease in humans. • Putative mechanisms by which *H. pylori* alters gastric physiology in humans include disruption of gastric mucosal barrier and alteration of gastric secretory activity. • *H. pylori* in humans has been associated with increased secretion of proinflammatory cytokines and nitric oxide. • Several *Helicobacter* spp. other than *H. pylori* have been isolated from stomachs of dogs and cats; typically, multiple species are present. • A possible cause–effect relationship of *Helicobacter* spp. and gastric inflammation in cats and dogs remains unresolved; inflammation or glandular degeneration accompanies infection in some but not all. • Experiments to determine pathogenicity of *H. pylori* in specific pathogen free (SPF) cats and *H. pylori* and *H. felis* in gnotobiotic dogs demonstrated gastritis, lymphoid follicle proliferation, and humoral immune responses after infection.

Helicobacter Spp. in the Liver and Intestines

• Role in intestinal and hepatic disease is unclear. • Several *Helicobacter*-like organisms (HLOs) have been identified in large intestine and feces from normal and diarrheic dogs and cats. • *H. canis* has been isolated from liver of a dog with active, multifocal hepatitis.

SYSTEMS AFFECTED

Gastrointestinal (GI)—*Helicobacter* spp. may lead to gastritis in some dogs and cats, diarrhea in some dogs with *H. canis*, possible acute hepatitis.

GENETICS

N/A

INCIDENCE/PREVALENCE

Gastric *Helicobacter* spp.

• Gastric HLOs are prevalent in dogs and cats—86–90% of clinically healthy cats, 67–86% of clinically healthy pet dogs. • HLOs demonstrated in gastric biopsy specimens in 57–76% of cats and 61–82% of dogs presented for investigation of recurrent vomiting. • To date *H. pylori* has been identified only in a single colony of laboratory cats.

Enterohepatic *Helicobacter* spp.

• *H. canis* isolated in 4% of 1,000 dogs evaluated. • A single case of *H. canis*–associated hepatitis reported in 2-month-old puppy. • Prevalence of *H. fennelliae* and *H. cinaedi* undetermined.

GEOGRAPHIC DISTRIBUTION

N/A

SIGNALMENT

Species

Dog and cat.

Mean Age and Range

Gastric infection acquired at a young age.

SIGNS

Historical Findings

• Asymptomatic presence of *Helicobacter* spp. common. • Vomiting, anorexia, abdominal pain, weight loss, and/or borborygmus have all been reported in dogs and cats with gastric *Helicobacter* spp. • *H. canis* in dogs may be associated with diarrhea. • Vomiting, weakness, and sudden death reported in puppy with hepatic *H. canis*.

Physical Examination Findings

• Usually unremarkable. • Dehydration due to vomiting or diarrhea.

CAUSES

Gastric *Helicobacter* spp.

• *H. felis*, *H. heilmannii*, and *H. baculiformis* have been identified in cats. • *H. felis*, *H. bizzozeronii*, *H. salomonis*, *H. heilmannii*, *H. bilis*, *H. cynogastricus*, and *Flexispira rappini* identified in dogs.

Enterohepatic *Helicobacter* spp.

• *H. bilis*, *H. canis*, *H. cinaedi*, and *Flexispira rappini* identified in feces from normal and diarrheic dogs. • *H. cinaedi* identified in one cat; its significance is unknown. • *H. canis* reported in one dog with acute hepatitis.

RISK FACTORS

Poor sanitary conditions and overcrowding may facilitate spread.

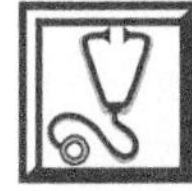

DIAGNOSIS

DIFFERENTIAL DIAGNOSIS

• High prevalence of *Helicobacter* spp. in dogs and cats. Therefore, exclusion of other causes of gastric disease and a positive identification of *Helicobacter* spp. are crucial before a diagnosis of GI disease due to *Helicobacter* spp. can be suspected. • Gastric helicobacteriosis—distinguish from other causes of vomiting. • Intestinal helicobacteriosis—distinguish from other causes of diarrhea. • Hepatic helicobacteriosis—distinguish from other causes of hepatobiliary disease.

CBC/BIOCHEMISTRY/URINALYSIS

• May reflect fluid and electrolyte abnormalities secondary to vomiting and/or diarrhea. • May indicate hepatic disease in patients with *H. canis*–associated hepatitis.

OTHER LABORATORY TESTS

• Examination of impression smears of gastric mucosa or gastric washings using May-Grünwald-Giemsa, Gram, or Diff-Quik® stain is sensitive for *Helicobacter* spp.; cannot distinguish between different HLOs. • Rapid urease test—requires gastric biopsy specimen. • ^{13}C-urea breath or blood test reliable in identifying infected dogs; not commercially available. • Bacterial culture requires special techniques and media and is impractical. • PCR of DNA extracted from biopsy specimens or from gastric juice. • Serologic tests (ELISA) measure circulating immunoglobulin (Ig) G in serum; cannot distinguish between HLOs. • Histopathology enables definitive diagnosis of infection, but cannot distinguish between different HLOs.

H

IMAGING

Abdominal radiography, ultrasonography usually normal.

DIAGNOSTIC PROCEDURES

• Gastric helicobacteriosis—in cases of *Helicobacter* spp.–associated gastritis, endoscopy may reveal superficial nodules that suggest hyperplasia of lymphoid follicles, diffuse gastric rugal thickening, punctate hemorrhages, erosions. • Hepatic helicobacteriosis—hepatic biopsy/histopathology (Warthin-Starry staining) and culture.

PATHOLOGIC FINDINGS

• Identification of HLOs requires special staining of tissue samples with Warthin-Starry or modified Steiner stain; routine H&E staining may reveal larger HLOs, but smaller organisms are often missed. • In cases of *Helicobacter* spp.–associated gastric disease—lymphocytic-plasmacytic gastritis and lymphoid follicle hyperplasia; rarely neutrophilic infiltrates; gastric ulcers have not been reported in dogs and cats. • In cases of *H. canis*–associated hepatitis—hepatocellular necrosis; infiltration of hepatic parenchyma with mononuclear cells, and spiral-shaped to curved bacteria predominantly in biliary canaliculi.

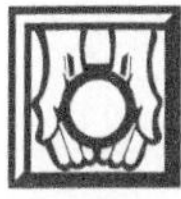

TREATMENT

APPROPRIATE HEALTH CARE

• Pathogenicity of *Helicobacter* spp. in dogs and cats is unclear; therefore, there are no generally accepted guidelines for treatment of HLO infections in dogs and cats. • Currently there is no indication for treating asymptomatic infected animals. • Eradication of gastric HLO should only be considered in infected dogs and cats that have compatible clinical signs that cannot be attributed to another disease process.

NURSING CARE

Fluid therapy in dehydrated patients.

HELICOBACTER SPP. (CONTINUED)

DIET

Easily digestible diets in patients with GI disease signs.

CLIENT EDUCATION

Explain difficulty of establishing a definitive diagnosis, high prevalence of infections with HLOs in normal dogs and cats, potential for recurrence, and zoonotic potential, though minimal, of these infections.

H

MEDICATIONS

- A triple therapy (combination of two antibiotics and one antisecretory drug) is effective in humans with *H. pylori* infection, with cure rates of approximately 90%.
- Combination therapy may eliminate *Helicobacter* spp. infections in dogs and cats less effectively than in humans. • Treat for 2–3 weeks.

DRUG(S) OF CHOICE

Antibiotics (Two Antibiotics with One Antisecretory Agent)

- Clarithromycin (dogs: 5 mg/kg PO q12h; cats: 62.5 mg/cat PO q12h). • Metronidazole (dogs: 11–15 mg/kg PO q12h; cats: 12.5 mg/kg PO q12h). • Amoxicillin (22 mg/kg PO q12h). • Azithromycin (5 mg/kg PO q24h). • Tetracycline (20 mg/kg PO q8h). • Bismuth subsalicylate has mucosal protectant, anti-endotoxemic, and weak antibacterial properties; it remains unclear which property is responsible for its beneficial effects in HLO infections (0.22 mL/kg of 130 mg/15 mL solution of Pepto-Bismol PO q4–6h).

Antisecretory Agents (One with Two Antibiotics)

- Omeprazole (0.7–1 mg/kg PO q12h).
- Famotidine (0.5 mg/kg PO q12–24h).
- Ranitidine (1–2 mg/kg PO q12h).

Intestinal and Hepatic Helicobacter spp. in Dogs

Combination of amoxicillin and metronidazole may be effective.

CONTRAINDICATIONS

Hypersensitivity to drug therapy.

ALTERNATIVE DRUG(S)

Patients with HLO infections and gastritis that do not respond to antibiotic therapy usually are given immunosuppressive therapy for inflammatory bowel disease with gastric involvement.

FOLLOW-UP

PATIENT MONITORING

- Serologic tests not useful to confirm eradication of gastric HLOs—serum IgG titers may not decrease for up to 6 months after infection cleared. • If vomiting persists or recurs after cessation of combination therapy, endoscopic biopsy to determine whether infection has been successfully eradicated indicated.

PREVENTION/AVOIDANCE

Avoid overcrowding and poor sanitation.

EXPECTED COURSE AND PROGNOSIS

- Efficacy of therapeutic regimens currently employed in dogs and cats for eradicating *Helicobacter* spp. infections is questionable.
- Metronidazole (20 mg/kg PO q12h), amoxicillin (20 mg/kg PO q12h), and famotidine (0.5 mg/kg PO q12h) for 14 days eradicated *Helicobacter* spp. in 6 of 8 dogs when evaluated 3 days post treatment; all dogs were recolonized by day 28 after treatment.
- Clarithromycin (30 mg/cat PO q12h), metronidazole (30 mg/cat PO q12h), ranitidine (20 mg/cat PO q12h), and bismuth subsalicylate (40 mg PO q12h) for 4 days were effective in eradicating *H. heilmannii* in 11 of 11 cats by 10 days; 2 cats were reinfected 42 days post treatment. • Amoxicillin (20 mg/kg PO q8h), metronidazole (20 mg/kg PO q8h), and omeprazole (0.7 mg/kg PO q24h) for 21 days transiently eradicated *H. pylori* in 6 cats; all were reinfected 6 weeks post treatment. (*Note:* this dose of metronidazole has potential for toxicity.)

MISCELLANEOUS

ASSOCIATED CONDITIONS

Other gastric diseases.

AGE-RELATED FACTORS

Gastric HLOs appear to be acquired at a young age.

ZOONOTIC POTENTIAL

- High prevalence of *Helicobacter* spp. in dogs and cats raises the possibility that household pets may serve as a reservoir for transmission of *Helicobacter* spp. to human beings. • *H. pylori*, *H. heilmannii*, and *H. felis* have been isolated from humans with gastritis. • *H. fennelliae* and *H. cinaedi* have been isolated from immunocompromised humans with proctitis and colitis.
- *H. cinaedi* and *H. canis* have been associated with septicemia in humans.
- *H. pylori* has not been identified in pet dogs or cats.

PREGNANCY/FERTILITY/BREEDING

Avoid metronidazole and tetracycline in pregnant animals.

SYNONYMS

- Gastric spiral bacterial. • Gastrospirillum.

SEE ALSO

- Gastritis, Chronic.
- Vomiting, Chronic.

ABBREVIATIONS

- GI = gastrointestinal.
- HLO = *Helicobacter*-like organism.
- Ig = immunoglobulin.
- SPF = specific pathogen free.

Suggested Reading

Leib MS, Duncan RB, Ward DL. Triple antimicrobial therapy and acid suppression in dogs with chronic vomiting and gastric *Helicobacter* spp. J Vet Intern Med 2007, 21:1185–1192.

Simpson KW, Neiger R, DeNovo R, et al. The relationship of *Helicobacter* spp. infection to gastric disease in dogs and cats. J Vet Intern Med 2000, 14:223–227.

Author Jan S. Suchodolski

Consulting Editor Amie Koenig

Acknowledgment The author and book editors acknowledge the prior contribution of Jörg M. Steiner.

Client Education Handout available online

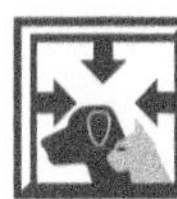

BASICS

OVERVIEW

• A soft tissue sarcoma (STS) arising around blood vessels in subcutaneous tissue. • Also known as perivascular wall tumor. • Locally invasive—microscopic disease often extending beyond gross visible tumor margins.
• Metastasizes in less than 15% of patients with grade I/II (low/intermediate-grade) STS and less than 44% of patients with grade III (high-grade) STS.

SIGNALMENT

• Common in dogs, rare in cats. • More common in large-breed than small-breed dogs. • Middle-aged to older dogs and cats.

SIGNS

Historical Findings

• Typically, slow-growing, nonpainful, fluctuant to firm mass (weeks to months).
• Rapid growth uncommon unless high-grade or associated with hemorrhage. • Local tumor growth can interfere with limb function.

Physical Examination Findings

• Subcutaneous soft tissue mass, more frequently located on extremity than on trunk. • Soft, fluctuant, or firm.
• Nonpainful unless ulcerated or invading into deeper structures (muscle, nerve, bone).
• Generally adhered to underlying tissue.
• Regional lymph node metastasis uncommon.

CAUSES & RISK FACTORS

Large-breed dogs at increased risk.

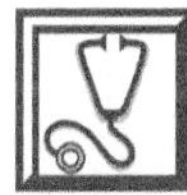

DIAGNOSIS

DIFFERENTIAL DIAGNOSIS

• Other sarcomas such as fibrosarcoma, peripheral nerve sheath tumor, myxosarcoma, malignant fibrous histiocytoma, histiocytic sarcoma, hemangiosarcoma. • Lipoma and other subcutaneous tumors—benign and malignant.

CBC/BIOCHEMISTRY/URINALYSIS

Usually normal.

IMAGING

• Thoracic radiographs recommended before treatment, although metastasis uncommonly identified. • Contrast-enhanced CT or MRI may be recommended to determine local extent of disease and optimize surgical treatment and radiation therapy planning.

DIAGNOSTIC PROCEDURES

• Fine-needle aspiration and cytology may provide tentative diagnosis, though cells do not exfoliate well given mesenchymal origin.
• Incisional biopsy and histopathology may be used to confirm diagnosis, determine grade of tumor, and plan treatment approach. • Immunohistochemistry evaluation of biopsy can aid in differentiation from other mesenchymal tumors. • Regional lymph node evaluation (cytology or histopathology) appropriate for high-grade tumors or if regional lymphadenomegaly detected.

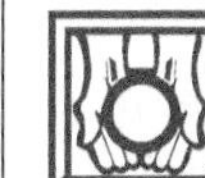

TREATMENT

Surgical Considerations

• Early, aggressive, en bloc surgical excision is treatment of choice. • Microscopically, cancer cells extend beyond gross tumor borders.
• Pseudocapsule composed of compressed cancer cells is common. • Excise tumor en bloc; if peeled out, healthy bed of cancer cells (pseudocapsule) is left as residual disease.
• Submit entire sample to pathologist for surgical margin evaluation; applying ink to surgical borders is advised. • Limb amputation may be necessary with tumors affecting appendicular extremities that may be otherwise unresectable. • Rib resection or abdominal wall resection may be required for tumors of trunk.

Radiation Therapy Considerations

• Adjuvant radiation therapy should be considered following either planned marginal resection or unplanned incomplete resection. • Radiation therapy most effective when directed at microscopic disease—either preoperatively or as postoperative full-course fractionated protocol. • As single modality treatment for macroscopic disease, radiation therapy considered palliative—may be used to decrease pain and slow tumor growth.

MEDICATIONS

DRUG(S) OF CHOICE

• Doxorubicin-based chemotherapy not consistently reported as beneficial, but remains recommended after excision of high-grade (grade III) tumor. • Low-dose chemotherapy (metronomic) with piroxicam and cyclophosphamide may help delay local recurrence when sarcoma incompletely resected. • Novel therapeutic options may be available—contact veterinary oncologist for potential updated treatments. • Analgesic therapy should be administered as needed if pain or discomfort present.

CONTRAINDICATIONS/POSSIBLE INTERACTIONS

N/A

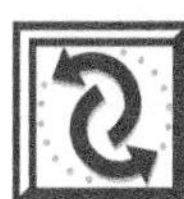

FOLLOW-UP

PATIENT MONITORING

• If complete surgical resection achievable and tumor categorized as low-grade, tumor regrowth or metastases unlikely and continued patient monitoring may not be necessity. • If surgical resection incomplete or tumor categorized as high-grade, further treatment should be considered and patient should be monitored for local regrowth and distant metastases, with repeat physical exam and thoracic radiographs every 3 months.

EXPECTED COURSE AND PROGNOSIS

• Local recurrence, metastasis, and overall survival time greatly affected by surgical margin assessment and histological grade. • Cure from disease possible when surgery aggressive and surgical margins tumor-free, especially with grade I and II tumors—median survival approaches 2 years with low-grade (I) STSs of extremities treated with surgery alone. • Local recurrence considered inevitable if treatment not aggressive; increased risk for metastatic disease especially with high-grade (III) tumors. • Long-term tumor control with radiation therapy after surgically debulking tumor gives 1–5-year control rates of 60–85%. • Incomplete surgical excision should be managed with either second aggressive surgery or radiation therapy as soon as possible; low-dosage chemotherapy (metronomic) is another option.

MISCELLANEOUS

ABBREVIATIONS

• STS = soft tissue sarcoma.

Suggested Reading

Bray JP. Soft tissue sarcoma in the dog – part 1: a current review. J Small Anim Pract 2016, 57:510–519.
Elmslie RE, Glawe P, Dow SW. Metronomic therapy with cyclophosphamide and piroxicam effectively delays tumor recurrence in dogs with incompletely resected soft tissue sarcomas. J Vet Intern Med 2008, 22:1373–1379.
Kuntz CA, Dernell WS, Poswers BE, et al. Prognostic factors for surgical treatment of soft tissue sarcomas in dogs: 75 cases (1986–1996). J Am Vet Med Assoc 1997, 211:1147–1151.
Stefanello D, Morello E, Roccabianca P, et al. Marginal excision of low-grade spindle cell sarcoma of canine extremities: 35 dogs (1996–2006). Vet Surg 2008, 37:461–465.

Author Matthew R. Berry
Consulting Editor Timothy M. Fan
Acknowledgement The author and book editors acknowledge the prior contributions of Phyllis Glawe and Louis-Philippe de Lorimier.

HEMANGIOSARCOMA, BONE

BASICS

OVERVIEW

• A highly metastatic malignant tumor of endothelial cell precursors. • Primary bone hemangiosarcoma (HSA) is rare and accounts for <5% of all canine bone tumors. • Can arise from various appendicular and axial sites—hind limb more common (78% tibial origin); rib most common axial location.

SIGNALMENT

• Dogs, rarely cats. • Typically middle-aged to older dogs, older cats. • Predisposition for male dogs. • Golden retrievers, Labrador retrievers, and German shepherds predisposed.

SIGNS

• Appendicular: ○ Pain/lameness. ○ Soft tissue swelling/mass effect. ○ Pathologic fracture. ○ Axial: ○ Thoracic wall mass. ○ Hemothorax. ○ Spinal pain. ○ Myelopathy (from vertebral body collapse, spinal cord compression).

CAUSES & RISK FACTORS

• Dogs—genetic abnormalities including inactivation of the tumor suppressor gene *PTEN*; overexpression of growth and apoptosis-related proteins RB, cyclin D1, Bcl2, and survivin; and overexpression of angiogenic factors such as vascular endothelial growth factor (VEGF) and angiopoietins.
• Cats—none identified.

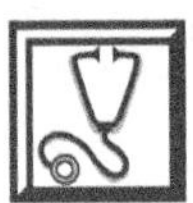

DIAGNOSIS

DIFFERENTIAL DIAGNOSIS

• *Radiography*—lesions may appear similar to other primary or metastatic bone tumors or osteomyelitis (bacterial or fungal).
• *Histopathology*—can be difficult to differentiate from telangiectatic subtype of osteosarcoma (OSA).

CBC/BIOCHEMISTRY/URINALYSIS

• Regenerative anemia. • Thrombocytopenia.
• Neutrophilic leukocytosis.

IMAGING

• *Musculoskeletal radiography*—may reveal poorly marginated osteolytic lesion, often with minimal periosteal reaction; pathologic fractures possible; can be difficult to differentiate primary vs. metastatic lesions.
• *Thoracic radiography*—used to screen for pulmonary metastasis, which typically appears as miliary to diffuse nodular pattern.
• *Abdominal and cardiac ultrasonography*—used to screen for primary and metastatic visceral tumors (spleen, liver, heart). • *CT scan*—can better define extent of bone tumor for surgical excision (especially axial lesions), more sensitive screening for pulmonary metastasis.

DIAGNOSTIC PROCEDURES

• Excisional biopsy is preferred method for diagnosis. • Incisional biopsy may yield a diagnosis, but due to the vascular nature of the tumor, blood contamination within the specimen may preclude a diagnosis or prevent differentiation between HSA and telangiectatic OSA.

PATHOLOGIC FINDINGS

• *Gross findings*—a dark, friable mass often within the medullary cavity of the bone; metastasis can be multifocal, including lungs, spleen, liver, kidneys, muscle, peritoneum.
• *Histopathology*—anaplastic mesenchymal cells arranged in chords forming vascular channels and spaces filled with red blood cells, thrombi, and necrotic debris.

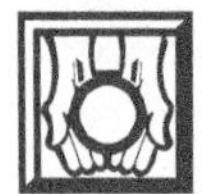

TREATMENT

• Wide margin surgical excision is treatment of choice. • Amputation recommended for appendicular lesions. • Axial tumors may be more difficult to resect. • Palliative (hypofractionated) radiation therapy may be used to control pain and swelling. • Adjuvant doxorubicin chemotherapy is indicated due to high metastatic potential.

MEDICATIONS

DRUG(S) OF CHOICE

• Doxorubicin—dogs: 30 mg/m^2 IV >15 kg; 1 mg/kg IV <15 kg, q2–3 weeks for 5 cycles; cats: 1 mg/kg IV q3 weeks for 5 cycles.
• Metronomic cyclophosphamide (12.5–15 mg/m^2 PO q24h) in combination with a nonsteroidal anti-inflammatory drugs (NSAID; e.g., piroxicam 0.3 mg/kg PO q24h) may be used concurrent to doxorubicin and/or as long-term maintenance therapy following doxorubicin. • Vincristine (0.5–0.7 mg/m^2) and cyclophosphamide (200–250 mg/m^2) q21 days can be used in rescue settings.

Alternative Drug(s)

• Bioactive extract (polysaccharide peptide) made from *Coriolus versicolor* mushroom may have benefit in dogs with HSA. • Chinese herbal remedy yunnan baiyao may have anti-bleeding and anti-neoplastic benefit for patients with has; however, was proven ineffective for HSA effusions.

CONTRAINDICATIONS/POSSIBLE INTERACTIONS

• Doxorubicin administration can lead to acute gastrointestinal, bone marrow, cardiac, renal, hypersensitivity, and extravasation toxicities. • Doxorubicin can lead to cumulative cardiotoxicity in dogs; dogs with preexisting cardiac disease or breeds at risk for dilated cardiomyopathy should be screened with echocardiogram/ECG before, during, and after treatment with doxorubicin.
• Metronomic cyclophosphamide can lead to sterile hemorrhagic cystitis in ~22–58% of dogs, but risk can be significantly reduced (<10%) with use of concurrent furosemide.
• NSAIDs can lead to gastrointestinal and liver/kidney toxicity.

FOLLOW-UP

PATIENT MONITORING

• Periodic physical examination, labwork, thoracic radiography, and abdominal ultrasonography during and after completion of therapy. • If treated with metronomic cyclophosphamide chemotherapy, monthly urinalysis recommended to screen for sterile hemorrhagic cystitis.

POSSIBLE COMPLICATIONS

• Pathologic fracture. • Bone lesions (esp. within rib) and visceral metastatic lesions may rupture, resulting in clinical signs related to effusion and/or anemia.

EXPECTED COURSE AND PROGNOSIS

• Aggressive disease with high risk for metastasis. • Less than 10% of patients survive 1 year following surgery alone.
• Treatment with amputation and chemotherapy is associated with median overall survival of ~10 months (range: 4 months–2 years). • Younger age and more aggressive treatment are associated with longer survival.

MISCELLANEOUS

ABBREVIATIONS

• HSA = hemangiosarcoma. • NSAID = nonsteroidal anti-inflammatory drug. • OSA = osteosarcoma. • VEGF = vascular endothelial growth factor.

Suggested Reading

Giuffrida MA, Kamstock DA, Selmic LE, et al. Primary appendicular hemangiosarcoma and telangiectatic osteosarcoma in 70 dogs: a Veterinary Society of Surgical Oncology retrospective study. Vet Surg 2018, 47:774–783.

Mullin CM, Clifford CS. Hemangiosarcoma. In: Withrow SJ, Vail DM, Thamm DH, Liptak J, eds. Small Animal Clinical Oncology, 6th ed. St. Louis, MO: Saunders/Elsevier, 2019, pp. 773–777.

Authors Christine Mullin and Craig A. Clifford
Consulting Editor Timothy M. Fan

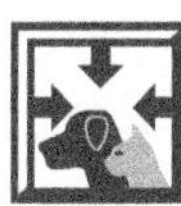

BASICS

OVERVIEW

• Highly metastatic malignant tumor of endothelial cell precursors • Most common cardiac tumor in dogs. • Can be primary or, less commonly, metastatic site. • Most tumors involve right atrium or right auricular appendage.

SIGNALMENT

• Dogs, rarely cats. • German shepherds, Labrador retrievers, golden retrievers predisposed. • Typically middle-aged to older animals. • Predisposition for male dogs.

SIGNS

• Signs most commonly related to pericardial effusion, cardiac tamponade, secondary right-sided congestive heart failure. • *Historical findings*—collapse, lethargy, weakness, exercise intolerance, anorexia, cough, dyspnea, vomiting. • *Physical examination findings*—muffled heart and lung sounds, arrhythmias, pulse deficits, pulsus paradoxus, pale mucous membranes, jugular vein distention, abdominal distension with effusion, hepatomegaly.

CAUSES & RISK FACTORS

Dogs—genetic abnormalities including inactivation of tumor suppressor gene *PTEN*; overexpression of growth and apoptosis-related proteins RB, cyclin D1, Bcl2, survivin; overexpression of angiogenic factors such as vascular endothelial growth factor (VEGF) and angiopoietins.

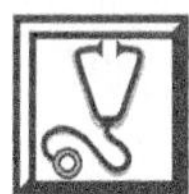

DIAGNOSIS

DIFFERENTIAL DIAGNOSIS

• Other cardiac neoplasia. • Idiopathic hemorrhagic pericardial effusion. • Other causes of right heart failure and arrhythmias.

CBC/BIOCHEMISTRY/URINALYSIS

• Regenerative anemia. • Thrombocytopenia. • Poikilocytosis—acanthocytes, schistocytes, spherocytes. • Neutrophilic leukocytosis.

OTHER LABORATORY TESTS

• Coagulation panel (prothrombin time [PT], partial thromboplastin time [PTT], D-dimers, fibrinogen)—criteria for disseminated intravascular coagulation (DIC) present in up to 50% of patients. • Plasma cardiac troponin (cTnI) levels elevated in dogs with pericardial effusion secondary to hemangiosarcoma (HSA) and can help differentiate from pericardial effusion not caused by HSA.

IMAGING

• *Thoracic radiography*—may reveal presence of globoid cardiac silhouette, pleural effusion, pulmonary metastasis, characterized by miliary to diffuse nodular pattern. • *Abdominal ultrasonography*—can screen for primary or metastatic hepatosplenic lesions, omental nodules, free abdominal fluid (hemoabdomen). • *Echocardiography*—useful for identifying and guiding removal of pericardial effusion and determining location and extent of tumor involvement (tumor better visualized when effusion present).

DIAGNOSTIC PROCEDURES

• Definitive diagnosis requires tissue biopsy. • Thoracoscopy can be used to perform pericardiectomy and obtain biopsies; thoracoscopic tumor resection also infrequently performed. • Cytologic evaluation of pericardial fluid rarely provides definitive diagnosis due to hemodilution and lack of tumor cell exfoliation. • ECG may reveal arrhythmias and electrical alternans.

PATHOLOGIC FINDINGS

• *Gross findings*—hemorrhagic friable mass in right side of heart; metastasis can be multifocal, including lungs, spleen, liver, kidneys, muscle, peritoneum. • *Histopathology findings*—anaplastic mesenchymal cells arranged in chords forming vascular channels and spaces filled with red blood cells, thrombi, necrotic debris.

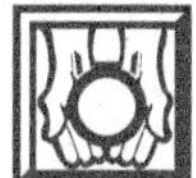

TREATMENT

• Periodic pericardiocentesis can provide temporary symptomatic relief from cardiac tamponade. • Thoracoscopic pericardectomy (pericardial window) can be performed as palliative procedure to lower risk of life-threatening cardiac tamponade. • Surgical tumor excision provides best chance of long-term tumor control, but restricted to tumors on atrial appendage and/or small areas of right atrial wall. • Use of doxorubicin chemotherapy in measurable disease setting associated with >40% objective tumor response rate and provides clinical benefit in almost 70%.

MEDICATIONS

DRUG(S) OF CHOICE

• Doxorubicin (30 mg/m^2 IV for dogs >15 kg; 1 mg/kg IV for dogs <15 kg) q2–3 weeks for 5 cycles. • Metronomic cyclophosphamide (12.5–15 mg/m^2 PO q24h) in combination with nonsteroidal anti-inflammatory drug (NSAID; e.g., piroxicam 0.3 mg/kg PO q24h) may be used concurrent to or as alternative to doxorubicin.

Alternative Drug(s)

Bioactive extract (polysaccharide peptide) from *Coriolus versicolor* mushroom may have benefit in dogs with HSA.

CONTRAINDICATIONS/POSSIBLE INTERACTIONS

• Doxorubicin administration can lead to acute gastrointestinal, bone marrow, cardiac, renal, hypersensitivity, extravasation toxicities. • Doxorubicin can lead to cumulative cardiotoxicity in dogs; those with preexisting cardiac disease or at risk for dilated cardiomyopathy should be screened with echocardiogram/ECG before, during, and after treatment with doxorubicin. • Metronomic cyclophosphamide can lead to sterile hemorrhagic cystitis in ~22–58% of dogs, but risk can be significantly reduced (<10%) with use of concurrent furosemide. • NSAIDs can lead to gastrointestinal toxicity and liver/kidney toxicity.

FOLLOW-UP

PATIENT MONITORING

• Periodic physical examination, labwork, thoracic radiography, abdominal ultrasonography during and after completion of therapy. • If treated with metronomic cyclophosphamide chemotherapy, monthly urinalysis recommended to screen for sterile hemorrhagic cystitis.

EXPECTED COURSE AND PROGNOSIS

• Prognosis guarded to poor, high risk of acute death due to cardiac tamponade or fatal arrhythmias. • Median survival ~2 weeks without treatment, ~4 months with doxorubicin, possibly longer if tumor resection performed.

MISCELLANEOUS

ABBREVIATIONS

• cTnI = cardiac troponin. • DIC = disseminated intravascular coagulation. • HSA = hemangiosarcoma. • NSAID = nonsteroidal anti-inflammatory drug. • PT = prothrombin time. • PTT = partial thromboplastin time. • VEGF = vascular endothelial growth factor.

Suggested Reading

Mullin CM, Arkans MA, Sammarco CD, et al. Doxorubicin chemotherapy for presumptive cardiac hemangiosarcoma in dogs. Vet Comp Oncol 2016, 14(4):e171–e183.

Mullin CM, Clifford CS. Hemangiosarcoma. In: Withrow SJ, Vail DM, Thamm DH, Liptak J, eds. Small Animal Clinical Oncology, 6th ed. St. Louis, MO: Saunders/Elsevier, 2019, pp. 773–777.

Authors Christine Mullin and Craig A. Clifford

Consulting Editor Timothy M. Fan

H

HEMANGIOSARCOMA, SKIN

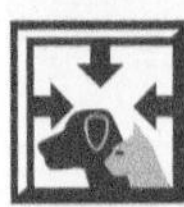

BASICS

DEFINITION

- A highly metastatic malignant tumor of endothelial cell precursors.
- Primary tumor develops within dermal or subcutaneous/intramuscular tissues.
- Accounts for ~14% of all hemangiosarcomas (HSAs) in dogs.
- Metastatic risk dependent upon grade and location within the tissues (stage).
- Subcutaneous/intramuscular lesions may represent metastasis from a primary visceral tumor.

SIGNALMENT

- Dogs and cats.
- Pit bulls, boxers, and German shepherds.
- Dermal hemangiosarcoma—whippet, greyhound, and related breeds.
- Median age 9 years.

SIGNS

Dermal

- Firm, raised, dark nodules on the limbs, head, face, nasal planum, ears, ventral abdomen, and inguinal region.
- When caused by UV radiation, lesions often appear as multiple small blood blisters on the ventral abdomen/inguinal region.

Subcutaneous/Intramuscular

- Usually solitary lesions.
- Firm to fluctuant masses with associated discoloration and/or bruising from intratumoral bleeding.
- Pelvic limbs are commonly affected, but tumors may arise in any location.
- In cats—the flank, ventral abdomen, inguinal region, and cervical region are most commonly affected sites.

CAUSES & RISK FACTORS

- Dermal HSA is associated with UV radiation via induction of actinic keratosis, especially along the ventral abdomen/inguinal region in sparsely haired and lightly pigmented dogs that sunbathe.
- Subcutaneous HSA may be secondary to prior ionizing radiation therapy.

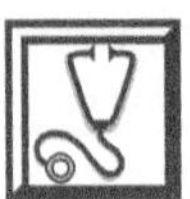

DIAGNOSIS

DIFFERENTIAL DIAGNOSIS

- Trauma-induced subcutaneous hematoma.
- Other sarcomas.
- Mast cell tumor.

CBC/BIOCHEMISTRY/URINALYSIS

- Regenerative anemia.
- Thrombocytopenia.
- Neutrophilic leukocytosis.

OTHER LABORATORY TESTS

Coagulation panel (prothrombin time [PT], partial thromboplastin time [PTT], D-dimers, fibrinogen)—may see changes compatible with disseminated intravascular coagulation (DIC) if large, bleeding subcutaneous/ intramuscular tumor.

IMAGING

- *Thoracic radiography*— used to screen for pulmonary metastasis, which typically appears as a miliary to diffuse nodular pattern.
- *Ultrasonography*—abdominal ultrasonography should be performed to screen for metastatic (or primary) hepatosplenic lesions, omental nodules, and free abdominal fluid (hemoabdomen); focal ultrasound of the mass may reveal cavitations.
- *Echocardiography*—can be used to identify right atrial masses.
- *Advanced imaging*—MRI/CT can be used for staging and surgical planning purposes, particularly for larger subcutaneous/ intramuscular tumors.

DIAGNOSTIC PROCEDURES

Cytology

- Often unrewarding due to insufficient cell numbers and blood contamination.
- Neoplastic cells are spindle to stellate with anisocytosis and anisokaryosis, single round, oval, pleomorphic nuclei with prominent nucleoli, low nuclear cytoplasmic ratio, and moderate to abundant basophilic and usually vacuolated cytoplasm.

PATHOLOGIC FINDINGS

- *Gross findings*—well-circumscribed, blood blister–like lesions confined to the dermis or more invasive, poorly circumscribed hemorrhagic tumors within the subcutaneous and intramuscular space; metastasis can be multifocal including lungs, spleen, liver, kidneys, muscle, peritoneum.
- *Histopathologic findings*—anaplastic mesenchymal cells arranged in chords forming vascular channels and spaces filled with red blood cells, thrombi, and necrotic debris.
    - o Allows differentiation between hemangioma and HSA and dermal versus subcutaneous/intramuscular origin.
    - o Immunohistochemistry for von Willebrand factor (factor VIII–related antigen) or CD31/platelet endothelial cell adhesion molecule (PECAM) can be used to confirm endothelial cell origin.

Histologic Staging System

- Stage I—confined to dermis.
- Stage II—subcutaneous involvement.
- Stage III—intramuscular involvement.

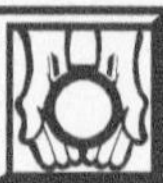

TREATMENT

- Wide margin surgical excision is the treatment of choice.
- Definitive radiation therapy may be used for the control of microscopic residual disease (incomplete margins after resection of subcutaneous/intramuscular tumors).
- Palliative (hypofractionated) radiation may be used for treatment of nonresectable tumors and ~60% of patients will have a positive response for a median of 3 months.
- Doxorubicin chemotherapy has been associated with a moderate response rate (~40%) for a median of ~2 months, but in some cases may allow for complete tumor resection and longer remission/survival.
- Metronomic (daily low-dose) chemotherapy can be used to delay time to locoregional recurrence after surgery given its anti-angiogenic effect.

MEDICATIONS

DRUG(S) OF CHOICE

- Doxorubicin—dogs: 30 mg/m^2 IV >15 kg; 1 mg/kg IV <15 kg, q2–3 weeks for 5 cycles; cats: 1 mg/kg IV q3 weeks for 5 cycles.
- Metronomic cyclophosphamide (12.5–15 mg/m^2 PO q24h) in combination with a nonsteroidal anti-inflammatory drug (NSAID; e.g., piroxicam 0.3 mg/kg PO q24h) may be used concurrent to doxorubicin and/or as a long-term maintenance therapy following doxorubicin.
- Vincristine (0.5–0.7 mg/m^2) and cyclophosphamide (200–250 mg/m^2) q21 days can be used in rescue settings.

CONTRAINDICATIONS

- Doxorubicin administration can lead to acute gastrointestinal, bone marrow, cardiac, renal, hypersensitivity, and extravasation toxicities.
- Doxorubicin can lead to cumulative cardiotoxicity in dogs; dogs with preexisting cardiac disease or those breeds at risk for dilated cardiomyopathy should be screened with echocardiogram/ECG before, during, and after treatment with doxorubicin.
- Metronomic cyclophosphamide can lead to sterile hemorrhagic cystitis in ~22–58% of dogs, but the risk can be significantly reduced (<10%) with the use of concurrent furosemide.
- NSAIDs can lead to gastrointestinal and liver/kidney toxicity.

ALTERNATIVE DRUG(S)

- A bioactive extract (polysaccharide peptide) made from the *Coriolus versicolor* mushroom may have benefit in dogs with HSA.

• The Chinese herbal remedy yunnan baiyao may have anti-bleeding and anti-neoplastic benefit for patients with HSA; however, this was proven ineffective for HSA effusions.

FOLLOW-UP

PATIENT MONITORING

• Periodic physical examination, labwork, thoracic radiography, and abdominal ultrasonography during and after completion of therapy.
• If treated with metronomic cyclophosphamide chemotherapy, monthly urinalysis recommended to screen for sterile hemorrhagic cystitis.

PREVENTION/AVOIDANCE

N/A

POSSIBLE COMPLICATIONS

Tumor hemorrhage.

EXPECTED COURSE AND PROGNOSIS

• Dermal HSA—prognosis very good with treatment; median survival time (MST) of 780–987 days for dogs undergoing surgery alone; disease-free interval >450 days for cats undergoing surgery alone.
• Higher risk of locoregional recurrence and distant metastasis with stage II (SC) and III (IM) HSA.
• Subcutaneous HSA—prognosis can be good with aggressive treatment; MST of 172 days for dogs undergoing surgery alone versus >1,100 days with surgery and adjuvant doxorubicin chemotherapy.
• Intramuscular HSA—MST of 272 days for dogs undergoing surgery and doxorubicin chemotherapy.

MISCELLANEOUS

ASSOCIATED CONDITIONS

Other UV-induced skin tumors such as squamous cell carcinoma.

PREGNANCY/FERTILITY/BREEDING

Chemotherapy drugs may be carcinogenic and mutagenic.

ZOONOTIC POTENTIAL

N/A

PREGNANCY/FERTILITY/BREEDING

Chemotherapy drugs may be carcinogenic and mutagenic.

ABBREVIATIONS

• DIC = disseminated intravascular coagulation.
• HSA = hemangiosarcoma.
• MST = median survival time.
• NSAIDs = nonsteroidal anti-inflammatory drugs.
• PECAM = platelet endothelial cell adhesion molecule.
• PT = prothrombin time.
• PTT = partial thromboplastin time.

Suggested Reading

Bulakowski EJ, Philibert JC, Siegel S, et al. Evaluation of outcome associated with subcutaneous and intramuscular hemangiosarcoma treated with adjuvant doxorubicin in dogs: 21 cases (2001–2006). J Am Vet Med Assoc 2008, 233:122–128.

Johannes CM, Henry CJ, Turnquist SE, et al. Hemangiosarcoma in cats: 53 cases (1992–2002). J Am Vet Med Assoc 2007, 231:1851–1856.

Mullin CM, Clifford CS. Hemangiosarcoma. In: Withrow SJ, Vail DM, Thamm DH, Liptak J, eds. Small Animal Clinical Oncology, 6th ed. St. Louis, MO: Saunders/Elsevier, 2019, pp. 773–777.

Ward H, Fox LE, Calderwood-Mays MB, et al. Cutaneous hemangiosarcoma in 25 dogs: a retrospective study. J Vet Intern Med 1994, 8:345–348.

Authors Christine Mullin and Craig A. Clifford

Consulting Editor Timothy M. Fan

HEMANGIOSARCOMA, SPLEEN AND LIVER

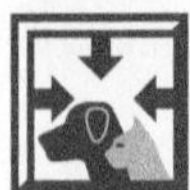

BASICS

DEFINITION

A highly metastatic malignant tumor of endothelial cell precursors.

PATHOPHYSIOLOGY

- Spleen is most common primary tumor location; liver is fourth most common location.
- Primary tumor rupture leads to acute hemorrhage, collapse, and often sudden death.
- Highly metastatic tumor that spreads early in the course of disease via hematogenous and intra-abdominal implantation routes.
- Metastasis can be to any organ including lungs, kidneys, muscle, peritoneum, omentum, lymph nodes, mesentery, adrenal glands, spinal cord, brain, subcutaneous tissue, and diaphragm.

SYSTEMS AFFECTED

- Cardiovascular.
- Hepatobiliary.
- Respiratory.
- Musculoskeletal.
- Nervous.
- Renal.

GENETICS

N/A

INCIDENCE/PREVALENCE

Accounts for 50–70% of all canine splenic tumors.

GEOGRAPHIC DISTRIBUTION

N/A

SIGNALMENT

- Dogs, rarely cats.
- German shepherd, Labrador retriever, golden retriever predisposed.
- Typically middle-aged to older animals.
- Possible slight predisposition for male dogs.

SIGNS

- *Historical findings*—can be variable and include weakness, lethargy, dyspnea, cough, inappetance, and weight loss.
- *Physical examination findings*—pale mucous membranes, arrhythmias, tachypnea, abdominal distension, and palpable cranial abdominal mass.

CAUSES

N/A

RISK FACTORS

- Dogs—genetic abnormalities including inactivation of the tumor suppressor gene *PTEN*; overexpression of growth and apoptosis-related proteins RB, cyclin D1, Bcl2, and survivin; and overexpression of angiogenic factors such as vascular endothelial growth factor (VEGF), endothlein-1, and angiopoietins.
- Cats—none identified.

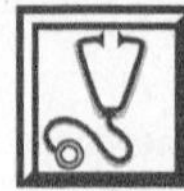

DIAGNOSIS

DIFFERENTIAL DIAGNOSIS

- Anticoagulant rodenticide ingestion.
- Other splenic and hepatic masses—hematoma, hemangioma, hepatoma, lymphoma, leiomyosarcoma, liposarcoma, splenic cyst, hepatocellular carcinoma, hepatic cyst, hepatic abscess.

CBC/BIOCHEMISTRY/URINALYSIS

- Regenerative anemia with nucleated red blood cells.
- Poikilocytosis—acanthocytes, schistocytes, spherocytes.
- Thrombocytopenia.
- Neutrophilic leukocytosis.
- Elevated liver enzymes.

OTHER LABORATORY TESTS

Coagulation panel (prothrombin time [PT], partial thromboplastin time [PTT], D-dimers, fibrinogen)—criteria for disseminated intravascular coagulation (DIC) present in up to 50% of patients.

IMAGING

Radiography

- Abdominal radiographs may identify a cranial abdominal mass and loss of serosal detail consistent with peritoneal effusion.
- Thoracic radiographs are used to screen for pulmonary metastasis, which typically appears as a miliary to diffuse nodular pattern.

Ultrasonography

- Abdominal ultrasonography is used for the detection of hepatosplenic lesions, omental nodules, and free abdominal fluid (hemoabdomen).
- Echocardiography is used to identify right atrial masses (better visualized when pericardial effusion is present).

Advanced Imaging

- MRI/CT provide high sensitivity and specificity in determining benign from malignant processes of the liver and spleen; more sensitive method of screening for metastasis.

DIAGNOSTIC PROCEDURES

- *Abdominocentesis*—usually a serosanguineous or hemorrhagic nonclotting effusion; can compare packed cell volume (PCV) of effusion to peripheral blood PCV to confirm hemorrhage.
- *Cytology*—often unrewarding due to insufficient cell numbers and blood contamination; neoplastic cells are spindle to stellate with anisocytosis and anisokaryosis, single round, oval, pleomorphic nuclei with prominent nucleoli, low nuclear cytoplasmic ratio, and moderate to abundant basophilic and usually vacuolated cytoplasm.

PATHOLOGIC FINDINGS

- *Gross findings*—solitary or multiple hemorrhagic, friable masses or nodules within the spleen and/or liver.
  - Stage I—tumor confined to one organ, no rupture.
  - Stage II—ruptured tumor.
  - Stage III—measurable metastatic disease.
- *Histopathology findings*— anaplastic mesenchymal cells arranged in chords forming vascular channels and spaces filled with red blood cells, thrombi, and necrotic debris; immunohistochemistry for von Willebrand factor (factor VIII–related antigen) or CD31/platelet endothelial cell adhesion molecule (PECAM) can be used to confirm endothelial cell origin.

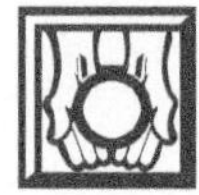

TREATMENT

APPROPRIATE HEALTH CARE

- Balanced isotonic electrolyte solutions ± colloids to correct hypovolemic shock and reduced cardiac output.
- Fresh whole blood or packed red blood cell transfusions to replace reduced oxygen-carrying capacity lost by acute hemorrhage.
- Fresh frozen plasma if coagulopathy or signs of DIC present.

NURSING CARE

N/A

ACTIVITY

N/A

DIET

N/A

CLIENT EDUCATION

N/A

SURGICAL CONSIDERATIONS

- Splenectomy or liver lobectomy is the standard of care surgical procedure and initial treatment of choice; removes macroscopic tumor burden and lessens the ongoing risk of acute death from hemorrhage.
- The use of adjuvant doxorubicin-based chemotherapy has been consistently shown to improve remission duration and survival times.
- Adjuvant metronomic chemotherapy appears to prolong survival vs. surgery alone. Added benefit when given concurrent to or following doxorubicin chemotherapy remains unclear.

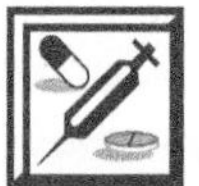

MEDICATIONS

DRUG(S) OF CHOICE

- Doxorubicin (30 mg/m^2 IV for dogs >15 kg, 1 mg/kg IV for dogs <15 kg, q2–3 weeks for 5 cycles) alone or as part of a

protocol with weekly vincristine (0.5–7 mg/m^2 IV) and cytoxan (250 mg/m^2 PO) or dacarbazine (200–250 mg/m^2 IV q24h for 5 days or 600–1000 mg/m^2 IV bolus q3 weeks)
• Metronomic cyclophosphamide (12.5–15 mg/m^2 PO q24h) in combination with a nonsteroidal anti-inflammatory drug (NSAID; e.g., piroxicam 0.3 mg/kg PO q24h) may be used concurrent to or as an alternative to doxorubicin.

CONTRAINDICATIONS

N/A

PRECAUTIONS

• Doxorubicin administration can lead to acute gastrointestinal, bone marrow, cardiac, renal, hypersensitivity, and extravasation toxicities.
• Doxorubicin can lead to cumulative cardiotoxicity in dogs; those with preexisting cardiac disease or breeds at risk for dilated cardiomyopathy should be screened with echocardiogram/ECG before, during, and after treatment with doxorubicin.
• Vincristine and dacarbazine administration can lead to acute gastrointestinal, bone marrow, and extravasation toxicities
• Metronomic cyclophosphamide can lead to sterile hemorrhagic cystitis in ~22–58% of dogs, but the risk can be significantly reduced (<10%) with the use of concurrent furosemide.
• NSAIDs can lead to gastrointestinal toxicity and liver/kidney toxicity.

POSSIBLE INTERACTIONS

N/A

ALTERNATIVE DRUG(S)

• A bioactive extract (polysaccharide peptide) made from the *Coriolus versicolor* mushroom may have benefit in dogs with hemangiosarcoma (HSA).
• The Chinese herbal remedy yunnan baiyao may have anti-bleeding and anti-neoplastic benefit for patients with HSA; however, this was proven ineffective for HSA effusions.

FOLLOW-UP

PATIENT MONITORING

• Periodic physical examination, labwork, thoracic radiography, and abdominal ultrasonography during and after the completion of therapy.
• If treated with metronomic chemotherapy, routine monthly urinalysis recommended to screen for sterile hemorrhagic cystitis.

PREVENTION/AVOIDANCE

N/A

POSSIBLE COMPLICATIONS

Death due to acute hemorrhage or fatal tachyarrhythmias.

EXPECTED COURSE AND PROGNOSIS

• Prognosis poor to grave.
• Less than 10% of dogs will live 1 year or longer from diagnosis.
• Median survival time with surgery alone (dogs): 1–3 months.
• Median survival time with surgery plus chemotherapy (dogs): 4.5–8 months.

MISCELLANEOUS

ASSOCIATED CONDITIONS

N/A

AGE-RELATED FACTORS

N/A

ZOONOTIC POTENTIAL

N/A

PREGNANCY/FERTILITY/BREEDING

Chemotherapy drugs may be carcinogenic and mutagenic.

SYNONYMS

N/A

ABBREVIATIONS

• DIC = disseminated intravascular coagulation.
• HSA = hemangiosarcoma.
• NSAIDs = nonsteroidal anti-inflammatory drugs.
• PCV = packed cell volume.
• PECAM = platelet endothelial cell adhesion molecule.
• PT = prothrombin time.
• PTT = partial thromboplastin time.
• VEGF = vascular endothelial growth factor.

Suggested Reading

Alvarez FJ, Hosoya K, Lara-Garcia A, et al. VAC protocol for treatment of dogs with stage III hemangiosarcoma. J Am Anim Hosp 2013, 49:370–377.

Finotello R, Stefanello D, Zini E, et al. Comparison of doxorubicin-cyclophosphamide with doxorubicin-dacarbazine for the adjuvant treatment of canine hemangiosarcoma. Vet Comp Oncol 2017, 15:25–35.

Mullin CM, Clifford CS. Hemangiosarcoma. In: Withrow SJ, Vail DM, Thamm DH, Liptak J, eds. Small Animal Clinical Oncology, 6th ed. St. Louis, MO: Saunders/Elsevier, 2019, pp. 773–777.

Authors Christine Mullin and Craig A. Clifford

Consulting Editor Timothy M. Fan

HEMATEMESIS

BASICS

DEFINITION

Vomiting of blood.

PATHOPHYSIOLOGY

A disruption in the gastric or upper small intestinal mucosal barrier leading to inflammation and bleeding. Coagulopathies can also present with hematemesis. An animal may also vomit blood that originated in the oral cavity or respiratory system and was swallowed.

SYSTEMS AFFECTED

• Gastrointestinal (GI)—inflammation, trauma, ulceration, neoplasia, and/or foreign body in oral cavity, pharyngeal area, esophagus, stomach, and/or duodenum. • Cardiovascular—acute, severe hemorrhage may result in tachycardia and hypotension. • Hematologic—coagulopathy with GI hemorrhage can lead to hematemesis. • Respiratory—respiratory hemorrhage with ingestion can lead to hematemesis.

GENETICS

N/A

INCIDENCE/PREVALENCE

Unknown

SIGNALMENT

Species

Dog and cat.

Breed Predilections

None

Mean Age and Range

Any age.

Predominant Sex

Male dogs have increased incidence of gastric carcinoma.

SIGNS

Historical Findings

• Vomiting with blood, which may appear as fresh blood, blood clots, or digested blood (looks like coffee grounds). • Melena.
• Anorexia. • Abdominal pain.

Physical Examination Findings

• Abdominal pain. • Melena. • If patient is anemic—tachycardia, heart murmur, pallor, weakness.

CAUSES

Coagulopathies

• Thrombocytopenia. • Thrombocytopathia.
• Von Willebrand's disease. • Hyperviscosity syndrome. • Disseminated intravascular coagulation. • Anticoagulant rodenticide toxicity. • Coagulation factor deficiency.
• Liver failure.

Drugs

Nonsteroidal anti-inflammatory drugs (NSAIDs), glucocorticoids, toceranib phosphate.

GI Diseases

• Inflammatory bowel disease. • Gastric or duodenal neoplasia. • Gastric or duodenal foreign body. • Gastric or intestinal volvulus.
• Hemorrhagic gastroenteritis. • Gastroduodenal ulcer. • Gastroesophageal intussusception.

Toxicity

• Heavy metal poisoning (arsenic, zinc, thallium, iron, or lead). • Plant intoxication (dieffenbachia, sago palm, mushroom, castor bean). • Chemical intoxication (phenol, ethylene glycol, corrosive agents, psoriasis creams—vitamin D analogues). • Pesticide/rodenticide toxicity (cholecalciferol). • Snake bite. • Aflatoxins. • Bee sting.

Infectious Diseases

• GI parasitism. • Pythiosis. • Viral, fungal, or bacterial gastroenteritis. • Virulent systemic feline calicivirus. • Rickettsial infections.

Metabolic Diseases

• Renal failure. • Liver disease. • Hypoadrenocorticism. • Pancreatitis.

Neoplasia

• Mastocytosis. • Gastrinoma. • Oral, nasal, respiratory, or GI tumors. • Amine precursor uptake decarboxylase cells (APUDomas).

Neurologic Diseases

• Head trauma. • Spinal cord disease.

Respiratory Diseases

• Nasal disease. • Pulmonary disease.
• Mediastinal neoplasia.

Stress/Major Medical Illness

• Shock. • Severe illness. • Burns. • Heat stroke. • Major surgery. • Sustained strenuous exercise. • Trauma. • Systemic hypertension. • Thromboembolic disease.
• Hypotension.

RISK FACTORS

• Administration of ulcerogenic drugs.
• Critically ill patients. • Shock. • Thrombocytopenia. • Concurrent administration of NSAIDs and glucocorticoids.

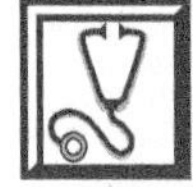

DIAGNOSIS

DIFFERENTIAL DIAGNOSIS

• Hemoptysis—thoracic radiographs may reveal presence of pulmonary disease.
• Regurgitation or vomiting of swallowed blood from extra-GI diseases (e.g., oropharyngeal, nasopharyngeal, cutaneous).
• Vomiting materials that look like fresh or digested blood (e.g., oral iron).

CBC/BIOCHEMISTRY/URINALYSIS

• If acute (3–5 days) blood loss—nonregenerative anemia. • If blood loss >5–7 days in duration—regenerative anemia. • If chronic blood loss—iron-deficiency anemia (microcytic, hypochromic, variable reticulocytosis, with or without thrombocytosis). • ± thrombocytopenia.
• ± panhypoproteinemia. • ± mature neutrophilia or left-shift neutrophilia with sepsis and/or gastroduodenal ulcer perforation. • Blood urea nitrogen (BUN) : creatinine ratio may be elevated with GI hemorrhage.

OTHER LABORATORY TESTS

• Fecal occult blood test—often false positive if not on nonmeat diet for 3 days prior to test.
• Fecal flotation—screen for GI parasitism.
• Coagulation profile—if coagulopathy is suspected. • Bile acids—if liver disease is suspected. • Adrenocorticotropic hormone (ACTH) stimulation—if hypoadrenocorticism suspected.

IMAGING

• Abdominal radiographs may identify gastric or duodenal foreign body or mass, pneumoperitoneum, effusion, or changes consistent with kidney, pancreas, or liver disease. • Thoracic radiographs may reveal esophageal foreign body or mass, gastroesophageal intussusception, mediastinal mass, pulmonary disease, or pulmonary metastasis. • Abdominal ultrasonography may identify gastric or duodenal mass, gastric or duodenal wall thickening or altered layering, gastric ulcer, and/or abdominal lymphadenopathy. • Abdominal ultrasonography can also screen for abnormalities in pancreas, liver, kidneys, and other abdominal organs as source of hematemesis. • GI scintigraphy may be used to localize blood loss.

DIAGNOSTIC PROCEDURES

• Endoscopy to evaluate mucosal appearance of esophagus, stomach, and upper small intestinal tract once extra-GI causes ruled out. • Capsule endoscopy may be useful to identify sites of GI hemorrhage. • Biopsy mucosal lesions to determine nature of underlying GI disease. • Abdominocentesis may identify septic peritonitis. • Fine-needle aspirates or biopsy of organs or masses to identify neoplasia/disease.

PATHOLOGIC FINDINGS

• Gastroduodenal inflammation and hemorrhage. • Ulcers may have necrosis, microthrombi, and hemorrhage.

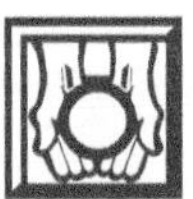

TREATMENT

APPROPRIATE HEALTH CARE

• Treat underlying cause. • Outpatient—those in which the cause is identified and removed, vomiting is not excessive, and gastroduodenal bleeding is minimal.
• Inpatients—those with severe gastroduodenal bleeding, ulcer perforation, excessive vomiting, and/or shock.

NURSING CARE

• IV fluids to maintain volume and hydration. • Hypoproteinemic patients may require colloids and/or albumin to increase oncotic pressure. • Anemic or coagulopathic patients may require transfusion. • In severe cases—to stop the GI bleeding, ice water lavage (10–20 mL/kg remaining in stomach for 15–30 min) or lavage with norepinephrine (8 mg/500 mL) diluted in ice water can be attempted.

ACTIVITY

Restriction is indicated until resolution.

DIET

• Discontinue oral intake if vomiting. • When feeding is resumed, feed small, frequent meals.

CLIENT EDUCATION

• NSAIDs should be administered to pets only under the guidance of a veterinarian. • NSAIDs and glucocorticoids should not be administered together. • Adverse effects of NSAIDs can be reduced by giving drug with food and concurrent administration of a synthetic prostaglandin E_1 analogue (e.g., misoprostol).

SURGICAL CONSIDERATIONS

Surgery is indicated if medical treatment fails after 5–7 days, hemorrhage is uncontrolled, gastroduodenal ulcer perforates, and/or potentially resectable tumor is identified.

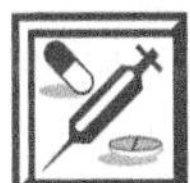

MEDICATIONS

DRUG(S) OF CHOICE

• Proton pump inhibitors (PPIs)—most potent inhibitors of gastric acid secretion and treatment of choice for gastroduodenal ulcer (dog and cat: omeprazole 1 mg/kg PO q12h; pantoprazole or esomeprazole 1 mg/kg IV q12h - esomeprazole may be superior for first 72 hours of therapy. • Histamine (H2) receptor antagonists also inhibit gastric acid secretion (dog and cat: famotidine 0.5–1 mg/kg PO/IV q12–24h); famotidine with a loading dose of 1 mg/kg followed by 8 mg/kg IV CRI daily for 3 consecutive days may be superior to pantoprazole. • H2 receptor antagonists are less potent than PPIs. • Sucralfate suspension (dog and cat: 0.25–1 g PO q6–8h) protects ulcerated tissue by binding to ulcer sites, adsorbing pepsin and bile salts, and stimulating prostaglandin synthesis; binding is greater in duodenal than gastric ulcers. • Antibiotic(s) with activity against enteric Gram-negative bacteria and anaerobes should be given parenterally if a break in GI mucosal barrier is suspected or aspiration pneumonia is present. • Antiemetics—dog and cat: chlorpromazine 0.5 mg/kg q6–8h SC/IM/IV, prochlorperazine 0.1–0.5 mg/kg q6–8h SC/IM, ondansetron 0.2–0.5 mg/kg IV q12h, maropitant 1 mg/kg SC/IV q24h; dog: metoclopramide 1–2 mg/kg/24h CRI, administered if vomiting occurs frequently or results in significant fluid losses.

CONTRAINDICATIONS

Avoid ulcerogenic drugs such as NSAIDs and corticosteroids.

PRECAUTIONS

Continued famotidine therapy can lead to tachyphylaxis.

POSSIBLE INTERACTIONS

• H2 blockers prevent uptake of omeprazole by oxyntic cells. • Sucralfate may alter absorption of other drugs and should be given 2 hours before or after other oral drugs. • Antacids may alter oral absorption and renal elimination of other drugs.

ALTERNATIVE DRUG(S)

Misoprostol, synthetic prostaglandin analogue (3 µg/kg PO q12h) with antisecretory and cytoprotective actions helps prevent NSAID-induced ulcers. There may be some efficacy in treating gastroduodenal ulcerations from other causes.

FOLLOW-UP

PATIENT MONITORING

• Improvement in some cases may be assessed on resolution of clinical signs; packed cell volume, total protein, fecal occult blood, and BUN may help detect continued blood loss. • Depending on the underlying cause of the hematemesis, specific laboratory or imaging tests may be necessary to monitor response to therapy.

PREVENTION/AVOIDANCE

• Avoid gastric irritants (e.g., NSAIDs, corticosteroids). • Concurrent use of misoprostol or PPI with NSAIDs; PPIs may be preferable because they are therapeutic as well. • Administer NSAIDs with food. • Cyclooxygenase (COX)-2 selective or dual lipoxygenase/COX inhibitors may have fewer adverse GI effects than nonselective NSAIDs.

POSSIBLE COMPLICATIONS

• Anemia. • Hypovolemia. • Ulcer perforation. • Sepsis.

EXPECTED COURSE AND PROGNOSIS

• Varies with underlying cause. • Patients with malignant gastric neoplasia, renal failure, liver failure, pythiosis, systemic mastocytosis, sepsis, and/or gastric perforation—guarded to poor prognosis. • Hematemesis secondary to NSAID administration, coagulopathies, inflammatory bowel disease, or hypoadrenocorticism—prognosis may be good to excellent, depending on severity of disease. • Hematemesis secondary to heat stroke, toxicities, and snake bites can have variable prognoses.

MISCELLANEOUS

ASSOCIATED CONDITIONS

Anemia

PREGNANCY/FERTILITY/BREEDING

Synthetic prostaglandins (e.g., misoprostol) cause abortion.

SEE ALSO

• Gastroduodenal Ulceration/Erosion. • Gastroenteritis, Acute Hemorrhagic Diarrhea Syndrome. • Melena.

ABBREVIATIONS

• ACTH = adrenocorticotropic hormone. • APUDoma = amine precursor uptake decarboxylase cells. • BUN = blood urea nitrogen. • COX = cyclooxygenase. • GI = gastrointestinal. • NSAID = nonsteroidal anti-inflammatory drug. • PPI = proton pump inhibitor.

Suggested Reading

Case V. Melena and hematochezia. In: Ettinger SJ, Feldman EC, eds. Textbook of Veterinary Internal Medicine Diseases of the Dog and Cat, 7th ed. St. Louis, MO: Saunders Elsevier, 2010, pp. 203–206.

Kuhl A, Odunayo A, Price J, et al. Comparative analysis of the effect of IV administered acid suppressants on gastric pH in dogs. J Vet Intern Med.2020:1–6. https://doi.org/10.1111/jvim.15718

Neiger R. Gastric ulceration. In: Bongura JD, Twedt DC, eds. Kirk's Current Veterinary Therapy XV. St. Louis, MO: Elsevier Saunders, 2014, e251–e255.

Tolbert K, Bissett S, King A, et al. Efficacy of oral famotidine and 2 omeprazole formulations for the control of intragastric pH in dogs. J Vet Intern Med 2011, 25:47–54.

Tolbert K, Odunayo A, Howell RS, et al. Efficacy of intravenous administration of combined acid suppressants in healthy dogs. J Vet Intern Med 2015, 29:556–560.

Author Jocelyn Mott
Consulting Editor Mark P. Rondeau

HEMATURIA

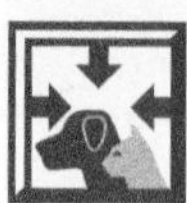

BASICS

DEFINITION

Blood in urine.

PATHOPHYSIOLOGY

Secondary to loss of endothelial integrity in urinary tract, clotting factor deficiency, or thrombocytopenia/cytopathia.

SYSTEMS AFFECTED

• Renal/urologic. • Reproductive. • Hemic/lymphatic/immune.

SIGNALMENT

• Dog and cat. • Familial hematuria in young animals; neoplasia in older animals. • Females at greater risk for urinary tract infection (UTI).

SIGNS

Historical Findings

Red-tinged urine with or without pollakiuria.

Physical Examination Findings

• Palpable mass in patients with neoplasia.
• Abdominal pain in some patients.
• Enlarged and/or painful prostate gland in males. • Petechiae or ecchymoses in patients with coagulopathy.

CAUSES

Systemic

• Coagulopathy. • Thrombocytopenia.
• Vasculitis.

Upper Urinary Tract

• Anatomic—cystic kidney disease and familial malformations. • Metabolic—nephrolithiasis. • Neoplastic—renal lymphoma, adenocarcinoma, and hemangiosarcoma. • Infectious—leptospirosis, feline infectious peritonitis (FIP), and bacterial or fungal UTI.
• Inflammatory—glomerulonephritis.
• Idiopathic renal hematuria. • Trauma.

Lower Urinary Tract

• Anatomic—bladder malformations.
• Metabolic—uroliths. • Neoplasia—transitional cell carcinoma and lymphosarcoma.
• Infectious—bacterial, fungal, and viral UTI. • Idiopathic—cats (idiopathic cystitis).
• Traumatic. • Cyclophosphamide-induced hemorrhagic cystitis.

Genitalia

• Metabolic—estrus, benign prostatic hyperplasia. • Neoplastic—transmissible venereal tumor (TVT), leiomyoma, and prostatic adenocarcinoma. • Infectious—bacterial and fungal disease. • Inflammatory—prostatitis. • Trauma.

RISK FACTORS

Breed predisposed to urolithiasis, coagulopathy, or neoplasia.

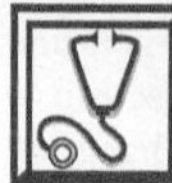

DIAGNOSIS

See Figure 1.

DIFFERENTIAL DIAGNOSIS

Other causes of discolored urine (myoglobinuria, hemoglobinuria, and bilirubinuria).

LABORATORY FINDINGS

Drugs That May Alter Laboratory Results

Substantial doses of vitamin C (ascorbic acid) may cause false-negative reagent test strip results; newer generations of reagent strips are more resistant to interference by reducing substances such as ascorbic acid.

Disorders That May Alter Laboratory Results

• Common urine reagent strip tests for blood are designed to detect red blood cells, hemoglobin, or myoglobin. • Low urine specific gravity (polyuric syndromes) lyses red blood cells (RBCs). • Bacteriuria (bacterial peroxidase) causes false-positive reagent test strip results. • Formalin preservative causes false-negative reagent test strip results.

Valid if Run in a Human Laboratory?

Yes

CBC/BIOCHEMISTRY/URINALYSIS

• Thrombocytopenia and severe anemia in some patients. • Azotemia in some patients with bilateral renal disease. • RBCs (>5–10 RBC/hpf) and possibly infectious agents seen in urine sediment. • Crystalluria in some patients with urolithiasis.

OTHER LABORATORY TESTS

• Coagulation testing to rule out coagulopathy.
• Bacterial culture of urine to identify UTI.
• Examination of ejaculate to identify prostatic disease.

IMAGING

Ultrasonography, radiography, and possibly contrast radiography are useful in localizing the underlying cause. Cystoscopy often required to diagnose renal hematuria.

DIAGNOSTIC PROCEDURES

• Biopsy of mass lesion.
• Vaginourethrocystoscopy in females or urethrocystoscopy in males and females.

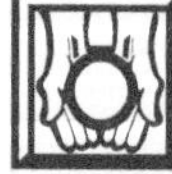

TREATMENT

• Hematuria may indicate a serious disease process. • Urolithiasis and renal failure may require diet modification. • UTI may be associated with another disease that also requires treatment—local (e.g., neoplasia and urolithiasis) or systemic (e.g., hyperadrenocorticism and diabetes mellitus). • Renal hematuria may be treated via endoscopic sclerotherapy; nephrectomy should not be performed.

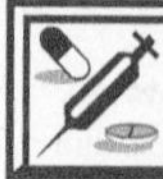

MEDICATIONS

DRUG(S) OF CHOICE

• Blood transfusion if patient is severely anemic. • Antibiotics to treat UTI and septicemia. • Heparin for disseminated intravascular coagulation (DIC).

CONTRAINDICATIONS

Immunosuppressive drugs, except to treat immune-mediated disease.

POSSIBLE INTERACTIONS

Intravenous contrast media may cause acute kidney injury.

FOLLOW-UP

PATIENT MONITORING

Depends on primary or associated diseases.

POSSIBLE COMPLICATIONS

• Anemia. • Hypovolemia if severe hemorrhage. • Ureteral or urethral obstruction due to blood clots.

MISCELLANEOUS

AGE-RELATED FACTORS

• Neoplasia tends to occur in older animals.
• Immune-mediated diseases tend to occur in young adult animals.

ZOONOTIC POTENTIAL

Leptospirosis

SEE ALSO

• Coagulation Factor Deficiency. • Crystalluria.
• Cylindruria. • Dysuria, Pollakiuria, and Stranguria. • Feline Idiopathic Lower Urinary Tract Disease. • Glomerulonephritis.
• Hemoglobinuria and Myoglobinuria.
• Lower Urinary Tract Infection, Bacterial.
• Lower Urinary Tract Infection, Fungal.
• Nephrolithiasis. • Prostatitis and Prostatic Abscess. • Prostatomegaly. • Proteinuria.
• Pyelonephritis. • Thrombocytopenia.

ABBREVIATIONS

• DIC = disseminated intravascular coagulation.
• FIP = feline infectious peritonitis. • RBC = red blood cell. • TVT= transmissible venereal tumor. • UTI = urinary tract infection.

Suggested Reading

Bartges JW. Discolored urine. In: Ettinger SJ, Feldman EC, eds., Textbook of Veterinary Internal Medicine, 7th ed. St. Louis, MO: Elsevier, 2008, pp. 164–168.

Author Joseph W. Bartges
Consulting Editor J.D. Foster

Client Education Handout available online

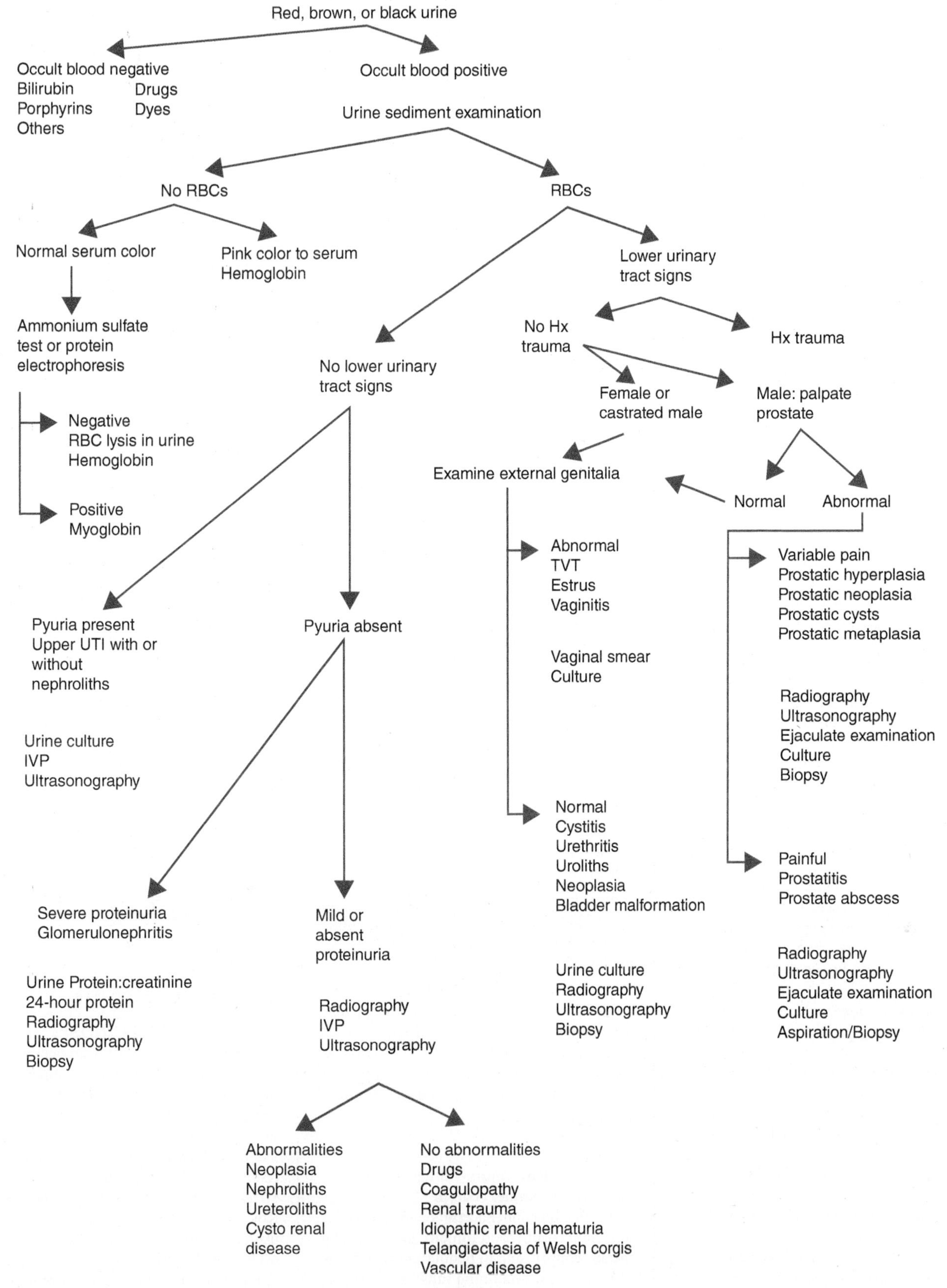

Figure 1.

Algorithm for the diagnosis of red, brown, or black urine.

HEMOGLOBINURIA AND MYOGLOBINURIA

BASICS

DEFINITION

Hemoglobinuria—presence of free hemoglobin (HGB) within urine secondary to intravascular hemolysis. Myoglobinuria—presence of myoglobin (MGB) within urine secondary to myocyte injury or death. Presence of either protein causes discoloration of urine (pigmenturia) as well as positive blood result during reagent test strip analysis of urine, a semiquantitative measurement of heme.

H

PATHOPHYSIOLOGY

- *Hemoglobinuria*—intravascular hemolysis or destruction of RBCs within vessels releases HGB from damaged red blood cells (RBCs). HGB, if free within plasma, can cause tissue injury. Haptoglobin, protein made by the liver, acts as HGB recovery system and binds free HGB. Resulting HGB–haptoglobin complexes too large to be cleared by glomerular filtration and so are removed primarily by splenic macrophages. Excessive intravascular hemolysis can saturate haptoglobin, resulting in free HGB in plasma, known as hemoglobinemia. Free HGB (4 heme-containing chains, 64,000 daltons) rapidly dissociates into unstable dimers (32,000 daltons) and passes freely through glomerular basement membrane leading to hemoglobinuria. Hemoglobinuria imparts pink, dark amber, red, or red-brown discoloration to urine. Methemoglobinemia causes analogous disease process.
- *Myoglobinuria*—MGB is single heme-containing chain (approximately 17,500 daltons). MGB able to carry oxygen without oxidation of ferrous (Fe^{2+}) to ferric (Fe^{3+}) iron due to interaction of heme with protein portion (globin). Myocyte injury and/or death releases MGB. Unlike free HGB, MGB is freely and rapidly cleared by glomerulus given its small size and absence of carrier protein, so plasma remains colorless even in face of significant myocyte death. Myoglobinuria causes brown or red-brown discoloration to urine.
- *Renal tubular injury*—presence of excess HGB or MGB in renal tubular fluid may result in kidney injury. Within tubules, acidic environment favors HGB or MGB precipitation, cast formation, and tubular obstruction. Both HGB and MGB are endocytosed by renal tubular epithelial cells. Globin, from HGB, is degraded within the cell, while free heme is catabolized by heme oxygenase, resulting in lipid peroxidation and Fe deposition. MGB also causes lipid peroxidation, but without release of free iron (via redox cycling of heme center). Alkaline conditions reported to prevent MGB-induced lipid peroxidation by stabilizing reactive ferryl MGB complex and also decreasing MGB precipitation in renal tubules. Free HGB also scavenges nitric oxide, leading to vasoconstriction of afferent renal arteriole and secondary hypoperfusion and ischemic injury.

SYSTEMS AFFECTED

Renal/urologic—HGB, methemoglobin, and MGB can result in tubular injury, especially with concurrent decreased renal perfusion and acidic conditions.

GENETICS

Some predispositions relating to breeds; see Signalment.

INCIDENCE/PREVALENCE

N/A

GEOGRAPHIC DISTRIBUTION

N/A

SIGNALMENT

Dog

- Hemoglobinuria secondary to phosphofructokinase (PFK) deficiency in affected English springer spaniel, American cocker spaniel, English cocker spaniel, cocker spaniel, wachtelhund, whippet.
- Hemoglobinuria uncommonly seen in Bedlington terriers with inherited copper toxicosis and copper release from hepatocytes causing hemolysis.
- Myoglobinuria secondary to exertional myopathy or rhabdomyolysis in racing sled dogs and greyhounds.
- Pigmenturia rarely reported secondary to exertional lactic acidosis in English sheepdog.

Cat

Hemoglobinuria secondary to neonatal isoerythrolysis in neonatal blood type A or AB kittens born to blood type B queens.

SIGNS

General Comments

Clinical signs diverse and related to specific causes; see Causes.

Historical Findings

Patient breed, exposure to certain drugs or foreign objects, and recent exertion particularly important; see Causes.

Physical Examination Findings

- Findings associated with hemolytic anemia may include pale mucous membranes, tachycardia, icterus.
- Findings associated with muscle damage may include muscle tenderness, swelling, bruising.

CAUSES

Hemoglobinuria

- Oxidative RBC injury—drugs (acetaminophen, benzocaine, vitamin K_3, new methylene blue, phenacetin, phenazopyridine, monensin); food (onions, garlic); heavy metals (copper, zinc in pennies minted before 1982 and zinc-containing sunscreens, diaper cream, hardware or toys).
- Physical RBC injury—severe burns, heat stroke, crush injury, electric shock, IV hypotonic fluid administration, shearing or microangiopathy due to disseminated intravascular coagulopathy, *D. immitis* caval syndrome.
- Toxin-induced RBC membrane damage—snake or spider venom; *Shiga* toxin in hemolytic uremic syndrome.
- Infection of RBCs—dogs: babesiosis; cats: *Mycoplasma hemofelis* infection, *Cytauxzoon felis*.
- Systemic infection—leptospirosis, *E. coli* or other *Shiga* toxin-producing bacteria causing hemolytic uremic syndrome, bacterial endocarditis.
- Immune-mediated RBC destruction—idiopathic or secondary immune-mediated hemolytic anemia, incompatible blood transfusions in dogs or cats, neonatal isoerythrolysis.
- Deficiencies—hypophosphatemia.
- Genetic associated—PFK deficiency, copper toxicity.
- Other—retroperitoneal hemorrhage, transfusion of inappropriately stored RBC units.

Myoglobinuria

- Exertional—extreme exercise.
- Myositis—infectious (e.g., toxoplasmosis, neosporosis), eosinophilic inflammatory (German shepherd dog, other breeds), immune mediated.
- Genetics-associated—X-linked muscular dystrophy; glycogenoses (storage diseases); mitochondrial abnormalities.
- Toxins (loss of membrane integrity)—snake or spider venom.
- Physical—ischemia, crush injury, compartment syndrome.
- Excessive body temperature (e.g., heat stroke, prolonged seizures).

RISK FACTORS

- Genetic predisposition (see Signalment).
- Exposure to specific drugs, toxins.
- Certain infectious agents.
- Extreme physical exertion.
- Heat stroke.
- Snake or spider venom.

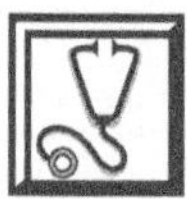

DIAGNOSIS

DIFFERENTIAL DIAGNOSIS

- Pigmenturia can result from hematuria, hemoglobinuria, methemoglobinuria, or myoglobinuria. Positive heme reaction of urine reagent test strip detects heme portion in intact RBCs, free HGB, and free MGB. Use of CBC, biochemical, and urinalysis results can aid in differentiation.
- Hematuria—supported by increased (>5/hpf) RBCs in urine sediment examination and clear plasma or serum.
- Hemoglobinuria—supported by <5/hpf RBCs in urine sediment, red or pink plasma or serum, indicating hemoglobinemia, anemia, RBC inclusions, or poikilocytes, supporting cause for hemolytic anemia,

hyperbilirubinemia, and bilirubinuria.

- Methemoglobinuria—supported by dark brown or chocolate-colored whole blood; often accompanies hemoglobinemia and hemoglobinuria.
- Myoglobinuria—supported by absence of RBCs in urine sediment, clear plasma or serum, increased creatine kinase (CK) and aspartate aminotransferase (AST), often normal packed cell volume (PCV), normal bilirubin.
- False-positive results.

LABORATORY FINDINGS

False-Positive Heme Urine Reagent Strip (Dipstick) Results

- Urine contact with bleach or hydrogen peroxide.
- Highly pigmented urine or marked bilirubinuria.
- Large amounts of bromide or iodide.
- Bacteriuria.

False-Negative Heme Urine Reagent Strip (Dipstick) Results

- Urine exposure to formalin.
- Patients taking captopril or ascorbic acid (Vitamin C).
- Failure to mix urine specimen prior to chemical/dipstick reagent testing or using supernatant for testing.

Disorders That May Alter Laboratory Results

Hyposthenuria or exposure of urine to extreme cold or heat in patients with hematuria may cause in vitro RBC lysis (no intact RBCs in sediment) with positive heme urine reagent dipstick reaction; could be misinterpreted as hemoglobinuria or myoglobinuria.

Valid if Run in Human Laboratory?

Yes

CBC/BIOCHEMISTRY/URINALYSIS

- Intravascular hemolysis and hemoglobinuria:
  - CBC support includes anemia, which may be preregenerative or regenerative depending on onset of hemolysis, RBC ghost cells, RBC inclusions (Heinz bodies to support oxidative injury, infectious agents), RBC poikilocytes (eccentrocytes and pyknocytes support oxidative injury, spherocytes support immune-mediated mechanisms, schistocytes support microangiopathic causes, some toxins), possibly increased mean cell HGB concentration (MCHC) or discrepant increase in HGB concentration from hemoglobinemia, red-colored plasma.
  - Chemistry support includes red-colored serum or plasma, hyperbilirubinemia.
  - Urinalysis support includes absence of hematuria, possible proteinuria.
- Rhabdomyolysis and myoglobinuria:
  - CBC changes not expected.
  - Chemistry findings include markedly increased (>4–5 × upper reference limit [URL]) CK with slower increases in AST; plasma and serum expected to be clear.
  - Urinalysis findings include absence of hematuria, possible proteinuria.

OTHER LABORATORY TESTS

- Ammonium sulfate precipitation test unreliable and recommendation to use CBC and chemistry changes for differentiation.
- Incubation of whole blood with new methylene blue to detect Heinz bodies.
- Methemoglobin detection confirms toxin as oxidant.
- Increased serum copper or zinc concentration.
- DNA test for PFK deficiency.

IMAGING

Abdominal radiographs or ultrasound—metallic objects in gastrointestinal tract.

DIAGNOSTIC PROCEDURES

- Liver biopsy and copper quantification.
- Genetic testing for PFK.

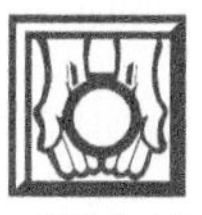

TREATMENT

- IV fluid therapy to maintain renal perfusion.
- Avoid hyperventilation in PFK-deficient patients.
- See Causes for specific treatments.

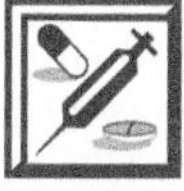

MEDICATIONS

DRUG(S) OF CHOICE

Vary with underlying cause.

ALTERNATIVE DRUGS

N/A

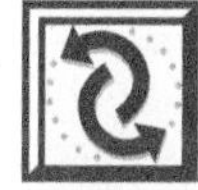

FOLLOW-UP

PATIENT MONITORING

PCV, urinalysis and urine sediment, serum creatinine, CK, urine production.

POSSIBLE COMPLICATIONS

Renal tubular injury may develop.

MISCELLANEOUS

AGE-RELATED FACTORS

Neonatal isoerythrolysis.

ZOONOTIC POTENTIAL

- Leptospirosis.
- Toxoplasmosis.

PREGNANCY/FERTILITY/BREEDING

N/A

SYNONYMS

Pigmenturia

SEE ALSO

See Causes.

ABBREVIATIONS

- AST = aspartate aminotransferase
- CK = creatine kinase
- HGB = hemoglobin
- MCHC = mean cell HGB concentration
- MGB = myoglobin
- PCV = packed cell volume
- PFK = phosphofructokinase
- RBC = red blood cell
- URL = upper reference limit.

Suggested Reading

Bartges JW. Hematuria and other conditions causing discolored urine. In: Ettinger SJ, Feldman EC, eds., Textbook of Veterinary Internal Medicine, 7th ed. St. Louis, MO: Elsevier, 2010, pp. 164–168.

Owen JL, Harvey JW. Hemolytic anemia in dogs and cats due to erythrocyte enzyme deficiencies. Vet Clin North Am Small Anim Pract 2012, 42(1):73–84.

Shelton DG. Rhabdomyolysis, myoglobinuria, and necrotizing myopathies. Vet Clin North Am Small Anim Pract 2004, 34:1469–1482.

Sink C, Weinstein NM. Routine urinalysis: chemical analysis. In: Sink C, Weinstein NM, Practical Veterinary Urinalysis. Ames, IA: Wiley Blackwell, 2012, pp. 42–45.

Stockham SL, Scott SA. Erythrocytes. In: Fundamentals of Veterinary Clinical Pathology, 2nd ed. Ames, IA: Blackwell, 2008, pp. 112–192.

Author Nicole M. Weinstein
Consulting Editor J.D. Foster

Acknowledgment The author and book editors acknowledge the prior contributions of Cheryl L. Swenson, Carl A. Osborne, and Eugene E. Nwaokorie.

H

HEMOTHORAX

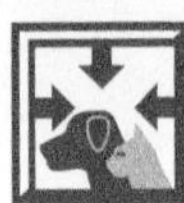

BASICS

OVERVIEW

• Accumulation of blood in pleural space. • Can develop acutely due to trauma or a coagulopathy, or neoplasia; may also be chronic. • Cardiovascular and respiratory systems commonly affected.

SIGNALMENT

Any age, breed, or sex of dog and cat; younger dogs more commonly affected with anticoagulant rodenticide and trauma, older dogs more commonly affected with cancer.

SIGNS

• Peracute to acute onset—hypovolemic signs can occur before sufficient blood volume accumulates in the pleural space to impair respiration. • In chronic cases, larger volumes of blood may accumulate. • Respiratory distress, tachypnea; honking cough is possible in dogs with rodenticide poisoning; ecchymoses along ventral cervical and thoracic inlet areas. • Pale mucous membranes. • Weakness and collapse. • Weak, rapid pulse.

CAUSES & RISK FACTORS

• Trauma—bleeding artery or vein of the thoracic wall, mediastinum, or thoracic spine; damaged heart, lungs, thymus, or diaphragm; herniated abdominal viscera (liver or spleen). • Neoplasia—involving any structure adjacent to the pleural cavity; rib tumors are particularly common. • Coagulopathies—can be congenital or acquired; rodenticide ingestion common. • Lung lobe torsion. • Acute thymic hemorrhage in young animals. • *Dirofilaria immitis, Spirocerca lupi, Angiostrongylus vasorum.*

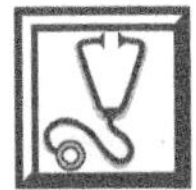

DIAGNOSIS

DIFFERENTIAL DIAGNOSIS

• Nonhemorrhagic pleural effusions—chylothorax; pyothorax; modified transudates; transudates. • Congestive heart failure.

CBC/BIOCHEMISTRY/URINALYSIS

• PCV and hemoglobin—reflect blood loss after initial fluid compartment shifts have occurred. • Platelet count may be low (~100,000) with acute blood loss. • Very low platelet count (<20,000) consistent with spontaneous bleeding, although thrombocytopenia alone rarely represents in hemothorax.

OTHER LABORATORY TESTS

Fluid Analysis

• Hemorrhage-produced effusion—packed cell volume (PCV) and protein content similar to that of peripheral blood; platelets commonly seen on cytology. • Inflammation- or vascular-congestion related effusion—PCV <8%. • Neoplasia or lung lobe torsion—PCV can be low or mid-range. • Cytologic examination—often fails to identify malignant causes, but is recommended.

Coagulation Tests

• Prolonged prothrombin time (PT)/partial thromboplastin time (PTT) suggestive of coagulopathy. • Specific factor analysis—needed to diagnose congenital defect or acquired coagulopathy. • Buccal mucosal bleeding time—identifies platelet function defect or vasculitis.

IMAGING

• Radiology—reveals pleural effusion varying from diffuse increase in radiopacity to ventral leafing, interlobar fissures, and localized pleural densities. • Can see associated lesions (e.g., rib fractures or tumors, pneumothorax or pneumomediastinum, mediastinal hemorrhage, pulmonary contusions, diaphragmatic lesions, and masses). • Lobar consolidation with vesicular gas pattern suggestive of lung lobe torsion. • In stable patients without coagulopathy—evacuation of pleural space may allow better radiographic visualization of masses or other pathology.

DIAGNOSTIC PROCEDURES

• Thoracentesis (contraindicated if clotting abnormality). • CT to evaluate for neoplasia or lung lobe torsion.

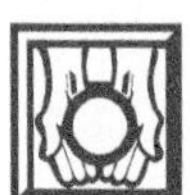

TREATMENT

• Acute—judicious use of IV fluids; try to get systolic blood pressure above 90 mmHg using crystalloids and/or hypertonic saline to correct hypovolemia. • Coexisting pneumothorax—generally requires needle thoracentesis or tube thoracostomy. • Plasma, specific clotting factors, and/or blood transfusion can be needed to restore clotting factors or provide red blood cells (RBCs) for oxygen transport. • Pulmonary contusion—may require ventilator support. • Severe or recurrent thoracic hemorrhage—may require surgical exploration. • Oxygen therapy. • Most coagulopathic cases have respiratory difficulty associated with soft tissue bleeding rather than pleural hemorrhage and therefore rarely require evacuation of pleural fluid to resolve tachypnea. • Autotransfusion.

MEDICATIONS

DRUG(S) OF CHOICE

• Hypovolemia—see Shock, Hypovolemic. • Vitamin K_1—5 mg/kg SC loading dose (using small-gauge needle) followed by 1.5–2.5 mg/kg PO q12h for 21–30 days; takes 12 hours or more to carboxylate clotting factors and restore activity. • Analgesics—systemically or as nerve blocks for trauma. • Broad-spectrum antibiotics— when indicated.

CONTRAINDICATIONS/POSSIBLE INTERACTIONS

Avoid aspirin and other nonsteroidal anti-inflammatory drugs (NSAIDs).

FOLLOW-UP

PATIENT MONITORING

• Clinical signs, respiratory rate and effort, heart rate. • Temperature. • Urine production. • Relief from pain. • Follow-up radiographs at 48-hour intervals until stable. • Coagulation panel in 48 hours if coagulopathy due to anticoagulant rodenticide toxicity diagnosed, and 48 hours after discontinuing vitamin K supplementation.

POSSIBLE COMPLICATIONS

• Pyothorax. • Sepsis. • Entrapment and constriction of lungs by scar tissue and fibrosis.

MISCELLANEOUS

ASSOCIATED CONDITIONS

• Peritonitis—with penetrating wounds (e.g., gunshot) into the abdomen. • Esophageal perforation.

SEE ALSO

- Disseminated Intravascular Coagulation.
- Lung Lobe Torsion.
- Pleural Effusion.
- Pulmonary Contusions.
- Rodenticide Toxicosis—Anticoagulants.

ABBREVIATIONS

• NSAID = nonsteroidal anti-inflammatory drug. • PCV = packed cell volume. • PT = prothrombin time. • PTT = partial thromboplastin time. • RBC = red blood cell.

Suggested Reading

Berry CR, Gallaway A, Thrall DE, Carlisle C. Thoracic radiographic features of anticoagulant rodenticide toxicity in fourteen dogs. Vet Radiol Ultrasound 1993, 34:391–396.

Nakamura RK, Rozanski EA, Rush JE. Non-coagulopathic spontaneous hemothorax in dogs. J Vet Emerg Crit Care 2008, 18:292–297.

Author Bradley L. Moses

Consulting Editor Elizabeth Rozanski

BASICS

OVERVIEW

Red blood cell (RBC) destruction and anemia caused by bacterial attachment to the external surface of RBCs, nutrient scavenging by bacteria from RBC, and immune response by the host.

SIGNALMENT

- Dog and cat.
- Acute disease most common in young cats, chronic form most common in adults.
- More common in outdoor and male cats.
- Acute disease in splenectomized dogs, chronic disease in nonsplenectomized dogs.
- Kennel-raised beagles at increased risk for infection.
- No sex prevalence in dogs.

SIGNS

Cats

- For *Mycoplasma haemofelis* infection:
  - Variable disease severity ranging from inapparent infection (chronic disease) to marked anemia and death (acute disease).
  - Intermittent fever (50% of the time) during the acute phase, depression, weakness, anorexia, anemia, pale mucous membranes, splenomegaly, and (occasionally) icterus.
- For *Candidatus M. haemominutum* infection:
  - Usually results in inapparent infection.
  - Minimal or no decrease in hematocrit.
- For *Candidatus M. turicensis*:
  - Limited information regarding natural infection.
  - Mild anemia following experimental infection.

Dogs

- Mild or inapparent signs (e.g., pale mucous membranes and listlessness)—except when dogs have been splenectomized or splenic function is altered.
- High prevalence of chronic, inapparent infection in kennel-raised beagles, which may threaten validity of research results.

CAUSES & RISK FACTORS

- Caused by bacteria previously classified in the genus *Haemobartonella*, these organisms are now recognized to be mycoplasmas (hemotropic mycoplasmas or hemoplasmas) based on genetic determination,
- *M. haemofelis* (previously classified as large form of *H. felis*), *M. haemominutum* (previously classified as small form of *H. felis*), and *M. haemocanis* (previously classified as *H. canis*).
- *M. haemofelis* infection in cats generally causes more severe disease than *M. haemominutum* or *Candidatus M. turicensis* infection.
- Cats—anemia more severe if feline leukemia virus (FeLV) infected.
- Dogs—likelihood of severe anemia greatly increased if splenectomized or with pathologic changes in the spleen.

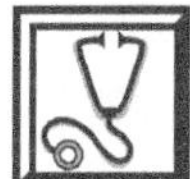

DIAGNOSIS

DIFFERENTIAL DIAGNOSIS

- Other causes of hemolytic anemia, including immune-mediated hemolytic anemia (IMHA), babesiosis (not in cats in the United States), cytauxzoonosis (cats only), Heinz body hemolytic anemia (new methylene blue can be used to identify Heinz bodies), microangiopathic hemolytic anemia, pyruvate kinase deficiency, and phosphofructokinase deficiency (dogs only).
- Differentiated from IMHA only by recognition of parasites in blood (stained blood film or species-specific PCR-based assays); both disorders (IMHA and/or *M. haemofelis* infection) may be Coombs' test positive.
- *Babesia* and *Cytauxzoon* species are protozoal organisms that differ in morphology from mycoplasma.
- Enzyme assays or specialized DNA tests can be used to diagnose pyruvate kinase and phosphofructokinase deficiencies.

CBC/BIOCHEMISTRY/URINALYSIS

- Anemia most often present with reticulocytosis in animals with clinically important infections—may appear poorly regenerative if precipitous decrease in packed cell volume (PCV) has occurred early in the disease or if there are other concurrent disorders (e.g., FeLV or feline immunodeficiency virus [FIV] infection in cats).
- Autoagglutination may be seen in feline blood samples after they cool to below body temperature.
- Hyperbilirubinemia may be measured and/or seen clinically at times but is seldom severe.
- Substantial bilirubinuria seen in some dogs.
- Abnormalities related to anemic hypoxia may be shown by clinical chemistry profiles, but profile can be normal.
- Hypoglycemia possible in moribund cats or if slow to separate blood cells from plasma or serum.

OTHER LABORATORY TESTS

- Routine blood stains (e.g., Wright-Giemsa) to identify organisms in blood films.
- Organism may detach from RBCs in stored blood anticoagulated with EDTA.
- Reticulocyte stains cannot be used to identify *Mycoplasma* organisms because punctate reticulocytes in cats appear similar to the parasites.
- Organisms must be differentiated from precipitated stain, refractile drying, or fixation artifacts, poorly staining Howell-Jolly bodies, and basophilic stippling.
- Feline organisms—small blue-staining cocci, rings, or rods on RBCs, often many parasites for *M. haemofelis*; small rods or coccoid organisms in low numbers for *Candidatus M. haemominutum*; parasites not conclusively seen in blood for *Candidatus M. turicensis*.
- Canine organisms—commonly form chains of organisms that appear as filamentous structures on the surface of RBCs.
- Infection is cyclic and thus organisms are not always identifiable in blood (especially in cats).
- PCR-based assays can detect parasites in blood below the number required to make a diagnosis by a stained blood film.

H

DIAGNOSTIC PROCEDURES

- In patients with nonregenerative anemia, bone marrow biopsy should be performed to detect other disorders.
- PCR testing of blood donor cats and dogs is strongly recommended.

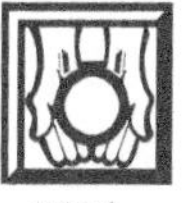

TREATMENT

- Without therapy, mortality with *M. haemofelis* infection may reach 30% in cats.
- Outpatient treatment unless severely anemic or moribund.
- Blood transfusions required when anemia is considered life-threatening.
- Shock should be treated with IV administration of isotonic crystalloid fluids, with or without glucose supplementation.

MEDICATIONS

DRUG(S) OF CHOICE

- Doxycycline (5 mg/kg PO q12h) should be given for minimum of 4 weeks.
- If PCR remains positive or bacteremia reoccurs after doxycycline therapy, antibiotic treatment should be switched to marbofloxacin (2 mg/kg PO q24h) for 2 weeks.

CONTRAINDICATIONS/POSSIBLE INTERACTIONS

- Esophageal strictures and gastrointestinal disease have been reported in cats following doxycycline administration.
- Fluroquinolones, including marbofloxacin, may cause arthropathy in young dogs and retinotoxicity in cats.

FOLLOW-UP

- Examine animal after 1 week of treatment to confirm that PCV has risen.
- Alert owners that cats may remain carriers even after completion of treatment, but seldom relapse with disease once PCV returns to normal.

HEMOTROPIC MYCOPLASMOSIS (CONTINUED)

- Cats have protective immunity against *M. haemofelis* reinfection for some period of time.

MISCELLANEOUS

SEE ALSO

- Anemia, Heinz Body.
- Anemia, Immune-Mediated.
- Anemia, Regenerative.
- Babesiosis.
- Cytauxzoonosis.
- Phosphofructokinase Deficiency.
- Pyruvate Kinase Deficiency.

ABBREVIATIONS

- FeLV = feline leukemia virus.
- FIV = feline immunodeficiency virus.
- IMHA = immune-mediated hemolytic anemia.
- PCV = packed cell volume.
- RBC = red blood cell.

Suggested Reading

Barker E. Tasker S. Haemoplasmas: lessons learnt from cats. N Z Vet J 2013, 61:184–192.

Messick JB, Harvey JW. Hemotrophic mycoplasmosis (haembartonellosis). In: Green CE, Infectious Diseases of the Dog and Cat. St. Louis, MO: Elsevier Sanders, 2012, pp. 310–319.

Novacco M, Sugiarto S, Willi B, et al. Consecutive antibiotic treatment with doxycycline and marbofloxacin clears bacteremia in *Mycoplasma felis*-infected cats. Vet Microbiol 2018, 217:112–120.

Author John W. Harvey

Consulting Editor Melinda S. Camus

Acknowledgment The author and book editors acknowledge the prior contribution of Joanne B. Messick.

H

HEPATIC AMYLOID

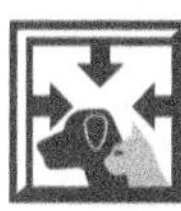

BASICS

OVERVIEW

- Amyloidosis—disorders of diverse etiology sharing common feature of deposition of extracellular insoluble fibrillar beta-pleated proteinaceous matrix with distinctive staining properties and fibrillar ultrastructure.
- Amyloid—derived from diverse primary proteins, sometimes an acute phase reactant.
- Serum amyloid A (SAA), an acute phase protein produced by hepatocytes, is produced during inflammation and is associated with the most commonly reported generalized form of amyloidosis in small animals.
- Amyloid AL, which is a monoclonal immunoglobulin G light chain and is associated with plasma cell dyscrasia, is not commonly reported in small animals and is not the form associated with hepatic amyloidosis.
- Amyloid may accumulate as a focal or systemic process secondary to inflammatory or lymphoproliferative disorders or as a familial genetic disorder.
- Liver and kidneys are most commonly affected.
- Familial amyloidosis—certain kindreds of purebred cats; certain breeds and kindreds of dogs; syndromic inflammatory disorders.
- Multiple organs commonly involved; clinical signs often reflect renal involvement.
- Liver amyloid accumulation—insidious; associated with variable liver enzymes, severe hepatomegaly, coagulopathies, liver rupture leading to hemoabdomen (cats), or liver failure.

SIGNALMENT

- Dogs—Chinese Shar-Pei, with cyclic "shar-pei fever syndrome"; Akita with cyclic fever and polyarthropathy; collie with "gray collie syndrome"; usually develop renal signs first, although some develop hepatic insufficiency.
- Cats—oriental shorthair, Siamese, Devon Rex, domestic shorthair cats; usually <5 years of age when first symptomatic (hepatic signs and coagulopathies predominate); familial in Abyssinians (renal signs predominate). Upper respiratory viral infection proposed to trigger amyloidosis in Siamese. Cats naturally infected with feline immunodeficiency virus (FIV) have been described to have systemic amyloid deposition, with kidneys, liver, and spleen most affected.

SIGNS

Historical Findings

- Episodic fever and swollen hocks—shar-pei.
- Episodic polyarthropathy, pain, and signs of meningitis—Akita.
- Acute lethargy, cyclic.
- Anorexia and vomiting, episodic.
- Polyuria and polydipsia.

Physical Examination Findings

- Pallor.
- Abdominal effusion—hemorrhage or ascites.
- Jaundice—unusual.
- Hepatomegaly with amyloid deposition.
- Edema—due to hypoalbuminemia secondary to pathologic proteinuria.
- Joint pain—Akita, shar-pei syndromes.
- Nonlocalized pain, meningeal pain, and abdominal discomfort—with different inflammatory disorders promoting amyloid.

CAUSES & RISK FACTORS

- Familial immunoregulatory disorders.
- Chronic infections—coccidioidomycosis; blastomycosis; tick-borne diseases; FIV.
- Cyclic neutropenia—gray collie syndrome.
- Bacterial endocarditis.
- Chronic inflammation (e.g., systemic lupus erythematosus [SLE]).
- Neoplasia.

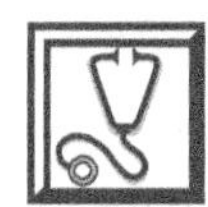

DIAGNOSIS

DIFFERENTIAL DIAGNOSIS

- Chronic hepatic inflammation.
- Infiltrative hepatic neoplasia.
- Primary or rodenticide-induced coagulopathy.
- Glomerulonephritis.
- Pyelonephritis.
- SLE.
- Abdominal trauma.
- Peritonitis.
- Meningitis.
- Immune-mediated or infectious polyarthropathy.

CBC/BIOCHEMISTRY/URINALYSIS

- Anemia secondary to hepatic hemorrhage or liver lobe rupture or chronic inflammation.
- Leukocytosis with a left shift during febrile episodes in shar-pei and Akita.
- Normal or high—liver enzymes, total bilirubin, and serum bile acids; may be normal with severe hepatic amyloid deposition.
- Azotemia with severe renal infiltration—glomeruli targeted in dogs (proteinuria), renal interstitium targeted in cats (azotemia).
- Proteinuria—dogs: glomerular amyloid.
- Dilute urine—renal involvement or failure.
- Feline systemic amyloidosis—involves multiple organ systems: thyroid, cardiac, renal, intestine, pancreatic, bone marrow, lymph nodes, adrenals.

OTHER LABORATORY TESTS

- Coagulation tests—normal to prolonged clotting times, hyperfibrinogenemia.
- Synovial fluid—dogs with joint swelling or pain: suppurative nonseptic inflammation.
- Cerebrospinal fluid (CSF)—if meningeal pain, increased protein, and suppurative inflammation.
- Lyme disease testing—ELISA for C6 antibody presence in dogs with joint swelling/pain/fever.
- FIV—cats with hepatic, renal, or respiratory symptoms.

IMAGING

- Abdominal radiography—hepatomegaly; variable renal size; abdominal effusion.
- Abdominal ultrasonography—hepatomegaly: hypoechoic parenchyma (diffuse amyloid); variable renal size with normal or equivocally hypoechoic parenchyma (renal amyloid); inconsistent mesenteric lymphadenopathy; thickened gut wall (amyloid deposition); abdominal effusion.

DIAGNOSTIC PROCEDURES

- Fine-needle aspiration cytology—may disclose amorphous fibrillar material.
- Liver or other tissue biopsy.
- Abdominocentesis—hemorrhagic (esp. cats) or transudative effusion (diffuse hepatopathy).

PATHOLOGIC FINDINGS

Gross

Liver—normal to pale color; large, firm to friable; hemorrhages (subcapsular hematomas, capsular tears) to overt rupture.

Microscopic

- Liver—diffuse acellular amorphous material in the space of Disse, associated with hepatic cord atrophy; may primarily involve blood vessels in portal triads (Abyssinian cats).
- Cats with systemic amyloidosis may have amyloid deposited in many organs and endocrine tissue.
- Amyloid stains amorphous pink with routine hematoxylin and eosin; may stain turquoise blue with Masson's trichrome; Congo red staining with bright field: amyloid is salmon pink but with polarized light is birefringent (beta-pleated sheet structure refracts polarized light) and apple green.

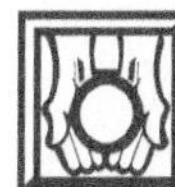

TREATMENT

- Warn client that hepatic amyloidosis is difficult to treat; guarded to poor prognosis.
- Dictated by severity of clinical signs.
- No curative treatment; manage underlying disease; colchicine as described below may reduce organ amyloid deposition.
- Fluids—for dehydration.
- Blood transfusion—for acute blood loss; essential in cats with hepatic amyloid-induced liver lobe rupture.
- Diet—individually tailored to organ function.
- Liver failure—consider measures appropriate for hepatic encephalopathy as appropriate.
- Pathologic proteinuria—see Nephrotic Syndrome.

HEPATIC AMYLOID (CONTINUED)

- Surgical intervention—hepatic lobe resection as emergency measure for catastrophic bleeding from fractured liver lobe in cats; histologic features may describe centrilobular necrosis due to anemia-induced hypoxia; amyloid may be overlooked without special stains.

MEDICATIONS

DRUG(S) OF CHOICE

- Colchicine—dogs: 0.03 mg/kg PO q24h; may block amyloid deposition in early disease or control deposition in chronic disorders in dogs; modulates expression of adhesion molecules and chemotactic factors; causes microtubule polymerization by binding to tubulin blocking cell mitosis in cells such as neutrophils. Effects attenuate inflammatory response, triggering acute phase protein (amyloid precursor) production. Monitor CBC for bone marrow toxicity; observe patient for enteric side effects (vomiting, diarrhea [bloody]), beware of toxicity if coadministered with p450 blocking drugs (e.g., ketoconazole, omeprazole, cimetidine). Use colchicine without added probenecid. Limited experience in cats.
- Dimethyl sulfoxide (DMSO)—controversial treatment; use medical grade only; dogs: 80 mg/kg given as no more than a 33% solution in sterile water PO three times a week; may promote dissolution of amyloid fibrils or provide anti-inflammatory or anti-amyloid effect. Side effects: garlic odor and objectionable taste. Sterile solutions have also been prepared and administered SC. In humans this treatment given PO daily (3–20 g/patient) has benefit in polysystemic amyloidosis, but not renal amyloidosis associated with renal failure.
- Lactulose—dogs: 2.5–15 mL PO q8h; cats: 2.5–5.0 mL PO q8–12h; for patients with suspected hepatic encephalopathy. If oral administration is not tolerated this may be given as a retention enema.
- Nonsteroidal anti-inflammatory drugs (NSAIDs)—in dogs (shar-pei fever syndrome) to reduce pain and fever if present.
- Vitamin K_1—dogs and cats: initially at three doses of 0.5–1.5 mg/kg SC/IM. Subsequent dosing may be necessary, especially in cats. Monitor prothrombin time (PT); dosing interval should be determined by resolution of prolongation of PT.
- Medications as indicated for concurrent renal disease and/or proteinuria if present.

CONTRAINDICATIONS/POSSIBLE INTERACTIONS

- Colchicine combined with probenecid may cause vomiting, as probenecid prolongs residence time of colchicine.
- Colchicine toxicity if coadministered with p450 cytochrome inhibitor drugs.
- Colchicine may cause/enhance bone marrow suppression if administered with antineoplastics, immunosuppressive medications, chloramphenicol, or amphotericin B.

FOLLOW-UP

- Shar-pei—with hepatic amyloid may survive >2 years; most have episodes of fever and cholestasis; some resolve clinical signs and diminish hepatic amyloid with colchicine.
- Akitas with cyclic clinical signs—grave prognosis.
- Cats surviving liver hemorrhage eventually succumb to renal failure and other polysystemic effects of deposited amyloid.

MISCELLANEOUS

SEE ALSO

Amyloidosis

ABBREVIATIONS

- CSF = cerebrospinal fluid.
- DMSO = dimethyl sulfoxide.
- FIV = feline immunodeficiency virus.
- NSAID = nonsteroidal anti-inflammatory drug.
- PT = prothrombin time.
- SLE = systemic lupus erythematosus.

Suggested Reading

Amemori S, Iwakiri R, Endo H, et al. Oral dimethyl sulfoxide for systemic amyloid A amyloidosis complication in chronic inflammatory disease: a retrospective patient chart review. J Gastroenterol 2006, 41:444–449.

Beatty JA, Barrs VR, Martin PA. Spontaneous hepatic rupture in six cats with systemic amyloidosis. J Small Anim Pract 2002, 43:355–363.

Hoffman HM. Therapy of autoinflammatory syndromes. J Allergy Clin Immunol 2009, 124:1129–1138.

Loevan KO. Hepatic amyloidosis in two Chinese Shar Pei dogs. J Am Vet Med Assoc 1994, 204:1212–1216.

Merlini G, Bellotti V. Molecular mechanisms of amyloidosis. N Engl J Med 2003, 349:583–596.

Author Kate Holan

Consulting Editor Kate Holan

Acknowledgment The author and book editors acknowledge the prior contribution of Sharon A. Center.

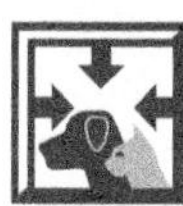

BASICS

DEFINITION

- Hepatic encephalopathy (HE) defines broad spectrum of neurobehavioral signs caused by failure of liver to remove endogenous toxins, including ammonia, acquired from alimentary canal (predominantly from colon) into splanchnic portal venous circulation.
- Associated with acute liver failure; portosystemic shunting: congenital (portosystemic vascular anomaly [PSVA]) or multiple acquired portosystemic shunts (APSSs); or severe liver injury: critical loss of functional hepatic mass or cirrhosis where loss of functional mass combines with hepatic fibrosis, leading to portal hypertension and development of APSS.
- Metabolic/physiologic dysregulations causal to HE potentially reversible; pathologic changes in neural tissue may become permanent in chronic HE.
- Acute brain edema associated with high central spinal fluid pressure may lead to lethal brain herniation.

PATHOPHYSIOLOGY

- Neurobehavioral and neurocognitive abnormalities—largely attributed to gut-derived substances (bacterial and protein metabolites), with ammonia considered predominant toxin.
- Neurologic signs—reflect impact of neurotoxic molecules on cortical, basal ganglia, pontine, cerebellum, increased permeability of blood–brain barrier (BBB); astrocyte type II Alzheimer change, microglial activation, axonal demyelination, decreased cerebellar inhibition.
- Multifactorial process with numerous etiopathogenic mechanisms.
- Ammonia—best-studied toxin with neurotoxic impact on astrocytes; high ammonia associated with astrocyte swelling and brain oxidative stress.
- Complex multifactorial pathophysiology contributes to electrophysiologic derangements—energy failure (neuroglycopenia), altered cerebral pH (lactate accumulation), calcium ion flux, abnormalities involving glutamatergic, GABAergic and catecholaminergic neurotransmission; perturbed aromatic amino acid metabolism, increased cerebral concentrations of endogenous benzodiazepine-like substances and neurosteroids; local accumulation of inflammatory cytokines and bile acids, altered cerebral blood flow, and oxidative injury. Altered BBB permeability increases access of toxic factors to brain.

SYSTEMS AFFECTED

- Nervous—abnormal cerebral function predominates; decreased awareness and function progress to stereotypic pacing, somnolence, coma, or agitation progresses to seizures; aggression and seizures more likely in cats with PSVA.
- Gastrointestinal (GI)—vomiting, diarrhea, anorexia, or constipation.
- Renal/urologic—ammonium biurate urolithiasis involving bladder, renal pelvis; may cause urethral obstruction.

GENETICS

- PSVA—see Portosystemic Vascular Anomaly, Congenital.
- See Hepatitis, Chronic; Copper Associated Hepatopathy.

INCIDENCE/PREVALENCE

Uncommon disorder.

SIGNALMENT

Species

Dog and cat.

Breed Predilections

PSVA—usually purebred small dogs and mixes of these.

Mean Age and Range

- PSVA—usually young animals.
- Acquired liver disease with APSS—any age.

SIGNS

General Comments

- Neurologic—usually coordinate with meal ingestion (esp. high protein, e.g., red meat, fish, dogs consuming cat foods); systemic infection; dehydration; azotemia; constipation; any cause of catabolism; increased heme turnover: hemolysis, enteric bleeding, eruption of adult teeth in juveniles, blood transfusion; certain drugs.
- Temporary resolution of HE signs following dietary protein restriction, modification of enteric flora or enteric contents (e.g., certain oral antibiotics, administration of cathartics such as lactulose, or use of cleansing enema), ± resolution of provocative conditions.
- Prolonged recovery from sedation or anesthesia.
- Ammonium biurate obstructive uropathy.

Historical Findings

- Episodic neurobehavioral signs or neurocognitive impairment—slow onset and resolution.
- Learning disabilities (difficult to train).
- Lethargy/somnolence may progress to coma.
- Anorexia/vomiting.
- Ptyalism—especially cats.
- Polyuria/polydipsia (PU/PD).
- Disorientation—aimless wandering; compulsive pacing; head pressing.
- Amaurotic blindness.
- Focal or generalized seizures—neurologic signs of lethargy or somnolence as prodrome.
- Signs more frequent in cats—ptyalism, seizure, aggression disorientation; ataxic stupor.
- Signs more frequent in dogs—compulsive behavior, e.g., head pressing, circling, aimless wandering, vocalizing; GI signs: vomiting; diarrhea; PU/PD; signs associated with ammonium biurate urolithiasis: hematuria, pollakiuria, stranguria, dysuria males > females.

Physical Examination Findings

- PSVA—see Portosystemic Vascular Anomaly, Congenital.
- Ascites common in dogs with HE secondary to acquired liver disease; variable coagulopathies.
- May have distended bladder if obstructive uropathy; may pass small dark green uroliths.
- Neurologic signs.

CAUSES

- PSVA—congenital malformations.
- APSS—see Hypertension, Portal; Portosystemic Shunting, Acquired.
- See Hepatic Failure, Acute; Hepatotoxins.

RISK FACTORS

- Feeding high-protein foods to dogs; dogs consuming cat foods.
- Enteric bleeding—most common acute cause of HE.
- Disorders increasing heme turnover—enteric bleeding; hemolysis; oral bleeding: tooth eruption in juvenile with PSVA; blood transfusions: stored blood products may contain high concentrations of ammonia, incompatible blood transfusions.
- Alkalosis, hypokalemia, hypoglycemia.
- Certain anesthetics (alfaxalone), sedatives (benzodiazepines).
- Drugs, e.g., methionine, tetracycline, antihistamines.
- Constipation.
- Catabolism.
- Infections or severe inflammation.

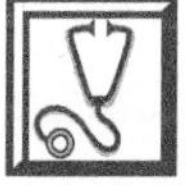

DIAGNOSIS

DIFFERENTIAL DIAGNOSIS

- Lead toxicosis.
- Urinary tract infection, urolithiasis.
- Intestinal parasitism.
- Primary GI disease.
- Hypoglycemia.
- Toxoplasmosis.
- Congenital CNS disease or malformation—hydrocephalus; storage diseases.
- CNS neoplasia.
- Acute ethylene glycol, xylitol, other toxicoses.
- Infectious—rabies; canine distemper; neurologic dissemination of toxoplasmosis or other.
- Thiamin deficiency.
- Drug intoxications—human recreational drugs.

HEPATIC ENCEPHALOPATHY (CONTINUED)

H

CBC/BIOCHEMISTRY/URINALYSIS

CBC

PSVA and APSS—red blood cell microcytosis; variable mild nonregenerative anemia; poikilocytosis (cats); target cells (dogs); ± jaundiced plasma.

Biochemistry

- Variable low blood urea nitrogen and creatinine.
- Hypoglycemia.
- Low cholesterol.
- Liver enzymes—variable depending on cause.
- Bilirubin—normal to high depending on cause.
- Hypoalbuminemia.

Urinalysis

- Low concentration—common with PSVA; variable with APSS.
- Ammonium urate crystalluria—causing hematuria, pyuria, proteinuria; may also cause secondary infection; crystalluria imparts orange/brown color to urine.

OTHER LABORATORY TESTS

- Blood ammonia—sensitive but unreliable indicator of HE; fasting hyperammonemia unreliably associated with HE; lability of blood ammonia makes ammonia determinations less reliable than total serum bile acids (TSBA); ammonia tolerance testing—most reliable method of demonstrating ammonia intolerance (administer NH_4Cl PO or per rectum) but *caution*: may induce HE.
- TSBA—confirms hepatic insufficiency or shunting associated with HE; hepatobiliary jaundice renders TSBA testing superfluous.
- Coagulation tests—variable depending on underlying cause.
- Protein C—low activity in dogs with substantial shunting, liver failure, protein-losing enteropathy, disseminated intravascular coagulation.
- Abdominal effusion—effusions pure or modified transudates.

IMAGING

See Portosystemic Vascular Anomaly, Congenital; Portosystemic Shunting, Acquired.

DIAGNOSTIC PROCEDURES

- Hepatic aspiration—cannot differentiate disorders causing portosystemic shunting.
- Liver biopsy—open surgical wedge biopsy or laparoscopic sampling; essential to collect tissue from several liver lobes.
- Tru-Cut® needle biopsy—may inadequately sample tissue.

PATHOLOGIC FINDINGS

- Gross—liver appearance reflects underlying disorder; rare brain herniation in acute HE.
- Microscopic—liver lesions define causal hepatic disorder; CNS lesions: may include polymicrocavitation and Alzheimer type II astrocyte changes; inconsistent in dogs and cats.

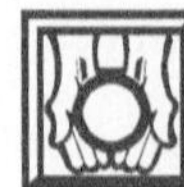

TREATMENT

APPROPRIATE HEALTH CARE

- Depends on underlying cause.
- See Portosystemic Vascular Anomaly, Congenital.

NURSING CARE

- Avoid risk factors.
- Treatment depends on underlying condition(s); essential to eliminate factors provoking HE.
- Improve dietary protein tolerance by concurrent oral or rectal (enema) treatments (see Medications) and altering protein type and quantity (see Diet).
- If hepatic coma—discontinue oral medications; ensure euglycemia; provide fluid, electrolyte, and water-soluble vitamin support.
- Fluids—balanced crystalloids; avoid lactate if fulminant hepatic failure, if hypoglycemic supplement fluids with 2.5–5.0% dextrose; provide 20–30 mEq/L potassium chloride (not to exceed 0.5 mEq/kg/h) titrated to need; sodium-restricted fluids used in patients with ascites with APSS (esp. cirrhosis) and patients with marked hypoalbuminemia.
- B-soluble vitamins supplemented in fluids (2 mL/L); ensure adequate B_{12}.

ACTIVITY

- Keep patient warm, inactive, hydrated, euglycemic.
- Protect animal from environmental injury secondary to propulsive or aimless pacing, obtundation, amaurosis, generalized seizures.

DIET

- Adequate calories—avoid catabolism; important to maintain muscle mass.
- Dietary protein modification and restriction—cornerstone of medical management; use commercially formulated liver diets or diets for moderate renal insufficiency. Dog: use dairy and soy protein sources with initial 2.2–2.5 g protein/kg bodyweight per day allowance. Cat: pure carnivores must have meat-derived protein restricted to ~3.5 g protein/kg bodyweight per day.
- Dogs: after initial observed response to restricted protein allowance (1–2 weeks) gradually titrate allowance upward (0.25 g protein/kg bodyweight per day for 5–10-day observational increments) using dairy quality protein (e.g., shredded cheddar or mixed cheeses, often effective); increase up to 1.5 g protein /kg bodyweight per day depending on individual tolerance (no signs of HE, no ammonium biurate crystalluria).
- Good-quality vitamin supplements.
- Ensure thiamin repletion—50–100 mg daily for 3 days in cats and dogs, with water-soluble vitamins added in fluids; follow with dietary supplementation; *caution*: anaphylactoid reactions may occur with injectable (IM/SC) thiamin.
- *S*-adenosylmethionine—20 mg/kg PO/day on empty stomach.
- Partial parenteral nutrition—*only* for short-term inappetence.
- Total parenteral nutrition considered if >5 days inappetence and enteral route unavailable.
- No benefit shown for specific supplementation of oral branched-chain amino acids.
- No need to restrict fat.

CLIENT EDUCATION

- HE—usually episodic; relapse risk exists if underlying cause cannot be eliminated.
- Train owner to administer enemas to abate acute-onset HE and judiciously adjust medications used to control ammonia formation and absorption PRN.
- APSS—see Portosystemic Shunting, Acquired.
- PSVA—see Portosystemic Vascular Anomaly, Congenital.

SURGICAL CONSIDERATIONS

- PSVA—medically treat HE *before* anesthesia and surgery.
- APSS—do not ligate this vasculature.

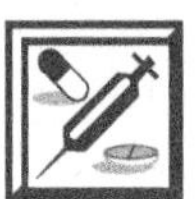

MEDICATIONS

DRUG(S) OF CHOICE

- Treatment goals include increasing dietary protein tolerance; altering enteric environment and microbiome to modify generation of encephalogenic toxins (e.g., endotoxin and ammonia); reduce bioavailability or colonic dwell time of substances provoking HE.
- Antibiotics—first choice: systemic metronidazole (7.5 mg/kg q12h) or amoxicillin (esp. cats, 12.5–25 mg/kg PO q8–12h); *caution* if using neomycin (10–22 mg/kg PO q12h) chronically as enteric absorption may cause renal and otic toxicity.
- Local instillation of antimicrobials used in retention enemas—same dosages as oral but *do not* administer by both oral and rectal routes.
- In humans, rifaximin is as effective as single agent or combined lactulose and neomycin in management of HE and has favorable safety and tolerability profile; is expensive; no data regarding utility for management of HE in animals; suggested dose in dogs 5 mg/kg PO q24h or q12h.
- Nonabsorbable-fermentable carbohydrates—lactulose, lactitol, or lactose in milk products if patient is lactase deficient; lactulose most commonly used: start at 0.5 mL/kg q8–12h

and titrate up to therapeutic goal of 2 or 3 soft stools/day; may also administer as enema for acute HE or patients in coma *after* cleansing enemas remove debris; *note*: concurrent use of neomycin may suppress bacterial fermentation of lactulose thereby diminishing its benefit.

- Probiotics combined with nonabsorbable-fermented carbohydrates may be advantageous for altering gut flora and provoking cathartic effect.
- Enemas—*cleansing enemas* (warmed polyionic fluids) mechanically cleanse the colon (10–15 mL/kg, until clear return); *retention enemas* deliver fermentable substrates, antimicrobials, or solution directly altering colonic pH: diluted lactulose, lactitol, or lactose (1 : 2 in water); antimicrobials mixed with water: metronidazole or neomycin but do not exceed PO dose, do not dose PO *and* rectally; diluted betadine (1 : 10 in water, *rinse well in 15 min*); diluted vinegar (1 : 10 in water) modifies colonic pH, alters colonic flora.
- Zinc supplementation—two urea cycle enzymes require zinc and portosystemic shunting may deplete body zinc reserves (shown in humans); measure baseline plasma zinc (dose 1–3 mg/kg elemental zinc PO using zinc acetate) then titrate dose using sequential plasma zinc measurements to avoid >800 µg/dL (causes hemolysis), but document an increase in baseline plasma zinc concentration inferring positive zinc balance; *note*: plasma zinc does not reflect liver zinc concentration.
- Cerebral edema—complicates acute HE; head-up posture (15–20° incline); mannitol (1 g/kg diluted in saline, over 30 min); nasal oxygen; *N*-acetylcysteine (140 mg/kg IV diluted 1 : 2 in saline given through nonpyrogenic filter unless sterile IV form used, then 70 mg/kg q8h); glucocorticoids controversial, may promote enteric bleeding but some evidence supports reduced astrocyte swelling.
- Salvage therapies for intractable HE (experimental)—L-ornithine-L-aspartate (humans, rats: 180–300 mg/kg/day divided into three doses); L-carnitine (100 mg/kg PO/IV) may attenuate HE-associated hyperammonemia.
- If epileptic seizure activity—Keppra® (levetiracetam; dose 20–60 mg/kg IV given 1 : 1 dilution over 15 min) is preferred anticonvulsant; secondary anticonvulsants include zonisamide (caution: rare idiopathic hepatotoxicity) or KBr (complicates fluid therapy) as preferred anticonvulsants to phenobarbital; avoid benzodiazepines in HE.

CONTRAINDICATIONS

- Avoid drugs metabolized by the liver or rapidly removed by first-pass extraction—or if used, judiciously reduce dose.
- Avoid alfaxalone.
- Avoid benzodiazepines.

PRECAUTIONS

- Consider altered drug pharmacokinetics—reduced first-pass extraction due to portosystemic shunting; reduced protein binding if hypoalbuminemia, and compromised hepatic metabolism.
- Use anesthetics, sedatives, tranquilizers, potassium-wasting diuretics, analgesics, highly protein-bound drugs (if hypoalbuminemic) cautiously; reduce dose.
- If possible, avoid drugs predominantly reliant on hepatic metabolism, biotransformation, and excretion in patients with acquired chronic liver disease associated with APSS vs. those with PSVA or ductal plate malformation-associated APSS where metabolic or synthetic failure less likely.
- Avoid drugs or reduce dose if highly reliant on first-pass hepatic extraction if PSVA or APSS.

POSSIBLE INTERACTIONS

Drugs that influence p450 cytochrome hepatic metabolism, e.g., cimetidine, chloramphenicol, barbiturates, ketoconazole, may provoke adverse drug interactions.

FOLLOW-UP

PATIENT MONITORING

- Reevaluate patient at-home behavior and cognitive function, body condition, muscle mass, and weight; owner should record diary of progress and video abnormal behaviors.
- Monitor albumin and glucose.
- Adjust nutrition to optimize protein allowance and avoid sarcopenia.
- Monitor electrolytes—especially potassium if PU/PD or if diuretics prescribed.

PREVENTION/AVOIDANCE

Avoid provocative conditions—dehydration, azotemia, constipation, endoparasitism, enteric or oral bleeding, infusion of stored blood, hemolysis, meal-related ammonia challenge, urinary tract infections, hypokalemia, hypomagnesemia, alkalemia; and manage systemic infection or inflammation.

POSSIBLE COMPLICATIONS

Permanent neurologic damage may develop in chronic recurrent HE but uncommon; most often encountered in PSVA with acute severe HE.

EXPECTED COURSE AND PROGNOSIS

- Depends on underlying disorder.
- Acute or chronic hepatic failure—may be fully or partially reversible, or patient may die.

H

MISCELLANEOUS

AGE-RELATED FACTORS

PSVA—surgical outcome may be good in young and old patients.

SYNONYMS

- Hepatic coma.
- Portosystemic encephalopathy.

SEE ALSO

- Arteriovenous Malformation of the Liver.
- Ductal Plate Malformation (Congenital Hepatic Fibrosis).
- Hepatic Failure, Acute.
- Hepatitis, Chronic.
- Portosystemic Shunting, Acquired.
- Portosystemic Vascular Anomaly, Congenital.

ABBREVIATIONS

- APSS = acquired portosystemic shunt.
- BBB = blood–brain barrier.
- GI = gastrointestinal.
- HE = hepatic encephalopathy.
- PSVA = portosystemic vascular anomaly.
- PU/PD = polyuria/polydipsia.
- TSBA = total serum bile acids.

Suggested Reading

Hajihambi A, Arias N, Sheikh M, et al. Hepatic encephalopathy: a critical current review. Hepatol Int 2018, 12 (Suppl 1):S135–S147.

Lidbury JA, Cook AK, Steiner JM. Hepatic encephalopathy in dogs and cats. J Vet Emerg Crit Care 2016, 26:471–487.

Author Sharon A. Center

Editor Kate Holan

Client Education Handout available online

HEPATIC FAILURE, ACUTE

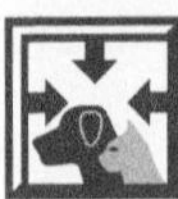

BASICS

DEFINITION

- Severe acute hepatic injury incapacitating ability to meet synthetic, metabolic, detoxification needs.
- Sudden loss of >75% of functional hepatic mass due to acute, massive hepatic necrosis.
- May lead to catastrophic multiorgan dysfunction/failure in previously healthy individual; may rapidly progress to death.

PATHOPHYSIOLOGY

- Necrosis—secondary to insufficient perfusion, hypoxia, hepatotoxins (drugs, other xenobiotics, toxins), heat excess, infectious agents.
- Severity of hepatic dysfunction depends on insult type and lobular (zonal) distribution.
- Reduced perfusion or hypoxia usually affects zone 3 (pericentral or centrilobular region).
- Ingested toxins—affect zone where toxin metabolized or toxic product formed, or where specific organelle tropism or propensity for oxidative injury (copper accumulation increases zone 3 vulnerability).
- Panlobular hepatic necrosis leading to acute liver failure uncommon; e.g., idiosyncratic drug toxicity: dogs—zonisamide, phenobarbital, primidone, diphenylhydantoin, nonsteroidal anti-inflammatory drugs (NSAIDs, e.g., carprofen), xylitol; cats—diazepam; dogs or cats—sulfa-antibiotics; primary toxins: dogs and cats—primary copper accumulation, acetaminophen; dogs—zonisamide, xylitol, cycad (sago palm), cheese tree (*Glochidion ferdinandi*) roots, blue-green algae, *Amanita* mushrooms, aflatoxin; infectious disease: dogs—leptospirosis, infectious canine hepatitis.
- Accompanied by enzyme leakage and markers of impaired liver function, hyperbilirubinemia, acute-onset splanchnic hypertension due to sinusoidal or centrilobular collapse.
- Lethal organ failure associated with coagulopathy, enteric hemorrhage, acute-onset hepatic encephalopathy (HE).
- Hepatic failure—associates with myriad metabolic derangements: altered glucose homeostasis, protein synthesis (albumin, transport proteins, procoagulants, anticoagulants), detoxification capabilities.

SYSTEMS AFFECTED

- Hepatobiliary—hepatocellular necrosis; hepatic failure, jaundice.
- Nervous—HE; cerebral edema.
- Gastrointestinal (GI)—vomiting; diarrhea; melena; hematochezia due to acute splanchnic hypertension ± coagulopathy.
- Hemic/lymphatic/immune—pro- and anticoagulant factor imbalances; disseminated intravascular coagulation (DIC).
- Renal/urologic—renal tubule damage from certain toxins or physiologic vasoconstriction; tubular injury: copper associated hepatopathy, leptospirosis, xylitol toxicity, NSAID toxicity.
- Hyperdynamic circulatory status—low systemic and pulmonary vascular resistance, increased cardiac output and metabolic rate, systemic hypotension; associates with endotoxemia, TNF-α, dehydration, and splanchnic hypertension.

INCIDENCE/PREVALENCE

Variable depending on preexistent liver disease: hepatocellular copper accumulation, chronic immune-mediated hepatitis, cholangitis.

SIGNALMENT

Species

More common in dog than cat.

Breed Predilections

Breeds with apparent predisposition to chronic hepatitis and copper associated hepatopathy (e.g., Labrador retriever, Doberman pinscher, Bedlington terrier) may have higher risk, e.g., Labrador retrievers and NSAID toxicity enhanced by copper associated hepatopathy.

SIGNS

- Acute-onset nonspecific clinical signs; lethargy, inappetence, GI disturbances (vomiting, small intestinal diarrhea may be bloody), polyuria/polydipsia (PU/PD).
- Tender hepatomegaly.
- Bleeding tendencies.
- Jaundice.
- HE.
- Seizures.

CAUSES

Drugs

- See Hepatotoxins.
- Drug-related toxicities *intrinsic* (direct) or *idiosyncratic* (unpredictable, unrelated to dose) consequent to immune-mediated hypersensitivity or metabolic injury.

Thermal Injury

- Heat stroke.
- Whole-body hyperthermia cancer treatment.

Hepatic Hypoxia

- Thromboembolic disease, shock, DIC.
- Acute circulatory failure from any cause.
- Acute centrilobular necrosis (zone 3).

RISK FACTORS

- Administration of potentially hepatotoxic substance or drug.
- Exposure to environmental toxins (e.g., *Amanita* mushroom, foodborne aflatoxin, cycad, cheese tree roots, blue-green algae), artificial sweetener—xylitol (gum, candy): dogs).
- Enzyme inducers (e.g., phenobarbital)—may increase risk for toxicities by enhancing xenobiotic toxin formation, e.g., acetaminophen toxicity greatly enhanced by phenobarbital.
- Indiscriminate substance ingestion—puppies; polyphagic animals.

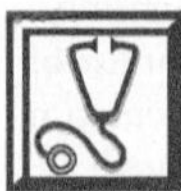

DIAGNOSIS

DIFFERENTIAL DIAGNOSIS

- Severe acute pancreatitis or gastroenteritis—differentiated via laboratory tests and imaging.
- Acutely decompensated chronic liver disease—distinguished by review of medical records, blood tests, abdominal US, liver biopsy.

CBC/BIOCHEMISTRY/URINALYSIS

- Anemia and panhypoproteinemia—bleeding, marrow toxicity, direct enteric toxicity.
- Thrombocytopenia—bleeding, DIC, portal hypertension.
- Liver enzyme activity—high acute alanine aminotransferase, and aspartate aminotransferase; smaller increases in alkaline phosphatase and γ-glutamyltransferase.
- Hypoglycemia—grave prognosis (esp. cats).
- Hypocholesterolemia—impaired synthesis or enteric loss with hemorrhage.
- Normal to low blood urea nitrogen concentration—reduced urea cycle function, PU/PD.
- Hyperbilirubinemia—initially absent.
- Bilirubinuria may precede hyperbilirubinemia—always abnormal in cats.
- Ammonium urate crystalluria signifies hyperammonemia, hepatic insufficiency, or portosystemic shunting.
- Acquired Fanconi syndrome—granular casts and renal glucosuria indicate proximal tubule injury (e.g., carprofen, copper, leptospirosis, other toxicities esp. in dogs).

OTHER LABORATORY TESTS

- Total serum bile acids (TSBA)—high values indicate hepatic dysfunction, cholestasis, or portosystemic shunting.
- Plasma ammonia concentration—high values coincide with high TSBA, confirm hepatic insufficiency; hyperammonemia inconsistent but reflected by ammonium biurate crystalluria; hyperammonemia may reflect concurrent myonecrosis.
- Coagulation tests—coagulation factor deficiencies, platelet dysfunction, low fibrinogen, low antithrombin or protein C activity, and DIC suggest severe liver failure, decompensated DIC, or enteric losses with hemorrhage.

IMAGING

- Abdominal radiography—may identify normal to slightly enlarged liver ± effusion.
- Abdominal US—may disclose nonhepatic disorders (e.g., pancreatitis), altered circulation (ratio hepatic vein : portal vein), altered liver echogenicity or surface contour reflecting chronic injury (e.g., remodeling

implicated by heterogeneous liver texture, nodularity, or hepatofugal portal blood flow); rule out biliary obstruction as source of hyperbilirubinemia.
• Brain MRI—may disclose early cerebral edema (not commonly done).

DIAGNOSTIC PROCEDURES

• Liver biopsy—confirms necrosis, characterizes lesion zonal distribution.
• Fine-needle liver aspirate may identify hepatocellular degeneration, copper accumulation, dysplastic hepatocytes observed with cycad or aflatoxin ingestion; canalicular cholestasis; many toxins lead to microvesicular hepatocellular lipid vacuolation.

PATHOLOGIC FINDINGS

• Gross—slightly enlarged, mottled liver.
• Microscopic—confirms necrosis; zonal involvement; may assist in determining underlying cause: hypoxia leading to zone 3 necrosis; certain toxins cause zone 1 or 3 necrosis; reticulin staining confirms zonal involvement, retention, or loss of reticulin substructure that orchestrates organized regeneration.

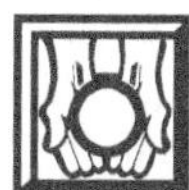

TREATMENT

APPROPRIATE HEALTH CARE

Inpatient—intensive care needed.

NURSING CARE

• *Caution*: delay inserting central catheters until bleeding diatheses controlled with vitamin K_1, fresh frozen plasma (FFP), or fresh whole blood; no advantage to prophylactic FFP administration as may contribute to onset of HE and cerebral edema.
• Fluids—non–lactate-containing; initially at resuscitation rate; monitor peripheral BP, pulse oximetry; mixed acid-base disturbances common.
• Colloid replacement—when low oncotic pressure from bleeding and protein loss; plasma always preferred; synthetic colloids second line; avoid dextran 70 and hetastarch (may promote bleeding) and human albumin (may induce fatal acute allergic reaction).
• Potassium, phosphate, glucose—supplement as appropriate; low phosphate, potassium, glucose aggravate HE and other clinical signs, complicating critical supportive care.
• Fluid regimen—adjust for maintenance needs after achieving euvolemia; typically provide ⅓ normal maintenance rate with polyionic crystalloids if concurrently giving slow CRI of synthetic colloid; avoid colloids if possible as leak from microvasculature (exacerbated with some toxicities that affect endothelium) and disturb signaling that triggers albumin and transporter protein synthesis.
• Supplemental oxygen—if pulse oximetry ≤94% saturation.
• If suspect cerebral edema—use 30° head-up elevation, consider mannitol, other interventions.
• Predisposition to infection from enteric bacterial translocation—cover with broad-spectrum antimicrobials; patient may not manifest fever or leukocytosis with infection; sepsis/systemic inflammatory response syndrome—major risks for cerebral edema.
• Early administration of *N*-acetylcysteine may improve microvascular perfusion, tissue oxygenation, and mitigate oxidative damage (see below).

ACTIVITY

Restricted activity—conserves energy and metabolites for healing and regeneration.

DIET

• Intractable vomiting—withhold PO food until controlled; antiemetics (see below).
• When enteric nutrition contraindicated (somnolent patient) use partial or total parenteral nutrition (TPN) until enteral feeding route established; <5 days advised.
• If enteric nutrition chronically compromised, establish TPN feeding catheter; use TPN formula with normal nitrogen content unless HE; branched-chain amino acids still controversial.
• Enteral feeding—small-volume, frequent meals; optimize digestion and assimilation, minimize enteric toxin formation contributing to HE.
• Diet composition—use normal protein (nitrogen) content in tolerant patients; moderate protein restriction if HE (2.5 g protein/kg bodyweight) but strive to maintain positive nitrogen balance for hepatic regeneration.
• Supplemental vitamins essential—water-soluble (twice normal); vitamin K_1 (0.5–1.5 mg/kg SC/IM, three doses at 12h intervals, then once to twice weekly); vitamin E (10 IU/kg PO or by injection q24h).
• Pro-/prebiotic yogurt—may protect against enteric bacterial translocation; tolerated dairy protein source if HE; controversial.

CLIENT EDUCATION

• Acute hepatic failure is serious condition.
• Some patients succumb despite optimal treatment.
• Cause of panlobular injury (e.g., exposure to drug or toxin) should be investigated but may remain unconfirmed.

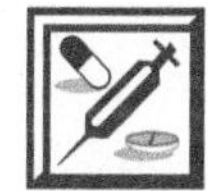

MEDICATIONS

DRUG(S) OF CHOICE

Drugs for Vomiting

• Metoclopramide—1–2 mg/kg/day CRI for intermittent mild vomiting; contraindicated if spironolactone used for ascites mobilization.
• Ondansetron—0.5–1.0 mg/kg IV q12h.
• Maropitant—1.0 mg/kg IV/SC q24h (some suggest decreasing dose by 50% in patients with hepatic dysfunction due to hepatic metabolism).
• Omeprazole (0.5–1.0 mg/kg PO q12–24h) or pantoprazole (0.7–1.0 mg/kg IV q12h) may induce P450 cytochrome–associated drug interactions; 24–48h delay in onset of action; preferred over H2 blockers for gastric ulceration.
• Histamine H2 blocker—famotidine (0.5–1.0 mg/kg IM/SC q12–24h) if enteric bleeding; reserve cimetidine (0.5 mg/kg q8–12h) for purposeful P450 cytochrome inhibition.
• Chlorpromazine—0.5 mg/kg SC/IM/rectally q8–24h for severe vomiting; ensure volume expansion first as causes alpha blockade vasodilation.

Drugs for HE

• Lactulose—0.5–2.0 mL/kg PO q8h or rectally if PO hazardous; goal is soft feces.
• Probiotic yogurt (see above).
• Metronidazole—7.5 mg/kg PO q12h or rectally if PO hazardous.
• Ampicillin/amoxicillin (esp. cats) —12.5–25 mg/kg IV/PO q8–12h.
• Rifaximin—5–10 mg/kg PO or rectally q12h (nonabsorbed antibiotic alters enteric flora).
• Neomycin—22 mg/kg PO or rectally q12h; *caution*: may be ototoxic and renal toxic if increased absorption with reduced gut integrity.

Treatment of Cerebral Edema Associated with HE

• Mannitol—1 g/kg over 10–20 min, filtered; if brisk diuresis does not occur (~1h), check for excessive volume expansion (plasma osmolality, BP) and renal function.
• Furosemide—0.5–1.0 mg/kg IV q8–24h increases free water excretion and reduces cerebrospinal fluid (CSF) production; monitor hydration and serum potassium; avoid dehydration and hypokalemia that provoke or worsen HE.
• Vasopressin V_2 antagonists (aquaretics) *may* assist with management of diuretic resistant ascites; tolvaptan successful in dogs with experimentally induced (rapid pacing) congestive heart failure (see Hypertension, Portal).

Drugs for Coagulopathy

Fresh whole blood or FFP—if clinically significant bleeding.

Free Radical Scavengers and Antioxidants

• For ongoing damage (membrane injury), reperfusion injury, and hypoxia.
• Vitamin E—10 IU/kg PO q24h.
• *N*-acetylcysteine—140 mg/kg IV/PO loading dose; IV use 10% solution diluted 1 : 2 in saline, administer via 0.25 μm nonpyrogenic filter; follow with 70 mg/kg q6–12h.
• *S*-adenosylmethionine as glutathione (GSH) donor, use proven bioavailable product—

H

20 mg/kg PO q24h on empty stomach; multiple benefits: essential intermediary metabolites, GSH synthesis, promotes liver regeneration, antifibrotic, anti-inflammatory.

Hepatoprotectants

- Silybin (milk thistle), efficacy reported for *Amanita* toxicity and certain other toxins; use complexed with polyunsaturated phosphatidylcholine, 2–5 mg/kg PO q24h.
- Ursodeoxycholic acid—if chronic liver injury or high bile acids persist, 10–15 mg/kg PO q24h or divided q12h, best absorbed with food.

Blocking Enterohepatic Circulation

Cholestyramine—30–40 mg/kg mixed with water PO q24h; bile acid–binding resin that can absorb certain toxins in alimentary canal that undergo enterohepatic circulation, diminishing systemic availability, e.g., sago palm (cycad toxin).

CONTRAINDICATIONS

- Ideally avoid drugs biotransformed primarily in liver, altering liver perfusion, or metabolizing enzyme activity; may be difficult as many drugs metabolized in hepatic pathways or eliminated in bile.
- Vitamin C—100–500 mg q24h, *avoid* if high liver iron or copper concentrations; ascorbate may augment transition metal–associated oxidative injury; no substantiation for vitamin C administration in liver failure.

PRECAUTIONS

Administration of stored whole blood or packed red blood cells may precipitate or exacerbate HE in dogs with hepatic failure because of spontaneously generated ammonia during storage.

POSSIBLE INTERACTIONS

Compromised hepatic metabolism.

ALTERNATIVE DRUG(S)

Case-based considerations.

FOLLOW-UP

PATIENT MONITORING

- Temperature, pulse, respiration, mental status—q1–2h until stable.
- Maintain vigilance for infection, especially catheter-induced.
- Bodyweight—twice daily guides fluid therapy; bodyweight and condition used to assess nitrogen and energy allowances.
- Acid-base, electrolyte balances (especially potassium and phosphate), glucose—q12–24h for first 72h.
- Sequential measurements of liver enzymes, bilirubin, cholesterol, fibrinogen q2–3 days provide evidence of recovery.

PREVENTION/AVOIDANCE

- Vaccinate dogs against infectious canine hepatitis virus.
- Avoid indiscriminate ingestion of hepatotoxins and environmental exposure.
- Consider drugs as potential toxins.

POSSIBLE COMPLICATIONS

- Hypoglycemia.
- Uncontrolled GI bleeding and DIC.
- HE, cerebral edema, brain herniation.
- Chronic hepatic insufficiency, cirrhosis, fibrosis from postnecrotic scarring.
- Acute renal failure.
- Death.

EXPECTED COURSE AND PROGNOSIS

Prognosis—depends on extent of liver injury, etiopathogenesis, supportive nursing care.

MISCELLANEOUS

ASSOCIATED CONDITIONS

- Pancreatitis.
- Sepsis/endotoxemia/shock.
- Bleeding diathesis; severe enteric hemorrhage; DIC.
- Renal failure.
- HE.

ZOONOTIC POTENTIAL

- Toxins (?).
- Leptospirosis.

SYNONYMS

- Acute hepatic necrosis.
- Fulminant hepatic failure.

SEE ALSO

- Acute Kidney Injury.
- Ascites.
- Coagulopathy of Liver Disease.
- Hepatic Encephalopathy.
- Hepatitis, Infectious (Viral) Canine.
- Hepatotoxins.
- Icterus.

ABBREVIATIONS

- CSF = cerebrospinal fluid.
- DIC = disseminated intravascular coagulation.
- FFP = fresh frozen plasma.
- GI = gastrointestinal.
- GSH = glutathione.
- HE = hepatic encephalopathy.
- NSAID = nonsteroidal anti-inflammatory drug.
- PU/PD = polyuria, polydipsia.
- TPN = total parenteral nutrition.
- TSBA = total serum bile acids.

Suggested Reading

Center SA. Acute hepatic injury: hepatic necrosis and fulminant hepatic failure. In: Guilford GW, Center SA, Strombeck DR, et al. Small Animal Gastroenterology. Philadelphia, PA: Saunders, 1996, pp. 654–704.

Center SA, Elston TH, Rowland PH, et al. Fulminant hepatic failure associated with oral administration of diazepam in 11 cats. J Am Vet Med Assoc 1996, 209:618–625.

Dunayer EK, Gwaltney-Brant SM. Acute hepatic failure and coagulopathy associated with xylitol ingestion in eight dogs. J Am Vet Med Assoc 2006, 229:1113–1117.

Hughes D, King LG. The diagnosis and management of acute liver failure in dogs and cats. Vet Clin North Am Small Anim Pract 1995, 25:437–460.

MacPhail CM, Lappin MR, Meyer DJ, et al. Hepatocellular toxicosis associated with administration of carprofen in 21 dogs. J Am Vet Med Assoc 1998, 212(12):1895–1901.

Miller ML, Center SA, Randolph JF, et al. Apparent acute idiosyncratic hepatic necrosis associated with zonisamide administration in a dog. J Vet Intern Med 2011, 25:1156–1160.

Authors Linda K. Okonkowski and Kate Holan

Consulting Editor Kate Holan

Acknowledgment The author and book editors acknowledge the prior contribution of Sharon A. Center

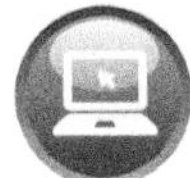

Client Education Handout available online

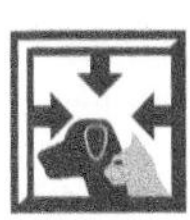

BASICS

DEFINITION

- Feline hepatic lipidosis (HL)—lipid vacuolation distends the cytosolic compartment in >80% of hepatocytes.
- Untreated—leads to progressive metabolic dysregulation, hepatic failure, and death.
- Develops secondary to a primary disease or condition causing anorexia or catabolism; idiopathic HL is uncommon: a cause is usually discoverable.

PATHOPHYSIOLOGY

- Cats have a unique propensity to accumulate triglyceride-filled hepatocellular vacuoles.
- Causal factors—negative energy and protein balance with increased peripheral fat mobilization.
- Cytosolic triglyceride vacuoles cause severe cholestasis and jaundice via canalicular compression and associated hepatic organelle dysfunction.
- Hepatic failure—with rare evidence of hepatic encephalopathy (HE).

SYSTEMS AFFECTED

- Hepatobiliary.
- Gastrointestinal—anorexia; vomiting.
- Musculoskeletal—peripheral muscle wasting (sarcopenia) and fat mobilization.
- Nervous—HE, ptyalism, moribund status.
- Hemic/lymphatic/immune—abnormal red blood cell (RBC) shapes (poikilocytes), Heinz body hemolysis.
- Renal/urologic—potassium wasting; renal tubule triglyceride accumulation.

INCIDENCE/PREVALENCE

Most common severe hepatopathy in North America causing jaundice in pet cats.

GEOGRAPHIC DISTRIBUTION

Worldwide

SIGNALMENT

Species

Cats, rarely dogs (toy-breed failure-to-thrive puppies), juveniles with lysosomal or glycogen storage disease; may develop in small-breed puppies with portosystemic vascular anomaly (PSVA).

Breed Predilection

N/A

Mean Age and Range

Middle-aged adult cats—median age 8 (range: 1–16 years).

Predominant Sex

N/A

SIGNS

Historical Findings

- Anorexia or hyporexia, weight loss, sarcopenia.
- Vomiting, diarrhea or constipation, jaundice.
- Lethargy, with gradual onset of weakness progressing to collapse.
- Ptyalism.
- Neck ventriflexion—weakness, electrolyte depletions (potassium, phosphate), thiamine deficiency.
- Underlying disease or illness causing hyporexia/anorexia → hepatic lipidosis.

Physical Examination Findings

- Jaundice.
- Hepatomegaly.
- Dehydration.
- Weakness—neck ventriflexion, recumbency.
- Ptyalism.
- Collapse ←→ obtunded (signs of HE).
- Others, depending on underlying primary disease.

CAUSES

"Idiopathic" Hepatic Lipidosis

Idiopathic = uncommon; antecedent health problems discoverable in >85% of cases causing anorexia or malassimilation; remainder have food deprivation often attributable to adverse social interactions, environmental cause.

Secondary Hepatic Lipidosis

- Primary liver disease—PSVA; cholangitis/cholangiohepatitis syndrome (CCHS); extrahepatic bile duct obstruction (EHBDO); cholelithiasis; neoplasia.
- Gastrointestinal—obstruction; neoplasia; inflammatory bowel disease (IBD); pancreatitis.
- Urogenital disease—renal failure, chronic interstitial nephritis (CIN), lower urinary tract syndromes.
- Neurologic conditions—cannot eat.
- Infectious diseases—toxoplasmosis; feline infectious peritonitis (FIP); feline immunodeficiency virus (FIV)– or feline leukemia virus (FeLV)–related disorders.
- Hyperthyroidism.
- Vitamin B_{12} deficiency and deficiency of other water-soluble vitamins may predispose cats to HL as a result of disrupted metabolism as one factor.
- Many other systemic conditions or toxins can provoke anorexia and lead to HL.
- Rapid weight loss protocols or change to restricted-calorie diet the cat refuses to eat.

RISK FACTORS

- Obesity.
- Anorexia, negative nitrogen balance.
- Catabolism or rapid weight loss.
- Water-soluble vitamin deficiency.

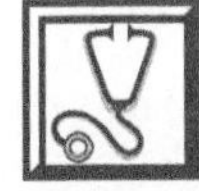

DIAGNOSIS

DIFFERENTIAL DIAGNOSIS

- Primary liver disease—CCHS, cholelithiasis, EHBDO, or neoplasia (esp. lymphosarcoma) differentiated by abdominal US, liver aspiration, and liver biopsy.
- PSVA—diagnosis by US or colorectal scintigraphy, lab testing.
- Hepatic toxoplasmosis or FIP—liver biopsy, serology, immunohistochemistry.
- Pancreatitis—differentiated by US, serum tests, pancreatic aspiration cytology, gross inspection, biopsy.
- Gastrointestinal disease—IBD differentiated by bowel biopsies; obstruction differentiated by abdominal survey or contrast radiography and US.
- Toxicities—suspected based on history (e.g., oral diazepam, acetaminophen, methimazole).
- Hyperthyroidism—serum thyroid panel, absence of jaundice.

H

CBC/BIOCHEMISTRY/URINALYSIS

- Hematology—poikilocytes common; nonregenerative anemia; hemolytic anemia (severe hypophosphatemia or Heinz bodies).
- Biochemistry—hyperbilirubinemia; high alkaline phosphatase (ALP), alanine aminotransferase (ALT), ± aspartate aminotransferase (AST) activity; normal or mild increase in γ-glutamyltransferase (GGT) if no primary necro-inflammatory ductal disorder (i.e., biliary, pancreatic); low blood urea nitrogen (BUN); normal creatinine; variable glucose (hypoglycemia rare); variable cholesterol, albumin, globulins; hypokalemia; hypophosphatemia, increased ketones (beta-hydroxybutyrate); lactic acidosis.
- Urinalysis—bilirubinuria, lipiduria, and unconcentrated urine common.

OTHER LABORATORY TESTS

- Prolonged coagulation times—prothrombin time (PT), activated partial thromboplastin time (APTT), activated clotting time (ACT); fibrinogen usually normal.
- Hyperammonemia—uncommon.
- Serum bile acids—high before hyperbilirubinemic; redundant test if hepatobiliary jaundice.
- B_{12} deficiency.

IMAGING

Survey Abdominal Radiography

- Hepatomegaly.
- May note features of underlying disorder.

Abdominal US

- Diffuse hyperechoic hepatic parenchyma, hepatomegaly.
- Look for primary disease causing HL.

DIAGNOSTIC PROCEDURES

- Fine-needle liver aspiration cytology—>80% hepatocytes display severe cytosolic lipid vacuolation; biopsy rarely needed to confirm HL.
- Definitive diagnosis HL—based on history, clinical features, high ALP, diffuse hyperechoic hepatic parenchyma, severe hepatocyte lipid

HEPATIC LIPIDOSIS (CONTINUED)

vacuolation on aspiration cytology; however, cannot rule out primary hepatic disorders (e.g., CCHS, EHBDO, PSVA) with these tests.
- Liver biopsy—definitive diagnosis of underlying "primary" liver disorders; *done only if poor response to therapy or high GGT*; *caution*: stabilize cat before anesthesia and liver biopsy.
- Vitamin K_1 (0.5–1.5 mg/kg SC/IM) three doses at 12h intervals, *before* aspiration sampling, liver biopsy, jugular vein catheterization, cystocentesis, or feeding appliance insertion.

H

PATHOLOGIC FINDINGS

- Gross—diffuse hepatomegaly, smooth surface, friable greasy consistency, yellow/pale color with reticulated appearance; sample floats in formalin.
- Microscopic—diffuse, severe hepatocellular lipid vacuolation; large (macrovesicular) or small (microvesicular) vacuolation; type of vacuolation lacks prognostic value.

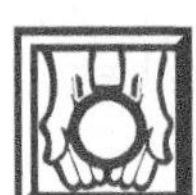

TREATMENT

APPROPRIATE HEALTH CARE

- Inpatient—recumbent cats or those with neck ventriflexion and anorectic.
- Discharge for home care—see Patient Monitoring.
- Frequent reevaluations imperative.
- Outpatient—reduces stress and thereby facilitates recovery in some cats.

NURSING CARE

- Balanced polyionic fluids—*avoid* lactate and dextrose supplementation; 0.9% NaCl preferred.
- Potassium chloride supplementation essential (see Hypokalemia).
- Phosphate supplements usually needed (see Hypophosphatemia) at initial feeding; often started prophylactically, see below.
- Magnesium supplements rarely needed.

Correct Hypophosphatemia

- Serum phosphate <2.0 mg/dL reflects refeeding syndrome; may provoke anorexia, vomiting, weakness, myonecrosis, ileus, hemolysis, coagulopathy, neurologic signs confused with HE.
- Treatment—potassium phosphate initial dose 0.01–0.03 mmol/kg/h IV; monitor serum phosphate q6h; discontinue when stable phosphate >2 mg/dL; *caution*: judiciously reduce IV potassium chloride supplements concurrently given in fluids; monitor potassium.

Correct Hepatic and Circulating GSH Depletion

- Low liver glutathione (GSH) confirmed in HL; routine GSH measurements not available.
- Crisis intervention for low hepatic GSH or Heinz body anemia—*N*-acetylcysteine (NAC) 140 mg/kg IV, then 70 mg/kg IV, 10% solution diluted 1 : 2 in saline; administered over 20 min otherwise may provoke hyperammonemia.
- When enteral feeding established, change to *S*-adenosylmethionine (SAMe) 200 mg/cat PO q24h; need for dosing on empty stomach complicates use.

ACTIVITY

Physical activity (walking), when possible, may increase gastric motility when gastroparesis complicates feeding (chronic vomiting).

DIET

- Nutritional support—cornerstone of recovery.
- High-protein, high-calorie balanced feline diet essential.
- Energy—50–60 kcal/kg ideal weight/day; gradual transition to full energy requirement over 3–7 days; feed multiple small meals/day or trickle feed through esophageal feeding tube (E-tube).
- Forced alimentation usually required; *caution*: *oral* forced feeding may provoke food aversion syndrome.
- Correct hypokalemia and hydration before commencing feeding; associated gastroparesis may lead to vomiting and potential for aspiration pneumonia.
- Tube feeding—initially by nasogastric tube (first 1–2 days *after* electrolyte and vitamin deficiency improved), transition to E-tube after hydration and electrolyte status improves, and vitamin K_1 protocol administered.
- Avoid laparotomy for gastric feeding tube insertion; cats with HL have high risk for mortality with general anesthesia and surgery; E-tube preferable.
- Cautiously offer PO food daily to assess interest.
- Human stress formula enteral diets (not recommended)—require supplemental arginine (or citrulline), and taurine; use feline formulated liquified diet with vitamin supplements.

Supplements

- Supplements improve survival in severely affected cats.
- Water-soluble vitamins—in IV fluids; generally 2 mL/L.
- Thiamin—50–100 mg/day, give PO rather than SC/IM, also add via water-soluble vitamins mixed in IV fluids.
- Vitamin B_{12}—initially 0.25–1 mg IM/SC once): determine chronic vitamin B_{12} needs by sequential B_{12} values (weekly, q2 weeks, to monthly then quarterly intervals).
- Medical-grade L-carnitine (250–500 mg/day); over-the-counter carnitine supplements have wide variability in bioavailability; Carnitor® (liquid medical-grade carnitine) recommended.
- Taurine 250–500 mg/day PO.
- Vitamin E 10 IU/kg/day PO in food- use water-soluble form initially.
- Thiol donors IV NAC, PO SAMe—as above.
- Potassium gluconate (for hypokalemia) PO, reduce fluid potassium supplements.
- Marine oil in food 2000 mg q24h.

CLIENT EDUCATION

- Warn client—sequential biochemical assessments needed to monitor recovery.
- Educate client about feeding tube use/care and need for chronic use (up to 4–6 months).
- Advise client—recurrence unlikely; liver function will not be chronically compromised.

SURGICAL CONSIDERATIONS

- Avoid surgical interventions until normalization of hydration, electrolyte depletions, and supplements of vitamins provided, Heinz body anemia alleviated.
- Exploratory laparotomy and liver biopsy—*only* indicated if failure to improve on described interventions or marked increase in GGT activity to identify underlying disorders; biopsy liver, pancreas, stomach, and small bowel if explored; lymph nodes if enlarged.

MEDICATIONS

DRUG(S) OF CHOICE

- Vitamin K_1—recommended for all cats with suspected HL; see above, avoid overdosage.
- Drugs to ameliorate HE (see Hepatic Encephalopathy), rarely.
- Emesis control—metoclopramide: for vomiting, nausea, gastroparesis (0.2–0.5 mg/kg SC q8h 30 min before feeding, or as CRI IV drip at 0.01–0.02 mg/kg/h or 1–2 mg/kg/day); dolasetron or ondansetron; or maropitant (1 mg/kg IV/SC/PO q24h 5 days max); pantoprazole to avert esophageal damage secondary to vomiting (0.5–1.0 mg/kg q12–24h).
- Systemic antibiotics—as appropriate for suspected infection.

CONTRAINDICATIONS/PRECAUTIONS

- Downward adjust dosages of medications relying on hepatic metabolism or excretion.
- Avoid benzodiazepines and barbiturates—may provoke HE.
- Appetite stimulants do not provide dependable energy intake in cats with HL; some produce sedation; diazepam may cause rare fulminant hepatic failure.
- Avoid injectable medications with propylene glycol carrier; may lead to hemolysis in cats with low GSH.
- Ursodeoxycholic acid—likely not beneficial; may promote taurine deficiency.
- Dextrose supplements—may provoke hepatic triglyceride accumulation.

- Avoid tetracyclines or stanozolol—promote hepatocyte triglyceride vacuolation.
- Avoid recurrent or prolonged use of propofol—may provoke hemolysis (12h after infusion) esp. in cats with Heinz body anemia; HL cats may recover slowly; alternatively use gas anesthesia.

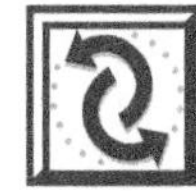

FOLLOW-UP

PATIENT MONITORING

- Bodyweight and condition, hydration, electrolytes; judicious adjustment of energy, fluid, electrolyte, and vitamin provisions essential.
- Serum bilirubin—predicts recovery.
- Reduced lactate and ketones reconcile with metabolic improvement.
- Liver enzyme activity—do not predict recovery.
- Discharge for home care—when vomiting controlled, gastroparesis resolved, bilirubin declining, patient ambulatory, and tube-feeding apparatus problem-free.
- Tube feeding—discontinued only after confirmed voluntary food consumption.

PREVENTION/AVOIDANCE

- Obesity—prevent; weight reduction must not exceed 2% bodyweight per week.
- Caution owner to verify food intake during weight loss regimens and at-home stress.

POSSIBLE COMPLICATIONS

- Feeding tube malfunction or obstruction—tube obstructions relieved with papaya juice, carbonated soft drink, or pancreatic enzyme slurry; 15 min dwell time, warm water flush.
- Rare HE after dietary support introduced.
- Unremitting HL can lead to lethal hepatic failure.
- Untreatable underlying causal disorder.

EXPECTED COURSE AND PROGNOSIS

- Optimal response to tube feeding and nutritional supplements—recovery in 3–6 weeks.
- Therapy as described—85% recovery in severely affected animals with controllable primary disease process that provoked HL.
- Underlying disease influences outcome.
- HL rarely recurs.
- HL does not cause chronic liver dysfunction, hepatitis, persistent remodeling.

MISCELLANEOUS

ASSOCIATED CONDITIONS

- Primary liver disorders.
- Pancreatitis.
- Malassimilation—various causes but IBD predominant.
- Diabetes mellitus—relatively uncommon.
- Neoplasia—hepatic and systemic.
- HE (rare).
- Systemic illness limiting food intake.

SYNONYMS

- Fatty liver syndrome.
- Hepatosteatosis.
- Feline hepatic vacuolation.
- Vacuolar hepatopathy.
- Vacuolar degeneration.

SEE ALSO

- Cholangitis/Cholangiohepatitis Syndrome.
- Hepatic Encephalopathy.

ABBREVIATIONS

- ACT = activated clotting time.
- ALP = alkaline phosphatase.
- ALT = alanine aminotransferase.
- APTT = activated partial thromboplastin time.
- AST = aspartate aminotransferase.
- BUN = blood urea nitrogen.
- CCHS = cholangitis/cholangiohepatitis syndrome.
- CIN = chronic interstitial nephritis.
- EHBDO = extrahepatic bile duct obstruction.
- FeLV = feline leukemia virus.
- FIV = feline immunodeficiency virus.
- GGT = gamma glutamyltransferase.
- GSH = glutathione.
- HE = hepatic encephalopathy.
- HL = hepatic lipidosis.
- IBD = inflammatory bowel disease.
- NAC = *N*-acetylcysteine.
- PSVA = portosystemic vascular anomaly.
- PT = prothrombin time.
- RBC = red blood cell.
- SAMe = *S*-adenosylmethionine.

Suggested Reading

Center SA. Feline hepatic lipidosis. Vet Clin North Am Small Anim Pract 2005, 35:225–269.

Center SA, Warner KL, Randolph JF, et al. Influence of dietary supplementation with (L)-carnitine on metabolic rate, fatty acid oxidation, body condition, and weight loss in overweight cats. Am J Vet Res 2012, 73:1002–1015.

Kuzi S, Segev G, Kedar S, et al. Prognostic markers in feline hepatic lipidosis: a retrospective study of 71 cats. Vet Rec. 2017, 181(19):512. doi: 10.1136/vr.104252

Author Sharon A. Center
Consulting Editor Kate Holan

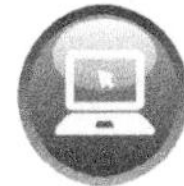

Client Education Handout available online

HEPATIC NODULAR HYPERPLASIA AND DYSPLASTIC HYPERPLASIA

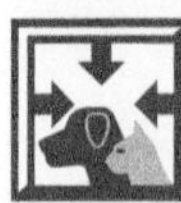

BASICS

OVERVIEW

Hepatic Nodular Hyperplasia (HNH)

• Benign parenchymal feature in middle-aged to older dogs; nonencapsulated, ≤2 cm (rarely up to 5 cm), expansile nodule of hepatocellular hyperplasia, maintaining a modified lobular architecture with recognizable central and portal elements that are irregularly spaced, organized hepatic cord structure 1 cell wide, without marginal parenchymal collapse or fibrosis (is not a regenerative nodule), smooth margins; hepatocyte phenotype may be similar to surrounding parenchyma but may contain glycogen of lipid vacuoles.
• May associate with increased liver enzymes in elderly dogs, especially alkaline phosphatase (ALP).
• Clinical concern derives from association with increased liver enzyme activity and US detection of hepatic nodules or hepatic nodularity during exploratory surgery.
• Variable US appearance.
• Biopsy specimens must include affected and unaffected liver for appropriate interpretation.
• Nodular hyperplasia may be mistaken for regeneration secondary to chronic hepatitis or hepatocellular neoplasia (adenoma) with needle core biopsies or when only nodular tissue without normal hepatic tissue is sampled.

Hepatocellular Dysplastic Hyperplasia (HDH)

• Potentially preneoplastic proliferative hepatocellular foci in dogs with glycogen-type vacuolar hepatopathy (VH); nonencapsulated, variably sized, reduced reticulin substructure, expansile nodules of nonvacuolated hepatocytes forming wide (2 cells wide, normal = 1 cell width) disorganized hepatic cords, an irregular (serrated) margin interfacing with adjacent "normal VH" affected hepatocytes, and lacking remodeled marginal lesions (fibrosis, parenchymal collapse).
• Associates with VH-related increased liver enzymes, dominated by increased ALP activity.
• Recognized as an antecedent hepatic lesion in dogs developing hepatocellular carcinoma (e.g., Scottish terriers, also other breeds) and is seemingly associated with increased sex hormone concentrations (androgens, progestins).
• Variable US appearance depending on size, number, distribution.
• May be mistaken for nodular regeneration without special stains to detail reticulin substructure and collagen fibril deposition.

SIGNALMENT

HNH

• Age-related lesion.
• Nodules develop by 6–8 years of age; one study documented lesions in all geriatric dogs >14 years of age.

HDH

• Associated with glycogen-type VH.
• Reflects adrenal hyperplasia syndromes.

SIGNS

Physical Examination Findings

• HNH does not cause clinical illness.
• Large nodules that rupture and bleed or nodules impairing hepatic sinusoidal perfusion likely represent misdiagnosed hepatic adenomas or well-differentiated hepatocellular carcinoma.
• HDH is associated with glycogen-type VH syndromes (see Glycogen-Type Vacuolar Hepatopathy).

CAUSES & RISK FACTORS

• HNH etiology—unknown; metabolic factors, prior injurious events. In humans associated with infarcts, but no evidence of this in dogs.
• HDH etiology—may represent hormonal influence promoting neoplastic transformation (sex hormone–related adrenal hyperplasia).

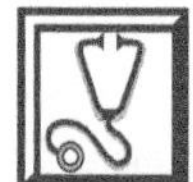

DIAGNOSIS

DIFFERENTIAL DIAGNOSIS

• Necroinflammatory liver disease—regenerative nodular hyperplasia involves the entire liver; formation of irregular nodules of variable size that are segregated by parenchymal collapse, often marginated by fibrous connective tissue; demonstrate loss of lobular architecture, sinusoidal fibrosis, reduced reticulin substructure, and wide disorganized hepatic cords.
• Neoplasia—hepatic adenoma: mass lesions with margins reflecting expansile compression on normal adjacent liver, encapsulated, hepatic cords double wide, disorganized, reduced reticulin substructure, and minimal atypia. Hepatocellular carcinoma: single or multiple confluent or separate mass lesions, margins reflecting irregular expansile compression on normal adjacent liver, partially encapsulated, variable width of disorganized hepatic cords >2 cells, multiple phenotypes differing from adjacent normal tissue, variable atypia (may be well differentiated), may display pseudoglandular pattern associated with giant canaliculi, well-vascularized with arterial twigs; retention of some normal lobular elements possible (primarily at the periphery).

CBC/BIOCHEMISTRY/URINALYSIS

• CBC—no association with HNH; for HDH see Glycogen-Type Vacuolar Hepatopathy.
• Biochemistry profile—increased serum ALP activity may be encountered with HNH and HDH; may range from 2.5- to 16-fold normal; higher with HDH and VH syndrome, see Glycogen-Type Vacuolar Hepatopathy; usually normal total protein, albumin, bilirubin, and cholesterol.
• Urinalysis—no consistent findings.

OTHER LABORATORY TESTS

Total serum bile acids (TSBA)—usually normal, unless lesions are diffuse and severe.

IMAGING

• Abdominal radiography—no abnormalities except hepatomegaly with HDH due to VH.
• Abdominal US—variable echogenicity relating to histologic features, nodule number and size, and associated VH. HNH often not noted until liver grossly inspected at surgery or laparoscopy.

DIAGNOSTIC PROCEDURES

• Aspiration cytology—may yield normal hepatocytes, hepatocytes with cytosolic rarefication and fragility consistent with VH (glycogen retention), or cells with discrete lipid (triglyceride) vacuoles (HNH); occasional binucleate hepatocytes may reflect cell proliferation or other concurrent disease (common in portosystemic vascular anomalies/ microvascular dysplasia); hepatocytes may be small with size variation in HDH. Liver biopsy—collection of a needle biopsy specimen may not clearly differentiate HNH lesion because of small specimen size; definitive diagnosis requires targeted sampling of a large enough tissue specimen to include lesion and adjacent normal hepatic tissue. HDH may be recognized on needle samples.
• Recommended biopsy methods—laparoscopy, open-wedge biopsy during laparotomy, or multiple 14-G needle samples.
• Special stains—reticulin staining illustrates hepatocyte reticulin substructure, lobular collapse/remodeling, and changes associated with nodule margins. Masson's trichrome staining illustrates collagen deposition and remodeling typical of regenerative nodules secondary to chronic liver injury; periodic acid-Schiff staining with and without amylase predigestion confirms excess glycogen in vacuolated hepatocytes (see Glycogen-Type Vacuolar Hepatopathy).

PATHOLOGIC FINDINGS

• HNH gross—single or multiple mass lesions, rarely >2 cm in diameter; color similar to adjacent normal hepatic tissue or paler if vacuolated with glycogen or lipid.
• HDH gross—single or multiple lesions, usually small, may appear darker colored compared to adjacent tissue. Microscopic—see above.

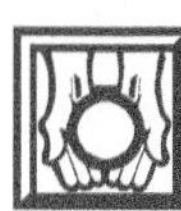

TREATMENT

- Usually none required; rupture of large nodules indicates hepatocellular carcinoma misdiagnosis; may necessitate blood transfusion and emergency mass excision. Palliate or alleviate underlying cause of VH.
- HDH—recommend biochemical assessments for rising ALP or alanine aminotransferase (ALT) that may indicate transformation of mass lesion to a neoplastic phenotype; US inspection of adrenal glands for adrenomegaly or nodules, US surveillance for expanding mass lesions that should be surgically removed; assess pituitary adrenal axis for typical or atypical hyperadrenocorticism; if increased sex hormones >2.5 × upper reference interval consider adrenal modulation with agent that does not increase sex hormones.

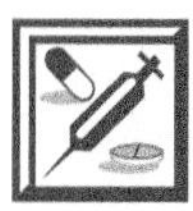

MEDICATIONS

DRUG(S) OF CHOICE

- HDH—if increased sex hormones, progressive VH, nodule formation, increasing ALP, or confirmed hepatocellular carcinoma (after mass resection), consider adrenal modulation with a drug that does not increase sex hormone concentrations (Lysodren® or mitotane); trilostane increases sex hormone concentrations and would be inappropriate.
- Scottish terrier syndrome does not respond to adrenal modulation; instead use surveillance to detect emerging hepatocellular carcinoma.

FOLLOW-UP

PATIENT MONITORING

- Quarterly biochemical profiles.
- Sequential abdominal US to evaluate progression of hepatic nodules.
- See Glycogen-Type Vacuolar Hepatopathy for related disorders.

POSSIBLE COMPLICATIONS

Distinction of HNH from neoplastic foci is not possible based only on clinical, laboratory, or imaging data, although lesions >2 cm are unlikely to be this diagnosis.

EXPECTED COURSE AND PROGNOSIS

More extensive numbers of nodules may develop in some dogs with HNH and HDH; HDH predicts risk for primary hepatocellular neoplasia, which requires surveillance and surgical treatment.

MISCELLANEOUS

SEE ALSO

- Cirrhosis and Fibrosis of the Liver.
- Glycogen-Type Vacuolar Hepatopathy.
- Hepatitis, Chronic.
- Hepatocellular Adenoma.
- Hepatocellular Carcinoma.

ABBREVIATIONS

- ALP = alkaline phosphatase.
- ALT = alanine aminotransferase.
- HDH = hepatic dysplastic hyperplasia.
- HNH = hepatic nodular hyperplasia.
- TSBA = total serum bile acids.
- VH = vacuolar hepatopathy.

Suggested Reading

Cortright CC, Center SA, Randolph JF, et al. Clinical features of progressive vacuolar hepatopathy in Scottish Terriers with and without hepatocellular carcinoma: 114 cases (1980–2013). J Am Vet Med Assoc 2014, 245:797–808.

Sepesy LM, Center SA, Randolph JF, et al. Vacuolar hepatopathy in dogs: 336 cases (1993–2005). J Am Vet Med Assoc 2006, 229:246–252.

Stowater JL, Lamb CR, Schelling SH. Ultrasonographic features of canine hepatic nodular hyperplasia. Vet Radiol 1990, 31:268–272.

Author Sharon A. Center

Consulting Editor Kate Holan

Acknowledgment The author and book editors acknowledge the prior contribution of Sean P. McDonough.

HEPATITIS, CHRONIC

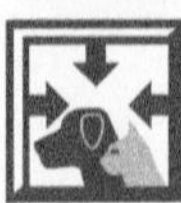

BASICS

DEFINITION

• Hepatic injury associated with active chronic necroinflammatory liver injury; "chronic active hepatitis" should not be used.
• Nonsuppurative inflammation—most common; lymphocytes, plasma cells, macrophages, occasional neutrophils.
• Chronicity—progressive remodeling, regenerative nodule formation, evolving sinusoidal fibrosis with location dependent on zonal tropism of inflammation; changes eventuate in cirrhosis.

PATHOPHYSIOLOGY

• A multitude of initiating events or agents cause hepatic injury; damage to cell and/or organelle membranes usually involves oxidative injury; activated cytokines and cell-mediated immune responses widen and perpetuate inflammation; hepatic neoepitopes may become targeted foci.
• Initial injury may include infectious agents, toxins, xenobiotics, or pathologic Cu accumulation; with exception of Cu-mediated injury, cause often remains undetermined.
• Inflammatory cells—predominantly lymphocytes, fewer Kupffer cells (resident hepatic sinusoidal macrophages), and variable neutrophils are initial effectors.
• Injury zone demarcates area of predominant necroinflammatory damage—zone 1 (periportal) common to idiopathic hepatitis or inflammation involving portal tract structures; zone 3 incriminates Cu, nonsteroidal anti-inflammatory drug (NSAID), other xenobiotic or toxin-mediated injury, or repeated ischemic/hypoxic insult; panlobular inflammation common.
• Lesion progression—variable, may include portal and periportal lymphoplasmacytic infiltrates with interface hepatitis (inflammation breaching limiting plate of portal tract), and otherwise variable lobular injury; chronic inflammation: leads to progressive fibrosis with bridging of involved zones.
• Bridging fibrosis and regenerative nodules distort lobular architecture; fibrosis, intrahepatic sinusoidal hypertension, neovascularization, and impaired hepatic function evolve into cirrhosis.
• Progressive cholestasis due to mechanical compression/distortion of bile ducts may occur.
• Cirrhosis and hepatic failure—late stage.
• Fibrosis—usually reflects chronic injury from sustained inflammation.
• Cirrhosis—associated with hepatic dysfunction, sinusoidal hypertension; intrahepatic shunting through collagenized sinusoids or neovascular pathways in fibrotic partitions that segregate regenerative nodules.
• Sinusoidal hypertension—leads to hepatofugal portal circulation (flow away from liver); mesenteric splanchnic hypertension; development of acquired portosystemic shunt(s) (APSS); episodic hepatic encephalopathy (HE); ascites; portal hypertensive enteric vasculopathy predisposes to enteric bleeding.

SYSTEMS AFFECTED

• Hepatobiliary—inflammation; necrosis; cholestasis; fibrosis.
• Gastrointestinal (GI)—emesis; diarrhea; anorexia, portal hypertension, ascites, and propensity for enteric bleeding.
• Neurologic—HE (advanced stage, associated with APSS).
• Hemic—red blood cell (RBC) microcytosis reflects APSS; bleeding or thrombotic tendencies: failed factor or anticoagulant synthesis or activation, thrombocytopenia or thrombopathia; coagulopathies typically observed with advanced injury or severe diffuse hepatic necrosis.
• Renal/urologic—polyuria/polydipsia (PU/PD); isosthenuria; ammonium biurate crystalluria (advanced stage with APSS and HE).
• Endocrine/metabolic—hypoglycemia if end-stage liver failure.
• Respiratory—tachypnea if tense ascites; bicavitary effusion or pulmonary edema.

GENETICS

• Breed or familial predisposition for chronic hepatitis—Doberman pinscher, Labrador retriever, West Highland white terrier, and Dalmatian may develop chronic hepatitis secondary to pathologic Cu accumulation; cocker spaniel hepatopathy, anecdotal in other breeds or breeding lines.
• Inherited Cu associated hepatopathy only proven in Bedlington terrier— autosomal recessive, genetic test available.

SIGNALMENT

Species

Dog

Breed Predilection

See Genetics.

Mean Age and Range

Average age 6–8 years (range: 2–14 years).

Predominant Gender

Inconsistent among reports for any breed.

SIGNS

General Comments

• Initially—vague and nonspecific, often includes lethargy and inappetence.
• Later—relate to complications of portal hypertension; impaired hepatic function including cholestasis.

Historical Findings

• May be no signs in early disease or mild lethargy.
• Anorexia, vomiting, weight loss, reduced body condition.
• PU/PD.
• Jaundice—later stage unless portal hepatitis involves bile duct injury.
• Ascites—late stage.
• HE—late stage, infers APSS with cirrhosis.

Physical Examination Findings

• May be no signs in early disease.
• Lethargy, poor coat, declining body condition.
• Variable jaundice.
• Liver size—normal to small, depends on chronicity.

Late-Stage Physical Findings

• Ascites.
• HE.
• Obstructive uropathy—ammonium biurates.
• Bleeding or thrombotic tendencies.

CAUSES

• Chronic necroinflammatory, oxidant, and immune-mediated liver injury has many causes.
• Infectious—canine hepatitis virus; leptospirosis, enteric-portal bacteremia or endotoxemia affiliated with inflammatory bowel disease; accidental parenteral administration of intranasal *Bordetella* vaccine.
• Immune-mediated—autoimmune with positive antinuclear antibody (ANA); acquired immune sensitization, nonsuppurative inflammation.
• Toxic—Cu associated hepatopathy; acute or chronic exposure to drugs—predictable or idiosyncratic toxicity: e.g., azole antifungals, trimethoprim-sulfa, zonisamide, phenobarbital, primidone, phenytoin, CCNU, NSAIDs (esp. carprofen); repeat exposure to environmental or food-borne toxins, e.g., dimethylnitrosamine, aflatoxin, cycad, cyanobacteria.

RISK FACTORS

• Immunostimulants (vaccinations?) and molecular mimicry of cell epitopes by infectious agents or infection of sinusoidal endothelium.
• Cu associated hepatopathy.
• Hepatic iron accumulation—from inappropriate supplementation.
• Xenobiotics (drugs, herbal, holistic, or Chinese remedies), inducers or inhibitors of microsomal enzymes, impaired hepatic antioxidant status; xenobiotic metabolites foster inflammation or augment direct initial liver injury.

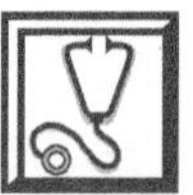

DIAGNOSIS

DIFFERENTIAL DIAGNOSIS

• Acute hepatitis—history, sequential biochemistry profiles or liver biopsy.
• Congenital portosystemic shunt (portosystemic vascular anomaly [PSVA]).

- Primary hepatic neoplasia.
- Metastatic neoplasia or carcinomatosis.
- Chronic pancreatitis.
- Other causes of abdominal effusion—hypoalbuminemia; passive congestion; carcinomatosis; chemical peritonitis (bile, urine, pancreatitis), hepatic or nonhepatic causes of portal hypertension: see Hypertension, Portal.
- Jaundice—extrahepatic bile duct occlusion (EHBDO); bile peritonitis, cholangitis/cholangiohepatitis syndrome, ductopenia, hemolysis.

CBC/BIOCHEMISTRY/URINALYSIS

Hemogram

CBC—nonregenerative anemia; RBC microcytosis if APSS; variable leukogram, occasional thrombocytopenia; low total protein if chronic disease with synthetic failure and portal hypertension causing enteric protein loss.

Biochemistry

High liver enzymes; variable bilirubin, albumin, blood urea nitrogen (BUN), glucose, cholesterol; hepatic failure—suggested by low albumin, BUN, glucose, and cholesterol in absence of alternative causes.

Urinalysis

Variable urine concentration; escalated bilirubinuria; ammonium biurate crystalluria if APSS.

OTHER LABORATORY TESTS

- Total serum bile acids (TSBA)—variable; depends on extent of hepatic remodeling, sinusoidal hypertension, and cholestasis; *superfluous test if hepatic hyperbilirubinemia.*
- Ammonia intolerance—reflects APSS; insensitive to cholestasis, lability impairs accuracy.
- Coagulation tests—reflect panlobular injury, chronicity, vascular injury, impaired synthetic capacity or vitamin K adequacy; early disease: few abnormalities except possible high fibrinogen; advanced stage or severe panlobular injury: single or multiple abnormalities including prolonged prothrombin, activated partial thromboplastin time, low fibrinogen, increased D-dimers.
- Low protein C or antithrombin activity—may reflect PSVA, APSS, hepatic failure, or consumptive coagulopathy.
- Abdominal effusion—chronic liver disease portal hypertension: pure or modified transudate.
- Liver tissue zinc—low with chronic disease and APSS.
- Serologic or PCR tests—possible infectious agents, e.g., leptospirosis, rickettsial diseases, *Borrelia*, *Bartonella*, endemic fungal agents.
- ANA titer—if potential for autoimmune disease; *note*: low-level positive titers nonspecific and more common with advanced age.
- Immunohistochemical staining of liver biopsy—can confirm infectious agents or phenotype of infiltrating cells (inflammatory or neoplastic).

IMAGING

Abdominal Radiography

- Microhepatia—suggests late-stage disease or APSS causing lobular atrophy.
- Abdominal effusion—obscures image.
- Ammonium biurate calculi—radiolucent unless combined with radiodense minerals.

US

- Liver size depends on disease stage.
- Normal to variable parenchymal and biliary tract echogenicity; may note nodularity and irregular liver margins with chronicity due to regenerative nodules.
- APSS—tortuous vessels most commonly identified caudal to left kidney or near splenic vein.
- Abdominal effusion—US facilitates fluid sampling.
- Uroliths—renal pelvis or urinary bladder; may signify ammonium biurate urolithiasis but cannot differentiate mineral composition without stone analysis.
- Rule out—EHBDO; identify mass lesions; cholelithiasis; gallbladder mucocele (GBM); cholecystitis; choledochitis; cystic lesions (abscess or ductal plate malformation–related).
- Enables fine-needle aspiration—cytology and cholecystocentesis for bile collection.

Colorectal/Splenoportal Scintigraphy (CRS/SPS)

- ^{99M}Technicium pertechnetate isotope time activity curve displays chronologic isotope distribution: delivery to liver first = no shunting, delivery to heart first = shunting.
- CRS—sensitive, noninvasive; cannot differentiate PSVA from APSS.
- SPS—no diagnostic advantage, US-guided splenic injection, uses a lower isotope dose and therefore has faster discharge from hospital.

DIAGNOSTIC PROCEDURES

Aspiration Cytology

- Fine-needle aspiration cytology—*cannot define* fibrosis or nonsuppurative inflammation*; cannot* recommend therapy.
- Cannot definitively diagnose chronic hepatitis, hepatic fibrosis, or Cu associated hepatopathy.

Liver Biopsy

- Liver biopsy—needed for definitive diagnosis; acquire biopsies from multiple liver lobes.
- Tru-Cut® needle biopsy—use 14–16 G.
- Laparoscopy—best biopsy method; lower morbidity and faster recovery vs. exploratory laparotomy.

Bacterial Culture

Aerobic and anaerobic bacterial culture and sensitivity of liver and bile; use particulate biliary debris if possible.

Metal Analyses

- Measure Cu, iron, and zinc concentrations in liver (dry matter basis).
- Low hepatic zinc associated with portosystemic shunting requires supplementation.
- Iron commonly accumulates in necroinflammatory disorders; must be reconciled with distribution for relevance: e.g., Prussian blue staining defines distribution in macrophages (chronic inflammation) vs. predominantly in hepatocytes (hemochromatosis).
- Cu quantification and rhodanine staining—ascertains relevance to parenchymal injury.

PATHOLOGIC FINDINGS

- Gross—early: no gross change; late stage: irregular surface contours, microhepatica, ± tortuous APSS varices.
- Microscopic—nonsuppurative inflammation in zone(s) of necroinflammatory injury; variable cholestasis and biliary hyperplasia; interface hepatitis: invasion of limiting plate; late-stage disease: fibrotic bridging partitions between or within involved zones and marginating regenerative nodules, sinusoidal dissecting fibrosis; final transition to cirrhosis.

Histopathology

- Immune-mediated hepatitis—periportal, lobular, centrilobular, or panlobular with lymphoplasmacytic infiltrates, hepatic cord injury causing disorganization, sinusoidal fibrosis, biliary hyperplasia.
- Cu associated hepatopathy—initially centrilobular, may evolve panlobular immune-mediated hepatitis.
- Cirrhosis—diffuse, unresolvable; fibrosis, nodular regeneration distorting lobular architecture.

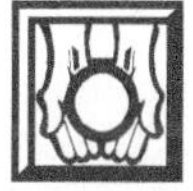

TREATMENT

APPROPRIATE HEALTH CARE

- Inpatient—for diagnostic testing, supportive care, treatment initiation in severe illness.
- Outpatient—if condition stable at diagnosis; slowly titrated onto medical therapy.

NURSING CARE

- Depends on underlying condition.
- Fluid therapy—balanced polyionic fluids supplemented to correct hydration, electrolyte aberrations, or hypoglycemia; restricted sodium if ascites, may require fresh frozen plasma, avoid synthetic colloids.
- Water-soluble vitamins—2 mL/L fluids.
- Ascites (see Cirrhosis and Fibrosis of the Liver).

ACTIVITY

Keep patient warm and hydrated; restricted activity may improve hepatic regeneration, euglycemia, and ascites mobilization.

HEPATITIS, CHRONIC (CONTINUED)

DIET

- Conserve body condition and muscle mass.
- Adequate calories and protein—to avoid negative nitrogen balance and catabolism.
- Dietary protein—restrict protein quantity *only* if signs of HE or observe ammonium biurate crystalluria; feed balanced species-specific diet; if HE, avoid fish and red meat source protein (dogs).
- Fat restriction rarely needed.
- If Cu associated liver injury, see Copper Associated Hepatopathy.
- Meal frequency—feed several small meals per day.
- Sodium restriction—with ascites or severe hypoalbuminemia: <100 mg/100 kcal or <0.2% dry matter basis formula.
- Balanced vitamin supplements (water soluble, fat soluble)— increased urinary water-soluble vitamin loss if PU/PD or diuretic therapy.
- Thiamin—ensure repletion to avoid metabolic complications and neurologic signs; 50–100 mg PO q24h; *caution*: anaphylactoid reactions may occur with injectable thiamin.
- Partial parenteral nutrition—may consider, insufficient to meet energy requirements.
- Total parenteral nutrition—if inappetence >7 days; branched-chain amino acids remain controversial in dogs with liver dysfunction.

CLIENT EDUCATION

- Control rather than cure is expected goal; medications usually required for life; chronic hepatitis is cyclic and will minimally require reevaluations q4–6 months after initial control.
- Antifibrotics—best control of fibrosis through control of inflammation and underlying primary process.
- Attenuate factors provoking HE—dehydration; azotemia, infection; catabolism; constipation; hypokalemia; alkalemia; high-protein meals; endoparasitism; enteric bleeding; certain drugs.

SURGICAL CONSIDERATIONS

- APSS—do not ligate APSS or band vena cava.
- Cirrhosis—high anesthetic risk; gas anesthesia preferred: isoflurane or sevoflurane.

MEDICATIONS

DRUG(S) OF CHOICE

- Treatments for specific etiologies.
- Withdraw plausible hepatotoxic drugs.
- No clinical trials prove efficacy of specific therapeutic regimens at this time.

Immunomodulation

- *Prednisolone/prednisone*—1–2 mg/kg daily PO; taper to lowest effective dose (0.25–0.5 mg/kg PO q48h); if ascites: use dexamethasone to avoid mineralocorticoid effects (divide prednisone dose by 7–10 for dexamethasone dose), SID q2–3 days.
- *Azathioprine*—dogs: 2 mg/kg (50 mg/m^2) PO q24h × 14 days *then* titrate to q48h; contraindicated in cats (toxic); dogs: combine with prednisone, antioxidants, antifibrotic polyunsaturated phosphatidylcholine (PPC); during chronic therapy, titrate by 25–50% dose reduction after 2–6 months based on sequential biochemistries showing improvements (e.g., normalization of total bilirubin and marked decline in liver enzyme activity); monitor CBC and biochemistry profile q7–14 days for first 2 months to ensure absence of hematopoietic, hepatic, or pancreatic toxicity; if acute hematopoietic toxicity, stop therapy, allow recovery, then reintroduce with 25% dose reduction; if insidious chronic hematopoietic toxicity (after months) or acute cholestatic liver or pancreatic injury, discontinue therapy and change to different drug (e.g., mycophenolate or cyclosporin); risk for neoplasia with chronic use.
- *Mycophenolate mofetil*—10–15 mg/kg PO q12h; doses ≥10 mg/kg PO BID may lead to diarrhea' start lower initial dose and/or divide total daily dose into 3–4 doses to reduce toxic effects; monitor as for azathioprine and adjust similarly; fewer bone marrow side effects than azathioprine but more GI toxicity; avoid dosing with food or after administration of proton pump inhibitor as these factors reduce drug bioavailability; if failure to respond to azathioprine go to cyclosporin vs. mycophenolate; if azathioprine toxicity go to mycophenolate.
- *Microemulsified cyclosporine* (Atopica®)—2.5–5 mg/kg PO q24h; use with glucocorticoids may increase drug efficacy and permit lower dose; side effects: gingival hyperplasia (managed with azithromycin), rare cholestatic liver injury, hyperlipidemia, hypercholesterolemia, worsening preexistent hypertension, risk for GB disease, risk for opportunistic infections; high dose can lead to nephrotoxicity; risk for neoplasia with chronic use; avoid concurrent use of p450 inhibitors unless cyclosporin dose substantially reduced.

Ursodeoxycholic Acid

Hepatomembranoprotectant, immunomodulatory, antifibrotic, choleretic, anti-endotoxic, and antioxidant effects; 10–15 mg/kg PO SID or divided q12h; administer with food for best bioavailability; may use as aqueous solution; no deleterious side effects; maintain indefinitely.

Antifibrotics

- Immunomodulators, *S*-adenosylmethionine (SAMe), vitamin E.
- *Polyunsaturated phosphatidylcholine* (PPC, dilinolylphosphatidylcholine [DLPC])—PPC containing DLPC antifibrotic, has immunomodulatory, antioxidant, hepatoprotectant effects, and improves membrane fluidity; 25–50 mg/kg/day PO with food; PhosChol® with preformed DLPC (52%) has benefit in some forms of liver disease (humans, animal models); may have corticosteroid-sparing effect (allows reduced glucocorticoid dosing); safely prescribed without liver biopsy.
- *Colchicine*—not recommended.
- *Silybin with PPC* (milk thistle)—experimental studies suggest potential hepatoprotectant (against numerous toxins), antifibrotic, antioxidant effects, and possibly promoting hepatocyte regeneration; low bioavailability of oral forms significantly limits biologic effect at traditional oral dosing: 2–5 mg/kg/day PO (PPC complexed form); only bioavailable form IV formulation (Legalon® SIL) used for *Amanita* death cap mushroom toxicity with high dose protocol; orphan drug.

Antioxidants

- Vitamin E—α-tocopherol, 10 IU/kg PO q24h with food.
- SAMe—20 mg/kg/day enteric-coated tablet PO, give on empty stomach for best bioavailability, 1–2h before feeding.
- Avoid vitamin C (ascorbate).
- Zinc (zinc acetate)—has antioxidant and antifibrotic benefits, supplementation may improve control of HE if low liver zinc concentration documented, unreliable for limiting enteric Cu uptake; elemental zinc 1.5–3 mg/kg PO daily as supplement if low liver zinc concentration (<120 µg/g dry weight liver); adjust dose using sequential plasma zinc concentrations that show increased concentrations; avoid plasma concentrations ≥800 µg/dL to prevent hemolysis; plasma zinc levels do not correlate with tissue levels.

Hepatoprotectants

- Ursodeoxycholate, vitamin E, SAMe, PPC—provide hepatoprotectant effects in addition to other benefits.
- Silybin—see above.

Bleeding Tendencies

See Coagulopathy of Liver Disease.

GI Signs/Vomiting/Hematemesis

- HCl pump inhibitors—omeprazole 0.5–1.0 mg/kg q12–24h PO or pantoprazole 0.7–1 mg/kg q12h IV, better long-term control vs. famotidine.
- Sucralfate—gastroprotectant dose 0.25–1.0 g/10 kg PO q8–12h; titrated to effect; beware of drug interactions as sucralfate may bind other medications, reducing bioavailability.
- Eliminate endoparasitism.

CONTRAINDICATIONS

- NSAIDs—avoid; may provoke enteric ulceration and bleeding; may worsen ascites; metabolites cause centrilobular hepatocyte injury.

• Avoid drugs requiring extensive hepatic metabolism or judiciously adjust dose if APSS, HE, jaundice, or hepatic failure evident.

PRECAUTIONS

• Diuretics—dehydration, hypokalemia, alkalosis, constipation: provoke or worsen HE.
• Glucocorticoids—increase susceptibility to infection, enteric bleeding, sodium and water retention (those with mineralocorticoid effects), PU/PD, protein catabolism, HE.
• Avoid drugs or reduce dose for those dependent on first-pass hepatic extraction if APSS or those requiring hepatic conjugation or biotransformation for detoxification, e.g., metronidazole—reduce conventional dose to 7.5 mg/kg PO q12h (often used for HE).
• Zinc overdose may cause hemolysis.

POSSIBLE INTERACTIONS

• Avoid medications altering hepatic p450 cytochrome biotransformation/elimination pathways (cimetidine, quinidine, ketoconazole).
• Avoid concurrent treatment with metoclopramide if spironolactone used for diuresis (causes aldosterone release).
• Adjust dose of immunomodulators if used in combination to avoid immunodeficiency.

ALTERNATIVE DRUG(S)

• Dexamethasone—if ascites, replace prednisone or prednisolone with this drug to avoid mineralocorticoid effect; divide dose by 7–10, administer q3 days.
• Mycophenolate—alternative if azathioprine intolerance, see above.

FOLLOW-UP

PATIENT MONITORING

• At-home behavior/cognitive function, bodyweight, body condition, and muscle mass scores monitored.
• CBC, biochemistry, urinalysis—depending on immunosuppressive medications (see above), initially q2 weeks for 2 months, then monthly or quarterly; depends on patient status and drugs administered; monitor for opportunistic infections.
• Serial monitoring of TSBA—usually does not add prognostic or diagnostic information.
• Abdominal girth—reflects ascites volume; important to standardize measurement site, method, and operator determining circumference.
• Azathioprine—monitor for possible bone marrow toxicity (serial CBCs q2 weeks for 2 months then quarterly); leukopenia may develop acutely or after chronic use; GI or pancreatic toxicity; hepatotoxicity (alanine aminotransferase activity), other effects and opportunistic infectious complications.
• Mycophenolate—monitor for GI toxicity, rare bone marrow toxicity, opportunistic infectious complications; diarrhea most common complication, manage by dividing daily drug dose into 3–4.
• Cyclosporine—renal function, infectious complications, avoid cytochrome p450 inhibitor drugs; remain aware of possible drug-provoked hyperlipidemia, hypercholesterolemia, related GB disease (dysmotility, GBM, cholelithiasis).

POSSIBLE COMPLICATIONS

HE, septicemia, bleeding—may be life-threatening; disseminated intravascular coagulation—may be terminal event.

EXPECTED COURSE AND PROGNOSIS

• Chronic hepatitis often cyclic; occasional flare-ups inconsistently associated with clinical illness, more consistently associated with vacillating liver enzymes or hyperbilirubinemia.
• Some dogs achieve solid long-term remission.
• Some dogs with Cu associated hepatopathy achieve permanent remission of apparent "immune-mediated" inflammation with Cu chelation and lifelong dietary Cu restriction.
• Development of ascites—severe liver injury, APSS, potential for HE, shorter survival.
• Severe disease—with APSS, HE, and ascites may require occasional hospitalizations to adjust nutritional and medical interventions.

MISCELLANEOUS

ZOONOTIC POTENTIAL

• Dogs with leptospirosis-associated chronic liver disease (rare) may shed organisms.
• *Bartonella* and rickettsial infections are sentinels for endemic vectors.

SEE ALSO

• Ascites.
• Cirrhosis and Fibrosis of the Liver.
• Copper Associated Hepatopathy.
• Glycogen-Type Vacuolar Hepatopathy.
• Hepatic Encephalopathy.
• Hepatic Failure, Acute.
• Hypertension, Portal.
• Portosystemic Shunting, Acquired.

ABBREVIATIONS

• ANA = antinuclear antibody.
• APSS = acquired portosystemic shunt.
• BUN = blood urea nitrogen.
• CRS = colorectal scintigraphy.
• DLPC = dilinolylphosphatidylcholine.
• EHBDO = extrahepatic bile duct occlusion.
• GBM = gallbladder mucocele.
• GI = gastrointestinal.
• HE = hepatic encephalopathy.
• NSAID = nonsteroidal anti-inflammatory drug.
• PPC = polyunsaturated phosphatidylcholine.
• PSVA = portosystemic vascular anomaly.
• PU/PD = polyuria/polydipsia.
• RBC = red blood cell.
• SAMe = S-adenosylmethionine.
• SPS = splenoportal scintigraphy.
• TSBA = total serum bile acids.

Suggested Reading

Webster CRL, Center SA, Cullen JM, et al. ACVIM consensus statement on the diagnosis and treatment of chronic hepatitis in dogs. J Vet Intern Med 2019, 33(3):1173–1200.

Author Sharon A. Center
Consulting Editor Kate Holan
Acknowledgment The author and book editors acknowledge the prior contribution of Sean P. McDonough.

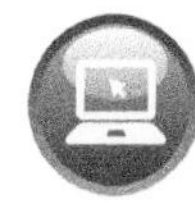
Client Education Handout available online

H

HEPATITIS, GRANULOMATOUS

BASICS

DEFINITION

- Uncommon necroinflammatory hepatitis.
- Characterized by histiocytes/macrophages, lymphocytes, plasma cells, and variable neutrophilic infiltrates forming granulomas that efface normal hepatic structure.
- May reflect infectious agents, immune-mediated or immunoregulatory disorders, or proliferative/neoplastic histiocytic syndrome.
- May localize to liver or be multisystemic (spleen, lymph nodes, bone marrow, lungs).
- Copper associated hepatopathy—involves unique small "copper granulomas" distinct from this syndrome.

PATHOPHYSIOLOGY

- Inflammatory process may be initiated by infection—bacteria (eubacterial, mycobacterial, chlamydial), viral, parasitic, protozoal, or fungal agents.
- May reflect immune-mediated or immunoregulatory disorders.
- May be initiated by adverse drug or xenobiotic interaction including herbal, holistic, or Chinese traditional remedies, or toxin exposure.
- May reflect proliferative histiocytic syndromes or histiocytic neoplasia.
- Hepatocyte necrosis—reflects insufficient regional perfusion and hypoxia, cytokine-mediated cytotoxic cell injury (histiocytes, lymphocytes), initial direct or indirect hepatotoxic injury.
- Severity of hepatic dysfunction—reflects density and lobular distribution of injury.
- Toxins—affect zone where bioactivated or metabolized as initial site of lesion distribution.
- Zone 3 copper accumulation—may augment zone 3 (centrilobular region) injury.
- Liver injury associated with enzyme leakage reflecting regional involvement; hyperbilirubinemia occurs with diffuse injury, canalicular damage, biliary tree involvement; sinusoidal injury leads to sinusoidal hypertension, splanchnic hypertension, ascites, acquired portosystemic shunt (APSS).
- Severe diffuse lobular involvement can lead to liver failure associated with complex coagulopathies; enteric hemorrhage may reflect acute splanchnic portal hypertension and lead to acute-onset hepatic encephalopathy (HE).
- Hepatic failure—associates numerous metabolic derangements and detoxification capabilities; may be lethal.

SIGNALMENT

- No breed, sex, or age predilection.
- More common in dogs than cats.

SIGNS

Historical Findings

- Nonspecific clinical signs, lethargy; abrupt or gradual onset of illness.
- Anorexia, vomiting, diarrhea, weight loss.
- Polyuria/polydipsia.

Physical Examination Findings

- Normal liver size or severe hepatomegaly.
- Abdominal pain—vague, due to hepatic capsule stretching.
- Distended abdomen—ascites; hepatomegaly.
- ± Splenomegaly—granulomatous process.
- ± Lymphadenopathy—granulomatous inflammation.
- ± Jaundice.
- ± Fever.
- ± Tachypnea—abdominal distention due to ascites or pulmonary involvement.
- Late stage—bleeding tendencies, ascites, HE.

CAUSES & RISK FACTORS

- Systemic fungal infection—histoplasmosis; blastomycosis; coccidioidomycosis; pythiosis.
- Bacterial infection—*Brucella, Nocardia, Borrelia, Propionibacterium acnes*, mycobacteria species; *Bartonella, Staphylococcus, Leptospirosis*, many other organisms.
- Rickettsial infections.
- Parasitism—visceral larval migrans; liver flukes, schistosomiasis; dirofilariasis.
- Virus—feline infectious peritonitis.
- Protozoal—*Toxoplasma*; visceral *Leishmania*.
- Neoplasia—histiocytic neoplasia, lymphoma.
- Hemophagocytic histiocytic sarcoma.
- Reactive or proliferative histiocytosis.
- Immune-mediated inflammation; may be autoimmune lupus like syndrome.
- Drug reactions (e.g., ketoconazole).
- Xenobiotics—holistic, herbal, Chinese traditional remedies.
- Toxins or infectious agents disseminated in treats or food products from countries with unregulated manufacturing processes.
- Idiopathic—no recognized cause after meticulous investigations; may be autoimmune.

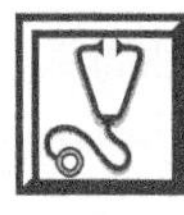

DIAGNOSIS

DIFFERENTIAL DIAGNOSIS

Widely disparate features initiate pursuit of diagnostic considerations; drug history must be carefully reviewed; consideration of splenic and/or bone marrow involvement necessary to rule out histiocytic neoplasia if biopsy discloses mitotically active dysplastic-appearing histiocytes.

CBC/BIOCHEMISTRY/URINALYSIS

- CBC—inflammatory or stress leukogram; nonregenerative anemia; spherocytes: microangiopathic shearing, immune-mediated anemia, or histiocytic hemophagocytic syndrome; monocytosis with chronic inflammation/infection.
- Biochemistry—high liver enzymes; variable: bilirubin, hypoglycemia; hypoalbuminemia, low blood urea nitrogen; high or low total proteins; high globulins; may note electrolyte abnormalities with fluid and acid-base disturbances, hypocholesterolemia with hemophagocytic histiocytic sarcoma.
- Urinalysis—may be normal or demonstrate: bilirubinuria, proteinuria, red blood cells, white blood cells, cellular and other casts.

OTHER LABORATORY TESTS

- Serum bile acid concentrations—often high with massive hepatic involvement or APSS.
- Coagulation assays—normal, except with end-stage liver failure.
- Acute-phase proteins may increase—certain globulins, fibrinogen, C-reactive protein, protein C, antithrombin.
- Serologic tests—evaluate titers with caution in regard to infectious agents; important to consider convalescent titers; increased immunoglobulin M titers to toxoplasmosis or leptospirosis support active infection, consider serology for *Bartonella*; test according to plausible exposures considering travel history and other variables (e.g., raw meat diet).
- Molecular diagnostic tests—PCR or fluorescent in situ hybridization (FISH) for eubacterial organisms or other infectious agents not visualized on microscopy of liver biopsy; mycobacterial PCR and *Bartonella* PCR may warrant investigation.
- Antinuclear antibody titer—positive with systemic lupus erythematosus but low positive titers nonspecific.
- Bacterial cultures—liver tissue, bile (use particulate debris), or blood; mycobacterial cultures grow slowly (months) thus mycobacteria may be more promptly detected using PCR and tissue staining (Ziehl-Neelsen, Fite Faraco); however, tissue staining with granulomatous inflammation and mycobacteria may be negative (as shown in humans).

IMAGING

- Abdominal radiography—may identify normal to large sized liver, abdominal mass(es), or ascites obscuring regional detail.
- Abdominal ultrasonography—discloses liver size and abnormal nodular parenchymal pattern, mass lesions, splenomegaly and lymphadenopathy; confirms abdominal effusion; enables diagnostic needle sampling of tissue for cytology or core liver biopsy.

DIAGNOSTIC PROCEDURES

- Aspiration sampling—hepatic parenchyma, spleen, bone marrow, and abdominal effusion.
- Liver biopsy—definitive diagnosis of granulomatous reaction but often does not define cause. Copper-specific stain and copper quantification in liver (dry weight basis) should be done to rule out, as copper granulomas misinterpreted as "pyogranulomatous" that

may lead to needless evaluations; copper concentration can be qualitatively estimated from liver stained with rhodanine; see Copper Associated Hepatopathy.
- Special staining for infectious agents—Gram stain, modified Steiner's, Ziehl-Neelsen and Fite Faraco (mycobacteria), periodic acid–Schiff (fungi, amoeba, protozoa), Grocott's methenamine silver (fungi, certain bacteria, e.g., *Norcardia, Actinomyces*).
- Consider bone marrow aspirate/core if histiocytic neoplasm or lymphoma suspected or to confirm certain infectious diseases (e.g., mycobacteria, brucellosis, toxoplasmosis).

PATHOLOGIC FINDINGS

- Gross—hepatomegaly; normal, finely irregular surface, indented circular or dimpled pale lesions; firm texture; may have blunted margins and abdominal effusion.
- Microscopic—pyogranulomatous reaction, random or variable zonal infiltrate distribution.

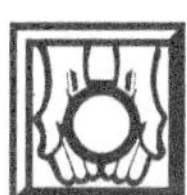

TREATMENT

- Inpatient vs. outpatient—dictated by severity of clinical signs.
- Fluid therapy—balanced polyionic solution for rehydration and maintenance needs, may require dextrose (2.5–5%) if hypoglycemic.
- Nutritional support essential; do not restrict protein if lacking signs of HE.
- Inform client that causes of this syndrome may be difficult to confirm and treat.
- If granulomatous response associates with copper, see Copper Associated Hepatopathy.

MEDICATIONS

DRUG(S) OF CHOICE

- Discontinue exposure to suspected causal xenobiotics, raw diets, rawhide products, jerky treats, or other consumables from foreign countries lacking enforced surveillance policies for pet care product manufacture.
- Depends on cause; see specific chapters for infectious disorders.
- Immunomodulation—if immune-mediated injury suspected with negative survey for infectious etiology; some injuries may transform to immune-mediated process.
- Idiopathic disease—glucocorticoids combined with azathioprine or mycophenolate or cyclosporin.
- Vomiting—antiemetics (e.g., metoclopramide 0.2–0.5 mg/kg PO/SC q6–8h; ondansetron 0.5–1.0 mg/kg 30 min before feeding q12–24h); or maropitant 1.0 mg/kg SC/PO.
- Gastrointestinal bleeding—omeprazole 1.0 mg/kg PO q12–24h or pantoprazole; sucralfate for gastroesophageal protection.

POSSIBLE INTERACTIONS

- Consider potential drug interactions because of broad spectrum of possible interventions.
- Consider adjusting drugs requiring hepatic activation, biotransformation, or elimination.
- Immunosuppression—may worsen clinical signs if cause is infectious disorder.

FOLLOW-UP

PATIENT MONITORING

- Routine monitoring of supportive care in hospital—fluids, acid-base and electrolyte balance, and general response to interventional medications.
- Sequential hematologic, biochemical, imaging, and relevant serologic titer/PCR evaluations.
- Sequential physical assessments and clinicopathologic monitoring especially important with immunomodulation because infectious causes may have been overlooked.

POSSIBLE COMPLICATIONS

- Chronic hepatitis, hepatic fibrosis, cirrhosis.
- Hepatic failure.
- Coagulopathy.
- Dissemination of undiagnosed infectious cause.

EXPECTED COURSE AND PROGNOSIS

Depend on primary cause.

MISCELLANEOUS

ZOONOTIC POTENTIAL

- Brucellosis, mycobacterial, leptospirosis infections—concern for zoonotic potential.
- Blastomycosis, coccidioidomycosis, bartonellosis, leishmaniosis, toxoplasmosis—not directly contagious but pet may serve as environmental exposure sentinel.

SEE ALSO

- Bartonellosis.
- Blastomycosis.
- Brucellosis.
- Coccidioidomycosis.
- Feline Infectious Peritonitis (FIP).
- Histoplasmosis.
- Leishmaniosis.
- Leptospirosis.
- Lupus Erythematosus, Systemic (SLE).
- Mycobacterial Infections.
- Pythiosis.

ABBREVIATIONS

- APSS = acquired portosystemic shunt.
- HE = hepatic encephalopathy.

Suggested Reading

Chapman BL, Hendrick MJ, Washabau RJ. Granulomatous hepatitis in dogs: nine cases (1987–1990). J Am Vet Med Assoc 1993, 203:680.

Hutchins RG, Breitschwerdt EB, Cullen JM, et al. Limited yield of diagnoses of intrahepatic infectious causes of canine granulomatous hepatitis from archival liver tissue. J Vet Diagn Invest 2012, 24:888–894.

Macho LP, Center SA, Randolph JF, et al. Clinical, clinicopathologic, and hepatic histologic features associated with probable ketoconazole drug-induced liver injury in dogs: 15 cases (2015–2018). J Am Vet Med Assoc 2020 256(11):1245–1256.

Author Sharon A. Center

Consulting Editor Kate Holan

HEPATITIS, INFECTIOUS (VIRAL) CANINE

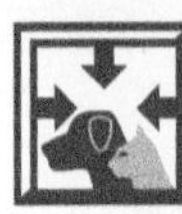

BASICS

OVERVIEW

- Viral disease of dogs (*Canidae*) caused by canine adenovirus-1 (CAV-1). It is serologically homogeneous and antigenically distinct from respiratory CAV-2, the causative agent of canine infectious laryngotracheitis.
- CAV-1 has worldwide geographic distribution and it also causes disease in wolves, coyotes, skunks, and bears. It causes encephalitis in foxes.
- Virus is spread via direct dog-to-dog oronasal contact or via contact of contaminated fomites. Airborne transmission is not an important means of contracting the virus.
- Virus initially replicates in tonsils, then spreads to regional lymph nodes and bloodstream via lymphatics.
- Infection—targets parenchymal organs (especially liver), eyes, endothelium, lung, spleen, kidneys, and brain.
- Oronasal exposure—viremia (4–8 days); virus shed in saliva and feces; initial dispersal to hepatic macrophages (hepatic Kupffer cells) and endothelium; replicates in Kupffer cells; damages adjacent hepatocytes producing massive viremia when released.
- Adequate antibody response clears organs in 10–14 days; virus can persist in renal tubules, glomeruli, iris, ciliary body, and cornea. Virus can be shed in urine for 6–9 months.
- Chronic hepatitis—after infection in dogs with only partial neutralizing antibody response.
- Cytotoxic ocular injury—anterior uveitis; leads to classic "hepatitis blue eye" and can cause glaucoma. Develops in ~1% of dogs after modified live virus (MLV) vaccine.
- Glomerulonephritis can develop 1–2 weeks after acute signs resolve and produce proteinuria and interstitial nephritis; chronic renal failure has not been described.

SIGNALMENT

- Dogs and other *Canidae.*
- No breed or sex predilections.
- Most common in dogs <1 year of age.
- Any dog not vaccinated is susceptible.

SIGNS

- Depend on immunologic status of host and degree of initial cytotoxic injury.
- Peracute—fever; CNS signs; vascular collapse; disseminated intravascular coagulation (DIC); death within hours.
- Acute—fever; anorexia; lethargy; vomiting; diarrhea; hepatomegaly; abdominal pain; abdominal effusion; vasculitis (petechia, bruising); DIC; lymphadenopathy; rarely, nonsuppurative encephalitis.
- Uncomplicated—lethargy; anorexia; transient fever; tonsillitis; vomiting; diarrhea; lymphadenopathy; hepatomegaly; abdominal pain.
- Late—20% of cases develop anterior uveitis and corneal edema 4–6 days post infection; recover within 21 days; may progress to glaucoma and corneal ulceration. May be the only clinical feature of inapparent infection.

CAUSES & RISK FACTORS

- CAV-1.
- Unvaccinated dogs susceptible.

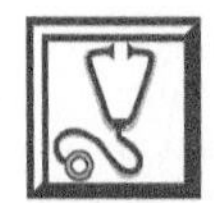

DIAGNOSIS

DIFFERENTIAL DIAGNOSIS

- Canine herpesvirus (neonatal).
- Other infectious hepatopathies.
- Leptospirosis.
- Granulomatous hepatitis.
- Toxic hepatitis.
- Fulminant infectious disease—e.g., parvovirus, canine distemper.

CBC/BIOCHEMISTRY/URINALYSIS

- CBC—schistocytes; leukopenia during acute viremia, followed by leukocytosis with reactive lymphocytosis and nucleated red blood cells (RBCs); thrombocytopenia.
- Biochemistry—liver enzyme activity high initially, begins to decline within 14 days; low glucose and albumin reflect fulminant hepatic failure, vasculitis, and endotoxemia; low sodium and potassium levels reflect GI losses; hyperbilirubinemia if survive several days.
- Urinalysis—proteinuria (glomerular injury); granular casts (renal tubule damage); bilirubinuria consistent with jaundice.

OTHER LABORATORY TESTS

- Coagulation tests—reflect severity of liver injury and DIC.
- Serology for antibodies to CAV-1—fourfold rise in immunoglobulin IgM and IgG; recent vaccine-induced antibodies confuse interpretation.
- PCR—real-time PCR not currently available; conventional PCR is able to differentiate between virulent CAV-1 and vaccine virus, which is CAV-2 in all current vaccines. Nasal, rectal, or ocular swabs or blood can be submitted as well as tissue at necropsy; positive results from urine can be difficult to interpret due to potential shedding from asymptomatic dogs.
- Viral isolation—anterior segment of eye, kidney, tonsil, and urine; difficult in parenchymal organs (especially liver) unless first week of infection.

IMAGING

- Abdominal radiography—normal or large liver; poor detail due to effusion.
- Abdominal ultrasonography—may observe hepatomegaly, hypoechoic parenchyma (multifocal or diffuse pattern), and effusion.

DIAGNOSTIC PROCEDURES

- Liver cytology via aspiration or biopsy may identify intranuclear hepatocyte inclusions.
- Viral culture.
- Acute and convalescent serology.
- Necropsy.

PATHOLOGIC FINDINGS

- Acute—edema and hemorrhage of lymph nodes; serosal visceral hemorrhages; liver large, dark-mottled; edematous gallbladder; fibrinous exudate on liver, gallbladder, and other viscera; splenomegaly; renal infarcts; abdominal effusion. Perivascular necrosis in liver and other organs; widespread centrilobular to panlobular necrosis. Liver is discolored; abdominal effusion also observed in canine herpesvirus in neonates.
- Chronic—small, fibrotic or cirrhotic liver.

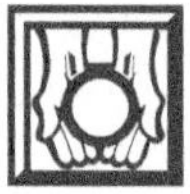

TREATMENT

- Usually inpatient.
- Fluid therapy—balanced polyionic fluids; avoid lactate if fulminant hepatic failure; carefully monitor fluids to avoid overhydration in context of increased vascular permeability.
- Judicious potassium (and other electrolyte) supplementation since electrolyte depletion may augment hepatic encephalopathy (HE).
- Avoid neuroglycopenia—supplement fluids with dextrose (2.5–5.0%) as necessary.
- Blood component therapy for coagulopathy; blood component preferred to synthetic colloids for support of colloidal osmotic pressure; widespread vasculitis and DIC allow rapid systemic third-space colloid dispersal.
- Overt DIC—fresh blood products and low molecular weight heparin, e.g., enoxaparin 100 U/kg (1 mg/kg) q24h. See Coagulopathy of Liver Disease.
- Nutritional support—frequent small meals as tolerated; optimize nitrogen intake; inappropriate protein restriction may impair tissue repair and regeneration; nitrogen restriction advised only if overt signs of HE. A feeding tube may be necessary initially.
- If oral feeding not tolerated, provide partial parenteral nutrition (maximum 5 days) or, preferably, total parenteral nutrition.

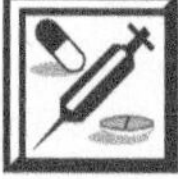

MEDICATIONS

DRUG(S) OF CHOICE

- Prophylactic antimicrobials—transmural passage of enteric bacteria and endotoxemia

with hepatic failure; e.g., ticarcillin (33–50 mg/kg q6–8h) combined with metronidazole (reduce conventional dose to 7.5 mg/kg IV q8–12h) and fluoroquinolone.
- Antiemetics—metoclopramide (0.2–0.5 mg/kg PO/SC q6–8h or CRI); ondansetron (0.5–1.0 mg/kg PO q12h); maropitant (1 mg/kg/day SC).
- Gastroprotection—proton pump inhibitors (omeprazole 0.5–1.0 mg/kg PO q12–24h, pantoprazole 0.7–1.0 mg/kg IV q12–24h); H2 receptor antagonists (e.g., famotidine 0.5 mg/kg PO/IV/SC q12–24h) and sucralfate (0.25–1.0 g PO q8–12h).
- Manage HE (see Hepatic Encephalopathy).
- Ursodeoxycholic acid—choleretic and hepatoprotectant (10–15 mg/kg daily in two divided doses, with food); give indefinitely if chronic hepatitis.
- Antioxidants—vitamin E (10 IU/kg/day PO), *N*-acetylcysteine IV (140 mg/kg load, then 70 mg/kg q8h) until PO route possible; transition to *S*-adenosylmethionine (20 mg/kg/day PO, dose on empty stomach) when patient can tolerate oral medications until liver enzymes normalize or indefinitely if chronic hepatitis.

CONTRAINDICATIONS/POSSIBLE INTERACTIONS

- Consider severity of liver injury, protein depletion, and age in calculating drug dosages.
- Sucralfate may impair oral absorption of certain medications (fluoroquinolones, tetracycline, doxycycline, and fat-soluble vitamins, e.g., vitamin E).

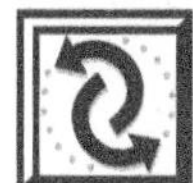

FOLLOW-UP

PATIENT MONITORING

- Monitor fluid, electrolyte, acid-base, and coagulation status to adjust supportive measures.
- Monitor for acute renal failure.

PREVENTION/AVOIDANCE

MLV vaccination—at 6–8 weeks of age; two boosters 3–4 weeks apart until 16 weeks of age; booster at 1 year; highly effective vaccine; boosters may not be needed.

POSSIBLE COMPLICATIONS

- Fulminant hepatic failure.
- HE.
- Septicemia.
- Acute renal failure.
- Glomerulonephritis.
- DIC.
- Glaucoma.
- Chronic hepatitis.

EXPECTED COURSE AND PROGNOSIS

- Peracute—poor prognosis; death within hours.
- Acute—variable: guarded to good prognosis.
- Poor antibody response (titer 1 : 16–1 : 50)— chronic hepatitis may develop.
- Good antibody response (titer >1 : 500 IgG)—complete recovery in 5–7 days possible.
- Recovered patients—may develop chronic liver or renal disease.

MISCELLANEOUS

AGE-RELATED FACTORS

- Maternal antibody—may protect some pups for first 8 weeks; depends on maternal antibody concentration and efficacy of passive transfer.
- Vaccination of pups with high levels of passively acquired antibodies—successful at 14–16 weeks of age.

SEE ALSO

- Acute Kidney Injury.
- Anterior Uveitis—Dogs.
- Disseminated Intravascular Coagulation.
- Hepatic Encephalopathy.
- Hepatic Failure, Acute.
- Hepatitis, Chronic.

ABBREVIATIONS

- CAV-1 = canine adenovirus-1.
- DIC = disseminated intravascular coagulation.
- HE = hepatic encephalopathy.
- Ig = immunoglobulin.
- MLV = modified live virus.
- RBC = red blood cells.

Suggested Reading

Greene, CE. Infectious canine hepatitis and canine acidophil cell hepatitis. In: Greene CE, ed. Infectious Diseases of the Dog and Cat, 3rd ed. Philadelphia, PA: Saunders, 2012, pp. 42–47.

Author Kate Holan

Consulting Editor Kate Holan

Acknowledgment The author and book editors acknowledge the prior contribution of Sharon A. Center.

H

HEPATITIS, SUPPURATIVE AND HEPATIC ABSCESS

BASICS

OVERVIEW

- Bacterial infection involving the hepatobiliary system.
- Distribution and lobular involvement—variable; multifocal microabscessation; diffuse suppurative cholangitis/cholangiohepatitis; cholecystitis; choledochitis, or discrete focal lesions; lesions associate with pyogenic bacteria.
- Large abscesses associated with hepatocellular carcinoma (HCA) in dogs.

SIGNALMENT

- Dog and cat.
- No breed predilection.
- Hepatic abscesses—most common: old dogs with HCA, or secondary to immunosuppression or diabetes mellitus; in neonates subsequent to omphalitis.
- Suppurative septic cholangitis/cholangiohepatitis—most common in young to middle-aged male cats.
- Cholestatic disorders predispose to enteric bacterial translocation and impair canalicular bacterial egress from the liver.

SIGNS

Historical Findings

- Anorexia.
- Lethargy.
- Gastrointestinal signs—vomiting, diarrhea.
- Weight loss.
- Polyuria and polydipsia.
- Trembling.
- Fever.
- May become jaundiced.

Physical Examination Findings

- Fever or hypothermia (cats).
- Abdominal pain—cranial abdomen.
- Dehydration.
- Hepatomegaly—focal, with large abscess or mass.
- Coagulopathy.
- Effusion—abdominal distention or fluid wave.
- May develop jaundice.
- Endotoxemia—tachycardia, tachypnea, hypotension, hypoglycemic collapse.

CAUSES & RISK FACTORS

- Hematogenous infection via the portal vein, hepatic artery, or umbilical vein.
- Biliary tree obstruction, preexisting hepatobiliary or pancreatic disease, and inflammatory bowel disease.
- Ascending biliary tract infection.
- Cholecystoenterostomy.
- HCA with necrotic foci.
- Compromised immune responses: diabetes mellitus, glucocorticoid administration, hyperadrenocorticism, hypothyroidism, chemotherapy, immune-mediated disorders managed with immunosuppressives.
- Recurrent urinary tract infections; pyelonephritis.
- Penetrating wounds.
- Complication of hepatic biopsy or other surgery.

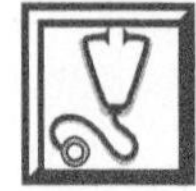

DIAGNOSIS

DIFFERENTIAL DIAGNOSIS

- Infectious or necroinflammatory disease.
- Pancreatitis or pancreatic abscess.
- Hepatobiliary neoplasia.
- Hematoma.
- Metastatic neoplasia.
- Biliary cystadenoma.
- Gastrointestinal obstruction or perforation.
- Peritonitis, other intra-abdominal abscess.
- Cholecystitis, choledochitis, cholelithiasis.

CBC/BIOCHEMISTRY/URINALYSIS

- CBC—neutrophilic leukocytosis with left shift and toxic white blood cell (WBC) changes; monocytosis; thrombocytopenia; nonregenerative anemia, schistocytes (disseminated intravascular coagulation [DIC]).
- Biochemistry—variably increased alanine aminotransferase (ALT) > alkaline phosphatase (ALP) activity, increased aspartate aminotransferase (AST), hypoglobulinemia, hyperglobulinemia, inconsistent hyperbilirubinemia and hypoglycemia, inconsistent hypocalcemia (cats).
- Urinalysis—usually normal; bilirubinuria; proteinuria.

OTHER LABORATORY TESTS

- Serum bile acids—normal or high.
- Coagulation tests: changes consistent with DIC.
- Urine culture may or may not disclose hematogenously dispersed organisms.

IMAGING

Abdominal Radiography

- Hepatomegaly; irregular or rounded liver margins: diffuse or single lobe if isolated abscess.
- Hepatic mass effect.
- Reduced abdominal detail—effusion or peritonitis.
- Gas pattern in hepatic parenchyma or biliary tree.
- Thoracic radiographs—normal, or consistent with pneumonia or chronic bronchitis.

Ultrasonography

- Best noninvasive method of abscess detection (>0.5 cm lesions); solitary, variably echogenic, cavitated, hyperechoic rim.
- Dystrophic tissue mineralization or entrapped gas.
- Highly echogenic interface with cavitated mass—may be gas; combination with an abdominal effusion and hyperechoic perilesional effect supports an abscess.
- Multiple masses, may be complex.
- Miliary abscesses—cannot discern from other parenchymal hepatic disorders.
- Suppurative septic cholangitis/cholangiohepatitis syndrome (CCHS)—image not unique from nonsuppurative CCHS.
- Inconsistent regional lymphadenopathy.

DIAGNOSTIC PROCEDURES

Cytology

- Cytology is essential; histologic specimens may not reveal bacterial organisms.
- Samples—effusion; hepatic parenchyma, discrete lesions; cholecystocentesis: transhepatic approach, liquid bile and biliary debris.
- Stains—Wright-Giemsa for bacterial detection; Gram stain for morphology.
- Look for bacteria within biliary debris, in WBCs; primary or predisposing disease (e.g., neoplasia, VH reflecting adrenal disease or diabetes mellitus).

Culture and Sensitivity Testing

- If suppurative or pyogranulomatous—culture for aerobic, anaerobic bacteria, fungal organisms.
- Blood—aerobic and anaerobic culture.
- Polymicrobial infections ~30%.

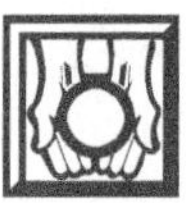

TREATMENT

- Inpatient—if signs of sepsis.
- IV fluids and antibiotics—essential.
- Fluid support—correct dehydration; rectify acid-base and electrolyte disturbances.
- Abscess—drain via lobectomy during laparotomy or under ultrasound guidance before surgery; if endotoxic shock, ultrasound facilitated drainage is best; after drainage, monitor body temperature, liver enzymes, WBC count, and sequentially image with ultrasound (monitor abscess size, focal or diffuse peritonitis); judiciously repeat drainage (may require insertion of an indwelling catheter for short-term continuous drainage); consider alcoholization of abscess after drainage.
- In middle-aged/older dogs—lobectomy for abscess removal and possible wide-margin resection of an HCA.
- If extrahepatic bile duct obstruction (EHBDO)—see Bile Duct Obstruction (Extrahepatic).

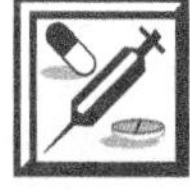

MEDICATIONS

DRUG(S) OF CHOICE

- Antibiotics—initially based on cytology and Gram stain, then adjusted based on culture and sensitivity results; continue for 2–4 months, perhaps longer.
- Initial treatment—combine antimicrobials for possible polymicrobial infection; common effective empirical combination includes

ticarcillin (25–50 mg/kg over 15 min CRI) or amoxicillin clavulanate (13.75–20 mg/kg PO q12h), enrofloxacin (5–10 mg/kg PO/IV/SC q12h in dogs or cats), and metronidazole (15 mg/kg IV q12h; reduce dose by 50% if hepatic dysfunction or severe cholestasis) or clindamycin (10–16 mg/kg SC per day; reduce dose if hepatic dysfunction or severe cholestasis to 5 mg/kg SC per day).
- Choleretics advised if biliary tree involved, but if EHBDO *not until* biliary decompression; see Bile Duct Obstruction (Extrahepatic); Cholangitis/Cholangiohepatitis Syndrome.
- Antioxidants advised (see Hepatitis, Chronic).

CONTRAINDICATIONS/POSSIBLE INTERACTIONS

- Aminoglycosides—do not use until normal hydration.
- Avoid drugs metabolized or excreted by the liver or those known to be hepatotoxic if compromised liver function; adjust dosages or frequency of drugs if suspect reduced hepatic elimination, cholestasis, or hepatic dysfunction.

FOLLOW-UP

PATIENT MONITORING

- Assess vital signs, labwork abnormalities, and physical condition.
- Sequential ultrasound examinations—monitor for abscess recrudescence or suppurative peritonitis.
- If percutaneous drainage and alcoholization of an abscess—ultrasound monitoring at 24 and 48 hours post procedure and 15, 30, 60, and 120 days is recommended.

POSSIBLE COMPLICATIONS

- DIC.
- Septicemia/endotoxemia.
- Fulminant hepatic failure.
- Septic peritonitis.
- Acute renal failure.

EXPECTED COURSE AND PROGNOSIS

- Favorable prognosis—early detection and aggressive antimicrobial treatment, with judicious surgical intervention.
- Guarded prognosis—concurrent disorders, especially hepatic neoplasia.

MISCELLANEOUS

ABBREVIATIONS

- ALP = alkaline phosphatase.
- ALT = alanine aminotransferase.
- AST = aspartate aminotransferase.
- CCHS = cholangitis/cholangiohepatitis syndrome.
- DIC = disseminated intravascular coagulation.
- EHBDO = extrahepatic bile duct obstruction.
- HCA = hepatocellular carcinoma.
- WBC = white blood cell.

Suggested Reading

Schwarz LA, Penninck DG, Leveille-Webster C. Hepatic abscesses in 13 dogs: a review of the ultrasonographic findings, clinical data, and therapeutic options. Vet Radiol Ultrasound 1998, 39:357–365.

Sergeeff JS, Armstrong PJ, Bunch SE. Hepatic abscesses in cats: 14 cases (1985–2002). J Vet Intern Med 2004, 18:295–300.

Zatelli A, Bonfanti U, Zini E, et al. Percutaneous drainage and alcoholization of hepatic abscesses in five dogs and a cat. J Am Anim Hosp Assoc 2005, 41:34–38.

Author Ashleigh Seigneur

Consulting Editor Kate Holan

Acknowledgment The author and book editors acknowledge the prior contribution of Sharon A. Center.

H

HEPATOCELLULAR ADENOMA

BASICS

OVERVIEW

- A benign liver tumor of epithelial origin.
- May be more common than primary malignant liver tumors.

SIGNALMENT

- Rare in dog and very rare in cat.
- Affected dogs commonly >10 years of age.
- Breed predispositions unknown.

SIGNS

- Usually asymptomatic; when clinical signs present, symptoms may be nonspecific; typically incidental finding.
- Acute tumor rupture may cause hemoperitoneum with resultant weakness and hypovolemic shock-like symptoms.
- Occasionally, large tumors may cause cranial abdominal pain, vomiting, and inappetance.

CAUSES & RISK FACTORS

Definitive cause or risk factors for tumor development are unknown.

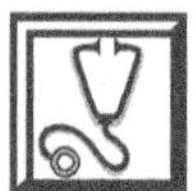

DIAGNOSIS

DIFFERENTIAL DIAGNOSIS

- Hepatocellular carcinoma.
- Hepatic nodular hyperplasia.
- Hepatic abscess.
- Abdominal mass.
- Splenomegaly.

CBC/BIOCHEMISTRY/URINALYSIS

CBC

- Usually unremarkable.
- Anemia—regenerative anemia if tumor is bleeding, or anemia of chronic disease.
- Leukocytosis with a left shift—large tumors with necrotic centers (rare).

Biochemistry

- Liver enzymes variable.
- Serum total bilirubin values—usually normal.

Urinalysis

Unremarkable

OTHER LABORATORY TESTS

- Serum bile acids are usually normal unless tumor growth compromises hepatic perfusion and biliary flow.
- Coagulation abnormalities consistent with disseminated intravascular coagulation (DIC) occur rarely with large necrotic or hemorrhagic tumors.

IMAGING

Radiography

- May demonstrate a single mass lesion or apparent asymmetry of hepatic silhouette.
- Rarely, gas in necrotic center of tumor.

Abdominal Ultrasonography

May identify discrete mass effect with variable echogenicity, ranging from normal liver echogenicity to mixed echogenicity, presence of multiple nodules, or cystic mass appearance.

Abdominal CT

- May allow for improved assessment regarding surgical feasibility, especially for large tumors, or tumors associated with critical structures, such as the gallbladder.
- May detect additional lesions, depending on the contrast enhancement protocol.

DIAGNOSTIC PROCEDURES

- Hepatic aspiration cytology with ultrasonographic guidance may allow the identification of normal hepatocytes or cells with mild atypia; this diagnostic will not be useful to differentiate between benign and low-grade malignant hepatic tumors, but will be useful to exclude other neoplastic diseases.
- Hepatic biopsy with Tru-Cut® needle—several core biopsies are necessary to provide enough tissue for histopathologic characterization; due to the overlap between the hepatocellular adenoma and the low-grade hepatocellular carcinoma, it may be difficult to obtain a definitive diagnosis.
- Abdominal exploratory surgery followed by mass resection (liver lobectomy) and histopathology is the best way to obtain a definitive diagnosis and treat the disease.

PATHOLOGIC FINDINGS

Gross Pathology

- Usually well-circumscribed single nodules <10 cm in diameter.
- May be yellow-brown.
- Often soft, highly vascular, and friable.
- Occasionally multiple.
- Occasionally very large (>20 cm).

Microscopic Findings

- May be difficult to distinguish from nodular hyperplasia, normal liver tissue, or low-grade hepatocellular carcinoma.
- Usually well-defined trabecular pattern; not necessarily encapsulated.
- Compression of adjacent hepatic parenchyma common.
- Mitotic figures infrequent.

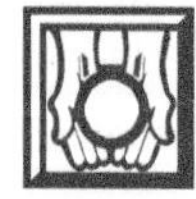

TREATMENT

- Surgical resection for large tumors, or tumors that cause clinical signs or organ dysfunction.
- Bleeding tumor—requires immediate emergency care: hemodynamic stabilization, blood transfusion, and exploratory surgery.

Surgical Considerations

- Excision recommended for large, single-mass lesions.
- Between 60% and 70% of the liver can be resected if the patient is healthy, and appropriate postoperative supportive care is available.
- Biopsy of local lymph nodes, normal-appearing liver, and any abnormal tissue identified during the exploratory surgery is of paramount importance.

MEDICATIONS

None

FOLLOW-UP

PATIENT MONITORING

- Liver enzymes—serial evaluation, especially if they were elevated at the time of diagnosis.
- Abdominal ultrasonography— every 3–4 months for the first year; preferred method of reevaluation.

POSSIBLE COMPLICATIONS

Risk of tumor necrosis and massive abdominal hemorrhage if not resected.

EXPECTED COURSE AND PROGNOSIS

Excellent

MISCELLANEOUS

SYNONYMS

Hepatoma—should be avoided; refers to hepatocellular carcinoma in human medicine and hepatocellular adenoma in veterinary medicine.

SEE ALSO

Hepatocellular Carcinoma

ABBREVIATIONS

- DIC = disseminated intravascular coagulation.

Suggested Reading

Cave TA, Johnson V, Beths T, et al. Treatment of unresectable hepatocellular adenoma in dogs with transarterial iodized oil and chemotherapy with and without an embolic agent: a report of two cases. J Vet Comp Oncol 2004, 1:191–199.

Warren-Smith CM, Andrew S, Mantis P, Lamb CR. Lack of associations between ultrasonographic appearance of parenchymal lesions of the canine liver and histological diagnosis. J Small Anim Pract 2012, 53(3):168–173.

Author Nick Dervisis

Consulting Editor Timothy M. Fan

BASICS

OVERVIEW

• Malignant epithelial liver tumor. • Accounts for about 50% of malignant hepatic tumors. • Metastasis to regional lymph nodes, lungs, and peritoneal cavity in dogs is associated with the nodular and diffuse forms of hepatocellular carcinoma.

SIGNALMENT

• Uncommon in dogs and rare in cats. • Affected dogs commonly >10 years of age. • No breed predispositions, although golden retrievers, miniature schnauzers, and male dogs are overrepresented in some studies.

SIGNS

• Typically absent until disease is advanced, unless it causes biliary obstruction. • Many times incidental finding. • Lethargy. • Weakness. • Anorexia. • Weight loss. • Polydipsia. • Diarrhea. • Vomiting. • Hepatomegaly (asymmetric)—consistent; precedes development of overt clinical signs. • Abdominal hemorrhage.

CAUSES & RISK FACTORS

• Unknown. • May be associated with chronic inflammation or hepatotoxicity.

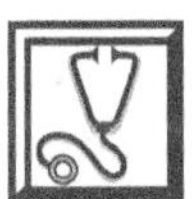

DIAGNOSIS

DIFFERENTIAL DIAGNOSIS

• Hepatic adenoma. • Nodular hyperplasia. • Biliary cystadenoma. • Bile duct adenoma/carcinoma. • Metastatic neoplasia. • Polycystic liver disease—less common form; fibrous stroma hyperplasia with anaplastic duct cells; few cysts. • Hepatic lymphoma, hemangiosarcoma, carcinoid.

CBC/BIOCHEMISTRY/URINALYSIS

CBC

• Usually unremarkable. • Anemia in >50% of cases with massive hepatocellular carcinoma in one study. • Anemia may be regenerative if tumor is bleeding. • Leukocytosis with a left shift—tumors with necrotic centers.

Biochemistry

• Liver enzymes variable. • Serum total bilirubin values—usually normal. • May note hypoalbuminemia, hypoglycemia, and hypocholesterolemia.

OTHER LABORATORY TESTS

• Serum bile acids—normal unless tumor impairs hepatic perfusion and biliary flow. • Coagulation parameters— consistent with disseminated intravascular coagulation (DIC) in patients with massive or necrotic tumors, or intra-abdominal bleeding.

IMAGING

Radiography

• May demonstrate a single-mass lesion, apparent asymmetry of hepatic silhouette, or hepatomegaly. • Rarely, gas in necrotic center of tumor. • Loss of serosal detail in case of hemoabdomen.

Abdominal Ultrasonography

• Discrete mass lesion with variable echogenicity, depending on the presence of intratumoral necrosis, hemorrhage, gas, or cystic cavities. • Massive enlargement of a single liver lobe is occasionally observed. • Mixed echogenic pattern—most common. • Nodular pattern of lesions.

CT/MRI

CT is indicated for surgical planning (determine divisional or lobar origin), or when tumor involves/close proximity to critical anatomic structures, such as major vessels and the bile duct.

DIAGNOSTIC PROCEDURES

• Aspiration cytology—to exclude other types of neoplasia (lymphoma, sarcoma, etc.); aspirate cytology cannot reliably differentiate between hepatocellular carcinoma and benign hepatocellular proliferation (adenoma, hyperplasia). • Surgical hepatic biopsy for confirmation. • If tumor is not surgically resectable, ultrasound-guided needle biopsy may be useful in obtaining definitive diagnosis.

PATHOLOGIC FINDINGS

• Three clinical subtypes of this tumor are described—massive, nodular, and diffuse. • Nodular forms account for 30% and diffuse types account for 10% of all reported hepatocellular carcinomas in dogs, and both types involve multiple liver lobes. • Massive form that is confined to one lobe accounts for about 60% of canine hepatocellular carcinoma cases. • Presence of necrotic areas. • Diffusely infiltrated tumors may not be grossly apparent other than hepatomegaly.

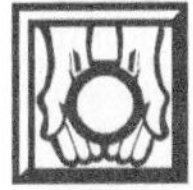

TREATMENT

Surgical Considerations

• Complete excision (liver lobectomy) recommended when possible; excision with microscopically dirty margins can still afford durable tumor control and long survival times. • Massive form is often amenable to surgical resection. • Nodular and diffuse forms are often not amenable to surgery. • Between 60% and 70% of the liver lobes can be resected if the patient is healthy and is given appropriate postoperative care.

MEDICATIONS

DRUG(S) OF CHOICE

While toceranib administration has resulted in short-term tumor control for some dogs, no medical treatment options have been successful in reducing tumor recurrence or risk for metastasis.

FOLLOW-UP

PATIENT MONITORING

• Abdominal ultrasonography—2 weeks postoperative for baseline and every 3–4 months for the first year. • Abdominal CT appears more sensitive than ultrasonography for detection of small, recurrent lesions. • Monitor liver enzymes serially.

POSSIBLE COMPLICATIONS

Risk of tumor necrosis and massive abdominal hemorrhage if unresected.

EXPECTED COURSE AND PROGNOSIS

• Massive forms treated with surgery have a better prognosis than do the nodular or diffuse forms. • Median survival of dogs with massive form treated with surgery may be >1,460 days. • Local tumor recurrence or de novo tumor growth is not uncommon.

MISCELLANEOUS

ASSOCIATED CONDITIONS

Polycystic liver disease in cats.

ABBREVIATIONS

• DIC = disseminated intravascular coagulation.

Suggested Reading

Goussev SA, Center SA, Randolph JF, et al. Clinical characteristics of hepatocellular carcinoma in 19 cats from a single institution (1980–2013). J Am Anim Hosp Assoc 2016, 52(1):36–41.

Liptak JM, Dernell WS, Withrow SJ. Liver tumors in cats and dogs. Compend Contin Educ Pract Vet 2004, 26:50–56.

Author Nick Dervisis

Consulting Editor Timothy M. Fan

HEPATOCUTANEOUS SYNDROME

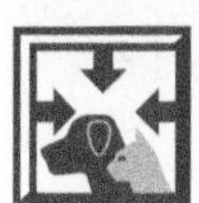

BASICS

OVERVIEW

- Liver lesion—severe degenerative vacuolar hepatopathy, hepatocyte degeneration leads to parenchymal collapse associated with marked proliferative hepatocyte response; this process leads to severe hepatic nodularity; hepatocutaneous syndrome (HCS) hepatopathy often associated with syndromic pressure point crusting, painful dermatosis, and diabetes mellitus (DM).
- Liver lesions—may precede cutaneous lesions and DM.
- Hepatopathy—recognized on abdominal US, pursued because of marked alkaline phosphatase (ALP) increase.
- Occasionally HCS hepatopathy develops in dogs treated chronically with phenobarbital.

SIGNALMENT

- Middle-aged to older dogs.
- Males may have a greater predilection.
- Familial syndrome in shih tzu dogs described.

SIGNS

Historical Findings

- Acute to subacute onset; may be few initial signs.
- Common signs— anorexia, weight loss, lethargy, polyuria/polydipsia, diarrhea, vomiting, ± jaundice, often with prominent cutaneous pressure point and painful foot pad lesions characterized as fissured crusted oozing wounds.

Physical Examination Findings

- Lethargy, poor body condition, with foot pad and elbow lesions causing pain in standing and recumbent postures, may be jaundiced.
- Cutaneous lesions—see Superficial Necrolytic Dermatitis.
- Normal, small to large hepatic size.
- Rare abdominal effusion—signifies late-stage HCS hepatopathy.

CAUSES & RISK FACTORS

- Etiology—associated with pathologic hypoaminoacidemia and aminoaciduria; low amino acid (AA) concentrations seemingly have causal association with cutaneous and liver lesions. Most significantly low AA affiliated with urea cycle and synthesis of glutathione and collagen.
- Hyperglucagonemia associated with glucagonoma—originally proposed as causal mechanism but that remains unproven; ~30–40% of tested dogs have increased plasma glucagon concentrations; glucagonoma confirmed in <15% of reported cases.
- Insulin-resistant DM—commonly associated with HCS; may reflect increased glucagon.
- Contributing role hypothesized for ill-defined deficiencies of zinc, fatty acids, or niacin.
- Similar cutaneous lesions described with primary hepatopathies caused by phenobarbital or rarely chronic mycotoxicosis.

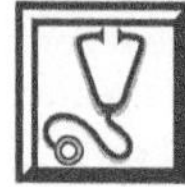

DIAGNOSIS

DIFFERENTIAL DIAGNOSIS

- Cirrhosis—unresolvable architectural remodeling with fibrosis, sinusoidal hypertension, and regenerative nodules.
- Chronic hepatitis—inflammatory infiltrates and individual hepatocyte necrosis.
- Copper associated hepatopathy—pathologic copper accumulation initially with zone 3 associated with oxidative necroinflammatory hepatocyte injury.
- Diffuse nodular hyperplasia—rare cause of hepatic nodularity of similar magnitude.
- Degenerative glycogen-type vacuolar hepatopathy (VH)—may evolve similar nodular hepatic US pattern.

CBC/BIOCHEMISTRY/URINALYSIS

- CBC—mild to moderate nonregenerative to mild regenerative anemia; red blood cell microcytosis; neutrophilic leukocytosis reflecting cutaneous lesion inflammation or infection.
- Biochemistry—high liver enzymes (especially ALP); variable hypoproteinemia with hypoalbuminemia, low cholesterol and blood urea nitrogen; euglycemic to fasting hyperglycemia.
- Urinalysis—ammonium biurate crystalluria reflects hepatic insufficiency in end-stage hepatopathy; occasionally develop acquired portosystemic shunts, with shunting contributing to hyperammonemia.

OTHER LABORATORY TESTS

- Total serum bile acids—normal or increased.
- Insulin—inappropriately increased before development of diabetes mellitus.
- Plasma glucagon—inconsistently increased.
- Plasma AA profile—30–50% reduction in AA concentrations of healthy dogs; dogs with cutaneous lesions have more severe AA deficiencies than dogs with only HCS hepatopathy.
- Urine AA profile—prodigious renal wasting of lysine and proline; profile of urine AA concentrations must be normalized with urine creatinine concentration for interpretation.

IMAGING

- Abdominal radiography—variable liver size (small, normal, to large); rare effusion.
- Abdominal US—may disclose irregular liver margin; characteristic nodular pattern: hypoechoic foci (proliferative nodules) with background hyperechoic parenchyma (glycogen-type VH and lipid-type VH) typified as "Swiss cheese pattern"; although suggested as pathognomonic, other causes of severe degenerative VH also may demonstrate this pattern; occasional diffuse nodularity cannot be imaged in HCS; pancreatic mass <15% of dogs.

DIAGNOSTIC PROCEDURES

- Aspiration sampling—hepatocytes display glycogen- and lipid-type vacuolation.
- Liver biopsy—needle biopsy may compromise definitive diagnosis due to limited sampling of distinctive proliferative hepatocyte foci between regions with massive degenerative VH; needle biopsy may be best option for dogs with extensive skin lesions; larger laparoscopic samples preferred; avoid laparotomy as dogs with cutaneous lesions may not promptly heal.
- Skin biopsy—see Superficial Necrolytic Dermatitis; usually diagnostic for HCS.
- AA profiles in plasma and urine with urine AA normalized using urine creatinine disclose profound reduction of plasma AA and severe aminoaciduria with prominent losses of lysine and proline.
- Glucagonomas often express somatostatin receptors; these might be identified using radioisotope somatostatin label; however, prohibitively expensive for most clients.
- If pancreatic mass discovered, should be resected, submitted for routine and special stains (request immunohistochemical stains for neuroendocrine neoplasia); like other islet cell tumors, glucagonomas may produce other hormones (see Suggested Reading). *Note*: positive immunohistochemical staining does not confirm pathologic hormone secretion.

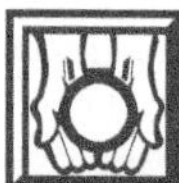

TREATMENT

- Diet—use high-quality/high-quantity protein, energy-dense diets; enteral or parenteral feeding may be required for some dogs at initial diagnosis.
- If hepatic encephalopathy (HE) observed—improve nitrogen tolerance with lactulose and metronidazole (see Hepatic Encephalopathy) and use liver-specific diet as baseline formula.
- Supplemental AA therapy is cornerstone of treatment—IV route superior to oral route.
- Oral AA supplementation—historically done with egg yolk (3–6 yolks per day) but *not* very effective; dietary supplementation with anabolic whey protein powder increases protein intake, but alone *not* very effective; oral treatment may lack efficacy due to reduced enteral AA uptake.
- IV AA infusion with IV lipid infusion—*most* effective therapy (lesion resolution and survival).

- IV AA infusion—8.5–10% solution of crystalline AA (Aminosyn®); using 10% solution (100 mL delivers 10 g AA) dose: 25 mL/kg bodyweight over 6–8h through peripheral vein.
- IV 20% Intralipid® (or generic 20% IV fat emulsion)—dose: 7 ml/kg bodyweight over 6–8h; given concurrently with IV AA using Y-adaptor for combined infusions through one line; combined therapy achieves best response to date.
- IV infusion treatment interval—initially q7–10 days until evidence of improvement: skin easiest to appraise with photo documentation and evidence of foot pad pain resolution; hepatic lesions require US imaging for assessment: these take months to improve; liver enzymes may be used to infer improvement but do not normalize (remain vacillating). RBC microcytosis resolves with significant recovery. After initial strong response, frequency of IV AA and IV Intralipid determined based on dog's physical and lesional status and trends in hematologic and biochemical profiles. Chronically managed patients typically receive IV infusions at 6-week intervals, titrated frequency achieved by gradually lengthening intervals between infusions while monitoring for relapse.
- Essential fatty acid supplementation—omega-3 fatty acids; double normal dose.
- Metastatic pancreatic tumors secreting glucagon may be controlled with longacting somatostatin analogue (octreotide: 2–3.7 μg/kg q6–12h); prohibitively expensive.
- Manage DM with insulin and judicious dose titration to response.
- Other supplements—see Medications.

MEDICATIONS

DRUG(S) OF CHOICE

- Insulin for DM management; may demonstrate insulin resistance.
- AA infusion and lipid infusions and diet—see above.
- Cutaneous or nail bed infections—systemic antimicrobials or antifungals; germicidal baths.
- Ketoconazole—for secondary yeast infection; anti-inflammatory and antipruritic effects: monitor liver enzymes for drug-induced liver injury warranting drug discontinuation.
- Zinc supplementation—2–4 mg/kg elemental zinc q24h; avoid zinc methionine if HE.
- Niacinamide—250–300 mg/dog q12h (500 mg for dogs >10 kg); watch for toxic effects; avoid extended-release form.
- Topical glucocorticoids—if unresponsive inflammatory skin lesions, after infection managed (*caution*: systemic glucocorticoids may promote HE, enteric ulceration, infection, may complicate DM management).
- Ursodeoxycholic acid—10–15 mg/kg PO daily, divided dose given with food; hepatoprotectant against bile acid mediated membrane injury.
- Antioxidants—vitamin E (10 IU/kg daily PO with food); *S*-adenosylmethionine (20 mg/kg PO daily, empty stomach) provides additional metabolic and hepatoprotective influences.
- If associated with phenobarbital, discontinue this drug.

CONTRAINDICATIONS/POSSIBLE INTERACTIONS

- HE induction—high-protein diet supplements and AA infusions.
- Toxic effects of ketoconazole and its interference with p450 drug metabolism.
- Toxic effects of niacinamide and zinc.

FOLLOW-UP

PATIENT MONITORING

- Weekly to monthly physical exam, CBC, biochemistry, and urinalysis to assess need for IV AA and lipid infusions and treatments for secondary infections.
- As needed for management of DM.

POSSIBLE COMPLICATIONS

- With HCS, IV infusions may cause thrombophlebitis and risk for thromboembolism.
- Ketoacidosis—uncommon.
- Hepatic encephalopathy.
- Sepsis—due to diabetes and skin lesions or IV catheter-related infections.
- Pain—from skin lesions may require analgesics.

EXPECTED COURSE AND PROGNOSIS

- Liver and skin lesions often improve with IV infusions.
- Some dogs achieve cutaneous remission ≥3 years with described therapies.
- Some dogs have unremitting HCS progression, necessitating euthanasia.

MISCELLANEOUS

SYNONYMS

- Superficial necrolytic dermatitis.
- Necrolytic migratory erythema.
- Metabolic epidermal necrosis.
- Glucagonoma syndrome.

ABBREVIATIONS

- AA = amino acids
- ALP = alkaline phosphatase.
- DM = diabetes mellitus
- HE = hepatic encephalopathy
- HCS = hepatocutaneous syndrome
- VH = vacuolar hepatopathy

Suggested Reading

Bach JF, Glasser SA. A case of necrolytic migratory erythema managed for 24 months with intravenous amino acid and lipid infusions. Can Vet J 2013, 54:873–875.

Hall-Fonte DL, Center SA, McDonough SP, et al. Hepatocutaneous syndrome in Shih Tzus: 31 cases (1996–2014). J Am Vet Med Assoc 2016, 248(7):802–813.

Oberkirchner U, Linder KE, Zadronzny L, et al. Successful treatment of canine necrolytic migratory erythema (superficial necrolytic dermatitis) due to metastatic glucagonoma with octreotide. Vet Dermatol 2010, 21:510–516.

Authors Sharon A. Center and John P. Loftus
Consulting Editor Kate Holan

HEPATOMEGALY

BASICS

DEFINITION

Large liver detected on physical examination, abdominal radiography, US, or direct visualization.

PATHOPHYSIOLOGY

• Liver size—influenced by hepatotropic factors produced by splanchnic viscera (insulin dominates); delivered in portal blood. • Enlargement may reflect sinusoidal capacitance (blood pooling), parenchymal or sinusoidal accumulation of cells or substrates, or storage products expanding hepatocytes.

Diffuse or Generalized

• Inflammatory—immune-mediated, infectious, pyogranulomatous hepatitis; classified by infiltrative cell type. • Lymphoreticular hyperplasia—response to antigens or accelerated erythrocyte destruction.
• Congestion—impaired drainage through hepatic vein (cardiac, pericardial, thrombotic, neoplastic causes); sinusoidal occlusion syndrome or Budd Chiari syndrome.
• Infiltration—cellular (neoplastic: primary hepatocellular, metastatic); excessive glycogen, lipid, or, rarely, metabolic products (genetic diseases) expanding hepatocytes or space of Disse (amyloid). • Cystic lesions as observed in ductal plate malformations (DPMs).
• Cholestasis—most commonly with extrahepatic bile duct obstruction (EHBDO); rarely, intrahepatic cholestasis causing bile duct distention. • Extramedullary hematopoiesis (EMH)—diffuse, severe, or obstructing perfusion.

Nodular, Focal, or Asymmetric Hepatic Enlargement

• Neoplasia—hepatocellular carcinoma (HCA), hemangiosarcoma, lymphoma, metastatic carcinoma, other. • Hemorrhage.
• Infection or inflammation. • Hepatic nodular hyperplasia (uncommon cause).
• Nodular regeneration (uncommonly associated with hepatomegaly). • Arteriovenous malformation—involved lobe larger than other lobes; other lobes atrophied. • Asymmetric regeneration after large-volume resection or panlobular necrosis. • Biliary cystic lesions (DPM). • Other DPM malformations—large liver lobes usually with some atretic liver lobes or even atretic gallbladder; proliferative-like biliary epithelium with fibrotic bridging portal trabeculae (congenital hepatic fibrosis: DPM phenotype). • Liver lobe torsion—acute venous congestion.

SYSTEMS AFFECTED

• Gastrointestinal—gastric compression or displacement by large liver. • Peritoneal effusion—sinusoidal or postsinusoidal hepatic hypertension weeping lymph. • Pulmonary—reduced ventilatory space from diaphragmatic compression. • General/vague pain—stretching of liver capsule, compression of adjacent viscera.

SIGNALMENT

• Dog and cat. • Old animals more commonly; younger if DPM related.

SIGNS

Historical Findings

• Abdominal distention or palpable mass.
• Abdominal discomfort—vague location.
• Depends on underlying cause.

Physical Examination Findings

• Dogs—liver palpable beyond costal margin (normal liver palpable in some breeds).
• Cats—liver palpable >1.5 cm beyond costal margin (normal liver palpable in some cats). • May be undetected in obese animals.

CAUSES

Inflammation

• Infectious or chronic (early) hepatitis.
• Acute toxic hepatopathy. • Feline cholangitis/cholangiohepatitis syndrome (CCHS). • EHBDO. • Lymphoreticular/pyogranulomatous—immune-mediated disease (hemolytic anemia, hemophagocytic syndrome, systemic lupus erythematosus, idiopathic), infectious disorders. • Venous outflow obstruction—sinusoidal occlusion syndrome or Budd Chiari syndrome.

Congestive Hepatopathy

• Increased central venous pressure—right-sided congestive heart failure: tricuspid valve disease; cardiomyopathy; congenital anomaly (cor triatriatum dexter); neoplasia; pericardial disease; heartworm disease; pulmonary hypertension; severe arrhythmias or bradycardia reducing cardiac output. • Vena caval or hepatic vein occlusion—thrombosis; tumor invasion or extramural caval occlusion; heartworm vena cava syndrome; vena caval stenosis or congenital kink (rare); diaphragmatic hernia; vena caval or large hepatic vein thrombosis (Budd Chiari syndrome); intrahepatic hepatic vein occlusion (thrombi, neoplasia, centrilobular parenchymal collapse causing sinusoidal occlusion syndrome).
• Sinusoidal occlusion syndrome—collapsed centrilobular parenchyma and/or damage to hepatic venules impairing circulatory egress; causes include xenobiotic or herbal toxicity (e.g., pyrrolizidine alkaloids), severe non-steroidal inflammatory drug–induced injury, severe copper hepatopathy. • Liver lobe torsion (acute).

Infiltration

• Neoplasia. • Metabolic abnormalities—amyloid; lipid (see Hepatic Lipidosis [cats]), glycogen (see Glycogen-Type Vacuolar Hepatopathy [dogs]); cats and dogs: diabetes mellitus (DM), hyperlipidemic syndromes; neonatal metabolic storage disorders.
• Lymphohistiocytic/pyogranulomatous—infectious disease, immune response, antigen stimulation, neoplasia (histiocytic/dendritic cells: histiocytic sarcoma), hemophagocytic syndrome.

Extramedullary Hematopoiesis

Regenerative anemias—hemolytic (immune-mediated, congenital, metabolic, infectious); oxidant injury; erythroparasitism; severe blood loss, bone marrow failure; idiopathic.

Neoplasia

• Infiltrative, diffuse, or large focal tumors—primary or metastatic. • Primary hepatic—lymphoma; massive HCA; cholangiocarcinoma (bile duct carcinoma ± EHBDO); hemangiosarcoma. • Metastatic—lymphosarcoma, hemangiosarcoma, histiocytic sarcoma, fibrosarcoma, leiomyoma/sarcoma, neuroendocrine, osteosarcoma, others.

Major Bile Duct Obstruction

• Pancreatitis; pancreatic neoplasia. • Neoplasms in porta hepatis—bile duct carcinoma, lymphoma. • Granuloma/fibrosis of common bile duct. • Inspissated bile syndrome, choledochal cyst (DPM phenotype), or gallbladder mucocele. • Cholelithiasis.
• Proximal duodenitis; duodenal foreign body.
• Fluke migration (cats).

Cystic Lesions

• Primary single hepatic or biliary cysts.
• Acquired cysts within neoplastic masses.
• DPM—may associate with renal cysts (common in Persian cats). • Biliary cystadenoma (cats; DPM phenotype).
• Hepatic abscesses (cystic cavitation); hepatocellular carcinoma housing abscess.
• Parasitic—echinococcus (hydatid cyst).

Other

• Drugs—corticosteroids (see Glycogen-Type Vacuolar Hepatopathy), phenobarbital (dogs).
• Hepatic nodular hyperplasia (rare cause).
• Acromegaly—cats.

RISK FACTORS

• Cardiac disease. • Heartworm disease.
• Neoplasia. • Primary hepatic disease—inflammatory, neoplastic, cystic, or other DPM phenotypes. • Corticosteroids—exogenous or endogenous. • Phenobarbital treatment. • Poorly controlled DM.
• Anorexia in obese cats—hepatic lipidosis.
• EHBDO. • Cystic malformations—DPM. • Certain anemias—diffuse hepatic EMH.

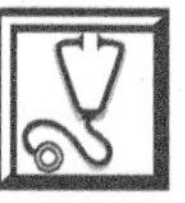

DIAGNOSIS

DIFFERENTIAL DIAGNOSIS

Similar Signs

Distinguish from other disorders causing visceromegaly (gastric, splenic), cranial abdominal masses, or effusions via radiography and US.

Differential Causes

• Cardiac disorders—heart murmur, weak femoral pulses, hepatojugular reflex, jugular distention and jugular pulses, muffled heart sounds, arrhythmias, cough, dyspnea/tachypnea. • Symptomatic anemia—pallor ± jaundice; tachycardia; tachypnea; exercise intolerance; bounding pulses. • Parenchymal liver disease—lethargy, anorexia, vomiting, diarrhea, weight loss, variable liver enzymes ± jaundice, coagulopathies, polyuria/polydipsia (PU/PD), if advanced may see hepatic encephalopathy (HE) or ascites. • Glycogen-type vacuolar hepatopathy (VH; dog)—signs of hyperadrenocorticism or adrenal hyperplasia or other chronic disease imposing stress; DM—persistent hyperglycemia; PU/PD, signs of underlying endocrinopathy. • Hepatic lipidosis—jaundice in obese hyporexic cat, poorly controlled DM (dog or cat); failure-to-thrive puppies or kittens; congenital lysosomal or glycogen storage disorders.

CBC/BIOCHEMISTRY/URINALYSIS

CBC

• Identify anemia and cause; spherocytes (immune-mediated hemolytic anemia, microangiopathic anemia); schistocytes (vascular shearing-microangiopathic, vena cava syndrome, hemangiosarcoma, disseminated intravascular coagulation (DIC), Heinz bodies (oxidant injury); erythroparasitism (*Mycoplasma haemofelis* or *haemominutum*, *Babesia*). • Circulating blast cells—myeloproliferative or lymphoproliferative disorders. • Nucleated red cells—EMH, splenic disease, regenerative anemia. • Macrocytosis and nonregenerative anemia—feline immunodeficiency virus (FIV), feline leukemia virus (FeLV), myelophthisis. • Thrombocytopenia—increased consumption, destruction, or reduced platelet production. • Thrombocytosis—neoplasia; inflammation; hyperadrenocorticism; splenic disease.

Biochemistry

• Inflammatory hepatic disorders—usually high liver enzyme activity; variable hyperglobulinemia, bilirubin, and albumin concentrations. • Reticuloendothelial hyperplasia—variable liver enzyme activity. • Primary hepatic neoplasia—moderate to marked increases in liver enzyme activity (alkaline phosphatase [ALP] and γ-glutamyltransferase [GGT] usually predominate with HCA, variable alanine aminotransferase [ALT]. • Metastatic neoplasia—variable liver enzymes; occasional high calcium or globulin. • Infiltrative disorders—minor liver enzyme change; variable bilirubin concentration. • Glycogen-type VH (dogs)—markedly high ALP; high cholesterol ± triglycerides with increased glucocorticoids or sex steroids; DM—high ALP, cholesterol, hyperglycemia. • Hepatic lipidosis (cats)—high ALP, aspartate aminotransferase (AST), ALT; minor increase in GGT unless concurrent pancreatitis, CCHS, or EHBDO. • Storage diseases—may display few abnormalities. • EHBDO—markedly high ALP, GGT, other enzymes; high bilirubin and cholesterol. • Cystic lesions—normal, except with hepatic abscess (markedly high ALT and AST) or CCHS (high ALP, ALT, GGT, variable bilirubin); DPM often presents with suppurative CCHS. • Phenobarbital-associated—high liver enzymes (especially ALP in dogs). • Nodular hyperplasia—normal to moderately high ALP, elderly dogs: rare cause of hepatomegaly.

OTHER LABORATORY TESTS

• FeLV and FIV testing—cats. • Buffy coat—circulating blasts with neoplasia or uncommon cell type observed. • Coagulation panel—DIC common with hemangiosarcoma or diffuse lymphoma; prolonged coagulation times common with EHBDO >5 days esp. in cats. • Total serum bile acids (TSBA)—high in diffuse disorders or EHBDO; *redundant test if nonhemolytic jaundice*. • Pituitary-adrenal axis testing (dogs)—see Glycogen-Type Vacuolar Hepatopathy; Hyperadrenocorticism (Cushing's Syndrome)—Dogs. • Insulin-like growth factor-1 (IGF-1) in acromegalic cats; typically males with DM. • Heartworm testing—in endemic areas. • Fungal serology—in endemic areas. • Other serology—e.g., Rickettsial, *Bartonella*, *Leishmania*, *Toxoplasmosis*.

IMAGING

Abdominal Radiography

• Hepatomegaly—rounded margins extending beyond costal arch; caudal-dorsal gastric displacement; caudal displacement: cranial duodenal flexure, right kidney, transverse colon. • May suggest cause.

Thoracic Radiography

• Three views (lateral [right, left], dorsal-ventral)—metastasis, other disorders, cranial displacement of diaphragm, wide vena cava if passive congestion. • Cardiac, pulmonary, pericardial, and vena caval disorders usually need US imaging. • Sternal lymphadenopathy—reflects abdominal inflammation or neoplasia. • Puppies, kittens, deep inspiration, and certain canine breeds—spurious hepatomegaly.

Abdominal US

• Liver size and surface contour. • Diffuse enlargement with normal echogenicity—congestion; cellular infiltration (lymphoma); inflammation; EMH; reticuloendothelial hyperplasia, diffuse amyloid deposition expanding space of Disse. • Diffuse enlargement with hypoechoic parenchyma—normal variation; congestion, lymphoma, diffuse sarcoma; amyloidosis expanding space of Disse. • Diffuse enlargement with hyperechoic parenchymal (minor nodularity)—lipid or glycogen; inflammation; fibrosis; lymphoma; DPM fibrotic bridging portal trabeculae. • Diffuse enlargement with hypoechoic nodules—neoplasia; abscess; degenerative glycogen-type VH (dog); HCS, cystic lesions (DPM). • Identify EHBDO. • Identify concurrent abdominal diseases—kidneys; intestines; lymph nodes; effusion; interrogation of porta hepatis for obstructions and lymphadenopathy. • Identify portal or vena caval thrombi. • Identify abdominal effusion—distribution and echogenic patterns. • Cannot distinguish benign from malignant disease.

H

DIAGNOSTIC PROCEDURES

ECG/Echocardiography

Characterize cardiac rhythm, structure, function, pulmonary pressure gradient.

Fine-Needle Aspiration

• Procedure—22-G, 2.5–3.75 cm (1–1.5 in) needle; diffusely large liver directly aspirated without US; focal lesions aspirated under US guidance. • Cytology—may disclose infectious agents, vacuolar change, neoplasia, inflammation, or EMH; definitive diagnosis seldom confidently confirmed (false-positive and -negative results). • Hepatic biopsy—if US rules out EHBDO, cytology does not indicate septic inflammation or neoplasia, and no obvious diagnoses made; percutaneous ultrasound–guided Tru-Cut® needle biopsy for suspected neoplasia or amyloid (avoid if abscess or EHBDO possible); otherwise, best sampling with laparoscopic or surgical exploratory approaches. • Microbial culture—aerobic and anaerobic bacterial; fungal as appropriate. • Staining—H&E (routine); reticulin (architectural substructural remodeling, infiltration, compression), Masson's trichrome (collagen deposition, amyloid detection); rhodanine (copper); periodic acid–Schiff (glycogen ± amylase predigestion); acid-fast stain (mycobacteria if granulomatous inflammation); Congo red (amyloid); Oil Red O (lipid, requires frozen section), infectious disease stains (see Hepatitis, Granulomatous). • Coagulation testing—before liver sampling, consider measurement of prothrombin time, activated partial thromboplastin time, fibrinogen, buccal mucosal bleeding time (BMBT); prediction of iatrogenic hemorrhage poor with bench tests; BMBT may be more relevant. • Abdominal effusion—cytology; protein content; culture; evaluate before tissue sampling. • Pericardiocentesis—if pericardial tamponade. • Cyst aspiration sampling—if possible infectious cause when plausible treatment might be recommended; risk for abdominal contamination if hepatic abscess.

HEPATOMEGALY (CONTINUED)

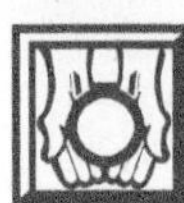

TREATMENT

APPROPRIATE HEALTH CARE

• Outpatient—except cardiac/pericardial causes or hepatic failure. • General supportive goals—eliminate or manage inciting cause; prevent complications; palliate derangements reflecting hepatic failure. • Important derangements—dehydration and hypovolemia; HE; hypoglycemia; acid-base and electrolyte abnormalities; coagulopathies; enteric hemorrhage; sepsis; endotoxemia.

NURSING CARE

• Heart failure or ascites—impose sodium restriction: fluids and food (<100 mg/100 kcal, <0.2% dry matter basis food), prescribe appropriate cardiac medications or diuretics.
• Supplement potassium chloride if IV fluids—sliding scale (maintenance = 20 mEq/L fluid). • Supplement B-soluble vitamins in IV fluids. • If jaundiced—parenteral vitamin K before invasive procedures.

ACTIVITY

Restricted; initial cage rest in some disorders.

DIET

• Dietary protein—restrict only if evidence of HE. • Well-balanced, adequate energy, positive nitrogen balance essential; adequate vitamins and micronutrients for most disorders; fat restriction only if hypertriglyceridemia or steatorrhea. • May need feeding tube (e.g., esophagostomy tube) in cats with HL (see Hepatic Lipidosis). • Sodium—restrict if cardiac failure or ascites.

CLIENT EDUCATION

• Treatment depends on underlying cause.
• Many causes life-threatening; some less serious and amenable to treatment.
• Thorough diagnostic evaluations essential for determining definitive cause and interventions.

SURGICAL CONSIDERATIONS

• Resection of primary or focal hepatic mass lesions (neoplasia, abscess, compromising cyst)—biliary decompression if EHBDO.
• Pericardiectomy (thoracoscopic procedure)—if effusion recurs after initial pericardiocentesis.

MEDICATIONS

DRUG(S) OF CHOICE

Vary with underlying cause.

CONTRAINDICATIONS

• Avoid hepatotoxic drugs. • Glycogen-type VH (dogs)—avoid glucocorticoids. • Hepatic lipidosis (cats)—avoid catabolism or drugs that promote it; avoid fasting.

FOLLOW-UP

PATIENT MONITORING

• Physical assessment and hepatic imaging—reassess liver size. • CBC, biochemistry, TSBA—serial assessments of lab abnormalities and liver function; packed cell volume and reticulocyte count with anemia.
• Thoracic radiography, ECG, and echocardiography—reassess status.
• Pituitary-adrenal axis—adrenal disorders.
• Adjust drug dosages according to status of liver function, body condition, and weight.

POSSIBLE COMPLICATIONS

Many causes are life-threatening.

MISCELLANEOUS

ZOONOTIC POTENTIAL

Certain infectious agents of concern.

SEE ALSO

• Amyloidosis.
• Anemia, Immune-Mediated.
• Bile Duct Obstruction (Extrahepatic).
• Cholangitis/Cholangiohepatitis Syndrome.
• Congestive Heart Failure, Right-Sided.
• Ductal Plate Malformation (Congenital Hepatic Fibrosis).
• Glycogen Storage Disease.
• Glycogen-Type Vacuolar Hepatopathy.
• Hepatic Lipidosis.
• Hepatitis, Granulomatous.
• Hepatitis, Suppurative and Hepatic Abscess.
• Hepatocellular Carcinoma.

ABBREVIATIONS

• ALP = alkaline phosphatase.
• ALT = alanine aminotransferase.
• AST = aspartate aminotransferase.
• BMBT = buccal mucosal bleeding time.
• CCHS = cholangitis/cholangiohepatitis syndrome.
• DIC = disseminated intravascular coagulation.
• DM = diabetes mellitus.
• DPM= ductal plate malformation.
• EHBDO = extrahepatic bile duct obstruction.
• EMH = extramedullary hematopoiesis.
• FeLV = feline leukemia virus.
• FIV = feline immunodeficiency virus.
• GGT = γ-glutamyltransferase.
• IGF-1 = Insulin-like growth factor-1.
• HCA = hepatocellular carcinoma.
• HE = hepatic encephalopathy.
• PU/PD= polyuria/polydipsia.
• TSBA = total serum bile acids.
• VH = vacuolar hepatopathy.

Author Sharon A. Center
Consulting Editor Kate Holan

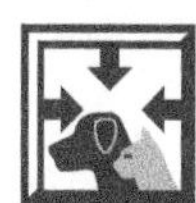

BASICS

DEFINITION

• Microvascular dysplasia (MVD) describes intrahepatic microscopic vascular malformations diminishing intrahepatic perfusion within tertiary portal vein branches; this is accompanied by a compensatory increase in hepatic arterial perfusion (hepatic arterial buffer response); MVD lacks macroscopic portosystemic shunting but genetically associates with congenital portosystemic vascular anomalies (PSVA, shunts) as an apparent complex polygenic autosomal syndrome.
• Occurs as an isolated malformation *or* associated with PSVA.
• Clinically distinct from severe intrahepatic portal vein atresia that causes formation of acquired portosystemic shunts (APSS).
• Histologic features—stereotypic histologic responses reflect portal venous hypoperfusion, of which MVD is one of many causes; often misdiagnosed as portal hypoplasia.
• Clinicopathologic hallmark—increased total serum bile acid (TSBA) concentrations in the absence of other abnormalities observed in PSVA or disorders associated with APSS.
• Coexistence of MVD with PSVA explains failure of TSBA to normalize after complete PSVA attenuation, and inability to fully attenuate PSVA (some dogs).

PATHOPHYSIOLOGY

• Malformations impairing intrahepatic portal venous perfusion reduce hepatocyte exposure to splanchnic-derived hepatotropic factors—this leads to lobular atrophy and impairs expedient hepatocyte extraction of bile acids from the enterohepatic circulation.
• Compensatory hepatic arterial buffer response maintains liver viability.
• Absence of macroscopic portosystemic shunting explains absence of clinical signs—there is no hepatic encephalopathy (HE) or ammonium biurate uroliths or crystalluria in dogs with MVD.

SYSTEMS AFFECTED

• Usually asymptomatic.
• May observe slow recovery from sedatives or anesthetics requiring first-pass hepatic extraction and apparent adverse drug reactions with other medications undergoing first-pass hepatic extraction or hepatic metabolism.
• If concurrent inflammatory bowel disease (IBD)—vacillating signs include vomiting, diarrhea, inappetence, increased liver enzymes (often alanine aminotransferase [ALT]).

GENETICS

• Compelling evidence supports inheritance of PSVA/MVD as a complex polygenic autosomal trait in many small pure-breed dogs.
• Unaffected parents may produce affected progeny due to polygenic inheritance.

INCIDENCE/PREVALENCE

• Prevalence of PSVA/MVD trait in small pure-breed dogs 30–80%—varies with breed.
• Genetic association of MVD and PSVA in kindreds of certain breeds confirms that MVD is most common—10–30 : 1 of MVD : PSVA.

GEOGRAPHIC DISTRIBUTION

Worldwide

SIGNALMENT

Species

Dog

Breed Predilections

• Small-breed dogs.
• Commonly affected breeds—Yorkshire terriers, Maltese, Cairn terriers, Tibetan spaniels, shih tzu, Havanese, miniature schnauzers, pugs, papillon, Norfolk terriers, bichon frisé, West Highland white terriers.
• Not identified in large-breed dogs.
• Not identified in cats.

Age and Range

MVD bile acid testing best done at 4–6 months of age; use paired TSBA tests (pre and 2h post meal); neonatal testing not advised.

SIGNS

Historical Findings

• Asymptomatic—unremarkable history; occasional delayed anesthetic recovery or drug intolerance reported.
• MVD often recognized serendipitously during routine screening tests or diagnostics for nonhepatic health problems, or during TSBA testing in breeds with high PSVA/MVD prevalence.
• Concurrent illnesses may complicate TSBA interpretation (e.g., gastrointestinal [GI] malabsorption or diarrhea may cause erroneously low TSBA values), cholestasis (causes high TSBA values).

Physical Examination Findings

Unremarkable.

CAUSES

Congenital inherited disorder.

RISK FACTORS

Purebred small-dog breeds and mixes of these breeds.

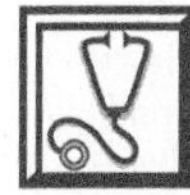

DIAGNOSIS

DIFFERENTIAL DIAGNOSIS

• PSVA—suspected in symptomatic young dog with increased TSBA or HE; however, 20% of PSVA dogs are asymptomatic or minimally symptomatic.
• Other causes of increased ALT or high TSBA values (e.g., GI disease, cholestasis).

CBC/BIOCHEMISTRY/URINALYSIS

• CBC—normal.
• Biochemistry—generally unremarkable; hepatic enzyme activities normal (expect high alkaline phosphatase in young patients due to bone growth); vacillating ALT if coexistent IBD or degenerative/inflammatory centrilobular hepatic lesion (dogs with eosinophilic IBD); mild hypoglobulinemia or hypoalbuminemia noted in ~50% of young dogs.
• Urinalysis—normal.
• Hyperammonemia *not* documented in dogs with MVD without severe portal atresia, PSVA, severe ductal plate malformation congenital hepatic fibrosis phenotype, arteriovenous malformation (fistula), or some other acquired liver disorder.

OTHER LABORATORY TESTS

TSBA

• Paired pre- and post-meal TSBA—recommended diagnostic test; pre- and post-meal TSBA >25 µmol/L reflect abnormal liver function or perfusion in absence of cholestasis.
• No need to fast patient before meal-provoked enterohepatic bile acid challenge.
• Random single TSBA in normal reference range not reliable assessment.
• Paired samples essential to evaluate bile acid enterohepatic circulation.
• Important TSBA testing strategy—food-initiated enterohepatic bile acid challenge essential; verify meal consumption; feed typical size meal; feed dog's regular diet for testing.
• Approximately 15–20% of dogs and ~10% of cats have pre-meal TSBA > post-meal TSBA; this reflects individual differences in physiologic coordination of gallbladder contraction, and gastric and enteric transit rate relative to food intake; thus, *do not* apply fasting TSBA reference ranges.
• "Shunting pattern"—common: higher post-meal TSBA; post-meal TSBA concentration usually 0.5- to 3-fold > pre-meal TSBA.
• Best assessments—young small breed dogs at 6 months; avoids serendipitous discovery of high TSBA when dog later presents for nonhepatic illnesses, when inappropriate testing may be pursued chasing abnormal TSBA values.
• Magnitude of increased TSBA—typically lower for MVD vs. PSVA; but wide overlapping of values invalidates utility of TSBA as standalone test to distinguish MVD from PSVA; however, TSBA values ≥200 µM/L usually associate with PSVA or APSS.
• Quantitative abnormal TSBA values cannot discriminate severity of MVD between dogs; sequential testing demonstrates vacillating abnormal values (reflects physiologic variables).
• Avoid qualitative TSBA tests.

Protein C

- Protein C reflects severity of portosystemic shunting in dogs; not valid for this use in cats.
- Generalities—MVD: protein C *usually* ≥70%; symptomatic PSVA: protein C <70%; asymptomatic PSVA: protein C *may be* ≥70% more common in portoazygous PSVA.

IMAGING

- Abdominal radiography—normal.
- Abdominal US—no macroscopic shunting vessel; liver size subjectively normal or slightly small.
- Mesenteric portovenography—subtle abnormalities of blunted small portal vein branches, protracted contrast "blush" in liver lobes; *caution*: PSVA may be overlooked if radiographic portography only completed in single recumbent posture; CT angiograms lack definition to display MVD hypoperfusion.
- Colorectal (CRS) or splenoportal scintigraphy—normal or slightly increased shunt fraction in MVD; scintigraphy may reveal irregular distribution of isotope among liver lobes.

DIAGNOSTIC PROCEDURES

- Liver biopsy—sample several liver lobes (at least 3) as MVD does not uniformly affect liver lobes; *avoid* sampling caudate lobe as this lobe receives perfusion from first portal vein branch and is often best-perfused liver lobe in dogs with PSVA or MVD; surgical wedge or laparoscopic biopsies recommended.
- US-guided needle biopsy—may not sample enough tissue for definitive diagnosis.

PATHOLOGIC FINDINGS

Gross

- Normal appearance and liver size.
- Some liver lobes comparatively small, coordinating with histologic severity of MVD.

Microscopic

- *Cannot* discriminate MVD, PSVA, noncirrhotic portal hypertension (NCPH), or extrahepatic portal venous thromboembolism (TE)/occlusion without history, clinical findings, and imaging details; *cannot* conclude portal vein hypoplasia.
- Histologic evaluation—required for definitive diagnosis of portal venous hypoperfusion but must be considered in context of clinical, clinicopathologic, and imaging details; rules out most acquired hepatobiliary disorders causing increased TSBA except portal TE and NCPH; histopathologic features of all disorders causing portal venous hypoperfusion are similar; impossible to differentiate MVD from PSVA based only on liver biopsies in most cases.
- MVD diagnosis confused by inappropriate terminology, where "portal hypoplasia" has been used to characterize histologic features of portal venous hypoperfusion; "hypoplasia" defines lack of development—impossible to ascertain from liver biopsy without clinical features and vascular imaging details; MVD one of many causes of portal venous hypoperfusion.
- Stereotypic histologic features of portal venous hypoperfusion:
  - Lobular atrophy—small hepatocytes, closely approximated portal tracts and centrilobular regions, increased appearance of miniaturized (or juvenile) portal tracts (tiny, too many, too close).
  - Increased number of binucleated hepatocytes in portal regions reflecting focal proliferative response induced by restricted portal venous perfusion (proven in experimental models).
  - Increased arteriolar profiles with thick muscular walls, occasional single orphaned arterioles in hepatic parenchyma—findings reflect physiologic compensatory hepatic arterial buffer response increasing perfusion to peribiliary arterial plexus (vasa vasorum for bile ducts and portal veins); serpiginous arteries reflect increased pressure and flow, angiogenic formation of new arterial twigs, and branching architecture of peribiliary arterial plexus.
  - Small nonperfused or absent portal vein silhouettes or vascular silhouettes with malformative sacculated profiles (see below).
  - Prominent perivenular smooth muscle "throttling apparatus" of hepatic veins/venules in dogs (influences transhepatic perfusion) hypothesized to reflect physiologic response to arterialized transhepatic perfusion.
  - Distended lymphatics—in portal tracts, adjacent to hepatic veins, and variably beneath liver capsule reflect increased ultralymph formation from arterialized sinusoidal perfusion.
  - Variable scattered lipogranulomas (coalesced foamy macrophages) inconsistently associate with hemosiderin-iron aggregates, represent foci of historic parenchymal injury.
  - Some dogs display obscured hepatic vein profiles by perivenular aggregates of lipid engorged macrophages (lipogranulomas) ± variable nonsuppurative inflammation, obscuring, or shrouding of venular profiles coordinates; if concurrent PSVA these may be intolerant of complete ligation.
- MVD malformative features in small-breed dogs:
  - Maldevelopment of tertiary portal vein branches—inconsistent identification of portal veins, portal vein silhouettes with dilated, thin-walled unusual-appearing vessels consistent with inlet veins (direct sinusoidal-portal tract interconnections).
  - Malposition of hepatic venules adjacent to portal triads sharing supportive adventitia termed "fusion complexes."
  - Randomly distributed, aberrant wide irregular hepatic sinusoids (microvascular malformation).
  - Disorganized centrilobular hepatic cords with malformative web-like reticulin substructure (reticulin staining).
  - Unusual longitudinal hepatic venule profiles—demonstrating prominent throttling muscle contraction in dog.
  - Variation in histologic features among hepatic lobes.
- *Note*: animals ≤4 months of age demonstrate increased juvenile or small portal triads.

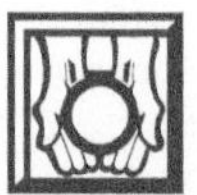

TREATMENT

APPROPRIATE HEALTH CARE

- Asymptomatic—requires no medical interventions except avoidance or dose reduction of drugs dependent on hepatic first-pass extraction.
- *Do not need* ursodeoxycholic acid, *S*-adenosylmethionine (SAMe; unless chronically increased liver enzymes implicating oxidative injury), silibinin extracts (milk thistle), or dietary protein restriction.
- Rarely, some dogs develop centrilobular (zone 3) hepatocyte degeneration that may lead to chronic progressive hepatopathy; diagnosis requires hepatic imaging *and* liver biopsy; may require management for hepatic insufficiency and ascites; more common in Maltese, shih tzu, bichon frisé, Yorkshire terriers; US imaging may disclose attenuated hepatic vein profiles.
- Confirmed MVD associated with nonsuppurative zone 3 inflammation (especially involving eosinophils) and IBD—usually managed with low-dose dexamethasone (0.05 mg/kg PO q48–72h) rather than prednisone to avoid mineralocorticoid supplementation that may provoke ascites, hypoallergenic or hydrolyzed diet (protein restriction only if HE; usually no protein restriction in MVD), or Vivonex® HN, and low-dose metronidazole 7.5 mg/kg PO q12h; if low protein C or increased D-dimers confirmed, add mini-dose aspirin 0.5 mg/kg PO q12–24h or clopidogrel; *must have liver biopsy* confirming need for glucocorticoid and anticoagulants.

DIET

Dogs with only MVD do not require protein-restricted diet.

CLIENT EDUCATION

- Parents with normal TSBA may produce progeny with MVD or PSVA; examination of TSBA in F1 and F2 progeny is only method of recognizing optimal breeding strategy.
- Counsel clients and breed enthusiasts that TSBA values *cannot* grade severity of MVD.
- TSBA testing should be used to identify MVD in juvenile dogs (6 months of age) to avoid future diagnostic confusion as might

occur in adult dogs with nonhepatic illnesses.

- Protein C—*should not be used* as screening test without TSBA to rule out PSVA.

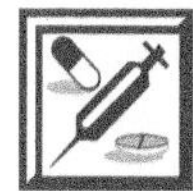

MEDICATIONS

DRUG(S) OF CHOICE

SAMe when chronically elevated liver enzyme activity (esp. ALT) indicates oxidative injury.

PRECAUTIONS

Beware of adverse reactions to drugs reliant on hepatic first-pass extraction or metabolism.

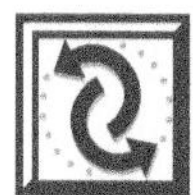

FOLLOW-UP

PATIENT MONITORING

- Asymptomatic dogs—no specific treatment/long-term follow-up has confirmed normal lifespan, no chronic illness, no progressive hepatic degeneration with exception noted above.
- Repeated TSBA tests not advised as values remain abnormal and fluctuate.

PREVENTION/AVOIDANCE

Specific recommendations to eliminate MVD from a particular genetic line or breed possible at present. Based on information from large pedigrees of multiple dog breeds, simply breeding unaffected parents does not eliminate MVD from kindred. In high-incidence kindreds, important to remain vigilant for vaguely ill dogs that may have PSVA; surgical exploration can miss PSVA as can portovenography if only single recumbent position evaluated; rather, CT angiography considered imaging gold standard; CRS definitively detects hepatofugal circulation (portosystemic shunting) and provides quick yes/no test to detect portosystemic shunting; protein C activity assists in differentiating dogs with PSVA from MVD to advise further expensive imaging, but is *not* definitive as standalone test.

EXPECTED COURSE AND PROGNOSIS

- Most dogs with MVD remain asymptomatic and have normal lifespan.
- Progressive increase in magnitude of TSBA values with age (juvenile to adult) has been documented in MVD; this does not coordinate with ill health.
- Generally, TSBA tests in MVD dogs not quantitatively related to histologic severity.
- Dogs with zone 3 degenerative lesions (described above) may develop progressive hepatopathy leading to HE, portal hypertension, APSS, ascites, and rarely portal venous TE; *rare* syndrome.

MISCELLANEOUS

ASSOCIATED CONDITIONS

Small-breed dogs with high incidence of PSVA affected.

AGE-RELATED FACTORS

TSBA can be used to screen young dogs (≥16 weeks of age) in breeds known to have high prevalence of PSVA/MVD.

PREGNANCY/FERTILITY/BREEDING

Bitches with MVD and even minimally symptomatic PSVA carry litters to term.

SYNONYMS

- Congenital portal hypoperfusion.
- Hepatic microvascular dysplasia.
- Microscopic portovascular dysplasia.
- Portal venous hypoplasia.

Confused Terminology

- Intrahepatic portal venous atresia not synonymous with MVD.
- Portal venous hypoplasia not interchangeable as histologic diagnostic term for MVD.

SEE ALSO

- Ductal Plate Malformation (Congenital Hepatic Fibrosis).
- Hepatic Encephalopathy.
- Portosystemic Shunting, Acquired.
- Portosystemic Vascular Anomaly, Congenital.

ABBREVIATIONS

- ALT = alanine aminotransferase.
- APSS = acquired portosystemic shunt.
- CRS = colorectal scintigraphy.
- GI = gastrointestinal.
- HE = hepatic encephalopathy.
- IBD = inflammatory bowel disease.
- MVD = microvascular dysplasia.
- NCPH = noncirrhotic portal hypertension.
- PSVA = portosystemic vascular anomaly.
- SAMe = *S*-adenosylmethionine.
- TE = thromboembolism.
- TSBA = total serum bile acids.

Suggested Reading

Allen L, Stobie D, Mauldin GN, Baer KE. Clinicopathological features of dogs with hepatic microvascular dysplasia with and without portosystemic shunts: 42 cases (1991–1996). J Am Vet Med Assoc 2000, 214:218–220.

Schermerhorn, T, Center SA, Dykes NL, et al. Characterization of hepatoportal microvascular dysplasia in a kindred of cairn terriers. J Vet Intern Med 1996, 10:219–230.

Toulza O, Center SA, Brooks MB, et al. Protein C deficiency in dogs with liver disease. J Am Vet Med Assoc 2006, 229:1761–1771.

Author Sharon A. Center
Consulting Editor Kate Holan

Acknowledgment The author and book editors acknowledge the prior contribution of Sean P. McDonough.

H

HEPATOSUPPORTIVE THERAPIES

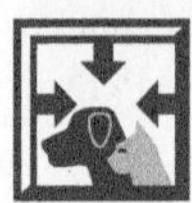

BASICS

OVERVIEW

- Goals of treatment of hepatobiliary disease involve identifying and treating the underlying cause and attenuating pathophysiologic mechanisms common to many hepatobiliary diseases, including inflammation, oxidative damage, and fibrosis.
- Hepatosupportive agents, including prescription drugs and dietary supplements (vitamins, minerals, and nutraceuticals), have received much attention for their concomitant role in treatment of hepatic disease.
- These medications purportedly enhance natural defense mechanisms to inhibit inflammation and fibrosis, prevent hepatocyte apoptosis, and protect against oxidant injury.

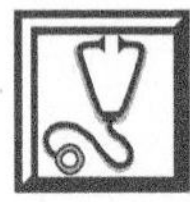

DIAGNOSIS

N/A

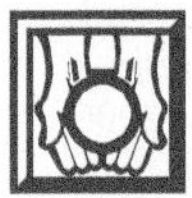

TREATMENT

See Medications.

MEDICATIONS

DRUG(S) OF CHOICE

S-adenosylmethionine (SAMe)

- Endogenous molecule produced from the amino acid methionine and ATP by the enzyme methionine adenosyltransferase synthetase.
- Mechanisms of action—anti-apoptotic, stabilization of cell membranes, modulates cytokine expression, antioxidant activity through enhancement of glutathione levels.
- Indications—necroinflammatory, cholestatic, metabolic, toxic, and ischemic hepatopathies.
- Dosage—20 mg/kg/day PO (dogs and cats).
- Dosage information and comments—best administered in *fasted* state; enteric-coated tablets should not be broken or crushed; lack of bioavailability may be issue in over-the-counter human products.
- Adverse effects and precautions—side effects are rare; post-pill nausea and lack of appetite have been reported in dogs (typically transient); some cats may develop post-pill vomiting.
- Notes—despite lack of supporting evidence, SAMe is frequently prescribed for a variety of hepatobiliary disorders, as it is generally considered safe and has the potential for benefit.

N-acetylcysteine (NAC)

- Stable formulation of the amino acid L-cysteine.
- Mechanisms of action—blocks polymorphonuclear leukocyte (PMN)–endothelial cell adhesion, PMN activation, and cytokine release (anti-inflammatory); improves tissue oxygen delivery; antioxidant activity.
- Indications—acute liver failure, toxic hepatopathies (acetaminophen), and severe feline hepatic lipidosis.
- Dosage—140 mg/kg IV once, then 70 mg/kg IV q6h or 100 mg/kg/day CRI (dogs and cats).
- Dosage information and comments—administer through a nonpyrogenic filter using a 10% solution diluted 1 : 2 or more with saline.
- Adverse effects and precautions—vomiting if given orally (use oral SAMe instead).
- Notes—use of NAC should be considered in any veterinary patient fitting criteria for *acute* liver failure.

Ursodeoxycholic Acid

- Cytoprotective hydrophilic dihydroxylated bile acid.
- Mechanisms of action—replaces hepatotoxic bile acids, stabilization of mitochondrial function, immunomodulatory, anti-apoptotic, stimulation of choleresis.
- Indications—cholestatic, necroinflammatory, metabolic hepatopathies; asymptomatic or mildly symptomatic dogs with gallbladder mucocele.
- Dosage—15 mg/kg PO q24h (dogs and cats).
- Dosage information and comments—absorption enhanced *with food*; can increase to q12h dosing with severe cholestasis.
- Adverse effects and precautions—rare vomiting and diarrhea; avoid in cases of complete bile duct obstruction; may increase bioavailability of vitamin E and cyclosporine.

Silymarin

- Group of flavonoids of which silybin is the major active component.
- Mechanisms of action—antioxidant (reactive oxygen species scavenger), anti-inflammatory, modulates hepatocyte transport, increases hepatic protein synthesis, antifibrotic, choleretic.
- Indications—toxic (*Amanita* mushroom), cholestatic, and necroinflammatory hepatopathies.
- Dosage—silymarin: 20–50 mg/kg/day divided q6–8h PO (dogs and cats); Siliphos®: 3–6 mg/kg/day PO.
- Dosage information and comments—bioavailability is variable.
- Adverse effects and precautions—no side effects; silymarin may inhibit the activity of drug-metabolizing enzymes.

Vitamin E

- Nutritional antioxidant found in all cell membranes.
- Mechanisms of action—antioxidant, anti-inflammatory.
- Indications—cholestatic and necroinflammatory hepatopathies.
- Dosage—10–15 IU/kg/day PO of alpha-tocopherol acetate (dogs and cats).
- Dosage information and comments—may need higher doses with severe cholestasis; parental formulation available and should be considered in animals with severe cholestasis.
- Adverse effects and precautions—none.

FOLLOW-UP

N/A

MISCELLANEOUS

ABBREVIATIONS

- NAC = *N*-acetylcysteine.
- PMN = polymorphonuclear leukocyte.
- SAMe = *S*-adenosylmethionine,

Suggested Reading

Webster CR, Cooper J. Therapeutic use of cytoprotective agents in canine and feline hepatobiliary disease. Vet Clin North Am Small Animal Pract 2009, 39:631–652.

Author Sara A. Wennogle
Consulting Editor Kate Holan

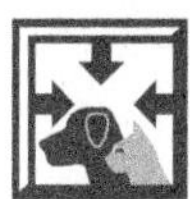

BASICS

DEFINITION

• Endogenous or exogenous substances (drugs, xenobiotics, toxins) that cause hepatic injury. • Direct—(dose dependent): causes predictable injury. • Idiosyncratic—(dose independent): unpredictable.

PATHOPHYSIOLOGY

• Liver highly susceptible because of location and central role in metabolism and detoxification; liver most commonly reported organ associated with true adverse drug reactions. • Mechanisms of damage are direct (active metabolic byproducts) or indirect (oxidative injury from free radical metabolites). • May cause hepatocellular or cytolytic injury (necrosis and apoptosis), cholestasis, immunologic (innocent bystander or hapten-mediated), or mixed histopathologic patterns of injury.

SYSTEMS AFFECTED

• Hepatobiliary. • Nervous—hepatic encephalopathy (HE). • Hemic/lymphatic/immune—disseminated intravascular coagulation (DIC). • Renal—proximal tubular necrosis or renal tubular acidosis/Fanconi syndrome; hepatorenal syndrome (rare).

GENETICS

See Breed Predilections.

INCIDENCE/PREVALENCE

Etiology dependent.

GEOGRAPHIC DISTRIBUTION

Etiology dependent.

SIGNALMENT

Species

Dog and cat.

Breed Predilections

• Siamese cats—some kindreds have high risk (reduced glucuronide formation). • Dog breeds at risk for selected drug toxicity—Doberman, Samoyed: sulfonamide antibiotics; Doberman: amiodarone; Labrador retriever: nonsteroidal anti-inflammatory drugs (NSAIDs); cocker spaniel, German shepherd: phenobarbital; herding breeds: *ABCB1* substrates (ATP-binding cassette subfamily B member 1 gene, encodes for P-glycoprotein).

Mean Age and Range

Any age.

Predominant Sex

No sex predilection.

SIGNS

General Comments

• May reflect chronic long-term or single acute exposure. • Detailed history essential—environmental, drug, and past medical history.

Historical Findings

• Malaise to moribund state. • Hyporexia, vomiting, diarrhea, jaundice, neurologic signs.

Physical Examination Findings

• May be clinically normal if intoxication observed. • Variable body temperature (hypothermic to febrile), vomiting, diarrhea, weakness. • Icterus—overt or progressive (48–96 hours post exposure). • Ascites—rare (grave sign). • HE or coma. • Hemorrhage; petechia; ecchymosis (if DIC present).

CAUSES

Any drug, toxin, or xenobiotic may cause hepatotoxicity, variable severity, any individual.

Common Drugs

• Acetaminophen. • Amiodarone. • Azathioprine. • Azole antifungals. • Beta-lactam antibiotics. • Cyclosporine. • Diazepam (cat, oral only). • Glipizide (cat). • Glucocorticoids (dog). • Glucosamine-based joint supplements (dog). • Griseofulvin (cat). • Imidocarb. • Lomustine (dog). • Methimazole (cat). • Mitotane (dog). • NSAIDs (dog). • Phenobarbital (dog). • Sulfonamide antibiotics (dog). • Tetracyclines. • Toceranib (cat). • Zonisamide (dog).

Common Environmental Toxins

• *Amanita* mushrooms (amanitin-containing mushrooms). • Aflatoxins/mycotoxins. • Blue-green algae (*Cyanobacteria*). • Chlorinated compounds. • Cycad (sago palm nuts). • Heavy metals (Pb, Zn, Mn, Ar, Fe, Cu). • Phenolic chemicals (especially cats). • Gossypol from cottonseed.

Endotoxins

• Enteric organisms—*Clostridium perfringens*; Gram-negative organisms. • Food poisoning—*Staphylococcus*; *Escherichia coli*; *Salmonella*.

Nutritional/Herbal

• *Atractylis gummifera*. • Black cohosh. • *Callilepis laureola*. • Chaparral. • Chinese herbal medicines (certain constituents, contents difficult to characterize). • Comfrey extracts (pyrrolizidine alkaloids). • Germander. • Greater celandine. • Green tea extract. • Kava kava (dogs). • Licorice. • Lipoic acid (cats). • Mistletoe. • Pennyroyal. • Senna. • Usnic acid. • Valerian. • Xylitol (sugar substitute; dogs).

RISK FACTORS

• Medications influencing hepatic metabolism. • Antecedent hepatic disease. • Nutritional and antioxidant status. • Hepatic copper accumulation. • Prior exposure to hepatotoxic compounds.

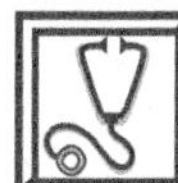

DIAGNOSIS

DIFFERENTIAL DIAGNOSIS

• Infectious disorders affecting liver/biliary tract—leptospirosis, cholangitis/cholecystitis, feline infectious peritonitis, toxoplasmosis, rickettsial diseases, histoplasmosis. • Acute necrotizing pancreatitis. • Traumatic or hypoxic liver injury. • Chronic hepatitis. • Hepatic neoplasia. • Diagnosis of hepatotoxicity requires integration of history, environment, food, medications, and temporal relationship(s).

CBC/BIOCHEMISTRY/URINALYSIS

• PCV and total solids—often normal or high in acute hepatotoxicosis (shock or dehydration). • Alanine aminotransferase (ALT)—reflects cellular membrane damage and leakage; may be 10- to 100-fold normal; prognosis not correlated with magnitude of increase. Increased ALT may precede increases in bilirubin and alkaline phosphatase (ALP). Some toxins suppress hepatic enzyme synthesis, impairing clinical recognition of hepatic injury (e.g., blue-green algae, aflatoxin). • ALP—usually continues to rise for days/weeks while ALT falls. • Aspartate aminotransferase (AST)—may reflect more severe injury (mitochondrial) than ALT; use creatine kinase to differentiate hepatic damage from myonecrosis. • Bilirubin, albumin, blood urea nitrogen, cholesterol, glucose—variable.

OTHER LABORATORY TESTS

• Coagulation profile—monitor for DIC. • Pre- and post-prandial total serum bile acids—assess hepatic function in nonicteric patients. • Low protein C activity—biomarker for blocked protein transcription in aflatoxicosis.

IMAGING

• Abdominal radiography—acute toxicity: normal to large liver; chronic injury: variable liver size. • Abdominal US—variable echogenicity, hepatic size, margins; assess for presence of ascites.

DIAGNOSTIC PROCEDURES

• Hepatic biopsy—seldom indicated in acute toxicity; helpful in chronic hepatic injury without obvious cause; laparoscopy yields better samples than needle biopsies. • Fine-needle aspiration—helpful if neoplasia or infectious agents visualized; no pathognomonic findings for toxicity.

PATHOLOGIC FINDINGS

Variable; depends on toxin, mechanism of cell injury, acinar zone of metabolism or product accumulation, vascular injury, and chronicity.

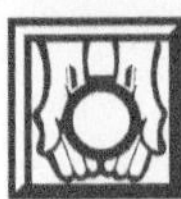

TREATMENT

APPROPRIATE HEALTH CARE

Inpatient—critical care setting.

NURSING CARE

• Decontamination—if intoxication observed and animal presented promptly, decontamination with emetics, adsorbents, and cathartics can be beneficial. • Prevention/correction of shock imperative. • Crystalloid therapy—maintain hepatic perfusion to improve oxygenation and toxin removal; administer maintenance requirements; avoid lactate-containing fluids in fulminant hepatic failure; provide adequate potassium supplementation and monitor, hypokalemia potentiates clinical signs of HE. • Colloid administration—plasma initially preferred for delivery of clotting and anticoagulant factors followed by cautious use of synthetic colloid, if oncotic pressure low.
• Coagulopathy—vitamin K_1 (0.5–1.5 mg/kg SC/IM q12–24h); fresh whole blood or fresh frozen plasma as needed (*caution*: stored blood products may have high ammonia concentration, causing HE). • Nasal oxygen—if compromised peripheral perfusion (hypotension) or pulmonary edema; may improve oxygen delivery to hepatic tissue. • Monitor urine output—diuretics as appropriate (see Acute Kidney Injury). • Hypoglycemia—administer dextrose as needed.

ACTIVITY

Restricted

DIET

• Protein—normal, unless overt HE.
• Nutritional support—if normal body condition score and acute disease, can wait up to 48h for patient to voluntarily ingest food; then consider nasoesophageal/esophageal tube feeding. Parenteral only if unable to feed enterally; can cause severe complications.
• Energy—begin with ~20–30% resting energy requirement (RER), then gradually increase to full RER over 3–5 days.

CLIENT EDUCATION

• Potential for 3–10 days of ICU. • Many recover but postnecrotic cirrhosis, acquired shunting, and chronic hepatitis can develop later.

SURGICAL CONSIDERATIONS

Surgical/laparoscopic liver biopsies—generally not indicated.

MEDICATIONS

DRUG(S) OF CHOICE

• *Discontinue* offending drug, if present.
• See Hepatic Failure, Acute. • Antioxidant therapy—*N*-acetylcysteine (140 mg/kg IV load, followed by 70 mg/kg IV q6–8h, give over 20 min); *S*-adenosylmethionine (20 mg/kg enteric-coated tablet PO q24h, on empty stomach). • Silybin—active component of silymarin/milk thistle extract (2–5 mg/kg q24h PO); may augment liver regeneration; antioxidant, hepatoprotective, antifibrotic effects. • Ursodeoxycholic acid—primarily for chronic hepatopathies (15 mg/kg/day PO with food). • B-complex vitamins—parenteral; cofactors for hepatic metabolism. • Antiemetics—if indicated.
• Antacids—if portal hypertension/gastric ulceration suspected. • Antibiotics—ampicillin/metronidazole, if HE or bacterial translocation suspected. • Lactulose—orally (0.5 mL/kg q8h) or retention enema (diluted 1 : 2 following cleansing enema) if HE suspected.

CONTRAINDICATIONS

Avoid known hepatotoxic drugs.

PRECAUTIONS

Caution when catheterizing large vessels or diagnostic needle aspirates/biopsies if coagulopathic.

POSSIBLE INTERACTIONS

Avoid drugs that require or inhibit hepatic metabolism.

ALTERNATIVE DRUG(S)

Alternative antioxidants—vitamin E (d-α-tocopherol acetate 10 IU/kg q24h PO); vitamin C (ascorbic acid 500–1000 mg/dog q24h PO, 125 mg/cat q12h PO).

FOLLOW-UP

PATIENT MONITORING

• Prevent hypothermia. • Blood glucose, electrolytes, packed cell volume—frequently; fluctuations occur rapidly in critically ill patients.
• CBC, serum biochemical analyses, coagulation tests—monitor q48h or as warranted.

PREVENTION/AVOIDANCE

Close scrutiny of environment and future medications.

POSSIBLE COMPLICATIONS

• DIC, hemorrhage. • HE. • Progressive hepatic failure. • Postnecrotic cirrhosis with acquired shunting/ascites.

EXPECTED COURSE AND PROGNOSIS

• 2–5 days to estimate prognosis. • Negative indicators—intractable emesis, hematemesis, intolerance to supportive treatments, oliguria, DIC, HE, decline of ALT with increasing bilirubin and/or decreasing serum albumin/cholesterol. • Positive indicator—ALT declining by 20–30% or more every 48–72 hours, with other evidence of improvement.
• Postnecrotic cirrhosis—possible in 2–6 months.

MISCELLANEOUS

ASSOCIATED CONDITIONS

• Hepatitis. • Fibrosis. • HE. • Hepatic lipidosis (cats). • Icterus. • Ascites.
• Hypoglycemia. • Sepsis.

AGE-RELATED FACTORS

• Young animals may have greater exposure risk for toxin ingestion; <16 weeks of age: immature hepatic metabolic and excretory pathways. • Older animals may have diseases requiring drug therapies, increasing their risk.

ZOONOTIC POTENTIAL

None

SEE ALSO

• Acetaminophen (APAP) Toxicosis.
• Cirrhosis and Fibrosis of the Liver.
• Hepatic Encephalopathy.
• Hepatic Failure, Acute.
• Poisoning (Intoxication) Therapy.

ABBREVIATIONS

• ALP = alkaline phosphatase.
• ALT = alanine aminotransferase.
• AST = aspartate aminotransferase.
• DIC = disseminated intravascular coagulation.
• HE = hepatic encephalopathy.
• NSAID = nonsteroidal anti-inflammatory drug.
• RER = resting energy requirement.

INTERNET RESOURCES

• https://www.aspca.org/pet-care/animal-poison-control •https://www.petpoisonhelpline.com

Suggested Reading

Peterson ME, Talcott PA. Small Animal Toxicology. St. Louis, MO: Saunders, 2006.

Trepanier LA. Drug-associated liver disease. In: Bonagura JD, Twedt DC, eds., Kirk's Current Veterinary Therapy XV. St. Louis, MO: Saunders, 2014, pp. 575–579.

Author Jennifer M. Reinhart

Consulting Editor Kate Holan

Acknowledgment The author and book editors acknowledge the prior contributions of Michael D. Willard and Sharon A. Center.

Client Education Handout available online

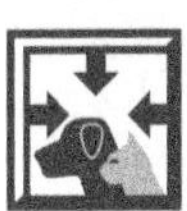

BASICS

OVERVIEW

- Disease caused by infection with the protozoan *Hepatozoon americanum* or *Hepatozoon canis*; here the focus is on systemic infection with *Hepatozoon americanum*—the primary cause of American canine hepatozoonosis.
- *Hepatozoon canis* is less prevalent in the United States than *Hepatozoon americanum*; it is also less virulent and infections are typically subclinical.
- Infection typically involves muscle and bone.
- Dogs—more common in the southern and southeastern United States.
- Cats—uncommon in the United States.

SIGNALMENT

- Dogs and rarely cats.
- No age, breed, or sex predilections.

SIGNS

- Lameness and stiff gait.
- Waxing and waning fever.
- Mucopurulent ocular discharge.
- Hyperesthesia.
- Weight loss and cachexia.
- Polyuria and polydipsia in some cases if glomerulonephritis is present.

CAUSES & RISK FACTORS

- *Amblyomma maculatum*—tick ingestion.
- Ingestion of infected paratenic hosts (predation or scavenging).

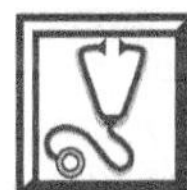

DIAGNOSIS

DIFFERENTIAL DIAGNOSIS

- Neoplasia.
- Endocarditis.
- Immune-mediated polyarthritis or polymyositis.
- Chagas disease.
- Leishmaniasis.
- Meningitis/meningoencephalitis.
- Hypertrophic osteopathy.
- Ehrlichiosis.
- Discospondylitis.
- Hepatic failure.

CBC/BIOCHEMISTRY/URINALYSIS

- Neutrophilic leukocytosis, usually profound (20,000–200,000 white blood cells [WBC]/μL), sometimes with a left shift.
- Anemia—mild to moderate, usually nonregenerative.
- Usually have a normal platelet count unless there is a coinfection.
- High serum alkaline phosphatase (ALP) activity.
- Decreased serum urea nitrogen concentration.
- Despite severe myositis, creatinine kinase concentrations are often within reference range.
- Hyperglobulinemia.
- Hypoalbuminemia.

OTHER LABORATORY TESTS

Blood smear—in rare cases identify organisms in circulating neutrophils and monocytes.

IMAGING

Radiographs—pelvis, lumbar vertebrae, and long bones; periosteal proliferation.

DIAGNOSTIC PROCEDURES

- Muscle biopsy.
- PCR on blood or muscle.

PATHOLOGIC FINDINGS

- Cachexia.
- Muscle atrophy—"onion-skin" meronts and pyogranulomatous myositis.
- Enlarged liver and spleen—may contain meront stages on histopathology.
- Periosteal proliferation of bone.

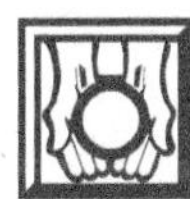

TREATMENT

- Inpatient—for severe pain; provide symptomatic relief.
- Pain management—as for any musculoskeletal disease.
- General activity level and appetite—depend on pain level.
- Most dogs will require lifelong treatment to maintain clinical remission.

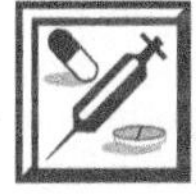

MEDICATIONS

DRUG(S) OF CHOICE

- Mostly palliative, as no treatments have been shown to clear infection.
- Combination therapy (TCP) initially:
  - Trimethoprim/sulfadiazine—15 mg/kg PO q12h for 14 days.
  - Clindamycin—10 mg/kg PO q8h for 14 days.
  - Pyrimethamine—0.25 mg/kg PO q24h for 14 days.
- Followed with long-term therapy—decoquinate 10–20 mg/kg PO q12h for up to 33 months (possibly indefinite).
- Ponazuril 10 mg/mg PO q12h for 28 days has shown promise as an alternative initial treatment; long-term therapy with decoquinate is still necessary.
- Glucocorticoids—may give temporary relief, but are not routinely recommended.
- Nonsteroidal anti-inflammatory drugs (NSAIDs) may provide analgesia.

CONTRAINDICATIONS/POSSIBLE INTERACTIONS

None

FOLLOW-UP

PATIENT MONITORING

- Difficult to monitor organisms in chronically infected dogs.
- Best to monitor for clinical improvement.

PREVENTION/AVOIDANCE

- Control ticks within the household or kennel.
- Avoid predation and scavenging.

POSSIBLE COMPLICATIONS

- Glucocorticoids—may exacerbate clinical disease.
- Radiographic changes may never occur.

EXPECTED COURSE AND PROGNOSIS

- Treatment typically results in improvement of clinical signs and quality of life, but does not cure the infection.
- Treatment is likely to be needed for the remainder of the patient's life.
- If clinical relapse occurs, repeat of both initial and long-term treatments is recommended.

MISCELLANEOUS

ZOONOTIC POTENTIAL

No reported risk to humans.

ABBREVIATIONS

- ALP = alkaline phosphatase.
- NSAID = nonsteroidal anti-inflammatory drug.
- TCP = trimethoprim-sulfa, clindamycin, pyrimethamine.
- WBC = white blood count.

Suggested Reading

Allen KE, Johnson EM, Little SE. Hepatozoon spp infections in the United States. Vet Clin North Am Small Anim Pract 2011, 41(6):1221–1238.

Baneth G. Perspectives on canine and feline hepatozoonosis. Vet Parasitol 2011, 181(1):3–11.

Author Adam J. Birkenheuer

Consulting Editor Amie Koenig

H

HIATAL HERNIA

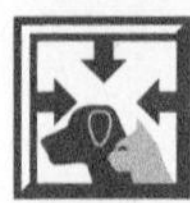

BASICS

OVERVIEW

- Herniation of abdominal contents (most commonly the stomach) cranial to the diaphragm into the thorax through the esophageal hiatus. Four types have been described:
  - Type I (sliding; most common).
  - Type II (paraesophageal).
  - Type III (includes elements of both types I and II).
  - Type IV (herniation of organs other than the stomach).
- May be congenital or acquired—acquired most commonly associated with upper respiratory disease (brachycephalic syndrome, laryngeal paralysis).

SIGNALMENT

- Dogs > cats.
- Congenital reported in English and French bulldogs, shar-peis and chow chows; acquired common in brachycephalic breeds.

SIGNS

- Most signs secondary to gastroesophageal reflux (GER) and esophagitis.
- Regurgitation.
- Dysphagia.
- Hypersalivation.
- Lip smacking.
- Inability to gain weight.
- Vomiting.
- Respiratory distress.
- Anorexia.
- Weight loss.

CAUSES & RISK FACTORS

Congenital. Acquired— traumatic event ± severe upper respiratory disease; brachycephalic airway syndrome.

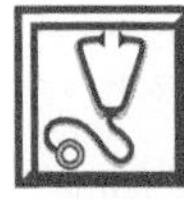

DIAGNOSIS

DIFFERENTIAL DIAGNOSIS

Other causes of weight loss or regurgitation such as megaesophagus, esophagitis, vascular ring anomaly, etc.

CBC/BIOCHEMISTRY/URINALYSIS

No specific abnormalities. May find inflammatory leukogram secondary to associated pneumonia.

OTHER LABORATORY TESTS

N/A

IMAGING

Thoracic Radiography

Cranial displacement of stomach. Soft tissue mass in caudal thorax adjacent to diaphragm. Gas-filled viscera in thorax. Infrequently diagnosed on survey thoracic radiographs alone.

Positive Contrast Esophagram

Preferably performed using videofluoroscopy. Helps to confirm diagnosis and differentiate between types I and II hernias. Can also diagnose associated GER and esophageal dysmotility. False-negative studies common due to highly intermittent and dynamic nature of hiatal herniation.

DIAGNOSTIC PROCEDURES

Upper gastrointestinal endoscopy can occasionally document herniation. However, effects of herniation such as esophagitis or stricture may be detectable if herniation does not occur during study.

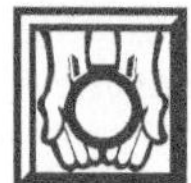

TREATMENT

Not all dogs that have radiographic evidence require treatment. Conservative therapy can be successful in controlling clinical signs in dogs with mild hiatal herniation.

Medical Management

- Can often be managed as outpatient unless animal has severe aspiration pneumonia.
- Reduce gastric acid secretion (proton pump inhibitors are superior to H2 receptor antagonists).
- Increase rate of gastric emptying and increase lower esophageal sphincter (LES) tone (prokinetic agents such as cisapride).
- Provide esophageal mucosal protection (sucralfate).
- Feed a low-fat diet in an elevated position.
- 30-day trial of medical management before surgery often recommended; not all patients require surgery.

Surgical Management

- Patients nonresponsive to medical therapy.
- Treat with antacids and prokinetics prior to surgery.
- Surgical procedures (used alone or in combination)—phrenoplasty; esophagopexy; left-sided gastropexy.

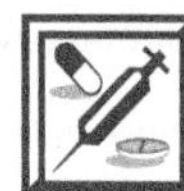

MEDICATIONS

DRUG(S) OF CHOICE

- H2 receptor antagonists—increase gastric pH and reduce esophagitis secondary to GER:
  - Famotidine 0.5–1 mg/kg PO/IV q12h.
  - Ranitidine 1–2 mg/kg PO/IV q8–12h.
- Proton pump inhibitors—more potent than H2 receptor antagonists:
  - Omeprazole 0.7–1.5 mg/kg PO q12h.
  - Pantoprazole 0.7–1.5 mg/kg IV q12h.
- Prokinetics—increase gastric emptying:
  - Metoclopramide 0.2–0.5 mg/kg PO q6–8h or 1–2 mg/kg/24h IV as CRI.
  - Cisapride 0.2–0.5 mg/kg PO q8–12h.

FOLLOW-UP

PATIENT MONITORING

- Long-term medical therapy may be indicated in both surgically and conservatively managed patients.
- Postoperative—monitor for dyspnea, worsening regurgitation (may require second surgery), abdominal distension that could result from overtightening of hiatus resulting in inability to eructate.

POSSIBLE COMPLICATIONS

Continuation of clinical signs, bloat episodes.

EXPECTED COURSE AND PROGNOSIS

- Overall prognosis is good.
- When medical management fails, surgical intervention leads to positive outcome in majority of cases.

MISCELLANEOUS

ASSOCIATED CONDITIONS

Often found in dogs with brachycephalic airway syndrome or other upper airway obstructive diseases. Hypothesized that decreases in intrathoracic pressures generated may pull the stomach into the thorax through the hiatus. Gastroesophageal reflux can worsen clinical signs of upper respiratory disease due to irritation of upper respiratory area or associated bronchospasm of the lower airway.

ABBREVIATIONS

- GER = Gastroesophageal reflux.
- LES = Lower esophageal sphincter.

Suggested Reading

Callan MB, Washabau RJ, Saunders HM, et al. Medical treatment versus surgery for hiatal hernias. J Am Vet Med Assoc 1998, 213:800.

Lorinson D, Bright RM. Long-term outcome of medical and surgical treatment of hiatal hernias in dogs and cats: 27 cases (1978–1996). J Am Vet Med Assoc 1998, 213:381–384.

Sivacolundhu RK, Read RA, Marchevsky AM. Hiatal hernia controversies: a review of pathophysiology and treatment options. Aust Vet J 2002, 80:48–53.

Authors Kathryn A. Pitt and Philipp D. Mayhew

Consulting Editor Mark P. Rondeau

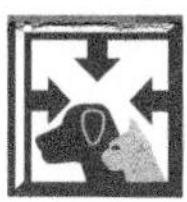

BASICS

DEFINITION

A developmental syndrome characterized in growing animals by excessive laxity of the coxofemoral joint that results in secondary osteoarthritis (OA) of the coxofemoral joints in the adult animal.

PATHOPHYSIOLOGY

- Developmental defect initiated by genetic predisposition to subluxation of immature hip joint.
- Poor congruence between femoral head and acetabulum; creates abnormal forces across joint; interferes with normal development (leading to irregularly shaped acetabula and femoral heads); overloads articular cartilage (causing microfractures and OA).

SYSTEMS AFFECTED

Musculoskeletal

GENETICS

- Complicated, polygenetic transmission. Genetic markers for diagnosis and prevention are under development but are not standardized or routinely used.
- Expression is determined by interaction of genetic and environmental factors, the latter including overall excess caloric consumption and excess calcium during growth.
- Heritability index—depends on breed, but generally estimated at 0.3.

INCIDENCE/PREVALENCE

- One of most common skeletal diseases encountered clinically in dogs.
- Actual incidence unknown; depends on breed.
- Incidence in cats significantly lower than dogs.

SIGNALMENT

Species

Dog, rarely cat.

Breed Predilections

- Large-breed dogs—Saint Bernard, German shepherd, Labrador retriever, golden retriever, Rottweiler.
- Smaller-breed dogs—may be affected; in fact, incidence of disease in pugs is highest of all breeds, approaching 70%; small-breed dogs less likely to exhibit clinical signs.
- Cats—more commonly affects purebred cats; reportedly affects ~18% of Maine coon cats.

Mean Age and Range

- Onset of clinical signs varies with severity of hip laxity in immature dog and with worsening secondary OA in mature dog.
- Clinical signs—may develop after 4 months of age in dogs with severe laxity; may also develop at any age after onset of secondary OA.
- Clinical signs are biphasic in dogs; young dogs often exhibit most severe clinical signs between 6 and 12 months of age; clinical signs often diminish in animals 12–18 months of age, worsening again in older dogs in 4–8-year age period.

Predominant Sex

- Dogs—none.
- Cats—more common in female cats.

SIGNS

General Comments

- Severity of signs depends on degree of joint laxity, degree of OA, and chronicity of disease.
- Early—related to joint laxity.
- Later—related to severity of OA.

Historical Findings

- Decreased activity.
- Difficulty or slow rising.
- Reluctance to run, jump, or climb stairs.
- Intermittent or persistent hind limb lameness—often worse after exercise.
- Pelvic limb lameness may be unilateral or bilateral.
- Bunny-hopping or swaying gait.
- Narrow stance in hind limbs.

Physical Examination Findings

- Pain on palpation or manipulation of hip joint(s); particularly extension.
- Increased joint laxity (positive Ortolani sign)—characteristic of early disease; may not be finding in chronic cases owing to periarticular fibrosis.
- Crepitus during hip motion.
- Decreased range of motion in hip joints.
- Atrophy of thigh muscles.

CAUSES

- Genetic predisposition for hip laxity.
- Rapid weight gain may be associated with onset of clinical signs due to increased demands on joint.
- Nutritional influences, particularly excess caloric intake in young dog and calcium >1.6% in diet on dry-matter basis, increase phenotypic expression, development of hip dysplasia (HD), and progression of disease.
- Decreased gluteal and caudal thigh muscle mass—increase expression and progression.

RISK FACTORS

- Overweight puppies fed in excess of caloric requirements for normal growth at risk for increased incidence of HD.
- Additional calcium supplementation in diet of young large-breed dogs contraindicated and may predispose to development of HD.

DIAGNOSIS

DIFFERENTIAL DIAGNOSIS

- Cranial cruciate ligament rupture—up to ⅓ of dogs referred for treatment of HD actually suffer from concurrent cranial cruciate rupture; cranial cruciate ligament rupture must remain alternative diagnosis for lameness in large-breed dogs until definitively eliminated from consideration.
- Degenerative myelopathy.
- Lumbosacral instability.
- Unilateral or bilateral stifle disease.
- Panosteitis.
- Polyarthropathies.

IMAGING

- Ventrodorsal hip-extended radiographs—commonly used for diagnosis; may need sedation or general anesthesia for accurate positioning.
- Early radiographic signs—subluxation of hip joint with poor congruence between femoral head and acetabulum; initially normally shaped acetabulum and femoral head; with disease progression, shallow acetabulum and flattened femoral head.
- Radiographic evidence of OA—flattening of femoral head; shallow acetabulum; periarticular osteophyte production; thickening of femoral neck; sclerosis of subchondral bone; periarticular soft tissue fibrosis. Remodeling of femoral neck is uncommon in cats.
- Distraction radiographs—quantify joint laxity; may accentuate laxity for more accurate diagnosis. Distraction radiographic procedures such as PennHip® have been standardized and allow better prediction of dogs likely to develop secondary hip OA and better selection of dogs for breeding potential.
- Dorsal acetabular rim view radiographs—evaluate acetabular rim; assess dorsal coverage of femoral head. Clinical efficacy of such views in diagnosis and treatment of HD has not been definitively established.

DIAGNOSTIC PROCEDURES

- Commercial genetic markers are under development but not in widespread use at this time.
- Arthroscopy of hip joint has been described in diagnosis of HD, but does not add useful clinical information regarding treatment.

PATHOLOGIC FINDINGS

- Early—normal conformation of femoral head and acetabulum; may note joint laxity and excess synovial fluid.
- With progression—malformed acetabulum and femoral head; synovitis; articular cartilage degeneration. Formation of periarticular osteophytes leads to radiographic formation of "Morgan's line," linear formation of enthesiophytes at origin of joint capsule on femoral neck.
- Chronic—may note full-thickness cartilage erosion.

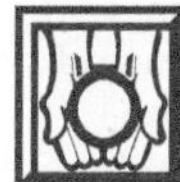

TREATMENT

APPROPRIATE HEALTH CARE

- May treat with conservative medical therapy or surgery.

- Depends on patient's size, age, and intended function; severity of joint laxity; degree of OA; clinician's preference; financial considerations of owner.

NURSING CARE

- Physical therapy (passive joint motion)—decreases joint stiffness; helps maintain muscle integrity.
- Swimming (hydrotherapy)—excellent nonconcussive form of physical therapy; encourages joint and muscle activity without exacerbating joint injury.

ACTIVITY

- As tolerated.
- Swimming—recommended to maintain joint mobility while minimizing weight-bearing activities.

DIET

- Weight control—important and first goal of therapy; decrease load applied to painful joint; minimize weight gain associated with reduced exercise.
- Supplementation with omega-3 fatty acids (in commercial diets or as food additive) beneficial to decrease pain and inflammation and improve function. While optimum dosage/feeding of omega-3 fatty acids yet to be determined, clinical efficacy of commercial diets containing 1.7–3.4% of omega-3 fatty acids and precursors has been established.

CLIENT EDUCATION

- Discuss heritability of the disease, recommend neutering of affected animals and elimination as breeding sources.
- Explain that medical therapy is palliative.
- Warn client that joint degeneration often progresses unless corrective osteotomy procedure is performed early in disease.
- Explain that surgical procedures can salvage joint function once severe joint degeneration occurs.

SURGICAL CONSIDERATIONS

Triple, Double, or 2.5 Pelvic Osteotomy

- Corrective procedure; designed to reestablish congruity between femoral head and acetabulum.
- Immature patient (6–10 months of age) without signs of OA.
- Rotate acetabulum—improve dorsal coverage of femoral head; correct forces acting on joint; minimizes progression of OA, but OA frequently progresses on radiographs even though progression not clinically apparent.
- Surgical procedure necessitates implantation of surgical implants, commonly bone plate and screws specially designed for procedure; large dogs may necessitate use of two bone plates; outcomes improved and complication rates decreased with use of locking implants.

Juvenile Pubic Symphysiodesis

- Pubic symphysis is fused at early age (8–16 weeks) using electrocautery.
- Requires extremely early diagnosis of condition, or use as preventative in nonbreeding animals to decrease need for more aggressive surgical procedure in dogs likely to develop secondary OA or more several clinical signs.
- Causes ventroversion of acetabulum during growth to better cover femoral head.
- Improves joint congruence and stability—similar effects to triple pelvic osteotomy without osteotomy and surgical implants.
- Minimal morbidity; easy to perform—must be performed very early (ideally 3–4 months of age) to achieve effect; minimal effect achieved if performed after 5 months of age.

Total Hip Replacement

- Indicated to salvage function in mature dogs with severe degenerative disease unresponsive to medical therapy.
- Multiple systems exist to replace both acetabular and femoral head surfaces and comprising both cemented and noncemented (ingrowth) implants; noncemented implants have best prognosis for long-term use and implant stability.
- Pain-free joint function—reported in >90% of cases.
- Unilateral joint replacement—provides acceptable function in ~80% of cases.
- Staged bilateral joint replacement now chosen by 50% of owners.
- Complications—luxation; femoral fracture, sciatic neuropraxia; infection; incidence of infection decreased with use of noncemented implant systems compared to cemented systems.

Excision Arthroplasty

- Removal of femoral head and neck to eliminate joint pain.
- Extremely important to achieve smooth osteotomy close to femoral shaft.
- Primarily a salvage procedure—for significant OA; when pain cannot be controlled medically; when total hip replacement is cost-prohibitive.
- Best results—small, light dogs (<20 kg); patients with good hip musculature.
- Can provide good results in larger dogs.
- Slightly abnormal gait often persists and consistently seen on objective gait analysis of patients, despite lack of lameness detection by owners or veterinarians on casual observation.
- Postoperative muscle atrophy—common, particularly in large dogs.

Denervation Procedure

- Surgical procedure described in anecdotal and research literature to reduce pain associated with HD.
- Does not improve joint conformation or OA.
- Little objective scientific evidence exists for this procedure's effectiveness despite numerous clinical reports.
- Recent blinded studies suggest the treatment does not improve the treated hip, but may slow development of further clinical signs.

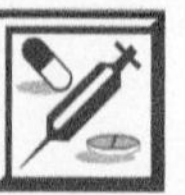

MEDICATIONS

DRUG(S) OF CHOICE

- Analgesics and anti-inflammatory drugs—minimize joint pain (and thus stiffness and muscle atrophy caused by limited usage); decrease synovitis.
- Medical therapy—does not correct biomechanical abnormality; degenerative process likely to progress; often provides only temporary relief of signs.
- Agents—carprofen (2.2 mg/kg POq12h or 4.4 mg/kg PO q24h); etodolac (10–15 mg/kg PO q24h); deracoxib (3–4 mg/kg PO q12h for 1 week, then 2 mg/kg PO q12h); firocoxib (4 mg/kg PO q24h).
- Diet supplementation with omega-3 fatty acids (fish oils) decreases joint inflammation and provides pain relief; commercial diets containing 1.7–3.4% omega-3 fatty acids and precursors are most consistent and easiest method of administration.

CONTRAINDICATIONS

Avoid corticosteroids—potential side effects; articular cartilage damage associated with long-term use.

PRECAUTIONS

- Nonsteroidal anti-inflammatory drugs—gastrointestinal upset may preclude use in some patients.
- Carprofen—reported to cause acute hepatotoxicity in some dogs.

ALTERNATIVE DRUG(S)

- Polysulfated glycosaminoglycan injections, or oral glucosamine, and chondroitin sulfate—may have chondroprotective effect in OA, but recent evidence suggests are not or are only minimally efficacious.
- There are single reports of agents such as elk antler velvet suggesting their efficacy for OA, but no confirmation or widespread acceptance for efficacy.
- Prophylactic laser therapy, extracorporeal pulse therapy, and acupuncture have been suggested for treatment, but no documented evidence demonstrating efficacy of these modalities for OA despite numerous research studies.
- Stem cell therapy, primarily mesenchymal stromal cell extractions, have been investigated in research studies and individual clinical patients, but show no clinical benefit at present.

FOLLOW-UP

PATIENT MONITORING

- Clinical and radiographic monitoring—assess progression.
- Medical treatment—clinical deterioration suggests alternative dosage or medication or

surgical intervention; weight management is important continuing consideration in management of HD.

- Triple pelvic osteotomy—monitored radiographically; assess healing, implant stability, joint congruence, and progression of OA; over 50% of dogs may develop radiographic signs of OA after pelvic osteotomy, but clinical signs or their lack remain stable in spite of OA.
- Hip replacement—monitored radiographically on annual basis; assess implant stability.

PREVENTION/AVOIDANCE

- Best prevented by not breeding affected dogs.
- Pelvic radiographs—may help identify phenotypically abnormal dogs; may not identify all dogs carrying the disease.
- Do not repeat dam–sire breedings that result in affected offspring.
- Special diets designed for rapidly growing large-breed dogs—may decrease severity.

EXPECTED COURSE AND PROGNOSIS

Joint degeneration usually progresses—most patients lead normal lives with proper medical or surgical management.

MISCELLANEOUS

PREGNANCY/FERTILITY/BREEDING

Do not breed affected dogs; added weight owing to pregnancy may exacerbate clinical signs.

ABBREVIATIONS

- HD = hip dysplasia.
- OA = osteoarthritis.

Suggested Reading

Lister SA, Roush JK, Renberg WC, Stephens CL. Ground reaction force analysis of unilateral coxofemoral denervation for the treatment of canine hip dysplasia. Vet Comp Orthop Traumatol 2009, 22(2):137–141.

Smith GK, Leighton EA, Karbe GT, McDonald-Lynch MB. Pathogenesis, diagnosis, and control of canine hip dysplasia. In: Johnston SA, Tobias KM, eds. Veterinary Surgery: Small Animal, 2nd ed. St. Louis, MO: Elsevier, 2018, pp. 964–992.

Upchurch DA, Renberg WC, Roush JK, et al. Administration of adipose-derived stromal vascular fraction and platelet rich plasma in dogs with coxofemoral osteoarthritis. Am J Vet Res 2016, 77:940–951.

Vezzoni A, Peck JN. Surgical management of hip dysplasia. In: Johnston SA, Tobias KM, eds. Veterinary Surgery: Small Animal, 2nd ed. St. Louis, MO: Elsevier, 2018, pp. 992–1018.

Author James K. Roush
Consulting Editor Mathieu M. Glassman

Client Education Handout available online

HISTIOCYTIC DISEASES—DOGS AND CATS

BASICS

DEFINITION

Histiocytic diseases encompass a wide spectrum of heterogenous dendritic or macrophage-derived proliferative disorders. Most of these histiocytic diseases are of dendritic cell lineage and in dogs include cutaneous histiocytoma, Langerhans cell histiocytosis (LCH), reactive histiocytoses (cutaneous histiocytosis [CH] and systemic histiocytosis [SH]), and histiocytic sarcoma (HS) complex, with hemophagocytic HS representing the only macrophage-derived disease entity. In cats, histiocytic diseases are limited to feline progressive histiocytosis (FPH), HS, and feline pulmonary Langerhans cell histiocytosis (FPLCH). All of these disorders represent neoplastic processes, except for the canine reactive histiocytoses, which are inflammatory diseases associated with underlying immune dysregulation.

SIGNALMENT

Canine

Cutaneous Histiocytoma

- Most common in young dogs; 50% of affected patients <2–3 years of age.
- Occurs in all breeds; predisposition in purebred dogs, particularly boxers and dachshunds, cocker spaniels, Great Danes, and bobtails.

Cutaneous LCH

- Rare entity in dogs, with similar signalment as for cutaneous histiocytoma.
- Occurs in many breeds.

CH

- Only described in the dog; age range: 2–13 years.
- Most common in collies, border collies, Shetland sheepdogs, briards, Bernese mountain dogs (BMDs), and golden retrievers, with no clear age or sex predilection.

SH

- Disease predominantly affecting young to middle-aged dogs (2–8 years).
- Familial association in BMDs (male predilection), but other large-breed dogs are affected (e.g., Rottweiler, Labrador retriever, basset hound, Irish wolfhound).

HS

- Middle-aged or older dogs, uncommon in cats.
- Strong breed predilections in BMD and flat-coated retrievers (FCRs), with other predisposed breeds including Rottweiler, golden retriever, Labrador retriever, and miniature schnauzer.

Hemophagocytic Histiocytic Sarcoma (HHS)

- Dogs, very rarely cats.
- Similar signalment to HS.

Feline

FPH

- Most common histiocytic disease in middle-aged to older cats (7–17 years).
- No sex or breed predilection.

FPLCH

Aged cats (10–15 years).

SIGNS

Canine

Cutaneous Histiocytoma

- Benign, solitary "button-like," raised, well-circumscribed, hairless dermal neoplasm that typically spontaneously regresses within 2–3 months.
- Common sites—head and limbs.
- Extremely low recurrence rates; de novo development or local metastasis rare.

Cutaneous LCH

- Multiple cutaneous histiocytomas with possible metastasis to lymph nodes and internal organs is a distinguishing feature from cutaneous histiocytoma.
- Delayed lesion regression common.

CH

- Multiple cutaneous/subcutaneous nodules that may wax and wane and spontaneously disappear, with new lesions appearing at different sites.
- Limited to the skin, subcutis, and local draining lymph node(s); lack of systemic extension beyond peripheral lymph nodes is a distinguishing factor from SH.

SH

- Cutaneous/subcutaneous lesions are similar to CH, with spontaneous remissions and relapses.
- Involvement of lymph nodes, bone marrow, spleen, liver, lung, kidneys, testes, and mucous membranes.
- Clinical signs include depression, anorexia, weight loss, conjunctivitis and respiratory difficulty.

HS

- Primary tumor sites include skin and subcutis, lung, lymph node, liver, spleen, and other sites; secondary sites of involvement commonly include liver, lung, and lymph node.
- Periarticular mass with synovial tissue involvement also reported.
- Clinical signs vary depending on organ involvement.

HHS

- Similar but more severe clinical signs to HS (e.g., marked anemia and thrombocytopenia).
- Subtype tends to present in a more infiltrative manner, causing hepatosplenomegaly and myelophthisis.

Feline

FPH

- Begins as nonpainful, nonpruritic, low-grade HS with indolent behavior initially.
- Some cats develop invasive masses in lymph nodes and internal organs in the terminal stage.

FPLCH

Acute or chronic presentation of respiratory failure due to extensive obliteration of all lung lobes by ill-defined coalescing nodular masses extending from peribronchiolar locations with enlargement of tracheobronchial lymph nodes and other draining lymph nodes.

CAUSES & RISK FACTORS

- Cutaneous histiocytoma is believed to represent a benign neoplasm with unique biologic behavior.
- SH/CH are believed to have an element of immune dysregulation.
- SH has probable familial causation in BMD.
- HS and HHS likely have a genetic origin due to breed predilections (specifically in BMD); abnormalities in tumor suppressor gene loci are potentially correlated to the development of HS in BMD and FCR.
- FPH—chronic antigenic stimulation is a possible triggering factor.

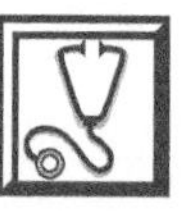

DIAGNOSIS

DIFFERENTIAL DIAGNOSIS

- Differentiate from focal granulomatous diseases, other sarcomas, other round cell tumors, and each distinctive subtype of the histiocytic disease.
- Differentiate HHS from immune-mediated anemia/thrombocytopenia, myelodysplastic syndromes, leukemias, and tick-borne diseases.

CBC/BIOCHEMISTRY/URINALYSIS

HHS—moderate to severe anemia (often regenerative), thrombocytopenia, neutrophilic/monocytic leukocytosis, increased liver enzymes, hypoalbuminemia, hypocholesterolemia.

OTHER LABORATORY TESTS

- Immunohistochemistry—used to differentiate cutaneous reactive histiocytosis from inflamed nonepitheliotropic T-cell lymphoma and HS from other sarcomas and round cell tumors.
- Serum ferritin—hyperferritinemia has been documented in dogs with HS and has potential as a biomarker for early screening.

IMAGING

- Thoracic radiography—pulmonary parenchymal involvement commonly observed:
  - LCH—peribronchial.
  - SH—perihilar/sternal lymphadenopathy, pulmonary infiltrates.
  - HS/HHS—diffuse interstitial infiltrate, patchy consolidated areas, focal or multifocal nodules or mass lesions.
  - Feline LCH—diffuse bronchointerstitial pattern of miliary to nodular opacities throughout all lung lobes.

- Extremity radiography—soft tissue mass ± lytic lesions may be noted for periarticular HS.
- Abdominal ultrasonography—hepatosplenic masses and lymphadenopathy characteristic of HS; diffuse hepatosplenomegaly with mottling and mild lymphadenopathy more common with HHS.

DIAGNOSTIC PROCEDURES

Cytology and histopathology of lesions—provides definitive diagnosis based upon specific cellular morphologic criteria.

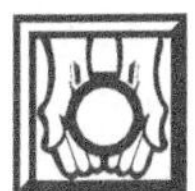

TREATMENT

Canine

Cutaneous Histiocytoma

- Surgical excision or cryosurgery is generally curative.
- Cutaneous histiocytomas usually spontaneously regress within 2–3 months.

Cutaneous LCH

- If localized, surgical removal may be curative.
- If multifocal or lymph node involvement, consider treatment with immunosuppressive drugs.

CH/SH

Cutaneous lesions may wax and wane or spontaneously regress, but both diseases are usually progressive and require treatment with immunosuppressive drugs.

HS/HHS

- Localized HS can be treated with wide-margin surgical excision or palliative radiation therapy.
- Due to high metastatic risk, adjuvant chemotherapy (CCNU) is indicated following surgery or radiation for localized HS.
- Disseminated HS and HHS treated with chemotherapy (CCNU), corticosteroids, and other immunosuppressive drugs.

FPH/Feline HS

- If localized, surgical removal or radiation therapy can provide long-term control.
- Due to high metastatic risk, adjuvant chemotherapy is indicated following surgery or radiation for localized feline HS.
- Disseminated FPH/HS typically treated with chemotherapy and corticosteroids.

FPLCH

Treated with corticosteroids and other immunosuppressive drugs.

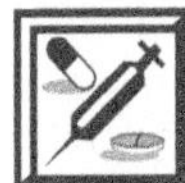

MEDICATIONS

DRUG(S) OF CHOICE

HS/HHS

Lomustine (CCNU)—dogs: 60–90 mg/m^2 q3 weeks; cats: 40–60 mg/ m^2 q3–4 weeks.

CH/SH

- Prednisone/prednisolone—1–2 mg/kg/day continuously.
- Leflunomide—dogs: 3–4 mg/kg/day.
- Cyclosporine—dogs: 5 mg/kg q12–24h.

CONTRAINDICATIONS

N/A

PRECAUTIONS

Lomustine can lead to severe myelosuppression and hepatotoxicity.

ALTERNATIVE DRUG(S)

Doxorubicin, vincristine, Doxil®, paclitaxel, cyclophosphamide, mitoxantrone, dacarbazine, epirubicin, vinorelbine, and vinblastine have all been used for HS/HHS with marginal success.

FOLLOW-UP

POSSIBLE COMPLICATIONS

Bleeding due to thrombocytopenia.

EXPECTED COURSE AND PROGNOSIS

Canine Cutaneous Histiocytoma

- Spontaneous regression is likely within 2–3 months.
- If required, surgical removal is typically curative.

LCH/CH/SH

- Rarely imminently fatal.
- Cutaneous lesions may wax and wane or spontaneously regress, but are usually progressive and require treatment with immunomodulatory drugs or surgical excision (if localized).
- SH is associated with a poorer prognosis; dogs are often ill from the disease and relapses are common.

HS/HHS

- Localized HS—long-term (>12 months) survival has been documented for dogs that undergo surgery/radiation therapy and chemotherapy.
- Disseminated HS—reported response rates to CCNU are 40–50% for median remission duration of 3–6 months.
- HHS is associated with rapid progression and a grave prognosis (median 7 weeks) even with treatment.

FPH

An indolent cutaneous disease initially, but may spread internally and become life-threatening.

FPLCH

Aggressive disease course; most cats succumb to respiratory failure and illness due to other organ involvement.

MISCELLANEOUS

PREGNANCY/FERTILITY/BREEDING

Chemotherapy drugs may be carcinogenic and mutagenic.

SYNONYMS

N/A

ABBREVIATIONS

- BMD = Bernese mountain dog.
- CH = cutaneous histiocytosis.
- FCR = flat-coated retriever.
- FPH = feline progressive histiocytosis.
- FPLCH = feline pulmonary Langerhans cell histiocytosis.
- HHS = hemophagocytic histiocytic sarcoma.
- HS = histiocytic sarcoma.
- LCH= Langerhans cell histiocytosis.
- SH = systemic histiocytosis.

Suggested Reading

Clifford CA, Skorupski KS. Tumors of the skin, subcutis and soft tissue; histiocytic diseases. In: Henry CJ, Higginbotham ML, eds., Cancer Management in Small Animal Practice. St. Louis, MO: Saunders Elsevier, 2010, pp. 326–330.

Moore, PF. A review of histiocytic diseases of dogs and cats. Vet Pathol 2014, 51:167–184.

Moore PF, Affolter VK. Feline progressive histiocytosis. Vet Pathol 2006, 43:646–655.

Skorupski KA, Clifford CA, Paoloni MC, et al. CCNU for the treatment of dogs with histiocytic sarcoma. J Vet Intern Med 2007, 21:121–126.

Authors Sophie Aschenbroich, Christine Mullin, and Craig A. Clifford

Consulting Editor Timothy M. Fan

HISTIOCYTOSIS, CUTANEOUS

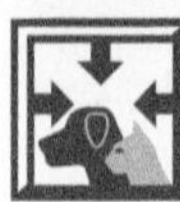

BASICS

OVERVIEW

Skin diseases characterized by infiltration of histiocytic cells.

SIGNALMENT

Histiocytoma

- Most common in dogs <3 years of age.
- Boxers, dachshunds, cocker spaniels, Great Danes, Shetland sheepdogs, bull terriers.
- Shar peis—Langerhans cell histiocytosis (LCH): multiple cutaneous histiocytoma syndrome.

Reactive Histiocytosis (RH)

- Cutaneous (cRH)—middle-aged to older dogs. • Systemic (sRH)—middle-aged dogs; male Bernese mountain dogs, Rottweilers, golden retrievers, Labrador retrievers.

Histiocytic Sarcoma (HS)

Middle-aged to older dogs—Bernese mountain dogs, flat-coated retrievers, Rottweilers, golden retrievers.

Feline Progressive Histiocytosis (fPH)

Middle-aged to older cats; female predisposition.

SIGNS

Histiocytoma

Solitary erythematous and/or ulcerated cutaneous nodule usually on head, extremities, and ears.

Cutaneous LCH

- Multiple histiocytomas; may persist for prolonged period or may never regress.
- Lymphadenopathy with metastasis—affects lungs and other organs.

cRH

- Erythematous or ulcerated nodules or plaques affecting the face, nose, neck, trunk, extremities, footpads, perineum; no systemic involvement. • Depigmentation of mucous membranes and nasal planum (with ulceration).

sRH

- Similar to cRH but with systemic organ involvement. • Peripheral lymphadenopathy.
- Stertor due to nasal mucosal infiltration.
- Ocular manifestations.

HS

- Cutaneous lesions uncommon; subcutaneous nodules develop. • Systemic signs depend on organ system involved.

fPH

- Initial solitary skin nodule with slow progression to multifocal alopecic or ulcerated nodules and plaques; nonpruritic and nonpainful. • Lesions wax and wane, do not regress on their own.

DIAGNOSIS

DIFFERENTIAL DIAGNOSIS

- Histiocytoma and RH—other causes of nodular lesions; solitary round cell tumors: plasmacytoma, mast cell tumor, epitheliotropic cutaneous T-cell lymphoma (CTCL)
- With depigmentation or ulceration—immune-mediated or neoplastic diseases.

CBC/BIOCHEMISTRY/URINALYSIS

Normal with cutaneous histiocytic diseases.

IMAGING

Chest radiographs/abdominal ultrasound—differentiate cRH from sRH; may provide evidence of metastasis: HS, disseminated HS, or fPH.

DIAGNOSTIC PROCEDURES

- Histopathology required for diagnosis of LCH, RH, HS, fPH, and nonregressing histiocytoma. • Fine-needle aspirates may be diagnostic for histiocytoma—cytology from lymph nodes or internal organs may provide evidence of sRH or HS.

PATHOLOGIC FINDINGS

Histiocytoma

- Top-heavy appearance; histiocytic cells invade dermis with occasional nests of cells in epidermis.
- Cellular atypia uncommon; mitotic index often high. • Lymphocytic infiltrate associated with tumor regression. • Immunophenotype—CD1a, CD11c/CD18, E-cadherin positive.

Cutaneous LCH

- Similar to histiocytomas, with more anisokaryosis and multinucleated giant cells.
- Immunophenotype same as histiocytoma.

RH

- Bottom-heavy appearance; cells invade mid to deep dermis, or extend into subcutis; composed primarily of lymphocytes and histiocytes; frequent vessel wall invasion. • Similar to inflamed nonepitheliotropic CTCL; definitive diagnosis requires T-cell receptor γ gene rearrangement analysis to detect clonal T-cell population. • Immunophenotype—CD1a, CD4, CD11c/CD18, CD90 positive.
- Histopathology identical for cRH and sRH.

HS

- Sheets of large, pleomorphic, mononuclear cells; cellular and nuclear atypia with mitotic figures and giant cells.
- Immunophenotype—CD1a, CD11c/CD18 positive.

fPH

- Infiltration of dermis with well-differentiated histiocytic cells; occasionally extends to subcutis. • Epitheliotropism common; single cells or aggregates of histiocytic cells within epidermis. • Cellular and nuclear atypia increase with progression.
- Immunophenotype—CD1a, CD11b/CD18 positive, CD5 positive in 50% of cases.

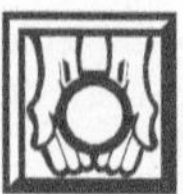

TREATMENT

Histiocytoma

- No treatment necessary; lesions usually regress within 3 months. • Surgical excision curative for persistent lesions.

HS

- Surgical excision of localized lesions recommended. • Variable response to medical therapy. • Poor prognosis—majority of patients survive a few months after diagnosis.

fPH

- Poor response to medical therapy. • Guarded prognosis—cats usually succumb to metastasis beyond the skin.

Cutaneous LCH

- Poor response to medical therapy; short-term improvement reported with lomustine.
- Guarded prognosis—cutaneous lesions as well as metastatic lesions progress, with 50% of patients euthanized.

RH

- Clinical signs wax and wane and may not necessitate therapy. • cRH or sRH—variable prognosis: some dogs respond to long-term therapy. • 50–100% response rate to steroids.
- Other drugs—azathioprine, modified cyclosporine, mycophenolate, leflunomide, and doxycycline/niacinamide. • Localized cutaneous lesions—topical tacrolimus or steroids.

MEDICATIONS

See Treatment.

FOLLOW-UP

Depends on disease.

MISCELLANEOUS

ABBREVIATIONS

- cRH = cutaneous RH. • CTCL = cutaneous T-cell lymphoma. • fPH = feline progressive histiocytosis. • HS = histiocytic sarcoma.
- LCH = Langerhans cell histiocytosis. • RH = reactive histiocytosis. • sRH = systemic RH.

Suggested Reading

Moore PF. A review of histiocytic diseases of dogs and cats. Vet Pathol 2014, 51:167–184.

Author Kathryn A. Rook
Contributing Editor Alexander H. Werner Resnick

BASICS

DEFINITION

Systemic fungal infection caused by *Histoplasma capsulatum.*

PATHOPHYSIOLOGY

• Soil-borne dimorphic fungus; mycelial form grows best in bird manure or organically enriched soil. • Mycelium in the soil—produces infectious spores (microconidia); inhaled into terminal airways. • Spores—germinate in the lungs, develop into yeast form at mammalian body temperature, reproduce by budding. • Yeast are phagocytized by mononuclear phagocytes that distribute the organisms throughout the body. • Ingested organisms may directly infect intestinal tract. • Immune response—determines whether disease develops; affected animals often develop transient, asymptomatic infection.

SYSTEMS AFFECTED

• Cats—respiratory tract, musculoskeletal, hepatobiliary, spleen, skin, and lymphatics; gastrointestinal, ophthalmic, renal, and nervous systems less frequent. • Dogs—gastrointestinal system, hepatobiliary, respiratory, spleen, and lymphatics; musculoskeletal, renal, ophthalmic, and reproductive systems less frequent.

GENETICS

N/A

INCIDENCE/PREVALENCE

Prevalence of clinically relevant histoplasmosis low in cats and dogs.

GEOGRAPHIC DISTRIBUTION

• Endemic areas—Ohio, Missouri, Mississippi, Tennessee, and St. Lawrence river basins. • Also Texas, southeastern United States, Great Lakes region, and California. • Has been isolated from the soil of 31 US states.

SIGNALMENT

Species

Dog and cat.

Breed Predilections

N/A

Mean Age and Range

• Cats—young (many <1 year of age); all ages can be infected. • Dogs—young to middle-aged; all ages can be infected.

Predominant Sex

• Cats—females may be overrepresented.
• Dogs—N/A.

SIGNS

Historical Findings

Cat

• Insidious onset (days–weeks). • Anorexia, weight loss, and dyspnea. • Occasional cough. • Lameness. • Ocular discharge. • Diarrhea.

Dogs

• Weight loss, depression, diarrhea with straining. • Coughing. • Dyspnea. • Exercise intolerance. • Lymphadenopathy. • Lameness and eye and skin changes less common.

Physical Examination Findings

Cats

• Fever to 104 °F (40 °C). • Increased respiratory effort, harsh lung sounds.
• Mucous membranes pale. • Enlarged lymph nodes. • Lameness, ocular changes, and skin lesions possible.

Dogs

• Thin to emaciated. • Fever to 104 °F (40 °C). • Hepatosplenomegaly. • Mucous membranes pale. • Icterus and ascites possible. • Coughing and dyspnea, harsh lung sounds. • Ocular and skin lesions less common.

CAUSES

Histoplasma capsulatum.

RISK FACTORS

• Bird roosts where the soil is enriched with bird or bat droppings are high-risk environments; old chicken coops and caves have been implicated. • Exposure to airborne dust contaminated with fungal spores (especially indoor cats). • Tissue samples from nearly half of stray dogs and cats from an endemic area were positive for *Histoplasma*; many animals are infected but few develop clinical disease.

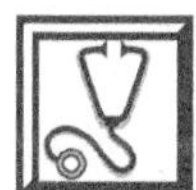

DIAGNOSIS

DIFFERENTIAL DIAGNOSIS

Cats

• Dyspnea—differentiate from heart failure, feline asthma, lymphoma, other infectious pneumonia, pleural effusion. • Lameness—trauma, neoplasia. • Ocular changes—differentiate from lymphoma, toxoplasmosis, and feline infectious peritonitis.

Dogs

• Severe chronic diarrhea, weight loss, and anemia—consider lymphocytic plasmacytic or eosinophilic enteritis, protein intolerance, lymphoma or other intestinal neoplasia, chronic parasitism, and hypoadrenocorticism.
• Hepatosplenomegaly and peripheral lymphadenopathy—consider lymphoma or other neoplasia. • Respiratory signs—differentiate from infectious causes (distemper, bacterial, or other fungal pneumonia), chronic bronchitis, pleural effusion, heart failure, and pulmonary hypertension.

CBC/BIOCHEMISTRY/URINALYSIS

• Moderate to severe nonregenerative anemia.
• Leukogram—usually normal; some have leukocytosis; leukopenia with bone marrow involvement. • *Histoplasma* organisms—may be found in circulating neutrophils and monocytes; 2–4 µm round body with basophilic center and lighter halo. • Liver involvement—may see hyperbilirubinemia and high alanine aminotransferase (ALT) enzyme activity. • Panhypoproteinemia in dogs with severe intestinal histoplasmosis.

OTHER LABORATORY TESTS

• Agar gel immunodiffusion (AGID) test—for antibodies; supports diagnosis; positive results indicate active disease; previous infections may produce false-positive results; many animals with active disease are negative on serology. • Urine antigen test—highly sensitive and specific test for diagnosis in dogs and cats. • Coombs' test—may be positive because antibodies to *Histoplasma* can cross-react with red blood cells; caution before diagnosing immune-mediated disease.

IMAGING

Thoracic Radiography

• Dogs—diffuse interstitial to nodular pneumonia, enlarged tracheobronchial lymph nodes; chronic lesions may be calcified, coin-like opacities that appear like metastatic tumors. • Cats—diffuse interstitial pulmonary pattern; calcification and tracheobronchial lymphadenopathy uncommon.

Abdominal Radiography and Ultrasonography

Dogs—hepatosplenomegaly, mesenteric lymphadenopathy, potentially ascites.

Bone Radiography

Cats and less often dogs—bone lesions predominantly osteolytic and usually distal to elbows and stifles.

DIAGNOSTIC PROCEDURES

• Identification of organisms on cytology, histopathology, or culture—definitive. • Tissue samples: ○ Needle aspiration of enlarged lymph nodes, liver, and spleen. ○ Rectal scrapings may be rich in organisms (yeast form packed in macrophages). ○ Bone marrow or lung aspirates (when less invasive procedures are not diagnostic); tracheal washes inconsistent.

PATHOLOGIC FINDINGS

• Multifocal, granulomatous lesions in reticuloendothelial organs (e.g., spleen, liver, lymph nodes, lungs, and bone marrow).
• Dogs—gastrointestinal tract is primary site; enlarged tracheobronchial lymph nodes.
• Cats—predominantly respiratory lesions.

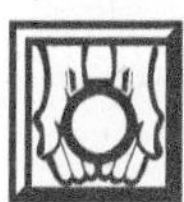

TREATMENT

APPROPRIATE HEALTH CARE

• Usually outpatient with oral itraconazole.
• Inpatient with IV amphotericin B—dogs with severe intestinal disease and

malabsorption, dogs or cats with severe respiratory disease.

NURSING CARE

• Amphotericin B therapy—keep well hydrated to decrease potential for nephrotoxicity. • Emaciated animals with malabsorption—consider parenteral nutrition until intestinal disease sufficiently resolves.
• Animals with severe dyspnea—oxygen supplementation.

ACTIVITY

Animals with dyspnea—reduce.

DIET

N/A

CLIENT EDUCATION

• Discuss possible areas of exposure in the home environment.
• Both pets and family members may have been exposed to the same source, but pet is not a hazard to the family.

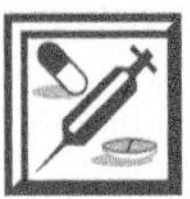

MEDICATIONS

DRUG(S) OF CHOICE

Azole Antifungal Drugs

• No differences reported between itraconazole and fluconazole in survival, clinical remission, or disease relapse rates.
• Duration of therapy depends on clinical response; minimum treatment 90 days.

Itraconazole

• Dogs and cats—5 mg/kg PO q12h; with high-fat meal. • Absorption of compounded itraconazole is inconsistent and these formulations are not recommended.

Fluconazole

• May be preferred for animals with eye or nervous system involvement (penetrates the blood–brain barrier). • Injectable (5 mg/kg IV q12h) for animals unable to take oral form and high risk for amphotericin B.

Intravenous Amphotericin B

Dogs

• With severe intestinal disease and malabsorption—use until intestinal absorption improves, then start on itraconazole. • Patient must be well hydrated before starting treatment. • Usual dose—0.5–1.0 mg/kg IV q48h. ○ Reconstitute in 5% dextrose and dilute for administration. ○ Dilution in electrolyte solution may precipitate drug.
○ Patients with normal renal function—dilute in 60–120 mL 5% dextrose and give over 2 hours. ○ Patients with renal compromise—dilute in 0.5–1 L 5% dextrose and give over 3–4 hours. • Liposomal amphotericin (Abelcet®) can reduce risk of renal toxicity.

Cats

• Use cautiously. • Usual dose—0.25 mg/kg IV in 5% dextrose over 3–4 hours q48h.
• More sensitive to drug than dogs.

CONTRAINDICATIONS

Amphotericin B—caution with azotemic patients (in life-threatening situation, may still consider); monitor creatinine: elevation above normal or 20% greater than baseline considered significant.

PRECAUTIONS

• Corticosteroids—use with caution; may be useful in patients with severe pulmonary disease; dexamethasone 0.1 mg/kg IV q24h for 2–3 days. • Itraconazole and fluconazole—hepatic toxicity; temporarily discontinue if patient becomes anorexic or if serum ALT activity >300 U/L; restart at half dose after appetite improves.

POSSIBLE INTERACTIONS

Itraconazole—can increase concentrations of cyclosporine, digoxin, and midazolam (P450 inhibition).

ALTERNATIVE DRUG(S)

N/A

FOLLOW-UP

PATIENT MONITORING

• Serum ALT—with itraconazole treatment; check monthly or as needed. • Thoracic radiographs—with pulmonary involvement; check after 60 days of treatment and repeat monthly until infiltrates are clear or remaining lesions are static (likely scarring); continue treatment for 1 month after all signs of active disease resolved. • Urinary antigen levels sensitive for monitoring remission in cats.

PREVENTION/AVOIDANCE

• Avoid suspected areas of exposure (e.g., bird roosts). • Recovered dogs may be immune.

POSSIBLE COMPLICATIONS

Recurrence possible.

EXPECTED COURSE AND PROGNOSIS

• Treatment—duration usually 4–6 months; drugs are expensive; some dogs require longer therapy. • Prognosis—good for stable patients without severe dyspnea; influenced by severity of lung involvement and debility of patient.
• Negative prognostic factors include Great Pyrenees breed, dyspnea, oxygen dependency, icterus/hyperbilirubinemia, palpable abdominal organomegaly, anemia, thrombocytopenia, hypercalcemia, high serum alkaline phosphatase activity.

MISCELLANEOUS

ASSOCIATED CONDITIONS

N/A

AGE-RELATED FACTORS

N/A

ZOONOTIC POTENTIAL

• Yeast form is not spread from animals to humans. • Avoid needlestick injury when collecting aspirates. • Infection can occur from cuts during necropsies on infected animals.

PREGNANCY/FERTILITY/BREEDING

Azole drugs can be teratogenic, use with caution in pregnant animals.

ABBREVIATIONS

• AGID = agar gel immunodiffusion.
• ALT = alanine aminotransferase.

Suggested Reading

Cunningham L, Cook A, Hanzlicek A, et al. Sensitivity and specificity of Histoplasma antigen detection by enzyme immunoassay. J Am Anim Hosp Assoc 2015, 51:306–310.

Hanzlicek AS, Meinkoth JH, Renschler JS, et al. Antigen concentrations as an indicator of clinical remission and disease relapse in cats with histoplasmosis. J Vet Intern Med 2016, 30:1065–1073.

Lin Blache J, Ryan K, Arceneaux K. Histoplasmosis. Compend Contin Educ Vet 2011, 33:E1–E10.

Schulman RL, McKiernan BC, Schaeffer DJ. Use of corticosteroids for treating dogs with airway obstruction secondary to hilar lymphadenopathy caused by chronic histoplasmosis: 16 cases (1979–1997). J Am Vet Med Assoc 1999, 214:1345–1448.

Wilson AG, KuKanich KS, Hanzlicek AS, et al. Clinical signs, treatment, and prognostic factors for dogs with histoplasmosis. J Am Vet Med Assoc 2018, 252:201–209.

Author Daniel S. Foy
Consulting Editor Amie Koenig

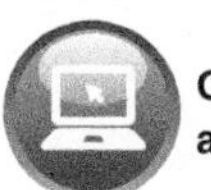

Client Education Handout available online

HOOKWORMS (ANCYLOSTOMIASIS)

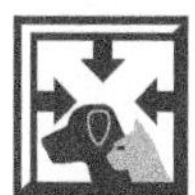

BASICS

OVERVIEW

• Nematode parasites of small intestine—dogs: *Ancylostoma caninum, A. braziliense, Uncinaria stenocephala*; cats: *A. tubaeforme, A. braziliense, U. stenocephala*. • Eggs larvate, hatch, develop into third-stage larvae (L3) in environment; transmitted by ingestion of infective larvae in food, water, or transport hosts and by larval skin penetration; *A. caninum* is transmitted via colostrum/milk to pups. • Some L3 migrate through lungs, enter somatic tissue, and become dormant; pregnancy and removal of adults from intestine can reactivate these larvae; many ingested larvae remain in gastrointestinal (GI) tract and mature. • Blood-sucking adults and fourth-stage larvae of *A. caninum* and *A. tubaeforme* cause blood-loss anemia and enteritis; leave bite sites with ongoing hemorrhage.
• Disease severity: ∘ Peracute—neonates; results from transmammary infection. ∘ Acute disease—older pups. ∘ Acute, chronic compensatory—adults. ∘ Chronic noncompensatory—immunosuppressed or debilitated dog. • *Uncinaria*—of little clinical concern.
• *A. braziliense*—major cause of cutaneous larval migrans (CLM) in humans.
• Respiratory disease may result from larval migration in lungs.

SIGNALMENT

• Peracute to acute disease (young animals); asymptomatic or chronic (mature animals). • More severe clinical disease in dogs than cats.

SIGNS

Historical Findings

• Pallor, melena, diarrhea, constipation, loss of condition, poor appetite, and/or dry cough. • Sudden death.

Physical Examination Findings

• Poor body condition, ill-thrift, poor hair coat. • Pallor. • Erythematous, pruritic lesions, papules on feet (especially between toes). • Shock—tachycardia, weak pulse, prolonged/absent capillary refill time.

CAUSES & RISK FACTORS

• Neonatal animals at highest risk. • Infected bitch or queen. • Environmental contamination.
• Concurrent enteric infections.
• Immunocompromise.

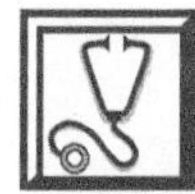

DIAGNOSIS

DIFFERENTIAL DIAGNOSIS

• Causes of anemia and hypovolemic/hemorrhagic shock; trichuriasis. • Ascariasis, coccidiosis, strongyloidosis—similar signs *without* significant anemia. • Physalopterosis—melena, mild anemia.

CBC/BIOCHEMISTRY/URINALYSIS

• Eosinophilia. • Anemia—normochromic, normocytic, regenerative; chronically microcytic, hypochromic (iron deficiency).

DIAGNOSTIC PROCEDURES

• Disease/death may occur prior to egg shedding. • Fecal flotation with centrifugation—morulated strongylid eggs; minor size differences among species. • Fecal ELISA—detects antigen from adult and immature worms, can detect prepatent infection. • Necropsy of littermates with similar clinical signs.

PATHOLOGIC FINDINGS

• Gross—hookworms attached to small intestinal mucosa, multifocal hemorrhagic ulcerations (bite sites) on mucosa, blood in intestinal lumen. • Microscopic—eosinophilic enteritis.

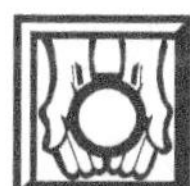

TREATMENT

• Peracute and severe acute cases treated as inpatients—anthelmintic, fluid therapy, blood transfusion, supplemental oxygen, symptomatic/supportive care as indicated.
• Chronic compensatory cases—anthelmintic, iron supplement.

MEDICATIONS

DRUG(S) OF CHOICE

Adulticide/Larvicide Anthelmintics

• Fenbendazole 50 mg/kg PO q24h for 3 consecutive days (dogs). • Milbemycin oxime 0.5 mg/kg (dogs) or 2 mg/kg (cats) PO q30 days. • Emodepside 3 mg/kg/praziquantel 12 mg/kg topically once (cats). • Moxidectin 0.17 mg/kg SC q6 months (dogs). • Moxidectin 2.5 mg/kg (dogs) or 1.0 mg/kg (cats)/imidocloprimide 10 mg/kg, topically q30 days. • Ivermectin 24 µg/kg PO q30 days (cats).

Adulticide Activity (Label Dose unless Stated)

• Pyrantel pamoate (dogs) 10–20 mg/kg PO (cats: extra-label). • Praziquantel/pyrantel pamoate/febantel (dogs).
• Praziquantel/pyrantel pamoate (cats).
• Ivermectin/pyrantel pamoate or ivermectin/pyrantel pamoate/praziquantel (dogs). • Selamectin 6 mg/kg topically q30 days (cats).

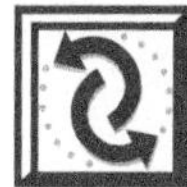

FOLLOW-UP

Monitor fecal egg counts and hematocrit after treatment.

PREVENTION/AVOIDANCE

• Routine deworming does not eliminate dormant L3; eliminate intestinal stages and reactivated larvae in breeding bitch using fenbendazole (50 mg/kg/day PO from day 40 of gestation to day 14 of lactation) or ivermectin (0.5 mg/kg PO 4–9 days prior to whelping, again 10 days later). • Begin biweekly anthelmintic treatment of pups at 2 weeks; continue until weaned, especially high-risk pups; treat monthly after weaning. • Treat queen with adulticide/larvicide anthelmintic prior to breeding, after queening. • Begin anthelmintic treatment of kittens at 3–4 weeks of age; treat monthly thereafter. • Promptly remove, dispose of feces to prevent environmental contamination. • Prevent hunting and ingestion of potential transport hosts.

EXPECTED COURSE AND PROGNOSIS

• Puppies (and rarely adults) with peracute/acute *A. caninum* infection may die despite treatment.
• Early recognition, anthelmintic treatment, prompt treatment of anemia, nutritional support necessary for successful outcome. • Anthelmintic treatment of adults can result in larval reactivation, repopulation of small intestine.

MISCELLANEOUS

AGE-RELATED FACTORS

• Disease more acute in young, usually chronic in adults. • Transmission of *A. caninum* from bitch to offspring results in high rate of infection in pups.

ZOONOTIC POTENTIAL

• All hookworms, especially *A. braziliense*, cause human CLM. • *A. caninum* larvae can cause visceral larva migrans or migrate to GI tract, causing abdominal pain and eosinophilia without becoming patent.

ABBREVIATIONS

• CLM = cutaneous larva migrans.
• GI = gastrointestinal.
• L3 = third-stage larvae.

INTERNET RESOURCES

• https://capcvet.org • https://www.cdc.gov/parasites/zoonotichookworm

Suggested Reading

Bowman DD. Georgis' Parasitology for Veterinarians, 9th ed. St. Louis, MO: Saunders, 2008, pp. 179–185.

Author Matt Brewer and Katy A. Martin
Consulting Editor Amie Koenig

H

HORNER'S SYNDROME

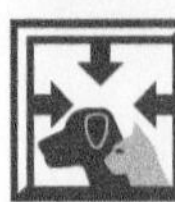

BASICS

OVERVIEW

- Sympathetic denervation to the eye.
- Anatomic pathway very important.
- Affects the ophthalmic and nervous systems (see Figure 1).

SIGNALMENT

- Idiopathic—one study suggests male golden retrievers 4–13 years of age at increased risk. Most of these localize to a postganglionic lesion. • Idiopathic—50–93% of Horner's syndrome in dogs; 45% in cats.

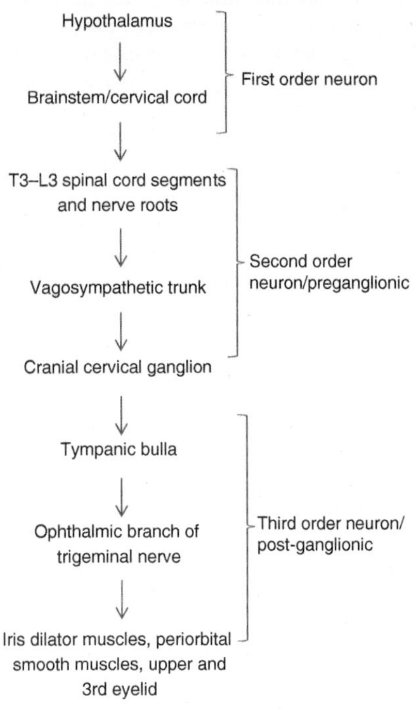

Figure 1.

SIGNS

- Miosis. • Protruding third eyelid. • Ptosis (drooping) of upper eyelid. • Enophthalmos.
- Other neurologic and non-neurologic signs dependent on the underlying cause.

CAUSES & RISK FACTORS

See Table 1.

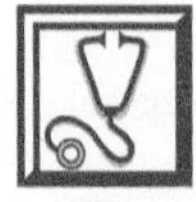

DIAGNOSIS

DIFFERENTIAL DIAGNOSIS

Anterior uveitis—intraocular pressure (IOP) usually low; aqueous flare present.

CBC/BIOCHEMISTRY/URINALYSIS

N/A

OTHER LABORATORY TESTS

N/A

IMAGING

- See Table 1. • Thoracic radiographs—may reveal cause of injury to the sympathetic trunk (e.g., trauma or mediastinal tumor).
- CT to image skull and middle ear.
- MRI—may help identify brainstem lesion, retrobulbar mass, cervical spinal cord problem, or jugular groove lesions.
- Ultrasonography—orbit; may reveal retrobulbar mass; jugular groove; may reveal jugular groove mass.

DIAGNOSTIC PROCEDURES

- See Table 1. • Cerebral spinal fluid (CSF) tap—identify brain and spinal cord inflammation. • Electromyography— look for brachial plexus denervation consistent with avulsion. • Pharmacologic testing—see Anisocoria.

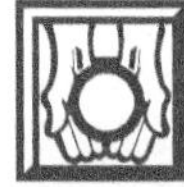

TREATMENT

Treat underlying disease.

MEDICATIONS

DRUG(S) OF CHOICE

- Depends on underlying disease.
- Idiopathic—none.

CONTRAINDICATIONS/POSSIBLE INTERACTIONS

Do not use drugs that alter the autonomic nervous system prior to referral for lesion localization.

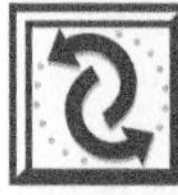

FOLLOW-UP

- Depends on severity of underlying disease.
- Idiopathic—may take up to 4 months for a partial or complete recovery.

MISCELLANEOUS

ABBREVIATIONS

- CN = cranial nerve. • CSF = cerebrospinal fluid. • FCE = fibrocartilaginous embolism.
- IOP = intraocular pressure. • IVDH = intervertebral disc herniation.

Suggested Reading

Cottrill NB. Differential diagnosis of anisocoria. In: Kirk's Current Veterinary Therapy, 14th ed. St. Louis, MO: Saunders, 2009, pp. 1168–1174.

Simpson KM, Williams DL, Cherubini GB. Neuropharmacological lesion localization in idiopathic Horner's syndrome in Golden Retrievers and dogs of other breeds. Vet Ophthalmol 2015, 18(1):1–5.

Author Heidi L. Barnes Heller

Consulting Editor Kathern E. Myrna

Table 1

Summary of lesions resulting in Horner's syndrome.

Lesion Location	*Causes*	*Common Concurrent Neurologic Abnormalities*	*Diagnostic Plan*
Brainstem	Neoplasia, encephalitis, vascular, trauma	Altered mental status, ipsilateral hemiparesis, ipsilateral postural reaction deficits	MRI; CSF analysis
C1–T3 spinal cord	IVDH, trauma, neoplasia, FCE	Ipsilateral or bilateral paresis/plegia, ± reduced reflexes to thoracic limbs, normal mentation	MRI preferred, myelogram also may show lesion. CSF analysis
T1–T3 nerve roots	Brachial plexus avulsion, peripheral nerve tumor (lymphoma, nerve sheath tumor most common)	Ipsilateral loss of thoracic limb reflexes, ipsilateral loss of cutaneous trunci, ipsilateral monoparesis/plegai, absent postural reactions in affected thoracic limb only	MRI, electrodiagnostic testing
Sympathetic trunk, cranial cervical ganglion	Trauma, iatrogenic following jugular venipuncture, mediastinal or thyroid neoplasia	Possibly laryngeal dysfunction	Neck ultrasound, MRI, thoracic radiographs
Tympanic bulla	Otitis media, polyp (cat), neoplasia, trauma	Ipsilateral vestibular disease, ipsilateral facial nerve paralysis	MRI, CT, bulla radiographs, myringotomy
Retrobulbar	Neoplasia, abscess, trauma	None, or dysfunction of CN II, III, IV, and VI.	MRI, orbital ultrasound

BASICS

DEFINITION

• Deposition of urine or feces outside the litter box.
• Urine housesoiling (also called periuria) includes toileting, a behavior in which urine is found on horizontal surfaces outside the litter box, and urine marking, in which urine is sprayed on vertical (occasionally horizontal) surfaces as part of a ritualistic tail-up display.
• Fecal housesoiling includes both toileting, a behavior characterized by feces deposited outside the litter box, and fecal marking, called middening, characterized by feces deposited in prominent locations.
• Marking behavior serves a normal communicative function in cats, particularly in response to other cats inside or outside the home.
• Housesoiling will negatively impact the human–animal bond and can lead to relegation outside, rehoming, relinquishment, or euthanasia.

PATHOPHYSIOLOGY

• Toileting—may be dissatisfaction with the litter box environment or preference for an alternative location or substrate, or may reflect an underlying pathophysiologic state such as a negative (pain) association with the litter box secondary to feline idiopathic cystitis (FIC) or feline lower urinary tract disease (FLUTD), uroliths, constipation, or orthopedic pain.
• Urine marking—a normal behavior observed in free-ranging and confined cats; significant individual differences exist in the propensity to urine mark in a given environment. Cat density is correlated to probability of urine marking. Cats who urine mark also commonly use a litter box for toileting (both urine and feces).
• Fecal marking (middening) is rarely observed; it should be a diagnosis of exclusion.
• Social or environmental stressors may contribute to housesoiling, primarily marking.

SYSTEMS AFFECTED

• Behavioral.
• Endocrine.
• Gastrointestinal (GI).
• Neurologic/musculoskeletal.
• Renal/urologic.

GENETICS

• Not specifically identified.
• Persians and Himalayans who exhibit toileting should be DNA tested for the genetic disorder polycystic kidney disease.

INCIDENCE/PREVALENCE

• Housesoiling is the most common behavioral problem for which cat owners seek veterinary advice and the second most common reason for relinquishment of cats to animal shelters.
• Toileting—in one survey, 11% of indoor cat owners reported toileting outside the litter box as a problem.
• Urine marking—exhibited by approximately 10% of castrated male and 5% of ovariectomized female house cats.

GEOGRAPHIC DISTRIBUTION

Housesoiling may be more problematic where cats are restricted indoors.

SIGNALMENT

Species

Cat

Breed Predilections

Housesoiling may occur in any breed, although Persians, Himalayans, and relatives are overrepresented in some studies.

Mean Age and Range

Toileting can occur at any age. Marking behaviors are typically seen in cats >6 months.

Predominant Sex

• Housesoiling can occur in either sex, intact or altered.
• Urine marking is more common in males (intact and neutered) than females (intact and neutered).

SIGNS

General Comments

Identify the Affected Cat in a Multicat Household

• Direct observation—although if punished, cats may become secretive.
• Videotaping or video monitoring.
• Separate the cats to identify the culprit. Note that this protocol may alter the social milieu sufficiently to inhibit toileting behavior.
• Add a urine indicator. Administer the dye fluorescein (6 fluorescein test strips in a gel capsule PO or 10 mg/cat). Urine outside the litter box will fluoresce under a Wood's light for approximately 24 hours. If negative, the test can be repeated on another cat. Negative results are common in households in which the frequency of urine housesoiling is low. Fluorescein may stain fabrics. If urine PH is alkaline, urine is more likely to fluoresce.
• Add a feces indicator. Small shavings of nontoxic crayons may be mixed into food, with different colors fed to each cat.

Identify the Locations of Housesoiling within the House

The owner should draw a diagram of the home layout, indicating the locations of urine and fecal housesoiling and locations of litter boxes. Location of housesoiling can provide insight into the type of housesoiling and etiology.

Historical Findings

Toileting Behavior

• Abnormal pattern of urination (incontinence, polyuria, hematuria, stranguria, dysuria) suggests an underlying congenital or medical problem.
• History of straining to defecate; vocalizing or running away when defecating; hard, dry, or bulky feces suggest painful defecations.
• Painful elimination or increases in volume or frequency of elimination could lead to soiling, conditioned avoidance, and new location or surface preferences.
• History of polydipsia, anorexia, vomiting, or diarrhea suggests an underlying medical etiology.

Urine Marking

• History of conflict, aggression, or avoidance behavior between cats in a multicat household.
• Observation of the posture of spraying urine—the cat orients caudally to a vertical surface, stiffens its posture, raises and quivers its tail, and directs a small burst of urine caudally.
• Observation of urine marks on vertical surfaces or puddled at the bottom of a wall.
• Urine marks can be found on prominent furniture or other objects, or on new objects brought into the house.
• Horizontal urine marks may be found on clothing or bedding associated with a particular person, cat, or dog, or in response to visitors or novel objects.

Fecal Marking

Feces deposited on prominent, conspicuous locations.

Physical Examination Findings

• If strictly behavioral, physical examination will be normal.
• Apparently neutered males that urine mark should be examined for the presence of penile spines, indicating the presence of endogenous testosterone, or quantify serum testosterone.

CAUSES

Medical Causes

• Any metabolic or GI condition that causes polyuria (e.g. diabetes mellitus), diarrhea, or constipation.
• Lower urinary tract disease including interstitial cystitis (may be associated with environmental stressors).
• Urolithiasis.
• Hyperthyroidism.
• Feline leukemia virus (FeLV).
• Feline immunodeficiency virus (FIV).
• Liver disease.
• CNS disease/cognitive dysfunction (senility).
• Iatrogenic—administration of fluids, corticosteroids, diuretics, laxatives.
• Musculoskeletal pain that makes entry to/exit from the litter box or elimination

postures difficult can contribute to litter box aversion.

- Hormonal influences may contribute to urine marking.

Behavioral Causes

Toileting Behavior

- Inadequate cleaning of litter box.
- Inadequate number of boxes or locations (one box per cat plus one is recommended).
- Box located in remote or unpleasant surroundings or subject to interference by dogs or children.
- Inappropriate type of box—covered or uncovered, too small; or allows other cats, pet dogs, and young children to target the cat as it exits.
- Time factors—daily or weekly temporal patterns of toileting suggest an environmental cause; acute onset in a cat who has previously used the litter box suggests a medical or social problem.
- Substrate—unacceptable litter type; preference tests indicate that most cats prefer unscented, fine-grained (clumping) litter, but individual variability; coincident change in litter box habits with new litter type suggests an association; sudden shift from one substrate (e.g., litter) to an unusual substrate (e.g., porcelain sink) suggests a lower urinary tract disorder.
- Location—urination outside the litter box may suggest a location preference or social factors; urination in the vicinity of the litter box may suggest dissatisfaction with qualities of the litter box, including litter box hygiene.
- Social dynamics—consider social conflicts between cats at the time the problem started (e.g., addition of a new cat).

Marking

- Marking is associated with arousal, anxiety, or territorial behavior.
- The probability of urine marking is directly proportional to the number of cats in the household.
- Marking can be a response to household disruption or another cat(s) in or outside the home; urine marks around windows and doors to the outside suggest a response to the presence of an outdoor cat.
- Urine marking grocery bags or new furniture suggests arousal in response to new stimuli.

RISK FACTORS

Toileting

- Inadequate litter box hygiene.
- Litter box features (litter type or scent, box size or style).

Urine Marking

- Male.
- Sexually intact.
- Multicat household.
- History of urine marking by a parent.

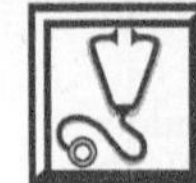

DIAGNOSIS

DIFFERENTIAL DIAGNOSIS

- Must identify if a medical problem underlies the behavioral problem.
- If behavioral, must differentiate toileting from urine/fecal marking.

CBC/BIOCHEMISTRY/URINALYSIS

Usually normal when urine marking and toileting are strictly behavioral; urinalysis via cystocentesis is the minimum database in any cat with toileting behavior; collect serial samples from cats whose behavioral signs wax and wane; CBC and biochemistry are recommended prior to administration of medication and to evaluate medical status.

OTHER LABORATORY TESTS

Cats with refractory toileting behavior or progressive signs should be tested for hyperthyroidism, FeLV, and FIV.

IMAGING

Abdominal ultrasonography, abdominal radiographs, and contrast studies if indicated to rule out urolithiasis and medical causes for toileting behavior.

DIAGNOSTIC PROCEDURES

Helpful historical information—map of the house with litter boxes and urine/fecal housesoiling identified; behavioral diary with daily frequency of urinations/ defecations inside each litter box and outside the litter boxes. Requires daily household monitoring.

PATHOLOGIC FINDINGS

None, unless an underlying medical etiology.

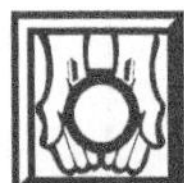

TREATMENT

APPROPRIATE HEALTH CARE

- Use environmental and behavioral therapies before or concomitant with pharmacologic treatment.
- The environment for indoor cats should include safe resting places, separated and plentiful resources, and positive and predictable human–cat interactions.
- Restrict the cat from rooms or areas in which housesoiling occurs.
- For immediate management and in cases of agonistic relationships between cats in a multicat household, it may be necessary to confine the cat to one room in the owner's absence. Provide a litter box (see specifications below), water, food, and resting sites. The cat can be let out of the room when the owner returns and is available for strict supervision. Initiate other, more permanent treatments.
- Clean urine "accidents" with an enzymatic cleaner specific for this purpose.

Toileting Behavior

- Scoop out litter boxes daily. Clean out and wash litter box and refill regularly.
- Avoid deodorizers, scented litters, or other strong odors in the vicinity of the litter box.
- Move food bowls away from litter boxes.
- Provide one litter box per cat, plus one, distributed in more than one location; positioned away from high traffic or noisy areas and with adequate opportunity for entry and exit to avoid conflict with other pets.
- If the litter box is covered, provide an additional large, plain, uncovered litter box filled with unscented, fine-grained, clumping litter, with no liner, and quantify cat use in a behavioral diary.
- Additional boxes may be provided ("litter box buffet") to determine preference for litter box type and substrate. Insure box is large enough for cat's needs for elimination and scratching.
- If one site in the home is preferred for toileting urination, place another litter box over this site. After it is in regular use, move very gradually each day to a site more acceptable to the owner.

Urine Marking

- If there are signs that the cat is marking in response to cats outside the home, use mechanical or olfactory products to deter outside animals, or trap and remove.
- Reduce cat numbers to lessen conflicts if possible.
- Synthetic feline F3 facial pheromone (Feliway® Classic) is commercially available as a treatment for urine marking. The product is sprayed on marked locations or diffused in the environment. For intraspecific social conflict, consider use of feline maternal-appeasing pheromone diffuser (Feliway Multi-cat or Feliway Friends).
- Litter box management, as described above, has been shown to decrease urine marking.
- Pharmacotherapy plays an important role in the control of urine marking.

ACTIVITY

Opportunities for active play that incorporate behavioral patterns of predatory stalking and pouncing should be provided daily.

DIET

No specific diet unless underlying medical etiology, such as urolithiasis or constipation. Consider use of urinary stress diets for stress-related cystitis.

CLIENT EDUCATION

- Cats do not housesoil to be spiteful.
- Scolding and punishment are contra-indicated—they may increase cat anxiety and avoidance or fear of the owner.

• Understanding the underlying motivation for housesoiling is critical for treatment success.
• Creating a predictable environment will decrease anxiety and arousal that may contribute to housesoiling.
• Work to resolve cat conflicts within the home (see Aggression, Intercat Aggression).
• Meet the cat's behavioral needs for play, sufficient resources, and safe elevated resting sites.

SURGICAL CONSIDERATIONS

Castration reduces urine marking in up to 90% of males and 95% of females.

MEDICATIONS

DRUG(S) OF CHOICE

Toileting

Psychotropic medication not usually indicated, except in treatment-resistant cases or when associated with generalized anxiety or heightened arousal.

Urine Marking

• Medication to decrease arousal is often needed for treatment success.
• Drugs from a number of drug classes may be used. All have the general effect of decreasing arousal and anxiety. Side effects can be sedation and/or altered social behavior (see Table 1). Drugs commonly used include fluoxetine, paroxetine, clomipramine, amitriptyline, buspirone.

Fecal Marking

Medication may be needed to decrease the arousal that drives this behavior.

CONTRAINDICATIONS

• Benzodiazepines—use cautiously or avoid because of rare cases of fatal idiopathic hepatic necrosis in cats receiving oral diazepam.
• Tricyclic antidepressants—cats with a history of cardiac conduction disturbances, urinary or fecal retention, megacolon, lower urinary tract blockages, seizures, and glaucoma.
• Transdermal route does not appear to consistently produce satisfactory drug levels.

PRECAUTIONS

All drugs listed are extra-label. Inform the client of extra-label use and potential side effects; document the discussion in the medical record or use a release form. Start psychotropic drugs when the owner is present to monitor the patient.

POSSIBLE INTERACTIONS

Do not use monoamine oxidase inhibitors (e.g., selegiline) concurrently with tricyclic antidepressants (TCAs) or selective serotonin reuptake inhibitors (SSRIs).

ALTERNATIVE DRUG(S)

• Synthetic progestins—the risk of serious side effects, including blood dyscrasias, pyometra, mammary hyperplasia, mammary carcinoma, diabetes mellitus, and obesity, has diminished their once-common use.
• Pheromone therapy (Feliway Classic) may reduce urine spraying.
• L-theanine (Anxitane®) or alpha-casozepine (Zylkene®) may reduce cat anxiety.
• L-tryptophan and alpha-casozepine supplemented diets (Multifunction Urinary + Calm Diet, Royal Canin, Hill's® Prescription Diet® c/d® Multicare Stress) may reduce cat anxiety and urine housesoiling.

FOLLOW-UP

PATIENT MONITORING

• Regular follow-up is essential.
• The owner should keep a daily log of elimination patterns so that treatment success can be evaluated and appropriate adjustments can be made. Number the litter boxes and request that client count and record the number of urinations/defecations in each box and outside the litter boxes each day.
• For marking behavior, after 2 months of successful medication management, medication might be withdrawn gradually over 2 weeks. However, if the social features that underlie the behavior are still present, medication may need to be continued for treatment success.
• For medication monitoring, an annual CBC, chemistry profile, urinalysis, and physical examination are recommended as a minimum.

PREVENTION/AVOIDANCE

• Neuter cats.
• Restrict cat numbers to decrease the probability of urine marking.
• Counsel clients on appropriate litter box selection, location, and hygiene.
• Veterinary practitioners should inquire about housesoiling at each veterinary visit. Early identification and treatment optimize treatment success.

POSSIBLE COMPLICATIONS

Client expectations must be realistic. Immediate control of a longstanding problem of housesoiling is unlikely; the goal is gradual improvement over time.

EXPECTED COURSE AND PROGNOSIS

• Prognosis for improvement is good if underlying etiology is identified and managed.
• Housesoiling is destructive to household belongings and erosive to the human–animal bond, which can lead to abandonment, relegation outside, relinquishment, and euthanasia.

MISCELLANEOUS

ASSOCIATED CONDITIONS

Aggression between cats may be associated with urine marking.

AGE-RELATED FACTORS

• Older cats might find litter box access difficult and seek alternative locations. Low-rise litter boxes in accessible areas can provide better access for these cats.
• Failure to use the litter box could be associated with age-related cognitive decline.

ZOONOTIC POTENTIAL

Pregnant women should avoid or take appropriate precautions when cleaning cat feces because of the risk of toxoplasmosis.

PREGNANCY/FERTILITY/BREEDING

TCAs are contraindicated in animals used for breeding.

SYNONYMS

• General—feline housesoiling.
• Urine—feline inappropriate elimination, urine marking, urine spraying, periuria.

H

Table 1

Drugs and dosages used to manage feline urine marking.

Drug	*Drug Class*	*Oral Dosage in Cats*	*Frequency*	*Side Effects (Usually Transient)*
Fluoxetine	SSRI	0.5–1.0 mg/kg	q24h	Decreased appetite, sleepiness
Paroxetine	SSRI	0.25–0.50 mg/kg	q24h	Constipation
Clomipramine	TCA	0.25–1.0 mg/kg	q24h	Sleepiness
Amitriptyline	TCA	0.25–1.0 mg/kg	q24h	Sleepiness
Buspirone	Azapirone	0.5–1.0 mg/kg	q12h	GI tract side effects (rare)

HOUSESOILING—CATS (CONTINUED)

• Feces—feline inappropriate defecation, fecal marking, middening.

SEE ALSO

• Aggression, Intercat Aggression.
• Fears, Phobias, and Anxieties—Cats.
• Kitten Behavior Problems.
• Marking, Roaming, and Mounting Behavior—Cats.

ABBREVIATIONS

• FeLV = feline leukemia virus.
• FIC = feline idiopathic cystitis.
• FIV = feline immunodeficiency virus.
• FLUTD = feline lower urinary tract disease.
• GI = gastrointestinal.
• SSRI = selective serotonin reuptake inhibitor.
• TCA = tricyclic antidepressant.

INTERNET RESOURCES

• https://www.catvets.com/guidelines/practice-guidelines/house-soiling
• https://indoorpet.osu.edu/cats/problem-solving

Suggested Reading

de Souza Dantas LM. Vertical or horizontal? Diagnosing and treating cats who urinate outside the box. Vet Clin Small Anim 2018; 48:403–417.

Herron, M. E., Horwitz, D., Siracusa, C., & Dale, S. (2020). Decoding your cat: The ultimate experts explain common cat behaviors and reveal how to prevent or change unwanted ones. New York: Houghton Mifflin Harcourt.

Landsberg G. Feline housesoiling. In: Landsberg G, Hunthausen W, Ackerman L. Behavior Problems of the Dog and Cat, 3rd ed. New York: Saunders/Elsevier, 2013, pp. 281–295.

Neilson JC. House soiling by cats. In: Horwitz DF, Mills D, eds. BSAVA Manual of Canine and Feline Behavioural Medicine, 2nd ed. Gloucester: BSAVA, 2009, pp. 117–126.

Authors Margaret E. Gruen and Barbara L. Sherman

Consulting Editor Gary M. Landsberg

Client Education Handout available online

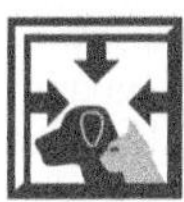

BASICS

DEFINITION

Urination and/or defecation, for elimination or marking of territory, in locations that owners consider inappropriate.

PATHOPHYSIOLOGY

• Improper or incomplete housetraining.
• Submissive or excitement urination.
• Marking behavior, due to territoriality, anxiety, testosterone influence. • Anxiety.
• Cognitive dysfunction.

SYSTEMS AFFECTED

Behavioral—shelter relinquishment, euthanasia, or rehoming.

GENETICS

Some breeds appear to be more easily housetrained than others.

INCIDENCE/PREVALENCE

• Approximately 15%. • Almost 20% of owners relinquishing a dog to a shelter did so because it soiled in the house. • 37% of owners who reported talking to their veterinarian about a behavior problem reported housesoiling. • Housesoiling is a common reason to see a veterinary behaviorist.

GEOGRAPHIC DISTRIBUTION

None described.

SIGNALMENT

Species

Dog

Breed Predilections

Potential genetic breed predisposition for ease of housetraining and submissive or excitement urination. Dogs obtained from a commercial breeding establishment are more likely to urinate vertically or submissively urinate than those obtained from a noncommercial breeder.

Mean Age and Range

• Inappropriate elimination due to improper or incomplete housetraining, primarily in younger dogs. • Submissive and excitement urination, primarily in younger dogs. • Urine marking begins as the dog reaches sexual maturity. • Housesoiling is a common complaint from owners of elderly dogs.

Predominant Sex

The incidence of inappropriate elimination, including marking, in intact male dogs is almost 60% higher than in castrated male dogs and intact or spayed female dogs.

SIGNS

General Comments

• Inappropriate elimination is the most common individual reason for shelter relinquishment. • Proper housetraining must be discussed with clients. • Housesoiling can be associated with medical problems.

Historical Findings

• History of urination and/or defecation in inappropriate areas. • May be associated with signs of other behavioral disorders (such as separation anxiety). • May be associated with lack of time or knowledge to properly housetrain. • May be associated with punishment. • A complete history will help determine potential triggers, including when, where, and how frequently the elimination occurs, and reliability of outdoor elimination training.

Physical Examination Findings

• If examination findings and laboratory results are normal, housesoiling is more likely due to a behavioral cause. • There may have been an inciting medical cause that has been resolved but the animal continues to eliminate inappropriately.

CAUSES

Canine inappropriate elimination can be due to a primary behavioral problem or secondary to/concurrent with a medical disorder. Medical causes should be ruled out if a previously housetrained dog begins to soil, in dogs that are refractory to training, and when volume or frequency of elimination is increased.

Behavioral

• Lack of, improper, or incomplete housetraining. • Marking behavior. • Submissive urination. • Excitement urination.
• Separation anxiety. • Cognitive dysfunction syndrome. • Noise phobia. • Fear induced.
• Psychogenic polydipsia/polyuria.

Medical Causes

Degenerative

• Osteoarthritis. • Renal failure. • Neuromuscular.

Anatomic

Ectopic ureters

Metabolic/Endocrine

• Incontinence. • Diabetes mellitus.
• Diabetes insipidus. • Hepatic insufficiency.
• Hyperadrenocorticism. • Hypoadrenocorticism. • Neurologic.

Neoplastic

• Genitourinary neoplasia. • Neurologic.
• Other neoplastic diseases causing weakness.

Infectious/Inflammatory

• Urinary tract infection or inflammation.
• Crystalluria with cystitis. • Inflammatory bowel disorder. • Pancreatic disease. • Intestinal parasites.

RISK FACTORS

• Intact male. • Greater number of hours worked. • Concurrent behavioral problem, such as separation anxiety. • Owners unable to properly housetrain. • Owner using punishment or aversive training methods.

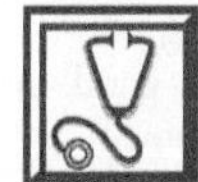

DIAGNOSIS

DIFFERENTIAL DIAGNOSIS

Differentiate behavioral causes of inappropriate elimination from medical causes (see Causes) with a proper workup.

CBC/BIOCHEMISTRY/URINALYSIS

Indicated to rule out medical causes.

IMAGING

Not indicated except to diagnose or rule out medical causes.

DIAGNOSTIC PROCEDURES

• Complete behavioral and medical history, including household layout and locations soiled. • Videorecording when the owner is present to view household interactions with the dog. • Journal to monitor potential causal factors, as well as to monitor improvement of the problem. • Videorecording when the owner is gone from the home to rule in/out separation anxiety or other anxiety disorders.

PATHOLOGIC FINDINGS

None for behavioral causes.

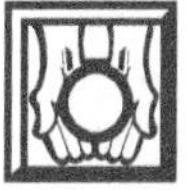

TREATMENT

APPROPRIATE HEALTH CARE

Appropriate measures to assure continued good health of the dog.

ACTIVITY

• Take dog outside often on a schedule to ensure enough access to eliminate outside, or provide acceptable access to the outside, e.g., via a dog door if the dog is trained properly.
• Increase activity level to potentially help in the treatment of other problem behaviors, as well as to improve the dog's mental and physical health.

DIET

• If the dog is inappropriately eliminating stool, feeding scheduled meals may help to maintain the dog on a schedule of elimination.
• Feeding a diet of higher caloric density may help decrease the urge to defecate as frequently.
• Water should not be withheld.

CLIENT EDUCATION

General Comments

• Counsel the owner as to the cause(s) of the inappropriate elimination, as well as potential long-term management of the problem. • Treat underlying/contributing medical problems.
• Treat other underlying/contributing behavioral problems. • Counsel owners on proper housetraining techniques that focus on reinforcing desirable and preventing undesirable behavior through supervision and confinement/safe haven training. • Counsel owners not to use punishment-based or aversive training methods—punishment creates fear, anxiety, and stress, which can increase housesoiling. • Do not use punishment to housetrain a dog, such as rubbing its nose in the soiled area, or verbally or physically reprimanding. • Clean the soiled areas with an enzymatic cleaner to help eliminate any odor that may attract the dog to eliminate there again; if the soiled object is a piece of clothing or other smaller cloth object, such as a throw rug, wash it. • Change the

HOUSESOILING—DOGS (CONTINUED)

significance of the soiled area, such as by feeding the dog in the area.

Incomplete Housetraining

• Supervise the dog at all times. Monitor for pre-elimination signs to immediately take to the appropriate site. • If not supervised, keep confined to an area where the dog will not eliminate or where an elimination site is offered (indoor elimination area); confinement areas should be in a room, behind a barricade (safety gate), or a crate or pen where the dog is comfortably housed (safe haven; see Puppy Behavior Problems); do not confine to an area that causes panic, destruction, and/or injury to the dog. • In some cases, tethering the dog to owners or nearby allows better supervision; never tether without supervision. • Take the dog outside frequently to eliminate; schedule outdoor times to meet the frequency and timing of elimination. • Accompany the pet to the appropriate elimination site and immediately reward elimination. • Use a consistent "key phrase" to help associate the act with the location and timing of elimination. • Feed on a set schedule, with water always available.

Submissive or Excitement Urination

• Do not punish the behavior, as this will contribute to further fear and conflict.
• People should ignore the dog when they enter the house (no verbal or physical interactions or eye contact). • The dog should go outside to urinate before greeting. • The dog should be greeted in a nonconfrontational and quiet manner; do not lean over the dog or institute interactive play at the time of greeting. • Tossing treats or a toy or teaching an alternate behavior at homecoming such as "sit" may change the dog's greeting response.

Urine Marking Behavior

• Educate owners on effectiveness of neutering to decrease urine marking. • Determine all triggers to the behavior, including anxiety-provoking stimuli. • Address those triggers with desensitization and counter-conditioning and/or avoidance of the trigger where appropriate. • Prevent access to the preferred marking locations. • Medications may be indicated to treat underlying anxiety disorder.

SURGICAL CONSIDERATIONS

Neutering intact male dogs decreases urine marking rapidly in 30% of dogs, with a gradual decline in 20% of dogs, and no change in 50%. The results are the same regardless of age of neutering.

MEDICATIONS

DRUG(S) OF CHOICE

• Negligible effect in animals if displaying submissive or excitement urination; not indicated unless anxiety is part of the problem behavior. • If urine marking or inappropriate elimination is anxiety induced, medications may be helpful, in conjunction with behavior modification. • Selective serotonin reuptake inhibitors (SSRIs), tricyclic antidepressants (TCAs)/anti-anxiety medications, or other anti-anxiety medications may be helpful, especially with underlying anxiety—SSRI: fluoxetine at 1–2 mg/kg PO q24h; TCA: clomipramine at 1–3 mg/kg PO q12h. • For SSRIs and TCAs, the full onset of action can be 4–6 weeks after initiation of treatment; inform owners of time required for response to be noted. • Side effects of SSRIs and TCAs can include nausea, vomiting, diarrhea, and lethargy. • Additional side effects of TCAs can include potentiation of seizure activity.

CONTRAINDICATIONS

• Medication without concurrent behavior modification. • Tricyclic antianxiety medications are contraindicated in seizures and cardiac disease, and may interfere with thyroid medications.

PRECAUTIONS

Based on drug chosen.

POSSIBLE INTERACTIONS

Do not use an SSRI and TCA together or in conjunction with a monoamine oxidase (MAO) inhibitor or opioid.

ALTERNATIVE DRUG(S)

Pheromones, or supplements containing alpha-casozepine, L-theanine, or a calming probiotic may help to decrease anxiety.

FOLLOW-UP

PATIENT MONITORING

Monitor with owner by follow-up visits or telephone calls. The owner should keep a journal of incidents, inciting factors, and treatments instituted to have an objective view of improvement.

PREVENTION/AVOIDANCE

• Properly housetrain. • Neuter male dogs.
• Monitor for signs and treat any underlying medical condition. • Treat any underlying behavioral condition.

POSSIBLE COMPLICATIONS

Recurrence if owner relapses in treatment, perhaps pet relinquishment.

EXPECTED COURSE AND PROGNOSIS

• Prognosis for any behavioral problem is highly dependent on an owner's ability and willingness to follow guidance—the following estimations of prognosis are based on the owner's ability and commitment to follow instructions. • Prognosis for decreasing submissive and excitement urination is good.
• Prognosis for managing incomplete housetraining is good. • Prognosis for marking in previously intact male: 50% improve (30% quickly, 20% more slowly) with neutering, even without complementary behavior modification. • Prognosis for managing urine marking in spayed or neutered dogs is good if the triggers are identified and managed with avoidance or other forms of behavior modification. • Some animals with a medical cause of inappropriate elimination will still eliminate inappropriately after the medical cause has been treated due to learning (e.g., self-reinforcing, new location preferences).

MISCELLANEOUS

AGE-RELATED FACTORS

• Puppies are more likely to present for lack of or incomplete housetraining, as well as for submissive and excitement urination.
• Cognitive dysfunction becomes more likely as the dog ages.

ZOONOTIC POTENTIAL

Low unless potentially zoonotic organisms in urine or feces.

SYNONYMS

• Inappropriate defecation. • Inappropriate elimination. • Inappropriate urination.
• Urine marking.

SEE ALSO

• Cognitive Dysfunction Syndrome.
• Separation Anxiety Syndrome.
• Submissive and Excitement Urination—Dogs.

ABBREVIATIONS

• MAO = monoamine oxidase.
• SSRI = selected serotonin reuptake inhibitor.
• TCA = tricyclic antidepressant.

INTERNET RESOURCES

• https://www.dacvb.org • https://avsab.org

Suggested Reading

Col R, Day C, Phillips CJC. An epidemiological analysis of dog behavior problems presented to an Australian behavior clinic, with associated risk factors. J Vet Behav 2016, 15:1–11.

Horwitz D, ed. Blackwell's Five-Minute Veterinary Consult Clinical Companion: Canine and Feline Behavior, 2nd ed. Ames, IA: Wiley-Blackwell, 2018, pp. 655–667.

Horwitz DF, Ciribassi J, Dale S, eds. Decoding Your Dog: The Ultimate Experts Explain Common Dog Behaviors and Reveal How to Prevent or Change Unwanted Ones. Boston, MA: Houghton Mifflin Harcourt, 2014.

Landsberg G, Hunthausen W, Ackerman L. Handbook of Behavior Problems of the Dog and Cat, 3rd ed. Philadelphia, PA: Saunders, 2012.

Author Melissa J. Bain
Consulting Editor Gary M. Landsberg

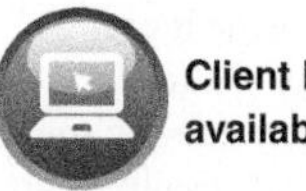

Client Education Handout available online

BASICS

DEFINITION

• Abnormal dilation of the ventricular system within the cranium.
• May be symmetric or asymmetric.
• May involve the entire ventricular system or partial elements secondary to underlying cause.

PATHOPHYSIOLOGY

• Obstructive—cerebrospinal fluid (CSF) accumulates in front of an obstruction along the normal CSF circulatory pattern (noncommunicating) or at its resorption site by the meningeal arachnoid villi (communicating); depending on the balance between production of CSF (which is constant and independent of intracranial pressure [ICP]) and the capacity for absorption of CSF, ICP may be high or normal; clinical signs may be noted in either case.
• Congenital obstruction—primary obstructive hydrocephalus; most common site is at the level of the mesencephalic aqueduct due to fusion of the rostral colliculi; prenatal infections (especially parainfluenza virus) may cause aqueductal stenosis with subsequent hydrocephalus; may result in considerable disruption of the architecture of the brain; diffuse ventricular enlargement may also suggest congenital ventricular dilation or obstruction at the level of the lateral apertures or foramen magnum; it is not uncommon to have asymmetric ventricular enlargement.
• Acquired obstruction—secondary obstructive hydrocephalus; sites include the interventricular foramina, mesencephalic aqueduct, or lateral apertures of the fourth ventricle.
• Overproduction of CSF (communicating)—rare; caused, e.g., by a choroid plexus tumor.
• "Compensatory hydrocephalus"—condition wherein CSF fills the space where the neural parenchyma was destroyed; not true hydrocephalus; terminology obsolete (hydrocephalus ex vacuo).
• External hydrocephalus—condition where CSF accumulates on the surface of the brain.
• Clinical signs of neurologic dysfunction result from damage to neural parenchyma, loss of neurons, and abnormal neuronal function.
• May also be associated with abnormalities in the spinal cord such as syringohydromyelia.

SYSTEMS AFFECTED

Nervous system.

GENETICS

Siamese cats—autosomal recessive.

INCIDENCE/PREVALENCE

Unknown

SIGNALMENT

Species

Dog and cat.

Breed Predilections

• Congenital—small and brachycephalic dogs: bulldogs, Chihuahuas, Maltese, Pomeranians, toy poodles, Yorkshire terriers, Lhasa apsos, Cairn terriers, Boston terriers, pug dogs, and Pekingese.
• Inherited—Siamese cats and Yorkshire terriers; high incidence of clinically asymptomatic ventriculomegaly in normal adult beagles.
• Acquired—any breed of cat or dog.

Mean Age and Range

• Congenital—usually becomes apparent at a few weeks up to 1 year of age; acute onset of signs can occur in dogs with previously undiagnosed congenital hydrocephalus; exact cause of this decompensation is uncertain.
• Acquired—any age.

Predominant Sex

None

SIGNS

General Comments

• Congenital—may occur without clinical signs, especially in dogs of toy breeds; other malformations or anomalies of the CNS may be noted (e.g., malformations of the cerebellum or syringomyelia), which may further contribute to the constellation of signs.
• Acquired—signs attributable to the underlying disease may be as or more prominent than the signs attributable to the hydrocephalus.
• Severity of the clinical signs may not correspond to the degree of ventricular enlargement.

Historical Findings

• Behavioral—decreased awareness; lack of or loss of training ability (including housetraining); excessive sleepiness; vocalization; sometimes hyperexcitability.
• Visual deficits including blindness.
• Seizures—may be noted.

Physical Examination Findings

• Head—may appear large and dome-shaped with an exaggerated "stop"; open sutures and/or persistent fontanelles often present, but these may be present without hydrocephalus and vice versa; bilaterally divergent strabismus in some dogs with severe congenital hydrocephalus: due to malformation of the orbit or to brainstem dysfunction.

Neurologic Examination Findings

• Signs may be acute or gradual in onset, and may be static or progressive.
• A wide variety of signs of brain dysfunction can occur.
• Cerebral disease—abnormal behavior (obtundation and drowsiness), cortical blindness (loss of vision with normal eyes and pupillary light reflexes), inappropriate vocalization, sometimes hyperexcitable, circling.
• Gait abnormalities—incoordination, ataxia, and decreased postural reactions.
• Seizures—may occur.
• Congenital form—malformation of the orbit during growth may result in a ventrolateral strabismus with normal oculocephalic movements; oculocephalic movements may be abnormal if brainstem dysfunction is the cause of strabismus.
• Severely increased ICP—stupor or coma, pinpoint or dilated fixed pupils, loss of normal oculocephalic movements (physiologic nystagmus), abnormal respiratory patterns, decerebrate posture; may lead to fatal tentorial herniation.
• Severity of clinical signs may not correlate with ventricular size, although there is a tendency for worse clinical signs with greater enlargement of the ventricles.

CAUSES

• Congenital—numerous congenital malformations cause obstruction of the ventricular system and result in hydrocephalus; heritable malformation, prenatal infection (e.g., dogs: parainfluenza virus; cats: coronavirus), exposure to teratogens, brain hemorrhage secondary to dystocia, nutritional deficiency (vitamin A), other.
• Acquired—tumors, abscesses, and inflammatory diseases (including inflammation resulting from hemorrhage caused by traumatic injuries or other causes of bleeding).

RISK FACTORS

Animals with compensated hydrocephalus may decompensate in the face of an insult such as infection or trauma, resulting in development of clinical signs.

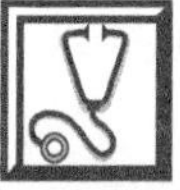

DIAGNOSIS

DIFFERENTIAL DIAGNOSIS

• Other congenital brain anomalies.
• Metabolic or toxic diseases resulting in cerebral dysfunction.
• Brain mass lesions or infectious diseases resulting in high ICP (hydrocephalus may coexist).
• Traumatic injury to the brain (hydrocephalus may coexist).

CBC/BIOCHEMISTRY/URINALYSIS

Usually normal.

IMAGING

• Skull radiography (congenital)—enlarged domed cranium with open sutures and persistent fontanelles; cranial vault may have a ground-glass appearance; also may reveal calvarial thinning.
• CT and MRI—provide definite diagnosis.
• Ultrasonography through fontanelles may reveal enlarged ventricles.

HYDROCEPHALUS (CONTINUED)

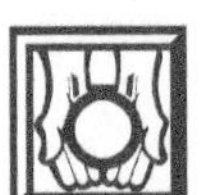

DIAGNOSTIC PROCEDURES

- CSF—use caution when collecting sample if patient has high ICP (may lead to fatal brain herniation through the foramen magnum and/or beneath the tentorium cerebelli); composition normal if no other intracranial disease (e.g., neoplasia, inflammation), but frequently abnormal when acquired underlying disease is present.
- Electroencephalography (EEG)—congenital: usually characteristic, including hypersynchrony, high amplitude (25–300 μV), and low frequency (1–7 Hz); acquired: varies.

PATHOLOGIC FINDINGS

- Brain—may be large with loss of the normal pattern of sulci and gyri; may see distortion of the parenchyma, including thinning of the cerebral cortex, rupture of the septum pellucidum, and atrophy of other adjacent structures; with severe disease, brain herniation may occur, either of the cerebrum and midbrain under the tentorium cerebelli or of the cerebellum and caudal medulla oblongata through the foramen magnum.
- Ventricular system—mildly to severely distended (either entirely or only the part rostral to the obstructive lesion); with noncommunicating form, narrowing or blockage of the ventricular system due to inflammation or mass lesions.

TREATMENT

APPROPRIATE HEALTH CARE

- Inpatient—intensive care for patients with severe signs or when undergoing surgical therapy.
- Outpatient—patients with mild to moderate signs that can be treated medically.

NURSING CARE

Prevent secondary complications of recumbency for stuporous or comatose patients—avoid pressure sores; drying eyes; hypostatic lung congestion.

CLIENT EDUCATION

Advise client to observe for deterioration in mental alertness, vision, and behavior, which may signal worsening of the problem.

SURGICAL CONSIDERATIONS

- Surgical shunting of the CSF from the ventricles to the peritoneal cavity or right atrium—definitive treatment.
- Surgery should be considered only when medical management is ineffective or results in adverse side effects.
- Complications—shunt blockage occurs in up to 50% of patients; infection is less common; shunt revision commonly needed; overshunting may result in severe and potentially fatal complications (collapse of the cerebral mantle).
- Clinical signs may not resolve completely; residual signs usually indicate irreversible brain damage.
- Surgery for a brain tumor or other mass lesion—consider if it is the underlying cause.

MEDICATIONS

DRUG(S) OF CHOICE

- Reduce CSF production—data on the efficacy of corticosteroids in reducing CSF production are conflicting, but beneficial clinical effects usually are seen (prednisone 0.25–0.5 mg/kg PO q12h or dexamethasone 0.1 mg/kg PO q12h); should be tapered to an alternate-day regimen and the dose lowered as far as possible.
    - Carbonic anhydrase inhibitors: acetazolamide (10 mg/kg PO q8h) with or without furosemide (1 mg/kg q24h); electrolytes must be monitored frequently; long-term use is unlikely to be beneficial and may lead to adverse consequences.
    - Omeprazole has been reported to reduce CSF production in normal dogs in an experimental model, but no data are available on the usefulness of this drug in the clinical setting; anecdotal reports have been disappointing.
- Reduce ICP—osmotic diuretics: mannitol (1 g/kg slow IV infusion over 20 min, may repeat twice at 6-hour intervals) and/or loop diuretics: furosemide (dogs: 2–8 mg/kg IV/IM/SC q12h; cats: 1–2 mg/kg IV/IM/SC q12h); these are short-term treatments only, helpful for acute treatment of severe cases.
- Treat underlying cause—administer specific drugs when possible (e.g., antibiotics for bacterial infection, irradiation, or surgery for neoplasia).

PRECAUTIONS

- Corticosteroids—long-term treatment may cause iatrogenic hyperadrenocorticism or hypoadrenocorticism if drug is suddenly withdrawn.
- Diuretics—may cause shock or electrolyte imbalances, especially hypokalemia with furosemide administration.

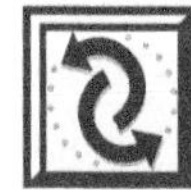

FOLLOW-UP

PATIENT MONITORING

Monitor for exacerbation of the hydrocephalus and for signs attributable to an underlying cause (e.g., intracranial neoplasia).

POSSIBLE COMPLICATIONS

- Brain herniation and death.
- Infection and blockage when ventriculoperitoneal shunting is carried out; shunt revision and specific treatment for bacterial infection are then indicated.

EXPECTED COURSE AND PROGNOSIS

- Good to poor—depend on cause and severity.
- Mild congenital form—good prognosis; may require only occasional medical treatment.

MISCELLANEOUS

ASSOCIATED CONDITIONS

Cerebellar hypoplasia in kittens congenitally infected with feline panleukopenia virus.

AGE-RELATED FACTORS

Congenital—usually seen in animals <1 year old.

SEE ALSO

Stupor and Coma.

ABBREVIATIONS

- CSF = cerebrospinal fluid.
- EEG = electroencephalography.
- ICP = intracranial pressure.

Suggested Reading

De Lahunta A, Glass E, Kent M. Veterinary Neuroanatomy and Clinical Neurology, 4th ed. St. Louis, MO: Elsevier Saunders, 2015, pp. 91–101.

Dewey CW. Encephalopathies: disorders of the brain. In: Dewey CW, ed., A Practical Guide to Canine and Feline Neurology, 2nd ed. Ames, IA: Wiley-Blackwell, 2008, pp. 126–129, 193.

Kawasaki Y, Tsuruta T, Setogawa Y, Sakamoto H. Hydrocephalus with visual deficits in a cat. J Vet Med Sci 2006, 65:1361–1364.

Thomas WB. Hydrocephalus in dogs and cats. Vet Clin North Am Small Anim Pract 2010, 40:143–159.

Author Stephanie Kube

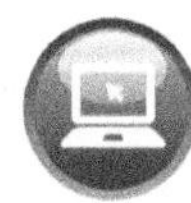

Client Education Handout available online

BASICS

OVERVIEW

• Hydronephrosis is progressive distention of the renal pelvis resulting in compression and atrophy of the renal parenchyma secondary to ureteral outflow tract obstruction and associated increased hydrostatic pressure.
• Most often hydronephrosis is unilateral (~80–85%) and occurs secondary to complete or partial obstruction of the ureter by uroliths, ureteral strictures, ureteral or trigonal neoplasia, retroperitoneal disease causing extraluminal compression, spay stump granuloma, trauma, radiotherapy, and accidental ligation of the ureter during ovariohysterectomy, cryptorchectomy, or after ectopic ureter surgery.
• Bilateral hydronephrosis is less common, resulting from ureteral stone disease, congenital ureteral strictures, trigonal neoplasia, or a urethral outflow obstruction. Severe hydronephrosis can also be seen in dogs with ectopic ureters (commonly males) associated with a ureterovesical junction (UVJ) stenosis.

SIGNALMENT

Dog and cat.

SIGNS

Historical Findings

• Subclinical in some dogs/cats.
• Inappetence.
• Weight loss.
• Polyuria and/or polydipsia (PU/PD).
• Hematuria.
• Depression, diarrhea, vomiting associated with uremia in patients with bilateral hydronephrosis or with compromised function in the contralateral kidney.
• May be referable to the cause of the obstruction (e.g., abdominal pain).
• Most dogs and cats with a ureteral obstruction will continue to produce urine due to the unilateral nature of the condition or the presence of a partial, rather than complete, ureteral obstruction.

Physical Examination Findings

• Normal in some patients.
• Renomegaly.
• Big kidney–little kidney syndrome associated with a previous ureteral obstruction.
• Renal, abdominal, or lumbar pain.
• Abdominal mass—bladder or prostate.
• Trigonal, prostatic, vaginal or urethral mass palpable on rectal exam.

CAUSES & RISK FACTORS

Ureteral Diseases

• Ureteroliths.
• Congenital ureteral stricture or circumcaval ureter.
• Acquired ureteral stricture/fibrosis.
• Pyonephrosis/pyoureter.
• Neoplasia.
• Ureteral ligation during ovariohysterectomy.
• Secondary to congenital ectopic ureter.
• Complication from previous ectopic ureter surgery.

Lower Urogenital Tract Diseases

• Urinary bladder neoplasia (e.g., transitional cell carcinoma).
• Prostatic disease (e.g., neoplasia).
• Vaginal mass.
• Cryptorchectomy resulting in inadvertent prostatectomy.

Retroperitoneal Disease

• Masses—granuloma, neoplasm, cyst, abscess, hematoma.
• Perineal hernia.
• Post-radiotherapy-induced fibrosis.

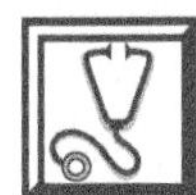

DIAGNOSIS

DIFFERENTIAL DIAGNOSIS

• Other causes for renal pelvic dilation—e.g., ureteral obstruction (stone, stricture, tumor), pyelonephritis, pyelonephrosis, IV fluid therapy, chronic kidney disease, PU/PD.
• Other causes of renomegaly—e.g., neoplasia, cysts, and perinephric pseudocysts (cats).
• Other causes of abdominal pain—e.g., pancreatitis and peritonitis.
• Intervertebral disc disease leading to lumbar pain.
• Other causes for azotemia—e.g., acute kidney injury, chronic kidney disease, dehydration, urethral obstruction.

CBC/BIOCHEMISTRY/URINALYSIS

• Normal in some patients.
• Loss of urine-concentrating ability (first abnormality detected), hematuria, pyuria.
• Azotemia, hyperphosphatemia, hyperkalemia, thrombocytopenia, and acidemia with either bilateral ureteral obstructions, concurrent renal parenchymal disease, or obstructive pyonephrosis.

IMAGING

• Abdominal radiographs may be normal or show nephroliths, ureteroliths, cystoliths, urethroliths, renomegaly, prostatomegaly, reduced retroperitoneal contrast, ureteral distension, or urinary bladder distension.
• Ultrasonography reveals dilation of the renal pelvis and diverticula, with thinning of the renal parenchyma; proximal dilation of affected ureter is detected in some dogs/cats if the hydronephrosis is associated with a ureteral obstruction (most common cause). If ureteral dilation is present, evaluation for cause (UVJ tumor, stenosis; ureteral stones; ureteral stricture).
• Injection of radiographic contrast material via either excretory urography (not recommended) or by nephropyelocentesis and ureteropyelography/retrograde ureterogram may be required to determine the location and cause of obstruction.
• CT can be helpful in cases where ultrasound and radiographs cannot determine cause.

DIAGNOSTIC PROCEDURES

Cystoscopy or vaginoscopy may help determine the location and cause of lower urinary tract obstruction or presence of ureteral ectopia, UVJ stenosis.

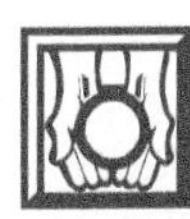

TREATMENT

• Emergency intervention is required for ureteral obstruction; metabolic and electrolyte abnormalities should be corrected prior to intervention. If severe enough then hemodialysis may be indicated.
• Treat as an inpatient.
• Start supportive care (e.g., fluids ± antibiotics) while performing diagnostic tests.
• Correct fluid and electrolyte deficits conservatively with IV fluid therapy over 12–24 hours, followed by maintenance fluids as needed. Patients with extreme PU may need higher maintenance fluid rates to maintain hydration. Do not fluid overload patients.
• Pending reestablishment of urinary patency, relieve lower urinary tract obstruction by catheterization, serial cystocentesis, or tube cystostomy as soon as possible.
• Specific treatment (e.g., interventional or surgical) depends on the cause and whether there is concurrent kidney disease or other disease processes (e.g., bilateral uroliths affecting contralateral kidney and/or ureter, metastatic neoplasia, etc.).
• Nephrectomy is rarely ever indicated (e.g., neoplasia).

MEDICATIONS

DRUG(S) OF CHOICE

• Success rate for medical management of obstruction is 8–13%.
• For a ureteral obstruction caused by uroliths—alpha-adrenergic blockade should be considered (cat: prazosin 0.25 mg/cat q12h; dog: 1 mg/15 kg q8–12h).
• IV fluid diuresis—being careful to avoid overhydration.
• Diuretics, e.g., mannitol 0.25 g/kg bolus over 30 min; consider CRI (1 mg/kg/min) if effective.

HYDRONEPHROSIS (CONTINUED)

• Hyperkalemia is often absent. Mild to moderate hyperkalemia often resolves with fluid replacement and/or bicarbonate administration unless bilateral obstruction and/or oliguria is present. Severe, symptomatic hyperkalemia requires prompt and aggressive medical or surgical management for emergent decompression.

CONTRAINDICATIONS/POSSIBLE INTERACTIONS

• Do not add or mix sodium bicarbonate with calcium-containing fluids.
• Do not give radiographic contrast material intravenously until the patient is rehydrated. Use radiographic contrast material with caution in azotemic patients.

Special Considerations

A patient with ureteral obstruction(s) should be considered an emergency and referred to colleagues who are highly experienced in managing this condition.

FOLLOW-UP

PATIENT MONITORING

• Ultrasonography—can repeat at 2–4-week intervals after relief of obstruction to assess improvement. Often some signs of resolution appear within days after relief of obstruction, but can take up to 3–4 months.
• Monitor serum chemistries and electrolytes as needed. Symmetric dimethylarginine (SDMA) likely has a place in the months following obstruction to track chronic kidney disease development.
• After relief of obstruction— PU and postobstructive diuresis may lead to hypokalemia, weight loss, dehydration, and possibly permanent renal injury, so care should be taken to monitor these patients carefully.

POSSIBLE COMPLICATIONS

Rupture of the excretory system and irreversible renal damage. Decompression should be considered when medical management fails to relieve obstruction.

EXPECTED COURSE AND PROGNOSIS

• Variable depending on the cause, duration of obstruction, and presence or absence of concurrent infection.
• Irreversible damage to the kidney usually begins 15–45 days after obstruction.
• If the obstruction is relieved within 2–4 weeks, some renal damage is reversible. If the obstruction is partial (over 80% of cases), the time before irreversible damage is prolonged.
• Concurrent infection accelerates the severity of renal damage. Antimicrobial therapy is often initiated empirically, however recent research recommends performing ultrasound guided pyelocentesis followed by anterograde pyelographic contrast study to confirm or rule-out ureteral obstruction.

MISCELLANEOUS

SEE ALSO

• Acidosis, Metabolic.
• Acute Kidney Injury.
• Chronic Kidney Disease.
• Hyperkalemia.

ABBREVIATIONS

• PU/PD = polyuria/polydipsia.
• SDMA = symmetric dimethylarginine.
• UVJ = ureterovesicular junction.

Author Ewan D.S. Wolff
Consulting Editor J.D. Foster
Acknowledgment The authors and book editors acknowledge the prior contributions of Allyson C. Berent and Cathy E. Langston.

HYPERADRENOCORTICISM (CUSHING'S SYNDROME)—CATS

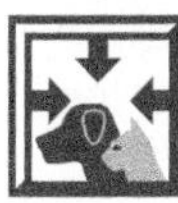

BASICS

OVERVIEW

Feline Cushing's syndrome (FCS) or hyperadrenocorticism is a consequence of abnormally increased functional activity of the adrenal cortex.

Pathophysiology

- Caused by increased glucocorticoid secretion by the adrenal gland(s).
- Approximately 85% of cases due to bilateral adrenocortical hyperplasia from pituitary hyperplasia or tumor— pituitary-dependent hyperadrenocorticism (PDH).
- Remaining 15% caused by adrenal tumor (AT), half of which are benign.
- Regardless of etiology, concurrent unregulated diabetes mellitus (DM) is frequent (90%) and other concurrent diseases (e.g., pancreatitis, chronic kidney, or cardiac disease) are reported.

SIGNALMENT

- Middle-aged to old cat.
- No known breed or sex predisposition.

SIGNS

- Dermatologic abnormalities (alopecia; unkempt hair coat; thin, fragile skin that is easily bruised or torn), polyuria, polydipsia, polyphagia, weight loss, muscle wasting, and pot-bellied appearance.
- Weight gain (unless concurrent DM causes weight loss), hepatomegaly, and curled pinnae also seen.
- Lethargy (dullness) secondary to muscle weakness or effects of pituitary mass.
- Excess sex hormones can cause signs such as penile barbs and behavioral changes (sexual).

CAUSES & RISK FACTORS

- Pituitary adenoma with subsequent corticotropic hyperplasia and excess glucocorticoid secretion.
- Autonomously functioning benign adrenal adenoma (50%) or malignant adenocarcinoma (50%).
- Iatrogenic from glucocorticoid administration (rare).

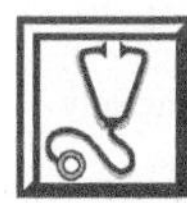

DIAGNOSIS

DIFFERENTIAL DIAGNOSIS

- Insulin-resistant DM.
- Acromegaly.
- Hepatopathy.
- Renal disease.
- Sex hormone–secreting adrenal tumor.
- Hyperprogesteronism.
- Dermatologic disease.

CBC/BIOCHEMISTRY/URINALYSIS

- Lymphopenia, anemia.
- Hyperglycemia, hypercholesterolemia, hypertriglyceridemia, hypochloremia.
- Elevated urine cortisol : creatinine (UC : Cr) ratio, proteinuria.
- Azotemia, hyperglobulinemia (less common).
- Elevated serum alkaline phosphatase uncommon.

OTHER LABORATORY TESTS

Screening Tests

- UC : Cr—sensitive (good negative predictive value).
- Low-dose dexamethasone-suppression test—good sensitivity. Dose: 0.1 mg/kg IV. Failure to suppress consistent with FCS.
- Adrenocorticotropic hormone (ACTH) stimulation test—specific but poorly sensitive, not recommended as initial diagnostic test.
- Assays for plasma sex hormone and progesterone concentrations may rule out differentials.

Differentiating Tests

- Plasma endogenous ACTH concentration high normal or greater with PDH compared to low plasma ACTH levels with AT (<10 pg/mL). Reference ranges vary with laboratories.
- Imaging.

IMAGING

- Abdominal ultrasound—accurate to differentiate PDH from AT in most cases; operator dependent. Symmetric adrenal glands of normal or enlarged size are suggestive of PDH; unilateral enlargement or asymmetric adrenal glands support AT.
- CT and MRI—visualization and measurement of pituitary tumors or characterization of adrenal tumors.

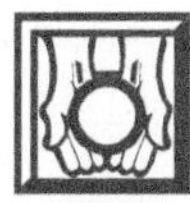

TREATMENT

- FCS is a debilitating disease. Prognosis is guarded due to severity of complications and concurrent diseases.
- Presurgical medical treatment is beneficial to prevent complications from fragile skin and infections.
- Radiation therapy of macroadenomas allows better control of the disease and insulin resistance.
- Unilateral adrenalectomy for AT and medical therapy for PDH are the most readily available effective treatment options.
- Hypophysectomy (microsurgical transsphenoidal) is effective and available at some institutions.

MEDICATIONS

DRUG(S) OF CHOICE

- Trilostane reversibly blocks steroid synthesis. In most patients with FCS from PDH, trilostane reduces clinical signs and improves endocrine test results. A starting dose of 5–10 mg/cat PO q12h is recommended.
- Mitotane (Lysodren®; o,p′-DDD) is not recommended for treatment of FCS.
- Other medications have limited efficacy (ketoconazole, metyrapone, and aminoglutethimide).

FOLLOW-UP

- Clinical improvement and improved diabetic control are indicative of successful drug therapy.
- ACTH stimulation tests are recommended for dose adjustments of trilostane.

MISCELLANEOUS

ABBREVIATIONS

- ACTH = adrenocorticotropic hormone.
- AT = adrenal tumor.
- DM = diabetes mellitus.
- FCS = feline Cushing's syndrome.
- PDH = pituitary-dependent hyperadrenocorticism.
- UC : Cr = urine cortisol : creatinine.

Suggested Reading

Feldman EC, Nelson RW. Hyperadrenocorticism in cats (Cushing's syndrome). In: Feldman EC, Nelson RW, eds., Canine and Feline Endocrinology and Reproduction, 3rd ed. Philadelphia, PA: Saunders, 2004, pp. 358–393.

Mellet, K, Bruyette, D, Stanley, S. Trilostane therapy for treatment of spontaneous hyperadrenocorticism in cats: 15 cases (2004–2012). J Vet Intern Med 2013, 27:1471–1477.

Valentin SY, Cortright CC, Nelson RH, et al. Clinical findings, diagnostic test results and treatment outcome in cats with spontaneous hyperadrenocorticism: 30 cases. J Vet Intern Med 2014, 28:481–487.

Author Suzy Y.M. Valentin

Consulting Editor Patty A. Lathan

Acknowledgment The author and book editors acknowledge the prior contribution of Deirdre Chiaramonte.

H

HYPERADRENOCORTICISM (CUSHING'S SYNDROME)—DOGS

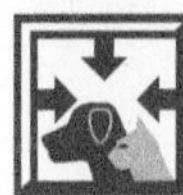

BASICS

DEFINITION

- Spontaneous hyperadrenocorticism (HAC)—disorder due to excessive production of cortisol by adrenal cortex.
- Iatrogenic HAC—from excessive exogenous administration of glucocorticoids by any route.
- Clinical signs due to effects of elevated circulating glucocorticoid concentrations.

PATHOPHYSIOLOGY

- ~80–85% of cases of naturally occurring HAC due to bilateral adrenocortical hyperplasia resulting from pituitary corticotroph adenoma or hyperplasia with oversecretion of adrenocorticotropic hormone (ACTH).
- In remaining 15–20%, cortisol-secreting adrenocortical neoplasia (AN) present; ~50% malignant.
- Rarely caused by ectopic ACTH secretion from nonpituitary tumor.
- One case of food-dependent hypercortisolemia reported, with increased cortisol concentration after meal; likely due to aberrant gastric inhibitory peptide receptors stimulating adrenal steroidogenesis.
- Iatrogenic HAC from excessive administration of exogenous glucocorticoids.

SYSTEMS AFFECTED

- Variable.
- Signs referable to urinary tract or skin common.
- Skin—bilaterally symmetric alopecia, comedones, hyperpigmentation, recurrent pyoderma.
- Renal/urologic—polyuria/polydipsia (PU/PD; 85–90% of cases), proteinuria, urinary tract infections (UTIs).
- Endocrine/metabolic—hyperglycemia; diabetes mellitus (DM) in 10%.
- Cardiovascular—hypertension (usually mild).
- Gastrointestinal—polyphagia.
- Hemic/lymphatic/immune—stress leukogram, immunosuppression, mild erythrocytosis and thrombocytosis, occasional nucleated red blood cells.
- Hepatobiliary—hepatopathy due to glycogen deposition, increased serum alkaline phosphatase (ALP) activity due to corticosteroid-induced isoenzyme; alanine aminotransferase (ALT) activity also increased, but by less.
- Neuromuscular—muscle weakness; CNS signs from macroadenoma may include anorexia, abnormal mentation, blindness, rarely seizures.
- Reproductive—testicular atrophy, anestrus.
- Respiratory—panting, pulmonary thromboembolism possible.

INCIDENCE/PREVALENCE

One of most common endocrine disorders in dogs.

SIGNALMENT

Species

Dog

Breed Predilections

Poodle, dachshund, Boston terrier, German shepherd dog, beagle.

Mean Age and Range

Generally, middle-aged to older animals; pituitary-dependent HAC (PDH) rarely seen in dogs as young as 1 year.

SIGNS

General Comments

- Severity varies greatly, depending on duration and extent of cortisol excess.
- In some cases physical presence of neoplastic process (pituitary or adrenal) contributes to illness.

Historical and Physical Examination Findings

PU/PD, polyphagia, pendulous abdomen, increased panting, hepatomegaly, hair loss, cutaneous hyperpigmentation, thin skin, muscle weakness, obesity, lethargy, muscle atrophy, comedones, bruising, testicular atrophy, anestrus, calcinosis cutis, facial nerve palsy.

CAUSES

- PDH—adenoma most common; adenocarcinomas rare; anterior pituitary involved in ~80% of cases, intermediate lobe in remainder; exact incidence of pituitary macroadenomas (tumors >1 cm diameter) unknown, may be 10–25%.
- AN—adenoma or carcinoma (50%).
- Ectopic ACTH secretion and food-dependent hypercortisolism—rare.
- Iatrogenic—due to glucocorticoid administration.

RISK FACTORS

- None known for spontaneous disease.
- Administration of exogenous glucocorticoids (risk for iatrogenic HAC).

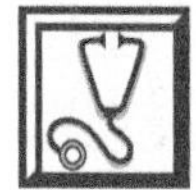

DIAGNOSIS

DIFFERENTIAL DIAGNOSIS

- Depends on clinical and laboratory abnormalities.
- Hypothyroidism, sex hormone dermatoses, alopecia X, sex hormone–secreting tumors, acromegaly, DM, hepatopathies, renal disease, other causes of PU/PD.
- Cortisol can decrease concentration of total T_4; important to check for HAC in dogs with weight gain or dermatologic disease that could be misdiagnosed as hypothyroidism.

CBC/BIOCHEMISTRY/URINALYSIS

- Hemogram may show eosinopenia, lymphopenia, leukocytosis, neutrophilia, erythrocytosis, thrombocytosis.
- Serum chemistry may show elevated cholesterol concentration; ALP activity high in ~85–90% and elevations proportionately greater than for ALT.
- Mild hyperglycemia common but only ~10% of dogs with HAC have concurrent DM.
- Urinalysis may reveal low specific gravity, proteinuria, hematuria, pyuria, and/or bacteriuria.

OTHER LABORATORY TESTS

- Endocrine testing required in dogs with history, clinical signs, and laboratory abnormalities suggestive of HAC; see Appendix II.
- Do not perform HAC testing in sick dogs unless clinical signs consistent with HAC.
- *Screening tests* determine if HAC present or not.
- Once diagnosis of HAC made, perform *differentiation test* to determine if PDH or AN present; differentiation crucial for therapeutic decisions and prognosis.
- To convert cortisol concentration in nmol/L to μg/dL, divide by 27.6.
- All cortisol concentrations below for illustration; normal ranges and cut-off values vary with lab.

Screening Tests

Urine Cortisol : Creatinine Ratio (UC : Cr)

- Urine cortisol excretion increases with augmented adrenal secretion of cortisol, whether due to PDH or AN.
- Should be measured in urine sample collected at home when pet not stressed.
- Elevated UC : Cr is sensitive marker of HAC, present in 90–100% of affected dogs; normal ratio makes diagnosis of HAC very unlikely.
- False-positive results common; only ~20% of dogs with elevated UC : Cr have HAC.
- Due to chance of false-positive, always do ACTH stimulation test or low-dose dexamethasone suppression test to confirm presence of HAC.

Low-Dose Dexamethasone Suppression Test (LDDST)

- Lack of suppression 8h after injection of low dose of dexamethasone consistent with diagnosis of HAC.
- Sensitivity ~95% in dogs.
- In dogs with nonadrenal illness, relatively high chance of false-positive.
- Lack of suppression at 4h but full suppression at 8h technically not consistent with HAC, but suspicious for its presence; further testing warranted.
- LDDST may also serve as differentiation test; if 8h sample >1.4 μg/dL, result consistent with HAC; if also suppression to <1.4 μg/dL at 4h post dexamethasone (i.e., "escape" at 8h post dexamethasone) or 4h and/or 8h post-dexamethasone samples <50% of baseline, results consistent with

PDH; if criteria for PDH not met, chances still ~⅔ for PDH vs. AN.
- If baseline values close to 1.4 µg/dL or suppression just at 50%, confirm presence of PDH by other means.
- Protocol exists in Utrecht, Netherlands, where min 2 morning urine samples collected and then dexamethasone administered (3 doses over 24h) for differentiating purposes and another urine sample collected; protocol reportedly has high sensitivity and specificity, but urinary cortisol assay proprietary and not commercially available; accuracy of protocol using cortisol assays commercially available in United States not established, so method not recommended in North America.

ACTH Stimulation Test
- Response > normal consistent with diagnosis of spontaneous HAC, but cannot differentiate between PDH and AN.
- Overall sensitivity of test ~80%; for PDH, sensitivity ~87%; for HAC due to AN sensitivity ~61%.
- More specific in dogs than LDDST (only 15% chance of false-positive with nonadrenal illness).
- Only test that can diagnose iatrogenic HAC; diagnosis made with history of glucocorticoid exposure by any route, consistent clinical signs, and post-ACTH cortisol concentration < reference range.
- Cosyntropin (or tetracosactrin) recommended form; if using compounded ACTH, collect samples before and at 1h and 2h post ACTH administration so peak response not missed.

Differentiating Tests

High-Dose Dexamethasone Suppression Test (HDDST)
- Two responses consistent with PDH—suppression to <1.4 µg/dL at 4h and/or 8h post dexamethasone; or 4h and/or 8h post-dexamethasone samples <50% of baseline.
- If baseline values close to 1.4 µg/dL or suppression just at 50%, confirm presence of PDH by other means.
- Can *never* confirm presence of AN; if criteria for diagnosis of PDH not met, 50/50 chance patient has PDH or AN; since HDDST does not significantly increase ability to differentiate PDH from AN, endogenous ACTH (eACTH) and/or abdominal US used instead.

eACTH Concentration
- Requires only single blood sample, but inappropriate handling can lead to decreased eACTH concentrations due to degradation.
- In patients with PDH, eACTH concentration usually normal to increased; with AN, eACTH concentration < normal.
- If concentration increased, consistent with PDH, but due to episodic secretion of ACTH even in patients with PDH, low value does not always confirm AN.
- If eACTH concentration falls in gray zone, results not diagnostic.

IMAGING
- Abdominal radiographs—~40–50% of canine ANs seen; adrenal mineralization suspicious for AN.
- Thoracic radiographs indicated in patients with AN to check for metastases.
- US—useful for staging AN, but poor screening test (adrenal enlargement occurs with chronic nonadrenal illness, AN may be difficult to see with US); adrenal atrophy can be difficult to determine with US, but bilaterally enlarged adrenal glands consistent with PDH; vena caval invasion and metastasis may be present with AN.
- CT and MRI—can show pituitary macroadenomas and assess AN invasion into adjacent structures; follow-up and treatment recommendations (e.g., radiation therapy) may vary with tumor size.

DIAGNOSTIC PROCEDURES
Adrenal histopathology following adrenalectomy for AN often needed to differentiate benign vs. malignant tumor; biopsy prior to removal may result in complications.

PATHOLOGIC FINDINGS
- PDH—normal to enlarged pituitary and bilateral adrenocortical enlargement.
- Microscopically, pituitary adenoma, adenocarcinoma, or corticotroph hyperplasia of pars distalis or pars intermedia and adrenocortical hyperplasia.
- AN—variable-sized adrenal mass, atrophy of contralateral gland (rarely bilateral tumors), metastasis and invasion into vena cava with thrombosis possible.
- Microscopically, adrenocortical adenoma or carcinoma.

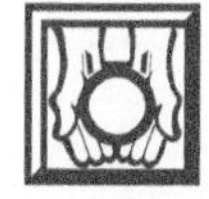

TREATMENT

APPROPRIATE HEALTH CARE
Dictated by severity of clinical signs, patient's overall condition, any complicating factors (e.g., DM, pulmonary thromboembolism).

CLIENT EDUCATION
- For medical therapy, lifelong therapy required.
- If adverse reaction to mitotane or trilostane occurs—discontinue drug, give dexamethisone, have veterinarian reevaluate next day; if no response noted in few hours, veterinarian should evaluate immediately.

SURGICAL CONSIDERATIONS
- Hypophysectomy—described, but limited availability.
- Bilateral adrenalectomy not used for treatment of PDH.
- Surgery treatment of choice in dogs with adrenocortical adenomas and carcinomas unless patient poor surgical candidate.
- Appropriate personnel and facilities required as adrenalectomy (especially with vena caval thrombi) is technically demanding and intensive postoperative management required.
- Surgery not curative, but long-term survival possible
- Medical control of HAC may be desirable prior to surgery.

H

MEDICATIONS

DRUG(S) OF CHOICE

Trilostane
- Trilostane (Vetoryl®) inhibits adrenocortical enzyme 3-β-hydroxysteroid dehydrogenase and maybe others, thereby suppressing production of progesterone and its end-products, including cortisol and aldosterone (less than cortisol); efficacy and survival time for treatment of PDH excellent.
- Initial dose 2–3 mg/kg PO q24h (in morning) or divided q12h with food; twice-daily dosing more expensive, but quicker resolution of clinical signs, fewer dose changes and monitoring tests; if q24h dosing elected and patient controlled during day but has more clinical signs at night, splitting daily dose ½ morning and ½ evening may improve clinical signs.
- Side effects include lethargy, decreased appetite, vomiting, diarrhea; sometimes occur within first few days of therapy and associated with gastrointestinal upset due to administration of oral medication; hypocortisolemia can also occur due to oversuppression of cortisol production and cause same clinical signs; rarely, idiosyncratic adrenal necrosis with hypocortisolemia and hypoaldosteronism, but less common with lower doses (as recommended above).
- Monitoring—primary goals to control clinical signs and avoid complications (especially hypocortisolemia); should include assessment of clinical signs (PU/PD, polyphagia, panting) and cortisol testing (see below) to ensure cortisol not suppressed excessively; obtaining detailed history and evidence of potential oversuppression of cortisol imperative.
- Historically, ACTH stimulation test used to monitor trilostane therapy, 4–6h post trilostane administration; 1 µg/kg cosyntropin IV effective for monitoring, but *not* for diagnosis (must use 5 µg/kg); ideal post-ACTH cortisol concentration 2–6 µg/dL, but must consider clinical signs; e.g., if patient clinically controlled with post-ACTH cortisol of 7.2 µg/dL, no need to increase dose; if clinical signs persist, dose increase recommended.

- Studies show post-ACTH stimulation cortisol values do not always correlate well with clinical signs, measuring cortisol concentration before morning dose of trilostane may correlate better; assessing clinical signs imperative when using pre-pill cortisol concentration for monitoring; if patient showing signs of hypocortisolemia (vomiting, diarrhea, decreased appetite), must use ACTH stimulation test; data lacking on decision-making using pre-pill cortisol, but some guidelines: cortisol concentration used to confirm patient not cortisol deficient (<1.4-2 μg/dL), clinical signs used to determine whether dose adequate; if patient clinically controlled and cortisol 2–6 μg/dL, appropriate to continue current dose; if <2 μg/dL, perform ACTH stimulation test or decrease dose; if patient still clinical (PU/PD, polyphagic, panting) and pre-pill cortisol >6 μg/dL, safe to increase dose; in clinically uncontrolled patient, cortisol concentration 2–6 μg/dL is gray zone: probably safe to increase dose if pre-pill cortisol 5 μg/dL, but probably not at 2.5 μg/dL; perform ACTH stimulation test in this situation.
- Perform either ACTH stimulation test or pre-pill cortisol at 10–14 days, 30 days, and 90 days after each dose change; if at 10–14-day recheck any improvement seen, do not increase dose even if cortisol concentration above ideal; wait until 30-day recheck and change dose then if necessary, as effect of trilostane often increases between 2 and 4 weeks; assess renal profile, including electrolytes, at 14- or 30-day exam; once clinical condition and dose stabilized, perform pre-pill cortisol or ACTH stimulation test, and electrolyte panel, q3–6 months.
- If lethargy, decreased appetite, vomiting, or diarrhea occurs, ACTH stimulation test to confirm dog not hypocortisolemic (post-ACTH stimulation cortisol <2 μg/dL); if hypocortisolemia confirmed, assess electrolyte panel to ensure hyponatremia and hyperkalemia not present; discontinue trilostane until clinical signs of HAC recur and baseline and/or post-ACTH cortisol concentrations >5-6 μg/dL.
- If signs of hypocortisolemia more severe than mild lethargy, vomiting, decreased appetite, give dexamethasone 0.1 mg/kg/day PO/IV, then taper to lowest effective dose to control signs; if signs of HAC recur, taper dexamethasone and discontinue, then perform baseline cortisol and/or ACTH stimulation test interpreted as above; if dexamethasone unavailable and prednisone used instead, delay cortisol testing until at least 24h after last prednisone dose, as prednisone can cross-react with cortisol assay.
- If more severe signs occur, hospitalization with IV fluids, dexamethasone, and other supportive therapy necessary.
- Hypocortisolemia secondary to trilostane administration usually resolves within 48–72h of drug discontinuation, but temporary cortisol suppression of weeks to months and even permanent suppression can occur.
- Trilostane can be used to treat hypercortisolemia from AN and usually controls clinical signs; although mitotane theoretically preferred due to chemotherapeutic properties, no difference shown between survival of patients with AN treated with mitotane or trilostane.

Mitotane

- Mitotane (o,p′-DDD, Lysodren®) selectively destroys glucocorticoid-secreting cells of adrenal cortex; in patients with AN may destroy tumor cells as well as controlling cortisol secretion, but no difference in survival between dogs with AN receiving mitotane vs. trilostane.
- PDH—initial loading dose 40–50 mg/kg PO divided twice daily; evaluate efficacy with ACTH stimulation test after 8 days, or sooner if decreased appetite, vomiting, diarrhea, listlessness, decreased water intake (<60 mL/kg/day); target for both basal and post-ACTH cortisol concentration 1–5 μg/dL; continue induction with repeat testing as necessary until adequate response, then initiate maintenance therapy at 50 mg/kg/week PO divided in 2–3 doses; adjust dosage based on ACTH stimulation testing (to maintain basal and post-ACTH cortisol levels in ideal range); if serum cortisol concentration pre- or post-ACTH <1 μg/dL, measure electrolyte concentrations, stop administering mitotane, and give physiologic doses of prednisone (0.1 mg/kg PO q12h; do not give within 24h before ACTH stimulation test); cortisol secretion usually recovers in weeks to months but can take longer; once cortisol concentration in ideal range, discontinue prednisone and begin maintenance therapy; if dog was on maintenance therapy when became cortisol deficient, restart maintenance at 25% lower dose; if relapse occurs at any time on maintenance therapy (as indicated by cortisol levels above ideal range), dose adjustment required; if post-ACTH serum cortisol concentration 5–10 μg/dL, increase maintenance mitotane dose by 25% and reevaluate in 4 weeks; if post-ACTH serum cortisol concentration >10 μg/dL, repeat loading sequence for 5–7 days and repeat ACTH stimulation test; continue loading until cortisol concentration in ideal range, then reinitiate weekly maintenance dose at ~50% higher dose.
- AN—goal of mitotane to achieve low to nondetectable (<1 μg/dL) basal and post-ACTH cortisol concentrations; starting dose 50–75 mg/kg PO divided daily; perform ACTH stimulation test after 10–14 days of therapy to evaluate efficacy, sooner if decreased appetite, vomiting, diarrhea, lethargy, decreased water intake (<60 mL/kg/day); induction typically requires higher doses and longer duration than for treatment of PDH and dose should be increased by 50 mg/kg/day q10–14 days if control not achieved (based on ACTH stimulation test); if adverse effects develop, continue administration at highest tolerable dose; once control achieved, begin maintenance therapy at 75–100 mg/kg/week PO divided into 2–3 doses; if cortisol levels pre- and post-ACTH rise into normal resting range (1–5 μg/dL), increase maintenance dose by 50%; if cortisol levels rise above normal resting range pre- and post-ACTH, reload until control achieved and increase weekly maintenance dose ~50%; because goal of induction and maintenance is to create glucocorticoid insufficiency, prednisone should be administered at 0.2 mg/kg/day PO.
- Aldosterone deficiency possible from mitotane therapy; if it occurs, patient will likely have permanent complete adrenocortical insufficiency and treatment for hypoadrenocorticism should be initiated.

l-Deprenyl

- l-Deprenyl (selegiline hydrochloride); FDA approved for treatment of PDH; decreases pituitary ACTH secretion, thus decreasing serum cortisol concentration.
- Questionable efficacy; not currently recommended.

Ketoconazole

Ketoconazole (10 mg/kg PO q12h initially; up to 20 mg/kg PO q12h in some dogs) inhibits cortisol synthesis; no longer recommended (trilostane causes fewer side effects).

CONTRAINDICATIONS

- Do not use ketoconazole with trilostane therapy (increased potential for hypocortisolism)
- Monitor for hyperkalemia if concurrent angiotensin-converting enzyme inhibitor therapy.

PRECAUTIONS

- Side effects of trilostane include anorexia, lethargy, vomiting, diarrhea; usually mild and resolve with discontinuation and dose adjustment; Addisonian crisis and adrenocortical necrosis reported.
- Use trilostane and mitotane with caution in patients with renal insufficiency and hepatic disease; trilostane contraindicated in pregnancy.
- Side effects of mitotane mild in most dogs; include lethargy, anorexia, vomiting, diarrhea, ataxia, iatrogenic hypoadrenocorticism.
- Side effects more common in dogs with AN given high dose mitotane.
- In diabetic patients, insulin requirement can decrease with control of HAC.

ALTERNATIVE DRUG(S)

Radiation therapy possible to treat pituitary macroadenomas. Treatment with trilostane or mitotane still usually required afterwards. ACTH levels may take several months to decrease and HAC controlled with drugs in interim.

FOLLOW-UP

PATIENT MONITORING

- Response to therapy—use periodic ACTH stimulation and/or cortisol testing to assess trilostane and mitotane efficacy (see above); once on maintenance mitotane therapy, test at 1, 3, and 6 months and q3–6 months thereafter or if clinical signs of HAC recur.
- Adequacy of any mitotane reloading period checked with ACTH stimulation test before higher maintenance dose initiated.
- Adequacy of trilostane dose alterations checked with ACTH stimulation test performed 4–6h after dosing.

PREVENTION/AVOIDANCE

For prevention of recurrence and hypocortisolemia, regular administration of medications with appropriate follow-up required.

POSSIBLE COMPLICATIONS

- Hypertension.
- Proteinuria.
- Recurrent infections.
- Urinary calculi (calcium oxalate).
- DM.
- Pulmonary thromboembolism.
- Neurologic signs secondary to pituitary macroadenoma.
- Hypoadrenocorticism secondary to treatment.

EXPECTED COURSE AND PROGNOSIS

- Untreated HAC—progressive disorder with survival of 6–18 months.
- Treated PDH—usually good prognosis; median survival time with mitotane or trilostane treatment ~2 years; at least 10% survive 4 years; dogs living >6 months tend to die of causes unrelated to HAC.
- Macroadenomas in animals with no or mild neurologic abnormalities have fair to good prognosis with radiation and medical therapy; in patients with significant neurologic abnormalities, prognosis poor to grave.
- Adrenal adenomas—usually good to excellent prognosis; small carcinomas (not metastasized) fair to good prognosis overall, good to excellent with surgical resection.
- Large carcinomas and AN with widespread metastasis—generally poor to fair prognosis, but impressive responses to high doses of mitotane occasionally seen.

MISCELLANEOUS

ASSOCIATED CONDITIONS

Neurologic signs in dogs with pituitary tumors; glucose intolerance or concurrent DM; pulmonary thromboembolism; increased incidence of infections, especially UTI and skin; hypertension; proteinuria/ glomerulopathy.

ABBREVIATIONS

- ACTH = adrenocorticotropic hormone.
- ALP = alkaline phosphatase.
- ALT = alanine aminotransferase.
- AN = adrenal neoplasia.
- DM = diabetes mellitus.
- eACTH = endogenous ACTH.
- HAC = hyperadrenocorticism.
- HDDST = high-dose dexamethasone-suppression test.
- LDDST = low-dose dexamethasone-suppression test.
- PDH = pituitary-dependent HAC.
- PU/PD = polyuria/polydipsia.
- UC : Cr = urine cortisol : creatinine.
- UTI = urinary tract infection.

Suggested Reading

Behrend EN, Kooistra HS, Nelson R, et al. Diagnosis of spontaneous canine hyperadrenocorticism: 2012 ACVIM consensus statement (small animal). J Vet Intern Med 2013, 27:1292–1304.

Braddock JA, Church DB, Robertson ID, et al. Trilostane treatment in dogs with pituitary-dependent hyperadrenocorticism. Aust Vet J 2003, 81:600–607.

Kintzer PP, Peterson ME. Mitotane (o,p′-ddd) treatment of 200 dogs with pituitary-dependent hyperadenocorticism. J Vet Intern Med 1991, 5:182–190.

Nagata N, Kokima K, Yuki M. Comparison of survival times for dogs with pituitary-dependent hyperadrenocorticism in a primary-care hospital: treated with trilostane versus untreated. J Vet Intern Med 2017, 31:22–28.

Vaughn MA, Feldman EC, Hoar BR, Nelson RW. Evaluation of twice-daily, low-dose trilostane treatment administered orally in dogs with naturally occurring hyperadrenocorticism. J Am Vet Med Assoc 2008, 232:1321–1328.

Author Patty A. Lathan

Consulting Editor Patty A. Lathan

Acknowledgment The author and book editors acknowledge the prior contribution of Deborah S. Greco

Client Education Handout available online

H

HYPERCALCEMIA

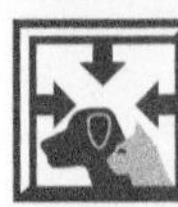

BASICS

DEFINITION

- Serum total calcium >11.5 mg/dL (dogs).
- Serum total calcium >10.5 mg/dL (cats).
- Serum ionized calcium >1.45 mmol/L (dogs).
- Serum ionized calcium >1.4 mmol/L (cats).
- Hypercalcemia must be confirmed by demonstration of increased concentrations of *ionized* calcium.
- Total calcium concentrations and correction formulas do not accurately predict ionized calcium and their use is discouraged.

PATHOPHYSIOLOGY

- Control of calcium is complex, tightly regulated, and influenced by the actions of parathyroid hormone (PTH), vitamin D, and the interaction of these hormones with the gastrointestinal tract, bone, kidneys, and parathyroid glands.
- Derangement in the function of these can lead to hypercalcemia.
- Secretory products of some neoplastic cells can also disturb calcium homeostasis.

SYSTEMS AFFECTED

- Cardiovascular—hypertension and altered cardiac contractility.
- Gastrointestinal—reduced smooth muscle excitability and potentially altered gastrointestinal function.
- Neuromuscular—depressed skeletal muscle contractility causes weakness.
- Renal/urologic—high calcium concentrations are toxic to the renal tubules and can cause polyuria and polydipsia (PU/PD) and renal failure; can also lead to urolithiasis and associated lower urinary tract disease.

SIGNALMENT

- Dog and cat.
- Primary hyperparathyroidism in the keeshond and Siamese cats.
- Primary hyperparathyroidism and neoplasia are more likely in geriatric dogs.

SIGNS

General Comments

- Depend on the cause of hypercalcemia.
- Patients with underlying neoplasia, renal failure, or hypoadrenocorticism generally appear ill.
- Patients with primary hyperparathyroidism show mild clinical signs, if any.
- Signs become apparent when hypercalcemia is severe and chronic.

Historical Findings

- Many asymptomatic.
- PU/PD—most common in dogs.
- Lethargy—most common in cats.
- Anorexia.
- Vomiting.
- Constipation.
- Weakness.
- Stupor and coma—severe cases.
- Lower urinary tract signs (e.g., stranguria) in animals with secondary calcium-containing uroliths.

Physical Examination Findings

- Lymphadenomegaly or abdominal organomegaly (patients with lymphoma).
- Rectal or mammary masses.
- Fundic examination may reveal evidence for granulomatous disease.
- Unremarkable in dogs with primary hyperparathyroidism.
- Parathyroid gland adenoma may be palpable in cats with primary hyperparathyroidism, but can be confused with the thyroid gland.

CAUSES

- Neoplasia—lymphoma (most common in dogs, less common in cats), anal sac apocrine gland adenocarcinoma (dogs), multiple myeloma, lymphocytic leukemia, metastatic bone tumor, fibrosarcoma (cats), other carcinomas.
- Primary hyperparathyroidism.
- Renal failure (acute or chronic).
- Granulomatous diseases (blastomycosis, histoplasmosis, schistosomiasis).
- Hypoadrenocorticism.
- Vitamin D intoxication from ingestion of human psoriasis medication or cholecalciferol rodenticide, or from plant or food sources.
- Osteolytic diseases.
- Idiopathic (most common cause in cats).
- Laboratory error.
- Occasionally observed in cats with hyperthyroidism.

RISK FACTORS

- Keeshond breed (hyperparathyroidism).
- Renal failure.
- Neoplasia.
- Use of calcium supplements or calcium-containing intestinal phosphate binders.
- Use of calcitriol or other vitamin D preparations.

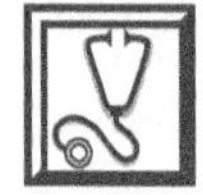

DIAGNOSIS

DIFFERENTIAL DIAGNOSIS

- History should include questions regarding exposure to exogenous vitamin D sources and any previous response to corticosteroids.
- History of waxing/waning illness suggests hypoadrenocorticism, renal failure, or emerging neoplasia.
- Complete lymph node, rectal, and abdominal palpation may raise index of suspicion for lymphoma or other neoplasia.
- Assessment of hydration status, renal palpation, and urinary history may point toward renal or lower urinary tract disease.

LABORATORY FINDINGS

Drugs That May Alter Laboratory Results

- Oxalate, citrate, and EDTA anticoagulants bind calcium and falsely lower calcium measurement.
- Thiazide diuretics can raise serum calcium concentrations.

Disorders That May Alter Laboratory Results

- Hemolysis and lipemia can falsely raise calcium concentrations.
- Hypoalbuminemia can lower total calcium concentration.

Valid if Run in Human Laboratory?

Yes

CBC/BIOCHEMISTRY/URINALYSIS

- Serum calcium—total calcium concentrations reflect the combination of protein-bound calcium, complexed calcium, and biologically active ionized calcium; elevations in total calcium should prompt clinicians to evaluate ionized calcium concentrations.
- Azotemia and urine specific gravity help to define degree of renal impairment.
- Serum phosphorus is usually low or low-normal in patients with primary hyperparathyroidism or hypercalcemia associated with malignancy.
- Hyperphosphatemia in the absence of azotemia suggests a nonparathyroid cause of hypercalcemia.
- Combination of hyperphosphatemia and azotemia is difficult to interpret because renal failure can be the cause or effect of hypercalcemia.
- Hyperkalemia and hyponatremia suggest hypoadrenocorticism.
- Hyperglobulinemia is associated with multiple myeloma.
- Cytopenias are seen in patients with myelophthisic disease.

OTHER LABORATORY TESTS

- Serum ionized calcium is high in patients with primary hyperparathyroidism or hypercalcemia associated with malignancy; usually normal or low in patients with hypercalcemia associated with renal failure.
- Serum PTH measurement—intact molecule and two-site assay methods have the greatest specificity; high-normal or high concentration suggests primary hyperparathyroidism; can be high in patients with chronic renal failure; low concentration makes neoplasia more likely; normal PTH concentrations do *not* exclude a diagnosis of primary hyperparathyroidism.
- Serum PTH-related peptide (PTH-rp) measurement is often high in patients with hypercalcemia associated with malignancy; lack of elevation in PTH-rp concentration does *not* exclude neoplasia as a possible cause of hypercalcemia.

• Serum Vitamin D assays are available at specific laboratories.
• Fecal PCR testing for schistosomiasis.

IMAGING

• Radiography is useful for assessing renal size and shape, urolithiasis, bone lysis, pulmonary infiltration, lymphadenomegaly, and occult neoplasia.
• Ultrasonography is valuable for assessing renal architecture, abdominal lymphadenomegaly, parathyroid tumors, and urolithiasis.

DIAGNOSTIC PROCEDURES

• Cytologic examination of fine-needle aspirate of lymph nodes, liver, spleen, anal glands, or other tumors or masses to diagnose neoplasia.
• Bone marrow aspirate or biopsy—to identify occult hematopoietic neoplasia.
• Adrenocorticotropic hormone (ACTH) stimulation testing to confirm hypoadrenocorticism.

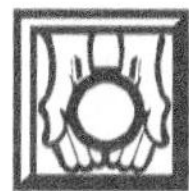

TREATMENT

• Definitive treatment of hypercalcemia is achieved by identification and correction of the primary cause.
• Inpatient care may be necessary because of the deleterious effects of hypercalcemia and the need for fluid therapy (diuresis).
• Consider severe hypercalcemia (ionized calcium >2.2 mmol/L) a medical emergency.

MEDICATIONS

DRUG(S) OF CHOICE

• Normal saline—fluid of choice (sodium promotes calcium excretion).
• Diuretics (furosemide) and corticosteroids promote calciuresis.
• Pamidronate or other bisphosphonate drugs (e.g., alendronate) have been used successfully for treatment of hypercalcemia of various causes in dogs and cats.

CONTRAINDICATIONS

• Do not use glucocorticoids until the diagnosis of lymphoma or other round cell neoplasia is excluded; they can obfuscate the diagnosis; if hypoadrenocorticism is suspected, do not give glucocorticoids until after ACTH stimulation testing, or use dexamethasone, which will not interfere with the serum cortisol assay.
• Thiazide diuretics can cause calcium retention.
• Oral bisphosphonates can cause esophageal erosions and should be used with caution.

PRECAUTIONS

Do not give diuretics to a dehydrated patient.

POSSIBLE INTERACTIONS

Avoid the use of calcium or phosphorus-containing compounds; they can cause soft tissue mineralization in severely hypercalcemic and hyperphosphatemic patients.

ALTERNATIVE DRUG(S)

• Sodium bicarbonate (1–4 mEq/kg) may be useful in combination with other treatments when metabolic acidosis is present.
• Calcitonin may be useful in the treatment of hypervitaminosis D.
• Hemodialysis and peritoneal dialysis are alternative treatments for some causes of hypercalcemia, but cost and availability limit their use.
• Novel therapies like calcimimetic drugs may hold potential for certain causes of hypercalcemia such as idiopathic hypercalcemia or primary hyperparathyroidism; cost is currently a deterrent, as is lack of routine efficacy.
• Mithramycin has been used in severe hypercalcemic crises; avoid its use because of associated nephrotoxicity and hepatotoxicity.

FOLLOW-UP

PATIENT MONITORING

• Serum calcium every 12 hours (ionized calcium if possible).
• Renal function assessment—the first sign of tubular damage may be casts in the urine sediment.
• Must closely monitor urine output, particularly if oligo-anuric renal failure is present.
• Hydration status must be monitored; indicators of overhydration include increased bodyweight, chemosis, and edema (pulmonary or subcutaneous).

POSSIBLE COMPLICATIONS

• Irreversible renal failure.
• Soft tissue mineralization.

MISCELLANEOUS

ASSOCIATED CONDITIONS

Calcium-containing urolithiasis.

AGE-RELATED FACTORS

• Mild elevations in calcium and phosphorus may be normal in growing animals.
• Middle-aged and older dogs and cats are at increased risk for cancer.

PREGNANCY/FERTILITY/BREEDING

A fetus is at the same risk as the dam; do not alter treatment because of pregnancy.

SEE ALSO

• Acute Kidney Injury.
• Chronic Kidney Disease.
• Hyperparathyroidism.
• Lymphoma—Dogs.
• Paraneoplastic Syndromes.

ABBREVIATIONS

• ACTH = adrenocorticotropic hormone.
• PTH = parathyroid hormone.
• PTH-rp = parathyroid hormone–related peptide.
• PU/PD = polyuria/polydipsia.

Suggested Reading

Daniels E, Sakakeeny C. Hypercalcemia: pathophysiology, clinical signs, and emergent treatment. J Am Anim Hosp Assoc 2015, 51(5):291–299.
de Brito Galvao JF, Parker V, Schenck PA, Chew DJ. Update on feline ionized hypercalcemia. Vet Clin North Am Small Anim Pract 2017, 47(2):273–292.
Greco DS. Endocrine causes of calcium disorders. Top Companion Anim Med 2012, 27(4):150–155.
Hostutler RA, Chew DJ, Jaeger JQ, et al. Uses and effectiveness of pamidronate disodium for treatment of dogs and cats with hypercalcemia. J Vet Intern Med 2005, 19(1):29–33.
Schenck PA, Chew DJ. Calcium: total or ionized? Vet Clin North Am Small Anim Pract 2008, 38(3):497–502.

Author Brett A. Wasik
Consulting Editor Patty A. Lathan
Acknowledgment The author and book editors acknowledge the prior contribution of Thomas K. Graves

Client Education Handout available online

HYPERCAPNIA

BASICS

DEFINITION

- An increase in the partial pressure of carbon dioxide in arterial blood ($PaCO_2$).
- Normal $PaCO_2$ values—35–45 mmHg.
- Hypercapnia is synonymous with hypercarbia.

PATHOPHYSIOLOGY

- CO_2—end product of aerobic cellular metabolism; considered the primary drive for ventilation by stimulation of central chemoreceptors in the medulla oblongata; carried in the blood in three forms: bicarbonate (65%), bound to hemoglobin (30%), and dissolved in plasma (5%; the source of $PaCO_2$ values); constantly being added to alveolar gas from the pulmonary circulation and removed by alveolar ventilation.
- Uncommonly encountered in nonanesthetized, clinically normal patient; result of alveolar hypoventilation.

SYSTEMS AFFECTED

- Cardiovascular—may result in endogenous catecholamine release, which may induce cardiac arrhythmias; may cause vasodilation leading to hypotension.
- Hemic/lymphatic/immune—may alter acid-base balance; acute increase results in production of excess hydrogen ions and decrease in pH (respiratory acidosis).
- Nervous—brain is primary affected organ; cerebral blood flow related to $PaCO_2$ in a linear fashion; hypercapnia results in increased cerebral blood flow and intracranial pressure; $PaCO_2$ >90 mmHg may lead to CO_2 narcosis and unconsciousness.

SIGNALMENT

Any breed, age, and sex of dog and cat.

SIGNS

Historical Findings

- Abnormal breathing pattern.
- Weakness—secondary to concurrent hypoxemia or primary neuromuscular disease.

Physical Examination Findings

- Anesthetized patients—usually no obvious signs; severe condition may lead to tachypnea, hypotension, and tachycardia.
- Hypoventilation owing to muscle weakness or neuropathy—weak respiratory efforts; decreased thoracic excursion; excessive abdominal effort; exaggerated movement of facial muscles during inspiration; possibly generalized weakness as a result of primary neuromuscular disorder (myasthenia gravis, polyradiculoneuropathy).
- Upper airway obstruction—marked, prolonged inspiratory efforts with variable expirations, depending on whether the obstruction is fixed (e.g., mass) or nonfixed (e.g., laryngeal paralysis); stertor or stridor common.
- Pleural effusion—may have shallow rapid respirations; may note a marked abdominal component; lung sounds decreased in ventral thorax.
- Pulmonary parenchymal disease—increased bronchovesicular sounds; crackles (edema, infection, contusions).

CAUSES

- Hypoventilation can result from anesthesia, muscular paralysis, upper airway obstruction, air or fluid in the pleural space, restriction in movement of the thoracic cage, diaphragmatic hernia, pulmonary parenchymal disease, drug therapy to control seizures, opioid and alpha-2 agonist use for analgesia, and CNS disease. Can occur in spontaneously breathing patients during inhalation anesthesia (isoflurane or sevoflurane).
- Increased inspired CO_2—rebreathing of expired gases because of accumulation of exhausted CO_2 absorbent in an anesthesia machine most common cause; also inadequate fresh gas flow in a non-rebreathing anesthesia circuit (e.g., Bain and Ayres T-Piece).
- Exogenous administration of sodium bicarbonate, which dissociates into CO_2, with inadequate ventilation.

RISK FACTORS

- Use of inhalation agent (isoflurane or sevoflurane) as sole anesthetic, since inhalation anesthetics are potent respiratory depressants.
- Use of opioid or alpha-2 agonist analgesia.
- Deep planes of inhalation anesthesia.
- Inadequate fresh flow of oxygen with non-rebreathing anesthesia circuits.
- Bronchial or alveolar disease.
- Upper airway obstruction.
- Pleural disease.
- Inadequate ventilation during administration of sodium bicarbonate.
- Severe cervical spinal cord compression.
- Severe lower motor neuron disease.

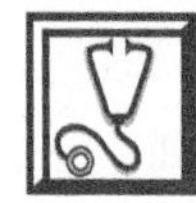

DIAGNOSIS

DIFFERENTIAL DIAGNOSIS

- Conscious patient—hyperthermia; hypoxemia; head trauma.
- Anesthetized patient—hypoxemia.

LABORATORY FINDINGS

Drugs That May Alter Laboratory Results

N/A

Disorders That May Alter Laboratory Results

Air bubbles in the arterial blood sample and/or improper packaging of the arterial blood sample—falsely low $PaCO_2$ values after approximately 30 min.

Valid if Run in Human Laboratory?

Yes

CBC/BIOCHEMISTRY/URINALYSIS

N/A

OTHER LABORATORY TESTS

- Arterial blood gas analysis—diagnosis determined from a blood sample collected in an anaerobic manner, as follows: use enough heparin to coat the needle and the inside of the syringe; obtain sample from femoral or dorsal pedal artery; place a rubber stopper on the needle or cover the hub of the syringe to prevent room air from entering the sample.
- Analyze sample within 15 minutes if left at room temperature; place sample on ice to extend time for safe and accurate analysis to 2–4 hours.
- Bedside or portable blood gas analyzers—several models available; make analysis more convenient.

IMAGING

Thoracic radiography—may reveal bronchial, alveolar, or pleural space disease. Cervical radiography can suggest a large airway obstruction.

DIAGNOSTIC PROCEDURES

- Upper airway endoscopy used to rule out laryngeal mass or paralysis.
- Alternative method of analysis—capnometer (see Figures 1 and 2).
- End-tidal gas ($PetCO_2$) is almost entirely alveolar gas and provides nearly the same value

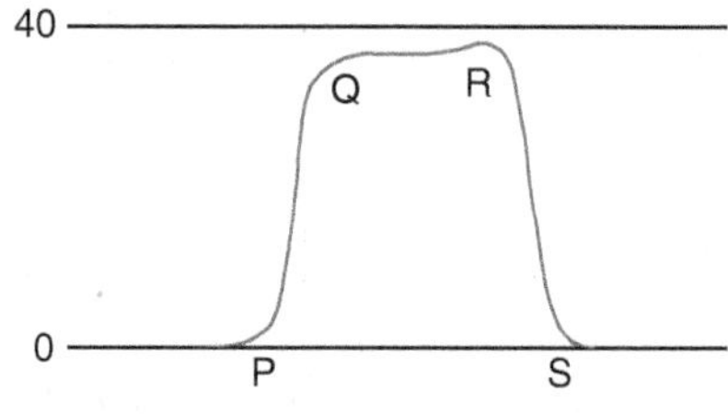

Figure 1.

Normal capnogram. The wave segment from P to Q is exhalation; Q to R is the plateau after exhalation; point R is the end tidal CO_2; R to S is inhalation.

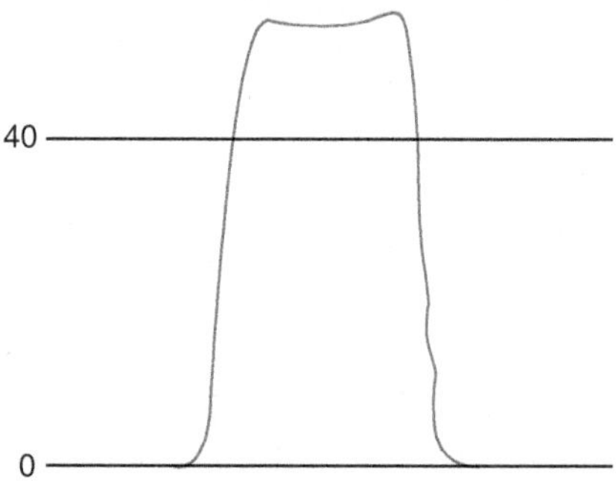

Figure 2.

Capnogram with hypercapnia. The plateau and end tidal CO_2 are above normal.

for CO_2 as $PaCO_2$, which closely approximates the mean value of perfused alveoli.
• Advantage of capnometry—can monitor $PaCO_2$ on a breath-by-breath basis, whereas a blood gas sample is a finite value at a finite time.
• Disadvantages—tachypnea and insufficient tidal volume will result in falsely low $PetCO_2$; $PaCO_2$ much higher than $PetCO_2$ with pulmonary thromboembolism; open thoracic cavity (surgery) reports falsely low $PetCO_2$ due to excessive dead space.

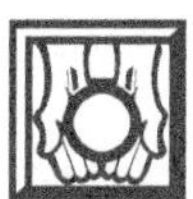

TREATMENT

• Provide adequate alveolar ventilation.
• Anesthesia—ventilation accomplished manually or mechanically with anesthesia ventilator.
• Nonanesthetized patient with severe pulmonary or CNS disease—mechanical ventilation with critical care ventilator; generally requires heavy sedation.
• Supplemental oxygen—need determined by primary disease; providing supplemental oxygen without providing ventilation will likely not correct hypercapnia.
• Definitive treatment—treat primary cause; discontinue inhalation anesthesia or provide ventilation during anesthesia; diagnostics for neuromuscular disease.

MEDICATIONS

DRUG(S) OF CHOICE

Respiratory stimulants not indicated and rarely reverse hypoventilation.

CONTRAINDICATIONS

Anesthetic drugs or other respiratory depressants—contraindicated with CNS disease if adequate ventilatory support cannot be provided; increased $PaCO_2$ may result in dangerous elevations of intracranial pressure and predispose patient to herniation of the brainstem.

PRECAUTIONS

N/A

POSSIBLE INTERACTIONS

N/A

FOLLOW-UP

PATIENT MONITORING

• Assess effectiveness of supportive therapy (ventilation) and definitive treatment—should result in decreased respiratory effort.
• Reevaluate arterial blood gas or capnometry—determine improvement; assess adequacy of ventilation.

POSSIBLE COMPLICATIONS

Concurrent CNS disease may cause high intracranial pressure and predispose the patient to herniation of the brainstem and death.

MISCELLANEOUS

ASSOCIATED CONDITIONS

N/A

AGE-RELATED FACTORS

N/A

PREGNANCY/FERTILITY/BREEDING

N/A

SYNONYMS

• Hypercarbia.
• Hypoventilation.

SEE ALSO

• Dyspnea and Respiratory Distress.
• Panting and Tachypnea.

ABBREVIATIONS

• $PaCO_2$ = partial pressure of carbon dioxide in arterial blood.
• $PetCO_2$ = end-tidal carbon dioxide.

Suggested Reading

Daly ML. Hypoventilation. In: Silverstein DC, Hopper K, eds. Small Animal Critical Care Medicine, 2nd ed. St. Louis, MO: Elsevier Saunders, 2015, pp. 86–92.
Haskins SC. Monitoring anesthetized patients. In: Grimm KA, Lamont LA, Tranquilli WJ, et al., eds. Veterinary Anesthesia and Analgesia, 5th ed. Ames, IA: Wiley-Blackwell, 2015, pp. 100–102.
McDonell WN, Kerr CL. Respiratory system. In: Grimm KA, Lamont LA, Tranquilli WJ, et al., eds. Veterinary Anesthesia and Analgesia, 5th ed. Ames, IA: Wiley-Blackwell, 2015, pp. 513–543.

Author Thomas K. Day
Consulting Editor Elizabeth Rozanski

HYPERCHLOREMIA

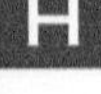

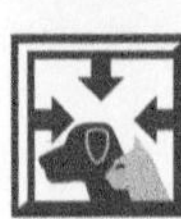

BASICS

DEFINITION

Serum chloride concentration above reference interval (generally >122 mEq/L in dogs and >129 mEq/L in cats).

PATHOPHYSIOLOGY

- Chloride is the most abundant anion in extracellular fluid.
- Hyperchloremia is associated with free water loss or excessive NaCl intake (oral or parenteral).
- Serum chloride concentration varies inversely to bicarbonate concentration; high bicarbonate loss (i.e., vomiting or renal wasting) is followed by renal chloride resorption and hyperchloremia.

SYSTEMS AFFECTED

Relate to underlying cause.

SIGNALMENT

Species

Dog and cat.

SIGNS

General Comments

- Related to concurrent hypernatremia (i.e., free water loss) or underlying disorder, or both.
- Severity of neurologic signs related to degree of hypernatremia and rate of development.

Historical and Physical Examination Findings

- Polydipsia.
- Disorientation.
- Seizures.
- Coma.

CAUSES

High Total Body Chloride

- Oral ingestion (salt or salt water)—rare.
- NaCl (0.9% or hypertonic) or other chloride salts administered IV.

Normal Total Body Chloride with Water Deficit

- High urinary water loss (e.g., diabetes insipidus).
- Low intake (e.g., no access to water).
- Insensible water loss (e.g., panting).

Low Total Body Chloride with Hypotonic Fluid Loss

- Urinary loss—diabetes mellitus, hypoadrenocorticism, osmotic diuresis, postobstructive diuresis.
- Drugs that interfere with ability to concentrate urine—lithium, demeclocycline, and amphotericin.
- Drugs that cause renal chloride retention—acetazolamide, ammonium chloride, androgens, cholestyramine, and spironolactone.

Hyperchloremic Metabolic Acidosis

- Normal anion gap.
- Renal tubular acidosis—renal tubular disorders causing wasting of bicarbonate or low hydrogen ion secretion.
- Diarrhea causing gastrointestinal loss of bicarbonate and renal resorption of chloride.
- Chronic respiratory alkalosis.

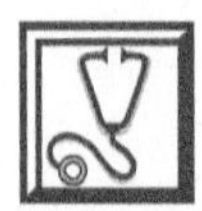

DIAGNOSIS

DIFFERENTIAL DIAGNOSIS

- Diabetes insipidus.
- Dehydration.
- Renal tubular acidosis.
- Diabetic ketoacidosis.
- Salt or salt water ingestion—rare.

LABORATORY FINDINGS

Drugs That May Alter Laboratory Results

A falsely high chloride concentration can occur with high serum concentrations of iodide or bromide (e.g., patients treated with potassium bromide) if ion-selective electrodes are used for measurement.

Disorders That May Alter Laboratory Results

Hemoglobin and bilirubin cause falsely high chloride readings if colorimetric tests are used. Lipemia may result in an artifactual hyperchloremia.

Valid if Run in Human Laboratory?

Yes

CBC/BIOCHEMISTRY/URINALYSIS

- Often coupled with hypernatremia.
- Diabetes insipidus—hyposthenuria, azotemia.
- Diabetic ketoacidosis—hyperglycemia, ketonemia, and ketonuria.
- Dehydration—urine specific gravity >1.030, prerenal azotemia.
- Renal tubular acidosis—metabolic acidosis in the presence of alkaline urine, hypokalemia, other causes of metabolic acidosis (e.g., azotemia, hyperlactatemia, ketonemia) not present.

OTHER LABORATORY TESTS

- Blood-gas analysis—metabolic acidosis, may have respiratory compensation.
- Anion gap—normal if primary hyperchloremia or bicarbonate loss.

IMAGING

CT or MRI in patients with diabetes insipidus to rule out pituitary tumor.

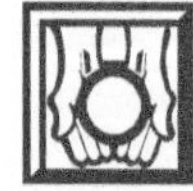

TREATMENT

APPROPRIATE HEALTH CARE

- If hyperchloremia and hypernatremia due to free water loss, administer free water either orally or IV (see below); target a sodium concentration decrease of 12 mEq/day; serum sodium concentration should be rechecked every 4–6 hours and fluids adjusted as necessary to maintain appropriate rate.
- If renal tubular acidosis, treat underlying cause (usually pyelonephritis).
- If renal or gastrointestinal bicarbonate loss, administration of $NaHCO_3$ can be considered.

MEDICATIONS

DRUG(S) OF CHOICE

- Sodium bicarbonate—calculate bicarbonate deficit (0.3 * bodyweight (kg) * [24 mEq – current [$HCO3^-$]]) and give ⅓–½ of this dose slowly IV.
- 5% dextrose in water—calculate free water deficit (see hypernatremia) and administer so that serum sodium does not decrease by more than 0.5 mEq/h (or 12 mEq/day).

PRECAUTIONS

- Rapid correction of hypernatremia can cause cerebral edema.
- Hypocalcemia may develop during correction of serum pH, in patients with borderline low serum ionized calcium concentrations.

FOLLOW-UP

PATIENT MONITORING

Electrolytes, bodyweight, and hydration status.

PREVENTION/AVOIDANCE

Animals should always have access to water.

POSSIBLE COMPLICATIONS

Rapid correction of hypernatremia can lead to cerebral edema.

EXPECTED COURSE AND PROGNOSIS

Vary with underlying cause.

MISCELLANEOUS

SEE ALSO

Hypernatremia

Suggested Reading

DiBartola SP. Fluid, Electrolyte and Acid-Base Disorders in Small Animal Practice, 3rd ed. Philadelphia, PA: Saunders, 2005.
Rose DB, Post T. Clinical Physiology of Acid-Base and Electrolyte Disorders, 5th ed. New York: McGraw-Hill, 2000.

Author Patty A. Lathan
Consulting Editor Patty A. Lathan
Acknowledgment The author and book editors acknowledge the prior contribution of Melinda Fleming.

HYPERCOAGULABILITY

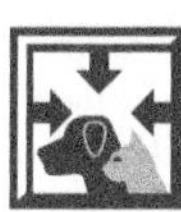

BASICS

OVERVIEW

- Hypercoagulability (aka thrombophilia) is an imbalance between procoagulant and anticoagulant factors that favors thrombosis.
- Thrombus formation occurs in the presence of endothelial injury, altered blood flow, and/or hypercoagulability (Virchow's triad).
- Hypercoagulability may result from platelet hyperaggregability, increased amounts or activation of clotting factors, reduced or inhibited anticoagulant proteins, or defective fibrinolysis.
- Common sites of thrombosis—pulmonary arteries, distal aorta, cranial vena cava, intestinal/mesenteric vessels, portal vein.

SIGNALMENT

Depends on underlying condition.

SIGNS

- Hypercoagulability is symptomless; thrombosis causes site-dependent signs.
- Pulmonary thromboembolism (PTE)—acute severe dyspnea and tachypnea.
- Arterial thromboembolism (ATE)—acute paresis/paralysis, limb pain (ischemic myopathy), decreased pulse and cold limbs; onset in dogs may be gradual vs. peracute in cats.
- Portal vein or caudal vena cava thrombosis—ascites.

CAUSES & RISK FACTORS

- Immune-mediated hemolytic anemia (IMHA).
- Protein-losing nephropathy.
- Hypoproteinemia.
- Systemic inflammation.
- Neoplasia.
- Cardiac disease.
- Hyperadrenocorticism or corticosteroid therapy.

DIAGNOSIS

DIFFERENTIAL DIAGNOSIS

- PTE may mimic pneumonia, pulmonary edema, dirofilariasis.
- Distal ATE—other causes of paraparesis and paraplegia (e.g., neurologic).

CBC/BIOCHEMISTRY/URINALYSIS

Reflect underlying disease or effects of thrombosis in specific organs. Animals with protein-losing nephropathy have proteinuria and elevated urine protein : creatinine ratio, possibly signs of nephrotic syndrome.

OTHER LABORATORY TESTS

- D-dimer—sensitive for fibrinolysis; thrombosis unlikely if normal; nonspecific for cause.
- Antithrombin (AT)—decreased activity increases risk of thrombosis.
- Prothrombin time (PT), activated partial thromboplastin time (APTT)—shortened clotting times are unreliable markers for thrombophilia.
- Thromboelastography, thromboelastometry, rotational thromboelastometry—can potentially identify hypercoagulability.
- Arterial blood gas, pulse oximetry—hypoxemia.

IMAGING

- Ultrasonography—confirm presence of arterial or venous thrombi.
- Echocardiography—identify cardiac disease, intracardiac thrombi, or spontaneous echocontrast ("smoke"); pulmonary hypertension associated with PTE.

DIAGNOSTIC PROCEDURES

- Angiography (standard or CT angiography).
- Nuclear perfusion scintigraphy—can support diagnosis of PTE.

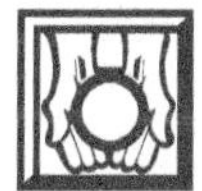

TREATMENT

- Inpatient—supportive care, analgesia, anticoagulation.
- Supportive care—ensure hydration, maintain perfusion, minimize vascular stasis, correct and monitor acid-base and electrolyte abnormalities, use venous catheters appropriately.
- Oxygen therapy for hypoxemia.

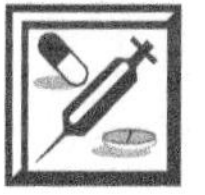

MEDICATIONS

DRUG(S) OF CHOICE

Anticoagulants

- Unfractionated heparin for initial therapy, starting dose: 150–200 IU/kg SC q6-8h; titrate to achieve 1.5-fold increase in APTT; check APTT daily (4h post heparin dose).
- Low molecular weight heparin—enoxaparin: 1 mg/kg (1,000 U/kg) SC q6–12h; dalteparin: 150 mg/kg SC q 6–8h. Monitor anti-Xa activity.
- Rivaroxaban—0.5 mg/kg PO q24h for chronic therapy; no reversal agents available.
- Warfarin for chronic therapy, starting dose: 0.1–0.2 mg/kg PO q24h; adjust dose based on international normalized ratio.

Platelet Inhibition

- Clopidogrel—prophylaxis, prevents repeat thrombosis; dogs: 0.5–1 mg/kg PO q24h; cats: 18.75 mg PO q24h; more effective than aspirin in preventing recurrence of ATE in cats.
- Aspirin—prophylaxis, after thrombosis; dogs: 0.5–5.0 mg/kg PO q12–24h.

Thrombolysis

- Severe side effects possible. Reperfusion injury is common.
- Tissue plasminogen activator (tPA)—1 mg/kg incrementally IV once; most effective in first 3–6 hours after thromboembolism.

CONTRAINDICATIONS/POSSIBLE INTERACTIONS

- Do not treat with warfarin initially; overlap with heparin therapy for 2 days.
- Reassess coagulation with any medication changes.
- If bleeding occurs, discontinue and administer protamine or vitamin K and plasma as indicated to correct hemorrhage.

FOLLOW-UP

- Monitor patients for clinical signs or imaging evidence of resolution of thrombosis.
- Risk of future thromboembolic events.

MISCELLANEOUS

SEE ALSO

- Amyloidosis.
- Anemia, Immune-Mediated.
- Aortic Thromboembolism.
- Disseminated Intravascular Coagulation.
- Pulmonary Thromboembolism.

ABBREVIATIONS

- APTT = activated partial thromboplastin time.
- AT = antithrombin.
- ATE = arterial thromboembolism.
- IMHA = immune-mediated hemolytic anemia.
- PT = prothrombin time.
- PTE = pulmonary thromboembolism.
- tPA = tissue plasminogen activator.

Suggested Reading

deLaforcade A, Bacek L, Blais MC, et al. Consensus on the Rational Use of Antithrombotics in Veterinary Critical Care (CURATIVE): domain 1—defining populations at risk. J Vet Emerg Crit Care 2019, 29(1):37–48.

Wiinberg B, Kristensen AT. Hypercoagulable states. In: Bonagura JD, Twedt DC, eds. Kirk's Current Veterinary Therapy XV. St. Louis, MO: Elsevier Saunders, 2014, pp. 297–301.

Author John A. Christian
Consulting Editor Melinda S. Camus

HYPEREOSINOPHILIC SYNDROME (HES)

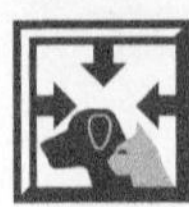

BASICS

OVERVIEW

- Idiopathic, persistent eosinophilia with infiltration of organs causing dysfunction, often leading to death.
- May be caused by a severe reaction to an unidentified antigen and/or dysregulation of immunologic control of eosinophilopoiesis.
- Organ damage caused by effects of eosinophil granule products and eosinophil-derived cytokines that are released in tissues from activated and/or necrotic cells.
- Common sites of infiltration: gastrointestinal (GI) tract (especially intestine and liver), spleen, bone marrow, lung (dogs), and lymph nodes (especially mesenteric).
- More common in cats than dogs.
- Unclear whether HES is a distinct entity from eosinophilic leukemia.
- Generally poor prognosis, especially cats.

SIGNALMENT

- Cats—occurs more frequently in female, middle-aged domestic shorthairs.
- Dogs—Rottweilers may be overrepresented.

SIGNS

- Lethargy.
- Anorexia.
- Intermittent vomiting and diarrhea.
- Hepatosplenomegaly.
- Weight loss.
- Thickened (diffuse or segmental) intestine that is often nonpainful.
- Lymphadenopathy (especially mesenteric).
- Dyspnea.
- Mass lesions caused by eosinophilic granulomatous inflammation and infiltration.
- Less frequently—fever, pruritus, seizures, thromboembolic events.

CAUSES & RISK FACTORS

- Unknown; probably severe reaction to unidentified antigen.
- Cats—eosinophilic enteritis may be early form.

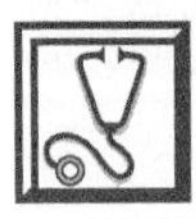

DIAGNOSIS

DIFFERENTIAL DIAGNOSIS

- Reactive eosinophilia—parasitism, allergic/hypersensitivity reactions, infectious disease, immune-mediated disease, fungal infections, neoplasia; with these conditions, eosinophilia usually limited in magnitude and remains confined to specific organ.
- Eosinophilic leukemia—differentiating criteria: eosinophilic leukemia tends to have immature eosinophils seen in higher numbers in circulation, constituting higher percentage of leukocyte differential; anemia more common and often more severe; myeloid : erythroid (M : E) ratio in bone marrow higher (>10 : 1) with more immature/blast forms and disorderly maturation; tissue infiltrates consist of immature eosinophils and may show sinusoidal pattern in liver without fibrosis; in cats, chloroma-like masses in kidneys are reported.

CBC/BIOCHEMISTRY/URINALYSIS

- Leukocytosis with marked eosinophilia, possibly with left shift in eosinophil series; mature eosinophil count from 5,000 to >130,000/μL.
- Basophilia.
- Mild anemia.
- With organ damage or dysfunction, associated abnormalities seen.

OTHER LABORATORY TESTS

Rule out identifiable etiologies—fecal flotation, heartworm test, biopsy.

IMAGING

- Organ enlargement/infiltration may be visualized with survey radiographs and/or ultrasound.
- Intestinal mucosal irregularities and thickening seen on ultrasound or contrast radiography.

DIAGNOSTIC PROCEDURES

- Bone marrow aspiration and/or core biopsy.
- Fine-needle aspirate or biopsy of affected tissues.

PATHOLOGIC FINDINGS

- Spleen—eosinophilic infiltrates in red pulp, sometimes white.
- GI tract—mucosal and submucosal eosinophilic infiltrates in small intestine, sometimes in colon and stomach.
- Bone marrow—hypercellularity, eosinophilic hyperplasia (up to 40% of all nucleated cells), unremarkable maturation and morphology with high M : E ratio (mean 7.27 : 1).
- Lymph nodes—reactive with eosinophilic infiltration.
- Other (less frequent)—eosinophilic infiltrates in skin, myocardium, body cavity effusions.

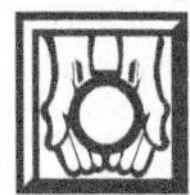

TREATMENT

- Eliminate identifiable primary disease.
- Address any specific organ dysfunction/failure.

MEDICATIONS

DRUG(S) OF CHOICE

- Corticosteroids—prednisone 1–2 mg/kg/day PO initially, then taper therapy if eosinophilia suppressed; if eosinophilia returns, resume higher daily dose.
- Imatinib mesylate approved in humans to treat chronic myelogenous leukemia as well as HES, used with possible efficacy in cats at 9.6 mg/kg PO q24h.
- Hydroxyurea—to reduce eosinophil count if not normal or near normal after 7–14 days of steroid treatment; used long term if effective in conjunction with steroids.
- Cyclosporine A—suppresses production of eosinophilopoietic factors by T cells.
- Vincristine and alkylating agents such as chlorambucil effective in humans.
- Reduce dosage or discontinue drugs if bone marrow suppression or thrombocytopenia develops.

CONTRAINDICATIONS/POSSIBLE INTERACTIONS

- Specific drug toxicities for each agent, most notably myelosuppression.
- Imatinib mesylate may lead to protein-losing nephropathy, although association uncertain.

FOLLOW-UP

- Serial CBC monitoring of eosinophil count (not always indicative of tissue infiltrates) and to detect myelosuppression if myelotoxic drugs used.
- Monitor clinical signs and any physical abnormalities.
- Other testing for specific organ function.

MISCELLANEOUS

SEE ALSO

Eosinophilia

ABBREVIATIONS

- GI = gastrointestinal.
- HES = hypereosinophilic syndrome.
- M : E = myeloid : erythroid.

Suggested Reading

Lilliehook I, Tvedten H. Investigation of hypereosinophilia and potential treatment. Vet Clin North Am Small Anim Pract 2003, 33:1359–1378.

Author Craig A. Thompson
Consulting Editor Melinda S. Camus

HYPERESTROGENISM (ESTROGEN TOXICITY)

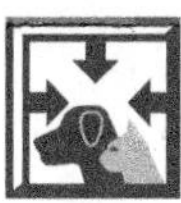

BASICS

OVERVIEW

• A syndrome characterized by high serum concentration of estrogen (estradiol, estriol, or estrone).
• Can occur secondary to endogenous estrogen secretion or exogenous administration of estrogens, such as diethylstilbestrol or estriol.
• Sites of endogenous estrogen production include ovarian follicles, follicular ovarian cysts, Leydig cells, and the adrenal cortex (zona fasciculata and reticularis); can also occur as a result of peripheral conversion of excessive androgens.
• Endogenous estrogens in females are responsible for normal sexual behavior and development and function of the reproductive tract; in the male, estrogens are responsible for Leydig cell function.
• In females, estrogens potentiate the stimulatory effect of progesterone in the endometrium and permit cervical relaxation; these two effects increase the risk of cystic endometrial hyperplasia and pyometra. In the male, estrogens potentiate the action of androgens in the prostate. Estrogens also increase osteoblastic activity, retention of calcium and phosphorus, total body protein, and metabolic rate.
• High serum concentration of estrogen provides a source of negative feedback in the hypothalamic-pituitary axis, suppressing gonadotropin secretion, and interferes with stem cell differentiation in the bone marrow and erythrocyte iron metabolism.

SIGNALMENT

Endogenous Hyperestrogenism

• Older male dog (secondary to functional testicular tumors).
• Older female dog (secondary to granulosa cell or other functional ovarian tumors, follicular ovarian cysts).
• Young female dog (follicular ovarian cysts).

Exogenous Hyperestrogenism

• All breeds, genders, and ages, associated with estrogen administration or exposure.
• Toy breed dogs are at increased risk for exposure to human transdermal hormone medications.

SIGNS

Historical Findings

• Attractive to intact male dogs.
• Infertility.
• Prolonged proestrus and estrus (female).
• Decreased libido (male).
• Nymphomania (female).
• Variable vulvar bleeding and enlargement, excessive vulvar licking.
• Epistaxis, hematuria (thrombocytopenia); lethargic, febrile (neutropenia); lethargic (anemia).

Physical Examination Findings

• Skin/endocrine—nonpruritic, symmetric alopecia (endocrine alopecia), hyperpigmentation.
• Reproductive (male)—palpable testicular mass, testicular asymmetry (tumor and/or atrophy), cryptorchidism (unilateral or bilateral), prostatomegaly (squamous metaplasia), gynecomastia.
• Reproductive (female)—vulvar edema and enlargement, vulvar discharge, gynecomastia mammary gland enlargement.
• Hemic/lymphatic/immune—pale mucous membranes, petechia, fever, lethargy (blood loss).

CAUSES & RISK FACTORS

• Follicular ovarian cysts.
• Functional ovarian tumor (granulosa cell tumor and other ovarian tumors).
• Testicular tumor (specifically Sertoli cell tumor, but also Leydig and interstitial cell tumors).
• Exogenous estrogen exposure.

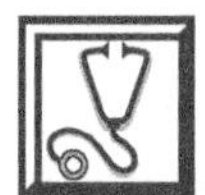

DIAGNOSIS

DIFFERENTIAL DIAGNOSIS

Nonpruritic, Symmetric Alopecia

• Hypothyroidism—diagnose on clinical signs, biochemistry, CBC, and thyroid function testing.
• Hyperadrenocorticism—diagnose on clinical signs (polyuria, polydipsia, exercise intolerance), CBC, serum biochemistry, specific testing (urine cortisol : creatinine ratio, adrenal function testing).
• Growth hormone–responsive dermatosis (breed risk: Pomeranian).

Attractive to Male Dogs

• Vaginitis, perivulvar dermatitis (differentiate from hyperestrogenism by lack of vaginal superficial epithelial cell predominance on vaginal cytology), lack of evidence of ovarian abnormalities, or confirmation of complete ovariohysterectomy or ovariectomy.
• Genitourinary tract infection, inflammation, foreign body, or neoplasia.

Infertility

• Testicular degeneration/atrophy/immune-mediated orchitis—diagnosis based on physical examination, lack of testicular or intra-abdominal masses, semen evaluation, and testicular biopsy or fine-needle aspirate.
• Intersex abnormalities—uncommon; diagnosis supported by abnormal external genitalia, abnormal karyotype, and histologic examination of the reproductive tract, when available.

CBC/BIOCHEMISTRY/URINALYSIS

• CBC—variable; initially characterized by thrombocytopenia or thrombocytosis, progressive anemia, and leukocytosis (may exceed 100,000 white blood cells [WBCs]/μL); after 3 weeks, pancytopenia and aplastic anemia seen.
• Chemistry panel and urinalysis are usually unremarkable, but hematuria can be present with thrombocytopenia.

OTHER LABORATORY TESTS

• Serum estrogen (estradiol) concentrations—prolonged (>30 days) elevation at levels above baseline is responsible for clinical signs rather than the actual concentration; serum concentrations may be within normal limits, and accuracy of radioimmunoassay is variable.
• Vaginal and preputial cytology—extremely reliable as a bioassay for estrogen; under the influence of estrogen, cytology reveals a predominance of superficial epithelial cells that are anuclear or have pyknotic nuclei; preputial cytology with greater than 20% superficial cells is consistent with elevated serum estrogen.
• Evaluation for ovarian remnant syndrome (ORS)—anti-Müllerian hormone (AMH) testing: a positive test in a bitch >6 months of age or >30 days from ovariohysterectomy supports the presence of ovarian tissue; in cases with negative AMH but convincing clinical evidence supporting ORS, some investigators advise measurement of serum progesterone to identify persistent luteal structures lacking AMH; the AMH test will differentiate between ORS and exogenous estrogen exposure.
• The semi-quantitative luteinizing hormone (LH) assay (Zoetis), if elevated, suggests a lack of ovaries, but cannot differentiate exogenous vs. endogenous estrogen exposure if low.

IMAGING

• Thoracic radiography—to evaluate for metastatic neoplasia.
• Ultrasonography of the abdomen, inguinal canal, and testes—to assess for testicular masses, cystic or enlarged ovarian structures, intra-abdominal masses, lymphadenopathy, and prostatomegaly.
• Vaginoscopy to evaluate the vaginal mucosa; under the influence of estrogen, the vaginal mucosa should appear edematous and pink.

DIAGNOSTIC PROCEDURES

• Fine-needle aspiration of testicular masses—cytologic diagnosis prior to surgery.
• Percutaneous ultrasound-guided aspiration of large ovarian follicular cysts—rarely results in clinical resolution (cystic structure persists); hormone concentration can be measured in the cystic fluid.

HYPERESTROGENISM (ESTROGEN TOXICITY) (CONTINUED)

- Examination and aspiration/biopsy of local lymph nodes—for evaluation of metastatic disease (via ultrasound or surgical biopsy).
- Bone marrow aspirate or core biopsy—assess myelosuppression.
- Skin biopsy—may reveal nonspecific changes associated with endocrine alopecia such as orthokeratotic hyperkeratosis, epidermal atrophy and melanosis, follicular keratosis, predominance of telogen hair follicles, and sebaceous gland atrophy.

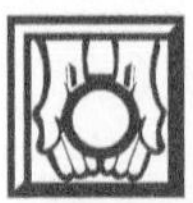

TREATMENT

- Treatment of choice in the intact or partially neutered female and male is surgical neutering; the prognosis is good if residual or malignant gonadal tissue can be completely removed.
- Unilateral orchiectomy or ovariectomy of the affected neoplastic testicle or cystic or neoplastic ovary may be considered in valuable breeding animals; use of testicular prosthetic devices is neither advised nor ethical; contralateral testicular changes (male) or endometrial changes (female) secondary to prolonged estrogen exposure can contribute to subfertility even if the abnormal gonad has been removed, with a guarded prognosis for fertility; histopathology should always be performed to evaluate for neoplasia and local lymphatic metastasis.
- Discontinue estrogen exposure in cases of exogenous hyperestrogenism; discontinue or reduce the dose of exogenous estrogen if used therapeutically; prognosis is good.

MEDICATIONS

DRUG(S) OF CHOICE

- Supportive care—including administration of appropriate antimicrobial therapy, IV fluids, and blood products to treat febrile neutropenia or anemia.
- Synthetic erythropoietin, darbopoietin, granulocyte colony-stimulating factor (G-CSF), granulocyte-macrophage colony-stimulating factor (GM-CSF)—may be considered to stimulate erythroid and granulocytic production at the level of the bone marrow; lithium has reportedly been of benefit in cases of estrogen-induced bone marrow aplasia.
- Gonadotropin-releasing hormone (GnRH)—unlikely to induce ovulation in cases of follicular cysts.
- Iron dextran to support erythrocyte regeneration—dog: 10–20 mg/kg (max 300 mg/dog) IM monthly PRN; cat: 10 mg/kg IM monthly PRN.

CONTRAINDICATIONS/POSSIBLE INTERACTIONS

Chemotherapeutic agents for treatment of metastatic testicular or ovarian neoplasia should be used cautiously due to increased risk of bone marrow suppression. Consult with a veterinary oncologist.

FOLLOW-UP

- Serial CBC analysis to evaluate response to therapy and progression of disease.
- Serial bone marrow cytology—to evaluate bone marrow response and erythroid, myeloid, and megakaryocytic regeneration when myelosuppression is chronic; peripheral signs of regeneration may not occur for weeks to months after initial insult.
- Clinical signs of male feminization syndrome should resolve 2–6 weeks after testicular tumor removal.
- Lack of resolving pancytopenia and continued bone marrow hypoplasia 3 weeks after surgical removal of ovarian or testicular neoplasia or removal of follicular cysts is associated with a grave prognosis.

MISCELLANEOUS

ASSOCIATED CONDITIONS

- ORS.
- Prostatomegaly.
- Cystic endometrial hyperplasia and subfertility/infertility.
- Hepatic insufficiency.
- Bone marrow aplasia, pancytopenia.
- Sepsis.

ABBREVIATIONS

- AMH = anti-Müllerian hormone.
- G-CSF = granulocyte colony-stimulating factor.
- GM-CSF = granulocyte-macrophage colony-stimulating factor.
- GnRH = gonadotropin-releasing hormone.
- LH = luteinizing hormone.
- ORS = ovarian remnant syndrome.
- WBC = white blood cell.

Suggested Reading

Davidson AP. Reproductive system disorders. In: Nelson RW, Couto GC, eds., Small Animal Internal Medicine, 5th ed. St. Louis, MO: Elsevier, 2014, pp. 897–966.

Authors Autumn P. Davidson and Sophie A. Grundy
Consulting Editor Patty A. Lathan

Client Education Handout available online

Hyperglycemia

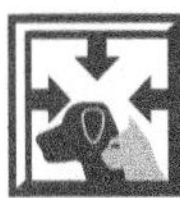

BASICS

DEFINITION

- Blood glucose (BG) concentration above the reference interval: >130 mg/dL (>7 mmol/L).
- For cats >8 years of age, BG concentration >189 mg/dL (10.5 mmol/L).

PATHOPHYSIOLOGY

- Physiologic (stress hyperglycemia)—normal, transient response to stress, especially in cats.
- Laboratory or portable glucometer error—anemia results in artificially high BG concentration with some portable glucometers.
- IV infusion of dextrose-containing fluids.
- Drugs that inhibit insulin secretion (e.g., dexmedetomidine).
- Diabetes mellitus (DM)—absolute or relative insulin deficiency.

SYSTEMS AFFECTED

- Endocrine/metabolic—insulin deficiency causes disorders of carbohydrate, protein, and fat metabolism; insulin resistance occurs via various mechanisms.
- Renal/urologic—osmotic diuresis from BG exceeding renal threshold causes polyuria (PU) with secondary polydipsia.
- Pancreas/hepatobiliary—beta cell loss; endocrine hepatopathy, hepatomegaly.
- Ophthalmic—persistent hyperglycemia can cause cataracts in dogs.
- Nervous—severe hyperglycemia may cause CNS dehydration from high serum osmolality; diabetic neuropathy in cats causes hind limb weakness and plantigrade, ± palmigrade, gait; other neuropathies are also possible (e.g., Horner's syndrome).

GENETICS

Breed predispositions indicate likely genetic influences for DM in dogs and cats.

INCIDENCE/PREVALENCE

Prevalence of DM in hospital populations is 6 in 1,000 cats and 3 in 1,000 dogs.

SIGNALMENT

Species

Dog and cat.

Mean Age and Range

Onset of DM typically occurs after 5 years of age; highest prevalence from 8–12 years of age.

Predominant Sex

Neutered males (cats and dogs) and intact females (dogs) are predisposed to DM.

SIGNS

General Comments

- DM—signs have insidious onset over weeks to months.
- Animals with concurrent disease, such as pancreatitis, might not show "classic" signs of hyperglycemia.

Historical Findings

- Polydipsia and PU—PU might manifest as inappropriate urination or urinary incontinence.
- Weight loss with normal or increased appetite.
- Lethargy.
- Vision loss due to diabetic cataracts (dogs).
- Weak plantigrade gait due to diabetic neuropathy (cats).
- Previous overweight/obesity (especially cats and intact female dogs).
- Severe hyperglycemia can cause decreased mentation, coma.

Physical Examination Findings

- May be normal.
- Obese, normal, or underweight.
- Sarcopenia.
- Lethargy.
- Dehydration.
- Plantigrade ± palmigrade gait (cats).
- Cataracts (dogs).
- Hepatomegaly.
- Chronic infections—respiratory, skin, urinary tract.
- Poor hair coat.
- Ketotic or sweet odor to breath.
- Separation of incisors, broadening of the face, and organomegaly in cats with hypersomatotropism.

CAUSES

- DM—a heterogeneous group of diseases characterized by hyperglycemia resulting from inadequate insulin secretion, inadequate insulin action, or both.
- Inadequate insulin action (insulin resistance) is associated with hyperadrenocorticism, pheochromocytoma, glucagonoma, hypersomatotropism, hyper- and hypothyroidism, high progesterone during diestrus (dogs), and drugs (e.g., thiazide diuretics, progestogens [e.g., megestrol acetate], growth hormone, topical and systemic corticosteroids, and dexmedetomidine.
- Chronic hyperglycemia (glucose toxicity) can cause insulin resistance.

RISK FACTORS

- Breed predispositions for DM vary with geographic region.
- Older age.
- Obesity.
- Sedentary/indoor lifestyle.
- Stress.
- Concurrent disease, particularly hyperadrenocorticism, hypersomatotropism, pancreatitis.
- Diestrus in dogs.
- Diabetogenic drugs—corticosteroids, progestogens.
- Dextrose-containing fluids.

DIAGNOSIS

DIFFERENTIAL DIAGNOSIS

- Stress hyperglycemia—differentiated from DM by documentation of persistent fasting hyperglycemia for more than 24 hours, or increased serum glycated protein concentrations.
- DM.
- Diagnosis of DM in cats:
  - Random (fasted or unfasted) BG ≥270 mg/dL (15 mmol/L) with clinical signs of hyperglycemia (with no other plausible cause) or hyperglycemic crisis *and* at least one of the following: increased serum glycated protein concentrations; glycosuria on more than one occasion on a voided sample acquired in a home environment at least 2 days after any stressful events.
  - Random (fasted or unfasted) BG between 130 and 270 mg/dL (7–15 mmol/L) *and* at least two of the following: clinical signs of hyperglycemia or hyperglycemic crisis; increased serum glycated protein concentrations; glycosuria on more than one occasion on a voided sample acquired in a home environment at least 2 days after any stressful events.
- Diagnosis of DM in dogs:
  - Fasted or unfasted BG ≥200 mg/dL (11 mmol/L) with clinical signs of hyperglycemia or hyperglycemic crisis.
  - Fasting BG 130–200 mg/dL (7–11 mmol/L) with or without clinical signs of hyperglycemia or hyperglycemic crisis.
- DM is likely when hyperglycemia occurs in combination with ketosis and/or ketonuria.

LABORATORY FINDINGS

Factors That May Alter Laboratory Results

- Delayed serum or plasma separation lowers glucose concentration; glucose concentration should be measured within 30 minutes of collection; whole blood samples collected in fluoride oxalate anticoagulant may be stored.
- Lipemia, hemolysis, and icterus may interfere with spectrophotometric assays.
- Glucometers intended for human use tend to underestimate the true BG in cats and dogs; wide variability in the accuracy of different meters necessitates correlation of results from each meter with results from a veterinary diagnostic laboratory prior to use.
- Veterinary-specific glucometers provide more accurate results than human glucometers.
- BG reagent strips require whole blood, must be stored correctly, and be in date.

CBC/BIOCHEMISTRY/URINALYSIS

- Hyperglycemia might be the only abnormal finding.
- For findings associated with DM, see specific chapters.

HYPERGLYCEMIA

OTHER LABORATORY TESTS

- Fructosamine concentration identifies degree of glycemia over the previous 2–3 weeks; results are assay dependent and may be affected by hemolysis or lipemia; provides no information on variability of BG concentrations.
- Glycosylated hemoglobin concentration identifies degree of glycemia over the previous 10 weeks (cats) or 16 weeks (dogs); provides no information on variability of BG concentrations.
- Adrenocorticotropic hormone (ACTH) stimulation test or low-dose dexamethasone-suppression test to diagnose hyperadrenocorticism in dogs; false-positive results might be obtained if there is poor diabetic control.
- Serum insulin-like growth factor 1 (IGF-1) assay to diagnose hypersomatotropism in cats; false-negative results are more likely when there is severe insulin deficiency; cats should be treated with insulin for 4–6 weeks prior to testing.

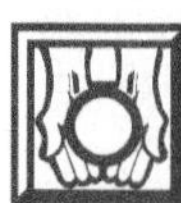

TREATMENT

APPROPRIATE HEALTH CARE

- Stress hyperglycemia is self-limiting.
- Diabetic cats and dogs that are eating well—outpatient management.
- Those that are unwell, inappetent, or have other signs such as vomiting require inpatient management with insulin and IV fluids.
- Concurrent disease can compromise DM management and should be promptly diagnosed and treated.

NURSING CARE

Glucose monitoring is recommended for all hospitalized hyperglycemic patients. Venous or capillary blood testing using a veterinary glucometer is appropriate. Real-time continuous glucose monitoring systems (CGMS) or flash glucose monitoring systems (FGMS) can simplify glucose monitoring of hospitalized patients.

ACTIVITY

Activity does not need to be limited in dogs and cats with DM and may decrease insulin requirement in working diabetic dogs.

DIET

- See relevant chapters on DM.
- Nutritional requirements for concurrent diseases take precedence over nutritional requirements for DM; good diabetic control can be achieved with insulin treatment regardless of diet.

CLIENT EDUCATION

- Client education is critical, because most treatment and monitoring of a diabetic patient will be done by the owner at home, and clinical signs will guide treatment decisions.
- Owner concerns relating to the impact that treating their pet will have on their lifestyle should be addressed.

SURGICAL CONSIDERATIONS

- Approximately 8% chance of diabetic remission following neutering and insulin therapy in female dogs; those that do not achieve remission generally have improved diabetic control.
- Improved diabetic control and possibly remission will occur following hypophysectomy in cats with hypersomatotropism; however, this treatment is expensive with limited availability.

MEDICATIONS

DRUG(S) OF CHOICE

- Exogenous insulin is the mainstay of treatment of DM.
- See chapters on DM.

PRECAUTIONS

- See chapters on DM.
- Drugs that cause insulin resistance (e.g., systemic or topical corticosteroids) should be used with caution in hyperglycemic animals; an increased insulin dose may be necessary.

POSSIBLE INTERACTIONS

Concurrent use of insulin and oral hypoglycemic agents might lead to hypoglycemia.

ALTERNATIVE DRUG(S)

- Glipizide and acarbose.
- See chapters on DM.

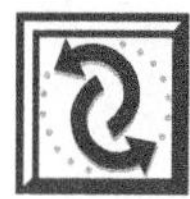

FOLLOW-UP

PATIENT MONITORING

- See chapters on DM.
- Animals in diabetic remission require ongoing monitoring for recurrence of hyperglycemia.

PREVENTION/AVOIDANCE

- Minimize use of diabetogenic drugs, particularly in susceptible individuals.
- Prevent obesity in cats and intact female dogs.
- Neuter female dogs at risk of developing DM.

POSSIBLE COMPLICATIONS

- Severe hyperglycemia may be associated with CNS depression and coma because of hyperosmolality.
- Diabetic cataracts (dogs).
- Diabetic neuropathy in cats with poor diabetic control.
- Insulin-induced hypoglycemia.

EXPECTED COURSE AND PROGNOSIS

- Transient stress hyperglycemia is self-limiting.
- Treatment of DM often is associated with an excellent prognosis, and typically results in a very good quality of life and similar life expectancy to animals without diabetes.

MISCELLANEOUS

ASSOCIATED CONDITIONS

- Hyperosmolality.
- Diabetic ketoacidosis.
- Hyperadrenocorticism.
- Hypersomatropism.
- Pancreatitis.

PREGNANCY/FERTILITY/BREEDING

- In intact bitches, a form of diabetes analogous to human gestational diabetes can occur during diestrus or pregnancy; if insulin therapy is initiated promptly, diabetic remission can sometimes be achieved following spay or whelping.
- Increased incidence of dystocia (large fetal size) and hypoglycemia in neonates when hyperglycemia has been present during pregnancy.

SYNONYMS

High blood sugar.

SEE ALSO

- Diabetes Mellitus with Ketoacidosis.
- Diabetes Mellitus Without Complication—Cats.
- Diabetes Mellitus Without Complication—Dogs.
- Hyperosmolality.

ABBREVIATIONS

- ACTH = adrenocorticotropic hormone.
- BG = blood glucose.
- CGMS = continuous glucose monitoring system.
- DM = diabetes mellitus.
- FGMS = flash glucose monitoring system.
- IGF-1 = insulin-like growth factor 1.
- PU = polyuria.

INTERNET RESOURCES

https://esve.org/alive/search.aspx

Suggested Reading

Behrend E, Holford A, Lathan P, et al. AAHA diabetes management guidelines for dogs and cats. J Am Anim Hosp Assoc 2018, 54(1):1–21.

Reeve-Johnson MK, Rand JS, Vankan D, et al. Cutpoints for screening BG concentrations in healthy cats. J Fel Med Surg 2017, 19(12):1181–1191.

Sparkes AH, Cannon M, Church D, et al. ISFM consensus guidelines on the practical management of diabetes mellitus in cats. J Fel Med Surg 2015, 17:235–250.

Thompson A, Lathan P, Fleeman L. Update on insulin treatments for dogs and cats: insulin dosing pens and more. Vet Med Res Reports 2015, 6:129–142.

Authors Linda M. Fleeman and Sarah B. Pierard

Consulting Editor Patty A. Lathan

HYPERKALEMIA

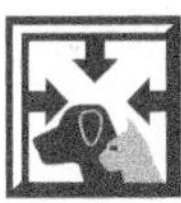

BASICS

DEFINITION

Serum potassium concentration higher than the testing laboratory's upper limit of normal, generally >5.7 mEq/L (mmol/L).

PATHOPHYSIOLOGY

• Potassium is primarily intracellular; serum concentrations do not accurately reflect tissue concentrations. • Hyperkalemia is often associated with cellular injury (e.g., trauma and ischemia) and other causes of translocation of potassium out of the intracellular space (e.g., acidosis). • Potassium is eliminated in the kidneys and elimination is enhanced by aldosterone; conditions that inhibit renal elimination of potassium will cause hyperkalemia.

SYSTEMS AFFECTED

• Cardiovascular—potassium affects cardiac conduction, and changes are reflected on the ECG; as potassium rises, the T waves become tall and spiked with a narrow base, the QRS complexes widen, and the P–R intervals lengthen; the P waves become smaller and wider and, in animals with severe hyperkalemia, disappear (atrial standstill); higher concentrations of potassium cause fusion of the QRS–T, which causes a wide complex idioventricular bradyarrhythmia followed by ventricular fibrillation or asystole; ECG changes in animals with hyperkalemia vary and are diminished by hypernatremia, hypercalcemia, and alkalosis.
• Nervous—neuromuscular weakness.

SIGNALMENT

• Dog and cat. • Pseudohyperkalemia in certain East Asian dog breeds (e.g., Akita, Shiba, Jindo, and Chinese Shar-Pei).

SIGNS

Historical Findings

• Weakness. • Collapse. • Stranguria, pollakiuria, pigmenturia (animals with urethral obstruction). • Flaccid paralysis. • Death.

Physical Examination Findings

• In addition to historical findings, arrhythmias, especially bradyarrhythmias. • Firm, non-expressible urinary bladder, abdominal pain in animals with urethral obstruction. • Abdominal fluid wave, distended abdomen in patients with urinary bladder rupture.

CAUSES

• Pseudohyperkalemia—some blood cells (generally reported in red blood cells [RBCs] of East Asian dog breeds including Akita, Shiba, Jindo, and Chinese Shar-Pei; also platelets and white blood cells [WBCs] in any breed) contain high concentrations of potassium; if the blood sample is not analyzed or separated promptly, this intracellular potassium is released into the serum, causing the potassium concentration to be artificially high (pseudohyperkalemia); seen in patients with thrombocytosis or severe leukocytosis. • Low potassium elimination—anuric or oliguric renal failure; hypoadrenocorticism; renal hypoperfusion; urinary tract rupture or urethral obstruction; administration of potassium-sparing diuretics, angiotensin-converting enzyme (ACE) inhibitors, trimethoprim, nonsteroidal anti-inflammatory drugs, or heparin (causing hypoaldosteronism); some gastrointestinal diseases (e.g., salmonellosis, trichuriasis).
• Translocation of potassium—metabolic acidosis, reperfusion syndrome, thrombolysis in feline aortic thromboembolism, tumor lysis syndrome, muscle injury (trauma, phosphofructokinase deficiency), digitalis overdose, infusion of mannitol and hyperglycemia (causing hyperosmolality). • High potassium intake—oral or parenteral potassium supplements or potassium bromide toxicosis. • Miscellaneous—third space fluid accumulation (e.g., pleural effusion, ascites).

RISK FACTORS

• IV fluid therapy with excessive potassium supplementation. • Administration of potassium-sparing diuretics (e.g., spironolactone) and ACE inhibitors (e.g., enalapril, benazepril), primarily in patients with renal disease.
• Hypoadrenocorticism. • Trauma. • Renal disease. • Lower urinary tract disease including cystic calculi. • Thrombocytosis and leukemia.
• Akita, Shiba, Jindo, and Chinese Shar-Pei—pseudohyperkalemia; not all animals within a breed are at risk for pseudohyperkalemia; approximately 20% of Akitas have the high potassium phenotype. • Phosphofructokinase deficiency.

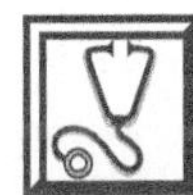

DIAGNOSIS

DIFFERENTIAL DIAGNOSIS

• Waxing and waning history of gastrointestinal complaints, weakness, collapse—consider hypoadrenocorticism. • Straining to urinate or low urine output—consider urinary obstruction or oliguric/anuric renal failure.

LABORATORY FINDINGS

Disorders That May Alter Laboratory Results

Thrombocytosis (>1,000,000 cells/mm^3), leukocytosis (>200,000 cells/mm^3), and abnormal (leukemic) leukocytes can cause release of large amounts of potassium into the serum.

CBC/BIOCHEMISTRY/URINALYSIS

• In patients with Na : K ratio <27, consider hypoadrenocorticism; some patients with metabolic acidosis due to diarrhea or renal tubular acidosis, ascites, chylothorax, or pregnancy may also have a low Na : K ratio.
• In patients with azotemia, consider hypoadrenocorticism, anuric or oliguric renal failure, and ruptured or obstructed urinary tract. • In patients with high creatine kinase, aspartate aminotransferase, and lactic dehydrogenase, consider muscle injury. • In patients with severe thrombocytosis or leukocytosis or if the patient is an East Asian dog breed, consider pseudohyperkalemia.

OTHER LABORATORY TESTS

Adrenocorticotropic hormone (ACTH) stimulation test—patients with hypoadrenocorticism generally have undetectable (<0.2 μg/dL) baseline and poststimulation serum cortisol concentration.

IMAGING

• Radiographic contrast studies or ultrasound to rule out urinary tract rupture or obstruction.
• Ultrasonography to evaluate urinary tract, adrenal gland size, presence of third-space fluid accumulation.

H

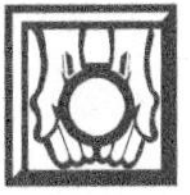

TREATMENT

• Varies, depending on the underlying cause of hyperkalemia. • Aggressiveness is dictated by patient's appearance and severity of ECG abnormalities. • Initiate supportive measures to lower potassium while pursuing definitive diagnosis. • Isotonic crystalloid fluids can be used to treat hypovolemia and will help decrease serum potassium; however, other treatments (see below) more rapidly decrease potassium concentration or blunt the effects on the heart; fluids can be administered in bolus doses of 20–30 mL/kg to effect; patients with primary cardiac disease or anuric renal failure may not tolerate large volumes of IV fluids (susceptible to volume overload). • Reduced potassium diet in animals with hyperkalemia secondary to chronic renal disease. • In patients with renal or postrenal oligo-anuria, urine flow must be restored emergently, either through relief of obstruction or restoration of urine production (see Urinary Tract Obstruction). • Hemodialysis may be necessary in patients with oligo-anuric renal failure.

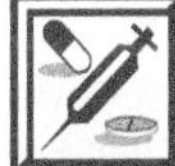

MEDICATIONS

DRUG(S) OF CHOICE

• For patients with life-threatening hyperkalemia, administer calcium gluconate 10% (0.5–1 mL/kg slow IV over 10 min) while monitoring the ECG; calcium antagonizes the effect of potassium on cardiac conduction without lowering the serum potassium concentration. • To decrease serum potassium: ◦ Regular insulin (0.25–0.5 U/kg IV) with dextrose (0.5 g/kg IV) activates Na^+/K^+ ATPase to move potassium into cells; may require additional supplementation of dextrose (e.g., 2.5% dextrose added to IV fluids). ◦ Dextrose (0.5 g/kg IV) can be used without insulin for mild hyperkalemia. ◦ Sodium bicarbonate (1 mEq/kg slow IV) induces exchange of potassium for hydrogen ions, moving potassium into cells. ◦ Albuterol (1–2 puffs from inhaler) activates beta receptors and Na^+/K^+ ATPase to move potassium into cells.

HYPERKALEMIA (CONTINUED)

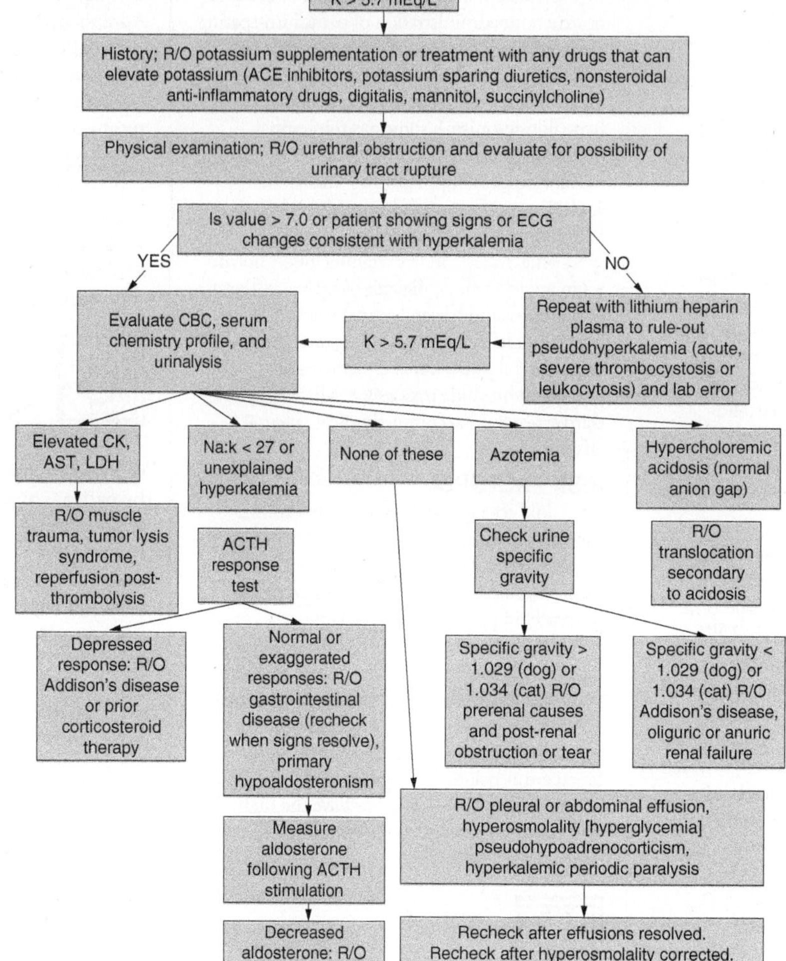

Figure 1.

Algorithm for diagnosing hyperkalemia.

CONTRAINDICATIONS

• Avoid IV fluids with high concentrations (>10 mEq/L) of potassium and fluids that cause hyponatremia, acidosis, or hypocalcemia. • Avoid drugs that contain potassium or interfere with potassium elimination (e.g., ACE inhibitors, trimethoprim antibiotics, potassium-sparing diuretics) or interfere with renal function (e.g., nonsteroidal anti-inflammatory drugs).

PRECAUTIONS

• Kayexalate and sodium bicarbonate cause a sodium load that may lead to fluid retention in patients with cardiac or renal failure. • Sodium bicarbonate lowers ionized calcium levels—use cautiously in hypocalcemic patients. • Sodium bicarbonate elevates blood carbon dioxide concentration—use cautiously in patients with hypoventilation.

ALTERNATIVE DRUG(S)

Patiromer and sodium zirconium cyclosilicate are recently approved agents that bind potassium within the intestinal tract, limiting absorption and reabsorption; rarely used in veterinary practice; may have application in chronic hyperkalemia.

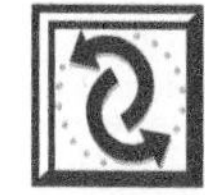

FOLLOW-UP

PATIENT MONITORING

• Recheck potassium at frequency dictated by the underlying disease. • Continuous ECG monitoring until rhythm disturbances resolve.

PREVENTION/AVOIDANCE

• Monitor potassium in patients receiving drugs that alter potassium elimination. • The maximum rate of IV potassium administration is 0.5 mEq/kg/h, and should be used only in the face of severe hypokalemia (average supplementation rate is between 0.05 and 0.2 mEq/kg/h in patients without acute renal disease).

POSSIBLE COMPLICATIONS

• Prolonged hypoglycemia following insulin administration. • Death of animals with severe hyperkalemia.

MISCELLANEOUS

PREGNANCY/FERTILITY/BREEDING

Combined hyperkalemia and hyponatremia may be seen in pregnant dogs due to third-space fluid accumulation in the uterus.

SEE ALSO

• Acidosis, Metabolic. • Acute Kidney Injury. • Atrial Standstill. • Hypoadrenocorticism (Addison's Disease). • Phosphofructokinase Deficiency. • Urinary Tract Obstruction.

ABBREVIATIONS

• ACE = angiotensin-converting enzyme.
• ACTH = adrenocorticotropic hormone.
• RBC = red blood cell.
• WBC = white blood cell.

Suggested Reading

Kogika MM, deMorais HA. A quick reference on hyperkalemia. Vet Clin North Am Small Anim Pract 2017, 47(2):223–228.

Author Francis W.K. Smith, Jr.
Consulting Editor Patty A. Lathan

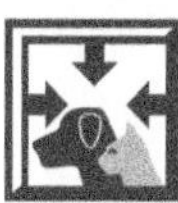

BASICS

DEFINITION

• Increased concentration of lipid in the blood of a fasted (>12 hours) patient; includes hypercholesterolemia, hypertriglyceridemia, or both.
• Lipemia—serum or plasma separated from blood that contains an excess concentration of triglycerides (>200 mg/dL).
• Lactescence—opaque, milk-like appearance of serum or plasma that contains an even higher concentration of triglycerides (>1,000 mg/dL) than lipemic serum.

PATHOPHYSIOLOGY

Primary Hyperlipidemia

• Primary (idiopathic) hyperlipidemia—defect in lipid metabolism causing hypertriglyceridemia with or without hyperchylomicronemia; likely hereditary in miniature schnauzer, but the genetic defect has yet to be determined.
• Idiopathic hyperchylomicronemia in cats—familial, autosomal recessive defect in lipoprotein lipase activity.
• Primary hypercholesterolemia—occurs in some families of briard, rough collie, Shetland sheepdog, Doberman pinscher, and Rottweiler; low-density lipoprotein (LDL) cholesterol is high.

Secondary Hyperlipidemia

• Postprandial—absorption of chylomicrons from the gastrointestinal tract occurs 30–60 minutes after ingestion of a meal containing fat; may increase serum triglycerides for up to 12 hours.
• Diabetes mellitus—low lipoprotein lipase (LPL) activity; high synthesis of very-low-density lipoprotein (VLDL) by the liver.
• Hypothyroidism—low LPL activity and lipolytic activity by other hormones (e.g., catecholamines); reduced hepatic degradation of cholesterol to bile acids.
• Hyperadrenocorticism—increased synthesis of VLDL by the liver and low LPL activity causes both hypercholesterolemia and hypertriglyceridemia.
• Cholestatic liver disease—hypercholesterolemia caused by reduced excretion of cholesterol in the bile.
• Nephrotic syndrome—upregulation of common synthetic pathway for albumin and cholesterol and possibly low oncotic pressure lead to increased cholesterol synthesis.
• Pancreatitis—associated with hypertriglyceridemia in dogs, especially miniature schnauzers.
• Obesity—excessive hepatic synthesis of VLDL.

Drug-Induced Hyperlipidemia

• Glucocorticoids.
• Megestrol acetate (cat).

SYSTEMS AFFECTED

• Endocrine/metabolic.
• Gastrointestinal.
• Hepatobiliary.
• Nervous.
• Ophthalmic.

SIGNALMENT

• Dog and cat.
• Variable, depending on the cause.
• Hereditary hyperlipidemias—age of onset is >8 months in cats and >4 years in predisposed breeds of dog such as the miniature schnauzer.

SIGNS

Historical Findings

• Asymptomatic.
• Recent ingestion of a meal.
• Seizures, neurologic signs.
• Abdominal pain and distress.
• Neuropathies.

Physical Examination Findings

• Lipemia retinalis.
• Lipemic aqueous.
• Neuropathy.
• Cutaneous xanthomata.
• Lipid granulomas in abdominal organs.

CAUSES

Increased Absorption of Triglycerides or Cholesterol

Postprandial

Increased Production of Triglycerides or Cholesterol

• Idiopathic.
• Nephrotic syndrome.
• Pregnancy.
• Defects in lipid clearance enzymes or lipid carrier proteins.
• Idiopathic hyperchylomicronemia.
• Hyperchylomicronemia in cats.

Decreased Clearance of Triglycerides or Cholesterol

• Hypothyroidism.
• Hyperadrenocorticism.
• Diabetes mellitus.
• Pancreatitis.
• Cholestasis.

RISK FACTORS

• Obesity.
• High dietary intake of fats.
• Genetic predisposition in miniature schnauzer and Himalayan cat.
• Idiopathic hypercholesterolemia observed in families of briard, rough collie, Shetland sheepdog, Doberman pinscher, and Rottweiler.

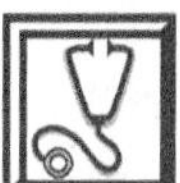

DIAGNOSIS

DIFFERENTIAL DIAGNOSIS

Fasting Hyperlipidemia

Rule out postprandial lipemia with a 12-hour fast.

Primary Hyperlipoproteinemia

• Idiopathic hyperlipidemia is observed most commonly in the miniature schnauzer breed.
• Hyperchylomicronemia in cats often manifests as polyneuropathies and lipogranulomas.
• Idiopathic hypercholesterolemia is observed in a variety of breeds; animals are often asymptomatic.

Secondary Hyperlipidemia

• Diabetes mellitus.
• Hypothyroidism.
• Pancreatitis.
• Hyperadrenocorticism.
• Hepatic disease and cholestatic disorders.
• Nephrotic syndrome.

LABORATORY FINDINGS

Sample Handling

• Submit serum.
• Lipemia causes hemolysis if serum remains with red blood cells for a long time; inquire about the laboratory method of clearing lipemic samples before submission.
• Two samples may be submitted—one for biochemical analysis, which may be cleared, and one for triglycerides and cholesterol concentrations.

Drugs That May Alter Laboratory Results

• Corticosteroids.
• Phenytoin.
• Prochlorperazine.
• Thiazides.
• Phenothiazines.

Disorders That May Alter Laboratory Results

• Falsely high cholesterol.
• Nonfasted samples (<12 hours).
• Icterus—spectrophotometric techniques.
• Fluoride and oxalate anticoagulants—enzymatic techniques.
• Lipemia.

Valid If Run in Human Laboratory?

Yes

CBC/BIOCHEMISTRY/URINALYSIS

• Results of hemogram usually normal.
• High serum triglyceride concentration—dogs: >150 mg/dL; cats: >100 mg/dL.
• High serum cholesterol concentration—dogs: >300 mg/dL; cats: >200 mg/dL.
• Serum biochemistry may reveal abnormalities consistent with causes of secondary hyperlipidemia.

HYPERLIPIDEMIA (CONTINUED)

- Results of urinalysis often normal; proteinuria if nephrotic syndrome present.

OTHER LABORATORY TESTS

- High-density lipoprotein (HDL) and LDL determinations—used in human medicine; values reported for HDL and LDL in dogs and cats cannot be assumed to be reliable.
- Chylomicron test—obtain serum sample after a 12-hour fast and refrigerate for 12–14 hours; do not freeze; chylomicrons rise to the surface and form a creamy layer.
- Lipoprotein electrophoresis—separates LDL, VLDL, and HDL1 and HDL2 subfractions.
- LPL activity—collect serum for triglycerides and cholesterol concentrations and lipoprotein electrophoresis before and 15 minutes after administration of heparin (90 IU/kg, IV); if there is no change in values before and after heparin administration, a defective LPL enzyme system should be suspected.
- Definitive diagnostics for hypothyroidism or hyperadrenocorticism, if suspected.

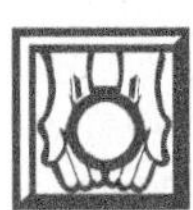

TREATMENT

Diet should contain <10% fat (e.g., Royal Canin® Low Fat; Hill's Prescription Diet r/d®, w/d®, and i/d® Low Fat; Purina® OM).

MEDICATIONS

DRUG(S) OF CHOICE

Initial management is dietary; omega-3 fatty acids, fibrates, and then niacin are added to refractory cases.

ALTERNATIVE DRUG(S)

- Gemfibrozil 10 mg/kg PO q12h; cats and dogs.
- Bezafibrate 4–10 mg/kg PO q12h; dogs only.
- Fish oils—omega-3 polyunsaturated fat 50–300 mg/kg PO q24h; dogs only.
- Niacin 50–200 mg/dog/day PO (slow release); dogs only.

FOLLOW-UP

PATIENT MONITORING

- Keep serum triglyceride concentrations <500 mg/dL to avoid possibly fatal episodes of acute pancreatitis.
- Monitoring serum cholesterol concentrations often is not necessary because hypercholesterolemia is not associated with clinical signs.
- Monitor alanine aminotransferase (ALT) and alkaline phosphatase (ALP) enzyme activities when using a fibrate and/or niacin, as toxicity may occur.

POSSIBLE COMPLICATIONS

- Pancreatitis and seizures are common complications of hyperlipidemia in the miniature schnauzer.
- In cats with hereditary chylomicronemia, xanthoma formation, lipemia retinalis, and neuropathies have been reported; peripheral neuropathies usually resolve 2–3 months after institution of a low-fat diet.

MISCELLANEOUS

ASSOCIATED CONDITIONS

- Pancreatitis.
- Seizures.
- Neuropathies.

AGE-RELATED FACTORS

None

PREGNANCY/FERTILITY/BREEDING

Potential cause of high cholesterol.

SYNONYMS

- Lipemia—turbid serum or plasma secondary to significant hypertriglyceridemia.
- Hyperlipoproteinemia—increased blood concentration of lipoproteins.

SEE ALSO

- Diabetes Mellitus Without Complication—Cats.
- Diabetes Mellitus Without Complication—Dogs.
- Hyperadrenocorticism (Cushing's Syndrome)—Cats.
- Hyperadrenocorticism (Cushing's Syndrome)—Dogs.
- Hypothyroidism.
- Nephrotic Syndrome.

ABBREVIATIONS

- ALP = alkaline phosphatase.
- ALT = alanine aminotransferase.
- HDL = high-density lipoprotein.
- LDL = low-density lipoprotein.
- LPL = lipoprotein lipase.
- VLDL = very-low-density lipoprotein.

Suggested Reading

Barrie J, Watson TOG. Hyperlipidemia. In: Bonagura JD, ed., Kirk's Current Veterinary Therapy XII. Philadelphia, PA: Saunders, 1995, pp. 430–434.

Ford R. Canine hyperlipidemias. In: Ettinger SJ, Feldman EC, eds., Textbook of Veterinary Internal Medicine, 4th ed. Philadelphia, PA: Saunders, 1994, pp. 1414–1418.

Jones B. Feline hyperlipidemias. In: Ettinger SJ, Feldman EC, eds., Textbook of Veterinary Internal Medicine, 4th ed. Philadelphia, PA: Saunders, 1994, pp. 1410–1413.

Xenoulis PG, Steiner JM. Lipid metabolism and hyperlipidemia in dogs. Vet J 2010, 183(1):12–21.

Author Patty A. Lathan

Consulting Editor Patty A. Lathan

Acknowledgment The author and book editors acknowledge the prior contribution of Melinda Fleming.

Client Education Handout available online

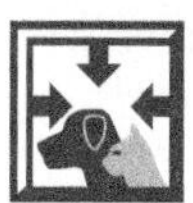

BASICS

DEFINITION

- Dogs—serum magnesium >2.51 mg/dL; ionized magnesium >0.58 mmol/L.
- Cats—serum magnesium >2.99 mg/dL; ionized magnesium >0.65 mmol/L.

PATHOPHYSIOLOGY

- Hypermagnesemia is less clinically significant than low total body magnesium in veterinary patients.
- Magnesium is second only to potassium as the most abundant intracellular cation. Found primarily in bone and muscle, it is required for many metabolic functions.
- Serum magnesium is present in three forms—protein-bound form (approximately 25–30%) and chelated and ionized forms (together account for 70–75%).
- Magnesium absorption occurs primarily in the ileum, but also in the jejunum and colon.
- Magnesium is an important cofactor in the sodium-potassium ATPase pump that maintains electrical gradients across membranes.
- Interference with the electrical gradient can change resting membrane potentials; repolarization disturbances result in neuromuscular and cardiac abnormalities.
- The kidneys maintain magnesium balance with 10–15% reabsorbed in the proximal tubule, 60–70% in the thick ascending limb of the loop of Henle, and 10–15% reabsorbed in the distal convoluted tubule. Reabsorption within the distal convoluted tubule is under hormonal and neurohormonal control and determines the final urine concentration of magnesium.
- Any condition that severely lowers the glomerular filtration rate can elicit hypermagnesemia because magnesium homeostasis is largely controlled by renal elimination.
- Clinically significant hypermagnesemia is more commonly associated with acute kidney injury, and the degree of hypermagnesemia is proportional to the severity of renal failure.
- Exuberant supplementation of magnesium can lead to iatrogenic hypermagnesemia, especially in patients with decreased renal function.
- High magnesium concentration impairs transmission of nerve impulses and decreases postsynaptic responses at the neuromuscular junction. When magnesium was given to anesthetized dogs at 0.12 mEq/kg/min, cardiovascular effects were not noted until plasma levels exceeded 12.2 mEq/L. The total dose of magnesium required to reach that level was 1–2 mEq/kg. It took cumulative doses of 5.9–10.9 mEq/kg to cause fatal cardiac arrhythmias (ventricular fibrillation).
- Magnesium has been called nature's calcium blocker; the most serious complications of hypermagnesemia result from calcium antagonism in the cardiac conduction system.

SYSTEMS AFFECTED

- Cardiovascular.
- Musculoskeletal.
- Nervous.

INCIDENCE/PREVALENCE

Increased plasma ionized magnesium concentration was found in 2% of 9,950 canine submissions to a clinical laboratory. In that study, 40% of the cases were caused by azotemia, 19% were iatrogenic, 11% had tissue damage, and 6% had endocrine disease. In another study, hypermagnesemia was found in 18% of hospitalized cats and 13% of hospitalized dogs. Most of these patients also had renal insufficiency or postrenal azotemia.

GEOGRAPHIC DISTRIBUTION

N/A

SIGNALMENT

Species

Dog and cat.

Breed Predilections

N/A

SIGNS

General Comments

- Usually caused by renal failure; clinical signs might be referable to azotemia and renal insufficiency. Clinical hypermagnesemia is reported most often in patients with preexisting renal disease that are oversupplemented with parenteral magnesium salts.
- Characterized by progressive loss of neuromuscular, respiratory, and cardiovascular function.

Historical and Physical Examination Findings

- Nausea, vomiting, weakness, bradycardia, flaccid paralysis, mental depression, and hyporeflexia (including menace and palpebral reflex).
- Hypotension and ECG changes, including delayed intraventricular conduction and prolonged QT interval.
- Atrioventricular block, respiratory depression, coma, and cardiac arrest have been observed in humans with serum magnesium concentrations >16 mg/dL.

CAUSES

- Renal failure.
- Intestinal hypomotility disorders and constipation.
- Endocrine disorders including hypoadrenocorticism, hypothyroidism, and hyperparathyroidism.
- Combined angiotensin-converting enzyme inhibitors and spironolactone administration.
- Excessive magnesium administration from magnesium-containing cathartic solutions given in conjunction with activated charcoal, magnesium-containing laxatives, and excess magnesium in peritoneal dialysis solutions.
- Iatrogenic oversupplementation, especially in patients with concurrent renal disease.

RISK FACTORS

- Dehydration.
- Renal disease.
- Intestinal hypomotility.
- Massive hemolysis.
- Hypoadrenocorticism.
- Hyperparathyroidism.
- Hypothyroidism.
- Patients receiving angiotensin-converting enzyme inhibitors and spironolactone concurrently.
- Excessive use of magnesium-containing cathartic solutions, especially in patients with renal insufficiency.

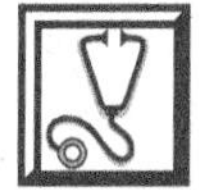

DIAGNOSIS

DIFFERENTIAL DIAGNOSIS

- Signs are most similar to those of hypocalcemia, which often occurs simultaneously.
- Bradycardia can be caused by neurologic disease, hyperkalemia, hypertension, hypothyroidism, sick sinus syndrome, and various drugs.

LABORATORY FINDINGS

Note: 12 mg of magnesium = 1 mEq of magnesium; to convert from mg/dL to mEq/L, divide by 1.2.

Drugs That May Alter Laboratory Results

- Serum is favored over plasma because the anticoagulant used for plasma samples can contain citrate or other ions that bind magnesium.
- EDTA, sodium fluoride-oxalate, sodium citrate, and intravenous calcium gluconate can cause falsely low serum magnesium values.

Disorders That May Alter Laboratory Results

- Hemolysis can result in falsely increased serum magnesium; the magnesium concentration in erythrocytes is approximately three times that in serum.
- Storage of serum or urine in metal containers can falsely elevate magnesium values.
- Hyperbilirubinemia can cause falsely decreased serum magnesium.

Valid if Run in Human Laboratory?

Yes

CBC/BIOCHEMISTRY/URINALYSIS

- Serum magnesium—dogs: >2.5 mg/dL; cats: >2.99 mg/dL.
- Hypocalcemia is common.
- Azotemia in some patients.

OTHER LABORATORY TESTS

- Ionized magnesium can be measured with an ion-selective electrode or by ultrafiltration of plasma; alternative methods of evaluating magnesium status include mononuclear blood cell magnesium levels or quantifying retention from a loading dose.
- Ionized hypermagnesemia is characterized as >0.58 mmol/L in dogs and >0.65 mmol/L in cats, but may vary slightly with the analyzer.

DIAGNOSTIC PROCEDURES

- Electrodiagnostics (e.g., electromyelography and electrocardiography) reveal effects of hypermagnesemia but do not differentiate the cause.
- Though not described in critically ill veterinary patients, hypermagnesemia can cause prolonged PR intervals and QRS duration in humans.

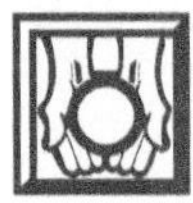

TREATMENT

APPROPRIATE HEALTH CARE

- Management involves enhancing elimination from the body and symptomatic therapy.
- Discontinue all magnesium-containing medications and nutritional supplements.
- Saline diuresis and loop diuretics enhance renal clearance of magnesium.
- Fluid therapy with 0.9% NaCl provides fluid volume to address hypovolemia, hypotension, and azotemia.
- Patients with oliguria might require peritoneal dialysis to treat severe hypermagnesemia.
- Parenteral calcium supplementation directly antagonizes the effects of magnesium, reversing respiratory depression, cardiac arrhythmias, and hypotension; calcium also enhances magnesium excretion.
- Hypermagnesemia associated with combined angiotensin-converting enzyme inhibitors and spironolactone is rare, mild, and unlikely to be clinically significant.
- Physostigmine, an anticholinesterase, can be used to treat severe neurotoxic effects.

NURSING CARE

Patients with neurologic manifestations of hypermagnesemia might require intensive nursing care to prevent aspiration pneumonitis, pulmonary atelectasis, pressure necrosis (bed sores), and urine and fecal scalding.

ACTIVITY

Patient activity is dependent on underlying conditions and response to therapy.

DIET

Any magnesium supplementation should be discontinued.

CLIENT EDUCATION

Clients should be advised if preexisting conditions contributed to hypermagnesemia.

MEDICATIONS

DRUG(S) OF CHOICE

- Furosemide promotes renal excretion of magnesium by decreasing absorption of magnesium in the loop of Henle.
- Enteral and parenteral calcium administration helps reverse clinical manifestations of hypermagnesemia and correct concurrent hypocalcemia; oral supplementation with any preparation can be given at a dosage of 25–50 mg/kg/day; severe hypermagnesemia can be treated with 10% calcium gluconate: 1–2 mL/kg (diluted 1 : 1 with saline) IV or SC q8h, administered slowly (may cause bradycardia).

CONTRAINDICATIONS

Magnesium-containing compounds and fluids.

PRECAUTIONS

Monitor ECG during calcium infusion.

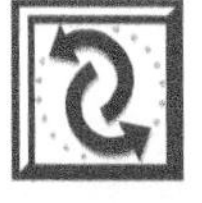

FOLLOW-UP

PATIENT MONITORING

- Serum magnesium and calcium concentrations.
- Renal function—azotemia and urine output.
- Continuous ECG if possible.

PREVENTION/AVOIDANCE

Magnesium supplementation should be approached cautiously in patients with renal insufficiency.

POSSIBLE COMPLICATIONS

- Severe hypermagnesemia and hypocalcemia can be fatal.
- Hypermagnesemic dogs were 2.6 times less likely to survive their illness than patients with normal serum magnesium levels.

EXPECTED COURSE AND PROGNOSIS

- Veterinary patients with iatrogenic overdose can have a good outcome with prompt recognition and supportive care.
- Increased ionized magnesium is rare and indicative of severe disease in noniatrogenic cases, particularly patients with acute renal disease, and can be associated with increased mortality.

MISCELLANEOUS

ASSOCIATED CONDITIONS

- Hypocalcemia.
- Hyperphosphatemia.
- Azotemia.

PREGNANCY/FERTILITY/BREEDING

Effects on the fetus are identical to effects on the dam.

SEE ALSO

Hypocalcemia

Suggested Reading

Bateman SW. Disorders of magnesium: magnesium deficit and excess. In: DiBartola SP, ed., Fluid, Electrolyte and Acid-Base Disorders in Small Animal Practice, 4th ed. Philadelphia, PA: Elsevier, 2011, pp. 212–229.

Humphrey S, Kirby R, Rudloff E. Magnesium physiology and clinical therapy in veterinary critical care. J Vet Emerg Crit Care 2015, 25(2):210–225.

Jackson CB, Drobatz KJ. Iatrogenic magnesium overdose: 2 case reports. J Vet Emerg Crit Care 2004, 14(2):115–123.

Martin LG, Allen-Durrance AE. Magnesium and phosphate disorders. In: Silverstein DC and Hopper K, eds., Small Animal Critical Care Medicine, 2nd ed. Philadelphia, PA: Elsevier, 2015, pp. 283–284.

Nakayama T, Nakayama H, Hiyamoto M, Hamlin RL. Hemodynamic and electrocardiographic effects of magnesium sulfate in healthy dogs. J Vet Intern Med 1999, 13:485–490.

Author Timothy B. Hackett

Consulting Editor Patty A. Lathan

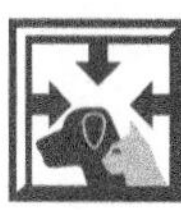

BASICS

DEFINITION

- Dysmetria—incoordination of the limbs during voluntary movement because of an inability to judge the rate, range, and force of movements.
- Hypermetria—overreaching limb movements giving a characteristic goose-stepping gait; the term dysmetria includes both hypo- and hypermetria.

PATHOPHYSIOLOGY

- The cerebellum plays a central role in generating skilled movements and maintaining muscle tone and body posture; it does not initiate but coordinates and smoothes movements.
- Damage to the cerebellum results in inaccurate gauging of voluntary movements; motor strength is preserved; conscious proprioception is unaffected.
- Rarely, compression of the spinocerebellar tracts in spinal cord disorders can produce dysmetria; this is more likely to occur with dorsally located lesions.

SYSTEMS AFFECTED

Nervous system.

GENETICS

- The hereditary ataxias are an important group of diseases in which cerebellar degenerations causes dysmetria and hypermetria in dogs.
- The majority of breed-related hereditary ataxias are autosomal recessive, highly penetrant traits.
- An X–linked hereditary ataxia has been described in pointers.
- Lysosomal storage diseases are genetic disorders, typically autosomal recessive in both dogs and cats.
- Immune-mediated encephalitis likely has a hereditary component—the mode of inheritance has not been described but is complex.

INCIDENCE/PREVALENCE

The incidence and prevalence of this presenting problem have not been reported.

GEOGRAPHIC DISTRIBUTION

There are no data on geographic distribution.

SIGNALMENT

Dog and cat of any age, breed, or sex.

SIGNS

Other signs of cerebellar disease that may be present include truncal sway, intention tremor, wide-based stance, head tilt, opsoclonus, spontaneous nystagmus, loss of menace response with normal vision, and anisocoria.

CAUSES

Cerebellar

- Dogs—hypoplasia (inherited or secondary to infection with canine herpesvirus in the perinatal period); hereditary ataxia (cerebellar abiotrophy or cerebellar cortical degeneration); lysosomal storage diseases; canine distemper virus (CDV); protozoal infections (*Neospora caninum* is most common, *Toxoplasma gondii* is possible but rare); rickettsial infections (*Ehrlichia canis* and Rocky Mountain spotted fever); *Cryptococcus* and other fungal infections; granulomatous meningoencephalitis; meningoencephalitis of unknown etiology; steroid-responsive tremor syndrome; neoplasia; trauma; infarct; hemorrhage; metronidazole toxicity.
- Cats—hypoplasia secondary to in utero infection with feline panleukopenia virus; lysosomal storage diseases; feline infectious peritonitis (FIP), feline leukemia virus (FeLV), feline immunodeficiency virus (FIV; associated immunosuppression predisposes to other encephalitides and to neoplasia); protozoal infections (*Toxoplasma gondii*); *Cryptococcus* and other fungal infections; neoplasia; hemorrhage; trauma.

Spinal

- While there are many causes of spinal cord disease, centro-dorsally located cervical lesions are more likely to produce hypermetria.
- Dogs—subarachnoid diverticula; neoplasia; vertebral malformation (atlantoaxial subluxation); and calcinosis circumscripta.

RISK FACTORS

Cerebellar

- Hereditary ataxia reported in Gordon and Irish setters, Kerry blue terriers, Airedale terriers, Finnish harriers and hounds, Samoyeds, Bern running dogs, cocker spaniels, Cairn terriers, Australian kelpies, bull mastiffs, Italian spinones, the terrier group, Lagotto-Romangolos, Old English sheepdogs, Rhodesian ridgebacks, border and rough-coated collies, Brittany spaniels, beagles, and Scottish terriers.
- Cerebellar hypoplasia has been reported in chow chows, Irish setters, and wire fox terriers.
- Lysosomal storage diseases causing dysmetria have been reported in Siamese, Balinese, Persian, and domestic shorthair cats, and in English springer spaniels, American Staffordshire terriers, Portuguese water dogs, German shorthaired pointers, Australian silky terriers, schipperkes, English setters, border collies, salukis, Chihuahuas, Queensland blue heelers, dachshunds, Yugoslavian shepherds, and Tibetan terriers.
- Small-breed dogs, such as Maltese, Yorkshire and West Highland white terriers, miniature pinschers, and Chihuahuas, are predisposed to immune-mediated encephalitis, including meningoencephalitis of unknown etiology and steroid-responsive tremor syndrome.
- Metronidazole at dosages >60 mg/kg/day can induce cerebello-vestibular signs in dogs; signs are induced in some dogs at lower doses.
- Vascular events, both thromboembolic and hemorrhagic, can cause cerebellar signs, typically due to thrombosis of the rostral cerebellar artery; disorders that cause a hypercoagulable state (such as hyperadrenocorticism) or hypertension (such as hyperthyroidism in cats, or chronic renal disease) can predispose to stroke; hypothyroidism has also been associated with cerebellar stroke; thrombosis of the rostral cerebellar artery occurs in older dogs—an underlying cause is not always identified.

Spinal

- Giant-breed dogs are predisposed to vertebral malformation.
- Toy-breed dogs are predisposed to atlanto-axial instability.
- Young large-breed dogs are predisposed to subarachnoid diverticula and calcinosis circumscripta.

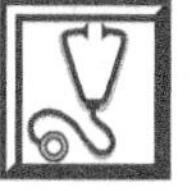

DIAGNOSIS

DIFFERENTIAL DIAGNOSIS

Some dogs, especially small breeds, have a high-stepping gait in their thoracic limbs as a normal finding. If there are no other signs of cerebellar disease, establish with the owners whether a high-stepping thoracic limb gait is normal for the dog.

CBC/BIOCHEMISTRY/URINALYSIS

- CBC may reflect infectious/inflammatory disease.
- Storage products may be present in leukocytes in some lysosomal storage diseases.

OTHER LABORATORY TESTS

- Acute and convalescent serologic titers—to diagnose rickettsial, protozoal, fungal, and viral diseases.
- Cerebrospinal fluid (CSF) antibody or antigen (*Cryptococcus*) titers—for some infections (e.g., *Toxoplasma, Cryptococcus*), measure in addition to serologic titers.
- PCR on CSF and serum—to diagnose rickettsial, bacterial, protozoal, fungal, and viral diseases; sensitive and specific if the infectious agent is present in the CSF or serum.
- Genetic tests available for hereditary ataxia in beagles, Finnish hounds, Italian spinones, Gordon setters, Old English sheepdogs, Lagotto-Romangolos, and the terrier group (Jack and Parson Russell terriers).

IMAGING

- Thoracic radiography—to identify metastatic disease in older patients.
- Abdominal ultrasonography—if intra-abdominal neoplasia is suspected.
- Brain CT or MRI—to diagnose neoplasia, vascular disease, encephalitis, cerebellar atrophy due to hypoplasia or abiotrophy; MRI is the preferred modality for evaluating the caudal fossa.

HYPERMETRIA AND DYSMETRIA (CONTINUED)

- Survey spinal radiography—if spinal cord disease is suspected; may be helpful in identifying vertebral malformations and calcinosis circumscripta.
- Spinal MRI—noninvasive and informative about spinal cord parenchyma.

DIAGNOSTIC PROCEDURES

- Fundic examination—to identify chorioretinitis (evidence of infectious/inflammatory disease) and vascular lesions associated with vasculitis or hypertension.
- CSF—to diagnose encephalitis; storage products may be present in CSF leukocytes in some lysosomal storage diseases.
- Liver biopsy—may be helpful in diagnosing certain lysosomal storage diseases in animals with hepatomegaly.

PATHOLOGIC FINDINGS

- These will depend on the underlying condition.
- Hereditary ataxias are associated with loss of neurons of the cerebellar cortex, as well as axonal pathology and gliosis.
- Lyososomal storage diseases are associated with accumulation of storage product within neurons and glial cells; frequently the Purkinje neuron is most severely affected.
- Infectious encephalitis is associated with infiltration of the cerebellum with inflammatory cells, and infectious organisms may be present (e.g., *Neospora caninum*; *Cryptococcal* infections); meningitis and perivascular cuffing may be present and there is frequently multifocal involvement of the CNS; there is profound cerebellar atrophy associated with *Neospora caninum* infections.
- Immune-mediated encephalitis is associated with infiltration of the CNS by inflammatory cells.

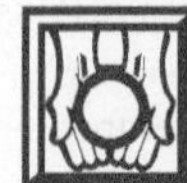

TREATMENT

APPROPRIATE HEALTH CARE

- Severe and/or rapidly progressive clinical signs—hospitalization for diagnostic workup and treatment.
- Mild and slowly progressive clinical signs—outpatient, but diagnostic tests requiring anesthesia necessitate hospitalization.
- Appropriate treatment of the underlying cause should be undertaken once a diagnosis has been established.

NURSING CARE

Severe intention tremors may make hand-feeding and IV fluids necessary.

ACTIVITY

Patients should be restricted to areas and activities where they are unlikely to fall and injure themselves.

DIET

No change. Dogs may benefit from a raised feeding bowl or hand-feeding.

SURGICAL CONSIDERATIONS

Surgical decompression of the spinal cord indicated for compressive myelopathies.

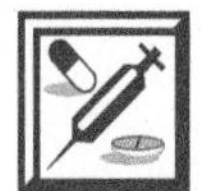

MEDICATIONS

DRUG(S) OF CHOICE

Discontinue metronidazole, regardless of the dose rate, to see if signs improve.

FOLLOW-UP

PATIENT MONITORING

- Periodic repeat neurologic examinations.
- Additional monitoring will depend on the underlying cause (e.g., serial monitoring of blood pressure in hypertensive patients).

MISCELLANEOUS

ZOONOTIC POTENTIAL

Fungal infections can be zoonotic.

ABBREVIATIONS

- CDV = canine distemper virus.
- CSF = cerebrospinal fluid.
- FeLV = feline leukemia virus.
- FIP = feline infectious peritonitis.
- FIV = feline immunodeficiency virus.

Suggested Reading

de Lahunta A, Glass E, Kent M. Veterinary Neuroanatomy and Clinical Neurology, 4th ed. St. Louis, MO: Elsevier Saunders, 2015, pp. 368–390.

Urkasemsin G, Olby NJ. Canine hereditary ataxia. Vet Clin North Am Small Anim Pract 2014, 44:1075–1089.

Author Natasha J. Olby

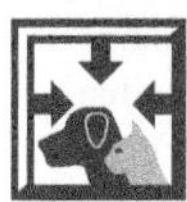

BASICS

DEFINITION

Serum sodium (Na^+) concentration >158 mEq/L in dogs or >165 mEq/L in cats.

PATHOPHYSIOLOGY

- Na^+ is the most abundant cation in the extracellular fluid, so hypernatremia usually results in hyperosmolality.
- Hypernatremia can be caused by excessive free water loss, increased intake of Na^+, or a combination of both.
- Common causes of hypernatremia include renal or gastrointestinal loss of water in excess of sodium loss and low water intake. Excessive Na^+ ingestion is a rare cause.

SYSTEMS AFFECTED

- Endocrine/metabolic.
- Nervous.

SIGNALMENT

Dog and cat.

SIGNS

- Polydipsia.
- Disorientation.
- Coma.
- Seizures.
- Other findings depend on underlying cause.
- Severity of signs usually correlates to the degree of hypernatremia.

CAUSES

- Free water deficit (most common cause)—low water intake (e.g., no access to water, adipsia, or hypodipsia); high urinary water loss; high insensible water loss (e.g., panting, hyperthermia).
    - Urinary loss (e.g., diabetes insipidus, diabetes mellitus, osmotic diuresis, diuresis after acute urinary obstruction).
    - Gastrointestinal sodium loss (e.g., administration of osmotic cathartic, vomiting, diarrhea).
    - A wide variety of drugs interfere with renal capacity to concentrate urine, leading to water loss in excess of Na^+; these drugs include lithium, demeclocycline, and amphotericin.
- Oral sodium ingestion (rare); IV administration of 0.9% or 7% NaCl; hyperaldosteronism (rarely hypernatremic); hyperadrenocorticism (mild).

DIAGNOSIS

DIFFERENTIAL DIAGNOSIS

- Central diabetes insipidus (due to neoplasia or head trauma).
- Alterations in thirst reaction pathway—rare.
- Salt ingestion—rare.

LABORATORY FINDINGS

Disorders That May Alter Laboratory Results

Lipemia or hyperproteinemia (>11 g/dL) can artifactually raise Na^+ concentration when the flame photometry method is used.

Valid if Run in a Human Laboratory?

Yes

CBC/BIOCHEMISTRY/URINALYSIS

- Consistent with underlying disease, if applicable.
- Diabetes insipidus—polyuria, hyposthenuria, and low urinary Na^+ concentration.
- Diabetes mellitus—hyperglycemia, isosthenuria.

IMAGING

CT scan or MRI in patients with diabetes insipidus to rule out pituitary tumor.

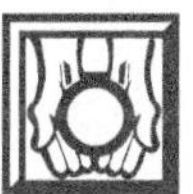

TREATMENT

- Fluid therapy and treatment of underlying disease.
- Water must be available at all times for patients with diabetes insipidus.

MEDICATIONS

DRUG(S) OF CHOICE

- If hypovolemia is present, replace volume with an isotonic crystalloid with a Na^+ concentration within 10 mEq/L of the patient's Na^+ concentration (0.9% saline has a Na^+ of 154 mEq/L, while lactated Ringer's has 130 mEq/L and Normosol®-R has 140 mEq/L). Volume replacement with this fluid may be continued as the free water deficit is replaced (below).
- Following volume resuscitation, administer hypotonic fluids (e.g., 5% dextrose in water or 5% dextrose with 0.45% saline) to reduce serum sodium by 0.5 mEq/h (12 mEq/L/day); supplement with potassium and phosphate if needed.
- Free water deficit—Wt (kg) × $\{[Na_{(presentation)}]/[Na_{(previous\ or\ normal)}] - 1\}$: administer this amount to achieve an ideal decrease of 0.5 mEq/h (i.e., if the sodium is 20 mEq above reference range, this should be administered over 40 hours).
- Formula to estimate how much each L of fluids will decrease the patient's serum Na^+—Δ in patient $[Na^+]$ = ($[Na^+]$ + $[K^+]$ in 1 L of solution – patient $[Na^+]$) / (0.6 × Wt (kg) +1).
- If the patient has oral water intake, this should be calculated as part of the free water restoration.

PRECAUTIONS

- Rapid correction of hypernatremia can cause cerebral edema. More rapid correction is only recommended if the hypernatremia is acute (<12 hours) or if the patient has neurologic abnormalities; correction should be slowed once signs abate.
- Cerebral edema is generally manifest as decreased mentation, and can be treated using hyperosmolar fluids (e.g., 7% NaCl, mannitol).

FOLLOW-UP

PATIENT MONITORING

- Acute setting—electrolytes, urine output, and bodyweight.
- Check sodium q4–6h initially and adjust fluid therapy as required to limit rapid changes.

POSSIBLE COMPLICATIONS

- CNS thrombosis or hemorrhage.
- Hyperactivity.
- Seizures.
- Serum sodium >180 mEq/L often associated with residual CNS damage.

MISCELLANEOUS

AGE-RELATED FACTORS

None

SYNONYMS

None

SEE ALSO

- Diabetes Insipidus.
- Hyposthenuria.

Suggested Reading

DiBartola SP. Fluid, Electrolyte, and Acid-Base Disorders in Small Animal Practice, 4th ed. Philadelphia, PA: Saunders, 2012.

Rose BD. Clinical Physiology of Acid-Base and Electrolyte Disorders, 5th ed. New York: McGraw-Hill, 2001.

Author Patty A. Lathan

Consulting Editor Patty A. Lathan

Acknowledgment The author and book editors acknowledge the prior contribution of Melinda Fleming.

HYPEROSMOLARITY

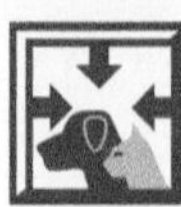

BASICS

DEFINITION

- Osmolarity—mOsm/L: the number of solute particles per liter of solution.
- Osmolality—mOsm/kg: the number of solute particles per kilogram of solution.
- Hyperosmolarity—a high concentration of solute particles per liter of solution.
- Serum concentrations >310 mOsm/L in dogs and >330 mOsm/L in cats are considered hyperosmolar.
- Morbidity from hyperosmolarity is related more to rapid changes in osmolarity than to the actual amount of change.

PATHOPHYSIOLOGY

- Serum sodium is responsible for most of the osmotically active particles that contribute to serum osmolarity; serum glucose and urea also contribute.
- Anything that causes free water loss increases concentrations of solutes in plasma or serum, thereby increasing serum osmolarity.
- Blood volume, hydration status, and anti-diuretic hormone (ADH) are intimately involved in controlling extracellular fluid volume.
- Low circulating blood volume and low blood pressure stimulates carotid and aortic baroreceptors to cause ADH secretion.
- Hyperosmolarity affects the osmoreceptors in the hypothalamus and stimulates ADH secretion from the posterior pituitary; the hypothalamic thirst center is also stimulated and causes an increase in water consumption.
- Rapid increases in serum osmolarity cause water movement along its concentration gradient from intracellular to extracellular spaces, resulting in neuronal dehydration, cell shrinkage, and cell death; cerebral vessels may weaken and hemorrhage.

SYSTEMS AFFECTED

- Cardiovascular—hypovolemia, hypotension, decreased ventricular contractility.
- Nervous—excessive thirst may be the first sign of hyperosmolarity. CNS depression may lead to coma.
- Renal/urologic—low urine output unless kidneys are source of free water loss.

SIGNALMENT

- Dog and cat.
- Hypodipsia and hyperosmolarity have been reported in young female miniature schnauzers.

SIGNS

General Comments

- Primarily neurologic or behavioral.
- Severity is related more to how quickly hyperosmolarity occurs than to the absolute magnitude of change.
- Clinical signs most likely if serum osmolarity is >350 mOsm/L and severe if >375 mOsm/L.

Historical Findings

Anorexia, lethargy, vomiting, weakness, disorientation, ataxia, seizures, and coma; polydipsia followed by hypodipsia.

Physical Examination Findings

- Normal, or abnormalities may reflect underlying disease.
- In addition to historical findings, dehydration, tachycardia, hypotension, weak pulses, and fever may be detected.

CAUSES

Increased Solute Concentrations

Hypernatremia, hyperglycemia, severe azotemia, ethylene glycol toxicosis, salt poisoning, sodium phosphate enemas in cats and small dogs, mannitol, radiographic contrast solution, administration of ethanol, aspirin toxicosis, shock, and parenteral nutrition solutions.

Decreased Extracellular Fluid Volume

Dehydration—gastrointestinal loss, cutaneous loss, third-space loss, low water consumption, polyuria without adequate compensatory polydipsia, excessive losses from panting.

RISK FACTORS

- Medical conditions that predispose—renal failure, diabetes insipidus (DI), diabetes mellitus (DM), hyperadrenocorticism, hyperaldosteronism, and heat stroke.
- Therapeutic hyperosmolar solutions—hypertonic saline, sodium bicarbonate, sodium phosphate enemas in cats and small dogs, mannitol, and parenteral nutrition solutions.
- High environmental temperatures, pain.
- Fever.

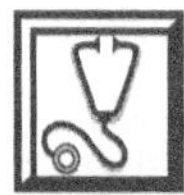

DIAGNOSIS

DIFFERENTIAL DIAGNOSIS

- Primary CNS disease and neoplasia may be characterized by altered mentation, but serum osmolarity is usually normal.
- Physical evidence or history of injury usually helps to rule out CNS depression caused by cranial trauma.
- Perform a thorough physical examination to assess hydration status and obtain information regarding previous therapy that may have included sodium-containing fluids or hyperosmolar solutions.

LABORATORY FINDINGS

Drugs That May Alter Laboratory Results

N/A

Disorders That May Alter Laboratory Results

N/A

Valid if Run in Human Laboratory?

Yes

CBC/BIOCHEMISTRY/URINALYSIS

High hematocrit, hemoglobin, and plasma proteins in dehydrated patients; serum electrolytes may also be increased.

OTHER LABORATORY TESTS

- Osmolarity is generally measured in the laboratory using freezing point depression but can be estimated from serum chemistry results (assuming the absence of unmeasured osmoles) using the formula: $2(Na^+ + K^+)$ + glucose/18 + BUN/2.8 = mOsm/L. Na^+ and K^+ concentrations are in mEq/L, glucose and blood urea nitrogen (BUN) concentrations are in mg/dL.
- Hyperosmolarity is an indication to evaluate serum sodium and glucose concentrations.
- Calculated osmolarity should not exceed measured osmolarity; if it does, consider laboratory error.
  - If measured osmolarity exceeds calculated osmolarity, determine the osmolar gap.
  - Osmolar gap = measured osmolarity – calculated osmolarity.
  - High measured osmolarity and normal calculated osmolarity with a high osmolar gap indicate the presence of unmeasured solutes (not Na^+, K^+, glucose, BUN).
  - High measured osmolarity and high calculated osmolarity with a normal osmolar gap usually indicate that the hyperosmolarity is caused by hyperglycemia or hypernatremia.
- Serum sodium concentration may be low in patients with severe hyperglycemia.
- Fasting hyperglycemia and glucosuria support a diagnosis of DM.
- Calcium oxalate monohydrate crystalluria suggests ethylene glycol toxicosis.
- High urine specific gravity (USG) rules out DI.
- Low USG, especially hyposthenuria, suggests DI.
- Urinary osmolarity lower than serum osmolarity suggests DI; concentrated urine rules out DI.

IMAGING

Renal ultrasonography may reveal bright hyperechoic kidneys in patients with ethylene glycol toxicosis.

TREATMENT

- Mild hyperosmolarity without clinical signs may not warrant specific treatment, but underlying disease(s) should be diagnosed and treated.
- Hospitalize patients with moderate to high osmolarity (>350 mOsm/L) and patients exhibiting clinical signs, and gradually lower serum osmolarity with IV fluids while a definitive diagnosis is pursued.
- Free water deficit can be calculated by the following formula: Free water deficit = 0.4 × lean bodyweight (kg) × [(Plasma Na/140) – 1].

- Administer 5% dextrose in water (D_5W) or 0.45% saline to slowly replace free water deficit.
- The goal is to not drop sodium more than 12 mEq/L in an 24-hour period. For example, if the free water deficit is 1 L and serum sodium concentration is 180 mEq/L, to normalize serum sodium concentration (to 145 mEq/L), the sodium concentration should drop over 35 hours (0.5 mEq/h). Thus, the 1 L of free water deficit should be given over 35 hours, or a rate of 28.5 mL/h (1000 mL/35h) if using D_5W. Maintenance isotonic IV fluids should be administered concurrently.
- Initially, 0.9% saline may be used to restore vascular volume; once hemodynamically stable, D_5W or 0.45% saline therapy may be initiated.
- If hyperosmolarity is acute (e.g. in patients with salt intoxication) and the duration is less than 6-8 hours, the free water deficit can be replaced more rapidly, through a combination of oral and IV water.
- If the patient is able to drink, free water deficit may be replaced orally; however, care must be taken to prevent excessive water ingestion.

MEDICATIONS

DRUG(S) OF CHOICE

- Intravenous free water replacement is best performed using D_5W or 0.45% NaCl.
- Seizures can be controlled with benzodiazepines or phenobarbital.

CONTRAINDICATIONS

Hypertonic saline and hyperosmolar solutions.

PRECAUTIONS

- Initial volume replacement should use a fluid with a Na^+ concentration closest to that of the patient.
- Rapid administration of hypotonic fluids (e.g., D_5W and 0.45% saline) may cause cerebral edema and worsen neurologic signs due to acute fluid shifts in the brain.

ALTERNATIVE DRUG(S)

Regular insulin 0.1 unit/kg IM/IV can be administered if a hyperglycemic crisis occurs secondary to parenteral nutrition administration.

FOLLOW-UP

PATIENT MONITORING

- Hydration status; avoid overhydration.
- Bladder size, urine output, serial bodyweight, and breathing patterns during IV fluid administration.
- Anuria, irregular breathing patterns, worsening depression, coma, or seizures are signs of deterioration.

POSSIBLE COMPLICATIONS

Altered consciousness and abnormal behavior.

MISCELLANEOUS

ASSOCIATED CONDITIONS

Hypernatremia and hyperglycemia.

AGE-RELATED FACTORS

None

PREGNANCY/FERTILITY/BREEDING

N/A

SEE ALSO

- Diabetes Mellitus with Hyperosmolar Hyperglycemic State.
- Hyperglycemia.
- Hypernatremia.

ABBREVIATIONS

- ADH = antidiuretic hormone.
- BUN = blood urea nitrogen.
- D_5W = 5% dextrose in water.
- DI = diabetes insipidus.
- DM =diabetes mellitus.
- USG = urine specific gravity.

Suggested Reding

DiBartola SP, ed. Fluid Therapy in Small Animal Practice. Philadelphia, PA: Saunders, 1992.

DiBartola SP, Green RA, Autran de Morais HS. Osmolality and osmolal gap. In: Willard MD, Tvedten H, Turnwald GH, eds., Small Animal Clinical Diagnosis by Laboratory Methods, 2nd ed. Philadelphia, PA: Saunders, 1994, pp. 106–107.

Goldcamp C, Schaer M. Hypernatremia in dogs. Compend Contin Educ Pract Vet 2007, 29(3):148–152.

Koenig A, Drobatz KJ, Beale AB, King LG. Hyperglycemic, hyperosmolar syndrome in feline diabetics: 17 cases (1995–2001). J Vet Emerg Crit Care 2004, 14:30–40.

Schermerhorn T, Barr SC. Relationships between glucose, sodium, and effective osmolality in dogs and cats. J Vet Emerg Crit Care 2006, 16:19–24.

Author Patty A. Lathan

Consulting Editor Patty A. Lathan

Acknowledgment The author and book editors acknowledge the prior contribution of Melinda Fleming.

HYPERPARATHYROIDISM

BASICS

DEFINITION

A pathologic, sustained, high, circulating concentration of parathyroid hormone (PTH).

PATHOPHYSIOLOGY

- PTH is secreted by the parathyroid glands in response to changes in the concentration of ionized calcium in the serum, and causes an increase in serum calcium concentration through direct effects on bone and renal tubular calcium resorption and indirectly by vitamin D–dependent intestinal calcium absorption.
- Hyperparathyroidism can develop as a primary condition or be secondary to a disorder of calcium homeostasis; primary hyperparathyroidism is usually associated with benign adenoma of the parathyroid gland(s), although adenocarcinoma and hyperplasia are possible; secondary hyperparathyroidism can be caused by a deficiency of calcium and vitamin D associated with malnutrition or chronic renal disease.

SYSTEMS AFFECTED

- Cardiovascular.
- Gastrointestinal.
- Neuromuscular.
- Renal/urologic.

GENETICS

- Autosomal dominant with possible age-dependent penetrance in the keeshond; genetic test available from Cornell.
- Secondary hyperparathyroidism can develop in association with hereditary nephropathy.

INCIDENCE/PREVALENCE

- Prevalence of primary form is unknown.
- More common in dogs than in cats.
- Common among causes of hypercalcemia, but less common than hypercalcemia of malignancy in dogs; more common in middle-aged to geriatric dogs.
- Chronic renal failure with secondary hyperparathyroidism is extremely common, more so in cats than in dogs.
- Nutritional secondary hyperparathyroidism is decreasing in prevalence as the public becomes more educated in pet nutrition.

SIGNALMENT

Species

Cat and dog.

Breed Predilections

- Keeshond, but seen in almost any breed.
- Siamese and domestic shorthair cats.

Mean Age and Range

- Cats—mean age 13 years; range: 8–20 years.
- Dogs—mean age 10 years; range: 4–17 years.

Predominant Sex

None

SIGNS

General Comments

- Most dogs and cats with primary hyperparathyroidism do not appear ill.
- Signs are usually mild and due to the effects of hypercalcemia, or lower urinary tract signs if urolithiasis is present.
- Signs become apparent when hypercalcemia is severe and chronic.

Historical Findings

- Polyuria.
- Polydipsia.
- Anorexia.
- Lethargy.
- Vomiting.
- Weakness.
- Urolithiasis.
- Stupor and coma.

Physical Examination Findings

- Often unremarkable.
- Parathyroid adenoma is not palpable in dogs but often is in cats.
- Nutritional secondary disease is sometimes associated with pathologic bone fractures and general poor body condition.

CAUSES

- Primary hyperparathyroidism—PTH-secreting adenoma of the parathyroid gland; in most cases only one gland is adenomatous; malignant tumors of the parathyroid glands are uncommon and usually noninvasive.
- Renal secondary hyperparathyroidism—renal calcium loss and reduced gut absorption of calcium due to deficiency in calcitriol production by the renal tubular cells.
- Nutritional secondary hyperparathyroidism—a nutritional deficiency of calcium and vitamin D.

RISK FACTORS

- Primary hyperparathyroidism—unknown.
- Secondary hyperparathyroidism—renal tubular disease or calcium/vitamin D malnutrition.

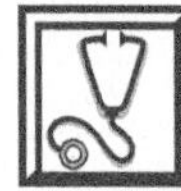

DIAGNOSIS

DIFFERENTIAL DIAGNOSIS

- The differential list includes causes of hypercalcemia.
- Lymphoma—common to cause hypercalcemia in dogs, rare to do so in cats.
- Anal sac apocrine gland adenocarcinoma—dogs.
- Other miscellaneous carcinomas—dogs and cats.
- Myeloproliferative disease—cats.
- Fibrosarcoma—cats.
- Chronic kidney disease.
- Hypoadrenocorticism.
- Vitamin D intoxication—cholecalciferol-containing rodenticides, plant sources, human anti-psoriasis topical creams, and vitamin supplements.
- Granulomatous diseases.
- Idiopathic hypercalcemia in cats.

CBC/BIOCHEMISTRY/URINALYSIS

- High serum total and ionized calcium concentrations.
- Low or low-normal serum phosphorus concentration in primary hyperparathyroidism.
- Hyperphosphatemia in renal secondary hyperparathyroidism or hypervitaminosis D.
- Serum blood urea nitrogen (BUN) and creatinine concentrations are usually normal in patients with primary hyperparathyroidism, except those with hypercalcemia-induced renal failure.

OTHER LABORATORY TESTS

- Serum ionized calcium determination is often normal (or low) in patients with chronic renal failure and high in patients with primary hyperparathyroidism or hypercalcemia associated with malignancy.
- High serum intact PTH concentration is diagnostic for primary hyperparathyroidism in the absence of azotemia; a serum PTH concentration within the normal reference range in an animal with ionized hypercalcemia should be considered *abnormal* and can signal parathyroid-dependent hypercalcemia.
- Measurement of PTH-related peptide (PTH-rp) may detect hyperparathyroidism related to neoplasia.

IMAGING

- Radiography can be useful to identify urolithiasis and occult neoplasia, as well as to assess renal morphology and bone density.
- Ultrasonography of the ventral cervical area sometimes reveals a parathyroid gland adenoma.
- Ultrasound of the abdomen can reveal lymphadenomegaly, urolithiasis, or renal morphologic abnormalities.

DIAGNOSTIC PROCEDURES

Surgical exploration of the ventral cervical area.

PATHOLOGIC FINDINGS

- Parathyroid adenoma is usually a solitary, small (≈1 cm), round, light brown or reddish mass located in the proximity of the thyroid gland.
- Occasionally multiple adenomas are found.
- The histologic distinctions between adenomas, hyperplasia, and carcinomas of the parathyroid gland are often unclear.

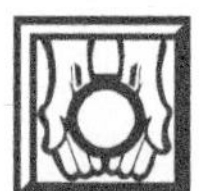

TREATMENT

APPROPRIATE HEALTH CARE

- Primary hyperparathyroidism generally requires inpatient care and surgery.
- Nutritional or renal secondary hyperparathyroidism in noncritical patients can be managed on an outpatient basis.

ACTIVITY

No alterations recommended.

DIET

Calcium supplementation for secondary forms.

CLIENT EDUCATION

Explain signs referable to changes in calcium status, because hypocalcemia is a potential complication of parathyroidectomy.

SURGICAL CONSIDERATIONS

- Surgery is the treatment of choice for primary hyperparathyroidism and is often important in establishing the diagnosis.
- Percutaneous ultrasound-guided heat ablation has been used successfully for treatment of parathyroid adenomas, and may be recommended if available.
- Percutaneous ultrasound-guided ethanol ablation has been reported to be less successful than surgery or heat ablation.

MEDICATIONS

DRUG(S) OF CHOICE

- Normal saline is the fluid of choice for treatment of hypercalcemia.
- Diuretics (furosemide) and corticosteroids can be useful in treating hypercalcemia.
- No medical treatment exists for primary hyperparathyroidism per se.
- Renal secondary hyperparathyroidism is sometimes treated with calcitriol, but its use has not gained uniform acceptance.
- A new class of calcimimetic drugs is being used to treat renal secondary hyperparathyroidism in human patients, but studies of these drugs in dogs and cats have not been reported and expense limits their use.

CONTRAINDICATIONS

Do not use glucocorticoids until the diagnosis of lymphoma has been excluded; they can obfuscate the diagnosis.

PRECAUTIONS

Use furosemide only in patients with adequate hydration.

ALTERNATIVE DRUG(S)

Pamidronate and other bisphosphonate drugs have been used to treat hypercalcemia of various causes in dogs and cats.

FOLLOW-UP

PATIENT MONITORING

- Postoperative hypocalcemia is relatively common after treatment of primary hyperparathyroidism; recent studies have shown that preoperative ionized calcium and PTH concentrations are poor predictors of postsurgical hypocalcemia, so monitoring is essential in all cases.
- Postoperative hypocalcemia requires treatment with vitamin D (calcitriol is recommended) and calcium supplements (see treatment of hypoparathyroidism), and ionized calcium should be monitored to guide dosage adjustments; contradictory evidence exists with respect to preoperative administration of calcitriol.
- In patients with renal impairment, check serum concentrations of BUN and creatinine.

PREVENTION/AVOIDANCE

- Avoid breeding affected keeshonden.
- Nutritional secondary hyperparathyroidism is prevented by proper nutrition.

POSSIBLE COMPLICATIONS

- Irreversible renal failure secondary to hypercalcemia.
- Fractures due to decreased bone density with chronic hyperparathyroidism.

EXPECTED COURSE AND PROGNOSIS

- Untreated primary hyperparathyroidism may progresses to end-stage kidney or neuromuscular disease depending on severity; many dogs clinically seem to do well even with no treatment, provided urolithiasis does not develop.
- Prognosis for surgical treatment of parathyroid adenoma is excellent.
- Recurrence is seen in a small percentage of cases.
- In animals that develop postoperative hypoparathyroidism, the return of normal parathyroid function is unpredictable and can take weeks to months.

MISCELLANEOUS

ASSOCIATED CONDITIONS

Calcium-containing urolithiasis.

AGE-RELATED FACTORS

N/A

PREGNANCY/FERTILITY/BREEDING

N/A

SEE ALSO

- Chronic Kidney Disease.
- Hypercalcemia.
- Hyperparathyroidism, Renal Secondary.

ABBREVIATIONS

- BUN = blood urea nitrogen.
- PTH = parathyroid hormone.
- PTH-rp = PTH-related peptide.

Suggested Reading

Dear JD, Kass PH, Della Maggiore AM, Feldman EC. Association of hypercalcemia before treatment with hypocalcemia after treatment in dogs with primary hyperparathyroidism. J Vet Intern Med 2017, 31(2):349–354.

Feldman EC, Hoar B, Pollard R, Nelson RW. Pretreatment clinical and laboratory findings in dogs with primary hyperparathyroidism: 210 cases (1987–2004). J Am Vet Med Assoc 2005, 227(5):756–761.

Milovancev M, Schmiedt CW. Preoperative factors associated with postoperative hypocalcemia in dogs with primary hyperparathyroidism that underwent parathyroidectomy: 62 cases (2004–2009). J Am Vet Med Assoc 2013, 242(4):507–515.

Richter KP, Kallet AJ, Feldman EC, Brum DE. Primary hyperparathyroidism in cats: seven cases (1984–1989). J Am Vet Med Assoc 1991, 199(12):1767–1771.

Schaefer C, Goldstein RE. Canine primary hyperparathyroidism. Compend Contin Educ Vet 2009, 31(8):382–389.

Author Brett A. Wasik

Consulting Editor Patty A. Lathan

Acknowledgment The author and book editors acknowledge the prior contribution of Thomas K. Graves.

Client Education Handout available online

H

HYPERPARATHYROIDISM, RENAL SECONDARY

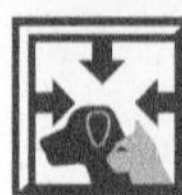

BASICS

OVERVIEW

- Syndrome characterized by a high parathyroid hormone (PTH) concentration secondary to chronic kidney disease (CKD); results from impaired renal excretion of phosphorus leading to hyperphosphatemia and ionized hypocalcemia, elevation of FGF-23, and suppression of renal calcitriol synthesis.
- In advanced CKD the diminished renal tubular mass produces less calcitriol. Calcitriol exerts negative feedback on PTH synthesis within the parathyroid gland. Low calcitriol, ionized hypocalcemia, and hyperphosphatemia result in increased PTH production and parathyroid gland hyperplasia.
- PTH may act as a uremic toxin, promoting nephrocalcinosis and progression of CKD.

SIGNALMENT

Dog and cat; see Chronic Kidney Disease for age and breed predilections.

SIGNS

- Uremia due to underlying CKD.
- Renal osteodystrophy or "rubber jaw" most commonly occurs in young dogs with severe renal secondary hyperparathyroidism (RSHPT).
- Pain around the head or long bones.

CAUSES & RISK FACTORS

- Any disease that causes CKD.
- Excess consumption of phosphorus.

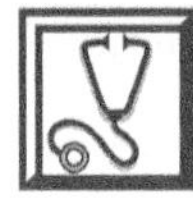

DIAGNOSIS

DIFFERENTIAL DIAGNOSIS

- Hypercalcemic nephropathy—kidney disease caused by ionized hypercalcemia; can be difficult to differentiate from longstanding RSHPT, in which hyperplasia of the parathyroid glands disrupts the normal feedback arc between PTH release and ionized calcium (tertiary hyperparathyroidism).
- Ionized serum calcium concentration is usually low or normal with RSHPT, but high with hypercalcemic nephropathy.
- Low serum PTH and PTH-related protein (PTHrP) high in animals with hypercalcemia of malignancy.
- Primary hyperparathyroidism—characterized by hypercalcemia, normal or low serum phosphorus, and inappropriate PTH concentration; kidney function is initially normal but may become compromised later.

CBC/BIOCHEMISTRY/URINALYSIS

- Azotemia.
- Hyperphosphatemia.
- Dilute urine.
- Total serum calcium does not reliably predict ionized calcium.

OTHER LABORATORY TESTS

Definitive diagnosis and therapeutic monitoring of RSHPT require measurement of serum PTH concentration using validated assay.

IMAGING

Radiographs may reveal low bone density, loss of the lamina dura around the teeth, and soft tissue mineralization of the gastric mucosa or other tissues.

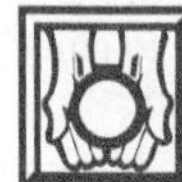

TREATMENT

- See Chronic Kidney Disease for general treatment principles.
- Minimize hyperphosphatemia by feeding a low phosphorus diet formulated for kidney disease and intestinal phosphate binders in order to achieve IRIS phosphorus goals.

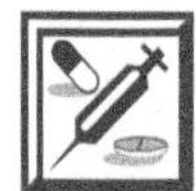

MEDICATIONS

DRUG(S) OF CHOICE

Intestinal Phosphate Binders

- If dietary management alone does not achieve the IRIS target serum phosphorus concentration, phosphorus binders can be used to further reduce serum phosphorus. Serum phosphorus targets based on the IRIS stages are stages 1 and 2: >2.7 to <4.6 mg/dL; Stage 3: >2.7 to <5.1 mg/dL; and Stage 4: >2.7 to <6.0 mg/dL.
- Aluminum hydroxide (60–90 mg/kg/day), calcium carbonate (90–150 mg/kg/day), calcium acetate (60–90 mg/kg/day), or lanthanum carbonate (60–90 mg/kg/day)—dose to achieve target serum phosphorus concentration, but do not exceed max dosage. All must be given with meals.
- Calcium-containing phosphate binders should be avoided with calcitriol therapy as hypercalcemia may occur. Combine different phosphate binders to reduce the dosage of each and minimize the risk of hypercalcemia or aluminum toxicity.

Calcitriol

- Low-dose calcitriol (2.0–3.5 ng/kg PO q24h)—may use after serum phosphorus is controlled, should be administered on an empty stomach and before bedtime (no food for 6–8 hours after administration).
- Maintain serum phosphorus concentration within the recommended IRIS target ranges before and during calcitriol therapy.

CONTRAINDICATIONS/POSSIBLE INTERACTIONS

- Calcitriol therapy may result in hypercalcemia, especially if combined with a calcium-containing phosphate binder. Increased total calcium concentration may develop in patients with long-standing CKD, but is unrelated to calcitriol treatment. Ionized calcium concentration is normal or low in these patients.
- Do not use calcium-containing intestinal phosphate binders in patients with a calcium × phosphorus product >70. Use aluminum- or lanthanum-containing intestinal phosphate binders initially to correct hyperphosphatemia. Calcium-containing phosphate binders can be used once the serum phosphorus concentration is within the target range.

FOLLOW-UP

PATIENT MONITORING

- Initially and in unstable patients, serum concentrations of calcium, phosphorus, creatinine, and urea nitrogen—monitor weekly to monthly depending on therapy and the severity of CKD.
- Patients receiving calcitriol should be monitored for hypercalcemia and hyperphosphatemia weekly for 4 weeks, then every 3–4 months.
- Serial evaluations of PTH concentration—most treated with low-dose calcitriol achieve near-normal levels of PTH within 3 months; it may be necessary to increase the dose in those with severe parathyroid gland hyperplasia.
- If hypercalcemia develops discontinue calcitriol; calcium should normalize within 5 days of discontinuation. Measurement of ionized calcium is recommended—animals with CKD may develop nonionized hypercalcemia that is unrelated to calcitriol treatment.

PREVENTION/AVOIDANCE

Dietary phosphorus restriction may delay the onset of RSHPT.

POSSIBLE COMPLICATIONS

Renal osteodystrophy and pathologic fractures (rare).

EXPECTED COURSE AND PROGNOSIS

- Progression of the underlying CKD may be slowed by minimizing phosphorus retention and RSHPT.
- Long-term prognosis is guarded to poor for patients with CKD and RSHPT.

MISCELLANEOUS

AGE-RELATED FACTORS

Young animals can develop severe renal osteodystrophy; calcitriol may be beneficial.

ABBREVIATIONS

- CKD = chronic kidney disease.
- PTH = parathyroid hormone.
- PTHrP = PTH-related protein.
- RSHPT = renal secondary hyperparathyroidism.

Suggested Reading

Foster J. Update on mineral and bone disorders in chronic kidney disease. Vet Clin North Am Small Anim Pract 2016, 46(6):1131–1149.

Polzin D. Chronic kidney disease. In: Ettinger SJ, Feldman EC, eds., Textbook of Veterinary Internal Medicine, 7th ed. St. Louis, MO: Elsevier, 2009, pp. 2036–2067.

Polzin DJ, Ross SJ, Osborne CA. Calcitriol therapy in chronic kidney disease. In: Bonagura J, ed., Current Veterinary Therapy XIV. Philadelphia, PA: Saunders, 2008, pp. 892–895.

Author David J. Polzin

Consulting Editor J.D. Foster

HYPERPHOSPHATEMIA

BASICS

DEFINITION

- Serum total phosphorus >5.5 mg/dL (dogs).
- Serum total phosphorus >6 mg/dL (cats).

PATHOPHYSIOLOGY

- Control of phosphorus is complex and is influenced by the actions of parathyroid hormone (PTH) and vitamin D and the interaction of these hormones with the gastrointestinal tract, bone, kidneys, and parathyroid glands. The phosphatonin fibroblast growth factor-23 (FGF-23) also regulates phosphorus levels.
- High serum phosphorus results from excessive gastrointestinal absorption of phosphorus, excessive bone resorption of phosphorus, and/or reduced renal excretion of phosphorus.

SYSTEMS AFFECTED

- Endocrine.
- Metabolic.
- Renal.

GENETICS

N/A

INCIDENCE/PREVALENCE

N/A

GEOGRAPHIC DISTRIBUTION

N/A

SIGNALMENT

- Dogs and cats.
- Any age, but commonly young, growing animals or older animals with renal insufficiency.

SIGNS

Historical Findings

- Depends on the underlying cause of hyperphosphatemia.
- No specific signs directly attributable to hyperphosphatemia.
- Acute hyperphosphatemia causes hypocalcemic tetany, seizures, or vascular collapse.

Physical Examination Findings

Chronic hyperphosphatemia causes calcification of soft tissues, resulting in chronic renal failure and tumoral calcinosis.

CAUSES

- Reduced glomerular filtration rate.
- Renal hypoperfusion (e.g., hypovolemia, systolic cardiac disease).
- Renal disease.
- Postrenal urinary tract disease (e.g., obstruction, ruptured urinary bladder).
- Metabolic acidosis.
- Excessive bone resorption.
- Rhabdomyolysis or massive tissue trauma.
- Young growing dogs.
- Hypoparathyroidism.
- Hypersomatotropism.
- Excessive gastrointestinal absorption of phosphorus.
- Osteolysis.
- Disuse osteoporosis.
- Osseous neoplasia.
- Hyperthyroidism.
- Phosphorus-containing enemas.
- Vitamin D toxicosis.
- Dietary supplementation.
- Nutritional secondary hyperparathyroidism.

RISK FACTORS

- Renal disease.
- Use of phosphorus-containing enemas, especially in smaller animals.
- Massive tissue injury.

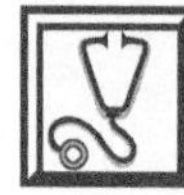

DIAGNOSIS

DIFFERENTIAL DIAGNOSIS

- Hypoparathyroidism—also characterized by clinical signs of hypocalcemia such as seizures and tetany.
- Prerenal azotemia as a cause of hyperphosphatemia—associated with disease states that result in low cardiac output such as congestive heart failure, hypovolemia, hypoadrenocorticism, and shock.
- Renal insufficiency, either acute or chronic renal failure—attended by azotemia and abnormal findings on urinalysis (low urinary specific gravity).
- Postrenal azotemia—associated with urinary obstruction or uroabdomen.
- Young, growing animals—can have serum phosphorus concentrations twice those of adults.
- Vitamin D intoxication—history of vitamin D supplementation or ingestion of rodenticides (e.g., Rampage® and D-CON®) or calcipotriene.
- Nutritional secondary hyperparathyroidism—history of dietary calcium–phosphorus imbalance.
- Hyperthyroidism in cats—clinical signs of weight loss, polyphagia, and polydipsia and polyuria.
- Hypersomatotropism—attended by a history of progesterone administration in dogs and insulin-resistant diabetes mellitus in cats.
- Nonazotemia tumoral calcinosis—observed in human beings as an autosomal dominant disorder; rare cause of hyperphosphatemia associated with large bone lesions.
- Jasmine toxicity—history of plant ingestion.
- Massive tissue injury.
- Rhabdomyolysis.
- Tumor lysis syndrome.
- Spurious.

LABORATORY FINDINGS

Drugs That May Alter Laboratory Results

Intravenous potassium phosphate.

Disorders That May Alter Laboratory Results

- Hemolysis, hyperbilirubinemia, and lipemia can falsely raise phosphorus concentrations.
- Collection in citrate, oxalate, or EDTA.

Valid If Run in Human Laboratory?

Yes

CBC/BIOCHEMISTRY/URINALYSIS

- Serum phosphorus >6 mg/dL.
- Low serum calcium in patients with primary hypoparathyroidism.
- High serum calcium in patients with vitamin D intoxication.
- Degree of azotemia and urine specific gravity help define level renal impairment.
- Hyperkalemia and hyponatremia suggest hypoadrenocorticism.

OTHER LABORATORY TESTS

- Serum PTH measurement—intact molecule and two-site assay methods have the greatest specificity; high-normal or high concentrations with concurrent hyperphosphatemia suggest primary hyperparathyroidism; low concentrations with concurrent hypocalcemia and hyperphosphatemia suggest neoplasia.
- Thyroxine concentrations—indicated in cats with hyperphosphatemia and clinical signs consistent with hyperthyroidism.
- Insulin-like growth factor 1 (IGF-1) concentrations—indicated in dogs or cats with unexplained hyperphosphatemia and clinical signs consistent with acromegaly; IGF-1 concentrations are elevated in animals with hypersomatotropism.
- Vitamin D assays are not readily available.
- Adrenocorticotropic hormone (ACTH) stimulation testing to confirm hypoadrenocorticism.

IMAGING

- Abdominal radiography to assess renal size and symmetry.
- Renal ultrasonography to detect soft tissue mineralization.
- Nuclear scintigraphy to rule out hyperthyroidism.
- Radiography of long bones to detect osteoporosis or neoplasia.

DIAGNOSTIC PROCEDURES

Renal biopsy.

PATHOLOGIC FINDINGS

Mineralization of soft tissues may be noted radiographically or histopathologically.

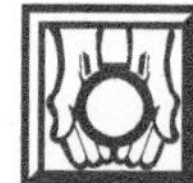

TREATMENT

APPROPRIATE HEALTH CARE

Inpatient, because of the deleterious effects of hyperphosphatemia and the need for fluid therapy; consider severe hyperphosphatemia a medical emergency. Long-term monitoring and management may be necessary.

NURSING CARE

Isotonic crystalloid fluids to increase glomerular filtration rate and promote phosphorus excretion.

ACTIVITY

N/A

DIET

Restrict dietary phosphorus.

CLIENT EDUCATION

Long-term monitoring and management may be necessary with phosphorus-restricted diets and/or oral phosphate binders.

SURGICAL CONSIDERATIONS

N/A

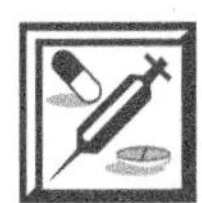

MEDICATIONS

DRUG(S) OF CHOICE

Acute Hyperphosphatemia

- Dextrose (0.5–1 g/kg IV) and regular insulin (0.25–0.5 U/kg IV), to shift phosphorus intracellularly.
- Avoid phosphorus-containing fluids.

Chronic Hyperphosphatemia

Oral administration of phosphorus binders (e.g., aluminum hydroxide or aluminum carbonate, 30–100 mg/kg/day PO, or calcium carbonate at 90–150 mg/kg/day PO, both with meals).

CONTRAINDICATIONS

N/A

PRECAUTIONS

Calcium carbonate should be avoided with hypercalcemia.

POSSIBLE INTERACTIONS

N/A

ALTERNATIVE DRUG(S)

The oral phosphate binders sevelamer hydrochloride and lanthanum carbonate may be used as oral phosphate binders, but relatively little information is available in the veterinary literature.

FOLLOW-UP

PATIENT MONITORING

- Serum calcium every 12 hours.
- Renal function tests—urine output must be monitored, particularly if oliguric renal failure is suspected, in which case urine output should be measured carefully; oliguria cannot be determined unless the patient is fully hydrated.
- Hydration status—indicators of over-hydration include increased bodyweight, chemosis, increased central venous pressure, and edema (pulmonary or subcutaneous).
- Long-term serial monitoring of phosphorus is used to make dose adjustments in oral phosphate binders.

PREVENTION/AVOIDANCE

- Avoid ingestion of cholecalciferol rodenticides, calcipotriene, or Vitamin D supplementation.
- Avoid phosphate-containing enemas.
- Well-balanced veterinary diets prevent nutritional secondary hyperparathyroidism.

POSSIBLE COMPLICATIONS

- Hypophosphatemia resulting in hemolysis.
- Soft tissue mineralization.

EXPECTED COURSE AND PROGNOSIS

Depends on the underlying cause. Chronic kidney disease often causes chronic hyperphosphatemia and has a poor to guarded prognosis in dogs.

MISCELLANEOUS

ASSOCIATED CONDITIONS

Hypocalcemia

AGE-RELATED FACTORS

Mild elevations in phosphorus may be normal in growing animals.

ZOONOTIC POTENTIAL

N/A

PREGNANCY/FERTILITY/BREEDING

N/A

SYNONYMS

N/A

SEE ALSO

- Acute Kidney Injury.
- Chronic Kidney Disease.
- Hypoparathyroidism.

ABBREVIATIONS

- ACTH = adrenocorticotropic hormone.
- FGF-23 = fibroblast growth factor-23.
- IGF-1 = insulin-like growth factor I.
- PTH = parathyroid hormone.

Suggested Reading

Allen-Durrance AE. A quick reference on phosphorus. Vet Clin North Am Small Anim Pract 2017, 47:257–262.

Aurbach GD, Marx SJ, Spiegel AM. Parathyroid hormone, calcitonin, and the calciferols. In: Wilson JD, Foster DW, eds., Williams Textbook of Endocrinology, 7th ed. Philadelphia, PA: Saunders, 1985, pp. 1208–1209.

Willard MD, Tvedten H, Turnwald GH. Clinical Diagnosis by Laboratory Methods. Philadelphia, PA: Saunders, 1989.

Author Alyssa M. Sullivant

Consulting Editor Patty A. Lathan

Acknowledgment The author and book editors acknowledge the prior contribution of Deborah S. Greco.

HYPERSOMATOTROPISM/ACROMEGALY IN CATS

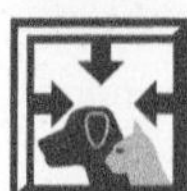

BASICS

OVERVIEW

- Caused by excessive growth hormone (GH) secretion from the anterior pituitary by an adenoma or somatotroph hyperplasia.
- GH induces hepatic insulin-like growth factor-1 (IGF-1) secretion. The combination of increased GH and IGF-1 causes lipolysis, protein synthesis, impaired carbohydrate metabolism, and insulin resistance (IR).
- Prevalence in Europe ranges from 1 : 3 to 1 : 5.5 diabetic cats.

SIGNALMENT

- Median age—11 years (range: 9.5–13 years).
- Male : female ratio is 2 : 1.
- No breed predisposition.

SIGNS

- Clinical signs of diabetes mellitus (DM; e.g., polyuria, polydipsia, and polyphagia) occur from GH-induced IR. IR can be variable or persistent, which makes the DM difficult to control.
- Many (~40%) diabetics with hypersomatotropism (HST) lose weight due to poorly controlled DM; a small proportion (~17%) gain weight.
- Anabolic state—patients may present with polyphagia (without DM), or soft tissue growth resulting in upper airway obstruction, broad facial features, or clubbed feet.
- A small proportion (~2%) develop neurologic signs due to pituitary adenoma.

CAUSES & RISK FACTORS

- GH-secreting pituitary adenoma or somatotroph hyperplasia.
- In dogs, but not cats, progestins can result in increased GH concentration.

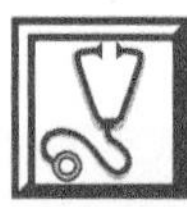

DIAGNOSIS

DIFFERENTIAL DIAGNOSIS

- Uncomplicated DM.
- Pituitary-dependent hyperadrenocorticism.
- Causes of polyphagia such as exocrine pancreatic insufficiency, gastrointestinal inflammatory diseases, hyperthyroidism, and inflammatory liver diseases. Cats with HST and polyphagia but without DM typically gain weight, unlike other differentials.

CBC/BIOCHEMISTRY/URINALYSIS

- Consistent with DM.
- Diabetic ketoacidosis uncommon.

OTHER LABORATORY TESTS

- Serum IGF-1 concentration using validated assays is test of choice.
  - Positive predictive value of IGF-1 >1000 ng/mL (131 nmol/L) of 95%.
  - Roughly one-third of cats with HST have a low IGF-1 at diagnosis, which increases to >1000 ng/mL after insulin therapy.
  - IGF-1 concentrations between 700 and 1000 ng/mL (92–131 nmol/L) is a "gray" zone—many non-HST diabetic cats are in this range.
- There is no commercially available GH assay.

IMAGING

- Abdominal ultrasound might identify organomegaly.
- Contrast-enhanced CT can assess pituitary size.
- Echocardiographic findings—increased left ventricular wall thickness, left atrial enlargement, aortic insufficiency.

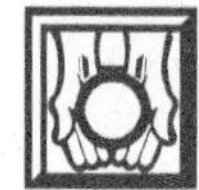

TREATMENT

Surgery

Hypophysectomy most consistently normalizes IGF-1 concentration (80% of cases) and results in highest diabetic remission rates (50% achieve long-term remission).

Medical Management

- Somatostatins (SSTs) are primary negative regulatory hormones of GH secretion.
- Pasireotide is an SST analogue. Short-acting pasireotide (0.03 mg/kg SC q12h) decreased IGF-1 in 12 cats after 3 days of treatment, while long-acting pasireotide (8 mg/kg SC monthly) resulted in normalization of IGF-1 in 2/8 cats; all cats experienced increased insulin sensitivity and 3/8 cats achieved diabetic remission.
- Octreotide is an SST analogue with a different binding profile that temporarily decreases GH without improvement in clinical control of HST or DM.
- Dopamine receptor 2 inhibits GH secretion. Cabergoline, a dopamine receptor 2 agonist, decreases IGF-1 and increases insulin sensitivity in some cats with HST.

Radiotherapy

Fractionated radiotherapy improves neurologic signs and may improve diabetic control. Stereotactic radiotherapy might be more favorable as improved diabetic control and diabetic remission is more likely.

Palliative Treatment

- Maximizing diabetic control (e.g. with insulin and diet) is recommended but may be challenging.
- Comorbidities (e.g., osteoarthritis, cardiac disease) should be managed.
- Controlling polyphagia in some cats with HST is challenging. Despite lack of endocrine improvement after cabergoline, many owners reported normalization of appetite.

MEDICATIONS

See Medical Management.

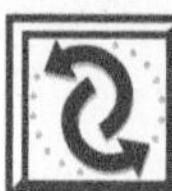

FOLLOW-UP

- Depends on treatment modality.
- Survival varies from months to years; most euthanized due to poor quality of life or causes unrelated to HST.
- Diabetic control should be monitored as for an uncomplicated diabetic. A small proportion of cats gain weight despite poor diabetic control and have persistent polyphagia despite good diabetic control.

MISCELLANEOUS

ABBREVIATIONS

- DM = diabetes mellitus.
- GH = growth hormone.
- HST = hypersomatotropism.
- IGF-1 = insulin like growth factor-1.
- IR = insulin resistance.
- SST = somatostatin.

Suggested Reading

Berg RI, Nelson RW, Feldman EC, et al. Serum insulin-like growth factor-I concentration in cats with diabetes mellitus and acromegaly. J Vet Intern Med 2007, 21(5):892–898.

Gostelow R, Scudder C, Keyte S, et al. Pasireotide long-acting release treatment for diabetic cats with underlying hypersomatotropism. J Vet Int Med 2017, 31(2):355–364.

Wormhoudt TL, Boss M-K, Lunn K, et al. Stereotactic radiation therapy for the treatment of functional pituitary adenomas associated with feline acromegaly. J Vet Int Med 2018, 32(4):1383–1389.

Author Christopher J. Scudder

Consulting Editor Patty A. Lathan

Acknowledgment The author and book editors acknowledge the prior contributions of Deborah S. Greco and David Church.

HYPERTENSION, PORTAL

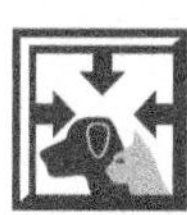

BASICS

DEFINITION

Portal pressure >13 cm H_2O (10 mmHg).

PATHOPHYSIOLOGY

- Causes—increased portal blood flow (arterialized system), increased resistance to portal blood flow, or combination.
- Increased portal flow—arterialization of portal circulation occurs in arteriovenous (AV) malformation or subsequent to increased hepatic resistance causing retrograde blood flow into valveless splanchnic portal circulation.
- Hepatofugal—portal splanchnic circulation away from liver.

Increased Resistance Relative to Liver

- Prehepatic—abdominal portion of portal vein.
- Hepatic—within liver.
- Posthepatic—cranial to liver: terminal hepatic veins, vena cava, heart, pericardium.

Intrahepatic Increase in Resistance

- Presinusoidal—within portal tract.
- Sinusoidal—within sinusoid or space of Disse.
- Postsinusoidal—hepatic venular outflow tract causing sinusoidal occlusion or Budd Chiari syndrome.
- Consequences—development of multiple acquired portosystemic shunts (APSS), abdominal effusion due to increased lymph formation, predisposition to hepatic encephalopathy (HE).
- Acquired portosystemic shunts (APSS)—develop within 1–2 months of acquired portal hypertension (PH).

Effusion Protein Content

- Hepatic causes—pure transudate reflects concurrent PH and hypoalbuminemia (protein <1.5 g/dL).
- Posthepatic causes—modified transudate (protein >2.5 g/dL).
- Prehepatic causes—pure or modified transudate, low cellularity.

SYSTEMS AFFECTED

- Hepatobiliary disorders—obstructed blood flow in any zone or diffusely across sinusoids causes intrahepatic PH, splanchnic PH, ± passive splenic congestion (splenomegaly).
- Posthepatic disorders—hepatic passive congestion, hepatomegaly, variable PH; *APSS usually absent.*
- Prehepatic disorders—cause splanchnic PH, splenic congestion, APSS; portal venous thrombi, stenosis, stricture, entrapment in porta hepatis (e.g., pancreatitis, neoplasia), mass compression (pancreatic inflammation; neoplasia).
- Nervous—HE due to APSS.
- Cardiovascular—APSS and ascites may develop with vena caval/hepatic vein obstruction (at level of diaphragm), *but not* with congestive heart failure or pericardial tamponade.
- Portal thrombi—caused by gastrointestinal (GI) inflammation/necrosis and splanchnic vasculitis, neoplasia, disseminated intravascular coagulation, loss of anticoagulants, accelerated thrombosis.
- GI—splanchnic hypertension can provoke enteric edema, increased gut wall permeability provoking transmural bacterial translocation (endotoxemia, bacteremia), hypertensive enteric vasculopathy (enteric bleeding, ulceration), diapedesis blood loss, protein malassimilation.

GENETICS

- Vascular malformations causing portal atresia (intrahepatic, prehepatic) are congenital and represent severe phenotype of polygenic portal venous malformations in small-breed dogs.
- Ductal plate malformation (DPM)—congenital hepatic fibrosis (CHF) phenotype causes APSS; occurs in numerous dog breeds and Persian-related cats; increased frequency in boxers.
- Noncirrhotic PH—adult-onset diminution of tertiary portal branches, affects individual dogs of many breeds, described in Doberman pinschers (rare).
- Acquired sinusoidal PH due to necroinflammatory liver injury—immune-mediated chronic hepatitis (anecdotal in some breeds).
- Copper associated hepatopathy—Bedlington terrier *COMMD1* mutation, predisposition for copper associated hepatopathy in Labrador retrievers, Dalmatian, Doberman pinscher, and numerous other dogs may reflect pharmacogenetic breed differences in copper transporters.

SIGNALMENT

Species

Dog > cat.

Breed Predilections

Familial hepatic vascular disorders—Doberman pinschers (noncirrhotic PH); Saint Bernard (AV malformation); cocker spaniel hepatopathy; copper associated hepatopathy: Bedlington terriers, Doberman pinschers, Labrador retriever, others; DPM with CHF phenotype: boxers predisposed, any large or small dog breed, cats.

Mean Age and Range

- Juveniles—inherited or congenital disorders; vena caval and cardiac malformations.
- Young dogs and cats <1.5 years of age—congenital hepatic vascular malformations with portal venous atresia: may be more common in Yorkshire terriers, Maltese, pugs, cats.
- Juvenile and young adult dogs and cats—DPM with CHF phenotype.
- Young dogs and cats—hepatic AV malformations, onset of signs <1.5 years of age.
- Middle-aged and older animals—acquired hepatobiliary disorders and portal thrombi.

SIGNS

General Comments

- Depend on site, degree, rate of onset of PH, and causal factors.
- Acquired disorders—slowly progressive, chronic in onset.

Historical Findings

- Portal thromboembolism may acutely appear but remain unnoticed until APSS form; vague GI signs at occurrence including bloody diarrhea, ileus, abdominal pain, lethargy, inappetence.
- Abdominal distention—ascites.
- HE—secondary to APSS.
- Cardiac disorders or pericardial restriction—cough; exercise intolerance; dyspnea, jugular pulse, weak femoral pulses or pulsus alternans, reduced heart sounds on auscultation.

Physical Examination Findings

- Abdominal effusion.
- Hepatomegaly—posthepatic causes only.
- Splenomegaly—reflects splanchnic congestion or venous thrombi, inconsistent.
- Jugular vein distention—posthepatic cardiac or pericardial causes.
- Muffled heart sounds—pericardial or pleural effusion.
- Cardiac arrhythmias or murmur—cardiac disease.
- Pulmonary "crackles" (edema)—cardiac or pericardial causes.
- Confusion, stupor, coma, blindness, other neurobehavioral abnormalities—HE.
- Jaundice—hepatic causes.
- Hepatic bruit (hepatic AV malformation).
- Signs consequent to surgical ligation of portosystemic venous anomaly (PSVA).

CAUSES

Prehepatic

- Portal vein thrombosis, stenosis, or neoplasia.
- Portal vein compression—large lymph nodes; neoplasia, granuloma; abscess; pancreatitis, entrapment in diaphragmatic hernia.
- Postoperative complication of PSVA ligation.
- Congenital portal vein atresia.

Intrahepatic

- Hepatic fibrosis/cirrhosis.
- Chronic inflammatory liver disease.
- Chronic extrahepatic bile duct obstruction (EHBDO) >6 weeks.
- DPM with CHF phenotype.
- Hepatic neoplasia—porta hepatis location.
- Liver entrapment—in diaphragmatic hernia.
- Sinusoidal occlusion syndrome.
- Veno-occlusive disease (zone 3 lesion).
- Noncirrhotic portal hypertension.
- Portal vein atresia (intra- or extrahepatic).
- Hepatic AV malformation.

HYPERTENSION, PORTAL (CONTINUED)

Posthepatic

- Right-sided congestive heart failure.
- Heartworm disease.
- Pericardial tamponade.
- Pericarditis—restrictive or constrictive.
- Cardiac neoplasia.
- Cor triatriatum dexter.
- Pulmonary thromboemboli (TE).
- Disorders affecting supradiaphragmatic caudal vena cava— thrombosis; congenital kink or web; heartworm vena cava syndrome; occlusion by neoplasia; entrapment in diaphragmatic hernia; trauma.
- Budd Chiari syndrome.

H

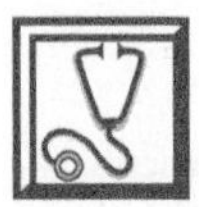

DIAGNOSIS

DIFFERENTIAL DIAGNOSIS

- Physicochemical analysis of abdominal effusion—helps narrow diagnoses.
- Pure transudate—hypoalbuminemia secondary to protein-losing enteropathy (PLE), protein-losing nephropathy (PLN), liver failure.
- Modified transudate with normal or low albumin—PLE, PLN, liver failure (chronic effusion), neoplasia, splanchnic TE, liver (visceral) entrapment in diaphragmatic hernia.
- Modified transudate with large liver and jugular distention—cardiac or pericardial abnormalities; heartworm; right atrial tumor.
- Modified transudate with large liver without jugular distention, muffled heart, or pulmonary edema—kinked vena cava; Budd Chiari–like or sinusoidal occlusion syndrome.
- HE— liver fibrosis; cirrhosis; CHF; hepatic AV malformation; any cause of APSS.
- Jaundice—chronic hepatitis, cholangitis; EHBDO; infiltrative hepatic neoplasm.
- Bloody diarrhea, abdominal pain, ileus, signs of endotoxemia—acute splanchnic portal TE.

CBC/BIOCHEMISTRY/URINALYSIS

- CBC—schistocytes with TE; red blood cell microcytosis with PSVA or APSS; icteric plasma with liver disease or microangiopathic shearing anemia.
- Biochemistry—liver disease associated with variable liver enzymes, low blood urea nitrogen, creatinine, cholesterol, and/or glucose concentrations, hyperbilirubinemia, coagulation abnormalities; posthepatic disorders associated with high liver enzymes, ± azotemia, normal plasma color.
- Urinalysis—ammonium biurate crystalluria with APSS; may note granular casts with TE affecting renal perfusion; may note proteinuria with heartworm disease.

OTHER LABORATORY TESTS

- Total serum bile acids (TSBA)—variable fasting and high 2h postprandial concentrations with APSS or hepatobiliary disease; shunting pattern (normal fasting and markedly high postprandial values) common.
- Blood ammonia—hyperammonemia with APSS or inferred by finding ammonium biurate crystalluria; less reliable compared to TSBA.
- Physicochemical characterization of abdominal effusion—high serum : effusion albumin ratio (>1.1) consistent with PH.

IMAGING

Radiography

- Thoracic radiography—may reveal cause of posthepatic PH.
- Abdominal radiography—may reveal effusion, splenomegaly, hepatomegaly; microhepatica in most hepatic disorders and portal atresia causing APSS.

ABDOMINAL US

- Identify abnormalities involving abdominal or extrahepatic portal vein—atresia, stricture, thrombi, occlusive lesions in porta hepatis.
- Identify lobe(s) containing AV malformations.
- Inspect splanchnic circulation using Doppler color flow; document hepatofugal circulation, identify portal thrombi, APSS, PSVA.
- Evaluate echogenicity of nonhepatic viscera, identify lymphadenomegaly, mass lesions, adhesions.
- Estimate hepatic venous distention—intrahepatic and supradiaphragmatic segments.

Echocardiography

Detects congenital and acquired cardiac and pericardial disorders, neoplasia, thrombi, heartworms, pleural effusion, malformed or thrombosed vena cava, diaphragmatic hernia.

Angiography and Nuclear Imaging

- Colorectal or splenoportal scintigraphy—confirms portosystemic shunting but not anatomic details.
- Radiographic angiography—celiac trunk and hepatic artery contrast studies confirm hepatic AV malformation; nonselective or selective studies: congenital cardiac disease, TE, hepatic vein disorders, AV malformation.
- Portovenography—confirms APSS.
- Multisector CT—displays arterial and venous phases.

DIAGNOSTIC PROCEDURES

- ECG and central venous pressure—with cardiac disease, cranial mediastinal obstructions.
- Liver biopsy—required for diagnosis of hepatobiliary disorders.
- Portal pressure—may be measured during laparotomy but not recommended; PH adequately confirmed with imaging studies and on gross inspection.

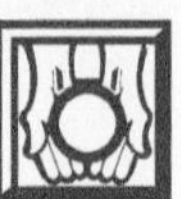

TREATMENT

APPROPRIATE HEALTH CARE

Inpatient—for severe HE, amelioration of tense ascites by therapeutic abdominocentesis, supportive care for acute TE.

NURSING CARE

- Fluid therapy—restrict sodium concentration (avoid 0.9% NaCl); avoid iatrogenic pulmonary edema during fluid therapy (*caution*: if hypoalbuminemia, monitor respiration rate/effort).
- Monitor bodyweight and condition, girth circumference, plasma proteins, packed cell volume—assess hydration status, volume of abdominal effusion, IV fluid tolerance.
- Low oncotic pressure—may require plasma or colloid administration (plasma preferred for liver patient); Voluven® or VetStarch® (6%; 130 MW/0.4 molar substitution) 10–20 mL/kg/day IV CRI) may be necessary for acute adjustments; avoid hetastarch as can reduce platelet function.
- Glucose supplementation—with hepatic dysfunction and hypoglycemia; 2.5–5.0% dextrose with half-strength polyionic fluids initially; avoid hyperglycemia.

Mobilization of Ascites

- *Abdominal effusion*—sequentially assess: bodyweight, girth, body condition score; initially exercise restrict; enforce dietary sodium restriction.
- *Conventional diuretics*—combine furosemide and spironolactone; furosemide (0.5–2 mg/kg PO q12–24h) and spironolactone (0.5–2 mg/kg PO q12h, use single doubled dose for loading one time): dose titrations based on response q4 days; adjust using incremental 25–50% dose increase; serum : effusion albumin ratio (>1.1) may predict response to diuretics.
- *Vasopressin V_2 antagonists* (aquaretics) *may* assist with management of diuretic-resistant ascites; tolvaptan successful in dogs with experimentally induced (rapid pacing) congestive heart failure; human dose in cirrhosis 7.5 mg/day; metabolized exclusively in liver primarily by cytochrome P450; dose undetermined in dogs with liver disease.
- *Telmisartan*—angiotensin receptor blocker is alternative diuretic worthy of consideration; administration PO at 1.0 mg/kg/day significantly increased urine volume and sodium excretion in healthy dogs in one study.
- Taper diuretic dose after initial positive response; individualize chronic treatment to response; may be used intermittently for recurring ascites.
- Avoid dehydration, can lead to HE.
- Avoid hypokalemia, can provoke HE.
- If ascites due to right-sided congestive heart failure, treat accordingly.

• *Diuretic-resistant ascites*—large-volume (therapeutic) abdominocentesis if ascites resistant to medical intervention or compromises food intake, ventilation, or sleep: requires aseptic technique, fluid removal over 45–90 min, concurrently provide polyionic fluids in moderation with colloids to reduce risk for postcentesis hypotension and acute renal failure (ARF); repeated large-volume fluid removal may result in hypovolemia, hypoproteinemia, electrolyte depletion; iatrogenic infection; postcentesis hypovolemia/hypoperfusion syndrome, ARF; general rule in humans: provide 4–8 g albumin per L of ascites removed (consider colloids, discussed above).
• If ascites fails to mobilize, consider measuring urine sodium output vs. sodium intake (dietary) to determine whether intake requires restriction or diuretics upward titration; urine output should be measured over min 12h.

ACTIVITY

Depends on cause—restrict activity if ascites.

DIET

• Ascites—restrict dietary sodium <100 mg/100 kcal.
• If HE—restrict dietary protein; *caution*: only do so if nitrogen intolerance suspected.

CLIENT EDUCATION

Inform client definitive diagnosis requires logical diagnostic strategies and no prediction for cure or chronic amelioration until diagnosis definitive.

SURGICAL CONSIDERATIONS

• Ligation of APSS or vena caval banding strongly contraindicated.
• If acute symptomatic PH after surgical ligation of PSVA—ligature removal imperative.
• Embolectomy of thrombi not recommended; emboli may recanalize with supportive care; clot dissolution (streptokinase, tissue plasminogen activator) complicated, expensive, requires ICU hospitalization and monitoring, warrants grave prognosis.
• Low molecular weight heparin—see Coagulopathy of Liver Disease.
• Correction of chronic diaphragmatic hernia—release of entrapped viscera may provoke perioperative/postoperative endotoxemia, hypotension, shock, ARF.
• Surgical correction and cure of cor triatriatum and kinked vena cava possible.
• Pericardectomy—pericardial restriction or tamponade; thoracoscopic procedure least invasive, with lowest mortality and best outcome.
• Removal of tumor or fibrous adhesions causing hepatic vein occlusion may be difficult.
• Removal (lobectomy) or embolization (acrylamide) of hepatic AV malformation may not be curative as microscopic intrahepatic AV shunting usually continues PH and APSS.

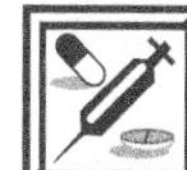

MEDICATIONS

DRUG(S) OF CHOICE

Treatment of abdominal effusion—sodium restriction (see Diet); combined diuretic therapy (spironolactone and furosemide), consider tolvaptan or telmisartan (see above), use large-volume paracentesis sparingly.

POSSIBLE INTERACTIONS

• Avoid drugs relying on first-pass hepatic extraction, biotransformation, or hepatic elimination; if not possible, adjust dosage based on available information.
• Reduce dose of highly protein-bound drugs if patient hypoalbuminemic.
• Avoid nonsteroidal anti-inflammatory drugs—may provoke ARF, sodium retention, and enteric bleeding that may augment HE.

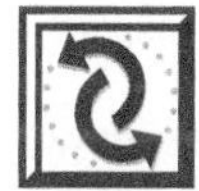

FOLLOW-UP

PATIENT MONITORING

• Sequentially monitor bodyweight, condition, abdominal girth.
• Sequentially assess hydration, electrolytes, acid-base, BP as necessary.
• Monitor albumin and glucose—with liver disease or APSS.
• Monitor lung sounds, pulse oximetry, ventilatory effort—in cardiovascular disorders.

POSSIBLE COMPLICATIONS

• Thrombosis.
• Endotoxemia.
• Hypotension.
• Hepatic encephalopathy.
• Acute renal failure.

MISCELLANEOUS

ASSOCIATED CONDITIONS

• Chronic liver disease.
• Numerous disorders may cause prehepatic or posthepatic portal hypertension.

PREGNANCY/FERTILITY/BREEDING

Affects uterine perfusion and likely leads to abortion or stillbirths.

SEE ALSO

• Ascites.
• Cirrhosis and Fibrosis of the Liver.
• Congestive Heart Failure, Right-Sided.
• Hepatic Encephalopathy.
• Pericardial Disease.
• Portosystemic Shunt, Acquired.
• Portosystemic Vascular Anomaly, Congenital.

ABBREVIATIONS

• ARF = acute renal failure.
• APSS = acquired portosystemic shunt(s).
• AV = arteriovenous.
• CHF = congenital hepatic fibrosis.
• DPM = ductal plate malformation.
• EHBDO = extrahepatic bile duct obstruction.
• GI = gastrointestinal.
• HE = hepatic encephalopathy.
• PH = portal hypertension.
• PLE = protein-losing enteropathy.
• PLN = protein-losing nephropathy.
• PSVA = portosystemic venous anomaly.
• TE = thromboembolism.
• TSBA = total serum bile acids.

Suggested Reading

Bunch SE, Johnson SE, Cullen JM. Idiopathic noncirrhotic portal hypertension in dogs: 33 cases (1982–1998). J Am Vet Med Assoc 2000, 218:392–399.

Buob S, Johnston AN, Webster CR. Portal hypertension: pathophysiology, diagnosis, and treatment. J Vet Intern Med 2011, 25:169–186.

Author Kate Holan

Consulting Editor Kate Holan

Acknowledgment The author/book editors acknowledge the prior contribution of Sharon A. Center.

HYPERTENSION, PULMONARY

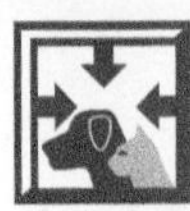

BASICS

DEFINITION

Peak systolic pulmonary artery (PA) pressure >35 mmHg and/or peak diastolic PA pressure >15 mmHg.

PATHOPHYSIOLOGY

• Causes of elevated PA pressure: ◦ PA vasoconstriction. ◦ PA obstruction. ◦ High left atrial (LA) pressure. ◦ Excessive pulmonary blood flow. • As a result of pulmonary hypertension (PH) right heart pressures increase to maintain pulmonary blood flow. ◦ May result in dysfunction of right ventricle RV and decreased pulmonary blood flow, which interferes with left heart filling and can lead to reduced cardiac output. ◦ High right heart pressures can cause venous congestion, tricuspid regurgitation (TR), and right-sided CHF.

SYSTEMS AFFECTED

• Cardiovascular. • Respiratory.
• Hepatobiliary (if right-sided CHF).

GENETICS

• No specific genetic basis found. • Causes of primary disease (congenital heart disease [CHD], left heart disease, pulmonary disease) may have a genetic basis.

GEOGRAPHIC DISTRIBUTION

Unknown; higher prevalence in heartworm-endemic areas and high altitudes.

SIGNALMENT

Species

Dog and cat.

Breed Predilections

• Possibly based on underlying cause of PH.
• Increased incidence suggested in terrier breeds.

Predominant Sex

Increased incidence reported in females.

SIGNS

General Comments

Signs due to hypoxia and cardiac dysfunction.

Historical Findings

• Exercise intolerance. • Dyspnea/tachypnea.
• Coughing/hemoptysis. • Syncope.
• Abdominal distention. • Weight loss.
• Lethargy. • Sudden death.

Physical Examination Findings

• Dyspnea/tachypnea. • Coughing/hemoptysis. • Loud and/or split second heart sound. • Pulmonary crackles and/or increased bronchovesicular sounds.
• Cyanosis. • Heart murmur. • Abdominal distention. • Jugular distention.
• Subcutaneous edema. • Weight loss.

CAUSES

Primary/Idiopathic/Familial PH

• Congenital disorders of the pulmonary vasculature identified in humans. • Abnormalities in endothelial derived vasodilator/vasoconstrictor substances result in vascular obstruction and vasoconstriction. • Not reported in companion animals.

Pulmonary Parenchymal Disease

• *Vascular obstruction*—resulting from pulmonary lesions (e.g., fibrosis, neoplasia), vascular hypertrophy/inflammation.
• *Vasoconstriction*—secondary to hypoxia and acidemia. • *Causes*—pneumonia (bacterial, viral, fungal, parasitic); chronic bronchitis; pulmonary fibrosis; eosinophilic bronchitis; pulmonary neoplasia; acute respiratory distress syndrome.

Pulmonary Thromboembolism (PTE)

• *Vascular obstruction*—secondary to thrombus. • *Vasoconstriction*—secondary to hypoxia and vasoconstrictive substances released from the thrombus. • *Causes*—hyperadrenocorticism; protein-losing nephropathy/enteropathy; sepsis; immune-mediated hemolytic anemia; neoplasia; pancreatitis; endocarditis; disseminated intravascular coagulation; primary cardiac disease (typically right-sided).

Heartworm Disease (HWD)

• *Vascular obstruction*—vascular hypertrophy, inflammation, thromboembolism, and presence of heartworms. • *Vasoconstriction*—secondary to hypoxia/thrombi.

Left-to-Right-Shunting CHD

• *Excessive pulmonary blood flow*—results in damage to pulmonary vasculature.
• *Vasoconstriction/vascular obstruction*—due to vascular damage and hypertrophy. • *Causes*—patent ductus arteriosus; ventricular septal defect; atrial septal defect; atrioventricular septal defect.

Left Heart Disease

• *High LA pressure*—results in pulmonary venous hypertension. • *Vasoconstriction/vascular obstruction*—result of elevated pressure and vascular hypertrophy. • *Causes*—mitral regurgitation; cardiomyopathy (dilated, hypertrophic, restrictive, unclassified); mitral stenosis; congenital pulmonary venous obstruction; LA tumors.

Extrapulmonary Causes of Chronic Hypoxia

• *Vasoconstriction and secondary vascular hypertrophy*—due to environmental/extrapulmonary factors that result in hypoxia and acidemia. • *Causes*—hypoventilation (Pickwickian syndrome, neuromuscular disorders); high altitude disease.

RISK FACTORS

• Cardiac and pulmonary disease. • HWD.
• Diseases causing hypercoagulability.
• Obesity. • High altitude.

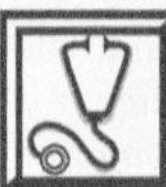

DIAGNOSIS

DIFFERENTIAL DIAGNOSIS

• Left-sided CHF*. • Tracheal collapse.
• Right-sided CHF*. • Primary pulmonary disease*. • HWD*. • Pneumothorax.
• Pleural effusion (pyothorax, chylothorax, hemothorax, hydrothorax). • Laryngeal disease. * = without concurrent PH.

CBC/BIOCHEMISTRY/URINALYSIS

• Polycythemia if hypoxemic. • Leukocytosis with infectious lung disease. • Possible evidence of hypercoagulability.

OTHER LABORATORY TESTS

• Arterial blood gases (hypoxemia). • Occult heartworm test. • Workup for PTE (urine protein : creatinine ratio, antithrombin III level, D-dimer, coagulation profile, urine cortisol : creatinine ratio, adrenocorticotropic hormone stimulation test, dexamethasone suppression test). • Cytology of effusions.

IMAGING

Radiography

• Dilated PA and/or torturous pulmonary vessels. • Enlarged RV and right atrium (RA).
• Dilated caudal vena cava. • Pleural effusion.
• Hepatomegaly. • Ascites. • Evidence of primary pulmonary disease, PTE, or HWD.

Echocardiography

• RV concentric/eccentric hypertrophy.
• Flattening of interventricular septum and/or paradoxical septal motion. • RA dilation. • PA dilation with decreased distensibility. • Pleural/pericardial effusion. • Evidence of left heart disease, HWD, CHD, or PTE. • Asymmetric, notched pulmonary outflow tracing. • TR gradient, if present without pulmonic stenosis or PA stenosis, estimates systolic PH severity. ◦ *Systolic pressure gradient* between PA and RA estimated with spectral Doppler using modified Bernoulli equation: $4 \times (\text{peak TR velocity})^2$. ◦ Pressure gradient >35 mmHg (TR velocity ≥3.0 m/s) suggestive of PH. ◦ Gradient determines severity—mild: 35–50 mmHg; moderate 51–80 mmHg; severe: >80–mmHg.
• Pulmonary valve insufficiency (PI), if present without PA stenosis, estimates diastolic PH severity. ◦ Diastolic pressure gradient between PA and RV estimated with spectral Doppler using modified Bernoulli equation: $4 \times (\text{end PI velocity})^2$. ◦ Pressure gradient >15 mmHg (end PI velocity >2.0 m/s) suggestive of PH.

CT/MRI

May be of value if pulmonary neoplasia or other infiltrative/obstructive disease.

DIAGNOSTIC PROCEDURES

Transtracheal wash, bronchoscopy/bronchoalveolar lavage, or lung aspirate/biopsy may be of value if evidence of primary pulmonary disease.

ECG

• Right mean electrical axis deviation. • Deep S waves (leads I, II, III, and aVF), • Widened QRS complex. • P-pulmonale. • ST segment depression/elevation. • Hypoxia-induced arrhythmias (ventricular premature complexes [VPCs]).

Cardiac Catheterization and Pulmonary Angiography

• Gold standard for diagnosis. • Uncommonly performed due to risk and usefulness of echocardiography. • Indicated if necessary to confirm diagnosis or cause.

PATHOLOGIC FINDINGS

Depend on underlying disease and severity—primary pulmonary lesions; PTE; dilated PA/RV/RA/vena cava; heartworms; pleural/pericardial/abdominal effusions; medial hypertrophy, intimal proliferation, and sclerosis of pulmonary vessels; necrotizing arteritis.

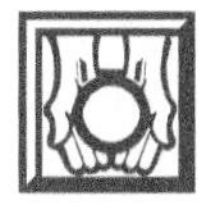

TREATMENT

APPROPRIATE HEALTH CARE

• Hospitalize patients in severe respiratory distress. • Perform diagnostics based on patient stability.

NURSING CARE

• Judicious fluid therapy may help improve pulmonary blood flow. • Risk of CHF must be considered. • Maintain low-stress environment.

CLIENT EDUCATION

• Prognosis varies with the underlying disease but generally very guarded. • Avoid respiratory triggers—heat/humidity extremes, secondhand smoke, high altitudes.

SURGICAL CONSIDERATIONS

Surgical heartworm extraction is a consideration in patients with severe infestation.

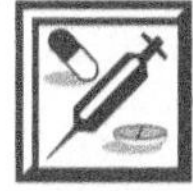

MEDICATIONS

DRUG(S) OF CHOICE

• Treat the primary underlying disease whenever possible. • The ideal therapeutic agent for PH causes pulmonary vasodilation without causing significant systemic hypotension.

Oxygen

• Treatment of choice but long-term administration unfeasible. • Useful in acute setting to correct hypoxia and cause pulmonary vasodilation.

Phosphodiesterase Type V (PDE5) Inhibitors

• Inhibit the breakdown of cyclic guanosine monophosphate (cGMP) causing increased nitric oxide and pulmonary vasodilation. • Avoid other drugs with similar effects (nitrates). • Sildenafil (1–2 mg/kg q8–12h)—drug of choice for most causes of PH in dogs. • Tadalafil—limited studies suggest benefit in dogs.

Phosphodiesterase Type III (PDE3) Inhibitor

• Pimobendan. • Causes pulmonary and systemic vasodilation. • Positive inotropic effect supports right heart dysfunction. • Indicated if PH secondary to left heart disease. • Unclear if useful with other causes of PH.

Other Vasodilators

• Limited benefit due to concurrent systemic vasodilation and hypotension. • Important in PH due to left heart disease. • Amlodipine, hydralazine, and angiotensin-converting enzyme (ACE) inhibitors.

Bronchodilators

• May help patients with pulmonary disease.
• Sympathomimetics (e.g., terbutaline).
• Methylxanthines (e.g., theophylline)—may also cause mild PA vasodilation.

Anticoagulants

• Common therapy for all causes of PH due to primary and/or secondary thromboembolism in humans. • Use in companion animals unclear except in patients with PTE.

Thrombolytics

• Streptokinase and tissue plasminogen activator indications and effectiveness debated in companion animals. • Likely only indicated if acute PTE with significant cardiac compromise.

Anti-inflammatories and Antibiotics

• Steroids may help if cause of PH has inflammatory component (e.g., HWD or primary pulmonary disease). • Antibiotics if bacterial component.

Other Therapies

• No large veterinary clinical trials to support use. • Endothelin receptor antagonists (Bosentan®)—pulmonary vasodilator that improves outcome in humans; cost prohibitive in veterinary patients. • Platelet-derived growth factor antagonists (toceranib, sorafenib, imatinib)—shown to decrease right heart pressure in rat PH model; preliminary studies of imatanib in dogs is promising. • L-arginine—possible benefit due to conversion to nitric oxide.

CONTRAINDICATIONS

• Respiratory depressants. • Cardiac myocardial depressants (e.g., beta blockers).
• Bronchoconstrictors (e.g., nonspecific beta blockers). • Vasoconstrictors.

PRECAUTIONS

• Vasodilators can cause systemic hypotension.
• Pulmonary vasodilation in patients with left heart disease may induce pulmonary edema.
• Bronchodilators can cause tachycardia and hyperexcitability. • Hypovolemia may reduce pulmonary blood flow.

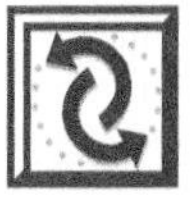

FOLLOW-UP

PATIENT MONITORING

• Serial echocardiography to assess improvement/progression. • Repeat thoracic radiographs, ECG, labwork, blood pressure as needed.

POSSIBLE COMPLICATIONS

• Right-sided CHF. • Syncope.
• Arrhythmias. • Sudden death.

EXPECTED COURSE AND PROGNOSIS

• Based on ability to reverse underlying disease. • Often very guarded prognosis.

MISCELLANEOUS

ABBREVIATIONS

• ACE = angiotensin-converting enzyme.
• cGMP = cyclic guanosine monophosphate.
• CHD = congenital heart disease.
• CHF = congestive heart failure.
• HWD = heartworm disease.
• LA = left atrium.
• PA = pulmonary artery.
• PH = pulmonary hypertension.
• PI = pulmonary valve insufficiency.
• PTE = pulmonary thromboembolism.
• RA = right atrium.
• RV = right ventricle.
• TR = tricuspid valve regurgitation.
• VPCs = ventricular premature complexes.

Suggested Reading

Poser H, Guglielmini C. Pulmonary hypertension in the dog. Acta Veterinaria-Beograd 2016, 66:1–25.

Authors Donald P. Schrope and Jennifer M. Mulz

Consulting Editor Michael Aherne

Client Education Handout available online

H

HYPERTENSION, SYSTEMIC ARTERIAL

BASICS

DEFINITION

Sustained increase in arterial blood pressure, corresponding to systolic BP (SBP) ≥160 mmHg confirmed during multiple measurement sessions. BP increases may be transient and related to the measurement process (situational or "white-coat" hypertension), or sustained and pathologic. In veterinary patients, systemic arterial hypertension (HT) usually occurs in association with a clinical disease or treatment known to cause HT and is categorized as secondary. If an underlying disease is not present or able to be determined, HT is considered idiopathic.

PATHOPHYSIOLOGY

- BP is the force exerted by a blood column against the vessel wall, and is determined by cardiac output, aortic impedance and systemic vascular resistance.
- Normally, BP is under close regulation, such that rapid or wide swings are avoided.
- Factors that favor BP increases by augmenting cardiac output (e.g., increases in intravascular volume, heart rate, or myocardial contractility) or systemic vascular resistance (e.g., arteriolar vasoconstriction, increased blood viscosity) are usually balanced by autonomic, renal, and local vascular responses that restore normal BP.
- Systemic HT may develop in association with diseases or pharmacologic agents that overwhelm or interfere with normal homeostatic mechanisms or with vascular responsiveness to these mechanisms.
- Chronic, sustained BP increases may cause injury to several organs, referred to as target organ damage (TOD).

SYSTEMS AFFECTED

- Renal/urologic.
- Cardiovascular.
- Ophthalmic.
- Nervous.

GENETICS

Rare instances of familial idiopathic HT are reported.

INCIDENCE/PREVALENCE

- Prevalence estimates are difficult to interpret due to differences in HT definitions, inclusion criteria, and measurement techniques among studies.
- Pathologic HT are rare in young, healthy dogs and cats.
- Reported prevalence in HT-associated diseases—chronic kidney disease (CKD), 9–93% (dogs) and 19–65% (cats); diabetes mellitus, 24–67% (dogs) and 0–15% (cats); hyperadrenocorticism, 20–80% (dogs); hyperthyroidism, 5–25% (cats); pheochromocytoma, 43–86% (dogs).

SIGNALMENT

Species

Dog and cat.

Breed Predilections

None

Mean Age and Range

- Usually older animals; median age 13–15 years (cats).
- May be noted in younger animals, especially those affected by infectious (e.g., leptospirosis) or heritable (e.g., polycystic kidney disease, renal dysplasia) disease.

SIGNS

General Comments

Clinical signs vary with affected target organ and underlying disease; may be apparently asymptomatic or display signs that are acute, severe, or rapidly progressive.

Historical Findings

- Signs attributable to underlying disease (e.g., polyuria/polydipsia, anorexia, vomiting, weight loss with CKD; hindlimb weakness, cervical ventroflexion with hyperaldosteronism).
- Acute-onset or progressive blindness.
- Altered mental state, lethargy, seizures (generalized or focal), or ataxia.
- Rarely, respiratory signs due to congestive heart failure (CHF), e.g., dyspnea/orthopnea (cats/dogs), cough (dogs).
- Epistaxis (rare).
- Headaches, blurred vision, and anxiety, reported by people with HT, may manifest as nonspecific signs in dogs and cats.

Physical Examination Findings

- Ocular—blindness, mydriasis, exudative retinal detachment, retinal hemorrhage/ edema, retinal vascular tortuosity or perivascular edema, vitreal hemorrhage, bullous retinal detachment, hyphema, glaucoma, retinal degeneration.
- Neurologic—abnormal mentation, central blindness, nystagmus, ataxia.
- Renal—palpable renal abnormalities.
- Cardiovascular—heart murmur, arrhythmia, gallop sound, pulmonary crackles.

CAUSES

Idiopathic

Subclinical CKD thought to contribute in some cases.

Secondary Hypertension

- CKD.
- Acute kidney injury (AKI).
- Hyperadrenocorticism.
- Hyperthyroidism.
- Diabetes mellitus.
- Pheochromocytoma.
- Primary hyperaldosteronism.
- Hypothyroidism.
- Polycythemia.
- Drug-related—glucocorticoids (uncommon), mineralocorticoids (high dosages), erythropoietin/darbepoetin, phenylpropanolamine, phenylephrine, ephedrine, toceranib phosphate.
- Intoxicants—cocaine, methamphetamine/ amphetamine, 5-hydroxytryptophan.

RISK FACTORS

Renal disease or endocrinopathy.

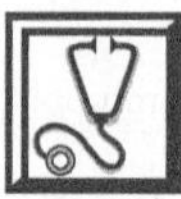

DIAGNOSIS

DIFFERENTIAL DIAGNOSIS

Differential signs—differentiate from other causes of acute-onset blindness, central neurologic signs, CHF, or epistaxis, depending on presenting signs and clinical findings.

CBC/BIOCHEMISTRY/URINALYSIS

- Abnormalities vary depending on underlying disease.
- Packed cell volume may be decreased (CKD) or mildly increased (hyperthyroidism).
- CBC may reveal stress leukogram and/or thrombocytosis (hyperadrenocorticism).
- May note azotemia, hyperphosphatemia, hyperkalemia (AKI, CKD); hyperglycemia (diabetes mellitus); increased serum alkaline phosphatase (hyperadrenocorticism); increased serum alanine aminotransferase (hyperthyroidism); hypokalemia (hyperaldosteronism).
- Urinalysis may reveal low urine specific gravity, proteinuria, hematuria, pyuria, bactiuria (AKI, CKD, hyperadrenocorticism); glucosuria (diabetes mellitus).

OTHER LABORATORY TESTS

- Assessment of glomerular filtration rate may detect early renal dysfunction.
- Urinary protein : creatinine ratio may disclose proteinuria.
- Serum total T_4 concentration, T_3 suppression test to evaluate for hyperthyroidism (cats).
- Serum T_3, T_4, free T_3, free T_4, and thyroid-stimulating hormone concentrations; T_3 and T_4 autoantibodies to evaluate for hypothyroidism (dogs).
- Screening tests for hyperadrenocorticism in dogs with other suggestive findings.
- Plasma aldosterone concentration if primary hyperaldosteronism suspected (cats).
- Plasma and urinary catecholamine concentrations if pheochromocytoma suspected.

IMAGING

- Abdominal ultrasonography to evaluate kidneys, liver, and adrenal glands.
- Echocardiography to evaluate for cardiac TOD—may be normal, or disclose left ventricular concentric and/or eccentric hypertrophy, diastolic dysfunction, left atrial enlargement.
- CT or MRI if cerebral hemorrhage, hyperadrenocorticism suspected.
- Thyroid scintigraphy to evaluate hyperthyroidism.

DIAGNOSTIC PROCEDURES

- Diagnosis requires documentation of persistently (i.e., during ≥2 sessions, performed on different days) high SBP, using reliable direct or indirect measurement methods.
- Methods should be standardized to avoid inaccuracies caused by common technical errors.
- Substantial effort should be made to minimize patient stress to reduce risk of falsely diagnosing "true" HT in patient with situational HT.
- See Suggested Reading to consult detailed published guidelines for BP measurement.

Direct (Invasive) BP Measurement Methods

- Gold standard—involve catheterization or needle puncture of peripheral artery.
- Reserved for monitoring under anesthesia or during emergency management of severe HT.

Indirect (Noninvasive) BP Measurement Methods

- More clinically useful than direct methods for outpatient setting.
- Utilize devices that rely on Doppler ultrasonography or oscillometry.
- Require placement of inflatable cuff to temporarily occlude arterial blood flow in extremity by applying external, compressive force.

Ancillary Diagnostics

Fundoscopic examination to evaluate for retinal lesions.

PATHOLOGIC FINDINGS

- Widespread, multisystemic arteriolosclerosis.
- Increased cardiac mass due to left ventricular hypertrophy.
- Aortic aneurysm/dissection (rare).
- Lesions associated with underlying disease.

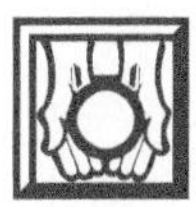

TREATMENT

Treatment Guidelines for Dogs and Cats

- General goal to reverse/limit ongoing TOD and prevent future TOD.
- If identified, treatment of underlying disease may resolve HT.
- Antihypertensive therapy indicated in dogs and cats with:
  - SBP ≥160 mmHg on two or more occasions for which situational hypertension considered unlikely.
  - SBP ≥160 mmHg on single occasion if clear evidence of ongoing neurologic or ocular TOD.
- Animals without evidence of TOD and mildly increased SBP (140–159 mmHg, "prehypertensive"), or suspected situational HT, should not be treated.
- Therapeutic targets—ideally, normotension (SBP 120–140 mmHg); SBP <160 mmHg at minimum.
- Gradual (i.e., over several weeks) reduction in BP should be targeted.
- HT considered an emergency if severe neurologic or ocular TOD is present; in these cases, goal is to cautiously reduce SBP to approximately 160 mmHg over 3–6 hours and to <140 mmHg over 1–2 days, with continuous/frequent BP monitoring.

APPROPRIATE HEALTH CARE

Usually managed on outpatient basis. Inpatient care may be necessary depending on underlying condition and severity of target organ damage.

ACTIVITY

No restrictions.

DIET

- Dietary sodium restriction is controversial.
- Avoid high sodium intake.

CLIENT EDUCATION

- Unless underlying cause is curable or controllable, patient is likely to require lifelong antihypertensive therapy.
- HT may persist or develop even with control of underlying disease (e.g., hyperthyroidism).
- Multiple agents and periodic dosage adjustments may be required for adequate control of HT.
- Frequent monitoring necessary until adequate BP control is achieved.

SURGICAL CONSIDERATIONS

May be indicated for pheochromocytoma, primary hyperaldosteronism, hyperthyroidism, and some forms of hyperadrenocorticism.

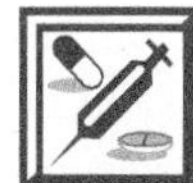

MEDICATIONS

DRUG(S) OF CHOICE

- Depend on underlying disease (e.g., adrenergic antagonists preferred in patients with pheochromocytoma, aldosterone antagonists in those with primary aldosteronism).
- Cats—amlodipine or telmisartan first line for SBP 160–200 mmHg; amlodipine first line if SBP >200 mmHg or ocular/neurologic TOD; angiotensin-converting enzyme (ACE) inhibitor or telmisartan may be added if proteinuria or poor control with amlodipine alone.
- Dogs—ACE inhibitor or angiotensin receptor blocker (ARB) first line; amlodipine coadministered as first line if SBP >200 mmHg, or added if SBP 160–200 mmHg and poor control with ACE inhibitor or ARB.
- In hypertensive emergency (HT with severe ocular or neurologic TOD), parenteral hydralazine, sodium nitroprusside, or fenoldopam can be used; continuous direct BP monitoring is necessary in these cases.

Dihydropyridine Calcium Channel Blocker

Amlodipine—dogs: 0.1–0.5 mg/kg PO q24h; cats: 0.625–1.25 mg/cat PO q24h (consider 1.25 mg/cat if SBP >200 mmHg; may be increased to 2.5 mg/cat if necessary).

ACE Inhibitor

Enalapril or benazepril—dogs: 0.5–1.0 mg/kg PO q12h; cats: 0.5 mg/kg PO q12–24h.

ARB

Telmisartan—dogs: 1.0 mg/kg PO q24h; cats: 2.0 mg/kg PO q 24h; in United States labeled to start with 1.5 mg/kg PO BID protocol for 2 weeks and then adjust to 2.0 mg/kg q24h.

Direct-Acting Vasodilator

Hydralazine—dogs: 0.5 mg/kg PO q12h, stepwise increase to 3 mg/kg PO q12h if needed; cats: 2.5 mg/cat q12–24h.

Alpha-Adrenergic Receptor Antagonist

Phenoxybenzamine—dogs: 0.25 mg/kg PO q8–12h; cats: 2.5 mg/cat PO q8–12h.

Aldosterone Antagonist

Spironolactone—dogs and cats: 1.0–2.0 mg/kg PO q12h.

CONTRAINDICATIONS

Decrease or discontinue vasoconstricting drugs (e.g., phenylpropanolamine).

PRECAUTIONS

- Abrupt BP reduction and hypotension (SBP <120 mmHg) should be avoided; use of rapidly acting drugs or combinations of vasodilators increases this risk.
- Direct arteriolar vasodilators and IV antihypertensives may cause reflex tachycardia.

POSSIBLE INTERACTIONS

- Use of antihypertensives in combination increases risk of hypotension.
- Hyperkalemia may result from coadministration of any combination of ACE inhibitor, ARB, and spironolactone.

ALTERNATIVE DRUG(S)

For Hypertensive Emergency

- Sodium nitroprusside (inorganic nitrate)—dogs and cats: 0.5–5 μg/kg/min IV, start low and increase by increments of 0.1–0.5 μg/kg/min to effect.
- Hydralazine (direct arteriolar vasodilator)—dogs: 0.5–2 mg/kg SC/IM q8–12h *or* 0.1–0.5 mg/kg IV q2–8h, CRI 1.5–5.0 μg/kg/min; cats: 1.0–2.5 mg/cat SC.
- Fenoldopam (dopamine-1 antagonist)—dogs and cats: 0.1–1.6 μg/kg/min; start low, increase by increments of 0.1 μg/kg/min to effect.

HYPERTENSION, SYSTEMIC ARTERIAL (CONTINUED)

FOLLOW-UP

PATIENT MONITORING

- BP and manifestations of ocular or neurologic TOD should be checked weekly (or every 1–3 days if severe TOD) until normotension (SBP 120–140 mmHg) achieved (ideally), or SBP <160 mmHg (at minimum).
- Periodic monitoring of laboratory tests to evaluate for side effects of medications and clinical response (e.g., proteinuria, hematuria, anemia, thrombocytopenia, potassium balance, sodium balance, azotemia).

POSSIBLE COMPLICATIONS

- Progression of underlying renal disease.
- Retinopathy, choroidopathy.
- Encephalopathy, cerebral vascular accident.
- CHF (uncommon), aortic aneurysm/dissection/rupture (rare).
- Gingival hyperplasia may develop with amlodipine treatment in dogs.
- Facial dermatitis/excoriation may develop with spironolactone treatment in cats (uncommon).

EXPECTED COURSE AND PROGNOSIS

- Treatment of systemic hypertension may reverse or slow progression of TOD.
- Rapid and complete improvement of neurologic signs (usually within 24–48 hours) is expected with adequate BP control.
- Improvement/resolution of visual deficits may take weeks with BP control; most blind eyes do not regain normal vision.

MISCELLANEOUS

ASSOCIATED CONDITIONS

- CKD.
- Endocrinopathies.

AGE-RELATED FACTORS

- CKD.
- Hyperthyroidism.
- Hyperadrenocorticism.

ZOONOTIC POTENTIAL

None, unless underlying leptospirosis.

PREGNANCY/FERTILITY/BREEDING

Pregnancy may exacerbate HT.

SYNONYMS

- High blood pressure.
- Systemic hypertension.

SEE ALSO

- Diabetes Mellitus Without Complication—Cats.
- Diabetes Mellitus Without Complication—Dogs.
- Glomerulonephritis.
- Hyperadrenocorticism (Cushing's Syndrome)—Cats.
- Hyperadrenocorticism (Cushing's Syndrome)—Dogs.
- Hyperthyroidism.
- Pheochromocytoma.

ABBREVIATIONS

- ACE = angiotensin-converting enzyme.
- AKI = acute kidney injury.
- ARB = angiotensin receptor blocker.
- CHF = congestive heart failure.
- CKD = chronic kidney disease.
- HT = systemic arterial hypertension.
- SBP = systolic arterial blood pressure.
- TOD = target organ damage.

INTERNET RESOURCES

https://icatcare.org/vets/guidelines/hypertension-cats

Suggested Reading

Acierno MJ, Brown S, Coleman AE, et al. ACVIM consensus statement: guidelines for the identification, evaluation, and management of systemic hypertension in dogs and cats. J Vet Intern Med 2018, 32(6):1803–1822.

Carter J. Hypertensive ocular disease in cats: a guide to fundic lesions to facilitate early diagnosis. J Feline Med Surg 2019, 21:35–45.

Jepson RE, Feline systemic hypertension: classification and pathogenesis. J Feline Med Surg 2011, 13(1):25–34.

Taylor SS, Sparkes AH, Briscoe K, et al. ISFM consensus guidelines on the diagnosis and management of hypertension in cats. J Feline Med Surg 2017, 19(3):288–303.

Author Amanda E. Coleman

Consulting Editor Michael Aherne

Acknowledgment The author and book editors acknowledge the prior contribution of Rosie A. Henik

Client Education Handout available online

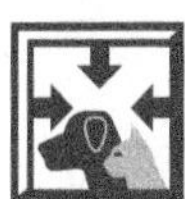

BASICS

DEFINITION

A state of increased metabolism caused by increased circulating concentrations of thyroid hormone.

PATHOPHYSIOLOGY

- Feline hyperthyroidism most often caused by benign adenomatous hyperplasia or follicular cell adenoma, causing increased secretion of thyroxine (T_4) and triiodothyronine (T_3).
- Naturally occurring hyperthyroidism rare in dogs; most often malignant carcinoma (<2% of cats have malignant thyroid carcinoma).
- Oversupplementation with exogenous thyroid hormone may cause hyperthyroidism in dogs.

SYSTEMS AFFECTED

- Cardiovascular—systemic hypertension, thyrotoxic cardiomyopathy. • Gastrointestinal (GI)—malabsorption, hypermotility.
- Nervous/behavioral—restlessness, irritability, aggression, vocalization, pacing. • Urologic—increased glomerular filtration rate (GFR).
- Musculoskeletal—catabolism, cachexia.

GENETICS

None known.

INCIDENCE/PREVALENCE

- Most common feline endocrinopathy; affects 3–8% of cats >10 years old. • Rare in dogs.

SIGNALMENT

- Cats 4–22 years old; mean age of onset is 13 years. • <5% of affected cats <8 years old.
- Most common in dogs >10 years old.

SIGNS

General Comments

- Signs related to increased metabolism.
- Small number of cats show atypical signs; the human term "apathetic hyperthyroidism" is characterized by lethargy, decreased appetite, and muscle weakness; signs may be more common with advanced hyperthyroidism.

Historical Findings

- Weight loss. • Polyphagia. • Hyperactivity/irritability/restlessness. • Polyuria/polydipsia.
- Vomiting. • Diarrhea. • Increased vocalization. • Tachypnea. • Muscle weakness.

Physical Examination Findings

- Cachexia/muscle loss. • Palpable thyroid gland (unilateral or bilateral). • Tachycardia/heart murmur/gallop rhythm. • Systemic hypertension/retinopathy. • Unkempt hair/hair loss. • Thickened nails. • Ventroflexion of neck (advanced disease).

CAUSES

- In cats, benign adenomatous hyperplasia and follicular cell adenoma lead to oversecretion of T_4 and T_3; thyroid carcinoma is rare.
- In dogs, thyroid carcinoma is more likely; hyperthyroidism in dogs may be secondary to oversupplementation of T_4.

RISK FACTORS

- Increased risk with aging. • Decreased risk in Burmese, Tonkinese, Persian, Siamese, Abyssinian, and British shorthair cats; possible increased risk in domestic longhair cats. • Multifactorial environmental contributors are possible, including bisphenol A (BPA) associated with canned food diets, and polybrominated diphenyl ether (PBDE) flame retardants, but further study is needed.

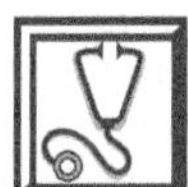

DIAGNOSIS

DIFFERENTIAL DIAGNOSIS

- Any of the differentials for hyperthyroidism can reflect concurrent disease. • Neoplasia.
- Inflammatory bowel conditions. • Diabetes mellitus. • Chronic kidney disease.
- Cardiomyopathy.

CBC/BIOCHEMISTRY/URINALYSIS

- CBC—mild packed cell volume (PCV) elevation or stress leukogram. • Elevated alanine aminotransferase (ALT) activity is common. • Elevated alkaline phosphatase (ALP), aspartate aminotransferase (AST) activities, and blood urea nitrogen, creatinine, phosphorus, bilirubin, and glucose concentrations may be seen. • Urinalysis (UA) shows variable urine specific gravity; pre-treatment specific gravity does not predict post-treatment renal function.
- Glucosuria and evidence of urinary tract infection possible.

OTHER LABORATORY TESTS

- Elevated serum total T_4 (TT_4) concentration is diagnostic for hyperthyroidism in cats with clinical signs.
  - T_4 concentrations naturally decrease with age; early hyperthyroid cats may have T_4 levels in high-normal range.
  - T_4 concentration may be decreased by concurrent disease. • Free T_4 concentration measured by equilibrium dialysis may be helpful in cats with concurrent disease or early hyperthyroidism, but is not a screening test. • T_3 concentration is not useful for diagnosis in cats. • Thyroid-stimulating hormone (TSH) concentration should not be used for diagnosis in cats. • T_3 suppression test or thyrotropin-releasing hormone (TRH) stimulation test can help to confirm diagnosis in mild cases. • Fructosamine concentration may be decreased by concurrent hyperthyroidism. • Cardiac biomarker concentrations (*N*-terminal pro brain natriuretic peptide, cardiac toponin I) may be elevated; myocardial disease and biomarkers may return to normal after control of hyperthyroidism.

IMAGING

- Thoracic and abdominal radiography helpful to evaluate for neoplasia and cardiac disease. • Abdominal ultrasound helpful in determining concurrent disease.
- Echocardiography to evaluate cardiac function. • Thyroid scintigraphy can determine location of abnormal and ectopic thyroid tissues.

DIAGNOSTIC PROCEDURES

- BP measurement is part of baseline database. • GFR measurement is possible but not always practical.

PATHOLOGIC FINDINGS

- Multinodular adenomatous hyperplasia can be unilateral or bilateral (98% of cats).
- Thyroid carcinoma in dogs and <2% of hyperthyroid cats.

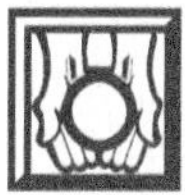

TREATMENT

APPROPRIATE HEALTH CARE

- Advanced hyperthyroidism with concurrent congestive heart failure requires hospitalization for stabilization. • Most cases managed on an outpatient basis. • Radioactive iodine and surgical treatments require hospitalization.

ACTIVITY

No activity restrictions.

DIET

- Because of increased metabolism and hypermotility of intestinal tract, highly digestible diets preferred. • Malabsorption improves with resolution of hyperthyroid state.
- Vitamin B_{12} supplementation may be helpful. • An iodine-deficient therapeutic diet is available and effective in appropriate situations.

CLIENT EDUCATION

- Hyperthyroidism in cats is common and treatable. • Treatment with medication or diet restriction is lifelong. • Medication dosing needs to be monitored regularly and adjusted accordingly. • Comorbidities are possible. • Hyperthyroidism in dogs is usually a malignancy and carries a poor long-term prognosis. • Possible side effects of medication. • Surgical thyroidectomy—anesthetic risks, risk of damage to parathyroid glands. • In some cases, radioactive iodine (I-131) treatment may need to be repeated.
- Resolution of thyrotoxicosis may reveal other, previously masked conditions (e.g., renal disease).

SURGICAL CONSIDERATIONS

- Surgical thyroidectomy is an accepted treatment option. • Thyroidectomy for carcinoma is not curative, but may be helpful with or without subsequent radioactive iodine treatment.

HYPERTHYROIDISM (CONTINUED)

MEDICATIONS

DRUG(S) OF CHOICE

• I-131 is treatment of choice for hyperthyroidism. • Methimazole (2.5–5 mg/cat PO q12–24h) is most common medication. ○ Methimazole should be dosed below expected therapeutic dose and titrated upward to minimize side effects. ○ Transdermal methimazole is available and effective; ideally, initial management with oral methimazole will stabilize patient, then transition to transdermal; resolution may be prolonged if treatment initiated with transdermal medication. ○ Methimazole may cause anorexia, vomiting, skin excoriations, thrombocytopenia, hepatopathy, and hypothyroidism; side effects occur within first weeks to months of treatment. ○ Anorexia, vomiting, and skin excoriations can be mitigated by starting at very low doses of methimazole and increasing to therapeutic levels; cessation of drug can resolve these issues, and restarting with transdermal methimazole may avoid recurrence of GI side effects. ○ Bleeding disorders, bone marrow dyscrasias, and hepatic issues require discontinuation of methimazole and choosing an alternative therapy. ○ Severe blood dyscrasias may require hospitalization and supportive care, but should resolve with appropriate treatment. • Atenolol may be used for severe tachycardia.

POSSIBLE INTERACTIONS

Concurrent use of phenobarbital may reduce effectiveness of methimazole.

ALTERNATIVE DRUG(S)

• Carbimazole—converted to methimazole after absorption; effective, may have fewer side effects than methimazole; not available in United States. • Propylthiouracil—not recommended. • Ipodate—for short-term treatment only, not effective for most hyperthyroid cats; not recommended in most cases.

FOLLOW-UP

PATIENT MONITORING

• Regardless of treatment option, GFR and renal function may decline after treatment, but will stabilize within 1 month of thyroid control. • I-131—physical exam (PE), BP, T_4, serum chemistry, and UA at 1, 3, 6, and 12 months post treatment.
• Methimazole—PE, CBC, serum chemistry, T_4, and UA every 2–4 weeks after starting treatment and after every dose change until T_4 is stabilized between 1 and 2.5 μg/L.
• In cats with renal insufficiency, serum T_4 should be maintained in upper half of reference interval. • Thyroidectomy—hypocalcemia can occur within several days post surgery; monitor for postoperative laryngeal paralysis; PE, T_4, serum chemistry, and UA 2–4 weeks post surgery, then every 3–6 months; supplementation should not be started postsurgically unless T_4 levels remain low after 3 months; hypothyroidism may be transient with subtotal thyroidectomy. • Therapeutic diet—PE, BP, serum chemistry, CBC, T_4, and UA every 4–6 months; may take as long as 6 months for cats with severe T_4 elevations to become euthyroid, if at all.

PREVENTION/AVOIDANCE

N/A

POSSIBLE COMPLICATIONS

• Fatal, if untreated. • Complications of thyroidectomy include hypothyroidism, hypoparathyroidism, laryngeal paralysis.
• I-131, antithyroid drugs, and thyroidectomy can all lead to hypothyroidism; proper dosing of I-131 and methimazole is imperative. • Iatrogenic hypothyroidism associated with worsening renal function and decreased survival.

EXPECTED COURSE AND PROGNOSIS

• Prognosis is excellent in cats without concurrent disease. • Cats on methimazole are likely to relapse if medication is not administered correctly. • Cats eating a therapeutic diet who do not strictly follow diet will not be successful. • Post I-131 treatment—mean survival time is 4 years.
• Treatment with methimazole—mean survival time is 2 years. • Overall mean survival time can be up to 5.3 years. • Cats with preexisting renal disease have a poorer prognosis. • Cats and dogs with carcinoma have a poor prognosis—best option for treatment may be surgical debulking of tumor followed by high dose I-131; recurrence is common.

MISCELLANEOUS

ASSOCIATED CONTITIONS

• Because hyperthyroidism is life-threatening, treatment of all hyperthyroid cats is recommended, with concurrent management of any comorbidities. • Less aggressive treatment options should be considered for cats with advanced (IRIS stage 3–4) renal disease.

AGE-RELATED FACTORS

Mature to geriatric cats and dogs.

ZOONOTIC POTENTIAL

N/A

PREGNANCY/FERTILITY/BREEDING

N/A

SYNONYMS

• Thyrotoxicosis. • Plummer's disease.

SEE ALSO

• Cardiomyopathy, Hypertrophic—Cats.
• Chronic Kidney Disease.
• Congestive Heart Failure, Right-Sided.
• Hypertension, Systemic Arterial.
• Hypoparathyroidism.

ABBREVIATIONS

• ALT = alanine aminotransferase.
• ALP = alkaline phosphatase.
• AST = aspartate aminotransferase.
• BPA = bisphenol A.
• GFR = glomerular filtration rate.
• GI = gastrointestinal.
• I-121 = radioactive iodine.
• PBDE = polybrominated diphenyl ether.
• PCV = packed cell volume.
• PE = Physical exam.
• T_3 = triiodothyronine.
• T_4 = thyroxine.
• TRH = thyrotropin-releasing hormone.
• TSH = thyroid-stimulating hormone.
• TT_4 = total thyroxine.
• UA = urinalysis.

INTERNET RESOURCES

https://www.catvets.com/public/PDFs/ClientBrochures/Hyperthyroidism-WebView.pdf

Suggested Reading

Carney HC, Ward CR, Bailey SJ, et al. 2016 AAFP guidelines for the management of feline hyperthyroidism. J Fel Med Surg 2016, 18:400–416.

Scott-Moncrief JC. Feline hyperthyroidism. In: Feldman EC, Nelson RW, Reusch CE, et al., eds., Canine and Feline Endocrinology and Reproduction, 4th ed. St. Louis, MO: Elsevier, 2015, pp. 136–195.

Stock E, Daminet S, Paepe D, et al. Evaluation of renal perfusion in hyperthyroid cats before and after radioiodine treatment. J Vet Intern Med 2017, 31:1658–1663.

Walter KM, Lin YP, Kass PH, Puschner B. Association of polybrominated diphenyl ethers (PBDEs) and polychlorinated biphenyls (PCBs) with hyperthyroidism in domestic felines: sentinels for thyroid hormone disruption. BMC Vet Res 2017, 13:120.

Author Renee Rucinsky
Consulting Editor Patty A. Lathan

Client Education Handout available online

HYPERTROPHIC OSTEODYSTROPHY

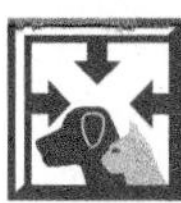

BASICS

DEFINITION

An inflammatory disease of bone that affects rapidly growing giant- and large-breed puppies.

PATHOPHYSIOLOGY

- Characterized by nonseptic, suppurative inflammation within metaphyseal trabeculae of long bones.
- Rapidly growing bones more severely affected (distal radius, ulna, and tibia).
- Metaphysis—widened owing to perimetaphyseal swelling and bone deposition.
- Trabecular microfracture and metaphyseal separation—occur adjacent and parallel to the physis.
- Bone formation defective.
- Ossifying periostitis—may be extensive and in some cases may bridge the physis, hindering growth.
- Etiology unknown.

SYSTEMS AFFECTED

- Gastrointestinal—diarrhea.
- Musculoskeletal—symmetric distribution; distal forelimbs most severely affected; may note soft tissue mineralization in other organs; widened costochondral junctions.
- Respiratory—interstitial pneumonia.

GENETICS

Suspect hyperreactivity to immune stimulation (vaccination).

INCIDENCE/PREVALENCE

Low

GEOGRAPHIC DISTRIBUTION

Northeastern United States—highest in fall; lowest in winter.

SIGNALMENT

Species

Dog

Breed Predilections

- Large and giant breeds.
- Great Danes; Weimaraners—most common.
- Reported—Irish wolfhounds; Saint Bernards; kuvaszes; Irish setters; Doberman pinschers; German shepherds; Labrador retrievers; boxers; Chesapeake Bay retriever; golden retriever; Irish setter; others.

Mean Age and Range

- Affects puppies 3–6 months old.
- Range of onset—2–8 months of age.

Predominant Sex

Males 2.3 times more than females.

SIGNS

General Comments

Lameness—may be episodic; degree varies from mild to non-weight-bearing; initial episode may resolve with or without relapse.

Historical Findings

- Depend on severity of the episode.
- Owners often describe a depressed puppy that is reluctant to move.
- Inappetence—common.
- Painful.
- Shifting leg lameness.

Physical Examination Findings

- Lameness—symmetric, more severe in forelimbs.
- Metaphyses—painful; warm; swollen distal metaphyses of radius, ulna, and tibia.
- Pyrexia—as high as 41.1 °C (106 °F).
- Inappetence.
- Depression.
- Weight loss.
- Dehydration.
- Diarrhea.
- Cachexia.
- Debilitation.
- Manifestations of systemic illness—respiratory or gastrointestinal.
- Foot pad hyperkeratosis.
- Anemia.

CAUSES

Unknown; the following hypotheses have been proposed.

Metabolic

- Hypovitaminosis C—discounted; may be seen as a result of overuse of available vitamin C in hyperactive bone formation.
- Hypocuprosis—in rats but not in dogs.

Nutritional

- Overnutrition and oversupplementation—association inconsistent.
- Incomplete occurrence in litters.
- Correcting diet does not always alter the course of the disease or eliminate relapses.

Infectious

- Bacterial or fungal organisms—may be secondary when found.
- Not transmissible.
- Temporal association with canine distemper virus vaccination.
- Secondary development may depend on the timing of the neonate's exposure.

RISK FACTORS

Vaccination against canine distemper virus may precipitate an uncontrolled inflammatory reaction in the osteogenic centers.

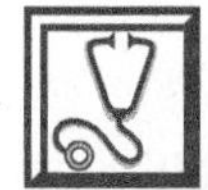

DIAGNOSIS

DIFFERENTIAL DIAGNOSIS

- Panosteitis—no metaphyseal swelling; cottony intramedullary densities in long bones on radiographs.
- Septic metaphysitis/epiphysitis—radiographs of the extremities not typical of hypertrophic osteodystrophy; asymmetric; may note septic suppurative inflammation on needle aspiration of metaphyseal/epiphyseal lesions; hematologic findings implicate bacterial infection (neutrophilia plus left shift).
- Elbow dysplasia—no metaphyseal swelling; no fever; pain localized to the elbow(s); typical radiographic signs.
- Osteochondritis dissecans—no metaphyseal swelling or fever; pain localized to shoulder or elbow; subchondral defects on radiographs.
- Septic polyarthritis—septic suppurative inflammation on arthrocentesis; culture.
- Nonseptic polyarthritis—nonseptic suppurative inflammation on arthrocentesis.

CBC/BIOCHEMISTRY/URINALYSIS

- Do not positively contribute to diagnosis.
- Stress leukogram.
- Normal serum parameters.
- Hypocalcemia uncommon.

OTHER LABORATORY TESTS

N/A

IMAGING

- Distal extremity radiographs—irregular radiolucent zones within metaphyses, parallel and adjacent to physes; flared metaphyses; extraperiosteal new bone extending up the diaphyses; mineralization of perimetaphyseal soft tissues; asynchronous growth in paired bones; cranial bowing; valgus deformity; usually bilaterally symmetric.
- Vertebrae, metacarpal bones, metatarsal bones, ribs, scapula, humerus, and mandible—rarely affected.
- Thoracic radiographs—may reveal interstitial infiltrates.

PATHOLOGIC FINDINGS

- Distal metaphysis of the radius and ulna—most severe changes; similar abnormalities in all long bones.
- Gross—wide metaphysis; peripheral mineralization; soft tissue swelling.

Histologic

- Nonseptic suppurative inflammation of the metaphysis (osteochondritis), especially adjacent to growth plates.
- Necrosis and probable secondary failure of osseous tissue deposition onto the calcified cartilage lattice of the primary spongiosa.
- Trabecular microfractures and impaction.
- Mineralization of perimetaphyseal soft tissues and soft tissues in other regions of the body.
- Interstitial pneumonia.

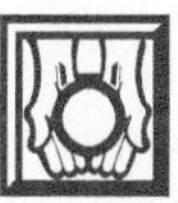

TREATMENT

APPROPRIATE HEALTH CARE

- None specific.
- Supportive—from none to intensive care for severely affected puppies.
- Depends on the severity of the episode, pyrexia, and the patient's ability to maintain normal hydration and willingness to eat.

HYPERTROPHIC OSTEODYSTROPHY (CONTINUED)

NURSING CARE

- Some patients will not stand or move—prone to develop pressure sores; turn every 2–4 hours to prevent sores and hypostatic congestion of the dependent lung.
- Intravenous fluid therapy—for dehydration; maintenance fluid thereafter.

ACTIVITY

- Restricted—running and jumping may exacerbate metaphyseal injury and result in further inflammation.
- Confine to a small well-padded area—recommended.
- Leash-walking only.

DIET

- Normal commercial puppy ration.
- Avoid supplements.

CLIENT EDUCATION

- Warn the client of the disease's relapsing nature.
- Inform client that bony deformities will remodel to some degree with time, but that bowing and valgus deformations are permanent.
- Warn client that the more severe the disease, the more severe the bowing deformity.

SURGICAL CONSIDERATIONS

- None specific.
- May implement surgical methods of alimentation (pharyngostomy tube, esophagostomy tube, gastrostomy tube)—in debilitated puppies that will not eat or drink and have frequently relapsing episodes of acute clinical signs.
- Corrective osteotomy if growth deformity develops from physeal disruption.

MEDICATIONS

DRUG(S) OF CHOICE

- Anti-inflammatory drugs—for pain and antipyretic effects; may try:
  - Aspirin 10 mg/kg PO q12h.
  - Carprofen 2.2 mg/kg IM/PO q12h.
  - Deracoxib 1–2 mg/kg PO q24h; 3–4 mg/kg PO q24h, 7-day limit.
  - Firocoxib 5 mg/kg PO q24h,
  - Grapiprant 2 mg/kg PO q24h, to animals >3.6 kg.
  - Meloxicam—dogs: load 0.2 mg/kg PO, then 0.1 mg/kg PO q24h; cats: 0.1 mg/kg PO q24h—liquid.
- Analgesics—can be used in conjunction with anti-inflammatory medication:
  - Tramadol 1–4 mg/kg PO q8–12h.
  - Prednisone 0.5–1 mg/kg PO q24h; may cause physeal growth disturbances.
  - Opiates may be needed in severe cases.

CONTRAINDICATIONS

Vitamin C—may be contraindicated; may accelerate dystrophic calcification and decrease bone remodeling.

PRECAUTIONS

- Avoid immunosuppressive drugs if secondary infection is present.
- Nonsteroidal anti-inflammatory drugs (NSAIDs)—may cause gastric ulceration; watch for hematemesis or melena; *never* use in conjunction with other NSAIDs or steroids.

POSSIBLE INTERACTIONS

None

ALTERNATIVE DRUG(S)

None

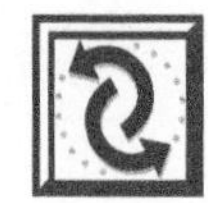

FOLLOW-UP

PATIENT MONITORING

Signs of improvement—less metaphyseal sensitivity; patient gets up; appetite improves; pyrexia resolves.

PREVENTION/AVOIDANCE

N/A

POSSIBLE COMPLICATIONS

- Cachexia.
- Permanent bowing deformities due to premature asymmetric physeal closure.
- Secondary bacterial infection.
- Pressure sores.
- Muscle fasciculations, seizure—with hypocalcemia.
- May see secondary septicemia.
- Recurrence.
- Death.

EXPECTED COURSE AND PROGNOSIS

- Course—days to weeks.
- Most patients—one or two episodes and recover.
- Some patients—seem to have intractable relapsing episodes of pain and pyrexia; rarely die or are euthanized.
- Prognosis—usually good; guarded with multiple relapses or complicating secondary problems.
- Persistent bowing deformity—eliminates many purebred puppies from the show ring.

MISCELLANEOUS

ASSOCIATED CONDITIONS

None proven.

AGE-RELATED FACTORS

Vaccination (canine distemper virus).

ZOONOTIC POTENTIAL

None

PREGNANCY/FERTILITY/BREEDING

Occurs only in juveniles.

SYNONYMS

- Metaphyseal osteopathy.
- Vitamin C deficiency.
- Scurvy.
- Moller Barlow's disease.
- Osteodystrophy II.

SEE ALSO

- Elbow Dysplasia.
- Osteochondrosis.
- Panosteitis.

ABBREVIATIONS

- NSAID = nonsteroidal anti-inflammatory drug.

Suggested Reading

Abeles V, Harrus S, Amgles JM. Hypertrophic osteodystrophy in six Weimaramer puppies associated with systemic signs. Vet Record 1999, 145(5):130–134.

Crumlish PT, Sweeney T, Jones B, Angles JM. Hypertrophic osteodystrophy in the Weimaraner dog: lack of association between DQA1 alleles of the canine MHC and hypertrophic osteodystrophy. Vet J 2006, 171:308–313.

Demko J, McLaughlin R. Developmental orthopedic disease. Vet Clin North Am Small Anim Pract 2005, 35(5):1111–1135.

Foale RD, Herrtgae ME, Day MJ. Retrospective study of 25 young Weimaraners with low serum immunoglobulin concentrations and inflammatory disease. Vet Record 2003, 153:553–558.

Franklin MA, Rochat MC, Broaddus KD. Hypertrophic osteodystrophy of the proximal humerus in two dogs. J Am Anim Hosp Assoc 2008, 44(6):342–346.

Harrus S, Waner T, Aizenberg I, et al. Development of hypertrophic osteodystrophy and antibody response in a litter of vaccinated Weimaraner puppies. J Small Anim Pract 2002, 43:27–31.

Author Steven M. Cogar

Consulting Editor Mathieu M. Glassman

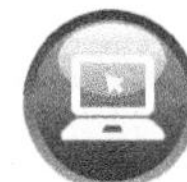

Client Education Handout available online

HYPERTROPHIC OSTEOPATHY

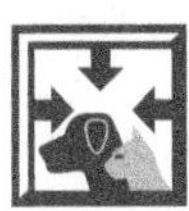

BASICS

OVERVIEW

• Disease of the distal extremities resulting from peripheral blood flow changes that stimulate an overgrowth of vascular connective tissue and subsequent periosteal proliferation.
• Pathogenesis—speculative; increased blood circulation in the limb due to neural or humoral mechanisms is likely secondary to an underlying disease process: most notably intra-thoracic or intra-abdominal neoplasia.
• Predominantly affects the diaphyseal region of phalanges, metacarpals, and metatarsals.

SIGNALMENT

• More common in dogs than cats.
• Age of highest frequency >8 years; coincides with the peak incidence of neoplasia.

SIGNS

Historical Findings

• Chronic or acute lameness with pain in one or more limbs.
• Reluctance to move or use affected limb(s).
• Large firm swelling of affected limb(s).
• Respiratory clinical signs if intra-thoracic disease present (rare).

Physical Examination Findings

• Long bone or distal extremities—enlarged, firm, taut, thickened; not edematous.
• Single or multiple limbs.
• Firm swelling may extend proximally with progression of disease.
• Lameness and pain noted in affected limb(s).

CAUSES & RISK FACTORS

• Primary and metastatic neoplasia—lung tumors; esophageal sarcoma; rhabdomyosarcoma; adenocarcinoma of the adrenal gland, liver, or prostate; nephroblastoma; renal cell carcinoma; thoracic and abdominal mesotheliomas.
• Non-neoplastic conditions—pneumonia, lung abscess/granulomas, dirofilariasis; congenital or acquired heart disease, bronchial foreign bodies; *Spirocerca lupi* infestation of the esophagus; focal lung atelectasis; obscure toxins; hypertension; hyperestrogenism; congenital idiopathic megaesophagus.

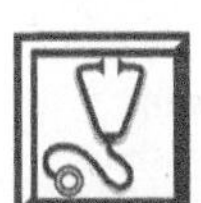

DIAGNOSIS

DIFFERENTIAL DIAGNOSIS

• Osteomyelitis—asymmetric; edematous; lytic bone lesions; history of penetrating trauma or systemic infection.
• Metastatic neoplasia—asymmetric.
• Hypervitaminosis A (feline)—asymmetric; generally involves joint surface.
• Hypertrophic osteodystrophy—metaphyseal abnormality, young dogs.
• Multiple cartilaginous exostosis—metaphyseal abnormality, young dogs.
• Degenerative joint disease—involves articular surface changes in multiple joints.

CBC/BIOCHEMISTRY/URINALYSIS

Dependent on underlying cause and concurrent conditions.

OTHER LABORATORY TESTS

Fecal examination—rule out gastrointestinal and respiratory parasitism.

IMAGING

• Radiographs of affected long bones—bilaterally symmetric extensive, aggressive, or nonaggressive periosteal new bone formation on diaphysis; palisading periosteal reaction; joints not affected.
• Thoracic and abdominal imaging (radiographs, ultrasound, and/or CT)—identify and differentiate primary lesions.

DIAGNOSTIC PROCEDURES

Bone biopsy and culture (bacterial and fungal)—in atypical cases to rule out neoplasia and osteomyelitis.

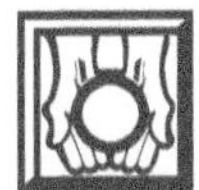

TREATMENT

• Directed at managing, treating, or removing the underlying cause.
• Options in selected cases—unilateral vagotomy on the side of a lung lesion or bilateral cervical vagotomy; incising through parietal pleura; subperiosteal rib resection.

MEDICATIONS

DRUG(S) OF CHOICE

• Dictated by underlying cause.
• Analgesics/anti-inflammatories—as needed.
• No known clinically proven benefit for steroid therapy.

FOLLOW-UP

PATIENT MONITORING

Condition indicates other disease processes—identify the primary cause.

EXPECTED COURSE AND PROGNOSIS

• Clinical signs and bone changes may resolve with treatment of underlying disease.
• Bone changes may take several months to regress.
• Prognosis—guarded to poor due to the common occurrence of neoplastic causes; non-neoplastic lesions may resolve with appropriate treatment of primary cause.
• Tumor recurrence or metastasis may result in recurrence of osteopathy.
• No relationship between size, site, or histologic type of primary lesion, the development of or recurrence of hypertrophic osteopathy postoperatively.

MISCELLANEOUS

SYNONYMS

• Hypertrophic pulmonary osteopathy/osteoarthropathy (HPO/HPOA).
• Hypertrophic osteoarthropathy (HOA).

Suggested Reading

Crumlish PT, Sweeney T, Jones B, Angles JM. Hypertrophic osteodystrophy in the Weimaraner dog: lack of association between DQA1 alleles of the canine MHC and hypertrophic osteodystrophy. Vet J 2006, 171(2):308–313.

Dunn ME, Blond L, Letard D, Difruscia R. Hypertrophic osteopathy associated with infective endocarditis in an adult boxer dog. J Small Anim Pract 2007, 48(2):99–103.

Foster SF. Idiopathic hypertrophic osteopathy in a cat. J Feline Med Surg 2007, 9(2):172–173.

Huang C-H, Jeng C-R, Lin C-T, Yeh L-S. Feline hypertrophic osteopathy: a collection of seven cases in Taiwan. JAAHA 2010, 46:346–352.

Liptak JM, Monnet E, Dernell WS, Withrow SJ. Pulmonary metastatectomy in the management of four dogs with hypertrophic osteopathy. Vet Comp Onc 2004, 2(1):1–12.

Author Marian E. Benitez

Consulting Editor Mathieu M. Glassman

HYPERTROPHIC PYLORIC GASTROPATHY, CHRONIC

BASICS

DEFINITION

Pyloric stenosis or chronic hypertrophic pyloric gastropathy is an obstructive narrowing of the pyloric canal resulting from varying degrees of muscular hypertrophy or mucosal hyperplasia.

PATHOPHYSIOLOGY

- Can result from a congenital lesion composed primarily of hypertrophy of the smooth muscle or be one of three types of acquired form—primarily circular muscle hypertrophy (type 1), a combination of muscular hypertrophy and mucosal hyperplasia (type 2), or primarily mucosal hyperplasia (type 3).
- The cause is unknown; proposed factors include increased gastrin concentrations (which have a trophic effect on the muscle and mucosa) or changes in the myenteric plexus that lead to chronic antral distension and its associated effects.

SYSTEMS AFFECTED

- Gastrointestinal (GI)—chronic intermittent vomiting; regurgitation has also been reported.
- Musculoskeletal—weight loss.
- Respiratory—possible aspiration pneumonia.

GENETICS

Inheritance pattern unknown.

INCIDENCE/PREVALENCE

Uncommon

GEOGRAPHIC DISTRIBUTION

N/A

SIGNALMENT

Species

- More common in the dog.
- Rare in the cat.

Breed Predilections

- Congenital—brachycephalic breeds (boxer, Boston terrier, bulldog); Siamese cats.
- Acquired—Lhasa apso, shih tzu, Pekingese, poodle.

Mean Age and Range

- Congenital—shortly after weaning (introduction of solid food) and up to 1 year of age.
- Acquired—typically middle-aged to older (average 9.8 years of age).

Predominant Sex

Twice as many males as females.

SIGNS

General Comments

- Clinical signs are related to the degree of pyloric narrowing.
- Projectile vomiting is generally not a presenting complaint.

Historical Findings

- Chronic intermittent vomiting of undigested or partially digested food (rarely containing bile), often several hours after eating.
- Congenital lesions associated with clinical signs shortly after weaning.
- Frequency of vomiting increases with time.
- Lack of response to antiemetic agents or motility modifying agents.
- Occasional anorexia with weight loss.
- Regurgitation.

Physical Examination Findings

Most dogs are generally in good physical condition.

CAUSES

- Congenital or acquired.
- May be influenced by infiltrative mural diseases.
- Chronic elevations in gastrin concentrations may play a role.
- Neuroendocrine factors may play a role.

RISK FACTORS

Chronic stress, inflammatory disorders, chronic gastritis, gastric ulcers, and genetic predispositions influence the disease process in humans and may play a role in small animals.

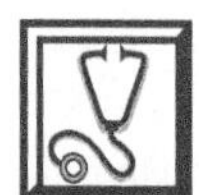

DIAGNOSIS

DIFFERENTIAL DIAGNOSIS

- Gastric neoplasia.
- Gastric foreign body.
- Granulomatous infectious disease (e.g., pythiosis).
- Eosinophilic granuloma.
- Motility disorders.
- Cranial abdominal mass—pancreatic or duodenal.

CBC/BIOCHEMISTRY/URINALYSIS

- Findings vary, depending on degree and chronicity of obstruction.
- Hypochloremic metabolic alkalosis (characteristic of pyloric outflow obstruction), metabolic acidosis, or mixed acid-base imbalance.
- Hypokalemia.
- Anemia—if concurrent GI ulceration.
- Prerenal azotemia—if dehydration present.

OTHER LABORATORY TESTS

N/A

IMAGING

Abdominal Radiographs

Normal to markedly distended stomach.

Upper GI Barium Contrast Study

- May display a "beak" sign created by pyloric narrowing, allowing minimal barium to pass into the pyloric antrum.
- Retention of most of the barium in the stomach after 6 hours indicates delayed gastric emptying.
- Intraluminal filling defects or pyloric wall thickening.

Fluoroscopic Barium Contrast Study

- Normal gastric contractility.
- Delayed passage of barium through the pylorus.

Abdominal Ultrasound

Measurable thickening of the wall of the pylorus and antrum.

DIAGNOSTIC PROCEDURES

Endoscopy—allows evaluation of the mucosa for ulceration, hyperplasia, and mass lesions; specimens can be obtained for histopathologic evaluation.

PATHOLOGIC FINDINGS

- Include focal to multifocal mucosal polyps, diffuse mucosal thickening, and pyloric wall thickening, with variable degree of pyloric narrowing.
- Changes range from hypertrophy of the circular smooth muscle to hyperplasia of the mucosa and associated glandular structures; a wide spectrum of inflammatory cell infiltration exists.

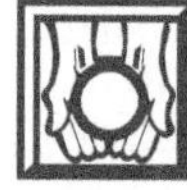

TREATMENT

APPROPRIATE HEALTH CARE

- Depends on severity of clinical signs.
- Patients should be evaluated and surgery scheduled at the earliest convenience.

NURSING CARE

- Appropriate parenteral fluids to correct any electrolyte imbalances and metabolic alkalosis or acidosis.
- Isotonic saline (with potassium supplementation) is the fluid of choice for hypochloremic metabolic alkalosis.
- Consideration of postoperative nutritional support is important.
- In severe cases treated with gastroduodenostomy or gastrojejunostomy, surgical placement of a jejunostomy tube for enteral nutrition may be advantageous.

ACTIVITY

Restrict as needed.

DIET

Highly digestible, low fat—until surgical intervention is feasible.

CLIENT EDUCATION

- Surgical treatment is highly successful.
- If clinical signs recur postoperatively, more aggressive surgical procedures may be indicated.

SURGICAL CONSIDERATIONS

- Surgical intervention is the treatment of choice.
- Goals involve establishing a diagnosis with histopathologic samples, excising abnormal tissue, and restoring GI function with the least invasive procedure.

- Surgical procedures depend on the extent of obstruction—pyloromyotomy (Fredet-Ramstedt), pyloroplasty (Heineke-Mikulicz or antral advancement flap), gastroduodenostomy (Billroth 1), gastrojejunostomy (Billroth 2).

MEDICATIONS

DRUG(S) OF CHOICE

- Antiemetics and motility modifiers are generally ineffective.
- H2 antagonists and proton pump inhibitors may provide symptomatic relief.

CONTRAINDICATIONS

- Evidence of complete pyloric obstruction precludes the use of promotility drugs.
- Avoid anticholinergic agents because of their inhibitory effects on GI motility.

PRECAUTIONS

N/A

POSSIBLE INTERACTIONS

N/A

ALTERNATIVE DRUG(S)

N/A

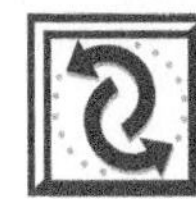

FOLLOW-UP

PATIENT MONITORING

Postoperatively for recurrence of clinical signs because of poor choice of surgical procedure.

PREVENTION/AVOIDANCE

N/A

POSSIBLE COMPLICATIONS

Postoperative surgical complications include recurrence of clinical signs, gastric ulceration, pancreatitis, bile duct obstruction, and incisional dehiscence with peritonitis.

EXPECTED COURSE AND PROGNOSIS

- 85% of dogs show good to excellent results with resolution of clinical signs on proper surgical intervention.
- Poor prognosis if gastric neoplasia (especially adenocarcinoma) is an underlying cause.

MISCELLANEOUS

ASSOCIATED CONDITIONS

Gastric ulceration.

AGE-RELATED FACTORS

Intermittent vomiting in young brachycephalic breeds on weaning is suggestive of congenital stenosis.

ZOONOTIC POTENTIAL

None

PREGNANCY/FERTILITY/BREEDING

High gastrin concentrations in pregnant females may predispose to development of the syndrome.

SYNONYMS

- Chronic hypertrophic antral gastropathy.
- Hypertrophic gastritis.
- Antral pyloric hypertrophy.
- Congenital pyloric stenosis.

ABBREVIATIONS

- GI = gastrointestinal.

Suggested Reading

Bellenger CR, Maddison JE, Macpherson GC, Ilkiw JE. Chronic hypertrophic pyloric gastropathy in 14 dogs. Aust Vet J 1990, 67:317–320.

Radlinsky M, Fossum TW. Surgery of the digestive system. In: Fossum TW, ed., Small Animal Surgery, 5th ed. Philadelphia, PA: Elsevier, 2019, pp. 425–427.

Author Steven L. Marks
Consulting Editor Mark P. Rondeau

HYPERVISCOSITY SYNDROME

BASICS

OVERVIEW

- An assortment of clinical signs caused by high blood viscosity.
- Typically results from markedly high concentration of plasma proteins, although can result (rarely) from extremely high erythrocyte or leukocyte counts.
- Most frequently seen as paraneoplastic syndrome, often associated with multiple myeloma or other lymphoid neoplasms.
- Total plasma protein may exceed 10 g/dL (100 g/L), with serum protein electrophoresis showing monoclonal gammopathy or rarely biclonal gammopathy.
- Clinical signs caused by reduced blood flow through smaller vessels, high plasma volume, and associated coagulopathy.
- Systems affected include hemic/lymphatic/immune, ophthalmic, and nervous; in rare cases, pulmonary thromboembolism may occur.

SIGNALMENT

- Dogs more frequently affected than cats.
- No sex or breed predilections.
- More common in older animals due to increased incidence of malignancy.

SIGNS

Historical Findings

- No consistent signs.
- Anorexia.
- Lethargy.
- Depression.
- Polyuria and polydipsia.
- Blindness, ataxia, seizures, syncope.
- Bleeding tendencies.
- Respiratory distress.
- Congestive heart failure.

Physical Examination Findings

- Neurologic deficits, including seizures and disorientation.
- Tachycardia and tachypnea due to volume overload (e.g., congestive heart failure) or pulmonary thromboembolism.
- Epistaxis or other mucosal bleeding.
- Hepatomegaly, splenomegaly, lymphadenopathy.
- Visual deficits associated with engorged retinal vessels, retinal hemorrhage or detachment, and papilledema.

CAUSES & RISK FACTORS

- Multiple myeloma and plasma cell tumors—immunoglobulin (Ig) M > IgA > IgG.
- Lymphocytic leukemia or lymphoma.
- Marked polycythemia—hematocrit (HCT) >65%, usually >75%.
- Chronic atypical inflammation with monoclonal gammopathy (e.g., ehrlichiosis or leishmaniasis in dogs).
- Chronic autoimmune disease (e.g., systemic lupus erythematosus and rheumatoid arthritis)—very rare.

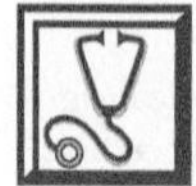

DIAGNOSIS

DIFFERENTIAL DIAGNOSIS

- Other unexplained neurologic disease or bleeding disorders.
- Hyperviscosity is a syndrome, not a final diagnosis.

CBC/BIOCHEMISTRY/URINALYSIS

- Nonregenerative anemia (in patients without erythrocytosis as a cause of hyperviscosity), thrombocytopenia, or leukopenia.
- Hyperproteinemia (total plasma protein >9 g/dL; 90 g/L) and hyperglobulinemia (>5 g/dL; 50 gm/L).
- Azotemia and hypercalcemia, if hyperviscosity caused by paraneoplastic syndrome.
- Isosthenuria and marked proteinuria.

OTHER LABORATORY TESTS

- High concentration of IgG, IgA, or IgM, as detected by radial immunodiffusion.
- High plasma or serum viscosity (>3× greater than water).
- Prolonged prothrombin time or activated partial thromboplastin time, abnormal platelet function testing.
- Other testing as indicated by primary disease.
- Bence-Jones proteinuria in patients with multiple myeloma.

IMAGING

Hepatosplenomegaly, cardiomegaly, and osteolytic lesions (in association with multiple myeloma) are possible.

DIAGNOSTIC PROCEDURES

Bone marrow aspirate or core biopsy—plasma cell or lymphoid infiltrate.

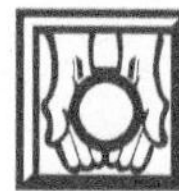

TREATMENT

Appropriate Health Care

- Generally treat as inpatient.
- Treat underlying disease.
- Phlebotomy (15–20 mL/kg) with isotonic crystalloid fluid volume replacement.
- Plasmapheresis, either manual or automated.

Nursing Care

As dictated by underlying disease.

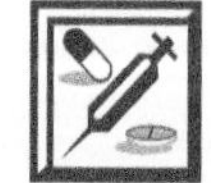

MEDICATIONS

DRUG(S) OF CHOICE

Provide treatment for underlying neoplastic or inflammatory condition.

CONTRAINDICATIONS/POSSIBLE INTERACTIONS

- Avoid use of medications that might increase vascular volume, including synthetic colloids (e.g., hetastarch); do not try to correct compensatory low albumin.
- Avoid medications that alter platelet function.

FOLLOW-UP

- Monitor serum or plasma proteins frequently as marker of treatment efficacy.
- CBC, biochemistry panel, and urinalysis to monitor other laboratory abnormalities.

MISCELLANEOUS

SEE ALSO

- Ehrlichiosis and Anaplasmosis.
- Erythrocytosis.
- Leukemia, Chronic Lymphocytic.
- Lymphoma—Cats.
- Lymphoma—Dogs.
- Multiple Myeloma.
- Plasmacytoma, Mucocutaneous.

ABBREVIATIONS

- HCT = hematocrit.
- Ig = immunoglobulin.

Suggested Reading

Hohenhaus AE. Syndromes of hyperglobulinemia: diagnosis and therapy. In: Kirk RW, ed., Current Veterinary Therapy XII. Philadelphia, PA: Saunders, 1995, pp. 523–530.

Author Elizabeth Rozanski
Consulting Editor Melinda S. Camus

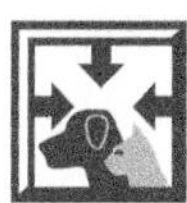

BASICS

DEFINITION

Blood inside the anterior chamber in the form of a blood clot, settled blood in the ventral anterior chamber, or red blood cells suspended throughout the aqueous.

PATHOPHYSIOLOGY

- Breakdown of the blood–aqueous barrier and/or direct injury to the iris and ciliary body blood vessels; causes include direct trauma to the cornea or anterior uvea (iris and ciliary body), inflammation, and damage to blood vessel walls (e.g., caused by systemic hypertension, antigen-antibody complexes, or circulating infectious organisms or neoplastic cells).
- Abnormal hemostasis due to a coagulopathy or thrombocytopenia.
- Bleeding from abnormal vessels within the eye; this is most commonly due to pre-iridal fibrovascular membranes (PIFMs), which form in response to chronic intraocular disease (uveitis, retinal detachment, glaucoma, neoplasia); rarely, abnormal congenital blood vessels in the eye such as persistent pupillary membranes, tunica vasculosa lentis, or hyaloid artery may bleed, causing hyphema.

SYSTEMS AFFECTED

Ophthalmic

INCIDENCE/PREVALENCE

Not uncommon ophthalmic finding and one that is important to recognize, as it may be the presenting clinical sign for serious underlying systemic disease.

SIGNALMENT

Species

Dog and cat.

Breed Predilections

Collies with collie eye anomaly.

SIGNS

Historical Findings—Primary Ophthalmic Causes

- Usually a unilateral presentation in an otherwise systemically normal patient.
- Blunt globe trauma will often have a compatible history.
- Corneal perforation may have a history of a corneal ulcer, or preceding encounter with a cat resulting in a cat claw laceration, especially in puppies.

Historical Findings—Systemic Causes

- Unilateral or bilateral presentation; bilateral presentation is strongly supportive of systemic etiology.
- Weight loss, anorexia, lethargy, decreased vision, or loss of vision may accompany some systemic causes.
- Ocular pain usually accompanies infectious and neoplastic causes due to accompanying uveitis.

Physical Examination Findings—Primary Ophthalmic Causes

- Except in cases of generalized trauma, the physical exam will be unremarkable with abnormalities restricted to the globe and periorbital soft tissues.
- Blunt trauma patients will have painful periorbital soft tissue swelling and uncommonly orbital rim fractures; there is often total hyphema obscuring other intraocular structures.
- Perforating trauma is associated with severe pain, a bloody or clear (aqueous) ocular discharge, varying degrees of hyphema, miosis, and anterior synechia, and a shallow anterior chamber; corneal edema will surround the perforation site and an iris prolapse may be present through the perforation.
- Hyphema due to PIFMs, retinal detachment, neoplasia, or congenital vasculature is usually nonpainful with very little intraocular inflammation (absent aqueous flare, miosis).
- Hypermature cataract supports the development of either PIFM or retinal detachment as a cause of hyphema.

Physical Examination Findings—Systemic Disease Causes

- Ophthalmic examination findings will vary depending on the etiology of the hyphema.
- When an underlying systemic disease is suspected, a thorough physical exam is warranted; the exam may be unremarkable or have significant findings such as lymphadenopathy, fever, or petechiae.
- Hyphema due to noninflammatory etiologies such as hypertension, thrombocytopenia, and coagulopathies will usually manifest minimal discomfort and uveitis (trace or no aqueous flare, no miosis, no conjunctival hyperemia); hypertension is almost always associated with retinal involvement such as retinal hemorrhages and/or retinal detachment.
- Patients with coagulopathies may have bleeding elsewhere, including the subconjunctival tissue and retrobulbar space; thrombocytopenia may create petechia on the palpebral or nictitans conjunctiva.
- Infectious and neoplastic etiologies often cause significant pain, anterior uveitis (miosis, aqueous flare, fibrin, iridal hyperemia and swelling), chorioretinitis with retinal detachment, and possible secondary glaucoma.

CAUSES

See Table 1.

RISK FACTORS

- Ophthalmic—hypermature cataract, retinal detachment, chronic anterior uveitis.
- Systemic—any disease or disorder predisposing to the systemic diseases known to cause uveitis or direct vascular damage

Table 1

Causes of hyphema.

Primary Ophthalmic Etiologies	*Systemic Disease Etiologies*
Trauma (blunt or perforating)	Hypertension
Extraocular vascular compression (choking, chest compression)	Hyperviscosity syndrome
PIFM	Thrombocytopenia
Retinal detachment	Coagulopathy
Primary intraocular neoplasia (iris melanoma, ciliary body adenoma/adenocarcinoma)	Metastatic neoplasia (especially lymphoma)
Golden retriever pigmentary uveitis	Rickettsial disease
Patent anomalous congenital blood vessels (persistent pupillary membranes, tunica vasculosa lentis, hyaloid artery)	FIP
	Fungal disease
	Prototheca
	Parasitic (aberrant intraocular larval migration)

HYPHEMA (CONTINUED)

(e.g., chronic renal disease, hyperthyroidism, systemic hypertension); living in geographic areas with endemic tick-borne disease.

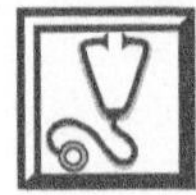

DIAGNOSIS

DIFFERENTIAL DIAGNOSIS

Deep corneal vascularization, along the ventral limbus, can be mistaken for hyphema.

CBC/BIOCHEMISTRY/URINALYSIS

Abnormal findings may help support a diagnosis of systemic disease.

OTHER LABORATORY TESTS

Based on history and physical examination findings, coagulation profile and serology (rickettsial, fungal) may be indicated if systemic disease is suspected.

IMAGING

- Ocular ultrasound is indicated to evaluate for retinal detachment or uveal tumors when not visible on the ophthalmic examination.
- Based on history and physical examination findings, thoracic radiographs, abdominal radiographs, and abdominal ultrasound may be indicated if systemic disease is suspected.

DIAGNOSTIC PROCEDURES

- Systemic arterial blood pressure measurement using Doppler ultrasonic flow probe or oscillometric techniques, if hypertension is suspected.
- Lymph node aspirates if lymphadenopathy is present or if neoplasia or fungal disease is suspected.

PATHOLOGIC FINDINGS

Gross hemorrhage in the anterior chamber.

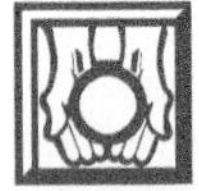

TREATMENT

APPROPRIATE HEALTH CARE

Outpatient medical care is appropriate unless an underlying systemic disease is identified that requires hospitalization.

ACTIVITY

No restricted activity is required unless the patient is blind (restrict environment to fenced yards, no in-ground pools, leash walks, etc.) or the hyphema is due to thrombocytopenia or coagulopathy (avoid rough play, unrestricted running, etc.).

CLIENT EDUCATION

- Hyphema itself, although it appears dramatic, is not painful.
- It is very important to identify the underlying cause of the hyphema, as some etiologies pose a serious health threat.
- Ophthalmic treatment should be initiated immediately to try to prevent painful and sometimes irreversible and blinding sequelae like glaucoma.

SURGICAL CONSIDERATIONS

- Hyphema secondary to a perforating corneal laceration or ulceration should be surgically repaired by direct suturing of the cornea (laceration) or corneal graft (perforated ulcer) when a visual outcome is expected; for a severe perforation with extensive iris prolapse and loss of the pupil, enucleation is recommended.
- Permanently blind and painful eyes should be enucleated (with histopathology) for permanent comfort.
- Surgical irrigation/removal of the hyphema is not successful, as the trauma of the surgery results in exacerbation of the hyphema and intraocular inflammation.

MEDICATIONS

DRUG(S) OF CHOICE

- Topical prednisolone acetate 1% or dexamethasone 0.1% q4–8h to help stabilize the blood–aqueous barrier; *do not use if a corneal ulcer or perforation is present.*
- Atropine 1% q6–24h to help prevent posterior synechia; *atropine is contraindicated if secondary glaucoma is present.*
- Systemic nonsteroidal anti-inflammatory drug (NSAID—carprofen, meloxicam, deracoxib) for analgesia in patients with perforating trauma; may help stabilize blood–aqueous barrier.
- Systemic prednisone/prednisolone with known or suspected choroidal/retinal involvement, *depending on the underlying cause*; anti-inflammatory dose (0.5–1.0 mg/kg PO q24h) can be used for blunt trauma, feline infectious peritonitis (FIP), and rickettsial and fungal disease with proper antimicrobial therapy.
- Topical carbonic anhydrase inhibitors (dorzolamide 2%, brinzolamide 1%, q8h), beta blocker (timolol 0.5% q8–12h), and/or sympathomimetic (dipivefrin 0.1% q8–12h) can be used if secondary glaucoma is present.

CONTRAINDICATIONS

- Topical NSAIDs (flurbiprofen, diclofenac, ketorolac, etc.) are generally considered contraindicated with hyphema.
- Topical prostaglandin analogues (latanoprost, travoprost, bimatoprost) are contraindicated in secondary glaucomas.

FOLLOW-UP

PATIENT MONITORING

- Tonometry should be used to monitor for secondary glaucoma, which lowers the prognosis for a visual outcome.
- Perform tonometry every 1–2 days if the intraocular pressure (IOP) is high normal or greater, or if risk factors such as fibrin and/or posterior synechia are present.
- Perform tonometry weekly if the IOP is low, or if the hyphema and anterior uveitis are mild to moderate in severity.
- *Tonometry is contraindicated with a corneal perforation.*

POSSIBLE COMPLICATIONS

Secondary glaucoma, posterior synechia/dyscoria, cataract formation, loss of vision, possible loss of the eye if the eye becomes permanently blind and painful.

EXPECTED COURSE AND PROGNOSIS

- If the underlying cause of the hyphema can be successfully treated, such as repair of a corneal laceration or control of hypertension, and intraocular damage is not extensive, the prognosis is good for complete resolution of the hyphema.
- If trauma to the eye is severe or if the underlying disease is not controlled, the hyphema will persist and blindness can result; no improvement in hyphema after 2 weeks following blunt trauma has a poor prognosis for return of vision; enucleation should be performed in any cat with permanent blindness from trauma due to the risk of developing traumatic ocular sarcoma.
- Hyphema caused by bleeding from PIFMs usually does not resolve or will resolve and recur.
- If the eye is painful due to a perforated globe or secondary glaucoma, with no reasonable hope of regaining vision, enucleation is recommended.

MISCELLANEOUS

ABBREVIATIONS

- FIP = feline infectious peritonitis.
- IOP = intraocular pressure.
- NSAID = nonsteroidal anti-inflammatory drug.
- PIFM = pre-iridal fibrovascular membrane.

Author Margi A. Gilmour
Consulting Editor Kathern E. Myrna

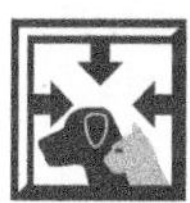

BASICS

DEFINITION

- Endocrine disorder resulting from deficient production of glucocorticoids and, usually, mineralocorticoids.
- Primary hypoadrenocorticism (Addison's disease) is due to destruction of the adrenal cortices resulting in glucocorticoid and mineralocorticoid deficiency.
- The term atypical hypoadrenocorticism has been applied to the subset of dogs with primary hypoadrenocorticism and normal electrolyte concentrations.
- Secondary hypoadrenocorticism results from pituitary adrenocorticotropic hormone (ACTH) insufficiency, resulting in inadequate glucocorticoid production by the adrenal cortices.

PATHOPHYSIOLOGY

- Mineralocorticoid (aldosterone) deficiency results in a diminished ability to excrete potassium and retain sodium, disrupting sodium and potassium balance in the body.
- Sodium loss leads to diminished effective circulating volume; this contributes to pathophysiologic changes and clinical abnormalities, including prerenal azotemia, hypotension, dehydration, weakness, and depression.
- Hyperkalemia can result in weakness, lethargy, and anorexia; it may result in bradyarryhthmias.
- Glucocorticoid (cortisol) deficiency contributes to anorexia, vomiting, diarrhea, melena, lethargy, and weight loss; due to its role in glucose homeostasis, hypocortisolemia predisposes to hypoglycemia.

SYSTEMS AFFECTED

- Gastrointestinal.
- Musculoskeletal.
- Cardiovascular.
- Renal/urologic.

GENETICS

A genetic basis has been determined in standard poodles, bearded collies, Nova Scotia duck tolling retrievers, and Leonbergers.

INCIDENCE/PREVALENCE

Unknown; considered uncommon in dogs and very rare in cats.

SIGNALMENT

Species

Dog and cat.

Breed Predilections

- Great Danes, Rottweilers, Portuguese water dogs, standard poodles, bearded collies, Leonbergers, West Highland white terriers, Novia Scotia duck tolling retrievers and soft coated wheaten terriers have increased relative risk; golden retrievers and Chihuahuas have decreased relative risk.
- No predilection in cats.

Mean Age and Range

- Dogs—range: <1 to >12 years; median: 4 years; young to middle-aged.
- Cats—range: 1–9 years; middle-aged.

Predominant Sex

Female dogs at increased relative risk; no predilection in cats.

SIGNS

General Comments

- Signs vary from mild in patients with chronic hypoadrenocorticism to severe and life-threatening in an acute Addisonian crisis.
- Multiple organ systems may be involved; type and extent of involvement vary with case.

Historical Findings

- Dogs—lethargy, anorexia, vomiting, weakness, weight loss, diarrhea, waxing/waning course, previous response to therapy, polyuria/polydipsia (PU/PD), melena.
- Cats—lethargy, anorexia, weight loss, vomiting, waxing/waning course, previous response to therapy, PU/PD.

Physical Examination Findings

- Dogs—depression, weakness, hypovolemia, dehydration, collapse, hypothermia, melena, hypotension, bradycardia, painful abdomen, hair loss.
- Cats—dehydration, hypovolemia, weakness, hypothermia, depression, hypotension, bradycardia, collapse.

CAUSES

- Primary hypoadrenocorticism—idiopathic (immune-mediated), mitotane or trilostane overdose, granulomatous disease, metastatic tumors, fungal disease, coagulopathy, adrenal hemorrhage or necrosis.
- Secondary hypoadrenocorticism—iatrogenic following withdrawal of long-term glucocorticoid administration, ACTH deficiency, panhypopituitarism, pituitary or hypothalamic lesions.

RISK FACTORS

N/A

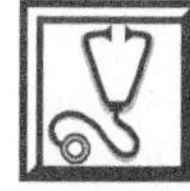

DIAGNOSIS

DIFFERENTIAL DIAGNOSIS

- Signs are nonspecific and often mimic gastrointestinal and renal diseases; differential diagnoses for gastrointestinal distress include intestinal obstruction (e.g., foreign body, intussusception, neoplasia), gastrointestinal perforation, pancreatitis, infectious disease, and others (see Acute Vomiting).
- Differential diagnoses for hyperkalemia include acute kidney injury, urinary tract obstruction, third-space fluid loss (e.g., peritoneal or pleural effusion, uroabdomen), and Trichuriasis.
- Although no signs are pathognomonic, a waxing and waning course and previous response to nonspecific medical intervention should alert the clinician.

CBC/BIOCHEMISTRY/URINALYSIS

- Hematologic abnormalities may include anemia, eosinophilia, and lymphocytosis.
- The absence of a stress leukogram in a sick patient should prompt consideration of hypoadrenocorticism.
- Serum biochemical findings may include hyperkalemia, azotemia, hyponatremia, hypochloremia, hyperphosphatemia, hypercalcemia, hypoalbuminemia, increased alanine aminotransferase (ALT) activity, and hypoglycemia.
- Urinalysis often reveals impaired urine-concentrating ability and in some cases isothenuria; some patients with isothenuria are also azotemic, potentially causing confusion with primary renal disease.
- Some patients with hypoadrenocorticism exhibit normal electrolyte levels (so-called atypical hypoadrenocorticism).

OTHER LABORATORY TESTS

- Definitive diagnosis is by demonstration of undetectable to low (<2 µg/dL) baseline serum cortisol concentrations that fail to increase above 2 µg/dL following ACTH administration.
- Cortisol concentrations should be measured before and 1 hour after administration of synthetic ACTH (1 µg/kg, IV in dogs and 5 µg/kg, IV in cats).
- The ACTH stimulation test can be performed during initial stabilization and treatment if dexamethasone is used (does not cross-react with the cortisol assay).
- If prednisone, prednisolone, or hydrocortisone has been administered, the treatment must be discontinued, and the ACTH stimulation test performed at least 24 hours after changing the glucocorticoid to dexamethasone (do not withhold corticosteroids from a patient in acute crisis).
- A low resting cortisol does not confirm hypoadrenocorticism; an ACTH stimulation test is required.
- Plasma ACTH concentration can be measured in patients with normal electrolyte concentrations to differentiate primary from secondary hypoadrenocorticism; must collect sample before initiating therapy, especially glucocorticoids; carefully follow sample handling instructions from the laboratory; plasma ACTH concentrations are high with primary hypoadrenocorticism and undetectable to low with secondary hypoadrenocorticism.

IMAGING

- Radiographs may reveal microcardia, narrowed vena cava or descending aorta, hypoperfused lung fields, less commonly microhepatica, and very rarely megaesophagus.

H

• Abdominal ultrasound may reveal small adrenal glands.
• Imaging is not usually necessary for diagnosis, but is often performed during the diagnostic workup in patients with gastrointestinal signs.

PATHOLOGIC FINDINGS

• Gross examination—atrophy of the adrenal glands.
• Microscopically—lymphocytic-plasmocytic adrenalitis and/or adrenocortical atrophy; other abnormalities may be present depending on etiology (neoplasia, fungal disease, etc.).

TREATMENT

APPROPRIATE HEALTH CARE

• An acute Addisonian crisis is a medical emergency requiring intensive therapy and 24-hour observation and care; the diagnostic workup is performed while initial treatment and stabilization are ongoing; cats often respond more slowly than dogs.
• The intensity of treatment for patients with chronic hypoadrenocorticism depends on the severity of clinical signs; usually initial stabilization and therapy are conducted on an inpatient basis.

NURSING CARE

• Treat acute Addisonian crisis with rapid correction of hypovolemia and restoration of volume status using isotonic fluids, preferably Plasma-Lyte® or lactated Ringer's solution; although normal saline (0.9% NaCl) was historically recommended, it can exacerbate existing acidosis, but can be used in the absence of other isotonic crystalloid fluids.
• Do not increase sodium concentration by more than 12 mEq/L every 24 hours to prevent CNS myelinolysis; this is more likely to occur when the initial sodium concentration is <120 mEq/L; lactated Ringer's solution has a sodium content of 130 mEq/L and will increase the sodium concentration more slowly than Plasma-Lyte (140 mEq/L) and 0.9% saline (154 mEq/L).
• Although most cases respond to fluid resuscitation alone, severe hyperkalemia (>8.5–9.0 mEq/L and/or bradycardia or other ECG abnormalities) may require additional therapy; see Hyperkalemia.
• If necessary, a colloid fluid also can be given to treat hypotension and hypovolemia.
• Treat hypoglycemia, if present, with IV dextrose; due to hyperosmolarity, 50% dextrose should be diluted a minimum of 1 : 3 prior to IV administration.
• Monitor hydration status, blood pressure, urine output, rectal temperature, and heart rate and rhythm.

ACTIVITY

Avoid unnecessary stress and exertion during an Addisonian crisis.

DIET

No need to alter.

CLIENT EDUCATION

• Lifelong glucocorticoid and/or mineralocorticoid replacement therapy is required.
• Increased dosages of glucocorticoid (above maintenance requirements) are required during periods of stress such as travel, boarding, hospitalization, and surgery.

MEDICATIONS

DRUG(S) OF CHOICE

• In an Addisonian crisis, parenteral administration of a rapidly acting glucocorticoid such as dexamethasone sodium phosphate is indicated; dexamethasone sodium phosphate is given at a dose of 0.25 mg/kg IV on the first day, and 0.15 mg/kg on the second day; glucocorticoid is gradually tapered and changed to oral prednisone or prednisolone as the condition improves.
• Alternatively, hydrocortisone (0.5–0.625 mg/kg/h) has both mineralocorticoid and glucocorticoid properties, and prednisolone sodium succinate (2 mg/kg IV initially, and then 0.5 mg/kg IV q12h) is also an option; since both of these cross-react with cortisol assays (dexamethasone does not), they should be administered after the ACTH stimulation test is complete, or ACTH stimulation testing should be delayed at least 24 hours after administration.
• During an Addisonian crisis, supportive therapy, including gastroprotectants and anti-emetics, is often necessary.
• Chronic primary hypoadrenocorticism—most patients will need daily glucocorticoid replacement (prednisone 0.1–0.2 mg/kg/day PO), as well as mineralocorticoid replacement (desoxycorticosterone [DOCP], 2.2 mg/kg IM/SC, typically given monthly and adjusted as needed on the basis of serial electrolyte determinations); the initial monthly DOCP dose for an average-sized cat is 12.5 mg IM/SC; though not preferred, an alternative means of administering glucocorticoid replacement to cats is Depo-Medrol® (10 mg IM monthly).
• Prednisone dose is adjusted based on clinical signs and side effects; the dose is decreased if PU/PD, polyphagia, and muscle wasting are present, but increased if vomiting, diarrhea, or lethargy occurs; some dogs, particularly large breeds, require less than 0.1 mg/kg/day, but all dogs with hypoadrenocorticism require some prednisone, but all dogs with hypoadrenocorticism require some glucocorticoid.
• The label dose of DOCP is 2.2 mg/kg, but this author routinely begins at 1.5 mg/kg with owner consent to use an off-label dose.
• Alternatively, an oral mineralocorticoid replacement can be used (fludrocortisone acetate 5–10 µg/kg PO q12h, adjusted by 0.05–0.1 mg increments on the basis of serial electrolyte determinations); fludrocortisone has some glucocorticoid activity and the maintenance dose of prednisone for patients receiving fludrocortisone may be lower than for dogs receiving DOCP; a few dogs develop PU/PD and/or polyphagia from fludrocortisone.
• Patients with confirmed atypical and secondary hypoadrenocorticism require only glucocorticoid supplementation (prednisone 0.1–0.2 mg/kg/day PO), adjusted as described above.

PRECAUTIONS

N/A

ALTERNATIVE DRUG(S)

See Hyperkalemia; Hyponatremia.

FOLLOW-UP

PATIENT MONITORING

• Depending on clinical presentation, patients hospitalized for treatment of hypoadrenocorticism may require intensive monitoring and frequent laboratory evaluations; monitor clinical status, urine output, CBC, blood chemistry, and ECG as needed; blood glucose and electrolytes may need to be evaluated several times daily during initial therapy; arterial or venous blood gas analysis may be of benefit.
• Monitor for melena, as some dogs experience severe gastrointestinal blood loss during and following a crisis, sometimes requiring blood transfusion.
• Measure electrolyte concentrations 2 and 4 weeks following the first injection of DOCP, to determine whether the dose (2 weeks) and the dosing interval (4 weeks, prior to next injection) are appropriate; recheck electrolytes prior to next injection and each time the dose or dosing interval is adjusted; then check electrolyte concentrations every 6 months, or when the patient is sick.
• DOCP is usually required at monthly intervals; rare patients need injections as often as every 3 weeks; some dogs may require DOCP less than every 28–30 days; however, the author prefers to adjust the dose instead of extending the dosing interval, and does not decrease the dose (as directed below) and extend the dosing interval in the same dog.
• The majority of dogs with hypoadrenocorticism will be well controlled on a maintenance DOCP dose of 1.5 mg/kg/injection every month; if necessary based on expense, the DOCP dosage can be sequentially decreased by 10% each month

based on electrolyte determinations, as some dogs can be controlled on a monthly dosage that is less than 1.5 mg/kg; make sure that the owner is aware that this is off-label use.

- Adjust the daily dose of fludrocortisone by 0.05–0.1 mg increments as needed, based on serial electrolyte determinations; following initiation of therapy, check electrolyte levels weekly until they stabilize in the normal range; thereafter, check electrolyte concentrations monthly for the first 3–6 months and then every 3–12 months.
- In many dogs given fludrocortisone, the daily dose required to control the disorder increases incrementally, usually during the first 6–24 months of therapy; in most dogs, the final fludrocortisone dosage needed is 20–30 μg/kg/day PO; very few can be controlled on 10 μg/kg/day or less.
- In patients that were initially azotemic, monitor creatinine concentrations as needed following discharge from the hospital.

PREVENTION/AVOIDANCE

- Continue hormone replacement therapy for the lifetime of the patient.
- Increase the dosage of replacement glucocorticoid during periods of stress such as travel, boarding, hospitalization, and surgery.

POSSIBLE COMPLICATIONS

- PU/PD may occur from prednisone administration, but this usually resolves with a decrease in dosage; rarely, it is necessary to try an alternative glucocorticoid, such as methylprednisolone, when the dog's clinical signs are not controlled on a dose of prednisone that is low enough to eliminate side effects.
- PU/PD may occur from fludrocortisone administration.
- Side effects from DOCP are uncommon; rarely weight gain and PU/PD are seen.

EXPECTED COURSE AND PROGNOSIS

- Except for patients with primary hypoadrenocorticism caused by granulomatous or metastatic disease and secondary hypoadrenocorticism caused by a pituitary mass, the vast majority of patients have a good to excellent prognosis following proper stabilization, treatment, and monitoring.
- Owners must be reminded that they should not skip DOCP injections, as this could precipitate a potentially fatal, and inevitably costly, Addisonian crisis.

MISCELLANEOUS

ASSOCIATED CONDITIONS

Concurrent endocrine gland failure occurs in up to 5% of dogs—hypothyroidism, diabetes mellitus, and/or hypoparathyroidism.

AGE-RELATED FACTORS

N/A

ZOONOTIC POTENTIAL

None

SYNONYMS

Addison's disease.

SEE ALSO

- Hyperkalemia.
- Hyponatremia.

ABBREVIATIONS

- ACTH = adrenocorticotropic hormone.
- ALT = alanine aminotransferase.
- DOCP = desoxycorticosterone.
- PU/PD = polyuria/polydipsia.

Suggested Reading

Bates JA, Shott S, Schall WD. Lower initial dose desoxycorticosterone pivalate for treatment of canine primary hypoadrenocorticism. Aust Vet J 2013, 91:77–82.

Lennon EM, Boyle TE, Hutchins RG, et al. Use of basal serum or plasma cortisol concentrations to rule out a diagnosis of hypoadrenocorticism in dogs: 123 cases (2000–2005). J Am Vet Med Assoc 2007, 231:413.

Peterson ME, Kintzer PP, Kass PH. Pretreatment clinical and laboratory findings in dogs with hypoadrenocorticism: 225 cases (1979–1993). J Am Vet Med Assoc 1996, 208:85–91.

Scott-Moncrieff JCR. Hypoadrenocorticism. In: Ettinger SJ, Feldman EC, eds., Textbook of Veterinary Internal Medicine, 7th ed. St. Louis, MO: Elsevier, 2010, pp. 1847–1757.

Author Patty A. Lathan

Consulting Editor Patty A. Lathan

Acknowledgment The author and book editors acknowledge the prior contribution of Deborah S. Greco.

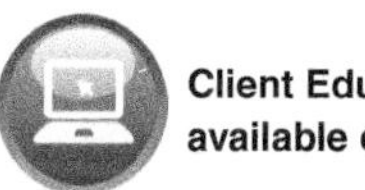

H

HYPOALBUMINEMIA

BASICS

DEFINITION

Hypoalbuminemia defined as measured serum albumin value less than reference range.

PATHOPHYSIOLOGY

• Albumin—constitutive protein exclusively synthesized in liver. • Provides 75–80% of plasma colloid oncotic pressure. • Low oncotic pressure due to serum albumin <1.5 g/dL permits fluid extravasation into interstitial and third-space compartments, causing edema and body cavity effusion.

SYSTEMS AFFECTED

Cardiovascular and respiratory—transudative effusions (pleural effusion, ascites); peripheral edema; pulmonary edema.

INCIDENCE/PREVALENCE

Accompanies many primary diseases that cause hepatic insufficiency, protein-losing enteropathy (PLE), protein-losing nephropathy (PLN), hemorrhage, negative acute-phase response in chronic disease.

SIGNALMENT

Species

Dog and cat.

Breed Predilections

Underlying disease may have breed predilection.

Mean Age and Range

Varies with syndrome association.

Predominant Sex

N/A

SIGNS

General Comments

• Reflect primary disease leading to hypoalbuminemia. • Hypoalbuminemia influences metabolite and xenobiotic protein binding, plasma oncotic pressure, third-space fluid distribution, acid-base balance, and ability to maintain intravascular perfusion pressure.

Historical Findings

• Vary with underlying disease. • Increased drug-related effects due to reduced protein binding.

Physical Examination Findings

• Vary with underlying primary disease.
• Serum albumin ≤1.5 g/dL often associated with pitting edema, decreased heart/lung sounds, and/or abdominal fluid wave.

CAUSES

Decreased Albumin Production

• Chronic hepatic insufficiency—chronic hepatitis; cirrhosis; idiopathic hepatic fibrosis; granulomatous hepatitis; congenital portosystemic shunt (PSS; dogs).
• Inadequate nutritional intake/absorption (modest effect).

Extracorporeal Albumin Loss

• PLN—amyloidosis; glomerulonephritis.
• PLE—lymphangiectasia; lymphoma; severe inflammatory bowel disease (IBD); histoplasmosis; pythiosis; chronic intussusception; Addison's disease. • Severely exudative cutaneous lesions. • Chronic severe blood loss—usually enteric. • Repeated large-volume paracentesis of abdominal or pleural effusion.

Sequestration: Body Cavities/Tissues

• Inflammatory effusions—pancreatitis; septic or aseptic peritoneal or pleural effusions; chylous effusions (modest effect).
• Vasculopathies—immune-mediated (systemic lupus erythematosus [SLE]); infectious (Ehrlichia, Rocky Mountain spotted fever); sepsis syndrome; other (modest effect).

Miscellaneous

Downregulated albumin synthesis—hyperglobulinemia, negative acute-phase response, negative nitrogen intake, catabolism (modest effect).

RISK FACTORS

• Diseases of the liver, kidney, intestines, and blood vessels.
• Negative nitrogen balance; poor nutrition.

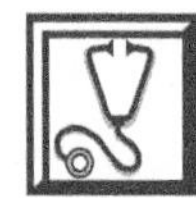

DIAGNOSIS

DIFFERENTIAL DIAGNOSIS

• Severe hepatic disease—may see jaundice; hepatic encephalopathy (HE); ascites. • PLE—diarrhea common but inconsistent. • Cutaneous lesions—must be severe and exudative (burns, toxic epidermal necrolysis [TEN], vasculitis, tumors, trauma). • External blood loss—hemorrhage (enteric, urinary, other).
• Malnutrition—mild hypoalbuminemia.
• Aggressive fluid therapy—exacerbates low albumin.

CBC/BIOCHEMISTRY/URINALYSIS

CBC

• Depends on underlying disease. • Severe hepatic disease—red blood cell (RBC) microcytosis suggests PSS. • Severe blood loss—regenerative anemia or microcytic/hypochromic anemia.

Biochemistry

• Chronic hepatic disease—low albumin; normal to high globulin. • PLE—low albumin; variable globulin. • PLN—low albumin; globulin usually normal but may be low with severe PLN. • Exudative losses—low albumin; variable globulin. • Malnutrition—low albumin; normal globulin. • Severe blood loss—low albumin; low to normal globulin.
• Cholesterol—low with chronic hepatic disease, severe PLE, Addison's disease, and severe malnutrition; high with PLN and pancreatitis. • Hepatic enzymes—alanine aminotransferase (ALT) may be high with chronic hepatitis, IBD causing PLE; high alkaline phosphatase (ALP) often seen with systemic inflammation as well as hepatic disease. • Bilirubin—sometimes high with hepatic disease. • Blood urea nitrogen (BUN)—often low with hepatic insufficiency or patients undergoing diuresis; high with reduced renal function or dehydration.
• Hyperkalemia and hyponatremia—suggest hypoadrenocorticism, third-space effusions, or pseudohypoadrenocorticism (endoparasitism).
• Spurious hypocalcemia—due to low protein.

Urinalysis

• Rules out PLN and urologic blood loss.
• Obtain urine by cystocentesis to avoid lower-tract contamination; *caution*: beware cystocentesis-induced microhematuria.
• Proteinuria—confirm dipstick detection with chemical determination. • Urine protein : creatinine (UP : UCr) ratio—important; >3.0 compatible with nephrotic range proteinuria; must evaluate urine sediment: spurious positive values with active sediment (i.e., substantial pyuria, macroscopic hematuria, bacteriuria); many dogs with glomerulonephritis have hyaline, waxy, or granular casts; bacterial culture of urine necessary to rule out bacteriuria as cause of increased urine protein. • Microalbuminuria—not helpful. • Ammonium biurate crystalluria—hepatic insufficiency, PSS, or acquired portosystemic shunt (APSS).

OTHER LABORATORY TESTS

• Total serum bile acids (TSBA)—usually high with severe hepatic disease; sometimes spurious low values with PLE (fat malabsorption).
• Physicochemical evaluation of effusion—transudate (usually pure) if hypoalbuminemia is the major causal factor. • Antithrombin (AT)—may be low with PLE, PLN, and hepatic synthetic failure. • Protein C (PC)—may be low with severe hepatic disease/failure, PSS, sepsis.

IMAGING

• Thoracic radiography—pleural effusion; pulmonary edema; lymphadenopathy, metastatic disease, cardiac or pulmonary disorders. • Abdominal radiographs—effusion; altered hepatic size; mass lesions; pancreatic disease. • Abdominal ultrasonography—small liver, lymphangiectasia in intestinal wall/mucosa, mass lesions, fluid pockets, altered portal blood flow, mesenteric lymphadenopathy, biliary tree abnormalities, renal abnormalities.

DIAGNOSTIC PROCEDURES

• Hepatic biopsy—after evaluating coagulation (mucosal bleeding time, platelet count) status. • Renal biopsy—differentiates amyloidosis from glomerulonephritis; submit samples for special renal panel staining and electron microscopy. • Intestinal biopsy—endoscopic or surgical.

PATHOLOGIC FINDINGS

Depend on underlying causal disease.

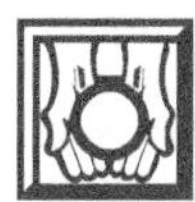

TREATMENT

APPROPRIATE HEALTH CARE

• Diverse, depends on cause. • Pleural/peritoneal effusion restricting ventilation—perform centesis.

NURSING CARE

Provide physical therapy and walk patient to improve mobilization of peripheral edema.

DIET

• Achieve positive energy and nitrogen balance. • HE—control protein intake (see Hepatic Encephalopathy). • PLE with IBD component—novel/hydrolyzed protein (see Inflammatory Bowel Disease). • PLE due to lymphangiectasia—feed ultra-low-fat diet. • PLN – feed high-quality/reduced-protein diet.

SURGICAL CONSIDERATIONS

Severe hypoalbuminemia delays healing, anesthetic drug metabolism, body cavity effusions may complicate drug dosing and dispersal, surgical approach, patient ventilation.

MEDICATIONS

DRUG(S) OF CHOICE

• Depend on underlying disease.
• Glucocorticoids—for some types of chronic hepatitis and some PLEs; prednisolone is preferred if it is effective; dexamethasone lacks mineralocorticoid effects that lessens sodium and water retention, but has greater potential for ulceration/erosion. • Diuretics—furosemide (1–4 mg/kg IV/IM/PO q4–12h) in combination with spironolactone (1–4 mg/kg q12h) in patients with hepatic or cardiac disease, combine with low-salt diet, use judiciously to avoid intravascular volume contraction; for body cavity effusion mobilization, taper diuretic dose after initial positive response; diuretics may be used intermittently to mobilize recurring ascites.
• Antithrombotic treatment (low AT, PC, evidence of thrombi)—clopidogrel (0.5–1.0 mg/kg PO q24h), especially in PLN.
• Enalapril (0.5 mg/kg PO q12–24h)—for dogs with PLN; alternatives are benazepril or the angiotensin receptor blocker telmisartan (1 mg/kg PO q24h).

CONTRAINDICATIONS

Synthetic colloids—avoid with anuria, renal failure, congestive heart failure, severe coagulopathy, or von Willebrand disease.

PRECAUTIONS

• Fluid therapy—avoid overdosing crystalloid fluids, especially when administered with synthetic colloids as these are rapidly distributed into interstitial spaces (70% volume within 1 hour), aggravating antecedent pulmonary or limb edema, and body cavity effusions; restrict maintenance fluid volume of crystalloids to one-third normal (depending on contemporary losses) when used with colloids.
• Transfusion of canine plasma or human albumin—may be complicated by transfusion or allergic reactions; plasma and albumin transfusions of dubious value if severe ongoing protein loss due to PLN, PLE, vasculitis.
• Diuretic therapy—high doses may cause severe intravascular volume contraction leading to azotemia, hypotension, and electrolyte and acid-base derangements. • Unanticipated drug side effects—due to reduced albumin drug binding. • Use of 1 desamino-8-darginine vasopressin (DDAVP) for bleeding—may aggravate fluid retention and associated complications. • Glucocorticoids—mineralocorticoid effects of some drugs may worsen fluid accumulation; prefer synthetic glucocorticoids without mineralocorticoid effects.

POSSIBLE INTERACTIONS

Inadvertent overdosing of drugs with high-protein binding.

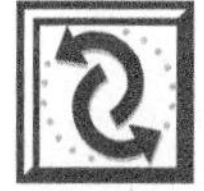

FOLLOW-UP

PATIENT MONITORING

• Bodyweight—especially during fluid therapy; monitors fluid retention. • Vital signs, thoracic auscultation for crackles—monitor for pulmonary edema. • Sequential serum albumin concentrations. • Blood pressure—monitors vascular expansion. • Abdominal girth—monitors ascites. • Central venous pressure—unreliable; potentially dangerous in patients with bleeding or thrombotic tendencies.

PREVENTION/AVOIDANCE

Limit glucocorticoid exposure as much as possible; use alternative medications to control primary illness if possible.

POSSIBLE COMPLICATIONS

• PLN/PLE—may be complicated by thromboembolism; minimize IV catheterization and trauma. • Hypovolemia—from dehydration, Addisonian crisis, blood loss, or diuretic overdose predisposes to acute renal failure, disseminated intravascular coagulation (DIC), or HE.

EXPECTED COURSE AND PROGNOSIS

Depend on underlying cause.

MISCELLANEOUS

ASSOCIATED CONDITIONS

Numerous diverse diseases or syndromes.

PREGNANCY/FERTILITY/BREEDING

Condition complicates pregnancy.

SEE ALSO

• Amyloidosis.
• Cirrhosis and Fibrosis of the Liver.
• Ductal Plate Malformation (Congenital Hepatic Fibrosis).
• Glomerulonephritis.
• Lymphangiectasia.
• Portosystemic Shunting, Acquired.
• Portosystemic Vascular Anomaly, Congenital.
• Protein-Losing Enteropathy.

ABBREVIATIONS

• ALP = alkaline phosphatase.
• ALT = alanine aminotransferase.
• APSS = acquired portosystemic shunt.
• AT = antithrombin.
• BUN = blood urea nitrogen.
• DDAVP = 1 desamino-8-darginine vasopressin.
• DIC = disseminated intravascular coagulation.
• HE = hepatic encephalopathy.
• IBD = inflammatory bowel disease.
• PC = protein C.
• PLE = protein-losing enteropathy.
• PLN = protein-losing nephropathy.
• PSS = portosystemic shunt.
• RBC = red blood cell.
• SLE = systemic lupus erythematosus.
• TEN = toxic epidermal necrolysis.
• TSBA = total serum bile acids.
• UP : UCr = urine protein : urine creatinine ratio.

Suggested Reading

Center SA. Fluid accumulation disorders. In: Willard MD, Tvedten H, eds, Small Animal Clinical Diagnosis by Laboratory Methods, 5th ed. St. Louis, MO: Saunders, 2012, pp. 226–259.

Author Michael D. Willard
Consulting Editor Kate Holan

HYPOCALCEMIA

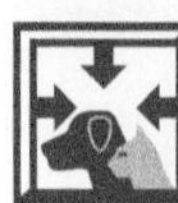

BASICS

DEFINITION

Serum total and ionized calcium concentration below the reference range.

PATHOPHYSIOLOGY

- Of total circulating serum calcium, 40–50% is protein-bound, 40–50% is ionized, and 10% is complexed with other substances. Protein-bound and complexed calcium are unavailable for use by tissues. Only ionized calcium is available to tissues and is responsible for clinical problems (hypo and hypercalcemia).
- Mechanisms of hypocalcemia include:
  - Low concentrations of binding proteins—hypoalbuminemia.
  - Reduced intestinal absorption—deficient vitamin D (renal disease, severe intestinal disease, rickets, chronic glucocorticoid treatment).
  - Reduced renal and bone resorption—hypoparathyroidism.
  - Inadequate dietary intake.
  - Excessive loss—lactation (eclampsia).
  - Sequestration—saponification (acute pancreatitis).
  - Binding/complexing with administered, ingested, or endogenous chemicals—phosphate-containing enemas, citrate toxicosis (multiple citrate-containing anticoagulant transfusions), ethylene glycol toxicosis, oxalate toxicosis, low calcium/high phosphorus diet (nutritional secondary hyperparathyroidism), acute tumor lysis syndrome (hyperphosphatemia from cancer therapy-induced rapid destruction of tumor cells).
  - Impaired synthesis or refractoriness to parathyroid hormone (PTH)—hypomagnesemia.
  - Target organ calcitriol (vitamin D) resistance (vitamin D–dependent rickets type 2).
  - Multifactorial—ionized hypocalcemia in critically ill patients.

SYSTEMS AFFECTED

- Cardiovascular—ECG changes and bradycardia.
- Gastrointestinal—anorexia and vomiting (especially cats).
- Nervous/neuromuscular—seizures, tetany, ataxia, and weakness.
- Ophthalmic—posterior lenticular cataracts.
- Respiratory—panting.

SIGNALMENT

Species

Dog and cat.

Breed Predilections

Small-breed bitches predisposed to eclampsia.

Mean Age and Range

Variable

Predominant Sex

Variable

SIGNS

General Comments

Signs of underlying disease may occur without clinical signs of hypocalcemia, because the latter do not occur until total serum calcium falls below 6.7 mg/dL. Severity of signs at a given calcium concentration are also dependent on rate of decrease; dogs with chronic hypocalcemia are less likely to show signs than dogs with acute hypocalcemia.

Historical Findings

- Facial rubbing.
- Muscle trembling, twitching, or fasciculations.
- Seizures.
- Ataxia or stiff gait.
- Weakness.
- Panting.
- Vomiting.
- Anorexia.

Physical Examination Findings

- Ataxia, stiff gait, weakness, muscle fasciculation, trembling, twitching.
- Hyperthermia.
- Posterior lenticular cataracts in patients with primary hypoparathyroidism.

CAUSES

Nonpathologic Hypocalcemia

- Laboratory error—confirm true hypocalcemia, especially if clinical signs are not present.
- Hypoalbuminemia—most common cause (>50% of patients); reduction of protein-bound calcium but not ionized calcium; not associated with clinical signs.
- Alkalosis—causes a reduction in ionized calcium while total can remain normal; not associated with clinical signs except in cases of borderline low serum ionized calcium concentrations.

Pathologic Hypocalcemia

- Primary hypoparathyroidism.
- Hypoparathyroidism secondary to bilateral thyroidectomy (or other corrective hyperthyroid therapies) causing parathyroid damage.
- Posthyperparathyroid correction due to prolonged negative feedback–induced hypofunction of normal parathyroid glands.
- Renal disease—acute or chronic.
- Ethylene glycol toxicosis.
- Oxalate toxicosis (lily, philodendron, etc.).
- Acute pancreatitis.
- Puerperal tetany—eclampsia.
- Phosphate-containing enemas.
- Nutritional secondary hyperparathyroidism.
- Hypomagnesemia.
- Intestinal malabsorption.
- Citrate toxicosis—multiple blood transfusions or improper citrate–blood ratio.
- Rickets (rare)–hypovitaminosis D, decreased plasma calcitriol, target organ calcitriol receptor resistance (vitamin D–dependent rickets type 2).
- Acute tumor lysis syndrome.
- Ionized hypocalcemia in critically ill patients. Multifactorial: parathyroid dysfunction; cytokine suppression of parathyroid function; vitamin D deficiency; hypomagnesemia; calcium chelation; accumulation of calcium in soft tissues, body fluids, and cells.

RISK FACTORS

- Puerperal tetany—small-breed bitches during first 21 days of nursing, but can affect large breeds. Preparturient eclampsia reported in cats, rarely in dogs.
- Postcorrective procedures for hyperthyroidism and hyperparathyroidism.

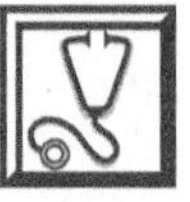

DIAGNOSIS

DIFFERENTIAL DIAGNOSIS

- Clinical signs of hypocalcemia—primary or secondary hypoparathyroidism, eclampsia, intoxication leading to rapid calcium binding/complexing (e.g., phosphate-containing enemas, ethylene glycol); other causes rarely lower serum calcium enough to cause clinical signs.
- Neurologic signs—ethylene glycol toxicosis, primary neurologic disease.
- Vomiting—acute pancreatitis, intestinal malabsorption, renal failure, ethylene glycol toxicosis.
- Bone pain or fractures—nutritional secondary hyperparathyroidism, neoplasia.

LABORATORY FINDINGS

Drugs That May Alter Laboratory Results

- Sodium bicarbonate causes alkalosis and lowers ionized calcium concentration.
- Samples collected in or contaminated by EDTA or citrate will be hypocalcemic.

Disorders That May Alter Laboratory Results

Hypoalbuminemia can lower total calcium concentration and is generally not associated with decreased ionized calcium. Patients with concurrent hypoalbuminemia and ionized hypocalcemia likely have a concurrent condition causing ionized hypocalcemia.

CBC/BIOCHEMISTRY/URINALYSIS

- Hypocalcemia.
- Hypoalbuminemia with conditions causing protein loss, translocation, or decreased production.
- High total CO_2 with metabolic alkalosis.
- Azotemia—with acute and chronic kidney injury.
- Hyperphosphatemia with acute and chronic kidney injury, primary or secondary hypoparathyroidism, acute tumor lysis syndrome, or in

patients receiving phosphate-containing enemas.

- High amylase and lipase in many, but not all, patients with acute pancreatitis or renal disease.
- Mild to moderate anemia possible with chronic renal failure, nutritional secondary hyperparathyroidism, or intestinal malabsorption.
- Leukocytosis possible with acute pancreatitis.
- Isosthenuria with chronic kidney injury, moderate to advanced acute kidney injury.
- Glucosuria in some patients with acute kidney injury, diabetes with acute pancreatitis, ethylene glycol toxicosis, or oxalate toxicosis.

OTHER LABORATORY TESTS

- Ionized calcium—helps determine if clinical signs are due to hypocalcemia.
- Ethylene glycol test—in patients suspected of ingesting ethylene glycol within previous 12–16 hours (questionable reliability).
- Pancreatic lipase immunoreactivity—in patients suspected of having acute pancreatitis (questionable reliability if only test used).
- Intact PTH assay—if primary hypoparathyroidism is suspected.
- Serum magnesium concentration—hypomagnesemia is rare cause of hypocalcemia.
- Plasma calcitriol (vitamin D, 1,25 dihydroxycholecalciferol) concentration—to screen for rickets or vitamin D–dependent rickets type 2 (rare).

IMAGING

- Radiography usually normal.
- Small kidneys with chronic renal disease and large kidneys with acute kidney injury.
- Osteopenia and pathologic fractures with nutritional secondary hyperparathyroidism.
- Ultrasound—hyperechoic renal parenchyma with ethylene glycol or oxalate toxicosis, may identify pancreatitis or abdominal effusion.

DIAGNOSTIC PROCEDURES

ECG—prolongation of ST and QT segments; sinus bradycardia and wide T waves or T wave alternans in some patients.

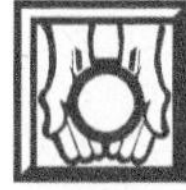

TREATMENT

APPROPRIATE HEALTH CARE

- Inpatient treatment for clinical hypocalcemia.
- Emergency treatment indicated for primary or secondary hypoparathyroidism, eclampsia, hyperphosphatemia, citrate and ethylene glycol toxicosis.
- Long-term treatment for primary hypoparathyroidism and sometimes post-thyroidectomy-associated PTH deficiency.
- Eclampsia—remove puppies from bitch and hand-nurse until weaned.

DIET

Diet change recommended for nutritional secondary hyperparathyroidism (to a balanced diet) and renal failure (see Chronic Kidney Disease).

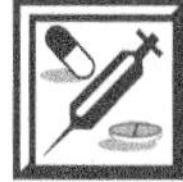

MEDICATIONS

DRUG(S) OF CHOICE

Emergency Treatment

- Calcium gluconate 10% solution—5–15 mg/kg (0.5–1.5 mL/kg); give IV slowly to effect over 10 min; monitor heart rate and stop temporarily if bradycardia occurs; if ECG monitoring is possible, QT interval shortening is an indication to temporarily stop administration. Vomiting can indicate excessive calcium administration.
- Calcium chloride 10% solution—also effective but not recommended in small animals because it is extremely caustic if administered extravascularly. Three times more potent than calcium gluconate; mg/kg dosage is the same, but only one-third the volume is needed (0.15–0.5 mL/kg).

Short-Term Treatment Immediately after Correction of Tetany for Hypoparathyroidism

- Relapse of clinical signs can be prevented by use of IV CRI of calcium gluconate 10% solution (60–90 mg/kg/day [6.5–9.75 mL/kg/day]) added to fluids that do not contain bicarbonate. Rarely necessary for postparturient eclampsia.
- Subcutaneous calcium gluconate 10% diluted 2–4 times with saline can be administered 3 or 4 times daily for initial control of tetany (reported to be safe in most patients, but there have been reports of marked and disabling inflammatory calcinosis cutis associated with subcutaneous use).

Long-Term Treatment

See Hypoparathyroidism.

CONTRAINDICATIONS

Avoid bicarbonate, as alkalinization may further decrease serum ionized calcium levels.

POSSIBLE INTERACTIONS

Calcium salts may precipitate if added to solutions containing bicarbonate, lactate, acetate, or phosphates.

FOLLOW-UP

PATIENT MONITORING

- For patients requiring long-term therapy, serum calcium should be assessed 4–7 days following initial treatment, then (if normocalcemic) monthly for first 6 months, then every 2–4 months.
- Goal—maintain serum calcium concentration between 8 and 10 mg/dL.

EXPECTED COURSE AND PROGNOSIS

- Vary dependent on underlying cause.
- Recurrence of hypocalcemia following calcium administration for primary hypoparathyroidism is common if calcitriol is not also administered; monitoring is advised.

H

MISCELLANEOUS

PREGNANCY/FERTILITY/BREEDING

- Hypocalcemia can lead to weakness and dystocia.
- Eclampsia in dogs is usually seen in first 21 days of nursing a litter.

SEE ALSO

- Acute Kidney Injury.
- Chronic Kidney Disease.
- Eclampsia.
- Ethylene Glycol Toxicosis.
- Hypoalbuminemia.
- Hypomagnesemia.
- Hypoparathyroidism.
- Lily Toxicosis.
- Pancreatitis—Cats.
- Pancreatitis—Dogs.

ABBREVIATIONS

- PTH = parathyroid hormone.

Suggested Reading

Drobatz K, Casey KK. Eclampsia in dogs: 31 cases (1995–1998). J Am Vet Med Assoc 2000, 217:216–219.

Feldman EC. Hypocalcemia and primary hypoparathyroidism. In: Feldman EC, Nelson RW, Reusch CE, et al., eds., Canine and Feline Endocrinology and Reproduction, 4th ed. St. Louis, MO: Saunders, 2015, pp. 625–648.

Waters CB, Scott-Moncrieff JCR. Hypocalcemia in cats. Compend Contin Educ Pract Vet 1992, 14:497–507.

Author Michael Schaer
Consulting Editor Patty A. Lathan

Client Education Handout available online

HYPOCHLOREMIA

BASICS

DEFINITION

Serum chloride concentration below the lower limit of reference interval—dogs: <105 mEq/L; cats: <117 mEq/L (reference intervals may vary from laboratory to laboratory).

H

PATHOPHYSIOLOGY

- Chloride is the most abundant anion in the extracellular fluid.
- Chloride concentration is controlled by electrochemical gradients resulting from the active transport of sodium.
- In general, chloride concentration varies directly with sodium concentration and inversely with bicarbonate concentration.

SYSTEMS AFFECTED

Depends on underlying disorder.

GENETICS

N/A

INCIDENCE/PREVALENCE

N/A

SIGNALMENT

Species

Dog and cat.

Breed Predilections

N/A

Predominant Sex

N/A

SIGNS

Depends on underlying disorder.

CAUSES

- Gastric vomiting.
- Hypoadrenocorticism.
- Metabolic alkalosis.
- Chronic respiratory acidosis.
- Excessive nasogastric suctioning.
- Excess total body water.
- Salt-losing nephropathy.
- Diuretic therapy (especially loop and thiazide diuretics).
- Treatment with bicarbonate.
- Treatment with laxatives.

RISK FACTORS

N/A

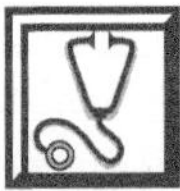

DIAGNOSIS

DIFFERENTIAL DIAGNOSIS

If the degree of hypochloremia exceeds that of hyponatremia, it suggests selective chloride loss, as seen in patients with gastric vomiting or metabolic alkalosis.

LABORATORY FINDINGS

Drugs That May Alter Laboratory Results

Potassium bromide therapy can cause pseudohyperchloremia, as many chemistry analyzers cannot differentiate bromide from chloride.

Disorders That May Alter Laboratory Results

Lipemia and hyperproteinemia can falsely lower chloride concentration if ion-specific electrodes are not used.

Valid if Run in Human Laboratory?

Yes

CBC/BIOCHEMISTRY/URINALYSIS

- Low chloride.
- Other abnormalities depend on underlying disorder, possibly hyponatremia, hyperkalemia, and high bicarbonate concentration.

OTHER LABORATORY TESTS

- Measurement of urine fractional excretion of chloride may demonstrate high excretion.
- Blood gas measurement may reveal metabolic alkalosis.

DIAGNOSTIC PROCEDURES

N/A

PATHOLOGIC FINDINGS

N/A

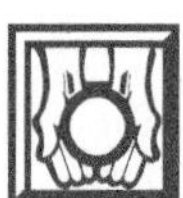

TREATMENT

APPROPRIATE HEALTH CARE

- Depends on underlying disorder.
- When choosing IV fluids, 0.9% NaCl has 154 mEq/L of chloride, Normosol®-R and Plasma-Lyte-148® have 98 mEq/L of chloride, and lactated Ringer's solution has 109 mEq/L of chloride; if fluid administration is indicated, 0.9% NaCl may increase chloride faster than the others; if both sodium and chloride concentrations are low due to excess free water, intravenous fluids may be contraindicated.
- If performing frequent nasogastric suctioning and removing large volumes of gastric residual volume, reinstallation of 2–3 mL/kg of aspirated volume may be considered. One study in dogs receiving routine nasogastric suctioning every 4 hours (average of 0.9 ± 1.2 mL/kg/h of gastric volume removed) did not identify the development of hypochloremia over the course of 36 hours.

NURSING CARE

N/A

DIET

No need to alter.

CLIENT EDUCATION

Depends on underlying disorder.

SURGICAL CONSIDERATIONS

N/A

MEDICATIONS

DRUG(S) OF CHOICE

Other fluid therapy and medication as dictated by underlying cause.

PRECAUTIONS

N/A

ALTERNATIVE DRUG(S)

N/A

FOLLOW-UP

PATIENT MONITORING

Serum electrolyte concentrations as needed to ensure appropriate response.

POSSIBLE COMPLICATIONS

Depends on underlying disorder.

PREVENTION/AVOIDANCE

Depends on underlying disorder.

EXPECTED COURSE AND PROGNOSIS

Depends on underlying cause.

MISCELLANEOUS

ASSOCIATED CONDITIONS

Often accompanied by hyponatremia.

AGE-RELATED FACTORS

N/A

PREGNANCY/FERTILITY/BREEDING

N/A

SEE ALSO

Hyponatremia

Suggested Reading

DiBartola SP. Fluid, Electrolyte and Acid-Base Disorders in Small Animal Practice, 3rd ed. Philadelphia, PA: Saunders, 2005.

Rose DB, Post T. Clinical Physiology of Acid-Base and Electrolyte Disorders, 5th ed. New York: McGraw-Hill, 2000.

Author Patty A. Lathan

Consulting Editor Patty A. Lathan

Acknowledgment The author and book editors acknowledge the prior contribution of Melinda Fleming.

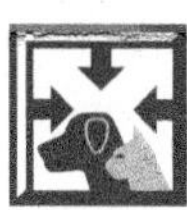

BASICS

DEFINITION

Blood glucose concentration below the lower reference interval (generally <60 mg/dL).

PATHOPHYSIOLOGY

Mechanisms responsible for hypoglycemia:
- Excess insulin or insulin-like factors (e.g., insulinoma, extrapancreatic paraneoplasia [insulin-like growth factor-2 (IGF-2)], xylitol toxicosis, iatrogenic insulin overdose).
- Reduced hepatic gluconeogenesis and glycogenolysis (e.g., hepatic disease, glycogen storage diseases, hypoadrenocorticism, sepsis).
- Excessive metabolic use of glucose (e.g., in hunting dogs, pregnancy, neoplasia, polycythemia, and sepsis).
- Reduced intake or underproduction of glucose (e.g., in puppies and kittens, toy breeds, glycogen storage disease, and severe malnutrition or starvation).

SYSTEMS AFFECTED

- Musculoskeletal.
- Nervous.

SIGNALMENT

- Dog and cat.
- Variable, depending on the underlying cause.

SIGNS

- Seizures.
- Posterior paresis.
- Weakness.
- Collapse.
- Muscle fasciculations.
- Abnormal behavior.
- Lethargy and depression.
- Ataxia.
- Polyphagia.
- Weight gain.
- Exercise intolerance.
- Some animals appear normal aside from findings associated with underlying disease.
- Many animals have episodic signs.
- Polyneuropathy.

CAUSES

Endocrine

- Insulinoma.
- Extrapancreatic neoplasia associated with IGF-2 overproduction (e.g., hepatocellular carcinoma, hepatocellular adenoma, intestinal leiomyoma or leiomyosarcoma).
- Iatrogenic insulin overdose.
- Hypoadrenocorticism.
- Islet cell hyperplasia (nesidioblastosis).

Hepatic Disease

- Portosystemic shunt.
- Cirrhosis.
- Severe hepatitis (e.g., toxic and inflammatory).
- Glycogen storage diseases.

Overuse

- Hunting dog (exertional) hypoglycemia.
- Pregnancy.
- Polycythemia.
- Neoplasia.
- Sepsis—increased glucose utilization induced by cytokine production in macrophage-rich tissues.

Reduced Intake/Underproduction

- Young puppies and kittens.
- Toy-breed dogs.
- Severe malnutrition or starvation.
- In sepsis there is also cytokine-induced inhibition of gluconeogenesis in the setting of nutritional glycogen depletion.

Toxicosis

- Iatrogenic insulin overdose.
- Xylitol toxicosis.
- Antihyperglycemic agent toxicosis (e.g., sulfonylureas).

RISK FACTORS

- Low energy intake predisposes to hypoglycemia in patients with conditions causing overuse and underproduction.
- Fasting, excitement, exercise, and eating may or may not increase the risk of hypoglycemic episodes in patients with insulinoma.

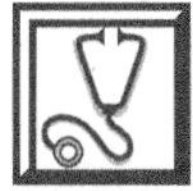

DIAGNOSIS

DIFFERENTIAL DIAGNOSIS

- Patients with hyperinsulinism—signs of hypoglycemia or a normal physical examination.
- Patients with hypoadrenocorticism—waxing, waning, nonspecific signs (e.g., vomiting, diarrhea, melena, weakness); Addisonian patients that present in a crisis usually display hypovolemia and hyperkalemia rather than hypoglycemia (e.g., shock, bradycardia, dehydration).
- Patients with portosystemic shunts—usually young to middle-aged; often thin or appear to have stunted growth; rarely, they have ascites or edema.
- Patients with cirrhosis and severe hepatitis usually have other signs of their disease (e.g., gastrointestinal abnormalities, icterus, and ascites or edema).
- Patients with sepsis—critical; usually in shock; pyrexia or hypothermia revealed by examination; may have gastrointestinal abnormalities.
- Glycogen storage diseases—rare; usually younger animals.
- Extrapancreatic neoplasia and large neoplastic processes (hepatoma) that cause hypoglycemia may be detected by physical examination.

LABORATORY FINDINGS

Drugs That May Alter Laboratory Results

None

Procedures That May Alter Laboratory Results

Delayed separation of serum causes falsely low serum glucose values; if serum cannot be separated within 30 minutes of collection, it should be collected in a sodium fluoride (gray-stoppered) tube. Polycythemia may result in false hypoglycemia if measured on a point-of-care glucometer.

Valid if Run in Human Laboratory?

Yes

CBC/BIOCHEMISTRY/URINALYSIS

- Patients with hyperinsulinism may have normal results.
- Patients with hypoadrenocorticism may have hypocholesterolemia, hypoalbuminemia, lymphocytosis, eosinophilia, hyperkalemia, hyponatremia, azotemia, or hypercalcemia.
- Patients with congenital portosystemic shunts may have microcytosis, hypoalbuminemia, low blood urea nitrogen, slightly elevated liver enzyme activities, ammonium biurate crystalluria, and hyposthenuria. Serum bilirubin concentration sometimes increased.
- Patients with cirrhosis, severe hepatitis, and hepatic neoplasia may have anemia associated with chronic disease, high liver enzyme activities, hyperbilirubinemia, hypoalbuminemia, bilirubinuria, and hyposthenuria.
- Patients with xylitol toxicosis may have hypokalemia and later signs of hepatic failure.

OTHER LABORATORY TESTS

- Simultaneous fasting glucose/insulin determination—indicated when insulinoma is suspected; plasma insulin concentration within the upper end or above reference range in the face of hypoglycemia (glucose <60 mg/dL) suggests insulinoma.
- Baseline cortisol ± adrenocorticotropic hormone stimulation test—to diagnose hypoadrenocorticism.
- Fasting and postprandial serum bile acids—diagnose portosystemic shunt or functional hepatic disease.
- Free abdominal fluid should be collected and analyzed.
- Fructosamine—chronic hypoglycemia will result in low fructosamine concentrations.

IMAGING

- Abdominal radiography and ultrasonography—useful in patients with extrapancreatic neoplasia and large neoplastic processes (may see organomegaly or masses), as well as portosystemic shunt (microhepatica), cirrhosis (microhepatica, hyperechogenicity), and severe hepatopathy. Not very sensitive nor specific for detecting insulinoma. Abdominal CT more accurately detects pancreatic endocrine tumors.

HYPOGLYCEMIA (CONTINUED)

- Ultrasound-guided, laparoscopic, or surgical hepatic biopsy—useful to evaluate hepatic parenchymal disease.
- Technetium-99m quantitative hepatic scintigraphy—to detect portosystemic shunt.
- Mesenteric portography—to detect portosystemic shunt (requires surgery).

DIAGNOSTIC PROCEDURES

Ultrasound-guided or surgical tissue biopsy—useful to evaluate hepatic parenchymal disorders and extrapancreatic neoplasia.

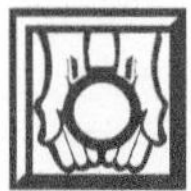

TREATMENT

- Animals with clinical hypoglycemia should be treated as inpatients.
- If able to eat (i.e., responsive, no vomiting), feeding should be part or all of initial treatment.
- If unable to eat, start continuous IV fluid therapy with 2.5–5% dextrose solution.
- Surgery is indicated if a portosystemic shunt or neoplasia is the cause of hypoglycemia.

MEDICATIONS

DRUG(S) OF CHOICE

Emergency/Acute Treatment

- In hospital—administer 50% dextrose 0.5 g/kg IV, diluted 1 : 3 as slow bolus. Glucagon as IV CRI at 5–10 ng/kg/min is transiently effective in cases of insulin-secreting tumors.
- At home—client should not administer medication orally during a seizure; hypoglycemic seizures usually abate within 1–2 min; if a seizure is prolonged, recommend transport to hospital; if a short seizure has ended or other signs of a hypoglycemic crisis exist, recommend rubbing corn syrup or 50% dextrose on the buccal mucosa, followed by 2 mL/kg of the same solution orally once the patient can swallow; then seek immediate attention.
- Owners of diabetic animals can be taught to inject prescribed glucagon 0.03 mg/kg IM.
- Initiate frequent feeding of a diet low in simple sugars or, if patient is unable to eat, continuous fluid therapy with 2.5 or 5% dextrose solution.

Long-Term Treatment

- See Insulinoma for treatment considerations.
- Hunting dog hypoglycemia—feed moderate meal of fat, protein, and complex carbohydrates a few hours before hunting; can feed snacks (e.g., dog biscuits) every 3–5 hours during the hunt.
- Toy-breed hypoglycemia—increase frequency of feeding.
- Puppy and kitten hypoglycemia—increase frequency of feeding.
- Other causes of hypoglycemia require treating the underlying disease and do not usually need long-term treatment (exception: glycogen storage disease type 1).

CONTRAINDICATIONS

- Insulin.
- Barbiturates and diazepam do not treat cause in patients with hypoglycemic seizures; may potentially worsen hepatoencephalopathy in patients with hepatic disease.

PRECAUTIONS

- 50% dextrose causes tissue necrosis and sloughing if given extravascularly; may cause phlebitis at concentrations above 5%.
- Administration of a dextrose bolus without subsequent frequent feedings or IV fluids with dextrose can predispose to hypoglycemic episodes.

ALTERNATIVE DRUG(S)

N/A

FOLLOW-UP

PATIENT MONITORING

- Based on underlying disease.
- At home—for return or progression of clinical signs of hypoglycemia; assess serum glucose if signs recur.
- Single, intermittent serum glucose determinations may not reflect true glycemic status of patient because of counter-regulatory hormones.
- If due to insulin overdose in the diabetic (or postinsulinoma resection diabetes), reassess response to insulin with a blood glucose curve and adjust the insulin dose accordingly. Check for metastatic insulinoma.

POSSIBLE COMPLICATIONS

Recurrent, progressive episodes of hypoglycemia.

MISCELLANEOUS

ASSOCIATED CONDITIONS

Prolonged hypoglycemia can cause transient (hours to days) to permanent dementia and blindness.

AGE-RELATED FACTORS

Neonatal animals have poor glycogen storage capacity and reduced capacity for gluconeogenesis; thus, short periods of fasting (6–12 hours) can cause hypoglycemia. Important to remember when fasting prior to and following anesthesia.

PREGNANCY/FERTILITY/BREEDING

Hypoglycemia can lead to weakness and dystocia.

SEE ALSO

- Cirrhosis and Fibrosis of the Liver.
- Glycogen Storage Disease.
- Hepatocellular Adenoma.
- Hepatocellular Carcinoma.
- Hypoadrenocorticism.
- Insulinoma.
- Leiomyoma, Stomach, Small and Large Intestine.
- Leiomyosarcoma, Stomach, Small and Large Intestine.
- Paraneoplastic Syndromes.
- Portosystemic Shunting, Acquired.
- Portosystemic Vascular Anomaly, Congenital.
- Sepsis and Bacteremia.
- Xylitol Toxicosis.

ABBREVIATIONS

- IGF = insulin-like growth factor.

Suggested Reading

Caywood DC, Klausner JS, O'Leary, et al. Pancreatic insulin-secreting neoplasms: clinical diagnostic, and prognostic features in 73 dogs. J Am Anim Hosp Assoc 1988, 24:577–584.

Cryer PE, Davis SN. Hypoglycemia. In: Longo DL, Fuaci AS, Kasper DL, et al. Harrison's Principles of Internal Medicine, 20th ed. New York: McGraw-Hill, 2018, pp. 2883–2889.

Lane SL, Koenig A, Brainard BM. Formulation and validation of a predictive model to correct blood glucose concentrations obtained with a veterinary point-of-care glucometer in hemodiluted and hemoconcentrated canine blood samples. J Am Vet Med Assoc. 2015, 246(3):307–312.

Nelson RW. Beta-cell neoplasia: insulinoma. In: Feldman E, Nelson R, Reusch C, Scott-Moncrieff JC, eds., Canine and Feline Endocrinology and Reproduction, 4th ed. St. Louis, MO: Saunders, 2015, pp. 348–375.

Author Michael Schaer

Consulting Editor Patty A. Lathan

Client Education Handout available online

HYPOKALEMIA

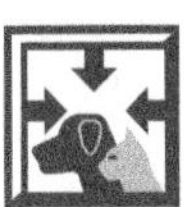

BASICS

DEFINITION

Serum potassium concentration <3.5 mEq/L (normal range: 3.5–5.5 mEq/L).

PATHOPHYSIOLOGY

- Potassium is primarily an intracellular electrolyte (98% of total body potassium is intracellular); serum levels, however, may not accurately reflect total body stores.
- It is predominantly responsible for the maintenance of intracellular fluid volume and required for normal function of many enzymes.
- Resting cellular membrane potential is determined by the ratio of intracellular to extracellular potassium concentration and maintained by the Na^+/K^+–adenosine triphosphate (ATPase) pump. Conduction disturbances in susceptible tissues (cardiac, nerve, muscle) are caused by rapid shifts in this ratio causing myoneural membrane hyperpolarization.
- Hypokalemia can be caused by decreased intake, loss (via the gastrointestinal tract or kidneys), or translocation of potassium from the extracellular to the intracellular fluid space.

SYSTEMS AFFECTED

- Neuromuscular—muscle weakness, including skeletal and muscles of respiration.
- Cardiac—electrocardiac changes and arrhythmias.
- Renal—hyposthenuria, nephropathy, and renal failure.
- Metabolic—acid-base balance (metabolic alkalosis); glucose homeostasis.

SIGNALMENT

- Dogs and cats with predispositions to increased potassium loss, translocation of potassium, or decreased intake of potassium.
- Young Burmese cats with recurrent hypokalemic periodic paralysis episodes.

SIGNS

- Generalized muscle weakness or paralysis.
- Muscle cramps.
- Lethargy and confusion.
- Vomiting.
- Anorexia.
- Carbohydrate intolerance and weight loss.
- Polyuria (PU).
- Polydipsia (PD).
- Decreased bowel motility (humans; maybe dogs and cats).
- Hyposthenuria.
- Ventroflexion of the neck.
- Respiratory muscle failure.

CAUSES

Decreased Intake

- Anorexia or starvation.
- Potassium deficient diet.
- Administration of potassium-deficient or potassium-free intravenous fluids.
- Bentonite clay ingestion (e.g., clumping cat litter).

Gastrointestinal Loss

- Vomiting.
- Diarrhea.
- Both upper and lower gastrointestinal obstruction, especially pyloric outflow obstruction.

Urinary Loss

- Chronic kidney disease (CKD).
- Renal tubular acidosis.
- Hypokalemic nephropathy.
- Postobstructive diuresis.
- Dialysis (hemodialysis or peritoneal).
- Intravenous fluid diuresis.
- Hyperaldosteronism.
- Hypochloremia.
- Drugs (loop diuretics, amphotericin B, penicillins, fludrocortisone, desoxycorticosterone pivalate).

Translocation (Extracellular to Intracellular Fluid)

- Glucose administration.
- Insulin administration or release.
- Sodium bicarbonate administration.
- Catecholamines.
- Alkalemia.
- Beta2-adrenergic agonist overdose (e.g., albuterol, terbutaline).
- Hypokalemic periodic paralysis (Burmese cats).
- Rattlesnake envenomation (presumably from catecholamine release).

RISK FACTORS

- Acidifying diets with negligible potassium.
- Diuresis or dialysis with potassium-deficient fluids.
- Chronic illness (sustained anorexia and muscle wasting).
- Hypomagnesemia.

DIAGNOSIS

DIFFERENTIAL DIAGNOSIS

- PU/PD, hyperglycemia, and glucosuria—rule out diabetes mellitus.
- PU/PD, azotemia, and isosthenuria—rule out CKD and nephropathy, especially in cats.
- Vomiting, metabolic alkalosis, and hypochloremia—rule out upper gastrointestinal obstruction.
- Metabolic acidosis with urine pH >6.5—rule out renal tubular acidosis.
- Urethral obstruction—rule out postobstructive diuresis.
- Hypertension with or without azotemia—rule out hyperaldosteronism
- Young Burmese cat with episodic muscle weakness—rule out hypokalemic periodic paralysis.

LABORATORY FINDINGS

Chemicals That May Alter Laboratory Results

Falsely elevated potassium measurement can be caused by excessive K_3EDTA relative to the blood sample, as found in "purple-top" blood tube for hematology; not a problem with additive-free "red-top" tubes for serum).

Valid if Run in Human Laboratory?

Yes

H

CBC/BIOCHEMISTRY/URINALYSIS

- Hyperglycemia, glucosuria, ± ketonuria, ± ketoacidosis in patients with diabetes mellitus.
- Normocytic, normochromic, nonregenerative anemia in patients with CKD.
- Elevated blood urea nitrogen (BUN) and creatinine concentrations, with isosthenuria in patients with CKD or hypokalemic nephropathy.
- Low total CO_2 or HCO_3^-—in patients with renal tubular acidosis (RTA) or renal failure.
- Normal anion gap metabolic acidosis in RTA.
- Urine pH >6.5 in patients with distal tubular acidosis.
- High total CO_2 or HCO_3^-—in patients with metabolic alkalosis.
- High PCO_2 with hypoventilation.

OTHER LABORATORY TESTS

- Increased aldosterone and decreased renin in patients with primary hyperaldosteronism.
- Elevated urinary fractional excretion of potassium in patients with CKD, hypokalemic nephropathy, and primary hyperaldosteronism.
- Adrenocorticotropic hormone (ACTH) stimulation tests are used to diagnose adrenal gland disorders.

IMAGING

- Radiography, ultrasonography are helpful to diagnose gastrointestinal tract obstructions (mass or foreign bodies), pancreatitis, CKD workup, adrenal gland diseases (adrenocortical hyperplasia, adrenocortical neoplasia).
- Upper gastrointestinal barium study to additionally diagnose gastrointestinal obstructions (anatomic or functional).
- CT to further diagnose adrenal gland, renal, and gastroenteric disorders.

DIAGNOSTIC PROCEDURES

Upper gastrointestinal endoscopy to diagnose upper gastrointestinal disorders.

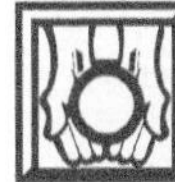

TREATMENT

- Mild hypokalemia (3.0–3.5 mEq/L) can be treated by oral supplementation.
- Moderate hypokalemia (2.5–3.0 mEq/L) is best treated by inpatient administration of oral ± intravenous supplementation and carefully monitored.
- Patients with severe hypokalemia (<2.5 mEq/L) should be hospitalized for intensive intravenous potassium supplementation.

HYPOKALEMIA

H

Table 1

Patient's K⁺ Concentration	*KCl/L (mEq)*	*Dosage (mEq K⁺/kg/h, IV)*
3.5–4.5	20	0.05–0.1
3.0–3.5	30	0.1–0.2
2.5–3.0	40	0.2–0.3
2.0–2.5	60	0.3–0.4
<2.0	80	0.5–1.5

Note: do not exceed an intravenous supplementation rate of 0.5 mEq/kg/h unless continually monitoring and on the verge of ventilator muscle failure. With severe life-threatening hypokalemia (serum potassium <2.0 mEq/L), potassium chloride can be administered at a rate of 1.0–1.5 mEq/kg/h with ECG monitoring.

Patients, especially cats, should be carefully monitored for cardiac arrhythmias, rhabdomyolysis and impaired ventilation.

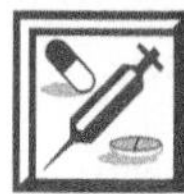

MEDICATIONS

DRUG(S) OF CHOICE

- Oral supplementation with potassium gluconate (e.g., Tumil-K®) is effective in mildly affected patients. The initial dosage is 2 mEq/4.5 kg bodyweight in food twice daily.
- Parenteral supplementation is required in anorectic or vomiting patients or in patients with moderate to severe hypokalemia (<3.0 mEq/L). Potassium chloride is added to intravenous fluids and delivered according to Table 1, best administered via infusion pump or with a pediatric fluid administration set (60 drops/mL). Monitor and taper accordingly.
- Provide magnesium sulfate, if hypomagnesemic; 1.0 mEq/kg/24h by CRI, or a 0.25 mEq/kg slow IV bolus.

CONTRAINDICATIONS

- Glucose supplementation.
- Insulin administration.
- Sodium bicarbonate administration.
- Untreated hypoadrenocorticism.
- Hyperkalemia.
- Oliguric or anuric renal failure or severe renal impairment.
- Rapid rehydration to correct severe dehydration (i.e., potassium-supplemented fluids should not be bolused IV).

PRECAUTIONS

Administer with caution, avoid over-supplementation, do not bolus, monitor frequently.

POSSIBLE INTERACTIONS

Concurrent potassium supplementation with angiotensin-converting enzyme (ACE) inhibitors (e.g., enalapril), potassium-sparing diuretics (e.g., spironolactone), prostaglandin inhibitors (e.g., nonsteroidal anti-inflammatory drugs), beta blockers (e.g., atenolol), or cardiac glycosides (e.g., digoxin) can cause adverse effects.

ALTERNATIVE DRUG(S)

Potassium phosphate can be used in patients with concurrent hypophosphatemia where one-half of the potassium dose (in mEq) is administered in the form of potassium phosphate solution.

FOLLOW-UP

PATIENT MONITORING

Check serum potassium every 6–24 hours based on severity of hypokalemia.

POSSIBLE COMPLICATIONS

Electrolyte disturbances and severe bradyarrhythmias. It is essential to close the IV fluid outflow valve and thoroughly mix the fluid contents when adding potassium chloride solution to the parenteral fluid bag.

MISCELLANEOUS

ASSOCIATED CONDITIONS

- Hypokalemic nephropathy.
- Hypophosphatemia.
- Hypomagnesemia.
- Metabolic alkalosis.

AGE-RELATED FACTORS

None

ZOONOTIC POTENTIAL

None

PREGNANCY/FERTILITY/BREEDING

N/A

SEE ALSO

- Alkalosis, Metabolic.
- Chronic Kidney Disease.
- Diarrhea, Chronic—Cats.
- Diarrhea, Chronic—Dogs.
- Hypochloremia.
- Renal Tubular Acidosis.
- Vomiting, Chronic.

ABBREVIATIONS

- ACE = angiotensin-converting enzyme.
- ACTH = adrenocorticotropic hormone.
- ATPase = adenosine triphosphate.
- BUN = blood urea nitrogen.
- CKD = chronic kidney disease.
- PD = polydipsia.
- PU = polyuria.
- RTA = renal tubular acidosis.

Suggested Reading

Boag AK, Coe RJ, Martinez TA, et al. Acid-base and electrolyte abnormalities in dogs with gastrointestinal foreign bodies. J Vet Intern Med 2005, 19:816–821.

DiBartola SP, Autran de Morais H. Disorders of potassium: hypokalemia and hyperkalemia. In: DiBartola SP, ed., Fluid Therapy in Small Animal Practice, 4th ed. Philadelphia, PA: Saunders, 2012, pp. 92–120.

Greenlee M, Wingo CS, McDonough AA, et al. Narrative review: evolving concepts in potassium homeostasis and hypokalemia. Ann Intern Med 2009, 150: 619–625.

Nager AL. Fluid and electrolyte therapy in infants and children. In: Tintinalli JE, Stapczynski JS, Ma OJ, eds., Emergency Medicine: A Comprehensive Study Guide, 7th ed. New York: McGraw-Hill, 2011, pp. 971–976.

Author Michael Schaer

Consulting Editor Patty A. Lathan

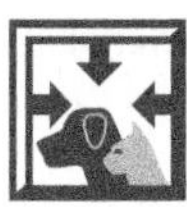

BASICS

DEFINITION

- Dogs—serum magnesium <1.89 mg/dL, ionized magnesium <0.43 mmol/L.
- Cats—serum magnesium <1.75 mg/dL, ionized magnesium <0.48 mmol/L.

PATHOPHYSIOLOGY

- Magnesium is the second most abundant intracellular cation, found primarily in bone (60%) and soft tissues (38%).
- Hypomagnesemia has many causes; incidence rates >50% have been reported in critically ill humans.
- Serum magnesium is present in three forms—protein-bound form (approximately 25–30%) and chelated and ionized forms (together 70–75%).
- Serum magnesium concentration does not always reflect whole-body magnesium status.
- Magnesium absorption occurs primarily in the ileum as well as the jejunum and colon.
- Kidneys maintain magnesium balance, with 10–15% reabsorbed in the proximal tubule, 60–70% in the thick ascending limb of the loop of Henle, and 10–15% reabsorbed in the distal convoluted tubule. Reabsorption within the distal convoluted tubule is under hormonal and neurohormonal control and determines the final urine concentration of magnesium.
- Magnesium is an important cofactor in the sodium–potassium adenosine triphosphate (ATPase) pump that maintains a membrane electrical gradient. Magnesium is also important in the production and elimination of acetylcholine; hypomagnesemia can increase acetylcholine at motor endplates and cause tetany.
- Interference with membrane potentials can result in neuromuscular and cardiac abnormalities.
- Magnesium regulates calcium movement into smooth muscle cells and is important for cardiac contractile strength, conduction, and peripheral vascular tone.
- Hypomagnesemia alters function of skeletal muscle, resulting in tetany and myopathies.
- Magnesium depletion affects membrane pumps on cardiac cells, resulting in depolarization and tachyarrhythmias; cardiac arrhythmias associated with hypomagnesemia include ventricular arrhythmias, torsades de pointes, QT prolongation, ST segment shortening, and widening of T waves; hypomagnesemia increases the risk of digoxin toxicity because both inhibit the membrane pump.
- Hypomagnesemia causes resistance to the effects of parathyroid hormone (PTH) and can increase the uptake of calcium into bone.

SYSTEMS AFFECTED

- Cardiovascular.
- Endocrine.
- Gastrointestinal.
- Neuromuscular.
- Renal.

INCIDENCE/PREVALENCE

Reported in 28–54% of critically ill dogs and cats, may have increased incidence in bulldogs.

SIGNALMENT

Dog and cat.

SIGNS

- Weakness.
- Muscle fibrillation.
- Ataxia and depression.
- Hyperreflexia.
- Tetany.
- Behavior changes.
- Cardiac arrhythmias.

CAUSES

- Gastrointestinal—severe malnutrition or significant intestinal malabsorptive disease, following excessive loss of body fluids (e.g., severe, prolonged diarrhea), secretory large-bowel diarrhea.
- Renal—nephrotoxic drugs (e.g., cisplatin, aminoglycosides, amphotericin B), osmotic diuresis (e.g., with diabetes mellitus), loop diuretics, chronic thiazide diuretic therapy, hypercalciuria, postobstructive diuresis, and renal tubular acidosis.
- Other drugs associated with hypomagnesemia include cyclosporine, ticarcillin, carbenicillin, and proton pump inhibitors.
- Endocrine diseases associated with hypomagnesemia include hyperaldosteronism, hyperthyroidism, and primary hypoparathyroidism. Hypomagnesemia is found in 32% of dogs and 85% of cats with hypoparathyroidism, and can be seen following surgical parathyroidectomy.
- Lactation, pancreatitis, insulin administration, and catecholamine excess can cause excessive magnesium loss.
- Magnesium can be redistributed by refeeding after starvation and insulin therapy in diabetic patients.
- Causes of hypomagnesemia in the critically ill include decreased intake, lack of magnesium in parenteral fluids (long-term fluid therapy or hemodialysis), use of a total parenteral nutrition formulation with inadequate magnesium content, excessive gastrointestinal loss, redistribution, and sequestration.
- Hypomagnesemia is associated with diabetes mellitus in humans, with nearly 25% of human diabetic outpatients having low serum magnesium, and may occur during therapy for diabetic ketoacidosis in dogs and cats.

RISK FACTORS

- Gastrointestinal malabsorption syndromes.
- Polyuric renal disease.
- Diuretic administration.
- Diabetes mellitus and diabetic ketoacidosis.
- Total parenteral nutrition.
- Peritoneal dialysis.
- Lactation.

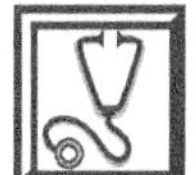

DIAGNOSIS

DIFFERENTIAL DIAGNOSIS

- Signs of hypomagnesemia are vague and multisystemic; therefore, other causes of neuromuscular abnormalities, especially other electrolyte abnormalities, must be investigated.
- Consider cardiac abnormalities, intoxications, and renal diseases.

LABORATORY FINDINGS

Note: 12 mg of magnesium = 1 mEq of magnesium; to convert from mg/dL to mEq/L, divide by 1.2.

Drugs That May Alter Laboratory Results

- Serum is favored over plasma because EDTA, sodium fluoride-oxalate, and sodium citrate anticoagulants used for plasma samples can contain citrate or other ions that bind magnesium. Heparinized whole blood or plasma may be used to determine ionized magnesium concentration
- Intravenous calcium gluconate can falsely decrease serum magnesium values.

Disorders That May Alter Laboratory Results

- Hemolysis can falsely elevate serum magnesium.
- Hypercalcemia (>16 mg/dL) and hyperproteinemia (>10 g/dL) can falsely elevate serum magnesium.
- Hyperbilirubinemia and lipemia can falsely decrease serum magnesium.

Valid if Run in Human Laboratory?

Yes

CBC/BIOCHEMISTRY/URINALYSIS

- Low serum magnesium.
- If patient is azotemic, consider renal causes.
- Tubular casts in urinary sediment might indicate nephrotoxicity.
- Hypokalemia, hyponatremia, and hypocalcemia are common findings with hypomagnesemia and should alert the clinician to the possibility of hypomagnesemia.

OTHER LABORATORY TESTS

- Diagnosis of magnesium depletion can be difficult since <1% of total body magnesium is located in serum; only 55% of the magnesium in plasma is in the active (ionized) form; 33% is bound to plasma proteins and 12% is chelated with divalent anions such as phosphate and sulfate; magnesium assays (spectrophotometry) measure all three fractions.
- Ionized magnesium can be measured with an ion-selective electrode or by ultrafiltration of plasma; alternative methods of evaluating magnesium status include measurement of

HYPOMAGNESEMIA (CONTINUED)

mononuclear blood cell magnesium levels or quantifying retention from a loading dose.
- Urinary magnesium determination might help differentiate conditions associated with high urinary magnesium loss from conditions of low intake or absorption.
- Human studies suggest that retention of >40–50% of an administered magnesium load indicates magnesium depletion, while retention of <20% indicates adequate magnesium stores.

DIAGNOSTIC PROCEDURES

- Electrodiagnostics (e.g., electromyelography and electrocardiography) might reveal effects of hypomagnesemia, but will not differentiate the cause.
- Hypomagnesemia can cause prolongation of the PR interval, widening of the QRS complex, depression of the ST segment, and peaking of the T wave, in addition to ventricular arrhythmias.

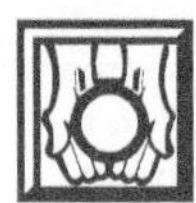

TREATMENT

APPROPRIATE HEALTH CARE

- Treatment depends on underlying cause and severity.
- Management includes treatment of the underlying condition(s) and magnesium replacement.
- Mild hypomagnesemia might resolve with treatment of the underlying disorder; however, if hypomagnesemia is severe, intensive care and magnesium replacement are needed.

NURSING CARE

Hypomagnesemia is a common finding in critically ill, hospitalized veterinary patients. Nursing should focus on the underlying disorder(s).

ACTIVITY

Based on concurrent conditions.

DIET

A balanced diet that takes into account all concurrent problems is appropriate.

MEDICATIONS

DRUG(S) OF CHOICE

- Magnesium sulfate or magnesium chloride.
  - Emergency loading—0.15–0.3 mEq/kg IV over 15–60 min.
  - Rapid replacement—0.75–1 mEq/kg/day (0.03 mEq/kg/h) IV.
  - Slow replacement—0.3–0.5 mEq/kg/day (0.013–0.02 mEq/kg/h) IV.
- Magnesium sulfate can be diluted in 5% dextrose in water or 0.9% saline; the solution of magnesium salts should be <20% and should use a separate IV port to minimize drug interactions

CONTRAINDICATIONS

- Hypomagnesemia potentiates nephrotoxicity of aminoglycosides.
- Avoid cisplatin chemotherapy.

PRECAUTIONS

- Discontinue digoxin if possible.
- Use diuretics with caution.
- Hypermagnesemia is possible with overzealous supplementation.
- Azotemic patients should receive a lower dose of magnesium and more frequent monitoring than patients with normal kidney function.

POSSIBLE INTERACTIONS

- Magnesium sulfate is incompatible with sodium bicarbonate, hydrocortisone, and dobutamine HCl.
- Calcium-containing compounds lower serum magnesium concentration.
- Additive CNS depression can occur when parenteral magnesium is used with CNS depressant sedatives, neuromuscular blocking agents, and anesthetics.
- Combined use of parenteral magnesium sulfate and nondepolarizing neuromuscular blocking agents is contraindicated.
- Use magnesium supplementation cautiously with digitalis compounds to avoid conduction disturbances.
- Calcium supplements might negate the effects of parenteral magnesium.

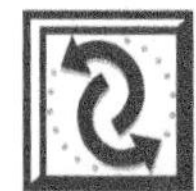

FOLLOW-UP

PATIENT MONITORING

- Measure serum magnesium and calcium concentrations daily.
- Continuous ECG and blood pressure monitoring, especially during magnesium infusion.

POSSIBLE COMPLICATIONS

- Severe hypomagnesemia can be fatal.
- Magnesium is inversely associated with fibroblast growth factor 23 (FGF23), an important prognostic factor in CKD in cats.

EXPECTED COURSE AND PROGNOSIS

Outcome is dependent on resolution of the underlying disease(s).

MISCELLANEOUS

ASSOCIATED CONDITIONS

- Hyperthyroidism.
- Hypocalcemia.
- Hypokalemia.
- Hyponatremia.
- Hypoparathyroidism.
- Hypophosphatemia.

PREGNANCY/FERTILITY/BREEDING

Effects on fetus are identical to effects on the dam.

SEE ALSO

Hypocalcemia

ABBREVIATIONS

- ATP = adenosine triphosphate.
- PTH = parathyroid hormone.

Suggested Reading

Bateman SW. Disorders of magnesium: magnesium deficit and excess. In: DiBartola SP, ed., Fluid, Electrolyte and Acid-Base Disorders in Small Animal Practice, 4th ed. Philadelphia, PA: Elsevier, 2011, pp. 212–229.

Della Maggiore AM, Differential diagnosis for clinicopathologic abnormalities: potassium and magnesium. In: Ettinger SJ, Feldman EC, Cote E, eds., Veterinary Internal Medicine, 8th ed. Philadelphia, PA: Elsevier, 2017, pp. 270–275.

Hendrick D, van den Broek N, Chang Y, et. al. Prognostic importance of plasma total magnesium in a cohort of cats with azotemic chronic kidney disease. J Vet Intern Med 2018, 32(4):1359–1371.

Humphrey S, Kirby R, Rudloff E. Magnesium physiology and clinical therapy in veterinary critical care. J Vet Emerg Crit Care 2015, 25(2):210–225.

Khanna C, Lund EM, Raffe M, et al. Hypomagnesemia in 188 dogs: a hospital population-based prevalence study. J Vet Intern Med 1998, 12(4):304–309.

Author Timothy B. Hackett

Consulting Editor Patty A. Lathan

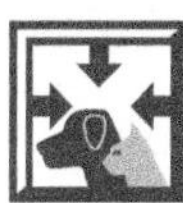

BASICS

OVERVIEW

• Also known as "shaking puppies." • Congenital deficit in myelin deposition caused by either delayed myelination or a permanent lack of myelin at birth. • Axons >1–2 mm in diameter have a myelin cover produced by oligodendrocytes in the central nervous system (CNS) and Schwann cells in the peripheral nervous system (PNS); myelin insulates axons and facilitates propagation of action potentials. • Affected axons with deficit in myelin deposition can alter impulse conduction or trigger spontaneous discharges and then generate tremors; the degree of tremor is usually correlated with the severity of the abnormal myelin deposition.

SIGNALMENT

CNS

• Clinical signs appear at birth or when the puppy starts to ambulate. • Dog—springer spaniel, Samoyed, chow chow, Weimaraner, Bernese mountain dog, Dalmatian, Catahoula, rat terrier, border terriers, and lurcher. • Cat—Siamese and presumed in domestic shorthair and Birman cats. • Predominant sex (X-linked)—springer spaniel and Samoyed male puppies clinically affected, whereas females remain largely asymptomatic carriers; no sex differences reported in other breeds.

PNS

• Dog. • Golden retriever—reported in both sexes.

SIGNS

CNS

• Action-related repetitive myoclonus—rapid contractions and relaxation of diffuse skeletal muscles manifested as generalized body tremors that worsen with exercise and subside during rest or sleep; some affected dogs and cats appear to be "bouncing." • The tremors diminish with time in the majority of affected dogs and usually resolve by 12 months of age or earlier; however, some dogs can retain a persistent fine tremor of the pelvic limbs. • Some dogs also present with head bobbing and nystagmus. • In rat terriers, associated with goiter and clinical signs of congenital hypothyroidism. • Springer spaniels and Samoyeds are usually affected for life.

PNS

• Clinical signs appear at 5–7 weeks of age. • Generalized weakness, pelvic limb ataxia and paresis, muscle wasting, and hyporeflexia that improve with age. • Tremors are not present.

CAUSES & RISK FACTORS

• Genetic—X-linked recessive condition for CNS disease in springer spaniels and autosomal recessive gene in rat terriers, Weimaraners, and border terriers. • Genetic basis speculative for other breeds. • Mutation identified in Weimaraners and rat terriers. • The carrier frequency in Weimaraners has been estimated to be 4.3%. • Viral or toxic—possible in some breeds. • PNS—undetermined; possibly genetic.

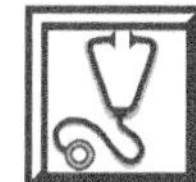

DIAGNOSIS

DIFFERENTIAL DIAGNOSIS

CNS

• Cerebellar hypoplasia or abiotrophy—tremors in neonates; but cerebellar ataxia (hypermetric gait) and intention tremors more prominent. • Storage diseases—associated with tremors; neonates are normal. • Generalized tremor syndrome in dogs (historically identified as "white shakers" but other hair coat colors can be affected)—affected dogs are usually >8 months old. • Metabolic diseases (hypocalcemia, hypernatremia, hyponatremia, hypoglycemia). • Feline polioencephalomyelitis—young to middle-aged cats; other neurologic signs are present (paresis, seizures, hyperesthesia). • Toxic—organophosphates, permethrins, mycotoxins: history of exposure to a toxic product.

PNS

• Muscular dystrophy—serum creatine kinase highly elevated. • Congenital myasthenia gravis. • Other polyneuropathies or myopathies.

CBC/BIOCHEMISTRY/URINALYSIS

Usually normal.

IMAGING

MRI—may detect white matter changes on CNS form.

DIAGNOSTIC PROCEDURES

CNS

• Presumed diagnosis based on signalment, clinical signs, and evolution. • Histopathology (necropsy). • DNA test for causative genetic mutation (currently available for Weimaraners and rat terriers).

PNS

• Electromyography—usually normal to mild diffuse spontaneous activity. • Motor nerve conduction velocity—small or no evoked potentials and slowed conduction. • Nerve biopsy—insufficient myelin surrounding peripheral axons.

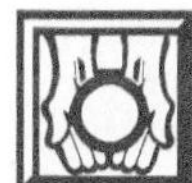

TREATMENT

None effective for either form.

MEDICATIONS

DRUG(S) OF CHOICE

N/A

FOLLOW-UP

PREVENTION/AVOIDANCE

Avoid breeding from affected animals in which a genetic cause is suspected.

EXPECTED COURSE AND PROGNOSIS

• CNS—Springer spaniels and Samoyeds affected for life; other breeds usually improve by 1 year of age. • PNS—dogs have normal lifespan.

H

MISCELLANEOUS

ABBREVIATIONS

• CNS = central nervous system.
• PNS = peripheral nervous system.

INTERNET RESOURCES

Genetic Tests

• https://www.vgl.ucdavis.edu/services/Weimaraner.php • https://www.centerforanimalgenetics.com/services/dog-genetic-testing/hereditary-disease-testing-for-dogs/congenital-hypothyroidism • http://www.laboklin.co.uk/laboklin/showGeneticTest.jsp?testID=8443

Video

http://www.neurovideos.vet.cornell.edu/Video.aspx?vid=20-39

Suggested Reading

Duncan ID. Abnormalities of myelination of the central nervous system associated with congenital tremor. J Vet Intern Med 1987, 1:10–23.

Lowrie M, Garosi L. Classification of involuntary movements in dogs: tremors and twitches. Vet J 2016, 214:109–116.

Martin-Vaquero P, da Costa RC, Simmons JK, et al. A novel spongiform leukoencephalomyelopathy in Border Terrier puppies. J Vet Intern Med 2012, 26:402–406.

Millán Y, Mascort J, Blanco A, et al. Hypomyelination in three Weimaraner dogs. J Small Anim Pract 2010, 51:594–598.

Pemberton TJ, Choi S, Mayer JA, et al. A mutation in the canine gene encoding folliculin-interacting protein 2 (FNIP2) associated with a unique disruption in spinal cord myelination. Glia 2014, 62:39–51.

Stoffregen DA, Huxtable CR, Cummings JF, et al. Hypomyelination of the central nervous system of two Siamese kitten littermates. Vet Pathol 1993, 30:388–391.

Author Elsa Beltran

HYPONATREMIA

BASICS

DEFINITION

Serum sodium concentration below the lower limit of the reference range.

PATHOPHYSIOLOGY

Sodium is the most abundant cation in the extracellular fluid. Hyponatremia usually reflects hypo-osmolality and is typically associated with a decreased total body sodium content. Either water retention or solute loss can cause hyponatremia. Most solute loss occurs in iso-osmotic solutions (e.g., vomit and diarrhea) and, as a result, water retention in relation to solute is the underlying cause in almost all patients with hyponatremia. In general, hyponatremia occurs only when a defect in renal water excretion is present.

SYSTEMS AFFECTED

- Nervous—severe neurologic dysfunction is not usually seen until serum sodium concentration falls below 110–115 mEq/L. Clinical signs may be more related to the rate of decline in serum sodium concentration than the actual nadir. Dogs with chronic hyponatremia often have mild, if any, clinical signs.
- Overly rapid correction of hyponatremia can also cause neurologic damage.

SIGNALMENT

Species

Dog and cat.

SIGNS

- Lethargy.
- Weakness.
- Confusion.
- Nausea/vomiting.
- Seizures.
- Obtundation.
- Coma.
- Other signs depend on the underlying cause.

CAUSES

Normal Osmolar Hyponatremia

- Hyperlipidemia (pseudohyponatremia).
- Hyperproteinemia (pseudohyponatremia).

Hyperosmolar Hyponatremia

- Hyperglycemia.
- Mannitol administration.

Hypo-osmolar Hyponatremia

Normovolemic

- Primary polydipsia.
- Hypothyroid myxedema coma.
- Hypotonic fluid infusion.
- Syndrome of inappropriate antidiuretic hormone secretion (SIADH).

Hypervolemic

- Congestive heart failure.
- Hepatic cirrhosis.
- Nephrotic syndrome.
- Severe renal failure.

Hypovolemic

- Gastrointestinal losses.
- Renal failure.
- Third-space losses.
- Cutaneous losses (e.g., burns).
- Diuresis.
- Hypoadrenocorticism.

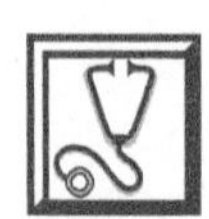

DIAGNOSIS

DIFFERENTIAL DIAGNOSIS

- Hypoadrenocorticism.
- Severe gastrointestinal disease.
- Metabolic or respiratory acidosis.
- Congestive heart failure.
- Primary polydipsia.

LABORATORY FINDINGS

Drugs That May Alter Lab Results

Mannitol can cause pseudohyponatremia by solvent drag.

Disorders That May Alter Lab Results

Hyperlipidemia and hyperproteinemia can cause pseudohyponatremia on analyzers that use indirect potentiometry or flame photometry. Hyperglycemia can cause pseudohyponatremia through solvent drag, and serum sodium concentration normalizes with correction of hyperglycemia (e.g., with IV fluid or insulin therapy in patients with diabetes mellitus).

Valid if Run in a Human Laboratory?

Yes

CBC/BIOCHEMISTRY/URINALYSIS

- Low serum sodium concentration.
- Other abnormalities may point to the underlying cause.

OTHER LABORATORY TESTS

- Plasma osmolality is usually low; if plasma osmolality is normal or high, exclude hyperlipidemia, hyperglycemia, hyperproteinemia, and mannitol administration.
- Urine osmolality <100–150 mOsmol/kg indicates primary polydipsia or reset osmostat. Urine osmolality >150–200 mOsmol/kg indicates impaired renal water excretion.
- Urine sodium concentration <15–20 mEq/L indicates low effective circulating volume, pure cortisol deficiency, or primary polydipsia with high urine output. Urine sodium concentration >20–25 mEq/L indicates SIADH, adrenal insufficiency, renal failure, reset osmostat, diuretic administration, or vomiting with marked bicarbonate loss.

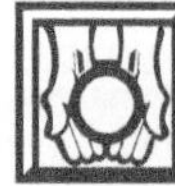

TREATMENT

Generally inpatient, depending on severity of hyponatremia, associated neurologic dysfunction, and underlying disorder.

MEDICATIONS

DRUG(S) OF CHOICE

- Treatment consists of addressing the underlying cause and increasing the serum sodium concentration if necessary. Overly rapid normalization (>10-12 mEq/L in 24 hours) of chronic hyponatremia can have potentially severe neurologic sequelae (myelinolysis) and may be more detrimental than the hyponatremia itself. Therefore, an isotonic crystalloid is the fluid of choice in most cases. More aggressive correction of serum sodium with hypertonic or normal saline in patients with chronic hyponatremia is not recommended.
- Acute hyponatremia (occurring over 24–48 hours) can be corrected more quickly, but is rare in small animals. Unless an acute cause of hyponatremia can be identified, or severe clinical signs of hyponatremia are present (seizures, cerebral edema), slower correction is recommended.
- Hypervolemic (edematous) patients are typically managed with diuretics and salt restriction, or hemodialysis if necessary (e.g., acute renal failure).
- Hypovolemic patients are managed by replacing the volume deficit with isotonic crystalloids. Isotonic (0.9%) saline, Normosol®-R, and lactated Ringer's solution (LRS) may be used. LRS has a sodium concentration of 130 mEq/L and is helpful in slowly increasing sodium concentrations in dogs with severe hyponatremia (<120 mEq/L).
- Other therapeutic interventions are dictated by the underlying cause of the hyponatremia.

PRECAUTIONS

Overly rapid correction of hyponatremia can result in neurologic damage (demyelination); avoid increasing serum sodium concentration by more than 10–12 mEq/L/day (0.5 mEq/L/h).

FOLLOW-UP

PATIENT MONITORING

- Serial serum sodium determinations (generally q4–6h) to avoid overly rapid correction of the serum sodium concentration and to assure appropriate response to other therapies.
- Monitor hydration status.
- Monitor other serum electrolyte concentrations as indicated by the patient's clinical condition and underlying disorder.

PREVENTION/AVOIDANCE

Depends on the underlying disorder.

POSSIBLE COMPLICATIONS

Depends on the underlying disorder.

EXPECTED COURSE AND PROGNOSIS

Depends on the underlying disorder.

MISCELLANEOUS

ASSOCIATED CONDITIONS

Other electrolyte and acid-base abnormalities are often associated with the clinical disorders that cause hyponatremia.

SEE ALSO

- Acute Kidney Injury.
- Chronic Kidney Disease.
- Cirrhosis and Fibrosis of the Liver.
- Congestive Heart Failure, Left-Sided.
- Hyperglycemia.
- Hyperlipemia.
- Hypoadrenocorticism (Addison's Disease).
- Myxedema and Myxedema Coma.
- Nephrotic Syndrome.
- Polyuria and Polydipsia.

ABBREVIATIONS

- LRS = lactated Ringer's solution.
- SIADH = syndrome of inappropriate ADH secretion.

Suggested Reading

DiBartola SP. Fluid, Electrolyte, and Acid-Base Disorders in Small Animal Practice, 4th ed. Philadelphia, PA: Saunders, 2012.

Author Patty A. Lathan

Consulting Editor Patty A. Lathan

Acknowledgment The author and book editors acknowledge the prior contribution of Melinda Fleming.

HYPOPARATHYROIDISM

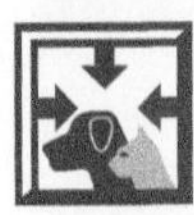

BASICS

DEFINITION

Absolute or relative deficiency of parathyroid hormone (PTH) secretion leading to hypocalcemia.

PATHOPHYSIOLOGY

• Dogs—most commonly idiopathic immune-mediated parathyroiditis, rarely following bilateral thyroidectomy or following severe cervical trauma. • Cats—most commonly iatrogenic secondary to damaged or removed parathyroid glands during thyroidectomy; idiopathic atrophy and immune-mediated parathyroiditis uncommon.

SYSTEMS AFFECTED

• Cardiovascular—ECG changes and bradycardia. • Gastrointestinal—anorexia and vomiting, possibly (altered gastrointestinal muscular activity). • Nervous/neuromuscular—seizures, tetany, ataxia, weakness (diminished neuronal membrane stability). • Ophthalmic—posterior lenticular cataracts. • Respiratory—panting (neuromuscular weakness, anxiety).

INCIDENCE/PREVALENCE

• Dog—uncommon. • Cat—common (10–82%) following bilateral thyroidectomy; spontaneous occurrence rare.

SIGNALMENT

Species

Dog and cat.

Breed Predilections

Toy poodle, miniature schnauzer, German shepherd dog, Labrador retriever, terrier breeds; mixed-breed cats.

Mean Age and Range

• Dogs—mean 4.8 years; range: 6 weeks–13 years. • Cats—secondary to thyroidectomy, mean 12–13 years; range: 4–22 years. • Cats—spontaneous, mean 2.25 years; range: 6 months–7 years.

Predominant Sex

Dogs—female (60%); cats—male (64%).

SIGNS

Historical Findings

Dogs

• Seizures (49–86%). • Ataxia/stiff gait (43–62%). • Facial rubbing (62%). • Muscle trembling, twitching, and fasciculations (57%). • Growling (57%). • Panting (35%). • Weakness. • Vomiting. • Anorexia.

Cats

• Lethargy, anorexia, and depression (100%). • Seizures (50%). • Muscle trembling, twitching, and fasciculations (83%). • Panting (33%). • Bradycardia (17%).

Physical Examination Findings

Dogs

• Tense, splinted abdomen (50–65%). • Ataxia/stiff gait (43–62%). • Fever (30–70%). • Muscle trembling, twitching, and fasciculations (57%). • Panting (35%). • Posterior lenticular cataracts (15–32%). • Weakness. • Normal physical examination (20%).

Cats

• Muscle trembling, twitching, and fasciculations (83%). • Panting (33%). • Posterior lenticular cataracts (33%). • Bradycardia (17%). • Fever (17%). • Hypothermia (17%).

CAUSES

See Pathophysiology.

RISK FACTORS

Dogs, cats—bilateral thyroidectomy.

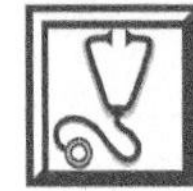

DIAGNOSIS

DIFFERENTIAL DIAGNOSIS

Seizures

• Cardiovascular—syncope. • Metabolic—hepatoencephalopathy, hypoglycemia, other causes of hypocalcemia. • Neurologic—epilepsy, neoplasia, toxin, inflammatory disease.

Weakness

• Cardiovascular—congenital defects, arrhythmias, heart failure, pericardial effusion. • Metabolic—hypoadrenocorticism, hypoglycemia, anemia, hypokalemia (especially cats), hypothyroidism. • Neurologic/neuromuscular—myasthenia gravis, polymyositis, polyradiculoneuropathy, spinal cord disease. • Toxic—tick paralysis, botulism, chronic organophosphate exposure, snake envenomation (Eastern coral snake and other elapids, Mojave and certain other pit vipers), lead poisoning.

Muscle Trembling, Twitching, and Fasciculations

• Metabolic—puerperal tetany (i.e., eclampsia), other causes of hypocalcemia. • Toxic—tetanus, strychnine, permethrin, snake envenomation.

CBC/BIOCHEMISTRY/URINALYSIS

• Hemogram and urinalysis usually normal; perform to rule out other differential diagnoses. • Hypocalcemia (usually <6.5 mg/dL) and normal or mild to moderate hyperphosphatemia. • Evaluate serum albumin carefully in all patients with hypocalcemia; hypoalbuminemia is most common asymptomatic cause of hypocalcemia (assuming ionized fraction is adequate). • The only other intrinsic disease process besides hypoparathyroidism that reduces serum calcium and raises serum phosphorus is renal failure, which is easily distinguished from hypoparathyroidism by presence of azotemia; highly concentrated phosphate enema solutions can also cause hyperphosphatemia and hypocalcemia, as can excessive potassium phosphate parenteral fluid supplementation.

OTHER LABORATORY TESTS

Serum PTH—undetectable or very low PTH concentration; patients with other processes causing hypocalcemia (e.g., renal failure) have normal to high serum PTH concentration.

IMAGING

Atrophic parathyroid glands will not be visible with ultrasonography (normally 2–3 mm).

DIAGNOSTIC PROCEDURES

• ECG changes from hypocalcemia include prolongation of ST and QT segments; sinus bradycardia and wide T waves; occasionally T wave alternans. • Cervical surgical exploration reveals absence or atrophy of parathyroid glands.

PATHOLOGIC FINDINGS

• Dogs—normal or diminished tissue with mature lymphocytes, plasma cells, and fibrous connective tissue along with chief cell degeneration. • Cats—parathyroid gland atrophy more common, although histopathologic findings similar to dogs also found.

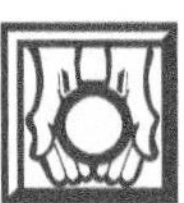

TREATMENT

APPROPRIATE HEALTH CARE

• Hospitalize for medical management of hypocalcemia until clinical signs of hypocalcemia are controlled and serum total calcium concentration is >7 mg/dL. • See Hypocalcemia for emergency inpatient management and appropriate fluid therapy

NURSING CARE

No specific care other than seizure watch.

DIET

Avoid calcium-poor diets; for dogs, puppy diets generally higher in calcium than adult dog food.

CLIENT EDUCATION

• Naturally occurring primary hypoparathyroidism requires lifelong therapy and monitoring. • Most cases of iatrogenic hypoparathyroidism (e.g., bilateral thyroidectomy) will recover over days to months and only require transient management and monitoring.

MEDICATIONS

DRUG(S) OF CHOICE

Emergency/Acute Therapy

See Hypocalcemia.

Short-Term Post-tetany Therapy

See Hypocalcemia.

Table 1

Vitamin D preparations.

Preparation	*Dose*	*Maximal Effect*	*Size*
1,25 Dihydroxycholecalciferol (active vitamin D_3, calcitriol)	0.03–0.06 µg/kg/day	1–4 days	0.25 and 0.5 µg capsules, 1.0 µg/mL oral solution, and 1 and 2 µg/mL injectable
Dihydrotachysterol	Initial—0.02–0.03 mg/kg/day Maintenance—0.01–0.02 mg/kg/24–48h	1–7 days	Currently unavailable in United States; formerly available as 0.125 mg, 0.2 mg, 0.4 mg tablets and 0.2 mg/mL syrup
Ergocalciferol (vitamin D_2)	Initial—4000–6000 U/kg/day Maintenance—1000–2000 U/kg/day–week	5–21 days	25,000 and 50,000 U capsules and 8000 U/mL syrup

Table 2

Calcium preparations.

Preparation	*Dose of Elemental Calcium*	*Available Calcium*	*Size Available (Needs to Be Converted to Elemental Calcium)*
Calcium carbonate	Canine—1–4 g/day Feline—0.5–1 g/day	40%	Tablets—500, 600, 650, 1250, 1500 mg Chewable tablets—400, 420, 500, 750, 50, 1000, 1250 mg Capsules—1250 mg Oral suspension—250 mg/mL
Calcium gluconate	Canine—1–4 g/day Feline—0.5–1 g/day	10%	Tablets—500, 650, 975 mg Chewable tablets—500 mg Capsules—500, 700 mg Powder for suspension—70 mg/mL
Calcium lactate	Canine—1–4 g/day Feline—0.5–1 g/day	13%	Tablets—650, 770 mg Capsules—500 mg
Calcium acetate	Canine—1–4 g/day Feline—0.5–1 g/day	25%	Tablets, gelcaps, and capsules—667 mg
Calcium citrate	Canine—1–4 g/day Feline—0.5–1 g/day	21%	Tablets—950, 1150 mg Effervescent tablets—2,380 mg Capsules—850, 1070 mg Powder for oral suspension—725 mg/mL
Calcium glubionate	Canine—1–4 g/day Feline—0.5–1 g/day	30%	Syrup—360 mg/mL

Long-Term Therapy

• Vitamin D administration is needed indefinitely for primary hypoparathyroidism and total parathyroidectomy; dosage should be adjusted based on serum calcium concentration. • Shorter-acting preparations of vitamin D are preferred so that overdosage (causing hypercalcemia) can be quickly corrected (see Table 1). • A more economical approach to treatment is to maximize oral administration of calcium and reduce oral administration of vitamin D (see Table 2); calcium is usually less expensive than vitamin D; dosage is influenced by each product's available elemental calcium content.

CONTRAINDICATIONS

Hypercalcemia

PRECAUTIONS

All calcium preparations given orally can cause nausea and constipation; calcium carbonate may be less irritating because of its high calcium availability and lower dosage requirement.

POSSIBLE INTERACTIONS

• Injectable and sometimes oral calcium solutions and tablets are incompatible with tetracycline drugs, cephalothin, methylprednisolone sodium succinate, dobutamine, metoclopramide, and amphotericin B.
• Thiazide diuretics used in conjunction with large doses of calcium may cause hypercalcemia.
• Patients on digitalis are more likely to develop arrhythmias if calcium is administered intravenously. • Calcium administration may antagonize effects of calcium channel blocking agents.

FOLLOW-UP

PATIENT MONITORING

• Hypocalcemia and hypercalcemia are both concerns with long-term management. • Once serum calcium is stable and normal, assess

HYPOPARATHYROIDISM (CONTINUED)

serum calcium concentration monthly for the first 6 months, then every 2–4 months; goal is to maintain serum total calcium between 8 and 10 mg/dL. • Inform clients about clinical signs of hypo- and hypercalcemia.

POSSIBLE COMPLICATIONS

• Hypocalcemia if undertreated. • Hypercalcemia, which can lead to nephrocalcinosis and kidney injury (see Hypercalcemia) and resistance to antidiuretic hormone.

EXPECTED COURSE AND PROGNOSIS

• With close monitoring of serum calcium and client dedication, the prognosis for long-term survival is excellent. • Adjustments in vitamin D and oral calcium administration can be expected during the course of management, especially during the initial 2–6 months.
• Cats with hypoparathyroidism secondary to thyroidectomy usually require only transient treatment because they typically regain normal parathyroid function within 4–6 months, often within 2–3 weeks.

MISCELLANEOUS

ASSOCIATED CONDITIONS

Excess muscular activity can lead to hyperthermia, which may necessitate treatment.

PREGNANCY/FERTILITY/BREEDING

Hypocalcemia can lead to weakness and dystocia.

SEE ALSO

- Hypercalcemia.
- Hyperthyroidism.
- Hypocalcemia.

ABBREVIATIONS

- PTH = parathyroid hormone.

Suggested Reading

Feldman EC, Nelson RW. Hypocalcemia and primary hypoparathyroidism. In: Feldman EC, Nelson RW, Reusch CE, et al., eds., Canine and Feline Endocrinology, 4th ed. St. Louis, MO: Saunders, 2015, pp. 625–646.

Henderson AK, Mahony O. Hypoparathyroidism: pathophysiology and diagnosis. Compend Contin Educ Pract Vet 2005, 27(4):270–279.

Henderson AK, Mahony O. Hypoparathyroidism: treatment. Compend Contin Educ Pract Vet 2005, 27(4): 280–287.

Peterson ME, James KM, Wallace M, et al. Idiopathic hypoparathyroidism in five cats. J Vet Intern Med 1991, 5:47–51.

Waters CB, Scott-Moncrieff JCR. Hypocalcemia in cats. Compend Contin Educ Pract Vet 1992, 14:497–507.

Author Michael Schaer
Consulting Editor Patty A. Lathan

Client Education Handout available online

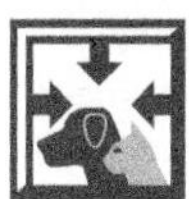

BASICS

DEFINITION

Serum phosphorus concentration <2.5 mg/dL.

PATHOPHYSIOLOGY

- Control of phosphorus is influenced by the actions and interactions of PTH and vitamin D with the gastrointestinal tract, bone, kidneys, and parathyroid glands.
- Decreased serum phosphorus concentration can be caused by translocation of phosphorus from the extracellular fluid into cells, decreased renal reabsorption, or decreased intestinal absorption of phosphorus.
- Low serum phosphorus can lead to adenosine triphosphate (ATP) depletion, which affects cells with high ATP energy demands (skeletal muscle, cardiac muscle, nerve tissue, and red blood cells).
- Many important enzyme systems are dependent on adequate phosphorus levels, including glycolysis, ammoniagenesis, 1-hydroxylation of 25(OH)-cholecalciferol, and 2,3-diphosphoglycerate, which are essential for energy production, acid excretion, calcium balance, and tissue oxygenation, respectively.
- Phosphorus is also required for maintenance of cell membrane integrity, playing an essential role in the production of ATP, guanosine triphosphate, cyclic adenosine monophosphate (AMP), and phosphocreatinine.
- Diabetic (ketototic and nonketotic) patients are at increased risk for hypophosphatemia due to depleted phosphorus stores, lost muscle mass, and urinary losses. Insulin administration yields ATP from glycolysis, causing translocation of phosphorus.

SYSTEMS AFFECTED

- Hemic/lymphatic/immune—hemolysis, impaired oxygen delivery to tissues, impaired leukocyte and platelet function.
- Neurologic—impaired glucose uptake leads to encephalopathy, seizures, and coma.
- Musculoskeletal—rhabdomyolysis, weakness, pain, ventilatory failure, and gastrointestinal ileus.
- Cardiac—impaired contractility.

SIGNALMENT

- Older dog and cat.
- Diabetic patient.
- Keeshonden have genetic predisposition to hyperparathyroidism.

SIGNS

Historical Findings

Usually consistent with the primary condition responsible for the hypophosphatemia; however, evidence of severe hypophosphatemia (e.g., hemolysis) is usually not observed unless serum concentrations decrease to 1.0 mg/dL or less.

Physical Examination Findings

- Hemolytic anemia (especially in cats) causes pallor, tachypnea, dyspnea, and/or hemoglobinuria.
- Skeletal and respiratory muscle weakness.
- Mental dullness.

CAUSES

- Maldistribution (translocation)—treatment of diabetic ketoacidosis, insulin administration or carbohydrate load, total parenteral nutrition or nutritional recovery, hyperventilation or respiratory alkalosis.
- Reduced renal reabsorption (increased renal loss)—primary hyperparathyroidism, renal tubular disorders (e.g., Fanconi syndrome), proximal tubule diuretics (e.g., carbonic anhydrase inhibitors), eclampsia (puerperal tetany), hyperadrenocorticism (corticosteroids promote renal phosphate loss), sodium bicarbonate administration.
- Reduced intestinal absorption (decreased intake)—phosphorus-deficient diets, vitamin D deficiency, malabsorption disorders, phosphate binders.
- Laboratory error—hemolysis, icterus, osmotic diuretic administration.

RISK FACTORS

- Phosphorus-deficient diets or parenteral nutrition (refeeding syndrome).
- Diabetes mellitus.
- Prolonged anorexia, malnutrition, or starvation.
- Primary hyperparathyroidism.

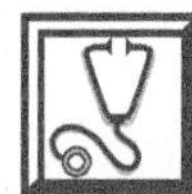

DIAGNOSIS

DIFFERENTIAL DIAGNOSIS

- Concurrent hyperglycemia, glucosuria, ketonuria, and high anion gap metabolic acidosis—rule out diabetic ketoacidosis.
- Concurrent glucosuria, normoglycemia, isosthenuria with or without azotemia—rule out renal tubular defects.
- Concurrent hypercalcemia and proteinuria, hematuria, with or without bacteria—rule out primary hyperparathyroidism with cystic calculi or nephroliths.
- Concurrent hypocalcemia—rule out puerperal tetany.
- Concurrent panhypoproteinemia—rule out intestinal malabsorption.

LABORATORY FINDINGS

Drugs That May Alter Laboratory Results

Liposomal amphotericin B (depending on assay).

Disorders That May Alter Laboratory Results

Monoclonal gammopathy may falsely lower serum phosphorus concentrations by binding to inorganic phosphorus.

Valid If Run In Human Laboratory?

Yes

CBC/BIOCHEMISTRY/URINALYSIS

- Serum phosphorus <2.5 mg/dL.
- Hyperglycemia, glucosuria, ketonuria, and high anion gap metabolic acidosis with diabetic ketoacidosis.
- Glucosuria, normoglycemia, isosthenuria, or azotemia with renal tubular defects.
- Hypercalcemia with primary hyperparathyroidism.
- Hypocalcemia with puerperal tetany.
- High serum alkaline phosphatase, proteinuria with hyperadrenocorticism.
- Panhypoproteinemia with intestinal malabsorption.

OTHER LABORATORY TESTS

- Serum fructosamine, ketone concentration—to diagnose or rule out diabetes mellitus or diabetic ketoacidosis, respectively.
- Parathyroid hormone (PTH) assay—to diagnose or rule out hyperparathyroidism.
- PTH-related peptide (PTH-rp)—for hypercalcemia of malignancy.
- Vitamin D metabolite measurement—to diagnose or rule out vitamin D deficiency.

IMAGING

- Radiography may reveal urolithiasis in cases of primary hyperparathyroidism or poor bone quality/pathologic fractures with disorders of vitamin D metabolism.
- Ultrasonography or CT may reveal parathyroid mass.

DIAGNOSTIC PROCEDURES

Surgical exploration of the cervical area may reveal a parathyroid mass. Urine anion gap can reveal renal tubular secretory defect.

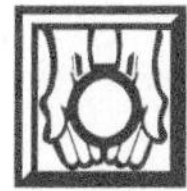

TREATMENT

- Prevention is preferred.
- Asymptomatic patients with low (1.5–2.5 mg/dL), but not depleted, phosphorus concentrations may not need phosphate treatment. Cats are more likely to have hemolysis with marked hypophosphatemia.
- If caused by insulin administration or hyperalimentation, administer supplemental phosphorus.
- Severe hypophosphatemia (<1.5 mg/dL)—patients need hospitalization and monitoring for hemolysis or hemolytic crisis. Administer isotonic crystalloid solution without calcium, IV, supplemented with potassium phosphate.
- Packed red blood cell transfusion for severe hemolytic crisis.

HYPOPHOSPHATEMIA (CONTINUED)

MEDICATIONS

DRUG(S) OF CHOICE

- Phosphate—0.01–0.12 mMol/kg/h IV. Monitor serum phosphorus every 6–8 hours.
  - Potassium phosphate (3 mMol phosphate/mL and 4.4 mEq potassium/mL) IV.
  - Sodium phosphate (3 mMol phosphate/mL and 4 mEq sodium/mL) IV.
- Discontinue therapy when serum phosphorus concentration reaches 2 mg/dL in order to avoid iatrogenic hyperphosphatemia and hypocalcemia.

CONTRAINDICATIONS

- Hyperphosphatemia.
- Hypocalcemia.
- Hypercalcemia.
- Renal failure.
- Hyperkalemia.

PRECAUTIONS

- Concurrent diuretic administration, especially carbonic anhydrase inhibitors.
- Renal disease.
- Iatrogenic hyperphosphatemia causes hypocalcemia and soft tissue (especially blood vessels) mineralization.

POSSIBLE INTERACTIONS

- Potassium phosphate may precipitate in IV line if coadministered with calcium-containing fluids, dobutamine, fluoroquinolones.
- Angiotensin-converting enzyme (ACE) inhibitor (e.g., enalapril) administration.
- Cardiac glycoside (e.g., digoxin) administration.
- Potassium-sparing diuretics (e.g., spironolactone).

ALTERNATIVE DRUG(S)

Oral phosphate supplement (e.g., phospho-soda) if not vomiting.

FOLLOW-UP

- Measure serum phosphorus levels every 6–8 hours until within normal range.
- Monitor patients for hyperphosphatemia and discontinue treatment immediately.
- Check serum potassium level daily until stable.

POSSIBLE COMPLICATIONS

- Hemolysis.
- Respiratory depression and failure.
- Cardiac arrest.

MISCELLANEOUS

ASSOCIATED CONDITIONS

Concurrent hypokalemia is common in patients with diabetic ketoacidosis.

AGE-RELATED FACTORS

Usually presents in older dogs.

PREGNANCY/FERTILITY/BREEDING

Concurrent hypocalcemia in the periparturient animal increases PTH-promoted renal excretion of phosphorus, causing hypophosphatemia.

SEE ALSO

- Diabetes Mellitus with Ketoacidosis.
- Hyperparathyroidism.

INTERNET RESOURCES

http://eclinpath.com/chemistry/minerals/phosphate

ABBREVIATIONS

- ACE = angiotensin-converting enzyme.
- AMP = adenosine monophosphate.
- ATP = adenosine triphosphate.
- PTH = parathyroid hormone.
- PTH-rp = PHT-related peptide.

Suggested Reading

DiBartola SP, Autran de Morais H. Disorders of phosphorus: hypophosphatemia and hyperphosphatemia. In: DiBartola SP, ed., Fluid Therapy in Small Animal Practice, 4th ed. Philadelphia, PA: Saunders, 2012, pp. 195–211.

Hooft KV, Drobatz KJ, Ward CR. Hypophosphatemia. Compend Cont Edu Vet 2005, 27:900–911.

Martin LG, Allen-Durrance AE. Magnesium and phosphate disorders. In: Silverstein DC, Hopper K. eds., Small Animal Critical Care Medicine, 2nd ed. St. Louis, MO: Elsevier Saunders, 2015, pp. 281–288.

Author Michael Schaer

Consulting Editor Patty A. Lathan

Hypopituitarism

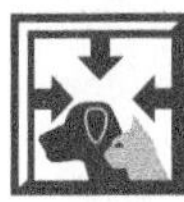

BASICS

OVERVIEW

- A condition resulting from a defect in pituitary hormone synthesis; most frequently due to a genetic mutation.
- Associated with low production of pituitary hormones including thyroid-stimulating hormone (TSH), luteinizing hormone, follicle-stimulating hormone, and growth hormone (GH). Adrenocorticotropic hormone (ACTH) synthesis is usually preserved in dogs with congenital hyposomatotropism (pituitary dwarfism).
- Hypopituitarism due to transsphenoidal hypophysectomy to treat pituitary-dependent hypercortisolism can result in hypothyroidism, hypocortisolism, and possible GH deficiency.

SIGNALMENT

- Dogs.
- Age—2–6 months.
- Breeds—German shepherd dog, Karelian bear dog, Saarloos wolfhound, spitz, miniature pinscher, and Weimaraner.
- Simple autosomal recessive in German shepherd dog and Karelian bear dog; mutation of the *LHX3* gene.

SIGNS

Historical Findings

- Mental retardation manifested as difficulty in housebreaking.
- Slow growth noticed in first 2–3 months of life.
- Proportionate dwarfism.

Physical Examination Findings

- Retained puppy hair coat.
- Thin, hypotonic skin.
- Shrill bark.
- Truncal alopecia.
- Cutaneous hyperpigmentation.
- Infantile genitalia.
- Delayed dental eruption.

CAUSES & RISK FACTORS

Congenital

- Mutation of *LHX3* gene.
- Isolated GH deficiency.

Acquired

- Pituitary tumor.
- Trauma.
- Radiotherapy.
- Hypophysectomy.

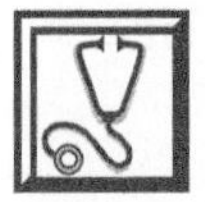

DIAGNOSIS

DIFFERENTIAL DIAGNOSIS

- Hypothyroid dwarfism.
- Portosystemic shunt, diabetes mellitus, hyperadrenocorticism, malnutrition, parasitism (all result in stunted growth).

CBC/BIOCHEMISTRY/URINALYSIS

- Mild anemia.
- Hypophosphatemia.
- Azotemia.

OTHER LABORATORY TESTS

- GH and insulin-like growth factor (IGF) assays; GH assay not currently available in the United States; recommend measurement of IGF-1, which is low.
- Adrenal function is usually preserved in dogs with the *LHX3* mutation.
- TSH response test; subnormal response to TSH.
- Ghrelin-stimulation test—monitors changes in GH levels in response to ghrelin; requires GH assay.
- DNA testing.

IMAGING

Radiography may reveal epiphyseal dysgenesis and abnormal retention of physeal growth plates.

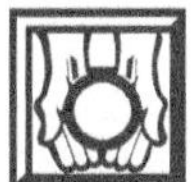

TREATMENT

Manage medically on an outpatient basis.

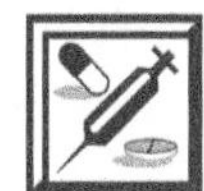

MEDICATIONS

DRUG(S) OF CHOICE

- GH—porcine GH, if available; has the same structure as canine GH: 0.1 IU/kg SC three times weekly for 4–6 weeks. Dose adjustments based on IGF-1 measurements every 4–6 weeks initially.
- The author is currently using the following source for porcine GH in the United States: http://www.humc.edu/hormones/material.html. This is not an FDA-approved drug in any species and requires client consent and special preparation and handling by a veterinary pharmacist.
- Medroxyprogesterone acetate (2.5–5 mg/kg IM q3 weeks, then q6 weeks after normal stature is achieved).
- Treat hypothyroidism with levothyroxine (22 µg/kg PO q24h).
- Glucocorticoids (e.g., prednisone: 0.2 mg/kg PO q24h) if ACTH response test results are consistent with hypoadrenocorticism; higher dosage of steroids is needed during periods of stress.

CONTRAINDICATIONS/POSSIBLE INTERACTIONS

Hypersensitivity reactions and carbohydrate intolerance may develop with growth hormone supplementation.

FOLLOW-UP

PATIENT MONITORING

- IGF-1 every 4–6 weeks initially, and then less frequently.
- Blood and urinary glucose concentration.
- Stop GH supplementation if glucosuria develops or blood glucose is >150 mg/dL.

POSSIBLE COMPLICATIONS

Acromegaly and diabetes mellitus; pyometra in female dogs treated with progestins.

EXPECTED COURSE AND PROGNOSIS

- Skin and hair coat improve within 6–8 weeks of initiating GH and thyroid supplementation.
- Generally no increase in stature because growth plates have usually closed by the time of diagnosis.
- Dogs often die at a young age (3–4 years) because of neurologic complications, renal failure, or infections.
- Poor long-term prognosis.

MISCELLANEOUS

SEE ALSO

- Hypoadrenocorticism (Addison's Disease).
- Hypothyroidism.

ABBREVIATIONS

- ACTH = adrenocorticotropic hormone.
- GH = growth hormone.
- IGF-1 = insulin-like growth factor-I.
- TSH = thyroid-stimulating hormone.

Suggested Reading

Campbell KL. Growth hormone-related disorders in dogs. Compend Cont Educ Pract Vet 1988, 10:477–482.

Voorbij AMWY, Leegwater PA, Kooistra HS. Pituitary dwarfism in Saarloos and Czechoslovakian wolfdogs is associated with a mutation in LHX3. J Vet Int Med 2014, 28(6):1770–1774.

Author Patty A. Lathan

Consulting Editor Patty A. Lathan

Acknowledgment The author and book editors acknowledge the prior contribution of Deborah S. Greco.

HYPOPYON AND LIPID FLARE

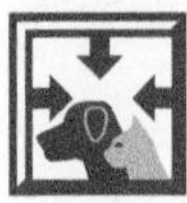

BASICS

OVERVIEW

Hypopyon

Accumulation of white blood cells in anterior chamber of eye; inflammatory breakdown of blood–aqueous barrier allows entry of cells into anterior chamber; chemoattractants mediate influx; cells settle in ventral anterior chamber due to gravity.

Lipid Flare

Resembles hypopyon but turbidity of anterior chamber is caused by lipids in aqueous humor; requires breakdown of blood–aqueous barrier and concurrent hyperlipidemia.

SIGNALMENT

Dogs and cats; no age or sex predilection.

SIGNS

Hypopyon

• White to yellow opacity within anterior chamber—may be a ventral accumulation of cells or may completely fill anterior chamber; fibrin accumulation in anterior chamber may prevent discrete settling of white blood cells, resulting in cells suspended within fibrin matrix. • Concurrent ophthalmic signs include blepharospasm, epiphora, diffuse corneal edema, aqueous flare, miosis, iridal swelling, and vision loss.

Lipid Flare

• Diffuse milky appearance to anterior chamber. • Concurrent ophthalmic signs may include vision loss, mild blepharospasm, and mild to moderate diffuse corneal edema.

CAUSES & RISK FACTORS

Hypopyon

Any cause of uveitis can result in hypopyon—most commonly associated with severe uveitis. Hypopyon can also result from neoplastic cell accumulation in ocular lymphoma.

Lipid Flare

Lipid flare results from hyperlipidemia and concurrent uveitis; hyperlipidemia may also destabilize blood–aqueous barrier directly. Postprandial lipemia may occasionally result in lipemic aqueous if uveitis is present.

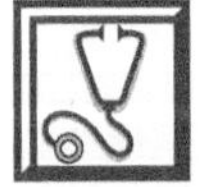

DIAGNOSIS

DIFFERENTIAL DIAGNOSIS

Hypopyon

Fibrin in anterior chamber—generally forms an irregular clot, not ventral horizontal line.

Lipid Flare

• Severe aqueous flare—does not appear as milky white as lipid flare; animals with aqueous flare generally exhibit more ocular pain. • Diffuse corneal edema—severe corneal edema may be confused with anterior chamber opacity, but corneal stromal thickening, keratoconus, and corneal bullae are noted with the former.

CBC/BIOCHEMISTRY/URINALYSIS

Hypopyon

Often normal; abnormalities relate to underlying cause of uveitis.

Lipid Flare

Elevated serum triglycerides and cholesterol; abnormalities reflect underlying metabolic disorder(s).

OTHER LABORATORY TESTS

Hypopyon

None if hypopyon is related to obvious corneal disease; if related to uveitis, look for underlying cause of uveitis (e.g., anterior uveitis).

Lipid Flare

See Hyperlipidemia.

DIAGNOSTIC PROCEDURES

Anterior chamber centesis indicated with suspicion of neoplastic hypopyon; otherwise unrewarding.

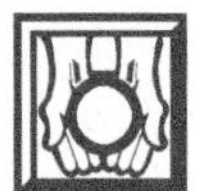

TREATMENT

• Hypopyon requires aggressive treatment for uveitis and underlying cause.
• Lipid flare requires treatment for uveitis and underlying metabolic disorder.

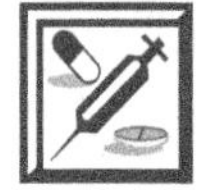

MEDICATIONS

DRUG(S) OF CHOICE

Hypopyon

Corticosteroids

• *Topical*—prednisolone acetate 1% or dexamethasone 0.1%: apply 2–6 times daily, depending on disease severity; taper medication as condition resolves.
• *Subconjunctival*—triamcinolone acetonide (dog: 4–6 mg; cat: 4 mg) or methylprednisolone (dog: 3–10 mg; cat: 4 mg) by subconjunctival injection; one-time injection followed by topical and/or systemic anti-inflammatories. • *Systemic*—prednisone (dog: 0.5–2.2 mg/kg/day; cat: 1–3 mg/kg/day); taper dose after 7–10 days; only if infectious causes of uveitis have been ruled out.

Nonsteroidal Anti-inflammatory Drugs (NSAIDs)

• *Topical*—flurbiprofen, diclofenac, or kerorolac: 2–4 times daily, depending on severity of disease; less effective than corticosteroids. • *Systemic*—carprofen (dog: 2.2 mg/kg PO q12h); meloxicam (dog: 0.2 mg/kg PO q24h); robenacoxib (cat: 1 mg/kg PO q24h; limit duration of use to 3 days); meloxicam (cat: 0.2 mg/kg IV/SC/PO once, then 0.05 mg/kg IV/SC/PO q24h for 2 days, then 0.025 mg/kg q24–48h; limit duration of use to 4 days); do not use NSAIDs concurrently with systemic corticosteroids.

Topical Mydriatic/Cycloplegic

Atropine sulfate 1%—1–4 times daily, depending on severity of disease; use ointment instead of solution in cats to minimize salivation.

Lipid Flare

Topical Corticosteroids

Prednisolone acetate 1% or dexamethasone 0.1%—2–4 times daily, depending on severity of disease; taper medication as condition resolves.

Topical Mydriatic/Cycloplegic

Atropine sulfate 1%—1–2 times daily, for ocular discomfort.

CONTRAINDICATIONS/POSSIBLE INTERACTIONS

• Avoid topical miotic medications. • Topical and subconjunctival corticosteroids contraindicated if ulcerative keratitis present. • Out of concern for secondary glaucoma, topical atropine should be used judiciously with intraocular pressure (IOP) monitoring.

FOLLOW-UP

PATIENT MONITORING

Recheck in 2–3 days. IOP should be monitored to detect secondary glaucoma. Frequency of subsequent rechecks dictated by response to treatment.

EXPECTED COURSE AND PROGNOSIS

• Hypopyon—prognosis guarded to good; depends on underlying disease and response to treatment. • Lipid flare—prognosis good; generally responds quickly (within 24–72 hours) to moderate anti-inflammatory therapy; recurrence possible.

MISCELLANEOUS

ABBREVIATIONS

• IOP = intraocular pressure.
• NSAID = nonsteroidal anti-inflammatory drug.

Author Ian P. Herring
Consulting Editor Kathern E. Myrna

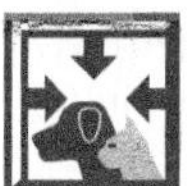

BASICS

OVERVIEW

- Spontaneous decrease in food intake, and implies inadequate caloric intake.
- Triggered by numerous conditions and reflects a derangement in hypothalamic processes that govern satiety and hunger.
- Prolonged hyporexia results in weight loss and contributes to sarcopenia and cachexia.

SIGNALMENT

Dogs and cats of all ages; no breed or sex predilections.

SIGNS

- Patients may refuse all food (anorexia) or consume a portion of their caloric needs.
- Preferential appetite may be reported for treats or highly desirable foods, but not a balanced diet.
- Signs suggesting nausea (e.g., drooling or gagging) may be reported, and severely affected animals may avoid food or try to hide it.
- Sustained hyporexia results in weight loss, and may be accompanied by a decrease in lean muscle mass as well as fat.

CAUSES & RISK FACTORS

- Any metabolic derangement (endocrine, renal, hepatic) or organic compromise (e.g., respiratory or cardiovascular or gastrointestinal disease).
- Systemic inflammation (infectious, sterile, neoplastic).
- Medications, pain/discomfort, or psychologic issues (fear, anxiety).
- Lesions in the hypothalamus or affecting smell.

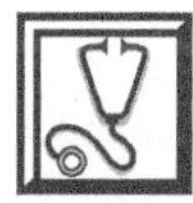

DIAGNOSIS

DIFFERENTIAL DIAGNOSIS

Must be differentiated from 'pseudo-inappetence', i.e., limited intake due to oral pathology, prehension disorders or palatability issues.

CBC/BIOCHEMISTRY/URINALYSIS

- Influenced by underlying cause(s), but can be normal despite inadequate intake.
- Sustained and severe hyporexia in cats may result in hepatic lipidosis, characterized by an increase in alkaline phosphatase activity and hyperbilirubinemia.

OTHER LABORATORY TESTS

As necessary to identify underlying cause(s).

IMAGING

As necessary to identify underlying cause(s).

DIAGNOSTIC PROCEDURES

As necessary to identify underlying cause(s).

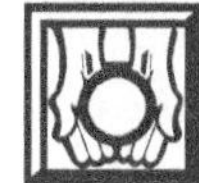

TREATMENT

- Underlying disorders, vomiting/nausea, pain, and anxiety should be addressed promptly.
- Medications contributing to poor intake should be withdrawn if possible.
- Offering warmed food or more palatable options may be helpful.
- Sustained hyporexia should be addressed with an enteral feeding device (e.g., esophageal feeding tube) or parenterally in patients with substantial gastrointestinal compromise.

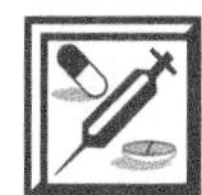

MEDICATIONS

- Numerous medications are anecdotally reported to improve food intake in companion animals, but most are not licensed for this purpose and there are limited efficacy and safety data.
- Practitioners are encouraged to use FDA-approved appetite stimulants before considering alternative approaches.
- The administration of an appetite stimulant should not delay efforts to identify and address the underlying cause(s) of hyporexia.

DRUG(S) OF CHOICE

- Capromorelin—dogs: 3 mg/kg PO q24h; a ghrelin receptor agonist, FDA-approved as an appetite stimulant for dogs (feline product under development).
  - Mimics actions of ghrelin, the "hunger hormone," a peptide secreted by gastric mucosa.
  - Receptors located in hypothalamus; activation promotes feelings of hunger and food-seeking behavior.
  - Ghrelin also triggers release of growth hormone, increasing muscle mass and lean weight gain.
- Mirtazapine—dogs: 3.75–30 mg/dog PO q24h; cats: 1.9 mg/cat PO q48h; used off-label for many years as an appetite stimulant; mechanism is likely related to increased central norepinephrine levels. Transdermal formulation approved for cats (2 mg/cat q24h).

CONTRAINDICATIONS/POSSIBLE INTERACTIONS

- Mirtazapine has relatively narrow therapeutic window; should be dosed cautiously in small patients and those with renal compromise. Side effects can include vocalization, behavior changes, and tremors.
- Serotonin syndrome may occur with concurrent administration of monoamine oxidase inhibitors, metoclopramide, ondansetron, or tramadol.

FOLLOW-UP

PATIENT MONITORING

Monitor food intake and bodyweight carefully, and modify therapy for both underlying disease and hyporexia as necessary.

PREVENTION/AVOIDANCE

Prompt recognition and management of conditions that may impact food intake.

POSSIBLE COMPLICATIONS

- Cats with sustained, substantial hyporexia may develop hepatic lipidosis.
- Hyporexia impacts outcome and mortality in hospitalized people and it likely has a similar impact in companion animals.

EXPECTED COURSE AND PROGNOSIS

- Response to appetite stimulants is variable; some animals require enteral feeding devices.
- Underlying cause(s) of hyporexia ultimately determines prognosis.

MISCELLANEOUS

ASSOCIATED CONDITIONS

Sarcopenia (i.e., age-related loss of muscle) and cachexia (i.e., rapid/extreme weight loss and muscle wasting) are associated with or exacerbated by hyporexia.

AGE-RELATED FACTORS

None (unless related to underlying cause).

INTERNET RESOURCES

- https://entyce.aratana.com
- https://kindredbio.com/mirataz-mirtazapine-transdermal-ointment

Suggested Reading

Rhodes L, Zollers B, Wofford JA, Heinen E. Capromorelin: a ghrelin receptor agonist and novel therapy for stimulation of appetite in dogs. Vet Med Sci 2017, 4(1):3–16.

Author Audrey K. Cook

Consulting Editor Patty A. Lathan

HYPOSTHENURIA

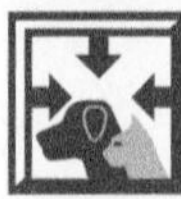

BASICS

DEFINITION

Urine specific gravity (USG) between 1.000 and 1.006.

PATHOPHYSIOLOGY

The ability to concentrate urine normally (dogs: >1.030; cats: >1.035) depends on a complex interaction between antidiuretic hormone (ADH), the protein receptor for ADH on the renal tubule, and a hypertonic renal medullary interstitium; interference with the synthesis, release, or actions of ADH, damage to the renal tubule, or altered tonicity of the medullary interstitium (medullary washout) can cause hyposthenuria.

SYSTEMS AFFECTED

Depends on the underlying disorder.

SIGNALMENT

Species

Dog and cat.

Breed Predilections

None

Mean Age and Range

None

Predominant Sex

None

SIGNS

- Polyuria and polydipsia.
- Urinary incontinence—occasional.
- Other signs depend on the underlying disorder.

CAUSES

Any disorder or drug that interferes with the release or action of ADH, damages the renal tubule, causes medullary washout, or causes a primary thirst disorder (see Differential Diagnosis).

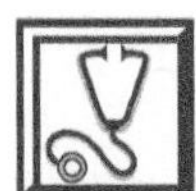

DIAGNOSIS

DIFFERENTIAL DIAGNOSIS

- Central diabetes insipidus (little or no ADH produced).
- Nephrogenic diabetes insipidus (resistance to ADH).
- Pyometra.
- Pyelonephritis.
- Hyperadrenocorticism.
- Hypoadrenocorticism.
- Hyperthyroidism.
- Hypercalcemia.
- Primary liver disease.
- Hypokalemia.
- Primary polydipsia—compulsive water drinking.

LABORATORY FINDINGS

Drugs That May Alter Laboratory Results

Cortisone, lithium, demeclocycline, methoxyflurane, thiazide diuretics, and intravenous administration of fluids can all lower USG into the hyposthenuric range.

Valid if Run in a Human Laboratory?

Yes

CBC/BIOCHEMISTRY/URINALYSIS

- Low USG (1.000–1.006); other abnormalities may point to the underlying cause.
- High serum alkaline phosphatase (ALP) enzyme activity suggests hyperadrenocorticism or primary liver disease.
- High cholesterol common in patients with hyperadrenocorticism.
- Leukocytosis with a left shift in some patients with pyometra or pyelonephritis.
- Hyperkalemia and hyponatremia suggest hypoadrenocorticism.
- Low serum potassium concentration confirms hypokalemia.
- Inflammatory sediment or bacteriuria and positive urine culture consistent with pyelonephritis.
- Proteinuria common in patients with pyelonephritis, pyometra, and hyperadrenocorticism.

OTHER LABORATORY TESTS

- Adrenocorticotropic hormone (ACTH) stimulation test to screen for hyperadrenocorticism and hypoadrenocorticism.
- Low-dose dexamethasone suppression test and urine : cortisol creatinine test to screen for hyperadrenocorticism.
- Serum bile acids concentration to evaluate liver function (*note*: dogs with hyperadrenocorticism often have mild elevations of bile acid concentration).

IMAGING

- Radiography to assess renal size and shape and to detect calcified adrenal tumor or large uterus.
- Ultrasonography to assess adrenal size, renal and hepatic size and architecture, and uterine size. Dilated renal pelves may indicate pyelonephritis or be an artifact of IV fluid therapy.
- MRI or CT may identify pituitary or hypothalamic mass that may be the cause of central diabetes insipidus or hyperadrenocorticism.

DIAGNOSTIC PROCEDURES

- Desmopressin response test to differentiate primary central diabetes insipidus from primary nephrogenic diabetes insipidus.
- Reassessment of USG following change of environment in a dog suspected of having primary polydipsia. For example, some dogs hospitalized with free access to water will drink less and concentrate urine by the end of the day, suggesting a diagnosis of primary polydipsia.

TREATMENT

- Depends on the underlying disorder.
- Do not restrict patient's water intake unless appropriate to the definitive diagnosis.
- Depends on the underlying disorder.

MEDICATIONS

DRUG(S) OF CHOICE

Depend on the underlying disorder.

FOLLOW-UP

PATIENT MONITORING

USG, hydration status, renal function, and electrolytes.

POSSIBLE COMPLICATIONS

Dehydration

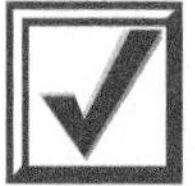

MISCELLANEOUS

ASSOCIATED CONDITIONS

See Differential Diagnosis.

ZOONOTIC POTENTIAL

None

SEE ALSO

- Diabetes Insipidus.
- Hyperadrenocorticism (Cushing's Syndrome)—Cats.
- Hyperadrenocorticism (Cushing's Syndrome)—Dogs.

ABBREVIATIONS

- ACTH = adrenocorticotropic hormone.
- ADH = antidiuretic hormone.
- ALP = alkaline phosphatase.
- USG = urine specific gravity.

Suggested Reading

DiBartola SP. Fluid, Electrolyte and Acid-Base Disorders in Small Animal Practice, 3rd ed. Philadelphia, PA: Saunders, 2005.

Rose DB, Post T. Clinical Physiology of Acid-Base and Electrolyte Disorders, 5th ed. New York: McGraw-Hill, 2000.

Author Patty A. Lathan

Consulting Editor Patty A. Lathan

Acknowledgment The author and book editors acknowledge the prior contribution of Melinda Fleming.

HYPOTHERMIA

BASICS

Due to limited clinical literature in veterinary science, much of the information below has been extrapolated from human medical literature and experimental animal studies.

DEFINITION

• Core body temperature drops below that required for normal metabolism. In primary hypothermia, the healthy individual's compensatory responses to heat loss are overwhelmed by exposure, whereas secondary hypothermia complicates many systemic diseases. • Stage I—90–95 °F (32–35 °C). • Stage II—82–90 °F (28–32 °C). • Stage III—75–82 °F (24–28 °C). • Stage IV—<75 °F (24 °C).

PATHOPHYSIOLOGY

• Normal thermoregulation balances heat gained or lost to the environment with heat produced via central thermogenesis; it is controlled by the hypothalamus with input from thermoreceptors; heat can be gained or lost to the environment via four mechanisms: evaporation, radiation, convection, and conduction; central thermogenesis generates heat via basal metabolism, muscle activity, and uncoupling of brown fat (neonates). • Heat production can be augmented via shivering and increased basal metabolic rate; activation of both sympathetic nervous and endocrine systems results in increased circulating levels of thyroid-releasing hormone, catecholamines, growth hormone, and glucocorticoids, which all contribute to increased glucose utilization and basal metabolic rate. • Adaptations to minimize heat loss include cutaneous vasoconstriction, piloerection, and behavioral responses such as curling up, sharing body heat, and seeking shelter.

SYSTEMS AFFECTED

• Cardiovascular—in mild hypothermia, sympathetic stimulation induces tachycardia and peripheral vasoconstriction with normal or elevated cardiac output (CO) and BP; as the patient becomes colder, cardiac pacemaker cell depolarization is slowed, resulting in bradycardia resistant to treatment with atropine; the resultant fall in CO is balanced by increased systemic vascular resistance; at lower temperatures, bradycardia becomes progressively extreme and systemic vascular resistance falls as catecholamine release and adrenergic receptor responsiveness are blunted.
• Endocrine—sympathetic activation and release of counter-regulatory hormones trigger increased glycogenolysis, gluconeogenesis, and lipolysis as well as inhibit the release and uptake of insulin resulting in hyperglycemia; when hypothermia develops slowly or is longlasting, glycogen stores become depleted and hypoglycemia develops. • Gastrointestinal—increased gastric acid production and reduced duodenal bicarbonate secretion may predispose to gastrointestinal ulceration; ileus is common.
• Hemic—plasma shifts and consequent hemoconcentration may lead to hyper- and hypocoagulopathy; depressed enzymatic activity of clotting factors and platelet hyporeactivity may exacerbate hypocoagulability.
• Hepatobiliary/pancreatic—hypoxia leads to hepatocellular damage and pancreatitis.
• Musculoskeletal—increased joint fluid viscosity and muscle stiffness. • Nervous—CNS metabolism and level of consciousness decrease and nerve conduction velocity progressively slows; mild incoordination is followed by lethargy, obtundation, and coma.
• Renal—peripheral vasoconstriction increases renal blood flow and glomerular filtration rate resulting in increased urine production; progressive tubular dysfunction and antidiuretic hormone resistance contribute further to cold diuresis; later, urine output decreases as result of falling CO; acute kidney injury may ensue.
• Respiratory—initial tachypnea replaced by decreased respiratory rate and tidal volume and increased airway secretions; as temperature falls, protective airway reflexes are reduced; below 93.2 °F (34 °C) ventilatory drive is attenuated and increased pulmonary vascular resistance leads to ventilation–perfusion mismatch; progressive hypoventilation, apnea, and, more rarely, pulmonary edema may develop; hypothermia shifts the oxyhemoglobin dissociation curve to the left; this may be masked by concurrent lactic and respiratory acidosis that may become so profound the overall result is a right shift. • Skin—edema secondary to increased vascular permeability.

GENETICS

Unknown

INCIDENCE/PREVALENCE

Varies with geographic location.

GEOGRAPHIC DISTRIBUTION

Most common in cold climates.

SIGNALMENT

Species

Dog and cat.

Breed Predilections

Smaller breeds with increased surface area.

Mean Age and Range

More common in neonates and geriatrics.

Predominant Sex

None

SIGNS

General Comments

A thorough search should be made to find precipitating, comorbid conditions.

Historical Findings

• Known prolonged exposure to cold ambient temperatures. • Possibly, disappearance from home or a history of trauma.

Physical Examination Findings

Stage I: 90–95 °F (32–35 °C)

• Lethargy and weakness. • Vigorous shivering (variable). • Variable heart rate, rhythm, and BP. • Light pink to pale mucous membranes. • Confusion, agitation, or obtundation. • Variable respiratory rate.

STAGE II: 82–90 °F (28–32 °C)

• Collapse. • Reduced shivering (variable).
• Bradyarrhythmia with hypotension. • Pale mucous membranes. • Muscle and joint stiffness. • Obtundation, stupor, or coma.
• Ataxia and hyporeflexia. • Reduced depth and rate of respiration.

STAGE III: 75–82 °F (24–28 °C)

• Moribund with cold, edematous skin. • Loss of shivering (variable). • Bradyarrhythmia with hypotension. • Pale mucous membranes.
• Muscle and joint stiffness. • Coma with fixed, dilated pupils. • Areflexia. • Reduced depth and rate of respiration or respiratory arrest. • Pulmonary edema.

STAGE IV: <75 °F (<24 °C)

• No vital signs. • Cardiac arrest.

CAUSES

• Inadequate thermogenesis: ○ Normal thermogenesis is overwhelmed. ○ Serious illness. • Extreme heat loss: ○ Excessive evaporation, conduction, convection, and radiation. ○ Inability to vasoconstrict blood vessels or piloerect hair. ○ Loss of behavioral adaptations. • Thermoregulatory center failure: ○ Hypothalamic injury or disease.

RISK FACTORS

• Extremes of age. • Low body fat and glycogen stores. • Burn injury. • Intracranial injury or disease. • Hypothyroidism.
• Diabetic ketoacidosis. • Sepsis. • Trauma.
• General anesthesia. • Medications including but not limited to beta blockers, barbiturates, narcotics, phenothiazines.

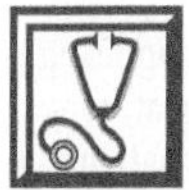

DIAGNOSIS

DIFFERENTIAL DIAGNOSIS

• Primary CNS disease, hypoglycemia, anemia, hepatic encephalopathy, myxedema, electrolyte disturbances, sepsis, intoxication, neoplasia, and death. • Bradyarrhythmia—cardiac disease, medication side effects, and toxicities.

CBC/BIOCHEMISTRY/URINALYSIS

• Results depend on severity and presence of comorbidities. • CBC—hemoconcentration, leukopenia, and thrombocytopenia.
• Biochemistry—azotemia, hyper- and hypoglycemia, variable electrolyte abnormalities, elevated liver enzyme activity, hyperbilirubinemia. • Urinalysis—isosthenuria and glucosuria.

HYPOTHERMIA (CONTINUED)

H

OTHER LABORATORY TESTS

• Blood gas—variable; metabolic and respiratory acidosis is common.
• Hyperlactatemia—shivering, reduced tissue perfusion, and impaired hepatic clearance.
• Coagulation—hyperfibrinogenemia and disseminated intravascular coagulation; in vivo prolongation of clotting times may not be reflected by in vitro assays and should correct with rewarming. • Thyroid hormone evaluation may confirm underlying hypothyroidism.

IMAGING

To investigate recovery complications or comorbid conditions.

DIAGNOSTIC PROCEDURES

ECG

Classic findings include presence of Osborn or J-waves, atrial and ventricular dysrhythmias, and prolongation of PR, QRS, and QT intervals with progression from sinus bradycardia through atrial fibrillation to ventricular fibrillation and ultimately asystole.

PATHOLOGIC FINDINGS

• Findings in patients who succumb to primary hypothermia are variable and nonspecific; if body cooling and death occur rapidly, necropsy findings are minimal but may include reddish discoloration of skin, hemorrhagic gastric erosions, and lipid deposits in epithelial cells of renal proximal tubules and other organs. • Patients who die from secondary hypothermia may have similar findings; however, they will also have evidence of a separate and significant disease process.

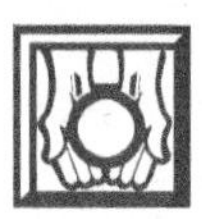

TREATMENT

APPROPRIATE HEALTH CARE

Emergency inpatient intensive care until normothermic and stable.

NURSING CARE

• Warming: ○ Active external rewarming using warm blankets, heating pads, radiant heat, forced warm air, and administration of warm parenteral fluids (stage II) is used in patients with stage I–II hypothermia; complications include core temperature after-drop whereby return of cold blood from periphery to central circulation causes further core cooling; rewarming of the trunk should be performed before the extremities to minimize this risk. ○ Techniques to warm patients with stage III–IV hypothermia include administration of warm humidified oxygen, warmed IV fluids, and bladder or gastric lavage with warm saline; more invasive and technically demanding methods include closed thoracic and peritoneal lavage, and extracorporeal rewarming. ○ Whole-body immersion in hot water is contraindicated, as it will cause massive vasodilatation and hypotension and is likely to provoke dysrhythmias and cardiovascular collapse. • Fluid therapy: ○ IV crystalloid fluids warmed to 104 °F (40 °C). ○ During rewarming, these patients have significant IV fluid requirements as vasoconstriction relaxes and cold diuresis is reversed. ○ Patients must be closely monitored for volume overload during resuscitation. • Consider inotropic drugs in patients unresponsive to volume resuscitation.
• Mechanically ventilate patients with respiratory failure.

ACTIVITY

Minimally affected patients should be encouraged to be active, as muscle activity will generate more endogenous body heat.

DIET

Withhold oral intake until patient is alert.

CLIENT EDUCATION

Prevention of exposure to cold temperatures is imperative in preventing primary hypothermia. Clients with very young and very old patients as well as those with serious medical conditions or taking medications that inhibit thermoregulatory ability should be counseled to keep their pets indoors and to take protective measures if they are to be exposed to cold temperatures.

SURGICAL CONSIDERATIONS

N/A

MEDICATIONS

DRUG(S) OF CHOICE

• Hypoglycemic patients warrant dextrose supplementation. • Antiarrhythmic agents generally not warranted as most arrhythmias will resolve with rewarming.

CONTRAINDICATIONS

No evidence to support routine use of steroids or antibiotics.

PRECAUTIONS

Systemic clearance of metabolized drugs is slowed proportionally—consider dose reduction to minimize likelihood of unanticipated toxicity.

POSSIBLE INTERACTIONS

N/A

ALTERNATIVE DRUG(S)

N/A

FOLLOW-UP

PATIENT MONITORING

• Continuous core body temperature.
• Continuous ECG and frequent BP during rewarming. • Frequent assessment (q6–12h) of electrolytes, acid-base status, packed cell volume, total protein, and blood glucose.
• Daily monitoring of blood urea nitrogen, urine specific gravity, coagulation indices, and liver enzymes in severely affected patients.

PREVENTION/AVOIDANCE

• Avoid prolonged exposure to cold. • Monitor and maintain body temperature in anesthetized animals.

POSSIBLE COMPLICATIONS

• Peripheral vasodilation during rewarming may further drop BP and body temperature.
• Iatrogenic burns. • Return of cool peripheral blood to the heart may precipitate cardiac arrhythmias. • Cardiac arrest. • Gastric lavage increases the risk of aspiration pneumonia and fluid and electrolyte shifts. • Thoracic and/or peritoneal lavage increases the risk for hemorrhage, lung or bowel trauma, and fluid and electrolyte shifts. • Extracorporeal rewarming techniques have increased risk for local vascular complications, air embolism, hypotension, hemorrhage, thrombosis, and hemolysis.

EXPECTED COURSE AND PROGNOSIS

Variable—depend on severity, underlying cause, and patient health status.

MISCELLANEOUS

ASSOCIATED CONDITIONS

None

AGE-RELATED FACTORS

Sick or hypoglycemic neonates can become markedly hypothermic in normal environments.

ZOONOTIC POTENTIAL

N/A

PREGNANCY/FERTILITY/BREEDING

N/A

SYNONYMS

None

SEE ALSO

Shock, Cardiogenic.

ABBREVIATIONS

• CO = cardiac output.

Suggested Reading

Brodeur A, Wright A, Cortes Y. Hypothermia and targeted temperature management in cats and dogs. JVECC 2017, 27(2):151–163.

Brown DJA, Brugger H, Boyd J, Paal P. Accidental hypothermia. NEJM 2012, 367:1930–1980.

Paal P, Gordon L, Strapazzon G, et al. Accidental hypothermia – an update. Scand J Trauma Resusc Emerg Med 2016, 24:111–130.

Author Gretchen L. Schoeffler
Consulting Editor Michael Aherne

Client Education Handout available online

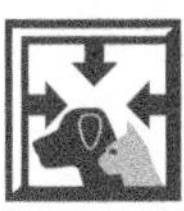

BASICS

DEFINITION

Clinical manifestations that result from inadequate production of thyroxine (T_4) and 3,5,3′-triiodothyronine (T_3) by the thyroid gland. Characterized by a generalized decrease in cellular metabolic activity.

PATHOPHYSIOLOGY

Acquired Hypothyroidism

- In dogs, acquired hypothyroidism can be primary, secondary, or tertiary.
- Primary hypothyroidism is associated with a defect localized to the thyroid gland. The thyroid tissue has been destroyed or replaced and thus becomes less responsive to thyroid-stimulating hormone (TSH). T_3 and T_4 levels gradually decline, with a compensatory increase in TSH.
  - Lymphocytic thyroiditis is an immune-mediated process characterized by chronic and progressive lymphocytic infiltration and destruction of the thyroid gland. This process is gradual and accounts for the slow onset of clinical signs associated with hypothyroidism. The immune-mediated process is associated with production of autoantibodies, predominantly against thyroglobulin; however, autoantibodies against T_3 and T_4 have been reported.
  - Idiopathic thyroid atrophy does not demonstrate an inflammatory component and is caused by the replacement of normal thyroid tissue with adipose tissue.
  - Together, these processes account for 95% of the clinical cases of hypothyroidism in dogs; each accounts for 50% of reported cases.
  - Rare causes of primary hypothyroidism include neoplastic destruction of thyroid tissue, iodine deficiency, infection, and iatrogenic destruction secondary to drugs, surgery, or radioiodine treatment.
- Secondary acquired hypothyroidism is rare. The defect is localized to the pituitary, where the ability to synthesize and secrete TSH is impaired. Secondary hypothyroidism may be caused by pituitary tumors, congenital malformation of the pituitary, infection, or TSH suppression. Drugs, hormones, or concurrent illness can cause TSH suppression.
- Tertiary hypothyroidism (not reported in the veterinary literature) is hypothalamic in origin, and production of thyrotropin-releasing hormone (TRH) is either decreased or nonexistent.
- Hypothyroidism may occur following radioactive iodine (I-131) therapy for hyperthyroidism in cats.

Congenital Hypothyroidism

- Congenital hypothyroidism is a rare disease that is categorized as goitrous or nongoitrous. Goiter (enlargement of the thyroid gland) develops when there is increased release of TSH, along with an intact thyroid TSH receptor.
- An autosomal recessive form of congenital hypothyroidism has been reported in specific dog and cat breeds. Affected animals have a thyroid peroxidase deficiency.
- Congenital hypothyroidism is also noted as an element of panhypopituitarism.

SYSTEMS AFFECTED

- Behavioral.
- Cardiovascular.
- Endocrine/metabolic.
- Gastrointestinal (GI).
- Nervous.
- Neuromuscular.
- Ophthalmic.
- Reproductive.
- Skin/exocrine.

GENETICS

- No known genetic basis for heritability associated with adult-onset primary hypothyroidism in dogs, although some breeds appear to be predisposed to thyroiditis.
- An autosomal recessive form of congenital hypothyroidism has been reported in toy fox terriers, giant schnauzers, Tenterfield terriers, and Abyssinian cats.

INCIDENCE/PREVALENCE

- Primary hypothyroidism is the most common endocrinopathy in dogs. Prevalence appears to average about 1 : 250.
- Hypothyroidism is rare in cats.

GEOGRAPHIC DISTRIBUTION

Worldwide

SIGNALMENT

Species

Dog, rarely cat.

Breed Predilections

Larger-breed dogs are more likely to develop hypothyroidism (golden retriever, Doberman pinscher, Great Dane, Irish setter), though several smaller-breed dogs do appear to also be predisposed (miniature schnauzer, cocker spaniel, poodle, dachshund).

Mean Age and Range

Most commonly seen in middle-aged dogs, with the average age of onset being 7 years.

Predominant Sex

None

SIGNS

General Comments

Clinical signs associated with hypothyroidism are vague and involve many different systems.

Historical Findings

- Lethargy, weight gain, and hair loss are the most common signs (40–50% of all cases).
- Pyoderma (often recurrent), hyperpigmentation of the skin, and a dry, brittle hair coat (10% of cases).
- Rarely (<5% of cases), facial paralysis, weakness, or conjunctivitis.

Physical Examination Findings

- Most changes appear to be secondary to decreased metabolism due to a lack of circulating thyroid hormones.
- The most common findings include dermatologic abnormalities (88% of hypothyroid dogs):
  - Bilateral symmetric nonpruritic truncal alopecia; hair loss is noted in areas of increased wear and usually includes the ventral thorax and neck, ventral abdomen, elbows, and tail. Loss of primary hair is most common, with retention of guard hairs, resulting in a short, fine hair coat.
  - Dry, lackluster hair coat.
  - Seborrhea is common and may be localized or have a more generalized distribution pattern.
  - Pyoderma is noted in 14% of hypothyroid dogs and may be recurrent in nature. Generalized demodicosis and *Malassezia* spp. infections are common. Though primary dermatologic conditions are nonpruritic, pruritis may accompany secondary parasitic, yeast, or bacterial infections. Chronic changes to the skin can result in thickening and hyperpigmentation.
- Otitis externa.
- Weight gain.
- Decreased activity/lethargy.
- Most neurologic signs are associated with polyneuropathy and include weakness, facial nerve paralysis, vestibular signs (usually peripheral), and hyporeflexia. No data support a direct association between megaesophagus or laryngeal paralysis and hypothyroidism.
- CNS signs, including seizures, ataxia, and coma (myxedema coma), are rare.
- In females, hypothyroidism is associated with increased periparturient mortality and lower birth rate in pups. In males, decreased fertility has been reported, but not confirmed, in hypothyroid dogs.
- Cardiovascular abnormalities are rare. Bradycardia, arrhythmias, decreased conduction, decreased contractility, and diastolic dysfunction have been reported.
- Ocular changes including corneal cholesterol deposits, keratoconjunctivitis sicca (KCS), and conjunctivitis are seen in less than 1% of hypothyroid dogs.

Congenital Hypothyroidism

- Lethargy and general inactivity.
- Dwarfism.
- Alopecia.
- Constipation (more common in cats).

CAUSES

- Lymphocytic thyroiditis.
- Idiopathic thyroid atrophy.
- Neoplasia.
- Pituitary disease.
- Congenital abnormalities.

HYPOTHYROIDISM (CONTINUED)

- Iodine deficiency (dietary).
- Iatrogenic (secondary to surgery or radiation).

RISK FACTORS

- Surgical removal (bilateral) of the thyroid gland.
- I-131 therapy for hyperthyroidism in cats.

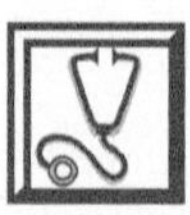

DIAGNOSIS

DIFFERENTIAL DIAGNOSIS

- Primary dermatologic disease.
- Other endocrinopathies (hyperadrenocorticism, diabetes mellitus, growth hormone deficiency).
- Pancreatitis.
- Nephrotic syndrome.
- Hepatobiliary disease.

CBC/BIOCHEMISTRY/URINALYSIS

- Useful to rule out nonthyroidal illness.
- Normochromic, normocytic, and nonregenerative anemia is a common finding (28–32% of hypothyroid dogs).
- Hyponatremia.
- Hypercholesterolemia (present in over 75% of hypothyroid dogs).
- Hypertriglyceridemia.
- Elevated levels of cholesterol and triglycerides have been associated with atherosclerosis in dogs, although this is rare.
- No specific changes are noted on urinalysis.

OTHER LABORATORY TESTS

- Diagnosing hypothyroidism is complex. The TSH stimulation test is a reliable single test used to diagnose hypothyroidism and is considered the gold standard. However, there is limited access to test reagents and the cost is often prohibitive.
- Several tests are available to assess thyroid function, thyroid hormone levels, and antithyroglobulin antibody levels. These tests include total T_4, free T_4, endogenous TSH, antithyroglobulin antibodies, anti-T_3 antibodies, anti-T_4 antibodies, total T_3, reverse T_3, and free T_3.
- Combination testing will yield a reliable result.

Total T_4

- Initial screening (high sensitivity) test of thyroid function.
- This test measures both protein-bound and free T_4 levels.
- The test is a direct assessment of the ability of the thyroid gland to produce hormone.
- A decreased total T_4 level is a common finding in hypothyroid animals, but is not diagnostic of hypothyroidism as concurrent illness can cause an artificial decrease in total T_4 level.

Free T_4

- Measures metabolically active portion of total T_4 level.
- Hypothyroid animals would be expected to have a low free T_4 level.
- Concurrent illness has less effect on the free T_4 level compared with the total T_4 level.
- Measurement by equilibrium dialysis (fT_4ED) has been demonstrated to be more reliable than radioimmunoassay, because it mitigates the influence of antithyroglobulin antibodies.
- Newer methods of free T_4 analysis utilize chemiluminescent technology with comparable sensitivity and specificity to fT_4ED, but the effect of antibodies on this assay is unclear, and the fT_4ED is still the gold standard.

Endogenous TSH Level

- Measurement of canine endogenous TSH is available.
- Cross-reactivity allows this assay to be used in cats; however, it may be accurate only 50% of the time in cats.
- This test has high specificity and low sensitivity; best used as a confirmatory test and not as a screening test.
- TSH level is expected to be elevated in primary hypothyroid animals due to loss of negative feedback, however, 20–40% of hypothyroid dogs have TSH values in the reference range.
- Interpretation of the TSH level requires knowledge of the total or free T_4 level.
- Methods of assessing TSH levels are less sensitive at low levels and evaluation of endogenous TSH cannot be used to diagnose secondary hypothyroidism.

Antithyroglobulin Antibodies

- Antithyroglobulin antibodies include antithyroglobulin, anti-T_3, and anti-T_4 antibodies.
- A positive titer is predictive of immune-mediated thyroiditis, and suggestive of hypothyroidism, but only 20% of euthyroid dogs with antibodies develop hypothyroidism within 1 year.
- Anti-T_3 and -T_4 antibodies are similar to T_3 and T_4 and can cross-react to falsely elevate these assay levels. In animals who are slightly hypothyroid (as measured by total T_4), the presence of anti-T_4 antibodies may make it appear as if these animals are euthyroid, leading to a delay in the diagnosis and treatment of hypothyroidism.

TSH Stimulation Test

- Historically considered the gold standard for diagnosing hypothyroidism.
- Pharmaceutical-grade bovine TSH was used to conduct this test; however, this is no longer available.
- Recombinant human TSH can be used safely in both dogs and cats to effectively conduct the test, but is expensive. Therefore, this test is unlikely to become routine.

Total T_3, Reverse T_3, and Free T_3

- Total T_3 measurement is an unreliable indicator of thyroid function.
- The total T_3 level has been demonstrated to be normal in up to 90% of hypothyroid dogs.
- The reverse T_3 level has not been validated in companion animals.
- Evaluation of total T_3, reverse T_3, and free T_3 levels is not recommended to assess thyroid function.

Nonthyroid Factors That Alter Thyroid Function Tests

- In addition to sick euthyroid syndrome, other factors alter the results of thyroid function tests, which may result in a misdiagnosis.
- Most nonthyroid factors cause an artificial *decrease* in thyroid hormone levels.
- Some drugs can decrease thyroid hormone levels, but do not usually result in an animal developing clinical signs of hypothyroidism. Glucocorticoids, phenobarbital, and nonsteroidal anti-inflammatory drugs (NSAIDs) can decrease circulating thyroid hormone levels.
- Sulfonamides can decrease thyroid hormone levels and lead to clinical disease. This effect is noted to occur within weeks of initiation of therapy and disappears 2 weeks after therapy has been discontinued.
- Glucocorticoids inhibit the entire hypothalamic-pituitary-thyroid axis and have a direct effect against thyroid hormone.
- Phenobarbital causes a decrease in thyroid levels only in animals receiving long-term treatment. Phenobarbital should not be administered for 4 weeks prior to thyroid function testing.
- The influence of NSAIDs is variable and evaluation of thyroid function should be made with caution, and preferably after stopping NSAIDs well in advance of testing.
- Well-conditioned and athletic dogs consistently have lower total and free T_4 levels. Certain breeds have normal ranges of thyroid hormones that are different from other breeds. The greyhound, Scottish deerhound, saluki, and whippet have total T_4 concentrations that are well below the mean concentrations for other dogs. Alaskan sled dogs have serum T_4, T_3, and free T_4 concentrations below the normal reference range.
- Vaccination causes a transient increase in circulating autoantibody levels, which may cause a truly hypothyroid animal to appear euthyroid. Thyroid function testing should not be conducted if a patient has been vaccinated within the previous 2 weeks.

IMAGING

Radiographic Findings

Developmental bone problems (delayed epiphyseal ossification or dysgenesis) are usually noted with congenital hypothyroidism.

Ultrasonographic Findings

- Significant differences in thyroid gland volume and echogenicity exist between hypothyroid and euthyroid patients, but interpretation is highly user dependent.
- No significant difference is noted between euthyroid and sick euthyroid subjects.

PATHOLOGIC FINDINGS

- Lymphocytic thyroiditis is characterized by chronic and progressive lymphocytic infiltration and destruction of the thyroid gland. Cytotoxic T cells initiate inflammation, leading to thyrocyte destruction and parenchymal fibrosis.
- Idiopathic thyroid atrophy is characterized by the replacement of normal thyroid parenchyma with adipose and connective tissue.
- Many cutaneous changes are nonspecific. However, certain findings, including dermal thickening, myxedema, and vacuolation of arrector pili muscles, are most characteristic.

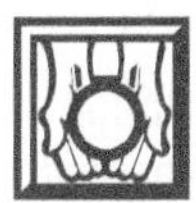

TREATMENT

APPROPRIATE HEALTH CARE

Outpatient medical management.

CLIENT EDUCATION

- Lifelong therapy required.
- Easily managed with oral thyroid hormone supplementation.
- Dose adjustments are common in the early stages of treatment.
- Most clinical signs will resolve over time with appropriate thyroid hormone supplementation.

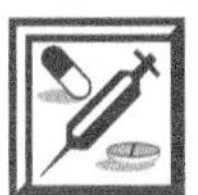

MEDICATIONS

DRUG(S) OF CHOICE

- Synthetic thyroid hormone supplementation easily treats hypothyroidism.
- Levothyroxine sodium is available as both human and veterinary products.
- Generic forms of the drug should be avoided, as human studies have demonstrated wide variability in the bioavailability of generic forms. If a generic form is used, always prescribe the same formulation.
- Hormone supplementation is initiated at 0.02 mg/kg PO q12h.
- Supplementation can often eventually be decreased to once daily after proper control is achieved.
- Levothyroxine doses for dogs exceed those for humans and may confuse pharmacists or human endocrinologists.
- Humans are instructed to take the medication on an empty stomach and proton pump inhibitors can impede absorption. This should be considered if a dog is difficult to regulate.

PRECAUTIONS

Patients with concurrent metabolic conditions (hepatic disease, endocrinopathies, renal disease, cardiac disease) should have supplementation started slowly (about 25% of recommended dose) and slowly increased over time (3 months) to the recommended maintenance level.

POSSIBLE INTERACTIONS

- Glucocorticoids, NSAIDs, furosemide may increase metabolism of levothyroxine.
- GI protectants can decrease absorption and administration should be separated from thyroid hormone supplementation by 2 hours.

ALTERNATIVE DRUG(S)

- If T_4 levels do not normalize after attempting monitoring and treatment, treatment can be attempted with liothyronine (4–6 mg/kg PO q8–12h).
- Monitoring is based on T_3 levels. However, there is no reliable method by which to measure T_3.

FOLLOW-UP

PATIENT MONITORING

- Assessment of clinical signs, weight, and thyroid function testing is recommended 6–8 weeks after therapy has begun, 2–4 weeks after each dose change, and then once to twice yearly. Patients should also be monitored if signs of thyroid toxicosis (e.g., polyuria/polydipsia [PU/PD], polyphagia) occur.
- The total T_4 level should be monitored and timed so that blood is taken 4–6 hours after pill administration.
- Once stable and well controlled, the total treatment dose may be given once daily in some dogs.
- For animals receiving supplementation once daily, blood should be taken immediately before the medication is given and then again 4–6 hours later, to measure trough and peak concentrations.
- When supplementation therapy is appropriate, the total postdose T_4 level should be in the upper half of the reference range, or slightly above it.
- If the total T_4 level is significantly increased above normal, the medication dose should be decreased or the frequency of administration reduced.
- If the total T_4 level is low, an increase in the dose may be necessary.
- Before increasing dose, assess client compliance, evaluate GI status to ensure there is no impact on absorption, and confirm there has been no change in the levothyroxine formulation.

PREVENTION/AVOIDANCE

Adequate hormone supplementation with routine monitoring should avoid recurrence of this condition.

POSSIBLE COMPLICATIONS

- If untreated hypothyroid animals are at increased risk of developing myxedema, myxedema coma, and atherosclerosis.
- Oversupplementation of thyroid hormone can result in iatrogenic hyperthyroidism.

EXPECTED COURSE AND PROGNOSIS

- Primary hypothyroidism can be easily and successfully controlled; the prognosis for affected animals, when appropriately treated, is excellent. Resolution of clinical signs is an important predictor of adequate supplementation therapy.
- Significant improvement in attitude, activity level, and alertness should occur within 1 week of starting therapy.
- Dermatologic abnormalities improve slowly, with complete resolution taking up to 3 months.
- Polyneuropathies usually begin improving quickly; complete resolution may take several months.
- Anemia and serum cholesterol levels gradually resolve in the first weeks of therapy.
- Life expectancy usually normal.
- Congenital hypothyroidism has a guarded to poor prognosis.

MISCELLANEOUS

ASSOCIATED CONDITIONS

May rarely be associated with other endocrinopathies.

PREGNANCY/FERTILITY/BREEDING

Increased periparturient mortality and lower birthweight pups.

SEE ALSO

Myxedema and Myxedema Coma

ABBREVIATIONS

- fT_4ED = Free T4 measured by equilibrium dialysis.
- GI = gastrointestinal.
- I-131 = radioactive iodine.
- KCS = keratoconjunctivitis sicca.
- NSAID = nonsteroidal anti-inflammatory drug.
- PU/PD = polyuria/polydipsia.
- TRH = thyrotropin-releasing hormone.
- TSH = thyroid-stimulating hormone.

Suggested Reading

Bellumori TP, Farnula TR, Bannasch DL, et al. Prevalence of inherited disorders among mixed-breed and purebred dogs; 27,254 cases (1995–2010). J Am Vet Assoc 2013, 242(11):1549–1555.

Scott-Moncrieff JCR. Hypothyroidism. In: Ettinger SJ, Feldman EC, eds., Textbook of Veterinary Internal Medicine, 7th ed. St. Louis, MO: Elsevier, 2010, pp. 1751–1761.

Author Patty A. Lathan

Consulting Editor Patty A. Lathan

Acknowledgment The author and book editors acknowledge the prior contribution of Deborah S. Greco.

Client Education Handout available online

HYPOXEMIA

BASICS

DEFINITION

- A decrease in partial pressure of arterial oxygen (PaO_2), resulting in marked desaturation of hemoglobin.
- PaO_2 at sea level ranges from 80 to 100 mmHg in normal animals.

H

PATHOPHYSIOLOGY

Six physiologic causes:

- Low partial pressure of inspired oxygen (PIO_2).
- Hypoventilation (increase in partial pressure of carbon dioxide in arterial blood [$PaCO_2$]).
- Mismatching of alveolar ventilation and perfusion so that areas of the lung that are not ventilated properly are still perfused adequately.
- Alveolar–capillary membrane diffusion defect.
- Right-to-left cardiac or pulmonary shunting.

SYSTEMS AFFECTED

- All organs—oxygen essential for normal cellular function; individual tissue oxygen requirements vary by organ.
- Cardiovascular—can result in focal or global ischemia; if prolonged, can develop arrhythmias and cardiac failure.
- Nervous—brain and CNS most important; hypoxemia can result in irreversible brain damage because there are no large oxygen stores in brain tissue.

SIGNALMENT

Any breed, age, and sex of dog and cat.

SIGNS

Historical Findings

- Breathing problems—especially open-mouth breathing.
- Trauma.
- Episodes of coughing.
- Gagging.
- Exercise intolerance.
- Cyanosis.
- Collapse.

Physical Examination Findings

- Tachypnea.
- Dyspnea.
- Orthopnea.
- Pale mucous membranes.
- Cyanosis.
- Coughing.
- Open-mouth breathing.
- Tachycardia.
- Poor peripheral pulse.
- Abnormal thoracic auscultation.

CAUSES

- Low PIO_2—high altitude (the higher the elevation, the lower the barometric pressure, which results in a decrease in PIO_2; fraction of oxygen in inspired air (FIO_2) is fixed at 0.21); suffocation; enclosure in small areas with improper ventilation.
- Hypoventilation—result of inadequate alveolar ventilation; muscular paralysis; upper airway obstruction; air or fluid in the pleural space; restriction of the thoracic cage, diaphragmatic hernia; CNS disease; anesthetics.
- Mismatching of alveolar ventilation and perfusion—most common cause of hypoxemia and occurs with virtually any lung disease: pulmonary thromboembolism; pulmonary parenchymal disease (infectious or neoplastic); lower airway disease; pneumonia; pulmonary contusions; pulmonary edema; also during anesthesia or prolonged recumbency when a large region of lung becomes atelectatic.
- Alveolar–capillary membrane diffusion impairment—rarely clinically important.
- Right-to-left cardiac or pulmonary shunting—tetralogy of Fallot; ventricular septal defect; reversed patent ductus arteriosus; intrapulmonary arteriovenous shunt.

RISK FACTORS

- Move to higher elevation.
- Trauma.
- Bronchopneumonia of any cause.
- Pleural disease.
- Anesthesia.
- Cardiac disease.
- Bronchial disease—chronic bronchitis, feline asthma.
- Diseases associated with risk of emboli-zation, e.g., immune-mediated hemolytic anemia, hyperadrenocorticism, neoplasia, pancreatitis, sepsis.

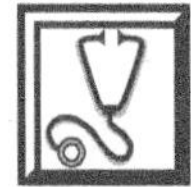

DIAGNOSIS

DIFFERENTIAL DIAGNOSIS

- Signs of tachypnea and/or dyspnea.
- Excitement or anxiety.
- Hyperthermia.
- Pyrexia.
- Head trauma.
- Pain.

LABORATORY FINDINGS

Drugs That May Alter Laboratory Results

N/A

Disorders That May Alter Laboratory Results

- Air bubbles in the arterial blood sample—falsely high PaO_2 values.
- Improper packaging of the arterial blood sample—falsely high PaO_2 values after approximately 30 min at room temperature.

Valid if Run in Human Laboratory?

Yes

CBC/BIOCHEMISTRY/URINALYSIS

- Packed cell volume (PCV)—can be high with chronic condition; can be low if inflammatory or neoplastic.
- Liver enzyme elevation common with organ hypoxia.

OTHER LABORATORY TESTS

Arterial Blood Gases

- Collect arterial blood sample in an anaerobic manner, as follows: use enough heparin to coat the needle and the inside of the syringe; collect sample from femoral or dorsal pedal artery; place a rubber stopper on the needle or covering the hub of the syringe, to prevent room air from entering the sample; analyze sample within 15 min if left at room temperature; place sample on ice to extend safe time for analysis to 2–4 hours.
- Bedside or portable blood gas analyzers—several models available; make analysis more convenient.

IMAGING

Thoracic radiographs and echocardiography— evaluate intrathoracic disease; differentiate pulmonary and cardiac disease.

DIAGNOSTIC PROCEDURES

Pulse Oximetry

- Indirectly determines saturation of arterial blood with oxygen (SaO_2); relation between PaO_2 and SaO_2 based on oxyhemoglobin dissociation curve: SaO_2 >90% when PaO_2 >60 mmHg.
- SaO_2 <95%—considered abnormal, indicates PaO_2 <80 mmHg.
- Best results when probe used on animal's tongue; thus may be limited to anesthetized, heavily sedated, or seriously ill patients with low level of consciousness; keep tongue moistened for most accurate readings.
- Other potentially successful probe sites—lip, ear; vulva (female), prepuce (male); skin between toes; thin skin in the flank area. Interpret values with caution.
- Poor results—using sites that have hair or poor perfusion; least accurate in low-flow states such as hypotension (global low flow) or hypothermia (low flow to skin); falsely low values (usually <85%) during carboxyhemo-globinemia (smoke inhalation).
- Rectal probes will allow readings in awake patients.

Endoscopy or Lung Biopsy

Airway sampling often required to determine primary abnormality resulting in hypoxemia.

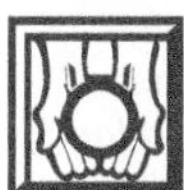

TREATMENT

Must identify and correct the primary cause.

Oxygen Therapy

- Most common supportive treatment.
- Corrects low-inspired oxygen, hypoventilation, and alveolar–capillary membrane diffusion defects; may not fully correct mismatching of ventilation and perfusion; does not correct right-to-left cardiac or pulmonary shunts and low cardiac output.
- May not be completely beneficial until adequate blood volume is established or alveolar contents are removed (e.g., pulmonary edema, purulent material).
- Delivery—directly from an oxygen source from the anesthetic machine via a face mask placed securely around the muzzle or from an E-tank fitted with an oxygen regulator through a face mask, intranasal catheter placed in the oropharynx, or oxygen cage.
- Increase in FIO_2—determined by the oxygen flow rate and the amount of oxygen mixed with room air.
- Positive pressure ventilation—may be needed for severe hypoxemia of any cause.
- High flow oxygen therapy (HFOT) has been shown to increase arterial oxygen in dogs with severe hypoxemia.

Fluid Therapy

- Low cardiac output—fluid administration and inotropic support (e.g., pimobendan, dobutamine, or dopamine) important.
- Cardiac failure—requires aggressive medical treatment; diuretics; afterload and preload reduction; inotropic support; oxygen administration; cautious amounts of fluids may be indicated after institution of primary treatment; use caution with type and rate of fluids after initial stabilization.
- Hypovolemic, hemorrhagic, traumatic, or septic shock—requires end point fluid administration; crystalloids (20–30 mL/kg), hypertonic solutions (7% NaCl, 4 mL/kg), or blood products (packed red blood cells [pRBC], whole blood, plasma), or a combination.
- Severe pulmonary contusion—hypertonic fluids or low dose crystalloids (5–10 mL/kg).

MEDICATIONS

DRUG(S) OF CHOICE

For bronchospasm—bronchodilators; terbutaline (0.01 mg/kg SC/IM/IV q8h) or albuterol inhaler.

CONTRAINDICATIONS

- Aggressive fluid administration—not indicated for cardiac failure and pulmonary edema.
- Diuretics—not indicated for shock, low PIO_2, alveolar–capillary membrane diffusion defects, mismatching of alveolar ventilation and perfusion, and right-to-left shunts.

PRECAUTIONS

- Inotropic drugs—arrhythmias may develop.
- Oxygen toxicity—prolonged (>12 hour) exposure to high-concentration (>70%) oxygen can result in pulmonary edema, seizures, and death.

POSSIBLE INTERACTIONS

N/A

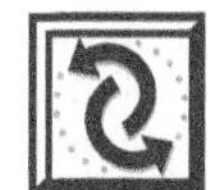

FOLLOW-UP

PATIENT MONITORING

- Decrease in respiratory effort and decrease in cyanosis (if initially noted)—check efficacy of treatment and support.
- Arterial blood gas—determine resolution.
- Pulse oximetry—alternative; interpret results cautiously with hypotension, hypothermia, smoke inhalation, and non-tongue probe site. Trend in the actual number being produced is important.

POSSIBLE COMPLICATIONS

- Brain damage—depends on severity and duration of hypoxemia; partial or complete loss of neuronal function; dementia; seizures; loss of consciousness.
- Arrhythmias—may develop secondary to myocardial hypoxia; may be very difficult to treat effectively.
- Respiratory arrest requiring intubation and positive pressure ventilation.

MISCELLANEOUS

ASSOCIATED CONDITIONS

N/A

AGE-RELATED FACTORS

N/A

PREGNANCY/FERTILITY/BREEDING

May adversely affect fetuses, especially during first trimester of pregnancy.

SEE ALSO

- Cyanosis.
- Dyspnea and Respiratory Distress.
- Panting and Tachypnea.

ABBREVIATIONS

- FIO_2 = fraction of oxygen in inspired air.
- HFOT = High flow oxygen therapy.
- $PaCO_2$ = partial pressure of carbon dioxide in arterial blood.
- PaO_2 = partial pressure of arterial oxygen.
- PCV = packed cell volume.
- PIO_2 = partial pressure of inspired oxygen.
- pRBC = packed red blood cells.
- SaO_2 = saturation of arterial blood with oxygen.

Suggested Reading

Guenther CL. Oxygen therapy. In: Drobatz KJ, Hopper K, Rozanski E, Silverstein DC. Textbook of Small Animal Emergency Medicine. Ames, IA: Wiley-Blackwell, 2019, pp. 1177–1182.

Haskins SC. Hypoxemia. In: Silverstein DC, Hooper K, eds. Small Animal Critical Care Medicine. St. Louis, MO: Elsevier Saunders, 2015, pp. 81–86.

Haskins SC. Monitoring anesthetized patients. In: Grimm KA, Lamont LA, Tranquilli WJ, et al., eds. Veterinary Anesthesia and Analgesia, 5th ed. Ames, IA: Wiley-Blackwell, 2015, pp. 102–108.

Mazzaferro EM. Oxygen therapy. In: Silverstein DC, Hooper K, eds. Small Animal Critical Care Medicine. St. Louis, MO: Elsevier Saunders, 2015, pp. 77–80.

McDonell WN, Kerr CL. Respiratory system. In: Grimm KA, Lamont LA, Tranquilli WJ, et al., eds. Veterinary Anesthesia and Analgesia, 5th ed. Ames, IA: Wiley-Blackwell, 2015, pp. 513–543.

Author Thomas K. Day
Consulting Editor Elizabeth Rozanski

ICTERUS

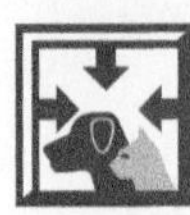

BASICS

DEFINITION

Increased total bilirubin concentration causing yellow tissue discoloration.

PATHOPHYSIOLOGY

• Bilirubin—derived from degradation of heme-containing proteins; most (80%) from senescent erythrocytes; remainder from other heme-containing proteins (e.g., P450 cytochromes, myoglobin). • Unconjugated bilirubin—transported in plasma bound to albumin; diglucuronide conjugated after hepatocellular uptake. • Conjugated bilirubin—transported in bile, expelled into intestines where most converted to other products, e.g., urobilinogen can undergo enterohepatic circulation, stercobilin colors feces brown.
• Hyperbilirubinemia—caused by increased bilirubin production (increased red blood cell [RBC] destruction; *hemolytic jaundice*); heme exceeding hepatic capacity for uptake, conjugation, or biliary excretion (*hepatic jaundice*), or interrupted biliary elimination (*posthepatic jaundice*). • Nonhemolytic jaundice caused by hepatobiliary disease or bile peritonitis.

SYSTEMS AFFECTED

• Skin/exocrine—skin discoloration (jaundice) reflects serum bilirubin >2.5 mg/dL. • Hepatobiliary—retained bile acids and markedly increased bilirubin may contribute to hepatocellular injury. • Renal/urologic—extreme hyperbilirubinemia may cause renal tubular injury. • Nervous—extreme unconjugated hyperbilirubinemia may cause degenerative brain lesions (rare, kernicterus).

SIGNALMENT

Species

Dog and cat.

Mean Age and Range

• Most causes—diseases of adult animals.
• Young, unvaccinated dogs—at risk for infectious canine hepatitis.

Predominant Sex

Adult female pure-bred dogs—at risk for immune-mediated hemolytic anemia.

SIGNS

Historical Findings

Increased Formation: Hemolysis

• Vague signs—lethargy, weakness.
• Gastrointestinal (GI) signs—anorexia, constipation, vomiting, weight loss. • Jaundice.
• Recent blood transfusion. • Severe trauma—bleeding into muscle, abdomen, or hematoma formation. • Rhabdomyolysis (rare cause).

Decreased Elimination: Cholestasis

• Vague GI signs—anorexia, vomiting, diarrhea, change in fecal color: nonobstructive jaundice green, orange; obstructed jaundice acholic. • Jaundice. • Change in urine color—orange. • Abdominal enlargement—if ascites. • Polyuria and polydipsia. • Altered mentation—if hepatic encephalopathy (HE).

Physical Examination Findings

Increased Formation: Hemolysis

• Pallor, tachycardia, tachypnea, weakness, bounding femoral pulses, anemic heart murmur.
• Jaundice. • Hepatomegaly/splenomegaly—extramedullary hematopoiesis, reticuloendothelial hyperplasia. • Lymphadenopathy.
• Bleeding tendencies—if thrombocytopenic.
• Orange feces. • Fever. • "Gelatinous" feel to skin (vasculopathy). • Rhabdomyolysis—weakness, pain.

Decreased Elimination: Cholestasis

• Weight loss. • Jaundice. • Hepatomegaly/splenomegaly. • Abdominal effusion/mass/pain.
• Melenic, orange, green, or acholic feces. • Fever.

CAUSES

Prehepatic Jaundice

• Hemolytic disorders—immune-mediated hemolysis; certain drugs (propylene glycol carriers in cats, trimethoprim sulfa); systemic lupus erythematosus; infectious disorders; toxins (e.g., oxidative injury: zinc, onions; phenols); severe hypophosphatemia. • Incompatible blood transfusion. • Infections—feline leukemia virus (FeLV); *Mycoplasma haemofelis*; heartworm; *Babesia*; *Ehrlichia*; *Cytauxzoon*. • Large-volume blood resorption—hematomas, body cavities (e.g., hemangiosarcoma, warfarin).

Hepatic Jaundice

• Chronic idiopathic or familial hepatitis.
• Adverse drug reactions—e.g., anticonvulsants; acetaminophen; trimethoprim sulfate; carprofen; stanozolol (cats); benzodiazepines (cats); see Hepatotoxins. • Cholangitis/cholangiohepatitis. • Infiltrative neoplasia—lymphoma. • Cirrhosis (dogs). • Hepatic lipidosis (cats). • Massive liver necrosis—e.g., aflatoxin, cycad, nonsteroidal anti-inflammatory drugs (carprofen), copper associated injury.
• Systemic illnesses with hepatic involvement—leptospirosis (dogs); histoplasmosis; feline infectious peritonitis; hyperthyroidism (cats); toxoplasmosis (cats). • Bacterial sepsis—originating anywhere in body; may elaborate bacterial products that impair hepatic bilirubin processing/elimination.

Posthepatic Jaundice

Transient or persistent mechanical bile duct obstruction—pancreatitis (transient obstruction); neoplasia: bile duct, pancreas, duodenum; intraluminal duct occlusion: cholelithiasis, sludged bile, liver flukes (cats), immune-mediated duct destruction (sclerosing cholangitis in cats), gall bladder mucocele (dogs); ruptured biliary tree causing bile peritonitis.

RISK FACTORS

• Young unvaccinated dogs—infectious disease, canine infectious hepatitis. • Breed predisposition for familial hepatic disease—Labrador retriever, Doberman pinscher, Bedlington terrier, cocker spaniel, Dalmatian. • Middle-aged, obese dogs—pancreatitis. • Anorectic, obese cats—hepatic lipidosis. • Hepatotoxic drugs. • Blunt abdominal trauma, chronic biliary tract disease, gallbladder mucocele—bile peritonitis.
• Hemolytic anemia.

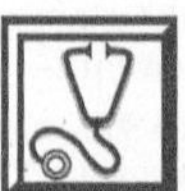

DIAGNOSIS

DIFFERENTIAL DIAGNOSIS

• Prehepatic jaundice—usually abrupt onset; mucous membrane pallor; mild to moderate jaundice; weakness; tachypnea; cardiac murmur with severe anemia. • Hepatic jaundice—breed risk for familial hepatitis; variable jaundice; otherwise normal mucous membranes; alteration in liver size (large or small); abdominal effusion (pure or modified transudate); polyuria and polydipsia; behavioral abnormalities of HE; coagulopathy.
• Posthepatic jaundice—chronic and/or recurrent bouts of apparent GI signs or pancreatitis with cholelithiasis; moderate or marked jaundice; otherwise normal mucous membranes; diffuse or cranial abdominal pain; cranial abdominal mass; abdominal effusion (septic, nonseptic, or bile peritonitis); bleeding tendencies; acholic feces unless melena.

LABORATORY FINDINGS

• Bilirubin assay—based on diazo reaction; assesses direct-reacting and total serum bilirubin; most yield reasonable total bilirubin results; values for direct bilirubin vary.
• Higher readings in heparinized plasma.
• Sample management—important; total bilirubin may decrease by 50% per hour with direct exposure to sunlight or artificial lighting.
• Hemolysis—variable effects on total bilirubin measured by spectrophotometry.
• Lipemia—falsely increases total bilirubin values measured by endpoint assays.
• Fractionation into conjugated and unconjugated—*unable to define causes of jaundice*, contrary to dogma.

CBC/BIOCHEMISTRY/URINALYSIS

Prehepatic Jaundice

• CBC—severe anemia (usually regenerative); blood smear may reveal autoagglutination, spherocytes, Heinz bodies, parasites; hemoglobinemia with intravascular hemolysis, normal to low platelets, normal to high WBCs, with left shift. • Biochemistry—normal to high alanine aminotransferase (ALT) and alkaline phosphatase (ALP) activity, blood urea nitrogen (BUN) concentration; normal to low albumin; normal to high globulin; normal glucose and cholesterol; high bilirubin.

Hepatic Jaundice

• CBC—mild nonregenerative anemia; low mean corpuscular volume (MCV) with chronic liver disease and portosystemic shunting; variable white blood cell (WBC) count. • Biochemistry—mildly to markedly high ALT ± ALP; normal to low albumin, BUN, glucose, cholesterol. • Urinalysis—normal to dilute urine; bilirubinuria precedes hyperbilirubinemia; bilirubinuria important in cats.

Posthepatic Jaundice

• CBC—± mild nonregenerative anemia; variable WBC count. • Biochemistry—increased ALT, moderate to markedly increased ALP; usually normal albumin, BUN, glucose concentrations; normal to high cholesterol.

OTHER LABORATORY TESTS

• In-saline autoagglutination slide test—with suspected RBC agglutination; may have reported high MCV. • Direct Coombs' test—submit if no evidence of autoagglutination. • Osmotic fragility test—detects likelihood of RBC hemolysis tonicity challenge. • Blood smears—hemoparasites, spherocytes, schistocytes, anisocytosis (regenerative). • Plasma zinc—if hemolytic anemia. • Antinuclear antibodies—with hemolytic anemia. • Serum bile acids—redundant if nonhemolytic jaundice already suspected. • Serology—for infectious diseases (e.g., FeLV, leptospirosis, mycoses) with signs of multisystemic illness and hepatic jaundice. • PCR for acute leptospirosis—within first few days, urine and/or serum; before appropriate antibiotic therapy. • Abdominal effusion—characterize cell and protein content. • Coagulation tests—prolonged values, esp. proteins invoked by vitamin K absence or antagonism and prothrombin time, with bile duct occlusion; vitamin K_1 responsive. • Microbial culture and sensitivity—blood ± other specimens if inflammatory leukon and suspected bacterial infection (e.g., urinary tract, biliary tract, liver).

IMAGING

• Abdominal radiography—obscured by effusion; may reveal hepatomegaly, mass effect, mineral or gas interface in liver (emphysematous cholecystitis, choleliths); splenomegaly (hemolytic anemia, portal hypertension, abdominal neoplasia); metallic foreign body with zinc-induced hemolysis. • Thoracic radiography—may reveal metastatic disease; sternal lymphadenopathy (reflecting abdominal disease); general lymphadenopathy (lymphosarcoma, systemic infection [fungal]). • Abdominal US—may distinguish parenchymal liver disease from extrahepatic biliary obstruction; characterizes hepatic parenchymal lesions; may disclose abdominal neoplasia; may determine cause of abdominal effusion; used to target lesions, fluid, or cystocentesis sampling (aspirates or needle biopsy).

DIAGNOSTIC PROCEDURES

• Fine-needle aspiration—cytology of mass, lymph node, hepatic parenchyma, bile. • Liver biopsy—bacterial culture of liver, bile, other specimens obtained via celiotomy, blind percutaneous, keyhole, laparoscopic, or US-guided techniques. • Surgical intervention—required for diagnosis and treatment of posthepatic disorders.

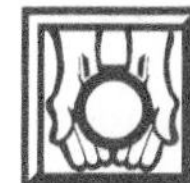

TREATMENT

• Depends on underlying cause. • Inpatient—for initial medical care. • Cage rest—to facilitate liver regeneration or reduce oxygen requirements if severe anemia. • Diet—important for hepatic and posthepatic jaundice; nutritionally balanced with maximum protein tolerated; carbohydrate based (dogs) with restricted protein for hepatic encephalopathy; restrict sodium if ascites. • Vitamin supplementation—water-soluble vitamins in all patients; parenteral vitamin K_1 for bile duct obstruction or severe cholestasis.

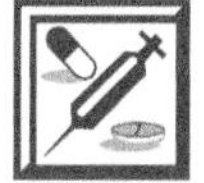

MEDICATIONS

DRUG(S) OF CHOICE

• Prehepatic jaundice—eliminate inciting cause; see Anemia, Immune-Mediated; whole blood transfusion for life-threatening anemia. • Hepatic/posthepatic jaundice—treat specific disorders based on imaging, biopsy, culture.

CONTRAINDICATIONS

• Avoid known hepatotoxic drugs. • Avoid tetracyclines unless clearly indicated—suppress hepatic protein synthesis, promote hepatic lipidosis. • Avoid analgesics, anesthetics, barbiturates—with hepatic failure.

PRECAUTIONS

• Sedatives—may precipitate HE. • Corticosteroids—for nonseptic inflammation; increase risk for infection; may aggravate ascites (water and sodium retention), promote vacuolar hepatopathy (dogs) and hepatic lipidosis (cats).

POSSIBLE INTERACTIONS

Consider influence of altered hepatic metabolism on drug therapy; hypoalbuminemia influences potency of protein-bound drugs, enhancing effects (may lead to toxicity).

FOLLOW-UP

PATIENT MONITORING

• Prehepatic jaundice—recheck packed cell volume and blood smears as needed; may require repeat transfusions; taper immunosuppressive drugs. • Hepatic and posthepatic jaundice—recheck serum biochemical profile as dictated by underlying disease; continue symptomatic and specific treatments until remission, varies with disease process.

MISCELLANEOUS

ASSOCIATED CONDITIONS

• Patients with immune-mediated hemolysis treated with immunosuppressive doses of corticosteroids predisposed to thromboembolism, GI ulcers, and infection. • Patients in hepatic failure susceptible to infections, enteric bleeding, ascites. • Patients with reconstructive biliary surgery have risk of recurrent bacterial cholangitis.

SYNONYMS

Jaundice

SEE ALSO

- Anemia, Heinz Body.
- Anemia, Immune-Mediated.
- Anemia, Regenerative.
- Babesiosis.
- Bartonellosis.
- Blood Transfusion Reactions.
- Cholangitis/Cholangiohepatitis Syndrome.
- Cholelithiasis.
- Cirrhosis and Fibrosis of the Liver.
- Copper Associated Hepatopathy.
- Gallbladder Mucocele.
- Hepatic Failure, Acute.
- Hepatic Lipidosis.
- Hepatitis, Chronic.
- Hepatitis, Infectious (Viral) Canine.
- Hepatitis, Suppurative and Hepatic Abscess.
- Hepatotoxins.
- Liver Fluke Infestation.
- Lupus Erythematosus, Systemic (SLE).
- Pancreatitis—Cats.
- Pancreatitis—Dogs.
- Zinc Toxicosis.

ABBREVIATIONS

• ALP = alkaline phosphatase. • ALT = alanine aminotransferase. • BUN = blood urea nitrogen. • FeLV = feline leukemia virus. • GI = gastrointestinal. • HE = hepatic encephalopathy. • MCV = mean corpuscular volume. • RBC = red blood cell. • WBC = white blood cell.

Suggested Reading

Willard MD, Twedt DC. Gastrointestinal, pancreatic, and hepatic disorders. In: Willard M, Tvedten H, eds., Small Animal Clinical Diagnosis by Laboratory Methods, 5th ed. St. Louis, MO: Saunders, 2012, pp. 212–214.

Author Sharon A. Center

Consulting Editor Kate Holan

Client Education Handout available online

I

IDIOVENTRICULAR RHYTHM

BASICS

DEFINITION

If conduction of sinus node pacemaker impulses to the ventricles is blocked or the impulses decrease in frequency, the lower regions of the heart automatically take over the role of pacemaker for the ventricles, which results in ventricular escape complexes (Figure 1) or an idioventricular rhythm (Figure 2).

ECG Features

- P waves may be absent or may precede, be hidden within, or follow the ectopic QRS complex.
- P waves are unrelated to the QRS complexes.
- QRS configuration—wide and bizarre; similar to that of a ventricular premature complex.

PATHOPHYSIOLOGY

- May be hemodynamically important with slow ventricular rates.
- Does not occur in healthy animals.
- Subsidiary pacemakers seem to discharge more rapidly in cats than in dogs.

SYSTEMS AFFECTED

Cardiovascular

GENETICS

N/A

INCIDENCE/PREVALENCE

Unknown

SIGNALMENT

Species

Dog and cat.

Breed Predilections

- Atrial standstill in English springer spaniels and Siamese cats.
- Pugs, miniature schnauzers, and Dalmatians prone to conduction abnormalities.

Mean Age and Range

N/A

Predominant Sex

N/A

SIGNS

Historical Findings

- Some animals asymptomatic.
- Weakness.
- Lethargy.
- Exercise intolerance.
- Syncope.
- Heart failure.

Physical Examination Findings

- Irregular rhythm associated with pulse deficits.
- Variation in heart sounds.
- Possible intermittent "cannon" waves in the jugular venous pulses (with atrioventricular [AV] block).

CAUSES

- Not a primary disease—a secondary result of a primary disease.
- The escape rhythm is a safety mechanism to maintain cardiac output.

Causes of Sinus Bradycardia and Sinus Arrest

- Increased vagal tone (high intracranial pressure, high ocular pressure).
- Drugs—digoxin, tranquilizers, propranolol, quinidine, and anesthetics.
- Addison's disease.
- Hypoglycemia.
- Renal failure.
- Hypothermia.
- Hyperkalemia.
- Hypothyroidism.

Causes of AV Block

- Congenital.
- Neoplasia.
- Fibrosis.
- Lyme disease.

RISK FACTORS

N/A

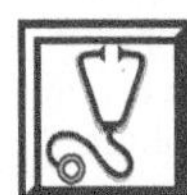

DIAGNOSIS

DIFFERENTIAL DIAGNOSIS

- A series of ventricular escape beats with a heart rate <65 bpm in dogs and <100 bpm in cats; heart rates of 65–160 bpm in dogs and 100–180 bpm in cats are often termed accelerated idioventricular rhythms.
- Ventricular tachycardia—dogs have a cardiac rate >160 bpm; cats >180 bpm.
- Slow heart rate in animals with right bundle branch block, left bundle branch block, or left anterior fascicular block; animals with these disturbances have the P waves associated with the QRS complexes.

CBC/BIOCHEMISTRY/URINALYSIS

- No specific findings.
- Complete blood testing may suggest a metabolic abnormality.

OTHER LABORATORY TESTS

- Drug toxicity.
- Lyme titer in animals with complete AV block.

IMAGING

Echocardiogram may show structural heart disease.

DIAGNOSTIC PROCEDURES

ECG

PATHOLOGIC FINDINGS

Depend on underlying cause.

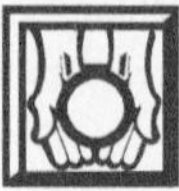

TREATMENT

APPROPRIATE HEALTH CARE

- Rhythm is an escape or safety mechanism for maintaining cardiac output; do *not* direct treatment toward suppressing this escape rhythm, but toward the primary disease process that allows the escape rhythm to assume pacemaker control of the heart.
- Symptomatic treatment is directed toward increasing the heart rate.

NURSING CARE

May be required for underlying disease.

ACTIVITY

Symptomatic animals may require cage rest.

DIET

No modifications or restrictions unless required for management of the underlying condition.

CLIENT EDUCATION

Inform of the need to seek and specifically treat an underlying cause.

SURGICAL CONSIDERATIONS

Pacemaker implantation may be necessary.

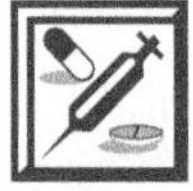

MEDICATIONS

DRUG(S) OF CHOICE

- Atropine or glycopyrrolate usually indicated to block vagal tone or increase the heart rate.
- If those drugs are ineffective, isoproterenol, dopamine, dobutamine, or artificial pacing may be needed.

CONTRAINDICATIONS

Lidocaine, procainamide, quinidine, propranolol, diltiazem, or any other drug that slows the cardiac rate or reduces contractility.

PRECAUTIONS

Atropine is briefly vagotonic immediately post injection and can temporarily exacerbate the condition.

POSSIBLE INTERACTIONS

N/A

ALTERNATIVE DRUG(S)

N/A

FOLLOW-UP

PATIENT MONITORING

- Serial ECG may show clearing of the lesion or progression to complete heart block.
- Serial blood profiles may be needed to monitor progress of the primary disease process.

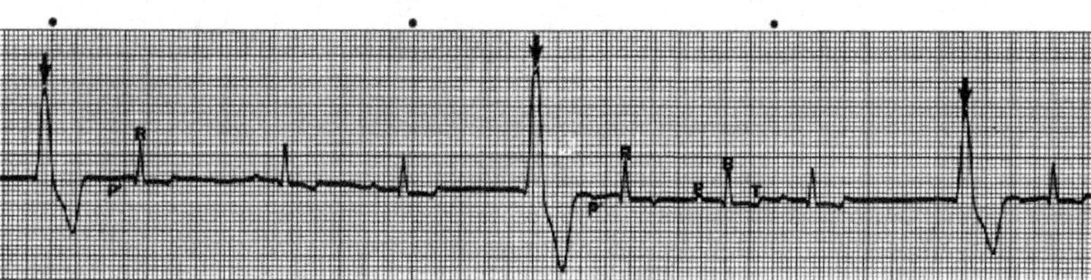

Figure 1.

Ventricular escape complexes (arrows) during various phases in the dominant sinus rhythm in a dog during anesthesia. The sinus rate increased (not shown) after anesthesia was stopped; ½ cm–1 mv. (Source: From Tilley LP. Essentials of Canine and Feline Electrocardiography, 3rd ed. Baltimore, MD: Williams & Wilkins, 1992. Reprinted with permission of Wolters Kluwer.)

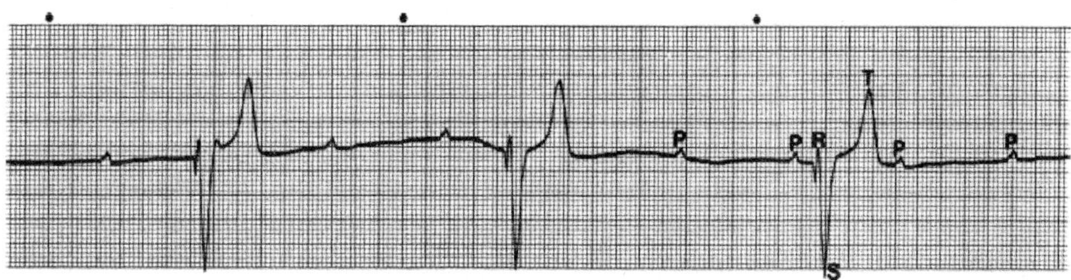

Figure 2.

Complete heart block. The P waves occur at a rate of 120, independent of the ventricular rate of 50. The QRS configuration is a right bundle branch block pattern. The heart rate and QRS shape suggest that the rescuing focus is probably near the AV junction. (Source: From Tilley LP. Essentials of Canine and Feline Electrocardiography, 3rd ed. Baltimore, MD: Williams & Wilkins, 1992. Reprinted with permission of Wolters Kluwer.)

- Serial echocardiograms may show improvement or progressive changes in cardiac structure.

PREVENTION/AVOIDANCE

N/A

POSSIBLE COMPLICATIONS

Prolonged bradycardia may cause secondary congestive heart failure or inadequate renal perfusion.

EXPECTED COURSE AND PROGNOSIS

- Arrhythmia may abate when the primary disorder is corrected.
- Guarded if condition is associated with cardiac or metabolic disorder; poor if the rate is not increased pharmacologically or if underlying cause cannot be identified and treated.

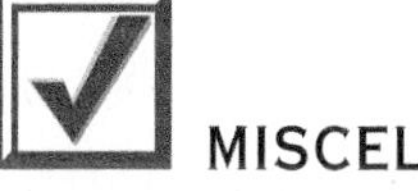

MISCELLANEOUS

ASSOCIATED CONDITIONS

N/A

AGE-RELATED FACTORS

N/A

SEE ALSO

- Atrial Standstill.
- Atrioventricular Block, Complete (Third Degree).

ABBREVIATIONS

- AV = atrioventricular.

Suggested Reading

Kittleson MD. Electrocardiography. In: Kittleson MD, Kienle RD, eds. Small Animal Cardiovascular Medicine. St. Louis, MO: Mosby, 1998, pp. 72–94.

Santilli R, Moïse NS, Pariaut R, Perego M. Electrocardiography of the Dog and Cat: Diagnosis of Arrhythmias, 2nd ed. Milan: Edra, 2018.

Tilley LP, Smith FWK, Jr. Electrocardiography. In: Smith FWK, Tilley LP, Oyama MA, Sleeper MM, eds. Manual of Canine and Feline Cardiology, 5th ed. St. Louis, MO: Saunders Elsevier, 2016, pp. 49–76.

Tilley LP, Smith FWK, Jr. Essentials of Canine and Feline Electrocardiography: Interpretation and Treatment, 4th ed. Ames, IA: Wiley-Blackwell, 2021 (in preparation).

Willis R, Oliveira P, Mavropoulou A. Guide to Canine and Feline Electrocardiography. Ames, IA: Wiley-Blackwell, 2018.

Author Larry P. Tilley
Consulting Editor Michael Aherne

ILEUS

BASICS

OVERVIEW

- Adynamic (paralytic, functional) ileus is defined as a transient and reversible intestinal obstruction resulting from inhibition of bowel motility.
- Lack of peristalsis of stomach, small bowel, or large bowel causes functional obstruction, as intestinal contents accumulate in the dependent areas of the gastrointestinal tract instead of being propelled in an aborad direction.
- Ileus is not a primary disease but a secondary complication of a number of disorders.
- Adynamic ileus is thought to occur secondary to electromechanical dissociation of the intestinal musculature due to increased sympathetic tone, release of humoral inhibitory factors (catecholamines, vasopressin, endogenous opiates), impaired release of prokinetic hormones (neurotensin, motilin), or hypokalemia.
- Secondary causes of intestinal pseudo-obstruction have been subclassified into developmental, infectious, inflammatory, autoimmune, metabolic, paraneoplastic, endocrine, and toxic etiologies.
- Lymphocytic leiomyositis represents a visceral myopathic form of chronic intestinal pseudo-obstruction that has been described in humans, dogs, horses, and cats; it is defined as lymphocytic infiltration of the muscularis propria and is thought to represent an autoimmune response to the myofibers of the muscularis propria layer of the bowel by T lymphocytes.
- Systems affected—gastrointestinal; autonomic nervous system.

SIGNALMENT

Cat and dog.

SIGNS

- Anorexia.
- Vomiting.
- Regurgitation.
- Lethargy.
- Diarrhea.
- Weight loss.
- Coughing secondary to aspiration pneumonia from gastroesophageal reflux.
- Mild abdominal distention or discomfort secondary to accumulation of gas in hypomotile bowel.
- Failure to auscultate gut sounds after 2–3 minutes suggests ileus.
- Gut sounds can be increased during initial state (partial loss of motility).

CAUSES & RISK FACTORS

- Surgery (especially gastrointestinal surgery).
- Pain.
- Electrolyte imbalance (hypokalemia, hypomagnesemia, hypocalcemia).
- Acute inflammatory lesions of bowel, peritoneal cavity, pancreas, or other abdominal organs.
- Unrelieved mechanical obstruction.
- Intestinal ischemia.
- Gram-negative sepsis.
- Endotoxemia.
- Shock.
- Retroperitoneal injury.
- Uremia.
- Autonomic neuropathies (dysautonomia, spinal cord injury).
- Visceral myopathies associated with autoimmune disease.
- Use of anticholinergic drugs.
- Intestinal overdistension (aerophagia).
- Lead poisoning.
- Stress (cold and noise).

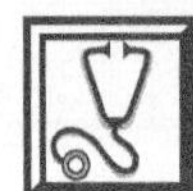

DIAGNOSIS

DIFFERENTIAL DIAGNOSIS

Adynamic ileus must be differentiated from mechanical obstruction caused by:

- Intestinal foreign bodies.
- Inflammatory bowel disease.
- Intussusception.
- Intramural abscess.
- Incarcerated or strangulated hernia.
- Volvulus.
- Mesenteric infarction.
- Parasites.
- Adhesions.
- Postoperative stricture.
- Impaction.
- Congenital malformation.
- Inflammatory or traumatic lesions.
- Neoplasia.

CBC/BIOCHEMISTRY/URINALYSIS

- Hemogram changes depend on primary cause of ileus.
- Serum chemistry profiles and urinalysis help assess electrolyte disturbances (especially hypokalemia) and presence of azotemia.

OTHER LABORATORY TESTS

- Measurement of pancreatic lipase concentration (Spec or SNAP cPL or fPL) to assess for pancreatitis.
- Fecal parvovirus ELISA test in puppies with ileus and diarrhea.

IMAGING

Abdominal Radiographic Findings

- Stomach and/or intestinal loops are distended with gas and fluid.
- Common radiographic patterns include:
  - Generalized gas ileus—consider aerophagia, smooth muscle paralyzing drugs, generalized peritonitis, or enteritis.
  - Generalized fluid ileus—consider enteritis, diffuse intestinal neoplasia.
  - Localized gas ileus—consider localized peritonitis (pancreatitis), early bowel obstruction, disruption of arterial supply.
  - Localized fluid ileus—consider foreign body, neoplastic obstruction, intussusception.

Ultrasonography

- Differentiate adynamic ileus from mechanical intestinal obstructions.
- Identify pancreatitis or peritonitis.
- Ultrasound has been used to assess frequency and contraction of pyloric antrum in dogs.
- Careful evaluation of intestinal layers for loss of normal layering associated with infiltrative neoplasia, thickening of muscularis propria layer and/or submucosal layer associated with inflammatory bowel disease or small cell lymphoma, and attenuation of muscularis layer associated with fibrosis secondary to leiomyositis.

DIAGNOSTIC PROCEDURES

Barium-Impregnated Polyethylene Spheres (BIPS)

- Confirm adynamic ileus.
- Delayed gastrointestinal transit along with retention of BIPS in the stomach.
- Scattering of BIPS throughout the upper gastrointestinal tract.

Upper Gastrointestinal Series

- Upper gastrointestinal series can be performed to help assess for presence of partial intestinal obstructions or delayed gastric and intestinal motility.
- Gastric and intestinal transit times must be interpreted cautiously following administration of liquid barium in light of marked variation in emptying times from animal to animal, and the stress of hospitalization can delay gastric and intestinal transit times.

Other Procedures to Consider

- Noninvasive electrogastrography is used experimentally to assess gastric myoelectrical activity in dogs.
- Abdominocentesis with peritoneal effusion to confirm peritonitis.
- Gastrointestinal endoscopy or exploratory laparotomy to rule out mechanical obstruction.
- Full-thickness intestinal biopsies are necessary to diagnose intestinal leiomyositis because the disorder affects the muscularis propria layer of the bowel, which is typically not accessible via endoscopic biopsy.
- Spinal radiographs, myelogram, spinal MRI, CT, cerebrospinal fluid (CSF) analysis to identify spinal cord injury.
- Ocular response test with 0.1% pilocarpine and 0.25% physostigmine for dysautonomia.

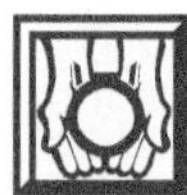

TREATMENT

- Identify and treat primary underlying cause.
- Correct electrolyte abnormalities (especially hypokalemia) if present.

• Use of prokinetic drugs such as cisapride, metoclopramide, or erythromycin should be considered, depending on underlying cause.
• Gastrointestinal decompression of stomach via nasogastric tube is beneficial in select cases.
• Fat-restricted diets should be implemented in dogs with delayed gastric emptying because higher-fat diets can delay gastric emptying in this species.

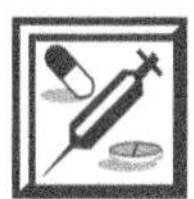

MEDICATIONS

DRUG(S) OF CHOICE

• Metoclopramide is most effective when administered as CRI (1–2 mg/kg/24h); bolus injections (0.4 mg/kg IV q6h) are less effective in light of relatively short half-life (90 min) in dogs; metoclopramide does not affect colonic motility and should be avoided in animals with colonic ileus or megacolon.
• Cisapride (0.5–0.75 mg/kg q8–12h) is a far more potent and effective prokinetic compared to metoclopramide and affects gastric, small intestinal, and colonic motility.
• Erythromycin (1–2 mg/kg PO q12h) has prokinetic activity in stomach and small intestine.
• Cyclosporine (5 mg/kg q12–24h) can be administered for management of intestinal leiomyositis or other immune-mediated disorders affecting intestinal tract.
• Prednisone (1 mg/kg q12h with progressive tapering over 10–12 weeks) can be administered for management of leiomyositis or inflammatory bowel disease.

CONTRAINDICATIONS/POSSIBLE INTERACTIONS

• Anticholinergic drugs (e.g., atropine, glycopyrrolate).
• Opiates (e.g., morphine, hydromorphone, oxymorphone, butorphanol).
• Opiate antidiarrheals (e.g., paregoric, diphenoxylate hydrochloride/atropine sulfate, loperamide hydrochloride).

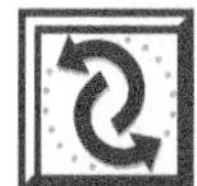

FOLLOW-UP

PATIENT MONITORING

• Monitor and correct electrolyte imbalance if present.
• Abdominal auscultation to evaluate gastrointestinal motility.
• Survey abdominal radiographs to evaluate gastric and intestinal distension.

PREVENTION/AVOIDANCE

Avoid anticholinergic drugs and opiates if not indicated.

POSSIBLE COMPLICATIONS

Animals with adynamic ileus are predisposed to development of intestinal dysbiosis, bacterial translocation, and sepsis.

EXPECTED COURSE AND PROGNOSIS

Prognosis depends on successful resolution of primary disease process.

MISCELLANEOUS

SYNONYMS

• Adynamic ileus—functional ileus, paralytic ileus.
• Pseudo-obstruction—chronic, more segmental adynamic ileus.
• Mechanical ileus—generally addressed in current literature as mechanical obstruction.

PREGNANCY/FERTILITY/BREEDING

Ileus has been reported in a lactating bitch with hypomagnesemia and hypocalcemia.

ABBREVIATIONS

• BIPS = barium-impregnated polyethylene spheres.
• CSF = cerebrospinal fluid

Suggested Reading

Choi M, Seo M, Jung J, et al. Evaluation of canine gastric motility with ultrasonography. J Vet Med Sci 2002, 64(1):17–21.
Couraud L, Jermyn K, Yam PS, et al. Intestinal pseudo-obstruction, lymphocytic leiomyositis and atrophy of the muscularis externa in a dog. Vet Rec 2006, 159(3):86–87.
Guilford WG. Motility disorders of the bowel. In: Guilford WG, Center SA, Strombeck DR, et al. Strombeck's Small Animal Gastroenterology, 3rd ed. Philadelphia, PA: Saunders, 1996, pp. 335–336.
Novellas R, Simpson KE, Gunn-Moore DA, Hammond GJ. Imaging findings in 11 cats with feline dysautonomia. J Feline Med Surg 2010, 12(8):584–591.

Author Stanley L. Marks
Consulting Editor Mark P. Rondeau

ILLICIT/CLUB DRUG TOXICOSIS

BASICS

OVERVIEW

Intoxication with illicit/club drugs includes various pharmaceuticals—barbiturates, benzodiazepines, cocaine, gamma hydroxybutyric acid (GHB), lysergic acid diethylamide (LSD), marijuana, methylenedioxymethamphetamine (MDMA: ecstasy), methamphetamine and other designer amphetamines, opioids, and phencyclidine (PCP).

Pathophysiology

• Barbiturates—sedative hypnotics causing CNS depression. • Cocaine—myocardial stimulant and increases catecholamine and serotonin levels, causing CNS stimulation. • GHB—synthetic γ-aminobutyric acid (GABA) derivative causing CNS depression. • LSD—CNS stimulation and hallucinations by increasing serotonin and glutamate in CNS, binds dopamine and α-adrenergic receptors. • MDMA—increases serotonin and catecholamines in CNS, leading to CNS stimulation and hallucinations. • Opioids—bind to opioid receptors causing CNS depression. • PCP—inhibits glutamate and stimulates α-adrenergic receptors; potentiates effects of norepinephrine, epinephrine, and serotonin; sympathomimetic and hallucinogen.

Systems Affected

• Cardiovascular—cocaine, GHB, LSD, MDMA, PCP: arrhythmias, hypertension; barbiturates, opioids: arrhythmias, hypotension. • Musculoskeletal—cocaine, PCP: tremors. • Nervous—cocaine, LSD, MDMA: stimulation; barbiturates, GHB: depression; opioids, PCP: sedative to stimulatory effects, ataxia. • Ophthalmic—cocaine, LSD, MDMA: mydriasis; opioids: miosis. • Respiratory—barbiturates, opioids: respiratory depression (rare).

SIGNS

• Barbiturates—sedation (rarely agitation), ataxia, bradycardia, hypotension, respiratory depression (rare), coma. • Cocaine—agitation, mydriasis, tachycardia, hypertension, tremors, seizures. • GHB, opioids—lethargy, weakness, coma, respiratory depression. • LSD—mydriasis, disorientation, hallucinations, agitation (rarely sedation), tachycardia. • MDMA—agitation, mydriasis, hyperthermia, tachycardia, tremors, hallucinations, seizures. • PCP—depression to agitation, hypertension, tachycardia, tremors, seizures.

CAUSES & RISK FACTORS

Ingestion of club drugs may occur in animals that live with people who take these pharmaceuticals or in police dogs.

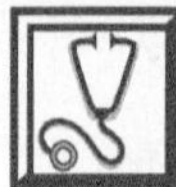

DIAGNOSIS

DIFFERENTIAL DIAGNOSIS

• Barbiturates, GHB, opioids—meningitis, hepatic encephalopathy, ethanol, ethylene glycol, phenothiazines. • Cocaine—amphetamines, caffeine, metaldehyde, MDMA. • LSD, MDMA, PCP—meningitis, hepatic encephalopathy, amphetamines, cocaine, ketamine, psilocybin, serotoninergic medications (selective serotonin reuptake inhibitors, etc.).

CBC/BIOCHEMISTRY/URINALYSIS

No direct abnormalities. May see creatine kinase and K elevation (rhabdomyolysis) and myoglobinuria secondary to tremors.

OTHER LABORATORY TESTS

Over-the-counter illicit urine drug screens available; not approved for use in animals, but appear to be reliable except for marijuana (false negative). GC/MS can detect all, but turnaround time decreases usefulness.

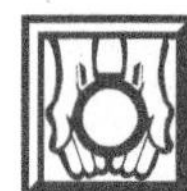

TREATMENT

• Inpatient care in dark quiet place; thermoregulation and fluid therapy to maintain body temperature and BP; fluids will also help to protect kidneys from myoglobinuria. • Monitor for respiratory depression (barbiturates, opioids); intubate and ventilate if needed. • Emesis (if asymptomatic and recent ingestion) or gastric lavage (if large amount ingested).

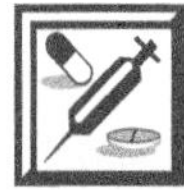

MEDICATIONS

DRUG(S) OF CHOICE

• Activated charcoal (1–2 g/kg PO) with cathartic (if severe signs expected). • Agitation—phenothiazines (acepromazine 0.025–0.05 mg/kg IV, titrate up as needed); cyproheptadine (dog: 1.1 mg/kg; cat: 2–4 mg PO q4–6h or can be given rectally if vomiting). • Agitation, seizures—benzodiazepines (diazepam 0.5–2 mg/kg IV); see Contraindications. • Tremors—methocarbamol (50–150 mg/kg IV). • Tachycardia—propranolol (0.02 mg/kg IV). • Naloxone—reversal for opioids (0.01–0.1 mg/kg IV).

CONTRAINDICATIONS/POSSIBLE INTERACTIONS

Do not use diazepam with MDMA (increases dysphoria and morbidity).

FOLLOW-UP

PATIENT MONITORING

BP, heart rate, urine color—q1h, then less frequently if patient remains stable.

EXPECTED COURSE AND PROGNOSIS

Signs occur within minutes. Most will have a good prognosis if treated and recover in 24–36 hours.

MISCELLANEOUS

PREGNANCY/FERTILITY/BREEDING

• Barbiturates, LSD, cocaine, and MDMA have been associated with severe birth defects. • Opioids and PCP have been associated with fetal intoxication and low birthweight.

SEE ALSO

• Amphetamine and ADD/ADHD Medication Toxicosis.
• Antidepressant Toxicosis—SSRIs and SNRIs.
• Benzodiazepine and Other Sleep Aids Toxicosis.
• Marijuana Toxicosis.

ABBREVIATIONS

• GABA = γ-aminobutyric acid.
• GHB = gamma hydroxybutyric acid.
• LSD = lysergic acid diethylamide.
• MDMA = methylenedioxymethamphetamine, ecstasy.
• PCP = phencyclidine.

Suggested Reading

Klatt CA. Club drugs (MDMA, GHB, flunitrazepam, and bath salts). In: Hovda L, Brutlag A, Poppenga RH, Peterson K, eds., Blackwell's Five-Minute Veterinary Consult Clinical Companion: Small Animal Toxicology, 2nd ed. Ames, IA: Wiley-Blackwell, 2011, pp. 245–252.

Author Tina Wismer
Consulting Editor Lynn R. Hovda

IMIDAZOLINE TOXICOSIS

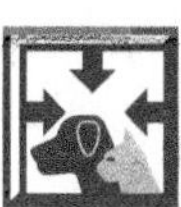

OVERVIEW

- Sympathomimetic drugs used for topical vasoconstrictive effects in ophthalmic anti-redness drops and nasal decongestant sprays.
- Oxymetazoline, naphazoline, tetrahydrozoline, brimonidine, and xylometazoline are imidazolines commonly used in prescription and over-the-counter ophthalmic and nasal products.

Pathophysiology

- Central and peripheral alpha$_2$ adrenergic agonist activity. In overdose, central activity predominates, resulting in norepinephrine release and clinical signs of hypotension, bradycardia, and sedation.
- Companion animal pharmacokinetic data limited. Imidazolines considered to have narrow margin of safety, with no known therapeutic dose in veterinary medicine.
- Absorption rapid and nearly complete when ingested.
- Imidazolines partially metabolized in liver and eliminated mostly unchanged in urine.

Systems Affected

- Cardiovascular—early transient tachycardia and hypertension followed by prolonged bradycardia and hypotension, arrhythmias, pallor, slow capillary refill time.
- Gastrointestinal—vomiting.
- Nervous—sedation, lethargy, ataxia, weakness, tremors, rare seizures, rare paradoxical agitation, coma.
- Ophthalmic—miosis.

SIGNALMENT

Dogs primarily; cats rarely.

SIGNS

- Lethargy and sedation.
- Early transient hypertension and tachycardia transitioning to prolonged bradycardia and hypotension.
- Pallor with prolonged capillary refill time.
- Ataxia.
- Hyperactivity.
- Arrhythmias.
- Vomiting.
- Weakness.
- Miosis.
- Tremors.
- Seizures.
- Coma.
- Death.

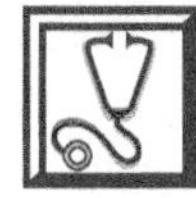

DIAGNOSIS

DIFFERENTIAL DIAGNOSIS

- Other alpha agonist drugs—clonidine, tizanidine, medetomidine, dexmedetomidine, xylazine, amitraz.
- Marijuana, methanol, ethanol.
- Beta adrenergic blocker toxicosis—metoprolol, atenolol, propranolol.
- Calcium channel blocker toxicosis—diltiazem, amlodipine, verapamil.
- Primary cardiac disease with signs of bradycardia and hypotension.

CBC/CHEMISTRY/URINALYSIS

Consider monitoring blood glucose and electrolytes in symptomatic patients.

OTHER LABORATORY TESTS

N/A

DIAGNOSTIC PROCEDURES

- ECG monitoring—arrhythmias, bradycardia vs. tachycardia depending on stage of presentation.
- Blood pressure monitoring—early hypertension vs. later prolonged hypotension.

PATHOLOGIC FINDINGS

N/A

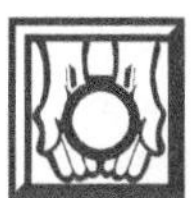

TREATMENT

- Emergency care with any exposure—narrow margin of safety, signs develop at low doses.
- Decontamination—emesis induction is *not* recommended: rapid absorption and early onset of clinical signs; activated charcoal only in asymptomatic animals presenting early.
- IV fluid therapy to correct dehydration and hypotension; IV fluid diuresis not expected to enhance excretion; colloids if no response to crystalloid IV fluid therapy.

MEDICATIONS

DRUG(S) OF CHOICE

- Activated charcoal (1 g/kg PO) with cathartic × 1 dose in asymptomatic patients presenting early (<1–2 hours after ingestion); avoid use in symptomatic patients.
- Alpha$_2$ adrenergic antagonists—atipamezole 50 µg/kg IV/IM may be used to reverse severe sedation and bradycardia; give ¼ dose IV and remainder IM to avoid worsening hypotension; administer additional doses PRN based on clinical signs; alternatively, yohimbine 0.1 mg/kg IV may be used.
- Bradycardia—atropine 0.01–0.02 mg/kg IV PRN; avoid use if hypertensive.
- Hyperactivity—diazepam (0.5–1 mg/kg IV) or butorphanol (0.2–0.8 mg/kg IM/IV) PRN.
- Seizures—diazepam (0.5–1 mg/kg IV) PRN.
- Tremors—diazepam (0.5–1 mg/kg IV) or methocarbamol (50–220 mg/kg IV slowly, up to a daily dose of 330 mg/kg)
- Vomiting—maropitant (1 mg/kg SC/IV q24h) PRN.

Alternative Drugs

Naloxone 0.011–0.022 mg/kg IV/IM PRN may be tried if atipamezole and yohimbine are unavailable. Mechanism of action is unknown, and results may be variable.

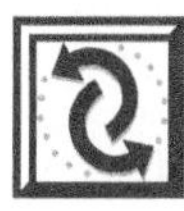

FOLLOW-UP

PATIENT MONITORING

Monitor heart rate, blood pressure, ECG, and temperature closely.

PREVENTION/AVOIDANCE

Keep imidazoline medications secured out of reach to prevent dogs from chewing and ingesting them.

EXPECTED COURSE AND PROGNOSIS

- Expected course—up to 24–36 hours depending on specific product ingested.
- Prognosis is good with appropriate treatment; successfully treated patients are expected to make a full recovery.

MISCELLANEOUS

AGE-RELATED FACTORS

- Animals with decreased renal function may experience prolonged duration of signs.
- Neonates and geriatric pets may be more sensitive.

PREGNANCY/FERTILITY/BREEDING

- Limited data available, but some imidazolines have been shown to pass into milk.
- Very high doses of oxymetazoline have resulted in fetal abnormalities in rats.

Suggested Reading

Waratuke KE. Imidazoline decongestants. In: Hovda LR, Brutlag AG, Osweiler G, Peterson K. The 5 Minute Veterinary Clinical Companion Consult: Small Animal Toxicology, 2nd ed. Ames, IA: Wiley-Blackwell, 2016, pp. 333–338.

Author Charlotte Flint

Consulting Editor Lynn R. Hovda

IMMUNODEFICIENCY DISORDERS, PRIMARY

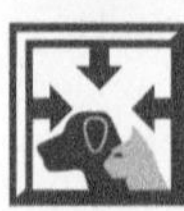

BASICS

DEFINITION

Diminished ability to mount an effective immune response due to heritable defects in the immune system.

PATHOPHYSIOLOGY

- Defects in the cell-mediated, humoral, complement, and phagocytic systems have all been described.
- Defects involving the humoral immune response—associated with a high susceptibility to bacterial infection.
- Defects involving the cell-mediated immune response—associated with a high susceptibility to viral, fungal, and protozoal infections.
- Defects in the phagocytic or complement system—associated with disseminated infection.

SYSTEMS AFFECTED

- Hemic/lymphatic/immune—defect in a specific cell population in lymphoid tissue.
- Skin/exocrine/respiratory/gastrointestinal—chronic or recurrent infections.
- Other organ systems—dissemination of infection, failure to thrive.

GENETICS

Typically breed specific with variable modes of inheritance.

INCIDENCE/PREVALENCE

Rare

SIGNALMENT

Species

Dog and cat.

Breed Predilections

- X-linked severe combined immunodeficiency—basset hounds, Cardigan Welsh corgis.
- Severe combined immunodeficiency disease—Parson Russell terriers.
- Immunoglobulin (Ig) A deficiency—beagles, German shepherd dogs, and Chinese Shar-Peis.
- IgM deficiency—Doberman pinschers
- Thymic hypoplasia—dwarfed Weimaraners.
- Cyclic hematopoiesis—gray collies.
- Chediak-Higashi syndrome—Persian cats.
- Leukocyte adhesion deficiency—Irish setters.
- Complement deficiency—Brittanys.
- Bactericidal defect—Doberman pinschers.
- Transient hypogammaglobulinemia—Samoyeds.

Mean Age and Range

Primary immunodeficiency diseases typically expressed in the first year of life.

Predominant Sex

X-linked recessive severe combined immunodeficiency disease of basset hounds—males affected and females are carriers.

SIGNS

General Comments

Depends on the level at which the immune response is defective; ranges from chronic respiratory and gastrointestinal signs and skin infections to life-threatening conditions.

Historical Findings

- High susceptibility to infection and failure to respond to appropriate conventional antibiotic therapy.
- Lethargy.
- Anorexia.
- Skin infection.
- Failure to thrive.
- Signs often appear when maternal antibody concentrations decline.
- Vaccine-induced disease by modified live virus preparation.

Physical Examination Findings

- Hallmark—failure to thrive.
- Clinical signs attributable to infections.

CAUSES

Congenital

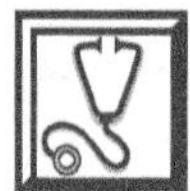

DIAGNOSIS

DIFFERENTIAL DIAGNOSIS

Patients must be rigorously evaluated for underlying disease process that may cause secondary (acquired) immunodeficient state (e.g., hyperadrenocorticism, feline leukemia virus [FeLV], feline immunodeficiency virus [FIV]).

CBC/BIOCHEMISTRY/URINALYSIS

CBC may indicate deficiencies in specifically affected cell lines or show chronic inflammation.

OTHER LABORATORY TESTS

- Serum protein electrophoresis—demonstrate gross deficiency in immunoglobulin concentration.
- Serum immunoglobulin quantitation—evaluate humoral immune system, identify selective immunoglobulin deficiency, support diagnosis of agammaglobulinemia.
- Lymphocyte transformation test—evaluate the cell-mediated immune system and identify animals with T-lymphocyte deficiency.
- Bactericidal assays—evaluate neutrophil function.
- Serum concentration of complement components—diagnose complement deficiency.
- Enumeration of lymphocyte subsets by immunofluorescence with monoclonal antibodies—identify deficiency of specific cell lines.
- Other more specific tests to evaluate immune function in veterinary species are available, but obtaining reliable results generally requires access to research laboratories that perform these tests.

DIAGNOSTIC PROCEDURES

In some patients, bone marrow and lymph node biopsy aids in classifying the type of immune deficiency.

PATHOLOGIC FINDINGS

- Lesions vary depending on the specific defect; most are the result of recurrent or opportunistic infection involving the skin, ear canal, and respiratory and gastrointestinal systems.
- Septicemia common in animals with severe defects.
- T-lymphocyte defects—hypoplastic or dysplastic lesions of the thymus and T-lymphocyte-dependent areas of secondary lymphoid tissues.
- B-lymphocyte defects—hypoplastic or dysplastic lesions of the bone marrow or B-lymphocyte-dependent areas of secondary lymphoid tissues.
- Lymphoid hypoplasia or hyperplasia may be seen, depending on the overall defect and the occurrence of infection.

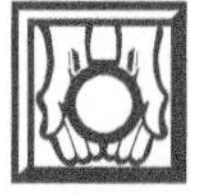

TREATMENT

APPROPRIATE HEALTH CARE

- Hospitalization may be necessary to control life-threatening infection.
- Outpatient management possible for some patients.

NURSING CARE

Supportive care appropriate to the nature of the infection.

ACTIVITY

Determined largely by the severity of the defect and the occurrence of infection.

DIET

- Dietary management may be required to ensure that the patient is maintained at an adequate level of nutrition.
- Potential sources of infectious agents such as raw meat diets must be avoided.

CLIENT EDUCATION

- Inform client that the condition is incurable.
- Discuss why the patient has high susceptibility to infection.
- Discuss and advise as to the heritability of the disease.
- Discuss the possibility of littermates being affected.
- Avoid/limit exposure to animals with infections or kennel situations.

MEDICATIONS

DRUG(S) OF CHOICE

- Antibiotics to control infections; culture and sensitivity testing important in patients with chronic recurrent infections.

- γ-globulin or plasma preparations can be used in conjunction with antibiotics to control infection in patients with humoral defect.
- Symptomatic treatment for secondary diseases.

CONTRAINDICATIONS

γ-globulin or plasma preparations should not be administered to patients with selective IgA deficiency because many affected patients have high concentrations of anti-IgA antibodies and may develop anaphylaxis.

PRECAUTIONS

Modified live virus vaccines should not be administered to patients with suspected T-lymphocyte deficiencies because they may induce disease in these patients.

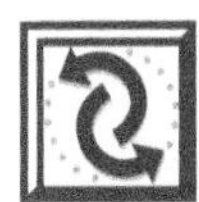

FOLLOW-UP

PATIENT MONITORING

- For clinical signs of secondary infection.
- Routine physical examination to assess efficacy of antibiotic therapy.

PREVENTION/AVOIDANCE

- Do not breed affected animals.
- Pedigree analysis to determine the mode of inheritance and prevent propagating the defect.

POSSIBLE COMPLICATIONS

Infection

EXPECTED COURSE AND PROGNOSIS

- The severity of the defect determines the course and prognosis.
- Patients with minor defects can be successfully managed.

MISCELLANEOUS

ABBREVIATIONS

- FeLV = feline leukemia virus.
- FIV = feline immunodeficiency virus.
- Ig = immunoglobulin.

SEE ALSO

Anaphylaxis

Suggested Reading

Datz CA. Noninfectious causes of immunosuppression in dogs and cats. Vet Clin North Am Small Anim Pract 2010, 40(3):459–467.

Felsburg PJ. Overview of the immune system and immunodeficiency diseases. Vet Clin North Am Small Anim Pract 1994, 24(4):629–653.

Gershwin LJ. Autoimmune diseases in small animals. Vet Clin North Am Small Anim Pract 2010, 40(3):439–457.

Author Paul W. Snyder

Consulting Editor Melinda S. Camus

IMMUNOPROLIFERATIVE ENTEROPATHY OF BASENJIS

BASICS

OVERVIEW

• Immune-mediated disease characterized by progressive, chronic intermittent diarrhea, anorexia, and weight loss, associated with intense lymphoplasmacytic, infiltrative gastroenteritis or enteritis and concurrent evidence of protein-losing enteropathy, malabsorption, and maldigestion.
• Hypergammaglobulinemia present due to increased concentrations of serum immunoglobulin (Ig) A. • Systems affected include gastrointestinal, immune, skin, renal, endocrine.

SIGNALMENT

• Young to middle-aged Basenji—usually <3 years of age. • No sex predilection.
• Related dogs often affected.

SIGNS

Historical Findings

• Chronic intermittent diarrhea. • Severe progressive weight loss. • Anorexia often preceding diarrhea. • Variable vomiting.

Physical Examination Findings

• Attitude—usually bright and alert.
• Bilaterally symmetric alopecia, ulceration of pinna. • Decreased body condition score.
• Ascites, peripheral edema with severe disease.

CAUSES & RISK FACTORS

• Pathogenesis unclear, but interaction between abnormal immune regulation, genetic predisposition, and possibly contribution by environmental factors is hypothesized. • Mode of inheritance not known, but autosomal recessive is suspected.
• Stressful events may exacerbate clinical signs.

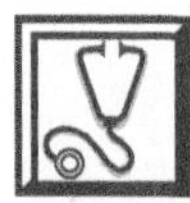

DIAGNOSIS

DIFFERENTIAL DIAGNOSIS

• Lymphangiectasia. • Lymphoplasmacytic enteritis. • Intestinal lymphoma.
• Eosinophilic enteritis. • Antibiotic-responsive diarrhea. • Diet-responsive enteropathy. • Histoplasmosis. • Intestinal parasitism. • Giardiasis. • Exocrine pancreatic insufficiency. • Hypoadrenocorticism. • Hepatobiliary disease.

CBC/BIOCHEMISTRY/URINALYSIS

• Severe hypoalbuminemia.
• Hyperglobulinemia. • Decreased albumin : globulin ratio. • Mature neutrophilia—more severe with advanced disease. • Mild, nonregenerative anemia of chronic disease.
• Moderately increased hepatic enzymes (alanine transaminase [ALT] and aspartate transaminase [AST]) due to reactive hepatopathy.

OTHER LABORATORY TESTS

• Hypergammaglobulinemia due to increased serum IgA. • May have hypergastrinemia and hyperchlorhydria. • May see changes in serum folate or hypocobalaminemia. • No one test or histologic finding definitive or pathognomonic.

IMAGING

Abdominal ultrasound may demonstrate generalized small bowel thickening (4–6 mm) with abnormal gastrointestinal wall layering and a lack of other visceral abnormalities.

DIAGNOSTIC PROCEDURES

• Endoscopic appearance of small bowel usually abnormal, but may be normal; biopsies always required for accurate diagnosis. • Genetic testing (DNA) not available at this time.

PATHOLOGIC FINDINGS

• Consistent pathologic lesions include uniform thickening of small bowel, generalized lymphoplasmacytic infiltration of intestinal lamina propria, lacteal dilation, crypt abscesses, and blunting and fusion of villous tips. • May be gastric rugal fold hypertrophy, lymphocytic gastritis, oxyntic gland hyperplasia, and/or gastric mucosal atrophy. • Presence and severity of gastric lesions do not correlate with severity of intestinal lesions. • Other associated lesions include thyroid parafollicular cell atrophy, ulceration of pinna, gastric acinar atrophy, and glomerulonephritis.

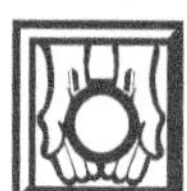

TREATMENT

• Outpatient medical management unless dehydration or other severe complications exist. • Advise clients not to breed affected dogs or their littermates. • Minimize stressful episodes. • Use dietary trials (ideally fat-restricted, highly digestible diets) to determine what diet is best tolerated.

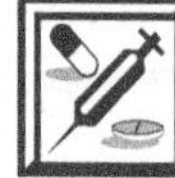

MEDICATIONS

DRUG(S) OF CHOICE

Immunosuppressive/Anti-inflammatory Drugs

• Variable success reported, but considered mainstay of treatment. • Prednisone—2 mg/kg PO q24h for 2–4 weeks, then slowly taper over 3–4 months to achieve 0.5–1 mg/kg PO q48h or lowest effective dose.
• Chlorambucil—0.25 mg/kg PO q72h with monitoring for adverse effects, or other immunosuppressive medications can be tried.

Antibiotics

• Trials of antibiotics are variably helpful for affected individuals that may have antibiotic-responsive diarrhea.
• Metronidazole—10 mg/kg PO q12h.
• Tylosin—10–20 mg/kg PO q12h.

Nutritional Supplements/Adjunctive Treatment

Use of probiotics is commonly advised and may favor reduced risk of dysbiosis and lowered state of inflammatory responses by gut-associated lymphoid tissues, but no specific data available to support this hypothesis.

CONTRAINDICATIONS/POSSIBLE INTERACTIONS

Anticholinergics contraindicated.

FOLLOW-UP

• Diarrhea and weight loss usually show initial improvement with treatment, but recurrence of signs is common. • Long-term prognosis is poor over course of months to a few years.

MISCELLANEOUS

ABBREVIATIONS

• ALT = alanine transaminase.
• AST = aspartate transaminase.
• Ig = immunoglobulin.

Suggested Reading

MacLachlan NJ, Breitschwerdt EB, Chambers JM, et al. Gastroenteritis of Basenji dogs. Vet Pathol 1988, 25(1):36–41.
Spohr A, Koch J, Jensen AL. Ultrasonographic findings in a Basenji with immunoproliferative enteropathy. J Small Anim Pract 1995, 36:79–82.

Author Megan McClosky
Consulting Editor Mark P. Rondeau

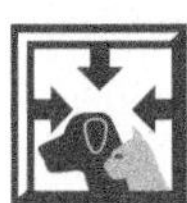

BASICS

DEFINITION

Inability to retain feces or generate a coordinated and appropriate act of defecation.

PATHOPHYSIOLOGY

• The colon, rectum, and anus are primary sites of function in normal defecation.
• Coordinated contractions of the circular and longitudinal smooth muscle of the colon result in orderly accumulation of fecal matter, which is stored in the descending colon. • Intense propulsive activity down the length of the colon, called mass movement, is stimulated by the autonomic nervous system and moves fecal matter toward the anus. • The internal anal sphincter is composed of smooth muscles while the external anal sphincter is composed of striated muscle; parasympathetic innervation to the internal sphincter is provided by the pelvic nerves via the sacral segments (S1–S3); sympathetic innervation is provided by the hypogastric nerves via the lumbar segments (L1–L4); parasympathetic stimulation leads to relaxation of the internal sphincter and contraction of the rectum, whereas sympathetic stimulation leads to contraction of the internal sphincter and relaxation of the rectum; the striated muscles of the external anal sphincter are under conscious control via the caudal rectal nerve (a branch of the pudendal nerve).
• Neurogenic sphincter incompetence can be caused by damage or denervation of the pudendal nerve, lesions that cause lumbar or sacral spinal segment dysfunction, autonomic dysfunction, or generalized peripheral neuropathy or myopathy. • Non-neurogenic sphincter incompetence is caused by damage to the anal sphincters. • Damage to, or degeneration of, the levator ani and coccygeus muscles may also contribute to fecal incontinence. • Reservoir fecal incontinence develops when disease processes reduce the capacity or compliance of the rectum; the patient is aware of the need to defecate, but sphincter control is overwhelmed by fecal volume or spastic colorectal/anal disease.

SYSTEMS AFFECTED

• Gastrointestinal (GI).
• Neurologic.

GENETICS

N/A

INCIDENCE/PREVALENCE

Unknown

GEOGRAPHIC DISTRIBUTION

N/A

SIGNALMENT

Species

Dog and cat.

Breed Predilections

N/A

Mean Age and Range

Increased incidence in older patients.

Predominant Sex

N/A

SIGNS

Historical Findings

• Reservoir incontinence—urge to defecate; frequent, conscious defecation; defecation may be associated with tenesmus or dyschezia.
• Sphincter incontinence—involuntary expulsion or dribbling of fecal material, especially during excitement or barking and coughing. • History of neurologic signs, anorectal surgery, and/or trauma. • Concurrent urinary incontinence suggests neurogenic sphincter incontinence.

Physical Examination Findings

• Reservoir incontinence—anorectal sensitivity or pain on digital palpation, rectal mass or thickening of rectal mucosa; external anal sphincter tone and perineal reflex are normal.
• Non-neurogenic sphincter incontinence—evidence of perineal trauma or perianal fistulae; anal reflex is present, but external anal sphincter may not be completely closed if sphincter has been anatomically disrupted.
• Neurogenic sphincter incontinence—loss of tone to external anal sphincter; perineal reflex is absent or diminished. • Neurologic examination findings may include lumbosacral pain, paraparesis, paraplegia, decreased postural reactions, hopping, paw placements, normal to decreased reflexes (patellar, withdrawal, perineal reflex), or absent nociception in perineum or tail. • Diffuse lower motor neuron (LMN) signs suggest generalized peripheral neuropathy or myopathy; these are rare causes of fecal incontinence in small animals.

CAUSES

Reservoir Incontinence

• Colorectal disease—colitis, irritable bowel syndrome, and neoplasia. • Diarrhea—large volumes of feces from any cause can overwhelm the absorptive and storage capacity of the colon.

Non-neurogenic Sphincter Incontinence

• Traumatic anal injuries. • Neoplasia.
• Iatrogenic—complication of anorectal surgery. • Anorectal or perianal diseases—e.g., perianal fistulae. • Mucocutaneous diseases—e.g., immune-mediated, infectious.

Neurogenic Sphincter Incontinence

• Iatrogenic—traumatic nerve injury as postoperative complication. • Diseases affecting dorsal funiculus (L4 and cranial). • Spinal cord—arachnoid diverticulum, arachnoid cysts, spinal malformations, syringomyelia, trauma, intervertebral disc disease, neoplasia, infectious or inflammatory meningomyelitis, fibrocartilaginous embolism, myelomalacia.
• Degenerative lumbosacral stenosis—L6–L7 or L7–S1, intervertebral disc disease, severe spondylosis deformans, synovial cysts, ligamentous hypertrophy, lumbosacral instability, neoplasia. • Peripheral neuropathy—infectious, endocrine/metabolic, immune-mediated, drug-induced (e.g., vincristine), dysautonomia, idiopathic. • Diffuse neuromuscular diseases—neuropathies, junctionopathies, myopathies (LMN unit).
• Degeneration (aging)—multiple factors likely involved, including atrophy of muscles involved in fecal continence, weakness, degenerative neuropathy, cognitive dysfunction.

RISK FACTORS

• Colonic disease. • Anorectal disease and surgery. • Neurologic disease.

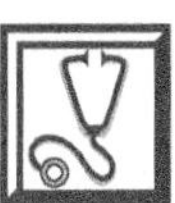

DIAGNOSIS

DIFFERENTIAL DIAGNOSIS

• Primary GI disease can increase urge to defecate; these animals typically attempt to go outside to defecate, or posture to defecate.
• Behavioral disorders (e.g., separation anxiety) often associated with destructive activities or excessive vocalization. • Inadequate house training usually occurs in young dogs or dogs recently introduced to indoor environment or in cats with litter box aversion.

CBC/BIOCHEMISTRY/URINALYSIS

Usually unremarkable.

OTHER LABORATORY TESTS

• Thyroid testing. • If junctionopathy suspected, consider submitting acetylcholine receptor antibody titers. • If polymyositis suspected, submit *Toxoplasma* and *Neospora* titers. • Rectal scraping for cytology is indicated in regions where *Heterobilharzia*, histoplasmosis, or pythiosis is endemic; rectal cytology may also indicate presence of neoplasia. • Zinc sulfate flotation tests and fecal PCR, ELISA, or culture to detect *Giardia* sp., *Tritrichomonas* (cats), and other parasitic, bacterial, viral, and protozoal infections. • Serum trypsin-like immunoreactivity to rule out exocrine pancreatic insufficiency. • Serum cobalamin and folate concentrations to investigate small intestinal malabsorptive disease.

IMAGING

• Lateral and ventrodorsal survey radiography of lumbosacral spine may show evidence of intervertebral disc extrusion, spondylosis deformans, discospondylitis, vertebral neoplasia, lumbosacral trauma, or vertebral malformations. • Abdominal ultrasound, barium radiographic studies, and CT may help identify masses or intestinal lining abnormalities. • MRI is optimum diagnostic tool to demonstrate specific spinal cord and brain lesions. • CT with IV contrast or CT with myelography may also demonstrate compressive lesions within spinal canal.

INCONTINENCE, FECAL (CONTINUED)

DIAGNOSTIC PROCEDURES

• Full-thickness or endoscopic GI biopsies if diarrhea present. • Colonoscopy and colorectal mucosal biopsy if reservoir incontinence suspected. • Electromyography/nerve conduction studies. • Muscle and nerve biopsy for myopathy and peripheral neuropathy. • Analysis of cerebrospinal fluid (CSF) may reveal evidence of CNS infectious or inflammatory process, neoplasia, or trauma.

PATHOLOGIC FINDINGS

Dependent on underlying disease.

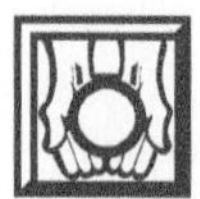

TREATMENT

APPROPRIATE HEALTH CARE

Inpatient vs. outpatient depends on underlying disease.

NURSING CARE

• In recumbent patients or patients with difficulty ambulating and fecal incontinence, nursing care is of paramount importance. • To prevent decubital ulcers, rotate recumbency every 2–4 hours and utilize a water bed. • Soiled bed should be changed immediately, and soiled hair coat and skin should be washed with gentle soap and warm water and dried thoroughly. • Occasional warm water enemas will diminish volume of feces in colon and may decrease incidence of inappropriate defecation. • Reflex defecation may be stimulated by applying warm washcloth to anus or perineum. • Physical therapy options include massage, passive range of motion exercises, and assisted walking; hydrotherapy, thermal therapies, and acupuncture may be considered when appropriate.

ACTIVITY

Animal should be encouraged to go outside to urinate and defecate every 4–6 hours. Sling walking may be necessary.

DIET

Fecal volume can be reduced by feeding low-residue commercial diets or foods such as cottage cheese and rice. Feed pet at established times to better control times needed to defecate.

CLIENT EDUCATION

• Prognosis for recovery of function is poor if underlying cause cannot be identified and successfully corrected; discuss prognosis with client early in evaluation to avoid unrealistic expectations. • Environmental changes (e.g., providing designated area that is easy to clean) may increase client satisfaction and thus avoid euthanasia of otherwise healthy animal.

SURGICAL CONSIDERATIONS

Fascial slings, silicone elastomer slings, and other surgical techniques to repair external anal sphincter or improve anorectal angulation have been attempted with low success rates.

MEDICATIONS

DRUG(S) OF CHOICE

• Diphenoxylate (0.1–0.2 mg/kg PO q12h) and loperamide (0.1–0.2 mg/kg PO q8–12h) are opiate motility-modifying drugs; they inhibit GI motility, thus increasing the amount of water absorbed from the feces. • Anti-inflammatory agents, such as glucocorticoids, metronidazole, and sulfasalazine (dogs only), may benefit patients with suspected reservoir incontinence due to inflammatory bowel disease or colitis. • Improvement in signs may be achieved if specific therapy for perianal fistulae, colitis, or other reservoir or non-neurogenic causes of incontinence can be given, but there are no specific drugs effective in patients with neurogenic incontinence.

CONTRAINDICATIONS

• Do not use motility-modifying drugs in patients if infectious or toxigenic cause of diarrhea is suspected. • Do not use opiate motility modifiers in debilitated patients, or patients with impaired liver or renal function. • Do not use diets containing high concentrations of insoluble fibers as this will produce large, bulky stool that is difficult to pass or may cause obstipation.

PRECAUTIONS

• Opiate motility-modifying drugs may cause sedation. • Use loperamide with caution in patients with p-glycoprotein defects.

POSSIBLE INTERACTIONS

Increased sedation and respiratory depression are possible when opiates are used concurrently with other CNS depressants (e.g., barbiturates, tranquilizers).

ALTERNATIVE DRUG(S)

N/A

FOLLOW-UP

PATIENT MONITORING

• If fecal incontinence is due to underlying neurologic cause, use serial neurologic examinations to monitor patient progress. • Radiographic procedures, electromyography, CSF analysis, and MRI can also be used to follow progress. • Check fecal consistency and volume and make sure pet does not become constipated or obstipated. • Examine perianal skin and hair coat to ensure there is no fecal matter and secondary inflammation or infection. • Adjust diet to find appropriate therapy for each individual patient.

PREVENTION/AVOIDANCE

N/A

POSSIBLE COMPLICATIONS

Neurogenic sphincter incontinence is often unresponsive despite appropriate dietary, medical, and surgical treatment.

EXPECTED COURSE AND PROGNOSIS

50% of pets with fecal incontinence were euthanized in a recent study.

MISCELLANEOUS

ASSOCIATED CONDITIONS

N/A

AGE-RELATED FACTORS

N/A

ZOONOTIC POTENTIAL

• Exposure to animal feces increases risk of exposure to zoonotic parasites. • Advise clients about zoonotic diseases (e.g., salmonellosis, cutaneous and visceral larval migrans, and toxoplasmosis).

PREGNANCY/FERTILITY/BREEDING

N/A

SYNONYMS

N/A

ABBREVIATIONS

• CSF = cerebrospinal fluid.
• GI = gastrointestinal.
• LMN = lower motor neuron.

Suggested Reading

de Lahunta A, Glass E, Kent M. Lower motor neuron: spinal nerve general somatic efferent system. In: de Lahunta A, Glass E, Kent M, Veterinary Neuroanatomy and Clinical Neurology, 4th ed. St. Louis, MO: Elsevier Saunders, 2015, pp. 102–161.

Foley P. Constipation, tenesmus, dyschezia, and fecal incontinence. In: Ettinger SJ, Feldman EC, Côté E, eds. Textbook of Veterinary Internal Medicine, 8th ed. St. Louis, MO: Elsevier Saunders, 2017, pp. 171–174.

Schermerhorn T. Gastrointestinal endocrinology. In: Ettinger SJ, Feldman EC, Côté E, eds. Textbook of Veterinary Internal Medicine, 8th ed. St. Louis, MO: Elsevier Saunders, 2017, pp. 1833–1838.

Washabau RJ. Dysmotility/fecal incontinence. In: Washabau RJ, Day MJ, eds., Canine and Feline Gastroenterology. St. Louis, MO: Elsevier Saunders, 2013, pp. 791–798.

Author Andrea Wang Munk

Consulting Editor Mark P. Rondeau

Acknowledgment The author and book editors acknowledge the prior contribution of Debra L. Zoran.

Client Education Handout available online

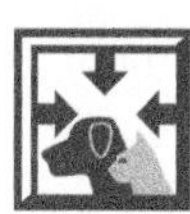

BASICS

DEFINITION

Loss of voluntary control of micturition, usually observed as involuntary urine leakage.

PATHOPHYSIOLOGY

Most commonly a disorder of the storage phase of micturition, resulting from impaired urethral sphincter mechanism, detrusor hyperreflexia, or poor bladder compliance. Congenital malformations such as ectopic ureters or urethral malformation can also cause incontinence. Overflow incontinence can result from partial or complete functional urethral obstruction or bladder atony.

SYSTEMS AFFECTED

- Renal/urogenital.
- Nervous.
- Skin—urine scald, perineal and ventral dermatitis.

INCIDENCE/PREVALENCE

Urinary incontinence may affect up to 20% of female spayed dogs and up to 30% of those weighing over 20 kg.

SIGNALMENT

- Dog and rarely cat.
- Most common in spayed female dogs.
- More common in dogs >20 kg.
- Overflow incontinence most common in young to middle-aged, large- to giant-breed male dogs.

CAUSES

Anatomic

- Congenital abnormality of the urethral sphincter mechanism.
- Ectopic ureters that terminate in the bladder neck, urethra, vestibule, or vagina.
- Shortened (hypoplastic) urethra.
- Ureterovaginal hypoplasia/aplasia (cats).
- Cystic hypoplasia.
- Patent urachal remnant.
- Intrapelvic bladder interfering with abdominal pressure transmission to the proximal urethra.
- Vestibular or vulvar conformational abnormalities contributing to urine pooling and leakage.

Neurologic

- Central or peripheral lower motor neuron injury to the sacral spinal cord and pudendal nerve leading to weak urethral closure and flaccid bladder.
- Overflow incontinence secondary to upper motor injury of the thoracolumbar spinal cord and loss of inhibitory signaling to the urethral sphincter.
- Dysautonomia leading to urine retention and overflow incontinence.
- Damage to local reflex arc allowing for relaxation of the urethral sphincter when the detrusor contracts.
- Lesions of the cerebellum or cerebral micturition center affecting inhibition and voluntary control of voiding, resulting in frequent involuntary urination or leakage of small amounts of urine.
- Feline leukemia virus–associated myelopathy leading to progressive paresis or paralysis.

Urinary Bladder Dysfunction

- Bladder atony leading to incomplete voiding and overflow incontinence.
- Bladder overdistension with loss of cellular tight junctions and incomplete contractile signal transmission.
- Bladder fibrosis leading to poor compliance and decreased storage capacity.
- Detrusor hyperreflexia (overactive bladder) and poor compliance.

Urethral Disorders

- Congenital or acquired urethral sphincter mechanism incompetence (most common).
- Functional outlet obstruction leading to overflow incontinence (detrusor urethral dyssynergia).
- Mechanical outflow obstruction from enlarged prostate, benign or malignant neoplasia, urolith, foreign body, or external compression.

Urine Retention

Overflow incontinence when intravesicular pressure exceeds outlet resistance.

Mixed Urinary Incontinence

Any combination of factors in dogs and cats leading to involuntary urine loss. Not typically defined in the way human mixed urinary incontinence is (overactive bladder and stress incontinence).

RISK FACTORS

- Large-breed (>20 kg) spayed female dog.
- Early spay (<12 weeks).
- Breed predispositions are possible.
- Intrapelvic bladder.
- Urogenital conformational abnormalities affecting bladder neck, urethral length, or vestibule.
- Other possible risk factors include obesity, tail-docking, and polyuria.

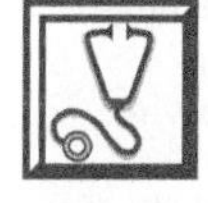

DIAGNOSIS

DIFFERENTIAL DIAGNOSIS

- Voluntary inappropriate urination.
- Pollakiuria.
- Prostatic or vaginal discharge.
- Polyuria—may worsen minor incontinence because of increased pressure on already weakened urethral sphincter mechanism.

CBC/BIOCHEMISTRY/URINALYSIS

- Hematology and serum biochemistry are indicated in patients with polyuria and polydipsia.
- CBC and serum biochemistry are usually normal unless comorbidities exist.
- Urinalysis frequently normal.
- Urine sediment may indicate urinary tract infection or polyuria.

OTHER LABORATORY TESTS

- Urine culture may be indicated if clinical signs (straining to urinate, pollakiuria) and urine sediment (pyuria, bacteriuria, hematuria) are consistent with urinary tract infection.
- Cats should be tested for feline leukemia virus.
- Additional testing for causes of polyuria and polydipsia may be indicated based on serum biochemistry and urinalysis results.

IMAGING

Radiographic Findings

- Plain radiography may identify a pelvically placed bladder.
- Intravenous contrast excretory urography may identify dilated or ectopic ureters; however, careful attention must be paid to proper technique and the sensitivity of the imaging is inferior to other methods.
- Retrograde contrast vaginourethrography may reveal congenital abnormalities of the vagina, urethra, and vestibule, and occasionally ectopic ureters.
- Single- or double-contrast cystourethrography allows for accurate assessment of bladder position and urethral length.
- Imaging of the dog or cat with acquired urethral sphincter mechanism incompetence, the most common cause of acquired urinary incontinence, is usually normal.

Ultrasonographic Findings

- Ultrasound assessment may detect ureteral dilation or ectopic ureters; however, the sensitivity is very operator dependent.
- Allows for evaluation of kidneys, bladder, and prostate.

CT Findings

CT excretory urography is currently the imaging modality of choice to diagnose ectopic ureters.

DIAGNOSTIC PROCEDURES

- Neurologic examination—tail tone, anal tone, perineal reflexes and sensation, and bulbospongiosus reflexes.
- Orthopedic examination—determination of pain or difficulty posturing to urinate, which can lead to urine retention.
- Urethral catheterization—to determine patency of urethra and residual urine volume in patients with suspected urine retention and overflow incontinence.
- Cystoscopy—evaluates urethra and bladder as well as visualization of position and shape of ureteral openings.
- Urodynamic assessment—may document decreased urethral pressure or detrusor hyperreflexia; limited availability at some specialty clinics.

INCONTINENCE, URINARY (CONTINUED)

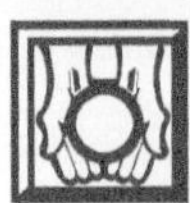

TREATMENT

APPROPRIATE HEALTH CARE

- Usually outpatient.
- Medical therapy is primary treatment for patients with urethral sphincter mechanism incompetence.
- Urinary tract infection should be treated appropriately if identified.
- Address partial urethral obstructive and neurologic disorders if identified.
- Ectopic ureters should be corrected either by cystoscopic laser ablation if intramural (common) or surgery if extramural (rare).
- Anatomic disorders should be identified and corrected if possible.
- Functional abnormalities of the bladder or urethra may require medical treatment.
- Bulking agents such as bovine cross-linked collagen may be injected into urethral submucosa, or surgical salvage procedures such as placement of urethral hydraulic occluder if urethral sphincter incompetence not responsive to medical therapy.

MEDICATIONS

DRUG(S) OF CHOICE

Urethral Sphincter Mechanism Incompetence

- Alpha-adrenergic agonist treatment (e.g., phenylpropanolamine 1–2 mg/kg PO q8–12h) or estrogen compounds (e.g., estriol 2 mg/dog PO q24h for 2 weeks, then decrease dose q2 weeks to lowest effective dose; diethylstilbestrol 0.1–1 mg/dog PO q24h for 5–7 days, then 0.1–1 mg/dog q5–7 days PRN).
- Phenylpropanolamine and estrogens may be used in combination in spayed females and may have a synergistic effect.
- Imipramine (5–15 mg/dog PO q12h), a tricyclic antidepressant with cholinergic and alpha-agonist effects, may be of use if other medical therapy fails, especially if detrusor hyperreflexia is suspected as well.
- Testosterone cypionate (2.2 mg/kg IM q30–45 days) may be used in males with urethral sphincter mechanism incompetence; however, its efficacy is far below phenylpropanolamine.

Detrusor Hyperreflexia

Antimuscarinic agents (oxybutynin chloride 0.2–0.3 mg/kg PO q8–12h or 1.25–5 mg/dog PO q8–12h; imipramine 5–15 mg/dog PO q12h).

Functional Outflow Obstruction

See Urinary Tract Obstruction.

CONTRAINDICATIONS

- Do not use estrogens in males or intact females.
- Do not use alpha agonists in patients with hypertension, and use with caution in patients with conditions that predispose to hypertension.
- Do not use anticholinergics in patients with glaucoma or cardiac disease.

PRECAUTIONS

- Adrenergic agonists can cause hypertension, changes in appetite, and restlessness.
- Adverse effects of estrogen use include vulvar swelling, mammary development, and attractiveness to males; these are usually dose dependent and will subside with dose reduction; always use the lowest effective dose.
- Bone marrow suppression is extremely rare secondary to estrogen use at the recommended doses.
- Testosterone use can lead to signs of aggression and increased libido in males.
- Anticholinergic agents can cause nausea, vomiting, and constipation.

POSSIBLE INTERACTIONS

- Do not administer tricyclic antidepressants concurrently with monoamine oxidase inhibitors (e.g., amitriptyline, clomipramine, imipramine).
- Hypertensive risk increases with concurrent use of alpha agonists and tricyclic antidepressants.

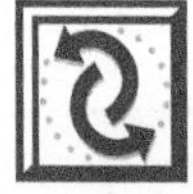

FOLLOW-UP

PATIENT MONITORING

- Monitor blood pressure periodically in patients receiving alpha agonists.
- Monitor vulvar and mammary swelling in patients receiving estrogen treatment.
- Monitor prostate size in males receiving testosterone.
- Once continence is achieved, gradually reduce to lowest effective dose.
- Perform urine cultures to guide treatment and prevent resistance of symptomatic urinary tract infections.

POSSIBLE COMPLICATIONS

- Hypertension.
- Recurrent and resistant urinary tract infections.
- Urine scald and perineal (females) or ventral abdominal (males) dermatitis.
- Refractory incontinence.

MISCELLANEOUS

ASSOCIATED CONDITIONS

- Urinary tract infection.
- Hydroureter and hydronephrosis in some ectopic ureter patients, even after correction.

PREGNANCY/FERTILITY/BREEDING

Dogs with congenital anomalies such as ectopic ureters should be removed from the breeding population.

SYNONYMS

- Hormone-responsive incontinence.
- Enuresis.

SEE ALSO

- Polyuria and Polydipsia.
- Urinary Retention, Functional.
- Urinary Tract Obstruction.

Suggested Reading

Acierno M, Labato M. Canine incontinence. Vet Clin North Am Small Anim Pract 2019, 49(2):125–140.

Byron J, Taylor K, Phillips G, Stahl M. Urethral sphincter mechanism incompetence in 163 neutered female dogs: diagnosis, treatment, and relationship of weight and age at neuter to development of disease. J Vet Intern Med 2017, 31(2):442–448.

Author Julie K. Byron

Consulting Editor J.D. Foster

Acknowledgment The author and book editors acknowledge the prior contribution of Jo R. Smith.

Client Education Handout available online

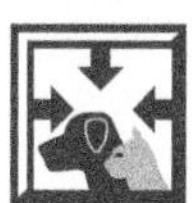

BASICS

DEFINITION

Abnormal cycling, copulation failure, conception failure, or pregnancy loss in bitches.

PATHOPHYSIOLOGY

- Normal fertility—requires normal estrous cyclicity with ovulation of normal ova into a patent, healthy reproductive tract; fertilization by normal spermatozoa; implantation of the conceptus into the endometrium; formation of the normal placenta; and maintenance of pregnancy in the presence of high progesterone concentration throughout the approximately 2-month gestation.
- Breakdown in any of these processes causes infertility.

SYSTEMS AFFECTED

Reproductive

SIGNALMENT

- Animals of all ages; more common in old animals.
- Dogs >6 years old—more likely to have underlying cystic endometrial hyperplasia; may be predisposed to uterine infection and failure of conception or implantation.
- Breeds predisposed to hypothyroidism—may have higher prevalence; include golden retrievers, Doberman pinschers, dachshunds, Irish setters, miniature schnauzers, Great Danes, poodles, and boxers.

SIGNS

Historical Findings

- Failure to cycle.
- Failure to cycle normally—shortened interestrous interval (interval of 4 months or less).
- Failure to copulate, poor semen quality, or lack of functional spermatozoa in the male.
- Failure to become pregnant and/or maintain pregnancy after normal copulation.
- Persistent estrus (>3 weeks).

Physical Examination Findings

- Negative pregnancy exam after mating.
- Positive pregnancy with no subsequent parturition.

CAUSES

- Insemination at the improper time in the estrous cycle—most common.
- Subclinical uterine infection.
- Cystic endometrial hyperplasia.
- Male infertility factors.
- Hypothyroidism.
- Hypercortisolism.
- Anatomic abnormality.
- Chromosomal abnormality.
- Abnormal ovarian function.
- Previous ovariectomy, hysterectomy, or ovariohysterectomy.
- *Brucella canis* infection.
- Silent estrus.

RISK FACTORS

- *B. canis.*
- Hypothyroidism.
- Hypercortisolism—endogenous or exogenous.
- Systemic viral infection—canine herpesvirus.
- Any chronic, debilitating disease.
- Congenital vaginal anomaly.
- Old age.

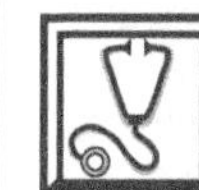

DIAGNOSIS

DIFFERENTIAL DIAGNOSIS

Historical Information

- Extremely useful in distinguishing causes.
- Is the patient cycling?
  - Primary anestrus = no overt estrous cycle by 2 years of age.
  - Secondary anestrus = no overt estrous cycle within 1 year of a normal cycle.
- Has the patient conceived or given birth in the past? If so, how recently? Litter size? Percentage of stillbirths? Percentage of litter weaned?
- Is the patient free of systemic viral or protozoal infection?
- Is the patient capable of normal copulation?
- Was the patient bred to a male of proven fertility (i.e., litter whelped within previous 6 months) at the proper time of the estrous cycle?
- Did the patient ovulate during the estrous cycle and maintain progesterone concentration consistent with pregnancy during the entire gestation?
- Is the bitch euthyroid?

CBC/BIOCHEMISTRY/URINALYSIS

Usually normal.

OTHER LABORATORY TESTS

Serologic Test for *B. canis* (Dogs)

- Rapid slide agglutination test—used as a screen; sensitive but not specific.
- If positive results—recommend recheck by an agar gel immunodiffusion test, bacterial culture, or PCR of whole blood or lymph node aspirate.

Serum Progesterone Measurement

- Should remain high throughout gestation.
- If concentration <2 ng/mL in mid-gestation and pregnancy loss occurs, insufficient luteal function indicated (hypoluteodism); see Abortion, Spontaneous (Early Pregnancy Loss)—Dogs, and Premature Labor.
- Concentration >2 ng/mL—may indicate diestrus, silent heat (estrus with no overt behavioral or physical changes), or pathologic production of progesterone from a luteal ovarian structure, functional ovarian neoplasm, or the adrenal gland.
- Quantitative (chemiluminescence, fluorescence, enzyme immunoassay) progesterone assay is important to detect levels <2.0 ng/mL; rapid in-hospital assays are least accurate between 2 and 5 ng/mL.
- Progesterone may be measured during proestrus and estrus to predict ovulation time and optimize breeding management.
- Concentration and ovulation:
  - 1–1.9 ng/mL, probable ovulation in 3 days (recheck).
  - 2–2.9 ng/mL, ovulation in 2 days.
  - 3–3.9 ng/mL, ovulation in 1 day.
  - 4–10 ng/mL, ovulation that day.
- Optimal breeding day for single breeding to produce maximum litter size—2 days after ovulation.
- Day of ovulation from onset of proestrus or estrus extremely variable; not well correlated with standing behavior (see Breeding, Timing).

Other Tests

- Bacterial culture for uterine organisms—vaginal discharge originating in the uterus during proestrus or estrus is collected directly by hysterotomy or transcervical catheterization, or indirectly from the anterior vagina using a guarded swab.
- Thyroid hormone testing—resting serum concentration of T_3 or T_4 and thyroid stimulating hormone (TSH).
- Serologic testing—canine herpesvirus; see Abortion, Spontaneous (Early Pregnancy Loss)—Dogs.
- Karyotype—performed on patients with primary or persistent anestrus; can identify chromosomal abnormalities that can cause abnormal sexual differentiation.
- Serum cortisol concentration—if the resting serum cortisol is high, the underlying cause should be identified; see Hyperadrenocorticism (Cushing's Syndrome)—Dogs.
- Semen evaluation—direct evaluation to rule out oligospermia or azoospermia; alternatively, may test-breed the male to another female to prove fertility; rule out azoospermia in tomcat by finding spermatozoa in a vaginal flush or swab specimens from the queen or in urine collected by cystocentesis from the tom; see Infertility, Male—Dogs.
- Serum anti-Müllerian hormone/progesterone, luteinizing hormone (LH)/estrogen for determination of ovarian presence; see Ovarian Remnant Syndrome.

IMAGING

- Radiography—normal ovaries and a nongravid uterus usually not visible with radiography; large ovaries may indicate cystic ovarian disease or neoplasia; visible uterus may indicate cystic endometrial hyperplasia.
- Ultrasound—may diagnose pregnancy as early as 20–24 days after ovulation; useful for documenting pregnancy loss; useful for detecting suspected cystic ovarian or neoplastic ovarian disease, cystic endometrial hyperplasia,

and intraluminal fluid; may be difficult to image normal ovaries and nongravid uterus—operator dependent.

• Positive-contrast procedures—vaginography; hysterography; performed prepuberally or when the patient is in estrus; may reveal anatomic abnormality (e.g., abnormal structure and impatency); see Vaginal Malformations and Acquired Lesions.

DIAGNOSTIC PROCEDURES

I

• Laparotomy—assess anatomy of the tubular tract and gonads.

• Hysterotomy—to obtain a direct uterine culture specimen; biopsy of the uterus or ovaries.

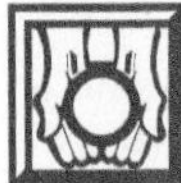

TREATMENT

• Heritable cause (e.g., thyroid insufficiency)—counsel owner regarding removing the patient from the breeding program.

• Surgical resection of vaginal anomalies—may ease natural service and vaginal delivery of pups.

• Surgical repair of impatent tubular tract—difficult procedure; prognosis for future fertility guarded.

• Surgical drainage of ovarian cysts—efficacy unknown.

• Unilateral ovariectomy of neoplastic ovary—future fertility depends on resumption of normal function of the remaining ovary and lack of metastasis.

• Estrus suppression for one to two estrous cycles may benefit bitches with short interestrous interval (4 months or less).

• Better breeding management—good prognosis for future fertility, unless other condition present (more guarded prognosis).

MEDICATIONS

DRUG(S) OF CHOICE

• Antibiotics—for uterine infection; choice depends on bacterial culture and sensitivity of the uterus or of vaginal discharge during proestrus or estrus.

• L-thyroxine—for thyroid insufficiency; dogs: 0.01–0.02 mg/kg PO q12h; prognosis for future fertility with return to euthyroid state guarded.

Gonadotropin Therapy

• For induction of ovulation.

• Gonadotropin-releasing hormone (GnRH), which causes release of endogenous LH from the pituitary, or human chorionic gonadotropin (hCG), which has LH-like activity.

• Ovarian cystic disease—GnRH (50 μg/dog IM) or hCG (1,000 IU/dog half IV/half IM); causes ovulation or luteinization of cystic ovarian tissue.

• Estrus induction—diethylstilbestrol (5 mg PO q24h for 9 days or until signs of proestrus induced); bromocriptine (20 μg/kg PO q12h for 21 days); cabergoline (5 μg/kg PO q24h for up to 30 days or until signs of proestrus induced); deslorelin (2.1 mg implant, Ovuplant®; placed in vestibule): must have serum progesterone <0.5 mg/mL at start; implant removed after ovulation confirmed with serum progesterone >10 ng/mL.

• Estrus suppression—megestrol acetate (2 mg/kg PO q24h for 8 days if begun within first 3 days of proestrus, or 0.5 mg/kg PO q24h for 32 days if begun in anestrus) or mibolerone (dose dependent on bodyweight; 30 μg PO q24h for dogs weighing 0.5–12 kg; 60 μg PO q24h for 12–23 kg; 120 μg PO q24h for weight 23–45 kg; 180 μg PO q24h daily for dogs weighing >45 kg and for German shepherd dogs and related breeds and crossbreds).

CONTRAINDICATIONS

• Treatment with progestins, including megestrol acetate, contraindicated in bitches with cystic endometrial hyperplasia or history of progesterone-dependent disease.

• Treatment with mibolerone contraindicated in Bedlington terriers and other breeds with familial liver disease.

• All hormonal therapies contraindicated in potentially pregnant bitches.

FOLLOW-UP

PATIENT MONITORING

• Hypothyroid dogs—recheck thyroid function after 1 month of supplementation.

• Ultrasonography—to definitively diagnose pregnancy; monitor gestation.

• Progesterone assay.

MISCELLANEOUS

Karotype testing can be performed by Molecular Cytogenetics Laboratory, Texas A&M University, or Veterinary Genetics Laboratory, UC Davis.

ASSOCIATED CONDITIONS

• Infertility caused by endocrinopathy—hypothyroidism, hyperadrenocorticism.

• Bitches with vaginal anatomic abnormality—persistent or recurrent urinary tract disease or vaginitis.

ZOONOTIC POTENTIAL

B. canis infection—organism is less readily shed if affected animals are gonadectomized; stress good hygiene.

SEE ALSO

• Abortion, Spontaneous (Early Pregnancy Loss)—Dogs.
• Breeding, Timing.
• Brucellosis.
• Hyperadrenocorticism (Cushing's Syndrome)—Dogs.
• Hypothyroidism.
• Infertility, Male—Dogs.
• Ovarian Remnant Syndrome.
• Vaginal Hyperplasia and Prolapse.
• Vaginal Malformations and Acquired Lesions.

ABBREVIATIONS

• GnRH = gonadotropin-releasing hormone.
• hCG = human chorionic gonadotropin.
• LH = luteinizing hormone.
• TSH = thyroid-stimulating hormone.

Suggested Reading

Johnston SD, Root Kustritz MV, Olson PN. Clinical approach to infertility in the bitch. In: Johnston SD, Root Kustritz MV, Olson-Schultz PN, Canine and Feline Theriogenology. Philadelphia, PA: Saunders, 2001, pp. 257–273.

Meyers-Wallen VN. Abnormal and unusual estrous cycles. Theriogenology 2007, 68:1205–1210.

Authors Lynda M.J. Miller and Maria Soledad Ferrer

Consulting Editor Erin E. Runcan

Client Education Handout available online

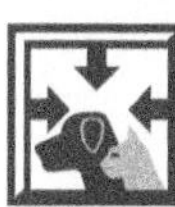

BASICS

DEFINITION

- Diminished or absent fertility; does not imply sterility.
- Results from wide range of problems that prevent delivery of sufficient numbers of normal spermatozoa to fertilize ovulated, mature oocytes in the bitch.

PATHOPHYSIOLOGY

- Spermatogenesis—formation and development of spermatozoa from spermatogonia to mature spermatozoa; coordinated, hormonally controlled, cyclic process; testicular problems require at least 70 days for recovery; epididymal problems require up to 10–14 days.
- Azoospermia—no spermatozoa in ejaculate.
- Oligozoospermia—low number of spermatozoa.
- Teratospermia—high number of abnormally shaped spermatozoa.
- Asthenospermia—reduced motility.
- Primary causes—impaired or arrested spermatogenesis, blockage of excurrent ducts, genitourinary inflammation, testicular neoplasia, environmental stress, congenital abnormality, endocrine abnormality.

SYSTEMS AFFECTED

- Reproductive.
- Endocrine/metabolic.
- Musculoskeletal.
- Nervous.

GENETICS

- Heritable component should be considered for autoimmune orchitis as cause of azoospermic infertility.
- Cryptorchidism—heritable, sex-limited polygenic autosomal recessive trait in dogs; associated with increased frequency of inguinal/umbilical hernias, patellar luxation, preputial and penile problems.
- Alpha-L-fucosidase deficiency—storage disorder causing acrosomal dysgenesis.
- Primary ciliary dyskinesia—congenital abnormality of ciliary ultrastructure; absent, irregular, or asynchronous motility patterns of all ciliated cells; diagnosed by electron microscopy of spermatozoa.
- Hypothyroidism—effect on male fertility probably minimal.

INCIDENCE/PREVALENCE

True incidence unknown; likely increased with inbreeding.

SIGNALMENT

Species

Dog

Breed Predilections

Relatively higher prevalence of specific problems in breeds with small genetic pool or intensive inbreeding.

Mean Age and Range

Prevalence increases with age.

SIGNS

General Comments

General complaint—no puppies produced; whelping rate <75% when bred with correct timing to fertile bitches.

Historical Findings

- Age of testicular descent.
- Age at first attempted mating.
- Temperament (high-strung).
- Libido and breeding behavior.
- Frequency and number of matings.
- Method used to time breedings.
- Type of semen used for breeding (fresh, fresh-extended, chilled-extended, frozen).
- Handling of semen and route of insemination.
- Litter size(s).
- Familial history of infertility.
- Coefficient of inbreeding.
- Fertility status of bitches.
- *Brucella canis* status of all breeding animals.
- Current and previous drug and dietary therapies, especially corticosteroids and steroid hormones.
- Previous medical or surgical illnesses.

Physical Examination Findings

- Sheath and penis—palpate to identify masses or adhesions.
- Nonerect penis—exteriorize to identify lesions of superficial mucosa and damage to os penis.
- Testes and epididymides—palpate and examine, note size and symmetry of epididymides relative to testes.
- Internal urethra and prostate—digital rectal palpation to determine location, size, and symmetry.

CAUSES

Incorrect timing of breeding—most common cause.

Congenital

- Chromosomal abnormalities: XXY syndrome and XX disorder of sexual development (see Sexual Development Disorders).
- Germinal cell aplasia—biopsy reveals "Sertoli cell only" syndrome.
- Segmental aplasia of epididymis or vas deferens—oligospermia (unilateral) or azoospermia (bilateral).

Acquired

- Incomplete ejaculation—unfamiliar surroundings; slippery flooring; no estrous bitch; dominant owner or bitch present.
- Obstruction of efferent ducts, epididymides, or ductus deferens—azoospermia if bilateral; sperm granuloma, spermatocele, acute inflammation, chronic inflammatory stenosis, segmental aplasia, neoplasia, vasectomy, attempts to tack testes into scrotal location.
- Hyperthermia/heat stroke.
- Inflammation or infection of testes—especially *Escherichia coli*; requires prompt and aggressive treatment to prevent infertility.
- Hypothyroidism—role unclear; may be associated with decreased libido.
- Hyperprolactinemia—role unclear; associated with azoospermia.
- Hyperadrenocorticism—testicular atrophy and oligospermia; probably reversible.
- Drugs—parasiticides, corticosteroids, anabolic steroids, estrogens, androgens, progestogens, gonadotropin-releasing hormone (GnRH) agonists/antagonists, ketoconazole, amphotericin B: may interfere with or interrupt spermatogenesis.
- Environmental toxins—endocrine-disrupting contaminants can affect hypothalamic-pituitary-gonadal axis and gonadal steroidogenesis.
- Trauma, testicular neoplasia, systemic disease, and ischemia—may cause transient infertility or sterility.
- Prostatic disease—can markedly reduce semen quality and libido.
- Inbreeding—reduces fertility; reduced-fertility lines might only be salvaged by concerted breeding program and out-crosses with highly fertile animals.
- Lymphocytic orchitis—familial in some breeds (e.g., beagle and borzoi); affected animals may be fertile when young; accelerated rate of fertility loss with age.
- Retrograde ejaculation—some retrograde flow into bladder normal.

RISK FACTORS

- Congenital disorders affecting reproductive function—occur in specific breeds.
- Teaser bitches and stud dogs not tested for infectious diseases (e.g., *B. canis* and bacterial culture of genital tract) before clinical use.

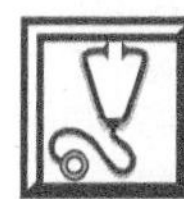

DIAGNOSIS

DIFFERENTIAL DIAGNOSIS

Before extensive diagnostic work on male, determine that bitches are fertile (previous litters) and breedings optimally timed (see Infertility, Female—Dogs, and Breeding, Timing).

CBC/BIOCHEMISTRY/URINALYSIS

- Usually normal.
- Brucellosis or prostatitis—variable changes in leukogram (normal or leukocytosis) and urinalysis (high numbers of leukocytes); depends on time course of infection; false-negative Brucellosis test possible, antibiotic therapy may cause false negative.
- Systemic illness—may impair reproductive function, but infertility usually not primary complaint.

INFERTILITY, MALE—DOGS (CONTINUED)

I

OTHER LABORATORY TESTS

Endocrine Profile

- Resting testosterone—normal, intact dogs, 0.4–10 ng/mL (1–4 ng/mL common range).
- Primary testicular failure—low testosterone and high follicle-stimulating hormone (FSH) and luteinizing hormone (LH).
- Germinal compartment failure—normal testosterone and high FSH; FSH high due to loss of inhibin secretion from Sertoli cells.
- Hypogonadism—low testosterone, FSH, and LH.
- Thyroid function—evaluated by baseline T_3, T_4, thyroid-stimulating hormone concentration (see Hypothyroidism).
- *B. canis*—screen with 2-mercaptoethanol rapid slide agglutination test (2-ME-RSAT); confirm with agar gel immunodiffusion test (AGID).

IMAGING

Ultrasonography—identify lesions that alter testicular and epididymal architecture (e.g., neoplasia, spermatocele, orchitis, epididymitis); evaluate prostate gland for hyperplasia, chronic prostatitis, cyst, abscess, or neoplasia (see Prostate Disease in the Breeding Male Dog).

DIAGNOSTIC PROCEDURES

Breeding Soundness Examination

- Must always consist of two semen collections.
- Sperm-rich and prostatic portions of ejaculate—collect as separate fractions by use of sterile artificial vagina and sterile, graduated, nontoxic plastic tubes, in presence of estrous bitch.
- Sperm-rich fraction—assess volume, concentration, motility, and morphologic characteristics of sperm cells; qualitative and quantitative cultures.
- Prostatic fraction and urine—cytologic examination; qualitative and quantitative cultures.
- Culture results—must be correlated with clinical and cytologic evidence of active infection; inflammation present if >3–5 white blood cells/hpf observed (especially sperm-rich fraction).
- If prostatic fraction indicates infection—reevaluate by other sampling techniques that avoid contamination from penile mucosa and prepuce; negative cytology possible with chronic prostatitis.
- Azoospermic or oligospermic ejaculate—recollect 1 hour later and again on several occasions before confirming infertility.

Epididymal Markers

Alkaline phosphatase (ALP) activity in seminal fluid—normal 8,000–40,000 U/mL; epididymal in origin; may indicate obstruction if <5,000 U/mL and complete ejaculate obtained; pathologic effects of obstruction more easily seen from ALP concentration if ALP performed on two ejaculates collected 1 hour apart.

PATHOLOGIC FINDINGS

Testicular biopsy—determines degree of spermatogenesis and integrity of blood–testis barrier; differentiates obstruction of efferent ducts from testicular hypoplasia and degeneration; allows informed prognosis.

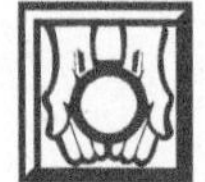

TREATMENT

ACTIVITY

- Restrict if activity results in hyperthermia.
- No restriction for other causes.

DIET

Ensure adequate diet and mineral supplementation; avoid supplementation of products containing excessive or undefined amounts of steroid hormones, e.g., extracts of testes, ovaries, and adrenals; phytoestrogens.

CLIENT EDUCATION

- Return to function may require at least 70 days from correction of identified cause(s).
- Stress patience and check patient regularly to ensure condition is not worsening.
- Emphasize potential role of heritable infertility.

SURGICAL CONSIDERATIONS

Re-anastomosis of blocked excurrent epididymal ducts (vasectomies) has been successful for reestablishment of sperm production.

MEDICATIONS

DRUG(S) OF CHOICE

- Antibiotics as indicated by culture and sensitivity.
- Pseudoephedrine—to treat retrograde ejaculation (used with limited success in men): 4–5 mg/kg PO q8h, or 1h and 3h before collection.
- Phenylpropanolamine—4–8 mg/kg PO q24h starting 5 days prior to collection.

CONTRAINDICATIONS

- Trimethoprim-sulfas—contraindicated if predisposed to keratoconjunctivitis sicca, can induce thrombocytopenia.
- Chloramphenicol—associated with anorexia and vomiting.

FOLLOW-UP

PATIENT MONITORING

Recheck at intervals that take into account length of spermatogenic cycle (70 days) but frequent enough to allow detection of deteriorating condition.

PREVENTION/AVOIDANCE

Avoid exposure to environmental temperature extremes.

POSSIBLE COMPLICATIONS

50–60% return to fertility after diagnosis and appropriate treatment.

MISCELLANEOUS

ASSOCIATED CONDITIONS

- Brucellosis—discospondylitis, polyarthritis, posterior paresis, fever, uveitis.
- Prostatic disease—obstipation, locomotor difficulties, fever, hematuria, pollakiuria, dysuria.
- Lymphocytic orchitis—lymphocytic thyroiditis.

AGE-RELATED FACTORS

- Daily sperm output and morphologically normal sperm cells decline with age.
- Difficult to assess effect of age alone on fertility.
- Most old, infertile dogs have concurrent diseases (e.g., systemic or prostatic disease, testicular neoplasia, osteoarthritis) that have documented effects on fertility or libido.

ABBREVIATIONS

- 2-ME-RSAT = 2-mercaptoethanol rapid slide agglutination test.
- AGID = agar gel immunodiffusion test.
- ALP = alkaline phosphatase.
- FSH = follicle-stimulating hormone.
- GnRH = gonadotropin-releasing hormone.
- LH = luteinizing hormone.

Suggested Reading

Kolster K. Evaluation of canine sperm and management of semen disorders. Vet Clin Small Anim Pract 2018, 48:533–545.

Author Richard A. Fayrer-Hosken
Consulting Editor Erin E. Runcan

Client Education Handout available online

BASICS

DEFINITION

A group of chronic enteropathies characterized by persistent or intermittent gastrointestinal (GI) signs with histopathologic evidence of intestinal inflammation. Inflammatory bowel disease (IBD) is generally categorized by the predominant mucosal cellular infiltrate, such as lymphocytic-plasmacytic, eosinophilic, or granulomatous enteritis.

PATHOPHYSIOLOGY

- Poorly understood but likely due to complex interplay between mucosal immunity and environmental factors (i.e., dietary and bacterial antigens) in genetically susceptible dogs; aberrant host immune responses are likely triggered by antigens derived from resident microbiota.
- Damage results from elaboration of cytokines, release of proteolytic and lysosomal enzymes, complement activation secondary to immune complex deposition, and generation of oxygen free radicals. • Host genetic susceptibility involving defects in innate immunity is suspected in dogs, and possibly cats.

SYSTEMS AFFECTED

- GI. • Hepatobiliary. • Hemic/lymphatic/immune—rarely. • Musculoskeletal—rarely.
- Ophthalmic—rarely. • Respiratory—rarely.
- Skin/exocrine—rarely.

GENETICS

Defects in host susceptibility genes have been identified in German shepherd dog, boxer, and soft-coated wheaten terrier.

INCIDENCE/PREVALENCE

IBD is most common histopathologic diagnosis in dogs and cats with chronic GI signs in which other causes have been eliminated through clinical trials and diagnostic testing.

GEOGRAPHIC DISTRIBUTION

N/A

SIGNALMENT

Species

Dog and cat.

Breed Predilections

- Increased risk in German shepherd, boxer, and soft-coated wheaten terrier, in addition to breed-specific forms described elsewhere.
- Siamese cats may be predisposed.

Mean Age and Range

Most common in middle-aged animals, but younger animals may be affected.

Predominant Sex

N/A

SIGNS

Historical Findings

- Intermittent or persistent chronic GI signs (>3 weeks' duration). • May include vomiting, small/large bowel diarrhea, decreased appetite, and/or weight loss. • Severe IBD may cause protein-losing enteropathy (PLE) in dogs.

Physical Examination Findings

- Vary from apparently healthy to a thin, lethargic animal. • Poor hair coat with chronic disease and nutritional deficiencies. • Abdominal palpation may reveal pain, thickened bowel loops, and mesenteric lymphadenopathy (especially in cats). • Ascites may occur in dogs with PLE. • Hematochezia, fecal mucus, and tenesmus seen with colonic involvement.

CAUSES

Pathogenesis unknown but most likely multifactorial, involving complex interactions between host genetics, mucosal immunity, and environmental (diet, intestinal bacteria) factors.

Infectious Agents

- Adherent and invasive *Escherichia coli* has been associated with granulomatous colitis in dogs.
- *Giardia*, *Salmonella*, *Campylobacter*, and resident microbiota have been implicated.

Dietary Agents

Meat proteins, milk proteins, gluten (wheat), and additives are all proposed causative agents, likely playing an important role.

Genetic Factors

- Some forms of IBD more common in certain breeds. • Defects in innate immunity (e.g., mutations in *TLR2*, *TLR5*, and *nod2* as seen in German shepherd dogs) that perturb mucosal homeostasis may predispose individual to IBD.

RISK FACTORS

Current hypotheses suggest that IBD is multifactorial disorder conditioned by genetic, immunologic, and environmental factors.

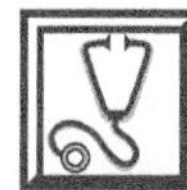

DIAGNOSIS

DIFFERENTIAL DIAGNOSIS

- Cats—hyperthyroidism, intestinal neoplasia (especially small cell lymphoma), adverse food reactions, feline infectious peritonitis and other viral infections (e.g., feline leukemia virus [FeLV] and feline immunodeficiency virus [FIV]), renal and hepatic insufficiency, exocrine pancreatic insufficiency, intestinal parasitism, and antibiotic-responsive diarrhea (ARD) are primary differentials.
- Dogs—intestinal neoplasia, motility disorders, adverse food reactions, lymphangiectasia, exocrine pancreatic insufficiency, intestinal parasitism, and ARD are primary differentials.

CBC/BIOCHEMISTRY/URINALYSIS

- Often unremarkable; these tests more often serve to eliminate other differential diagnoses.
- Anemia of chronic disease; mild leukocytosis ± left shift sometimes seen with mucosal disruption (e.g., erosions); mild eosinophilia may be seen with eosinophilic enteritis, food allergy, and intestinal parasites among other causes. • Cats may show alterations in serum total protein (i.e., hyperproteinemia) and albumin concentrations, with increased liver enzyme activities.
- Hypoproteinemia more common in dogs than cats. • Cobalamin deficiency in both dogs and cats with involvement of ileum.

OTHER LABORATORY TESTS

- Useful to eliminate other differentials.
- Dogs—evaluation of exocrine pancreatic function: canine trypsin-like immunoreactivity (cTLI); serology for pancreatitis: canine pancreatic lipase activity (Spec cPL), and serum cobalamin and folate assays to localize small intestinal disease. • Cats—T_4 and FeLV/FIV serology; fasting serum TLI (if exocrine pancreatic insufficiency suspected); serology for pancreatitis (Spec fPL), and serum cobalamin and folate assays to localize small intestinal disease.

I

IMAGING

- Survey abdominal radiographs—usually unremarkable. • Barium contrast studies—may reveal mucosal abnormalities and thickened bowel loops; normal findings do not eliminate possibility of IBD.
- Ultrasonography—may indicate increased intestinal wall thickness (particularly muscularis propria and submucosal layers) and mesenteric lymphadenopathy; however, these abnormalities not specific for IBD.

DIAGNOSTIC PROCEDURES

- Perform elimination dietary trial to rule out adverse food reactions; if GI signs resolve within 2 weeks, then diagnosis of adverse food reaction is made. • Perform fecal testing for nematode and protozoal parasites; treat for *Giardia* spp. and endoparasitic infection with fenbendazole (50 mg/kg for 5 days). • Definitive diagnosis of IBD requires intestinal biopsy and histopathology, usually obtained via GI endoscopy; WSAVA guidelines should be used to define severity of mucosal inflammation. • Laparotomy indicated if GI endoscopy unavailable or to collect full-thickness mucosal specimens; *always be sure to collect ileal biopsies.* • Use scoring indices (canine inflammatory bowel disease activity index) to define clinical severity and assess response to therapy.

PATHOLOGIC FINDINGS

Morphologic evidence of mucosal inflammation including epithelial changes, architectural distortion (e.g., erosion/ulceration, crypt hyperplasia, fibrosis, loss of colonic goblet cells), and increased lamina propria cellularity. Histopathologic guidelines for defining severity of GI inflammation have been described.

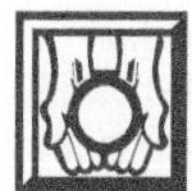

TREATMENT

APPROPRIATE HEALTH CARE

Outpatient, unless patient is debilitated from dehydration, hypoproteinemia, or cachexia.

INFLAMMATORY BOWEL DISEASE (CONTINUED)

NURSING CARE

- If patient is dehydrated or must have food restricted because of intractable vomiting, any balanced crystalloid fluid is adequate (for a patient without concurrent disease); otherwise, select fluids on basis of secondary diseases.
- If severe hypoalbuminemia from PLE, consider use of colloids.

ACTIVITY

No restrictions.

DIET

- Feed novel intact protein or hydrolysate elimination diet to help reduce intestinal inflammation. • Fiber supplementation (e.g., fermentable fiber such as pumpkin, Metamucil®) suggested in dogs and cats with colitis. • Fish oil (n-3 fatty acids) as free radical scavenger to reduce inflammation.
- Probiotics may be of benefit in some animals but clinically unproven at this time; must be given continuously over several weeks for potential benefit to be realized.

CLIENT EDUCATION

- Emphasize that IBD is not cured but is controllable in most instances. • Relapses are common; clients should be patient during the various food and medication trials that are often necessary to control the disease.

SURGICAL CONSIDERATIONS

Surgery only indicated for collection of intestinal biopsies in dogs and intestinal and/or liver, pancreatic and/or mesenteric biopsies in cats.

MEDICATIONS

DRUG(S) OF CHOICE

- Evidence-based data indicate glucocorticoids are effective drugs for inducing remission in majority of dogs and cats; use prednisone or prednisolone in dogs at 1–2 mg/kg PO daily for 21 days to induce remission, then taper dose by 25% every 2 weeks.
- Dogs weighing >30 kg will require lower steroid dosage to provide comparable clinical efficacy; this will also reduce adverse effects; *dose large dogs by body surface area.* • Treat cats with oral prednisolone at 1–2 mg/kg for 14–21 days, then taper as above; avoid glucocorticoids in cats with diabetes mellitus and those with history of adverse effects.
- Budesonide may be used to minimize adverse steroid effects and maintain remission in some dogs and cats; dosage ranges dogs: 1–3 mg/m^2 daily; cats: 1 mg/day. • Correct hypocobalaminemia by weekly parenteral cobalamin injections for first 6 weeks and thereafter every 2–3 weeks or as needed based on repeat testing of cobalamin concentrations; oral cobalamin therapy requires daily administration; antibiotics (metronidazole, tylosin) generally *not* indicated for treatment of IBD; these drugs may cause significant disruption to gut microbiota even after administration discontinued. • Some evidence that oral cyclosporine is of value in dogs with steroid-refractory disease and PLE; dose at 5 mg/kg PO daily for 4–6 weeks or as needed to induce remission. • Use of other immunosuppressive drugs, including azathioprine, chlorambucil, leflunomide, or mycophenolate, has been reported. • Empirical deworming with fenbendazole (50 mg/kg PO q24h for 5 days).
- Fecal microbiota transplant anecdotally effective in cases of refractory IBD; however, clinical trial data yet to be reported.

CONTRAINDICATIONS

Based on concurrent disease.

PRECAUTIONS

See Drug(s) of Choice.

POSSIBLE INTERACTIONS

See Drug(s) of Choice.

ALTERNATIVE DRUG(S)

See Drug(s) of Choice.

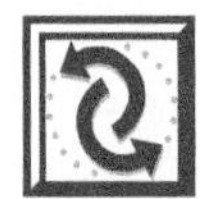

FOLLOW-UP

PATIENT MONITORING

- Periodic (q2–4 weeks) physical and laboratory evaluations may be necessary until the patient's condition stabilizes; serum albumin provides important prognostic information in dogs; serum cobalamin deficiency will delay complete clinical recovery in both dogs and cats.
- Monitor serum cobalamin concentrations in hypocobalaminemic dogs and cats. • No other follow-up may be required except yearly physical examinations and assessment during relapse.

PREVENTION/AVOIDANCE

N/A

POSSIBLE COMPLICATIONS

Dehydration, malnutrition, adverse drug reactions, hypoproteinemia, hypocobalaminemia, anemia, and diseases secondary to therapy.

EXPECTED COURSE AND PROGNOSIS

- Generally good to excellent short-term prognosis. • Poor long-term prognosis in dogs with IBD has been associated with severe clinical disease, marked endoscopic (duodenal) abnormalities, ascites, and hypoalbuminemia; long-term prognosis worse compared to food-responsive diarrhea and ARD, other forms of canine chronic enteropathy.

MISCELLANEOUS

ASSOCIATED CONDITIONS

- See discussion under specific diseases.
- Cats may demonstrate concurrent inflammatory lesions in the liver and/or pancreas ("triaditis").

AGE-RELATED FACTORS

Some differentials more likely in younger individuals (i.e., intestinal parasitism vs. neoplasia).

ZOONOTIC POTENTIAL

N/A

PREGNANCY/FERTILITY/BREEDING

Counsel clients about breeding and monitoring for appearance of other diseases.

SYNONYMS

None

SEE ALSO

- Colitis, Histiocytic Ulcerative.
- Diarrhea, Chronic—Cats.
- Diarrhea, Chronic—Dogs.
- Food Reactions (Gastrointestinal), Adverse.
- Gastroenteritis, Eosinophilic.
- Immunoproliferative Enteropathy of Basenjis.
- Protein-Losing Enteropathy.
- Small Intestinal Dysbiosis.
- Vomiting, Chronic.

ABBREVIATIONS

- ARD = antibiotic-responsive diarrhea.
- cPL = canine pancreatic lipase. • FeLV = feline leukemia virus. • FIV = feline immunodeficiency virus. • fPL = feline pancreatic lipase. • GI = gastrointestinal.
- IBD = inflammatory bowel disease. • PLE = protein-losing enteropathy. • TLI = trypsin-like immunoreactivity.

INTERNET RESOURCES

http://www.vin.com/VIN.plx

Suggested Reading

Allenspach K, Culverwell C, Chan D. Long-term outcome in dogs with chronic enteropathies: 203 cases. Vet Rec 2016, 178:368.

Day MJ, Bilzer T, Mansell J, et al. International standards for the histopathological diagnosis of gastrointestinal inflammation in the dog and cat: a report from the World Small Animal Veterinary Association Gastrointestinal Standardization Group. J Comp Pathol 2008, Suppl 1:S1–S43.

Makielski K, Cullen J, O'Connor A, Jergens AE. Narrative review of therapies for chronic enteropathies in dogs and cats. J Vet Intern Med 2019, 33(1):11–22.

Simpson KW, Jergens AE. Pitfalls and progress in the diagnosis and management of canine inflammatory bowel disease. Vet Clin North Am Small Anim Pract 2011, 41(2):381–398.

Author Albert E. Jergens

Consulting Editor Mark P. Rondeau

Client Education Handout available online

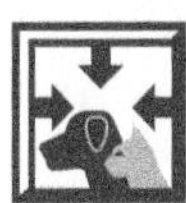

BASICS

OVERVIEW

- An acute to subacute contagious viral disease with an almost exclusive respiratory manifestation caused by influenza viruses.
- Canine influenza viruses (CIV) are influenza type A viruses that developed from equine (H3N8, USA) or avian (H3N2; East Asia) influenza viruses. Although the viruses originated in other species, the H3 viruses are considered "canine influenza viruses" as they are now transmissible dog to dog. Influenza H7N2 is an avian influenza A virus that was documented in shelter cats. H1N1 human pandemic influenza is also capable of infecting dogs and cats, but there is no evidence of transmission.
- Natural route of infection is airborne particles or oral contact with contaminated surfaces. Replication of the virus appears to be restricted to epithelial cells of the upper and lower airways, with possible involvement of alveolar macrophages. Antibody response detectable by 8 days post infection and titers remain detectable for >1 year. Protective immune responses have not been defined.
- H3N8 CIV activity was first detected in racing greyhounds in the United States in 2004 and has subsequently been identified in dogs across the country.
- H3N2 CIV was detected in South Korea in 2007, but existed in China several years earlier; genetic lineage is of avian origin and probably arose in East Asia.
- H3N2 CIV infection causes more severe clinical signs, is more easily transmissible, and is shed for a longer period than H3N8 CIV.

SIGNALMENT

- Natural infections of H3N8 CIV currently limited to dogs; H3N2 virus is capable of infecting dogs and cats; H7N2 has infected shelter cats.
- All dogs and cats are susceptible to infection; there are no known age, breed, or sex restrictions on susceptibility.

SIGNS

- 60–80% of infected dogs develop clinical signs.
- Incubation period 2–4 days post infection.
- Modest febrile response 39.4–40 °C (103–104 °F) 3–6 days post infection.
- Clear nasal discharge, which can progress to thick, mucoid discharge, most frequently caused by secondary bacterial colonization.
- More severe form of disease shows higher body temperatures with development of pneumonia and tachypnea 6–10 days post infection.
- Many dogs develop a cough that can last for several weeks.

CAUSES & RISK FACTORS

- Respiratory infection caused by influenza viruses.
- Most cases have a history of group housing in kennels, day care centers, and rescue shelters, or contact with animals that have recently been in group housing or social settings such as dog shows.

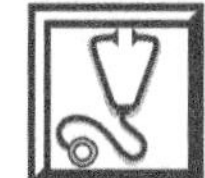

DIAGNOSIS

DIFFERENTIAL DIAGNOSIS

- On an individual basis, early signs of influenza are indistinguishable from signs of kennel cough complex.
- Distinction from typical respiratory pathogens of dogs is found in group settings in which 60–80% of dogs can show clinical signs.
- Later in disease course—pneumonia may develop with or without secondary bacterial infections.

CBC/BIOCHEMISTRY/URINALYSIS

- Generally unremarkable.
- CBC may reflect stress initially, then bacterial pneumonia later in disease (leukocytosis, left shift).

OTHER LABORATORY TESTS

N/A

DIAGNOSTIC PROCEDURES

- Matrix gene reverse transcriptase polymerase chain reaction (RT-PCR) test—most reliable and preferred test; can detect agent in acute phase of disease (1–7 days post onset of clinical signs) in nasal swab.
- Viral isolation—possible early (~first 3 days) in infection.
  - PCR and viral isolation can be negative if collected too late in infection.
  - Serologic tests for H3N8 will not detect H3N2 and vice versa; must test for each separately.
- Hemagglutination inhibition test—preferred serologic test; acute and convalescent titers optimal; since most dogs have no circulating CIV antibodies, antibodies detected in serum more than 7 days post onset of clinical signs determine exposure to CIV.
- Antigen-capture ELISA tests gave unacceptable levels of false negatives with H3N8 infections, but higher viral loads with H3N2 give acceptable results if testing done early in course of infection.

PATHOLOGIC FINDINGS

Primary lesion caused by infection is destruction of ciliated epithelial cell layer in upper airways with extension into lungs. Areas of lung consolidation can be found 6–10 days post infection.

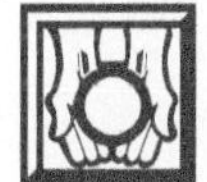

TREATMENT

- Infected animals should be isolated to prevent infection of other animals.
- Contagious period for H3N2 CIV extends approximately 2 weeks after onset of clinical signs.
- Continued coughing of affected animal is not a sign of virus shedding.
- Strongly recommend treating uncomplicated cases as outpatients to prevent hospital contamination.
- Only hospitalize those with pneumonia that require IV fluid or oxygen support.
- Enforced rest—for at least 14–21 days (uncomplicated cases); 2 months in cases of pneumonia.

MEDICATIONS

- Antiviral drugs have not been tested for efficacy.
- Antibiotics to control secondary bacterial infections recommended if fever, lethargy, or inappetence accompany mucopurulent nasal discharge—amoxicillin, amoxicillin–clavulanic acid, and doxycycline are empiric first-line options for mild cases.
- Clinical pneumonia—first-line recommendations include parenteral administration of fluoroquinolone and penicillin (ampicillin) or clindamycin initially until antimicrobial culture and sensitivity available.
  - Resistant bacteria—important to culture and establish bacterial sensitivity; consider inherent resistance of Mycoplasma to penicillins and cephalosporins; for organisms resistant to first-choice antibiotic therapies above, consider aminoglycosides (gentamicin or amikacin, contraindicated in animals with renal dysfunction, dehydration), cephalosporins (cephalexin, cefazolin, cefadroxil, cefoxitin, cefovecin); see Suggested Reading.
  - In absence of controlled studies on efficacy, inhalational antimicrobial therapy not recommended.
- In animals treated for pneumonia—recheck patient and radiographs after 10–14 days to decide whether continued antibiotic therapy indicated; optimal duration of therapy for pneumonia unknown; shorter courses of antibiotics (as used in humans with pneumonia) than traditionally recommended 4–6 weeks may be effective.
- Cough suppressants (butorphanol or hydrocodone bitartrate)—often effective in suppressing dry nonproductive cough; cough suppression counterproductive in animals with pneumonia.
- Bronchodilators (theophylline or aminophylline)—may relieve wheezing.

FOLLOW-UP

- If infection established in a kennel, evacuate kennel for 1–2 weeks and disinfect with sodium hypochlorite (1 : 30 dilution), chlorhexidine, or benzalkonium; influenza virus can live on hard surfaces for up to 24 hours.

INFLUENZA (CONTINUED)

- Uncomplicated cases should resolve within 10–14 days; if patient continues to cough beyond 14 days, further diagnostics indicated.
- Mortality rate highly variable and likely linked to degree of secondary bacterial infection, strain of virus, and intensity of veterinary care.
- Currently there are licensed influenza vaccines for use in dogs that cover H3N8, H3N2, or both. There are no licensed vaccines for cats.

I

MISCELLANEOUS

ZOONOTIC POTENTIAL

- Risk thought to be low; however, influenza viruses mutate rapidly and outbreaks in dogs and cats monitored for this potential; one person documented to develop infection with H7N2 working with cats in shelter outbreak.
- Cats can be experimentally infected with H3N8 CIV; H7N2 virus was isolated from cats in an animal shelter.
- H3N2 virus can also infect ferrets, guinea pigs, and mice.

ABBREVIATIONS

- CIV = canine influenza virus.
- RT-PCR = reverse transcriptase polymerase chain reaction.

INTERNET RESOURCES

https://www.avma.org/resources-tools/animal-health-and-welfare/canine-influenza

Suggested Reading

Dubovi EJ, Njaa BL. Canine influenza. Vet Clin Small Anim 2008, 38:827–836.

Lappin MR, Blondeau J, Boothe D, et al. Antimicrobial use guidelines for treatment of respiratory tract disease in dogs and cats: Antimicrobial Guidelines Working Group of the International Society for Companion Animal Infectious Diseases. J Vet Intern Med 2017, 31:279–294.

Author Edward J. Dubovi

Consulting Editor Amie Koenig

INSOLUBLE OXALATE PLANT TOXICOSIS

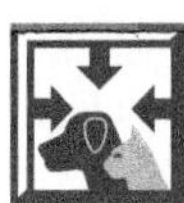

BASICS

OVERVIEW

- Over 200 species of plants contain insoluble oxalate crystals.
- Most houseplants are in the Araceae family; many are found in homes and offices.
- Common names vary; scientific names must be used for accurate identification.
- Insoluble oxalate crystals are not absorbed systemically, and signs are often self-limiting.
- Signs are generally limited to irritation of oral mucosa; other signs occur more rarely.
- *Dieffenbachia* spp. (dumbcane) ingestion by dogs and cats has been associated with more serious outcomes, including death.
- Cats ingesting *Philodendron* spp. may exhibit more severe clinical signs.
- Common plants include:
  - *Aglaonema commutatum* (Chinese evergreen).
  - *Anthurium* spp. (flamingo flower).
  - *Arisaema amurense* (Jack-in-the-pulpit).
  - *Dieffenbachia* spp. (dumbcane).
  - *Epipremnum* spp. (pothos, devil's ivy, variegated philodendron).
  - *Monstera deliciosa* (fruit salad plant).
  - *Philodendron* spp. (sweetheart vine, fiddle leaf).
  - *Schefflera actionphylla* (umbrella plant).
  - *Spathiphyllum* spp. (peace lily).
  - *Syngonium* spp. (arrowhead vine).
  - *Zantedeschia* spp. (calla lily).

SIGNALMENT

- Indoor cats and dogs primarily, although pets may be exposed by houseplants moved outside during summer months.
- Dogs tend to chew and destroy the entire plant; cats nibble on leaves.
- May occur more often in younger pets that are bored or inquisitive.

SIGNS

- Rapid onset, often within minutes of exposure.
- Oral—vocalization, pawing at muzzle, head shaking, hypersalivation, edema of lips, tongue or pharynx; rarely gagging, choking, and vomiting.
- Ocular—pawing at eyes, photophobia, conjunctival swelling.
- Respiratory—*rarely*, dyspnea from pharyngeal swelling and inflammation.

CAUSES & RISK FACTORS

- Plants in environment.
- Insoluble oxalate crystals are arranged in bundles called raphides that are contained in idioblasts within plant stems and leaves.
- Chewing or biting on plant material releases crystals from stems and leaves until idioblast is emptied.
- Crystals act as miniature pins or mechanical irritants to mucous membranes, but are not absorbed systemically.
- Potential for chemical irritation with release of prostaglandins, histamine, proteolytic enzymes.

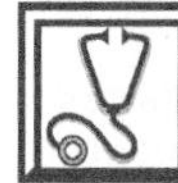

DIAGNOSIS

DIFFERENTIAL DIAGNOSIS

- Caustic agents (alkalis and acids in household products; drain cleaners).
- Other agents causing oral irritation (capsaicin, detergents, topical spot-on flea and tick products.
- Quaternary ammonium compounds (>2% in cats).
- Stinging nettle (*Urtica dioica*) ingestion.
- Systemic disease-causing oral lesions.

CBC/BIOCHEMISTRY/URINALYSIS

- Rarely performed unless prolonged vomiting.
- CBC, electrolytes, serum chemistry.

OTHER LABORATORY TESTS

N/A

IMAGING

N/A

DIAGNOSTIC PROCEDURES

- Exam of oral cavity including visualization of pharynx.
- Fluorescein ophthalmic stain if ocular signs are present.

PATHOLOGIC FINDINGS

- Death rarely occurs.
- Few cases with severe erosive, ulcerative glossitis; oropharyngeal edema.

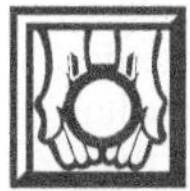

TREATMENT

- Generally limited to supportive care.
- IV fluids if dehydrated from excessive salivation or vomiting.
- Oral—irrigation of oral cavity with copious amounts of cool fluids; small amounts of calcium-containing product (milk, yogurt, etc.) to bind oxalate crystals.
- Ocular—lavage for 15 min with tepid water.
- Respiratory—endotracheal tube or temporary tracheostomy if dyspnea severe.

MEDICATIONS

No specific antidote available.

DRUG(S) OF CHOICE

- Antiemetics as needed:
  - Maropitant 1 mg/kg SC/PO/IV q24h.
  - Ondansetron 0.1–1mg/kg IV q8–12h.
- GI protectants as needed:
  - H2 blockers (famotidine, ranitidine).
  - Omeprazole 0.5–1 mg/kg PO daily.
  - Sucralfate 0.25–1 g PO q8h.
- Pain medication as needed:
  - Butorphanol 0.1–0.5 mg/kg IV/IM/SC.

CONTRAINDICATIONS/POSSIBLE INTERACTIONS

Corticosteroids—use is controversial, but dexamethasone phosphate 0.125–0.5 mg/kg IV/IM/SC may be useful in severe inflammatory conditions.

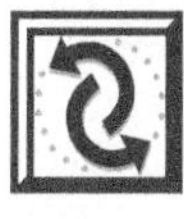

FOLLOW-UP

PATIENT MONITORING

Monitor for signs of dyspnea and respiratory difficulty.

PREVENTION/AVOIDANCE

Identify plants in household and keep away from pets.

POSSIBLE COMPLICATIONS

- Corneal abrasion or ulcer from pawing at eyes.
- Erosive ulcers in mouth and gastrointestinal tract.
- Pharyngeal edema and death (rare).

EXPECTED COURSE AND PROGNOSIS

- Most signs are mild to moderate and of short duration, generally lasting 2–4 hours; less often signs last 12–24 hours.
- Excellent prognosis as signs are generally self-limiting.

MISCELLANEOUS

AGE-RELATED FACTORS

Young pets are more frequently represented; likely due to boredom and inquisitive nature.

INTERNET RESOURCES

- http://www.petpoisonhelpline.com/poisons
- http://www.aspca.org/pet-care/animal-poison-control/toxic-and-non-toxic-plants

Suggested Reading

Hovda LR. Oxalates – insoluble. In: Hovda LR, Brutlag A, Poppenga RH, Peterson K, eds. Blackwell's Five-Minute Veterinary Consults Clinical Companion: Small Animal Toxicology, 2nd ed. Ames, IA: Wiley-Blackwell, 2016, pp. 787–796.

Author Lynn R. Hovda
Consulting Editor Lynn R. Hovda

Client Education Handout available online

I

INSULINOMA

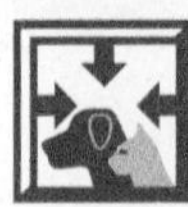

BASICS

DEFINITION

Functional pancreatic islet beta-cell tumor that secretes insulin, independent of systemic glucose concentration.

PATHOPHYSIOLOGY

- Excessive insulin secretion leads to glucose uptake and use by insulin-sensitive tissues and reduced hepatic production of glucose, resulting in hypoglycemia and associated clinical signs.
- Insulinomas can secrete other hormones, such as somatostatin, glucagon, gastrin, pancreatic polypeptide, insulin-like growth factor 1 (somatomedin), and serotonin; however, clinical signs are typically associated with hypoglycemia.
- Nervous system abnormalities are typically the first clinical signs seen due to the brain's dependence on glucose for energy and lack of glycogen stores.
- Hypoglycemia stimulates release of counter-regulatory hormones (e.g., glucocorticoids, growth hormone, catecholamines, and glucagon) that cause adrenal stimulation in an effort to raise plasma glucose levels.
- Release of counter-regulatory hormones and adrenal stimulation can lead to muscle tremors, restlessness, nervousness, and hunger.

SYSTEMS AFFECTED

- Nervous—seizures, disorientation, abnormal behavior, collapse, polyneuropathy/peripheral neuropathy, posterior paresis, ataxia.
- Musculoskeletal—weakness, muscle fasciculations.
- Gastrointestinal—variable appetite and weight.
- Urinary—polyuria, polydipsia.

INCIDENCE/PREVALENCE

- Dogs—uncommon.
- Cats—rare.

SIGNALMENT

Species

Dog and cat.

Breed Predilections

- Dogs—Labrador retrievers, standard poodles, boxers, fox terriers, Irish setters, German shepherd dogs, golden retrievers, collies.
- Cats—possibly Siamese.

Mean Age and Range

- Dogs—middle-aged to old; mean: 10 years, range: 3–14 years.
- Cats—mean: 15 years, range: 12–17 years.

SIGNS

General Comments

- Often episodic and vague.
- May be related to fasting, excitement, exercise, and/or eating.

Historical Findings

- Dogs—generalized or focal seizures; historical findings may include weakness, posterior paresis, collapse, muscle fasciculations, bizarre behavior, lethargy and depression, ataxia, polyphagia or inappetance, weight gain or loss, polyuria and polydipsia, and exercise intolerance.
- Cats—seizures, ataxia, muscle fasciculations, weakness, lethargy and depression, anorexia, weight loss, and polydipsia.

Physical Examination Findings

- Usually within normal limits unless in a hypoglycemic crisis.
- Obesity may be noted.
- Polyneuropathy is seen rarely in dogs (paresis to paralysis, muscle atrophy, and/or hyporeflexia).

CAUSES

Many dogs and cats have single insulin-producing beta-islet cell carcinoma or adenocarcinoma of the pancreas, but 50% or more will develop or present with metastasis.

RISK FACTORS

For hypoglycemic episodes—fasting, excitement, exercise, and eating.

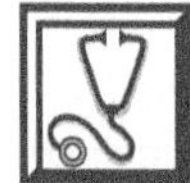

DIAGNOSIS

DIFFERENTIAL DIAGNOSIS

- Extrapancreatic tumor hypoglycemia—paraneoplastic hypoglycemia has been documented in dogs with tumors including leiomyosarcoma and hepatocellular, mammary, and pulmonary carcinomas, among others; these tumors secrete insulin or insulin-like substances.
- Rule out causes such as insulin overdose, neonatal/toy breed hypoglycemia, ingestion of oral hypoglycemic agents, hepatic failure, sepsis, hypoadrenocorticism, hunting dog (exertional) hypoglycemia, and glycogen storage diseases.
- Seizures and collapse—consider a variety of differentials including cardiovascular, metabolic, and neurologic disease.

CBC/BIOCHEMISTRY/URINALYSIS

- Often within normal limits except for hypoglycemia (<65–70 mg/dL in majority of patients).
- Normoglycemia does not rule out the presence of an insulinoma; a small percentage of patients may be intermittently normoglycemic, which is thought to be due to counter-regulatory hormone production (e.g., epinephrine, glucocorticoids, glucagon).

OTHER LABORATORY TESTS

Simultaneous Fasting Glucose and Insulin Determinations

- Paired glucose and insulin can often be measured without fasting, since hypoglycemia is commonly identified at presentation.
- If a patient presents for hypoglycemia, obtain additional serum for possible insulin level evaluation prior to administering exogenous dextrose.
- If necessary, patients may be fasted (and hospitalized and monitored closely due to the risk for hypoglycemia), and serial (q1–2h) blood samples collected; when serum glucose drops below 60 mg/dL, that sample should be analyzed for simultaneous glucose and insulin concentrations.
  - Elevated insulin concentration (>20 μU/mL) in the face of hypoglycemia—insulinoma highly likely.
  - Insulin concentration within reference range (5–20 μU/mL) in the face of hypoglycemia—insulinoma probable
  - Any insulin concentration within reference range with concurrent hypoglycemia is abnormal; if insulin concentration below normal limits with hypoglycemia then an insulinoma is unlikely, but repeated sampling may be necessary.
- Formulas utilizing simultaneous hypoglycemic glucose and insulin concentrations such as the insulin : glucose ratio and the amended insulin : glucose ratio have poor specificity.

IMAGING

- Thoracic and abdominal radiography—helpful for identification of metastatic disease and/or extrapancreatic tumor-induced causes of hypoglycemia as well as some other differential diagnoses.
- Ultrasonography—30–75% of pancreatic masses are clearly identified through ultrasonography; can be used for screening for metastatic disease, but relatively insensitive.
- CT—superior technique for detection of primary insulinomas in dogs; however, false-positive lymph node metastases are common.
- Scintigraphy and single proton emission computed tomography (SPECT)—intermittently successful in detecting insulinomas.
- Intraoperative ultrasound—widely used for gross occult tumor detection in human insulinomas; rarely reported in veterinary medicine.

DIAGNOSTIC PROCEDURES

Exploratory laparotomy—indicated when insulinoma is suspected based on the aforementioned physical, biochemical, and/or imaging results, but imaging is inconclusive.

PATHOLOGIC FINDINGS

- Histopathologically, primary pancreatic insulinomas in dogs are either beta-islet cell carcinomas or adenocarcinomas and occasionally adenomas, although dogs with adenomas may subsequently develop metastasis.
- In cats, most insulinomas are malignant with metastasis common.

• In both species, metastatic disease is frequently noted in the liver, mesentery, and regional lymph nodes, and appears histopathologically similar to the primary tumor.

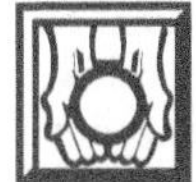

TREATMENT

APPROPRIATE HEALTH CARE

• Hospitalize for workup and surgery.
• Outpatient if the owner declines surgery and the patient is not clinically hypoglycemic.

NURSING CARE

Close monitoring for recurrence of signs associated with hypoglycemia is indicated, especially as most hospitalized patients become refractory to glucose supplementation and require increasing dosages.

ACTIVITY

Restricted

DIET

• Feed four to six (or more) small meals a day.
• Food should be high in protein, fat, and complex carbohydrates and low in simple sugars.

CLIENT EDUCATION

Client should be educated about the signs of hypoglycemia and seek immediate attention if they occur.

SURGICAL CONSIDERATIONS

• Surgical management improves prognosis over medical therapy alone.
• Medical management is important before exploratory laparotomy; most patients respond well to frequent small feedings and corticosteroids; in refractory cases, IV fluids containing 2.5–5% dextrose and/or glucagon may be necessary.
• Objectives include confirmation of diagnosis, identification of extrapancreatic metastases or other disease, and removal of as much cancerous tissue as possible.
• At surgery, most insulinomas can be visualized and/or palpated; if a pancreatic mass cannot be found, intraoperative ultrasound may be beneficial.
• Approximately 15% of dogs have multiple primary insulinomas, so always examine the entire pancreas.
• Biopsy regional lymph nodes and carefully evaluate the liver (and other abdominal contents) with biopsy of any abnormalities; 40–50% of dogs will have metastasis; in one study, of 14 dogs suspected to have extrapancreatic metastasis from a primary pancreatic insulinoma, only 8 (57%) had histologic evidence of metastasis; therefore, the presence of what appears to be metastasis should be biopsied and not automatically lead to intraoperative euthanasia.
• Insulinoma can be classified as stage I (confined to the pancreas); stage II (regional lymph node metastasis present); or stage III (distant metastasis present).
• Postoperative complications include pancreatitis, persistent hypoglycemia secondary to incomplete removal of the primary tumor or metastatic disease, and diabetes mellitus (DM). DM is thought to occur secondary to atrophy of remaining normal beta-islet cells.

MEDICATIONS

DRUG(S) OF CHOICE

Emergency/Acute Therapy

• 50% dextrose (0.5 g/kg IV diluted 1 : 3, slowly over 1–3 min)—for emergency control of hypoglycemic episodes; once hypoglycemic signs abate, IV fluid therapy with 2.5–5% dextrose added to an isotonic crystalloid solution should be administered (dextrose may be increased to 7.5% if needed to control clinical signs, but should be administered through a central venous catheter to prevent phlebitis).
• Glucagon (1–5 ng/kg/min IV as CRI) is gluconeogenic and may be used to effect to treat clinical signs associated with severe refractory hypoglycemia, in preparation for surgery.

Long-Term Therapy

• If exploratory laparotomy is pursued and complete excision of the tumor is obtained, long-term therapy may not be needed.
• If dietary therapy is ineffective for controlling hypoglycemia, glucocorticoids (e.g., prednisone 0.25 mg/kg PO q12h, increased as necessary up to 2 mg/kg PO q12h) may be given.
• Diazoxide (Proglycem®) stimulates hepatic gluconeogenesis/glycogenolysis and inhibits insulin secretion—dosage is 5–60 mg/kg PO q12h, starting at the low end and increasing as needed; should be used in addition to dietary modifications and glucocorticoids when they become less effective for controlling clinical signs.
• Streptozotocin is a nitrosourea that semi-selectively targets pancreatic beta-cells; may be given at 500 mg/m^2 slow IV over 2h, after a 3h IV diuresis with isotonic crystalloid and followed by a 2h diuresis; this protocol may be repeated every 3 weeks until normoglycemia is achieved. Streptozotocin is emetogenic and can be hepatotoxic and/or nephrotoxic; it can also cause DM secondary to cytotoxic effects on pancreatic beta-islet cells; is currently difficult to obtain.
• The synthetic somatostatin analogues octreotide (10–20 µg SC q8–12h) or lantreotide (no determined dose in veterinary species) may be utilized to prevent hypoglycemia in dogs refractory to conventional treatments.
• Anecdotal reports of the use of toceranib phosphate (Palladia®) exist for medical management in nonsurgical cases and/or postoperative treatment in patients with metastatic disease.

CONTRAINDICATIONS

Insulin

PRECAUTIONS

• Dextrose boluses, when given alone, may precipitate further hypoglycemic crises.
• Glucocorticoids used at high dosages for prolonged periods can cause iatrogenic hyperadrenocorticism.
• Diazoxide may cause bone marrow suppression, gastrointestinal irritation, aplastic anemia, cataracts, thrombocytopenia, and tachycardia in humans.
• Streptozocin can cause emesis, hepatic failure, renal failure, DM, and pancreatitis.
• Neither diazoxide nor streptozotocin has been evaluated in cats.
• Glucagon is indicated for short-term therapy to stabilize refractory patients, but is not a definitive or long-term therapy.

POSSIBLE INTERACTIONS

Hydrochlorothiazide can potentiate diazoxide.

FOLLOW-UP

PATIENT MONITORING

• Teach client to monitor for return and/or progression of signs of hypoglycemia.
• Serum glucose determinations are important for monitoring for return and/or progression of insulinoma-associated hypoglycemia.
• Abdominal ultrasound may be used for postoperative long-term monitoring.

POSSIBLE COMPLICATIONS

Recurrent or progressive episodes of hypoglycemia.

EXPECTED COURSE AND PROGNOSIS

• Dogs that undergo exploratory laparotomy are more likely to become and remain euglycemic and have longer survivals than dogs managed by medical means.
• Even in the presence of local metastatic disease, any reduction of tumor burden is likely to improve glycemic control with medical therapies; the median length of euglycemic control after surgery is inversely correlated with the stage of disease and varies from 14 months for dogs without evidence of metastasis to 2–3 months for dogs with nodal and/or distant metastasis.
• Median survival time is inversely correlated with the stage of disease and varies from 16–19 months (range: 2–60 months) for dogs without evidence of metastasis to 7–9 months in dogs with evidence of nodal and/or distant metastasis; more recent studies have documented even longer median survival times of

17–18 months for all dogs with insulinoma and 25–42 months for those dogs undergoing surgery and surgery followed by prednisone therapy at time of relapse, respectively.
• Cats—mean survival time about 6.5 months; range: 0–32 months. Too few cases to accurately predict prognosis.

MISCELLANEOUS

ASSOCIATED CONDITIONS

Obesity due to hyperinsulinemia.

AGE-RELATED FACTORS

Younger dogs have shorter survival times.

SYNONYMS

• Beta-cell tumor.
• Hyperinsulinism.
• Insulin-producing pancreatic tumor.
• Insulin-secreting tumor.
• Islet or beta-cell (adeno)carcinoma.
• Islet cell tumor.

SEE ALSO

Hypoglycemia

ABBREVIATIONS

• DM = diabetes mellitus.
• SPECT = single proton emission computed tomography.

Suggested Reading

Grant ER, Burgess KE. Canine insulinoma: diagnosis, treatment, & staging. Today Vet Pract 2016, 6(6): 60–64.

Moore AS, Nelson RW, Henry CJ, et al. Streptozocin for treatment of pancreatic islet cell tumors in dogs: 17 cases (1989–1999). J Am Vet Med Assoc 2002, 221(6):811–818.

Polton GA, White RN, Brearley MJ, et al. Improved survival in a retrospective cohort of 28 dogs with insulinoma. J Small Anim Pract 2007, 48(3):151–156.

Author Virginia L. Gill

Consulting Editor Patty A. Lathan

Client Education Handout available online

INTERSTITIAL CELL TUMOR, TESTICLE

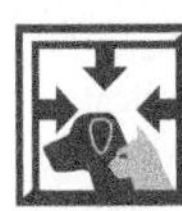

BASICS

OVERVIEW

Benign tumor of the testicle that arises from interstitial (Leydig) cells.

SIGNALMENT

- 33–50% of all testicular tumors in dogs, but rare in cats.
- Median age, 10 years.
- Boxer, German shepherd, Afghan hound, Weimaraner, Shetland sheepdog, collie, and Maltese may be at increased risk.

SIGNS

- Usually incidental finding.
- Fertility issues in breeding dogs.
- May be associated with testosterone secretion and perianal gland hyperplasia or adenomas.
- 4–20% of dogs will have more than one type of testicular tumor. Up to 50% of dogs will have bilateral tumors; only 12% of contralateral tumors will be palpable.

CAUSES & RISK FACTORS

- Generally unknown.
- Cryptorchidism—may predispose.

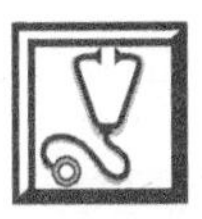

DIAGNOSIS

DIFFERENTIAL DIAGNOSIS

- Sertoli cell tumor.
- Seminoma.
- Hyperadrenocorticism—with feminization.
- Hypothyroidism—with feminization.

CBC/BIOCHEMISTRY/URINALYSIS

- Usually normal, unless estrogen excess causes bone marrow hypoplasia (rare).
- Various cytopenias—with estrogen excess (rare).

OTHER LABORATORY TESTS

- High serum estradiol concentration.
- Low serum testosterone concentration.
- Immunohistochemical evaluation with inhibin-α and calretinin.

IMAGING

- Testicular sonography may aid in differential diagnoses.
- Abdominal ultrasonography for retained testicles and to evaluate for concurrent malignancies.

DIAGNOSTIC PROCEDURES

N/A

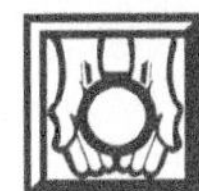

TREATMENT

- Bilateral orchiectomy and scrotal ablation is the treatment of choice; exploratory laparotomy for retained testicles.
- Histopathologic examination of appropriate tissue.
- Immunohistochemistry may be necessary to identify cell of origin in some cases.

MEDICATIONS

DRUG(S) OF CHOICE

None, unless bone marrow hypoplasia induces a dangerous cytopenia.

CONTRAINDICATIONS/POSSIBLE INTERACTIONS

N/A

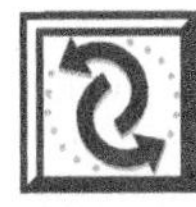

FOLLOW-UP

PATIENT MONITORING

None required, unless bone marrow hypoplasia.

POSSIBLE COMPLICATIONS

Cytopenias caused by estrogen excess.

EXPECTED COURSE AND PROGNOSIS

Bilateral orchiectomy and scrotal ablation are often curative; cutaneous and muscle metastases have been reported.

MISCELLANEOUS

ASSOCIATED CONDITIONS

- Prostate disease—with testicular tumor.
- Perianal gland hyperplasia/adenomas.

SEE ALSO

- Seminoma.
- Sertoli Cell Tumor.

Suggested Reading

Lawrence JA, Saba C. Tumors of the male reproductive system. In: Withrow SJ, ed., Small Animal Clinical Oncology. St. Louis, MO: Elsevier Saunders, 2013, pp. 557–571.

Morrison WB. Cancers of the reproductive tract. In: Morrison WB, ed., Cancer in Dogs and Cats: Medical and Surgical Management. Jackson, WY: Teton NewMedia, 2002, pp. 555–564.

Author Shawna L. Klahn
Consulting Editor Timothy M. Fan

I

INTERVERTEBRAL DISC DISEASE—CATS

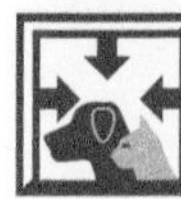

BASICS

OVERVIEW

• Disc extrusion or protrusion causing myelopathy is more common in dogs; both Hansen's type I and type II disc disease, and acute, noncompressive nucleus pulposus extrusion (ANNPE) are reported in cats.
• Type I disc disease is secondary to chondroid metaplasia and mineralization of the nucleus pulposus. • Type II disc disease is secondary to fibroid degeneration and protrusion of the annulus fibrosus. • With ANNPE, normal nucleus pulposus is extruded through a tear in the dorsal annulus, resulting in a concussive or contusive injury, with minimal to no ongoing compression of the spinal cord.

SIGNALMENT

• For all reported cats with myelopathy secondary to disc disease—mean age 8.4 years, range: 1.5–17 years. • Cats with mineralized type I disc disease—mean age 7.3 years, range: 2–13 years. • Predominantly domestic breeds, several purebred (Oriental) breeds reported; rare exotic large cat (tiger) reported. • No sex predisposition.

SIGNS

• Majority of cats have thoracolumbar or lumbosacral disc disease—clinical signs confined to pelvic limbs; cervical disc disease also described, in which case all four limbs may be affected; sacrocaudal disc disease can result in urinary and/or fecal retention or incontinence, lower lumbar pain. • Signs frequently acute or peracute, but may be chronic. • Paresis/ paralysis. • Ataxia. • Gait abnormality, lameness, reluctance to jump. • Spinal/back pain. • Urinary/fecal incontinence.
• Abnormalities of tail carriage or tone. • Loss of pain perception (if severe lesion).
• Hypoventilation (if severe cervical lesion).

CAUSES & RISK FACTORS

• Majority of cats reported had type I disc degeneration, with extrusion of mineralized nucleus pulposus into vertebral canal resulting in spinal cord trauma and compression.
• Unlike dogs, where chondrodystrophic breeds (e.g., dachshunds) predisposed to type I disc disease and subsequent extrusion, no obvious risk factors apparent in cats. • Most cats reported had clinically significant disc protrusions or extrusions between T11 and S1; similar to dogs, presence of the intercapital ligament from T1 to T10 may make disc protrusions in that region less likely.

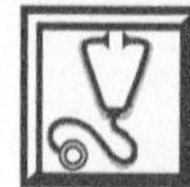

DIAGNOSIS

DIFFERENTIAL DIAGNOSIS

• Trauma. • Vascular—ischemic neuromyopathy ("saddle thrombus"), ischemic myelopathy. • Neoplasia, especially lymphoma. • Vascular—ischemia to spinal cord. • Infectious—feline infectious peritonitis (FIP), *Cryptococcus*, etc.

CBC/BIOCHEMISTRY/URINALYSIS

USUALLY NORMAL.

IMAGING

• Vertebral column radiographs—narrowed disc space(s), mineralized discs in situ, mineralized disc material within vertebral canal or overlying intervertebral foraminae.
• Myelography—extradural compressive lesion at affected disc. • CT—extradural compression; mineralization of compressive material may be apparent. • MRI—T2 hyperintensity within injured cord; mineralized disc material appears hypointense on all imaging sequences; extradural compression may be apparent; with ANNPE, decreased T2 intensity of nucleus pulposus of likely extruded disc, hyperintensity in overlying spinal cord with minimal to no compressive epidural material.

DIAGNOSTIC PROCEDURES

• Cerebrospinal fluid—unremarkable or contaminated with blood in most cats; neutrophilic pleocytosis noted in three cats.
• Histopathology of material removed at surgery—consistent with degenerative disc material (type I or II).

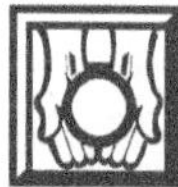

TREATMENT

• Surgical spinal cord decompression likely most effective treatment for compressive disc disease; cats with noncompressive disc extrusions had successful outcomes with physical rehabilitation alone. • Risks of spinal surgery should be discussed with owner—hemorrhage, iatrogenic injury to spinal cord, instability. • Hemilaminectomy, ventral slot, lateral corpectomy, and lumbosacral dorsal laminectomy surgeries are described in the cat. • Postoperative care—good recumbent patient care, pain management, bladder management if incontinent cat (indwelling urinary catheter or manual expression), and appropriate physical therapy. • Fenestration of adjacent mineralized discs should be considered to avoid recurrence. • Medical management (cage rest, pain management) may be considered in ambulatory cats, but more aggressive diagnostics and treatment should be considered in nonambulatory cats and those with progressive neurologic signs.

MEDICATIONS

DRUG(S) OF CHOICE

• Pain management, preferably opiates, if cat tolerates them. • Efficacy of corticosteroids in feline disc disease has not been evaluated.

FOLLOW-UP

• Repeat neurologic examinations (at least 1–2 times/day) during hospitalization to monitor postoperative and medically managed patients for improvement or decline in neurologic status. • Strict cage rest for medically managed and postoperative patients for 4–6 weeks, then gradual increase in activity and physical therapy, as needed.
• Unknown whether long-term activity restriction beneficial. • Because disc disease uncommon in cats, possible recurrence rate unknown, but in one cat that recovered well after hemilaminectomy, additional mineralized disc extrusion caused paraplegia and necessitated second surgery (unpublished data). • A few cats had persistent urinary retention in spite of good recovery of ambulation, requiring routine bladder expression by owner. • Majority of cats managed surgically (even two without pain perception) had good to excellent outcome.

MISCELLANEOUS

ABBREVIATIONS

• ANNPE = acute, noncompressive nucleus pulposus extrusion.
• FIP = feline infectious peritonitis.

Suggested Reading

Rayward RM. Feline intervertebral disc disease: a review of the literature. Vet Comp Orthop Traumatol 2002, 15:137–144.

Author Marguerite F. Knipe

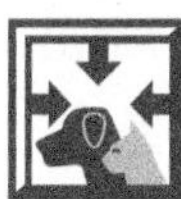

BASICS

DEFINITION

Degeneration of the cervical intervertebral discs that may result in protrusion or extrusion of disc material into the spinal canal. The protruded or extruded disc material causes spinal cord compression (myelopathy) and/or nerve root compression (radiculopathy), as well as concussive spinal cord injury in varying degrees.

PATHOPHYSIOLOGY

- Traditionally classified as acute disc herniation (Hansen type I disc) or chronic disc protrusion (Hansen type II disc); other types include extrusion of apparently healthy, hydrated nucleus pulposus with or without spinal cord compression, the latter termed acute noncompressive nucleus pulposus extrusion (ANNPE).
- Hansen type I—degeneration of the nucleus pulposus and acute rupture of the annulus fibrosus with extrusion of the nucleus pulposus into the spinal canal.
- Hansen type II—fibrinoid degeneration and protrusion of the dorsal annulus fibrosus into the vertebral canal (can involve a dynamic component).
- Disc extrusion or protrusion into the spinal canal causes focal compression of the spinal cord (myelopathy) and/or focal compression of a nerve root (radiculopathy) in addition to a variable degree of contusion injury; ANNPE primarily results in a contusion injury.
- Consequences of spinal cord compression are ischemia and demyelination.
- Consequences of spinal cord contusion include axonal and vascular injury as well as secondary cellular injury.
- Disc extrusion may be secondary to trauma, but this rarely occurs aside from those patients with hydrated disc herniations.
- Surgical fusion of cervical vertebrae may alter the biomechanics of adjacent vertebral bodies and therefore predispose discs to protrusion or extrusion; this is termed the domino effect.

SYSTEMS AFFECTED

Nervous system—either focal myelopathy or focal radiculopathy.

GENETICS

- Not known.
- Chondrodystrophic breeds (e.g., dachshund) are most commonly affected with Hansen type I disc extrusion.
- Large-breed dogs are most commonly affected with Hansen type II disc extrusion.

SIGNALMENT

Species

Dogs, rarely cats.

Breed Predisposition

- Hansen type I—dachshund, poodle, beagle, cocker spaniel, French bulldog, shih tzu; chondrodystrophic breeds.
- Hansen type II—Doberman pinscher, Labrador retriever.

Mean Age and Range

- Hansen type I—3–6 years of age.
- Hansen type II—8–10 years of age.

Predominant Sex

None recognized.

SIGNS

- Severity of clinical signs and spinal cord injury is dependent on several factors, including the rate and volume of disc protrusion or extrusion, spinal cord diameter relative to vertebral canal diameter, and the velocity of disc material that is extruded.
- Herniation in the cervical region can result in fewer neurologic deficits compared to similar lesions in the thoracolumbar region, because the spinal canal area is greater and can accommodate more disc material before spinal cord compression.

Historical Findings

- Neck pain—most common owner complaint.
- Stiff, stilted gait, lameness, or reluctance to move the head and neck.
- Lowered head stance and muscle spasms of the head, neck, and shoulder.
- Inability to rise or falling forward frequently.

Physical Examination Findings

- Neck pain—elicited upon slow manipulation of the neck or by deep palpation of the cervical muscles.
- Apparent forelimb lameness or nerve root signature (e.g., a thoracic limb that knuckles, appears lame, or is held in partial flexion).
- Paresis with or without general proprioceptive deficits involving one or both thoracic and pelvic limbs may be present.
- Pelvic limb paresis may be more severe than thoracic limb paresis.
- Pelvic limb spinal reflexes may be normal to exaggerated.
- Thoracic limb spinal reflexes may be normal to exaggerated when lesions are located in the C1–C6 spinal cord segment, and may be normal to decreased when the C6–T2 spinal cord segment is affected, although this finding is not reliable in some patients.
- Severity of clinical signs and degree of compression are not always correlated.
- Bladder function may be upper motor neuron in nature or normal.

CAUSES

- Degeneration of the intervertebral disc material and subsequent herniation or protrusion.
- Trauma may lead to extrusion of healthy material or otherwise degenerative material.

RISK FACTORS

Obesity and repeated traumatic events in those breeds predisposed to intervertebral disc disease.

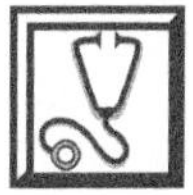

DIAGNOSIS

DIFFERENTIAL DIAGNOSIS

- Neoplasia.
- Atlantoaxial instability.
- Spinal fracture/luxation.
- Discospondylitis.
- Meningitis.
- Fibrocartilaginous embolism.
- Cervical vertebral instability.
- Systemic illness—hypoadrenocorticism, hypothyroidism.
- Spondylomyelopathy.

CBC/BIOCHEMISTRY/URINALYSIS

Often performed in anticipation of medication administration, general anesthesia, and/or surgery.

OTHER LABORATORY TESTS

- Cerebrospinal fluid (CSF) analysis—performed under general anesthesia (prior to myelography if performed).
- CSF analysis reveals nonspecific changes such as mild to moderate elevation in protein levels and mild to moderate pleocytosis, which is more pronounced in Hansen type I disc extrusion.
- Electromyography may be useful if the underlying cause is associated with denervation.

IMAGING

Cross-sectional Imaging

- MRI and CT are most sensitive for diagnosis of cervical intervertebral disc disease and intervertebral disc herniation (IVDH) as well as for surgical planning.
- MRI is the best available method for early recognition of intervertebral disc degeneration (IVDD) in dogs and is capable of the most complete evaluation of the spinal cord parenchyma.
- CT is also useful in diagnosis of spinal cord compression, especially by degenerative disc material; the spinal cord parenchyma is not as well assessed with this modality compared with MRI.

Cervical Spinal Radiography

- Well-positioned lateral and ventrodorsal survey radiographs of the cervical spine aid in excluding other differentials (i.e., discospondylitis, fracture/luxation, atlantoaxial instability, or lytic vertebrae suggestive of a bone tumor), but are not reliable for many patients with IVDH.
- Classic findings include narrowed intervertebral disc space or disc space wedging, collapse of the articular facets, or calcified disc material present in the

intervertebral foramen or in the spinal canal, although many of these findings can be seen without clinical signs, especially in over-represented breeds.
• Hansen type II disc disease may be associated with spondylosis deformans.

Myelography

• Survey cervical radiographs may be misleading; therefore, myelography is more sensitive compared to survey radiographs, although cross-sectional imaging has replaced this modality in most practices.
• Lateral radiographs reveal dorsal deviation of the ventral contrast column over the intervertebral disc space consistent with extradural compression; intraforaminal or dorsolateral disc herniation is best seen on an oblique views.
• Acute cases with spinal cord swelling can cause blockage of contrast material and prevent it from flowing past the obstruction, limiting the diagnostic capabilities of the image.

DIAGNOSTIC PROCEDURES

CSF analysis.

PATHOLOGIC FINDINGS

Gross Findings

• Hansen type I disc—white extruded disc material that has a granular consistency and is usually easily removed from the spinal canal.
• Hansen type II disc—firm protrusion of the dorsal annulus fibrosus that is adherent to the floor of the spinal canal and to the dura of the spinal cord; type II discs are much more difficult to remove from the spinal canal.
• Spinal cord—in acute disc extrusion the spinal cord may appear bruised or swollen or may appear grossly normal; in chronic disc protrusion, the spinal cord may appear to be atrophied but is often normal in appearance.

Histopathologic Findings

• Hansen type I disc—shifting concentration of glycosaminoglycans, loss of water and proteoglycan content, and increased collagen content; the disc becomes more cartilaginous and undergoes dystrophic calcification.
• Hansen type II disc—a gradual fibroid metaplasia leaves the disc with increased glycosaminoglycan levels and lower collagen content; the nucleus does not undergo cartilaginous metaplasia.
• Spinal cord—dependent on the severity of the disease and type of disc disease; Hansen type II: demyelination and gliosis are seen; Hansen type I: hemorrhage and edema can be seen; with severe disease, myelomalacia can be observed.

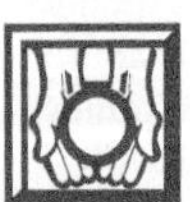

TREATMENT

APPROPRIATE HEALTH CARE

• Conservative or surgical management dependent on patient's history and presenting neurologic status.
• In general, conservative management can be considered with a gradual onset of clinical signs or clinical signs that are limited to hyperpathia or mild ataxia.
• Surgical management is often indicated in patients with repeated episodes of neck pain, severe neck pain and neurologic deficits, or a lack of response to conservative management.
• Patients with hydrated intervertebral disc herniations may perform similarly with conservative and surgical treatment.
• ANNPE is treated conservatively as there is no compression to address surgically.

NURSING CARE

• Level of nursing care needed depends on the severity of the injury; if unable to be cared for at home, patients should be monitored as inpatients.
• Minimal manipulation of the head and neck to avoid worsening discomfort.
• Urination—monitor patients for complete emptying of the bladder; patients may need to have bladder manually expressed or intermittent bladder catheterization; in some cases, indwelling urinary catheter may need to be placed.
• Defecation—patients typically defecate normally, although frequent cleaning and management of any soft stool are important.
• Recumbent patients—should be kept on a well-padded mat and turned frequently (often every 4 hours); should be checked for pressure sores over bony prominences; should be diligently cleaned and kept dry.
• Physical therapy—passive range of motion of all joints should be performed as often as possible to prevent severe muscle atrophy, especially in patients with minimal voluntary motor ability; hydrotherapy can be considered in tetraparetic patients as well.

ACTIVITY

• Activity should be very limited; no running or jumping, and confined to a crate-sized space; when patients are being walked, a harness should be used instead of a collar.
• With conservative or postoperative management, patients should be strictly confined to cage rest for 4 weeks, followed by a gradual return to normal activity over the course of another 4 weeks.

DIET

For obese patients, a decrease in caloric intake should be instituted.

CLIENT EDUCATION

• Appropriate expectations for clinical improvement or signs of worsening should be discussed.
• Confinement is very important for recovery.
• Weight loss if the animal is obese.

SURGICAL CONSIDERATIONS

• The goal of surgery is to remove disc material from the spinal canal and therefore decompress the spinal cord and/or nerve root.
• Surgery usually provides rapid pain relief and significantly improved motor function.
• A ventral cervical slot is the most common surgical approach for the removal of disc material; disc material that has extruded dorsolaterally into the intervertebral foramen or dorsally is removed via a lateral approach or through a dorsal laminectomy.
• Fenestration alone for dogs with neck pain usually does not resolve clinical signs and is no longer recommended.

MEDICATIONS

DRUG(S) OF CHOICE

• Anti-inflammatory therapy (low-dose glucocorticoid or nonsteroidal anti-inflammatory drugs [NSAIDs]) is often beneficial in order to decrease the pain in animals that are being treated conservatively as well as those recovering from surgery; use of high-dose glucocorticoids is not well supported by the literature and is generally not recommended.
• Analgesic medications such as gabapentin and muscle relaxants such as methocarbamol can also be used in conjunction with anti-inflammatories to improve pain control in both conservative as well as surgical treatment.

CONTRAINDICATIONS

Systemic status should be considered when choosing medications.

PRECAUTIONS

Anti-inflammatories or analgesic medications given to animals without simultaneous strict cage confinement could exacerbate disc extrusion by encouraging activity.

POSSIBLE INTERACTIONS

Using glucocorticoids with NSAIDs can cause severe gastrointestinal irritation and possibly intestinal perforation.

FOLLOW-UP

PATIENT MONITORING

• Weekly evaluations should be performed until resolution of clinical signs or until clinical progress plateaus.
• All patients should be fitted with a harness, and neck collars should be avoided.

PREVENTION/AVOIDANCE

• Inherent in particular breeds.
• Keeping patients at an ideal weight may help.

POSSIBLE COMPLICATIONS

• Complications are uncommon.
• Conservative management—continued neck pain, deteriorating motor status.
• Surgical management—hemorrhage, infection, neurologic deterioration,

respiratory compromise, subluxation/luxation of vertebral bodies, collapse of intervertebral disc space, and foraminal collapse.

EXPECTED COURSE AND PROGNOSIS

• Prognosis for patients treated surgically or conservatively depends on neurologic signs at the time of presentation; lack of nociception leads to a poor prognosis for recovery of function long term (<50%) and duration of clinical signs beyond days likely worsens the prognosis.
• Prognosis is generally favorable for most patients; surgical treatment often leads to rapid improvement in pain control, especially in patients undergoing a ventral slot procedure.
• Some patients treated conservatively have recurrence of disease or deterioration and may require surgical intervention.
• Patients who experience IVDH may be predisposed to IVDH at other sites in the future due to the underlying pathology (IVDD).

MISCELLANEOUS

ASSOCIATED CONDITIONS

Animals predisposed to cervical disc disease are also the same breeds that are predisposed to thoracolumbar disc disease.

SEE ALSO

Intervertebral Disc Disease, Thoracolumbar.

ABBREVIATIONS

• ANNPE = acute noncompressive nucleus pulposus extrusion.
• CSF = cerebrospinal fluid.
• IVDD = intervertebral disc degeneration.
• IVDH = intervertebral disc herniation.
• NSAID = nonsteroidal anti-inflammatory drug.

Suggested Reading

Jeffery ND, Levine JM, Olby NJ, Stein VM. Intervertebral disc degeneration in dogs: consequences, diagnosis, treatment and future directions. J Vet Intern Med 2013, 27(6):1318–1333.
Lorenz MD, Coates J, Kent M. Handbook of Veterinary Neurology, 5th ed. St. Louis, MO: Saunders, 2011.

Author Lindsay Boozer
Consulting Editor Mathieu M. Glassman
Acknowledgment The author and book editors acknowledge the prior contribution of Otto I. Lanz

Client Education Handout available online

INTERVERTEBRAL DISC DISEASE, THORACOLUMBAR

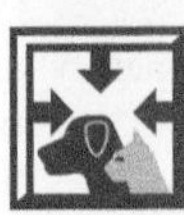

BASICS

DEFINITION

Intervertebral disc disease (IVDD) is an acute traumatic or chronic degenerative condition that causes loss of normal neurologic function to the pelvic limbs, bladder, and anal sphincter. Intervertebral discs chronically degenerate by loss of water, cellular necrosis, and dystrophic calcification. In the chronic condition, biomechanical properties of the disc deteriorate, and subsequently protrusion (Hansen type II) or extrusion (Hansen type I) of disc material occurs.

PATHOPHYSIOLOGY

• Intervertebral disc degeneration is initiated by one or more factors including trauma, chronic overload, decreased spinal mobility, age-related deterioration in collagen and cartilage, and hypermobility. • Hansen type I refers to acute extrusion of nucleus pulposus through the annulus fibrosis into the vertebral canal; Hansen type I lesions typically occur in chondrodystrophic dogs, but may occur in larger nonchondrodystrophic dogs as well; onset of neurologic signs is usually acute and often severe; acute disc extrusion results in extruded material causing direct trauma to the spinal cord and residual disc mass leading to extradural spinal cord compression; trauma and spinal cord compression results in ischemia and spinal cord changes that vary from mild demyelination to necrosis of both gray and white matter; events at the cellular level include release of vasoactive substances, increased intracellular calcium, and increased free radical formation and lipid peroxides. • Hansen type II lesions involve gradual protrusion (bulging) of the dorsal annular fibers into the vertebral canal associated with fibroid degeneration of the disc; Hansen type II lesions typically occur in nonchondrodystrophic dogs; the most common case presentation is of gradual onset of neurologic dysfunction and slow progression. • Hansen type III injuries occur when the nucleus pulposus herniates with such force as to enter the spinal cord by penetration of the dura; Hansen type III injuries are rare, but carry a poor prognosis because they are commonly associated with subsequent myelomalacia and loss of deep pain response.• Affected animals exhibit pain due to dural irritation, nerve root impingement, or possibly discogenic (annular pain receptors) in origin. • Disc herniation is rare between T3 and T10 owing to the barrier of the intercapital ligament between dorsal annulus and spinal cord.

SYSTEMS AFFECTED

• Nervous. • Neuromuscular. • Renal/urologic (loss of voluntary urethral sphincter control). • Digestive (loss of voluntary anal sphincter control). • Musculoskeletal (muscle atrophy in chronic disease).

GENETICS

Early studies suggest a polygenetic model with no dominance or sex linkage.

INCIDENCE/PREVALENCE

• Most common neurologic dysfunction in small animals; affects 2% of the canine population. • Occurs less commonly in cats, but the exact incidence is unknown, and the disease is likely underdiagnosed or reported due to lack of suspicion as a differential diagnosis. • In specific breeds, such as dachshunds, affected prevalence as high as 20% has been reported. • Thoracolumbar disc disease comprises 85% of all disc herniations; 70% occur from T11 to L3.

SIGNALMENT

Species

Dog and occasionally cat.

Breed Predilections

• Type I—dachshund; shih tzu, Lhaso apso; Pekingese, cocker spaniel, Welsh corgi; toy and miniature poodle. • Type II—large breeds, but may occur in any breed. • Type III—active agility, racing, or working breeds; greyhound; border collie; Australian shepherd.

Mean Age and Range

• Type I—3–6 years of age. • Type II—8–10 years of age; cats: mean age of 10 years. • Type III—any age; occurs during exertion or trauma.

SIGNS

General Comments

The severity of clinical signs depends on the type of herniation, velocity of disc contact with the spinal cord, amount and duration of cord compression, location (upper motor neuron [UMN] or lower motor neuron [LMN]), and regional spinal canal/spinal cord diameter ratio (cervical vs. thoracolumbar).

Historical Findings

• Onset may be peracute or acute in chondrodystrophoid dogs (type I disease) and may occur during vigorous activity. • Larger dogs or smaller dogs with type II disease have a more insidious onset and tend to worsen with time. • Dogs with type III disease have a history of active exertion followed by sudden loss of function, or of severe traumatic origin such as vehicular trauma or racing injury.

Physical Examination Findings

• Thoracolumbar pain is a common finding in dogs; reluctant to ambulate and hunched posture; careful palpation of spinous processes and epaxial musculature produces distinct localized pain; often some degree of paraparesis with decreased or absent proprioception or decreased motor ability in the pelvic limbs. • Myotactic spinal reflexes in the pelvic limbs are exaggerated (hyperreflexive) when the lesion is between T3 and L3; reflexes are decreased (hyporeflexive) when lesion is caudal to L3. • Superficial and deep pain perception may be decreased or absent in the pelvic limbs. • Presence of deep pain sensation is the single most reliable prognostic factor for return to acceptable function; pain perception should be conscious in nature and not confused with a withdrawal reflex (local spinal reflex); in animals with diminished conscious deep pain response, observation of mydriasis or tachycardia may be useful in confirming the presence of deep pain. • Forelimb function is normal with thoracolumbar disc rupture; occasionally Schiff–Sherrington phenomena may cause increased muscle tone in the forelimbs, but this clinical sign is location related only and does not indicate a poor prognosis. • Urinary incontinence or retention is common when the lesion affects motor function. • Pain is less obvious in cats; the site of herniation is often lumbar.

CAUSES

• Chondroid or fibroid degeneration of the thoracolumbar intervertebral discs. • Acute trauma that overloads the capacity of the intervertebral disc to absorb force and ruptures the dorsal annulus. • 15% of animals with spinal fractures have been reported to have disc extrusions in addition to the fracture/luxation.

RISK FACTORS

• Type I disease most often affects chondrodystrophic breeds. • Racing and breeds used for agility competition are at risk for Type III disk disease.

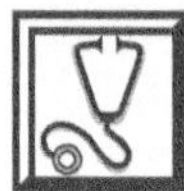

DIAGNOSIS

DIFFERENTIAL DIAGNOSIS

• Type I—trauma causing fracture/luxation, neoplasia, discospondylitis, fibrocartilaginous embolism; differentiated by history, survey radiography, myelography, CT, or MRI. • Type II—degenerative myelopathy, spinal neoplasia, discospondylitis, orthopedic disease; differentiated by history, radiographic modalities, and careful orthopedic and neurologic examination. • Type III—trauma causing spinal fracture or subluxation/luxation of vertebrae in the thoracolumbar region, fibrocartilaginous embolism, or Type I disk disease; differentiated by survey radiography, myelography, CT, or MRI.

CBC/BIOCHEMISTRY/URINALYSIS

• Elevation of liver enzymes is common if the patient has received previous corticosteroids for pain or neurologic disease. • Urine retention/incontinence increases risk of urinary tract infection characterized by leukocytes, protein, and bacteriuria on urinalysis.

OTHER LABORATORY TESTS

Cerebrospinal fluid (CSF) analysis performed routinely in conjunction with myelography if there is high suspicion of another disease process; may be normal, but more typically shows mild to moderate increase in protein with or without pleocytosis when IVDD occurs.

IMAGING

• Thoracolumbar spinal radiography with the patient anesthetized; unanesthetized radiographs can be used to rule out neoplasia and other processes, but can be misleading for thoracolumbar disc disease. • Survey radiographs rule out some other disease processes.
• Diagnostic radiographs taken under general anesthesia may reveal a narrowed or wedged disc space, collapsed articular facet space, and small intervertebral foramen with increased or mineralized density within the spinal canal.
• Accuracy and sensitivity of survey radiographs for determining a specific site of disc herniation are low; in conjunction with careful neurologic examination, the exact location can often be narrowed down to a small vertebral area, but the extent of herniation and pressure on the meninges from herniation of disc material may extend over more than one space.

DIAGNOSTIC PROCEDURES

• MRI is now considered the diagnostic mode of choice when available due to the noninvasive nature and superior information regarding location and extent of disease; presence of a hyperintense spinal cord lesion as long as the body of L2 on a T2-weighted image in deep-pain-negative dogs is associated with a poorer prognosis.
• CT with or without contrast is often diagnostic in chondrodystrophic dogs; dystrophic calcification of extruded material is easily visualized and lateralization can be easily determined; contrast enhancement can different disc disease from neoplastic or granulomatous processes. • Myelography performed with iohexol was previously the method of choice and is still indicated when CT or MRI is not available; the contrast agent is usually introduced at L5–L6; positive diagnosis is an extradural mass lesion causing spinal cord compression adjacent to the affected disc; spinal cord swelling may be evidenced by thinning of contrast columns over several intervertebral spaces.
• Lateralization is more consistent when determined from both oblique and dorsoventral myelogram views. • CSF analysis is an important addition when alternative causes of neuropathy are likely differential diagnoses or when imaging findings are equivocal or nondiagnostic.

PATHOLOGIC FINDINGS

Gross

• Extruded disc material (type I disease)—white to yellow and "toothpaste" consistency seen on laminectomy; if chronic, may be hardened and adhered to surrounding structures; extradural hemorrhage is usually present and mixed with extruded disc material; the ventral sinus may be ruptured and actively bleeding; subdural hemorrhage may be visible. • Protruded disc material (type II disease)—usually firm, grayish-white, and may be adherent to surrounding structures; compression of the spinal cord is apparent, but usually without evidence of recent hemorrhage or trauma visible.
• Extradural or intradural hemorrhage without or with minimal extruded disc material (type III disease); the dural membrane may be penetrated and extruded material may be present within the spinal cord parenchyma; myelomalacia may be detectable as loss of dural and parenchymal integrity at the affected site. • Spinal cord may appear normal or be swollen and discolored in acute severe disease.

Histopathologic

• Degenerated discs have decreased amounts of proteoglycans, glycosaminoglycans, and water; discs may become mineralized or cartilaginous. • Spinal cord lesion depends upon type and severity of disc extrusion or protrusion; acute, severe disease may cause hemorrhage, edema, tissue necrosis; chronic disease demyelination of white and in some cases gray matter.

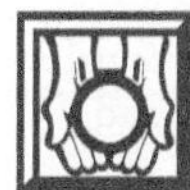

TREATMENT

APPROPRIATE HEALTH CARE

Guidelines for Therapy Based on Classification of Clinical Condition

• Class 1—back pain only, first episode.
• Class 2—recurrent back pain, ataxia, mild paraparesis, motor ability good. • Class 3—severe paraparesis, proprioceptive deficits, motor ability affected but still present; voluntary control of urination may be diminished; bladder many be easy to manually express or difficult due to detrusor dysfunction. • Class 4A—complete paralysis (no motor ability) with deep pain perception present; voluntary control of urination and defecation absent, bladder usually easy to express manually. • Class 4B—complete paralysis, no deep pain perception present.

Treatment Recommendations Based on Classification of Clinical Condition

• Class 1—treated medically unless pain persists. • Class 2—treated medically initially with serial neurologic exam; surgery is performed if patient remains static or condition declines. • Classes 3 and 4A—immediate surgical decompression recommended; prognosis good. • Class 4B—surgical decompression and fair prognosis if within the first 12–48 hours of occurrence or for slower onset of clinical signs (clinical signs progressive over 12 hours); poor prognosis if deep pain perception has been absent for >48 hours or if the clinical signs progressed rapidly (<6 hours) from normal to loss of deep pain. • Serial neurologic examination important for all affected animals.

I

NURSING CARE

• Absolute restricted confinement for 2–4 weeks or until ambulatory. • Minimize spinal manipulation and support spine when handling patient. • Ensure ability to urinate or consider bladder expression, intermittent catheterization, or indwelling urinary catheter for patients in classes 3–4B. • Recumbent patients should be kept clean on padded bedding placed on elevated cage racks and turned frequently to prevent formation of decubital ulcers. • Manual evacuation of the bowel or enemas may be necessary to promote defecation. • Physical therapy with passive manipulation of pelvic limbs begun early followed by more intense therapy (hydrotherapy) for animals with neurologic deficits but regaining motor function; rehabilitation protocols are not contraindicated, but recent research suggests that they may not be beneficial in improving the speed of return to function. • Carts useful in many patients in promoting return to function; patient tolerance is limiting factor.

ACTIVITY

• Restricted movement most important part of medical management. • Cage rest in hospital or enforced cage rest as an outpatient for 2–4 weeks for class 1 patients or postoperative animals.

DIET

Weight reduction if patient is obese.

CLIENT EDUCATION

• Some degree of restricted activity may be important for the remainder of the animal's life since it has disc disease. • Most animals in classes 1–4A have a good to excellent prognosis for return to function, i.e., ambulation with bowel and bladder continence; patients in class 4B have a poorer but not hopeless prognosis;

INTERVERTEBRAL DISC DISEASE, THORACOLUMBAR (CONTINUED)

percentages vary, but up to approximately 50% may regain deep pain and some function, especially if appropriate surgical decompression occurs early in the disease process.

SURGICAL CONSIDERATIONS

• Surgery strongly indicated for animals in classes 3 and 4, also within the first 12–48 hours for class 4B dogs; also indicated for static or worsening class 1 and 2 dogs. • Primary surgical goal is to relieve spinal cord compression by disc mass removal via hemilaminectomy, dorsal laminectomy, or pediculectomy; disc fenestration alone is not effective for treating acute disc extrusions, but is frequently recommended as an adjunct to decompression at the primary site. • Hemilaminectomy on the side of predominant disc extrusion is the surgical procedure of choice for most thoracolumbar discs; studies indicate improved return to function, minimized spinal destabilization, and decreased formation of compressive laminectomy scars in the long-term postoperative period. • Foramenotomy and pediculectomy are similar to hemilaminectomy and may allow a more limited approach and decreased cord manipulation. • Dorsal laminectomy is the procedure of choice for disc herniation in the region of the lumbosacral plexus or where extensive examination of the spinal cord is necessary. • Recurrence of clinical signs in animals in the immediate postoperative period may be due to further extrusion of disc from the original site if fenestration is not adjunctively performed at the site of disc disease during hemilaminectomy or dorsal laminectomy; later recurrence of clinical signs after recovery is usually due to protrusion/extrusion at adjacent sites; several studies document approximately 8% long-term recurrence of clinical signs in dogs after initial hemilaminectomy and active site fenestration due to protrusion/extrusion at other sites. • Controversy remains over the efficacy of multiple site prophylactic disc fenestrations performed during the decompressive surgery, because evidence that fenestration prevents recurrence of clinical signs is not definitive and fenestration causes osteoarthritis to form at the intervertebral space of each site of fenestration, leading to potential chronic patient discomfort and pain.

MEDICATIONS

DRUG(S) OF CHOICE

• Nonsteroidal anti-inflammatory drugs (NSAIDs) or narcotics may be used as analgesics in class 1 cases to alleviate patient discomfort during recovery; use of analgesics is not a substitute for the cage rest period required of all patients.
• Narcotic analgesics may be necessary postoperatively; hydromorphone (0.05–0.2 mg/kg IV/IM/SC q4h) or similar narcotic injectable used at appropriate doses are the treatment of choice in the immediate postoperative period; oral narcotics such as codeine (1–2 mg/kg PO q8h) or tramadol (5–8 mg/kg PO q8h) are useful to alleviate patient discomfort within the first week after decompression; transdermal lidocaine or fentanyl may be useful modes of analgesic administration in some animals, particularly those intractable to frequent dosing of injectable or oral agents.
• Gabapentin (5–10 mg/kg PO q12h), an NMDA receptor antagonist in dogs with chronic pain sensitization, is not an appropriate analgesic used alone in the immediate postoperative period.
• Methocarbamol (25–45 mg/kg q8h) may be useful in cases where muscle spasm is contributing to pain; more applicable with cervical disease. • Bethanechol (5–15 mg/dog PO) and phenoxybenzamine (0.25 mg/kg PO q8–12h) or prazosin (1 mg/15 kg PO q8–12h) are variably helpful in managing bladder dysfunction associated with spinal cord lesion. • Previous indications for methylprednisolone sodium succinate for treatment of acute pain are now controversial for efficacy; the high potential for side effects may outweigh the small gains from the drug.
• Corticosteroids are no longer commonly recommended in the treatment of acute intervertebral disc disease due to lack of demonstrated clinical efficacy.

PRECAUTIONS

• Glucocorticoid use is discouraged in cases of IVDD where drug side effects such as gastrointestinal hemorrhage and intestinal perforation often far outweigh benefits; potent glucocorticoids such as dexamethasone should never be used. • Glucocorticoids are contraindicated within 48 hours of using an NSAID in dogs. • Use of glucocorticoids without cage confinement may decrease pain, thereby encouraging excessive activity and leading to further disc herniation and deterioration of clinical condition.

ALTERNATIVE DRUG(S)

Alternative Therapies

• Acupuncture use has been described, but consistent efficacy has not been demonstrated.
• Chiropractic therapy has no proven benefits for IVDD and may potentially be harmful to the animal. • Percutaneous therapeutic lasers do not reach the site of inflammation and are not efficacious; one recent study did demonstrate slightly more rapid recovery from IVDD if laser therapy regimens occurred as an adjunct to surgical decompression procedures. • Discolysis by enzymatic injection or laser ablation has been described but is not proven therapy in dogs.

FOLLOW-UP

PATIENT MONITORING

• Patients treated medically should be reevaluated two to three times daily for worsening neurologic signs for the first 48 hours after onset. • If stable, reevaluate daily, then weekly, until clinical signs have resolved.
• Patients treated surgically are evaluated twice daily until improvement is noted; urinary bladder function or awaiting development of an autonomic bladder are the limiting factors for hospitalization.

POSSIBLE COMPLICATIONS

• Recurrence of signs associated with disc herniation at original or at new site.
• Deterioration of clinical signs with or without surgery; continued inflammatory processes initiated by the initial extrusion may result in myelomalacia or diminished function. • Rarely, development of ascending or descending myelomalacia; occurs in class 4A or 4B dogs 3–5 days following injury and is characterized by variable and progressive neurologic deterioration, possible fever, possible dyspnea, and extreme pain, with the cranial movement of the inflammation; careful monitoring of the anatomic position of detection of the panniculus reflex is recommended; cranial movement of the reflex can indicate ascending myelomalacia and provide early warning of a grave condition; such animals are often euthanized when diagnosed.

EXPECTED COURSE AND PROGNOSIS

• Overall prognosis for dogs in classes 1–4A good to excellent (85–95%); those treated conservatively may experience recurrence of clinical signs. • Recurrence rates of dogs without fenestration at the time of laminectomy range from 5–30%. • Dogs in class 4B have a variable (10–75%) chance of recovery; overall a guarded but seemingly favorable prognosis if surgery is performed within 48 hours and the animal is allowed sufficient time to recover.
• Dogs with type III disc extrusions often exhibit severe initial clinical signs and carry a grave prognosis for full recovery.

MISCELLANEOUS

ABBREVIATIONS

• CSF = cerebrospinal fluid.
• IVDD = intervertebral disc disease.
• LMN = lower motor neuron.
• NSAID = nonsteroidal anti-inflammatory drug.
• UMN = upper motor neuron.

Suggested Reading

Dewey CW. Surgery of the thoracolumbar spine. In: Fossum TW, ed., Small Animal Surgery, 4th ed. St. Louis, MO: Elsevier Mosby, 2013, pp. 1508–1528.

Kerwin SC, Levine JM, Mankin JM. Thoracolumbar vertebral column. In: Johnston SA, Toias KM, eds., Veterinary Surgery: Small Animal, 2nd ed. St. Louis, MO: Elsevier, 2018, pp. 485–513.

Zidan N, Sims C, Fenn J, et al. A randomized, blinded, prospective clinical trial of postoperative rehabilitation in dogs after surgical decompression of acute thoracolumbar intervertebral disc herniation. J Vet Int Med 2018, 32:1133–1144.

Author James K. Roush

Consulting Editor Mathieu M. Glassman

Client Education Handout available online

INTUSSUSCEPTION

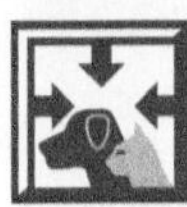

BASICS

DEFINITION

• Invagination of one gastrointestinal (GI) segment into the lumen of the adjacent segment. • Intussusceptions are classified according to their localization within the GI tract—ileocolic and jejunojejunal intussusceptions are the most common; other types include gastroesophageal, duodenojejunal, and cecocolic.

I

PATHOPHYSIOLOGY

• The mechanism is unknown—GI irritation and hypermotility may cause the orad segment to invaginate into the aborad segment; uncoupling of coordinated peristaltic rhythm may be a contributing factor. • Intussusception often leads to a partial or complete mechanical obstruction of the GI tract. • Compromise of venous and lymphatic drainage of the affected bowel leads to marked edema and intramural hemorrhage, and, if left untreated, loss of segmental arterial supply and necrosis; full-thickness compromise of the integrity of the bowel may occur leading to septic peritonitis. • The segment entrapped within the lumen is the intussusceptum; the engulfing segment is the intussuscipiens.

SYSTEMS AFFECTED

• GI—partial or complete mechanical obstruction, bowel wall necrosis, hematochezia, melena, hypermotility followed by ileus, vomiting, and diarrhea.
• Cardiovascular—distributive and hypovolemic shock (vomiting and diarrhea, intraluminal hemorrhage, peritonitis).

GENETICS

N/A

INCIDENCE/PREVALENCE

Uncommon

GEOGRAPHIC DISTRIBUTION

N/A

SIGNALMENT

Species

Dog > cat.

Breed Predilections

• German shepherd—gastroesophageal intussusceptions (60% of reported cases) and other types of intussusceptions. • Siamese cats are overrepresented.

Mean Age and Range

• Most commonly younger animals. • Older affected animals should be evaluated for underlying disease such as chronic enteropathy and intestinal neoplasia.

Predominant Sex

None

SIGNS

General Comments

• Clinical signs depend on the inciting cause, location and type of intussusception, completeness of obstruction, degree of bowel wall compromise and presence of peritonitis.
• Gastroesophageal intussusceptions present with the most acute and severe clinical signs compared to more aborad locations.

Historical Findings

• Recent foreign body ingestion. • Previous or current enteropathy. • Vomiting. • Diarrhea.
• Hematochezia. • Hematemesis. • Melena.
• Abdominal pain. • Abdominal distention.
• Decreased appetite or anorexia. • Weight loss. • Historical findings are typically acute in onset, but chronic cases are reported.

Physical Examination Findings

• Abdominal pain. • Palpation of thickened tube of bowel. • Tachycardia from hypovolemia and pain. • Bradycardia if significant vagal nerve stimulation has occurred.
• Prolonged or rapid capillary refill time.
• Thin body condition. • Fever. • Ileocolic intussusceptions may present with protrusion of the intussusceptum from the rectum; this can be differentiated from a rectal prolapse via probing along the side of the protruding tissue; the presence of a blind-ending fornix indicates the existence of a rectal prolapse.

CAUSES

• Any disease that alters GI motility. • Acute or chronic enteropathy and enteritis.
• Recent abdominal surgery. • Intestinal mural disease or intraluminal foreign body.
• Intestinal parasitism. • Less common causes include renal allograft transplantation (8–33% incidence) and hematopoietic cell grafts (5% incidence) in dogs. The reason for this relationship is unclear.

RISK FACTORS

Presence of any condition listed under Causes.

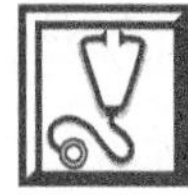

DIAGNOSIS

DIFFERENTIAL DIAGNOSIS

Any disease that can cause vomiting and diarrhea, including intestinal parasites; viral enteritis; bacterial enteritis; intraluminal foreign bodies; chronic enteropathy; mesenteric volvulus; GI neoplasia.

CBC/BIOCHEMISTRY/URINALYSIS

• Leukogram—leukopenia: especially with sepsis or parvoviral infection; leukocytosis: either stress response, acute inflammation, or sepsis. • Hematocrit—elevated if dehydration or underlying hemorrhagic gastroenteritis; decreased: GI hemorrhage. • Biochemical analysis—derangements of electrolytes due to loss through vomiting or diarrhea (may include hyponatremia, hypochloridemia, hypokalemia); azotemia (prerenal) if significantly dehydrated; hypoalbuminemia due to intestinal luminal loss from chronic protein-losing enteropathy or acute changes in bowel wall integrity and permeability.
• Urinalysis—may reveal elevated specific gravity in response to dehydration.

OTHER LABORATORY TESTS

• May see hyperlactatemia secondary to vascular compromise to intestinal segment.
• Blood gas evaluation may reveal a metabolic acidosis secondary to dehydration and hypoperfusion. • Alternately, if the obstruction results in primarily gastric vomiting (pyloric obstruction), a hypochloremic, hypokalemic, metabolic alkalosis may be present.

IMAGING

• Plain abdominal radiographs may reveal an obstructive intestinal pattern—the degree of intestinal distention may be related to the degree of obstruction; may or may not reveal a soft tissue mass consistent with the intussusception. • With gastroesophageal intussusception, a soft tissue mass may be seen within the lumen of the esophagus near the esophageal hiatus of the diaphragm—may be confused with a hiatal hernia, but the severity of the clinical signs typically associated with a hiatal hernia is less severe compared to the often peracute presentation associated with gastroesophageal intussusception.
• Abdominal ultrasound is useful in the diagnosis of intussusceptions—the small intestinal intussusception appears as a target patterned mass on transverse sections, and as a multitude of parallel lines on longitudinal sections. • Upper GI contrast studies or barium enemas can be helpful in supporting the diagnosis of an intussusception.

DIAGNOSTIC PROCEDURES

Upper GI endoscopy will definitively identify gastroesophageal intussusception and differentiate it from hiatal hernia.

PATHOLOGIC FINDINGS

• Gross examination of the intussusception reveals telescoping of a segment of bowel into the adjacent segment. • Histopathologic examination reveals variable degrees of venous and lymphatic congestion, vascular compromise, bowel wall necrosis, and peritonitis.

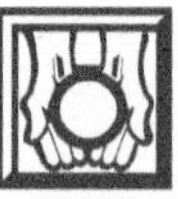

TREATMENT

APPROPRIATE HEALTH CARE

• Initial efforts should be focused on patient stabilization as well as correction of dehydration and existing electrolyte abnormalities. • GI obstruction caused by intussusception is a surgical emergency; proceed with surgery once patient is stabilized.

NURSING CARE

• IV fluid administration to correct dehydration as well as replace anticipated ongoing losses through vomiting and diarrhea. • Specific rate of administration and choice of fluid type are dictated by patient status and electrolyte derangements.

ACTIVITY

Recommend controlled activity for 10–14 days postoperatively.

DIET

• Postoperative anorexia may be due to pain, nausea, and/or esophagitis. • Nasal-esophageal, esophageal, or gastric feeding tubes may be indicated—enteral nutrition is required for intestinal mucosal healing and is preferred; enteral nutrition should be provided within the first 24 hours after surgery, once the patient is awake from anesthesia, at normal body temperature, and treatment of pain, ileus, nausea, and vomiting have been initiated. • If patient is vomiting, a postpyloric feeding tube may be indicated.

CLIENT EDUCATION

• Communication centered on the importance of the identification and treatment of an underlying cause.
• Complications may include perioperative mortality, septic peritonitis, or protracted hospital stay related to dehydration, hypovolemia, regurgitation, vomiting, blood loss, and peritonitis. • Recurrence rates have been reported to be 6–27%.

SURGICAL CONSIDERATIONS

• Surgical correction should be performed as soon as the patient is stable enough to undergo anesthesia and surgery. • Once identified, all intussusceptions are a surgical emergency. • A full abdominal exploratory is always performed for the identification of any potential underlying causes; full-thickness biopsy of the bowel is recommended.
• Multiple intussusceptions may be present.
• Some intussusceptions can be manually reduced by gently milking the intussusceptum from within the intussuscipiens; upon reduction, the bowel may or may not be viable. • In the event that manual reduction is not possible, or the bowel has questionable viability, an intestinal resection and anastomosis is necessary. • Surgical enteroplication has been proposed as a procedure for preventing recurrence. ◦ The rate of side effects and complications associated with enteroplication may be higher than the recurrence rate. ◦ It is important to exercise care when performing this procedure.
◦ Briefly, the loops created in the bowel should be gentle, and sharp turns in the bowel loops are to be avoided; the submucosal layer of the adjacent loops of bowel should be included in the sutures, but the lumen should not be entered.

MEDICATIONS

DRUG(S) OF CHOICE

• Perioperative antibiotics are recommended—manual reduction of an intussusception is considered a clean surgical procedure, while an intestinal resection and anastomosis is considered a clean contaminated procedure; septic peritonitis is considered a dirty/infected procedure.
• Long-term antibiotic administration is not recommended, except in cases in which septic peritonitis is present either preoperatively or postoperatively.

CONTRAINDICATIONS

Some surgeons believe that drugs with promotility properties are contraindicated postoperatively in patients with intussusception, but reports of such drugs causing recurrence is lacking.

PRECAUTIONS

N/A

POSSIBLE INTERACTIONS

N/A

ALTERNATIVE DRUG(S)

N/A

FOLLOW-UP

PATIENT MONITORING

• Postoperatively, patients should be maintained on IV fluids. • Pain ileus, nausea, and vomiting should be treated. • Most recurrences occur within the first few days of surgery, but recurrences have been reported up to 3 weeks after surgery. • Intestinal dehiscence typically occurs 3–5 days postoperatively, as collagenase and matrix metalloproteinase levels rapidly increase at the anastomosis site.

PREVENTION/AVOIDANCE

Prevention of many of the underlying causes can be achieved through such actions as vaccination, intestinal parasite control, and limiting situations in which patients can be exposed to dietary indiscretion or foreign body ingestion.

POSSIBLE COMPLICATIONS

• Recurrence—6–27% of patients. • Septic peritonitis—may result from postoperative intestinal dehiscence or intraoperative contamination. • Short bowel syndrome is a rare complication that can occur with massive resections (generally >70% in dogs) of the small intestine.

EXPECTED COURSE AND PROGNOSIS

Highly dependent upon underlying cause, location of intussusception, and condition at presentation. • In general, the prognosis improves as the location of the intussusception moves more aborad. • Gastroesophageal intussusceptions have a grave prognosis with mortality rates approaching 95%, while intestinal intussusceptions have a good prognosis.

MISCELLANEOUS

ASSOCIATED CONDITIONS

• Intestinal parasites. • Viral enteritis.
• Intestinal mural diseases. • Gastroesophageal intussusceptions are typically associated with an underlying esophageal disorder or gastric motility disorders.

I

AGE-RELATED FACTORS

• Younger patients are typically affected with underlying enteritis (viral or bacterial) or intestinal parasitism. • Older patients are more commonly affected with intestinal neoplasia.

ZOONOTIC POTENTIAL

Some underlying causes may be zoonotic (parasitic, bacterial, and protozoal causes of enteritis).

PREGNANCY/FERTILITY/BREEDING

N/A

SYNONYMS

N/A

SEE ALSO

• Gastrointestinal Obstruction. • Peritonitis.

ABBREVIATIONS

• GI = gastrointestinal.

Suggested Reading

Applewhite AA, Cornell KK, Selcer BA. Diagnosis and treatment of intussusceptions in dogs. Compend Contin Educ Pract Vet 2002, 24:110–127.

Burkitt JM, Drobatz KJ, Saunders HM, Washabau RJ. Signalment, history, and outcome of cats with gastrointestinal tract intussusception: 20 cases (1986–2000). J Am Vet Med Assoc 2009, 234:771–776.

Nordquist B, Culp W. Focal and linear gastrointestinal obstructions. In: Monnet E, ed., Small Animal Soft Tissue Surgery. Ames, IA: Wiley-Blackwell, 2013, p. 360.

Oaks MG, Lewis DD, Hosgood G, et al. Enteroplication for the prevention of intussusception recurrence in dogs: 31 cases. J Am Vet Med Assoc 1994, 205:72–75.

Patsikas MN, Jakovljevic S. Moustardas N. Ultrasonographic signs of intestinal intussusception associated with acute enteritis or gastroenteritis in 19 young dogs. J Am Anim Hosp Assoc 2003, 39:57–66.

Author Stephen Mehler
Consulting Editor Mark P. Rondeau

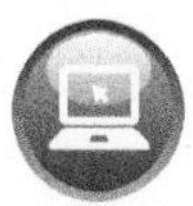

Client Education Handout available online

IRIS ATROPHY

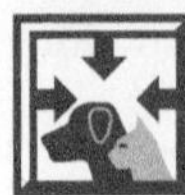

BASICS

OVERVIEW

- Degeneration of iris tissues; both the iris stroma and posterior iris epithelium can be affected, resulting in loss of iris sphincter and dilator muscle function, atrophy of iris vessels, and loss of iris pigment.
- Both the pupillary margin and more peripheral portions of the iris can be affected, resulting in an iris that is thin or has areas of full-thickness tissue loss.
- Senile or secondary change.
- Secondary iris atrophy is usually a result of chronic inflammation (uveitis).
- Iris sphincter muscle is frequently affected by atrophy, resulting in incomplete pupillary constriction, unequal pupil size (anisocoria), and possibly abnormal pupil shape (dyscoria).
- Irregular scalloped, moth-eaten pupil margin is a common manifestation.
- Pupil margin may remain unaffected; peripheral loss of iris tissue can cause large holes in the iris that resemble multiple pupillary openings.
- Vision largely unaffected.

SIGNALMENT

- Dog—common aging change; all breeds, but affects small breeds (e.g., miniature and toy poodles, miniature schnauzers, Chihuahuas) more commonly.
- Cat—uncommon; most common with blue irides.
- Secondary—any breed of dog or cat.

SIGNS

Historical Findings

- Large or dyscoric pupil in one or both eyes.
- Photophobia.
- Previous episodes of uveitis.

Physical Examination Findings

- Incomplete or absent pupillary light reflex accompanied by normal menace response and dazzle reflex.
- Anisocoria may be present with unilateral or asymmetric presentation.
- Irregular, scalloped edge to pupillary margin; dyscoria (see Web Figures 1 and 2).
- Tapetal reflex visible through thin or absent areas of the iris on transillumination—translucent patches or holes within the iris stroma: may resemble additional pupils.
- Strands of iris arising from free pupillary margin occasionally remain, spanning across portions of the pupil (Web Figures 1 and 2).
- Secondary—may be accompanied by any sign associated with chronic uveitis.

CAUSES & RISK FACTORS

- Normal aging.
- Uveitis.
- Glaucoma.

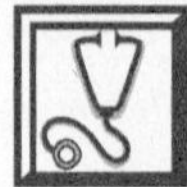

DIAGNOSIS

DIFFERENTIAL DIAGNOSIS

- Must differentiate from congenital iris anomalies:
  - Iris aplasia—rare in dog and cats.
  - Iris hypoplasia—differentiate based on age at first presentation of signs.
  - Iris coloboma—complete, full-thickness area of lack of development of all layers of the iris; frequently associated with the merle condition; may also see associated lack of lens zonules and indentation of the lens posterior to the colobomatous iris area; differentiate based on age and presence of associated abnormalities.
  - Polycoria—more than one pupil, each with ability to constrict due to presence of an iris sphincter.
  - Persistent pupillary membranes—arise from collarette (midportion) of the iris, not from the free pupillary margin.
- Pupil dilation due to glaucoma—elevated intraocular pressure (IOP), corneal edema, conjunctival ± episcleral vascular injection, enlargement of globe may also be present; may also be blind.
- Adhesions of iris to lens or cornea (posterior or anterior synechia) as a result of uveitis or trauma—differentiate based on associated abnormalities consistent with uveitis or perforating trauma (e.g., full-thickness corneal scar).

CBC/BIOCHEMISTRY/URINALYSIS

N/A

OTHER LABORATORY TESTS

N/A

IMAGING

N/A

DIAGNOSTIC PROCEDURES

Tonometry—low IOP possible if secondary to uveitis; high IOP if secondary to glaucoma or if uveitis has also caused secondary glaucoma; normal IOP if primary senile iris atrophy.

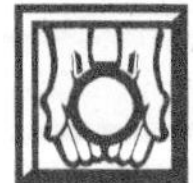

TREATMENT

- Irreversible.
- Secondary—successful treatment aimed at controlling the underlying disease may halt progression of the condition.
- Patient may exhibit photophobia because of inability to constrict the pupil; provide adequate shade.

MEDICATIONS

DRUG(S) OF CHOICE

- Senile—none.
- Secondary—depending on underlying disease.

CONTRAINDICATIONS/POSSIBLE INTERACTIONS

Topical atropine—exacerbates pupillary dilation and photophobia.

FOLLOW-UP

- Senile—may continue to progress with age.
- Secondary—usually does not progress once primary disease is controlled.

MISCELLANEOUS

SEE ALSO

- Anterior Uveitis—Cats.
- Anterior Uveitis—Dogs.
- Glaucoma.

ABBREVIATIONS

- IOP = intraocular pressure.

Suggested Reading

Hendrix DVH. Diseases and surgery of the canine anterior uvea. In: Gelatt KN, Gilger BC, Kern TJ, eds., Veterinary Ophthalmology, 5th ed. Ames, IA: Wiley-Blackwell, 2013, pp. 1146–1198.

Author Simon A. Pot

Consulting Editor Kathern E. Myrna

IRON TOXICOSIS

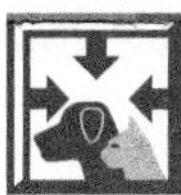

BASICS

OVERVIEW

• Iron is an essential metal for mammals; overdose results in clinical signs and potential death. • Absorption increases with readily ionized and soluble iron. • Oral sources may include dietary supplements (multivitamin, prenatal), snail and slug baits, single-use heat-producing packs (hand warmers), fertilizers, most oxygen absorber packets; overdoses of injectable iron may occur.
• Oral overdose leads to disruption of gastrointestinal (GI) mucosa allowing greater iron absorption, resulting in possible systemic toxicity. • Potential organ systems involved include GI, cardiovascular (CV), hepatobiliary, nervous, hemic, and renal.
• Tissue damage occurs due to free radical/reactive oxygen species formation resulting in direct or secondary damage through processes such as lipid peroxidation.
• Disrupts mitochondrial function and interferes with cellular respiration.

SIGNALMENT

• Predominantly dogs, uncommon in other species. • All ages susceptible.

SIGNS

• History of iron ingestion or injectable overdose. • Initial signs related to GI irritation and mucosal damage; onset of signs occurs within 6–8 hours post ingestion; may include vomiting, diarrhea, mucosal damage (hematemesis, melena), abdominal pain and depression; signs with mild to moderate ingestions may not progress beyond GI. • In absence of significant initial GI signs, systemic toxicity unlikely. • A quiet/latent period may follow initial GI signs and last up to 24 hours post ingestion. • In severe cases, recurrence of clinical signs occurs 12–96 hours post ingestion and can include ongoing vomiting/diarrhea ± mucosal damage, tachycardia, hypotension, CV collapse, metabolic acidosis, shock, hepatic necrosis, coagulopathy/disseminated intravascular coagulation (DIC), acute kidney injury, seizures, death. • Following GI involvement, scarring and stricture formation may occur during healing.

CAUSES & RISK FACTORS

• Ingestion of iron-containing medication or other materials. • Majority of cases due to canine dietary indiscretion. • Elemental/absorbable iron results in mild signs at 20 mg/kg PO and severe signs at 60 mg/kg; other forms of iron including iron salts require conversion to elemental iron for dose calculations. • Metallic iron and iron oxide (rust)not readily ionizable/absorbable and toxicity not expected.

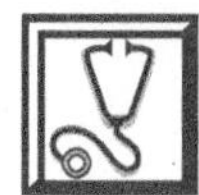

DIAGNOSIS

DIFFERENTIAL DIAGNOSIS

Other causes of severe gastroenteritis and shock, viral/bacterial enteritis, caustic/corrosive ingestion, other dietary indiscretion, gastric torsion, heatstroke, snake bite.

CBC/BIOCHEMISTRY/URINALYSIS

• Leukocytosis. • Anemia (blood loss) or hemoconcentration. • Normal to high aspartate aminotransferase (AST), alanine aminotransferase (ALT), alkaline phosphatase (ALP), serum bilirubin.

OTHER LABORATORY TESTS

• Blood gas to monitor for metabolic acidosis. • Serum iron levels ± total iron binding capacity (TIBC); serum iron level more commonly performed and drawn 4–6 hours post ingestion with capsule or tablet ingestion and 2–3 hours post ingestion with liquid or chewable tablets; repeat q2–4h until peak level if able. • Hemolyzed serum samples increase iron content and should be avoided. • ECG/blood pressure.
• Coagulation profile for DIC.

IMAGING

Abdominal radiography—iron-containing material may be radiopaque; adherence to mucosa may be visible.

DIAGNOSTIC PROCEDURES

Analysis of GI or stomach contents may aid in documenting high iron exposures.

PATHOLOGIC FINDINGS

• Primary gross lesions—hemorrhage in GI tract and liver; hepatomegaly.
• Histopathologic lesions—GI necrosis with potential of hepatocellular and vascular endothelial necrosis.

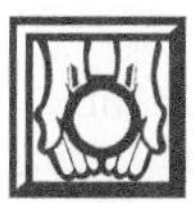

TREATMENT

• Inpatient monitoring with toxic doses; home monitoring if patient remains asymptomatic during initial 8 hours post ingestion; continue inpatient care if symptomatic. • Correct hypovolemic shock with IV fluids. • Correct severe acidosis with IV sodium bicarbonate. • Feed patient bland diet depending on GI status.

Decontamination

• Oral milk of magnesia or aluminum hydroxide (precipitates iron in GI tract) at 5–30 mL PO q8–12h × 24h; may cause diarrhea. • Induce emesis or gastric lavage (if emesis contraindicated). • Emergency gastrotomy if lavage fails to remove adherent pills or bezoars. • Whole bowel irrigation or enema.

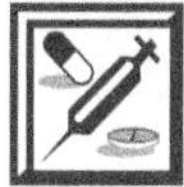

MEDICATIONS

DRUG(S) OF CHOICE

Chelation

• Chelate when serum iron >350–500 μg/dL or serum iron >TIBC. • Deferoxamine mesylate (40 mg/kg IM q4–8h) until urine no longer becomes reddish brown after treatment; IV administration at 15 mg/kg/h CRI reserved for critical patients. • Continue therapy until signs resolved and serum iron below 300 μg/dL.

Other

• Antiemetic (maropitant 1 mg/kg SC/IV q24h). • GI protectant—proton pump inhibitor (omeprazole 1 mg/kg PO q24h); sucralfate (0.5–1 g PO q8–12h). • Ascorbic acid once iron fully removed from GI tract to enhance excretion (10–15 mg/kg q4–6h PO/SC/IM/IV).

CONTRAINDICATIONS/POSSIBLE INTERACTIONS

• Activated charcoal does not bind iron.
• Avoid gastric lavage in presence of hematemesis due to increased risk of perforation. • Administer IV deferoxamine slowly or may precipitate cardiac arrhythmias.

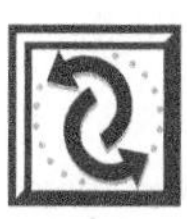

FOLLOW-UP

• Liver enzymes—monitor up to 24 hours after excess circulating iron controlled. • Watch for evidence of GI stricture formation/obstruction.
• Prognosis generally good with early treatment; decreases once signs of iron toxicosis develop or with very large ingestions.

MISCELLANEOUS

SEE ALSO

Poisoning (Intoxication) Therapy.

ABBREVIATIONS

• ALP = alkaline phosphatase. • ALT = alanine aminotransferase. • AST = aspartate aminotransferase. • CV = cardiovascular.
• DIC = disseminated intravascular coagulation. • GI = gastrointestinal. • TIBC = total iron binding capacity.

Suggested Reading

Hall JO. Iron. In: Peterson ME, Talcott PA, eds., Small Animal Toxicology, 3rd ed. Philadelphia, PA: W.B. Saunders, 2012, pp. 595–600.

Author Sarah R. Alpert
Consulting Editor Lynn R. Hovda
Acknowledgment The author and book editors acknowledge the prior contribution of Jeffery O. Hall.

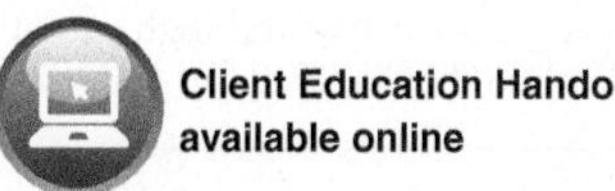
Client Education Handout available online

I

IVERMECTIN AND OTHER MACROCYCLIC LACTONES TOXICOSIS

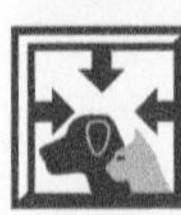

BASICS

OVERVIEW

• Ivermectin, milbemycin, moxidectin, selamectin, others. • Toxicity—dogs given large extra-label dosages (>10–15 times recommended dosage). • Ivermectin—binds to glutamate-gated chloride ion channels in invertebrate nerve and muscle cells causing subsequent paralysis and death of the parasite. Also interacts with other ligand-gated chloride channels, including those gated by γ-aminobutyric acid (GABA).
• Sensitivity—collies and certain other breeds are more sensitive to high doses of ivermectin. This sensitivity has been associated with an inherited deletion of the ABCB1-1Δ gene that encodes a transmembrane protein pump called P-glycoprotein. P-glycoprotein is believed to transport ivermectin out of brain tissue and into circulation.

SIGNALMENT

• Dogs. • Collies—most commonly affected.
• Dogs homozygous for the ABCB1-1Δ gene deletion also affected; heterozygous dogs can react at higher doses. The ABCB1-1Δ gene mutation has been found in Shetland sheepdogs, Australian shepherds, Old English sheepdogs, German shepherds, English shepherds, longhaired whippets, silken windhounds, and a variety of mixed-breed dogs.
• No age or sex predilections.

SIGNS

• Mydriasis. • Depression. • Drooling/salivation. • Vomiting. • Ataxia. • Tremors.
• Disorientation. • Weakness, recumbency.
• Nonresponsiveness. • Transient blindness.
• Bradycardia. • Hypoventilation. • Coma.
• Death.

CAUSES & RISK FACTORS

• Extra-label use at high dosage. • Breed sensitivity—see above. • Treating demodicosis with high-dose ivermectin while patient is on spinosad.

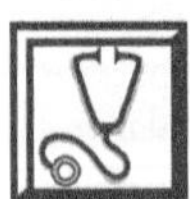

DIAGNOSIS

• History and clinical signs. • No specific tests useful.

DIFFERENTIAL DIAGNOSIS

• Overdoses of other insecticides such as pyrethrins, pyrethroids, organophosphorus, and carbamate compounds. • Other toxicants, such as loperamide or diseases affecting CNS.

CBC/BIOCHEMISTRY/URINALYSIS

N/A

OTHER LABORATORY TESTS

Arterial blood gases—may reveal high partial pressure of carbon dioxide ($PaCO_2$) and low partial pressure of oxygen (PaO_2) from respiratory depression and hypoventilation.

DIAGNOSTIC PROCEDURES

Physostigmine 1 mg IV; temporary (30–40 min) return to consciousness or resumed alertness and muscle activity after administration supports but does not confirm diagnosis; does not speed recovery; not indicated for treatment; glycopyrrolate administered first may prevent severe bradycardia.

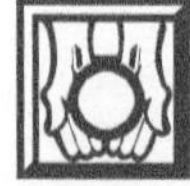

TREATMENT

• Supportive and symptomatic care. • If patient alert and able to swallow, activated charcoal repeated every 6–8 hours; monitor for hypernatremia. • Use of IV lipid emulsion has been successful in ameliorating clinical signs in many cases; recent literature has conflicting data on effectiveness in dogs with ABCB1-1Δ homozygous mutations.
• Important goals—proper fluid therapy, maintenance of electrolyte balance, nutritional support, and prevention of secondary complications. • Nutritional support—institute early, preferably within 2–3 days of exposure; severe CNS depression or coma may last for days or weeks depending on severity of exposure. • Good nursing care for recumbent patient. • Ocular lubricants.
• Mechanical ventilation—may be required with respiratory depression.

MEDICATIONS

DRUG(S) OF CHOICE

• No known reversal agent. • Atropine or glycopyrrolate—may be administered as needed to treat bradycardia. • 20% intravenous lipid emulsions—bolus dose 1.5 mL/kg over 2–3 min; CRI of 0.25 mL/kg/min for 30–60 min; check serum q2h and if not lipemic; repeat as needed; if no clinical improvement after three doses, discontinue.

CONTRAINDICATIONS/POSSIBLE INTERACTIONS

• Other drugs known to cause toxicity in dogs with ABCB1 mutation—loperamide, doxorubicin, vincristine, vinblastine, acepromazine, butorphanol, emopside, and erythromycin. • Do not use ivermectin concurrently with ketoconazole.
• Concomitant extra-label use of ivermectin and spinosad may produce clinical signs.

FOLLOW-UP

• Prognosis and eventual outcome—depends on individual and breed sensitivity, amount of drug ingested or injected, how rapidly clinical signs develop, response to supportive treatment, and overall health of patient.
• Convalescence may be prolonged (several weeks); good supportive care in many seemingly hopeless cases has resulted in complete recovery.

MISCELLANEOUS

SEE ALSO

• Heartworm Disease—Dogs.
• Poisoning (Intoxication) Therapy.

ABBREVIATIONS

• GABA = γ-aminobutyric acid.
• PaCO2 = partial pressure of carbon dioxide.
• PaO_2 = partial pressure of oxygen.

Suggested Reading

Crandell DE, Weinberg GI. Moxidectin toxicosis in a puppy successfully treated with intravenous lipids. J Vet Emerg Crit Care 2009, 19(2):181–186.

Gupta, Ramesh C., ed. Veterinary Toxicology: Basic and Clinical Principles, 3rd ed. San Diego, CA: Elsevier, 2018, pp. 539–550.

Mealy KL. Canine ABCB1 and macrocyclic lactones: heartworm prevention and pharmacogenetics. Vet Parasitol 2008, 158:215–222.

Author Dominic A. Tauer

Consulting Editor Lynn R. Hovda

Acknowledgment The author and book editors acknowledge the prior contribution of Allan J. Paul

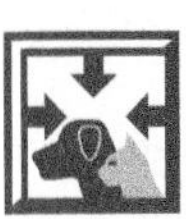

BASICS

DEFINITION

Luxation is the complete disruption of the contiguous articular surfaces of a joint when the supporting structures around the joint are damaged or missing. Subluxation is a partial disruption.

PATHOPHYSIOLOGY

• Synovial joints have a joint capsule that joins the articulating bones together. The fibrous layer of this capsule is a primary stabilizer of the joint. Most joints have additional ligaments that reinforce the joint capsule to improve the resistance to movement outside of the normal range of motion of that joint. All motion joints also have a system of muscles and tendons that exert forces on the joint to control movement and prevent subluxation of the joint. The co-contraction forces around a joint are very influential on the stability of the joint. Instability occurs when the stabilizing system is damaged, disrupted, or does not develop normally. • If laxity is clinically apparent, then the instability is generally described as luxation or subluxation of the joint. • Luxation may occur as a result of traumatic forces causing the joint to move beyond the elastic limits of the supporting tissues. • Secondary changes are set in motion by damage to the tissues that creates early, and then later, more chronic joint damage.

SYSTEMS AFFECTED

• Musculoskeletal—primarily the intra-articular environment and the support structures around the joint, including joint capsule, fibrocartilage, collateral ligaments, and supporting muscle/tendon units.
• Neurologic—neurologic feedback and supply to the support system may also be affected.

GENETICS

• Hyperlaxity syndrome is an inherited trait in humans. Puppies may show temporary hyperlaxity when confined or when housed on poor substrates.
• Hip dysplasia is a form of inherited laxity of the coxofemoral joint. • Shoulder luxation is an inherited predisposition in small breeds, such as miniature poodles. • Femoropatellar instability leading to medial patellar luxation is a common inherited disease in small-breed dogs. • Ehlers–Danlos syndrome is a congenital collagen disorder that leads to generalized joint laxity.

INCIDENCE/PREVALENCE

Various forms of laxity/luxation (specifically hip dysplasia and medial patella luxation) are very common. Other forms such as Ehlers–Danlos syndrome are extremely uncommon.

SIGNALMENT

Species

All species.

Breed Predilections

• Traumatic luxation has not been shown to be breed specific in any joint. • Breed predilection for nontraumatic luxations varies with the joint affected. • Hip—large breeds show clinical signs of hip dysplasia more frequently than smaller breeds, but breeds of all sizes can have radiographic signs. • Congenital shoulder luxation occurs most commonly in miniature breeds (miniature poodle). • Medial patella luxation is more common in small-breed dogs.

Mean Age and Range

• Traumatic—any age. • Congenital laxity/luxation is typically seen in the juvenile dog, with secondary degenerative joint disease showing later in life.

SIGNS

• Acute swelling, pain, and non-use of the limb are usually seen with acute luxation. Partial weight-bearing may occur with subluxation or chronic luxation. • Abnormal anatomic position of one bone in relation to the adjoining bone. • Hip luxation is commonly craniodorsal (the displacement of the femoral head in relation to the acetabulum). • Shoulder luxation is commonly medial. • Elbow luxation is commonly proximolateral. • Carpal and tarsal luxations commonly result in varus, valgus, or hyperextension when stressed.

CAUSES

• Traumatic overstress of normal soft tissues beyond their elastic limit. • Fracture of the bone attaching the origin or insertion of a tendon or ligament to the body of the bone.
• Minimal stress on abnormally unstable joints of congenital etiology.

RISK FACTORS

• Abnormal congenital conformation, causing altered joint stresses. • Fatigue, causing muscle weakness and incoordination.
• Neurologic derangement. • Environments conducive to traumatic events.

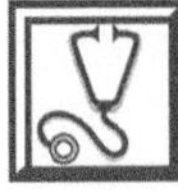

DIAGNOSIS

DIFFERENTIAL DIAGNOSIS

• Fractures. • Joint disease—immune-mediated, septic, or degenerative.

CBC/BIOCHEMISTRY/URINALYSIS

• No abnormalities expected that are directly related to the luxation. • Trauma-induced abnormalities in traumatic situations.

OTHER LABORATORY TESTS

Arthrocentesis may help to rule out nontraumatic joint disease.

IMAGING

• Radiographs confirm the diagnosis by documenting the anatomic malalignment.
• Radiographs to rule out other pathology, such as intra- or extra-articular fractures that could affect the decision to perform closed reduction. • Stress views may be needed in some situations.

DIAGNOSTIC PROCEDURES

• Palpation of the laxity/luxation (ex. ortolani, cranial drawer, medial patella luxation, stress-induced laxity/instability).
• Palpation of the position of the displaced bone.

PATHOLOGIC FINDINGS

• Trauma-induced hemorrhage, edema, and disruption of ligaments and joint capsule.
• Secondary changes related to degenerative joint disease.

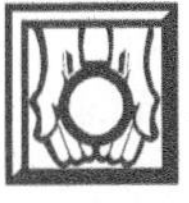

TREATMENT

APPROPRIATE HEALTH CARE

Closed Reduction

• Closed reduction is attempted if: there is no underlying intraarticular pathology (fracture); there is adequate intact support structures to maintain marginal stability immediately after reduction; there is no underlying dysplasia that predisposes the joint to luxation (as this would increase the chance of reduction failure); there is no additional pathology in other limbs that would require immediate weight-bearing of the affected limb. • Closed reduction is often considered the first line of treatment (when appropriate) for hip luxations (craniodorsal and caudoventral), shoulder luxation, and elbow luxations.
• Surgical stabilization is often required with carpal, tarsal, and stifle luxations. • Surgical intervention (arthrodesis) or long-term brace (orthotic) are required for palmar or plantar instability due to the excessive stresses placed on palmar and plantar ligaments and fibrocartilage in the dog and cat.

Immobilization

Immobilize the joint with a bandage/splint if the affected joint is distal to the inguinal or axial areas.

External Coaptation (Maintenance Period)

• Craniodorsal hip luxation—ehmer sling (~14 days). • Caudoventral hip luxation—hobbles (~14 days). • Elbow luxation—spica splint (~14 days). • Shoulder luxation (medial)—valpeau sling (~14 days).
• Shoulder luxation (lateral)—spica splint (~14–21 days). • Tarsocrural and radiocarpal instability (except palmar and plantar instability)—cast or medial/lateral splint (6–10 weeks depending on degree of injury).
• Medial, lateral, or dorsal pes and manus instability caudal spoon splint or cast (6–10 weeks depending on degree of injury).

JOINT LUXATIONS

NURSING CARE

• Rest, exercise restriction, pain control, and maintenance of external coaptation. • Cold compresses for 5–10 minutes four or five times a day initially to reduce inflammation.

ACTIVITY

Cage rest for joint stabilization period, then slow return to function to encourage healing and strengthening of soft tissue support of the limb.

DIET

Normal

CLIENT EDUCATION

Activity and weight gain increase the likelihood of degenerative changes in the long term.

SURGICAL CONSIDERATIONS

• Surgery is typically required for spinal luxations. • For appendicular skeleton for which closed reduction is ideal, an open surgical approach is preferred if: closed reduction fails; there is evidence of predisposing joint dysplasia; there is evidence of an intra-articular fracture; there is concurrent pathology that requires early stability and weight-bearing on the affected limb. • With open reduction, stabilization via prosthetic ligament placement, ligament reconstruction, or temporary transarticular stabilization is considered. • Salvage procedures include prosthetic joint replacement, surgical removal of bone-to-bone contact points (femoral head and neck ostectomy), arthrodesis, and amputation. Arthrodesis is the first line of treatment for all palmar and plantar luxations of the pes or manus.

MEDICATIONS

DRUG(S) OF CHOICE

• Nonsteroidal anti-inflammatory drugs (NSAIDs) decrease prostaglandin synthesis by inhibiting cyclooxygenase enzymes:
∘ Carprofen 2.2 mg/kg PO or SC q12h, or 4.4 mg/kg PO or SC q24h. ∘ Deracoxib 1–2 mg/kg PO q24h. ∘ Firocoxib 5 mg/kg PO q24h. ∘ Grapiprant 2 mg/kg PO q24h—for canines. ∘ Meloxicam 0.1 mg/kg PO or SC q24h. ∘ Robenacoxib 1–2 tablets PO depending on weight q24h for 3 days—for felines. • Tramadol 1–4 mg/kg PO q8–12h. • Gabapentin 5–10 mg/kg PO q8–12h.

CONTRAINDICATIONS

• NSAIDs and gastrointestinal sensitivity.
• NSAIDs and liver or renal pathology.

PRECAUTIONS

Stop medications if diarrhea or vomiting is seen.

POSSIBLE INTERACTIONS

• Other NSAIDs. • Steroids.

ALTERNATIVE DRUG(S)

• Analgesics (opioids). • Fish oil supplementation to decrease inflammatory mediator production.

FOLLOW-UP

PATIENT MONITORING

• Always take a radiograph after reduction.
• Some clinicians will evaluate reduction 3–5 days after initial stabilization via radiographs to ensure surgical stabilization is not warranted (note—do not remove coaptation for radiographs as this will increase risk of reluxation). • Take follow-up radiographs when the splint/sling is removed (typically 2–10 weeks post stabilization).

PREVENTION/AVOIDANCE

• Fenced-in yards. • Keep pets on a leash when outside. • Keep the sling in place for the duration of planned stabilization (for coaptation that is maintained for <3 weeks).

POSSIBLE COMPLICATIONS

• Reluxation. • Pressure sores from bandages and coaptation. • Clinical osteoarthritis.
• Infection after surgery. • Implant failure of joint prosthetic.

EXPECTED COURSE AND PROGNOSIS

• Return of function is expected unless a complication occurs. • Progressive degenerative joint disease.

MISCELLANEOUS

ASSOCIATED CONDITIONS

Osteoarthritis

AGE-RELATED FACTORS

None

PREGNANCY/FERTILITY/BREEDING

If patient is pregnant, care should be taken to prescribe appropriate pain management.

SYNONYMS

Dislocation

SEE ALSO

• Arthritis (Osteoarthritis).
• Hip Dysplasia.

ABBREVIATIONS

• NSAID = nonsteroidal anti-inflammatory drug.

Suggested Reading

Alam MR, Lee JI, Kang HS, et al. Frequency and distribution of patellar luxation in dogs: 134 cases (2000 to 2005). Vet Comp Orthop Traumatol 2007, 20(1):59–64.

DeCamp CE. Brinker, Piermattei and Flo's Handbook of Small Animal Orthopedics and Fracture Repair, 5th ed. St. Louis, MO: Elsevier Health Sciences, 2016.

Evers P, Johnston GR, Wallace LJ, Lipowitz AJ, King VL. Long-term results of treatment of traumatic coxofemoral joint dislocation in dogs: 64 cases (1973–1992). J Am Vet Med Assoc 1997, 210(1):59–64.

Kieves NR, Lotsikas PJ, Schulz KS, Canapp SO. Hip toggle stabilization using the TightRope® system in 17 dogs: technique and long-term outcome. Vet Surg 2014, 43:515–522.

McLaughlin RM. Traumatic joint luxations in small animals. Vet Clin North Am Small Anim Pract 1995, 25(5):1175–1196.

Authors Victoria A. DeMello and Wesley J. Roach

Consulting Editor Mathieu M. Glassman

Acknowledgments The authors and editor acknowledge the prior contributions of Spencer A. Johnston and Caitlyn F. Connor.

Client Education Handout available online

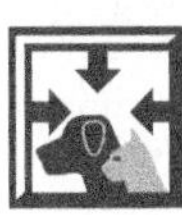

BASICS

OVERVIEW

- Presumed immune-mediated inflammation of the cornea characterized by perilimbal corneal vascularization, white-pink corneal infiltrate, and corneal edema.
- Synonym—proliferative keratitis.

SIGNALMENT

Young adult to middle-aged cats.

SIGNS

- Unilateral or bilateral.
- Variable ocular pain, often minimal.
- Serous to mucoid ocular discharge.
- Limbal superficial corneal vascularization 90–360° (temporal or inferior nasal quadrants are first affected).
- White to pink, flat or raised granular corneal infiltrate.
- Multifocal, small, white gritty corneal deposits.
- Corneal edema.
- Corneal ulceration may be present.
- Conjunctival and third eyelid hyperemia, chemosis, and thickening with possible cobblestone surface texture.

CAUSES & RISK FACTORS

- Feline herpesvirus-1 (FHV-1) may be associated, but exact role is unclear.
- Exact etiopathogenesis unknown; proposed theories are: (1) type I hypersensitivity with IgE-mediated mast cell and eosinophil degranulation, (2) type IV reaction where sensitized T-lymphocytes stimulate eosinophil-mediated corneal damage.
- Bacterial and fungal infection are not consistent etiologic causes, although secondary bacterial keratitis may occur.

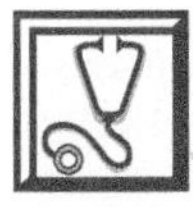

DIAGNOSIS

DIFFERENTIAL DIAGNOSIS

- Chronic corneal ulceration with secondary corneal vascularization (granulation tissue).
- FHV-1 stromal keratitis—appears similar, but lacks proliferative component, with more severe ocular pain and corneal ulceration.
- Corneal neoplasia: (1) lymphoma—concurrent conjunctival and/or uveal infiltration is common, (2) squamous cell carcinoma—rarely involves cornea in cats.
- *Chlamydia psittaci* or *Mycoplasma felis*—usually conjunctival diseases without corneal involvement.

CBC/BIOCHEMISTRY/URINALYSIS

Peripheral eosinophilia may be present.

OTHER LABORATORY TESTS

- PCR for FHV-1 has limited diagnostic value since healthy cats may have positive results.
- Immunofluorescent antibody test (IFA) testing for *Chlamydia psittaci.*

DIAGNOSTIC PROCEDURES

- Corneal cytology provides definitive diagnosis and should be done first. Typically numerous eosinophils, free eosinophil granules and/or mast cells, neutrophils, lymphocytes, plasma cells, and epithelial cells are seen.
- Cytology helps rule out chlamydia and mycoplasma.
- Fluorescein staining to evaluate for corneal ulceration.
- Keratectomy and histopathology may confirm diagnosis in chronic or nonresponsive cases.

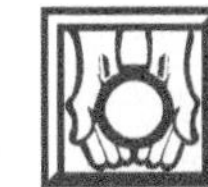

TREATMENT

Outpatient

MEDICATIONS

DRUG(S) OF CHOICE

- Topical corticosteroids—1% prednisolone acetate or 0.1% dexamethasone sodium phosphate q6–12h for 5–7 days, then gradually taper to the lowest effective frequency of application or discontinue.
- Topical 1–2% cyclosporine A q8–12h, then tapered to lowest effective frequency of application or discontinued. Can use in cats in which oral megestrol acetate and topical corticosteroids are contraindicated. May be irritating or cause blepharitis.
- Topical 0.5% megestrol acetate q8–12h initially, then tapered to lowest effective frequency or discontinued.
- Adjunctive topical or systemic antiviral therapy may be warranted in cases with history or clinical signs compatible with FHV-1 infection.
- Subconjunctival corticosteroids—triamcinolone acetonide (0.1–0.2 mL q3–7 days); only in cats that are difficult to treat with topical medications.
- Systemic prednisolone—2.2 mg/kg PO q12h and taper. Use only if a cat will not tolerate topical therapy or oral megestrol acetate.
- Megestrol acetate—2.5 mg PO q24h for 3–5 days, then 2.5 mg PO q48h for 3–5 days, then gradually decrease frequency to the lowest effective frequency or discontinue.

CONTRAINDICATIONS/POSSIBLE INTERACTIONS

- Topical corticosteroid administration may be associated with recrudescence of FHV-1 keratoconjunctivitis and should be used and monitored carefully. Client should be advised to immediately report any adverse change in the condition of the eye (blepharospasm, corneal edema, increased ocular discharge, etc.).
- Megestrol acetate causes adrenal cortical suppression and may result in diabetes mellitus, polyphagia, temperament change, mammary gland hyperplasia, or neoplasia and pyometra. It should not be used in cats with hepatic disease or other illness.

FOLLOW-UP

- Response to therapy is usually rapid.
- Complete resolution may take several days to months. May require long-term therapy.
- Corneal vascularization and infiltrate may resolve completely with minimal corneal scarring.
- Recurrences in both the short and long term are common.

MISCELLANEOUS

Not typically associated with dermatologic eosinophilic granuloma complex.

ABBREVIATIONS

- FHV-1 = feline herpesvirus-1.
- IFA = immunofluorescent antibody test.

Suggested Reading

Stiles J. Feline ophthalmology. In: Gelatt KN, Gilger BC, Kern TJ, eds., Veterinary Ophthalmology, 5th ed. Ames, IA: John Wiley & Sons, 2013, pp. 1496–1498.

Stiles J, Coster M. Use of an ophthalmic formulation of megestrol acetate for the treatment of eosinophilic keratitis in cats. Vet Ophthalmol 2016, 19(Suppl 1):86–90.

Author Anne J. Gemensky Metzler

Consulting Editor Kathern E. Myrna

KERATITIS, NONULCERATIVE

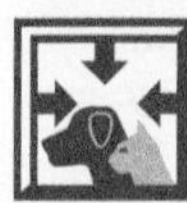

BASICS

DEFINITION

An inflammatory disorder of the cornea that does not retain fluorescein stain.

PATHOPHYSIOLOGY

A pathologic response resulting in reduced corneal clarity secondary to edema, inflammatory cell infiltration, vascularization, pigmentation, lipid or calcium deposition, or scarring.

SYSTEMS AFFECTED

K

Ophthalmic

GENETICS

• No proven genetic basis in dogs or cats.
• Chronic superficial keratitis (pannus)—inherited predisposition in German shepherd dogs.

INCIDENCE/PREVALENCE

Common in dogs and cats.

GEOGRAPHIC DISTRIBUTION

Chronic superficial keratitis is more common in regions of high UV light exposure.

SIGNALMENT

Species

• Dog—chronic superficial keratitis (pannus); pigmentary keratitis; pigmentary keratopathy of pugs; nodular granulomatous episcleritis (NGE; see Episcleritis); keratoconjunctivitis sicca (KCS; see Keratoconjunctivitis Sicca).
• Cat—eosinophilic keratitis (see Keratitis, Eosinophilic—Cats); herpesvirus (stromal form); corneal sequestrum; KCS uncommon, usually secondary to chronic herpesvirus infection.

Breed Predilections

Dogs

• Chronic superficial keratitis (pannus)—highest prevalence in German shepherd dogs and sighthounds. • Pigmentary keratitis—notably brachycephalic breeds with exposure keratopathy from lagophthalmia, tear film deficiencies, and trichiasis. • Pigmentary keratopathy of pugs—suspected genetic condition that results in progressive corneal pigmentation, cause currently unknown.
• NGE—prevalent in cocker spaniels, collies, and Shetland sheepdogs. • KCS—brachycephalic breeds, cocker spaniels, English bulldogs, West Highland white terriers, cavalier King Charles spaniels.

Cats

• Eosinophilic keratitis—most prevalent in domestic shorthair. • Corneal sequestration—most prevalent in brachycephalic breeds.

Mean Age and Range

• Dogs: chronic superficial keratitis—any age, usually between 3-6 years (younger in sighthounds); pigmentary keratitis and pigmentary keratopathy of pugs may occur at any age; NGE—any age, mean 3.8 years in Collies; KCS—middle-aged to older dogs.
• Cats: herpesvirus, eosinophilic keratitis, and corneal sequestrum—any age.

Predominant Sex

• Dogs—female predisposition reported for pannus and KCS. • Cats—castrated male predisposition reported for eosinophilic keratitis.

SIGNS

Historical Findings

Corneal discoloration and ocular discomfort.

Physical Examination Findings

Dogs

• Chronic superficial keratitis—usually bilateral, corneal vascularization range from superficial vessels to dense granulation tissue with variable pigmentation; lateral or ventrolateral cornea (entire cornea affected in advanced cases); thickened and depigmented third eyelids; white deposits (corneal degeneration) may be present at the leading edge of corneal lesion; may lead to blindness.
• Pigmentary keratitis—Focal to diffuse brown discoloration of the cornea; often with corneal vascularization or scarring.
• Pigmentary keratopathy of pugs—brown corneal pigmentation originating from medial cornea and progressing towards central cornea. • NGE—bilateral or unilateral; raised, fleshy masses affecting the lateral limbus and cornea; corneal deposits, edema, and vascularization may occur in adjacent corneal stroma; slow to rapidly progressive; third eyelids may appear thickened. • KCS—unilateral or bilateral; mucoid ocular discharge, conjunctival hyperemia, corneal vascularization, pigmentation, and scarring; corneal ulceration may occur.

Cats

• Herpesvirus (stromal form)—unilateral or bilateral; stromal edema, infiltrates, deep vascularization and scarring; ulceration may occur; severe scarring may threaten vision.
• Eosinophilic keratitis—usually unilateral; raised vascularized lesion with pink-white infiltrates forming gritty plaques; may retain fluorescein stain at the lesion's periphery.
• Corneal sequestrum—usually unilateral (can be bilateral); amber, brown, or black plaques on the central or paracentral cornea; vary in size and depth; edges may appear raised; corneal vascularization is variable; may retain fluorescein at periphery of lesion.

CAUSES

Dogs

• Chronic superficial keratitis—presumed to be immune-mediated; high altitude (increased UV radiation exposure) increases the prevalence and severity of disease.
• Pigmentary keratitis—secondary to chronic corneal irritation; evaluate for primary underlying ocular conditions; frequently associated with exposure keratopathy and KCS. • Pigmentary keratopathy of pugs—unknown, may have genetic basis. • NGE—presumed to be immune mediated.
• KCS—bilateral: usually immune-mediated or drug-induced; unilateral: congenital, iatrogenic, neurogenic.

Cats

• Herpesvirus (stromal form)—immune-mediated T-cell lymphocyte reaction to herpesvirus antigen (vs. cytopathic effect of the virus). • Eosinophilic keratitis—possible hypersensitivity reaction; high incidence of animals PCR positive for feline herpesvirus type 1 (FHV-1); fewer positive for *Chlamydia*-like agents. • Corneal sequestrum—unknown; likely due to chronic corneal irritation or ulceration; suggested relationship with herpesvirus.

RISK FACTORS

Dogs—chronic superficial keratitis more likely to occur at high altitudes.

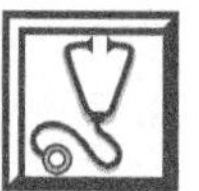

DIAGNOSIS

DIFFERENTIAL DIAGNOSIS

• Infectious keratitis is usually ulcerative and painful; cytology of the cornea reveals white blood cells, infectious organisms. In cats, stromal herpesvirus may be associated with ulcerative keratitis and secondary bacterial infection. • Neoplasia—rare involvement of sclera or cornea; distinguish based on color, age of animal, breed predilection; usually unilateral; lack of response to topical anti-inflammatory therapy. Very rare in cats.

DIAGNOSTIC PROCEDURES

Dogs

• Schirmer tear test—values <15 mm/min suggest KCS but should be interpreted with breed and ocular findings. • Cytologic examination of corneal or conjunctival scrapings—chronic superficial keratitis characterized by lymphocytes, plasma cells, and mast cells. • Biopsy of episcleral nodular mass or cornea (superficial keratectomy)—for NGE diagnosis, can be considered for patients with chronic superficial keratitis.

Cats

• Conjunctival or corneal scraping—PCR most successful for diagnosis for herpesvirus (IFA or viral culture of limited value). Eosinophilic keratitis: eosinophils on cytology. • Superficial keratectomy—consider for diagnosis of eosinophilic keratitis or sequestrum but usually unnecessary.

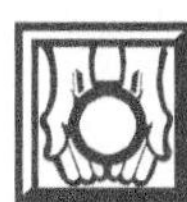

TREATMENT

APPROPRIATE HEALTH CARE

- Outpatient—generally sufficient.
- Inpatient—cases that warrant surgery due to inadequate response to medical therapy.

CLIENT EDUCATION

Dogs

Typically lifelong treatment; disease is controlled rather than cured.

Cats

- Herpesvirus—ocular discomfort and keratitis often recur. • Eosinophilic keratitis—disease controlled rather than cured. • Corneal sequestrum—may slough spontaneously, however cornea may rupture; clinical course often protracted without surgery; removal of sequestrum by superficial keratectomy may be curative, although recurrence possible.

SURGICAL CONSIDERATIONS

Dogs

- Chronic superficial keratitis—superficial keratectomy for severe disease in which vision is impaired due to corneal pigmentation; patients still require indefinite medical treatment to prevent recurrence; β-irradiation with a strontium-90 probe is noninvasive and may be performed in severe cases.
- Pigmentary keratitis—superficial keratectomy may be performed only after initial underlying cause is corrected; only in severe cases that threaten vision. • Pigmentary keratopathy of pugs—high likelihood of recurrence after superficial keratectomy.
- NGE—superficial keratectomy is diagnostic; medical treatment is still required. • KCS—parotid duct transposition or permanent partial tarsorrhaphy to reduce exposure.

Cats

- Eosinophilic keratitis—superficial keratectomy is diagnostic but not curative; medical treatment is preferred. • Corneal sequestrum—superficial keratectomy may be curative; recurrence is possible.

MEDICATIONS

DRUG(S) OF CHOICE

Dogs

- Chronic superficial keratitis—topical corticosteroids (1% prednisolone or 0.1% dexamethasone q6–12h); topical 0.2–2% cyclosporine, 1% pimecrolimus, or 0.03% tacrolimus q8–12h; agents can be used alone or in combination for more severe cases; subconjunctival corticosteroid injection (triamcinolone acetonide, 2–8 mg) can be used as an adjunct to topical therapy in severe cases. • Pigmentary keratitis—treatment directed at underlying cause; topical corticosteroids if primary cause is inflammatory; lubricants and cyclosporine or tacrolimus if primary condition is KCS; cyclosporine or tacrolimus may reduce pigmentation in all cases. • Pigmentary keratopathy of pugs—topical cyclosporine 0.2–2% or tacrolimus 0.02–0.03% may arrest progression of corneal pigmentation; topical corticosteroids may temporarily reduce density of corneal pigment. • NGE—topical corticosteroids and/or cyclosporine as described above; systemic azathioprine (2 mg/kg/day PO, initially, then gradually reduce) may be effective when used alone or in combination with topical medications.
- KCS—topical 0.2–2% cyclosporine, or 0.02–0.03% tacrolimus q8–12h (see Keratoconjunctivitis Sicca).

Cats

- Herpesvirus—topical antiviral agents recommended: cidofovir 0.5% q12h or trifluridine q4–6h for 2 days, then taper. Systemic antiviral agents include: famciclovir 90 mg/kg PO q12h. For inflammation, topical nonsteroidal anti-inflammatory drugs or cyclosporine q12h may be used.
- Eosinophilic keratitis—topical corticosteroids (1% prednisolone or 0.1% dexamethasone) q6–12h; patient monitored for ulceration or worsening of clinical signs; topical antivirals can be used in combination with corticosteroids if concurrent herpesvirus; use of topical cyclosporine reported (0.2–1.5%) with variable results; megestrol acetate (5 mg PO q24h for 5 days, then 5 mg PO q48h for 1 week, then 5 mg PO weekly for maintenance) is highly effective, but associated with side effects. • Corneal sequestrum—topical antibiotic (terramycin or erythromycin) q8–12h for associated corneal ulceration; artificial tear lubrication may relieve discomfort; topical antivirals can be used if herpesvirus infection is suspected; topical 1% atropine ointment q12–24h for pain from concurrent uveitis if present.

CONTRAINDICATIONS

Topical corticosteroids contraindicated with corneal ulcers; topical atropine contraindicated with KCS, glaucoma, or lens luxation. Topical neomycin and polymixin may cause anaphylactic reactions in cats.

PRECAUTIONS

- Azathioprine may cause gastrointestinal signs, pancreatitis, hepatotoxicity, and myelosuppression. • Megestrol acetate—not FDA-approved for use in cats; possible side effects include polyphagia, diabetes mellitus, mammary hyperplasia, mammary neoplasia, and pyometra. • Famciclovir— anorexia, polydipsia.

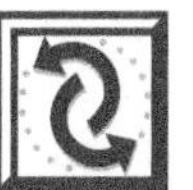

FOLLOW-UP

PATIENT MONITORING

Periodic ocular examination recommended to evaluate efficacy of treatment; examine at 1- to 2-week intervals, gradually lengthening the interval with remission or resolution of clinical signs; taper medications based on resolution of clinical signs; complete resolution of pigmentation may not occur. UV light protection (tinted goggles) is recommended for pannus.

POSSIBLE COMPLICATIONS

All of the above may lead to continued ocular discomfort, visual defects, or blindness in severe cases.

MISCELLANEOUS

SEE ALSO

- Corneal Sequestrum—Cats.
- Episcleritis.
- Keratitis, Eosinophilic—Cats.
- Keratitis, Ulcerative.
- Keratoconjunctivitis Sicca.

ABBREVIATIONS

- FHV-1 = feline herpesvirus type 1.
- IFA = immunofluorescent antibody test.
- KCS = keratoconjunctivitis sicca.
- NGE = nodular granulomatous episcleritis.

Suggested Reading

Andrew SE. Immune-mediated canine and feline keratitis. Vet Clin Small Anim 2008, 38:269–290.

Chavkin MJ, Roberts SM, Salman MD, et al. Risk factors for development of chronic superficial keratitis in dogs. J Am Vet Med Assoc 1994, 204:1630–1634.

Labelle AL, Dresser CB, Hamor RE, et al. Characteristics of, prevalence of and risk factors for corneal pigmentation (pigmentary keratopathy) in pugs. J Am Vet Med Assoc 2013, 243:667–674.

Author Kathern E. Myrna

Consulting Editor Kathern E. Myrna

Acknowledgments The author/editor acknowledges the prior contribution of Amber L. Labelle.

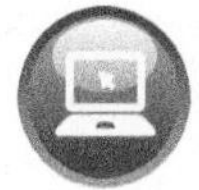

Client Education Handout available online

KERATITIS, ULCERATIVE

BASICS

DEFINITION

Inflammation of the cornea associated with loss of corneal epithelium (corneal erosion) or loss of variable amounts of underlying corneal stroma (corneal ulcer).

PATHOPHYSIOLOGY

• May be caused by any condition (traumatic or nontraumatic) that disrupts corneal epithelium or stroma. • Ulcers—superficial or deep, uncomplicated or complicated: ○ Superficial—involves epithelium and possibly superficial stroma. ○ Deep—involves a greater thickness of stroma and may extend to Descemet's membrane (descemetocele), possibly leading to rupture of globe. ○ Complicated—persistence of underlying/inciting cause, microbial infection, or production of degradative enzymes (melting). • Epithelial wound healing—adjacent corneal epithelial cells loosen and begin migration over the defect within a few hours; mitosis occurs within a few days to restore normal epithelial thickness; healing process complete in 5–7 days in uncomplicated, superficial ulcers.
• Stromal wound healing—slower, more complex; can be in an avascular or vascular manner; in shallow wounds, epithelial migration may be sufficient to fill defect; epithelium may cover some deeper ulcers even when epithelium and stromal regeneration are insufficient to restore normal corneal thickness (nonulcerated divot defect is called a facet); stroma usually heals by fibrovascular infiltration, resulting in scarring.
• Stromal ulcers—often complicated by microbial infection or enzymatic destruction initiated by microbial organisms, host inflammatory cells, or corneal epithelial or stromal cells; enzymatic destruction may result in gelatinous appearance of corneal stroma ("melting" or "malacic" ulcer).

K

SYSTEMS AFFECTED

Ophthalmic

GENETICS

• No proven basis; breed predilections exist.
• May be secondary to other corneal diseases with breed predispositions and genetic basis, such as corneal epithelial dystrophy in Shetland sheepdogs and corneal endothelial dystrophy in Boston terriers.

INCIDENCE/PREVALENCE

Common

SIGNALMENT

Species

Dog and cat.

Breed Predilections

• Dogs—brachycephalic breeds predisposed.
• Spontaneous chronic corneal epithelial defects (SCCED)/indolent erosion—any breed. • Cats—Persian, Himalayans, Siamese, and Burmese predisposed to corneal sequestrums (see Corneal Sequestrum—Cats).

Mean Age and Range

• Age of onset—variable; determined by cause.
• SCCED—middle-aged and older dogs.

SIGNS

Historical Findings

• May be acute or chronic (SCCED).
• Tearing, squinting, rubbing at eyes.
• Owners may report a "film" over the eye (often corneal edema); prolapsed third eyelid.
• Herpetic ulcers (cats)—may have history of respiratory disease.

Physical Examination Findings

• Nonspecific—serous to mucopurulent ocular discharge, blepharospasm, nictitans prolapse, conjunctival hyperemia. • Superficial—may note one or more circumscribed, linear, or geographic defects in cornea. • Deep stromal ulcer or descemetocele—may appear as a crater-like defect. • Depending on cause and duration—may see neovascularization, pigmentation, scarring, inflammatory cell infiltrate (yellow to cream-colored opacity with indistinct margins, often surrounded by corneal edema), collagenolytic activity (melting) of corneal stroma. • SCCED—loose or redundant epithelial edges; may demonstrate fluorescein stain extending into areas with seemingly intact epithelium (ring of less intense staining). • Reflex anterior uveitis—mild or severe, secondary to ulceration; severe may result in hypopyon; severe suggests concurrent bacterial infection.

CAUSES

• Trauma—blunt; penetrating; perforating.
• Adnexal disease—ectopic cilia, entropion, ectropion, eyelid mass, distichiasis.
• Lagophthalmos (inability to close eyelids completely)—results in exposure keratitis; may be breed-related in brachycephalic dogs and cats; may be caused by exophthalmos, buphthalmos, or may be neuroparalytic from facial nerve paralysis. • Tear-film abnormality—quantitative tear deficiency (keratoconjunctivitis sicca [KCS]); qualitative tear film deficiency caused by mucin deficiency or some other unidentified tear abnormality.
• Infection—usually secondary in dogs; can be primary herpesvirus infection in cats.
• Primary corneal disease—endothelial dystrophy; other endothelial disease.
• Miscellaneous—foreign body (corneal or conjunctival), chemical burns, neurotrophic keratitis (loss of trigeminal sensation), immune-mediated disease.

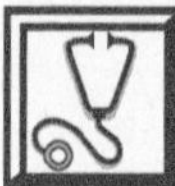

DIAGNOSIS

DIFFERENTIAL DIAGNOSIS

• Other causes of a red and painful eye—conjunctivitis, uveitis, KCS, glaucoma (see Red Eye). • May develop concurrently with other causes of a red eye (e.g., secondary to KCS).

OTHER LABORATORY TESTS

• Corneal culture and sensitivity—aerobic culture; particularly for complicated, deep, or rapidly progressive corneal ulcers.
• Herpesvirus (cats)—PCR or immunofluorescent antibody test (IFA) for herpesvirus available; negative test does not rule out herpesvirus infection.

DIAGNOSTIC PROCEDURES

Fluorescein Staining

• Homogeneous stain uptake—superficial or stromal ulcer; may be circular to geographic, linear, or combination; location and shape may help determine cause (e.g., linear may indicate foreign body or rubbing of ectopic cilia); interpretation of depth subjective. • SCCED—may have leakage of stain under surrounding loose epithelium.
• Descemetocele—crater-like defect that retains stain at periphery but is clear at center; may see Descemet's membrane bulging if large defect. • Previous stromal ulcer that has epithelialized (facet)—crater-like defect with transient pooling of stain that is easily rinsed; must distinguish from descemetocele.

Other

• Cytologic evaluation of cornea and Gram, Giemsa, or Wright staining may reveal microbial or fungal organisms and help direct initial antimicrobial therapy. • Schirmer tear test may identify ulceration associated with KCS; contraindicated in very deep ulcers or descemetoceles.

PATHOLOGIC FINDINGS

• Ulcers—suppurative inflammation, possibly neovascularization, loss of epithelium and basement membrane; possibly organisms.
• SCCEDs—superficial hylanized zone in stroma; epithelial lipping around erosions; varying degrees and types of leukocytic infiltrate and fibrosis.

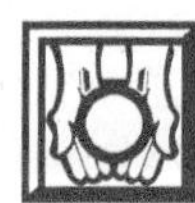

TREATMENT

APPROPRIATE HEALTH CARE

Hospitalize deep or rapidly progressive ulcers; these may require surgery and/or frequent medical treatments.

NURSING CARE

Keep facial hair out of eyes and clean.

ACTIVITY

• Restrict with deep stromal ulcer or descemetocele to prevent rupture. • Prevent self-trauma with Elizabethan collar.

CLIENT EDUCATION

• Instruct client to wait at least 5 minutes between medications if more than one ophthalmic drop is prescribed; wait longer between ointments. • Advise client to contact veterinarian if patient appears more painful or the eye markedly changes in appearance.
• SCCED—discuss protracted course with client; usually achieve healing within 2–6 weeks but may require weekly rechecks and multiple procedures.

SURGICAL CONSIDERATIONS

• Superficial ulcers do not usually require surgery if inciting cause has been eliminated.
• Ulcer that extends one-half or greater corneal thickness and particularly to Descemet's membrane may benefit from surgery.
• Descemetocele or full-thickness corneal laceration—surgical emergency, possible referral.

Procedures

• SCCED—debridement of loose epithelium with a dry, sterile, cotton-tipped swab after application of topical anesthesia (50% success rate); punctate or grid keratotomy easily performed after epithelial debridement with topical anesthesia (80% success rate); superficial keratectomy is more invasive and may cause more scarring but has 100% success rate; application of a contact lens or nictitans flap after any of these procedures may improve comfort and aid healing. • Diamond burr keratotomy for SCCED/indolent erosion only; use gently over surface of erosion; may be associated with increased risk of infection.
• Rotational pedicle conjunctival flap, corneoscleral transposition, corneal transplant—surgical procedures for ulcers >50% stromal thickness and descemetoceles. • Cyanoacrylate repair (corneal glue)—can be used for deep ulcers; promotes corneal vascularization and stabilizes cornea, but has lower success rate compared to other corneal surgeries.

MEDICATIONS

DRUG(S) OF CHOICE

Antibiotics

• Topical agents—indicated for all patients.
• Frequency of application—determined by severity and preparation; ointments have relatively long contact time and are applied q6–12h; solutions are applied more frequently (q2–6h) in initial treatment of complicated ulcers; solutions probably more appropriate in deep ulcers. • Commonly used agents—erythromycin (cats); triple antibiotic, gentamicin, and tobramycin.
• Uncomplicated ulcers or superficial erosions—combination of neomycin, polymyxin B, and bacitracin an excellent first choice; broad spectrum of antimicrobial activity; often used 2–3 times/day for prophylactic therapy. • Complicated ulcers—often use combination therapy of cefazolin (use IV solution to make 33–50 mg solution in saline or artificial tears for topical use) with a fluoroquinolone (ciprofloxacin, ofloxacin); particularly in rapidly progressive, deep, or melting ulcers; frequency depends on severity but usually a minimum of q3–4h.

Atropine

• 1% ointment or solution. • Indicated for reflex anterior uveitis; frequency—usually q8–24h to effect (mydriasis).

Antiviral Agents

• Indicated for herpetic ulcers in cats.
• Trifluridine (Viroptic) solution—q4–6h until clinical response is observed; then reduce for 1–2 weeks after clinical signs have subsided. • Famciclovir—90 mg/kg PO q12h for 2–4 weeks.

Nonsteroidal Anti-inflammatory Drugs (NSAIDs)

• Flurbiprofen, diclofenac. • For anti-inflammatory and analgesic properties.

CONTRAINDICATIONS

• Topical corticosteroids—contraindicated with any corneal erosion or ulcer. • Topical NSAIDs—contraindicated with herpetic ulcers. • Topical atropine—contraindicated with glaucoma, KCS.

PRECAUTIONS

• Topical NSAIDs may delay corneal healing, may potentiate corneal melting.
• Trifluridine, neomycin—may be irritating. • Topical cyclosporine can be used safely in KCS patients with uncomplicated ulcers.

POSSIBLE INTERACTIONS

Combining antibiotics in solution may inactivate some antibiotics.

ALTERNATIVE DRUG(S)

• Acetylcysteine—anticollagenolytic agent used for treatment of melting ulcers; efficacy is controversial; dilute 20% stock solution to 5–10% with artificial tears; apply q2–4h.
• Serum—anticollagenolytic agent; keep refrigerated; avoid contamination; discard after 48 hours.

FOLLOW-UP

PATIENT MONITORING

• Superficial ulcers—repeat fluorescein stain in 3–6 days; if it persists 7 days or longer, either inciting cause has not been eliminated or patient has an SCCED. • Deep stromal or rapidly progressive ulcers—assess every 24 hours initially if outpatient until improvement is seen; many of these patients are hospitalized or undergo surgery; decrease frequency of antibiotic therapy as condition improves.

PREVENTION/AVOIDANCE

• Brachycephalic dogs—lubricant ointment administration, permanent partial tarsorrhaphy surgery, or both may prevent recurrent ulceration. • KCS-related ulcers—lifelong treatment of KCS (cyclosporine) or parotid duct transposition surgery. • Herpesvirus (cats)—oral lysine (250 mg PO q12h) may prevent viral replication; may decrease severity and/or frequency of outbreaks.

POSSIBLE COMPLICATIONS

Progressive corneal ulceration—rupture of globe, endophthalmitis, secondary glaucoma, phthisis bulbi, blindness, blind and painful eye (may require enucleation).

EXPECTED COURSE AND PROGNOSIS

• Uncomplicated superficial ulcer—usually heals in 5–7 days. • SCCED—may persist for weeks to months; may require multiple procedures. • Deep corneal ulcer treated medically—may require several weeks for fibrovascular repair of defect; does not always granulate satisfactorily; continued deterioration of ulcer and globe rupture are possible.
• Deep ulcer treated with conjunctival flap—frequently results in more comfort within a few days after surgery; blood supply to flap can be cut in 4–6 weeks to decrease scarring.

MISCELLANEOUS

ABBREVIATIONS

• IFA = immunofluorescent antibody test.
• KCS = keratoconjunctivitis sicca.
• NSAID = nonsteroidal anti-inflammatory drug.
• SCCED = spontaneous chronic corneal epithelial defect.

Author Ellison Bentley
Consulting Editor Kathern E. Myrna

Client Education Handout available online

K

KERATOCONJUNCTIVITIS SICCA

BASICS

OVERVIEW

- Deficiency of the aqueous layer of precorneal tear film.
- Causes corneal/conjunctival drying and resultant surface inflammation.

SIGNALMENT

- Common in dog; rare in cat.
- Predisposed dog breeds—many brachycephalic and spaniel breeds, miniature schnauzers, poodles, bloodhounds, Samoyeds, West Highland white terriers, and Yorkshire terriers.
- Inheritance—undefined.
- Age of onset—variable and depends on inciting cause.

SIGNS

- Conjunctival hyperemia.
- Mucoid to mucopurulent ocular discharge—intermittent to persistent depending on severity.
- Blepharospasm.
- Corneal changes—dryness, superficial vascularization, pigmentation, fibrosis, ulceration.
- Blepharitis due to ocular exudates.
- Severe disease—impaired vision or blindness.
- Cats are less symptomatic than dogs.

CAUSES & RISK FACTORS

- Immune-mediated/idiopathic—most common, possibly associated with other immune-mediated diseases (e.g., atopy).
- Infectious—canine distemper virus; leishmaniasis; chronic blepharoconjunctivitis (e.g., feline herpesvirus).
- Iatrogenic—removal of third eyelid gland (especially in at-risk breeds), radiation therapy.
- Congenital—Yorkshire terriers overrepresented.
- Neurologic—loss of parasympathetic innervation to lacrimal gland, trigeminal nerve deficit, or dysautonomia; neurogenic parasympathetic loss may have ipsilateral dry nose.
- Traumatic—after ocular proptosis or orbit inflammation.
- Systemic disease—diabetes mellitus, hyperadrenocorticism, hypothyroidism, or any debilitating disease.
- Drug-induced—systemic sulfonamides (e.g., trimethoprim-sulfadiazine).
- Transient—general anesthesia and atropine.

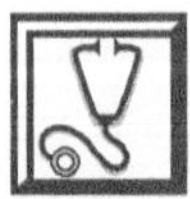

DIAGNOSIS

DIFFERENTIAL DIAGNOSIS

- Often confused with allergic or bacterial conjunctivitis.
- Dogs with keratoconjunctivitis sicca (KCS) may have concurrent bacterial overgrowth.
- Differentiate with Schirmer tear test.

DIAGNOSTIC PROCEDURES

- Schirmer tear test—normal value at least 9 mm/min (cat) or 15 mm/min (dog) of wetting; symptomatic patients usually <10 mm/min of wetting; lower values combined with clinical signs suggest KCS.
- Fluorescein staining—may show corneal ulcers.
- Conjunctival cytology—may demonstrate bacterial overgrowth.

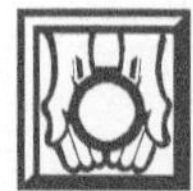

TREATMENT

- Outpatient—unless severe corneal ulceration.
- Instruct client to use solution(s) before ointment(s) and wait 5 minutes between treatments.
- Advise client to call at once if ocular pain increases (patients are predisposed to corneal ulceration).
- Parotid duct transposition—surgical option for dogs and cats that reroutes parotid duct to deliver saliva to ocular surface if KCS is refractory to lacrimostimulant therapy.
    - More common with congenital KCS.
    - Saliva can irritate cornea and result in mineral deposits; some patients require ongoing topical therapy.
- Episcleral cyclosporine implant—for dogs responsive to topical cyclosporine but with poor owner compliance.

MEDICATIONS

DRUG(S) OF CHOICE

- Lacrimostimulants—cyclosporine 0.2% ointment or 1–2% solution; tacrolimus 0.02–0.03% solution or ointment—therapy q12h recommended (q8h if severe or refractory).
- For neurogenic KCS—pilocarpine 0.1–0.2% topically q8h or very careful oral pilocarpine (narrow therapeutic window; see Suggested Reading).
- For feline KCS—antiviral therapy (see Conjunctivitis—Cats); hyaluronate-based artificial tear in short term; consider lacrimostimulant therapy.
- Lacrimomimetics—artificial tears to moisten ocular surface to improve comfort; use viscous solutions or gels q2–12h depending on severity and ointment before bedtime; can reduce frequency once patient responds to lacrimostimulants.
- Broad-spectrum antibiotics—topical ointment q6–8h for 3–4 weeks; indicated for secondary bacterial overgrowth or concurrent corneal ulceration.
- Ocular cleansing—use eye wash to remove discharge and debris prior to administering medications; if mucoid discharge is very tenacious, 5% *N*-acetylcysteine can be used q6–12h as a mucinolytic agent prior to eye rinsing.
- Corticosteroids—topical; minimize inflammation; can reduce corneal vascularization and pigmentation once aqueous tears improve; not commonly used (corneal ulcer risk).

CONTRAINDICATIONS/POSSIBLE INTERACTIONS

- Topical cyclosporine or tacrolimus—rarely irritating, but if noted consider compounded aqueous preparation.
- Pilocarpine—initially irritating topically; systemic side effect risk.
- Topical corticosteroids—avoid with ulcerative keratitis or severe KCS (corneal ulcer risk).

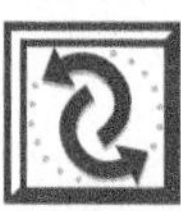

FOLLOW-UP

- Regular rechecks—monitor response and progress.
- Schirmer tear test—4–6 weeks after initiating cyclosporine or tacrolimus (patient should receive drug as prescribed on day of visit).
- Usually requires life-long treatment.
- Good prognosis but refractory cases may require more aggressive therapy (e.g., up to 1% tacrolimus) or surgery (e.g., parotid duct transposition).

MISCELLANEOUS

ABBREVIATIONS

- KCS = keratoconjunctivitis sicca.

Suggested Reading

Maggs DJ, Miller PE, Ofri R. Diseases of the lacrimal system. In: Slatter's Fundamentals of Veterinary Ophthalmology, 6th ed. St. Louis, MO: Elsevier, 2018, pp. 186–212.

Author Rachel A. Allbaugh
Consulting Editor Kathern E. Myrna

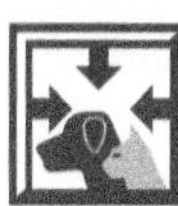

BASICS

DEFINITION

Undesirable behaviors exhibited by kittens between birth and puberty.

PATHOPHYSIOLOGY

• Most pediatric behavior problems are normal, species-typical behaviors. • Lack of appropriate social interactions and environmental stimulation and genetics can contribute to abnormal or unwanted behaviors.

SYSTEMS AFFECTED

Behavioral

GENETICS

Paternal influences on friendliness to people and boldness to unfamiliar or novel objects have been supported.

SIGNALMENT

Species

Cats

Mean Age and Range

Generally 6–48 weeks.

SIGNS

General Comments

Play Aggression

• Elements of predation including stalking, chasing, attacking, pouncing, swatting, and biting. Play can be solitary, with objects, or social to another kitten, animal or person.
• With normal play, bites are inhibited and claws retracted. Vocalizations are rare compared to other forms of feline aggression.
• Inappropriate play behaviors may be uninhibited, leading to bite and scratch injuries.

Excessive Play/Activity and/or Destructive Play

High level of solitary play (running, jumping, climbing, object play) may result in household damage and disruption.

Scratching

• Use of claws to scratch on household items and/or people.
• Scratching is a normal behavior for claw maintenance, territorial marking, and defense but becomes problematic when scratched objects include walls, furniture, carpets, and other household items.

Fearful Behaviors

Includes hiding, hissing, scratching, and unsocial behaviors and can include varying manifestations of aggression to another animal or person.

Historical Findings

Aggressive Play Directed toward People or Other Pets in the Household

• Attacks directed toward people or other pets in the household. • Ambushes are common and lack vocalizations. Bites are generally inhibited but may puncture the skin and light scratches with claws may occur. Can be more serious in the elderly owner.

Uninhibited Aggressive Play Directed toward People

• Signs similar to above except more intense.
• Bites and scratches are not as inhibited and can break skin.

Play Directed toward Household Objects

• Bursts of solitary play that include intense running, climbing across and up household furnishings. • Knocks or swipes objects from surfaces.

Scratching

Household items and family members.

Fear and Defensive Behaviors Due to Lack of Socialization

• Insufficient exposure to people before 7–9 weeks of age. • Behaviors associated with fear, e.g., dilated pupils, piloerection, defensive postures, hissing, hiding, fleeing, aggression.

Fear and Defensive Behaviors Related to Early Trauma

Normal until experience traumatic event, e.g., abuse, attack by another animal.

Fear and Defensive Behaviors Related to Correction Techniques

• History of punishment by owner(s).
• Kitten shows defensive postures including hissing, fleeing, hiding, dilated pupils, piloerection in presence of owner or in response to corrections.

CAUSES

Aggressive Play Directed toward People or Other Cats in the Household

• Normal species-typical behavior but without appropriate social interaction with conspecifics, the behavior can become uninhibited and injurious. • Owners may encourage inappropriate interactive play by promoting play with human body parts (fingers, hands, feet). • Lack of outlets for appropriate play.

Play Directed toward Objects in the Household

Normal species-typical behavior beginning at 7–8 weeks of age.

Fear and Defensive Behaviors Due to Lack of Early Socialization

No or minimal amount of exposure to people before 7–9 weeks of age.

Fear and Defensive Behaviors Related to Early Trauma

Early traumatic event.

Fear and Defensive Behaviors Related to Correction Techniques

Normal until "corrected" by person, e.g., spanked, swatted, flicked on nose, yelled at, chased.

RISK FACTORS

Aggressive Play Directed toward People

• Only cat in household, hand-reared kitten, or adoption prior to 6 weeks of age. • Insufficient appropriate outlets for normal play and exploration. • Encouragement of inappropriate play (e.g., with hands, fingers, feet).

Play Directed toward Objects in the Household

• Lack of sufficient/appropriate enrichment including toys and interactive play with people or other animals. • Only pet in household.

Scratching

Lack of appropriate/inadequate scratching outlets.

Fear and Defensive Behaviors

• Lack of appropriate socialization with people, use of punishment and other traumatic experience(s). • Removing kittens less than 2 weeks of age from queen may result in fearful and aggressive kittens towards humans and other cats.

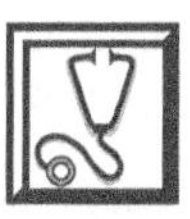

DIAGNOSIS

DIFFERENTIAL DIAGNOSIS

Play Aggression toward People

Differentiate normal play from the more serious, uninhibited play aggression.

Excessive Play/Destructive Behaviors

None.

Scratching

Nail maintenance, marking, play-related, or defense.

Fearful and Defensive Behaviors

CNS diseases, pain, metabolic disorders, pain.

CBC/BIOCHEMISTRY/URINALYSIS

Frightened kittens may have elevated glucose levels, stress leukogram.

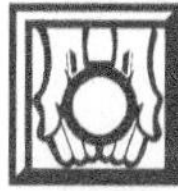

TREATMENT

ACTIVITY

Many kitten behavior problems can be alleviated or reduced by enriching kitten's environment (e.g., provide movable toys, variety of toys, rotating them regularly). Engage the kitten in interactive play directed away from the owner's body parts. Provide access to window sills and perches. Offer a variety of enticing scratching surfaces. Possibly get second kitten.

DIET

Provide multiple small meals. Use food delivery toys.

CLIENT EDUCATION

Most of these problems are normal kitten behaviors that owners perceive as abnormal or excessive and inappropriate for their lifestyle. Most kittens will mature out of these problem behaviors with appropriate management and by providing for behavioral needs.

Aggressive Play Directed toward People

• Owner needs to initiate regular interactive play that allows for hunt, stalk and attack behaviors directed at appropriate toys or objects.

KITTEN BEHAVIOR PROBLEMS (CONTINUED)

Ensure owners never use hands, fingers, or feet to encourage play. • Effective treatment may be to acquire another kitten, if size and temperament are compatible. • Redirection: Identify situations in which the attacks may occur. Watch for signs of dilated pupils, stalking, crouching, tail swishing. Be prepared to redirect the play to another object (e.g., tossing a wadded piece of paper or chasing a toy) or to cue and reward alternative desirable behaviors that the kitten has learned (e.g., go to mat, sit/watch, let's eat, let's play). • Educate the client to not hit or swat or punish. • Immediately stop any attention or play for inappropriate behaviors. • Interrupt to redirect into alternative acceptable behaviors with trained cues (sit, go to mat) or with a noise to reorient into desirable play. • Frequent trimming of claws helps reduce damage caused by nails. • For humane and welfare reasons declawing is strongly discouraged and prohibited in many countries and jurisdictions. Where legally permissible it should be a last resort only if owners have been fully counselled on behavior management, modification and alternative options.

Aggressive Play Directed toward Other Cats in the Household

• Acquire additional kitten of the same size and temperament as the problem kitten. • Watch for signs and redirect into alternative acceptable behaviors (sit/watch, go to mat). • Problem kitten and other cat should have restricted access to each other at times when problems might arise. • Startling, punitive techniques may aversively affect the other cat and are not recommended. • Provide appropriate outlets for predatory behaviors with the problem kitten on a regular, daily basis using toys or objects.

Play That Is Excessive and/or Destructive, and Scratching

• Put valuable, breakable, or dangerous objects away. • Provide a variety of appropriate toys for batting and food delivery and rotate every few days to maintain novelty and interest. • Interactive play with kitten using toys or objects on a daily basis. • Provide scratching posts using materials that are cat's preferred substrates and assure they are long enough and stable enough for the cat to stretch and scratch. • Place scratching stations in commonly used areas and encourage use with catnip, treats, and integrating perches and resting areas. • Decrease the appeal of the targeted objects, e.g., with sticky tape, unpleasant taste or odor, or less appealing substrate. • Frequent trimming of claws. • Declawing is a humane concern and in many places prohibited.

Fear and Defensive Behaviors Due to Lack of Early Socialization or from Early Trauma

• Gradual exposure to people without forcing interactions, provided no negative outcome/endpoint. • House kitten where it is comfortable, where it can remove itself from view but be aware of people. • Counter-conditioning generally required. Highly enticing food and treats should be offered. Initially, food can be put in or near hiding area. Gradually food is given with increasing proximity to the people, ending each session at a distance or location where the cat remains calm and will take food. No attempt should be made to grab or hold the kitten. Progress gradually until the kitten takes food that is tossed toward it, given by hand, or given while the kitten is on the person's lap. Counter-conditioning can also include play with toys that can tossed or chased, such as those on wands or ropes. • Important: Let the kitten make the advances—not the person—and avoid any fearful endpoint by forcing interaction, preventing escape, or progressing too quickly.

Fear and Defensive Behaviors Related to Correction Techniques

Identify and cease inappropriate punishment.

MEDICATIONS

DRUG(S) OF CHOICE

• None needed except as indicated for fear and anxiety. See also Fears, Phobias, and Anxieties—Cats. • May consider use of feline pheromones and nutritional supplements with alpha-casozepine or L-theanine for mild fear and anxiety.

FOLLOW-UP

PATIENT MONITORING

• Telephone follow-up support is helpful.
• Be sure clients are not using aversive techniques that may induce fear and aggression in the kitten and/or exacerbate intensity of play aggression.

PREVENTION/AVOIDANCE

• Kitten behavior problems are often a result of owner's unrealistic expectations and misunderstanding of normal kitten behavior, as well as lack of enrichment and appropriate predatory play outlets. • Between 3 and 7 weeks of age, kittens should experience positive interactions with people to reduce fear and develop appropriate social bonds with humans.
• Between 4 and 18 weeks, it is helpful to have exposure to tolerant (and playful) conspecifics to learn effective bite and play inhibition.
• Advise family members to avoid rough-housing and body part play with kittens.
• Discourage punitive corrections.

EXPECTED COURSE AND PROGNOSIS

Normal Play Behaviors Directed toward People, Other Cats, and Household Objects

Reduction or resolution of problem when appropriate treatment protocols are followed. Many behaviors may begin to wane with maturity.

Uninhibited Aggressive Play Directed toward People

• Guarded prognosis. • Aggression may become more severe with maturity. A better prognosis is given to those cases that are caught early and appropriately counseled or by obtaining a second compatible cat.

Scratching

If measures to prevent, divert, and reward for using appropriate scratching surfaces are successful, the prognosis is good, and as the kitten matures, the behaviors wane. Some cats may need long-term management.

Fear and Defensive Behaviors Due to Lack of Early Socialization or Related to Early Trauma

Kittens vary in the degree to which they acclimate to people; improvement may take months to years; some may never be comfortable around people.
• The longer the interval from 3 weeks of age to exposure to people, the poorer the prognosis.
• The more intense the early trauma, the poorer the prognosis.

Fear and Defensive Behaviors Related to Correction Techniques

These can resolve if corrections have not been too frequent or too intense, and the clients follow advice to replace these techniques with reward-based, avoidance, and redirection procedures.

MISCELLANEOUS

AGE-RELATED FACTORS

Fear and Defensive Behaviors Due to Lack of Early Socialization

During the sensitive period, between 3 and 7 weeks, the kitten must be exposed to people to prevent fearful and defensive responses to them.

INTERNET RESOURCES

• https://indoorpet.osu.edu/cats • https://catvets.com/guidelines/practice-guidelines—environmental needs, lifestyle, enrichment

Suggested Reading

Bradshaw J, Ellis S. The Trainable Cat—A Practical Guide to Making Life Happier for You and Your Cat. New York, NY: Basic Books, 2016.

Herron ME, Horwitz D, Siracusa C, et al. Decoding your cat: The ultimate experts explain common cat behaviors and reveal how to prevent or change unwanted ones. New York, Houghton Mifflin Harcourt, 2020.

Author Kelly Moffat
Consulting Editor Gary M. Landsberg

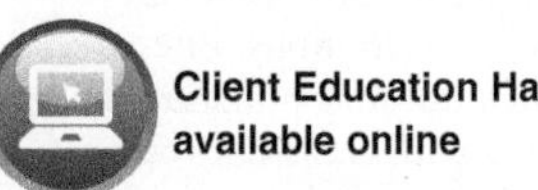
Client Education Handout available online

KITTEN SOCIALIZATION AND KITTEN CLASSES

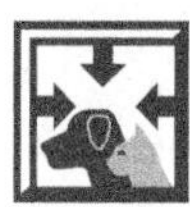

BASICS

OVERVIEW

• Early experiences set the foundation for future behavior, having long lasting effects on social behavior, temperament, and the ability to learn and relate to various stimuli and to cope in various environmental contexts.
• For a kitten to grow up into a well-adjusted adult cat, adequate socialization and environmental exposure is needed during the socialization period and beyond into the first year of life.

Definitions

• Socialization—a process of learning normal behavior, communication, and social skills for appropriate interactions with other individuals in various contexts. • Socialization period—a sensitive window of development whereby a cat learns to communicate and relate to other cats, humans, and the environment. • Kitten classes—also called kitten "kindy" or kindergarten. Allow cats to socialize with other cats, a variety of people, and to be exposed to multiple and varied environmental stimuli in a positive and nonthreatening manner.

Pathophysiology

Potential effects on behavioral and neurological development.

SIGNALMENT

Genetics

Genetics or the paternity of the kittens, with kittens sired from friendly toms being friendlier toward people.

Mean Age

• The sensitive socialization period is between 2 weeks and 7 weeks, yet socialization is a continuous process. During the socialization period, less experience is necessary to produce profound effects on future behavior. Handling only 15 minutes per day from 2 to 6 weeks of age has been shown to produce more friendly kittens. • For kitten classes—healthy dewormed kittens should begin attending group classes 10 days after receiving the first vaccination of their kitten immunization series. Typically begin classes between 8 and 12 weeks and conclude by 14 weeks.

Predominant Sex

• Male kittens play more with objects than females. • No sex differences in social play.

SIGNS

• Lack of adequate socialization experiences during sensitive periods of development.
• Cat-directed fear and/or aggression—lack of early familiarity and positive exposure with other cats. • Human-directed fear and/or aggression—early positive social experiences with humans prior to 7 weeks, otherwise fear, avoidance, aggression, and behaving as if "feral." • Predatory aggression—exposure to future prey species, starting at 4 weeks, can improve predatory behavior and hunting ability, whereas exposure to non-prey species may reduce aggression later in life. • Fear and anxiety in unfamiliar environments.
• Attendance at group kitten classes at an early age can prevent future behavior problems and/or allow for the early identification of abnormal and problematic behavior. • Kitten classes—age-specific (8 and 12 weeks at start and finished by 14 weeks) for group-controlled interactions. Focus is education regarding normal behavior, the prevention of behavior problems, and addressing normal problematic behaviors through management, supervision, and positive reinforcement training.

CAUSES & RISK FACTORS

• Avoiding environmental and social experiences prior to the completion of kitten vaccination series increases the risk of future behavior problems. • The risk of exposure to infectious disease with socialization and environmental exposure needs to be considered along with the risk of being undersocialized and not suitable as a pet because of lifelong fear, anxiety, and aggressive issues. • A clean bill of health and initial vaccinations must have been administered at least 10 days prior to class. • Kittens should be dewormed according to the Companion Animal Parasite Council guidelines. https://capcvet.org/guidelines/general-guidelines/
• Kittens should be screened for contagious diseases, such as upper respiratory infection and ringworm, prior to each class. • Kitten classes "vaccinate" the kitten against behavior problems later in life. • Genetics and a lack of socialization can render some kittens intolerant to human handling and behaving as if feral. • Kittens removed from the queen and exclusively hand raised by humans are more fearful and aggressive toward cats and humans, tend to be hyperactive, have difficulty forming social attachments with other cats, and display poor learning ability.
• Removal from the queen and littermates prior to 10 weeks of age may increase the risk of inter-cat aggression with a lack of learned social skills. • Kittens weaned too early are more likely to perform non-nutritive suckling and kneading of objects. • Experiences at the veterinary clinic should employ Fear Free and/or Low Stress handling techniques.
• Traumatic experiences that induce fear during sensitive fear periods when the kitten is between 6 and 8 weeks of age should be avoided. • Avoiding exposure to other species during socialization may result in fear toward the species, whereas experience with species that might normally have a predator–prey relationship may increase predatory behavior toward that species. • Early exposure of kittens to dogs living within the household improves the likelihood of successful cohabitation. • Kitten socialization with people and cats is only beneficial to behavioral development if the kitten finds human and/or cat contact enjoyable. Continued exposure when it induces fear is unlikely to result in habituation to the stimulus and is likely to exacerbate fear and/or aggression.

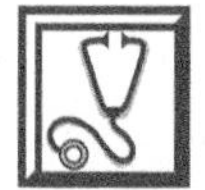

DIAGNOSIS

DIFFERENTIAL DIAGNOSIS

Identify abnormal and/or problematic behavior and make a behavioral diagnosis or schedule or refer for a behavior consultation.

Possible Behavioral Manifestations of a Lack of Socialization

• Global fears, encompassing fears of people, cats, other animals, objects, sounds, and environments. • Generalized anxiety and situational anxiety in unfamiliar environments.
• Specific fears, neophobia and failure to habituate to novelty or stimuli. • Noise sensitivity, aversions, and phobias.
• Hyperexcitability and hypervigilance with an inability to settle due to a lack of early environmental enrichment. • Aggression toward people and cats in various contexts with various motivations (e.g., fear, predatory).

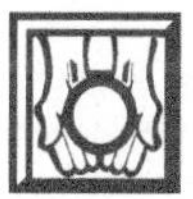

TREATMENT

Recommendations for Socialization

• Socialization "vaccinates" the kitten against the development of future behavioral problems and should begin concurrently with the kitten immunization series. • Food treats and social play should be used liberally with new and repeated kitten socialization experiences while keeping the kitten safe.
• Social play and exploration should be encouraged using toys in various contexts and environments while keeping the kitten safe.
• Healthy kittens usually have good appetites. If the kitten is not consuming food treats in specific contexts, it suggests the kitten is fearful and the experience is not positive or beneficial for socialization.
• Healthy and well-adjusted kittens play. If the kitten will not engage in play, it suggests the kitten is fearful and the experience is not positive or beneficial for socialization.
• Socialization by the breeder—gentle handling should occur daily, shortly after birth, and include exposure to multiple

KITTEN SOCIALIZATION AND KITTEN CLASSES (CONTINUED)

people, various smells and different surfaces with mild fluctuations in temperature.
• Socialization at the owner's home—allow the kitten to choose to interact and make exposure positive with the liberal use of food treats. Meet people of different ages, stature, gait and complexion. Meet other pets to potentially prevent fear and aggression.
• Attendance at group kitten classes and social exposure is recommended for all healthy kittens prior to 14 weeks of age and prior to being fully vaccinated.

Recommendations for Kitten Classes

• All healthy kittens between 8 and 12 weeks should be enrolled into group classes.
• Kittens attending are deemed healthy by a veterinary examination, have been dewormed, and have started their vaccination series. The first class might be attended by owners only, particularly if scheduled to begin within the first 10 days after vaccination. • Group classes are often held at veterinary clinics, allowing for positive interactions with other kittens, people, and objects. • Classes are attended by kittens and their owners at least weekly and are typically about an hour in length.
• Rotating classes cover the following topics: ○ Play sessions—controlled and monitored play (5–10 minutes) with other kittens in a secure environment, typically at the start and end of class. ○ Health and handling—instruction and positive handling for routine health and grooming procedures in the veterinary clinic, at the grooming facility, and at home. ○ Sights and sounds—exposure to novel environments, objects, surfaces, and sounds in a positive and fun manner. Various people attending interact with kittens in a positive manner. ○ Rearing advice—education on normal cat body language, learning, behavior problem solving and prevention, and kitten rearing. ○ Basic manners—positive reinforcement training to address mouthing/biting/scratching, jumping on furniture/counters, chewing and scratching objects, stealing objects, carrier, collar/harness/leash, and litterbox training. ○ Kitten classes offered at the veterinary hospital can also insure a focus on positive exposures to the veterinary facility, equipment, and procedures.

MEDICATIONS

DRUG(S) OF CHOICE

• A selective serotonin reuptake inhibitor or tricyclic antidepressant may be indicated for fear, anxiety, and aggression-related problems when combined with behavior and environmental modification for the specific diagnosis. • May "in effect" chemically place the kitten back into its socialization state and aid socialization. • Consider daily or situational behavior medications for cats 12 weeks of age or greater who demonstrate abnormal fear, anxiety, or aggression.

Nutraceuticals/Supplements

• Alpha-casozepine, a bovine-sourced hydrolyzed milk protein, may have calming properties. • L-Theanine, an extract of green tea, may reduce fear, anxiety, and stress.

Pheromones

• Feliway Classic (CEVA), a synthetic cheek gland pheromone, may have calming properties and facilitate adaptation to new environments. • Feliway Multicat (CEVA), a synthetic mammary pheromone, can mediate social tension between cats.
• FeliScratch (CEVA), a synthetic interdigital pheromone, may promote scratching in specific locations.

CONTRAINDICATIONS/POSSIBLE INTERACTIONS

Avoid selective serotonin reuptake inhibitors and tricyclic antidepressants in combination and use with caution with other serotonin-influencing drugs.

FOLLOW-UP

PATIENT MONITORING

Kitten owners should be questioned during routine heath examinations and encouraged to bring concerns regarding problematic behavior to their veterinarian's attention as soon as the problem is identified.

PREVENTION/AVOIDANCE

• Prevention of problems is preferable and easier than treatment. • Socialization experiences must be positive for the kitten to benefit from those experiences. • Avoid exposure which induces negative emotions as it is difficult to habituate to stimuli that induce fear, anxiety, and stress.
• Preventive counseling at the first kitten visit reduces the risk of undesirable climbing on furniture and curtains, undesirable vocalization, and increases amenability to body handling.

POSSIBLE COMPLICATIONS

• Kittens obtained after their socialization period with little prior socialization and those that have been raised in suboptimal environments may be resistant to socialization.
• Unwillingness to consume treats, explore, and/or play in socialization contexts suggest that the exposure is not positive for the kitten.

EXPECTED COURSE AND PROGNOSIS

Early identification and intervention gives the best prognostic outcome and chance for cure.

MISCELLANEOUS

ASSOCIATED CONDITIONS

Behavioral conditions associated with fear, anxiety, and aggression contexts.

INTERNET RESOURCES

• www.stevedalepetworld.com/blog/kitty-k/
• dacvb.org • catvets.com • indoorpet.osu.edu/cats

Suggested Reading

Bradshaw J, Ellis S. The Trainable Cat—A Practical Guide to Making Life Happier for You and Your Cat. New York, NY: Basic Books, 2016.

Herron, M. E., Horwitz, D., Siracusa, C., & Dale, S. (2020). Decoding your cat: The ultimate experts explain common cat behaviors and reveal how to prevent or change unwanted ones. Boston: Houghton Mifflin Harcourt.

Houpt, K. Domestic Animal Behavior for Veterinarians and Animal Scientists, 6th ed. Hoboken, NJ: John Wiley & Sons, 2018.

Shaw, JK, Martin D. Canine and Feline Behavior for Veterinary Technicians and Nurses. Ames, IA: John Wiley & Sons, 2015.

Authors Kenneth M. Martin and Debbie Martin
Consulting Editor Gary M. Landsberg

LACTIC ACIDOSIS (HYPERLACTATEMIA)

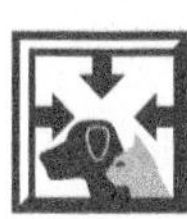

BASICS

DEFINITION

• Blood lactate concentration >1.5 mmol/L in dogs and >1.8 mmol/L in cats.
• Lactic acidosis is hyperlactatemia with concurrent metabolic acidosis.

PATHOPHYSIOLOGY

• Plasma lactate is a late but quantitative indicator of tissue hypoperfusion. Hypoperfusion and tissue hypoxia occur before a rise in blood lactate is detectable.
• Lactic acid is the end product of anaerobic glucose metabolism; at physiologic pH, lactic acid immediately dissociates to lactate and hydrogen ions. Clinically significant lactate accumulation can be due to anaerobic glycolysis occurring during normal physiologic (e.g., exercise) or pathologic processes (e.g., shock, seizures).
• Lactate exists as levorotatory (L-lactate) and dextrorotatory (D-lactate) stereoisomers. L-Lactate predominates in mammalian cells and is the only form detectable by routine analysis.
• Hepatic and renal lactate metabolism maintains a balance between lactate production and clearance.
• In most critically ill or injured patients, hyperlactatemia and lactic acidosis are due to conditions that cause tissue hypoxia, with a shift to anaerobic glycolysis.
• Inadequate perfusion, severe hypoxemia, increased oxygen demand, decreased hemoglobin concentration, or combinations of these factors can cause tissue hypoxia.
• Clinically evident tissue hypoperfusion does not usually occur in patients with hyperlactatemia alone, but hyperlactatemia from "occult" hypoperfusion (not detectable by routine monitoring) might be a precursor to overt hypoperfusion.
• Lactic acidosis can occur secondary to marked tissue hypoxia and hypoperfusion, certain drugs or toxins, or congenital defects in carbohydrate metabolism.
• Blood lactate measurement is a useful tool for assessing severity of tissue hypoxia, response to therapy, and prognosis:
  ○ In human trauma and shock patients, lactate predicts outcome, and mortality is correlated with severity of lactic acidosis.
  ○ Lactate concentrations are increased in critically ill and injured dogs; severity of hyperlactatemia is associated with outcome.
• Serial lactate measurement allows the clinician to assess the response of critically ill patients to resuscitative therapy (decreasing lactate concentration indicates restoration of tissue oxygen delivery).

SYSTEMS AFFECTED

• Cardiovascular—persistent lactic acidosis associated with impaired cardiac contractility, impaired pressor response to catecholamines, increased sensitivity of myocardium to ventricular arrhythmias, and reduced cardiac output. These changes may worsen organ hypoperfusion, leading to further tissue hypoxia.
• As acidosis and tissue hypoxia become severe, failure of multiple organ systems and death can occur.

SIGNALMENT

Dog and cat.

SIGNS

General Comments

Signs relate more to underlying disorder than to direct effects of acidosis. As tissue hypoperfusion, hypoxia, and acidosis worsen, signs of dysfunction can occur in any organ system.

Historical Findings

Disorders causing lactic acidosis are common; historical facts should prompt suspicion of an underlying acidosis.

Physical Examination Findings

• Tachypnea is usually present due to attempted respiratory compensation.
• Most patients with acidosis are hypovolemic and demonstrate poor tissue perfusion or dehydration—dark mucous membranes, prolonged capillary refill time, or increased skin turgor.
• Severely acidotic patients might have cardiac dysrhythmias and weak pulses.

CAUSES

• Two types of hyperlactatemia, A and B, based on presence or absence of hypoperfusion or tissue hypoxia.
• Type A hyperlactatemia—more common; due to decreased or inadequate oxygen delivery or increased oxygen demand. Causes of type A hyperlactatemia include shock, regional hypoperfusion, arterial obstruction, severe hypoxemia or anemia, carbon monoxide poisoning, and severe motor seizures.
• Increased oxygen demand can be caused by increased muscle activity (e.g., exercise, tremors, struggling, fever, seizure activity).
• Type B hyperlactatemia—all other causes of lactic acidosis; subdivided into three subsets (B_1, B_2, B_3); characterized by absence of hypoxemia or poor tissue perfusion. Many causes of type B lactic acidosis might be "occult" hypoperfusion not detectable by routine monitoring parameters or possibly combinations of types A and B lactic acidosis.
  ○ Type B_1 hyperlactatemia is associated with diseases such as sepsis, neoplasia, liver disease and diabetes mellitus.
  ○ Type B_2 hyperlactatemia is associated with a wide variety of drugs or toxins including corticosteroids, activated charcoal, propofol, lactulose, morphine, terbutaline, theophylline, xylitol, and parenteral nutrition.
  ○ Type B_3 hyperlactatemias are caused by congenital metabolic diseases, mitochondrial myopathies, and enzyme deficiencies.
• Most common causes of type B lactic acidosis in veterinary medicine include neoplasia, alkalosis, sepsis, renal failure, liver disease, catecholamine use (norepinephrine, epinephrine), and intoxications (strychnine, cyanide, ethylene glycol, salicylates, acetaminophen, propylene glycol).
• Elevated blood lactate has been observed in patients with lymphoma and meningioma. Though the type and cause of hyperlactatemia in these animals is not clearly understood, the presence of a high lactate should prompt the clinician to evaluate other markers of perfusion (heart rate, mucous membrane color, pulse quality, capillary refill, serum creatinine) before attempting aggressive fluid resuscitation.
• Metformin intoxication is associated with severe lactic acidosis and hypoglycemia in people and dogs.

RISK FACTORS

Risk factors for hyperlactatemia are risk factors for specific disorders that cause tissue hypoxia.

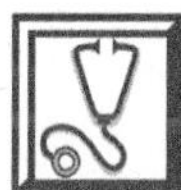

DIAGNOSIS

DIFFERENTIAL DIAGNOSIS

Differential diagnoses for hyperlactatemia and lactic acidosis include those disorders described under Causes.

LABORATORY FINDINGS

Drugs That May Alter Laboratory Results

• Activated charcoal, catecholamines, salicylates, acetaminophen, terbutaline, nitroprusside, halothane, bicarbonate, and propylene glycol can cause mild-to-moderate hyperlactatemia in the absence of true tissue hypoperfusion and hypoxia.
• Lower lactate concentrations are found in blood samples with sodium citrate anticoagulant than in those with heparin and EDTA.
• Even small amounts of lactate-containing intravenous fluids (e.g., lactated Ringer's solution) can cause false increases in measured blood lactate concentration if not properly cleared from the catheter prior to sampling.

Disorders That May Alter Laboratory Results

• Stress, trembling, resisting restraint, excitement, and venous stasis can increase

LACTIC ACIDOSIS (HYPERLACTATEMIA) (CONTINUED)

lactate to 2.5–5.0 mmol/L, but lactate usually normalizes in ≤2 hours.

- Seizures or extreme muscular exertion can increase lactate to 4–10 mmol/L, but lactate usually normalizes in ≤2 hours.
- Several types of neoplasia increase lactate concentrations because tumor cells preferentially use anaerobic glucose metabolism.
- Alkalosis, sepsis, liver disease, and renal failure can also increase lactate concentrations by mechanisms other than poor tissue perfusion and hypoxia.
- Failure to detect hyperlactatemia does not ensure adequate perfusion to all organs; significant organ hypoperfusion can still exist that might ultimately lead to multiple organ failure.
- Regional hypoperfusion, especially splanchnic, occurs in the absence of, or before, increases in systemic lactate and often despite therapy that successfully maintains blood pressure, cardiac output, and respiratory parameters.
- D-Lactate is not detected by routine analysis. Although D-lactate normally only exists at 1–5% the concentration of L-lactate, D-lactate elevation has been associated with short bowel syndrome and exocrine pancreatic insufficiency in humans. In cats, D-lactate has been associated with gastrointestinal disease, diabetic ketoacidosis, and propylene glycol intoxication.
- D-Lactate hyperlactatemia is a rare cause of high anion gap acidosis.

Valid if Run in Human Laboratory?

- Yes; semiautomated and automated techniques are available for rapid measurement of lactate concentration in microliter samples of whole blood, serum, and plasma.
- Lactate should be sampled from comparable sites (e.g., all venous or arterial) for serial measurement.

CBC/BIOCHEMISTRY/URINALYSIS

- CBC generally reflects underlying cause(s).
- Biochemical and urinalysis findings can help determine underlying cause of acidosis; examples include renal azotemia and increased serum osmolality seen with ethylene glycol intoxication; renal azotemia, hyperkalemia, and tubular casts seen with acute renal failure; and increased total protein and increased hematocrit with hemoconcentration and poor tissue perfusion in a hypovolemic patient.

OTHER LABORATORY TESTS

- Blood gas analysis (arterial preferred to assess blood oxygen) might define extent of a concurrent respiratory disorder or a mixed acid–base disorder.
- Additional tests (e.g., ethylene glycol, serum and urine glucose and ketones) might be helpful, depending on suspected cause.

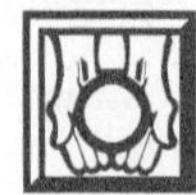

TREATMENT

- Hyperlactatemia is more important as a marker of severe or developing systemic problems. Aggressive treatment is not recommended for elevated blood lactate in the absence of other signs of circulatory shock. Fluid resuscitation is also not indicated if cardiogenic shock is the cause.
- Hyperlactatemia, with or without acidosis, should drive the clinician to seek causes of hypoperfusion and should focus early therapeutic interventions to improve tissue oxygen delivery.
- If lactic acidosis is severe, aggressive therapy to correct underlying cause(s) and specifically treat acidosis or hypoperfusion is indicated.

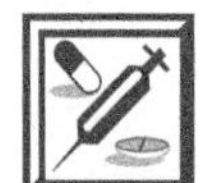

MEDICATIONS

DRUG(S) OF CHOICE

- Specific drug and fluid use depends on underlying cause.
- Many causes of hyperlactatemia and lactic acidosis are characterized by hypovolemia; thus, IV fluid therapy is generally first step in treatment (unless cardiogenic).
- Alkalinizing and pH-neutral isotonic crystalloid fluids might be preferred (vs. 0.9% NaCl) in cases of hypovolemic lactic acidosis to more rapidly normalize blood pH.
- Though controversial, sodium bicarbonate therapy to correct blood pH <7.1 might be indicated when the pH fails to increase in response to aggressive fluid resuscitation or when cardiovascular collapse is suspected to be due to low blood pH.

PRECAUTIONS

- Sodium bicarbonate should only be used to correct pH to 7.2. This can be accomplished by calculating the bicarbonate deficit or giving an empirical dose of 1 mEq/kg IV and rechecking blood pH.
- Sodium bicarbonate is more likely to be effective in patients with a normal anion gap metabolic acidosis (normal lactate) than patients with high anion gap metabolic acidosis, as the latter will correct acidemia when organic anions (lactate or ketoacids) are converted to bicarbonate during hemodynamic recovery.
- 10–15% of administered bicarbonate is converted to CO_2; it is important that only patients with adequate ventilation are treated.
- Complications of sodium bicarbonate therapy can include volume overload, paradoxic central nervous system acidosis, hypocalcemic tetany and a left-shift of oxygen–hemoglobin dissociation curve (iatrogenic alkalosis).

FOLLOW-UP

PATIENT MONITORING

- Serial lactate determinations are more valuable than single measurements; monitor lactate over time in critical patients.
- The ability of a patient to clear lactate predicts response to therapy and survival.
- Monitor other parameters that gauge response to therapy of underlying cause.

PREVENTION/AVOIDANCE

Owners should understand early warning signs of condition(s) that led to lactic acidosis in their pet with instructions to seek prompt medical attention should they recur.

POSSIBLE COMPLICATIONS

- Dogs with hyperlactatemia and acidosis have poorer outcomes, similar to humans.
- Lactate >6–6.5 mmol/L suggests tissue hypoperfusion (e.g., shock) or local ischemia (e.g., gastric necrosis in patients with gastric dilatation and volvulus [GDV]).

EXPECTED COURSE AND PROGNOSIS

- Lactic acidosis should correct with resuscitation. Lactic acidosis that fails to respond is a grave prognostic indicator.
- Hypotensive dogs without hyperlactatemia have a better prognosis and chance of survival than do hypotensive dogs with hyperlactatemia.
- Hypotensive, normolactatemic cats in an intensive care unit have a significantly greater chance of survival to hospital discharge than their hyperlactatemic counterparts.

MISCELLANEOUS

ASSOCIATED CONDITIONS

- Lactic acidosis can be found with any condition causing tissue hypoxia.
- Hyperlactatemia in patients with lymphoma and meningioma may exist despite normal tissue oxygen delivery. In these patients, other parameters should be used to assess tissue perfusion as blood lactate can remain elevated despite adequate resuscitation.

SEE ALSO

Acidosis, Metabolic.

ABBREVIATIONS

- GDV = gastric dilatation and volvulus.

Suggested Reading

Ateca LB, Dombrowski SC, Silverstein DC. Survival analysis of critically ill dogs with hypotension with or without hyperlactatemia: 67 cases (2006–2011). J Am Vet Med Assoc 2015, 246(1):100–104.

Kohen CJ, Hopper K, Kass PH, et al. Retrospective evaluation of the prognostic utility of plasma lactate concentration, base deficit, pH, and anion gap in canine and feline emergency patients. J Vet Emerg Crit Care 2018, 28(1):54–61.

Rosenstein PG, Hughes D. Hyperlactatemia. In: Silverstein DC, Hopper K, eds., Small Animal Critical Care Medicine, 2nd ed. Philadelphia, PA: Elsevier, 2015, pp. 300–305.

Shea EK, Dombrowski SC, Silverstein DC. Survival analysis of hypotensive cats admitted to an intensive care unit with or without hyperlactatemia: 39 cases (2005–2011). J Am Vet Med Assoc 2017, 250(8):887–893.

Author Timothy B. Hackett
Consulting Editor Patty A. Lathan

LAMENESS

BASICS

DEFINITION

A disturbance in gait and locomotion in response to pain, anatomic disruption, or injury.

PATHOPHYSIOLOGY

- Severe, sharp pain—limited limb movement during all phases of locomotion, little to no load bearing in motion or at rest.
- Milder, dull, or aching pain—reduced loading and ground contact time during all phases of locomotion.
- Pain produced only during certain phases of movement—patient adjusts its motion and gait to minimize discomfort.
- Anatomic dysfunction resulting in certain normal motions being altered or impossible.

L

SYSTEMS AFFECTED

- Musculoskeletal.
- Nervous.

SIGNALMENT

- Any age or breed of dog.
- Age, breed, and sex predilection—depend on specific disease.

SIGNS

General Comments

- Unilateral forelimb—head and neck moves upward when the affected limb is placed on the ground and drops when the sound limb loads.
- Unilateral hind limb—pelvis drops when affected leg loads, rises when it unloads.
- Bilateral hind limb—thoracic limbs carried lower and shifted caudally at the stance, to shift weight forward.
- Always assess the patient's neurologic status, especially with a suspected proximal lesion.

Historical Findings

- Complete history—identify known trauma; alterations with weather, exercise tolerance, response to rest, effect of previous treatments.
- Determine speed of onset of lameness.
- Determine progression—static, slow, rapid.
- Determine consistency—intermittent, constant, associations with interventions, rest or activities.
- How does the patient show pain?

Physical Examination Findings

- Perform a complete routine examination.
- Observe posture—standing, getting up or lying down, sitting.
- Observe gait—walking; trotting; climbing stairs; tight turns or figure eights.
- Palpate—asymmetry of muscle mass (measure and compare); note bony prominences.
- Manipulate bones and joints, beginning distally and working proximally.
- Assess—instability; incongruency; pain; range of motion (measure); abnormal sounds or crepitus.
- Examine suspected area of involvement last—by starting with normal limbs, patient may relax, allowing comparison of normal to abnormal reactions.

CAUSES

Forelimb

Growing Dog (<12 Months of Age)

- Osteochondrosis of the shoulder.
- Shoulder luxation or subluxation—congenital.
- Osteochondrosis of the elbow.
- Ununited anconeal process.
- Medial coronoid disease.
- Elbow incongruity.
- Avulsion or calcification of the flexor muscles—elbow.
- Asymmetric growth of the radius and ulna.
- Panosteitis.
- Hypertrophic osteodystrophy.
- Trauma—soft tissue; bone; joint.
- Infection—local; systemic.
- Nutritional imbalances.
- Congenital anomalies.

Mature Dog (>12 Months of Age)

- Degenerative joint disease.
- Bicipital tenosynovitis.
- Calcification or mineralization of supraspinatus or infraspinatus tendon.
- Contracture of supraspinatus or infraspinatus muscle.
- Soft tissue or bone neoplasia—primary; metastatic.
- Trauma—soft tissue; bone; joint.
- Panosteitis.
- Polyarthropathies.
- Polymyositis.
- Polyneuritis.

Hind Limb

Growing Dog (<12 Months of Age)

- Hip laxity (hip dysplasia).
- Avascular necrosis of femoral head—Legg–Calvé–Perthes disease.
- Osteochondritis of stifle.
- Patella luxation—medial or lateral.
- Osteochondritis of hock.
- Panosteitis.
- Hypertrophic osteodystrophy.
- Trauma—soft tissue; bone; joint.
- Infection—local; systemic.
- Nutritional imbalances.
- Congenital anomalies.

Mature Dog (>12 Months of Age)

- Degenerative joint disease (hip dysplasia).
- Cruciate ligament disease.
- Avulsion of long digital extensor tendon.
- Soft tissue or bone neoplasia—primary; metastatic.
- Trauma—soft tissue; bone; joint.
- Panosteitis.
- Polyarthropathies.
- Polymyositis.
- Polyneuritis.

RISK FACTORS

Breed, size, overweight, strenuous activity, metabolic disease (Cushing's, hypothyrodism).

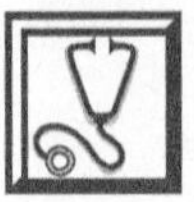

DIAGNOSIS

DIFFERENTIAL DIAGNOSIS

Must differentiate musculoskeletal from neurogenic and metabolic causes.

CBC/BIOCHEMISTRY/URINALYSIS

Muscle injury elevates creatine phosphokinase levels. General inflammatory disease such as infectious inflammatory arthropathies have been associated with elevations of C-reactive protein (CRP).

OTHER LABORATORY TESTS

Depends on suspected cause, however various tests available for infectious or inflammatory diseases.

IMAGING

- Radiographs—recommend two views of region of interest. Stressed views indicated if ligamentous injury is part of the differential list.
- CT, MRI, ultrasound, and nuclear scintigraphy where appropriate.

DIAGNOSTIC PROCEDURES

- Cytologic examination of joint fluid—identify and differentiate intra-articular disease.
- Electromyogram (EMG)—differentiate chronic neuromuscular from musculoskeletal disease.
- Muscle and/or nerve biopsy—reveal and identify neuromuscular disease.

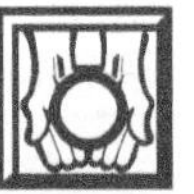

TREATMENT

Depends on underlying cause.

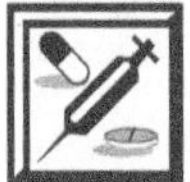

MEDICATIONS

DRUG(S) OF CHOICE

Nonsteroidal Anti-inflammatory Drugs (NSAIDs) and Analgesics

- May be used for symptomatic treatment; minimize pain, decrease inflammation.
- Carprofen 2.2 mg/kg PO q12h or 4.4 mg/kg PO q24h.
- Deracoxib 1–2 mg/kg PO q24h, chewable.
- Firocoxib 5 mg/kg PO q24h.
- Grapiprant 2 mg/kg PO q24h, to animals >3.6 kg.
- Meloxicam—load 0.2 mg/kg PO, then 0.1 mg/kg PO q24h—liquid.
- Tepoxalin—load 20 mg/kg, then 10 mg/kg PO q24h.

PRECAUTIONS

NSAIDs—gastrointestinal irritation or renal/hepatic toxicity may preclude use in some patients.

ALTERNATIVE DRUG(S)

- Chondroprotective drugs, such as polysulfated glycosaminoglycans, green-lipped mussel extract, and glucosamine/chondroitin sulfate (limited supportive data), may help limit associated cartilage damage and degeneration.
- Nonspecific anti-inflammatory supplements—e.g. green-lipped muscle extract and omega 3 fatty acid supplementation.

FOLLOW-UP

PATIENT MONITORING

Depends on underlying cause.

MISCELLANEOUS

SEE ALSO

Chapters covering musculoskeletal and neuromuscular disorders.

ABBREVIATIONS

- CRP = C-reactive protein.
- EMG = electromyogram.
- NSAID = nonsteroidal anti-inflammatory drug.

Suggested Reading

Brinker WO, Piermattei DL, Flo GL. Physical examination for lameness. In: Handbook of Small Animal Orthopedics and Fracture Repair, 3rd ed. Philadelphia, PA: Saunders, 1997, pp. 228–230.

Renberg WC, Roush JK. Lameness. Vet Clin North Am Small Anim Pract 2001, 31:1.

Author Mathieu M. Glassman

Consulting Editor Mathieu M. Glassman

Acknowledgment The author/editor acknowledges the prior contribution of Walter C. Renberg.

Client Education Handout available online

LARYNGEAL AND TRACHEAL PERFORATION

BASICS

OVERVIEW

Tracheal perforation is a loss of integrity of the tracheal wall, allowing leakage of air to create subcutaneous (SC) emphysema, pneumomediastinum, pneumopericardium, pneumothorax, and pneumoretroperitoneum. Caused by penetrating, intraluminal, or blunt cervical or thoracic trauma. Severity ranges from small perforation to complete avulsion. With complete avulsion, mediastinal tissues can form a pseudomembrane to maintain airway patency. Laryngeal perforation is disruption of laryngeal structures (thyroid, cricoid, and arytenoid cartilages) and can create similar leakage of air and may result in upper airway obstruction.

L

Systems Affected

- Respiratory—compromise of airway, possible pneumomediastinum and pneumothorax. Laryngeal swelling may result in upper airway obstruction.
- Cardiovascular—pneumothorax and tension pneumothorax can decrease venous return and cardiac output.
- Nervous, musculoskeletal—depends on severity of hypoxia.
- Skin—SC emphysema, initially cervical but can affect entire body.

SIGNALMENT

Dog and cat—no breed, age, or sex predilection.

SIGNS

- Onset: immediate or up to 1 week after injury.
- SC emphysema and respiratory distress are most common.
- Other signs—respiratory distress, may have stridor, anorexia, lethargy, exercise intolerance, gagging, ptyalism, vomiting, coughing, hemoptysis, upper airway obstruction, and shock. May have dysphonia (voice change) and/or dysphagia.

CAUSES & RISK FACTORS

- Access to outside while unsupervised causing increased risk of all types of trauma.
- Exposure to other animals causing increased risk of bite wounds.
- Penetrating cervical wounds—bite wounds, impalement, projectile missiles, foreign bodies.
- Iatrogenic perforation during endotracheal intubation, transtracheal wash, jugular venipuncture, cervical surgery, radiation therapy, tracheal stent fracture, or failure to deflate cuff or to stabilize the tube while repositioning patient. Overinflation of endotracheal cuff can cause a linear tear in the trachealis muscle at thoracic inlet or intrathoracic trachea. Occurs most often with dental procedures.
- Blunt trauma can cause intrathoracic tracheal avulsion.
- Blunt trauma to the cervical region can cause laryngeal avulsion or fracture.

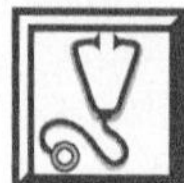

DIAGNOSIS

DIFFERENTIAL DIAGNOSIS

- Anesthesia—barotrauma resulting in alveolar rupture and pneumothorax.
- Penetrating wounds—perforation of esophagus or cervical bite.
- After blunt trauma—pulmonary contusions, pneumothorax, rib fractures.
- Differentials for tracheal perforation include intrathoracic tracheal compression by mediastinal mass, spontaneous pneumothorax, pleural effusion, and bronchoesophageal fistula.
- Differentials for laryngeal perforation include trauma to caudal pharynx or larynx, pharyngeal or laryngeal mass (such as squamous cell carcinoma, lymphoma, granuloma, other), laryngeal paralysis, abscess, pharyngeal mucocele, foreign body in airway.

CBC/BIOCHEMISTRY/URINALYSIS

Usually normal.

OTHER LABORATORY TESTS

Arterial blood gas analysis can show hypoxemia, hypercarbia, and respiratory acidosis.

IMAGING

- Lateral cervical and thoracic radiographs are essential. SC emphysema, pneumomediastinum, pneumopericardium, and pneumothorax can be seen. Also evaluate for concurrent thoracic trauma (e.g., rib fractures), and noncardiogenic pulmonary edema.
- In cases of tracheal avulsion, site of disruption may be visible.
- In cases of laryngeal trauma may observe disruption of the hyoid apparatus.
- Abdominal radiographs occasionally show pneumoretroperitoneum.
- CT can be useful to identify location and extent of laryngeal and tracheal damage. Laryngeal and hyoid fractures and dislocations can be visualized.

DIAGNOSTIC PROCEDURES

- Laryngoscopy and tracheoscopy used to confirm laryngeal or tracheal perforation or avulsion and characterize severity; false negatives can occur.
- If patient does not have a patent airway, can be stabilized with general anesthesia and a temporary tracheostomy. Laryngoscopy can then be performed.
- Larynx should be evaluated for symmetry and function of laryngeal structures, presence of
- hematomas, exposed cartilage, foreign body, or flaps of laryngeal mucosa.
- Esophagoscopy performed to rule out concurrent esophageal injury.

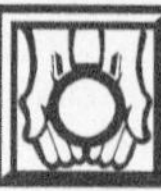

TREATMENT

- Hospitalization is indicated.
- Oxygen supplementation with 95% O_2 for 4 hours will decrease SC emphysema.
- Minimal handling to reduce stress; most cases of iatrogenic perforation will heal.
- If pneumothorax develops, thoracocentesis ± thoracostomy tubes may be required.
- Intubation if needed.
- If patient decompensates, surgical exploration is indicated.
- Tracheal rupture secondary to blunt trauma or penetrating injury requires surgical repair.
- If tracheal avulsion is present, intubate only the proximal segment using an undersized endotracheal tube. Avoid positive-pressure ventilation to prevent disruption of pseudomembrane.
- Cervical tracheal perforation—approach via ventral midline; may require a partial median sternotomy. Damaged areas of trachea are often on the dorsolateral surface: debride and repair with 3-0 to 5-0 monofilament absorbable suture.
- Tracheal resection and anastomosis indicated for severe tracheal damage or tracheal avulsion.
- Intrathoracic tracheal avulsion—approach via a right lateral 3rd or 4th intercostal thoracotomy. Open the pseudomembrane and intubate the caudal segment. Preplace sutures, guide an endotracheal tube from the cranial segment into the caudal segment, and complete repair.
- If upper airway obstruction or unable to intubate, an emergency temporary tracheostomy is indicated. Temporary tracheostomy is performed at approximately the 4th tracheal ring and tube is sized to about 50% of tracheal lumen.
- Laryngeal repair indicated if avulsed/exposed arytenoid cartilage with debridement or partial arytenoidectomy or tieback procedure. If there is collapse or fracture of the cricothyroid cartilages, laryngeal exploration via ventral laryngotomy may be needed to stabilize laryngeal structures to reduce stenosis.
- Hyoid bone avulsion and laryngotracheal avulsion should be repaired with apposition via ventral approach.
- Mucosal flaps should be trimmed and edges apposed with 4-0 or 5-0 absorbable suture.
- Intraluminal stents can be used for preventing adhesions, collapse, and other complications.
- Stents will require second procedures 3–4 weeks later for removal.
- Unilateral arytenoid lateralization (tieback) if traumatic laryngeal paralysis without fractures or if arytenoid avulsion.

- Permanent tracheostomy may be indicated if unable to restore patent airway or with severe laryngeal damage.
- Exercise restriction for 3–4 weeks post trauma and surgical repair.
- No neck leads and harness only when leash walking.

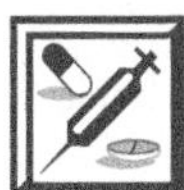

MEDICATIONS

DRUG(S) OF CHOICE

- Broad-spectrum antibiotic therapy if caused by bite wounds.
- Antibiotics after obtaining cultures from contaminated wounds; continue 1–2 weeks in the postoperative period. Empirical selections while awaiting culture results could include:
  - Ampicillin 22 mg/kg IV q8h (both dogs and cats) and enrofloxacin 10–15 mg/kg diluted and given slowly IV or PO q24h in dogs (5 mg/kg q24h in cats).
  - Clindamycin 10 mg/kg IV or PO q8h and either amoxicillin/clavulanic acid 15 mg/kg PO q12h or enrofloxacin, as listed above.
  - Corticosteroids (dexamethasone sodium phosphate 0.1–0.2 mg/kg IV) at time of surgery to reduce inflammation; may repeat at a dose of 0.05–0.1 mg/kg IV q24h for first 24–48 hours.

CONTRAINDICATIONS/POSSIBLE INTERACTIONS

- Sedation—use with caution, can decrease respiratory drive.
- Corticosteroids are not indicated unless there is a large degree of upper airway swelling or concern for postoperative swelling.

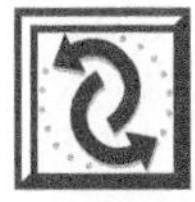

FOLLOW-UP

PATIENT MONITORING

- Monitor respiratory rate and effort, mucous membrane color, capillary refill time, pulse quality, and heart rate, and auscult frequently.
- Pulse oximetry and/or arterial blood gases.
- Thoracic radiographs to monitor pneumomediastinum, pneumothorax, and help detect tracheal stenosis. Tracheoscopy required in some cases.
- Tracheostomy care if tracheostomy is needed.
- Respiratory rate and effort, respiratory noise, and exercise tolerance, during and after the recovery stage.

PREVENTION/AVOIDANCE

- Use of 3 mL syringe for cuff inflation for cats and small dogs to prevent overinflation of cuff.
- High-volume low-pressure endotracheal tube cuff may also reduce risk of tracheal damage.
- Disconnect endotracheal tube from anesthetic circuit when repositioning animal during anesthesia.
- Selection of appropriate endotracheal tube and endoscope size along with use of lubrication will reduce iatrogenic tracheal and laryngeal trauma.
- Direct visualization of the larynx for intubation can reduce risk of iatrogenic trauma.
- Long-term intubation for positive-pressure ventilation can be maintained by temporary tracheostomy to prevent laryngeal damage.

POSSIBLE COMPLICATIONS

- Tracheal stricture and stenosis at site of perforation or repair.
- Laryngeal paralysis from damage to recurrent laryngeal nerve.
- Dehiscence of tracheal anastomosis site.
- Stenosis or stricture resulting in airway compromise.
- Infection from trauma, or post operatively.
- Sepsis (rare).
- Obstruction of temporary or permanent tracheostomy with mucus.
- Death, particularly at induction of anesthesia with complete tracheal avulsion, or with complete airway obstruction.

EXPECTED COURSE AND PROGNOSIS

- Most cases respond well to appropriate therapy.
- Complete tracheal avulsion—guarded prognosis. Without surgery—extremely poor prognosis due to stricture formation.
- Prognosis depends on severity of trauma, concurrent injuries, and treatment.
- If severe laryngeal trauma is present and veterinary care can be quickly obtained, permanent tracheostomy can allow for fair to good prognosis (with the exception of cats and very small dogs, where stoma obstruction with mucus may be recurrent and severe).

MISCELLANEOUS

ASSOCIATED CONDITIONS

With tracheal perforation caused by blunt trauma, can have pulmonary contusions, pneumothorax, rib fractures, and hemothorax.

PREGNANCY/FERTILITY/BREEDING

Hypoxia can result in fetal distress and death.

ABBREVIATIONS

- SC = subcutaneous.

Suggested Reading

Basdani EE, Papazoglou LG, Patsikas MN, et al. Upper airway injury in dogs secondary to trauma: 10 dogs (2000–2011). J Am Anim Hosp Assoc 2016, 52:291–296.

Jordan CJ, Halfacree ZJ, Tivers MS. Airway injury associated with cervical bite wounds in dogs and cats: 56 cases. Vet Comp Orthop Traumatol 2013, 26:89–93.

Mitchell SL, McCarthy R, Rudloff E, Pernell RT. Tracheal rupture associated with intubation in cats: 20 cases (1996–1998). J Am Vet Med Assoc 2000, 216:1592–1595.

Nelson AW. Laryngeal trauma and stenosis. In: Slatter D, ed., Textbook of Small Animal Surgery, 3rd ed. Philadelphia, PA: Saunders, 2003, pp. 845–857.

White RN, Burton CA. Surgical management of intrathoracic tracheal avulsion in cats: long-term results in 9 consecutive cases. Vet Surg 2000, 29:430–435.

Authors Lori S. Waddell and David A. Puerto
Consulting Editor Elizabeth Rozanski

LARYNGEAL DISEASES

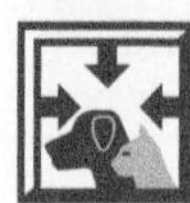

BASICS

DEFINITION

• The larynx is made of cartilage structures surrounding the rima glottis. The functions of the larynx are to control airflow during respiration, protect the lower airways from aspiration during swallowing, and control phonation. • Laryngeal diseases in dogs and cats include laryngeal paralysis, laryngitis, laryngeal collapse, foreign body obstruction, neoplasia, and trauma.

PATHOPHYSIOLOGY

• Decreased diameter of the laryngeal opening increases resistance to airflow during inspiration and results in stridor on inspiration. The decrease in airflow will lead to hypoxemia, cyanosis, and/or respiratory distress and a decrease in heat exchange (heat intolerance, hyperthermia). • Inflammation or lesions of the vocal cords can lead to aphonia or change in bark/meow.

L

SYSTEMS AFFECTED

• Respiratory—respiratory distress, often associated with airway obstruction. Aspiration pneumonia may develop. Stridor is common.
• Cardiovascular—hypoxemia/distress may lead to tachycardia; laryngeal stimulation may trigger vagal response (bradycardia).
• Gastrointestinal—retching, regurgitation, vomiting, and/or dysphagia can occur when polyneuropathy causes laryngeal paralysis and esophageal dysfunction; esophagitis is frequently associated with brachycephalic airway syndrome (BAS). • Nervous—depression, stupor, or coma may occur if severe laryngeal obstruction leads to severe hyperthermia. Older dogs with laryngeal paralysis often have geriatric-onset laryngeal paralysis polyneuropathy (GOLPP), which includes hind limb weakness.

GENETICS

• Juvenile laryngeal paralysis in the bouvier des Flandres is transmitted as a dominant trait. • In laryngeal paralysis associated with polyneuropathy in the Leonberger dog, X-linked inheritance is suggested. • No other laryngeal disorder has been proven to be genetic in the dog or cat, but familial conditions and breed predispositions have been reported.

INCIDENCE/PREVALENCE

• More common in dogs than in cats.
• Currently, congenital laryngeal paralysis is only sporadic in the bouvier des Flandres.
• Idiopathic laryngeal paralysis is a common disease of older large-breed dogs; exact prevalence unknown. • BAS is a common syndrome in French and English bulldogs.
• Laryngeal trauma may occur in conjunction with bite wounds; tracheal bite wounds may result in laryngeal paralysis/collapse due to damage to the recurrent laryngeal nerves.
• Neoplasia is rare in dogs, but fairly common in older cats, who are often initially thought to have lower airway disease due to "wheezing" that accompanies laryngeal masses.

SIGNALMENT

Species

Dog and cat.

Breed Predilections

• Familial laryngeal paralysis/polyneuropathy complex occurs in the Dalmatian, Rottweiler, Leonberger, and Pyrenean mountain dog (great Pyrenees). • Congenital laryngeal paralysis is found in bouviers des Flandres, huskies, husky crosses, white German shepherd dogs, and probably bull terriers.
• Idiopathic acquired laryngeal paralysis is most often found in large-breed dogs (especially Labrador and golden retrievers).
• BAS is found in brachycephalic breeds of dogs. • Upper airway obstruction due to laryngeal collapse or narrowed laryngeal opening occurs in Norwich terriers.

Mean Age and Range

• Congenital and familial laryngeal paralysis—onset of signs usually in the first months of life (2 and 8 months). Later in the Leonberger, 1–9 years, and white German shepherd dog, 2 years. • Acquired laryngeal paralysis—possible at any age but more frequent in older dogs.
• Neoplasia—middle-aged to old dogs.

SIGNS

Historical Findings

• Panting. • Exercise and heat intolerance.
• Noisy respiration. • Change of voice.
• Occasional cough. • Severe cases—inspiratory respiratory distress, collapse, syncope, or even sudden death.
• Polyneuropathy, polymyopathy, or myasthenia gravis—regurgitation, weakness, abnormal gait (pattern of abnormalities varies).
• Absence of signs is possible in Norwich terriers with upper airway obstruction.

Physical Examination Findings

• Panting, polypnea, and inspiratory stridor in canine cases. • Respiration is less noisy in cats with laryngeal disease. • Cyanosis.
• Hyperthermia frequent. • Aspiration pneumonia—fever, crackles on respiratory auscultation. • Polyneuropathy, polymyopathy, or myasthenia gravis—paraparesis or tetraparesis with decreased spinal reflexes. • Leonberger with familial polyneuropathy—high-stepping pelvic-limb gait with depressed spinal and cranial nerve reflexes. • Rottweilers with laryngeal paralysis/polyneuropathy complex—cataracts frequently observed. • Normal physical examination in some Norwich terriers with upper airway obstruction.

CAUSES

• Laryngeal paralysis: ∘ Congenital—(1) neuronal degeneration of the nucleus ambiguous (bouvier des Flandres and husky); (2) idiopathic. ∘ Acquired—(1) polyneuropathy: idiopathic; familial (laryngeal paralysis–polyneuropathy complex); immune-mediated; (2) myasthenia gravis; (3) polymyopathy: idiopathic; immune-mediated; infectious (toxoplasmosis, neosporosis); (4) ventral cervical or cranial thoracic lesion—neoplasia or trauma affecting one or both recurrent nerves; examples include lymphoma of the vagus nerve in the cat and traumatic neuropathy secondary to thyroidectomy. • Acute laryngitis: ∘ Cause often not found. ∘ Virus—canine parainfluenza virus, feline herpesvirus 1. ∘ Bacteria—*Bordetella bronchiseptica*. ∘ Gastroesophageal reflux.
• Idiopathic chronic obstructive laryngitis (lymphoplasmacytic, granulomatous).
• Laryngeal neoplasia: ∘ Dog—rhabdomyoma, rhabdomyosarcoma, adenocarcinoma, squamous cell carcinoma, lipoma, extramedullary plasmacytoma. ∘ Cat—lymphoma, squamous cell carcinoma. • Trauma: injuries caused by foreign bodies. • Neck trauma, bite wounds.
• Laryngeal collapse secondary to BAS.
• Idiopathic laryngeal malformation, collapse in Norwich terriers.

RISK FACTORS

Breed associations. Risk factors for developing severe or fatal clinical signs include obesity, dark coat, hot or humid temperature (especially in a closed environment), and concurrent lower airway or pulmonary disease.

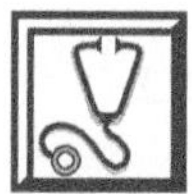

DIAGNOSIS

DIFFERENTIAL DIAGNOSIS

• Pharyngeal diseases—also cause gagging, stridor, and cough. Dysphagia is not seen with laryngeal disease but may be present in the case of pharyngeal lesion. • Tracheal diseases may be confused with laryngeal disease in some cases. Cough is more frequent in tracheal disease than in laryngeal disease, while inspiratory stridor is more frequent in laryngeal disease.

CBC/BIOCHEMISTRY/URINALYSIS

• No specific abnormalities. • Leukocytosis may be present in aspiration pneumonia.
• Mild-to-moderate increase in liver enzymes if chronic hypoxemia. • Hypercholesterolemia may be present if concurrent hypothyroidism is present.

OTHER LABORATORY TESTS

If laryngeal paralysis is secondary to polyneuropathy/polymyopathy, these may be considered, but are low yield:
• Thyroid panel in the dog. • Antibody titers against *Toxoplasma gondii* (dog and cat) and *Neospora caninum* (dog). • Anticholinesterase receptor antibody titer.

IMAGING

• Thoracic radiographs—to rule-out aspiration pneumonia as a complication, other lower airway conditions, and a mediastinal mass as a cause of laryngeal paralysis. • If vomiting/regurgitation present—barium swallow with fluoroscopy (to identify esophageal dysfunction, reflux esophagitis/hiatal hernia coexisting in some cases of brachycephalic airway syndrome). • Pharynx/larynx radiographs or ultrasonography—to identify potential mass.

DIAGNOSTIC PROCEDURES

Laryngoscopy

• Method of choice to identify laryngeal paralysis, collapse, mass, trauma, foreign body, or laryngitis. • General anesthesia or deep sedation is required. • Laryngeal paralysis: ◦ Diagnosis confirmed by loss of abduction of arytenoid cartilages during deep inspiration. ◦ Usually bilateral but unilateral paralysis is possible in the early course of the disease. ◦ Unilateral paralysis has been described in cats. ◦ False-positive result possible because of the influence of general anesthesia on laryngeal function. Intravenous doxapram HCl (1–2 mg/kg) to increase respiratory effort is advised if the diagnosis is in doubt.

Esophagoscopy

When vomiting/regurgitation is observed, to rule out reflux esophagitis or hiatal hernia.

Retrograde Rhinoscopy

When pharyngeal disease is suspected or in the case of BAS.

PATHOLOGIC FINDINGS

• Laryngeal paralysis: ◦ Gross findings—redness, swelling, and thickening of the arytenoid cartilages and the vocal folds. ◦ Histopathology—nonspecific edema and inflammation of laryngeal mucosa and submucosa; denervation atrophy of laryngeal muscles in the case of neuropathy of recurrent laryngeal nerve(s). • Idiopathic chronic obstructive laryngitis: ◦ Histopathology—lymphoplasmacytic, granulomatous, or pyogranulomatous inflammation of the laryngeal submucosa.

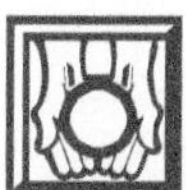

TREATMENT

APPROPRIATE HEALTH CARE

• Paralysis: ◦ Surgical palliation (arytenoid lateralization) is recommended for dogs with clinical signs but may be associated with postoperative aspiration. ◦ If signs are mild, avoidance of triggers is advised (e.g., heat, humidity). • Emergency: ◦ Sedation/anesthesia; supplemental oxygen; cooling therapy. ◦ Do not sedate to "look" with the thought to do surgery in the future as aspiration may occur on recovery. • Cats with suspected laryngeal masses may be very difficult to intubate; be sure to have surgical supplies for urgent tracheostomy readily available.

NURSING CARE

• Paralysis: ◦ Avoid warm, poorly ventilated environments, stress, and intense excitation as these further compromise normal cooling mechanisms and proper air exchange. ◦ Avoid cervical collars. ◦ Avoid weight gain.

ACTIVITY

Exercise should be severely restricted in animals suffering from laryngeal paralysis, especially in warm temperatures.

DIET

Loss of weight is advocated in overweight patients with any upper airway disorder.

CLIENT EDUCATION

• Paralysis: ◦ Discuss the importance of surgery and the risk of not performing surgery (chronic hypoxemia, heat stroke, risk of suffocation, and death) in moderately to severely affected dogs. ◦ Discuss potential complications of surgery including aspiration pneumonia. ◦ Discuss the potential progression of neuromuscular disease. ◦ Discuss the potential heritability of this condition in certain breeds. • Neoplasia: ◦ Discuss surgical/chemotherapeutical options.

SURGICAL CONSIDERATIONS

• Paralysis: ◦ Surgery (unilateral arytenoid lateralization) is the treatment of choice in both dogs and cats; bilateral surgical correction is not advised because it increases the risk of aspiration pneumonia. ◦ Cats that are breathing comfortably but have a voice change alone may be managed medically. • Neoplasia: ◦ Surgery, radiation or chemotherapy. ◦ Permanent tracheostomy in dogs may improve quality of life if surgical excision is not possible.

MEDICATIONS

DRUG(S) OF CHOICE

• Paralysis—if surgery is declined, anxiolytic may be considered. • Lymphoma (mainly in cats)—chemotherapy (see Lymphoma—Cats).

PRECAUTIONS

Usual safety precautions if chemotherapy is administered.

FOLLOW-UP

PATIENT MONITORING

• Immediate postsurgical period—check rectal temperature (should remain normal). • Monitor for aspiration pneumonia (short and long term). • If surgery is successful, exercise, stridor, and heat intolerance should decrease.

POSSIBLE COMPLICATIONS

• Paralysis—recurrence of clinical signs are uncommon if surgery is correctly performed; aspiration pneumonia is possible as the larynx is placed in a fixed open position; risk of aspiration pneumonia increased if bilateral arytenoid lateralization is performed or if dysphagia due to pharyngeal and/or esophageal dysfunction coexists. • Tumor—recurrence of clinical signs if complete resection is not possible; increased risk of aspiration pneumonia in the postoperative period.

EXPECTED COURSE AND PROGNOSIS

• Idiopathic paralysis—good with surgery; guarded to poor if surgery is declined. • Paralysis associated with esophageal dysfunction—poor. • Tumor—guarded to good in the case of successful resection of a benign tumor; poor in the case of carcinoma, even with radiation therapy; variable in the case of feline lymphoma.

MISCELLANEOUS

ASSOCIATED CONDITIONS

• Laryngeal paralysis is sometimes associated with a mass in the anterior mediastinum or the ventral cervical region. • Coexistence of megaesophagus, weakness, or abnormal gait with laryngeal paralysis suggests polyneuropathy, polymyopathy, or myasthenia gravis.

AGE-RELATED FACTORS

Congenital and familial laryngeal paralysis—onset of clinical signs in the first year of life.

PREGNANCY/FERTILITY/BREEDING

Dogs affected with congenital laryngeal paralysis or laryngeal paralysis/polyneuropathy complex should not be bred.

SEE ALSO

• Brachycephalic Airway Syndrome.
• Cyanosis.
• Myasthenia Gravis.

ABBREVIATIONS

• BAS = brachycephalic airway syndrome.
• GOLPP = geriatric-onset laryngeal paralysis polyneuropathy.

Author Elizabeth Rozanski
Consulting Editor Elizabeth Rozanski
Acknowledgment The author and editors acknowledge the prior contributions of Dominique Peeters and Cécile Clercx.

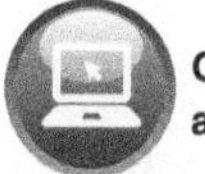

Client Education Handout available online

L

LEAD TOXICOSIS

BASICS

DEFINITION

Intoxication (blood lead >0.35 ppm, although somewhat variable) owing to acute or chronic exposure to some form of lead.

PATHOPHYSIOLOGY

• Cell damage is due to the ability of lead to substitute for other polyvalent cations (especially divalent cations such as Ca and Zn) important for cell homeostasis. • Diverse biological processes are affected, including metal transport, energy metabolism, apoptosis, ion conduction, cell adhesion, inter- and intracellular signaling, enzymatic processes, protein maturation, and genetic regulation.

L

SYSTEMS AFFECTED

• Gastrointestinal—unknown mechanism; likely damage to peripheral nerves.
• Nervous—capillary damage; alteration of membrane ionic channels and signaling molecules. • Renal/urologic—damage to proximal tubule cells due to enzyme disruption and oxidative damage. • Hemic/lymph/immune—interference with hemoglobin synthesis; increased fragility and decreased survival of red blood cells (RBCs); release of reticulocytes and nucleated RBCs from bone marrow; inhibition of 5′-pyrimidine nucleotidase causing retention of RNA degradation products; aggregation of ribosomes resulting in basophilic stippling.

INCIDENCE/PREVALENCE

• True incidence unknown. • Decreasing prevalence in dogs—owing to elimination of sources. • Steady to increasing prevalence in cats—increased awareness and diagnosis.
• Higher prevalence during warmer months.
• Higher prevalence in young animals—greater bioavailability of lead and more permeable blood–brain barrier.

GEOGRAPHIC DISTRIBUTION

• Low socioeconomic status of pet-owning family associated with high blood lead concentration in pets. • Areas with older homes/buildings.

SIGNALMENT

Species

Dogs and cats—dogs more commonly than cats.

Breed Predilections

N/A

Mean Age and Range

Mainly dogs <1 year of age.

Predominant Sex

N/A

SIGNS

General Comments

• Primarily gastrointestinal and neurologic.
• Gastrointestinal—often precede CNS signs; predominant with chronic, low-level exposure. • CNS—occur more often with acute exposure, more common in younger animals. • Renal—proximal tubular nephropathy has been reported.

Historical Findings

History of renovation of older house or building or ingestion of lead objects.

Physical Examination Findings

• Vomiting. • Diarrhea. • Anorexia.
• Abdominal pain. • Regurgitation due to megaesophagus. • Lethargy. • Hysteria.
• Seizures. • Blindness. • Cats—central vestibular abnormalities such as vertical nystagmus and ataxia reported.

CAUSES

• Ingestion of some form of lead—paint and paint residues or dust from sanding; car batteries; linoleum; solder; plumbing materials and supplies; lubricating compounds; putty; tar paper; lead foil; golf balls; lead object (e.g., shot, fishing sinkers, drapery weights); leaded glass. • Use of improperly glazed ceramic food or water bowl. • Lead paint or lead-contaminated dust or soil are common sources for exposure; cats ingest lead as a result of self-grooming.

RISK FACTORS

• Age <1 year. • Living in economically depressed areas. • Living in old house or building that is being renovated. • Feeding trimmings from lead-shot game.

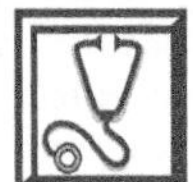

DIAGNOSIS

DIFFERENTIAL DIAGNOSIS

Dogs

• Canine distemper. • Infectious encephalitides.
• Epilepsy. • Bromethalin, methylxanthine, or tremorgenic mycotoxin toxicosis.
• Nonsteroidal anti-inflammatory drug (NSAID) toxicosis. • Heat stroke. • Intestinal parasitism. • Intussusception. • Foreign body.
• Pancreatitis. • Infectious canine hepatitis.

Cats

• Degenerative or storage diseases. • Hepatic encephalopathy. • Infectious encephalitides.
• Organophosphate, bromethalin, or methylxanthine toxicosis.

CBC/BIOCHEMISTRY/URINALYSIS

• Between 5 and 40 nucleated RBCs/100 white blood cells (WBCs) without anemia.
• Absence of nucleated RBCs does not rule out the diagnosis. • Anisocytosis, polychromasia, poikilocytosis, target cells, hypochromasia. • Basophilic stippling of RBCs; often difficult to detect.
• Neutrophilic leukocytosis. • Cats—elevated aspartate aminotransferase (AST) and alkaline phosphatase (ALP) reported.
• Urinalysis—mild nonspecific renal damage; glucosuria; proteinuria; hemoglobinuria.

OTHER LABORATORY TESTS

Lead Concentration

• Toxic—antemortem whole blood: >0.35 ppm (35 µg/dL); postmortem liver and/or kidney: >5 ppm (wet weight).
• Blood lead concentrations fluctuate and do not necessarily correlate with total body burden. • Lower values—must be interpreted in conjunction with history and clinical signs. • No normal "background" blood lead concentrations; typically less than 0.05 ppm. • Blood concentrations—do not correlate with occurrence or severity of clinical signs. • $CaNa_2EDTA$ mobilization test—collect one 24-hour urine sample; administer $CaNa_2EDTA$ (75 mg/kg IM); collect a second 24-hour urine sample; with toxicosis, urine lead increases 10- to 60-fold post-EDTA (succimer could conceivably be substituted for $CaNa_2EDTA$ but this has not been evaluated). • Point-of-care testing is available, but results might underestimate true blood lead concentrations; confirmation of results using other techniques such as GFAAS or ICP-MS is recommended.

IMAGING

May note radiopaque material in gastrointestinal tract; not diagnostic.

DIAGNOSTIC PROCEDURES

N/A

PATHOLOGIC FINDINGS

• Gross—may note paint chips or lead objects in gastrointestinal tract.
• Intranuclear inclusion bodies—may be noted in hepatocytes or renal tubular epithelial cells; intracellular storage form of lead; considered pathognomonic.
• Cerebrocortical lesions—spongiosis, vascular hypertrophy, gliosis, neuronal necrosis, demyelination.

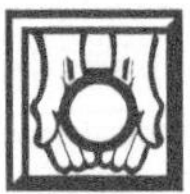

TREATMENT

APPROPRIATE HEALTH CARE

• Inpatient—first course of chelation, depending on severity of clinical signs.
• Outpatient—orally administered chelators.

NURSING CARE

• Balanced electrolyte fluids—Ringer's solution; replacement of hydration deficit.
• Gastric lavage or whole bowel irrigation—may be indicated.

ACTIVITY

N/A

DIET

N/A

CLIENT EDUCATION

• Inform client of the potential of adverse human health effects of lead. • Notify public health officials. • Determine the source of the lead.

SURGICAL CONSIDERATIONS

Removal of lead objects from the gastrointestinal tract.

MEDICATIONS

DRUG(S) OF CHOICE

• Evacuation of gastrointestinal tract—saline cathartics; sodium or magnesium sulfate (dogs 2–25 g; cats 2–5 g PO as 20% solution or less). • Control of seizures—diazepam (given to effect; dogs and cats 0.5 mg/kg IV) or phenobarbital sodium (administer in increments of 10–20 mg/kg IV to effect). • Alleviation of cerebral edema—mannitol (0.25–2 g/kg of 15–25% IV, slow infusion over 30–60 minutes) and dexamethasone (2.2–4.4 mg/kg IV).
• Some evidence that antioxidants or thiol-containing drugs may be useful—vitamins C and E, α-lipoic acid, *N*-acetylcysteine; optimal doses not determined. • B vitamins, especially thiamine, may also be useful; optimal doses not determined. • Reduction of lead body burden—chelation therapy: ○ $CaNa_2EDTA$ (dogs and cats, 25 mg/kg SC, IM, IV q6h for 2–5 days); dilute to a 1% solution with D_5W before administration; may need multiple treatment courses if blood lead concentration is high; allow 5-day rest period between treatment courses.
○ Succimer—alternative to $CaNa_2EDTA$; orally administered chelating agent; 10 mg/kg PO q8h for 5 days followed by 10 mg PO q12h for 2 weeks; allow 2-week rest period between treatments; may administer per rectum if clinical signs such as emesis preclude oral administration; cats successfully treated with 10 mg/kg PO q8h for 17 days. Advantages over other chelators: can be given PO, allowing for outpatient treatment; does not increase lead absorption from the gastrointestinal tract; not reported to be nephrotoxic; chelation of essential elements such as zinc and copper is not clinically significant.

CONTRAINDICATIONS

$CaNa_2EDTA$—do not administer to patients with renal impairment or anuria; establish urine flow before administration; do not administer orally.

PRECAUTIONS

• $CaNa_2EDTA$—safety in pregnancy not established; teratogenic at therapeutic doses although in human medicine is recommended over succimer for pregnant patients.
• Succimer—safety in pregnancy not established; fetotoxic at doses much higher (100–1000 mg/kg) than recommended therapeutic dose.

POSSIBLE INTERACTIONS

$CaNa_2EDTA$—depletion of zinc, iron, and manganese with long-term therapy.

ALTERNATIVE DRUG(S)

N/A

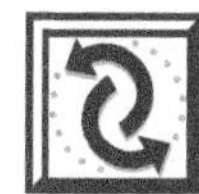

FOLLOW-UP

PATIENT MONITORING

Blood lead—should be <0.1 ppm; assess 10–14 days after cessation of chelation therapy.

PREVENTION/AVOIDANCE

• Test paint, dust, soil prior to animal access if likelihood of lead contamination.
• Determine source of lead and remove it from the patient's environment.

POSSIBLE COMPLICATIONS

Occasionally, permanent neurologic signs (e.g., blindness).

EXPECTED COURSE AND PROGNOSIS

• Signs should dramatically improve within 24–48 hours after initiating chelation therapy.
• Prognosis—favorable with treatment.
• Uncontrolled seizures—guarded prognosis.

MISCELLANEOUS

ASSOCIATED CONDITIONS

N/A

AGE-RELATED FACTORS

Dogs <1 year of age—more likely to be affected.

ZOONOTIC POTENTIAL

None; however, humans in the same environment may be at risk for exposure.

PREGNANCY/FERTILITY/BREEDING

• Transplacental passage—may cause neonatal poisoning.
• Lactation—lead mobilized from bones unlikely to poison nursing animals.

SYNONYMS

Plumbism

SEE ALSO

Poisoning (Intoxication) Therapy.

ABBREVIATIONS

• ALP = alkaline phosphatase.
• AST = aspartate aminotransferase.
• GFAAS = graphite furnace atomic absorption spectrometry
• ICP-MS = inductively coupled plasma mass spectrometry.
• NSAID = nonsteroidal anti-inflammatory drug.
• RBC = red blood cell.
• WBC = white blood cell

Suggested Reading

Braton R, Kowalczyk D. Lead poisoning. In: Kirk, R., ed. Current Veterinary Therapy X. Philadelphia, PA: Saunders, 1989, pp. 152–159.
Knight TE, Kent M, Junk JE. Succimer for treatment of lead toxicosis in two cats. J Am Vet Med Assoc 2001, 218:1946–1948.
Knight TE, Kumar MSA. Lead toxicosis in cats—a review. J Feline Med Surg 2003, 5(5):249–255.
Morgan RV. Lead poisoning in small companion animals: an update (1987–1992). Vet Hum Toxicol 1994, 36:18–22.
Morgan RV, Moore FM, Pearce LK, et al. Clinical and laboratory findings in small companion animals with lead poisoning: 347 cases (1977–1986). J Am Vet Med Assoc 1991, 199:93–97.
Morgan RV, Pearce LK, Moore FM, et al. Demographic data and treatment of small companion animals with lead poisoning: 347 cases (1977–1986). J Am Vet Med Assoc 1991, 199:98–102.
Ramsey DT, Casteel SW, Fagella AM, et al. Use of orally administered succimer (meso-2,3-dimercaptosuccinic acid) for treatment of lead poisoning in dogs. J Am Vet Med Assoc 1996, 208:371–375.
VanAlstine WG, Wickliffe LW, Everson RJ, et al. Acute lead toxicosis in a household of cats. J Vet Diagn Invest 1993, 5:496–498.

Author Robert H. Poppenga
Consulting Editor Lynn R. Hovda

LEFT ANTERIOR FASCICULAR BLOCK

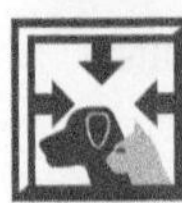

BASICS

DEFINITION

• Conduction delay or block in the anterior fascicle of the left bundle branch (Figures 1 and 2). • Left ventricle activation is altered or delayed toward the blocked fascicle and corresponding papillary muscle.
• Controversial terminology in veterinary cardiology because, in contrast to humans, dogs and cats do not appear to have an anatomic left anterior fascicle.

Electrocardiogram (ECG) Features

• QRS complex—normal duration. • Left axis deviation—dogs, <+40°; cats, <0°: ∘ Small q waves and tall R waves in leads I and aVL—small q not essential. • Deep S waves (exceeding the R waves) in leads II, III, and aVF.

PATHOPHYSIOLOGY

• Anatomic basis still speculative—anterior fascicle vulnerable because it has a single blood supply, is long and thin, and is located in the turbulent outflow tract of the left ventricle. • No hemodynamic compromise.

SYSTEMS AFFECTED

Cardiovascular

GENETICS

N/A

INCIDENCE/PREVALENCE

• Most commonly described form of bundle branch block in cats. • Uncommon in dogs.

GEOGRAPHIC DISTRIBUTION

N/A

SIGNALMENT

Species

Dog and cat.

Breed Predilections

N/A

Mean Age and Range

N/A

Predominant Sex

N/A

SIGNS

Historical Findings

• Signs usually associated with the underlying cause. • Usually an incidental ECG finding.

Physical Examination Findings

No associated signs or hemodynamic compromise.

CAUSES

• Hypertrophic cardiomyopathy (cats).
• Left ventricular hypertrophy (e.g., mitral insufficiency, aortic stenosis, aortic body tumor, hypertension, hyperthyroidism).
• Hyperkalemia (e.g., urethral obstruction, acute renal insufficiency, Addison's disease).
• Ischemic cardiomyopathy (e.g., arteriosclerosis of the coronary arteries, myocardial infarction, myocardial hypertrophy that obstructs coronary arteries). • Surgical repair of a cardiac defect (e.g., ventricular septal defect or aortic valvular disease).
• Restrictive cardiomyopathy (cats).
• Fibrosis. • Often noted in otherwise normal individuals.

RISK FACTORS

N/A

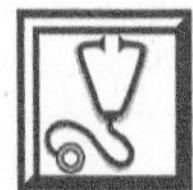

DIAGNOSIS

DIFFERENTIAL DIAGNOSIS

• Left ventricular enlargement—absence of left ventricular enlargement on thoracic radiograph or cardiac ultrasound supports a diagnosis of left anterior fascicular block.
• Right bundle branch block—deep, wide S waves in leads I, II, III, and aVF causing a right axis deviation; in patients with left anterior fascicular block, leads I and aVL are positive and leads II, III, and aVF have deep S waves resulting in a left axis deviation.
• Altered position of the heart within the thorax—thoracic radiographs help identify mass or foreign body that may be displacing the heart. • Suspect hyperkalemia if signs of urethral obstruction, renal insufficiency, or hypoadrenocorticism (Addison's disease); determine serum potassium concentration.

CBC/BIOCHEMISTRY/URINALYSIS

Hyperkalemia possible.

OTHER LABORATORY TESTS

N/A

IMAGING

• Echocardiogram may show structural heart disease. • Thoracic and abdominal radiographs may show mass, pulmonary metastatic lesion, foreign body, or abnormal cardiac position.

DIAGNOSTIC PROCEDURES

• Electrocardiography. • Long-term ambulatory monitoring (Holter) may reveal intermittent bundle branch block.

PATHOLOGIC FINDINGS

Possible lesions or scarring on endocardial surface in the path of the bundle branches; applying Lugol's iodine to the endocardial surface within 2 hours post mortem enables clear visualization of the conduction system.

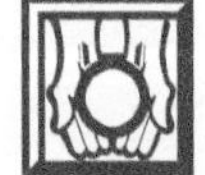

TREATMENT

APPROPRIATE HEALTH CARE

• Treatment unnecessary. • Treat underlying disease if present.

NURSING CARE

Unnecessary

ACTIVITY

Unrestricted unless indicated by underlying condition.

DIET

No modifications unless indicated by underlying condition.

CLIENT EDUCATION

Fascicular block per se does not cause hemodynamic compromise; combined with right bundle branch block it may develop into second- or third-degree AV block, making treatment essential; need to treat underlying cause if present.

SURGICAL CONSIDERATIONS

N/A

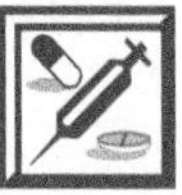

MEDICATIONS

DRUG(S) OF CHOICE

Treatment directed toward possible underlying primary disease (e.g., drugs to lower the serum potassium in hyperkalemia).

CONTRAINDICATIONS

N/A

PRECAUTIONS

N/A

POSSIBLE INTERACTIONS

N/A

FOLLOW-UP

PATIENT MONITORING

ECG regularly.

PREVENTION/AVOIDANCE

N/A

POSSIBLE COMPLICATIONS

Causative lesion could progress and lead to a more serious arrhythmia or complete heart block.

EXPECTED COURSE AND PROGNOSIS

No hemodynamic compromise.

MISCELLANEOUS

ASSOCIATED CONDITIONS

N/A

AGE-RELATED FACTORS

N/A

ZOONOTIC POTENTIAL

N/A

PREGNANCY/FERTILITY/BREEDING

N/A

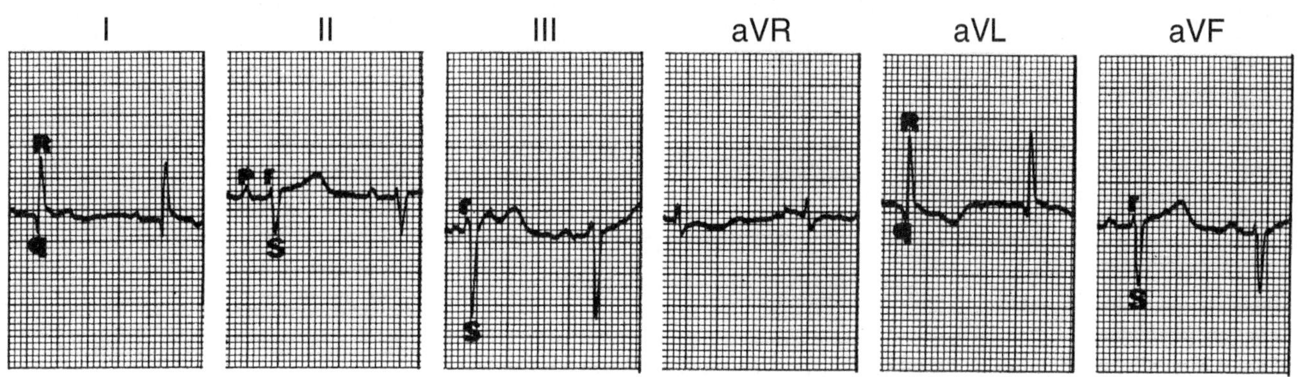

Figure 1.

Left anterior fascicular block in a dog with hyperkalemia (serum potassium, 5.3 mEq/L). There is abnormal left axis deviation (–60°) with a qR pattern in leads I and aVL and an rS pattern in leads II, III, and aVF. The large T waves are compatible with hyperkalemia. (Source: From Tilley LP. Essentials of Canine and Feline Electrocardiography, 3rd ed. Baltimore: Williams & Wilkins, 1992. Reprinted with permission of Wolters Kluwer.)

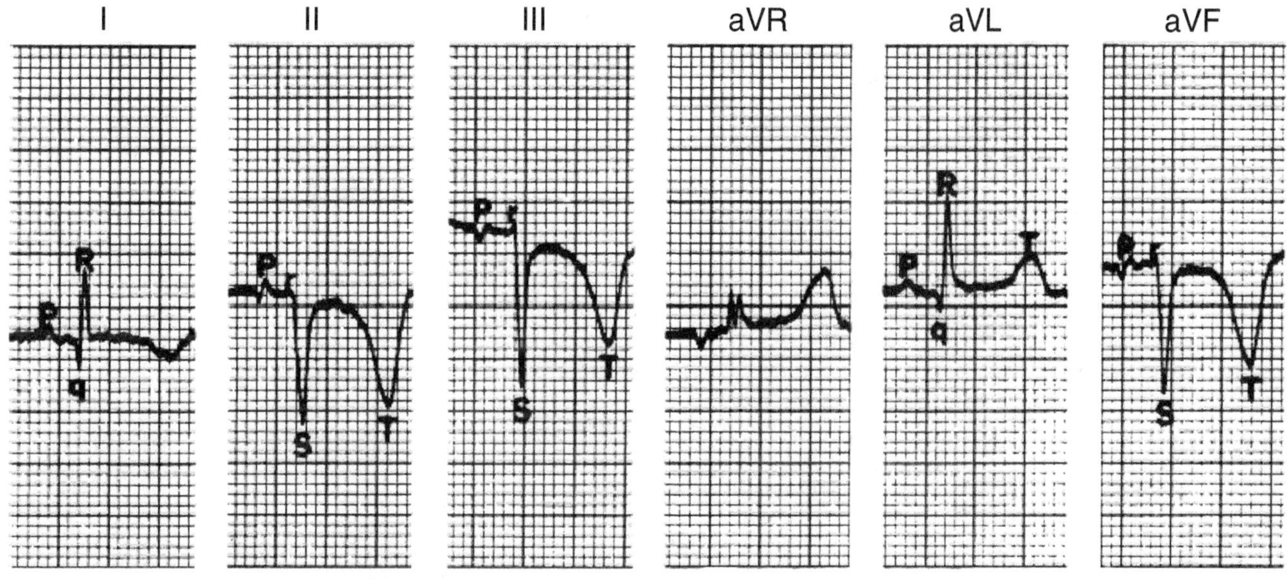

Figure 2.

Left anterior fascicular block in a cat with hypertrophic cardiomyopathy. Severe left axis deviation (–60°) with a qR pattern in leads I and aVL and an rS pattern in leads II, III, and aVF. The QRS complexes are of normal duration. (Source: From Tilley LP. Essentials of Canine and Feline Electrocardiography, 3rd ed. Baltimore: Williams & Wilkins, 1992. Reprinted with permission of Wolters Kluwer.)

SEE ALSO

- Atrioventricular Block, Complete (Third Degree).
- Atrioventricular Block, First Degree.
- Atrioventricular Block, Second Degree—Mobitz Type I.
- Atrioventricular Block, Second Degree—Mobitz Type II.
- Left Bundle Branch Block.
- Right Bundle Branch Block.

ABBREVIATIONS

- AV = atrioventricular.
- ECG = electrocardiogram.

Suggested Reading

Santilli R, Moise NS, Pariaut R, Perego M. Electrocardiography of the Dog and Cat: Diagnosis of Arrhythmias, 2nd ed. Milan, Italy: Edra S.P.A., 2018.

Tilley LP. Essentials of Canine and Feline Electrocardiography, Interpretation and Treatment, 3rd ed. Baltimore, MD: Williams and Wilkins, 1992.

Tilley LP, Smith FWK, Jr. Electrocardiography. In: Smith FWK, Tilley LP, Oyama M, Sleeper M, eds., Manual of Canine and Feline Cardiology, 5th ed. St. Louis, MO: Saunders Elsevier, 2016, pp. 49–76.

Willis R, Oliveira P., Mavropoulou A. Guide to Canine and Feline Electrocardiography. Ames, IA: Wiley-Blackwell, 2018.

Author Larry P. Tilley

Consulting Editor Michael Aherne

LEFT BUNDLE BRANCH BLOCK

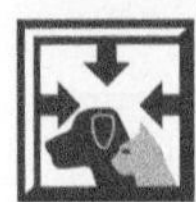

BASICS

DEFINITION

Conduction delay or block in both the left posterior and left anterior fascicles of the left bundle (Figures 1 and 2); a supraventricular impulse activates the right ventricle first through the right bundle branch; the left ventricle is activated late, causing the QRS to become wide and bizarre.

Electrocardiogram (ECG) Features

• QRS prolonged—dogs >0.08 seconds; cats >0.06 seconds. • QRS wide and positive in leads I, II, III, and aVF. • Block can be intermittent or constant.

PATHOPHYSIOLOGY

• Because the left bundle branch is thick and extensive, the lesion causing the block is often large. • Usually an incidental ECG finding—does not cause hemodynamic abnormalities.

SYSTEMS AFFECTED

Cardiovascular

GENETICS

N/A

INCIDENCE/PREVALENCE

Uncommon in cats and dogs. In cats with hypertrophic cardiomyopathy, left bundle branch block is not as commonly seen as left anterior fascicular block.

GEOGRAPHIC DISTRIBUTION

N/A

SIGNALMENT

Species

Dog and cat.

Breed Predilections

N/A

Mean Age and Range

N/A

Predominant Sex

N/A

SIGNS

Historical Findings

• Usually an incidental ECG finding—does not cause hemodynamic abnormalities.
• Signs may be associated with the underlying condition if present.

Physical Examination Findings

Does not cause signs or hemodynamic compromise.

CAUSES

• Cardiomyopathy. • Direct or indirect cardiac trauma (e.g., hit by car, cardiac needle puncture). • Neoplasia. • Subvalvular aortic stenosis. • Fibrosis. • Ischemic cardiomyopathy (e.g., arteriosclerosis of the coronary arteries, myocardial infarction, myocardial hypertrophy that obstructs coronary arteries).

RISK FACTORS

N/A

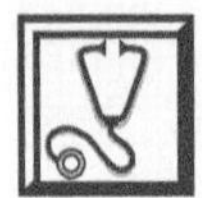

DIAGNOSIS

DIFFERENTIAL DIAGNOSIS

• Left ventricular enlargement.
• No left ventricular enlargement on thoracic radiograph or cardiac ultrasound studies supports diagnosis of isolated left bundle branch block. • Can also be confused with ventricular ectopic beats, but the PR interval is usually constant and left bundle branch block does not result in pulse deficits.

CBC/BIOCHEMISTRY/URINALYSIS

N/A

OTHER LABORATORY TESTS

N/A

IMAGING

• Echocardiography may reveal structural heart disease; absence of left heart enlargement supports a diagnosis of left bundle branch block. • Thoracic and abdominal radiographs may show masses or pulmonary metastatic lesions; traumatic injuries could result in localized or diffuse pulmonary densities.

DIAGNOSTIC PROCEDURES

• ECG. • Long-term ambulatory monitoring (Holter) may reveal intermittent left bundle branch block.

PATHOLOGIC FINDINGS

Possible lesions or scarring on endocardial surface in the path of the bundle branches; applying Lugol's iodine to the endocardial surface within 2 hours post mortem enables clear visualization of the conduction system.

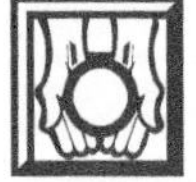

TREATMENT

APPROPRIATE HEALTH CARE

Directed toward the underlying cause if applicable.

NURSING CARE

Generally not necessary.

ACTIVITY

Unrestricted unless required for management of underlying condition.

DIET

No modifications unless required for management of underlying condition.

CLIENT EDUCATION

• Left bundle branch block per se does not cause hemodynamic abnormalities.
• Lesion causing the block could progress, leading to more serious arrhythmias or complete heart block.

SURGICAL CONSIDERATIONS

N/A

MEDICATIONS

DRUG(S) OF CHOICE

N/A (unless required for management of underlying condition).

CONTRAINDICATIONS

N/A

PRECAUTIONS

N/A

POSSIBLE INTERACTIONS

N/A

ALTERNATIVE DRUG(S)

N/A

FOLLOW-UP

PATIENT MONITORING

Serial ECG may show clearing or progression to complete heart block.

PREVENTION/AVOIDANCE

N/A

POSSIBLE COMPLICATIONS

• Causative lesion could progress, leading to a more serious arrhythmia or complete heart block. • First- or second-degree atrioventricular (AV) block may indicate involvement of the right bundle branch.

EXPECTED COURSE AND PROGNOSIS

No hemodynamic compromise.

MISCELLANEOUS

ASSOCIATED CONDITIONS

N/A

AGE-RELATED FACTORS

N/A

ZOONOTIC POTENTIAL

N/A

PREGNANCY/FERTILITY/BREEDING

N/A

SEE ALSO

• Atrioventricular Block, Complete (Third Degree).

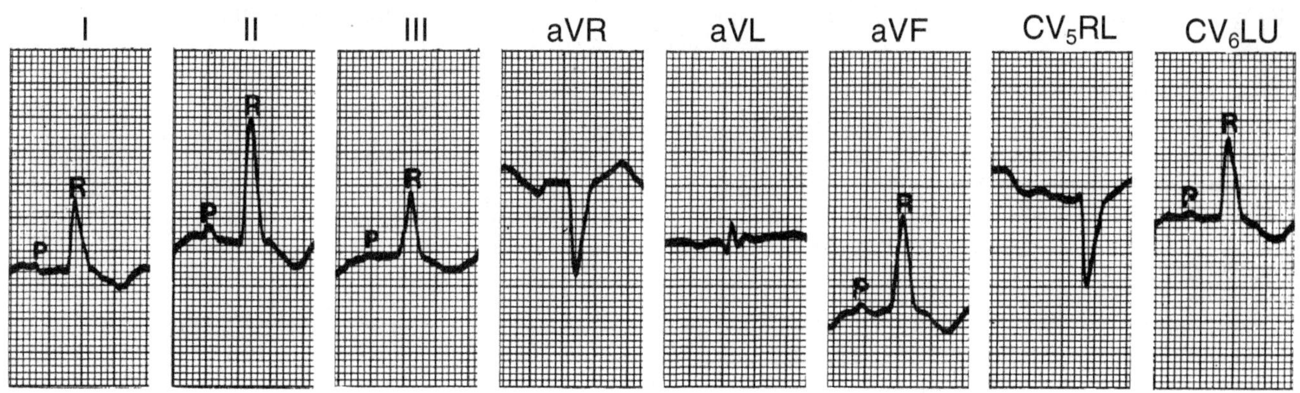

Figure 1.

Intermittent left bundle branch block in a Chihuahua. QRS complexes are wider (0.07–0.08 seconds) in the second, third, and fourth complexes and in the last three complexes. Consistent PR interval confirms a sinus origin for the abnormal-appearing QRS complexes (lead II, 50 mm/s, 1 cm = 1 mV). (Source: From Tilley LP. Essentials of Canine and Feline Electrocardiography, 3rd ed. Baltimore: Williams & Wilkins, 1992. Reprinted with permission of Wolters Kluwer.)

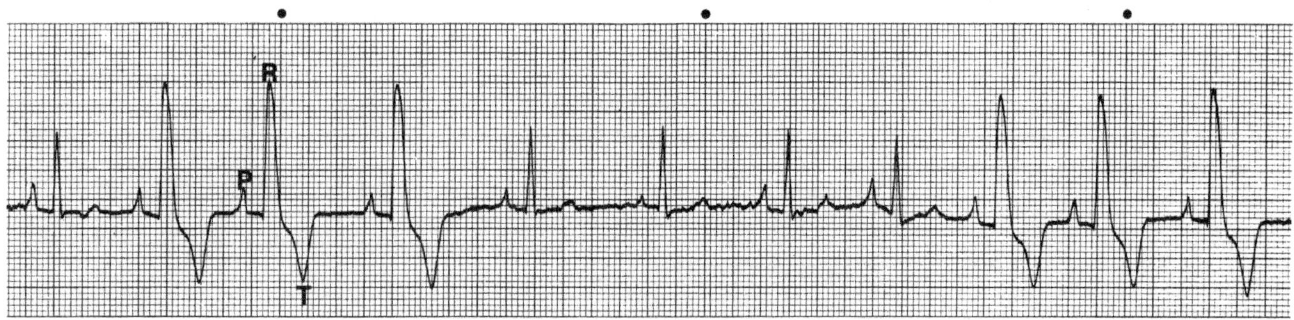

Figure 2.

Left bundle branch block in a cat with hypertrophic cardiomyopathy. The QRS complex is of 0.07-second duration and is positive in leads I, II, III, and aVF. Neither a Q wave nor an S wave occurs in these leads. The QRS complex is inverted in leads aVR. (Source: From Tilley LP. Essentials of Canine and Feline Electrocardiography, 3rd ed. Baltimore: Williams & Wilkins, 1992. Reprinted with permission of Wolters Kluwer.)

- Atrioventricular Block, First Degree.
- Atrioventricular Block, Second Degree—Mobitz Type I.
- Atrioventricular Block, Second Degree—Mobitz Type II.
- Left Anterior Fascicular Block.
- Right Bundle Branch Block.

ABBREVIATIONS

- AV = atrioventricular.
- ECG = electrocardiogram.

Suggested Reading

Santilli R, Moise NS, Pariaut R, Perego M. Electrocardiography of the Dog and Cat: Diagnosis of Arrhythmias, 2nd ed. Milan, Italy: Edra S.P.A., 2018.

Tilley LP. Essentials of Canine and Feline Electrocardiography, Interpretation and Treatment, 3rd ed. Baltimore, MD: Williams and Wilkins, 1992.

Tilley LP, Smith FWK, Jr. Electrocardiography. In: Smith FWK, Tilley LP, Oyama M, Sleeper M, eds., Manual of Canine and Feline Cardiology, 5th ed. St. Louis, MO: Saunders Elsevier, 2016, pp. 49–76.

Willis R, Oliveira P, Mavropoulou A. Guide to Canine and Feline Electrocardiography. Ames, IA: Wiley-Blackwell, 2018.

Author Larry P. Tilley

Consulting Editor Michael Aherne

LEGG-CALVÉ-PERTHES DISEASE

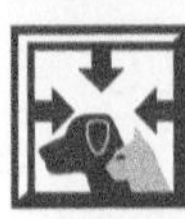

BASICS

DEFINITION

Spontaneous deterioration of the femoral head and neck, leading to an incongruent, malformed coxofemoral joint and secondary osteoarthritis.

PATHOPHYSIOLOGY

- Precise cause unknown; a specific vascular lesion not identified.
- Histologic evidence points to infarction of vessels supplying the proximal femur.
- Necrosis of subchondral bone leads to collapse of subchondral bone and deformation of the femoral head during normal loading.
- Articular cartilage becomes thickened, develops clefts, and undergoes superficial fraying.
- Simultaneous osseous degeneration and repair is characteristic of ischemia and revascularization of bone.
- No known association with hypercoagulability or other coagulopathy.

SYSTEMS AFFECTED

Musculoskeletal—causes a pelvic limb lameness; insidious in onset.

GENETICS

- Manchester terriers have multifactorial inheritance pattern with a high degree of heritability.
- Probable autosomal recessive inheritance in miniature poodles, West Highland white terriers, Yorkshire terriers, and pugs.
- Hereditary predisposition likely.

INCIDENCE/PREVALENCE

- Most common among adolescent dogs of miniature, toy, and small breeds.
- No accurate estimates available.

GEOGRAPHIC DISTRIBUTION

N/A

SIGNALMENT

Species

Dog

Breed Predilections

- Toy breeds and terriers are most susceptible.
- Manchester terriers, miniature pinschers, toy poodles, Lakeland terriers, West Highland white terriers, Yorkshire terriers, Cairn terriers, and pugs—higher than expected incidence.

Mean Age and Range

- Most patients are 5–8 months of age.
- Range 3–13 months.

Predominant Sex

None

SIGNS

General Comments

Usually unilateral; only 12–16% of cases are bilateral.

Historical Findings

Progressive pelvic limb lameness that is usually insidious in onset over 2–3 months; ranges from weight-bearing to non-weight-bearing lameness.

Physical Examination Findings

- Pain on manipulation of the hip—common.
- Atrophy of the thigh muscles—common.
- Decreased range of motion of hip—inconsistent.
- Crepitation of hip—inconsistent.
- Patient otherwise normal.

CAUSES

- Unknown.
- Tamponade of the epiphyseal intracapsular subsynovial vessels supplying the femoral head is suggested cause of ischemia leading to the pathologic changes.
- Other proposed causes include abnormal anatomic conformation, increased intracapsular pressure, hormonal influences, and hereditary factors.

RISK FACTORS

- Adolescent small, toy, and miniature breed dogs.
- Trauma to the hip region.

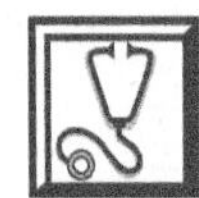

DIAGNOSIS

DIFFERENTIAL DIAGNOSIS

- Intracapsular hip trauma (e.g. femoral head or neck fracture).
- Severe hip dysplasia (but atypical breeds).
- Femoral head osteochondrosis.
- Infection and neoplasia considered less likely in patients with classic signalment, clinical findings, and radiographic lesions.
- Medial patellar luxation—differential for pelvic limb lameness in young toy breed dogs.
- Rupture of the cranial cruciate ligament—differential for pelvic limb lameness in older dogs.

CBC/BIOCHEMISTRY/URINALYSIS

N/A

OTHER LABORATORY TESTS

N/A

IMAGING

- Early radiographic changes—widening of the joint space; focal decreased or increased bone density of the epiphysis; sclerosis and thickening of the femoral neck.
- Later radiographic changes—lucent areas within the femoral head (apple-core or moth-eaten).
- End-stage radiographic changes—flattening and extreme deformation of the femoral head; severe osteoarthrosis; potential femoral neck fractures.
- Advanced imaging (computed tomography or magnetic resonance imaging) may be more sensitive than radiographs in early stages.

DIAGNOSTIC PROCEDURES

N/A

PATHOLOGIC FINDINGS

- Femoral head—removed during femoral head and neck excision (FHNE) or total hip replacement; usually deformed with a thickened, irregular articular surface.
- Early disease—histologically characterized by loss of lacunar osteocytes and necrosis of marrow elements; trabeculae surrounded by granulation tissue.
- Later disease—thickened metaphyseal trabeculae; mixture of necrosis and repair tissue typical of revascularization of bone.
- Advanced disease—osteoclastic activity; new bone formation.

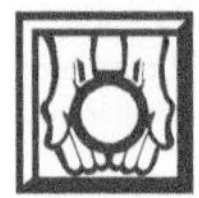

TREATMENT

APPROPRIATE HEALTH CARE

- Rest and analgesics—successful in alleviating lameness in less than 25% of patients.
- Ehmer sling—successful in one patient; maintained for 10 weeks; increased risk of ankylosis. Not widely recommended.
- Insidious onset often prevents early recognition and possibility of successful conservative treatment.
- FHNE with early and vigorous physical therapy after surgery—treatment of choice.
- Micro total hip replacement (THR) has been reported to successfully restore normal ground reaction forces.

NURSING CARE

Post Surgery

- Physical therapy—crucial for rehabilitating the affected limb.
- Analgesics, anti-inflammatory drugs, and cold packing—reduces pain and inflammation to increase limb use.
- Range-of-motion exercises initiated immediately—reduces risk of muscle contraction and limited range of motion.
- Small lead weights attached as ankle bracelets above the hock joint—encourages early use of the treated limb.

ACTIVITY

- Post surgery—early, low-impact activity encouraged to improve leg use.
- Conservative therapy—restricted activity recommended.

DIET

Avoid obesity.

CLIENT EDUCATION

- Warn owners of potential genetic basis of the disease in Manchester terriers, miniature poodles, Yorkshire terriers, West Highland white terriers, and pugs; discourage breeding affected dogs.

• Warn client that recovery after FHNE may take 3–6 months and requires early and vigorous physical therapy.

SURGICAL CONSIDERATIONS

FHNE or micro THR—treatment of choice.

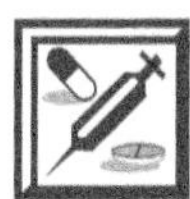

MEDICATIONS

DRUG(S) OF CHOICE

Nonsteroidal anti-inflammatory drugs (NSAIDs)—preoperative or postoperative; minimize joint pain; reduce synovitis; reduce soft tissue pain and inflammation to encourage postsurgery limb use:

• Carprofen 2.2 mg/kg PO q12h or 4.4 mg/kg PO q24h.
• Deracoxib 1–2 mg/kg PO q24h, chewable.
• Etodolac 10–15 mg/kg PO q24h.
• Firocoxib 5 mg/kg PO q24h.
• Grapiprant 2 mg/kg PO q24h, to animals >3.6 kg.
• Meloxicam—load 0.2 mg/kg PO, then 0.1 mg/kg PO q24h—liquid.
• Tepoxalin—load 20 mg/kg, then 10 mg/kg PO q24h.

CONTRAINDICATIONS

NSAIDs—gastrointestinal disease, liver disease, or renal disease may preclude use in some patients.

PRECAUTIONS

NSAIDs—can cause gastrointestinal tract ulceration, hepatotoxicity, or nephrotoxicity; inhibition of platelet activity may increase hemorrhage at surgery; discontinue aspirin for at least 1 week before surgery, if possible.

POSSIBLE INTERACTIONS

NSAIDs—do not use in conjunction with glucocorticoids; risk of gastrointestinal tract ulceration; consider appropriate wash-out times when switching from one NSAID to another.

ALTERNATIVE DRUG(S)

Chondroprotective drugs (e.g., polysulfated glycosaminoglycans, glucosamine, and chondroitin sulfate)—minimal benefit in advanced disease; no evidence to suggest that these drugs prevent or reverse the disease process.

FOLLOW-UP

PATIENT MONITORING

• Postsurgical progress checks—1- to 2-week intervals depending on progress with limb use; ensure compliance with exercise recommendations.
• Conservative therapy—reevaluate after 4–6 weeks of strict rest (physical examination, radiographs) to determine if surgery is needed.

PREVENTION/AVOIDANCE

• Discourage breeding of affected animals.
• Do not repeat dam–sire breeding that resulted in affected offspring.

POSSIBLE COMPLICATIONS

Noncompliance with postsurgical physical therapy exercises may result in less than optimal limb function.

EXPECTED COURSE AND PROGNOSIS

• FHNE—good to excellent prognosis for full recovery (84–100% success rate).
• Micro THR—excellent prognosis for full recovery.
• Conservative therapy—reported to alleviate lameness after 2–3 months in less than 25% of patients.

MISCELLANEOUS

ASSOCIATED CONDITIONS

N/A

AGE-RELATED FACTORS

Usually affects juvenile small-breed dogs, but mature dogs may be affected by chronic disease.

ZOONOTIC POTENTIAL

N/A

PREGNANCY/FERTILITY/BREEDING

N/A

SYNONYMS

• Aseptic necrosis of the femoral head.
• Avascular necrosis of the femoral head.
• Coxa magna.
• Coxa plana.
• Osteochondritis juvenilis.
• Perthes disease.

SEE ALSO

• Cruciate Ligament Disease, Cranial.
• Hip Dysplasia.
• Osteochondrosis.
• Patellar Luxation.

ABBREVIATIONS

• FHNE = femoral head and neck excision.
• NSAID = nonsteroidal anti-inflammatory drug.
• THR = total hip replacement.

Suggested Reading

Bowlus R, Armbrust L, Biller D. Magnetic resonance imaging of the femoral head of normal dogs and dogs with avascular necrosis. Vet Radiol Ultrasound 2008, 49:7–12.

Brenig B, Leeb T, Jansen S, Kopp T. Analysis of blood clotting factor activities in canine Legg-Calvé-Perthes disease. J Vet Intern Med 1999, 13:570–573.

Gambardella PC. Legg-Calvé-Perthes disease in dogs. In: Bojrab MJ, ed., Disease Mechanisms in Small Animal Surgery, 2nd ed. Philadelphia, PA: Saunders, 1993, pp. 804–807.

Gibson KL, Lewis DD, Perchman RD. Use of external coaptation for the treatment of avascular necrosis of the femoral head in a dog. J Am Vet Med Assoc 1990, 197:868–869.

Jankovits D, Liska W, Kalis R. Treatment of avascular necrosis of the femoral head in small dogs with micro total hip replacement. Vet Surg 2012, 41(1):143–147.

LaFond E, Breur GJ, Austin CC. Breed susceptibility for developmental orthopedic diseases in dogs. J Am Anim Hosp Assoc 2002, 38:467–477.

Peycke L. Femoral head and neck ostectomy. NAVC Clinician's Brief 2011, 9(2):55–59.

Piek CJ, Hazewinkel HAW, Wolvekamp WTC, et al. Long term follow-up of avascular necrosis of the femoral head in the dog. J Small Anim Pract 1996, 37:12–18.

Piermattei DL, Flo GL, DeCamp CE. Hip joint. In: Handbook of Small Animal Orthopedics and Fracture Repair, 4th ed. Philadelphia, PA: Saunders, 2006, pp. 507–508.

Towle-Millard HA, Breur GJ. Miscellaneous orthopedic conditions. In: Veterinary Surgery Small Animal, 2nd ed., Vol. 1. St. Louis, MO: Elsevier Saunders, 2018, pp. 1309.

Trostel CT, Pool RR, McLaughlin RM. Canine lameness caused by developmental orthopedic diseases: panosteitis, Legg-Calvé-Perthes disease, and hypertophic osteodystrophy. Compend Contin Educ Pract Vet 2003, 25(4):282–292.

Author Laura A. Barbur

Consulting Editor Mathieu M. Glassman

Acknowledgment The author and editors acknowledge the prior contribution of Larry Carpenter.

Client Education Handout available online

L

LEIOMYOMA, STOMACH, SMALL AND LARGE INTESTINE

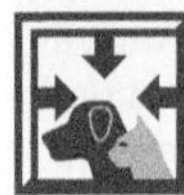

BASICS

OVERVIEW

Uncommon benign tumor arising from the smooth muscle of the stomach and intestinal tract; with immunohistochemistry these tumors may be reclassified as a gastrointestinal stromal tumor (GIST) or GIST-like.

SIGNALMENT

- Dog more commonly affected than cat.
- Middle-aged to older (>6 years) dogs and cats.
- No breed predisposition.

SIGNS

Historical Findings

- Relate to location in the gastrointestinal tract.
- Stomach—vomiting.
- Small intestine—vomiting; weight loss; borborygmus; flatulence.
- Large intestine and rectum—tenesmus; hematochezia; sometimes rectal prolapse.

Physical Examination Findings

- Stomach—no specific abnormalities; may have melena on rectal exam.
- Small intestine—often no abnormal findings; may feel mid-abdominal mass; occasionally distended, painful loops of small bowel; possible melena on rectal exam.
- Large intestine and rectum—may feel palpable mass per rectum; may have bright red blood on rectal exam.

CAUSES & RISK FACTORS

Unknown

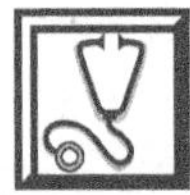

DIAGNOSIS

DIFFERENTIAL DIAGNOSIS

- Foreign body.
- Inflammatory bowel disease.
- Adenocarcinoma.
- Leiomyosarcoma.
- GIST.
- GIST-like.
- Lymphoma.
- Pancreatitis.

CBC/BIOCHEMISTRY/URINALYSIS

- Usually normal.
- Hypoglycemia—occasionally associated with paraneoplastic syndrome.
- Stomach and small intestine—may see microcytic hypochromic anemia (iron-deficiency anemia).

OTHER LABORATORY TESTS

N/A

IMAGING

- Abdominal ultrasonography—may reveal a thickened wall of stomach or bowel; gastric leiomyoma most common at esophageal–gastric junction.
- Contrast radiography (stomach and small intestine)—may reveal a space-occupying mass.
- Double-contrast radiography (large intestine and rectum)—reveals a space-occupying mass.
- Contrast-enhanced CT—highest details of gastrointestinal tract and abdominal lymph node visualization.

DIAGNOSTIC PROCEDURES

Fine-Needle Aspirates

If mass or thickening seen with ultrasound, fine-needle aspirate (FNA) with cytology may be performed to rule out other differentials; for leiomyomas cytology is generally low yield.

Upper Gastrointestinal Tract

Perform upper gastrointestinal tract endoscopy and mucosal biopsy; however, this is frequently nondiagnostic because tumors are deep to the mucosal surface or distal to scope length. Therefore surgical biopsy often required to confirm the diagnosis.

Large Intestine and Rectum

Colonoscopy may reveal a mass; mucosal biopsy may be nondiagnostic because of normal mucosal covering of the tumor; surgical biopsy often required. If mass can be palpated per rectum, transrectal biopsies may be obtained.

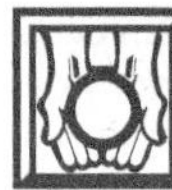

TREATMENT

- Surgical resection—treatment of choice; curative if tumor is resectable.
- Even large leiomyomas often can be removed successfully and cured with narrow margins.

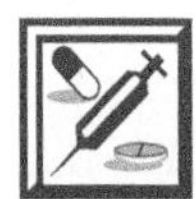

MEDICATIONS

DRUG(S) OF CHOICE

If reclassified as a GIST (c-KIT-positive), may consider a tyrosine kinase inhibitor (toceranib phosphate) as follow-up therapy.

CONTRAINDICATIONS/POSSIBLE INTERACTIONS

N/A

FOLLOW-UP

- Complete resection—normal postoperative care; no additional follow-up necessary.
- Monitor blood glucose postoperatively if hypoglycemic prior to surgery.

MISCELLANEOUS

ASSOCIATED CONDITIONS

Hypoglycemia—recognized as an associated paraneoplastic syndrome.

ABBREVIATIONS

- FNA = fine-needle aspirate.
- GIST = gastrointestinal stromal tumor.

Suggested Reading

Frost D, Lasota J, Miettinen M. Gastrointestinal stromal tumors and leiomyomas in the dog: a histopathologic, immunohistochemical, and molecular genetic study of 50 cases. Vet Pathol 2003, 40:42–54.

Gillespie V, Baer K, Farrelly J, et al. Canine gastrointestinal stromal tumors: immunohistochemical expression of CD34 and examination of prognostic indicators including proliferation markers Ki67 and AgNOR. Vet Pathol 2011, 48:283–291.

Maas CP, ter Haar G, Van Der Gaag I, et al. Reclassification of small intestinal and cecal smooth muscle tumors in 72 dogs: clinical, histologic, and immunohistochemical evaluation. Vet Surg 2007, 36:302–313.

McPherron MA, Withrow SJ, Seim HB, Powers BE. Colorectal leiomyoma in seven dogs. J Am Anim Hosp Assoc 1992, 28:43–46.

Tanaka T, Akiyoshi H, Mie K, et al. Contrast-enhanced computed tomography may be helpful for characterizing and staging canine gastric tumors. Vet Radiol Ultrasound 2019, 60(1):7–18.

Author Laura D. Garrett

Consulting Editor Timothy M. Fan

LEIOMYOSARCOMA, STOMACH, SMALL AND LARGE INTESTINE

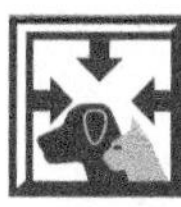

BASICS

OVERVIEW

- Uncommon malignant tumor arising from smooth muscle of stomach or intestines.
- Locally invasive; metastatic rate up to 50%, usually intra-abdominal sites, especially lymph nodes and liver.
- Prognosis fair to guarded.
- In large intestine the cecum is often affected.
- Analyses reclassified many leiomyosarcomas to gastrointestinal stromal tumors (GISTs) or GIST-like tumors; differentiate with immunohistochemistry.
- True leiomyosarcomas (LMS) rare; this chapter discusses GISTs with LMS.

SIGNALMENT

- Dog more commonly affected than cat.
- Mostly middle-aged to older (>6 years).
- No breed predisposition.

SIGNS

Historical Findings

- Relate to GI tract.
- Stomach—vomiting; weight loss.
- Small intestine—vomiting; weight loss; diarrhea; borborygmus; flatulence.
- Large intestine and rectum—tenesmus, may lead to rectal prolapse; hematochezia.

Physical Examination Findings

- Stomach—nonspecific.
- Small intestine—may feel mid-abdominal mass; sometimes distended, painful loops of small bowel.
- Large intestine and rectum—may feel mass per rectum.

CAUSES & RISK FACTORS

Unknown

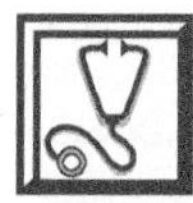

DIAGNOSIS

DIFFERENTIAL DIAGNOSIS

- Foreign body.
- Inflammatory bowel disease.
- Adenocarcinoma.
- Leiomyoma.
- GIST.
- GIST-like.
- Lymphoma.
- Pancreatitis.

CBC/BIOCHEMISTRY/URINALYSIS

- Usually normal.
- Anemia—may be hypochromic, microcytic (iron-deficiency anemia).
- Leukocytosis.
- Hypoglycemia— paraneoplastic syndrome.

IMAGING

- Abdominal ultrasonography—may reveal mass or mural thickening:
  - GISTs more likely to have abdominal effusion.
  - Contrast-enhanced CT—highest detail for GI tract and abdominal lymph node visualization.

DIAGNOSTIC PROCEDURES

Fine-Needle Aspirates (FNA)

- FNA and cytology of mass or GI thickening may show malignant mesenchymal cells supportive of sarcoma.
- FNA and cytology of intra-abdominal lymph nodes important for metastasis evaluation.

Upper Gastrointestinal Tract

- Endoscopy and mucosal biopsy—often nondiagnostic as tumors are deep to the mucosal surface; mass may be beyond reach of endoscope.
- Surgical biopsy—often required to confirm diagnosis.

Large Intestine and Rectum

- Colonoscopy—may allow a mass to be seen; mucosal biopsy may be nondiagnostic due to normal mucosa covering the tumor.
- Deep biopsy—perform if possible.

Immunohistochemistry on Biopsy

- Perform to differentiate LMS from GIST.
- c-KIT-positive; DOG1 is sensitive and specific marker.

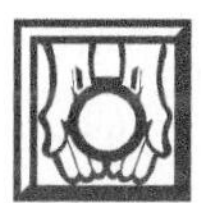

TREATMENT

- Surgical resection—treatment of choice.
- Evaluate for metastasis prior to surgery (e.g., mesenteric lymph nodes, liver, lungs).

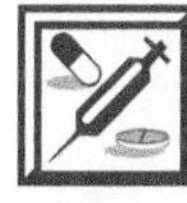

MEDICATIONS

DRUG(S) OF CHOICE

- If reclassified as a GIST (c-KIT-positive), consider a tyrosine kinase inhibitor (toceranib phosphate) as follow-up therapy:
  - 5/7 dogs with gross disease had clinical benefit (3 complete response, 1 partial response, 1 stable disease); median progression-free survival = 110 weeks.

FOLLOW-UP

EXPECTED COURSE AND PROGNOSIS

- LMS often metastasize to liver and regional lymph nodes.
- Older case series:
  - Small intestine: median survival time (MST) 12 months.
  - Cecum: MST 7.5 months, but most died of other diseases.
  - Gastric: rare, high rate of metastasis, short survival.
- Even dogs with metastasis can have prolonged survivals; MST 21.7 months in one study of dogs with metastatic LMS.
- One report showed similar survival times between dogs with leiomyoma, LMS, GIST, and GIST-like tumors:
  - 42 dogs, small intestinal tumors treated surgically: 1- and 2-year survivals of 62.6% and 52.3%.
  - 19 dogs, cecal tumors treated surgically: 1- and 2-year survivals of 84.2% and 66%.
- Mitotic index <9 and histological grade were prognostic for survival in abdominal visceral soft tissue sarcomas (mostly spleen and small intestine).

L

MISCELLANEOUS

ASSOCIATED CONDITIONS

Hypoglycemia—reported as paraneoplastic syndrome.

ABBREVIATIONS

- FNA = fine-needle aspirate.
- GIST = gastrointestinal stromal tumor.
- LMS = leiomyosarcomas.
- MST = median survival time.

Suggested Reading

Berger EP, Johannes CM, Jergens AE, et al. Retrospective evaluation of toceranib phosphate (Palladia®) use in the treatment of gastrointestinal stromal tumors of dogs. J Vet Intern Med 2018, 32(6):2045–2053.

Gillespie V, Baer K, Farrelly J, et al. Canine gastrointestinal stromal tumors: immunohistochemical expression of CD34 and examination of prognostic indicators including proliferation markers Ki67 and AgNOR. Vet Pathol 2011, 48:283–291.

Hobbs J, Sutherland-Smith J, Penninck D, et al. Ultrasonographic features of canine gastrointestinal stromal tumors compared to other gastrointestinal spindle cell tumors. Vet Radiol Ultrasound 2015, 56(4):432–438.

Maas CP, ter Haar G, Van Der Gaag I, et al. Reclassification of small intestinal and cecal smooth muscle tumors in 72 dogs: clinical, histologic, and immunohistochemical evaluation. Vet Surg 2007, 36:302–313.

Author Laura D. Garrett

Consulting Editor Timothy M. Fan

LEISHMANIOSIS

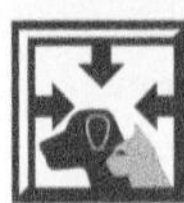

BASICS

OVERVIEW

• Primary species infecting dogs and cats is protozoan *Leishmania infantum* which is endemic in Mediterranean basin countries, the Middle East, Central Asia, China, and South and Central America. • Dogs in the United States may acquire infection in another country, or part of endemic foxhound population (vertical transmission). • Sand fly vectors transmit flagellated parasites (promastigotes) to skin of host. Other modes of transmission include vertical, venereal, and blood transfusion. • Dogs and cats—clinical manifestations range from subclinical to severe; main systems affected: lymphoid organs, skin, eyes, kidneys, liver; renal failure is most common cause of death.

L

SIGNALMENT

• Dogs—purebred dogs (except Ibizan hounds) more susceptible; no sex or age predilection. • Cats—no breed, sex, or age predilection.

SIGNS

• Similar in dogs and cats. • Lymphadenomegaly. • Nonpruritic, exfoliative, erosive–ulcerative, nodular, papular, or pustular dermal and mucocutaneous lesions. • Blepharitis, conjunctivitis, keratoconjunctivitis, uveitis. • Polyuria, polydipsia. • Hyporexia, weight loss, vomiting, diarrhea, melena. • Splenomegaly, hepatomegaly. • Lameness. • Epistaxis. • Fever (rare).

CAUSES & RISK FACTORS

• Travel to or acquisition from endemic regions. • Coinfections (e.g., *E. canis*, retroviruses), immunosuppression, or malnutrition predispose.

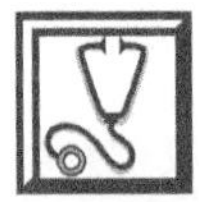

DIAGNOSIS

DIFFERENTIAL DIAGNOSIS

• Scaling and alopecia—infectious (bacterial, parasitic, fungal) or immune-mediated disease (lupus). • Renal disease—infection (pyelonephritis, Lyme nephritis), other glomerulonephropathy.

CBC/BIOCHEMISTRY/URINALYSIS

• Hyperproteinemia, hypergammaglobulinemia (polyclonal). • Hypoalbuminemia. • Nonregenerative normocytic normochromic anemia. • Proteinuria—quantitate with urine protein/creatinine ratio. • Leukocytosis or leukopenia with lymphopenia. • Increased hepatocellular enzyme activities. • Renal azotemia. • Thrombocytopenia.

OTHER LABORATORY TESTS

• Protein electrophoresis—differentiate polyclonal from monoclonal gammopathy. • Serologic diagnosis (IFA or ELISA)—most cross-react to *Trypanosoma cruzi*; differentiate based on clinical signs, history, and likelihood of exposure. In-house immunochromatographic tests available. • PCR—sensitive with aspirates of bone marrow, lymph nodes, spleen, skin; blood is less sensitive.

DIAGNOSTIC PROCEDURES

Fine-needle aspirates or biopsy of relevant tissues.

PATHOLOGIC FINDINGS

• Granulomatous, suppurative, or pyogranulomatous inflammation, lymphoplasmacellular inflammation in skin and hemolymphoid tissues. Reactive hyperplasia in lymphoid organs. • Visualization of amastigotes confirms diagnosis. Absence of amastigotes does not rule out. • Mucosal ulcerations—nasal, oral, gastrointestinal tract.

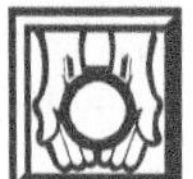

TREATMENT

• Medical management of infection. • Follow IRIS Guidelines for treatment of renal disease (see Internet Resources). • Diet—high-quality protein; renal diet as indicated.

MEDICATIONS

DRUG(S) OF CHOICE

• Dogs—meglumine antimoniate (100 mg/kg SC q24h or 50–75 mg/kg SC q12h for 1 month) or miltefosine (2 mg/kg PO q24h for 1 month). Best in combination with long-term allopurinol (10 mg/kg PO q12h for 12–24 months). Allopurinol may also be used alone. • Cats—allopurinol (10 mg/kg PO q12–24h) as monotherapy. Short-term meglumine antimoniate (20–50 mg/kg SC q24h) plus allopurinol is optional.

FOLLOW-UP

PATIENT MONITORING

• Monitor clinical signs, laboratory abnormalities, and antibody levels (quantitative serology) at day 30, 90, 180 and then every 6 months. • Relapses (rise in antibody or globulin concentrations and/or reappearance of clinical signs, laboratory abnormalities) may occur months to years after therapy or during therapy if drug resistance develops; recheck at least every 2 months after treatment completion. Drug resistance reported for allopurinol. • Monitor for urolithiasis and renal mineralization in dogs on long-term allopurinol.

PREVENTION/AVOIDANCE

• Topical pyrethroid-based repellents. • Canine vaccines available in Europe, parts of South America; reduces incidence of clinical disease but not subclinical infection.

EXPECTED COURSE AND PROGNOSIS

• Good (lymphadenomegaly, skin lesions) to poor (severe renal insufficiency) outcome, defined by clinical stage (LeishVet system outlines four stages). • Death usually from end-stage glomerulonephritis, nephrotic syndrome, and/or hypertension. • Infection may not be completely eliminated; in long-term treatment, monitoring required to prevent relapses.

MISCELLANEOUS

ZOONOTIC POTENTIAL

• Advise client of risk via exposure to sand flies in endemic areas. • Leishmaniosis is reportable in the United States and some other countries.

ABBREVIATIONS

• IFA = immunofluorescence antibody assay.

INTERNET RESOURCES

• LeishVet Staging: http://www.leishvet.org/fact-sheet/clinical-staging/• IRIS Guidelines: http://www.iris-kidney.com/guidelines/

Suggested Reading

Pennisi MG, Cardoso L, Baneth G, et al. LeishVet update and recommendations on feline leishmaniosis. Parasit Vectors 2015, 8:302.

Solano-Gallego L, Miró G, Koutinas A, et al. LeishVet guidelines for the practical management of canine leishmaniosis. Parasit. Vectors 2011, 4:86.

Authors Laia Solano-Gallego and Gad Baneth

Consulting Editor Amie Koenig

Acknowledgment The authors and editors acknowledge the prior contribution of Stephen C. Barr.

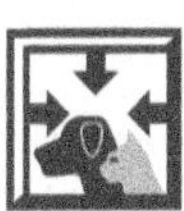

BASICS

DEFINITION

Leishmaniosis is a group of infectious diseases occurring throughout the Mediterranean region, the Middle East, parts of Asia, and Central and South America. It is caused by parasitic protozoa of the genus *Leishmania*, and *Leishmania infantum* is the most common cause of disease in the dog. It occurs infrequently in the cat.

PATHOPHYSIOLOGY

Infection is transmitted by the bite of female sand flies of the genus *Phlebotomus* in Europe and *Lutzomia* in the New World. Nonvectorial transmission modalities have been demonstrated (venereal, vertical, dog-to-dog, blood transfusion), but are much less common. Following inoculation of a small number of promastigotes into the dermis, the innate immune response (complement, neutrophils, macrophages) and then the adaptive response (T-cell-mediated) attempt to control the infection. A high percentage of dogs develop an effective T helper-1 response, resulting in subclinical infection and becoming seronegative or developing a low anti-*Leishmania* antibody titer. A smaller group of dogs develop a predominantly T helper-2 response, have elevated antibody titers (immunoglobulin G [IgGs]), and allow the progression of the infection causing lesions and clinical signs. Active infection causes lesions by different mechanisms, including an acute inflammatory response (fever, lethargy, asthenia) and granulomatous inflammatory lesions, by generating immunocomplexes that are deposited in different organs causing inflammation and tissue damage (glomerulonephritis, arthritis, uveitis).

SYSTEMS AFFECTED

Infection with *Leishmania infantum* (CanL) is considered systemic. Rarely (papulonodular cutaneous form), the infection is exclusively cutaneous. From the dermis, infection first spreads to the hematopoietic organs (bone marrow, lymph nodes, spleen) and then systemically. The spread of infection and the involvement of numerous organs and systems explains the clinical pleomorphism of the disease.

GENETICS

Several haplotypes, possibly associated with tendency to develop a T helper-2 response, are associated with increased susceptibility to the development of the disease. Some breeds, including German shepherd dog, boxer, Rottweiler, Alaskan Malamutes, appear to be susceptible. Conversely, some autochthonous Mediterranean breeds (e.g., Ibizian hound) respond with an effective cellular response and very rarely develop clinical signs.

INCIDENCE/PREVALENCE

In areas where CanL is endemic, the prevalence of infection is very high (over 50%) with seroprevalences ranging between 5% and 30%. However, less than 5% of dogs develop clinical signs. Isolated cases have been observed in non-endemic areas (Northern Europe, United States), most often in dogs that have visited areas where the disease is endemic.

GEOGRAPHIC DISTRIBUTION

Found in Mediterranean countries, Portugal, the Middle East, Central and South Asia, and Central and South America. Vertical transmission of CanL has been seen in hunting foxhounds in the United States.

SIGNALMENT

No breed or age predisposition.

SIGNS

Historical Findings

- Loss of body weight.
- Decreased or increased appetite.
- Lethargy.
- Polyuria/polydipsia.
- Vomiting.
- Diarrhea.

Physical Examination Findings

- Generalized lymphadenomegaly.
- Skin lesions:
  - Nonpruritic dermatitis.
  - Generalized exfoliative dermatitis with or without alopecia.
  - Erosive–ulcerative dermatitis (planum nasale, distal legs, paw pads).
  - Nodular dermatitis.
  - Pustular dermatitis.
  - Papular dermatitis (ventral pinnae, nose, abdomen).
- Onychogryphosis.
- Lethargy.
- Muscle atrophy.
- Mucous membranes pallor.
- Fever.
- Splenomegaly.
- Epistaxis.
- Arthritis/articular pain/lameness.
- Ocular lesions: keratoconjunctivitis, blepharitis, and uveitis.

CAUSES

Leishmania infantum (syn. *L. chagasi*) zymodeme MON1 is a protozoan parasite with two structural variants: the amastigote form found in mononuclear phagocytes within the mammalian host and the infective flagellated promastigote form found in the sand fly.

RISK FACTORS

Living in an endemic area and outdoors lifestyle. Immunosuppression can trigger disease progression in a previously infected dog.

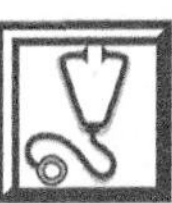

DIAGNOSIS

DIFFERENTIAL DIAGNOSIS

Any cause of cutaneous granulomatous disease with or without systemic symptoms. Leishmaniosis is considered one of the great imitators.

CBC/BIOCHEMISTRY/URINALYSIS

- Mild to moderate nonregenerative anemia.
- Leukocytosis or leukopenia—lymphopenia, neutrophilia, neutropenia.
- Thrombocytopathy.
- Thrombocytopenia.
- Impaired secondary hemostasis and fibrinolysis.
- Hyperproteinemia.
- Hyperglobulinemia (polyclonal beta- and/or gammaglobulinemia).
- Hypoalbuminemia.
- Decreased albumin/globulin ratio.
- Proteinuria.
- Renal azotemia.
- Elevated liver enzymes.

OTHER LABORATORY TESTS

Cytology—finding *Leishmania* amastigotes in lymph node or bone marrow smears is considered diagnostic with low sensitivity. Serum anti-*Leishmania* antibodies by immunofluorescence antibody test (IFAT) or ELISA. Main diagnostic test—dogs with clinical CanL usually have high antibody titers (>1:80 in IFAT). Biopsies (skin, lymph node) are recommended with low or borderline titers for histopathology and detection of *Leishmania* in the tissue with immunohistochemistry or PCR. Positive PCR for *Leishmania* DNA in sample of bone marrow, lymph node, or ocular conjunctiva is not definitive proof that clinical signs are the consequence of *Leishmania* infection.

IMAGING

Abdominal ultrasonography—splenomegaly.

DIAGNOSTIC PROCEDURES

N/A

PATHOLOGIC FINDINGS

Granulomatous inflammation in tissues (nodular to diffuse dermatitis, granulomatous colitis, granulomatous nephritis).

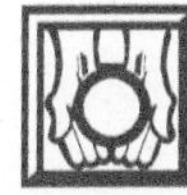

TREATMENT

APPROPRIATE HEALTH CARE

Outpatient medical management except in cases with severe organ involvement.

ACTIVITY

N/A

LEISHMANIOSIS, CUTANEOUS (CONTINUED)

DIET

During treatment with allopurinol, a low-purine diet is recommended to avoid xanthinuria and urolithiasis.

CLIENT EDUCATION

Treatment does not completely eliminate infection despite the clinical improvement. Dogs remain infected life-long. Regular examinations for early detection of disease relapses needed. Application of topical insecticides (pyrethroids) are necessary to minimize the risk of transmission to other animals.

SURGICAL CONSIDERATIONS

N/A

MEDICATIONS

DRUG(S) OF CHOICE

Meglumine antimoniate 100 mg/kg SC q24h for 4–6 weeks with allopurinol 10 mg/kg PO q12h for at least 6 months. Miltefosine 2 mg/kg PO q24h (with allopurinol) instead of meglumine antimoniate: This combination appears to be less effective. The use of immunostimulants (domperidone, nucleotides) may reduce the risk of disease relapses. Treatment with allopurinol and an immunostimulant (domperidone or nucleotides) alone effective in cases of mild or moderate disease, but it is generally not effective (not recommended) in severe cases.

CONTRAINDICATIONS

Meglumine antimoniate is contraindicated in patients with severe kidney disease due to potential nephrotoxicity.

PRECAUTIONS

Meglumine antimoniate causes pain and inflammation at injection site; vomiting and diarrhea are common side effects. Allopurinol can cause development of xanthine uroliths. Dogs on long treatment with allopurinol should be fed a low-purine diet.

POSSIBLE INTERACTIONS

Allopurinol may decrease the hepatic metabolism of azathioprine. If used concurrently the dosage of azathioprine should be reduced by one-third. Allopurinol may increase serum cyclosporine level.

ALTERNATIVE DRUG(S)

N/A

FOLLOW-UP

PATIENT MONITORING

Follow-up visits: 4–6 weeks after diagnosis, every 3 months during the first year, and then every 6 months. A complete physical examination, CBC, serum biochemistry including serum protein electrophoresis, urine analysis, and serology should be performed at each check-up.

PREVENTION/AVOIDANCE

Topical pyrethroids in collars (deltamethrine, flumethrin) or spot on (permethrin) have been demonstrated to reduce the risk of infection and to reduce the prevalence of the disease. All dogs living in endemic areas should be treated regularly with topical pyrethroids. Three protein vaccines are currently licensed for CanL: two in Europe and one in Brazil. These vaccines are safe and have protection efficacies close to 70%. They do not prevent infection, but reduce the risk of having clinical leishmaniosis if infected. They can be administered to dogs living in endemic areas along with topical insecticides/repellents to increase protection. Dogs visiting endemic areas should be treated with topical pyrethroids.

POSSIBLE COMPLICATIONS

N/A

EXPECTED COURSE AND PROGNOSIS

Four clinical stages have been defined based on clinical signs, serology, pathologic abnormalities, and renal disease. Prognosis depends on clinical stage: from good in mild disease (stage I) to poor in very severe disease (stage IV). Treatment causes clinical improvement in most dogs. However, dogs remain infected life-long.

MISCELLANEOUS

ASSOCIATED CONDITIONS

Coinfection with other vector-borne diseases (e.g., ehrlichiosis) are frequently diagnosed in dogs with leishmaniosis. It is recommended to test dogs with leishmaniosis for prevalent local vector-borne infectious diseases.

AGE-RELATED FACTORS

N/A.

ZOONOTIC POTENTIAL

Leishmaniosis is a zoonosis and dogs are considered the most important peri-domestic reservoir of *L. infantum* infection for humans. The ownership of an infected dog does not appear to greatly increase the risk of developing leishmaniosis. Dogs diagnosed with leishmaniosis must be treated and monitored, and topical pyrethroids used, to prevent transmission of infection. Reporting of infection to public health authorities is required in some countries.

PREGNANCY/FERTILITY/BREEDING

Leishmaniosis can be transmitted vertically and by venereal route. Infected dogs should not be used as breeders. Allopurinol is considered to be safe during pregnancy. Information regarding the risk of using meglumine antimoniate in pregnant or lactating animals is limited. Use should be avoided. Miltefosine is contraindicated in pregnant and lactating animals. Puppies born to a mother with leishmaniosis should be screened for *Leishmania* infection with serology or PCR of a bone marrow sample at 3–6 months of age.

SYNONYMS

Leishmaniasis.

ABBREVIATIONS

- CanL = canine leishmaniosis caused by *Leishmania infantum*.
- IFAT = immunofluorescence antibody test.

INTERNET RESOURCES

http://www.leishvet.org

Suggested Reading

Noli C, Saridomichelakis M. An update on the diagnosis and treatment of canine leishmaniosis caused by *Leishmania infantum* (syn. *L. chagasi*). Vet J 2014, 202:425–435.

Pennisi MG, Persichetti MF. Feline leishmaniosis. Is the cat a small dog? Vet Parasitol 2018, 251:131–137.

Reguera RM, Morán M, Pérez-Pertejo Y, et al. Current status on prevention and treatment of canine leishmaniasis. Vet Parasitol 2016, 227:98–114.

Solano-Gallego L, Miró G, Koutinas A, et al. LeishVet guidelines for the practical management of canine leishmaniosis. Parasites Vectors 2011, 4:86.

Author Lluís Ferrer
Consulting Editor Alexander H. Werner Resnick

BASICS

OVERVIEW

- Lens luxation—total dislocation of lens from its normal location; occurs when lens capsule separates 360° from the zonules that hold lens in place.
- Anterior—forward displacement through the pupil into anterior chamber.
- Posterior—backward displacement into vitreous.
- Subluxation—partial separation of lens from its zonular attachments; lens remains in a normal or near-normal position in pupil.
- Primary (hereditary) luxation—inherited zonular defect of dogs resulting in bilateral but often asymmetrical clinical signs.
- Congenital luxation—often associated with other congenital ocular anomalies.
- Secondary luxation—due to chronic inflammation, buphthalmia, intraocular neoplasia, senile zonular degeneration, or trauma.

SIGNALMENT

- Primary—usually adult dogs (typically 3–6 years); common breeds include terriers, Chinese crested and Chinese Shar-Pei. Rare in cats.
- Secondary—dog and cat; any age/breed.

SIGNS

- Fibrils of liquefied vitreous in anterior chamber.
- Abnormally shallow (anterior luxation) or deep anterior chamber (posterior luxation).
- Abnormal iris curvature secondary to tilting of lens.
- Phacodonesis (tremor of lens with globe movement).
- Iridodonesis (tremor of iris with globe movement).
- Aphakic crescent (crescent-shaped area of pupil lacking lens).
- Acute or chronic painful eye, episcleral injection, diffuse or central corneal edema.
- Glaucoma more common in anterior lens luxation but can be detected in any stage.
- Uveitis.
- Cataracts.
- Retinal detachment.

CAUSES & RISK FACTORS

- Primary—associated with *ADAMTS17* gene mutation in some canine breeds; inheritance pattern uncertain in others.
- Primary luxation and primary glaucoma—may occur simultaneously in some breeds.
- Chronic uveitis.
- Intraocular neoplasia—secondary to physical luxation or chronic inflammation.
- Trauma—rarely causes a normal lens to luxate without severe ocular injury.
- Cataracts—can cause tension and breakage of lens zonules.

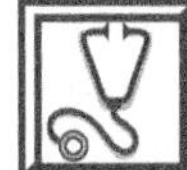

DIAGNOSIS

DIFFERENTIAL DIAGNOSIS

- Uveitis, glaucoma—painful, red eyes with corneal edema; may be concurrent.
- Buphthalmia may cause lens luxation.
- Corneal endothelial dystrophy or degeneration may also cause corneal edema.
- Diagnosis made by careful ophthalmic examination and history.

CBC/BIOCHEMISTRY/URINALYSIS

Normal, unless systemic disease present.

IMAGING

- Thoracic radiographs, abdominal ultrasonography—may be indicated if intraocular neoplasia.
- Ocular ultrasonography—useful if corneal edema or cloudy ocular media preclude examination.

DIAGNOSTIC PROCEDURES

- Complete ophthalmic examination, including tonometry.
- Genetic test available for some predisposed breeds.

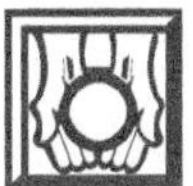

TREATMENT

- Potentially visual eyes—immediate referral to a veterinary ophthalmologist for possible intracapsular lens extraction is indicated.
- Manual trans-corneal reduction of anterior lens luxation and medical management of posterior luxation has been described.
- Topical miotic therapy may be used to keep a posteriorly luxated lens behind pupil and avoid surgery in some cases.
- Irreversibly blind eyes can be enucleated or eviscerated with intrascleral prosthesis; if secondary to neoplasia, enucleation is the best choice (therapeutic and diagnostic).

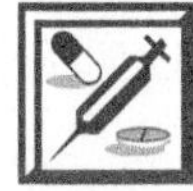

MEDICATIONS

DRUG(S) OF CHOICE

- Topical miotics—demecarium bromide or prostaglandin analogs (latanoprost) q12h indicated if the lens is primarily subluxated or posteriorly luxated.
- If the pupil is blocked due to anterior lens luxation, tropicamide may allow the pupil to dilate, releasing lens and decreasing risk for pupillary block glaucoma.
- Mannitol: 1 g/kg IV over 20 minutes indicated for intraocular pressure (IOP) >40 mmHg.
- Carbonic anhydrase inhibitors—topical dorzolamide q8h for high IOP.
- Topical anti-inflammatory—0.1% dexamethasone sodium phosphate or 1% prednisolone acetate (q6–24h) if inflammation present.

CONTRAINDICATIONS/POSSIBLE INTERACTIONS

- Topical miotics—contraindicated if lens in anterior chamber.
- Client must verify location of lens prior to applying a miotic
- Mannitol—contraindicated in patients with cardiac disease, dehydration, pulmonary edema, anuria and intracranial bleeding.

FOLLOW-UP

- Medically treated primary posterior luxation—recheck IOP 24 hours after starting treatment and frequently thereafter; once IOP is stable, re-examine patient 3 or 4 times/year.
- Monitor for secondary glaucoma and retinal detachment.
- If only one lens is involved at the time of examination, the other lens may eventually luxate as well; the ophthalmologist may choose to perform prophylactic phacoemulsification in the contralateral eye if not yet luxated.

MISCELLANEOUS

ABBREVIATIONS

- IOP = intraocular pressure.

Suggested Reading

Davidson MG, Nelms SR. Diseases of the lens and cataract formation. In: Veterinary Ophthalmology, 5th ed. Ames, IA: Wiley Blackwell, 2013, pp. 1199–1233.

Maggs DJ, Miller PE, Ofri R. Diseases of the lens. In: Slatter's Fundamentals of Veterinary Ophthalmology, 6th ed. St. Louis, MO: Saunders, 2018, pp. 306–333.

Author Renee T. Carter

Consulting Editor Kathern E. Myrna

Acknowledgment The author and editors acknowledge the prior contribution of Filipe Espinheira.

LEPTOSPIROSIS

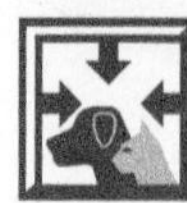

BASICS

DEFINITION

• Caused by pathogenic members of genus *Leptospira*; each serovar has own virulence factors, infectious dose, route of exposure.
• Acute and chronic diseases of dogs (mainly nephritis and hepatitis) and rarely cats.
• Dogs—serovars causing disease vary by geographic area; recent serovars of concern in the United States are *L. grippotyphosa*, *L. autumnalis*, and *L. pomona*; vaccines should include regional serovars.

PATHOPHYSIOLOGY

L

• *Leptospira* penetrate intact/cut skin/mucous membranes; rapidly invade bloodstream (4–7 days); disseminated spread (2–4 days).
• Invasion leads to transient fever, leukocytosis, mild hemolysis and hemoglobinuria, albuminuria. • Capillaries—endothelial cell damage. • Liver—hepatic necrosis.
• Kidney—leptospiruria; *Leptospira* localize in damaged renal tubules; organism replicates in tubular epithelium. • Serum antibodies appear as bacteremia decreases. • Death—usually due to interstitial nephritis, vascular damage, renal failure; may result from septicemia, disseminated intravascular coagulopathy (DIC), respiratory failure.

SYSTEMS AFFECTED

• Cardiovascular—endothelial cell damage, hemorrhage. • Hepatobiliary—hepatitis, necrosis. • Nervous—meningitis. • Renal/urologic—focal interstitial nephritis, hemoglobinuric nephrosis, tubular damage/failure.
• Respiratory—vasculitis, interstitial pneumonia, leptospiral pulmonary hemorrhage syndrome (LPHS).

Chronic Disease

• Ophthalmic—anterior uveitis. • Renal/urologic—chronic kidney disease.
• Reproductive—abortion; weak puppies; linked to feline stillbirth.

INCIDENCE/PREVALENCE

• Reported incidence (dogs)—falsely low due to inapparent and undiagnosed infections.
• Prevalence (dogs)—Increasing in urban dogs; hospital prevalence increasing since 1990s.

GEOGRAPHIC DISTRIBUTION

• Worldwide, especially in warm, wet climates. • Standing water, neutral or slightly alkaline soil promote presence in environment. • *L. canicola* most common worldwide; *L. icterohaemorrhagiae* most common in Australia. • *L. bratislava* has yet to be confirmed by culture as a serovar in dogs in the United States.

SIGNALMENT

Species

Dogs, rarely cats.

Mean Age and Range

• Young dogs without maternal antibodies and unvaccinated older dogs more likely to exhibit clincal disease. • Dogs with adequate antibody titers seldom exhibit clinical disease unless exposed to serovar not in vaccine.

Predominant Sex

N/A

SIGNS

General Comments

Signs vary with age/immune status, virulence of infecting serovar, host response.

Historical Findings

Peracute to Subacute Disease

• Fever. • Sore muscles/stiffness. • Weakness, lethargy. • Anorexia, vomiting. • Diarrhea—with/without blood. • Icterus. • Cough, dyspnea. • Polyuria/polydipsia (PU/PD) progressing to anuria. • Death.

Chronic Disease

• No apparent illness. • Fever. • PU/PD.

Physical Examination Findings

Peracute to Acute Disease

• Tachypnea. • Tachycardia, weak pulses.
• Hematemesis. • Hematochezia, melena.
• Epistaxis. • Injected mucous membranes.
• Widespread petechial and ecchymotic hemorrhages. • Reluctance to move, paraspinal hyperesthesia, stiff gait. • Conjunctivitis.
• Rhinitis. • Hematuria. • Mild lymphadenopathy.

CAUSES

• Dogs—*L. canicola, L. icterohaemorrhagiae, L. pomona, L. grippotyphosa, L. copenhagenii, L. australis, L. autumnalis, L. ballum*, and *L. bataviae*.
• Cats—*L. canicola, L. grippotyphosa, L. pomona*, and *L. bataviae*.

RISK FACTORS

Transmission

• Direct—via urine, post-abortion discharge, fetus, sexual contact (semen). • Indirect—exposure (via urine) to contaminated environment (vegetation, soil, food, water, bedding). • Disease in companion animals is often result of spillover from diseased wildlife maintenance hosts.

Host Factors

• Vaccine—protection is serovar-specific; may not prevent kidney colonization and urine shedding; new vaccines available of "subunit" type; newer panvalent antigen may cross-protect against many serovars. • Outdoor animals, hunting dogs—exposure of abraded or water-softened skin increases risk of infection.

Environmental Factors

• Warm, moist environment (low-lying areas, rainy season of temperate regions).
• Temperature range—44.6–50°F (7–10°C) to 93–96°F (34–36°C). • Organism survives best in stagnant water with neutral or slightly alkaline pH: ○ 180 days in wet soil; longer in standing water. • Dense animal population—kennels or urban settings. • Exposure to rodents, other wildlife (e.g., deer).

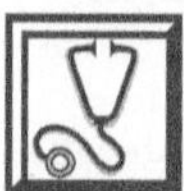

DIAGNOSIS

DIFFERENTIAL DIAGNOSIS

Subacute to Acute Disease

• Dogs—heartworm disease; hemolytic anemias; septicemia; viral infections (canine hepatitis, canine herpesvirus); neoplasia; trauma; lupus; tick-borne disease; toxoplasmosis; postrenal obstruction; renal toxins (e.g., ethylene glycol, aminoglycosides); causes of pulmonary interstitial/alveolar disease. • Cats—hemotropic mycoplasmosis; toxins (e.g., acetaminophen); septicemia; feline immunodeficiency virus (FIV)- and feline leukemia virus (FeLV)-associated diseases; cholangitis; toxoplasmosis; feline infectious peritonitis (FIP); neoplasia; trauma; postrenal obstruction.

Reproductive/Neonatal Disease

• Dogs—brucellosis, canine distemper, herpesviruses. • Cats—FIP, FeLV, panleukopenia, herpesvirus, toxoplasmosis, salmonellosis.

CBC/BIOCHEMISTRY/URINALYSIS

• CBC—leukocytosis with left shift; leukopenia during leptospiremic phase; thrombocytopenia. Hematocrit variable with hemoconcentration, bleeding, or hemolysis.
• Chemistry— azotemia; electrolyte alterations—depend on degree of renal and gastrointestinal dysfunction (hyponatremia, hyper/hypokalemia, hypochloremia, hyperphosphatemia); hypoalbuminemia; elevated hepatic enzyme activities; hyperbilirubinemia. • Prolonged prothrombin and partial thromboplastin times; increased d-dimer concentrations.
• Urinalysis—isosthenuria; proteinuria; glucosuria.

OTHER LABORATORY TESTS

Serology (Microscopic Agglutination Test [MAT])

• Test serum in acute stage and 3–4 weeks later (convalescent). • Unvaccinated patients—titers initially low (1:100–1:200), higher in convalescent sample (1:800–1:1,600 or higher) if homologous *Leptospira* serovar is tested; several serovars may cross-react in MAT test, especially if high titers to one serovar. • Vaccinated patients—high titers for up to 12–16 weeks post vaccination, then drop to <1:400; new subunit vaccines—titers rise to ≥1:1,600 for

12 weeks for serovars *L. canicola* and *L. icterohaemorrhagiae*; titers for other serovars (*L. pomona* and *L. grippotyphosa*) variable. • Run acute and convalescent samples at same time, if possible.

Darkfield Microscopy of Urine

Fresh urine, often inconclusive.

Fluorescent Antibody Test of Urine

• *Leptospira* viability not required; submit urine to lab on ice by overnight courier.
• More conclusive than microscopy.

PCR Test of Urine and Tissue

Only indicates genus *Leptospira*; may be useful with refinement and validation.

DIAGNOSTIC PROCEDURES

Culture (body fluids or tissues) not practical due to fastidiousness of leptospiras; require special culture/transport medium.

PATHOLOGIC FINDINGS

• Degree of kidney and liver disease depends on serovar and host immunity. • Cats—generally less severe lesions. • Dogs (acute disease)—lungs may be edematous; kidneys pale and enlarged; liver enlarged, may be friable with multifocal necrosis/hemorrhage; gastrointestinal tract may hemorrhage.
• Warthin–Starry silver stain; immunohistochemistry; fluorescent antibody test on formalin-fixed sections of kidney, liver, fetal/placental tissue.

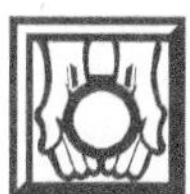

TREATMENT

NURSING CARE

• Shock—IV, balanced, isotonic replacement solution. • Dehydration—IV or oral maintenance solutions as indicated. • Severe hemorrhage—blood transfusion may be indicated. • Oliguria, anuria—restore circulating volume; then give intravenous osmotic diuretics or tubular diuretics; dialysis may be needed. • LPHS—oxygen supplementation or mechanical ventilation as indicated.

CLIENT EDUCATION

Inform client of zoonotic potential from contaminated urine of affected dogs and environment.

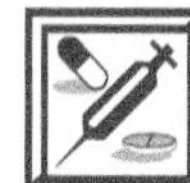

MEDICATIONS

DRUG(S) OF CHOICE

• Doxycycline 5 mg/kg PO or IV q12h for 2 weeks; use alone to clear both leptospiremia and leptospiruria. • Ampicillin 22 mg/kg IV q6–8h (or other penicillins as available); only clears leptospiremia; must be followed by course of doxycyline.

PRECAUTIONS

Doxycycline can cause esophagitis, esophageal stricture.

FOLLOW-UP

PREVENTION/AVOIDANCE

• Vaccine (dogs)—whole-cell bacterin vaccines contain serovars *L. canicola*/*icterohaemorrhagiae* (newer also include *L. pomona*/*grippotyphosa*): ○ Promotes immunity to homologous serovars and protection from overt clinical disease; may not prevent colonization of the kidneys, resulting in chronic carrier state. ○ Serovar-specific.
○ Newer subunit vaccine contains *L. pomona*, *L. icterohaemorrhagiae*, *L. grippotyphosa*, and *L. canicola*; possibly provides protection from clinical disease/prevents kidney colonization.
○ Bacteria-induced immunity lasts 6–8 months and is serovar-specific. ○ Revaccinate at least yearly. ○ Vaccinate high-risk dogs (hunter, show dogs, dogs with access to water/ponds) every 4–6 months, especially in endemic areas. • Kennels—strict sanitation to avoid contact with infected urine; control rodents; monitor/remove carrier dogs until treated; isolate infected animals during treatment. • Activity—limit access to marshy/muddy areas, ponds, low-lying areas with stagnant surface water, heavily irrigated pastures; limit access to wildlife. • Environmental contamination—leptospira shedding in urine is intermittent; leptospira survive but do not multiply in environment; cells survive until either drying, UV light exposure, or freeze-thaw has killed the leptospires.

POSSIBLE COMPLICATIONS

• DIC. • Permanent liver/kidney dysfunction. • Uveitis. • Abortion.

EXPECTED COURSE AND PROGNOSIS

• Most infections subclinical or chronic.
• Prognosis guarded for acute severe disease.

MISCELLANEOUS

AGE-RELATED FACTORS

Severe clinical disease in young dogs (nonvaccinated or lacking maternal antibody).

ZOONOTIC POTENTIAL

• High—spreads in urine of infected animals.
• Strict kennel hygiene and disinfection of premises.

PREGNANCY/FERTILITY/BREEDING

• Possible abortion. • Antimicrobial therapy—consider effect of drug on developing fetus.

ABBREVIATIONS

• DIC = disseminated intravascular coagulopathy.
• FeLV = feline leukemia virus.
• FIP = feline infectious peritonitis.
• FIV = feline immunodeficiency virus.
• LPHS = leptospiral pulmonary hemorrhage syndrome.
• MAT = microscopic agglutination test.
• PU/PD = polyuria/polydipsia.

INTERNET RESOURCES

http://www.cfsph.iastate.edu/DiseaseInfo/disease.php?name=leptospirosis&lang=en

Suggested Reading

Reagan KL, Sykes JE. Diagnosis of canine leptospirosis. Vet Clin North Am Small Anim Pract 2019, 49:719–731.

Sykes JE, Hartmann K, Lunn KF, et al. 2010 ACVIM small animal consensus statement on leptospirosis: diagnosis, epidemiology, treatment, and prevention. J Vet Intern Med 2011, 25(1):1–13.

Author Patrick L. McDonough

Consulting Editor Amie Koenig

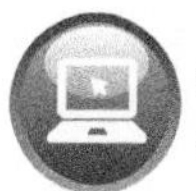

Client Education Handout available online

LEUKEMIA, CHRONIC LYMPHOCYTIC

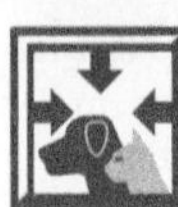

BASICS

OVERVIEW

- Uncommon, lymphoproliferative disorder.
- Slowly progressive over months to years.
- Circulating neoplastic lymphocytes are mature and well differentiated. • May originate in spleen or bone marrow.

SIGNALMENT

- More frequent in dog than cat. • No sex predilection reported. • Dogs—mean age 10 years (range 1.5–15 years). • Cats—median age 12.5 years (range 5–20 years).

SIGNS

- Nonspecific, often no clinical signs of illness. • Lethargy, decreased appetite, chronic weight loss. • Lymphadenomegaly, splenomegaly. • Fever. • Polydipsia/polyuria.

CAUSES & RISK FACTORS

Unknown

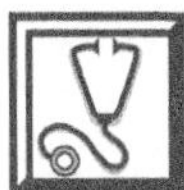

DIAGNOSIS

DIFFERENTIAL DIAGNOSIS

- Lymphoma—may have a leukemic phase (stage V). • Acute lymphoblastic leukemia.
- Immune-mediated hematologic diseases.
- Chronic antigenic stimulation (reactive lymphocytosis)—ehrlichiosis. • Acute viral infection-associated lymphocytosis.

CBC/BIOCHEMISTRY/URINALYSIS

- Lymphocytosis—range 5,000 to >500,000 cells/µL; typically small, mature lymphocytes.
- Larger size cells (intermediate-size or blasts) may be observed, especially with progression to blast crisis (advanced stage). • Mild-to-moderate normocytic, normochromic anemia (nonregenerative). • Normal-to-low platelet count (uncommon). • Normal-to-low neutrophil count (uncommon). • Normal-to-mildly increased serum globulins.

OTHER LABORATORY TESTS

- Immunophenotyping by flow cytometry (peripheral blood) is becoming more common practice for classification of leukemias (noninvasive)—affords prognostic information.
- Immunocytochemical staining (bone marrow samples), flow cytometry of bone marrow aspirates, or PCR for antigen receptor rearrangement (PARR) may be useful for classification of leukemias. • Cytologic examination (bone marrow aspirate or core biopsy) may show high numbers of mature lymphocytes (especially B-cell chronic lymphocytic leukemia [CLL]); crowding out of normal cell lines in advanced stages. • If hyperglobulinemia, serum protein electrophoresis to detect monoclonal gammopathy. • Direct Coombs' test may be positive with secondary immune-mediated hemolytic anemia.
- Serology for *Erlichia canis*.

IMAGING

Radiography and ultrasonography may reveal splenomegaly or internal lymphadenomegaly.

DIAGNOSTIC PROCEDURES

- Bone marrow aspiration (cytology) or marrow biopsy (histopathology) may be used for immunophenotyping. • Lymph node and spleen cytology or histopathology may help differentiate CLL from leukemic phase of lymphoma.

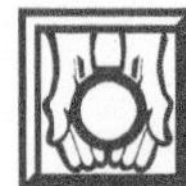

TREATMENT

- Usually outpatients treated with oral therapy.
- Treatment should be instituted when patient demonstrates clinical signs of illness (including weight loss, lethargy), lymphadenomegaly or organomegaly, cytopenias, or with lymphocyte count above 50,000/µL. • Consult a veterinary oncologist for updates in treatment options and regimens.

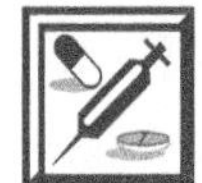

MEDICATIONS

DRUG(S) OF CHOICE

- Dogs—chlorambucil 6 mg/m^2 PO q24h for 7–14 days; then 3 mg/m^2 PO q24h; and eventually (maintenance) 2–4 mg/m^2 q48h, adjusted based on response and chronic hematologic tolerability. • Cats—chlorambucil 2 mg/patient regardless of body weight q2–4 days. • Prednisone 2 mg/kg (up to maximum of 60 mg) PO q24h (dogs); 5–10 mg/cat q24h (cats; use prednisolone); in combination with chlorambucil; may be tapered or discontinued when lymphocyte count normalizes. • Alternative chemotherapy agents and protocols to be considered when resistance or blast crisis develops over time—consult with an oncologist.

CONTRAINDICATIONS/POSSIBLE INTERACTIONS

Chemotherapy may have toxic side effects; seek advice with oncologist before starting treatment if you are unfamiliar with cytotoxic drugs.

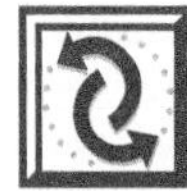

FOLLOW-UP

PATIENT MONITORING

Initially, examination of CBC every 2 weeks; response to treatment and disease progression.

POSSIBLE COMPLICATIONS

Chronic chemotherapy-induced myelosuppression; may need to alter dosage, depending on neutrophil and platelet counts.

EXPECTED COURSE AND PROGNOSIS

- Variable course, but eventually progressive to blast crisis or becomes resistant to therapy.
- Median survival time with therapy approaches 18 months in dogs with B-cell CLL, and surpasses 24 months in dogs with T-cell CLL. • Median survival time with therapy in cats was >14 months in one study.

MISCELLANEOUS

ABBREVIATIONS

- CLL = chronic lymphocytic leukemia.
- PARR = PCR for antigen receptor rearrangement.

Suggested Reading

Adam F, Villiers E, Watson S, et al. Clinical pathological and epidemiological assessment of morphologically and immunologically confirmed canine leukemia. Vet Comp Onc 2009, 7:181–195.

Bromberek JL, Rout ED, Agnew MR, et al. Breed distribution and clinical characteristics of B cell chronic lymphocytic leukemia in dogs. J Vet Intern Med 2016, 30:215–222.

Campbell MW, Hess PR, Williams LE. Chronic lymphocytic leukaemia in the cat: 18 cases (2000–2010). Vet Comp Oncol 2013, 11:256–264.

Comazzi S, Gelain ME, Martini V, et al. Immunophenotype predicts survival time in dogs with chronic lymphocytic leukemia. J Vet Intern Med 2011, 25:100–106.

Workman HC, Vernau W. Chronic lymphocytic leukemia in dogs and cats: the veterinary perspective. Vet Clin North Am Small Anim Pract 2003, 33:1379–1399.

Author Matthew R. Berry

Consulting Editor Timothy M. Fan

Acknowledgment The author and editors acknowledge the prior contribution of Louis-Philippe de Lorimier.

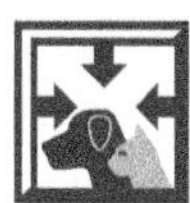

BASICS

DEFINITION

General term—white blood cell (WBC) count increased above reference interval; nonspecific to type of cell. Evaluation of individual leukocyte absolute numbers is needed to discern the cellular population(s) causing the overall increase in WBC count. Neutrophilia is the most common cause of a total WBC increase, and a left shift with toxic changes (e.g., Döhle bodies, cytoplasmic basophilia, foamy cytoplasmic vacuolation, and/or toxic granulation) may be present.

PATHOPHYSIOLOGY

One or more of the following mechanisms:

- Inflammation and increased tissue demand for leukocytes causing myeloid hyperplasia in the bone marrow.
- Translocation of cells from the marginating pool to the circulating pool of large vessels.
- Altered cytokine production resulting in increased release of cells from marrow storage pool.
- Decreased migration to tissues.
- Delayed apoptosis.

SYSTEMS AFFECTED

Chronic inflammation/leukocytosis may lead to nonspecific tissue damage and organ dysfunction.

GENETICS

Leukocyte adhesion deficiency (LAD) is an uncommon, autosomal recessive, primary immunodeficiency resulting in reduced neutrophil adhesion and inability to migrate to tissues.

SIGNALMENT

- Nothing specific for generalized causes.
- LAD reported in Irish setters and a domestic longhair cat.
- Young and nervous/anxious animals with a physiologic response.
- Rottweilers, Alaskan Malamutes, Siberian huskies, and cats with eosinophil dysregulation diseases.

SIGNS

- Animals with leukocytosis may exhibit fever, anorexia, weight loss, organomegaly, and other signs caused by the primary disease process.
- Affected animals with LAD can exhibit persistent marked leukocytosis/neutrophilia, impaired wound-healing, recurrent infections, and/or weight loss.

CAUSES

- Etiologies resulting in increased inflammatory cytokine production include infectious or sterile causes, immune-mediated diseases, paraneoplastic or inflammatory disease.
- Shifting of neutrophils from the marginating pool to the circulating pool (measured) can be caused by stress or fear.
- Increases in circulating leukocytes due to decreased margination to the tissues can be caused by excessive endogenous corticosteroid or in patients with LAD.
- Delayed apoptosis can lead to hypersegmentation of neutrophils.

Neutrophilia

- Mature neutrophil count above reference interval.
- Most common—stress/physiologic response or inflammation caused by infectious or noninfectious conditions.
- Metabolic disease, corticosteroid excess (endogenous or exogenous).
- Physiologic (shift) or stress response.
- Tissue necrosis or trauma (surgical or other).
- Neoplasia—chronic myelogenous leukemia (primary) and secondary to histiocytic sarcoma; leiomyosarcoma; lymphoma; and mammary, pancreatic, squamous cell, bronchogenic, and hepatocellular carcinomas.

Monocytosis

- Monocyte count above reference interval, usually accompanies a neutrophilia.
- Most common—corticosteroid-mediated stress response (dogs), or chronic inflammatory conditions (infectious and noninfectious).
- Metabolic disease, chemotherapeutic drugs.
- Recovery from acute marrow injury.
- Tissue necrosis or trauma.
- Acute or chronic myelomonocytic or monocytic leukemia.

Lymphocytosis

- Lymphocyte count above reference interval.
- Most common—physiologic response or young (<6 months) age.
- Infectious agents and inflammatory conditions.
- Post vaccine.
- Physiologic (epinephrine-mediated) anxiety, excitement, exercise, fright, pain.
- Neoplasia (dogs and cats)—acute or chronic lymphocytic leukemia (primary), and non-hemic, lymphoma, thymoma.

Eosinophilia

- Eosinophil count above reference interval.
- Most common—allergic or hypersensitivity reaction, inflammation in selected tissues, or parasitic infection.
- Infectious agents and inflammatory conditions.
- Hypereosinophilic syndrome.
- Neoplasia—chronic eosinophilic leukemia (primary/uncommon), and paraneoplastic syndrome (common) associated with lymphoma, mast cell tumor, and infrequently other neoplasms.

Basophilia

- Basophil count above reference interval.
- Rare cause of a leukocytosis, may accompany an eosinophilia (same differentials apply).
- Chronic basophilic leukemia (primary/uncommon) and paraneoplastic syndrome associated with chronic myeloid leukemia and essential thrombocythemia.

RISK FACTORS

- Breeds predisposed to hyperadrenocorticism, eosinophilic diseases, or immune-mediated diseases.
- Geographic areas with specific infectious agents.
- Drugs—adenocorticotropic hormone (ACTH); catecholamine injections; corticosteroids; granulocyte colony-stimulating factor (G-CSF); methimazole.

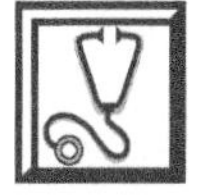

DIAGNOSIS

DIFFERENTIAL DIAGNOSIS

Based upon individual leukocyte population(s) causing the leukocytosis.

Leukogram Patterns

- Inflammatory leukogram resulting from inflammatory cytokines may include one or more of the following: neutrophilia, left shift, toxic change, monocytosis, eosinophilia, and/or basophilia.
- Stress leukogram induced by endogenous or exogenous corticosteroids presents with a neutrophilia without a significant left shift or toxic change, monocytosis, lymphopenia, and/or eosinopenia (dogs).
- Excitement/physiologic (shift) leukogram mediated by catecholamines resulting in a neutrophilia without a significant left shift and toxicity, lymphocytosis, and/or monocytosis.
- Neoplastic leukograms typically involve the uncontrolled proliferation of cells, typically lymphocytes. Leukemias of other origin (neutrophils/monocytes) occur less frequently and inflammation should be excluded first. Some non-hemic neoplasms can cause a paraneoplastic neutrophilia, eosinophilia, and/or basophilia.
- With intense inflammation, the neutrophil count can increase dramatically into a range more commonly seen with leukemia (>50,000/μL), sometimes referred to as a "leukemoid reaction."
- Consider causes of severe inflammation first (e.g., pyometra, peritonitis) as chronic myeloid leukemia comprising mature neutrophils is rare in veterinary medicine.

CBC/BIOCHEMISTRY/URINALYSIS

- CBC with leukocyte differential and absolute numbers with morphology review of a blood smear.
- Biochemical profile.
- Urinalysis with bacterial culture and sensitivity to evaluate for urinary tract infection, if indicated.

Factors That May Erroneously Alter Laboratory Results

Blood smear review may help exclude errors in automated cell counting that can occur in the presence of nucleated erythrocytes or parasites.

OTHER LABORATORY TESTS

- Culture, serology, and/or PCR for infectious agents.
- ACTH stimulation test—if clinical concern for hyperadrenocorticism.
- Coombs' test, saline agglutination test—if suspicion for immune-mediated anemia.
- Flow cytometry—if suspicion for hemic neoplasia, immune-mediated disease.
- PCR for antigen receptor rearrangement (PARR)—if suspicion for lymphoid neoplasia.

IMAGING

Radiography and ultrasonography can aid in identifying occult site(s) of infection or neoplasia.

DIAGNOSTIC PROCEDURES

- Bone marrow aspirate or biopsy if indicated.
- Biopsy any masses.
- Organ evaluation, as indicated.

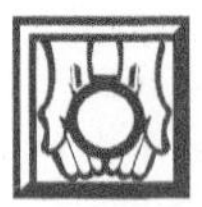

TREATMENT

APPROPRIATE HEALTH CARE

- Treatment should be based on the identified underlying etiology of the leukocytosis.
- Animals with infectious causes should receive appropriate antimicrobial medications.
- Suitable immunosuppression for immune-mediated diseases.
- Patients with extreme leukocytosis >50,000/μL require intensive management, including the possibility of hospitalization due to increased risk of mortality.

MEDICATIONS

N/A

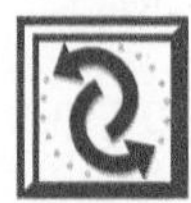

FOLLOW-UP

PATIENT MONITORING

- Determine if leukocytosis is persistent via repeat CBC to exclude physiologic response.
- In patients with extreme leukocytosis, serial CBCs every 24 hours, or as indicated, to assess the leukocyte response to medical therapy.

EXPECTED COURSE AND PROGNOSIS

- Leukocyte counts decrease after treatment of the inciting cause.
- Resolution can vary from a few hours (e.g., lymphocytes post stress) to a few days or weeks (e.g., inflammatory neutrophilia).
- Extreme leukocytosis >50,000/μL is associated with a poor prognosis and high mortality rate; patients with fever and neoplasia have the shortest survival times.

MISCELLANEOUS

AGE-RELATED FACTORS

Young animals (<6 months) have higher lymphocyte counts than adult animals and age-appropriate reference intervals are recommended.

PREGNANCY/FERTILITY/BREEDING

Mild leukocytosis characterized by a mature neutrophilia may be observed in pregnant animals.

SYNONYMS

None

SEE ALSO

- Anemia, Immune-Mediated.
- Eosinophilia.
- Leukemia, Chronic Lymphocytic.
- Lymphoma—Cats.
- Lymphoma—Dogs.
- Lymphoma, Cutaneous Epitheliotropic.
- Peritonitis.

ABBREVIATIONS

- ACTH = adenocorticotropic hormone.
- FeLV = feline leukemia virus.
- G-CSF = granulocyte colony-stimulating factor.
- LAD = leukocyte adhesion deficiency.
- PARR = PCR for antigen receptor rearrangement.
- WBC = white blood cell.

INTERNET RESOURCES

http://eclinpath.com/hematology/leukogram-changes/leukocytes/

Suggested Reading

Harvey JW. Veterinary Hematology: A Diagnostic Guide and Color Atlas. St. Louis, MO: Elsevier Saunders, 2012, pp. 122–176.

Stockham SL, Keeton KS, Szladovits B. Clinical assessment of leukocytosis: distinguishing leukocytoses caused by inflammatory, glucocorticoid, physiologic, and leukemic disorders or conditions. Vet Clin North Am Small Anim Pract 2003, 33:1335–1357.

Thrall MA, Weiser G, Allison RW, Campbell TW. Veterinary Hematology and Clinical Chemistry. Ames, IA: John Wiley & Sons, 2012, pp. 118–184.

Author Sarah S.K. Beatty

Consulting Editor Melinda S. Camus

LEUKOENCEPHALOMYELOPATHY IN ROTTWEILERS

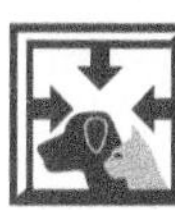

BASICS

OVERVIEW

- Neurodegenerative disorder that affects the white matter of young adult Rottweilers leading to chronic progressive ataxia of the limbs.
- The clinical signs are primarily associated to involvement of the cervical spinal cord, but white matter lesions are also present in the brainstem, cerebellum, and subcortical white matter.
- Occurs worldwide.
- Probably autosomal recessive inheritance.

SIGNALMENT

Rottweiler—either sex; onset in adult dogs 1.5–4 years old.

SIGNS

- Insidious, nonpainful, progressive onset.
- Cervical spinal cord signs prevail despite widespread demyelinating process.
- Proprioceptive ataxia of the thoracic (delayed protraction with overreaching of the limb) and pelvic limbs, with upper motor neuron weakness.
- Front limbs are more severely affected than hind limbs. Mild asymmetry between right and left limbs may be present.
- Nail scuffing in all limbs.
- Proprioceptive positioning and hopping delayed to absent in all limbs.
- Spinal reflexes normal to exaggerated.

CAUSES & RISK FACTORS

- Autosomal recessive inheritance suspected.
- Inbreeding.

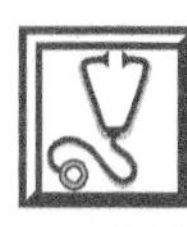

DIAGNOSIS

DIFFERENTIAL DIAGNOSIS

- Cervical compressive lesions such as cervical vertebral spondylomyelopathy (wobbler), cervical subarachnoid diverticula, fibrotic stenosis, spinal cord tumors—difficult to differentiate on clinical signs alone; all can have an insidious onset; MRI necessary for diagnosis.
- Neuroaxonal dystrophy and distal sensorimotor polyneuropathy—neurologic disorders reported in Rottweilers; differentiated on the basis of neurologic deficits; neuroaxonal dystrophy: deficits relate to the cerebellum; distal sensorimotor polyneuropathy: tetraparesis associated with lower motor neuron signs.
- Discospondylitis, fracture/luxation, intervertebral disc disease—neck pain; disc disease rarely seen in large-breed dogs at a young age.

CBC/BIOCHEMISTRY/URINALYSIS

Normal

OTHER LABORATORY TESTS

N/A

IMAGING

- Spinal cervical survey radiographs normal.
- MRI—on T2W transverse images of the cervical spine, bilateral and symmetrical well-demarcated, ovoid in shape, intra-axial hyperintensities in the white matter of the dorsolateral funiculi, extending contiguously from the cervicomedullary junction to the sixth cervical vertebral body. Symmetrical hyperintensities also observed in pyramids and ventral aspect of the crus cerebri in the brain. No contrast enhancement.

DIAGNOSTIC PROCEDURES

Cerebrospinal fluid (CSF) analysis normal.

PATHOLOGIC FINDINGS

- Although the most severe lesion is located in the white matter of the cervical spinal cord, it extends caudally into the thoracic spinal cord and rostrally into the brainstem.
- Macroscopic examination—in the dorsal aspect of the lateral funiculi of the cervical spinal cord and in the pyramidal tracts of the medulla oblongata, presence of well-demarcated whitish opaque foci located bilaterally and symmetrically, corresponding to myelin loss.
- Microscopy—in the cervical spinal cord, the lesion affects the cervical spinal cord white matter in the dorsal portion of the lateral funiculi (dorsal spinocerebellar, lateral corticospinal, reticulospinal, and rubrospinal tracts). In the brain, the lesion affects the pyramidal tracts, crus cerebri, medial lemniscus, caudal cerebellar peduncle, trapezoid body, spinal tracts of the trigeminal nerve, and optic tracts; multifocal lesions are also observed in the cerebellar folia.
- The myelin loss exceeds axon loss with extensive astrogliosis and astrocytosis. Normal-appearing axons observed in areas of severe demyelination.
- Lesion bilateral with some asymmetry.

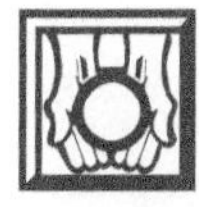

TREATMENT

- Outpatient, unless the severity of neurologic deficits precludes nursing care at home.
- Activity—whatever can be tolerated.
- Diet—ensure proper intake of food; patient may have difficulty reaching the feeding area.
- Neurologic status—slowly and progressively deteriorates; eventually, the patient is unable to walk or get up.

MEDICATIONS

DRUG(S) OF CHOICE

N/A

FOLLOW-UP

- Neurologic examination—monitor monthly to assess progression.
- Avoid bed sores and urine and fecal scalding by keeping the patient on a clean, dry, and cushioned pad (e.g., synthetic sheepskin).
- Severe tetraparesis—within 6–12 months after onset of clinical signs.
- Euthanasia—because of severe debility.

MISCELLANEOUS

ABBREVIATIONS

- CSF = cerebrospinal fluid.
- T2W = T2-weighted.

Suggested Reading

Davies DR, Irwin PJ. Degenerative neurological and neuromuscular disease in young rottweilers. J Small Anim Pract 2003, 44(9):388–394.

Eagleson JS, Kent M, Platt SR, et al. MRI findings in a rottweiler with leukoencephalomyelopathy. J Am Anim Hosp Assoc 2013, 49:255–261.

Hirschvogel K, Matiasek K, Flatz K, et al. Magnetic resonance imaging and genetic investigation of a case of Rottweiler leukoencephalomyelopathy. BMC Vet Res 2013, 9:57.

Author Joane M. Parent

LILY TOXICOSIS

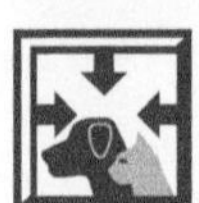

BASICS

OVERVIEW

• Plants in the *Lilium* and *Hemerocallis* genera—widely used ornamental plants—are very toxic to cats; *Lilium*—Easter lilies, tiger lilies, Japanese show lilies, rubrum lilies, numerous *Lilium* hybrids; *Hemerocallis*—daylilies. • Ingestion of leaves or flowers and, potentially, pollen or vase water—results in a severe nephrotoxic syndrome; as little as 1–2 leaves reported to be lethal. • Toxic principle(s) not elucidated but found to be in the water-soluble plant fraction.

SIGNALMENT

• Cats—systemic poisoning. • Dogs—only mild gastrointestinal upset, even after ingestion of large quantities of plant material.
• No age or breed predilections noted.

SIGNS

• Sudden onset of vomiting and drooling—gradually subsides within 4–6 hours.
• Depression and anorexia—typically within 12 hours of exposure; both persist throughout the syndrome. • Polyuria and dehydration; azotemia by 12–24 hours; progresses to anuric renal failure by 24–48 hours. • Vomiting—recurs by 36 hours; accompanied by progressive weakness. • Recumbency—by 2–4 days.
• Death—by 3–7 days post ingestion. • Severe pancreatitis has also been reported but is rare.

CAUSES & RISK FACTORS

• Plants—Easter lilies, tiger lilies, Asiatic hybrid lilies, Japanese show lilies, *Lilium* hybrids, daylily; primarily when used in cut-flower arrangements or as household potted plants. • All ingestions by cats of plant material from the *Lilium* and *Hemerocallis* genera should be considered potentially lethal.
• Primarily indoor cats—predisposed to ingestion of newly introduced flowers or plants.

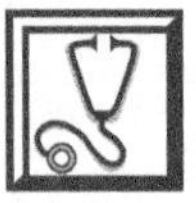

DIAGNOSIS

DIFFERENTIAL DIAGNOSIS

Nephrotoxins

• Aspirin and other nonsteroidal anti-inflammatory drug (NSAIDs).
• Cholecalciferol (vitamin D3); calcipotriene.
• Soluble oxalate-containing plants.
• Ethylene glycol. • Nephrotoxic antibiotics—aminoglycosides. • Melamine/cyanuric acid poisoning.

Systemic Diseases

• Acute presentation of chronic renal failure.
• Urinary obstruction. • Immune-mediated renal disease. • Leptospirosis.
• Pyelonephritis. • Lymphoma.

CBC/BIOCHEMISTRY/URINALYSIS

• Stress leukogram. • Increases in BUN, creatinine, phosphorous, and potassium.
• Creatinine—may be disproportionately elevated compared to BUN. • Increased aspartate aminotransferase (AST), alanine aminotransferase (ALT), and alkaline phosphatase (ALP) possible late in disease—likely secondary to prolonged anorexia and hepatic stress. • Proteinuria, glucosuria, and isosthenuria; numerous tubular epithelial casts. Early in the syndrome, tubular cell detail can be seen in the casts.
• Crystalluria—*not* caused by ingestion of these plants. • Increased amylase and lipase may occur with very large ingestions.

DIAGNOSTIC PROCEDURES

• If possible, examine plant to verify that it has been chewed. • Have plant positively identified by a professional horticulturist or other expert if necessary.

PATHOLOGIC FINDINGS

• Gross—swollen, edematous kidneys; systemic congestion; pancreatic necrosis may be seen. • Histologic—severe acute renal tubular necrosis with intact basement membranes; mild to severe interstitial edema; severe cast formation in the collecting ducts; later in the syndrome may note evidence of mitotic figures in the remaining tubular epithelium.

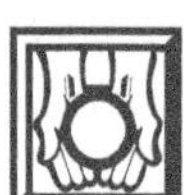

TREATMENT

• Early decontamination—lessens duration and severity of signs. Inducing emesis may be helpful if vomiting has not already occurred. Endoscopy has been used to remove plant pieces. Bathe cats if pollen is noted on the patient's face or fur.
• Fluid therapy—initiation within 18 hours of ingestion typically prevents anuric renal failure; intravenous balanced crystalloids at 2–3 times maintenance for 48–72 hours. • Anuric renal failure—peritoneal or hemodialysis is the only effective treatment; 7 days or more of therapy has resulted in a return of renal function in a few cases but does not guarantee recovery.

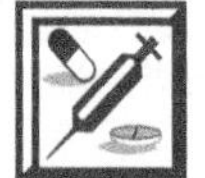

MEDICATIONS

DRUG(S) OF CHOICE

Decontamination

• Emetic agents for cats—xylazine 0.44 mg/kg IM or dexmedetomidine 7 µg/kg IM.
• Activated charcoal 1–2 g/kg PO.
• Cathartic—sorbitol 70% solution 1–2 mL/kg PO.

CONTRAINDICATIONS/POSSIBLE INTERACTIONS

• Avoid fluids containing potassium if hyperkalemic. • Avoid drugs eliminated by renal clearance. • Diuretics (mannitol, hypertonic fluids, furosemide, thiazides) are not effective at initiating urine production once anuric renal failure has occurred.

FOLLOW-UP

PATIENT MONITORING

• Monitor renal values and electrolytes every 12–24 hours during treatment with IV fluids.
• Repeat 2–3 days after discharge, then as needed based on results and signs.

EXPECTED COURSE AND PROGNOSIS

• Dehydration from polyuric renal failure is required for the disease to progress to anuria.
• Prevention of dehydration (early fluids)—prevents the progression of the syndrome to anuria. • Initiation of IV fluids within 18 hours of exposure and prior to development of renal failure carries a good prognosis.
• Without treatment or if treatment is delayed, the mortality rate of lily toxicosis in cats is reportedly as high as 100%.

MISCELLANEOUS

SEE ALSO

• Poisoning (Intoxication) Therapy.

ABBREVIATIONS

• ALP = alkaline phosphatase.
• ALT = alanine aminotransferase.
• AST = aspartate aminotransferase.
• NSAID = nonsteroidal anti-inflammatory drug.

Suggested Reading

Bennet AJ, Reineke EL. Outcome following gastrointestinal tract decontamination and intravenous fluid diuresis in cats with known lily ingestion: 25 cases (2001–2010). J Am Vet Med Assoc 2013, 242(8):1110–1116.

Hall JO. Lily poisoning. In: Peterson ME, Talcott PA, eds., Small Animal Toxicology, 3rd ed. Philadelphia: W.B. Saunders, 2013, pp. 617–620.

Author Amanda L. Poldoski
Consulting Editor Lynn R. Hovda
Acknowledgment The author and editors acknowledge the prior contribution of Jeffery O. Hall.

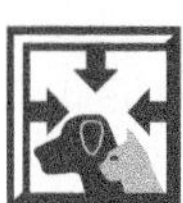

BASICS

OVERVIEW

- Invasive, non-encapsulated, lipoma variant that does not metastasize.
- A benign neoplasm that infiltrates soft tissues, particularly muscles, and including fasciae, tendons, nerves, blood vessels, salivary glands, lymph nodes, and joint capsules, and occasionally bones.
- Muscle infiltration typically extensive.
- Surgical cure—possible but difficult to obtain. Radiation therapy has utility to control growth.
- Occurs much less frequently than does lipoma.

SIGNALMENT

- Usually middle-aged dogs.
- No breed predilection definitively demonstrated; Labrador retrievers possibly overrepresented.
- May be more common in females than in males.

SIGNS

- Large, diffuse, soft tissue mass.
- Clinically appears as localized muscle swelling and/or distended abdomen if abdominal component.
- Infiltration of pelvic, thigh, shoulder, sternal, and lateral cervical musculature most common; recent evidence suggests no clear site prediction.

CAUSES & RISK FACTORS

Unknown

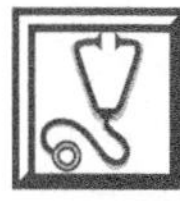

DIAGNOSIS

DIFFERENTIAL DIAGNOSIS

- Soft tissue sarcoma, particularly liposarcoma, hemangiopericytoma, myxosarcoma, rhabdomyosarcoma, and fibrosarcoma.
- Lipoma.
- Intermuscular lipoma.
- Mast cell neoplasia.

CBC/BIOCHEMISTRY/URINALYSIS

Normal

OTHER LABORATORY TESTS

N/A

IMAGING

- Radiography—reveals fat dense tissue between soft tissue dense structures.
- CT or MRI—fat-attenuating lesions allow adequate discrimination of tumor for surgery and/or radiation treatment planning; however, differentiation of normal fat from infiltrative lipoma can be problematic.

DIAGNOSTIC PROCEDURES

- Cytologic examination of aspirate reveals mature adipocytes with no cellular or nuclear atypia, identical to cells that form adult fat.
- Incisional biopsy can provide definitive histologic diagnosis if sufficient tissue representation of adipocytes and myocyte fibers can be identified.

PATHOLOGIC FINDINGS

- Histologic examination—well-differentiated adipocytes; may be indistinguishable from normal adipose tissue.
- Distinctive feature—tumor infiltration into and between muscle bundles and other tissues.

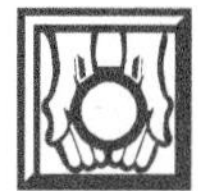

TREATMENT

Surgical Considerations

- Characteristic invasiveness makes excision extremely problematic; difficult to distinguish between tumor and normal adipose tissue.
- Poorly defined tumor margins—may contribute to the observed high recurrence rate after surgical excision.
- 36–50% of patients have recurrence within 3–16 months, except with limb amputation for appendicular tumor.
- Amputation of an affected limb is recommended only when quality of life is affected; tumor causes little inconvenience unless it interferes with movement (mechanical lameness), causes pressure-related pain, or develops in a vitally important anatomic site. However, amputation must be performed before growth of proximal extent of tumor crosses attainable surgical margin.

External Beam Radiotherapy

- Beneficial for long-term tumor control—median survival 40 months in a retrospective study of 13 dogs, with only 1 dog (7.7%) euthanized owing to tumor-related signs (vs. 26.7% with surgery alone).
- Dogs with measurable disease may only have stabilization of the tumor.
- Cytoreductive surgery to microscopic disease prior to radiation may result in long-term disease control.
- Unlikely to kill mitotically inactive mature adipocytes but may inhibit progressive infiltration by damaging tumor microcirculation.

MEDICATIONS

DRUG(S) OF CHOICE

N/A

CONTRAINDICATIONS/POSSIBLE INTERACTIONS

N/A

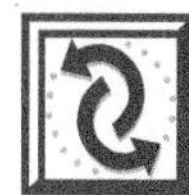

FOLLOW-UP

PATIENT MONITORING

- Therapeutic recommendations— guided by size, anatomic location and quality of life to determine whether and when to recommend surgery and adjunctive radiation therapy for incomplete surgical margins.
- Reevaluations—schedule as dictated by tumor growth and choice of therapy.

POSSIBLE COMPLICATIONS

Temporary acute side effects (e.g., moist dermatitis and alopecia) expected with radiation therapy; consultation with a radiation oncologist is recommended regarding specific, anatomic site-related side effects.

EXPECTED COURSE AND PROGNOSIS

- Surgical cure only possible if all affected tissues can be removed. Long-term control of tumor growth may be attained with external beam radiation therapy alone or in combination with surgery.
- Lack of metastatic potential affords a good prognosis if local tumor growth can be controlled.
- If liposarcoma diagnosed, behavior is similar to other soft tissue sarcomas, therefore consult relevant literature on these tumors.

MISCELLANEOUS

SYNONYMS

Lipomatosis

Suggested Reading

McEntee MC, Page RL, Mauldin GN, et al. Results of irradiation of infiltrative lipoma in 13 dogs. Vet Radiol Ultrasound 2000, 41:554–556.

Author Anthony J. Mutsaers
Consulting Editor Timothy M. Fan

LIVER FLUKE INFESTATION

BASICS

OVERVIEW

• Flukes reported in cats: *Platynosomum concinnum* (syn. *P. fastosum, P. illiciens*) (infection occurs in cats in Florida, Hawaii, Puerto Rico, and other tropical–semitropical areas); *Opisthorchis felineus* (Italy, Eastern Europe); *Opisthorchis viverrini* (southern Vietnam, Thailand, Laos, Malaysia, India); *Amphimerus pseudofelineus* (the Americas); *Clonorchis sinensis* (also known as Oriental liver fluke of people; northern Vietnam, China); *Metorchis albidus, M. conjunctus* (North America, Europe, Russia); *Eurytrema procyonis* (eastern United States). • Flukes reported in dogs: *Heterobilharzia americana* (southeastern United States); *Clonorchis conjunctus*; *Clonorchis sinensis* (China); *Schistosoma japonicum* (Philippines); *Schistosoma haematobium* (Zambia); *Metorchis bilis*, and *Opisthorchis felineus* (Germany) in sled dogs fed a diet including raw fish; *Opisthorchis viverrini* (southern Vietnam, Thailand, Laos, Malaysia, India).

• *Platynosomum concinnum* is the most common fluke infecting cats. One report of infection in a cat from Ohio and one from Illinois. It is the most common trematode infection affecting the liver of companion pets in North America. • Infestation acquired from ingestion of infected intermediate host (e.g., lizard or frog). • Estimated 15–85% of cats with intermediate host access are infected in endemic areas. • *Heterobilharzia americana*—raccoon is the natural definitive host and most important reservoir host; dogs can also serve as the definitive host.

SIGNALMENT

• *Platynosmum concinnum*—young (6–24 months) cat with access to local fauna.

• *Heterobilharzia americana*—dogs swimming or wading in contaminated freshwater sources; young adult dogs more commonly affected.

SIGNS

• Cats (*P. concinnum*)—depends on severity of infection. • Most infected cats lack clinical signs. • With severe infestation—jaundice, emaciation, anorexia, vomiting, mucoid diarrhea, hepatomegaly, abdominal distention, malaise, fever. • Dogs (*H. americana*)—lethargy, weight loss, vomiting, diarrhea, inappetence, hypercalcemia, polyuria/polydipsia (PU/PD), melena.

CAUSES & RISK FACTORS

P. concinnum

• Adults reside in bile ducts and gallbladder; life cycle requires two intermediate hosts and tropical or semitropical climate.

• Embryonated eggs pass in cat's feces; ingested by first intermediate host (a land snail). • Miracidia hatch from eggs in the snail penetrating host tissue and develop sporocysts. • Mature daughter sporocysts emerge from the snail and thereafter are ingested by a second intermediate host, usually an anole lizard (but also skinks, geckos, frogs, and toads); enter bile ducts where they reside until host ingested as prey by the cat. • Cercariae released in the upper digestive tract of the cat; migrate to the bile ducts where they mature and shed eggs within 8 weeks. • Risk factors for infection—tropical or subtropical climate; appropriate intermediate hosts; access to an outdoor or indoor/outdoor environment; successful hunting skills; consumption of infected intermediate host.

Metorchis conjunctus

• In cats—may infect the liver and biliary structures initially causing watery blood-tinged diarrhea and later evidence of biliary tree invasion; eggs are passed in feces 17 days from initial infection. • Infection typically associated with increased liver enzyme and may be associated with transient eosinophilia.

Heterobilharzia americana

• Eggs containing fully developed miracidium are passed in feces of definitive (final) host. In fresh water, eggs hatch, release miracidia that penetrate snail hosts, where sporocysts develop. Cercaria released from snail host 25 days after infection; these infect vertebrate host (dog, human) by skin penetration.

• Adult flukes develop in liver and migrate to mesenteric veins where eggs disseminate to various viscera, including liver, pancreas, mesenteric lymph nodes, spleen, and intestines; there they initiate granulomatous inflammation and sclerotic vascular lesions.

• Healing leads to scar formation and organ injury that can result in liver failure and gastrointestinal malabsorption. • Eggs appear in feces 68 days after infection.

Schistosoma haematobium

Adult fluke and eggs disperse to splanchnic organs, including liver and pancreas; in portal or hepatic veins eggs and adults associate with encapsulated fibrotic granulomatous foci.

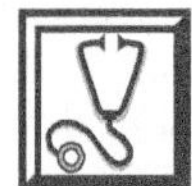

DIAGNOSIS

DIFFERENTIAL DIAGNOSIS

• Cholangiohepatitis; hepatic lipidosis; bile duct carcinoma; hepatic lymphoma; choleliths and any disorder causing major bile duct occlusion. • In dogs, primary gastrointestinal diseases and neoplasia (lymphoma) may be suspected. • Identified by finding trematode eggs in feces, rarely observing anechoic ovoid structures with echoic center in biliary tree by ultrasound, cytologic examination of bile or hepatic aspirates; most definitively from histopathology of biopsied liver, biliary structures, or pancreas.

CBC/BIOCHEMISTRY/URINALYSIS

• CBC—cats: variable; eosinophilia beginning 3 weeks after infection; persists for months; not all infected cats demonstrate eosinophilia; dogs: most common findings are lymphopenia and mild to marked thrombocytopenia; anemia; eosinophilia is uncommon.

• Biochemistry—cats: high liver enzyme activities, especially alanine aminotransferase (ALT) and aspartate aminotransferase (AST); alkaline phosphatase (ALP) may be normal or only slightly increased initially; bilirubin usually increased, markedly high in advanced cases; dogs: variable elevation in liver enzyme activities; hypercalcemia thought to be secondary to granulomatous inflammation; hypernatremia, hypercholesterolemia, hypo- or hyperalbuminemia, hyperglobulinemia, azotemia. • Bilirubin—cats: increased; markedly high in advanced severe disease; dogs: usually normal, may be increased.

• Urinalysis—cats: bilirubinuria.

OTHER LABORATORY TESTS

• Fasting/postprandial bile acid—increased.

• Fecal examination in cats—noninvasive definitive diagnostic test: *P. concinnum* eggs detected in only 25% of infected cats. • Fecal egg retrieval—cats: sedimentation most successful; formalin-ether or sodium acetate most reliable (demonstrates eightfold more eggs than direct fecal examination); dogs: sedimentation with saline recommended as miracidium will hatch in fresh water making identification difficult. Direct saline smear of feces may identify eggs. • Feline patients with few parasites (one to five flukes) may shed only 2–10 eggs/g of feces; eggs may not be discovered by fecal testing. • Serial fecal examinations may be necessary.

• Coagulation testing—dogs: prothombin time/partial thromboplastin time (PT/PTT) may be prolonged; antithrombin III (ATIII) decreased. • Parathyroid hormone/parathyroid-related hormone (PTH/PTHrp)—dogs: PTHrp may be elevated in hypercalcemic patients.

IMAGING

• Abdominal radiography—cats: may show mild hepatomegaly; dogs: may show hepatosplenomegaly, lymphadomegaly.

• Abdominal ultrasonography—cats: differentiates biliary obstruction from hepatocellular disease; shows one or more of the following: (1) biliary obstruction: dilated gallbladder, common bile duct (>2 mm), and intrahepatic ducts; (2) gallbladder sediment with flukes (oval hypoechoic structures with echoic center), mildly thick gallbladder wall with a double-layered appearance (cholecystitis); (3) hypoechoic hepatic parenchyma with prominent hyperechoic portal areas (ducts) associated with cholangiohepatitis; dogs: heterogeneous parenchyma, ascites, splenomegaly, lymphadomegaly, thickened gastric and intestinal walls.

DIAGNOSTIC PROCEDURES

- Fecal examination for trematode eggs.
- Cholecystocentesis—discloses fluke eggs in cats. • Liver biopsy (cats and dogs)—reveals signs of infection, ova.

PATHOLOGIC FINDINGS

Cats

- Gross—liver may appear large and yellow-green with dilated bile ducts; may see flukes in bile ducts or gallbladder; increased size and tortuosity of bile ducts on cut section. • Histologic lesions—depend on the number of flukes and duration of infestation; *early stage* (4–6 weeks): enlarged bile ducts and periductal areas infiltrated with inflammatory cells, especially eosinophils; *mid-stage* (4 months): severe adenomatous hyperplasia of bile duct epithelium and coincident periductal inflammation; *late stage* (6 months): extensive peribiliary fibrous connective tissue that may cause bile duct stenosis.

Dogs

- Gross—ulcerative gastritis, submucosal edema, red mucosal discoloration along intestinal tract, dystrophic mineralization of multiple organs. • Histologic lesions—trematode eggs in multiple organs; granulomatous inflammation and fibrosis throughout multiple organs; dystrophic mineralization of multiple organs.

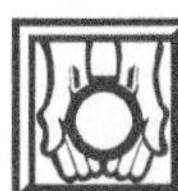

TREATMENT

Outpatient vs. inpatient—depends on severity of illness.

Inpatient

- Balanced polyionic fluids with supplemental potassium chloride 20–40 mEq/L; as appropriate; based on serum electrolytes. • Nutritional support—avoid development of hepatic lipidosis; feed high-protein calorically dense food and ensure food intake; use feeding tubes if needed to ensure adequate food intake in inappetent cats; rarely, severe clinical signs may require parenteral nutrition; rarely hepatic encephalopathy necessitates protein restriction. • B vitamin supplementation—important for anorectic and ill cats on fluid therapy; 2 mL B-soluble vitamins/L fluids.

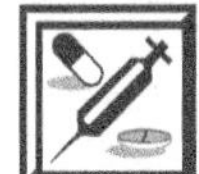

MEDICATIONS

DRUG(S) OF CHOICE

- Praziquantel 20 mg/kg SC q24h for 3–5 days is treatment of choice for cats; eggs may pass in feces for up to 2 months after treatment. For dogs, varying dosages have been reported. Praziquantel at 30 mg/kg PO once and 50 mg/kg SC once cleared a dog symptomatic for *H. americana*; more recently 25 mg/kg TID for 2 days and 3 days either orally or SQ, or 15–20 mg/kg PO q8h for 1–2 days is also reported. Some dogs were also treated concurrently with fenbendazole at 50 mg/kg PO q24h for 10 days. • Prednisolone—initial dose for cats showing eosinophilia, significant inflammation on biopsy or having severe clinical signs: 1–2 mg/kg/day for 2–4 weeks; then tapered in 50% decrements every 2 weeks. • Ursodeoxycholic acid 10–15 mg/kg q24h PO; tablet form and divided dose administered with feeding achieves best bioavailability; avoid if evidence of extrahepatic bile duct obstruction. • Broad-spectrum antibiotic coverage to protect against retrograde biliary tree infection with enteric organisms introduced by parasite; infection encouraged by fluke death in tissues.
- Antioxidant therapy—suggested by necro-inflammatory tissue injury; vitamin E (10 IU/kg day PO) and *S*-adenosyl-L-methionine (SAMe; Denosyl-SD4 has proven bioavailability in cats as a glutathione [GSH] donor): 20 mg/kg PO daily, enteric coated tablets, until liver enzymes normalize. • Antiemetic—metoclopramide (0.2–0.4 mg/kg PO, SC q6–8h or by constant rate infusion 1–2 mg/kg/day); ondansetron (0.5 mg/kg q12h IV or PO 30 minutes before feeding); maropitant (1.0 mg/kg [5 mg/cat] IV, SC or PO once per day; maximum of 5 days).

CONTRAINDICATIONS/POSSIBLE INTERACTIONS

Pregnancy—use caution with drug use.

FOLLOW-UP

PATIENT MONITORING

- Monitor clinical signs, appetite, body condition and weight, liver enzymes, bilirubin, and fecal sedimentation.
- Hypercalcemia in dogs usually resolves within 36–48 hours after praziquantel administration. • Watch for signs of biliary tree occlusion after administration of praziquantel. • Monitor fecal saline sedimentation for clearance of ova in dogs.

PREVENTION/AVOIDANCE

- Restrict outdoor access if endemic parasite.
- Praziquantel prophylaxis—every 3 months; for outdoor cats in endemic, tropical climates.

POSSIBLE COMPLICATIONS

- Death from liver failure; untreated symptomatic disease. • Biliary tree obstruction. • Pancreatitis. • Pancreatic exocrine insufficiency—with chronic infection. • Cholangitis/cholangiohepatitis (suppurative or nonsuppurative).

EXPECTED COURSE AND PROGNOSIS

Uncomplicated recovery with treatment expected in most patients.

L

MISCELLANEOUS

ZOONOTIC POTENTIAL

None

SEE ALSO

- Bile Duct Obstruction (Extrahepatic).
- Cholangitis/Cholangiohepatitis Syndrome.
- Hepatic Lipidosis.
- Hypercalcemia.

ABBREVIATIONS

- ALP = alkaline phosphatase.
- ALT = alanine aminotransferase.
- AST = aspartate aminotransferase.
- ATIII = antithrombin III.
- GSH = glutathione.
- PT = prothrombin time.
- PTH = parathyroid hormone.
- PTHrp = parathyroid-related hormone.
- PTT = partial thromboplastin time.
- PU/PD = polyuria/polydipsia.
- SAMe = *S*-adenosyl-L-methionine.

Suggested Reading

Fabrick C, Bugbee A, Fosgate G. Clinical features and outcome of *Heterobilharzia americana* infections in dogs, J Vet Intern Med 2010, 24:140–144.

Tams TR. Hepatobiliary parasites. In: Sherding RG, ed., The Cat: Disease and Management. Philadelphia, PA: Saunders, 1994, pp. 607–611.

Author Kate Holan

Consulting Editor Kate Holan

Acknowledgment The author/editor acknowledges the prior contribution of Julie R. Pembleton-Corbett.

LOWER URINARY TRACT INFECTION, BACTERIAL

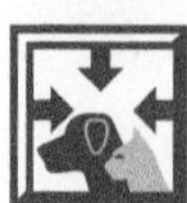

BASICS

DEFINITION

• Urinary tract infection (UTI)—bacterial adherence, replication, and persistence within the urinary tract associated with clinical signs and/or inflammation. • Sporadic cystitis (uncomplicated UTI): lower UTI that occurs no more than once every 6 months.
• Recurrent UTI—UTI that occurs ≥3 times in a year, or ≥2 times in 6 months. Subcategories include: ◦ Persistent—UTI that fails to resolve after appropriate antimicrobial therapy.
◦ Relapse—UTI that appears to resolve; however, subsequent urine cultures confirm persistence of the original bacterial isolate.
◦ Reinfection—UTI resolves with appropriate therapy but abnormal urinary defenses allow for recolonization of different bacterial species.
• Subclinical bacteriuria (asymptomatic bacteriuria)—bacterial presence within the urinary tract not associated with detectable clinical signs and/or inflammation.

L

PATHOPHYSIOLOGY

UTI development is dependent on the interplay between bacterial virulence factors and impairment of the anatomical, functional, environmental, and immunologic competency of the host. Most commonly, uropathogenic bacteria originate from the enteric flora and ascend from the distal urogenital tract into the proximal urethra and urinary bladder. Colonization may elicit a mucosal inflammatory response resulting in dysuria, pollakiuria, pyuria, and hematuria.

SYSTEMS AFFECTED

Renal/urologic.

INCIDENCE/PREVALENCE

• Bacteriuria is not equivalent to UTI. Current data identifies UTI prevalence given predisposing conditions. • Prevalence of bacteriuria in dogs: ◦ With subclinical bacteriuria: 2.1–8.9%. ◦ With diabetes mellitus: 37%. ◦ With hyperadrenocorticism, at diagnosis: 46%. ◦ With thoracolumbar intervertebral disc extrusion: 20.0–38.5%.
◦ With indwelling urinary catheters: 63.8%.
• Prevalence of bacteriuria in cats: ◦ With subclinical bacteriuria: 0.9–28.8%. ◦ With lower urinary tract-associated clinical signs: 3.4–12.0%. ◦ With ureteral calculi: 8.4%.
◦ With chronic kidney disease: 16.9–29.1%.
◦ With diabetes mellitus: 12.2–12.8%.
◦ With perineal urethrostomies: 22%.

GEOGRAPHIC DISTRIBUTION

N/A

SIGNALMENT

Species

More common in dogs than cats.

Breed Predilections

Breed-associated conditions (hyperadrenocorticism, urolithiasis, etc.) may promote bacteriuria.

Mean Age and Range

• UTIs occur at any age, but are more common in older dogs and cats. • Dogs—female: mean 7.7 ± 0.1 years; male: mean 8.0 ± 0.1 years. • Cats—female: mean 11.8 ± 4.4 years; male: mean 9.8 ± 4.8 years.

Predominant Sex

• Dogs—female dogs more commonly affected.
• Cats—female cats are slightly overrepresented.

SIGNS

Historical Findings

• Patients may be asymptomatic. • Pollakiuria, dysuria, hematuria, stranguria, inappropriate elimination, and excessive licking at or discharge from the genitalia may be present.
• Systemic clinical signs (anorexia, fever) are infrequent and suggest complicating factors (e.g., pyelonephritis).

Physical Examination Findings

• Unremarkable in most animals. • Abnormalities occasionally noted with urinary bladder palpation: ◦ Stimulation of micturition. ◦ Pain reactions.

CAUSES

• Uropathogenic bacteria commonly originate from enteric flora with rare hematogenous origins. • *Escherichia coli* is the most common bacterial isolate in dogs (45–55%) and cats (37.3%). • Eight species of bacteria (*E. coli*, *Staphylococcus*, *Proteus*, *Streptococcus*, *Klebsiella*, *Enterococcus*, *Pseudomonas*, and *Corynebacterium*) account for approximately 95% of UTIs.

RISK FACTORS

• Immune dysfunction/suppression (e.g., hyperadrenocorticism, feline leukemia virus [FeLV], feline immunodeficiency virus [FIV]).
• Nidus for bacterial adherence and harboring (e.g., indwelling urinary catheters, uroliths).
• Altered urine composition (e.g., persistently dilute urine, glucosuria). • Abnormal micturition/urine retention (e.g., loss of urethral tone, neurologic disease, urethral obstruction).
• Abnormal anatomy (e.g., ectopic ureters, hooded vulva). • Disrupted urinary tract mucosal defenses (e.g., mucosal trauma).

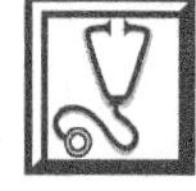

DIAGNOSIS

DIFFERENTIAL DIAGNOSIS

• UTI cannot be diagnosed or excluded based on the presence/absence of clinical signs. • Dysuria, pollakiuria, hematuria, and stranguria occur with lower urinary tract diseases including cystolithiasis, urinary tract neoplasia, prostatitis, obstructive uropathy, and feline idiopathic cystitis.

CBC/BIOCHEMISTRY/URINALYSIS

• CBC and biochemistry are unremarkable.
• Urinalysis: ◦ Proteinuria and hematuria indicate inflammation. ◦ Urine pH >7.5 may indicate the presence of urease-producing bacteria (*Proteus* spp., *Staphylococcus* spp., *Ureaplasma* spp., or *Corynebacterium* spp.). ◦ Pyuria is present in most animals with UTI but is not synonymous with infection. ◦ Bacteriuria identification increases UTI suspicion. Using a modified Wright–Giemsa stain (Diff-Quik) or Gram stain can improve bacterial detection.

OTHER LABORATORY TESTS

Urine Culture

• Definitive diagnosis requires aerobic urine culture. • In female dogs with limited antibiotic exposure forgoing a urine culture can be justified for uncomplicated UTI if the pathogen and local susceptibility patterns are known. In male dogs, cats, and animals with recurrent UTI urine culture is recommended. • Cystocentesis is the gold standard method for collecting urine culture specimens. Bacterial growth $>10^3$ cfu/mL is diagnostic. • Urine samples obtained by catheterization are often contaminated by the normal flora of the distal urethra. Bacterial growth $>10^4$ cfu/mL in male dogs, $>10^5$ cfu/mL in female dogs, and $>10^3$ cfu/mL in cats is diagnostic. Indwelling catheters may be colonized without concurrent UTI; therefore, sample collection from indwelling urinary catheters should be avoided. • Culturing voided midstream urine samples should be avoided unless other urine collection techniques are contraindicated or not possible. • Urine collected from nonsterile surfaces should not be cultured.

Antibiotic Sensitivity Testing

Antibiotic sensitivity is accurately predicted by use of the isolate's "susceptible" vs. "resistant" profiles.

IMAGING

Rarely is imaging necessary for uncomplicated infections. Radiographs, contrast studies, and ultrasound may help to identify recurrent UTI-predisposing causes.

DIAGNOSTIC PROCEDURES

Cystoscopy is used in patients with recurrent UTI to visualize abnormalities within the urinary bladder and urethra including uroliths, masses, polyps, ectopic ureters, etc.

PATHOLOGIC FINDINGS

N/A

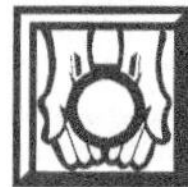

TREATMENT

APPROPRIATE HEALTH CARE

Outpatient treatment is appropriate; inpatient treatment may be necessary with UTI complications or associated conditions (e.g., acute pyelonephritis).

NURSING CARE
N/A

ACTIVITY
Unrestricted

DIET
N/A

CLIENT EDUCATION
N/A

SURGICAL CONSIDERATIONS
Management of uroliths, polypoid cystitis, and infection niduses may require surgical intervention.

MEDICATIONS

DRUG(S) OF CHOICE
• Given the morbidity associated with sporadic cystitis, empiric antimicrobial treatment is commonly started before receiving urine culture results. • When susceptibility data is available, the lowest tier antimicrobial should be selected. • "First-line" antimicrobials—should be selected when possible: ○ Amoxicillin (11–15 mg/kg PO q8h). ○ Trimethoprim-sulfadiazine (TMS) (15 mg/kg PO q12h). ○ Amoxicillin/clavulanic acid (12–25 mg/kg PO q12h).
• "Second-line" antimicrobials—reserved for resistant isolates based on culture and sensitivity or when patient factors prohibit the use of "first-line" therapies: ○ Floroquinolones (e.g., marbofloxacin 2.7–5.5 mg/kg PO q24h; enrofloxacin; ciprofloxacin). ○ Cefovecin (8 mg/kg SC). ○ Nitrofurantoin (4.4–5.0 mg/kg PO q8h).
• "Third-line" antimicrobials—reserved for multidrug resistant infections necessitating therapeutic intervention: ○ Amikacin (dogs 15–30 mg/kg IV or SC q24h; cats 10–14 mg/kg IV or SC q24h). ○ Chloramphenicol (dogs 40–50 mg/kg PO q8h; cats 12.5–20 mg/kg [not exceeding 50 mg/cat] PO q12h).
• Antibiotic treatment of uncomplicated infections is recommended for 3–10 days.
• Recurrent UTI treatment requires a urine culture and sensitivity. • Treatment durations are extended for persistent and relapse infections (up to 4 weeks).
• Reinfections are treated as multiple uncomplicated infections, however an attempt to identify an abnormality in host defenses should be pursued.

CONTRAINDICATIONS
N/A

PRECAUTIONS
Pyelonephritis or prostatitis necessitates therapies able to penetrate the respective tissues (see Pyelonephritis; Prostatitis and Prostatic Abscess).

POSSIBLE INTERACTIONS
N/A

ALTERNATE DRUGS
Nonsteroidal anti-inflammatory drugs (NSAIDs) may be used cautiously to reduce clinical signs in dogs with cystitis while awaiting urine culture results. They should not be used in dehydrated patients.

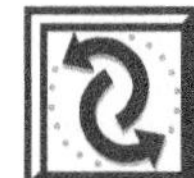

FOLLOW-UP

PATIENT MONITORING
• For uncomplicated UTIs clinical improvement should occur within 48 hours. If clinical signs remain for >48 hours, complicating factors should be investigated.
• Complicated UTIs—continue therapy for 7–10 days beyond resolution of clinical signs, pyuria, and bacteriuria. Confirm resolution via urine culture 7–10 days after end of therapy.

PREVENTION/AVOIDANCE
• Diagnosis and control of predisposing conditions is the most effective method for preventing UTIs. • Ancillary therapies can be considered to prevent recurrence: ○ Cranberry extract may inhibit *E. coli* attachment to the bladder mucosa. ○ Methenamine—converted into formalin when urine pH is <7.0. Concurrent administration of ascorbic acid (vitamin C) promotes urinary acidification. ○ Prophylactic antibiotics—once-daily administration of antibiotics may lengthen infection-free intervals; however, multidrug resistance is likely in subsequent isolates.

POSSIBLE COMPLICATIONS
UTIs may lead to pyelonephritis, struvite urolith formation, or polypoid cystitis.

EXPECTED COURSE AND PROGNOSIS
Prognosis for patients with uncomplicated UTIs is excellent. The prognosis for patients with complicated infections is determined by successful control or resolution of predisposing conditions.

MISCELLANEOUS

ASSOCIATED CONDITIONS
• Struvite urolithiasis. • Polypoid cystitis.
• Pyelonephritis. • Prostatitis.
• Emphysematous cystitis.

AGE-RELATED FACTORS
Juvenile animals with recurrent UTIs should be evaluated for urolithiasis or urinary tract malformations.

ZOONOTIC POTENTIAL
N/A

PREGNANCY/FERTILITY/BREEDING
N/A

SYNONYMS
Bacterial cystitis.

SEE ALSO
• Prostatitis and Prostatic Abscess.
• Pyelonephritis.
• Urolithiasis, Struvite—Dogs.

ABBREVIATIONS
• FeLV = feline leukemia virus.
• FIV = feline infectious virus.
• NSAID = nonsteroidal anti-inflammatory drug.
• TMS = trimethoprim-sulfadiazine.
• UTI = urinary tract infection.

Suggested Reading

Weese JS, Blondeau JM, Boothe D, et al. International Society for Companion Animal Infectious Diseases (ISCAID) guidelines for the diagnosis and management of bacterial urinary tract infections in dogs and cats. Vet J 2019, 247:8–25.

Wood MW. Lower urinary tract infections. In: Ettinger SJ, Feldman EC, Cote E, eds., Textbook of Veterinary Internal Medicine, 8th ed. St. Louis, MO: Saunders, 2016, pp. 1992–1996.

Author Michael W. Wood

Consulting Editor J.D. Foster

Acknowledgment The author and editors acknowledge the prior contribution of Barrak M. Pressler.

Client Education Handout available online

L

LOWER URINARY TRACT INFECTION, FUNGAL

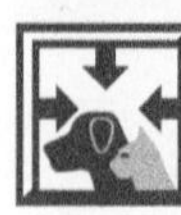

BASICS

OVERVIEW

- Funguria is usually due to ascending infection of normal commensal flora of the skin and mucosa, or environmentally ubiquitous organisms (primary funguria).
- *Candida albicans* is the most common isolate; other *Candida* spp. are less common, and non-*Candida* spp. fungi are rare.
- Urinary shedding may occur with systemic fungal infections (secondary funguria).
- Organ system affected—renal/urologic.

SIGNALMENT

- Dog and cat.
- German shepherd dogs and female dogs are overrepresented in systemic aspergillosis.

SIGNS

- Dysuria, stranguria, and pollakiuria; gross hematuria is rare.
- Many animals are asymptomatic.

CAUSES & RISK FACTORS

- Fungal urinary tract infections (UTIs) are associated with immunosuppression or immunocompromised disease states.
- Suspected risk factors—diabetes mellitus, urinary tract stomata (perineal urethrostomy, cystotomy tubes, indwelling urinary catheters), lower urinary tract disease (transitional cell carcinoma, chronic bacterial UTI), recent or chronic antibiotic or immunosuppressive therapy.

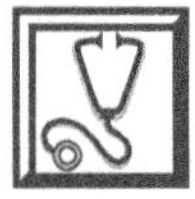

DIAGNOSIS

DIFFERENTIAL DIAGNOSIS

- Causes of lower urinary tract disease including bacterial UTI, cystolithiasis, sterile cystitis, urethritis, and bladder and urethral neoplasia.
- Primary funguria must be differentiated from systemic infections with secondary funguria.
- Contamination of urine samples during collection may occur in animals with cutaneous or mucocutaneous yeast overgrowth.

CBC/BIOCHEMISTRY/URINALYSIS

- Yeast/fungal elements are often visible within urine sediment. *Candida* spp. may appear as both budding yeast and filamentous structures.
- CBC and biochemistry usually unremarkable. With renal or systemic involvement, abnormalities will reflect those organs involved.

IMAGING

- Chest radiographs and abdominal ultrasound screen for diseases causing immunocompromise.
- Spinal radiographs may show diskospondylitis in cases of systemic aspergillosis.

DIAGNOSTIC PROCEDURES

Urine Culture

- *Candida* spp. grow within 3 days on standard blood agar.
- Other fungi grow more slowly and thus will not be detected by standard urine culture protocols.
- If fungal UTI is suspected or confirmed, fungal culture should be requested.

Antifungal Sensitivity Testing

- *C. albicans* is usually susceptible to fluconazole; antifungal sensitivity testing is typically unnecessary.
- Non-*albicans* species of *Candida* are more commonly resistant to fluconazole, and thus susceptibility testing should be considered.
- Susceptibility testing should be performed on non-*Candida* spp. and with persistent *Candida* spp. UTI despite 4–6 weeks of appropriate antifungal therapy.

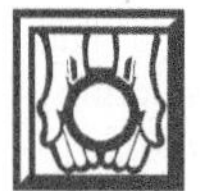

TREATMENT

- Identify and correct any risk factors.
- Patients with asymptomatic funguria and no risk factors for disease should have a repeat urine culture performed prior to starting therapy.

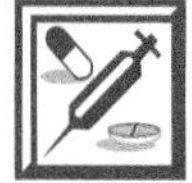

MEDICATIONS

DRUG(S) OF CHOICE

- Fluconazole 5–10 mg/kg PO q12h is the initial treatment of choice for *C. albicans*.
- Antifungal therapy for non-*C. albicans* spp. should be based on susceptibility testing.
- Drugs with poor urinary excretion of active drug, such as itraconazole, ketoconazole, posaconazole, and voriconazole, are not recommended.
- Patients with persistent infection after 4–8 weeks of fluconazole may benefit from intravesicular infusion of 1% clotrimazole.
- Amphotericin B (intravenous or intravesicular) can be used, but efficacy is unknown. Intravenous therapy is primarily used for systemic disease.

CONTRAINDICATIONS/POSSIBLE INTERACTIONS

Intravesicular clotrimazole should be avoided in animals with recent bladder surgery or urethral trauma.

FOLLOW-UP

- Repeat urine sediment and urine culture every 2–3 weeks to confirm treatment efficacy. Treatment should be continued for a minimum of 4–6 weeks.
- Urine sediment analysis and culture should be performed 1 and 2 months after cessation of therapy.
- 25% of dogs and cats with candiduria may have persistent and asymptomatic infections. Treatment should be reserved for symptomatic episodes in these patients.

MISCELLANEOUS

ASSOCIATED CONDITIONS

- Diabetes mellitus.
- Transitional cell carcinoma.

SEE ALSO

- Aspergillosis, Disseminated Invasive.
- Aspergillosis, Nasal.
- Cryptococcosis.
- Immunodeficiency Disorders, Primary.

ABBREVIATIONS

- UTI = urinary tract infection.

Suggested Reading

Jin Y, Lin D. Fungal urinary tract infections in the dog and cat: a retrospective study (2001–2004). J Am Anim Hosp Assoc 2005, 41:373–381.

Pressler B. Fungal urinary tract infection. In: Bartges J, Polzin DJ, eds., Nephrology and Urology of Small Animals. Ames, IA: Wiley Blackwell, 2011, pp. 717–724.

Pressler B, Vaden SL, Lane IF, et al. *Candida* spp. urinary tract infections in 13 dogs and seven cats: predisposing factors, treatment, and outcome. J Am Anim Hosp Assoc 2003, 39:263–270.

Schultz RM, Johnson EG, Wisner ER, et al. Clinicopathologic and diagnostic imaging characteristics of systemic aspergillosis in 30 dogs. J Vet Intern Med 2008, 22:851–859.

Author Nahvid M. Etedali

Consulting Editor J.D. Foster

Acknowledgment The author and editors acknowledge the prior contribution of Barrak M. Pressler.

LUMBOSACRAL STENOSIS AND CAUDA EQUINA SYNDROME

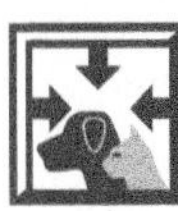

BASICS

DEFINITION

- Lumbosacral stenosis refers to narrowing of the lumbosacral vertebral canal and/or L7–sacral intervertebral foramina, causing compression of L7, sacral, or caudal nerves.
- Cauda equina syndrome implies pain or other clinical signs related to dysfunction of these nerves.

PATHOPHYSIOLOGY

- Congenital—abnormal vertebral development causing narrowing of the lumbosacral vertebral canal. Transitional vertebrae and other malformations are common at this site and may contribute to (early) disease progression.
- Acquired—bony and soft tissue degenerative changes, most commonly affecting the L7 intervertebral disc, that cause stenosis of the vertebral canal and/or intervertebral foramina. Specific syndrome of sacral osteochondrosis dissecans is recognized in young German shepherd dogs and other breeds.

SYSTEMS AFFECTED

Nervous—specifically nerves from L7 caudally.

GENETICS

No known genetic basis.

INCIDENCE/PREVALENCE

Unknown

SIGNALMENT

Species

- Reasonably common in dogs.
- Uncommonly reported in cats but suspected with increasing frequency.

Breed Predilections

- Congenital—small to medium dogs; border collies.
- Acquired—any medium–large dog; often suspected in working dogs, so frequently German shepherd dogs and Malinois but also common in boxers, Rottweilers.

Mean Age and Range

- Congenital—3–8 years.
- Acquired—mean age at onset 6–7 years. Sacral osteochondrosis signs often appear ~1 year old.

Predominant Sex

- Congenital—none.
- Acquired—male.

SIGNS

- Lumbosacral pain—salient feature; may be the only clinical sign; may be evident in reluctance to jump or climb stairs. Pain on pressure on, or dorsiflexion of, the lumbosacral vertebral column (often also induced during extension of hip joints).
- Pelvic limb lameness—caused by lumbar 7th and/or sacral nerve dysfunction; may progress to pelvic limb weakness, muscle wasting, and postural reaction deficits.
- Urinary and/or fecal incontinence—caused by S1–3 nerve dysfunction.
- Abnormal tail carriage, tail weakness or paralysis—results from dysfunction of caudal nerves.
- Self-inflicted lesions—most often associated with congenital lesions or cauda equina inflammation.

CAUSES

- Congenital vertebral malformation, including transitional vertebrae, or osteochondrosis of the cranial sacrum.
- Intervertebral disc herniation (types I and II).
- Hypertrophy or hyperplasia of the interarcuate ligament.
- Proliferation of the articular facets and/or periarticular soft tissues.
- Subluxation at the lumbosacral junction.
- Inflammatory or neoplastic disease of the vertebral canal can produce identical clinical signs (hence "cauda equina syndrome").

RISK FACTORS

Dogs with lumbosacral transitional vertebrae, especially German shepherd dogs, have increased risk to develop the syndrome.

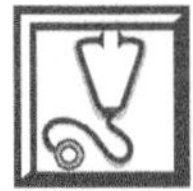

DIAGNOSIS

DIFFERENTIAL DIAGNOSIS

- Hip dysplasia or other orthopedic disease (notably iliopsoas injury)—distinguish via thorough orthopedic examination ± imaging.
- Chronic discospondylitis, osteomyelitis, neoplastic disease—cannot be differentiated by clinical signs alone.
- Vertebral fractures and subluxations—acute; characterized by more bilateral signs.
- Localized meningomyelitis or radiculoneuritis—usually more diffuse pain.

CBC/BIOCHEMISTRY/URINALYSIS

- Usually normal.
- Urinalysis—may reveal lower urinary tract infection secondary to urinary incontinence, or associated with discospondylitis.

OTHER LABORATORY TESTS

If images suggest the need, cerebrospinal fluid (CSF) analysis may aid in diagnosing inflammatory (or infectious or neoplastic) disease.

IMAGING

- Radiology—commonly exhibit spondylosis at the lumbosacral junction; narrowing of the L7–S1 disc space; ventral displacement of the sacrum relative to the lumbar vertebrae; *but* interpret with caution because all these can be observed in clinically normal animals.
- CT and MRI—modalities of choice. Apparent abnormalities must be interpreted with regard to the whole clinical picture because many are also observed in normal animals.

DIAGNOSTIC PROCEDURES

- Electromyography—denervation may be detected in muscles innervated by the nerves L7 to caudal; denervation confirms localization of the lesion but is not specific for compressive lesions.
- Slowed sciatic–tibial nerve conduction or prolongation of F wave latencies may be detected.

PATHOLOGIC FINDINGS

- May see one or more of the following features:
  - Type II disc disease with bulging of dorsal annulus.
  - Hypertrophy of the interarcuate ligament.
  - Stenosis of the intervertebral foramen by soft tissue or bony proliferation compressing L7 nerve(s) or as a congenital lesion.
  - Ventral displacement of the sacrum in relation to lumbar vertebrae.
  - Proliferation of articular facets and hypertrophy of joint capsule.
  - Congenitally shortened pedicles.
  - Thickened and sclerotic laminae and articular processes.
  - Various vertebral malformations (not only transitional vertebrae).
- Cauda equina syndrome can also be associated with neoplasia, inflammation, infection.

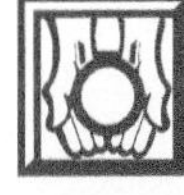

TREATMENT

APPROPRIATE HEALTH CARE

Urinary incontinence—inpatient for initial management.

NURSING CARE

Urinary incontinence—manual expression or catheterize the bladder until adequate voluntary control returns; monitor for urinary tract infection and administer appropriate antibiotics following culture and sensitivity.

ACTIVITY

- Nonsurgical treatment—confinement and restricted leash walks, alone or combined with systemic anti-inflammatory drugs or analgesics, or epidural injection of corticosteroids, frequently alleviate pain; clinical signs may return with increasing levels of exercise.
- If treated surgically, restrict for 6–12 weeks; then gradual return to athletic function.

LUMBOSACRAL STENOSIS AND CAUDA EQUINA SYNDROME (CONTINUED)

DIET

Avoid obesity; excess weight increases biomechanical stress on the spine.

CLIENT EDUCATION

- Inform client that there may be progressive neurologic impairment of the pelvic limbs, urinary and fecal incontinence, and paralysis of the tail.
- Inform client that pelvic limb lameness and self-inflicted lesions result from pain associated with nerve root irritation and/or compression.
- Discuss surgical treatment, which is appropriate for cases with severe pain and may be suitable for cases with neurologic deficits (especially incontinence, which may be difficult to reverse).
- Medical management is frequently successful for animals with mild pain and/or mild neurologic deficits only.

L

SURGICAL CONSIDERATIONS

Several options, each focused on alleviating the specific source of the problems defined by imaging; dorsal laminectomy, lateral foraminotomy, or fixation–fusion may all be effective in specifically selected cases.

MEDICATIONS

DRUG(S) OF CHOICE

- NSAIDs—e.g., carprofen 2 mg/kg q12h for 5–7 days then reducing doses until PRN.
- Gabapentin—frequently used at ~20–30 mg/kg q8h and may be effective (side effect: sedation; dizziness reported in humans).
- Epidural corticosteroid—methylprednisolone acetate 1 mg/kg (<0.5 mL total volume).

CONTRAINDICATIONS

N/A

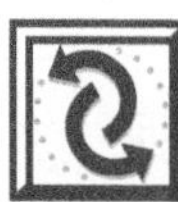

FOLLOW-UP

PREVENTION/AVOIDANCE

N/A

POSSIBLE COMPLICATIONS

- Syndrome progression, increasingly severe neurologic signs.
- Seroma formation—frequent sequela to surgery; can be effectively managed by cage rest and surgical drainage. Prevent by careful soft tissue closure.
- Adhesions between nerves and surrounding soft tissues after surgery.
- Recurrence of clinical signs following medical (commonly) or surgical (less commonly) intervention.
- Failure of fixation–fusion implant.
- Fracture of articular process after excessive lateral bone excision at surgery.
- Infection (especially if an implant is used for surgery).

EXPECTED COURSE AND PROGNOSIS

- Vary with the severity of neurologic injury.
- Majority are successfully managed medically, but need to ensure outcome matches requirements for dog's way of life; surgery remains an option.
- If low lumbar pain and mild neurologic deficits—good prognosis after surgery; 70–80% have an excellent or good outcome.
- If fecal and urinary incontinence—guarded prognosis.

MISCELLANEOUS

ASSOCIATED CONDITIONS

Lower urinary tract infections frequently accompany urinary incontinence.

AGE-RELATED FACTORS

- If a lumbosacral transitional vertebra is present, syndrome may develop 1–2 years earlier than the average dog.
- Older large-breed dogs may have concomitant diseases that also cause neurologic deficits: type II disc protrusions at other sites, degenerative peripheral nerve disease (especially Labrador retrievers), degenerative myelopathy (especially German shepherd dogs).

SYNONYMS

- Lumbosacral instability.
- Lumbosacral malarticulation or malformation.
- Lumbosacral spondylolisthesis.
- Lumbosacral spondylopathy.

SEE ALSO

- Discospondylitis.
- Intervertebral Disc Disease—Cats.
- Intervertebral Disc Disease, Thoracolumbar.

ABBREVIATIONS

- CSF = cerebrospinal fluid.
- NSAID = nonsteroidal anti-inflammatory drug.

INTERNET RESOURCES

http://veterinarymedicine.dvm360.com/vetmed/Medicine/Degenerative-lumbosacralstenosis-in-dogs/Article Standard/Article/detail/169902

Suggested Reading

De Risio L, Sharp NJ, Olby NJ, et al. Predictors of outcome after dorsal decompressive laminectomy for degenerative lumbosacral stenosis in dogs: 69 cases (1987–1997). J Am Vet Med Assoc 2001, 219(5):624–628.

Janssens L, Beosier Y, Daems R. Lumbosacral degenerative stenosis in the dog. The results of epidural infiltration with methylprednisolone acetate: a retrospective study. Vet Comp Orthop Traumatol 2009, 22(6):486–491.

Jeffery ND, Barker A, Harcourt-Brown T. What progress has been made in the understanding and treatment of degenerative lumbosacral stenosis in dogs during the past 30 years? Vet J 2014, 201(1):9–14.

Jones JC, Banfield CM, Ward DL. Association between postoperative outcome and results of magnetic resonance imaging and computed tomography in working dogs with degenerative lumbosacral stenosis. J Am Vet Med Assoc 2000, 216(11):1769–1774.

Linn L, Bartels K, Rochat M, et al. Lumbosacral stenosis in 29 military working dogs: Epidemiologic findings and outcome after surgical intervention (1990–1999). Vet Surg 2003, 32:21–29.

Meij BP, Bergknut N. Degenerative lumbosacral stenosis in dogs. Vet Clin North Am Small Anim Pract 2010, 40(5):983–1009.

Suwankong N, Voorhout G, Hazewinkle HA, Meij BP. Agreement between computed tomography, magnetic resonance imaging, and surgical findings in dogs with degenerative lumbosacral stenosis. J Am Vet Med Assoc 2006, 229(12):1924–1929.

Author Nick D. Jeffery

Client Education Handout available online

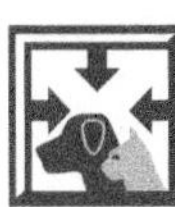

BASICS

OVERVIEW

• Twisting of lung lobe(s) at the hilus with occlusion or narrowing of the bronchus, lymphatics, vein, and (finally) arteries. • Affected lobes—right middle lobe most commonly affected (especially in large dogs) with preexisting pleural effusion; other lobes can twist singly or in pairs. Occasionally torsion occurs in midlobar area. Pugs are very commonly affected, with the left cranial lobe most common. • Initially, the lobe becomes engorged with blood and enlarges; infarction and necrosis may follow; hemorrhagic pleural effusion typically develops.

SIGNALMENT

• Dogs and less commonly cats. • Pugs are most commonly affected, although any dog may be affected. • Large-breed dogs more commonly have pleural effusion first, and then develop torsion. • Afghan hounds were initially reported as commonly affected due to chylothorax, but this is rarely seen. • Any age. • More common in males.

SIGNS

• Tachypnea, acute or chronic respiratory distress. • Lethargy. • Anorexia. • Fever. • Pain. • Orthopnea. • Cough, hemoptysis. • Retching. • Tachycardia. • Pale mucous membranes. • Cyanosis.

CAUSES & RISK FACTORS

• Inconsistently found with preexisting conditions (e.g., trauma, neoplasia, and chylothorax; asthma/bronchitis in the cat). Atelectasis and or pleural effusion seem to be predisposing factors. • Thoracic or diaphragmatic surgery. • Spontaneous or idiopathic.

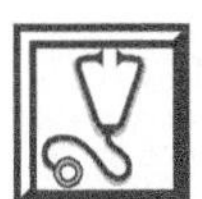

DIAGNOSIS

DIFFERENTIAL DIAGNOSIS

• Pulmonary contusion or atelectasis. • Diaphragmatic hernia. • Pulmonary abscess or infarction. • Neoplasia. • Coagulopathy. • Pneumonia, embolization, or thrombosis. • Congestive heart failure. • Pleural effusion and compression atelectasis. • Fungal or foreign body granuloma. • Lobar consolidation or bronchial obstruction from a foreign body.

CBC/BIOCHEMISTRY/URINALYSIS

Nonspecific abnormalities.

OTHER LABORATORY TESTS

Fluid analysis—pleural effusion can be hemorrhagic; with chronicity or preexisting effusions; the effusion may be a modified transudate or chylous.

IMAGING

Radiography

• Opacification of affected lobe with loss of visible lobar vessels and truncation of bronchus. • Initially may reveal air bronchograms with proximal narrowing or disorientation of the torsed bronchus. Small gas bubbles with "sponge appearance" can be scattered throughout affected lobe (vesicular gas pattern); seen in 87% of one series. • Progressive pleural effusion—suggested by ventral leafing and interlobar fissure lines. • Consolidation and occasional swelling of the torsed lobe with possible displacement or rotation of the heart, trachea, or carina. Mediastinal shift can be contralateral or ipsilateral. Other lobes can be displaced. • Thoracentesis provides therapeutic benefits and can improve visualization of intrathoracic structures.

Ultrasonography

• Thoracic ultrasound prior to fluid removal often allows better resolution of internal structures. • Hypoechoic periphery with scattered reverberating foci (bronchial cartilage) centrally. • Rounded edges of lobes.

CT

Very useful for confirmation of diagnosis.

DIAGNOSTIC PROCEDURES

• Thoracentesis—obtain pleural fluid for analysis (modified transudate, exudate, hemorrhage, or chylous effusion possible). • Bronchoscopy—may reveal occlusion or twist of the associated bronchus. • Surgical exploration—for definitive diagnosis and treatment.

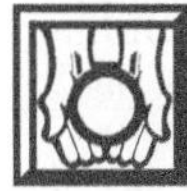

TREATMENT

• Thoracentesis or chest tube placement as needed. • Intravenous fluid administration for support. • Administer oxygen and treat for shock—when indicated. • Anesthesia—requires adequate ventilatory support; carefully monitor patient. • Surgical removal of the involved lobe(s)—only effective treatment; do not untwist lobe and attempt to salvage—may lead to recurrence or necrosis; in situ ligation of the vessels or clamping with noncrushing forceps has been advocated to avoid reperfusion problems such as acidosis; consider use of surgical stapling device; closely inspect remaining thoracic structures for any abnormalities; perform culture and pathologic examination of excised specimen. • Post surgery—monitoring; supportive care; tube drainage. Torsion of a second lung lobe may occur.

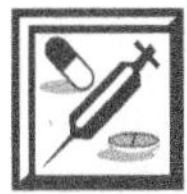

MEDICATIONS

DRUG(S) OF CHOICE

• Antibiotics—perioperatively. • Pain control.

CONTRAINDICATIONS/POSSIBLE INTERACTIONS

N/A

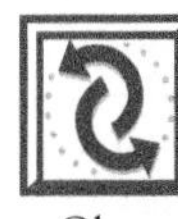

FOLLOW-UP

• Observe for recurrence of pleural effusion. • Reexpansion pulmonary edema—can be a serious problem (especially in cats) if large volumes of pleural fluid are withdrawn quickly or if chronically compressed lungs are acutely inflated at surgery. • Thoracic radiographs—before discharge; as needed thereafter. • Prognosis—fair to good if no underlying abnormality remains.

MISCELLANEOUS

Suggested Reading

Benavides KL, Rozanski EA, Oura TJ. Lung lobe torsion in 35 dogs and 4 cats. Can Vet J. 2019, 60(1):60–66.

D'Anjou M, Tidwell AS, Hecht S. Radiographic diagnosis of lung lobe torsion. Vet Radiol Ultrasound 2005, 46:478–484.

Park KM, Grimes JA, Wallace ML, et al. Lung lobe torsion in dogs: 52 cases (2005–2017). Vet Surg 2018, 47(8):1002–1008.

Wainberg SH, Brisson BA, Reabel SN, et al. Evaluation of risk factors for mortality in dogs with lung lobe torsion: a retrospective study of 66 dogs (2000–2015). Can Vet J 2019, 60(2):167–173.

Author Bradley L. Moses

Consulting Editor Elizabeth Rozanski

LUPUS ERYTHEMATOSUS, CUTANEOUS (DISCOID)

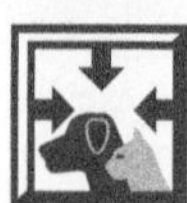

BASICS

OVERVIEW

• Considered to be a relatively benign variant of systemic lupus erythematosus (SLE). • Divided into facial discoid lupus erythematosus (FDLE) and generalized DLE (GDLE). • FDLE is one of the most common immune-mediated skin diseases in dogs. • FDLE predominantly involves the nasal planum, face, and ears. • GDLE—lesions progress beyond the head.

SIGNALMENT

• Dogs and cats. • Very uncommon in cats. • FDLE—collie, German shepherd dog, Siberian husky, Shetland sheepdog, Alaskan Malamute, chow chow, and their crosses. • GDLE—German shepherd dog and Chinese crested (predominantly). • FDLE—no age predilection; GDLE—older dogs.

SIGNS

FDLE

• Initial depigmentation of nasal planum and/or lips progresses to erosions and ulcerations. • Loss of normal "cobblestone" architecture of the nasal planum. • Tissue loss and scarring can occur. • Chronic lesions are fragile and may easily bleed; severe hemorrhage associated with arteriole damage. • May involve pinnae and periocular region.

GDLE

• Lesion behind the neck and/or on mucocutaneous junctions. • Initial lesion—annular hyperpigmented plaques with adherent crust, follicular plugging and central alopecia. • Advanced lesions—reticulated patterns of hyperpigmentation or hypertrophic scars.

CAUSES & RISK FACTORS

• Actinic radiation may alter antigenic nature of keratinocytes. • Seasonal and geographic exacerbation.

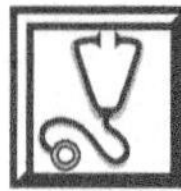

DIAGNOSIS

DIFFERENTIAL DIAGNOSIS

Major Considerations

• Other immune-mediated diseases (pemphigus foliaceus, pemphigus erythematosus, SLE, ischemic dermatitis, vasculitis). • Drug reaction. • Dermatomyositis. • Nasal dermatophytosis. • Mucocutaneous pyoderma. • Insect bite hypersensitivity.

Other (Rare) Considerations

• Contact allergy. • Zinc-responsive dermatosis. • Trauma. • Superficial necrolytic dermatitis. • Epitheliotropic lymphoma. • Squamous cell carcinoma.

CBC/BIOCHEMISTRY/URINALYSIS

Normal unless due to an underlying cause.

OTHER LABORATORY TESTS

Antinuclear antibody (ANA), LE preparation, and Coombs' tests—usually normal or negative except in SLE.

DIAGNOSTIC PROCEDURES

• Biopsy and histopathology will differentiate DLE from most other disorders; may be complicated by untreated mucocutaneous pyoderma. • Biopsy early lesions—depigmented areas, mild erosions, or mildly crusted lesions.

PATHOLOGIC FINDINGS

Interface-lichenoid dermatitis with prominent basal cell apoptosis, varying degrees of epidermal atrophy, and pigment incontinence;. chronic lesions may include scarring.

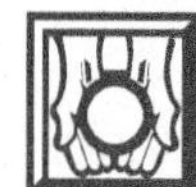

TREATMENT

• FDLE—good prognosis; may be disfiguring. • GDLE—guarded prognosis; depends on response to therapy. • Avoid sunlight/apply sunblock.

MEDICATIONS

DRUG(S) OF CHOICE

• Topical therapy (FDLE):
○ Glucocorticosteroids—potent fluorinated product initially; less potent product later if possible (q24h for 14 days; then q48–72h).
○ Tacrolimus ointment (0.1%) q12–24h initially then taper to q24–72h once in remission. ○ Use a soft muzzle for 10 minutes after applying topical therapy to prevent medication removal by the patient.
• Systemic therapy (GDLE; severe FDLE):
○ Tetracycline and niacinamide—250 mg each PO q8h for dogs <10 kg; 500 mg PO q8h for larger dogs (alternatives include doxycycline 10 mg/kg PO q24h and minocycline 5 mg/kg PO q12h).
○ Prednisolone—2–4 mg/kg/day either solely or in combination with azathioprine 2 mg/kg PO q48h; taper prednisone to 0.5–1 mg/kg PO q48h for long-term maintenance.
○ Cyclosporine—5–10 mg/kg PO q24h as alternative immunosuppressive therapy.
• Systemic antibiotic treatment for 3–4 weeks prior to systemic immunosuppressive therapy to differentiate from mucocutaneous pyoderma. • Vitamin E—10–20 IU/kg PO q12h may help reduce inflammation and protect the skin. • Hydroxychloroquine—5 mg/kg q24h; antimalarial drug that has been used in human cases.

FOLLOW-UP

PATIENT MONITORING

• Recheck 4 weeks after initiating treatment to evaluate for clinical response. • CBC and biochemistry—every 12 months (topical therapy); every 3–6 months (systemic therapy). • Azathioprine—CBC and platelet counts every 2 weeks for the first month, then every 3–6 months.

PREVENTION/AVOIDANCE

Affected animals should avoid UV light exposure.

POSSIBLE COMPLICATIONS

• Scarring. • Secondary pyoderma. • Hemorrhage. • Disfigurement.

EXPECTED COURSE AND PROGNOSIS

• FDLE—progressive but not usually life-threatening if left untreated. • With proper treatment, expect remission in majority of cases. • GDLE—prognosis is more guarded.

MISCELLANEOUS

ABBREVIATIONS

• ANA = antinuclear antibody.
• FDLE = facial discoid lupus erythematosus.
• GDLE = generalized discoid lupus erythematosus.
• LE = lupus erythematosus.
• SLE = systemic lupus erythematosus.

Suggested Reading

Banovic F. Canine cutaneous lupus erythematosus: newly discovered variants. Vet Clin Small Anim 2019, 49:37–45.

Thierry O, Linder KE, Banovic F. Cutaneous lupus erythematosus in the dogs: a comprehensive review. BMC Vet Res 2018, 14:132.

Author Dawn E. Logas

Consulting Editor Alexander H. Werner Resnick

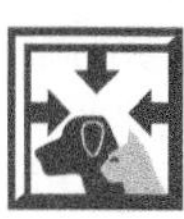

BASICS

DEFINITION

A systemic autoimmune disease characterized by the formation of antibodies against a wide array of self-antigens. Pathogenic antibodies, circulating immune complexes, and autoreactive T-cells are the primary mediators of tissue injury.

PATHOPHYSIOLOGY

- Antigen–antibody complexes are formed and deposited in a variety of sites, including blood vessels, glomeruli, synovial membranes, choroid plexus, and skin (type III hypersensitivity).
- Antibodies directed against a broad range of membrane, cytoplasmic, and nuclear antigens are produced, resulting in direct cytotoxic damage (type II hypersensitivity).
- Production of autoreactive T-cells causes cell-mediated damage (type IV hypersensitivity).
- Tissue injury is caused by immune-complex mediated activation of complement, infiltration of inflammatory cells, and direct cytotoxicity of autoantibodies against membrane-bound antigens.
- Clinical manifestations depend on localization of the immune complexes and specificity of the autoantibodies.
- Genetic, environmental, pharmacologic, and infectious factors may be triggers.

SYSTEMS AFFECTED

- Musculoskeletal—deposition of immune complexes in synovial membranes.
- Skin/exocrine—deposition of immune complexes in the skin.
- Renal/urologic—immune-complex glomerulonephritis.
- Hemic/lymphatic/immune—autoantibodies against red blood cells (RBCs), leukocytes, platelets, and bone marrow precursors.
- Other organ systems—associated with deposition of immune complexes or antibodies.

GENETICS

- In dogs, SLE has been positively associated with the presence of dog leukocyte antigen (DLA) A7 and negatively associated with the presence of DLA A1 and B5. Decreased serum IgA has been reported as a predisposing factor for SLE in dogs.
- An immune-mediated disease in the Nova Scotia duck tolling retriever characterized by immune-mediated arthropathy and steroid-responsive meningitis–arteritis has been reported and is termed SLE-related disease in this breed.

INCIDENCE/PREVALENCE

Uncommon in dog, rare in cat.

SIGNALMENT

Species

Dog and cat—male dogs overrepresented.

Breed Predilections

- Medium to large breeds; breed predispositions reported for the Finnish spitz, German Shepherd dog, Shetland sheepdog, collie, beagle, and poodle.
- Purebred cats, particularly Siamese and Persians, may be at increased risk.

Mean Age and Range

Mean age 5 years; range 6 months to 13 years.

SIGNS

Historical Findings

- Onset of clinical signs may be acute or insidious with waxing and waning course, and different clinical manifestations may occur sequentially:
  - Lethargy/weakness.
  - Anorexia.
  - Shifting-leg lameness.
  - Skin lesions.

Physical Examination Findings

- Swollen and/or painful joints are the major presenting sign. Joints are swollen but not deformed (nonerosive).
- Symmetric or focal skin lesions—erythema, scaling, ulceration, depigmentation, vesicles, ulcerated or draining nodules, and/or alopecia.
- Ulceration of mucocutaneous junctions and oral mucosa.
- Persistent or cyclic fever—especially in the acute phase.
- Lymphadenopathy.
- Hepatosplenomegaly.
- Muscle pain or atrophy.

CAUSES

Definitive cause not identified. T suppressor cells may be defective.

RISK FACTORS

Exposure to UV light may exacerbate cutaneous lesions.

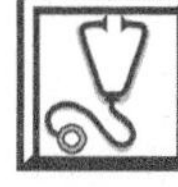

DIAGNOSIS

- Major signs—polyarthritis, glomerulonephritis, consistent dermatologic lesions, hemolytic anemia, thrombocytopenia, polymyositis, leukopenia.
- Minor signs—fever of unknown origin, oral ulcers, peripheral lymphadenopathy, pleuritis, pericarditis, myocarditis, neurologic abnormalities.
- Definitive diagnosis—positive antinuclear antibody (ANA) or lupus erythematosus (LE) test (or both), and two major signs or one major *and* two minor signs.
- Probable diagnosis—positive ANA or LE test (or both), and one major sign *or* two minor signs.

DIFFERENTIAL DIAGNOSIS

- Neoplasia.
- Infectious diseases (e.g., tick-borne disease, septic arthritis).
- Immune-mediated polyarthropathy.

CBC/BIOCHEMISTRY/URINALYSIS

- CBC—anemia, leukopenia, leukocytosis, or thrombocytopenia; anemia may be moderate and nonregenerative or severe and regenerative (hemolytic).
- Biochemistry—results vary widely, depending on the organ(s) affected.
- Urinalysis—repeatable elevated protein:creatinine ratio (>1) with benign sediment and negative culture.

OTHER LABORATORY TESTS

- ANA test—detects antibodies directed against nuclear antigens. False positive and false negatives occur.
- LE test on synovial fluid—identifies phagocytized nuclear material within neutrophils and macrophages; time-consuming.
- Direct antiglobulin (Coombs') test—identifies complement or antibody on the surface of RBCs; test should only be run in patients with anemia.

IMAGING

- Radiographs of affected joints reveal soft-tissue swelling consistent with nonerosive arthritis.
- Thoracic and abdominal radiographs may demonstrate hepatomegaly or splenomegaly.

DIAGNOSTIC PROCEDURES

- Arthrocentesis—high cell count with nondegenerate neutrophils and monocytes and low viscosity are characteristic findings.
- Bacterial culture of synovial fluid—negative.
- Blood culture in animals with fever—negative.
- Skin biopsy—in patients with skin lesions; save specimen in 10% buffered formalin (for histologic examination) and Michel's solution (for immunofluorescence).

PATHOLOGIC FINDINGS

- Nonerosive polyarthritis with infiltrations of synovial membrane by neutrophils and lymphocytes; no pannus formation.
- Membranous or membranoproliferative glomerulonephritis.
- Mononuclear interface dermatitis with hydropic degeneration of keratinocytes and eosinophilic round bodies representing apoptotic basal keratinocytes.
- Vasculitis and panniculitis in some patients.
- Deposition of immune complexes along the basement membrane of the dermal–epidermal junction (detected by immunofluorescence).
- Vasculitis may be seen in any organ.

LUPUS ERYTHEMATOSUS, SYSTEMIC (SLE) (CONTINUED)

- Reactive lymphoid hyperplasia in the lymph nodes and spleen.

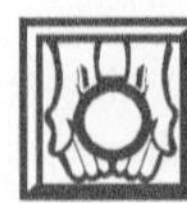

TREATMENT

APPROPRIATE HEALTH CARE

- Hospitalization—may be necessary for initial management.
- Outpatient management—often possible.

NURSING CARE

Supportive care varies with systems affected.

ACTIVITY

- Enforced rest—during episodes of acute polyarthritis.
- Avoid sunlight if photosensitization suspected.

DIET

Restricted protein, high-quality protein diet with *n*-3 fatty acid supplementation in animals with glomerulonephritis.

CLIENT EDUCATION

- Progressive, unpredictable disease course .
- Need for long-term, immunosuppressive therapy and its side effects.
- Heritability of the disease.

MEDICATIONS

DRUG(S) OF CHOICE

- Corticosteroids—to control the abnormal immune response and reduce inflammation (e.g., prednisone 1–2.2 mg/kg/day PO). Consider alternative steroids (equivalent doses) in cats; e.g., prednisolone, dexamethasone, triamcinolone, methylprednisolone.
- Cytotoxic immunosuppressive drugs—add when prednisone fails to improve the condition after 7–10 days or if the patient is steroid intolerant.
- Azathioprine (dogs only) 2 mg/kg PO q24h until remission, then q48h.
- Chlorambucil (cats and dogs) 0.1–0.2 mg/kg PO q24h initially, then q48h.
- Cyclosporine – microemulsion (e.g., Atopica); dogs: 5–10 mg/kg/day PO, divided twice daily; cats: 0.5–3 mg/kg PO q12h.
- Mycophenolate mofetil (dogs) 10 mg/kg PO q12h until remission, then taper.
- Gradually taper doses (no more often than every 3–4 weeks) once remission is achieved.

PRECAUTIONS

- Azathioprine should be avoided in cats.
- Azathioprine and chlorambucil may cause bone marrow suppression.
- Cyclosporine may cause gastrointestinal upset, papillomatosis, and gingival hyperplasia.
- Mycophenolate mofetil may cause GI upset, lymphopenia.
- Treatment with immunosuppressive drugs can increase the risk of severe infection.

POSSIBLE INTERACTIONS

- Concurrent use of aspirin (or other nonsteroidal anti-inflammotory drugs) and prednisone is contraindicated.
- Cyclosporine may have multiple drug interactions due to inhibition of cytochrome P450 enzymes.

ALTERNATIVE DRUG(S)

- Levamisole: dogs, 2–5 mg/kg PO, EOD for 4 months (maximum 150 mg per patient) combined with prednisone 0.5–1.0 mg/kg PO q12h. The prednisone is tapered over 1–2 months and the levamisole continued for 4 months.
- Other immunosuppressive drugs can be considered depending upon the clinical manifestations exhibited (leflunomide for immune-mediated hemolytic anemia, polyarthritis, and myasthenia gravis, topical tacrolimus for skin lesions).

FOLLOW-UP

PATIENT MONITORING

- Physical examination – weekly.
- CBC and biochemical analysis—to monitor for side effects of therapeutics; day 7 then every 2–4 weeks.
- ANA—often remains elevated during remission but may fall as patient improves.

PREVENTION/AVOIDANCE

Do not breed affected animals.

POSSIBLE COMPLICATIONS

- Renal failure and nephrotic syndrome secondary to glomerulonephritis.
- Bronchopneumonia, urinary tract infection, or sepsis secondary to immunosuppression.

EXPECTED COURSE AND PROGNOSIS

Prognosis is guarded. The presence of hemolytic anemia and glomerulonephritis and the development of bacterial infection warrant a poor prognosis. In up to 40% of cases, death occurs during the first year of treatment as a result of renal failure, poor response to therapy, drug complications, or secondary systemic infections.

MISCELLANEOUS

PREGNANCY/FERTILITY/BREEDING

The use of cytotoxic immunosuppressive drugs in pregnant animals is contraindicated.

SEE ALSO

- Anemia, Immune-Mediated.
- Glomerulonephritis.
- Polyarthritis, Nonerosive, Immune-Mediated, Dogs.
- Thrombocytopenia, Primary Immune-Mediated.

ABBREVIATIONS

- ANA = antinuclear antibody.
- DLA = dog leukocyte antigen.
- LE = lupus erythematosus.
- RBC = red blood cell.
- SLE = systemic lupus erythematosus.

Suggested Reading

Berent A, Cerundolo R. Systemic lupus erythematosus. Compend Stand Care Emerg Crit Care Med 2005, 7:7–11.

Chabanne L, Fournel C, Monier JC. Canine systemic lupus erythematosus: part 2: diagnosis and treatment. Compendium 1999, 21:402–421.

Gross TL, Ihrke PJ, Walder EJ, Affolter VK. Skin Diseases of the Dog and Cat: Clinical and Histopathological Diagnosis, 2nd ed. Ames, IA. Blackwell Science, 2005, pp. 55–57.

Stone M. Systemic lupus erythematosus. In: Ettinger S, Feldman E, eds., Textbook of Veterinary Internal Medicine, 7th ed. Vol. 1. St. Louis, MO: Saunders Elsevier, 2009, pp. 783–787.

Author Fiona L. Bateman

Consulting Editor Melinda S. Camus

BASICS

DEFINITION

- One of the most common tick-transmitted zoonotic diseases in the world.
- Caused by spirochetes of the *Borrelia burgdorferi* (*Bb*) sensu lato complex.
- Most seropositive dogs are nonclinical; 5% may show Lyme arthritis (LA), 1–2% may show Lyme nephritis (LN).
- Reported in humans, dogs, horses, and, sporadically, in cats.

PATHOPHYSIOLOGY

- Experimentally, 2–5 months incubation period.
- LA—self-limiting episodic arthritis/anorexia/fever due to interstitial migration of organisms and host immune responses.
- LN—associated with glomerular deposition of *Bb*-specific antigen–antibody complexes.
- In dogs, cardiac involvement rare.

SYSTEMS AFFECTED

- Organisms persist associated with collagen and fibroblasts in skin, joints, tendons, pericardium, peritoneum, meninges, muscle, heart, and lymph nodes; rarely found in body fluids.
- Pathologic changes—with few exceptions restricted to joints, draining lymph nodes; rarely, immune-complex glomerulonephritis (ICGN).

GENETICS

Genetic predisposition for infection (not illness) in beagles and Bernese mountain dogs. Labrador and golden retrievers are predisposed to LN, but it remains rare (proteinuria is not associated with seropositivity).

INCIDENCE/PREVALENCE

- Seroprevalence in dogs varies with exposure to infected ticks in endemic areas (5–30%). In some areas before tick control was common, seroprevalence was 70–90% in healthy dogs.
- Clinical Lyme borreliosis (LB) develops in small fraction of infected individuals; coinfections with other organisms (e.g., *Anaplasma phagocytophilum*) may impact outcome.

GEOGRAPHIC DISTRIBUTION

- Northern hemisphere:
  - North America—most cases reported in the Mid-Atlantic states, New England, Upper Midwest, adjacent Canada. Ecologic conditions supporting LB exist in adjacent states and on West Coast.
  - Europe—central; less frequent in areas bordering Mediterranean basin.

SIGNALMENT

Species

Dog and rarely cat.

Mean Age and Range

Experimentally, puppies are more susceptible than adult dogs.

SIGNS

- LA—acute or recurrent lameness in one or more legs; possible fever, anorexia, depression, local lymphadenopathy. Affected joints may be swollen, warm, painful. Self-limiting or responds well to antibiotic treatment.
- Experimentally—puppies developed acute self-limiting (3–4 days) form of LA in the leg closest to tick bite; may reoccur weeks later in the same or other leg. Older puppies had fewer signs; adult untreated dogs showed no clinical signs but had histologic changes of chronic nonerosive polyarthritis; 10–15% were persistent carriers despite antimicrobial therapy
- LN—protein-losing nephropathy (PLN) due to ICGN; may present for renal failure, thromboembolism, hypertension, or nephrotic syndrome.

CAUSES

- *Bb*—transmitted by three-host *Ixodes* ticks.
- Infection—usually after nymph or adult female tick attachment for 2–4 days.

Ixodes Ticks

- 2- to 3-year life cycle depending on availability of hosts.
- Summer—uninfected eggs laid, hatch in several weeks; become infected by feeding on infected host (small mammal or bird).
- Following spring—larvae molt into nymphs; stay or become infected by feeding on infected host.
- Fall—nymphs molt into adults which stay infected; females mate, feed on larger mammals (e.g., deer); drop off and hide under leaves until laying eggs following summer; males rarely attach or feed.

RISK FACTORS

Canine LB is a peridomestic disease due to expansion of housing into tick habitat; outdoor activities in endemic areas put dogs at risk.

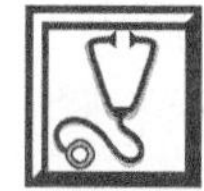

DIAGNOSIS

Diagnosis based on clinicopathologic signs, response to antibiotic therapy, exclusion of other diagnoses, serologic evidence of natural exposure antibodies, and history of exposure to ticks in endemic or emerging area.

DIFFERENTIAL DIAGNOSIS

- LA—infectious (anaplasmosis, ehrlichiosis, Rocky Mountain spotted fever), inflammatory (immune-mediated polyarthropathy, lupus, rheumatoid arthritis), and genetic (Akita, shar-pei) arthritides; degenerative joint disease; neuromuscular, traumatic, or other causes of lameness or weakness.
- LN—leptospirosis, ICGN caused by babesiosis, dirofilariasis, leishmaniasis, lupus, neoplasia; amyloidosis, glomerulosclerosis, genetic, toxic, and other causes of glomerular disease.

CBC/BIOCHEMISTRY/URINALYSIS

- LA—unremarkable.
- LN—proteinuria, hypoalbuminemia, hypercholesterolemia; later azotemia, hyperphosphatemia, thrombocytopenia, isosthenuria, glucosuria.

OTHER LABORATORY TESTS

- Joint tap cytology—hypercellular (up to 75,000 neutrophils/µL).
- Antibodies—VlsE, C_6, and OspF antibodies; OspA and OspC antibodies may be induced by vaccines or natural exposure.
- ELISA to detect a subgroup of antibodies against outer surface protein VlsE of *Bb* using C_6 peptide; C_6 antibodies wane 3–6 months after antibiotic therapy. Low to moderate pretherapy C_6 levels do not drop significantly.

IMAGING

- Thoracic radiographs, abdominal ultrasound—rule out other causes of proteinuria. Usually no ultrasonographic renal changes in LN dogs.
- Orthopedic radiographs—joint effusion, distinguish erosive from nonerosive joint disease; rule out trauma.

DIAGNOSTIC PROCEDURES

- Experimentally, organisms may be demonstrated in skin (tick bite site) or synovium with PCR or culture; these tests are time-consuming, unreliable, and not recommended.
- Blood samples typically test negative via PCR or culture.

PATHOLOGIC FINDINGS

Gross

- Swollen joints with joint effusion.
- Possible local lymphadenopathy.
- PLN: may include peripheral edema, effusions, thromboembolism, hypertensive organ damage (retinal hemorrhage/detachment, left ventricular hypertrophy, cerebrovascular disease).

Histopathology

- LA—acute arthritis, fibrinopurulent synovitis. Mild lymphoplasmacytic synovitis in other joints.
- Lymph nodes—possible cortical hyperplasia, multiple enlarged follicles, expanded parafollicular areas.
- Superficial dermis near tick bite site—perivascular lymphoplasmacytic infiltrate with some mast cells.

- LN—ICGN, diffuse tubular necrosis with regeneration, interstitial inflammation.

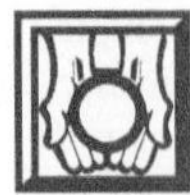

TREATMENT

APPROPRIATE HEALTH CARE

LA—outpatient; LN—may require hospitalization, IV fluids, colloids, and PLN therapy, antiemetics, etc.

NURSING CARE

Consider leptospirosis differential (isolation) for LN suspects.

DIET

LA—no change needed; LN—renal diets, omega-3 fatty acid supplement.

CLIENT EDUCATION

- Antibiotics should be administered as prescribed.
- Discuss the risk to humans in same environs.

SURGICAL CONSIDERATIONS

- Aspiration of synovial fluid—may be considered for diagnostic purposes.
- Renal biopsy may be indicated to differentiate ICGN from other causes of renal proteinuria.

MEDICATIONS

DRUG(S) OF CHOICE

- Antibiotics: may not clear infection completely; treatment significantly improves LA clinical signs and pathology:
    - Doxycycline 5–10 mg/kg PO q12h, with food; preferred.
    - Amoxicillin 20 mg/kg PO q8–12h.
    - Azithromycin 25 mg/kg PO q24h.
- Recommended treatment period—4 weeks for LA; LN may be treated until Quant C_6 level wanes.
- Additional therapy for PLN/ICGN may include renin–angiotensin–aldosterone system inhibitors, antithrombotics, antihypertensives, etc. (see consensus statement in Suggested Reading).
- Immunosuppressive drugs (e.g., mycophenolate, corticosteroids) indicated if biopsy-confirmed ICGN or rapid deterioration despite standard treatments.

CONTRAINDICATIONS

Consider potential drug side effects. Renal biopsy contraindicated in dogs with severe thrombocytopenia, unregulated hypertension, or end-stage renal failure.

PRECAUTIONS

Doxycycline can be used during growth without fear of dental harm; may cause esophagitis or gastritis.

ALTERNATIVE DRUG(S)

Nonsteroidal medications—not recommended initially; use caution with renal dysfunction or prior corticosteroid therapy.

FOLLOW-UP

PATIENT MONITORING

- Improvement—in acute LA seen within 1–3 days of antibiotic treatment.
- If no improvement or if signs exacerbate—consider other diagnoses.
- All seropositive dogs should be screened, monitored, and treated if proteinuria present.

PREVENTION/AVOIDANCE

- Mechanical removal of ticks.
- Prevention of tick attachment or fast kill—acaricides and repellents supplied as topicals, collars, or oral medications.
- Vaccines—5 currently available (nonadjuvanted recombinant OspA, 3 adjuvanted bacterins, and an adjuvanted recombinant chimeric OspA with 7 strains of OspC). All induce antibodies against spirochete's OspA to kill the spirochete within the tick while it feeds. Bacterins (produced from inactivated cultured *Bb* organisms) and the recombinant chimeric OspA/OspC also induce OspC antibodies to kill spirochetes within the host.
    - Efficacy is improved by booster immunizations at 6 months after an initial series; at least annual booster is needed thereafter.
    - Tick control still recommended because of inconsistent vaccinal efficacy and duration of immunity.
- Year-round tick population control in environment—restricted to small areas; clear leaf piles, difficult to reduce host mammal population.

POSSIBLE COMPLICATIONS

Renal failure.

EXPECTED COURSE AND PROGNOSIS

- Recovery from acute lameness expected 1–3 days after starting antibiotics.
- Recurrence of LA signs may be due to coinfection or reinfection, not necessarily relapse.
- Prognosis for LN is largely unknown but appears to vary as for other PLN/ICGN cases.

MISCELLANEOUS

ZOONOTIC POTENTIAL

- Infection in humans acquired only from infected ticks.
- Dogs can transport unattached ticks which can later attach to humans—however, ixodid ticks are not intermittent feeders; once feeding starts, they do not change hosts.

PREGNANCY/FERTILITY/BREEDING

- No convincing evidence that *Bb* infection is transmitted *in utero* in dogs.
- Avoid tetracyclines in pregnant animals.
- Maternal C_6 antibodies can be passed to puppies.

SYNONYMS

Lyme arthritis, Lyme nephritis, or Lyme disease.

ABBREVIATIONS

- *Bb* = *Borrelia burgdorferi.*
- ICGN = immune-complex glomerulonephritis.
- LA = Lyme arthritis.
- LB = Lyme borreliosis.
- LN = Lyme nephritis.
- PLN = protein-losing nephropathy.

INTERNET RESOURCES

- Centers for Disease Control and Prevention: http://www.cdc.gov/lyme
- Companion Animal Parasite Council: www.capcvet.org
- IRIS Glomerular Disease Study Group: https://onlinelibrary.wiley.com/toc/19391676/27/s1

Suggested Reading

Borys MA, Kass PH, Mohr FC, et al. Differences in clinicopathologic variables between *Borrelia* C6 antigen seroreactive and *Borrelia* C6 seronegative glomerulopathy in dogs. J Vet Intern Med 2019, 33:2096–2104.

Greene CE, Straubinger RK, Levy SA. Borreliosis. In: Greene CE, ed., Infectious Diseases of the Dog and Cat, 4th ed. St. Louis, MO: Saunders Elsevier, 2012, pp. 447–465.

IRIS Canine GN Study Group Standard Therapy Subgroup, Brown S, Elliott J, et al. Consensus recommendations for standard therapy of glomerular disease in dogs. J Vet Intern Med 2013, 27(S1):S27–S43.

Littman MP, Gerber B, Goldstein RE, et al. ACVIM consensus update on Lyme borreliosis in dogs and cats. J Vet Intern Med 2018, 32:887–903.

Author Meryl P. Littman

Consulting Editor Amie Koenig

Acknowledgment The author and editors acknowledges the prior contribution of Reinhard K. Straubinger.

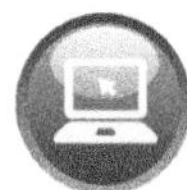

Client Education Handout available online

BASICS

DEFINITION

An obstructive disorder of the lymphatic system of the gastrointestinal (GI) tract, resulting in lymphatic hypertension and protein-losing enteropathy (PLE).

PATHOPHYSIOLOGY

- Lymphatic obstruction results in dilation and rupture of intestinal lacteals with subsequent loss of lymphatic contents (plasma proteins, lymphocytes, and chylomicrons) into the intestinal lumen.
- Although some of the proteins may be digested and reabsorbed, excessive enteric loss of plasma proteins will ultimately result in panhypoproteinemia.
- Hypoproteinemia causes a decrease in plasma oncotic pressure, which, if severe, will lead to ascites, pleural effusion, and/or (rarely) edema.
- Loss of antithrombin and other anticoagulants can cause a hypercoaguable state.

SYSTEMS AFFECTED

- GI—diarrhea.
- Respiratory—pleural effusion.
- Skin—subcutaneous edema.
- Systemic—ascites.
- Vascular—thromboembolic disease.

GENETICS

A familial tendency for PLE has been reported for soft-coated wheaten terriers, basenjis, Yorkshire terriers, and Norwegian lundehunds, but the actual genetic cause has not been identified for any of these breeds.

INCIDENCE/PREVALENCE

Uncommon

GEOGRAPHIC DISTRIBUTION

N/A

SIGNALMENT

Species

Dog

Breed Predilections

Soft-coated wheaten terrier, basenji, Norwegian lundehund, Yorkshire terrier.

Mean Age and Range

Any age; most common in middle-aged dogs.

Predominant Sex

Increased prevalence reported in female soft-coated wheaten terriers; no sex predilection reported for other breeds.

SIGNS

- Clinical signs are variable.
- Diarrhea—chronic; typically small bowel diarrhea; however, not all animals have diarrhea.
- Ascites.
- Subcutaneous edema.
- Dyspnea from pleural effusion.
- Weight loss and sarcopenia.
- Flatulence.
- Vomiting.

CAUSES

Primary or Congenital Lymphangiectasia

- Focal—intestinal only.
- Diffuse lymphatic abnormalities (e.g., chylothorax, lymphedema, chyloabdomen, thoracic duct obstruction).

Secondary Lymphangiectasia

- Right-sided congestive heart failure.
- Constrictive pericarditis.
- Budd–Chiari syndrome.
- Neoplasia (e.g., lymphoma, thymoma, mediastinal masses).
- Fungal disease.

RISK FACTORS

N/A

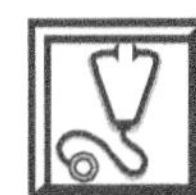

DIAGNOSIS

DIFFERENTIAL DIAGNOSIS

- Other causes of PLE.
- PLE must be differentiated from other causes of hypoalbuminemia.

CBC/BIOCHEMISTRY/URINALYSIS

- Panhypoproteinemia.
- Hypocholesterolemia.
- Hypocalcemia.
- Hypomagnesemia.
- Lymphopenia.

OTHER LABORATORY TESTS

Differentiate PLE from Other Causes of Hypoalbuminemia

- Serum chemistry and pre- and postprandial serum bile acids to rule out hepatic failure.
- Urine protein:creatinine ratio to rule out protein-losing nephropathy.
- Occult fecal blood test to rule out GI blood loss (*o*-toluidine-based tests are preferable as these tests are less likely to be falsely positive due to meat in the diet than guaiac-based tests).
- Fecal α_1-protease inhibitor to help confirm intestinal protein loss (most useful in dogs that do not yet have any GI signs).

Differentiate Other Causes of Excessive Protein Loss into the GI Tract

- Fecal smear and flotation to rule out intestinal parasites.
- Serum cobalamin and folate concentrations to rule out small intestinal dysbiosis or cobalamin deficiency. Cobalamin deficiency is an indicator of chronic severe distal small intestinal disease, which could be associated with excessive protein loss.
- Fecal culture for diagnosis of specific enteric pathogens (e.g., *Salmonella* spp.); PCR for enteropathogenic *Campylobacter* spp. and other enteropathogens.
- Fluid analysis of cavitary effusions—lymphangiectasia usually results in a transudate, but chyloabdomen and chylothorax may be observed.
- Chronic chylous effusions might be difficult to differentiate from modified transudates. In chylous effusions the triglyceride concentration is higher than in serum.

IMAGING

- Thoracic radiographs—survey to rule out cardiac disease and neoplasia.
- Abdominal radiographs—to rule out mechanical intestinal disease (obstruction or partial obstruction) and other causes of PLE. However, routine abdominal radiographs are less useful for assessment of these patients than abdominal ultrasound.
- Abdominal ultrasound—to rule out mechanical intestinal disease and other causes of PLE. Ultrasound often shows hyperechoic mucosal striations ("tiger stripe" effect), mucosal speckles, and/or a hyperechoic line within the mucosa running parallel to the submucosa. Corn oil 1–2 mL/kg given orally 60–90 minutes before the study may improve the diagnostic yield.
- Echocardiography—to rule out right-sided congestive heart failure.

DIAGNOSTIC PROCEDURES

- Endoscopy—allows intestinal mucosal visualization and biopsy. Ileal biopsies should be procured in hypocobalaminemic animals.
- Laparotomy—allows visualization of dilated intestinal lymphatics and biopsies of intestines (full thickness) and lymph nodes, but may be contraindicated in patients with hypoproteinemia due to increased complications (e.g., dehiscence).
- ECG and/or echocardiography—can aid in evaluating animals suspected of having right-sided congestive heart failure or arrhythmias.

PATHOLOGIC FINDINGS

- Dilated lymphatics may appear as a web-like network throughout the mesentery and serosal surface.
- Lipogranulomas may appear as yellow-white nodules and foamy granular deposits adjacent to lymphatics.
- Lacteal dilatation, villous blunting, and crypt lesions (i.e., dilatation, cysts, abscesses) are the most consistent findings on histopathology with lymphangiectasia and PLE.
- Often associated with mucosal edema or diffuse or multifocal accumulations of lymphocytes and plasma cells in the lamina propria.

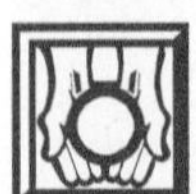

TREATMENT

APPROPRIATE HEALTH CARE

May need hospitalization if complications due to hypoalbuminemia develop.

NURSING CARE

Consider placement of an esophageal feeding tube in anorectic patients to meet increased caloric demands.

ACTIVITY

Normal

DIET

- Low-fat or ultra-low fat diets are the cornerstone of treatment.
- Commercial low fat diets contain 20 g fat/1000 kcal or less. A lower fat content with a novel protein source (if desired) can be achieved by a home-cooked diet. Protein sources may include chicken breast, tilapia, tuna, and/or fat-free cottage cheese. Possible carbohydrate sources are potato, rice, pasta, and/or egg noodles.
- Initially a simple home-cooked diet can be used, but long-term the diet must be balanced.
- Avoid high-fiber diets.
- Dogs with concurrent lymphangiectasia and inflammatory bowel disease may benefit from a commercial hydrolyzed protein diet that is moderately fat restricted.
- Long-chain triglycerides stimulate intestinal lymph flow and may lead to increased intestinal protein loss.
- Diets fortified with medium-chain triglycerides (MCTs) may be beneficial.
- May feed MCTs (e.g., MCT oil, Enfamil Portagen) to supplement fat and calorie intake.
- Supplement with fat-soluble vitamins—A, D, E, and K.
- Elemental diets can also be used.

CLIENT EDUCATION

Discuss unpredictable disease progression and response to therapy.

SURGICAL CONSIDERATIONS

- Patients that benefit from surgical intervention are rare.
- Consider surgery to relieve an identifiable lymphatic obstruction, if present.
- Pericardiectomy may be indicated with constrictive pericarditis.

MEDICATIONS

DRUG(S) OF CHOICE

- Clopidogrel 1–3 mg/kg PO q24h or ultra-low dose aspirin 0.5 mg/kg PO q24h to reduce the risk of thromboembolic events.
- Try corticosteroids if dietary therapy alone is unsuccessful (however, such therapy is not intended to treat lymphangiectasia but rather concurrent GI inflammation). Prednisone or prednisolone 1–2 mg/kg PO q12h for 5–7 days, followed by 1 mg/kg q12h for at least 6 weeks. In large-breed dogs the starting dose should be more conservative than in small-breed dogs. After remission, dosage can be slowly tapered to the lowest dose effective at controlling the disease. Alternatively, consider the use of a locally effective corticosteroid (e.g., budesonide), or other immunomodulators such as chlorambucil, azathioprine, or cyclosporine.
- In hypocobalaminemic patients, cobalamin must be supplemented parenterally or orally to achieve therapeutic response (see Cobalamin Deficiency for dosing).
- If secondary small intestinal dysbiosis is suspected, the patient should be treated with tylosin at 20 mg/kg q12h for 6 weeks.
- Magnesium sulfate should be supplemented parenterally (IV) at 1 mEq/kg/day in dogs that are hypomagnesemic before oral supplementation with magnesium oxide, magnesium citrate, or magnesium carbonate.
- Diuretics such as furosemide 1 mg/kg q12h or spironolactone 1 mg/kg q12h in animals with severe ascites to improve comfort.

CONTRAINDICATIONS

N/A

PRECAUTIONS

Steroids might increase the risk for thromboembolic events.

POSSIBLE INTERACTIONS

Clopidogrel should not be used with nonsteroidal anti-inflammatory drugs, phenytoin, torsemide, or warfarin.

ALTERNATIVE DRUG(S)

Some patients may respond to treatment with octreotide; dosing for this condition is empirical.

FOLLOW-UP

PATIENT MONITORING

- Body weight, serum total protein, albumin, and globulin concentrations, and clinical signs (pleural effusion, ascites, and/or edema).
- Patients need to be reevaluated depending on the severity of the disease process.

PREVENTION/AVOIDANCE

N/A

POSSIBLE COMPLICATIONS

- Thromboembolic disease.
- Hypocalcemia.
- Dyspnea from pleural effusion or pulmonary thromboembolism.
- Severe protein-calorie depletion.
- Intractable diarrhea.

EXPECTED COURSE AND PROGNOSIS

- Prognosis is guarded. More than 50% of patients die from the disease or from associated thromboembolic disease.
- Remissions of several months to more than 2 years can be achieved in some patients.

MISCELLANEOUS

ASSOCIATED CONDITIONS

Soft-coated wheaten terriers may have concurrent protein-losing nephropathy.

SEE ALSO

- Cobalamin Deficiency.
- Diarrhea, Chronic—Dogs.
- Protein-Losing Enteropathy.

ABBREVIATIONS

- ECG = electrocardiogram.
- GI = gastrointestinal.
- MCT = medium-chain triglycerides.
- PLE = protein-losing enteropathy.

Suggested Reading

Kull PA, Hess RS, Craig LE, et al. Clinical, clinicopathologic, radiographic, and ultrasonographic characteristics of intestinal lymphangiectasia in dogs: 17 cases (1996–1998). J Am Vet Med Assoc 2001, 219:197–202.

Larson RN, Ginn JA, Bell CM, et al. Duodenal endoscopic findings and histopathologic confirmation of intestinal lymphangiectasia in dogs. J Vet Intern Med 2012, 26:1087–1092.

Littman MP, Dambach DM, Vaden SL, et al. Familial protein-losing enteropathy and protein-losing nephropathy in soft coated wheaten terriers: 222 cases (1983–1997). J Vet Intern Med 2000, 14:68–80.

Okanishi H, Yoshioka R, Kagawa Y, et al. The clinical efficacy of dietary fat restriction in treatment of dogs with intestinal lymphangiectasia. J Vet Intern Med 2014, 28:809–817.

Pollard RE, Johnson EG, Pesavento PA, et al. Effects of corn oil administered orally on conspicuity of ultrasonographic small intestinal lesions in dogs with lymphangiectasia. Vet Radiol Ultrasound 2013, 54:390–397.

Authors Jörg M. Steiner and Sina Marsilio
Consulting Editor Mark P. Rondeau

Client Education Handout available online

BASICS

DEFINITION

• Lymphadenopathy—lymph node enlargement.
• Generalized lymphadenopathy—enlargement of multiple lymph nodes.
• Lymphoid hyperplasia/reactivity—benign, non-neoplastic, reactive response to immune stimulation; results in proliferation of plasma cells and lymphocytes of all sizes, which results in lymphadenopathy.
• Lymphadenitis—inflammation of the lymph node; can represent primary infection of the lymph node or drainage of regional inflammation.

PATHOPHYSIOLOGY

• Lymphoid hyperplasia/reactivity—can occur secondary to a localized process like dental disease or localized skin allergies (i.e., pododermatitis). Lymphoid hyperplasia can also be seen secondary to systemic inflammation. Lymph node enlargement can be singular or generalized.
• Lymphadenitis—inflammation within a lymph node can represent a primary process (inflammation or necrosis of the lymph node itself) or a secondary process (drainage of an area of inflammation or necrosis).
• Infectious lymphadenitis—the drainage function of lymph nodes increases their exposure to infectious agents within the node.
• Noninfectious lymphadenitis—often occurs secondary to drainage of areas of inflammation.
• Neoplasia—primary lymph node neoplasia (lymphoma) or metastatic disease. Lymph node enlargement can be singular or generalized.

SYSTEMS AFFECTED

• Hemic/lymphatic/immune.
• May be a component of more widespread systemic disease.

GENETICS

No known genetic basis for lymphoid hyperplasia/reactivity or lymphadenitis.

INCIDENCE/PREVALENCE

• Seen with a variety of systemic diseases.
• Overall incidence is unknown.

GEOGRAPHIC DISTRIBUTION

Geographic distribution should be considered in cases of lymphadenitis caused by fungal infection.

SIGNALMENT

Species

Dogs and cats.

Breed Predilections

None for lymphoid hyperplasia or lymphadenitis. Increased incidence of lymphoma can be seen in golden retrievers, basset hounds, St. Bernard, boxer, Scottish terrier, Airedale terrier, Rottweiler, Labrador retriever, bull mastiff, and bouvier des Flandres.

Mean Age and Range

None

Predominant Sex

None

SIGNS

General Comments

• Marked submandibular lymph node enlargement can result in difficulty swallowing.
• Clinical signs are often related to systemic disease.

Historical Findings

• Owners may report finding mass lesions, particularly when lymph node enlargement is marked.
• Systemic signs of inflammatory disease or organ dysfunction may be reported.

Physical Examination Findings

• Hyperplastic lymph nodes vary in size. In early stages, lymph nodes may be firm yet still mobile.
• Inflamed lymph nodes are typically large and firm and may be painful.
• Bacterial infection can result in abscess formation within the node, which may rupture and result in draining tracts. Patients may also have fever and other systemic signs of inflammation.
• Lymph nodes affected by lymphoma are often at least twice normal size and very firm.
• Lymph nodes with metastatic neoplasia can have a variable presentation.

CAUSES

Lymphoid Hyperplasia/Reactivity

• Hyperplastic lymph nodes represent a proliferation of lymphocytes in response to any source of antigenic stimulation.
• Stimulation can be localized where a lymph node drains an area of inflammation.
• Systemic disease can also result in hyperplastic/reactive lymph nodes.
• Chronic hyperplasia can occasionally lead to lymphadenitis.
• A benign condition has been reported in young cats, featuring generalized lymphadenopathy characterized by increased numbers of intermediate to large lymphocytes, which can mimic lymphoma. Care must be taken not to misdiagnose these patients with lymphoma.
• Generalized lymphadenopathy can occur in cats infected with *Bartonella* spp. or feline immunodeficiency virus (FIV).

Neutrophilic Lymphadenitis

• Commonly seen in lymph nodes draining a site of infection.
• Bacterial infection will also result in neutrophilic lymphadenitis, including *Streptococcus* spp., *Brucella* spp., *Francisella tularensis* (tularemia), and *Yersinia pestis* (bubonic plague). The latter two organisms are more likely to cause lymphadenitis in feline patients.

Eosinophilic Lymphadenitis

• Common with dermatitis and parasitic skin diseases.
• Can also be observed with drainage of mast cell tumors, some lymphomas, and with hypereosinophilic syndrome.

Granulomatous/Pyogranulomatous Lymphadenitis

• Indicative of chronic inflammation; can occur concurrently with neutrophilic lymphadenitis.
• Multinucleated giant cells with neutrophils indicate pyogranulomatous inflammation.
• Fungal, protozoal, and bacterial infections.

Neoplasia

• Lymphoma often results in generalized lymphadenopathy with marked lymph node enlargement.
• Metastatic neoplasia may cause a singular or generalized lymphadenopathy of variable size.

RISK FACTORS

• Patients with compromised immune function due to chronic illness or immunosuppressive therapy can be more susceptible to infection and lymphadenitis.
• Feline leukemia virus (FeLV) and FIV infection may also be associated with lymphoid neoplasia.

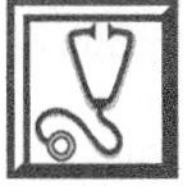

DIAGNOSIS

DIFFERENTIAL DIAGNOSIS

• It is essential to determine that a mass effect in the region of a lymph node is not a neoplastic mass or other regional structure (e.g., salivary gland).
• Differentiation between lymphoid hyperplasia, lymphadenitis, lymphoma, or metastatic neoplasia cannot be achieved by evaluating clinical signs alone.
• Fever and painful, enlarged lymph nodes are suggestive of lymphadenitis.
• Lymphoma and lymphoid hyperplasia are more common causes of generalized lymphadenopathy than lymphadenitis.

CBC/BIOCHEMISTRY/URINALYSIS

• Localized lymphoid hyperplasia secondary to local inflammation may not be associated with specific CBC/chemistry abnormalities.
• Patients with infectious causes of lymphadenitis may have marked hyperglobulinemia.

- Marked eosinophilia can be seen with hypereosinophilic syndrome or as a paraneoplastic phenomenon.
- Biochemistry results may reflect organ involvement from underlying disease process.
- Hypercalcemia can be seen in dogs with lymphoma, but this finding is uncommon in cats.

OTHER LABORATORY TESTS

Serologic or urine antigen tests for various systemic fungal diseases are available.

IMAGING

- Radiographs—evaluate for enlargement of internal organs or patterns associated with infectious or neoplastic disease.
- Ultrasound—evaluate intra-abdominal lymph nodes and organ architecture.

DIAGNOSTIC PROCEDURES

- Fine-needle aspiration cytology stained with a Romanowsky stain (e.g., Diff-Quik) in most cases is sufficient for diagnosis of the primary cause of lymph node enlargement.
- Culture of aspirated material or a fresh tissue sample obtained via tissue biopsy can be considered if an infectious etiology is suspected.
- Fine-needle aspiration/cytology results:
  - Lymphoid hyperplasia—increased numbers of intermediate and large lymphocytes (<50% of the total population); increased numbers of plasma cells.
  - Lymphadenitis—increased numbers of neutrophils, eosinophils, macrophages, or a combination of these types.
  - Infectious agents—bacterial, fungal, and protozoal organisms can be found free in the background or within the cytoplasm of macrophages and, rarely, neutrophils.
  - Lymphoma—over 50% of the lymphocyte population is made up of immature lymphocytes. Immature cells can be intermediate to large in size. Some forms of lymphoma (e.g., indolent lymphoma) cannot be diagnosed with cytology alone and may require advanced diagnostics including flow cytometry or PCR for antigen receptor rearrangement (PARR).
  - Metastatic neoplasia—findings include the presence of cells not normally observed in a lymph node and can range from rare nests of neoplastic cells to complete effacement of the lymph node.
- When a definitive diagnosis cannot be made with cytology alone, a lymph node biopsy may be required, particularly if cytology results are consistently inconclusive or if enlargement of a lymph node is persistent, progressive, or unexplained.

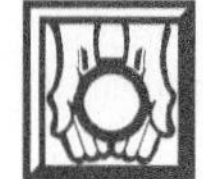

TREATMENT

APPROPRIATE HEALTH CARE

Treatments are aimed at the underlying etiology.

MEDICATIONS

DRUG(S) OF CHOICE

- Effective drug therapy involves identification and treatment of the underlying cause.
- Solitary enlarged lymph nodes with neutrophilic lymphadenitis are likely to have a bacterial component either within the node or the primary drainage area.
- Chemotherapeutic agents can be used to treat lymphoma.

FOLLOW-UP

EXPECTED COURSE AND PROGNOSIS

Variable

MISCELLANEOUS

AGE-RELATED FACTORS

None

ZOONOTIC POTENTIAL

- Bubonic plague, tularemia, and mycobacterial infections may present risk of human infection.
- Specimens from affected animals should be handled with appropriate caution.

ABBREVIATIONS

- FeLV = feline leukemia virus.
- FIV = feline immunodeficiency virus.
- PARR = PCR for antigen receptor rearrangement.

Suggested Reading

Cowell R, Dorsey K, Meinkoth J. Lymph node cytology. Vet Clin Small Anim 2003, 33:47–67.

Messick JB. The lymph nodes. In: Valenciano AC, Cowell RL, eds., Cowell and Tyler's Diagnostic Cytology and Hematology of the Dog and Cat, 4th ed. St. Louis, MO: Elsevier, 2014, pp. 180–194.

Raskin RE. Hemolymphatic System. In: Raskin RE, Meyer DJ, eds., Canine and Feline Cytology, 3rd ed. St. Louis, MO: Saunders, 2016, pp. 91–117.

Viall VEO, Kiupel M, Bienzle D. Hematopoietic system: lymph nodes. In: Maxie, G, ed., Pathology of Domestic Animals, 6th ed. Vol. 3. St. Louis, MO: Elsevier, 2016, pp. 196–215.

Author Corry K. Yeuroukis

Consulting Editor Melinda S. Camus

Acknowledgment The author and editors acknowledge the prior contributions of Kenneth M. Rassnick and Alan H. Rebar.

LYMPHEDEMA

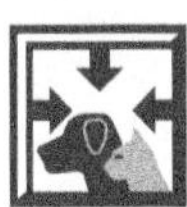

BASICS

OVERVIEW

• Pathologic accumulation of protein-rich lymph into interstitial spaces, especially subcutaneous fat due to primary/secondary failure of lymphatic drainage. • If chronic, causes tissue fibrosis. • May be congenital or acquired.

SIGNALMENT

• Dog (more common) and cat. • Congenital in bulldogs. • Hereditary/congenital in a family of poodles and whippets. • Possible breed predilection in Labrador retrievers and Old English sheepdogs.

SIGNS

Historical Findings

• Primary/congenital—peripheral limb swelling/pitting edema at birth or develops within the first several months. • Progressive, nonpainful swelling starting at distal extremity and slowly advances proximally.

Physical Examination Findings

• Most common in limbs, especially pelvic limbs; unilateral or bilateral. • Less common in ventral thorax, abdomen, ears, and tail.
• Nonpainful pitting; affected area is normothermic. • Pitting quality lost with chronicity as fibrosis occurs. • Lameness and pain uncommon unless cellulitis develops.

CAUSES & RISK FACTORS

• Hereditary/congenital malformation of lymphatics—aplasia of thoracic duct, cisterna chyli or peripheral lymphatics, valvular incompetence, and lymph node fibrosis.
• Excessive interstitial fluid production due to venous hypertension (e.g., congestive heart failure, venous obstruction) or increased vascular permeability (e.g., infection, trauma, heat, irradiation). • Secondary damage to lymphatic vessels or lymph nodes—associated with trauma, infection (e.g., *Brugia pahangi* lymphatic filarial infection—Southeast Asia), neoplasia (e.g., lymphoma, lymphangiosarcoma [rare]), radiation therapy and thoracic duct ligation (rare).

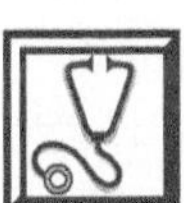

DIAGNOSIS

DIFFERENTIAL DIAGNOSIS

• Edema due to venous stasis (e.g., congestive heart failure, cirrhosis); look for varices, hyperpigmentation, and ulceration.
• Arteriovenous fistulae—listen for machinery murmur; feel for pulsatile vessels; confirm with angiogram. • Edema due to hypoproteinemia—protein-losing nephropathy or enteropathy, hepatic failure, serum loss from burns or hemorrhage; check serum protein concentration. • Trauma—review history; look for bruising and lacerations.
• Neoplasia—if swelling is firm, obtain aspirate for cytology. • Cellulitis—fever, pain, and warm swelling. • Insect bites.

CBC/BIOCHEMISTRY/URINALYSIS

Normal

OTHER LABORATORY TESTS

Serologic tests for tick-borne infections, including *Bartonella* spp.

IMAGING

• Radiography and ultrasound to rule out obvious masses. • Lymphangiography ± computed tomography allows evaluation of lymphatic abnormalities; best results obtained with direct injection of water-based contrast media into a lymphatic vessel (see Suggested Reading).

DIAGNOSTIC PROCEDURES

• Biopsy of affected tissues to rule out lymphangiosarcoma. • Culture and sensitivity when lymphangitis present.

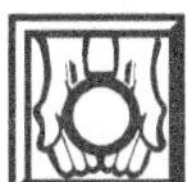

TREATMENT

• No curative therapy—a number of surgical and medical treatments may be tried. • Rest and massage of the affected limbs do not help.
• Conservative care—long-term use of pressure wraps, coupled with skin care and use of antibiotics to treat cellulitis and lymphangitis; may be successful in some patients.
• Surgical procedures—attempted when conservative care and medications fail; two main categories: (1) Facilitate lymph drainage (lymphangioplasty, bridging techniques, lymphaticovenous shunts, superficial and deep lymphatic anastomosis). (2) Excisional procedures to remove abnormal tissue; no treatment consistently beneficial; excisional procedures reported in dogs only. • In humans—microwave heating of affected areas appears beneficial and adds to the effect of benzopyrones (see Drugs of Choice). • Diets severely restricted in long-chain triglycerides are being investigated in humans.

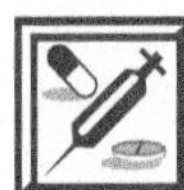

MEDICATIONS

DRUG(S) OF CHOICE

• Benzopyrones reduce high-protein edema by stimulating macrophages to release proteases with resulting fragmented proteins reabsorbed into the blood; beneficial effects have been recorded in experimental studies in dogs (e.g., rutin 50 mg/kg PO q8h). A study in humans showed combined usage of oral and topical benzopyrones to be more effective than either alone. • Diuretics, steroids, anticoagulants, and fibrinolytic agents have been used, but no confirmed benefit. • Treat underlying cause where possible (e.g., ivermectin for *Brugia pahangi* infection).

CONTRAINDICATIONS/POSSIBLE INTERACTIONS

Diuretics—initially reduce swelling but increase protein content of interstitial fluid, resulting in further tissue damage and fibrosis.

FOLLOW-UP

• Puppies with severe lymphedema may die.
• Spontaneous resolution may be seen in some puppies with pelvic limb involvement.
• Prognosis with lymphangiosarcoma is poor.

L

MISCELLANEOUS

Suggested Reading

Fossum TW, King LA, Miller MW, et al. Lymphedema: clinical signs, diagnosis, and treatment. J Vet Intern Med 1992, 6:312–319.
Fossum TW, Miller MW. Lymphedema: etiopathogenesis. J Vet Intern Med 1992, 6:283–293.

Author Stuart A. Walton
Consulting Editor Michael Aherne
Acknowledgment The author and editors acknowledge the prior contribution of Francis W.K. Smith, Jr.

LYMPHOMA—CATS

BASICS

DEFINITION

Malignant transformation of lymphocytes.

PATHOPHYSIOLOGY

Viral (feline leukemia virus [FeLV]) or chemical (tobacco smoke) oncogenesis.

SYSTEMS AFFECTED

• Gastrointestinal. • Hemic/lymphatic/ immune. • Nervous—most common spinal cord tumor in cats. • Ophthalmic. • Renal (high rate of relapse in CNS).
• Respiratory—nasal, thoracic cavities.

L

GENETICS

N/A

INCIDENCE/PREVALENCE

• About 90% of hematopoietic tumors and 33% of all tumors in cats. • Prevalence—41.6–200 per 100,000 cats.

GEOGRAPHIC DISTRIBUTION

Regional differences may relate to differences in FeLV prevalence.

Breed Predilections

Siamese/Oriental breeds overrepresented in some studies.

Mean Age and Range

• FeLV-positive cats—3 years. • FeLV-negative cats—7 years. • Median age of cats with localized extranodal lymphoma—13 years. • Most cats with Hodgkin's-like lymphoma are older than 6 years.

Predominant Sex

None

SIGNS

General Comments

Depend on anatomic form.

Historical Findings

• Mediastinal form—open-mouthed breathing, coughing, regurgitation, anorexia, weight loss. • Alimentary form—anorexia, weight loss, lethargy, vomiting, constipation, diarrhea, melena, hematochezia. Small cell lymphoma (SCL) typically more chronic signs compared to large cell lymphoma (LCL).
• Renal form—consistent with renal failure.
• Nasal form—nasal discharge or epistaxis, facial swelling, ocular signs, respiratory noise, sneezing, anorexia. • Multicentric form—possibly none except for swellings in areas of lymph nodes in early stages; anorexia, weight loss, and depression with progression of disease. • Spinal form—quickly progressing posterior paresis may be seen. • Cutaneous form—pruritic, hemorrhagic, or alopecic dermal masses may be seen.

Physical Examination Findings

• Mediastinal form—non-compressible cranial thorax, dyspnea, tachypnea. • Alimentary form—thickened intestines or abdominal masses. • Renal form—large, irregular kidneys.
• Nasal form—purulent or mucoid nasal discharge, facial deformity, epiphora, exophthalmos, poor globe retropulsion.
• Multicentric form—generalized lymphadenomegaly, possible hepatosplenomegaly. • All forms—fever; dehydration; depression; cachexia in some patients.

CAUSES

FeLV

RISK FACTORS

• FeLV exposure. • Exposure to environmental tobacco smoke (relative risk 2.4, increases linearly with duration and quantity of exposure). • Feline immunodeficiency virus (FIV) infection.

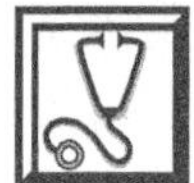

DIAGNOSIS

DIFFERENTIAL DIAGNOSIS

• Mediastinal form—congestive heart failure; cardiomyopathy; chylothorax; pyothorax; hemothorax; pneumothorax; diaphragmatic hernia; allergic lung disease; thymoma; ectopic thyroid carcinoma; pleural carcinomatosis; acetaminophen toxicity. • Alimentary form—foreign body ingestion; intestinal ulceration; intestinal fungal infection; inflammatory bowel disease; intussusception; lymphangiectasia; other gastrointestinal tumor. • Renal form—pyelonephritis; amyloidosis; glomerulonephritis; chronic renal failure; polycystic kidneys; feline infectious peritonitis. • Multicentric form—systemic mycotic infection; immune-mediated disease; toxoplasmosis; lymphoid hyperplasia; hypersensitivity reaction; plague (specifically if prominent cervical lymphadenopathy as with Hodgkin's-like form).

CBC/BIOCHEMISTRY/URINALYSIS

• May see anemia (negative prognostic factor), leukocytosis, and lymphoblastosis.
• May find high creatinine, high serum urea nitrogen, high hepatic enzyme activity, hypercalcemia (rare), and monoclonal gammopathy.

OTHER LABORATORY TESTS

FeLV testing—usually negative in older cats and in cats with large granular lymphocyte lymphoma (LGLL), usually positive in younger cats and those with mediastinal (85%) or CNS lymphoma, renal (45% positive), multicentric (20%), intestinal (15%).

IMAGING

• Thoracic radiography—may see mediastinal mass, pleural effusion, abnormal pulmonary parenchymal patterns (rare), perihilar or retrosternal lymphadenomegaly.
• Abdominal ultrasonography—may see diffuse echotexture changes in the liver, spleen, and kidneys, focal or diffuse thickening of the intestines and the gastric wall, abdominal lymphadenopathy, intestinal/gastric mass: ○ Hypoechoic subcapsular thickening is associated with renal lymphoma. ○ Despite thickening of intestines, layering may be preserved.
• Computed tomography—space-occupying mass effect in affected area, especially used for nasal lymphoma.

DIAGNOSTIC PROCEDURES

• Aspiration or biopsy of a mass or lymph node. • Aspirate often sufficient to diagnose LCL; biopsy often required for SCL. • Can be challenging to distinguish SCL from inflammatory bowel disease (IBD).
• Immunohistochemistry (IHC) ± PCR for antigen receptor rearrangement (PARR) testing can be done to distinguish between IBD and SCL; sensitivity of IHC for detecting lymphoma 78% vs. 83% for IHC + PARR; sensitivity of PARR for detecting T-cell and B-cell lymphoma is 78% and 50%, respectively. • Staging—CBC/chemistry profile/urinalysis/FeLV/FIV testing, thoracic radiographs, abdominal ultrasound, regional lymph node aspirates for localized lesions, ± bone marrow aspirate depending on CBC findings; serum cobalamin level in SCL.

PATHOLOGIC FINDINGS

• Gross—usually white to gray in color with areas of hemorrhage and necrosis.
• Cytologic—monomorphic population of intermediate to large sized immature lymphocytes (lymphoblasts) in LCL vs monomorphic population of small mature lymphocytes in SCL. • Histopathologic—vary; several morphologic classification schemes in use: ○ Nasal lymphoma is most often immunoblastic B-cell origin. ○ Hodgkin's-like lymphoma is characterized by Reed–Sternberg cells and few neoplastic cells in a background of a reactive T-cell population with histiocytes and granulocytes. ○ LGL lymphoma most commonly affects the intestine and mesenteric lymph nodes. ○ B-cell most common in stomach (100%) and large intestine (88%); T-cell most common in small intestine (52%). ○ In gastrointestinal (GI) lymphoma, LCL more common than SCL when both cytologic and histopathologic samples are evaluated.

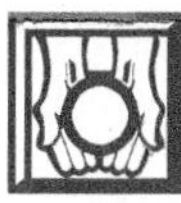

TREATMENT

APPROPRIATE HEALTH CARE

Outpatient whenever possible, supportive care if needed.

NURSING CARE

Fluid therapy, antiemetics, appetite stimulants, analgesia, thoracocentesis, etc. when indicated.

ACTIVITY

Normal

DIET

No change, can add *n*-3 fatty acids to diet (fish oil origin).

CLIENT EDUCATION

- Emphasize that side effects are treatable and should be addressed promptly. • Inform client that the goal is to induce remission and achieve a good quality of life for as long as possible.

SURGICAL CONSIDERATIONS

- To relieve intestinal obstructions or perforations and remove solitary masses. • To obtain specimens for histopathologic examination.

RADIATION THERAPY

Possible option for localized lesions, such as nasal cavity or mediastinum, as well as rescue treatment for GI LCL.

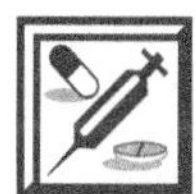

MEDICATIONS

DRUG(S) OF CHOICE

- Chemotherapy—there are many variations of similar combination protocols, all with similar efficacy. • High-grade lymphoma can respond to CHOP-based protocols (cyclophosphamide, doxorubicin, vincristine, prednisone/prednisolone) such as the University of Wisconsin–Madison protocol (alternating drugs in repeated sequence) or COP-based protocols (cyclophosphamide, vincristine, prednisone/prednisolone).
- Vinblastine has similar efficacy but less GI toxicity compared to vincristine. • SCL can respond to oral chlorambucil (either low dose daily/every other day or high dose pulsed) and prednisone/prednisolone. • Consult a veterinary oncologist for doses, schedules, and to help assess best option(s) for treatment.

CONTRAINDICATIONS

Avoid doxorubicin in cats with preexisting renal failure as high-cumulative dosages have been demonstrated to potentially be nephrotoxic.

PRECAUTIONS

- Myelosuppression secondary to chemotherapy—more in FeLV-positive cats. • Seek advice before initiating treatment if you are unfamiliar with cytotoxic drugs. Some drugs such as vincristine and doxorubicin are vesicants and can cause severe tissue sloughing if leaked outside the vein.

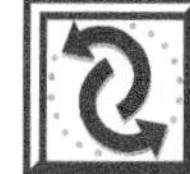

FOLLOW-UP

PATIENT MONITORING

- Physical examination and CBC—before each chemotherapy treatment and 1 week after each new drug is administered, or if there are concerns about low cell counts.
- Diagnostic imaging—as necessary depending on location to assess response to therapy.

PREVENTION/AVOIDANCE

Avoid exposure to or breeding FeLV-positive cats.

POSSIBLE COMPLICATIONS

- Leukopenia/neutropenia. • Sepsis.
- Anorexia, vomiting, weight loss; may need imaging tests to distinguish between chemotherapy side effects and lymphoma progression.

EXPECTED COURSE AND PROGNOSIS

- Depends on initial response to chemotherapy, anatomic type, FeLV status, and tumor burden.
- Median survival according to treatment (overall 50–70% response rate): ○ Prednisone alone—1.5–2 months. ○ COP/CHOP-based chemotherapy—6–9 months. • Doxorubicin-based, lomustine, MOMP (mechlorethamine, vincristine, melphalan, prednisone), and DMAC (dexamethasone, melphalan, actinomycin-D, cytarabine) rescue therapy reported for refractory lymphoma. • Median survival according to FeLV status: ○ Negative—7 months (17.5 months if low tumor burden). ○ Positive—3.5 months (4 months if low tumor burden). • Median survival according to anatomic location: ○ Renal—FeLV-negative, 11.5 months; FeLV-positive, 6.5 months. ○ Nasal—1.5–2.5 years with radiation and chemotherapy. • Chemotherapy may not improve survival over radiation alone. • Higher radiation doses (>32 Gy) result in longer survival. • Mediastinal—about 10% of patients live >2 years. • Alimentary—8 months.
- Peripheral multicentric—23.5 months. • If localized (median remission time)—114 weeks.
- Median survival according to histology (tumor grade or subtype): ○ SCL of GI tract with or without additional visceral involvement—95% overall response to chlorambucil and prednisone for median survival of approximately 2 years (longer in complete vs. partial remission). ○ LGLL—~30% response for median survival 57 days. • Cats with Hodgkin's-like lymphoma can do well for extended periods of time, even without treatment (months to years). • Weight loss during first month of treatment of LCL associated with shorter survival. • Clinical response after 1 cycle of COP chemotherapy associated with longer survival.

MISCELLANEOUS

ASSOCIATED CONDITIONS

- Hypoglycemia (rare). • Monoclonal gammopathy (rare). • Hypercalcemia (10–15%).

AGE-RELATED FACTORS

Young cats with lymphoma are generally FeLV-positive.

ZOONOTIC POTENTIAL

None

PREGNANCY/FERTILITY/BREEDING

Do not use chemotherapy in pregnant animals.

SYNONYMS

- Lymphosarcoma. • Malignant lymphoma.

ABBREVIATIONS

- FeLV = feline leukemia virus.
- GI = gastrointestinal.
- IBD = inflammatory bowel disease.
- IHC = immunohistochemistry.
- LCL = large cell lymphoma.
- LGLL = large granular lymphocyte lymphoma.
- PARR = PCR for antigen receptor rearrangement.
- SCL = small cell lymphoma.

Suggested Reading

Kiupel M, Smedley RC, Pfent C, et al. Diagnostic algorithm to differentiate lymphoma from inflammation in feline small intestinal biopsy samples. Vet Pathol 2011, 48(1):212–222.

Vail DM. Feline lymphoma and leukemia. In: Withrow SJ, Vail DM, Page RL, eds., Withrow and MacEwen's Small Animal Clinical Oncology, 5th ed. St. Louis, MO: Saunders Elsevier, 2013, pp. 638–653.

Wilson HM. Feline alimentary lymphoma: demystifying the enigma. Top Companion Anim Med 2008, 23(4):177–184.

Author Erika L. Krick

Consulting Editor Timothy M. Fan

Acknowledgment The author and editors acknowledge the prior contribution of Kim A. Selting.

Client Education Handout available online

LYMPHOMA—DOGS

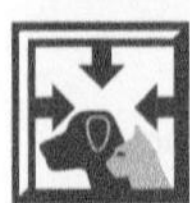

BASICS

DEFINITION

• Clonal proliferation of B-, T-, or non-B-/non-T-type (null cell) lymphoblasts found primarily in enlarged peripheral lymph nodes. • Cells can spread systemically to invade bone marrow, peripheral blood, CNS, and visceral organs.

PATHOPHYSIOLOGY

• ~85% of cases are multicentric (involving more than one lymph node). • ~75% are B-cell in origin and ~25% are T-cell in origin. • B-cell lymphoma (LSA) includes mainly multicentric B-cell lymphoma (80% of cases) which is an aggressive disease similar to human diffuse, large B-cell lymphoma (DLBCL), and marginal zone lymphoma (MZL, 20% of cases). Follicular lymphoma (FL) is rare. • Multicentric T-cell LSA includes aggressive (peripheral T-cell LSA—not otherwise specified [PTCL-NOS]) and indolent (T-zone LSA [TZL]) subtypes. T-cell LSAs are most commonly associated with hypercalcemia. • Aggressive lymphomas respond to treatment quickly, but have shorter overall survivals.

SYSTEMS AFFECTED

• Lymphatic (~85%)—generalized peripheral lymphadenopathy with or without splenic, hepatic, peripheral blood, and/or bone marrow involvement. • Gastrointestinal (~5–7%)—focal or diffuse infiltration of intestines, and associated lymph nodes. • Mediastinal (~5%)—proliferation of neoplastic lymphocytes in mediastinal lymph nodes, thymus, or both. • Skin—divided into cutaneous non-epitheliotropic B- and T-cell LSA and mycosis fungoides (epitheleiotropic T-cell LSA). • Hepatosplenic γδ T-cell LSA (rare)—liver/spleen sinusoidal infiltration of T-cells with eventual bone marrow infiltration. Erythrophagia commonly seen. • Intravascular LSA (rare)—typically T- or null cell proliferation in lumen or wall of blood vessel.

GENETICS

• Some chromosome copy number aberrations are shared between human and canine lymphomas. • Gene expression profiling can be used to separate distinct subtypes of human and canine lymphoma. • Canine DLBCL and MZL may be a continuum of the same disease.

INCIDENCE/PREVALENCE

• 20–107 LSA cases per 100,000 dogs. • LSA comprises up to 24% of all canine neoplasms and 83% of all canine hematopoietic malignancies.

SIGNALMENT

Breed Predilections

• Boxer, basset hound, golden retriever, Saint Bernard, Scottish terrier, Airedale terrier, and bulldog—reported high-risk breeds. • Dachshund and Pomeranian—reported low-risk breeds. • Breed determines relative risk for B-cell or T-cell disease: ~85% of boxer LSAs are T-cell in origin (>50% are CD3+CD4+ in origin), while golden retrievers develop both B- and T-cell LSA in an ~50:50 ratio.

Median Age

Historically, 6–9 years.

SIGNS

History

• Multicentric—from no clinical signs to anorexia, lethargy, vomiting, diarrhea, weight loss, fever, polydipsia and polyuria secondary to hypercalcemia. • Gastrointestinal—vomiting, diarrhea, anorexia, weight loss, malabsorption. • Mediastinal—respiratory distress, pleural effusion, coughing, difficulty swallowing, caval syndrome. • Skin: ○ Cutaneous LSA—lesions usually generalized or multifocal: nodules, plaques, ulcers, focal alopecia and hypopigmentation. ○ Mycosis fungoides—initial scaling, alopecia, pruritus progressing to thickened, ulcerated, exudative lesions. Later stages include proliferative plaques and nodules with progressive ulceration. Oral mucosa many times involved. • Extranodal—vary with the anatomic site: ocular—photophobia and conjunctivitis; CNS—neurologic deficits, paresis, paralysis, seizures; hepatosplenic—lethargy, inappetance, weakness, icterus.

Physical Examination Findings

• Multicentric—generalized, painless, enlarged peripheral lymph node(s) with or without hepatosplenomegaly. • Gastrointestinal—unremarkable to palpable thickened gut loops and/or abdominal mass, rectal mucosal irregularities, ascites. • Mediastinal—dyspnea; tachypnea; muffled heart sounds secondary to pleural effusion, pitting edema of head, neck, forelimbs. • Skin—raised plaques that may coalesce, patch lesions, and erythematous, exudative lesions. • Extranodal—ocular—anterior uveitis, retinal hemorrhages, and hyphema; CNS—dementia, seizures, and paralysis.

CAUSES

Suggested causes include heritable breed risks, chromosomal aberrations, increased telomerase activity, germline and somatic genetic mutations, epigenetic changes, retroviral infection, Epstein–Barr virus infection, and environmental factors.

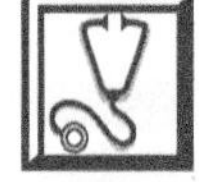

DIAGNOSIS

DIFFERENTIAL DIAGNOSIS

• Multicentric—disseminated infections, metastatic disease, immune-mediated disorders, other hematopoietic tumors. • Gastrointestinal—other GI tumors, foreign body, enteritis, GI ulceration, systemic mycosis. • Mediastinal—other tumors (thymoma, chemodectoma, ectopic thyroid), infectious disease. • Skin—infectious dermatitis, pyoderma, immune-mediated dermatitis, histiocytic or mast cell disease. • Extranodal—depends on affected site.

CBC/BIOCHEMISTRY/URINALYSIS

• Anemia of chronic disease, thrombocytopenia, lymphocytosis, lymphopenia, neutrophilia, monocytosis, circulating blasts, hypoproteinemia (GI). • Hypercalcemia, increased liver enzymes with hepatic involvement, increased creatinine or blood urea nitrogen with renal involvement. • Urinalysis usually normal.

OTHER LABORATORY TESTS

• Immunohistochemistry (lymph node [LN] biopsy/resection)—to determine immunophenotype. • Flow cytometry or PCR for antigen receptor rearrangements (PARR) (LN or affected organ fine-needle aspirates)—to determine immunophenotype.

IMAGING

• Thoracic radiography—sternal or tracheobronchial lymphadenopathy, widened mediastinum, pulmonary densities, and pleural effusion. • Abdominal ultrasonography—abdominal lymphadenopathy, hepatosplenic involvement, thickened bowel loops, other visceral organ involvement, ascites.

DIAGNOSTIC PROCEDURES

• Fine-needle aspirate cytology of enlarged lymph nodes or other affected organs—for cytopathologic confirmation. • LN biopsy or resection—for accurate histopathologic classification. • Bone marrow cytology—for accurate prognosis. • CSF analysis—if patient has neurologic signs. • ECG—identify arrhythmias before doxorubicin administration.

PATHOLOGIC FINDINGS

• Multicentric— effacement of LN parenchyma with large, neoplastic CD79a+ B-cells (high-grade DLBCL) or perifollicular proliferation of CD79a+ cells (MZL) or CD79a+ cell proliferation that maintains follicle architecture (FL). Effacement of LN parenchyma with large, neoplastic CD3+ T-cells (PTCL-NOS) or small, CD3+ cell proliferation between fading follicles (indolent TZL). • Gastrointestinal—infiltration of neoplastic lymphocytes throughout mucosa and submucosa, with occasional transmural infiltration. • Skin—CD79a+ B-cells infiltrating mucosa and submucosa, but sparing the epidermis (non-epitheliotrophic) LSA or CD3+ T-cells invading the epidermis: Pautrier's microabscesses (mycosis fungoides). Hepatosplenic—sinusoidal infiltration of erythrophagocytic CD3+ T-cells.

Staging

• I—one enlarged LN. • II—regionally enlarged LNs. • III—generalized LN involvement. • IV—visceral organ involvement.

• V—blood or bone marrow involvement.
• Substage a—not sick. • Substage b—sick.

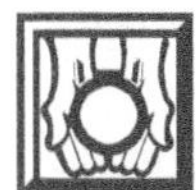

TREATMENT

APPROPRIATE HEALTH CARE

• High-grade LSAs are exquisitely sensitive to both chemotherapy and radiation. • Systemic multiagent chemotherapy—therapy of choice. • Radiation therapy—for refractory lymphadenopathy, large mediastinal masses, and solitary cutaneous areas. Half-body irradiation has been included into some chemotherapy protocols. • Surgery—rarely used unless an acutely obstructive GI mass is identified or to remove a refractory lymphadenopathy. • Autologous and allogeneic bone marrow transplantation (BMT)—after total body irradiation can be considered. • Fluid therapy—for advanced disease to treat clinically ill, azotemic, and/or dehydrated patients. Fluid therapy, steroids, ±calcitonin—to treat hypercalcemia. • Consider aggressive fluid therapy—to prevent tumor lysis syndrome when inducing dogs with a high tumor burden or dogs with peripheral blood lymphoblasts.

CLIENT EDUCATION

• Canine LSA is a treatable, but rarely curable disease. • Side effects of chemotherapy drugs include reversible GI tract and bone marrow toxicities. • Most dogs will not experience alopecia, but, dogs who need grooming will. • The vast majority of dogs receiving chemotherapy enjoy an excellent quality of life.

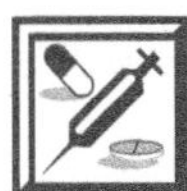

MEDICATIONS

DRUG(S) OF CHOICE

• Consider combination chemotherapy protocols to treat intermediate and high-grade diseases and single-agent protocols to treat indolent diseases. • Most multiagent protocols have superior remission and survival times when compared to single-agent protocols. • Corticosteroids alone can induce significant multidrug resistance.

Intermediate and High-Grade Lymphomas

• L-CHOP—L-asparaginase 10,000 IU/m^2, vincristine (Onvcovin) 0.7 mg/m^2 IV, cyclophosphamide (Cytoxan) 250 mg/m^2 IV or PO, doxorubicin (Adriamycin) 30 mg/m^2 IV, prednisone 30, 20, 10 mg/m^2 PO q24h tapering for 3 weeks. Consult a veterinary oncologist concerning the treatment schedule. • COP—vincristine 0.7 mg/m^2 IV, cyclophosphamide (Cytoxan) 250 mg/m^2 IV or PO, prednisone 30, 20, 10 mg/m^2 PO q24h tapering for 3 weeks. Each drug given weekly.

Single Agent

• Any drug of L-CHOP can be used as a single agent, but expect shorter overall survival than multiagent. • Doxorubicin (Adriamycin) 30 mg/m^2 IV every 3 weeks (1 mg/kg for dog <15 kg) 5–6 treatments. • CCNU (lomustine) 70 mg/m^2 PO every 3 weeks, prednisone 2 mg/kg PO daily. • Tanovea (rabacfosadine) 1 mg/kg IV every 3 weeks, prednisone 1 mg/kg PO EOD.

Low-Grade Lymphomas

• Chlorambucil (Leukeran) 6 mg/m^2 PO daily for 7–14 days, prednisone 2 mg/kg PO daily. Consider reducing chlorambucil dose to 3 mg/m^2 for maintenance. • CCNU (lomustine) as above.

PRECAUTIONS

• Doxorubicin—use dexrazoxane (Zinecard) in conjunction with doxorubicin or substitute epirubicin for dogs with cardiac issues. Always use a freshly placed catheter when administering IV doxorubicin. • L-Asparaginase and doxorubicin—pretreat with diphenhydramine 1–2 mg/kg SC, 15 minutes before administration. • Cytoxan—pretreat with furosemide 2 mg/kg to prevent sterile hemorrhagic cystitis.

POSSIBLE INTERACTIONS

Most chemotherapy drugs have overlapping GI and bone marrow toxicities. Consider antidiarrheals (metronidazole, loperamide) and antiemetics (metoclopramide, maropitant, ondansetron) to abrogate these effects.

ALTERNATIVE DRUG(S)

• Many published rescue protocols have been reported; therefore, always consult with a medical oncologist. • MOPP—mechlorethamine (Mustargen), vincristine, procarbazine, and prednisone. • DMAC—dexamethasone, melphalan, actinomycin-D, and cytosine arabinoside. • CCNU ± L-asparaginase, prednisone, or DTIC (dacarbazine). • Mitoxantrone alone or doxorubicin/DTIC.

FOLLOW-UP

PATIENT MONITORING

• Weekly physical examination to assess response and CBC to gauge bone marrow toxicities. • If neutropenia (neutrophils <1,500 cells/mm^3) is noted, reduce dosage (20–25%) of drug when given again.

POSSIBLE COMPLICATIONS

• Reversible neutropenia 7–10 days after chemotherapy. • Temporary vomiting, diarrhea, and anorexia 3–5 days after chemotherapy. • Alopecia in certain dog breeds that require grooming (poodle, shih tzu, etc.). • Febrile neutropenia (treated with broad-spectrum antibiotics).

EXPECTED COURSE AND PROGNOSIS

• >80% of dogs will go into clinical remission during the first month of induction chemotherapy. • Stage, substage, and immunophenotype are important prognostic indicators. • Expect median survivals of ~12–14 months and ~6–9 months in dogs with high-grade multicentric B- and T-cell LSA, respectively, when treated with a multiagent protocol. Dogs with indolent disease can live years. GI, mediastinal (T-cell ± hypercalcemia), and mycosis fungoides are associated with poorer response to treatment and an overall shorter survival time. • Autologous BMT can cure ~33% of dogs with B-cell LSA and ~15% of dogs with T-cell LSA. The cure rate of allogeneic BMT is currently unknown.

MISCELLANEOUS

PREGNANCY/FERTILITY/BREEDING

Treatment of pregnant dogs is usually contraindicated.

SYNONYMS

• Lymphosarcoma. • Malignant lymphoma.

SEE ALSO

• Hypercalcemia.
• Leukemia, Chronic Lymphocytic.

ABBREVIATIONS

• DLBCL = diffuse, large B-cell lymphoma.
• FL = follicular lymphoma.
• GI = gastrointestinal.
• LN = lymph node.
• LSA = lymphoma.
• MZL = marginal zone lymphoma.
• PTCL-NOS = peripheral T-cell lymphoma—not otherwise specified.
• TZL = T-zone lymphoma.

Suggested Reading

Bienzle D, Vernau W. The diagnostic assessment of canine lymphoma: implications for treatment. Clin Lab Med 2011, 31(1):21–39.

Rassnick KM, McEntee MC, Erb HN, et al. Comparison of 3 protocols for treatment after induction of remission in dogs with lymphoma. J Vet Intern Med 2007, 21(6):1364–1373.

Author Steven E. Suter

Consulting Editor Timothy M. Fan

Acknowledgment The author and editors acknowledge the prior contribution of Wallace B. Morrison.

Client Education Handout available online

LYMPHOMA, CUTANEOUS EPITHELIOTROPIC

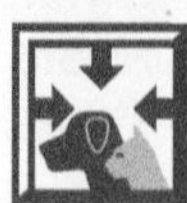

BASICS

OVERVIEW

- Cutaneous epitheliotropic lymphoma—most common form of cutaneous T-cell lymphoma.
- An uncommon malignant neoplasia of dogs and cats.
- Sézary syndrome—rare; cutaneous lesions, invasion of peripheral lymph nodes by neoplastic lymphocytes, and leukemia occur simultaneously.
- Pagetoid reticulosis—rare; the lymphoid infiltrate is confined to the epidermis and adnexal structures in the early stages of the disease and extends to the dermis in the late stages.
- Systems affected—hemic/lymphatic/immune; skin/exocrine.
- Synonyms—mycosis fungoides, lymphoma epidermotropic.

SIGNALMENT

- Dogs and cats—most common in dogs.
- Age range 6–14 years; mean 8.6 years.
- No apparent breed or sex predilection.

SIGNS

Historical Findings

- Chronic skin disease—months before diagnosis.
- Rarely acute.
- Mimics other inflammatory dermatoses.
- Typically pruritic in dogs and variably pruritic in cats.

Physical Examination Findings

- Four clinical categories of presentation:
  - Exfoliative erythroderma—generalized erythema, scaling, depigmentation, alopecia.
  - Mucocutaneous—depigmentation, erythema, erosion, and ulceration affecting mucocutaneous junctions.
  - Tumoral—solitary or multiple erythematous and scaly plaques, nodules, and masses.
  - Oral mucosal ulceration of gingiva, palate, and/or tongue.
- Lesions—typically throughout the skin; marked tendency for involvement of mucocutaneous junctions or oral cavity; lesions can be limited to the mucocutaneous junctions or oral mucosa.
- Exfoliative erythroderma; progression to the tumor stage is very rapid in dogs compared to humans.
- Mucocutaneous form and oral mucosa form: tend to merge with chronicity.
- Rarely nodules develop without a preexisting patch or plaque stage (d'emblee form).
- Nodular stage may occasionally progress to a disseminated form with lymph node involvement, leukemia, and rarely other organs.

CAUSES & RISK FACTORS

Risk of development from chronic antigenic stimulation (including allergy) theorized.

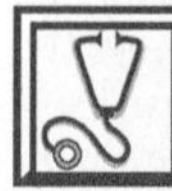

DIAGNOSIS

DIFFERENTIAL DIAGNOSIS

- Dermatophytosis.
- Demodicosis.
- Feline thymoma-associated exfoliative dermatitis.
- Allergic or parasitic dermatitis.
- Discoid lupus erythematosus.
- Erythema multiforme.
- Mucocutaneous pyoderma.
- Non-neoplastic stomatitis.
- Cutaneous neoplasia.

CBC/BIOCHEMISTRY/URINALYSIS

- Generally unremarkable if only the skin or mucosa is affected.
- Sézary cells—neoplastic lymphocytes (8–20 μm) with convoluted nucleus and cerebriform appearance are present in peripheral blood of Sézary syndrome patients.

DIAGNOSTIC PROCEDURES

Skin biopsy—definitive diagnosis; sample multiple different-appearing lesions, avoid eroded/ulcerated and infected lesions.

PATHOLOGIC FINDINGS

- Infiltrate of neoplastic lymphocytes—into epidermis, hair follicle epithelium, and adnexa; distributed diffusely or as discrete Pautrier microaggregates.
- Dermal infiltrate—polymorphous; malignant lymphocytes may obscure the dermoepidermal junction; patch and plaque stages, limited to the superficial dermis; nodular stage, extends to the deep dermis and subcutis.
- Immunohistochemical tissue staining reveals a predominance of CD8+ cytotoxic T-cells (dogs).

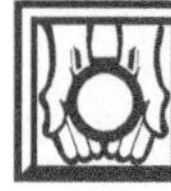

TREATMENT

- Grave prognosis—goal is to maintain a good quality of life.
- Therapy is rarely curative.
- Rarely, solitary nodules can be surgically excised.
- Total skin electron therapy or orthovoltage radiation: well tolerated, may be beneficial in some cases.

MEDICATIONS

DRUG(S) OF CHOICE

- Lomustine (CCNU)—overall response rate of 82% with remission achieved in about 32% of cases (initial dose 60 mg/m^2 PO; range 30–90 mg/m^2 every 3–4 weeks for a mean of 3–5 treatments).
- Dacarbazine 1000 mg/m^2—3 cycles report of remission in one dog with nodal involvement.
- Pegylated liposomal doxorubicin—44% response rate in dogs (average dose, 1 mg/kg IV every 3 weeks).
- Combination protocol (cyclophosphamide, doxorubicin, vincristine, and prednisolone)—partial to complete response in dogs that failed lomustine therapy.
- High-dose linoleic acid (e.g., safflower oil)—3 mL/kg orally twice weekly; good improvement in 7/10 dogs for up to 2 years.
- Topical chemotherapy—mechlorethamine (nitrogen mustard); some success in managing early lesions.
- Corticosteroids—topical and/or systemic may result in some symptomatic relief.
- Retinoids—isotretinoin 3 mg/kg/day or acitretin 2 mg/kg/day may be beneficial.
- Rabacfosadine—45% of dogs (5/11) had either complete remission or partial remission.

CONTRAINDICATIONS/POSSIBLE INTERACTIONS

Management by veterinary oncologist or dermatologist recommended.

FOLLOW-UP

- Average survival time for dogs depends upon stage of disease at diagnosis, therapeutic choice, and response to therapy; median 6 months (range 1 month–2 years).
- Death is usually the result of euthanasia.

MISCELLANEOUS

Suggested Reading

Rook KA. Canine and feline cutaneous epitheliotropic lymphoma and cutaneous lymphocytosis. Vet Clin North Am Small Anim Pract 2019, 49:67–81.

Author Sheila M.F. Torres

Consulting Editor Alexander H. Werner Resnick

LYSOSOMAL STORAGE DISEASES

BASICS

OVERVIEW

• Inherited disorders caused by partial or complete deficiency of a lysosomal enzyme or an enzyme-activator protein, which leads to intracellular accumulation (storage) of the substrate of that enzyme. • Storage products—proteins, carbohydrates, lipids, or a combination. • Classes of diseases—proteinoses, glycoproteinoses, oligosaccharidoses, sphingolipidoses, mucopolysaccharidoses. • Many different types reported in dogs and cats. • Inheritance is autosomal recessive.

SIGNALMENT

• Dog—German shepherd dog, German shorthaired pointer, English setter, beagle, Cairn terrier, bluetick hound, West Highland white terrier, Sydney silky terrier, English springer spaniel, Portuguese water dog, Japanese spaniel, Labrador retriever, American bulldog, Irish setter, mixed-breed dogs, many others. • Cat—Persian, Siamese, Korat, Balinese, domestic shorthair. • Most affected animals <1 year old; a few adult-onset diseases described, with onset as late as 2 years old, or older.

SIGNS

General Comments

• Vary with severity of the enzyme deficiency. • In certain diseases, carrier animals can be affected with a milder form of the disease. • Many organ systems are affected, but neurologic signs tend to predominate.

Historical Findings

• Affected animals are normal at birth. • Fail to thrive and may manifest skeletal malformations, particularly in the mucopolysaccharidoses. • Neurologic signs within the first few months of life suggest multifocal neurologic disease.

Physical/Neurologic Examination

• Cerebellar dysfunction common—intention tremors, nystagmus, dysmetria. • Peripheral neuropathy occurs in some diseases—weakness, hyporeflexia or areflexia, muscle wasting. • Other neurologic signs—ataxia; exercise intolerance; seizures; behavioral changes; visual deficits, deafness, stereotypical behaviors, proprioceptive deficits, tremors. • Non-neurologic signs—may see organomegaly or skeletal malformations. • Ocular pathology in some diseases—corneal opacification, cataract formation.

CAUSES & RISK FACTORS

• Genetic—deletion or mutation involving a single gene that causes an absolute or partial deficiency of a lysosomal enzyme or activator protein; deficient production of enzymes that do not have normal biologic activity. • Susceptible breed.

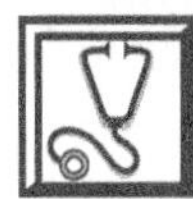

DIAGNOSIS

DIFFERENTIAL DIAGNOSIS

• Metabolic encephalopathy—usually episodic clinical signs; results of CBC, biochemistry, and urinalysis often diagnostic. • Toxicities—acute onset of clinical signs; history of exposure. • Cerebellar hypoplasia—onset at 3–6 weeks of age; nonprogressive. • Cerebellar abiotrophy—deficits limited to the cerebellum; may be difficult to differentiate in the early stages without specific tests. • Prenatal or neonatal infections (especially viral) resulting in meningoencephalomyelitis—differentiated by CSF analysis; may be other signs, such as chorioretinitis. • Metabolic diseases—especially organic and amino acidurias.

CBC/BIOCHEMISTRY/URINALYSIS

• Regular blood smears and CSF analysis—cytoplasmic vacuolation of leukocytes caused by accumulation of storage products is present in some cases. • Urine—may find abnormal accumulation of substances (e.g., oligosaccharide in α-mannosidosis).

IMAGING

• Radiography—bony malformation may be present in diseases in which skeletal pathology is a feature (e.g., mucopolysaccharidoses). • MRI—used in one case to reveal diffuse white matter pathology in the brain of a dog with globoid cell leukodystrophy.

DIAGNOSTIC PROCEDURES

• Molecular genetic testing—available for the diagnosis of many lysosomal storage diseases; may be used to identify potential carriers. • Aspirates or biopsies of parenchymal organs, particularly the liver and spleen—may reveal intracellular storage material. • Biochemical tests—diagnosis may be made by demonstrating low enzyme activity or presence of accumulated substrate or metabolic intermediates in preparations of serum, brain, viscera, leukocytes, or skin fibroblasts. • Electromyography and nerve conduction studies—abnormal in diseases in which peripheral neuropathy or myopathy is a feature. • Biopsy of peripheral nerve or skeletal muscle—may demonstrate specific pathology.

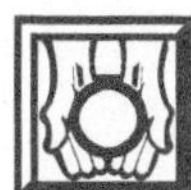

TREATMENT

• Outpatient—unless severe deficits preclude nursing care at home. • Activity—restrict to safe areas; avoid stairs. • Diet and fluids—ensure proper intake in patients often debilitated; parenteral fluid therapy and enteral or parenteral nutritional support may be needed with severe disease. • Bone marrow transplantation—used experimentally with some success. • Gene therapy—area of intense research that may offer hope for specific treatment. • Enzyme replacement therapy—intrathecal enzyme replacement has shown some efficacy in an experimental setting. • Primary treatment—preventive; control of breeding; genetic counseling. • Patients may be at risk of developing secondary infection; initiate appropriate treatment if infection develops.

MEDICATIONS

DRUG(S) OF CHOICE

N/A

FOLLOW-UP

• Progressive; ultimately fatal. • Pedigree analysis—useful in diagnosis; important for identification of potential carrier animals.

MISCELLANEOUS

Suggested Reading

Bradbury AM, Gurda BL, Casal ML, et al. A review of gene therapy in canine and feline models of lysosomal storage disorders. Hum Gene Ther Clin Dev 2015, Feb 11.

Dewey CW. Encephalopathies: disorders of the brain. In: Dewey CW, ed., A Practical Guide to Canine and Feline Neurology, 2nd ed. Ames, IA: Wiley-Blackwell, 2008, pp. 115–121.

Mellersh C. Inherited neurologic disorders in the dog: the science behind the solutions. Vet Clin North Am Small Anim Pract 2014, 44:1223–1234.

Skelly BJ, Franklin RJM. Recognition and diagnosis of lysosomal storage diseases in the cat and dog. J Vet Intern Med 2002, 16:133–141.

Author Stephanie Kube

MALASSEZIA DERMATITIS

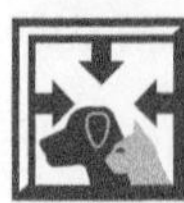

BASICS

OVERVIEW

- *Malassezia pachydermatis* is a lipid-loving commensal of the skin, ears, and mucocutaneous areas; can overgrow causing dermatitis, cheilitis, and otitis externa.
- Transformation from harmless commensal to pathogen related to allergy, seborrheic conditions, and congenital and hormonal factors.
- Systems affected—skin/exocrine.

SIGNALMENT

- Dog—any breed; West Highland white terrier, poodle, basset hound, cocker spaniel, and dachshund predisposed.
- Cat—less common; associated with internal neoplasia in aged cats; affects all breeds; young Rex cats predisposed.

M

SIGNS

- Pruritus variable; erythema, alopecia, scale, and greasiness of lips, ears, feet, axillae, inguinal area, and ventral neck; malodor.
- Hyperpigmentation and lichenification—chronic cases.
- Concurrent black waxy to seborrheic otitis—frequent.
- Frenzied facial pruritus—uncommon but characteristic.
- Often an allergy history that worsens and develops glucocorticoid tachyphylaxis.
- Concurrent bacterial folliculitis, hypersensitivity, endocrine and seborrheic dermatitis.

CAUSES & RISK FACTORS

- High humidity and temperature—may increase the frequency.
- Concurrent hypersensitivity disease predisposing factor.
- Seborrheic dermatitis (young dogs)—in predisposed breeds.
- Endocrinopathy—suspected predisposing factor.
- Genetic factors—in predisposed dog breeds. In Rex cats: genetic factors of the skin and/or their predisposition to a mast cell abnormality called urticaria pigmentosa are speculative risk factors.
- Concurrent increase of *Staphylococcus pseudintermedius* folliculitis—with overgrowth of both; treatment of one produces partial resolution and unmasks the other.
- Cats have a young and an adult-age disease that can be allergy-associated. Aged cats—*Malassezia* dermatitis associated with thymomas and carcinomas of the pancreas and liver.

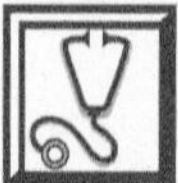

DIAGNOSIS

Demonstration of excessive numbers of the organism on diseased skin, and significant improvement following removal of the yeast.

DIFFERENTIAL DIAGNOSIS

- Allergic dermatitis—including flea allergy, atopy, and cutaneous adverse reaction to food.
- Superficial bacterial folliculitis.
- Primary and secondary seborrhea (keratinization defect).
- Acanthosis nigricans—dachshund.

CBC/BIOCHEMISTRY/URINALYSIS

Normal unless affected by underlying cause.

OTHER LABORATORY TESTS

- Fungal culture—press contact plates onto the affected skin surface; incubate for 3–7 days; count the distinctive yellow or buff, round, domed colonies (1–1.5 mm); provides semi-qualitative data.
- Nonquantitative culture methods—no value because *Malassezia* is a normal commensal.

DIAGNOSTIC PROCEDURES

- Skin cytology—touch, cotton swab, or cellophane tape preparation; apply stain as a drop directly onto the slide (yeast may wash off during staining); pass a flame under the slide to improve stain penetration and visualization.
- Greasy and/or scaly areas most likely to produce positive results.

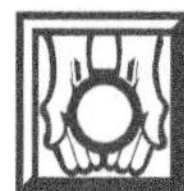

TREATMENT

- Identify and treat predisposing factors or diseases.
- Topical therapy—yeast is principally located in the stratum corneum.
- Shampoo treatment—to remove scale and exudation: miconazole and chlorhexidine shampoo most effective; selenium sulfide shampoo less effective but useful; twice-weekly treatments.
- Other topical antifungal agents (e.g., ketoconazole) also of value if given with suitable systemic medications.
- Alternative combinations—topical keratolytic shampoo treatment with systemic antiyeast and antibacterial drugs.

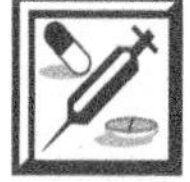

MEDICATIONS

DRUG(S) OF CHOICE

- Localized cases—may respond to lotions containing imidazole compounds.
- Ketoconazole 10 mg/kg q24h, fluconazole 10 mg/kg q24h, or itraconazole 5 mg/kg q24h for 2–4 weeks in widespread or chronic lichenified cases.
- Other imidazoles also effective.
- Topical antimicrobial antibacterial shampoo—to maintain remission in chronic cases.

CONTRAINDICATIONS/POSSIBLE INTERACTIONS

Ketoconazole may cause hepatic reaction; masks signs of hyperadrenocorticism and interferes with adrenal function tests due to blocking of cortisol production (via inhibition of P450) in the adrenal gland; may affect metabolism of other medications; contraindicated in cats. Azole-tolerant strains of Malassezia pachydermatis have been described.

FOLLOW-UP

- Physical examination and skin cytology—after 2–4 weeks, to monitor therapy.
- Treat until only rare organisms can be demonstrated or 7 days after a complete response is achieved.
- Pruritus and odor—usually noticeably improved within 1 week.
- Recurrences—common when underlying dermatoses are not well controlled; regular bathing with antifungal antibacterial shampoo combinations helps decrease recurrence.

MISCELLANEOUS

PREGNANCY/FERTILITY/BREEDING

Ketoconazole contraindicated.

Suggested Reading

Bond R, Morris DO, Guillot J, et al. Biology, diagnosis and treatment of *Malassezia* dermatitis in dogs and cats: Clinical Consensus Guidelines of the World Association for Veterinary Dermatology. Vet Dermatol 2020, 31:73–77.

Helton Rhodes KA, Werner A. Blackwell's Five-Minute Veterinary Consult: Clinical Companion: Small Animal Dermatology, 3rd ed. Hoboken, NJ: Wiley-Blackwell, 2018.

Author Kenneth V. Mason

Consulting Editor Alexander H. Werner Resnick

MALIGNANT FIBROUS HISTIOCYTOMA

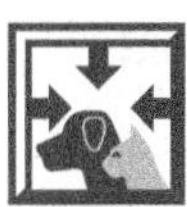

BASICS

OVERVIEW

- Name based on histologic features of fibroblast- and histiocyte-like cells.
- A group of primitive pleomorphic mesenchymal neoplasms, but definitive cellular origin unknown; likely possibilities include fibroblasts, histiocytes, and undifferentiated mesenchymal cells.
- Several histologic variants.
- Storiform-pleomorphic and giant cell—two major variants; both locally invasive; firm, subcutaneous, or visceral masses on examination.
- Despite previous reports to the contrary, metastatic potential in dogs appears to be moderate to high.
- Have been reported as injection site-related sarcomas of cats.

SIGNALMENT

- More commonly reported in cats than in dogs.
- Similar biologic behavior in both species.
- Mean age—cats: 9 years (range 2–12 years); dogs: 8 years (range <1–10 years).
- No proven breed or sex predilection, although flat-coated retrievers, Rottweilers, and golden retrievers appear overrepresented and may be predisposed.

SIGNS

Historical Findings

- Anorexia, weight loss, and lethargy may occur.
- Depend on site of involvement.

Physical Examination Findings

- Firm, invasive tumor arising in subcutaneous tissue.
- May exhibit deep extension into underlying skeletal muscle.
- May develop adjacent to bone and induce bone destruction and proliferation.
- Most common sites—dorsal thoracic and scapular area, limbs, and pelvic region.
- May also be a primary splenic tumor in dogs; palpable splenomegaly may be found.
- Distant metastasis—common.

CAUSES & RISK FACTORS

- Unknown.
- Can be induced with carcinogens in laboratory animal species.
- Injection sites in cats.

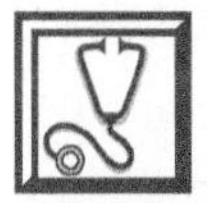

DIAGNOSIS

DIFFERENTIAL DIAGNOSIS

- Other forms of soft tissue sarcoma (e.g., fibrosarcoma, leiomyosarcoma).
- Chondrosarcoma.
- Osteosarcoma (extraskeletal).
- Liposarcoma.
- Peripheral nerve sheath tumors.
- Histiocytic diseases, such as histiocytic sarcoma or systemic histiocytosis.
- Mast cell neoplasia.

CBC/BIOCHEMISTRY/URINALYSIS

- CBC—may vary; may be normal; may see regenerative or nonregenerative anemia.
- Biochemistry—variably abnormal.
- Urinalysis—usually normal.

OTHER LABORATORY TESTS

Cytologic examination of aspirate—may reveal histiocyte- and fibroblast-like cells.

IMAGING

- Radiography—reveals soft tissue dense mass; may note bone proliferation or destruction.
- Three-view thoracic radiography to check for lung metastasis.
- MRI or CT may be superior for delineating extent of tumor invasion into surrounding tissues.
- Ultrasonography may detect abnormalities consistent with abdominal metastasis (most common in lymph nodes and liver).

DIAGNOSTIC PROCEDURES

Histologic examination of biopsy specimen—necessary for definitive diagnosis.

PATHOLOGIC FINDINGS

- Classification—considerable debate exists among pathologists regarding use of the term malignant fibrous histiocytoma, which may account for the apparent differences in behavior reported in the literature.
- Storiform-pleomorphic (may be called inflammatory) and giant cell (also called osteoclast-like) are the two major variants reported. Myxoid variant also described.
- Many are histologically high grade.
- Specialized immunohistologic stains, such as CD18, vimentin, desmin, alpha-smooth muscle actin, extra domain 1 (ED1), and/or azan (for collagen) may aid classification. Definitive staining patterns have not been clearly identified.
- Recent report of considerable overlapping histopathologic characteristics with histiocytic diseases in the splenic form.

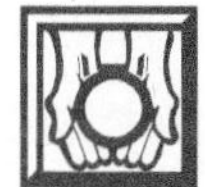

TREATMENT

- Surgical excision—difficult owing to local invasive nature; recurrence rate is high.
- Amputation of an affected limb—may be appropriate, however considerable metastatic risk; thoracic and abdominal radiographs and abdominal ultrasound critical for evaluating detectable metastasis before surgical treatment.
- Radiotherapy may be helpful as adjuvant treatment for localized tumor not amenable to complete surgical resection. Expected local tumor control rates may be similar to other high-grade soft tissue sarcomas.

MEDICATIONS

DRUG(S) OF CHOICE

Chemotherapy—may be helpful in residual, high-grade tumor or metastatic disease setting; doxorubicin-based protocols are most popular (dose for canine patients >10 kg, 30 mg/m^2 IV every 3 weeks; patients <10 kg, 1 mg/kg IV every 3 weeks).

CONTRAINDICATIONS/POSSIBLE INTERACTIONS

N/A

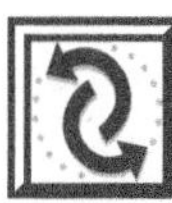

FOLLOW-UP

PATIENT MONITORING

Reexamination—metastatic potential would suggest physical examination and possible imaging; monthly for 3 months, then every 3 months thereafter.

POSSIBLE COMPLICATIONS

Temporary acute side effects (e.g., moist dermatitis and alopecia) may be expected with radiation therapy, and consultation with a radiation oncologist is recommended regarding specific, anatomic site-related side effects.

MISCELLANEOUS

Suggested Reading

Fulmer AK, Mauldin GE. Canine histiocytic neoplasia: an overview. Can Vet J 2007, 48:1041–1050.

Author Anthony J. Mutsaers
Consulting Editor Timothy M. Fan

M

MALOCCLUSIONS—SKELETAL AND DENTAL

BASICS

OVERVIEW

- Malocclusion is any deviation from normal occlusion due to abnormal positioning of a tooth (dental malocclusion) or due to asymmetry or deviation of bones that support the dentition (skeletal malocclusion).
- Ideal occlusion:
  - Maxillary incisors positioned rostral to the mandibular incisors.
  - Mandibular canine is inclined labially and bisects the space between the opposing maxillary third incisor and canine.
  - Maxillary premolars do not contact the mandibular premolars; mandibular premolar crowns are positioned lingual to the maxillary premolars; mandibular premolar crown cusps bisect the inter-dental spaces rostral to the corresponding maxillary premolar.
  - Maxillary fourth premolar mesial cusp is lateral to the space between the mandibular fourth premolar and first molar.

Terms of Malocclusion (American Veterinary Dental College Nomenclature)

- Neutroclusion (Class 1)—a normal rostral–caudal relationship of the maxillary and mandibular dental arches with malposition of one or more individual teeth (dental malocclusion); rostral (anterior) crossbite; mesioversion ("lance tooth"), linguoversion ("base-narrow" mandibular canine), and caudal (posterior) crossbite.
- Mandibular distoclusion (Class 2)—an abnormal rostral–caudal relationship in which the mandibular arch occludes caudal to its normal position relative to the maxillary arch (skeletal malocclusion).
- Mandibular mesioclusion (Class 3)—an abnormal rostral–caudal relationship in which the mandibular arch occludes rostral to its normal position relative to the maxillary (skeletal malocclusion).
- Asymmetrical skeletal malocclusion—maxillary–mandibular asymmetry that can occur in a rostro-caudal direction (unilateral abnormal relationship), in a side-to-side direction (loss of midline alignment), or in a dorso-ventral direction with abnormal vertical space between opposing dental arches (open bite).

SIGNALMENT

Species

Dogs and cats.

Breed Predilections

Breed predilection for certain malocclusions, some within breed standards.

Mean Age and Range

Malocclusion usually apparent after eruption of teeth (permanent or deciduous).

SIGNS

- Vary greatly according to type, extent, and consequent injuries caused by the malocclusion.
- May be associated with open or closed bites or overcrowding of the teeth.
- Periodontal disease—from crowding or misalignment of teeth.
- Soft tissue defects—from traumatic tooth contact; may be seen in the floor of the mouth and palate; palatal trauma may eventually result in oronasal fistula formation.
- Fractures or attrition (wear) of teeth—may result from improper tooth contact.

Class 1 Malocclusions

- Rostral crossbite—palatally displaced maxillary incisor(s) or labially displaced mandibular incisor(s); level bite—maxillary and mandibular cusps contact directly.
- Linguoversion base-narrow canines—tips of mandibular canines touch palate lingual to normal contact point, just labial to the diastema between corner incisor and maxillary canine (linguoversion).
- Lance teeth—mesioversion of maxillary canine(s); the diastema between the corner incisor and this canine is often diminished and may force the mandibular canine into an abnormal position. Dolichocephalic breeds (e.g., shelties and collies).
- Caudal crossbite—one or more mandibular cheek teeth buccal to maxillary teeth; more common in dolichocephalic breeds (e.g., collies, shelties, some sight hounds).

CAUSES & RISK FACTORS

- Congenital or hereditary factors—skeletal malocclusions (Classes 2, 3, and 4) and breed predilection.
- Impediment to tooth eruption—operculum; retention of soft tissue covering.
- Delayed eruption of deciduous or permanent teeth.
- Retention (persistent) or delayed loss of deciduous teeth; permanent mandibular canines (and most other teeth) will erupt lingual to persistent deciduous teeth; the permanent maxillary canine will erupt rostral to the deciduous tooth.
- Traumatic injury affecting the jaws or teeth.

Risk Factors

Hereditary predispositions.

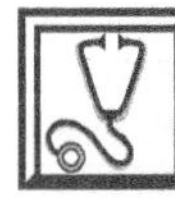

DIAGNOSIS

DIFFERENTIAL DIAGNOSIS

- Tooth displacement—due to trauma, oral masses, or other causes.
- Mechanical block—due to jaw fractures, luxated or subluxated teeth, or foreign bodies causing open bite.
- Examine breed standards to determine what might be acceptable for the breed.

CBC/BIOCHEMISTRY/URINALYSIS

Generally normal.

IMAGING

- Oral photography—pre-, peri-, and post-therapy.
- Intraoral radiography—to evaluate roots and abnormalities, jaw anatomy, root maturity.

DIAGNOSTIC PROCEDURES

- Complete oral examination to assess other oral abnormalities, including persistent deciduous teeth.
- Impressions and models—for evaluation and appliance production.

TREATMENT

Appropriate Health Care

- The accurate assessment of abnormalities of occlusion will help determine if treatment is warranted and what treatment is appropriate.
- Extraction of affected teeth can many times be an effective alternative to more classic orthodontic treatments.
- If the bite is functional and nontraumatic to the animal, treatment may not be necessary. Extraction (or crown reduction with pulp capping) of offending teeth can often be an effective alternative to more classic orthodontic treatments. Orthodontic treatment is usually based on prevention of improper contact trauma, wear, or injury to hard or soft tissues, and should only be performed by a trained individual.

Diet

Soft diet with appliances.

Client Education

Home Care with Appliance

- Examine the appliance twice daily.
- Flush the mouth with an oral hygiene solution or gel.
- Prevent chewing of items and provide a soft diet until the appliance is removed.

Surgical Considerations

Permanent Tooth Class 1 Malocclusion

- Treatment primarily involves tipping movements of the teeth, although extrusion may be required to provide proper retention.
- Rostral crossbite—correction for esthetics not recommended.
- Linguoversion mandibular canine teeth—prevention of contact trauma, pain and discomfort, and oronasal fistula formation.
  - The maxillary diastema must be sufficient for the mandibular canine to fit; natural retention once corrected.
  - Early intervention with manual manipulation or "ball therapy" for newly

erupting teeth may influence a more buccal position.
 - A hard rubber ball is placed in the mouth to help "slide" the canines laterally; two to three times daily, a few minutes at a time.
 - Gingivoplasty in the diastema may release the tooth if there is minimal maxillary mucosal contact.
 - A composite crown extension can help splay the tip buccal to the gingival margin.
 - More severe cases may require an orthodontic appliance (incline plane), to be handled by a specialist.
 - Mandibular canine extraction or crown reduction with vital pulp therapy.

- Maxillary canine mesioversion (Lance tooth): complicated movement; handled by specialist.
- Caudal crossbite—in traumatic situations, extraction of one of the offending teeth; orthodontic correction would be long and tedious.

Permanent Tooth Class 2, 3, and Asymmetrical Malocclusion

- If malocclusion is functional and nontraumatic, treatment may not be necessary.
- May require advanced orthodontic and surgical procedures by a specialist.

Deciduous Tooth Class 1 Malocclusion

Careful and gentle extraction of the maloccluded deciduous tooth (interceptive orthodontics) in hopes that the permanent tooth will erupt in the appropriate position; when performed at least 4 weeks prior to permanent tooth eruption, success rate >80% is not uncommon.

Deciduous Tooth Class 2, 3, and 4 Malocclusion

Careful and gentle extraction of the maloccluded deciduous tooth in hopes that the short jaws will be released from the bite interlock, allowing it to grow (if the genetic potential is present), performed at least 6 weeks prior to permanent tooth eruption, success rate <20% is common.

FOLLOW-UP

PATIENT MONITORING

- For the corrected occlusion to be stable, it needs to be self-retaining, or it may tend to revert to malocclusion; examine at 2 weeks, 2 months, and 6 months after the treatment is complete to see if desired outcome is stable.
- Radiographs at 6 months post therapy for radiographs to evaluate roots and teeth for any changes.

PREVENTION/AVOIDANCE

- Selective breeding based on preferred breed characteristics.
- Careful monitoring of deciduous and permanent tooth eruption for early detection and treatment, if required.

POSSIBLE COMPLICATIONS

- Deciduous tooth extractions—potential injury to underlying permanent tooth buds; injuries may result in tooth buds dying, teeth becoming nonvital as they erupt, root dysplasia or dilaceration, crown enamel hypoplasia, or hypomineralization.
- Orthodontic movement of permanent teeth—several conditions may result, including movement of anchor teeth, root resorption, root ankylosis, or nonvitality of the tooth; these conditions are uncommon in properly managed orthodontic procedures.

EXPECTED COURSE AND PROGNOSIS

- Course of treatment may vary with the type of malocclusion and the animal's nature and habits (e.g., inappropriate chewing).
- Generally, most cases take 1–7 months for movement and retention phase, depending on severity and if extrusion of tooth/teeth is required for stabilization of the bite. Prognosis is good to excellent in most treated patients.
- Prognosis is fair to good in most untreated malocclusions.
- Complications in untreated cases—periodontal disease; attrition or fractures of teeth; trauma to soft tissues; oronasal fistula formation; drying or desiccation of exposed tooth surfaces, resulting in beige to brown discoloration.
- Some cases do *not* need or require orthodontic intervention; only routine observation for early detection and treatment of any secondary complications (e.g., periodontal disease, worn or chipped teeth) is advised.

MISCELLANEOUS

ASSOCIATED CONDITIONS

- Lack of head symmetry.
- Oral soft tissue trauma.
- Chipped teeth.
- Desiccation of exposed tooth surfaces.
- Periodontal disease.

PREGNANCY/FERTILITY/BREEDING

Although animals have the medical right to as functional and correct an occlusion as can be reasonably provided by therapy, animal club rules, professional association principles, and state and national laws may conflict with an animal's right to proper medical therapy. Some kennel club rules disqualify animals with modification to natural appearance (with certain exceptions), and owners should be made aware of this. If hereditary involvement is suspected, inform the owner. If treatment is being considered, the owner or agent should acknowledge his or her responsibility to inform anyone who has the right to know of such alterations. Additionally, the possibility of removing the animal from the genetic pool by appropriate methods should be discussed.

INTERNET RESOURCES

hthttps://avdc.org/avdc-nomenclature/ (Accessed July 27, 2020).

Suggested Reading

Lobprise HB, Dodd JR. Wiggs' Veterinary Dentistry Principles and Practice. Hoboken, NJ: Wiley-Blackwell, 2019.

Author Heidi B. Lobprise

Consulting Editor Heidi B. Lobprise

Client Education Handout available online

MAMMARY GLAND HYPERPLASIA—CATS

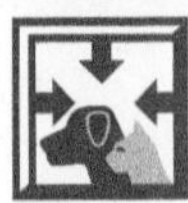

BASICS

OVERVIEW

Benign enlargement of one or more mammary glands.

SIGNALMENT

- Young, intact, cycling, or pregnant queens.
- Cats of either gender after gonadectomy (rare in tom).
- Cats of either gender that are receiving exogenous progestogen (e.g., megestrol acetate).
- Less often in older (9–12 years) pregnant queens.

SIGNS

- Localized or diffuse rapid (2–5 weeks) enlargement of one or more mammary glands.
- Firm and nonpainful masses in uncomplicated cases.
- No concurrent signs of systemic illness.

CAUSES & RISK FACTORS

- Exaggerated proliferation secondary to an endogenous progesterone influence (pregnancy, pseudopregnancy) or exogenous progestogens (megestrol or medroxyprogesterone acetate).
- May develop after gonadectomy; pathogenesis may involve progesterone, growth hormone, prolactin, insulin-like growth factors. Suspect ovarian remnant syndrome.
- Reported in one male with adrenocortical carcinoma producing steroid hormones.

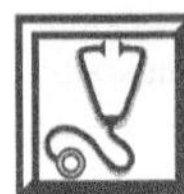

DIAGNOSIS

DIFFERENTIAL DIAGNOSIS

- Mastitis—lactating queen; mammary glands erythematous and painful; systemic illness with fever and immature neutrophilia; inflammatory cells and bacteria in fluid expressed from the affected gland(s).
- Mammary neoplasia—old queens (>6 years); gross appearance may be indistinguishable; irregular shape and margins, heterogeneous echogenicity on ultrasound; differentiated by biopsy or fine-needle aspirate of affected tissue.

CBC/BIOCHEMISTRY/URINALYSIS

Normal; leukocytosis possible if secondary mastitis present.

OTHER LABORATORY TESTS

Progesterone analysis—confirm exposure or ovarian remnant syndrome.

IMAGING

- Transabdominal ultrasonography—to rule out pregnancy.
- Ultrasonography of affected gland(s)—homogeneous parenchyma, round or oval with regular margins.

DIAGNOSTIC PROCEDURES

- Cytologic examination of fluid expressed from affected glands—noninflammatory.
- Fine-needle aspirates of affected glands may help to diagnose neoplasia and inflammation.
- Excisional biopsy—benign fibroglandular proliferation with no inflammation or necrosis.

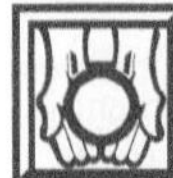

TREATMENT

- Hyperplasia owing to high endogenous progesterone—regresses when progesterone falls at the end of false pregnancy or gestation; consider ovariohysterectomy if preservation of fertility is not desired.
- Hyperplasia owing to exogenous progestagens—regresses when medication is withdrawn.
- Hyperplasia developing after gonadectomy—suspect ovarian remnant; surgical removal of remnants indicated.
- In uncomfortable animals, may attempt progesterone receptor blockers (aglepristone), prolactin inhibitors (bromocriptine, cabergoline), testosterone.
- Mastectomy, systemic antibiotics, or supportive care may be needed with complications.

MEDICATIONS

DRUG(S) OF CHOICE

- Bromocriptine mesylate 0.25 mg (per cat) PO q24h for 5–7 days; not approved for use in cats; may cause nausea. Can divide daily dose q12h to decrease nausea.
- Metoclopramide 0.2 mg/kg PO q6–8h for nausea.
- Cabergoline 5 µg/kg PO q24h for 5–7 days.
- Aglepristone 10–15 mg/kg SC on 2 consecutive days or 20 mg/kg SC once a week until resolution; not approved for use in cats, not readily available in the United States.
- Testosterone cypionate or testosterone enanthate 2 mg/kg IM once; not approved for use in cats.

CONTRAINDICATIONS/POSSIBLE INTERACTIONS

- Aglepristone—pregnant animals will abort. May see dermatitis at the site of injection.
- Dopamine agonists—pregnant animals will abort; may cause vomiting.

FOLLOW-UP

EXPECTED COURSE AND PROGNOSIS

- Remission within 4 weeks after the end of pseudopregnancy or gestation, withdrawal of progestins, ovariectomy, or aglepristone treatment.
- Unknown likelihood of recurrence in cats left intact.
- Unknown correlation with other abnormal conditions of the reproductive tract.

MISCELLANEOUS

PREGNANCY/FERTILITY/BREEDING

Fertility not affected after aglepristone treatment.

SEE ALSO

Ovarian Remnant Syndrome.

Suggested Reading

Burstyn U. Management of mastitis and abscessation of mammary glands secondary to fibroadenomatous hyperplasia in a primiparturient cat. J Am Vet Med Assoc 2010, 236:326–329.

Gimenz F, Hecht S, Craig LE, et al. Early detection, aggressive therapy: Optimizing the management of feline mammary masses. J Feline Med Surg 2010, 12:214–224.

Görlinger S, Kooistra HS, van den Borek A, et al. Treatment of fibroadenomatous hyperplasia in cats with aglepristone. J Vet Intern Med 2002, 16:710–713.

Hayden DW, Johnston SD, Krang DT, et al. Feline mammary hypertrophy/fibroadenoma complex: clinical and hormonal aspects. Am J Vet Res 1981, 42:1699–1703.

Johnston SD, Root Kustritz MV, Olson PN. Disorders of the mammary glands of the queen. In: Canine and Feline Theriogenology. Philadelphia, PA: Saunders, 2001, pp. 474–485.

Authors Maria Soledad Ferrer and Lynda M.J. Miller

Consulting Editor Erin E. Runcan

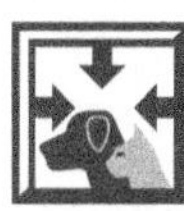

BASICS

DEFINITION

Malignant and benign tumors of the mammary glands in cats.

PATHOPHYSIOLOGY

• The majority of mammary gland tumors are malignant (85–95%) and tend to have an aggressive biologic behavior. Most malignant mammary tumors are adenocarcinomas; sarcomas are rare. • Exposure to ovarian hormones and exogenous progestin increases risk of mammary tumor development. Intact cats have a 7-fold increased risk of developing mammary tumors as compared to spayed cats. Spaying cats prior to 1 year of age greatly reduces risk of mammary tumor development. • While less common at diagnosis, pulmonary metastasis occurs in up to 80% of cats. Regional lymph node metastasis is common at diagnosis and may occur in up to 45% of cats. At necropsy, metastasis is identified in >90% of cats; other sites of metastasis may include liver, spleen, kidney, adrenal gland, pleura, peritoneum, and bone. • Inflammatory mammary carcinomas are rare. These are anaplastic carcinomas with considerable inflammatory cell infiltrates, and are associated with extensive local ulceration, edema, and pain, as well as rapid metastasis.

SYSTEMS AFFECTED

• Reproductive—mammary glands.
• Metastasis can affect any organ system, especially the respiratory and lymphatic systems.

GENETICS

The high incidence of mammary tumors in Siamese cats suggests a genetic component to this disease, but specific genes have not been identified to date.

INCIDENCE/PREVALENCE

• Third most common neoplasia in cats (after lymphoma and skin tumors). • The estimated incidence rate is 12.8–25.4 per 100,000 cats.

SIGNALMENT

Species

Cat

Breed Predilections

• Domestic shorthair and longhair breeds are affected most commonly, but likely reflects the popularity of these breeds rather than a true predilection. • Siamese cats have twice the risk of other breeds for developing mammary tumors.

Mean Age and Range

• Mean—10–12 years. • Range—9 months to 23 years; most are >5 years of age.
• Siamese cats tend to be diagnosed with mammary tumors at a younger age (mean of 9 years). • Male cats tend to be diagnosed with mammary tumors at an older age (mean of 12.8 years).

Predominant Sex

• Females predominate with only 1–5% of mammary carcinomas occurring in male cats.
• While being intact increases the risk of mammary tumors (see Risk Factors), most cats diagnosed with mammary tumors are spayed.

SIGNS

Historical Findings

• Most cats present for evaluation of a palpable ventral abdominal mass. • Cats with advanced metastatic disease may present for general signs of illness (e.g., lethargy or anorexia) or for signs attributable to a specific site of metastasis (e.g., dyspnea due to pulmonary metastasis or pleural effusion).
• The duration of clinical signs can vary from days to several months.

Physical Examination Findings

• Mammary masses can be discrete or infiltrative, soft or firm. Smaller masses often are freely moveable, whereas larger masses can adhere to the underlying abdominal musculature. • The overlying skin is often intact for smaller tumors, but larger tumors may be ulcerated and inflamed. • The associated nipple may be inflamed and exude serous fluid. • Any gland can be affected, although the caudal two glands are affected more commonly. Left and right sides are affected with equal frequency. • Up to 60% of cats will have multiple tumors on the same and/or opposite mammary chain. • Axillary or inguinal lymphadenopathy (reactive or metastatic) may be present. • Cats with inflammatory carcinomas present with severe ulceration, erythema, pain, and edema in the ventral abdomen and pelvic limbs.

CAUSES

Unknown

RISK FACTORS

• Compared to intact cats, those spayed at <6 months of age or 6–12 months had a 91% and 86% risk reduction, respectively, for mammary carcinoma development, suggesting that hormonal influence is significant.
• There is no obvious protective effect when cats are spayed at >12 months of age.
• Exogenous progestins (e.g., medroxyprogesterone acetate) increase the risk of benign and malignant mammary tumor development in female and male cats. In one study, 8 of 22 male cats with mammary carcinomas had a history of exogenous progestin therapy. • Parity has not been shown to affect mammary tumor development.

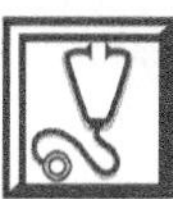

DIAGNOSIS

DIFFERENTIAL DIAGNOSIS

• Fibroepithelial hyperplasia—especially in young (<2 years) intact female cats, and older or spayed cats receiving exogenous progestins.
• Mastitis. • Other cutaneous or subcutaneous tumors. • Inguinal or axillary lymphadenopathy (reactive or neoplastic). • Inguinal hernia. • Large/prominent inguinal fat pad.

CBC/BIOCHEMISTRY/URINALYSIS

Usually unremarkable.

OTHER LABORATORY TESTS

Coagulation profile recommended for cats with suspected inflammatory carcinomas due to the high incidence of secondary disseminated intravascular coagulopathy.

M

IMAGING

• Three-view thoracic radiographs are recommended to screen for pulmonary metastasis, pleural effusion, and/or sternal lymphadenomegaly. Pulmonary metastases commonly appear as ill-defined interstitial nodules or a diffuse pulmonary pattern, although well-defined interstitial nodules are seen occasionally. Malignant pleural effusion is common and can obstruct adequate visualization of pulmonary parenchyma.
• Abdominal ultrasound is recommended to screen the medial iliac lymph nodes and other abdominal viscera for metastases. • Ultrasound also can be used to visualize nonpalpable axillary or inguinal lymph nodes, as well as to look for additional small masses within the mammary glands.

DIAGNOSTIC PROCEDURES

• Cytology can be useful for ruling out other nonmammary malignancies. However, it is not useful for distinguishing between benign and malignant mammary masses.
• Histopathologic evaluation is needed to reach a definitive diagnosis. Since most mammary tumors are malignant, this is usually performed on tissue removed during radical mastectomy (see Treatment). While not contraindicated, incisional biopsies are routinely recommended only for cats with advanced-stage disease that are not candidates for aggressive local surgery. • All tissue removed must be submitted for histopathologic evaluation. This allows for the most accurate diagnosis, and also allows for evaluation of surgical margins for completeness of excision. • The ipsilateral draining lymph nodes (axillary and inguinal) should be removed whenever possible and submitted separately for histopathologic evaluation, even if grossly normal. • Cytology of pleural fluid

can be useful for confirming intrathoracic metastasis.

PATHOLOGIC FINDINGS

• The most common histologic subtypes are tubulopapillary, cribriform, and solid carcinomas. • Histologic subtype has not consistently been shown to affect prognosis, but there is some evidence that tubulopapillary carcinomas carry a better prognosis. • Tumor grade, based on degree of tubule formation, nuclear and cellular pleomorphism, and mitotic index, is predictive of survival after surgery. • Vascular and lymphatic invasion is associated with more advanced clinical stage and shorter disease-free interval after treatment. • Mammary sarcomas are rare but potentially slow to metastasize. • Benign histologic subtypes are uncommon and may include mammary adenomas, ductal adenomas, fibroadenomas, and intraductal papillary adenomas.

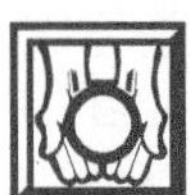

TREATMENT

APPROPRIATE HEALTH CARE

• Surgery is recommended for cats with gross disease confined to the mammary glands with or without regional lymph node involvement. • Adjuvant chemotherapy is recommended after the cat has recovered from surgery. • Chemotherapy can be used as a sole treatment modality for cats with nonsurgical local disease and/or distant metastasis, although long-term control would not be expected to be durable. • Radiation therapy has not been evaluated. • Palliative pain therapy is recommended for cats with nonresectable local disease or gross metastasis, or when definitive therapy is declined.

CLIENT EDUCATION

• Stress the benefits of early ovariohysterectomy (<6 months of age) in nonbreeding cats. • Stress the importance of early detection and aggressive treatment as small tumors (<2 cm) have a better prognosis.

SURGICAL CONSIDERATIONS

• Radical mastectomy of the affected mammary chain(s) is recommended. This significantly reduces the risk of local tumor recurrence as well as recurrence in the lymphatic vessels coursing through the mammary tissue. • Bilateral radical mastectomy, regardless of tumor location, has been shown to lead to deceased rates of local tumor recurrence, new mammary tumor development, and metastasis as well as increased survival time as compared unilateral mastectomy. Mastectomies are usually staged 2–4 weeks apart as performing bilateral mastectomies in a single surgical procedure is associated with increased risk of incisional dehiscence and/or infections and, less commonly, respiratory difficulty. • The inguinal and (if possible) axillary lymph nodes should be removed at the same time, regardless if they are normal in size. • In cats with advanced metastatic disease, palliative local mastectomy can be considered to remove an ulcerated or infected tumor.

MEDICATIONS

DRUG(S) OF CHOICE

• Doxorubicin 25 mg/m² IV every 3 weeks, alone or in combination with cyclophosphamide 100 mg/m² IV or PO divided over 4 days. • Mitoxantrone, carboplatin, and docetaxel might have activity. • Consult with an oncologist for current chemotherapy recommendations. • Palliative analgesics and antibiotics should be considered for cats with tumors that are painful and/or ulcerated.

CONTRAINDICATIONS

Use doxorubicin with caution in cats with renal or hepatic insufficiency.

PRECAUTIONS

If you are unfamiliar with chemotherapy, consult an oncologist before administering.

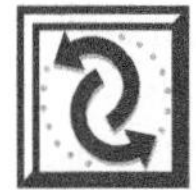

FOLLOW-UP

PATIENT MONITORING

• Thorough physical examination conducted monthly for the first 3 months, then every 2–3 months thereafter is recommended. Palpation of the previous incision line, the remaining mammary glands (if only unilateral radical mastectomy performed), and regional lymph nodes should be emphasized during examination. • Three-view thoracic radiographs every 2–3 months for detection of metastases. • Consider abdominal ultrasound every 2–3 months to monitor for local lymph node metastasis.

PREVENTION/AVOIDANCE

Ovariohysterectomy prior to 6 months of age is associated with a 91% risk reduction in the development of mammary carcinoma.

POSSIBLE COMPLICATIONS

Malignant pleural effusion may develop rapidly causing life-threatening dyspnea.

EXPECTED COURSE AND PROGNOSIS

• Most cats die from local recurrence and/or metastasis. • Tumor size is strongly predictive of prognosis. For tumors ≤2 cm in diameter median survival is >4.5 years (14 months in males), for tumors 2–3 cm it is 1–2 years (5–6 months in males), for tumors >3 cm it is 4–6 months (1–2 months in males). • Radical mastectomy significantly reduces the risk for local tumor recurrence. The impact on survival is not as consistent because of the high metastatic rate associated with this tumor. • In retrospective studies, adjuvant chemotherapy (doxorubicin with or without cyclophosphamide) has not consistently improved disease-free interval or survival. However, chemotherapy has proven efficacy against nonresectable and metastatic feline mammary tumors (gross disease), and given the high metastatic rate of these tumors adjuvant chemotherapy is still strongly recommended. • For cats with advanced-stage disease treated with chemotherapy alone, response rates are around 50%. Survival times are 6–12 months for cats that do have a positive response to treatment, <6 months for those that do not.

MISCELLANEOUS

PREGNANCY/FERTILITY/BREEDING

• Given the possible genetic contribution to this disease, particularly in Siamese cats, breeding affected cats is not recommended. • Chemotherapy is not recommended in pregnant queens, particularly during the early stages of pregnancy.

Suggested Reading

Gemignani F, Mayhew PD, Giuffrida MA, et al. Association of surgical approach with complication rate, progression-free survival time, and disease-specific survival time in cats with mammary adenocarcinoma: 107 cases (1991–2014). J Am Vet Med Assoc 2018, 252(11):1393–1402.

Morris J. Mammary tumours in the cat: size matters, so early intervention saves lives. J Feline Med Surg 2013, 15(5):391–400.

Novosad CA, O'Brien MG, McKnight JA, et al. Retrospective evaluation of adjunctive doxorubicin for the treatment of feline mammary gland adenocarcinoma: 67 cases. J Am Anim Hosp Assoc 2006, 42:110–120.

Overley B, Shofer FS, Goldschmidt MH, et al. Association between ovarihysterectomy and feline mammary carcinoma. J Vet Intern Med 2005, 19:560–563.

Author Jenna H. Burton

Consulting Editor Timothy M. Fan

Acknowledgment The author and editors acknowledge the prior contribution of Dennis B. Bailey.

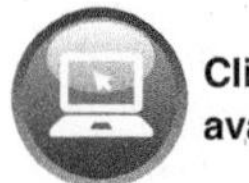

Client Education Handout available online

MAMMARY GLAND TUMORS—DOGS

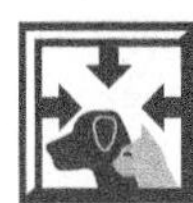

BASICS

DEFINITION

Benign or malignant tumors of the mammary glands in dogs.

PATHOPHYSIOLOGY

- Estrogen can exert direct genotoxic effects on mammary epithelium leading to mutations and aneuploidy.
- Progesterone may increase growth hormone and growth hormone receptor expression by the mammary gland, leading to increased insulin-like growth factor-1 (IGF-1) which is associated with proliferation and survival.
- Most dogs develop multiple tumors due to entire mammary tissue exposed to sex hormones during puberty, i.e., "field carcinogenesis."
- Mammary gland tumors are a continuum from benign to malignant.
- Obesity decreases sex hormone-binding globulin, leading to increased concentration of free estrogen.

SYSTEMS AFFECTED

- Reproductive.
- Metastasis—lymphatic, respiratory, skeletal, nervous, and other systems.

GENETICS

Germline mutations of *BRCA-1* and *-2* and *CDK5RAP2* genes reported in English springer spaniels.

INCIDENCE/PREVALENCE

Constitute 50–70% of all tumors in female dogs; 71% of all female beagles developed at least one mammary neoplasm.

SIGNALMENT

Breed Predilections

Toy and miniature poodle, English springer spaniel, Brittany spaniel, cocker spaniel, English setter, boxer, English pointer, German shepherd dog, Maltese, Samoyed, schnauzer, Doberman pinscher, shih tzu, and Yorkshire terrier.

Mean Age and Range

Uncommon in dogs <5 years; mean age 9–11 years (malignant) and 7–9 years (benign).

SIGNS

- 70% of patients have multiple tumors.
- Caudal mammary glands more commonly affected.
- Discrete, well-circumscribed mass in systemically healthy patient.
- Inflammatory carcinoma—diffuse edematous, warm, painful mammary chains.
- Inflammatory carcinoma associated with distant metastasis and systemic illness.

CAUSES

Unknown; likely hormonal.

RISK FACTORS

- Age.
- Breed—more common in small breeds than in large breeds.
- Hormone influence (see Prevention/Avoidance).
- Obesity during puberty increases risk. Underweight at 9–12 months of age associated with protective effect.

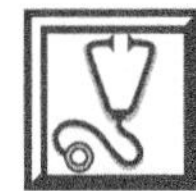

DIAGNOSIS

DIFFERENTIAL DIAGNOSIS

- Lipoma.
- Mast cell tumor.
- Mammary hyperplasia.
- Mastitis.
- Soft tissue sarcoma.

CBC/BIOCHEMISTRY/URINALYSIS

Usually normal.

OTHER LABORATORY TESTS

N/A

IMAGING

- Thoracic radiography may detect metastasis and three views are advised.
- CT is more sensitive for detection of pulmonary metastasis than are plain radiographs.
- CT lymphography could aid in the assessment of sentinel lymph node metastasis.
- Abdominal radiography may detect metastasis to regional lymph nodes or vertebrae.
- Abdominal sonography to evaluate for regional or distant metastasis.

DIAGNOSTIC PROCEDURES

- Fine-needle aspirate cytology—67.5–93% correlation with histopathology; 88% sensitivity and 96% specificity for malignancy.
- Fine-needle aspirate cytology of local lymph node(s).
- Histologic evaluation for definitive diagnosis. Request margin evaluation.

PATHOLOGIC FINDINGS

- There is a wide histologic spectrum of mammary tumors. Dogs may have concurrent benign and malignant tumors. Histologic examination of all excised masses is indicated.
- Histologic grading 1 (well-differentiated) to 3 (poorly differentiated) based on tubule formation, nuclear pleomorphism, and mitotic index valid for epithelial tumors only.
- Stromal invasion, vascular/lymphatic invasion, and lymph node status important.
- Complex carcinoma is more common than simple carcinoma.

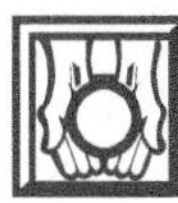

TREATMENT

APPROPRIATE HEALTH CARE

- Surgery—primary mode of treatment. Completeness of excision is prognostic.
- Chemotherapy—may be effective and indicated for patients with high risk of metastasis or recurrence: histologic high grade or subtype, lymphatic/vascular invasion, stage III or higher.

CLIENT EDUCATION

- Advise client that a mammary lump should be evaluated by a veterinary health professional.
- Inform client that early surgical intervention is best.
- Advise ovariohysterectomy at time of tumor removal.

SURGICAL CONSIDERATIONS

- Type of surgery determined by therapeutic intent: curative intent with wide excision; preventative with chain mastectomy; palliative intent for advanced disease.
- Consider age, tumor size, number of tumors, history of prior tumors, and clinical stage.
- Most patients with inflammatory carcinoma are poor surgical candidates due to profound diffuse microscopic disease, advanced stage, systemic illness, and local coagulopathies.
- 58% of dogs treated with regional mastectomy will develop a new tumor in the ipsilateral chain; increased risk if initial tumor is malignant (>70%).
- Current recommendations for single tumor of unknown histology: wide excision to achieve complete removal is the adequate surgical "dose," i.e., 2 cm lateral margins and 1 fascial plane deep.
- Extirpation of the draining lymph node is advised. Immunohistochemistry may be indicated to detect occult metastasis.
- Ovariohysterectomy (OHE) concurrent with tumor removal may decrease the risk of relapse in dogs with grade 2, estrogen receptor-positive tumors, or dogs with increased presurgical serum estradiol.
- Remove tumor following abdominal closure if performing concurrent OHE to avoid tumor seeding of abdomen or incision.

MEDICATIONS

DRUG(S) OF CHOICE

- Always consult a veterinary oncologist for updated information.
- Nonsteroidal anti-inflammatory drug (NSAID) as sole adjuvant therapy.
- Doxorubicin 30 mg/m^2 IV (dogs >15 kg)

MAMMARY GLAND TUMORS—DOGS (CONTINUED)

every 21 days (maximum 6 treatments).
- NSAID ± chemotherapy for inflammatory carcinoma.

CONTRAINDICATIONS

Doxorubicin—myocardial failure.

PRECAUTIONS

Chemotherapy may be toxic; seek advice before treatment if you are unfamiliar with cytotoxic drugs.

POSSIBLE INTERACTIONS

Doxorubicin—potential side effects include myelotoxicity, vomiting, diarrhea, and cardiac damage.

ALTERNATIVE DRUG(S)

- Carboplatin, mitoxantrone, gemcitabine, fluorouracil (5-FU), cyclophosphamide have been reported with varying impact on clinical outcome.
- Perioperative desmospressin for grade 2–3 carcinoma may improve survival.
- Tamoxifen—helpful in some humans with breast cancer; ineffective in dogs and has serious side effects (e.g., pyometra); do not use in dogs.

FOLLOW-UP

PATIENT MONITORING

Physical examination, abdominal sonography, and thoracic radiographs—1, 3, 6, 9, 12, 15, 18 months after treatment, then every 6 months thereafter.

PREVENTION/AVOIDANCE

- Spayed before first estrous cycle—0.5% lifetime risk of developing tumor.
- Spayed before second estrous cycle—8.0% lifetime risk.
- Spayed after second estrus—26% lifetime risk.
- Spayed after 2.5 years of age—no sparing effect on risk.

POSSIBLE COMPLICATIONS

- Infection or dehiscence with surgery.
- Myelosuppression with chemotherapy.
- Disseminated intravascular coagulation (DIC) with some (especially inflammatory carcinomas) types.

EXPECTED COURSE AND PROGNOSIS

- 50–70% of canine mammary tumors are malignant.
- 50% of malignant tumors metastasize.
- 58–70% of dogs will develop another tumor in the ipsilateral chain.
- Tumor diameter is strong predictor of local recurrence and distant metastasis and is a negative, independent prognosticator of survival.
- Lymph node status, histologic grade, and proposed World Health Organization (WHO) clinical stage (I–V) are most consistent prognostic factors.
    - Stage I: Tumor size <3 cm, no regional or distant metastasis—complete excision has excellent prognosis.
    - Stage II: Tumor 3–5 cm, no regional or distant metastasis—complete excision has excellent prognosis.
    - Stage III: Tumor >5 cm, no regional or distant metastasis—median survival 10 months with surgery alone.
    - Stage IV: Any tumor size, lymph node metastasis, no distant metastasis—median survival time 5–10 months with surgery.
    - Stage V: Any tumor size, any lymph node status, evidence of distant metastasis—median survival time <6 months.
- Clinical stage, presence of lymphatic invasion, ulceration, and incomplete surgical margins are reported as independent negative prognostic factors.
- Complex carcinoma and simple tubular carcinoma associated with prolonged survival
- Simple tubulopapillary carcinoma, intraductal papillary carcinoma, and malignant myoepithelialoma carries 10-fold higher risk of tumor-related death
- Adenosquamous carcinoma may have a high recurrence rate (50%).
- Anaplastic carcinoma and carcinosarcoma carry worst prognosis (<3 months) with >90% metastatic rate.
- Inflammatory carcinoma median survival time <3 months.
- WHO clinical stage may be applicable to noninflammatory epithelial tumors.
- Simple carcinoma and grade 1 tumors more commonly associated with stages I, II, or III.
- Lymph node invasion and less cellular differentiation more common in complex carcinoma than simple carcinoma.
- High COX2/CD31 or high COX2/VEGF coexpression have been associated with a decreased survival.

MISCELLANEOUS

ASSOCIATED CONDITIONS

- Paraneoplastic glomerulopathy and proteinuria.
- Hypertrophic osteopathy.
- Metastasis to lymph nodes, lungs, and CNS.

PREGNANCY/FERTILITY/BREEDING

- Treatment with progestin increases the chance of tumor development at a younger age.
- Treatment with progestin increases risk of development of benign tumor.
- Treatment with progestin and estrogen increases risk of malignant tumor development.

ABBREVIATIONS

- 5-FU = fluorouracil.
- DIC = disseminated intravascular coagulation.
- IGF-1 = insulin-like growth factor-1.
- NSAID = nonsteroidal anti-inflammatory drug.
- OHE = ovariohysterectomy.
- WHO = World Health Organization.

Suggested Reading

Henry, CJ. Mammary tumors. In: Henry CJ, Higginbotham ML, eds., Cancer Management in Small Animal Practice. Maryland Heights, MO: Elsevier Saunders, 2010, pp. 275–282.

Marconato L, Romanelli G, Stefanello D, et al. Prognostic factors for dogs with mammary inflammatory carcinoma: 43 cases (2003–2008). J Am Vet Med Assoc 2009, 235:967–972.

Rasotto R, Berlato D, Goldschmidt MH, Zappulli V. Prognostic significance of canine mammary tumor histologic subtypes: an observational cohort study of 229 cases. Vet Pathol 2017, 54:571–578.

Sorenmo KU, Rasotto R, Zappulli V, Goldschmidt MH. Development, anatomy, histology, lymphatic drainage, clinical features, and cell differentiation markers of canine mammary gland neoplasms. Vet Pathol 2011, 48:85–97.

Sorenmo KU, Worley DR, Goldschmidt MH. Tumors of the mammary gland. In: Withrow SJ, Vail DM, Page RL, eds., Small Animal Clinical Oncology, 5th ed. St. Louis, MO: Elsevier Saunders, 2013, pp. 538–556.

Tran CM, Moore AS, Frimberger AE. Surgical treatment of mammary carcinomas in dogs with or without postoperative chemotherapy. Vet Comp Oncol 2014, Apr 16.

Author Shawna L. Klahn

Consulting Editor Timothy M. Fan

Client Education Handout available online

MARIJUANA TOXICOSIS

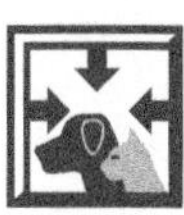

BASICS

OVERVIEW

• Marijuana is a general term that typically refers to *Cannabis sativa* or *C. indica* plants and is synonymous with cannabis. Its legal status in North America has changed substantially in the past decade and varies based on the country and state. • Of the 100+ cannabinoids in marijuana, the primary psychoactive compound (i.e., induces a "high") is δ-9-tetrahydrocannabinol (THC). THC is likely responsible for the clinical signs of poisoning in pets. • THC extracts can be added to foods or sold in a wide variety of products such as tinctures, capsules, oils, sublingual sprays, topical creams, bath bombs, even suppositories, or made into "concentrates"—wax-like formulations which are smoked or vaped. • The minimum lethal dose of marijuana plant material is greater than 3 g/kg for dogs. • THC binds to endocannabinoid receptors CB1 and CB2. • Cannabidiol (CBD), a cannabinoid commonly used in medical cannabis or sold as a "supplement" for pets and people, is not psychoactive although, depending on the quality of the product, some may inadvertently contain THC.
• Commonly affected organ systems are cardiovascular, gastrointestinal, nervous, ophthalmic, respiratory, renal/urologic.

SIGNALMENT

Younger animals may be overrepresented due to an increased tendency to ingest foreign items.

SIGNS

• Often begin 0.5–2 hours after ingestion; may begin in minutes following inhalation.
• Lethargy, ataxia, vomiting, glazed eyes, mydriasis, depression, hypothermia, trembling, urinary incontinence. • Higher doses may cause bradycardia, hypotension, and coma. Nystagmus, vocalization, sinus tachycardia, seizures, and hyperthermia may also occur.

CAUSES & RISK FACTORS

• Intoxication occurs via ingestion of foods containing THC, medical cannabis products, marijuana "concentrates," or inhalation of marijuana smoke. Pets in homes of recreational or medical marijuana users are at greater risk for exposure. • Of the cases reported to Pet Poison Helpline, an animal poison control center, about 65% involve food products, the majority of which also contain chocolate. Such foods may contain other toxic ingredients such as raisins, macadamia nuts, xylitol, etc. • Regions with marijuana dispensaries correlate to increased exposures.

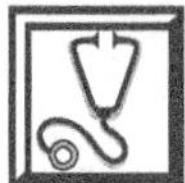

DIAGNOSIS

DIFFERENTIAL DIAGNOSIS

• Other illicit drugs—LSD (lysergic acid diethylamide), PCP (phencyclidine), hallucinogenic mushrooms. • Opioids (greater cardiac/respiratory depression, miosis, reversed with naloxone), benzodiazepines, muscle relaxants, ethanol, ethylene glycol (metabolic acidosis, crystalluria), methanol, diethylene glycol, propylene glycol, tranquilizers, depressants, xylitol (hypoglycemia).

CBC/BIOCHEMISTRY/URINALYSIS

No specific abnormalities but should be used to rule out other causes.

OTHER LABORATORY TESTS

• Human urine drug tests are generally unreliable and may result in false negatives. A positive result can typically be considered a true positive. • Serum, stomach contents and/or urine can be submitted to diagnostic labs for confirmatory testing.

IMAGING

No specific abnormalities but abdominal radiography is useful if an obstruction is suspected (e.g., ingestion of a baggie containing marijuana, packaging of a food product).

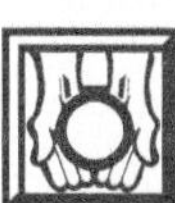

TREATMENT

• Mildly affected patients may not require intervention and can be kept in a low-stimulatory, protective environment. • Treatment is focused on decontamination and supportive care. Induce emesis following recent (<2 hours) ingestion in asymptomatic patients if they have not already vomited. If symptomatic, gastric lavage should be considered for large ingestions or if concentrated products were ingested. • Activated charcoal q8h for 2–3 doses if severe signs.
• Warming/cooling measures as needed. • IV fluid support if poor perfusion parameters or dehydration. • Oxygen if respiratory depression. • Provide ocular lubricant and rotation to comatose animals.

MEDICATIONS

DRUG(S) OF CHOICE

• Antiemetics (e.g., maropitant 1 mg/kg SQ, IV q24h dogs or cats) as needed. • Diazepam (0.5–1 mg/kg IV PRN dogs or cats) or butorphanol (0.1–0.4 mg/kg IM or IV dogs or cats) for CNS stimulation, anxiety, agitation.

CONTRAINDICATIONS/POSSIBLE INTERACTIONS

• Use acepromazine cautiously due to risk of hypotension. • Use phenobarbital cautiously due to the risk of severe sedation and respiratory depression.

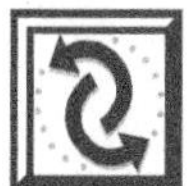

FOLLOW-UP

PATIENT MONITORING

Monitor temperature, pulse, and respiration q2–3h until normal. Monitor blood pressure in severe cases (hypotension).

PREVENTION/AVOIDANCE

• Educate pet owners about the risks of leaving cannabis products, especially food, accessible to pets. Stress that pets will readily consume such products. • Keep pets confined during parties.

EXPECTED COURSE AND PROGNOSIS

• Clinical signs may last up to 24 hours in mild cases and may be monitored at home.
• Clinical signs may persist for several days in severe cases, especially if a large dose were ingested. • The prognosis is excellent with appropriate care. • Death is rare but has been reported in dogs ingesting foods made with marijuana butter.

MISCELLANEOUS

ABBREVIATIONS

• CBD = cannabidiol.
• THC = δ-9-tetrahydrocannabinol.

Suggested Reading

Brutlag, A., Hommerding, H. Toxicology of marijuana, synthetic cannabinoids, and cannabidiol in dogs and cats. Vet Clin Small Anim 2018, 48:1087–1102.

Author Ahna G. Brutlag
Consulting Editor Lynn R. Hovda

Client Education Handout available online

MARKING, ROAMING, AND MOUNTING BEHAVIOR—CATS

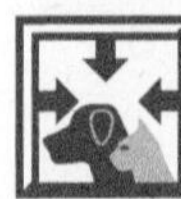

BASICS

OVERVIEW

- Urine marking—depositing of urine on vertical (spraying) or horizontal (especially novel) surfaces for communication (territorial, sexual, or agonistic situations).
- Roaming—escape or wandering for the purpose of seeking mates, defining territory, obtaining food, or sensory stimulation/enrichment.
- Urine marking and roaming behavior are normal but undesirable behaviors in companion cats.
- Mounting—mating behavior; mounting of inanimate objects for the purpose of masturbation.

M

SIGNALMENT

- Common in intact males, especially if estrus females are present.
- Can also occur in intact females or neutered individuals; marking reported in 10% of neutered males and 5% of spayed females.
- Roaming and mounting may be seen in 5–10% of neutered males.
- No age or breed predilection for marking or roaming.
- Mounting may be more common in sexually deprived, intact male cats mounting other males, females, kittens, people, and inanimate objects.

SIGNS

- Urine marking—characterized by the cat backing up to vertical object with an erect and quivering tail and projecting a stream of urine backward; may also occur with the cat assuming a squatting posture and depositing urine on horizontal surfaces, notably personal or novel items in the environment; urine deposited on multiple surface types in conjunction with normal litter box use for toileting of urine and feces.
- Mounting—of other cats, people, or objects.

CAUSES & RISK FACTORS

- Urine marking may function to delineate territory, aggressive intent, or reproductive communication between cats or as a response to anxiety.
- Likelihood of urine marking increases with density of cats in the household; however, urine marking may occur in households with only 1 or 2 cats.
- Marking associated with social conflict between cats in the same household, introduction of new cats, new furniture, or novel objects.
- Roaming is a normal exploratory behavior for enrichment, food, or sexual activity.
- Roaming is more likely in outdoor cats being housed indoors, intact male cats, and cats with a barren indoor environment (resulting in increased motivation to explore outdoors).
- Mounting can be seen in deprived males or isolated males or if males are housed in pairs.

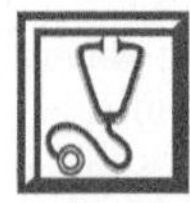

DIAGNOSIS

DIFFERENTIAL DIAGNOSIS

- Rule out causes of lower urinary tract disease and systemic diseases that might increase irritability including hyperthyroidism.
- Urine marking must be distinguished from inappropriate urination for the purpose of emptying the bladder. The latter problem is characterized by elimination on a consistent surface or location, may involve feces, and is usually associated with a decrease in use or avoidance of the litter box use. Cats that urine mark continue to use the litter box for toileting of urine and feces.
- Roaming behavior may occur due to any disease process that might cause a cat to seek isolation due to illness.
- For marking and mounting also consider neonatal testosterone exposure, treatment with anabolic steroids or testosterone, or retained or residual testicular tissue.

CBC/BIOCHEMISTRY/URINALYSIS

- Rarely do cats with roaming or mounting behaviors display abnormalities in lab work.
- CBC/biochemistry tests and thyroid evaluation can provide helpful information to rule out coexisting conditions and provide baseline data prior to initiating drug therapy.
- Urinalysis required to rule out underlying urinary tract disorders.

OTHER LABORATORY TESTS

- Unless indicated from baseline data, no further lab tests are necessary.
- In neutered and spayed females, rule out potential hormonal effects from retained or residual testicular tissue which might be associated with secondary sexual characteristics such as penile barbs and elevated testosterone in males or estrus-like behaviors in females.

IMAGING

Radiographs and ultrasound if exam, signs, and/or laboratory results indicate a need to further explore the urinary tract.

DIAGNOSTIC PROCEDURES

None indicated.

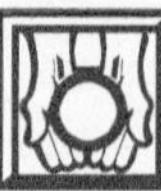

TREATMENT

Marking

- Neuter and spay intact animals.
- Provide alternate marking options such as scratching posts and facial marking combs (Cat-A-Comb). For some cats the use of a urine marking station (empty litter box placed vertically at location where marking occurs) may be appropriate.
- Multiple resources including feeding stations, water bowls, climbing and perching stations, and litter boxes in multiple locations (one litter box per cat plus one additional).
- Manage litter hygiene so that boxes are scooped daily and completely cleaned weekly (clay litters) or monthly (clumping litters) using hot water only (no cleansers).
- Increase perching and hiding opportunities (especially elevated locations) in each room of the home.
- Prevent access or supervise access to area being marked.
- Make marked areas less appealing by using double-sided tape or bubble wrap, or unpleasant odors (e.g., mothballs).
- Manage stress factors in the household (address relationship issues between cats in the home, provide for each cat's behavioral needs, manage interactions between cats and people in home to increase positive relationships by encouraging play and reinforcement-based training).
- Reduce exposure to outdoor cats by blocking visual access; decrease number of cats in yard (use of fencing, motion-activated sprinkler, remove bird feeders, etc.).
- Consider increasing (or decreasing) time allowed outdoors.
- Use synthetic facial pheromone (F3 fraction) spray or diffuser.
- Consider cat-appeasing pheromone for intraspecific social conflict.
- If necessary, reduce numbers of cats in the household to reduce density if intraspecific conflict due to overcrowding or social incompatibilities are an issue.

Roaming

- Neuter if intact.
- Use double barriers at exits (for example, screen doors) or confine away from doors (e.g., room).
- Alternately, allow controlled access to outdoors using cat fencing or screened areas or outdoor access on a leash and harness.
- Enrich environment with multiple small meals, random treats, and increased play opportunities. Feed the cat as soon as it returns home.

- Remove outdoor reinforcements such as outdoor cats through the use of fencing, motion-activated water sprinklers, removing bird feeders, and insuring neighbors not feeding.
- ID cat (tags, tattoo, or microchips).
- Synthetic facial pheromone (F3) diffuser in home.

Mounting

- Neuter if intact.
- Interrupt the behavior and redirect to more desirable behaviors such as play.
- Identify and remove any triggers which initiate the behavior.
- Provide alternative outlets for play/ enrichment.

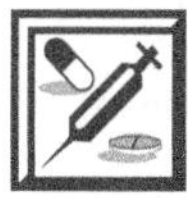

MEDICATIONS

DRUG(S) OF CHOICE

Marking

- Selective serotonin reuptake inhibitors (SSRIs)—fluoxetine or paroxetine 0.25–1.0 mg/kg PO q24h; side effects include sedation, anorexia, irritability, urine retention, constipation.
- Tricyclic antidepressants (TCAs)—clomipramine 0.25–1.0 mg/kg PO q24h; side effects include sedation, anticholinergic effects, arrhythmias, and gastrointestinal disturbances.
- Natural products that might aid in reducing anxiety—pheromones; L-theanine alone or in combination products; alpha-casozepine alone or in stress/calming diets (e.g., with L-tryptophan).

Roaming

No medications are recommended for roaming behavior.

Mounting

- Medications might be a consideration if a stress/anxiety component identified.
- Fluoxetine or clomipramine as in urine marking.
- Lorazepam 0.125–0.5 mg per cat PO q12–24h; side effects include sedation, hyperphagia, and rare hepatic toxicity (as reported with diazepam).

CONTRAINDICATIONS/POSSIBLE INTERACTIONS

- Do not use fluoxetine or clomipramine with monoamine oxidase (MAO) inhibitors such as selegiline.
- Caution in using TCAs when treating cats with diabetes, glaucoma, cardiac disease, or seizures.
- Do not combine a TCA with an SSRI or other drugs that might increase serotonin.

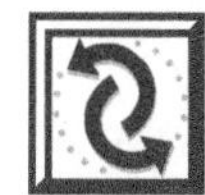

FOLLOW-UP

PATIENT MONITORING

- Telephone follow-up within 2 weeks after consultation, repeat as needed to monitor progress and assess response to treatment.
- ECG if concerns about cardiac status.
- CBC and biochemistry profile 3–4 weeks after initiating medical therapy and then q6–12 months.

EXPECTED COURSE AND PROGNOSIS

- Response to therapy within 4 weeks.
- Continue drug therapy for minimum 8 weeks if response noted; continue 1 month beyond resolution.
- When behavior is stable, wean dose by 25% per week.
- If behavior recurs, reinstitute lowest effective dose.
- Some cats may need to be maintained on medication indefinitely.

MISCELLANEOUS

SEE ALSO

Housesoiling—Cats.

ABBREVIATIONS

- MAO = monoamine oxidase.
- SSRI = selective serotonin reuptake inhibitor.
- TCA = tricyclic antidepressant.

Suggested Reading

Hart BL, Cliff KD, Tynes VV, et al. Control of urine marking by use of long-term treatment with fluoxetine or clomipramine in cats. J Am Vet Med Assoc 2005, 226:378–382.

Horwitz D, ed. Blackwell's Five-Minute Veterinary Consult Clinical Companion: Canine and Feline Behavior, 2nd ed. Hoboken, NJ: John Wiley & Sons, 2018, pp. 700–711.

Pryor PA, Hart BL, Bain MJ, et al. Causes of urine marking in cats and the effects of environmental management on the frequency of marking. J Am Vet Med Assoc 2001, 219:1709–1713.

Author John J. Ciribassi

Consulting Editor Gary M. Landsberg

MARKING, ROAMING, AND MOUNTING BEHAVIOR—DOGS

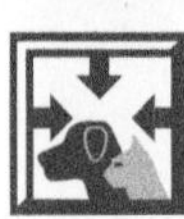

BASICS

DEFINITION

• Marking, roaming, and mounting fall within the normal behavioral repertoire for the dog. However, they are objectionable to owners if shown to excess or in an inappropriate context, particularly in a sexually altered dog. • Normal behaviors with multiple causes—may be maladaptive owing to stimuli in the environment. • Marking—generates a signal for conspecifics with a visual mark, scent (urine, feces, anal sacs, or sebaceous glands) or both on an object or to define territory. • Roaming—wandering from territory for exploration or in search of mates, food, or social contact. • Mounting—primarily a component of mating behavior but also shown in social contexts and play (especially in prepubertal dogs).

GENETICS

None; however, may be more common in familial lines.

INCIDENCE/PREVALENCE

• Mounting—approximately 11%; running away—approximately 11%. • Marking—unknown; estimates up to 8%.

SIGNALMENT

Breed Predilections

Any breed.

Mean Age and Range

• Age at onset—sexual maturity (between 6 and 18 months of age). • Mounting may occur in prepubertal puppies.

Predominant Sex

• Most common in intact males. • May be seen in intact females in estrus, castrated males, and spayed females.

SIGNS

Historical Findings

• Marking—deposition of urine and/or feces in locations unacceptable to owners; occurs inside and outside of the home.
• Roaming—wandering behavior that takes the dog away from its home territory.
• Mounting—a behavior in which a dog places the cranial part of its body onto other dogs, animals, people, or objects while wrapping forelimbs around the target often with pelvic thrusting.

Physical Examination Findings

• Typically unremarkable unless a medical etiology is suspected (especially for marking behavior). • For inappropriate mounting of other dogs, it is advisable to also perform a physical examination on the target animal.

CAUSES

• Normal behaviors. Urine marking occurs most commonly in novel areas. Female dogs rarely mark in the home. • Hormonally regulated; intact males likely to roam, mark, and mount; prenatal testosterone surge leads to the brain's response to testosterone at puberty (i.e., sexual dimorphic behavior).
• Learned components possible; reproductive status not sole variable.

Roaming

• Anxiety. • Curiosity. • Reproduction.
• Social contact and play.

Marking

• Medical. • Communication with conspecifics; communicates social rank, sexual status, territorial boundaries, or general information not related to the need to empty the bladder or bowel. • Anxiety if excessive or in the home.

Mounting

• Sexual (including courtship and masturbation).
• Play. • Social status or cohesion. • Attention-seeking. • Anxiety. • Displacement behavior/compulsive disorder.

RISK FACTORS

• Intact males more likely to roam, mark, and mount. • Marking on walks; learned behavior. • Mounting only in front of owners; attention-seeking. • Intact bitches, or females spayed after first heat.

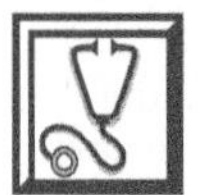

DIAGNOSIS

DIFFERENTIAL DIAGNOSIS

Normal or a sign of another diagnosis.

Roaming

• Sexually motivated. • Testosterone-producing tumors. • Searching for food.
• Separation anxiety—escape/avoidance.
• Noise phobias—escape/avoidance.
• Territorial behavior. • Social seeking.
• Social conflict in home territory.
• Predatory behavior. • Escaping from enclosure—play/investigative behavior.

Marking

• Sexually motivated. • Testosterone-producing tumors. • Territorial behavior.
• Social status behavior. • Conflict behavior.
• Anxiety. • Cognitive dysfunction syndrome.
• Housesoiling. • Excitement/submissive urination. • Urinary tract disease. • Any medical condition that causes polyuria/polydipsia (PU/PD). • Constipation or diarrhea. • Anal sac disease.

Mounting

• Sexually motivated. • Testosterone-producing tumors. • Social status behavior.
• Endocrine disease. • Urinary tract disease.
• If target is another dog, look at target for:
◦ Estrogen-producing tumors. ◦ Infections of anal sacs, uterus, vagina, or urinary tract.

OTHER LABORATORY TESTS

• If indicated, based on physical exam, clinical signs, sex, and age. • Thyroid testing if roaming for food. • In neutered males showing intact male behavior, consider baseline testosterone then administer gonadotropin-releasing hormone (GnRH) followed by a post-injection blood sample to rule out retained testicular tissue. • Urine culture and sensitivity. • Vaginal cytology to determine estrus status. • If target of mounting is another dog, exam target for:
◦ Blood estrogen levels (reproductive tumors). ◦ Urine culture and sensitivity.
◦ Vaginal cytology, culture and sensitivity.

DIAGNOSTIC PROCEDURES

• Behavioral history and clinical signs. • Rule out medical differentials.

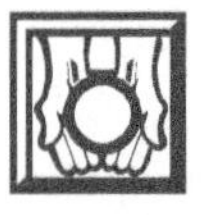

TREATMENT

ACTIVITY

See Client Education.

DIET

No special dietary considerations.

CLIENT EDUCATION

Roaming

• Secure enclosure to prevent escape. • Leash walk. • Adequate exercise, attention, supervision, stimulation. • Doggie daycare.

Marking

• Restrict access to targeted areas with confinement training or barricades. • Provide indoor supervision when the owner is present.
• Remove stimuli or triggers. • Express anal sacs if necessary. • Use Bellyband (male) or Puppy Pants (female). • Clean marked areas with effective enzymatic cleaners. • Cue/reward-based interaction with dog. • Avoid confrontation or punishment. • Counter-conditioning and desensitization to trigger stimuli or for anxiety conditions.

Mounting

• Obedience training. • Cue/reward-based interaction with dog. • Counter-conditioning or systematic desensitization to trigger stimuli or for anxiety conditions. • Adequate exercise, attention, and stimulation. • Ignore behavior if attention seeking - reorient or redirect into alternative desirable. • Avoid confrontation that adds to anxiety and conflict.

SURGICAL CONSIDERATIONS

• Neuter intact males. • Remove retained testicular tissue if indicated. • Spay marking females.

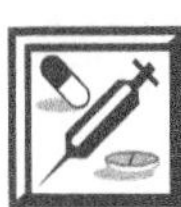

MEDICATIONS

DRUG(S) OF CHOICE

• Medication is not necessary for roaming unless the primary problem (separation anxiety or noise phobias) warrants its use. Medical etiologies should be treated accordingly. • No drug is approved for the treatment of marking or mounting; medication use is *only* indicated if anxiety is a contributing motivation. • Medication should *only* be used in combination with a sound behavior modification plan.

Tricyclic Antidepressants (TCAs)

• Amitriptyline 2–4 mg/kg PO q12h.
• Clomipramine 1–3 mg/kg PO q12h. • Side effects include sedation, anticholinergic effects, cardiac conduction disturbances, and gastrointestinal (GI) signs.

Selective Serotonin Reuptake Inhibitors (SSRIs)

• Fluoxetine 0.5–2 mg/kg PO q24h.
• Paroxetine 1–2 mg/kg PO q24h.
• Sertraline 1–3 mg/kg PO q24h or divided q12h. • Side effects include inappetence, lethargy, irritability, urine retention and anticholinergic effects with paroxetine.

Azapirone

• Buspirone 0.5–2 mg/kg PO q8–12h.
• Side effects—GI signs.

Benzodiazepines

In dogs with concurrent anxiety diagnoses—alprazolam 0.01–0.1 mg/kg PO q8–12h.

CONTRAINDICATIONS

TCAs are contraindicated in animals with cardiac conduction disturbances or glaucoma.

PRECAUTIONS

• Clients should be advised that occasional cases of increased aggression have been reported with TCAs and SSRIs. • Use caution with all drugs if dog has hepatic or renal compromise. • Use benzodiazepines with caution in aggressive dogs because of potential for disinhibition.

POSSIBLE INTERACTIONS

• TCAs and SSRIs should not be used together. • Do not use TCAs or SSRIs with monoamine oxidase inhibitors, including amitraz products and selegiline.

ALTERNATIVE DRUG(S)

• For anxiety, consider dog-appeasing pheromones and natural supplements containing alpha-casozepine (Zylkene) alone or in a diet in combination with L-tryptophan (Canine Calm diet); L-theanine alone (Anxitane) or in combination products containing whey protein, *Phellodendron amurense* and *Magnolia officinalis* (Solliquin); *Souroubea* and *Plantanus* (Zentrol) or probiotics (Calming Care). • In intact males, when the behavior is suspected to be hormonally modulated, consider the use of medications that decrease blood testosterone levels.

GnRH Agonists

• Do not use in breeding animals during the breeding season. • Effect is reversible when GnRH agonist is discontinued.

Megestrol Acetate

• Outdated treatment. • Side effects include obesity, pyometra, PU/PD, diabetes mellitus, mammary hyperplasia, and carcinoma.

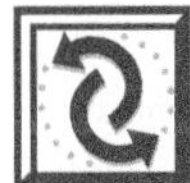

FOLLOW-UP

PATIENT MONITORING

Follow-up is variable depending on the severity of the problem and whether medication is prescribed. Help may be needed implementing changes to the environment and behavior modification. Owners should be encouraged to keep logs or journals detailing episodes of marking, roaming, or mounting to assess treatment success or nonresponse. If medication is prescribed, follow-up and journals are essential to assess response. In urine marking, owners should be encouraged to supervise the dog indoors and to inspect areas daily for urine marks.

PREVENTION/AVOIDANCE

• Neutering males and spaying females reduces likelihood of marking, roaming, and mounting behavior. • Provide client education for prevention and management with proper husbandry and reward-based training.

POSSIBLE COMPLICATIONS

• Roaming—becoming lost or picked up by animal control; possible injury from car accidents or fighting with other animals.
• Marking—property damage when it occurs inside the home. • Mounting—disruption of relationship with familiar dogs; possible fighting with other animals. • Pet relinquishment.

EXPECTED COURSE AND PROGNOSIS

• Prognosis is good if the correct cause is determined and the owner is compliant with the behavior protocols. • Castration will decrease house marking by 90% or better in 40% of male dogs, while 80% of dogs will decrease marking by at least 50%. Castration has little to no effect on urine marking in outdoor areas. • Castration decreases mounting in more than 65% of dogs but relatively few stop completely. Castration has its greatest effect when the target of mounting is human rather than dog.

MISCELLANEOUS

AGE-RELATED FACTORS

Intact animals older than sexual maturity.

ZOONOTIC POTENTIAL

Roaming exposes pet to other animals, including wildlife—rabies exposure possible.

PREGNANCY/FERTILITY/BREEDING

Listed medications should be avoided in pregnant animals.

SEE ALSO

Housesoiling—Dogs.

ABBREVIATIONS

• GI = gastrointestinal.
• GnRH = gonadotropin-releasing hormone.
• PU/PD = polyuria/polydipsia.
• SSRI = selective serotonin reuptake inhibitor.
• TCA = tricyclic antidepressant.

Suggested Reading

Connolly PB. Reproductive behavior problems. In: Horwitz DF, Mills DS, Heath S, eds., BSAVA Manual of Canine and Feline Behavioural Medicine. Gloucester: British Small Animal Veterinary Association, 2002, pp. 128–143.

Horwitz D, ed. Blackwell's Five-Minute Veterinary Consult Clinical Companion: Canine and Feline Behavior, 2nd ed. Hoboken, NJ: John Wiley & Sons, 2018, pp. 690–699, 795–804, 847–853.

Author Gerrard Flannigan
Consulting Editor Gary M. Landsberg

M

MAST CELL TUMORS

BASICS

DEFINITION

• Malignant round cells derived of hematopoietic origin containing granules packed with many vasoactive substances, including histamine, heparin, serotonin, dopamine, tryptase, and chymase. • Tumors may affect dermis, subcutis, spleen, liver, intestines as well as other connective and mucosal sites.

PATHOPHYSIOLOGY

• Histamine release from mast cell tumors (MCTs) affects a multitude of tissues.
• Histamine (H2) receptors are primarily located within the stomach and histamine is thought to be one of the most significant stimulants of gastric acid secretion in addition to gastrin and acetylcholine. • In extreme cases, perforation of the gastrointestinal (GI) tract may occur, leading to peritonitis.
• Histamine release around a tumor leads to the production of wheals, hives, and erythema (Darier's flare). • Local release of heparin is also common, resulting in bleeding and subsequent bruising, which can be seen around the tumor.

SYSTEMS AFFECTED

• Skin—MCTs are the most common malignant cutaneous tumor of the dog.
• GI—on necropsy evaluation, 35–83% of dogs with MCTs have evidence of GI ulceration. • Hemic/lymph/immune—regional lymph node metastasis is common in high-grade tumors. • Hepatobiliary—liver and spleen are common distant sites of metastasis for high-grade MCTs.

GENETICS

The specific breed predilections indicate that a genetic predisposition exists.

INCIDENCE/PREVALENCE

• Most common malignant skin tumor in the dog, representing approximately 7–21% of all canine skin tumors. • Primary visceral and intestinal MCTs are rare in the dog (small/toy breeds affected). • Second most common malignant skin tumor in the cat, accounting for 20% of cutaneous tumors. • Most common splenic tumors of cats, comprising half of the MCTs diagnosed in cats.

SIGNALMENT

Species

Dog and cat.

Breed Predilections

• Dogs—brachycephalic breeds, as well as golden retriever, Labrador retriever, Rhodesian ridgeback, beagle, Staffordshire terrier, Weimaraner, shar-pei, and Australian cattle dog. • Cats—Siamese.

Mean Age and Range

• Dogs—middle-aged, range 4 months–18 years. • Cats—middle-aged (8–9 for cutaneous mastocytic types) and older cats (intestinal and splenic); however, the histiocytic form of cutaneous MCTs affects young cats (Siamese) with a mean age of 2.4 years.

Predominant Sex

Dogs—no predilection; cats—male Siamese.

SIGNS

Dogs

• Mass is found in the subcutis or on the skin and may also be present within lipomas.
• Regional edema or a Darier's sign may be seen in the region around a tumor that has degranulated. • Lymphadenopathy of regional lymph nodes may be seen in dogs with metastatic disease. • History of intermittent progression and regression in size. • Systemic illness with advanced local or systemic disease; vomiting, anorexia, weight loss, and melena.

Cats

• Visceral disease manifests as chronic weight loss, anorexia, diarrhea, and lethargy. • Focal mass lesion may be palpated with primary intestinal MCT. • Cutaneous masses tend to be epidermal and on the face or feet.

CAUSES

• Up to 30% of canine MCTs have been shown to contain a mutation in the c-*kit* oncogene, leading to constitutively activated receptor and unchecked cell division. • Up to 56% of feline MCTs have a c-*kit* mutation though these mutations do not appear to have any bearing on prognosis.

RISK FACTORS

See Breed Predilections and Causes.

DIAGNOSIS

DIFFERENTIAL DIAGNOSIS

• Cutaneous/subcutaneous forms—adenexal tumors, basal cell tumors, histiocytoma, lipoma, and soft tissue sarcoma. • Visceral forms—lymphoma, histiocytic tumors, malignant fibrous histiocytomas, multiple myeloma, hemangiosarcoma, hemangioma, and erythroid myeloid hyperplasia.
• Intestinal forms—lymphoma, adenocarcinoma, leiomyoma, leiomyosarcoma, GI stromal tumors, and fungal infections.

CBC/BIOCHEMISTRY/URINALYSIS

• Anemia (initially regenerative secondary to GI blood loss, but can progress to microcytic, hypochromic, nonregenerative anemia).
• Eosinophilia. • Identification of circulating mast cells is more common in the cat with visceral MCT than the dog. • Increased BUN secondary to GI bleeding.

OTHER LABORATORY TESTS

• Regional lymph node aspiration and cytology. • Liver and splenic aspiration and cytology. • MCT prognostic panel. • c-*kit* PCR and immunohistochemistry staining.

IMAGING

Abdominal ultrasound—viscera assessment with emphasis on liver, spleen, and mesenteric lymph nodes.

DIAGNOSTIC PROCEDURES

• Fine-needle aspirate and cytology for definitive diagnosis. • Biopsy (incisional or excisional) for definitive diagnosis and histologic grading.

PATHOLOGIC FINDINGS

Dogs

• Two tiered grading system for cutaneous MCTs: ∘ Low grade—mitotic index of <7, <3 multinucleated cells per 10 HPFs, <3 bizarre nuclei per 10 HPFs, mild to moderate karyomegaly. ∘ High grade—mitotic index of at least 7, 3 or more multinucleated cells per 10 HPFs, 3 or more bizarre nuclei per 10 HPFs, significant karyomegaly. • No validated grading system for subcutaneous MCTs currently exist. • Intestinal MCTs tend to be high grade in the dog.

Cats

• Histologic forms of cutaneous MCTs: ∘ Mastocytic form—single tumor and is the most common (compact or diffuse). ∘ There are two histologic varieties of mastocytic MCTs in the cat: compact—more benign behavior; diffuse—more undifferentiated and aggressive. • Histiocytic form—multiple lesions on the head and neck with relatively benign behavior.

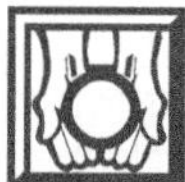

TREATMENT

ACTIVITY

Limit for animals with heavy tumor burdens (such as cats with visceral MCTs or dogs with large tumors) until the mass has been treated appropriately.

DIET

N/A

CLIENT EDUCATION

Owners of dogs with MCTs should be informed that 14–17% of dogs will develop additional MCTs.

SURGICAL CONSIDERATIONS

• Conventional recommendations (dogs)—2–3 cm margins and one fascial plane deep, may be unnecessary with low-grade MCTs in dogs as many of "dirty" margins fail to locally regrow. • Narrow margins (cats)—majority of tumors will not regrow following narrow surgical margins. • Splenectomy (cats)—recommended in cats with massive visceral tumor burden despite the presence of metastases.

RADIATION THERAPY

• For incompletely excised MCTs in locations that are not amenable to surgical re-excision or in cases where another surgery is not possible (dogs). • Treatment of regional lymph node beds for high-grade tumors
• Can be used in a gross disease setting, but severe systemic degranulation reactions (including death) are possible. Pretreatment with ancillary medications is indicated.

MEDICATIONS

DRUG(S) OF CHOICE

Dogs

• Vinblastine 2–3 mg/m² IV q7 days for 4 treatments, then q14 days for 4 treatments and prednisone 1 mg/kg PO q24h.
• Vinblastine only 3.5 mg/m² IV q14 days.
• Lomustine 50–70 mg/m² PO q21 days.
• Toceranib phosphate (Palladia) 2.75 mg/kg PO Monday, Wednesday, Friday.

Cats

• Lomustine 32–60 mg/m² PO q4–6 weeks.
• Vinblastine 2 mg/m² IV q7 days for 4 treatments, then q14 days for 4 treatments and prednisone 1 mg/kg PO q24h.

CONTRAINDICATIONS AND PRECAUTIONS

• Vinblastine—use with caution in animals with liver disease; drug is also myelo-suppressive and possesses vesicant properties.
• Lomustine is hepatotoxic and should be avoided in dogs with underlying liver disease;
• drug is extremely myelosuppressive and associated with refractory thrombocytopenia. Administer with Denamarin. Unknown time to white blood cell nadir in cats. • Toceranib can cause GI ulcers, myelosuppression, muscle pain, hypertension, proteinuria and GI upset.

POSSIBLE INTERACTIONS

• Toceranib should be used with caution with other drugs that induce gastric ulcers such as prednisone or nonsteroidal anti-inflammatory drugs (NSAIDs), or in patients with gastric ulceration secondary to MCT. • Lomustine should be used with caution with other hepatotoxic drugs such as NSAIDs.

ALTERNATIVE DRUG(S)

Symptomatic treatment—diphenhydramine, prednisone famotidine or other H2 inhibitors, omeprazole, and sucralfate should be considered for any dog or cat with gross mast cell disease and clinical symptoms consistent with GI bleeding.

FOLLOW-UP

PATIENT MONITORING

Dogs

• Low-grade cutaneous—complete surgical resection should be curative in the majority of patients. Median survival time greater than 2 years. Follow-up should include evaluation every 3 months for 1 year with physical examination and lymph node assessment.
• High-grade—complete surgical resection evaluate every 3 months for 1.5 years with physical examination, blood work, abdominal ultrasound, and lymph node assessment then every 6 months for another 1.5 years.

Cats

Visceral or intestinal—abdominal ultrasound and blood work every 3 months for 1 year.

PREVENTION/AVOIDANCE

N/A

POSSIBLE COMPLICATIONS

Chemotherapy-related myelotoxicity or hepatotoxicity.

EXPECTED COURSE AND PROGNOSIS

• Complete excision of low-grade MCTs in most locations is curative. • Complete excision of high-grade MCTs even with aggressive treatment is associated with eventual tumor progression/relapse.
• Incomplete excision of a low-grade MCT may require additional local therapy with another surgery (often cured) or radiation therapy (93% disease-free at 3 years).
• Incomplete excision of a high-grade MCT requires additional local therapy in addition to systemic chemotherapy. • Regional metastasis to a lymph node should be treated with surgical excision at the time of the primary tumor removal. Systemic chemo-therapy is necessary. • Evidence of distant metastasis is often treated with systemic chemotherapy or ancillary therapies alone with a median survival of 4 months or less.

MISCELLANEOUS

ASSOCIATED CONDITIONS

Progressive and metastatic disease has the potential to cause excessive parietal cell production of hydrochloric acid with associated gastric ulceration, melena, and iron-deficiency anemia and gastric perforation.

AGE-RELATED FACTORS

N/A

ZOONOTIC POTENTIAL

N/A

PREGNANCY/FERTILITY/BREEDING

While on chemotherapy dogs should not be bred. There are no long-term studies regarding fertility in dogs or cats previously treated with lomustine, vinblastine, or receptor tyrosine kinase inhibitors (RTKIs).

SYNONYMS

• Mastocytoma. • Systemic mastocytosis.

ABBREVIATIONS

• GI = gastrointestinal.
• MCT = mast cell tumor.
• NSAID = nonsteroidal anti-inflammatory drug.
• RTKI = receptor tyrosine kinase inhibitor.

INTERNET RESOURCES

www.merckvetmanual.com/mvm/index

Suggested Reading

Kiupel M, Webster JD, Bailey KL, et al. Proposal of a 2-tier histologic grading system for canine cutaneous mast cell tumors to more accurately predict biological behavior. Vet Pathol 2011, 48(1):147–155.

London CA, Kisseberth WC, Galli SJ, et al. Expression of stem cell factor receptor (c-kit) by the malignant mast cells from spontaneous canine mast cell tumours. J Comp Pathol 1996, 115(4):399–414.

Wilcock BP, Yager JA, Zink MC.The morphology and behavior of feline cutaneous mastocytomas. Vet Pathol 1986, 23(3):320–324.

Author Heather M. Wilson-Robles

Consulting Editor Timothy M. Fan

Client Education Handout available online

MASTITIS

BASICS

OVERVIEW

- Bacterial infection of one or more lactating mammary glands.
- Result of ascending infection, trauma to the gland, or hematogenous spread.
- *Escherichia coli*, staphylococci, and β-hemolytic streptococci most commonly involved; *Mycobacterium* and blastomycosis reported.
- Potentially life-threatening infection; may lead to sepsis if systemic involvement.

SIGNALMENT

- Postpartum bitch and queen.
- Pseudopregnant lactating bitch or queen (rare).

SIGNS

Historical Findings

- Anorexia.
- Lethargy.
- Neglect of puppies or kittens.
- Failure of puppies or kittens to thrive.

Physical Examination Findings

- Firm, swollen, warm, and painful mammary gland(s) from which purulent or hemorrhagic fluid can be expressed.
- Fever, dehydration, and shock—with systemic involvement.
- Abscessation or gangrene of gland(s) can result.

CAUSES & RISK FACTORS

- Ascending infection via teat canals.
- Trauma inflicted by puppy or kitten toenails and teeth.
- Poor hygiene.
- Systemic infection originating elsewhere (e.g., metritis).
- Rarely secondary to fibroadenomatous hyperplasia in queens.

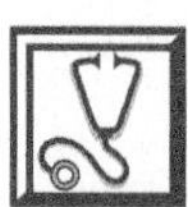

DIAGNOSIS

DIFFERENTIAL DIAGNOSIS

- Galactostasis—no systemic illness; cytologic examination and culture of milk aid differentiation.
- Inflammatory mammary adenocarcinoma—affected gland does not produce milk; differentiated by biopsy.

CBC/BIOCHEMISTRY/URINALYSIS

- Leukocytosis with left shift, or leukopenia with sepsis.
- Hemoconcentration (increased packed cell volume, total plasma protein concentration), and azotemia from dehydration or prerenal effects.

OTHER LABORATORY TESTS

N/A

IMAGING

Ultrasonography reveals loss of distinct layering of normal tissue in glands, decreased echogenicity, increased heterogeneity, and altered blood vessel density on color Doppler.

DIAGNOSTIC PROCEDURES

- Cytology—neutrophils, macrophages, and other mononuclear cells can be observed in normal milk; the presence of large numbers of free and phagocytosed bacteria and degenerative neutrophils occurs with mastitis.
- Microbial culture—identification and sensitivity of microorganisms from milk of affected glands; screening for methicillin-resistant *Staphylococcus aureus* recommended.

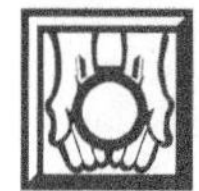

TREATMENT

- Inpatient until stable.
- Puppies and kittens—neonates may be allowed to continue nursing unless glands are necrotic or dam is systemically ill; affects choice of antibiotics; monitor weight gain in neonates: pups should gain 10% of birth weight per day, kittens should gain a minimum of 7–10 g/day.
- IV isotonic crystalloid fluid to treat dehydration, hypovolemia, shock.
- Correct electrolyte imbalances, hypovolemia, hypoglycemia.
- Apply warm compress and milk out affected gland(s) several times daily.
- Cover friable glands to prevent excoriation if nursing is allowed.
- Application of cabbage leaf wraps to affected glands may speed resolution.
- Abscessed or gangrenous glands—require surgical debridement.
- Open wound management or negative pressure wound therapy may be needed after surgery in some cases; negative pressure therapy may also be used for conservatively managed cases.

MEDICATIONS

DRUG(S) OF CHOICE

- Acidic milk—weak bases; erythromycin 10 mg/kg PO q8h, lincomycin 15 mg/kg PO q8h, or trimethoprim-sulfadiazine 15–30 mg/kg PO q12h for 21 days.
- Alkaline milk—weak acids; amoxicillin or cephalosporin 20 mg/kg PO q8h, dogs and cats; amoxicillin/clavulanic acid 13.75 mg/kg PO q12h (dogs); 62.5 mg/cat PO q12h (cats) for 21 days.
- Either alkaline or acidic milk—chloramphenicol 40–50 mg/kg PO q8h or enrofloxacin 5–20 mg/kg/day PO for 21 days.
- May infuse affected gland(s) with 1% betadine solution by lacrimal cannula.
- Cabergoline 5 µg/kg PO q24h for 5–7 days to suppress lactation in unaffected glands in patients with sepsis; neonates must be hand-reared.

CONTRAINDICATIONS/POSSIBLE INTERACTIONS

Patient allowed to nurse—avoid tetracycline and chloramphenicol; may use cephalosporins, amoxicillin, and amoxicillin with clavulanic acid. Enrofloxacin may be used in dogs up to 3 weeks of age.

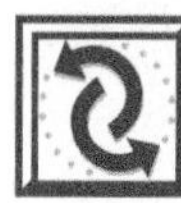

FOLLOW-UP

PATIENT MONITORING

- Physical examination and CBC.
- Repeated ultrasonographic evaluation helps assess healing—normal distinct layering of tissues will appear with recovery.

PREVENTION/AVOIDANCE

- Clean environment.
- Hair shaved from around mammary glands.
- Toenails of puppies and kittens clipped.
- Ensure neonates nurse from all glands.
- Probiotic administration.

POSSIBLE COMPLICATIONS

- Abscessation or gangrene—may cause loss of gland(s).
- Hand-raising puppies and kittens—requires considerable commitment by the owner; may affect behavioral outcome of offspring.

EXPECTED COURSE AND PROGNOSIS

Prognosis—good with treatment.

MISCELLANEOUS

Suggested Reading

Johnston SD, Root Kustritz MV, Olson PNS. Periparturient disorders in the bitch. In: Johnston SD, Root Kustritz MV, Olson PNS, eds., Canine and Feline Theriogenology. Philadelphia, PA: Saunders, 2001, pp. 131–134.

Author Tessa Fiamengo

Consulting Editor Erin E. Runcan

Acknowledgment The author and editors acknowledge the prior contribution of Joni L. Freshman.

BASICS

DEFINITION

Abnormal maternal behavior is either excessive maternal behavior in the absence of neonates or deficient maternal behavior in the presence of the dam's own neonates. The latter is more common in dogs, the former in cats.

PATHOPHYSIOLOGY

The pathophysiology of one type of excessive maternal behavior, pseudocyesis, appears to be elevated progesterone levels following estrus in unbred bitches followed by an abrupt drop in progesterone levels. The pathophysiology of the refusal to accept puppies by females after caesarean section is the waning of factors, including oxytocin, needed during the sensitive period for acceptance of the neonate. The pathophysiology of other types of deficient maternal behavior is unknown. The impairment or absence of mother–infant bonding strongly affects the offspring's sociability or affiliative behavior throughout the animal's lifespan.

SYSTEMS AFFECTED

• Behavioral. • Reproductive.

GENETICS

There is no identified genetic predisposition, but a breed disposition for deficient maternal behavior in Jack Russell terriers indicates there may be a genetic component. There are genetic models in mice. The genes responsible for deficient maternal behavior in mice are paternally imprinted. If this is true in dogs and cats, one would expect that rejecting mothers were normally mothered themselves, but their paternal grandmother may have been deficient.

INCIDENCE/PREVALENCE

The incidence of deficient maternal behavior has not been determined but seems to be low, less than 1% of cases in a behavior practice. Pseudopregnancy is more common. Cannibalism of offspring is more common in cats and may account for approximately 12.5% of all kitten deaths.

SIGNALMENT

Species

Dogs and cats.

Breed Predilections

Poor maternal behavior may be more common in Jack Russell terriers and cocker spaniels, but there has been no quantitative study.

Mean Age and Range

Primiparous females and older bitches seem to be at risk of deficient maternal behavior. Lower ranking females that have not bred successfully have a higher likelihood of entering pseudocyesis, which may allow for them to help raise the offspring.

Predominant Sex

Female generally, but some males may allow suckling behavior.

SIGNS

Deficient Maternal Behavior

Absent maternal behavior; the mother simply abandons her offspring. This is most apt to occur after caesarean section.

Poor Maternal Behavior

• The mother stays with her offspring but will not allow them to nurse. • The mother may show inadequate retrieval of young, insufficient cleaning of the young, or failure to stimulate elimination. • The bitch carries the puppies from place to place without settling down. • In the most extreme form, the mother kills some or all of her litter.

Abnormal Maternal Behavior

• The bitch or queen may allow her offspring to suckle but kills her offspring either at birth or over a period of days. Occasionally the bitch, or more rarely the queen, will abandon or attack her offspring if it has changed in odor or appearance. A female may be disturbed by another animal or by people and can redirect her aggression to her offspring. • Cannibalism of kittens may occur as a result of too large a litter or overcrowding. • A bitch may accidentally disembowel or even consume offspring completely while eating the fetal membranes and umbilical cord. This should be distinguished from normal licking, which can be quite vigorous, even dislodging the pup from a teat.

Maternal Aggression

Cats with kittens may be aggressive to other animals, especially dogs in the same household. Bitches may be aggressive to unfamiliar humans or even to familiar humans, especially if they are hypocalcemic or painful (i.e., mastitis).

Excessive Maternal Behavior

• The pseudopregnant bitch or a bitch spayed during the late luteal phase of the estrous cycle adopts, attempts to nurse, and guards inanimate objects (stuffed animals or even leashes). The pseudopregnant bitch may have mammary development and may lactate.
• The newly spayed queen may steal kittens from a lactating queen. Queens post-spaying may also lactate if suckled.

CAUSES

• Genetics—offspring of poor mothers.
• Sick/unhealthy offspring. • Environmental (see Risk Factors).

RISK FACTORS

• The presence of kittens in the environment of the recently spayed cat may prompt excessive maternal behavior and kitten stealing. • The risk of excessive carrying of pups, redirected aggression, or even cannibalism is increased if there are other dogs or too many people present in the nest area. • Primiparous females or those subjected to caesarian section are at higher risk than multiparous or naturally delivering females. • A large litter of kittens or sick offspring. • Queens fed low protein diets during late gestation and lactation may show decreased mother–kitten social interactions and retarded attachment formation. • Other risk factors include individual differences, lack of experience, pain, discomfort, and suboptimal conditions. • Inability to perform species-specific behavior before, during, and after parturition increases the possibility of infanticide or ingestion of offspring.

M

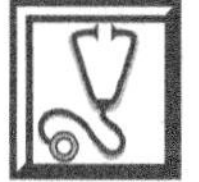

DIAGNOSIS

DIFFERENTIAL DIAGNOSIS

• The most important differential is between primary abnormal maternal behavior and poor maternal behavior secondary to mastitis or metritis. • Lactation tetany can result in aggressive behavior, although this behavior is rarely directed at the puppies and occurs later in lactation, not at parturition.

CBC/BIOCHEMISTRY/URINALYSIS

Usually normal unless other medical conditions are present. Blood calcium levels will be low if the bitch is suffering from lactation tetany.

OTHER LABORATORY TESTS

Only as indicated by metabolic conditions of the bitch or queen.

PATHOLOGIC FINDINGS

Presence of milk in the mammary glands of females with excessive maternal behavior.

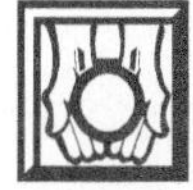

TREATMENT

APPROPRIATE HEALTH CARE

Normal health care.

DIET

• Adequate diet for nursing bitches and queens to meet protein, energy and calcium demands. • Restricted diets for pseudocyesis to discourage lactation and diminish milk production. • In the case of deficient maternal behavior, the bitch or queen should be fed ad libitum to encourage lactation.

MATERNAL BEHAVIOR PROBLEMS (CONTINUED)

CLIENT EDUCATION

Abnormal or Poor Maternal Behavior

• The bitch that is carrying her pups or exhibiting redirected aggression to them should be isolated in a quiet, dark area. The bitch that bites her pups should be muzzled and mildly sedated. The owner must stimulate elimination of the puppies or kittens because the muzzled female cannot. An Elizabethan collar inhibits cannibalism in queens. • The bitch should be attended at parturition and the pups removed temporarily if she is biting the pups themselves in addition to the umbilical cord. • Bitches and queens with poor maternal behavior may exhibit the same behavior with subsequent litters. • Some mothers reject specific offspring that are cold or inactive, which indicates a problem with the individual offspring and warrants veterinary intervention. • If the mother rejects the entire litter, abnormality is with the dam.

M

Excessive Maternal Behavior

• Cats that have stolen kittens should be separated from the biologic mother and kittens. • The mothered objects should be removed from the pseudopregnant bitch. However, some bitches will compulsively search for the object or transfer maternal behavior to another. In which case, it is in the bitch's best interest to allow her to remain with the object. • Food intake should be restricted to inhibit lactation.

Maternal Aggression toward Animals or Humans

The best treatment for maternal aggression beyond weaning is to separate the kittens; weaning alone may not suffice because the presence of the kittens alone may sustain or even reinstate maternal aggression in a queen separated from her kittens for several weeks.

SURGICAL CONSIDERATIONS

• Delay spaying for 4 months post estrus to avoid post-spaying maternal behavior and its accompanying aggression. • Spaying avoids future excessive maternal behavior in the absence of young.

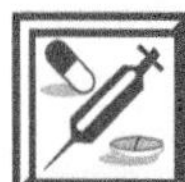

MEDICATIONS

DRUG(S) OF CHOICE

Excessive Maternal Behavior

• Mibolerone was the drug of choice for pseudopregnant bitches or those exhibiting maternal behavior and lactation following spaying. The dose is 16 μg/kg PO once daily for 5 days. Mibolerone is a potent anabolic–androgenic steroid which inhibits prolactin and thereby inhibits lactation. The drug is no longer available except through some compounding pharmacies. • Bromocriptine (Parlodel) can be used to inhibit prolactin. The dose is 10 μg/kg for 10 days. Should not be administered to pregnant animals.
• Cabergoline is a dopamine agonist shown to be effective for the treatment of pseudopregnancy in dogs by lowering prolactin. Dosage is 5 μg/kg PO q24h for 4–6 days. Some animals may require more than one course of treatment. Not commercially available in North America.

Deficient Maternal Behavior

• Oxytocin may be administered either parenterally 1–5 units or by nasal spray (Syntocinon). • Because prolactin appears to be necessary for maternal behavior in other species, a dopamine blocker, acepromazine (0.55–2.2 mg/kg PO), can be used. Dopamine inhibits prolactin release.

CONTRAINDICATIONS

• Do not use mibolerone in cats because it has a narrow margin of safety in that species. It should not be administered to Bedlington terriers due to their predisposition for chronic hepatitis. • Do not give oxytocin to pregnant animals or in combination with sympathomimetic agents.

PRECAUTIONS

Mibolerone can cause masculinization that may include male sexual behavior, clitoral hypertrophy, vulvovaginitis, and urinary incontinence in females. Bromocriptine can cause gastrointestinal vomiting, sedation, and hypotension as well as abortion.

POSSIBLE INTERACTIONS

• If tranquilizers are administered, care must be taken that the puppies or kittens are not sedated. • Do not use estrogen or progesterones at the same time as mibolerone.

FOLLOW-UP

PATIENT MONITORING

Puppies or kittens of females with deficient or poor maternal behavior should be monitored daily to ensure they are gaining weight.

PREVENTION/AVOIDANCE

• Place a nursing female in quiet, comfortable quarters away from noise and disturbance by other animals or people. • Do not rebreed females with poor maternal behavior. Determine whether any female offspring of the female with abnormal behavior have also exhibited poor maternal behavior. In other species, poor maternal behavior is a paternally imprinted gene; the father must contribute the gene for poor maternal behavior. The daughters of rejecting mothers will not reject, but the daughters of their sons may. • Allow species-specific behavior before, during, and after parturition.

POSSIBLE COMPLICATIONS

• Loss of offspring. • Hand-reared puppies and kittens frequently have abnormal or deficient social behavior. This is due in part to insufficient suckling time and to the consequences of lack of maternal licking, which adversely affects response to stress and reproductive behavior. • Absent maternal environment during the first 8 weeks has been associated with increased anxiety and aggression in puppies.

EXPECTED COURSE AND PROGNOSIS

• Excessive maternal behavior usually wanes around the time of normal weaning (6–8 weeks). • Poor and deficient maternal behavior can occur with each litter.
• Maternal aggression by the bitch may begin as early as nest building behavior, reaches its height during the first 2 weeks after parturition and may last for 3 weeks post parturition. • Kittens from queens with poor maternal behavior can be cross-fostered to another lactating queen. Puppies may also be cross-fostered to another lactating bitch, but this is best accomplished within the first week of life. Best success of cross-fostering occurs between related dams.

MISCELLANEOUS

AGE-RELATED FACTORS

Poor maternal behavior is more likely in very young and very old mothers.

PREGNANCY/FERTILITY/BREEDING

• Consider especially drug use and effect of disease on the fetus. • Do not breed dogs with history of poor maternal behavior.

SYNONYMS

Mismothering

Suggested Reading

Connolly PB. Reproductive behaviour problems. In: Horwitz D, Mills D, Heath S, eds., BSAVA Manual of Canine and Feline Behavioural Medicine. Gloucestershire, UK: BSAVA, 2002, pp. 128–143.

Houpt KA. Maternal behavior. In: Domestic Animal Behavior, 5th ed. Ames, IA: Wiley-Blackwell, 2011, pp 235–270.

Root Kustritz MV. Reproductive behavior of small animals. Theriogenology 2005, 64(3): 734–746.

Authors Amy L. Pike and Amy Learn

Consulting Editor Gary M. Landsberg

Acknowledgment The authors and editors acknowledge the prior contribution of Katherine A. Houpt.

Client Education Handout available online

BASICS

DEFINITION

Fractures of the mandibles, maxillae, and associated structures are described according to location, severity (i.e., tooth involvement, soft tissue tears, and type of bone fracture), and effects of the muscles of mastication on reduction.

PATHOPHYSIOLOGY

Effects of the Muscles of Mastication

The muscles that open and close the mouth may help reduce (favorable) or displace (nonfavorable) a fracture.

Classification of Jaw Fracture by Location

• Rostral mandible—including the canines and incisors. • Mandibular horizontal ramus. • Mandibular vertical ramus. • Temporomandibular joint. • Rostral maxillary/incisive bone. • Maxillary/facial fractures. • Maxillary symphysis. • Combination fractures.

SIGNALMENT

Species

Dog and cat.

SIGNS

• Vary greatly according to the location, type, extent, cause, and underlying risk factors resulting in the injury. • Facial deformity, malocclusion, fractured teeth, oral or nasal bleeding, and inability to properly close the jaw are common signs.

CAUSES

Injury, trauma, and predisposing factors.

RISK FACTORS

• High-risk environment or temperament. • Oral infections (e.g., periodontal disease, osteomyelitis), neoplasia, or certain metabolic diseases (e.g., hypoparathyroidism)—may result in weaker jaws that are more prone to injury. • Traumatic injury affecting the jaws or teeth. • Congenital or hereditary factors resulting in weakened or deformed jaw bone.

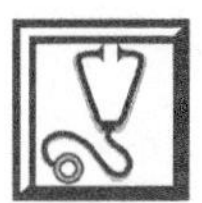

DIAGNOSIS

A thorough and complete physical examination is very important in traumatic jaw injuries as many unseen or multiple injuries and complications are possible.

DIFFERENTIAL DIAGNOSIS

• Temporomandibular joint (TMJ) conditions—see Temporomandibular Joint Disorders. • Tooth subluxation or luxation (i.e., interference with jaw closure). • Endodontic disease (e.g., tooth abscess). • Foreign body lodged in or near the oral cavity. • Maxillary or mandibular nerve injury or disease. • Masticatory muscle myositis. • Craniomandibular osteopathy. • Neoplasia.

CBC/BIOCHEMISTRY/URINALYSIS

As required—to assess and treat shock from initial injury; to assess animal prior to surgery.

IMAGING

Radiography—intraoral and extraoral; CT and MRI.

DIAGNOSTIC PROCEDURES

• Oral examination. • Neurologic examination. • Biopsy for histopathology, if indicated. • Bacterial culture and sensitivity, if indicated.

PATHOLOGIC FINDINGS

• Non-unions. • Neoplasia. • Osteomyelitis. • Periodontal and/or endodontic disease.

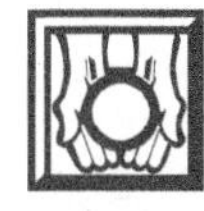

TREATMENT

APPROPRIATE HEALTH CARE

Typical Types of Treatments for Classes of Fractures

• Interarch stabilization (caudal fractures or severely comminuted combination fractures including the TMJ)—tape muzzle; maxillomandibular fixation (MMF) with dental composites or acrylic materials; cross-arch wiring or buttons (maxilla to mandible). • Intra-arch stabilization (symphyseal and parasymphyseal injuries)—pin and wire combination, dental wiring, acrylic or composite splint. • Intraoral stabilization with splint (mandibular body fractures, useful in edentulous patients)—composite or acrylic splint. • Intraoral stabilization with wire (mandibular body, maxillary fractures)—interdental wiring (Ivy loop, Stout's multiple loop, Essig and Risdon techniques); dental wiring: circumdental for splint anchorage (pig tails, cerclage or twists); osseous wiring (circumferential, transosseous, transcircumferential). • Internal fixation (most types of fractures, used selectively with consideration of teeth and roots): orthopedic wire; mini-plates; screws; intramedullary pins (*not* within the mandibular canal). • External fixation (most types of fractures, used selectively with consideration of teeth and roots)—intramedullary pins with bars (stainless steel or carbon) or tubing (e.g., Penrose) reinforced with composite or acrylic. • Salvage surgery (fractures with large defects, non-unions)—condylectomy (nonrepairable fractures of the TMJ); cheiloplasty (salvage procedure to maintain reasonable mandibular support in certain nonunion conditions); rostral (or other) mandibulectomy (used in certain non-union cases or with massive injury).

Initial Treatment

• Awareness of occlusion, tooth roots, and anatomy during treatment is critical. • Patient should be intubated, pharyngostomy or transmylohyoid placement aids in occlusal checks intraoperatively. • Teeth in the fracture line should be assessed and maintained by appropriate treatment until the fracture heals, if possible, as removal may result in instability. • Bone graft to reestablish structural stability—autograft (harvested from individual); allograft (same species); alloplast (artificial material). • Treatment with composite/acrylic splints in association with wiring (Ivy loop, Stout's multiple loop) is generally very effective. • Assess soft tissue damage; debride and suture where appropriate.

Procedure

• Disinfect with dilute chlorhexidine and clean and polish teeth (flour pumice without fluoride). • Reduce fracture in proper occlusion. • Before applying splint materials, coat adjacent teeth and soft tissue with petroleum jelly. Acid etch the teeth with a 37% phosphoric acid gel; leave on for 30–60 seconds; rinse off thoroughly and air dry the teeth. Spot bonding of the teeth with light-cured unfilled resin if desired to increase adherence of dental materials to teeth.

Materials

Acrylics

• Warning: Use acrylics in well-ventiliated areas. They also generate heat can result in thermal injury to the teeth. • Place the powder and liquid in a salt-and-pepper fashion in small increments (to avoid hyperthermic reaction) until the desired shape and density of splint attained. • Finish and smooth with acrylic bur on high-speed handpiece.

Composites (Protemp Garant, Maxitemp)

• Little exothermal reaction and fumes; more expensive. • After acid-etching, use a dentinal bonding agent and apply a separator agent to opposing arcade to prevent composite from bonding to these teeth during occlusion check. • With a new mixing tip, apply product to splint area, shaping it as it hardens. • Finish and smooth with white stone bur and place a final layer of unfilled resin.

Circumferential Osseous Wiring or Suturing

• Wiring around the bone—used most commonly for symphyseal separations. • 20- or 18-gauge needle—to pass wire. • 24- to 28-gauge wire—in neonates, small dogs or cats, absorbable (long-acting, e.g., PDS) or nonabsorbable 1- to 2-0 suture

MAXILLARY AND MANDIBULAR FRACTURES (CONTINUED)

material can sometimes be substituted for wire. • Run wire from stab incision (ventral intermandibular space) to vestibule; pass behind canines, down through vestibule on opposite side, and back down through the ventral incision. • Tighten wire to reduce fracture, but do not overtighten the wire ends or the teeth may be pulled too far medially (lingually displaced) and hit the palate. If this happens, either loosen the wire ends or place a figure-eight wire looped around the canine teeth and under the jaw.

Homecare

• Orthodontic wax—soft, pliable wax sent with owner to periodically cover irritating wires, or can cover wire twists and ends with dental composite materials. • Oral irrigants—use twice daily for oral hygiene and to reduce bacteria; chlorhexidine solutions help reduce bacteria; zinc and ascorbic acid solutions (Maxi-Guard Gel) help reduce bacteria and stimulate soft tissue healing. • Diet—soft food or gruel may be required during healing.
• Nutritional and fluid maintenance required. • Chewing exercise—avoid hard chew items during healing process.

SURGICAL CONSIDERATIONS

• Based on type of fracture, available equipment, supplies, and the doctor's knowledge, experience, and comfort level.
• Treatment selection is based on four major points: (1) Reduction of fracture and reasonable contact of fracture ends, if possible. (2) Reestablishment of natural occlusion, and avoidance of causing a malocclusion when the fracture is reduced. (3) Stabilization sufficient for proper healing. (4) Salvage condition (nonrepairable or nonstabilizable condition).

MEDICATIONS

DRUG(S) OF CHOICE

Pain Management

• Local anesthesia—intraoral local blocks; regional nerve blocks: mental n., mandibular n., infraorbital n., and maxillary n. • Injectables—hydromorphone, buprenorphine, fentanyl, CRI, certain drug combinations. • Transdermal patches—fentanyl. • Oral—nonsteroidal anti-inflammatory drugs (NSAIDs); gabapentin, tramadol, hydrocodone.

Antibiotics

Limit usage to cases with suspected osteomyelitis; bacterial culture and sensitivity should be performed to prescribe appropriate drug.

FOLLOW-UP

PATIENT MONITORING

• Physical—recheck every 2 weeks postoperatively until appliance is removed.
• Radiographic—recheck 4–6 weeks postoperatively, then every 2 weeks until fracture is healed and/or appliance is removed. • Fracture site may temporarily (1–2 weeks) be more at risk to refracture after the support of the appliance is removed. • Once the fracture line is stable, compromised teeth may need additional endodontic treatment (e.g., root canal) or careful extraction. • If the healing process results in a malocclusion—orthodontics, endodontics, and/or selective exodontia (extraction) may be required. • Other considerations—stability of fracture and appliance; oral hygiene; oral intake of food and water; maintenance of weight; appropriate urination and defecation; indications of pain or swelling.

PREVENTION/AVOIDANCE

Try to minimize risk of trauma.

POSSIBLE COMPLICATIONS

• Malocclusion. • Endodontic disease.
• Osteomyelitis. • Non-union.
• Sequestrum. • Dehiscence. • Neurologic defects. • Facial pain syndrome.
• Impaired mastication. • Temporary weight loss. • Soft tissue trauma due to appliance or wires.

Possible Sequelae

Impaired Mastication

• TMJ arthritis—chronic or intermittent TMJ pain; may require condylectomy.
• Malocclusion—dental attrition; may require extractions. • Non-union—may require partial or complete mandibulectomy or maxillectomy. • Ankylosis or pseudoankylosis of the mandible at the TMJ or zygomatic arch region.

Facial Pain Syndrome

• Acute or chronic. • Due to nerve trauma from injury or as a complication of surgery.

Nerve Damage

Affecting motor function

EXPECTED COURSE AND PROGNOSIS

• Generally good; however, predisposing factors, initiating force, location, type of fracture, quality of homecare, and selection of treatment modality all affect the healing outcome. • 4–12 weeks to bony union.

MISCELLANEOUS

ASSOCIATED CONDITIONS

• Malocclusion. • Mastication difficulty.
• Lack of head symmetry. • Soft tissue trauma. • Periodontal disease. • Chipped, broken, luxated, or avulsed teeth.

AGE-RELATED FACTORS

Fracture healing may be faster in younger animals.

SEE ALSO

Temporomandibular Joint Disorders.

ABBREVIATIONS

• MMF = maxillomandibular fixation.
• NSAID = nonsteroidal anti-inflammatory drug.
• TMJ = temporomandibular joint.

INTERNET RESOURCES

https://avdc.org/avdc-nomenclature/

Suggested Reading

Taney K, Smithson CW. Oral surgery—fracture and trauma repair. In: Lobprise HB, Dodd JR, eds., Wigg's Veterinary Dentistry: Principles and Practice, 2nd ed. Hoboken, NJ: John Wiley & Sons, 2019, pp. 265–288.

Author Kendall Taney
Consulting Editor Heidi B. Lobprise

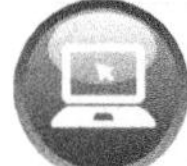

Client Education Handout available online

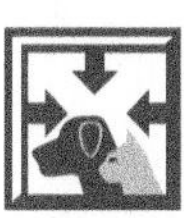

BASICS

DEFINITION

A disorder characterized by persistent, irreversible dilation of the colon that is often the result of chronic constipation/obstipation.

PATHOPHYSIOLOGY

• Idiopathic dilated megacolon is the most common cause of chronic constipation in cats and occurs due to generalized colonic smooth muscle dysfunction. • The diagnosis of idiopathic dilated megacolon is often preceded by chronic, recurrent constipation so it is unclear whether a primary disorder of colonic smooth muscle occurs first or whether smooth muscle dysfunction results from prolonged colonic distension. • Megacolon can also occur secondary to abnormal neurologic function of the colon, including dysautonomia, spinal cord injury or deformities, pelvic nerve injury, and autonomic ganglioneuritis. • Colonic aganglionosis/hypoganglionosis (Hirschsprung's disease in humans) is a congenital absence of ganglia in the colonic smooth muscle; affected segments are unable to relax, resulting in megacolon. • Hypertrophic megacolon can develop as a consequence of obstructive lesions and will progress to dilated megacolon if the obstruction is not corrected.

SYSTEMS AFFECTED

• Gastrointestinal. • Neuromuscular—concurrent neurologic abnormalities may be seen when megacolon has a neurogenic cause. • Musculoskeletal—megacolon can occur secondary to pelvic fractures. • Endocrine/metabolic—megacolon can result in electrolyte derangements due to prolonged vomiting. Electrolyte and endocrine abnormalities (hypercalcemia, hypokalemia, hypothyroidism) can promote constipation and possibly lead to or exacerbate megacolon.

GENETICS

N/A

INCIDENCE/PREVALENCE

Unknown

GEOGRAPHIC DISTRIBUTION

N/A

SIGNALMENT

Species

Cat > dog.

Breed Predilections

Possible increased risk in Manx cat.

Mean Age and Range

• Idiopathic megacolon—young adult cats most commonly (mean 6 years) although cats of any age can be affected. • Acquired megacolon—none.

Predominant Sex

Male

SIGNS

Historical Findings

• Idiopathic megacolon—typically a chronic/recurrent problem; signs often present for months to years. • Acquired megacolon—signs may be acute or chronic. • Constipation/obstipation. • Tenesmus with small or no fecal volume. • Hard, dry feces. • Infrequent defecation. • Small amount of diarrhea (often mucoid) may occur after prolonged tenesmus. • Occasional vomiting, anorexia, and/or lethargy with chronic fecal impaction. • Weight loss.

Physical Examination Findings

• Abdominal palpation reveals an enlarged colon with hard feces. • Digital rectal examination may indicate an underlying (obstructive) cause and confirms fecal impaction. • Dehydration. • Unkempt hair coat. • Weight loss with chronicity. • Neurologic examination may reveal underlying neurologic disease.

CAUSES

• Mechanical obstruction—pelvic fractures, neoplasia, rectal foreign body, rectal stricture, atresia ani, prostatomegaly. • Neurologic disease—dysautonomia, sacral spinal cord deformities (Manx cat), cauda equina syndrome, pelvic nerve injury or dysfunction. • Endocrine/metabolic—hypercalcemia, hypokalemia, hypothyroidism, severe dehydration. • Drugs—opioids, anticholinergics, phenothiazines.

RISK FACTORS

• Chronic constipation. • Conditions leading to obstruction or difficulty defecating, including prior trauma and spinal cord injury or deformity. • Possible association with low physical activity and obesity as well as consumption of bone meal in dogs.

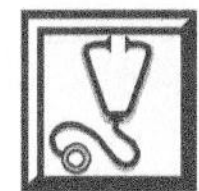

DIAGNOSIS

DIFFERENTIAL DIAGNOSIS

• Other causes of palpable colonic masses (e.g., lymphoma, carcinoma, intussusception)—distinguish on the basis of texture, rectal examination, imaging, and mucosal biopsy. • Dysuria/stranguria—exclude by palpation of the bladder and colon, and by urinalysis. • Tenesmus due to inflammation of the colonic mucosa (colitis)—exclude by palpation, rectal examination, and colonoscopy with mucosal biopsy.

CBC/BIOCHEMISTRY/URINALYSIS

• Often normal. • May show evidence of dehydration and stress leukogram. • Electrolyte abnormalities may develop; may be prerenal azotemia with dehydration. • Urinalysis—typically unremarkable.

OTHER LABORATORY TESTS

Total thyroxine (T_4) to assess thyroid function.

IMAGING

• Abdominal/pelvic radiographs to identify underlying causes. • Can easily visualize an enlarged, fecal-filled colon on survey abdominal radiographs. • Abdominal ultrasound may identify mural or obstructive masses.

DIAGNOSTIC PROCEDURES

Rarely need colonoscopy to rule out mural or intraluminal obstructive lesions.

PATHOLOGIC FINDINGS

• Feline idiopathic megacolon has no defining histologic changes. Smooth muscle typically appears normal with evidence of normal innervation. Mucosal and submucosal ulceration, fibrosis, and inflammation can be variably present and are secondary to chronic fecal impaction. • Megacolon resulting from other etiologies may have features such as abnormalities in or reduced numbers of ganglia (ganglioneuritis or hypogangliosis), or smooth muscle hypertrophy (hypertrophic megacolon).

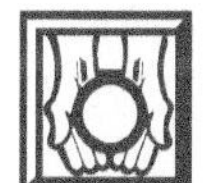

TREATMENT

APPROPRIATE HEALTH CARE

• If administration of laxatives or enemas fails to resolve fecal impaction, inpatient management and manual evacuation of feces will be necessary. • For manual evacuation of feces, the patient should be placed under general anesthesia and intubated to prevent aspiration should manipulation of the colon trigger vomiting or regurgitation: ○ Warm water combined with a water-based lubricant can be administered during the procedure to help facilitate removal of feces. Feces are then removed manually while providing gentle assistance with abdominal palpation of the colon. ○ Periprocedural administration of an IV antibiotic with a good anaerobic spectrum can be considered in case manipulation of the compromised colon results in bacterial translocation. ○ This procedure may need to be repeated if the impaction is too severe to safely accomplish removal of all feces under one anesthetic event. • Trickle administration of polyethylene glycol 3350 via nasogastric tube for 24–48 hours prior to manual extraction will result in better fecal hydration and may facilitate stool removal.

NURSING CARE

• Most patients require parenteral fluid support to correct dehydration. • IV administration of balanced electrolyte solutions is the preferred route. • Control nausea and vomiting with antiemetic medications.

ACTIVITY

• Encourage activity and exercise. • Restriction indicated postoperatively if surgery is performed.

MEGACOLON (CONTINUED)

DIET

• Many patients require a low-residue producing diet; bulk-forming fiber diets can worsen or lead to recurrence of colonic fecal distension. • A soluble fiber-rich diet may be helpful. • A maintenance-type diet can be supplemented with fiber-enriched foods (pumpkin) or products containing fermentable fiber such as Metamucil.

CLIENT EDUCATION

• Following treatment for constipation, medical therapy, including dietary management, laxatives, and/or colonic prokinetics, may be required long term and has the potential to fail.
• Subtotal colectomy is indicated in cases of medical treatment failure.

SURGICAL CONSIDERATIONS

• An underlying obstructive cause should be surgically corrected, if possible. Alternatively, subtotal colectomy has been described in the successful management of megacolon occurring secondary to pelvic fracture malunion. • For patients that do not respond favorably to medical treatment, subtotal colectomy is the treatment of choice. • Subtotal colectomy may be required with obstructive megacolon even if the obstruction is corrected if irreversible changes in colonic motility have already occurred. • Avoid enema administration or attempts at colonic evacuation prior to surgery. These efforts result in increased likelihood of fecal contamination of the abdomen during surgery. • Subtotal colectomy can be performed with either ileorectal or colorectal anastomosis. Preservation of the ileocolic junction is recommended as this results in more formed stool compared to cats in which it is excised.

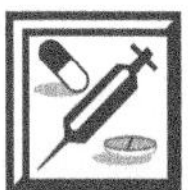

MEDICATIONS

DRUG(S) OF CHOICE

• Colonic prokinetic agents—cisapride (5-HT receptor agonist) has been shown to stimulate colonic smooth muscle motility in cats and dogs with constipation. The dose is 0.1–0.5 mg/kg PO q8–12h, but may be increased up to 1 mg/kg if well tolerated. Metoclopramide is not effective for constipation. • Hyperosmotic laxatives—polyethylene glycol 3350 powder (Miralax®) 1/8–¼ tsp with food q12h; lactulose 0.5 mL/kg PO q8–12h to effect. In cats with severe constipation, polyethylene glycol electrolyte solution (GoLytely®, Colyte®) can be given via nasogastric or nasoesophageal feeding tube at 6–10 mL/kg/h for 12–48 hours in a 24-hour care hospital setting to facilitate passage of feces, either as an alternative to or in preparation for manual evacuation of feces.
• Enemas—5–10 mL/kg warm water or a 50–50 mixture of warm water and water-soluble lubricant administered slowly via a lubricated 10–12 Fr red rubber catheter gently passed into the rectum. Lactulose can also be administered as an enema at a dose of 5–10 mL/kg.

CONTRAINDICATIONS

• Sodium phosphate retention enemas (e.g., Fleet by C.B. Fleet Co., Inc.)—because of their association with severe hypocalcemia.
• Mineral oil and white petrolatum—because of danger of fatal lipoid aspiration pneumonia due to lack of taste.

PRECAUTIONS

Common hairball laxatives (e.g., Laxatone, Cat-a-Lax) are typically ineffective.

POSSIBLE INTERACTIONS

N/A

ALTERNATIVE DRUG(S)

• Docusate sodium can be used as a stool softener in place of lactulose. • Psyllium can be added to food at a dose of ¼–1 tsp twice a day. Fiber may be beneficial in early stages but may exacerbate clinical signs in cats with loss of colonic muscle function. • Dioctyl sodium sulfosuccinate (Colace®) is an emollient laxative that can be given as an alternative to lactulose or polyethylene glycol.
• Ranitidine, a member of the H_2-receptor antagonist drug class, may stimulate colonic motility and can be given if cisapride is unavailable. The dose is 1–3 mg/kg PO q12h.
• One recent pilot study using multistrain probiotic SLAB51™ showed clinical improvement in some cats with chronic constipation and idiopathic megacolon.

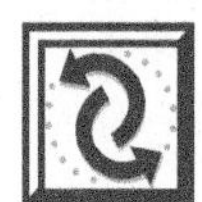

FOLLOW-UP

PATIENT MONITORING

• Following colonic resection and anastomosis—for 3–5 days check for signs of dehiscence and peritonitis. • Clinical deterioration warrants abdominocentesis and/or peritoneal lavage to detect anastomotic leakage. • Continue fluid support until the patient is willing to eat and drink.

PREVENTION/AVOIDANCE

• Repair pelvic fractures that narrow the pelvic canal. • Avoid exposure to foreign bodies and feeding bones. • Encourage physical activity.

POSSIBLE COMPLICATIONS

• Recurrence or persistence—most common.
• Potential surgical complications include peritonitis, persistent diarrhea, fecal incontinence, stricture formation, and recurrence of obstipation. • Traumatic perforation of the colon is a serious complication of overzealous fecal evacuation.

EXPECTED COURSE AND PROGNOSIS

• Historically, medical management has been unrewarding for the long term. • Cisapride appears to improve the prognosis with medical management in some patients, but may not suffice in severe or long-standing cases. • Postoperative diarrhea—expected; typically resolves within 6 weeks (80% of cats with idiopathic megacolon undergoing subtotal colectomy) but can persist for several months; stools become more formed as the ileum adapts by increasing reservoir capacity and water absorption. • Subtotal colectomy is well tolerated by cats; constipation recurrence rates are typically low.

MISCELLANEOUS

ASSOCIATED CONDITIONS

Perineal hernia.

AGE-RELATED FACTORS

Concurrent medical conditions (e.g., chronic renal insufficiency, hyperthyroidism) may occur with idiopathic megacolon, because many cats are old.

ZOONOTIC POTENTIAL

N/A

PREGNANCY/FERTILITY/BREEDING

• The effect of cisapride on the fetus is unknown. • Patients would be at increased risk for dystocia if they carried a pregnancy to term.

SYNONYMS

None

SEE ALSO

• Constipation and Obstipation.
• Dyschezia and Hematochezia.
• Perineal Hernia.

ABBREVIATIONS

• T_4 = thyroxine.

Suggested Reading

Carr AP, Gaunt MC. Constipation resolution with administration of polyethylene-glycol solution in cats (abstract). J Vet Intern Med 2010, 24:753.

Nemeth T, Solymosi N, Balka G. Long-term results of subtotal colectomy for acquired hypertrophic mega- colon in eight dogs. J Small Anim Pract 2008, 49:618–624.

Rosin E, Walshaw R, Mehlhaff C, et al. Subtotal colectomy for treatment of chronic constipation associated with idiopathic megacolon in cats: 38 cases (1979–1985). J Am Vet Med Assoc 1988, 193:850–853.

Rossi G, Jergens A, Cerquetella M, et al. Effects of a probiotic (SLAB51™) on clinical and histologic variables and microbiota of cats with chronic constipation/megacolon: a pilot study. Benef Microbes 2018, 9:101–110.

Washabau RJ. Large intestine dysmotility. In: Washabau RJ, Day MJ, eds., Canine and Feline Gastroenterology. St. Louis, MO: Elsevier, 2013, pp. 757–764.

Author Albert E. Jergens
Consulting Editor Mark P. Rondeau

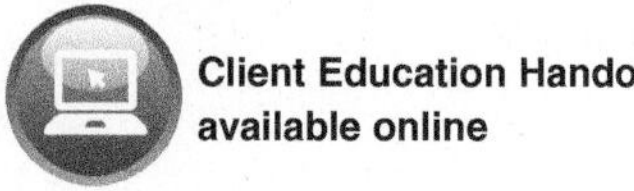

BASICS

DEFINITION

A focal or generalized, diffuse dilation of the esophagus with decreased to absent peristalsis.

PATHOPHYSIOLOGY

• In the normal esophagus, the presence of a food bolus in the proximal esophagus stimulates afferent sensory neurons. • Signals are transferred centrally, via the vagus and glossopharyngeal nerves to the tractus solitarius and nucleus ambiguus. • Motor impulses travel back via the efferent neurons of the vagus nerve to stimulate striated muscle (canine) and striated and smooth muscle (feline) esophageal contraction. • Lesions anywhere along this pathway may lead to megaesophagus and resultant retention of food and liquids. • Approximately 60% of dogs with megaesophagus have an "achalasia-like" syndrome of the lower esophageal sphincter (LES), that is a well-documented cause of megaesophagus in people.
• Functional obstruction of the LES results in esophageal dilatation, retention of ingesta, loss of esophageal motility, and associated clinical signs of esophageal dysphagia. • Dogs with evidence of esophageal achalasia may respond to targeted therapy with subsequent improvement in esophageal dysphagia.
• Focal megaesophagus is typically caused by esophageal obstruction secondary to strictures or a vascular ring anomaly with dilation of the esophagus proximal to the obstruction.

SYSTEMS AFFECTED

• Gastrointestinal—dysphagia, regurgitation, weight loss. • Musculoskeletal—weakness, weight loss, exercise intolerance, dysphonia.
• Nervous—possible manifestation of systemic neurologic/neuromuscular disorder.
• Respiratory—aspiration pneumonia, coughing.

GENETICS

• Congenital form—megaesophagus can be inherited in smooth fox terriers (autosomal recessive) and miniature schnauzers (autosomal dominant or 60% penetrance autosomal recessive). In addition, Jack Russell terriers, springer spaniels, long-haired miniature dachshunds, golden retrievers, Labrador retrievers, and Samoyeds are predisposed to the congenital form of myasthenia gravis.
• Other breeds in which acquired megaesophagus is more commonly reported include German shepherd dog, Great Dane, Irish setter, Labrador retriever, pug, and Chinese Shar-Pei.
• Acquired form—many diseases, especially neuromuscular diseases, may have an association with megaesophagus. Genetic predispositions for such diseases are listed under each disease separately.

INCIDENCE/PREVALENCE

• Congenital forms—relatively uncommon.
• Acquired disease—increasingly recognized in the dog and rare in the cat.

SIGNALMENT

Species

Dogs are more commonly affected than cats.

Breed Predilections

• Dogs—see Genetics. • Cats—Siamese and Siamese-related cats.

Mean Age and Range

• Congenital cases present soon after birth or at weaning during transition from liquid diets to solid foods. • Acquired cases may be seen at any age, depending on the etiology.

SIGNS

Historical Findings

• Owners often report vomiting; the veterinarian must differentiate vomiting from regurgitation. • Regurgitation (considered the hallmark sign); dysphagia; coughing/nasal discharge with aspiration pneumonia; ravenous appetite or inappetence; weight loss or poor growth; ptyalism, and halitosis. Dysphonia may occur secondary to neuromuscular disease. • Other signs depend upon underlying etiology.

Physical Examination Findings

• Cervical swelling may be noted, representing a distended cervical esophagus; ptyalism; halitosis; increased respiratory noises, nasal discharge, and fever (if concurrent pneumonia); cachexia; weakness; weight loss. • Assess for concurrent neurologic deficits that may indicate generalized disease. Special attention should be paid to cranial nerves IX, X, and XI. Muscle atrophy (if present) may be focal or generalized.

CAUSES

Congenital

Idiopathic megaesophagus; congenital myasthenia gravis (MG) (rare).

Acquired/Adult Onset

• Idiopathic (most common).
• Neuromuscular disease—MG, focal or generalized (25% of cases in dogs); systemic lupus erythematosus (SLE); myositis/myopathic disease; dysautonomia (more common in cats); botulism; vagal dysfunction/damage (bilateral); a possible association between laryngeal paralysis and esophageal dysmotility secondary to polyneuropathy has been identified. • Brainstem disease—disease involving cranial nerves IX, X nuclei or peripheral nerves. • Esophageal obstruction—vascular ring anomaly; esophageal or periesophageal neoplasia (e.g., lymphoma, thymoma, leiomyoma); stricture; foreign body; granuloma. • Toxicity—lead, thallium, anticholinesterase; acrylamide. • Endocrine disease—hypoadrenocorticism, hypothyroidism (controversial). Thymoma is associated with MG and megaesophagus in approximately 25% of cats. • Miscellaneous—gastric dilatation volvulus, hiatal hernia, gastroesophageal intussusception; esophagitis (gastroesophageal reflux, parasitic infection).

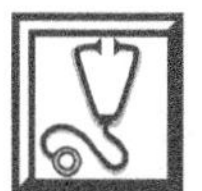

DIAGNOSIS

DIFFERENTIAL DIAGNOSIS

• Must distinguish regurgitation from vomiting. • Regurgitation—passive; little to no abdominal effort; no prodromal phase; regurgitated material has increased amounts of thick mucus. Regurgitation often occurs many hours after a meal has been consumed due to retention of the food bolus within the esophagus. • Vomiting—active process; prodromal phase; vomited material may have increased bile staining. • The shape of the expelled material, presence of undigested food, and length of time from ingestion to regurgitation or vomiting are less helpful to differentiate.

CBC/BIOCHEMISTRY/URINALYSIS

• May be unremarkable. • Inflammatory leukogram may be seen with pneumonia.
• Other changes may identify underlying etiology—basophilic stippling on red blood cells with lead toxicity; electrolyte disturbances with hypoadrenocorticism, although lack of electrolyte changes does not rule out hypoadrenocorticism; hypercholesterolemia with hypothyroidism; elevated creatine kinase with myopathic disease, particularly during the acute phase.

OTHER LABORATORY TESTS

• Acetylcholine receptor (AchR) antibody titer in all cases of acquired megaesophagus (screen for MG). Approximately 2% of dogs with generalized MG are seronegative; testing should be repeated 2–3 months later, particularly if initial antibody titer is only slightly below the reference interval. Dogs with congenital MG do not have an autoimmune disorder associated with circulating AchR antibodies, but instead have a deficiency of the AchR receptor itself. Serologic testing of antibodies to the AchR in puppies or dogs suspected of the congenital form of MG is thus of no diagnostic value and is a waste of money. • Adrenocorticotropic hormone (ACTH) stimulation test or baseline cortisol level for hypoadrenocorticism. • Thyroid panel for hypothyroidism (may be affected by concurrent disease). • Blood and urine lead levels. • Antinuclear antibody (ANA) titers for SLE. • Blood cholinesterase levels for organophosphate toxicity.

IMAGING

Survey Thoracic Radiographs

• Dilated esophagus filled with air, fluid, or food. Interpret thoracic radiographs in anesthetized animals and anxious or painful animals with caution in light of aerophagia that can cause distention of the esophagus with air. • Evidence of aspiration pneumonia may be evident. • Ventral displacement of the trachea on lateral radiographs. • Ventrodorsal radiographs may show lateral tracheal displacement. • Evidence of underlying etiology: mediastinal mass (thymoma), hiatal hernia, neoplasia, etc. • Radiographs do not differentiate dogs with megaesophagus due to MG from dogs with megaesophagus due to other etiologies.

Contrast Esophagram and Videofluoroscopy

• Barium liquid and barium meal may demonstrate abnormal pooling, poor motility, or structural lesions. Iohexol may be used if perforation is a concern. • Use with caution in animals with megaesophagus due to risk of aspiration of contrast material. • Exercise extreme caution in animals with radiographic evidence of pneumonia. • Monitor animals closely after radiographs for signs of aspiration. • Videofluoroscopy—may be used to assess primary and secondary esophageal peristalsis. May help determine the best food consistency for long-term management. Videofluoroscopy commonly demonstrates marked retention of the food bolus within the esophagus for hours, despite gravity-assisted feeding in a Bailey chair. A bird-beak effect of the lower esophageal sphincter may be evident due to esophageal achalasia.

DIAGNOSTIC PROCEDURES

• Esophagoscopy—may be used for foreign body retrieval, evaluation of suspected obstructive lesions, neoplasia, or esophagitis. Distal esophageal neoplasia or stricture of the lower esophageal sphincter may mimic idiopathic megaesophagus and may require endoscopy for diagnosis. • Electrophysiology—in cases of suspected neuromuscular disease, may be used in conjunction with muscle and nerve biopsies. • Additional tests—may be indicated in cases of CNS disease: CSF analysis, distemper titers, brain CT or MRI. • Fecal exam—may indicate *Spirocerca lupi* infection.

PATHOLOGIC FINDINGS

Depend upon underlying etiology and presence of complicating factors.

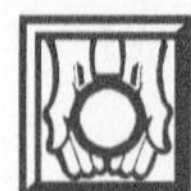

TREATMENT

APPROPRIATE HEALTH CARE

• Treat underlying etiology (when applicable). • Most important aspects are meeting nutritional requirements and treating or preventing aspiration pneumonia.

NURSING CARE

• Aspiration pneumonia may require oxygen therapy, nebulization/coupage, fluid therapy with balanced electrolyte solution. • These animals may be recumbent and require soft bedding and should be maintained in sternal recumbency or turned to alternate down side every 4 hours.

ACTIVITY

Depending on etiology, restricted activity is not necessary.

DIET

• Calculate precise nutritional requirements, including degree of debilitation.
• Experimentation with different food consistencies is essential (e.g., liquid gruel, small meatballs, blenderized slurries).
• Many cases benefit from gastrostomy tube placement for feeding; however, this does not prevent gastroesophageal reflux and potential aspiration or aspiration of saliva.
• Feeding and drinking should be from an elevated position (45–90° from floor) and the upright position should be maintained for 10–15 minutes after eating or drinking. An upright position may be easier to attain with the use of a specific "chair" (e.g., Bailey chair).

CLIENT EDUCATION

• Most cases of megaesophagus require life-long therapy. Even if an underlying etiology is found and treated, prognosis for resolution of idiopathic acquired megaesophagus is unlikely. Client dedication is important for long-term management.
• Most animals succumb to or are euthanized because of aspiration pneumonia, malnutrition, or progression of underlying disease.

SURGICAL CONSIDERATIONS

• Surgery is indicated for vascular ring anomalies, bronchoesophageal fistula, some foreign bodies and other obstructive lesions, or thymectomy. • Balloon dilation is indicated for cases of esophageal stricture.
• Surgical management of esophageal achalasia (Heller's myotomy followed by fundoplication) has been well documented in people with acquired megaesophagus secondary to esophageal achalasia and in a recent publication evaluating acquired megaesophagus in dogs.

MEDICATIONS

DRUG(S) OF CHOICE

• Antibiotics for aspiration pneumonia (ideally based on culture and sensitivity from transtracheal wash or bronchoalveolar lavage). • Therapy for underlying etiology if indicated—immunosuppressives (use with caution if pneumonia present) for immune-mediated disease; pyridostigmine for MG, prednisone supplementation for hypoadrenocorticism. • Proton pump inhibitors (PPIs) are superior acid suppressants to H_2-receptor antagonists (H2RAs) for the management of moderate to severe esophagitis, and are not susceptible to tolerance (tachyphylaxis) that has been well documented in people, dogs, and cats within 3–5 days following the implementation of H2RA therapy. PPIs such as omeprazole or pantoprazole must always be given twice daily for optimal benefit (1 mg/kg PO or IV q12h). In addition, PPIs should be gradually tapered before discontinuing to avoid acid rebound hypersecretion.

Prokinetics

The use of prokinetics such as cisapride and metoclopramide in dogs and cats with diffuse megaesophagus is contraindicated and should be avoided because they will tighten the LES (which already has increased tone in most dogs with megaesophagus as a consequence of achalasia) and possibly increase the risk of aspiration pneumonia. Prokinetics such as metoclopramide (1.0–2.0 mg/kg/day IV CRI or PO q6–8h) or cisapride (0.5 mg/kg PO q8–12h) are more effective for minimizing gastroesophageal reflux and subsequent esophagitis in dogs that do not have megaesophagus. Cisapride is more potent and effective than metoclopramide for increasing LES tone and enhancing gastric emptying, and can be used in animals with evidence of esophagitis but no evidence of megaesophagus, or in cats with esophageal dysmotility affecting the smooth muscle in the distal 1/3 of the esophagus.

PRECAUTIONS

• Absorption of orally administered drugs may be compromised. • Injectable forms should be used when applicable.
• Immunosuppression, if indicated, must be used with caution due to risk of aspiration pneumonia.

FOLLOW-UP

PATIENT MONITORING

• Thoracic radiographs when aspiration pneumonia is suspected (fever, cough, lethargy). • Cases of pneumonia may require CBC, blood gas analysis, and bronchoalveolar lavage. Repeat thoracic radiographs in animals with congenital megaesophagus as spontaneous resolution may occur. • Examine and weigh patients regularly to evaluate disease progression and ensure adequate nutritional intake.

PREVENTION/AVOIDANCE

If an esophageal foreign body is identified, remove as quickly as possible.

POSSIBLE COMPLICATIONS

• Aspiration pneumonia. • Others, depending on etiology.

EXPECTED COURSE AND PROGNOSIS

• Congenital cases have a guarded prognosis (20–46% recovery). • Miniature schnauzers may have better prognosis. • Prognosis may be improved with identification and treatment of specific etiology (e.g., hypoadrenocorticism, vascular ring anomaly). • Roughly 50% cases of MG respond to therapy; however, megaesophagus may persist even if other signs of MG resolve. • Prognosis for idiopathic, adult-onset disease is poor. • Owner dedication is crucial.

MISCELLANEOUS

ASSOCIATED CONDITIONS

Aspiration pneumonia.

AGE-RELATED FACTORS

• Signs of regurgitation in very young animal or at weaning may indicate congenital lesion.
• Prognosis may be better in young animals.

ZOONOTIC POTENTIAL

• None for megaesophagus. • Rabies vaccination status should be determined in any animal with possible neurologic disease.

SYNONYMS

• Esophageal aperistalsis. • Esophageal dilatation.

SEE ALSO

- Dysphagia.
- Esophageal Foreign Bodies.
- Myasthenia Gravis.
- Pneumonia, Aspiration.
- Pneumonia, Bacterial.
- Regurgitation.

ABBREVIATIONS

- AchR = acetylcholine receptor.
- ACTH = adrenocorticotropic hormone.
- ANA = antinuclear antibody.
- H2RAs = H_2-receptor antagonists.
- LES = lower esophageal sphincter.
- MG = myasthenia gravis.
- PPI = proton pump inhibitor.
- SLE = systemic lupus erythematosus.

INTERNET RESOURCES

• https://www.marvistavet.com/megaesophagus.pml • http://www.baileychairs4dogs.com/

Suggested Reading

Grobman ME, Hutcheson KD, Lever TE, et al. Mechanical dilation, botulinum toxin A injection, and surgical myotomy with fundoplication for treatment of lower esophageal sphincter achalasia-like syndrome in dogs. J Vet Intern Med 2019, 33(3):1423–1433.

Mace S, Shelton GD, Eddlestone S. Megaesophagus. Compend Contin Educ Vet 2012, 34(2):E1.

McBrearty AR, Ramsey IK, Courcier EA, et al. Clinical factors associated with death before discharge and overall survival time in dogs with generalized megaesophagus. J Am Vet Med Assoc 2011, 238(12):1622–1628.

Authors Stanley L. Marks and Marguerite F. Knipe

Consulting Editor Mark P. Rondeau

Client Education Handout available online

MELANOCYTIC TUMORS, ORAL

BASICS

DEFINITION

Tumor of melanocytes arising in the oral cavity (gingiva, palate, tongue), most frequently malignant.

PATHOPHYSIOLOGY

• Locally invasive, may invade into underlying bone. • Metastatic in >75% cases in dogs. • Immunohistochemical evaluation may be required for the diagnosis of amelanotic melanomas.

SYSTEMS AFFECTED

• Oral cavity (gingiva, palate, tongue).
• Metastatic sites—regional lymph nodes and lungs most common; liver, spleen, bones, meninges, other.

GENETICS

Unknown

INCIDENCE/PREVALENCE

• Dogs—most common malignant oral tumor, accounting for ~40% of oral malignancies.
• Cats—third most common oral malignancy.

SIGNALMENT

Species

Dog more than cat.

Breed Predilections

• Dogs—cocker spaniel, miniature poodle, retriever breed, dachshunds, chow chow (tongue). • Cats—no predilection reported.

Mean Age and Range

• Dogs—11 years (5–18 years). • Cats—12 years (11–15 years).

Predominant Sex

• Dogs—male predisposed (in some studies).
• Cats—not reported.

SIGNS

Historical Findings

• Excessive salivation. • Halitosis.
• Dysphagia. • Hyporexia. • Bloody oral discharge. • Weight loss.

Physical Examination Findings

• Oral mass (up to a third are poorly pigmented or amelanotic), often friable and ulcerated. • Loose teeth if involvement of mandibular or maxillary bone. • Facial deformity (including exophthalmos).
• Regional lymphadenomegaly. • Pain or discomfort.

RISK FACTORS

Overrepresented breeds of dogs.

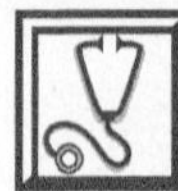

DIAGNOSIS

DIFFERENTIAL DIAGNOSIS

• Other oral malignancy (squamous cell carcinoma, fibrosarcoma). • Acanthomatous ameloblastoma/peripheral odontogenic fibroma. • Gingival hyperplasia. • Tooth root abscess. • Foreign body reaction.

CBC/BIOCHEMISTRY/URINALYSIS

Usually normal.

IMAGING

• High-detail skull radiography or dental radiographs—evaluate for osteolytic changes.
• Advanced imaging (contrast-enhanced CT or MRI) affords better detail and helps with therapeutic planning (surgery or radiation therapy). • Three-view thoracic imaging (radiography or CT)—evaluate lungs for metastasis. • Abdominal imaging (ultrasonography or CT)—to complete clinical staging; occasional distant metastasis in abdominal visceral organs.

DIAGNOSTIC PROCEDURES

• Carefully measure primary tumor—important prognostic information. • Fine-needle aspiration and cytology of ipsilateral and contralateral mandibular lymph nodes recommended to evaluate for regional metastases, regardless of their size and consistency upon palpation—up to 40% of normal-sized regional lymph nodes have metastasis. • Carefully palpate other regional lymph nodes (retropharyngeal, parotid, superficial cervical) and perform fine-needle aspiration and cytology if abnormal. • Large and deep-tissue biopsies may be required to obtain definitive diagnosis (via histopathology) and gather prognostic information.
• Fine-needle aspiration or biopsies of primary tumor should always be taken from inside the mouth, not through the skin (could compromise local control with surgery due to needle or biopsy track seeding).

PATHOLOGIC FINDINGS

Gross

• Masses may be ulcerated and friable; often bleed when large and malignant.
• Amelanotic to dark brown, gray, or black.
• Vary greatly in size; often invasive in surrounding tissues.

Cytologic Findings

• Brown, rod-like intracellular granules (melanin) of various size and shapes.
• Pigment may be absent with amelanotic tumors. • May see melanophages (phagocytic macrophages) with large intracytoplasmic vacuoles containing melanin, especially in lymph nodes. • More cellular atypia observed in malignant tumors.

Histopathologic Findings

• Cells may vary in shape (e.g., epithelioid, fusiform, dendritic, and mixed), degree of pigmentation, and cytoplasmic morphology.
• Malignant—generally high mitotic index; nuclear and nucleolar pleomorphism (more atypia, less differentiation); invasive into surrounding tissues; amelanotic may pose a diagnostic challenge; immunohistochemistry and special stains may be particularly useful; proliferation markers may help predict behavior. • Immunohistochemistry (e.g., Melan-A, S100, PNL2, HMB-45, vimentin)—may help confirm a diagnosis, especially if amelanotic (approximately one-third of cases).
• Histopathology report should include mitotic index (mitoses per 10 HPF), degree of atypia/differentiation, invasiveness, and surgical margins if excisional biopsy.

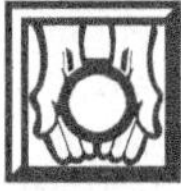

TREATMENT

APPROPRIATE HEALTH CARE

Inpatient if undergoing aggressive oral surgery.

NURSING CARE

Pain management—multimodal analgesia (preemptive, intra- and postoperative) is mandatory with aggressive surgeries.

ACTIVITY

Restrict until sutures are removed and all surgical wounds healed.

DIET

• Soft food recommended to prevent tumor ulceration or following aggressive oral surgery.
• Avoid toys and hard treats until oral tissues are healed completely.

CLIENT EDUCATION

• Discuss importance of clinical staging.
• Discuss need for early aggressive approach with surgical removal • Warn caretaker that malignant melanoma frequently metastasizes early in the course of the disease, resulting in a guarded prognosis. • Adjuvant therapy is recommended to improve survival time and delay metastasis. • Repeat clinical staging recommended after therapy.

SURGICAL CONSIDERATIONS

• Goal should be to remove all macroscopic tumor burden and obtain complete margins in order to improve overall prognosis.
• Radical *en bloc* surgical excision—required (e.g., mandibulectomy or maxillectomy); well

M

tolerated by most patients; surgical margins of at least 2 cm; improved survival when margins are free of neoplastic cells. • Surgical removal of the draining lymph node(s) is recommended when metastasis confirmed or suspected and no evidence of distant (e.g., lung) metastatic disease.

RADIATION THERAPY

• May be used to improve local disease control following unplanned incomplete resection. • As single modality treatment for macroscopic disease, radiation therapy affords a good response rate (>80%) and may offer long-term control with inoperable tumors; 3–6, weekly to twice weekly, large fractions of megavoltage radiation therapy.

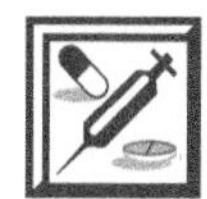

MEDICATIONS

DRUG(S) OF CHOICE

• Carboplatin has been described for oral melanoma in dogs and remains recommended following surgical excision of macroscopic disease (primary tumor, metastatic regional lymph nodes). • Carboplatin may still be advised if surgical excision is not possible, with a response rate approximating 30% on measurable disease, and may be coupled with palliative radiation therapy protocols.
• Contact a veterinary oncologist for any updated treatments that may be available.
• No effective chemotherapy described in cats. • Pain management with multimodal analgesia therapy is mandatory (nonsteroidal anti-inflammatory drugs, opioid, adjuvant analgesia medications, aminobisphosphonates if osteolysis is present).

Immunotherapy

• Many immunotherapies have been attempted with varied success. • A therapeutic vaccine is available (Oncept™) that involves the injection of human cDNA (xenogeneic) coding for a melanocyte-specific protein, tyrosinase, and results in a measurable immune response in some patients. • The tyrosinase vaccine is approved for the postoperative treatment of stage II and III oral malignant melanomas and some reports suggest improved survival times in comparison with historical control studies.

CONTRAINDICATIONS

Avoid the use of cisplatin in cats.

PRECAUTIONS

Seek advice from an oncologist before initiating treatment if you are unfamiliar with cytotoxic drugs (myelosuppression, specific toxicities, etc.).

POSSIBLE INTERACTIONS

Drugs with overlapping toxicities should be avoided.

ALTERNATIVE DRUG(S)

Novel therapeutics or treatment regimens may be available. Contact a veterinary oncologist for any updated treatments that may be available.

FOLLOW-UP

PATIENT MONITORING

• Evaluate for local recurrence and regional metastasis every 2–3 months following surgery or earlier if the owner believes the mass is returning; or if the patient is otherwise not normal. • Recommend three-view thoracic radiography at the time of rechecks (every 3 months).

POSSIBLE COMPLICATIONS

• Poor wound healing, dehiscence, infection possible after aggressive surgery. • Early radiation side effects, such as mucositis or dermatitis, may result from hypofractionated protocols.

EXPECTED COURSE AND PROGNOSIS

• Poor prognosis when untreated (median 2 months). • Depends upon disease stage; better prognosis with stage I. • Complete surgical excision (local and regional lymph node when positive) is essential to improve the prognosis—median survival time with surgery alone varies with stage: ◦ Stage I—over 18 months. ◦ Stage II and III—5–12 months. ◦ Stage IV—less than 3 months. • Adjuvant carboplatin chemotherapy is not consistently reported as beneficial but remains recommended. • Prognosis of stage II and III canine oral melanoma may be improved to over 18 months with the adjuvant use of the recombinant xenogeneic tyrosinase vaccine. • Survival with radiotherapy treatment alone (dogs)—6–10 months. • Cause of death in dogs may be metastatic disease or local tumor recurrence. • Overall prognosis in cats is poor; most tumors are locally invasive and diagnosed late in the course of the disease; cause of death is often due to local disease progression—median survival time of 146 days in 5 cats treated with hypofractionated radiation therapy.

MISCELLANEOUS

AGE-RELATED FACTORS

Older age at diagnosis (>12 years) might predict a poorer prognosis in dogs.

SEE ALSO

Melanocytic Tumors, Skin and Digit.

Suggested Reading

Boston SE, Lu X, Culp WT, et al. Efficacy of adjuvant therapies administered to dogs after excision of oral malignant melanomas: 151 cases (2001–2012). J Am Vet Med Assoc 2014, 245:401–407.

Brockley LK, Cooper MA, Bennett PF. Malignant melanoma in 63 dogs (2001–2011): the effect of carboplatin chemotherapy on survival. N Z Vet J 2013, 61:25–31.

Farrelly J, Denman DL, Hohenhaus AE, et al. Hypofractionated radiation therapy of oral melanoma in five cats. Vet Radiol Ultrasound 2004, 45:91–93.

Grosenbaugh DA, Leard AT, Bergman PJ, et al. Safety and efficacy of a xenogeneic DNA vaccine encoding for human tyrosinase as adjunctive treatment for oral malignant melanoma in dogs following surgical excision of the primary tumor. Am J Vet Res 2011, 72:1631–1638.

Proulx DR, Ruslander DM, Dodge RK, et al. A retrospective analysis of 140 dogs with oral melanoma treated with external beam radiation. Vet Radiol Ultrasound 2003, 44:352–359.

Rassnick KM, Ruslander DM, Cotter SM, et al. Use of carboplatin for treatment of dogs with malignant melanoma: 27 cases (1989–2000). J Am Vet Med Assoc 2001, 218:1444–1448.

Smedley RC, Spangler WL, Esplin DG, et al. Prognostic markers for canine melanocytic neoplasms: a comparative review of the literature and goals for future investigation. Vet Pathol 2011, 48:54–72.

Verganti S, Berlato D, Blackwood L, et al. Use of Oncept melanoma vaccine in 69 canine oral malignant melanoma in the UK. J Small Anim Pract 2017, 58:10–16.

Author Matthew R. Berry

Consulting Editor Timothy M. Fan

Acknowledgment The author and editors acknowledge the prior contribution of Louis-Philippe de Lorimier.

MELANOCYTIC TUMORS, SKIN AND DIGIT

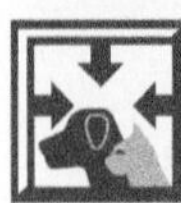

BASICS

OVERVIEW

• Benign or malignant neoplasm arising from melanocytes within the epidermis or the nail bed. • Anatomic site is highly predictive of invasiveness and metastatic propensity: ○ Digit and mucocutaneous junction melanomas tend to be malignant. ○ Melanomas of haired-skin tend to behave in benign manner. • When malignant—occasionally invades bone (e.g., third phalanx) and metastasizes (lymph node, lungs, and other sites).

SIGNALMENT

• Dogs—around 5% of all skin tumors.
• Cats—<5% of all skin tumors. • Dogs, mean age 9 years, certain breeds more common—terriers (Scottish, Boston, and Airedale), schnauzers, cocker and springer spaniels, Irish setter, chow chow, retriever breeds, poodles, Doberman pinschers. • Cats, mean age 10–13 years, no breed predilection.

M

SIGNS

• Skin mass with variable growth rates, may be ulcerated and friable, usually solitary.
• Develops anywhere; in dogs more common on face, trunk, feet, and scrotum; in cats more common on head, digit, pinna, and nose.
• Benign—brown to black; varies from macules and plaques to firm, dome-shaped nodules, 0.5–2 cm in diameter, well demarcated. • Malignant—amelanotic to dark brown, gray, or black, often >2 cm in diameter and more invasive in surrounding tissues.
• Lameness and pain if digit is involved and associated with infection or bone lysis.
• Regional lymphadenomegaly possible.

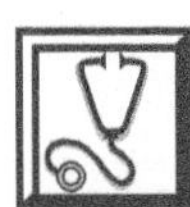

DIAGNOSIS

DIFFERENTIAL DIAGNOSIS

Distinguish amelanotic melanoma from poorly differentiated discrete cell tumors (mast cell tumor, lymphoma), various sarcomas (e.g., histiocytic, soft tissue sarcoma), carcinomas (especially basal cell), other benign changes (pyogranulomatous inflammation).

CBC/BIOCHEMISTRY/URINALYSIS

Usually normal.

IMAGING

• Thoracic radiography recommended for evaluation of distant metastasis. • Advanced imaging (CT scan) is more sensitive to detect smaller distant metastases. • With digital melanoma, radiography of the lesion is recommended to determine if underlying bone (P3) is involved; bone lysis is less common with nailbed melanoma (approximately 10%) compared with squamous cell carcinoma (approximately 75%).

DIAGNOSTIC PROCEDURES

• Cytologic examination of fine-needle aspirates (primary mass, draining lymph nodes). • Draining lymph nodes should be evaluated with cytology, regardless of their size and consistency upon palpation. • Tissue biopsies may be required to obtain definitive diagnosis (via histopathology).
• Immunohistochemical markers—may help differentiate melanoma (especially amelanotic) from other tumors; may stain positive with Melan-A, S100, PNL2, HMB-45, vimentin; proliferation markers may help predict behavior (e.g., Ki67).

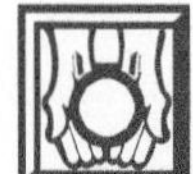

TREATMENT

Surgical Considerations

• Wide surgical excision—treatment of choice. • Amputation of digit (P3 and P2) with nailbed localization.
• Lymphadenectomy of the draining lymph node might be indicated when regional metastasis confirmed or suspected and no evidence of detectable distant dissemination.

Radiation Therapy Considerations

• May be used to improve local disease control following unplanned incomplete resection. • Palliative radiation therapy may be considered for inoperable tumors.

MEDICATIONS

DRUG(S) OF CHOICE

• Adjuvant chemotherapy (often carboplatin) recommended following excision of macroscopic malignant melanoma (primary tumor, metastatic regional lymph nodes).
• Chemotherapy may still be advised if surgical excision is not possible, with a response rate approximating 30% on measurable disease, and may be coupled with palliative radiation therapy protocols.
• Contact a veterinary oncologist for updates on novel therapeutic options or treatment regimens. • Multimodal analgesia recommended to control pain and discomfort.

Immunotherapy

• Many immunotherapies have been attempted with varied success. • Therapeutic vaccination—injection of cDNA coding for a melanocyte-specific protein, tyrosinase, is considered safe and results in a measurable immune response in some patients.

CONTRAINDICATIONS/POSSIBLE INTERACTIONS

• Cisplatin is contraindicated in cats. • Seek advice from an oncologist before initiating treatment if you are unfamiliar with cytotoxic drugs (myelosuppression, specific toxicities, etc.).

FOLLOW-UP

PATIENT MONITORING

• Evaluate for local recurrence and regional metastasis—every 2–3 months following surgery or earlier if the owner believes the mass is returning; or if the patient is otherwise not normal. • 3-view thoracic radiography—at the time of rechecks and periodically thereafter.

EXPECTED COURSE AND PROGNOSIS

Dogs

• Melanomas on the digit, footpad, scrotum, and mucocutaneous junctions are more frequently malignant. • Prognosis with benign cutaneous melanomas is excellent. • Median survival with malignant cutaneous or digit melanoma is 12 months. • Breed differences in prognosis in some studies—majority of cutaneous melanomas in Doberman pinschers and miniature schnauzers behave in a benign fashion, and a majority of cutaneous melanomas in miniature poodles behave in a malignant fashion.

Cats

• 35–50% of melanomas reported to be malignant. • Median survival with melanoma of the skin or digit not well documented and reported to be 4.5 months after surgery. • Cats with auricular melanoma may have a more favorable prognosis compared to melanomas of other cutaneous sites or oral cavity.

MISCELLANEOUS

SEE ALSO

Melanocytic Tumors, Oral.

Suggested Reading

Chamel G, Abadie J, Albaric O, et al. Non-ocular melanomas in cats: a retrospective study of 30 cases. J Feline Med Surg 2017, 19:351–357.

Henry CJ, Brewer WG Jr., Whitley EM, et al. Canine digital tumors: a veterinary cooperative oncology group retrospective study of 64 dogs. J Vet Intern Med 2005, 19(5):720–724.

Smedley RC, Spangler WL, Esplin DG, et al. Prognostic markers for canine melanocytic neoplasms: a comparative review of the literature and goals for future investigation. Vet Pathol 2011, 48:54–72.

Author Matthew R. Berry

Consulting Editor Timothy M. Fan

Acknowledgment The author and editors acknowledge the prior contribution of Louis-Philippe de Lorimier.

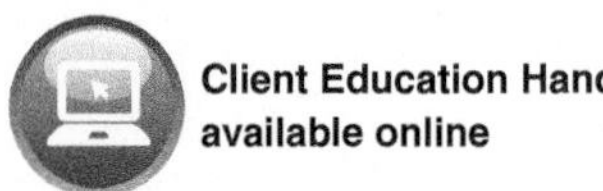

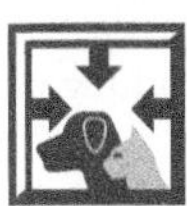

BASICS

DEFINITION

Black, tarry appearance of feces caused by the presence of digested or oxidized blood.

PATHOPHYSIOLOGY

Usually results from upper gastrointestinal (GI) bleeding (esophagus, stomach, small intestine), but can be associated with ingested blood from the oral cavity or respiratory tract. Rarely can be caused by bleeding in the cecum or colon.

SYSTEMS AFFECTED

- GI.
- Respiratory.
- Coagulation.
- Cardiovascular.

GENETICS

N/A

INCIDENCE/PREVALENCE

Unknown

GEOGRAPHIC DISTRIBUTION

Worldwide

SIGNALMENT

Species

- More common in dog than cat.

Breed Predilections

None

Mean Age and Range

Any age.

Predominant Sex

None

SIGNS

Historical Findings

- Patients with clinically significant anemia may demonstrate lethargy, inappetence, weakness, collapse, mucous membrane pallor, and/or dyspnea.
- Patients with primary GI disease may demonstrate hypersalivation, dysphagia, regurgitation, vomiting with or without blood (frank blood or "coffee grounds" appearance), inappetence, weight loss, increased borborygmi, or diarrhea.
- Patients with respiratory tract hemorrhage may demonstrate epistaxis, sneezing, hemoptysis, mucous membrane pallor, weakness, and/or dyspnea.
- Patients with abnormal coagulation may demonstrate petechiae, ecchymoses, mucous membrane pallor, epistaxis, hematuria, hematochezia, hyphema, and/or weakness.

Physical Examination Findings

Depends on the underlying cause.

CAUSES

Primary GI Ulceration/Erosion

- Neoplasia—adenocarcinoma, lymphoma, sarcoma.
- Inflammatory bowel disease (IBD)—lymphoplasmacytic, eosinophilic, granulomatous, and/or histiocytic gastritis/enteritis.
- Benign polyps.
- Infectious—Bacterial (*Salmonella* spp., *Clostridium perfringens, C. difficile*); fungal or fungal-like (pythiosis, histoplasmosis), parasitic (*Physaloptera, Ollulanus,* hookworms), viral (parvovirus, circovirus, distemper).
- Mechanical—foreign body.
- Inflammatory—acute and chronic gastritis; acute hemorrhagic diarrhea syndrome.
- Drugs—nonsteroidal anti-inflammatory drugs (NSAIDs), corticosteroids.
- Toxins—ingestion of heavy metals, some plants, cleaners, etc.

Metabolic/Other Diseases That Cause GI Ulceration

- Hypoadrenocorticism.
- Neoplasia—gastrinoma, mast cell tumor.
- Shock, poor perfusion.
- Pancreatitis.
- Acute kidney injury or advanced chronic kidney disease.
- Hepatic disease/failure, intrahepatic portosystemic shunts.

Ingestion of Blood

- Diet (raw foods).
- Esophageal lesion—neoplasia, esophagitis.
- Oral or pharyngeal lesion—neoplasia, abscess.
- Nasal lesion—neoplasia, fungal rhinitis, inflammatory rhinitis, trauma.
- Respiratory lesion—lung lobe torsion, neoplasia, pneumonia, trauma (causing hemoptysis).

Coagulopathy

- Thrombocytopenia.
- Thrombocytopathia—congenital vs. acquired.
- von Willebrand disease.
- Clotting factor abnormalities—anticoagulant rodenticide ingestion, selected clotting factor deficiencies.
- Disseminated intravascular coagulation.

RISK FACTORS

Arthritis, intervertebral disc disease or other conditions requiring use of NSAIDs or corticosteroids.

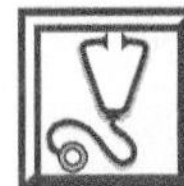

DIAGNOSIS

DIFFERENTIAL DIAGNOSIS

- Medications that cause dark stool—bismuth subsalicylate, oral iron therapy, sucralfate, barium sulfate, activated charcoal.
- Must distinguish primary intestinal from extraintestinal disease.

CBC/BIOCHEMISTRY/URINALYSIS

- Microcytic, hypochromic, poorly regenerative anemia if chronic blood loss.
- Regenerative anemia in early blood loss—may be pre-regenerative if <3–5 days.
- Panhypoproteinemia, hypocholesterolemia if significant blood loss or diffuse GI disease
- Thrombocytopenia—may be mild from consumption with GI bleeding; severe thrombocytopenia may be primary cause of bleeding.
- Neutrophilia in some patients.
- Biochemistry analysis may reveal extraintestinal cause of melena—renal failure, hepatic disease, hypoadrenocorticism. Increased blood urea nitrogen (BUN):creatinine ratio can be seen secondary to GI bleeding.
- Urinalysis may demonstrate hematuria in patients with coagulation defects.

OTHER LABORATORY TESTS

- Prothrobin time/activated partial thromboplastin time (PT/aPTT) may be prolonged with coagulopathy.
- Buccal mucosal bleeding time tests primary hemostasis. Will be prolonged with thrombocytopenia and anemia.
- Fecal centrifugation flotation may reveal parasites.
- Diarrhea PCR panels for bacterial DNA and toxin genes in combination with ELISA testing for *C. perfringens* enterotoxin and *C. difficile* toxins A and B may be helpful but should be interpreted based on history, physical examination findings, environment, and risk factors.
- Parvo antigen testing.
- Serum cobalamin and folate may be useful to screen for diffuse GI disease.
- Rectal scraping may demonstrate fungal organisms (*Histoplasma* spp.).
- Resting cortisol and/or adrenocorticotropic hormone (ACTH) stimulation test abnormally low with hypoadrenocorticism.

IMAGING

- Abdominal radiography may reveal a mass or foreign body, or abnormalities in renal or hepatic size/shape.
- Thoracic radiographs may identify esophageal foreign bodies, pulmonary or tracheobronchial lesions or metastatic disease.
- Nasal CT may demonstrate intranasal lesions.
- Ultrasonography may reveal a GI mass, loss of intestinal layering, evidence of GI ulceration (mucosal defect, intramural gas), alterations in hepatic echotexture and size, pancreatic changes suggestive of pancreatitis, or changes supportive of renal disease or hypoadrenocorticism.
- Upper GI barium series may delineate gastric or proximal small intestinal masses, ulceration, or filling defects; however, upper GI series is insensitive for detection of gastric and intestinal ulceration.

MELENA (CONTINUED)

DIAGNOSTIC PROCEDURES

- Endoscopy allows visualization of masses and/or ulcers (esophageal, gastric, and/or duodenal), retrieval of esophageal or gastric foreign bodies, and procurement of biopsy samples.
- Retroflex and/or anterograde rhinoscopy may allow visualization of nasal lesions.
- Tracheobronchoscopy allows visualization of large airway lesions.
- Capsule endoscopy may be useful for delineating sites of intestinal bleeding that cannot be visualized via flexible endoscopy.

PATHOLOGIC FINDINGS

Vary with underlying disease.

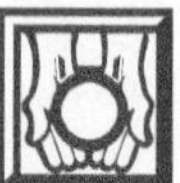

TREATMENT

APPROPRIATE HEALTH CARE

- Inpatient—most patients admitted for work-up and management with exception of animals with melena secondary to intestinal parasites.
- Treat underlying disease—renal failure, hepatic disease, hypoadrenocorticism, respiratory disease, etc.

NURSING CARE

- Fluid replacement with balanced electrolyte solutions and potassium supplementation.
- Whole blood or packed red blood cell transfusions if anemia is severe.
- Whole blood, platelet concentrate or plasma transfusion if the patient has a coagulopathy.

ACTIVITY

Need for restriction varies with underlying disease.

DIET

Temporarily discontinue oral intake if vomiting is intractable.

CLIENT EDUCATION

Depends on underlying disease.

SURGICAL CONSIDERATIONS

Surgery may be required for severe gastroduodenal ulceration, neoplasia, or foreign bodies.

MEDICATIONS

DRUG(S) OF CHOICE

- Varies with underlying disease.
- For known or suspected gastric ulceration:
  - Proton pump inhibitors (PPI; e.g., omeprazole 1 mg/kg PO q12h, pantoprazole 1 mg/kg IV q12h, esomeprazole 0.7 mg/kg IV q12h) are superior to H_2 antagonists for acid suppression. PPIs should be tapered following chronic use >3–4 weeks (50% reduction weekly).
  - Misoprostol (3–5 µg/kg PO q12h) for cases of NSAID-induced gastric ulcers.
  - Sucralfate (0.5–1 g PO q6–8h as a suspension) for esophagitis or gastric ulceration.

CONTRAINDICATIONS

Avoid corticosteroids and NSAIDs in patients with gastroduodenal ulceration/erosion.

PRECAUTIONS

Misoprostol should not be used in pregnant animals.

POSSIBLE INTERACTIONS

- Antacids may cause decreased absorption of medications that require an acid pH for absorption.
- Sucralfate should be separated from meals or other medications by 2 hours.

ALTERNATIVE DRUG(S)

H_2-receptor antagonists (e.g., ranitidine 1–2 mg/kg IV, SC, or PO q12h or famotidine 0.5–1 mg/kg IV, SC, or PO q12h) may be used for acid suppression if PPIs are not available.

FOLLOW-UP

PATIENT MONITORING

- Packed cell volume (PCV) 2–3 times daily until anemia stabilized, then weekly.
- Hydration daily if patient vomiting.

PREVENTION/AVOIDANCE

Use ulcerogenic drugs with caution. Avoid concurrent use of NSAIDs and glucocorticoids.

POSSIBLE COMPLICATIONS

- Gastric or duodenal perforation resulting in peritonitis.
- Hypovolemic shock and death if severe, acute blood loss.

EXPECTED COURSE AND PROGNOSIS

Varies with underlying disease.

MISCELLANEOUS

ASSOCIATED CONDITIONS

N/A

AGE-RELATED FACTORS

N/A

ZOONOTIC POTENTIAL

Bacterial (*Clostridium* spp., *Salmonella* spp.) and parasitic infectious causes are potentially zoonotic.

PREGNANCY/FERTILITY/BREEDING

Misoprostol should not be used in pregnant animals.

SYNONYMS

N/A

SEE ALSO

- Gastroduodenal Ulceration/Erosion.
- Gastroenteritis, Acute Hemorrhagic Diarrhea Syndrome.

ABBREVIATIONS

- ACTH = adrenocorticotropic hormone.
- BUN = blood urea nitrogen.
- GI = gastrointestinal.
- IBD = inflammatory bowel disease.
- NSAID = nonsteroidal anti-inflammatory drug.
- PCV = packed cell volume.
- PPI = proton pump inhibitor.
- PT/aPTT = prothrobin time/activated partial thromboplastin time.

Author Megan McClosky
Consulting Editor Mark P. Rondeau
Acknowledgment The author and editors acknowledge the prior contribution of Lisa E. Moore.

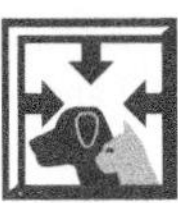

BASICS

DEFINITION

• Tumor of the meninges. Most commonly affects meninges overlying the cerebrum.
• Most common tumor of the canine brain and spinal cord. • Most common tumor of the feline brain; second most common tumor of the feline spinal cord (most common being lymphoma).

PATHOPHYSIOLOGY

• Primary tumor arising from the arachnoid cap cells. • Intradural–extramedullary location. • Usually solitary masses; occasionally multiple (cats > dogs). • May occur as plaque-like masses on the floor of the calvaria, paranasally, or retrobulbar space (rare, more common in dogs than in cats).
• Causes neurologic deficits secondary to compression of the adjacent tissue. Progresses slowly, causing vasogenic edema and, occasionally, obstructive hydrocephalus or infarction. • Most are *cytologically* benign. In dogs, tend to be more invasive into brain parenchyma or surrounding vasculature, and can be considered *biologically* malignant, unless aggressive surgical resection is possible (e.g., within the olfactory bulb).

SYSTEMS AFFECTED

Nervous—primary effects (e.g., infiltration and compression of adjacent structures) and secondary effects (e.g., edema, increased intracranial pressure [ICP], brain herniation).

INCIDENCE/PREVALENCE

• Reported incidence of brain tumors is 14.5/100,000 dogs and 3.5/100,000 cats. Meningiomas account for approximately 22% of all canine brain tumors, and 59% of all feline brain tumors. • 17% of cats with intracranial meningioma have >1 tumor of the same type. • Incidence of spinal tumors in dogs and cats—unknown; considerably less than that of brain tumors. Spinal meningiomas account for 14% of all canine meningiomas and 4% of all feline meningiomas.

SIGNALMENT

Dog and cat.

Dogs

• Boxers and golden retrievers most commonly affected; dolichocephalic breeds may have an increased risk of intracranial meningioma; mesocephalic breeds may have a higher incidence of paranasal meningioma.
• Most >7 years of age; median 9 years, range 11 weeks–14 years; a spinal meningeal sarcoma was diagnosed in an 11-week-old Rottweiler. • Slight predominance for females. • Cystic meningiomas reported.

Cats

• Domestic shorthair cats overrepresented.
• Most >9 years of age; mean 12 years, range 1–24 years; slight predominance for males.

SIGNS

General Comments

• Vary with tumor location. • Typically chronic and insidiously progressive over weeks to months. • May be acute if vascular invasion results in focal ischemia or if edema develops rapidly. • Lateralizing deficits predominate. • Elevated ICP, cerebral edema, or brain herniation may cause multifocal deficits, making localization of a focal mass/lesion difficult based on clinical signs.

Historical Findings

May be prolonged history of vague signs until compensatory mechanisms (e.g., decreased cerebrospinal fluid [CSF] and blood volume) are overwhelmed, followed by rapid progression of clinical signs.

Intracranial

• Dogs—late-onset seizures is the most common presenting sign. • Cats—abnormal behavior and mentation are the most common presenting signs. Nonspecific signs include lethargy, inappetence, and anorexia. Seizures less common than in dogs.

Intraspinal

• Neck or back pain. • Progressive incoordination and weakness, which may worsen with exercise.

Physical Examination Findings

Intracranial

• Cerebral disease is most common, causing abnormal behavior and mentation; circling or head-pressing; contralateral hemi-neglect, hemianopsia, facial paresis, facial and thoracic hypesthesia and conscious proprioceptive deficits; seizures. • Brainstem—alterations of consciousness; abnormal gait; ipsilateral proprioceptive and cranial nerve deficits in cranial nerves III to XII; central vestibular abnormalities. • Cerebellum—ataxia and dysmetria; intention tremors; truncal sway; broad-based stance; lack of menace responses with normal vision, and pupillary light and palpebral reflexes.
• Orbital—exophthalmos, orbital swelling, prolapsed globe; blindness in the affected eye; fundic abnormalities.

Intraspinal

• Paraspinal or radicular pain referable to the region of spinal column affected. • Ataxia and paresis caudal to the level of the lesion.

CAUSES

• Unknown. • Documentation in young cats with mucopolysaccharidosis type I suggests a causal relationship.

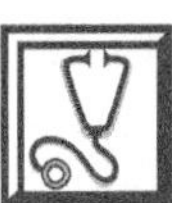

DIAGNOSIS

DIFFERENTIAL DIAGNOSIS

• Metabolic or toxic encephalopathy—may also present with seizures or mentation changes and normal neurologic exam; differentiate with brain imaging. • Other primary CNS (e.g., glioma, pituitary, nephroblastoma) or secondary (e.g., lymphoma, extensional, metastatic) tumors—may have more rapid onset and progression of signs; differentiate with brain or spinal imaging. • Granulomatous meningoencephalitis—may cause progressive focal deficits in dogs; differentiate based on age and further diagnostics, such as imaging and CSF analysis. • Nerve sheath tumors, gliomas, lymphoma, focal meningomyelitis, type II intervertebral disc disease, degenerative myelopathy—differentiate by spinal cord imaging. • *Cryptococcus* granuloma—reported to have same appearance on CT as a meningioma in a cat.

CBC/BIOCHEMISTRY/URINALYSIS

Usually normal.

IMAGING

• MRI—preferred imaging modality for intracranial and spinal disease. • MRI—often hyperintense on T2-weighted images (T2WI), isointense on T1-weighted images (T1WI), and uniformly contrast-enhancing mass lesion of the brain or spinal cord; broad-based, with extra-axial attachment. A 'dural tail' is a characteristic feature. If present, 'dural tail' helps to differentiate an intraventricular meningioma from a choroid plexus tumor. Spinal cord swelling may make the distinction between intradural/extramedullary and intramedullary difficult. • CT—often homogeneous contrast enhancement of well-circumscribed mass lesion. • Skull radiography and CT—may reveal hyperostosis of the calvaria adjacent to the meningioma. Calcification of the mass causes increased tissue density. Hyperostosis may be seen in cats.
• Spinal radiography—usually normal with intraspinal meningioma; can be helpful to rule out bony lesions. • Myelography—typically reveals an intradural–extramedullary mass and interruption of the normal flow of contrast at the tumor. 'Golf tee' appearance can be present with both nerve sheath tumor and meningioma. Differentiation requires biopsy.

DIAGNOSTIC PROCEDURES

• CSF analysis—infrequently performed because diagnostic imaging is diagnostic. If performed, normal-to-high protein concentration with possible neutrophilic or mixed pleocytosis. Should not be considered unless CT or MRI have been performed. Contraindicated with increased ICP, as collection of CSF increases risk of brain herniation and consequent neurologic decompensation. • Electroencephalography—reveals slow-wave, medium--to-high-voltage activity, indicating cortical depression. Paroxysmal waveforms characteristic of seizure activity may be evident. • Biopsy—necessary for definitive diagnosis; perform intraoperatively or, for intracranial tumors, using a CT-guided stereotactic system.

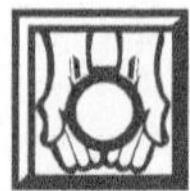

TREATMENT

APPROPRIATE HEALTH CARE

M

• Inpatient—necessary if dehydration, anorexia, disequilibrium, and/or frequent or life-threatening seizures. • Surgical excision—for definitive management; usually successful if the tumor is accessible. Incomplete excision is common, particularly for intracranial meningiomas in dogs, intraspinal meningiomas in cats, and in tumors ventral to the spinal cord.
• Fractionated conventional radiation therapy—15–20 treatments over 3–4 weeks, following incomplete excision, if excision not possible, or if a less invasive approach is desired. When combined with surgery, radiation is associated with prolonged survival time in canine intracranial and intraspinal meningiomas compared to surgery alone, and delays or prevents local recurrence of disease. Given the success of complete surgical excision of intracranial meningiomas in cats, radiation is rarely necessary. Feline intracranial meningiomas are likely radiation sensitive, but data are lacking. It should be considered when surgery is not an option • Stereotactic radiosurgery (SRS)—high dose of radiation delivered to tumor with sub-millimeter accuracy. A steep dose-gradient limits exposure of normal tissue and reduces side effects of radiation. Can be conducted on an outpatient basis in 1–5 treatments delivered on consecutive days. The best candidates are those who are stable or able to be stabilized with steroids prior to the procedure. SRS significantly decreases tumor volume, but occurs slowly. SRS should be distinguished from intensity modulated radiation therapy (IMRT) delivered in 3–5 fractions (hypo-fractionated IMRT), the former being more accurate. • Chemotherapy—may be associated with prolonged survival after incomplete excision, post-radiation, or as sole agent. Hydroxyurea inhibits DNA synthesis, leading to cell death during the S phase of the cell cycle. Hydroxyurea shows effectiveness in humans with intracranial meningiomas and is commonly used in veterinary medicine, but controlled studies are lacking. • Medical management—antiepileptic drugs and corticosteroids are palliative, without effect on the primary disease process. Neither radiation or chemotherapy aid directly in control of edema or of neurologic signs such as seizures.

NURSING CARE

• Fluids—avoid overzealous fluid administration, as this may exacerbate cerebral edema and neurologic deficits. • Use caution with jugular compression during venipuncture or when positioning for surgery to avoid increases in ICP.

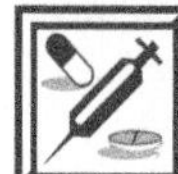

MEDICATIONS

DRUG(S) OF CHOICE

Cerebral Edema

• Corticosteroids—improve neurologic deficits associated with vasogenic edema.
• Stuporous, severely ataxic, or showing signs of herniation—methylprednisolone sodium succinate 30 mg/kg IV or dexamethasone sodium phosphate 0.1 mg/kg IV. • Continued deterioration or no improvement—20% mannitol solution 0.5–1 g/kg IV over 15–20 minutes. Furosemide 2 mg/kg IV acts synergistically with mannitol and can be added if needed. Hypertonic saline 3–5 mL/kg may be used as an alternative or in addition to mannitol. Dexamethasone 0.05–0.1 mg/kg q24h IV.
• Once patient is stable—dexamethasone 0.05–0.1 mg/kg q24h or in divided daily doses PO or prednisone 0.25–0.5 mg/kg PO q12h; then taper to lowest effective dose.

Seizures

• Antiepileptic drugs—mandatory if isolated seizures >1/month, cluster seizures, or status; recommended if any seizure activity in animal with meningioma, and possibly prophylactically in animals with forebrain meningioma.
• Maintenance treatment—phenobarbital (first choice in dogs and cats) 2–3 mg/kg IV or PO q12h; or zonisamide 5–10 mg/kg q12h PO (dogs or cats); or levetiracetam 20–30 mg/kg q8h IV or PO as starting dose; if extended release levetiracetam q12h PO (dogs or cats). • Cluster seizures or status—diazepam 0.25–5 mg/kg/h CRI; or phenobarbital 4 mg/kg IV q2–6h until 12–16 mg/kg total loading dose; or midazolam 0.2–0.4 mg/kg/h CRI; or levetiracetam 60 mg/kg IV.

Chemotherapy

Hydroxyurea—150 mg/kg/week (dogs) and 75 mg/kg/week (cats).

FOLLOW-UP

PATIENT MONITORING

• Mannitol—monitor serum osmolality and electrolytes, particularly with repeated administration. Maintain osmolality at or below 320 mOsm/L to reduce risk of renal failure due to renal vasoconstriction.
• Corticosteroids—perform serial neurologic examinations; marked neurologic improvement is possible within 24–48 hours after initiation of treatment with corticosteroids. • Antiepileptic drugs—evaluate serum phenobarbital levels 3 weeks after initiation of therapy; evaluate liver enzymes every 6 months while on phenobarbital. • Hydroxyurea—monitor CBC with platelet count before starting, at 2 weeks, 6 weeks then CBC, chemistry profile every 3–4 months. May lead to vomiting or diarrhea, stomatitis, sloughing of nails, alopecia, and dysuria; most serious effects are bone marrow depression and pulmonary fibrosis.

EXPECTED COURSE AND PROGNOSIS

Dogs

Intracranial

• Surgical excision—outcome depends on surgical technique. Reported median survival time is 6.7 months (3 dogs). Survival increased with regional cerebral resection (16.5 months in 6 dogs), or with the use of a surgical aspirator (41.8 months in 17 dogs) or with endoscopy-assisted tumor removal (70.1 months with forebrain and 23.4 months with caudal brain meningioma in 33 dogs). • Surgical excision with postoperative fractionated radiation therapy—reported median survival times of 16.5 months–3 years. • Radiation therapy alone—reported median survival times of 5–12.5 months with conventional radiation.
• Chemotherapy using hydroxyurea—reported mean survival time of 7–8 months. • SRS (e.g., Frameless SRS, Varian Trilogy/TruBeam, Cyberknife)—reported mean survival time of 16.4 months in 38 dogs, and 19.8 months in 20 dogs. • Medical management—reported median survival time of 3–4 months in dogs treated with palliative therapy alone.

Intraspinal

• Surgical excision—reported mean survival time of 19 months in 8 dogs. • Surgical excision with postoperative radiation therapy—reported median survival time of 13.5 months in 6 dogs.

Cats

Intracranial

• Surgical excision—good prognosis. Surgery is curative in 75–80% of patients that undergo surgical excision. Reported mean survival time 22–27 months. Seizure activity may persist despite successful excision. Recurrence, if it occurs, is usually in same location. • Medical management—neurologic deficits become more severe with time. Progression is often slow because meningiomas are slow growing.

Intraspinal

• Surgical excision—survival time is shorter than that of cats with cerebral meningiomas: reported median survival times of 14.2 months in 16 cats and 17.3 months in 26 cats. • Corticosteroids—palliative in the short term. Thoracolumbar disease progresses to paralysis and inability to control urination (urinary retention and possibly bladder atony and cystitis).

MISCELLANEOUS

AGE-RELATED FACTORS

Brain tumor should be suspected in dogs and cats >5 years with recent onset of seizures and unremarkable extracranial diagnostic workup for seizures.

ABBREVIATIONS

• CSF = cerebrospinal fluid.
• GI = gastrointestinal.
• ICP = intracranial pressure.
• IMRT = intensity modulated radiation therapy.
• SRS = stereotactic radiosurgery.
• T1WI = T1-weighted images.
• T2WI = T2-weighted images.

Suggested Reading

Dewey CW, da Costa RC. A Practical Guide to Canine and Feline Neurology, 3rd ed. Ames, IA: Wiley-Blackwell, 2016, pp. 183–191.

Larue SM, Gordon IK. Radiation therapy. In: Withrow SJ, Vail DM, Page RL, eds., Withrow and MacEwen's Small Animal Clinical Oncology, 5th ed. St. Louis, MO: W.B. Saunders, 2013, pp. 180–197.

Motta L, Mandara MT, Skerritt GC. Canine and feline intracranial meningiomas: an updated review. Vet J 2012, 192(2):153–165.

Petersen SA, Sturges BK, Dickinson PJ, et al. Canine intraspinal meningiomas: imaging features, histopathologic classification, and long-term outcome in 34 dogs. J Vet Intern Med 2008, 22:946–953.

Sessums K, Mariani C. Intracranial meningioma in dogs and cats: a comparative review. Compend Cont Educ Vet 2009, 7:330–339.

Authors Richard J. Joseph and Anne E. Buglione

MENINGITIS/MENINGOENCEPHALITIS/MENINGOMYELITIS, BACTERIAL

BASICS

DEFINITION

- Meningitis—inflammation of the meninges.
- Meningoencephalitis—inflammation of the meninges and brain.
- Meningomyelitis—inflammation of the meninges and spinal cord.

PATHOPHYSIOLOGY

- Bacterial infection of the CNS can occur by direct extension from an infected extraneural site or when bacteria are introduced by penetrating trauma or a migrating foreign body.
- Hematogenous spread of bacteria to the CNS from mucous membrane colonization or a distant pyogenic focus can occur. This is the most common cause in septicemic neonates and immunocompromised patients.
- Neurological deficits often develop from secondary inflammation but may be from bacterial invasion of the brain or spinal cord parenchyma.
- Inflammatory debris and adhesions can obstruct cerebrospinal fluid (CSF) flow, leading to secondary hydrocephalus.

M

SYSTEMS AFFECTED

- Nervous—meninges, brain, or spinal cord.
- Multisystemic signs—may be present when the infection originates in an extraneural site or when the systemic inflammatory response is severe.

INCIDENCE/PREVALENCE

Rare

SIGNALMENT

Species

Dog and cat.

Mean Age and Range

Any age.

Predominant Sex

Males and females affected equally.

SIGNS

General Comments

- Patients are often systemically ill.
- Shock, hypotension, and disseminated intravascular coagulation (DIC) are often found in septicemic patients.
- CNS signs may be profound and rapidly progressive.

Physical Examination Findings

- Pyrexia in approximately 50%.
- Cervical rigidity and hyperesthesia—especially with meningitis.
- Neurologic deficits—reflect the location of the involved spinal cord or brain parenchyma (e.g., altered mentation, cranial nerve deficits, postural reaction deficits, ataxia, paresis, seizures).
- May find an extraneural site of underlying bacterial infection.
- Vomiting.
- Bradycardia with systemic hypertension suggests increased intracranial pressure.

CAUSES

- Meningoencephalitis—can be secondary to local extension from otitis media/interna or infection of the eye, retrobulbar space, sinuses, or nasal passages or due to direct inoculation by traumatic skull fractures or migrating foreign bodies.
- Meningomyelitis—can be secondary to discospondylitis or vertebral osteomyelitis.
- Hematogenous spread of bacterial infection to the CNS can occur in neonates with omphalophlebitis, immunocompromised patients, or in dogs with bacterial endocarditis, prostatitis, discospondylitis, pneumonia, urinary tract infections or severe gastroenteritis.
- The point of origin is not always found.

RISK FACTORS

- Untreated bacterial infection.
- Immunocompromised state.
- Injury involving the CNS or adjacent structures.

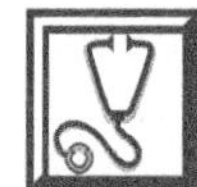

DIAGNOSIS

DIFFERENTIAL DIAGNOSIS

Infectious Meningitis (Nonbacterial)

- Canine distemper, toxoplasmosis, neosporosis, cryptococcosis, blastomycosis, rickettsial organisms, West Nile virus, and feline infectious peritonitis all cause meningitis/meningoencephalitis that can be difficult to distinguish from bacterial disease.
- CSF—inflammatory with a variable lymphocytic, mixed mononuclear or neutrophilic pleocytosis depending on the specific infectious etiology.
- Antemortem diagnosis suspected based on typical clinical findings and identification of affected extraneural sites.
- Diagnosis is by identifying organisms in the CSF or in extraneural sites (using cytology, culture, or PCR) and by serology.

Steroid-Responsive Meningitis–Arteritis (Aseptic Meningitis)

- Observed mainly in young (6–19 months) adult large-breed dogs.
- Beagles, boxers, Bernese mountain dogs, German shorthaired pointers, Weimaraners, and Nova Scotia duck tolling retrievers are predisposed; any breed can be affected.
- Cervical pain without neurologic deficits is most common.
- Fever occurs in 60–80% of affected dogs. Signs may wax and wane initially.
- Affected dogs are systemically normal.
- CSF—increased nucleated cell count and protein. Neutrophilic pleocytosis in acute cases, mononuclear cells may predominate in chronic cases. Negative bacterial culture.
- Serum and CSF IgA increased.
- Dramatic response to corticosteroid administration.

Meningoencephalitis of Unknown Origin (MUO)

- Idiopathic noninfectious inflammatory diseases of the brain, spinal cord, and meninges in dogs including granulomatous meningoencephalomyelitis (GME), necrotizing meningoencephalitis (NME), and necrotizing leukoencephalitis (NLE). A definitive diagnosis requires histopathology.
- Young adult (3–7 years), female, small-breed dogs are most commonly affected.
- Neurologic abnormalities reflect the location of the lesion(s).
- MRI—usually multifocal parenchymal lesions with variable contrast enhancement.
- CSF— pleocytosis with >50% mononuclear cells and increased protein concentrations.
- CSF culture—negative.

Primary CNS Neoplasia

- History protracted; neurologic signs limited to the CNS; standard laboratory tests normal.
- Diagnosis by CT, MRI, CSF analysis, and biopsy.

CBC/BIOCHEMISTRY/URINALYSIS

- Leukocytosis is common; left-shift or toxicity may be seen. Thrombocytopenia may be present in septicemic patients.
- Biochemical changes are variable and often nonspecific.
- Pyuria and bacteriuria occur in patients with underlying urinary tract or prostatic infection and in some bacteremic animals.

OTHER LABORATORY TESTS

- Serologic tests—may differentiate bacterial from other infectious diseases; in cats, toxoplasma titer may be positive without clinical disease.
- Cytology of infected tissues—skin, eyes, nasal discharge, lymph node, tracheal wash; helps identify nonbacterial causative organisms, especially in patients with fungal disease.
- Blood culture—positive in 30% of dogs with bacterial meningitis.

IMAGING

- Thorax radiography and abdominal ultrasound—to identify underlying infection or other significant disease.
- Vertebral column radiography—discospondylitis may be identified as a focus of infection.
- Head CT—may identify infected sinus, nasal cavity, or middle and inner ear as initiating site. Inflamed regions of brain parenchyma and meninges usually enhance with contrast.

- Echocardiography—performed when valvular endocarditis suspected based on murmur/arrhythmia.
- MRI with contrast—documents brain, spinal cord and meningeal inflammation and can identify extraneural sites of infection (sinus, nasal, ear).

DIAGNOSTIC PROCEDURES

CSF Analysis

- Collection—a concern in animals with altered mentation suggesting high intracranial pressure, because the procedure may precipitate brain herniation. Pretreat with mannitol.
- Analysis—neutrophilic pleocytosis with high protein concentration; neutrophils may appear toxic or degenerated and intracellular bacteria are occasionally seen; often difficult to differentiate aseptic from bacterial meningitis cytologically.
- Culture—aerobic or anaerobic; may be positive (<40%)—inoculation of CSF into broth enrichment media improves diagnostic yield.
- Universal bacterial PCR assay of CSF can be used to identify DNA from causative organisms when bacterial culture is negative.

PATHOLOGIC FINDINGS

- May note subdural empyema, or purulent material on the surface of the brain or spinal cord.
- Asymmetric diffuse or multifocal brain or spinal cord and meningeal suppurative inflammation common.
- Culture of affected neurologic tissue—positive in >75% of patients.

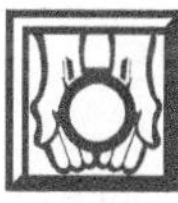

TREATMENT

APPROPRIATE HEALTH CARE

Inpatient—treat aggressively; intensive care monitoring often necessary.

NURSING CARE

Fluid therapy and supportive care.

CLIENT EDUCATION

Inform client that rapid and aggressive treatment is important and that the prognosis for recovery is guarded.

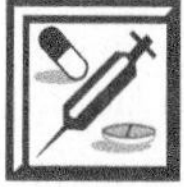

MEDICATIONS

DRUG(S) OF CHOICE

Antibiotics

- Bactericidal agents that achieve therapeutic concentrations within CSF are most desirable—lipid-soluble drugs with small molecular size, low protein binding, and a low degree of ionization at physiologic pH recommended.
- Cultures—CSF, blood, urine, primary site; determine drug sensitivity; until cultures identify the organism choose a broad-spectrum agent that penetrates the blood–brain barrier (BBB).
- Recommended drugs include third-generation cephalosporins (moxalactam, ceftriaxone, cefotaxime), fluoroquinolones, trimethoprim-sulfonamides, doxycycline and metronidazole.
- Penicillin, ampicillin, amoxicillin-clavulanate, and carbapenems enter the CNS when there is inflammation and are a good choice to use in combination with another antibiotic that will continue to cross the BBB as inflammation resolves, such as trimethoprim-sulfonamides. Ampicillin may achieve high CSF concentrations even without inflammation.
- Metronidazole reaches high levels in CSF, brain parenchyma, and abscesses and demonstrates the best bactericidal activity against anaerobes.
- Clindamycin is lipid soluble but does not readily cross the BBB. Concentrations in brain and spinal cord are adequate for treatment of *Toxoplasma* and *Neospora* infections but insufficient for treating most CNS bacterial infections.
- Administer antibiotics intravenously for 3–5 days to achieve high CSF concentrations rapidly, then maintain on oral therapy.
- Immediate IV therapy can be based on cytology; penicillin for Gram-positive infections, fluoroquinolone or third-generation cephalosporin for Gram-negative infections.

Antiepileptic Drugs

- Indicated for seizures.
- Long-term use may be needed.

Corticosteroids

- Most CNS dysfunction is due to inflammation.
- May administer dexamethasone 0.1 mg/kg q24h for several days but use is somewhat controversial.

CONTRAINDICATIONS

Aminoglycosides and first-generation cephalosporins—do not penetrate the BBB even in the presence of inflamed meninges.

FOLLOW-UP

PATIENT MONITORING

Monitor for nervous system signs, fever, leukocytosis, and systemic signs.

PREVENTION/AVOIDANCE

Treat local infections adjacent to the CNS (e.g., infections of the eyes, ears, sinuses, nose, and vertebral column) early and aggressively to prevent extension to the CNS.

POSSIBLE COMPLICATIONS

Damage to the brain and spinal cord may be irreversible.

EXPECTED COURSE AND PROGNOSIS

- Response to antibiotics—variable; prognosis guarded.
- Many patients die despite treatment
- Residual neurologic deficits are possible.
- Treatment for at least 4 weeks after resolution of all signs is recommended.

MISCELLANEOUS

M

SEE ALSO

- Encephalitis.
- Meningoencephalomyelitis of Unknown Etiology (MUE).
- Steroid-Responsive Meningitis–Arteritis—Dogs.

ABBREVIATIONS

- BBB = blood–brain barrier.
- CSF = cerebrospinal fluid.
- DIC = disseminated intravascular coagulation.
- GME = granulomatous meningoencephalomyelitis.
- NLE = necrotizing leukoencephalitis.
- NME = necrotizing meningoencephalitis.

Suggested Reading

Greene CE. Bacterial meningits. In: Sykes JE, ed., Canine and Feline Infectious Diseases. St. Louis, MO: Saunders Elsevier, 2014, pp. 886–892.

Radaelli ST, Platt SR. Bacterial menigoencephalomyelitis in dogs: a retrospective study in 23 cases (1990–1999). J Vet Intern Med 2002, 16:159–163.

Tipold A, Stein VM. Inflammatory diseases of the spine in small animals. Vet Clin Small Anim 2010, 40:871–879.

Authors Danielle Zwueste and Susan M. Taylor

MENINGOENCEPHALOMYELITIS, EOSINOPHILIC

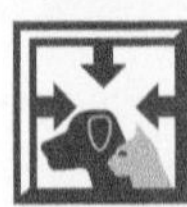

BASICS

OVERVIEW

Although eosinophilic meningoencephalomyelitis (EME) can be associated with meningitis, encephalitis, and myelitis as a result of CNS infection or parasitic migration, in most cases, no underlying cause can be found. Idiopathic EME occurs in young to middle-aged large-breed dogs and resolves in many cases following steroid treatment.

SIGNALMENT

• Dog and rarely cat. • Idiopathic EME—often larger dogs (>25 kg); Rottweilers and golden retrievers predisposed. • Mean age—4 years (2 months–13 years).

M

SIGNS

• Vary with CNS location and severity.
• Neurologic deficits—most frequently associated with cranium, infrequently with spinal cord and rarely with cranial nerve involvement.

CAUSES & RISK FACTORS

• Idiopathic EME (unknown cause)—majority of reported cases. • Infectious—*Dirofilaria immitis* and cuterebra myiasis in cats; *Toxoplasma gondii, Neospora* spp., *Prototheca* spp., *Cryptococcus* spp., and nematode migration with *Baylisascaris procyonis* in dogs. • *Angiostrongylus*—dogs in Australia. • Intervertebral disc disease probably as allergic response to disc material.

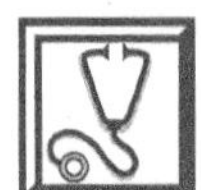

DIAGNOSIS

DIFFERENTIAL DIAGNOSIS

• Cannot be differentiated from other encephalitides solely on clinical signs; CSF analysis must be done. • Idiopathic EME—negative serologic test results; marked CSF eosinophilic pleocytosis (20–95%); usually steroid-responsive. • Infectious diseases—identified on presence of systemic signs, blood work, fecal sample, CSF, serum/CSF serology, and imaging.

CBC/BIOCHEMISTRY/URINALYSIS

• Peripheral eosinophilia—may or may not be present. • Biochemistry and urinalysis—usually normal with idiopathic disease; eosinophilia, liver enzyme activity, and creatine kinase may be elevated in infectious diseases.

OTHER LABORATORY TESTS

• Serology—to rule out suspected infectious diseases. • Fecal flotation and sedimentation—to rule out migratory parasite.

IMAGING

• Thoracic radiography and abdominal ultrasound—to rule out systemic involvement.
• MRI—variable; focal mass lesions, diffuse parenchymal abnormalities, postcontrast diffuse meningeal enhancement; abnormalities depend on cause and location of lesion.

DIAGNOSTIC PROCEDURES

CSF Analysis

• Eosinophilic pleocytosis significant when >10%. • Presence of eosinophilic pleocytosis by itself cannot differentiate idiopathic EME from infection causing CSF eosinophilic pleocytosis.
• Idiopathic EME—total nucleated cell count 4–3880 cells/μL (median 99 cells/mL; reference <0.003) with 22–95% eosinophils.
• Infections—62–4740 cells/mL (median 875 cells/mL) with 30–95% eosinophils.

CSF Serologic Testing

• If CSF eosinophils >10%, look for parasitic and fungal disease. • Test for heartworm, *Neospora caninum, Toxoplasma gondii*, and *Cryptococcus neoformans*.

PATHOLOGIC FINDINGS

• CSF eosinophilic pleocytosis does not necessarily correlate with eosinophils observed in CNS parenchyma. • Wide variety of pathologic findings may indicate multiple causes, or the same disease taken at different times.

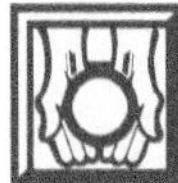

TREATMENT

• Usually inpatient, because of severity of clinical signs. • Activity—as tolerated. • Regular diet.

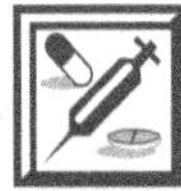

MEDICATIONS

DRUG(S) OF CHOICE

• Idiopathic disease—steroid administration; dexamethasone (0.2 mg/kg q24h for 1 day; then 0.15 mg/kg q24h for 6 days); follow with prednisone (0.5 mg/kg q24h for 8 weeks); then slowly wean patient off prednisone over 8 weeks–6 months depending on clinical response.
• Protozoal disease—clindamycin, sulfonamides, and pyrimethamine. • Heartworm—microfilarial migration to the CNS is rare; no available treatment other than supportive.

CONTRAINDICATIONS/POSSIBLE INTERACTIONS

• Important to differentiate idiopathic EME from infection as treatment greatly differs—immunosuppressive dose of steroids vs. anti-organism treatment. • Steroid should be used with caution if diagnosis has not been substantiated.

FOLLOW-UP

PATIENT MONITORING

Inpatient—repeat neurologic examination every 6 hours to monitor progress.

PREVENTION/AVOIDANCE

Steroid treatment should not be stopped even if the animal is back to normal within a few days. A minimum of 8 weeks followed by tapering of the medication over as many weeks is mandatory.

POSSIBLE COMPLICATIONS

• Recurrence may occur following cessation of medication. • Ensure treatment dosage is adequate and reinstate for a longer period.

EXPECTED COURSE AND PROGNOSIS

• Idiopathic disease—good prognosis in most cases with early treatment; improvement usually seen in the first 72 hours; full recovery in 2–6 months. Some patients continue to deteriorate despite steroids, and die.
• Protozoal and fungal diseases—poor-to-grave prognosis. • Larval migration—prognosis guarded to poor and depends on location of the lesion; signs may resolve, but larvae often continue to migrate and death may ensue. • Degradation of eosinophils is toxic to nervous tissue; patient may have permanent deficits from not only the primary disease but also cell death.

MISCELLANEOUS

AGE-RELATED FACTORS

Idiopathic EME is more frequent in young to middle-aged larger dog breeds (>25 kg).

SEE ALSO

Encephalitis

ABBREVIATIONS

• EME = eosinophilic meningoencephomyelitis.

Suggested Reading

Cardy TJA, Cornelis I. Clinical presentation and magnetic resonance imaging findings in 11 dogs with eosinophilic meningoencephalitis of unknown aetiology. J Small Anim Pract. 2018, 59(7):422–431.

Williams JH, Köster LS, Naidoo V, et al. Review of idiopathic eosinophilic meningitis in dogs and cats, with a detailed description of two recent cases in dogs. J S Afr Vet Assoc 2008, 79(4):194–204.

Windsor RC, Sturges BK, Vernau KM, et al. Cerebrospinal fluid eosinophilia in dogs. J Vet Intern Med 2009, 23(2):275–281.

Author Joane M. Parent

Meningoencephalomyelitis of Unknown Etiology (MUE)

BASICS

DEFINITION

Meningoencephalomyelitis of unknown etiology (MUE) is a broad term used to describe inflammatory disorders that affect the CNS focally, diffusely, or multifocally. In the past, the majority of CNS inflammatory disorders were categorized as granulomatous meningoencephalomyelitis (GME). As a result, multiple less serious viral and idiopathic disorders were frequently erroneously diagnosed as GME. The appropriate clinical term to describe cases in which CNS inflammation is suspected is now considered MUE or meningioencephalitis of unknown etiology (MUO).

PATHOPHYSIOLOGY

• Unknown. Although a specific etiologic agent is not recognized, in the majority of cases, viral and immune causes are strongly suspected. • Three clinicopathologic forms are recognized: ocular, multifocal (brain or brain and spinal cord), and focal (single focus in the brain or spinal cord).

SYSTEMS AFFECTED

• Nervous. • Ophthalmic.

GENETICS

Not proven.

INCIDENCE/PREVALENCE

Unknown. Since brain biopsies are rarely obtained, a presumptive diagnosis is made in most cases.

GEOGRAPHIC DISTRIBUTION

Worldwide

SIGNALMENT

Breed Predilections

Any breed can develop MUE. Smaller toy breeds may be overrepresented and can be less responsive to therapy. However, the condition also occurs in medium and large-breed dogs.

Mean Age and Range

• Mean—5 years. • Range—6 months–10 years.

Predominant Sex

Slightly higher prevalence in females.

SIGNS

• Depend on the form of the disease and neuroanatomic localization. • Cerebral form—frequently results in seizure activity. • Ocular form—acute onset of blindness with dilated, unresponsive pupils. • Focal form—*cerebral lesion*: disorientation, behavioral changes, seizures, cortical blindness, compulsive circling, head pressing; *brainstem lesion*: somnolence, cranial nerve deficits (most commonly facial and vestibular dysfunction), ipsilateral hemiparesis; *spinal cord*: neck pain, tetraparesis (C1–C5 or C6–T2 lesions) or paraparesis (T3–L3 or L4–S2 lesions) and proprioceptive ataxia. In some patients the clinical signs can be unspecific and vague, delaying a prompt diagnosis and timely therapy.

CAUSES

Unknown

RISK FACTORS

• Unknown. • Some dogs develop clinical signs within 5–15 days of vaccination.

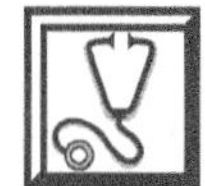

DIAGNOSIS

DIFFERENTIAL DIAGNOSIS

• The combination of history, neurologic examination, CSF analysis, and MRI results usually lead to a presumptive diagnosis of inflammatory disease, but defining the cause of the inflammation can be problematic. • It is possible that some dogs surviving inflammatory CNS disease have lesions compatible with GME, but post-mortem studies are not available to prove it. Alternatively, dogs who survive CNS inflammatory disease could have been suffering from other type of less serious viral or idiopathic inflammatory disease. Therefore the current accepted medical term to group these categories is MUE. • Infectious inflammatory diseases—viral (distemper virus, other viruses); fungal (*Blastomyces dermatitidis*, *Coccidioides* spp., *Cryptococcus neoformans*); rickettsial (*Rickettsia rickettsii*); bacterial (*Ehrlichia* spp., *E. coli*, *Streptococcus*); protozoal (*Neospora caninum*, *Toxoplasma gondii*). • Other inflammatory disease—necrotizing encephalitis of the Yorkshire terrier, Maltese, and pug; immune-mediated steroid-responsive meningitis (beagles, Bernese mountain dogs, Nova Scotia duck tolling retrievers, Weimaraners, boxers). • Sudden acquired retinal degeneration. • Brain tumor—meningioma, glioma, choroids plexus papilloma, lymphoma. • Subatlantoaxial luxation. • Caudo-occipital malformation syndrome (COMS).

CBC/BIOCHEMISTRY/URINALYSIS

Usually normal.

OTHER LABORATORY TESTS

Serologic testing to rule out infectious CNS diseases.

IMAGING

MRI—method of choice; abnormalities are variable and consist of solitary, multiple, or circumscribed mass lesions. Multiple areas of heterogeneous contrast enhancement are frequent in the multifocal form of the disease. Other findings include mass effect with midline shift, obstructive hydrocephalus, white matter edema, and effacement of the sulci. Usually MRI lesions are characterized as hypointense in T1-weighted and hyperintense in T2-weighted images. Necrotic lesions are recognized by a center of hypointensity with a peripheral ring of enhancement.

DIAGNOSTIC PROCEDURES

CSF Analysis

• Reference range—white cell count (0–3 cells/μL); protein concentration (0–30 mg/dL). • Helps confirm presence of inflammatory disease but rarely demonstrates a definitive cause. The following are only guidelines, as significant overlap exists regarding CSF cytology of different inflammatory disorders. • Inflammatory diseases—white cell count and protein concentration usually increased. Even with a normal cell count, presence of an abnormal cell population (e.g., macrophages) should be taken into consideration as evidence of pathology. • Usually, mononuclear pleocytosis; however, polymorphonuclear pleocytosis, or a normal CSF can be present. • Bacterial (rare in dogs)—marked polymorphonuclear pleocytosis. • Fungal, protozoal infections—mixed pleocytosis (mononuclear and polymorphonuclear); rarely a fungal organism (*Cryptococcus neoformans* or *Blastomyces dermatitidis*) is identified. • Viral infections—mononuclear pleocytosis.

Brain Biopsy

Brain biopsy is the only procedure that can confirm conclusively a diagnosis of MUE. Due to morbidity, mortality, and cost associated with brain biopsy the test is not performed routinely. It is important to note that GME is *not* a clinical diagnosis but a term to describe findings at post-mortem. The term should not be used as clinical diagnosis, to avoid confusion.

PATHOLOGIC FINDINGS

• Hallmark feature—dense perivascular distribution of mononuclear infiltrates (lymphocytes, monocytes, and plasma cells). • Macroscopically, discoloration and softening of affected tissue sometimes evident.

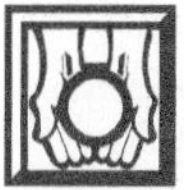

TREATMENT

APPROPRIATE HEALTH CARE

• Stable patients can be discharged with recommended treatment. • Inpatient—for severely affected dogs; monitor patient closely for progression of neurologic deficits. • In severe cases, sequential assessment of pupil size and reaction to light, and mentation are helpful to determine risk of herniation.

NURSING CARE

• IV fluids for the anorexic patient. Take care not to overhydrate to exacerbate cerebral edema. • Provide a padded cage for dogs with vestibular ataxia, severe dementia, or seizure

MENINGOENCEPHALOMYELITIS OF UNKNOWN ETIOLOGY (MUE) (CONTINUED)

activity. • Recumbent patients should be turned frequently (every 4 hours).

ACTIVITY

• Depends on severity of disease and lesion localization. • Ataxic patients should be confined to a padded cage to avoid injury.

DIET

Ensure adequate caloric intake.

CLIENT EDUCATION

• Explain to the client that there is significant overlap of clinical signs among different inflammatory diseases. Insist on the importance of a diagnostic workup.
• Mortality rate is variable but clearly biased by older literature describing the severe cases that went to post-mortem as suffering from GME. Brain biopsies are rarely conducted. Clinical experience suggests that up to 70% of patients can respond to therapy, especially if initiated early in the course of the disease. However, treatment may be prolonged or could be required for life. • Corticosteroid therapy may be necessary indefinitely.

M

MEDICATIONS

DRUG(S) OF CHOICE

• Dexamethasone 0.2 mg/kg IV or PO q24h for 4 days followed by prednisone 0.5–1.0 mg/kg PO q24h for 2 weeks. Dose is adjusted according to response and side effects. The goal is to find dosage that keeps the clinical signs controlled with minimal side effects. If deterioration of clinical signs noted when tapering steroids, immediately go back to previous dose that controlled the signs or consider adding other immunosuppressant listed below. • To prevent gastrointestinal ulceration, combine steroid therapy with omeprazole 0.5 mg/kg PO q24h, famotidine 0.5–1 mg/kg IV or PO q12h. • Azathioprine 2 mg/kg PO q24h can be added if the patient is not tolerating the steroids well, to allow reduction of the prednisone dose. Usually, the dose of azathioprine is reduced to 1 mg/kg PO q 24 after 7 days of initiating the medication.
• Cytosine arabinoside 100 mg/m^2 body surface area as a CRI over 12 hours. Alternatively 6 doses of cytosine arabinoside can be given q12h via SC injection. Repeat treatment every 3 weeks to 8 weeks pending clinical response. • Mycophenolate mofetil has been recently advocated at a dose of 7–20 mg/kg PO q12h for 3–4 weeks, then 10 mg/kg q24h. This medication can cause vomiting and diarrhea. • If there is seizure activity—phenobarbital 2 mg/kg PO q12h, levetiracetam 20–30 mg/kg PO (ideally q8h but may be attempted q12h), or zonisamide 5–10 mg/kg PO q12h. • Gabapentin 2–5 mg/kg PO q8–12h if compulsive circling is present.

CONTRAINDICATIONS

• Fungal, bacterial, and protozoal conditions can be exacerbated by the use of steroids. It is important to rule out these infectious disorders with proper diagnostic workup.
• Steroid should not be used in a patient treated or recently treated with nonsteroidal anti-inflammatory drugs (NSAIDs).

PRECAUTIONS

Reduction in corticosteroid therapy can result in recrudescence of clinical signs that may not be controlled again as initially.

ALTERNATIVE DRUG(S)

• Cyclosporine 3–7 mg/kg PO q12h.
• Leflunomide 4 mg/kg PO q24h.

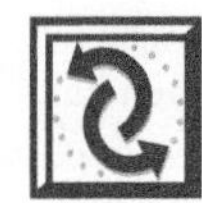

FOLLOW-UP

PATIENT MONITORING

• Repeat neurologic examination periodically (every 2–4 weeks). • Evaluate CBC and biochemical profile regularly to monitor for leukopenia, thrombocytopenia, and liver and kidney function if alternative drugs are used.
• Monitor urine in patients on long-term steroid treatment—proteinuria or infection are frequent consequences. Patients receiving zonisamide may be at risk for keratoconjunctivitis sicca and immune-mediated conditions—hemolytic anemia, immune thrombocytopenia, and polyarthritis.

POSSIBLE COMPLICATIONS

• Deterioration of clinical signs despite aggressive treatment. • Status epilepticus, dementia, brain herniation, and death.

EXPECTED COURSE AND PROGNOSIS

• Not all patients with CNS inflammatory disease have a poor prognosis. • GME has been stereotyped as fatal without enough evidence. Uncertain if surviving dogs had GME as brain biopsies are rarely done.

MISCELLANEOUS

PREGNANCY/FERTILITY/BREEDING

Corticosteroid therapy can affect gestation.

SYNONYMS

• Granulomatous encephalitis.
• Granulomatous meningoencephalitis.
• Meningoencephalitis of unknown etiology.
• Meningomyelitis. • Encephalitis. • Myelitis.

SEE ALSO

• Encephalitis. • Encephalitis Secondary to Parasitic Migration. • Meningitis/Meningoencephalitis/Meningomyelitis, Bacterial. • Meningoencephalomyelitis, Eosinophilic. • Necrotizing Encephalitis.
• Steroid-Responsive Meningitis–Arteritis—Dogs.

ABBREVIATIONS

• COMS = caudo-occipital malformation syndrome. • GME = granulomatous meningoencephalomyelitis. • MUE = meningoencephalomyelitis of unknown etiology. • MUO = meningoencephalomyelitis of unknown origin. • NSAID = nonsteroidal anti-inflammatory drug.

INTERNET RESOURCES

• http://www.ivis.org • http://www.vin.com

Suggested Reading

Adamo PF, Rylaner H, Adams WM. Cyclosporine use in multi-drug therapy for meningoencephalomyelitis of unknown etiology in dogs. J Small Anim Pract 2007, 48(9):486–496.

Coates JR, Jeffery ND. Perspectives on meningoencephalomyelitis of unknown origin. Vet Clin North Am Small Anim Pract 2014, 44:1157–1185.

Demierre S, Tipold A, Griot-Wenk ME, et al. Correlation between the clinical course of granulomatous meningoencephalomyelitis in dogs and the extent of mast cell infiltration. Vet Record 2001, 148:467–472.

Granger N, Smith PM, Jeffery ND. Clinical findings and treatment of non-infectious meningoencephalomyelitis in dogs: a systematic review of 457 published cases from 1962 to 2008. Vet J 2010, 184(3):290–297.

Lowrie M, Thomson S, Smith P, Garosi L. Effect of a constant rate infusion of cytosine arabinoside on mortality in dogs with meningoencephalitis of unknown origin. Vet J 2016, 213:1–5.

Smith PM, Stalin CE, Shaw D, et al. Comparison of two regimens for the treatment of meningoencephalomyelitis of unknown etiology. J Vet Intern Med 2009, 23(3):520–526.

Talarico LR, Schatzberg SJ. Idiopathic granulomatous and necrotizing inflammatory disorders of the canine central nervous system: a review and future perspectives. J Small Anim Pract 2010, 51(3):138–149.

Woolcock AD, Wang A, Haley A, et al. Treatment of canine meningoencephalomyelitis of unknown aetiology with mycophenolate mofetil and corticosteroids: 25 cases (2007–2012). Vet Med Sci 2016, 10(2):125–135.

Author Carolina Duque

Client Education Handout available online

BASICS

OVERVIEW

- Rare tumor in dogs and cats arising from the mesothelial cells of the serosal lining of the pleural, pericardial, or peritoneal cavities.
- Also has been reported in dogs to arise from the tunica vaginalis of the testes.

SIGNALMENT

- Older animals—dog and cat.
- Sclerosing subtype more common in males.
- German shepherd dogs overrepresented.

SIGNS

- Pleural effusion—dyspnea, tachypnea, exercise intolerance, coughing, gagging, cyanosis.
- Pericardial effusion—lethargy, anorexia, weakness, collapse, respiratory distress, exercise intolerance, distended abdomen, vomiting.
- Ascites—distended abdomen, anorexia, vomiting, lethargy, abdominal discomfort.
- Swollen testes.
- Sclerosing subtype signs are secondary to restriction around affected organs—vomiting, urinary issues.

CAUSES & RISK FACTORS

- Increased risk with asbestos exposure.
- Possible increased risk in golden retrievers with idiopathic hemorrhagic pericardial effusion.

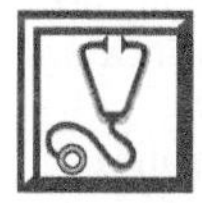

DIAGNOSIS

DIFFERENTIAL DIAGNOSIS

Other causes of effusions—hypoproteinemia, vasculitis, neoplasia (e.g., lymphoma, chemodectomas, hemangiosarcoma, carcinomatosis), idiopathic, congestive heart failure, liver disease, infectious/inflammatory.

CBC/BIOCHEMISTRY/URINALYSIS

N/A

IMAGING

- Thoracic radiography—identification of pleural effusion, evaluation of cardiac silhouette (i.e., globoid heart consistent with pericardial effusion).
- Echocardiography—identification of pericardial effusion; rule out primary cardiac neoplasia.
- Thoracic and abdominal ultrasonography—evaluation of effusions.
- CT—identification of mass lesions and evaluation of lungs in the face of pleural effusion.

DIAGNOSTIC PROCEDURES

- Cytology of effusions to rule out infectious causes or lymphoma—difficult to diagnose mesothelioma on cytology as mesothelial cells are typically shed into effusions and can be highly reactive.
- Exploratory surgery (open or via thoracoscopic or laparoscopic examination) with biopsies.
- Fibronectin levels in effusions—not specific for mesothelioma but typically elevated in neoplastic effusions.

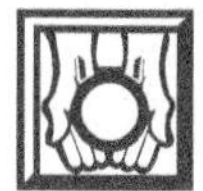

TREATMENT

- Pericardiectomy or mass removal if possible.
- Symptomatic pericardiocentesis or thoracocentesis.

MEDICATIONS

DRUG(S) OF CHOICE

- Intracavitary chemotherapy:
  - Cisplatin (dog only) 50–70 mg/m^2 every 3 weeks with saline diuresis.
  - Carboplatin (cat) 180–200 mg/m^2 every 3–4 weeks.
  - Carboplatin (dog) 300 mg/m^2 every 3 weeks.
  - Mitoxantrone (dog) 5.0–5.5 mg/m^2 every 3 weeks.
- IV chemotherapy—doxorubicin 30 mg/m^2 (dog >10 kg) or 1 mg/kg (dog <10 kg or cat), or mitoxantrone (4.5–5.5 mg/m^2 dog and cat) once every 3 weeks.

CONTRAINDICATIONS/POSSIBLE INTERACTIONS

- Chemotherapy can cause gastrointestinal, bone marrow, cardiac, and other toxicities—seek advice if unfamiliar with cytotoxic drugs.
- Cisplatin in particular is nephrotoxic. Do not use in cats; causes fatal pulmonary edema.

FOLLOW-UP

PATIENT MONITORING

- Blood tests—especially CBC to monitor for bone marrow suppression secondary to chemotherapy and renal values to monitor for renal toxicity if treating with cisplatin.
- Serial thoracic radiography and/or ultrasounds of heart, thoracic cavity, or abdominal cavity to monitor for recurrence of effusions and to monitor tumor response.

EXPECTED COURSE AND PROGNOSIS

- Prognosis—variable and anecdotal:
  - Intracavitary cisplatin (dogs)—range 8 months to >3 years.
  - Intracavitary carboplatin (cats) with piroxicam—6 months.
  - Surgery and intracavitary cisplatin and IV doxorubicin—>27 months.
  - Reported survival with surgery alone—4–9 months.

MISCELLANEOUS

It is not recommended to breed animals with cancer. Chemotherapy is teratogenic—do not give to pregnant animals.

Suggested Reading

Garrett LD. Mesothelioma. In: Withrow SJ, Vail DM, Page RL, eds., Small Animal Clinical Oncology, 5th ed. Philadelphia, PA: Saunders, 2013, pp. 696–700.

Author Rebecca G. Newman

Consulting Editor Timothy M. Fan

M

METABOLIC, NUTRITIONAL, AND ENDOCRINE BONE DISORDERS

BASICS

DEFINITION

• Osteochoendrodysplasia, osteogenesis imperfecta (OI), and growth hormone (GH) anomalies include many metabolic, nutritional, and endocrine bone disorders. • Osteochondrodysplasia (OCDP) is a growth and developmental abnormality resulting in the lack of normal bone growth and bone deformities. • OI is a hereditary disease characterized by extremely fragile bones and teeth caused by defects in the structure of type I collagen. • GH anomalies include, among others: ○ Acromegaly (ACM)—results from excessive pituitary GH production or excessive production of female sex GH. ○ Dwarfism (DW)—results from congenital lack of pituitary GH production.

M

PATHOPHYSIOLOGY

• OCDP—genetic defect affecting all cartilage in the entire body. • OI—genetic defect of type I collagen formation. Type I collagen is the most abundant structural component of skin, bone, cartilage, tendons, and ligaments. • ACM—endogenous progesterone or exogenous progestins may give rise to GH hypersecretion of mammary origin. Mammary-derived (with or without mammary tumors) GH is biochemically identical to pituitary GH. Pituitary adenoma-related increased progesterone production is also possible. Hypothyroidism can also lead to ACM. • DW—congenital GH deficiency.

SYSTEMS AFFECTED

• Cardiovascular. • Endocrine/metabolic. • Musculoskeletal. • Respiratory. • Skin/exocrine.

GENETICS

• OCDP—autosomal dominant inheritance. • OI—autosomal recessive; collagen type I-encoding genes *COL1A1* and *COL1A2* are affected. • ACM—abnormalities in the anterior pituitary gland; inherited in the Saint Bernard. • DW—autosomal recessive inheritance.

INCIDENCE/PREVALENCE

All conditions discussed are rare.

GEOGRAPHIC DISTRIBUTION

N/A

SIGNALMENT

Species

• OCDP, ACM—dog and cat. • OI—dog; rare in cat. • DW—dog.

Breed Predilections

• OCPD—Scottish fold cat; great Pyrenees, Alaskan Malamute, Samoyed, Scottish deerhound, Labrador retriever, basset hound, and Norwegian elkhound. • OI—golden retriever, collie, poodle, beagle, Bedlington terrier, wirehaired dachshund, Norwegian elkhound; domestic shorthair cats. • ACM—Saint Bernard, cats. • DW—German shepherd dogs.

Mean Age and Range

• OCDP—immature animals. • OI—3–18 weeks. • ACM—middle-aged to elderly females. • DW—2–5 months.

Predominant Sex

• OCPD—N/A. • OI—N/A. • ACM—dogs: female; cats: male or female.

SIGNS

• OCDP—short, thickened, and hard, movable tail; short, buckled legs. Severity of the clinical signs most likely influenced by level of expression of dominant gene carrier of the mutation (homo- or heterozygous). • OI—signs range from perinatal death to mild bone fragility, severe bone deformity, and innumerable fractures following minor trauma. • ACM—soft tissue swelling of the face and abdomen; severe hypertrophy of soft tissues of the mouth, tongue, and pharynx (latter may cause stridor); polyuria; occasionally polyphagia. • DW—proportionate growth retardation and an abnormally soft and woolly hair coat without guard hair.

General Comments

Signs frequently reported by the owner: • OCDP—difficult and decreased mobility, jumping, climbing, lameness; signs progressing. • OI—sudden onset or progressive lameness. • ACM, DW—similar to physical examination findings.

Physical Examination Findings

• OCDP: ○ Cats—pain of long bones; unwillingness to rise. ○ Dogs—larger than normal head, shorter jaw and resulting malaligned teeth, shortened bones, joint enlargement, lateral deviation of thoracic limbs, spinal deviation to either side. • OI—pain and lameness secondary to fractures. Dentinogenesis imperfecta (secondary to abnormal collagen I) can be noted in addition to or as single entity: severe thinning of the dentine layer, leading to a translucent appearance, pink discoloration, and multiple tooth fractures. Sudden death due to rupture of chordae tendineae (also affected by abnormal cartilage), has been reported. • ACM—inspiratory stridor, thick skin folds (mainly neck), prognathism, wide interdental spaces. Visceromegaly, if generalized, can result in abdominal enlargement. • DW—profound dwarfism, retention of puppy hairs, lack of guard hairs. Hairs can be epilated easily. Gradual progressive truncal alopecia can be noted. Progressive dermal hyperpigmentation, scaly skin, and dermatitis is possible. In males, cryptorchidism is common; in females, persistent estrus is frequent. Continuous heart murmur secondary to a patent ductus arteriosus has been reported.

CAUSES

See Genetics.

RISK FACTORS

N/A for any discussed diseases; except ACM if exogenous progesterone is administered.

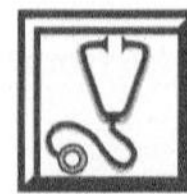

DIAGNOSIS

DIFFERENTIAL DIAGNOSIS

• OCDP, OI—metabolic disease, physical abuse, alimentary secondary hyperparathyroidism, hypovitaminosis D, hypothyroidism. • ACM—Pituitary gland tumor; long-term use of progesterone (older dogs, infertile bitches, aggressive dogs). • DW—malnutrition.

CBC/BIOCHEMISTRY/URINALYSIS

• The following should be specifically evaluated for all discussed diseases: serum concentrations of ionized calcium, phosphorus, vitamin D, and parathormone. • OCDP, OI, DW—N/A. • ACM—hyperglycemia, hyperphosphatemia, hypercholesterolemia, hyperproteinemia, increases in liver enzymes (specifically elevated alkaline phosphate), decreased thyroid hormone. • DW—elevated plasma creatinine concentration.

OTHER LABORATORY TESTS

• OCDP, OI—N/A. • ACM—prolactin, cortisol, basal plasma GH levels elevated with disease progression. Elevated plasma insulin-like growth factor I (IGF-I) levels (however, increased GH and IGF can also be seen in healthy animals). Free thyroxine, thyroid-stimulating hormone (TSH), and adrenocorticotropic hormone (ACTH) stimulation tests recommended. GH test recommended to evaluate the pituitary gland function. Follicle-stimulating hormone (FSH) and luteinizing hormone (LH) tests are recommended. Diabetes mellitus has been reported to develop secondary to insulin resistance, thus urinalysis with ACM can reveal glucosuria. • DW—basal plasma concentrations of GH and IGF-I, prolactin, thyrotropin, and LH are low. With combined anterior pituitary function test, often no response of GH, TSH, and prolactin, but minor response of LH and FSH.

IMAGING

• OCDP—radiographic changes more prominent in pelvic limbs (size and shape of the tarsal, carpal, metatarsal, metacarpal bones, phalanges), sacrum (articular spaces decreased), exostoses with diffuse osteopenia, zones of rarefication. Spine may show scoliosis, lordosis, or kyphosis. • OI—radiographs reveal less opaque than normal long bone cortices, frequently pathologic fractures or evidence of chronic healing fractures.

• ACM—radiographs of thorax (in case of mammary tumor metastasis; also 85% cardiomegaly reported in cats); MRI of brain (pituitary); ultrasound of abdomen (assess organomegaly—specifically liver and kidneys). • DW—MRI (brain), echocardiography.

DIAGNOSTIC PROCEDURES

• OCDP—bone histology. • OI—analysis of type I collagen obtained from cultured skin fibroblasts. • ACM/DW—N/A.

PATHOLOGIC FINDINGS

• OCDP, DW—N/A. • OI—bone: absence of secondary spongiosa, irregular woven bone with absence of Haversian canals. • ACM—pituitary or mammary gland changes depend on tumor. • DW—aplasia of the hypophysis/pituitary gland.

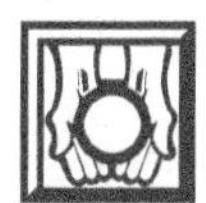

TREATMENT

NURSING CARE

N/A

ACTIVITY

• OCDP, OI—decrease activity to reduce discomfort. • ACM—N/A. Rest 3 weeks if surgery (ovariohysterectomy) done. Specific care based on specialist's recommendation following pituitary gland radiation. • DW—N/A.

DIET

OCDP, OI, ACM, DW—healthy diet.

CLIENT EDUCATION

• OCDP, OI—N/A; no cure. • ACM, DW—N/A.

SURGICAL CONSIDERATIONS

• OCDP—N/A; corrective osteotomies are not rewarding. • OI—surgical treatment of fractures. • ACM—withdrawal of exogenous progestagens and/or ovario(hyster)ectomy. If pituitary, consider hypophysectomy. Radiation of the hypophysis can also be considered. • DW—N/A.

MEDICATIONS

DRUG(S) OF CHOICE

• OCDP—dogs: nonsteroidal anti-inflammatory drugs (NSAIDs); cats: robenacoxib 1 mg/kg PO once a day for 3 days. • OI—vitamin C 75 mg/kg PO once a day; bisphosphonate supplementation (alendronate sodium): dogs: 0.5–1 mg/kg PO once a day on empty stomach; cats: 10 mg/cat PO on empty stomach once a week. Note: effectiveness of bisphosphonates to treat OI in dogs and cats has not been evaluated. • ACM: ○ If progestagen-induced—aglepristone (progesterone-receptor blocker) 15 mg/kg SQ on 2 consecutive days, repeat weekly until effect of progestagen ceases; surgery (see Surgical Considerations). ○ If hypothyroidism-induced—levothyroxine sodium 0.02 mg/kg (dog) or 0.01 mg/kg (cat) PO once a day. Adjust dose based on the serum total thyroxine concentrations 4–6 hours post tablet administration, along with clinical response. • DW—porcine GH 0.1–0.3 IU/kg SQ, 3 times a week. Thyroid hormone replacement if evidence of secondary hypothyroidism (see ACM dosing recommendation above).

CONTRAINDICATIONS

N/A

PRECAUTIONS

• OCDP, OI—N/A. If NSAIDs are used, monitor for possible side effects as listed in package inserts. • ACM—N/A.

POSSIBLE INTERACTIONS

• OCDP—must not use other NSAIDs. • OI—none. • ACM—theoretically, the following interactions may occur with aglepristone: efficacy of glucocorticoids and progestins might be reduced. Manufacturer states that despite lack of data, the following medications may interact with aglepristone: ketoconazole, itraconazole, erythromycin. Drug interactions when using levothyroxine sodium can include: amiodarone, antidepressants, antidiabetics, cholestyramine, corticosteroids, digoxin, ferrous sulfate, ketamine, phenobarbital, propylthiouracil, rifampin, sertraline, sucralfate, sympathicomimetic agents, warfarin.

ALTERNATIVE DRUG(S)

• OCDP, OI—N/A. • ACM—aglepristone; may be difficult to obtain in the United States.

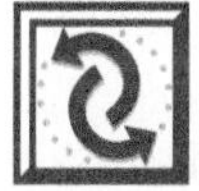

FOLLOW-UP

PATIENT MONITORING

• OCDP—2 weeks, then as needed. Note that osteoarthritis can develop long term. • OI—4–8 weeks for bone healing and improvement of bone density. • ACM—initially weekly, then every month to monitor until stable. • DW—weekly.

PREVENTION/AVOIDANCE

N/A

POSSIBLE COMPLICATIONS

• OCDP, DW—N/A. • OI—other fractures. • ACM—if tumorous cause, metastasis and worsening of disease.

EXPECTED COURSE AND PROGNOSIS

• OCDP—recurrence of signs and discomfort from arthritis. • OI—development of other fractures. • ACM—regression of clinical signs over time is expected; if GH did not completely exhaust pancreatic beta cells, diabetes mellitus might resolve. • DW—significant increase in body size often not seen (due to closure of epiphyseal plates); growth of primary hair is expected, while growth of guard hairs is variable.

MISCELLANEOUS

ASSOCIATED CONDITIONS

• OCDP—N/A. • OI—can be accompanied by blue sclera, hearing loss, dwarfism, pulmonary pathology. • ACM—diabetes mellitus, cardiac disease, decreased hepatic and renal function, peripheral neuropathies. • DW—secondary bacterial dermatitis. Due to combined pituitary hormone deficiency, secondary hypothyroidism is frequent. GH administration might result in development of diabetes mellitus.

PREGNANCY/FERTILITY/BREEDING

Affected animals for all discussed topics are not to be used for breeding. To treat ACM, ovario(hyster)ectomy is often needed.

ABBREVIATIONS

• ACM = acromegaly. • ACTH = adrenocorticotropic hormone. • DW = dwarfism. • FSH = follicle-stimulating hormone. • GH = growth hormone. • IGF = insulin-like growth factor. • LH = luteinizing hormone. • OCDP = osteochondrodysplasia. • OI = osteogenesis imperfecta. • TSH = thyroid-stimulating hormone.

Suggested Reading

Hazewinkel HAW. Metabolic, nutritional, and endocrine bone disorders. In: Bojrab MJ, Monnet E, eds., Mechanisms of Disease in Small Animal Surgery, 3rd ed. Jackson, WY: Teton NewMedia, 2010, pp. 601–610.

Kooistra H.S. Acromegaly in dogs. In: Rand J., ed., Clinical Endocrinology of Companion Animals. Hoboken, NJ: Wiley-Blackwell, 2014, pp. 421–426.

Montgomery R. Miscellaneous orthopedic diseases. In: Bojrab MJ, Monnet E., eds., Mechanisms of Disease in Small Animal Surgery, 3rd ed. Jackson, WY: Teton NewMedia, 2010, pp. 590–600.

Seeliger F, Leeb T, Peters M, et al. Osteogenesis imperfecta in two litters of dachshunds. Vet Pathol 2003, 40:530–539.

Von Pfeil DJF, DeCamp CE, Abood SK. The epiphyseal plate: nutritional and hormonal influences; hereditary and other disorders. Compend Contin Educ Vet 2009, 31(7):E1–E14.

Author Dirsko J.F. von Pfeil

Consulting Editor Mathieu M. Glassman

M

METALDEHYDE TOXICOSIS

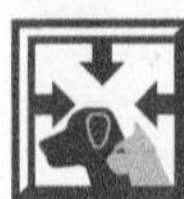

BASICS

OVERVIEW

- Form of acetaldehyde; primarily affects the nervous system.
- Mainly found in slug and snail baits; sometimes in solid fuel for camp stoves.
- Crosses the blood–brain barrier and disrupts GABAergic inhibitory action, facilitating neuronal excitation and increasing potential for convulsions.
- Systems affected include: neuromuscular (seizures and muscle tremors), hepatobiliary (delayed hepatotoxicosis reported in dogs only), and multiple organ failure (secondary to seizures and hyperthermia).
- Incidence/prevalence—depends on presence and accessibility; weather resistant: persists in the environment for >14 days.
- More frequent in coastal, low-lying, temperate and subtropical regions of United States. Snails and slugs are common pests in those locations.

SIGNALMENT

Species

Dogs; much less often in cats.

SIGNS

- Generally, within 3-4 hours but may occur in <30 minutes.
- Anxiety, panting, restlessness.
- Salivation, gastrointestinal upset.
- Tachycardia.
- Tachypnea, dyspnea.
- Hyperthermia up to 108°F (42.2°C).
- Hyperesthesia.
- Ataxia, tremors, seizures (intermittent then continuous).
- Mydriasis, nystagmus (especially in cats).

CAUSES

Ingestion of metaldehyde.

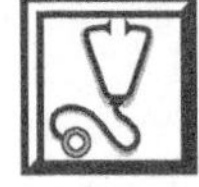

DIAGNOSIS

DIFFERENTIAL DIAGNOSIS

- Toxins capable of neurologic signs—amphetamines, bromethalin, blue-green algae, chocolate, hops, ivermectin, lead, neurotoxic mushrooms, organophosphate and some carbamate insecticides, pyrethroids, salt (ornaments, playdough), strychnine, tremorgenic mycotoxins, xylitol, and zinc phosphide.
- Nontoxic causes.

CBC/BIOCHEMISTRY/URINALYSIS

- No specific diagnostic features.
- Metabolic acidosis.
- Delayed changes in hepatic or renal values from uncontrolled hyperthermia/seizures.

OTHER LABORATORY TESTS

Presence in gastric contents, serum, urine, brain, or liver. Testing capabilities vary by lab; call to see what samples are recommended.

PATHOLOGIC FINDINGS

- Lesions neither consistent nor pathognomonic on necropsy (gross or histopathology).
- Gastric contents may have a formaldehyde odor.

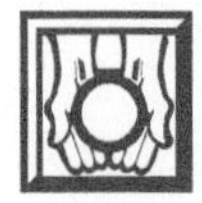

TREATMENT

- Appropriate health care consists of emergency exam, decontamination, intensive care until signs resolve (24–72 hours).
- Full recovery may take several weeks with hepatotoxicosis.
- Nursing care involves controling hyperthermia with cooling measures until reaching 103.5°F (39.7°C). Do not overcool. Monitor to prevent aspiration of vomitus.
- Monitor CNS status.
- Do not feed vomiting, convulsing, or heavily sedated patients.

MEDICATIONS

DRUG(S) OF CHOICE

- No antidote available.
- Emetics if minutes after ingestion or gastric lavage with intubation (preferred with large ingestions or symptomatic patient).
- Activated charcoal with cathartic if no contraindications.
- Crystalloids to prevent/correct dehydration or acidosis.
- Seizures—benzodiazepines (first choice), barbiturates, levetiracetam, propofol, or inhalant anesthetics. Consider CRIs.
- Tremors—methocarbamol 55–220 mg/kg IV; do not exceed 330 mg/kg/day.
- Hepatoprotectants as needed.
- Warm water enemas if toxicant seen in the stool.

CONTRAINDICATIONS/POSSIBLE INTERACTIONS

Do not induce vomiting or give activated charcoal to a patient that is convulsing or heavily sedated.

Precautions

Use depressant drugs cautiously in an already depressed patient, and only if other options are unavailable or ineffective. Use anticonvulsants at lowest effective doses.

FOLLOW-UP

PATIENT MONITORING

- Periodically allow anticonvulsants to wear off to reevaluate seizure condition.
- Once acute phase has passed, monitor hepatic/renal function. Hepatic damage may develop 48–72 hours later. Rhabdomyolysis-induced acute renal failure rare but possible.

PREVENTION/AVOIDANCE

- Do not apply in areas accessible to pets.
- Manufacturers may add green/blue dye to assist with identification. Can cause confusion with rodenticides.
- Added bittering agents do not reliably discourage ingestion. New products contain iron phosphate instead (less toxic).

POSSIBLE COMPLICATIONS

- Liver or renal dysfunction after initial signs (sequelae to seizures and hyperthermia).
- Aspiration pneumonia secondary to seizures.
- Hyperthermia may lead to disseminated intravascular coagulation (DIC) or multiple organ failure.

EXPECTED COURSE AND PROGNOSIS

- Good to excellent if treated early and aggressively.
- Guarded to poor if large ingestion or if treatment delayed or inadequate.
- Fatalities can be seen secondary to DIC or respiratory failure.
- Survival beyond the first 24 hours is positive prognostic indicator.

MISCELLANEOUS

ABBREVIATIONS

- DIC = disseminated intravascular coagulation.

Suggested Reading

Hovda L, Brutlag A, Poppenga R, et al. Five-Minute Veterinary Consult Clinical Companion Small Animal Toxicology, 2rd ed. Ames, IA: Wiley-Blackwell, 2016, pp. 672–677.

Peterson M, Talcott, P. Small Animal Toxicology, 3rd ed. St. Louis, MO: Elsevier, 2013, pp. 635–642.

Author Kia Benson

Consulting Editor Lynn R. Hovda

Acknowledgment The author and editors acknowledge the prior contribution of James N. Eucher.

Client Education Handout available online

METFORMIN TOXICOSIS

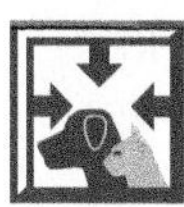

BASICS

OVERVIEW

• Metformin (Glucophage) is a biguanide antihyperglycemic prescription medication labeled for the treatment of non-insulin-dependent (type 2) diabetes mellitus in humans.
• Available as single or extended release formulation (Glucophage XR).
• Formulated as a single ingredient and in combination with other antidiabetic medications.
• The agent potentially could be useful in the adjunctive treatment of non-insulin-dependent diabetes mellitus in cats; use is controversial.
• Toxicity causes gastrointestinal signs and lethargy.
• 578 exposures to metformin were reported to the American Society for the Prevention of Cruelty to Animals (ASPCA) Animal Poison Control Center (APCC) during 2015–2018. Of these, 96.1% dogs, 3.7% cats, 0.3% birds. Common findings recorded are vomiting 9.3%, lethargy 3.1%, hypoglycemia 1.9%, trembling 1.5%, diarrhea 1.2%.
• Vomiting developed from doses as low as 15.3 mg/kg with hypoglycemia at 48 mg/kg.

SIGNALMENT

• Dogs and cats.
• No breed, age, or sex predilections.

SIGNS

Dogs

• Common sign—vomiting.
• Possible signs—lethargy, hypoglycemia, trembling and diarrhea.

Cats

• Frequent sign—vomiting.
• Possible signs—lethargy, diarrhea, and vocalization.

CAUSES & RISK FACTORS

Ingestion of metformin in single-ingredient preparations as well as in combination with other antidiabetic agents.

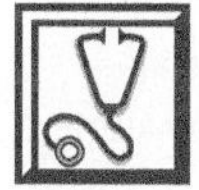

DIAGNOSIS

DIFFERENTIAL DIAGNOSIS

Other gastrointestinal tract irritants.

CBC/BIOCHEMISTRY/URINALYSIS

Azotemia reported in humans due to acute renal failure in cases of biguanide lactic acidosis; not reported in animal toxicities.

OTHER LABORATORY TESTS

• Blood gases—lactic acidosis rare but possible with large ingestions (a shih tzu ingesting 167.2 mg/kg of metformin developed lactic acidosis, vomiting, and hypothermia; no hypoglycemia developed and the dog fully recovered with treatment).
• High-performance liquid chromatography may identify presence of metformin in plasma; drug levels are not clinically useful.

DIAGNOSTIC PROCEDURES

N/A

PATHOLOGIC FINDINGS

N/A

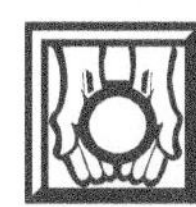

TREATMENT

• Induce emesis within the first 2–3 hours of exposure.
• Activated charcoal should only be considered with very large exposure.
• Treat gastrointestinal signs supportively.
• Treat lactic acidosis if present.

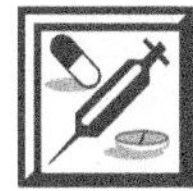

MEDICATIONS

DRUG(S) OF CHOICE

• Metoclopramide 0.2–0.5 mg/kg PO, SC, or IM q6h.
• Sucralfate 0.5–1 g PO q8–12h for dogs and 0.25–0.5 g PO q8–12h for cats.
• Famotidine 0.5–1.1 mg/kg orally q12–24h for dogs and cats.
• Ranitidine 1–2 mg/kg PO, SC, or IM q8–12h for dogs and 2.5 mg/kg IV q12h or 3.5 mg/kg PO q12h for cats.
• Omeprazole 0.5–1 mg/kg PO q24h for dogs and cats.
• Bicarbonate—if serum bicarbonate or total CO_2 is unavailable: 2–3 mEq/kg IV over 30 minutes if patient has decreased tissue perfusion or renal failure and does not have diabetic ketoacidosis. Must be used judiciously.

CONTRAINDICATIONS/POSSIBLE INTERACTIONS

• Concurrent administration of cimetidine may reduce the urinary excretion of metformin by competing for renal tubular organic cationic transport systems.
• The manufacturer states that other cationic drugs that undergo substantial tubular secretion (e.g., amiloride, digoxin, morphine, procainamide, quinidine, quinine, ranitidine, triamterene, trimethoprim, and vancomycin) may possibly decrease the urinary excretion of metformin.

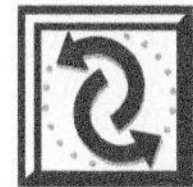

FOLLOW-UP

PATIENT MONITORING

N/A

EXPECTED COURSE AND PROGNOSIS

Good prognosis assuming lactic acidosis does not occur.

MISCELLANEOUS

ASSOCIATED CONDITIONS

N/A

PREGNANCY/FERTILITY/BREEDING

• No evidence of harm to the fetus or impaired fertility during reproduction studies in rats and rabbits given metformin hydrochloride dosages of 600 mg/kg daily.
• No adequate and controlled studies to date using metformin hydrochloride in pregnant women.
• Excreted in milk in levels similar to plasma. Caution advised in lactating queens.

SEE ALSO

Poisoning (Intoxication) Therapy.

ABBREVIATIONS

• APCC = Animal Poison Control Center.
• ASPCA = American Society for the Prevention of Cruelty to Animals.

INTERNET RESOURCES

• http://chem.sis.nlm.nih.gov/chemidplus/rn/657-24-9
• http://www.aspcapro.org/search/index/METFORMIN

Suggested Reading

Heller JB. Metformin overdose in dogs and cats. Vet Med 2007, 231–234.
Plumb DC. Metformin. In: Plumb DC, ed., Veterinary Drug Handbook, 8th ed. Ames, IA: Wiley-Blackwell, 2018, pp. 762–763.

Author Hany Youssef
Consulting Editor Lynn R. Hovda

METHEMOGLOBINEMIA

BASICS

DEFINITION

- Methemoglobin content in blood >1.5% of total hemoglobin.
- Methemoglobin differs from hemoglobin in that the iron moiety of heme groups has been oxidized from the ferrous (2+) to the ferric (3+) state.

PATHOPHYSIOLOGY

- About 3% of hemoglobin is oxidized to methemoglobin each day in normal animals as a result of autoxidation of hemoglobin or secondary to oxidants produced in normal metabolic reactions.
- Methemoglobin usually accounts for <1% of total hemoglobin, because it is constantly reduced back to hemoglobin by an NADH-dependent cytochrome b_5 reductase (methemoglobin reductase) enzyme reaction within red blood cells (RBCs).
- Caused by either increased production of methemoglobin by oxidants or decreased reduction of methemoglobin associated with a deficiency of the RBC cytochrome b_5 reductase enzyme or defective cytochrome b_5.

SYSTEMS AFFECTED

- Hemic/lymphatic/immune—reduced oxygen-carrying capacity of blood, because methemoglobin cannot bind oxygen; if methemoglobin content reaches high values (e.g., >50% of total hemoglobin), organs may suffer hypoxic injury.
- Hepatobiliary—in addition to hypoxic injury, the liver may be damaged directly by oxidant drugs that it metabolizes.
- Renal/urologic—in addition to hypoxic injury, the kidneys may be damaged if intravascular hemolysis occurs (pigmentary nephropathy).

SIGNALMENT

- Dogs and cats.
- Deficiency in RBC cytochrome b_5 reductase has been recognized in the Chihuahua, borzoi, English setter, mixed-breed dog, coonhound, poodle, corgi, Pomeranian, Staffordshire bull terrier, Parson Russell terrier, Australian shepherd dog, and American Eskimo dog, and in domestic shorthair cats. A defect in cytochrome b_5 has been described in a mixed-breed dog.

SIGNS

Caused Directly

- Possibly none in animals with mild to moderate methemoglobinemia.
- Cyanotic-appearing mucous membranes—may be difficult to recognize in heavily pigmented animals.
- Lethargy, tachycardia, tachypnea, ataxia, and stupor caused by hypoxemia when methemoglobin content exceeds 50%.
- Coma-like state and death when methemoglobin content reaches 80%.

Caused by Associated Diseases

- Vomiting, anorexia, and diarrhea possible in patients with drug toxicity.
- Hemoglobinuria secondary to severe intravascular hemolysis in some patients with Heinz body hemolytic anemia.
- Subcutaneous edema, especially involving the face, and salivation in animals with acetaminophen toxicity.

CAUSES

- Toxicity—acetaminophen, benzocaine, phenazopyridine, and skunk musk cause Heinz body hemolytic anemia; excess nitrite in pet food and hydroxycarbamide toxicity are reported to cause methemoglobinemia without Heinz body hemolytic anemia.
- Deficiency in RBC cytochrome b_5 reductase or a defect in RBC cytochrome b_5.

RISK FACTORS

- Application of benzocaine or prilocaine to traumatized skin or mucous membranes increases the likelihood of systemic absorption and methemoglobinemia.
- Cats are much more likely to develop clinically significant methemoglobinemia than are dogs after acetaminophen administration; this drug is not recommended for use in cats.
- Methemoglobinemia secondary to cytochrome b_5 reductase deficiency and a defect in cytochrome b are inherited disorders.

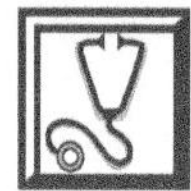

DIAGNOSIS

DIFFERENTIAL DIAGNOSIS

- Both low blood oxygen tension and methemoglobinemia can cause cyanotic-appearing mucous membranes and dark-colored blood samples; hypoxemia is documented by measuring PaO_2 <80 mmHg in an arterial blood sample, or an SpO_2 <95% measured via pulse oximetry.
- Methemoglobinemia is suspected when arterial blood with normal or high PO_2 is dark colored.

LABORATORY FINDINGS

Drugs That Alter Laboratory Results

None

Disorders That May Alter Laboratory Results

Hemolysis in the sample may raise the methemoglobin value, especially if the methemoglobin assay is not conducted soon after sample collection.

Valid If Run in Human Laboratory?

- Valid, as long as the method to lyse RBCs does not cause methemoglobin formation in the animal being tested.
- Saponin should not be used to lyse RBCs, because it raises the methemoglobin value in some species.

CBC/BIOCHEMISTRY/URINALYSIS

- Chronic methemoglobinemia secondary to cytochrome b_5 reductase deficiency can result in an elevated hematocrit (HCT); in contrast, hemolytic anemia may accompany methemoglobinemia caused by oxidant drugs.
- If severe or induced by oxidant drugs, evidence of injury to various organs (e.g., high serum creatinine concentration or alanine aminotransferase [ALT] activity) may be seen.

OTHER LABORATORY TESTS

- Spot test—determine if the patient's methemoglobin content is clinically important: one drop of blood from the patient is placed on a piece of absorbent white paper and a drop of normal control blood is placed next to it. If the methemoglobin content is ≥10%, the patient's blood will be noticeably browner than the bright red of the control blood.
- Co-oximetry is the method of choice for accurate measurement of methemoglobin content in whole blood samples.
- Methemoglobin content in dogs with cytochrome b_5 reductase deficiency reportedly varies from 13 to 51%; the methemoglobin content in six deficient cats ranged from 44 to 52%.
- A definitive diagnosis of cytochrome b_5 reductase deficiency is made by measuring enzyme activity in RBCs; this assay is done in a few research laboratories and requires that arrangements be made before blood samples are submitted. Genetic testing may become available now that mutations have been documented in the cytochrome b_5 reductase gene (*CYB5R3*) in dogs and a cat. Genetic testing is required to diagnose a cytochrome b_5 defect.

IMAGING

N/A

DIAGNOSTIC PROCEDURES

- Blood smears should be stained with methylene blue for detection of Heinz bodies.
- The presence of Heinz bodies indicates exposure to an oxidant drug that may also cause hemolytic anemia.

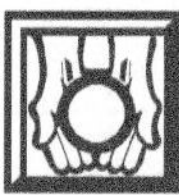

TREATMENT

- Mild to moderate—does not require specific treatment to reduce the methemoglobin content.
- Drug-induced—the use of the drug should be discontinued; RBCs can convert much of the methemoglobin back to hemoglobin

within 24 hours after elimination of drug exposure.

- Inherited cytochrome b_5 reductase deficiency—animals have normal life expectancy and generally do not require treatment, although veterinarians may wish to give a single IV injection of methylene blue 1 hour before a deficient animal is anesthetized for surgery to maximize the amount of hemoglobin that is capable of binding oxygen.
- Whole blood or packed RBC transfusions should be given to patients with severe anemia and those with rapidly decreasing HCT and clinical signs suggesting a deteriorating condition.
- Severe intravascular hemolysis—IV fluid administration recommended in addition to blood products.
- Treatment of electrolyte or acid–base imbalances may also be indicated in patients with severe vomiting or diarrhea, concomitant renal injury, or shock.
- Administration of oxygen is of limited value because methemoglobin cannot bind oxygen, and an increase in dissolved oxygen results in only a small increase in blood oxygen content.

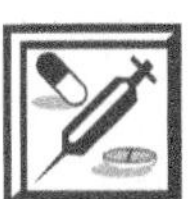

MEDICATIONS

DRUG(S) OF CHOICE

- Methylene blue—given slowly over several minutes as a 1% solution (1 mg/kg IV), may be administered in patients with severe methemoglobinemia; a dramatic response should occur during the first 30 minutes of treatment.
- *N*-Acetylcysteine is efficacious in the treatment of acetaminophen toxicity if given within a few hours after exposure; recommended dosage is 140 mg/kg PO, IV followed by 70 mg/kg PO, IV q6h for seven treatments.

CONTRAINDICATIONS

None

PRECAUTIONS

Methylene blue treatment can potentiate the formation of Heinz bodies and cause anemia. In patients that have been given drugs that cause substantial Heinz body formation, it is prudent to measure the HCT for 3 days after methylene blue treatment to ensure that clinically important anemia does not develop.

POSSIBLE INTERACTIONS

Methylene blue treatment will interfere with monitoring of Spo_2 by pulse oximetry.

ALTERNATIVE DRUG(S)

None

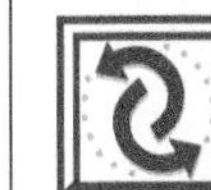

FOLLOW-UP

PATIENT MONITORING

- The cyanotic appearance of skin and mucous membranes should disappear after reduction of methemoglobin to an amount that does not produce clinical signs.
- Blood on the spot test should appear bright red after reduction of methemoglobin to values <10% of total hemoglobin.
- HCT should be monitored in patients with Heinz body anemia or following methylene blue administration for at least 3 days after initial exposure.

POSSIBLE COMPLICATIONS

Coma and death can occur if methemoglobin content reaches 80% of total hemoglobin.

MISCELLANEOUS

ASSOCIATED CONDITIONS

Heinz body anemia.

ZOONOTIC POTENTIAL

None

SEE ALSO

- Acetaminophen (APAP) Toxicosis.
- Anemia, Heinz Body.

ABBREVIATIONS

- ALT = alanine aminotransferase.
- HCT = hematocrit.
- RBC = red blood cell.

Suggested Readings

Harvey JW. Veterinary Hematology. A Diagnostic Guide and Color Atlas. St. Louis, MO: Elsevier Saunders, 2012, pp. 12–13, 96–97.

Jaffe JA, Harmon MR, Villani NA, et al. Long-term treatment with methylene blue in a dog with hereditary methemoglobinemia caused by cytochrome b5 reductase deficiency. J Vet Intern Med 2017, 31:1860–1865.

McKenna JA, Sacco J, Son TT, et al. Congenital methemoglobinemia in a dog with a promoter deletion and a nonsynonymous coding variant in the gene encoding cytochrome b_5. J Vet Intern Med 2014, 28:1626–1631.

Tani A, Yamazaki J, Nakamura K, et al. Congenital methemoglobinemia in a cat with reduced NADH-cytochrome b5 reductase 3 activity and missense mutations in CYB5R3. Jpn J Vet Res 2017, 65:201–206.

Author John W. Harvey

Consulting Editor Melinda S. Camus

METRITIS

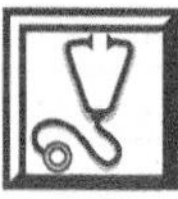

BASICS

OVERVIEW

- Bacterial uterine infection that develops in the immediate postpartum period (usually within the first week); occasionally develops after an abortion or nonsterile artificial insemination—rarely after natural breeding.
- Bacteria—ascend through the open cervix to the uterus; postpartum uterus provides an ideal environment for growth; Gram-negative bacteria (e.g., *Escherichia coli*) commonly isolated.
- Potentially life-threatening infection; may lead to septic shock.
- Can become chronic and lead to infertility.

M

SIGNALMENT

- Postpartum bitch and queen.
- No age or breed predilection.

SIGNS

Historical Findings

- Malodorous, purulent, sanguinopurulent, or dark green vulvar discharge.
- Depression.
- Anorexia.
- Neglect of puppies and kittens.
- Reduced milk production.
- Polyuria/polydipsia.

Physical Examination Findings

- Fever.
- Large uterus on abdominal palpation.
- Dehydration.
- Injected mucous membranes (septic shock).
- Tachycardia, hypotension, other signs of shock.

CAUSES & RISK FACTORS

- Dystocia.
- Obstetric manipulation.
- Retained fetuses or placentas.
- Prolonged delivery (large litter).
- Post abortion, and post natural or artificial insemination (rare).

DIAGNOSIS

DIFFERENTIAL DIAGNOSIS

- Subinvolution of placental sites—no sign of infection on cytologic examination of vagina.
- Eclampsia—differentiated by serum calcium concentration.

CBC/BIOCHEMISTRY/URINALYSIS

- Neutrophilia with left shift, although neutropenia and leukopenia are occasionally seen, especially in patients with septic shock.
- High packed cell volume and total plasma protein concentration; azotemia secondary to dehydration/hypovolemia. Normocytic, normochromic nonregenerative anemia may also occur.
- With endotoxemia or sepsis, hypoalbuminemia, elevation of C-reactive protein concentration, and other acute phase changes may occur. Elevated liver enzyme activities may be seen.
- Urine specific gravity may be elevated (from dehydration) or decreased (isosthenuria).
- Urinalysis (obtain via ultrasound-guided cystocentesis) may reveal bacteriuria.

OTHER LABORATORY TESTS

N/A

IMAGING

- Radiography—reveals a large uterus and possibly retained fetus(es).
- Ultrasonography—intrauterine fluid accumulation and increased horn width, retained placenta(s), and retained fetus(es); abdominal effusion may be present if uterine rupture.

DIAGNOSTIC PROCEDURES

- Vaginal cytologic examination—detect degenerative neutrophils with intracellular bacteria.
- Guarded anterior vaginal or transcervical culture—aerobes and anaerobes; culture and sensitivity recommended.

TREATMENT

- Inpatient until systemic signs resolve.
- Treat shock—IV balanced electrolyte solution.
- Correct electrolyte imbalances and hypoglycemia.
- Ovariohysterectomy—treatment of choice for uterine rupture or severe sepsis, and if future breeding is not desired; the uterus is friable; pack off and handle gently at surgery.

MEDICATIONS

DRUG(S) OF CHOICE

- Antibiotics—start broad-spectrum agents (oral if patient is stable; IV if patient is in shock); choice confirmed by bacterial culture and sensitivity; continued at least 14 days. Give at separate time from prostaglandin F2α (PGF2α) administration due to risk of vomiting.
- Nursing planned—amoxicillin–clavulanic acid 22 mg/kg PO q12h; can administer q8h to treat Gram-negative infections, enrofloxacin 10 mg/kg PO, IV q24h (dogs); 5 mg/kg PO q24h (cats), if puppies <3 weeks of age and susceptibility indicates.
- If ovariohysterectomy not performed and cervix is open—oxytocin 0.5–1 U/kg IM, SC (do not exceed 5 IU total); then repeat in 1–2 hours; may require increased dose to attain similar degree of uterine contraction if >48 hours since parturition.
- PGF2α 10–50 μg/kg SC q3–5h for 3–5 days or 100 μg/kg SC q12h for 3–5 days; to evacuate uterus, ultrasound prior to cessation of treatment to ensure resolution of fluid accumulation in uterine lumen.

CONTRAINDICATIONS/POSSIBLE INTERACTIONS

- Prostaglandin—may induce uterine rupture if the tissue is devitalized.
- Oxytocin—reduced efficacy beyond 48 hours post partum.

FOLLOW-UP

PATIENT MONITORING

- Physical exam, CBC, vaginal cytologic examination.
- Ultrasonography—monitor evacuation of uterine fluid.

POSSIBLE COMPLICATIONS

- Ovariohysterectomy—when medical treatment is ineffective.
- Uterine rupture and peritonitis—may occur with medical treatment.
- Owners may need to foster or hand-raise puppies and kittens.

EXPECTED COURSE AND PROGNOSIS

- Ovariohysterectomy—prognosis for recovery good.
- Medical treatment—prognosis for recovery dependent on early recognition of problem by owner; good if early, but may adversely affect future reproduction.

MISCELLANEOUS

ABBREVIATIONS

- PGF2α = prostaglandin F2α.

Suggested Reading

Johnston SD, Root Kustritz MV, Olson PNS. Periparturient disorders in the bitch. In: Johnston SD, Root Kustritz MV, Olson PNS, eds., Canine and Feline Theriogenology. Philadelphia, PA: Saunders, 2001, pp. 129–145.

Author Tessa Fiamengo

Consulting Editor Erin E. Runcan

Acknowledgment The author and editors acknowledge the prior contribution of Joni L. Freshman.

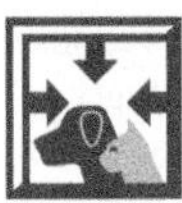

BASICS

OVERVIEW

• Non-epileptic CNS disorders. • Characterized by the occurrence of continuous or episodic involuntary movements in a conscious, responsive animal. • Unrelated to epileptic activity. • Movements may involve the whole body or be restricted to one body part, e.g., one or two limbs or one side of the body. • Hyperkinetic movement disorders often occur as paroxysmal dyskinesias with long episodes of abnormal movements and increased muscle tone (dystonia) alternating with normal neurologic function. • Hypokinetic movement disorders manifest as bradykinesia or collapse. • Pathophysiology—abnormal CNS neural transmission, unrelated to epilepsy, dysfunction of basal nuclei, altered dopaminergic or serotinergic neurotransmission.

SIGNALMENT

• Dogs; less common in cats. • Breed-related syndromes. • Age of onset variable; often <3 years.

SIGNS

• Physical examination—unremarkable. • Neurologic examination—unremarkable between episodes. • Cardiologic examination—unremarkable between and during episodes. • Signs may include—repeated flexion or kicking, excessive lifting of one or more limbs, episodic muscle rigidity, muscle hypertonicity, difficulty initiating movements, episodic ataxia, kyphosis, scoliosis, backward gait, falling, collapse. • Description of episodes may vary between dog breeds. See specific references for detailed information on breed-specific syndromes. • Frequently long duration—minutes to hours. • Differentiated from epileptic seizures—no autonomic signs: no salivation, urination, normal pupils, no postictal period, responsive during episode. • Triggers are frequent—excitement, stress, excessive exercise, heat. • In some dog breeds there are gastrointestinal signs in association with episodes (Border terriers, paroxysmal gluten-sensitive dyskinesia).

CAUSES & RISK FACTORS

• Frequently breed-specific syndromes—Norwich terrier, chinook (paroxysmal dyskinesia), border collie/Australian shepherd dog (collapse), Scottish terrier (collapse). • Gluten hypersensitivity—border terrier, possibly also other dog breeds. • Gene mutations—cavalier King Charles spaniel (*BCAN*, episodic falling), Irish wolfhound puppies (*SLGA5*; glycine receptor, startle disease), Russell terrier (*KCNJ10*, hereditary cerebellar ataxia associated with myokymia), soft-coated wheaten terrier (*PIGN*); Labrador retriever collapse (*DNM1*); Chinese-crested dog, Kerry blue terrier (multisystem degeneration, *SERAC1*), Sheltie (PCK2).

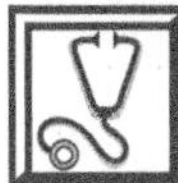

DIAGNOSIS

DIFFERENTIAL DIAGNOSIS

• Epilepsy—autonomous signs: salivation, urination, mydriasis; typically short duration <1–2 minutes; postictal period. • Cardiac disease—bradyarrhythmias, ventricular tachycardia. • Metabolic, electrolyte disorders—hypoglycemia, hypocalcemia, hypokalemia, hyperkalemia, hepatic encephalopathy. • Drugs—phenobarbital, propofol, potassium bromide, dopamine antagonists, metoclopramide. • Toxins—lead, copper, psychoactive drugs, environmental toxins. • Obsessive compulsive behavior—complex behavior, responsive, interruptible. • Episodes of spinal pain. • Vestibular attacks. • Rapid eye movement (REM) sleep disorder. • Myotonic myopathies—inherited, acquired. • Feline hyperesthesia syndrome, feline orofacial pain syndrome—cats, unknown etiology.

CBC/BIOCHEMISTRY/URINALYSIS

• Unremarkable. • Specific consideration—glucose (fasted, during episode), potassium, sodium, ionized calcium, creatine kinase.

OTHER LABORATORY TESTS

• Specific genetic tests—based on availability for the breed. • Ammonia, fasted and postprandial bile acids. • T_4. • Serologic testing for gluten hypersensitivity—border terriers; other breeds if gastrointestinal signs. • Neurometabolic screening—lactate, pyruvate, urinary organic acids, amino acids.

IMAGING

MRI brain, spinal cord—exclude structural disease, frequently unremarkable.

DIAGNOSTIC PROCEDURES

• Video documentation of episodes. • Electrocardiography (ECG)—long-term, ambulatory (Holter); exclude arrhythmias. • Electroencephalography (EEG)—ambulatory video-EEG to exclude epilepsy. • CSF—to exclude CNS inflammation; frequently normal.

PATHOLOGIC FINDINGS

Frequently unremarkable.

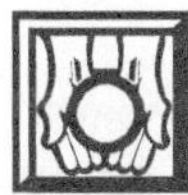

TREATMENT

• Avoid triggers—stress, excitement; exercise, heat (Jack Russell terrier). • Treat underlying cause if any identified. • Gluten-free diet in border terriers. • Trial therapy with anti-epileptic drugs, • Dietary trials (gluten-free, hypoallergenic) in other dog breeds.

MEDICATIONS

DRUG(S) OF CHOICE

• Use based on low levels of evidence. • Diazepam 0.25–0.5 mg/kg q8h; clonazepam 0.5 mg/kg q8–12h; acetazolamide 4–8 mg/kg q8–12h; 4-aminopyridine 0.25–0.5 mg/kg q12h; fluoxetine 1–2 mg/kg q24h. • Trial therapy with antiepileptic drugs—gabapentin 10–20 mg/kg q8h; levetiracetam 10–20 mg/kg q8h; phenobarbital 2.5 mg/kg q12h.

CONTRAINDICATIONS/POSSIBLE INTERACTIONS

4-aminopyridine - may cause seizures; acetazolamide - metabolic acidosis; fluoxetine - drug interactions, hyperthermia.

FOLLOW-UP

PATIENT MONITORING

Acetazolamide—hypokalemia, acidosis.

PREVENTION/AVOIDANCE

Avoid potential triggers. Avoid heat in Jack Russell terriers.

POSSIBLE COMPLICATIONS

Rarely hyperthermia (death) described in association with collapse.

EXPECTED COURSE AND PROGNOSIS

Unpredictable frequency and clinical course, lifelong or may spontaneously resolve.

MISCELLANEOUS

AGE-RELATED FACTORS

Often appears in dogs <3 years old.

PREGNANCY/FERTILITY/BREEDING

Breeding not recommended. Genetic testing recommended.

SEE ALSO

• Exercise-Induced Weakness/Collapse in Labradors Retrievers. • Head Tremors (Bobbing), Idiopathic—Dogs. • Myoclonus. • Shaker/Tremor Syndrome, Corticosteroid Responsive.

ABBREVIATIONS

• ECG = electrocardiography. • EEG = electroencephalography. • REM = rapid eye movement.

INTERNET RESOURCES

• www.omia.org • www.aht.org.uk/cms-display/genetics_canine.html • www.caninegeneticdiseases.net/CGD_main.htm • www.ofa.org/browse-by-breed

Suggested Reading

Lowrie M, Garosi L. Classification of involuntary movements in dogs: paroxysmal dyskinesias. Vet J 2017, 220:65–71.

Author Andrea Fischer

Client Education Handout available online

MUCOPOLYSACCHARIDOSES

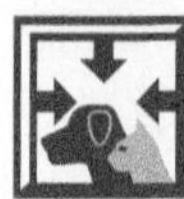

BASICS

OVERVIEW

• Mucopolysaccharidoses (MPS) are characterized by the accumulation of glycosaminoglycans (GAGs) in cells, and result from the impaired function of 1 of 11 enzymes required for normal GAG degradation.
• Undegraded GAGs are stored in lysosomes, resulting in progressive tissue and organ dysfunction.

Types of MPS Reported in Dogs and Cats

• MPS I—α-L-iduronidase deficiency: dermatan and heparan sulfate stored.
• MPS II—iduronate sulfatase deficiency: dermatan and heparan sulfate stored.
• MPS IIIA—heparan *N*-sulfatase deficiency: heparan sulfate stored.
• MPS VI—arylsulfatase B deficiency: dermatan sulfate stored.
• MPS VII—β-glucuronidase deficiency: dermatan, heparan, and chondroitin sulfate stored.

SIGNALMENT

• Cats—MPS I and VII (domestic shorthair [DSH]); MPS VI (Siamese and DSH).
• Dogs—MPS I, Plott hounds; MPS II, Labrador retrievers; MPS IIIA, wire-haired dachshunds and Huntaways; MPS VI, miniature pinschers, miniature schnauzers, miniature poodles, and Welsh corgis; MPS VII, mixed breeds and Belgian, White Swiss, and German shepherd dogs.
• Both sexes equally affected by MPS I, III, VI, and VII; primarily males affected by MPS II.

SIGNS

• Clinical signs apparent at 2–4 months of age.
• Affected animals may live several years, but locomotor difficulty is progressive.
• Skeletal abnormalities more severe in cats with MPS VI than in those with MPS I; some MPS VI cats develop posterior paresis from spinal cord compression.
• Dwarfism (except cats with MPS I).
• Severe bone disease (dysostosis multiplex), degenerative joint disease, facial dysmorphia.
• Hepatomegaly (except cats with MPS VI).
• Corneal clouding—~8 weeks of age.
• Enlarged tongue (dogs).
• Heart valve thickening, resulting in left- or right-sided heart failure.
• Excess urinary excretion of GAG.
• Manipulation of the head or neck usually painful.

CAUSES & RISK FACTORS

• MPS transmission is autosomal recessive, except MPS II, which is X-linked recessive.
• In-breeding increases risk.

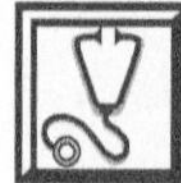

DIAGNOSIS

DIFFERENTIAL DIAGNOSIS

• Metachromatic granules within neutrophils and lymphocytes–suggest MPS; also observed with GM_2 gangliosidosis, which, unlike MPS, is characterized by progressive neurologic disease and early death.
• Corneal clouding—also observed in other storage diseases, including acid lipase deficiency, GM_1 and GM_2 gangliosidosis, and mannosidosis; lysosomal enzyme panels can be performed to definitively diagnose the type of disorder.
• Radiographic appearance of MPS is characteristic; other disorders with similarities include congenital hypothyroidism, epiphyseal dysplasia, and hypervitaminosis A.

CBC/BIOCHEMISTRY/URINALYSIS

• Wright's-stained blood films reveal neutrophils and monocytes containing numerous distinctive metachromatic granules (Alder–Reilly bodies).
• Granules indistinct in animals with MPS I.
• Granules usually inapparent when stained with Diff-Quik.
• Occasional lymphocytes have vacuoles with metachromatic granules, particularly in MPS VII.

OTHER LABORATORY TESTS

• Wright's stained cytologic preparations of lymph node, liver, bone marrow, and joint fluid specimens reveal Alder–Reilly bodies within cells.
• Presence of excess GAG in urine usually indicates MPS.
• Definitive diagnosis made by measuring lysosomal enzyme activity in serum, leukocyte pellets, or frozen liver.

IMAGING

• Radiography—low bone density with thin cortices.
• Epiphyseal abnormalities.
• Degenerative joint disease.
• In some cats, proliferative bone is present around all articular facets of vertebrae, causing fusion of cervical vertebrae.

DIAGNOSTIC PROCEDURES

Specialized laboratories can measure lysosomal enzyme activity in leukocyte pellets and detect specific gene mutations for some disorders.

PATHOLOGIC FINDINGS

Distended lysosomes seen in cells of many tissues examined by light and electron microscopy.

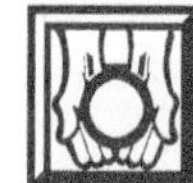

TREATMENT

• Bone marrow transplant (BMT)—after successful engraftment, donor-derived normal leukocytes provide missing enzyme to various tissues; when performed at a very early age, affected animals lead near-normal lives; not as helpful when performed after skeletal maturity; unaffected sibling is needed as a donor.
• Gene therapy has been effective in some animal models.

MEDICATIONS

DRUG(S) OF CHOICE

Affected animals are susceptible to viral and bacterial respiratory infection. Antibiotics may be indicated.

FOLLOW-UP

PREVENTION/AVOIDANCE

• Avoid in-breeding.
• Enzyme assays should be performed to diagnose heterozygotes.

EXPECTED COURSE AND PROGNOSIS

• Prognosis reasonably good in animals treated with BMT.
• Untreated animals usually develop severe skeletal and joint disease and may become nonambulatory at 3–5 years of age or earlier.

MISCELLANEOUS

ABBREVIATIONS

• BMT = bone marrow transplant.
• DSH = domestic shorthair cat.
• GAG = glycosaminoglycan.
• MPS = mucopolysaccharidoses.

Suggested Reading

Haskins M, Casal M, Ellinwood NM, et al. Animal models for mucopolysaccharidoses and their clinical relevance. Acta Paediatr Suppl 2002, 91:88–97.

Author Mary Anna Thrall
Consulting Editor Melinda S. Camus

M

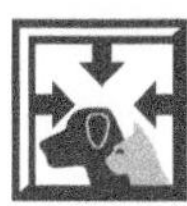

BASICS

DEFINITION

Antimicrobial resistance (AMR) is the ability of microbes to grow in the presence of antimicrobial agents that would normally kill them or inhibit their growth. Multidrug-resistant (MDR) infections are those that are resistant to more than one class of antimicrobials.

PATHOPHYSIOLOGY

AMR can develop in several ways:

- Use of antimicrobials creates selection pressure, allowing growth of bacteria resistant to a specific drug by decreasing competition with susceptible organisms.
- Antimicrobial-resistant bacteria can share genetic elements, conferring resistance to other bacteria.
- Spontaneous new mutations can develop that allow bacterial survival in the face of antimicrobials.
- MDR infections occur through any of these mechanisms; resistance is often additive with antimicrobial use over time.

SYSTEMS AFFECTED

Any tissue affected by bacterial infections may be affected by antimicrobial-resistant bacterial infections. Some examples are:

- Renal/urologic—recurrent urinary tract infections.
- Skin—abscesses, pyoderma.
- Respiratory—pneumonia.
- Musculoskeletal—surgical site infections.
- Gastrointestinal—gastrointestinal pathogens such as *Campylobacter* spp., *Salmonella* spp., *Escherichia coli*, *Enterococcus* spp.
- Hepatobiliary—ascending cholangitis/cholecystitis.
- Cardiovascular—endocarditis.

GENETICS

N/A

INCIDENCE/PREVALENCE

Due to a lack of robust surveillance, prevalence of MDR infections in dogs and cats is unknown; however, studies suggest between <1 and 50% of bacteria cultured from companion animals are MDR, depending on geographic region.

GEOGRAPHIC DISTRIBUTION

N/A

SIGNALMENT

Species

Dog and cat.

Breed Predilections

N/A

Mean Age and Range

N/A

Predominant Sex

N/A

SIGNS

General Comments

Bacterial infections that do not resolve with first-line empiric antimicrobial therapy should cause suspicion for AMR.

Historical Findings

- No or minimal response to antimicrobial therapy.
- History of previous course(s) of anti-microbial therapy.
- Exposure to humans or animals with MDR infections.
- Recent hospitalization and/or surgery.
- Raw food diet.

Physical Examination Findings

Depends on site of infection.

CAUSES

Any bacteria can become resistant to antimicrobials. Common AMR bacterial pathogens include:

- Methicillin-resistant *Staphylococcus pseudintermedius* (MRSP).
- Methicillin-resistant *Staphylococcus aureus* (MRSA).
- MDR *Enterococcus faecalis* and *Enterococcus faecium.*
- Extended-spectrum beta-lactamase (ESBL) producing Gram-negative bacteria including:
    - *E. coli.*
    - *Salmonella enterica.*
    - *Klebsiella pneumoniae.*
    - *Pseudomonas aeruginosa.*
    - *Proteus mirabilis.*
    - *Enterobacter* spp.

RISK FACTORS

- Antimicrobial use.
- Hospitalization.
- Surgery.
- Co-habitation with health care worker.
- Co-habitation with human colonized with MRSA.
- Co-habitation with animal or human infected or colonized with AMR organism.

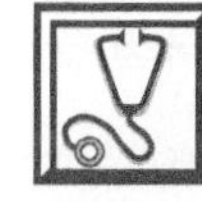

DIAGNOSIS

DIFFERENTIAL DIAGNOSIS

Bacterial infections, nonbacterial infections and other inflammatory diseases can mimic AMR bacterial infections, in that clinical response is not achieved with empiric antimicrobial therapy.

- Treating a microbe inherently resistant to empiric drug chosen (e.g., treating anaerobic infection with a drug ineffective against anaerobes) or using drug that does not penetrate site of infection.
- Viral, fungal, or protozoal infections.
- Immune-mediated disease.
- Neoplasia.

CBC/BIOCHEMISTRY/URINALYSIS

Findings are dependent on location of infection.

- CBC may lack abnormalities or range from leukocytosis and neutrophilia to neutropenia with degenerative left shift.
- Chemistry abnormalities associated with site of infection (e.g., azotemia with pyelonephritis).
- Urinalysis may reveal bacteriuria and pyuria in patients with urinary tract infections.

OTHER LABORATORY TESTS

- Quantitative bacterial culture and susceptibility testing are required for identification of AMR and MDR infections.
- Cytologic examination using a Romanowsky-type stain (e.g., Diff-Quik) and/or Gram stain of samples obtained for culture may help with culture interpretation, especially if more than one organism is cultured or suspected.

IMAGING

Imaging studies should identify source of infection and guide sampling for bacterial culture and susceptibility testing.

DIAGNOSTIC PROCEDURES

Sampling of site of infection is required for diagnosis and for guiding therapy; such procedures may include swabs of skin wounds or lesions, cystocentesis, thoracocentesis, abdominocentesis, pyelocentesis, airway samples (transtracheal, endotracheal wash or bronchoalveolar lavage).

PATHOLOGIC FINDINGS

Findings are dependent on site of infection. In general, active infections would be expected to contain innate immune cells and intracellular bacteria.

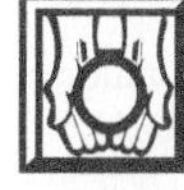

TREATMENT

APPROPRIATE HEALTH CARE

- If hospitalization is required, patient should be isolated and proper personal protective equipment (gloves, gowns, eye or face shield, as indicated) utilized to prevent nosocomial infections of other patients and colonization of caregivers.
- Therapy dependent on location and type of infection.
- Treatment of underlying disease and addressing predisposing risk factor(s) is critical to clear infection and prevent recurrence (e.g., removal of urinary cystoliths to resolve bladder infection).
- Surgical debridement of wound infections may be necessary.

MULTIDRUG-RESISTANT INFECTIONS (CONTINUED)

- Topical antiseptic therapy for localized cutaneous infections, such as MRSP and MRSA, is recommended in lieu of systemic antimicrobials, when possible.

NURSING CARE

- For cutaneous wounds, bandaging is recommended to protect wound and prevent spread of AMR organisms.
- For patients with urinary or gastrointestinal infections, patients should eliminate in areas amenable to disinfection.

ACTIVITY

Social activities such as daycare, boarding, grooming, dog parks, should be avoided until infection is resolved.

DIET

Raw food diets are discouraged due to risk of bacterial pathogen contamination.

M

CLIENT EDUCATION

- Educate clients on potential side effects of antimicrobials.
- Ethical dilemmas regarding using drugs critically important to human medicine should be discussed.
- Educate clients on handwashing and cleaning environment to protect themselves and household from MDR pathogens.

SURGICAL CONSIDERATIONS

N/A

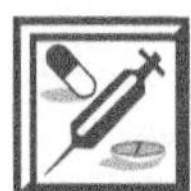

MEDICATIONS

DRUG(S) OF CHOICE

- Antimicrobial therapy should be based upon bacterial culture and susceptibility (C&S) testing.
- Use of highest priority drugs of critical importance for human health is controversial in veterinary medicine. If antimicrobial selection choices are limited to drugs of highest priority (e.g., 3rd and 4th generation cephalosporins, carbapenems) at a minimum, the following criteria should be applied: (1) Use is supported by C&S testing. (2) There is no other reasonable alternative or alternatives are contraindicated for the patient (e.g., aminoglycosides for animal with renal disease). (3) Infection is not improving with current management (e.g., topical therapy, wound debridement, bandaging). (4) There is good chance that treatment will be curative; these drugs should not be used in pets likely to have recurrent infections. (5) A specialist in infectious disease, microbiology, and infectious disease pharmacology should be consulted.

CONTRAINDICATIONS

Immunosuppressive drugs.

PRECAUTIONS

Ensure that bacterial C&S-based antimicrobial decisions are appropriate for site of infection (e.g., choose lipophilic drugs with good tissue penetration if treating parenchymal disease such as pyelonephritis). Inadequate drug concentration at site of infection may lead to further AMR.

POSSIBLE INTERACTIONS

N/A

ALTERNATIVE DRUG(S)

For localized and/or mild superficial pyoderma, topical antiseptics are encouraged in lieu of antimicrobials. These may include chlorhexidine or benzoyl peroxide shampoos, lotions and sprays; acetic, lactic and malic acids, benzoyl peroxide and silver sulfadiazine gels, creams and wipes. Mupirocin ointment may be appropriate topical antimicrobial for MRSA infections if supported by bacterial C&S.

FOLLOW-UP

PATIENT MONITORING

- Confirmation of effective antimicrobial treatment via repeated bacterial culture and cytology should be performed during therapy and after cessation of therapy to ensure resolution.
- Consider reevaluation of patient 72 hours after initiation of therapy to evaluate for expected response.

PREVENTION/AVOIDANCE

- Prevention of AMR infections involves judicious use of antimicrobials. In patients likely to have recurrent infections (e.g., aspiration pneumonia in patients with megaesophagus) using the minimal effective duration of therapy is recommended.
- As nosocomial infections are likely to exhibit AMR, appropriate infection control protocols should be used in veterinary hospital settings.

POSSIBLE COMPLICATIONS

In some cases, side effects of antimicrobial therapy required to treat AMR and MDR infections may result in morbidity, precluding clearance of infection.

EXPECTED COURSE AND PROGNOSIS

AMR and MDR infections are not necessarily more virulent than antimicrobial-susceptible infections. With appropriate antimicrobial selection, dose, and duration of therapy, patients without unresolved predisposing factors are expected to have similar prognosis as those with antimicrobial-susceptible infections.

MISCELLANEOUS

ASSOCIATED CONDITIONS

- Risk factors that break down immune barrier of urinary bladder (e.g., ectopic ureters, urinary calculi, urachal diverticulum, transitional cell carcinoma) are associated with AMR and MDR urinary tract infections.
- Atopy (chronic or recurrent pyoderma).
- Megaesophagus and chronic bronchitis (chronic or recurrent upper and lower respiratory infections).
- Implants (e.g., bone plates) may be associated with surgical site infections.

AGE-RELATED FACTORS

N/A

ZOONOTIC POTENTIAL

There have been sporadic reports of both zoonotic and reverse-zoonotic transmission of AMR and MDR pathogens between animals and humans.

PREGNANCY/FERTILITY/BREEDING

Female dams or bitches can pass AMR bacteria to their offspring, thus causing colonization or infection with AMR organisms despite a lack of previous antimicrobial exposure.

SYNONYMS

- Antibiotic-resistant infection.
- Antimicrobial-resistant infection.

SEE ALSO

Methicillin-Resistant *Staphylococcus*.

ABBREVIATIONS

- AMR = antimicrobial resistance.
- C&S = culture and susceptibility.
- ESBL = extended-spectrum beta-lactamase.
- MDR = multidrug-resistant.
- MRSA = methicillin-resistant *Staphylococcus aureus*.
- MSRP = methicillin-resistant *Staphylococcus pseudintermedius*.

INTERNET RESOURCES

- International Society for Companion Animal Infectious Diseases: www.iscaid.org
- Antimicrobial Resistance and Stewardship Initiative: https://arsi.umn.edu/

Suggested Reading

Weese JS, Giguere S, Guardabassi L, et al. ACVIM consensus statement on therapeutic antimicrobial use in animals and antimicrobial resistance. J Vet Intern Med 2015, 29:487–498.

Author Jennifer L. Granick

Consulting Editor Amie Koenig

MULTIPLE MYELOMA

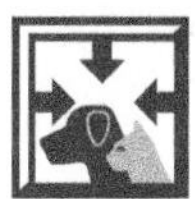

BASICS

OVERVIEW

• Defined as malignant plasma cells in the bone marrow. • Diagnosis requires documentation of bone marrow plasmacytosis, osteolytic bone lesions, and serum or urine myeloma proteins (M-component).

PATHOPHYSIOLOGY

• Proliferation of malignant plasma cells that produce immunoglobulins or subunits.
• Immunoglobulins may polymerize and increase serum viscosity. • Bleeding disorders due to paraprotein coating of platelets, thrombocytopenia, hyperviscosity, or interference with coagulation factors.
• Nephrotoxicity due to protein deposition of amyloid or direct effect of the protein on renal tubular epithelial cells. • Hypercalcemia due to osteoclast activation and bone lysis.

Systems Affected

• Musculoskeletal—multiple punctate areas of bone lysis in the absence of bony proliferation.
• Nervous, cardiovascular, and respiratory—abnormalities secondary to hyperviscosity.
• Soft tissues—neoplastic infiltration.

Incidence/Prevalence

• Dogs—1% of all malignancies; <8% of hematopoietic malignancies; 3.6% of all bone tumors. • Cats—<1% of hematopoietic tumors.

SIGNALMENT

Dogs and cats; 6–13 years.

SIGNS

Due to bone infiltration and lysis, immunoglobulins produced, and infiltration of organ(s).

Dogs

• Lethargy, weakness (62%). • Lameness (47%). • Bleeding diathesis (37%): gingiva and epistaxis. • Funduscopic abnormalities including retinal hemorrhage or detachment and tortuous vessels (35%).

Cats

Anorexia, weight loss, malaise, polydipsia, polyuria.

DIAGNOSIS

DIFFERENTIAL DIAGNOSIS

• Ehrlichiosis, leishmaniosis. • Metastatic bone lesions. • Rheumatoid arthritis.

CBC/BIOCHEMISTRY/URINALYSIS

Dogs

• Hemogram—nonregenerative anemia (66%); neutropenia (25%); thrombocytopenia (33%). • Chemistry—hyperglobulinemia, hypercalcemia (10–25%), azotemia (33%).
• Urinalysis: proteinuria, isosthenuria, cylindruria, pyuria, hematuria, or bacteriuria.

OTHER LABORATORY TESTS

• Serum protein electrophoresis—monoclonal gammopathy in the beta or gamma region, and occasionally a biclonal gammopathy will be present. • Urine protein electrophoresis—Bence-Jones proteins in 25–40%. • Coagulation profile—~50% will have abnormal coagulation values.

IMAGING

• Radiography (dogs)—25–66% have multifocal, lytic lesions or diffuse osteoporosis.
• Radiography (cats)—bony lesions rare, more common for visceral organ infiltration (myeloma-related disorder). • Ultrasonography—detect changes in visceral organs.

DIAGNOSTIC PROCEDURES

• Diagnosis depends on identifying at least 3 of 4 pathologies: ○ Monoclonal gammopathy. ○ Lytic bone lesions. ○ Bence Jones proteinuria. ○ Bone marrow cytology: >20% plasma cells or >5% malignant plasma cells. • For cats—bone marrow involvement is rare, and hence diagnosis is based upon the identification of malignant plasma cells within the visceral organs (myeloma-related disorder).

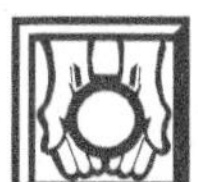

TREATMENT

Appropriate Health Care

• Hospitalization if azotemia, hypercalcemia, bleeding disorder, or bacterial infection.
• Plasmapheresis lowers protein burden—for symptomatic patient, withdraw a volume of venous blood, centrifuge, discard plasma, and return red blood cells to patient in IV crystalloid fluids. • Phlebotomy for hyperviscosity; replace with an equal volume of isotonic fluids IV.
• Always consult a veterinary oncologist for latest information regarding treatment.

Client Education

• Inform client that chemotherapy is palliative but long remissions are possible. • Warn client that relapse will occur. • Discuss side effects, which depend on the drugs used.

Surgical Considerations

Areas nonresponsive to chemotherapy or solitary lesions can be removed surgically.

Radiation Therapy

Radiation therapy can be palliative and highly effective for managing osteolytic bone cancer pain. Indications include painful bone lesions, spinal cord compression, pathologic fractures (after fracture stabilization), or a large soft tissue mass. Consult with a radiation oncologist.

MEDICATIONS

DRUG(S) OF CHOICE

• Dogs—melphalan and prednisone; cyclophosphamide can be used in addition to or in place of melphalan. • Cats—melphalan and prednisone. • IV aminobisphosphonate drugs for management of hypercalcemia and palliation of bone pain. • Consult a veterinary oncologist or reliable drug resource for dosages.

Precautions

• Melphalan—delayed thrombocytopenia.
• Cyclophosphamide—sterile hemorrhagic cystitis.

FOLLOW-UP

PATIENT MONITORING

• CBC and chemistry every 2 weeks for 2 months, then monthly. • Serum electrophoresis and/or Bence Jones proteinuria monthly until at least 50% decrease in baseline values, then once every 2–3 months.

POSSIBLE COMPLICATIONS

Chemotherapy may cause leukopenia or thrombocytopenia, anorexia, alopecia, hemorrhagic cystitis, and/or pancreatitis.

EXPECTED COURSE AND PROGNOSIS

• Improvement in clinical signs and laboratory abnormalities expected within 3–6 weeks. • Radiographic abnormalities could take longer and be partial.

Dogs

• Median survival with alkylating agent and prednisone—18–30 months. • Overall response rate >90%. • Hypercalcemia, extensive bone lysis, or Bence-Jones proteinuria may have shorter survival.
• Death typically due to kidney failure, secondary infections, or bone/spinal pain.

Cats

Survival with alkylating agents and prednisone—2–9 months.

MISCELLANEOUS

SEE ALSO

Hypercalcemia

Suggested Reading

Vail D. Myeloma-related disorders. In: Withrow SJ, Vail DM, Page RL, eds., Small Animal Clinical Oncology, 5th ed. St. Louis, MO: Elsevier Saunders, 2013, pp. 665–678.

Author Shawna L. Klahn
Consulting Editor Timothy M. Fan

Client Education Handout available online

MURMURS, HEART

BASICS

DEFINITION

Vibrations caused by disturbed blood flow.

Timing of Murmurs

- Systolic murmurs occur between S1 and S2 (systole).
- Diastolic murmurs occur between S2 and S1 (diastole).
- Continuous and to-and-fro murmurs occur throughout all or most of the cardiac cycle (systole and diastole).
- Continuous murmurs are usually accentuated near S2 and to-and-fro murmurs are usually absent near S2.

Grading Scale for Murmurs

M

- Grade I—barely audible.
- Grade II—soft, but easily auscultated. Does not radiate far from point of maximal intensity.
- Grade III—intermediate loudness; heard easily some distance from point of maximal intensity (PMI), but not to opposite side of chest; most hemodynamically important murmurs are at least grade III.
- Grade IV—loud murmur radiating widely, often including opposite side of chest.
- Grade V—very loud, audible with stethoscope barely touching the chest; palpable thrill.
- Grade VI—very loud, audible without the stethoscope touching the chest; palpable thrill.

Configuration

- Plateau murmurs have uniform loudness and are typical of atrioventricular (AV) valve regurgitant murmurs such as mitral and tricuspid insufficiency and also ventricular septal defect.
- Crescendo–decrescendo murmurs get louder and then softer and are typical of ejection murmurs such as pulmonic and aortic stenosis and also atrial septal defect.
- Decrescendo murmurs start loud and then get softer and are typical of diastolic murmurs such as aortic or pulmonic insufficiency and mitral or tricuspid stenosis.

Location

Dogs

- Mitral area—left fifth intercostal space at costochondral junction.
- Aortic area—left fourth intercostal space above costochondral junction.
- Pulmonic area—left second to fourth intercostal space at sternal border.
- Tricuspid area—right third to fifth intercostal space near costochondral junction.

Cats

- Mitral area—left fifth to sixth intercostal adjacent to the sterum.
- Aortic area—left second to third intercostal space just above the pulmonic area.
- Pulmonic area—left second to third intercostal space adjacent to the sterum.
- Tricuspid area—right fourth to fifth intercostal space adjacent to the sterum.

PATHOPHYSIOLOGY

- Disturbed blood flow associated with high flow through normal or abnormal valves or with structures vibrating in the blood flow.
- Flow disturbances associated with outflow obstruction or forward flow through stenosed valves or into a dilated great vessel. Intensity of the murmur generally correlates with the severity of the stenosis.
- Flow disturbances associated with regurgitant flow through an incompetent valve, septal defect, or patent ductus arteriosus.

SYSTEMS AFFECTED

Cardiovascular

SIGNALMENT

Dogs and cats.

SIGNS

Relate to cause of the murmur.

CAUSES

Systolic Murmurs

- Myxomatous valve disease (mitral and tricuspid valves).
- Cardiomyopathy and AV valve insufficiency.
- Physiologic flow murmurs.
- Anemia.
- Mitral and tricuspid valve dysplasia.
- Systolic anterior mitral motion.
- Dynamic right ventricular outflow obstruction.
- Dynamic subaortic stenosis.
- Atrial septal defect.
- Ventricular septal defect (VSD).
- Pulmonic stenosis.
- Aortic stenosis.
- Tetralogy of Fallot.
- Mitral and tricuspid valve endocarditis.
- Hyperthyroidism.
- Heartworm disease.

Continuous and To-and-Fro Murmurs

- Patent ductus arteriosus (continuous).
- VSD with aortic regurgitation (to-and-fro).
- Aortic stenosis with aortic regurgitation (to-and-fro).

Diastolic Murmurs

- Mitral and tricuspid valve stenosis.
- Aortic and pulmonic valve endocarditis.

RISK FACTORS

Cardiac disease.

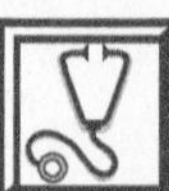

DIAGNOSIS

DIFFERENTIAL DIAGNOSIS

Differential Signs

- Must differentiate from other abnormal heart sounds—split sounds, ejection sounds, gallop sounds, and clicks.
- Must differentiate from abnormal lung sounds and pleural rubs; listen to see if timing of abnormal sound is correlated with respiration or heartbeat.

Differential Causes

- Pale mucous membranes support diagnosis of anemic murmur.
- Location and radiation of murmur and timing during cardiac cycle can help determine cause (see Figure 1).

CBC/BIOCHEMISTRY/URINALYSIS

- Anemia in animals with anemic murmurs.
- Polycythemia in animals with right-to-left shunting congenital defects.
- Leukocytosis with left-shift in animals with endocarditis.

OTHER LABORATORY TESTS

N/A

IMAGING

- Thoracic radiography—useful for evaluating heart size and pulmonary vasculature to help determine cause and significance of murmur.
- Echocardiography—allows definitive diagnosis of cause of murmur.
- Doppler studies sometimes required to confirm cause of murmur.

DIAGNOSTIC PROCEDURES

- Electrocardiography may be useful in assessing heart enlargement patterns in animals with murmurs.
- Blood cultures and serology for *Bartonella* if suspect endocarditis.

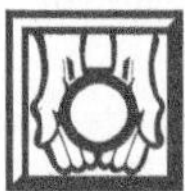

TREATMENT

- Outpatient unless heart failure is evident.
- Base decisions on the cause of the murmur and associated clinical signs.
- None indicated for murmur alone.

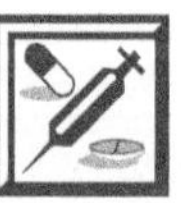

MEDICATIONS

DRUG(S) OF CHOICE

N/A

CONTRAINDICATIONS

N/A

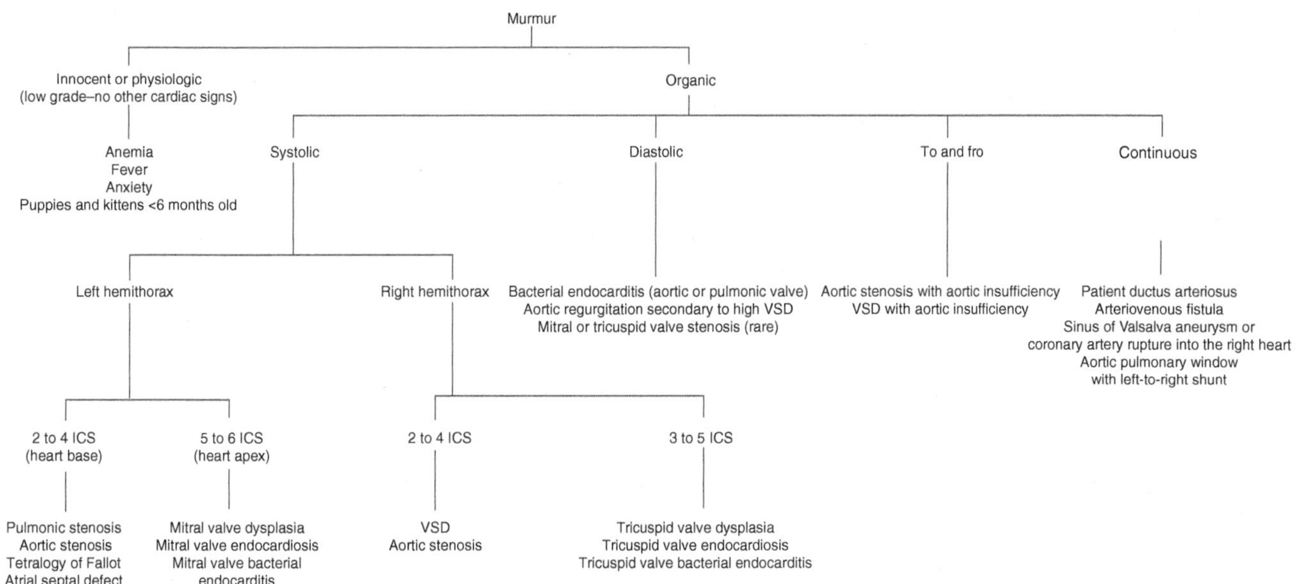

Figure 1.

Algorithm for differential diagnosis of murmurs.

PRECAUTIONS

N/A

POSSIBLE INTERACTIONS

N/A

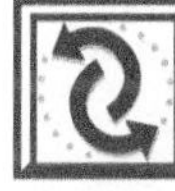

FOLLOW-UP

PATIENT MONITORING

Low-grade systolic ejection murmurs in puppies may be physiologic; most resolve by 6 months of age. If murmur still present after 6 months, include diagnostic imaging.

POSSIBLE COMPLICATIONS

If murmur is associated with structural heart disease, may see signs of congestive heart failure (e.g., coughing, dyspnea, and ascites) or exercise intolerance.

MISCELLANEOUS

ASSOCIATED CONDITIONS

N/A

AGE-RELATED FACTORS

- Murmurs present since birth generally associated with a congenital defect or physiologic flow murmur.
- Acquired murmurs in geriatric, small-breed dogs usually associated with degenerative valve disease.
- Acquired murmurs in large-breed dogs usually associated with dilated cardiomyopathy.
- Acquired murmurs in geriatric cats can be associated with cardiomyopathy, hyperthyroidism or innocent.

ZOONOTIC POTENTIAL

None

PREGNANCY/FERTILITY/BREEDING

Murmurs in puppies and kittens may reflect a congenital defect and thereby influence decisions on breeding that animal or repeating the mating.

ABBREVIATIONS

- AV = atrioventricular.
- PMI = point of maximal intensity.
- S1 = first heart sound.
- S2 = second heart sound.
- VSD = ventricular septal defect.

Suggested Reading

Caivano D, Dickson D, Martin M, Rishniw M. Murmur intensity in adult dogs with pulmonic and subaortic stenosis reflects disease severity. J Small Anim Pract 2018, 59(3):161–166.

Gompf RE. The history and physical examination. In: Smith FWK, Tilley LP, Oyama MA, Sleeper MM, eds, Manual of Canine and Feline Cardiology, 5th ed. St. Louis, MO: Saunders Elsevier, 2016.

Keene B, Smith FWK, Tilley LP, Hansen B. Rapid Interpretation of Heart Sounds, Murmurs, Arrhythmias, and Lung Sounds: A Guide to Cardiac Auscultation in Dogs and Cats, 3rd ed. CD-ROM and Manual. Philadelphia, PA: Elsevier, 2015.

Author Francis W.K. Smith, Jr.
Consulting Editor Michael Aherne

MUSCLE RUPTURE (MUSCLE TEAR)

BASICS

OVERVIEW

A normal muscle may be stretched, pinched, or injured directly, resulting in fiber disruption, weakening, and immediate or delayed separation of the uninjured portions. Alternatively, the muscle structure may be compromised by systemic or iatrogenic conditions, and normal activity may cause muscle disruption. The rupture may be complete or incomplete, and it may be mid-substance or at the muscle–tendon junction. The acute stage is characterized by a typical inflammatory reaction that becomes chronic with collagen maturation, cross-linking, fibrosis, and adhesion development over time. Frequently the acute phase is overlooked, as the signs may be temporary and respond well to rest. The chronic effects are often progressive and unresponsive to support therapies.

M

SIGNALMENT

- Limb and masticatory muscles are the primary structures affected.
- Traumatic injury is indiscriminate, although certain activities may predispose because of exposure.
- The ruptures that are apparently unrelated to trauma seem to affect middle-aged to older working dogs, with no reported sex predilection.
- Cats are affected less frequently than dogs.

SIGNS

Acute Injury

- Immediate lameness that is characterized by the specific muscle affected.
- Localized swelling, heat, and pain.
- Generally present for a few days to a week.
- Animals may experience re-injury.

Chronic Phase (If It Develops)

- Progressive.
- Painless.
- Usually associated with scar tissue that impedes normal function of an extremity.

CAUSES & RISK FACTORS

- Trauma.
- Repeated overuse.
- Overextension.
- Myositis.
- Degenerative (unknown etiology).
- Myopathy secondary to medical conditions such as Cushing disease.
- Apparent risk factor for dogs is involvement in hunting, tracking, or similar activities in the outdoors.

Gait Analysis and Physical Examination Findings

Various disorders will result in characteristic gait abnormalities and pain elicited on specific limb manipulation—a few of which are listed here.

- Psoas muscle injury:
  - Pain on internal rotation with extension or abduction of the pelvic limb.
  - Pain on palpation of the lesser trochanter of the affected femur.
  - Short, choppy gait.
- Gracilis, semimembranosus, and semitendinosus muscle contractures:
  - In late stages, these animals are typically not painful on palpation of the gracilis, semitendinosus or semimembranosus muscles.
  - Palpation of a fibrous band in the area of the affected muscle is also apparent.
  - Shortened stride with medial rotation of the paw, internal rotation of the hock, and external rotation of the calcaneus, with internal rotation of the stifle in late phase of the forward stride.
- Infraspinatus muscle contracture:
  - Significant forelimb lameness with circumduction of the affected limb.
  - Marked elbow adduction/foot abduction; upon flexion of the elbow, the distal antebrachium will deviate laterally.
  - Fibrous band will be apparent on palpation of the infraspinatus muscle.
- Quadriceps contracture:
  - Typically occurs with limb disuse/immobilization after femur fracture fixation in young dogs without appropriate physical therapy.
  - Patient will be unable to flex stifle.
- Achilles mechanism injuries:
  - Non-weight-bearing lameness with soft tissue swelling proximal to the calcaneous for tendinous avulsions (mid-substance tears will present with mid gastroc pain and swelling).
  - Hyperflexion of the tarsus.
  - Hyperflexion of the digits, if superficial digital flexor is unaffected (crab claw).
- Sartorius muscle injury/fibrosis:
  - Scant reports in the veterinary literature.
  - Nonpainful, non-weight-bearing pelvic limb.
  - Palpable fibrous band in the area of the sartorius muscle.
  - Short, choppy gait, characterized by an inability to extend the hip.

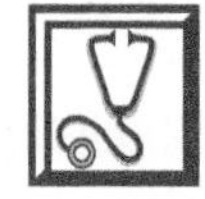

DIAGNOSIS

DIFFERENTIAL DIAGNOSIS

- Neurologic dysfunction—recognized by neurologic abnormalities.
- Tendon rupture—visible or palpable disruption in the tendon.
- Origin/insertion avulsion fracture—radiographic evidence of bone fragment defect and translocation.
- Luxation/subluxation—palpable or radiographic evidence of joint instability or malalignment.

CBC/BIOCHEMISTRY/URINALYSIS

No injury-specific findings.

OTHER LABORATORY TESTS

- Creatine phosphokinase (CPK) may be elevated in acute cases.
- No known specific tests available.

IMAGING

Radiographic Findings

- Soft tissue swelling may be evident in the early stages.
- Calcification of muscle can occur in the traumatized area in chronic situations.
- Avulsion fractures and calcification of the tendon of insertion or origin may be noted on radiographs.

Ultrasonographic Findings

- Local swelling and disorganization of the normal muscle fiber orientation may be seen at the site of injury in acute cases.
- Scar tissue and contracted areas of fibrous tissue can be seen in the muscle in chronic cases—noted as hyperechoic foci in the muscle belly of concern.
- Measurable differences between normal and abnormal sides may be useful in documenting the affected muscle site.

Cross-Sectional Imaging Studies

- CT findings—produces better tissue contrast than the above but still constrained to an axial plane of view.
- MRI findings—edema and hemorrhage cause a change in the signal that can be differentiated from changes due to fibrous tissue replacement of muscle. This allows localization of the problem and helps to identify the type of problem.

DIAGNOSTIC PROCEDURES

Muscle Biopsy

The presence of fibrous tissue and the loss of muscle cells may be documented. Differentiating disuse atrophy from neurologic atrophy and from injury-induced fibrosis may be impossible without corroborating evidence.

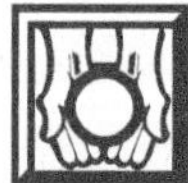

TREATMENT

- There is no documented evidence to support a single "best" way to treat acute muscle injuries, preventing fibrous contracture and adhesions. It is generally believed that immediate post-injury care should involve rest, local cold application followed within hours (24–48 hours) by heat, and passive physical therapy (movement). Severe, strict immobilization (via cast or cage) is potentially contraindicated as it may encourage muscle contracture and muscle fibrosis, leading to irreversible long-term debilitation. Light or non-weight-bearing activity is appropriate for an extended period of time (4–6 weeks). Analgesics and anti-inflammatory drugs should be recommended for several days to weeks. Surgery may be performed within a few days of the injury to repair obvious, acute muscle rupture that results in a separation of the uninjured muscle segments. An essential part of muscle repair is effective tension relief for the injured muscle so that healing can occur without disruption as function returns. Internal or external orthopedic devices may be necessary to provide effective tension relief (transarticular orthopedic implants or orthotics). Owners should be made aware of the possibility of scar-related problems affecting the patient's gait in the long term.

- Once the muscle injury becomes chronic and associated with contracture or adhesions, treatment is aimed at function salvage. Surgical release of the adhesions or fibrous tissue bands is often accompanied by instantaneous symptomatic relief. The prevention of readhesion and progressive contracture is much less rewarding.
- Specific muscle injuries have widely disparate prognoses. Infraspinatus and psoas muscle contractures respond well to surgical excision of the tendon of insertion. Gracilis, semimembranosus, and semitendinosus contractures have a 100% recurrence rate after surgical resection. Quadriceps contracture has a similarly dismal failure rate after surgery.
- Muscle injuries that have healed in an elongated state have a better prognosis for surgical improvement of function than contracted muscles. The most common elongation injury affects the muscles of the calcaneus (Achilles) group. Hock hyperflexion can be surgically reconstructed to return these animals to relatively normal function. This is usually accomplished by shortening the Achilles tendon rather than the injured muscle or musculotendinous junction.

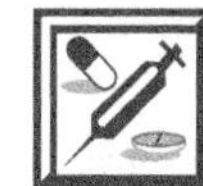

MEDICATIONS

DRUG(S) OF CHOICE

None are specific. Anti-inflammatory drugs may be indicated in acute situations.

CONTRAINDICATIONS/POSSIBLE INTERACTIONS

Immobilization of the injured muscle in a position that allows adhesions to develop to nearby bone will often result in "tie down" contractures.

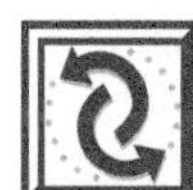

FOLLOW-UP

PATIENT MONITORING

Repetitive range-of-motion monitoring and recheck examination.

PREVENTION/AVOIDANCE

Early inflammation control and non-weight-bearing passive physical therapy accompanied by strict cage rest may be beneficial.

POSSIBLE COMPLICATIONS

Contracture of the muscle and fibrous replacement of muscle tissue.

EXPECTED COURSE AND PROGNOSIS

Specific to the muscle and the type of injury.

MISCELLANEOUS

ASSOCIATED CONDITIONS

Joint hypermobility, angular limb deformities, flexion/extension joint abnormalities.

AGE-RELATED FACTORS

Growth plate fractures in young dogs, particularly distal femoral Salter–Harris fractures, are associated with quadriceps contracture.

ABBREVIATIONS

- CPK = creatine phosphokinase.

Suggested Reading

Vaughan LC. Muscle and tendon injuries in dogs. J Small Anim Pract 1979, 20:711–736.

Author Mathieu M. Glassman
Consulting Editor Mathieu M. Glassman

MUSHROOM TOXICOSES

BASICS

DEFINITION

Cytotoxic Mushroom Poisoning

• *Amanita verna* (European springtime destroying angel), *A. virosa* (destroying angel), *A. phalloides* (death cap, green death cap), *A. bisporigera* (destroying angel), *A. ocreata*, *A. farinosa* and likely many others in the *Amanita* genus. Other important species include *Galerina autumnalis*, *G. marginata* (white rot fungus), *G. venenata* (deadly lawn galerina), *G. sulciceps*, *G. venenata*, *Lepiota helveola*, *L. brunneoincanata*, *L. castanea*, *L. citrophylla*, and *L. subincarnata*. • A number of *Conocybe* species (notably *C. filaris*), which are very commonly found in urban lawns and other urban environments, have been implicated in many cases of fulminant hepatic failure in dogs.

M

Primary Acute Nephrotoxic Mushroom Poisoning

Amanita proxima, *A. pseudoporphyria*, *A. smithiana*.

Delayed Nephrotoxic Mushroom Poisoning

Cortinarius gentilis (deadly cort), *C. orellanus* (fool's webcap), *C. speciosissimus*, *C. splendens*.

Hallucinogenic Mushroom Poisoning

• *Psilocybe* genus (most species). • *Panaeolus foenisecii* (haymaker mushroom), *P. fimicola*, *P. subbalteatus*. • *Conocybe smithii* (bog conocybe). • *Gymnopilus junonius* (big laughing gym). • *Copelandia* genus. • *Pluteus* genus. • Possibly *Stropharia* genus. • Liquid extracts are commonly sold.

Autonomic Toxicity Mushroom Poisoning

• *Clitocybe* genus (most species). • *Inocybe* genus (most species).

Psychoactive *Isoxazole* Mushroom Poisoning

Amanita cokeri (Coker's amanita), *A. cothurnata*, *A. gemmate*, *A. muscaria* (fly agaric, fly mushroom, fly amanita, Satan's mushroom, sacred mushroom), *A. pantherina*.

Rapid-Onset Myotoxic Mushroom Poisoning

Russula subnigricans.

Delayed-Onset Myotoxic Mushroom Poisoning

Tricholoma equestre.

Gamma-Aminobutyric Acid (GABA) Antagonist Mushroom Poisoning

Gyrometra genus (many species; false morels).

Gastrointestinal (GI) Irritant Mushroom Poisoning

A wide variety of mushrooms can induce GI irritation when ingested.

• Paxillus syndrome: *Paxillus involutus* (brown roll-rim, poisonous paxillus, brown chantarelle, roll-rim fungus).

PATHOPHYSIOLOGY

Cytotoxic Mushroom Poisoning

• Major toxins are amatoxins (bicyclic octapeptides with an indole-(*R*)-sulfoxide bridge), phallotoxins (cyclic heptapeptides with an indole/thio-etherbridge), and/or virotoxins (heptapeptides have a monocyclic structure, this includes 2-methylsulfonyltryptophan or 2-methylsulfoxytryptophan and dihydroxyproline). • Critically, amatoxins are heat stable and not inactivated by cooking. • Phallotoxins do not cause poisoning when ingested. • The major mode of action is inhibition of RNA polymerase II, resulting in cell death.

Primary Acute Nephrotoxic Mushroom Poisoning

Major toxin is aminohexadienoic acid, which produces rapid-onset (latent period of 30 minutes to 12 hours), fulminant nephrotoxicity.

Delayed Nephrotoxic Mushroom Poisoning

• Major toxins are orellanine and orelline. • Inhibit DNA and RNA polymerases. • A typical *C. orellanus* mushroom contains 15–20 mg of orellanine.

Hallucinogenic Mushroom Poisoning

• Major toxins are psilocybin and psilocin; psilocybin is a pro-toxin which is metabolized to the active toxin psilocin. • Purchased hallucinogenic mushrooms may be laced with LSD (lysergic acid diethylamide), phencyclidine, and/or ketamine. • Hallucinogenic mushrooms are often incorporated into bars of chocolate to aid ingestion (the mushrooms often have an astringent taste).

Autonomic Toxicity Mushroom Poisoning

• Major toxin is L-(+)-muscarine. • Other muscarine enantiomers are commonly present but are much less potent and less important in cases of poisoning. • L-(+)-Muscarine forms a very stable chlorine salt. • Heating, boiling, and drying does not inactivate the toxin. • Clinical signs reflect muscarinic parasympathetic nervous system stimulation and a muscarinic cholinergic crisis.

Psychoactive Isoxazole Mushroom Poisoning

• Major toxins are ibotenic acid and its decarboxylated derivative muscimol. • Act as GABA antagonists. • Muscarine is present in small amounts. • *A. pantherina* may also contain amatoxins; however, hepatotoxicity with this species appears to be very rare.

Rapid-Onset Myotoxic Mushroom Poisoning

• The major myotoxin is cycloprop-2-ene carboxylic acid. • A number of other cytotoxic toxins (russuphelins) have been identified. • Mushroom also contains a gastrointestinal toxin and cadmium.

Delayed-Onset Myotoxic Mushroom Poisoning

Major toxins are unknown.

GABA Antagonist Mushroom Poisoning

• Major pro-toxin is gyromitrin. • In the digestive tract gyromitrin forms monomethylhydrazine, the ultimate toxin. • Monomethylhydrazine reacts with pyridoxal-5-phosphate forming a hydrozone, which decreases glutamic acid decarboxylase activity and decreases formation of GABA. • Gyromitrin also forms methyl-*N*-formylhydrazine, which is hepatotoxic. • Gyromitrin is a carcinogen. • Uncooked or partially cooked mushrooms have a higher toxicity than fully cooked mushrooms (gyromitrin is volatile).

GI Irritant Mushroom Poisoning

A diverse array of toxins is involved but they produce clinically similar effects.

Paxillus Syndrome

• Major toxins include involutin (a diphenylcyclopenteneone compound). • An antigen of an unknown structure in the fungus stimulates the formation of IgG antibodies in the blood serum. In subsequent meals the antigen–antibody complexes are formed and become attached to the surface of erythrocytes, causing their agglutination and hemolysis.

SYSTEMS AFFECTED

Cytotoxic Mushroom Poisoning

Intestine, liver and kidneys; pancreatitis reported with *A. phalloides*; cellular injury is widespread, but typically the liver is the major target organ.

Primary Acute Nephrotoxic Mushroom Poisoning

Kidneys

Delayed Nephrotoxic Mushroom Poisoning

Kidneys

Hallucinogenic Mushroom Poisoning

• CNS. • Liver, kidneys, and GI systems with mistaken ingestion of other toxic species

Autonomic Toxicity Mushroom Poisoning

Muscarinic parasympathetic nervous system.

Psychoactive Isoxazole Mushroom Poisoning

CNS

Rapid-Onset Myotoxic Mushroom Poisoning

Musculoskeletal system.

Delayed-Onset Myotoxic Mushroom Poisoning

Musculoskeletal system.

GABA Antagonist Mushroom Poisoning

CNS

GI Irritant Mushroom Poisoning

GI tract.

Paxillus Syndrome

- GI tract.
- Erythron.

GEOGRAPHIC DISTRIBUTION

Worldwide; classically fruiting occurs during spring to autumn.

SIGNS

Cytotoxic Mushroom Poisoning

Patients commonly presented with fulminant hepatic failure or found dead with fulminant hepatic failure of "unknown origin" identified during necropsy. The classical clinical course occurs over a 7-day period:

• Day 1: Mushroom meal and symptom-free interval (6–12 hours). • Day 2: GI phase with vomiting, abdominal pain, diarrhea. • Day 3: Apparent symptomatic remission, but laboratory evidence of developing liver damage. • Day 4: Coagulopathy develops and GI bleeding commences. • Day 5: Onset of hepatic encephalopathy, onset of hepatic coma. • Day 6: Renal failure. • Day 7: Death.

Primary Acute Nephrotoxic Mushroom Poisoning

• Rapid-onset, acute, fulminant renal failure with a 30-minute to 12-hour post-ingestion latency period. • Clinical presentation resembles nonspecific acute renal failure.

Delayed Nephrotoxic Mushroom Poisoning

Delayed-onset, acute, fulminant renal failure with a 36-hour to 17-day post-ingestion latency period.

Hallucinogenic Mushroom Poisoning

• Latency is typically 10–30 minutes post ingestion. • Clinical signs reflect auditory, visual (e.g., biting at invisible flies) or tactile hallucinations with the degree of clinical signs being dose-dependent. • Most CNS reactions are euphoric or excitatory; however, aggression can be enhanced in some cases. • Clinical signs attributable to anxiety, agitation, and ataxia may occur. • Other effects include pupillary dilation, nausea, abdominal pain, vomiting, yawning, parasthesiae, hyperreflexia, tachycardia, hypertension, cardiac arrhythmias, and myocardial ischemic effects. • Convulsions can occur, but are more likely in young animals.
• CNS depression can occur late in the clinical course. • For unadulterated mushrooms the clinical course is typically less than 1 hour; if longer than this ingestion of LSD and/or phencyclidine (effects may last >12 hours) should be considered. • *Beware*—ongoing convulsive episodes, myocardial ischemia, hyperthermia, and rhabdomyolysis are possible, particularly with adulterated mushrooms.

Autonomic Toxicity Mushroom Poisoning

• Onset is typically 15 minutes to 2 hours post ingestion. • The clinical course is dose-dependent: about 2 hours in mild cases and up to 1 day in more severe cases. • *Remember*: DUMBELS—diarrhea, urination, miosis, bradycardia/bronchorrhea/bronchoconstriction, emesis, lacrimation, and salivation. • Impaired sight due to impaired accommodation. • Hypotension, vasodilation, and circulatory shock may occur.

Psychoactive Isoxazole Mushroom Poisoning

• Onset is typically within minutes to 3 hours post ingestion. • The typical clinical course is an initial period of drowsiness followed by a period of manic excitement with visual hallucinations (e.g. biting at invisible flies) and bizarre behavior lasting up to 48 hours. This is then followed by a period of deep CNS depression during which intense dreaming has been reported in humans. • Ataxia, incoordination, dizziness, mydriasis, myoclonus, muscle fasciculation/tremors, hyporeflexia, coma, and convulsions (in severe poisoning) can occur.
• Rarely vomiting and/or diarrhea can occur

Rapid-Onset Myotoxic Mushroom Poisoning

• Onset is typically within 2 hours post ingestion. • The initial phase (2–24 hours post ingestion) consists of acute gastroenteritis which may resolve over the next 24 hours. • The later phase, developing around 6–12 hours post ingestion, consists of muscle pain, myalgias, rhabdomyolysis, myoglobinuria, hypertension, dehydration, renal failure, hyperkalemia, arrhythmias, myocarditis, and cardiovascular collapse. • Respiratory failure, acute renal failure, pulmonary edema, ventricular tachycardia, and circulatory shock have been recorded in humans. • In fatal cases, death ensues within 12–24 hours post ingestion.

Delayed-Onset Myotoxic Mushroom Poisoning

Resembles acute myotoxic poisoning except onset is delayed typically for 24 hours with resolution over about 15 days in survivors.

GABA Antagonist Mushroom Poisoning

• Onset is unpredictable.
• Most cases result in mild, self-limiting GI disturbance starting 6–12 hours post ingestion. • Cases of severe poisoning may or may not present with an initial GI upset phase followed by hepatorenal toxicity plus neurological disturbance (seizures, mydriasis, muscle fasciculations progressing to coma). Multiorgan failure is common in severe cases.
• Methemoglobinemia and hemoglobinuria occurs in some cases. • Hydrazines also affect the cross-linking of collagen and have been associated with dissecting aortic aneurysms.

GI Irritant Mushroom Poisoning

• Onset is typically 1–3 hours post ingestion.
• Clinical signs include vomiting, abdominal pain and diarrhea. • Fluid and electrolyte disturbances can be severe, particularly in small animals. • Disseminated intravascular coagulation and renal failure can occur.
• GI upset is usually short and self-limiting.

Paxillus Syndrome

• Self-limiting GI upset. • Immune mediate hemolytic anemia. • Sensitivity to the mushroom builds up with repeated ingestion over a period of years.

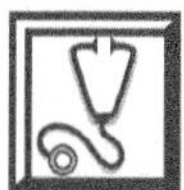

DIAGNOSIS

CBC/BIOCHEMISTRY/URINALYSIS

Cytotoxic Mushroom Poisoning

• Early stages—resembles per-acute/acute gastroenteritis (fluid loss, hypovolemia, serum ion disturbances). • Later stages—typically reflect fulminant hepatic failure with massive increases in serum liver enzymes, hyperbilirubinemia, and coagulopathy.

M

Primary Acute Nephrotoxic Mushroom Poisoning

Reflects acute oliguric/anuric renal failure following acute renal tubular necrosis.

Delayed Nephrotoxic Mushroom Poisoning

Reflects acute oliguric/anuric renal failure following acute renal tubular necrosis.

Hallucinogenic Mushroom Poisoning

Nonspecific

Autonomic Toxicity Mushroom Poisoning

Nonspecific

Psychoactive Isoxazole Mushroom Poisoning

Nonspecific

Rapid-Onset Myotoxic Mushroom Poisoning

• Serum chemistry results may reflect acute renal failure with massively elevated serum creatine kinase; other serum chemistry changes may include increased lactate dehydrogenase and increased transaminases. • Hyperkalemia and hypocalcemia are often prominent.
• Urinalysis may indicate myoglobinuria.

Delayed-Onset Myotoxic Mushroom Poisoning

As per rapid-onset myotoxic mushroom poisoning.

GABA Antagonist Mushroom Poisoning

• CBC may indicate oxidative damage to erythrocytes (e.g., Heinz body formation) and hemolysis. • Methemoglobinemia is present in some cases. • Evidence of liver damage (increased serum transaminases) may occur in some cases. • Hyper- and hypoglycemia can occur. • Hypovolemia and serum ion

MUSHROOM TOXICOSES (CONTINUED)

abnormalities may occur following GI damage. • Coagulopathies occur in some cases.

GI Irritant Mushroom Poisoning
Reflect fluid loss and serum ion disturbances.

Paxillus Syndrome
Reflect fluid loss and serum ion disturbances and immune-mediated anemia.

OTHER LABORATORY TESTS

Uneaten mushrooms should be placed in a dry paper bag for transport to an expert mycologist.

DIAGNOSTIC PROCEDURES

Identification of uneaten mushrooms or spores in gastric contents by an experienced mycologist

Cytotoxic Mushroom Poisoning
• Meixner test is unreliable. • Serum and urine amatoxins have no clinical value.

M

Primary Acute Nephrotoxic Mushroom Poisoning
Aminohexadienoic acid determination in body fluids and kidney is possible but rarely performed.

Delayed Nephrotoxic Mushroom Poisoning
In renal biopsy tissue, orellanine is detectable by thin-layer chromatography up to 6 months after poisoning.

Hallucinogenic Mushroom Poisoning
Psilocybin and psilocin can be measured in blood, plasma, serum, and urine; detection period in urine is typically about 3 days.

Autonomic Toxicity Mushroom Poisoning
Response to low-dose treatment with atropine can be considered.

Psychoactive Isoxazole Mushroom Poisoning
Nonspecific

Rapid-Onset Myotoxic Mushroom Poisoning
Nonspecific

Delayed-Onset Myotoxic Mushroom Poisoning
Nonspecific

GABA Antagonist Mushroom Poisoning
Nonspecific

GI Irritant Mushroom Poisoning
Nonspecific

Paxillus Syndrome
Nonspecific.

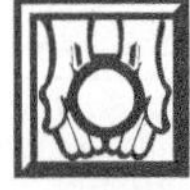

TREATMENT

APPROPRIATE HEALTH CARE

Cytotoxic Mushroom Poisoning
• Early euthanasia in confirmed cases should be considered. • Cases of suspect ingestion should be hospitalized for observation for at least 3–4 days.

Primary Acute Nephrotoxic Mushroom Poisoning
Cases of suspect ingestion should be hospitalized for observation for at least 3–4 days

Delayed Nephrotoxic Mushroom Poisoning
Cases of suspect ingestion require careful and repeated assessment of renal status for up to 17 days.

Hallucinogenic Mushroom Poisoning
Cases of suspect ingestion should be hospitalized for observation.

Autonomic Toxicity Mushroom Poisoning
Cases of suspect ingestion should be hospitalized for observation.

Psychoactive Isoxazole Mushroom Poisoning
Cases of suspect ingestion should be hospitalized for observation.

Rapid-Onset Myotoxic Mushroom Poisoning
• Early euthanasia in confirmed cases should be considered. • Cases of suspect ingestion should be hospitalized and may require urgent treatment.

Delayed-Onset Myotoxic Mushroom Poisoning
As per rapid-onset myotoxic mushroom poisoning.

GABA Antagonist Mushroom Poisoning
Cases of suspect ingestion should be hospitalized for observation.

GI Irritant Mushroom Poisoning
Cases of suspect ingestion should be hospitalized for observation.

Paxillus Syndrome
Cases of suspect ingestion should be hospitalized for observation.

NURSING CARE

Cytotoxic Mushroom Poisoning
• Observation, fluid resuscitation, and electrolyte replacement as required. • If a confirmed case presents within 1-4 hours post ingestion (very unusual), gastric lavage and oral activated charcoal treatment (for up to the first 36 hours) could be considered. • Hemoperfusion and plasmapheresis are ineffective. • Therapeutic total plasma exchange could be considered.

Primary Acute Nephrotoxic Mushroom Poisoning
• If a confirmed case presents within 1–4 hours post ingestion (very unusual), gastric lavage could be considered. • Treatment as per any form of acute renal failure.

Delayed Nephrotoxic Mushroom Poisoning
• Given the long latency period, patients are unlikely to be presented early enough for GI decontamination to be of any benefit. • Treatment as per any form of acute renal failure.

Hallucinogenic Mushroom Poisoning
• Simple supportive care consisting of placement in a dark, quiet room with the owner is often effective for simple hallucinogenic mushroom poisoning. • *Beware*—risk of self-injury is present.

Autonomic Toxicity Mushroom Poisoning
• If a confirmed case presents within 1–4 hours post ingestion (very unusual), gastric lavage and/or single-dose activated charcoal treatment could be considered. • Careful hemodynamic and electrocardiographic monitoring is recommended. • Fluid resuscitation and careful electrolyte monitoring may be required if diarrhea is severe.

Psychoactive Isoxazole Mushroom Poisoning
• Treatment is primarily supportive. • Placing in a dark, quiet environment in the presence of the owner may be helpful. • *Beware*—risk of self-injury is present.

Rapid-Onset Myotoxic Mushroom Poisoning
• If a confirmed case presents within 1–4 hours post ingestion (very unusual), gastric lavage and/or single-dose activated charcoal treatment could be considered. • Fluid resuscitation and careful electrolyte monitoring and management is required.

Delayed-Onset Myotoxic Mushroom Poisoning
As per rapid-onset myotoxic mushroom poisoning.

GABA Antagonist Mushroom Poisoning
Fluid resuscitation and careful electrolyte monitoring may be required.

GI Irritant Mushroom Poisoning
Fluid resuscitation and careful electrolyte monitoring are the mainstays of treatment.

Paxillus Syndrome
Fluid resuscitation and careful electrolyte monitoring are the mainstays of treatment.

ACTIVITY

As needed and clinically justifiable.

MEDICATIONS

DRUG(S) OF CHOICE

Cytotoxic Mushroom Poisoning
• There are no specific antidotes. • Silibinin (20–40 mg/kg/day in divided doses) may have

limited value. • Penicillin G (300,000–1 million U/kg/day) may have limited value. • IV glucose during hepatic failure phase. • Fresh frozen plasma and vitamin K if coagulopathy is present.

Primary Acute Nephrotoxic Mushroom Poisoning

As per any form of acute renal failure.

Delayed Nephrotoxic Mushroom Poisoning

As per any form of acute renal failure.

Hallucinogenic Mushroom Poisoning

• For severe reactions, longer acting benzodiazepines such as diazepam may be useful.
• Convulsions can be managed by the use of barbiturates. • *Beware*—reactions lasting longer than an hour or so may indicate LSD, ketamine, or phencyclidine poisoning.

Autonomic Toxicity Mushroom Poisoning

• Mild cases may not require drug treatment.
• In moderate to severe cases the drug of choice (and antidote) is atropine administered slowly and carefully to effect (the key clinical endpoint is the drying of respiratory secretions, not pupil size). • Fluid resuscitation and careful electrolyte monitoring may be required if diarrhea is severe.

Psychoactive Isoxazole Mushroom Poisoning

• Typically monitoring and prevention of self-injury is sufficient. • Benzodiazepines such as diazepam could be considered during the manic phase.

Rapid-Onset Myotoxic Mushroom Poisoning

• Nonspecific symptomatic and supportive care is required. • The major priorities are fluid and electrolyte management. • Dantrolene could be considered.

Delayed-Onset Myotoxic Mushroom Poisoning

As per rapid-onset myotoxic mushroom poisoning.

GABA Antagonist Mushroom Poisoning

• Pyridoxine (vitamin B6) can be used as an "antidote" in treatment of convulsions or coma at about 25 mg/kg IV over 15–20 minutes.
• Methylene blue 1 mg/kg IV over 5–30 minutes; if the methemoglobin level remains greater than 30% or if symptoms persist, a repeat dose of 1 mg/kg IV may be given 1 hour after the first dose; if methemoglobinemia does not resolve after 2 doses, consider alternative interventions if methemoglobinemia is clinically significant. • Benzodiazepines and barbiturates may be useful if CNS excitation is present.

GI Irritant Mushroom Poisoning

Mainstay of treatment is fluid resuscitation and electrolyte management.

Paxillus Syndrome

Mainstay of treatment is fluid resuscitation and electrolyte management.

FOLLOW-UP

PATIENT MONITORING

Cytotoxic Mushroom Poisoning

• Survival is unlikely following clinically significant ingestions. • Survivors of fulminant liver failure require ongoing monitoring of liver and kidney functions and monitoring of the coagulation system.

Primary Acute Nephrotoxic Mushroom Poisoning

• Survival is possible. • Ongoing monitoring of renal function is recommended.

Delayed Nephrotoxic Mushroom Poisoning

• Survival is possible. • Ongoing monitoring of renal function is recommended.

Hallucinogenic Mushroom Poisoning

Risk of reexposure if owners are consumers of hallucinogens.

Autonomic Toxicity Mushroom Poisoning

Outcome is typically good when supportive care is provided.

Psychoactive Isoxazole Mushroom Poisoning

Outcome is typically good when supportive care is provided.

Rapid-Onset Myotoxic Mushroom Poisoning

• Survival is rare. • Severe muscle damage is likely in survivors.

Delayed-Onset Myotoxic Mushroom Poisoning

As per rapid-onset myotoxic mushroom poisoning.

GABA Antagonist Mushroom Poisoning

• Poisoning is often severe.
• Multiorgan failure (primary, or secondary to hemolysis or hepatorenal failure) occurs in severe cases.

GI Irritant Mushroom Poisoning

GI damage can be severe, but recovery is usual.

Paxillus Syndrome

• GI damage is typically mild and self-limiting. • Require monitoring for immune mediated anemia.

PREVENTION/AVOIDANCE

Prevent dogs roaming, control mushrooms in areas where animals are kept.

EXPECTED COURSE AND PROGNOSIS

Cytotoxic Mushroom Poisoning

Survival following clinically significant ingestion is unlikely; the major determinant of survival is the amount of amatoxins ingested.

Primary Acute Nephrotoxic Mushroom Poisoning

• Poorly documented in veterinary species.
• Survival is possible with appropriate treatment.

Delayed Nephrotoxic Mushroom Poisoning

• Poorly documented in veterinary species.
• Survival is possible with appropriate treatment.

Hallucinogenic Mushroom Poisoning

Prognosis is typically good provided misadventure is prevented.

Autonomic Toxicity Mushroom Poisoning

Prognosis is typically good with symptomatic and supportive care.

Psychoactive Isoxazole Mushroom Poisoning

Outcome is typically good when supportive care is provided.

Rapid-Onset Myotoxic Mushroom Poisoning

Survival is rare.

Delayed-Onset Myotoxic Mushroom Poisoning

Survival is rare.

GABA Antagonist Mushroom Poisoning

• Many cases are mild. • Evidence of hepatorenal failure indicates a poor prognosis.

GI Irritant Mushroom Poisoning

Prognosis is typically good with symptomatic and supportive care.

Paxillus Syndrome

Prognosis is reasonable provided reexposure to the mushrooms does not reoccur.

MISCELLANEOUS

AGE-RELATED FACTORS

Young animals or animals that are inexperienced with a specific location are possibly more likely to be poisoned.

SYNONYMS

Mushroom poisoning; shroom poisoning.

ABBREVIATIONS

• GABA = γ-aminobutyric acid.
• GI = gastrointestinal.
• LSD = lysergic acid diethylamide.

INTERNET RESOURCES

http://www.toxinology.com/index.cfm

Author Rhian Cope
Consulting Editor Lynn R. Hovda

MYASTHENIA GRAVIS

BASICS

DEFINITION

A disorder of neuromuscular transmission characterized by muscular weakness and excessive fatigability.

PATHOPHYSIOLOGY

Transmission failure at the neuromuscular junction—results from structural or functional abnormalities of the nicotinic acetylcholine receptors (AChRs) or other end-plate proteins and enzymes (congenital form) and from autoantibody-mediated destruction of AChRs and postsynaptic membranes (acquired form).

SYSTEMS AFFECTED

- Neuromuscular—result of abnormalities or destruction of AChRs, choline acetyltransferase or end-plate cholinesterase.
- Respiratory—may find aspiration pneumonia secondary to megaesophagus.

GENETICS

- Congenital familial forms—Jack Russell terrier, springer spaniel, smooth fox terrier; smooth-haired miniature dachshund, Gammel Dansk hønsehund, Labrador retriever; autosomal recessive mode of inheritance.
- Acquired—as with other autoimmune diseases, requires appropriate genetic background for disease to occur; multifactorial, involving environmental, infectious, and hormonal influences.
- Familial forms of acquired myasthenia gravis (MG) occur in the Newfoundland and Great Dane breeds.

INCIDENCE/PREVALENCE

- Congenital—rare.
- Acquired—not uncommon in dogs; uncommon in cats.

GEOGRAPHIC DISTRIBUTION

Worldwide

SIGNALMENT

Species

Dogs and cats.

Breed Predilections

- Congenital—Jack Russell terriers; springer spaniels; smooth fox terriers; smooth-haired miniature dachshunds, Gammel Dansk hønsehund. Labrador retriever.
- Acquired—several breeds: golden retrievers; German shepherd dogs; Labrador retrievers; dachshunds; Scottish terriers; Akitas; and Abyssinian and Somali cats.

Mean Age and Range

- Congenital—6–8 weeks of age.
- Acquired—bimodal age of onset; dogs: 1–4 years of age and 9–13 years of age.

Predominant Sex

- Congenital—none.
- Acquired—may be a slight predilection for females in the young age group; none in the old age group.

SIGNS

General Comments

- Acquired—may have several clinical presentations ranging from focal involvement of the esophageal, pharyngeal, and extraocular muscles to acute generalized collapse.
- Should be on the differential diagnosis of any dog with acquired megaesophagus, lower motor neuron weakness, or a cranial mediastinal mass.

Historical Findings

- Regurgitation—common; important to differentiate between vomiting and regurgitation.
- Voice change.
- Exercise-related weakness.
- Acute collapse.
- Progressive weakness.
- Sleep with eyes open.

Physical Examination Findings

- Patient may look normal at rest.
- Excessive drooling, regurgitation, and repeated attempts at swallowing.
- Muscle atrophy—usually not found.
- Dyspnea—with aspiration pneumonia.
- Fatigue or cramping—with mild exercise.
- Careful neurologic examination—subtle findings: decreased or absent palpebral reflex (may be fatigable); may note a poor or absent gag reflex; spinal reflexes usually normal but fatigable (rarely absent and dog unable to support its weight).
- Ventroflexion of the neck (cats, uncommon in dogs).

CAUSES

- Congenital.
- Immune-mediated.
- Paraneoplastic.

RISK FACTORS

- Appropriate genetic background.
- Neoplasia—particularly thymoma.
- Methimazole treatment (cats)—may result in reversible disease.
- Vaccination can exacerbate active MG.
- Intact female.

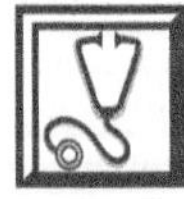

DIAGNOSIS

DIFFERENTIAL DIAGNOSIS

- Other disorders of neuromuscular transmission—tick paralysis; botulism; cholinesterase toxicity.
- Acute or chronic polyneuropathies.
- Polymyopathies—including polymyositis.
- Diagnosis depends upon a careful history, thorough physical and neurologic examinations, and specialized laboratory testing.

CBC/BIOCHEMISTRY/URINALYSIS

- Normal.
- Serum creatine kinase activity—usually normal; may be elevated if MG is associated with polymyositis and concurrent thymoma.

OTHER LABORATORY TESTS

- Serum AChR antibody titer—diagnostic for acquired form.
- Thyroid and adrenal function—may see abnormalities associated with acquired form.

IMAGING

Thoracic radiographs—megaesophagus; cranial mediastinal mass, aspiration pneumonia.

DIAGNOSTIC PROCEDURES

- Ultrasound-guided biopsy of cranial mediastinal mass—may support diagnosis of thymoma.
- Dramatic increase in muscle strength after administration of edrophonium chloride 0.1 mg/kg IV—may see false-negative and false-positive responses.
- Decreased or absent palpebral reflex—may return after edrophonium chloride administration.
- Electrophysiologic evaluation—necessity questionable with increased availability of AChR antibody testing; many patients with acquired form are poor anesthetic risks.
- Electrocardiogram—with bradycardia; third-degree heart block has been documented in some patients with acquired disease.

PATHOLOGIC FINDINGS

Biopsy of a cranial mediastinal mass may reveal thymoma, thymic hyperplasia, or thymic atrophy.

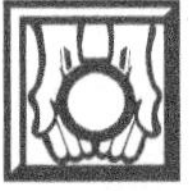

TREATMENT

APPROPRIATE HEALTH CARE

- Inpatient—until adequate dosages of anticholinesterase drugs are achieved.
- Aspiration pneumonia—may require intensive care.
- Gastrostomy tube—may be required if patient is unable to eat or drink without significant regurgitation.

NURSING CARE

- Oxygen therapy, intensive antibiotic therapy, IV fluid therapy, and supportive care—generally required for aspiration pneumonia.
- Nutritional maintenance with a gastrostomy tube—multiple feedings of a high-caloric diet; good hygiene care.
- Elevation of food and water.

ACTIVITY

Self-limited owing to the severity of muscle weakness and extent of aspiration pneumonia.

DIET

May try different consistencies of food—gruel; hard food; soft food; evaluate what is best tolerated.

CLIENT EDUCATION

- Warn client that, although the acquired disease is treatable, most patients require months of special feeding and medication.
- Inform client that a dedicated owner is important to a favorable outcome for acquired myasthenia.
- Prognosis is poor for congenital myasthenic syndrome.

SURGICAL CONSIDERATIONS

- Cranial mediastinal mass—thymoma.
- Before attempting surgical removal, stabilize patient with anticholinesterase drugs and treat aspiration pneumonia.
- Weakness may not be clinically evident initially.
- Suspected thymoma—test all patients for acquired MG before surgery.

MEDICATIONS

DRUG(S) OF CHOICE

- Anticholinesterase drugs—prolong the action of acetylcholine at the neuromuscular junction; pyridostigmine bromide tablets or syrup (Mestinon syrup, diluted half and half in water) at 1–3 mg/kg PO q8–12h.
- Corticosteroids 0.5 mg/kg q24h; initiated if there is a poor response to pyridostigmine or if there is no response to the edrophonium chloride challenge.

CONTRAINDICATIONS

Avoid drugs that may reduce the safety margin of neuromuscular transmission—aminoglycoside antibiotics; antiarrhythmic agents; phenothiazines; anesthetics; narcotics; muscle relaxants; magnesium.

PRECAUTIONS

- Avoid large volumes of barium for evaluating megaesophagus.
- Large air-filled esophagus seen on survey radiographs—barium study not indicated.
- Avoid immunosuppressive dosages of prednisone—may worsen muscle weakness.
- Avoid unnecessary vaccinations.

POSSIBLE INTERACTIONS

N/A

ALTERNATIVE DRUG(S)

- Azathioprine 2 mg/kg PO through gastrostomy tube q24h. Taper to q48h when clinical remission of the disease.
- Mycophenolate 20 mg/kg PO q12h. Reduce dosage by 50% once significant improvement or resolution of clinical signs is noted.

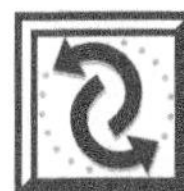

FOLLOW-UP

PATIENT MONITORING

- Return of muscle strength should be evident.
- Thoracic radiographs—evaluated every 4–6 weeks for resolution of megaesophagus.
- AChR antibody titers—evaluated every 8–12 weeks; decrease to the normal range with immune remission.

PREVENTION/AVOIDANCE

N/A

POSSIBLE COMPLICATIONS

- Aspiration pneumonia.
- Respiratory arrest.

EXPECTED COURSE AND PROGNOSIS

- No severe aspiration pneumonia or pharyngeal weakness—good prognosis for complete recovery; resolution usually within 6–8 months.
- Thymoma present—guarded prognosis unless complete surgical removal and control of myasthenic signs are achieved.

MISCELLANEOUS

ASSOCIATED CONDITIONS

- Other autoimmune disorders—thyroiditis; skin disorders; hypoadrenocorticism, thrombocytopenia, hemolytic anemia, inflammatory bowel disease.
- Disorders of the thymus—thymoma; thymic hyperplasia.
- Other neoplasias.

AGE-RELATED FACTORS

Bimodal age of onset—1–4 years of age and 9–13 years of age.

ZOONOTIC POTENTIAL

N/A

PREGNANCY/FERTILITY/BREEDING

- In humans, weakness may improve during pregnancy but worsens after delivery; some neonates of affected mothers have a temporary MG-like weakness that lasts several days to weeks that is due to *in utero* transfer of autoantibodies from the mother.
- Documented in dogs after whelping.

SEE ALSO

- Chapters covering autoimmune diseases.
- Megaesophagus.

ABBREVIATIONS

- AChR = acetylcholine receptor.
- MG = myasthenia gravis.

INTERNET RESOURCES

Comparative Neuromuscular Laboratory: http://vetneuromuscular.ucsd.edu

Suggested Reading

Khorzad R, Whelan M, Sisson A, Shelton GD. Myasthenia gravis in dogs with an emphasis on treatment and critical care management. Vet Emerg Crit Care 2011, 21:193–208.

Mace S, Shelton GD, Eddlestone S. Megaesophagus. Compend Contin Edu Vet 2012, 34:E1–8.

Shelton GD. Myasthenia gravis and disorders of neuromuscular transmission. Vet Clin North Am 2002, 31:189–200.

Shelton GD. Routine and specialized laboratory testing for the diagnosis of neuromuscular diseases in dogs and cats. Vet Clin Pathol 2010, 39:278–295.

Shelton GD. Treatment of autoimmune myasthenia gravis. In: Bonagura JD, Twedt DC, eds., Current Veterinary Therapy XIV. Philadelphia, PA: Saunders, 2009, pp. 1108–1111.

Shelton GD, Lindstrom JM. Spontaneous remission in canine myasthenia gravis: implications for assessing human MG therapies. Neurology 2001, 57:2139–2141.

Author Lauren Talarico

Consulting Editor Mathieu M. Glassman

Acknowledgment The author and editors acknowledge the prior contribution of G. Diane Shelton.

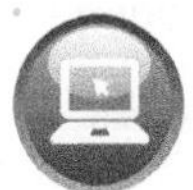

Client Education Handout available online

M

MYCOBACTERIAL INFECTIONS

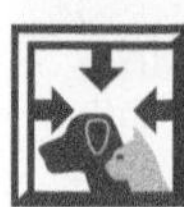

BASICS

OVERVIEW

- Mycobacteria—Gram-positive, acid-fast higher bacteria (genus *Mycobacterium*); obligate or sporadic pathogens in humans and animals.
- Tuberculosis—rare in dogs and cats.
- Leprosy:
  - Cats—two syndromes.
  - Dogs—canine leproid granuloma syndrome.
- Systemic or noncutaneous infection with nontuberculous mycobacteria.
- Cutaneous/subcutaneous infections due to rapidly growing mycobacteria (e.g., mycobacterial panniculitis):
  - Dogs and cats—caused by saprophytic mycobacteria.
- Systems affected—respiratory, skin/exocrine; determined by cause.

M

SIGNALMENT

Tuberculosis

- Cats and dogs of any age.
- Basset hound and Siamese cat reported as possibly more susceptible.

Feline Leprosy

- Syndome 1—free-roaming kittens and young adult cats.
- Syndrome 2—older cats (average 9 years).

Canine Leproid Granuloma

Shorthaired outdoor-housed large-breed dogs, especially boxers and German shepherd dogs.

Systemic Nontuberculous Mycobacteriosis

Sporadic disease that can affect dogs and cats of any age.

Mycobacterial Panniculitis

Adult dogs and cats.

SIGNS

Tuberculosis

- Organism—*Mycobacterium tuberculosis* (humans), *M. bovis* (cattle, wild mammals), and *M. microti* (voles), and *M. microti*-like.
- Dogs and cats exposed to infected primary hosts sporadically infected.
- Disseminated or multiorgan disease caused by intracellular facultative organism.
- Correlated with the route of exposure.
- Major sites of involvement—oropharyngeal lymph nodes, cutaneous and subcutaneous tissues of the head and extremities; pulmonary system; gastrointestinal system.
- Dogs—respiratory, especially coughing.
- Cats—from contaminated milk: weight loss, chronic diarrhea, and thickened intestines; from predation: cutaneous nodules, ulcers, and draining tracts.
- Most dogs and many cats—pharyngeal and cervical lymphadenopathy; unproductive vomiting, ptyalism, or tonsillar abscess; lymphadenopathy; may ulcerate and drain.
- Pyrexia.
- Depression.
- Anorexia and weight loss.
- Hypertrophic osteopathy or hypercalcemia.
- Disseminated disease—body cavity effusion; visceral masses; bone or joint lesions; dermal and subcutaneous masses and ulcers; lymphadenopathy and/or abscesses; CNS signs; sudden death.

Feline Leprosy

- Organisms—*M. lepraemurium* (from rodents) and two unnamed leprosy organisms (*M. visibilis* [provisional]).
- Syndrome 1—*M. lepraemurium*: young cats with localized nodular disease, affecting limbs with sparse to moderate numbers of acid-fast bacilli present in lesions initially; progress rapidly, may ulcerate; aggressive clinical course; recurrence after surgical excision; widespread lesions develop in several weeks.
- Syndrome 2—unnamed species with affinity to *M. malmoense*: older cats with generalized skin lesions and large numbers of acid-fast bacilli in lesions; initial skin nodules that do not ulcerate, progressive over months to years.
- Feline multisystemic granulomatous mycobacteriosis—diffuse cutaneous thickening and multiple organ involvement.

Canine Leproid Granuloma

- Organism—*Mycobacterium* sp. Murphy identified by DNA sequencing.
- Well-circumscribed painless nodules (2 mm–5 cm) in dermis or subcutis; head or ear, but may be anywhere on the body; only large lesions ulcerate.
- No systemic signs of illness.

Systemic Nontuberculous Mycobacteriosis

- Organisms—*M. chelonae-abscessus* group, *M. avium* complex, *M. fortuitum*, *M. genavense*, *M. kansasii*, *M. massiliense*, *M. simiae*, *M. smegmatis*, *M. thermoresistable*, *M. xenopi*.
- Sporadic infections in dogs and cats; associated in patients with concurrent disease immunosuppression or as a result of traumatic tissue introduction of saprophytic organism; syndromes include pleuritis, granulomas, disseminated disease, neuritis, or bronchopneumonia.
- Pulmonary and systemic infections with atypical mycobacteriosis are rare in dogs, in which case the signs are as for tuberculosis.
- *M. avium* infection—disease most often disseminated.

Mycobacterial Panniculitis

- Organisms—*M. fortuitum* group, *M. chelonae-abscessus* group, *M. smegmati* groups, *M. phlei*, *M. terrae* complex, *M. thermoresistable*, *M. ulcerans*.
- Cutaneous—traumatic lesion that fails to heal with therapy; spreads locally in the subcutaneous tissue (panniculitis); original lesion enlarges, forming a deep ulcer that drains hemorrhagic exudate; surrounding tissue becomes firm; satellite pinpoint ulcerations open and drain.
- Wound dehiscence at surgery sites.

CAUSES & RISK FACTORS

Tuberculosis

- Source of exposure—always an infected typical host.
- Dogs—usually from an infected person in the household (*M. tuberculosis*); route is ingestion of expectorated infectious material; aerosol exposure; patients often found in urban areas with newly arrived immigrants.
- Cats—classically exposed by drinking unpasteurized milk of infected cattle (*M. bovis*); much less common now; may be exposed by predation on infected small mammals (*M. bovis*, undefined tuberculosis species).

Feline Leprosy

- Syndrome 1—cases have been reported from temperate coastal areas and port cities; cool climate may facilitate growth of the organism in extremities.
- Syndrome 2—cases are from rural environments; old age or immune-incompetence may be a risk factor; exact risk factors remain undefined; exposure to rodents postulated.

Canine Leproid Granuloma

- Associated with fly bites and may fluctuate seasonally; short coats may predispose.
- Disease likely to be worldwide; most cases reported from Australia, Asia, and Brazil.
- In the United States, reported in California, Hawaii, and Florida.

Systemic Nontuberculous Mycobacteriosis

- Patients are immunosuppressed or have concurrent systemic disease.
- Routes of exposure in pulmonary and systemic disease are uncertain.

Mycobacterial Panniculitis

- Infections usually have antecedent trauma or surgical wound; most patients are immune-competent.
- Trauma and accidental inoculation of the subcutaneous fat results in infection; history of bite wound possible (subcutaneous disease).
- Overweight of obese animals are more at risk.

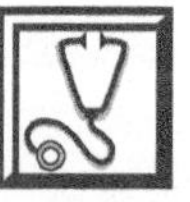

DIAGNOSIS

DIFFERENTIAL DIAGNOSIS

- All manifestations—fungal and other actinomycotic infections.

- Panniculitis: nocardiosis.

OTHER LABORATORY TESTS

Tuberculosis

Tuberculosis (dogs)—intradermal skin testing with PPD (purified protein derivative) or BCG (bacillus Calmette–Guérin) on inner pinna; may produce false-positive.

IMAGING

Radiography

- Thoracic, abdominal, or skeletal lesions—suggest granulomatous infectious disease.
- No specific lesions for the mycobacterioses.
- Pulmonary tuberculosis lesions—may become calcified or cavitated.

DIAGNOSTIC PROCEDURES

- Biopsy material from affected tissue.
- Aspiration of purulent material—used for microbiological identification; ultrasound-guided aspiration techniques may be warranted.
- Biopsy specimens—sterile collection; incorporate center of a granulomatous focus.
- Exudate from infected tissues—detection with acid-fast carbolfuchsin or auramine-rhodamine fluorochromes; on routine staining, organisms are negatively stained, showing "ghosts" of bacilli within macrophages; swabs or aspirations of draining cutaneous lesions or lymph nodes, transtracheal wash; endoscopic brushings; rectal cytology; impressions taken at surgical biopsy; heat-fixed exudate should be submitted with tissue for culture.
- Culture—special media and techniques required; referral to specialized laboratories may be required for nontuberculous organisms.
- PCR methodologies—useful for any of the mycobacterial infections using tissue specimens or fluids; for canine leproid granuloma and the two feline leprosy syndromes, primers are not commercially available, but can be used to identify the suspect organisms.

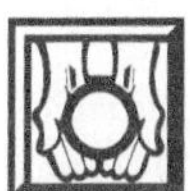

TREATMENT

TUBERCULOSIS

- Obtain permission of health authorities in cases of *M. tuberculosis* infection; zoonotic potential should be considered.
- Multiple agent chemotherapy with drugs used to treat human tuberculosis have been successful; *M. avium* complex infections are difficult to treat.

Feline Leprosy

- Individual lesions may be excised with aggressive margins.
- Surgical treatment should be preceded by systemic therapy.

Canine Leproid Granuloma

Excision is curative; lesions may self-cure; antimicrobial therapy may assist healing.

Subcutaneous and Systemic Nontuberculous Infections

- Treatment should be based on organism identification and antibiotic sensitivity testing.
- Multiple drug therapy is often warranted.
- Aggressive surgical debulking may aid resolution; antimicrobial therapy pre- and intraoperatively is recommended.

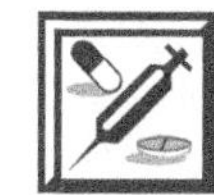

MEDICATIONS

DRUG(S) OF CHOICE

Tuberculosis

- Multidrug oral therapy mandatory.
- Current recommendation—fluoroquinolones, clarithromycin, and doxycycline for 6–9 months.
- Marbofloxacin 5.5 mg/kg PO q24h, pradofloxacin 5–7.5 mg/kg PO q24h.
- Clarithromycin 5–10 mg/kg PO q24h.
- Isoniazid and rifampin—combinations have been used; single report of use in cats.
- Isoniazid 10–20 mg/kg (up to 300 mg total) PO q24h.
- Ethambutol 15 mg/kg PO q24h.
- Pyrazinamide—instead of ethambutol 15–40 mg/kg PO q24h.

Feline Leprosy

- Pradofloxacin 5–7.5 mg/kg PO q24h.
- Clarithromycin 5–10 mg/kg PO q24h.

Subcutaneous and Systemic Nontuberculous Infections

- *In vitro* sensitivity testing may be used to choose chemotherapy.
- Antibiotics reported to be effective: macrolide, trimethoprim-potentiated sulfonamide, tetracycline, aminoglycoside, and fluoroquinolone antibiotics.
- Antituberculosis drugs are not generally effective.
- Single-agent therapy not recommended due to poor long-term response; double-agent therapy recommended.
- Long-term therapy should be based on sensitivity testing.
- Treatment should be continued for 2–6 months.
- Relapses are common.

FOLLOW-UP

PATIENT MONITORING

- Antituberculosis and antileprosy drugs—examine monthly; monitor for anorexia and weight loss.
- Liver profile monthly.
- Instruct owners to report cutaneous lesions immediately.

EXPECTED COURSE AND PROGNOSIS

Tuberculosis

Guarded; but undefined as experience with modern drugs is limited.

Feline Leprosy

- Guarded to poor—syndrome 1.
- Fair—syndrome 2, especially if lesions are amenable to surgical excision.

Canine Leproid Granuloma

Good

Subcutaneous and Systemic Nontuberculous Infections

Relapses are common; aggressive surgical approaches and multiple drug therapy may improve outlook.

MISCELLANEOUS

ZOONOTIC POTENTIAL

- Tuberculosis—reverse zoonosis possible.
- Affected domestic pets are potential serious zoonotic threats to owners; do not attempt treatment without agreement of public health authorities.
- *M. tuberculosis*—greatest potential for zoonosis, especially with draining cutaneous lesions.
- Disease transmission from dogs and cats to humans—rarely recorded.

Suggested Reading

Malik R, Smits B, Reppas G, et al. Ulcerated and nonulcerated nontuberculous cutaneous mycobacterial granulomas in cats and dogs. Vet Dermatol 2013, 24(1):146–153. e32–33.

O'Halloran C, Gunn-Moore DA. Mycobacteria in cats: an update. In Pract 2017, 39(9):399–406.

Author Mitchell D. Song

Consulting Editor Alexander H. Werner Resnick

MYCOPLASMOSIS

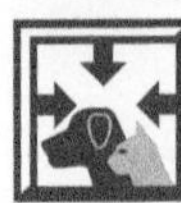

BASICS

DEFINITION

- Class Mollicutes.
- Divided into hemotropic (formerly Haemobartonella and Eperythrozoon, see: Hemotropic Mycoplasmosis) and nonhemotropic types (discussed here).
- More than 80 genera, three families: Mycoplasmas, Ureaplasmas, and Acholeplasmas.
- Smallest (0.2–0.3 µm) and simplest prokaryotic cells capable of self-replication.
- Fastidious, facultative anaerobic, Gram-negative rods.
- Lack cell wall; thus plastic, highly pleomorphic, fragile and sensitive to lysis by osmotic shock, detergents, alcohols, and specific antibody plus complement. Enclosed by a trilayered cell membrane built of amphipathic lipids and proteins; therefore resistant to lysozyme and cell wall-inhibiting antibacterials; most require sterols for growth.
- Reproduce by binary fission; genome replication not necessarily synchronized with cell division, resulting in budding forms and chains of beads.
- Small genome (0.6–1.6 Mb), believed to be result of reductive evolution from a common Gram-positive ancestor adapting to obligate parasitic life.
- Ubiquitous in nature as parasites, commensals, or saprophytes in animals, plants, and insects; many are pathogens of humans, animals, plants, and insects.

PATHOPHYSIOLOGY

- Often part of the resident flora as commensals on mucous membranes of the upper respiratory, digestive, and genital tracts; pathogenicity and role in disease often controversial.
- Species show considerable host specificity.
- Mechanisms by which disease is caused are poorly understood.
- Some species attach to cells by specific receptors; small size and plastic nature enable them to adapt to the shape and contours of host cell surfaces.
- Intimate contact with host cells—necessary for assimilation of vital nutrients and growth factors which organism cannot synthesize. This, along with the tendency of exogenous proteins to bind to mycoplasmal membrane may allow organism to evade the host's immune response. May incorporate host cell antigen onto mycoplasma membrane (capping) because of lack of cell wall. Conversely, mycoplasmal protein antigen may become incorporated onto surface of host cell, involving host cell in deleterious immunologic reactions intended against the organism.
- Products produced during growth—capsular carbohydrate, hemolysins, proteolytic enzymes, ammonia, and endonucleases; accumulation of *Mycoplasma* metabolites (i.e., H_2O_2, NH_3) may contribute to cytopathic effects and tissue damage; cytotoxic glycoproteins and proteins have been isolated from the membranes of several species.
- Immune response—predominantly humoral; as with bacterial infections, IgM and IgA are first antibodies to appear, followed by IgG.
- Fibrinous exudate accompanying infections—protects organism from antibodies and antimicrobial drugs; contributes to chronicity.
- Secondary bacterial invaders—common (e.g., attachment to respiratory tract cells results in destruction of cilia, which predisposes patient to secondary bacterial infection).
- Sialidase, a virulence factor that promotes colonization, tissue invasion, and damage to host cells—varies in expression among strains of canine mycoplasma species.

SYSTEMS AFFECTED

Dogs

- Gastrointestinal—associated with colitis.
- Musculoskeletal—arthritis; from *Mycoplasma spumans*.
- Renal/urologic—urinary and genital tract infections (e.g., balanoposthitis, urethritis, prostatitis, cystitis, nephritis, vaginitis, endometritis); caused by *M. canis* and *M. spumans*.
- Reproductive—*Mycoplasma* and *Ureaplasma*; associated with infertility, early embryonic death, abortion, stillbirths or weak newborns, and neonatal mortality.
- Respiratory—pneumonia and upper respiratory infections; caused by *M. cynos*; associated with *M. canis*, *M. spumans*, *M. edwardii*, *M. feliminutum*, *M. gateae*, and *M. bovigenitalium*.
- Nervous—meningitis, associated with *M. edwardii*.

Cats

- Musculoskeletal—chronic fibrinopurulent polyarthritis and tenosynovitis; associated with *M. gateae* and unspecified mycoplasmal organisms.
- Ophthalmic—conjunctivitis; associated with *M. felis* (5–25%).
- Renal/urologic—urinary tract infections.
- Reproductive—abortions and fetal deaths; associated with *M. gateae* and ureaplasmas.
- Respiratory—pneumonia, associated with *M. gateae*, *M. feliminutum*, and *M. felis*; upper respiratory infections, associated with *M. felis*.
- Skin/exocrine—chronic cutaneous abscesses.
- Nervous—meningoencephalitis, associated with *M. felis*.

INCIDENCE/PREVALENCE

- Frequent inhabitants of mucosal membranes; *M. gateae* and/or *M. felis* found in oral cavity or urogenital tract of 70–80% of healthy cats.
- Rate of isolation in diseased dogs much higher than in normal dogs.

GEOGRAPHIC DISTRIBUTION

Ubiquitous

SIGNALMENT

Species

Dogs and cats.

Mean Age and Range

All ages.

SIGNS

General Comments

Pathogenic role controversial, can be identified in asymptomatic animals.

Historical Findings

- Polyarthritis—chronic intermittent lameness; reluctance to move; joint pain.
- Fever.
- Malaise.
- Conjunctivitis—unilateral or bilateral.
- Cough.

Physical Examination Findings

- Polyarthritis—diffuse limb edema, joint swelling, pain.
- Conjunctivitis—blepharospasm; chemosis, conjunctival hyperemia, epiphora, and serous or purulent ocular discharge.
- Mild rhinitis—sneezing.

CAUSES

- *Mycoplasma* flora of dogs—*M. canis*, *M. spumans*, *M. maculosum*, *M. edwardii*, *M. cynos*, *M. molare*, *M. opalescens*, *M. felis*, *M. feliminutum*, *M. gateae*, *M. arginini*, *M. bovigenitalium*, *M. mucosicanis*, *Acholeplasma laidlawii*, and ureaplasmas.
- *Mycoplasma* flora of cats—*M. felis*, *M. gateae*, *M. feliminutum*, *M. arginini*, *M. pulmonis*, *M. arthritidis*, *M. gallisepticum*, *Acholeplasma laidlawi*, and ureaplasmas.

RISK FACTORS

- Commensals—occasionally cause systemic infection associated with immunodeficiency, immunosuppression, or cancer.
- Impaired resistance of the host—may allow organism to cross the mucosal barrier and disseminate (e.g., primary ciliary dyskinesia).
- Organism may be opportunistic—one factor in a multifactorial causal complex (e.g., impaired pulmonary clearance from viral infection may allow organism to establish infection in lungs as secondary opportunistic pathogen).
- Predisposing factors—stresses (e.g., reproductive problems associated with overcrowded operations) and other factors (e.g., urinary tumors and urinary calculi).

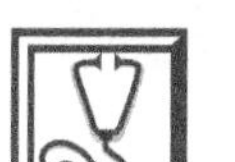

DIAGNOSIS

DIFFERENTIAL DIAGNOSIS

- Upper respiratory infection (dogs and cats)—viruses (parainfluenza virus, canine distemper, canine influenza virus, herpesvirus, feline calcivirus, reovirus); *Chlamydia psittaci*; bacteria (*Bordetella bronchiseptica*, staphylococci, streptococci, coliforms).
- Urinary tract infection (dogs and cats)—bacteria (staphylococci, streptococci, coliforms); fungus (*Candida*); parasites.
- Infertility, early embryonic death, abortion, stillbirths or weak newborns, and neonatal mortality (dogs)—bacteria (*Brucella, Salmonella, Campylobacter, E. coli, Streptococcus*); viruses (canine herpesvirus, canine distemper, canine adenovirus); *Toxoplasma gondii*; endocrinopathies (progesterone deficiency, hypothyroidism).
- Prostatitis (dogs)—bacteria (*E. coli, Brucella canis*); fungi (*Blastomyces, Cryptococcus*).
- Arthritis (dogs and cats)—immune-mediated; bacteria (staphylococci, streptococci, coliforms, anaerobes); L-form bacteria; *Rickettsia* (*Ehrlichia*); *Borrelia burgdorferi*; fungi (*Coccidioides, Cryptococcus, Blastomyces*); protozoa (*Leishmania*); viruses (feline calicivirus).
- Conjunctivitis (cats)—feline herpesvirus; feline calicivirus; feline reovirus; *Chlamydia psittaci*; bacteria.

CBC/BIOCHEMISTRY/URINALYSIS

With Polyarthritis

- Mild anemia.
- Neutrophilic leukocytosis.
- Hypoalbuminemia.
- Hypoglobulinemia.
- Proteinuria, resulting from immune-complex glomerulonephritis.

OTHER LABORATORY TESTS

- Difficult to demonstrate in and from tissues.
- PCR of 16S rRNA.
    - PCR denaturing gradient gel electrophoresis (PCR-DGGE)—used to identify difficult-to culture or difficult-to-differentiate mycoplasma.
- Fluorescent antibody test—definitive diagnosis; isolate and identify or detect the organism in tissues:
    - Submit cotton swabs placed in Hayflick broth medium or commercially available swabs; organisms fragile; refrigerate specimens and deliver to the laboratory within 48 hours; freeze (–80°C) to preserve longer.
- Extremely pleomorphic—in smears (e.g., conjunctival scrapings) seen as coccobacilli, coccal forms, ring forms, spirals, and filaments.
- Stains—stain poorly (Gram-negative); preferred: Giemsa or other Romanowsky stain.
- Culture—fastidious, require complex growth media; form microcolonies having characteristic "fried egg" appearance.

IMAGING

Polyarthritis—no radiographic changes.

DIAGNOSTIC PROCEDURES

- Arthrocentesis—polyarthritis, high numbers of nondegenerative neutrophils in synovial fluid.
- Prostatic wash/urine —inflammatory cells with negative routine bacterial culture.
- Transtracheal or endotracheal wash—high numbers of nondegenerate neutrophils with no organisms seen.

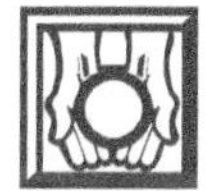

TREATMENT

APPROPRIATE HEALTH CARE

Outpatient

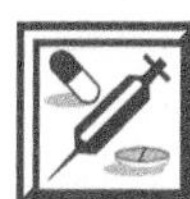

MEDICATIONS

DRUG(S) OF CHOICE

- Doxycycline 5 mg/kg PO q12h.
- Tetracyclines 22 mg/kg PO q8h.
- Pradofloxacin 5 mg/kg PO q12h.
- Chloramphenicol 40–50 mg/kg IV, IM, SC, PO q8–12h.
- No standardized procedure for *in vitro* antimicrobial susceptibility tests.
- Topical antibiotic—conjunctivitis.

ALTERNATIVE DRUG(S)

- Gentamicin.
- Kanamycin.
- Spectinomycin.
- Spiramycin.
- Tylosin.
- Erythromycin.
- Nitrofurans.
- Fluoroquinolones.

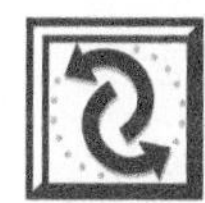

FOLLOW-UP

PATIENT MONITORING

Treat for an extended period of time.

PREVENTION/AVOIDANCE

- No vaccines are available.
- Organism readily killed by drying, sunshine, and chemical disinfection.

EXPECTED COURSE AND PROGNOSIS

Prognosis good in animals with competent immune systems and given appropriate antibiotic therapy.

MISCELLANEOUS

ASSOCIATED CONDITIONS

M. pneumoniae—infects respiratory tracts in humans worldwide; causes mycoplasmal pneumonia, bronchitis, or upper respiratory infection; usually self-limited; rarely fatal.

ZOONOTIC POTENTIAL

- Not generally considered zoonotic unless person is immunosuppressed.
- Host specificity of mycoplasmas has been questioned by some, particularly between closely related species of mammals.

SYNONYMS

Pleuropneumonia-like organisms.

ABBREVIATIONS

- PCR-DGGE = polymerase chain reaction denaturing gradient gel electrophoresis.

Suggested Reading

Lee-Fowler T. Feline respiratory disease: what is the role of Mycoplasma species? J Feline Med Surg 2014, 16:563–571.

Reed N. Respiratory and ocular mycoplasmal infections: significance, diagnosis, and management. In: Little SE, ed., August's Consultations in Feline Internal Medicine, 7th ed. St. Louis, MO: Elsevier, 2016, pp. 23–33.

Sykes JE. Mycoplasma infections. In: Sykes JE, ed., Canine and Feline Infectious Diseases. St. Louis, MO: Elsevier, 2014, pp. 382–389.

Author J. Paul Woods

Consulting Editor Amie Koenig

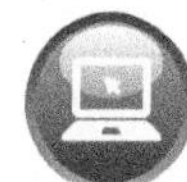

Client Education Handout available online

M

MYCOTOXICOSIS—AFLATOXIN

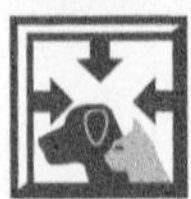

BASICS

OVERVIEW

Aflatoxins are hepatotoxic mycotoxins (mold toxins) and are the most commonly reported cause of mycotoxicosis associated with pet food. The four major forms of aflatoxin in feedstuffs are aflatoxin B1, B2, G1, and G2. Aflatoxin B1 is the most common and most toxic.

SIGNALMENT

- Rarely reported in dogs but occurs periodically in large outbreaks associated with pet foods.
- Reported experimentally in cats, rarely as field cases.

SIGNS

M

Acute Onset

- Most common presentation in small animals.
- Refusal of contaminated feeds.
- Rapid onset of signs may develop up to 3 weeks post exposure.
- Vomiting and diarrhea.
- Icterus.
- Coagulopathy and gastrointestinal hemorrhage.

Chronic

- Anorexia or feed refusal.
- Vomiting.
- Diarrhea.
- Liver failure.
- Ascites.

CAUSES & RISK FACTORS

- Common in various cereal grains, peanuts, other nuts, and potatoes.
- Postproduction contamination of improperly stored pet foods; foods with obvious mold spoilage; garbage ingestion.
- Mycotoxin-producing molds grow at temperatures of 24–35°C, moisture of 18–20%.
- Acute signs have been seen in dogs ingesting food containing 60 ppb aflatoxin.
- Activated to toxic epoxide by liver cytochrome P450 enzymes.
- Depletes glutathione.
- Binds with nucleic acids, proteins, and cell and organelle membranes.

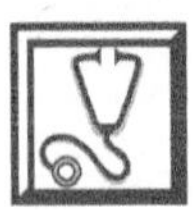

DIAGNOSIS

DIFFERENTIAL DIAGNOSIS

- Leptospirosis:
  - Serology.
- Parvovirus:
  - ELISA.
  - Serology.
  - Viral isolation.
- Anticoagulant rodenticide toxicosis:
  - Anticoagulant rodenticide screen.
- Other causes of subacute to chronic liver disease and associated disseminated intravascular coagulation.

CBC/BIOCHEMISTRY/URINALYSIS

- Decreased serum protein C, antithrombin III, and cholesterol.
- Hyperbilirubinemia.
- Hypoalbuminemia.
- Elevated alanine aminotransferase.
- Variable elevations in γ-glutamyltransferase, aspartate aminotransferase, and alkaline phosphatase.

OTHER LABORATORY TESTS

Prolonged activated partial thromboplastin time (aPTT) and prothrombin time (PT).

DIAGNOSTIC PROCEDURES

- Liver biopsy.
- Histopathology.
- Assay suspect food samples for aflatoxin:
  - Contaminated food is often gone due to delayed clinical signs.

PATHOLOGIC FINDINGS

- Hepatomegaly with fatty change.
- Icterus.
- Ascites.
- Multifocal hemorrhage, especially gastrointestinal.
- Microvesicular fatty change in hepatocytes.
- Centrilobular hepatocellular necrosis.
- Canalicular cholestasis.
- Bridging portal fibrosis, proliferation of bile ducts.

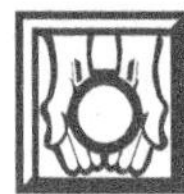

TREATMENT

- Transfusion of whole blood or plasma.
- Correct fluid and electrolyte imbalances.
- Activated charcoal for recent, high-dose exposure.
- B vitamins, vitamin K1, vitamin E, antioxidants, and hepatoprotectants.
- Gastroprotectants.
- Clean, uncontaminated diet:
  - High-quality protein source.

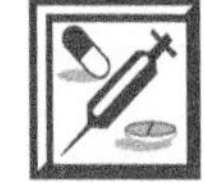

MEDICATIONS

DRUG(S) OF CHOICE

- No specific antidotal therapy.
- Limited success with hepatoprotectants.
- Parenteral *N*-acetylcysteine in severely affected dogs—20% solution diluted 1:4 in sterile saline slow IV at a loading dose of 140 mg/kg, follow with maintenance dose of 70 mg/kg IV q8h × 7 doses.
- Oral *S*-adenosylmethionine—20 mg/kg PO daily as enteric-coated tablets given on empty stomach × 1–2 weeks.

CONTRAINDICATIONS/POSSIBLE INTERACTIONS

Avoid drugs metabolized by the liver.

FOLLOW-UP

PATIENT MONITORING

- Daily serum enzymes and chemistry, including cholesterol.
- PT and aPTT.
- Protein C.

PREVENTION/AVOIDANCE

- Consider as a cause of food refusal.
- Avoid using moldy feedstuff.
- Store food in cool, clean, dry area.
- Clean food containers and feed bowls regularly.

POSSIBLE COMPLICATIONS

Chronic liver disease possible.

EXPECTED COURSE AND PROGNOSIS

Prognosis—poor, even with treatment. Improved prognosis if treatment initiated before onset of signs.

MISCELLANEOUS

AGE-RELATED FACTORS

Young animals more susceptible to aflatoxin.

PREGNANCY/FERTILITY/BREEDING

- Indirect effects on uterus.
- Potentially teratogenic.
- Pregnant animals may be more susceptible.

ABBREVIATIONS

- aPTT = activated partial thromboplastin time.
- PT = prothrombin time.

Suggested Reading

Arnot LF, Duncan NM, Coetzer H, et al. An outbreak of canine aflatoxicosis in Gauteng Province, South Africa. J S Afr Vet Assoc 2012, 83(1):1–4.

Bischoff K, Garland T. Aflatoxicosis in dogs. In: Bonagura JD, Twedt DC, eds., Kirk's Current Veterinary Therapy, 14th ed. St. Louis, MO: Saunders, 2009, pp. 156–159.

Bruchim Y, Segev G, Sela U, et al. Accidental fatal aflatoxicosis due to contaminated commercial diet in 50 dogs. Res Vet Sci 2012, 93(1):279–287.

Author Karyn Bischoff

Consulting Editor Lynn R. Hovda

MYCOTOXICOSIS—TREMORGENIC TOXINS

BASICS

OVERVIEW

- Penitrem A—produced by the fungus *Penicillium crustosum* (and perhaps other *Penicillium* spp.); poisoning by this toxin has been reported in dogs ingesting moldy bread, cheese, and English walnuts.
- Roquefortine—produced by *Penicillium roquefortii* (and perhaps other *Penicillium* spp.); has been reported to cause poisoning in dogs through ingestion of moldy cheese or decaying organic material (compost).

SIGNALMENT

- Dogs and rarely cats.
- Poisoning by penitrem A and roquefortine has been reported in dogs of various ages and breeds soon after the ingestion of moldy foods or compost.

SIGNS

- Moderate to severe muscle tremors and seizures—begin minutes to hours (0.5–4 hours in case reports) after ingestion of moldy food or compost.
- Affected dogs may be hyperresponsive to external stimuli.
- Early signs—may include panting, hyperactivity, vomiting, ataxia, incoordination, weakness, tachycardia, and/or rigidity.
- Prolonged muscle tremors or seizures—may lead to hyperthermia, hypoglycemia, dehydration, and anorexia.
- Severe cases—may result in death.
- Liver necrosis—has been reported experimentally.

CAUSES & RISK FACTORS

- Dogs (and potentially cats) are exposed to penitrem A and roquefortine when they ingest moldy food or decomposing organic matter (compost).
- Experimentally, doses of 0.125 mg/kg penitrem A produced tremors within 30 minutes. Doses of 0.5 mg/kg of penitrem A resulted in acute onset of tremors, severe liver necrosis, and death.

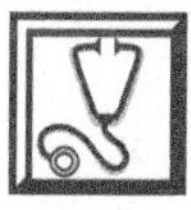

DIAGNOSIS

DIFFERENTIAL DIAGNOSIS

- Toxic causes of seizures—strychnine; insecticides (e.g., organophosphate, carbamate, organochlorine, nicotine, pyrethroid); metaldehyde; zinc phosphide; bromethalin; methylxanthines (theobromine and caffeine); amphetamines; cocaine; sago palm; xylitol.
- Nontoxic causes of seizures—inflammation; congenital abnormal myelin formation; metabolic conditions (e.g., hepatic or uremic encephalopathy).

CBC/BIOCHEMISTRY/URINALYSIS

CBC, biochemistry, and urinalysis to assess the patient's status and to help rule out other causes of tremors and seizures.

OTHER LABORATORY TESTS

N/A

IMAGING

N/A

DIAGNOSTIC PROCEDURES

- High-pressure liquid chromatography/mass spectroscopy—analysis of vomitus, stomach contents, and gastric lavage washings for penitrem A or roquefortine.
- The presence of roquefortine C in vomitus or stomach contents can serve as a sensitive biomarker for penitrem A intoxication.
- Bile analysis—reported to be of value.

PATHOLOGIC FINDINGS

- There are no pathognomonic lesions associated with penitrem A or roquefortine toxicosis.
- High doses of penitrem A have been reported to cause severe liver damage experimentally.

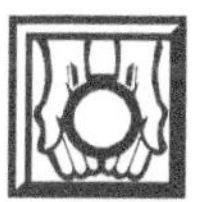

TREATMENT

- Remove contaminated food or organic material.
- Induce vomiting (if patient is not at risk of aspirating vomitus) or institute gastric lavage followed by administration of activated charcoal.
- Control seizures.
- Thermoregulation as indicated.

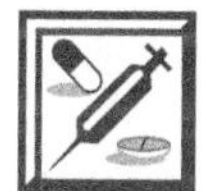

MEDICATIONS

DRUG(S) OF CHOICE

- Diazepam 0.25–1 mg/kg IV PRN—to control tremors/seizures.
- Methocarbamol 50–220 mg/kg IV to control tremors/seizures; do not exceed 330 mg/kg/day. Give 1/2 rapidly and administer rest to effect.
- Barbiturates phenobarbital 2–5 mg/kg IV PRN—if tremors and seizures cannot be controlled with diazepam.
- Sodium bicarbonate—may be required if an acid–base imbalance exists.
- Other symptomatic and supportive therapy—as indicated.

CONTRAINDICATIONS/POSSIBLE INTERACTIONS

N/A

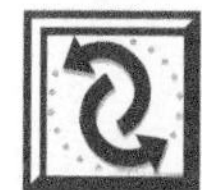

FOLLOW-UP

PATIENT MONITORING

Patients should be monitored for occurrence of tremors or seizures, hyperthermia, dehydration, acid–base imbalances, liver damage, rhabdomyolysis, and respiratory difficulties.

PREVENTION/AVOIDANCE

Prevent animals from eating moldy food items, garbage, or compost.

POSSIBLE COMPLICATIONS

- Seizures—may not be controlled with diazepam.
- Acid–base imbalances—may develop.
- Hepatic damage and rhabdomyolysis—may occur.
- Aspiration pneumonia has been reported as a sequelae to vomiting and/or gastric lavage.
- Exposure can be fatal if lethal doses are consumed and are absorbed before gastrointestinal decontamination and therapy are instituted.

EXPECTED COURSE AND PROGNOSIS

- Very good if appropriate therapy is promptly instituted, the toxin is removed from the gastrointestinal tract, and the seizures are controlled with diazepam, methocarbamol or barbiturates.
- Recovery in most clinical cases is reported to be complete within 24–48 hours.
- In a few reported cases, signs of weakness, muscle rigidity, and incoordination were persistent and slowly resolved over 1–2 weeks.
- A few severe cases have been reported to be fatal.

M

MISCELLANEOUS

Suggested Reading

Barker AK, Stahl C, Ensley SM, et al. Tremorgenic mycotoxicosis in dogs. Compend Contin Educ Vet 2013, 35(2):E1–E6.

Puschner B. Mycotoxins. Vet Clin North Am Small Anim Pract 2002, 32:409–419.

Young KL, Villar D, Carson TL, et al. Tremorgenic mycotoxin intoxication with penitrem A and roquefortine in two dogs. J Am Vet Med Assoc 2003, 222:52–53.

Author Stephen B. Hooser

Consulting Editor Lynn R. Hovda

MYELODYSPLASTIC SYNDROMES

BASICS

OVERVIEW

• Category of diseases characterized by nonregenerative anemias or cytopenias and dysplastic features in the blood or bone marrow.
• Primary myelodysplastic syndromes (MDS) result from a clonal expansion of a genetically altered pluripotent stem cell resulting in a hypercellular bone marrow with maturation arrest as a consequence of apoptosis.
• Subcategorized as MDS with excessive blasts, which may progress to acute myeloid leukemia, MDS with refractory cytopenia, and MDS with erythroid predominance.
• Secondary MDS in dogs is associated with neoplasia (lymphoma, multiple myeloma), drug or toxin exposure, immune-mediated disease, infections, or ionizing radiation exposure.
• Secondary MDS in cats is typically associated with feline leukemia virus (FeLV) infection.

SIGNALMENT

• Dog and less commonly cat.
• Primary MDS typically older dogs.

SIGNS

• Lethargy.
• Exercise intolerance.
• Depression.
• Anorexia.
• Fever.
• Pale mucous membranes.
• Petechiation.
• Heart murmur due to anemia.

CAUSES & RISK FACTORS

• Viral—FeLV, feline immunodeficiency virus (FIV), parvovirus.
• Neoplasia—lymphoma, multiple myeloma.
• Autoimmune—immune-mediated hemolytic anemia, immune-mediated thrombocytopenia.
• Drugs—chemotherapeutics, estrogen, chloramphenicol, cephalosporins, phenylbutazone, trimethoprim-sulfadiazine, quinidine, thiacetarsamide, griseofulvin, albendazole.
• Iron deficiency, folic acid deficiency.
• Lead toxicity.
• Infectious—ehrlichiosis, bacterial septicemia, and endotoxemia.

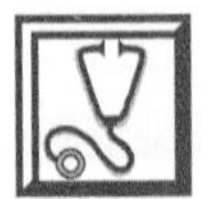

DIAGNOSIS

DIFFERENTIAL DIAGNOSIS

• Need to differentiate between primary and secondary MDS.
• Other causes of nonregenerative anemias—anemia of chronic disease, chronic renal failure, myeloproliferative diseases, lymphoproliferative diseases, myelofibrosis.

CBC/BIOCHEMISTRY/URINALYSIS

Nonregenerative anemia, cytopenias.

OTHER LABORATORY TESTS

To diagnose underlying causes of secondary MDS—viral antigen/antibody titers, iron levels, tick titers, Coombs' test.

IMAGING

• As needed to rule out secondary causes of MDS.
• Abdominal radiography—evaluate for lead foreign bodies.
• Abdominal ultrasonography—evaluate for abdominal masses consistent with retained testes and Sertoli cell tumors associated with estrogen secretion.

DIAGNOSTIC PROCEDURES

Bone marrow aspirate or biopsy.

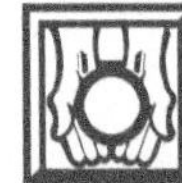

TREATMENT

• Inpatient or outpatient.
• If secondary MDS—treat underlying disease (e.g., discontinue drug, treat underlying infection).
• If neutropenic—limit exposure to other sick animals.
• Blood transfusions for anemic patients.

MEDICATIONS

DRUG(S) OF CHOICE

• For neutropenia—broad-spectrum antibiotics and filgrastim 3–5 μg/kg SC q24h in dogs and cats.
• For anemia—erythropoietin 35–50 U/kg SC 3 times a week or darbepoetin 0.45 μg/kg once a week.
• Chemotherapy for primary MDS has been reported—hydroxyurea, cytosine arabinoside, prednisone, cyclosporine A, vincristine.
• Interferon α (cats with FeLV).

FOLLOW-UP

• Serial monitoring of CBC for resolution of cytopenias.
• Prognosis dependent on primary vs. secondary.
• Increasing blast percentage, multiple cytopenias, marked cellular atypia are poor prognostic factors for patients with primary MDS.

MISCELLANEOUS

PREGNANCY/FERTILITY/BREEDING

• Do not use chemotherapy in pregnant or nursing animals.
• It is not recommended to breed animals with cancer.

SEE ALSO

• Feline Immunodeficiency Virus (FIV) Infection.
• Feline Leukemia Virus (FeLV) Infection.
• Myeloproliferative Disorders.

ABBREVIATIONS

• FeLV = feline leukemia virus.
• FIV = feline immunodeficiency virus.
• MDS = myelodysplastic syndromes.

Suggested Reading

Juopperi TA, Bienzle D, Bernreuter DC, et al. Prognostic markers for myeloid neoplasms: a comparative review of the literature and goals for future investigation. Vet Pathol 2011, 48(1):182–197.

Author Rebecca G. Newman
Consulting Editor Timothy M. Fan

MYELOMALACIA, SPINAL CORD (ASCENDING, DESCENDING, PROGRESSIVE)

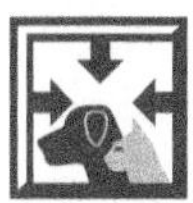

BASICS

OVERVIEW

- Acute, progressive, ischemic and hemorrhagic necrosis of the spinal cord after acute spinal cord injury (SCI).
- First appears at the site of injury; then may progress cranially and caudally.
- Overall prevalence: 2% in dogs with acute thoracolumbar intervertebral disc herniation (IVDH), up to about 15% in more severely affected cases with paraplegia and loss of pain perception.
- Death usually caused by respiratory paralysis.

SIGNALMENT

- Any age or breed.
- Because of the close association between acute (type I) IVDH and myelomalacia, chondrodystrophic breeds, particularly dachshunds, are more commonly affected because of their predisposition to the former.
- French bulldogs were at higher risk than dachshunds in one study.

SIGNS

- Not clinically recognizable in acute phase of SCI—suggestive clinical signs usually seen within 48 hours after presentation, but a delayed onset up to 2 weeks after injury has been reported.
- Acute onset of paraplegia—initial clinical sign.
- Pain perception—usually absent caudal to the lesion (i.e., pelvic limbs and tail).
- Thoracolumbar injury—pelvic limbs paralysis with normal to exaggerated spinal reflexes in the pelvic limbs; some dogs might present with absent spinal reflexes (lesion at the lumbosacral intumescence or secondary to spinal shock).
- Involvement of the lumbosacral spinal cord segments within 12–72 hours, causing pelvic limb areflexia and atonia, loss of abdominal and anal tone and flaccid urinary bladder.
- Thoracic and cervical spinal cord segments may be involved within 24 hours to 10 days after initial injury, causing loss of cutaneous trunci muscle reflex, progression to tetraplegia, bilateral Horner syndrome, hypoventilation, and death.
- Extensive subarachnoid hemorrhage may cause hyperthermia and diffuse meningeal pain.

CAUSES & RISK FACTORS

- Acute intervertebral disc herniation — herniation at the lumbosacral intumescence associated with higher risk.
- Acute, severe, spinal cord trauma.
- Fibrocartilaginous embolism or acute noncompressive nucleus pulposus extrusion.

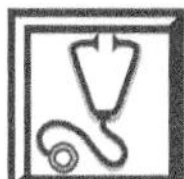

DIAGNOSIS

DIFFERENTIAL DIAGNOSIS

- On presentation, cannot be differentiated from spinal shock (acute paralysis with initial areflexia improving after a few hours to days post injury) following acute SCI.
- Diagnosis based on hind limb upper motor neuron paralysis with absent nociception progressing to a lower motor neuron paralysis and rostrally advancing line of analgesia and cutaneous trunci reflex.

CBC/BIOCHEMISTRY/URINALYSIS

- Usually normal.
- Possible degenerative left-shift caused by massive spinal cord necrosis.

OTHER LABORATORY TESTS

Serum glial fibrillary acidic protein (GFAP)—elevated; experimental only.

IMAGING

- Spinal survey radiographs—evidence of calcified, herniated disc, narrowed intervertebral disc space; vertebral fracture or luxation.
- Myelography—cord compression; edema; contrast medium infiltration into the spinal parenchyma.
- MRI—extensive parenchymal T2 hyperintensity and spinal cord swelling; associated with other evidence of SCI.

DIAGNOSTIC PROCEDURES

CSF—unspecific results; hemorrhagic, neutrophilic pleocytosis and high protein concentration.

PATHOLOGIC FINDINGS

Extensive, multifocal, necrosis of the spinal cord parenchyma with ischemic changes and multifocal hemorrhages.

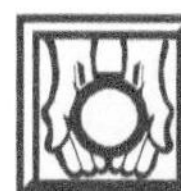

TREATMENT

- None to reverse spinal cord damage and stop disease progression.
- Rapid spinal cord decompression—indicated for IVDH as delayed surgical treatment on dogs with complete sensorimotor loss can alter chances of recovery; if performed less than 12 hours following loss of ambulation the risk of myelomalacia is decreased.
- Surgery does not always prevent its occurrence, especially if delayed: inform the owners of the risk of myelomalacia postoperatively despite rapid intervention.
- Strong suspicion of myelomalacia—poor outcome, consider euthanasia.

MEDICATIONS

DRUG(S) OF CHOICE

For palliative care—gabapentin 10 mg/kg PO q8h, opioids (fentanyl, hydromorphone) to relieve pain associated with SCI.

CONTRAINDICATIONS/POSSIBLE INTERACTIONS

- Gabapentin may cause sedation.
- Opioids side effects include sedation, nausea, constipation, dysphoria.

FOLLOW-UP

In rare cases, condition progresses only caudally; paralysis is permanent, but respiratory compromise does not occur.

MISCELLANEOUS

SEE ALSO

Intervertebral Disc Disease, Thoracolumbar.

ABBREVIATIONS

- GFAP = glial fibrillary acidic protein.
- IVDH = intervertebral disc herniation.
- SCI = spinal cord injury.

Suggested Reading

Balducci F, Canal S, Contiero B, et al. Prevalence and risk factors for presumptive ascending/descending myelomalacia in dogs after thoracolumbar intervertebral disk herniation. J Vet Intern Med 2017, 31:498–504.

Castel A, Olby NJ, Mariani CL, et al. Clinical characteristics of dogs with progressive myelomalacia following acute intervertebral disc extrusion. J Vet Intern Med 2017, 31:1782–1789.

Author Aude M.H. Castel

MYELOPATHY—PARESIS/PARALYSIS—CATS

BASICS

DEFINITION

• Myelopathy—any disease affecting the spinal cord; can cause paralysis (complete loss of voluntary movements) or paresis (weakness) that may affect all limbs (tetraparesis/plegia), the pelvic limbs (para-) only, the ipsilateral thoracic and pelvic limbs (hemi-), or one limb (mono-). • Paresis/paralysis can also be caused by neuromuscular disorders.

PATHOPHYSIOLOGY

• Myelopathy—can affect gray or white matter of the spinal cord or, most often, both.
• Lesions of the ascending white matter tracts—affect sensory modalities such as touch, pressure, proprioception, pain, and temperature sensation below the level of the lesion. • Lesions of the descending white matter tracts—affect the motor pathways producing signs of upper motor neuron disorder. The upper motor neuron cell bodies are located in the brain; they control voluntary activity and have inhibitory function on the lower motor neurons. Signs of upper motor neuron disease include paresis/paralysis, normal to increased muscle tone (hypertonia), and normal to exaggerated spinal reflexes (hyperreflexia) below the level of the lesion.
• Lesions in the gray matter of the spinal cord—affect sensory and motor functions of the region innervated by the nerves whose cell bodies are located in the gray matter. The motor nerves in the gray matter of the spinal cord are also called lower motor neurons. Signs of lower motor neuron disease include paresis/paralysis, decreased or absent muscle tone (hypo- or atonia), atrophy of the muscles innervated by that segment, and reduced or absent spinal reflexes (hypo- or areflexia).

GENETICS

• Lysosomal storage diseases—gangliosidosis GM1/GM2, sphingomyelinosis (Niemann-Pick disease), mucopolysaccharidosis VI (MPS VI), and glycogenosis type IV cause paresis or paralysis in cats; autosomal recessive pattern of inheritance. • Neuroaxonal dystrophy and spinal muscular atrophy—degenerative diseases of the spinal cord reported as autosomal recessive conditions.
• Syringohydromyelia/myelodysplasia may be associated with sacrocaudal (sacrocoggygeal) dysgenesis—autosomal dominant condition in Manx cats.

SIGNALMENT

Breed Predilections

• Gangliosidosis GM1/GM2—Siamese, Burmese, Korat cats, and domestic shorthair (DSH). • Glycogen storage disease type IV—Norwegian forest cats.
• Spinal muscular atrophy—Maine coon.
• Syringohydromyelia/myelodysplasia—Manx and Manx crosses with sacrocaudal dysgenesis. • Sphyngomyelinosis (Niemann-Pick disease)—Siamese, Balinese, and DSH. • Mucopolysaccharidosis type VI—Siamese and DSH. • Mucopolysaccharidosis type VII—DSH. • Idiopathic complex polysaccharide storage disease—Abyssinians.
• Neuroaxonal dystrophy—Siamese and DSH.

SIGNS

• Signs vary with location and severity of lesion. • Cervical lesion (spinal cord segments C1–5)—all limbs or ipsilateral limbs affected with proprioceptive ataxia and tetraparesis/plegia, hemiparesis/plegia; normal to increased reflexes and tone; ± neck pain; ± ipsi-/bilateral Horner's syndrome; ± urinary incontinence with bladder difficult to express; increased urethral sphincter tone and tense bladder. • Cervicothoracic lesion (C6–T2)—all limbs or ipsilateral limbs affected with proprioceptive ataxia and tetraparesis/plegia, hemiparesis/plegia; hypo-/areflexia, hypo-/atonia and muscle atrophy in thoracic limbs with normal to increased reflexes and tone in pelvic limbs; ± neck pain; ± ipsi-/bilateral Horner's syndrome; ipsi-/bilateral decreased/absent cutaneous trunci reflex; ± urinary incontinence with bladder difficult to express; increased urethral sphincter tone and tense bladder. • Thoracolumbar lesion (T3–L3)—normal thoracic limbs; both pelvic limbs or ipsilateral pelvic limb affected with proprioceptive ataxia and paraparesis/plegia; normal to increased reflexes and tone; ± thoracolumbar pain; ± decreased/absent cutaneous trunci reflex below the lesion; ± decreased/absent sensation below lesion; ± Schiff–Sherrington posture; ± urinary incontinence with bladder difficult to express, increased urethral sphincter tone and tense bladder. • Lumbosacral lesion (L4–S3) — normal thoracic limbs; both pelvic limbs or ipsilateral limb affected with proprioceptive ataxia and paraparesis/plegia or monoparesis/plegia; hypo-/areflexia; hypo-/atonia; muscle atrophy; ± regional pain; ± urinary and fecal incontinence, large and flaccid bladder easy to express, decreased urethral sphincter tone; ± decreased or absent tail and anal tone; ± decreased or absent sensation below lesion.

CAUSES

• Degenerative and/or inherited—neuroaxonal or neuronal dystrophy, spinal muscular atrophy, storage diseases (gangliosidosis GM1/GM2, sphingomyelinosis, glycogenosis type IV, idiopathic complex polysaccharide storage disease, and mucopolysaccharidosis type VI) and spinal dural ossification. • Anomalous—syringohydromyelia, myelodysplasia, meningocele or meningomyelocele, and tethered spinal cord often associated with sacrocaudal dysgenesis, spinal arachnoid cyst, spinal intradural epithelial cyst, spinal dermoid cyst/sinus. • Metabolic—hypervitaminosis A, nutritional secondary hyperparathyroidism, cobalamine deficiency-associated myelopathy. • Neoplastic—lymphoma, vertebral column neoplasia (osteosarcoma, fibrosarcoma, plasma cell tumor, and chondrosarcoma), meningiomas, sarcomas, histiocytic tumors, glial tumors (astrocytoma, oligodendroglioma, gliomatosis cerebri), primitive neuroectodermal tumors, peripheral nerve sheath tumors, and metastatic tumors. • Inflammatory or infectious—feline infectious peritonitis (FIP), Borna virus (Europe), bacterial meningomyelitis, fungal meningomyelitis (*Cryptococcus neoformans*, *Coccidioides immitis*, *Histoplasma capsulatum*), *Toxoplasma gondii* meningomyelitis, eosinophilic meningomyelitis, idiopathic poliomyelitis, and feline leukemia virus (FeLV)-associated myelopathy. • Traumatic—vertebral fractures/luxations and penetrating wounds (bite wounds, BB pellets, microchips); intervertebral disc disease. • Vascular—ischemia or infarct of unknown etiology, fibrocartilaginous embolisms, ischemic myelopathy secondary to hyaline arteriopathy, intraosseous vascular malformations, and myelopathy secondary to aortocaval fistula.

RISK FACTORS

• Outdoor cats—at risk for traumatic and infectious myelitis.
• FeLV-positive cats—at risk for lymphoma and FeLV-associated myelopathy.

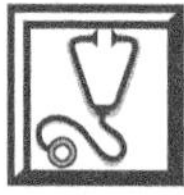

DIAGNOSIS

DIFFERENTIAL DIAGNOSIS

Differentiate from other disease processes that can cause paresis/paralysis—ischemic neuromyopathy caused by arterial thromboembolism, and peripheral neuromuscular diseases such as diabetic neuropathy, polyradiculoneuritis, hypokalemic myopathy, muscular dystrophy, polymyositis, and myasthenia gravis.

CBC/BIOCHEMISTRY/URINALYSIS

• Often normal. • Various nonspecific abnormalities can be found associated with infectious myelitis and lymphoma.
• Lysosomal storage diseases—abnormal accumulation of products of cell metabolism can be seen within the cytoplasm of peripheral leukocytes.

OTHER LABORATORY TESTS

• Serology—FeLV/FIV, Cryptococcus neoformans, Coccidioides immitis, Histoplasma capsulatum, and Toxoplasma gondii. • Latex agglutination test—

Cryptococcus neoformans (serum or CSF). • α-Acid glycoprotein (AGP) can be used as a discriminating marker for FIP when coupled with other high-risk factors. • Urine metabolic screening for lysosomal storage diseases. • Genetic tests for inherited myelopathies—see a frequently updated list of tests available worldwide and genetic testing laboratories in Internet Resources.

IMAGING

• Spinal radiography—may reveal congenital or acquired (MPS VI) vertebral malformations, discospondylitis, vertebral fractures and luxations, bony tumors, and radiographic signs suggestive of intervertebral disc disease. • Myelography—may reveal extradural compression consistent with intervertebral disc disease or tumor, or intradural–extramedullary tumors. • CT—more sensitive than radiography for diagnosis of discospondylitis, vertebral fractures, and bony tumors; may reveal syringomyelia and intramedullary tumors. • MRI—more sensitive than CT for diagnosis of intramedullary tumors, inflammatory/infectious and vascular diseases, and anomalies, such as syringomyelia, myelodysplasia, meningocele or meningomyelocele, tethered spinal cord, spinal arachnoid cyst, spinal intradural epithelial cyst, and spinal dermoid cyst/sinus.

DIAGNOSTIC PROCEDURES

CSF Analysis

• To confirm an inflammatory process affecting meninges and/or spinal cord. • Elevated total nucleated cell count and proteins suggest an inflammatory process affecting meninges and/or spinal cord; should be examined for fungal and bacterial organisms. • Other laboratory tests performed on CSF—latex agglutination test for *Cryptococcus neoformans*; ELISA for *Cryptococcus neoformans* and *Histoplasma capsulatum*; PCR for feline coronavirus and *Toxoplasma gondii*; bacterial and fungal culture.

Electrodiagnostics

Electromyography, nerve conduction velocity, repetitive stimulations—help differentiating paresis/paralysis caused by a myelopathy from peripheral neuromuscular disorders.

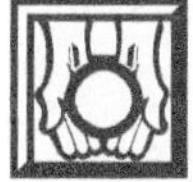

TREATMENT

APPROPRIATE HEALTH CARE

• Emergency evaluation and possible surgery—when a traumatic cause of paresis/paralysis is suspected. • Inpatient medical management—for severe neurologic deficits such as paralysis and urinary incontinence.

NURSING CARE

• Non-ambulatory cats should be confined to a soft padded crate or enclosed area, kept dry and clean, and turned every 6 hours if they are not able to assume a sternal position. • If there is urinary incontinence, the bladder should be expressed every 8 hours. • Prevent/treat decubital ulcers and urine scalding. • Treat constipation. • Physical therapy is useful to prevent muscle atrophy and contractures and to keep the joints flexible, especially for postoperative rehabilitation in vertebral trauma or intervertebral disc disease.

CLIENT EDUCATION

If the cat is treated as an outpatient, discuss all aspects of nursing care and possible complications with the client.

SURGICAL CONSIDERATIONS

Surgical management—for vertebral fractures and luxations, intervertebral disc disease, and some neoplasms. The objectives of surgical management should be decompression of the spinal cord, and/or reduction and stabilization of the fracture/luxation.

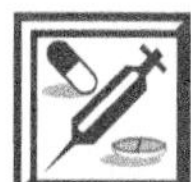

MEDICATIONS

DRUG(S) OF CHOICE

• Not recommended until a diagnosis has been established. • Spinal trauma—controversial: in experimental studies of acute spinal cord injury (ASCI) in cats, the administration of methylprednisolone sodium succinate (MPSS) within 8 hours from injury (30 mg/kg initial bolus, followed by MPSS CRI of 5.4 mg/kg/h for 24 hours or 15 mg/kg q6h for 2 doses) led to improved neurologic function; however, these studies have not been replicated in a clinical setting. Please note that the use of high-dose glucocorticoids in trauma patients has been associated with hyperglycemia, pneumonia, urinary tract infection, gastrointestinal ulceration, and increased mortality. Dexamethasone was not found to improve neurologic outcome in experimental cat models of ASCI.

CONTRAINDICATIONS

Glucocorticoids—contraindicated when an infectious disease is suspected; may also alter CSF, MRI, or CT results, precluding reaching a diagnosis.

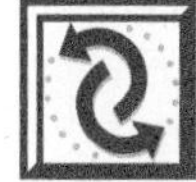

FOLLOW-UP

POSSIBLE COMPLICATIONS

• Urinary infection. • Urine scalding. • Constipation or fecal incontinence. • Muscle atrophy and contractures. • Decubital ulcers.

MISCELLANEOUS

AGE-RELATED FACTORS

• Cats <2 years—myelopathies often caused by anomalous or inherited, inflammatory, or infectious, metabolic, and traumatic diseases. FIP is the most important cause of myelopathy in this age group. • Cats 2–8 years—lymphoma (LSA), FIP, and trauma are important causes of myelopathy. • Cats >8 years—vascular and neoplastic diseases more common, especially LSA and vertebral tumors.

ZOONOTIC POTENTIAL

Toxoplasma gondii infections represent a zoonotic potential.

SEE ALSO

Schiff–Sherrington Phenomenon.

ABBREVIATIONS

- AGP = α-Acid glycoprotein.
- DSH = domestic shorthair.
- FeLV = feline leukemia virus.
- FIP = feline infectious peritonitis.
- FIV = feline immunodeficiency virus.
- LSA = lymphoma.
- MPS = mucopolysaccharidosis.

INTERNET RESOURCES

PennGen DNA Tests Available Worldwide for Canine and Feline Hereditary Diseases: https://www.vet.upenn.edu/research/academic-departments/clinical-sciences-advanced-medicine/research-labs-centers/penngen/tests-worldwide

Suggested Reading

Aharon MA, Prittie JE, Buriko KA. review of associated controversies surrounding glucocorticoid use in veterinary emergency and critical care. J Vet Emerg Crit Care 2017, 27:267–77.

Marioni-Henry K, Van Winkle TJ, Smith SH, et al. Tumors affecting the spinal cord of cats: 85 cases (1980–2005). J Am Vet Med Assoc 2008, 232:237–243.

Marioni-Henry K, Vite CH, Newton AL, et al. Prevalence of diseases of the spinal cord of cats. J Vet Intern Med 2004, 8:851–858.

Sharp B. Feline physiotherapy and rehabilitation: 2. clinical applications. J Feline Med Surg 2012, 14:633–645.

Author Katia Marioni-Henry

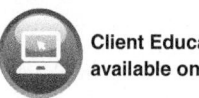

Client Education Handout available online

MYELOPROLIFERATIVE DISORDERS

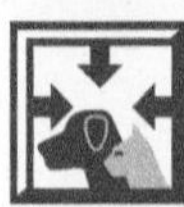

BASICS

OVERVIEW

- Unregulated neoplastic proliferation of nonlymphoid cells originating in the bone marrow (granulocytic, monocytic, erythrocytic, and megakaryocytic cells) resulting in accumulations of differentiated cells.
- Includes polycythemia vera, chronic myelogenous leukemia, essential thrombocythemia, and possibly primary myelofibrosis.
- Believed to represent a spectrum of disorders in which the stem cell involved is a hematopoietic precursor capable of differentiating into all blood cell types except lymphocytes.

SIGNALMENT

- Cats and dogs—more common in cats.
- May be more common in large-breed dogs than small-breed dogs.

SIGNS

- Pale mucous membranes.
- Petechiation.
- Lethargy.
- Inappetance.
- Weight loss.
- Hepatosplenomegaly.
- Peripheral lymphadenomegaly—occasionally.
- Neurologic signs—disorientation, ataxia, seizure.

CAUSES & RISK FACTORS

- Cats—most commonly associated with feline leukemia virus (FeLV) infection; when recovering from panleukopenia or hemobartonellosis, may be a relatively higher risk of developing a mutant cell line induced by FeLV.
- Dogs—has been experimentally induced with chronic low-dose radiation exposure.

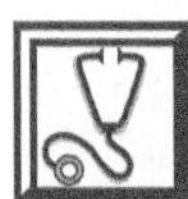

DIAGNOSIS

DIFFERENTIAL DIAGNOSIS

- Acute lymphocytic leukemia—usually differentiated by special staining techniques (immunohistochemistry or immunocytochemistry for lymphoid markers) or PCR for antigen receptor rearrangement (PARR).
- Leukemoid response secondary to inflammation.
- Other causes of eosinophilia—parasitism; allergic disease; eosinophilic gastroenteritis; mast cell neoplasia; differentiate from eosinophilic leukemia.
- Relative and secondary absolute polycythemia.
- Reactive thrombocytosis—secondary to inflammation, hemolytic or iron-deficiency anemia, splenectomy, rebound from immune-mediated thrombocytopenia, and drug-induced (e.g., vincristine).

CBC/BIOCHEMISTRY/URINALYSIS

- Severe, nonregenerative anemia.
- Severe elevated hematocrit in cases of primary polycythemia vera.
- Circulating nucleated red blood cells.
- Megaloblastic erythrocytes.
- Leukocytosis or leukopenia.
- Thrombocytopenia with abnormal platelet morphology.
- Thrombocytosis in cases of essential thrombocythemia.
- Circulation of immature myeloid cells.

OTHER LABORATORY TESTS

- Examination of bone marrow aspirate or core biopsy—reveals hypercellular bone marrow with abnormal morphology in all cell lines; neoplastic proliferation or absence of one cell line.
- Immunohistochemical or other special stains—may be necessary to determine cell lineage.

IMAGING

Abdominal radiography and ultrasonography—hepatomegaly and splenomegaly common.

DIAGNOSTIC PROCEDURES

Examination of bone marrow aspirates or core biopsy.

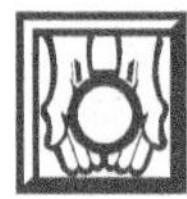

TREATMENT

- Outpatient or inpatient.
- Supportive care—blood transfusions and fluid administration to correct dehydration.
- Therapeutic phlebotomies.
- Radiophosphorus (^{32}P) has been effective in cases of polycythemia vera and essential thrombocythemia but there are limited facilities that can offer this therapy.
- Seek consultation from a veterinary oncologist regarding treatment.

MEDICATIONS

DRUG(S) OF CHOICE

- Little information available in the literature regarding treatment.
- Cytosine arabinoside—may be used; 100 mg/m^2 SC divided q12h 4 days per week, or as a constant rate infusion over 6–8 hours at a dose of 400 mg/m^2.
- Hydroxyurea 30–45 mg/kg q24h for 7–10 days; then 30–45 mg/kg q48h or 15 mg/kg q24h; initially, titrate dosage to patient response.
- Antibiotics—may be indicated to combat secondary infection.

CONTRAINDICATIONS/POSSIBLE INTERACTIONS

Chemotherapy can be toxic; seek advice before treatment if unfamiliar with cytotoxic drugs.

FOLLOW-UP

- Complete blood count and examination of bone marrow aspirate—determine response to treatment and progression of disease.
- Prognosis—guarded.

MISCELLANEOUS

PREGNANCY/FERTILITY/BREEDING

- Chemotherapy drugs are contraindicated in pregnant animals.
- It is not recommended to breed animals with neoplasia.

ABBREVIATIONS

- FeLV = feline leukemia virus.
- PARR = polymerase chain reaction for antigen receptor rearrangement.

Suggested Reading

Young KM, Vail DM. Canine acute myeloid leukemia, myeloproliferative neoplasms, and myelodysplasia. In: Withrow SJ, Vail DM, Page RL, eds., Small Animal Clinical Oncology, 5th ed. Philadelphia, PA: Saunders, 2013, pp. 653–665.

Author Rebecca G. Newman
Consulting Editor Timothy M. Fan

M

MYOCARDIAL INFARCTION

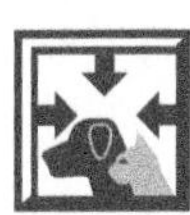

BASICS

OVERVIEW

• Rapid development of myocardial necrosis resulting from sustained, complete reduction of blood flow to a portion of the myocardium, caused by thrombus formation.
• Uncommon as a naturally occurring disease in dogs. • Microscopic intramural myocardial infarctions and focal areas of myocardial fibrosis are common in dogs with acquired cardiovascular disease. • Consistent electrocardiogram (ECG) characteristics of spontaneous myocardial infarction are not well characterized in dogs and cats.

SIGNALMENT

Rare in dog and cat

SIGNS

Historical Findings

• Lethargy. • Anorexia. • Weakness.
• Dyspnea. • Collapse. • Vomiting.
• Obesity. • Unexpected death.

Physical Examination Findings

• Lameness. • Tachycardia. • Heart murmur.
• Cardiac rhythm disturbances. • Low-grade fever.

CAUSES & RISK FACTORS

Dogs

• Atherosclerosis and coronary artery disease.
• Nephrotic syndrome. • Vasculitis.
• Hypothyroidism. • Bacterial endocarditis.
• Neoplasia. • Septicemia. • Intramural coronary arteriosclerosis in old dogs.
• Subvalvular aortic stenosis.

Cats

• Cardiomyopathy. • Thromboembolism.

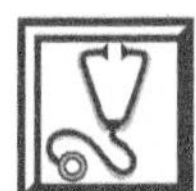

DIAGNOSIS

Generally presumptive, based on acute onset of signs in a patient with predisposing factors, consistent ECG changes (ST segment changes) and elevated circulating biomarkers (cardiac troponin I [cTnI]).

DIFFERENTIAL DIAGNOSIS

Other Causes of ST Segment Changes

• Normal variation. • Myocardial ischemia/hypoxia. • Hyperkalemia or hypokalemia.
• Digitalis toxicity. • Trauma to the heart.
• Pericarditis. • Artifact—wandering baseline.

Other Causes of Weakness and Collapse

• Trauma. • Neurologic disease.
• Thromboembolism. • Pericardial effusion.
• Arrhythmia.

CBC/BIOCHEMISTRY/URINALYSIS

• Mild leukocytosis. • High liver enzymes.
• Hyperlipidemia—if animal is hypothyroid.
• High amylase. • High creatine kinase and cardiac isoenzymes. • High cTnI.

OTHER LABORATORY TESTS

Low triiodothyronine (T_3) and thyroxine (T_4).

IMAGING

Echocardiography—2D and M-mode echocardiography useful in evaluating wall motion abnormalities and overall left ventricular function.

DIAGNOSTIC PROCEDURES

Electrocardiographic Findings

• Sudden deviation of the ST segment (Figure 1). • Tall peaked T waves—first few hours. • Sudden development of Q waves or a change in direction of the T wave. • Axis shift of the frontal plane. • Low-voltage QRS complexes. • Sudden development of bundle branch block or heart block. • Sudden onset of ventricular arrhythmias because of myocardial ischemia. • Sloppy "R" wave descent may be associated with intramural myocardial infarction.

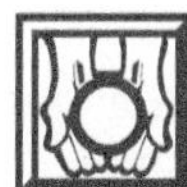

TREATMENT

• Treat the underlying disorder; likewise the symptomatic therapy (e.g., congestive heart failure [CHF]). • Must identify and immediately treat life-threatening arrhythmias.

MEDICATIONS

DRUG(S) OF CHOICE

• IV thrombolytic agents—(e.g., streptokinase); cost prohibitive and lack of experience with myocardial infarction in veterinary medicine with dosage and use.
• Lidocaine for ventricular arrhythmias.
• Beta-blockers—use cautiously with dilated cardiomyopathy because of possible development of low-output CHF.
• Antithrombotic agents (e.g., dalteparin; low molecular weight heparin, heparin and aspirin).

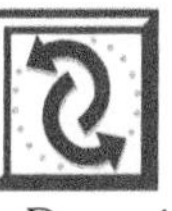

FOLLOW-UP

• Determined by clinical status and diagnosis of underlying disorder. • Monitor anticoagulated patient; CBC and bleeding profiles, including fibrinogen.

MISCELLANEOUS

ABBREVIATIONS

• CHF = congestive heart failure. • cTnI = cardiac troponin I. • ECG = electrocardiogram.
• T_3 = triiodothyronine. • T_4 = thyroxine.

Suggested Reading

Driehuys E, Van Winkle TJ, Sammarco CD, Drobatz KJ. Myocardial infarction in dogs and cats: 37 cases (1985–1994). J Am Vet Med Assoc 1998, 213:1444–1448.

Kidd L, Stepien RL, Amoheim DP. Clinical findings and coronary artery disease in dogs and cats with acute & subacute myocardial necrosis: 28 cases. J Am Anim Hosp Assoc 2000, 36:199–208.

Author Larry P. Tilley
Consulting Editor Michael Aherne

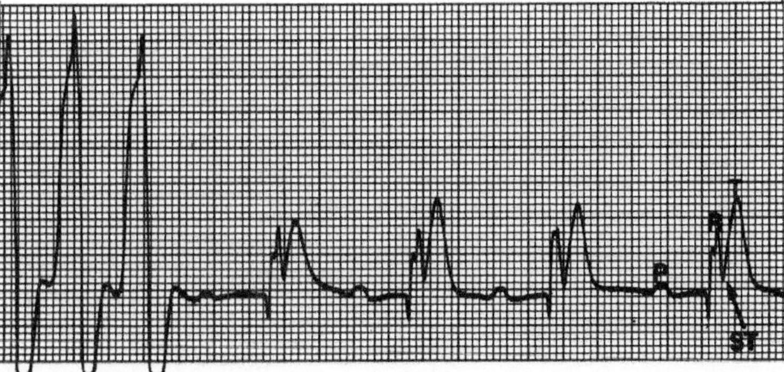

Figure 1.

Transmural infarction of the left ventricle in a dog with arteriosclerosis and hypothyroidism. The first three rapid successive complexes represent ventricular tachycardia. The sinus rhythm that follows illustrates small complexes, marked elevation of the ST segment, and first-degree atrioventricular block (prolonged PR interval). (Source: From Tilley LP. Essentials of Canine and Feline Electrocardiography, 3rd ed. Baltimore: Williams & Wilkins, 1992. Reprinted with permission of Wolters Kluwer.)

MYOCARDIAL TUMORS

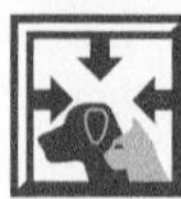

BASICS

OVERVIEW

- Primary and metastatic myocardial tumors are rare tumors in dogs and cats; incidence 0.19% in dogs and 0.03% in cats.
- Reported primary tumors include hemangiosarcoma, ectopic thyroid carcinoma, lymphoma, with less frequently documented rhabdomyoma, rhabdomyosarcoma, thymoma, mesothelioma, chondrosarcoma, osteosarcoma, fibrosarcoma, myxoma, myxosarcoma, lipoma, peripheral nerve sheath tumor, and granular cell tumor.

SIGNALMENT

- Dogs and cats—but less common in cats.
- In dogs—any age but more common between 7 and 15 years.
- Possible increased incidence in neutered animals.
- Increased incidence in Saluki, French bulldog, Irish water spaniel, flat-coated retriever, golden retriever, boxer, Afghan hound, English Setter, Scottish terrier, Boston terrier, bulldog, German shepherd dog.

SIGNS

- Sudden collapse.
- Abdominal distention.
- Exercise intolerance.
- Dyspnea.
- Anorexia.
- Vomiting.
- Diarrhea.
- Acute death.

CAUSES & RISK FACTORS

Unknown

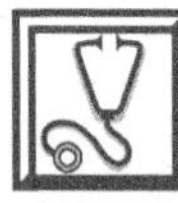

DIAGNOSIS

DIFFERENTIAL DIAGNOSIS

- Idiopathic pericardial effusion.
- Pericarditis.
- Cardiomyopathy.
- Heart failure.
- Valvular disease.
- Heart base tumors.

CBC/BIOCHEMISTRY/URINALYSIS

Anemia in some patients.

OTHER LABORATORY TESTS

Serum/plasma cardiac troponin I levels are increased in patients with cardiac hemangiosarcoma and might have utility for the detection of other myocardial neoplasms.

IMAGING

- Thoracic radiography—may reveal a globoid heart suggestive of pericardial effusion, masses in the area of the atria, or metastatic lesions in the lungs.
- Echocardiography—helpful in finding primary masses; positive predictive value of 92%, negative predictive values 64%.
- Advanced imaging such as CT, positron emission tomography (PET) scan, and MRI may be helpful in defining mass lesions.

DIAGNOSTIC PROCEDURES

- Pericardiocentesis and fluid evaluation—helpful in diagnosis of lymphoma.
- Cytology of pericardial effusion limited in usefulness in differentiating neoplastic from non-neoplastic effusions.
- ECG—may be normal or display a variety of arrhythmias; may see electrical alternans and small complexes with pericardial effusion.
- Surgical biopsy of mass—if possible.

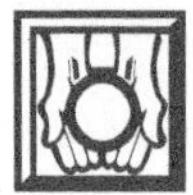

TREATMENT

- Surgical removal of mass—if possible.
- Pericardectomy—may offer relief of pericardial effusion.
- Address concern for sudden death with owner.

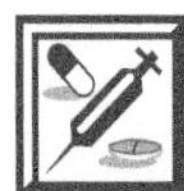

MEDICATIONS

DRUG(S) OF CHOICE

- Management of arrhythmias—lidocaine (dogs) 2–4 mg/kg IV (to a maximum 8 mg/kg over 10-minute period), CRI—25–75 μg/kg/minute IV, mexiletine (dogs) 5–8 mg/kg PO q8–12h, sotalol 1–2 mg/kg PO q12h.
- Chemotherapy dependent on tumor type (see Lymphoma—Cats, Lymphoma—Dogs, and Hemangiosarcoma, Heart).

CONTRAINDICATIONS/POSSIBLE INTERACTIONS

Chemotherapy can cause gastrointestinal, bone marrow, cardiac, and other toxicities—seek advice if unfamiliar with cytotoxic drugs.

FOLLOW-UP

- Serial echocardiograms—to monitor tumor response to chemotherapy.
- Thoracic radiography and abdominal ultrasonography—to monitor for metastatic disease progression.
- ECG—to monitor response to antiarrhythmogenic medications.
- Blood tests—especially CBC to monitor for bone marrow suppression secondary to chemotherapy.
- Prognosis—guarded to poor.

MISCELLANEOUS

PREGNANCY/FERTILITY/BREEDING

- It is not recommended to breed animals with cancer.
- Chemotherapy is teratogenic—do not give to pregnant animals.

SEE ALSO

- Chemodectoma.
- Hemangiosarcoma, Heart.
- Lymphoma—Cats.
- Lymphoma—Dogs.

ABBREVIATIONS

- PET = positron emission tomography.

Suggested Reading

Treggiari E, Pedro B, Dukes-McEwan J, et al. A descriptive review of cardiac tumours in dogs and cats. Vet Comp Oncol 2017, 15(2):273–288.

Author Rebecca G. Newman
Consulting Editor Timothy M. Fan

M

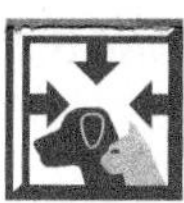

BASICS

DEFINITION

• Inflammation of the myocardium, definitive identification of which requires histologic examination. • In humans, the widely accepted Dallas criteria specify that necrosis and/or degeneration of myocytes adjacent to inflammatory infiltrates is a requisite for diagnosis. • Causes are diverse and include infective (viral, bacterial, protozoal, mycotic) pathogens and noninfective (toxic, possibly immune) disease agents. • Traumatic myocarditis is a term applied to the syndrome of arrhythmias that sometimes complicates blunt trauma. The term is a misnomer because myocardial lesions (if present) are more likely to take the form of necrosis than inflammation.

PATHOPHYSIOLOGY

• Numerous mechanisms, determined partly by the nature of the causative agent, are implicated. • Microbial agents and toxins can result in direct cellular damage causing cell death, activation of the immune system, and inflammation. • Though incompletely described in veterinary patients, chronic myocarditis, immune myocarditis and autoreactive myocarditis—the latter occurring in the absence of microbial agents—as well as dilated cardiomyopathy (DCM) are potential sequelae of acute myocarditis. • The cellular character of inflammation is partly determined by the nature of the pathologic insult; protozoal and mycotic agents result in pyogranulomatous infiltrates, while viral myocarditis is generally lymphocytic.
• Myocardial involvement may be focal or diffuse. • Canine parvoviral infection can result in myocarditis in pups, and has been implicated as a cause of DCM. The virus has tropism for dividing cells, and adult myocytes do not replicate. Parvovirus myocarditis is most likely to occur in unvaccinated pups from immunologically naïve dams.
• Protozoal myocarditis resulting from *Trypanosoma cruzi* infection causes Chagas disease. Acute phase illness is characterized primarily by electrocardiogram (ECG) abnormalities. Chronic infection can result in myocardial dysfunction and development of heart failure. • It has been hypothesized that feline endomyocarditis might be a precursor of restrictive cardiomyopathy; recent findings implicate infection by *Bartonella* spp.
• Bacterial myocarditis can be observed in patients with overwhelming sepsis.
• Bacterial, protozoal, and mycotic myocarditis may reflect immunosuppression.
• An apparently rare, as yet idiopathic, atrial myocarditis might be important in the pathogenesis of persistent canine atrial standstill. • The pathogenetic importance of myocardial inflammation in canine arrhythmogenic right ventricular cardiomyopathy is unresolved; however, myocarditis is observed in a substantial proportion of cases. • The pathogenesis of traumatic myocarditis is incompletely defined; direct trauma resulting in necrosis is likely responsible in some cases, but extracardiac factors including electrolyte derangements, hypoxia, acid–base disturbances, and altered function of the autonomic nervous system might contribute.

SYSTEMS AFFECTED

• Systemic involvement depends on the causative agent. • Cardiovascular—myocardial dysfunction and/or arrhythmias.
• Respiratory—if pulmonary edema develops.

INCIDENCE/PREVALENCE

• Histologically confirmed myocarditis is rarely identified in veterinary patients, therefore epidemiology of myocarditis is incompletely described. • Viral myocarditis is seemingly rare. • Chagas disease is uncommon and occurs primarily in the southern United States. • Fungal myocarditis—primarily seen in association with systemic fungal infection—is rare and occurs regionally, where mycoses are endemic.
• Spirochetal myocarditis and atrioventricular (AV) block resulting from *Borrelia burgdorferi* infection has been reported, but seemingly is rare. • Infection by *Bartonella* spp. has been associated with canine and feline myocarditis.

GEOGRAPHIC DISTRIBUTION

Myocarditis can result from infectious agents that have distinct geographic distributions.

SIGNALMENT

Species

Dog and cat.

Mean Age and Range

Largely unknown.

SIGNS

General Comments

• Related to the extent and duration of myocardial involvement. • Signs relating to arrhythmias or heart failure are most common.
• Onset of cardiac dysfunction in association with systemic illness should prompt consideration of myocarditis and, because myocardial disease in veterinary patients is often familial, development of cardiac dysfunction in patients with atypical signalment suggests the possibility of myocarditis.

Historical Findings

• Coughing, exercise intolerance, dyspnea—associated with congestive heart failure (CHF).
• Syncope and weakness—associated with arrhythmias. • Concurrent manifestations of systemic disease reflective of the etiologic agent. • Road traffic or other accidents often precede the development of traumatic myocarditis.

Physical Examination Findings

• Gallop sounds or murmurs may be heard.
• Arrhythmias—may be auscultated.
• Fever—potentially observed in patients with infective myocarditis. • Evidence of injury in those with traumatic myocarditis.

CAUSES

• Virus (e.g., parvovirus, distemper virus, herpesvirus, West Nile virus). • Protozoa (e.g., *T. cruzi*, *Toxoplasma gondii*, *Neospora caninum*, *Hepatozoon canis*, *Babesia* spp., and *Leishmania* spp.). • Bacteria (e.g., *Bartonella vinsonii* subsp. *berkhoffii*). • Fungi (e.g., *Cryptococcus neoformans*, *Coccidioides immitis*, *Blastomyces dermatitidis*, and *Aspergillus terreus*). • Algae (e.g., *Prototheca* spp.).
• Blunt trauma can result in the syndrome of traumatic myocarditis.

RISK FACTORS

• Exposure to infectious agents.
• Immunosuppression. • Debilitating diseases. • Trauma.

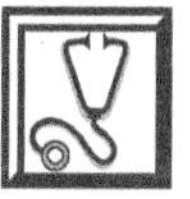

DIAGNOSIS

DIFFERENTIAL DIAGNOSIS

• Consider the possibility that preexisting heart disease such as congenital defects, cardiomyopathy, and acquired valvular disease are responsible for clinical findings. • History of a heart murmur or the presence of arrhythmias before onset of systemic illness helps differentiate from other diseases.
• Extracardiac organ involvement and identification of infectious agents may aid in the diagnosis. • History of road traffic accident generally makes the diagnosis of traumatic myocarditis obvious.

CBC/BIOCHEMISTRY/URINALYSIS

Abnormalities—vary, depending on organ involvement.

OTHER LABORATORY TESTS

• Serologic tests can be used to detect exposure to infectious agents. • Cytologic examination of pericardial, pleural, and peritoneal effusions to identify the infectious organism. • Blood culture to identify bacteremia. • Troponin—concentrations might be high and reflect myocyte necrosis.

IMAGING

Thoracic Radiography

• Cardiac silhouette may be enlarged if myocarditis has resulted in cardiac dysfunction; potential consequences of cardiac dysfunction include: pulmonary edema and/or pleural effusion. • Pulmonary granuloma may be found in animals with granulomatous myocardial infection.
• Evidence of trauma potentially including pulmonary contusions or pneumothorax.

MYOCARDITIS (CONTINUED)

Echocardiography

• Reflects the extent of myocardial damage; may be normal if lesions are small or primarily affect the conduction system. • Evaluation of systolic myocardial function might reveal minor segmental abnormalities, or global dysfunction associated with chamber enlargement. • In humans and experimental models, an increase in wall thickness has been associated with inflammatory infiltrates/edema; this observation might be relevant to the syndrome of "transient wall thickening" observed in cats. • Pericardial effusion in patients with pancarditis. • In exceptional cases granulomas result in echocardiographically evident masses.

DIAGNOSTIC PROCEDURES

ECG

• Arrhythmias of all types—supraventricular tachyarrhythmias, ventricular tachyarrhythmias, and bradyarrhythmias, perhaps particularly AV block—can be observed in association with inflammatory myocardial disease. • Arrhythmias associated with trauma—ventricular tachyarrhythmias occur in most affected patients; supraventricular arrhythmias and bradyarrhythmias are rare. Ventricular rhythms that complicate blunt trauma often have relatively slow rates detected only during pauses in the sinus rhythm; they are most appropriately referred to as accelerated idioventricular rhythms (AIVRs). The QRS complexes are wide and bizarre; the rate is >100 bpm but <160 bpm. Usually, these rhythms are electrically and hemodynamically benign. However, dangerous ventricular tachycardias can complicate blunt trauma and evolve from seemingly benign AIVRs, compromising perfusion and placing the patient at risk for sudden death.

Endomyocardial Biopsy

A minimally invasive technique that is required for definitive ante-mortem diagnosis but rarely performed in veterinary patients.

Pericardiocentesis

• Alleviates tamponade caused by pericardial effusion. • Submit fluid for cytologic examination and, possibly, bacterial culture.

Holter Monitoring

• To define the burden of arrhythmia in terms of frequency and character over a 24-48 hour period. • To monitor antiarrhythmic therapy.

PATHOLOGIC FINDINGS

• Dilated cardiac chambers with patchy areas of hyperemia, necrosis, or fibrosis.
• Granulomas seen grossly in some patients.
• Histologic examination of the myocardium or pericardium may reveal inflammatory cells (e.g., lymphocytes, plasma cells, and macrophages), patchy fibrosis, or the infectious agents themselves.

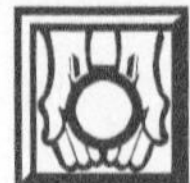

TREATMENT

APPROPRIATE HEALTH CARE

• Hospitalize patients with decompensated heart failure for initial medical management.
• Hospitalize patients with hemodynamically consequential ventricular arrhythmias for initial, parenteral antiarrhythmic therapy.
• Hospitalize patients with severe systemic manifestations for appropriate medical therapy.

ACTIVITY

Restricted

DIET

Sodium restriction if CHF.

CLIENT EDUCATION

• Cardiac manifestations may persist even after resolution of systemic illness. • Certain arrhythmias (e.g., ventricular tachycardia, third-degree AV block) may predispose to sudden death. • Antemortem diagnosis may be difficult. • Some infectious agents may pose a public health risk.

SURGICAL CONSIDERATIONS

Complete AV block may require pacemaker implantation.

MEDICATIONS

DRUG(S) OF CHOICE

• If a specific pathogenetic agent is identified, appropriate, etiologically targeted therapy.
• Tailor antiarrhythmic therapy based on ECG findings.

CONTRAINDICATIONS

N/A.

PRECAUTIONS

• All antiarrhythmic drugs potentially have proarrhythmic properties and their effects should be closely monitored. • Systemic organ involvement (e.g., renal involvement) may necessitate modifying drug dosages. • Some agents that result in canine or feline myocarditis can also affect humans, so potentially there are public health considerations.

FOLLOW-UP

PATIENT MONITORING

• Antiarrhythmic therapy—frequent auscultation and ECG. • Serologic titers when appropriate. • Auscultation and follow-up radiographs—treatment of heart failure. • Hemograms and serum biochemical analysis—systemic effects.

PREVENTION/AVOIDANCE

• Avoid breeding animals that have not been immunized. • Avoid endemic areas if possible.

EXPECTED COURSE AND PROGNOSIS

• Depend on the extent and severity of myocardial involvement. • Many systemic fungal and protozoal diseases do not respond well to medical management. • Patients with extensive myocardial inflammation, degeneration, and signs of heart failure have a very poor prognosis. • Good prognosis if the underlying cause can be treated successfully.

MISCELLANEOUS

ASSOCIATED CONDITIONS

Often accompanies systemic illness.

AGE-RELATED FACTORS

Viral myocarditis—most often seen in animals <1 year old.

ZOONOTIC POTENTIAL

• Varies with infectious agent involved.
• May be high with protozoal and mycotic infections.

PREGNANCY/FERTILITY/BREEDING

Some viral diseases (e.g., canine herpesvirus and parvovirus) have been passed to the fetus during pregnancy.

SEE ALSO

• Aspergillosis, Disseminated Invasive.
• Babesiosis. • Bartonellosis. • Blastomycosis.
• Canine Distemper. • Canine Parvovirus.
• Chagas Disease (American Trypanosomiasis).
• Coccidioidomycosis. • Cryptococcosis.
• Hepatozoonosis. • Idioventricular Rhythm.
• Leishmaniosis. • Neosporosis.
• Protothecosis. • Toxoplasmosis. • Ventricular Premature Complexes. • Ventricular Tachycardia.

ABBREVIATIONS

• AIVR = accelerated idioventricular rhythm.
• AV = atrioventricular. • CHF = congestive heart failure. • DCM = dilated cardiomyopathy. • ECG = electrocardiogram

Suggested Reading

Breitschwerdt EB, Atkins CE, Brown TT, et al. *Bartonella vinsonii* subsp. *berkhoffii* and related members of the alpha subdivision of the Proteobacteria in dogs with cardiac arrhythmias, endocarditis, or myocarditis. J Clin Microbiol 1999, 37(11):3618–3626.

Donovan TA, Balakrishnan N, Carvalho Barbosa I, et al. *Bartonella* spp. as a possible cause or cofactor of feline endomyocarditis–left ventricular endocardial fibrosis complex. J Comp Pathol 2018, 162:29–42.

Janus I, Noszczyk-Nowak A, Nowak M, et al. Myocarditis in dogs: etiology, clinical and histopathological features (11 cases, 2007–2013). Ir Vet J 2014, 67:1–8.

Author Jonathan A. Abbott
Consulting Editor Michael Aherne
Acknowledgment The author and editors acknowledge the prior contribution of Larry P. Tilley.

MYOCLONUS

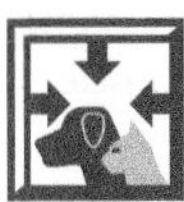

BASICS

OVERVIEW

• Involuntary, rhythmic, or irregular muscle jerks. Can involve only a few adjacent muscles (focal), many or most muscles of the body (generalized), or many muscles in different jerks (multifocal) synchronously or asynchronously. • The myoclonic movements are spontaneous or activated by sensory stimulation (reflex myoclonus). • May persist during sleep. • CNS dysfunction involving segmental lower motor neurons and interneurons of the spinal cord or the brainstem. • Canine distemper virus infection—most frequent cause of myoclonus in dogs; thought to be secondary to some pacemaker activity in neurons damaged by the virus. May be caused by other encephalitides and degenerative processes affecting motor neurons.

SIGNALMENT

Acquired

• Dog and rarely cat. • No breed, sex, or age predispositions.

Congenital

• Familial reflex myoclonus—Labrador retriever and Dalmatian; develops in the first 3 weeks of life. • Spongy degeneration of either gray and/or white matter—dogs: myoclonus of the paravertebral muscles in neonate silky terrier; Samoyed at 2 weeks; Saluki at 3 months; Labrador retriever at 4–6 months. Cats—Egyptian mau at 7 weeks. Rare syndromes.

SIGNS

Historical Findings

• Canine distemper—after a bout of gastrointestinal signs, cough, and/or ocular or nasal purulent discharge; persists at rest and even during sleep or light anesthesia; consistent frequency in a given patient; distemper diagnosis may precede the myoclonus by months to years; occurs more frequently in chronic phase of distemper. • Familial reflex myoclonus—observed when the patient starts walking; intermittent muscle contractions induced by auditory or tactile stimulus and by exercise; involves all limbs, neck, and head (e.g., the facial and masticatory muscles); patient unable to rise without assistance. • With spongy degeneration—variety of signs observed such as tremor, spasticity, opisthotonos, and myoclonus. • Chlorambucil-induced myoclonus reported in a cat with lymphoma.

Physical Examination Findings

• The patient may be otherwise healthy. • Masticatory and appendicular muscles—most frequent affected muscles in distemper virus-induced myoclonus; may be paresis of the affected limb. • May see other signs suggesting distemper (e.g., hard pads, ocular and nasal purulent discharge, and chorioretinitis). • Neurologic deficits suggest multifocal lesions in some patients.

CAUSES & RISK FACTORS

Congenital

• Familial in Labrador retrievers. • Spongy degeneration of unknown cause but likely inherited.

Acquired

• Canine distemper virus—the only CNS disease repeatedly associated with myoclonus in dogs; unvaccinated dogs at risk. • Encephalitis of any cause—dogs and cats. • Degenerative disease—especially spongy degeneration.
• Described in a dog with lead poisoning.
• Total IV anesthesia with propofol.
• Intrathecal administration of morphine.
• Treatment with chlorambucil in cats.

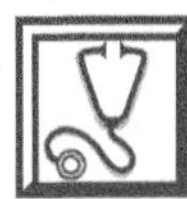

DIAGNOSIS

DIFFERENTIAL DIAGNOSIS

• The quickness of the jerks and the absence of voluntary influence help differentiating myoclonus from other movement disorders. • Congenital myoclonus—in neonates or during the first months of life in otherwise healthy dogs. Excitement, voluntary activity, and tactile/auditory stimuli often increase the myoclonus. • Canine distemper virus—unvaccinated dog; observed before, during, or after the acute CNS disease; more frequently observed later when the animal is otherwise healthy. Myoclonus involves one limb, more than one limb, the facial or the masticatory muscles. • Lafora disease (progressive myoclonic epilepsy)—neurodegenerative disease that can cause myoclonic jerks. Differentiated on presence of other seizure types (generalized tonic–clonic seizures) and altered mentation. • Myoclonic epilepsy—jerks usually generalized, proximal more than distal, and flexor more than extensor; exacerbated by sensory stimulus (light, noise) and voluntary movements. Other types of seizures may be present concomitantly.

CBC/BIOCHEMISTRY/URINALYSIS

• Congenital or post canine distemper virus infection—normal. • Other acquired forms—may suggest a specific cause if the patient has infectious encephalomyelitis; otherwise, normal.

IMAGING

MRI—may help determine diagnosis in acute acquired disease.

DIAGNOSTIC PROCEDURES

Acute onset—CSF analysis, serologic testing, imaging to determine the cause if other physical or neurologic signs present. Electroencephalography and electromyography—may help differentiate myoclonic epilepsy and peripheral nervous system disease from myoclonus.

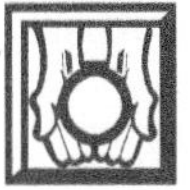

TREATMENT

• Active encephalomyelitis—inpatient; establish a diagnosis and initiate treatment. • Exercise—as tolerated. • Diet—ensure proper nutrition with active CNS disease; modify, if necessary, with vomiting or diarrhea. • Familial reflex myoclonus—clinical signs in Labrador retriever and Dalmatian are severe and usually not compatible with quality of life.

M

MEDICATIONS

DRUG(S) OF CHOICE

• With chronic, inactive canine distemper—treatment often unnecessary; alleviation may be obtained with procainamide 125–250 mg/dog PO q6–12h. • Gabapentin 10–20 mg/kg q8h reported beneficial in tremor syndrome. • Clorazepate 0.6–2 mg/kg PO q8h—familial reflex myoclonus; may see improvement. • Active encephalomyelitis—treat accordingly.

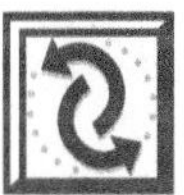

FOLLOW-UP

• Monitor CNS disease. • Myoclonus usually persists indefinitely; spontaneous remission may occur. • Active distemper virus infection—poor-to-grave prognosis. • Chronic distemper—myoclonus persists but patient otherwise healthy.

MISCELLANEOUS

Suggested Reading

Cattai A, Rabozzi R, Natale V, et al. The incidence of spontaneous movements (myoclonus) in dogs undergoing total intravenous anaesthesia with propofol. Vet Anaesth Analg 2015, 42(1):93–98.

Lowrie M, Garosi L. Classification of involuntary movements in dogs: myoclonus and myotonia. J Vet Intern Med 2017, 31(4)979–987.

Author Joane M. Parent

MYOPATHY—HEREDITARY X-LINKED MUSCULAR DYSTROPHY

BASICS

OVERVIEW

• Muscular dystrophy is an inherited, progressive and degenerative, generalized myopathy. Most muscular dystrophies are due to mutations in genes that code for muscle membrane associated proteins in the dystrophin–glycoprotein (DAG) complex. • Most common form in dogs occurs as a result of a deficiency of the protein dystrophin.
• Muscular dystrophy due to dystrophin deficiency has an X-linked mode of inheritance and affected animals are predominantly male.
• Dystrophin deficiency—identified first in golden retrievers. Subsequently, cases have been reported in many other dog breeds. Sporadic cases in other breeds are likely. • The dystrophin gene is large and new mutations are likely to occur. • Hypertrophic muscular dystrophy associated with dystrophin deficiency also occurs in domestic shorthair cats. • Deficiency of other muscle-associated proteins, e.g., alpha2 laminin (merosin) and sarcoglycan, has been identified more recently in dogs and cats and is not necessarily X-linked (females affected). • A myopathy associated with loss of alpha-dystroglycan with an autosomal recessive mode of inheritance occurs in young Devon Rex and Sphynx cats. Alpha-dystroglycan expression, which is associated with *COLQ* anchorage at the motor end-plate, has been shown to be deficient in affected cats, resulting in a congenital myasthenic syndrome.
• Unclassified muscular dystrophies have also been reported in other dogs (males and females).

SIGNALMENT

• Seen primarily in neonate and young dogs (<1 year). • Described in cats. • Muscular dystrophy due to dystrophin deficiency primarily affects males. • Several dog breeds known to be affected. Best described in golden retrievers.
• Females—usually carriers of dystrophin gene defect, but dystrophin-deficient females may exhibit muscle weakness, tremors, limb deformities, and exercise intolerance. • Muscular dystrophy due to other muscle protein or unclassified defects may be seen in young male or female dogs and cats of any breed.

SIGNS

Dogs

• Golden retrievers—exercise intolerance; stilted gait; bunny-hopping pelvic limb gait; plantigrade stance; partial trismus; muscle atrophy (especially the truncal and temporalis muscles); hypertrophy of some muscles (especially the tongue); kyphosis; lordosis; drooling; dysphagia; aspiration pneumonia (due to pharyngeal and/or esophageal involvement).
• Other breeds—similar; include vomiting and megaesophagus. • Abnormalities vary in severity, onset, and progression; may be seen as early as 6 weeks; tend to stabilize by 6 months.
• Stunting and ineffective suckling—may be evident in younger pups. • Cardiac failure—may occur owing to cardiomyopathy. • Severe muscle contractures may develop. • Spinal reflexes—normal initially; may become hypoactive.

Cats

• Dystrophin deficient—muscle hypertrophy; stiff gait; cervical rigidity; exercise intolerance; vomiting; may see calcified nodules on the tongue. • Usually young animals but not apparent in one cat until 21 months of age.
• Other hereditary myopathies in cats may cause muscle atrophy; weakness; ventroflexion of the head and neck; dorsal protrusion of the scapulae with triceps brachii and dorsal cervical muscles most severely affected.

CAUSES & RISK FACTORS

• Dystrophin deficiency—inherited defect of the X chromosome. • Other muscular dystrophies may not be X-linked. • Devon Rex/Sphynx myopathy—autosomal recessive.

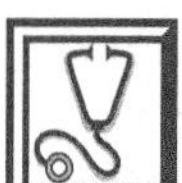

DIAGNOSIS

DIFFERENTIAL DIAGNOSIS

Other inherited myopathies such as centronuclear X-linked myotubular myopathies, infectious (especially protozoal), immune-mediated, or metabolic myopathies. Distinguished by muscle histology and demonstration of dystrophin deficiency or other muscle membrane protein associated deficiency.

CBC/BIOCHEMISTRY/URINALYSIS

• Dystrophin deficiency—normal except for marked elevation in serum creatine kinase (may be >10,000 U/L; further increased after exercise). Aspartate aminotransferase also likely to be elevated. • Other muscular dystrophies—creatine kinase may be normal.

OTHER LABORATORY TESTS

• Muscle biopsy—dystrophin deficiency demonstrated by immunohistochemical evaluation of fresh frozen muscle; diagnostic.
• Immunohistochemistry and immunoblotting analysis of muscle biopsy specimens can also assess abnormalities of other muscle proteins including dystrophin-associated proteins, laminin, sarcoglycan. • DNA tests available for specific genetic abnormalities in some breeds. • Serologic testing—may be warranted to rule out infectious and immune-mediated causes.

DIAGNOSTIC PROCEDURES

Electromyography—shows complex repetitive discharges.

PATHOLOGIC FINDINGS

Histologic examination of muscle—muscle fiber necrosis and regeneration; myofiber mineralization (may be dramatic); myofiber hypertrophy (may be variation in myofiber size); fibrosis.

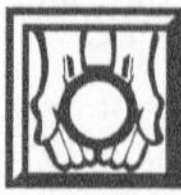

TREATMENT

None proven effective.

MEDICATIONS

DRUG(S) OF CHOICE

Glucocorticosteriods—may provide some improvement; reason unknown. However, myofiber calcification increases, which may be deleterious.

FOLLOW-UP

PATIENT MONITORING

Monitor periodically for aspiration pneumonia or cardiomyopathy.

PREVENTION/AVOIDANCE

• Discourage breeding of affected animals.
• Do not repeat dam–sire matings that result in affected offspring. • Consider DNA testing of breeding animals where tests are available.

EXPECTED COURSE AND PROGNOSIS

• Overall prognosis—guarded to poor as no effective palliative treatment. • Golden retrievers—signs tend to stabilize at 6 months. • Other dog breeds and cats—progression variable.

MISCELLANEOUS

Suggested Reading

Dickinson PJ, LeCouteur RA. Feline neuromuscular disorders. Vet Clin North Am Small Anim Pract 2004, 34(6):1307–1359.

Gandolfi B, Grahn RA, Creighton EK, et al. COLQ variant associated with Devon Rex and Sphynx feline hereditary myopathy. Anim Genet 2015, 46:711–715.

Shelton GD, Engvall E. Muscular dystrophies and other inherited myopathies. Vet Clin North Am Small Anim Pract 2002, 32(1):103–124.

Author Georgina Child

Consulting Editor Mathieu M. Glassman

M

MYOPATHY—MASTICATORY AND EXTRAOCULAR MYOSITIS

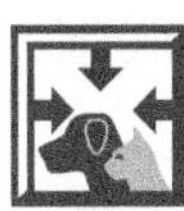

BASICS

DEFINITION

- Masticatory—focal inflammatory myopathy affecting the muscles of mastication (temporalis, masseter, and pterygoid muscles) and sparing the limb muscles.
- Extraocular—selectively affects the extraocular muscles, sparing limb and masticatory muscles.

PATHOPHYSIOLOGY

- Masticatory—suspected immune-mediated cause owing to autoantibodies against type 2M fibers and a positive clinical response to immunosuppressive doses of corticosteroids.
- Extraocular—suspected immune-mediated cause owing to positive clinical response to corticosteroids.

SYSTEMS AFFECTED

Neuromuscular—muscles of mastication; extraocular muscles.

GENETICS

- Unknown.
- As with autoimmune diseases in general, the appropriate genetic background must exist.
- Masticatory—cavalier King Charles spaniels have a familial form and may be affected at less than 6 months of age.
- Extraocular—golden retrievers may have a genetic predisposition.

INCIDENCE/PREVALENCE

- Unknown.
- Masticatory—relatively common.

GEOGRAPHIC DISTRIBUTION

Probably worldwide.

SIGNALMENT

Species

- Dog (common).
- Cat (rare).

Breed Predilections

- Various.
- Masticatory—Rottweiler, Doberman, Samoyed, and cavalier King Charles spaniel develop severe forms.
- Extraocular—golden retriever.

Mean Age and Range

No obvious age predisposition.

Predominant Sex

None obvious.

SIGNS

General Comments

Masticatory—usually related to abnormalities of jaw movement, jaw pain, and masticatory muscle atrophy; not a "tabletop" diagnosis; usually requires laboratory testing to confirm diagnosis.

Historical Findings

- Masticatory—acute or chronic pain when opening the jaw; inability to pick up a ball or get food into the mouth; acutely swollen muscles; progressive muscle atrophy.
- Extraocular—bilateral exophthalmos.

Physical Examination Findings

- Masticatory—marked jaw pain with manipulation and/or trismus; acute muscle swelling with exophthalmos; muscle atrophy with enophthalmos; inability to open the jaw under anesthesia.
- Extraocular—bilateral exophthalmos; impaired vision.

CAUSES

Immune-mediated.

RISK FACTORS

- Appropriate genetic background.
- Possible previous bacterial or viral infection.
- Vaccination may exacerbate active disease.

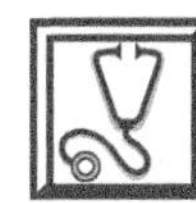

DIAGNOSIS

DIFFERENTIAL DIAGNOSIS

- Retro-orbital abscess—probe behind last upper molar.
- Temporomandibular joint disease—radiographically abnormal joint.
- Polymyositis—high serum creatine kinase activity; generalized electromyogram (EMG) abnormalities; diagnostic muscle biopsies.
- Neurogenic atrophy of temporalis muscles—determined by EMG and muscle biopsy.
- Atrophy of masticatory muscles from corticosteroids—history of corticosteroid use; characteristic changes on muscle biopsy.
- Atrophy of masticatory muscles from endocrine disorders—test for thyroid and adrenal disorders.

CBC/BIOCHEMISTRY/URINALYSIS

Serum creatine kinase activity—normal or mildly elevated.

OTHER LABORATORY TESTS

- Muscle biopsy—diagnostic test of choice for masticatory muscle disease.
- Immunohistochemical assay—demonstrate autoantibodies against masticatory muscle type 2M fibers in frozen muscle biopsy sections; negative in polymyositis and extraocular disease.
- ELISA—demonstrate autoantibodies against masticatory muscle type 2M fiber proteins.

IMAGING

- Radiography of the temporomandibular joints.
- Orbital sonogram—for extraorbital disease; demonstrate swollen extraocular muscles.
- MRI—for demonstration of inflammation/myonecrosis in muscles.

DIAGNOSTIC PROCEDURES

EMG—differentiate between extraocular disease and polymyositis; abnormal masticatory muscles in masticatory myositis only; generalized abnormalities including masticatory muscles in polymyositis.

PATHOLOGIC FINDINGS

Masticatory

- Swelling or atrophy of the masticatory muscles.
- Biopsy specimen—may see myofiber necrosis, phagocytosis, mononuclear cell infiltration with a multifocal and perivascular distribution; may see myofiber atrophy and fibrosis with chronic condition; eosinophils rare.

Extraocular

Mononuclear cell infiltration—restricted to extraocular muscles

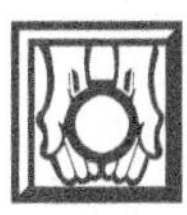

TREATMENT

APPROPRIATE HEALTH CARE

Outpatient

NURSING CARE

Gastrostomy tube—may be required with severe restrictions in jaw mobility; requires good hygiene and supportive care.

ACTIVITY

N/A

DIET

Masticatory—may require liquid food or gruel until jaw mobility is regained; may need a gastric feeding tube to facilitate fluid and caloric intake.

CLIENT EDUCATION

- Warn client that long-term corticosteroid therapy may be required.
- Inform client that residual muscle atrophy and restricted jaw movement may occur with chronic masticatory muscle disease.

SURGICAL CONSIDERATIONS

Not indicated.

MEDICATIONS

DRUG(S) OF CHOICE

Corticosteroids—immunosuppressive dosages, tapered as jaw mobility, swelling, and serum creatine kinase activity return to normal; maintained at lowest alternate-day dosage that prevents restricted jaw mobility; treated for a minimum of 6 months.

CONTRAINDICATIONS

N/A

PRECAUTIONS

- Corticosteroids—watch for infection and undesirable side effects.
- Clinical signs may recur if treatment is stopped too soon.

POSSIBLE INTERACTIONS

N/A

ALTERNATIVE DRUG(S)

Intolerable side effects of corticosteroids—institute a lower dose of corticosteroids and combine with another drug (e.g., azathioprine).

MYOPATHY—MASTICATORY AND EXTRAOCULAR MYOSITIS (CONTINUED)

FOLLOW-UP

PATIENT MONITORING

- Masticatory—return of jaw mobility and decreased serum creatine kinase activity.
- Extraocular—decreased swelling of extraocular muscles.

PREVENTION/AVOIDANCE

N/A

POSSIBLE COMPLICATIONS

- Corticosteroids—undesirable side effects.
- Recurrence of clinical signs—treatment stopped too early.
- Poor clinical response—inadequate dosages of corticosteroids.
- Restrictive strabismus (extraocular myositis).
- Note position of tongue—venous congestion and tongue protrusion may occur under anesthesia.

M

EXPECTED COURSE AND PROGNOSIS

- Masticatory—jaw mobility should return to normal unless the condition is chronic and severe fibrosis develops; good prognosis if treated early with adequate dosages of corticosteroids.
- Extraocular—good response to corticosteroids; good prognosis unless chronic with restrictive strabismus.

MISCELLANEOUS

ASSOCIATED CONDITIONS

Other concurrent autoimmune disorders.

AGE-RELATED FACTORS

N/A

ZOONOTIC POTENTIAL

N/A

PREGNANCY/FERTILITY/BREEDING

Unknown

SYNONYMS

- Atrophic myositis.
- Eosinophilic myositis.

SEE ALSO

- Myopathy—Polymyositis and Dermatomyositis.
- Myopathy, Noninflammatory—Endocrine.

ABBREVIATIONS

- EMG = electromyogram.

INTERNET RESOURCES

Comparative Neuromuscular Laboratory: http://vetneuromuscular.ucsd.edu

Suggested Reading

Allgoewer I, Blair M, Basher T, Davidson M. Extraocular myositis and restrictive strabismus in 10 dogs. Vet Ophthalmol 2000, 3:21–26.

Carpenter JL, Schmidt GM, Moore FM, et al. Canine bilateral extraocular polymyositis. Vet Pathol 1989, 26:510–512.

Melmed C, Shelton GD, Bergman R, Barton C. Masticatory muscle myositis: Pathogenesis, diagnosis, and treatment. Compend Contin Educ Pract Vet 2004, 26:590–605.

Nanai B, Phillips L, Christiansen J, Shelton GD. Life threatening complication associated with anesthesia in a dog with masticatory muscle myositis. Vet Surg 2009, 38:645–649.

Orvis JS, Cardinet GH III. Canine muscle fiber types and susceptibility of masticatory muscles to myositis. Muscle Nerve 1981, 4:354–359.

Pitcher GDC, Hahn CN. Atypical masticatory muscle myositis in three cavalier King Charles spaniel littermates. J Small Anim Pract 2007, 48:226–228.

Podell M. Inflammatory myopathies. Vet Clin North Am 2002, 31:147–167.

Shelton GD. Routine and specialized laboratory testing for the diagnosis of neurouscular diseases in dogs and cats. Vet Clin Pathol 2010, 39:278–295.

Shelton GD, Cardinet GH III, Bandman E. Canine masticatory muscle disorders: a clinicopathological and immunochemical study of 29 cases. Muscle Nerve 1987, 10:753–766.

Author Lauren Talarico

Consulting Editor Mathieu M. Glassman

Acknowledgment The author and editors acknowledge the prior contribution of G. Diane Shelton.

Client Education Handout available online

MYOPATHY, NONINFLAMMATORY—ENDOCRINE

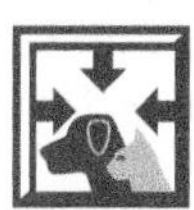

BASICS

DEFINITION

Myopathies associated with various endocrinopathies (including hypothyroidism, hyperthyroidism, hypoadrenocorticism, hyperadrenocorticism) and associated with exogenous corticosteroid use (steroid myopathy).

PATHOPHYSIOLOGY

With Adrenal Dysfunction

- Glucocorticoid excess—impaired muscle protein metabolism; may accelerate degradation of myofibrillar and soluble protein in skeletal muscle; impairment of carbohydrate metabolism owing to induction of an insulin-resistant state; may note elevated adrenocorticotropic hormone (ACTH) levels.
- Adrenal insufficiency—circulatory insufficiency; fluid and electrolyte imbalance; impaired carbohydrate metabolism.

With Thyroid Disease

- Hyperthyroidism—increased mitochondrial respiration; accelerated protein degradation and lipid oxidation; glycogen depletion; impaired glucose uptake.
- Hypothyroidism—impaired muscle energy metabolism by reduced glycogen breakdown, gluconeogenesis, and oxidative and glycolytic capacity; impaired insulin-stimulated carbohydrate metabolism.

SYSTEMS AFFECTED

- Neuromuscular—impaired energy metabolism.
- Cardiovascular—impaired energy metabolism; circulatory disorders.

GENETICS

N/A

INCIDENCE/PREVALENCE

- Exact incidence unknown.
- Myopathies related to exogenous corticosteroids—common.
- Myopathies associated with Cushing syndrome and hypothyroidism—not uncommon.

GEOGRAPHIC DISTRIBUTION

Probably worldwide.

SIGNALMENT

Species

- Dog—steroid myopathy; weakness associated with hyperadrenocorticism and hypoadrenocorticism; hypothyroidism.
- Cat—weakness associated with hyperthyroidism.

Breed Predilections

Affects several breeds.

Mean Age and Range

- Steroid myopathy—dogs of any age.
- Other disorders—see specific disease.

Predominant Sex

None found.

SIGNS

General Comments

Corticosteroid use in dogs—muscles very susceptible; muscle atrophy (particularly the masticatory muscles) is not uncommon with prolonged corticosteroid use.

Historical Findings

- Muscle weakness, atrophy, and stiffness.
- Regurgitation.
- Dysphagia.
- Dysphonia.

Physical Examination Findings

- Muscle weakness, stiffness, cramping, and myalgia.
- Muscle hypertrophy or atrophy.
- May not note other clinical signs of an endocrine disorder.

CAUSES

- Endocrine dysfunction.
- Autoimmune.
- Neoplastic.

RISK FACTORS

N/A

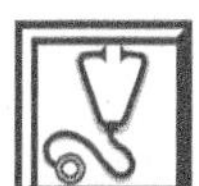

DIAGNOSIS

DIFFERENTIAL DIAGNOSIS

- Inflammatory myopathies—distinguished by muscle biopsy.
- Noninflammatory myopathies—distinguished by muscle biopsy.

CBC/BIOCHEMISTRY/URINALYSIS

- Baseline testing—abnormalities consistent with endocrine disorder.
- Serum creatine kinase activity—usually normal, but may be mildly elevated if necrotic muscle fibers.

OTHER LABORATORY TESTS

Thyroid and adrenal function tests—should be diagnostic.

IMAGING

- Dynamic studies—evaluate pharyngeal and esophageal function; with regurgitation and dysphagia.
- Cardiac evaluation—for cats with hyperthyroidism.

DIAGNOSTIC PROCEDURES

- Muscle biopsy—fiber typing in fresh frozen muscle biopsy sections important, paraffin sections will not be diagnostic.
- Electromyography.

PATHOLOGIC FINDINGS

- Hyperadrenocorticism and steroid myopathies—selective atrophy of type 2 muscle fibers; may see lobulated or ragged-red fibers with associated myotonia.
- Hypoadrenocorticism—muscle biopsies normal.
- Hyperthyroidism (cats)—muscle biopsies normal.
- Hypothyroidism—atrophy of type 2 fibers; may see an increase in type 1 fibers; may see periodic acid–Schiff (PAS)-positive deposits and nemaline rod bodies.

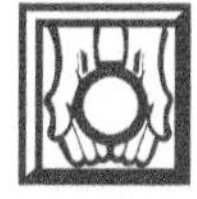

TREATMENT

APPROPRIATE HEALTH CARE

Depends on specific endocrine disorder.

NURSING CARE

Physical therapy—with musculoskeletal manifestations.

ACTIVITY

- Clinical corticosteroid myopathy (humans)—inactivity worsens condition; increased muscle activity may partially prevent atrophy.
- Physical therapy—may help prevent and treat muscle weakness and wasting in dogs receiving glucocorticoids.

DIET

- Regurgitation and megaesophagus—feed from an elevation.
- Dysphagia and esophageal dilation—give food with the best-tolerated consistency.
- Gastric feeding tube—if oral feeding is not tolerated.

CLIENT EDUCATION

Depends on specific endocrine disorder.

SURGICAL CONSIDERATIONS

Removal of neoplasia.

MEDICATIONS

DRUG(S) OF CHOICE

- Depends on specific endocrine disorder.
- Corticosteroid myopathy—decrease corticosteroid dosage to the lowest possible level; use a nonfluorinated corticosteroid and alternate-day dosing.
- Intramyofiber lipid storage with steroid myopathy—L-carnitine 50 mg/kg PO q12h may improve muscle strength.

CONTRAINDICATIONS

N/A

PRECAUTIONS

Depend on specific endocrine disorder.

POSSIBLE INTERACTIONS

N/A

ALTERNATIVE DRUG(S)

Fluorinated corticosteroids, triamcinolone, betamethasone, and dexamethasone—most likely to produce muscle weakness; use an equivalent dose of another corticosteroid.

MYOPATHY, NONINFLAMMATORY—ENDOCRINE (CONTINUED)

FOLLOW-UP

PATIENT MONITORING

- Depends on specific endocrine disorder.
- Steroid myopathy—should note return of muscle strength and mass with decreased steroid use.

PREVENTION/AVOIDANCE

N/A

POSSIBLE COMPLICATIONS

Depend on specific endocrine disorders.

EXPECTED COURSE AND PROGNOSIS

- Myotonia associated with hyperadrenocorticism—poor prognosis for resolution.
- Steroid myopathy—good prognosis for return of muscle strength and mass; recovery may take weeks.
- Hypothyroid myopathy—improvement in muscle pain and stiffness common.
- Hyperthyroidism (cats)—good prognosis for return of muscle strength following reversion to euthyroid state.
- Hypoadrenocorticism—good prognosis for return of muscle strength.
- Dysphagia and regurgitation—may resolve with adequate treatment.

MISCELLANEOUS

ASSOCIATED CONDITIONS

- May note multiple endocrinopathies.
- Hypothyroidism (dogs)—concurrent myasthenia gravis.

AGE-RELATED FACTORS

N/A

ZOONOTIC POTENTIAL

N/A

PREGNANCY/FERTILITY/BREEDING

Unknown

ABBREVIATIONS

- ACTH = adrenocorticotropic hormone.
- PAS = periodic acid–Schiff.

INTERNET RESOURCES

Comparative Neuromuscular Laboratory: http://vetneuromuscular.ucsd.edu

Suggested Reading

Jaggy A, Oliver JE, Ferguson DC, et al. Neurological manifestations of hypothyroidism: a retrospective study of 29 cases. J Vet Intern Med 1994; 8:328–330.

LeCouteur RA, Dow SW, Sisson AF. Metabolic and endocrine myopathies of dogs and cats. Semin Vet Med Surg Small Anim 1989, 4:146–155.

Platt SR. Neuromuscular complications in endocrine and metabolic disorders. Vet Clin North Am 2002, 31:125–146.

Rossmeisl JH, Duncan RB, Inzana KD, et al. Longitudinal study of the effects of chronic hypothyroidism on skeletal muscle in dogs. Am J Vet Res 2009, 70:879–889.

Author Lauren Talarico

Consulting Editor Mathieu M. Glassman

Acknowledgment The author and editors acknowledge the prior contribution of G. Diane Shelton.

MYOPATHY, NONINFLAMMATORY—HEREDITARY LABRADOR RETRIEVER

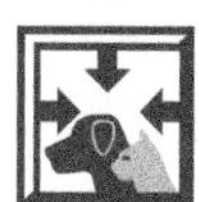

BASICS

OVERVIEW

• An inherited myopathy of Labrador retrievers. • Recognized worldwide. • Autosomal recessive mode of inheritance; severity of clinical signs varies. • More recently classified as a centronuclear myopathy (CNM). • The causative genetic mutation has been identified—called protein tyrosine phosphatase-like A gene (*PTPLA*). CNM-causing genes, including *PTPLA*, interact to build a functional muscle and to maintain its homeostasis. • Loss of tendon reflexes and muscle histology—may be more suggestive clinically of a neurogenic than a myopathic cause without further testing. No histologic abnormalities found in CNS or peripheral nervous system (PNS). • Studies suggest *PTPLA* mutation may have arisen spontaneously in one popular sire and is now disseminated widely in the Labrador population.

SIGNALMENT

• Occurs in black and yellow Labrador retrievers. • Age of onset—variable (6 weeks–7 months); most commonly recognized at 3–4 months. • Affects males and females. • A similar inherited CNM has been identified in young male and female Great Danes.

SIGNS

• Severity ranges from stilted gait and exercise intolerance to severe muscle weakness, bunny-hopping pelvic limb gait, ventroflexion of the head and neck, arched back, and abnormal joint posture (cow-hocked stance, hyperextended carpi). • Worsen with exercise, excitement, and cold weather. • Patient may collapse with forced exercise. • Some improvement with rest. • Generalized muscle atrophy—mild to severe. • Atrophy of proximal limb and masticatory muscles often most prominent. • Tendon reflexes—normal, hypoactive, or absent. • Occasionally, patients become recumbent or develop megaesophagus.

CAUSES & RISK FACTORS

Autosomal recessive mode of inheritance.

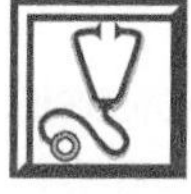

DIAGNOSIS

DIFFERENTIAL DIAGNOSIS

• With little muscle atrophy—exercise intolerance may mimic signs of myasthenia gravis, cardiac or orthopedic disease. • Exercise-induced collapse syndrome also recognized in this breed; however, not associated with muscle atrophy and collapse seen only after strenuous exercise. • With marked muscle atrophy—consider other myopathies (infectious, immune-mediated, metabolic, congenital) and generalized lower motor neuron disorders. • Infectious myopathy due to congenital neospora caninum infection has a higher incidence in Labrador retrievers. • Congenital muscular dystrophy in a male due to dystrophin deficiency and in a female due to sarcolemmal collagen deficiency myopathy have also been reported in Labrador retrievers. • An X-linked myotubular myopathy (XLMTM), which is an unrelated CNM, due to a mutation in *MTM1* gene, has also been identified in young male Labrador retrievers. Affected dogs show progressive and severe weakness and muscle atrophy in the first 2 months of life resulting in euthanasia before 6 months of age.

CBC/BIOCHEMISTRY/URINALYSIS

Creatine kinase—normal or mildly or moderately elevated.

OTHER LABORATORY TESTS

A DNA test is available for the causative genetic mutation.

IMAGING

N/A

DIAGNOSTIC PROCEDURES

• Electromyogram (EMG)—spontaneous activity, including complex repetitive discharges, especially in proximal limb and masticatory muscles; may reveal no abnormalities with mild disease. • Muscle histology—reveals variation in fiber size, angular atrophy of both type 1 and 2 myofibers, grouped atrophy, increase in central nuclei, muscle degeneration and regeneration, and fibrosis; may note deficiency in type 2 myofibers or predominance of type 1 myofibers. • DNA test for causative genetic mutation.

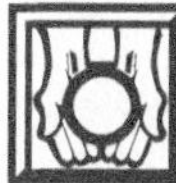

TREATMENT

• None specific. • Avoid cold, because it exacerbates clinical signs. • DNA testing of breeding animals recommended. • Discourage breeding of affected animals and parents and littermates of affected dogs. • Do not repeat dam–sire matings that result in affected offspring.

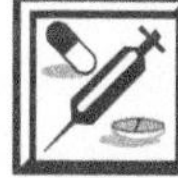

MEDICATIONS

DRUG(S) OF CHOICE

Supplementation with L-carnitine 50 mg/kg PO q12h may be of benefit in improving muscle strength.

CONTRAINDICATIONS/POSSIBLE INTERACTIONS

None known.

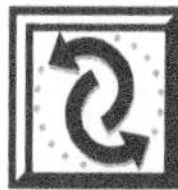

FOLLOW-UP

• Clinical signs generally stabilize at approximately 1 year of age. • Mild disease—may be an acceptable pet; may show some improvement in exercise tolerance. • Aspiration pneumonia—a risk in dogs with megaesophagus.

MISCELLANEOUS

ASSOCIATED CONDITIONS

N/A

AGE-RELATED FACTORS

N/A

ZOONOTIC POTENTIAL

N/A

PREGNANCY/FERTILITY/BREEDING

N/A

ABBREVIATIONS

• CNM = centronuclear myopathy.
• EMG = electromyogram.
• PNS = peripheral nervous system.
• *PTPLA* = protein tyrosine phosphatase-like A gene.
• XLMTM = X-linked myotubular myopathy.

Suggested Reading

Cosford KL, Taylor SM, Thompson L, Shelton GD. A possible new inherited myopathy in a young Labrador retriever. Can Vet J 2008, 49(4):393–397.

Maurer M, Mary J, Guillaud L, et al. Centronuclear myopathy in Labrador retrievers: a recent founder mutation in the PTPLA gene has rapidly disseminated worldwide. PLoS ONE 2012, 7(10): e46408.

McKerrell RE, Braund KG. Hereditary myopathy of Labrador retrievers. In: Kirk RW, Bonagura JD, eds., Current Veterinary Therapy X. Philadelphia, PA: Saunders, 1989, pp. 820–821.

Schatzberg SJ, Shelton GD. Newly identified neuromuscular disorders. Vet Clin North Am Small Anim Pract 2004, 34(6):1497–1524.

Shelton GD, Engvall E. Muscular dystrophies and other inherited myopathies. Vet Clin North Am Small Anim Pract 2002, 32(1):103–124.

Author Georgina Child

Consulting Editor Mathieu M. Glassman

MYOPATHY, NONINFLAMMATORY—HEREDITARY MYOTONIA

BASICS

OVERVIEW

- Myotonia characterized by persistent contraction or delayed relaxation of muscle fibers on initiation of movement or when stimulated to contract.
- May affect all skeletal muscles.
- Myotonia may be congenital or acquired.
- A genetic basis has been determined in some breeds.
- Acquired myotonia may be associated with noninflammatory or inflammatory myopathy.
- Neuromyotonia and myokymia, characterized by continuous muscle fiber activity, are believed to be due to hyperexcitability of terminal nerve branches (neuromyotonia) or hyperexcitability of the motor nerve axon at any level (myokymia) rather than a primary muscle disorder.
- Neuromyotonia is characterized by muscle stiffness and delayed relaxation.
- Myokymia describes rhythmic undulating muscle movements that produce a rippling movement of the skin.
- The cause of neuromyotonia and myokymia (continuous muscle fiber activity [CMFA]) in all reported cases remains unclear.
- CMFA and spinocerebellar ataxia may occur concurrently in Jack Russell terriers (JRTs) (and related breeds) and both are associated with a genetic mutation causing neuronal ion channel dysfunction.

M

SIGNALMENT

- Congenital myotonia—chow chows, miniature schnauzers and Australian cattledogs; rarely seen in other dog breeds.
- Clinical signs seen when affected puppies begin to walk.
- Acquired myotonia—all breeds of any age potentially susceptible.
- Myotonia reported in young domestic cats.
- Neuromyotonia and myokymia (CMFA)—described in predominantly young JRTs worldwide, rarely in other breeds, and a cat.

SIGNS

- Difficulty rising.
- Stiffness after rest or initiation of activity.
- May note dyspnea, voice change, dysphagia, and/or regurgitation, especially after eating.
- May improve with exercise.
- May be exacerbated by cold.
- Muscle stiffness and myokymia observed in young JRTs may result in life-threatening hyperthermia. In this breed clinical signs are episodic but dogs may have continuous ataxia.

Physical Examination Findings

- Hypertrophy of proximal limb muscles, neck muscles, and tongue.
- Tongue may protrude from the mouth.
- Abduction of thoracic limbs.
- Stiff, stilted, pelvic limb gait.
- Patient may fall and remain rigid in lateral recumbency for short periods. May become cyanotic.
- Affected miniature schnauzers may have craniofacial abnormalities such as mandibular shortening.

CAUSES & RISK FACTORS

- Chow chows—suspected autosomal recessive mode of inheritance.
- Miniature schnauzers, Australian cattledogs—autosomal recessive mode of inheritance (*CLCN1* gene).
- JRT group CMFA and spinocerebellar ataxia—autosomal recessive mode of inheritance (*KCNJ10* gene).

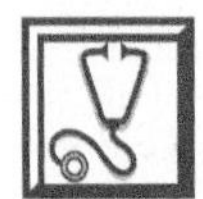

DIAGNOSIS

DIFFERENTIAL DIAGNOSIS

- Other myopathies—distinguished by signalment and clinical, electromyographic, and histologic findings.
- Hypertonicity disorders or other movement disorders—recognized breed association.

CBC/BIOCHEMISTRY/URINALYSIS

Creatine kinase—may be normal or slightly elevated.

OTHER LABORATORY TESTS

DNA testing for known genetic mutations.

DIAGNOSTIC PROCEDURES

- Percussion of muscles and tongue—causes sustained dimpling.
- Electromyography—myotonia characterized by multifocal or generalized high-frequency discharges that wax and wane in amplitude and frequency (dive bomber sounding potentials) and are increased after muscle percussion. Myokymic discharges—rhythmic high-frequency bursts of single motor unit potentials are characteristic findings in myokymia.

PATHOLOGIC FINDINGS

- Muscle histology—congenital myotonia: normal or mild changes.
- Degenerative and/or inflammatory changes on muscle histology may be seen in cases of acquired myotonia.
- No abnormalities found on muscle biopsy in JRTs with neuromyotonia and myokymia (CMFA).

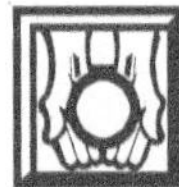

TREATMENT

- None specific.
- Discourage activities that result in hyperventilation.
- Avoid strenuous exercise and excitement.
- Avoid cold.
- Anesthesia (induction and recovery)—possible risk of respiratory obstruction owing to adduction of vocal cords or regurgitation.

MEDICATIONS

DRUG(S) OF CHOICE

- Membrane-stabilizing drugs—procainamide, quinidine, phenytoin, and mexiletine; may decrease severity of clinical signs.
- Procainamide reported to be most effective in chow chows. Treatment may decrease stiffness, stridor, and regurgitation, but gait remains abnormal.
- Extended-release procainamide 40–50 mg/kg q8–12h or mexiletine 8.3 mg/kg q8h reported to be effective in miniature schnauzers.
- Procainamide 10 mg/kg q8h or mexiletine 4 mg/kg q12h or sustained-release phenytoin at an increasing dose 50–100 mg/kg for 6 weeks then on serum concentration monitoring 2–8 mg/L reported to reduce frequency of episodes of CMFA in approximately half of affected JRTs, but response is generally temporary.
- Anesthesia and cooling to treat hyperthermia may be required to treat episodes of CMFA in JRTs.

CONTRAINDICATIONS/POSSIBLE INTERACTIONS

Myotonia in humans is worsened with treatment with dantrolene, beta-adrenergic blocking agents, diuretics, and neuromuscular blocking agents. Bromide-containing agents such as potassium bromide may be contraindicated.

FOLLOW-UP

PREVENTION/AVOIDANCE

- Chow chows, miniature schnauzers, Australian cattledogs—inherited condition; advise owner regarding breeding.
- DNA testing for carrier dogs prior to breeding.
- Discourage breeding of affected animals.
- Do not repeat dam–sire matings that resulted in affected offspring.

POSSIBLE COMPLICATIONS

- Respiratory obstruction and/or aspiration of regurgitated food—may be life-threatening; advise owners of the clinical symptoms and treatment.
- Hyperthermia associated with CMFA in JRTs is life-threatening.

EXPECTED COURSE AND PROGNOSIS

Prognosis guarded.

ABBREVIATIONS

- CMFA = continuous muscle fiber activity.
- JRT = Jack Russell terrier.

Suggested Reading

Vite CH. Myotonia and disorders of altered muscle cell membrane excitability. Vet Clin North Am Small Anim Pract 2002, 32(1):169–187.

Author Georgina Child
Consulting Editor Mathieu M. Glassman

MYOPATHY, NONINFLAMMATORY—HEREDITARY SCOTTIE CRAMP

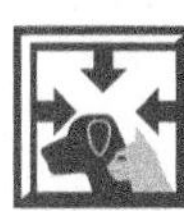

BASICS

OVERVIEW

- Inherited disorder in Scottish terriers characterized by episodic muscle hypertonicity or cramping.
- Not associated with any morphologic changes in muscle, peripheral nerve, or the CNS.
- Is better characterized as a hypertonicity disorder than a myopathy.
- Thought to be the result of a disorder in serotonin metabolism within the CNS.
- Similar condition (reflex myoclonus) reported in young Dalmatians and Labrador retrievers—may be result of low numbers of neurotransmitter glycine receptors in the CNS.
- Episodic muscle hypertonicity syndromes also occur in cavalier King Charles spaniels (episodic falling syndrome), Norwich terriers, bichon frises, border terriers (Spike's disease or canine epileptoid cramping syndrome), Wheaten terriers, springer spaniels, and sporadically in other breeds.

SIGNALMENT

- Young Scottish terriers, typically <1 year of age. Clinical signs may be seen in puppies as early as 6–8 weeks of age.
- No known sex predilection. Females may be overrepresented.

SIGNS

- Normal at rest and on initial exercise.
- Further exercise or excitement—abduction of the thoracic limbs; arching (kyphosis) of the thoracolumbar vertebral column; stiffening or overflexion of the pelvic limbs (goose-stepping gait).
- Patient may fall, with tail and pelvic limbs flexed tightly against the body.
- Respiration—may cease for a short time.
- Facial muscles—may be contracted.
- No loss of consciousness.
- Severity varies. Generalized spasticity may be seen during episodes or only hind limb spasticity and skipping.
- Episodes—may last up to 30 minutes.

CAUSES & RISK FACTORS

Inherited condition with probable autosomal recessive mode of transmission. Presence of dogs with cerebellar degeneration in the same pedigrees may suggest a more complex mode of inheritance than previously reported.

DIAGNOSIS

DIFFERENTIAL DIAGNOSIS

- Seizure disorder—distinguished on basis of family history, typical clinical signs with no loss of consciousness, and induction of signs with serotonin antagonists.
- Cerebellar cortical degeneration described in Scottish terriers—clinical signs are not episodic and neurologic abnormalities are slowly progressive.

CBC/BIOCHEMISTRY/URINALYSIS

Normal

OTHER LABORATORY TESTS

DNA test available for episodic falling syndrome in cavalier King Charles spaniels. Genetic abnormality associated with other hypertonicity disorders not yet determined.

IMAGING

N/A

DIAGNOSTIC PROCEDURES

Diagnosis usually made on clinical presentation. Clinical signs may be induced by giving the serotonin antagonist methysergide (0.3 mg/kg PO). Cramping is evident in 2 hours and may last for 8 hours.

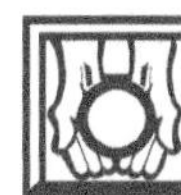

TREATMENT

Behavioral modification and/or environmental changes—eliminate triggering situations (excitement, stress); may be adequate in controlling episodes.

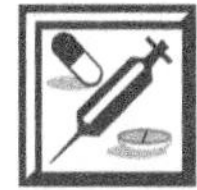

MEDICATIONS

DRUG(S) OF CHOICE

- Acepromazine maleate 0.1–0.75 mg/kg IM or PO, diazepam 0.5–1.5 mg/kg PO q8h, or vitamin E >125 U/kg q24h—may reduce the incidence and severity of Scottie cramp.
- Fluoxetine, a selective serotonin-reuptake inhibitor, may result in reduction in clinical signs. Recommended dose 1.2 mg/kg q12h initially followed by 0.8 mg/kg q12h. Clinical improvement has been maintained for >1 year in some dogs.
- Clonazepam 0.5 mg/kg q8h may result in improvement in cavalier King Charles spaniels with hypertonicity syndrome (episodic falling syndrome).

CONTRAINDICATIONS/POSSIBLE INTERACTIONS

- Serotonin antagonists—increase severity of clinical signs.
- Aspirin, indomethacin, phenylbutazone, flunixin meglumine (Banamine), and penicillin—may exacerbate clinical signs.

FOLLOW-UP

PATIENT MONITORING

Nonprogressive

PREVENTION/AVOIDANCE

- Discourage breeding of affected and related animals.
- Do not repeat dam–sire matings that result in affected offspring.

EXPECTED COURSE AND PROGNOSIS

- Mild to moderate—fair to good long-term prognosis; usually manageable disability by owners; nonprogressive.
- Severe—guarded prognosis.

MISCELLANEOUS

ASSOCIATED CONDITIONS

N/A

AGE-RELATED FACTORS

N/A

ZOONOTIC POTENTIAL

N/A

PREGNANCY/FERTILITY/BREEDING

N/A

Suggested Reading

Geiger KM, Klopp LS. Use of a selective serotonin reuptake inhibitor for treatment of episodes of hypertonia and kyphosis in a young adult Scottish terrier. J Am Vet Med Assoc 2009, 235:168–171.

Meyers KM, Clemmons RM. Scotty cramp. In: Kirk RW, ed., Current Veterinary Therapy VIII. Philadelphia, PA: Saunders, 1983, pp. 702–704.

Shelton GD. Muscle pain, cramps and hypertonicity. Vet Clin North Am Small Anim Pract 2004, 34(6):1483–1496.

Urkasemsin G, Olby NJ. Clinical characteristics of Scottie cramp in 31 cases. J Small Anim Pract 2015, 56:276–280.

Author Georgina Child

Consulting Editor Mathieu M. Glassman

M

MYOPATHY, NONINFLAMMATORY—METABOLIC

BASICS

DEFINITION

- Myopathy associated with disorders of glycogen metabolism, lipid metabolism, or oxidative phosphorylation and mitochondrial metabolism.
- Currently poorly characterized in veterinary medicine.

PATHOPHYSIOLOGY

- Usually associated with inherited or acquired enzyme defects involving major metabolic pathways.
- May result in storage of the abnormal metabolic byproduct or morphologic abnormalities of mitochondria.

SYSTEMS AFFECTED

- Cardiovascular—dependent on oxidative metabolism for energy.
- Hemic/lymphatic/immune—red blood cells (RBCs) depend on glycolytic metabolism.
- Nervous—dependent on glycolytic and oxidative metabolism for energy.
- Neuromuscular—dependent on oxidative metabolism for energy.
- Storage products in other organs—liver, spleen.

GENETICS

Undetermined

INCIDENCE/PREVALENCE

Rare, except lipid-storage myopathies.

GEOGRAPHIC DISTRIBUTION

Unknown; probably worldwide.

SIGNALMENT

Species

Dog and cat.

Breed Predilections

- Muscle phosphofructokinase deficiency—English springer spaniel, American cocker spaniel, whippet.
- Acid maltase deficiency—Lapland dog.
- Branching enzyme deficiency—Norwegian forest cat.
- Debranching enzyme deficiency—German shepherd dog, Akita, curly-coated retrievers.
- Pyrvuate dehydrogenase phosphatase 1 deficiency—Clumber spaniel, Sussex spaniel.
- Mitochondrial myopathy—Old English sheepdog, Yorkshire terrier, possibly Jack Russell terrier.

Mean Age and Range

- Inherited metabolic defects—2–3 months.
- Acquired metabolic defects—adults.

Predominant Sex

None found.

SIGNS

General Comments

Very few of these conditions have been adequately described.

Historical Findings

- Muscular weakness.
- Exercise intolerance.
- Cramping.
- Collapse.
- Regurgitation and/or dysphagia.
- Esophageal and/or pharyngeal abnormalities.
- Dark urine; myoglobinuria, hemoglobinuria.
- Encephalopathy.
- Vomiting.

Physical Examination Findings

- Exercise-related weakness, stiffness, and/or cramping.
- Abnormal neurologic examination—disorientation; stupor; coma.
- Abdominal distention—storage product accumulation in liver.
- May appear normal, with fluctuating clinical signs.

CAUSES

- Inborn error of metabolism.
- Acquired metabolic defect.
- Viral infections.
- Drug-induced.
- Environmental factors.

RISK FACTORS

- Inherited disorders.
- Appropriate genetic background.
- Others unknown.

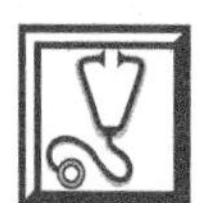

DIAGNOSIS

DIFFERENTIAL DIAGNOSIS

- Inflammatory myopathies—differentiated by muscle biopsy.
- Other noninflammatory myopathies—differentiated by muscle biopsy.
- Other metabolic encephalopathies—differentiated by laboratory evaluation.

CBC/BIOCHEMISTRY/URINALYSIS

- Plasma lactate and pyruvate levels—elevated resting or post exercise with disorders of fatty acid oxidation or oxidative phosphorylation; no elevation with glycolytic disorders.
- Serum creatine kinase activity—may be elevated with exercise and normal at rest; may be persistently elevated.
- Hypoglycemia—may occur with some glycolytic and oxidative disorders.
- Hyperammonemia—may occur with urea cycle defects.

OTHER LABORATORY TESTS

- Quantitation of plasma amino acids—abnormal accumulations.
- Quantitation of urine organic acids—demonstrate abnormal organic acid production.
- Quantitation of plasma, urine, and muscle carnitine—may be low with primary or secondary disorders of carnitine; low with primary organic acidurias.
- Specific enzyme assays—depend on suspected metabolic defect.
- Fibroblast cultures—study metabolic defect.
- DNA-based tests to identify affected dogs and carriers when available.

IMAGING

MRI—evaluate the CNS; reveals abnormalities in humans.

DIAGNOSTIC PROCEDURES

- Light microscopy—fresh frozen muscle sections; demonstrates storage products (glycogen, lipid) or abnormal mitochondria.
- Electron microscopy of muscle reveals abnormal mitochondria, paracrystalline inclusions, and glycogen or lipid accumulation.
- Cardiovascular system evaluation—may have concurrent cardiomyopathy.
- Other organ biopsies—with organomegaly.

PATHOLOGIC FINDINGS

- Triglyceride droplets in muscle—lipid storage myopathy.
- Ragged-red fibers in muscle—mitochondrial myopathy.
- Glycogen deposition in muscle—glycogen storage disorder.

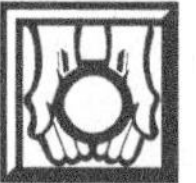

TREATMENT

APPROPRIATE HEALTH CARE

- Inpatient—may require intensive care for severe encephalopathy, seizures, lactic acidemia, hypoglycemia, or hyperammonemia.
- Outpatient—clinical signs related only to neuromuscular system.

NURSING CARE

Depends on type and severity of disorder.

ACTIVITY

Exercise restriction—with muscle weakness, stiffness, or exercise-induced collapse.

DIET

- Avoid prolonged periods of fasting.
- Restrictions—depend on underlying defect.
- Vitamin and co-factor therapy—determined by underlying defect.

CLIENT EDUCATION

- Warn client that most inherited metabolic defects cannot be cured, although some can be treated.
- Advise against breeding affected individuals.

SURGICAL CONSIDERATIONS

N/A

MEDICATIONS

DRUG(S) OF CHOICE

- Depend on the abnormality and clinical signs.

M

- Lipid storage myopathies—L-carnitine 50 mg/kg PO q12h; riboflavin 50–100 mg PO q24h; coenzyme Q10 1 mg/kg PO q24h.
- Mitochondrial myopathies—may benefit from therapy similar to that listed for lipid storage myopathies.

CONTRAINDICATIONS

None known.

PRECAUTIONS

Avoid fasting and strenuous exercise if they precipitate clinical signs.

POSSIBLE INTERACTIONS

N/A

ALTERNATIVE DRUG(S)

N/A

FOLLOW-UP

PATIENT MONITORING

- Lipid storage myopathies—return of muscle strength; elimination of muscle pain.
- Elevated serum creatine kinase—should return to normal.

PREVENTION/AVOIDANCE

N/A

POSSIBLE COMPLICATIONS

Severe neurologic impairment.

EXPECTED COURSE AND PROGNOSIS

- Untreatable disorder—poor prognosis.
- Lipid storage myopathies—good prognosis if no underlying organic academia.

MISCELLANEOUS

ASSOCIATED CONDITIONS

- Iatrogenic and naturally occurring Cushing syndrome.
- Lipid storage myopathies—found in some dogs.
- Hemolytic anemia—due to underlying metabolic defect.

AGE-RELATED FACTORS

- Inborn errors—usually found in young dogs.
- Acquired defects—found in adult dogs.

ZOONOTIC POTENTIAL

N/A

PREGNANCY/FERTILITY/BREEDING

Unknown

SYNONYMS

- Acid maltase deficiency—glycogenosis type II.
- Cori disease—glycogenosis type III.
- Glycogen storage disorders.
- Lipid storage myopathies.
- Mitochondrial myopathies.
- Phosphofructokinase deficiency—glycogenosis type VII.

ABBREVIATIONS

- RBC = red blood cell.

INTERNET RESOURCES

- Comparative Neuromuscular Laboratory: http://vetneuromuscular.ucsd.edu
- PennGen: http://vet.upenn.edu/researchcenters/penngen
- VetGenLLC: http://www.vetgen.com/

Suggested Reading

Cameron JM, Maj MC, Levandovskiy V, et al. Identification of a canine model of pyruvate dehydrogenase phosphatase 1 deficiency. Mol Genet Metab 2007, 90:15–23.

Fyfe JC. Molecular diagnosis of inherited neuromuscular disease. Vet Clin North Am 2002, 31:287–300.

Gerber K, Harvey JW, D'Agorne S, et al. Hemolysis, myopathy, and cardiac disease associated with hereditary phosphofructokinase deficiency in two Whippets. Vet Clin Path 2009, 38:46–51.

Platt SR. Neuromuscular complications in endocrine and metabolic disorders. Vet Clin North Am 2002, 31:125–146.

Shelton GD. Canine lipid storage myopathies. In: Bonagura JD, Kirk RW, eds., Current Veterinary Therapy XII. Philadelphia, PA: Saunders, 1995, pp. 1161–1163.

Shelton GD, Engvall E. Muscular dystrophies and other inherited myopathies. Vet Clin North Am 2002, 31:103–124.

Author Lauren Talarico

Consulting Editor Mathieu M. Glassman

Acknowledgment The author and editors acknowledge the prior contribution of G. Diane Shelton.

MYOPATHY—POLYMYOSITIS AND DERMATOMOSITIS

BASICS

DEFINITION

• Polymyositis—a condition in which skeletal muscles are damaged by a nonsuppurative inflammatory process dominated by lymphocytic infiltration. Terminology restricted to the immune-mediated form.
• Dermatomyositis—polymyositis is associated with characteristic skin lesions.

PATHOPHYSIOLOGY

• Inflammation of skeletal muscles—results in muscle weakness, stiffness, myalgia, and atrophy.
• Muscle inflammation—may be a result of immune-mediated, infectious, or paraneoplastic disorders; may be a sequela to certain drug therapies.

SYSTEMS AFFECTED

• Gastrointestinal—particularly the pharyngeal and esophageal muscles, because they are composed predominantly of skeletal muscle in dogs.
• Neuromuscular—generalized muscle involvement including masticatory and limb muscles.
• Skin/exocrine—particularly if related to a generalized immune-mediated connective tissue disorder. Skin lesions predominate over neuromuscular signs in canine dermatomyositis.

GENETICS

• Unknown.
• As for autoimmune diseases in general, the appropriate genetic background must exist.
• Familial form of autoimmune polymyositis in Newfoundland and vizsla.
• Dermatomyositis—reported to have an autosomal dominant inheritance pattern in rough-coated collie and Shetland sheepdog.

INCIDENCE/PREVALENCE

• Unknown.
• Generalized inflammatory myopathies—not common but recognition may be increasing.

GEOGRAPHIC DISTRIBUTION

Probably worldwide.

SIGNALMENT

Species

Dog and rarely cat.

Breed Predilections

• Polymyositis—various breeds of dogs and cats may be affected; breed-associated in Newfoundland, boxer, and vizsla.
• Dermatomyositis—reported in rough-coated collie, Shetland sheepdog, and Australian cattle dog.

Mean Age and Range

• Polymyositis—none obvious.
• Dermatomyositis—3–5 months of age.

Predominant Sex

None obvious.

SIGNS

General Comments

• Polymyositis—usually associated with a stiff-stilted gait, variable myalgia, and/or muscle weakness. May see regurgitation and megaesophagus.
• Elevated serum creatine kinase activity—supports but does not make the diagnosis of myositis. Do not rule out polymyositis if creatine kinase activity normal.
• Muscle biopsy—needed to confirm the diagnosis.

Historical Findings

• Stiff-stilted gait—acute or chronic.
• Muscle swelling and/or atrophy.
• Variable muscle pain.
• Generalized muscle weakness and exercise intolerance.
• Regurgitation of food or difficulty swallowing.

Physical Examination Findings

• Variable pain upon palpation of muscle groups.
• Generalized muscle atrophy, including the muscles of mastication.
• Gait abnormalities, including a stiff-stilted gait.
• Neurologic examination—not abnormal; may be a decreased gag reflex if the pharyngeal muscles are affected.
• Dermatomyositis (dogs)—typical skin lesions.

CAUSES

• Immune-mediated.
• Infections—*Toxoplasma gondii*; *Neospora canis*; *Sarcocystis* spp.; tick-related diseases, bacterial infection uncommon.
• Drug-induced.
• Paraneoplastic or pre-neoplastic syndrome.

RISK FACTORS

• Appropriate genetic background.
• Possibly previous bacterial or viral infection.
• Neoplasia, possibly occult.
• Exposure to ticks.

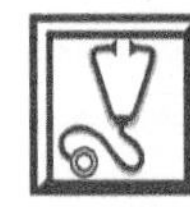

DIAGNOSIS

DIFFERENTIAL DIAGNOSIS

• Polyarthritis—differentiated by physical examination and evaluation of joint fluid.
• Noninflammatory muscle disorders—differentiated by muscle biopsy.
• Polyneuropathy—differentiated by neurologic examination, electrophysiology, and muscle and peripheral nerve biopsies.
• Chronic intervertebral disc disease—differentiated by neurologic examination and serum creatine kinase activity.
• Myasthenia gravis—differentiated by positive acetylcholine receptor (AChR) antibody titer.

CBC/BIOCHEMISTRY/URINALYSIS

Serum creatine kinase activity—variably elevated.

OTHER LABORATORY TESTS

• Serum antinuclear antibody titer—may be positive in connective tissue disorders.
• May see concurrent hypothyroidism.
• Cardiac troponin I—may have concurrent myocarditis.

IMAGING

• Regurgitation—evaluate thoracic radiography for esophageal dilatation, neoplasia.
• Cardiac silhouette—evaluate myocardial size and shape.
• Pharyngeal weakness—perform a dynamic study for the evaluation of the swallowing process.

DIAGNOSTIC PROCEDURES

• Muscle biopsy—single most important test for diagnosing polymyositis; sample multiple muscles, because condition may be missed if distribution is patchy.
• Echocardiograph—evaluate myocardial function.
• Electrodiagnostic evaluation (electromyogram [EMG], measurement of nerve conduction velocity)—performed to determine the distribution of muscle involvement and the muscles to be biopsied; should help differentiate myopathic from neuropathic causes of muscle weakness.

PATHOLOGIC FINDINGS

• Muscle swelling or atrophy.
• Biopsy specimens—usually contain mononuclear cell infiltrates.
• Rare neutrophils or eosinophils—may be noted.
• Regenerating myofibers—may be observed.
• Intramyofiber parasite cyst—rare.
• Chronic condition—may see extensive myofiber atrophy and fibrosis.

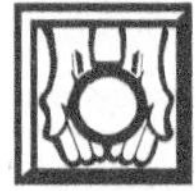

TREATMENT

APPROPRIATE HEALTH CARE

Outpatient

NURSING CARE

Supportive care—may be required to prevent skin wounds and decubital ulcers in nonambulatory, severely affected patients.

ACTIVITY

Should increase, along with muscle strength, as muscle inflammation decreases.

DIET

- Megaesophagus—may require feeding from an elevation; try foods of different consistencies.
- Severe regurgitation—may need to place a gastric feeding tube to maintain hydration and nutrition.

CLIENT EDUCATION

- Warn client that long-term immunosuppressive therapy may be required for an immune-mediated condition.
- Inform client that residual muscle atrophy and contractures may occur with chronic disease and extensive fibrosis.
- Suggest genetic counseling for familial disorders.

SURGICAL CONSIDERATIONS

Only for concurrent neoplasia.

MEDICATIONS

DRUG(S) OF CHOICE

- Corticosteroids—immunosuppressive dosages usually result in clinical improvement of immune-mediated condition; decrease to the lowest alternate-day dosage that maintains normal creatine kinase activity and improved muscle strength and mobility; may require long-term therapy.
- Identified infectious agent—initiate specific therapy.
- Identified myocardial failure—initiate specific therapy.

CONTRAINDICATIONS

N/A

PRECAUTIONS

Corticosteroids—observe for infection and undesirable side effects; remember that chronic therapy may lead to muscle atrophy (steroid myopathy).

POSSIBLE INTERACTIONS

N/A

ALTERNATIVE DRUG(S)

Intolerable side effects of corticosteroids—institute a lower dose of corticosteroids combined with another drug (e.g., azathioprine, cyclosporine).

FOLLOW-UP

PATIENT MONITORING

- Serum creatine kinase activity—periodic evaluation; if elevated, should decrease into the normal range.
- Corticosteroids—side effects.

PREVENTION/AVOIDANCE

N/A

POSSIBLE COMPLICATIONS

- Corticosteroids—undesirable side effects.
- Recurrence of clinical signs—treatment stopped too early.
- Poor clinical response—inadequate dosages of corticosteroids. May need additional or alternative immunosuppressant.

EXPECTED COURSE AND PROGNOSIS

- Immune-mediated condition—good to fair prognosis.
- Paraneoplastic disorder associated with occult neoplasia—guarded prognosis.

MISCELLANEOUS

ASSOCIATED CONDITIONS

- Other concurrent autoimmune disorders.
- Neoplasia.

AGE-RELATED FACTORS

N/A

ZOONOTIC POTENTIAL

N/A

PREGNANCY/FERTILITY/BREEDING

Unknown

SEE ALSO

Myopathy, Noninflammatory—Endocrine.

ABBREVIATIONS

- AChR = acetylcholine receptor.
- EMG = electromyogram.

INTERNET RESOURCES

Comparative Neuromuscular Laboratory: http://vetneuromuscular.ucsd.edu

Suggested Reading

Evans J, Levesque D, Shelton GD. Canine inflammatory myopathies: a clinicopathologic review of 200 cases. J Vet Intern Med 2004, 18:679–691.

Haley AC, Platt SR, Kent M, et al. Breed-specific polymyositis in Hungarian Vizla dogs. J Vet Intern Med 2011, 25:393–397.

Hargis AM, Haupt KH, Prieur DJ, Moore MP. A skin disorder in three Shetland sheepdogs: Comparison with familial canine dermatomyositis of collies. Compend Contin Educ Pract Vet 1985, 7:306–318.

Neravanda D, Kent M, Platt SR, et al. Lymphoma-associated polymyositis in dogs. J Vet Intern Med 2009, 23:1293–1298.

Podell M. Inflammatory myopathies. Vet Clin North Am 2002, 31:147–167.

Shelton GD. From dog to man: the broad spectrum of inflammatory myopathies. Neuromusc Disord 2007, 17:663–670.

Warman S, Pearson G, Barrett E, Shelton GD. Dilatation of the right atrium in a dog with polymyositis and myocarditis. J Small Anim Pract 2008, 49:302–305.

Author Lauren Talarico

Consulting Editor Mathieu M. Glassman

Acknowledgment The author and editors acknowledge the prior contribution of G. Diane Shelton.

Client Education Handout available online

M

MYXEDEMA AND MYXEDEMA COMA

BASICS

OVERVIEW

- Myxedema coma is a rare, life-threatening manifestation of severe hypothyroidism and an endocrine emergency.
- The development of myxedema coma requires a precipitating event (often infection) that overwhelms normal homeostatic mechanisms.
- The greatest challenge with myxedema coma is recognition. Once recognized, immediate and intensive supportive care is necessary. Successful treatment requires treatment of the underlying cause, if present. Mortality rates can be high.

M

SIGNALMENT

- Dogs.
- Median age—6 years.
- Female dogs predisposed.
- Not reported in cats.

SIGNS

Historical Findings

- The most common findings are changes in mental status, altered thermoregulation, and nonpitting skin edema.
- Mentation changes are due to brain edema, ranging from altered alertness to obtundation. Mental depression is the most common mental status. Coma is rarely reported.
- Other signs consistent with hypothyroidism.
- Prior diagnosis of hypothyroidism.

Physical Examination Findings

- Hypothermia, nonpitting edema, tachypnea, alopecia, dehydration, dermatitis, otitis.
- Mental dullness is common and decreased postural reactions may be present.
- In humans, classic signs of myxedema coma include mental dullness, bradycardia, hypothermia, hypoventilation, and hypotension. These signs have been reported in dogs, but most do not present with all of them.

CAUSES & RISK FACTORS

- Myxedema coma results from chronic untreated severe primary hypothyroidism.
- Both forms of primary hypothyroidism (lymphocytic thyroiditis and idiopathic thyroid atrophy) have been associated with the development of myxedema coma.
- A secondary precipitating event is usually associated with the onset of a myxedema crisis.
- Precipitating events can include infections, respiratory disease, heart failure, and hypovolemia.
- Exposure to cold temperatures may be a precipitating event.

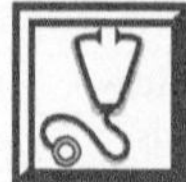

DIAGNOSIS

DIFFERENTIAL DIAGNOSIS

Weakness may be associated with cardiovascular disease, neurologic disease, and other endocrinopathies.

CBC/BIOCHEMISTRY/URINALYSIS

- Mild nonregenerative anemia.
- Hypercholesterolemia.
- Hypertriglyceridemia.
- Hypoglycemia.
- Hyponatremia.
- Urinalysis is normal.

OTHER LABORATORY TESTS

- Thyroid function tests—severe hypothyroidism with low total thyroxine (T_4), low free T_4, and elevated thyroid-stimulating hormone (TSH) levels.
- Blood gas analysis may note hypoxemia or hypercarbia.
- Diagnostics are aimed at identifying an underlying cause.

IMAGING

Thoracic radiographs/ultrasound—pulmonary alveolar pattern, pleural effusion (modified transudate).

PATHOLOGIC FINDINGS

Skin biopsies show dermal thickening, myxedema, and vacuolation of arrector pili muscles.

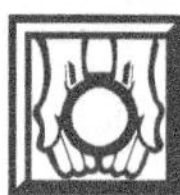

TREATMENT

- Myxedema coma is a medical emergency.
- Once a presumptive diagnosis is made, immediate inpatient treatment is necessary.
- Due to the critical nature of myxedema coma, treatment must be initiated before thyroid function test results confirm diagnosis.
- Immediate provision of a patent airway and resuscitation of hypotension are necessary.
- Mechanical ventilation may be necessary.
- IV fluid therapy to support blood pressure and to address hyponatremia. Patients with myxedema have a decreased ability to excrete free water.
- Replacement isotonic crystalloids (Normosol-R or lactated Ringer's solution, 20–30 mL/kg, IV initial bolus) are first-line therapy. Reassess and continue IV fluids (2.5–7 mL/kg/h) as necessary to maintain blood pressure and heart rate.
- IV administration of synthetic thyroid hormone.
- Rapid rewarming may cause peripheral vasodilatation, hypotension, and potential cardiovascular collapse; correction of hypothermia should be passive and occur over a number of hours.

MEDICATIONS

DRUG(S) OF CHOICE

- Definitive immediate treatment—levothyroxine 5 µg/kg (0.005 mg/kg) IV q12h.
- A more conservative dose should be used when there is concern about cardiac function, and the heart's ability to deal with a rapid increase in metabolic rate. Decrease levothyroxine dose by 50–75% in these cases.
- Once the patient's condition has stabilized and the patient is able to swallow, oral levothyroxine therapy should be initiated at 0.02 mg/kg PO q12h.

CONTRAINDICATIONS/POSSIBLE INTERACTIONS

- Lower IV levothyroxine dose in patients with cardiac disease.
- Avoid rapid rewarming.

FOLLOW-UP

- Prognosis is guarded to grave.
- If patient survives initial treatment, treat and monitor as recommended for hypothyroidism.

MISCELLANEOUS

SEE ALSO

Hypothyroidism.

ABBREVIATIONS

- T_4 = thyroxine, tetraiodothyronine.
- TSH = thyroid-stimulating hormone.

Suggested Reading

Finora K, Greco DS. Hypothyroidism and myxedema coma in veterinary medicine—physiology, diagnosis and treatment. Compend Contin Educ Pract Vet 2007, 29:19–32.

Koenig A. Endocrine emergencies in dogs and cats. Vet Clin North Am 2013, 43:869–897.

Pullen WH, Hess RS. Hypothyroid dogs treated with intravenous levothyroxine. J Vet Intern Med 2006, 20:32–37.

Author Patty A. Lathan

Consulting Editor Patty A. Lathan

Acknowledgment The author/editor acknowledges the prior contribution of Deborah S. Greco.

MYXOMATOUS MITRAL VALVE DISEASE

BASICS

DEFINITION

Myxomatous mitral valve disease (MMVD) is characterized by progressive myxomatous degeneration, which refers to a characteristic pathologic weakening and disorganization of valvular connective tissue. Although myxomatous degeneration most commonly affects the mitral valve, any of the four intracardiac valves can be affected, and the most commonly used descriptor "mitral" does not exclude involvement of other valves.

PATHOPHYSIOLOGY

• Pathologic weakened and disorganized valvular connective tissue, in which the spongiosa component is unusually prominent with accumulation of mucopolysaccarides and glycosaminoglycans. • Valve leaflets become thickened and elongated with disease progression. • Degenerative changes in chordae tendineae lead to thickening and elongation of these structures, thus contributing to valve flattening and prolapse.
• With progression, valve lesions cause insufficient systolic coaptation of the leaflets, leading to backward regurgitation of blood from the ventricle into the atrium. • Severity of mitral regurgitation depends on severity of valve lesions (leaflets and/or chordae tendineae).
• Compensatory mechanisms include cardiac dilation and eccentric hypertrophy, increased force of contraction, increased heart rate, increased pulmonary lymphatic drainage, fluid retention, and neurohormonal modulation of cardiovascular function.
• With progression, valvular regurgitation eventually may not be compensated, leading to reduced cardiac output and increased venous pressures, leading to pulmonary edema if left-sided congestive heart failure (CHF) and ascites if right-sided CHF.
• Acute cardiac tamponade may result from atrial tear.

SYSTEMS AFFECTED

• Cardiovascular—myxomatous degeneration most commonly affects the mitral valve but any intracardiac valve can be affected.
• Hepatobiliary—passive congestion at advanced stages. • Renal/urologic—prerenal azotemia at advanced stages. • Respiratory—if edema and/or pulmonary hypertension (PH) develops.

GENETICS

Etiology currently unknown, but the current leading scientific hypothesis is that a genetically determined dystrophic process initiates valve degeneration. Age of onset is inherited as a polygenetic threshold trait (i.e., multiple genes influence the trait and a certain threshold has to be reached before the disease develops). This mode of inheritance means that a combination of a sire and a dam that both have an early onset of MMVD will give offspring that have, on average, an early onset of the disease. A combination of dogs with late onset will give offspring that manifest the disease at old age or never.

INCIDENCE/PREVALENCE

The most common cardiac disease in dogs. Prevalence is strongly influenced by age: it is uncommon in young dogs but common in old dogs. MMVD is encountered in all breeds, but the highest prevalence is seen in small to medium-sized dog breeds. The prevalence reaches >90% in some affected dog breeds >10 years.

SIGNALMENT

Species

Dogs; extremely rare in cats.

Breed Predilections

Typically small breeds (<20 kg, but may be encountered in larger dogs), such as cavalier King Charles spaniel (CKCS), Chihuahua, miniature schnauzer, Maltese terrier, Pomeranian, cocker spaniel, Pekingese, poodle, and others.

Mean Age and Range

Murmur may be detected from 2 years of age with a peak incidence for detection at 6–8 years in widely affected breeds such as the CKCS. Onset of CHF from 8–12 years.

Predominant Sex

Males develop the disease at a younger age than females, which means higher prevalence at a given age in males,

SIGNS

Signs depend on the stage of disease. The descriptions here align with the grading system described in the American College of Veterinary Internal Medicine (ACVIM) consensus statement on MMVD.

Clinically Healthy Patients but at a Higher Risk of Developing the Disease (ACVIM Stage A)

No abnormal findings.

Dogs Diagnosed with the Disease but with No Overt Clinical Signs (ACVIM Stage B)

• Systolic click (early stage). • Systolic murmur best heard over the mitral or tricuspid areas. • Murmurs may range from soft low-intensity to loud holosystolic.
• With progression, murmurs typically get louder and radiate more widely. • Initially, patients have no obvious radiographic or echocardiographic changes in cardiac chamber size or have mild cardiomegaly and do not meet the so called "EPIC trial criteria" (see ACVIM stage B1). Stage B2 is defined as dogs with cardiac enlargement meeting EPIC trial criteria, i.e., presenting a moderate or loud intensity murmur (≥3/6), VHS >10.5, bodyweight normalized left ventricular end-diastolic diameter (LVIDDn) ≥1,7, and a left atrial to aortic root ratio (LA/Ao) ≥1.6.

Dogs with Overt Clinical Signs of CHF or with Clinical Signs Stabilized by CHF Therapy (ACVIM stages C and D)

• Usually a loud holosystolic heart murmur.
• Tachypnea/dyspnea/orthopnea if decompensated CHF. • Tachycardia and loss of respiratory sinus arrhythmia if decompensated CHF. • Arrhythmia, such as supraventricular premature beats, ventricular premature beats, or atrial fibrillation, may be present.
• Respiratory crackles if decompensated CHF.
• Weak femoral pulse, prolonged capillary refill time and pale mucous membranes in low output failure. • Pink froth, i.e., pulmonary edema, may be evident in the nares and oropharynx in severe decompensated CHF.
• Ascites if right-sided CHF (caused by myxomatous tricuspid lesions and/or pulmonary hypertension [PH]).

CAUSES

Primary (inciting) factor unknown but the disease is influenced by genetic factors in affected breeds.

RISK FACTORS

• Breed. • Sex (males have earlier onset).

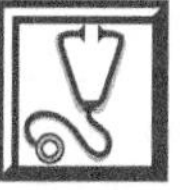

DIAGNOSIS

DIFFERENTIAL DIAGNOSIS

• Bacterial endocarditis. • Congenital heart disease. • Dilated cardiomyopathy.
• Chronic airway or interstitial lung disease.
• Pneumonia. • Pulmonary embolism.
• Pulmonary neoplasia. • Heartworm disease.

CBC/BIOCHEMISTRY/URINALYSIS

• CBC/biochemistry usually unremarkable unless severe disease and ongoing CHF therapy. • Prerenal azotemia secondary to impaired renal perfusion; high urine specific gravity unless complicated by underlying kidney disease or recent/ongoing diuretics.
• High liver enzyme activity in many patients with right-sided CHF.

OTHER LABORATORY TESTS

• Natriuretic peptides—often unremarkable unless moderate to severe disease. • Serum troponin I—unremarkable unless severe disease.

IMAGING

Radiography

• Heart size ranges from normal to left-sided or generalized cardiomegaly. • LA enlargement is usually the earliest finding. • LV may be enlarged. • Left-sided CHF—pulmonary congestion; increased interstitial pattern ± alveolar pattern with air bronchograms.

MYXOMATOUS MITRAL VALVE DISEASE (CONTINUED)

Initially, congestion and edema are perihilar, but all lungfields may eventually show changes.

Echocardiography

• Thickened and distorted mitral valve leaflets. • Elongated and ruptured chordae tendineae, causing mitral valve prolapse. • Normal to severely dilated atrium (uni- or bilateral). • LV may be dilated and is hyperdynamic if regurgitant flow is significant and myocardial function intact; as LV becomes more grossly distended, it may become normo- or, uncommonly, hypodynamic because of myocardial failure. • Pericardial effusion (usually mild) may be present in severe disease. • Doppler studies show a jet of regurgitation into the atrium. • Doppler evaluation for the presence of PH should be routinely performed.

M

DIAGNOSTIC PROCEDURES

• Arterial/venous blood gases can be used to quantify hypoxemia and monitor treatment response. • Systemic blood pressure should be monitored; especially patients receiving diuretics and other cardiovascular drugs to check for hypotension; hypertension is not associated with the disease, but if concurrent can exacerbate the disease.

Electrocardiographic Findings

• Sinus tachycardia common in patients with CHF. • May show evidence of LA enlargement (P mitrale) or LV enlargement (tall and wide R waves). • Supraventricular, or ventricular arrhythmias may develop in severe disease.

PATHOLOGIC FINDINGS

• Gross valvular changes range from only a few discrete nodules at the line of closure to gross distortion by gray-white nodules and plaques causing contraction of the cusps and rolling of the free edge; the chordae are irregularly thickened, with regions of tapering and rupture. • Mild disease—normal cardiac size. More progressed cases—LA and LV dilation. Degree of right-sided dilatation variable. • Degree of LV hypertrophy may be apparent only when weighing the heart. • Jet lesions—irregular thickening and opacity of the atrial endocardium. • LA splits or tears in some cases.

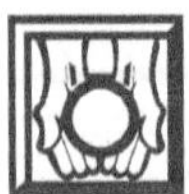

TREATMENT

APPROPRIATE HEALTH CARE

Dogs with preclinical MMVD can be managed at home with scheduled rechecks to identify dogs that meet EPIC trial criteria for initiation of pimobendan. Some dogs with mild to moderate signs of CHF may be managed at home, whereas dogs with more severe signs should be hospitalized initially for intensive CHF therapy.

NURSING CARE

Oxygen therapy as needed for hypoxemic dogs with moderate to severe CHF. Dogs receiving diuretics must be given the opportunity to urinate. Dyspnea-associated anxiety should be treated. Carefully monitor blood pressure and respiratory response to narcotics and tranquilizers in the setting of acute decompensated CHF. Butorphanol 0.2–0.25 mg/kg IM or IV is commonly used for sedation, but combinations of buprenorphine 0.0075–0.01 mg/kg and acepromazine 0.01–0.03 mg/kg IV, IM, or SQ can also be used.

ACTIVITY

• Exercise restriction for symptomatic patients in acute decompensated CHF. • Exercise recommended for stable CHF patients on medical therapy, but avoid strenuous exercise.

DIET

• Prevent cardiac cachexia by ensuring adequate calorie intake. • Avoid high sodium diets.

CLIENT EDUCATION

• Discuss the progressive nature of the disease. • Mild disease severity is suggestive of a long period without clinical signs; moderate to severe disease indicates a shorter period until signs of CHF may develop. • If a breeder, inform about the disease genetics and impact for future breeding. • Pimobendan therapy prolongs preclinical period and survival times in dogs meeting the EPIC criteria. • Appropriate level of exercise, but at the same time maintain quality of life. • Common signs of CHF listed earlier. • How to medicate (if indicated)—information about consistent dosing and that diuretic doses should be adjusted in consultation with the veterinarian. • Possible adverse side reactions of medications. • How to monitor resting and/or sleeping respiratory rates at home, and at which rate new contact with the clinician should be initiated. • Diet (if indicated)—emphasize importance of avoiding cardiac cachexia by paying close attention to appetite and using an appropriate diet. Salt loads should be avoided.

SURGICAL CONSIDERATIONS

Surgical valve repair can be performed at a few sites in the world.

MEDICATIONS

DRUG(S) OF CHOICE

Recommended treatment depends on disease stage; these recommendations follow the guidelines set by the consensus statement developed by the ACVIM.

Patients without Overt Clinical Signs (ACVIM Stage B)

• If no cardiomegaly, no treatment currently recommended. • Pimobendan 0.25–0.3 mg/kg q12h PO prolongs preclinical period (by a median of approximately 15 months) and survival in Stage B2 dogs. • Administering angiotensin-converting enzyme inhibitors (ACEIs) to Stage B patients has been shown to be ineffective in two clinical trials.

Patients Showing Overt Clinical Signs (ACVIM Stages C and D)

Acute Decompensated CHF

• Furosemide IV, SC, IM, or PO; dose is dependent on severity of CHF: ◦ Mild to moderate CHF: 2–4 mg/kg q8–24h. ◦ Severe or fulminant CHF: 4–8 mg/kg q2–6h, preferably IV, IM, or SC. ◦ Monitor outcome of treatment by respiratory rate and general clinical status. ◦ Dose can often be reduced once the patient is stabilized. • Oxygen supplementation and cage rest to patients with significant dyspnea: 40% in O_2 cage (can intermittently go as high as 100%) up to 24 hours; nasal O_2 may be used in large-breed dogs, 50–100 mL/kg/min through humidifier. • Pimobendan 0.25–0.3 mg/kg q12h PO. In many countries outside of the United States, IV pimobendan is available and used as an initial single-dose treatment before oral medication. • Additional options in severe fulminant CHF: ◦ Nitroglycerin: ointment (one-fourth inch/5 kg up to 2 inches percutaneously), sublingual spray (one puff/10 kg) or injectable (1–5 µg/kg/min CRI). ◦ Arterial vasodilator to decrease afterload rapidly, e.g., hydralazine 0.5 mg/kg q12h (titrate up to 2 mg/kg if necessary) or sodium nitroprusside 1–10 µg/kg/min (expensive drug and difficult to obtain). Both drugs require blood pressure monitoring and should be considered only in hospitalized dogs under care of a specialist. ◦ Dobutamine—dogs: 1–10 µg/kg/min; cats: 1–5 µg/kg/min. • Antiarrhythmics—as needed. • Severe ascites may require abdominocentesis.

Chronic CHF (Typically Treated as an Outpatient)

• Exact composition of medical therapy depends on disease severity and clinical signs. All dogs with CHF require life-long treatment with a diuretic, such as furosemide: ◦ Mild to moderate CHF: 1 mg/kg q12h to 2 mg/kg q8h PO. ◦ Moderate to severe CHF: 2–3 mg/kg q12h or higher. • Pimobendan at 0.25–0.3 mg/kg q12h PO. • ACEI (e.g., enalapril, benazepril, ramipril)—dose and frequency depend on ACEI used, e.g., enalapril 0.5 mg/kg q12–24h; benazepril 0.25–0.5 mg/kg q24h. • Spironolactone 2 mg/kg q12–24h PO and/or hydrochlorothiazide at 2–4 mg/kg q12h PO. • Digoxin 0.22 mg/m^2 q12h PO, or lower. • Antiarrhythmics—as needed. • Sildenafil 1–2 mg/kg q8–12h if PH present.

PRECAUTIONS

• Use digoxin, diuretics, and ACEIs cautiously in patients with renal disease.
• Beta blockers are negative inotropes and may have an acute adverse effect on myocardial function and clinical status.

POSSIBLE INTERACTIONS

• Furosemide potentiates the effects of ACEIs, spironolactone, or thiazides. • Use nonsteroidal anti-inflammatory drugs cautiously in patients receiving furosemide or ACEIs.

ALTERNATIVE DRUG(S)

• Diuretics—add thiazide and/or spironolactone in refractory animals.
• Torsemide—administered at approximately 1/10th of the furosemide dose, or 0.1–0.6 mg/kg once to twice daily is an alternative to furosemide. • Vasodilators—isosorbide dinitrate can be used in place of nitroglycerin ointment in patients requiring long-term nitrate administration.

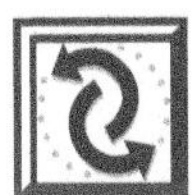

FOLLOW-UP

PATIENT MONITORING

• Frequency of rechecks depends on stage of MMVD and severity of CHF (if present).
• Dogs without signs of CHF: ○ Mild to moderate disease—perform echocardiography when a murmur is first detected and every 6–12 months (interval depends on findings of previous echocardiogram) thereafter to document progressive cardiomegaly. Baseline radiographs may be useful. ○ Owners are instructed to regulary measure respiratory rates at home during rest or sleep and contact the veterinarian should rates be consistently higher than 30 breaths/minute. • Dogs with signs of CHF: ○ Once acute CHF has been successfully treated, dogs can be treated at home. ○ Follow-up with owner, by phone or email, should be conducted after 1–3 days at home, to monitor for maintained treatment effect. A change in the furosemide dose (partly based on respiratory rates during sleep or deep rest and amount of side effects of the treatment initiated) may be performed. ○ Reexamine after 1–2 weeks (check for signs of decompensated CHF, dehydration, electrolyte imbalance, renal dysfunction, and presence of complications) or sooner if treatment response is unsatisfactory. ○ Thereafter once every 3–6 months if the patient is stable on the medications. More severe cases may require more frequent monitoring. • Monitor BUN and creatinine especially when high doses of diuretics and ACEIs are used. • Monitor potassium, especially if combinations of spironolactone, ACEIs, and digoxin are used.

POSSIBLE COMPLICATIONS

• Preclinical patients may develop acute CHF.
• Recurrent decompensated CHF in patients stabilized by medical therapy. • PH.
• Biventricular CHF in dogs with initial left-sided CHF. • Mild pleural and/or pericardial effusion. • Arrhythmia. • Rupture of major chordae tendineae, leading to a flail valve leaflet and acute decompensation.
• Atrial tear leading to acquired atrial septal defect or cardiac tamponade.

EXPECTED COURSE AND PROGNOSIS

Valve lesions are progressive in nature and myocardial function may worsen, requiring increased drug dosages. Long-term prognosis depends on response to therapy and stage of heart disease.

MISCELLANEOUS

SYNONYMS

• Chronic valvular disease (CVD). • Chronic mitral valve disease. • Degenerative valvular disease. • Degenerative mitral valve disease (DMVD). • Degenerative valve disease.

SEE ALSO

• Atrial Wall Tear.
• Congestive Heart Failure, Left-Sided.
• Congestive Heart Failure, Right-Sided.

ABBREVIATIONS

• ACEI = angiotensin-converting enzyme inhibitor.
• ACVIM = American College of Veterinary Internal Medicine.
• CHF = congestive heart failure.
• LA = left atrium.
• LV = left ventricle.
• MMVD = myxomatous mitral valve disease.
• PH = pulmonary hypertension.

Suggested Reading

Keene BW, Atkins CE, Bonagura JD, et al. ACVIM consensus guidelines for the diagnosis and treatment of myxomatous mitral valve disease. J Vet Intern Med 2019, 33(3):1127–1140.

Authors Ingrid Ljungvall and Jens Häggström
Consulting Editor Michael Aherne

NARCOLEPSY AND CATAPLEXY

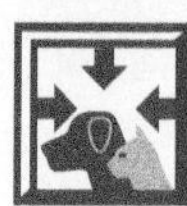

BASICS

OVERVIEW

Narcolepsy/cataplexy refer to the same disorder, cataplexy being the clinical sign easiest to recognize in domestic animals.

Narcolepsy

• Sleep disorders. • Syndrome characterized by excessive sleepiness, cataplexy sleep paralysis, and hypnagogic hallucinations (humans). Sudden episodes of paradoxical sleep without a preceding period of slow-wave sleep.

Cataplexy

• Sudden, episodic, and spontaneous collapse secondary to complete atonia of skeletal muscles (flaccid paralysis) caused by inhibition of spinal cord lower motor neurons. • Patient stays alert and will follow with its eyes.• Most common clinical sign of narcolepsy in small animals.

N

SIGNALMENT

• Dog and rarely cat. • Proven hereditary—Labrador retriever, dachshund, and Doberman pinscher. • Autosomal recessive gene mutation—*canarc-1* gene found on chromosome 12, which codes for a hypocretin (orexin) receptor. Mutations of *OxR2* (type II orexin receptor gene). Increased microglial expression of MHC II in Doberman pinscher. • Assumed genetic basis for miniature poodle—mode of inheritance unknown. • For inherited disease, clinical signs appear between 2 and 4 months of age with escalation of signs around 1 year of age. Possible disappearance of clinical signs later in life. • Acquired form may develop in older animals (possible depletion of hypocretin production by hypothalamus) and can occur in any dog breed or mixed breed, at any age.
• Clinical signs in acquired form will usually remain for life.

SIGNS

• Physical and neurologic examinations—normal except during an episode. • Onset—peracute. • Excessive daytime sleepiness and fragmented sleep patterns reported in domestic animals, but cataplexy is usually the clinical sign recognized by owners.
• Cataplexy episodes—acute onset of flaccid paralysis without loss of consciousness lasting a few seconds to minutes (up to 20 minutes) with sudden return to normal; multiple episodes in 1 day. • Narcolepsy—eye movements, muscular twitching, and whining (as in REM sleep) frequently observed during episodes. • Patients are usually aroused by loud noises, petting, or other external stimuli.

CAUSES & RISK FACTORS

• Hereditary in some breeds. • Possible immune system involvement in acquired disease.
• Neurotransmitter abnormalities—serotonin, dopamine, norepinephrine, neuropeptide hypocretin (orexin). • Rarely reported with pontomedullary (brainstem) lesions.
• Excitement, emotions, feeding, and general anesthesia may induce narcoleptic episodes.

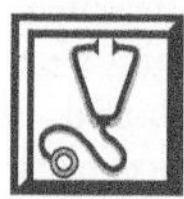

DIAGNOSIS

DIFFERENTIAL DIAGNOSIS

• Syncope. • Seizure activity—urinary or fecal incontinence, excessive salivation and muscle rigidity are not characteristic of narcolepsy in which atonia predominates. Recovery after a narcoleptic event is immediate. • Nonconvulsive seizure (drop attack). • Neuromuscular disorders—onset of clinical signs usually not as sudden and recovery not immediate as in narcolepsy.

CBC/BIOCHEMISTRY/URINALYSIS

Normal

OTHER LABORATORY TESTS

• DNA test for specific breeds (Labrador retriever, dachshund, and Doberman pinscher). • CSF—normal. Low levels of orexin A in CSF. • Standardized food-elicited cataplexy test; play-elicited cataplexy.

IMAGING

Brain MRI—normal.

DIAGNOSTIC PROCEDURES

• Observe an episode—if a consistent activity (feeding, excitement, etc.) elicits attacks, attempt to simulate the activity. • Food-elicited cataplexy test—place 10 pieces of food in a row 12–24 inches apart; record the time required for the patient to eat all the pieces and the number, type, and duration of any attacks that occur; normal dogs eat all food in <45 seconds and have no attacks; affected dogs take >2 minutes to eat the food and can have 2–20 attacks. • Play-elicited cataplexy—2 dogs are left in a room and allowed to interact together and with toys.
• Physostigmine (cholinesterase inhibitor) challenge to induce cataplexy in an affected dog—administer 0.025–0.1 mg/kg IV; repeat the food-elicited test 5–15 minutes after the injection; increase dosage if necessary (0.05 mg/kg, 0.075 mg/kg, 0.10 mg/kg); effects of each dose last 15–45 minutes.

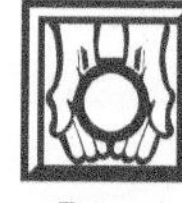

TREATMENT

• Primary goal—reduce the severity and frequency of cataplectic episodes. • Inform client that cataplexy is not a fatal disease, choking on food and airway obstruction do not occur, and the pet is not suffering.
• Inform client that activities such as hunting, swimming, and unleashed exercise put the patient at risk. • If episodes are infrequent and quality of life is preserved, treatment should be postponed and environment adapted to avoid specific stimulations.

MEDICATIONS

DRUG(S) OF CHOICE

• Imipramine 0.5 mg/kg PO q8h.
• Methylphenidate 0.25 mg/kg PO q12–24h. • Selegiline 2 mg/kg PO q24h.
• Yohimbine 50–100 µg/kg SC or PO q8–12h. • Combination also possible—imipramine and methylphenidate.

CONTRAINDICATIONS/POSSIBLE INTERACTIONS

• Many patients develop drug tolerance; change of drug may become necessary.
• Increased heart and respiratory rates, anorexia, tremors, exercise-induced hyperthermia.

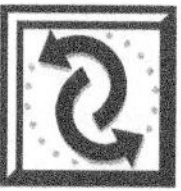

FOLLOW-UP

• Avoiding inciting activities may reduce episodes so that medication is not needed.
• Patients with the inherited form may improve with age. • Prognosis varies even with treatment; some patients remain symptomatic.

MISCELLANEOUS

Suggested Reading

De Lahunta A, Glass EN, Kent M. Veterinary Neuroanatomy and Clinical Neurology, 4th ed. St. Louis, MO: Elsevier Saunders, 2015, pp. 491–496.

Author Mylène-Kim Leclerc

NASAL AND NASOPHARYNGEAL POLYPS

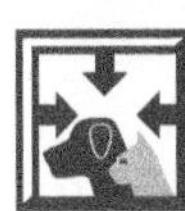

BASICS

OVERVIEW

• Non-neoplastic, inflammatory growths arising from epithelium, usually originate from a stalk.
• Nasal—uncommon; originate from the mucosa of the nasal turbinates and are inflammatory in dogs and cats.
• Nasopharyngeal—relatively common; originate from the base of the epithelial lining of the tympanic bulla or eustachian tube; when polyps extend into the nasopharynx they are referred to as nasopharyngeal polyps; when extending into the ear, they are known as middle ear polyps, aural or auricular polyps, or benign, inflammatory polyps.

SIGNALMENT

• Nasal polyps—middle-aged to older dogs and cats.
• Nasopharyngeal polyps—typically kittens and young adult cats, but can be seen in older cats (months—15 years), rarely seen in dogs.

SIGNS

Nasal Polyps

• Chronic mucopurulent nasal discharge.
• Noisy breathing—stertor.
• Nasal congestion and/or discharge.
• Sneezing or epistaxis.
• Decreased nasal airflow, generally unilateral.
• Generally nonresponsive to antibiotics.

Nasopharyngeal or Aural Polyps

• Inspiratory stridor.
• Gagging.
• Cyanosis.
• Voice change.
• Dysphagia.
• Chronic otitis externa/otitis media.
• Head tilt.
• Nystagmus.
• Ataxia.
• Horner's syndrome.

CAUSES & RISK FACTORS

Unknown—suspect congenital or response to chronic inflammatory processes.

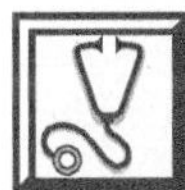

DIAGNOSIS

DIFFERENTIAL DIAGNOSIS

• Feline upper respiratory disease complex.
• Nasopharyngeal stenosis.
• Chronic otitis externa or media.
• Nasal or nasopharyngeal foreign body.
• Laryngeal paralysis.
• Nasal neoplasia—lymphoma, nasal adenocarcinoma.
• Laryngeal neoplasia—squamous cell carcinoma, lymphoma, adenocarcinoma.
• Aural neoplasia—ceruminous adenocarcinoma.

CBC/BIOCHEMISTRY/URINALYSIS

N/A

OTHER LABORATORY TESTS

Feline leukemia virus/feline immunodeficiency virus (FeLV/FIV)—general retroviral screening.

IMAGING

• Skull radiographs—soft tissue density within nasal cavity, nasopharynx, tympanic bulla, external ear canal; 25% false-negative rate.
• CT and MRI—better sensitivity for nasal, nasopharyngeal, and aural masses.

DIAGNOSTIC PROCEDURES

• Digital palpation of soft palate, visual examination of the nasopharynx and larynx under general anesthesia utilizing spay hook, dental mirror, and laryngoscope.
• Flexible fiber-optic caudal rhinoscopy to examine the dorsal nasopharynx, choanae, and caudal nasal cavity.
• Rigid rostral rhinoscopy to examine the nasal cavity.
• Deep otoscopic examination.
• Fine-needle aspirate and/or biopsy.
• Cytology and histopathology.

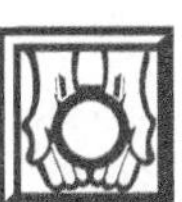

TREATMENT

• Excisional biopsy for nasal polyps.
• Traction removal of nasopharyngeal polyps via oral cavity.
• Ventral bulla osteotomy for nasopharyngeal polyps to release stalk and remove epithelial lining; may decrease rate of recurrence of polyps. Recommended if bullous involvement (clinical evidence of otitis media) is apparent.

MEDICATIONS

DRUG(S) OF CHOICE

• Consider anti-inflammatory course of corticosteroids following traction removal of nasopharyngeal polyps; decreased recurrence rate reported.
• Appropriate antimicrobial medications if secondary nasal or otic infection present.

FOLLOW-UP

• Incomplete removal of polyp and stalk may result in recurrence.
• Horner's syndrome can occur following removal by traction or ventral bulla osteotomy; usually transient but can be permanent.
• Facial paresis or paralysis or vestibular syndrome may develop after bulla osteotomy but is generally transient.
• Prognosis excellent with complete removal.

MISCELLANEOUS

ABBREVIATIONS

• FeLV = feline leukemia.
• FIV = feline immunodeficiency virus.

Suggested Reading

Greci V, Mortellaro CM. Management of otic and nasopharyngeal, and nasal polyps in cats and dogs. Vet Clin North Am Small Anim Pract 2016, 46(4):643–561.

Holt DE, Goldschmidt MH. Nasal polyps in dogs: five cases (2005 to 2011). J Small Anim Pract 2011, 52(12):660–663.

Klose TC, MacPhail CM, Schultheiss PC, et al. Prevalence of select infectious agents in inflammatory aural and nasopharyngeal polyps from client-owned cats. J Feline Med Surg 2010, 12(10):769–774.

Reed N, Gunn-Moore D. Nasopharyngeal disease in cats: diagnostic investigation and specific conditions and their management. J Feline Med Surg 2012, 14(5):306–326.

Author Catriona M. MacPhail
Consulting Editor Elizabeth Rozanski

NASAL DERMATOSES—CANINE

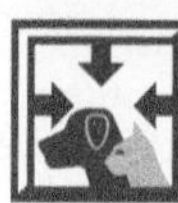

BASICS

DEFINITION

Pathologic condition of the nasal skin involving either the haired portion (bridge of the nose/dorsal muzzle) or non-haired portion (nasal planum).

PATHOPHYSIOLOGY

Dependent on cause.

SYSTEMS AFFECTED

Skin/exocrine.

SIGNALMENT

• Dogs <1 year of age—dermatophytosis, zinc-responsive dermatosis, dermatomyositis, demodicosis, eosinophilic folliculitis and furunculosis (often insect trigger; also seen in adult patients). • Zinc-responsive dermatosis—Siberian husky, Alaskan Malamute.
• Dermatomyositis—collie, Shetland sheepdog. • Uveodermatologic syndrome—Akita, Samoyed, Siberian husky. • Systemic lupus erythematosus (SLE) and discoid lupus erythematosus (DLE)—collie, Shetland sheepdog, German shepherd dog. • DLE may occur more often in females.
• Epitheliotropic lymphoma—older dogs.
• Dermal arteritis of the nasal philtrum—Saint Bernard and other large breeds. • Nasal solar dermatosis—lightly pigmented breeds.
• Nasal parakeratosis—Labrador retriever.
• Senile idiopathic nasal hyperkeratosis—cocker spaniel, Boston terrier, bulldogs.
• Seasonal nasal hypopigmentation—Labrador retriever, golden retriever, Siberian husky, Bernese mountain dog. • Idiopathic leukoderma/leukotrichia (vitiligo)—Doberman pinscher, Rottweiler, dachshund.
• Reactive histiocytosis ("clown nose")—Bernese mountain dog, golden retriever.
• Mucocutaneous pyoderma – German shepherd dog.

SIGNS

• Depigmentation. • Erythema. • Erosion/ulceration. • Vesicles/pustules. • Crusts.
• Scarring. • Alopecia. • Nodules/plaques.
• Hyperkeratosis.

CAUSES

• Nasal pyoderma/furunculosis; mucocutaneous pyoderma. • Demodicosis.
• Dermatophytosis, cryptococcosis, sporotrichosis, aspergillosis. • DLE and SLE.
• Eosinophilic folliculitis and furunculosis.
• Mosquito-bite hypersensitivity.
• Pemphigus foliaceus (PF) and erythematosus (PE). • Pemphigus vulgaris (PV). • Nasal philtrum arteritis. • Nasal solar dermatitis.
• Dermatomyositis. • Zinc-responsive dermatosis. • Uveodermatologic syndrome.
• Superficial necrolytic dermatitis. • Vitiligo.
• Idiopathic nasal depigmentation. • Contact dermatitis— irritant or hypersensitivity; plastic dish dermatitis, topical drug hypersensitivity (neomycin). • Neoplasia—squamous cell carcinoma, basal cell carcinoma, epitheliotropic lymphoma, cutaneous histiocytosis. • Trauma.
• Idiopathic sterile granuloma. • Idiopathic nasal hyperkeratosis. • Distemper virus dermatitis. • Xeromycteria – otitis media compromising sympathetic nerve supply/ parasympathetic function or lacrimal gland damaged, cause drying of nasal tissues.

RISK FACTORS

• Adult cats—may be inapparent carriers of dermatophytes. • Rooting behavior—pyoderma, dermatophytosis. • Sun exposure—nasal solar dermatitis, DLE, SLE, PE.
• Poorly pigmented nose—nasal solar dermatitis, squamous cell carcinoma. • Large, rapidly growing breeds—zinc-responsive dermatosis. • Immunosuppression—demodicosis, pyoderma, dermatophytosis.
• Insect exposure—mosquito-bite dermatitis, eosinophilic folliculitis and furunculosis.

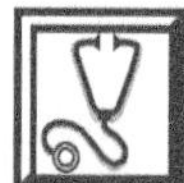

DIAGNOSIS

DIFFERENTIAL DIAGNOSIS

Nasal Solar Dermatitis

• Lesions—confined to nose; precipitated by heavy sunlight exposure. • Begins in poorly pigmented skin at junction of nasal planum and dorsal muzzle. • Lightly pigmented eyelid margins may also be affected.

DLE

• Primarily affects nasal area. • May affect mucocutaneous margins of the lips and eyelids. • Exacerbated by sunlight.
• Dermatitis often preceded by depigmentation. • Biopsy—interface dermatitis with pigmentary incontinence.

SLE

• Multisystemic disease. • Skin lesions—often involve nose, face, mucocutaneous junctions; multifocal or generalized.

Pemphigus Foliaceus

• Lesions—usually start on face and ears; commonly involve footpads and pinnae; eventually generalize. • Biopsy—subcorneal pustules with acantholysis.

Pemphigus Erythematosus

• Lesions—primarily confined to face and ears; features of both PF and DLE; typically more severe than lesions of DLE. • Dermatitis often preceded by depigmentation. • Biopsy—intraepidermal pustules with acantholysis and pigmentary incontinence.

Demodicosis

• Often starts on face or forelimbs; affects only haired skin of the dorsal muzzle.
• Juvenile-onset frequently facial at first.
• May generalize.

Contact Dermatitis: Plastic (or Rubber) Dish Dermatitis

• Depigmentation and erythema of anterior nasal planum and lips. • No ulceration or crusting. • Uncommon; overly suspected—lesions more often due to trauma from roughened bowl edges. Similar symptoms seen with trauma from rubber toys.

Dermatomyositis

• Breeds at increased risk. • Young age of onset. • Nasal, facial, and extremity lesions—erosion, alopecia, scarring, and hyperpigmentation. • Lesions especially noted at points of trauma or pressure.
• Polymyositis and megaesophagus may be seen. • Biopsy—interface dermatitis with follicular atrophy.

Uveodermatologic Syndrome

• Breeds at increased risk. • Dermatitis often preceded by ocular symptoms (uveitis).
• Striking leukotrichia and leukoderma on nose, lips and eyelids. • Biopsy of early lesions—interface dermatitis, pigmentary incontinence.

Zinc-Responsive Dermatosis

• Breeds at increased risk. • Typical signalment or diet (i.e., high-fiber or calcium supplementation). • Crusted lesions—face, mucocutaneous junctions, pressure points, footpads. • Biopsy—parakeratotic hyperkeratosis.

Eosinophilic Folliculitis and Furunculosis

• Rapid progression from popular papular/nodular pattern to ulcers and plaques.
• Highly pruritic. • Acute reaction to insect or arthropod bite and stings.

Mucocutaneous Pyoderma

• Crusting and fissures on mucocutaneous junctions of lateral aspects of the nares, lips and perioral skin.

Mosquito Bite Hypersensitivity

• Seasonal pruritic dermatitis. • Erythema, papules, crusts affecting face and nasal planum, occasionally lesions on pinnae and feet. • Biopsy—eosinophilic inflammation, collagen necrosis around the hair follicles.

Other

• Dermatophytosis—haired portion of the nose; diagnosed by culture or biopsy.
• Vitiligo—cutaneous macular depigmentation without inflammation on nose, lips, eyelids, footpads, and claws; leukotrichia with leukoderma may be seen; diagnosed by biopsy. • Nasal hypopigmentation—normal black coloration of nasal planum fades to light brown or whitish light pink color; loss of pigment is usually symmetrical and often becomes complete; in some individuals may be seasonal or wax and wane; considered cosmetic and not pathologic. • Idiopathic

N

nasal hyperkeratosis—dry, horny growths of keratin localized to nasal planum; may or may not be associated with digital hyperkeratosis, possibly associated with senility. • Other diseases—differentiate by history or biopsy (i.e., neoplastic cell infiltrate).

CBC/BIOCHEMISTRY/URINALYSIS

• Usually normal. • SLE—may see hemolytic anemia, thrombocytopenia, evidence of glomerulonephritis (high BUN, proteinuria), joint disease, or other symptoms based on body system(s) affected.

DIAGNOSTIC PROCEDURES

• Skin scrapings—*Demodex*. • Cytology—fungal organisms, bacteria, eosinophils (eosinophilic folliculitis and furunculosis), or acantholytic keratinocytes (pemphigus).
• Dermatophyte test medium (fungal culture)—dermatophytosis. • Culture on Sabouraud agar—other fungal infections.
• Bacterial culture and sensitivity or cytologic evaluation—pyoderma. • Joint tap—evidence of polyarthritis in SLE. • Antinuclear antibody (ANA)—positive in cases of SLE.
• Ocular examination—uveitis in uveodermatologic syndrome. • Electrocardiogram (ECG)—evidence of myocarditis in SLE.
• Electromyography (EMG)—evidence of polymyositis in SLE and dermatomyositis.
• Direct immunofluorescence—deposition of immunoglobulin at the basement membrane zone in DLE, SLE, and PE, and intercellular spaces of epidermis in PF, PE, and PV.
• Neoplasia—cytology or biopsy.

PATHOLOGIC FINDINGS

Histopathology

• Folliculitis/furunculosis (± mites, bacteria, fungal elements)—demodicosis, dermatophytosis, nasal pyoderma/furunculosis.
• Eosinophilic predominance—mosquito-bite dermatitis, eosinophilic folliculitis and furunculosis. • Follicular atrophy and perifollicular fibrosis—dermatomyositis.
• Interface dermatitis—DLE, SLE, dermatomyositis, uveodermatologic syndrome.
• Intraepidermal pustules with acantholysis—PF and PE. • Suprabasilar acantholysis—PV.
• Parakeratotic hyperkeratosis—zinc-responsive dermatosis. • Hypomelanosis—vitiligo, uveodermatologic syndrome. • Granulomatous/pyogranulomatous dermatitis—pyoderma, fungal, foreign body, idiopathic sterile granuloma. • Neoplastic cell infiltrate—cutaneous histiocytosis, other neoplasia.

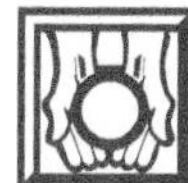

TREATMENT

• Outpatient, except SLE with multiorgan dysfunction or tumors requiring surgical excision or radiation therapy. • Reduce exposure to sunlight—DLE, SLE, PE, nasal solar dermatitis, squamous cell carcinoma.
• Discourage rooting behavior—pyoderma, dermatophytosis. • Protection from insects (mosquito-bite dermatitis; eosinophilic folliculitis furunculosis). • Warm soaks—aid removal of exudate and crusts. • Replace plastic or rubber dish and avoid contact with topical drug or other agent causing hypersensitivity reaction.

MEDICATIONS

DRUG(S) OF CHOICE

• Fungal infections—systemic antifungals: ketoconazole, itraconazole; surgical excision of early discrete lesions (deep fungal infections). • Nasal solar dermatitis—topical corticosteroids; antibiotics for secondary infection; sunscreens; firocoxib. • DLE and PE—topical corticosteroids or tacrolimus 0.1% (Protopic); cyclosporine (Atopica); tetracycline and niacinamide; oral therapy (as for PF) if temporarily needed in severe cases. • PF, PV, SLE—immunosuppressive therapy with prednisolone ± azathioprine (dogs), chlorambucil.
• Vitiligo/nasal depigmentation—no treatment. • Neoplasia—surgical excision; chemotherapy; radiation therapy. • Idiopathic nasal hyperkeratosis—topical antibiotic-corticosteroid cream, topical keratolytic and humectant; topical tacrolimus. • Other diseases—see specific cause.

PRECAUTIONS

Ketoconazole—caution in animals with liver disease or thrombocytopenia; avoid use in cats.

FOLLOW-UP

PATIENT MONITORING

Varies with specific disease and treatment prescribed.

MISCELLANEOUS

ZOONOTIC POTENTIAL

Dermatophytosis

PREGNANCY/FERTILITY/BREEDING

Ketoconazole may cause infertility in male dogs.

SYNONYMS

• Superficial necrolytic dermatitis = superficial necrolytic migratory erythema and hepatocutaneous syndrome.
• Uveodermatologic syndrome = Vogt–Koyanagi–Harada-like syndrome.

ABBREVIATIONS

• ANA = antinuclear antibody.
• DLE = discoid lupus erythematosus.
• ECG = electrocardiogram.
• EMG = electromyography.
• PE = pemphigus erythematosus.
• PF = pemphigus foliaceus.
• PV = pemphigus vulgaris.
• SLE = systemic lupus erythematosus.

Suggested Reading

Harvey RG, Haar G. Ear, Nose and Throat Diseases of the Dog and Cat. Boca Raton, FL: CRC Press, 2017, pp. 225–288.

Helton Rhodes KA, Werner A. Blackwell's Five Minute Veterinary Consult: Clinical Companion; Small Animal Dermatology, 2nd ed. Chichester: Wiley-Blackwell, 2011.

Author Clarissa P. Souza

Consulting Editor Alexander H. Werner Resnick

Acknowledgment The author and editors acknowledge the prior contribution of Karen Helton Rhodes.

Client Education Handout available online

N

NASAL DISCHARGE

BASICS

DEFINITION

May be serous, mucoid, mucopurulent, purulent, blood tinged, or frank blood (epistaxis); may contain food debris, from one or both nasal cavitiy(ies), may be permanent or in variable amount or consistency over time.

PATHOPHYSIOLOGY

• Secretions—produced by mucous cells of the epithelium and submucosal glands; increased production from glandular hypertrophy and hyperplasia owing to irritation of the nasal mucosa by infectious, mechanical, chemical, or inflammatory stimuli. • Blood from vascular leakage related to infectious, mechanical, chemical, inflammatory, or tumoral stimuli. • Xeromycteria—"dry nose"; facial nerve damage secondary to middle ear disease may decrease serous secretions from the lateral nasal glands leading to compensatory mucoid secretion; usually unilateral with unilateral nasal planum hyperkeratosis, ± keratoconjunctivitis sicca (KCS).

SYSTEMS AFFECTED

• Respiratory—mucosa of the upper tract, including the nasal cavities, sinuses, and nasopharynx; lower tract disease can also result in secretions from the upper airways. • Gastrointestinal—signs may be observed with swallowing disorders or esophageal or gastrointestinal diseases when secretions are forced into the nasopharynx. • Hemic/lymphatic/immune—blood-tinged discharge or epistaxis owing to platelet or hemostatic defects. • Ophthalmic—may have KCS ipsilaterally if there is nerve damage due to middle ear disease.

SIGNALMENT

• Dogs and cats. • Young animals—cleft palate; nasal polyp, ciliary dyskinesia; immunoglobulin deficiency. • Older animals—nasal tumors; primary dental disease (tooth root abscess). • Hunting dogs—foreign body. • Dolichocephalic dogs—aspergillosis, nasal neoplasia.

SIGNS

Historical Findings

• Sneezing—often found concurrently. • Reverse sneezing—can be found concurrently, if nasopharyngeal involvement or passage of nasal secretions through the choanae towards the nasopharynx. • Important to know both the initial and current character of the discharge as well as whether it originally started unilaterally or bilaterally. • Stertor—owners frequently report noisy breathing, especially when animal is sleeping. • Response to previous antibiotic therapy common due to secondary bacterial infection.

Physical Examination Findings

• Secretions or dried discharge on the hair of the muzzle or forelimbs. • May note reduction in nasal air flow, particularly with nasal neoplasia. • Concurrent dental, nasopharyngeal, or lower airway disease. • Bony involvement—with a tumor or fourth premolar abscess; may be detected as facial or hard palate swelling or as pain secondary to fungal or bacterial osteomyelitis or neoplasia. • Mucosal depigmentation of the nasal alar cartilage—observed with canine nasal aspergillosis. • Mandibular lymphadenomegaly—neoplasia, fungal infection, dental disease. • Polyp—may be visible on otoscopic exam, or pushing the soft palate down on oral exam. • Chorioretinitis—may be seen with canine distemper or cryptococcosis. • Eyeball deviation (abscess, sino-orbital aspergillosis in cats, tumors).

CAUSES

• Unilateral—often associated with non-systemic processes; foreign body; dental-related disease; fungal infections; nasal tumor; facial nerve damage leading to xeromycteria, nasopharyngeal stenosis, or atresia. • Bilateral—infectious agents (e.g., feline viral rhinotracheitis or calicivirus, canine herpesvirus, canine distemper, secondary bacterial infection); IgA deficiency; airborne irritant; allergy; ciliary dyskinesia; lymphoplasmacytic or hyperplastic rhinitis. • Unilateral progressing to bilateral—*Aspergillus*; nasal tumor. • Either unilateral or bilateral—epistaxis; foreign body; extranasal disease; nasal parasites, inflammatory rhinitis. • Extranasal diseases—chronic pneumonia, chronic vomiting, nasopharyngeal diseases.

RISK FACTORS

• Dental disease. • Foreign bodies. • Infectious—poorly vaccinated animal; kennel situations, exposure to other animals. • Nasal aspergillosis. • Thrombocyte disorder—thrombocytopenia or thrombocytopathy: primary immune or secondary to infectious (i.e., rickettsial) disease or neoplasia. • Coagulation defect due to rodenticide intoxication. • Nasal mites—kennel-raised dogs. • Immunosuppression, chronic corticosteroid use; feline leukemia virus (FeLV) or feline immunodeficiency virus (FIV) infection. • Chronic, low-grade pneumonia. • Chronic vomiting. • Chronic otitis (facial nerve damage).

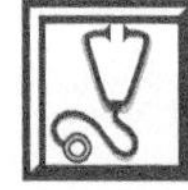

DIAGNOSIS

DIFFERENTIAL DIAGNOSIS

Important to differentiate nasal discharge, secretions, or crusting from diseases that occur at mucocutaneous junctions, such as pemphigus, vasculitis, or leishmaniosis.

Differential Diagnosis Causes

• Serous—mild irritation; viral and parasitic (e.g., nasal mites) disorders. • Mucoid—allergy; nonspecific airborne irritants; early neoplasia. • Purulent (or mucopurulent)—secondary bacterial or fungal infection, neoplasia. • Serosanguinous to epistaxis—nasal tumor and aspergillosis; after violent or paroxysmal sneezing episodes; coagulopathy, platelet disorder, angiostrongylosis and systemic hypertension.

CBC/BIOCHEMISTRY/URINALYSIS

Results not specific for any particular cause but can detect concurrent problems; part of a thorough evaluation before general anesthesia for diagnostic procedures.

OTHER LABORATORY TESTS

• Serologic tests—help to diagnose fungal or rickettsial disease. • Coagulation studies—determine platelet numbers and function, coagulation panel.

IMAGING

Skull Imaging

• Anesthetize and carefully position patient. • Perform before rhinoscopy and periodontal probing, which may cause nasal bleeding and alter imaging findings. • Radiography (not performed when CT is available): ○ Lateral view—detect any periosteal reaction; note gross changes in the maxillary teeth, nasal cavity, and frontal sinuses; evaluate air column outlining the nasopharynx for filling defects. ○ Open-mouth ventrodorsal and intraoral views (using sheet film)—excellent for evaluating nasal cavities and turbinates. ○ Rostrocaudal view—evaluate each frontal sinus (periosteal reaction and filling). • CT and MRI—CT superior to radiography in making diagnosis; CT and MRI help detect the extent of bony changes or CNS involvement associated with nasal tumors, fungal rhinitis, or chronic otitis.

Thoracic Radiography

May reveal areas of alveolar infiltrates in patient with chronic pneumonia, or situs inversus in some dogs with primary ciliary dyskinesia.

DIAGNOSTIC PROCEDURES

• Rhinoscopy—indicated with chronic or recurrent nasal discharge; acute epistaxis; evaluate both anterior and posterior; may be contraindicated with bleeding disorders. • Nasal cytologic examination—nonspecific inflammation most commonly found. • Fungal culture—difficult to interpret; false positives and negatives common. • Bacterial culture may be useful when resistant organisms are suspected, but requires deep nasal sampling under anesthesia. • Biopsy of the nasal cavity—indicated with chronic nasal discharge or visualized abnormalities; multiple samples required to ensure adequate representation; may perform electron microscopy for suspected ciliary dyskinesia. • Bronchoscopy—indicated if there has been a history of coughing with nasal discharge. • Periodontal probing of all upper teeth—perform after rhinoscopy; the normal gingival sulcus: dogs, ≤4 mm; cats, ≤1 mm. • Blood pressure, platelets, and coagulation profile for epistaxis. • Angiostrongylosis rapid detection test or PCR. • Schirmer tear test, otoscopic exam, or CT—to evaluate for possible facial nerve damage from chronic otitis. • Tracheal/bronchial scintigraphy and electron transmission microscopy—to confirm primary ciliary dyskinesia.

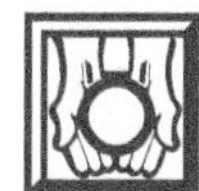

TREATMENT

• Outpatient—adequate hydration, nutrition, warmth, and hygiene (keeping nares clean)—important with chronic sneezing and nasal discharge. Prioritize local therapy (nasal drops, nasal nebulization). • Inpatient—any surgical treatment, topical therapy for aspergillosis.

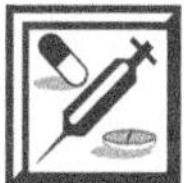

MEDICATIONS

DRUG(S) OF CHOICE

• Secondary bacterial infection—antibiotics; choose a good Gram-positive spectrum of activity (e.g., amoxicillin, clavamox, clindamycin, azithromycin, cephalosporins). • Attempt to dry up serous nasal secretions—decongestants (dogs: ephedrine at 10–50 mg total PO q8–12h, to a maximum of 4 mg/kg; cats: 2–4 mg/kg q8–12h); topical vasoconstrictors (neosynephrine at 0.25–0.5% q8–24h or oxymetazoline at 0.25% q24h) but for a limited period of time—less than 1 week—since they do not treat any cause and could induce damage to the nasal mucosa. • Dental-associated rhinitis—antibiotics; dental surgery as indicated. • Foreign body—removal, antibiotics. • Nasal parasites—ivermectin 300 µg/kg PO or SC weekly for 3 weeks or milbemycin 1 mg/kg PO weekly for 3 weeks (in collie and similar breeds) to treat *Pneumonyssoides*; fenbendazole 50 mg/kg PO q24h for 10 days to treat *Eucoleus* (nasal nematode). • Nonspecific inflammation—prednisolone 1–2 mg/kg PO q12–24h or piroxicam 0.3 mg/kg PO q24–48h. • Canine nasal aspergillosis—topical treatment with enilconazole or clotrimazole. • Feline cryptococcosis or sporothricosis—itraconazole 5–10 mg/kg PO q24h or fluconazole 50 mg/cat q12h. • Feline aspergillosis—topical therapy, itraconazole. • Canine angiostrongylosis—antiparasitic (e.g., fenbendazole 50 mg/kg PO q24h for 3 weeks), • Neoplasia—radiotherapy and chemotherapy. • Xeromycteria—oral administration of ophthalmic pilocarpine in attempt to stimulate nasal secretions.

CONTRAINDICATIONS

• Ephedrine—in cardiac patients.
• Ivermectin—in collies and similar breeds.

PRECAUTIONS

• Itraconazole—anorexia, nausea, vomiting, and high liver enzymes. • Rebound phenomenon—reported with overuse of topical nasal vasoconstrictors.

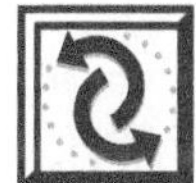

FOLLOW-UP

PATIENT MONITORING

• Nasal discharge and sneezing—note changes in frequency, volume, and character. • Repeat rhinoscopy—indicated to ensure adequate response to treatment of fungal rhinitis. • Recheck thoracic radiographs or bronchoscopy—monitor response to treatment for chronic pneumonia.

POSSIBLE COMPLICATIONS

• Loss of appetite—especially in cats. • Extension of primary disease (e.g., fungal infection, tumor) into the mouth, eye, or brain. • Respiratory distress—with nasal obstruction. • Involvement of the cribriform plate in dogs with aspergillosis—CNS damage during topical drug therapy is a risk.

MISCELLANEOUS

ASSOCIATED CONDITIONS

• Sinusitis. • Dental disease. • Secondary causes—coagulopathy, pneumonia, cricopharyngeal disease, megaesophagus.

AGE-RELATED FACTORS

Middle-aged to old patients—often associated with dental or neoplastic conditions.

ZOONOTIC POTENTIAL

N/A

PREGNANCY/FERTILITY/BREEDING

The safety of most recommended drugs has not been established in pregnant animals.

SEE ALSO

- Aspergillosis, Nasal.
- Cryptococcosis.
- Epistaxis.
- Nasal and Nasopharyngeal Polyps.
- Nasal tumor chapters.
- Nasopharyngeal Stenosis.
- Primary Ciliary Dyskinesia.
- Rhinitis and Sinusitis.

ABBREVIATIONS

- FeLV = feline leukemia virus.
- FIV = feline immunodeficiency virus.
- KCS = keratoconjunctivitis sicca.

Suggested Reading

Cohn LA. Canine nasal disease: An update. Vet Clin North Am Small Anim Pract 2020;50(2):359–374.

Lopez J. Sneezing and nasal discharge. In: Ettinger SJ, Feldmann EC, Cote E, eds., Textbook of Veterinary Internal Medicine, 8th ed. Philadelphia, PA: Elsevier, 2017, pp. 111–115.

Author Cécile Clercx

Consulting Editor Elizabeth Rozanski

Client Education Handout available online

NASOPHARYNGEAL STENOSIS

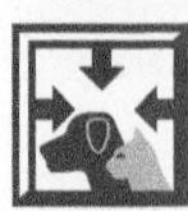

BASICS

OVERVIEW

- Formation of a thin soft tissue membrane or a fibrous band of tissue at the choanae or anywhere above the soft palate, resulting in the occlusion of the caudal nasopharyngeal openings or narrowing of the orifice from a 1+ cm oval opening to a 1- to 2-mm opening or less.
- Inflammation secondary to chronic rhinitis, or from regurgitation or vomiting of material into the nasopharynx, particularly after anesthesia, should be considered as possible causes. Might also occur secondary to lodging of a foreign body in the choana.
- Congenital narrowing or dysgenesis of the region can also be encountered; thickened palatopharyngeal muscles have been reported as a cause of nasopharyngeal stenosis in the dachshund.

SIGNALMENT

- Cats of any breed or sex.
- Less commonly seen in dogs.
- Age—any age as long as ample time has passed since exposure to the inciting cause; congenital cases may present early or late in life.

SIGNS

- Evidence of upper respiratory obstruction.
- Whistling, stridorous, or snoring sounds during respiration.
- Open-mouth breathing.
- Minimal nasal discharge in many cases.
- Duration of signs for at least several months.
- Aggravation of obstruction during eating or drinking.
- Failure to respond to antibiotics or corticosteroids.
- Absence of nasal airflow from one or both nares.

CAUSES & RISK FACTORS

- Chronic upper respiratory disease.
- Foreign body or irritant contacting the affected area (perianesthetic regurgitation, reflux of gastric contents secondary to esophageal or gastric disease).

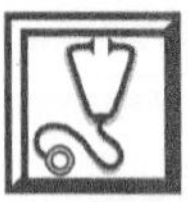

DIAGNOSIS

DIFFERENTIAL DIAGNOSIS

- Nasopharyngeal polyps—seen during oral examination or by radiography or endoscopy.
- Chronic rhinitis or sinusitis—moderate to severe nasal discharge and sneezing; obvious radiographic changes in the rostral nasal cavity commonly seen.
- Foreign body—unilateral mucopurulent nasal discharge; radiographic abnormalities.
- Intranasal neoplasia—unilateral obstruction; nasal discharge often bloody; radiographic changes.
- Mycotic rhinitis—moderate-to-severe nasal discharge, often hemorrhagic; radiographic changes.
- Laryngeal disease—no improvement with open-mouth breathing; lack of snoring or nasal discharge; abnormalities on laryngeal examination.

CBC/BIOCHEMISTRY/URINALYSIS

N/A

IMAGING

- Near-normal radiographic findings rostrally.
- Lateral neck radiograph will occasionally show a tissue obstruction.
- Nasopharyngeal stenosis sometimes can be visualized on CT. Sagittal reconstruction of the images can be required.

DIAGNOSTIC PROCEDURES

- Inability to pass a 3.5 French catheter through the ventral nasal meatus into the pharynx in a cat.
- Visualization of the stenosis by use of a retroflexed pediatric bronchoscope into the nasopharynx or use of an illuminated dental mirror.

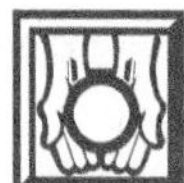

TREATMENT

- Balloon dilatation—noninvasive; fluoroscopy simplifies procedure; repeat episodes can be required (more often needed in the dog than cat).
- Stent placement can be required for cases with recurrent stenosis. Temporary red rubber stents have shown promise in reestablishing airway openings.

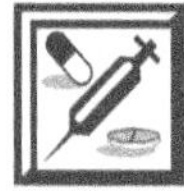

MEDICATIONS

DRUG(S) OF CHOICE

Antibiotics and steroids sometimes used post balloon dilation.

CONTRAINDICATIONS/POSSIBLE INTERACTIONS

N/A

FOLLOW-UP

Have owners evaluate nasal airflow at home and warn that recurrence is possible.

MISCELLANEOUS

Suggested Reading

Berent AC, Kinns J, Weisse C. Balloon dilatation of nasopharyngeal stenosis in a dog. J Am Vet Med Assoc 2006, 229:385–388.

Glaus TM, Gerber B, Tomsa K, Keiser M. Reproducible and long-lasting success of balloon dilation of nasopharyngeal stenosis in cats. Vet Rec 2005, 157:257–259.

Unterer S, Kirberger RM, Steenkamp G, et al. Stenotic nasopharyngeal dysgenesis in the dachshund: Seven cases (2002–2004). J Am Anim Hosp Assoc 2006, 42:290–297.

Author Lynelle R. Johnson

Consulting Editor Elizabeth Rozanski

NECK AND BACK PAIN

BASICS

DEFINITION

Discomfort along the vertebral column.

PATHOPHYSIOLOGY

Caused by multiple neurologic or non-neurologic diseases (e.g., polyarthritis). Secondary to stimulation of nociceptors located in meninges, nerve roots, spinal nerves, vertebrae and associated structures (e.g., periosteum, joint capsules), and epaxial musculature. An intra-cranial disease can develop referred neck pain when intracranial pressure is elevated.

SYSTEMS AFFECTED

• Nervous. • Musculoskeletal. • Neuromuscular.

SIGNALMENT

Species

Dog and cat.

Breed Predilections

• Intervertebral disc herniation (IVDH)—dogs; extrusion chondrodystrophic breeds, protrusion large breeds. Less common in cats. • Cervical spondylomyelopathy (CSM)—Doberman, Great Dane, Bernese mountain dog, Rottweiler, Dalmatian. • Atlantoaxial (AA) instability—small and miniature canine breeds (e.g., Yorkshire terrier, Chihuahua). • Steroid-responsive meningitis-arteritis (SRMA)—Bernese mountain dog, Boxer, Beagle. • Caudal occipital malformation syndrome and syringomyelia—cavalier King Charles spaniel. • Immune-mediated polymyositis—Newfoundland, boxer.

Mean Age and Range

• IVDH extrusion—unusual <2 years, peak 3–8 years. • IVDH protrusion—>5 years. • CSM—middle-aged to older Dobermans (mean: 6 years), young Great Danes (<3 years). • AA instability—young to middle-aged. • SRMA—<2 years (6–18 months). • Lumbosacral syndrome—middle-aged large dogs; German shepherd dogs.

SIGNS

Historical Findings

Primary complaint—relates to perceived discomfort; e.g., vocalization, decreased activity, reluctance to get up or lie down, reluctance to go up or down stairs, inability to drink or eat from bowls on the floor (neck), neck muscle spasms. Neck pain may be intermittent.

Physical Examination Findings

• Abnormal neck carriage, reluctance to move the head, stiff neck posture. • Arched back (kyphosis). • Pain on spinal palpation and/or neck manipulation. • Abdominal rigidity (referred from back pain). • Increased epaxial muscle tone. • Intermittent neck muscle spasms. • Reluctance to walk, stilted gait, limb stiffness, guarded short stride. • Non-weight-bearing lameness (nerve root signature). • Autonomic signs (e.g., tachycardia, pupillary dilation). • Neurologic deficits possible (e.g., paresis, ataxia). • Pyrexia (SRMA, infectious diseases).

CAUSES

Degenerative

• IVDH—most common cause of spinal pain in dogs. • CSM. • Spinal synovial cysts. • Vertebral facet hypertrophy. • Calcinosis circumscripta.

Anomalous/Developmental

• AA instability. • Caudal occipital malformation syndrome (COMS) and syringomyelia. • Vertebral malformations: e.g., hemivertebra (usually asymptomatic). • Osteochondromatosis. • Dermoid sinus.

Neoplastic

• Spinal (primary or secondary), nerve root–peripheral nerve (e.g., peripheral nerve sheath tumor), muscle. • Intracranial tumors with secondary increased intracranial pressure (ICP) (referred neck pain).

Nutritional

Feline hypervitaminosis A.

Inflammatory

• Discospondylitis, vertebral osteomyelitis, vertebral physitis. • Infectious meningitis/meningomyelitis—viral (e.g., feline infectious peritonitis [FIP]), bacterial, rickettsial, fungal, protozoal, parasitic, algae. • Noninfectious meningitis/meningomyelitis—SRMA, meningoencephalomyelitis of unknown origin (MUO). • Spinal epidural empyema. • Paraspinal abscess. • Polyarthritis—immune-mediated, infectious. • Polymyositis—immune-mediated polymyositis, infectious, exertional rhabdomyolysis.

Idiopathic

Subarachnoid diverticulum (rarely painful).

Traumatic

• Spinal fracture, luxation. • Traumatic intervertebral disc herniation.

Vascular

Spinal hemorrhage.

RISK FACTORS

• Breed—chondrodystrophic (IVDH), miniature dog (AA instability). • Trauma. • Previous surgical procedure (discospondylitis, subluxation). • Malignant neoplasm. • Bite wound, foreign body, urinary tract infection (UTI), endocarditis. • Coagulopathy. • Liver diet (hypervitaminosis A). • Feline leukemia virus (FeLV) infection (spinal lymphoma).

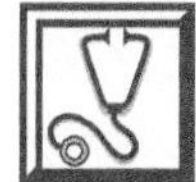

DIAGNOSIS

DIFFERENTIAL DIAGNOSIS

• Orthopedic disease. • Abdominal pain (back). • Behavioral or abnormal mentation (delirium). • Increased ICP (referred neck pain). • Nonpainful myelopathy—e.g., degenerative myelopathy, fibrocartilaginous embolic myelopathy. • Paroxysmal disorders. • Feline hyperesthesia syndrome.

CBC/BIOCHEMISTRY/URINALYSIS

• CBC usually normal. May see neutrophilia (SRMA, dyscospondylitis), thrombocytopenia (rickettsial disease, malignant neoplasm). • Elevated creatine kinase (CK), aspartate aminotransferase (AST)—myositis, recumbence, trauma, anorexia (cat). • Hyperproteinemia—neoplastic, infectious. • UTI— primary focus for discospondylitis, with urinary retention. • Myoglobinuria—myositis.

OTHER LABORATORY TESTS

• Serologic titers, PCRs (blood, CSF) for infectious diseases. • Blood/urine cultures—discospondylitis. • IgA and acute phase proteins levels (blood, CSF) in SRMA. • Serum protein electrophoresis. • Coagulation panel.

IMAGING

Survey Spinal Radiography

• Not able to identify spinal cord compression. • IVDH—may detect narrowed and/or mineralized intervertebral disc space. • Detects discospondylitis but potentially normal first 3 weeks. • Spinal neoplasms—osteolysis, bony proliferation, wider vertebral canal. • Detects fractures, luxations, AA instability, vertebral facet hypertrophy, malformations, calcinosis circumscripta, osteochondromatosis.

Thoracic Radiography and Ultrasonography

Detect neoplasms (primary or metastatic), disseminated infections, endocarditis, trauma-related lesions.

Myelography

Detects and delineates spinal cord lesions as extradural, intradural–extramedullary and intramedullary. Low sensitivity in detecting parenchymal lesions.

CT

• More sensitive than radiographs for discospondylitis, vertebral fractures, bone tumors. Clearly defines bony lesions but less soft tissue contrast than MRI. Can be useful to diagnose IVDH extrusion if mineralized material. • CT-myelogram—more sensitive to assess spinal cord compressive lesions.

MRI

More sensitive than CT for soft tissue. Most rewarding imaging technique for identifying location and extent of spinal cord parenchymal lesion, nerve roots, nerves, and muscle.

DIAGNOSTIC PROCEDURES

CSF

• Useful in meningitis/meningomyelitis, but normal or nonspecific in many other situations. Rarely, neoplastic cells can be detected (spinal lymphoma). • Consider measuring IgA levels, acute phase proteins, serologic titers, PCRs, bacterial culture.

Arthrocentesis and Synovial Fluid Analysis

Polyarthritis

NECK AND BACK PAIN (CONTINUED)

Electrodiagnostics

EMG, nerve conduction studies—detect and localize neuromuscular disease (e.g., polymyositis).

Fluoroscopy or CT-Guided Percutaneous Fine-Needle Aspiration (FNA)

Discospondylitis, neoplasms.

Biopsy

Bone (e.g., neoplasia, osteomyelitis), muscle (e.g., polymyositis).

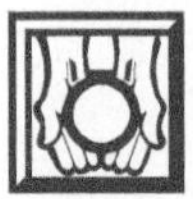

TREATMENT

APPROPRIATE HEALTH CARE

• Inpatient—when severe clinical signs; emergency intensive care due to severe pain or neurologic deficit. • Outpatient—when medical treatment is pursued (restricted exercise can be done). • Emergency surgery—if traumatic spinal instability or severe neurologic deficit (nonambulatory paraparesis, tetraplegia) due to an acute spinal cord compression.

N

NURSING CARE

• Nonambulatory patients—soft bedding, alternate recumbence site, urinary bladder voiding. • Vertebral instability—extreme care on manipulation to avoid exacerbating injury.

ACTIVITY

Restrict exercise at least 3–4 weeks in medically treated patients.

DIET

Change diet in case of hypervitaminosis A.

CLIENT EDUCATION

• Monitor pain, response to treatment and possible gait abnormalities. Relapses common in many diseases. • Most common cause of spinal pain in dogs is IVDH. Inform that restricted activity and cage confinement for 3–4 weeks are necessary when medical treatment is pursued; recurrence frequent. If pain persists or neurologic status deteriorates, surgical treatment is recommended, even as an emergency procedure.

SURGICAL CONSIDERATIONS

Vary according to disease. Generally, deep pain perception is considered the most important prognostic indicator for functional recovery in neurologic disease. AA instability correction is associated with high perioperative morbidity and mortality.

MEDICATIONS

DRUG(S) OF CHOICE

• Opioids—morphine 0.1–1.0 mg/kg q4h (dog), hydromorphone 0.05–0.2 mg/kg q4h (dog), buprenorphine 0.005–0.02 mg/kg q8h (dog); SR 0.03–0.06 mg/kg q72h (dog), fentanyl(transdermalpatch).• Glucocorticoids—Use of glucocorticoids in acute spinal cord trauma is controversial as no benefits in outcome are proven. Medical management of acute IVDH should focus on cage confinement. Prednisone 0.5–1 mg/kg q24h (dog) in decreasing dosage could be used in many noninfectious chronic and compressive conditions (IVDH protrusion, CSM, etc.) but never in combination with nonsteroidal anti-inflammatory drugs (NSAIDs). Higher doses required in immune-mediated disease (2–4 mg/kg q24h). • NSAIDs—potentially more effective in acute cervical IVDH. Meloxicam 0.1 mg/kg q24h (dog), carprofen 2.2 mg/kg q12h (dog). • Gabapentin 10–15 mg/kg q8h PO (dog); chronic neuropathic pain (syringomyelia, nerve root disease). • According to disease—antimicrobials (e.g., discospondylitis), immunosuppressive drugs, chemotherapy (neoplasms).

CONTRAINDICATIONS

• Glucocorticoids, immunosuppressive agents—infections. • Opioids—diarrhea caused by a toxic ingestion, constipation.

PRECAUTIONS

• Concurrent administration of NSAIDs and glucocorticoids is strongly contraindicated.
• Glucocorticoids, NSAIDs—may cause gastrointestinal ulceration/hemorrhage.
• Glucocorticoids—may cause UTI.
• Vertebral instability or IVDH—strict cage rest mandatory while on anti-inflammatory and analgesic drugs; increased activity can exacerbate the problem. • Opioids—caution if respiratory dysfunction, increased ICP, CNS depression, bradyarrhythmias.
• Gabapentin—caution if renal insufficiency.

POSSIBLE INTERACTIONS

• Opioids—increased CNS and respiratory depression when combined with other CNS depressants. • Gabapentin—oral antacids may decrease oral bioavailability 20%.

ALTERNATIVE DRUG(S)

• NMDA antagonists (e.g., ketamine)—analgesics. • Pregabalin—chronic neuropathic pain. • Furosemide, omeprazol—COMS/syringomyelia. • Azathioprine, cyclosporine, cytosine arabinoside—immune-mediated diseases.

FOLLOW-UP

PATIENT MONITORING

• Primarily based on clinical signs and response to treatment. Initially, monitor at least once a week. If acute severe pain and/or neurologic deficit present, inpatient or daily monitoring recommended. Make adjustments or consider surgery when medical treatment is not effective. • CSF analysis (e.g., SRMA), spinal radiographs (e.g., discospondylitis), acute phase proteins levels, bloodwork/thoracic radiographs/ultrasound (e.g., neoplasms, infectious diseases).

PREVENTION/AVOIDANCE

Avoid excessive activity, jumping, going up-/downstairs, and excess weight. Avoid neck collars (harness preferred).

POSSIBLE COMPLICATIONS

• Recurrences or deterioration. Surgical treatment can be recommended on an emergency basis according to disease.
• Chronic unresponsive pain. • Permanent neurologic dysfunction. • Spread to other locations, pathological vertebral fracture/luxation (discospondylitis, neoplasms).
• Degenerative joint disease (polyarthritis).

EXPECTED COURSE AND PROGNOSIS

• Varies with disease, severity of clinical signs, and neurologic deficit. • IVDH extrusion—success with medical treatment in dogs with only pain or mild deficits is about 50%.

MISCELLANEOUS

ASSOCIATED CONDITIONS

• Immune-mediated non-erosive polyarthritis and SRMA. • Discospondylitis and UTI.
• FeLV and feline spinal lymphoma.
• Polymyositis and lymphoma.
• Polymyopathies/myositis—megaesophagus/dysphagia and aspiration pneumonia.

ABBREVIATIONS

• AA = atlantoaxial. • AST = aspartate aminotransferase. • CK = creatine kinase.
• COMS = caudal occipital malformation syndrome. • CSM = cervical spondylomyelopathy (wobbler). • EMG = electromyography. • FeLV = feline leukemia virus. • FIP = feline infectious peritonitis.
• FNA = fine-needle aspiration. • GME = granulomatous meningoencephalomyelitis.
• ICP = intracranial pressure. • IVDH = intervertebral disc herniation. • MUO = meningoencephalomyelitis of unknown origin.
• NSAID = nonsteroidal anti-inflammatory drug. • SR = slow release (drug formulation).
• SRMA = steroid-responsive meningitis-arteritis. • UTI = urinary tract infection.

Suggested Reading

Dewey CW, da Costa RC. A Practical Guide to Canine and Feline Neurology, 3rd ed. Ames, IA: Wiley-Blackwell, 2016, pp. 329–436.

Platt S, Olby N. BSAVA Manual of Canine and Feline Neurology, 4th ed. Gloucester, UK: British Small Animal Veterinary Association, 2012.

Author Luis Gaitero

NECROTIZING ENCEPHALITIS

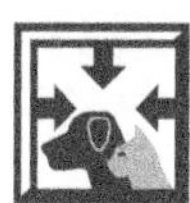

BASICS

OVERVIEW

• Historically restricted to a few breeds such as the pug, Yorkshire terrier, and Maltese dog. Described nowadays also in other breeds such as the Chihuahua, the shih tzu, and others. Even described in large-breed dogs. The disease includes necrotizing meningoencephalitis (NME) and necrotizing leukoencephalitis (NLE), since an overlap of clinical signs and histopathologic findings occurs.
• Systems affected—nervous.
• Genetics—a genetic basis (genetic risk loci) detected in pug dogs, Maltese dogs, and toy dog breeds; multifactorial disorder suspected.
• Incidence/prevalence—not determined but disease occurring regularly.
• Geographic distribution—occurs worldwide, mostly seen in toy breeds.

SIGNALMENT

Breed Predilections

Maltese, pugs, Yorkshire terriers, French bulldogs, Chihuahuas, shih tzus, Pekingese, and other toy breeds.

Mean Age and Range

Mostly young adult dogs (range 4 months–10 years).

Predominant Sex

No sex predilection.

SIGNS

Progressive signs related to a forebrain lesion (abnormal behavior, seizures, circling, blindness), brainstem lesions with central vestibular signs, or a multifocal lesion.

CAUSES & RISK FACTORS

• Genetic risk factors.
• An infectious agent might be suspected, but was never confirmed; multifactorial disorder, autoimmune disease.

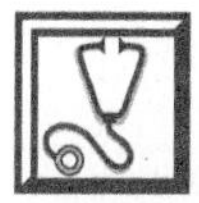

DIAGNOSIS

DIFFERENTIAL DIAGNOSIS

• Other CNS inflammatory/infectious diseases—differentiated on serology, CSF, MRI, and brain biopsy results.
• Neoplasia—differentiated on MRI findings and brain biopsy results.

CBC/BIOCHEMISTRY/URINALYSIS

Results are usually normal.

OTHER LABORATORY TESTS

Genetic test for predisposition.

IMAGING

MRI—results help support the clinical diagnosis considering breed, age, clinical signs, and course of the disease. Lesions may be asymmetric, multifocal prosencephalic with varying contrast enhancement, and can include multiple cystic areas of necrosis.

DIAGNOSTIC PROCEDURES

• CSF—pleocytosis with predominantly mononuclear cells; mild to marked protein elevation.
• Brain biopsy—to confirm diagnosis.

PATHOLOGIC FINDINGS

• Necrosis and nonsuppurative inflammation of the cerebral gray and white matter; multifocal lesions; active lesions consist of a large malacic gliotic center surrounded by a wall of severe mononuclear inflammation.
• Old lesions consist of rarefied or cystic areas surrounded by intense astroglial sclerosis.

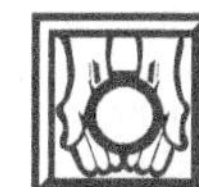

TREATMENT

• Inpatient or outpatient based on the neurologic status.
• Symptomatic treatment recommended.

Client Education

• Disease cannot be treated specifically; improvement with anti-inflammatory or immunosuppressive drugs.
• Seizures may be the only sign at onset of the disease in pug dogs; diagnostic workup including MRI in pug dogs presented with seizures is recommended.

MEDICATIONS

DRUG(S) OF CHOICE

• Symptomatic treatment.
• To control seizures, phenobarbital 2–6 mg/kg PO q12h.
• Corticosteroids can reduce the inflammatory response and improve clinical signs (e.g., prednisolone or prednisone 1–2 mg/kg PO q24h for the first 1–2 weeks; then the dosage can be tapered slowly); frequently used medication: cytosine arabinoside 50 mg/m^2 SQ q12h for 2-4 days, repeat about every 4 weeks (other dosage regimens possible); other immunosuppressive drugs are used successfully.

CONTRAINDICATIONS/POSSIBLE INTERACTIONS

N/A

Alternative Drug(s)

Procarbazine, azathioprine, cyclosporine, leflunomide, lomustine, mycophenolate mofetil.

FOLLOW-UP

PATIENT MONITORING

• Regular clinical and neurologic examinations to monitor response to symptomatic treatment.
• Monitoring of seizures and phenobarbital serum levels.

PREVENTION/AVOIDANCE

N/A

EXPECTED COURSE AND PROGNOSIS

• The course of the disease is chronic for months or even years; in every confirmed case, the neurologic signs have been progressive.
• Prognosis is guarded, survival with good quality of life in part of the cases.

N

MISCELLANEOUS

ASSOCIATED CONDITIONS

In one pug dog, myocardial necrosis was seen in addition to the encephalitic lesions.

ZOONOTIC POTENTIAL

N/A

PREGNANCY/FERTILITY/BREEDING

Three pugs described in Japan had a history of pregnancy before onset of clinical signs.

ABBREVIATIONS

• NLE = necrotizing leukoencephalitis.
• NME = necrotizing meningoencephalitis.

Suggested Reading

Flegel T. Breed-specific magnetic resonance imaging characteristics of necrotizing encephalitis in dogs. Front Vet Sci 2017, 864:203.

Hoon-Hanks LL, McGrath S, Tyler KL, et al. Metagenomic investigation of idiopathic meningoencephalomyelitis in dogs. J Vet Intern Med 2018, 32:324–330.

Schrauwen I, Barber RM, Schatzberg SJ, et al. Identification of novel genetic risk loci in Maltese dogs with necrotizing meningoencephalitis and evidence of a shared genetic risk across toy dog breeds. Plos ONE 2014, 9:e112755.

Author Andrea Tipold

NEONATAL MORTALITY AND CANINE HERPESVIRUS

BASICS

DEFINITION

• Death occurring between birth and 2–3 weeks of age. • Fading syndrome describes a clinical presentation rather than a specific etiology.

PATHOPHYSIOLOGY

• Four major factors lead to vulnerability of neonates—poorly developed thermoregulatory mechanisms; increased risk of dehydration (immature kidney function); increased risk of hypoglycemia (small reserve of glycogen); and immunologic immaturity (95% of antibodies from derived from colostrum). • Highly susceptible to environmental, infectious, nutritional, and metabolic factors.

SYSTEMS AFFECTED

N

All systems.

SIGNALMENT

• Puppies and kittens. • Pedigree puppies, kittens—more prone to congenital and hereditary defects, higher overall incidence of stillbirth and neonatal mortality.

SIGNS

General Comments

• Preweaning mortality —typically 10–30%; about 65% occur during first week; greater losses in a cattery or kennel should be considered abnormal. • Thorough history vital to identify potential causes; attention should be given to signalment, breeding history, vaccination, deworming history, exposure to toxins, problems during parturition, size of litter, feeding regimen, whelping environment, mothering abilities.

Historical Findings

• Low birth weight, loss of weight, failure to gain weight. • Decreased activity, appetite. • Weakness. • Poor suckling response. • Constantly vocal or restless early, quiet and inactive later. • Separation from dam and rest of litter. • Low Apgar scores at birth (see Neonatal Resuscitation and Early Neonatal Care).

Physical Examination Findings

• Nonspecific. • Dark red or bluish ventral abdominal skin indicates sepsis or cyanosis. • Red to purple toes, swollen red and/or purulent umbilical stump may indicate sepsis. • Gross anatomic defects—e.g., cleft palate, imperforate anus, pectus excavatum, asymmetry of limbs; abnormal haircoat over dorsum may indicate spina bifida. • Weakness, hypothermia (newborn temperature is 34.7–37.2°C [94.5–99°F], rising to 36.1–37.8°C [99–100°F] during first week of life); hypoglycemia and dehydration are common interrelated findings. • Respiratory distress, diarrhea, hemoglobinuria.

CAUSES

Infection, poor maternal management, low birthweight and congenital abnormalities most common.

Noninfectious

• Dam-related—dystocia or prolonged labor, cannibalism, lactation failure, trauma, inattention or overattention, inadequate nutrition (e.g., taurine deficiency in kittens). • Signalment—breed, older dam, larger litters associated with mortality rate. • Environmental—factors that discourage nursing and allow hypothermia including temperature or humidity extremes, inadequate sanitation, overcrowding, stress. • Nutritional—inadequate, ineffective nursing, hypoglycemia, hypothermia-induced digestive dysfunction. • Neonatal isoerythrolysis—queen with blood type B, kitten with blood type A.

Birth Defects

• Gross anatomic defects—more frequent in kittens than puppies. • Alimentary—cleft palate, segmental intestinal agenesis/atresia, imperforate anus, congenital megaesophagus, portosystemic shunt, mucopolysaccharide storage disease. • Cardiac defects—valvular dysplasia, ventricular septal defect, atrio-ventricular fistula, tetralogy of Fallot, patent ductus arteriosis, congenital rhythm disorders. • Respiratory defects—thoracic wall abnormalities, pectus excavatum, ciliary dyskinesia, surfactant deficiency. • Renal defects—agenesis, dysplasia, fanconi syndrome, polycystic kidney disease, ureteral abnormalities. • Endocrine—diabetes mellitus, hypothyroidism, hyposomatrotropism, central diabetes insipidus. • CNS—cerebellar hypoplasia and abiotrophy, hydrocephalus, spinal dysraphism, neuronopathies, lysosomal storage disease. • Hematologic—coagulopathies, von Willebrand disease, pyruvate kinase deficiency, hemolytic anemia, phosphofructokinase deficiency. • Immune system—thymus dysfunction, atrophy. • Miscellaneous—anasarca, skin or ocular defects.

Infectious

• Viral: ◦ Kittens—feline calicivirus; feline leukemia virus (FeLV); feline immunodeficiency virus (FIV); feline herpesvirus type 1, feline panleukopenia virus. ◦ Puppies—canine adenovirus type 1; canine distemper virus; canine herpesvirus-1 (CHV-1); canine parvovirus type 1 (minute virus) and type 2; canine influenza virus, canine coronavirus. • Bacterial—acquired mainly across placenta or via umbilicus but also through gastrointestinal tract, respiratory tract, urinary tract, skin wounds: ◦ *E. coli*, β-hemolytic *Streptococcus*, coagulase-positive *Staphylococcus*, *Salmonella* spp., *Campylobacter* spp., *Bordetella bronchiseptica*, *Pasteurella multocida*, *Brucella canis*, *Leptospirosis*. • Parasitic: ◦ Helminths—*Toxocara* spp., *Ancylostoma* spp. ◦ Protozoal—*Toxoplasma*, *Neospora*, *Cryptosporidium*, *Giardia*. ◦ Coccidia—*Isospora*.

RISK FACTORS

• Low birth weight, failure to gain weight; gain of 5–10% body weight per day acceptable: ◦ Kittens: minimum daily gain of 7–10 g. ◦ Puppies: should double in weight by 10–12 days. • Dystocia or prolonged labor. • Inbreeding—higher incidence of homozygous recessive genotype. • Blood type mismatch (cats). • Increased litter size, older dam, certain breeds. • CHV-1 is temperature sensitive; cold puppies more susceptible.

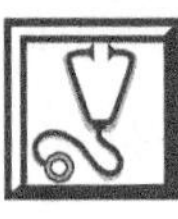

DIAGNOSIS

DIFFERENTIAL DIAGNOSIS

Excessive losses often due to combination of environmental, immunologic, nutritional, infectious, and metabolic factors; detection and correction of all necessary to prevent ongoing losses.

CBC/BIOCHEMISTRY/URINALYSIS

CBC

• Hydration status and age influence results. • Mild normocytic, normochromic anemia (normal packed cell volume at 1 week 33–52%, at 2 weeks 29–34%). • White blood cell concentration variable; thrombocytopenia and neutrophilia (with left shift) if septic.

Biochemistry

• Hypoglycemia. • Hypocholestrolemia, hypertriglyceridemia. • Low alkaline phosphatase activity, hypophosphatemia. • Low gamma-glutamyltransferase activity—indicates failure to receive colostrum. • Other changes depend on organ system.

Urinalysis

• Hemoglobinuria—with neonatal isoerythrolysis. • Bacteria—with infection. • Urine specific gravity >1.017 suggests inadequate hydration.

OTHER LABORATORY TESTS

• FeLV/FIV tests. • Serology—*Brucella canis*; CHV-1; canine influenza virus; *Toxoplasma*; *Neospora*; *Leptospirosis*.

IMAGING

• Abdominal ultrasound. • Thoracic and abdominal radiographs can show aspiration pneumonia, gastrointestinal obstruction, but difficult to obtain diagnostic films (low contrast).

DIAGNOSTIC PROCEDURES

• Histopathologic—tissues collected at necropsy. • Metabolic urine screening—rule out inborn errors of metabolism. • Virus isolation. • Bacterial culture. • PCR of placenta or fetal tissues—*Brucella canis*; CHV-1; *Toxoplasma*; *Neospora*; *Leptospirosis*.
• Blood typing in cats (dam and kitten).
• Fecal examination.

PATHOLOGIC FINDINGS

• Post-mortem—important; examine as soon after death as possible to minimize autolysis: ◦ Stomach—empty: lack of nursing; consider dam-related causes or neonatal problems; filled with milk: suggests sudden death or digestive dysfunction. ◦ Thymus small—not necessarily thymic dysfunction; atrophy can be a result of multiple causes (e.g., viral infection, stress, toxins, nutrition, defective immune system). ◦ Petechiation—common; suggests coagulopathy or septicemia. ◦ Urine in urinary bladder—implies renal dysfunction or inadequate care by dam. ◦ Lungs—homogeneous dark red color typical of a stillborn animal that has not taken a breath; hemorrhage, edema, congestion, mottled color abnormal but nonspecific. ◦ CHV-1—renal hemorrhage, multifocal areas of necrosis in lungs and liver are pathognomonic findings. • Note malformations. • Multiple tissue samples—submit to diagnostic laboratory; virus isolation, bacterial culture and sensitivity, PCR, histopathology; check with laboratory for proper submission.

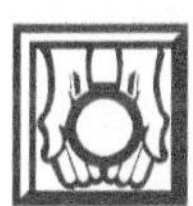

TREATMENT

• Correct deficiencies in husbandry or breeding selection. • Warmth—slowly warm neonate to 36–37.2°C (97–99°F) by 1°C per hour, if necessary; provide ambient temperature of 29–35°C (85–95°F) and relative humidity of 55%–65%. • Oxygen—supplement at 30–40%, if necessary. (Difficult to detect hypoxia as puppies and kittens do not always hyperventilate; clinical signs can include increased respiratory effort, bradycardia, hypotension, distended abdomen due to aerophagia.) • Fluid therapy—IV via jugular or cephalic vein; intraosseous in femur or humerus.
• Fluid requirements: 80–100 mL/kg/day, or 3-6 mL/kg/h using balanced isotonic replacement crystalloid; volume overload can occur due to immature kidney function
• Dextrose supplementation—0.5–1.0 g/kg IV/IO, given as a bolus, diluted to 5% dextrose in isotonic replacement crystalloid; then administered as CRI (2.5–5% dextrose in crystalloids) as needed. • Do not attempt to feed if body temperature <35°C (95°F) and no sucking reflex; once warmed, encourage nursing.
• Neonatal isoerythrolysis—prevent nursing for first 24 hours after birth; provide alternative colostrum, strip dam's colostrum before allowing kittens to nurse. • CHV-1—prevention is key; antiviral medication has not proven effective; CHV-1 vaccine available in Europe.

MEDICATIONS

DRUG(S) OF CHOICE

• Antibiotics—penicillins (penicillin G, ampicillin, amoxicillin, amoxicillin with clavulanic acid) and first-generation cephalosporins preferred; reduce adult dose by one-half and use same dosage interval.
• Supplement—milk replacer; serum or plasma can be provided (10–20 mL/kg PO, split in 2–4 feedings in first 24 hours of life) as colostrum supplement. • Vitamin K1 0.01–0.1 mg SC or IM, once.

CONTRAINDICATIONS

Aminoglycosides, tetracyclines, fluoroquinolones, trimethoprim/sulfonamide, chloramphenicol—avoid during neonatal period.

PRECAUTIONS

Drug absorption, distribution, metabolism, and excretion during first 5 weeks of life differs from adults.

POSSIBLE INTERACTIONS

N/A

ALTERNATIVE DRUG(S)

N/A

FOLLOW-UP

PATIENT MONITORING

• Hydration—monitor regularly (mucous membranes, urine specific gravity, nursing and urination). • Body weight—monitor daily or every other day. • Dam—monitor mothering abilities and milk production; supplement nutrition to neonates if required.

POSSIBLE COMPLICATIONS

N/A

MISCELLANEOUS

ZOONOTIC POTENTIAL

Some infectious agents have zoonotic potential (e.g., *Toxoplasma*, *Leptospira*, *Brucella*).

PREGNANCY/FERTILITY/BREEDING

Do not breed individuals with congenital defects.

SYNONYMS

• Fading puppy or kitten syndrome.
• Wasting syndrome.

ABBREVIATIONS

• CHV-1 = canine herpesvirus-1.
• FeLV = feline leukemia virus.
• FIV = feline immunodeficiency virus.

INTERNET RESOURCES

http://veterinarymedicine.dvm360.com/vetmed/article/articleDetail.jsp?id=197161

Suggested Reading:

Davidson AP. Canine herpesvirus infection. In: Sykes JE, ed., Canine and Feline Infectious Diseases. Philadelphia, PA: Saunders, 2014, pp. 166–169.

Lamm CG. Clinical approach to abortion, stillbirth and neonatal death in dogs and cats. Vet Clin North Am Small Anim Pract 2012, 42:501–513.

Tonneessen R, Sverdrup Borge K, et al. Canine perinatal mortality: a cohort study of 224 breeds. Theriogenology 2012, 77:1788–1801.

Wilborn RR. Small animal neonatal health. Vet Clin North Am Small Anim Pract 2018, 48:683–699.

Author Robyn Ellerbrock
Consulting Editor Amie Koenig
Acknowledgment The author and editors acknowledge the prior contribution of Hannah N. Pipe-Martin.

Client Education Handout available online

N

NEONATAL RESUSCITATION AND EARLY NEONATAL CARE

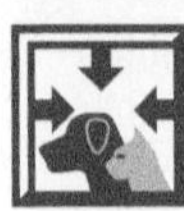

BASICS

DEFINITION

The neonatal period is defined as the first 3 weeks of extrauterine life. It is a delicate period where neonates are particularly susceptible to disease as well as congenital pathology. Neonatal organ systems including renal and hepatic function, gastrointestinal disease, and basic reflexes such as gagging, shivering, and thermoregulation are undeveloped or absent. Efforts to assist the neonate with cardiopulmonary function and consciousness during the immediate period following birth is referred to as neonatal resuscitation.

SIGNALMENT

Young puppies and kittens less than 3 weeks of age.

N

SIGNS

- Poor weight gain (<5–10% of body weight per day) is the earliest sign of failure to thrive.
- Hypothermia (normal body temperature for 1st week of life is 35–36°C [95–97°F]).
- Hypoglycemia.
- Hypovolemia (concentrated urine, dry or tacky mucous membranes).
- Bradycardia (normal 200–250 bpm at birth, 180–200 bpm until 2 weeks).
- Excessive crying.
- Weak or absent suckle reflex.

RISK FACTORS

- Dystocia.
- Prolonged stage 2 labor >5 hours.
- Decreased Apgar score within 8 hours of life (6 or lower on a 10-point scale; see Table 1).
- Low birth weight (less than 50% of average litter weight).
- Agalactia.
- Failure of passive transfer.
- Improper hygiene.
- Bacterial or viral infections.

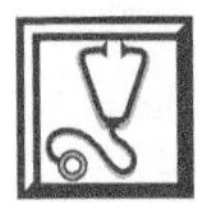

DIAGNOSIS

DIFFERENTIAL DIAGNOSIS

- Congenital defects.
- Bacterial sepsis.
- Failure of passive transfer.
- Viral infections.

CBC/BIOCHEMISTRY/URINALYSIS

- Alkaline phosphatase and gamma-glutamyltransferase enzyme activities—markedly elevated in neonates that have ingested colostrum.
- Urine—color is best indication of hydration status; should be nearly colorless in healthy neonate; brown color may indicate hemoglobinuria in kittens with neonatal isoerythrolysis.

OTHER LABORATORY TESTS

N/A

IMAGING

Thoracic radiography—helpful in diagnosis of aspiration pneumonia, a common cause of neonatal mortality.

PATHOLOGIC FINDINGS

- Congenital abnormalities such as cleft palate, atresia ani, omphalocele, anasarca, etc. may be noted at the time of birth. Many breeders will opt for euthanasia in these instances.
- Renal petechiation may indicate herpesvirus infection.
- On necropsy, clotted milk in the stomach often indicates intestinal ileus secondary to hypothermia. Only saliva in the stomach may indicate death secondary to starvation and failure of the bitch to produce milk.
- If possible, submit both deceased neonate and placenta for necropsy.

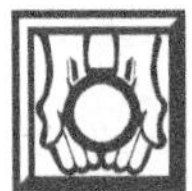

TREATMENT

- Vigorous external rubbing with a warm dry towel is sufficient for neonatal resuscitation at birth. Suction may be warranted to clear secretions from airway. "Swinging" neonates to clear airways is contraindicated and may result in cerebral hemorrhage.
- Cyanotic or pale mucous membranes at birth necessitate oxygen administration or mouth-to-mouth resuscitation.
- Bradycardia during the first 4 days is not vagally mediated and is indicative of hypoxemia.
- Warm slowly if body temperature is below 34.5°C (94°F). External heat sources are best, or warmed interosseous or IV fluids may be used.
- Do not feed unless body temperature is greater than 34.5°C (94°F) due to presence of intestinal ileus.
- Milk should be given in the form of commercially available milk replacer. Homemade formula and goat's milk are deficient in arginine and may result in cataract formation.
- Only feed neonates via a bottle if they are warm and have a strong suckle reflex. As neonates cannot gag during the first week of life, it is the author's preference that all neonates be fed via orogastric intubation until strong enough to nurse due to the risk of aspiration pneumonia. Droppers, cosmetic sponges, and syringe feeding are not recommended feeding methods due to excessive swallowing of air and high risk of aspiration.
- IV or intraosseous fluids are treatment of choice for hypovolemia. Neonates poorly absorb SQ fluids due to lack of fat. All fluids should be warmed before administration to avoid hypothermia.

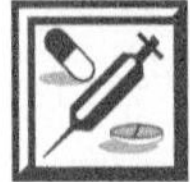

MEDICATIONS

DRUG(S) OF CHOICE

Neonatal Resuscitation Drugs

- Epinephrine 0.2 mg/kg IV, in umbilical vein or intraosseous route if cardiac arrest.
- Naloxone 0.1 mg/kg IM, only if opioids used during anesthesia of bitch.
- Doxapram—unlikely to be beneficial due to lack of efficacy in stimulating hypoxic neonates.

Antibiotics for Neonatal Sepsis

- Ceftiofur sodium (Naxcel) 2.5 mg/kg SQ q12h.
- Amoxicillin/clavulanic Acid (Clavamox) 13.75 mg/kg PO q12h.

Plasma or Serum for Failure of Passive Transfer

- Live donor can be used or commercially-available fresh frozen plasma at body temperature.
- For puppies: 22 mL/kg divided and administered SQ. Half dose can be administered PO if neonate is less than 12 hours old.
- For kittens: 15 mL per kitten, SQ, in 5 mL boluses given at birth, at 12 hours, and 24 hours of age.

Pain Control

- Opioids (fentanyl, buprenorphine) may be used with careful monitoring.

CONTRAINDICATIONS

- Fluoroquinolones may be used safely in neonates until 3 weeks of age. Afterwards there is a risk of cartilage defects with use.
- Tetracyclines (doxycycline), aminoglycocides (amikacin), and chloramphenicol should not be used unless absolutely necessary due to systemic effects.
- Metronidazole is contraindicated in patients younger than 2 weeks of age.
- Atropine is contraindicated during neonatal resuscitation due to exacerbation of myocardial hypoxemia.
- Nonsteroidal anti-inflammatory drugs should not be used in neonates due to potential for renal injury.

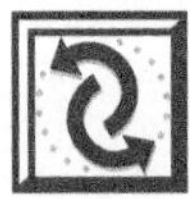

FOLLOW-UP

PATIENT MONITORING

Weight gain should be monitored daily at home using a scale capable of measuring

Table 1

Apgar scoring: each row is scored based on newborn activity and scores added together to obtain full Apgar score. A score of 7–10 indicates no distress, 4–6 indicates moderate distress, and 0–3 severe distress. Scoring should be performed at 5 minutes, 30 minutes, and 2 hours after birth.

	0	*1*	*2*	*Score:*
Mucous membrane color	Cyanotic	Pale	Pink	
Heart rate	<180 bpm	180–220 bpm	>220 bpm	
Respiratory effort/rate	No crying/<6 rpm	Mild crying/6–15 rpm	Crying/>15 rpm	
Reflex irritability	Absent	Feeble reaction (grimace)	Vigorous reaction (grimace/vocalization)	
Mobility, muscle tone	Flaccid	Some tone in extremities	Active movements	
Suckling (scored as –, +, ++)				
Rooting (scored as –, +, ++)				

Source: From Wilborn (2018). Reprinted with permission of Elsevier.

grams or ounces (kitchen scale). Failure to gain weight is the first clinical sign of a problem and should not be ignored.

PREVENTION/AVOIDANCE

- Neonates should be kept separate from other animals for the first 3 weeks postpartum to avoid disease transmission.
- Good environmental hygiene is imperative.
- Environmental temperatures should be kept warm yet comfortable (19.5–24°/67–75°F) and free of drafts in order to prevent the dam from leaving the whelping box. Increased temperatures of 27–32°C (80–90°F) are only required if puppies are orphaned.
- Ensure colostrum ingestion during the first 12 hours of life. If dam is not producing milk, or neonate is orphaned, serum or plasma should be given to provide immunoglobulins, but colostrum should be the first line of defense.
- Ensure the umbilicus is clamped and cleaned with a tincture of iodine solution immediately following birth to prevent ascending umbilical infections.
- Dam's mammary glands should be inspected daily for cleanliness and early signs of mastitis. Neonatal septicemia has been reported to occur secondary to bacterial exposure via the dam's milk.
- Probiotics can be given to minimize diarrhea associated with antibiotic use. Pastes and powders can be mixed into milk replacer or dabbed under the tongue to provide dosage without a risk of aspiration.

POSSIBLE COMPLICATIONS

Highest mortality rate occurs within the first 7 days of life (17–30% in dogs).

EXPECTED COURSE AND PROGNOSIS

- Depends on underlying cause—many "fading puppies/kittens" can be saved with early recognition and intervention.
- Bacterial sepsis and herpesvirus infections in puppies have fair to poor prognosis.

MISCELLANEOUS

Suggested Reading

Wilborn RR. Small animal neonatal health. Vet Clin North Am Small Anim Pract 2018, 48:683–699.

Authors Erin E. Runcan and Tessa Fiamengo
Consulting Editor Erin E. Runcan

N

NEONICOTINOID TOXICOSIS

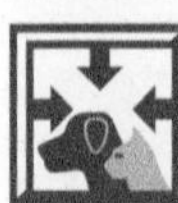

BASICS

OVERVIEW

• Neonicotinoids are a class of insecticides referred to as nitroguanidines, neonicotinyl, chloronicotines, and most recently as chloronicotinyls. Neonicotinoids are chemically similar to nicotine.
• Like nicotine, neonicotinoid insecticides act as agonists to nicotinic acetylcholine receptors.
• They act on insects at three different postsynaptic nicotinic receptors found in CNS.
• Wide safety margin in mammals due to high selectivity for specific subtypes of nicotinic receptors in insects.
• Compounds used in veterinary products include imidacloprid, nitenpyram and dinotefuran. Other common neonicotinoid products on the parket include acetamiprid, clothianidin, nithiazine, sulfoxaflor, and thiamethoxam.
• Widespread use in veterinary medicine for flea control. Used as oral tablets and in collars and topical spot on products.
• Used in termite and grub control and crop production against sucking and chewing pests in a variety of formulationsas well as ant and roach baits.

SIGNALMENT

• Primarily dogs—chewing up ant bait containers, collars, boxes of tablets, bags, liquid products.
• Rarely reported in cats.

SIGNS

• Imidacloprid has low toxicity in mammals. Results of a chronic feeding study revealed no adverse effects in dogs given imidacloprid at a dose of 15 mg/kg/day for a year. Topical application in dogs and cats at a dose of 50 mg/kg also caused no adverse effects.
• Most common adverse effects observed were decreased activity, tremors, mydriasis or miosis and uncoordinated gait; hypothermia was observed at higher doses.
• Alopecia and erythema have been reported following dermal application.
• Due to the large safety margin of safety margin in mammals, CNS signs are rarely seen.
• Oral toxicity is possible if the concentration or dose is excessively high.

CAUSES & RISK FACTORS

• Dietary indiscretion in dogs increases risk of exposure.
• Wide availability and frequent access to products.

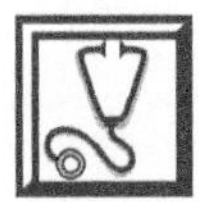

DIAGNOSIS

History of exposure and clinical signs.

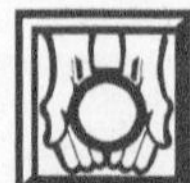

TREATMENT

• Dermal exposure—bathe with liquid dishwashing detergent.
• Oral exposure—dilute with cool water, emesis, gastric lavage, activated charcoal, depending on amount ingested, time of ingestion, and clinical signs.
• Baseline CBC, chemistry profile, and urinalysis to rule out any preexisting organ dysfunction, which could increase the risk for toxicosis.
• Antihistamines and/or dexamethasone SP for signs of dermal hypersensitivity.
• Methocarbamol for tremors.
• IV or SC fluids (crystalloid) as needed for dehydration.

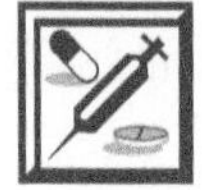

MEDICATIONS

• Dog emesis—apomorphine 0.04 mg/kg IV.
• Cat emesis—dexmedetomidine 7 mcg/kg IM or IV; or xylazine 0.44 mg/kg IM or SC. Avoid hydrogen peroxide due to risk for hemorrhagic gastroenteritis.
• Activated charcoal with a cathartic (sorbitol), 1 g/kg × one dose.
• Methocarbamol 50–220 mg/kg IV. Max daily dose 330 mg/kg/day (cats and dogs). Give 1/2 dose rapidly, wait until animal relaxes, and give remainder of dose to effect.
• Diphenhydramine (dog and cat): 2–4 mg/kg IM, PO q8–12 hours; 0.5–2 mg/kg IM, IV, SC.
• Dexamethasone sodium phosphate: 0.5 mg/kg IV (dog); 0.125–0.5 mg per cat IM or IV.

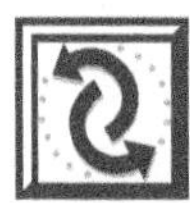

FOLLOW-UP

Patients usually recover with symptomatic and supportive care; no long-term organ damage is expected.

MISCELLANEOUS

ASSOCIATED CONDITIONS

N/A

AGE-RELATED FACTORS

• Puppies/young dogs are less discriminating and more likely to chew up product containers.
• Young and geriatric animals may have lower detoxification capabilities.

ZOONOTIC POTENTIAL

N/A

PREGNANCY/FERTILITY/BREEDING

Studies confirmed that imidacloprid is not mutagenic, non-embryotoxic, and nonteratogenic.

INTERNET RESOURCES

• Extension Toxicology Network, Imidacloprid, Cornell PMEP: http://pmep.cce.cornell.edu/profiles/extoxnet/haloxyfop-methylparathion/imidacloprid-ext.html
• National Pesticide Information Center, Imidacloprid fact sheet: http://npic.orst.edu/factsheets/imidagen.html
• Wismer T, Small Animal Toxicosis, Insecticides, VSPN: http://www.vspn.org/Library/misc/VSPN_M01289.htm

Suggested Reading

Dryden MW, Ectoparasiticides used in small animals. Neonicotinoids. In: Merck Veterinary Manual, revised 2015

Ensley SM. Neonicotinoids. In: Gupta RC, ed., Veterinary Toxicology Basic and Clinical Principles, 2nd ed. Waltham, MA: Elsevier, 2012, pp. 596–598.

Hovda LR, Hooser SB. Toxicology of new pesticides for use in dogs and cats. Vet Clinics of North America, Small Animal Practice 32:455–467, 2002.

Author Sharon L. Rippel
Consulting Editor Lynn R. Hovda

NEOSPOROSIS

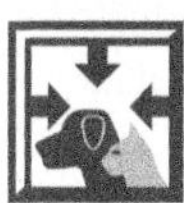

BASICS

OVERVIEW

- *Neospora caninum*—obligate, intracellular, coccidial, protozoan.
- Domestic and wild canids excrete infective oocysts in feces; numerous ruminant intermediate hosts.
- Transmission—vertical (transplacental or transmammary), ingestion of sporulated oocysts in dog feces, or ingestion of infected tissues from intermediate hosts.
- Disease caused by necrosis and inflammation from cyst rupture and tachyzoite invasion.
- Neurologic disease in dogs; other organ systems less commonly affected.

SIGNALMENT

- Dogs—puppies and adults.
- Cats—experimentally infected; antibodies in domestic and wild cats without known disease; *N. caninum* myocarditis reported in adult lion.

SIGNS

- Young dogs (4 weeks to 6 months of age)—ascending lower motor neuron paralysis, myositis, muscle atrophy, fibrous muscle contracture, and arthrogryposis; may progress to tetraparesis/plegia, trismus, dysphagia, hypoventilation; subclinical disease of other organ systems possible; less common: meningoencephalomyelitis, hepatitis, myocarditis, pneumonia, acute dyspnea, sudden death.
- Adult dogs—meningoencephalomyelitis and/or polymyositis; lesions can be found anywhere in CNS but have predilection for the cerebellum, resulting in slowly progressive cerebellar ataxia ± other cerebellovestibular signs; uncommonly affects other organs.
- Nodular dermatitis, particularly in immunosuppressed dogs.

CAUSES & RISK FACTORS

Raw meat may be a risk factor; should be avoided.

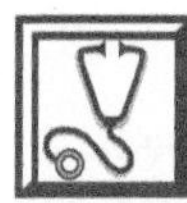

DIAGNOSIS

DIFFERENTIAL DIAGNOSIS

Other infectious disease (toxoplasmosis, sarcocystosis, hepatozoonosis, mycoses, rabies, canine distemper), neuronal storage diseases, noninfectious meningoencephalomyelitis or polymyositis, or immune-mediated neuromuscular disease, neoplasia.

CBC/BIOCHEMISTRY/URINALYSIS

- Dependent on the organ system involved.
- Muscle involvement—creatine phosphokinase and aspartate aminotransferase activities increased.

OTHER LABORATORY TESTS

- CSF analysis—normal to markedly increased total nucleated cell count; mononuclear pleocytosis more common than neutrophilic or eosinophilic; elevated total protein.
- Serologic testing (IFA, ELISA, and immunoprecipitation)—CSF or serum.
- Antibodies do not crossreact with *Toxoplasma gondii*, but do with *Neospora hughesi*, an equine protozoan.
- Organism detection—oocysts in feces; must distinguish from *Hammondia* spp.
- Tachyzoites in aspirates, smears, or biopsies need to be differentiated from those of *Toxoplasma* (immunohistochemistry).
- PCR—diagnostic tool, distinguishes between other parasites.

IMAGING

MRI of adult dogs—moderate to marked cerebellar atrophy with or without meningeal contrast enhancement; single or multifocal T2-weighted hyperintensities that contrast enhance within the CNS or muscles.

DIAGNOSTIC PROCEDURES

Muscle biopsy in dogs with myositis can identify organism by microscopy or PCR.

PATHOLOGIC FINDINGS

- Nonsuppurative encephalomyelitis.
- Severe nonsuppurative inflammation of cerebellar leptomeninges and cortex (more severe than that caused by *T. gondii*); cerebellar atrophy.
- Myositis, myofibrosis.
- Polyradiculoneuritis.
- Pneumonia, cerebellar atrophy, multifocal necrotizing myocarditis, and nodular dermatitis possible.
- Ulcerative and pyogranulomatous dermatitis.
- Histology—differentiate by location in host cell cytoplasm (*T. gondii* within a parasitophorous vacuole).
- Tissue cysts—those of *N. caninum* have thicker walls; differentiated from *T. gondii* by immunohistochemistry.
- Electron microscopy—rhoptries of *N. caninum* tachyzoites electron dense; those of *T. gondii* honeycomb.

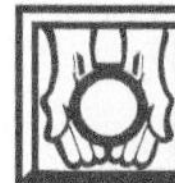

TREATMENT

- Long treatment period (min. 8 weeks); continue treatment 2 weeks beyond plateau of clinical improvement.
- Consider treatment of all puppies with infected littermates.
- Avoid immunosuppression if possible.

MEDICATIONS

DRUG(S) OF CHOICE

- Ideal treatment unknown; clindamycin most commonly used but bradyzoites persist despite treatment.
- Clindamycin 10–20 mg/kg PO q12h.
- Trimethoprim-sulfadiazine (TMS) 15 mg/kg PO q12h.
- Combination therapy—clindamycin and TMS, clindamycin and pyrimethamine (1 mg/kg PO q24h), or TMS and pyrimethamine.

CONTRAINDICATIONS/POSSIBLE INTERACTIONS

N/A

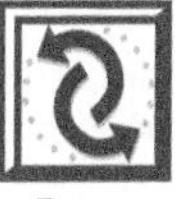

FOLLOW-UP

- Progression of clinical disease might cease with treatment.
- Once muscle contracture or ascending paralysis has occurred, prognosis for clinical improvement is poor.
- Serologically test dam or other in-contact dogs and cattle.

MISCELLANEOUS

ZOONOTIC POTENTIAL

N/A

SEE ALSO

Toxoplasmosis

ABBREVIATIONS

- TMS = trimethoprim-sulfadiazine.

Suggested Reading

Dubey JP, Lappin MR. Toxoplasmosis and neosporosis. In: Greene CE, ed., Infectious Diseases of the Dog and Cat, 4th ed. St. Louis, MO: Saunders Elsevier, 2012, pp. 806–827.

Silva RC, Machado GP. Canine neosporosis: perspectives on pathogenesis and management. Vet Med 2016, 7:59–70.

Author Renee Barber

Consulting Editor Amie Koenig

Acknowledgment The author and editors acknowledge the prior contribution of Stephen C. Barr.

NEPHROLITHIASIS

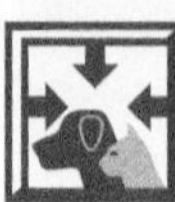

BASICS

DEFINITION

• Nephroliths—uroliths located in the renal pelvis or collecting diverticula of the kidney.
• Nephroliths or nephrolith fragments may pass into the ureters (ureteroliths).
• Nephroliths that are not infected, causing obstruction or clinical signs, or progressively enlarging are termed *incidental* nephroliths.

PATHOPHYSIOLOGY

Nephroliths can obstruct the renal pelvis or ureter, predispose to pyelonephritis, and lead to compressive injury of the renal parenchyma and chronic kidney disease (CKD); see urolithiasis chapters for pathophysiology.

SYSTEMS AFFECTED

• Renal/urologic—affects the urinary tract, with potential for obstruction, recurrent urinary tract infection (UTI), or progressive CKD.
• Obstruction of the renal pelvis or ureter with pyelonephritis may result in septicemia and affect any body system.

GENETICS

See specific chapter on type of stone.

INCIDENCE/PREVALENCE

• Nephroliths comprise 1–1.5% of uroliths submitted to the Minnesota Urolith Center for analysis. The true incidence of nephroliths is likely higher. Many animals with nephroliths are asymptomatic, or are not treated by methods that allow retrieval of uroliths for analysis.
• Composition of canine nephroliths submitted for analysis, in descending frequency: calcium oxalate, struvite, compound, purines, calcium phosphate, cystine, and silica. Composition of nephroliths in cats (descending frequency): calcium oxalate, dried solidified blood calculi, compound, struvite, calcium phosphate, and purine.

SIGNALMENT

Species

Dog and cat.

Breed Predilections

Dogs
• Calcium oxalate—shih tzu, Yorkshire terrier, bichon frise, miniature schnauzer, and Maltese.
• Struvite—miniature schnauzer, shih tzu, pug, and miniature poodle.
• Purine—English bulldog, Dalmatian, Yorkshire terrier, and shih tzu.
• Cystine—Newfoundland, English bulldog, and French bulldog.

Cats
Domestic shorthair, European and American shorthair, domestic longhair, Persian, Siamese and Scottish fold.

Mean Age and Range

• Dogs—mean age 10 years (range 2 months–21.5 years).
• Cats—mean age 7.7 years (range 5 months–19.5 years).

Predominant Sex

• Dogs—nephroliths slightly more common in females than males; struvite nephroliths, females > males; however, calcium oxalate, cystine, and urate nephroliths males > females.
• Cat— nephroliths slightly more common in females than males; for calcium oxalate females > males; however, noncrystalline matrix (includes dried blood), and urate nephroliths males > females.

SIGNS

General Comments

Many patients are asymptomatic, and the nephroliths are diagnosed during evaluation of other problems.

Historical Findings

• None or hematuria, vomiting, and recurrent UTI; dysuria and pollakiuria in animals with UTI or concomitant urocystoliths.
• Uremia in animals with bilateral obstruction or nonfunctional contralateral kidney.
• Signs referable to lower urinary tract urolithiasis if uroliths are present in the upper and lower urinary tract.
• Renal colic with acute abdominal/lumbar pain and vomiting is possible.

Physical Examination Findings

Abdominal or lumbar pain upon palpation of kidneys or no significant findings.

CAUSES

See chapters on each urolithiasis. Oversaturation of the urine with calculogenic minerals is a risk factor for urolithiasis.

RISK FACTORS

• Alkaluria—struvite and calcium phosphate uroliths.
• Aciduria—calcium oxalate, cystine, urate, and xanthine uroliths.
• Urine retention and formation of highly concentrated urine.
• Lower UTI—ascending infection and pyelonephritis.
• Conditions that predispose to UTI.

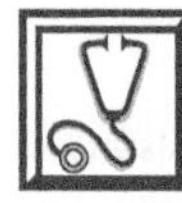

DIAGNOSIS

DIFFERENTIAL DIAGNOSIS

• Consider nephroliths in any patient with CKD, recurrent UTI, acute vomiting (pancreatitis, gastroenteritis, intestinal or gastric obstruction, etc.), or abdominal or lumbar pain (e.g., intervertebral disc protrusion, peritonitis).
• Nephroliths are usually confirmed by radiographs or ultrasonography; differentiate mineralization of the renal pelvis or collecting diverticula from true nephrolithiasis.

CBC/BIOCHEMISTRY/URINALYSIS

• CBC—usually normal; patients with pyelonephritis may have leukocytosis, immature neutrophilia, and thrombocytopenia.
• Serum biochemistry—usually normal unless bilateral obstruction, pyelonephritis, or compressive renal injury leads to acute kidney injury (AKI) or CKD; hypercalcemia may contribute to formation of calcium oxalate or calcium phosphate nephroliths.
• Urinalysis—may reveal hematuria and crystalluria; crystal type may suggest mineral composition; pyuria, proteinuria, and bacteriuria may also be seen with UTI.

OTHER LABORATORY TESTS

• Submit nephroliths or nephrolith fragments for quantitative analysis.
• Urine culture may confirm UTI or concurrent pyelonephritis.

IMAGING

• Can detect radiopaque nephroliths (e.g., calcium phosphate, calcium oxalate, struvite) by survey radiography; cystine and silica are slightly radiopaque.
• Purines (urate or xanthine) are often radiolucent or faintly radiopaque when large unless they contain other radiodense minerals.
• Use ultrasonography or contrast CT to confirm, size and number of nephroliths or ureteroliths.

DIAGNOSTIC PROCEDURES

After extracorporeal shock wave lithotripsy (ESWL), fragments can be retrieved for quantitative analysis by voiding, cystoscopic basket retrieval, or voiding urohydropropulsion.

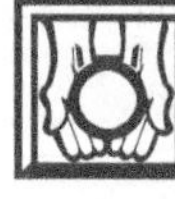

TREATMENT

APPROPRIATE HEALTH CARE

Manage patients with incidental nephroliths as outpatients. When appropriate, medical dissolution protocols can be administered to outpatients. Removal of nephroliths by surgery or ESWL requires hospitalization.

DIET

Medical dissolution of nephroliths requires a diet appropriate for the specific nephrolith type. See Medications.

CLIENT EDUCATION

- Incidental nephroliths—may not require removal but should be monitored periodically by urinalysis, urine culture, and radiography. Nephroliths may cause obstruction at any time, which can result in hydronephrosis without clinical signs. Conservative management and monitoring carries a risk of undetected and potentially irreversible renal damage, which must be weighed against the potential renal damage from nephrotomy.
- Nephroliths often recur after removal; monitor the patient every 3–6 months.

SURGICAL CONSIDERATIONS

- Indications for removal of canine nephroliths—obstruction, recurrent infection, progressive nephrolith enlargement, and a nonfunctional contralateral kidney. In cats, only obstructive uroliths in the renal pelvis or ureters are treated (see Ureterolithiasis).
- Treatment options for nephroliths—medical dissolution, surgery, and ESWL. Calcium oxalate is the most common nephrolith in dogs and cats, and is not amenable to medical dissolution. Medical dissolution of nephroliths causing outflow obstruction requires endoscopic or surgical placement of a ureteral stent.
- Surgical options—nephrotomy, percutaneous endoscopic nephrolithotomy, or surgically assisted endoscopic nephrolithotomy. Endoscopic nephrolithotomy may be preferred over ESWL for nephroliths >1.5 cm in diameter.
- ESWL—safe and effective method of treating canine nephroliths and ureteroliths; nephrolith fragments pass down the ureter into the bladder and are voided with urine or removed by voiding urohydropropulsion. Large (1–1.5 cm) nephroliths may be managed by endoscopic placement of ureteral stent to induce ureteral dilatation followed by ESWL 2–4 weeks later.
- ESWL is not effective for treatment of nephroureteroliths in cats.

MEDICATIONS

DRUG(S) OF CHOICE

- Antibiotics selected on the basis of urine culture and sensitivity testing as needed; periprocedural antibiotics are recommended when infected nephroliths are treated by ESWL or surgical removal.
- Medical dissolution protocols are limited to struvite, purine, and cystine uroliths.
- When feasible, consumption of water in high moisture (canned) foods should be incorporated into dissolution protocol. Target urine specific gravity <1.020 (dogs), <1.025 (cats).
- Medical dissolution protocols for canine struvite nephroliths include struvite-preventative or -dissolution diets and culture-guided antibiotic therapy for the duration of dissolution.
- Medical dissolution of canine purine nephroliths can be attempted by a purine-restricted diet, allopurinol 15 mg/kg PO q12h, and supplemental potassium citrate as needed to maintain urine pH ~7.0.
- Medical dissolution of canine cystine nephrolithiasis can be attempted using a therapeutic diet, 2-mercaptopropionylglycine (2-MPG, tiopronin) 15 mg/kg PO q12h, and supplemental potassium citrate as needed to maintain urine pH ~7.5.

CONTRAINDICATIONS

- Do not use allopurinol without dietary purine restriction; this combination may cause xanthine nephrolithiasis in dogs predisposed to urate urolithiasis.
- Do not give acidifying diets to azotemic patients unless blood pH and total CO_2 are monitored for development of metabolic acidosis.

FOLLOW-UP

PATIENT MONITORING

Abdominal radiographs or ultrasonography, urinalysis, and urine culture every 3–6 months to detect nephrolith recurrence. Dogs treated with ESWL—check every 2–4 weeks by radiographs and ultrasonography until nephrolith fragments have passed.

PREVENTION/AVOIDANCE

Eliminate factors predisposing to individual urolith type, augment urine volume, and correct factors contributing to urine retention. Dietary therapy is indicated for prevention of calcium oxalate, urate and cystine nephroliths. Castration of male dogs with cystine uroliths aids in prevention.

POSSIBLE COMPLICATIONS

Hydronephrosis, AKI, CKD, recurrent UTI, and pyelonephritis.

EXPECTED COURSE AND PROGNOSIS

- Highly variable; depends on nephrolith type, location, and size, secondary complications (e.g., obstruction, infection, CKD), and owner compliance with treatment and prevention protocol.
- Incidental nephroliths may remain inactive for years, resulting in an excellent prognosis.
- Return to normal health and good prognosis have been observed with ESWL for treatment of dogs with nephroliths.
- The prognosis for patients with CKD caused by nephrolithiasis depends on the severity and rate of progression of CKD.
- Nephroliths causing outflow obstruction should not be dissolved medically without placement of a ureteral stent.

MISCELLANEOUS

ASSOCIATED CONDITIONS

Hyperadrenocorticism and glucocorticoid administration are associated with calcium oxalate uroliths, and UTI resulting in struvite urolithiasis.

PREGNANCY/FERTILITY/BREEDING

ESWL is contraindicated in pregnant animals.

SYNONYMS

- Kidney stones.
- Nephroureteroliths
- Renal calculi.
- Renoliths.
- Kidney calculi.

SEE ALSO

- Chronic Kidney Disease.
- Hydronephrosis.
- Pyelonephritis.
- Ureterolithiasis.
- Urinary Tract Obstruction.
- Urolithiasis, specific types.

ABBREVIATIONS

- 2-MPG = 2-mercaptopropionylglycine.
- AKI = acute kidney injury.
- CKD = chronic kidney disease.
- ESWL = extracorporeal shock wave lithotripsy.
- UTI = urinary tract infection.

Suggested Reading

Adams LG, Goldman CK. Extracorporeal shock wave lithotripsy. In: Polzin DJ, Bartges JB, eds. Nephrology and Urology of Small Animals. Ames, IA: Blackwell Publishing, 2011, pp. 340–348.

Berent AC, Adams LG. Interventional management of complicated nephrolithiasis. In: Weisse CW, Berent AC, eds., Veterinary Imaging-Guided Interventions. Ames, IA: Wiley-Blackwell, 2015, pp. 289–300.

Author Larry G. Adams

Consulting Editor J.D. Foster

Acknowledgment The author and editors acknowledge the prior contributions of Carl A. Osborne, Jody P. Lulich, and Lori A. Koehler.

Client Education Handout available online

N

NEPHROTIC SYNDROME

BASICS

DEFINITION

Concurrent proteinuria, hypoalbuminemia, hypercholesterolemia, and third-space fluid accumulation (i.e., ascites, subcutaneous edema, etc.). Partial nephrotic syndrome refers to proteinuria, hypoalbuminemia, hypercholesterolemia without fluid accumulation.

PATHOPHYSIOLOGY

• Magnitude of hypoalbuminemia and proteinuria causing nephrotic syndrome in dogs and cats is unknown; although affected patients usually have very low serum albumin concentrations, not all hypoalbuminemic patients will develop nephrotic syndrome. • Reduced plasma oncotic pressure may result in hyperaldosteronism, which induces sodium and water retention, leading to edema and ascites. • Hypercholesterolemia is a consequence of decreased catabolism and increased hepatic synthesis of lipoproteins. • Complications include hypertension, hypercoagulability, muscle wasting, and weight loss. • Thromboembolism is a consequence of a generalized procoagulative state, due to increased platelet number and sensitivity, urinary loss of antithrombin, and increased concentrations of clotting factors.

SYSTEMS AFFECTED

• Renal/urologic—persistent proteinuria. With progressive disease and nephron loss, azotemia chronic kidney disease and uremia may occur. • Cardiovascular—edema, ascites, hypercholesterolemia/hyperlipidemia, hypertension, hypercoagulability, and thromboembolic disease.

GENETICS

Familial glomerular diseases have been reported (see Glomerulonephritis and Amyloidosis), but may be less likely to result in nephrotic syndrome than nonfamilial disease.

INCIDENCE/PREVALENCE

• Nephrotic syndrome is an uncommon complication of glomerular disease, with a median of 0.5 new cases per year diagnosed at 8 veterinary teaching hospitals. • Nephrotic syndrome has not been associated with histologic subtype of glomerular disease. Amyloidosis and immune-complex mediated glomerulonephritis have the highest magnitude of proteinuria and might be expected to have a higher prevalence of nephrotic syndrome.

SIGNALMENT

Species

Dog and cat.

Breed Predilections

None

Mean Age and Range

Dogs with nephrotic syndrome are typically younger than those with non-nephrotic glomerular disease (mean, 6.2 years vs. 8.4 years).

Predominant Sex

None

SIGNS

Historical Findings

• Pitting subcutaneous edema and/or ascites. • Clinical signs associated with an underlying infectious, inflammatory, or neoplastic disease may be the primary reason for seeking veterinary care. • Rarely, acute dyspnea, severe panting, weakness, or collapse due to pleural or pericardial effusion, pulmonary edema, or pulmonary thromboembolism.

Physical Examination Findings

• Dependent pitting, subcutaneous edema, or ascites. • Complications of hypertension: retinal hemorrhage or detachment, papilledema, arrhythmia and/or murmur secondary to left ventricular hypertrophy. • Dyspnea and/or cyanosis with pleural effusion or pulmonary thromboembolism.

CAUSES

• Glomerular disease may be a consequence of chronic inflammatory conditions (e.g., infection, neoplasia, or immune-mediated diseases). • Nephrotic syndrome is unlikely to be solely a consequence of severe proteinuria; additional unidentified factors appear to be necessary.

RISK FACTORS

See Causes.

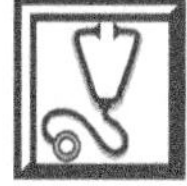

DIAGNOSIS

DIFFERENTIAL DIAGNOSIS

Proteinuria

• Rule out inflammatory or hemorrhagic postglomerular urinary tract disease (e.g., bacterial cystitis/pyelonephritis, urolithiasis, tubular renal failure, or lower urinary tract neoplasia). Inflammation of the urinary tract is usually associated with active urine sediment. • Protein-losing nephropathies typically associated with inactive urine sediment (although hyaline casts may be present); renal biopsy is the only accurate way to distinguish the various types of glomerular disease.

Hypoalbuminemia

Rule out decreased albumin production (severe liver disease) and gastrointestinal albumin loss (protein-losing enteropathy).

CBC/BIOCHEMISTRY/URINALYSIS

• Persistent, significant proteinuria with inactive urine sediment. • Hypoalbuminemia and hypercholesterolemia. • Renal failure may occur with advanced disease. Azotemia may precede loss of urine concentrating ability.

OTHER LABORATORY TESTS

Urine protein:creatinine ratio (UPC)—confirms and quantifies the severity of proteinuria and can be used to assess response to therapy or progression of disease.

IMAGING

• Radiography—loss of abdominal detail due to ascites, pleural effusion (uncommon), pulmonary edema, or pericardial effusion (very uncommon) may be present. • Abdominal ultrasonography—confirms peritoneal and retroperitoneal fluid. Mild renomegaly may be observed with glomerular diseases.

DIAGNOSTIC PROCEDURES

Renal biopsy is indicated if significant and persistent proteinuria with inactive urine sediment exists. Microscopic evaluation of renal tissue will establish subtype of glomerular disease and help in formulating a prognosis. Consider renal biopsy after CBC, serum biochemistry profile, urinalysis, UPC, and coagulation testing are completed.

PATHOLOGIC FINDINGS

Renal biopsy specimens should be evaluated by light, fluorescent, and electron microscopy by a pathologist with expertise in nephropathology. Some of the more common glomerular diseases include glomerulonephritis (e.g., immune-complex mediated, membranous, membranoproliferative, proliferative), minimal change disease, hereditary nephritis, amyloidosis, podocyopathy, focal segmental glomerulosclerosis, glomerulosclerosis.

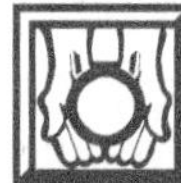

TREATMENT

APPROPRIATE HEALTH CARE

• Most can be treated as outpatient. • Severely azotemic or hypertensive patients, or those with thromboembolic disease may require hospitalization.

NURSING CARE

• Abdominocentesis—reserve for patients with respiratory distress or abdominal discomfort caused by ascites. Excessive fluid removal will promote fluid accumulation and electrolyte abnormalities. • Plasma transfusion is not indicated for treatment of hypoalbuminemia. Very large volumes of plasma are required to significantly increase serum albumin concentration, and transfused proteins have short half-lives. • IV albumin can be used in patients with life-threatening complications due to fluid accumulation (e.g., pulmonary edema; pleural effusion). • Hypotonic "maintenance"-type fluids (e.g., 0.45%

N

NaCl) as IV fluid therapy may minimize extravascular fluid accumulation. • Synthetic colloids may exacerbate fluid extravasation in patients with nephrotic syndrome. These fluids should therefore be limited to patients with immediate, life-threatening needs for oncotic pressure support.

ACTIVITY

Activity restriction may increase likelihood of thromboembolic disease; activity promotes fluid mobilization and lymphatic uptake.

DIET

• Sodium-reduced, high-quality, low-quantity protein diets are recommended, such as prescription "renal diets." • Normal or high dietary protein may contribute to renal disease progression by exacerbating glomerular hyperfiltration, proteinuria, and glomerulosclerosis. However, dogs that have persistent and severe hypoalbuminemia may benefit from amino acid supplementation.

CLIENT EDUCATION

• Identifying and correcting underlying disease may slow or stop the progression of kidney disease. • Renal biopsy is required to differentiate between the various subtypes of glomerular disease and to optimize treatment protocols. • Nephrotic syndrome is associated with shortened survival time. In one canine study, median survival time of nephrotic syndrome was 12.5 (range 0–2,783 days), vs. 104.5 (range 0–3,124 days) with non-nephrotic glomerular disease. Azotemia and uremia are associated with shorter survival.

SURGICAL CONSIDERATIONS

Animals with severe hypoalbuminemia (i.e., <2 g/dL) present unique challenges to anesthesia. Consideration should be given to referral of these patients to a secondary or tertiary care facility if anesthesia and/or surgery are indicated.

MEDICATIONS

DRUG(S) OF CHOICE

See Glomerulonephritis.

Edema and Ascites

• Dietary sodium reduction. • Reserve abdominocentesis and diuretics for patients with respiratory distress or abdominal discomfort. Overzealous diuretic use may result in dehydration and acute renal decompensation. • Severe, persistent extravascular fluid accumulation should be treated with an aldosterone antagonist (spironolactone 1–2 mg/kg PO q12h), and low doses of loop diuretics (i.e., furosemide 0.5–2 mg/kg PO q8–12h). • Plasma or albumin transfusions provide only temporary benefit.

Proteinuria

• Angiotensin receptor blocker (ARB) (e.g., telmisartan 1 mg/kg PO q24h) or an angiotensin-converting enzyme (ACE) inhibitor (e.g., enalapril 0.5 mg/kg PO q12h) decrease severity of proteinuria. Because proteinuria is toxic to renal tubules, therapy should be initiated at the time of diagnosis, unless severe azotemia is present. • Aspirin (1–5 mg/kg PO q24h) or clopidogrel (1.1 mg/kg PO q24h) decreases thromboembolism risk.

CONTRAINDICATIONS

Highly protein bound drugs may be contraindicated if their margin of safety is small.

PRECAUTIONS

• Dose adjustment may be needed for highly protein-bound drugs that have a wider margin of safety. • Use ACE inhibitors or ARBs cautiously in patients with serum creatinine >5.0 mg/dL. • Diuretics should be used cautiously in nephrotic syndrome because of the risk of causing or worsening azotemia.

POSSIBLE INTERACTIONS

See Precautions.

FOLLOW-UP

PATIENT MONITORING

UPC; serum urea nitrogen, creatinine, albumin, and electrolyte concentrations; blood pressure; and body weight. Nephrotic syndrome is a dynamic condition and affected animals may require frequent reevaluation to address new symptoms or evaluate changes in medications.

PREVENTION/AVOIDANCE

N/A

POSSIBLE COMPLICATIONS

• See Glomerulonephritis for complications unassociated with nephrotic syndrome.
• Complications more likely to develop include: thrombosis (e.g., pulmonary thromboembolism), electrolyte disturbances, particularly with repeated abdominocenteses or high doses of diuretics.

EXPECTED COURSE AND PROGNOSIS

Nephrotic syndrome is associated with a faster progression to azotemia and uremia, and decreased median survival time when compared to dogs that have glomerular disease without nephrotic syndrome.

MISCELLANEOUS

ASSOCIATED CONDITIONS

• Amyloidosis. • Glomerulonephritis.
• Glomerulopathy. • Hypercoagulability.
• Hypertension.

AGE-RELATED FACTORS

Familial glomerular diseases should be considered in young animals with nephrotic syndrome.

ZOONOTIC POTENTIAL

Glomerular diseases can occur with some zoonotic infectious diseases.

PREGNANCY/FERTILITY/BREEDING

Likely high risk in those patients with severe hypoalbuminemia and/or hypertension.

SYNONYMS

N/A

SEE ALSO

- Amyloidosis.
- Glomerulonephritis.
- Proteinuria.

ABBREVIATIONS

- ACE = angiotensin-converting enzyme.
- ARB = angiotensin receptor blocker.
- UPC = urine protein:creatinine ratio.

INTERNET RESOURCES

Atlas of Renal Lesions in Proteinuric Dogs: https://ohiostate.pressbooks.pub/vetrenalpathatlas/

Suggested Reading

Brown S, Elliot J, Francey T, et al. Consensus recommendations for standard therapy of glomerular disease in dogs. J Vet Intern Med 2013, 27(Suppl.1):S27–S43.

Klosterman ES, Moore GE, de Brito Galvao JF, et al. Comparison of signalment, clinicopathologic findings, histologic diagnosis, and prognosis in dogs with glomerular disease with or without nephrotic syndrome. J Vet Intern Med 2011, 25:206–214.

Author Shelly Vaden

Consulting Editor J.D. Foster

Acknowledgment The author and editors acknowledge the prior contribution of Barrak M. Pressler.

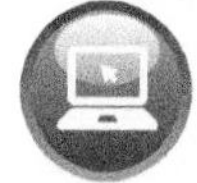

Client Education Handout available online

N

NEPHROTOXICITY, DRUG-INDUCED

BASICS

DEFINITION

Renal injury caused by a pharmacologic agent used to diagnose or treat a medical disorder.

PATHOPHYSIOLOGY

- Drugs can cause nephrotoxicosis by interfering with renal blood flow, glomerular function, tubular function, or inducing interstitial inflammation.
- Many drugs are nephrotoxic because they are excreted primarily by the kidneys.
- Most nephrotoxic drugs cause proximal renal tubular necrosis.
- If renal injury is severe, acute kidney injury develops.

SYSTEMS AFFECTED

N

- Renal/urologic.
- Gastrointestinal—inappetence, vomiting, diarrhea, or melena due to gastrointestinal irritation or uremic ulceration.
- Endocrine/metabolic—metabolic acidosis due to decreased elimination of acid by kidneys and inability to reclaim bicarbonate filtered into tubules by glomeruli.
- Hemic/lymphatic/immune—anemia due to blood loss or decreased red blood cell survival in patients with uremia; increased susceptibility to infections because of immune dysfunction in patients with uremia.
- Nervous—depression, lethargy associated with effect of uremic toxins on the CNS.
- Neuromuscular—weakness due to systemic effects of uremia.
- Respiratory—tachypnea or respiratory distress due to uremic pneumonitis or compensatory response for metabolic acidosis.

SIGNALMENT

Species

Dog and cat.

Breed Predilections

N/A

Mean Age and Range

Any age; older patients are more susceptible.

Predominant Sex

N/A

SIGNS

Historical Findings

- Polyuria and polydipsia; sometimes oliguria.
- Inappetence.
- Depression.
- Vomiting.
- Diarrhea.

Physical Examination Findings

- Dehydration.
- Oral ulcers.
- Uremic halitosis.

CAUSES

Antimicrobial Drugs

- Aminoglycosides—all drugs in this class are potentially nephrotoxic, including neomycin, gentamicin, amikacin, kanamycin, and streptomycin. Due to frequent use in the past, nephrotoxicosis associated with aminoglycoside treatment was most often associated with gentamicin.
- Tetracyclines—outdated products can cause acquired Fanconi-like syndrome characterized by glucosuria, proteinuria, and renal tubular acidosis; IV administration to dogs at high dosages (>30 mg/kg) can cause acute kidney injury.
- Administration of sulfa drugs (e.g., trimethoprim–sulfadiazine) has been associated with acute kidney injury in dogs, but no causal relationship has been proven.

Antifungal Drugs

Amphotericin B.

Antineoplastic Drugs

- Cisplatin—clinically important cause of nephrotoxicosis in dogs.
- Doxorubicin—possible cause of nephrotoxicosis in cats but not well documented.

Nonsteroidal Anti-inflammatory Drugs (NSAIDs)

- Aspirin, ibuprofen, naproxen, carprofen, piroxicam, meloxicam, flunixin meglumine, and others may cause nephrotoxicosis.
- Most likely to cause renal injury in patients with preexisting kidney disease or patients with concomitant dehydration or other causes of hypovolemia.

Angiotensin-Converting Enzyme (ACE) Inhibitors

- Enalapril, benazepril, and others.
- Most likely to cause acute kidney injury in patients with hyponatremia, dehydration, or congestive heart failure.

Radiographic Contrast Agents

IV administration of ionic radiographic contrast agents can cause acute kidney injury, especially in patients with dehydration, hypovolemia, or hypotension associated with inhalational anesthesia.

RISK FACTORS

- Dehydration.
- Advanced age, probably because older patients have preexisting kidney disease.
- Kidney disease, inactive or active.
- Renal hypoperfusion; potential causes include any disorder associated with hypovolemia (e.g., vomiting, hemorrhage, hypoadrenocorticism), low cardiac output (e.g., congestive heart failure, pericardial disease, cardiac arrhythmias, inhalational anesthesia), or renal vasoconstriction (e.g., NSAID administration).
- Electrolyte and acid–base abnormalities including hypokalemia, hyponatremia, hypocalcemia, hypomagnesemia, and metabolic acidosis.
- Concurrent drug therapy—administration of furosemide increases nephrotoxicosis of aminoglycosides; treatment with cytotoxic drugs (e.g., cyclophosphamide) may increase nephrotoxic potential of drugs.
- Fever.
- Sepsis.

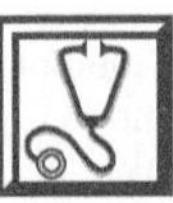

DIAGNOSIS

DIFFERENTIAL DIAGNOSIS

- Must differentiate from other causes of acute kidney injury (e.g., ethylene glycol toxicosis, raisin/grape ingestion [dogs], lily toxicosis [cats], renal ischemia, leptospirosis).
- Most patients have a history of recent treatment (i.e., within the previous 2 weeks) with a potentially nephrotoxic drug; acute kidney injury may occur several days after discontinuation of an aminoglycoside.
- Accidental ingestion of large doses of medications may occur, especially with palatable chewable formulations (prescribed for this patient or other animals).
- Determine all drugs that have been administered to the patient, including over-the-counter preparations (e.g., aspirin, ibuprofen, and naproxen) and medications prescribed for human use (e.g., NSAID or ACE inhibitor).

CBC/BIOCHEMISTRY/URINALYSIS

- Hemogram—usually normal unless concomitant problems exist (e.g., gastrointestinal hemorrhage associated with administration of NSAIDs).
- Biochemistry—normal in early stages of drug-induced nephrotoxicosis or reveals signs consistent with acute kidney injury including azotemia, hyperphosphatemia, and metabolic acidosis.
- Urinalysis—may reveal inadequately concentrated urinary specific gravity (often <1.025), proteinuria, glucosuria, or cylindruria. Casts may be one of the earliest indicators of acute kidney injury.

OTHER LABORATORY TESTS

N/A

IMAGING

N/A

DIAGNOSTIC PROCEDURES

Renal biopsy may be indicated to determine cause of acute kidney injury and potential for reversibility, especially in patients that do not favorably respond to treatment as expected. The magnitude of renal morphologic changes may appear mild compared to the magnitude of azotemia.

PATHOLOGIC FINDINGS

Most nephrotoxic drugs cause proximal renal tubular necrosis.

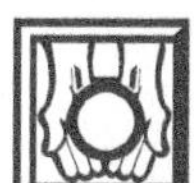

TREATMENT

APPROPRIATE HEALTH CARE

- Manage patients with acute kidney injury as inpatients.
- Manage patients without azotemia that can eat, and drink enough to maintain hydration, as outpatients.

NURSING CARE

- Administer balanced polyionic fluid (e.g., lactated Ringer's solution).
- Correct hydration deficits rapidly (i.e., over 6–8 hours) to minimize further renal injury. Calculate volume of fluid to administer as follows: volume (mL) = body weight (kg) ×% dehydration × 1,000 mL.
- In addition to correcting hydration deficits, administer maintenance requirements (~66 mL/kg/day) unless the patient is oliguric or anuric, and replace any ongoing losses caused by vomiting and diarrhea or polyuria.
- Extracorporeal therapies such as hemodialysis, charcoal hemoperfusion, or therapeutic plasma exchange may be indicated for certain drugs before toxicity has manifest.

ACTIVITY

Reduce

DIET

- Outpatients can be fed their regular food.
- Avoid oral feeding until vomiting is controlled, but initiate nutritional support as early as possible with acute kidney injury.
- If oral feeding is not possible initially, consider total or partial parenteral nutrition.
- The appropriate nutritional composition for patients with severe acute kidney injury has not been determined.
- Patients that recover from drug-induced nephrotoxicosis may develop chronic kidney disease, which should be managed by feeding a therapeutic renal diet indefinitely.

CLIENT EDUCATION

- Provide unlimited access to clean, fresh water at all times.
- If any signs of illness such as inappetence, vomiting, or diarrhea develop, return the patient immediately for veterinary care to minimize worsening of renal function.

SURGICAL CONSIDERATIONS

- Avoid elective surgery until kidney disease is resolved.
- If surgery is necessary, administer fluids (5–20 mL/kg/h) during anesthesia to maintain adequate mean arterial blood pressure (>60 mmHg) and renal perfusion. Monitor urine output and adjust rate of fluid administration to maintain urine production of 1–2 mL/kg/h.

MEDICATIONS

DRUG(S) OF CHOICE

None

CONTRAINDICATIONS

Do not use furosemide to promote diuresis in patients with aminoglycoside nephrotoxicosis.

PRECAUTIONS

- Avoid drugs that may worsen renal injury in patients with nephrotoxicosis, including NSAIDs, vasodilators, and ACE inhibitors.
- Use less toxic drugs when possible (e.g., carboplatin instead of cisplatin, other effective antimicrobials instead of aminoglycosides).

POSSIBLE INTERACTIONS

N/A

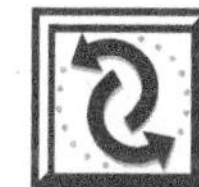

FOLLOW-UP

PATIENT MONITORING

- Weigh hospitalized patients several times daily to detect changes in fluid balance and adjust fluid therapy accordingly.
- Perform biochemical analysis, including electrolytes, every 1–2 days to evaluate severity of azotemia and to detect electrolyte and acid/base abnormalities.
- Patients receiving aminoglycosides—perform urinalysis every 1–2 days to detect early signs of nephrotoxicosis such as glucosuria, increased proteinuria, and cylindruria; discontinue aminoglycoside if any of these signs are observed.
- Measure urine output to determine if patient is polyuric or oliguric; adjust fluid therapy on the basis of these findings and determine need for additional treatment to stimulate urine production. Do not overhydrate patient with parenteral fluids.

PREVENTION/AVOIDANCE

- Avoid or correct risk factors that predispose to development of drug-induced nephrotoxicosis.
- Initiate saline diuresis to all dogs receiving cisplatin.
- Avoid using nephrotoxic drugs unless they are necessary (e.g., use aminoglycosides only if patient has overwhelming sepsis and culture results indicate aminoglycosides are the only effective antimicrobial).
- Monitor serum aminoglycoside concentration and perform frequent urinalyses while administering an aminoglycoside; cylindruria may precede changes to urine concentration.
- Do not administer furosemide with an aminoglycoside as this combination is likely to enhance nephrotoxicity of the aminoglycoside.

POSSIBLE COMPLICATIONS

- Acute kidney injury.
- Chronic kidney disease.

EXPECTED COURSE AND PROGNOSIS

- Patients without azotemia may develop acute kidney injury after several days of exposure, especially to aminoglycosides.
- Renal injury caused by nephrotoxic drugs may lead to development of chronic kidney disease months to years after recovery from drug-induced renal injury.

MISCELLANEOUS

ASSOCIATED CONDITIONS

N/A

AGE-RELATED FACTORS

N/A

PREGNANCY/FERTILITY/BREEDING

N/A

SEE ALSO

Acute Kidney Injury.

ABBREVIATIONS

- ACE = angiotensin-converting enzyme.
- NSAID = nonsteroidal anti-inflammatory drug.

Suggested Reading

Behrend EN, Grauer GF, Mani I, et al. Hospital-acquired acute renal failure in dogs: 29 cases (1983–1992). J Am Vet Med Assoc 1996, 208:537–541.

Cowgill L, Langston C. Acute kidney insufficiency. In: Bartges J, Polzin D, eds., Nephrology and Urology of Small Animals. Ames, IA: John Wiley & Sons, 2011, pp. 472–523.

Langston C. Acute uremia. In: Ettinger SJ, Feldman EC, eds., Textbook of Veterinary Internal Medicine, 7th ed. Philadelphia, PA: Elsevier, 2009, pp. 1969–1985.

Vaden SL, Levine J, Breitschewerdt EB. A retrospective case-control of acute renal failure in 99 dogs. J Vet Intern Med 1997, 11:58–64.

Author Cathy E. Langston

Consulting Editor J.D. Foster

Acknowledgment The author and editors acknowledge the prior contribution of Allyson C. Berent.

NERVE SHEATH TUMORS

BASICS

OVERVIEW

• Tumors of the peripheral nerves, spinal nerves, or nerve roots. • Malignant peripheral nerve sheath tumor is the recommended denomination for these tumors, instead of schwannoma, neurilemmoma, or neurofibroma, since determination of the cell of origin is often impossible. • Most tumors (80%) occur in the thoracic limb of dogs. • Approximately 50% of the tumors are located in the plexus or peripheral nerve region and 50% in the nerve root region.

SIGNALMENT

• Dogs—no breed or gender predisposition. • Mean age in dogs—7.9 years; uncommon in dogs younger than 3 years. • Rare in cats.

SIGNS

• Chronic progressive thoracic limb lameness. • Muscle atrophy (neurogenic atrophy) often present, more severe than that observed with orthopedic disorders. • Decreased muscle tone and decreased flexor reflex can be observed. • Axillary palpation detects a mass in less than 30% of cases. • Axillary pain upon palpation occasionally. • Horner's syndrome can be seen in tumors involving the T1–T3 nerve roots. • Ataxia, paresis, and asymmetric proprioceptive deficits can be seen if the tumor compresses the spinal cord. • Cutaneous trunci reflex may be poor to absent on the affected side. • In lumbosacral tumors, rectal palpation can be useful for mass detection. • Self-mutilation is occasionally observed.

CAUSES & RISK FACTORS

Mutation of the *neu* oncogene was identified in some cases.

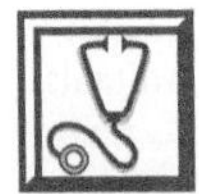

DIAGNOSIS

DIFFERENTIAL DIAGNOSIS

• Orthopedic conditions causing thoracic or pelvic limb lameness. Differentiate by orthopedic examination, radiographs, scintigraphy, CT, or MRI and response to rest and anti-inflammatory drugs. The severity of muscle atrophy also useful. • Lateralized nerve root compression by intervertebral disc disease, lumbosacral disease (cauda equina syndrome), or spinal neoplasia. Intervertebral disc disease and lumbosacral disease are usually associated with spinal pain. Advanced imaging (CT or MRI) is required to distinguish these diseases. • Secondary nerve neoplasia—lymphoma, histiocytic sarcoma, chondrosarcoma. Fine-needle or core biopsy needed to differentiate these conditions.

OTHER LABORATORY TESTS

• CSF analysis—nonspecific findings. • Cytology—ultrasound (US)-guided fine-needle biopsy can provide diagnostic sample. Cytologic features of malignant peripheral nerve sheath tumor (MPNST) are characteristics of a soft tissue sarcoma.

IMAGING

• Survey radiographs—well-positioned survey radiographs may allow visualization of an enlarged intervertebral foramen; most often unrewarding. • US—can identify a mass in cases where axillary palpation is unrewarding in distally located tumors. Patient sedation allows better positioning and US-guided fine-needle aspiration biopsy. Tumor echogenicity is variable. • Myelography—if the neoplasm has invaded the vertebral canal, an intradural extramedullary pattern can be seen. Due to the location of neoplasms, myelography is diagnostic in approximately 50% of dogs. • CT and MRI—to visualize proximal or distal limb tumors. Hyperintensity on T2-weighted images is the most common MRI pattern. MPNSTs usually show contrast enhancement on both CT and MRI. Due to the high soft tissue characterization, MRI is the diagnostic modality of choice.

DIAGNOSTIC PROCEDURES

• Electromyography (EMG)—to differentiate neurogenic from disuse muscle atrophy. Fibrillation potentials and positive sharp waves are suggestive of neurogenic muscle atrophy. EMG changes found in 96% of dogs with confirmed or suspected nerve sheath tumors. Epaxial muscle EMG changes predictive of vertebral canal invasion in cases of proximal tumors. • Nerve conduction velocity—conduction velocities may be prolonged with amplitude reduced. • F-wave, H-wave, cord dorsum potentials—evaluate the root portion of the nerve and can be useful to differentiate a lesion affecting predominantly the sensory or motor root.

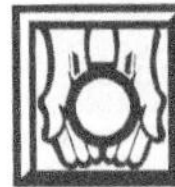

TREATMENT

• Surgical resection following the principles of oncologic surgery is the recommended treatment. • Local resection with clean margins was recently shown to yield very long survival times. • Amputation is also an option for large size tumors. • Hemilaminectomy or dorsal laminectomy may be required to allow resection of the nerve root region. • Oral corticosteroids may allow clinical improvement by reduction of peritumoral edema. • Radiation therapy—can be used for nonresectable tumors or in cases where surgery is contraindicated. It can also be used postoperatively to decrease the chance of local recurrence.

MEDICATIONS

DRUG(S) OF CHOICE

• Chemotherapy—metronomic therapy (cyclophosphamide 10 mg/m^2 and piroxicam 0.3 mg/kg) can be used for incompletely resected nerve sheath tumors in dogs. • Dexamethasone 0.1–0.25 mg/kg q24h or prednisone 0.5–1 mg/kg q12–24h can be used to provide short-term improvement. • Gabapentin 5–20 mg/kg q8–12h can be used for analgesia in cases of neuropathic pain. • Pregabalin 2–4 mg/kg q12h can be used in cases refractory to gabapentin.

FOLLOW-UP

• Nerve sheath tumors are locally invasive and rarely metastasize. • Postoperative local recurrence is common (up to 72% of cases).

MISCELLANEOUS

ABBREVIATIONS

• EMG = electromyography.
• MPNST = malignant peripheral nerve sheath tumor.
• US = ultrasonography.

Suggested Reading

da Costa RC, Parent JM, Dobson H, et al. Ultrasound-guided fine needle aspiration in the diagnosis of peripheral nerve sheath tumors in 4 dogs. Can Vet J 2008, 49:77–81.

Lacassagne K, Hearon K, Berg J, et al. Canine spinal meningiomas and nerve sheath tumours in 34 dogs (2008-2016): distribution and long-term outcome based upon histopathology and treatment modality. Vet Comp Oncol 2018, 16(3):344–351.

van Stee L, Boston S, Teske E, Meij B. Compartmental resection of peripheral nerve tumours with limb preservation in 16 dogs (1995–2011). Vet J 2017, 226:40–45.

Author Ronaldo Casimiro da Costa

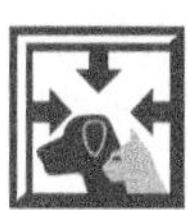

BASICS

OVERVIEW

- Inherited degenerative diseases of neurons in diverse regions of the CNS, particularly the cerebellum and associated pathways.
- Primary neuroaxonal dystrophy disorders are sometimes classified as abiotrophies.
- Inheritance—autosomal recessive in breeds where heritability is proven.
- The main pathologic feature of neuroaxonal dystrophy, axonal spheroids, also occurs in normal aging, as well as secondary to a number of other diseases, such as acquired or inherited metabolic diseases, and toxicities.

SIGNALMENT

- Dog and cat.
- Breeds predisposed—domestic and Siamese cats, Rottweilers, collies, papillons, Chihuahuas, German shepherd dogs, Jack Russell terriers, and boxers.
- Age at onset—breed-specific, ranging from under 2 months of age in cats, Chihuahuas, and papillons, to 1–2 years in Rottweilers.

SIGNS

- Cerebellar ataxia—progressive dysmetria and hypermetria of the limbs (rarely hypometria) with patellar hyperreflexia.
- Strength and proprioception normal in most cases. Rottweilers may have extensive involvement of the dorsal columns of the cervical spinal cord and may exhibit proprioceptive deficits.
- Loss of menace responses despite normal vision and facial nerves.
- Progressive signs of brainstem involvement may be a feature, especially in papillons, including loss of swallowing reflex and abnormal tongue movement; tetraplegia may develop in the final stages.
- Mild intention tremors or head and neck dysmetria in some patients.
- Primarily cerebellar signs in Rottweilers, collies, Chihuahuas, and domestic cats; predominantly spinal cord lesions in German shepherd dogs and boxers; tremors and cerebellar ataxia present in all affected animals.

CAUSES & RISK FACTORS

- Unknown.
- Usually classified as neuronal abiotrophy.
- Autosomal recessive inheritance proven in some breeds.
- Breed predisposition.

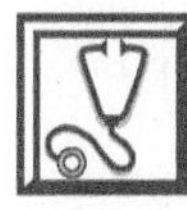

DIAGNOSIS

- Suspicion is based on clinical signs in a predisposed breed, usually in juvenile animals.
- Definitive diagnosis requires histopathologic examination of CNS tissue, usually post-mortem.

DIFFERENTIAL DIAGNOSIS

- Other congenital cerebellar anomalies, abiotrophies, and degenerative disorders. Reported occasionally in cats, and in a number of breeds of dog including border collie, Brittany, coton de Tulear, Gordon setter, Jack Russell (Parson Russell) terrier, Labrador retriever, Old English sheepdog, and many others.
- Other structural anomalies of the caudal brainstem, including caudal occipital malformation syndrome and Dandy–Walker syndrome. Differentiated by imaging studies, particularly MRI. Certain breeds are predisposed, e.g., caudal occipital malformation syndrome in the cavalier King Charles spaniel.
- Cerebellar hypoplasia caused by *in utero* infection of kittens with feline panleukopenia virus—apparent by 3–6 weeks of age; nonprogressive.
- Distemper encephalitis—differentiated on the basis of systemic signs preceding or accompanying the neurologic deficits and on results of CSF analysis (normal with neuro-axonal dystrophy).
- Other infectious encephalitides—fungal, rickettsial, and protozoal; differentiated on the basis of multisystemic signs in some patients, serologic testing, and CSF analysis.
- Noninfectious inflammatory encephalitides, particularly granulomatous meningoencephalomyelitis. Breed-specific encephalitides (pug, Maltese terrier, Yorkshire terrier) usually cause forebrain signs (seizures), but cerebellar involvement may occur. Differentiated by the presence of inflammatory changes in CSF and, in some cases, by contrast-enhancing lesions in the brain apparent with MRI.
- Neoplasia affecting the cerebellum—primary, metastatic, or locally invasive. Occurs in older dogs and cats, usually over 5 years of age. Differentiated on the basis of imaging studies (particularly MRI), CSF analysis in some cases, and systemic involvement in the case of metastatic neoplasia.
- Cervical spinal cord disease—proprioceptive deficits and tetraparesis.
- Diagnosis of neuraxonal dystrophy is by exclusion; it may not be possible to reach an antemortem diagnosis.

CBC/BIOCHEMISTRY/URINALYSIS

Normal

IMAGING

Atrophy of the cerebellum may be appreciable on MRI in certain patients (e.g., papillons).

PATHOLOGIC FINDINGS

- Axonal spheroids—present throughout the CNS gray or white matter, depending on the breed affected. Spheroids contain abnormal accumulations of intracellular proteins, particularly several associated with axonal transport and synaptic function.
- Myelin degeneration may occur secondary to axonal pathology.

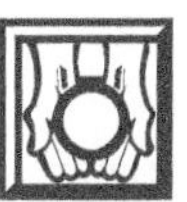

TREATMENT

- None available that alters the course of the disease.
- Activity—restrict activity to areas where a fall can be avoided (avoid stairs, swimming pools, etc.).

MEDICATIONS

DRUG(S) OF CHOICE

N/A

FOLLOW-UP

- Rottweilers—worsen over 1–5 years; develop clonic patellar and crossed extensor reflexes.
- Not fatal, but severely incapacitating.

MISCELLANEOUS

Suggested Reading

Diaz JV, Duque C, Geisel R. Neuroaxonal dystrophy in dogs: case report in 2 litters of papillon puppies. J Vet Intern Med 2007, 21:531–534.

Nibe K, Kita C, Morozumi M, et al. Clinicopathological features of canine neuroaxonal dystrophy and cerebellar cortical abiotrophy in papillon and papillon-related dogs. J Vet Med Sci 2007, 69:1047–1052.

Sanders SG, Bagley RS. Cerebellar diseases and tremor syndromes. In: Dewey CW, ed., A Practical Guide to Canine and Feline Neurology, 2nd ed. Ames, IA: Wiley-Blackwell, 2008, pp. 300–301.

Author Stephanie Kube

NEUTROPENIA

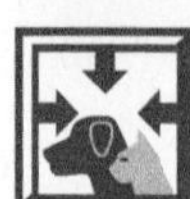

BASICS

DEFINITION

- Neutrophil count below the reference interval.
- Can occur alone or as a component of bi- or pancytopenia.
- Often accompanied by a left shift and toxic change (e.g., cytoplasmic basophilia, Döhle bodies, foamy cytoplasmic vacuolation, and/or toxic granulation).
- Certain breeds (e.g., greyhound, Belgian Tervuren) can have a neutrophil count below the reference interval for other breeds.

PATHOPHYSIOLOGY

Results from one of four mechanisms: (1) decreased production or release of neutrophils from the bone marrow, (2) a shift from the circulating pool within the large vessels to the marginating pool, (3) increased migration from blood into the tissues due to severe inflammation/tissue consumption, and (4) immune-mediated destruction.

SYSTEMS AFFECTED

Predisposes to infections, affecting many body systems in any combination, depending on the site(s) of infection.

GENETICS

- Cyclic hematopoiesis can result in intermittent neutropenia.
- A genetic trait with delayed penetrance results in age-related neutropenia in Belgian Tervuren dogs.
- Selective cobalamin malabsorption is an autosomal recessive trait in many breeds that results in neutropenia, including Imerslund–Gräsbeck syndrome in border collies.
- An autosomal recessive neutropenia (trapped neutrophil syndrome) in border collies from Australia and New Zealand is characterized by a deficiency of circulating segmented neutrophils and myeloid cell hyperplasia in the bone marrow.

SIGNALMENT

- Not specific for secondary infections.
- Schnauzers, beagles, Australian shepherd dogs, shar-peis, Komondorok, and border collies can have heritable cobalamin malabsorption.
- Grey collies and possibly border collies and Basset hounds may exhibit cyclic hematopoiesis.
- Aged Belgian Tervurens.
- Related border collies in Australia and New Zealand can have chronic neutropenia.
- Rottweiler dogs overrepresented for granulocyte colony-stimulating factor (G-CSF) deficiency.

SIGNS

- Septic animals usually have nonspecific signs. Fever is common, but normothermia does not exclude infection. Septic shock may be present.
- Grey collies with cyclic hematopoiesis exhibit severe neutropenia every 12–14 days. Episodes of fever, diarrhea, gingivitis, respiratory infection, lymphadenitis, and arthritis occur in association with the neutropenia.
- No clinical signs in Belgian Tervurens.

CAUSES

Deficient Neutrophil Production, Stem Cell Death, or Inhibition

- Infectious agents—parvovirus, bacteria-induced myelonecrosis, systemic mycosis (dogs and cats); feline leukemia virus (FeLV) and feline immunodeficiency virus (FIV) (cats); monocytic and granulocytic ehrlichiosis, babesiosis (dogs).
- Drugs, chemicals, and toxins—chemotherapy agents and cephalosporins (dogs and cats); T-2 mycotoxin ingestion, chloramphenicol and benzene-ring compounds, methimazole, and griseofulvin (cats); estrogen, phenylbutazone, trimethoprim–sulfadiazine, phenobarbital (dogs).
- Lack of trophic factors—inherited malabsorption of cobalamin/vitamin B12.
- Ionizing radiation.

Reduced Hematopoietic Space (Myelophthisis)

- Myelonecrosis.
- Myelofibrosis.
- Disseminated neoplasia, leukemia, or myelodysplastic syndrome.
- Disseminated infectious disease (e.g., histoplasmosis, cryptococcosis, leishmaniasis).

Cyclic Stem Cell Proliferation

- Inherited cyclic hematopoiesis.
- Cyclophosphamide treatment.
- Idiopathic disease.
- Immune-mediated suppression of granulopoiesis.

Neutrophil Migration

A shift in neutrophils from the circulating pool to the marginating pool can occur in patients with endotoxemia or anaphylaxis.

Reduced Survival

- Severe bacterial infection—sepsis, pneumonia, peritonitis, pyothorax, pyometra.
- Immune-mediated destruction.
- Drug-induced destruction.
- Hypersplenism (sequestration).
- Heat stroke.

RISK FACTORS

- Inherited disease—cyclic hematopoiesis, cobalamin malabsorption as noted earlier.
- Drug or toxin exposure.
- Infectious agents exposure (e.g., in kennels or catteries): *Ehrlichia canis*, parvovirus, *Bordetella bronchiseptica* (causing secondary pneumonia) (dogs); panleukopenia, FIV, and FeLV infection (cats).

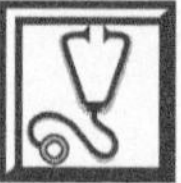

DIAGNOSIS

DIFFERENTIAL DIAGNOSIS

- Most neutropenias are due to nonbacterial infectious diseases (e.g., FeLV, FIV, systemic mycoses, parvoviruses).
- Acute bacterial infection with marked inflammation and/or endotoxemia.
- Direct cytotoxic effects of drugs or toxins on myeloid stem cells.
- Primary bone marrow disease.
- Immune-mediated destruction (diagnosis of exclusion).
- Inherited disease (more likely in younger animals unless adult-onset).

CBC/BIOCHEMISTRY/URINALYSIS

- Diagnosis is verified by CBC with blood smear evaluation.
- Serial CBCs may be necessary to confirm neutropenia or detect cyclic hematopoiesis.
- Urinalysis to identify urinary tract infection.

Factors That May Erroneously Alter Laboratory Results

- Inadequately mixed blood sample.
- Partial clotting of the specimen.
- Leukergy/leukocyte agglutination caused by antibody-related factors, leading to incorrect counting by automated machines. May rarely occur as a temperature-dependent phenomenon, resolved by warming the sample to 37°C (98.5°F).

OTHER LABORATORY TESTS

- Infectious disease screening—serologic or molecular testing for infectious organisms.
- Detection of antineutrophil antibodies by flow cytometry and observation of leuko-agglutination identifies immune-mediated neutropenia (IMN).
- Aerobic or anaerobic microbial culture of blood or areas of bacterial infection when indicated.

IMAGING

Survey radiography or ultrasonography may identify sites of infection or inflammation.

DIAGNOSTIC PROCEDURES/ PATHOLOGIC FINDINGS

- Bone marrow aspirate and core biopsy—to evaluate neutrophil precursors; a higher percentage of myeloblasts may be seen in animals rebounding from neutropenia, and should not be misdiagnosed as acute leukemia. Patients with IMN have myeloid hyperplasia with a left-shift, but hypoplasia can be seen if antibodies are precursor-directed.
- Cytologic examination of tissues—to verify neutrophil presence in body cavity effusions or tissues, confirm bacterial infections.

- Genetic testing or identification of abnormal urine metabolites may identify dogs with cobalamin malabsorption.

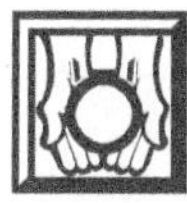

TREATMENT

APPROPRIATE HEALTH CARE

- Primary concern is the presence or development of infection.
- Nonfebrile patients—prophylactic broad-spectrum oral antibiotics that spare normal gastrointestinal flora are indicated.
- Febrile patients—suggests infection; inpatient treatment recommended for further diagnostic testing and therapy with IV broad-spectrum antibiotics and other therapies (e.g., IV fluids, surgery) as indicated.

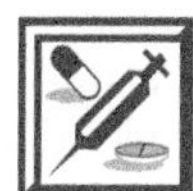

MEDICATIONS

DRUG(S) OF CHOICE

- Nonfebrile patients—cephalexin 30 mg/kg PO q12h or enrofloxacin 10 mg/kg PO q24h; cephalosporins or other classes of antimicrobials are contraindicated if thought to be the trigger for neutropenia.
- Febrile patients—ampicillin 22 mg/kg IV q6–8h or ampicillin + sulbactam 22–30 mg/kg IV q8h and enrofloxacin 10 mg/kg IV q24h (caution in cats) or cefotaxime 50 mg/kg IV q6–8h (dogs), 20–60 mg/kg IV q6–8h (cats).
- If clinically warranted, metronidazole 10 mg/kg IV q12h provides anerobic bacterial coverage.
- Recombinant human G-CSF (rhG-CSF) 5–10 µg/kg/day SC for 3–6 doses may stimulate short-term neutrophil production, but can result in production of neutralizing antibodies in 14–21 days, which may crossreact with endogenous G-CSF; ineffective in canine parvovirus.
- IMN—prednis(ol)one 1 mg/kg PO q12h, additional immunosuppression from either azathioprine 1–2 mg/kg PO q24h (dogs), 0.3 mg/kg PO q24h (cats), cyclosporine 3.3–6.7 mg/kg PO q24h, or mycophenolate 7–20 mg/kg PO q12h (dogs), 7–10 mg/kg PO (cats) may be necessary.

FOLLOW-UP

PATIENT MONITORING

- Neutropenia is likely to occur 7–10 days after administration of most chemotherapeutic drugs but may develop as late as 2–3 weeks following lomustine (CCNU) or carboplatin administration.
- Improvement is generally denoted by a rising leukocyte or neutrophil count, resolution of left shift, and disappearance of toxic changes on CBC analysis.
- Rebound neutrophilic leukocytosis is expected during recovery from neutropenia.
- The accelerated neutrophil production following rhG-CSF therapy can result in toxic-appearing and left-shifted neutrophils in circulation.

POSSIBLE COMPLICATIONS

Secondary infections.

MISCELLANEOUS

ASSOCIATED CONDITIONS

Viral or bacterial infection, sepsis, chemotherapy.

AGE-RELATED FACTORS

Middle-aged and older animals are less effective at repopulating the bone marrow with hematopoietic cells after an insult, due to age-related reduction in stem cell numbers.

PREGNANCY/FERTILITY/BREEDING

Pregnant Animals

- Drugs listed should be used only if the benefits supersede the inherent risks.
- Adequately controlled safety studies of rhG-CSF have not been performed in dogs and cats (including pregnant animals).

SEE ALSO

- Canine Parvovirus.
- Cobalamin deficiency.
- Cyclic Hematopoiesis.
- Ehrlichiosis and Anaplasmosis.
- Feline Immunodeficiency Virus (FIV) Infection.
- Feline Leukemia Virus (FeLV) Infection.
- Feline Panleukopenia.
- Sepsis and Bacteremia.

ABBREVIATIONS

- FeLV = feline leukemia virus.
- FIV = feline immunodeficiency virus.
- G-CSF = granulocyte colony-stimulating factor.
- IMN = immune-mediated neutropenia.
- rhG-CSF = recombinant human granulocyte colony-stimulating factor.

N

Suggested Reading

Devine L, Armstrong PJ, Whittemore JC, et al. Presumed primary immune-mediated neutropenia in 35 dogs: a retrospective study. J Small Anim Pract 2017, 58:307–313.

Schnelle AN, Barger AM. Neutropenia in dogs and cats: causes and consequences. Vet Clin North Am Small Anim Pract 2012, 42:111–122.

Thrall MA, Weiser G, Allison R, Campbell TW. Veterinary Hematology and Clinical Chemistry, 2nd ed. Ames, IA: John Wiley & Sons, 2012.

Vail DM. Supporting the veterinary cancer patient on chemotherapy: neutropenia and gastrointestinal toxicity. Top Companion Anim Med 2009, 24:122–129.

Authors Francisco O. Conrado and Jennifer L. Owen

Consulting Editor Melinda S. Camus

NOCARDIOSIS/ACTINOMYCOSIS—CUTANEOUS

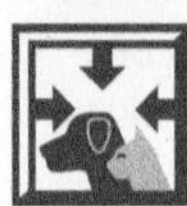

BASICS

OVERVIEW

Nocardiosis and actinomycosis are deep suppurative or pyogranulomatous cutaneous infections caused by bacteria of the genera *Nocardia* or *Actinomyces* and *Arcanobacteria* (respectively). Infection arises from direct inoculation of the organisms into the skin. *Nocardia* spp are ubiquitous soil and water saprophytes: Infection is usually a consequence of inoculation via scratch, bite or foreign body penetrating wound. *Actinomyces* and *Arcanobacteria* are normal inhabitants of the oropharynx and infection frequently follows a bite wound. Infection typically remains restricted to the skin, but dissemination to internal organs (lungs) can occur in both diseases.

N

SIGNALMENT

Dogs and cats with access to the outdoors are predisposed.

SIGNS

Cutaneous lesions in both infections consist of nodules, subcutaneous swellings or abscesses that often develop draining sinuses. Diffuse cellulitis with numerous draining tracts may occur. In actinomycosis, draining tracts discharge a thick yellow-gray or hemorrhagic exudate that may contain sulfur granules. In nocardiosis the discharge is less abundant. Lesions are typically located on areas of wounds as limbs, feet, thorax, or abdomen. Regional lymphadenopathy is common.

CAUSES & RISK FACTORS

Nocardia (most commonly *N. cyriacigeorgica*, *N. nova*, *N. abscessus*, *N. farcinica*, and *N. otitisdiscaviarum*) are Gram-positive, partially acid-fast, branching filamentous aerobic bacteria with worldwide distribution. *Actinomyces* (most commonly *A. bowdenii*, *A. canis*, *A. viscosus*, *A. odontolyticus*, A. *meyeri*, and *Arcanobacterium pyogenes*) are Gram-positive, non-acid fast, filamentous anaerobic rods that are opportunistic commensals of the oral cavity and bowel. Most *Actinomyces* infections are complicated by mixed infections with other bacteria.

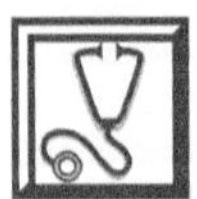

DIAGNOSIS

Diagnosis is by skin biopsy obtained for culture and histopathology. *Nocardia* is easily cultured under aerobic conditions. *Actinomyces* has fastidious growth requirements and may be slow-growing and/or difficult to grow. Species identification may require a specialized laboratory. Fine-needle aspiration for cytology and culture may also be useful.

DIFFERENTIAL DIAGNOSIS

Other systemic fungal infections, subcutaneous mycosis, panniculitis (sterile or due to mycobacterial infection), bacterial pseudomycetoma, and foreign body reactions.

CBC/BIOCHEMISTRY/URINALYSIS

Usually subtle. May vary according to the extent and duration of disease. Extensive, chronic, or disseminated disease may cause a mild to moderate nonregenerative anemia, leukocytosis, neutrophilia, and monocytosis. Hypercalcemia due to granulomatous disease can be present.

IMAGING

Thoracic radiography and abdominal ultrasound are recommended to assess for dissemination of infection.

PATHOLOGIC FINDINGS

Histopathologic lesions consist of granulomatous to pyogranulomatous dermatitis and panniculitis accompanied by extensive fibrosis. Special stains are used to identify microorganisms in tissues. Granules of actinomycosis are basophilic with an eosinophilic periphery (Splendore–Hoepli phenomenon).

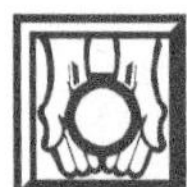

TREATMENT

Surgical drainage of abscesses or surgical debridement followed by long-term antibiotic administration is recommended. Treatment must be continued at least 1 month after clinical cure.

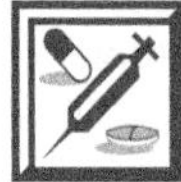

MEDICATIONS

Nocardiosis

Sulfonamides (trimethoprim-sulfonamide 30 mg/kg q12h). Clinical improvement should be observed within 2 weeks. Susceptibility testing is strongly recommended in cases that fail to respond to empirical treatment or in cases of relapse. Treatment success with alternative antibiotics, including amikacin, cephalosporins, clarithromycin, and doxycycline, has been reported.

Actinomycosis

High-dose penicillin (penicillin G 40 mg/kg q8h). Strains of *Actimomyces* spp. have not shown resistance to penicillin. For animals not tolerating penicillin, alternative antibiotics include clindamycin, erythromycin, and doxycycline.

CONTRAINDICATIONS

Caution advised with use of sulfonamides in Doberman pinschers.

FOLLOW-UP

Prolonged treatment with monitoring is required. Prognosis is guarded, although most immunocompetent animals with only cutaneous infection and properly treated are usually cured.

MISCELLANEOUS

ZOONOTIC POTENTIAL

No cases of human of actinomycosis or nocardiosis acquired from direct contact with a dog or cat with clinical disease have been reported. Rare cases of cutaneous actinomycosis or nocardiosis in humans as a consequence of a scratch or bite from a cat or dog have been reported. Pet owners, veterinarians, and nurses should wear protective gloves when handling infected dogs and cats to avoid inadvertent infection through damaged skin.

Suggested Reading

Sykes JE. Actinomycosis and nocardiosis. In: Greene CG, ed., Infectious Diseases of the Dog and Cat, 4th ed. St. Louis, MO: Elsevier, 2012, pp. 484–495.

Author Lluís Ferrer

Consulting Editor Alexander H. Werner Resnick

NONSTEROIDAL ANTI-INFLAMMATORY DRUG TOXICOSIS

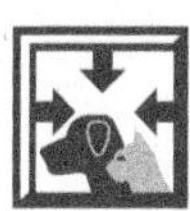

BASICS

DEFINITION

• Toxicosis secondary to the acute or chronic ingestion of a nonsteroidal anti-inflammatory drug (NSAID). • NSAIDs—classed as carboxylic acids (aspirin, indomethacin, sulindac, ibuprofen, naproxen, carprofen, meclofenamic acid, etodolac, flunixin meglumine) or enolic acids (phenylbutazone, dipyrone, meloxicam, tepoxalin, and piroxicam); selective cyclooxygenase-2 (COX-2) inhibitors (deracoxib, firocoxib, mavacoxib (Europe), and robenacoxib).
• Newer selective COX-2 inhibitors and NSAIDs with preferential activity against COX-2 may have fewer adverse reactions than older COX-1 inhibitors, though both pathways may be inhibited following overdose.

PATHOPHYSIOLOGY

• Action—analgesic, antipyretic, and anti-inflammatory due to the inhibition of cyclooxygenase; decreases production of prostaglandins that act as mediators of inflammation. • Well absorbed orally.
• Clearance—varies greatly among species; eliminated slowly in dogs and cats; half-life varies significantly among NSAIDs.
• Metabolized in the liver to active or inactive metabolites. • Excreted in the kidney via glomerular filtration and tubular secretion, and/or biliary excretion.

SYSTEMS AFFECTED

• Gastrointestinal (GI)—irritation, erosions, and ulcerations. • Renal/urologic—acute kidney injury; acute interstitial nephritis.
• Hepatobiliary—idiosyncratic hepatocellular damage. • Hemic/lymphatic/immune—bleeding disorders from decreased platelet aggregation.
• Nervous – ataxia, seizures, CNS depression, and coma may occur with very large doses.

GENETICS

• Very large species differences in absorption, excretion, and metabolism of different agents; avoid extrapolation of data from other species or dosages. • Off-label use of NSAIDs can result in significant, potentially life-threatening adverse effects in all species, especially cats. • Over-the-counter NSAIDs (especially ibuprofen and naproxen) are common causes of NSAID toxicosis in dogs and cats. Naproxen has an extremely long half-life in domestic animals and exposures carry a high risk of significant adverse effects.

INCIDENCE/PREVALENCE

Among the 10 most common toxicoses reported to both the Pet Poison Helpline (PPH) and the American Society for the Prevention of Cruelty to Animals (ASPCA) Animal Poison Control Center (APCC).

GEOGRAPHIC DISTRIBUTION

N/A

SIGNALMENT

• Dogs and cats. • Cats are more sensitive.
• No breed or gender predilections.

SIGNS

General Comments

• GI irritation—within a few hours. • Renal involvement or GI ulceration—may be delayed several days.

Historical Findings

• Evidence of accidental consumption of medication or reported administration of an NSAID (either prescribed or unprescribed).
• Lethargy. • Anorexia. • Vomiting—with or without blood. • Diarrhea. • Icterus.
• Melena. • Polyuria, polydipsia, and oliguria.
• Ataxia, seizures, coma—may occur with large ingestions. • Collapse and sudden death—may occur from a perforated gastric ulcer.

Physical Examination Findings

• Depression. • Pale mucous membranes.
• Painful abdomen. • Dehydration. • Fever.
• Tachycardia. • Icterus.

CAUSES

Accidental exposure or inappropriate administration.

Toxic Doses for Common NSAIDs

• Carprofen: ○ Dogs: 20 mg/kg—GI ulceration; 40 mg/kg—renal injury. ○ Cats: 4 mg/kg—GI ulceration; 8 mg/kg—renal injury. • Ibuprofen: ○ Dogs: 50 mg/kg—GI ulceration; 100–175 mg/kg—renal injury; 400 mg/kg—CNS signs. ○ Cats: considered about twice as sensitive as dogs. • Naproxen: ○ Dogs: 5 mg/kg—GI ulceration; 25 mg/kg—severe renal injury (may occur at lower doses); 50 mg/kg—CNS signs. ○ Cats: considered at least twice as sensitive as dogs.

RISK FACTORS

• Age—neonatal or geriatric. • Previous history of GI disease, ulcer, or bleeding. • Preexisting renal, hepatic, or cardiovascular disease.
• Hypotension; dehydration or hypovolemia.
• Other concurrent illness and/or medications (especially other NSAIDs or corticosteroids).

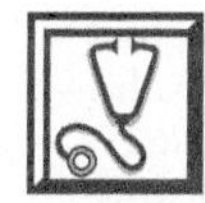

DIAGNOSIS

DIFFERENTIAL DIAGNOSIS

Other conditions that cause GI and/or renal effects:
• Inflammatory bowel disease, hemorrhagic gastroenteritis, hypoadrenocorticism, GI foreign body, neoplasia, ethylene glycol toxicosis, lily ingestion (cats), grape/raisin ingestion (dogs), renal failure (acute or chronic), urinary tract obstruction, pyelonephritis. • Diagnosis based on history of exposure and compatible clinical signs.

CBC/BIOCHEMISTRY/URINALYSIS

• Anemia—regenerative or nonregenerative, depending on duration of bleeding.
• Leukocytosis with left shift—associated with perforated gastric ulcer and accompanying peritonitis. • BUN and creatinine—may be elevated secondary to prerenal azotemia or primary renal insult.
• Panhypoproteinemia – secondary to GI bleeding. • Liver enzymes—occasionally elevated. • Monitor urine output for evidence of oliguria; monitor for isosthenuria, glucosuria, proteinuria, and casts.

OTHER LABORATORY TESTS

N/A

IMAGING

N/A

DIAGNOSTIC PROCEDURES

Endoscopy—verify GI ulceration.

PATHOLOGIC FINDINGS

• GI irritation, ulceration, or hemorrhage with possible perforation and peritonitis.
• Renal tubular or papillary necrosis or interstitial nephritis.

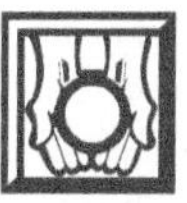

TREATMENT

APPROPRIATE HEALTH CARE

• Outpatient—mild clinical signs (with low ingested dose); managed at home with appropriate medication and dietary and symptomatic measures. • Inpatient—high ingested dose; potential for renal toxicosis; more serious clinical signs (frequent vomiting, bloody vomitus, melena, anemia, or evidence of renal involvement); aggressive treatment to avoid life-threatening complications.

Recent Ingestion

• Ingestion within 2 hours and no vomiting—induce emesis (apomorphine or hydrogen peroxide), only if patient not at-risk for aspiration. • After emesis—activated charcoal (1–2 g/kg PO) with a cathartic ×1 dose.
• Repeat activated charcoal without a cathartic q6–8h ×2 doses for NSAIDs that undergo enterohepatic recirculation.

NURSING CARE

• Fluid therapy—restore hydration when moderate to severe vomiting; twice maintenance rates with known or potential renal involvement. Titrate fluids as needed based on clinical signs and blood work results. Use caution in patients with underlying cardiac disease to avoid fluid overload. • If severely anemic, a blood transfusion may be indicated.

NONSTEROIDAL ANTI-INFLAMMATORY DRUG TOXICOSIS (CONTINUED)

ACTIVITY

N/A

DIET

• Vomiting—NPO. • Vomiting resolved—begin with a bland, low-protein diet.

CLIENT EDUCATION

• Stress the importance of contacting a veterinarian or animal poison control center (PPH or ASPCA APCC) whenever an animal is exposed to a nonprescribed NSAID or an overdose of a prescribed NSAID. • Inform client that dogs and particularly cats have a low tolerance to NSAIDs. • With a prescribed NSAID, instruct client to look for adverse or idiosyncratic effects and to stop the drug and contact the clinic if they occur.

SURGICAL CONSIDERATIONS

Surgical intervention may be required for a perforated GI ulcer.

N

MEDICATIONS

DRUG(S) OF CHOICE

H_2-Receptor Antagonists

• For GI upset or ulceration.
• Primarily effective for treating ulcers from acute overdose or from chronic administration after the drug withdrawn.
• Famotidine or ranitidine may be best choices as cimetidine may inhibit microsomal enzymes that metabolize some NSAIDs.
• Famotidine—dogs: 0.5–1.0 mg/kg PO, SC, IV, or IM q12–24h; cats: 0.5 mg/kg PO, SC, IV, or IM q12–24h. • Ranitidine—dogs: 2 mg/kg PO, IV q8h; cats: 2.5 mg/kg IV q12h or 3.5 mg/kg PO q12h.

Proton Pump Inhibitors

• Omeprazole 0.5–1 mg/kg PO q24h.
• Pantoprazole 0.7–1 mg/kg IV over 15 minutes q24h.

Other

• Sucralfate—dogs: 0.5–1 g PO q8–12h; cats: 0.25 g PO q8h; binds to proteins in the ulcer base; stimulates mucus and bicarbonate secretion. • Misoprostol 1–3 µg/kg PO q8h; prostaglandin E2 analogue; prevents GI bleeding and ulceration; promotes healing during chronic use in humans and dogs treated with aspirin.• Dopamine—may be indicated for acute renal failure. • Standard anticonvulsant therapy—diazepam, phenobarbital, levetiracetam, etc. if needed. • Naloxone may be useful in comatose patients.

Duration of Treatment

Depends on the dose and half-life of the NSAID ingested.

CONTRAINDICATIONS

Avoid concomitant use of corticosteroids or multiple NSAIDs; contraindicated in pregnancy (abortifacient effect).

PRECAUTIONS

Patients using other nephrotoxic drugs (e.g., aminoglycosides and angiotensin-converting enzyme [ACE] inhibitors)—at higher risk for developing NSAID nephropathy.

POSSIBLE INTERACTIONS

NSAIDs are highly protein-bound; may be affected by concurrent use of other highly protein-bound drugs.

FOLLOW-UP

PATIENT MONITORING

• Urine output—monitor for oliguria; examine for casts, protein, and glucose.
• Stool and vomitus—check for GI bleeding (may not develop for several days). • BUN and creatinine—daily for several days (full extent of renal damage may not be immediately evident); recheck 2–3 days after discharge if hospitalized. • Packed cell volume/total solids—check q12–24h while hospitalized, then 2–3 days after discharge to monitor for GI bleeding.

PREVENTION/AVOIDANCE

• Store medications out of the reach of pets.
• Discourage owners from medicating pet without veterinary supervision. • Appropriate laboratory tests for high-risk patients before beginning NSAID therapy.

POSSIBLE COMPLICATIONS

• Perforation of a GI ulcer and peritonitis.
• Irreversible acute and chronic renal failure.

EXPECTED COURSE AND PROGNOSIS

• GI upset or ulceration—usually complete recovery with appropriate treatment. • Renal effects—generally reversible with early and aggressive treatment. • Acute hepatopathies—generally resolve with early symptomatic treatment and discontinuation of the drug.

MISCELLANEOUS

PREGNANCY/FERTILITY/BREEDING

• Exposure during pregnancy—risk for fetal cardiopulmonary and renal effects. • May prolong pregnancy, especially if administered during the third trimester and before the onset of labor.

SEE ALSO

• Acute Kidney Injury.
• Aspirin Toxicosis.
• Poisoning (Intoxication) Therapy.

ABBREVIATIONS

• ACE = angiotensin-converting enzyme.
• APCC = Animal Poison Control Center.
• ASPCA = American Society for the Prevention of Cruelty to Animals.
• COX-2 = cyclooxygenase-2.
• GI = gastrointestinal.
• NSAID = nonsteroidal anti-inflammatory drug.
• PPH = Pet Poison Helpline.

INTERNET RESOURCES

https://www.petpoisonhelpline.com/poison/nsaids

Suggested Reading

Enberg TB, Braun LD, Kuzma AB. Gastrointestinal perforation in five dogs associated with the administration of meloxicam. J Vet Emerg Crit Care 2006, 16(1):34–43.

KuKanich B, Bidgood T, Knesl O. Clinical pharmacology of nonsteroidal anti-inflammatory drugs in dogs. Vet Anaes Analg 2012, 39(1):69–90.

McLean MK, Khan SA. Toxicology of frequently encountered nonsteroidal anti-inflammatory drugs in dogs and cats. Vet Clin North Am Small Anim Pract 2012, 42(2):289–306.

Talcott PA, Gwaltney-Brant SM. Nonsteroidal anti-inflammatories. In: Peterson ME, Talcott PA, eds., Small Animal Toxicology, 3rd ed. Philadelphia, PA: W.B. Saunders, 2013, pp. 687–708.

Author Amanda L. Poldoski

Consulting Editor Lynn R. Hovda

Acknowledgment The author and editors acknowledge the prior contribution of Judy Holding.

NOTOEDRIC MANGE

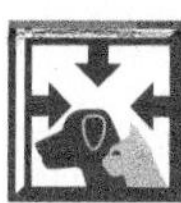

BASICS

OVERVIEW

- A nonseasonal, intensely pruritic, highly contagious parasitic skin disease of cats caused by *Notoedres cati*.
- Mites burrow through the superficial skin between follicles causing intense pruritus.
- Can cause transient pruritus in humans.

SIGNALMENT

- Domestic cats of all ages and both sexes.
- Fairly host-specific, but can also produce symptoms in dogs, cheetahs, raccoons, rabbits, coatis, palm civets, bobcats, ocelots, foxes, and humans.
- All in-contact cats usually develop clinical signs.
- Epizootic in localized areas.
- Endemic in large feral cat populations.
- Transmission by direct contact: mite is very short-lived when off the host.

SIGNS

- Nonseasonal intense pruritus.
- Following exposure, initial pruritus may be mild, but progresses to severe.
- Change from mild pruritus to onset of severe pruritus (incubation period) of 3–6 weeks may indicate eventual seroconversion and the development of hypersensitivity (IgG as well as humoral response).
- Rare individuals do not seroconvert, and therefore may not develop severe pruritus.
- Papules and crusts develop on pinnae and spread to eyelids, face, and neck (also known as "head mange").
- Progresses to the legs, feet and perineum.
- Severe self-trauma leads to secondary lesions.
- Skin becomes thickened, lichenified, and covered with gray-yellow crust.
- Large patches of lesions and alopecia develop over the entire body if untreated.
- Unlike canine scabies, large numbers of mites are present on the skin.
- Peripheral lymphadenopathy often develops.
- Causes significant debilitation in severe cases.

CAUSES & RISK FACTORS

Close contact with other cats.

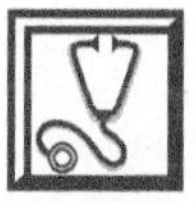

DIAGNOSIS

DIFFERENTIAL DIAGNOSIS

- Atopy.
- Cutaneous adverse reaction to food.
- Bacterial folliculitis.
- Dermatophytosis.
- Demodicosis.
- *Malassezia* dermatitis.
- *Cheyletiellosis*.
- Trombiculosis (chiggers).
- Otodectic dermatitis.
- Pemphigus foliaceus.
- Pemphigus erythematosus.
- Systemic lupus erythematosus.

CBC/BIOCHEMISTRY/URINALYSIS

N/A

OTHER LABORATORY TESTS

N/A

DIAGNOSTIC PROCEDURES

- Superficial skin scraping—relatively easy to find mites.
- Mite smaller than *S. scabiei*, with dorsal anus, typical dorsal concentric "finger print" striae, and only two pairs of forelegs protruding from the body line.
- Serum testing (ELISA) for mite antibody not available.
- Acetate tape impression—as sensitive as skin scraping.

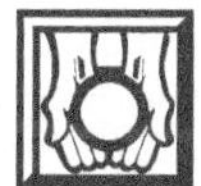

TREATMENT

- When scabicidal dips are used, the entire cat must be treated.
- Treatment failures occur if product is not applied to the face and ears.
- All in-contact cats should be treated.
- Response is usually quick if all in-contact animals are treated.
- Thorough cleaning of the cat's environment may be helpful if severely contaminated.
- Systemic antibiotics—may be needed to resolve secondary bacterial folliculitis.

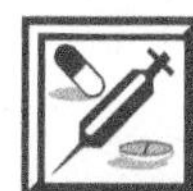

MEDICATIONS

DRUG(S) OF CHOICE

- Lime sulfur rinses 2–3%; apply to entire body weekly for 6–8 applications; clipping might be necessary to permit adequate contact with the skin.
- Ivermectin—effective; 0.2–0.3 mg/kg SC every 2 weeks for 2–3 treatments.
- Doramectin 0.2–0.3 mg/kg SC once.
- Selamectin—off-label; applied every 2 weeks for three applications.
- Imidacloprid/moxidectin spot-on applied once or twice as directed on the label.
- Isoxazoline parasiticides—not FDA approved: single administration.

CONTRAINDICATIONS/POSSIBLE INTERACTIONS

- Amitraz rinse may cause sedation.
- Lime sulfur has unpleasant odor and is staining.

FOLLOW-UP

PREVENTION/AVOIDANCE

Reinfestation may occur if contact with infested animals continues; the source of infestation must be determined (if possible) as well as all in-contact cats must be treated.

POSSIBLE COMPLICATIONS

- Topical scabicidal treatments are more prone to failure because of incomplete application of the treatment solution.
- Persistent infection if not all in-contact animals are treated.

EXPECTED COURSE AND PROGNOSIS

- Response to therapy is rapid providing all in-contact animals are treated; symptoms should significantly reduce within 2 weeks of treatment.
- There is no immunity from repeat infestation; clinical signs following a reinfestation are likely to be more rapid due to previous exposure and sensitization.

MISCELLANEOUS

ZOONOTIC POTENTIAL

- Humans in close contact with an affected cat may develop a pruritic, papular rash (often on arms, chest, or abdomen).
- Human lesions are usually transient and resolve spontaneously following treatment of affected animals.

Suggested Reading

Hellman K, Petry G, Capari B, et al. Treatment of naturally *Notoedres cati*-infested cats with combination of imidacloprid 10%/moxidectin 1% spot-on (Advocate/Advantage multi, Bayer). Parasitol Res 2013, 112:S57–S66.

Sampio KO, de Oliveira LM, Burmann PM, et al. Acetate tape impression test for diagnosis of notoedric mange in cats. J Feline Med Surg. 2017, 19(6):702–705.

Author Liora Waldman

Consulting Editor Alexander H. Werner Resnick

N

NYSTAGMUS

BASICS

DEFINITION

- Involuntary, rhythmic oscillation of the eyeballs.
- Jerk nystagmus—most common; slow eye movements in one direction with a rapid recovery phase in the opposite direction.
- Pendular nystagmus—seen less frequently; characterized by slow oscillations of the eyes in a trajectory that resembles that of a pendulum, with no fast phase.

PATHOPHYSIOLOGY

- Neural projections traverse in the brainstem from the vestibular nuclei to cranial nerve (CN) III, IV, and VI nuclei, which innervate the extraocular muscles. This pathway is part of the vestibular system, and provides coordinated conjugate eye movements in association with changes in head position.
- Physiologic nystagmus (ocular–vestibular reflex)—normal finding, induced by rotating the head from side to side; characterized by a jerk nystagmus with a slow drifting of the eye in the opposite direction of the head rotation followed by a fast compensatory phase in the same direction as the head movement. Decreased to absent physiologic nystagmus is indicative of vestibular disease.
- Pathologic nystagmus—a sign of vestibular dysfunction; characterized by a jerk nystagmus that develops independent of head movement. The nystagmus is described according to the axis of movement of the globe (horizontal, rotary, or vertical), and the direction of the fast phase of movement.
- Spontaneous or resting nystagmus—pathologic nystagmus that occurs when the head is in a normal position and not moving; frequently resolves after several days.
- Positional nystagmus—pathologic nystagmus, elicited only when the head is placed in unusual position; can often be seen in more chronic conditions.
- Jerk nystagmus must be differentiated from pendular nystagmus and from opsoclonus.
- Pendular nystagmus—congenital abnormality in which a larger-than-usual portion of the optic nerve fibers crosses in the chiasm; most often observed as an incidental finding in Siamese, Birman, and Himalayan cats but can also be seen with cerebellar disease and with visual deficits.
- Opsoclonus—involuntary, rapid, random eye movements in multiple directions that can be seen with cerebellar disease; can be differentiated from jerk nystagmus by the lack of a slow phase and its chaotic nature.

SYSTEMS AFFECTED

Nervous

GENETICS

N/A

INCIDENCE/PREVALENCE

Nystagmus, as a sign of vestibular disease, is a relatively common clinical presentation in dogs and cats.

SIGNALMENT

Species

Dog and cat.

Breed Predilections

None

Mean Age and Range

Varies, depending on underlying cause; neoplastic and vascular conditions and canine geriatric vestibular disease more common in older animals.

Predominant Sex

None

CAUSES

Peripheral Vestibular Disease

- Metabolic—hypothyroidism.
- Neoplastic—nerve sheath tumor or tumor involving surrounding bone or soft tissues.
- Inflammatory—otitis media-interna; nasopharyngeal polyps (cats).
- Idiopathic—canine geriatric vestibular disease; feline idiopathic vestibular disease.
- Toxic—e.g., aminoglycosides, topical iodophors, topical chlorhexidine.
- Trauma.

Central Vestibular Disease

- Degenerative—storage disorders; neuronal degeneration; demyelinating disease.
- Neoplastic—primary or metastatic tumors.
- Nutritional—thiamine deficiency.
- Inflammatory/infectious—viral (canine distemper, feline infectious peritonitis); bacterial; protozoal (toxoplasmosis, neosporosis); fungal (cryptococcosis, blastomycosis, histoplasmosis, coccidioidomycosis, aspergillosis); rickettsial (ehrlichiosis, Rocky Mountain spotted fever); inflammatory, noninfectious (meningoencephalitis of unknown etiology; includes granulomatous meningoencephalomyelitis and the necrotizing meningoencephalitides).
- Toxic—lead; hexachlorophene; metronidazole.
- Trauma.
- Vascular—cerebrovascular disease (hemorrhage, infarction).

RISK FACTORS

Systemic administration of certain antibiotics (metronidazole, aminoglycoside), otic administration of iodophors and chlorhexidine solutions.

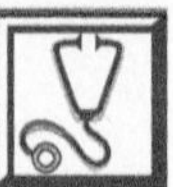

DIAGNOSIS

DIFFERENTIAL DIAGNOSIS

Peripheral Vestibular Disease

- Nystagmus—either rotary or horizontal in character, with the fast phase directed away from the side of the lesion; does not change direction with different head positions.
- Other signs of vestibular disease—head tilt, ataxia, circling, falling or rolling, and vestibular strabismus often present and occur ipsilateral to the lesion.
- Ipsilateral facial nerve deficits and/or Horner's syndrome—can be seen due to the close association of CN VII and sympathetic nerve to CN VIII as they course through the petrous temporal bone.

Central Vestibular Disease

- Nystagmus—horizontal, rotary, or vertical; can change direction with different head positions.
- Other signs of vestibular disease—head tilt, ataxia, circling, falling or rolling, and vestibular strabismus often present.
- Involvement of other brainstem structures—alterations in level of consciousness, paresis, postural reaction deficits, and other CN deficits (V and VII most common); deficits are typically ipsilateral to the lesion.
- Paradoxical vestibular disease—with certain lesions of the cerebellum; in these cases, postural reaction deficits occur ipsilateral to the lesion whereas the head tilt and other vestibular signs are contralateral to the lesion.

CBC/BIOCHEMISTRY/URINALYSIS

Results usually normal

OTHER LABORATORY TESTS

- Thyroid profile—if hypothyroidism is suspected.
- Bacterial culture of sample obtained via myringotomy—if otitis media-interna is likely.
- Serologic testing—for potential infectious agents.

IMAGING

- Imaging of the tympanic bullae to assess for otitis media-interna—survey radiographs of limited value; CT and MRI are more sensitive.
- Brain imaging (CT or MRI)—indicated in animals with central vestibular disease to evaluate for structural brain abnormalities. MRI is superior to CT for imaging the brain.

DIAGNOSTIC PROCEDURES

CSF—if central disease, to evaluate for inflammation.

PATHOLOGIC FINDINGS

Variable, depending of the underlying cause

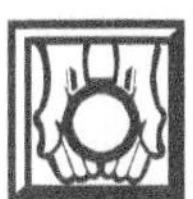

TREATMENT

APPROPRIATE HEALTH CARE

- The cause of the disease and the severity of signs determine whether the animal is best treated on an inpatient or an outpatient basis.
- In general, animals with central disease require more intensive care than those with peripheral disease.

NURSING CARE

- Fluid therapy is indicated in the acute stages of disease for animals that experience anorexia and vomiting.
- Animals with severe vestibular dysfunction should be confined to a well-padded area in the acute stage of the disease to minimize self-trauma secondary to disorientation.

ACTIVITY

- Animals should be housed on nonslippery surfaces; stairs should be avoided.
- Exercise should be supervised, with assistance provided until signs of imbalance resolve.

DIET

N/A

CLIENT EDUCATION

- Many animals show improvement over the first several days; the nervous system is able to compensate for vestibular disturbances that remain static or are slowly progressive regardless of cause.
- Compensation involves visual and somatosensory (tactile) cues and is dependent on feedback from vestibular pathways; return to normal activity should be encouraged to enhance compensatory mechanisms.

SURGICAL CONSIDERATIONS

Signs of vestibular dysfunction can transiently worsen after an anesthetic episode; most likely reflects a loss of compensation.

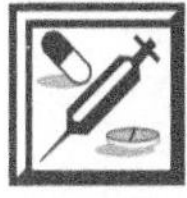

MEDICATIONS

DRUG(S) OF CHOICE

- Meclizine (dogs: 4 mg/kg PO q24h) or maropitant (dogs: 1 mg/kg SC or 2 mg/kg PO q24h; cats: 1 mg/kg SC q24h)—used to treat motion sickness; can alleviate nausea and vomiting associated with acute disease.
- Diazepam (dogs: 0.5 mg/kg PO q8h)—recommended in cases of metronidazole toxicity; can help decrease acute vestibular signs from other causes by decreasing the resting activity of vestibular neurons and alleviating the imbalance in vestibular input to the brain.
- Specific medical therapy is directed at the underlying cause, if one can be identified.

CONTRAINDICATIONS

- Avoid potential ototoxic drugs, such as aminoglycosides. Toxicity is more likely in animals with renal impairment.
- Avoid instilling topical medications into the ear of an animal with suspected otitis media-interna, especially if the tympanic membrane cannot be visualized or is not intact. Such agents can exacerbate vestibular signs and cause deafness.

PRECAUTIONS

- Avoid the use of metronidazole at daily doses greater than 60 mg/kg, as this has been associated with vestibular dysfunction in dogs.
- Vestibular dysfunction can develop after administration of metronidazole at lower dosages but is less likely.

FOLLOW-UP

PATIENT MONITORING

Repeat neurologic examination—perform 2 weeks after initial diagnosis to monitor for improvement or progression of disease.

PREVENTION/AVOIDANCE

N/A

POSSIBLE COMPLICATIONS

- Dehydration and electrolyte imbalance associated with anorexia and vomiting.
- Rare extension of otitis media-interna into the adjacent brainstem.

EXPECTED COURSE AND PROGNOSIS

- Prognosis varies, depending on the cause of the vestibular disturbance.
- In general, animals with peripheral vestibular disease have a better prognosis than those with central involvement.
- Residual deficits can remain after resolution of the underlying disease process due to irreversible damage to the neural structures.
- Recurrence is possible with some of the conditions (otitis media-interna, canine geriatric vestibular disease, feline idiopathic vestibular disease).

MISCELLANEOUS

ASSOCIATED CONDITIONS

N/A

AGE-RELATED FACTORS

N/A

PREGNANCY/FERTILITY/BREEDING

N/A

SEE ALSO

- Ataxia.
- Head Tilt.
- Otitis Media and Interna.

ABBREVIATIONS

- CN = cranial nerve.

INTERNET RESOURCES

- http://www.vetfolio.com/neurology/vestibular-disease-diseases-causing-vestibular-signs-compendium
- https://vestibular.org/sites/default/files/page_files/Vestibular%20disease%20in%20dogs%20and%20cats.pdf

Suggested Reading

Lowrie M. Vestibular disease: anatomy, physiology, and clinical signs. Compend Contin Educ Vet 2012, 34(7):E1–E5.

Rossmeisl JH Jr. Vestibular disease in dogs and cats. Vet Clin North Am Small Anim Pract 2010, 40:81–100.

Author Karen R. Muñana

OBESITY

BASICS

DEFINITION

Obesity is the unhealthy accumulation of body fat. Precise definitions are debated but it is widely accepted that dogs or cats with body condition score (BCS) 6 or 7 on a 9-point scale are overweight, and those with BCS 8 or 9 are obese.

PATHOPHYSIOLOGY

• Animals gain weight when energy intake from food chronically exceeds energy expended to maintain basic homeostatic processes and during exercise. • Homeostatic neuroendocrine responses ensure food intake meets energy requirements and establish modest energy reserves in case of a period of fasting. • Energy homeostasis may be disrupted by: ready availability of highly palatable energy-dense food (which elicits hedonic responses that override homeostatic satiation); genetic variation in appetite; neutering; and limits to a pet's ability to exercise.

SYSTEMS AFFECTED

• Endocrine—insulin resistance develops secondary to obesity and can lead to diabetes mellitus in cats. • Immune—adipose tissue dysfunction in obesity causes a proinflammatory state. • Other organ systems may be affected by the mechanical effect of increased body fat and/or endocrine and metabolic disruption.

GENETICS

• Breed variation in obesity predisposition suggests obesity susceptibility is in part heritable with a polygenic mode of inheritance. • Mutations in the genes *POMC* (Labrador and flatcoat retrievers) and *MC4R* (beagles) are associated with obesity and/or food motivation.

INCIDENCE/PREVALENCE

Common. As many as 65% of dogs and 25% cats are overweight or obese.

GEOGRAPHIC DISTRIBUTION

Widespread

SIGNALMENT

Species

Dog and cat.

Breed Predilections

• Domestic shorthair cats. • Labrador retriever, Cairn terrier, cavalier King Charles spaniel, Scottish terrier, cocker spaniel.

Mean Age and Range

Obesity prevalence is highest in middle age but can occur throughout life.

Predominant Sex

Neutered pets of either sex are predisposed.

SIGNS

Historical Findings

• Weight gain. • Change in BCS. • A full diet and exercise history and understanding of concurrent medical problems is essential to formulating a treatment plan.

Physical Examination Findings

Excess body fat and BCS (see Diagnostic Procedures).

CAUSES

Energy intake chronically exceeding energy output.

RISK FACTORS

• Neutering. • Middle age. • Feeding highly palatable, energy-dense foods without adequate restriction. • Restricted exercise (e.g., following injury, indoor cats, or leash-only exercise). • High drive for food, driven by genetic variation (e.g. Labrador retriever *POMC* mutation). • Uncommonly, endocrinopathies can cause obesity (hypothyroidism, insulinoma), or mimic obesity (as with the abdominal enlargement of hyperadrenocorticism).

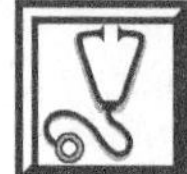

DIAGNOSIS

DIFFERENTIAL DIAGNOSIS

Abdominal distention from pregnancy, ascites, hyperadrenocorticism, or neoplasia.

CBC/BIOCHEMISTRY/URINALYSIS

Normal or may reflect endocrine disruption (hyperglycemia, dyslipidemia) or concurrent disease.

OTHER LABORATORY TESTS

N/A

IMAGING

Ultrasound, MRI, or dual-energy x-ray absorptiometry can measure body fat more accurately.

DIAGNOSTIC PROCEDURES

• BCS is a semi-quantitative, ordinal measure of body composition. Observation and palpation are used to assign a score based on how findings best match a series of descriptors. The best validated 9-point scale assigns BCS 4–5 as ideal, 6–7 as overweight, and 8–9 as obese. • Serial measurement of body weight is more sensitive for monitoring.

PATHOLOGIC FINDINGS

N/A

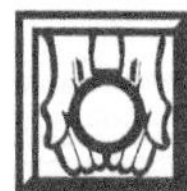

TREATMENT

APPROPRIATE HEALTH CARE

• Outpatient. • Calorie restriction is the mainstay of successful weight loss. • Changes in owner management behavior are critical to success. • Energy requirements for maintenance are lower after weight loss so long-term vigilance and food restriction are required to prevent recurrence.

NURSING CARE

N/A

ACTIVITY

• Increasing exercise is ineffective to induce weight loss alone so if owners are reluctant to make management changes, focus should be on food restriction. • However, exercise is encouraged because it promotes retention of lean mass (muscle) during weight loss.

DIET

• Reducing daily energy intake in food to below maintenance requirements is essential. • Target weight is estimated from current weight and BCS—every 1 unit increase over BCS 5/9 equates to 10% excess body mass; e.g., to calculate the target weight of a dog in BCS 7, divide current weight by 1.2. • The amount of food required to promote weight loss can be estimated from calculated maintenance energy requirements (MER) or by reducing current food intake by 10–20%. • To calculate MER, use estimated target weight (MER (kJ) = 440 × body weight $[BW]_{kg}^{0.75}$) and feed 50–65% of MER as a starting point. • Feeding recommendations should be altered from baseline to maintain weight loss at 0.5–1% per week until target weight is reached. • For weight loss of <20% (i.e., starting BCS ≤6), food restriction is moderate and a conventional diet is adequate, although specialized diets may be advantageous. Where energy restriction is greater (starting BCS ≥7), the density of essential nutrients in maintenance diets may be inadequate so a specialized diet is recommended. • Specialized diets improve the success of weight loss programs and improve satiety, which itself may improve compliance because owners are subjected to less begging behavior. • Specialized diets are commonly formulated to provide: high essential nutrient density; low energy density (added water in canned food or air in kibble); high protein (improves satiety and promotes lean mass retention); and high fiber (promotes satiety). Canned (compared to dry) food may improve weight loss in cats. • Accurate feeding using weighed portions is important. Treats are ideally excluded but if owners feel they are essential, factor them into the diet plan.

CLIENT EDUCATION

• Owners of obese pets often do not follow advice to reduce their pets' weight because they do not recognize obesity, do not see it as a problem, or struggle to follow the advice. By definition, they have already failed to make the small adjustments needed to keep their dog slim; it follows that they are likely to find making the major changes required to reduce their dog's weight difficult. • Although it might sound simple to "feed less and exercise more," the reality is that owners are being asked to change established habits, spend more time caring for their pets, and perhaps work to motivate other family members. • Promoting those behavior changes requires us to motivate owners, to understand their barriers to change, and to offer practical and simple advice on how to overcome those barriers. Information does not automatically lead to motivation; it is more likely if the actions required are consistent with their existing values and beliefs. • Owners may not recognize obesity. Being overweight is regarded as the norm for some breeds. Regular recording of body weight and BCS can objectively identify a problem early ("I see she's gained a pound—it would be good to cut the food down before that becomes a problem"). • Owners may not appreciate that obesity causes health problems. Positive motivation ("slimming him down could really improve his mobility") is more effective than negative ("if he doesn't lose weight he'll never walk properly again"). • Lack of motivation may be difficult to modify ("his breeder says his weight is fine") or challenge ("everyone in our family carries a little extra weight—it's cuddly"). • Owners often find food restriction difficult. Reducing intake in highly food-motivated animals may require constant vigilance to reduce scavenging, stealing, or hunting. Ignoring begging requires a strong will because of the importance of food-giving in maintaining the human–animal bond. Owners may not feel confident in how or what to feed. Practical problems may limit the exercise they offer their pet. • Practical advice to overcome those barriers should ideally be tailored to each owner. If owners complain their pets are always hungry, a satiety-promoting diet or trickle feeding using toys or frequent small meals may help. If owners insist on treat feeding, suggest low-calorie treats or factor planned treats into the daily ration. If owner mobility restricts dog walks, suggest ball play or longer time in the yard to increase activity. • Human behavior change is also improved by goal-setting, action planning, and monitoring. For instance, the aim for a weight loss consultation could be that owners leave with written plans formulated in the session: "my goal is to slim her down to 18 kg"; "I have chosen to make these 3 management changes from the list of suggestions…"; and "I will bring her back once a month to be weighed." • Fostering a nonjudgmental and supportive veterinary practice culture regarding pet obesity should encourage owners to seek support and act early.

SURGICAL CONSIDERATIONS

N/A

MEDICATIONS

DRUG(S) OF CHOICE

No approved medications for use in United States or Europe.

CONTRAINDICATIONS

N/A

PRECAUTIONS

N/A

POSSIBLE INTERACTIONS

N/A

ALTERNATIVE DRUGS

N/A

FOLLOW-UP

PATIENT MONITORING

• Monitoring progress is important. After initiating a diet change, check progress after 2 weeks and alter food ration to aim for 0.5–1% body weight loss per week. Regular monthly visits promote owner compliance and allow ration changes to maintain progress. • Once target weight is achieved, ongoing monitoring is essential to minimize rebound weight gain. Weighing at veterinary visits is ideally supplemented by owners becoming more adept at noticing weight gain and acting to reverse it.

PREVENTION/AVOIDANCE

• Prevention should be a central aim of routine vet visits. Veterinary teams should work to empower owners to recognize a healthy weight and to intervene effectively when obesity occurs. • Weight and BCS should be recorded at every practice visit.
• Incorporating weight management advice into waiting room displays will establish the importance of maintaining a healthy weight to the client population.

POSSIBLE COMPLICATIONS

See Associated Conditions.

EXPECTED COURSE AND PROGNOSIS

• Food restriction leads to weight loss in research settings but in client-owned dogs has lower success rates. Compliance is frequently poor and total weight loss often falls short of the target. Rebound weight gain is common.
• Encouragingly, however, even modest weight loss (of approximately 10%) can produce clinically significant improvement.

MISCELLANEOUS

ASSOCIATED CONDITIONS

Endocrine and Metabolic

• Dyslipidemia.* • Insulin resistance (dogs and cats), diabetes mellitus (cats).* • Hepatic lipidosis (cats).* • Hypothyroidism.**
• Insulinoma.**

Orthopedic

• Osteoarthritis. • Humeral condylar fractures. • Cranial cruciate ligament rupture.
• Intervertebral disc disease.

Cardiorespiratory Disease

• Tracheal collapse.* • Brachycephalic obstructive airway syndrome.* • Laryngeal paralysis.* • Increased blood pressure.*

Urogenital System

• Urethral sphincter mechanism incompetence.*
• Feline lower urinary tract disease.* • Dystocia.*

Neoplasia

• General incidence and specifically mammary neoplasia and transitional cell carcinoma.*

Other

• Heat intolerance/heat stroke.*
• Increased anesthetic risk.*
• Decreased lifespan.*

*Conditions where obesity is proven or implicated in causing or exacerbating disease. **Conditions implicated in causing obesity. Where unspecified, obesity association is likely to be both cause and effect or is unknown.

AGE-RELATED FACTORS

Obesity is most common in middle-aged dogs and middle-aged to old cats.

ZOONOTIC POTENTIAL

N/A

PREGNANCY/FERTILITY/BREEDING

Obesity is associated with reduced fertility and dystocia. Food restriction is contraindicated during pregnancy.

SYNONYMS

Overweight

SEE ALSO

Diabetes Mellitus.

ABBREVIATIONS

• BCS = body condition score.
• MER = maintenance energy requirement.

INTERNET RESOURCES

• https://www.wsava.org/nutrition-toolkit
• https://petnutritionalliance.org/

Suggested Reading

Flanagan J, Bissot T, Hours M-A, et al. Success of a weight loss plan for overweight dogs: the results of an international weight loss study. PLoS ONE 2017, 12(9):e0184199.

Laflamme DP. Development and validation of a body condition score system for cats: a clinical tool. Feline Pract 1997, 25:13–18.

Laflamme DP. Development and validation of a body condition score system for dogs: a clinical tool. Canine Pract 1997, 22:10–15.

Linder DE, Parker VJ. Dietary aspects of weight management in cats and dogs. Vet Clin North Am Small Anim Pract 2016, 46:869–882.

Raffan E, Dennis RJ, O'Donovan CJ, et al. A deletion in the canine POMC gene is associated with weight and appetite in obesity-prone Labrador retriever dogs. Cell Metab 2016, 23(5):893–900.

Author Eleanor Raffan
Consulting Editor Mark P. Rondeau

Client Education Handout available online

O

ODONTOGENIC TUMORS

BASICS

OVERVIEW

- Odontogenic tumors are defined by the World Health Organization (WHO) as "lesions derived from epithelial, ectomesenchymal and/or mesenchymal elements that still are, or have been, part of the tooth-forming apparatus".
- *Epulis* (Greek *epi-oulon* meaning "on the gum") is a nonspecific, clinical term used to describe tumors and tumor-like masses of the gingiva.
- Odontogenic tumors are categorized into three broad groups with specific tumor types in each category:
  - Tumors of odontogenic epithelium: conventional ameloblastoma; canine acanthomatous ameloblastoma; amyloid-producing odontogenic tumor.
  - Tumors of odontogenic epithelium with odontogenic ectomesenchyme: ameloblastic fibroma, ameloblastic fibro-dentinoma, and ameloblastic fibro-odontoma; feline inductive odontogenic tumor; odontoma.
  - Tumors of mesenchyme and/or odontogenic ectomesenchyme: peripheral odontogenic fibroma; feline "epulides"; odontogenic myxoma/myxofibroma.

We focus here on the most common odontogenic tumors:

- Conventional ameloblastoma (CA):
  - Benign but expansile, locular to multilocular tumor of the jaws in dogs and cats.
  - Differs in biological behavior from the more common CAA.
- Canine acanthomatous ameloblastoma (CAA):
  - Benign but invasive tumor of the jaws.
  - Typically more invasive than expansile.
  - No apparent human analogue.
- Amyloid-producing odontogenic tumor (APOT):
  - Benign but expansile tumor of the jaws affecting primarily dogs.
  - Similar biological behavior to the CA with a propensity to produce amyloid.
- Feline inductive odontogenic tumor (FIOT):
  - Benign odontogenic tumor unique to cats.
  - Generally expansile and locular with epicenter at an impacted and/or malformed maxillary canine tooth.
- Peripheral odontogenic fibroma (POF):
  - Benign tumor primarily composed of periodontal ligament-like stroma arising from tissue near the alveolar margin.
  - Current debate as to whether this is a tumor or a reactive lesion.
- Feline "epulides":
  - Clinically presents as a typical epulis.
  - Not clear whether this lesion is analogous to POF of dogs.
  - Most cats are presented with multifocal lesions distributed throughout the entire oral cavity.

SIGNALMENT

- Dog—odontogenic tumors are generally considered uncommon but CAA has been reported to be the fourth most common oral tumor in dogs. POF may be even more common.
- Cat—odontogenic tumors are rare in cats.
- CAA is more common in golden retrievers and possibly cocker spaniels.
- Boxers may have higher incidence of POF.

SIGNS

Historical Findings

- Often minimal—incidental finding detected on routine physical examination.
- If severe—excessive salivation, halitosis, dysphagia, bloody oral discharge, weight loss.

Physical Examination Findings

- Oral mass—in early cases, may appear as small, pedunculated masses.
- Displacement of tooth structures due to the expansile nature of the mass.
- Possible facial deformity due to asymmetry of the maxilla or mandible.
- Occasionally cervical lymphadenopathy.
- CA—generally an intraosseous cystic lesion with osseous expansion.
- CAA—generally an extraosseous lesion with an irregular surface that arises within the gingiva; more common in rostral mandible.
- APOT—generally an expansile mass, similar to the CA; when the amyloid deposits become mineralized a mixed radiolucent–radiopaque appearance may be seen.
- FIOT—a central tumor typically presenting as a large swelling of the rostral maxilla in young cats.
- POF—typically a firm, sessile to pedunculated, nonulcerated lesion that is most often associated with the free gingiva. Infrequently seen primarily as a broad-based mass in the attached gingiva.
- Feline "epulides"—most cats present with multifocal lesions distributed throughout the entire oral cavity.

CAUSES & RISK FACTORS

None identified.

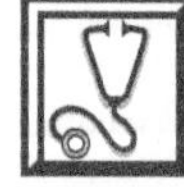

DIAGNOSIS

DIFFERENTIAL DIAGNOSIS

- Benign oral tumor.
- Malignant oral tumor.
- Focal fibrous hyperplasia.
- Pyogenic granuloma.
- Gingival hyperplasia/enlargement.
- Differentiated from other types of masses by incisional biopsy coupled with radiographic appearance.

CBC/BIOCHEMISTRY/URINALYSIS

Results usually normal.

OTHER LABORATORY TESTS

Cytologic preparations are rarely diagnostic.

IMAGING

- Determine tumor borders by CT or intraoral radiographs.
- Radiographs of CA, APOT and FIOT typically demonstrate significant expansion with loculated appearance; APOT may exhibit mixed radiopacity due to mineralization of amyloid; CAA is typically infiltrative into bone; POF and feline "epulides" generally do not invade bone but can displace tooth structures and may have ossified component.
- CT scan is best modality for surgical planning.

DIAGNOSTIC PROCEDURES

A large, deep tissue biopsy (down to and including bone) is required to definitively diagnose.

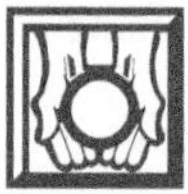

TREATMENT

Surgical Considerations

- Ameloblastomas and APOT—complete surgical excision is realistic and prognosis with clean margins is good to excellent, making wide surgical excision the treatment of choice. Radiation therapy has been utilized in dogs and cats with variable results. CA is located primarily within bone and is, as such, more radioresistant.
- POF—POFs arise from periodontal-like stroma in the gingiva or underlying periosteum at or near the cementoenamel junction. Local conservative excision of the tumor with particular attention paid to removing the entire lesion, excising down to and including the affected periosteum, should be anticipated to be curative. Such an approach may, however, require reconstruction of the gingiva surrounding the remaining tooth. Recurrence is likely if the entire lesion is not excised. More aggressive treatments may be reserved for recurrent lesions or those that have a more regional, broad-based presentation.
- FIOT—similar to most odontogenic tumors, no case-controlled studies have been performed to evaluate the appropriate treatment for FIOTs. However, similar to most odontogenic tumors, it appears that if the tumor is surgically resected in its entirety (0.5–1 cm intended surgical margins), the tumor is unlikely to recur.
- Feline "epulides"—it is clear that surgical management of feline epulides, while recommended, is not as straightforward as is the case with canine POF. This is because most cats are presented with multifocal lesions, making local surgical excision alone

challenging. Recurrence with such a conservative approach is likely and some cases require multiple extractions and gingivectomy to achieve complete resolution.

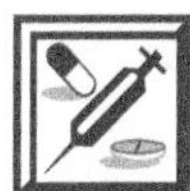

MEDICATIONS

DRUG(S) OF CHOICE

- Efficacy of outpatient chemotherapy is unreported; most tumors of mesenchymal origin respond poorly.
- Intralesional bleomycin has been reported for CAA.

FOLLOW-UP

PATIENT MONITORING

- Thorough oral, head, and neck examination regularly after treatment.
- Medical surveillance with CT or intraoral radiographs every 3–6 months.

EXPECTED COURSE AND PROGNOSIS

- CA, CAA, APOT, and FIOT are highly invasive/expansile in bone.
- No known metastasis.
- Good to excellent prognosis/surgical cure can be expected when excisional margins are free of neoplastic cells.
- Mean survival after radiotherapy in dogs with CAA ranges from 1 to 102 months (median, 37 months); 1-year survival rate 85%; 2-year survival rate 67%.

MISCELLANEOUS

ABBREVIATIONS

- APOT = amyloid-producing odontogenic tumor.
- CA = conventional ameloblastoma.
- CAA = canine acanthomatous ameloblastoma.
- FIOT = feline inductive odontogenic tumor.
- POF = peripheral odontogenic fibroma.
- WHO = World Health Organization.

INTERNET RESOURCES

https://avdc.org/avdc-nomenclature/

Suggested Reading

Amory JT, Reetz JA, Sanchez MD, et al. Computed tomographic characteristics of odontogenic neoplasms in dogs. Vet Radiol Ultrasound 2014, 55:147–158.

Fiani N, Verstraete FMJ, Kass PH, Cos DP. Clinicopathological characterization of odontogenic tumors and focal fibrous hyperplasia in dogs: 152 cases (1995–2005). J Am Vet Med Assoc 2011, 238(4):495–500.

Goldschmidt SL, Bell CM, Hetzel S, Soukup JW. Clinical characterization of canine acanthomatous ameloblastoma (CAA) in 263 dogs and the influence of postsurgical histopathological margins on local recurrence. J Vet Dent 2017, 34(4):241–247.

Thrall DE. Orthovoltage radiotherapy of acanthomatous epulis in 39 dogs. J Am Vet Med Assoc 1984, 184:826–829.

Author Jason W. Soukup

Consulting Editor Heidi B. Lobprise

ODONTOMA

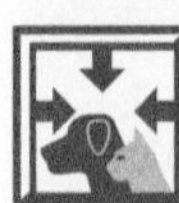

BASICS

OVERVIEW

- Odontoma—oral mass that arises from odontogenic epithelial and mesenchymal origin:
  - Ameloblastic fibro-odontoma (AFO) (formerly ameloblastic odontoma)—radiolucent, mass with osteolysis and varying amounts of intralesional mineralization.
  - Complex odontoma—radiodense mass with fully differentiated dental components (more organized than AFO), but unorganized at the cellular level with no tooth-like structures.
  - Compound odontoma—mass with fully differentiated dental components resulting in the presence of denticles (tooth-like structures).
- Hamartoma—proliferation of normal cellular components with an abnormal organization; not a true neoplasm (applicable to complex and compound odontoma types).
  - A definition to help delineate the three types of odontoma, not a type in itself.

SIGNALMENT

Typically found in young animals.

SIGNS

- Oral swelling or mass.
- Delayed deciduous tooth exfoliation or delayed or abnormal tooth eruption at site.
- AFO:
  - Most lesions are radiolucent with single or multiple (multilocular) expansile lesions of irregular configurations of dental components.
  - Some lesions are associated with impacted teeth.
  - Neoplastic mechanism, may recur (World Health Organization [WHO]—benign neoplasm).
- Complex:
  - Disorganized tissues within a thin, fibrous capsule.
  - Radiographically, often a radial structure of hard tissue particles inside a radiolucent zone, embedded in the maxilla or mandible.
  - Erupted teeth in that area may allow for communication between the odontoma and oral cavity, with a potential for bacterial contamination and infection.
- Compound:
  - The presence of denticles is pathognomonic.
  - Small, rudimentary teeth with crown formed, but the roots are often misshapen (dilacerated).
  - Denticles often associated with radiolucency.
  - May be embedded or have some extent of eruption.

CAUSES & RISK FACTORS

AFO

- Mixed odontogenic tumor with differentiation of odontoblasts, ameloblasts and cementoblasts embedded in cellular mesenchymal tissue.
- Reciprocal inductive interaction of epithelial and mesenchymal tissues.
- WHO classification as a benign neoplasm with possible reoccurrence.

Complex Odontoma

Inductive processes resulting in dental components but not fully organized.

Compound Odontoma

Differentiation of dental components into varying levels of organization—denticles.

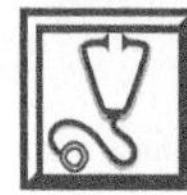

DIAGNOSIS

DIFFERENTIAL DIAGNOSIS

- Infection.
- Foreign body.
- Dentigerous cyst.
- Other oral masses:
  - Ameloblastic fibroma—similar to AFO but would contain no hard tissue.
  - Calcifying epithelial odontogenic tumor (CEOT)—osteolysis but no mineralization or dental (mesenchymal) aspect; slow, not inductive, noninvasive.
  - Amyloid producing odontogenic tumor (APOT)—similar to CEOT, but amyloid producing; shares biologic features with ameloblastoma.
  - Peripheral odontoma (4 human cases diagnosed)—develops in gingiva or alveolar mucosa with no attachment to bone; associated with impacted or retained teeth; similar to erupted odontoma.

CBC/BIOCHEMISTRY/URINALYSIS

Typically not affected.

IMAGING

- Intraoral radiography.
- Advanced imaging typically not warranted.

DIAGNOSTIC PROCEDURES

- Histopathology.
- Complete oral examination.

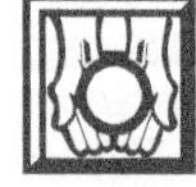

TREATMENT

Surgical Considerations

- Appropriate antimicrobial and pain management therapy when indicated.
- Appropriate patient monitoring and support during anesthetic procedures.
- AFO:
  - More aggressive excision may be necessary due to neoplastic classification; consider obtaining a 1 cm surgical margin.
  - Monitor for local recurrence.
- Complex and compound odontoma:
  - Enucleation and intracapsular excision with aggressive debridement of cyst; more aggressive surgical excision can decrease the chance of recurrence.
  - No chemotherapeutic regimens recommended.
  - Rarely radiotherapy may be beneficial by treating microscopically recurring disease.

MEDICATIONS

None indicated.

FOLLOW-UP

PATIENT MONITORING

Typical postoperative—pain management, nutrition.

POSSIBLE COMPLICATIONS

Recurrence, local infection, fragile jaw structure.

EXPECTED COURSE AND PROGNOSIS

- AFO—fair to guarded prognosis, as there is a chance of recurrence.
- Complex and compound odontoma—short- and long-term prognosis good with adequate therapy.

MISCELLANEOUS

ABBREVIATIONS

- AFO = ameloblastic fibro-odontoma.
- APOT = amyloid-producing odontogenic tumor.
- CEOT = calcifying epithelial odontogenic tumor.
- WHO = World Health Organization.

Suggested Reading

Felizzola CR, Martins MT, Stopiglia A, et al. Compound odontoma in three dogs. J Vet Dent 2003, 20(2):79.

Sowers J, Gengler W. Diagnosis and treatment of maxillary compound odontoma. J Vet Dent 2005, 21(1):26.

Walker KS, Lewis JR, Durham AC, Reiter AM. Diagnostic imaging in dental practice. Odontoma and impacted premolar. J Am Vet Med Assoc 2009, 235(11):1279–1281.

Author Matthew S. Lemmons

Consulting Editor Heidi B. Lobprise

BASICS

DEFINITION

- Oliguria—production of an abnormally small amount of urine. Several proposed definitions; in hydrated patients with good perfusion, urine output (UOP) <1.0 mL/kg/h = absolute oliguria. Acute kidney injury (AKI) is typically polyuric, where UOP >2 mL/kg/h is expected.
- Anuria—limited/no urine formation (UOP <0.08 mL/kg/h).

PATHOPHYSIOLOGY

- Physiologic (prerenal) oliguria—kidneys limit water loss during state of reduced renal perfusion to preserve fluid and electrolyte balance. High plasma osmolality or low circulating fluid volume stimulate antidiuretic hormone (ADH) synthesis and release, which induces formation of small quantity of concentrated urine.
- Pathologic (renal) oliguria—severe renal parenchymal impairment. Factors include: high resistance in afferent glomerular vessels, low glomerular permeability, back leak of filtrate from damaged renal tubules, renal intratubular obstruction, and extensive loss of nephrons resulting in marked reduction of glomerular filtrate produced.
- Anuria—may be renal or postrenal origin. Severe renal disease occasionally causes anuria. Mechanisms are the same as for pathologic oliguria (e.g., urinary tract obstruction (UTO) or excretory pathway rupture).

SYSTEMS AFFECTED

- Renal—inability to adequately eliminate wastes and water; hyperkalemia.
- Urologic—obstruction-induced distension of the collecting system. Increased risk of urinary tract infection (UTI) due to failure to empty bladder.

SIGNALMENT

- Dog and cat.
- Young adult cats—higher incidence of anuria associated with UTO.

SIGNS

- Reduction in quantity of urine voided.
- Enlarged urinary bladder, stranguria, pollakiuria with urethral obstruction.
- Systemic signs of uremia if oliguria/anuria persists.

CAUSES

- Physiologic oliguria—renal hypoperfusion or serum hyperosmolality.
- Pathologic oliguria—AKI or advanced chronic kidney disease (CKD).
- Anuria—complete UTO, urinary tract rupture, or severe primary kidney disease.

RISK FACTORS

- Physiologic oliguria—dehydration, decreased cardiac output, hypotension.
- Pathologic oliguria and anuria—primary kidney disease, nephrotoxin exposure, dehydration, low cardiac output, hypotension, electrolyte imbalance, acidosis, fever, sepsis, liver disease, multiple organ failure, trauma, hypoalbuminemia, hyperviscosity syndrome.
- Anuria—caused by urolithiasis, urinary tract neoplasia, idiopathic feline lower urinary tract disease, functional micturition disorder, trauma, gross hematuria.

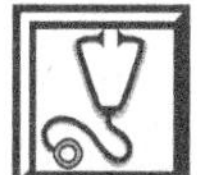

DIAGNOSIS

DIFFERENTIAL DIAGNOSIS

- Physiologic oliguria—poor tissue perfusion, history of recent fluid loss, signs of uremia are typically absent. Oliguria resolves rapidly when renal hypoperfusion is corrected.
- Pathologic oliguria—caused by CKD have a history of progressive kidney disease (polyuria, polydipsia, poor appetite, weight loss). Patients with CKD are at risk for AKI. Signs of uremia are commonly observed; fluid therapy and other measures to restore adequate renal perfusion often fail to increase urine flow.
- Suspect anuria due to UTO or rupture of the excretory pathway with repeated stranguria and inability to produce urine. Patients may have a history of pollakiuria, dysuria, hematuria, urolithiasis, trauma, instrumentation of the urinary tract. Physical exam may reveal enlarged urinary bladder, painful posterior abdomen, masses or uroliths in the urethra or bladder. Patients with rupture of the urinary tract may have ascites, fluid infiltration in tissues, painful caudal abdomen, masses or uroliths in the bladder or urethra, or evidence of trauma. UTO caused by functional urinary obstruction: suspect in patients with urinary bladder enlargement, increased resistance to manual bladder expression, and neurologic signs affecting the hind limbs and/or tail. Signs of uremia may develop. Restoring urinary flow/correcting rents in the excretory pathway rapidly restores adequate urine flow.

CBC/BIOCHEMISTRY/URINALYSIS

- Serum urea nitrogen, creatinine concentration—elevated unless onset of oliguria or anuria is very recent.
- Hyperkalemia—common with pathologic oliguria and anuria, less common/less severe in animals with physiologic oliguria (except with hypoadrenocorticism).
- Physiologic oliguria—characterized by high urine specific gravity (USG) (dogs >1.030, cats >1.035). Oliguria associated with lower USG suggests renal parenchymal disease or UTO. Patients with urine concentrating defects due to other diseases or drugs are the exception to this rule.
- Renal parenchymal anuria is typically characterized by USG <1.030 (dogs) or <1.035 (cats). USG varies in patients with post-renal anuria. Adequate urine-concentrating ability often lost after UTO.

IMAGING

- Abdominal radiographs and ultrasound are useful to rule out UTO/excretory pathway rupture.
- Excretory urography, retrograde urethrocystography, pyelography, or vaginourethrocystography may provide definitive proof of UTO/excretory pathway rupture.
- Distension of the excretory pathway or detection of uroliths in the ureters, bladder neck, urethra suggest UTO.
- Detection of fluid within the peritoneum supports a diagnosis of excretory pathway rupture. Contrast media leakage confirms a rupture.

DIAGNOSTIC PROCEDURES

- Electrocardiography—to identify significant arrhythmia (see Hyperkalemia).
- Urethrocystoscopy—may provide evidence for UTO/urinary tract rupture.
- Urinary catheterization—may provide information about the integrity of the lower urinary tract. Not recommended as a diagnostic procedure because it may be misleading and may cause additional trauma; iatrogenic UTI.

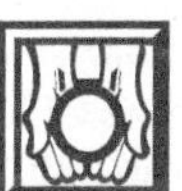

TREATMENT

- Oliguria and anuria are emergencies. Untreated, may lead to death within hours to days from uremia, hyperkalemia, acidosis, sepsis.
- Persistent hypovolemia may lead to ischemic renal injury.
- Correct renal hypoperfusion rapidly by intravenous administration of balanced isotonic crystalloid.
- Therapy for primary renal oliguria/anuria is limited to symptomatic, supportive care while awaiting spontaneous renal function recovery. Elimination of causative factors may slow or stop further renal injury (e.g., terminating aminoglycoside therapy, correcting hypercalcemia, or restoring adequate renal perfusion); however, once pathologic oliguria/anuria has developed, few kidney diseases will be amenable to specific treatment (exception = leptospirosis).
- Correct postrenal causes for anuria by nonsurgical/surgical methods including retrogradeurohydropropulsion of uroliths/urethral plugs; placement of transurethral catheters to restore low-pressure urinary flow; removal of uroliths, polyps, neoplastic tissue; or surgical repair of rents, strictures, malposition of kidneys, ureters, bladder, urethra.

OLIGURIA AND ANURIA (CONTINUED)

MEDICATIONS

DRUG(S) OF CHOICE

• Diuretics—indicated after establishing euvolemia in patients with renal oliguria. Diuretic-induced UOP facilitates fluid and electrolyte therapy and may imply less severe kidney injury.
• Administration of diuretics before restoring adequate renal perfusion is counterproductive and may promote renal injury.
• Avoid diuretic-induced dehydration.
• Furosemide 2–4 mg/kg IV—often used first in patients with renal oliguria. Urinary flow should increase within 1 hour; if not, repeat at the same or double dosage. If diuresis ensues, administer to sustain diuresis (0.25–1 mg/kg/h or 2–4 mg/kg IV q8h). Reduction in glomerular filtration rate (GFR) may be seen with therapy.
• Mannitol 0.25–1 g/kg IV can be given as a 10% or 20% solution over 15–20 minutes. Urinary flow should increase within 1 hour. Do not repeat if diuresis does not ensue; may cause excessive volume expansion. If diuresis ensues, mannitol may be continued as continuous infusion (1–2 mg/kg/h) or intermittent IV doses (0.25–0.5 g/kg every 4–6 hours) to sustain diuresis. Avoid mannitol when overhydration, pulmonary edema, or congestive heart failure present.
• Fenoldopam 0.1–0.8 µg/kg/min, a selective dopamine A1 receptor antagonist, promotes diuresis in healthy animals and increases GFR in dogs. Evidence of efficacy in animals with renal disease is lacking.

CONTRAINDICATIONS

Nephrotoxic drugs.

PRECAUTIONS

• Administer fluids carefully to patients that are persistently oligoanuric to avoid overhydration. Do not continue to administer fluids to oligoanuric patients after their fluid volume deficit has been restored in the absence of a plan to prevent development of overhydration. In patients with unresponsive renal oliguria, peritoneal dialysis/hemodialysis may be required to correct iatrogenic fluid-induced volume overexpansion.
• Failure to correct fluid deficits before initiating diuretic administration may cause further renal hypoperfusion and ischemic renal injury.
• Use drugs requiring renal excretion with caution.
• Avoid electrolyte solutions containing >4 mEq of potassium/L. Some hypokalemic patients may require cautious administration of higher doses of potassium.
• Dopamine can cause arrhythmias, particularly in animals with hyperkalemia. Its use is no longer recommended.

POSSIBLE INTERACTIONS

Furosemide may promote the nephrotoxicity associated with aminoglycoside antibiotics.

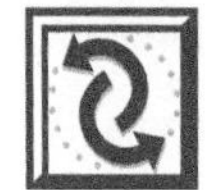

FOLLOW-UP

PATIENT MONITORING

• UOP—determine early during the course of management. When unclear, consider transurethral catheterization to accurately determine UOP. Place catheters using aseptic technique. Short indwelling time lowers the risk of UTI. Properly placed/managed indwelling catheters are usually safe for at least 48 hours. Use a closed, sterile drainage system.
• Creatinine, serum urea nitrogen, and potassium concentrations should be reevaluated q12–24 hours; patients with severe hyperkalemia need more frequent monitoring.
• ECG should be performed at appropriate intervals to assess cardiac effects of drugs and hyperkalemia and to monitor response to therapy.

PREVENTION/AVOIDANCE

• Avoid nephrotoxic drugs.
• Avoid dehydration and hypoperfusion.

POSSIBLE COMPLICATIONS

• Hyperkalemia and arrhythmia.
• Uremia.
• Dehydration.
• Overhydration.

EXPECTED COURSE AND PROGNOSIS

• Oliguria and anuria are poor prognostic signs in AKI or CKD; unless urine outflow can be corrected, survival is not expected.
• Anuria associated with UTO is often reversible if urethral patency is restored.

MISCELLANEOUS

SEE ALSO

• Acute Kidney Injury.
• Azotemia and Uremia.
• Chronic Kidney Disease.
• Hyperkalemia.
• Nephrotoxicity, Drug-Induced.
• Urinary Tract Obstruction.

ABBREVIATIONS

• ADH = antidiuretic hormone.
• AKI = acute kidney injury.
• CKD = chronic kidney disease.
• GFR = glomerular filtration rate.
• UOP = urine output.
• USG = urine specific gravity.
• UTI = urinary tract infection.
• UTO = urinary tract obstruction.

Suggested Reading

Cowgill LD, Langston C. Acute kidney disease. In: Bartges J, Polzin DJ, eds., Nephrology and Urology of Small Animals. Ames, IA: Wiley-Blackwell, 2011, pp. 472–523.

Ross L. Acute renal failure. In: Bonagura JD, Twedt DC, eds., Kirk's Current Veterinary Therapy XIV. St. Louis, MO: Saunders, 2009, pp. 879–882.

Author David J. Polzin
Consulting Editor J.D. Foster

O

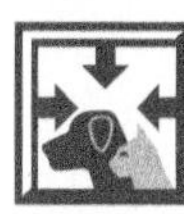

BASICS

OVERVIEW

- *Ollulanus* adult worms are found in stomach of cats.
- Infection causes chronic gastritis resulting in anorexia, vomiting, weight loss.
- No intermediate hosts required to complete lifecycle; transmission is mainly by contact with vomitus of infected cats.
- Eggs develop into larvae within female worm; released larvae may mature to adults without leaving stomach.

SIGNALMENT

- Colony cats—predisposed, probably because of access to other cats' vomitus.
- Stray cats living in urban areas heavily populated with cats—high incidence of infection.
- Captive cheetahs, lions, tigers, cougars—susceptible.

SIGNS

- Chronic vomiting, anorexia, weight loss.
- Death from chronic gastritis.

CAUSES & RISK FACTORS

- *Ollulanus tricuspis*—adults (only up to 1 mm in length) coil into gastric mucosa, causing superficial erosions.
- Over time, gastric erosions can become severe with marked inflammation, accumulation of lymphoid aggregates, and fibrous changes in mucosa and submucosa.
- Eggs—hatch within female worms; larvae develop to infective L3 larvae within stomach.
- L3 larvae and adults—vomited and infective to other cats; internal autoinfection also occurs.
- No fecal transmission known.
- Distributed throughout North America, Australia, New Zealand, Europe, Argentina, Chile.

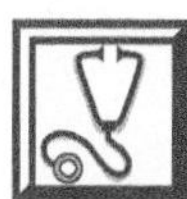

DIAGNOSIS

DIFFERENTIAL DIAGNOSIS

Other causes of vomiting including:

- Dietary.
- Intoxications.
- Metabolic—diabetes mellitus, renal disease, liver disease, acidosis, heat stroke, hypoadrenocorticism, hyperthyroidism.
- Gastric abnormalities—inflammatory bowel disease, neoplasia, obstruction, atrophic gastritis, ulcers, dilatation/volvulus, parasitic such as *Physaloptera*.
- Gastroesophageal junction disorders—hiatal hernia.
- Small intestinal disorders—inflammatory bowel disease, neoplasia, fungal, viral, obstruction, paralytic ileus.
- Large intestinal disorders—colitis, obstipation, inflammatory bowel disease.
- Abdominal disorders—pancreatitis, gastrinoma, peritonitis, steatitis, pyometra, diaphragmatic hernia, other neoplasia.
- Neurologic disorders—psychogenic, motion sickness, vestibular lesions, head trauma, neoplasia.
- Miscellaneous—heartworm disease and heart disease.

CBC/BIOCHEMISTRY/URINALYSIS

Reflects vomiting—dehydration, hypovolemia.

OTHER LABORATORY TESTS

- Baermann—examine vomitus for L3 larvae.
- Fecal examination, direct or flotation—larvae or eggs seldom found in feces as they are digested within the gastrointestinal tract.

IMAGING

Abdominal ultrasound—may show gastric thickening; rarely see parasites.

DIAGNOSTIC PROCEDURES

- View worms through an endoscope—difficult due to size of worms.
- Gastric lavage—using saline collection followed by centrifugation to precipitate L3 larvae, or use Baermann technique.
- Histopathology—gastric biopsy occasionally shows parasites.

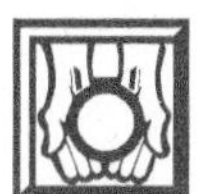

TREATMENT

Anthelmintic use is extra-label and anecdotal.

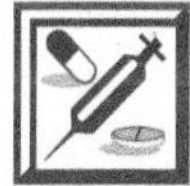

MEDICATIONS

DRUG(S) OF CHOICE

- Fenbendazole 50 mg/kg PO q24h for 5 days, oxfendazole 10 mg/kg q24h for 5 days, and pyrantel pamoate 10 mg/kg PO q24h for 3 days are recommended but there is little information available regarding treatment success.
- Tetramisole—give as a 2.5% formulation at 5 mg/kg PO once; effective but not available in the United States.

CONTRAINDICATIONS/POSSIBLE INTERACTIONS

Tetramisole—at this dose should not cause any side effects in cats.

FOLLOW-UP

Warn owner to watch for further vomiting—retreatment may be required.

MISCELLANEOUS

Ollulanus infection has been identified in a cat with concurrent gastric adenocarcinoma.

Suggested Reading

Barr SC, Bowman DD. *Ollulanus* infection. In: Canine and Feline Infectious Diseases and Parasitology. Ames, IA: Blackwell, 2006, pp. 385–387.

Bowman DD, Hendrix CM, Lindsay DS, et al. *Ollulanus tricuspis*. In: Feline Clinical Parasitology. Ames, IA: Iowa State University Press, 2002, pp. 262–265.

Cecchi R, Wills SJ, Dean R, et al. Demonstration of *Ollulanus tricuspis* in the stomach of domestic cats by biopsy. J Comp Pathol 2006, 134:374–377.

Dennis MM, Bennett N, Ehrhart EJ. Gastric adenocarcinoma and chronic gastritis in two related Persian cats. Vet Pathol 2006, 43:358–362.

Authors Matt Brewer and Jeba R.J. Jesudoss Chelladurai

Consulting Editor Amie Koenig

OPHTHALMIA NEONATORUM

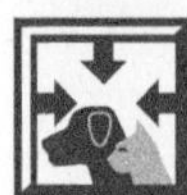

BASICS

OVERVIEW

- Infection of the conjunctiva and/or cornea before or just after the separation of the eyelids in the neonate.
- Occurs in puppies and kittens.
- Associated with *Staphylococcus* spp. or *Streptococcus* spp. in dogs and cats, and with herpesvirus in cats.
- Potentially vision threatening.
- Source of infection—believed to be from an intrauterine infection, a vaginal infection of the dam at the time of birth, or from a nonhygienic environment.

SIGNALMENT

- Affects all breeds of cats and dogs.
- Neonates before the time that the eyelids open (10–14 days postpartum).

O

SIGNS

- Upper and lower eyelid margins are fused (physiologic ankyloblepharon) and lids bulge outward because of the accumulation of debris and discharge within the conjunctival sac (Figure 1).
- Mucous to mucopurulent discharge may extrude through a patent opening at the medial canthus.
- Cornea and conjunctiva may be ulcerated.
- May note adhesions (symblepharon) of the conjunctiva to the cornea or to other areas of the conjunctiva (including that of the nictitans).
- Perforation of the cornea with iris prolapse and collapse of the globe is occasionally seen.

CAUSES & RISK FACTORS

- Intrauterine or vaginal infections in the dam near the time of birth.
- Unclean environment for the neonates.

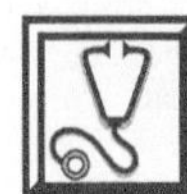

DIAGNOSIS

DIFFERENTIAL DIAGNOSIS

Neonates with entropion in which the eyelids have already separated—mucus to mucopurulent discharge may be present; view of the cornea may be obscured; may have appearance of ankyloblepharon; differentiated by age (patients older than 10–14 days) and ability to separate the eyelids.

CBC/BIOCHEMISTRY/URINALYSIS

Normal unless there is a concurrent systemic infection.

OTHER LABORATORY TESTS

- Cultures of neonate's ocular discharge and/or dam's vaginal discharge—may help diagnose bacterial infection and guide antibacterial therapy.
- Cytology of the affected tissues—may help diagnose bacterial infection and guide antibacterial therapy.
- Immunofluorescent antibody or PCR tests (cats)—feline herpesvirus.

IMAGING

N/A

DIAGNOSTIC PROCEDURES

- Full physical examination of the dam and neonate.
- Fluorescein staining—corneal or conjunctival ulceration.

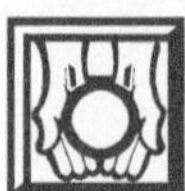

TREATMENT

- Separation of the eyelids—cornerstone of treatment; can be accomplished by careful massage and manual traction beginning at the medial canthus or introduction of a closed hemostat, small blunt scissor blade or the blunt, butt end of a scalpel blade into the patent opening or groove of the future lid fissure at the medial canthus and gently separating (not cutting) the eyelids.
- Lavage of conjunctival sac and cornea with warm saline or a 1:50 diluted povidone–iodine aqueous solution to remove the discharge.
- Warm compresses may aid in separating the eyelids and preventing readherence.
- Systemic support as needed.

MEDICATIONS

DRUG(S) OF CHOICE

- Broad-spectrum, topical antibiotics—e.g., neomycin/bacitracin/polymyxin B; applied 4 times daily for at least 1 week; antibiotic chosen on basis of bacterial culture and sensitivity, if available.
- Antiviral therapy in the case of herpesvirus infection in cats.

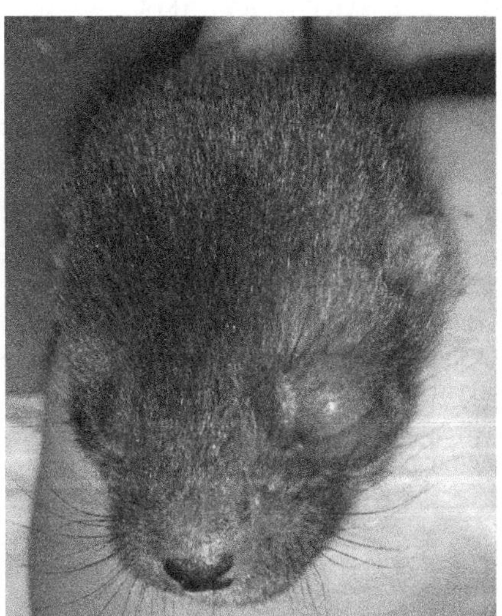

Figure 1.

Ophthalmia neonatorum. Typical outward-bulging lids due to accumulation of debris and discharge within the conjunctival sac. Source: Ophthalmology Section, Vetsuisse Faculty, University of Zurich.

CONTRAINDICATIONS/POSSIBLE INTERACTIONS

• Tetracyclines—do not use in neonates because of the risk of affecting bone or teeth; topical ofloxacin or ciprofloxacin is drug of choice for *Chlamydophila*.
• Topical corticosteroids—contraindicated.

FOLLOW-UP

PATIENT MONITORING

• Warm compresses—may be necessary for a few days to keep the eyelids from readhering.
• Topical antibiotics—continued for a minimum of 7 days.
• Observe littermates that are not initially affected.
• Treat vaginal infections in the dam with appropriate medications.

PREVENTION/AVOIDANCE

• Keep the external environment and the dam's nipples clean.
• Treat vaginal infection in the dam before delivery, if possible.

POSSIBLE COMPLICATIONS

• Severe keratitis with scarring and symblepharon.
• Rupture of the cornea with secondary phthisis; blindness may be irreversible.

EXPECTED COURSE AND PROGNOSIS

Favorable with correct and timely diagnosis and treatment and if no major complications occur.

MISCELLANEOUS

Suggested Reading

Stades FC, van der Woerdt A. Diseases and surgery of the canine eyelid. In: Gelatt KN, Gilger BC, Kern TJ, eds., Veterinary Ophthalmology, 5th ed. Ames, IA: Wiley Blackwell, 2013, pp. 832–893.

Author Simon A. Pot
Consulting Editor Kathern E. Myrna

OPIATES/OPIOIDS TOXICOSIS

BASICS

DEFINITION

- Opiates are derived from opium; opioids are synthetic.
- Opium was initially obtained from unripe seed capsules of the *Papaver somniferum* (poppy plant). Raw opium powder contains 24 alkaloids including ~10% morphine, 0.5% codeine, and thebaine (codeine methyl enol ether).
- Opioids have been used for millennia, but human use and abuse of opioids has drastically increased the last several years and has been increasing overall for the prior 20 years. This corresponds to an increase in accidental canine oral exposures.
- In dogs, opioids generally act as CNS, respiratory, and cardiovascular depressants, however thebaine has stimulatory properties.
- In cats, CNS stimulation often occurs following opioid toxicosis.
- Range of opioids and opiates includes:
  - Agonists—morphine, codeine, hydromorphone, oxycodone, fentanyl, heroin, desomorphine, alfentanil, tramadol (also a serotonin reuptake inhibitor), loperamide (relatively low concentrations achieved in the CNS).
  - Partial agonists or agonists/antagonists—butorphanol, buprenorphine.
- Toxic dose is highly variable depending on specific opioid. Cats have an increased susceptibility to morphine due to the lack of glucuronyl transferase and therefore glucuronidation.

PATHOPHYSIOLOGY

- Opioids are weakly acidic and well absorbed by oral and transmucosal route.
- Significant hepatic metabolism and first pass effect.
- Oral exposure to cut or chewed transdermal patches can result in increased and rapid absorption compared to that of the intended transdermal route. The amount of fentanyl remaining in used patches is highly variable and can be between 28 and 84%.
- Opioid receptors are found in the CNS, autonomic nervous system (ANS), gastrointestinal (GI) tract, heart, kidney, adipocytes, lymphocytes, vas deferens, and adrenal gland. The receptor types present and the clinical significance in toxicosis varies widely between tissue type.
- Major opioid receptors include:
  - mu—2 specific types. Agonist stimulation of mu_1 results in supraspinal analgesia while mu_2 results in spinal analgesia, respiratory suppression and decreased GI motility.
  - delta—equivocal role; possibly potentiates mu receptor agonists or has increased selectivity for enkephalins compared to mu receptors. Results in spinal analgesia and possibly decreased GI motility, decreased cardiovascular function, and altered behavior.
  - kappa—agonist stimulation results in analgesia, sedation, and dysphoria.
  - sigma—does not mediate analgesia significantly; no longer classified as an opioid receptor.
- Minor receptors include: epsilon and zeta.

SYSTEMS AFFECTED

- Respiratory—respiratory depression, hypoxia, apnea.
- Cardiovascular—bradycardia, hypotension, cardiovascular collapse, vasodilation, hypertension.
- Nervous—dog: CNS depression, ataxia, seizures, coma; cat: CNS stimulation, aggression, vocalization, ataxia.
- Gastrointestinal—vomiting, hypersalivation, ileus, constipation.
- Behavioral—aggression.
- Ophthalmic—miosis initially; mydriasis more commonly in cats and in dogs if hypoxia occurs.
- Hemic/lymphatic/immune—immune suppression reported in humans and potential in canines/felines with chronic exposures.
- Other—hypothermia, hyperthermia.

GENETICS

Dogs with the *MDR1/ABCB1* genetic mutation have an increased sensitivity to loperamide. Clinical signs may occur at approximately 0.06 mg/kg, compared to 0.65 mg/kg in dogs with no mutation.

INCIDENCE/PREVALENCE

- Opioid exposures are underreported by animal owners due to stigma and fear of law enforcement.
- Increased incidence of exposure among police or narcotic working dogs.

GEOGRAPHIC DISTRIBUTION

N/A

SIGNALMENT

Species

Dog and cat.

Breed Predilections

Collies, and other breeds prone to the *MDR1/ABCB1* gene mutation have a greater sensitivity to loperamide.

Mean Age and Range

Increased risk of exposure with puppies and younger adult dogs due to general increased incidence of dietary indiscretions.

SIGNS

- Dogs—analgesia, lethargy, ataxia, hypotension, bradycardia, arrhythmia, bradypnea, vomiting, ileus, early excitation and tachypnea, hypothermia, miosis, hypersalivation, defecation, cyanosis, coma.
- Cats—analgesia, CNS excitation, aggression, depression, hypotension, arrhythmia, seizures, mydriasis, ileus, bradypnea (tachypnea possible early), hypothermia, miosis, hyperthermia.

CAUSES

- Primarily dietary indiscretion of prescription medications or illicit opioids.
- Other possible exposures include iatrogenic exposure, malicious intent, and severe exposures in dogs that have been used to transport drugs illicitly ("pack dogs" or "mule dogs") where the packages have ruptured while inside the dog.

RISK FACTORS

- Access to opioids/opiates.
- Police or narcotic working dogs.

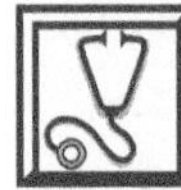

DIAGNOSIS

DIFFERENTIAL DIAGNOSIS

- Depressants—other possible intoxicants including benzodiazepines, barbiturates, marijuana/tetrahydrocannabinol (THC), rodenticide (bromethalin), ivermectin, alcohol, ethylene glycol, xylitol; trauma; infection (encephalitis); other causes of encephalopathy or hypoglycemia.
- Stimulants—amphetamines and amphetamine-like medications/drugs, cocaine, caffeine, metaldehyde, strychnine.

CBC/CHEMISTRY/URINALYSIS

No alterations expected directly from opioid exposure, though secondary alterations may occur depending on presence and degree of clinical signs.

OTHER LABORATORY TESTS

- Over-the-counter urine drug tests may have positive results following an exposure to opioids/opiates depending on the specific drug, dose ingested, and time frame. Possible false positives include rifampin, quinolone antibiotics, and poppy seeds.
- Serum or urine gas chromatography–mass spectrometry (GC/MS) or liquid chromatography tandem mass spectrometry (LC/MS-MS) may be performed, but results are unlikely to be available in a timely fashion to help guide treatment.

IMAGING

None

DIAGNOSTIC PROCEDURES

None

PATHOLOGIC FINDINGS

No specific findings.

TREATMENT

APPROPRIATE HEALTH CARE

- Inpatient vs. outpatient medical management depends largely on the dose ingested, time

frame, and clinical signs. Typically, inpatient medical management is recommended with a recent ingestion significantly above therapeutic doses (if available).
- For inpatient care, monitor for development or worsening of clinical signs and treat as needed. If there is severe respiratory depression, intubation and ventilation may be required and may necessitate transfer to a referral center depending on locally available facilities.

NURSING CARE

Monitor neurological status, temperature, respiratory rate, heart rate/electrocardiogram, blood pressure, hydration, and evidence of normal GI motility. Correct abnormalities as needed.

ACTIVITY

Prevent self-trauma while the patient has CNS depression or agitation.

DIET

Feed normally if the patient can protect their airway.

CLIENT EDUCATION

- Minimize potential future exposures.
- Keep medications/drugs out of reach of pets and pets away from gatherings where exposure is possible.

SURGICAL CONSIDERATIONS

If packets containing drugs have been surgically placed in a "pack dog" or ingested whole by a police or narcotic working dog, surgical removal of the intact packets is prudent.

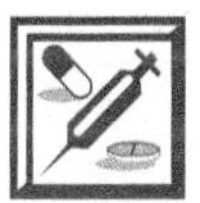

MEDICATIONS

DRUG(S) OF CHOICE

- Decontamination:
  - If asymptomatic, induce emesis in dogs within 1–2 hours post ingestion with apomorphine (0.03 mg/kg IV) or H_2O_2 (1 mL/kg PO first dose, 2 mL/kg (up to 50 mL) PO second dose if the dog does not vomit within 10–15 minutes). Do not induce emesis if there is risk of aspiration.
  - Gastric lavage may be performed within 1–2 hours of an ingestion if unable to induce emesis due to clinical signs or large dose was ingested.
- Activated charcoal with a cathartic (sorbitol) ×1 dose. Administer activated charcoal without a cathartic q6–8h × 2 additional doses for medications/drugs that undergo enterohepatic recirculation (e.g., morphine) or extended release products.
- IV fluids to maintain hydration and perfusion; adjust rate as needed based on cardiovascular and hydration status.
- Naloxone (reversal agent with a high affinity for the mu receptor) 0.01–0.04 mg/kg IV, IM, or SQ. Depending on response, may need to increase dose (0.1–0.2 mg/kg) to reach an effective dose in cats or with opioids such as buprenorphine that have a strong mu bonds and/or also bind the delta or kappa receptors. The duration of action is short (<2–3 hours in dogs; <1 hour in cats); redose as needed based on recurrence of clinical signs.
- Ileus—metoclopramide 0.1–0.5 mg/kg IM, SQ, PO q6h or 1–2 mg/kg/day IV CRI.
- Seizures—diazepam 0.5–1 mg/kg IV or phenobarbital 3–10 mg/kg IV to effect.

CONTRAINDICATIONS

None

PRECAUTIONS

Naloxone is not effective for reversing seizures resulting from meperidine, tramadol, or propoxyphene toxicosis.

POSSIBLE INTERACTIONS

None

ALTERNATIVE DRUG(S)

Butorphanol 0.05–0.1 mg/kg IV, IM PRN to partially reverse pure mu agonists.

FOLLOW-UP

PATIENT MONITORING

- Discharge when asymptomatic. No further monitoring is expected to be required if severe clinical signs such as persistent poor perfusion, hyperthermia, seizures did not occur.
- If severe signs occurred, secondary renal or hepatic elevations are possible (though unlikely), and ongoing monitoring is recommended as needed based on the clinical signs. Acute kidney injury may occur if there is prolonged hypotension present; hepatic and creatine kinase elevations with persistent seizures/hyperthermia.

PREVENTION/AVOIDANCE

- Minimize access for ingestion of opioids/opiates. Additional training, supervision, and use of basket muzzles for working police or narcotic dogs.
- Verify dose and concentration prior to administration of opioids therapeutically.

POSSIBLE COMPLICATIONS

- None routinely expected.
- Possibility for secondary complications in rare cases with severe clinical signs.

EXPECTED COURSE AND PROGNOSIS

Prognosis is dose dependent, though generally good if clinical signs are controlled.

MISCELLANEOUS

ASSOCIATED CONDITIONS

Potential for co-ingestion of other medications/drugs (illicit or prescription).

AGE-RELATED FACTORS

Neonatal patients may have an increased risk of CNS signs due to incomplete blood–brain barrier formation.

ZOONOTIC POTENTIAL

None

PREGNANCY/FERTILITY/BREEDING

Potential for exposure to fetus, embryos, and nursing young.

SYNONYMS

- Codeine—schoolboy, T-3.
- Desomorphine—krokodil.
- Fentanyl—cash, China white, tango, TNT.
- Heroin—brown sugar, H, hell dust, junk, smack, [black] tar.
- Morphine—M, Miss Emma, dreamer.

ABBREVIATIONS

- ANS = autonomic nervous system.
- GC/MS = gas chromatography–mass spectrometry.
- GI = gastrointestinal.
- LC/MS-MS = liquid chromatography tandem mass spectrometry.

Suggested Reading

Bischoff K. Toxicity of drugs of abuse. In: Veterinary Toxicology: Basic and Clinical Principles, 3rd ed. Hopkinsville, KY: Elsevier, 2018, pp. 385–408.

Volmer PA. "Recreational" drugs. In: Peterson ME, Talcott PA, eds., Small Animal Toxicology, 3rd ed. Philadelphia, PA: W.B. Saunders, 2012, pp. 309–335.

Author Sarah R. Alpert

Consulting Editor Lynn R. Hovda

OPTIC NEURITIS AND PAPILLEDEMA

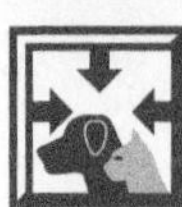

BASICS

DEFINITION

• Optic neuritis—inflammation of one or both optic nerves, resulting in reduction of visual function.
• Papilledema is edema of the optic nerve head that does not obviously affect the function of the optic nerve.

PATHOPHYSIOLOGY

• Optic neuritis may be a primary disease or secondary to CNS disease because the optic nerve communicates with the subarachnoid space.
• Papilledema occurs when intracranial pressure (ICP) is elevated.
• Papilledema may occur separately from optic neuritis.
• Optic neuritis may also feature papilledema.

SYSTEMS AFFECTED

• Nervous.
• Ophthalmic.

GENETICS

No genetic basis.

INCIDENCE/PREVALENCE

Occasional cause of blindness in dogs; rare in cats.

GEOGRAPHIC DISTRIBUTION

N/A

SIGNALMENT

Species

Dog and cat.

Breed Predilections

None

Mean Age and Range

Middle-aged.

Predominant Sex

None

SIGNS

Historical Findings

• Optic neuritis—acute blindness, may report other neurologic abnormalities such as ataxia, seizures, or behavior changes.
• Papilledema—no clinically detectable visual abnormalities but may report other neurologic abnormalities attributable to increased ICP.

Physical Examination Findings

• Optic neuritis—may be unilateral or bilateral; absent menace response, absent dazzle, mydriatic and nonresponsive pupil; may have anisocoria if unilaterally affected. Usually, the anterior segment appears normal, but hyperemia, congestion, and hemorrhages of the optic nerve head are seen. The retina surrounding the optic nerve may be detached; chorioretinitis can occur concurrently.
• Papilledema—usually bilateral, menace response is present, dazzle is present, normal pupillary light reflexes. The anterior segment appears normal, but there is swelling and elevation of optic nerve head with loss of the physiologic cup in the center of the optic nerve head. The retina usually appears normal.

CAUSES

Optic Neuritis

• Idiopathic (dogs).
• Systemic mycoses.
• Canine distemper (dogs).
• Feline infectious peritonitis (FIP) (cats).
• Neoplasia—primary or metastatic.
• Toxoplasmosis.
• *Neosporum caninum.*
• Granulomatous meningoencephalomyelitis.
• Ehrlichiosis.
• Orbital cellulitis.
• Hepatozoonosis.
• Toxicity—lead.
• Tick-borne encephalitis virus.

Papilledema

• CNS neoplasia (primary or metastatic).
• Hepatic encephalopathy.
• Hydrocephalus.
• Distemper (dogs).
• FIP (cats).
• Systemic mycoses.
• Toxoplasmosis.
• Granulomatous mengingoencephalitis.
• Trauma.

RISK FACTORS

None

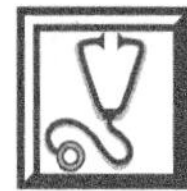

DIAGNOSIS

DIFFERENTIAL DIAGNOSIS

• Papilledema is differentiated from optic neuritis by the presence of normal pupillary light reflexes and no obvious visual deficits.
• Cortical blindness—normal pupillary light reflex; normal fundus examination; possibly other neurologic deficits; normal electroretinogram.
• Sudden acquired retinal degeneration syndrome (SARDS, dogs)—normal to absent pupillary light reflex; normal fundus (early in course); flat electroretinogram.

CBC/BIOCHEMISTRY/URINALYSIS

No specific abnormalities.

OTHER LABORATORY TESTS

Specific viral, protozoal, or fungal serologic tests as indicated.

IMAGING

Neuroimaging—MRI and/or CT may demonstrate intracranial disease.

DIAGNOSTIC PROCEDURES

• CSF analysis.
• Electroretinogram—investigate retinal function; normal in patients with optic neuritis and papilledema, flat in those with SARDS.
• Measure ICP.

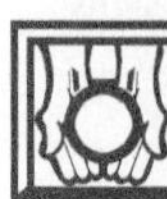

TREATMENT

APPROPRIATE HEALTH CARE

Inpatient—most cases will need to be hospitalized for workup and medical therapy depending on the primary disease process.

NURSING CARE

Depending on degree of neurologic impairment, special attention to patient cleanliness.

ACTIVITY

Activity may need to be restricted if visual deficits are present and depending on degree of neurologic impairment.

DIET

May need to be altered depending on degree of neurologic impairment.

CLIENT EDUCATION

Optic neuritis—important to emphasize that vision may not return, particularly in idiopathic cases, and treatment may be life-long (immunosuppressive therapy).

SURGICAL CONSIDERATIONS

Surgery infrequently indicated.

MEDICATIONS

DRUG(S) OF CHOICE

Optic Neuritis

• Depends on primary disease process when identifiable, treat any infectious process identified.
• Idiopathic—prednisone 2 mg/kg PO q12h for 14 days; then 1 mg/kg PO q12h for 14 days; then gradual reduction to maintenance dosage.

Papilledema

• Mannitol 1 g/kg IV over 20 minutes; repeated as necessary to treat elevated ICP.
• Hypertonic saline 3 mL/kg IV over 10 minutes as alternative therapy for elevated ICP.
• Corticosteroids—prednisone 0.5 mg/kg PO q12h or dexamethasone SP 0.025 mg/kg IV q12h; not indicated for head trauma.

CONTRAINDICATIONS

Immunosuppressive drugs may be contraindicated in patients where etiology is unknown.

PRECAUTIONS

Ensure patients receiving mannitol can urinate; immunosuppressive agents should be used cautiously in patients with infectious disease.

POSSIBLE INTERACTIONS

None

FOLLOW-UP

PATIENT MONITORING

Serial ophthalmic examinations should be performed, including fundic exam. Careful attention should be paid to visual deficits; resolution of deficits indicates improvement in disease, but may also reflect the patient's adaptation to vision loss, making client's reports of vision unreliable.

PREVENTION/AVOIDANCE

None

POSSIBLE COMPLICATIONS

- Optic neuritis—vision loss may be permanent.
- Papilledema—increased ICP may result in brain herniation if not treated emergently.

EXPECTED COURSE AND PROGNOSIS

- Optic neuritis—guarded to poor prognosis for return of vision, but idiopathic cases have good prognosis for life.
- Papilledema—guarded to poor prognosis for life.

MISCELLANEOUS

ASSOCIATED CONDITIONS

- Optic neuritis—chorioretinitis, CNS disease.
- Papilledema—CNS disease.

AGE-RELATED FACTORS

None

ZOONOTIC POTENTIAL

Zoonotic infectious CNS disease is rare.

PREGNANCY/FERTILITY/BREEDING

Infectious diseases such as canine distemper may be associated with fetal disease and congenital abnormalities.

ABBREVIATIONS

- FIP = feline infectious peritonitis.
- ICP = intracranial pressure.
- SARDS = sudden acquired retinal degeneration syndrome.

Suggested Reading

Montgomery KW, van der Woerdt A, Cottrill NB. Acute blindness in dogs: sudden acquired retinal degeneration syndrome versus neurological disease (140 cases, 2000–2006). Vet Ophthalmol 2008, 11:314–320.

Nell, B. Optic neuritis in dogs and cats. Vet Clin North Am Small Anim Pract 2008, 38:403–415.

Author Kathern E. Myrna

Consulting Editor Kathern E. Myrna

Acknowledgement The author/editor acknowledges the prior contribution of Amber L. Labelle.

ORAL CAVITY TUMORS, UNDIFFERENTIATED MALIGNANT TUMORS

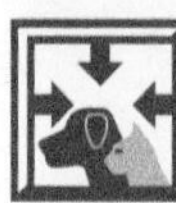

BASICS

OVERVIEW

- Uncommon, highly aggressive, rapidly growing tumor typically affecting the caudal maxilla and orbit of young dogs.
- Most are highly bone-invasive and are non-encapsulated with a smooth to slightly nodular surface (mistaken as benign); may become ulcerated.
- Biopsy—reveals undifferentiated malignancy of undetermined histogenesis.
- Highly metastatic—regional lymphatic spread and distant sites.
- Local disease often represents life-limiting issue despite the high metastatic propensity.

SIGNALMENT

- Dog.
- Primarily a disease of large breeds.
- All dogs <2 years old; range 6–22 months.
- No sex predilection reported.

O

SIGNS

Historical Findings

- Excessive salivation.
- Halitosis.
- Dysphagia.
- Hyporexia.
- Bloody oral discharge.
- Weight loss.

Physical Examination Findings

- Oral mass.
- Loose teeth.
- Facial deformity, exophthalmia.
- Regional lymphadenopathy.
- Pain upon palpating or opening the mouth.

CAUSES & RISK FACTORS

None identified.

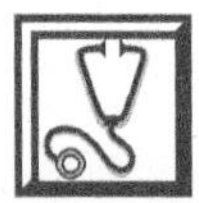

DIAGNOSIS

DIFFERENTIAL DIAGNOSIS

- Other aggressive oral malignancy such as oral melanoma, squamous cell carcinoma, or fibrosarcoma.
- Acanthomatous ameloblastoma/peripheral odontogenic fibroma.
- Foreign body reaction.
- Tooth root abscess.

CBC/BIOCHEMISTRY/URINALYSIS

Often normal.

OTHER LABORATORY TESTS

N/A

IMAGING

- High detail skull/dental radiography—evaluate for osteolytic changes.
- 3-view thoracic radiography—detect lung metastasis.
- Advanced sectional imaging (CT or MRI)—define local and regional/distant extent of disease, and facilitate therapeutic planning.

DIAGNOSTIC PROCEDURES

- Carefully palpate regional lymph nodes (mandibular, retropharyngeal, superficial cervical).
- Cytologic evaluation of primary tumor and regional lymph nodes may provide tentative diagnosis of malignancy.
- Large, deep-tissue biopsy required to differentiate from other oral malignancies.
- Fine-needle aspiration or biopsies of primary tumor should always be taken from inside the mouth, not through the overlying skin (could compromise local control with surgery).
- Histopathology consistent with an undifferentiated tumor without characteristic morphologic features of mesenchymal or epithelial origin.
- Immunocytochemistry (various markers) required to rule out other tumors, including rhabdomyosarcoma (aggressive tumor also seen in young dogs).

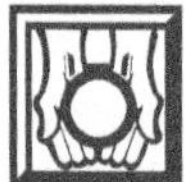

TREATMENT

Diet

Soft food recommended to prevent tumor ulceration or following radical oral excision.

Surgical Considerations

- Radical surgical excision—often ineffective because of extensive local disease or regional metastasis at diagnosis.
- If attempted, must have margins of at least 2 cm into normal bone and soft tissues and ideally be planned with the help of contrast-enhanced advanced sectional imaging.

Radiation Therapy

- Efficacy unreported.
- Undifferentiated tumors often poorly responsive to megavoltage radiation therapy.
- Considered for palliation (hypofractionated protocol).

MEDICATIONS

DRUG(S) OF CHOICE

- Chemotherapy—efficacy unreported; undifferentiated tumors often poorly responsive to systemic chemotherapy.
- Pain management with multimodal analgesic therapy is mandatory (nonsteroidal anti-inflammatory drug, opioid, adjuvant analgesic medications, aminobisphosphonate if osteolysis is present).

CONTRAINDICATIONS/POSSIBLE INTERACTIONS

Chemotherapy can be toxic; seek advice of a medical oncologist before initiating treatment if you are unfamiliar with cytotoxic drugs.

FOLLOW-UP

- Most dogs have detectable metastatic dissemination at diagnosis.
- Patients often euthanized within 30 days of diagnosis because tumor growth is progressive and uncontrolled, resulting in decreased quality of life and condition.

MISCELLANEOUS

Suggested Reading

Patnaik AL, Lieberman PH, Erlandson RA, et al. A clinicopathologic and ultrastructural study of undifferentiated malignant tumors of the oral cavity in dogs. Vet Pathol 1986, 23:170–175.

Author Matthew R. Berry

Consulting Editor Timothy M. Fan

Acknowledgment The author and editors acknowledge the prior contribution of Louis-Philippe de Lorimier.

ORBITAL DISEASES (EXOPHTHALMOS, ENOPHTHALMOS, STRABISMUS)

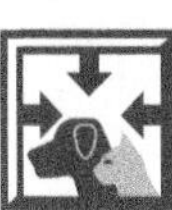

BASICS

DEFINITION

- Abnormal position of the globe.
- Exophthalmos—anterior displacement of the globe.
- Enophthalmos—posterior displacement of the globe.
- Strabismus—deviation of the globe from the correct position of fixation, which the patient cannot correct.

PATHOPHYSIOLOGY

- Orbit cannot be examined directly; orbital disease manifested by signs that alter the position, appearance, or function of the globe and adnexa.
- Malpositioned globe—caused by changes in volume (loss or gain) of the orbital contents or abnormal extraocular muscle function.
- Exophthalmos—caused by space-occupying lesions posterior to the equator of the globe.
- Enophthalmos—caused by loss of orbital volume, Horner's syndrome, or space-occupying lesions anterior to the equator of the globe.
- Strabismus—usually caused by an imbalance of extraocular muscle tone or lesions that restrict extraocular muscle mobility.

SYSTEMS AFFECTED

- Ophthalmic.
- Respiratory—because of proximity, the nasal cavity and frontal and maxillary sinuses may be involved.

SIGNALMENT

- Dog and cat.
- Orbital abscess or cellulitis and myositis—more common in young adult dogs.
- Myositis—predisposed breeds: German shepherd dog, golden retriever, Weimaraner.
- Orbital neoplasia—more common in middle-aged to old dogs.

SIGNS

Exophthalmos

- Secondary signs of space-occupying orbital disease.
- Difficulty in retropulsing the globe.
- Serous to mucopurulent ocular discharge.
- Chemosis.
- Eyelid swelling.
- Lagophthalmos—inability to close the eyelids over the cornea during blinking.
- Exposure keratitis—with or without ulceration.
- Pain on opening the mouth.
- Third eyelid protrusion due to extraconal mass or advanced intraconal mass.
- Visual impairment due to optic neuropathy.
- Fundic abnormalities, including retinal detachment, retinal vascular congestion, optic disc swelling.
- Focal inward deviation of the posterior globe.
- Neurotropic keratitis after damage to the ophthalmic branch of cranial nerve V.
- Fever and malaise—with orbital abscess or cellulitis.
- Intraocular pressure (IOP)—rarely high.

Enophthalmos

- Ptosis.
- Third eyelid protrusion.
- Extraocular muscle atrophy.
- Entropion—with severe disease.

Strabismus

- Deviation of one or both eyes from the normal position.
- May note exophthalmos or enophthalmos.

CAUSES

Exophthalmos

- Neoplasm—primary or secondary.
- Abscess or cellulitis—bacterial or fungal; fungal more likely in cats; look for foreign bodies:
  - Bacterial infections may be mixed; *Pasteurella multocida* and *Enterobacteriaceae* common.
- Zygomatic mucocele—not described in cats.
- Myositis—muscles of mastication or extraocular muscles (eosinophilic or extraocular polymyositis).
- Orbital hemorrhage secondary to trauma.
- Arteriovenous fistula or varix—rare.

Enophthalmos

- Ocular pain.
- Microphthalmia.
- Phthisis bulbi.
- Collapsed globe.
- Horner's syndrome.
- Dehydration.
- Loss of orbital fat or muscle.
- Conformational enophthalmos in dolichocephalic breeds.
- Neoplasia—especially if originating from rostral orbit.

Strabismus

- Abnormal innervation of extraocular muscle.
- Restriction of extraocular muscle mobility by scar tissue from previous trauma or inflammation.
- Destruction of extraocular muscle attachments after proptosis.
- Convergent strabismus—congenital; results from abnormal crossing of visual fibers in the CNS (Siamese cats).
- Shar-pei strabismus.

RISK FACTORS

Proptosis—more common in brachycephalic dogs with shallow orbits.

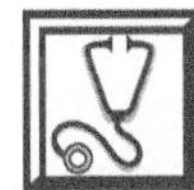

DIAGNOSIS

DIFFERENTIAL DIAGNOSIS

Similar Signs

- Buphthalmic globe—may simulate a space-occupying mass causing anterior displacement of the eye owing to its size in relationship to the orbital volume; IOP usually high; corneal diameter greater than normal, corneal edema, mydriatic pupil, optic nerve cupping (i.e., signs of glaucoma), blindness.
- Episcleritis—may cause severe diffuse or focal thickening of the fibrous tunic, imitating a buphthalmic globe; corneal edema; normal or low IOP; aqueous flare.

Causes

- Acute onset of exophthalmos—often with inflammatory orbital disease. Pain, especially on opening the mouth, is more likely inflammatory orbital disease than orbital neoplasia.
- Salivary mucoceles—more variable in speed of onset and degree of patient discomfort.
- Extraocular or eosinophilic myositis—bilateral diseases; *Neospora caninum* caused extraocular polymyositis in a litter of dogs.
- Neoplasia—usually slowly progressive, nonpainful, unilateral exophthalmos.

CBC/BIOCHEMISTRY/URINALYSIS

- Usually normal.
- Leukogram—may show inflammation (abscess, cellulitis, or myositis).
- Peripheral eosinophilia—occasionally seen in dogs with eosinophilic (masticatory muscle) myositis.

IMAGING

- Orbital ultrasonography, CT and MRI—define the extent of the lesion(s) and distinguish between types of myositis.
- Skull radiographs (especially of the frontal sinuses and nasal cavity).
- Thoracic radiographs—to identify metastatic disease.

DIAGNOSTIC PROCEDURES

- Lack of globe retropulsion—confirms space-occupying mass.
- Oral examination, ocular ultrasound, and fine-needle aspiration (FNA) of the orbit—may require anesthesia.
- FNA (18- to 20-gauge)—submit samples for aerobic and anaerobic bacterial cultures, Gram staining, and cytologic examination.
- Cytology—often diagnostic for abscess or cellulitis, zygomatic salivary gland mucocele, and neoplasia.
- Biopsy—indicated if FNA is nondiagnostic. Biopsy of masseter, temporal, or extraocular muscle if myositis suspected; assays for type 2M fibers may be helpful.
- Forced duction of the globe (strabismus)—grasp the conjunctiva with a fine pair of forceps following topical anesthesia; differentiates neurologic disease (globe moves freely) from restrictive condition (globe cannot be moved manually).

O

TREATMENT

Proptosis

See Proptosis.

Orbital Abscess or Cellulitis

- Drainage is seen in less than half of patients, usually because the lesion is just cellulitis and a true abscess has not yet formed.
- If an obvious swelling of the oral mucosa behind the last molar is not present and ultrasound does not show an abscess, it is best to avoid incising the oral mucosa and treat with systemic antibiotics and anti-inflammatory medications; the affected globe should also be kept moist with topical lubricants q6h.
- Severe cases may require IV fluids to restore and maintain hydration until patient is able to eat.
- If a swelling of the oral mucosa behind the last molar is evident, establish ventral orbital drainage:
  - Incise the surgically prepared mucosa approximately 1 cm behind the last molar.
  - Push blunt-tipped forceps (e.g., Kelly or Carmalt) into the orbital space and open; in general, advance the forceps until the abscess drains, to the level of the box lock, or until movement of the eye occurs with forceps opening.
  - Minimize retrobulbar trauma and optic nerve damage; use only blunt dissection; never cut or crush tissue.
  - Complications from aggressive dissection include damage to the optic and ciliary nerves.
  - Collect samples for bacterial culture and cytologic examination through this port.
- Feed soft food until globe is back in normal position and pain resolved.
- Hot packing—q6h; helps decrease swelling and cleans discharge.

Orbital Neoplasms

- Usually primary and malignant.
- Early exenteration or orbital exploratory surgery and mass debulking via a lateral approach to the orbit to save the globe are rational therapeutic choices.
- Adjunctive chemotherapy or radiotherapy—depending on neoplasm and extent of the lesion.
- Without adjunct therapy—survival is weeks to months if malignant (patients are usually presented late in the course of disease).
- Consultation with an oncologist is recommended once the diagnosis is made.

Zygomatic Mucocele

May resolve with antibiotic and corticosteroid administration; if not, surgical excision of the cyst and associated salivary gland is usually curative.

Strabismus

- Neurologic—Identify and treat the underlying cause, if possible.
- Restrictive or post-traumatic—may be treated surgically by repositioning or excising the attachments of extraocular muscles to relieve excessive tension on those muscles; usually a very difficult procedure.

MEDICATIONS

DRUG(S) OF CHOICE

- Exophthalmos (all patients)—lubricate cornea with artificial tear ointment or gel, q6h, to prevent desiccation and ulceration.
- Corneal ulceration—topical antibiotic (e.g., bacitracin, neomycin, polymyxin, q8h) and cycloplegic (e.g., 1% atropine, q12–24h), to prevent infection and reduce ciliary spasm, respectively.

Orbital Abscess or Cellulitis

- Oral or IV antibiotics—ampicillin 20 mg/kg q8h ×2–3 weeks or drugs with an anaerobic spectrum (amoxicillin with clavulanic acid or clindamycin) should be considered while awaiting results of bacterial culture and cytologic examination, or if client declines diagnostic testing.
- Fluconazole 2.5 mg/kg PO q12h or 5 mg/kg PO q24h or posaconazole 5 mg/kg PO q12h for orbital aspergillosis.
- Prednisone 1 mg/kg SC, IM q24h, once, to minimize optic neuritis and reduce orbital swelling and globe exposure (severe cases).
- Nonsteroidal anti-inflammatory drugs can be used in place of prednisone and administered for a longer period.

Acute Myositis

- Difficult prehension—systemic corticosteroids (prednisone 2 mg/kg SC, IM), then oral (prednisone 2 mg/kg q24h) for 4–6 weeks until swelling subsides; then taper.
- Azathioprine 1–2 mg/kg PO q24h for 3–7 days then q48h and taper, with or without corticosteroids. May be used chronically to manage recurrent disease.

PRECAUTIONS

- Systemic corticosteroids—extreme caution with deep fungal orbital disease.
- Azathioprine—may be hepatotoxic and cause myelosuppression. Follow CBC and liver enzyme activities every 1–2 weeks for 8 weeks, then periodically.

FOLLOW-UP

PATIENT MONITORING

- Inflammatory orbital disease—examine at least weekly until clinical signs abate.
- Advise client to watch for recurrence of signs, especially if an orbital foreign body likely.
- Treat fungal infections for 60 days after signs resolve.

POSSIBLE COMPLICATIONS

- Vision loss.
- Loss of the eye.
- Permanent malposition of the globe.
- Death.

MISCELLANEOUS

AGE-RELATED FACTORS

Give a course of antibiotic therapy first prior to attempting ventral orbital drainage.

PREGNANCY/FERTILITY/BREEDING

Avoid systemic corticosteroids, antifungals, and azathioprine in pregnant animals.

SEE ALSO

- Proptosis.
- Red Eye.

ABBREVIATIONS

- FNA = fine-needle aspiration.
- IOP = intraocular pressure.

Suggested Reading

Miller PE. Orbit. In: Maggs DJ, Miller PE, Ofri R, eds., Slatter's Fundamentals of Veterinary Ophthalmology, 5th ed. St. Louis, MO: Elsevier, 2013, pp. 352–373.

Author Kathern E. Myrna

Consulting Editor Kathern E. Myrna

O

ORGANOPHOSPHORUS AND CARBAMATE TOXICOSIS

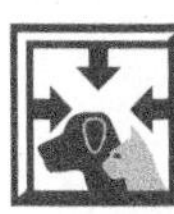

BASICS

DEFINITION

- Results from exposure to organophosphorus compounds or carbamates.
- Calls to the American Society for the Prevention of Cruelty to Animals (ASPCA) Animal Poison Control Center (APCC) regarding exposure to organophosphorus compounds continue to decrease. In 2017, organophosphate and carbamate exposures represented only 2.2% of insecticide-related exposure calls..
- The decrease is likely related to EPA cancellations of various registrations and approval of new, less hazardous compounds and delivery formulations. Canceled products, however, often remain in homes and businesses for years. In 2017 the most commonly reported exposures from most to least were to products containing propoxur, acephate, carbaryl, and tetrachlorvinphos.
- Animal products—organophosphate: chlorpyrifos, coumaphos, cythioate, diazinon, famphur, fenthion, phosmet, and tetrachlorvinphos; carbamate: carbaryl and propoxur. (Many animal products containing phosmet, tetrachlorvinphos, carbaryl, chlorpyrifos, diazinon [all] have been discontinued.)
- Agricultural, lawn, and garden products—organophosphate: acephate, chlorpyrifos, diazinon, disulfoton, fonofos, malathion, parathion, terbufos, and others; carbamate: carbofuran and methomyl. (Same comment as above for environmental products.)

PATHOPHYSIOLOGY

- Cause nervous system effects by inhibiting cholinesterase, which includes acetylcholinesterase, pseudocholinesterase, other esterases.
- Acetylcholinesterase—normally hydrolyzes the neurotransmitter acetylcholine in nervous tissue, red blood cells, and muscle, resulting in termination of nervous transmission.
- Pseudocholinesterase—found in plasma, liver, pancreas, nervous tissue; mainly in cats.
- Cholinesterase inhibition—allows acetylcholine accumulation at the postsynaptic receptor; causes stimulation of effector organs; spontaneous reactivation after organophosphorus compound binding is very slow and once aging occurs is virtually nonexistent; reversible after carbamate binding.

SYSTEMS AFFECTED

Nervous—results from overriding stimulation of parasympathetic pathways; may also result from sympathetic stimulation; acetylcholine stimulates nicotinic receptors of the somatic nervous system (skeletal muscle), parasympathetic preganglionic nicotinic and postganglionic muscarinic receptors (cardiac muscle, pupil, blood vessels, smooth muscles in lung and gastrointestinal tract, exocrine glands), and sympathetic preganglionic nicotinic receptors (adrenal and indirectly cardiac muscle, pupil, blood vessels, smooth muscles in lung and gastrointestinal tract, exocrine glands).

GENETICS

- Animals with inherently low cholinesterase activity—more susceptible to cholinesterase depression.
- Cholinesterase activity—more easily inhibited in cats than in dogs.

INCIDENCE/PREVALENCE

Uncommon in small animals.

GEOGRAPHIC DISTRIBUTION

Historically more common in areas of high flea prevalence and intense agricultural activity.

SIGNALMENT

Species

- Dog and cat.
- Cats most susceptible.

Breed Predilections

Lean dogs (e.g., sight hounds and racing breeds) and lean longhaired cats—more susceptible to cholinesterase inhibition because of lack of fat; many organophosphorus compounds and metabolites are stored in fat and slowly released into circulation.

Mean Age and Range

Young animals—more likely intoxicated due to lower detoxification capability.

Predominant Sex

Intact males more susceptible to some organophosphates.

SIGNS

General Comments

- Parasympathetic stimulation—usually predominates.
- Sympathetic stimulation—may result in lack of specific expected signs; may note signs opposite from expected.

Historical Findings

- Medical history—often discloses heavy or repeated applications of flea and tick insecticides; evidence of exposure to an agricultural or home and garden product.
- Carbamate insecticides (methomyl and carbofuran)—may cause rapid onset of seizures, respiratory failure, and death; treat aggressively without delay.
- Organophosphate insecticides (cats, especially chlorpyrifos)—chronic anorexia, muscle weakness and twitching, with or without episodes of acute toxicosis; may last days to weeks.

Physical Examination Findings

- Hypersalivation.
- Vomiting.
- Diarrhea.
- Miosis.
- Bradycardia.
- Depression.
- Ataxia.
- Muscle tremors.
- Seizures.
- Hyperthermia.
- Dyspnea.
- Respiratory failure.
- Death.
- Patient may not exhibit all signs.
- Sympathetic stimulation—signs reversed.

CAUSES

- Overuse, misuse, or use of multiple cholinesterase-inhibiting insecticides.
- Misuse of organophosphate insecticides in cats (e.g., organophosphate-containing dips labeled for dogs only, inappropriately applied to cats).
- Intentional dermal application of house or yard insecticides.

RISK FACTORS

- Concurrent exposure to multiple products containing organophosphate and/or carbamate.
- Exposure to floors that are damp with organophosphorus premise products.
- Incorrect dilution of insecticides.

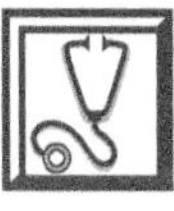

DIAGNOSIS

DIFFERENTIAL DIAGNOSIS

- Exposure to other insecticidal products—pyrethrin/pyrethroids (flea and tick); d-limonene (citrus flea and tick); fipronil (flea and tick); imidacloprid (flea).
- Other pesticides—strychnine; fluoroacetate (1080); 4-aminopyridine (avicide); metaldehyde (snail bait); zinc/aluminum phosphide (rodenticide); bromethalin (rodenticide).
- Other toxicants—chocolate; caffeine; cocaine; amphetamine; tremorgenic mycotoxins.

CBC/BIOCHEMISTRY/URINALYSIS

N/A

OTHER LABORATORY TESTS

Cholinesterase Activity

- Reduced to <25% of normal in whole blood, retina, or brain—suggests exposure to a cholinesterase-inhibiting compound; must compare to normal reference values in that species generated by the same laboratory.
- Test results—must be interpreted in context of the amount of exposure and the clinical signs and the time of their onset.
- Use laboratories experienced in handling animal samples.
- Chlorpyrifos—experimentally exposed animals may remain clinically normal with no detectable cholinesterase activity.

O

- Carbamate inhibition—reactivation can occur during sample transport, storage, and testing, giving false-negative results.

DIAGNOSTIC PROCEDURES

- Atropine response test—administer atropine at pre-anesthetic dose (0.02 mg/kg IV). Antimuscarinic response (tachycardia, mydriasis) suggests lack of anticholinesterase exposure.
- Detection of insecticides—tissue (e.g., brain, liver, kidney, and fat); stomach contents; gastrointestinal tract; fur or hair; negative results do not rule out toxicosis.
- May find pieces of chewed containers in the gastrointestinal tract.

PATHOLOGIC FINDINGS

- Histopathologic lesions—rare, no characteristic lesions likely in acute toxicosis.
- Delayed neuropathy—not usually associated with commercially available organophosphorus compounds.

O

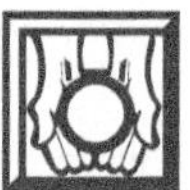

TREATMENT

APPROPRIATE HEALTH CARE

- Outpatient—mild signs from exposure to flea and tick collars and powders; treat by removing the collar or brushing excess powder from the coat.
- Inpatient—continued salivation, tremors, or dyspnea.

NURSING CARE

- Basics—stabilization; decontamination; antidotal treatment with atropine (and pralidoxime chloride for organophosphate toxicosis); supportive care.
- Control seizure activity, tremors.
- Oxygen—if necessary, until respiration returns to normal.
- Fluid therapy—may be needed in anorexic cats and dehydrated animals.
- Bathing (dermal exposure)—use hand dish-washing detergent; rinse with copious amounts of water.

DIET

Chronically anorexic cats—maintain nutritional and fluid requirements.

CLIENT EDUCATION

- Stress the importance of following insecticide label directions.
- Caution client that cats with chronic anorexia and weakness may need days to weeks of supportive care for full recovery.

MEDICATIONS

DRUG(S) OF CHOICE

- Emesis:
  - Ingestion of liquid insecticidal solution—avoid inducing emesis; risk of aspiration because many solutions contain hydrocarbon solvents.
  - Liquid solvent *not* ingested, no clinical signs, and very recent ingestion—induce emesis with 3% hydrogen peroxide (2.2 mL/kg PO to a maximum of 45 mL) after feeding a moist meal.
- Activated charcoal:
  - Evacuation of the stomach for patient with clinical signs—gastric lavage with the patient intubated, under anesthesia, with a large-bore stomach tube; then administration of activated charcoal (2 g/kg PO) containing sorbitol as a cathartic in a water slurry.
  - Diarrhea—do not administer sorbitol-containing products.
- Diazepam (0.5–1 mg/kg IV to effect) used initially for seizures. Pentobarbital (5–15 mg/kg IV to effect) added for persistent seizure activity. Phenobarbital (3–30 mg/kg IV to effect, low dosage in cats), propofol (3–6 mg/kg IV or 0.1 mg/kg/min CRI) or levetiracetam (30–60 mg/kg slow IV bolus in dogs; 20 mg/kg IV in cats) can be used for refractory seizures.
- Atropine sulfate—0.2 mg/kg one-quarter IV, remaining SC, as needed; administered immediately; repeated only as needed to control life-threatening clinical signs from muscarinic stimulation.
- Pralidoxime chloride (Protopam) 10–15 mg/kg IM, SC q8–12h until recovery; discontinue after 3 doses if no response; reduces muscle fasciculations; most beneficial against organophosphorus insecticides when started within 24 hours of exposure; even several days after dermal exposure may stimulate anorexic cats (with or without tremors) to resume eating; if refrigerated and wrapped in foil, reconstituted bottles may be successfully used for up to 2 weeks.

CONTRAINDICATIONS

Phenothiazine tranquilizers may potentiate organophosphate toxicosis.

PRECAUTIONS

Atropine—avoid overuse; may cause tachycardia, CNS stimulation, seizures, disorientation, drowsiness, and respiratory depression.

POSSIBLE INTERACTIONS

N/A

ALTERNATIVE DRUG(S)

N/A

FOLLOW-UP

PATIENT MONITORING

Monitor heart rate, respiration, and fluid and caloric intake.

PREVENTION/AVOIDANCE

- Follow directions on insecticide labels closely.
- Avoid use on sick or debilitated animals.
- Avoid simultaneous use of organophosphate and carbamate products.

POSSIBLE COMPLICATIONS

N/A

EXPECTED COURSE AND PROGNOSIS

- Chronic organophosphate insecticide-induced weakness and anorexia (cats, chlorpyrifos exposure)—may last 2–4 weeks; most patients fully recover with aggressive nursing care.
- Acute toxicosis treated promptly—good prognosis.

MISCELLANEOUS

ASSOCIATED CONDITIONS

N/A

AGE-RELATED FACTORS

Young animals have lower detoxification ability.

ZOONOTIC POTENTIAL

None

PREGNANCY/FERTILITY/BREEDING

N/A

SEE ALSO

Poisoning (Intoxication) Therapy.

ABBREVIATIONS

- APCC = Animal Poison Control Center.
- ASPCA = American Society for the Prevention of Cruelty to Animals.

Suggested Reading

Fikes JD. Organophosphate and carbamate insecticides. Vet Clin North Am Small Anim Pract 1990, 20:353–367.

Means C. Organophosphate and carbamate insecticides. In: Peterson ME, Talcott PA, eds., Small Animal Toxicology, 3rd ed. St. Louis, MO: Elsevier, 2013, pp. 715–723.

Authors Steven R. Hansen and Elizabeth A. Curry-Galvin

Consulting Editor Lynn R. Hovda

Client Education Handout available online

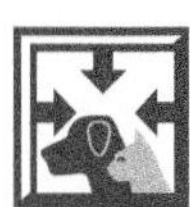

BASICS

OVERVIEW

- An oronasal fistula is an abnormal connection between the oral and nasal cavities.
- which can occur from pathology of any of the tissues surrounding the maxillary teeth or hard palate.
- The maxillary canines are most commonly involved.
- The palatal root of the maxillary fourth premolar is the next most common area involved.

SIGNALMENT

- Dogs—dolichocephalic head types are affected most often, especially dachshunds.
- Cats—rare

SIGNS

- Chronic rhinitis—with or without blood.
- Sneezing—common, especially when the maxillary canines are digitally palpated.

CAUSES & RISK FACTORS

- Usually associated with advanced-periodontitis (PD4) of the maxillary canine tooth, leading to destruction of the bone separating the nasal and oral cavities.
- Other causes include trauma, penetration of a foreign body, bite wounds, traumatic tooth extraction, electrical shock, or oral cancer.
- Fistula width can be related to the size of the tooth affected; fistula depth to the chronicity of the periodontal infection.
- Dogs with lingually displaced (mesioverted) mandibular canines, mandibular distoclusion (overbite) resulting in penetration of the hard palate are predisposed to oronasal fistulas.
- Dachshunds predisposed.

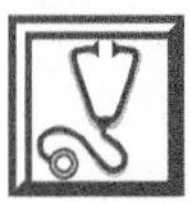

DIAGNOSIS

DIFFERENTIAL DIAGNOSIS

- Periodontal disease.
- Oral neoplasia.
- Trauma.
- Foreign body penetration.

CBC/BIOCHEMISTRY/URINALYSIS

N/A

OTHER LABORATORY TESTS

N/A

IMAGING

- Skull radiographs rarely helpful in diagnosing oronasal fistula because the lesions are generally isolated to the palatal surface.
- Intraoral radiographs are highly recommended to evaluate the periodontal status of the patient's teeth.
- Radiographs may show foreign body entrapment or lysis consistent with neoplasia.

DIAGNOSTIC PROCEDURES

Periodontal probing—results in direct extension into the nasal cavity or epistaxis in cases of oronasal fistula. Periodontal probing will also identify areas where significant palatal defects are present which can be treated to help prevent the occurrence of oronasal fistulas.

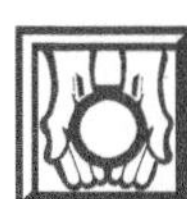

TREATMENT

- Extract the tooth and close the defect; after extraction, the goal of surgical closure is to place an epithelial layer in both the oral and nasal cavities.
- Full-thickness flap—after tooth extraction, a mucoperiosteal pedicle flap may be elevated from the dorsal aspect of the fistula, released, advanced to cover the defect, and sutured in place; a successful full-thickness flap requires at least 2 mm attached gingiva above the defect, with sutures at the edge of the defect (not over the void), without tension on the suture line.
- Double reposition flap—used for large fistulas or repair failures where no attached gingiva remains or where periosteal tissue cannot be included; after extraction, the first flap is harvested from the hard palate and inverted so that the oral epithelium is toward the nasal passage; the second flap is mucobuccal and harvested from the alveolar mucosa and underside of the lip rostral to the fistula; it is sutured over the first flap and donor site.
- Guided tissue regeneration of the maxillary canine—may be used for repair of a deep palatal pocket if not yet fistulated; a palatal flap is elevated to approach the infrabony defect; soft tissue and calculus are removed from the defect with a curette.
- In deep, infrabony pockets before fistulation, bone grafts such as PerioGlas, Consil, synthetic and natural hydroxyapatite, autogenous and heterologous bone, polylactic acid, and Osteoallograft (freeze-dried canine cadaver bone) have been used to exclude regrowth of gingival connective tissue and epithelium, promoting regeneration of bone and periodontal ligament. Implant materials should not be used if an oronasal fistula is present.
- Ear cartilage has been used as a membrane to cover the defect before closure.
- Oroantral fistulas located in the central portion of the hard palate may be surgically repaired with a transposition flap of the hard palate mucoperiosteum from tissue adjacent to the defect.

MEDICATIONS

DRUG(S) OF CHOICE

N/A

CONTRAINDICATIONS/POSSIBLE INTERACTIONS

N/A

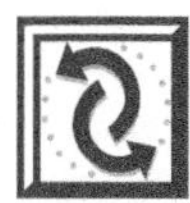

FOLLOW-UP

PATIENT MONITORING

Normal postoperative monitoring.

EXPECTED COURSE AND PROGNOSIS

Even with adequate tissue, excellent release of tension on the flap, and good technique, a persistent opening may occur due to constant tension on the site during each breath. With inadequate tissue or technique, the prognosis decreases, and additional surgeries with advanced flaps may be required.

MISCELLANEOUS

INTERNET RESOURCES

https://avdc.org/avdc-nomenclature/

Suggested Reading

Bellows JE, Small Animal Dental Equipment and Techniques 2nd ed, Ames, IA: Wiley Blackwell, 2019.

Lorrain RP, Legendre LF. Oronasal fistula repair using auricular cartilage. J Vet Dent 2012, 29(3):172–175.

Author Jan Bellows

Consulting Editor Heidi B. Lobprise

OSTEOCHONDRODYSPLASIA

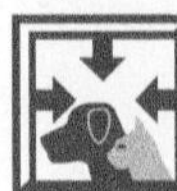

BASICS

OVERVIEW

• A developmental abnormality of cartilage and bone; encompasses many disorders involving bone growth. • Results from abnormal endochondral ossification.
• Skeletal defects—usually involve the appendicular skeleton; specifically the metaphyseal growth plates.
• Achondroplasia—failure of cartilage growth; characterized by a proportionate short-limbed dysplasia; evident soon after birth.
• Hypochondrodysplasia—less severe form of achondrodysplasia. • Characteristic breeds—result of selection of certain desirable traits. • Affects musculoskeletal and possibly ophthalmic systems.

SIGNALMENT

• Achondroplastic breeds—bulldog; Boston terrier; pug; Pekingese; Japanese spaniel; shih tzu.
• Hypochondroplastic breeds—dachshund; basset hound; beagle; Welsh corgi; Dandie Dinmont terrier; Scottish terrier; Skye terrier.
• Reported nonselected chondrodysplastic abnormalities—Alaskan Malamute; Samoyed; Labrador retriever; English pointer; Norwegian elkhound; Great Pyrenees; cocker spaniel; Scottish terrier; Scottish deerhound; beagle; miniature poodle; French bulldog; Scottish fold cat.
• Oculoskeletal dysplasia—diagnosed in Labrador retriever and Samoyed.

O

SIGNS

Historical Findings

Phenotypically normal at birth, retardation of growth recognized in first few months of life.

Physical Examination Findings

• Usually affects the appendicular skeleton; may affect axial skeleton. • Long bones—appear shorter than normal; often bowed.
• Major joints (elbow, stifle, carpus, tarsus)—appear enlarged. • Radius and ulna—often severely affected owing to asynchronous growth. • Lateral bowing of the forelimbs.
• Enlarged carpal joints. • Valgus deformity of the paws. • Shortened maxilla—relative mandibular prognathism. • Spinal deviations—due to vertebral abnormalities (hemi, wedge, block, transitional, etc.). • Retina—dysplasia; partial to complete detachment.

CAUSES & RISK FACTORS

• Achondrodysplastic and hypochondrodysplastic breeds—autosomal dominant trait.
• Nonselected chondrodysplastic breeds—autosomal recessive or polygenic trait.
• Littermates often affected. • Congenital hypothyroidism. • Autosomal incomplete dominant trait in Scottish folds.

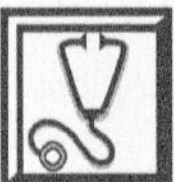

DIAGNOSIS

DIFFERENTIAL DIAGNOSIS

• Premature closure of the ulnar or radial physes—history of trauma; no other bones affected; unilateral or bilateral abnormalities.
• Pituitary dwarfism.

IMAGING

• Radiography of affected limbs—irregular flattening of the metaphysis; stippled appearance of epiphyses; widening of the physeal line; retained endochondral cores; irregularities in ossification of the affected long bone; degenerative joint disease and joint laxity owing to abnormal stress and weightbearing on the limbs. • Radiography of the spine—hemivertebrae; wedge-shaped vertebrae. Tail/caudal vertebrae—bony proliferation, shortened and malformed, reduced intervertebral spaces.

DIAGNOSTIC PROCEDURES

Bone biopsy of growth plate—definitive diagnosis.

PATHOLOGIC FINDINGS

Histologic findings—disorganization of the proliferative zone, abnormalities within the hypertrophic zone, abnormal formation of the primary and secondary spongiosa.

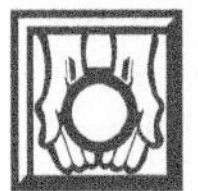

TREATMENT

• Achondrodysplasia—considered a normal abnormality in some (chondrodystrophic) breeds.
• Surgery—usually of little benefit for nonselected chondrodysplasia. • Corrective osteotomy to realign limb(s) or joint(s)—may have limited benefit. • Radiation therapy—pain relief for long periods in Scottish folds.

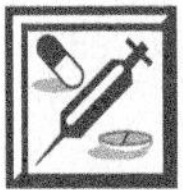

MEDICATIONS

DRUG(S) OF CHOICE

• Analgesics and anti-inflammatory agents—palliative use warranted. ○ Carprofen 2.2 mg/kg PO q12h or q24h. ○ Deracoxib 1–2 mg/kg PO q24h. ○ Firocoxib 5 mg/kg PO q24h. ○ Gabapentin 10–20 mg/kg PO q8h. ○ Gapiprant 2 mg/kg/day PO. ○ Meloxicam (load 0.2 mg/kg PO, then 0.1 mg/kg PO q24h—liquid). ○ Tramadol 4–10 mg/kg PO q8–12h. • Chondroprotective agents—polysulfated glycosaminoglycans, glucosamine, and chondroitin sulfate; may have limited benefit in preventing articular cartilage changes.

FOLLOW-UP

PREVENTION/AVOIDANCE

• Do not repeat dam–sire breedings that resulted in affected offspring. • Discourage breeding affected animals.

POSSIBLE COMPLICATIONS

Intra-articular and periarticular joint structures—degenerate owing to abnormal conformation of the appendicular skeleton; leads to altered biomechanics; results in poor quality of life.

MISCELLANEOUS

SYNONYMS

• Cherubism, • Dwarfism.

ABBREVIATIONS

• NSAID = nonsteroidal anti-inflammatory drug.

Suggested Reading

Franch J, Font J, Ramis A, et al. Multiple cartilaginous exostosis in a Golden retriever cross-bred puppy: clinical, radiographic and backscattered scanning microscopy findings. Vet Comp Orthop Traumatol 2005, 18(3):189–193.

Horton WA. The evolving definition of a chondrodysplasia. Pediatr Pathol Mol Med 2003, 22(1):47–52.

Jacobson LS, Kirberger RM. Canine multiple cartilaginous exostoses: unusual manifestations and a review of the literature. J Am Anim Hosp Assoc 1996, 32(1):45–51.

Kyostila K, Lappalainen KS, Lohi H. Canine chondrodysplasia caused by a truncating mutation in collagen-binding integrin alpha subunit 10. PLoS ONE 2013, 8(9):e75621.

Malik R, Allan GS, Howlett CR, et al. Osteochondrodysplasia in Scottish Fold cats. Aust Vet J 1999, 77(2):85–92.

Martinez S, Fajardo R, Valdes J, et al. Histopathologic study of long-bone growth plates confirms the basset hound as an osteochondrodysplastic breed. Can J Vet Res 2007, 71(1):66–69.

Neff MW, Beck JS, Koeman JM, et al. Partial deletion of the sulfate transporter *SLC13A1* is associated with an osteochondrodysplasia in the miniature poodle breed. PLoS ONE 2012, 7(12):e51917.

Rorvik AM, Teige J, Ottesen N, Lingass F. Clinical, radiographic, and pathologic abnormalities in dogs with multiple epiphyseal dysplasia: 19 cases (1991–2005). J Am Vet Med Assoc 2008, 233:600–606.

Authors Annika Sundby and Wesley J. Roach

Consulting Editor Mathieu M. Glassman

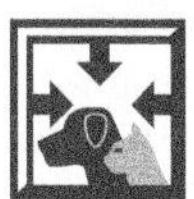

BASICS

DEFINITION

A pathologic process in growing cartilage, primarily characterized by a disturbance of endochondral ossification that leads to excessive retention of cartilage.

PATHOPHYSIOLOGY

- Cells of the immature articular joint cartilage and growth plates do not differentiate normally.
- For articular cartilage, the process of endochondral ossification is retarded, presumably due to localized, focal disruption of blood supply. If blood supply is reestablished, healing occurs. Alternatively, if blood supply is not reestablished, cartilage remains thick and there is separation between the cartilage and subchondral bone. Eventually a fissure occurs through the articular cartilage that allows communication with the joint cavity. The result is creation of a cartilage flap that is separated from the underlying subchondral bone; this condition is known as osteochondritis dissecans (OCD).
- Bilateral disease common.
- Most commonly affected joints—shoulder (caudocentral humeral head); elbow (medial aspect of the humeral condyle); stifle (femoral condyle, lateral more often than medial); hock (ridge of the talus, medial more common than lateral).
- Other reported locations—femoral head; dorsal rim of the acetabulum; glenoid cavity (scapula); patella; distal radius; medial malleolus; cranial end plate of the sacrum; vertebral articular facets; cervical vertebrae.

Immature Joint Cartilage

- Thickened cartilage results in impaired metabolism, leading to degeneration and necrosis of the poorly supplied cells.
- Fissure within the thickened cartilage—may result from mechanical stress; eventually leads to the formation of a cartilage flap or OCD; may cause lameness.
- Lameness (pain)—usually becomes evident once OCD develops; osteochondrosis is often asymptomatic.

Retention of Cartilage in Growth Plates

- Usually does not lead to necrosis, probably owing to nutrition provided by vessels within the cartilage.
- Failure of endochondral ossification can lead to decreased longitudinal bone growth. When this is severe and occurs in the distal ulnar physis, angular limb deformity may result.

SYSTEMS AFFECTED

Musculoskeletal

GENETICS

- Polygenetic transmission—expression determined by an interaction of genetic and environmental factors.
- Heritability index—depends on breed; 0.25–0.45.

INCIDENCE/PREVALENCE

Frequent and serious problem in many dog breeds.

GEOGRAPHIC DISTRIBUTION

N/A

SIGNALMENT

Species

Dog

Breed Predilections

Large and giant breeds—Great Dane, Labrador retriever, Newfoundland, Rottweiler, Bernese mountain dog, English setter, Old English sheepdog.

Mean Age and Range

- Onset of clinical signs—typically 4–8 months.
- Diagnosis—generally 4–18 months.
- Symptoms of osteoarthritis—any age.

Predominant Sex

- Shoulder—males (2:1).
- Elbow, stifle, and hock—none.

SIGNS

General Comments

Depend on the affected joint(s) and concurrent osteoarthritis.

Historical Findings

Lameness—most common; sudden or insidious in onset; one or more limbs; becomes worse after exercise; duration of several weeks to months; slight, moderate, or severe.

Physical Examination Findings

- Pain—usually elicited on palpation by flexing, extending, or rotating the involved joint.
- Generally a weight-bearing lameness.
- Joint effusion with capsular distention—common with OCD of elbow, stifle, and hock.
- Muscle atrophy—consistent finding with chronic lameness.
- Hock OCD—hyperextension of the tarsocrural joint.

CAUSES

- Developmental.
- Nutritional.

RISK FACTORS

- Diet containing 3 times the recommended calcium levels.
- Rapid growth and weight gain.
- Overfeeding.

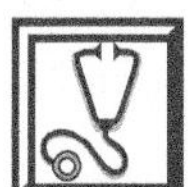

DIAGNOSIS

DIFFERENTIAL DIAGNOSIS

- Soft tissue trauma.
- Intra-articular (osteochondral) fractures.
- Elbow dysplasia.
- Panosteitis.

CBC/BIOCHEMISTRY/URINALYSIS

N/A

OTHER LABORATORY TESTS

N/A

IMAGING

Radiography

- Standard craniocaudal and mediolateral views—necessary for all involved joints.
- Failure of normal endochondral ossification results in radiolucency. Thus the normal bone contour is lost, which radiographically appears as flattening of the subchondral bone or as a subchondral lucency.
- Cannot be differentiated from OCD on plain radiographs unless the cartilage flap is mineralized.
- Sclerosis of the underlying bone—common in chronic OCD lesions.
- Calcified bodies within the joint (joint mice)—indicate dislodged cartilage flap.
- Contralateral joint—comparison; check for involvement.
- Oblique views—may improve visualization, especially for hock, elbow, and shoulder lesions.
- Skyline views of the talar ridges of the hock joint—help identify medial and lateral lesions.

CT and MRI

Useful for visualizing extent of subchondral lesions. MRI is the most accurate method of detecting osteochondrosis/OCD lesions, flaps, and fragments.

Ultrasonography

Can be used to detect lesions, but is very operator dependent and is the least accurate diagnostic imaging method.

Positive Contrast Arthrography

Useful for differentiating OCD of the shoulder from other conditions.

DIAGNOSTIC PROCEDURES

- Diagnosis most frequently made based on physical examination and diagnostic imaging.
- Arthrocentesis and analysis of synovial fluid—confirms involvement; should note straw-colored fluid with normal to decreased viscosity; from cytology, should note >90% mononuclear cells. Not specific for osteochondrosis.
- Arthroscopy—minimally invasive; excellent method for differentiating from OCD and for therapeutic treatment.

OSTEOCHONDROSIS (CONTINUED)

PATHOLOGIC FINDINGS

- Articular cartilage—initially may appear yellowish.
- Retention of articular cartilage extending into subchondral bone surrounded by increased amount of trabecular bone.
- Clefts between the underlying subchondral bone and the degenerated and necrotic deep layer of the overlying thickened (retained) cartilage.

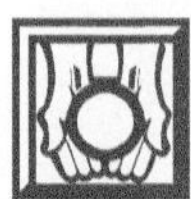

TREATMENT

APPROPRIATE HEALTH CARE

N/A

NURSING CARE

- Cryotherapy (ice packing) of affected joint—immediately post-surgery; 5–10 minutes q8h for 3–5 days.
- Range-of-motion exercises—initiated as soon as patient can tolerate.

ACTIVITY

- Restricted.
- Avoid hard concussive activities (e.g., running on concrete).

DIET

Weight control—important for decreasing load and, therefore, the stress on the affected joint(s).

CLIENT EDUCATION

- Discuss the heritability of the disease.
- Warn client that osteoarthritis is likely to develop.
- Discuss the influence of excessive intake of nutrients that promote rapid growth.

SURGICAL CONSIDERATIONS

- Osteochondrosis of articular cartilage is generally a nonsurgical condition..
- May progress to OCD as the patient grows. If OCD develops, surgery is generally recommended.
- Surgery is performed by arthrotomy or arthroscopy, and is indicated for most patients with OCD.
- Surgical treatment usually involves removal of the cartilage flap and subchondral bone debridement.
- Osteochondral autografts have been described for treatment of OCD of the caudal humeral head, medial aspect of the humeral condyle, and femoral condyles. Benefit beyond surgical debridement by flap removal requires further investigation.
- Synthetic osteochondral implants are available for resurfacing and have been described for use in the stifle joint of dogs.
- Shoulder—indicated for all OCD lesions; exploratory procedure indicated for pain and lameness with radiographic evidence of osteochondrosis.
- Elbow—indicated for all OCD lesions; indicated to assess for other conditions (see Elbow Dysplasia).
- Stifle—controversial; patients develop osteoarthritis even with procedure; arthroscopy may improve the recovery rate and long-term function.
- Hock—remove osteochondral flap; controversial; all patients develop severe osteoarthritis even with procedure. Arthrodesis is considered an option for patients with severe disease.
- Sacrum—remove fragment if impinging on the cauda equina.

MEDICATIONS

DRUG(S) OF CHOICE

Nonsteroidal anti-inflammatory drugs (NSAIDs) and analgesics—may be used to symptomatically treat osteoarthritis associated with OCD; does not promote healing of the cartilage flap (thus surgery is still indicated).

CONTRAINDICATIONS

Avoid corticosteroids owing to potential side effects and articular cartilage damage associated with long-term use.

PRECAUTIONS

NSAIDs—gastrointestinal irritation or renal/hepatic toxicity may preclude use in some patients.

POSSIBLE INTERACTIONS

N/A

ALTERNATIVE DRUG(S)

Chondroprotective drugs (e.g., polysulfated glycosaminoglycans, green-lipped mussel extract, and glucosamine/chondroitin sulfate)—may help limit cartilage damage and degeneration; may help alleviate pain and inflammation.

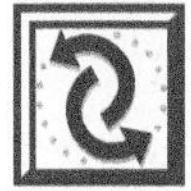

FOLLOW-UP

PATIENT MONITORING

- Periodic monitoring until patient is skeletally mature—recommended to assess progression to an OCD lesion.
- Post-surgery for OCD—limit activity for 4–6 weeks; encourage early, active movement of the affected joint(s).
- Yearly examinations—recommended to assess progression of osteoarthritis.

PREVENTION/AVOIDANCE

- Discourage breeding of patients.
- Do not repeat dam–sire breedings that resulted in affected offspring.
- Restricted weight gain and growth in young dogs—may decrease incidence.

POSSIBLE COMPLICATIONS

N/A

EXPECTED COURSE AND PROGNOSIS

- Shoulder—good to excellent prognosis for return to full function; minimal osteoarthritis development with osteochondrosis and after OCD surgery.
- Elbow, stifle, and hock—fair prognosis for osteochondrosis, guarded for OCD; depends on size of lesion (most important), osteoarthritis, and age at diagnosis and treatment; progressive osteoarthritis development, even after surgery.
- Sacrum—good after cartilage fragment removal.

MISCELLANEOUS

ASSOCIATED CONDITIONS

N/A

AGE-RELATED FACTORS

N/A

ZOONOTIC POTENTIAL

N/A

PREGNANCY/FERTILITY/BREEDING

N/A

SEE ALSO

Elbow Dysplasia.

ABBREVIATIONS

- NSAID = nonsteroidal anti-inflammatory drug.
- OCD = osteochondritis dissecans.

Suggested Reading

Breur GJ, Lambrechts NE. Osteochondrosis. In: Johnston SA, Tobias KM, eds., Veterinary Surgery Small Animal, 2nd ed. St. Louis, MO: Elsevier Saunders, 2018, pp. 1372–1385.

Egan P, Murphy S, Jovanovik J, et al. Treatment of osteochondrosis dissecans of the canine stifle using synthetic osteochondral resurfacing. Vet Comp Orthop Traumatol 2018, 31(2):144–152.

Kuroki K, Cook JL, Stoker AM, et al. Characterizing osteochondrosis in the dog: Potential roles for matrix metalloproteinases and mechanical load in pathogenesis and disease progression. Osteoarthritis Cartilage 2005, 13(3):225–234.

Wall CR, Cook CR, Cook JL. Diagnostic sensitivity of radiography, ultrasonography, and magnetic resonance imaging for detecting shoulder osteochondrosis/osteochondritis dissecans in dogs. Vet Radiol Ultrasound 2015, 56(1):3–11.

Author Spencer A. Johnston

Consulting Editor Mathieu M. Glassman

Client Education Handout available online

O

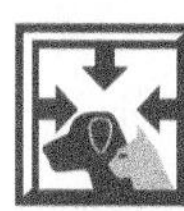

BASICS

DEFINITION

Acute or chronic inflammation of bone, usually caused by bacteria. Less common causes include fungi, parasites, viruses, foreign bodies, and corrosion of metallic implants.

PATHOPHYSIOLOGY

• Direct inoculation of bone with pathogenic bacteria—most common route of infection. May not initiate infection unless local tissue environment is affected (e.g., poor vascularity, necrotic bone or soft tissue, sequestration, altered tissue defenses or systemic immune response, foreign material, or surgical implants). • Hematogenously disseminated microorganisms from a distant site in the body localize in the metaphyseal region of long bones in young animals and vertebrae of adults. Inflammation and thrombus formation produce an ischemic environment that promotes bacterial proliferation. Mycotic infections are often due to hematogenous dissemination of inhaled spores. • Extension of soft tissue infections to bone—uncommon in small animals. • Biofilm formation protects bacteria from phagocytes, antibacterials and antibodies.

SYSTEMS AFFECTED

Musculoskeletal

GENETICS

Breeds with heritable immunodeficiency or hematogenous diseases.

INCIDENCE/PREVALENCE

• Hematogenous disease—rare. • Prevalence of fracture-associated osteomyelitis—radius/ulna 41.5%; femur 28.5%. • Discospondylitis in adult dogs and cats and fungal disease—not uncommon.

GEOGRAPHIC DISTRIBUTION

• Actinomycosis—migrating grass awns can cause soft tissue infections, which may extend to bone. • Blastomycosis—central and eastern regions of the United States, Canadian provinces of Quebec, Manitoba, and Ontario. • Coccidioidomycosis—southwestern United States, Mexico, and Central and South America. • Histoplasmosis—Ohio, Missouri, and Mississippi river valleys.

SIGNALMENT

Species

Dog and cat.

Breed Predilections

Breeds with immunodeficiency and hematogenous diseases.

Mean Age and Range

Hematogenous metaphyseal infection—immature dogs.

Predominant Sex

Male dogs—for post-traumatic infection; blastomycosis.

SIGNS

General Comments

• Acute postoperative wound infections after orthopedic surgery—may be indistinguishable from acute condition; may progress to chronic disease. • Most patients have chronic disease at time of examination and diagnosis.

Historical Findings

• Lameness. • Draining tracts. • Previous trauma. • Fracture or surgery. • Hind limb weakness and difficulty in rising—discospondylitis or vertebral osteomyelitis. • Travel to regions endemic for mycotic infections.

Physical Examination Findings

• Acute hematogenous disease (dogs)—sudden onset of systemic illness; soft tissue swelling over affected site; lameness; pyrexia; lethargy; limb pain. • Chronic condition—localized disease, usually no systemic component; chronic draining tracts, pain, muscle atrophy, muscle contracture.
• Infected non-union fracture—instability, crepitus, limb deformity. • Bone infections of the spine—pain and neurologic deficits.

CAUSES

• Trauma or orthopedic surgery. • Penetrating foreign body. • Extension to bone of soft tissue infection—periodontitis; rhinitis; otitis media; paronychia. • Hematogenous infection.
• *Staphylococcus pseudintermedius* common—almost 50% are methicillin-resistant strains; often monomicrobial infection. Polymicrobial infections are common—may include Gram-negative organisms: *E. coli*, *Pasteurella*, *Serratia*, *Pseudomonas*, *Proteus*, and *Klebsiella* spp. • Anaerobic bacteria—*Actinomyces*, *Clostridium*, *Peptostreptococcus*, *Bacteroides*, *Nocardia* and *Fusobacterium*. • Fungal infection—*Coccidioides*, *Blastomyces*, *Histoplasma*, *Candida*, *Cryptococcus*, *and Aspergillus* species.

RISK FACTORS

• Open fracture. • Soft tissue trauma.
• Penetrating wounds. • Migrating foreign body. • Orthopedic surgery/implants.
• Cortical bone allograft. • Immunodeficiency.
• Nosocomial infection.

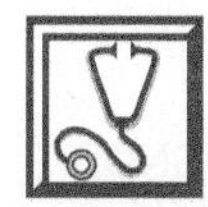

DIAGNOSIS

DIFFERENTIAL DIAGNOSIS

• Panosteitis. • Neoplasia. • Bone cysts.
• Delayed fracture union due to instability.
• Hypertrophic osteodystrophy.
• Hypertrophic osteopathy. • Medullary bone infarction.

CBC/BIOCHEMISTRY/URINALYSIS

• Hemogram—neutrophilia ± left shift with acute disease. • Fungal hyphae may be present in the urine of systemically ill patients with aspergillosis.

OTHER LABORATORY TESTS

• Serology—confirms some fungal infections.
• Blood cultures if hematogenous infection suspected. • Urine excretion of antigen for blastomycosis.

IMAGING

Radiographic Findings

• Acute disease—bone architecture normal; soft tissue swelling; gas may be evident if anaerobic infection. • Chronic disease—sequestrum (avascular segment of bone); periosteal new bone formation; involucrum formation (reactive bone surrounding sequestrum); bone resorption—widening of fracture gaps; cortical thinning; generalized osteopenia; implant loosening.
• Fistulogram—can help identify sequestra or radiolucent foreign bodies.

Other

• Ultrasonography—localize large fluid accumulations for needle aspiration or foreign bodies. • Contrast CT or MRI identification of sequestra, foreign material.
• Scintigraphy—uncommonly available and performed.

DIAGNOSTIC PROCEDURES

• Fluid aspirates of fluctuant areas or Jamshidi needle tissue biopsies for aerobic and anaerobic culture and *in vitro* antimicrobial drug susceptibility—collect by sterile techniques.
• Open surgical biopsy—indicated when needle aspirates are negative or when debridement is necessary for treatment; culture samples of necrotic tissue, sequestra, implants, and foreign material; histopathologic examination for suspected fungal infection and to rule out neoplasia. Request special fungal stains on pathology samples. • Samples for anaerobic culture—immediately place into appropriate transport medium. Avoid culturing purulent fluid from draining tracts—results misleading as often get contaminants from skin. • Blood cultures—indicated in acute hematogenous osteomyelitis or chronic disease with septicemia. • Urine culture to rule out urinary tract infection as a source for hematogenous disease.

PATHOLOGIC FINDINGS

• Bone sequestration—virtually diagnostic.
• Inflammation and necrosis of bone and the adjacent tissues. • Cytologic or histopathologic examination of smears or sections—can be helpful for identification of pathogenic organisms (especially fungal hyphae).

OSTEOMYELITIS (CONTINUED)

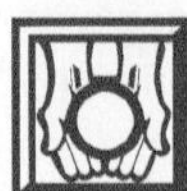

TREATMENT

APPROPRIATE HEALTH CARE

• Inpatient—surgical debridement, drainage, culturing, irrigation, and wound management until infection begins to resolve; infected fractures (surgical stabilization).
• Outpatient—long-term oral antimicrobial drug therapy.

NURSING CARE

• Depends on severity, location, and degree of associated soft tissue injury. • Avoid pathogen contamination to other patients.
• Physical rehabilitation therapy.

ACTIVITY

Restricted—to prevent pathologic fracture; with an unhealed fracture.

DIET

No restriction.

CLIENT EDUCATION

• Warn the client about cost of treatment, likelihood of recurrence, possibility of repeated surgical intervention, and long duration of therapy. • Discuss prognosis.

SURGICAL CONSIDERATIONS

• Chronic disease—surgical debridement; sequestrectomy; establish drainage. • Infected stable fracture—leave preexisting implants in place during healing. • Infected unstable fracture—remove implants; stabilize with external or internal skeletal fixation. • Bone deficits—graft with autologous cancellous bone either acutely or after infection has abated and granulation tissue is present.
• Large segmental deficits in long bones—bone regeneration by bone transport utilizing the Ilizarov technique or other bone segment transport mechanism. • Localized chronic infection—consider amputation or *en bloc* resection and primary wound closure.
• Remove all implants after the fracture has healed to eliminate biofilm. • Muscle flap coverage of exposed bone early in the course of treatment greatly reduces contamination of bone and promotes fracture healing.

MEDICATIONS

DRUG(S) OF CHOICE

• Administer a broad-spectrum bactericidal antimicrobial intravenously for 3–5 days while awaiting culture and susceptibility results, then switch to appropriate antimicrobial which must be given for 4–8 weeks; continue for at least 2 weeks beyond radiographic and clinical resolution of infection. • *S. pseudintermedius*—amoxicillin–clavulanate, cefazolin, oxacillin are reasonable empirical choices. • Antibiotics effective against anaerobes that are also available for parenteral administration—ampicillin sodium, metronidazole, clindamycin.
• Aminoglycosides and quinolones—effective against Gram-negative aerobic bacteria.
• Quinolones—may give orally; not nephrotoxic; to protect against resistance, use only for infections caused by Gram-negative organisms that are resistant to other oral antimicrobial drugs. • Chronic disease—continuous local delivery of antimicrobial drugs by antibiotic-impregnated bone cement (beads) or biodegradable material (gels).
• Fungal osteomyelitis—long-term therapy (months); treat at least a month beyond resolution of clinical signs; e.g., itraconazole 5–10 mg/kg PO q24h; given continuously may control disseminated aspergillosis long-term. • Analgesics— important to encourage limb use.

CONTRAINDICATIONS

Quinolones— potential for cartilage injury in immature dogs.

PRECAUTIONS

Aminoglycosides—may cause nephrotoxicity.

ALTERNATIVE DRUG(S)

Identify other antimicrobial drugs by repeating cultures and susceptibility determination if the infection becomes unresponsive to the initial agent.

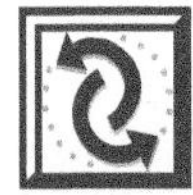

FOLLOW-UP

PATIENT MONITORING

• Radiography—2–3 weeks after intervention and then every 4–6 weeks to monitor bone healing. • Reculture bone—suspected persistent infection.

PREVENTION/AVOIDANCE

N/A

POSSIBLE COMPLICATIONS

• Recurrence. • Progression to chronic disease. • Malignant neoplasia—rare sequela to chronic infection of fractures repaired by internal fixation.

EXPECTED COURSE AND PROGNOSIS

• Acute infection—may be cured by 4–8 weeks of antimicrobial drug therapy if there is limited bone necrosis and no fracture.
• Chronic disease—resolution with antimicrobial drug therapy alone unlikely; provide appropriate surgical treatment.
• Recurrence of chronic infection may require repeated sequestrectomy. • Consider amputation in severe chronic cases with irreversible loss of limb function.

MISCELLANEOUS

ASSOCIATED CONDITIONS

N/A

AGE-RELATED FACTORS

N/A

ZOONOTIC POTENTIAL

Pets with multidrug-resistant bacterial infections can shed organisms that can colonize humans.

PREGNANCY/FERTILITY/BREEDING

N/A

SYNONYMS

Bone infection.

SEE ALSO

Discospondylitis

Suggested Reading

Fossum TW. Other diseases of bones and joints: osteomyelitis. In: Small Animal Surgery, 4th ed. St. Louis, MO: Elsevier Mosby, 2013, pp. 1407–1410.
Greene CE, Bennett D. Musculoskeletal infections. In: Greene CE, ed., Infectious Diseases of the Dog and Cat, 4th ed. St. Louis, MO: Saunders Elsevier, 2012, pp. 892–902.
Inzana JA, Schwarz EM, Kates SL, Awad HA. Biomaterials approaches to treating implant-associated osteomyelitis. Biomaterials 2016, 81:58–71.
Robinson D. Osteomyelitis and implant-associated infections. In: Johnston SA, Tobias KM, eds., Veterinary Surgery Small Animal, 2nd ed. St. Louis, MO: Elsevier, 2017, pp. 775–783.
Sykes JE, Kapatkin AS. Osteomyelitis, discospondylitis, and infectious arthritis. In: Sykes JE, ed., Canine and Feline Infectious Diseases. St. Louis, MO: Elsevier Saunders, 2013, pp. 814–829.

Author Tisha A.M. Harper
Consulting Editor Mathieu M. Glassman

Client Education Handout available online

BASICS

DEFINITION

Osteosarcoma (OS) is a cancer derived from a malignant osteoblast cell lineage within the endosteum, and is the most common primary bone tumor in dogs. Large- to giant-breed dogs most commonly develop appendicular OS, while axial OS tends to affect smaller breeds (<15 kg). The biologic behavior of OS is aggressive locally and distantly, with presumed microscopic lung metastases present in ≥85% of dogs at diagnosis. OS is rare in cats, and the biologic behavior is less malignant than in dogs.

PATHOPHYSIOLOGY

Genetic predisposition is likely a major contributor for the development of OS. Other factors contributing include chronic inflammation associated with metallic implants, history of prior radiation therapy to the site of tumorigenesis, and rapid bone turnover, all associated with the development of OS in dogs.

SYSTEMS AFFECTED

- Musculoskeletal—the appendicular skeleton (metaphyseal region of long bones) is most commonly affected in dogs. OS may also occur in the axial skeleton.
- Respiratory—the most common metastatic site is the lung parenchyma; however, other sites include bones, regional lymph node, skin, and visceral organs (liver, kidney).

GENETICS

There is a strong breed predilection, with some degree of heritability being identified in giant breeds such as Scottish deerhound, Rottweiler, greyhound, and Irish wolfhound.

INCIDENCE/PREVALENCE

- Dogs—OS accounts for up to 85% of primary bone tumors in dogs, representing ~5% of all reported malignancies in dogs.
- Cats—OS is the most common primary bone tumor in cats, accounting for <7% of all reported cancers in this species.

SIGNALMENT

Species

Dog and cat.

Breed Predilections

- Dogs—large to giant breed (>40 kg).
- Cats—domestic shorthair cats.

Mean Age and Range

- Dogs—bimodal peak at 2 years and 7 years, reported to occur as young as 6 months.
- Cats—average age 8.5 years (range 4–18 years).

Predominant Sex

Dogs and cats—no strong sex predilection.

SIGNS

General Comments

- Because OS occurs most commonly in the appendicular skeleton of dogs and cats, lameness and pain are common clinical findings.
- Clinical symptoms associated with OS affecting the axial skeleton can be variable depending upon the anatomic site involved.

Historical Findings

- Lameness (acute or chronic) is the most common presenting clinical sign.
- Signs of axial skeletal OS vary, depending on the site of the lesion.

Physical Examination Findings

- A firm, painful swelling of the affected site is common with either appendicular or axial skeletal OS.
- Degree of lameness varies from mild to non-weight-bearing.
- Soft tissue swelling secondary to tumor infiltration.

CAUSES

Unknown in both species.

RISK FACTORS

- Dogs—large- to giant-breed dogs at greater risk.
- Metallic implants at fracture repair sites.
- Exposure to ionizing radiation.
- Cats—unknown.

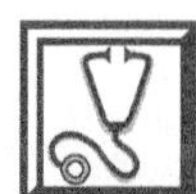

DIAGNOSIS

DIFFERENTIAL DIAGNOSIS

- Other primary bone tumor (i.e., fibrosarcoma, chondrosarcoma).
- Metastatic bone tumor (i.e., prostatic, mammary, other carcinoma).
- Infectious (i.e., fungal or bacterial osteomyelitis).

CBC/BIOCHEMISTRY/URINALYSIS

Elevated alkaline phosphatase is a poor prognostic factor.

IMAGING

Radiography of Primary Site

- At least two views of the primary lesion should be acquired.
- Radiographic findings include mixed osteolytic/osteoproductive effects involving the affected skeletal site.
- Soft tissue swelling overlying diseased bone.

Thoracic Radiography

- Three-view thoracic radiographs should be performed; although visible macroscopic metastatic disease is present in <10% of cases at the time of presentation.
- Pulmonary metastases at initial diagnosis is associated with an extremely poor prognosis.
- Metastatic lesions typically appear as discrete, round, soft tissue density nodules.

OTHER DIAGNOSTIC PROCEDURES

Bone Aspirate

- A relatively noninvasive, high-yield procedure using an 18-gauge needle to collect OS cells from the diseased skeletal site.
- Cytology can provide a diagnosis of malignant mesenchymal neoplasia.
- Concurrent alkaline phosphatase positivity on cytology is sensitive and specific for OS diagnosis.

Bone Biopsy

- Performed with the patient under light general anesthesia or moderate sedation.
- Samples should be taken through the center of the lesion; peripheral biopsies are often nondiagnostic and contain reactive osteoblasts.
- Biopsy may be performed using a Michele trephine, Jamshidi bone biopsy needle, or open biopsy technique.

PATHOLOGIC FINDINGS

- Gross—moderate to severe destruction of cortical bone with new bone proliferation.
- Histologic—malignant population of mesenchymal cells that are plump, polygonal to spindyloid in shape. The finding of osteoid production is necessary and diagnostic for OS.

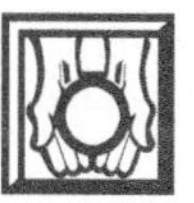

TREATMENT

DIET

No specific dietary management is required, although weight loss may benefit amputees in general.

CLIENT EDUCATION

- Long-term prognosis is poor; however, a subpopulation (15%) of patients achieve long-term survival (>2 years).
- Clients must understand that treatment goals are to relieve discomfort and prolong life; a cure is unlikely.

SURGICAL CONSIDERATIONS

Dogs—Appendicular Sites

- Surgical management involves amputation of the affected limb.
- Limb salvage therapy is available at a limited number of referral hospitals. This technique is appropriate only for locally confined and small distal radial lesions. The primary tumor is surgically removed, replaced by a commercially available metal endoprosthesis with modified bone plate.

Dogs—Axial Sites

- Depending on location, aggressive surgical excision or radiation therapy, in conjunction with adjuvant chemotherapy are recommended.

- If surgical resection is not possible, palliative radiation is effective for the alleviation of osteolytic bone pain.

Cats—Appendicular Sites

- Amputation alone is considered appropriate.
- Adjuvant chemotherapy not necessary.

Cats—Axial Sites

- Depending on site of lesion, aggressive surgical excision or radiation therapy should be instituted.
- Local recurrence appears to be the main reason for treatment failure.

Metastatectomy

- Pulmonary metastatectomy has been described for dogs with OS; however, is not routinely practiced.
- Selection criteria for dogs to undergo this procedure include a long disease-free interval (>300 days) and only 1–2 pulmonary nodules based on thoracic radiographs.

Inoperable Neoplasms

- Palliative (coarse fractionation) radiotherapy or stereotactic radiosurgery combined with systemic chemotherapy and aminobisphosphonate therapy can provide prolonged survival times with acceptable pain control (10–12 months).
- Pain management with nonsteroidal anti-inflammatory drugs, opioids, and/or bisphosphonates may improve quality of life and thus prolong survival.

MEDICATIONS

DRUG(S) OF CHOICE

Definitive Therapy

- Chemotherapy with either platinum-based drugs (cisplatin or carboplatin) or doxorubicin is the current standard of care; a minimum of four doses is recommended.
- Cisplatin 70 mg/m² IV q3 weeks. Must be given with a saline-induced diuresis to prevent nephrotoxocity: 18.3 mL/kg/h for 4 hours, administer chemotherapy over 20 minutes, then continue diuresis for another 2 hours. Antiemetics must be given before cisplatin, and the patient may need to be sent home with antiemetic therapy.
- Carboplatin 300 mg/m² IV q3 weeks.
- Doxorubicin 30 mg/m² IV q3 weeks for 5 doses.
- Chemotherapy or toceranib phosphate (Palladia) is not effective against gross disease; less than 5% expected response rate.
- Chemotherapy typically initiated within 2 weeks of surgery.

CONTRAINDICATIONS

- Patients with preexisting renal dysfunction should not be treated with platinum-based chemotherapy drugs.
- Do not give cisplatin to cats.

ALTERNATIVE DRUG(S)

Palliative Therapy

- Pain management must be addressed in patients whose owners decline definitive therapy.
- Manage pain with nonsteroidal anti-inflammatory drugs, ± tramadol (2–5 mg/kg q8–12h), ± acetaminophen with codeine (0.5–2 mg/kg q8–12h), ± transdermal fentanyl (as per package instructions) ± gabapentin (3–10 mg/kg q8–24h).
- Euthanasia when quality of life declines.

FOLLOW-UP

PATIENT MONITORING

- Monitor CBC for evidence of myelosuppression 7–14 days following chemotherapy.
- Doxorubicin—periodic echocardiography and ECGs as cumulative cardiotoxicity may occur at >180 mg/m².
- Three-view thoracic radiographs every 2–3 months after surgery to assess for metastasis.

POSSIBLE COMPLICATIONS

- Metastatic disease is very likely; sites of spread include lungs, other bones, soft tissue.
- Animals that undergo limb salvage may develop recurrent infections, local recurrence, or implant failure.
- Animals treated with systemic chemotherapy can develop adverse side effects, including bone marrow suppression and gastrointestinal upset. Symptomatic management is typically effective, however, life-threatening complications can occur infrequently.

EXPECTED COURSE AND PROGNOSIS

Dogs

- Without treatment, with amputation alone, or with palliative radiotherapy alone, median survival is approximately 4 months. When conventional palliative radiotherapy is combined with IV aminobisphosphonates and oral analgesics, acceptable quality of life can be extended up to 6–9 months. The use of stereotactic radiosurgery in combination with chemotherapy and aminobisphosphonates can extend survival times to 10–12 months.
- With surgery and chemotherapy, median survival is extended to a median of 10 months.

Cats

- Appendicular OS, with surgery, median survival of >2 years.
- Axial OS, with surgery, median survival of 5.5 months.

MISCELLANEOUS

PREGNANCY/FERTILITY/BREEDING

Do not breed animals that are undergoing chemotherapy.

SYNONYMS

Osteogenic sarcoma.

SEE ALSO

- Chondrosarcoma, Bone.
- Fibrosarcoma, Bone.
- Hemangiosarcoma, Bone.

ABBREVIATIONS

- ECG = electrocardiogram.
- OS = osteosarcoma.

Suggested Reading

Ehrhart NP, Ryan S, Fan TM. Tumors of the skeletal system. In: Withrow and MacEwen's Small Animal Clinical Oncology, 5th ed. St. Louis, MO: Elsevier, pp. 463–503.

Author Timothy M. Fan

Consulting Editor Timothy M. Fan

Client Education Handout available online

OTITIS EXTERNA AND MEDIA

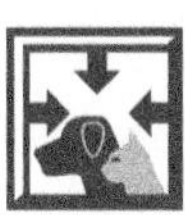

BASICS

DEFINITION

• Otitis externa—inflammation of the external ear canal; includes anatomic structures of the pinna, horizontal and vertical canals, and the external layer of the tympanic membrane.
• Otitis media—inflammation of the middle ear; includes anatomic structures of the tympanic membrane, bulla (tympanic cavity), auditory ossicles, and auditory tube.

PATHOPHYSIOLOGY

• Otitis externa—chronic inflammation results in alterations in the environment of the canal; with inflammation, cerumen glands enlarge and produce excessive wax; the epidermis and dermis thicken and become fibrotic; thickened canal folds reduce canal width; calcification/ossification of auricular cartilage is the end-stage result.
• Otitis media—often an extension of otitis externa through the tympanic membrane (dogs); a result of infection ascending through the auditory tube to the middle ear (cats). Chronic viral upper respiratory infection early in life may change the ability of the auditory tube to protect the bulla from infection. Otitis media can occur from polyps or neoplasia within the middle ear or auditory tube.

SYSTEMS AFFECTED

• Skin/exocrine.
• Nervous.

GEOGRAPHIC DISTRIBUTION

Environmental humidity may predispose to infection.

SIGNALMENT

Species

Dog and cat.

Breed Predilections

• Pendulous-eared dogs—especially spaniel and retriever.
• Dogs with hirsute external canals—terrier and poodle.
• Stenosis of the external ear canal—pug and bulldog; stenosis of the external orifice of ear canal—shar pei.
• Primary secretory otitis media—cavalier King Charles spaniel.

SIGNS

Historical Findings

• Pain—shying from touching of the head, refusing to open the mouth, dropping food.
• Head shaking.
• Scratching at the pinnae.
• Malodor from canals.
• Peripheral vestibular deficits or facial paralysis or paresis.

Physical Examination Findings

Otitis Externa

• Inflammation, pain, pruritus, and erythema of the pinnae and external canals.
• Stenosis of external orifices and/or ear canals.
• Deafness from obstruction.
• Purulent and malodorous exudates.
• Aural hematoma.
• Palpable scarring and calcification of the auricular cartilage.
• Holding of the pinna down and/or head tilt toward the affected side (if unilateral).

Otitis Media

• Vestibular signs—ipsilateral facial nerve paralysis and/or Horner's syndrome; uncommon in the cat, more common in the dog.
• Intact tympanic membrane—bulging pars flaccida.
• Evidence of fluid and/or gas behind the pars tensa; membrane may be opaque; fluid may be purulent or hemorrhagic.
• Ruptured tympanic membrane—discharge into canal or bullae filled with debris.
• Deafness (otitis media progressing to otitis interna).
• Pain on palpation or opening of the mouth.
• Xeromycteria (uni- or bilateral nasal planum hyperkeratosis—lack of nasal secretion due to parasympathetic nerve dysfunction).

CAUSES

• Predisposing factors—present prior to the development of ear disease:
  ◦ Conformation (see Breeds).
  ◦ Excessive moisture (high humidity, swimming).
  ◦ Obstructive ear disease (neoplasia, polyp).
  ◦ Primary otitis media.
• Perpetuating factors—changes in anatomy or physiology in response to otitis externa:
  ◦ Altered wax migration, excessive production of debris.
  ◦ Proliferative changes, stenosis.
  ◦ Calcification.
• Primary causes—directly initiate or cause inflammation within the ear canal:
  ◦ Parasites—*Otodectes cynotis*, *Demodex* spp., *Otobius megnini*, chiggers.
  ◦ Hypersensitivities—atopy, food, contact; recurrent otitis externa may be the only clinical sign of hypersensitivity.
  ◦ Foreign bodies—plant awns.
  ◦ Keratinization disorders and increased cerumen production.
  ◦ Endocrinopathy—immune-mediated; drug reaction (topical or systemic).
• Secondary causes—create disease in an abnormal ear:
  ◦ Bacterial or yeast infection.
  ◦ Excessive moisture and maceration (overcleaning, trauma).
  ◦ Topical irritants.

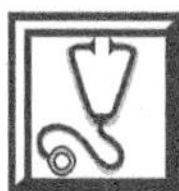

DIAGNOSIS

CBC/BIOCHEMISTRY/URINALYSIS

Usually normal.

OTHER LABORATORY TESTS

• Strict diet trial to diagnosis cutaneous adverse reaction to food.

IMAGING

• Bullae radiographs—may be normal; bullae may appear cloudy if filled with exudate; thickening of bulla and petrous temporal bone with chronic disease; presence of bone lysis with osteomyelitis or neoplastic disease.
• CT or MRI—detailed evidence of fluid or tissue density in the bulla, adjacent tissues, or auditory tube.

DIAGNOSTIC PROCEDURES

• Otoscopy or video-otoscopy—visualization of the external canal, tympanic membrane, and portions of the bulla (if tympanum ruptured).
• Cytologic examination of exudate—most important diagnostic tool after complete examination of the ear canal; otic discharge sample should be taken before cleaning or treatment are initiated; examine exudates from each ear canal:
  ◦ Morphologically describe and quantitate bacteria, yeast, inflammatory cells (0 to 4+ scale) for treatment monitoring.
  ◦ Type(s) of bacteria or yeast—assist in the choice of therapy .
• Infections within the canal can change with prolonged or recurrent therapy; repeat cytology is required in chronic cases.
• Myringotomy—spinal needle or sterile catheter is inserted through the tympanic membrane to sample fluid within the bulla for cytologic examination and culture.
• Culture of otic exudate—recommended in cases of otitis media and/or persistent infection.
• Parasites—*Otodectes*, *Otobius*, and chiggers are visualized on otoscopy; *Demodex* can be diagnosed on ear cytology.

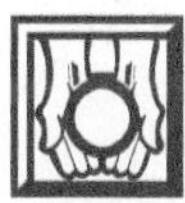

TREATMENT

CLIENT EDUCATION

Demonstrate proper method for cleaning and medicating ears (e.g., volume of medication to instill).

SURGICAL CONSIDERATIONS

• Lateral ear resection—disease affects primarily the vertical canal.
• Total ear ablation—entire canal is severely stenotic and oral glucocorticoids have failed to decrease stenosis or proliferative changes; tympanic bulla is diseased; or neoplasia affects the canal.

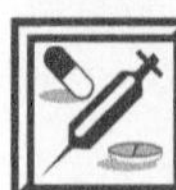

MEDICATIONS

DRUG(S) OF CHOICE

Cleansing Solutions

- Tympanum integrity should be assessed prior to introduction of solutions and/or medications into the external ear canal.
- At home cleaning:
  - Cleanser/dryer 2–3 times a week for mild to moderate amounts of wax. Combination cleanser/drying products—contain ceruminolytics (e.g., docusate sodium or dioctyl sodium sulfocuccinate, propylene glycol), drying agents (e.g., dimethicone), germicidals (e.g., acetic acid, boric acid)—contraindicated in cases of perforated tympanic membrane.
  - Acetic acid 5% (white vinegar) diluted 1:2 in water—good activity against bacteria including *Pseudomonas*, and yeast. Safe in middle/inner ear.
  - Tris-EDTA—antibacterial activity; enhances susceptibility of bacteria to various antibiotics. Low ototoxic potential; safe in middle ear.
  - Chlorhexidine—antiseptic, concentrations of less than 0.2% are safe within the middle ear.
  - *N*-Acetylcysteine—antimicrobial and mucolytic properties, and ability to disrupt bacterial biofilm.
- "In clinic" cleaning on awake animals:
  - Bulb syringe or trimmed French red rubber catheter used to flush in solution and remove debris.
  - Deep ear cleaning with general anesthesia when needed.

O

Systemic Antibiotics (Indications)

- Severe otitis and neutrophils are seen on cytology suggesting a deeper infection.
- Otitis media.
- Best chosen by culture and sensitivity test—empiric choices include cephalexin 30 mg/kg q12h, amoxicilin+clavulanic acid 13.75 mg/kg q12h, clindamycin 11 mg/kg q12h when cocci are seen cytologically; marbofloxacin 2.75 mg/kg q24h if rods are seen cytologically.

Systemic Antifungals (Indications)

- Refractory *Malassezia* infection or when owners are unable to apply topical treatment.
- Otitis media caused by *Malassezia* or other fungal organism.
- Dogs—ketoconazole 5–10 mg/kg q24h, terbinafine 20–30 mg/kg q24h.
- Cats—itraconazole 5 mg/kg q24h.

Systemic Glucocorticoids (Indications)

- Reduce inflammation and cerumen production associated with otitis externa.
- Reduce proliferative changes secondary to inflammation in ear canals.
- Starting dosages—prednisolone 1 mg/kg/day, dexamethasone 0.1 mg/kg/day, triamcinolone 0.1 mg/kg/day; higher dosages can be used for more severe inflammatory changes.
- Antiparasitic therapy against mites—avermectins, isoxazolines.
- *Otobius* (ear tick) should be removed from inside the ear canal.

Topical

- Continue cleanings until symptoms resolve and then routinely to maintain control.
- Apply appropriate topical medications in sufficient quantity to completely treat the entire canal: Amount used is determined by the size of ear—instilled once or twice daily.
- Antibiotic—based on cytologic evaluation and/or empiric choice. Gentamicin, neomycin—cocci infection; enrofloxacin and silver sulfadiazine—rods; amikacin—resistant *Pseudomonas*.
- Antifungal (anti-*Malassezia*)—clotrimazole, ketoconazole, miconazole, thiabendazole, nystatin, terbinafine; posaconazole—refractory *Malassezia* cases.
- Anti-inflammatory (glucocorticoid)—dexamethasone, fluocinolone, betamethasone, triamcinolone, hydrocortisone aceponate, and mometasone.
- Antiparasitic—ivermectin and thiabendazole.

CONTRAINDICATIONS

- Ruptured tympanum—use caution with topical cleansers other than sterile saline or dilute acetic acid; potential for ototoxicity; controversial.
- Ivermectin—non-FDA approved for use systemically; herding (dog) breeds have increased sensitivity (*MDR1/ABCB1* gene mutation).

PRECAUTIONS

- Use caution when cleaning the external ear canals of all animals with severe and chronic otitis externa; the tympanum can easily rupture.
- Post-flushing vestibular complications are more common in cats, although usually temporary; warn clients of possible complications and residual effects.

POSSIBLE INTERACTIONS

Topical medications infrequently induce contact irritation or allergic response; reevaluate all worsening cases.

FOLLOW-UP

PATIENT MONITORING

Cytology of ear canals should be repeated at each clinic visit.

PREVENTION/AVOIDANCE

- Routine ear cleaning at home.
- Control of underlying diseases.

POSSIBLE COMPLICATIONS

Deafness, vestibular disease, cellulitis, facial nerve paralysis, progression to otitis interna, and rarely meningoencephalitis.

EXPECTED COURSE AND PROGNOSIS

- Otitis externa—with proper therapy, most mild initial cases resolve in 3–4 weeks; failure to correct underlying primary cause results in recurrence.
- Otitis media—requires at least 6 weeks of systemic antibiotics until all signs resolve.
- Osteomyelitis of petrous temporal bone and bulla—may require 6–8 weeks of antibiotics.
- Vestibular signs may improve within 2–6 weeks; some animals may have residual symptoms.

MISCELLANEOUS

Suggested Reading

Harvey RG, Haar G. Ear, Nose and Throat Diseases of the Dog and Cat. Boca Raton, FL: CRC Press, 2017, pp. 1–223.

Author Clarissa P. Souza

Consulting Editor Alexander H. Werner Resnick

Acknowledgment The author acknowledges the prior contribution of Alexander H. Werner Resnick.

Client Education Handout available online

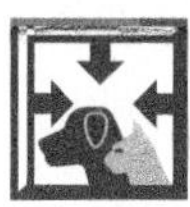

BASICS

DEFINITION

Inflammation of the middle (otitis media) and inner (otitis interna) ears, commonly caused by bacterial infection.

PATHOPHYSIOLOGY

• Media—from extension of infection of the external ear through the tympanic membrane; may extend from the oral and nasopharyngeal cavities via the eustachian tube. • Interna—may also result from hematogenous spread of a systemic infection.

SYSTEMS AFFECTED

Nervous

• Impaired balance due to damage to the vestibular apparatus in the inner ear or to the vestibular portion of vestibulocochlear nerve.
• Nausea from dizziness due to impaired balance. • Hearing loss due to damage to hair cells in the cochlea or to the cochlear portion of vestibulocochlear nerve. • CNS signs when spread of infection intracranially (otogenic intracranial infection).

Ophthalmic

• Keratoconjunctivitis sicca (KCS; dry eye)—from damage to parasympathetic branch of the facial nerve supplying the lacrimal gland.
• Corneal ulcer—as a consequence of inability to blink due to damage to facial nerve or from KCS. • Horner's syndrome—from damage to sympathetic nerve as they course through the middle ear.

SIGNALMENT

Breed Predilections

• Dogs more often affected than cats.
• Cocker spaniels and other long-ear breeds.
• Poodles with chronic otitis or pharyngitis from dental disease. • Primary secretory otitis media in cavalier King Charles spaniels.

SIGNS

Historical Findings

• Pain when opening the mouth; reluctance to chew; shaking the head; pawing at the affected ear. • Vestibular deficits, which may be persistent, transient, or episodic.
• Unilateral involvement causes head tilt, leaning, veering, or rolling. • Bilateral involvement causes wide head excursions, truncal ataxia; ± deafness. • Vomiting and nausea may occur during the acute phase.
• Saliva and food dropping from corner of the mouth; inability to blink; ocular discharge.
• Anisocoria (smaller pupil on affected side), protrusion of the third eyelid, enophthalmos and ptosis (Horner's syndrome) may be noted.

Physical Examination Findings

• The presence of aural erythema, discharge, and thickened and stenotic external canals support otitis externa. • Pain upon opening of the mouth or on bulla palpation. • Gray, dull, opaque, and bulging tympanic membrane on otoscopic examination indicates middle ear exudate. • Dental tartar, gingivitis, tonsillitis, or pharyngitis may be present and have a role in the pathogenesis. • With severe infections, the ipsilateral mandibular lymph nodes may be enlarged. • Corneal ulcer from inability to blink or KCS.

Neurologic Examination Findings

• Unilateral damage to vestibular portion of cranial nerve VIII—ipsilateral head tilt, leaning, veering, falling, or rolling.
• Nystagmus—resting or positional; rotary or horizontal; fast phase characteristically opposite the affected side, and does not change in direction with a change in head position. • Vestibular strabismus—ipsilateral ventral deviation of eyeball with neck extension. • Bilateral damage of vestibular portion of cranial nerve VIII—patient reluctant to move, may stay in a crouched posture, wide head excursions; physiologic nystagmus poor to absent. • Facial nerve damage—ipsilateral paresis/paralysis of the ear, eyelids, lips, and nares; reduced tear production (indicated by Schirmer tear test).
• Chronic facial paralysis—contracture of the affected face caused by fibrosis of denervated muscles. • Sympathetic nerve damage—ipsilateral Horner's syndrome; always miosis; may also note protrusion of third eyelid, ptosis, and enophthalmos.

CAUSES

• Bacteria—*Staphylococcus* spp., *Streptococcus* spp., *Proteus* spp., *Pseudomonas* spp., *Pasteurella* spp., and *E. coli* and obligate anaerobes. • Fungi—yeast (*Malassezia* spp., *Candida* spp.) and *Aspergillus*. • Ear mites predispose to secondary bacterial infections.
• Foreign bodies (e.g., grass awns, foxtail awns, or spear grass in endemic areas), trauma, polyps, tumors (e.g., fibromas, squamous cell carcinoma, ceruminous gland carcinoma, primary bone tumors).
• Iatrogenic damage during cleaning or flushing or in investigation of otitis externa.

RISK FACTORS

• Recurrent otitis externa. • Nasopharyngeal polyps and inner, middle, or outer ear neoplasia may predispose to bacterial infection. • Ear-cleaning solutions (e.g., chlorhexidine) may be irritating to middle/inner ear or be ototoxic. These should be avoided if tympanum is ruptured.

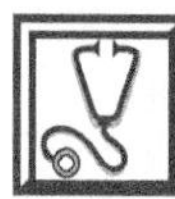

DIAGNOSIS

DIFFERENTIAL DIAGNOSIS

• Congenital vestibular anomalies—signs present from birth. • Hypothyroidism may be associated with cranial nerve VII and VIII deficits. Abnormal thyroid profile supports diagnosis. • Neoplasia and nasopharyngeal polyps are common causes of refractory and relapsing otitis media and interna. Diagnosed by oral and otic exam and imaging of the head.
• Idiopathic vestibular disease (old dogs and young to middle-aged cats), idiopathic facial paralysis, and idiopathic Horner's syndrome are diagnoses made by exclusion. • *Cryptococcus* is reported to be associated with peripheral vestibular disease in cats. • Traumatic causes may have physical external evidence of injury, and history supporting occurrence of a traumatic event. • Thiamine deficiency occurs in cats with a history of an all-fish diet or persistent anorexia; causes bilateral central vestibular signs.
• Metronidazole used for an extended duration and/or at a high dose damages the vestibular portion of the cerebellum. Signs of bilateral cerebellar disease and history of metronidazole use. • Central vestibular disease may cause lethargy, somnolence, vertical nystagmus, and other brainstem signs.

CBC/BIOCHEMISTRY/URINALYSIS

• Leukocytosis with left-shift may be noted.
• Globulins may be high if chronic infection.

OTHER LABORATORY TESTS

• Blood, urine cultures may show growth if hematogenous source of infection. • Low thyroxine (T_4), free T_4 with normal or high thyroid-stimulating hormone (TSH) level with hypothyroidism.

IMAGING

• Video-otoscopy—enables detailed examination of external ear canal and tympanic membrane. With middle ear exudate, the membrane may appear cloudy. Helpful in evaluating the integrity of the tympanic membrane, obtaining samples for cytology and culture/sensitivity, and performing therapeutic lavages of the ear canal and middle ear cavity. • Bullae radiographs—not sensitive. May show thickening of the bullae and petrous temporal bone with chronic disease, boney lysis with severe cases of osteomyelitis, evidence of neoplasia, or may be normal.
• CT or MRI—necessary to demonstrate fluid and soft tissue density within the middle ear and extent of involvement of adjacent structures. CT is better at revealing associated bony changes, MRI for evaluating soft tissue structures including brainstem and cerebellum.

OTITIS MEDIA AND INTERNA (CONTINUED)

DIAGNOSTIC PROCEDURES

• Myringotomy—insert a spinal needle (20-gauge; 2.5- to 3.5-inches) through the otoscope and tympanic membrane to aspirate middle ear fluid for cytologic examination and culture and sensitivity. Examine for bacterial and fungal causes of infection.
• Brainstem auditory evoked response (BAER)—tests the peripheral and central auditory pathways, detects hearing loss.
• CSF analysis—if evidence of intracranial extension, perform culture and sensitivity.

PATHOLOGIC FINDINGS

Purulent exudate within the middle ear cavity surrounded by a thickened bullae and microscopic evidence of degenerate neutrophils with intracellular bacteria or other microorganisms; other causes such as polyps or neoplasia.

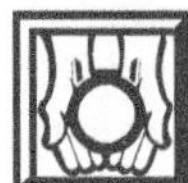

TREATMENT

APPROPRIATE HEALTH CARE

• Inpatient care is recommended with severe debilitating infection or if significantly compromising neurologic signs are present.
• Outpatient care is appropriate if the patient is stable, pending further diagnostics, if indicated.

DIET

• If vomiting, withhold food and water for 12–24 hours. • If unable to stand or severely disoriented, hand-feed and water small amounts frequently. Ensure that the patient is sternal during feeding to decrease risk of aspiration pneumonia.

CLIENT EDUCATION

• Inform client that most bacterial infections resolve without recurrence when treated early with an aggressive course of long-term, broad-spectrum antibiotics. • Warn client that relapsing signs may occur, that the patient may improve but may never be neurologically normal. • Warn client that the condition may require surgical intervention.

SURGICAL CONSIDERATIONS

• Severity of neurologic signs is not directly related to degree of pathology, and should not be used to make decisions regarding need for surgical intervention. • Surgical treatment is indicated for patients with evidence of middle ear exudate, osteomyelitis refractory to medical management, nasopharyngeal polyps, or neoplasia. • Bullae osteotomy allows drainage of the middle ear cavity. • Total ablation of ear canal is indicated when otitis media is associated with recurrent otitis externa or neoplasia. • Perform cytologic examination and culture of middle ear effusion and histopathology of abnormal tissue sampled at the time of surgery.

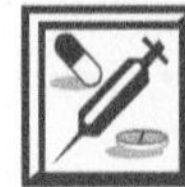

MEDICATIONS

DRUG(S) OF CHOICE

• Topical sterile water, saline, or TrizEDTA-based otic antimicrobial preparations if tympanum is ruptured. • Treat mites if present. • Long-term (6–8 weeks) topical and systemic antibiotics selected on basis of culture and sensitivity, if available.
• Amoxicillin/clavulanic acid (12.5–22 mg/kg q12h PO) is a good first-choice antibiotic.
• Fluoroquinolone or third-generation cephalosporins are good second alternatives or can be used in combination, if culture and sensitivity unavailable; enrofloxacin (Baytril) 5–10 mg/kg q24h (dogs), 5 mg/kg q24h (cats), or marbofloxacin (Zeniquin 5 mg/kg q24h), or cefpodoxime (Simplicef 10 mg/kg q12h); clindamycin (Cleocin 5–30 mg/kg q12h), if anaerobes are suspected. • In cats, where oral dosing is too challenging, consider using cefovecin (Convenia) 8 mg/kg SC every 2 weeks. This can also be used in combination with a fluoroquinolone. • Antiemetics to treat or prevent nausea, vomiting, and dizziness. Meclizine (Antivert, Antrizine, Bonine, Dramamine Less Drowsy Formula) 12.5 mg PO q24h (dogs <10 kg and cats), 25 mg PO q24h (dogs >10 kg); or maropitant citrate (Cerenia) 1 mg/kg SC or 2 mg/kg PO q24h (dogs), 1 mg/kg SC or 1 mg/kg PO q24h (cats); or dolasetron mesylate (Anzemet) 0.6 mg/kg IV q24h (dogs, cats).

CONTRAINDICATIONS

• If ruptured tympanum or associated neurologic deficits, avoid oil-based or irritating external ear preparations (e.g., chlorhexidine) and aminoglycosides, which are toxic to inner ear structures. • Use topical and systemic corticosteroids judiciously in treatment of otitis media or interna. May exacerbate infection. Reserve for cases in which flushing of the ear canal is prevented by inflammation, or to treat edema associated with intracranial spread of infection.

PRECAUTIONS

Avoid vigorous external ear flush.

FOLLOW-UP

PATIENT MONITORING

Evaluate for resolution of signs after 10–14 days or sooner if the patient is deteriorating.

POSSIBLE COMPLICATIONS

• Signs associated with vestibular (head tilt) and facial nerve damage or Horner's syndrome may not resolve. • Severe middle/inner ear infections may spread to brainstem or sometimes forebrain. Clinical signs indicate central vestibular lesion, typically preceded by peripheral vestibular or middle/inner ear signs. Aggressive surgical debridement and antibiotic therapy are required. • Osteomyelitis of the petrous temporal bone and middle ear effusion are common sequelae to severe, chronic otitis externa. • Complications following bulla osteotomy include Horner's syndrome, facial paralysis, onset or exacerbation of vestibular dysfunction, and deafness.

EXPECTED COURSE AND PROGNOSIS

• Otitis media-interna is usually responsive to medical management. To decrease likelihood of relapse, a 2- to 4-month course of antibiotic is recommended. • When medical management of otitis externa is ineffective, consider lateral ear resection. • Vestibular signs typically improve in 2–6 weeks.

MISCELLANEOUS

AGE-RELATED FACTORS

Ear mites more common in kittens and puppies.

SEE ALSO

• Facial Nerve Paresis and Paralysis.
• Head Tilt.
• Horner's Syndrome.
• Otitis Externa and Media.

ABBREVIATIONS

• BAER = brainstem auditory evoked response.
• KCS = keratoconjunctivitis sicca.
• T_4 = thyroxine.
• TSH = thyroid-stimulating hormone.

Suggested Reading

Negrin A, Cherubini GB, Lamb C, et al. Clinical signs, magnetic resonance imaging findings and outcome in 77 cats with vestibular disease: a retrospective study. J Feline Med Surg 2010, 12:291–299.

Sturges BK, Dickinson PJ, Kortz GD, et al. Clinical signs, magnetic resonance imaging features, and outcome after surgical and medical treatment of otogenic intracranial infection in 11 cats and 4 dogs. J Vet Intern Med 2006, 20:648–656.

Authors Richard J. Joseph and Anne E. Buglione

Client Education Handout available online

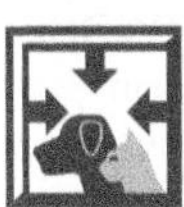

BASICS

OVERVIEW

• Ovarian remnant syndrome is the presence of behavioral and/or physical signs of estrus in a female dog or cat reported as having previously undergone ovariohysterectomy or ovariectomy (OVH/OE).
• It is caused by the presence of functional residual ovarian tissue.
• It is responsible for 17% of all post-OVH/OE complications.

SIGNALMENT

• Female dog and cat; more common in the cat.
• No breed predisposition or geographic distribution.
• Signs of an estrous cycle usually occur months to years after OVH/OE; can begin within days after surgery.

SIGNS

Bitches

Estrogen Influence

• Attraction of male dogs.
• Swelling of the vulva.
• Mucoid to sanguineous vaginal discharge.
• Flagging.
• May allow copulation.
• Signs of pro-estrus last an average of 9 days; signs of estrus last an average of 9 days; average interval between signs of estrous cycles is 7 months.
• Signs are typically cyclical (i.e., q6 months), unlike estrogen toxicity.

Progesterone Influence

• Prominent vulva compared to patients with complete OVH/OE.
• Enlargement of the uterine stump ultrasonographically.
• Uterine stump pyometra can develop due to progesterone effect.

Queens

Estrogen Influence

• Vocalization.
• Lordosis.
• Restlessness.
• Head rubbing.
• Rolling.
• Tail deviation and treading the hind limbs.
• May allow copulation.
• Demonstrate typical behavioral signs of estrus in a cyclical (seasonally polyestrous) fashion.
• Estrus lasts 2–19 days, followed by an interestrous interval that lasts for 8–10 days unless ovulation and luteinization occurred, in which case the interestrous interval is at least 45 days.

Progesterone Influence

• Enlargement of the uterine stump ultrasonographically.
• Uterine stump pyometra can develop due to progesterone effect.

CAUSES & RISK FACTORS

• Failure to remove both ovaries completely.
• No correlation with age at OVH/OE, difficulty of surgery, obesity of patient, or experience of surgeon.
• Presence of anatomically abnormal ovarian tissue (fragmentation into the broad ligament) is possible; more common in queens.
• Supernumerary ovary (rare).
• Experimentally, functionality returns to ovarian tissue removed from its vascular supply and replaced into or onto the lateral abdominal wall, mesentery, or serosal surface.

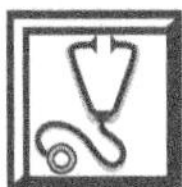

DIAGNOSIS

DIFFERENTIAL DIAGNOSIS

• Inflammation or infection of the genitourinary tract.
• Vaginal hemorrhage due to trauma, foreign body, or coagulopathy.
• Uterine stump granuloma secondary to local pathology (foreign body reaction to suture material or grass awn).
• Neoplasia of a remnant portion of the tubular tract (uterine stump leiomyoma or leiomyosarcoma).
• Neoplasia of an ovarian remnant (granulosa cell tumor, carcinoma, luteoma, functional teratoma), typically not cyclical.
• Neoplasia of the urinary tract (transitional cell carcinoma).
• Vascular anomalies of the genitourinary tract.
• Exogenous estrogen administration, typically not cyclical.
• Exposure to human transdermal hormone replacement therapy, typically not cyclical.
• Endogenous extra-ovarian source of estrogen—adrenal pathology (rare), typically not cyclical.

CBC/BIOCHEMISTRY/URINALYSIS

• Usually normal.
• Chronic blood loss anemia if vaginal hemorrhage is profound.
• Pancytopenia from estrogen toxicity is uncommon.
• An inflammatory leukogram and isosthenuria can occur subsequent to uterine stump pyometra.

OTHER LABORATORY TESTS

• Observation of behavioral and physical signs of estrus together with vaginal cytology and/or measurement of serum progesterone concentration confirming the presence of functional ovarian tissue.
• Vaginal cytology—vaginal mucosal cornification is an excellent bioassay for elevated plasma estradiol concentrations (see Breeding, Timing).
  ◦ Bitch—epithelial cell cornification is generally >90% during estrus (superficial and pyknotic or anuclear cells).
  ◦ Queen—epithelial cell cornification ranges from 10% to 40% (usually retain nucleus); clearing (absence of debris and clumping of cells) occurs in 90% of smears during estrus.
• Serum progesterone:
  ◦ Bitch—a serum progesterone concentration >2 ng/mL (measured 1–3 weeks after behavioral estrus) is consistent with functional luteal tissue. Gonadotropin-releasing hormone (GnRH, 50 μg, IM), human chorionic gonadotropin (hCG; 400 IU, IV, or 500 IU, IV and 500 IU, IM) can be used to attempt to induce ovulation/luteinization for diagnostic purposes; serum progesterone concentration is measured 2–3 weeks later. Note: both normal and pathologic ovarian tissue may fail to respond to either hormone.
  ◦ Queen—ovulation and luteinization is stimulated most commonly by coital stimulation during behavioral estrus, and serum progesterone concentration is measured 2–3 weeks later; post-stimulation serum progesterone concentrations >2 ng/mL are consistent with adequate coital stimulation and functional luteal tissue. Feline ovulation can occur spontaneously. GnRH (25 μg, IM) can be used to attempt to induce ovulation or luteinization for diagnostic purposes; serum progesterone concentration is measured 2–3 weeks later. Both normal and pathologic ovarian tissue may fail to respond.
• Luteinizing hormone (LH) assay (Witness LH, Zoetis)—should be positive (>1 ng/mL) in a completely gonadectomized bitch due to lack of pituitary feedback. When an unexpected positive result is obtained in a bitch suspected to have a remnant, consider repeating in >24 hours to rule out inadvertent detection of the LH surge in the estrual bitch (should also have representative vaginal cytology with superficial cells predominating). If both are positive, then the bitch has been spayed. A negative test (<1 ng/mL) is found in intact dogs unless performed at the moment of the natural LH surge. The assay is licensed for use in the bitch, but likely is applicable in male dogs, toms and queens, provided that the queen is exposed to >14 hours of light/day. Note: exogenous estrogen exposure in a gonadectomized dog can cause the LH to become misleadingly negative.
• Anti-Müllerian hormone (AMH) testing: A positive test in a bitch or queen >6 months of age supports the presence of ovarian tissue (UC Davis Clinical Endocrinology Laboratory, Animal Health Diagnostic Center, Cornell University). In cases with a negative AMH but convincing clinical evidence supporting remnant syndrome, investigators advise obtaining a progesterone to identify persistent

OVARIAN REMNANT SYNDROME (CONTINUED)

luteal structures lacking AMH. AMH differentiates exogenous estrogen exposure (negative) from the ovarian remnant (positive).
• Cytology of vulvar discharge can be suppurative if a uterine stump granuloma or pyometra exists.
• Provocative adrenal testing (pre- and post-adrenocorticotropin [ACTH] administration).

IMAGING

Ultrasonography

• Can be used to support a diagnosis of ovarian remnant syndrome that is based on cytology and hormonal profiles; guides the surgical approach.
• Remnant ovarian tissue is most visible during the follicular phase (anechoic, cystic structures) or the luteal phase (hypo- or isoechoic cystic structures).
• Ultrasonographic imaging of ectopic ovarian tissue requires technical expertise and is best accomplished with a higher frequency, linear transducer (8–10 mHz). Ovarian remnants containing follicular or luteal structures often cause distal enhancement due to their fluid content; this can be used to locate them caudolateral to the ipsilateral kidney (see Web Figure 1).
• Evaluate the region dorsal to the bladder for a uterine remnant, which can enlarge under hormonal influence or with pathology (see Web Figure 2a,b).
• Evaluate the adrenal glands for normal size and shape. Normal canine adrenal glands are <0.51–0.74 cm in sagittal (see Web Figures 3 and 4).

DIAGNOSTIC PROCEDURES

• Exploratory laparotomy/laparoscopy—removal of residual ovarian tissue confirms and resolves the problem.
• Identification of residual ovarian tissue is facilitated by the presence of follicles or corpora lutea; schedule procedure during times of elevated progesterone or during behavioral estrus.
• Histopathology—always submit visible ovarian tissue; if no visible ovarian tissue is identified, submit all residual tissue at the ovarian pedicles. This helps confirm the diagnosis and screens for malignancy. Submit revised abnormal uterine stump tissue for aerobic and anaerobic cultures and histopathology (hormone influence, inflammatory response, malignancy).

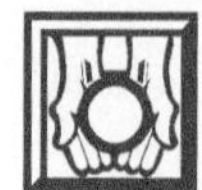

TREATMENT

• Surgical removal of residual ovarian tissue.
• Surgical removal of diseased uterine stump if present.
• Although not curative, restricting light exposure to <8 hours per day can suppress signs of estrus in some, but not all, cats with residual ovarian tissue.

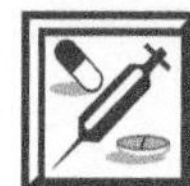

MEDICATIONS

DRUG(S) OF CHOICE

• Progestational or androgenic compounds to suppress follicular ovarian activity—not recommended because of undesirable side effects (mammary neoplasia, diabetes, undesirable behavior, hepatopathy, dermatopathy).
• GnRH agonist (Suprelorin) administration will offer a viable alternative or adjunctive therapy to laparotomy when perfected and commercially available in the United States.

FOLLOW-UP

POSSIBLE COMPLICATIONS

• Removal of functional luteal tissue may induce transient signs of pseudopregnancy in dogs and cats postoperatively (see False Pregnancy).
• The use of oral antiprolactin agents (cabergoline) can be considered for pseudopregnancy.

EXPECTED COURSE AND PROGNOSIS

• Successful removal of remnant ovarian tissue should result in cessation of clinical signs of estrus/diestrus.
• Adjunctive therapy for stump pyometra (systemic antibiotics, supportive care) as indicated.
• Adjunctive therapy for functional ovarian neoplasia as indicated.

MISCELLANEOUS

SEE ALSO

• Breeding, Timing.
• False Pregnancy.
• Hyperestrogenism (Estrogen Toxicity).

ABBREVIATIONS

• ACTH = adrenocorticotropic hormone.
• AMH = anti-Müllerian hormone.
• GnRH = gonadotropin-releasing hormone.
• hCG = human chorionic gonadotropin.
• LH = luteinizing hormone.
• OE = ovariectomy.
• OVH = ovariohysterectomy.

Suggested Reading

Davidson AP, Feldman EC. Ovarian and estrous cycle abnormalities. In: Ettinger SJ, Feldman EC, eds., Textbook of Veterinary Internal Medicine, 6th ed. St. Louis, MO: Elsevier, 2005, pp. 1649–1655.

Miller DM. Ovarian remnant syndrome in dogs and cats: 46 cases (1988–1992). J Vet Diagn Invest 1995, 7:572–574.

Place NJ, Hansen JL, Chereskin SE, et al. Measurement of serum anti-mullerian hormone concentration in female dogs and cats before and after ovariohysterectomy. J Vet Diagn Invest 2011, 23:524.

Authors Autumn P. Davidson and Tomas W. Baker

Consulting Editor Erin E. Runcan

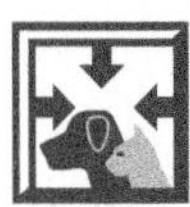

BASICS

OVERVIEW

• Epithelial (carcinoma), germ cell (dysgerminoma and teratoma), and sex cord stromal (granulosa cell tumor, Sertoli–Leydig cell tumor, thecoma, and luteoma) tumors.
• Dogs—rare (0.5–1.2% of tumors); 40% carcinomas, 10% germ cell, and 50% sex cord.
• Cats—rare (0.7–3.6% of tumors); 15% germ cell, and 85% sex cord.
• Metastasis common for malignant epithelial and germ cell tumors in the dog and all tumors in cats.
• Some tumors produce hormones resulting in paraneoplastic syndromes.

SIGNALMENT

• Dog and cat.
• Middle-aged to older animals.
• Teratoma may develop in young patients.

SIGNS

• Bilaterally symmetrical alopecia; pancytopenia; masculinization (hormone-secreting tumors with associated paraneoplastic manifestation).
• Malignant ascites or pleural.
• Effusion (carcinomatosis)—occasionally.
• Other signs associated with mass effects of the tumor (abdominal discomfort, compression of adjacent organs).

CAUSES & RISK FACTORS

• Intact sexual status.
• Dogs—pointer, English bulldog, boxer, German shepherd dog, and Yorkshire terrier at risk.

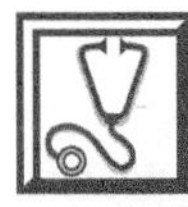

DIAGNOSIS

DIFFERENTIAL DIAGNOSIS

• Other causes of abdominal effusion including vasculitis and pancreatitis.
• Other mid-abdominal masses or gossypiboma (foreign body granuloma).
• Ovarian cysts, paraovarian cysts, cystic rete tubules, vascular hematomas, metastatic neoplasia.

CBC/BIOCHEMISTRY/URINALYSIS

• No consistent abnormalities.
• Pancytopenia in dogs with functional estrogen-secreting tumors.

OTHER LABORATORY TESTS

Serum progesterone—levels >2 mg/mL with functional tumors.

IMAGING

• Abdominal radiography—may reveal unilateral or bilateral mid-abdominal mass at the caudal pole of the kidney or effusion, mineralization of tumor may be seen.
• Abdominal ultrasonography—confirm abdominal radiographic findings and provide greater certainty for the origin of mass effect.
• Advanced imaging—CT or MRI can provide detailed assessment for origin and associated tissues that might be involved in disease process.
• Thoracic radiography—may reveal distant metastasis (rare).

DIAGNOSTIC PROCEDURES

• Cytologic evaluation of pleural or abdominal fluid—may be diagnostic for malignant effusion (carcinomatosis).
• Cytologic evaluation of tumor—tumor cells may readily implant on the body wall via fine-needle aspirate. Therefore, excisional biopsy is often recommended over fine-needle aspirate of the mass.
• Histopathologic examination—necessary for definitive diagnosis.

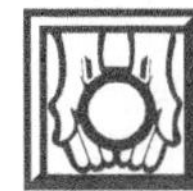

TREATMENT

• Ovariohysterectomy—treatment of choice for a solitary mass.
• Peritoneal transplantation during surgical removal is possible; change gloves and surgical instruments during procedure.
• Laparoscopic-assisted ovariohysterectomy may be possible for smaller tumors.

MEDICATIONS

DRUG(S) OF CHOICE

• Chemotherapy—little information for dogs and cats, no standard therapy.
• Cisplatin—successful treatment reported in three dogs and treatment of choice for comparative tumors in human beings.

CONTRAINDICATIONS/POSSIBLE INTERACTIONS

• Cisplatin—do not use in dogs with renal disease; do not use without appropriate and concurrent diuresis; do not use in cats (fatal).
• Chemotherapy may be toxic; seek advice if unfamiliar with these agents.

FOLLOW-UP

• Abdominal ultrasonography and thoracic radiography—every 3 months; monitor for recurrence and metastasis.
• Ovariohysterectomy—prevention.
• Prognosis—guarded.
• Chemotherapy—has potential to lengthen survival.

MISCELLANEOUS

ASSOCIATED CONDITIONS

• Pyometra.
• Ovarian cysts.
• Cystic endometrial hyperplasia.
• Ovarian remnant syndrome.

Suggested Reading

Morrison WB. Cancer of the reproductive tract. In: Morrison WB, ed., Cancer in Dogs and Cats: Medical and Surgical Management. Jackson, WY: Teton NewMedia, 2002, pp. 555–564.

Patnaik AK, Greenlee PG. Canine ovarian neoplasms: a clinicopathologic study of 71cases including histology of 12 granulosa cell tumors. Vet Pathol 1987, 24:509–514.

Author Heather M. Wilson-Robles

Consulting Editor Timothy M. Fan

Acknowledgment The author and editors acknowledge the prior contribution of Terrance A. Hamilton.

OVULATORY FAILURE

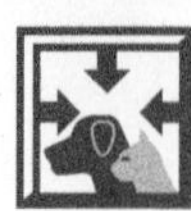

BASICS

OVERVIEW

- Breakdown in the process of ovulation, without normal corpus luteum formation and progesterone production.
- Clinical signs of prolonged estrogen production; may develop estrogen toxicity.

SIGNALMENT

- Intact bitch or queen of any age—greater predisposition in older females.
- Reported in 1.2% of bitches presented for breeding management.
- No breed predisposition for anovulation; follicular cysts reported more commonly in German shepherd dog, Malamute, golden retriever, bouvier des Flandres, and Labrador retriever.
- Heritability unknown.

SIGNS

- Prolonged proestrus or estrus.
- Edematous vulva.
- Sanguineous vulvar discharge (bitch).
- Anestrus.
- Decreased interestrous interval.
- Bilaterally symmetric alopecia (progressive, nonpruritic).
- If neoplasia—abdominal mass ± ascites.
- If chromosome abnormality—genitalia ranges from infantile or ambiguous to normal to enlarged clitoris or os clitoris; small stature; anestrus.

CAUSES & RISK FACTORS

- Failure of release of gonadotropin-releasing hormone (GnRH) or luteinizing hormone (LH).
- Failure of receptors on the follicular wall to respond to LH.
- Failure of the follicles to produce adequate estrogen to elicit GnRH surge.
- Functional follicular cysts—may mimic normal estrous cycle initially, but estrus persists and ovulation does not occur.
- Immune-mediated oophoritis.
- Cachexia or obesity.
- Stress (performance, travel, kennel).
- Adrenal disease.

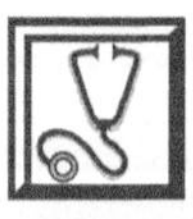

DIAGNOSIS

DIFFERENTIAL DIAGNOSIS

- Prolonged proestrus (up to 30 days) or estrus (up to 30 days).
- Split heat—anovulatory cycle will be followed by a normal, fertile, ovulatory cycle in 1–8 weeks.
- Hypoluteoidism.
- Granulosa cell tumor or serous cystadenoma—abdominal mass; enlarged ovary on ultrasound; ± ascites; ± bilaterally-symmetric alopecia.
- Ovarian senescence.
- Immune-mediated oophoritis.
- Chromosomal abnormality—may develop follicles that either ovulate or regress.
- Exogenous estrogen administration or exposure.

CBC/BIOCHEMISTRY/URINALYSIS

If estrogen toxicity—normocytic, normochromic anemia, thrombocytopenia, leukocytosis followed by leukopenia.

OTHER LABORATORY TESTS

- Serum progesterone concentration <4–10 ng/mL over multiple samplings once vaginal cytology exceeds 70% anucleated superficial cells. Often remains 3–5 ng/mL for prolonged period, never exceeding 10 ng/mL. Vaginal cytology eventually returns to proestrus/anestrus characteristics, confirming ovulatory failure.
- Karyotyping—diagnose chromosomal abnormality.

IMAGING

- Radiography—ovarian mass.
- Ultrasonography—multiple anechoic structures on the ovary may be considered follicles, anechoic structures >1 cm considered cystic; enlarged ovaries may be neoplastic; anechoic structures with thickened walls may indicate luteinization (partial or complete) of follicular structures. Daily ultrasonography to document ovulation; color Doppler can assess ovarian follicular blood flow (increased with follicles, minimal with luteal structures).

DIAGNOSTIC PROCEDURES

Exploratory laparotomy to examine the ovaries or to obtain ovarian biopsies—the ovarian bursa must be opened to visualize the ovary.

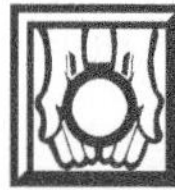

TREATMENT

N/A

MEDICATIONS

DRUG(S) OF CHOICE

- Ovulation induction may be attempted once cytology reaches >70% anucleated cells and follicles are >4–5 mm (toy to small-breed canine), 5–7 mm (medium to large-breed canine), 7–10 mm (giant-breed canine), or 2–3 mm (feline).
- Ovulation-inducing agents:
  - GnRH: 1.1–2.2 µg/kg IM or IV; 25 µg/cat IM; may repeat daily for 1–3 days in bitches, single dose for queens.
  - Human chorionic gonadotropin (hCG): 500–1,000 IU/dog IM; 500 IU/queen IM; may repeat in 2–3 days if ovulation does not occur.
  - GnRH and hCG may be given concurrently or alternating days.
  - Deslorelin implant (2.1 mg implant—Ovuplant® or 4.7 mg implant—Suprelorin®) placed subcutaneously. If breeding and ovulation is confirmed (progesterone >10 ng/mL), implant should be removed. If not breeding, leave implant in place.
  - In queens, cervical stimulation may be performed from initial induction several times daily for 24–48 hours.

FOLLOW-UP

- Monitor progesterone concentrations during pregnancy—luteal failure or hypoluteoidism more common with induced ovulation.
- Monitor progesterone after induction to confirm normal rise.
- Serial ultrasound exams (using color Doppler) may be useful to document ovulation.

MISCELLANEOUS

ASSOCIATED CONDITIONS

Bilaterally symmetric nonpruritic alopecia (with prolonged estrus).

PREGNANCY/FERTILITY/BREEDING

- Anovulation may be hereditary; discuss with owner prior to breeding.
- Subsequent cycles may be normal, necessitating no treatment, or abnormal again.

SEE ALSO

- Infertility, Female—Dogs.
- Sexual Development Disorders.

ABBREVIATIONS

- GnRH = gonadotropin-releasing hormone.
- hCG = human chorionic gonadotropin.
- LH = luteinizing hormone.

Suggested Reading

Meyers-Wallen VN. Unusual and abnormal canine estrous cycles. Theriogenology 2007, 68:1205–1210.

Author Cheryl Lopate

Consulting Editor Erin E. Runcan

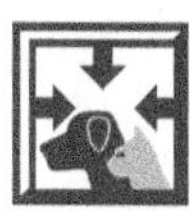

BASICS

DEFINITION

• Unpleasant sensory or emotional experience associated with actual or potential tissue damage (adaptive pain) or altered sensory neurobiology (chronic pain).
• The inability for the animal to communicate does not negate presence of pain and the need for appropriate pain-relieving treatment.

PATHOPHYSIOLOGY

• With physiologic pain, an application of a noxious stimulus activates specialized nerve endings called nociceptors; nociceptors transduce noxious chemical, mechanical, or thermal stimuli into electrochemical potentials that are transmitted via sensory nerves from the affected tissue to the spinal cord.
• In the dorsal horn of the spinal cord, the incoming first-order peripheral nerve synapses with ascending spinal neurons, which terminate in the brainstem. Incoming noxious information can be modulated in the dorsal horn by other incoming information, descending inhibitory nerve impulses, or pharmacologic inhibition by several classes of drugs. The ascending neurons synapse in the brainstem to form ascending tracts that end in the cortex, where sensation occurs. Neuroendocrine and physiologic responses (e.g., tachycardia, elevated cortisol) to noxious stimuli may originate from the brainstem and do not necessarily correlate with the perceived intensity of pain.
• Nociceptive processes (i.e., transduction, transmission, and modulation) appear to be similar anatomically and physiologically in most mammalian and many non-mammalian species. The perception of pain may vary between species and individuals of the same species since anatomic differences in cortical development exist and integration of past experiences and learned behaviors varies.
• Prolonged activity in nociceptive pathways (e.g., days, weeks, or months) from chronic injury or disease, or injury to nervous system tissues, may cause altered neuroprocessing resulting in sensitization of these pathways and hyperresponsiveness. This may cause an increased response to a stimulus not normally considered noxious (allodynia).

SYSTEMS AFFECTED

• Pain may originate from any tissue, including the nervous system itself. In humans, certain pain syndromes may be associated with fear, anxiety, or depression in the absence of any observable injury.
• The physiologic response to pain can include decreased immune function, increased catabolism, and elevated neuroendocrine markers of stress. Pain can result in a loss of function of affected tissues.

GENETICS

Age, sex, breeding strain, and species can influence responses to noxious stimuli. Genes have been described that modify individual behavioral responses to noxious stimuli in several species. Genes may also be variably expressed depending on stimulus intensity and duration, which can lead to altered neuroprocessing and maladaptive or chronic pain.

INCIDENCE/PREVALENCE

• Evolutionarily, aversion to noxious stimuli was protective to organisms, keeping them away from harm.
• While acute pain is beneficial to warn or teach an animal about potential harmful objects in its environment, persistent acute pain associated with surgery or injury does not benefit the patient and should be treated appropriately.
• Any form of chronic pain syndrome does not serve a protective function and should be treated.

SIGNS

• Behavioral signs of pain and distress vary considerably among individuals.
• Experience, environment, age, species, and other factors can modify the intensity of the reaction to noxious stimuli or to an altered neurobiology associated with maladaptive or chronic pain.
• The most obvious clinical signs of distress in the dog and cat can include vocalization, agitation, abnormal posture or gait, thrashing, hyperesthesia, or hyperalgesia.
• More subtle signs shared by many conditions include trembling, lethargy, reduced appetite, stupor, and biting.
• Tachypnea, tachycardia, mydriasis, and hypertension are signs observed with the stress response that may also accompany pain; these are nonspecific and present in many nonpainful conditions. The stress response is often not associated with chronic pain due to adaptation.
• Clinical signs associated with chronically painful conditions may be very subtle or difficult to evaluate since homeostatic mechanisms tend to help the animal compensate. Chronically painful conditions are often associated with decreased activity, lameness, and/or depression.

CAUSES

• Physiologic or adaptive pain can be caused by perceived or actual tissue disruption associated with trauma or surgery and also by chronic degenerative changes and inflammation associated with conditions such as osteoarthritis.
• Pain that extends beyond the initial tissue damage and healing processes is pathologic (maladaptive) and may indicate that the initiation of altered nervous system processing has occurred.

RISK FACTORS

• All animals that experience surgical or traumatic tissue damage or have recently altered behavior should be evaluated for the presence of pain.
• Due to the increasing prevalence of degenerative diseases in older patients, routine examination should include evaluation for pain.
• Pain intensity may not always correlate with the degree of tissue damage. However, more invasive soft tissue and orthopedic procedures or inflammatory disease progression in older patients are likely associated with greater pain.

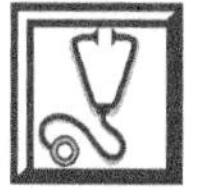

DIAGNOSIS

DIFFERENTIAL DIAGNOSIS

• Identifying pain in veterinary patients is a diagnosis, and the medical record should reflect the veterinarian's clinical diagnostic and treatment plan.
• Acute pain is almost always accompanied by tissue damage or disease, and diagnosis and treatment of the primary disorder should be done before or concomitantly with treatment of pain. The presence or absence of pain is sometimes used as a way of monitoring and diagnosing some conditions, and treatment should be in accordance with good medical practice. Pain should be differentiated from distress associated with other factors, such as restraint, restrictive bandaging, and separation from owners. Drugs used to treat pain, particularly opioids and dissociative anesthetics, may cause dysphoria, which often resembles and can be confused with signs of pain and distress.

CBC/BIOCHEMISTRY/URINALYSIS

• Cortisol release associated with acute pain may appear as a stress leukogram.
• Hyperglycemia may also be observed in some patients, but can also be seen with anesthesia in the absence of tissue trauma.
• Normal laboratory test values do not rule out the presence of pain.

OTHER LABORATORY TESTS

N/A

IMAGING

• Many painful patients have underlying changes in anatomic structures observable on ultrasound, radiography, CT or MRI.
• Chronic pathologic tissue changes such as the degree of osteophyte formation with osteoarthritis do not necessarily always correlate with the degree of pain and dysfunction experienced by the patient. Some patients can be painful without observable tissue or structural changes.

DIAGNOSTIC PROCEDURES

- Review patient signalment, obtain a thorough history, and include pain assessment as part of every physical examination. The pain score should be recorded in the patient's record along with temperature, pulse, and respiration.
- Thoroughly evaluate underlying conditions that may be contributing to pain and treat appropriately.
- Use a species-specific scoring tool for pain assessment to decrease subjectivity and observer bias. This will result in more effective pain management. Such tools are referred to as multifactorial clinical measurement instruments (CMIs) and are available for acute postoperative or chronic pain.
- CMIs for acute postoperative pain involve observing the patient without interaction; observing the patient while interacting with a caregiver; observing the patient's response to palpation of the surgical site; and assigning a numerical score using a dynamic interactive visual analogue scale. The reevaluation interval will depend on the procedure, duration of intervention chosen, and previous pain score.
- CMIs for chronic pain primarily involve owner observations of their pets regarding exercise tolerance and general activity; ability to stand, walk, do stairs, jump, or rise; grooming behavior; and urination or defecation habits.
- Complete abolishment of pain may not be possible or desirable if analgesic administration results in excessive adverse effects. Therapy should aim to make pain tolerable.

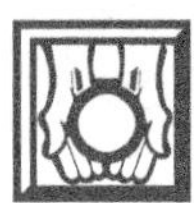

TREATMENT

APPROPRIATE HEALTH CARE

- Analgesic drug selection depends on species, pain intensity, and underlying cause.
- Treat the underlying cause at the same time if possible.
- Acupuncture, prescribed activity (e.g., physical therapy), mesenchymal stromal cell or platelet-rich plasma injection, and physical manipulation (massage, trigger point manipulation, chiropractic) may be useful adjunctive treatment modalities for certain types of painful musculoskeletal conditions.
- If the patient's quality of life is not acceptable after all reasonable therapeutic options have been explored, euthanasia may be the most humane option.

NURSING CARE

- General good nursing practices.
- Nonpharmacologic, including bandaging and hydrotherapy, may be appropriate.

ACTIVITY

- Rehabilitation medicine and weight loss is a useful adjunct for some musculoskeletal conditions.
- Cage rest or limited activity may be useful for certain types of pain.

DIET

- Dietary changes to help treat the underlying condition (e.g., weight reduction for hip dysplasia) may be beneficial.
- Many supplements have been marketed that may have beneficial effects on articular cartilage or modify inflammatory disease progression.
- Commercial veterinary diets are marketed specifically for animals with mobility issues.

CLIENT EDUCATION

- When pain medication is dispensed, educate clients on what to look for with effective treatment, as well as adverse effects. Use caution when dispensing opioids to clients for at-home administration and ensure they understand requirements for safe storage and disposal.
- Inform the client that analgesic effectiveness varies and several drugs may need to be tried before an effective treatment is found. Pain management must be individualized because of the neurobiologic complexity of pain perception.
- Clients should be asked to participate in evaluation of their pet's pain, especially chronic pain. Species-specific CMIs are available and can help document treatment effectiveness.

SURGICAL CONSIDERATIONS

- Surgical treatment of the underlying condition causing pain may be the best treatment in some circumstances.
- Ablative procedures (neurectomy) to halt pain transmission is not always associated with positive results and may result in worsening of the painful condition. These procedures are rarely performed in veterinary patients.

MEDICATIONS

DRUG(S) OF CHOICE (SEE ALSO APPENDIX VII)

- Opioids, alone or in combination with other classes of drugs, such as sedative/tranquilizers or nonsteroidal anti-inflammatory drugs (NSAIDs), are widely used for the management of acute postoperative pain.
- Full μ-opioid receptor agonists, such as morphine, hydromorphone, and fentanyl, are usually effective for moderate to severe pain. Partial agonist or agonist–antagonist drugs, such as buprenorphine and butorphanol, are usually reserved for mild to moderate pain.
- Opioids generally have poor oral bioavailability, and oral doses should be adjusted accordingly.
- Full μ-opioid receptor agonists can be used safely in cats; however, doses are usually reduced relative to dog doses.
- An SC injectable formulation of buprenorphine has been approved for 24-hour postoperative pain control in cats.
- Should dysphoria develop after opioid administration, tranquilization with an α_2-agonist or acepromazine may be beneficial.
- NSAIDs are used most commonly for the chronic treatment of painful conditions in dogs. They can be safe when administered chronically, but gastrointestinal (GI), hepatic, and renal adverse effects are possible. The best strategy appears to be reducing the dose to the lowest effective dose in an individual. If chronic administration is anticipated serum chemistries should be considered to monitor for hepatic and renal adverse effects.
- Veterinary-approved NSAIDs for dogs and cats have demonstrated acceptable safety profiles; however, there is no strong indication that any particular veterinary-approved NSAID is associated with a greater or lesser incidence or prevalence of adverse events.
- Long-term use of low-dose meloxicam is approved in cats in many countries other than the United States.
- Grapiprant is a non-cyclooxygenase (COX)-inhibiting NSAID that targets prostaglandin E2 (EP4 receptors) approved for osteoarthritic pain and inflammation in dogs.
- Liposome-encapsulated bupivacaine is approved for peri-incisional infiltration in dogs undergoing cranial cruciate ligament surgery and for peripheral nerve block in cats. Gradually released local anesthetic can provide analgesia for up to 72 hours. Extralabel use is also encountered frequently for other types of procedures.
- Additional information is available for many drugs and should be referred to when considering extralabel use. Owners should be informed of the risks of analgesic drug therapy in their pet before consenting to treatment.

Neuropathic Pain

Treatment of neuropathic pain is a subcategory of pathologic pain. It may originate from brain or spinal masses, injury (such as with intervertebral disc disease), inflammation, or the repetitive stimulation of the pain transmission system by a chronic injury outside the CNS. Classic signs that accompany neuropathic pain are allodynia and hyperalgesia. Neuropathic pain does not always respond well to traditional analgesics, such as NSAIDs and opioids, although these drugs are usually tried initially (except for NSAIDs when neurosurgery is imminent). Tricyclic antidepressants, antiepileptic drugs (e.g., gabapentin), *N*-methyl-D-aspartate (NMDA) receptor antagonists, and other alternative (complementary) therapies may be effective. Most of these treatments consist of extra- or off-label use of human medications and require careful client communication and approval.

CONTRAINDICATIONS

- Opioids may be associated with severe respiratory depression in human patients, but in most dogs and cats cause only minimal respiratory depression. In patients with severe respiratory compromise or intracranial hypertension, opioids may be contraindicated. Most μ-opioid receptor agonists can also alter GI and urinary tract motility, resulting in constipation, urinary retention, and vomiting.
- NSAIDs can cause GI ulceration, hepatopathies, and impaired renal function. Preexisting GI, hepatic, or renal disease may be a contraindication to their use. Concomitant glucocorticoid therapy, severe stress, or anorexia may predispose many animals to adverse effects. NSAIDs that significantly inhibit COX-1 may also alter platelet function and may result in increased surgical blood loss. Acetaminophen or acetaminophen-containing analgesics should not be used in cats.

PRECAUTIONS

- Carefully monitor patients for adverse effects and clinical effectiveness following administration of analgesic drugs.
- Opioid-induced hyperthermia has been reported in feline patients, most commonly after fentanyl patch application or hydromorphone administration.
- Opioid administration may result in altered GI motility (constipation), inappetence, and urine retention. These signs usually appear soon after initiation of opioid therapy and should resolve within 12–36 hours of stopping opioid administration. In the interim supportive care such as passing a urinary catheter may be necessary.
- In consultation with the pet owner, the veterinarian may feel the need to prescribe NSAIDs to a particular patient even if the risk for adverse events is deemed increased due to disease or preexisting conditions. The veterinarian should strive to ethically balance the long-term therapeutic risk of drugs such as NSAIDs against the benefit of improved quality of life.
- Opioid abuse has affected all health professions including veterinary medicine and veterinarians must play active roles in combating abuse and misuse of opioids. With new opioid prescribing guidelines now published in many jurisdictions, veterinarians must remain up to date on all relevant regulations.

POSSIBLE INTERACTIONS

- Opioids can reduce the anesthetic requirements for most species, especially when combined with α_2-agonists or acepromazine as a premedication before anesthesia. In humans the combination of certain opioids such as meperidine with serotonin-altering drugs may result in toxicity (e.g., L-deprenyl, amitriptyline, tramadol, trazadone) and are occasionally prescribed to veterinary patients.
- Concurrent glucocorticoid therapy may enhance NSAID toxicity.
- Other drugs that predispose animals to GI or renal impairment, such as aminoglycoside antimicrobials, should be used with caution when NSAIDs are also being administered.

ALTERNATIVE DRUG(S)

- Adjunctive analgesic drugs (e.g., gabapentin, amantadine, amitriptyline, tramadol) may be beneficial for patients that have altered neuroprocessing associated with chronic disease changes or nervous system injury. To select and administer an adjuvant analgesic properly, the veterinarian should be aware of the drug's clinical pharmacology. The following information about the drug is necessary: (1) approved indication, (2) unapproved indication (e.g., as an analgesic) widely accepted in veterinary medical practice, (3) common side effects and potentially serious adverse effects, (4) pharmacokinetic features, and (5) specific dosing guidelines for pain (see Appendix VII).
- Nontraditional medical treatments are common, but should be evaluated for safety and effectiveness before recommendation.
- A number of alternative treatments for chronic pain in dogs and/or cats are in various stages of development and marketing including mesenchymal stem cell therapy and anti-nerve growth factor (anti-NGF) monoclonal drugs.
- Potential novel approaches to chronic pain currently being investigated include cannabidiol (CBD) which is available commercially and from marijuana dispensaries in jurisdictions where allowed. The FDA has decided to regulate CBD as a food additive and the legality of recommending and producing CBD for veterinary patients is unclear at this time. More research is needed before such therapies can be routinely recommended.
- Low-level laser therapy has gained popularity as an adjunctive technique to manage postoperative pain and facilitate earlier return to function following cruciate surgery in dogs. While this therapy may prove beneficial in individual cases, controlled studies using force plate analysis have not documented efficacy to date.

FOLLOW-UP

PATIENT MONITORING

- Frequent evaluation of analgesic drug effectiveness should be performed.
- Patients receiving chronic analgesic medication, especially NSAIDs, should be evaluated periodically to monitor GI, liver, and renal function.
- It is the responsibility of the veterinarian to ensure that information about the effects of prescribed drugs is disseminated to clients.

PREVENTION/AVOIDANCE

Although some degree of pain is usually an unavoidable consequence of surgery or trauma, when possible, the preemptive administration of analgesic drugs may provide better pain control and reduce the potential for CNS wind-up. Use of proper anesthetic techniques incorporating analgesic premedications and local and regional analgesic techniques where appropriate, are effective ways of practicing preemptive analgesia.

EXPECTED COURSE AND PROGNOSIS

Acute pain associated with surgery or trauma usually resolves with tissue healing. Opioids may be most effective for the 12–24 hours following surgery, whereas NSAIDs may be better after that period. Some NSAIDs are effective analgesics immediately after surgery. When pain signs persist beyond the normal course of a few days to weeks, suspect persistent disease, injury, or CNS changes and consult an anesthesiologist or a board-certified specialist trained in pain management for suggestions about appropriate therapy.

MISCELLANEOUS

PREGNANCY/FERTILITY/BREEDING

- Opioids may cause fetal respiratory depression following delivery. NSAIDs may alter maternal or fetal prostaglandin production, resulting in pregnancy complications.
- The effects on the fetus of many of the analgesic drugs approved for use in dogs and cats are not widely reported.

ABBREVIATIONS

- CBD = cannabidiol.
- CMI = multifactorial clinical measurement instrument.
- COX = cyclooxygenase.
- GI = gastrointestinal.
- NGF = nerve growth factor.
- NMDA = *N*-methyl-D-aspartate.
- NSAID = nonsteroidal anti-inflammatory drug.

INTERNET RESOURCES

- American College of Veterinary Anesthesia and Analgesia's position paper on treatment of pain in animals: http://acvaa.org/docs/Pain_Treatment

- International Veterinary Academy of Pain Management: http://www.ivapm.org
- World Small Animal Veterinary Association (WSAVA) Global Pain Council Guidelines: https://wsava.org/global-guidelines/global-pain-council-guidelines/

Suggested Reading

Epstein M, Rodan I, Griffenhagen G, et al. AAHA/AAFP pain management guidelines for dogs and cats. J Am Anim Hosp Assoc 2015, 51(2):67–84.

Grimm KA, Tranquilli WJ, Lamont LA, et al. Veterinary Anesthesia and Analgesia: The Fifth Edition of Lumb and Jones. Ames, IA: Wiley-Blackwell, 2015.

Renwick SM, Renwick AI, Brodbelt DC, et al. Influence of class IV laser therapy on the outcomes of tibial plateau leveling osteotomy in dogs. Vet Surg 2018, 47(4):507–515.

Steagall P, Robertson SA, Taylor P. Feline Anesthesia and Pain Management, Ames, IA: Wiley-Blackwell, 2017.

Authors Leigh A. Lamont, Kurt A. Grimm, and William J. Tranquilli

Client Education Handout available online

P

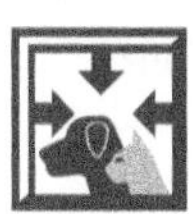

BASICS

DEFINITION

Communication between the nasal and oral cavities.

PATHOPHYSIOLOGY

- Secondary to congenital cleft of the secondary palate to include the hard and/or soft palate.
- Secondary to a traumatic injury causing disruption of the lateral maxilla and/or hard palate.
- Secondary to resective surgery for neoplasms of the lateral maxilla and/or hard palate.
- Secondary to extraction of maxillary canine and rostral premolar teeth (see Oronasal Fistula).

SYSTEMS AFFECTED

- Gastrointestinal (oral cavity).
- Respiratory.

GENETICS

May be inherited or secondary to intrauterine abnormality.

INCIDENCE/PREVALENCE

- Primary cleft palate is an abnormality of the lip and premaxilla and is rarely associated with a palatal defect communicating with the nasal cavity.
- Brachycephalic breeds are predisposed to primary cleft palate.
- Breed predilection for congenital cleft of the secondary palate.

SIGNALMENT

Species

Dogs more common than cats.

Breed Predilections

Brachycephalic breeds, miniature schnauzer, beagle, cocker spaniel, dachshund, and Siamese cats.

Mean Age and Range

At birth in dogs with primary or secondary cleft palate.

Predominant Sex

N/A

SIGNS

- Difficulty nursing.
- Regurgitation.
- Nasal discharge; often mucopurulent.
- Sneezing.
- Gagging when drinking water or eating.
- Poor growth.
- Lethargy and depression in chronic cases with severe secondary rhinitis.
- Cough in cases of secondary aspiration pneumonia.

General Comments

Dogs with primary or secondary cleft palate should be neutered since the condition is considered to be inherited.

Historical Findings

Signs reported by the owner as above; or following trauma or oncologic surgery.

Physical Examination Findings

- Hard and/or soft plate defect communicating with the nasal cavity.
- Nasal discharge.
- Thoracic auscultation for aspiration pneumonia.
- Patient is "poor doer."
- Check for other congenital abnormalities.

CAUSES

- Failure of the palatine shelves to fuse during development at 25–28 days of gestation.
- Foreign body, vehicular, or bite trauma.
- Oncologic surgery for neoplasms of the hard palate and/or lateral maxilla.
- Wound dehiscence following maxillofacial reconstructive surgery.

RISK FACTORS

- Inherited (recessive or irregular dominant, polygenic).
- Nutritional.
- Hormonal (steroids).
- *In utero* abnormality.
- Viral.

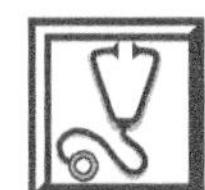

DIAGNOSIS

DIFFERENTIAL DIAGNOSIS

Fungal or bacterial rhinitis.

CBC/BIOCHEMISTRY/URINALYSIS

- Recommended as preoperative database.
- CBC may reflect secondary chronic rhinitis and/or secondary aspiration pneumonia.

OTHER LABORATORY TESTS

Consider aerobic bacterial culture and sensitivity of nasal tissue in cases of chronic rhinitis.

IMAGING

- Thoracic radiographs are recommended to rule out aspiration pneumonia.
- MRI or CT imaging is recommended prior to oncologic surgery for imaging of the maxillary/palatal lesion.
- Three-view thoracic radiographs are recommended to check for distant metastasis before operating patients with neoplasms.

DIAGNOSTIC PROCEDURES

Sedated oral examination.

PATHOLOGIC FINDINGS

- Secondary rhinitis is usually self-limiting and resolves following surgical repair.
- Long-term (4–6 weeks) antimicrobial therapy based on culture and sensitivity may be necessary to treat the chronic rhinitis.

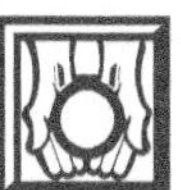

TREATMENT

APPROPRIATE HEALTH CARE

Inpatient

NURSING CARE

Supportive preoperative care.

ACTIVITY

N/A

DIET

- Preoperative diet should be small-dog food "meatballs" fed by hand or a diet with a consistency that does not cause potential aspiration pneumonia.
- Postoperative diet should be a thick liquid consistency for the first 2 weeks.

CLIENT EDUCATION

- A palatal defect requires surgery for repair.
- Multiple surgeries may be required to repair the palatal defect.
- Medical management is ineffective and is only indicated when multiple surgical attempts to repair the palatal defect have failed.
- There is a higher surgical success rate in older puppies.
- Tube feeding may be required for the neonate patient until surgery, or until the patient can eat a diet of appropriate consistency.
- Secondary rhinitis is expected and self-limiting with clinical signs more of a nuisance than pathologic.

SURGICAL CONSIDERATIONS

- The surgical goal is to provide a soft tissue barrier or layer to reestablish and segregate the oral and nasal cavities.
- Congenital secondary cleft palate—recommend using a sliding bipedicle flap repair technique or an overlapping flap repair technique.
- Traumatic palatal defect—recommend either a buccal mucosal flap repair technique or hard palate mucoperiosteal flap repair technique.
- Palatal defect following oncologic surgery—recommend either a buccal mucosal flap repair technique and/or hard palate mucoperiosteal flap repair technique.
- Palatal defect following maxillofacial reconstruction dehiscence—recommend either a buccal mucosal flap repair technique and/or hard palate mucoperiosteal flap repair technique.
- Lavage the nasal cavity before surgery to remove any foreign material or debris that may have accumulated in the nose.
- A permanent silastic obturator may used to occlude small palatal defects in refractory cases where surgery has failed multiple times.

PALATAL DEFECTS (CONTINUED)

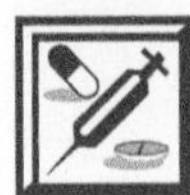

MEDICATIONS

DRUG(S) OF CHOICE

N/A unless treating preoperative rhinitis.

PRECAUTIONS

N/A

POSSIBLE INTERACTIONS

N/A

ALTERNATIVE DRUGS

N/A

FOLLOW-UP

PATIENT MONITORING

Recommend 2- and 4-week postoperative examinations to determine success of the surgical procedure.

PREVENTION/AVOIDANCE

- Diet should be a thick liquid consistency for 2 weeks postoperatively.
- Chew toys and other objects are prohibited for the first 8 weeks postoperatively.

POSSIBLE COMPLICATIONS

- Wound dehiscence and failure to repair the palatal defect.
- Chronic, preexisting rhinitis may require extended postoperative antimicrobial therapy.

EXPECTED COURSE AND PROGNOSIS

- Surgery is usually successful, however multiple surgical procedures may be required.
- The overall prognosis is "good."

MISCELLANEOUS

ASSOCIATED CONDITIONS

- Rhinitis.
- Aspiration pneumonia.

AGE-RELATED FACTORS

- There is a higher surgical success rate in older puppies.
- Tube feeding may be required for the neonate patient until surgery, or until the patient can eat a diet of appropriate consistency.
- Initial dietary management and feeding by the owner is labor intensive.

ZOONOTIC POTENTIAL

N/A

PREGNANCY/FERTILITY/BREEDING

Congenital cleft palate defects are considered inherited and affected dogs should be neutered.

SYNONYMS

N/A

INTERNET RESOURCES

Search oronasal communication, oronasal fistula, cleft palate.

Suggested Reading

Hedlund CS. Surgery of the oral cavity and oropharynx. In: Fossum TW, Hedlund CS, Hulse DA, et al., eds., Small Animal Surgery. St. Louis, MO: Mosby, 1997, pp. 210–215.

Manfra Marretta S, Grove TK, Grillo JF. Split palatal U-flap: a new technique for repair of caudal hard palate defects. J Vet Dent 1991, 8:5–8.

Smith MM. Island mucoperiosteal flap for repair of oronasal fistula in a dog. J Vet Dent 2001, 18:140–144.

Smith MM, Rockhill AD. Prosthodontic appliance for repair of oronasal fistula in a cat. J Am Vet Med Assoc 1996, 208:1410–1412.

Author Mark M. Smith

Consulting Editor Heidi B. Lobprise

P

BASICS

DEFINITION

• Inflammation of the pancreas most often of unknown cause(s). • Acute pancreatitis—inflammation of the pancreas that occurs abruptly with little or no permanent pathologic change. • Chronic pancreatitis—continuing inflammatory disease that is accompanied by irreversible morphologic change such as fibrosis.

PATHOPHYSIOLOGY

• Host defense mechanisms normally prevent pancreatic autodigestion by pancreatic enzymes, but under select circumstances these natural defenses fail; autodigestion occurs when these digestive enzymes are activated within acinar cells. • Local and systemic tissue injury is due to the activity of released pancreatic enzymes and a variety of inflammatory mediators such as kinins, free radicals, and complement factors that are released by infiltrating neutrophils and macrophages. The most common pathologies involving the feline pancreas include acute necrotizing pancreatitis (ANP), acute suppurative pancreatitis, and chronic nonsuppurative pancreatitis.

SYSTEMS AFFECTED

• Gastrointestinal (GI)—altered GI motility (ileus) due to regional chemical peritonitis; local or generalized peritonitis due to enhanced vascular permeability; concurrent inflammatory bowel disease (IBD) may be seen in some cats. • Hepatobiliary—lesions due to shock, pancreatic enzyme injury, inflammatory cellular infiltrates, hepatic lipidosis, and intra/extrahepatic cholestasis. Feline GI inflammatory disease (concurrent cholangitis ± IBD) may be seen in some cats. • Respiratory—pulmonary edema or pleural effusion. • Cardiovascular—cardiac arrhythmias may result from release of myocardial depressant factor. • Hematologic—activation of the coagulation cascade and systemic consumptive coagulopathy (disseminated intravascular coagulation [DIC]) may occur.

GENETICS

No genetic basis for disease pathogenesis in cats has been identified.

INCIDENCE/PREVALENCE

• True prevalence is unknown but this is a relatively common clinical disorder in cats. • Necropsy surveys suggest an increased prevalence in cats with cholangitis, and IBD. The unique feline pancreaticobiliary anatomy and intestinal microbiota likely contribute to multiorgan inflammatory disease in this species.

GEOGRAPHIC DISTRIBUTION

Worldwide

SIGNALMENT

Species

Cat

Breed Predilections

Siamese cats.

Mean Age and Range

Mean age for acute pancreatitis is 7.3 years; any age may be affected.

Predominant Sex

None

SIGNS

Historical Findings

• Vague, nonspecific, and nonlocalizing signs. • Anorexia, lethargy, and vomiting are reported most frequently. • Weakness. • Abdominal pain. • Diarrhea—small bowel and large bowel diarrhea and fever are less common in cats than in dogs.

Physical Examination Findings

• Severe lethargy. • Inappetance. • Dehydration—common; due to GI losses. • Abdominal pain—recognized much less frequently in cats than dogs. • Mass lesions may be palpable. • Fever—observed in 25% of cats.

CAUSES

Etiology is most often unknown; possibilities include: • Hepatobiliary disease—both inflammatory and degenerative (hepatic lipidosis). • Pancreatic trauma/ischemia. • Duodenal reflux. • Drugs/toxins (organophosphates). • Pancreatic duct obstruction. • Hypercalcemia. • Inflammatory GI disease. • Nutrition—excessively lean body mass is associated with ANP.

RISK FACTORS

• Breed? • Obesity? • Organophosphate poisoning. • Concurrent hepatic/intestinal inflammatory disease.

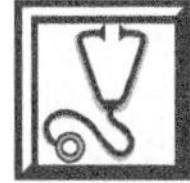

DIAGNOSIS

DIFFERENTIAL DIAGNOSIS

• GI disease (obstruction, foreign body, perforation, infectious gastroenteritis, ulcer disease)—exclude with CBC/biochemistry/urinalysis, diagnostic imaging, and paracentesis. • GI or hepatic neoplasia—exclude with tissue biopsy. • Urogenital disease (pyelonephritis, prostatitis or abscessation, pyometra, urinary tract rupture or obstruction, acute renal failure)—exclude with CBC/biochemistry/urinalysis, urine culture/sensitivity, and imaging. • Hepatobiliary disease (cholangitis and extrahepatic biliary obstruction [EHBO])—exclude with CBC/biochemistry/urinalysis, bile acids, imaging, and liver biopsy. • Abdominal neoplasia—exclude with imaging and cytology or biopsy.

CBC/BIOCHEMISTRY/URINALYSIS

• CBC—often reveals nonregenerative anemia (40%), leukocytosis (38%), and/or leukopenia (15%). • Serum biochemistries—often show prerenal azotemia; liver enzyme activities (alanine aminotransferase, alkaline phosphatase) are often elevated because of hepatic ischemia or exposure to pancreatic enzymes; hyperbilirubinemia with intra/extrahepatic biliary obstruction; hyperglycemia with necrotizing pancreatitis due to hyperglucagonemia; hypoalbuminemia, hypercholesterolemia, and hypertriglyceridemia are common. Hypocalcemia is more common in cats than dogs, and a low ionized calcium concentration is a negative prognostic indicator in cats. • Urinalysis—increased urine specific gravity associated with dehydration or can be unremarkable.

OTHER LABORATORY TESTS

• Serum amylase and lipase activities are unreliable serologic markers—may be elevated, but are nonspecific; can also increase with hepatic, renal, or neoplastic disease in the absence of pancreatitis. • Serum pancreatic lipase immunoreactivity (fPL) is a highly sensitive and specific serologic marker of acute pancreatic inflammation. A cage-side fPL assay (SNAP fPL) has been developed as a useful screening tool. Elevation in SNAP fPL should be followed up by laboratory measurement of serum Spec fPL to quantitate the degree of elevation.

IMAGING

• Abdominal radiographs—may include increased soft tissue opacity in the right cranial abdominal compartment; loss of visceral detail ("ground glass appearance") due to abdominal effusion; static gas pattern in the proximal duodenum. • Abdominal ultrasound—nonhomogeneous solid or cystic mass lesions suggest pancreatic abscess; may be a pancreatic mass or altered echogenicity (hypoechoic) in the area of the pancreas; pancreas is usually enlarged with irregular borders, surrounding mesentery may be hyperechoic due to focal peritonitis, may see peritoneal effusion and extrahepatic biliary obstruction. • fPL assay and pancreatic ultrasound in combination have the highest specificity for an antemortem diagnosis of acute pancreatitis.

DIAGNOSTIC PROCEDURES

• Ultrasound-guided needle aspiration may confirm inflammation (cytology), abscess, or cyst. • Laparoscopy with pancreatic forceps biopsy for histologic diagnosis. • Histopathologic evaluation may miss focal or segmental pancreatic inflammation and results should be interpreted with caution.

PATHOLOGIC FINDINGS

• Gross findings (acute pancreatitis)—mild swelling with edematous pancreatitis. • Gross findings (chronic pancreatitis)—pancreas is reduced in size, firm, gray, and irregular; may contain extensive adhesions to surrounding

viscera. • Microscopic changes (acute pancreatitis)—include edema, parenchymal necrosis, hemorrhage, and neutrophilic cellular infiltrate with acute lesions.
• Microscopic changes (chronic pancreatitis)—pancreatic fibrosis around ducts, ductal epithelial hyperplasia, atrophy, and mononuclear cellular infiltrate.

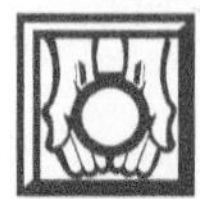

TREATMENT

APPROPRIATE HEALTH CARE

• Eliminate the inciting cause (if possible).
• Supportive care is most important.

NURSING CARE

• Aggressive IV fluid therapy. Fluid therapy goals—correct hypovolemia and maintain pancreatic microcirculation. • An isotonic crystalloid such as lactated Ringer's solution or Normosol-R® is the first-choice rehydration fluid. • Correct initial dehydration (mL = % dehydration × weight in kg × 1000) and give over 4–6 hours. • May need colloids to improve pancreatic circulatory needs and prevent ischemia. • Following replacement of deficits, give additional fluids to match maintenance requirements (2.5 × weight in kg = mL/kg/h) and ongoing losses (estimated). • Potassium chloride (KCl) supplementation usually needed because of potassium loss in the vomitus; base potassium supplementation on measured serum levels (use 20 mEq of KCl/L of IV fluid if serum potassium levels are not known; do not administer faster than 0.5 mEq/kg/h).

ACTIVITY

Restrict

DIET

• Continue to feed orally unless vomiting is intractable; feeding maintains intestinal epithelial integrity and minimizes bacterial translocation. • Initiate enteral feeding via esophagostomy, gastrostomy enteral feeding device, or nasoesophageal tube placement.
• NPO in animals with persistent vomiting for the shortest time possible; when there has been no vomiting for 12 hours, offer small volumes of water; if tolerated, begin small, frequent feedings of a diet that does not contain excessive amounts of dietary fat. Most nutritionists agree that excessive dietary fat restriction is not necessary in cats with pancreatitis.

CLIENT EDUCATION

• Discuss the need for extended hospitalization.
• Discuss the expense of diagnosis and treatment. • Discuss possible short-term and long-term complications (see Associated Conditions).

SURGICAL CONSIDERATIONS

• May need surgery to remove pseudocysts, abscesses, or devitalized tissue seen with necrotizing pancreatitis. • May need laparotomy and pancreatic biopsy to confirm pancreatitis and/or rule out other, nonpancreatic diseases such as cholangitis, lipidosis, and/or IBD. • EHBO from pancreatitis may require ductal decompression with surgical correction.

MEDICATIONS

DRUG(S) OF CHOICE

• Animals with intermittent vomiting should be treated with antiemetics. Maropitant 1 mg/kg SQ or PO q24h or ondansetron 0.1–0.5 mg/kg slow IV q8–12h are good first-choice options. • Analgesics to relieve abdominal pain, e.g., butorphanol 0.1–0.4 mg/kg SQ q6h, buprenorphine 0.005–0.015 mg/kg IM or IV q6–12h or fentanyl CRI 2–4 μg/kg/h as needed. • Antibiotics only if evidence of sepsis from bacterial translocation and to prevent pancreatic infection.

CONTRAINDICATIONS

Drugs reported to cause or exacerbate pancreatitis: • Anticholinergics (e.g., atropine).
• Azathioprine. • Chlorothiazide. • Estrogens.
• Furosemide. • Tetracycline. • L-Asparaginase.

PRECAUTIONS

Only use antibiotics if a clear clinical condition exists, such as infection.

FOLLOW-UP

PATIENT MONITORING

• Evaluate hydration status closely during first 24 hours of therapy; twice daily check physical examination, body weight, hematocrit, total plasma protein, BUN, and urine output. Evaluate the effectiveness of fluid therapy after 24 hours and adjust flow rates and fluid composition accordingly; repeat biochemistries to assess electrolyte/acid–base status. • Watch closely for systemic complications involving a variety of organ systems; perform appropriate diagnostic tests as needed (see Associated Conditions).
• Gradually taper fluids down to maintenance requirements if possible. Maintain oral alimentation or enteral nutrition as described above, being careful to feed diets that do not contain excessive amounts of dietary fat.
• Monitor for clinical evidence of IBD and treat accordingly. • Monitor for progression to diabetes mellitus, exocrine pancreatic insufficiency (EPI), and/or hepatic lipidosis in cats with ANP.

PREVENTION/AVOIDANCE

• Weight reduction if obese. • Avoid high-fat diets.

POSSIBLE COMPLICATIONS

• Failed response to supportive therapy.
• Associated conditions such as EPI, diabetes mellitus, and hepatic lipidosis. • Progression of acute pancreatitis to chronic pancreatitis.

EXPECTED COURSE AND PROGNOSIS

• Guarded for most patients with ANP; cats with multiorgan inflammation may be less responsive to treatment. • More guarded to poor for patients with severe necrotizing pancreatitis, decreased ionized calcium fraction, hyperkalemia, fPL >20 μg/L, and systemic conditions.

MISCELLANEOUS

ASSOCIATED CONDITIONS

Life-Threatening

• Pulmonary edema (e.g., adult respiratory distress syndrome). • Cardiac arrhythmias.
• Peritonitis. • DIC.

Non-Life-Threatening

• Diabetes mellitus. • EPI. • Chronic pancreatitis. • Cholangitis and hepatic lipidosis. • IBD.

SEE ALSO

• Acute Abdomen. • Cholangitis/Cholangiohepatitis Syndrome. • Exocrine Pancreatic Insufficiency. • Inflammatory Bowel Disease.

ABBREVIATIONS

• ANP = acute necrotizing pancreatitis.
• DIC = disseminated intravascular coagulation. • EHBO = extrahepatic biliary obstruction. • EPI = exocrine pancreatic insufficiency. • fPL = feline pancreatic lipase immunoreactivity. • GI = gastrointestinal.
• IBD = inflammatory bowel disease.

INTERNET RESOURCES

Veterinary Information Network: http://www.vin.com/VIN.plx

Suggested Reading

Simpson KS. Pancreatitis and triaditis in cats: causes and treatment. J Small Anim Pract 2015, 56(1):40–49.

Stockhaus C, Teske E, Schellenberger K, et al. Serial serum feline pancreatic lipase immunoreactivity concentrations and prognostic variables in 33 cats with pancreatitis. J Am Vet Med Assoc 2013, 243:1713–1718.

Xenoulis PG. Diagnosis of pancreatitis in dogs and cats. J Small Anim Pract 2015, 56(1):13–26.

Author Albert E. Jergens

Consulting Editor Mark P. Rondeau

Client Education Handout available online

P

BASICS

DEFINITION

Inflammation of the pancreas, which may occur abruptly with little or no permanent pathologic change (acute pancreatitis) or occur continuously or intermittently with irreversible morphologic change such as fibrosis and atrophy (chronic pancreatitis).

PATHOPHYSIOLOGY

• Premature intrapancreatic activation of zymogens results in local inflammation, edema, and necrosis of the pancreas and peripancreatic fat. • Pancreatic enzymes and inflammatory cytokines result in local (abdominal pain, vomiting) and possibly systemic effects (pyrexia, systemic inflammatory response syndrome [SIRS], multiple organ dysfunction syndrome [MODS], and acute kidney injury [AKI]). • An autoimmune mechanism is suspected in English cocker spaniels, but remains unproven.

SYSTEMS AFFECTED

• Gastrointestinal (GI)—altered GI motility (ileus) due to regional chemical peritonitis; local or generalized peritonitis due to enhanced vascular permeability.
• Cardiovascular—cardiac arrhythmias may result from release of myocardial depressant factor. • Hemic/lymphatic/immune—circulating proinflammatory cytokines and altered endothelial cell function can result in complications such as SIRS and/or disseminated intravascular coagulation (DIC).
• Hepatobiliary—hepatocellular damage can occur secondary to regional inflammation. Inflammation of the pancreas can also result in extrahepatic bile duct obstruction. • Renal/urologic—AKI can occur as a consequence of MODS. • Respiratory—regional vasculitis can cause pulmonary edema and/or pleural effusion. In severe cases, life-threatening acute respiratory distress syndrome can develop.

GENETICS

A possible genetic basis has been reported in miniature schnauzers where mutations in the *SPINK1* gene may confer increased susceptibility.

INCIDENCE/PREVALENCE

• Unknown, but it is a relatively common clinical disorder. • Up to 1% of normal dogs may have histologic evidence of pancreatitis.

GEOGRAPHIC DISTRIBUTION

Worldwide

SIGNALMENT

Species

Dog

Breed Predilections

• Acute—miniature schnauzer, Yorkshire terrier, other terriers. • Chronic—cocker spaniel and cavalier King Charles spaniel.

Mean Age and Range

Acute pancreatitis is most common in middle-aged and older (>7 years) dogs.

Predominant Sex

Females overrepresented in some reports.

SIGNS

Historical Findings

• Duration and severity of clinical signs can be variable, depending on the form of disease (acute vs. chronic). • Lethargy/anorexia.
• Vomiting. • Weakness. • Abdominal pain (may be absent in chronic disease).
• Diarrhea—small or large bowel type.

Physical Examination Findings

• Lethargy. • Dehydration—common; due to GI losses. • Abdominal pain—may adopt a "prayer position." • Mass lesions may be palpable. • Fever—common with more severe acute pancreatitis. • Less common—respiratory distress, bleeding, and cardiac arrhythmias.

CAUSES

Etiology is most often unknown; possibilities include: • Nutritional factors (e.g., dietary indiscretion, hyperlipoproteinemia).
• Pancreatic trauma/ischemia. • Duodenal reflux. • Drugs/toxins. • Pancreatic duct obstruction. • Hypercalcemia. • Infectious agents—babesiosis.

RISK FACTORS

• Breed—miniature schnauzers, terriers.
• Obesity. • Prior GI disease. • Endocrine disease. • Dietary indiscretion—access to garbage or fatty foods. • Hypertriglyceridemia—while an association exists between hypertriglyceridemia and pancreatitis, a causative link remains unclear. • Infectious—vector-borne diseases (babesiosis, ehrlichiosis, and leishmaniasis) have been identified in some cases of acute pancreatitis. • Drugs/toxins—idiosyncratic reactions to certain drugs (L-asparaginase, azathioprine, chlorpromazine, clomipramine, potassium bromide) have been described. Zinc toxicosis, mainly from ingestion of pennies minted after 1982, may cause pancreatitis.
• Hypercalcemia—not specifically documented in dogs, but shown in multiple species. • Surgery—possible; secondary to hypoperfusion or traumatic manipulation of the pancreas.

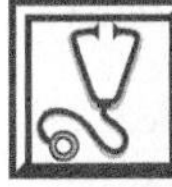

DIAGNOSIS

DIFFERENTIAL DIAGNOSIS

• GI (obstruction, septic peritonitis, ulcer, neoplasia)—differentiate via abdominal imaging. • Hepatobiliary (cholangiohepatitis, copper hepatopathy, mucocele, neoplasia, toxicity)—abdominal imaging showing significant gallbladder pathology, liver histopathology, hepatic copper quantification.
• Genitourinary (AKI, pyelonephritis, leptospirosis, uroabdomen, pyometra, prostatitis)—azotemia, hyperphosphatemia, hyperkalemia, isosthenuric urine, active urinary sediment; positive urine culture; leptospiral microscopic agglutination titers. Abdominal imaging showing uterine, prostatic or urinary bladder pathology. • Other:
  ○ Hypoadrenocorticism—concurrent hyponatremia and hyperkalemia, lack of a stress leukogram, post adrenocorticotropic hormone stimulation cortisol of <1 µg/dL. ○ Splenic torsion—splenomegaly with abnormal splenic positioning on abdominal imaging.

CBC/BIOCHEMISTRY/URINALYSIS

• CBC—hemoconcentration; inflammatory leukogram; thrombocytopenia.
• Biochemistry—azotemia; increased liver enzyme activities; hyperbilirubinemia; electrolyte abnormalities associated with vomiting; hyperglycemia; hypoalbuminemia; hypercholesterolemia and hypertriglyceridemia.
• Urinalysis—may show evidence of proteinuria or may be unremarkable.

OTHER LABORATORY TESTS

• Serum amylase and lipase activities are unreliable serologic markers. • Serum pancreatic lipase immunoreactivity (cPL) is a sensitive and specific marker of acute pancreatic inflammation, although is less sensitive for detecting chronic pancreatic inflammation. A cage-side cPL assay (SNAP cPL) is a useful screening tool. Elevation in SNAP cPL should be followed up by measurement of serum Spec cPL to obtain a quantitative value.

IMAGING

• Abdominal radiographs—increased soft tissue opacity in the right cranial abdomen; loss of visceral detail ("ground glass appearance") due to abdominal effusion; static gas pattern in the proximal duodenum; widened pyloroduodenal angle. • Abdominal radiographs are insensitive for pancreatitis and are of greater value for ruling out other causes of vomiting such as gastric or intestinal foreign bodies. • Thoracic radiographs—may be normal, reveal pleural effusion or pulmonary edema. • Abdominal ultrasound—imaging modality of choice; nonhomogeneous mass lesions suggest pancreatic abscess; pancreas is usually enlarged and irregular; may be a pancreatic mass or hypoechogenicity in the area of the pancreas due to edema; surrounding mesentery is typically hyperechoic due to peritonitis; may see peritoneal effusion and extrahepatic biliary obstruction. • cPL assay and ultrasound in combination have the highest sensitivity for an antemortem diagnosis of acute pancreatitis.

DIAGNOSTIC PROCEDURES

• Ultrasound-guided needle-aspiration cytology may confirm inflammation, abscess, or cyst. • Laparoscopy with pancreatic biopsy for histologic diagnosis. • Histopathologic evaluation may miss focal or segmental pancreatic inflammation and must be interpreted with caution.

PATHOLOGIC FINDINGS

• Gross findings (acute)—mild swelling with edema; gray-yellow areas of necrosis with varying amounts of hemorrhage with necrotizing pancreatitis. • Gross findings (chronic)—pancreas is reduced in size, firm, gray, and irregular; may contain extensive adhesions to surrounding viscera. • Microscopic changes (acute)—edema, parenchymal necrosis, hemorrhage, and neutrophilic cellular infiltrate. • Microscopic changes (chronic)— fibrosis around ducts, ductal epithelial hyperplasia, atrophy, and mononuclear cellular infiltrate.

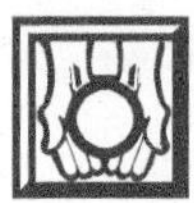

TREATMENT

APPROPRIATE HEALTH CARE

• Inpatient management typically required. • Identify and remove any predisposing causes.

P

NURSING CARE

• Patients are at increased risk of aspiration pneumonia because of the concurrent presence of vomiting and lethargy. Therefore, aggressive nursing care (maintain in sternal recumbency with elevated head) and management of vomiting (antiemetics and promotility drugs, suction of gastric contents with nasogastric tube) should be instituted. • Aggressive IV fluid resuscitation with isotonic crystalloids should be administered to correct dehydration and encourage perfusion of the pancreas. • In cases where hypoalbuminemia is present, colloid support with synthetic colloids may be needed (10–20 mL/kg/day). • Hypokalemia is common, so IV potassium supplementation (not to exceed 0.5 mEq/kg/h) is often required.

ACTIVITY

Clinical status will determine.

DIET

• Food should be withheld if patient has uncontrolled vomiting. • Enteral feeding should be encouraged as it supports enterocyte health, decreases bacterial translocation, and decreases incidence of vomiting episodes. • Feeding cranial to the duodenum (prepyloric) is safe. Therefore, if the patient is not eating voluntarily, nasoesophageal, nasogastric, or esophageal feeding tubes should be used to deliver low-fat diets.

CLIENT EDUCATION

Discuss possible complications, variable clinical severity, and risk of recurrence associated with pancreatitis.

SURGICAL CONSIDERATIONS

• Surgery should be avoided if possible; minimally invasive techniques (laparoscopy) or alternatives to surgery (ultrasound-guided percutaneous drainage) should be used. • Surgical intervention may be indicated if there is suspicion of an infected necrotic area of the pancreas, pancreatic abscess, or pancreatic enlargement causing extrahepatic biliary obstruction.

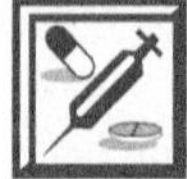

MEDICATIONS

DRUG(S) OF CHOICE (EMPHASIS ON ACUTE PANCREATITIS)

• Analgesic—fentanyl 2–5 μg/kg/h IV CRI; buprenorphine 0.01–0.02 mg/kg q6–8h IV or IM. • Antiemetics—maropitant 1 mg/kg SQ q24h; ondansetron 0.5–1.0 mg/kg IV or SQ q8h; metoclopramide 2 mg/kg/day IV CRI. • Antibiotics—usually not indicated. If bacterial translocation from the GI tract is suspected, broad-spectrum antibiotic therapy is recommended (e.g., ampicillin/sulbactam 30 mg/kg IV q8h). • Fresh frozen plasma—no clinical benefit has been shown. • Glucocorticoids—limited evidence to support benefit. Dogs with chronic autoimmune pancreatitis (English cocker spaniels are predisposed) may be treated with prednisone 2 mg/kg PO as induction therapy and then tapered as based on cPL levels and clinical signs.

CONTRAINDICATIONS

• Anticholinergics. • Azathioprine. • Chlorothiazide. • L-Asparaginase. • Meglumine antimonite. • Potassium bromide.

PRECAUTIONS

Use antimicrobials only if indicated.

ALTERNATIVE DRUG(S)

N/A

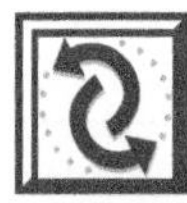

FOLLOW-UP

PATIENT MONITORING

• The patient's hydration status as well as electrolyte levels should be monitored frequently. Special attention should be paid to development of systemic signs suggestive of SIRS or MODS (increased respiratory rate, decreased urine production, bleeding). • The patient's need for more or less aggressive pain control should be frequently reassessed. • Since ultrasound findings can lag behind clinical improvement and circulating cPL levels can remain increased for extended periods, the decision of when a patient is ready to be discharged from veterinary care should be based on the overall clinical disease activity.

PREVENTION/AVOIDANCE

Patients with a history of pancreatitis should be fed a low-fat diet and medications known to be triggers for pancreatitis should be avoided.

POSSIBLE COMPLICATIONS

• Acute complications—extrahepatic biliary tract obstruction, aspiration pneumonia, SIRS, MODS. • Chronic complications—exocrine pancreatic insufficiency, diabetes mellitus.

EXPECTED COURSE AND PROGNOSIS

Prognosis is generally good for mild cases. Severe cases with development of SIRS/MODS have a more guarded prognosis. Negative prognostic factors—increases in blood urea/creatinine, thrombocytopenia, and marked increases in Spec cPL have been associated with increased mortality. Increased alanine aminotransferase has been associated with extended hospitalization in dogs with acute pancreatitis.

MISCELLANEOUS

ASSOCIATED CONDITIONS

• Endocrinopathy. • Epilepsy. • Prior GI disease.

AGE-RELATED FACTORS

N/A

ZOONOTIC POTENTIAL

N/A

PREGNANCY/FERTILITY/BREEDING

N/A

SYNONYMS

N/A

SEE ALSO

• Acute Vomiting. • Vomiting, Chronic

ABBREVIATIONS

• AKI = acute kidney injury. • cPL = canine pancreatic lipase immunoreactivity. • DIC = disseminated intravascular coagulation. • GI = gastrointestinal. • MODS = multiple organ dysfunction syndrome. • PLI = pancreatic lipase immunoreactivity. • SIRS = systemic inflammatory response syndrome.

INTERNET RESOURCES

Veterinary Information Network: http://www.vin.com/VIN.plx

Suggested Reading

Mansfield C. Pathophysiology of acute pancreatitis: potential applications from experimental models and human medicine to dogs. J Vet Intern Med 2012, 26:875–887.

Watson P. Chronic pancreatitis in dogs. Top Companion Anim Med 2012, 27:133–139.

Xenoulis PG, Steiner JM. Pancreas: necrosis and inflammation: canine. In: Washabau RJ, Day MJ, eds., Canine and Feline Gastroenterology. St. Louis, MO: Elsevier, 2013, pp. 812–821.

Author Albert E. Jergens

Consulting Editor Mark P. Rondeau

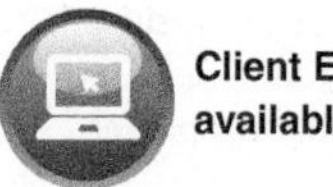

Client Education Handout available online

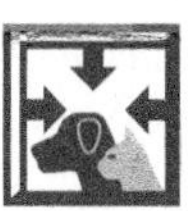

BASICS

DEFINITION

Simultaneous leukopenia, nonregenerative anemia, and thrombocytopenia; not a disease itself—rather, a group of laboratory findings that can result from multiple causes.

PATHOPHYSIOLOGY

- Mechanisms may include decreased production of cells in the bone marrow or increased peripheral use, destruction, or sequestration; one or more of these mechanisms may occur together.
- Decreased production occurs when pluripotent, multipotent, or committed stem cells are destroyed, their proliferation or differentiation is suppressed, or the maturation of differentiated cells is delayed or arrested.
- If pluripotent stem cells are affected, pancytopenia develops; if committed stem cells are involved, cytopenia of the specific cell type develops.
- Increased use and destruction of cells typically results in increased production in the bone marrow. At least 2–3 days are required before increased production begins to have an effect on peripheral blood cell counts, and peak output usually takes about a week; thus, the rate of use or destruction necessary to cause cytopenia is not as great during the first few days of disease as it is later.
- Sequestration of cells in the microcirculation, especially that of the spleen, intestine, and lungs, can cause cytopenia of the cell type involved.

SYSTEMS AFFECTED

Hemic/lymphatic/immune—bone marrow, spleen, lymph nodes, and other lymphocytic tissues; depending on the cause, these organs can be affected by cellular depletion, degeneration, necrosis, hyperplasia, dysplasia, or dyscrasia; changes may occur alone or in combination.

INCIDENCE/PREVALENCE

Pancytopenia is an uncommon occurrence and does not always occur with the causes listed (see Causes). The incidence is reported as 2.4% in dogs and 2.8% in cats.

GEOGRAPHIC DISTRIBUTION

Unless the cause of pancytopenia is an infectious agent that is localized to a certain region (e.g., leishmaniasis, histoplasmosis), no specific geographic distribution exists.

SIGNALMENT

- Dogs and cats.
- No age, sex, or breed predilection.

SIGNS

Historical Findings

- History reflects the underlying cause.
- Lethargy, weakness, or pallor from anemia.
- Petechial hemorrhage or mucosal bleeding from thrombocytopenia.
- Repeated febrile episodes or frequent or persistent infections from leukopenia.

Physical Examination Findings

- Lethargy, weakness.
- Pale mucous membranes.
- Petechial hemorrhages.
- Mucosal hemorrhage (e.g., hematuria, epistaxis, hemoptysis, melena).
- Fever.

CAUSES

Infectious Diseases/Agents

- Feline leukemia virus (FeLV).
- Feline immunodeficiency virus (FIV).
- Feline infectious peritonitis (FIP).
- Infectious canine hepatitis (ICH).
- Canine and feline parvovirus.
- Anaplasmosis.
- Histoplasmosis.
- Ehrlichiosis.
- Cytauxzoonosis.
- Leishmaniasis.
- Endotoxemia or septicemia.

Drugs, Chemicals, and Toxins

- Chloramphenicol.
- Second-generation cephalosporins.
- Trimethoprim–sulfadiazine.
- Albendazole.
- Fenbendazole.
- Griseofulvin.
- Angiotensin-converting enzyme inhibitors (e.g., enalapril).
- Methimazole.
- Phenobarbital.
- Phenylbutazone.
- Estrogen (exogenous administration, Sertoli cell tumor, interstitial cell tumor).
- Chemotherapeutic drugs (azathioprine, carboplatin, cyclophosphamide, cytosine arabinoside, doxorubicin, hydroxyurea, vinblastine).
- *Fusarium* T-2 toxin.
- Thallium.
- Ionizing radiation.

Proliferative and Infiltrative Diseases

- Hematopoietic neoplasia (e.g., leukemias, lymphoma, histiocytic tumors, myelodysplastic syndrome).
- Myelofibrosis.
- Osteosclerosis.

Immune-Mediated Diseases

- Aplastic anemia (also known as aplastic pancytopenia).
- Immune-mediated hemolytic anemia and thrombocytopenia (when precursor cells are targeted by the immune system).

RISK FACTORS

Vary with individual cause.

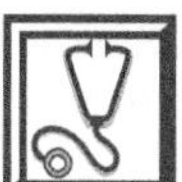

DIAGNOSIS

DIFFERENTIAL DIAGNOSIS

- Acute onset with severe clinical signs—more consistent with conditions that cause necrosis, destruction, or sequestration of cells.
- Slow, insidious onset—more consistent with conditions that cause bone marrow suppression.

LABORATORY FINDINGS

Drugs That May Alter Laboratory Results

Glucocorticoids often mildly to moderately increase the segmented neutrophil count, which may then obscure the presence of neutropenia.

Disorders That May Alter Laboratory Results

Phlebotomy technique may result in platelet clumping and hemolysis, leading to spuriously low platelet count and packed cell volume, respectively.

CBC/BIOCHEMISTRY/URINALYSIS

- Leukopenia—characterized by neutropenia with or without lymphopenia.
- Nonregenerative anemia—severity depends on duration and underlying cause.
- Thrombocytopenia.
- Blood smear evaluation—may reveal infectious agents (e.g., *Ehrlichia* spp., *Histoplasma capsulatum*); may reveal abnormal cells of any lineage, suggesting myeloproliferative or lymphoproliferative diseases.
- Toxic changes in leukocytes—may suggest bone marrow injury or early release.
- Biochemical alterations—depends on organ and degree of involvement (e.g., increased liver enzymes may be seen with certain infectious diseases, toxins, and infiltrative diseases).

OTHER LABORATORY TESTS

- Reticulocyte count—a regenerative response to anemia suggests destruction, use, or sequestration of red blood cells; a nonregenerative response suggests bone marrow suppression and merits bone marrow examination
- Immunologic tests for infectious diseases (e.g., FeLV, FIV, *Ehrlichia* spp.); FeLV may be detected on immunofluorescence assay of bone marrow aspirate, even with negative serology.
- PCR for infectious agents.

DIAGNOSTIC PROCEDURES

- Bone marrow examination (aspirate smear or biopsy)—indicated when cause of pancytopenia cannot be determined with other tests.
- Hypercellular bone marrow associated with myelodysplastic syndrome, leukemias, myelophthisis, or recovery from prior neutropenia.

PANCYTOPENIA (CONTINUED)

- Hypocellular bone marrow associated with necrosis, myelofibrosis, and suppression (e.g., drugs, estrogen).
- If a bone marrow aspirate cannot be obtained, myelofibrosis, necrosis, or marked hypocellularity should be suspected and a core biopsy should be evaluated.

PATHOLOGIC FINDINGS

Bone marrow core biopsy—may see replacement of normal hematopoietic tissue with necrotic, neoplastic, fibrous, or adipose tissue, depending on the specific underlying cause.

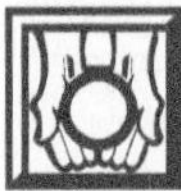

TREATMENT

- Supportive treatment depends on the clinical situation and includes aggressive antibiotic therapy and blood component transfusions.
- Treatment of the underlying condition is paramount.

P

MEDICATIONS

DRUG(S) OF CHOICE

Treatment should be appropriate for the clinical situation (i.e., the degree to which each cell population is decreased, presence of fever or infection, and established or suspected specific diagnoses); see specific causes.

CONTRAINDICATIONS

- Drugs that may suppress hematopoiesis or trigger immune-mediated destruction (see Causes).
- Nonsteroidal anti-inflammatory drugs, clopidogrel, or other drugs that may interfere with platelet function if thrombocytopenia present.

PRECAUTIONS

Because of the patient's potentially compromised immune status, glucocorticoids and other immunosuppressive drugs should be used only when necessary (e.g., when an immune component is suspected) and with extreme care and frequent monitoring.

ALTERNATIVE DRUG(S)

Recombinant Hematopoietic Growth Factors

- Recombinant human granulocyte colony-stimulating factor (rhG-CSF) 1–5 μg/kg/day SC; stimulates neutrophil production, may result in development of antibodies against endogenous G-CSF.
- Recombinant human erythropoietin (rhEPO)—initial dosage 100 U/kg SC, 3 times/week; stimulates erythropoiesis, may result in development of antibodies against endogenous EPO, darbepoetin may also be considered.

FOLLOW-UP

PATIENT MONITORING

- Daily physical examination, including frequent monitoring of body temperature.
- Periodic CBC—frequency depends on severity of cytopenia, age, general physical condition of the patient, and underlying cause.

PREVENTION/AVOIDANCE

- Castration of cryptorchid males (to prevent development of a Sertoli or interstitial cell tumor).
- Vaccination for infectious diseases.
- Frequent monitoring of CBC in cancer patients receiving chemotherapy or radiation therapy.

POSSIBLE COMPLICATIONS

- Hemorrhage.
- Sepsis.

EXPECTED COURSE AND PROGNOSIS

- Depends on the underlying cause.
- Often a guarded prognosis is warranted.

MISCELLANEOUS

ASSOCIATED CONDITIONS

Secondary infections—in patients with neutropenia.

ZOONOTIC POTENTIAL

- Tularemia, if this is the underlying cause.
- An owner can contract histoplasmosis from the same source as the patient.

PREGNANCY/FERTILITY/BREEDING

Stress of underlying disease may cause abortion; see respective topics for the effects of different causes on pregnancy.

SEE ALSO

- Anemia, Aplastic.
- Anemia, Immune-Mediated.
- Anemia, Nonregenerative.
- Anemia, Regenerative.
- Neutropenia.
- Thrombocytopenia.
- Thrombocytopenia, Primary Immune-Mediated.

ABBREVIATIONS

- FeLV = feline leukemia virus.
- FIP = feline infectious peritonitis.
- FIV = feline immunodeficiency virus.
- ICH = infectious canine hepatitis.
- rhEPO = recombinant human erythropoietin.
- rhG-CSF = recombinant human granulocyte colony-stimulating factor.

Suggested Reading

Brazzell JL, Weiss DJ. A retrospective study of aplastic pancytopenia in the dog: 9 cases (1996–2003). Vet Clin Pathol 2006, 35:413–417.

Weiss DJ. Aplastic anemia. In: Weiss DJ, Wardrop KJ, eds., Schalm's Veterinary Hematology, 6th ed. Ames, IA: Blackwell, 2010, pp. 256–260.

Weiss, DJ. New insights into the physiology and treatment of acquired myelodysplastic syndromes and aplastic pancytopenia. Vet Clin North Am Small Anim Pract 2003, 33(6):1317–1334.

Weiss DJ, Evanson OA. A retrospective study of feline pancytopenia. Comp Haematol Int 2000, 1:50–55.

Weiss DJ, Evanson OA, Sykes J. A retrospective study of canine pancytopenia. Vet Clin Pathol 1999, 28:83–88.

Author R. Darren Wood

Consulting Editor Melinda S. Camus

Client Education Handout available online

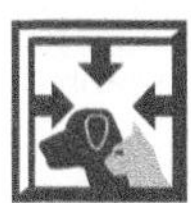

BASICS

OVERVIEW

Inflammation of the subcutaneous fat tissue.

SYSTEMS AFFECTED

Skin/exocrine.

SIGNALMENT

Species

Steatitis—predominantly cats, but can occur in dogs with concurrent diseases.

Mean Age and Range

• Panniculitis—any age. • Steatitis—young to middle-aged cats; older dogs.

SIGNS

• Uncommon in dogs and cats. • Single or multiple subcutaneous nodules or draining tracts. • May be painful and fluctuant to firm. • Nodules—few millimeters to several centimeters in diameter. • Involved fat may necrose. • Exudate—usually a small amount of oily discharge; yellow-brown to bloody.
• Multiple lesions (dogs and cats)—systemic signs common (e.g., anorexia, pyrexia, lethargy, and depression).

CAUSES & RISK FACTORS

• Infectious—bacterial, fungal (deep mycosis or dermatophyte), opportunistic mycobacteria, *Nocardia*, viral. • Immune-mediated—lupus panniculitis, erythema nodosum, vasculitis, or drug reaction. • Idiopathic—sterile nodular panniculitis, thromboembolism, sterile pyogranulomatous dermatitis and panniculitis.
• Trauma. • Neoplastic—multicentric mast cell tumors, cutaneous lymphoma, pancreatic carcinoma. • Foreign bodies. • Post-injection—corticosteroids, vaccines, other subcutaneous injections. • Nutritional—vitamin E deficiency in cats, oily fish-based diet (steatitis).

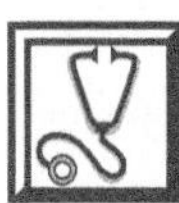

DIAGNOSIS

DIFFERENTIAL DIAGNOSIS

Infectious

• More common than sterile/immune-mediated panniculitis. • Deep pyoderma.
• Feline infectious peritonitis.

Cutaneous Cyst

• Usually nonpainful, noninflamed. • Well demarcated.

Lipoma

• Soft; usually well demarcated. • No inflammation or draining tracts. • Usually solitary.

Mast Cell Tumors/Epitheliotropic Lymphoma

• Multifocal. • Often erythematous.
• Variable presentations.

Sterile Nodular Panniculitis

Diagnosis made by ruling out other causes of panniculitis.

CBC/BIOCHEMISTRY/URINALYSIS

• Panniculitis—no abnormalities. • Steatitis and panniculitis (occasional)—moderate to severe neutrophilia with mild eosinophilia; mild to moderate leukocytosis; mild nonregenerative anemia; hypoalbuminemia and proteinuria, possible hypocalcemia.

OTHER LABORATORY TESTS

• Antinuclear antibody—lupus panniculitis.
• Serum protein electrophoresis. • Serum lipase/amylase levels. • Feline leukemia virus/ feline immunodeficiency virus.

IMAGING

• Abdominal ultrasound: ◦ Panniculitis—pancreatitis may be a contributing factor.
◦ Steatitis—may see mottled subcutaneous, inguinal, or falciform fat; loss of contrast in abdominal cavity.

DIAGNOSTIC PROCEDURES

• Aspirates and impression smears:
◦ Pyoderma—numerous neutrophils and variable numbers of mononuclear cells and bacteria. ◦ Fungal infections—fungal organisms and variable numbers of mononuclear cells may be noted.
• Blastomycosis—urine antigen testing.
• Bacterial culture and susceptibility testing (tissue)—identify primary or secondary bacterial infection. • Fungal and opportunistic mycobacteria culture (tissue).
• Biopsy with negative cultures for diagnosis of sterile nodular panniculitis. • Special stains of histopathologic samples—may help identify causative agent.

PATHOLOGIC FINDINGS

• Surgical excisional biopsies—more accurate than punch biopsy specimens in most cases.
• Panniculitis—lobular or diffuse infiltrate (granulomatous, pyogranulomatous, suppurative, eosinophilic, necrotizing, or fibrosing) of panniculus; may identify if vasculitis present. • Steatitis—lumpy, granular fat, normal to yellowish-orange coloration of body fat.

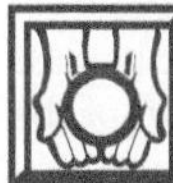

TREATMENT

Diet

Steatitis—remove fish products from diet; feed nutritionally complete, balanced, commercially prepared food; may require parenteral feeding (e.g., PEG tube, esophagostomy feeding tube).

MEDICATIONS

DRUG(S) OF CHOICE

Positive culture results require appropriate antibacterial, antifungal, or antimycobacterial treatment.

Sterile Nodular Panniculitis

• Systemic treatment with corticosteroids; prednisolone 2.2 mg/kg daily in dogs or 4.4 mg/kg daily in cats: taper based on response: may require low dose to maintain remission.
• Azathioprine (dogs: 1 mg/kg PO daily initially)—used with corticosteroids if insufficient response. • Oral vitamin E 200 IU q12h <10 kg, 400 IU q12h >10 kg.
• Cyclosporine beneficial in some dogs (initially 5 mg/kg q24h for 4–8 weeks, then tapered).

Steatitis

Oral vitamin E 200 IU q12h <10 kg, 400 IU q12h >10 kg; corticosteroids at an anti-inflammatory dosage; *S*-adenosylmethionine PO on an empty stomach.

P

FOLLOW-UP

• Depends on underlying etiology type and duration of treatment. • Monitor CBC, platelet count, chemistry profile, and urinalysis/urine bacterial culture and sensitivity if immunosuppressive agents or long-term corticosteroids prescribed.

MISCELLANEOUS

ASSOCIATED CONDITIONS

• Pancreatic carcinoma. • Chylous ascites.
• Peritonitis.

ABBREVIATIONS

• PEG tube = percutaneous endoscopically placed gastrostomy tube.

Suggested Reading

Helton Rhodes KA, Werner A. Blackwell's Five-Minute Veterinary Consult: Clinical Companion: Small Animal Dermatology, 3rd ed. Hoboken, NJ: Wiley-Blackwell, 2018.

Author Karen A. Kuhl

Consulting Editor Alexander H. Werner Resnick

PANOSTEITIS

BASICS

DEFINITION

A self-limiting, painful condition of uncertain etiology that typically affects juvenile dogs of large to giant breeds. It is characterized clinically by lameness and pain on palpation of one or more long bones, and radiographically by increased density of the marrow cavity of affected long bones.

PATHOPHYSIOLOGY

- Cause unknown.
- Attempts to isolate microorganisms have failed.
- Suggested metabolic, allergic, or endocrine aberrations are without support.
- Pain may be associated with the disturbance of endosteal and periosteal elements, vascular congestion, or high intramedullary pressure.

SYSTEMS AFFECTED

Musculoskeletal—causes lameness of variable intensity; may affect a single limb or progress to a shifting leg lameness.

GENETICS

- No proven transmission.
- Predominance of German shepherd dogs in the affected population strongly suggests an inheritable basis.

INCIDENCE/PREVALENCE

Estimated at 2.6 per 1000 patients.

GEOGRAPHIC DISTRIBUTION

N/A

SIGNALMENT

Species

Dog

Breed Predilections

- Large- to giant-breed dogs are more commonly affected.
- German shepherd dogs and German shepherd dog mixes are more commonly affected.

Mean Age and Range

- Usually 5–12 months of age.
- As young as 2 months and as old as 5 years.

Predominant Sex

Males affected more than females by a ratio of 4:1.

SIGNS

General Comments

Lameness evaluation—if no distinct abnormalities noted on physical examination or radiographs, repeat examination and radiographs 4–6 weeks later.

Historical Findings

- No associated trauma.
- Lameness of varying intensity; often involves the forelimbs initially; may affect the hind limbs; may see shifting leg lameness; may be non-weight-bearing.
- Mild depression, inappetence, fever, and weight loss may be seen with severe disease.

Physical Examination Findings

- Pain on deep palpation of the long bones (diaphysis) in an affected limb; distinguishing characteristic; palpate firmly along the entire shaft of each bone while carefully avoiding any pinching of nearby muscle.
- Bones—ulna most commonly affected; may affect radius, humerus, femur, and tibia (in decreasing order of frequency) either concurrently or subsequently.
- May note low-grade fever or lethargy with severe disease.
- May see muscle atrophy.

CAUSES

Unknown

RISK FACTORS

Purebred German shepherd dog or German shepherd dog mix.

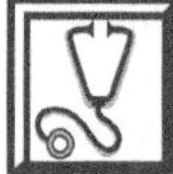

DIAGNOSIS

DIFFERENTIAL DIAGNOSIS

- Always consider the diagnosis with lameness in a young large- and giant-breed dogs; especially in German shepherd dog or German shepherd dog mix.
- May occur alone or with other juvenile orthopedic diseases.
- Hypertrophic osteodystrophy.
- Osteochondritis dissecans.
- Fragmented medial coronoid process.
- Un-united anconeal process.
- Hip dysplasia.
- Fractures and ligamentous injuries from unobserved trauma.
- Shifting leg lameness—immune-mediated arthropathy; Lyme disease; bacterial endocarditis.
- Coccidioidomycosis.
- Bacterial osteomyelitis.

CBC/BIOCHEMISTRY/URINALYSIS

- Usually normal.
- May note eosinophilia early in disease.

OTHER LABORATORY TESTS

N/A

IMAGING

- Radiographic densities within the medulla of long bones are characteristic finding.
- Early, middle, and late radiographic lesions.
- Early—trabecular pattern of the ends of the diaphysis becomes more prominent; may appear blurred; may see granular opacities.
- Middle—patchy sclerotic opacities first around the nutrient foramen and later throughout the diaphysis; widened cortex; thickened periosteum with increased opacity.
- Late—during resolution, diminished overall opacity of the medullary canal (toward normal); a coarse trabecular pattern and some granular opacity may remain; may be a period in which the medullary canal becomes more lucent than normal.
- Bone scintigraphy may reveal subtle lesions that later become more apparent on follow-up radiographs.

DIAGNOSTIC PROCEDURES

Bone biopsy is occasionally indicated to rule out neoplasia and bacterial or fungal osteomyelitis that have similar radiographic appearances.

PATHOLOGIC FINDINGS

- Biopsy or necropsy are rarely performed because of excellent prognosis for recovery.
- No gross pathologic lesions.
- Degeneration of the marrow adipocytes surrounding the nutrient foramen followed by proliferation of vascular stromal cells within the marrow sinusoids.
- Osteoid formation and endosteal new bone formation—progress proximally and distally.
- Vascular congestion—may accompany the proliferation of new bone, secondarily stimulating endosteal and periosteal reaction.
- Remodeling of the endosteum—occurs during resolution; reestablishes normal endosteal and marrow architecture.

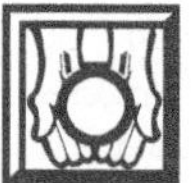

TREATMENT

APPROPRIATE HEALTH CARE

Typically treat as an outpatient.

NURSING CARE

Maintenance and replacement fluid therapy is occasionally needed if prolonged periods of inappetence and pyrexia.

ACTIVITY

- Limit activity to lessen pain; not shown to hasten recovery.
- Moderate to severe disease can cause pain that limits movement, leading to muscle atrophy.

CLIENT EDUCATION

- Warn client that patient may develop other juvenile orthopedic diseases.
- Inform client that signs of pain and lameness may last for several weeks.
- Warn client that recurrence of clinical signs is common up to 2 years of age.

SURGICAL CONSIDERATIONS

N/A

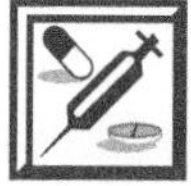

MEDICATIONS

DRUG(S) OF CHOICE

- Nonsteroidal anti-inflammatory drugs (NSAIDs):
    - Minimize pain; decrease inflammation.
    - Symptomatic therapy has no bearing on the duration of the disease.

- Carprofen 2.2 mg/kg PO q12h or 4.4 mg/kg PO q24h.
- Deracoxib 1–2 mg/kg PO q24h, chewable.
- Etodolac 10–15 mg/kg PO q24h.
- Firocoxib 5 mg/kg PO q24h.
- Grapiprant 2 mg/kg PO q24h, to animals >3.6 kg.
- Meloxicam—load 0.2 mg/kg PO, then 0.1 mg/kg PO q24h—liquid.
- Tepoxalin—load 20 mg/kg, then 10 mg/kg PO q24h.

• Glucocorticoids:
- May give anti-inflammatory dosage—prednisone 0.5–1 mg/kg PO.
- Potential side effects well documented.
- Goal for chronic use—low-dose and alternate-day therapy.

PRECAUTIONS

NSAIDs—can cause gastrointestinal tract ulceration, hepatotoxicity, or nephrotoxicity.

POSSIBLE INTERACTIONS

NSAIDs—do not use in conjunction with glucocorticoids; risk of gastrointestinal tract ulceration; consider appropriate washout times when switching from one NSAID to another.

ALTERNATIVE DRUG(S)

N/A

FOLLOW-UP

PATIENT MONITORING

Recheck lameness every 2–4 weeks to detect more serious concurrent orthopedic problems.

PREVENTION/AVOIDANCE

N/A

POSSIBLE COMPLICATIONS

N/A

EXPECTED COURSE AND PROGNOSIS

- Self-limiting disease.
- Treatment is symptomatic and appears to have no influence on duration of clinical signs.
- Multiple limb involvement is common.
- Lameness typically lasts from a few days to several weeks; may persist for months; may recur.
- Occasional case has unrelenting pain and lameness that is unresponsive to therapy. Euthanasia has been recommended in these dogs.

MISCELLANEOUS

ASSOCIATED CONDITIONS

N/A

AGE-RELATED FACTORS

Typically affects immature and young dogs

ZOONOTIC POTENTIAL

N/A

PREGNANCY/FERTILITY/BREEDING

Females reported to be more susceptible to panosteitis during estrus; no proven relationship to reproductive hormones or pregnancy.

SYNONYMS

- Enostosis.
- Eosinophilic panosteitis.
- Fibrous osteodystrophy.
- Juvenile osteomyelitis.

ABBREVIATIONS

- NSAID = nonsteroidal anti-inflammatory drug.

Suggested Reading

Halliwell WH. Tumorlike lesions of bone. In: Bojrab MJ, ed., Disease Mechanisms in Small Animal Surgery, 2nd ed. Philadelphia, PA: Saunders, 1993, pp. 932–933.

LaFond E, Bruer GJ, Austin CC. Breed susceptibility for developmental diseases in dogs. J Am Anim Hosp Assoc 2002, 38:467–477.

Muir P, Dubielzig RR, Johnson KA. Panosteitis. Compend Contin Educ Pract Vet 1996, 18:29–33.

Piermattei DL, Flo GL, DeCamp CE. Miscellaneous conditions of the musculoskeletal system. In: Handbook of Small Animal Orthopedics and Fracture Repair, 4th ed. Philadelphia, PA: Saunders, 2006, pp. 775–778.

Schwarz T, Johnson VS, Voute L, Sullivan M. Bone scintigraphy in the investigation of occult lameness in the dog. J Small Anim Pract 2004, 45:232–237.

Trostel CT, Pool RR, McLaughlin RM. Canine lameness caused by developmental orthopedic diseases: Panosteitis, Legg-Calvé-Perthes disease, and hypertophic osteodystrophy. Compend Contin Educ Pract Vet 2003, 25(4):282–292.

Author Laura A. Barbur

Consulting Editor Mathieu M. Glassman

Acknowledgment The author and editors acknowledge the prior contribution of Larry Carpenter.

Client Education Handout available online

PANTING AND TACHYPNEA

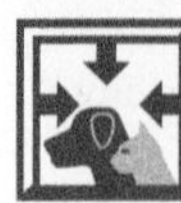

BASICS

DEFINITION

- Tachypnea—increased respiratory rate.
- Panting—rapid, shallow, open-mouth breathing that is usually not associated with gas exchange issues.

PATHOPHYSIOLOGY

- Respiratory rate, rhythm, and effort are controlled by the respiratory center in the brainstem in response to numerous afferent pathways, both central and peripheral in origin. These include the cerebral cortex, central chemoreceptors, peripheral chemoreceptors, stimulation of mechanoreceptors in the airways that sense lung inflation and deflation, stimulation of irritant receptors of the airways, stimulation of C-fibers in the alveoli and pulmonary blood vessels that sense interstitial congestion, and baroreceptors that sense changes in blood pressure.
- Tachypnea and panting can occur in response to stimulation of any of the above receptor pathways.

P

SYSTEMS AFFECTED

Respiratory

SIGNALMENT

- Dog and cat; no age, or sex predilection.
- Older, large-breed dogs predisposed to panting associated with laryngeal paralysis.
- Brachycephalic dogs prone to panting due to upper airway obstruction.

SIGNS

Historical Findings

- Patients with primary respiratory or cardiac disease usually have associated coughing or exercise intolerance.
- Nonrespiratory causes—clinical complaints associated with the primary disease, e.g., polyuria, polydipsia, polyphagia (PU/PD/PP) with hyperadrenocorticism, intermittent signs of systemic hypertension with pheochromocytoma.

Physical Examination Findings

- Brachycephalic syndrome (stenotic nares, stertorous respirations associated with soft palate elongation or saccular eversion) may be observed.
- Stridor can be evident with upper airway diseases.
- Lower airway disease—cough, expiratory wheezes on auscultation, abdominal effort.
- Pulmonary parenchymal disease—may have crackles on auscultation; harsh or moist lung sounds common, may be normal.
- Cardiogenic pulmonary edema—heart murmur or arrhythmia, tachycardia, gallop sound, hypothermia, pale mucous membranes, poor capillary refill time.
- Pleural space disease—diminished breath sounds: ventrally—fluid; dorsally—air; unilaterally—space-occupying lesions, pyothorax, chylothorax.
- Thoracic wall disease—can have paradoxical respiratory pattern, visible and/or palpable trauma.
- Nonrespiratory diseases—findings will depend on the other diseases, e.g., pale mucous membranes if anemic, hepatomegaly with hyperadrenocorticism.
- Other signs could indicate trauma.

CAUSES

Panting

- Pain, anxiety, hyperthermia, fever.
- Brachycephalic airway syndrome.
- Laryngeal disease.
- CNS disease causing abnormal ventilatory control.
- Cardiovascular compromise (shock), hypertension, arrhythmia.
- Drug therapy (opioids)
- Metabolic acidosis.
- Hyperadrenocorticism, corticosteroid therapy.
- Pheochromocytoma.
- Hyperthyroidism.
- Hypocalcemia.
- Can be a normal behavioral pattern in some dogs.

Tachypnea

- Hypoxemia, hypercapnia, hypotension, hyperthermia/fever, anemia, acidosis, systemic inflammatory response syndrome (SIRS)/sepsis, brainstem disease.
- Upper airway/larynx—elongated soft palate, laryngeal paralysis, edema, collapse, foreign body, neoplasia, granuloma, stenosis, inflammation, trauma, webbing.
- Trachea—collapse, stenosis, trauma, foreign body, neoplasia, parasites, extraluminal compression (lymphadenopathy, enlarged left atrium, heart-base tumors).
- Lower airway disease—allergic disease, inflammation, infection (*Mycoplasma*), parasites, neoplasia.
- Pulmonary parenchymal disease—edema (cardiogenic or noncardiogenic), pneumonia or pneumonitis, neoplasia (primary or metastatic), hemorrhage, fibrosis, lung lobe torsion, atelectasis.
- Pulmonary thromboembolism associated with—immune-mediated hemolytic anemia (IMHA), hyperadrenocorticism, pulmonary thromboembolism (PLE), protein-losing nephropathy (PLN), cardiac disease, neoplasia, heartworm disease.
- Pleural space disease—pleural effusion or pneumothorax, neoplasia, diaphragmatic hernia.
- Abdominal distention—organomegaly; neoplasia, pregnancy; obesity; ascites; gastric dilatation, torsion.
- CNS disease—compression or infarct near the respiratory center.
- Metabolic acidosis—diabetic ketoacidosis, lactic acidosis, uremia, renal tubular acidosis, diarrhea.

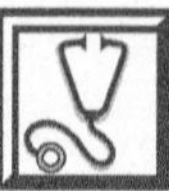

DIAGNOSIS

DIFFERENTIAL DIAGNOSIS

- Tachypnea without respiratory distress—may be a nonrespiratory problem.
- Stertor and stridor are features of upper airway disease—auscultation over the trachea can help delineate upper airway noises from lower airway noises.
- Thoracic auscultation and percussion—most useful for distinguishing pleural disease (dampened lung sounds, dull percussion) from parenchymal disease (normal, harsh or moist lung sounds, crackles on auscultation).
- Wheezes on auscultation are suggestive of narrowed lower airway (bronchi, bronchioles).
- Crackles on auscultation are features of pulmonary parenchymal diseases.
- Congestive heart failure—murmur, tachycardia, poor pulse quality, jugular pulses, hypothermia.

CBC/BIOCHEMISTRY/URINALYSIS

- Anemia—can cause nonrespiratory tachypnea.
- Polycythemia—chronic hypoxia.
- Inflammatory leukogram—pneumonia, pneumonitis, pyothorax, or nonrespiratory causes (SIRS, sepsis).
- Eosinophilia—hypersensitivity or parasitic airway disease.
- Thrombocytosis—hyperadrenocorticism predisposes to pulmonary thromboembolism (PTE); alternatively, could indicate iron-deficiency anemia.
- Sodium:potassium ratio <27—can be seen with pleural or abdominal effusions.
- High alkaline phosphatase—hyperadrenocorticism predisposes to panting and PTE.
- Hypoproteinemia—may suggest protein-losing disease that can predispose to PTE.
- Proteinuria—can predispose to PTE.
- Azotemia—if severe can lead to uremic pneumonitis.
- Hyperglycemia, glucosuria, and ketonuria—could indicate ketoacidosis as cause of tachypnea.

OTHER LABORATORY TESTS

- Fecal examinations for parasites if indicated.
- Low-dose dexamethasone suppression test or adrenocorticotropic hormone stimulation test to assess adrenal cortical function, if indicated.
- Pleural fluid analysis.
- Serum antigen or antibody titers—heartworm, toxoplasmosis, distemper, feline leukemia virus, feline immunodeficiency virus.
- Pulse oximetry or arterial blood gas—can help differentiate pulmonary from nonrespiratory causes.

- Hemoglobin saturation with oxygen <95% supportive of hypoxemia.
- $Pa\text{O}_2$—partial pressure of oxygen dissolved in arterial blood; normoxemia: $Pa\text{O}_2$ 80–120 mmHg (room air, sea level), hypoxemia: $Pa\text{O}_2$ <80 mmHg; $F_I\text{O}_2$—fraction of inspired oxygen ranges from 0.21 (room air) to 1.0; $Pa\text{O}_2/F_I\text{O}_2$ ratio—measure of lung efficiency during oxygen therapy; $Pa\text{O}_2/F_I\text{O}_2$ ≥400—normal lung efficiency; 300–400—mild insufficiency; 200–300—moderate insufficiency; <200—severe insufficiency. Reduction in lung efficiency can be due to venous admixture, hypoventilation, low inspired oxygen.
- $Pa\text{CO}_2$ or $Pv\text{CO}_2$—partial pressure of CO_2 dissolved in arterial or venous blood; measure of ventilation; normal 30 mmHg <$P\text{CO}_2$ <40 mmHg. Hypercapnia = hypoventilation = decreased alveolar minute ventilation. Hypocapnia = hyperventilation = increased alveolar minute ventilation. Hypoventilation can be due to airway obstruction, pleural space disease, thoracic wall disease and abdominal distention; respiratory muscle fatigue from a prolonged period of tachypnea can lead to hypoventilation.
- Blood gas may reveal metabolic acidosis as a cause.
- Coagulation testing—if suspect hemothorax and/or pulmonary hemorrhage.

IMAGING

Cervical and Thoracic Radiography

- Increased density could suggest edema or soft tissue mass lesion. Also can see soft palate elongation, large airway narrowing, lymphadenopathy, intraluminal abnormalities.
- Lower airway disease—bronchial thickening, middle lung lobe consolidation (cats), atelectasis, hyperinflation and diaphragmatic flattening (primarily cats).
- Pneumonia—alveolar infiltrates; aspiration pneumonia usually cranioventral distribution or middle lobe affected.
- Cardiogenic pulmonary edema—enlarged cardiac silhouette, pulmonary venous distention, enlarged left atrium with perihilar pulmonary infiltrates in dogs; infiltrates can be of any distribution in cats.
- Noncardiogenic pulmonary edema—usually caudodorsal distribution. Acute respiratory distress syndrome (ARDS)—diffuse, symmetrical alveolar infiltrates.
- Pulmonary vascular abnormalities—PTE, heartworm disease.
- Pleural space disease—pneumothorax, pleural effusion, mass lesions, diaphragmatic hernias.
- Thoracic wall disease—rib fractures, neoplasia.

Thoracic Ultrasonography

- Evaluation of distribution of pleural effusion (excellent as guide for thoracocentesis), pneumothorax (absence of "glide sign"), and parenchymal disease (presence of "comet tail" artifact).
- Pulmonary mass identification—guide fine-needle aspiration; mediastinal evaluation.

Echocardiography

Evaluate cardiac function and chamber size if cardiogenic pulmonary edema or pleural effusion suspected; elevated pulmonary artery pressure and right ventricular overload with ventricular septal flattening can support diagnosis of PTE; visualize heart-based masses, rule out pericardial effusion.

Abdominal Ultrasound

Evaluation of abdominal distension; assess adrenal gland size.

Fluoroscopy

Evaluate tracheal and bronchial collapse; evaluate diaphragmatic function.

CT

Airway, pulmonary parenchymal, and pleural space disease can be evaluated; can detect lesions not clearly defined on radiographs.

Pulmonary Vascular Angiography

Gold standard for diagnosis of PTE.

Ventilation Perfusion Scintigraphy

Abnormal perfusion scan is considered supportive of PTE.

Other

May need CNS imaging.

DIAGNOSTIC PROCEDURES

- Pulse oximetry—$Sp\text{O}_2$; peripheral capillary hemoglobin oxygen saturation. The relationship between $Pa\text{O}_2$ and $Sp\text{O}_2$ is defined by the oxygen hemoglobin dissociation curve; $Pa\text{O}_2$ of 60 mmHg = $Sp\text{O}_2$ of 90%; $Pa\text{O}_2$ of 80 mmHg = $Sp\text{O}_2$ of 95%; $Pa\text{O}_2$ of >100 mmHg = $Sp\text{O}_2$ of 100%. Below 95%, small changes in $Sp\text{O}_2$ signify large changes in $Pa\text{O}_2$. $Sp\text{O}_2$ measurements in animals on high inspired oxygen lack sensitivity.
- Thoracentesis—fluid analysis and culture.
- Laryngoscopy/nasopharyngoscopy/tracheoscopy—to evaluate laryngeal function and visualize foreign bodies and masses; visualize caudal nasopharyngeal region with flexible endoscope or spay hook and dental mirror.
- Bronchoscopy—evaluate upper and lower airways; take biopsies; perform bronchoalveolar lavage for cytology and culture.

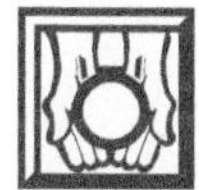

TREATMENT

APPROPRIATE HEALTH CARE

- Inpatient care if life-threatening; therapy depends on underlying cause.
- Administer oxygen and see if tachypnea resolves—this would be supportive of a primary respiratory problem.
- Upper airway disease—use sedation to reduce respiratory effort. Check body temperature frequently and actively cool patients as needed. Severe upper airway disease requires intubation to stabilize; if the problem cannot be immediately cured, placement of a temporary tracheostomy tube is indicated. Remove foreign bodies; perform surgical excision/biopsy of masses, surgical correction for laryngeal paralysis and brachycephalic syndrome; give anti-inflammatory medications for laryngeal edema.
- Lower airway disease—bronchodilators; systemic corticosteroids may be required to stabilize cats with acute bronchoconstriction.
- Pulmonary parenchymal disease—antibiotics if pneumonia; treat coagulation disorders; cardiogenic edema requires furosemide ± vasodilators. Noncardiogenic edema requires oxygen therapy, may require positive-pressure ventilation if oxygen therapy alone is not adequate to stabilize the patient.
- Pleural space disease—thoracentesis for air and fluid. Place a chest tube if repeated chest taps are needed to keep patient stable.
- Abdominal distention—drain ascites only as needed to keep the patient comfortable; relieve gastric distention.
- Nonrespiratory diseases—treat primary problem.

NURSING CARE

- Oxygen therapy via cage, nasal cannula, E-collar covered in plastic wrap, mask, or flow-by. Humidify oxygen source if giving oxygen therapy for more than a few hours.
- Monitor temperature regularly, as hyperthermia will worsen respiratory difficulty.

DIET

Weight-reducing diet if obesity is a contributing cause.

SURGICAL CONSIDERATIONS

- Anesthesia must be carefully tailored to the patient. Securing an airway is essential and rapid IV induction is important. Have multiple sizes of endotracheal tubes available if upper airway obstruction is suspected.
- If laryngeal paralysis or brachycephalic syndrome is suspected, prepare for surgical correction at the time of diagnosis. Warn owners of increased likelihood of aspiration pneumonia in dogs with laryngeal disease.

MEDICATIONS

DRUG(S) OF CHOICE

Varies with underlying cause (see Appropriate Health Care).

FOLLOW-UP

N/A

P

PANTING AND TACHYPNEA (CONTINUED)

MISCELLANEOUS

SEE ALSO

- Acidosis, Metabolic.
- Acute Respiratory Distress Syndrome.
- Asthma, Bronchitis—Cats.
- Brachycephalic Airway Syndrome.
- Congestive Heart Failure, Left-Sided.
- Hyperadrenocorticism (Cushing's Syndrome)—Cats.
- Hyperadrenocorticism (Cushing's Syndrome)—Dogs.
- Laryngeal Diseases.
- Pneumonia chapters.
- Pneumothorax.
- Pulmonary Edema, Noncardiogenic.

ABBREVIATIONS

- ARDS = acute respiratory distress syndrome.
- IMHA = immune-mediated hemolytic anemia.
- PLE = protein-losing enteropathy.
- PLN = protein-losing nephropathy.
- PTE = pulmonary thromboembolism.
- PU/PD/PP = polyuria, polydipsia, polyphagia.
- SIRS = systemic inflammatory response syndrome.

Suggested Reading

Hackner SG. Panting. In: King LG, ed., Textbook of Respiratory Disease in Dogs and Cats. Philadelphia, PA: Saunders, 2004, pp. 46–48.

Lee JA. Nonrespiratory look-alikes. In: Silverstein DC, Hopper K, eds., Small Animal Critical Care Medicine, 2nd ed. Philadelphia, PA: Saunders Elsevier, 2015, pp. 157–160.

Mandell DC. Respiratory distress in cats. In: King LG, Textbook of Respiratory Disease in Dogs and Cats. Philadelphia, PA: Saunders, 2004, pp. 12–17.

O'Sullivan ML. Tachypnea, dyspnea, and respiratory distress. In: Ettinger SJ, Feldman EC, Cote E, eds., Textbook of Small Animal Internal Medicine, 8th ed. Philadelphia, PA: Saunders Elsevier, 2017, pp. 115–119.

Author Yu Ueda

Consulting Editor Elizabeth Rozanski

Acknowledgement The author and editors acknowledge the prior contribution of Kate Hopper.

P

BASICS

OVERVIEW

Cutaneous mucous membrane lesions of dogs and cats caused by various papillomaviruses.

SIGNALMENT

Dogs

• Puppies and young adult dogs—oral papillomatosis, venereal papillomatosis, multiple papillomas of the footpad, cutaneous inverted papillomas, canine pigmented viral plaques (breed predisposition). • Older dogs—exophytic cutaneous papillomas, cutaneous inverted papillomas. • Miniature schnauzers and pugs—pigmented viral plaques; associated with immunosuppression in other breeds.

Cats

• More common in older cats; associated with immunocompromise (e.g., feline immunodeficiency virus [FIV]). • Feline sarcoids—younger cats, especially with outdoor exposure.

SIGNS

Dogs

• Cutaneous papillomas—pedunculated, fronds of epithelium, up to 1 cm in diameter. • Canine oral papillomatosis/papillomavirus (COPV)—oral mucosa, hard palate, epiglottis; may interfere with prehension, swallowing; trauma results in halitosis and ptyalism; may be confined to genital or eyelid regions. • Cutaneous inverted papillomas—less common, multiple lesions found with a central pore; on ventral abdomen; caused by distinctly different papillomavirus from COPV. • Multiple papillomas affecting footpads in younger dogs—firm, hyperkeratotic lesions causing discomfort, lameness. • Canine pigmented viral plaques—miniature schnauzers, pugs; Boston terriers, French bulldogs; rarely transform to squamous cell carcinoma (SCC); ventral abdomen, inner thigh region.

Cats

• Feline cutaneous papillomas—rare. • Feline viral plaques—more common; may progress to bowenoid *in situ* carcinoma (BISC) or invasive carcinoma. • Feline sarcoid lesions—uncommon. • Cats 10 years or older; other systemic disease causing immunosuppression (e.g., FIV).

CAUSES & RISK FACTORS

• Oral papillomas affecting naive dogs and recovered animals develop lifelong immunity. • Dogs—cutaneous papillomas may involve cell-mediated immunologic defects. • Older and/or immunosuppressed cats develop plaques and BISC. • Canine pigmented viral plaques—strong breed predisposition.

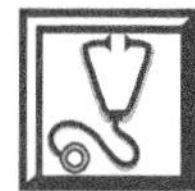

DIAGNOSIS

DIFFERENTIAL DIAGNOSIS

Dogs

• Oral cavity, oropharynx—fibromatous epulis, transmissible venereal tumor, SCC. • Cutaneous—sebaceous hyperplasia, acrochordon. • Pigmented plaque—melanocytoma. • Inverted—infundibular keratinizing acanthoma.

Cats

• Eosinophilic granuloma. • Actinic keratoses • Cutaneous feline leukemia virus (FeLV) lesions. • Multicentric SCC *in situ*. • SCC.

CBC/BIOCHEMISTRY/URINALYSIS

Normal

OTHER LABORATORY TESTS

Cats—FeLV, FIV.

DIAGNOSTIC PROCEDURES

• Gross lesions have a typical appearance. • Biopsy for histopathology; immunohistochemistry demonstrates viral antigens within lesions; PCR not definitive.

PATHOLOGIC FINDINGS

• Dependent upon syndrome; all lesions share cytopathic effects of papillomavirus infection: hyperkeratosis, acanthosis, koilocytes in stratum spinosum, abnormal, large keratohyalin granules in stratum granulosum. • Viral pigmented plaques may lack koilocytes and viral inclusion bodies.

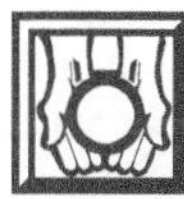

TREATMENT

• Usually regress spontaneously (especially oral forms). • Surgery if needed (excision, cryosurgery, or electrosurgery). • Persistent disease (dogs)—COPV vaccine reported to induce epithelial tumors and SCC at vaccination sites; latency period 11–34 months; autogenous vaccination: treatment controversial. • Cats—diagnosis for visceral diseases, causes of immunosuppression.

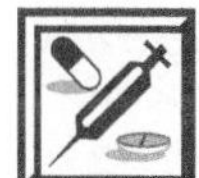

MEDICATIONS

DRUG(S) OF CHOICE

• α-Interferon—20,000iu PO q24h; various reports of efficacy for the treatment of persistent COPV but studies are lacking regarding dosage and protocol for administration. • Imiquimod—applied to lesions 3 times/week for 4 weeks. • Azithromycin 10 mg/kg PO q24h × 14 days.

CONTRAINDICATIONS/POSSIBLE INTERACTIONS

Imiquimod—human exposure potential; causes severe localized reaction; use with caution at mucocutaneous junctions.

FOLLOW-UP

PATIENT MONITORING

Monitor for signs of malignant transformation to SCC.

PREVENTION/AVOIDANCE

• Separate dogs with oral papillomas from susceptible animals. • Commercial kennels—may consider autogenous vaccination.

EXPECTED COURSE AND PROGNOSIS

• Dogs—prognosis good; incubation period 1–8 weeks; regression usually 1–5 months; lesions persist 24 months or more. • Cats—long-term prognosis for plaques and BISC depends on concurrent diseases.

MISCELLANEOUS

ASSOCIATED CONDITIONS

N/A

AGE-RELATED FACTORS

Viral strain dependent.

ZOONOTIC POTENTIAL

Papillomaviruses—species specific.

PREGNANCY/FERTILITY/BREEDING

• Venereal lesions may preclude breeding. • Transmission of viral infection likely; especially if active lesions present.

SYNONYMS

Bowen's disease = BISC.

SEE ALSO

Dermatoses, Viral (Nonpapillomatosis).

ABBREVIATIONS

• BISC = bowenoid *in situ* carcinoma. • COPV = canine oral papillomatosis/papillomavirus. • FeLV = feline leukemia virus. • FIV = feline immunodeficiency virus. • SCC = squamous cell carcinoma.

Suggested Reading

Helton Rhodes KA, Werner A. Blackwell's Five-Minute Veterinary Consult: Clinical Companion: Small Animal Dermatology, 3rd ed. Hoboken, NJ: Wiley-Blackwell, 2018.

Author Elizabeth R. Drake
Consulting Editor Alexander H. Werner Resnick

PARALYSIS

BASICS

DEFINITION

• Paresis—weakness of voluntary movement. • Paralysis—lack of voluntary movement. • Quadriparesis (tetraparesis)—weakness of voluntary movements in all limbs. • Quadriplegia (tetraplegia)—absence of all voluntary limb movement. • Paraparesis—weakness of voluntary movements in pelvic limbs. • Paraplegia—absence of all voluntary pelvic limb movement. • Schiff–Sherrington syndrome—may occur with severe spinal cord trauma below T2. Patient presents paraplegic, in lateral recumbency with extension of front limbs and neck. However front limb function is normal on neurologic examination. Prognosis based on presence or absence of pain perception in pelvic limbs. • Spinal shock—may occur with severe spinal cord trauma, usually near the thoracolumbar spine. Initially the paralyzed pelvic limbs are areflexic but become hyperreflexic (and more indicative of a T3–L3 lesion localization) within minutes to a few hours after the trauma.

PATHOPHYSIOLOGY

• Weakness—caused by lesions in the upper motor neuron (UMN) or lower motor neuron (LMN) systems. • UMN system—cell bodies or nuclei located within the brain are responsible for initiating voluntary movement; axons from these cell bodies form tracts (rubrospinal, corticospinal, vestibulospinal, reticulospinal) that descend from the brain to synapse on the interneurons in the spinal cord. Interneuronal axons synapse on large alpha motor neurons in the ventral gray matter of the spinal cord; these are cell bodies of origin for the LMN system, which is responsible for spinal reflexes. • LMN system—collections of lower motor neurons in the cervical and lumbar intumescences give rise to axons that form the ventral nerve roots, spinal nerves, and (ultimately) the peripheral nerves that innervate limb muscles. • Evaluation of limb reflexes—determines which system (UMN or LMN) is involved. • UMN and their axons—have inhibitory influence on the large alpha motor neurons of the LMN system; maintain normal muscle tone and normal spinal reflexes. • If UMN is injured, spinal reflexes are no longer inhibited or controlled and spinal reflexes become exaggerated or hyperreflexic. • If LMN system is injured, spinal reflexes cannot be elicited (areflexic) or are reduced (hyporeflexic). Large alpha motor neurons or their processes (peripheral nerves) also maintain normal muscle tone. With LMN injury, muscle wasting is usually severe and within 5–7 days of injury.

SYSTEMS AFFECTED

Nervous

SIGNALMENT

Dog and cat.

SIGNS

General Comments

Limb weakness—acute or gradual onset.

Historical Findings

• Owner may describe the patient as being "down," unable to move, walk, or get up. • Many focal compressive spinal cord diseases begin with ataxia and progress to weakness, then to paralysis.

Physical Examination Findings

• Usually normal, unless the disease is systemic. • If in pain, patient may resent handling and manipulation. • Aortic emboli (ischemic neuromyopathy)—patient may be paraplegic and areflexic or hyporeflexic; femoral pulses absent; limbs often cold; nail beds often blue.

Neurologic Examination Findings

• Confirm that the problem is weakness or paralysis. • If limbs are paralyzed—likely bladder is also paralyzed, negating voluntary urination. • Localize problem to either LMN or UMN system. • Tetraparesis with exaggerated spinal reflexes in all limbs—lesion located at C1–C5 spinal segments or in the brain. • Tetraparesis with normal or depressed front limb spinal reflexes and exaggerated pelvic limb spinal reflexes—lesion located at C6–T2 spinal segments. • Tetraparesis with depressed spinal reflexes and decreased muscle tone in all limbs—lesion is diffuse involving muscles or peripheral nerves, or both intumescences (cervical C6–T2 spinal cord segments and lumbar L4–S2 spinal segments). • Normal front limbs but paraparesis/paraplegia with exaggerated pelvic limb spinal reflexes—lesion located at T3–L3 spinal segments. • Normal front limbs but paraparesis/paraplegia with depressed to absent pelvic limb spinal reflexes—lesion located at L4 spinal segment and caudally. • Normal front limb and pelvic limb motor activity but flaccid tail/anus and urinary and/or fecal incontinence—lesion located at S2 spinal segment and caudally. • Normal front limbs but paraparesis/paraplegia and depressed patellar reflexes—lesion involves spinal segments L4–6, located in vertebral bodies L3–4. • Normal front limbs but paraparesis/paraplegia, exaggerated patellar reflexes, and weak flexor and sciatic reflexes—if only the spinal cord is affected (no root involvement), lesion involves spinal segments L6–S2, located in vertebral bodies L4–L6.

CAUSES

Quadriplegia

• If LMN system—acute onset: acute idiopathic polyradiculoneuritis (coonhound paralysis), botulism, tick paralysis, fulminating form of myasthenia gravis, protozoal myoneuritis. • If LMN system—more gradual onset: polyneuropathies and polymyopathies from toxicity, infection, inflammation, endocrinopathy, metabolic disease, or congenital/inherited disease. • If UMN system—acute onset: disc herniation; fibrocartilaginous embolism; trauma; neoplasia; myelitis of many causes. • If UMN system—gradual onset: disc herniation; discospondylitis; neoplasia; myelitis of many causes; malformations of the spine or spinal cord.

Paraplegia

• If UMN or LMN system—acute onset: disc herniation; fibrocartilaginous embolism; neoplasia; trauma. • If UMN or LMN system—gradual onset: disc herniation; congenital malformations of spine or spinal cord; degenerative myelopathy; lumbosacral instability; discospondylitis; neoplasia.

Quadriplegia with Cranial Nerve Deficits, Seizures, or Stupor

• UMN system—diseases of the brainstem: encephalitis; neoplasia; trauma; vascular accidents; congenital or inherited disorders.

RISK FACTORS

• Degenerative disc disease—dachshunds, poodles, cocker spaniels, beagles, others. • Hunting dogs—acute idiopathic polyradiculoneuritis (coonhound paralysis). • Roaming animals—spinal cord and vertebral trauma, tick paralysis, botulism. • Atlantoaxial luxation—toy and small breeds. • Lumbosacral instability—large breeds, working breeds, German shepherd dogs. • Cervical spondylomyelopathy (wobbler syndrome)—large breeds, Doberman pinschers, Great Danes. • Syringomyelia—cavalier King Charles spaniels, brachycephalic toy breeds and others. • Spinal arachnoid diverticulum: Rottweilers, pugs, small breeds.

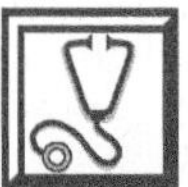

DIAGNOSIS

DIFFERENTIAL DIAGNOSIS

• Weak or paralyzed pelvic limbs—ensure femoral pulses are present and normal; aortic or femoral artery emboli may lead to LMN paraparesis or paraplegia. • Spinal reflexes—localize weakness to the cervical, thoracolumbar, or lower lumbar cord segments. • Acute onset—be careful when moving patient if possibility of trauma.

CBC/BIOCHEMISTRY/URINALYSIS

Usually normal, unless inflammatory diseases involved.

OTHER LABORATORY TESTS

• Urinary tract inflammation—urine culture may be positive in discospondylitis or in any dog that has had chronic bladder paralysis or repeated urinary catheterizations.

• Discospondylitis—diagnose by spinal radiography (intervertebral disc space lysis); perform *Brucella* titer; consider blood and urine bacterial cultures. • Exercise-induced weakness—determine acetylcholine receptor antibody titers (test for myasthenia gravis); check serum creatine kinase concentration (polymyositis or polymyopathy), red blood cell count (anemia or polycythemia), and blood glucose concentration (hypoglycemia); check for cardiac arrhythmia/hypoxia via electrocardiogram, thoracic radiography, Holter monitoring, echocardiography; muscle biopsy.
• LMN weakness or muscle pain, muscle atrophy, or hypertrophy—determine creatine kinase concentration (polymyositis or polymyopathy); evaluate *Neospora caninum* and *Toxoplasma gondii* serum titers; perform electromyography, nerve conduction, muscle and nerve biopsies. • Myelitis or meningitis—Dog: perform titers for *N. caninum*, *T. gondii*, canine distemper virus and/or fungal diseases; perform PCR for Rocky Mountain spotted fever, *Ehrlichia* spp., and canine distemper virus; evaluate spinal fluid for infectious diseases. Cat: evaluate for feline leukemia virus and feline immunodeficiency virus; perform serum titers for *T. gondii* and *Cryptococcus* spp.; evaluate spinal fluid for signs of feline infectious peritonitis virus and *Cryptococcus* spp.

IMAGING

• Spinal radiography—may reveal disc herniation, discospondylitis, bony tumor, congenital vertebral malformation, and fracture or luxation. • Myelography—required if survey radiography not diagnostic and if CT or MRI unavailable. • CT or MRI—has replaced myelography where technology is available.

DIAGNOSTIC PROCEDURES

• CSF—before myelography to detect myelitis and meningitis; if high protein value or inflammatory cells, consider infectious disease diagnostics (titers, PCR). • Needle electromyography and motor nerve conduction velocity—may help with diagnosis and characterization of generalized LMN. • Muscle and nerve biopsy—generalized LMN weakness. • Aspiration of intervertebral disc space under fluoroscopy if discospondylitis observed on imaging studies—perform cytology and culture to isolate an infectious agent.

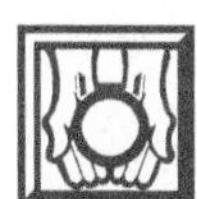

TREATMENT

• Inpatient—with severe weakness or paralysis until bladder function can be ascertained.
• Hand feeding if necesssary—with diffuse LMN, swallowing can be affected. • Feeding from an elevated platform or installation of a feeding tube if necessary—recommended for animals with megaesophagus. • Activity—restrict until spinal trauma and disc herniation can be ruled out. • Physical therapy—important for paralyzed patients; tone muscles and keep joints flexible. • Bedding—check and clean frequently to prevent urine scalding and superficial pyoderma; use padded bedding or waterbed to help prevent decubital ulcer formation. • Turn quadriplegic patients from side to side 4–8 times daily to prevent hypostatic lung congestion and decubital ulcer formation. • Surgery—for disc herniation, fracture, and some neoplasias and congenital conditions; often the quickest and most effective method to improve neurologic status.

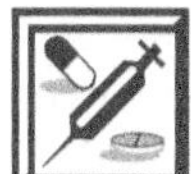

MEDICATIONS

DRUG(S) OF CHOICE

• Medications depend on underlying cause of weakness. • NSAIDs for spinal diseases associated with bone discomfort or pain.
• Corticosteroid use, even in known diseases like spinal trauma or disc herniation, is controversial. May help to allay pain associated with some causes of paralysis, but does not expedite spinal cord recovery. • Dexamethasone 0.1–0.2 mg/kg q48h for pain relief for 2–3 doses. Prednisolone 0.5–1 mg/kg q12–24h for pain relief for 3–5 days. • Antibiotics or antifungals—used for discospondylitis, protozoal myelitis/meningitis. • Pyridostigmine bromide 0.5–3 mg/kg PO q8–12h for suspected myasthenia gravis; administer cautiously at low dose while waiting for titer results. • If acute generalized LMN signs—check for ticks; use appropriate insecticides.

CONTRAINDICATIONS

Corticosteroids—do not use with discospondylitis or fungal or protozoal myelitis/meningitis; do not use with myasthenia gravis if aspiration pneumonia is present.

PRECAUTIONS

Corticosteroids—associated with GI ulceration and hemorrhage, delayed wound healing, and heightened susceptibility to infection.

ALTERNATIVE DRUG(S)

• Tramadol 2 mg/kg q12h PO (dogs or cats), up to 4–5 mg/kg q12h (dogs only) for pain relief. Avoid using with antidepressants.
• Gabapentin 3–10 mg/kg q12h PO for neuropathic pain. • Butorphanol 0.2–0.6 mg/kg q2–4h for pain control.

FOLLOW-UP

PATIENT MONITORING

• Neurologic examinations—daily to monitor status. • Bladder—evacuate (via manual expression or catheterization) 3–4 times a day to prevent overdistension and subsequent bladder atony; once bladder function has returned, patient can be managed at home.

POSSIBLE COMPLICATIONS

• Urinary tract infection, bladder atony, urine scalding and pyoderma, constipation, decubital ulcer formation. • Aspiration pneumonia—with generalized LMN disease or in any quadriplegic patient. • Myelomalacia—with severe spinal cord trauma or disc herniations.
• Respiratory compromise or paralysis—with myelomalacia or generalized LMN disease.

MISCELLANEOUS

SEE ALSO

• Exercise-Induced Weakness/Collapse in Labrador Retrievers.
• Fibrocartilaginous Embolic Myelopathy.
• Intervertebral Disc Disease—Cats.
• Intervertebral Disc Disease, Cervical.
• Lumbosacral Stenosis and Cauda Equine Syndrome.
• Myelopathy—Paresis/Paralysis—Cats.
• Neck and Back Pain.
• Pneumonia—Aspiration.
• Polyneuropathies (Peripheral Neuropathies).
• Schiff-Sherrington Phenomenon.
• Syringomyelia and Chiari-Like Malformation.
• Urinary Retention, Functional.

ABBREVIATIONS

• LMN = lower motor neuron.
• NSAID = nonsteroidal anti-inflammatory drug.
• UMN = upper motor neuron.

Suggested Reading

de Lahunta A, Glass EN, Kent M. Veterinary Neuroanatomy and Clinical Neurology, 4th ed. St. Louis, MO: Elsevier-Saunders, 2015.
Negrin A, Schatzberg S, Platt SR. The paralyzed cat: neuroanatomic diagnosis and specific spinal cord diseases. J Feline Med Surg 2009, 11:361–372.

Author Linda G. Shell

Client Education Handout available online

PARANEOPLASTIC SYNDROMES

BASICS

DEFINITION

Paraneoplastic syndromes (PNS) are a diverse group of systemic disorders resulting from the metabolic or physiologic effects of cancer on tissues remote from the tumor. These disorders are usually caused by production and release of substances not normally released by the cancerous cell of origin or in amounts not normally produced by those cells. Other etiologies of PNS aside from production of metabolically active substances include autoimmune disease stimulation, immune complex formation, immunosuppression, and ectopic receptor production/competitive blockade of normal signaling molecules.

PATHOPHYSIOLOGY

The pathophysiology depends on the specific PNS (see Table 1). Many PNS in veterinary medicine have an unknown pathophysiologic etiology.

P

SYSTEMS AFFECTED

Any body system can be affected by a PNS. Some of the more common systems include:
- Endocrine/metabolic—hypercalcemia.
- Hemic/lymphatic/immune—anemia, thrombocytopenia.

GENETICS

One known genetic cause of a PNS is the mutation H255R of the encoding folliculin gene (*FLCN*) leading to renal cystadenocarcinoma and nodular dermatofibrosis, predominantly seen in German shepherd dogs but rarely noted in non-shepherds.

SIGNALMENT

Any dog or cat with a histologically malignant (most common) or benign cancer (rare).

SIGNS

Vary with tumor type and organ systems affected but include:
- Alopecia (feline paraneoplastic syndrome).
- Anemia.
- Cutaneous flushing.
- Diencephalic syndrome.
- Disseminated intravascular coagulation.
- Eosinophilia.
- Gastroduodenal ulceration.
- Hypercalcemia.
- Hypertrophic osteopathy.
- Hypoglycemia.
- Myelofibrosis.
- Neutrophilic leukocytosis.
- Nodular dermatofibrosis.
- Polycythemia.
- Superficial necrolytic dermatitis.
- Thrombocytopathy.
- Thrombocytopenia.
- Thrombocytosis.

CAUSES

By definition, PNS are caused by an underlying neoplasia, and occur due to a wide range of tumor-related factors including substances secreted from the tumor or cells within the local microenvironment. Many PNS do not have a recognized etiology.

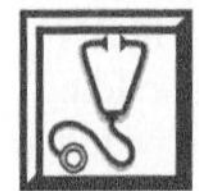

DIAGNOSIS

DIFFERENTIAL DIAGNOSIS

Varies with syndrome.

CBC/BIOCHEMISTRY/URINALYSIS

Helpful in identifying and monitoring several of the reported syndromes.

OTHER LABORATORY TESTS

Ionized calcium and parathormone levels—assess patients with hypercalcemia; hypercalcemia of malignancy usually characterized by high ionized calcium and inappropriate parathormone (PTH) levels; may have elevated parathyroid hormone-related protein (PTH-rP).

IMAGING

Imaging is crucial for the detection of many of the tumors that underlie the PNS:
- Radiography—assess thorax for masses, assess bones for lytic lesions, and detect hypertrophic osteopathy.
- Abdominal ultrasound—assess liver/spleen/kidneys/pancreas/GI tract for masses
- Ventral neck ultrasound—assess for parathyroid or thyroid masses.
- Advanced imaging (CT or MRI)—more sensitive detection of occult tumors within body cavities.

DIAGNOSTIC PROCEDURES

- Fine-needle aspirate and cytology—can provide diagnosis for several tumor types commonly associated with PNS, including lymphoma, multiple myeloma, and apocrine gland adenocarcinoma of the anal sac.
- Biopsy—may be needed for some tumor types; also use to diagnose paraneoplastic skin lesions.

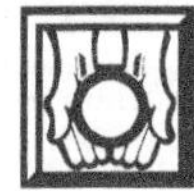

TREATMENT

- Varies based on the underlying tumor and the clinical manifestations of the paraneoplastic syndrome.
- The only definitive treatment is to address the underlying neoplasia rather than to try to control the clinical signs of the paraneoplastic syndrome. If the primary tumor cannot be treated, then management of clinical signs is indicated for palliation.

MEDICATIONS

DRUG(S) OF CHOICE

Depends on underlying tumor type.

FOLLOW-UP

PATIENT MONITORING

As for underlying tumor type.

MISCELLANEOUS

ABBREVIATIONS

- AGASACA = apocrine gland adenocarcinoma of the anal sac.
- PNS = paraneoplastic syndromes.
- PTH = parathormone.
- PTH-rP = parathyroid hormone-related protein.

Suggested Reading

Garneau MS, Price LL, Withrow SJ, et al. Perioperative mortality and long-term survival in 80 dogs and 32 cats undergoing excision of thymic epithelial tumors. Vet Surg 2015; 44:557–564

Lucas P, Lacoste H, de Lorimier LP, Fan TM. Treating paraneoplastic hypercalcemia in dogs and cats. Vet Med May 1, 2007.

Sternberg RA, Wypij J, Barger AM. An overview of multiple myeloma in dogs and cats. Vet Med Oct 1, 2009.

Tumielewicz KL, Hudak D, Kim J, et al. Review of oncological emergencies in small animal patients. Vet Med Sci 2019, 5(3):271–296.

Turek MM. Cutaneous paraneoplastic syndromes in dogs and cats: a review of the literature. Vet Dermatol 2003, 14:279–296.

Author Laura D. Garrett

Consulting Editor Timothy M. Fan

Table 1

Syndrome	*Primary Tumor Association (Dog)*	*Primary Tumor Association (Cat)*	*Primary Mechanism*
Alopecia	Adrenal carcinoma		Dogs: due to an excess of cortisol production; most often associated with hyperadrenocorticism
Alopecia (feline paraneoplastic alopecia)		Pancreatic carcinoma and carcinoma of the biliary tree	Cats: mechanism unknown. See Adenocarcinoma, Pancreas; Feline Paraneoplastic Alopecia; Hyperadrenocorticism (Cushing's Syndrome—Cats)
Cutaneous flushing syndrome	Pheochromocytoma; mast cell tumor	Not reported	Inappropriate release of vasoactive substances, such as histamine, causes paroxysmal flushing of the skin
Diencephalic syndrome	Astrocytoma, anaplastic ependymoma	Not reported	Tumor is present in the diencephalon region of the brain; excess of growth hormone results in dramatic weight loss (without acromegaly) despite adequate caloric intake
Disseminated intravascular coagulation	Hemangiosarcoma; many others	Myeloproliferative disease	See Disseminated Intravascular Coagulation
Eosinophilia	Assorted, including lymphoma and mast cell tumors	Assorted, including lymphoma and mast cell tumors	May be due to stimulation of eosinophil precursors by products such as interleukin-2, -3, and -5 and granulocyte–macrophage colony-stimulating factor
Exfoliative dermatitis (feline thymoma-associated exfoliative dermatitis)	Not reported	Thymoma	Not completely elucidated, likely due to the induction of autoreacting T-lymphocytes
Feminization syndrome	Testicular tumors—especially functional Sertoli cell and seminoma tumors	Not reported	Due to hyperestrogenism or a relative testosterone:estrotgen imbalance that is uncomplicated by myelosuppression
Gastroduodenal ulceration	Non-islet cell pancreatic neoplasia; mast cell tumor	Rare	Inappropriate gastrin secretion (non-islet cell tumor) or excess histamine secretion (mast cell tumor)
Hypercalcemia	Lymphoma; apocrine gland adenocarcinoma of the anal sac (AGASACA); multiple myeloma; others	Relatively rare; lymphoma; squamous cell carcinoma; others	Dogs: multiple secreted factors involved; AGASACA is the most likely tumor to lead to parathyroid hormone-related protein (PTHrP) production Cats: mechanisms unexplored. See Hypercalcemia
Hypertrophic osteopathy	Metastatic and primary tumors of the lung, also seen with intra-abdominal tumors	Metastatic and primary tumors of the lung, also seen with intra-abdominal tumors	Characterized by severe lameness and distal limb soft tissue swelling followed by periosteal new bone growth. The etiology is unknown. Several mechanisms likely play a role, including vagally mediated changes in limb perfusion, cytokine and growth factor secretion, immune mechanisms, vascular thrombi caused by platelets and antiphospholipid antibodies, and interaction between activated platelets and the endothelium
Hyperviscosity syndrome	Immunoglobulin-secreting tumor (e.g., multiple myeloma, lymphoma, and rarely plasma cell tumor)	Immunoglobulin-secreting tumor	Accumulation of large immunoglobulin proteins or polymerized small immunoglobulin proteins in the blood that result in decreased blood flow from increased viscosity. See Multiple Myeloma and Paraproteinemia

PARANEOPLASTIC SYNDROMES (CONTINUED)

Table 1

(Continued)

Syndrome	*Primary Tumor Association (Dog)*	*Primary Tumor Association (Cat)*	*Primary Mechanism*
Hypoglycemia	Insulinoma; benign and malignant smooth muscle tumors; large mesenchymal tumors; others	Rare; insulinoma	Involves the excess production of insulin or insulin-like factors or excessive glucose utilization. See Insulinoma
Immune complex disorders	Lymphocytic leukemia; primary erythrocytosis	Lymphoma	Secondary to antigen-antibody–immune complex activation; glomerulonephritis is most recognized problem
Myasthenia gravis	Thymoma; others	Very rare; thymoma	Exact mechanism is unknown, likely immune-mediated, may be due to effects of follicular helper T-cells. See Myasthenia Gravis
Myelofibrosis	Assorted	Assorted	See Myelodysplastic Syndromes
Neutrophilic leukocytosis	Hemangiosarcoma; lymphoma; others	Assorted; lymphoma, carcinomas and sarcomas	Production of a granulocyte–monocyte-stimulating cytokine is likely cause
Nodular dermatofibrosis	Renal cystadenoma or cystadenocarcinoma primarily in German shepherd dogs and shepherd crosses	Not reported	Mechanism is unknown but involves proliferation of fibroblasts. Propensity to develop is inherited in an autosomal dominant pattern. May be linked to chromosome 5. Loss of heterozygosity/function of the *FLCN* gene may contribute to neoplastic transformation of renal epithelial cells. Renal tumors are usually slowly progressive and almost always bilateral
Pemphigus	Rare; reported in one case of mediastinal lymphoma and one splenic sarcoma	Not reported	Autoimmunity to target antigens (periplakin and envoplakin) in the skin
Peripheral nerve syndromes	Various	Not reported	Unknown, but usually subclinical and secondary to changes in myelination
Polycythemia	Renal sarcoma and carcinoma; others	Renal carcinoma	Inappropriate secretion of erythropoietin or erythropoietin-like peptides. See Polycythemia Vera
Superficial necrolytic dermatitis (metabolic epidermal necrosis, hepatocutaneous syndrome, necrolytic migratory erythema)	Hepatic neoplasia; pancreatic neoplasia (glucagonoma)	Pancreatic neoplasia (glucagonoma)	Many names used to describe similar clinical entities; usually observed in patients with hepatic disease and less commonly with glucagon-secreting pancreatic tumors; sometimes referred to as glucagonoma syndrome; exact mechanism is unclear; may see associated glucose intolerance or diabetes mellitus
Thrombocytopathy	Immunoglobulin-secreting tumors	Immunoglobulin-secreting tumors	Immunoglobulin molecules inhibit normal platelet aggregation. See Thrombocytopathies
Thrombocytopenia	Lymphoma, multiple myeloma, hemangiosarcoma, others	Lymphoma, others	Thrombocytopenia, primary immune-mediated or secondary to myelophthisis. See Thrombocytopenia and Thrombocytopenia, Primary Immune-Mediated
Thrombocytosis	Myeloproliferative disorders	Myeloproliferative disorders	Overproduction of cytokines that stimulate thrombopoietin production (e.g., interleukin-1, -3, -6, -11)

PARAPHIMOSIS, PHIMOSIS, AND PRIAPISM

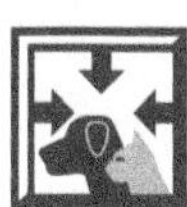

BASICS

OVERVIEW

• Phimosis—inability to protrude the penis beyond the preputial orifice.
• Paraphimosis—inability for exteriorized penis to retract into the sheath.
• Priapism—prolonged extrusion of an erect penis not associated with sexual arousal.

SIGNALMENT

• Dog and cat.
• German shepherd dog, Golden retriever (phimosis)—observed congenital preputial stenosis; possibly hereditary.
• Siamese cat—overrepresented.

SIGNS

• Phimosis—can go undetected until unsuccessful copulation attempts as an adult; severe cases in the neonate resulting in preputial urine pooling may lead to balanoposthitis and septicemia.
• Paraphimosis—initially: licking of an exteriorized penis; after hours of exposure: ischemic necrosis and urethral obstruction; edema and swelling may make differentiation from priapism difficult.
• Priapism—persistent penile erection lasting >4 hours; bulbus glandis firm and swollen.

CAUSES & RISK FACTORS

• Phimosis—abnormally small preputial orifice; congenital or acquired (e.g., caused by injury or disease); may be associated with persistent penile or preputial frenulum (thin band of connective tissue joining the penis and prepuce along the ventral glans).
• Paraphimosis—preputial hair rings; stenotic preputial orifice; injury; os penis fractures; neurologic disease (encephalomyelitis, intervertebral disc disease); penile swelling (neoplasia, balanoposthitis, strangulation with foreign body); incompetent preputial muscles.
• Priapism—ischemic (most common and serious in nature, veno-occlusive/low flow): cause often unknown, trauma during mating, chronic distemper encephalomyelitis, penile thromboembolism, amphetamine use, penile neoplasia, perineal abscess; nonischemic (arterial/high flow): trauma, vasoactive drugs, neurologic conditions, canine distemper; less likely to cause necrosis due to lack of venous obstruction.

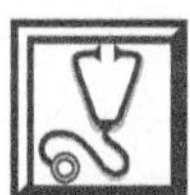

DIAGNOSIS

DIFFERENTIAL DIAGNOSIS

• Phimosis (cats)—inability for penis to exteriorize in prepubertal tom cats is normal as penile adhesion breakdown is androgen-dependent and occurs about 7–12 months of age; early neutered cats may continue to maintain penile adhesion.
• Paraphimosis—abnormality of the retractor penis muscles or prepuce muscles, large preputial opening, short prepuce, or priapism.
• Priapism—urethral obstruction.

CBC/BIOCHEMISTRY/URINALYSIS

• Usually normal.
• Phimosis in neonates—septicemia may result from preputial urine pooling.

OTHER LABORATORY TESTS

Penile blood-gas analysis differentiates forms of priapism:

- Ischemic (i.e., veno-occlusive)—pH <7.25, Po_2 <30 mmHg, Pco_2 >60 mmHg; may respond to phenylephrine therapy (see Medications).
- Nonischemic (i.e., arterial)—pH of 7.4, Po_2 >90 mmHg, Pco_2 <40 mmHg.

DIAGNOSTIC PROCEDURES

• Ultrasonography—visualization of engorged penile vessels.
• Neurologic exam, radiographs, magnetic resonance imaging—to evaluate spinal cord.

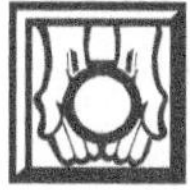

TREATMENT

Phimosis

• Surgical enlargement of the preputial orifice, if required, due to presenting clinical signs.
• Persistent penile frenulum (dogs)—remove band of tissue holding the glans penis to the parietal lamina of prepuce.

Paraphimosis and Priapism

• Main goal—detumesce (priapism) and replace the penis within the prepuce.
• Castration not effective; not testosterone-dependent.
• At times only lubrication required (paraphimosis).
• Penile amputation and urethrostomy required if excessive damage present.
• If urethral patency is in question place an indwelling urinary catheter.
• Under sedation, apply firm pressure wrap soaked with hypertonic glucose solution (decrease edema), firmly replace within prepuce once able; temporary preputial stay sutures may be required for continued reduction (preputial orifice patency for urine flow required if urinary catheter not maintained); surgically enlarge preputial orifice, if necessary.
• Recurrent paraphimosis may require phallopexy.
• Aspiration of penile blood may provide analgesia and prove diagnostic (blood gas analysis).
• Intrapenile phenylephrine may enhance venous outflow if veno-occlusive priapism.
• Penile amputation and perineal urethrostomy—indicated for cats with difficulty urinating.

MEDICATIONS

DRUG(S) OF CHOICE

• Antibiotic ointments—prevent penile adhesions with prepuce.
• Phenylephrine (priapism)—intracavernosal infusion of 100–500 µg diluted in 1 mL of 0.9% saline.

FOLLOW-UP

EXPECTED COURSE AND PROGNOSIS

• Phimosis—fair to good if identified prior to development of septicemia.
• Paraphimosis and priapism—depending on cause, may be guarded to poor for return to breeding activity; fair to good for life with successful medical and/or surgical management.

MISCELLANEOUS

Suggested Reading

Johnston SD, Root Kustritz MV, Olson PNS. Disorders of the feline penis and prepuce. In: Canine and Feline Theriogenology. Philadelphia, PA: Saunders, 2001, pp. 539–543.

Lavely JA. Priapism in dogs. Top Companion Anim Med 2009, 24:49–54.

Author Candace C. Lyman

Consulting Editor Erin E. Runcan

Acknowledgment The author and editors acknowledge the prior contribution of Carlos R.F. Pinto.

PARAPROTEINEMIA

BASICS

OVERVIEW

• The presence of excessive serum paraproteins. Paraproteins are produced by a single clone of cells and may be whole immunoglobulins, subunits, light chains, or heavy chains. Commonly seen with plasma cell neoplasms (multiple myeloma), chronic lymphocytic leukemia, or B-cell lymphoma.
• Primary signs are related to the underlying neoplasm and could be related to bone or bone marrow invasion with neoplastic cells.
• Markedly elevated paraprotein concentration can result in hyperviscosity syndrome (HVS).

SYSTEMS AFFECTED

• Musculoskeletal—bone lysis by neoplasia can cause pain, lameness and pathologic fractures. More common in dogs.
• Nervous—vertebral lysis and HVS can cause neurologic abnormalities including seizures, acute blindness, paraparesis. • Hemic/lymphatic/immune—myelophthisis and secondary immune-mediated destruction may cause cytopenias. Paraproteins may interfere with platelet and coagulation factor function; decreased production of normal immunoglobulins may increase susceptibility to infection. • Ophthalmic—dilated, tortuous retinal vessels, retinal detachment, or retinal hemorrhage from HVS. • Cardiovascular—HVS can cause hypervolemia and tachycardia, gallop rhythm, and cardiac failure (cats more than dogs). • Renal—failure due to antibody deposition in tubules.

P

SIGNALMENT

• Dogs—middle to old aged. • Cats (rare)—middle to old aged. • No sex predilection.

SIGNS

• Lethargy and weakness. • Lameness, paresis. • Bleeding. • Blindness or retinal hemorrhage. • Polyuria and polydipsia.
• Seizures.

CAUSES & RISK FACTORS

• Multiple myeloma—genetic predisposition, viral infections, chronic immune stimulation, and carcinogen exposure. • Lymphoma or leukemia linked to retroviral infections in cats.

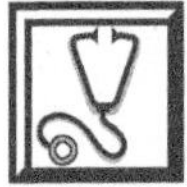

DIAGNOSIS

DIFFERENTIAL DIAGNOSIS

• Monoclonal gammopathy—extramedullary plasmacytoma, lymphoma, lymphocytic leukemia, ehrlichiosis, leishmaniasis, bartonellosis, dirofilariasis, plasmacytic gastroenteritis, feline stomatitis, feline infectious peritonitis (FIP). • Polyclonal gammopathy—chronic infectious/inflammatory disorders, stomatitis, chronic autoimmune disease, and neoplasia.
• Bleeding— thrombocytopenia, thrombocytopathy, other coagulopathy. • Neurologic or ophthalmologic signs of HVS—intracranial or spinal disease (neoplasia, meningitis, immune-mediated), hypertension.

CBC/BIOCHEMISTRY/URINALYSIS

• Anemia/leukopenia/thrombocytopenia—secondary to myelophthisis or autoimmune mechanisms; marked lymphocytosis associated with chronic lymphocytic leukemia or lymphoma. • Serum total protein and globulin concentrations—elevated. • Serum albumin concentration—may be low.
• Serum total or ionized calcium concentration—elevated secondary to malignancy, renal failure, or bone lysis. • Proteinuria—caused by light chains (i.e., Bence Jones protein) not detected on routine urinalysis; urine protein electrophoresis to identify.

OTHER LABORATORY TESTS

• Serum/urine protein electrophoresis—to further characterize immunoglobulins.
• Immunoelectrophoresis—helps define the type of gammopathy. • Infectious disease testing (serology or PCR as indicated). • Flow cytometry—characterization of leukemia, lymphoma.

IMAGING

• Skeletal survey radiographs or bone scan—identify lytic lesions and sites to aspirate or biopsy. Common locations for multiple myeloma lesions include vertebral bodies, ribs, pelvis, skull, and proximal long bones. • Thoracic and abdominal radiographs or ultrasound.

OTHER DIAGNOSTIC PROCEDURES

• Bone marrow aspiration/biopsy—plasmacytosis is often marked (>20%) in dogs with multiple myeloma (<5% is normal); in cats, presence of plasma cell atypia is more important than number.
• Biopsy of lytic bony lesions. • Organ or lymph node aspiration—to identify neoplastic populations of cells, *Leishmania* amastigotes, or amyloid. Relatively contraindicated with coagulopathy.

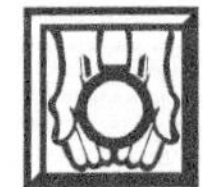

TREATMENT

• Supportive care—analgesia, anticonvulsant therapy, other therapy as indicated.
• Automated or manual plasmapheresis may rapidly decrease paraproteins.
• Chemotherapy for neoplasia.

MEDICATIONS

DRUG(S) OF CHOICE

See specific diseases.

FOLLOW-UP

• See specific diseases. • Electrophoresis may be monitored to assess response to therapy.

MISCELLANEOUS

SYNONYMS

• Monoclonal gammopathy. • M protein.

SEE ALSO

• Hyperviscosity Syndrome.
• Lymphoma—Cats.
• Lymphoma—Dogs.
• Multiple Myeloma.

ABBREVIATIONS

• FIP = feline infectious peritonitis.
• HVS = hyperviscosity syndrome.

Suggested Reading

Boyle TE, Holowaychuk MK, Adams AK, Marks SL. Treatment of three cats with hyperviscosity syndrome and congestive heart failure using plasmapheresis. J Am Anim Hosp Assoc 2011, 47:50–55.

Francey T, Schweighauser A. Membrane-based therapeutic plasma exchange in dogs. J Vet Intern Med 2019, 33(4):1635–1645.

Hohenhaus AE. Syndromes of hyperglobulinemia: diagnosis and therapy. In: Bonagura JD, Kirk RW, eds., Kirk's Current VeterinaryTherapy XII. Philadelphia, PA: Saunders, 1995, pp. 523–530.

Author Kristina Meichner
Consulting Editor Melinda S. Camus

Acknowledgment The author and editors acknowledge the prior contribution of Julie Armstrong.

PATELLAR LUXATION

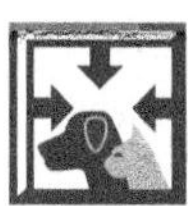

BASICS

DEFINITION

Medial or lateral displacement of the patella from its normal anatomic position in the femoral trochlea.

PATHOPHYSIOLOGY

• Clinical signs may be mild to severe; different degrees of clinical and pathologic changes; classified into grades I–IV (see Physical Examination Findings). • Common musculoskeletal changes occur secondary to abnormal forces on the femur and tibia and lack of normal patellar position during growth—tibial rotation on its long axis; bowing of the distal femur and proximal tibia; shallow to absent femoral trochlea; dysplasia of the femoral and tibial epiphysis; displacement of the quadriceps muscle group.

SYSTEMS AFFECTED

Musculoskeletal

GENETICS

• Recessive, polygenic, and multifocal inheritances proposed. Genetic markers are not yet identified to facilitate the choice of selective elimination of patella luxation from specific breeds. • Hereditary factor in Devon Rex cats.

INCIDENCE/PREVALENCE

• One of the most common stifle joint abnormalities in dogs. • Medial—>75% of cases (large and small dogs and cats).
• Bilateral involvement—50% of cases.
• Uncommon in cats, but may be more common than suspected because most affected cats are not lame.

SIGNALMENT

Species

• Predominantly dog.
• Rarely cat.

Breed Predilections

• Most common in toy and miniature dog breeds. • Dogs—miniature and toy poodles; Yorkshire terriers; Pomeranians; Pekingese; Chihuahuas; Boston terriers. In large-breed dogs, Great Pyrenees and Labrador retrievers are most commonly affected.

Mean Age and Range

Clinical signs—may develop soon after birth with severe luxation or secondary bone deformities; generally after 4 months of age. Mild clinical signs that are not interpreted by clients as lameness are often undetected until secondary osteoarthritis advances.

Predominant Sex

Risk for females 1.5 times that for males.

SIGNS

General Comments

Clinical expression depends on grade (severity), amount of degenerative arthritis, chronicity of disease, and occurrence of other stifle joint abnormalities (e.g., cruciate ligament rupture).

Historical Findings

• Persistent abnormal hind limb carriage and function in neonates and puppies. Clients may complain of "bowed legs" (genu varum) or crouched gait in small-breed dogs.
• Occasional skipping or intermittent hind limb lameness—worsens in young to mature dogs. • Sudden signs of lameness—owing to minor trauma or worsening degenerative joint disease in mature animals.

Physical Examination Findings

• Grade I—patella can be manually displaced from the trochlea, but immediately resumes a normal position when pressure is released. Usually an incidental finding on physical examination and is not normally associated with clinical lameness. • Grade II—patella can be manually displaced or can spontaneously do so with flexion of the stifle joint; patella remains malpositioned until it is manually reduced or the patient extends the stifle joint. Patient intermittently carries the affected limb with the stifle joint flexed, but ambulates normally at other times. • Grade III—patella remains luxated most of the time but can be manually reduced with the stifle joint in extension; movement of the stifle joint results in reluxation of the patella. • Grade IV—patella is permanently luxated and cannot be manually repositioned; may be up to 90° of rotation of the proximal tibial plateau; shallow or missing femoral trochlea. • Grades III and IV—crouching, bowlegged (genu varum) or knock-kneed (genu valgum) stance for medial or lateral luxations, respectively; more of the body weight is transferred to the front limbs.
• Pain—occurs as the patella relocates or if abrasion creates contact with exposed bone.

CAUSES

• Congenital due to polygenetic influences.
• Rarely, traumatic; clinical history will determine traumatic etiology and secondary bone malformations are not present in acute traumatic patella luxation.

RISK FACTORS

Coxa vara—lateral displacement of the proximal femur; vastus medialis and rectus femoris muscles pull the patella medially.

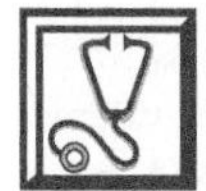

DIAGNOSIS

DIFFERENTIAL DIAGNOSIS

• Cranial cruciate ligament rupture—positive cranial drawer; concurrent in 15–20% of cases. • Avulsion of the tibial tubercle—patellar alta. • Rupture of the patellar tendon—patella alta. • Excessive tibial plateau angle—patella baja. • Malunion and malalignment of fractures of the femur or tibia—may result in displacement of the quadriceps muscle group.

LABORATORY FINDINGS

Not useful in the diagnosis of patella luxation in the dog.

IMAGING

Patella luxation is diagnosed based on clinical signs and physical examination. CT or orthogonal radiography of the femur and tibia may be indicated in grade III and IV luxations to assess bowing and torsion of the femur and tibia and evaluate the need for femoral or tibial osteotomy as an adjunct to correction.

DIAGNOSTIC PROCEDURES

• Palpation of patellar position and movement during flexion and extension of the stifle. Medial and lateral force exerted on patella to relocate the patella into the trochlear groove (if luxated) or luxate the patella (in grade I or II luxations).
• Calculation of the "Q-angle," or the angle of the direction of the quadriceps femoris muscle, under MRI may help to differentiate patella luxation from dogs with partial cranial cruciate ligament rupture. Q-angle (10.5° in normal dogs) increases with increasing grade of patella luxation, but should be only slightly increased in dogs with cranial cruciate rupture.

PATHOLOGIC FINDINGS

• Gross—cartilage wear lesions of the patella and femoral trochlea; joint capsule redundancy on the side opposite to luxation; fibrosis and contracture on the side of luxation. • Microscopic—cartilage fibrillation and loss of glycosaminoglycan content; synovitis.

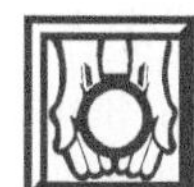

TREATMENT

APPROPRIATE HEALTH CARE

• Outpatient—all grade I and some grade II luxations. • Inpatient (surgery)—most grade II and all grade III and IV luxations.

NURSING CARE

• Cryotherapy (ice packing)—immediately after surgery; 5–10 minutes q8h for 3–5 days, followed by warm-packing, 5–10 minutes q8h for 3–5 additional days. • Passive stifle range-of-motion exercises—as soon as tolerated.

ACTIVITY

Normal to restricted, depending on severity and if surgical correction was performed.

PATELLAR LUXATION (CONTINUED)

DIET

Weight control—decreases the load and stress on the patella support mechanism.

CLIENT EDUCATION

• Discuss the heritability of the condition. • Warn about relapse potential after surgery. Retrospective studies indicate that 8–19.8% of patellas reluxate after surgery. Revision surgery is necessary in 13% of cases. • Inform about increased risk of cranial cruciate ligament disease. • Warn that the condition could worsen over time (e.g., from grade I to grade II).

SURGICAL CONSIDERATIONS

• Malalignment is the underlying cause—tibial crest transposition is the definitive realignment procedure, but often needs to be combined with other techniques such as sulcoplasty. • Retinacular and joint capsule tension on the side of luxation prevents realignment—medial capsulotomy (release) is essential. • Shallowness of the trochlea sulcus is assessed and managed with one of the following: ○ Trochleoplasty—rasp or burr to deepen the sulcus. Not recommended as a primary means of deepening the sulcus because of the poor quality of the fibrocartilage upon healing; often leads to increased secondary osteoarthritis of the stifle. ○ Trochlea chondroplasty—only indicated in very young dogs because of easy separation of the cartilage and subchondral bone in these dogs; lift the surface hyaline cartilage and curette out cancellous bone to deepen the sulcus; lay the cartilage back over exposed bone. ○ Recession sulcoplasty—remove a pie-shaped wedge; deepen the defect, replace the wedge; preferred technique for most patients since the surface cartilage is mostly intact. ○ Block recession sulcoplasty—remove a block instead of a wedge; increases surface area of cartilage in contact with patella. More difficult surgical procedure than simple recession sulcoplasty. ○ Transposition of the tibial tubercle—realign the longitudinal axis of the quadriceps mechanism so that it is centered over the femoral trochlea, in effect, deepening the Q-angle; osteotomize the tibia tubercle leaving it attached distally, transpose it opposite the direction of luxation, and stabilize it with K-wires and, in larger dogs, a tension band wire. ○ Imbricate the joint capsule and supporting soft tissues on the side opposite the luxation—to help keep the patella in the sulcus. Imbrication can occur by removal of a longitudinal full-thickness portion of the excess capsule and edge-to-edge tissue apposition during closure (strongest method), or by overlapping the joint capsule incision with a "vest-over-pants" surgical technique. Imbrication as a sole procedure is not sufficient to permanently correct the position. ○ Corrective osteotomies of the distal femur and proximal tibia—realigns the longitudinal axis of the hind limb; generally indicated most commonly for grade IV luxations with significant femoral or tibial bowing and torsion.

MEDICATIONS

DRUG(S) OF CHOICE

• Nonsteroidal anti-inflammatory drugs (NSAIDs)—minimize pain; decrease inflammation; meloxicam (load 0.2 mg/kg PO, then 0.1 mg/kg q24h PO—liquid), carprofen (2.2 mg/kg PO q12h), etodolac (10–15 mg/kg PO q24h), deracoxib (3–4 mg/kg PO q24h—chewable) for 7 days (for postoperative pain). • Food supplementation with omega-3 fatty acids to decrease inflammation and progression of secondary osteoarthritis. Commercial diets containing 1.7–3.4% omega-3 fatty acids or precursors are beneficial.

CONTRAINDICATIONS

Avoid corticosteroids because of potential side effects and articular cartilage damage associated with long-term use.

PRECAUTIONS

NSAIDs—gastrointestinal irritation may preclude their use.

ALTERNATIVE DRUG(S)

Chondroprotective drugs (e.g., polysulfated glycosaminoglycans, glucosamine, and chondroitin sulfate)—may help limit cartilage damage and degeneration, but recent evidence suggests they are not or are only minimally efficacious.

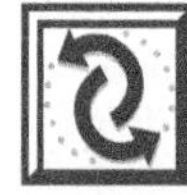

FOLLOW-UP

PATIENT MONITORING

• Post-trochleoplasty—encourage early, active use of the limb. Small-breed dogs are commonly reluctant to bear weight on the operated limb at an early period and are prime candidates for joint range of motion and other exercises to encourage early limb use. • Leash walk exercise for 4–8 weeks; prevent jumping. The duration of exercise restriction is variable depending on the surgical procedure with 4 weeks for only soft tissue corrections and 8 weeks for osteotomy procedures recommended. When corrected with tibial crest transposition, cage rest is indicated until follow-up radiographs indicate the crest is healed in its new position. • Yearly examinations—to assess progression of uncorrected patella luxation or to monitor progression of secondary osteoarthritis.

PREVENTION/AVOIDANCE

• Discourage breeding of affected animals.
• Do not repeat dam–sire breedings that result in affected offspring.

POSSIBLE COMPLICATIONS

Infection, recurrence, tibial crest avulsion, pin migration.

EXPECTED COURSE AND PROGNOSIS

• With surgical treatment—>90% of patients are free from lameness and clinical dysfunction.
• Osteoarthritis—radiographic evidence in almost all affected stifle joints after surgery. Clinical impact appears minimal in small dogs.

MISCELLANEOUS

ASSOCIATED CONDITIONS

Cranial cruciate ligament rupture.

SEE ALSO

Arthritis (Osteoarthritis).

ABBREVIATIONS

• NSAID = nonsteroidal anti-inflammatory drug.

Suggested Reading

Arthurs GI, Langley-Hobbs SJ. Complications associated with corrective surgery for patellar luxation in 109 dogs. Vet Surg 2006, 34:559–566.

Kowaleski MP, Boudrieau RJ, Pozzi A. Stifle joint. In: Johnston SA, Tobias KM, eds., Veterinary Srugery Small Animal, 2nd ed. St. Louis, MO: Elsevier, 2018, pp. 1141–1159.

Linney WR, Hammer DL, Shott S. Surgical treatment of medial patellar luxation without femoral trochlear groove deepening procedures in dogs: 91 cases (1998–2009). J Am Vet Med Assoc 2011, 238:1168–1172.

Roush JK. Canine patellar luxation. Vet Clin North Am 1993, 23:855–875.

Schultz KS. Diseases of the joints. In: Fossum TW, ed., Small Animal Surgery, 4th ed. St. Louis, MO: Elsevier Mosby, 2013, pp. 1353–1362.

Towle HA, Griffon DJ, Thomas MW, et al. Pre- and postoperative radiographic and computed tomographic evaluation of dogs with medial patellar luxation. Vet Surg 2005, 34(3):265–272.

Author James K. Roush
Consulting Editor Mathieu M. Glassman

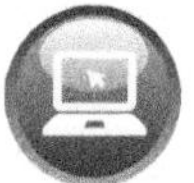

Client Education Handout available online

PATENT DUCTUS ARTERIOSUS

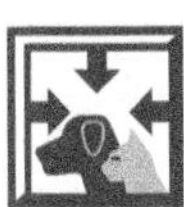

BASICS

DEFINITION

Persistent patency of this normal fetal structure.

PATHOPHYSIOLOGY

Due to insufficient vascular smooth muscle the ductus arteriosus fails to close after birth, maintaining a persistent communication between the low-pressure pulmonary artery (PA) and high-pressure aorta (see Web Figures 1 and 2). Blood typically shunts left to right, with hemodynamic consequences depending on the magnitude of the shunt, pulmonary vascular resistance, and concurrent heart defects. Moderate-to-large shunts cause left-sided congestive heart failure (CHF) from volume overload of the left ventricle (LV). Less often a large-diameter patent ductus arteriosus (PDA) induces severe pulmonary vascular injury, high pulmonary vascular resistance, and pulmonary hypertension (PH), causing shunt reversal from Eisenmenger's pathophysiology. This is termed a "reversed" PDA (rPDA), and leads to bidirectional shunting, arterial desaturation, and secondary erythrocytosis.

SYSTEMS AFFECTED

• Cardiovascular—volume overload or pulmonary vascular disease. • Hemic/lymph/immune—potential for erythrocytosis and hyperviscosity. • Respiratory—cough or labored breathing from pulmonary edema or PH.

GENETICS

"Polygenic" model defect in many canine breeds.

INCIDENCE/PREVALENCE

Estimated prevalence up to 2.5 cases/1,000 live canine births; less common in cats.

SIGNALMENT

Species

Dog and cat.

Breed Predilections

Bichon frise, cavalier King Charles spaniel, Chihuahua, cocker spaniel, collie, English springer spaniel, German shepherd dog, Labrador retriever, Maltese, miniature (and toy) poodle, Pomeranian, Shetland sheepdog, and others.

Mean Age and Range

• Vast majority identified during initial vaccination sequence. • Onset of signs—weeks to years.

Predominant Sex

Dogs—females predisposed in some breeds.

SIGNS

General Comments

• Signs vary by major hemodynamic effect at time of presentation—no signs vs. volume overload vs. increased pulmonary vascular resistance. • Onset of rPDA may be sudden in dogs (usually before 4–6 months of age); can develop gradually in cats but often before 1 year of age. • Signs related to rPDA can be overlooked for years.

Historical Findings

• Most have no clinical signs at initial evaluation. • Dyspnea, coughing, exercise intolerance with development of CHF. • Stunted growth in some. • Exertional rear limb weakness and complications of hyperviscosity (seizures or sudden death) with rPDA. • Signs usually precipitated by or worsened with exercise.

Physical Examination Findings

• Continuous, loud, machinery-type murmur loudest over PA at the left craniodorsal cardiac base; often a systolic mitral regurgitant murmur at the left apex. The murmur in puppies <6 weeks of age or cats of any age might resemble a long systolic and abbreviated diastolic murmur. • Precordial thrill. • Arterial pulses—hyperkinetic ("waterhammer"). • Caudoventral displacement of palpable LV apex. • Tachypnea, dyspnea, and inspiratory crackles—can indicate left-sided CHF or concurrent respiratory disease such as pneumonia. • Rapid, irregular cardiac rhythm with variable-intensity arterial pulses if atrial fibrillation develops—more common in large-breed dogs. • In rPDA findings differ— systolic ejection murmur with tympanic or split second heart sound; normal arterial pulses, prominent right ventricular impulse, and prominent jugular pulse. Differential cyanosis—blue discoloration limited to the caudal mucous membranes.

CAUSES

Genetic in most cases.

RISK FACTORS

Breed and sex in dogs; unknown for cats.

DIAGNOSIS

DIFFERENTIAL DIAGNOSIS

• Congenital aortic stenosis with aortic insufficiency (to-and-fro systolic/diastolic murmurs) and ventricular septal defect (VSD) with aortic valve prolapse (systolic murmur of VSD and diastolic murmur of aortic insufficiency). • Rare causes of continuous thoracic murmurs—pulmonary arteriovenous malformations, aortopulmonary communication, rupture of the aorta into the right atrium or ventricle, and coronary artery fistula. • Systemic arterial to PA vascular malformations can result in similar imaging findings to those of PDA but murmurs are often soft or absent. • Exertional rear limb weakness of rPDA often misdiagnosed as myasthenia gravis.

CBC/BIOCHEMISTRY/URINALYSIS

Usually normal unless rPDA (erythrocytosis with packed cell volume [PCV] 55–80%).

OTHER LABORATORY TESTS

Low femoral arterial PO_2 compared to brachial artery in rPDA (rarely necessary).

IMAGING

Thoracic Radiography

• Lateral projection—left cardiomegaly; pulmonary overcirculation; frequently the lobar pulmonary veins are slightly larger than attendant arteries (see Web Figure 3). • Dorsoventral projection—cardiac elongation (LV enlargement), left auricular enlargement, dilation of the descending aorta ("ductus bump") and the main PA. • Left-sided CHF—distended pulmonary veins; increased interstitial/alveolar densities. • With rPDA—heart normal sized but contour of the right ventricle (RV) is more prominent, the pulmonary circulation appears normal to reduced, and main PA and proximal lobar branches are dilated (see Web Figure 4); a ductus bump may be evident; lung fields are clear.

Echocardiography

• The left atrium (LA), LV, ascending aorta, and main PA are dilated and LV systolic dysfunction might be observed. The RV is normal, except in rPDA or in some animals with progressive PH. • Ductal ampulla and the entry to PA can be imaged; optimally with transesophageal echo (see Web Figure 5). • Doppler studies demonstrate continuous flow into the main PA (see Web Figure 6), usually with concurrent pulmonary insufficiency from dilation of that vessel, along with mitral regurgitation from LV and LA dilation. Transmitral flow velocity is increased from increased flow volume and LA pressure. Aortic outflow velocities are augmented substantially (often around 3 m/s), mimicking mild aortic stenosis. Trace aortic regurgitation is common from aortic dilation. • With rPDA—small left heart chambers, right atrial dilation, RV hypertrophy, and dilation of the main PA and branches. Saline contrast injected in peripheral vein is identified in the abdominal aorta. Color and spectral Doppler studies identify low velocity and bidirectional or right-to-left shunting across ductus (see Web Figure 7). High-velocity pulmonary and tricuspid regurgitation indicate PH.

PATENT DUCTUS ARTERIOSUS (CONTINUED)

Angiography

Fluoroscopic angiography or CT angiography can be useful for the differential diagnosis of rare aortic or coronary arterial malformations, abnormal aortic arch (with right-sided PDA), systemic to pulmonary arterial malformations, and during interventional catheterization procedures to demonstrate ductal morphology and guide catheter-based ductal occlusion.

DIAGNOSTIC PROCEDURES

Electrocardiogram

• Typical abnormalities are wide P-waves and tall R-waves in the caudal leads (II, aVF, III) and left precordial leads. • Atrial fibrillation—observed infrequently; related to marked dilatation of the LA; more common in large-breed dogs. • With rPDA—findings of RV hypertrophy with S-waves in leads I, II, III, and right axis deviation are more typical.

PATHOLOGIC FINDINGS

• Persistent patency of the ductus arteriosus between descending aorta and origin of the left PA. • Left-to-right shunting PDA—pulmonary edema, cardiomegaly (left-sided), and dilation of the aorta and PA. • rPDA—RV hypertrophy, PA dilation, and prominent bronchial arteries; ductal diameter is invariably very wide, similar to descending aorta. Histologic changes of pulmonary vascular disease (medial hypertrophy, plexiform lesions or necrotizing arteritis).

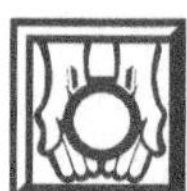

TREATMENT

APPROPRIATE HEALTH CARE

• Manage pulmonary edema with furosemide, pimobendan, and, if necessary, oxygen, nitrates, and cage rest; following stabilization, promptly occlude the PDA. If medical stabilization is ineffective, surgery can often relieve CHF.
• Ductal closure by surgical ligation or various catheter-based occlusion techniques (See Web Figure 8). These are referral procedures.
• Schedule stable animals for elective surgery or device closure without delay; dogs as young as 7–8 weeks of age show no higher operative mortality. • Treat dogs with erythrocytosis from rPDA with rehydration and salting of food to encourage water intake. If needed, consider periodic phlebotomy to maintain target PCV of 62–65%.

ACTIVITY

• Restrict activity until the ductus is closed and in all dogs with CHF. • After suture removal and first follow-up examination, resume normal activity.

DIET

Normal; restrict sodium intake if CHF.

CLIENT EDUCATION

• Do not delay treatment as mortality is higher and LV function impaired if clinical signs or atrial fibrillation develop.
• Following successful PDA closure and a 2 week convalescence, most dogs can be treated normally.

SURGICAL CONSIDERATIONS

• Smaller patient sizes (<2.5 kg) are a limiting factor with current intravascular PDA occlusion devices. • Surgery can generally proceed within 24–48 hours of medical stabilization. • Surgical therapy involves ductal ligation via left thoracotomy; surgical and perioperative mortality is <3% at the most experienced centers. • Mortality with devices is even lower, but complications including failure to achieve closure and device embolization infrequently occur. • Never close a true rPDA as the RV cannot eject against the pulmonary vascular resistance. PDA with moderate PH and predominately left-to-right shunting can often be closed, especially in cats, provided pulmonary vascular resistance is not fixed. Medication trial with sildenafil may be performed cautiously to determine degree of vascular reactivity in PDA with PH; monitor in-hospital for first 24 hours if pursued.

MEDICATIONS

DRUG(S) OF CHOICE

• Treat pulmonary edema with furosemide 2–4 mg/kg q6–12h PO, SC, IM, or IV as required; and pimobendan 0.2–0.3 mg/kg q12h PO. These are usually discontinued once the PDA is closed. • When closure is not an option—if CHF, prescribe furosemide, ACE inhibitor such as enalapril 0.5 mg/kg q12–24h PO, and pimobendan. • If atrial fibrillation develops add digoxin and diltiazem (see Atrial Fibrillation and Atrial Flutter). An alternative is electrical cardioversion—this is a reasonable therapy provided the ductus can be closed. Refer to a cardiologist. • To control severe, life-threatening CHF—can use direct vasodilators such as hydralazine 1–2 mg/kg q12h PO or sodium nitroprusside 1–5 µg/kg/min IV to reduce left-to-right shunting. Maintain systolic blood pressure at 85–90 mmHg. Artificial ventilation might be needed.
• Consider sildenafil at 1–2 mg/kg q8h PO if moderate to severe PH is present.

CONTRAINDICATIONS

• Left-to-right PDA—drugs that increase systemic vascular resistance and arterial blood pressure, except as needed for anesthesia and surgery. • rPDA—drugs that cause systemic arterial vasodilation and reduce systemic arterial blood pressure, including drugs with arterial vasodilating effects.

PRECAUTIONS

• Measure digoxin levels if prescribed.
• Monitor arterial blood pressure, renal function, and serum electrolytes to identify problems related to diuretic and vasodilator therapies.

POSSIBLE INTERACTIONS

Aggressive diuresis leading to dehydration or hypokalemia exacerbates the risk for digoxin toxicity. Sildenafil in a balanced PDA can increase pulmonary overcirculation and result in left-sided CHF.

ALTERNATIVE DRUG(S)

• Prostaglandin inhibitors (e.g., indomethacin) do *not* close PDAs effectively in dogs.
• Hydroxyurea—infrequently considered for treatment of severe erythrocytosis unresponsive to phlebotomy. Consult with internist or oncologist before using.

FOLLOW-UP

PATIENT MONITORING

• Intra- and postoperative pain management with opiates and regional blocks as appropriate for the procedure. Analgesic therapy following catheter-based closure is less aggressive but also continued for 24–48 hours. • Postoperative—vital signs and respiratory rate. • Cardiac auscultation postoperatively and at suture removal; if heart sounds are normal, no further follow-up or diagnostic studies are required unless preoperative echocardiography showed moderate to severe LV dysfunction. There is no basis for recommending annual cardiac reevaluation of uncomplicated cases.
• Persistent, continuous murmur indicates either incomplete closure of the ductus, recanalization (infection or device migration), or a concurrent cardiac or vascular defect.
• Systolic murmurs are variably heard postoperatively; these typically abate by the time of suture removal. Reinvestigate unexpected murmurs by Doppler echocardiography. When only partial surgical ligation is achieved, consider referral for device occlusion.

PREVENTION/AVOIDANCE

Do not breed.

POSSIBLE COMPLICATIONS

• Sudden illness, fever, or acute respiratory signs postoperatively—consider bacterial infection of the closure site with hematogenous pneumonia; aggressive antibiotic therapy needed. • An unusual complication is acquired stenosis of the main or branch PA following surgery to correct PDA.

EXPECTED COURSE AND PROGNOSIS

• Infrequently dogs remain asymptomatic for life. PDA closure adds an estimated 10 years to median lifespan in dogs (12 years with closure, 2 years without). In older reports, ~50–60% of dogs died from CHF within 1 year of diagnosis if the PDA was not closed. • Closure prior to onset of moderate-to-severe CHF—excellent prognosis. • Moderate-to-severe CHF is related to myocardial failure of LV or atrial fibrillation—guarded prognosis; referral to a cardiologist is advised. • Dogs with rPDA can live for several years but often die suddenly; occasionally, dogs live beyond 5 years of age (especially cocker spaniels). • Cats—varies from rapidly progressive left-sided CHF to gradual development of pulmonary vascular disease; even right-sided CHF can develop with PDA and PH.

MISCELLANEOUS

ASSOCIATED CONDITIONS

Typically an isolated defect, but is recognized with other congenital heart lesions—more likely in larger breeds. Occasionally a vascular ring anomaly is evident, such as persistent right fourth aortic arch.

AGE-RELATED FACTORS

Presentation is typically young animals; median age of presentation reported as 5 months in dogs.

PREGNANCY/FERTILITY/BREEDING

Greater risk for CHF in pregnant bitches; offspring have greater risk for large PDA or rPDA; do not breed affected dogs.

SYNONYMS

Duct of Botallo, ductus Botalli, patent arterial duct.

SEE ALSO

- Atrial Fibrillation and Atrial Flutter.
- Congestive Heart Failure, Left-Sided.
- Hypertension, Pulmonary.
- Murmurs, Heart.

ABBREVIATIONS

- CHF = congestive heart failure.
- LA = left atrium.
- LV = left ventricle.
- PA = pulmonary artery.
- PCV = packed cell volume.
- PDA = patent ductus arteriosus.
- PH = pulmonary hypertension.
- rPDA = reversed patent ductus arteriosus.
- RV = right ventricle.
- VSD = ventricular septal defect.

INTERNET RESOURCES

Dr. James Buchanan Cardiology Library: https://www.vin.com/doc/?id=2993158&pid=84

Suggested Reading

Beijerink NJ, Oyama MA, Bonagura JD. Congenital heart disease. In: Ettinger SJ, Feldman EC, Côté E, eds., Textbook of Veterinary Internal Medicine, 8th ed. St. Louis, MO: Elsevier, 2017, pp. 1207–1218.

Authors John D. Bonagura and Brian A. Scansen

Consulting Editor Michael Aherne

Client Education Handout available online

PECTUS EXCAVATUM

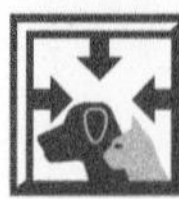

BASICS

OVERVIEW

- Deformity of the sternum and costal cartilages that results in a dorsal-to-ventral narrowing of the chest, primarily in the caudal aspect.
- Can have secondary abnormalities of respiratory and cardiovascular function from restriction of ventilation and cardiac compression.
- Considered congenital in origin although an acquired case has been reported.
- Upper respiratory obstruction at a young age could cause abnormal respiratory gradients and subsequent pectus excavatum.
- Uncommon defect.
- Concurrent cardiac defects common.
- Some patients demonstrate swimmer syndrome—neonatal dogs lack the ability to posture properly and remain in sternal recumbency, which can lead to invagination of the sternum.

P

Systems Affected

- Respiratory.
- Cardiovascular.

SIGNALMENT

- Dogs and cats.
- Brachycephalic breeds and Bengal cats are overrepresented.
- Most common age of presentation—4 weeks–3 months.
- Male cats more often reported than females, no sex predisposition noted in dogs.

SIGNS

- Thoracic defect, easily palpated or seen.
- Varying degrees of respiratory distress.
- Exercise intolerance.
- Weight loss.
- Recurrent respiratory infections.
- Cough.
- Vomiting.
- Cyanosis.
- Poor appetite.
- Cardiac murmurs associated with concurrent cardiac defects or compression of the heart.
- Muffled heart sounds.
- No correlation between severity of signs and severity of anatomic or physiologic abnormalities.
- Vertebral deformities.
- Swimmer syndrome—limbs not adducted properly; ambulation impaired.

CAUSES & RISK FACTORS

- Genetic predisposition—may exist.
- Unknown etiology—suspected causes include intrauterine pressure abnormalities, shortening of central tendon of the diaphragm, cranial abdominal muscle deficiency, and abnormal osteogenesis or chondrogenesis.
- Dogs predisposed to respiratory obstructive processes have a higher risk than others.
- Single report in a geriatric golden retriever with laryngeal paralysis.
- Puppies raised on surfaces causing poor footing may be predisposed to swimmer syndrome.

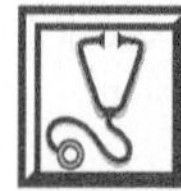

DIAGNOSIS

DIFFERENTIAL DIAGNOSIS

- Congenital diaphragmatic hernia (pleuroperitoneal or pericardioperitoneal).
- Tracheal malformations or collapse.
- Congenital heart defects.
- Pulmonary edema.
- Pleural effusion.
- Pneumonia.
- Tracheobronchitis/bronchitis.
- Brachycephalic obstructive airway syndrome.

IMAGING

Thoracic Radiography (see Web Figure 1)

- Confirm sternal and costal skeletal abnormalities.
- Decreased thoracic volume.
- Cardiac malpositioning—left and cranial displacement of cardiac silhouette.
- Concurrent secondary pulmonary disease.
- Measure frontosagittal and vertebral indices to characterize degree of deformity as mild, moderate, or severe and help predict response to treatment.
- The frontosagittal index is the ratio between the width of the chest at the 10th thoracic vertebra and the distance between the center of the ventral surface of the 10th thoracic vertebral body and the nearest point on the sternum.
- The vertebral index is the ratio between the distance from the center of the dorsal surface of the 10th vertebral body to the nearest point on the sternum and the dorsoventral diameter of the vertebral body at the same level.

Echocardiography

Rule out concurrent congenital cardiac defects or other cardiac disease.

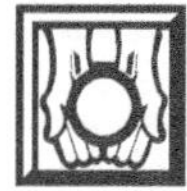

TREATMENT

- Decision to repair deformities is made on the basis of clinical signs. If it is an incidental finding with minimal to no clinical signs, then intervention may not be indicated.
- Treatment options include external coaptation, partial sternectomy, or both. Decision is based on age of the animal and degree of deformity.
- Surgery benefits patients with concurrent respiratory distress; benefits are unknown in patients with no respiratory distress but with moderate or severe deformity.
- Nonclinical patients can develop signs at a later date; patients with clinical signs of disease may show progression.
- For puppies with swimmer syndrome, place on surfaces with excellent footing; careful toggling of front and rear legs may improve adduction.
- Brachycephalic breeds with concurrent upper airway obstruction may benefit from surgery directed at these problems.
- Anesthesia—patients require constant monitoring; ventilatory support should be available.

MEDICATIONS

N/A

FOLLOW-UP

- Examinations—dictated by clinical signs or when surgical intervention has been precluded.
- No specific actions for avoiding disease; genetic factors may sometimes be involved.
- Progression of respiratory signs—can develop in nonclinical or mildly clinical patients.
- Prognosis—guarded to good depending on properly timed and expertly administered intervention.

MISCELLANEOUS

ASSOCIATED CONDITIONS

- Cardiac defects.
- Swimmer syndrome.

Suggested Reading

Charlesworth TM, Sturgess CP. Increased incidence of thoracic wall deformities in related Bengal kittens. J Feline Med Surg 2012, 14(6):365–368.

Hassan EA, Hassan MH, Torad FA. Correlation between clinical severity and type and degree of pectus excavatum in twelve brachycephalic dogs. J Vet Med Sci 2018, 80:766–771.

Kurosawa TA, Ruth JD, Steurer J, et al. Imaging diagnosis: acquired pectus excavatum secondary to laryngeal paralysis in a dog. Vet Radiol Ultrasound 2012, 53:329–332.

Mestrinho LA, Ferreira CA, Lopes AM, et al. Open surgical correction combined with an external splint for correction of a non-compliant pectus excavatum in a cat. J Feline Med Surg 2012, 14:151–154.

Author Catriona M. MacPhail

Consulting Editor Elizabeth Rozanski

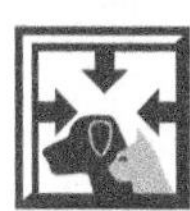

BASICS

OVERVIEW

- Congenital hereditary disorder that has been seen in several breeds of dogs and domestic shorthair cats.
- Results in nuclear hyposegmentation of many to all granulocytes (neutrophils, eosinophils, and basophils).
- Hypolobulation of monocytes and megakaryocytes has also been reported.
- Chromatin patterns of leukocytes are normochromatic, or occasionally hyperchromatic, rather than the open, immature chromatin of immature leukocytes.
- Cytoplasm of cells is unremarkable (i.e., no toxic changes are observed).
- Cell function is unaffected in heterozygotes; homozygotes are usually stillborn or die *in utero*.
- Care should be taken not to misinterpret as a severe left shift.

SIGNALMENT

- Dogs—Pelger–Huët anomaly (PHA) has been reported in mixed-breed dogs as well as numerous pure-breed animals. Overall the incidence is low; however, Australian shepherd dogs have been shown to have a 9.8% incidence rate.
- Cats—PHA has only been reported in domestic shorthair cats. The overall incidence in cats is unknown; however, it is likely rare when compared to dogs.
- An autosomal dominant mode of inheritance is likely; however, incomplete penetrance has been seen in Australian shepherd dogs.

SIGNS

No clinical signs are associated with heterozygous animals, as the leukocytes are fully functional.

CAUSES & RISK FACTORS

- In humans, caused by an inherited defect of the lamin B receptor.
- Australian shepherd dogs are over-represented in reported canine cases.

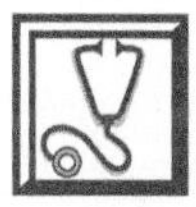

DIAGNOSIS

DIFFERENTIAL DIAGNOSES

- The primary differential diagnosis to rule out is a severe left shift, indicating severe inflammation or infection.
- An inflammatory leukogram may show a leukocytosis or leukopenia. Immature leukocytes exhibit an open, pale chromatin pattern.
- Toxic changes (Döhle bodies, blue foamy cytoplasm, toxic granulation, etc.) are frequently seen with severe inflammation, but not PHA.
- Pelger–Huët cells have a nucleus that shows a mature, condensed chromatin pattern and exhibit no toxic changes.
- Animals with PHA are clinically healthy, whereas animals with severe left shifts tend to be systemically ill.
- Pseudo- or acquired PHA is an acquired condition that results in granulocyte hyposegmentation, secondary to myelodysplastic conditions or drug therapy.

CBC/SERUM BIOCHEMISTRY/ URINALYSIS

- The blood smear reveals a persistent varying hyposegmentation of all granulocytes and often monocytes.
- Granulocyte nuclei have mature, condensed chromatin and may be round, oval, peanut, dumbbell, horseshoe, and bilobed in shape.
- The serum biochemistry profile and urinalysis are unremarkable.

OTHER LABORATORY TESTS

Examination of a peripheral blood smear which exhibits hyposegmentation of all granulatocytes is all that is needed to diagnose PHA.

IMAGING

Imaging is not useful in diagnosing PHA.

DIAGNOSTIC PROCEDURES

- Establishment of a hereditary pattern typically an academic exercise, but potentially useful.
- No additional diagnostic procedures are indicated to diagnose PHA.
- Additional diagnostics are warranted if an underlying disease is suspected to cause a severe left shift.

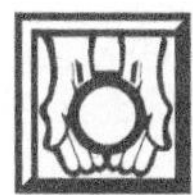

TREATMENT

No treatment is indicated for PHA.

MEDICATIONS

N/A

FOLLOW-UP

No follow-up is necessary.

MISCELLANEOUS

Affected animals should not be bred, as it is lethal *in utero*.

ABBREVIATIONS

- PHA = Pelger–Huët anomaly.

Suggested Reading

Latimer KS. Pelger-Huët anomaly. In: Feldman BF, Zinkle JG, Jain NC, eds., Schalm's Veterinary Hematology, 5th ed. Philadelphia, PA: Lippincott Williams & Williams, 2000, pp. 976–983.

Author Craig A. Thompson
Consulting Editor Melinda S. Camus

P

PELVIC BLADDER

BASICS

OVERVIEW

Pelvic bladder or "intrapelvic bladder" is characterized by abnormal position of the urinary bladder neck caudal to the pubic bone, causing the proximal urethra and a variable portion of the trigone or the body of the bladder to remain within the pelvic canal. It is commonly associated with a short urethral length and urethral sphincter mechanism incompetence (USMI).

SIGNALMENT

- Dogs and rarely cats.
- Primarily young female dogs (<1 year of age).

SIGNS

- May be asymptomatic.
- Incontinence can be continuous or intermittent.
- Conscious voiding patterns often present.
- Perineum stained/soaked with urine, urine scalding, wet vulva/prepuce.
- Urgency with small volume elimination may be seen.

CAUSES & RISK FACTORS

The position of the bladder in incontinent female dogs has been shown to be more intrapelvic and associated with a shorter urethral length, suggesting that an intrapelvic bladder neck and a short urethra together encourage urinary incontinence. It is hypothesized that this could result from an unbalanced distribution of the pressure exerted by the abdominal organs between the bladder and urethra.

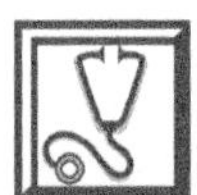

DIAGNOSIS

DIFFERENTIAL DIAGNOSIS

- Urinary incontinence—ectopic ureter, USMI, inappropriate urination, urge incontinence, urinary tract infection (UTI), neurogenic incontinence, overflow incontinence.
- Often associated with ectopic ureters.

CBC/BIOCHEMISTRY/URINALYSIS

- CBC and biochemistry typically unremarkable.
- Urinalysis may reveal evidence of a UTI (including pyuria, bacteriuria, and hematuria) or polyuria (urine specific gravity [USG] <1.035).
- Urine culture and sensitivity via a cystocentesis should be performed.

IMAGING

- Abdominal radiographs may reveal a caudally displaced bladder, but this should be interpreted carefully without bladder distension.
- Excretory urography may allow visualization of the kidneys, ureteral terminations, urinary bladder, and urethra but does not provide bladder distension. Without bladder distension, interpretation of bladder neck location should be made with caution.
- Retrograde vaginourethography or urethrocystography allows visualization of the vaginal vault, urethra, urethral length, prostate, urinary bladder shape, and bladder neck location.
- If the urinary bladder and urethra are inside the bony pelvis, double contrast cystourethrography may be required for full visualization.
- Ultrasonography of the kidneys, ureters, and urinary bladder can aid in documentation of concurrent urologic anomalies, hydronephrosis, pyelonephritis, or ectopic ureters.
- The diagnostic combination of choice is cystourethroscopy with contrast cystourethrography, allowing investigation of urethral, ureteral, urinary bladder, vaginal, and vestibular defects. It also allows measurement of urethral length and width and aids in formulating therapy.

DIAGNOSTIC PROCEDURES

- Neurologic exam should be normal.
- Urodynamic procedures—consider cystometrography and urethral pressure profilometry to evaluate urinary bladder and urethral function, as well as urethral length.

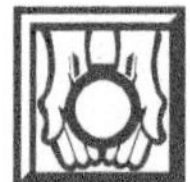

TREATMENT

- Identify UTI and treat appropriately.
- Goal is to increase urethral resistance (intraurethral injections of bulking agents, urethral hydraulic occluder, etc.), and/or relocate the bladder neck to an intra-abdominal position (colposuspension, urethropexy, prostatopexy, or vas deferensopexy).
- Detrusor relaxation may treat refractory incontinent dogs with an overactive bladder contributing to incontinence or urgency.
- Medical management for traditional USMI is typically successful in 75–90% of female dogs.

Surgical Considerations

- Colposuspension has a reported cure rate of 53%.
- Placement of a urethral hydraulic occluder, also termed "artificial urethral sphincter" has been successful and is currently the surgical treatment of choice if other minimally invasive or medical interventions fail. Experience with this procedure has been limited and the risk of urethral strictures can be up to 20%. Cystopexy can also be considered.

Minimally Invasive Treatment

Transurethral submucosal bulking agent (e.g., collagen) therapy has been described for patients refractory to medical management and is associated with good, but temporary success. While this may improve incontinence, it does not alter the location of the urinary bladder.

MEDICATIONS

DRUG(S) OF CHOICE

- All should be reduced to lowest effective dosage. Combination therapy may be more effective.
- Phenylpropanolamine (PPA)—an α-agonist (1–2 mg/kg PO q8–12h) will improve continence in a majority of USMI cases.
- Diethylstilbestrol (DES)—an estrogen (0.1–1 mg PO q24h for 3–5 days, then 0.1–1 mg per week thereafter). DES can be toxic to the bone marrow in dogs and cats and can cause blood dyscrasias. This can progress, in rare cases, to fatal aplastic anemia. Estrogenic effects may also be seen.
- Estriol—an estrogen (2 mg once daily per dog (regardless of body weight) for 14 days, then taper every 7 days). Estriol can be toxic to the bone marrow in dogs and cats and can cause blood dyscrasias, but is considered safer than DES. Estrogenic effects may also be seen.

FOLLOW-UP

PATIENT MONITORING

- Monitor for the development of lower urinary tract signs which could indicate UTI.
- Patients receiving an α-agonist should have serial blood pressure evaluations, as this is contraindicated in hypertensive patients or those with renal or heart disease.
- Patients receiving estrogen therapy (DES or estriol) should have serial CBC evaluations to monitor for bone marrow dyscrasia.
- Use all medications at the lowest effective dose.

MISCELLANEOUS

ABBREVIATIONS

- DES = diethylstilbestrol.
- PPA = phenylpropanolamine.
- USG = urine specific gravity.
- USMI = urethral sphincter mechanism incompetence.
- UTI = urinary tract infection.

Suggested Reading

Crawford JT, Adams WM. Influence of vestibulovaginal stenosis, pelvic bladder, and recessed vulva on response to treatment for clinical signs of lower urinary tract disease in dogs: 38 cases (1990–1999). J Am Vet Med Assoc 2002, 221(7):995–999.

Author Andreanne Cleroux
Consulting Editor J.D. Foster
Acknowledgment The author and editors acknowledge the prior contribution of Allyson C. Berent.

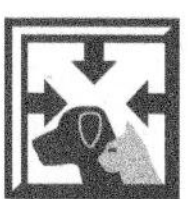

BASICS

DEFINITION

• A group of autoimmune dermatoses characterized by varying degrees of erosion, ulceration, crusting, pustule and vesicle formation. • Affects the skin and sometimes mucous membranes. • Forms identified in animals—pemphigus foliaceus (PF), pemphigus erythematosus (PE), pemphigus vulgaris (PV), paraneoplastic pemphigus (PP), and panepidermal pustular pemphigus (PEP)/ pemphigus vegetans (PVeg).

PATHOPHYSIOLOGY

• Tissue-bound autoantibody directed at intraepidermal cell antigens (desmoglein and desmocollin) and acetylcholine receptors is deposited within the intercellular spaces, causing epidermal cell separation and cell rounding (acantholysis). • Severity of ulceration and disease—related to depth of autoantibody deposition within the skin. • PF—autoantibody deposition in the superficial layers of the epidermis. • PV—lesions more severe; auto-antibody deposition just above the basement membrane zone; rapidly leads to ulcer formation. • The disease is typically considered to be idiopathic. Possible drug association has been proposed in dogs and cats with PF. Sunlight exposure is suspected to induce flares of PF and PE. Thymoma has been associated with pemphigus variants in dogs and cats.

SYSTEMS AFFECTED

Skin/exocrine

INCIDENCE/PREVALENCE

• PF—most common autoimmune skin disease in dogs and cats. • PE—relatively common. • PV/PP—more severe forms, much rarer than PF/PE. • PEP/PVeg—rarest form; may represent a more severe variant of PF.

SIGNALMENT

Species

Dogs and cats.

Breed Predilections

PF— Dogs: Akita, chow chow, dachshund, cocker spaniel, Labrador retriever, and English bulldog. Cats: possibly short-haired and Siamese.

Mean Age and Range

Usually middle-aged to old animals.

Predominant Sex

None reported.

SIGNS

PF

• Scales, crust, pustules, epidermal collarettes, erosions, erythema, alopecia, and footpad hyperkeratosis with fissuring. • Common involvement—head, face, ears, and footpads. • Most cases develop extensive disease within one month. • Nasal depigmentation may develop, but this is a late event. • Head and facial distribution is an important distinction from a staphylococcal pyoderma. • Cats—nipple and ungual fold involvement common. • Lymphadenopathy, edema, depression, fever, and lameness (if footpads involved) when severe or generalized. • Variable pain and pruritus. • Secondary bacterial infection possible.

PE

• May be a variant of PF or a crossover between PF and discoid lupus erythematosus (DLE). • Dogs and cats—pustules, erosions and crusts on face and pinnae. Along with depigmentation, erythema and erosion/ ulceration of the nasal planum and dorsal muzzle. Rare patients exhibit nonfacial lesions. • Depigmentation more common than with other pemphigus forms, often precedes crusting.

PV/PP

• Oral cavity lesions frequent and may precede skin lesions. • Initially vesiculobullous lesions rapidly progressing to ulcerations and erosions. • More severe than PF and PE. • Affects mucous membranes, mucocutaneous junctions, and skin; may become generalized. • Footpads and ungual folds may be involved, with resultant onychomadesis. • Positive Nikolsky sign (new or extended erosive lesion created when lateral pressure is applied to the skin near an existing lesion). • Variable pruritus and pain. • Anorexia, depression, and fever. • Secondary bacterial infections common.

PEP/PVeg

• Pustule groups become eruptive papillomatous lesions with exudation. • No oral involvement. • No systemic illness.

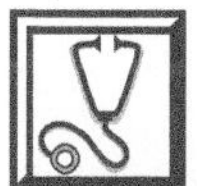

DIAGNOSIS

DIFFERENTIAL DIAGNOSIS

PF

• Superficial pyoderma. • Dermatophytosis. • Demodicosis. • Candidiasis. • Keratinization disorders. • Cutaneous lupus erythematosus or DLE. • PE. • Subcorneal pustular dermatosis. • Drug eruption. • Zinc-responsive dermatitis. • Dermatomyositis. • Tyrosinemia. • Mycosis fungoides. • Metabolic epidermal necrosis. • Linear IgA dermatosis.

PE

• PF. • DLE. • Mucocutaneous pyoderma. • Demodicosis. • Dermatophytosis. • Epidermolysis bullosa simplex. • Uveodermatologic syndrome.

PV/PP

• Subepidermal blistering diseases. • Systemic lupus erythematosus. • Toxic epidermal necrolysis. • Drug eruption. • Mycosis fungoides. • Ulcerative stomatitis causes. • Erythema multiforme.

PEP/PVeg

• PF. • PV. • Superficial pyoderma. • Lichenoid dermatoses.

CBC/BIOCHEMISTRY/URINALYSIS

• Abnormalities uncommon. • Leukocytosis and hyperglobulinemia with chronicity and/ or secondary infection.

OTHER LABORATORY TESTS

Antinuclear antibody—may be weakly positive in PE only.

DIAGNOSTIC PROCEDURES

• Cytology of pustules—aspirates or impression smears from pustules or under crusts: acantholytic keratinocytes (rounded and deeply staining isolated keratinocytes) and neutrophils; occasionally with eosinophils. • Biopsy of pustules or crusted lesions (submit crusts with the biopsy samples of the skin).

PATHOLOGIC FINDINGS

• Histopathology: ∘ PF—subcorneal pustules with acantholytic cells and neutrophils; eosinophils often present; follicles may be involved. ∘ PE—intragranular and subcorneal pustules, eosinophils, neutrophils, lichenoid interface dermatitis. ∘ PV—suprabasilar intraepidermal cleft with the remaining basal cells exhibiting a tombstone appearance. ∘ PP—suprabasilar clefting with interface dermatitis and apoptotic keratinocytes. ∘ PEP/PVeg—pustules present throughout the epidermal layers and includes follicular epithelium. • Immunopathology of biopsied skin via immunofluorescent antibody assays or immunohistochemical testing—may demonstrate positive staining in the intercellular spaces in 50–90% of cases; results can be affected by concurrent or previous corticosteroid (or other immuno-suppressive drug) administration; indirect immunofluorescence usually negative; PE may demonstrate staining of basement membranes and intercellular spaces.

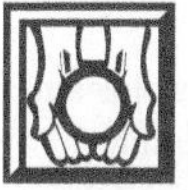

TREATMENT

APPROPRIATE HEALTH CARE

• Initial inpatient supportive therapy for severely affected patients. • Outpatient treatment with initial frequent hospital visits (every 1–3 weeks); taper to every 1–3 months when remission is achieved and the patient is on a maintenance medical regimen.

NURSING CARE

Severely affected patients may require antibiotics and hydrotherapy/soaks.

CLIENT EDUCATION

Sun avoidance/use of sunblock—ultraviolet light may exacerbate lesions (PF and PE).

MEDICATIONS

DRUG(S) OF CHOICE

PF

Corticosteroids—Dogs

• Prednisone or prednisolone 2 mg/kg/day PO divided q12h to initiate control. An attempt to reduce this dose should be made when the disease undergoes remission. • Minimum maintenance—0.5 mg/kg PO q48h to twice weekly. • High pulse therapy—10 mg/kg once daily for 3 consecutive days, followed by standard dosage (<2 mg/kg/day). Pulses can be repeated if new lesions continue to appear in spite of the lower doses. Pulse should not be repeated more than once weekly.

Corticosteroids—Cats

• Prednisolone—2 mg/kg/day until clinical resolution. Majority of cats achieve disease control with corticosteroids monotherapy.

P

Cytotoxic Agents

• Most patients require additional immunomodulating drugs. • Work synergistically with corticosteroids to allow reduction in dose and side effects. • Azathioprine 1.5–2.5 mg/kg PO q24h, then q48h. Recommended for canine cases that fail to achieve adequate control with glucocorticoids alone (dogs only; potential for marked bone marrow suppression in cats). • Chlorambucil 0.1–0.2 mg/kg every other day; best option for cats with disease control that is not achieved with corticosteroid monotherapy. • Cyclosporine 5–10 mg/kg PO q24h; variable efficacy in dogs and cats. • Mycophenolate mofetil 10–20 mg/kg twice daily.

PE

• Oral prednisone or prednisolone 1.1 mg/kg PO q24h; then q48h; then to the lowest maintenance dose possible; may be stopped when in remission. • Topical steroids may be sufficient in mild cases. • Topical tacrolimus.

PV

• Aggressive therapy with corticosteroids and azathioprine or chlorambucil + systemic antibiotic therapy.

PP

• Aggressive therapy with corticosteroids and azathioprine or chlorambucil + systemic antibiotic therapy. • Identification and treatment or removal of underlying neoplasia.

PEP/PVeg

• Treatment similar to PF. • Response more variable; some patients may achieve remission with conservative treatment.

PRECAUTIONS

• Corticosteroids—polyuria, polydipsia, polyphagia, temperament changes, diabetes mellitus, pancreatitis, and hepatotoxicity.
• Azathioprine—pancreatitis, bone marrow suppression. • Cytotoxic drugs—leukopenia, thrombocytopenia, nephrotoxicity, hepatotoxicity, and gastrointestinal upset.
• Immunosuppression—can predispose animal to demodicosis, cutaneous and systemic bacterial and fungal infection.

ALTERNATIVE DRUG(S)

Alternative Corticosteroids

• Use instead of prednisone if undesirable side effects or poor response noted.
• Methylprednisolone 0.8–1.5 mg/kg PO q12h; for patients that tolerate prednisone poorly. • Triamcinolone or dexamethasone 0.2–0.3 mg/kg PO q12h; then 0.05–0.1 mg/kg q48–72h.

Topical Steroids

• Hydrocortisone cream. • Potent topical corticosteroids—0.1% betamethasone valerate, fluocinolone acetonide, or 0.1% triamcinolone; q12h; then q24–48h.

Miscellaneous

• PE cases—doxycycline 5 mg/kg twice daily and niacinamide 500 mg twice daily for dogs >10 kg; 250 mg for dogs <10 kg.

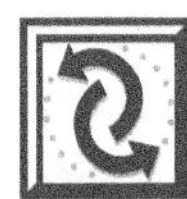

FOLLOW-UP

PATIENT MONITORING

• Monitor response to therapy. • Monitor for medication side effects—routine hematology and serum biochemistry, especially patients on high doses of corticosteroids and cytotoxic drugs; check every 1–3 weeks, then every 1–3 months when in remission.

EXPECTED COURSE AND PROGNOSIS

PV and PF

• Dogs—poor (PV/PP) to fair (PF/PEP): life-long or long-term therapy with corticosteroids and cytotoxic drugs usually needed; good (PE): relatively benign and self-limiting. • Cats—good (PF), but long-term treatment required, tendency to relapse spontaneously or with treatment changes. • Regular monitoring necessary.
• Side effects of medications may affect quality of life. • May be fatal if untreated (especially PV). • Secondary infections cause morbidity and possible mortality (especially PV).

MISCELLANEOUS

PREGNANCY/FERTILITY/BREEDING

Avoid steroids and cytotoxic drugs during pregnancy.

ABBREVIATIONS

• DLE = discoid lupus erythematosus.
• PE = pemphigus erythematosus.
• PEP/PVeg = panepidermal pustular pemphigus/pemphigus vegetans.
• PF = pemphigus foliaceus.
• PP = paraneoplastic pemphigus.
• PV = pemphigus vulgaris.

Suggested Reading

Ackermann AL, May ER, Frank LA. Use of mycophenolate mofetil to treat immune-mediated skin disease in 14 dogs: a retrospective evaluation. Vet Dermatol 2017, 28:195–e44.

Bizikova P, Burrows A. Feline pemphigus foliaceus: original case series and a comprehensive literature review. BMC Vet 2019, 15:22.

Bizikova P, Olivry T. Oral glucocorticoid pulse therapy for induction of treatment of canine pemphigus foliaceus—a comparative study. Vet Dermatol 2015, 26:354–e77.

Helton Rhodes KA, Werner A. Blackwell's Five-Minute Veterinary Consult: Clinical Companion: Small Animal Dermatology, 3rd ed. Hoboken, NJ: Wiley-Blackwell, 2018.

Author Clarissa P. Souza

Consulting Editor Alexander H. Werner Resnick

Acknowledgment The author and editors acknowledge the prior contribution of Karen Helton Rhodes.

Client Education Handout available online

BASICS

OVERVIEW

Chronic inflammatory condition characterized by multiple, painful, progressive, ulcerating sinuses or, less frequently, true fistulous tracts involving the perianal region.

SIGNALMENT

• Dog. • German shepherd dogs primarily; Irish setters. • Mean age 5–7 years; range 7 months–14 years. • Males more commonly affected.

SIGNS

• Dyschezia. • Tenesmus. • Hematochezia. • Constipation. • Diarrhea. • Malodorous mucopurulent anal discharge. • Ulceration of the perianal skin with sinus tract formation. • Licking and self-mutilation. • Reluctance to sit; posturing difficulties; personality changes. • Pain on manipulation of tail and examination of perianal area. • Fecal incontinence. • Anorexia. • Weight loss.

CAUSES & RISK FACTORS

• Multifactorial immune-mediated mechanism is suspected. • Appears to be an inappropriate T-cell mediated response. • An association with colitis has also been proposed, particularly in German shepherd dogs. • A genetic predisposition has been proposed but not proven. • Low tail carriage and a broad-based tail may contribute in German shepherd dogs. • High density of apocrine sweat glands in the cutaneous zone of the anal canal of German shepherd dogs.

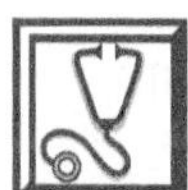

DIAGNOSIS

DIFFERENTIAL DIAGNOSIS

• Other inflammatory processes—e.g., anusitis, hydradenitis suppurativa. • Chronic anal sac abscess. • Perianal adenoma or adenocarcinoma with ulceration and drainage. • Squamous cell carcinoma. • Atypical bacterial infection. • Oomycosis. • Rectal fistula.

CBC/BIOCHEMISTRY/URINALYSIS

• Usually unremarkable. • May have an inflammatory leukogram.

DIAGNOSTIC PROCEDURES

• Presumptive diagnosis—clinical signs and physical examination. • Definitive diagnosis—biopsy of the affected area. • Colonoscopy with biopsy—may reveal associated colitis.

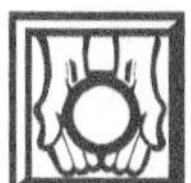

TREATMENT

• Outpatient medical therapy recommended initially in all cases. • Clipping and cleaning the perianal area facilitates local therapy. • Bathing with an antimicrobial shampoo may be helpful. • Dietary modification—strictly enforced hydrolyzed or novel protein elimination diet. • Stool softeners—with pain or tenesmus. • Surgery is considered for patients with incomplete resolution following appropriate medical therapy. • Anal sacculectomy—if anal sac involvement. • Surgical options—resection of inflammatory tissue and/or ablation of remaining sinuses with carbon dioxide laser is preferred. • Surgical debridement (deroofing) with fulguration by chemical cautery or electrocautery; surgical resection followed by primary closure or second intention healing are other options. • Radical excision of the rectal ring with modified rectal pull-through is rarely necessary and is associated with a higher risk of fecal incontinence.

MEDICATIONS

DRUG(S) OF CHOICE

• Cyclosporine (CsA) ± ketoconazole is treatment of choice but is expensive. Ketaconazole reduces dose of cyclosporine required by inhibiting CsA-metabolizing enzymes: ○ Give CsA orally at 1–5 mg/kg/day PO and ketoconazole at 5–10 mg/kg/day PO and then taper CsA as clinical signs resolve. ○ Continue treatment at least 4 weeks after complete resolution of fistula(e). Many patients require chronic treatment at reduced frequency to prevent recurrence. • Tacrolimus (0.1% ointment) topically as maintenance therapy may be sufficient to control lesions; begin application as dose of oral medications is reduced: ○ Apply q12h with gloved hand, then taper to q24–72h. • Oral prednisone and topical tacrolimus appears to be efficacious and economical in less severe cases: ○ Prednisone 2 mg/kg PO q24h for 2 weeks, decrease to 1 mg/kg q24h for 4 weeks and then 1 mg/kg q48h for 10 weeks. ○ Tacrolimus 0.1% ointment as above. ○ Chronic maintenance therapy with tacrolimus and possibly prednisone likely necessary for long-term control. • Azathioprine alone or combined with prednisone is another treatment option.

ALTERNATIVE DRUG(S)

• Analgesics may be necessary. • Metronidazole 10 mg/kg q12h for 2 weeks at initiation of therapy to control secondary infection.

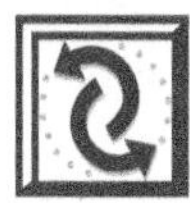

FOLLOW-UP

PATIENT MONITORING

• Assess CsA trough levels if improvement is not seen or if toxicity is suspected. • Reexamine to assess healing, signs of recurrence, and associated complications.

POSSIBLE COMPLICATIONS

• Reversible alopecia. • Vomiting, diarrhea, anorexia. • Weight loss. • Recurrence. • Failure to heal. • Surgical dehiscence. • Tenesmus. • Fecal incontinence. • Anal stricture. • Flatulence. • Iatrogenic Cushing's disease from corticosteroids. • Gingival hyperplasia from CsA.

EXPECTED COURSE AND PROGNOSIS

• Guarded for complete resolution except in mildly affected patients. • Chronic treatment may be necessary.

MISCELLANEOUS

ASSOCIATED CONDITIONS

• Colitis.
• Constipation and/or obstipation may develop.

ABBREVIATIONS

• CsA = cyclosporine.

Suggested Reading

Fallipowicz D. Nonsurgical management of perianal fistulae. In: Bojrab MJ, Waldron D, Tombs JR, eds., Currrent Techniques in Small Animal Surgery, 5th ed. Jackson, KY: Teton Newmedia, 2014, pp. 309–315.

Pieper J, McKay L. Perianal fistulas. Compend Contin Educ Vet 2011, 33(9):E4.

Author Eric R. Pope
Consulting Editor Mark P. Rondeau

P

PERICARDIAL DISEASE

BASICS

DEFINITION

Pericardial diseases include pericardial effusion (PE), constrictive pericardial disease, and space-occupying entities in the pericardial space. PE can be defined as an abnormally high volume of fluid within the pericardial sac; cardiac tamponade refers to the clinical syndrome that results from reduced cardiac output due to mechanical compression of the heart. Constrictive pericardial disease results when a markedly thickened and fibrotic pericardium limits the diastolic filling of the heart. Examples of space-occupying pericardial disease can include large masses in the pericardial space and peritoneopericardial diaphragmatic hernia (PPDH).

PATHOPHYSIOLOGY

- All pericardial diseases cause diastolic dysfunction, resulting in elevation and equalization of ventricular and venous pressures and reduced cardiac output.
- Accumulation of effusion exceeds the elastic capabilities of the pericardial sac, resulting in elevated intrapericardial pressure. Cardiac tamponade occurs when intrapericardial pressure exceeds cardiac diastolic filling pressures. The compliant right atrium and right ventricle normally have the lowest filling pressures and are thus predominantly affected. Cardiac tamponade is present when intrapericardial pressures exceed the central venous pressure. The resultant reduction in cardiac venous return diminishes cardiac output. Animals with acute effusions typically exhibit signs of weakness or collapse. If intrapericardial pressure exceeds central venous pressure continuously for more than a few minutes, death occurs.
- Constrictive pericardial disease directly restricts diastolic filling, causes dissociation of intracardiac and intrathoracic pressures and increases interventricular interdependence.
- In animals with chronic pericardial disease, low cardiac output activates compensatory mechanisms that lead to fluid accumulation, typically manifested as right-sided congestive heart failure (CHF).

SYSTEMS AFFECTED

- Cardiovascular—signs of low cardiac output and CHF.
- Hepatobiliary—chronic passive congestion with mildly to moderately high liver enzymes.
- Renal/urologic—prerenal azotemia.
- Respiratory—tachypnea or pleural effusion.
- Gastrointestinal—vomiting seen in some cases.

GENETICS

N/A

INCIDENCE/PREVALENCE

Pericardial disorders comprise approximately 4–8% of the canine cardiology caseload at referral institutions.

GEOGRAPHIC DISTRIBUTION

Worldwide distribution; increased incidence of coccidioidomycosis-induced effusive constrictive pericarditis in the southwestern United States, Mexico, and Central and South America.

SIGNALMENT

Species

Dog; PE in cat is often secondary to CHF.

Breed Predilections

- Golden retrievers and German shepherd dogs are predisposed to both right atrial hemangiosarcoma (HSA) and idiopathic effusion.
- Brachycephalic breeds are predisposed to aortic body tumors (chemodectoma common in Boston terrier, boxer and bulldogs).
- Idiopathic hemorrhagic pericarditis is more common in young to middle-aged, large-breed dogs (e.g., Great Pyrenees, Great Dane, Saint Bernard, golden retriever).

Mean Age and Range

Middle-aged to older dogs.

Predominant Sex

Male dogs may be predisposed to idiopathic effusion.

SIGNS

General Comments

Chronic PE often causes jugular distension and ascites without a murmur. Acute cardiac tamponade often results in collapse and signs of low cardiac output.

Historical Findings

- Lethargy.
- Anorexia.
- Weakness.
- Exercise intolerance.
- Abdominal distension.
- Respiratory distress; occasionally cough.
- Syncope or collapse.
- Vomiting.

Physical Examination Findings

- Jugular vein distension.
- Ascites (especially with chronic effusion).
- Muffled heart sounds.
- Weak arterial pulses.
- Pulsus paradoxus.
- Pallor or slow capillary refill time.
- Tachypnea and/or tachycardia.

CAUSES

- Neoplasia—HSA, heart base tumor, thyroid adenoma/carcinoma, mesothelioma, metastatic neoplasia, and lymphosarcoma (LSA) (especially cats).
- Idiopathic—pericarditis (benign hemorrhagic effusion vs. effusive constrictive pericarditis with pericardial fibrosis).
- Coagulopathy—anticoagulant rodenticide toxicity, other coagulopathies.
- CHF (especially cats).
- Infection—feline infectious peritonitis (FIP), coccidioidomycosis, bacterial pericarditis.
- Congenital disorders—PPDH, intrapericardial cysts.
- Left atrial tear or cardiac trauma.
- Pericardial foreign body.

RISK FACTORS

- Cardiac neoplasia.
- Advanced myxomatous mitral valve disease.
- Coagulopathy.

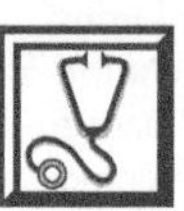

DIAGNOSIS

DIFFERENTIAL DIAGNOSIS

- CHF secondary to other causes (e.g., valvular disease, cardiomyopathy, congenital heart disease such as tricuspid valve dysplasia, myocarditis), hepatic failure, abdominal neoplasia with hemorrhage, protein-losing nephropathy or enteropathy, Budd–Chiari-like syndrome.
- Other causes of ascites (e.g., hepatic failure, hypoproteinemia, intraabdominal neoplasia, and hemorrhage)—characteristically result in remarkable abnormalities on CBC and biochemistry profile, with a lack of jugular venous distension.
- Other causes of collapse and shock with low cardiac output signs such as sepsis, trauma, cardiac arrhythmias, blood loss and tension pneumothorax.

CBC/BIOCHEMISTRY/URINALYSIS

- CBC—usually normal; anemia possible with HSA, LSA, or coagulopathy; red cell morphology may be abnormal; may see thrombocytopenia with neoplasia or disseminated intravascular coagulation (DIC).
- Biochemistry profile—often normal; may see mild to moderately elevated liver enzymes (hepatic congestion), mild azotemia (typically prerenal), hypoproteinemia, and mild electrolyte abnormalities (e.g., hyponatremia, hypochloremia, and hyperkalemia).
- Urinalysis—usually normal unless diuretics administered.

OTHER LABORATORY TESTS

- Elevated serum cardiac troponin I demonstrated in dogs with PE, especially with HSA.
- Clotting times (e.g., activated partial thromboplastin time and one-stage prothrombin time)—prolonged with anticoagulant rodenticide toxicity or DIC.

• Pericardial fluid analysis, although limited in diagnostic sensitivity and specificity, may be helpful in identifying certain neoplastic etiologies (e.g., LSA) or infectious causes.
• FIP testing or feline leukemia virus testing may be useful in cats.

IMAGING

Thoracic Radiography

• Mild-to-severe cardiomegaly; cardiac silhouette often globoid with very sharp edges most evident on the dorsoventral view due to lack of cardiac motion artifact. Cardiac size sometimes normal.
• Pleural effusion in some patients.
• Ascites in many patients.
• Large caudal vena cava in some patients.
• May see nodular pulmonary infiltrates with metastatic neoplasia.

Echocardiography

• Ideally prior to pericardiocentesis in stable patients to facilitate detection of intrapericardial masses.
• Superior diagnostic test to diagnose PE and evaluate for a cardiac mass (depends on operator skill); only moderate accuracy in predicting histopathologic diagnosis of masses.
• Echo-free space between the parietal pericardium and the epicardium.
• Often demonstrates the cause of PE in patients with neoplasia (e.g. right atrial HSA or heart base tumor) or PPDH.
• Left atrial rupture suspected based on concurrent findings of PE and advanced chronic valvular disease, especially if an intra-atrial or intra-pericardial thrombus is visualized.
• Diastolic collapse of the right atrium or ventricle indicates cardiac tamponade.

Advanced Imaging

Cardiac MRI has not been found to be superior to echocardiography in detecting cardiac neoplasia to date; CT may be helpful in detecting pulmonary, hepatic, or splenic metastases.

DIAGNOSTIC PROCEDURES

ECG

• Often sinus tachycardia; occasionally ventricular or supraventricular arrhythmias.
• May see low-voltage QRS complexes (<0.9 mV in leads I, II, III, aVR, aVL, and aVF).
• May see ST segment elevation in leads II, aVF, V3.
• May see electrical alternans, a regular (1:1 or 2:1) variation in QRS-T wave height or morphology, due to swinging of the heart within the pericardial sac.

Pericardial Fluid Analysis

Cytology of PE cannot reliably differentiate the common neoplastic (e.g., HSA, chemodectoma, mesothelioma) and idiopathic causes of effusion. Cytology can identify or rule out some potential causes of effusion (e.g., LSA, FIP, sepsis). If an infectious agent is suspected, aerobic and anaerobic cultures of the effusion are indicated.

PATHOLOGIC FINDINGS

• Vary based on the underlying cause of pericardial disease.
• Small masses may be identified that were not visible on antemortem testing.
• Dogs with left atrial tears will have advanced mitral degeneration with thickened and irregular mitral and/or tricuspid valve leaflets, left atrial enlargement and endocardial jet lesions, and possible ruptured chordae tendineae.
• Mesothelioma can be difficult to differentiate from idiopathic pericardial disease in some dogs, even with histopathology.

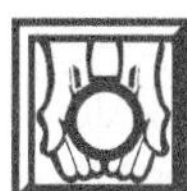

TREATMENT

APPROPRIATE HEALTH CARE

Cardiac tamponade warrants immediate pericardiocentesis. Repeated pericardiocentesis may be needed; surgery may be indicated in selected dogs. Pericardiocentesis is rarely required in the cat.

Pericardiocentesis

• Sedation with low-dose narcotic may be appropriate, except if moribund. Patient may be placed in sternal or lateral recumbency. Clip haircoat on the right or left thorax between the 3rd and 8th intercostal spaces from above the costochondral junction ventrally to the sternum. Simultaneous ECG and/or echocardiographic monitoring is ideal to confirm the presence of the catheter tip in the pericardium and detect arrhythmias caused by the catheter contacting the heart. If echocardiography is not available, perform pericardiocentesis at the 5th intercostal space (at the palpable apex beat) below the costochondral junction. Following aseptic skin preparation and local anesthetic block of the skin, subcutaneous tissues and pleura with lidocaine, advance a long, large-bore (~14–18 gauge), preferably fenestrated, over-the-needle catheter into the pericardial sac. In dogs, PE is usually hemorrhagic, but some patients have a serous, serosanguinous, or purulent effusion. If echocardiography is available, removal and reinjection of approximately 1 mL of pericardial fluid causes visible spontaneous echo contrast to appear in the pericardial space, confirming catheter placement. Remove as much effusion as possible (unless active bleeding is suspected). If ventricular arrhythmias develop, reposition the catheter and be prepared to administer IV lidocaine.
• Unless the patient has active hemorrhage into the pericardial sac, the effusion obtained by pericardiocentesis should not clot, and should have a packed cell volume that differs from that of peripheral blood. The supernatant of chronic effusions is often xanthochromic.

NURSING CARE

Unless there is marked dehydration, fluids are generally not required or recommended for chronic PE. Mild volume expansion may be useful in some animals with acute PE and signs of cardiovascular collapse. Administer oxygen if tachypneic or signs of hemodynamic instability.

ACTIVITY

Cage rest for animals with cardiac tamponade, followed by exercise restriction after pericardiocentesis.

DIET

N/A

CLIENT EDUCATION

Inform that PE is typically recurrent in nature, though prognosis may vary greatly depending on the underlying cause. Educate about the importance for close monitoring for recurrent effusion and warn of the potential for sudden death.

SURGICAL CONSIDERATIONS

• Pericardiectomy may be useful in the treatment of recurrent cardiac tamponade for PE accompanying heart base tumors and prolongs survival; this may also be considered for palliation of right atrial HSA but whether it has any impact on survival is unknown.
• Idiopathic PE may respond to pericardiocentesis; pericardiectomy is indicated for recurrent effusion.
• Infectious pericarditis due to bacterial cause, and pericardial foreign bodies, is usually best treated surgically to avoid subsequent constrictive pericardial disease.
• Right auricular appendage masses may be treated surgically but resection alone without adjuvant chemotherapy is unlikely to significantly prolong survival.
• Thoracoscopy allows for partial pericardiectomy with reduced risk and reduced postoperative pain. However some surgeons believe that extensive pericardiectomy is preferred in cases of benign PE to avoid the possibility of recurrent pleural effusion.
• Constrictive pericardial disease is usually best treated surgically.
• PPDH is treated surgically when clinical signs referable to the defect are clearly present; the diagnosis is sometimes established incidentally and the need for surgery is uncertain.
• Radiation therapy may also play a role in management of pericardial disease due to certain neoplastic causes, although concerns exist about the development of radiation-induced cardiac injury or cardiac arrhythmias.

PERICARDIAL DISEASE (CONTINUED)

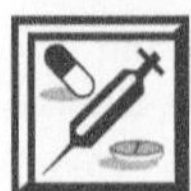

MEDICATIONS

DRUG(S) OF CHOICE

- Drugs should not be used in place of pericardiocentesis.
- Vitamin K—indicated for patients with anticoagulant rodenticide intoxication.
- Appropriate antibiotics or antifungals are indicated with infectious pericarditis.
- Chemotherapy—may be useful to treat effusion caused by LSA; partially effective in the treatment of atrial HSA and generally ineffective for heart-base tumor; adjuvant doxorubicin-based chemotherapy following right atrial mass resection has been shown to increase survival times but dogs rarely survive more than 6 months postoperatively.
- In a double blind, randomized study in dogs with splenic HSA, a mushroom extract delayed the progression of metastases and afforded the longest survival times reported in canine HSA.
- Some clinicians use antifibrinolytic drug (aminocaproic or tranexamic acid) or other possible clot-stabilizing drugs (Yunnan Baiyao) in an attempt to reduce recurrent bleeding, although the efficacy of these compounds is uncertain.

CONTRAINDICATIONS

Diuretics may worsen tamponade by reducing circulating blood volume, and hence intracardiac pressures, and can lead to progressive azotemia, patient weakness and collapse. Digitalis, vasodilators, and angiotensin-converting enzyme inhibitors are reported to be relatively or absolutely contraindicated. Corticosteroids or other immunosuppressive drugs may exacerbate infection, if present.

PRECAUTIONS

N/A

ALTERNATIVE DRUG(S)

- Intracavitary chemotherapy may be attempted to treat mesothelioma, especially in cases with recurrent pleural effusion after pericardiectomy.
- Anti-inflammatory, immunosuppressive, or antifibrotic strategies have been tried in dogs with idiopathic PE (e.g., corticosteroids, nonsteroidal anti-inflammatory drugs, azothiaprine, or colchicine); efficacy of these strategies for preventing recurrent effusion is unknown.

FOLLOW-UP

PATIENT MONITORING

PE may recur at any stage; examination and echocardiography at 10–14 days and every 2–4 months recommended to detect recurrent idiopathic PE.

POSSIBLE COMPLICATIONS

- Hypotension or shock.
- Pneumothorax, arrhythmias, and myocardial perforation or coronary laceration secondary to pericardiocentesis.

EXPECTED COURSE AND PROGNOSIS

- Right atrial HSA—poor; tumor is highly malignant, usually not resectable at the time of diagnosis; may respond transiently to doxorubicin-based chemotherapy; the benefit of palliative pericardiectomy is unproven.
- Chemodectoma—fair; slow-growing tumor, late to metastasize; pericardiectomy often resolves clinical signs; may respond to chemotherapy or radiation therapy; survival of up to 3 years has been reported following pericardiectomy alone. Large masses sometimes cause compression of cardiovascular structures that might be resolved with IV stent placement.
- Prognosis is good with idiopathic PE; approximately 50% of cases resolve after one or two pericardiocenteses; pericardiectomy is often curative in persistent cases, although recurrent pleural effusion is seen in some dogs after surgery.

MISCELLANEOUS

ASSOCIATED CONDITIONS

Splenic HSA.

AGE-RELATED FACTORS

- Idiopathic PE may be more common in middle-aged to elderly dogs.
- HSA and heart-base tumors more common in elderly dogs.

ZOONOTIC POTENTIAL

Coccidioidomycosis

SYNONYMS

- Cardiac tamponade.
- Pericardial tamponade.
- Pericarditis.

SEE ALSO

- Atrial Wall Tear.
- Chemodectoma.
- Coccidioidomycosis.
- Feline Infectious Peritonitis (FIP).
- Hemangiosarcoma, Heart.
- Myocardial Tumors.
- Rodenticide Toxicosis—Anticoagulants.

ABBREVIATIONS

- CHF = congestive heart failure.
- DIC = disseminated intravascular coagulation.
- ECG = electrocardiogram.
- FIP = feline infectious peritonitis.
- HSA = hemangiosarcoma.
- LSA = lymphosarcoma.
- PE = pericardial effusion.
- PPDH = peritoneopericardial diaphragmatic hernia.

Suggested Reading

Brown DC, Reetz J. Single agent polysaccharopeptide delays metastases and improves survival in naturally occurring hemangiosarcoma. Evid Based Complement Alternat Med 2012, 2012:384301.

Coleman AE, Rapoport GS. Pericardial disorders and cardiac tumors. In: Smith FWK, Tilley LP, Oyama MA, Sleeper MM, eds., Manual of Canine and Feline Cardiology, 5th ed. St. Louis, MO: Saunders Elsevier, 2016, pp. 198–217.

Nelson OL, Ware WA. Pericardial effusion. In: Bonagura JD, Twedt DC, eds., Kirk's Current Veterinary Therapy XV. St. Louis, MO: Saunders Elsevier, 2014, pp. 816–823.

Authors John E. Rush and Bruce W. Keene
Consulting Editor Michael Aherne

Client Education Handout available online

P

PERINEAL HERNIA

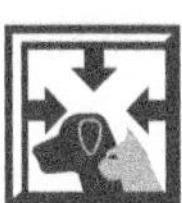

BASICS

OVERVIEW

- Perineal hernia (PH) refers to a spectrum of disorders in which the pelvic diaphragm is weakened, with rupture or atrophy of the muscles. Rectal sacculation and dilation often occur. This results in abnormal function during defecation and, if left untreated, leads to herniation of pelvic and abdominal viscera.
- Weakening of the pelvic diaphragm in male dogs is postulated to result from hormonal influences and by increased pressure secondary to enlargement of the prostate.
- Separation of the perineal muscles (levator ani and coccygeus) from the external anal sphincter (EAS) and rectum allows lateral and ventral bulging and sacculation of the rectum when caudal abdominal pressure increases during defecation. Feces become entrapped within the sacculated rectum, contributing to the uncoordinated defecation often presented in patients with PH. Separation and weakening of the muscles also allows pelvic and abdominal viscera to migrate caudally, enter the hernia sac, and eventually become incarcerated or strangulated.

SIGNALMENT

Intact male dogs are at highest risk. The disease occurs rarely in castrated male dogs, female dogs, and cats.

SIGNS

- Constipation is the main feature, although some patients present with diarrhea as looser stool escapes around the firmer stool.
- Unilateral or bilateral perineal bulge due to fecal impaction and/or herniation:
  - May be dynamic or static.
  - May become more obvious during events of increased intra-abdominal pressure—barking, coughing, defecation, and urination.
  - Often the only presenting sign in cats.
- Straining to urinate if bladder incarceration occurs.

CAUSES & RISK FACTORS

- Intact status in older male dogs and male dogs with unilateral or bilateral cryptorchidism.
- Underlying pathology leading to excessive straining:
  - Prostatomegaly in male dogs.
  - Megacolon and malunion of pelvic fractures in cats.
- Caudal neuropathy, malformation or injury such as tail traction or avulsion.
- Trauma (rare).

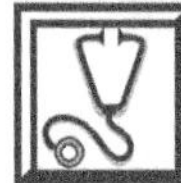

DIAGNOSIS

DIFFERENTIAL DIAGNOSIS

- Other causes of straining during defecation or urination include perineal or intrapelvic mass:
  - Neoplasia (adenoma, lipoma, adenocarcinoma, sarcoma).
  - Sublumbar lymphadenomegaly secondary to anal sac adenocarcinoma.
  - Rectal tumor.
  - Paraprostatic cyst or abscess.
  - Perineal abscess (e.g., anal sac).

CBC/BIOCHEMISTRY/URINALYSIS

No specific abnormalities. Azotemia if urinary obstruction occurs.

OTHER LABORATORY TESTS

N/A

IMAGING

- Abdominal radiography—evaluate constipation or obstipation, prostatomegaly, sublumbar lymphadenomegaly, location of urinary bladder and prostate, and megacolon in cats.
- Pelvic radiography—evaluate pelvic fracture malunion, intrapelvic mass, caudal displacement of the prostate and bladder, entrapment of bladder or bowel in hernia.
- Abdominal ultrasonography—evaluate the size and consistency of the prostate, location of urinary bladder and prostate, intrapelvic or caudal abdominal masses, sublumbar lymphadenomegaly, presence of abdominal cryptorchid testicle.
- Perineal ultrasonography—evaluate presence of abdominal viscera or masses.

DIAGNOSTIC PROCEDURES

- Visual perianal examination:
  - Normally the anus and EAS are held in position dorsal and slightly cranial to the caudal extent of the tuber ischii.
  - When the perineal diaphragm is weakened, the anus migrates caudally. May be severe in bilateral PH.
  - Eliciting a cough reflex by gentle tracheal palpation will increase intra-abdominal pressure and aid evaluation of the position and movement of the anus.
- Rectal examination:
  - Confirm accumulation of feces in the dilated and sacculated rectum and perineal laxity.
  - If the integrity of the pelvic diaphragm has been compromised, it will be possible to pinch the rectal mucosa and skin together between the tip of the forefinger and thumb without palpating a muscle shelf in between.
  - Evaluate both sides; bilateral PH is common especially in intact male dogs.
- Endoscopy or percutaneous fine-needle aspiration biopsy may be indicated if a mass lesion is present extra- or intraluminally.

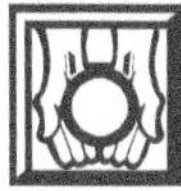

TREATMENT

- Surgical management required for definitive treatment:
  - Emergency if bladder retroflexion and entrapment, or intestinal entrapment have occurred.
- Conservative treatment may temporarily ameliorate clinical signs:
  - Low residue diet.
  - Stool softeners.

Nursing Care

- IV fluid therapy in the pre- and post-operative period.
- Incisional icing postoperatively.
- Elizabethan collar postoperatively.

Activity

Restrict for at least 3–4 weeks following surgical repair.

Diet

- Low-residue canned diet:
  - Part of conservative medical management.
  - Postoperatively.

Client Education

N/A

Surgical Considerations

- Castration of male dogs should always be performed simultaneously with herniorrhaphy, due to the high rate of recurrence in intact dogs regardless of surgical technique used.
- In patients with bladder retroflexion and entrapment, the urethra should be catheterized, and the bladder decompressed if possible:
  - Percutaneous perineal cystocentesis may be required to decompress and reposition the bladder before a urethral catheter can be passed.
  - If the bladder is able to be decompressed, correction of biochemical abnormalities is preferred prior to anesthesia and surgery in the urinary obstruction patient with PH.
- Prior to surgical correction, the author prefers the use of an epidural with local anesthetic and/or morphine.
- Impacted feces should be gently removed from the rectum prior to surgery:
  - Enemas are not recommended as liquid feces may not be completely evacuated, leading to excessive contamination during surgery and postoperatively.
- Primary repair of the weakened muscles alone often leads to recurrence and is not recommended as the only form of repair.
- The internal obturator muscle flap is the preferred local method of repair combined with primary bolstering of the perineal musculature. The author prefers to repair both sides of the pelvic diaphragm regardless of the unilateral nature of the hernia.
- It may be helpful in large dogs with large bilateral hernias, especially if bladder

retroflexion or visceral entrapment, to perform exploratory laparotomy, reposition the bladder and rectum, and perform incisional colopexy and cystopexy:
  - Herniorrhaphy can be performed at a later time (2–7 days), when the patient's condition has stabilized and the perineal edema has resolved.
  - In patients with poor perineal muscle development and in patients with large defects, the repair is often bolstered with the use of secondary local muscle flaps.
  - Absorbable and nonabsorbable mesh implants are needed in some severe cases.
  - A superficial gluteal muscle flap is recommended in cats and very small dogs to bolster the internal obturator muscle flap and primary repair techniques.

MEDICATIONS

DRUG(S) OF CHOICE

- Stool softeners may be considered as a component of conservative medical management or prior to surgery:
  - Lactulose 0.5–1 mL/kg PO q8–12h, adjusted to effect.
  - PEG 3350 (MiraLax®) ¼–1 tsp on food q12h, adjusted to effect.
  - Goal is 2–3 soft-formed stools per day.
- Intraoperative antibiotics may be given, but there is no indication to continue antibiotic treatment postoperatively unless significant contamination occurs during surgery.

P

CONTRAINDICATIONS/POSSIBLE INTERACTIONS

Avoid stool softeners postoperatively, as they may lead to diarrhea and fecal soiling in the first days after surgery, especially if a bilateral repair has been performed.

FOLLOW-UP

PATIENT MONITORING

- The patient should be evaluated frequently for the first 48 hours following surgery, with particular attention paid to urination and defecation regardless if bladder entrapment was present preoperatively.
- A rectal examination should be performed at the time of suture removal (10–14 days) if feasible.

PREVENTION/AVOIDANCE

- Castration.
- Address conditions causing straining during defecation and urination, if present.

POSSIBLE COMPLICATIONS

- Constipation, obstipation, and bladder retroflexion/obstruction, visceral entrapment, and strangulation.
- Postoperative complications include recurrence (greatly reduced by castration and use of internal obturator flap), and temporary or permanent dysfunction of the anal sphincter due to stretching following bilateral herniorrhaphy:
  - Fecal and urinary incontinence can occur if excessive dissection around the pudendal nerve, caudal rectal nerve, or peritoneal reflections are performed.

EXPECTED COURSE AND PROGNOSIS

- Excellent with surgery.
- There is a 10–50% risk of recurrence depending on presence of underlying conditions, surgical technique, and reproductive status of the dog.

MISCELLANEOUS

ASSOCIATED CONDITIONS

Primary conditions causing excessive straining (e.g., megacolon in cats).

ABBREVIATIONS

- EAS = external anal sphincter.
- PH = perineal hernia.

Suggested Reading

Gill SS, Barstad RD. A review of the surgical management of perineal hernias in dogs. J Am Anim Hosp Assoc 2018, 4:179–187.

Mann F. Serum testosterone and estradiol 17-beta concentrations in 15 dogs with perineal hernia. J Am Vet Med Assoc 1989, 194:1578–1580.

Souza CH, Mann T. Perineal hernias. In: Monnet E, ed., Small Animal Soft Tissue Surgery. Hoboken, NJ: Wiley Blackwell, 2013, pp. 286–296.

Szabo S, Wilkens B, Radasch, RM. Use of polypropylene mesh in addition to obturator transposition: a review of 59 cases (2000–2004). J Am Anim Hosp Assoc 2007, 43:136–142.

Author Stephen Mehler
Consulting Editor Mark P. Rondeau

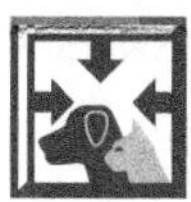

BASICS

DEFINITION

Inflammation and destruction of the periodontium (i.e., gingiva, cementum, periodontal ligament, and alveolar bone) secondary to the subgingival biofilm of bacteria.

PATHOPHYSIOLOGY

A pellicle of salivary glycoproteins adheres to the clean tooth and first colonizing Gram-positive aerobic bacteria attach; the plaque biofilm is created. The supragingival plaque biofilm matures and influences the development of the subgingival biofilm. The constituents of the biofilm progress to Gram-negative anaerobic, motile, and spirochete bacteria. Bacterial byproducts and proteolytic enzymes with the host inflammatory response cause destruction of the periodontium, resulting in the loss of attachment for the tooth. The biofilm forms within days. Calculus is the mineralization of plaque. It is rough, acts a surface area for more plaque development, and can be mechanically irritating to the tissues.

SYSTEMS AFFECTED

Gastrointestinal—oral cavity/dentition (primary); systemic inflammation/distant organ changes.

GENETICS

N/A

INCIDENCE/PREVALENCE

Common—estimated to be around 85%.

GEOGRAPHIC DISTRIBUTION

Worldwide

SIGNALMENT

Species

Dog and cat.

Breed Predilections

Toy, brachycephalic, sighthounds, long-facial haired, and purebred cats.

Mean Age and Range

Begins as juvenile and progresses through life.

Predominant Sex

None

SIGNS

Historical Findings

Hidden/no clinical signs to halitosis, head shyness, oral bleeding, dropping food, reluctance to chew, pawing at the mouth, exaggerated jaw movements, face rubbing, maxillofacial swellings, ptyalism, sneezing, and nasal discharge.

Physical Examination Findings

• Conscious examination—inflammation of the gingiva, plaque and/or calculus, root exposure, furcation exposure, mobile teeth, parulides, disproportionate plaque and calculus distribution, oral discharge, maxillofacial swellings, and mandibular lymphadenopathy. The conscious examination significantly underestimates the presence and severity of PD and therefore an anesthetized examination with periodontal probing and intraoral radiographs is required for complete assessment. • Anesthetized examination—the degree of severity of periodontal disease relates to a single tooth. • American Veterinary Dental College (AVDC) nomenclature: ◦ Normal (PD 0)—clinically normal; no gingival inflammation or periodontitis clinically evident. ◦ Stage 1 (PD 1)—gingivitis only without attachment loss. The height and architecture of the alveolar margin are normal. ◦ Stage 2 (PD 2)—early periodontitis; less than 25% of attachment loss,* or at most, there is a Stage 1 furcation involvement in multirooted teeth. ◦ Stage 3 (PD 3)—moderate periodontitis; 25–50% of attachment loss*, and/or there is a Stage 2 furcation involvement in multirooted teeth. ◦ Stage 4 (PD 4)—advanced periodontitis; more than 50% of attachment loss* or there is a Stage 3 furcation involvement in multirooted teeth. Furcation indices subjectively measure when the periodontal probe extends less than half way between the roots (F1), extends greater than half way (F2), or through and through from one side of the furcation and out the other under the crown (F3).

*Periodontal attachment loss is measured by probing of the clinical attachment level and radiographic determination of the distance of the alveolar margin from the tooth's cementoenamel junction relative to the length of the root.

CAUSES

Bacterial plaque biofilm and associated host inflammatory response.

RISK FACTORS

Lack of daily preventive home care and professional veterinary dental care, signalment, systemic health (e.g., immunosuppression from pharmaceuticals or metabolic disease), inappropriate chewing behavior, malocclusions, crowding of dentition, oral foreign bodies.

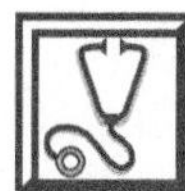

DIAGNOSIS

DIFFERENTIAL DIAGNOSIS

Oral neoplasia, drug-associated gingival enlargement (e.g., cyclosporine, amlodipine), oral autoimmune inflammatory conditions, viral ulcerative gingivitis/mucositis (e.g., calicivirus), oral trauma and foreign bodies, rare fungal. Clinical history, imaging (i.e., intraoral radiographs and/or advanced imaging), and histopathology for differentiation.

CBC/BIOCHEMISTRY/URINALYSIS

Overall systemic/metabolic health status and for preparation for anesthesia.

OTHER LABORATORY TESTS

N/A

IMAGING

• Intraoral radiography—required diagnostic instrument to assess attachment loss, to include marginal bone loss, loss of the lamina dura, widening of the periodontal ligament space, horizontal and vertical bone loss, inflammatory resorption of the tooth root surface, furcation bone loss, combined patterns of bone loss. Horizontal bone loss is a pattern where the cortical and alveolar bone surrounding the tooth and adjacent teeth are lost at a similar rate; the periodontal pocket is above the bone (i.e., suprabony pocket). Vertical bone loss is a pattern where there is bone loss around a tooth root where the adjacent supporting bone remains more coronal; the periodontal pocket is within the bone (i.e., infra(intra) bony pocket).
• Osteopermeative patterns mimicking neoplasia can be present in severe cases. Osteitis secondary to the inflammation may result in paradoxical proliferation of bone.
• Cone-beam CT has been reported to be of additional valuable in assessing periodontal attachment loss in brachycephalic breeds.

DIAGNOSTIC PROCEDURES

• Periodontal probing—the distance between free gingival margin and apical extent of the sulcus or pocket; probing depths <3 mm in dogs and <1 mm in cats are considered normal gingival sulcus; variations based on the range of breed sizes in dogs. • Measurement of root exposure, furcation exposures and tooth mobility are recorded. • Clinical probing information and intraoral radiographic assessment are used to assign periodontal score to each tooth (PD0–PD4).

PATHOLOGIC FINDINGS

Tissues may be edematous, exhibit gingival hyperplasia/enlargement, exocytosis of inflammatory cells such as lymphocytes, plasma cells, and polymorphonuclear leukocytes, abundant colonies of bacterial microorganisms, areas of fibrosis, edema, and hemorrhage; bone may demonstrate infiltration of inflammatory cells, and resorption with both osteoclastic and osteoblastic activity. Osteomyelitis/osteitis can result.

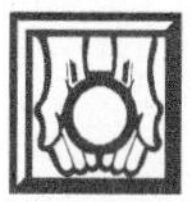

TREATMENT

APPROPRIATE HEALTH CARE

• Prevention of PD with daily home care and annual preventive cleaning, starting in first 1–2 years of life; oral examinations and periodontal treatments before excessive attachment loss. • Daily home care prevention should begin the first year of life. Daily tooth brushing is the best daily home care prevention. • Annual or semi-annual evaluations and periodontal cleanings/"prophylaxis" and treatment based on the patient signalment and progressive PD stage status. • Client communication and education throughout all patient life stages.

NURSING CARE

Acute-on-chronic periodontal abscessation—nonsteroidal anti-inflammatory medications, if not contraindicated; analgesia and appropriate antibiotic selection pending scheduling for anesthesia, assessment, and treatment.

ACTIVITY

No restrictions.

DIET

Dental diets with fiber arrangements and/or added dental products added for patients without other dietary restrictions, or needs, and who have teeth remaining to chew.

CLIENT EDUCATION

Daily home care, the necessity of general anesthesia, and the lifelong prevention, management, and treatment of PD.

SURGICAL CONSIDERATIONS

• Remove the plaque biofilm and calculus, eliminate periodontal pocket(s), prevent further attachment loss, extract hopelessly compromised teeth, address contributing dental factors, and treat oral/dental pain. Individualized general anesthetic management. • Periodontal surgery including, but not limited to, gingivectomy/gingivoplasty, periceutical treatment, closed root planing, open root planing, periodontal flaps, osseous resective surgery, osseous additive surgery including bone augmentation and guided tissue regeneration. Plans are based on PD stage, tooth/teeth involved, overall systemic health of the patient, ability for home care, ability to have further follow-up treatments and anesthetic procedures, and overall financial aspects for the client with the goal to have a pain- and infection-free oral cavity.

MEDICATIONS

DRUG(S) OF CHOICE

Systemic use of antimicrobials is *not* indicated in the treatment of PD without surgical attention to the underlying cause. Clindamycin, amoxicillin/clavulanic acid, and doxycycline may be chosen to augment periodontal surgical treatment. Metronidazole may be selected based on clinical findings and patient history.

CONTRAINDICATIONS

• Immunosuppressive drugs in untreated PD can cause acute-on-chronic exacerbations.
• Chronic use of bisphosphonates should be avoided unless the oral cavity and dentition have all active infection and inflammation treated.

PRECAUTIONS

Prolonged/increased dosages of immunosuppressive medications may contribute to acute on chronic exacerbations.

POSSIBLE INTERACTIONS

Oral chlorhexidine and oral fluoride inactivate with simultaneous use.

ALTERNATIVE DRUG(S)

N/A

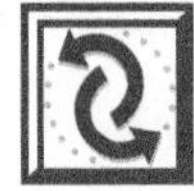

FOLLOW-UP

PATIENT MONITORING

The diagnosed PD stage guides the recheck interval; evaluation every 3–12 months.

PREVENTION/AVOIDANCE

Daily tooth brushing with pet toothpaste mechanically removes the supragingival plaque biofilm. Oral 0.1–0.12% chlorhexidine products target oral bacteria involved in the plaque biofilm. Dental diets, dental chews, barriers sealants, dental wipes, dental enzyme systems, dental gels, and water additives can be a part of a dental home care program based on individual patient and client needs. The Veterinary Oral Health Council can help guide selection of pet dental products.

POSSIBLE COMPLICATIONS

N/A

EXPECTED COURSE AND PROGNOSIS

Due to the multifactorial aspect of PD and individual patient response, the expected course and prognosis can be variable, but predicable with appropriate treatment.

MISCELLANEOUS

ASSOCIATED CONDITIONS

N/A

AGE-RELATED FACTORS

Progresses with age; Adult-onset periodontitis is most common; juvenile and aggressive forms of periodontitis occur.

ZOONOTIC POTENTIAL

Capnocytophaga spp. may cause serious opportunistic infections in immunosuppressed humans; *Pasteurella multocida* may cause severe infections in humans following cat bites. Scientific developments in the study of oral microbiomes suggest transmission/sharing of oral bacteria can occur between species.

PREGNANCY/FERTILITY/BREEDING

N/A

SYNONYMS

N/A

ABBREVIATIONS

• AVDC = American Veterinary Dental College.
• PD = periodontal disease.

INTERNET RESOURCES

• https://avdc.org/avdc-nomenclature/
• http://www.vohc.org

Suggested Reading

Lobprise H, Stepaniuk K. Oral surgery—periodontal surgery. In: Lobprise H, Dodd JR, eds., 'Wiggs' Veterinary Dentistry—Principles and Practice, 2nd ed. Hoboken, NJ: Wiley-Blackwell, 2019, pp. 193–228.

Author Kevin S. Stepaniuk
Consulting Editor Heidi B. Lobprise

Client Education Handout available online

PERIPHERAL EDEMA

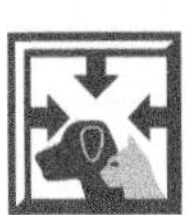

BASICS

DEFINITION

Edema is focal or diffuse excessive accumulation of tissue fluid within the interstitium; often at gravitative surfaces, whether localized or generalized.

PATHOPHYSIOLOGY

- High capillary hydrostatic pressure.
- Increased capillary permeability.
- Lymphatic drainage abnormality. • Low plasma colloid osmotic pressure.

SYSTEMS AFFECTED

- Musculoskeletal. • Skin/exocrine.

GENETICS

- Dominantly inherited primary lymphedema has been described in poodles.
- Lethal congenital edema has been documented in bulldogs.

INCIDENCE/PREVALENCE

Variable

GEOGRAPHIC DISTRIBUTION

Pertinent when considering infectious disease mechanisms.

SIGNALMENT

Species

Dog and cat.

Breed Predilections

Primary or congenital lymphedema has been reported in bulldogs, poodles, Old English sheepdogs, Labradors, and myriad other canine breeds as well as cats.

SIGNS

Historical Findings

- Allergic or other immune, cardiac, hepatic, or other organic disease. • Trauma.
- Exposure to infectious or toxic (venomous) agents such as ticks or other arachnids.

Physical Examination Findings

- Unexplained weight gain may be noted initially; otherwise, early detection is unlikely.
- Noninflammatory subcutaneous edema is often first recognized at the dependent thorax, abdomen, or distal limbs.
- Inflammatory edema may be noted in nondependent foci of the interstitium.

CAUSES

Localized or Single-Limb Edema

- High capillary hydrostatic pressure.
- Venous or arterial obstruction (e.g., thrombosis or postcaval syndrome).
- Arteriovenous fistula. • Increased capillary permeability. • Focal or multifocal immune, infectious, or toxic (chemical or biologic) insults (e.g., snake bite or bee sting).
- Trauma. • Burns. • Lymphatic obstruction.
- Sterile (juvenile pyoderma) or infectious lymphangitis. • Primary or metastatic neoplastic invasion of lymphatic tissue.
- Congenital aplasia or dysgenesis of the lymphatic system.

Regional or Generalized Edema

- High capillary hydrostatic pressure.
- Congestive heart failure (CHF). • Cardiac tamponade. • Cranial or caudal vena caval thrombosis. • Renal failure and hypernatremia (salt retention). • Paralysis or prolonged recumbency with subsequent failure of the venous pump. • Tourniquet effect of a bandage. • Increased capillary permeability.
- Systemic immune, infectious, or toxic insults (e.g., sepsis or vasculitis). • Lymphatic abnormalities. • Acquired regional traumatic, immune, infectious, or neoplastic process.
- Congenital aplasia or other lymphatic dysgenesis. • Low plasma colloid osmotic pressure. • Protein-losing disease (e.g., nephrotic syndrome or intestinal lymphangiectasia). • Failure to produce protein (e.g., cirrhosis). • Exudative protein loss (e.g., severe burn).

RISK FACTORS

Variable

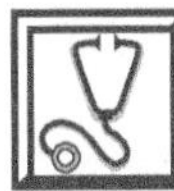

DIAGNOSIS

DIFFERENTIAL DIAGNOSIS

- Peripheral edema secondary to myxedema or inflammation is typically non-pitting.
- Bilateral forelimb edema with jugular venous distention implies cranial vena caval syndrome. • Bilateral rear limb edema with or without ascites implies either hypoalbuminemia or caudal vena caval obstruction. • Fore and/or rear limb edema with jugular venous distension, hydrothorax, and/or ascites implies cardiac disease. • Focal edema with bruit and fremitus implies an arteriovenous fistula. • Focal edema with erythema may be secondary to an insect or other bite. • Multifocal or diffuse edema with petechiation and/or ecchymosis may be associated with a coagulopathy or vasculitis.

CBC/BIOCHEMISTRY/URINALYSIS

- Leukocytosis suggests inflammatory or infectious disease. • Thrombocytopenia may be secondary to vasculitis (e.g., Rocky Mountain spotted fever [RMSF]), systemic lupus erythematosus, or a coagulopathy (e.g., disseminated intravascular coagulation [DIC]). • Panhypoproteinemia is consistent with gastrointestinal disease, but diarrhea is not an obligatory clinical sign.
- Panhypoproteinemia and hypocholesterolemia are seen with intestinal lymphangiectasia.
- Hypoalbuminemia may occur with hepatic failure. • Hypoalbuminemia with proteinuria suggests glomerular disease.
- Hypoalbuminemia with proteinuria and hypercholesterolemia in an edematous patient defines nephrotic syndrome.

OTHER LABORATORY TESTS

- Antithrombin III assay indicated in conditions with albumin loss. • Further delineate thrombocytopenia with a bone marrow biopsy, antinuclear antibody, screen for *Ehrlichia* and RMSF, and a coagulation profile. • Panhypoproteinemia may dictate a need for intestinal biopsy.
- Hypoalbuminemia may warrant liver function testing (e.g., bile acid test, hepatic biopsy). • Confirm proteinuria with a urine protein:creatinine ratio. • Bacterial and fungal cultures of blind fistulae may prove useful. • Fungal or other assays of infectious disease may be warranted; patient's primary residence and patient's travel history need to be considered. • Pleural or peritoneal fluid analysis is suggested, if effusion is present.
- Low resting thyroid hormone (T_4) should be elaborated with a thyrotropin-releasing hormone stimulation test, free T_4 by equilibrium dialysis, or thyroid-stimulating hormone (TSH) concentration.

IMAGING

- Suspected heart disease necessitates thoracic radiographs and/or echocardiogram.
- Angiography (e.g., venacavagram) may help to define a vascular obstruction. • Diagnostic ultrasound may help to delineate a vascular occlusion. • Thermography and perfusion scans (e.g., scintigraphy) are esoteric but have been used to diagnose occlusive vascular disease.

DIAGNOSTIC PROCEDURES

- Fine-needle aspiration of an affected area for cytology and culture may be helpful.
- Biopsy and deep culture may help define an underlying cause for edema.

PATHOLOGIC FINDINGS

Depend on cause of the edema.

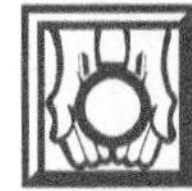

TREATMENT

APPROPRIATE HEALTH CARE

Depends on the cause of the edema and stability of the patient.

NURSING CARE

- Application of warm compresses is recommended for patients with edema secondary to infection. • Good nursing care required to prevent decubital ulceration in recumbent patients.

ACTIVITY

Depends on cause of edema—e.g., exercise restriction is recommended in patients with congestive heart failure.

PERIPHERAL EDEMA

DIET

Depends on the cause of edema—e.g., patients with protein-losing nephropathy require a restricted protein diet.

CLIENT EDUCATION

Depends on the cause of edema.

SURGICAL CONSIDERATIONS

• Surgery such as lymphangioplasty, thrombectomy, or lymphaticovenous shunt may be palliative. • Amputation of the edematous limb is sometimes indicated.
• Arteriovenous fistulae may be treated by various surgical methods.

MEDICATIONS

DRUG(S) OF CHOICE

• Anaphylaxis—epinephrine (1 mg/mL) at 0.01 mL/kg IM or SC to a maximum of 0.02–0.05 mL; prednisone sodium succinate 10–30 mg/kg IV; antihistamines are of equivocal benefit once anaphylaxis ensues.
• Lymphedema—benzopyrone use yields variable results in veterinary medicine; rutin 50 mg/kg PO q8h has been mixed with food for cats with chylothorax. • Cardiogenic edema—combinations of positive inotropes, vasodilators, and diuretics commonly used in patients with CHF. • Immune-mediated edema requires immunosuppressive therapy (e.g., prednisone). • Vasculitis and edema secondary to rickettsial disease typically responds to tetracycline 22 mg/kg PO q8h or doxycycline 5 mg/kg PO q12h. • Edema in association with other infectious agents requires antifungal therapy or antibiotic therapy. • Myxedema secondary to hypothyroidism should respond gradually to T_4 supplementation. • Edema associated with toxic insults may be slowed with antidotes (e.g., antivenom). • Anticoagulant therapy may benefit patients with DIC or antithrombin III deficiency. • Vascular volume expanders such as hydroxyethyl starch or plasma often benefit patients with low plasma oncotic pressure; very-low-dose furosemide in a constant-rate infusion of 0.1 mg/kg/h has been effective in conjunction with a volume expander.

CONTRAINDICATIONS

• Diuretics generally aggravate edema of noncardiogenic origin. • Steroids may worsen edema secondary to infectious disease. • Epinephrine—generally contraindicated in shock except in anaphylaxis. • Propranolol (beta-blocker)—contraindicated in patients predisposed to bronchospasm.

PRECAUTIONS

• Avoid intramuscular injections in patients with thrombocytopenia. • Taper patients on long-term steroid therapy so that endogenous steroid production resumes. • Use epinephrine cautiously in patients predisposed to ventricular fibrillation. • Use enalapril and other ACE inhibitors cautiously in patients with renal disease. • Long-term antibiotic therapy may facilitate a superinfection by a fungus (e.g., *Candida*) or resistant bacteria.
• Monitor anticoagulants closely to avoid fatal hemorrhage.

FOLLOW-UP

PATIENT MONITORING

• Repeat complete blood counts, chemistries, and urine protein:creatinine ratios for blood dyscrasias and serum and urine protein concentrations. • Weekly assessment of prothrombin or partial thromboplastin time for patients on warfarin or heparin. • Serial biopsies of affected tissue such as kidney with glomerulonephritis may help to prognosticate.
• Repeat cultures or acute and convalescing titers for patients suffering from an infectious disease. • Periodic T_4/TSH assay (4–6 hours post pill) for patients receiving thyroid supplementation.

PREVENTION/AVOIDANCE

Depends on the cause of the edema.

POSSIBLE COMPLICATIONS

• Decubital ulceration. • Fatal hemorrhage.
• Fatal thrombosis. • Refractory cardiac, gastrointestinal, hepatic, or renal failure.
• Malnutrition. • Cerebral edema and herniation. • Resistant infection and sepsis.

EXPECTED COURSE AND PROGNOSIS

Depends on cause of the edema.

MISCELLANEOUS

ASSOCIATED CONDITIONS

Pericardial, pleural, or peritoneal effusion.

AGE-RELATED FACTORS

Vascular anomalies or primary lymphedema are generally documented in juvenile patients (e.g., anasarca).

ZOONOTIC POTENTIAL

• Tick exposure is common in pets and their owners; both may suffer simultaneously from rickettsial disease. • Certain protozoal (*Leishmania*), fungal (*Sporothrix*), and bacterial (*Brucella*) organisms may transfer to people via direct contact.

PREGNANCY/FERTILITY/BREEDING

Brucellosis has been associated with vulvar edema, necrotizing vasculitis, and embryonic death or fetal abortion.

SYNONYMS

Anasarca

SEE ALSO

- Ascites.
- Chylothorax.
- Cirrhosis and Fibrosis of the Liver.
- Hyperlipidemia.
- Hypoalbuminemia.
- Lymphedema.
- Proteinuria.
- Thrombocytopenia.
- Vasculitis, Cutaneous.
- Vasculitis, Systemic (Including Phlebitis).

ABBREVIATIONS

- CHF = congestive heart failure.
- DIC = disseminated intravascular coagulation.
- RMSF = Rocky Mountain spotted fever.
- T_4 = thyroxine.
- TSH = thyroid-stimulating hormone.

Suggested Reading

Fossum TW, King LA, Miller MW, et al. Lymphedema: clinical signs, diagnosis and treatment. J Vet Intern Med 1992, 6:312–319.

Fossum TW, Miller MW. Lymphedema: etiopathogenesis. J Vet Intern Med 1992, 6:283–293.

Fox PR, Petrie JP, Hohenhaus AE. Peripheral vascular disease. In: Ettinger SJ, Feldman EC, eds., Textbook of Veterinary Internal Medicine, 6th ed. St. Louis, MO: Elsevier, 2005.

Jacobsen JO, Eggers C. Primary lymphedema in a kitten. J Small Anim Pract 1997, 18–20.

Author Marc Elie

Consulting Editor Michael Aherne

P

PERIRENAL PSEUDOCYSTS

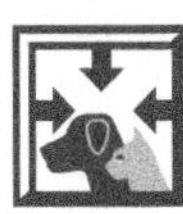

BASICS

OVERVIEW

• Capsulogenic renal cyst, capsular cyst, pararenal pseudocyst, capsular hydronephrosis, perirenal cyst, and perirenal pseudocyst are terms used to describe renomegaly caused by accumulation of fluid between the kidney and its surrounding capsule. One or both kidneys are affected. • The tissue sac in which the fluid accumulates is not lined with secretory epithelium; and thus the name "pseudo"-cyst is appropriate.

SIGNALMENT

• Primarily older male cats (>8 years).
• When detected in young cats, the disease is usually unilateral. • Rare in dogs; the difference in prevalence between species may be related to the prominent network of subcapsular veins that characterize feline kidneys.

SIGNS

• May be asymptomatic. • Nonpainful, enlarged abdomen is common. • Signs of concomitant renal failure in some patients.

CAUSES & RISK FACTORS

• Cause of perirenal accumulation of fluid is often not understood. • Accumulation of pseudocyst fluid is a dynamic, not a static, process. • Cytologic and biochemical evaluation of pseudocyst fluid may aid understanding of pathophysiologic mechanisms. • Fluid with characteristics of a transudate may accumulate because of high capillary hydrostatic pressure or lymphatic obstruction. Some cats have light microscopic evidence of renal fibrosis. However, it is not known whether progressive renal parenchymal contraction occludes lymphatics and blood vessels, promoting transudation of fluid.
• Perirenal accumulation of transudate can also result from rupture of renal cysts.
• Accumulation of perirenal urine may indicate disruption of the renal pelvis or the proximal ureter. • Accumulation of blood in pseudocysts can result from external trauma, surgery, neoplastic erosion of blood vessels, rupture of aneurysms, coagulopathies, or paracentesis of the urinary tract.

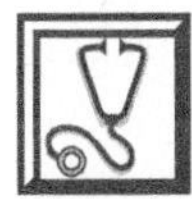

DIAGNOSIS

DIFFERENTIAL DIAGNOSIS

• Causes of renomegaly include renal neoplasia, hydronephrosis, polycystic kidney disease (common), feline infectious peritonitis, and mycotic or bacterial nephritis (less common).
• Ascites and enlargement of other abdominal organs can cause nonpainful distension of the abdomen.

CBC/BIOCHEMISTRY/URINALYSIS

• Results unremarkable until patient develops renal insufficiency. • Azotemia and inappropriately low urinary specific gravity (<1.035) indicate concomitant chronic kidney disease (CKD).

OTHER LABORATORY TESTS

N/A

IMAGING

• Renomegaly is commonly detected by abdominal radiography. • Excretory urography and ultrasonography can be used to determine whether the underlying renal parenchyma is normal or abnormal. Small kidneys beneath an abnormally wide fluid-filled intracapsular space is a common finding.

DIAGNOSTIC PROCEDURES

Cytologic examination of pseudocyst fluid may provide evidence of the underlying disease process resulting in fluid accumulation (e.g., transudation, hemorrhage, lymphatic obstruction, inflammation, urine, etc.) or secondary complications (e.g., infection). Creatinine concentrations that are higher in pseudocyst fluid compared to serum are consistent with urinary tract rupture.

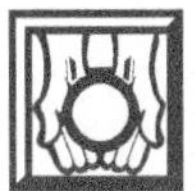

TREATMENT

• Perirenal pseudocysts are not immediately life-threatening. • Some patients need no treatment. • Many patients require further diagnostic evaluation and treatment of concomitant CKD. • Capsulectomy or pseudocyst fenestration (remove greater than 1 cm × 1 cm section of capsule to minimize spontaneous closure of the fenestration) is generally associated with amelioration of abdominal distention and abdominal organ displacement. Early stages of CKD may resolve; however, progression of CKD commonly occurs. • Long-term response is unknown. • Avoid nephrectomy to maximize remaining kidney function.
• Decompression by paracentesis with a needle and syringe provides temporary relief. • If pseudocysts refill with fluid (often in 1–2 weeks), paracentesis can then be repeated.

MEDICATIONS

DRUG(S) OF CHOICE

Consider appropriate antimicrobic (i.e., lipid-soluble antibiotic chosen on the basis of antimicrobial susceptibility) if pseudocysts become infected.

FOLLOW-UP

• Monitor patients periodically (every 2–6 months) for development and progression of CKD. • Short-term prognosis appears favorable with or without pseudocyst decompression in patients with no evidence of CKD. • Long-term prognosis is unknown because it has not been determined whether perirenal pseudocysts are associated with underlying lesions in the renal parenchyma that may be progressive. It is also unknown whether perirenal pseudocysts are associated with hypertension. • Survival is related to the severity and progression of CKD.

MISCELLANEOUS

ABBREVIATIONS

• CKD = chronic kidney disease.

Suggested Reading

Beck JA, Bellenger CR, Lamb WA, et al. Perirenal pseudocysts in 26 cats. Aust Vet J 2000, 78:166–171.

Lulich JP, Osborne CA, Polzin DJ. Cystic diseases of the kidney. In: Osborne CA, Finco DR, eds., Canine and Feline Nephrology and Urology. Philadelphia, PA: Williams & Wilkins, 1995, pp. 460–483.

Ochoa VB, DiBartola SP, Chew DJ, et al. Perinephric pseudocysts in the cat: a retrospective study and review of the literature. J Vet Intern Med 1999, 13:47–55.

Author Jody P. Lulich

Consulting Editor J.D. Foster

Acknowledgment The author and editors acknowledge the prior contribution of Carl A. Osborne.

PERITONEOPERICARDIAL DIAPHRAGMATIC HERNIA

BASICS

OVERVIEW

• Embryologic malformation of the ventral midline allowing communication between the pericardial and peritoneal cavities.
• May be associated with other congenital malformations including sternal deformities (especially in cats), cranial abdominal hernia, and ventricular septal defects.
• Signs may be due to large amounts of abdominal viscera compressing the heart or lungs and incarceration of abdominal organs (e.g., liver and small bowel). However, many affected animals remain asymptomatic.

SIGNALMENT

• Dog and cat.
• Age when clinical signs first occur varies; more than one-third of patients are 4 years of age or older.
• Weimaraners and Persians may be predisposed.
• No evidence that lesions are hereditary, but they have been reported in littermates.

P

SIGNS

General Comments

Depend on the nature and amount of abdominal contents that are herniated.

Historical Findings

• Vomiting.
• Diarrhea.
• Weight loss.
• Abdominal pain.
• Coughing.
• Dyspnea.

Physical Examination Findings

• Muffled heart sounds.
• Displaced or attenuated apical cardiac impulse.
• Palpable sternal deformity or cranial abdominal hernia.
• Cardiac tamponade and signs of right-sided congestive heart failure (rare).

CAUSES & RISK FACTORS

• Embryologic malformation.
• Prenatal injury of the septum transversum and pleuroperitoneal folds.

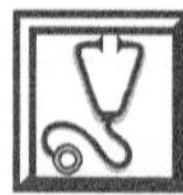

DIAGNOSIS

DIFFERENTIAL DIAGNOSIS

• Never an acquired traumatic defect because no natural direct communication exists between the peritoneal and pericardial cavities after birth.
• Pericardial effusion.

CBC/BIOCHEMISTRY/URINALYSIS

No associated hematologic or biochemical alterations.

OTHER LABORATORY TESTS

N/A

IMAGING

• Radiographic findings depend on size of defect and amount of herniated abdominal contents; caudal heart border and diaphragm usually overlap; thoracic radiographs may show an "empty" abdomen and possible multiple radiographic densities within the cardiac silhouette.
• Positive and negative contrast peritoneography have been used to evaluate the diaphragm. Injection of 1–2 mL/kg body weight of water-soluble positive contrast into the peritoneal cavity followed by right and left lateral, sternal, and dorsal recumbent radiographs allows complete evaluation of the diaphragm. Identification of contrast within the pleural space confirms the diagnosis of diaphragmatic rupture. Air, carbon dioxide, or nitrous oxide may also be used.
• Barium series may demonstrate bowel loops crossing the diaphragm and within the pericardial sac.
• Nonselective angiography outlines the cardiac chambers within the large cardiac silhouette.
• Echocardiography gives a definitive diagnosis.

DIAGNOSTIC PROCEDURES

Electrocardiogram may show small complexes if abdominal contents have herniated or if marked effusion is present.

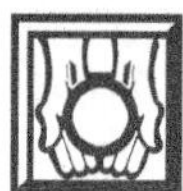

TREATMENT

Surgical closure of the hernia after returning viable organs to their normal location is usually curative. In asymptomatic adult patients, treatment may not be indicated.

MEDICATIONS

DRUG(S) OF CHOICE

• Myocardial contractility is unaffected in most patients; drugs for improving cardiac output are not indicated.
• Can give symptomatic treatment based on nature and amount of abdominal contents that are herniated.

CONTRAINDICATIONS/POSSIBLE INTERACTIONS

Drugs that reduce ventricular afterload (e.g., arteriolar vasodilators) or preload (e.g., venous dilators and diuretics) are not useful and can cause reduction of ventricular filling, hypotension, and low cardiac output.

FOLLOW-UP

Prognosis after surgery is excellent in animals with no other significant congenital anomalies or complicating factors. Some affected animals remain asymptomatic throughout life.

MISCELLANEOUS

Suggested Reading

Burns CG, Bergh MS, McLouhlin, MA. Surgical and nonsurgical treatment of peritoneopericardial diaphragmatic hernia in dogs and cats: 58 cases (1999–2008). J Am Vet Med Assoc 2011, 22:643–650.
Coleman AE, Rapoport GS. Pericardial disorders and cardiac tumors. In: Smith FWK, Tilley LP, Oyama M, Sleeper M, eds., Manual of Canine and Feline Cardiology, 5th ed. St. Louis, MO: Saunders Elsevier, 2016, pp. 198–217.
Kienle RD. Pericardial disease and cardiac neoplasia. In: Kittleson MD, Kienle RD, eds., Small Animal Cardiovascular Medicine. St. Louis, MO: Mosby, 1999, pp. 413–432.
Neiger R. Peritoneopericardial diaphragmatic hernia in cats. Compend Contin Educ Pract Vet 1996, 461–479.
Reimer SB, Kyles AE, Filipowicz DE, et al. Long-term outcome of cats treated conservatively or surgically for peritoneopericardial diaphragmatic hernia: 66 cases (1987–2002). J Am Vet Med Assoc 2004, 224:728–732.

Author Larry P. Tilley
Consulting Editor Michael Aherne

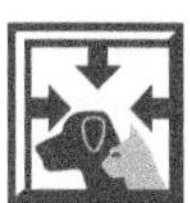

BASICS

DEFINITION

Inflammatory process involving the serous membrane of the abdominal cavity.

PATHOPHYSIOLOGY

• Insult to the peritoneal cavity (localized or generalized) leads to inflammation characterized by vasodilation, cellular infiltration, pain, and development of adhesions. Fluid production is eventually favored over absorption, and progresses from transudate to exudate. • Extent and severity depend on type and severity of insult.
• Response to bacterial peritonitis associated with lipopolysaccharide (LPS; Gram-negative bacteria) or peptidoglycans (Gram-positive bacteria), causing inflammatory cytokine and nitric oxide (NO) production. NO causes vasodilation, can lead to hypotension.
• Inflammation causes vasodilation and increased vascular permeability. Cytokine release from leukocytes results in chemotaxis and activation of complement. Activation of complement results in coagulation, fibrin production and decreased fibrinolysis, resulting in adhesion formation. • Result of significant abdominal inflammation can be systemic inflammatory response syndrome (SIRS) and sepsis. SIRS can progress to multiple organ dysfunction (MODS) and affect respiratory system (acute respiratory distress syndrome or pulmonary thromboembolism), or cause renal dysfunction, reduced cardiac function, and neurologic dysfunction.

SYSTEMS AFFECTED

• Cardiovascular. • Gastrointestinal (GI).
• Hemic/lymphatic/immune. • Renal/urologic hepatobiliary.

GENETICS

N/A

INCIDENCE/PREVALENCE

N/A

GEOGRAPHIC DISTRIBUTION

N/A

SIGNALMENT

Species

Dog and cat.

Breed Predilections

None

Mean Age and Range

None

Predominant Sex

None

SIGNS

General Comments

Signs may be vague and nonspecific and depend on timeline of evaluation in relation to inflammation and systemic response.

Historical Findings

Lethargy, depression, anorexia, vomiting (common), diarrhea, collapse.

Physical Examination Findings

• Abdominal discomfort or pain—localized or generalized. • Shock: ○ Compensatory—tachycardia, tachypnea, injected mucus membranes, rapid capillary refill time (CRT).
○ Early decompensatory—tachycardia, poor pulse quality, depressed mentation, pallor, prolonged CRT. Cats may show a normal to decreased heart rate (<140/min).
○ Decompensatory—bradycardia, weak or absent pulses, severely depressed mentation, pallor or cyanosis, prolonged CRT.
• Arrhythmias/pulse deficits may be detected.
• Fever. • Weight loss—reported in 1/3 of dogs and cats with secondary peritonitis.
• SIRS—tachycardia (dog >140/min, cat >240/min) or bradycardia (cat <130/min); tachypnea (dog >30/min, cat >40/min), hyperthermia (dog >102.5°F [39.1°C], cat >104.5°F [40.3°C]) or hypothermia (dog or cat <100°F [37.7°C]), leukocytosis (dog >19,000/µL, cat >18,000/µL), or leukopenia (dog <6000/µL, cat <5000/µL).

CAUSES

Primary Peritonitis

• Uncommon, no identifiable intraperitoneal source. More common in cats (14%). • May be monomicrobial, Gram-positive in 80% of dogs, 60% of cats. • Results from hematogenous or lymphatic spread or translocation from GI tract; may spread from oviduct. • Feline infectious peritonitis (FIP) in cats.

Secondary Peritonitis

• Most common. • Contamination of peritoneal cavity from abdominal organ: ○ GI source (up to 75%) from perforation (ulcerations, neoplasia, ischemia), leakage following GI surgery, penetrating trauma, biliary tract rupture (obstruction, trauma, mucocele), or pancreatitis. ○ Abscessation (liver, pancreas, kidney, prostate, lymph nodes, spleen). ○ Urogenital source (pyometra, urine leakage). ○ Uroabdomen and bile peritonitis may or may not be septic; regardless, chemical peritonitis is present.

RISK FACTORS

• Trauma. • Foreign body ingestion. • Biliary mucocele. • GI surgery. • Nonsteroidal anti-inflammatory drug (NSAID) use associated with GI perforation.

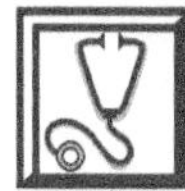

DIAGNOSIS

DIFFERENTIAL DIAGNOSIS

Other causes of abdominal pain or distention, sepsis, and shock.

CBC/BIOCHEMISTRY/URINALYSIS

• Neutrophilic leukocytosis common; possible left shift; degenerative left shift, or development of neutropenia may portend worsening prognosis. • Hemoconcentration or anemia. • Hypoproteinemia. • Hypo- or hyperkalemia; hyponatremia (fluid loss into peritoneum). • Azotemia—prerenal, renal, or post renal. • Metabolic acidosis. • Hypoglycemia—may indicate sepsis; hyperglycemia may be present in cats. • Liver enzyme activity elevations—hepatic causes of peritonitis or MODS. • Hyperlactatemia—poor tissue oxygen delivery.

OTHER LABORATORY TESTS

Coagulation testing—disseminated intravascular coagulation (DIC): prolonged activated partial thromboplastin time (aPTT) and thrombocytopenia initially, progress to prolonged prothrombin time (PT), aPTT, elevated D-dimers (>1,000 ng/mL).

IMAGING

Radiography

• Findings depend on cause; make right and left lateral projections of abdomen. • Loss of serosal detail (ground-glass appearance suggests fluid in abdominal cavity)—rule out lack of intra-abdominal fat (cachexia, neonates). • Generalized ileus. • Pneumoperitoneum—gas in abdomen may be slight, closely evaluate region near diaphragm; consider making lateral beam images with patient in a sternal or lateral recumbency.
• Can be diagnostic for gastric dilatation/volvulus, GI foreign bodies, mass lesions, organs enlargement (neoplasia, abscess).
• Contrast procedures—rarely warranted; may complicate management if contrast material enters abdominal cavity; avoid barium if GI perforation suspected.

Ultrasound

Identify (and aspirate) small volumes of peritoneal effusion, abscesses, gallbladder rupture or mucocele, tumors, obstructions, or mass lesions.

DIAGNOSTIC PROCEDURES

• Abdominocentesis and diagnostic peritoneal lavage—perform as soon as possible:
(1) Cytology—collect aliquot of sample into EDTA tube; note color and clarity and presence of fibrin. (2) Place second aliquot into red-top tube for biochemical testing if needed, based on suspected etiology. Chemical

peritonitis—analyze abdominal fluid for creatinine (for uroabdomen), specific pancreatic lipase (for pancreatitis), and bilirubin (for bile leakage). (3) Culture and sensitivity—next, aseptically place an aliquot of sample in a sterile-white top (no additive) tube. • Suspect FIP—submit abdominal fluid for protein electrophoresis and globulin determination.

PATHOLOGIC FINDINGS

• Intracellular bacteria, degenerative neutrophils, and plant material are diagnostic of septic peritonitis. • Normal peritoneal fluid contains <2,500 cells/μL. • Glucose concentration in abdominal fluid more than 20 mg/dL less than peripheral blood glucose concentration suggests septic peritonitis.
• Peritoneal lactate >4.2 mmol/L suggests peritonitis in dogs. • Recent surgery results in <10,000 cells/mL; primary peritonitis usually results in 7,000 cells/μL in dogs and 3,000 cells/μL in cats. • Fluid bilirubin or creatinine levels at least two times higher than that of peripheral blood indicate bile peritonitis or uroabdomen, respectively. Acellular homogenous, laminated, basophilic material on cytology may be mucoid material associated with bile peritonitis.

P

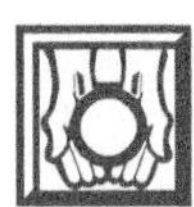

TREATMENT

APPROPRIATE HEALTH CARE

• Inpatient—intensive monitoring and supportive care are required. • Goals—blood pressure >90 mmHg (measured by Doppler), heart rate 80–140/min (dogs) and 160–225/min (cats), CRT 1.5–2 seconds, urine output >1–2 mL/kg/h, blood lactate <2.5 mmol/L. Blood lactate concentration should improve with resuscitation; inability to do so suggests poorer prognosis.

IV Fluid Therapy

• Critical for correction of hemodynamic disturbances, electrolyte and acid–base abnormalities prior to surgery. • Balanced isotonic replacement crystalloid solution—evaluate response to therapy frequently:
◦ Rate—may initially require multiple boluses of 10–30 mL/kg (depending on other patient parameters); reevaluate patient frequently, adjust fluid rate or repeat boluses as patient status changes. • Potassium and glucose supplementation as necessary: ◦ Rate of potassium supplementation should not exceed 0.5 mEq/kg/h of potassium.
• Synthetic colloids sometimes utilized (up to 20 mL/kg/d); concerns for acute kidney injury have decreased usage, especially in patients with sepsis. • Canine albumin transfusion indicated for severe hypoalbuminemia (<1.2 mg/dL). • Whole blood or packed red blood cells—as required for anemia. • Inadequate response to therapy may prompt vasopressor administration (norepinephrine, vasopressin, dopamine). Norepinephrine is recommended for animals with sepsis. • DIC—remove inciting cause, support coagulation with fresh frozen plasma transfusion.

NURSING CARE

• Significant; dependent upon severity of systemic signs.
• IV fluid therapy and maintenance of tissue oxygen delivery.

ACTIVITY

Decreased; depends on inciting cause and clinical signs.

DIET

• Dictated by cause and concurrent conditions (e.g., heart disease). • Feeding tube placement should be considered and placed at time of surgery for early nutritional support (e.g., esophagostomy, gastrostomy, jejunostomy). Nasogastric tube for feeding and gastric decompression if necessary.
• Adequate nutrition—essential to optimize outcome, attenuate hypermetabolic state, preserve hepatic antioxidant defenses, prevent protein-calorie malnutrition, maintain GI barrier function.

CLIENT EDUCATION

• Advise client of high rate of morbidity and (especially septic peritonitis) mortality.
• Extensive monitoring and intensive care may be costly, with prolonged hospitalization.

SURGICAL CONSIDERATIONS

• Decision to treat medically or surgically—dictated by etiology, patient's response to initial treatment, and owner's financial constraints. • Known bacterial contamination or suspected chemical peritonitis—surgical intervention necessary. • Perform surgery as soon as patient is stable. Prompt source control allows deescalation of antibosis, which may only be required for 4–8 days.
• Exploratory laparotomy—prepare for incision extending from xiphoid to pubis; goals of surgery are to remove source of contamination, debride and lavage abdomen, collect fluid or tissue for Gram stain and aerobic and anaerobic culture, and provide access for nutritional support; use monofilament absorbable or nonabsorbable suture within abdomen; before closing, thoroughly lavage abdomen with 200–300 mL/kg warm sterile saline. Do not add antimicrobials or other products to lavage solution; remove all lavage solution from abdomen. • Surgeon must assess organ viability and perform resections if necessary. Anastomosis of GI tract should utilize healthy tissue; consider serosal patching, perform omental patching if serosal patching not done. Stapled anastomoses may have a decreased risk of dehiscence in septic peritonitis. • Consider omentalization of pancreatic abscesses, perform omentalization for prostatic abscessation. Remove affected organ or part in other cases of abscessation (liver lobectomy, nephrectomy). • Consider abdominal drainage—based on degree of contamination, ability to debride abdomen, severity of illness, and anticipation of septic complications: ◦ Allows continued removal of fluid, bacteria, and toxins. ◦ Forms include closed suction drains, vacuum-assisted peritoneal drainage (VAPD), and closure of caudal abdomen with partial closure of cranial abdomen. Sterile bandaging is required in each form; less external materials for VAPD, but regulate suction and specialized foam and connections to suction required. ◦ Requires anesthesia for abdominal closure unless closed suction drains are used. Severe peritonitis may require repeated exploration, debridement, and lavage prior to closure.

MEDICATIONS

DRUG(S) OF CHOICE

• Antimicrobials—early and aggressive broad-spectrum therapy for suspected septic peritonitis; final therapy based on culture and susceptibility testing. • Initial therapy—Gram-negative (enrofloxacin, cefotaxime, amikacin); Gram-positive (ampicillin, clindamycin); anaerobes (metronidazole):
◦ Ampicillin 22 mg/kg IV q6–8h.
◦ Ampicillin/sulbactam 25–30 mg/kg IV q6–8h. ◦ Clindamycin 12 mg/kg IV q12h.
◦ Cefotaxime 20–80 mg/kg IV q8h.
◦ Enrofloxacin 10–20 mg/kg IV q24h (dogs); 5 mg/kg IV q24h (cats). ◦ Amikacin 15 mg/kg IV q24h. ◦ Metronidazole 10 mg/kg IV q12h. ◦ Analgesia—depends on pain severity; may be intermittent or via CRI; opioids recommended: ◦ Multimodal IV combinations for pain; dogs, morphine 0.05–0.2 mg/kg/h or fentanyl 2–5 μg/kg/h, ketamine 0.2–0.5 mg/kg/h, lidocaine 2–4 mg/kg/h; cats, fentanyl 2–5 μg/kg/h, ketamine 0.05–0.2 mg/kg/h. Lidocaine may improve outcome following surgery in dogs.
• GI protectants— if GI ulceration:
◦ Famotidine 0.5–1.0 mg/kg IV q12h.
◦ Pantoprazole 1 mg/kg IV q12–24h (more effective acid reduction). ◦ Sucralfate: dogs, 0.5–1.0 mg PO q8h; cats, 0.25–0.5 mg PO q8h.

CONTRAINDICATIONS

• Glucocorticoids—physiologic dose (0.5 mg/kg prednisone equivalent) may be indicated for hypotension unresponsive to fluids and pressors. • NSAIDs are not recommended due to risk of acute kidney injury and GI ulceration in poorly perfused patients.

PRECAUTIONS

• Aminoglycosides—use with caution if hypotensive, dehydrated, impaired renal function. • Adequate hydration—essential to enhance safety of these drugs.

POSSIBLE INTERACTIONS

Sucralfate works best at low pH; administration should be staggered with GI acid reducers, if both used. Avoid giving oral medications at same time as sucralfate.

ALTERNATIVE DRUG(S)

Fluoroquinolone—enrofloxacin or orbifloxacin; substitute for an aminoglycoside, especially with impaired renal function.

FOLLOW-UP

PATIENT MONITORING

• Fluid balance, electrolyte balance, acid–base status, blood lactate—as necessary depending on severity of condition. • Frequency of monitoring—varies with condition and response to treatment; generally q2h. • Urine output—target 1–2 mL/kg/h. • Quantify and replace fluid losses (vomiting, diarrhea).
• Change recumbency q4–6h. • Enteral nutrition as soon as possible via oral or tube feeding: promotes enterocyte health and decreases bacterial translocation. Does not increase risk of complications. • Repeat ultrasound and abdominal fluid cytologic evaluation depending on index of suspicion for leakage of intestinal surgery sites. • CBC, chemistry profile, urinalysis—every 1–2 days during periods of intensive monitoring, even in patients that are responding. • Coagulation testing q24–48h.

PREVENTION/AVOIDANCE

Prevention—difficult except with specific risk factors (e.g., pyometra, prostatic abscess can be avoided with sterilization).

POSSIBLE COMPLICATIONS

• If underlying cause is not identified and managed, patient is at risk for complications.
• Open peritoneal drainage—increased cost and required intensive care, repeated sedation or anesthesia for aseptic bandage changes, nosocomial infection, hypoproteinemia, electrolyte imbalances, enterocutaneous fistulation, and abdominal hernia formation.
• Adhesions, granuloma formation with barium peritonitis.

EXPECTED COURSE AND PROGNOSIS

• Prognosis—depends on rapid identification and successful management of underlying cause and appropriate follow-up care. • Septic peritonitis—mortality of 30–68%. Prognosis worse in animals with preexisting septic peritonitis, uncorrectable hypotension, low serum albumin and total protein concentrations, respiratory dysfunction, DIC, low concentrations of protein C, or antithrombin, MODS; better survival in patients with lower preoperative alanine aminotransferase, gamma-glutamyltransferase, packed cell volume, total solids, and albumin concentration. Open peritoneal drainage may improve survival. • Septic bile peritonitis—27% survival compared to 100% with nonseptic bile peritonitis. • Antibiotic treatment within first hour in cases of suspected septic peritonitis may significantly reduce mortality. • Blood lactate >2.5 mmol/L or inability to normalize plasma lactate—poorer survival. • Feeding tube complications depend on site of placement—esophagostomy (localized infection or abscessation); gastrostomy and jejunostomy (leakage or premature dislodgement associated peritonitis): nasoesophageal or nasogastric (sneezing, epistaxis). Refeeding syndrome—decreased magnesium, phosphorus, potassium; relatively rare but warrants close monitoring. • Bradycardia and hypothermia in cats with primary septic peritonitis associated with mortality.

MISCELLANEOUS

ASSOCIATED CONDITIONS

N/A

AGE-RELATED FACTORS

N/A

ZOONOTIC POTENTIAL

N/A

PREGNANCY/FERTILITY/BREEDING

N/A

SEE ALSO

Sepsis and Bacteremia.

ABBREVIATIONS

• aPTT = activated partial thromboplastin time.
• CRT = capillary refill time.
• FIP = feline infectious peritonitis.
• LPS = lipopolysaccharide.
• MODS = multiple organ dysfunction.
• NO = nitric oxide.
• NSAID = nonsteroidal anti-inflammatory drug.
• PT = prothrombin time.
• SIRS = systemic inflammatory response syndrome.
• VAPD = vacuum-assisted peritoneal drainage.

Suggested Reading

Cortellini S, Seth M, Kellett-Gregory LM. Plasma lactate concentrations in septic peritonitis: a retrospective study of 83 dogs (2007–2012). J Vet Emerg Crit Care 2015, 25:388–395.

Dickinson AE, Summers JF, Wignal J, et al. Impact of appropriate empirical antimicrobial therapy on outcome of dogs with septic peritonitis. J Vet Emerg Crit Care 2015, 25:152–259.

Grimes JA, Schmiedt CW, Cornell KK, Radlinsky MA. Identification of risk factors for septic peritonitis and failure to survive following gastrointestinal surgery in dogs. J Am Vet Med Assoc 2011, 238:486–494.

Hoffberg J, Koenigshof A. Evaluation of the safety of early compared to later enteral nutrition in canine septic peritonitis. J Am Anim Hosp Assoc 2017, 53:90–105.

Author MaryAnn G. Radlinsky

Consulting Editor Amie Koenig

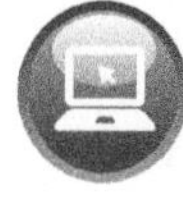

Client Education Handout available online

PETECHIAE, ECCHYMOSIS, BRUISING

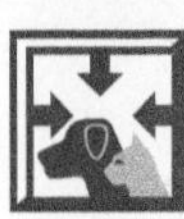

BASICS

DEFINITION

Pinpoint (petechia) or larger (ecchymosis) hemorrhage in the skin or mucous membranes most often secondary to abnormal primary hemostasis (platelet or vessel wall-mediated); may appear spontaneously or following trauma. Spontaneous development often occurs at sites of increased capillary trauma.

PATHOPHYSIOLOGY

- Thrombocytopenia results in impaired primary hemostasis and decreased production of platelet-derived trophic factors that maintain endothelial cell junction integrity.
- Platelet numbers below $50 \times 10^3/\mu L$ and more often below $25 \times 10^3/\mu L$ are associated with an increased risk of spontaneous hemorrhage.
- Thrombocytopathies are not generally associated with the development of petechiae. Some animals with von Willebrand disease (VWD) may develop petechiae.
- Vascular hemostatic defects—generally caused by systemic disease causing increased capillary permeability, vasculitis, or altered dermal vascular support (e.g., collagen alterations).

P

SYSTEMS AFFECTED

- Gastrointestinal—melena/hematochezia/hematemesis.
- Hemic/lymphatic/immune—anemia from bleeding.
- Neurologic—variable depending on location of bleeding.
- Ophthalmic—scleral/retinal hemorrhage, hyphema, secondary glaucoma, and uveitis.
- Renal/urologic—hematuria.
- Respiratory—epistaxis/hemoptysis.
- Skin/exocrine—petechia/ecchymosis/bruising.

GENETICS

Most etiologies are acquired; immune-mediated thrombocytopenia (ITP) has a possible genetic predisposition in cocker spaniels, poodles, Maltese, and Old English sheepdogs. Genetic associations exist for many thrombocytopathies. VWD is seen in Doberman pinschers, German shorthaired pointers, Shetland sheepdogs, Scottish terriers, and Chesapeake Bay retrievers.

INCIDENCE/PREVELENCE

Common in dogs. Uncommon in cats.

GEOGRAPHIC DISTRIBUTION

Applicable if associated with a vector-borne disease.

SIGNALMENT

- Middle-aged female dogs are at increased risk.
- Cats—primary ITP is rare.

CAUSES

- Thrombocytopenia—due to platelet consumption, destruction, or sequestration
- Vasculitis—secondary to inflammation, infection (e.g., *Rickettsia rickettsia*, sepsis), immune-mediated causes.

RISK FACTORS

- Nonsteroidal anti-inflammatory drug (NSAID) use.
- Geography/travel history (susceptibility to tick-borne disease).
- Certain drug exposures (e.g., sulfa-containing antimicrobials).

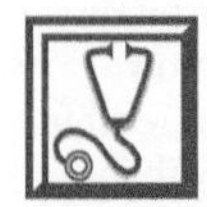

DIAGNOSIS

DIFFERENTIAL DIAGNOSIS

Some inflammatory skin lesions may look like petechiae. Vasculitis lesions may have associated edema. Trauma may cause ecchymoses/bruising.

CBC/BIOCHEMISTRY/URINALYSIS

- Thrombocytopenia.
- Red blood cell fragmentation (schistocytosis) is associated with disseminated intravascular coagulation or microangiopathies.
- *Ehrlichia* morulae or other hemoparasites may be seen on a peripheral blood smear.
- Patients with myeloproliferative or lymphoproliferative disease, myelofibrosis, or a history of chemotherapy or administration of drugs such as estrogens may be concurrently leukopenic or have other cytopenias. Excessive blood loss will result in anemia.
- Urinalysis (free catch or catheter sample instead of cystocentesis if animal may be coagulopathic)—may identify hematuria.

OTHER LABORATORY TESTS

- Coagulation studies (activated partial thromboplastin time [aPTT], prothrombin time [PT], D-dimer, antithrombin activity).
- von Willebrand's factor antigen assay.
- Platelet function tests (e.g., buccal mucosal bleeding time [BMBT], PFA-100) are inaccurate with thrombocytopenia, but may be necessary to rule out platelet function disorders, especially if platelet count is normal in animals with petechiae.
- Feline leukemia virus (FeLV)/feline immunodeficiency virus (FIV) testing—underlying cause of thrombocytopenia.
- Serology—to diagnose ehrlichiosis, *Anaplasma platys*, *Bartonella vinsonii*, or RMSF.
- PCR—for possible infections such as *Ehrlichia* spp., *Anaplasma platys* or *Babesia* spp., *Mycoplasma* spp.

IMAGING

Thoracic and abdominal radiography or abdominal ultrasonography may help to identify neoplasia, pulmonary or other hemorrhage, abnormal splenic or lymph node architecture.

DIAGNOSTIC PROCEDURES

- Animals with pancytopenia may benefit from bone marrow aspirate or biopsy.
- Invasive diagnostic or therapeutic procedures may be performed with less risk if platelet concentrate or fresh whole blood can be administered before or during the procedure.

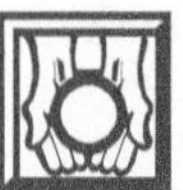

TREATMENT

- Minimize activity to reduce the risk of trauma.
- Discontinue any medications that may alter platelet function (e.g., NSAIDs).
- Discontinue medications that might be associated with ITP.
- Avoid jugular venipuncture.
- Fresh whole blood, platelet-rich plasma, or platelet concentrate transfusions may be necessary before a definitive diagnosis is made. Blood samples for diagnostic testing should be collected prior to transfusion if possible.
- Desmopressin acetate (DDAVP) may be an effective therapy to control bleeding in patients with VWD or NSAID-associated thrombocytopathia.
- Acquired thrombopathias and vascular disorders should have the underlying disease corrected.

MEDICATIONS

DRUG(S) OF CHOICE

Depends on the underlying diagnosis; see specific chapters.

CONTRAINDICATIONS

Avoid IM injectable medications whenever possible.

PRECAUTIONS

Avoid NSAIDs and other drugs that inhibit platelet function.

FOLLOW-UP

Serial platelet count for patients with thrombocytopenia until an adequate response to therapy is seen.

POSSIBLE COMPLICATIONS

- Death or morbidity caused by hemorrhage into critical organs.
- Shock caused by hemorrhagic shock.
- Blindness secondary to sequelae of hyphema.

MISCELLANEOUS

SYNONYMS

- Bleeding.
- Hemorrhagic diatheses.

SEE ALSO

- Disseminated Intravascular Coagulation.
- Myeloproliferative Disorders.
- Thrombocytopathies.
- Thrombocytopenia.
- Thrombocytopenia, Primary Immune-Mediated.
- Von Willebrand Disease.

ABBREVIATIONS

- aPTT = activated partial thromboplastin time.
- BMBT = buccal mucosal bleeding time.
- DDAVP = desmopressin acetate.
- FeLV = feline leukemia virus.
- FIP = feline infectious peritonitis.
- FIV = feline immunodeficiency virus.
- IMHA = immune-mediated hemolytic anemia.
- ITP = immune-mediated thrombocytopenia.
- NSAID = nonsteroidal anti-inflammatory drug.
- PT = prothrombin time.
- RMSF = Rocky Mountain spotted fever.
- VWD = von Willebrand disease.

Suggested Reading

Blois S. Petechiae and ecchymoses. In: Ettinger SJ, ed., Textbook of Veterinary Internal Medicine, 8th ed. Philadelphia, PA: Saunders, 2017, pp. 217–219.

Brooks M, Catalfamo JL. Immune-mediated thrombocytopenia, von Willebrand disease, and platelet disorders. In: Ettinger SJ, ed., Textbook of Veterinary Internal Medicine, 7th ed. Philadelphia, PA: Saunders, 2010, pp. 772–783.

Brooks M, Catalfamo JL. Platelet dysfunction. In: Bonagura JD, Twedt DC, eds., Kirk's Current Veterinary Therapy XIV: Small Animal Practice. Philadelphia, PA: Saunders, 2009, pp. 292–297.

Neel JA, Birkenheuer AJ, Grindem CB. Infectious and immune-mediated thrombocytopenia. In: Bonagura JD, Twedt DC, eds., Kirk's Current Veterinary Therapy XIV: Small Animal Practice. Philadelphia, PA: Saunders, 2009, pp. 281–287.

Russell KE, Grindem CB. Secondary thrombocytopenia. In: Feldman BF, Zinki JG, Jain NC, eds., Schalm's Veterinary Hematology. Philadelphia, PA: Lippincott Williams & Wilkins, 2000, pp. 469–477.

Authors Justin Farris and Benjamin M. Brainard

Consulting Editor Melinda S. Camus

Acknowledgment The author and editors acknowledge the prior contribution of Julie Armstrong.

Client Education Handout available online

PETROLEUM HYDROCARBON TOXICOSIS

BASICS

DEFINITION

- Petroleum hydrocarbons are a diverse group of products derived or synthesized from crude oil.
- Certain nonpetroleum-origin hydrocarbons, such as turpentine and linseed oil, are toxicologically similar enough to be considered with petroleum-origin products of similar molecular weight. Halogenated hydrocarbons, such as carbon tetrachloride or methylene chloride, are sufficiently unique to warrant separate consideration.
- Small animal poisoning most commonly results from exposure to refined commercial products including such disparate mixtures as fuels, solvents, lubricants, and waxes.
- Petroleum-based solvents are often used as "inert" carriers for other potential toxicants (e.g., pesticides, paints, medications).
- Most petroleum hydrocarbons can be "lumped" into a relatively few broad categories based on volatility, viscosity, and surface tension. Mixtures with high boiling points (low volatility), such as asphalt, mineral oil, and waxes, are relatively nontoxic. Products with relatively low boiling points and low viscosities, such as benzene or turpentine, are more readily aspirated, penetrate further into airways, and are more likely to cause chemical pneumonitis. In general, products that are more volatile also tend to be more lipophilic and more readily absorbed systemically. Products with high aromatic content are also predisposed to cause systemic toxicity.

P

PATHOPHYSIOLOGY

- In general, the most *acutely* life-threatening effects of hydrocarbon ingestion result from aspiration-induced pneumonitis.
- Viscosity and surface tension are reliable determinants of pneumotoxic potential. Low viscosity permits hydrocarbons to penetrate further into smaller airways. Low surface tension increases their tendency to "wet" pulmonary surfaces. For example, aspiration of as little as 0.1 mL of a low-viscosity hydrocarbon (e.g., hexane) may produce severe pneumonitis, whereas a high-viscosity product (e.g., motor oil) would not penetrate past the major airways.
- Inhalation of hydrocarbon vapors (as opposed to aspirating liquid) may compromise pulmonary immune function and displace oxygen.
- Topical exposure to hydrocarbon-based solvents (e.g., petroleum distillates, turpentine) may result in irritation and necrosis of skin and cornea.
- Systemic toxicity is possible after oral or topical exposure. Although there are no quantitative data readily applicable to small animals, systemic toxicity should be considered when evaluating pets that have received a heavy topical exposure if the hydrocarbon is aromatic (e.g., benzene) or a low molecular weight (e.g., hexane). Topical exposure is especially important in very small animals (e.g., puppies, kittens, rodents), which have a relatively high body surface area to mass ratio. Systemic uptake and thus toxicity are also enhanced by factors such as a long hair coat, which traps the product against the skin.

SYSTEMS AFFECTED

- Cardiac.
- Gastrointestinal.
- Nervous.
- Respiratory.
- Skin.
- Hematopoietic.

INCIDENCE/PREVALENCE

In the author's experience, the incidence of small animal poisonings has decreased in recent years.

SIGNALMENT

Species

Dogs and cats.

SIGNS

General Comments

- Pneumonitis is the most serious complication associated with ingestion of more volatile (e.g., gasoline) hydrocarbons. Respiratory signs usually occur within a few minutes to 1–2 hours post ingestion. The central nervous and gastrointestinal systems may also be affected; death usually results from respiratory failure.
- If aspiration occurs simultaneously with ingestion, choking, coughing, gagging, and varying degrees of dyspnea will occur. Direct damage of airway components and bronchospasm may result in hypoxia. Cyanosis may develop immediately as alveolar oxygen is displaced by hydrocarbon vapor.
- There is some evidence that *some* hydrocarbons sensitize the myocardium to both endogenous and exogenous catecholamines, precipitating arrhythmias; hemolytic anemia has been occasionally reported in children.

Historical Findings

- A history of (possible) exposure is essential to the diagnosis of hydrocarbon intoxication. Signs of hydrocarbon poisoning are seldom sufficiently characteristic to permit diagnosis.
- Respiratory involvement, when present, is usually progressive over the first 24–48 hours, then gradually resolves 3–10 days following exposure. Animals that remain completely asymptomatic for 6–12 hours after ingestion are unlikely to develop respiratory illness.

Physical Examination Findings

- Characteristic hydrocarbon odor on the animal's breath or coat.
- Animals appear to experience a burning sensation in the mouth and pharynx after ingesting hydrocarbons, evidenced by slobbering, champing the jaws, shaking the head, and pawing at the muzzle.
- Fever in 3–4 hours following aspiration; may occur in less than an hour or as much as 24 hours.
- Vomiting, colic, and diarrhea after oral exposure. The severity and presence of such signs are a function of the dose and the individual hydrocarbon. Heavy aliphatic hydrocarbons (e.g., mineral oil) may produce mild diarrhea but little else. Lighter hydrocarbons (e.g., gasoline) are more likely to produce colic and vomiting.
- Intoxicated animals may exhibit vertigo, ataxia, and mental confusion. Hydrocarbons produce depression and narcosis in most cases, but tremors and convulsions have also been reported in a few cases. If the dose is very high, the animal may become comatose and die prior to exhibiting signs of pneumonitis, although this is very rare.
- Arrhythmias and syncope may occur as a result of myocardial sensitization to endogenous catecholamines. Myocardial sensitization may persist for 24–48 hours after apparent recovery from the neurologic effects of intoxication.

CAUSES

- Storage in inappropriate containers and failure to clean up spills.
- Folk remedies using gasoline, kerosene, and other solvents as tonics or vermifuges.
- Use of gasoline or other solvents to remove sticky material from an animal's coat. Cats may ingest significant amounts of gasoline or other hydrocarbons by grooming themselves after topical contamination.

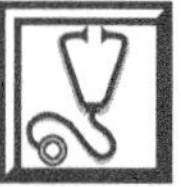

DIAGNOSIS

DIFFERENTIAL DIAGNOSIS

- Infectious diseases, toxins, and/or injuries may result in respiratory signs like hydrocarbon aspiration, but only very acute processes (e.g., trauma, chylothorax) exhibit a similar rapid onset.
- Acute ethylene glycol, ethanol, or drug intoxication.

CBC/BIOCHEMISTRY/URINALYSIS

- Urine and serum will be negative for ethylene glycol; serum osmolality will be normal.
- CBC may indicate stress, but this usually does not occur early in the process.

OTHER LABORATORY TESTS

- A simple spot test involves mixing vomitus or gastric contents vigorously with warm water. Gasoline or other petroleum distillates will float to the surface. Care must be taken to distinguish between petroleum products and dietary lipids. The former usually have a characteristic odor.

• Most petroleum products lighter than kerosene, if isolated and absorbed onto a paper towel, evaporate relatively quickly with little residue and have a characteristic odor.
• Chemical analysis of ingesta or post-mortem tissues is useful forensically but is not practical for clinical evaluation. If chemical analysis is conducted, samples must be taken quickly and frozen in airtight containers to prevent loss due to volatilization.

IMAGING

Radiographic findings are typical of aspiration pneumonia and consist of fine, perihilar densities and extensive infiltrates in ventral portions of the lungs. These are worst at 3–4 days, then gradually improve. Not all animals with radiographic signs of hydrocarbon aspiration develop respiratory signs, and radiographic changes usually persist past the resolution of clinical signs.

PATHOLOGIC FINDINGS

• If aspiration has occurred, the principle lesions will be in the respiratory tract. Pulmonary lesions are bilateral and typically involve caudoventral portions of the lung. The earliest lesions include hyperemia, edema, and hemorrhage into the airways. Foreign matter may be grossly visible in the smaller airways. Later, there is bronchospasm, emphysema, and atelectasis. Pneumatoceles, pneumothorax, and subcutaneous emphysema result from airway collapse. There may be ulcerations in the mucosa of the trachea and larger airways.
• Bacterial pneumonia occasionally supervenes and may result in abscesses.
• Systemic toxicity very occasionally results in hepatic, myocardial, and/or renal tubular necrosis if the animal survives >24 hours.

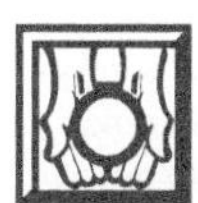

TREATMENT

APPROPRIATE HEALTH CARE

• In all cases of uncomplicated (i.e., not contaminated with some other, more toxic, substance) petroleum hydrocarbon ingestion, the primary goal is to minimize the risk of aspiration.
• If the amount ingested was small and the hydrocarbon ingested was one of the less volatile, more viscous products (e.g., motor oil, grease), cage rest and observation may be all that is required.
• Emetics and activated charcoal are not normally recommended due to potential vomiting and aspiration.
• If the volume ingested was substantial and the product involved known to cause systemic toxicity (e.g., gasoline) or if the product contains other, highly toxic substances (e.g., pesticides), gastric decontamination may be indicated, despite the risk of aspiration. It is essential that precautions (e.g., tracheal intubation) be taken to prevent possible aspiration of stomach contents. Emetics are contraindicated unless an absolute last resort.
• Respiratory effects should be treated symptomatically. Supplemental oxygen and mechanical ventilation should be used as needed. Pneumomediastinum, pneumatoceles, and pneumothorax are common complications so positive pressure systems must be used with caution. High-frequency jet ventilation reportedly results in fewer adverse sequelae than conventional mechanical ventilation. Since the lungs are the major route of systemic elimination for volatile hydrocarbons, closed or semi-closed systems should be purged frequently.
• Topical exposure may be treated by gently bathing with warm water and a mild detergent shampoo. If the hair coat is heavy or matted, it may be necessary to clip the contaminated areas.
• Symptomatic treatment of petroleum burns may involve topical antibacterials or other agents.
• Very viscous hydrocarbons (e.g., tar, waxes) may also be removed with mild detergents. They are not readily absorbed, pose only a cosmetic and skin irritation problem, and removal is not critical. Lipophilic materials (e.g., butter, lard, mechanic's hand cleaner) may also be useful, but the use of solvents is not recommended.

NURSING CARE

Cage rest is indicated, both for promotion of healing and to minimize the effects of excitement-induced catecholamines on a potentially sensitized myocardium.

CLIENT EDUCATION

Pet owners should be educated about proper storage and use of petroleum products.

MEDICATIONS

DRUG(S) OF CHOICE

• Historically, oral mineral or vegetable oil was recommended to increase the viscosity of petroleum hydrocarbons and decrease the risk of aspiration. Retrospective studies suggest that such treatment increases the likelihood of aspiration pneumonia, and the use of such oils is no longer recommended.
• The routine use of antibiotics is questionable. Hydrocarbon pneumonitis is largely nonbacterial in origin; however, given the potentially severe consequences and the relatively small downside to antibiotic use, it may be prudent to use antimicrobial prophylaxis if vomiting has occurred.
• Corticosteroids have been associated with increased numbers of positive lung cultures and are contraindicated.
• Bronchospasm may be treated with a beta-adrenergic agonist such as albuterol.

PRECAUTIONS

Emesis should only be used when there is a high degree of certainty that leaving the foreign material in the gut poses a greater hazard than aspiration.

FOLLOW-UP

PATIENT MONITORING

Monitor patients for 3–4 days to ensure that ingested hydrocarbons have cleared the gastrointestinal tract and no pulmonary sequelae will occur.

EXPECTED COURSE AND PROGNOSIS

The diversity of this class of products precludes absolute prediction, but most hydrocarbon exposures respond well to conservative, supportive therapy.

MISCELLANEOUS

Suggested Reading

Balme KH, Zar H, Swift DK, Mann MD. The efficacy of prophylactic antibiotics in the management of children with kerosene-associated pneumonitis: a double-blind randomized controlled trial. Clin Toxicol (Phila). 2015 Jun 26:1–8.

Reese E, Kimbrough RD. Acute toxicity of gasoline and some additives. Environ Health Perspect 1993, 101:115–131.

Seymour FK, Henry JA. Assessment and management of acute poisoning by petroleum products. Hum Exp Toxicol 2001, 20:551–562.

Author Merl F. Raisbeck
Consulting Editor Lynn R. Hovda

P

PHEOCHROMOCYTOMA

BASICS

DEFINITION

A tumor arising from catecholamine-producing chromaffin cells that originate from neural crest cells within the adrenal medulla.

PATHOPHYSIOLOGY

Clinical signs develop as a result of the space-occupying nature of the tumor and its metastases or from excessive secretion of catecholamines (e.g., causing hypertension or tachycardia). Signs of catecholamine release may be constant or intermittent. Paragangliomas are catecholamine-secreting tumors that arise from cells in the sympathetic ganglia.

SYSTEMS AFFECTED

- Cardiovascular.
- Neurologic.
- Renal.
- Respiratory.

INCIDENCE/PREVALENCE

Uncommon disease in dogs; rare in cats.

SIGNALMENT

Species

Dog and cat.

Breed Predilections

None

Mean Age and Range

- Median age in dogs is 11 years; range is 1–16 years.
- Older cats.

SIGNS

General Comments

- The predominant clinical signs result from alpha-mediated vasoconstriction and beta-mediated cardiac effects that cause systemic hypertension or tachyarrhythmias.
- Signs of hypertension may be constant or paroxysmal. Signs may be present for more than a year or develop suddenly, resulting in death.
- 30% of cases are asymptomatic and only identified at necropsy.

Historical Findings

- Clinical signs are often episodic or acute.
- Generalized weakness and lethargy are common.
- Collapse.
- Anorexia.
- Vomiting.
- Weight loss.
- Panting, dyspnea.
- Diarrhea.
- Whining, pacing.
- Ascites, edema.
- Polyuria and polydipsia.
- Shaking/shivering.
- Epistaxis.

Physical Examination Findings

- May be normal.
- Panting, tachypnea, dyspnea.
- Pale or hyperemic mucous membranes.
- Dehydration and/or hypovolemic shock.
- Thin, muscle wasting.
- Abdominal pain.
- Weakness.
- Blindness/retinal detachment.
- Cardiac arrhythmias.
- Peripheral edema.
- Ascites.
- Abdominal mass.

CAUSES

Chromaffin cell tumor.

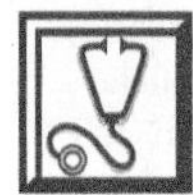

DIAGNOSIS

DIFFERENTIAL DIAGNOSIS

- Hyperadrenocorticism.
- Hyperaldosteronism.
- Essential hypertension (cats).
- Renal disease with secondary hypertension.
- Other abdominal neoplasia, especially adrenocortical tumor (adenoma vs. adenocarcinoma).
- Paraganglioma (rare).

CBC/BIOCHEMISTRY/URINALYSIS

- Nonregenerative anemia.
- Hemoconcentration.
- Leukocytosis.
- Mild hyperglycemia.
- Mild azotemia.
- Increased liver enzyme activities.
- Hypoalbuminemia.
- Proteinuria.

OTHER LABORATORY TESTS

Arterial Blood Pressure

Systolic >160 mmHg or diastolic >100 mmHg represents significant hypertension. Only 50% of animals with pheochromocytoma are hypertensive when blood pressure is measured because of the episodic nature of secretion of catecholamines from the tumor.

Electrocardiography

Sinus tachycardia is the most common arrhythmia; ventricular premature contractions or ventricular tachycardia less common.

IMAGING

Abdominal Radiography

- Abdominal mass.
- Mineralization of the adrenal mass (rare).
- Hepatomegaly.
- Renal displacement.
- Abnormal renal contour.
- Ascites.
- Enlargement of the caudal venal cava.

Thoracic Radiography

- Generalized cardiomegaly.
- Pulmonary congestion or edema.

Abdominal Ultrasonography

- Adrenal mass.
- Tumor invasion of the caudal vena cava and other adjacent structures (does not differentiate pheochromocytoma from other adrenocortical tumor).
- Intra-abdominal and liver metastasis.

Other Imaging Modalities

- CT scan and MRI to evaluate invasion of nearby structures; superior to ultrasound for surgical planning.
- Scintigraphy using ^{123}I-meta-iodobenzyl-guanidine scan.

DIAGNOSTIC PROCEDURES

- The plasma half-life of catecholamines is short (1–3 minutes), and release from pheochomocytomas is episodic. However, catecholamine metabolites (metanephrines—normetanephrine and metanephrine) constantly leak into peripheral circulation. Thus, measurement of metanephrines is preferred over measurement of catecholamines. Urinary normetanephrine:creatinine ratio is superior to the metanephrine:creatinine ratio for differentiating pheochromocytoma from hyperadrenocorticism (HAC). Additionally, using plasma normetanephrine concentrations is better than metanephrine concentrations.
- Urinary metanephrine:creatinine and normetanephrine:creatinine ratios:
  - Urine must be acidified soon after collection, and shipped cold. Follow the specific instructions of the laboratory used; laboratory may provide a special tube with acid for shipping.
  - In the United States, Marshfield Labs will run these ratios and provides canine reference ranges.
  - No vanilla ingestion, drugs (including phenoxybenzamine), or radiographic contrast agents prior to obtaining the urine sample.
  - Urine normetanephine:creatinine ratio greater than 4 times the upper limit of the reference range is consistent with a diagnosis of pheochromocytoma. Some cases may have ratios between (or below) 2 and 4 times the upper limit, but so do some cases of HAC.
- Inhibin concentration:
  - In one study, inhibin concentrations were found to be very low in neutered patients with and without pheochromocytoma, whereas the concentrations were higher in patients with adrenocortical tumors. Thus, it could be used to differentiate between pheochromocytoma and HAC in neutered dogs.
  - No longer commercially available.

PATHOLOGIC FINDINGS

Immunohistochemical staining of tumor tissues with chromogranin A or synaptophysin allows differentiation of pheochromocytomas from other tumor types.

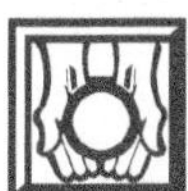

TREATMENT

APPROPRIATE HEALTH CARE

- Surgical removal of the tumor is the treatment of choice.
- Medical therapy is most commonly used to stabilize patients prior to surgery, but may be elected as the sole therapy if the patient is not a surgical candidate due to vascular invasion or other factors. If the patient is not a surgical candidate, phenoxybenzamine, with or without atenolol, is used, as described under Drug(s) of Choice.

CLIENT EDUCATION

Survival times may be as long as 3 years following successful resection of tumor. Perioperative mortality is 20–30%, and decreased survival is associated with larger tumors (>5 cm) and invasion of nearby structures (such as the vena cava). In cats, removal of tumor is often curative; these are often benign, in contrast to the malignant tumors seen in dogs.

SURGICAL CONSIDERATIONS

Preoperative Care

Medications as described under Drug(s) of Choice.

Complications and Patient Monitoring

Common complications—hypertension, severe tachycardia, other cardiac arrhythmias, and hypovolemia/hypotension. Postoperative thromboembolism has been reported.

Anesthesia

- A balanced anesthetic protocol should be used, with close monitoring of arterial blood pressure, urine output, patient volume status, and analgesia. Patients should have a blood type performed prior to surgery, and adequate blood products available in the event of perioperative hemorrhage.
- Anticipate cardiac arrhythmias (brady and tachyarrhythmias); ECG monitoring should be initiated prior to and during anesthetic induction.

Surgery

Unilateral adrenalectomy and often thrombectomy. Manipulation of the tumor may cause severe hypertension if patient is not properly premedicated.

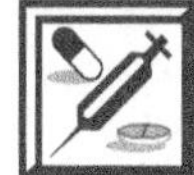

MEDICATIONS

DRUG(S) OF CHOICE

- Phenoxybenzamine 0.2–1.5 mg/kg PO q12h, should be given for 2 weeks prior to surgery. Start at 0.25 mg/kg twice daily and increase every 2–3 days to a final dose of 1 mg/kg twice daily. Monitor blood pressure and decrease dose if hypotension occurs.
- Atenolol, a β_1-selective antagonist 0.2–1 mg/kg PO q12–24h to control clinically significant supraventricular tachycardia. Do not use a beta-blocker prior to using an alpha-blocker for at least 2 days, as hypertension may become more severe.
- In the anesthetized patient or emergent patient with critical unresponsive supraventricular tachycardia—esmolol 0.05–0.5 mg/kg IV followed by 0.01–0.2 mg/kg/min IV may be used.
- In the anesthetized patient or emergent patient with critical unresponsive hypertension—nitroprusside 0.0005–0.005 mg/kg/min IV may be used.

CONTRAINDICATIONS

Severe hypertension can develop if a non-selective beta-blocker (e.g., propranolol) is used without prior alpha-adrenergic blockade (e.g., phentolamine, phenoxybenzamine).

PRECAUTIONS

Nonselective beta-blockade without alpha-blockade can lead to fatal hypertension.

ALTERNATIVE DRUG(S)

Prazosin 0.5–2.5 mg/dog PO q12h is an alpha-blocking drug that can be used if phenoxybenzamine is not available.

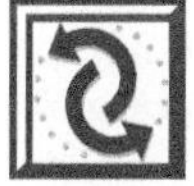

FOLLOW-UP

PATIENT MONITORING

Blood pressure, urine output, and ECG should be closely monitored in the immediate postoperative period (24–72 hours).

POSSIBLE COMPLICATIONS

Perioperative—intra-abdominal hemorrhage, hypotension, peritonitis, sepsis.

EXPECTED COURSE AND PROGNOSIS

Prognosis is guarded to fair. Dogs that survive the perioperative period may survive for 2–3 years or longer. Patients that are medically managed can live more than a year.

MISCELLANEOUS

ASSOCIATED CONDITIONS

Multiple endocrine neoplasia types II and III.

PREGNANCY/FERTILITY/BREEDING

N/A

SEE ALSO

Hypertension, Systemic Arterial.

ABBREVIATIONS

- ECG = electrocardiogram.
- HAC = hyperadrenocorticism.

Suggested Reading

Barrera J, Bernard F, Ehrhart J, et al. Evaluation of risk factors for outcome associated with adrenal gland tumors with or without invasion of the vena cava and treated via adrenalectomy in dogs: 86 cases (1993–2009). J Am Vet Med Assoc 2013, 242:1715–1721.

Bathez PY, Marks SL, Woo J, et al. Pheochromocytoma in dogs: 61 cases (1984–1995). J Vet Intern Med 1997, 11(5):272–278.

Kook PH, Grest P, Quante S, et al. Urinary catecholamine and metadrenaline to creatinine ratios in dogs with a phaeochromocytoma. Vet Rec 2010, 166(6):169–174.

Kyles AE, Feldman EC, De Cock HEV, et al. Surgical management of adrenal gland tumors with and without associated tumor thrombi in dogs: 40 cases (1994–2001). J Am Vet Med Assoc 2003, 223:654–662.

Reusch C. Pheochromocytoma and multiple endocrine neoplasia. In: Feldman EC, Nelson RW, Reusch CE, Scott-Moncrieff JCR, eds., Feline and Canine Endocrinology, 4th ed. Philadelphia, PA: Saunders, 2015, pp. 521–549.

Author Patty A. Lathan

Consulting Editor Patty A. Lathan

Acknowledgment The author/editor acknowledges the prior contribution of Deborah S. Greco.

PHOSPHOFRUCTOKINASE DEFICIENCY

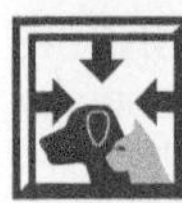

BASICS

OVERVIEW

• Phosphofructokinase is the most important rate-controlling enzyme in glycolysis, and red blood cells (RBCs) and intensely exercising skeletal muscles depend heavily on anaerobic glycolysis for energy.
• Affected dogs have compensated hemolytic anemia and mild myopathy caused by markedly reduced total phosphofructokinase activity in both tissues.
• Anemia develops because of insufficient generation of ATP to maintain normal RBC shape, ionic composition, and deformability and because RBCs from affected dogs are alkaline fragile and lyse when blood pH is slightly high.

SIGNALMENT

• English springer spaniel, American cocker spaniel, mixed-breed, whippet, and wachtelhund dogs are overrepresented.
• Transmitted as an autosomal recessive trait.
• Affected homozygous animals generally not recognized as abnormal before age 1.

SIGNS

• Some animals exhibit mild clinical signs that go unrecognized for years; others regularly exhibit episodes of severe illness.
• Depression or weakness concomitant with episodes of pigmenturia.
• Mild lethargy with slight fever during mild hemolytic episodes.
• Marked lethargy, weakness, pale or icteric mucous membranes, mild hepatosplenomegaly, and fever as high as 106°F (41°C) during severe hemolytic crises.
• Intravascular hemolysis can be caused by hyperventilation-induced alkalemia associated with exercise or excitement.
• Signs of muscle dysfunction—usually limited to exercise intolerance and slightly diminished muscle mass, but muscle cramping and severe progressive myopathy can occur.
• Two affected whippets had progressive cardiac disease in addition to muscle cramping after exercise.
• Heterozygous carrier animals appear clinically normal.

CAUSES & RISK FACTORS

Deficiency of the muscle-type subunit of phosphofructokinase—markedly reduced total activity in RBCs and skeletal muscle.

DIAGNOSIS

DIFFERENTIAL DIAGNOSIS

• Other causes of hemolytic anemia—immune-mediated hemolytic anemia, hemotropic mycoplasmosis, babesiosis, Heinz body anemia, microangiopathic hemolytic anemia, and pyruvate kinase deficiency.
• Affected dogs—negative Coombs' test, no parasites or Heinz bodies in stained blood films, seronegative for *Babesia* spp., and no evidence of disseminated intravascular coagulation or heartworm disease.
• Differentiated from pyruvate kinase deficiency by specific enzyme assays or DNA test.

CBC/BIOCHEMISTRY/URINALYSIS

• Persistent compensated hemolytic anemia.
• Mean cell volume usually 80–90 fL.
• Reticulocyte counts generally 10–30% of the total RBC number.
• Hematocrit values generally 30–40%; during hemolytic crises may decrease to ≤15%.
• Bilirubinuria—often markedly high in male dogs.
• Hemoglobinuria in association with episodes of intravascular hemolysis.
• Serum biochemical analysis—slight elevations of serum potassium, magnesium, calcium, urea, total protein, and globulin concentrations and aspartate aminotransferase activity; slight to moderate elevation of serum iron and bilirubin concentrations and lactate dehydrogenase and alkaline phosphatase activities; marked hyperbilirubinemia during hemolytic crisis; marked azotemia if renal failure develops secondary to pigmentary nephropathy or shock.

OTHER LABORATORY TESTS

• RBC phosphofructokinase activity—identifiable in affected animals older than 3 months; heterozygous carriers have approximately one-half normal activity.
• DNA testing to differentiate normal and carrier animals of any age. Wachtelhund dogs have a genetic mutation different from other dog breeds (http://research.vet.upenn.edu/penngen).

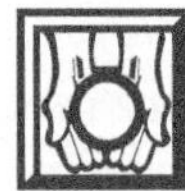

TREATMENT

• Bone marrow transplantation is the only cure.
• In patients with severe intravascular hemolysis, IV fluid therapy minimizes the chance of acute renal failure.
• Blood transfusions, if anemia becomes life-threatening.

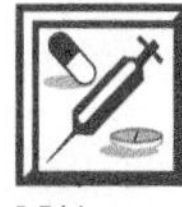

MEDICATIONS

N/A

FOLLOW-UP

• Infrequently, affected dogs may die during a hemolytic crisis because of anemia or renal failure.
• Affected animals can have a normal lifespan if properly managed.
• Owners should avoid placing affected dogs in stressful situations or subjecting them to strenuous exercise, excitement, or high environmental temperatures.

MISCELLANEOUS

ABBREVIATIONS

• RBC = red blood cell.

INTERNET RESOURCES

http://research.vet.upenn.edu/penngen

Suggested Reading

Inal Gultekin G, Raj K, Lehman S, et al. Missense mutation in PFKM associated with muscle-type phosphofructokinase deficiency in the Wachtelhund dog. Mol Cell Probes 2012, 26:243–247.

Owen JL, Harvey JW. Hemolytic anemia in dogs and cats due to erythrocyte enzyme deficiencies. Vet Clin North Am Small Anim Pract 2012, 42:73–84.

Author John W. Harvey
Consulting Editor Melinda S. Camus

BASICS

OVERVIEW

• *Physaloptera* spp. are parasitic nematodes that occur in dogs and cats; adults attach to stomach mucosa; no larval migration occurs outside the gastrointestinal tract.
• Infection can be asymptomatic or cause gastritis and vomiting.
• Typically, few worms are present; single-worm or all-female infections are common.
• Transmitted by ingestion of infective larvae in intermediate hosts (e.g., coprophagous grubs, beetles, cockroaches, crickets) or in paratenic hosts (e.g., birds, rodents, frogs, snakes, lizards).

SIGNALMENT

Dogs and cats; any breed, age, or sex. Infected animals often undergo extensive workups for suspected inflammatory bowel disease/ulcers, only for the nematodes to be discovered via endoscopy.

SIGNS

• Vomiting, often chronic and intermittent; occasionally find worms in vomitus.
• Weight loss can occur, especially with chronic infection.
• Signs can occur without egg production during prepatent period, single-worm, or female-only infections.
• Possible melena, especially in cats.

CAUSES & RISK FACTORS

• Outdoor exposure—access to insect intermediate hosts or small vertebrate transport hosts.
• Access to habitat occupied by wildlife species (raccoon, fox, coyote, bobcat, cougar, badger, skunk) infected with *Physaloptera*.

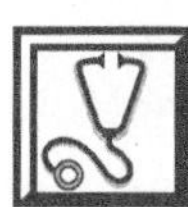

DIAGNOSIS

DIFFERENTIAL DIAGNOSIS

• Other infectious causes of vomiting including parasite, viral, or bacterial infections.
• *Spirocerca*, the esophageal worm—produces similar but smaller eggs (11–15 × 30–37 µm).
• *Ollulanus*, a trichostrongylid nematode, can cause chronic vomiting; seen mainly in colony and feral cats; larvae and adults (<1 mm long) but no eggs present in vomitus or feces.
• Roundworms (ascarids) in puppies and kittens—worms can be present in feces and vomitus; larger than *Physaloptera*; characterized by three lips and cervical alae.
• Other noninfectious causes of vomiting including dietary indiscretion, foreign objects in the stomach, noxious substances accidentally ingested, gastrointestinal neoplasia, metabolic diseases.

CBC/BIOCHEMISTRY/URINALYSIS

Mild anemia and eosinophilia can occur.

OTHER LABORATORY TESTS

N/A

IMAGING

Abdominal radiography and ultrasonography, to eliminate other causes of vomiting.

DIAGNOSTIC PROCEDURES

• Endoscopy (gastroscopy) to visualize and remove worms, usually attached to stomach or duodenal mucosa; careful, thorough exam necessary to detect all worms; typically few are present and they can be hidden by mucus, ingesta, stomach rugae; pinpoint hemorrhages from prior attachment sites can be seen:
  ◦ *Physaloptera* spp. are small (2.5–5 cm long), stout, white or pink, with an anterior cuticular collar; male and female *P. praeputialis* have a posterior prepuce-like cuticular sheath.
• Direct smear, wet mount, or fecal flotation to detect eggs in vomitus or feces; prepatent period is 2–5 months; eggs are dense and can be difficult to detect by fecal flotation using low specific gravity solutions; use flotation solution with specific gravity >1.25:
  ◦ Eggs are small (42–58 × 29–42 µm), thick-shelled, larvated, ovoid to ellipsoidal, often clear and colorless.

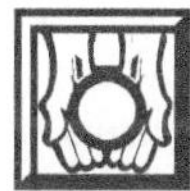

TREATMENT

• Outpatient treatment; anthelmintic with or without endoscopic removal of worms.
• Anthelmintic use is extra-label and anecdotal.

MEDICATIONS

DRUG(S) OF CHOICE

• Pyrantel pamoate (dogs/cats) 20 mg/kg PO every 2 weeks for at least 3 treatments; repeat if signs persist; treatment of choice.
• Fenbendazole (dogs) 50 mg/kg PO q24h for 3–5 days; repeat if signs persist.
• Ivermectin (cats) 0.2 mg/kg PO, SC, once.
• Medication to reduce gastritis—histamine H_2-antagonists (e.g., famotidine 0.5 mg/kg PO q12h); sucralfate 0.25–1 g PO q8–12h.

FOLLOW-UP

PATIENT MONITORING

Recheck 1–2 weeks post treatment and re-treat with anthelmintic if eggs still present on fecal exam and/or if vomiting persists.

PREVENTION/AVOIDANCE

• Prompt removal and disposal of feces to prevent infection of arthropod intermediate hosts.
• Prevent exposure to arthropod intermediate hosts.
• No products approved specifically for *Physaloptera* spp. prevention or control; monthly intestinal parasite control likely effective to limit infections.

EXPECTED COURSE AND PROGNOSIS

Clinical signs and/or shedding of eggs in feces should resolve within 2 weeks of treatment.

MISCELLANEOUS

INTERNET RESOURCES

http://www.capcvet.org

Suggested Reading

Campbell KL, Graham JC. Physaloptera infection in dogs and cats. Compend Contin Educ Pract Vet 1999, 21:299–314.

Authors Matt Brewer and Jeba R.J. Jesudoss Chelladurai

Consulting Editor Amie Koenig

PLAGUE

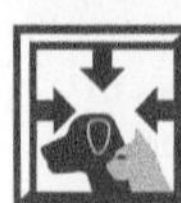

BASICS

OVERVIEW

• *Yersinia pestis*—Gram-negative, bipolar staining rod; reservoir: wild rodents (sylvatic), ground squirrels, prairie dogs, rabbits, bobcats, coyotes. • Occurs worldwide; movement of animals results in occurrence in non-endemic areas. • United States—Western states/Hawaii. • Common May–October. • Bacterium transmitted by infected fleas, also by ingestion of infected rodents; incubation period 2–7 days after infection. • Bacteria migrate from skin lymphatics to regional lymph nodes (LN), survive phagocytosis and multiply in LN; phagocytic cells rupture. • Fever and painful lymphadenopathy (bubo); intense local inflammation results in bubonic plague; intermittent bacteremia; LN rupture; may become septicemic with or without LN involvement. • Cats—severe fatal disease. • Dogs—naturally resistant. • Potential bioterrorist agent (beware of clusters of cases).

P

SIGNALMENT

Cat and rarely dog.

SIGNS

• Dogs—exhibit mild fever/depression. • Cats—exhibit bubonic/pneumonic/septicemic forms. • Bubonic (cats): ◦ Most common form. ◦ Buboes—head and neck; marked lymphadenopathy; if patient survives long enough, LN abscess, rupture, form fistulae to skin. ◦ Fever: 103–105°F (39.5–40.5°C). ◦ Lethargy, ataxia, coma. ◦ Enlarged tonsils, oral ulcers. ◦ Vomiting, diarrhea, anorexia. ◦ Dehydration. ◦ Ocular discharge. ◦ Weight loss. • Septicemic (cats): ◦ Rare. ◦ Septicemia without lymphadenopathy or abscess formation. ◦ Other signs same as bubonic. • Pneumonic (cats): ◦ Severe disease; greatest risk for spread to humans (euthanasia strongly recommended to prevent zoonotic spread).

CAUSES & RISK FACTORS

• Outdoor, hunting cats. • Travel to endemic areas. • Environment—heavy flea infestation, large nearby rodent populations. • More common as homes encroach on wildlife habitats in plague-endemic areas.

DIAGNOSIS

DIFFERENTIAL DIAGNOSIS

Infection (feline calicivirus, feline coronavirus, feline immunodeficiency virus, feline leukemia virus, cryptococcosis, histoplasmosis, toxoplasmosis, tularemia, leishmaniasis), neoplasia, drug eruption/skin hypersensitivity, epidermolysis bullosa, pemphigus, systemic lupus erythematosus, oropharyngeal foreign body, trauma, gingivitis, stomatitis, osteomyelitis, sequestrum.

CBC/BIOCHEMISTRY/URINALYSIS

• Leukocytosis: left shift/marked toxic change. • Thrombocytopenia. • High liver enzyme activity and hyperbilirubinemia.

OTHER LABORATORY TESTS

• Serology—Communicable Disease Center/state health department. • Fluorescent antibody test—presumptive identification. • Molecular testing—PCR of blood/tissues. • Coagulation profile—prolonged with consumptive coagulopathy.

DIAGNOSTIC PROCEDURES

• Culture is definitive; sample abscess, LN, peripheral blood before treatment is given or culture from post-mortem tissue (LN, abscess, liver, spleen). • Impression smears of tissue—large numbers of Gram-negative coccobacilli with bipolar staining. • Thoracic radiographs may show nodular lesions with pneumonic plague.

PATHOLOGIC FINDINGS

• Acutely ill cats—few lesions; enlarged head and neck LN; enlarged liver and spleen. • LN—destruction of normal architecture, hemorrhagic necrosis, extracellular bacteria.

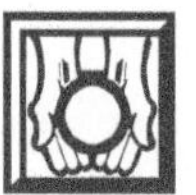

TREATMENT

• Inpatient. • High mortality if not treated early. • Treat sepsis aggressively (see Sepsis and Bacteremia). • Treat for fleas.

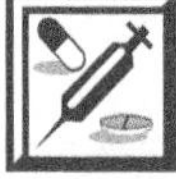

MEDICATIONS

DRUG(S) OF CHOICE

• Treat all suspect cases empirically pending confirmation. • Systemic antimicrobials: ◦ Tetracycline 20 mg/kg PO q8h for 21–42 days. ◦ Doxycycline 5–10 mg/kg PO q12h; likely effective (not definitively established). ◦ Chloramphenicol 30–50 mg/kg PO q8h. ◦ Aminoglycosides, trimethoprim-sulfamethoxazole—also likely effective. • Coordinate with public health officials; bioengineered strains may be drug resistant.

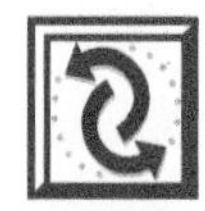

FOLLOW-UP

PATIENT MONITORING

Consumptive coagulopathy common later in infection.

PREVENTION/AVOIDANCE

• Avoid travel to endemic areas. • Endemic areas—keep pet on leash; use flea control on pet and home. • Limit cat hunting behavior/rodent exposure. • Eliminate rodents/habitats near houses/outbuildings; store food in rodent-proof containers.

EXPECTED COURSE AND PROGNOSIS

• Duration of illness variable. • Prognosis—poor if not treated early. • Pneumonic plague has greatest risk of death.

MISCELLANEOUS

ZOONOTIC POTENTIAL

High

CDC Recommendations

• Notify public health officials. • Avoid contact with infectious materials from patient, fleas. • Disinfect/autoclave/incinerate any material used in examination of patients. • Isolate patients and wear mask/gloves when handling. • Assess pulmonary involvement. • Use respirator/protective eye equipment during necropsies. • Monitor staff for 2 weeks post exposure; discuss postexposure prophylaxis/fever watch with health care provider.

ABBREVIATIONS

• LN = lymph node.

INTERNET RESOURCES

• http://www.cfsph.iastate.edu/DiseaseInfo/disease.php?name=plague&lang=en • https://www.cdc.gov/plague/prevention/index.html

Suggested Reading

Kassem AM, Tengelsen L, Atkins B, et al. Notes from the field: plague in domestic cats—Idaho, 2016. Morb Mortal Wkly Rep 2016, 65:1378–1379.

Pennisi MG, Egberink H, et al. *Yersina pestis* infection in cats: ABCD guidelines on prevention and management. J Feline Med Surg 2013, 15:582–584.

Author Patrick L. McDonough

Consulting Editor Amie Koenig

PLASMACYTOMA, MUCOCUTANEOUS

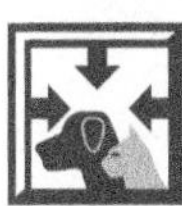

BASICS

OVERVIEW

- Tumor of plasma cell origin.
- Typically benign and local therapy can be curative.
- Rarely (<1%) part of multiple myeloma process.
- Gastrointestinal extramedullary plasmacytoma (GI EMP) may be more aggressive.

SIGNALMENT

- Dog, rarely cat.
- Cocker spaniel, West Highland white terrier, boxer, German shepherd dog, Airedale.
- Median age 9–10 years.

SIGNS

- 86% are cutaneous, 9% affect mucous membranes, 4% colorectal, 1% noncutaneous/non-oral.
- Solitary, smooth, raised pink nodules, typically 1–2 cm in diameter.
- Bleeding, hematochezia, tenesmus, rectal prolapse if colorectal form.
- Vague, nonspecific signs if GI EMP.

CAUSES & RISK FACTORS

Unknown

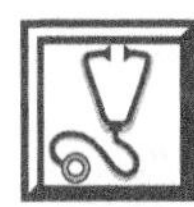

DIAGNOSIS

DIFFERENTIAL DIAGNOSIS

- Other round cell tumor types including lymphoma, mast cell tumor, histiocytoma, transmissible venereal tumor.
- Poorly differentiated carcinoma.
- Amelanotic melanoma.

CBC/BIOCHEMISTRY/URINALYSIS

Usually normal for EMP

OTHER LABORATORY TESTS

Bone marrow aspirate cytology and serum electrophoresis may be indicated for GI EMP.

IMAGING

- Colonoscopy recommended for colorectal EMP.
- Thoracic radiographs and abdominal ultrasound may be indicated for GI EMP.

DIAGNOSTIC PROCEDURES

- Cytologic examination of fine-needle aspirate reveals moderate to marked cellularity with round to polyhedral individual tumor cells with discrete margins, abundant royal blue cytoplasm, paranuclear clear zone, eccentric round nucleus, and clumped chromatin. Multinuclearity is common.
- Histologic evaluation—classified into mature, hyaline, cleaved, asynchronous, monomorphous blastic, and polymorphous blastic cell types. However, no prognostic significance has been associated with this classification.
- Immunohistochemistry may be necessary to distinguish from other neoplasms.

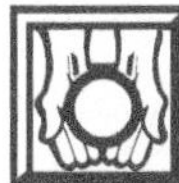

TREATMENT

- Conservative surgery.
- Radiation therapy if nonresectable.

MEDICATIONS

DRUG(S) OF CHOICE

Melphalan and prednisone or single-agent lomustine may be indicated in GI EMP or multiple tumors.

CONTRAINDICATIONS/POSSIBLE INTERACTIONS

N/A

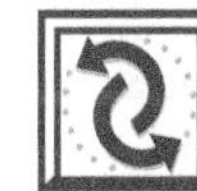

FOLLOW-UP

PATIENT MONITORING

Reevaluation every 3 months to monitor for local tumor control and metastases.

EXPECTED COURSE AND PROGNOSIS

- Excellent in most patients.
- Long-term survival expected for GI EMP treated with surgery ± chemotherapy.
- Reported 15-month median survival time for colorectal form with surgery alone.
- 5% local recurrence rate with conservative surgery for the majority of EMP.
- Metastasis reported in 2% of patients with EMP.
- 2% of patients will develop *de novo* EMP.

MISCELLANEOUS

ASSOCIATED CONDITIONS

- Multiple myeloma.
- Lymphoma—dogs.
- Cats—may note systemic amyloidosis.

SEE ALSO

- Amyloidosis.
- Lymphoma—Dogs.
- Multiple Myeloma.

ABBREVIATIONS

- EMP = extramedullary plasmacytoma.
- GI = gastrointestinal.

Suggested Reading

Cangul IT, Wijnen M, Van Garderen E, et al. Clinico-pathological aspects of canine cutaneous and mucocutaneous plasmacytomas. J Vet Med A Physiol Pathol Clin Med 2002, 49(6):307–312.

Morrison WB. Plasma cell neoplasms. In: Morrison WB, ed., Cancer in Dogs and Cats: Medical and Surgical Management. Jackson, WY: Teton NewMedia, 2002, pp. 671–677.

Vail D. Myeloma-Related Disorders. In: Withrow SJ, Vail DM, Page RL, eds., Small Animal Clinical Oncology, 5th ed. St. Louis, MO: Elsevier Saunders, 2013, pp. 665–678.

Author Shawna L. Klahn

Consulting Editor Timothy M. Fan

PLEURAL EFFUSION

BASICS

DEFINITION

Abnormal accumulation of fluid within the pleural cavity.

PATHOPHYSIOLOGY

• More than normal production or less than normal resorption of fluid. • Alterations in hydrostatic and oncotic pressures or vascular permeability and lymphatic function may contribute to fluid accumulation.

SYSTEMS AFFECTED

• Cardiovascular. • Respiratory.

SIGNALMENT

Species

Dog and cat.

Breed Predilections

Varies with underlying cause.

Mean Age and Range

• Young animals—more commonly infection.
• Old animals—more commonly cardiac or neoplastic.

Predominant Sex

Varies with underlying cause.

SIGNS

General Comments

Depend on the fluid volume, rapidity of fluid accumulation, and the underlying cause.

Historical Findings

• Dyspnea. • Tachypnea. • Orthopnea.
• Open-mouth breathing. • Cyanosis.
• Exercise intolerance. • Lethargy.
• Inappetence. • Cough.

Physical Examination Findings

• Dyspnea—respirations often shallow and rapid.
• Muffled or inaudible heart and lung sounds ventrally. • Preservation of breath sounds dorsally. • Dullness ventrally on thoracic percussion.

CAUSES

High Hydrostatic Pressure

• Congestive heart failure (CHF).
• Overhydration. • Intrathoracic neoplasia.

Low Oncotic Pressure

Hypoalbuminemia—occurs in protein-losing enteropathy, protein-losing nephropathy, and liver disease.

Vascular or Lymphatic Abnormality

• Infectious—bacterial, viral, or fungal.
• Neoplasia (e.g., mediastinal lymphoma, thymoma, mesothelioma, primary lung tumor, and metastatic disease). • Chylothorax (e.g., from lymphangiectasia, CHF, cranial vena caval obstruction [sometimes associated with transvenous pacemaker implantation], neoplasia, fungal infections, heartworms, diaphragmatic hernia, lung lobe torsion, trauma). • Diaphragmatic hernia.
• Hemothorax (e.g., from trauma, neoplasia, coagulopathy, *Angiostrongylus vasorum*).
• Lung lobe torsion. • Pulmonary thromboembolism. • Pancreatitis.

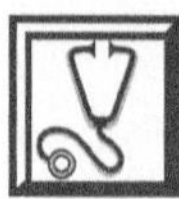

DIAGNOSIS

DIFFERENTIAL DIAGNOSIS

• Historical or physical evidence of external trauma—consider hemothorax or diaphragmatic hernia. • Fever suggests an inflammatory, infectious, or neoplastic cause.
• Murmurs, gallops, or arrhythmias combined with jugular venous distension or pulsation suggest an underlying cardiac cause.
• Concurrent ascites suggests feline infectious peritonitis (FIP), CHF (mainly dogs), severe hypoalbuminemia, diaphragmatic hernia, disseminated neoplasia, or pancreatitis. • In cats, decreased compressibility of the cranial thorax suggests a cranial mediastinal mass.
• Concurrent ocular changes (e.g., chorioretinitis and uveitis) suggest FIP or fungal disease. • Hypothermia often associated with cardiac cause.

CBC/BIOCHEMISTRY/URINALYSIS

• Hemogram results may be abnormal in patients with pyothorax, FIP, neoplasia, or lung lobe torsion. • Severe hypoalbuminemia (generally <1 g/dL to cause effusion) suggests protein-losing enteropathy, protein-losing nephropathy, or liver disease.
• Hyperglobulinemia (polyclonal) suggests FIP.

OTHER LABORATORY TESTS

• Fluid analysis should include physical characteristics (i.e., color, clarity, odor, clots), pH, glucose, total protein, total nucleated cell count, and cytologic examination; Table 1 provides characteristics of various pleural fluid types and their disease associations. • In cats the lactate dehydrogenase concentration in transudates is <200 IU/L and in exudates it is >200 IU/L. • Pleural fluid pH <6.9 suggests pyothorax in cats. • Glucose concentration in pleural fluid usually parallels levels in serum. In cats, pyothorax and malignancy lower pleural fluid glucose concentration relative to serum glucose concentration; thus, pleural fluid with a normal pH and low glucose concentration suggests malignancy in cats. • Serologic tests for feline leukemia virus (if patient has mediastinal lymphoma), feline immunodeficiency virus (if patient has pyothorax), and coronavirus (if FIP is suspected) are available. • Cardiac disease suspected—consider a heartworm test in dogs and cats; NT-proBNP and thyroid evaluation in cats.
• Infection suspected—obtain aerobic and anaerobic bacterial culture and sensitivity tests and consider special stains (e.g., Gram and acid-fast stains) of the fluid. • FIP suspected—consider protein electrophoresis of the fluid; gamma-globulin level >32% of total protein strongly suggests a diagnosis of FIP. • Chyle suspected—do an ether clearance test or Sudan stain of the pleural fluid, and triglyceride and cholesterol evaluations of the fluid and serum.

IMAGING

Radiographic Findings

• Used to confirm pleural effusion; should not be performed until after thoracocentesis in dyspneic patients with evidence of pleural effusion on physical examination. • Evidence of pleural effusion includes separation of lung borders away from the thoracic wall and sternum by fluid density in the pleural space, fluid-filled interlobar fissure lines, loss or blurring of the cardiac and diaphragmatic borders, blunting of the lung margins at the costophrenic angles (ventrodorsal view), and widening of the mediastinum (ventrodorsal view). • Rounding of the caudal lung lobe borders (lateral view)—most common in patients with fibrosing pleuritis caused by chylothorax, pyothorax, or FIP. • Unilateral effusion—most common in patients with chylothorax and pyothorax; hemothorax, pulmonary neoplasia, diaphragmatic hernia, and lung lobe torsion. • Evaluate post-thoracocentesis radiographs carefully for cardiomegaly, intrapulmonary lesions, mediastinal masses, diaphragmatic hernia, lung lobe torsion, and evidence of trauma (e.g., rib fractures). • Can diagnose a diaphragmatic hernia with positive-contrast peritoneography. • Can evaluate the thoracic duct by positive-contrast lymphangiography.
• CT imaging may help differentiate malignant from inflammatory effusions.

Echocardiographic Findings

• Ultrasonographic evaluation of the thorax is recommended whenever cardiac disease, diaphragmatic hernia, or cranial mediastinal mass is suspected. • Echocardiography is easiest to perform before thoracocentesis, provided the patient is stable.

DIAGNOSTIC PROCEDURES

• Thoracocentesis—allows characterization of the fluid type and determination of potential underlying cause. • Exploratory thoracotomy or thoracoscopy—to obtain biopsy specimens of lung, lymph nodes, or pleura, if indicated.

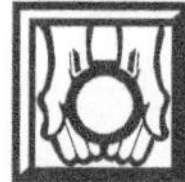

TREATMENT

• First, thoracocentesis to relieve respiratory distress; if the patient is stable after thoracocentesis, outpatient treatment may be possible for some diseases. Most patients are

Table 1

Characterization of pleural fluid.

	Transudate	*Modified Transudate*	*Nonseptic Exudate*	*Septic Exudate*	*Chyle*	*Hemorrhage*
Color	Colorless to pale yellow	Yellow or pink	Yellow or pink	Yellow to red-brown	Milky white	Red
Turbidity	Clear	Clear to cloudy	Clear to cloudy; fibrin	Cloudy to opaque; fibrin	Opaque	Opaque
Protein (g/dL)	<1.5	2.5–5.0	3.0–8.0	3.0–7.0	2.5–6.0	3.0
Nucleated cells/μL	<1,000	1,000–7,000 (LSA up to 100,000)	5,000–20,000 (LSA up to 100,000)	5,000–300,000	1,000–20,000	Similar to peripheral blood
Cytology	Mostly mesothelial cells and macrophages	Mostly macrophages and mesothelial cells; few nondegenerate PMNs; neoplastic cells in some cases	Mostly nondegenerate PMNs and macrophages; neoplastic cells in some cases	Mostly degenerate PMNs; also macrophages; bacteria	Small lymphocytes, PMNs, and macrophages	Mostly RBCs;with erythrophagocytosis
Disease associations	Hypoalbuminemia (protein-losing nephropathy, protein-losing enteropathy, or liver disease); early CHF	CHF; neoplasia; diaphragmatic hernia; pancreatitis	FIP; neoplasia; diaphragmatic hernia; lung lobe torsion	Pyothorax	Lymphangiectasia, CHF, cranial vena cava obstruction, neoplasia, fungal, dirofilariasias, diaphragmatic hernia, lung lobe torsion, trauma	Trauma, coagulopathy, neoplasia, lung lobe torsion

Source: Modified from Sherding RG. Diseases of the pleural cavity. In: Sherding RG, ed., The Cat: Diseases and Clinical Management, 2nd ed. New York: Churchill Livingstone, 1994, p. 1061.

hospitalized because they require intensive management such as indwelling chest tubes (e.g., patients with pyothorax) or thoracic surgery. • Preventing fluid reaccumulation requires treatment based on a definitive diagnosis. • Surgery is indicated for management of some neoplasias, diaphragmatic hernia repair, lymphangiectasia (i.e., thoracic duct ligation), foreign body removal, and lung lobe torsion (i.e., lung lobectomy).
• Pleuroperitoneal shunts may relieve clinical signs in animals with intractable pleural effusion.
• Vascular access ports attached to intrathoracic Jackson–Pratt drains can be tried for chronic effusions that are not responsive to the therapy of the underlying disorder.

MEDICATIONS

DRUG(S) OF CHOICE

• Treatment varies with specific disease.
• Diuretics generally reserved for patients with diseases causing fluid retention and volume overload (e.g., CHF).

PRECAUTIONS

• Avoid drugs that depress respiration or decrease blood pressure. • Inappropriate use of diuretics predisposes the patient to dehydration and electrolyte disturbances without eliminating the effusion.

FOLLOW-UP

PATIENT MONITORING

Radiographic evaluation is key to assessment of treatment in most patients.

POSSIBLE COMPLICATIONS

• Death due to respiratory compromise.
• Reexpansion pulmonary edema may develop after pleural effusion is manually removed.

EXPECTED COURSE AND PROGNOSIS

Varies with underlying cause, but usually guarded to poor. In a study of 81 cases of pleural effusion in dogs, 25% recovered completely and 33% died during or were euthanized immediately after completing diagnostic evaluation.

MISCELLANEOUS

SYNONYMS

• Hydrothorax = transudates and modified transudates. • Pyothorax = empyema, septic pleuritis.

ABBREVIATIONS

• CHF = congestive heart failure. • FIP = feline infectious peritonitis. • LSA = lymphoma. • PMN = polymorphonuclear cell. • RBC = red blood cell.

Suggested Reading

Epstein SE. Exudative pleural diseases in small animals. Vet Clin North Am Small Anim Pract 2014, 44(1):161–180.

König A, Hartmann K, Mueller RS, et al. Retrospective analysis of pleural effusion in cats. J Feline Med Surg 2019, 21(12):1102–1110.

Mellanby RJ, Villiers E, Herrtage ME. Canine pleural effusions: a retrospective study of 81 cases. J Small Anim Pract 2002, 43(10):447–451.

Ruiz MD, Vessieres F, Ragetly GR, Hernandez JL. Characterization of and factors associated with causes of pleural effusion in cats. J Am Vet Med Assoc 2018, 253(2):181–187.

Smeak DD, Birchard SJ, McLoughlin MA, et al. Treatment of chronic pleural effusion with pleuroperitoneal shunts in dogs: 14 cases (1985–1999). J Am Vet Med Assoc 2001, 219(11):1590–1597.

Author Francis W.K. Smith, Jr.
Consulting Editor Michael Aherne

Client Education Handout available online

PNEUMOCYSTOSIS

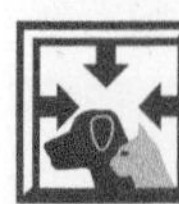

BASICS

OVERVIEW

• *Pneumocystis* spp.—saprophyte/commensal of low virulence; infect virtually all mammals worldwide. ○ *Pneumocystis carinii* f. sp. *canis*: organism infecting dogs (hereafter "*Pneumocystis canis*"). • Primary habitat is lung. • Atypical fungal organism, based on nucleic acid sequencing; exhibits behavior more typical of protozoa. • Subclinical infections in cats and dogs; clinical infections in dogs linked with immunodeficiency; clinical infection not reported in cats even with immunosuppression.

SIGNALMENT

• Young dogs (<1 year of age). • Miniature dachshunds and cavalier King Charles spaniels (CKCS, worldwide), Pomeranians (in Japan) predisposed (congenital immunodeficiencies).

P

SIGNS

• Progressive respiratory difficulty (weeks to months). • Dyspnea and tachypnea, cyanosis. • Exercise intolerance. • Cough. • Fever uncommon. • Inappetence, weight loss, and thin body condition. • Some dogs have concurrent generalized demodicosis.

CAUSES & RISK FACTORS

• Spread by airborne droplets. Neonates may be infected at birth. • Congenital or acquired immunodeficiency predisposes to development of clinical disease: ○ Severe immunosuppression—deficiency of IgA, IgG, IgM in dachshunds; immunoglobulin deficiency and decreased lymphocyte function in CKCS.

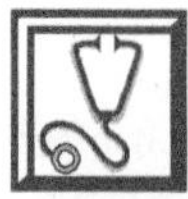

DIAGNOSIS

DIFFERENTIAL DIAGNOSIS

• Inflammatory (chronic pulmonary fibrosis, eosinophilic bronchopneumopathy, inhalational irritants). • Infection (viral, bacterial, fungal, protozoal or parasitic pneumonia). • Pulmonary edema (cardiogenic or noncardiogenic). • Thromboembolism. • Neoplasia.

CBC/BIOCHEMISTRY/URINALYSIS

• Usually nonspecific. • Leukocytosis with neutrophilia and a left shift. • Eosinophilia and monocytosis. • Erythrocytosis—secondary to chronic hypoxia. • Thrombocytopenia (CKCS) or thrombocytosis (dachshunds). • Variable hypoglobulinemia.

OTHER LABORATORY TESTS

• Arterial blood gas—hypoxemia; hypocapnia. • Immunoglobulin fraction quantification—hypogammaglobulinemia. • Indirect or direct fluorescent antibody test—detect organism in sputum, washes, and pulmonary tissues. • PCR of bronchoalveolar fluid and tissues.

IMAGING

Thoracic Radiography

• Diffuse miliary—interstitial to alveolar pattern with peribronchial opacification. • Middle lung lobes may be more severely affected. • Rarely cavitary lesions and pneumothorax.

CT

Diffuse to multifocal "ground-glass" appearance with variable bronchial bands; signs consistent with pulmonary hypertension.

DIAGNOSTIC PROCEDURES

• Transtracheal aspiration, bronchoalveolar lavage, transbronchoscopic and endobronchial brushing: ○ Direct visualization of *P. canis*. • Biopsy for histopathology (cytology not as sensitive or specific): ○ Invasive, potential complications of hemorrhage, pneumothorax. • PCR assays for *P. canis*—interpreted in light of consistent clinical signs and other diagnostic findings because of subclinical infection in dogs; assays designed to detect *P. jirovecii* may not detect *P. canis*.

PATHOLOGIC FINDINGS

• Lungs—firm, consolidated, pale brown or gray; fluid not expressed from cut surfaces; do not collapse when chest cavity opened; alveoli may be filled with amorphous, foamy, eosinophilic material with honeycomb appearance; trophozoites and cyst stages may be identified. • Pulmonary and mediastinal lymphadenopathy. • Right-sided cardiomegaly. • H&E only weakly stains internal structures of organism; methenamine silver, toluidine blue, Gram and periodic acid–Schiff will stain cyst walls.

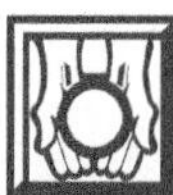

TREATMENT

• Inpatient—supportive care for pneumonia: oxygen, nebulization, bronchodilators, IV fluids as required. • Discontinue immunosuppressant agents. • Cage rest.

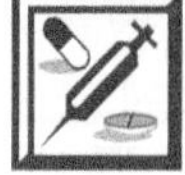

MEDICATIONS

DRUG(S) OF CHOICE

• Trimethoprim-sulfonamide 15–20 mg/kg PO q8h or 30 mg/kg PO q12h for 3 weeks—preferred therapy (IV may be more effective than PO in humans). • Alternative treatments—pentamidine isethionate 4 mg/kg IM q24h for 3 weeks; atovaquone 15 mg/kg PO q24h for 3 weeks (not as effective but less toxic); combination of clindamycin and primaquine or dapsone and trimethoprim. • Potential new drug options—caspofungin (no veterinary cases reported) and trimetrexate. • Short-term treatment with anti-inflammatory doses of glucocorticoids may be beneficial.

CONTRAINDICATIONS/POSSIBLE INTERACTIONS

• Pentamidine isethionate—renal and hepatic dysfunction (check renal parameters daily during therapy), hypoglycemia, hypotension, hypocalcemia, urticaria, and hematologic disorders. • Trimethoprim-sulfonamides—keratoconjunctivitis sicca, thrombocytopenia.

FOLLOW-UP

PATIENT MONITORING

• Monitor clinical signs, radiographs; may need months-long treatment. • For side effects of medications.

MISCELLANEOUS

ZOONOTIC POTENTIAL

Ubiquitous in environment; humans and animals are exposed to same sources.

ABBREVIATIONS

• CKCS = cavalier King Charles spaniel.

Suggested Reading

Danesi P, Ravagnan S, Johnson L, et al. Molecular diagnosis of *Pneumocystis* pneumonia in dogs. Med Mycol 2017, 55(8):828–842.

Weissenbacher-Lang C, Fuchs-Baumgartinger A, Guija-De-Arespacochaga, et al. Pneumocystosis in dogs: meta-analysis of 43 published cases including clinical signs, diagnostic procedures, and treatment. J Vet Diagn Invest 2018, 30(1):26–35.

Author Jane E. Sykes

Consulting Editor Amie Koenig

Acknowledgment The author and editors acknowledge the prior contribution of Hannah N. Pipe-Martin and Steven C. Barr.

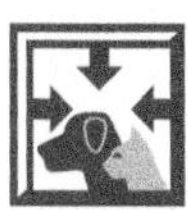

BASICS

OVERVIEW

• Inflammation of the lungs caused by inhalation of oral ingesta, regurgitated material, and vomitus with subsequent pulmonary dysfunction; develops when laryngeal reflexes function improperly or are overwhelmed. • Pulmonary dysfunction—caused by (1) direct obstruction of small airways and indirect obstruction from bronchospasm and production of mucus and exudate; (2) aspiration of gastric acid—damages respiratory epithelium; can cause bronchospasm and acute lung injury/acute respiratory distress syndrome (ALI/ARDS); (3) bacterial pneumonia—bacteria in aspirated material can initiate an immediate infection; or later infections occur secondary to lung damage.

SIGNALMENT

Dogs; less commonly cats.

SIGNS

• Peracute, acute, or chronic. • Cough, tachypnea, nasal discharge, or exercise intolerance. • Respiratory distress or cyanosis when severe. • Depending on underlying cause—regurgitation; vomiting; dysphagia; altered consciousness; stertor or stridor.

CAUSES & RISK FACTORS

• Pharyngeal abnormalities—local paralysis; generalized neuromuscular disease; cricopharyngeal motor dysfunction; anatomic malformations. • Esophageal abnormalities—megaesophagus; reflux esophagitis; esophageal dysmotility; esophageal obstruction; broncho-esophageal fistula. • Laryngeal paralysis, webbing, or obstruction; post-laryngeal surgery. •Altered consciousness—sedation, anesthesia; post-ictus; forebrain disease; metabolic disturbance. • Iatrogenic—force feeding; tube feeding, mineral oil administration.

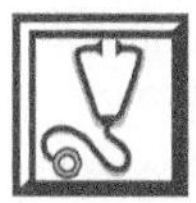

DIAGNOSIS

DIFFERENTIAL DIAGNOSIS

• Bacterial pneumonia. • Lung abscess.

CBC/BIOCHEMISTRY/URINALYSIS

Neutrophilic leukocytosis, left shift, although white blood cells may be normal.

OTHER LABORATORY TESTS

• Arterial blood gas analysis—hypoxemia; $P\text{aco}_2$ generally low. • Consider tests for predisposing problems—acetylcholine receptor antibodies, resting cortisol or adrenocorticotropic hormone stimulation, creatine kinase.

IMAGING

• Thoracic radiography—bronchoalveolar pattern usually most severe in the gravity-dependent lobes (right cranial and middle, left cranial); can take up to 24 hours for pattern to develop after aspiration; scrutinize for evidence of esophageal or mediastinal disease. • Videofluoroscopic swallowing study—provides evidence of swallowing or esophageal dysfunction that can predispose to aspiration. Caution: could result in aspiration of contrast medium.

DIAGNOSTIC PROCEDURES

• Tracheal wash—for bacterial culture and sensitivity testing before administering antibiotics; infection often caused by multiple organisms with unpredictable susceptibility.
• Bronchoscopy—rarely indicated.
• Laryngeal function examination—always perform if patient anesthetized for other purposes; otherwise, after resolution of pneumonia if supportive clinical signs.

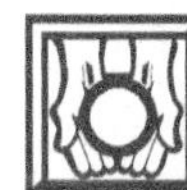

TREATMENT

• Oxygen and cage rest—respiratory distress.
• Ventilatory support—if not oxygen responsive. • IV fluids—avoid overhydration, which can exacerbate secondary edema.
• Oral intake—withhold until primary problem identified and managed. • Do not allow patient to remain laterally recumbent on one side for more than 2 hours. • Mild exercise and saline nebulization with coupage can facilitate airway clearance. • Airway suction—only if performed immediately following aspiration (such as during recovery from anesthesia). • Airway lavage—contraindicated.

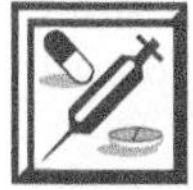

MEDICATIONS

DRUG(S) OF CHOICE

• Antibiotic therapy—if signs of sepsis or severe compromise, ampicillin with sulbactam (20 mg/kg IV q8h) plus a fluoroquinolone IV. Adjust antibiotic selection based on results of airway cytology, culture and sensitivity, and clinical response; continue for 10 days after resolution of clinical and radiographic signs; if no signs of sepsis, ampicillin with sulbactam pending results of culture.
• Beta-agonist bronchodilators—sometimes cause dramatic improvement but have the potential to worsen ventilation:perfusion mismatch; most often helpful in acute aspiration or with auscultable wheezes.
• Short-acting corticosteroids—consider for up to 48 hours to combat inflammation associated with life-threatening aspiration.

CONTRAINDICATIONS/POSSIBLE INTERACTIONS

• Diuretics—generally contraindicated; drying of airways reduces mucociliary clearance.
• Corticosteroids—contraindicated beyond initial stabilization; predispose patient to infection.
• Fluoroquinolones and chloramphenicol—can prolong clearance of theophylline-derivative bronchodilators; decrease theophylline dosage by 30–50% or prolong dosing interval.

FOLLOW-UP

PATIENT MONITORING

• Radiographs—evaluate every 2–7 days initially to determine appropriateness of treatment; then every 1–2 weeks. • If signs do not resolve or suddenly worsen—possible recurrence of aspiration or a secondary infection; repeat diagnostic evaluation, including tracheal wash or bronchoscopy.

PREVENTION/AVOIDANCE

• Predisposed patients undergoing anesthesia—cisapride (slow infusion, 1 mL/kg over 30 minutes) 1–2 hours pre-induction may decrease esophageal reflux. • Suction esophagus prior to extubation. • Antacids could decrease acid-related lung injury in predisposed patients; may also increase risk of infection.

POSSIBLE COMPLICATIONS

• Secondary infection common. • ALI/ARDS.
• Abscessation or granuloma formation rare.

EXPECTED COURSE AND PROGNOSIS

• Prognosis—depends on severity of signs and ability to correct underlying disease.
• Severe aspiration—can be fatal.
• Recurrence—likely if underlying cause not addressed.

MISCELLANEOUS

SEE ALSO

• Acute Respiratory Distress Syndrome.
• Megaesophagus. • Pneumonia, Bacterial.

ABBREVIATIONS

• ALI/ARDS = acute lung injury/acute respiratory distress syndrome.

Suggested Reading

Lappin MR, Blondeau J, Boothe D, et al. Antimicrobial use guidelines for the treatment of respiratory tract disease in dogs and cats: Antimicrobial Guidelines Working Group of the International Society for Companion Animal Infectious Diseases. J Vet Intern Med 2017, 31:279–294.

Author Eleanor C. Hawkins
Consulting Editor Elizabeth Rozanski

PNEUMONIA, BACTERIAL

BASICS

DEFINITION

Acquired inflammatory response to bacteria in lung parenchyma characterized by exudation of cells and fluid into conducting airways and alveolar spaces.

PATHOPHYSIOLOGY

• Bacteria—enter the lower respiratory tract primarily by inhalation or aspiration; less commonly by the hematogenous route. Infection incites an inflammatory reaction. • Tracheobronchial tree and carina—normally not sterile. • Oropharyngeal bacteria—frequently aspirated; may be present for an unknown time period in the normal tracheobronchial tree and lung; can cause or complicate respiratory infection; presence complicates interpretation of airway and lung cultures. • Respiratory infection—development depends on the complex interplay of many factors: inoculation site, number of organisms and their virulence, and age and resistance of the host. • Bacteria produce extracellular proteins called invasins that impair host defenses and assist in the spread of bacteria. • Viral infections—alter bacterial colonization patterns; increase bacterial adherence to respiratory epithelium; reduce mucociliary clearance and phagocytosis; allow resident bacteria to invade the lower respiratory tract. • Foreign body—inoculates bacteria into a focal lung region and leads to obstructive pneumonia. • Exudative phase—inflammatory hyperemia; extravasation of high-protein fluid into interstitial and alveolar spaces. • Leukocytic migration phase—leukocytes infiltrate the airways and alveoli; consolidation, ischemia, tissue necrosis, and atelectasis owing to bronchial occlusion, obstructive bronchiolitis, and impaired collateral ventilation.

SYSTEMS AFFECTED

Respiratory—primary or secondary infection.

GENETICS

Heritable rhinitis/bronchopneumonia syndrome of Irish wolfhounds, unknown pathogenesis.

INCIDENCE/PREVALENCE

Common in both young and old dogs, less common in cats.

GEOGRAPHIC DISTRIBUTION

Widespread

SIGNALMENT

Species

Dog and cat.

Breed Predilections

Dogs—sporting breeds, hounds, working breeds, and mixed breeds >12 kg.

Mean Age and Range

Dogs—range, 1 month–15 years.

Predominant Sex

Dogs—60% males.

SIGNS

Historical Findings

• Cough. • Labored breathing. • Recent vomiting/regurgitation (aspiration). • Anorexia. • Lethargy. • Nasal discharge.

Physical Examination Findings

• Cough. • Fever. • Difficult or rapid breathing. • Abnormal breath sounds on auscultation—increased intensity, crackles, and wheezes. • Nasal discharge. • Lethargy. • Dehydration.

CAUSES

Dogs

• Most common primary pathogens—*Bordetella bronchiseptica* and *Mycoplasma* spp. • Most common Gram-positive bacteria—*Staphylococcus*, *Streptococcus*, and *Enterococcus* spp. • Most common Gram-negative bacteria—*Escherichia coli*, *Klebsiella* spp., *Pseudomonas* spp., *Pasteurella* spp. • Anaerobic bacteria—found in pulmonary abscesses and various types of pneumonia (particularly with aspiration or foreign bodies); reported in ~20% of cases.

Cats

• Bacterial pathogens—poorly documented; *B. bronchiseptica*, *Pasteurella* spp., and *Moraxella* spp. most frequently reported. *Mycoplasma* spp. may be a primary pathogen in the lower respiratory tract. • Carrier state—may exist; periods of shedding *B. bronchiseptica* after stress; infected queens may not shed organism prepartum but begin shedding post partum, serving as a source of infection for kittens.

RISK FACTORS

• Prior viral infection. • Regurgitation, dysphagia, or vomiting. • Functional or anatomic defects—laryngeal paralysis, brachycephalic breed, megaesophagus, cleft palate, primary ciliary dyskinesia. • Reduced level of consciousness—stupor, coma, and anesthesia. • Bronchial foreign body. • Bronchiectasis. • Immunosuppressive therapy—chemotherapy, glucocorticoids. • Severe metabolic disorders—uremia, diabetes mellitus, hyperadrenocorticism. • Sepsis. • Age—very young more susceptible to fatal infections. • Immunization status. • Environment—housing, sanitation, ventilation. • Phagocyte dysfunction—feline leukemia virus and diabetes mellitus. • Complement deficiency—rare. • Selective IgA deficiency—rare. • Combined T-cell and B-cell dysfunction—rare.

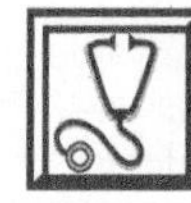

DIAGNOSIS

DIFFERENTIAL DIAGNOSIS

• Viral pneumonia (canine distemper virus, adenovirus, influenza virus, herpesvirus). • Protozoal pneumonia (*Toxoplasma*). • Parasitic pneumonia (capillariasis, filaroidiasis, lungworm). • Fungal pneumonia (*Histoplasma, Blastomyces, Coccidioides, Cryptococcus*). • Eosinophilic pneumonia. • Feline bronchial disease (asthma). • Pulmonary abscess. • Pleural infection (pyothorax). • Bronchial foreign body.

CBC/BIOCHEMISTRY/URINALYSIS

Inflammatory leukogram—neutrophilic leukocytosis with or without a left shift; absence does not rule out the diagnosis.

OTHER LABORATORY TESTS

• Arterial blood gas analysis—values correlate well with the degree of physiologic disruption; sensitive monitor of progress during treatment; $Pa{O_2}$ <80 mmHg on room air = mild or moderate hypoxemia; $Pa{O_2}$ <60mmHg on room air = severe hypoxemia. • Consider viral serology. • Molecular diagnostics also available for viral and bacterial presence.

IMAGING

Thoracic Radiography

• Variable—diffuse, bronchointerstitial pattern, partial or complete alveolar infiltrates, consolidation. • Most common—alveolar pattern characterized by increased pulmonary densities (margins indistinct; air bronchograms or lobar consolidation). • More variable lung patterns in cats such as multifocal, patchy interstitial and alveolar changes and/or a diffuse nodular pattern.

DIAGNOSTIC PROCEDURES

• Microbiologic (aerobic, anaerobic, and *Mycoplasma* culture) and cytology for definitive diagnosis. • Samples—transtracheal or endotracheal washing, bronchoscopy, bronchoalveolar lavage (with or without bronchoscope), or fine-needle lung aspiration. • Degenerate neutrophils with septic inflammation (intracellular bacteria) predominating. • Recent antibiotic administration—nonseptic inflammation likely. • Bacteria—not always obvious microscopically; always culture specimens even if no bacteria are seen on cytology.

PATHOLOGIC FINDINGS

• Irregular consolidation in cranioventral regions. • Consolidated lung—varies from dark red to gray-pink to more gray, depending on age of patient and nature of the process. • Palpable firmness of the tissue. • Nidus of inflammation—bronchiolar-alveolar junction. • Early—bronchioles and adjacent alveoli filled with neutrophils and an admixture of cell debris, fibrin, and macrophages; necrotic to hyperplastic epithelium. • Later—neutrophilic, fibrinous, hemorrhagic, or necrotizing inflammation depending on virulence of bacteria and host response.

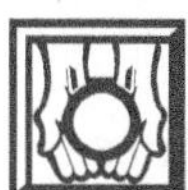

TREATMENT

APPROPRIATE HEALTH CARE

Inpatient—recommended with multisystemic signs (e.g., anorexia, fever) or in patients with respiratory compromise in the absence of multisystemic signs.

NURSING CARE

• Maintain normal systemic hydration—important to aid mucociliary clearance and secretion mobilization; use a balanced electrolyte solution. • Saline nebulization—results in more rapid resolution if used with physical therapy and systemic antimicrobials. • Physical therapy—chest wall coupage, tracheal manipulation to stimulate mild cough and postural drainage; may enhance clearance of secretions; always do immediately after nebulization; avoid allowing the patient to lie in one position for a prolonged time.
• Oxygen therapy—as warranted for patients with hypoxemia, signs of respiratory distress.

ACTIVITY

Restrict during treatment (inpatient or outpatient), except as part of physical therapy after aerosolization.

DIET

• Ensure normal intake with food high in protein and energy density. • Enteral or parenteral nutritional support—indicated in severely ill patients. • Use caution in feeding animals with megaesophagus, laryngeal dysfunction or surgery, pharyngeal disease, or recumbent patients.

CLIENT EDUCATION

Warn client that high morbidity and mortality are associated with severe hypoxemia and sepsis.

SURGICAL CONSIDERATIONS

Lung lobectomy may be required with pulmonary abscessation or bronchopulmonary foreign body with secondary pneumonia; may be indicated if patient is unresponsive to conventional treatment and disease is limited to one or two lobes.

MEDICATIONS

DRUG(S) OF CHOICE

Antimicrobials

• Antimicrobials are best selected based on results of culture and susceptibility testing from tracheal wash or other pulmonary specimens.
• Empiric antimicrobial therapy is justified when there is significant risk in obtaining adequate samples or if the time required to culture causes a life-threatening delay in treatment. • Recently administered antimicrobials should be avoided.
• Reasonable initial antimicrobial choices pending culture results include amoxicillin-clavulanic acid 15 mg/kg PO q12h or cephalexin 22–30 mg/kg PO q12h with enrofloxacin (dogs, 10–20 mg/kg q24h; cats, maximum 5 mg/kg q24h), or trimethoprim-sulfonamide 15 mg/kg PO q12h. • Gram-positive cocci—ampicillin 20–40 mg/kg IV q6–8h, ampicillin-sulbactam 22–30 mg/kg IV q6–8h; amoxicillin 22 mg/kg PO q12h; amoxicillin-clavulanic acid; azithromycin; chloramphenicol, erythromycin; trimethoprim-sulfonamide; first-generation cephalosporins. • Gram-negative rods—enrofloxacin or marbofloxacin; cefpodoxime; chloramphenicol; trimethoprim-sulfonamide; amikacin. • *Bordetella*—doxycycline 5 mg/kg PO q12h; chloramphenicol; enrofloxacin; azithromycin. • *Mycoplasma*—doxycycline, enrofloxacin, marbofloxacin, chloramphenicol.
• Anaerobes—amoxicillin–clavulanic acid; chloramphenicol; metronidazole; clindamycin; ticarcillin-clavulanic acid. • Antimicrobial nebulization for *Bordetella*—gentamicin nebulization 5 mg/kg q24h for 5–7 days, typically adjunctive with systemic antimicrobials.

Duration of Treatment

• Authors have traditionally recommended continued treatment for at least 10 days beyond clinical resolution and/or 1–2 weeks following radiographic resolution. • Total of ≤14 days of therapy is not associated with worse outcomes when compared to >14 days of therapy in dogs.

CONTRAINDICATIONS

• Anticholinergics and antihistamines—may thicken secretions and inhibit mucokinesis and exudate removal from airways.
• Antitussives—potent, centrally acting agents inhibit mucokinesis and exudate removal from airways; can potentiate pulmonary infection and inflammation.

POSSIBLE INTERACTIONS

Avoid use of theophylline and fluoroquinolones concurrently.

ALTERNATIVE DRUG(S)

• Expectorants—recommended by some clinicians; no objective evidence that they increase mucokinesis or mobilization of secretions. • Bronchodilators—recommended by some clinicians to alleviate bronchospasm.

FOLLOW-UP

PATIENT MONITORING

• Monitor respiratory rate and effort. • Complete blood count will normalize. • Arterial blood gases—sensitive monitor of progress, pulse oximetry can be helpful. • Frequent thoracic auscultation. • Thoracic radiographs—improve more slowly than the clinical appearance.

PREVENTION/AVOIDANCE

• Vaccination—against upper respiratory viruses and *Bordetella* if a dog is boarded or exposed to large numbers of other animals.
• Catteries—environmental strategies to lower population density and improve hygiene help control outbreaks of bordetellosis.

POSSIBLE COMPLICATIONS

• Sepsis can develop. • Severe respiratory compromise may require intubation/mechanical ventilation.

EXPECTED COURSE AND PROGNOSIS

• Prognosis—good with aggressive antibacterial and supportive therapy; more guarded in young animals, patients with immunodeficiency, and patients that are debilitated or have severe underlying disease. • Prolonged infection—potential for chronic bronchitis or bronchiectasis in any patient. • Mortality—associated with severe hypoxemia and sepsis.

MISCELLANEOUS

ASSOCIATED CONDITIONS

• Frequently develops secondary to underlying functional or anatomic abnormalities—cleft palate; tracheal hypoplasia; primary ciliary dyskinesia; laryngeal paralysis; megaesophagus or other esophageal dysmotility disorder.
• Bronchiectasis—both predisposing factor and potential complication.

AGE-RELATED FACTORS

• Young puppies and kittens—may have a poorer prognosis. • Underlying functional and anatomic problems and immunodeficiencies—suspect in young patients.

PREGNANCY/FERTILITY/BREEDING

Bitches or queens infected with *B. bronchiseptica*—may transmit infection to neonates.

Suggested Reading

Dear JD. Bacterial pneumonia in dogs and cats. Vet Clin North Am Small Anim Prac 2014, 44(1):143–159.

Jameson PH, King LA, Lappin MR, et al. Comparison of clinical signs, diagnostic findings, organisms isolated, and clinical outcome in dogs with bacterial pneumonia: 93 cases (1986–1991). J Am Vet Med Assoc 1995, 206:206–209.

Proulx A, Hume DZ, Drobatz KJ, et al. In vitro bacterial isolate susceptibility to empirically selected antimicrobials in 111 dogs with bacterial pneumonia. J Vet Emerg Crit Care 2013, 24(2):194–200.

Wayne AS, Davis M, Sinnott VB, et al. Outcomes in dogs with uncomplicated, presumptive bacterial pneumonia treated with short or long course antibiotics. Can Vet J 2017, 58:610–613.

Author Ian DeStefano

Consulting Editor Elizabeth Rozanski

Acknowledgment The author and editors acknowledge the prior contribution of Melissa A. Herrera.

Client Education Handout available online

P

PNEUMONIA, EOSINOPHILIC

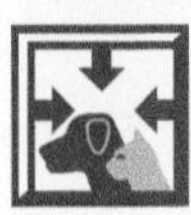

BASICS

DEFINITION

The fully developed inflammatory response to antigens in lung parenchyma characterized by exudation of eosinophils and fluid into lung interstitium, conducting airways, and alveolar spaces.

PATHOPHYSIOLOGY

• Immunologic basis—supporting evidence generally accepted; mechanisms involved not yet clarified. • Eosinophilic infiltration and a predominance of CD4+ T-cells in bronchoalveolar lavage fluid support the role of a dominant Th2 immune response in the lower airways. • Evolution of disease—likely determined by characteristics of antigens, host response, and regulation of that response.
• Antigens enter the lower respiratory tract by inhalation or hematogenous routes. • Chronic exposure to antigens—elicits a humoral and cellular immune response. • Allergic or hypersensitivity pulmonary disorders—associated with an abnormal humoral antibody response and a cell-mediated immunoregulatory defect. • Immunoglobulin classes involved—IgE, IgG, and others.
• High numbers of activated macrophages and T-lymphocytes and depressed suppressor T-cell activity—alter cell-mediated immunity.
• Collagenolytic enzyme activity—increased.
• Generally referred to as eosinophilic bronchopneumopathy although at least three disease patterns appear to exist: eosinophilic pneumonitis, eosinophilic bronchitis, and pulmonary eosinophilic granulomatosis.
• Severely affected dogs appear to develop marked granulomatous disease. • Heartworm disease with pneumonitis—microfilaria may become entrapped in the pulmonary circulation and trigger an immune response.
• Mortality—associated with severe hypoxemia (e.g., low arterial oxygen concentration) and (rarely) severe hemoptysis.

SYSTEMS AFFECTED

• Respiratory—lower respiratory tract primarily but nasal cavity can also be involved. • Cardiovascular—can develop cor pulmonale.

GENETICS

N/A

INCIDENCE/PREVALENCE

N/A

GEOGRAPHIC DISTRIBUTION

Widespread

SIGNALMENT

Species

Dog

Breed Predilections

Siberian husky, possibly.

Mean Age and Range

All ages but more often young adults (4–6 years of age).

Predominant Sex

None

SIGNS

General Comments

Extremely variable, depending on the severity.

Historical Findings

• Cough—unresponsive to antibacterial therapy. • Labored breathing. • Exercise intolerance. • Anorexia. • Lethargy. • Weight loss. • Nasal discharge. • Fever (uncommon).

Physical Examination Findings

• Harsh, moist cough. • Tachypnea or respiratory distress. • Abnormal breath sounds on auscultation—increased-intensity breath sounds; crackles; wheezes; decreased sounds can occur. • Weight loss. • Yellow-green or mucopurulent nasal discharge.
• Fever (uncommon).

CAUSES

• Purported aeroallergens—spores or hyphae from fungi and actinomycetes; pollen; insect antigens; dust or storage mites; unidentified triggers of the immune response. • Parasitic antigens—heartworm microfilaria, respiratory parasites.

RISK FACTORS

• Living in a heartworm-endemic area without receiving preventive medication. • Dusty or moldy environment. • Air pollution.

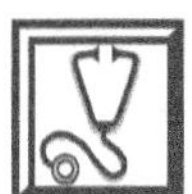

DIAGNOSIS

DIFFERENTIAL DIAGNOSIS

• Parasitic pneumonia—capillariasis; paragonimiasis; dirofilariasis. • Fungal pneumonia—histoplasmosis; blastomycosis; coccidioidomycosis; cryptococcosis. • For eosinophilic pneumonitis—bacterial pneumonia; viral pneumonia (e.g., canine distemper virus and canine adenovirus); rickettsial pneumonia (e.g., ehrlichiosis and Rocky Mountain spotted fever); protozoal pneumonia (e.g., toxoplasmosis); congestive heart failure; bartonellosis. • For eosinophilic bronchitis—infectious tracheobronchitis; chronic bronchitis. • For pulmonary eosinophilic granulomatosis—neoplasia (including lymphomatoid granulomatosis); pulmonary abscess; bronchial foreign body.

CBC/BIOCHEMISTRY/URINALYSIS

• Inflammatory leukogram—neutrophilic leukocytosis with or without a left shift, eosinophilia, basophilia, or monocytosis.
• Absence of eosinophilia does not exclude diagnosis. • Hyperglobulinemia—suggests chronic antigenic stimulus; rule out occult dirofilariasis.

OTHER LABORATORY TESTS

Arterial Blood Gas Analysis

• Values correlate well with the degree of physiologic disruption; sensitive monitor of patient's progress during treatment.
• Hypoxemia—mild or moderate, Pao_2 <80 mmHg on room air; severe, Pao_2 <60 mmHg on room air.

Other

• Heartworm microfilaria and antigen tests—positive results suggest dirofilariasis or eosinophilic pneumonitis associated with microfilaria trapped in the lung. Multiple tests can be required to rule out disease.
• Fecal flotation and Baermann sedimentation.
• Protein electrophoresis—β-globulin spike (hyperbetaglobulinemia) often found with occult dirofilariasis.

IMAGING

• Radiographic findings depend on extent and severity of disease. • Thoracic radiographs—help document the severity of pulmonary artery disease; reveal interstitial pneumonitis in dogs with dirofilariasis. • Eosinophilic pneumonitis—linear or miliary interstitial pattern that resembles changes seen with early pulmonary edema or fungal pneumonia; alveolar pattern characterized by increased pulmonary densities with indistinct margins in severely affected patients; tortuous, large pulmonary arteries and right-sided cardiomegaly in patients with dirofilariasis.
• Eosinophilic bronchitis—bronchial pattern with thickened bronchi extending into the periphery of the lung (tram/railroad track and donut signs); bronchiectasis in chronic cases.
• Eosinophilic granuloma—multiple nodular lesions of variable sizes in different lung lobes; patchy, focal alveolar densities; tracheobronchial lymphadenopathy possible.

DIAGNOSTIC PROCEDURES

• Transtracheal or endotracheal wash appropriate for sample collection.
• Bronchoscopy; yellow-green mucus, polypoid mucosal proliferation, partial airway collapse. Occlusive eosinophilic plaques or granulomas sometimes visible within airways.
• Bronchoalveolar lavage—with or without bronchoscope. • Bacterial and mycoplasmal culture of bronchoalveolar lavage fluid is recommended to rule-out bacterial infection. Occasionally, concurrent bacterial infection can be identified in dogs with eosinophilic lung disease. • Fine-needle lung aspiration and examination. • Cytologic examination of aspirates, washings, or brushings—definitive diagnosis: eosinophilic inflammation predominates; may note other types of inflammatory cells; carefully examine specimens for antigenic sources (e.g., parasites, fungi, or neoplasia). • Consider intradermal skin or serologic allergen testing—rarely may identify allergens. • Fecal

examinations—routine flotation, direct smear, sediment examination, and Baermann technique to rule out parasitic pneumonia; negative test can occur due to intermittent shedding and empirical therapy warranted in some cases.

PATHOLOGIC FINDINGS

• Gross—diffuse, patchy, or nodular firm lesions; usually pale or mottled.
• Histopathologic—eosinophilic, lymphocytic, and macrophagic infiltration of alveolar walls and alveolar spaces; as disease progresses, interstitial infiltrative process becomes fibrotic with obliteration of alveolar spaces, and granulomas can be dispersed within the interstitial fibrosis. Upper respiratory tract epithelium can also be involved with eosinophilic infiltration.

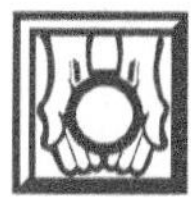

TREATMENT

APPROPRIATE HEALTH CARE

Inpatient—recommended with multisystemic signs (e.g., anorexia, weight loss, or lethargy).

NURSING CARE

• Dehydration—hinders mucociliary clearance and secretion mobilization; maintain normal systemic hydration with a balanced multielectrolyte solution.
• Supplemental oxygen—for respiratory distress.

ACTIVITY

Restricted during treatment (inpatient or outpatient).

DIET

Ensure normal intake.

CLIENT EDUCATION

Warn client that morbidity and mortality are associated with severe hypoxemia.

SURGICAL CONSIDERATIONS

Lung lobectomy can be required with large granulomas.

MEDICATIONS

DRUG(S) OF CHOICE

• Corticosteroids—prednisolone or prednisone at 2 mg/kg/day until clinical signs begin to resolve (typically 2–3 weeks); then taper slowly (over months). Maintenance dosages of prednisone are often required long term (0.125–0.5 mg/kg q48h or every 3 or 4 days for 4–6 months or longer). • Following adequate control of disease and/or due to side effects of systemic glucocorticoids, inhaled corticosteroids (e.g., fluticasone propionate) can be used in conjunction with a spacing chamber and facemask. • Antibiotic therapy indicated only if active infection documented on airway culture. Prophylactic therapy could lead to development of antimicrobial resistance. • Heartworm adulticidal therapy—for heartworm-positive patient; initiate after the patient has been stabilized with corticosteroids and rest. • Itraconazole or ketoconazole—use antifungal drugs only if the fungal infection is confirmed by cytologic examination or culture. • Hyposensitization—allergy shots based on results of intradermal skin or serologic testing can be attempted but is not the treatment of choice in most patients. Most dogs will still require steroid therapy.

CONTRAINDICATIONS

N/A

PRECAUTIONS

N/A

ALTERNATIVE DRUG(S)

Other immunosuppressive drugs (e.g., cyclosporine)—can use when corticosteroids are contraindicated or have been ineffective, although inhaled steroids are preferred. No trial results are available to date.

FOLLOW-UP

PATIENT MONITORING

• Complete blood count will show resolution of peripheral eosinophilia or neutrophilia.
• Arterial blood gases—most sensitive monitor of progress. Can remain abnormal even with successful management of disease.
• Auscultate patient thoroughly several times daily. • Thoracic radiographs—improve more slowly than the clinical appearance.

PREVENTION/AVOIDANCE

• Routine heartworm-prevention medication.
• Consider changing patient's environment if an aeroallergen is suspected.

POSSIBLE COMPLICATIONS

Pulmonary embolization—dogs treated with adulticidal therapy for dirofilariasis.

EXPECTED COURSE AND PROGNOSIS

• Prognosis good for mild-to-moderate cases; many patients require long-term treatment with steroids. • If allergen can be identified and eliminated—suspect improved prognosis. • Heartworm infection—prognosis depends on severity of pulmonary hypertension, cor pulmonale, and embolization.
• Eosinophilic granulomatosis—prognosis guarded; often disease is progressive.

MISCELLANEOUS

ASSOCIATED CONDITIONS

• Dirofilariasis. • Bronchopulmonary fungal infection.

AGE-RELATED FACTORS

N/A

ZOONOTIC POTENTIAL

N/A

PREGNANCY/FERTILITY/BREEDING

Corticosteroids and other immunosuppressive drugs are relatively contraindicated in pregnant animals.

SYNONYMS

• Allergic alveolitis. • Allergic bronchitis.
• Bronchitic pulmonary eosinophilia.
• Eosinophilic bronchitis or bronchopneumopathy. • Eosinophilic pneumonia/pneumonitis. • Eosinophilic pulmonary granulomatosis. • Extrinsic allergic alveolitis. • Hypersensitivity pneumonitis. • Occult heartworm pneumonia. • Parasitic pulmonary eosinophilia. • Pulmonary infiltrates with eosinophilia.

SEE ALSO

• Cough.
• Dyspnea and Respiratory Distress.
• Heartworm Disease—Dogs.
• Panting and Tachypnea.
• Respiratory Parasites.

Suggested Reading

Clercx C, Peeters D. Canine eosinophilic bronchopneumopathy. Vet Clin North Am Small Anim Pract 2007, 37:917–935.
Clercx C, Peeters D, German AJ, et al. An immunologic investigation of canine eosinophilic bronchopneumopathy. J Vet Intern Med 2002, 16:229–237.
Clercx C, Peeters D, Snaps F, et al. Eosinophilic bronchopneumopathy in dogs. J Vet Intern Med 2000, 14:282–291.
Cooper ES, Schober KE, Drost WT. Severe bronchoconstriction after bronchoalveolar lavage in a dog with eosinophilic airway disease. J Am Vet Med Assoc 2005, 227:1257–1262.

Author Elizabeth Rozanski
Consulting Editor Elizabeth Rozanski
Acknowledgment The author/editor acknowledges the prior contribution of Melissa A. Herrera.

PNEUMONIA, FUNGAL

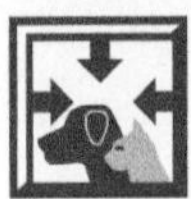

BASICS

DEFINITION

Inflammation of the pulmonary interstitial, lymphatic, and peribronchial tissues caused by deep mycotic infection.

PATHOPHYSIOLOGY

• Mycelial fungal elements—inhaled from contaminated soil or plant debris; organisms then colonize the lungs. • Dimorphic fungi such as *Blastomyces dermatitidis, Histoplasma capsulatum, Coccidioides immitis*—yeast phase at body temperature. Invasive fungal infections with *Aspergillus* spp. follow inhalation of airborne spores with growth as mycelia within tissue. • Systemic dissemination of yeast from the lungs common in dogs and cats.
• Pulmonary interstitial and alveolar involvement—can cause hypoxia. • Airway involvement—causes cough. • Cell-mediated immune response leads to pyogranulomatous inflammation. • Pulmonary complications include interstitial and/or bronchial pneumonia, pleural effusion, mediastinal granuloma formation, acute respiratory distress syndrome, and pulmonary thromboembolism.

SYSTEMS AFFECTED

• Depend on the specific fungal disease.
• Blastomycosis—respiratory involvement in ~85% of cases; diffuse interstitial, alveolar, or bronchial pneumonia most common; solitary mass lesions can be seen, especially in cats; tracheobronchial lymphadenopathy can contribute to cough; nasal infection rare. Multisystemic involvement of skin, lymph nodes, eyes, bone, reproductive tract, and CNS often seen. • Histoplasmosis—respiratory disease alone is only seen in 10% of cases; but multisystemic involvement with diffuse interstitial pneumonia is common, especially in cats; perihilar or mediastinal lymphadenopathy contributes to cough. Multisystemic involvement of gastrointestinal tract, liver, lymph nodes, spleen, bone marrow, eyes, bone, and CNS often seen. • Coccidioidomycosis—diffuse interstitial or bronchial pneumonia common in dogs but less common in cats; perihilar or mediastinal lymphadenopathy common. Multisystemic involvement of bone, skin, eyes, lymph nodes, heart, and CNS often seen. • Cryptococcosis—nasal cavity involvement most common in cats, neurologic system in dogs. Skin and other organs also affected. • Systemic aspergillosis—*Aspergillus terreus*: pneumonia less common, renal and bone (especially vertebral) involvement common.

GENETICS

Breed susceptibilities may be related to defects in cell-mediated immunity.

INCIDENCE/PREVALENCE

Depends on geographic distribution.

GEOGRAPHIC DISTRIBUTION

• Blastomycosis—endemic in US Southeast and Midwest along the Mississippi, Ohio, Missouri, and Tennessee rivers and southern Great Lakes; also in southern Mid-Atlantic States, Pacific Northwest, and southern Canada from east coast to prairie regions of southern Saskatchewan and Manitoba.
• Histoplasmosis—similar to but more widely distributed than blastomycosis; pockets of disease in Texas, Oklahoma, and California.
• Coccidioidomycosis—US Southwest from Texas to California. Northern Mexico and parts of South America. • Cryptococcosis and aspergillosis—worldwide.

SIGNALMENT

Species

Dog and less commonly cat (except cryptococcosis and histoplasmosis where the cat is affected more often than dogs).

Breed Predilections

• Systemic mycosis—large-breed, sporting, working, hunting or field trial dogs; Doberman pinschers and Rottweilers appear predisposed to disseminated disease. • Systemic aspergillosis—German shepherd dogs overrepresented. • Cryptococcosis—cocker spaniels overrepresented.

Mean Age and Range

• Young animals (<5 years) predisposed.
• Any age can be affected.

Predominant Sex

Males affected 2–4 times more often than females.

SIGNS

General Comments

Multisystemic illness depends on organ systems involved.

Historical Findings

• Chronic weight loss and inappetence.
• Oculonasal discharge. • Coughing—can be prominent but seen inconsistently even with marked pulmonary disease. • Tachypnea or exercise intolerance common. • Labored breathing—more common in cats; sign of severe disease in both dogs and cats. • Acute blindness or blepharospasm—if eyes are affected. • Papules and cutaneous nodules—common but often missed until draining tracts appear. • Lameness—if bones affected or if osteomyelitis develops. • Seizures, ataxia, behavior change—if CNS affected.

Physical Examination Findings

• Emaciation—in chronically affected patients. • Fever—about 50% of patients.
• Harsh, loud breath sounds, crackles in cats, cough on tracheal palpation.
• Dyspnea—at rest with severe disease.
• Lymphadenopathy—common in dogs with dimorphic fungal infections.
• Blastomycosis (dogs)—cutaneous and subcutaneous nodules with draining tracts; chorioretinitis; granulomatous retinal detachment common. • Coccidioidomycosis (dogs)—lameness and pain from osteomyelitis, pericardial disease; cats—skin lesions.
• Histoplasmosis (dogs)—emaciation and bloody diarrhea; cats—skin lesions.
• Cryptococcosis—nasal cavity and soft tissue infection common in cats; chorioretinitis in dogs and cats.

CAUSES

• Primary route of infection—*Blastomyces dermatitidis*: lungs, *Histoplasma capsulatum*: lungs and possibly gastrointestinal tract, *Coccidioides immitis*: lungs. • *Cryptococcus neoformans* and *C. gattii*—nasal cavity, with direct extension into the eyes or CNS, lungs (especially in dogs, less often in cats).
• *Aspergillus* spp.—nasal cavity and lungs.

RISK FACTORS

• Blastomycosis, histoplasmosis, and cryptococcosis—environmental exposure to soils rich in organic matter; blastomycosis and cryptococcosis—exposure to bird droppings or other fecal matter; blastomycosis—living near water. • Coccidioidomycosis—environmental exposure to sandy, alkaline soil after periods of rainfall; outdoor activities (hunting and field trials). • Feline leukemia virus does not appear to be a risk factor and feline immunodeficiency virus may be minor risk factor. • Prednisone—may worsen the disease. • Antineoplastic chemotherapy.
• Lymphoreticular neoplasia.

DIAGNOSIS

DIFFERENTIAL DIAGNOSIS

• Metastatic neoplasia. • Eosinophilic lung disease. • Lymphomatoid granulomatosis.
• Lymphoreticular and histiocytic neoplasia.
• Idiopathic pyogranulomatous disease.
• Feline infectious peritonitis or other vasculitic disease. • Parasitic pneumonia.
• Bacterial pneumonia. • Viral pneumonia.
• Chronic bronchial disease. • Pulmonary edema. • Pulmonary thromboembolism.

CBC/BIOCHEMISTRY/URINALYSIS

• Moderate leukocytosis with or without a left shift. • Lymphopenia common.
• Leukopenia, thrombocytopenia, nonregenerative anemia—with histoplasmosis.
• Hyperglobulinemia and hypoalbuminemia common. • Hypercalcemia—occasionally (most often in dogs with blastomycosis).
• Liver enzyme activities—more likely to be increased with histoplasmosis. • Urinalysis usually normal; proteinuria—occasionally seen. • Organisms—rarely can be seen in urine (common with *Aspergillus*) if kidneys or lower urinary tract are affected.

OTHER LABORATORY TESTS

• Antigen can be detected in serum or urine by enzyme immunoassay for diagnosis of *Blastomyces* or *Histoplasma*—sensitivity and specificity high, especially in urine. Cross-reaction occurs between *Blastomyces* and *Histoplasma*. Antigen testing for *Coccidioides* is insensitive. • Serologic (antibody) testing for blastomycosis and histoplasmosis—false-positive and false-negative results common. Positive titer for *Coccidioides* using heat-precipitated agar gel immunodiffusion consistent with infection with relevant clinical history and signs. • Latex agglutination test—for capsular antigen; highly reliable for cryptococcosis. • Cytologic or histologic identification of the organism—definitive diagnosis. • Culture—not usually necessary; can be difficult to isolate and risky due to zoonosis.

IMAGING

• Thoracic radiography—diffuse interstitial (histoplasmosis and coccidioidomycosis) to nodular interstitial and peribronchial infiltrates (blastomycosis); nodular densities can coalesce to granulomatous masses with indistinct edges; tracheobronchial lymphadenopathy common; large focal granulomas more likely in cats.
• Appendicular or axial skeleton radiography—osteolysis with periosteal proliferation; soft tissue swelling. • Abdominal ultrasonography—granulomas or large lymph nodes. • Ocular ultrasonography—retrobulbar mass, posterior uveitis.

DIAGNOSTIC PROCEDURES

• Impression smear or aspirate of a skin nodule—most likely to yield organisms. • Fine-needle lung aspirate—possibly more diagnostic than tracheal aspirate or bronchoalveolar lavage specimen. • Lymph node aspirate or biopsy.
• CSF tap—with cryptococcosis. • Bone marrow or liver/splenic aspirate—with histoplasmosis.
• Biopsy—may be needed.

PATHOLOGIC FINDINGS

• Pyogranulomatous inflammation.
• Organisms—usually seen with blastomycosis, histoplasmosis, cryptococcosis, and aspergillosis; difficult to find with coccidioidomycosis.

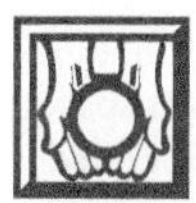

TREATMENT

APPROPRIATE HEALTH CARE

• Outpatient—if patient is stable. • Inpatient evaluation and treatment—dehydration, anorexia, and severe hypoxia.

NURSING CARE

Administration of fluids, oxygen, and antifungals as needed.

DIET

• Feed high-quality protein, calorically dense food. • Histoplasmosis accompanied by marked gastrointestinal involvement—feed highly digestible food.

CLIENT EDUCATION

• Complete response to treatment in <70% of dogs and a smaller percentage of cats.
• Relapse is common. • Treatment is expensive and will be long term (>2 months).
• Clean environmental areas of highly organic matter or feces.

SURGICAL CONSIDERATIONS

Focal granulomas or glaucomatous painful eyes can require removal.

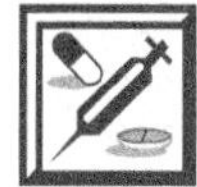

MEDICATIONS

DRUG(S) OF CHOICE

• Itraconazole 5–10 mg/kg PO daily; must be given with food. Liquid suspension more bioavailable in cats (dose 1–1.5 mg/kg/day PO). • Fluconazole 10 mg/kg PO q12h; drug of choice for cryptococcosis and patients with CNS or urinary tract involvement. Usually requires longer treatment. • Lipid-complex amphotericin B 1–2 mg/kg IV q48h for 12 treatments; nephrotoxicity low; diuresis not required. • Posaconazole 5 mg/kg PO q24h with food may be more effective for aspergillosis.

CONTRAINDICATIONS

Corticosteroids are relatively contraindicated but may be required to reduce inflammation during initial treatment in severely dyspneic patients or patients with CNS disease.

PRECAUTIONS

• Azole drugs—do not use with severe liver disease. • Amphotericin B—do not use in azotemic or dehydrated patients; stop use if BUN >50 mg/dL or creatinine >3 mg/dL.
• Itraconazole and the other azole drugs—anorexia; increase in liver enzymes; cutaneous vasculitis.

POSSIBLE INTERACTIONS

Antacids and anticonvulsants—can lower blood concentration of itraconazole.

ALTERNATIVE DRUG(S)

• Ketoconazole 10–30 mg/kg PO q12h; can be effective; higher incidence of side effects; longer treatment is necessary; relapse common. • Amphotericin B 0.5 mg/kg (dogs) or 0.25 mg/kg (cats) IV three times/week to a total dose of 8 mg/kg if used alone or 4 mg/kg if used with an azole drug; administer in 200–500 mL of D_5W after saline diuresis; best used with itraconazole or ketoconazole for severely affected patients.
• Amphotericin B—alternative: 0.5–0.8 mg/kg 2–3 times per week; to reduce nephrotoxicity, can give subcutaneously diluted in 0.45% saline/2.5% dextrose solution (400 mL for cats, 500 mL for dogs <20 kg, 1,000 mL for dogs >20 kg). • Voriconazole 3–4 mg/kg PO q12h for invasive aspergillosis; causes CNS signs in cats. • Terbinafine 30–40 mg/kg PO q12h can be added to azole treatment regimes in resistant infections. • Nikkomycin Z 250 mg PO q12h for dogs 5–15 kg; 500 mg PO q12h for dogs >15 kg for treatment of coccidioidomycosis.

FOLLOW-UP

PATIENT MONITORING

• Liver enzymes—evaluated monthly during azole therapy. • BUN and creatinine—measure before each dose of amphotericin B.
• Thoracic radiographs—reevaluate before discontinuing treatment. • Urine antigen testing for *Blastomyces*/*Histoplasma*—use to monitor therapy.

PREVENTION/AVOIDANCE

Reduce possible exposure.

POSSIBLE COMPLICATIONS

• Blindness is usually permanent. • Renal failure from amphotericin B.

EXPECTED COURSE AND PROGNOSIS

• Blastomycosis—requires a minimum of 2 months of treatment; 60–70% of dogs cured by itraconazole. Dogs with dyspnea or hypoxemia have poorer prognosis.
• Histoplasmosis, coccidioidomycosis—continue at least 1 month past remission (usually 6 months or more). • Systemic aspergillosis—poor prognosis. • Relapse—can occur up to 1 year after treatment.

P

MISCELLANEOUS

AGE-RELATED FACTORS

Young animals predisposed.

ZOONOTIC POTENTIAL

Infections in people—primarily from a common environmental source; no direct transmission from animals to humans, except by penetrating wounds contaminated by the organism; needle stick injury.

PREGNANCY/FERTILITY/BREEDING

• Fungal abortion possible. • Azole antifungals—teratogenic; do not use in pregnant animals.

SEE ALSO

• Aspergillosis, Disseminated Invasive.
• Aspergillosis, Nasal. • Blastomycosis.
• Coccidioidomycosis. • Cryptococcosis.
• Histoplasmosis.

Author Joseph Taboada
Consulting Editor Elizabeth Rozanski

Client Education Handout available online

PNEUMONIA, INTERSTITIAL

BASICS

DEFINITION

A form of pneumonia in which the inflammatory process occurs in alveolar walls and interstitial space.

PATHOPHYSIOLOGY

• Results from either aerogenous injury to the alveolar epithelium (type I or II pneumocytes) or hematogenous injury to the alveolar capillaries; may be triggered by infectious agents. • Alveolar wall damage often occurs secondary to inflammation and antigen–antibody complex deposition. • Progression from acute to chronic interstitial pneumonia can occur leading to alveolar fibrosis ± interstitial mononuclear cell accumulation and persistent type II pneumocyte hyperplasia.

SYSTEMS AFFECTED

• Respiratory. • Cardiovascular (if cor pulmonale develops).

P

GENETICS

Idiopathic pulmonary fibrosis (IPF) is breed-associated (West Highland white terriers/terrier breeds); a definitive genetic defect is not known.

INCIDENCE/PREVALENCE

Incompletely understood.

GEOGRAPHIC DISTRIBUTION

• Infectious organisms: *Aelurostrongylus abstrusus*—Europe, United States, Australia.
• *Angiostrongylus vasorum*—Europe, Africa, South America, North America. • *Leishmania chagasi*—South and Central America.
• H3N2/H3N8—China, USA. Pneumocystis and toxoplasmosis—worldwide.

SIGNALMENT

• Canine distemper virus—dogs 3–6 months of age. Greyhounds, Siberian huskies, Weimaraners, Samoyeds, and Alaskan Malamutes overrepresented.
• Endogenous lipid pneumonia (EnLP)—older cats of either sex. • Pulmonary interstitial lung disease—middle- to old-aged West Highland white terrier, ± Cairn terriers and bull terriers. • Feline IPF-like disease—middle-aged to older cats.
• *Pneumocystis jirovecii*—miniature dachshunds <1 year of age at risk, cavalier King Charles spaniels, any immunocompromised dog. • Toxoplasmosis—middle-aged male cats.

SIGNS

General Comments

Depends on severity of disease.

Historical Findings

Tachypnea, coughing, respiratory difficulty, exercise intolerance.

Physical Examination Findings

• Open-mouth breathing, end-inspiratory and early expiratory crackles, orthopnea, cyanosis, ± hemoptysis. • Animals with paraquat toxicity often display vomiting, oliguria, diarrhea, and oropharyngeal ulcers (± hyperexcitability and neurologic signs in the early phase). • Retinitis, uveitis, neurologic signs, and/or gastrointestinal signs can be seen with toxoplasmosis.

CAUSES

• Congenital—bronchiolitis obliterans with organizing pneumonia (BOOP) secondary to primary ciliary dyskinesia. • Metabolic—uremic pneumonitis ± BOOP, hepatic disease, or pancreatitis in cats. • Neoplastic—bronchiectasis or BOOP, pulmonary carcinoma associated with pulmonary fibrosis in cats. • Idiopathic—pulmonary interstitial fibrosis and desquamative interstitial pneumonitis (DIP), some cases of EnLP, BOOP, primary pulmonary alveolar proteinosis (PAP). • Inflammatory—EnLP most common in cats with bronchitis, bronchiectasis or necrotizing bronchiolitis.
• Infectious—Dogs: canine distemper virus, canine adenovirus-2, H3N2 or H3N8 influenza virus, *Leishmania chagasi, Pneumocystis jirovecii, Angiostrongylus vasorum, Mycoplasma* sp, Toxoplasma, Leptospirosis, *Babesia* sp, *Ehrlichia canis.* Cats: *Aelurostrongylus abstrusus, Toxoplasma*, feline immunodeficiency virus, influenza virus (anthroponotic transmission described).
• Toxic—inhalation of dusts, gases, or vapors, thiacetarsamide, aspiration of petroleum-based products in cats, secondary PAP, paraquat toxicity, silicosis, asbestosis. • Vascular—thromboembolism, circulating larval migrans.

RISK FACTORS

• Immunosuppression, inadequate vaccination or preventative, and exposure to other animals can predispose to viral or parasitic pulmonary disease. • Inhalation of toxic material or gases may predispose to pulmonary fibrosis.

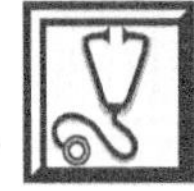

DIAGNOSIS

DIFFERENTIAL DIAGNOSIS

• Airway disease. • Bronchopneumonia.
• Heartworm disease. • Embolic pneumonia.
• Granulomatous pneumonia. • Neoplasia.
• Cardiac disease.

CBC/BIOCHEMISTRY/URINALYSIS

• Neutrophilia, eosinophilia, lymphocytosis, hyperglobulinemia possible; polycythemia if chronically hypoxemic. • Thrombocytopenia with *Angiostrongylus vasorum.* • Neutropenia or high liver enzymes and hyperbilirubinemia possible with *Toxoplasma.* • High liver enzymes and hyperbilirubinemia (dogs only) possible with hepatotoxicity due to thiacetarsemide therapy ± paraquat toxicity. • Severe azotemia and isosthenuria with uremic pneumonitis.

OTHER LABORATORY TESTS

• Arterial blood gas measurement and calculation of alveolar–arterial (A-a) gradient to assess degree of respiratory impairment; Pao_2 <80 mmHg indicates hypoxemia, A-a gradient >15 is abnormal. • Serologic and other tests for infectious causes. • Fecal Baermann examination for *Aelurostrongylus abstrusus* or *Angiostrongylus vasorum.*
• Toxicologic analysis of the urine or serum to diagnose paraquat toxicity in live animals.
• Coagulation testing with *Angiostrongylus.*
• Immunodiagnostic testing for exposure to *Leishmania.*

IMAGING

Thoracic Radiographic Findings

• A focal or diffuse, mild to severe interstitial to bronchial to alveolar pattern can be present, dilated bronchi with bronchiectasis or BOOP.
• Right heart ± PA enlargement and hepatosplenomegaly if secondary pulmonary hypertension. • Pleural effusion occasionally seen.

CT

CT characteristics include ground-glass opacification, peribronchovascular thickening, and parenchymal banding.

DIAGNOSTIC PROCEDURES

• Electrocardiography—arrhythmias can occur with severe hypoxia or systemic disease.
• Open lung biopsy required for definitive diagnostic test. • Endotracheal or transtracheal wash, bronchoscopy with bronchoalveolar lavage, and/or fine-needle aspirate of lungs might be useful (e.g., may visualize trophozoite or cysts of *Pneumocystis jirovecii* or *Toxoplasma* or see L1 larvae with *Aelurostrongylus abstrusus or Angiostrongylus vasorum*); cultures can reveal secondary bacterial infections. Viral testing (serology or swab). With PAP, an opaque white material is retrieved from airway wash. • Echocardiogram can document pulmonary hypertension.

PATHOLOGIC FINDINGS

• *Aelurostrongylus abstrusus*—greenish nodules in lungs, eggs and larvae in the alveolar spaces with foreign body type reaction (surrounded by mononuclear cells and giant cells), submucosal gland hypertrophy, and smooth muscle hypertrophy in airway and vessel walls. • *Angiostrongylus vasorum*—thrombosing arteritis and fibrotic peribronchitis, parasites in arterioles. • BOOP—polypoid plugs of loose, fibrous tissue fill bronchioles and alveoli, foamy macrophages within alveoli, variable inflammatory infiltrate with type II pneumocyte reactivity. • Interstitial lung disease in the West Highland white terrier—diffuse, mature pulmonary fibrosis (most common in caudal lung lobes),

multifocal areas of accentuated subpleural and peribronchiolar fibrosis, thickening of the alveolar septum due to excess collagen in the extracellular matrix. • IPF-like disease in the cat lacks inflammation and may be associated with pulmonary carcinoma. Typical changes include multifocal distribution of interstitial fibrosis with foci of fibroblast/myofibroblasts, alveolar epithelial metaplasia, and interstitial smooth muscle metaplasia/hyperplasia.
• *Leishmania chagasi* is characterized by chronic and diffuse interstitial pneumonitis and thickened interalveolar septae in some cases. • Lipid pneumonias—macroscopic lesions can include subpleural, parenchymal, or perivascular white, firm nodules. Mixed pattern of inflammation with accumulation of lipid-laden macrophages, cholesterol clefts, and multinucleated giant cells. • Paraquat toxicity—lungs are heavy, edematous, and hemorrhagic. Emphysematous bullae and pneumomediastinum are commonly present.
• PAP—alveolar spaces are distended with a periodic acid–Schiff staining eosinophilic proteinaceous material. Intra-alveolar cholesterol clefts and mucus-laden macrophages with mild mixed inflammatory infiltrates are common. • Uremic pneumonitis—pulmonary edema and calcification of smooth muscle and/or alveolar walls.

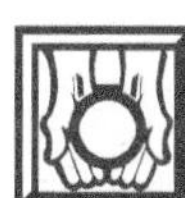

TREATMENT

APPROPRIATE HEALTH CARE

Inpatient care and monitoring for animals with evidence of respiratory distress.

NURSING CARE

• Oxygen therapy. • Minimize exposure to house dust, vapors, chemical fumes, or tobacco smoke. • Humidification of inspired air. • PAP—therapeutic bronchoalveolar lavage. • Antimicrobial therapy—as indicated by results of culture and susceptibility.

ACTIVITY

• Exercise restriction as needed. • Harness preferred to collar.

DIET

Weight loss if obese.

CLIENT EDUCATION

Palliative care employed.

SURGICAL CONSIDERATIONS

Definitive diagnosis of interstitial lung disease requires histopathology; it is best preceded by CT to determine an appropriate site for biopsy.

MEDICATIONS

DRUG(S) OF CHOICE

• Inhaled corticosteroids (e.g., fluticasone, 1 puff q12h) using a spacing chamber and facemask. • Bronchodilators can be helpful in reducing respiratory effort: extended-release theophylline (dog, 10 mg/kg PO q12h; cat, 15–19 mg/kg q24h in the evening), terbutaline sulfate (dog or cat, 0.01 mg/kg SC, IM, or IV q8–12h). Inhaled bronchodilators can also be used. • *Aelurostrongylus abstrusus*—fenbendazole 50 mg/kg PO q24h for 14 days (off-label), ivermectin (400 µg/kg SC twice at a 3-week interval), or spot-on selamectin 45 mg (once). • *Angiostrongylus vasorum*—levamisole 20–40 mg/kg PO q48h for 5 treatments ± aspirin ± corticosteroids. Alternative therapies include fenbendazole, mebendazole, and ivermectin. • BOOP—corticosteroid use has been reported. • IPF—no effective therapy. Anti-inflammatory steroid therapy with prednisolone (0.5–1 mg/kg PO q24–48h often used) and bronchodilators, antitussives, or antibiotics if indicated. Pirfenidone not yet investigated. • *Leishmania chagasi*—meglumine antimonate 100 mg/kg IV or SC q24h for 3–4 weeks or sodium stibogluconate 30–50 mg/kg IV or SC q24h for 3–4 weeks. • Paraquat toxicity—vomition and activated charcoal therapy is indicated if recent ingestion is known. Supportive care, diuresis using furosemide (most effective in the first 3 days following ingestion), ± immunosuppressive dexamethasone, cyclophosphamide, nicotinamide, superoxide dismutase, and vitamin A.

CONTRAINDICATIONS/PRECAUTIONS

Immunosuppressive therapy can exacerbate secondary infections.

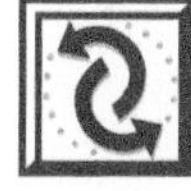

FOLLOW-UP

PATIENT MONITORING

• Have owners observe clinical response to therapy, monitor respiratory rate and effort.
• Repeat physical examination/chest auscultation, chest radiographs, lab test, and arterial blood gas analysis as indicated.

PREVENTION/AVOIDANCE

• Avoid proximity to toxic fumes or paraquat.
• Vaccinate and deworm animals. • Appropriate insect and rodent control. Avoid ingestion by pets of frogs, lizards, rodents, and birds.

POSSIBLE COMPLICATIONS

• Secondary pulmonary infections possible.
• Pulmonary hypertension can develop.

EXPECTED COURSE AND PROGNOSIS

• Guarded to poor with interstitial pneumonia caused by infectious agents or uremic pneumonitis. • Poor long-term prognosis with IPF (mean survival time is 17 months in dogs and 5.5 months in cats).
• Paraquat toxicity—commonly fatal in dogs.

MISCELLANEOUS

ASSOCIATED CONDITIONS

Pulmonary carcinoma—associated with IPF in cats.

AGE-RELATED FACTORS

Young, free-roaming animals are more likely to succumb to infectious diseases.

ZOONOTIC POTENTIAL

Toxoplasmosis, if animal is shedding oocysts.

PREGNANCY/FERTILITY/BREEDING

Transplacental infection with *Toxoplasma* and canine distemper virus is possible.

SEE ALSO

• Bronchiectasis. • Canine Distemper.
• Canine Infectious Respiratory Disease.
• Feline Immunodeficiency Virus (FIV) Infection. • Leishmaniosis. • Toxoplasmosis.

ABBREVIATIONS

• BOOP = bronchiolitis obliterans with organizing pneumonia. • DIP = desquamative interstitial pneumonitis.
• EnLP = endogenous lipid pneumonia.
• IPF = idiopathic pulmonary fibrosis. • PAP = pulmonary alveolar proteinosis.

Suggested Reading

Cohn LA, Norris CR, Hawkins EC, et al. Identification and characterization of an idiopathic pulmonary fibrosis-like condition in cats. J Vet Intern Med 2004, 18(5):632–641.

Corcoran BM, Cobb M, Martin WS, et al. Chronic pulmonary disease in West Highland white terriers. Vet Rec 1999, 144:611–616.

Heikkilä HP, Lappalainen AK, Day MJ, et al. Clinical, bronchoscopic, histopathologic, diagnostic imaging, and arterial oxygenation findings in West Highland white terriers with idiopathic pulmonary fibrosis. J Vet Intern Med 2011, 25(3):433–439.

Author Deborah C. Silverstein
Consulting Editor Elizabeth Rozanski

Client Education Handout available online

P

PNEUMOTHORAX

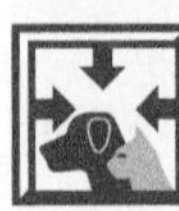

BASICS

DEFINITION

- Air accumulation in the pleural space (traumatic or spontaneous).
- Closed pneumothorax—no defects in the thoracic wall.
- Open pneumothorax—defect in the thoracic wall
- Tension pneumothorax—pleural pressure in a closed pneumothorax exceeds atmospheric pressure created by unidirectional transfer of air into the pleural space.

PATHOPHYSIOLOGY

- The pleural space is a potential space between the visceral and parietal pleura containing a thin layer of fluid that contributes to "tethering" of the lungs to the thoracic wall.
- Closed pneumothorax—air leakage from the pulmonary parenchyma, large airway, or esophagus.
- Tension pneumothorax—typically due to a pleural or pulmonary flap-like defect that opens on inspiration to allow leakage of air into the pleural space and closes during expiration. Development of high intrathoracic pressure can cause cardiovascular collapse.
- Open pneumothorax—pleural pressure equals atmospheric pressure, leading to lung collapse.
- Spontaneous pneumothorax—associated with underlying pulmonary disease that ruptures, allowing air leakage.
- Pneumothorax is usually bilateral disease due to mediastinal fenestrations.

P

SYSTEMS AFFECTED

- Respiratory.
- Cardiovascular.

INCIDENCE/PREVALENCE

Traumatic pneumothorax occurs in >40% of cases with chest trauma and 11–18% of dogs and cats presented for vehicular trauma. Pneumothorax has been reported in 25% of cases with intrathoracic grass awns and 70% of dogs with thoracic bite wounds.

SIGNALMENT

Species

Dog and cat.

Breed Predilections

Spontaneous pneumothorax—more common in large, deep-chested dogs. Siberian huskies may be overrepresented.

SIGNS

Historical Findings

- Traumatic—recent trauma, thoracocentesis, jugular venipuncture, lung aspirate, thoracotomy, mechanical ventilation, neck surgery, recent endotracheal intubation.
- Spontaneous—possible history of pulmonary disease; usually acute.

Physical Examination Findings

- Respiratory distress (tachypnea, increased respiratory effort, ± orthopnea).
- Shallow, rapid abdominal breathing.
- Decreased to absent breath sounds dorsally.
- Cyanosis.
- Tachycardia.

Traumatic Pneumothorax

- Signs of trauma (blunt or penetrating thoracic wall injury) or hypovolemic shock (pale mucous membranes, prolonged capillary refill time, altered mentation, poor pulse quality, tachycardia, decreased extremity compared to core temperature).
- Subcutaneous emphysema in some cases with pneumomediastinum and/or tracheal trauma.

CAUSES

- Traumatic—blunt trauma, penetrating thoracic or cervical injuries, post-thoracocentesis or thoracotomy, esophageal perforation, endotracheal tube-associated tracheal trauma, mechanical ventilation, pulmonary aspirate.
- Spontaneous—bullous emphysema (most common in dogs), pulmonary bullae or bleb.
- Migrating pulmonary foreign body, pulmonary neoplasia, pulmonary abscess, feline asthma, bronchopneumonia, mycotic pulmonary granuloma, parasitic pulmonary disease (*Paragonimus*), congenital pulmonary cyst, congenital lobar emphysema, secondary to lung lobe torsion.
- Extension of pneumomediastinum.

RISK FACTORS

- Trauma.
- Thoracocentesis.
- Thoracotomy.
- Overinflation of endotracheal cuff.
- Excessive airway pressure during ventilation.
- Pulmonary disease/pathology.
- Migrating grass awns.

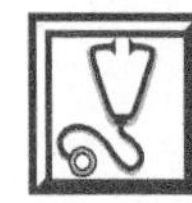

DIAGNOSIS

DIFFERENTIAL DIAGNOSIS

- Pleural effusion.
- Diaphragmatic hernia.
- Pulmonary parenchymal disease.

CBC/BIOCHEMISTRY/URINALYSIS

Neutrophilia with a left shift if infection or inflammation.

OTHER LABORATORY TESTS

- Arterial blood gases—hypoxemia; hypocapnia or hypercapnia.
- Fecal sedimentation or zinc sulfate flotation for *Paragonimus kellicotti*.

IMAGING

Thoracic Radiography

- Delay until patient is stable.
- Air in pleural space, pulmonary vascular pattern does not extend to the chest wall, cardiac silhouette elevated off the sternum.
- Pulmonary pathology can be obscured by lung lobe collapse.
- Traumatic pneumothorax—pulmonary contusions, rib fractures, diaphragmatic hernia, hemothorax, foreign bodies.
- Spontaneous pneumothorax—evaluate for any sign of parenchymal pathology.
- Right lateral horizontal beam results in the highest rate of detection and severity gradation while ventrodorsal/dorsoventral views have the lowest rate.

Thoracic Ultrasound

- Pneumothorax evidenced by loss of the "glide sign."
- Reverse sliding sign has a 100% specificity for detecting mild pneumothorax.
- Sensitivity of 78% and specificity of 93% compared to thoracic radiographs in identification of traumatic pneumothorax in dogs with higher sensitivity in penetrating trauma (93%) compared to blunt trauma (65%).
- CT has a higher diagnostic yield for detecting pneumothorax than thoracic-focused assessment with sonography for trauma.

Thoracic CT

- Used preoperatively to improve localization of pulmonary pathology in cases with spontaneous pneumothorax.
- CT can fail to detect pulmonary bullae prior to surgical exploration.

DIAGNOSTIC PROCEDURES

- Thoracocentesis.
- Bronchoscopy—consider if evidence of tracheal or large airway trauma.

PATHOLOGIC FINDINGS

- Varies depending on underlying disease.
- Gross evaluation—pulmonary blebs, pulmonary or airway tears, pulmonary parenchymal disease or masses.
- Histopathology—blebs are most commonly found at the apex and are contained entirely within the pleura; bullae are lined by pleura, fibrous pulmonary tissue, and emphysematous lung.

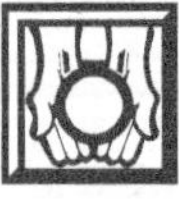

TREATMENT

APPROPRIATE HEALTH CARE

- Inpatient care until air accumulation has stopped or has stabilized.
- Thoracocentesis in patients with respiratory distress—can be performed with an IV catheter attached to an extension set and stopcock or via a butterfly needle.
- *Always* provide oxygen therapy until patient is stabilized.
- If large open chest wound—chest tube placement, cover with sterile airtight bandage; surgical closure once animal is stable.

- Tube thoracostomy—use if unable to stabilize with thoracocentesis or repeated thoracocentesis required for continued pneumothorax. A Seldinger technique allows chest tube placement under light sedation and may be preferable over other thoracostomy tube placement techniques.
- If pneumothorax is rapidly accumulating—use continuous chest tube suction via one-, two- or three-bottle drainage system with an underwater seal. If pneumothorax is not severe—use intermittent tube aspiration.
- Emergency thoracotomy in life-threatening pneumothorax.
- Open traumatic pneumothorax—surgery as soon as patient is stable.
- Closed traumatic pneumothorax—rarely requires surgical intervention.
- Spontaneous pneumothorax—early surgical intervention recommended in dogs (consider median sternotomy), ± pleural access port placed for medical management.
- Blood pleurodesis may be of benefit in refractory cases—blood is collected from the jugular vein and injected into the pleural cavity via a thoracostomy tube.

NURSING CARE

- Appropriate pain control.
- Chest tube maintenance—ensure all connections are airtight (cable ties for securing connections); ensure the tube is attached at two points. Clean tube site and change dressing once daily.

ACTIVITY

Strict rest for at least a week following resolution.

CLIENT EDUCATION

- Traumatic pneumothorax—discuss possibility of a chest tube, hospitalization; ± surgery.
- Spontaneous pneumothorax—early surgical intervention. Discuss possibility of underlying pulmonary disease that can make resolution challenging and recurrence possible. Warn owner that even with thoracotomy, the source of the pneumothorax may not be found and recurrent disease is possible.

SURGICAL CONSIDERATIONS

- Do not use positive-pressure ventilation for closed pneumothorax. Place chest tube prior to ventilation or await thoracotomy prior to ventilation.
- Thoracoscopy—may allow visualization of local lesion; allows instillation of substances for pleurodesis.
- Thoracotomy—if lesion is not evident, can fill thorax with saline and look for bubbles as sign of a leak. Partial or full lung lobectomy for localized lesions. Place thoracostomy tube.
- Pleurodesis with mechanical abrasion of the pleura or instillation of an inflammatory substance, such as talc, into the pleural space (success rate poor).
- Autologous blood-patch for persistent pneumothorax (simple and relatively safe procedure) in patients that have failed conservative or surgical management.

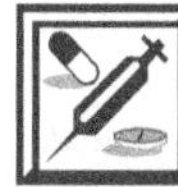

MEDICATIONS

DRUG(S) OF CHOICE

Judicious use of pain control.

PRECAUTIONS

Beware excess respiratory depression with opiates.

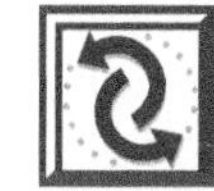

FOLLOW-UP

PATIENT MONITORING

- Respiratory rate—increased rate suggests recurrence.
- Serial thoracic radiographs to quantitate accumulation of air.
- Pulse oximetry and arterial blood gases may be considered.
- Central venous (jugular) blood gases to evaluate ventilation status ($P\text{vCO}_2$).
- Rate of air production from chest tube.

PREVENTION/AVOIDANCE

Keep pets confined—less likely to be injured.

POSSIBLE COMPLICATIONS

- Death from hypoxemia and cardiovascular compromise.
- Incorrect placement of chest tube or trauma associated with thoracocentesis—lung lobe laceration, cardiac puncture, diaphragmatic laceration, liver trauma.
- Pleural infection from thoracocentesis or thoracostomy tube. The risk of pyothorax associated with thoracostomy tube is higher between 4 and 6 days after placement.

EXPECTED COURSE AND PROGNOSIS

- Traumatic pneumothorax—good prognosis with mild trauma ± chest drain placement. Guarded prognosis with severe trauma usually because of severe pulmonary contusions.
- Spontaneous pneumothorax—prognosis depends on underlying cause. Good prognosis with focal lesion amenable to surgical resection. Poor prognosis with multiple lesions or neoplasia.

MISCELLANEOUS

SYNONYMS

Punctured lung.

SEE ALSO

- Dyspnea and Respiratory Distress.
- Panting and Tachypnea.

Suggested Reading

Lisciandro GR, Lagutchik MS, Mann KA, et al. Evaluation of a thoracic focused assessment with sonography for trauma (TFAST) protocol to detect pneumothorax and concurrent thoracic injury in 145 traumatized dogs. J Vet Emerg Crit Care 2008, 18:258–269.

Oppenheimer N, Klainbart S, Merbl Y, et al. Retrospective evaluation of the use of autologous blood-patch treatment for persistent pneumothorax in 8 dogs (2009–2012). J Vet Emerg Crit Care 2014, 24:215–220.

Puerto DA, Brockman DJ, Lindquist C, Drobatz K. Surgical and nonsurgical management of and selected risk factors for spontaneous pneumothorax in dogs: 64 cases (1986–1999). J Am Vet Med Assoc 2002, 220:1670–1674.

Reetz JA, Caceres AV, Suran JN, et al. Sensitivity, positive predictive value, and interobserver variability of computed tomography in the diagnosis of bullae associated with spontaneous pneumothorax in dogs: 19 cases (2003–2012). J Am Vet Med Assoc 2013, 243:244–251.

Scheepens ET, Peeters ME, L'Eplattenier HF, Kirpensteijn J. Thoracic bite trauma in dogs: A comparison of clinical and radiological parameters with surgical results. J Small Anim Pract 2006, 47:721–726.

Authors Laura Cagle and Kate Hopper
Consulting Editor Elizabeth Rozanski

Client Education Handout available online

PODODERMATITIS

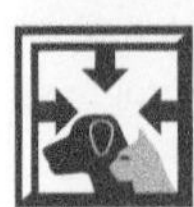

BASICS

DEFINITION

An inflammatory, multifaceted complex of diseases that involves the feet of dogs and cats.

PATHOPHYSIOLOGY

• Depends on the underlying cause.
• Psychogenic dermatosis (rare cause).

SYSTEMS AFFECTED

Skin/exocrine.

INCIDENCE/PREVALENCE

• Dogs—common. • Cats—uncommon.

SIGNALMENT

Breed Predilections

• Dogs, short-coated breeds—most commonly affected; English bulldog, Great Dane, basset hound, mastiff, bull terrier, boxer, dachshund, Dalmatian, German shorthaired pointer, and Weimaraner. • Dogs, long-coated breeds—German shepherd dog, Labrador retriever, golden retriever, Irish setter, and Pekingese. • Cats—none.

Mean Age and Range

• Any age. • Young dogs—hypersensitivity, demodicosis, infection, follicular cysts, autoimmune dermatoses. • Old dogs—also neoplasia or systemic diseases.

Predominant Sex

• Dogs—male. • Cats—none.

SIGNS

General Comments

History and physical findings vary considerably depending on the underlying cause.

Historical Findings

• Environment and general husbandry—indoor vs. outdoor, working dog, unsanitary conditions, contact irritants, hookworms. • Age of onset.
• Seasonality—atopic dermatitis, allergic contact dermatitis, or irritant contact dermatitis.
• Lesions elsewhere on the body or confined to just the feet; note which feet are affected and what parts of the feet are affected (entire foot, one area, or one digit). • Response to previous therapy—antibiotics, antifungals, and corticosteroids. • Diet, travel history, and other medical problems.

Physical Examination Findings

Infectious (Dogs)

• Erythema and edema, nodules, inflammatory plaques (fungal "kerions"), ulcers, fistulae, hemorrhagic bullae, or serosanguineous or seropurulent discharge.
• Feet—may be grossly swollen; often interdigital swellings that have a history of opening and draining, may have pitting edema of the metacarpal and metatarsal areas.
• Skin—may be alopecic and moist from constant licking; patient may have some degree of pain, pruritus, and paronychia.
• Regional lymph nodes may be enlarged.

Infectious (Cats)

• Painful paronychia, involving one or more claws. • Higher incidence of nodular, often ulcerated lesions, compared to dog.
• Footpads and periungual areas—commonly involved. • Interdigital spaces—seldom affected. • Scaly and crusted lesions—occasionally seen.

Allergic (Dogs)

• Salivary staining, erythema and alopecia (dorsal or ventral or both) secondary to pruritus; dorsal surfaces may be more severely affected than ventral surfaces. Hypersensitivities typically do not produce draining tracts. • Interdigital erythema. • Allergic contact dermatitis—uncommon; ventral interdigital surfaces most affected.

Allergic (Cats)

• Single or multiple, exudative or ulcerated, pruritic plaques of the digits, periungual, and interdigital spaces. • Eosinophilic granuloma complex lesions.

Immune-Mediated (Dogs)

• Crusts and ulcerations—most common lesions; occasional vesicles or bullae. • All feet affected, especially the ungual folds and footpads. • Hyperkeratotic and erosive dermatitis of the footpad margins—common finding in pemphigus foliaceus.

Immune-Mediated (Cats)

• Lesions—generally involve the footpad, including hyperkeratosis and ulceration.
• Lameness and paronychia with ungual fold exudate.

Endocrine/Metabolic (Dogs)

• Lesions—usually consistent with secondary infection. • Hepatocutaneous syndrome (superficial necrolytic dermatitis)—rare condition; skin disease precedes the onset of signs of internal disease; hyperkeratosis (with adherent crusts), fissures, and ulceration of the footpads. • Metastatic calcinosis cutis—seen with chronic renal disease; painful swollen footpads that ulcerate/discharge chalk-like material.

Endocrine/Metabolic (Cats)

• Cutaneous xanthomatosis—seen with diabetes mellitus; whitish nodules resembling candle wax. • Metastatic calcinosis cutis—seen with chronic renal disease; painful swollen footpads that ulcerate/discharge chalk-like material.

Neoplastic

• Dogs—nodules, variably ulcerated, scale, erythema, depigmentation of the footpads; may have only one digit involved (clawbed carcinoma, ungual keratoacanthoma); multiple feet involvement with clawbed squamous cell carcinoma, epitheliotropic lymphoma; pruritus variable. • Cats—nodules; variably ulcerated and painful; localized destruction variable, depends on tumor type foot pad tumors may develop *de novo* or be metastatic carcinoma.

Environmental (Dogs and Cats)

• Involve one digit or foot (foreign body, trauma) or multiple digits (irritant contact dermatitis, thallium toxicity, housing on rough surface or in moist environment).
• Chronic interdigital inflammation, ulceration, pyogranulomatous abscesses, draining tracts, or swelling, with or without pruritus.

Miscellaneous

• Hyperkeratosis of the footpads (dogs)—associated with several diseases (e.g., zinc-responsive dermatosis), and idiopathic digital hyperkeratosis. • Interdigital follicular cysts—interdigital nodules, fistulae and draining tracts dorsally; most often affects the lateral interdigital space of the front feet; history of recurrence and poor to no response to antibiotics, with an area of alopecic, thickened skin with comedones ventrally. • Nodules without draining tracts (dogs)—associated with sterile pyogranuloma in several breeds and nodular dermatofibrosis of German shepherd dogs and golden retrievers.
• Hypomelanosis of the footpads (cats)—associated with vitiligo. • Hypermelanosis of the footpads (cats)—associated with lentigo simplex. • Acral mutilation and analgesia—seen in pointers (English and German shorthaired) and spaniels (English springer and French)—cause unknown; often runts of the litter; no known treatment; dogs are usually euthanized within days to months of diagnosis.

CAUSES

Infectious (Dogs)

• Bacterial—*Staphylococcus pseudintermedius*, *Pseudomonas* spp., *Proteus* spp., *Mycobacterium* spp., *Nocardia* spp., *Actinomyces* spp.
• Fungal—dermatophytes, intermediate mycoses (sporotrichosis, mycetoma), deep mycoses (blastomycosis, cryptococcosis).
• Parasitic—*Demodex canis*, *Pelodera strongyloides*, hookworms.
• Protozoal—leishmaniasis.

Infectious (Cats)

• Bacterial—same as dog; *Pasteurella* spp.
• Fungal—same as dog, excluding blastomycosis. • Parasitic—*Neotrombicula autumnalis*, *Notoedres cati*, *Demodex* spp.
• Protozoal—*Anatrichosoma cutaneum*.

Allergic

• Dogs—atopy; food hypersensitivity; allergic contact dermatitis. • Cats—atopy; rare for flea allergic dermatitis, food hypersensitivity, or contact dermatitis to involve paws (except lesions of eosinophilic granuloma complex).

Immune-Mediated

- Dogs—pemphigus foliaceus; systemic lupus erythematosus; erythema multiforme; cold agglutinin disease; pemphigus vulgaris; bullous pemphigoid; epidermolysis bullosa acquisita, symmetrical lupoid onychodystrophy.
- Cats—pemphigus foliaceus; systemic lupus erythematosus; erythema multiforme; vasculitis; cold agglutinin disease; plasma cell pododermatitis.

Endocrine/Metabolic

- Dogs—hypothyroidism; hyperadrenocorticism; hepatocutaneous syndrome; chronic renal failure. • Cats—hyperthyroidism; hyperadrenocorticism; cutaneous xanthomatosis (secondary to diabetes mellitus); chronic renal failure; endocrine pododermatitis rare.

Neoplastic

- Higher incidence in cats than in dogs.
- Dogs—squamous cell carcinoma; epitheliotropic lymphoma, melanoma; mast cell tumor; keratoacanthoma; inverted papilloma; eccrine adenocarcinoma.
- Cats—papilloma; squamous cell carcinoma; trichoepithelioma; fibrosarcoma; malignant fibrous histiocytoma; metastatic primary adenocarcinoma or squamous cell carcinoma of the lung (feline lung-digit syndrome).

Environmental

- Dogs—irritant contact dermatitis; trauma; concrete and gravel dog runs; excessive exercise; clipper burn; foreign bodies; thallium toxicity. • Cats—irritant contact dermatitis; foreign bodies; thallium toxicity.

Miscellaneous

- Dogs—sterile interdigital granuloma; interdigital follicular cyst (see Physical Examination Findings). • Cats—see Physical Examination Findings.

RISK FACTORS

- Lifestyle and general husbandry conditions—influence development. • Excess exercise, abrasive or moist housing, poor grooming, and/or lack of preventive medical care may predispose an animal or exacerbate condition.
- Body size, foot conformation, and breed influence the development of interdigital follicular cysts.

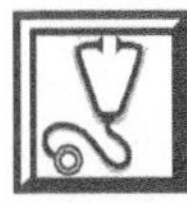

DIAGNOSIS

DIFFERENTIAL DIAGNOSIS

See Signs and Causes.

CBC/BIOCHEMISTRY/URINALYSIS

Depends on the underlying cause.

IMAGING

Depends on the underlying cause.

DIAGNOSTIC PROCEDURES

- Skin scrapings or hair plucks—demodicosis.
- Fungal culture—dermatophytosis.
- Exudate or pustule smear—bacterial or yeast infection. • Culture and sensitivity from exudates and/or biopsy tissues. • Dogs—biopsies indicated if skin scrapings are negative and lesions (nodules, draining tracts) are seen; samples from the ventral surface with draining tracts may reveal follicular cysts and pyogranulomatous inflammation leading to the dorsal surface. • Cats—biopsies may be indicated in all cases; pedal dermatosis is relatively rare. • Restricted-ingredient food trial—food hypersensitivity. • Intradermal testing—atopy. • Endocrine assays—hypothyroidism, hyperadrenocorticism, diabetes mellitus.

PATHOLOGIC FINDINGS

Depends on the underlying cause.

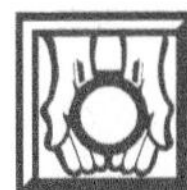

TREATMENT

APPROPRIATE HEALTH CARE

Outpatient, unless surgery is indicated.

NURSING CARE

Foot soaking and/or bandaging may be necessary, depending on cause.

CLIENT EDUCATION

- Depends on underlying cause and severity of condition. • Discuss husbandry and preventive medical practices. • Many etiologies can be managed but not cured.

SURGICAL CONSIDERATIONS

- Melanoma and squamous cell carcinoma—very poor prognosis; early diagnosis necessitates amputation of the digit(s) or paw.
- Infectious—may benefit from surgical debridement of devitalized tissue before medical therapy. • Recurrent draining tracts caused by interdigital follicular cysts may be cleared with laser ablation.

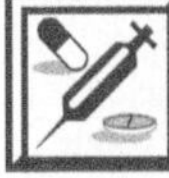

MEDICATIONS

DRUG(S) OF CHOICE

- Depend on the underlying cause and secondary infections; see related chapters for dosages of appropriate medications.
- Antibiotics based on culture and sensitivity; 4–6 weeks minimum.

PRECAUTIONS

Depend on the treatment protocol selected for the underlying cause; see specific drugs and their precautions.

POSSIBLE INTERACTIONS

Depends on the underlying cause and treatment protocol selected.

FOLLOW-UP

PATIENT MONITORING

Depends on the underlying cause and treatment protocol selected.

PREVENTION/AVOIDANCE

Environmental cause—good husbandry and preventive medical care.

POSSIBLE COMPLICATIONS

Depends on the underlying cause and treatment protocol selected.

EXPECTED COURSE AND PROGNOSIS

- Success of therapy depends on finding the underlying cause; often the cause is unknown; even when the cause is known, management can be frustrating owing to relapses or lack of affordable therapeutics. • Often the disease can only be managed and not cured.
- Referral to dermatologist often appropriate.
- Surgical intervention is sometimes necessary.

MISCELLANEOUS

ZOONOTIC POTENTIAL

Depends on the underlying cause; uncommon.

PREGNANCY/FERTILITY/BREEDING

Depends on treatment protocol selected.

Suggested Reading

Duclos DD. Canine pododermatitis. Vet Clin North Am Small Anim Pract 2013, 43(1):57–87.

Author David D. Duclos

Consulting Editor Alexander H. Werner Resnick

Client Education Handout available online

P

POISONING (INTOXICATION) THERAPY

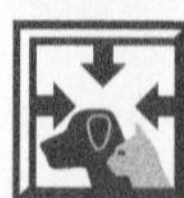

BASICS

DEFINITION

- Acutely ill patients are often diagnosed as poisoned when no other diagnosis is obvious.
- Direct initial efforts toward stabilizing the patient.
- Proper patient and toxicant assessment are critical in determining the appropriate decontamination and therapy needs for patient.
- Goals of treatment—provide emergency intervention; prevent further exposure; prevent additional absorption; apply specific antidotes; hasten elimination; provide supportive measures.
- Valuable time can be saved by applying the appropriate treatment for a suspected or known intoxicant.
- Suspected intentional intoxication—suspected toxic materials and specimens may be valuable from a medical–legal aspect; maintain a proper chain of physical evidence and keep excellent medical records if malicious intent is suspected.
- Initial patient evaluation includes the following:
  - Assess patient status and review signalment.
  - Determine any current or past medical conditions and current medications.
  - Determine the toxicant patient was exposed to as well as the route, dose, and time since exposure.
  - Determining location of exposure may be helpful at ruling in or out additional potential concerns.

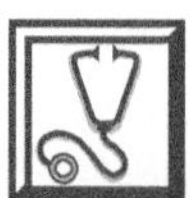

DIAGNOSIS

DIFFERENTIAL DIAGNOSIS

- Definitive diagnosis is often difficult; animals may come in contact with varying substances that pet owners are unaware of.
- Pet Poison Helpline, ASPCA Animal Poison Control Center, local poison control centers, and state diagnostic laboratories all offer support in determining toxicity risk and potential therapy needs for animal.
- When suspected exposure and clinical signs do not correlate—offer symptomatic and supportive care to treat current signs.
- Confirmation of diagnosis—most commonly achieved by finding remnants of exposed substance and animal's clinical status; chemical analysis (rarely done and is often after the fact).

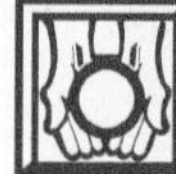

TREATMENT

APPROPRIATE HEALTH CARE

Supportive Care

- Control body temperature.
- Maintain respiratory and cardiovascular function.
- Control acid–base balance.
- Control CNS disorders—see specific chapters.
- Alleviate pain.

Emergency

- Establish a patent airway.
- Assisted ventilation, as needed.
- Cardiopulmonary resuscitation methods, as needed.
- After stabilization—proceed with more specific therapeutic measures.

Prevent Absorption

- Remove patient from the affected environment, especially with inhaled toxins.
- Protect caregivers as well from inhaled toxins.
- Decontamination methods include dermal, ocular, respiratory, and gastrointestinal.

Dermal Decontamination: Bathing Skin/Haircoat

- Indicated for external toxicants.
- Bathe to remove the noxious agent using liquid dishwashing detergent.
- *Caution*: Use protective measures to avoid contamination of those handling the patient.

Ocular Decontamination

- Irritants—rinse eye(s) with eye wash or tap water for 10–15 minutes. Monitor for signs of irritation.
- Corrosives—rinse eye(s) with eye wash or tap water for 15–20 minutes and perform fluorescein stain; treat as needed.

Respiratory Decontamination

- Removal from source is often sufficient.
- Oxygen and humidified oxygen therapy may be necessary in more affected patients.

Gastrointestinal Decontamination

- Emetics:
  - Of little value beyond 1–2 hours after ingestion of many toxicants. Exceptions include large ingestions, grapes/raisins, gum, chocolate, and plant material.
  - Do not induce in patients who have neurologic abnormalities including severe agitation or severe depression/sedation. Avoid emesis after ingestion of strong acids, alkalis, petroleum distillates or substances that may result in a rapid onset of neurologic abnormalities.
  - Apomorphine—most effective and reliable for use in dogs; dopaminergic agonist; 0.03–0.04 mg/kg IV or IM, crushed tablet for conjunctival administration; emesis occurs within 10 minutes.
  - 3% Hydrogen peroxide—emetic of choice for home use; 1–2 mL/kg PO, do not exceed 45 mL in most dogs, 60 mL in large dogs; ineffective and contraindicated in cats, not always effective in dogs.
  - Dexmedetomidine—most effective and reliable for use in cats; α_2 agonist; 5–10 µg/kg IM; emesis expected within 10–20 minutes; reverse with atipamezole (equal volume in mL).
  - Xylazine—α_2 agonist for use in cats 0.44–1 mg/kg IM or SQ. Can be reversed with an α_2-adrenergic antagonist such as atipamezole or yohimbine.
  - Hydromorphone- mu opioid agonist for use in cats; 0.1 mg/kg SQ; emesis expected within 5–15 minutes; reverse with naloxone (0.01–0.04 mg/kg Im or SQ).
  - Ipecac—not recommended.
  - Salt or salt solution—not recommended; may result in salt toxicity.
- Activated charcoal:
  - Adsorbant—prevents absorption of toxic substance for certain toxicants.
  - Highly adsorptive of many toxicants including rodenticides, insecticides, and most over-the-counter and prescription medications.
  - Ineffective against xylitol, alcohols, chlorate, cyanide, heavy metals, corrosive and caustic chemicals, and petroleum distillates.
  - Administered after emetic—increases efficacy of toxicant elimination.
  - Dosage 1–5 g/kg body weight; generally a single dose administration; multidose administration if substance undergoes enterohepatic circulation (1–2 g/kg PO q6-8h for 24 hours).
  - Generally administered with a cathartic such as sorbitol; only the first dose should contain a cathartic. Magnesium-containing cathartics should be avoided or used with caution.
  - Hypernatremia has been reported after administration of activated charcoal, especially when a cathartic (sorbitol) is used in a dehydrated patient. Sub q or IV fluids can help to minimize risk.
- Gastric lavage:
  - Indicated in patients who are not acceptable candidates for emesis, have ingested a potentially life-threatening toxin or if emesis was unsuccessful. Most effective if performed in the first 1–2 hours.
  - An appropriately sized cuffed endotracheal tube must be in place prior to starting the lavage procedure.
  - Orogastric (stomach) tube size—use the largest possible; a good rule: use the same size as the cuffed endotracheal tube (1 mm = 3 Fr), measured to the last rib.

- Volume of warm water or lavage solution for each washing—5–10 mL/kg body weight; avoid forceful administration.
- Agitate stomach and either aspirate or allow gravity drainage of stomach contents. Activated charcoal with a cathartic can be infused, if indicated, before removing orogastric tube; however, caution should be used to ensure patient maintains a protected airway in the event of regurgitation.
- Procedure should only be used in appropriate exposures and proper patient status.

- Surgery or endoscopic removal:
  - May be indicated for coins, metals, batteries, and drug-infused patches.
- Enemas:
  - May hasten the elimination of toxicants from the lower gastrointestinal tract.
  - Warm water ± lubricant.
  - Take care to avoid the induction of dehydration and electrolyte imbalances with overzealous treatment.

Enhance Elimination

- Absorbed toxicants—often excreted by the kidneys; may be excreted by other routes (e.g., bile, feces, lungs, and other body secretions).
- Renal excretion—may be manipulated in many animals.
- Urinary excretion—may be enhanced using diuretics or by altering the pH of the urine; not frequently performed.

Diuretics

- Enhance urinary excretion of some toxicants—requires maintenance of adequate renal function.
- If minimum urine flow cannot be established—must use peritoneal dialysis (normal urine output is 1–2 mL/kg/h).
- Agents of choice—furosemide 2 mg/kg IV q6–8h, if no response increase dose to 4–6 mg/kg IV q6–8h, or mannitol 1–2 g/kg IV slowly over 20–30 minutes q6h.
- Caution should be used as electrolyte abnormalities may occur.

Manipulating Urine pH

- Not routinely performed; elimination may not be enhanced to a level that improves clinical outcome and may cause or worsen metabolic acidosis.
- Acidic compounds remain ionized in alkaline urine; alkaline compounds remain ionized in acidic urine.
- IV 0.9% sodium chloride—rapid, urinary acidifying agent.
- IV sodium bicarbonate may be used as an alkalinizing agent.

Fluid Therapy

- Consider volume replacement with crystalloids and colloids if necessary.
- May enhance elimination of toxicants that undergo renal excretion.

Peritoneal Dialysis

- Potentially indicated for water-soluble, low-molecular-weight, poorly protein-bound compounds with a small volume of distribution such as alcohols, lithium, and salicylates.
- Indicated for simple removal of absorbed toxicants in patient with normal renal function.
- pH of the solution—may be altered to maintain the ionized state of the offending compound.

Lipid Emulsion Therapy

- Promising use as antidote for toxicosis from many fat-soluble drugs.
- Has been used successfully in veterinary medicine to treat toxicity from highly lipophilic drugs such as baclofen, beta antagonists, calcium channel antagonists, ivermectin, moxidectin, and other fat-soluble medications.
- Exact mechanism of action remains unknown, but may act as a lipid sink.
- Potential adverse effects, although rare, include hyperlipidemia, hepatosplenomegaly, jaundice, seizures, hemolytic anemia, prolonged clotting time, thrombocytopenia, and fat embolism.
- Dosage extrapolated from humans using the 20% commercially available fat emulsion product. Standard protocol: 1.5–4 mL/kg IV over 5–10 minutes followed by 0.25 mL/kg/min CRI over 30–60 minutes. Repeat approximately every 6 hours, as needed, for up to 3–5 doses. If serum lipemia is present, wait 1–2 hours before readministration. See Appendix V on Antidotes and Useful Drugs.

MEDICATIONS

Specific antidotes or procedures are available for the more common toxicants; see specific chapters and Appendix V.

FOLLOW-UP

Specific monitoring depends on the toxicant and the patient's signs and laboratory abnormalities.

P

MISCELLANEOUS

INTERNET RESOURCES

- Pet Poison Helpline: http://www.petpoisonhelpline.com/
- ASPCA Poison Control Center: http://www.aspca.org/pet-care/poison-control/

Suggested Reading

Peterson ME, Talcott PA, eds. Small Animal Toxicology, 3rd ed. Philadelphia, PA: Saunders, 2013.

Author Renee D. Schmid

Consulting Editor Lynn R. Hovda

Acknowledgment The author and editors acknowledge the prior contribution of Tam Garland and E. Murl Bailey.

POLIOENCEPHALOMYELITIS—CATS

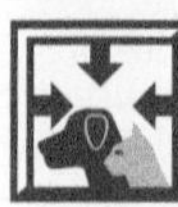

BASICS

OVERVIEW

- Subacute to chronic nonsuppurative encephalomyelitis with a predominance of pathologic changes in the gray matter, mainly affecting the medulla oblongata and the spinal cord.
- This disease is considered rare, with a prevalence of less than 1% in cats presented with spinal cord diseases.

SIGNALMENT

- There is no breed or sex predilection.
- Cats of any age can be affected.
- The disease is sporadic but has been observed worldwide, especially in northern Europe.

SIGNS

- Ataxia, paresis, and decreased postural reactions of pelvic or all four limbs.
- Lower motor neuron signs may be also possible (muscle atrophy and decreased to absent segmental spinal reflexes).
- Intracranial signs (seizures, cerebellar signs, and cranial nerve deficits) are uncommon.
- The progression is subacute to chronic (over weeks to months) but may also stabilize.

CAUSES & RISK FACTORS

The underlying cause remains still unknown but pathologic findings are highly suggestive of a viral agent.

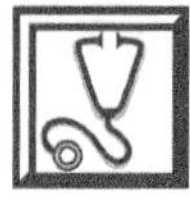

DIAGNOSIS

DIFFERENTIAL DIAGNOSIS

- Feline infectious peritonitis.
- Toxoplasmosis.
- Fungal infection.
- Bacterial infection.

CBC/BIOCHEMISTRY/URINALYSIS

- Laboratory changes not well characterized.
- Nonspecific changes (e.g., leukopenia and non-regenerative anemia) rare.

OTHER LABORATORY TESTS

N/A

DIAGNOSTIC PROCEDURES

- The presumptive diagnosis is based on history, clinical signs, and possibly CSF changes (mononuclear pleocytosis with or without moderate increased total protein levels).
- The final diagnosis is based on histopathology (disseminated inflammatory lesions in the brain and spinal cord and, as the disease progresses, there is extensive neuronal loss and astrogliosis with little inflammation).

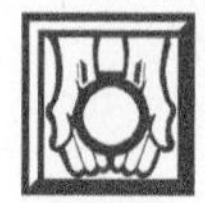

TREATMENT

No curative treatment has been found.

MEDICATIONS

DRUG(S) OF CHOICE

- No drug therapy used in reported cases.
- Because lesions are nonsuppurative, steroid therapy may palliate clinical signs, at least temporarily.
- Supportive treatment with antiepileptic medication to control seizures if indicated.

FOLLOW-UP

Prognosis can be good if the neurologic signs are mild and nonprogressive.

MISCELLANEOUS

Suggested Reading

Gunn-Moore D. Infectious diseases of the central nervous system. Vet Clin North Am Small Anim Pract 2005, 35:103–128.

Hoff EJ, Vandevelde M. Non-suppurative encephalomyelitis in cats suggestive of a viral origin. Vet Pathol 1981, 18:170–180.

Tipold A. Inflammatory diseases of the spine in small animals. Vet Clin North Am Small Anim Pract 2010, 40:871–879.

Tipold A, Vandevelde M. Neurological diseases of suspected infectious origin and prion disease. In: Greene CE, eds., Infectious Diseases of the Dog and Cat, 4th ed. St. Louis, MO: Elsevier, 2012, p. 860.

Author Elsa Beltran

P

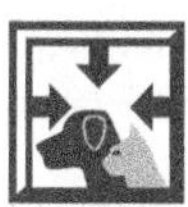

BASICS

DEFINITION

• An autoimmune disease of the joint that results in destruction of articular cartilage, subchondral bone and surrounding ligaments. This damage can result in joint instability, laxity and deformation with chronicity.
• Canine syndromes: ○ Rheumatoid arthritis—antibody response against rheumatoid factors or autoantibodies that results in severe damage to the articular cartilage, periarticular bone and ligaments. ○ Felty's syndrome—constellation of arthritis, neutropenia, and splenomegaly. ○ Erosive polyarthritis of greyhounds—minimal subchondral changes despite necrosis of the articular cartilage and proliferative synovitis; peripheral lymphadenopathy. • Feline erosive polyarthritis: ○ Periosteal proliferative polyarthritis—acute onset of pain and systemic manifestations (fever, lymphadenopathy) related to arthropathy with prolific periarticular periosteal bone formation. ○ Feline rheumatoid arthritis—insidious development of joint deformity accompanied by less systemic illness and periosteal bone formation.

PATHOPHYSIOLOGY

• Immune-complex deposition within the synovial membrane results in an inflammatory response (involving complement and cytokines) leading to cartilage erosion. Release of matrix-degrading enzymes (metalloproteases) responsible for cartilage destruction. • Chronic synovitis results in a pannus, or granulation tissue, across the articular cartilage that extends into subchondral bone, replacing areas of destruction. • Destruction of joint ligaments leads to joint instability and luxation.

SYSTEMS AFFECTED

Musculoskeletal

GENETICS

No genetic predisposition known.

INCIDENCE/PREVALENCE

• Uncommon to rare. • Nonerosive disease more common.

SIGNALMENT

Species

Dog and cat.

Breed Predilections

• More common in small-breed dogs; Shetland sheepdogs, cocker spaniels, collies appear more affected. • Siamese cats.

Mean Age and Range

• Canine—middle age (3–9.5 years).
• Feline—bimodal distribution of young adults and middle-aged to older cats.

Predominant Sex

• Feline—predominantly male. • Dogs—none.

SIGNS

General Comments

• Typically affects more distal joints (carpus, elbow, stifle and tarsal joints more frequently, digital joints and vertebral column may be affected). • Clinically, it can appear as though only one joint is affected.
• Evaluate cats for causes of reactive polyarthritis (septic arthritis, systemic infection and neoplasia).

Historical Findings

• Progressive, intermittent, or shifting-leg lameness. • Reluctance to walk or stand, inappetence and weight loss.

Physical Examination Findings

• Pain and/or effusion detected on palpation of one or more joints. • Deformation, instability, and luxation of the joint is unique to erosive (as compared to nonerosive) arthritis; occurs with chronicity. May be associated with cranial cruciate ligament rupture (CCLR). • Stiffness on gait evaluation, decreased range of motion and muscle atrophy. • Pyrexia and/or peripheral lymphadenopathy. • Cats may resent handling. May present with acute signs or may be more insidious over weeks to months.

CAUSES

• Underlying etiology has yet to be identified.
• Canine distemper virus within synovial fluid can result in sustained inflammation within the joint possibly predisposing a dog to erosive arthritis. • Feline leukemia virus (FeLV) and feline syncytium-forming virus are associated with feline periosteal proliferative polyarthritis (FPPP), but causation has not been shown.

RISK FACTORS

None currently known.

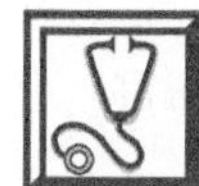

DIAGNOSIS

DIFFERENTIAL DIAGNOSIS

• Other causes of arthropathy—infectious arthritis, degenerative joint disease, neoplasia (e.g., synovial cell sarcoma), hemarthrosis, congenital arthropathies (elbow dysplasia, osteochondrosis dissecans), tick-borne disease. • Hypertrophic osteodystrophy.
• Panosteitis. • Polymyositis. • Steroid-responsive meningitis–arteritis. • Systemic lupus erythematosus (SLE). • Reactive polyarthritis due to antigenic stimulation from systemic disease. • Drug-induced polyarthritis (sulfa drugs, phenobarbital, erythropoietin, penicillins, cephalosporins, vaccines). • Trauma.

CBC/BIOCHEMISTRY/URINALYSIS

• Hemogram—a mild, non-regenerative anemia and mild leukocytosis may be present although hemogram can be unremarkable.
• Chemistry—hyperglobulinemia may be present. • Urinalysis and urine culture—generally unremarkable. Proteinuria should be quantified with a UPC.

OTHER LABORATORY TESTS

• Synovial fluid analysis—aseptic, neutrophilic, or mixed inflammation with greater than 10% non-degenerate neutrophils:
○ Protein concentration often >3.0 g/dL and total nucleated cell count (TNCC) usually >3,000 cells/μL (not associated with severity).
○ Make a direct smear prior to lab submission. • Synovial fluid culture (bacteria and mycoplasma)—negative results do not entirely rule out septic arthritis. • Antinuclear antibody titers—usually negative, unlikely to be clinically useful unless SLE suspected.
• Rheumatoid factor testing—positive test is supportive only when erosive disease is present; other causes of joint disease can elevate rheumatoid factor levels: ○ Positive results seen in cats with rheumatoid arthritis, not in FPPP. • Testing for infectious diseases (tick-borne disease (*Borrelia*, *Ehrlichia*, *Rickettsia*), FeLV/feline immunodeficiency virus (FIV) testing, systemic mycoses, *Leishmania* if endemic, blood and urine culture, ± echocardiogram for bacterial endocarditis). • CSF collection, serum creatine kinase, and direct Coombs' testing can be considered on an individual basis to evaluate for systemic diseases.

IMAGING

• Joints: ○ Imaging of multiple joints is recommended; initial radiographs may be unremarkable without obvious change for 6 or more months. ○ Progressive disease results in subchondral bone lysis, irregular joint surface, and narrowing or widening of the joint space, calcification of soft tissues around the joint, and extensive bone destruction.
○ Cats can have periosteal new bone formation and enthesophytes. • Thoracic and vertebral radiographs with abdominal ultrasound can help rule out reactive polyarthritis.

DIAGNOSTIC PROCEDURES

Arthrocentesis (joint tap): four joints should be sampled.

PATHOLOGIC FINDINGS

• Grossly, the synovium can be discolored, thickened, and ulcerated with extension of granulation tissue into the subchondral bone.
• Histopathology of synovial membrane is rarely necessary, but may reveal synovial hypertrophy and hyperplasia, necrosis, and mononuclear inflammation (often lymphoplasmacytic).

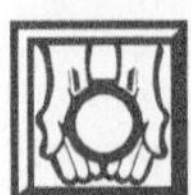

TREATMENT

APPROPRIATE HEALTH CARE

Outpatient

NURSING CARE

Larger dogs may require more assistance and support during treatment.

ACTIVITY

Strict rest is recommended while symptomatic and painful.

DIET

No dietary restrictions.

CLIENT EDUCATION

• Management is lifelong. • Erosive disease is often progressive and less responsive to treatment. • Importance of weight management.

SURGICAL CONSIDERATIONS

• Arthrodesis (primarily carpal) has been used for joint luxation to improve quality of life.
• Surgical repair of CCLR if necessary.
• Synovectomy, arthroplasty, or joint replacement can be considered.
• Splenectomy as last resort in Felty's syndrome.

P

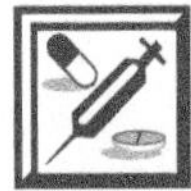

MEDICATIONS

DRUG(S) OF CHOICE

Antibiotics

• Doxycycline or minocycline recommended in cats and dogs while infectious disease testing is pending. • Tylosin trial in greyhounds for mycoplasma.

Dogs

Initial Therapy

• Prednisone or prednisolone 1–2 mg/kg/day or 50 mg/m^2, until remission encountered (often 4 weeks), then taper. • Cyclosporine 5 mg/kg PO q12—suitable alternative to corticosteroids.

Combination Therapy

Can be helpful to achieve remission, allow for tapering of corticosteroids and aid in refractory cases; each can be combined with corticosteroids:
• Mycophenolate mofetil 10 mg/kg PO q12h; taper by 50% after 2–3 weeks or if hemorrhagic gastrointestinal signs noted.
• Leflunomide 3–4 mg/kg PO q24h; allow 4–6 weeks before decreasing dose to every 48 hours then every 72 hours. • Azathioprine 1.6–2 mg/kg PO q24h for 2 weeks or until remission, then taper to every 48 hours.
• Other immunosuppressives to consider include chlorambucil, cyclophosphamide, levamisole, methotrexate.

Cats

• Prednisolone 2 mg/kg PO q12h followed by a taper; ~50% of cats with FPPP show improvement in signs and slowing of progression when used with analgesia. • 58% of cats improved using a protocol of methotrexate + leflunomide: methotrexate 2.5 mg/cat PO q12h for 3 consecutive doses (7.5 mg/24 hours) repeated weekly until improvement then 2.5 mg/cat PO weekly; leflunomide 10 mg/cat PO q24h until improvement then 10 mg/cat PO twice weekly. • Other immunosuppressive agents that can be considered include cyclosporine or chlorambucil.

Other

Omega-3 fatty acid supplementation.

Analgesia

Gabapentin 5–15 mg/kg PO q8–12h; amantadine 3–5 mg/kg PO q24h; nonsteroidal anti-inflammatory drug (NSAIDs) as appropriate if not using corticosteroids.

CONTRAINDICATIONS

Glucocorticoids should not be given with NSAIDs.

PRECAUTIONS

• Tapering immunosuppressive therapy too soon can lead to relapses. • Confirm aseptic inflammation prior to initiating immunosuppressive therapy. • Consider secondary immunosuppressive agent if unable to attain remission or if symptoms relapse while still on glucocorticoids. • Monitor for infectious diseases and opportunistic infections.

POSSIBLE INTERACTIONS

Concurrent use of multiple immunosuppressives with the same mechanism of action.

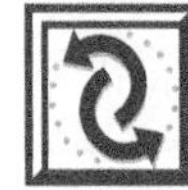

FOLLOW-UP

PATIENT MONITORING

• Monitor for potential side effects of treatments (liver enzymes, hyperglycemia, etc.) and concurrent disorders (e.g., hematologic abnormalities, proteinuria, etc.) as necessary, • Tapering of medications often possible after 4 weeks of therapy. A 50% taper every month or dose reduction of 25–30% every 2–3 weeks with a minimum of 4 months of therapy can be considered. • If relapse occurs during taper, increase corticosteroid to the most recent effective dose and/or consider a second agent, if not already utilized. • If relapse occurs after the taper, a short course of corticosteroid and the dose of the second agent that maintained clinical control can be utilized long term.
• Serial or repeated arthrocentesis can be performed to rule out poor control of immune-mediated disease in cases of ongoing or recurrent lameness. In some dogs, this may identify degenerative joint disease as the cause of lameness rather than relapse of polyarthritis.

EXPECTED COURSE AND PROGNOSIS

• Erosive disease is typically progressive; ~50% of cats will improve with good quality of life. • Monitoring recommended if initially nonerosive. • Tick-borne disease usually responds to appropriate antibiotic therapy within 7 days.

MISCELLANEOUS

ABBREVIATIONS

• CCLR = cranial cruciate ligament rupture.
• FeLV = feline leukemia virus.
• FIV = feline immunodeficiency virus.
• FPPP = feline periosteal proliferative polyarthritis.
• SLE = systemic lupus erythematosus.
• TNCC = total nucleated cell count.

Suggested Reading

Lemetayer J, Taylor S. Inflammatory joint disease in cats: diagnostic approach and treatment. J Feline Med Surg 2014, 16(7):547–562.

Shaughnessy M, Sample S, Abicht C, et al. Clinical features and pathological joint changes in dogs with erosive immune-mediated polyarthritis: 13 cases (2004–2012). J Am Vet Med Assoc 2016, 249(10):1156–1164.

Author J.D. Foster
Consulting Editor Mathieu M. Glassman

Client Education Handout available online

POLYARTHRITIS, NONEROSIVE, IMMUNE-MEDIATED, DOGS

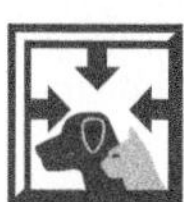

BASICS

DEFINITION

• Nonerosive polyarthritis—a non-infectious inflammatory disease of multiple (>2) joints without radiographic evidence of bone or cartilage involvement. • Most common polyarthropathy in dogs, idiopathic or type I immune-mediated polyarthritis (IMPA).
• Reactive polyarthropathy, where inflammation in the joints is secondary to distant disease, includes types II, III, and IV—disease is secondary to chronic inflammatory or infectious disease, chronic gastrointestinal disease, and neoplasia, respectively. • Systemic lupus erythematosus (SLE), familial shar-pei fever (FSF), and familial juvenile-onset polyarthritis of Akitas are less common nonerosive polyarthritides.

PATHOPHYSIOLOGY

• All causes of nonerosive polyarthritis are immune-mediated. • Immune complex deposition is the underlying mechanism in idiopathic IMPA (type I) and reactive polyarthropathy (types II, III, and IV). • Reactive polyarthropathy involves immune stimulus distant to the joints due to underlying infectious, inflammatory, or neoplastic disease, as well as adverse drug reactions, with subsequent immune complex deposition in the synovium. • SLE is the result of immune complex deposition secondary to autoantibodies (antinuclear antibodies [ANA]) formed against tissue proteins and DNA. • FSF is the result of amyloid deposition in the synovium.

SYSTEMS AFFECTED

• Musculoskeletal: ○ Appendicular joints are more commonly affected than axial joints. Intervertebral joints are not usually affected.
○ Distal joints (carpus, tarsus) are more commonly affected than proximal joints (stifle, shoulder, coxofemoral) in IMPA. ○ The hock joints are typically affected in FSF. • Hemic/lymphatic/immune: ○ Immune stimulus may result in fever, lethargy, and poor appetite.
○ Hemolytic anemia and thrombocytopenia may be present in SLE. • Skin/exocrine:
○ Immune-mediated skin disease targeting the mucocutaneous junctions is common in SLE.
• Renal/urologic: ○ Immune-complex deposition in the kidneys and protein-losing nephropathy may be present in SLE.
○ Glomerulonephropathy and proteinuria secondary to amyloidosis may occur in FSF.

GENETICS

MTBP gene missense mutation is believed to be responsible for FSF.

INCIDENCE/PREVALENCE

• Idiopathic IMPA is common in dogs.
• Reactive polyarthritis accounts for only 25% of nonerosive polyarthritis cases in dogs.
• IMPA is rare in cats.

SIGNALMENT

Species

Dog and cat.

Breed Predilections

• Large-breed dogs, such as Labrador retrievers, golden retrievers, Rottweilers, Irish setters, Shetland sheepdogs, cocker spaniels, and American Eskimo dogs are over-represented for idiopathic IMPA.
• Doberman pinschers are overreported in cases of polyarthropathy secondary to sulfonamide administration.

Mean Age and Range

Mean age 4–6 years old, range 6 months to 12 years.

Predominant Sex

None reported.

SIGNS

Historical Findings

• Shifting limb lameness. • Stiff gait. • Fever.
• Reluctance to walk. • Lethargy.
• Inappetence. • Exercise intolerance.
• Lymphadenopathy.

Physical Examination Findings

• Joint pain. • Joint effusion. • Fever.
• Lameness.

CAUSES

• Type I IMPA—idiopathic. • Immune-mediated dermatopathy and hepatopathy are among the most common noninfectious causes of type II IMPA. Infectious sources to consider include endocarditis, discospondylitis, prostatitis, deep pyoderma, and systemic infections (fungal, protozoal). • Type III IMPA occurs secondary to chronic gastrointestinal disease such as inflammatory bowel disease, but is rare. • Type IV IMPA has been reported secondary to renal carcinoma, mammary carcinoma, leiomyoma, Sertoli cell tumor, and seminoma. • Drugs implicated in adverse drug reaction-related polyarthropathy (type II) include human albumin, erythropoeitin, phenobarbital, and antibiotics such as sulfonamides, cephalosporins, penicillins, lincosamides, and macrolides. This should be considered a potential cause when administered 5–20 days prior to the onset of signs.
• Reports of postvaccinal polyarthropathy have included canine distemper and Lyme vaccines, typically within 30 days of vaccine administration.

RISK FACTORS

N/A

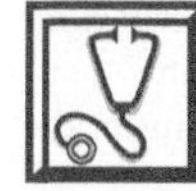

DIAGNOSIS

DIFFERENTIAL DIAGNOSIS

• Infectious polyarthritis, including rickettsial disease, *Mycoplasma*, bacterial, and fungal etiologies: ○ *Borrelia burgdorferi, Anaplasma phagocytophilum, Rickettsia rickettsii, Ehrlichia canis, E. ewingii*, and *E. chaffeensis* are among the rickettsial diseases that should be considered for polyarthropathy. • Leishmaniasis should be considered, particularly in instances of significant systemic involvement, presence of skin lesions, and/or history of travel to the Mediterranean/southern Europe, Africa, India, or South America within the past 7 years.
• Panosteitis and hypertrophic osteodystrophy should be considered, particularly in young dogs with lameness and fever. • Degenerative joint disease (DJD) should be considered in middle-age to older animals. • Viral etiologies have been implicated as a cause of polyarthritis in cats, including feline calicivirus and feline coronavirus associated with feline infectious peritonitis.

CBC/BIOCHEMISTRY/URINALYSIS

• CBC—mild non-regenerative anemia and mild leukocytosis; leukopenia is also possible. Presence of thrombocytopenia may be suggestive of tick-borne disease or when severe, SLE. • Chemistry—often normal, except when distant (reactive polyarthropathy) or polysystemic disease (SLE) is present.
• Urinalysis—proteinuria may be present and should prompt obtaining a UPC.

OTHER LABORATORY TESTS

• Definitive diagnosis can be obtained by arthrocentesis and cytology of multiple joints.
• Aerobic and anerobic joint culture to definitively exclude septic arthritis in all cases; sensitivity is ~50% and can be improved with broth-enrichment media and incubation prior to culture. • Fungal cultures of joint fluid may be considered, though direct joint involvement is rare. • Mycoplasmal PCR or culture of synovial fluid may be considered, with PCR being more sensitive. • Tick PCR panels to exclude rickettsial disease should be performed in all cases. Quantitative serology may be considered but positive results may lag behind onset of clinical signs, and false-negative results are common. Qualitative tests for antibody production, including SNAP ELISA tests, may be indicated in cases with high index of clinical suspicion for rickettsial diseases such as Lyme disease. • Serologic fungal titers may be considered where fungal disease is endemic or there has been travel history to rule it out as a cause of reactive polyarthropathy. • Blood and urine cultures should be considered to exclude bacterial causes of reactive polyarthropathy in cases where no obvious infectious or inflammatory focus is identified. Positive blood cultures may be indicative of primary septic polyarthritis of hematogenous origin given relatively low sensitivity of bacterial culture of synovial fluid.
• C-reactive protein (CRP) can be measured as a nonspecific indicator of inflammation and reassessed for response to therapy. • ANA titer may be submitted in cases where there is multisystemic immune-mediated involvement.

POLYARTHRITIS, NONEROSIVE, IMMUNE-MEDIATED, DOGS (CONTINUED)

IMAGING

• Appendicular radiographs including affected joints are necessary to exclude erosive causes of polyarthropathy, though these diseases are uncommon in dogs and may not be radiographically visible initially. Absence of palpable joint effusion should not preclude recommendation to obtain radiographs in cases where clinical suspicion is otherwise suggestive of polyarthritis and screening radiographs of multiple joints should be obtained. • Joint effusion is the main radiographic finding. Radiographic signs of osteoarthritis may be concurrently present and do not exclude nonerosive polyarthritis as a diagnosis. • Thoracic radiography, abdominal ultrasonography, and echocardiography should ideally be performed to assess for causes of reactive polyarthropathy.

DIAGNOSTIC PROCEDURES

• Arthrocentesis should be performed aseptically on 3–5 joints for synovial fluid collection, under sedation or general anesthesia. • Synovial biopsy can be used for confirmation in challenging cases.

P

PATHOLOGIC FINDINGS

• Turbid ± reduced viscosity of synovial fluid, ± voluminous fluid. • Synovial fluid cytology characterized by predominantly neutrophilic (>10%) inflammation without evidence of infectious agents in the synovial fluid.

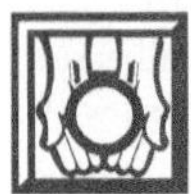

TREATMENT

APPROPRIATE HEALTH CARE

• Typically outpatient therapy.
• Systemic signs (i.e., fever, inappetence) may necessitate hospitalized supportive care.

ACTIVITY

Activity restriction to avoid exacerbation of pain and lameness.

DIET

Weight reduction as applicable to avoid undue stress on joints.

CLIENT EDUCATION

Discuss failure to control clinical signs, particularly in cases where underlying disease cannot be eliminated, and possibility or recurrence and/or need for lifelong medication and monitoring.

MEDICATIONS

DRUG(S) OF CHOICE

• Immunosuppressive dose of steroids, i.e., prednisone (dog) or prednisolone (cat): 2 mg/kg/day PO for 4 weeks, then gradually tapered over at least 4 months unless combination immunosuppressive protocols are used. • Nonsteroidal anti-inflammatory drugs (NSAIDs) for FSF, i.e., carprofen 2.2 mg/kg PO twice daily.

PRECAUTIONS

Consider risks and complications of prolonged steroid courses, including immunosuppression, diabetes mellitus, risk for congestive heart failure, and muscle-wasting.

POSSIBLE INTERACTIONS

NSAIDs and steroids should be not be given together due to increased risk of gastrointestinal ulceration; a 7-day washout period is indicated between medications.

ALTERNATIVE DRUG(S)

• Cyclosporine—dog: 5 mg/kg PO twice daily; cat: 4 mg/kg PO twice daily.
• Mycophenolate mofetil—dog: 10 mg/kg PO or IV twice daily. • Leflunomide—dog: 2–4 mg/kg PO once daily; cat: 10 mg/cat PO once daily. • Azathioprine—dog: 2 mg/kg PO once daily, tapered to 0.5–2 mg/kg PO every other day. • Chlorambucil—dog: 1–2 mg/m^2 PO once daily; cat: 15 mg/m^2 PO once daily for 4 days once every 3 weeks or 2 mg/cat every other day. • Cyclophosphamide—dog: 1.5 mg/kg PO when patient >25 kg, 2 mg/kg PO when patient 5–25 kg, 2.5 mg/kg PO when patient <5 kg every other day or 4 consecutive days of the week; cat: 2.5 mg/kg once daily. • Analgesics may be considered for additional pain control (e.g., gabapentin (dog), 5–10 mg/kg PO twice daily). • Given the disease is rare in cats, consider doxycycline 5 mg/kg PO twice daily for 14 days to treat infectious etiologies prior to initiating immunosuppression.

FOLLOW-UP

PATIENT MONITORING

• Repeat arthrocentesis may be considered for evaluation of response to treatment, especially prior to medication changes (i.e., at 4 weeks, prior to beginning steroid taper).
• CRP has a modest correlation to synovial fluid cytology and may be performed as a noninvasive means of patient monitoring.
• CRP and IL-6 may be used to distinguish recurrence of IMPA from osteoarthritis.

PREVENTION/AVOIDANCE

Avoid nonessential vaccination for prevention of recurrence. Canine distemper vaccine should not be given if seroprotective antibody titer levels are present.

POSSIBLE COMPLICATIONS

• Immunosuppression and risk of secondary infection, particularly when multiple immunosuppressive drugs are used.
• Subsequent DJD may occur following IMPA. Patients may show lameness when steroid therapy is tapered, however most are afebrile.

EXPECTED COURSE AND PROGNOSIS

• Good prognosis for idiopathic IMPA with expected improvement in clinical signs within 7 days. • Recurrence is possible and reported in almost 30% of cases. • 10% of cases fail to respond to immunosuppressive therapy.
• Variable prognosis for reactive polyarthropathy, depending on the ability to eliminate or control the underlying disease process.
• Guarded prognosis for SLE.

MISCELLANEOUS

ABBREVIATIONS

• ANA = antinuclear antibody. • CRP = C-reactive protein. • DJD = degenerative joint disease. • FSF = familial shar-pei fever.
• IL-6 = interleukin-6. • IMPA = immune-mediated polyarthritis. • NSAID = nonsteroidal anti-inflammatory drug.
• SLE = systemic lupus erythematosus.

Suggested Reading

Clements DN, Gear RNA, Tattersall J, et al. Type I immune-mediated polyarthritis in dogs: 39 cases (1997–2002). J Am Vet Med Assoc 2004, 224:1323–1327.

Hillstrom A, Bylin J, Hagman R, et al. Measurement of serum C-reactive protein concentration for discriminating between suppurative arthritis and osteoarthritis in dogs. BMC Vet Res 2016, 12:240–249.

Lemetayer J, Taylor S. Inflammatory joint disease in cats: diagnostic approach and treatment. J Feline Med Surg 2014, 16:547–562.

Stone M. Immune-mediated polyarthritis and other polyarthritides. In: Ettinger SJ, ed., Textbook of Veterinary Internal Medicine, 8th ed. St. Louis, MO: Elsevier, 2017, pp. 3055–3070.

Authors Ashley E. Bava and J.D. Foster

Consulting Editor Mathieu M. Glassman

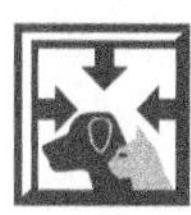

BASICS

OVERVIEW

Disorder in which large portions of normal renal parenchyma are displaced by multiple cysts; renal cysts develop in nephrons and collecting ducts; both kidneys are invariably affected. In most cases the disease is inherited, irreversible, and progressive.

SIGNALMENT

- Persian and related breeds (e.g., exotic shorthair, Himalayan, British shorthair) more commonly affected.
- Dog breeds affected include Cairn terriers and beagles.

SIGNS

- Cysts are clinically silent until their increasing size and number contribute to azotemia or abdominal enlargement.
- May detect bosselated (lumpy) kidneys by abdominal palpation.
- Most renal cysts are not painful when palpated, but acute secondary infection may cause rapid distension of the renal capsule and pain.

CAUSES & RISK FACTORS

- Autosomal-dominant inheritance in Persian cats.
- Cause of renal cyst formation remains obscure; genetic, endogenous, and environmental factors appear to influence the process.

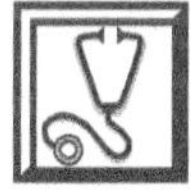

DIAGNOSIS

DIFFERENTIAL DIAGNOSIS

- Other multicystic diseases of the kidneys.
- Glomerulocystic disease of collies.
- Renal cystadenocarcinoma associated with nodular fibrosis in German shepherd dogs.
- Renal cysts associated with chronic kidney disease (CKD) or renal dysplasia.
- Renal neoplasia.
- Hydronephrosis.
- Perirenal pseudocysts.
- Mycotic or bacterial nephritis.

CBC/BIOCHEMISTRY/URINALYSIS

- Results unremarkable unless patient has CKD.
- Hematuria is rare.

OTHER LABORATORY TESTS

- Genetic tests are available to identify the autosomal dominant polycystic kidney disease (AD-PKD) type 1 mutation in cats. This test is useful to screen kittens less than 3–4 months old when ultrasonography may be less sensitive, as well as in breeding cats. Other mutations may also cause inherited kidney cysts.
- Cyst fluid can be clear, cloudy, or hemorrhagic, and the fluid from two cysts in the same kidney can differ.
- Bacterial culture of cyst fluid aids in diagnosing infection.

IMAGING

Radiography

Survey radiography and IV contrast urography are insensitive methods of confirming cystic disease.

Ultrasonography

- Reveals anechoic cavitating lesions characterized by sharply marginated smooth walls and distal enhancement.
- Can usually detect cysts >2 mm in diameter.
- Cysts have been detected in cats as young as 7 weeks; screening cats younger than 6 months is associated with higher false-negative results.
- Hypoechoic cystic cavities may be seen in some cysts infected with bacteria.
- Detection of cysts in other organs which helps to differentiate AD-PKD from other inherited or acquired multicystic disorders of the kidneys.

DIAGNOSTIC PROCEDURES

Evaluation of fine-needle aspirates of the kidney may allow differentiation of cystic disease from other diseases that cause renomegaly.

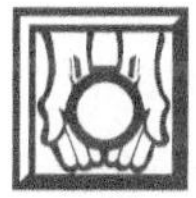

TREATMENT

- Usually not life-threatening, but pyelonephritis and cyst involvement warrant immediate measures to prevent sepsis and mortality.
- Most cysts increase in size and number, often impairing adjacent renal parenchyma.
- Elimination of renal cysts is not yet feasible; treatment is limited to minimizing the consequences of renal cyst formation (i.e., CKD, infection, hematuria, and pain).
- Removing fluid from large cysts may minimize pain and compression of adjacent renal parenchyma. This procedure is impractical in kidneys with multiple large cysts.
- A vasopressin antagonist (tolvaptan), has been shown to slow kidney enlargement and slow decline in kidney function in people with AD-PKD.
- Some patients require treatment for concomitant CKD.
- Consider nephrectomy only if infected cysts are associated with uncontrollable sepsis.
- Disease eradication by selective breeding of unaffected cats may be impossible because ~40% of Persians are affected.

MEDICATIONS

DRUG(S) OF CHOICE

- Bacterial infection of cysts is rare. Unless infection is accompanied by pyelonephritis, bacteria may not be observed in urine. Consider parenchymal infection when cysts are associated with renal pain and fever, even in absence of bacteriuria.
- The acidic cyst fluid and its epithelial barrier may reduce concentrations of acidic antibiotics (e.g., cephalosporins and penicillins) within cystic lumens. Alkaline, lipid-soluble antibiotics (e.g., trimethoprim–sulfonamide, fluoroquinolones, chloramphenicol, tetracycline, and clindamycin), which penetrate epithelial barriers and become ionized and trapped in cyst lumens, are recommended.

FOLLOW-UP

- Monitor every 2–6 months for progressive disease (e.g., CKD, renal infection, and pain).
- In the absence of sepsis, the short-term prognosis is favorable.

MISCELLANEOUS

ABBREVIATIONS

- AD-PKD = autosomal dominant-polycystic kidney disease.
- CKD = chronic kidney disease.

Suggested Reading

Bonazzi M, Volta A, Gnudi G, et al. Comparison between ultrasound and genetic testing for early diagnosis of polycystic kidney disease in Persian and Exotic Shorthair cats. J Feline Med Surg 2009, 11:430–434.

Author Jody P. Lulich

Consulting Editor J.D. Foster

Acknowledgment The author and editors acknowledge the prior contribution of Carl A. Osborne.

POLYCYTHEMIA VERA

BASICS

OVERVIEW

Myeloproliferative disorder of the chronic myelogenous leukemia (CML) spectrum, resulting in high blood viscosity secondary to an increased red blood cell (RBC) mass.

SIGNALMENT

- Dog and cat.
- Primarily old animals.

SIGNS

- Gradual in onset; may be incidental diagnosis.
- Depression.
- Anorexia.
- Weakness.
- Polydipsia and polyuria.
- Erythema of skin and mucous membranes.
- Dilated and tortuous retinal blood vessels.
- Uveitis.
- Acute blindness.
- Splenomegaly and hepatomegaly uncommon.

CAUSES & RISK FACTORS

A *JAK2* mutation has been implicated in the disease pathogenesis.

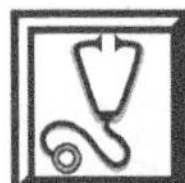

DIAGNOSIS

Diagnostic tests should exclude all other conditions that may lead to increased packed cell volume (PCV) and RBC mass.

DIFFERENTIAL DIAGNOSIS

- Severe dehydration.
- Renal neoplasia.
- Chronic pyelonephritis.
- Hyperadrenocorticism.
- Androgen stimulation.
- Chronic pulmonary disease.
- Cardiac disease with right-to-left shunts.

CBC/BIOCHEMISTRY/URINALYSIS

- High PCV.
- Absolute increase in RBC mass.
- Prerenal azotemia possible.
- Leukocytosis in 50% of dogs.

OTHER LABORATORY TESTS

- Pao_2—normal.
- Serum erythropoietin concentrations are usually low to zero and often overlap with those reported for other causes of polycythemia.
- Cytologic examination of bone marrow and core biopsy, in parallel with peripheral blood count analysis.

IMAGING

- Radiography—assess kidneys and cardiopulmonary system.
- Abdominal ultrasonography—assess kidneys and adrenal glands.
- Echocardiography—evaluate for right-to-left cardiac shunts.

DIAGNOSTIC PROCEDURES

- Bone marrow biopsy.
- Electrocardiography—assess heart disease.
- Retinal examination/ophthalmologic consult.
- Blood pressure measurement.

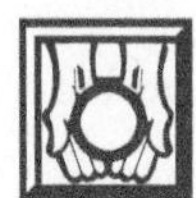

TREATMENT

- Phlebotomy and concurrent replacement with intravenous isotonic fluids—to provide relief of signs during clinical crisis.
- Hydroxyurea—may temporarily decrease the RBCs and provide disease control.
- Consult a veterinary medical oncologist for most current recommendations and disease management.

MEDICATIONS

DRUG(S) OF CHOICE

Hydroxyurea 40–50 mg/kg PO divided twice daily; titrate to response and toxicity (dog and cat).

CONTRAINDICATIONS/POSSIBLE INTERACTIONS

N/A

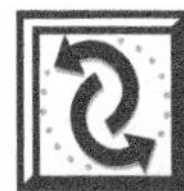

FOLLOW-UP

Periodic reexaminations with serial CBCs, retinal examinations, and serum biochemical profiles to monitor disease control and hydroxyurea side effects on bone marrow and other organs.

MISCELLANEOUS

ABBREVIATIONS

- CML = chronic myelogenous leukemia.
- PCV = packed cell volume.
- RBC = red blood cell.

Suggested Reading

Juopperi TA, Bienzle D, Bernreuter DC, et al. Prognostic markers for myeloid neoplasms: a comparative review of the literature and goals for future investigation. Vet Pathol 2011, 48(1):182–197.

Weiss DJ, Aird B. Cytologic evaluation of primary and secondary myelodysplastic syndromes in the dog. Vet Clin Pathol 2001, 30:67–75.

Author Nick Dervisis

Consulting Editor Timothy M. Fan

POLYNEUROPATHIES (PERIPHERAL NEUROPATHIES)

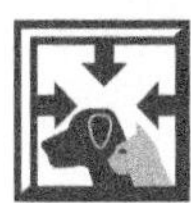

BASICS

DEFINITION

Diseases affecting peripheral motor, sensory, autonomic, and/or cranial nerves, in any combination.

PATHOPHYSIOLOGY

• Inherited or acquired (degenerative, idiopathic, metabolic/endocrine, neoplastic/paraneoplastic, immune-mediated inflammatory, infectious, drugs/toxic). • Primary pathologic process—(1) *axonal neuropathies*, caused by either destruction or degeneration of neuronal cell bodies in dorsal root ganglia, ventral horn cells, or autonomic ganglia (neuronopathies) or axonal degeneration with secondary demyelination (axonopathies), or (2) *demyelinating neuropathies* with primary demyelination due to disease of the Schwann cells or myelin sheath.

SYSTEMS AFFECTED

• Nervous—peripheral nervous system (occasionally also affecting CNS); possible involvement of the cranial nerves. • Other organ systems may be involved in the primary disease process.

GENETICS

• Most inherited—autosomal recessive disorders. • Spinal muscular atrophy in Brittany spaniels, laryngeal paralysis in bouvier des Flandres—autosomal dominant.

INCIDENCE/PREVALENCE

• Inherited—rare. • Peripheral nerve involvement in metabolic and neoplastic diseases—incidence unknown.
• Inflammatory—uncommon; coonhound paralysis (CHP) most frequent.

GEOGRAPHIC DISTRIBUTION

• CHP—North and Central America, parts of South America. • Distal denervating disease—dogs in UK; not reported elsewhere.
• Dysautonomia—mostly dogs (occasionally cats) in Missouri, Oklahoma, and Kansas; cats in Scandinavia and UK.

SIGNALMENT

Species

Dog and cat.

Breed Predilections—Inherited

Spinal Muscular Atrophy

• Brittany spaniel, Swedish Lapland dog, English pointer, German shepherd dog, Doberman pinscher, Rottweiler, griffon Briquet, Saluki, Maine Coon cats. • Progressive neuronopathy—Cairn terrier.

Axonopathies

• Giant axonal neuropathy—German shepherd dog. • Progressive axonopathy—boxer. • Laryngeal paralysis—bouvier des Flandres. • Laryngeal paralysis/polyneuropathy complex—Dalmatian, Rottweiler, Pyrenean mountain dog. • Distal sensorimotor polyneuropathy—Rottweiler, Alaskan Malamute, Great Dane, Leonberger dog, bouvier des Flandres. • Progressive central and peripheral sensorimotor axonopathy—golden retriever. • Central-peripheral distal axonopathy—Birman cat. • Axonal neuropathy—Snowshoe cat. • Primary hyperoxaluria—domestic shorthair cats.

Demyelination

• Hypertrophic neuropathy—Tibetan mastiff. • Congenital hypomyelination neuropathy—golden retriever.
• Demyelinating polyneuropathy–miniature schnauzers. • Recurrent demyelinating-remyelinating polyneuropathy—Bengal cat.

Lysosomal Storage Diseases

• Globoid cell leukodystrophy—West Highland white terrier, Cairn terrier, domestic shorthair cats • Alpha-L-fucosidosis—English Springer spaniel. • Mannosidosis—Persian and domestic shorthair cats. • G_{M1} gangliosidosis type II—Siamese and Korat cats. • Sphingomyelinosis (Niemann–Pick disease type A)—Siamese and Balinese cats. • Glycogenosis type IV—Norwegian forest cat.

Sensory Neuropathy

• Longhaired dachshund, English pointer, German shorthaired pointer, English springer spaniels, French spaniels, Jack Russell terrier, border collies. • Ganglioradiculitis—Siberian husky.

Breed Predilections—Acquired

• CHP—higher incidence in coonhounds.
• Clinical diabetic polyneuropathy—more common in cat than dog. • Insulinomas—German shepherd dog, boxer, Irish setter, standard poodle, collie.

Mean Age and Range

Inherited

• Often begin at <6 months of age. • Feline hyperchylomicronemia—1–8 months.
• Feline hyperoxaluria—5–9 months.
• Rottweiler, bouvier, Leonberger distal polyneuropathies—>1 year. • Giant axonal neuropathy in German shepherd dog—14–16 months. • Intermediate and chronic forms of spinal muscular atrophy in heterozygote Brittany spaniel—6–12 months.

Acquired

• Secondary to neoplasia and insulinoma-associated hypoglycemia—middle-aged to older animals. • *Neospora caninum* polyradiculoneuritis—usually dogs <6 months of age. • Ganglioradiculitis—>1 year.

SIGNS

Historical Findings

Inherited

• Most—progressive lower motor neuron (LMN) tetraparesis; generalized weakness, muscle tremors and atrophy, plantigrade/palmigrade stance; stridor/voice change if laryngeal paralysis. • Sensory neuropathies—self-mutilation (nociceptive deficits), mild to severe ataxia. • Lysosomal storage diseases—slowly progressive CNS involvement (head tremors, ataxia, dysmetria, seizures, blindness, dementia) occur in conjunction with the LMN signs. • Sphingomyelinosis in cats—often present only with progressive motor and sensory neuropathy. • Giant axonal neuropathy of German shepherd dogs—rapidly progressive generalized weakness (<3 weeks).

Acquired

• Rapid or slow progression. • Rapidly progressive course—initial stiff, stilted gait, leading to generalized LMN paresis or paralysis (CHP, distal denervating disease).
• Slowly progressive course—generalized weakness and muscle atrophy; in distal polyneuropathies (diabetic neuropathy especially in cats), plantigrade/palmigrade stance. • Dysautonomia—primarily acute onset (<48 hours) of depression, anorexia, regurgitation, vomiting, paralytic ileus, xerostomia, keratoconjunctivitis sicca (KCS), third eyelid protrusion, urinary incontinence.
• Metabolic—owner reports non-neurologic clinical signs associated with weakness.
• Paraneoplastic—primary tumor may be clinically silent at time of presentation or revealed on thoracic radiographs or abdominal ultrasound.

Physical Examination Findings

• Motor and sensorimotor—tetraparesis to tetraplegia, hyporeflexia to areflexia, hypotonia to atonia, and muscle atrophy classic; muscle tremors common. • Sensory—proprioceptive deficits, hypoesthesia to anesthesia, without muscle atrophy or hyporeflexia (except in boxers); sensory ataxia.
• Paraesthesia—feline diabetic neuropathy, sensory neuropathies. • Hypothyroidism—may be associated with generalized polyneuropathy, laryngeal and/or facial nerve paralysis, megaesophagus, and vestibular signs.
• Lysosomal storage diseases—hepatosplenomegaly common. • Paraneoplastic—may find evidence of neoplasia. • Dysautonomia—dry nose, KCS, bradycardia, anal areflexia.
• Primary hyperchylomicronemia (cats)—lipid granulomata, which can be palpated under the skin and abdomen. • Primary hyperoxaluria (cats)—enlarged, painful kidneys on palpation. • Cranial nerve abnormalities (including dysphonia/aphonia)—variable.

CAUSES

Acquired

• Immune-mediated—primary or secondary; may be seen with systemic lupus erythematosus (SLE), glomerulonephritis, polyarthritis.
• Metabolic/endocrine—diabetes mellitus (cats), hypothyroidism, hyperadrenocorticism.
• Neoplastic/paraneoplastic—insulinoma, carcinomas, malignant melanoma, mast cell tumor, osteosarcoma, multiple myeloma,

lymphosarcoma. • Infectious—*N. caninum,* feline leukemia virus (FeLV), feline immunodeficiency virus (FIV). • Chemotherapy drugs—vincristine, vinblastine, cisplatin. • Toxic—thallium, organophosphates, salinomycin (cats), lasalocid (dogs). • Idiopathic.

RISK FACTORS

Development of specific diseases (metabolic, immune, neoplastic) or exposure to specific drugs/toxins or causal factors (raccoon saliva).

DIAGNOSIS

DIFFERENTIAL DIAGNOSIS

• Acute—botulism; tick paralysis; fulminant myasthenia gravis; acute multifocal myelopathies. • Chronic—polymyopathy; chronic multifocal myelopathies.

CBC/BIOCHEMISTRY/URINALYSIS

• Standard laboratory tests—often normal; may indicate underlying metabolic or neoplastic disease. • High serum creatine kinase—indicates an accompanying myopathy or diagnosis of polymyopathy.

OTHER LABORATORY TESTS

• Antinuclear antibody, Coombs' test—if immune disease suspected. • Low total thyroxine (T_4), low free T_4, and high endogenous thyroid-stimulating hormone (TSH)—hypothyroidism. • Amended insulin: glucose ratio >30—supports the diagnosis of insulinoma. • Serology—assists in the diagnosis of *N. caninum,* FIV, FeLV infection. • Diminished lysosomal enzyme activity in leukocytes, cultured fibroblasts—lysosomal storage diseases. • Pharmacologic testing (pilocarpine ophthalmic drops, bethanechol challenge)—dysautonomia. • High serum cholesterol and triglycerides, low lipoprotein lipase—hyperchylomicronemia. • Oxalate and/or L-glyceric acid in urine—primary hyperoxaluria. • Monoclonal gammopathy—multiple myeloma.

IMAGING

Thoracic and abdominal radiographs—search for a neoplastic cause; megaesophagus, ileus, bladder atony, constipation, and delayed gastric emptying in dysautonomia.

DIAGNOSTIC PROCEDURES

• Electrophysiology (EMG, motor and sensory nerve conduction studies ventral and dorsal nerve root studies)—cornerstone for diagnosis. • Lumbar CSF analysis—valuable in diagnosing nerve root involvement. • Muscle biopsy—confirms denervation. • Peripheral nerve biopsy (distal)—further characterizes disease process.

PATHOLOGIC FINDINGS

Lesion distribution along peripheral nerves (proximal, distal, widespread) and degree of axonal degeneration, demyelination, and/or neuronal cell body degeneration depends on the specific condition present.

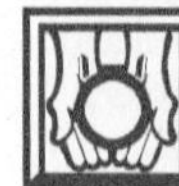

TREATMENT

APPROPRIATE HEALTH CARE

• Usually outpatient. • Inpatient—observe dogs with CHP closely for respiratory failure in early progressive phase of disease.

NURSING CARE

• Dysautonomia—may require IV fluid therapy and/or parenteral feeding. • Physical therapy.

DIET

• Generally no special management, unless megaesophagus or dysphagia occurs. • Hyperchylomicronemia—low-fat diet alone can resolve the polyneuropathy in 2–3 months. • Paralysis—ensure patient can reach food and water. • Regurgitation and/or vomiting—temporarily halt oral intake; consider gastrostomy tube. • Diabetes mellitus—monitor food intake; in cats, feed a low-carbohydrate, high-protein diet; diabetic neuropathy often reversible with treatment.

CLIENT EDUCATION

• Treatment of primary cause may not lead to reversal of signs; in some cases, deterioration will continue. • Canine axonal degeneration—progressive deterioration.

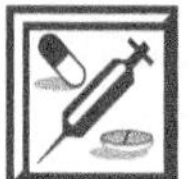

MEDICATIONS

DRUG(S) OF CHOICE

• Inherited—most untreatable. • Acquired—treat primary cause with the hope that the secondary polyneuropathy improves or resolves; not always successful. • Chronic relapsing demyelinating neuropathy—most likely of immune origin; may improve with long-term immunosuppressive therapy (prednisone, azathioprine, cyclophosphamide); response of individual patient variable. • SLE-related—treat as for chronic relapsing polyneuropathy. • Neoplasia—treat primary neoplasia. • *Neospora*-associated polyradiculoneuritis—clindamycin combined with pyrimethamine. • Dysautonomia—treat symptomatically with IV fluids, artificial tears, metoclopramide, bethanechol (cats, 0.5–2.5 mg SC q12h or 2.5–10 mg PO q6–8h; dogs, 0.5–15 mg SC q12h or 2.5–30 mg PO q6–8h), and pilocarpine eye drops.

CONTRAINDICATIONS

Corticosteroids—contraindicated in *Neospora*-associated polyradiculoneuritis, hyperadrenocorticism, and CHP.

FOLLOW-UP

PATIENT MONITORING

Repeat neurologic examinations.

PREVENTION/AVOIDANCE

• Avoid breeding patients with *Neospora* (placental transfer of the organism from the bitch). • Avoid contact with raccoons. • Avoid future vaccinations if suspected associated with vaccines.

POSSIBLE COMPLICATIONS

Continued neurologic deterioration leading to inability to ambulate, severe muscle atrophy, pressure sores, urinary tract infection, muscle fibrosis, aspiration pneumonia.

EXPECTED COURSE AND PROGNOSIS

• Demyelinating conditions—more rapid improvement than axonal neuropathies (majority), which can take months for partial or complete recovery, if at all. • Inherited—most have a poor prognosis (except hyperchylomicronemia in cats). • Acute polyradiculoneuritis (CHP)—good long-term prognosis; may take weeks to months to recover. • Metabolic—fair-to-good prognosis with successful treatment of primary metabolic abnormality; insulinomas have high recurrence rate. • Other acquired—most show continued deterioration despite treatment.

MISCELLANEOUS

PREGNANCY/FERTILITY/BREEDING

Immunosuppressive agents—contraindicated.

ABBREVIATIONS

• CHP = coonhound paralysis. • EMG = electromyography. • FeLV = feline leukemia virus. • FIV = feline immunodeficiency virus. • LMN = lower motor neuron. • KCS = keratoconjunctivitis sicca. • SLE = systemic lupus erythematosus. • T_4 = thyroxine. • TSH = thyroid-stimulating hormone.

INTERNET RESOURCES

vetneuromuscular.ucsd.edu

Suggested Reading

Dewey CW, Cerda-Gonzalez S. Disorders of the peripheral nervous system: mononeuropathies and polyneuropathies. 2nd ed. Ames, IA: Wiley-Blackwell, 2008, pp. 427–467.

Granger N. Canine inherited motor and sensory neuropathies: an updated classification in 22 breeds and comparison to Charcot-Marie-Tooth disease. Vet J 2011, 188:274–285.

Author Paula Martín Vaquero

Client Education Handout available online

BASICS

DEFINITION

Increased food intake.

PATHOPHYSIOLOGY

- Failure to assimilate or loss of nutrients (e.g., maldigestion/malabsorption syndromes such as exocrine pancreatic insufficiency).
- Inability to use nutrients (e.g., diabetes mellitus, poor-quality diets, gastrointestinal parasites).
- Hypoglycemia (e.g., insulinoma, insulin overdose).
- Increased metabolic rate or demand (e.g., hyperthyroidism, cold environments, pregnancy, lactation).
- Psychologic or learned behaviors (e.g., palatable diets, competition with other household pets).
- Iatrogenic (e.g., drugs such as anticonvulsants or glucocorticoids).
- Genetic (e.g., Labrador and flat-coated retrievers).

SYSTEMS AFFECTED

- Cardiovascular—obesity can worsen clinical cardiac disease.
- CNS—tumors of the brain, especially of the hypothalamus, can cause polyphagia.
- Integument—obese animals, especially cats, are susceptible to dermatitis.
- Musculoskeletal—overweight patients are susceptible to arthritis and other orthopedic problems.
- Respiratory—obesity exacerbates dyspnea in patients with respiratory disease.

SIGNALMENT

- Dogs and cats.
- Some dog breeds are prone to obesity: beagle, Rottweiler, cocker spaniel, dachshund, Shetland sheepdog, dalmation, and the retrievers.

SIGNS

Historical Findings

- Eating more frequently and/or a greater quantity than normal.
- Excessive food-seeking and food-stealing behaviors.
- Weight loss may occur with certain disease states (e.g., exocrine pancreatic insufficiency, diabetes mellitus, hyperthyroidism).
- Polyuria/polydipsia (PU/PD) occurs in some patients (diabetes mellitus, hyperthyroidism, hyperadrenocorticism).

Physical Examination Findings

Patients may have excessive body fat, but those with an underlying medical problem (e.g., exocrine pancreatic insufficiency, diabetes mellitus, hyperthyroidism) may be thin.

CAUSES

Physiologic

- Pregnancy.
- Lactation.
- Growth.
- Response to a cold environment.
- Increased exercise.
- Genetic predispositions:
  - 14-bp deletion in the pro-opiomelanocortin (*POMC*) gene of Labrador and flat-coated retrievers leading to increases in obesity, adiposity, and food motivation.
  - Polymorphism in the melanocortin 4 receptor gene (*MC4R*: c.92C>T) predisposing obese cats to development of diabetes mellitus.

Pathologic

- Diabetes mellitus.
- Hyperthyroidism—cats.
- Hyperadrenocorticism—dogs.
- Exocrine pancreatic insufficiency.
- Gastrointestinal parasites.
- Insulinoma.
- Insulin overdose.
- Lymphangiectasia.
- Growth hormone-secreting pituitary tumor.
- Megaesophagus.
- Lymphocytic plasmacytic enteritis in cats—uncommon.
- Neoplasms of the brain—rare.
- Gastrointestinal neoplasms—rare.
- Compulsive polyphagia—rare.

Iatrogenic

- Corticosteroids.
- Progestins.
- Benzodiazepines.
- Anticonvulsants.
- Palatable food.
- Free feeding/overfeeding.
- Poor diet.
- Competition for food.

RISK FACTORS

Environmental

- Lower income owners.
- Older age of the patient.
- Older age of the owner.
- Female spayed > male neutered > intact both sexes.

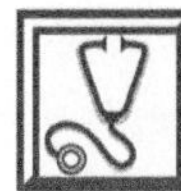

DIAGNOSIS

DIFFERENTIAL DIAGNOSIS

PU/PD (excessive trips to food/water area)—differentiate by observation.

CBC/BIOCHEMISTRY/URINALYSIS

- Neutrophilia, monocytosis, lymphopenia, and eosinopenia with hyperadrenocorticism, and in patients receiving corticosteroids.
- Hyperglycemia with diabetes mellitus, growth hormone-secreting pituitary tumors (cats, insulin-resistant diabetes mellitus), and hyperadrenocorticism (mild).
- Hypercholesterolemia with recent food intake, hyperadrenocorticism, and diabetes mellitus, and in patients receiving corticosteroids.
- High alkaline phosphatase and alanine aminotransferase activity with hyperadrenocorticism (dogs), hyperthyroidism (cats), and diabetes mellitus, and in patients receiving corticosteroids.
- Hypoproteinemia with protein-losing enteropathies (e.g., lymphangiectasia, inflammatory bowel disease).
- Hypoglycemia in patients with insulinoma or insulin overdose.
- Low urine specific gravity with diabetes mellitus, diabetes insipidus, hyperthyroidism, and hyperadrenocorticism, and in patients receiving corticosteroids.
- Glucosuria, possibly ketonuria, with diabetes mellitus.

OTHER LABORATORY TESTS

- Fecal examination to rule out gastrointestinal parasites.
- Serum trypsin-like immunoreactivity to diagnose exocrine pancreatic insufficiency.
- Total serum T_4 to rule out hyperthyroidism (cats); T_3 suppression testing if hyperthyroidism is suspected but serum total T_4 is normal.
- Low-dose dexamethasone suppression or adrenocorticotropic hormone (ACTH) stimulation test to diagnose hyperadrenocorticism; plasma ACTH level or high-dose dexamethasone suppression testing to differentiate pituitary-dependent hyperadrenocorticism from adrenal tumor if hyperadrenocorticism is confirmed with the low-dose dexamethasone suppression test or ACTH stimulation test.
- Serum insulin levels in hypoglycemic patients to rule out insulinoma.

IMAGING

- Abdominal radiology may demonstrate hepatomegaly associated with hyperadrenocorticism, diabetes mellitus, and corticosteroid administration.
- Abdominal ultrasonography may demonstrate an adrenal mass or bilateral adrenomegaly (hyperadrenocorticism), hepatomegaly (hyperadrenocorticism, diabetes mellitus, and corticosteroid administration), bowel wall thickening or bowel wall layering disruption (inflammatory bowel disease, lymphoma, lymphangiectasia), and pancreatic masses (insulinoma).
- MRI could be used to visualize a neoplasm of the hypothalamus.

DIAGNOSTIC PROCEDURES

Endoscopy with biopsy of the upper gastrointestinal tract to rule out gastrointestinal diseases.

POLYPHAGIA (CONTINUED)

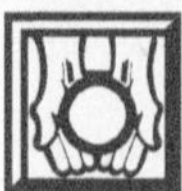

TREATMENT

- Usually outpatient medical management.
- Polyphagia without weight gain or with weight loss is more likely due to a medical problem; evaluate the animal prior to food restriction or manipulation.
- Once pathologic causes of polyphagia have been excluded, limit the amount of food available, feed a reduced-calorie diet, and/or increase exercise if obesity or weight gain is present:
    - Owners must measure food to accurately assess intake.
    - Gram scale measuring provides best accuracy.
    - Some dogs may benefit by the addition of low-calorie bulky foods such as canned or frozen green beans.
    - Feeding smaller meals 2–3 times daily may be beneficial for some patients, provided the total food provided remains the same as required by life stage and activity to promote weight loss or prevent weight gain.
    - Removing the pet during human meal preparation and consumption to reduce begging behavior and the pet obtaining additional food.
- Slowing down the rate of eating may be beneficial in some dogs, using food-dispensing toys that require manipulation to obtain daily ration.
- If social issues within the home influence intake these must be addressed:
    - Feed all dogs in separate locations, preferably without visual contact.
    - Have multiple feeding stations available in a multiple-cat home.
- The average animal's daily caloric need can be estimated by the formula 30 × weight (kg) + 70:
    - Alternatively, using the website https://petnutritionalliance.org/ can provide clinicians with the ability to quickly calculate necessary weight loss and feeding amounts based on specific diet being fed.
- Chew toys can be used as a substitute for food and desires for mastication.
- Dietary options:
    - High fiber, high protein diets provide greater satiety and reduce begging behavior (e.g., Royal Canin Veterinary Diet® Canine and Feline Satiety® Support).
    - Metabolism-increasing diets naturally increase metabolic rate (e.g., Hill's® Prescription Diet® Metabolic Canine and Feline).

MEDICATIONS

DRUG(S) OF CHOICE

- See specific diseases for detailed therapy.
- Drug-induced—attempt to taper or discontinue drug.
- If a compulsive eating disorder is suspected in dogs, clomipramine 1–3 mg/kg PO q12h or fluoxetine 1–2 mg/kg q24h may be used or in cats clomipramine 0.25–1.0 mg/kg q24h or fluoxetine 0.5–1.0 mg/kg q24h.

FOLLOW-UP

PATIENT MONITORING

- Monitor body weight in patients with nonpathologic causes of polyphagia.
- Assess compliance with feeding regime and food measurement to decrease intake and promote weight loss.

POSSIBLE COMPLICATIONS

- Obesity in nonpathologic polyphagia.
- Owner compliance:
    - Owner responds to begging behavior and caloric intake is not decreased.
    - Owner does not factor treats or additives into daily caloric count.
- Weight loss/emaciation in pathologic causes of polyphagia.
- Worsening of respiratory or cardiovascular disease processes in obese patient.
- Difficulty achieving level of appropriate exercise due to respiratory, cardiovascular, or musculoskeletal diseases.
- Decreased metabolic rate after spaying/neutering.
- Increased resource guarding behaviors.
- Increased irritability and aggression.
- Anesthetic complications associated with obesity and adiposity.

MISCELLANEOUS

ASSOCIATED CONDITIONS

Obesity

PREGNANCY/FERTILITY/BREEDING

A normal physiologic response to pregnancy.

SYNONYMS

- Eating disorder.
- Hyperphagia.

SEE ALSO

- Compulsive Disorders—Cats.
- Compulsive Disorders—Dogs.
- Coprophagia and Pica.
- Obesity.

ABBREVIATIONS

- ACTH = adrenocorticotropic hormone.
- PU/PD = polyuria/polydipsia.
- T_3 = triiodothyronine.
- T_4 = thyroxine.

Suggested Reading

Courcier EA, Thomson RM, Mellor DJ, Yam PS. An epidemiological study of environmental factors associated with canine obesity. J Small Anim Pract 2010, 51(7):362–367.

Houpt KA. Ingestive behavior: food and water intake. In: Domestic Animal Behavior, 5th ed. Ames, IA: Wiley-Blackwell, 2011, pp. 235–270.

Luescher AU. Diagnosis and management of compulsive disorders in dogs and cats. Vet Clin North Am Small Anim Pract 2003, 33(2):253–267.

Savidge C. Polyphagia. In: Cote E, ed., Clinical Veterinary Advisor Dogs and Cats, 3rd ed. St. Louis, MO: Mosby, 2014, pp. 826–828.

Authors Amy L. Pike and Amy Learn

Consulting Editor Gary M. Landsberg

Acknowledgment The authors and editors acknowledge the prior contribution of Katherine A. Houpt.

BASICS

OVERVIEW

A chronic inflammatory condition of the urinary bladder characterized by villous or polypoid protrusions from the mucosa and associated with chronic infectious or noninfectious causes. Also called proliferative cystitis. Polypoid projections are diffusely located over the luminal surface of the bladder. It is unclear if proliferative urethritis is a separate disease with different causes. If polyps erode and ulcerate, varying degrees of hematuria and dysuria occur. The gross appearance of polyps cannot be distinguished from that of bladder neoplasms, such as transitional cell carcinomas (TCCs), without histological evaluation.

SIGNALMENT

- Dogs with chronic urinary tract infection (UTI)s or urolithiasis.
- No cases reported in cats.

SIGNS

- Initially, may be asymptomatic.
- Hematuria is the most common sign.
- Gross hematuria often occurs at the end of the micturition stream during maximal bladder contraction.
- Pollakiuria and dysuria may also be present and are associated with irritation of the polyps.
- Urethral obstruction could occur if a sufficient number of bladder polyps are located in the trigone of the bladder. Polyps originating or in the urethra may also cause partial or total obstruction.
- Ureteral obstruction may occur if polyps surround the ureteral orifice.
- UTI may be present concurrently, which can predispose to upper UTI.

CAUSES & RISK FACTORS

- Causes of polypoid cystitis in dogs have not been well documented, but this disorder is commonly associated with UTI, urolithiasis, and other types of chronic irritation.
- Chronic infection and inflammation secondary to long-term indwelling transurethral urinary catheters and urinary stents have been associated with polypoid cystitis.

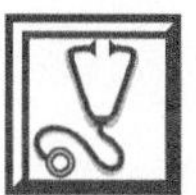

DIAGNOSIS

DIFFERENTIAL DIAGNOSIS

- Polypoid cystitis should be ruled out in cases of hematuria, pollakiuria, dysuria, and recurrent UTI.
- Bladder neoplasms (such as TCC), UTI, and urolithiasis are the most common rule-outs.

CBC/BIOCHEMISTRY/URINALYSIS

- Serum biochemistry profiles should be normal in most cases of polypoid cystitis unless azotemia occurs as a result of obstruction to urine outflow and/or concurrent pyelonephritis.
- Urinalysis may reveal hematuria, pyuria, and transitional epithelial cells.

OTHER LABORATORY TESTS

- Urine should be cultured by clean midstream collection, clean catheterization or at the time of cystoscopy. Culture by cystocentesis is also appropriate once TCC has been ruled out. This will prevent potential spread of TCC along the needle track.
- Representative polyps removed via cystoscopy or cystotomy should be preserved in formalin for light microscopic examination.
- An adequate sample of bladder tissue should be placed in culture media suitable for growth of microbes, preferably prior to antibiotic administration.
- Survey radiographs may reveal a normal bladder, an irregular thickening of the surface contour of the bladder, and/or concurrent urolithiasis.
- Double-contrast cystography or positive-contrast cystography may reveal irregular polypoid fronds projecting in the bladder lumen and/or a thickened bladder wall. The most common location of involvement is the cranioventral bladder wall. Single large polyps with a narrow or broad base may be observed scattered throughout the contrast puddle. Uroliths will migrate to the most dependent portion of the contrast puddle.
- Ultrasonography may show polyps scattered along the mucosal surface of the bladder, especially in the cranioventral aspect.

DIAGNOSTIC PROCEDURES

- Cystoscopic or ultrasound-guided biopsy may be used to obtain representative portions of the polyps for light microscopic examination of stained sections of the lesions.
- More invasive, full-thickness biopsy of the wall of the bladder via cystotomy may be required to include the base of the polyps with an adequate margin of healthy tissue.

PATHOLOGIC FINDINGS

- Gross changes involving the mucosal surface of the urinary bladder include single or multiple small masses ranging from 1 to 10 mm in size. The masses may be nodular with a broad base or attached to the bladder wall by a thin stalk.
- Light microscopic changes include polypoid projections of hyperplastic epithelium that surround a core of proliferative connective tissue mixed with acute and chronic inflammation (congestion, edema, and acute and chronic inflammatory cells). Findings characteristic of malignancy (e.g., disproportionate enlargement of nuclei in relation to the cytoplasm; increase in chromatin content causing hyperchromasia; structural changes such as aberrant chromatin patterns, lack of distinct cell boundaries, irregularity in cell outlines; enlargement and/or increase in number of nuclei; multinucleated cells with atypical nuclei; abnormal number of mitotic figures; cytoplasmic inclusions and vacuolization; invasion of basement membranes) are conspicuously absent. Eosinophils have been present; their significance is unknown. In some patients, changes typical of granulomatous inflammation predominate.
- Fluorescence in situ hybridization identifies bacteria when urine and tissue culture was negative.

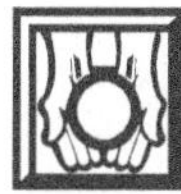

TREATMENT

- Elimination of bacteria that are a source of chronic irritation is a rational therapeutic goal.
- Nonsurgical removal of urocystoliths (voiding urohydropropulsion, lithotripsy, dietary management) that are causing chronic irritation may result in elimination of inflammatory polyps.
- The polyps can be removed nonsurgically (stone basket extraction, laser ablation, electrocautery via cystoscopy or surgically via cystotomy).
- Partial cystectomy may be required to remove polyps affecting large portions of the bladder. The remaining portion of the urinary bladder may return to normal size in 3–6 months.

MEDICATIONS

DRUG(S) OF CHOICE

- Select an antimicrobic based on culture of urine and polyp tissue. Optimal duration of antibiotic therapy is unknown. Post-therapy urine cultures can be used to determine if longer courses of antimicrobs are needed.
- Use of piroxicam and immunosuppressive drugs are suggested, but efficacy is variable.

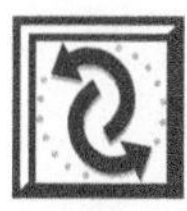

FOLLOW-UP

PATIENT MONITORING

- A urine culture should be performed 7–10 days after antimicrobial therapy is initiated, to confirm urine sterility. Follow-up urinalysis and urine cultures should also be performed by cystocentesis 7 days after antimicrobial therapy has ceased and 1 month post therapy.
- Ultrasonographic reevaluation of the urinary tract is recommended at 1, 3, and 6 months.
- Persistent asymptomatic polyps are not treated.

PREVENTION/AVOIDANCE

Control of predisposing factors such as UTI, urolithiasis, urinary stenting.

POLYPOID CYSTITIS (CONTINUED)

POSSIBLE COMPLICATIONS

- Chronic UTIs.
- Upper UTI.
- Complete obstruction of ureters or urethra.

EXPECTED COURSE AND PROGNOSIS

- The expected course is favorable and the prognosis good if the underlying cause is treated and eradicated.
- Rarely patients with polypoid cystitis develop TCC several years after initial diagnosis. It is unknown if some of these cases represent early carcinoma *in situ*.

MISCELLANEOUS

ASSOCIATED CONDITIONS

- Urinary tract infection.
- Urolithiasis.

AGE-RELATED FACTORS

No age-related factors have been reported, but usually not found in immature dogs.

SEE ALSO

- Hematuria.
- Transitional Cell Carcinoma.
- Urinary Tract Obstruction.
- Urolithiasis.

ABBREVIATIONS

- TCC = transitional cell carcinoma.
- UTI = urinary tract infection.

Suggested Reading

Cooper JE, Brearley MJ. Urothelial abnormalities in the dog. Vet Rec 1986, 118:513–514.

Johnston SD, Osborne CA, Stevens JB. Canine polyploid cystitis. J Am Vet Med Assoc 1975, 166:1155–1160.

Martinez I, Matton JS, Eaton KA, et al. Polypoid cystitis in 17 dogs (1978–2001). J Vet Intern Med 2003, 17:499–509.

Tagiguchi M, Inaba M. Diagnostic ultrasound of polypoid cystitis in dogs. J Vet Med Sci 2005, 67(1):57–61.

Author Jody P. Lulich

Consulting Editor J.D. Foster

Acknowledgment The author and editors acknowledge the prior contribution of Carl A. Osborne.

P

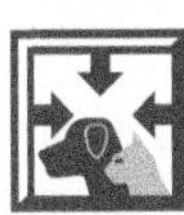

BASICS

DEFINITION

- Polyuria (PU)—increased urine production (dogs, >45 mL/kg/day; cats, >40 mL/kg/day).
- Polydipsia (PD)—increased water consumption (dogs, >90 mL/kg/day; cats, >45 mL/kg/day).

PATHOPHYSIOLOGY

- The volumes of urine produced and water consumed are controlled by interactions between the kidneys, pituitary gland, and hypothalamus through monitoring of plasma osmolality. Volume receptors within the atria and aortic arch also influence thirst and urine production. PU may occur when the quantity of functional antidiuretic hormone (ADH) synthesized in the hypothalamus or released from the posterior pituitary is limited, or when the kidneys fail to respond normally to ADH. PD occurs when the thirst center in the anterior hypothalamus is stimulated.
- In most PU patients, plasma becomes relatively hypertonic and activates thirst mechanisms; the PD maintains hydration as a compensatory response. Occasionally PD is the primary process and PU is compensatory. In this case, the patient's plasma becomes relatively hypotonic because of excessive water intake, ADH secretion is reduced, resulting in PU.

SYSTEMS AFFECTED

- Urologic—full bladder.
- Cardiovascular—circulating volume.
- Endocrine/metabolic—pituitary gland, hypothalamus play a role in compensation to PU or PD.

SIGNALMENT

- Dog and cat.
- Congenital diseases in many breeds (e.g., central diabetes insipidus [CDI], nephrogenic diabetes insipidus [NDI], portovascular anomaly, kidney disease).
- Kidney disease, hyperadrenocorticism (HAC), hyperthyroidism, neoplasia affecting the pituitary or hypothalamus predominantly affect middle-aged and older animals.

CAUSES

- Primary PU due to impaired kidney response to ADH—kidney disease, HAC, hyperthyroidism, pyelonephritis, leptospirosis, pyometra, hepatic failure, hypercalcemia, hypokalemia, kidney medullary solute washout, dietary protein restriction, drugs, congenital NDI.
- Primary PU caused by osmotic diuresis—diabetes mellitus (DM), primary kidney glucosuria, postobstructive diuresis, some diuretics (e.g., mannitol and furosemide), ingestion or administration of large quantities of solute (e.g., sodium chloride or glucose), and hypersomatotropism.
- Primary PU due to ADH deficiency—idiopathic, traumatic, neoplastic, or congenital CDI; some drugs (e.g., alcohol and phenytoin).
- Primary PD—behavioral, pyrexia, pain, organic disease of the anterior hypothalamic thirst center of neoplastic, traumatic, or inflammatory origin.

RISK FACTORS

- Kidney, liver and/or endocrine disease.
- Administration of diuretics, corticosteroids, anticonvulsants.
- Low-protein diets.

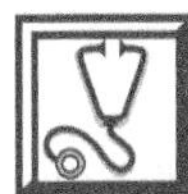

DIAGNOSIS

DIFFERENTIAL DIAGNOSIS

Differentiating Similar Signs

- Differentiate PU from pollakiuria. Pollakiuria: often associated with dysuria, stranguria, hematuria. Patients with PU void large quantities of urine; patients with pollakiuria frequently void small quantities of urine. Confirm PU/PD by measuring 24-hour water intake and urine output (3- to 5-day collection period preferred).
- Urine specific gravity (USG) measurement may provide evidence of hypersthenuria (dogs, >1.030; cats, >1.035), ruling out persistent PU/PD.

Differentiating Causes

- Kidney disease, HAC, DM, hyperthyroidism.
- Progressive weight loss—consider chronic kidney disease, DM, hyperthyroidism, hepatic failure, pyometra, pyelonephritis, hypoadrenocorticism, malignancy-induced hypercalcemia.
- Decreased appetite—consider kidney disease, pyelonephritis, malignancy-induced hypercalcemia, hepatic disease, hypoadrenocorticism.
- Polyphagia—consider DM, hyperthyroidism, HAC, acromegaly.
- Bilateral alopecia or other cutaneous problems—consider HAC, endocrinologic disorders
- Uremic breath and stomatitis—consider advanced kidney disease.
- Vomiting—consider kidney disease, hypoadrenocorticism, pyelonephritis, hepatic failure, hypercalcemia, hypokalemia, hyperthyroidism, DM.
- Malaise and/or weakness—kidney disease, hypoadrenocorticism, pyometra, hypercalcemia, DM, hepatic disease, hypokalemia, HAC.
- Palpable thyroid nodule—consider hyperthyroidism.
- Hypertensive retinopathy—consider chronic kidney disease (CKD), hyperthyroidism, DM, HAC.
- Recent estrus (previous 2 months) in a middle-aged intact female—consider pyometra.
- Abdominal distention—consider hepatic failure, HAC, pyometra, nephrotic syndrome.
- Lymphadenopathy, anal sac mass or other neoplastic process—consider hypercalcemia of malignancy.
- Behavioral or neurologic disorder—consider hepatic failure, primary PD, CDI.
- Marked PD (patients almost continuously seek and consume water)—consider primary PD, CDI, NDI.
- Consider drug-induced (steroids, diuretics, anticonvulsants) PU/PD.
- Consequence of urolith prevention/dissolution or high salt diet.

Key point: PU/PD may be the first symptom of many diseases.

CBC/BIOCHEMISTRY/URINALYSIS

- Urinalysis is useful to confirm PU, discriminate water diuresis from solute diuresis, and identify urinary tract infection (UTI).
- Serum sodium concentration or osmolality may help differentiate primary PU from PD. Measuring serum osmolality is preferred; calculated serum osmolality is not an acceptable alternative.
- Relative hypernatremia or high serum osmolarity suggests primary PU.
- Hyponatremia or low serum osmolarity suggests primary PD, except in animals with hypoadrenocorticism, which have hyponatremia and primary PU.
- Azotemia is typical of kidney causes for PU/PD, but may also indicate dehydration resulting from inadequate compensatory PD.
- Unexpectedly low BUN concentrations suggest hepatic failure.
- With high hepatic enzymes, consider HAC, hyperthyroidism, hepatic failure, pyometra, DM, or administration of drugs (e.g., anticonvulsants and corticosteroids).
- Persistent hyperglycemia suggests DM.
- Hyperkalemia, particularly if associated with hyponatremia, suggests hypoadrenocorticism or therapy with potassium-sparing diuretics.
- Hypercalcemia induces PU only when it results from increased ionized calcium (not protein-bound calcium) concentration.
- Hypoalbuminemia supports kidney or hepatic causes of PU/PD.
- Neutrophilia is consistent with pyelonephritis, pyometra, HAC, corticosteroid administration.
- USG values 1.001–1.003 suggest primary PD, CDI, and congenital NDI.
- Glucosuria supports a diagnosis of DM or kidney glucosuria.
- Pyuria, white blood cell casts, and/or bacteriuria should prompt consideration of pyelonephritis.

POLYURIA AND POLYDIPSIA (CONTINUED)

P

OTHER LABORATORY TESTS

- ACTH stimulation or dexamethasone suppression tests rule out HAC.
- Thyroxine concentration to rule out hyperthyroidism.
- Bile acids (fasting and postprandial) to rule out portosystemic shunt or hepatic failure.
- Urine culture—chronic pyelonephritis cannot be conclusively excluded by absence of pyuria or bacteriuria.
- Cytology from lymph node aspirate may diagnose lymphoma, which induces PU by hypercalcemic nephrotoxicity or direct infiltration of kidney tissues.
- Paired *Leptospira* titer to rule out leptospirosis.
- ADH response test to rule out CDI.
- Water deprivation testing (see Diagnostic Procedures) is controversial due to dehydration risk; use selectively.

IMAGING

Abdominal survey radiography, ultrasonography: may provide evidence of kidney, hepatic, adrenal, or uterine disorders that can cause PU/PD.

DIAGNOSTIC PROCEDURES

Modified Water Deprivation with ADH Response Test

- Differentiates CDI from primary PD and NDI. Rule out other causes for PU/PD before performing this test. Controversial, some suggest omitting water deprivation and proceeding directly to ADH administration to rule in CDI, however administration of ADH to patients with primary PD may be dangerous.
- Contraindicated in dehydrated and azotemic patients; ADH response testing may be performed safely in these patients.
- Patients that concentrate urine adequately in response to water deprivation have adequate ADH production and kidney response to ADH. If other causes have been ruled out, primary PD is presumed to be present.
- Failure to concentrate urine adequately in response to properly designed water deprivation tests, but forming concentrated urine in response to administration of exogenous ADH = CDI.
- Failure to concentrate urine adequately in response to water deprivation and also failure to further concentrate urine in response to administration of exogenous ADH = NDI.

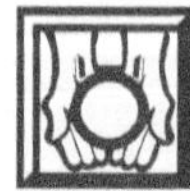

TREATMENT

- Serious medical consequences are rare if patient has free access to water and is able to drink. Until the mechanism of PU is understood, discourage owners from limiting access to water. Direct treatment at the underlying cause.
- Provide PU patients with free access to water unless they are vomiting. If vomiting, give replacement maintenance fluids parenterally after appropriate samples have been collected for initial diagnostics. Provide fluids parenterally when other conditions limit oral intake or dehydration persists despite PD.
- Base fluid selection on the underlying cause for fluid loss; lactated Ringer's solution is acceptable for most patients.
- When dehydration has resulted from withholding water, or when urine is hyposthenuric, providing oral water or parenteral administration of dextrose 5% in water may be preferred to lactated Ringer's solution.
- Primary PD—treat by gradually limiting water intake to a normal daily volume. May be necessary to reduce water intake over days–weeks to avoid undesirable behavior such as barking, urine consumption, or other bizarre behavior. Monitor patient closely to avoid iatrogenic dehydration. Salt (1 g/30 kg q12h) or sodium bicarbonate (0.6 g/30 kg q12h) may be given orally to help reestablish kidney medullary solute gradient. Consider behavior modification if water restriction alone is unsuccessful.

CLIENT EDUCATION

Do not withhold water from patients with PU because potentially dangerous dehydration may result.

MEDICATIONS

DRUG(S) OF CHOICE

Varies with underlying cause.

CONTRAINDICATIONS

Do not administer ADH to patients with primary PD due to risk of inducing water intoxication (hyponatremia, hypoosmolality, and neurologic complications).

PRECAUTIONS

Until kidney disease and hepatic failure have been excluded as potential causes for PU/PD, use caution in administering any drug eliminated via these pathways.

FOLLOW-UP

PATIENT MONITORING

- Hydration status—assessment of hydration, serial evaluation of body weight.
- Fluid intake and urine output provide a useful baseline for assessing response to therapy.

POSSIBLE COMPLICATIONS

Dehydration, hypovolemic shock, hypernatremia.

MISCELLANEOUS

ASSOCIATED CONDITIONS

- Bacterial UTI.
- Urinary incontinence may develop in dogs with concurrent urethral sphincter dysfunction, presumably because of increased bladder filling associated with PD.

SEE ALSO

- Acute Kidney Injury.
- Chronic Kidney Disease.
- Congenital and Developmental Renal Diseases.
- Diabetes Insipidus.
- Diabetes Mellitus.
- Fanconi Syndrome.
- Hepatic Failure, Acute.
- Hyperadrenocorticism.
- Hypercalcemia.
- Hyperthyroidism.
- Hypoadrenocorticism (Addison's Disease).
- Hypokalemia.
- Leptospirosis.
- Pyelonephritis.
- Pyometra.
- Urinary Tract Obstruction.

ABBREVIATIONS

- ACTH = adrenocorticotropic hormone.
- ADH = antidiuretic hormone.
- CDI = central diabetes insipidus.
- CKD = chronic kidney disease.
- DM = diabetes mellitus.
- HAC = hyperadrenocorticism.
- NDI = nephrogenic diabetes insipidus.
- PU/PD = polyuria/polydipsia.
- USG = urine specific gravity.
- UTI = urinary tract infection.

Author David J. Polzin

Consulting Editor J.D. Foster

Client Education Handout available online

PORTOSYSTEMIC SHUNTING, ACQUIRED

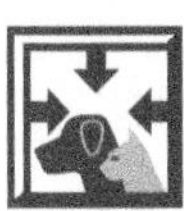

BASICS

OVERVIEW

- Acquired portosystemic shunts (APSS)—develop subsequent to portal hypertension (PH) and involve complex physiology aberrations and adaptations; experimentally form 5–14 weeks after onset of PH.
- Prehepatic PH—compromised perfusion through abdominal portion of the portal vein.
- Intrahepatic PH—classified as presinusoidal, sinusoidal, postsinusoidal causes.
- Posthepatic PH—rostral to hepatic vein; cardiac, pericardial, or major vein causes.
- APSS evolve from preexisting remnant vessels and the process of angiogenesis.
- APSS common in dogs and cats but differ in location from the clinically symptomatic esophageal APSS common in humans; common APSS in dogs and cats involve communications between left gonadal remnants vessels, the left renal vein, and splenic veins with the caudal vena cava.

SIGNALMENT

- Most common—in dogs with chronic necroinflammatory liver disease.
- Less common—in dogs with ductal plate malformations (DPM, congenital hepatic fibrosis [CHF] phenotype), rare noncirrhotic portal hypertension (NCPH), recovery from severe panlobular necrosis, dogs with porto-systemic vascular anomaly (PSVA) intolerant to surgical shunt attenuation, or dogs simply with severe portal vein hypoplasia/atresia.
- APSS in cats—DPM with CHF phenotype, severe CCHS (rare), or PSVA intolerant to surgical shunt attenuation (severe portal hypoplasia) or rarely just severe portal vein atresia.
- Extrahepatic bile duct obstruction (EHBDO) >6 weeks.
- Certain disorders—have age or breed incidence (see Ductal Plate Malformation (Congenital Hepatic Fibrosis); Cirrhosis and Fibrosis of the Liver; Hepatitis, Chronic).
- Breeds—DPM more common in domestic longhair, Persian and Himalayan cats, boxer dogs but may affect any pure- or mixed-breed dog.

SIGNS

- Clinical signs—sequelae of PH, impaired hepatic perfusion, and hepatofugal circulation (hepatofugal = splanchnic portal circulation away from the liver) with or without or reduced hepatic function depending on cause.
- Ascites—common but variable; often fluctuates in severity.
- APSS may associate with episodic hepatic encephalopathy (HE)— may manifest as neurobehavioral or neurocognitive abnormalities, amaurotic blindness, polyuria/polydipsia (PU/PD), anorexia, lethargy, vomiting; neurologic signs may localize to cerebrum, brainstem, or suggest transverse myelopathy.
- PH leads to hypertensive splanchnic vasculopathy—may provoke gastroduodenal bleeding/ulceration because of thin-walled dilated arterials; may progress to perforation and septic peritonitis, life-endangering blood loss if coexistent coagulopathy; can provoke severe HE; causes anorexia, vomiting, diarrhea, abdominal pain, anemia, and sometimes iron deficiency (if chronic blood loss).
- Urogenital—obstructive uropathy due to ammonium biurate urolithiasis, gross or microscopic hematuria, pollakiuria, dysuria, rare severe hematuria (ureteral APSS varices).

CAUSES & RISK FACTORS

- Multiple tortuous vessels—represent acquired vasculature interconnecting portal and systemic venous circulations.
- Lack of valves in main portal vein structure allows blood to follow "a path of least resistance" through APSS to vena cava (systemic circulation). Valves in portal tributaries influence hepatofugal circulatory routes.
- PH—results from many disease processes.
- Common causes of PH—diffuse hepatic fibrosis with or without cirrhosis; chronic unresolved EHBDO (>6 weeks); portal venous thromboembolism (TE), hepatic sinusoidal occlusion syndrome (zone 3, injury causing regional parenchymal collapse or vascular damage to hepatic venules, veins).
- Less common causes of PH involve idiopathic PH or NCPH (obliteration of tertiary portal venules), blockade of large hepatic veins or prehepatic vena cava (Budd–Chiari syndrome) by thrombi, neoplasia or vascular "kinking"; disorders constraining splanchnic portal circulation: vascular stricture or strangulation, severe portal vein atresia rare congenital or acquired hepatic AV malformation(s) causing arterialization of the portal circulation, or severe intrahepatic portal vein atresia.
- Episodic HE.
- Ammonium urate urolithiasis.

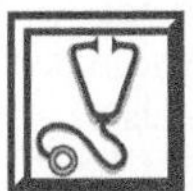

DIAGNOSIS

DIFFERENTIAL DIAGNOSIS

- CNS signs—infectious disorders (e.g., FIP, FeLV- or FIV-related infections or conditions, canine distemper, toxoplasmosis, other); toxicities (e.g., lead, mushrooms, drugs, acute hepatic failure); hydrocephalus; idiopathic epilepsy; metabolic disorders (e.g., severe hypoglycemia, hypo- or hyperkalemia, hypocalcemia, severe hypophosphatemia).
- Gastrointestinal signs—bowel obstruction; dietary indiscretion; foreign body ingestion; inflammatory bowel disease.
- Urinary tract signs—bacterial urinary tract infection; urolithiasis; obstructive uropathy.
- PU/PD—disorders of urine concentration (diabetes insipidus, diabetes mellitus, adrenal hyperplasia, hypercalcemia), primary PD, congenital or acquired renal disease.
- Causes of abdominal effusion—cardiopulmonary disorders causing right-sided heart failure; pericardial disease; primary inflammatory hepatopathies; infiltrative hepatic disease (e.g., neoplasia, amyloid); liver lobe torsion; nonhepatic abdominal disorders associated with effusions (e.g., splenic torsion, visceral neoplasia, carcinomatosis, pancreatitis); or peritonitis: chemical (e.g., bile, urine, chyle) or septic.

CBC/BIOCHEMISTRY/URINALYSIS

- CBC—microcytosis (reflects portosystemic shunting or iron deficiency); mild non-regenerative anemia common; poikilocytes (cats) and target cells (dogs).
- Biochemistry—low BUN, low to low-normal creatinine, glucose, albumin, and cholesterol are common; variable liver enzyme activity (ALP usually high in young animals), ALP induction by inflammatory cytokines or cholestasis, ALT normal or elevated; bilirubin variable; features depend on underlying cause and chronicity.
- Urinalysis—variable urine concentration; ammonium biurate crystalluria, hematuria, pyuria, and proteinuria reflect urolithiasis or infection.

OTHER LABORATORY TESTS

- Total serum bile acids (TSBA)—sensitive indicator of PSS; variable pre- with markedly increased post-meal values (>100 µmol/L); "shunting pattern" implicated by relatively low pre- and markedly increased post-meal values; *however*, 10–20% dogs and cats have higher pre- than post-meal TSBA reflecting slow gastric or enteric transit or delayed gallbladder contraction.
- Blood ammonia—fasting, sensitive but inconsistent indicator of HE and shunting; ammonium biurate crystalluria infers high blood ammonia (evaluate 3 urine specimens, 4–8 hours after eating); ammonia tolerance testing—(oral or rectal $NHCl_4$) best test for ammonia intolerance; *caution*: may induce HE.
- Coagulation tests—prolonged PT, aPTT, reflect severity of liver dysfunction, synthetic failure, DIC, or vitamin K_1 adequacy; low protein C activity reflects PSVA or APSS, enteric or renal losses or consumption.
- Abdominal effusion—usually pure or modified transudate.

IMAGING

Abdominal Radiography

- Liver size depends on underlying cause; microhepatia common in dogs with chronic liver disease with APSS, PSVA, or severe portal vein atresia. Some disorders associate with large liver size or large liver lobes: AV malformations, some DPM (cystic lesions).

PORTOSYSTEMIC SHUNTING, ACQUIRED (CONTINUED)

- Abdominal effusion—impairs visualization of visceral margins; ascites associated with severe portal atresia, some PSVA after surgical attenuation, some animals with DPM (CHF phenotype) with APSS, chronic liver disease with APSS, and other causes of PH.
- Ammonium biurate calculi—radiolucent unless radiodense mineral shell (infection).
- Size of post-hepatic vena cava may reflect pericardial or cardiac causes (distended vein).

Radiographic Portovenography

Demonstrates multiple APSS; not recommended due to complicating risks, see alternatives.

Abdominal Ultrasonography

- Liver size depends on underlying cause. May disclose change in size or absence of specific liver lobes or gallbladder in DPM or AV malformations.
- May disclose disease-related hepatic parenchymal or biliary changes.
- APSS—characterized by hepatofugal portal flow (unreliable US detection) and APSS using color-flow Doppler; tortuous APSS varices have turbulent blood flow; APSS often situated adjacent to left kidney or associated with splenic vasculature.
- Intrahepatic AV communication/fistula—pulsating arterialized vascular within enlarged liver lobe, abdominal effusion and APSS.
- Other causes of PH and APSS are detected using US color-flow Doppler: portal venous thrombi or stricture, hypoplastic portal vein at porta hepatis, diminished hepatic venule/vein filling (venoocclusive syndrome), or Budd–Chiari hepatic vein outflow obstruction.
- Abdominal effusion—common.
- Uroliths—renal pelvis, urinary bladder; rare ureteral.

Colorectal (CRS) or Splenoportal (SPS) Scintigraphy

- Sensitive noninvasive test that confirms PSS.
- Cannot definitively differentiate PSVA from APSS.
- CRS—administer Tc^{99m} pertechnetate into colon.
- SPS—isotope splenic injection via US guidance under heavy sedation or anesthesia; advantage in using less isotope, may miss caudal rectal PSVA.

Multisector CT

Noninvasive imaging of choice; details vascular anatomy, visceral abnormalities.

DIAGNOSTIC PROCEDURES

Fine-Needle Aspiration Cytology

- Hepatic aspiration—usually cannot differentiate disorders causing APSS.
- Liver biopsy—open surgical wedge biopsy or laparoscopic sampling best approach; obtain tissue from several ($n = 3$) liver lobes; Tru-Cut samples may not provide adequate tissue for definitive diagnosis.

PATHOLOGIC FINDINGS

- Gross—small, irregularly contoured liver with chronic liver disease (cirrhosis, fibrosis).
- Normal to large liver in early venous outflow obstruction: Budd–Chiari, sinusoidal occlusion syndrome.
- Isolated large liver lobe—intrahepatic AV malformation.
- Normal to small liver—DPM (CHF phenotype), NCPH, portal TE, portal atresia, PSVA.
- Normal to large liver in some cats with DPM.

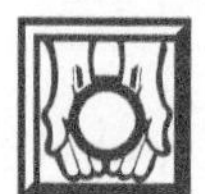

TREATMENT

Appropriate Health Care

Inpatient—severe signs of HE or tense abdominal effusion requiring therapeutic abdominocentesis and critical care.

Diet

- Nutritional support—essential to maintain body condition to optimize control of hyperammonemia-associated HE; species-specific balanced, restricted-protein diet (avoid red meat, organ meat, fish in dogs); protein allowance optimized to tolerance (see Hepatic Encephalopathy). Cats have different protein requirements compared to dogs.
- Protein allowance titrated to response with adjunctive treatment modulating production and absorption of enteric toxins contributing to HE (colonic products mainly); use commercial diets formulated for liver disease or moderate renal insufficiency as a baseline diet.
- Dogs—commercial liver diets provide 2.2–2.5 g protein/kg body weight when fed to meet energy requirements; titrate protein using 0.25 g/kg additional allocations q5–7 days until optimized tolerance determined: dairy and soy protein are best sources for dogs; if necessary white meat chicken can be introduced in small amounts to stimulate appetite.
- Cats—pure carnivores require meat-derived protein; use diets for renal insufficiency.
- Parenteral nutrition rarely used—see Hepatic Encephalopathy.
- Sodium restriction important in dogs with ascites; 50–100 mg sodium/100 kcal or <0.2% dry matter basis formula of sodium; initiate before or with start of diuretic therapy.

Client Education

- Depends on underlying cause.
- Educate client of HE and potential for ammonium biurate obstructive uropathy (males); permanent pre-scrotal urethrostomy may be needed (persistent ammonium biurate uroliths).
- Educate client how to adjust diuretics (as-needed basis) to mobilize abdominal effusion.
- Educate client how to adjust oral medications and use enemas (as-needed basis) to ameliorate HE.
- Emphasize importance of sodium restriction if ascites.

MEDICATIONS

DRUG(S) OF CHOICE

- Enteric hemorrhage—associated with hypertensive splanchnic vasculopathy and coagulopathy; some clinicians use *prophylactic* acid blockers or gastroprotectants to reduce risk, however, ulceration is not linked with hypergastrinemia; symptomatic animals treated with proton pump inhibitor (omeprazole; pantoprazole) and sucralfate; may require blood component therapy or DDAVP (see Coagulopathy of Liver Disease) if critical hemorrhage.
- Abdominal effusion—sequentially measure weight, girth (standardize measurements: location and operator) to monitor ascites; advise dietary sodium restriction combined with titrated dosing of furosemide with spironolactone.
- Conventional diuretics—combined use of furosemide and spironolactone is superior to single drugs alone; furosemide 0.5–2 mg/kg PO q12–24h and spironolactone 0.5–2 mg/kg PO q12h, single loading dose of spironolactone (doubled dose) followed by dose titrations based on response q4–5 days with close monitoring of serum electrolytes and renal function. Adjustments: incremental 25–50% dose increase. Spironolactone is potassium sparing and a less potent diuretic than furosemide. Furosemide is potassium wasting and typically initiates a brisk diuresis that can provoke RAAS response with effect attenuated by spironolactone.
- Vasopressin V_2 antagonists (aquaretics) *may* be superior for ascites control compared to conventional diuretics (proven in humans, e.g., tolvaptan); this class of drugs is not routinely available or affordable for veterinary patients; no relevant clinical experience.
- Diuretic-resistant ascites—may require therapeutic abdominocentesis (see Hypertension, Portal). May reflect insidious increased sodium intake or RAAS response to diuresis.
- Avoid dehydration or hypokalemia by frequent monitoring initially: these can provoke HE.

Precautions

- Remain aware of altered drug metabolism due to reduced first-pass extraction (PSS),

altered hepatic metabolism/biotransformation, and reduced protein binding.
- Remain vigilant for diuretic-induced dehydration and electrolyte dysregulation that may provoke HE and/or hepatorenal syndrome (acute renal failure due to severe vasoconstriction).
- Beware that aggressive therapeutic abdominocentesis may provoke hypotensive post-centesis syndrome (see Ascites).

CONTRAINDICATIONS/POSSIBLE INTERACTIONS

Avoid metoclopramide if using spironolactone (blocks effect); avoid NSAIDs as these may inhibit furosemide-induced diuresis, potentiate renal injury, or provoke sodium accumulation.

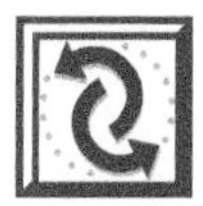

FOLLOW-UP

PATIENT MONITORING

- Reevaluate patient's at-home demeanor and appetite as a reflection of HE.
- Monitor clinical signs, appetite, body condition, muscle mass, weight, abdominal girth, CBC, serum biochemistry, and urine (concentration, ammonium biurate crystalluria); TSBA not useful for sequential evaluation as these are predictably increased with APSS and ursodeoxycholic acid (drug measured in assay) administration.
- Adjust medical management to alleviate episodic HE, ammonium biurate crystalluria, and abdominal effusion.
- Inspect patient carefully for evidence of clinical bleeding; determine need for intermittent chronic vitamin K_1 administration (parenteral route).

PREVENTION/AVOIDANCE

- Early treatment of acquired liver disease and EHBDO minimizes fibrosis/remodeling.
- Cautious PSVA attenuation.

POSSIBLE COMPLICATIONS

- Treat underlying disorder(s).
- Enteric hemorrhage associated with hypertensive vasculopathy; may require acute intensive care: manage hypovolemia, coagulopathy, and ensuing HE; may require surgical resection of involved gut (rare).
- Dehydration, contraction alkalosis, azotemia, acute renal failure—complications of diuretics.
- Death risk—from liver failure, HE complications, lethal enteric hemorrhage, or sepsis.

EXPECTED COURSE AND PROGNOSIS

- Varies with underlying cause.
- Management of chronic liver disease or hepatic fibrosis seemingly extends life.
- Animals with NCPH and DPM (CHF phenotype) may live >5 years if managed successfully during symptomatic illnesses.

MISCELLANEOUS

ASSOCIATED CONDITIONS

- Ammonium urate urolithiasis.
- Ascites.
- Coagulopathy.
- Hepatic encephalopathy.
- Enteric bleeding/ulceration.
- Obstructive uropathy.

SEE ALSO

- Ascites.
- Cirrhosis and Fibrosis of the Liver.
- Coagulopathy of Liver Disease.
- Ductal Plate Malformation (Congenital Hepatic Fibrosis).
- Hepatic Encephalopathy.
- Hepatitis, Chronic.
- Portal Hypertension.
- Portosystemic Vascular Anomaly, Congenital.

ABBREVIATIONS

- APSS = acquired portosystemic shunt.
- AV = arteriovenous.
- CCHS = cholangitis/cholangiohepatitis syndrome.
- CHF = congenital hepatic fibrosis.
- CRS = colorectal scintigraphy.
- DPM = ductal plate malformation.
- EHBDO = extrahepatic bile duct obstruction.
- HE = hepatic encephalopathy.
- NCPH = noncirrhotic portal hypertension.
- NSAID = nonsteroidal anti-inflammatory drug.
- PH = portal hypertension.
- PSVA = portosystemic vascular anomaly.
- PU/PD = polyuria/polydipsia.
- SPS = splenoportal scintigraphy.
- TE = thromboembolism.
- TSBA = total serum bile acids.

P

Suggested Reading

Buob S, Johnston AN, Webster CR. Portal hypertension: pathophysiology, diagnosis, and treatment. J Vet Intern Med 2011, 25:169–186.
Iwakiri Y. Pathophysiology of portal hypertension. Clin Liver Dis. 2014, 18(2):281–291.
Simonetto DA, Liu M, Kamath PS. Portal hypertension and related complications: diagnosis and management. Mayo Clinic Proc 2019, 94:714–726.

Author Sharon A. Center
Consulting Editor Kate Holan

PORTOSYSTEMIC VASCULAR ANOMALY, CONGENITAL

BASICS

DEFINITION

• Aberrant venous connections between the portal and systemic circulations; macroscopic shunts permit portal hepatofugal circulation (flow away from or around the liver).
• May be extrahepatic portosystemic vascular anomaly (E-PSVA) or intrahepatic (I-PSVA).
• Most are single vessels; occasionally two shunts may be identified.
• Most small-breed dogs with PSVA also have microscopic vascular abnormalities (see Hepatoportal Microvascular Dysplasia).

PATHOPHYSIOLOGY

• Clinical signs—reflect hepatofugal circulation that prohibits hepatic cleansing of enteric toxins, food-derived nitrogenous toxins, and other noxious colonic substances from portal blood.
• Microhepatia—deprivation of splanchnic hepatotrophic factors (e.g., insulin) causes hepatic atrophy.
• Episodic hepatic encephalopathy (HE)—associated with consumption of high-protein foods, gastrointestinal bleeding, other causes of increased heme turnover (blood transfusions, hemolysis), dehydration, azotemia, alkalosis, hypokalemia, infections, constipation, catabolism, and certain drugs.
• Ammonium biurate crystalluria/urolithiasis—reflect hyperammonemia and impaired conversion of uric acid to water-soluble allantoin; may be a presenting problem.
• Severity of clinical signs reflect the magnitude of macroscopic shunting.

SYSTEMS AFFECTED

• Nervous—episodic HE in most but not all.
• Gastrointestinal—intermittent inappetence; vomiting; diarrhea; pica; ptyalism (cats).
• Urogenital— "plump" kidneys; ammonium urate urolithiasis; 50% male dogs cryptorchid in one retrospective report.
• Asymptomatic—up to 20% of dogs with PSVA.

GENETICS

• E-PSVA—most common in small-breed dogs (e.g., Yorkshire terrier, Cairn terrier, Maltese, Tibetan spaniel, miniature schnauzer, Norfolk terrier, pug, shih tzu, Havanese, papillon.
• I-PSVA—most common in large-breed dogs (e.g., Irish wolfhound, Labrador retriever, Old English sheepdog, golden retrievers).
• Autosomal dominant complex polygenic inheritance suspected to cause PSVA/microvascular dysplasia (MVD) trait in small-breed dogs; MVD most common phenotype.
• I-PSVA—appears heritable in Irish wolfhounds patent ductus venosus type I-PSVA and kindred of Labrador retrievers, Old English sheepdogs, golden retrievers.

INCIDENCE/PREVALENCE

0.2–0.6% of large referral clinic.

GEOGRAPHIC DISTRIBUTION

Reported worldwide.

SIGNALMENT

Species

Dog and cat; most common in small-breed dogs.

Breed Predilections

Higher risk—purebred and mixed small "terrier" type dogs; cats—domestic shorthair, fewer pure breeds.

Mean Age and Range

• Usually identified in juveniles; some asymptomatic dogs as old as 13 years at initial diagnosis.
• Asymptomatic animals present older; miniature schnauzers and dogs with porto-azygous shunts.

Predominant Sex

N/A

SIGNS

Historical Findings

• Stunted growth—common.
• Signs often initiate with weaning of puppy or kitten to commercial growth foods.
• Gastrointestinal signs—inappetence, vomiting, diarrhea, pica.
• Cats—ptyalism.
• Episodic HE—most dramatic and predominating sign in many dogs, improves with fluids, broad-spectrum antibiotics, and lactulose.
• CNS signs—weakness, propulsive circling or pacing, vocalization, apparent hallucinations, ataxia, disorientation, head pressing, signs consistent with transverse myelopathy, vague hyperpathia, amaurotic blindness, behavioral changes (aggression in cats), twitching or trembling, focal or generalized seizures, or progressive obtundation to coma.
• Urinary signs—polyuria/polydipsia (PU/PD); ammonium biurate crystalluria: pollakiuria, dysuria; hematuria; urethral/ureteral ammonium biurate urolith obstruction.
• Asymptomatic—up to 20% of dogs.
• Affected bitches may produce viable litters.

Physical Examination Findings

• Normal appearance, but most have stunted stature; microhepatia; HE; copper-colored irises in non-blue-eyed cats (note: Persian, Russian blue, some others normally have copper-colored iris; iris color does not change with PSVA ligation).
• Neurologic signs.

CAUSES

Congenital developmental vascular malformations.

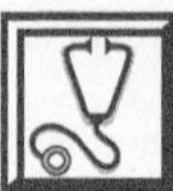

DIAGNOSIS

DIFFERENTIAL DIAGNOSES

• CNS signs—infectious disorders (FIP-, FeLV- or FIV-related infections in cats, canine distemper, toxoplasmosis); toxicities (lead, mushrooms, recreational drugs); congenital CNS malformations (hydrocephalus); congenital storage disorders; idiopathic epilepsy; metabolic disorders (severe hypoglycemia, hypokalemia, hyperkalemia, hypocalcemia); necrotizing meningoencephalitis or granulomatous meningoencephalitis—idiopathic inflammatory CNS syndromes in small-breed dogs (e.g., pug, Maltese, Yorkshire terriers).
• Gastrointestinal signs—bowel obstruction; dietary indiscretion; foreign body ingestion; inflammatory bowel disease.
• Urinary tract signs—bacterial urinary tract infection or other forms of urolithiasis.
• PU/PD—disorders of urine concentration (diabetes insipidus, diabetes mellitus, abnormal adrenal function, hypercalcemia), primary polydipsia.
• Primary liver disease.
• MVD—in asymptomatic PSVA animals.

CBC/BIOCHEMISTRY/URINALYSIS

• CBC—microcytosis; mild non-regenerative anemia; poikilocytosis (cats); target cells (dogs).
• Biochemistry—inconsistent low BUN, creatinine, cholesterol; hypoglycemia—in young tiny toy breeds, variable liver enzyme activity (ALP high in young patients), ALT normal or elevated; bilirubin normal; hypoalbuminemia inconsistent and mild.
• Urinalysis—normally concentrated or dilute urine; ammonium biurate crystalluria; hematuria, pyuria, and proteinuria: with urolithiasis or infection.

OTHER LABORATORY TESTS

• Total serum bile acid (TSBA)—sensitive indicator of portosystemic shunting (PSS); random fasting values may be within reference intervals; 2 hours post-meal values usually markedly high (>100 µmol/L); always use paired samples around confirmed meal ingestion; no need to fast before testing. TSBA often remain abnormal in small-breed dogs after PSVA attenuation due to concurrent MVD. Important TSBA testing strategy—food-initiated enterohepatic bile acid challenge essential; verify meal consumption; feed typical size meal; feed dog's regular diet for testing.
• Blood ammonia—fasting, sensitive but inconsistent indicator of HE and shunting; ammonia tolerance testing—oral or rectal $NHCl_4$ administration; may cause transient HE.
• Coagulation tests—prolonged clotting times compared to healthy dogs but not clinically significant; are not associated with increased risk for bleeding.

P

• Protein C—low values help differentiate PSVA from MVD; usually <70% in symptomatic PSVA, usually >70% in MVD, may be ≥70% in asymptomatic PSVA. Test reflects magnitude of macroscopic shunting. Protein C especially useful for postoperative assessment after PSVA ligation if initial activity subnormal; normalization coordinates with good surgical outcome despite sustained high TSBA values. Protein C is *not* similarly applicable in cats.

IMAGING

Abdominal Radiography

• Microhepatia—dogs > cats.
• Renomegaly—some dogs.
• Ammonium urate urolithiasis—radiolucent unless combined with radiodense mineral shell.

Radiographic Portovenography

• Mesenteric portography—old gold standard for PSVA diagnosis.
• Currently used as intraoperative assessment of hepatic portal perfusion via fluoroscopy, accurate PSVA localization and assesses postligation liver perfusion.

Abdominal Ultrasonography

• Subjective assessment of microhepatia and vascular profiles; difficult to identify some PSVA (portoazygos, splenophrenic, gastrophrenic); US identification of PSVA is highly operator dependent.
• Color-flow Doppler—assists in US PSVA verification.
• I-PSVA—usually more easily imaged with US than E-PSVA.
• Other US features—renomegaly, uroliths: bladder, renal pelvis, rare ureteral.
• US microbubble study—can confirm PSS; splenic injection of agitated heparinized blood (microbubbles).

Colorectal (CRS) or Splenoportal (SPS) Scintigraphy

• Tc^{99m} pertechnetate CRS or SPS measures shunt fraction; normal dog shunt fraction ≤15%; PSVA shunt fraction usually >60% but depends on severity of macroscopic shunting; shunt fraction in MVD is usually mildly increased above normal.
• CRS—sensitive noninvasive test confirming macroscopic shunting; cannot differentiate PSVA from acquired PSS (APSS) or E-PSVA from I-PSVA.
• SPS—may miss caudal PSVA; details insufficient to differentiate type of shunt (APSS vs. PSVA or I-PSVA, E-PSVA).

Multisector CT

Gold standard imaging modality defining arterial and venous circulations; definitively demonstrates PSVA and APSS.

DIAGNOSTIC PROCEDURES

• Vascular imaging provides definitive diagnosis of PSVA.
• Fine-needle aspiration cytology—cannot diagnose PSVA or MVD.
• Liver biopsy—required for definitive diagnosis of portal venous hypoperfusion; rules out most acquired hepatobiliary disorders causing increased TSBA except splanchnic portal thromboembolism (TE), noncirrhotic portal hypertension (NCPH) and cannot usually differentiate MVD from PSVA.
• Open surgical wedge or laparoscopic liver biopsies preferred with samples collected from several (n = 3) liver lobes; avoid sampling caudate lobe.
• Needle core samples may be inadequate for definitive diagnosis of portal venous hypoperfusion.

PATHOLOGIC FINDINGS

• Gross—small, smooth-surfaced liver; PSVA may be difficult to verify at autopsy due to collapse of portal vasculature.
• Histologic features—cannot discriminate MVD, PSVA, NCPH, or extrahepatic portal venous TE/occlusion without history, clinical findings, and imaging details. Note: dogs with MVD lacking PSVA have histologic features identical to PSVA but lack macroscopic shunting.
• Portal venous hypoplasia—invalid histologic diagnosis as failure to identify perfused portal veins can reflect any cause of portal venous hypoperfusion.
• Note: dogs ≤4 months of age demonstrate increased juvenile or small portal triads.

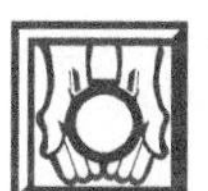

TREATMENT

APPROPRIATE HEALTH CARE

Inpatient—severe signs of HE; medical intervention prior to liver biopsy and PSVA ligation.

NURSING CARE

See Hepatic Encephalopathy.

DIET

• Nutritional support—essential to maintain body condition and muscle mass.
• Species-specific balanced protein-restricted diet—use commercial canine liver diet for dogs and feline renal diet for cats as a baseline diet. To these diets, additional protein allocations are titrated based on patient response, in combination with treatments ameliorating HE.
• Dogs—as tolerated, add an additional 0.25 g up to 1.0 g protein/kg body weight using dairy quality protein (e.g., cottage cheese, cheddar cheese, yogurt, scrambled eggs); incrementally adjust observing over 5–7 day intervals (see Hepatic Encephalopathy).
• Cats—as tolerated, additional white meat chicken may be used.
• Avoid organ meats, fish, and red meat as protein sources.
• Asymptomatic or minimally symptomatic animals can survive well with dietary and medical interventions.

CLIENT EDUCATION

• Explain therapeutic options: medical vs. surgical and risks of each managerial strategy.
• Surgical ligation—has potential to cure; expect improvement in all symptomatic dogs that tolerate some degree of shunt attenuation.
• Postoperative clinical signs—may persist despite PSVA attenuation requiring chronic nutritional and medical management; some dogs can have medical and dietary interventions withdrawn.
• Clinical improvement may occur after surgical ligation despite persistent high TSBA values.
• Surgical/anesthetic risks—influenced by surgeon skill and experience, hospital, supportive critical care, type of PSVA, and histologic liver features.
• Monitoring protein C—can document improved portal perfusion in dogs with sustained high TSBA values; protein C activity will increase and may normalize with successful surgery (if low preoperatively); retest 2–6 months after surgery. This test is useful in cats for this purpose.
• If surgery not pursued or ligation not tolerated: remain vigilant for ammonium biurate obstructive uropathy; urethral obstruction (males) may require permanent urethrostomy.

SURGICAL CONSIDERATIONS

• HE—should be mitigated with medical management before anesthesia and surgery.
• ICU monitoring—recommended postoperatively for 72–96 hours.
• Surgical PSVA ligation—optimal goal of complete ligation; may not be tolerated leading to APSS. APSS may develop with any method of shunt attenuation: direct silk ligation, ameroid device, cellophane banding, or IV coiling (I-PSVA).
• Partial PSVA ligation—improves patient health in most cases.
• Degree of tolerated PSVA closure judged at surgery—physiologic responses to temporary shunt occlusion but intraoperative assessments can still be inaccurate or misleading.
• Intraoperative portography advised—verifies correct PSVA identification and evaluates immediate change in hepatic portal perfusion as a real-time assessment.
• Ameroid constrictor, cellophane banding, IV coiling—gradual PSVA attenuation, reduce immediate postoperative surgical risk; *caution*: may later result in APSS in some patients, degree of PSVA attenuation is unknown with these methods without follow-up vascular imaging.
• Intrahepatic PSVA—more difficult to ligate than E-PSVA; right-sided I-PSVA most difficult, left-sided I-PSVA consistent with

PORTOSYSTEMIC VASCULAR ANOMALY, CONGENITAL (CONTINUED)

patent DV easiest; IV coiling an alternative method but may require multiple procedures for optimal response, is expensive, requires interventional training.
- Ammonium biurate urolith removal—bladder stones most common, ensure urethra is free of uroliths by retrograde catheterization/flushing.
- Occasional male dog may require permanent urethrostomy.

Postoperative Complications

- Prolonged postoperative recovery—small patients developing intraoperative hypothermia.
- Acute severe PH—may reflect intolerance to PSVA ligation, flipping of ameroid constrictor, portal vein thrombi; mesenteric ischemia characterized by acute enteric hemorrhage, abdominal pain, tachycardia, hyper- or hypothermia, pancreatitis, endotoxemia, sepsis, acute renal failure and hypovolemic shock.
- Seizures—usually develop within 96 hours of PSVA ligation; risk factors remain unclarified with no demonstrated association with presence or absence of preoperative seizures, type of PSVA, method or degree of shunt attenuation, or patient age. Postoperative seizure prevalence—recent large multihospital study of dogs with seizures within 7 days of surgery: 6.7% of 524 dogs without preoperative levetiracetam treatment and 8.3–11.2% of 416 dogs receiving different pre- and postoperative levetiracetam protocols. One study implicates greater risk for pugs. Postoperative seizures reported in ~22% of cats undergoing PSVA ligation.
- Management of postligation seizures—often unsuccessful with persistent neurologic deficits in survivors, especially cats. Treatment remains anecdotal and requires consideration of cerebral edema if protracted seizure activity and intensive supportive care; successful management protocols (dogs and cats) include: IM phenobarbital (4–6 mg/kg IM q12h) combined with propofol CRI (0.3–0.6 mg/kg/minute titrated to achieve heavy sedation to drug-induced coma), and in one dog additional medetomidine (CRI (0.016 μg/kg/min). Initial treatment with IV levetiracetam has variable short-term response; flumazenil has no effect. Follow-up at-home treatments with phenobarbital, KBr, and/or levetiracetam have been successfully used.
- Abdominal effusion—typically transient after shunt ligation resolving within 7 days; alone, does not indicate intolerable PSVA attenuation; serious PH indicated by signs of mesenteric ischemia; monitor girth and body weight postoperatively to evaluate effusion.
- Administration of hetastarch can increase perioperative bleeding.
- Blood component therapy containing acid citrate dextrose may provoke hypocalcemia and coagulopathy (hypercitratemia) in patients <5 kg.
- Emergency surgery—rarely required for ligature removal after PSVA attenuation; ameroid constrictors difficult to impossible to remove; IV coils nonretrievable.

MEDICATIONS

DRUG(S) OF CHOICE

See Hepatic Encephalopathy and previous description of postoperative seizure management.

PRECAUTIONS

Remain aware of altered drug metabolism related to reduced first-pass extraction, altered hepatic metabolism/biotransformation.

FOLLOW-UP

PATIENT MONITORING

- Reevaluate—at-home behavior, cognitive function, water consumption, body condition, weight, girth circumference; CBC for resolution of microcytosis, biochemistry for normalization of cholesterol, BUN, creatinine, urinalysis for resolution of ammonium biurate crystalluria.
- TSBA (small-breed dogs)—persistent high values do not substantiate surgical failure because of common coexistent MVD.
- If low preoperative protein C (<70%), reevaluate 2–4 months after surgery as evidence of improved liver perfusion—values will improve or normalize.

POSSIBLE COMPLICATIONS

See Surgical Considerations.

PREVENTION/AVOIDANCE

Multiple APSS—should be detected preoperatively by US imaging; if identified these indicate need for liver biopsy, contraindicate shunt ligation, and implicate severe portal atresia or another underlying disorder causing PH; PSVA is not associated with PH and APSS.

EXPECTED COURSE AND PROGNOSIS

- Cannot predict individual response to surgery but asymptomatic dogs with preoperative normal protein C activity have the best prognosis for curative ligation.
- Dogs—ligation improves signs in ~80% symptomatic patients.
- Cats—increased risk for development of APSS with full ligation.
- Post-surgery—continue HE management (especially diet) until reevaluation and observations confirm improvements.
- Some patients—require indefinite nutritional and medical support after surgical ligation.
- Partial ligation—may result achieve full shunt attenuation by granulation response to ligature.
- Ameroid constrictor—may result in full ligation within hours or a few days, may cause APSS; rare erosion of portal vein causes catastrophic hemorrhage.
- Cellophane banding—some procedures fail because wrong type of cellophane used.
- Increased risk for poor surgical outcome—small dogs with zone 3 lipogranulomas shrouding hepatic venules; cats generally have less predictable surgical outcome compared to dogs.
- Despite initial good response, recrudescent shunting may develop 3 years post ligation.
- Asymptomatic nonligated PSVA dogs can have normal life expectancy with optimized medical management.

MISCELLANEOUS

ASSOCIATED CONDITIONS

- Ammonium urate urolithiasis.
- Copper-colored iris (cats).
- Cryptorchidism (dogs).
- Hepatic encephalopathy.

AGE-RELATED FACTORS

- Surgical outcome may be good in young and old patients, especially those with minimal signs of HE (asymptomatic).
- Dogs with PSVA identified at older ages are usually asymptomatic for HE and may have easily attenuated shunts (portoazygous, splenophrenic, or gastrophrenic).

PREGNANCY/FERTILITY/BREEDING

- Asymptomatic bitches can carry viable litters to term.
- Asymptomatic dogs have been naively used for stud.
- Breeding PSVA dogs not advised (genetic disorder, especially small-breed dogs).

SYNONYMS

Portacaval shunt.

SEE ALSO

- Ductal Plate Malformation (Congenital Hepatic Fibrosis).
- Hepatic Encephalopathy.
- Hepatoportal Microvascular Dysplasia.
- Hypertension, Portal.
- Portosystemic Shunting, Acquired.

ABBREVIATIONS

- APSS = acquired portosystemic shunt.
- CRS = colorectal scintigraphy.
- DV = ductus venosus.
- E-PSVA = extrahepatic PSVA.
- HE = hepatic encephalopathy.
- I-PSVA = intrahepatic PSVA.
- MVD = microvascular dysplasia.
- NCPH= noncirrhotic portal hypertension.

- PH = portal hypertension.
- PSS = portosystemic shunting.
- PSVA = portosystemic vascular anomaly.
- PU/PD = polyuria/polydipsia.
- SPS = splenoportal scintigraphy.
- TSBA = total serum bile acids.

Suggested Reading

Heidenreich DC, Giordano P, Kirby BM. Successful treatment of refractory seizures with phenobarbital, propofol, and medetomidine following congenital portosystemic shunt ligation in a dog. J Vet Emerg Crit Care (San Antonio) 2016, 26:831–836.

Lipsomb VJ, Jones HJ, Brockman DJ. Complications and long-term outcomes of the ligation of congenital portosystemic shunts in 49 cats. Vet Rec 2007, 160:465–470.

Fukushima K, Kanemoto H, Ohno K, et al. Computed tomographic morphology and clinical features of extrahepatic portosystemic shunts in 172 dogs in Japan. Vet J 2014, 199:376–381.

Mehl ML, Kyles AE, Hardie EM, et al. Evaluation of ameroid ring constrictors for treatment for single extrahepatic portosystemic shunts in dogs: 168 cases (1995–2001). J Am Vet Med Assoc 2005, 226:2020–2030.

Mullins RA, Sanchez Villamil C, de Rooster H, et al. Effect of prophylactic treatment with levetiracetam on the incidence of postattenuation seizures in dogs undergoing surgical management of single congenital extrahepatic portosystemic shunts. Vet Surg. 2019, 48:164–172.

Weisse C, Berent AC, Todd K, et al. Endovascular evaluation and treatment of intrahepatic portosystemic shunts in dogs: 100 cases (2001–2011). J Am Vet Med Assoc 2014, 244:78–94.

Author Sharon A. Center

Consulting Editor Kate Holan

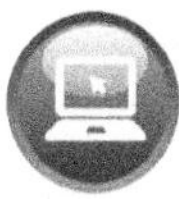

Client Education Handout available online

POXVIRUS INFECTION—CATS

BASICS

OVERVIEW

- Member of the genus *Orthopoxvirus*, family Poxviridae.
- Enveloped, double-stranded DNA virus, resistant to drying (viable for years) but readily inactivated by most disinfectants.
- Geographically limited to Eurasia.
- Relatively common.
- Serologic evidence of infection may approach 10% in cats in western Europe.

SIGNALMENT

- Cats—domestic and exotic.
- No age, sex, or breed predisposition.

SIGNS

- Skin lesions—multiple, circular; dominant feature; usually develop on head, neck, or forelimbs.
- Primary lesions—crusted papules, plaques, nodules, crateriform ulcers, or areas of cellulitis or abscesses.
- Secondary lesions—erythematous nodules that ulcerate and crust; often widespread; develop after 1–3 weeks.
- Oral lesions—erosions, ulcers either concurrently or alone (20% of cases).
- Pruritus variable.
- Systemic—20% of cases; anorexia, lethargy, pyrexia, vomiting, diarrhea, oculonasal discharge, conjunctivitis, pneumonia.

CAUSES & RISK FACTORS

- Reservoir host—wild rodents (voles, mice, gerbils, ground squirrels).
- Infection in cat thought to be acquired during hunting and being wounded by infected rodents; most common in young adults and active hunters, often from rural environment.
- Lesions—often develop at the site of a bite wound (presumably inflicted by the prey animal carrying the virus).
- Most cases occur between August and October, when small wild mammals are at maximum population and most active.
- Severe cutaneous and systemic signs with poor prognosis are frequently associated with immunosuppression (iatrogenic or coinfection with feline leukemia virus or feline immunodeficiency virus).
- Cat-to-cat transmission—rare; causes only subclinical infection.

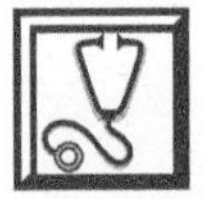

DIAGNOSIS

DIFFERENTIAL DIAGNOSIS

- Bacterial and fungal infections.
- Eosinophilic granuloma complex.
- Neoplasia—particularly mast cell tumor; lymphoma.
- Miliary dermatitis.

CBC/BIOCHEMISTRY/URINALYSIS

Noncontributory.

OTHER LABORATORY TESTS

Serologic testing—demonstrate rising titers; hemagglutination inhibition, virus neutralizing, complement fixation, or ELISA; titers may remain high for months or years.

DIAGNOSTIC PROCEDURES

- Virus isolation from scab material—definitive diagnosis; 90% positive.
- Electron microscopy of extracts of scab, biopsy, or exudate—rapid presumptive diagnosis; 70% positive.
- Skin biopsy—characteristic histologic changes of epidermal hyperplasia and hypertrophy, multilocular vesicle and ulceration, large eosinophilic intracytoplasmic inclusion bodies, immunofluorescence tests.
- PCR.
- Serologic assays: immunofluorescent antibody, ELISA, and virus neutralization assays.

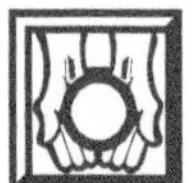

TREATMENT

- No specific treatment.
- Clean and treat ulcerated areas to prevent secondary infection.
- Supportive (antibiotics, fluids) when necessary.
- Elizabethan collar—to prevent self-induced damage.

MEDICATIONS

DRUG(S) OF CHOICE

Antibiotics—prevent secondary infections.

CONTRAINDICATIONS/POSSIBLE INTERACTIONS

Immunosuppressive agents (e.g., glucocorticoids, megestrol acetate)—absolutely contraindicated because they can induce fatal systemic disease.

FOLLOW-UP

PREVENTION/AVOIDANCE

- Natural reservoir hosts are probably small rodents, with cats infected incidentally; therefore, housing cats indoors should help prevent infection in cats.
- Vaccines—none available; vaccinia virus may be considered for valuable zoo collections, but its effects in nondomestic cats have not been investigated.

EXPECTED COURSE AND PROGNOSIS

- Most cats recover spontaneously in 1–2 months.
- Healing may be delayed by secondary bacterial skin infection.
- Prognosis is poor with severe respiratory or pulmonary involvement.

MISCELLANEOUS

ZOONOTIC POTENTIAL

- Rare human poxvirus infections have been linked to contact with infected cats with skin lesions; use basic hygiene precautions (disposable gloves) when handling infected cats.
- Infection is usually mild and transient in healthy humans, but severe and even lethal infections can occur in immunocompromised individuals.
- May cause painful skin lesions and severe systemic illness, particularly in the very young or elderly, people with a preexisting skin condition, and the immunodeficient.
- With discontinuation of vaccination against smallpox (with its cross-reactive immune effect) may expect increase in human poxvirus infections.
- Virus is hardy, can survive in scabs for weeks to months in environment where it can be source for human infection.

INTERNET RESOURCES

www.abcdcatsvets.org/cowpox-virus-infection

Suggested Reading

Bennett M. Feline poxvirus infections. In: Sykes JE, ed. Canine and Feline Infectious Diseases. St. Louis, MO: Elsevier, 2014, pp. 252–255.

Breheny CR, Fox V, Tamborini A, et al. Novel characteristics identified in two cases of feline cowpox virus infection. JFMS Open Rep 2017, 3:1–5.

Author J. Paul Woods

Consulting Editor Amie Koenig

P

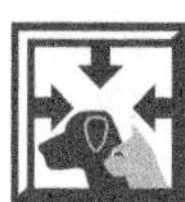

BASICS

DEFINITION

- Edema associated with pregnancy varies from mild to severe pitting edema of the distal pelvic limbs, the ventral abdomen, mammary glands, and perineal subcutaneous tissues; sometimes accompanied with an increase in intrauterine amniotic/allantoic fluid accumulation.
- Abnormal fluid accumulation in the fetus/neonate, hydrops fetalis, is a separate disorder, and not a comorbidity.
- Edema in canine pregnancy has been referred to as "hydrops" by breeders; there is no evidence that the condition is comparable to hydrops in humans. The pathophysiology of the pregnancy edema syndrome in the dog has not yet been established. Hydrops allantois and hydrops amnii have been reported in mares and cows.

PATHOPHYSIOLOGY

- Edema can occur secondary to venous/lymphatic compression from an enlarged, gravid uterus.
- In humans, pregnancy edema can be normal (80%), or can be associated with preeclampsia, pregnancy toxemia, and eclampsia (proteinuric hypertension); a placental trigger is suspected (immunologic).
- During normal pregnancy total body water increases both extracellularly and interstitially. There is also cumulative retention of sodium distributed between the maternal extracellular compartments and the fetus. Changes in factors governing renal sodium and water handling accompany alterations in local Starling forces whereby there is a moderate fall in interstitial fluid colloid osmotic pressure and a rise in capillary hydrostatic pressure, as well as changes in hydration of connective tissue.

SYSTEMS AFFECTED

- Cardiovascular.
- Endocrine/metabolic.
- Hemic/lymphatic/immune.
- Hepatobiliary.
- Musculoskeletal.
- Renal/urologic.
- Reproductive.

GENETICS

Heritability unknown, breed tendencies (see Signalment) support DNA sampling in confirmed cases for future genetic evaluation.

INCIDENCE/PREVALENCE

Uncommon

GEOGRAPHIC DISTRIBUTION

N/A

SIGNALMENT

Pregnancy edema occurs most commonly in bitches with very large litters in mid to late gestation. Many breeds have been affected, most commonly reported are golden retrievers, Labrador retrievers, pugs, Doberman pinschers, English bulldogs and French bulldogs, and bullmastiffs.

SIGNS

- Swelling/pitting edema of pelvic limbs, paws, mammary glands, perineum, ventrum, vulva.
- Marked abdominomegaly.
- Marked and sudden weight gain.
- Variable anorexia, nausea and lethargy; sometimes hemorrhagic gastroenterocolitis.
- Possible systemic hypertension.
- Possible increased allantoic/amniotic fluid volume.
- Possible ascites.

CAUSES

N/A

RISK FACTORS

- Large litter (10–12+).
- Occurs variably with previous/subsequent pregnancies.

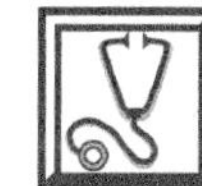

DIAGNOSIS

DIFFERENTIAL DIAGNOSIS

- Uteromegaly—closed pyometra, pregnancy.
- Edema—cardiogenic, secondary to electrolyte abnormalities, hypoalbuminemia, vasculitis, protein losing nephropathy or enteropathy, thrombosis, or hepatopathy.
- Abdominomegaly—ascites, hepato/splenomegaly, ruptured uterus, uterine torsion.
- Hypertension—primary, secondary to renal disease, endocrine disease.

CBC/BIOCHEMISTRY/URINALYSIS

- May be normal; anticipated anemia of pregnancy, stress leukogram, possible electrolyte abnormalities (e.g., hyponatremia, hyperkalemia, hypomagnesemia). Proteinuria possible.
- Hypomagnesemia is associated with preeclampsia in women.

OTHER LABORATORY TESTS

- Consider urine electrolyte evaluation if electrolyte abnormalities exist.
- Urine protein creatinine ratio if proteinuric.
- Adrenocorticotropic hormone stimulation test can identify hypo- or hyperadrenocorticism.

IMAGING

- Abdominal ultrasound with attention to fetal viability, and intra-abdominal, intrauterine, placental, allantoic and amniotic fluid volumes.
- Echocardiography for evaluation of dam for cardiac disorders.

DIAGNOSTIC PROCEDURES

- Blood pressure measurement, serial if hypertensive.
- Tocodynamometry to assess myometrial activity/irritability.
- Fetal heart rate determinations with Doppler or ultrasound to determine fetal wellbeing.

PATHOLOGIC FINDINGS

- Poorly characterized; collection of deceased fetuses, placentae encouraged for histopathologic evaluation.
- Consider uterine/placental biopsy during cesarean section.
- Complete necropsy with histopathology desirable in the event of maternal death to elucidate the cause.

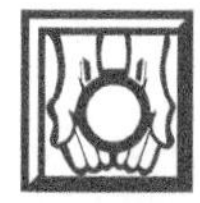

TREATMENT

APPROPRIATE HEALTH CARE

- Address life-threatening conditions (malignant hypertension, hypomagnesemia) first, then secondary conditions (edema, nausea).
- Medical pregnancy termination not advised due to the fragile condition of the bitch and likely myometrial hypocontractility.

NURSING CARE

Mild distal limb edema can benefit from mild walking, hydrotherapy, or massage. Elevating the limbs and avoiding further compression of the caudal abdominal veins/lymphatics can help disseminate edema.

ACTIVITY

Appropriate but not excessive restriction.

DIET

- Mild sodium restriction if advanced heart disease is present.
- Appropriate-for-pregnancy dietary protein, especially if hypoalbuminemia or significant proteinuria present.

CLIENT EDUCATION

Anticipate the likely need for cesarean section due to litter size, uterine wall distension, and vulvar edema contributing to an obstructive dystocia.

SURGICAL CONSIDERATIONS

Elective cesarean section at term, or pregnancy termination via ovariohysterectomy should be considered in cases of severe edema.

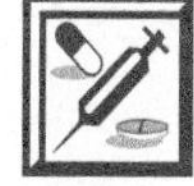

MEDICATIONS

DRUG(S) OF CHOICE

- Hypertension—hydralazine 0.5–2 mg/kg PO q12h, titrate up to effect; or 0.2 mg/kg IM; repeat q2h as needed; monitor for hypotension, hospitalize until normotensive. Continue blood pressure monitoring until normotension is maintained.
- Hypomagnesemia and related signs—magnesium sulfate 0.7–1 mEq/kg/ day IV CRI; 0.25 mEq/kg slow IV bolus (loading dose); reduce 50% if patient is azotemic.

PREGNANCY EDEMA IN THE BITCH (CONTINUED)

• Edema—medical treatment of edematous conditions in pregnancy in the bitch is controversial and without evidence-based data. In human medicine, diuretics are *not* advised to treat physiologic edema of pregnancy and do not prevent preeclampsia.
• Nausea/anorexia—metoclopramide (0.1–0.2 mg/kg SC or PO q12h, ondansetron [FDA pregnancy category B; 0.5–1 mg/kg PO q8–12h], maropitant [1 mg/kg SC or 2 mg/kg PO q 24h × 5d.] Note: safe use of maropitant in pregnant dogs has not been evaluated.)

CONTRAINDICATIONS

Furosemide can cause a significant decrease in placental intervillous blood flow. Diuretics are contraindicated with contracted IV volume. Caution must be exercised if diuretic therapy is implemented.

PRECAUTIONS

• Any drug used is likely to cross the placenta; fetal effects should be considered and informed consent acquired.
• The use of diuretics can exacerbate hypertension by promoting dehydration, and at this time, use of diuretics cannot be routinely recommended unless studies demonstrate benefit to the dam/fetuses (beyond anecdotal reports).
• In humans, the role of diuretics in obstetric practice is restricted to the management of pulmonary edema in preeclampsia.

POSSIBLE INTERACTIONS

N/A

ALTERNATIVE DRUGS

Anecdotal use of the aldosterone antagonist spironolactone (1–2 mg/kg PO q12h) or furosemide (1–2 mg/kg PO q12h) has occurred in veterinary practice. The effects of these drugs on the fetuses are unknown (spironolactone is an antiandrogen and can feminize male rats) and their use is not recommended.

FOLLOW-UP

POSSIBLE COMPLICATIONS

• Dystocia secondary to uterine inertia related to stretching of the uterine wall.
• Fetal and maternal mortality.

EXPECTED COURSE AND PROGNOSIS

Fair to guarded prognosis.

MISCELLANEOUS

ASSOCIATED CONDITIONS

N/A

AGE-RELATED FACTORS

N/A

ZOONOTIC POTENTIAL

N/A

PREGNANCY/FERTILITY/BREEDING

• Consider pedigree evaluation. If an increased incidence occurs in related bitches, removal from the breeding program should be strongly considered.
• Research litter size associated with various stud dogs/brood bitches; select away from large litter size (>8).

SYNONYMS

None, as they syndrome is not well defined; hydrops (allantois, amnion) has been suggested but not documented to be the equivalent disease in humans and dogs.

SEE ALSO

• Dystocia.
• Hypertension, Portal.
• Hypertension, Pulmonary.
• Hypertension, Systemic Arterial.

Suggested Reading

Davidson AP. Clinical approach to abnormal pregnancy. In: England G, ed., BSAVA Manual of Canine and Feline Reproduction, 13-1. Quedgeley, Glos: BSAVA, 2012.

Davidson AP. Clinical conditions in the bitch and queen. In: Nelson R, Couto C, ed., Small Animal Internal Medicine, 6th ed. St. Louis, MO: Elsevier, 2019, pp. 953–990.

Davison JM. Edema in pregnancy. Kidney Int Supp 1997, 59:90–96.

Root Kustritz, M. Pregnancy diagnosis and abnormalities in the pregnant dog. Theriogenology 2005, 64:755–765.

Weiner CP, Buhimschi C. Drugs for Pregnant and Lactating Women. Philadelphia, PA: Churchill Livingstone, 2004.

Author Autumn P. Davidson
Consulting Editor Erin E. Runcan

PREGNANCY TOXEMIA

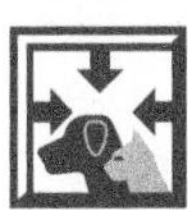

BASICS

OVERVIEW

Pregnancy toxemia is a rare condition in the bitch associated with an insufficient supply of carbohydrates to meet the increased energy demands of the late-gestational fetus. Sustained anorexia or carbohydrate-deficient diets result in a relative hypoglycemia and a negative energy balance. Prolonged negative energy balance causes hepatic lipolysis and the production of ketone bodies. Hypoglycemia and ketonemia are seen in bitches with pregnancy toxemia.

SYSTEMS AFFECTED

- Endocrine/metabolic.
- Gastrointestinal.
- Hepatobiliary.
- Nervous.
- Neuromuscular.
- Renal/urologic.
- Reproductive.

SIGNALMENT

Pregnant bitches, of any breed, typically late in gestation.

SIGNS

- Anorexia.
- Lethargy/malaise.
- Ataxia.
- Weakness.
- Collapse.
- Seizure.
- Coma.

CAUSES & RISK FACTORS

- Pregnancy.
- Large litters.
- Any event inciting sustained anorexia.
- Carbohydrate-deficient diets.

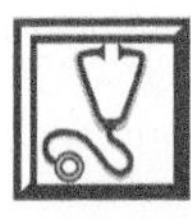

DIAGNOSIS

DIFFERENTIAL DIAGNOSIS

- Puerperal tetany (hypocalcemia).
- Gestational diabetes.
- Sepsis/septic shock.

CBC/CHEMISTRY/URINALYSIS

- Ketonuria (no glucosuria) or ketonemia.
- Hypoglycemia.
- Elevations in hepatocellular enzyme activities.

OTHER LABORATORY TESTS

Venous blood gas analysis: metabolic acidosis.

IMAGING

Abdominal ultrasonography of the bitch to assess fetal viability and fetal stability. Fetal stress is associated with fetal heart rate <160.

DIAGNOSTIC PROCEDURES

N/A

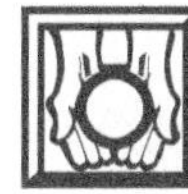

TREATMENT

- Mildly affected (alert and appetent)—may resolve with appropriate carbohydrate intake; feed an energy-dense diet ad libitum.
- Moderately affected (clinically ill)—dextrose IV (0.5 g/kg IV bolus, may also be added to isotonic crystalloid fluids to a total concentration of 2.5% or 5% dextrose, and administer as constant IV infusion); tailor therapy to maintain euglycemia and prevent swings in blood glucose; taper treatment slowly as patient oral intake increases.
- Severely affected (nonresponsive to above therapy)—termination of pregnancy or cesarean section.

MEDICATIONS

Supportive care.

CONTRAINDICATIONS/POSSIBLE INTERACTIONS

Concurrent hepatic lipidosis may decrease hepatic metabolism of certain drugs. Choose analgesics and anesthetics with caution.

FOLLOW-UP

PATIENT MONITORING

- Serial blood glucose concentration monitoring (q2–4h); adjust therapy as necessary.
- Serial urine or serum ketone measurements.
- Response to treatment (increased carbohydrate intake, euglycemia, and resolving ketonuria).

PREVENTION/AVOIDANCE

Feeding an energy-dense diet during pregnancy.

POSSIBLE COMPLICATIONS

Fetal mortality.

EXPECTED COURSE AND PROGNOSIS

Prognostic outcome depends on severity and response to treatment. If clinical signs are mild, the prognosis is good for dam and pups. Increased carbohydrate intake, alert mentation, and resolving ketonuria are good prognostic indicators in the dam. However, prolonged negative energy balance and ketonuria increase chances of fetal mortality. In severe cases pregnancy toxemia can be life-threatening for the dam and pups.

MISCELLANEOUS

ASSOCIATED CONDITIONS

Hypocalcemia

AGE-RELATED FACTORS

N/A

ZOONOTIC POTENTIAL

N/A

PREGNANCY/FERTILITY/BREEDING

- Incidence of recurrence, effects on fertility, and heritability not investigated.
- If underlying cause of pregnancy toxemia is identified and correctable (i.e., poor nutrition), bitch could theoretically be used for breeding in the future.

SEE ALSO

Hypocalcemia

Suggested Reading

Johnson CA. Glucose homeostasis during canine pregnancy: insulin resistance, ketosis, and hypoglycemia. Theriogenology 2008, 70:1418–1423.

Johnston SD, Root Kustritz MV, Olson PN. Canine pregnancy. In: Canine and Feline Theriogenology. Philadelphia, PA: W.B. Saunders, 2001, pp. 66–104.

Authors Samantha B. Souther and Victor J. Stora

Consulting Editor Erin E. Runcan

PREMATURE LABOR

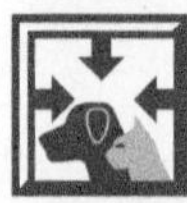

BASICS

OVERVIEW

Inappropriate myometrial activity preterm, which can lead to loss of pregnancy.

SIGNALMENT

Gravid female dog or cat; no age or breed predilection.

SIGNS

- Early—often no signs, fetal resorption evident ultrasonographically.
- Late—vulvar discharge: hemorrhagic or lochia, abortion.
- History of unexplained loss of pregnancy.

CAUSES & RISK FACTORS

- Often idiopathic; genetics can play a role. Secondary luteolysis results without intervention.
- Myometrial activity inappropriate for stage of pregnancy precedes luteolysis.
- Primary luteal insufficiency has not been documented.

P

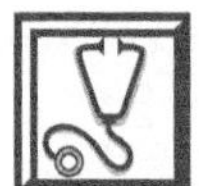

DIAGNOSIS

DIFFERENTIAL DIAGNOSIS

- Term gestation, onset of normal labor.
- Pathologic loss of pregnancy (see Miscellaneous).

CBC/BIOCHEMISTRY/URINALYSIS

- Usually normal.
- Anemia of pregnancy can be present, and rarely signs of hemorrhage.
- Inflammatory leukogram possible.

OTHER LABORATORY TESTS

Serum progesterone: will be <2 ng/mL when resorption/abortion occurs.

IMAGING

- Ultrasonographic evaluation of fetal heart rate (stress evidenced by heart rates consistently <170 bpm).
- Abnormal morphologic appearance of fetuses in uterus following death (see Web Figures 1 and 2).

DIAGNOSTIC PROCEDURES

- Tocodynamometry is diagnostic—finding >0–2 contractions/hour is not normal for preterm (earlier than 8th week) gestation.
- Progesterone measurement with a quantitative (chemiluminescence, fluorescence enzyme immunoassay) progesterone assay or accurate in house equipment should be performed to detect levels <2.0 ng/mL.

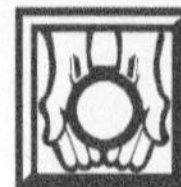

TREATMENT

- In humans, bed and pelvic rest and antibiotics do not contribute to a positive outcome, although frequently prescribed.
- Tocolytic agents are advised in veterinary cases (beta-agonists, calcium channel blockers, magnesium sulfate, prostaglandin synthetase inhibitors).

MEDICATIONS

DRUG(S) OF CHOICE

- Tocolytics (terbutaline 0.03 mg/kg PO q6–12h PRN); the dose is titrated based on uterine monitoring.
- Progestogens compounds—progesterone in oil (2 mg/kg IM q72h); altrenogest (Regu-Mate), a synthetic progestogen (0.088 mg/kg PO q24h); oral progesterone (Prometrium®; 10 mg/kg PO q24h) with monitoring of serum progesterone q24–48h for dosage adjustments. Clients should be informed of probable side effects with exogenous progesterone; it should only be used if the serum progesterone is <2 ng/mL and tocolytics have failed.
- Systemic antibiotics are rarely indicated.

CONTRAINDICATIONS/POSSIBLE INTERACTIONS

- Prolonged gestation if terbutaline or progestogen compounds are not withdrawn 24–48 hours before due date calculated from first progesterone rise, luteinizing hormone peak, or day 1 cytologic diestrus (see Breeding, Timing) if natural whelping is planned. Many successfully managed cases have ineffective labor despite drug discontinuation. If elective cesarean section is planned, medications can be continued until day of surgery.
- Poor lactation if progestogen compounds are used (inhibits normal prolactin elevation resulting from declining progesterone level).
- Masculinization of female fetuses if progestogen compounds are used, resulting in infertility and genitourinary abnormalities.
- Forced retention of a pathologic pregnancy if idiopathic premature labor is misdiagnosed.

FOLLOW-UP

- Serial abdominal ultrasound and/or fetal heart rate monitoring with Doppler to evaluate fetal viability.
- Serial tocodynamometry evaluating effective tocolysis.

MISCELLANEOUS

Usually a retrospective diagnosis by exclusion of all other causes of late-term abortion (see Abortion, Spontaneous) prompting midterm proactive tocodynamometry at the next pregnancy.

INTERNET RESOURCES

http://whelpwise.com/

Suggested Reading

Davidson AP. Tocodynamometry detects preterm labor in the bitch prior to luteolysis. Top Companion Anim Med 2015, 30(1):2–4.

Johnson CA. High-risk pregnancy and hypoluteoidism in the bitch. Theriogenology 2008, 70:1424–1430.

Root Kustritz MV. Use of supplemental progesterone in management of canine pregnancy. In: Concannon PW, England G, Verstegen III J, Linde-Forsberg C, eds., Recent Advances in Small Animal Reproduction. Ithaca NY: International Veterinary Information Service, 2001.

Scott-Moncrieff JC, Nelson RW, Bill RL, et al. Serum disposition of exogenous progesterone after intramuscular administration in bitches. Am J Vet Res 1990, 51:893–895.

Wilkens L. Masculinization of female fetuses due to the use of orally given progestins. J Am Med Assoc 1960, 172(10):1028–1032.

Authors Autumn P. Davidson and Tomas W. Baker

Consulting Editor Erin E. Runcan

PROLAPSED GLAND OF THE THIRD EYELID (CHERRY EYE)

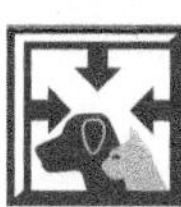

BASICS

OVERVIEW

• Definition—prolapsed gland of the third eyelid.
• Pathophysiology—the gland is normally anchored by a fibrous attachment to the periorbita beneath the third eyelid. In cases of prolapse these attachments are weak, resulting in dorsal movement of the gland. Commonly occurs in dogs and rarely in cats; animals may have unilateral or bilateral prolapse.

SIGNALMENT

• Dog and cat.
• Dog—usually in young dogs (6 months to 2 years of age); common breeds: American cocker spaniel, English bulldog, beagle, bloodhound, Lhasa apso, mastiff, shih tzu, other brachycephalic breeds.
• Cat—rare; occurs in Burmese, Persians, and has been reported in domestic shorthair cats.

SIGNS

• Oval, hyperemic mass protruding from behind the leading edge of the third eyelid in the medial canthus.
• May be unilateral or bilateral.
• May see signs of epiphora, hyperemic conjunctiva, keratitis, or blepharospasm.
• Additional swelling and hyperemia of the exposed gland can result from environmental exposure leading to irritation and desiccation.

CAUSES & RISK FACTORS

• Congenital weakness of the attachment of the gland of the third eyelid.
• Inheritance unknown but considered complex and multigenic.

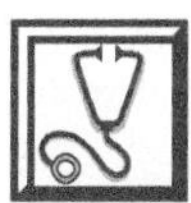

DIAGNOSIS

DIFFERENTIAL DIAGNOSIS

• Scrolled or everted cartilage of the third eyelid—seen in Weimaraner, Great Dane, German shorthaired pointer, and other breeds in which the T-shaped cartilage of the third eyelid is rolled away from the surface of the cornea instead of conforming to the surface of the cornea.
• Neoplasia of the third eyelid—usually seen in older animals. Most common third eyelid neoplasms in the dog are adenocarcinoma, adenoma, and squamous cell carcinoma. May also see lymphoma or fibrosarcoma. Most common third eyelid neoplasms in the cat are adenocarcinoma followed by squamous cell carcinoma. A small incisional biopsy is indicated to differentiate.
• Orbital fat prolapse—may dissect anteriorly between the conjunctiva and globe; occasionally occurs in the medial canthus.

CBC/BIOCHEMISTRY/URINALYSIS

N/A

OTHER LABORATORY TESTS

N/A

IMAGING

N/A

DIAGNOSTIC PROCEDURES

N/A

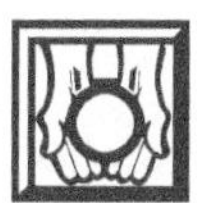

TREATMENT

• Surgical replacement of the gland (various techniques can be performed)—see Suggested Reading.
• Gland excision contraindicated; gland can produce up to 50% (or more) of the aqueous tear film; puts patient at substantial risk for developing keratoconjunctivitis sicca as the dog ages. Excision may be considered if neoplasia is confirmed, although potential complications and risks should be discussed.
• Elizabethan collar—to prevent self-trauma.

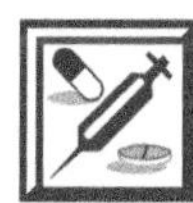

MEDICATIONS

DRUG(S) OF CHOICE

• Topical anti-inflammatory medications, such as corticosteroids (if no corneal ulceration) or nonsteroidal anti-inflammatory medications—may be used before and after surgery.
• Topical lubricating medications (ointments or gels)—may be used to reduce environmental exposure causing irritation and/or desiccation.

CONTRAINDICATIONS/POSSIBLE INTERACTIONS

N/A

FOLLOW-UP

• Recurrence—5–20%, depending on the breed, with large-breed dogs (e.g., mastiff) having the highest recurrence rates; re-replacement of the gland is encouraged.
• If unilateral, warn client that the other gland may also prolapse and that no preventive procedure or medication exists.

MISCELLANEOUS

SYNONYMS

Cherry eye.

Suggested Reading

Hendrix DVH. Diseases and surgery of the canine conjunctiva and nictitating membrane. In: Gelatt KN, Gilger BC, Kern T, eds., Veterinary Ophthalmology, 5th ed. Ames, IA: Wiley-Blackwell, 2013, pp. 945–975.

Multari D, Perazzi A, Contiero B, et al. Pocket technique or pocket technique combined with modified orbital rim anchorage for the replacement of a prolapsed gland of the third eyelid in dogs: 353 dogs. Vet Ophthalmol 2016, 19:214–219.

Peruccio C. Diseases of the third eyelid. In: Maggs DJ, Miller PE, Ofri R, Slatter's Fundamentals of Veterinary Ophthalmology, 6th Ed. St. Louis, MOL Elsevier, 2018, pp. 178–184.

Sapienza JS, Mayordomo A, Beyer AM. Suture anchor placement technique around the insertion of the ventral rectus muscle for the replacement of the prolapsed gland of the third eyelid in dogs: 100 cases. Vet Ophthalmol 2014, 17:81–86.

Stiles J. Feline ophthalmology. In: Gelatt KN, Gilger BC, Kerns T, eds., Veterinary Ophthalmology, 5th ed Ames, IA: Wiley-Blackwell, 2013, pp. 945–975.

Author Silvia G. Pryor
Consulting Editor Kathern E. Myrna
Acknowledgment The author and editors acknowledge the prior contribution of Brian C. Gilger.

PROPTOSIS

BASICS

OVERVIEW

- Forward displacement of globe, with eyelids trapped behind globe's equator (see Web Figures 1 and 2).
- Frequently acute and due to bite wounds, head trauma.
- Vision threatening.
- Immediate repositioning of globe critical.

SIGNALMENT

- More common in brachycephalic breeds (shallow orbit, large palpebral fissure).
- May occur in any species or breed with severe enough traumatic force.

SIGNS

Possible Accompanying Signs

- Subconjunctival or intraocular hemorrhage.
- Pupil dilated or constricted.
- Intraocular inflammation (uveitis).
- Globe deviation/strabismus/rupture.
- Corneal ulceration/desiccation.
- Periocular bite wounds.
- Fractures of bony orbit or skull.
- Systemic injuries.

CAUSES & RISK FACTORS

Trauma—primary cause; may be relatively minor force (e.g., restraint) in brachycephalic breeds; usually severe impact or trauma in other breeds.

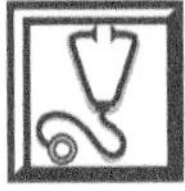

DIAGNOSIS

DIFFERENTIAL DIAGNOSIS

- Buphthalmia—globe enlargement; rarely acute.
- Exophthalmia—forward displacement of globe due to retrobulbar space-occupying lesion; may be acute, rarely peracute.

CBC/BIOCHEMISTRY/URINALYSIS

Normal, unless trauma-related abnormalities present.

IMAGING

Skull CT or radiographs—may show trauma-related fractures. Further diagnostic workup indicated if other systemic injuries.

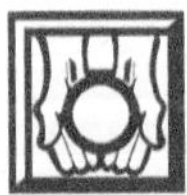

TREATMENT

- Prevent further trauma—lubricate cornea, Elizabethan collar.
- Stabilize patient and perform thorough systemic physical examination before surgery.

Repositioning the Globe

- As soon as safely possible.
- Performed under sedation and local anesthesia or general anesthesia.
- Fluorescein—stain cornea prior to replacing globe.
- Lateral canthotomy—may ease tension on eyelids and allow easier globe repositioning; not always necessary.
- Engage eyelid margins with eyelid forceps (e.g., Von Graefe or Allis forceps) or strabismus/muscle hooks, pull eyelids forward and away from globe while protecting and gently pushing globe back into orbit (e.g., with lubricated scalpel blade handle), preventing forward traction on globe and optic nerve.
- Place 2–3 temporary tarsorrhaphy mattress sutures (sutures emerge from eyelid margin in line with meibomian gland openings) with stents; suture lateral canthotomy wound.

Eye Removal

With extensive globe or periocular tissue damage (loss of shape and turgor of ruptured globe, most conjunctival and muscle attachments severed), enucleation may be best option.

MEDICATIONS

DRUG(S) OF CHOICE

- Systemic and topical broad-spectrum antibiotics—until suture removal.
- Systemic corticosteroids—use initially; may be continued if marked periorbital/retrobulbar swelling.
- Topical corticosteroids—treat uveitis or hyphema, if no corneal ulceration.
- Topical atropine—for intraocular inflammation or hemorrhage; relieve ciliary spasm and lower risk of synechiae.

CONTRAINDICATIONS/POSSIBLE INTERACTIONS

- Topical corticosteroids—do not use with corneal ulcerations.
- Systemic corticosteroids—do not use with peri- or retrobulbar infection.

FOLLOW-UP

PATIENT MONITORING

Suture removal—usually sequential, starting 10–14 days after surgery. Reassess integrity of globe and vision.

PREVENTION/AVOIDANCE

Bilateral medial and/or lateral canthoplasty to shorten palpebral fissure and prevent future proptosis in brachycephalic breeds.

POSSIBLE COMPLICATIONS

- Blindness.
- Most patients retain dorsolateral strabismus and slight forward displacement of medial side of globe due to rupture of inferior oblique and medial rectus muscles. May improve with time.
- Decreased tear production—perform Schirmer tear tests after suture removal.
- Corneal denervation causing neurotrophic keratitis with chronic ulceration, decreased corneal sensitivity.
- Exposure keratitis from forward displacement of globe, decreased tear production, facial nerve palsy and/or corneal denervation (decreased blink reflex).
- Phthisis bulbi.

EXPECTED COURSE AND PROGNOSIS

- Most affected eyes can be salvaged; if in doubt, reposition and try to salvage the globe; majority will be blind.
- Extensive tissue damage, avulsion of three or more extraocular muscles, facial and/or orbital fractures, and corneal or scleral rupture—grave prognosis for vision and globe salvage for cosmesis.
- Normal retinal vessels and optic nerve, normal intraocular pressure, and short time from occurrence to repair—relatively favorable prognosis for maintaining vision.
- Positive menace response, dazzle and/or pupillary light reflexes—good prognosis for maintaining vision (always observe indirect pupillary light reflex in healthy eye originating from injured eye!).
- Pupil size at time of injury—not an accurate prognostic indicator.

MISCELLANEOUS

SEE ALSO

Orbital Diseases (Exophthalmos, Enophthalmos, Strabismus).

Suggested Reading

Miller PE. Ophthalmic emergencies. In: Maggs DJ, Miller PE, Ofri R, eds., Slatter's Fundamentals of Veterinary Ophthalmology, 6th ed. St. Louis, MO: Saunders, 2017, pp. 432–441.

Spiess BM, Pot SA. Diseases and surgery of the canine orbit. In: Gelatt KN, Gilger BC, Kern TJ, eds., Veterinary Ophthalmology, 5th ed. Ames, IA: Wiley-Blackwell, 2013, pp. 793–831.

Author Simon A. Pot
Consulting Editor Kathern E. Myrna

PROSTATE DISEASE IN THE BREEDING MALE DOG

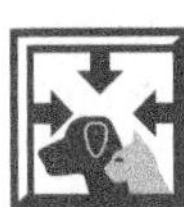

BASICS

OVERVIEW

• The prostate is the only accessory sex gland in the dog and is palpable per rectum as a bilobed oval gland with a median septum. • Dihydrotestosterone (DHT) stimulates growth of prostate gland; 5-α reductase in prostatic epithelial cells metabolizes serum testosterone to DHT.

Benign Prostatic Hyperplasia

• Commonly diagnosed in intact dogs—a result of diffuse, hormone-dependent, glandular, stromal hyperplasia and hypertrophy of prostate. • Cystic hyperplasia may occur later in disease process. • Contributing factors include age-associated changes in intraprostatic estrogen:androgen ratio, which potentiates hyperplastic response, and DHT-permissive growth of prostate. • Clinical effects minimal or absent in most dogs. • Renders prostate more susceptible to ascending infection and development of bacterial prostatitis.

Prostatitis/Prostatic Abscess

• Inflammation/infection of prostate. • Acute or chronic bacterial infection, abscess usually secondary to chronic bacterial prostatitis. • Also associated with benign prostatic hyperplasia (BPH) or retention cysts. • Bacterial colonization is typically via ascending urinary tract pathogens; hematogenous spread possible. • Common isolates include *Escherichia coli*, *Klebsiella*, *Pseudomonas*, *Pasteurella*, streptococci, and staphylococci species. • Concurrent bacterial urinary tract infection is not always noted with chronic bacterial prostatitis. • *Brucella canis* may be associated with acute or chronic prostatitis and has zoonotic potential. • Fungal prostatitis has been reported (*Blastomyces* and *Cryptococcus*).

Prostatic Cysts

• Within prostatic parenchyma, coalescing glandular/cystic hyperplasia and ductular occlusion (retention cysts) caused by estrogen effects (e.g., from Sertoli cell tumor) on prostatic epithelium. • Paraprostatic cysts are attached to prostate, lined by secretory epithelium, and variable in size; larger cysts may be transabdominally palpable; almost always sterile.

Prostatic Neoplasia

• Prostatic adenocarcinoma (ACA) is most common; other tumor types include fibrosarcoma, leiomyosarcoma, and squamous cell carcinoma (SCC). • Prostatic transitional cell carcinoma (TCC) arise from the prostatic urethra and invade the prostate gland. • BPH is not a risk factor for prostatic neoplasia. • Tumor development is androgen independent; castration is not protective. • Tumors typically detected after metastatic spread as clinical signs occur late and early screening is unavailable. • ACA bone metastasis is common, typically to spine or pelvis; intraprostatic fibrosis with some areas of ossification and hyperplasia is seen.

SIGNALMENT

• BPH—50% of intact dogs exhibit histologic evidence by 5 years of age, >95% by 9 years of age. • Prostatitis/prostatic abscess: common. • Prostatic cysts—prevalence around 14%; 42% of these had evidence of bacterial infection. • Neoplasia—prevalence 0.2–0.6% in general population, 5–7% of dogs with prostatic disease.

Mean Age and Range

• BPH—microscopic onset by 5 years of age. • Prostatitis/prostatic abscess—any age; more common in adults. • Prostatic cysts—more common after 8 years of age. • Neoplasia—mean age 10 years.

SIGNS

General Comments

• Dogs with prostatic disease display overlapping clinical signs. • Many dogs are asymptomatic. • Dyschezia, tenesmus, constipation, ribbon-like stool with advanced disease. • Sanguinous urethral/preputial discharge. • Dysuria, hematuria, stranguria. • Hemospermia.

Benign Prostatic Hyperplasia

• If mild, generally asymptomatic. • Hematuria and hemospermia are most common signs.

Prostatitis—Acute

• Systemic illness (vomiting, fever, inappetence). • Pyuria. • Stiff-legged gait.

Prostatitis—Chronic

• Recurrent/chronic urinary tract infection. • Stiff gait. • Infertility.

Prostatic Cyst

• If mild, generally asymptomatic. • If infected see signs associated with prostatitis.

Prostatic Neoplasia

• Emaciation. • Dyschezia. • Rear limb locomotory disturbance. • Lumbosacral pain.

Physical Examination Findings

Benign Prostatic Hyperplasia

Large, symmetrically enlarged, nonpainful prostate.

Prostatitis—Acute

• Fever. • Dehydration. • Sepsis/shock. • Caudal abdominal pain. • Normal to enlarged, asymmetric, painful prostate.

Prostatitis—Chronic

• Symmetric, nonpainful, firm, normal size prostate. • May have fluctuant areas (focal cysts) on palpation.

Prostatic Cyst

• Symmetric, enlarged prostate with fluctuant areas; large cysts may preclude rectal palpation, enlarged prostate may be transabdominally palpable. • External signs of feminization if cyst formation is due to estrogen exposure.

Prostatic Neoplasia

• Large, asymmetric, irregular painful prostate. • Rectal, abdominal, lumbosacral pain. • Palpable abdominal mass. • Lymphadenopathy (sublumbar).

CAUSES & RISK FACTORS

Benign Prostatic Hyperplasia

Older, intact males.

PROSTATITIS

• BPH and/or prostatic cysts. • Breeding dogs may have higher risk for *Brucella canis*.

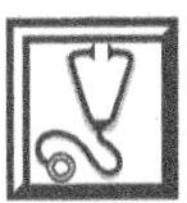

DIAGNOSIS

DIFFERENTIAL DIAGNOSIS

Hematuria

• Urinary tract infection. • Thrombocytopenia. • Trauma. • Neoplasia.

TENESMUS

Colonic or rectal disease.

Hind Limb Gait/Locomotory Disturbance

• Arthritis. • Degenerative disc disease. • Neuromuscular disease.

CBC/BIOCHEMISTRY/URINALYSIS

Benign Prostatic Hyperplasia

Typically normal, except hematuria.

Prostatitis—Acute

• Leukocytosis and neutrophilia (± immaturity and signs of toxicity). • Pyuria. • Bacteriuria. • Hematuria.

Prostatitis—Chronic

• Occasionally leukocytosis. • Pyuria. • Bacteriuria. • Hematuria.

Prostatic Cyst

• Anemia (if hyperestrogenism present). • Biochemistry and urinalysis typically normal.

Prostatic Neoplasia

• Leukocytosis and neutrophilia. • Elevated alkaline phosphatase. • Pyuria. • Hematuria. • Atypical cells may be noted in urine sediment.

OTHER LABORATORY TESTS

• Prostatic fluid culture—culture third ejaculate fraction or fine-needle aspirate of prostate; positive growth supports bacterial prostatitis. • Paired seminal fluid and urethral culture—prostatitis is confirmed when seminal fluid bacterial growth (in colony-forming units) is ≥100 times corresponding urethral/urine growth. • Semen evaluation—may be normal or hemospermic with BPH; neutrophils, phagocytized bacteria, variable degree of

P

PROSTATE DISEASE IN THE BREEDING MALE DOG (CONTINUED)

reduced sperm motility and teratospermia with bacterial prostatitis. • Prostate-specific antigen/canine prostatic-specific esterase are not of clinical use in dogs. • Positive urine screening for cells with *BRAF* gene mutations (CADET™ *BRAF*) is highly sensitive and specific for the presence of prostatic urethral TCC.

IMAGING

• Abdominal ultrasound—detects size, homogeneity of prostate. Identifies focal parenchymal abnormalities (cysts or abscesses); loss of tissue homogeneity (prostatitis or neoplasia); regional lymph nodes and paraprostatic structures (paraprostatic cysts). • Abdominal radiography—bony metastases; degree of prostatomegaly. • Lack of prostatic mineralization in intact dogs with prostatomegaly has a negative predictive value of 96% for neoplasia. • Retrograde cystourethrogram—evaluates urethral compression, identifies contrast leakage.

P

DIAGNOSTIC PROCEDURES

• Prostatic wash to obtain culture and cytologic evaluation of prostatic fluid. • Ultrasound-guided fine-needle aspirate—cytologic evaluation may distinguish between BPH, prostatitis, and neoplasia; aspiration of active infections may seed periprostatic and subcutaneous tissues; aspiration of cysts rarely provides clinical resolution • Ultrasound-guided transabdominal biopsy—provides definitive diagnosis for BPH, prostatitis, prostatic neoplasia.

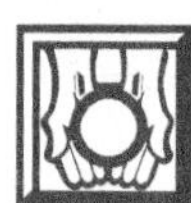

TREATMENT

• Temporary indwelling urethral catheter placement in animals with severe pain or urethral obstruction. • Analgesia. • Stool softeners and low-residue diets to ease defecation.

Benign Prostatic Hyperplasia

• Treat symptomatic dogs. • Castration is curative. • Finasteride is medical treatment of choice in breeding animals; decreases prostatic weight and diameter; prostate returns to pretreatment size 8 weeks after stopping therapy; typically used to reduce clinical signs permitting frozen semen stores to be generated; castrate when desired doses of semen are stored.

Prostatitis—Acute and Chronic

• Antimicrobials (based on culture and sensitivity) and that penetrate blood–prostate barrier (e.g., veterinary fluoroquinolone for Gram-negative organisms and clindamycin or a macrolide for Gram-positive organisms). Chloramphenicol and trimethoprim–sulfonamide are additional options. • Antimicrobials with poor penetration through an intact blood–prostate barrier should not be used. • Antimicrobials should be administered for a minimum of 4 weeks in acute cases, and up to 6 weeks for chronic cases. • Response to therapy should be monitored based on clinical signs, prostatic size and architecture, return of semen quality. Repeat cultures are not recommended unless poor initial response. • Finasteride may be considered to treat underlying prostatic pathology in dogs with future breeding intent. Castration is advised for nonbreeding animals and those that respond poorly to appropriate therapy.

Prostatic Abscess

Prostatic abscesses should be percutaneously drained with ultrasound guidance after administration of perioperative antimicrobials.

Prostatic Cyst

• Castration—treatment of choice. • Finasteride may be useful if associated with BPH. • Remove source of estrogen if squamous metaplasia. • Large solitary cysts—surgical marsupalization and castration. • Paraprostatic cysts—may be surgically excised. • Aspiration and drainage of cysts—not associated with resolution; fluid should be cultured.

Prostatic Neoplasia

• Differentiation between ACA and TCC will determine appropriate treatment (see specific chapters). • Urine culture. • A piroxicam trial should always be offered with or without chemotherapy.

Client Education

• Regular *B. canis* testing for breeding animals (minimum every 6 months). • Proactive semen freezing at young age prior to onset of prostatic disease/BPH.

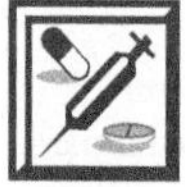

MEDICATIONS

DRUG(S) OF CHOICE

• Finasteride 0.1 mg/kg PO q24h to a maximum of 5 mg PO q24h. • Antimicrobials—drug used and duration will vary with culture results and disease process; chronic prostatitis requires lipid-soluble antibiotics to reach parenchyma (e.g., enrofloxacin 10–20 mg/kg PO q24h) for 4–6 weeks.

Precautions

• Estrogens and progestogens—decrease prostatic mass via negative feedback on serum testosterone concentrations; however, toxic side effects are common and their use is not recommended. • Nonsteroidal anti-inflammatory drugs—may be associated with hepatic and/or renal dysfunction, gastrointestinal ulceration. • Trimethoprim–sulfamethoxazole—may be associated with keratoconjunctivitis sicca, thrombocytopenia, and hepatic necrosis.

Alternative Drug(s)

Deslorelin (Suprelorin)—not approved for this use in United States; not recommended for dogs intended for breeding; dramatically suppresses hypothalamic–pituitary–gonadal axis and testosterone production.

FOLLOW-UP

PATIENT MONITORING

• Serial prostatic fluid cultures to document antimicrobial efficacy. • Semen evaluation should be performed 70 days after resolution of illness in any breeding dog. • Serial abdominal ultrasound to evaluate response to treatment. • Dogs testing positive for brucellosis should not be used for breeding.

EXPECTED COURSE AND PROGNOSIS

• BPH generally responsive to finasteride. • Chronic prostatitis more refractory to medical management; castration may be indicated. • Poor prognosis for prostatic neoplasia.

MISCELLANEOUS

ASSOCIATED CONDITIONS

• Sertoli cell tumor. • Infertility. • Recurrent urinary tract infection.

ABBREVIATIONS

- ACA = adenocarcinoma.
- BPH = benign prostatic hyperplasia.
- DHT = dihydrotestosterone.
- SCC = squamous cell carcinoma.
- TCC = transitional cell carcinoma.

Suggested Reading

Weese J, Blondeau J, Boothe D, et al. International Society for Companion Animal Infectious Diseases (ISCAID) guidelines for the diagnosis and management of bacterial urinary tract infections in dogs and cats. Vet J 2019, 247:8–25.

Author Sophie A. Grundy
Consulting Editor Erin E. Runcan

BASICS

OVERVIEW

- Prostatic cysts in dogs include those associated with diffuse epithelial cystic change from androgen-dependent benign prostatic hyperplasia (BPH), cavitating retention cysts within the prostatic parenchyma, fluid-filled lesions with a distinct capsule, and paraprostatic cysts that are cavitating, fluid-filled lesions with a distinct capsule located outside of the prostatic parenchyma. Prostatic cysts may range in diameter from a few millimeters to more than 20 cm.
- Paraprostatic cysts usually arise craniolateral to the prostate, displacing the bladder cranially and ventrally, or caudal to the prostate in the pelvis. Prostatic cysts may represent dilated embryonal remnants of the wolffian ducts.
- Pathogenesis is unknown, but the occurrence of retention cysts in dogs with estrogen-secreting Sertoli cell tumors causes speculation that these cysts are dilations of prostatic acini secondary to estrogen-induced squamous metaplasia.

SIGNALMENT

- Male intact dogs; rare occurrence in castrated dogs.
- Age range 2–12 years, mean age 8 years.
- Large dogs more commonly affected than small dogs.

SIGNS

- Asymptomatic.
- Lethargy and anorexia.
- Abdominal distention.
- Tenesmus if the cyst compresses the rectum.
- Dysuria if the cyst compresses the urethra.
- Sanguinous urethral discharge in the presence of BPH.

CAUSES & RISK FACTORS

- BPH.
- Androgenic hormones.
- Estrogenic hormones.

DIAGNOSIS

DIFFERENTIAL DIAGNOSIS

- BPH—distinguished by ultrasound.
- Prostatic abscess—distinguished by ultrasound and semen culture.
- Distended urinary bladder—distinguished by cystocentesis, imaging.
- Caudal abdominal mass of undetermined origin—distinguished by imaging.

CBC/BIOCHEMISTRY/URINALYSIS

No abnormalities.

OTHER LABORATORY TESTS

- Examination of prostatic fluid collected by ejaculation or prostatic massage confirms absence of infection.
- Culture and cytology of cyst fluid collected by ultrasound-guided fine-needle aspiration or by aspiration at surgical exploration reveals sterile clear or sanguineous fluid consistent with prostatic fluid.

IMAGING

Retrograde contrast urethrocystography followed by prostatic ultrasonography confirms presence, location, echo-texture, and size of prostatic cysts, and differentiates retention cysts from paraprostatic cysts.

DIAGNOSTIC PROCEDURES

Collection of prostatic fluid by ejaculation followed by prostatic imaging is recommended prior to fine-needle aspiration of cystic fluid to rule out bacterial infection.

PATHOLOGIC FINDINGS

Epithelial cysts within the prostatic parenchyma occur with parenchymal hypertrophy and hyperplasia; squamous metaplasia of the ducts and alveoli may be present. Retention cysts and paraprostatic cysts are lined by a single layer of prostatic epithelium or fibrous connective tissue and contain clear to sanguineous fluid with fibrin.

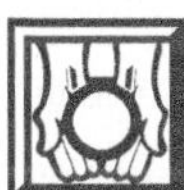

TREATMENT

- Intraprostatic cysts (epithelial, retention) respond to prostatic involution via castration or the 5α-reductase inhibitor finasteride. Large cysts may be drained percutaneously with ultrasound guidance prior to initiation of finasteride therapy.
- Large retention cysts and paraprostatic cysts should be partially or completely surgically resected, depending on adherence to surrounding structures, or marsupialized and drained for 1–2 months.
- Simple drainage of the cyst is not recommended as persistence of the capsule may result in recurrence.

MEDICATIONS

DRUG(S) OF CHOICE

Prostatic parenchyma and diffuse epithelial cysts involute following treatment with finasteride 0.1–1 mg/kg PO q 24 h, not to exceed 5 mg/dog, for 2–4 months or as long as the dog remains intact to treat BPH. Finasteride prevents conversion of testosterone to dihydrotestosterone, causing prostatic involution without adversely affecting libido or spermatogenesis. BPH recurs following cessation of finasteride therapy. Paraprostatic cysts do not respond to finasteride treatment.

CONTRAINDICATIONS/POSSIBLE INTERACTIONS

N/A

FOLLOW-UP

- Imaging assessment of cyst size at 4-week intervals following treatment.
- Standard postoperative monitoring of marsupialized stoma.

MISCELLANEOUS

ABBREVIATIONS

- BPH = benign prostatic hyperplasia.

Suggested Reading

Johnston SD, Root Kustritz MV, Olson PN. Disorders of the canine prostate. In: Canine and FelineTheriogenology. Philadelphia, PA: Saunders, 2001, pp. 337–355.

Rawlings CA, Mahaffey MB, Barsanti JA, et al. Use of partial prostatectomy for treatment of prostatic abscesses and cysts in dogs. J Am Vet Med Assoc 1997, 211:868–871.

Smith J. Canine prostatic disease: a review of anatomy, pathology, diagnosis, and treatment. Theriogenology 2008, 70:375–383.

Stowater JL, Lamb CR. Ultrasonographic features of paraprostatic cysts in nine dogs. Vet Radiol Ultrasound 1989, 30:232–239.

White RAS, Herrtage ME, Dennis R. The diagnosis and management of paraprostatic and prostatic retention cysts in the dog. J Small Anim Pract 1987, 28:551–574.

Author Bruce W. Christensen

Consulting Editor J.D. Foster

Acknowledgment The author and editors would like to acknowledge the prior contribution of Carl A. Osborne.

PROSTATITIS AND PROSTATIC ABSCESS

BASICS

DEFINITION

Acute Prostatitis

Infection of the canine prostate with bacteria, mycoplasmas, or fungi with systemic signs of fever, anorexia, lethargy, pain, and inflammatory exudate in prostatic fluid. Abscessation is variable, but occasionally rupture into the peritoneal cavity, causing sepsis, shock, and death.

Chronic Prostatitis

Subclinical infection of the canine prostate in absence of prostatic abscessation and polysystemic signs. Affected animals are asymptomatic except for inflammatory exudate in the prostatic fluid, which causes infertility. Chronic prostatitis may occur after or independently of acute prostatitis.

PATHOPHYSIOLOGY

P

- Predisposing pathology is benign prostatic hyperplasia (BPH), which occurs under the influence of dihydrotestosterone (DHT) in more than 80% of intact male dogs >5 years of age (see Benign Prostatic Hyperplasia).
- Infection of the hypertrophied canine prostate develops most commonly from ascending flora—rarely from blood-borne bacteria or from penetrating wounds. The prostate of intact dogs constantly secretes prostatic fluid, which is deposited into the prostatic urethra and then flows into the urinary bladder and out of the penile urethra. With prostatitis, prostatic fluid containing blood, inflammatory exudate, and microorganisms is deposited into the urinary bladder and discharged intermittently from the tip of the penis.

SYSTEMS AFFECTED

- Hemic/lymphatic/immune—mature or immature neutrophilia in acute prostatitis.
- Polysystemic—septic shock if prostatic abscesses rupture, fever, and focal or generalized peritonitis.
- Urinary—dysuria if the enlarged prostate compresses the urethra; deposition of prostatic fluid with inflammatory exudate into the urinary bladder.
- Reproductive—pain at copulation and reduction in libido; infertility from infected prostatic fluid in the ejaculate.

INCIDENCE/PREVALENCE

Intact male dogs >5 years of age are at highest risk, though overall incidence is low. Infection is reported in 40% of dogs with prostatic disease. Prostatitis in castrated males is exceedingly rare.

SIGNALMENT

Species

Dog

Breed Predilections

All breeds.

Mean Age and Range

Mean age range 7–11 years.

Predominant Sex

Intact male dogs; may occur secondary to prostatic neoplasia in castrated dogs.

SIGNS

Acute Prostatitis

- Lethargy/depression.
- Anorexia.
- Pyrexia.
- Pain at prostatic or caudal abdominal palpation.
- Sanguineous or purulent urethral discharge.
- Stiff hind limb gait.
- Septic shock.
- Tenesmus.
- Dysuria.

Chronic Prostatitis

- Asymptomatic.
- Sanguinous or purulent urethral discharge.
- Tenesmus.
- Dysuria.

CAUSES

- Infection of the hypertrophied prostate with ascending urethral flora (most commonly *E. coli*), anaerobic bacteria, or *Mycoplasma*.
- Infection of the hypertrophied prostate with systemic bacterial infection, including *Brucella canis*.
- Systemic or local puncture wound infection with *Blastomyces dermatitidis*.

RISK FACTORS

- Increasing age.
- Intact male.
- BPH and, less commonly, prostatic neoplasia.
- Historical androgen or estrogen administration.
- Impaired host defense mechanisms.

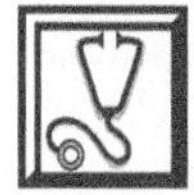

DIAGNOSIS

DIFFERENTIAL DIAGNOSIS

- BPH distinguished by prostatic cytology or semen culture.
- Prostatic cysts distinguished by ultrasound and semen culture.
- Prostatic neoplasia distinguished by ultrasound, tissue biopsy, and castrated state.
- Abdominal mass or abscess distinguished by abdominal imaging.

CBC/BIOCHEMISTRY/URINALYSIS

- CBC—include immature neutrophilia and toxic neutrophils; immature neutropenia may occur with sepsis. Most dogs with chronic prostatitis have a normal CBC.
- Serum chemistry—abnormalities are variable with acute prostatitis, normal in most chronic cases.
- Urinalysis—hematuria, pyuria, and causative microbes arise from deposition of infected prostatic fluid into the urinary bladder.

OTHER LABORATORY TESTS

- Cytology, and culture of whole semen or the prostatic fluid fraction of semen or fluid collected at prostatic massage yields inflammatory exudate with microorganisms. Normal prostatic fluid should contain <100,000 cfu/mL, and <5 leukocytes per hpf following fluid centrifugation.
- Although infection with *B. canis* is uncommon, because of the zoonotic potential of this infection, serology is recommended.

IMAGING

Survey radiography of the caudal abdomen, retrograde urethrocystography, and prostatic ultrasonography can evaluate prostatic size, echotexture, and detection of cavitating prostatic lesions.

DIAGNOSTIC PROCEDURES

- Collection and evaluation of prostatic fluid in seminal plasma or by prostatic massage.
- Ultrasound-guided percutaneous fine-needle aspirate of the prostate.

PATHOLOGIC FINDINGS

- Gross pathology of the infected prostate includes focal, multifocal, or diffuse enlargement, variable loss of symmetry of the dorsal median raphe, and variable presence of fluid-filled abscesses within or on the surface of the gland.
- Infection causes suppurative (bacterial) or granulomatous (fungal) inflammation, which may be focal, multifocal, or diffuse. Abscesses contain purulent fluid exudate.
- Biopsy of the infected prostate is not recommended because biopsy may result in the spread of infection to adjacent tissues.

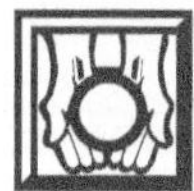

TREATMENT

APPROPRIATE HEALTH CARE

- Acute prostatitis, prostatic abscess, and rupture of prostatic abscesses into the peritoneal cavity are potentially life-threatening emergencies that can lead to septic shock and death. Hospitalize affected patients and collect diagnostic samples immediately.
- Chronic prostatitis patients may be seen as outpatients for diagnostic procedures and started on therapy when laboratory results are available.

NURSING CARE

- Dogs with acute prostatitis or prostatic abscess should receive IV antimicrobial drugs.
- If abscess rupture and peritonitis is suspected, administer therapy for septic shock.

ACTIVITY

Breeding should be avoided until bacteria have been cleared from the prostatic fluid.

CLIENT EDUCATION

- Castration is recommended for nonbreeding dogs with prostatitis and/or prostatic abscess, as castration induces permanent prostatic involution.
- If maintenance of breeding potential is desired, long-term treatment with finasteride (see Benign Prostatic Hyperplasia) is recommended to induce prostatic involution. BPH recurs over time in intact male dogs after treatment with finasteride is discontinued, and BPH increases risk of recurrence of prostatitis.

SURGICAL CONSIDERATIONS

- Surgical management of prostatic abscesses should be deferred until after initiation of antimicrobial therapy and prostatic involution; involution is associated with resolution of smaller abscesses, often making surgery unnecessary.
- Castration is recommended for induction of prostatic involution in nonbreeding dogs with prostatitis; castration should be deferred until after identification and treatment (for at least 1 week) of the causative bacterial/fungal agent.
- Surgical drainage with subsequent packing of the cavity with omentum has been associated with the fewest adverse sequelae among surgical treatments. Referral to a surgical specialist is recommended.

MEDICATIONS

DRUG(S) OF CHOICE

Eradicating Infection

- Choice of antimicrobial agent is based on culture of the prostatic fluid and the ability of the antibiotic to cross the blood–prostate barrier. Antibiotics should be lipophilic, not highly protein-bound, and be a weak base.
- Antibiotics of choice—fluoroquinolones, trimethoprim, chloramphenicol, and macrolides. In acute prostatitis, the blood–prostate barrier is disrupted and almost any antibiotic will penetrate the prostatic parenchyma initially, but once healing has begun one of the preferred antibiotics discussed should be used.
- Antibiotic therapy should be administered for 4 weeks with repeat culture of prostatic fluid performed 1–2 weeks after the end of antibiotic treatment.

Inducing Prostatic Involution

- Treatment of choice in nonbreeding dogs for inducing permanent prostatic involution is castration.
- Alternatively, the 5α-reductase inhibitor finasteride (0.1–1 mg/kg PO q 24 h; not to exceed 5 mg/dog) for 2–4 months induces involution of the prostatic parenchyma and diffuse epithelial cysts and abscesses.
- Finasteride prevents conversion of testosterone to DHT, thereby causing prostatic involution without adversely affecting libido or spermatogenesis.
- BPH recurs following cessation of finasteride therapy; intact males should be maintained on finasteride.

CONTRAINDICATIONS

Estrogens and androgens cause squamous metaplasia of the prostate and BPH, respectively.

PRECAUTIONS

Long-term therapy with trimethoprim may lead to keratoconjunctivitis sicca or hypothyroidism.

FOLLOW-UP

PATIENT MONITORING

- Serial evaluation of semen culture, cytology, and prostatic imaging.
- Intervals between reevaluations vary with severity of signs, presence of an abscess, selection of castration or finasteride therapy for prostatic involution, and use of the dog in a breeding program. Intervals between evaluations range from 1 to 8 weeks, with recheck recommended prior to breeding.
- Continue patient monitoring until the dog has been castrated.

PREVENTION/AVOIDANCE

Castration is recommended in nonbreeding, affected dogs to induce prostatic involution, resolution of BPH, and prevention of recurrent infection. Breeding males should be maintained on finasteride.

POSSIBLE COMPLICATIONS

- Recurrence of infection if prostatic involution is not induced or antibiotic therapy is discontinued prematurely.
- Surgical drainage of abscesses is associated with many complications, including urinary incontinence, recurrent abscessation, hypoproteinemia, scrotal edema, anemia, sepsis, and shock.

EXPECTED COURSE AND PROGNOSIS

- Prognosis is good to excellent except in the case of rupture of prostatic abscesses into the peritoneal cavity.
- Castration prevents recurrence and improves prognosis.
- Surgical management of prostatic abscesses is associated with complications and a poorer prognosis than medical/surgical induction of prostatic involution.

MISCELLANEOUS

ASSOCIATED CONDITIONS

When prostatic fluid is infected, blood, inflammatory exudate, and microbial organisms may reflux into the urinary bladder, which, if detected in a urine sample collected by cystocentesis, may be misinterpreted as primary urinary tract infection.

ZOONOTIC POTENTIAL

Rare; *B. canis* and *Blastomyces dermatitidis* have been isolated from the urine of dogs with prostatic infection, but human infection from these sources has not been reported.

SEE ALSO

- Benign Prostatic Hyperplasia.
- Dysuria, Pollakiuria, and Stranguria.
- Hematuria.
- Peritonitis.
- Prostatic Cysts.
- Shock, Septic.

ABBREVIATIONS

- BPH = benign prostatic hyperplasia.
- DHT = dihydrotestosterone.

Suggested Reading

Christensen, BW. Canine prostate disease. Vet Clin North Am Small Anim Pract 2018, 48(4):701–719.

Root Kustritz MV. Collection of tissue and culture samples from the canine reproductive tract. Theriogenology 2006, 66:567–574.

Smith J. Canine prostatic disease: a review of anatomy, pathology, diagnosis, and treatment. Theriogenology 2008, 70:375–383.

Author Bruce W. Christensen

Consulting Editor J.D. Foster

Acknowledgment The author and editors would like to acknowledge the prior contribution of Carl A. Osborne.

Client Education Handout available online

P

PROSTATOMEGALY

BASICS

DEFINITION

Abnormally large prostate gland determined by rectal or abdominal palpation, abdominal radiography, or prostatic ultrasonography. The enlargement can be symmetrical or asymmetrical, painful or nonpainful. Normal prostate size varies with age, body size, castration status, and breed so assessment of enlargement is subjective.

PATHOPHYSIOLOGY

Enlargement can result from epithelial cell hyperplasia or hypertrophy (e.g., benign prostatic hyperplasia [BPH]), neoplasia of prostatic epithelium or stroma, cystic change within the prostatic parenchyma, or inflammatory cell infiltration (e.g., acute and chronic bacterial prostatitis and prostatic abscess).

SYSTEMS AFFECTED

- Urinary.
- Reproductive.

P

SIGNALMENT

- Dog.
- Typically occurs in middle-aged to older males.

SIGNS

- May be none.
- Straining to defecate.
- Ribbon-like stools.
- Dysuria.
- Urethral outflow obstruction.

CAUSES

- BPH.
- Squamous metaplasia.
- Adenocarcinoma.
- Transitional cell carcinoma.
- Sarcoma.
- Metastatic neoplasia.
- Acute or chronic bacterial prostatitis.
- Prostatic abscess.
- Prostatic cyst.

RISK FACTORS

- Castration lowers the risk of BPH and bacterial prostatitis.
- Risk of adenocarcinoma may be increased threefold in castrated dogs.

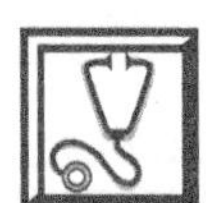

DIAGNOSIS

DIFFERENTIAL DIAGNOSIS

- BPH—typically causes nonpainful symmetrical enlargement of the prostate gland; not found in neutered dogs.
- Primary or metastatic neoplasia—typically causes painful, nonsymmetric enlargement of the prostate gland; weight loss, impaired appetite, rear limb weakness observed in some patients; suspect neoplasia in castrated dogs.
- Acute bacterial prostatitis—typically results in slight-to-moderate symmetric or nonsymmetric enlargement of the prostate gland with prostatic pain. Fever, impaired appetite, rear limb weakness, and painful abdomen observed in some patients.
- Chronic bacterial prostatitis—signs similar to those seen in dogs with acute prostatitis or those related to recurrent lower urinary tract infection (e.g., dysuria and hematuria). Systemic signs less common than in acute bacterial prostatitis; bacterial prostatitis uncommon in castrated dogs.
- Prostatic abscess—may result in signs similar to those in patients with acute or chronic prostatitis; abscess rupture causes fever and caudal abdominal pain.
- Prostatic cysts—may be associated with palpable caudal abdominal mass, straining to urinate, or straining to defecate; patient may also be asymptomatic.

CBC/BIOCHEMISTRY/URINALYSIS

- CBC normal in patients with BPH.
- Leukocytosis in patients with prostatic abscess and bacterial prostatitis, occasionally with chronic bacterial prostatitis and prostatic neoplasia.
- High bilirubin and alkaline phosphatase in some patients with prostatic abscess.
- Urinalysis—usually normal.
- Hematuria in patients with BPH.
- Pyuria, hematuria, proteinuria, and bacteriuria in patients with bacterial prostatitis
- Pyuria, hematuria, proteinuria, and, occasionally, neoplastic cells in dogs with prostatic neoplasia.

OTHER LABORATORY TESTS

Serum canine prostate-specific arginine esterase concentration may be high in dogs with BPH.

IMAGING

Radiographic Findings

Prostatomegaly

Ultrasonographic Findings

- Abscess or cyst—hypoechoic or anechoic lesions with distal enhancement.
- Acute bacterial prostatitis—uniform prostatic echogenicity.
- BPH—uniform prostatic echogenicity; small fluid-filled cysts in some patients.
- Chronic bacterial prostatitis—focal or diffuse hyperechogenicity.
- Prostatic neoplasia—focal to multifocal areas of coalescing echogenicity and acoustic shadowing (if dystrophic mineralization occurs).

DIAGNOSTIC PROCEDURES

- Examination of prostatic fluid obtained by ejaculation or prostatic massage may reveal red blood cells with BPH, neutrophils with prostate infection, or neoplastic cells with carcinoma
- Bacterial culture of prostatic fluid typically reveals >100,000 cfu/mL in dogs with bacterial prostatitis.
- Needle biopsy of the prostate with ultrasound guidance provides visualization of the area to be sampled and increases the likelihood of obtaining a diagnostic sample; take care to avoid iatrogenic rupture of a prostatic abscess.

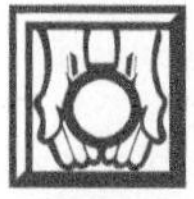

TREATMENT

- Varies with the cause of prostatomegaly.
- Surgical castration—indicated in symptomatic nonbreeding dogs with BPH and after acute infection resolves in dogs with bacterial prostatitis.
- Surgical drainage—indicated in dogs with prostatic abscess or large prostatic cysts.

MEDICATIONS

DRUG(S) OF CHOICE

BPH

If castration is not desired, the following drugs may produce a temporary response:

- Finasteride 0.1–0.5 mg/kg/day PO; not to exceed 5 mg/dog, for as long as the dog remains intact.
- Medroxyprogesterone 3 mg/kg SC once.
- Osaterone acetate 0.25 mg/kg PO once daily for 7 days.
- Delmadinone acetate 3 mg/kg SC once.
- Deslorelin acetate (SC implant administered every 6–12 months).

Bacterial Prostatitis

Choose antibiotics on the basis of anti-bacterial susceptibility testing of the isolated pathogen and ability of the antibiotic to diffuse into prostatic fluid in therapeutic concentrations. Good choices for the latter include fluoroquinolones, trimethoprim–sulfamethoxazole, chloramphenicol, and macrolides. Treatment should be for a minimum of 4 weeks.

Prostatic Carcinoma

Cox-2 inhibitors such as piroxicam and carprofen have been shown to prolong acceptable quality of life an average of 6 months compared to 3 weeks in nontreated dogs. These are used sometimes in combination with chemotherapeutic agents such as mitoxantrone, vinblastine, or metronomic chlorambucil. Referral to an oncologist is recommended.

PRECAUTIONS

Long-term administration of medroxyprogesterone and trimethoprim–sulfamethoxazole can cause diabetes mellitus and keratoconjuctivitis sicca, respectively.

FOLLOW-UP

PATIENT MONITORING

- Abdominal radiographs or prostatic ultrasonography to assess efficacy of treatment in BPH, prostatic carcinoma, or bacterial prostatitis.
- Urine and prostatic fluid culture to access efficacy of treatment in patients with bacterial prostatitis.

POSSIBLE COMPLICATIONS

- Metastatic disease.
- Subfertility.
- Dysuria.

MISCELLANEOUS

SEE ALSO

- Adenocarcinoma, Prostate.
- Benign Prostatic Hyperplasia.
- Prostatic Cysts.
- Prostatitis and Prostatic Abscess.

ABBREVIATIONS

- BPH = benign prostatic hyperplasia.

Suggested Reading

Christensen, BW. Canine prostate disease. Vet Clin North Am Small Anim Pract 2018, 48(4):701–719.

Smith J. Canine prostatic disease: a review of anatomy, pathology, diagnosis, and treatment. Theriogenology 2008, 70:375–383.

Author Bruce W. Christensen

Consulting Editor J.D. Foster

Acknowledgment The author and editors would like to acknowledge the prior contributions of Carl A. Osborne and Jeffrey S. Klausner.

P

PROTEIN-LOSING ENTEROPATHY

BASICS

DEFINITION

• A disease process characterized by excessive loss of protein into the gastrointestinal (GI) lumen. • Protein-losing enteropathy (PLE) may be associated with primary GI diseases (e.g., inflammatory bowel disease, intestinal lymphoma, or intestinal lymphangiectasia) and systemic disorders (e.g., fungal disease or congestive heart failure [CHF]).

PATHOPHYSIOLOGY

• Under physiologic conditions, two-thirds of normal protein loss in dogs occurs through the small intestine. • Plasma proteins that leak into the GI lumen are rapidly digested into constituent amino acids that can be reabsorbed and used for the synthesis of new proteins. • This normal loss of plasma proteins can be accelerated by GI mucosal disease or by increased leakage of lymph into the GI lumen. • GI protein loss is associated with loss of both albumin and globulin, often resulting in panhypoproteinemia. • In response to increased GI protein loss, the liver increases albumin synthesis. However, the liver cannot increase albumin synthesis to more than twice the normal output. • When protein loss exceeds protein synthesis, hypoproteinemia results. • Hypoproteinemia causes decreased plasma oncotic pressure, which may lead to hemodynamic changes, effusion into body cavities or peripheral edema.

P

SYSTEMS AFFECTED

• Coagulation—patients with PLE lose antithrombin and other anticoagulants, resulting in a hypercoagulable state which may lead to thromboembolic events such as pulmonary thromboembolism (PTE). • GI—primary GI disease may be associated with diarrhea, vomiting, or weight loss. • Hemodynamic—decreased oncotic pressure leading to cavitary effusion. • Lymphatic—lymphangiectasia. • Respiratory—dyspnea due to pleural effusion or PTE. • Skin—subcutaneous edema.

GENETICS

PLE due to specific underlying causes is suspected to be hereditary based on an increased prevalence in specific dog breeds.

INCIDENCE/PREVALENCE

• Unknown. • Many dogs with subacute or acute gastroenteritis have transient PLE.

GEOGRAPHIC DISTRIBUTION

N/A

SIGNALMENT

Species

Dog and cat.

Breed Predilections

Soft-coated wheaten terrier, Basenji, Yorkshire terrier, and Norwegian lundehund.

Mean Age and Range

Any age.

Predominant Sex

No predilection.

SIGNS

General Comments

Clinical signs are variable.

Historical Findings

• Chronic diarrhea, weight loss, sarcopenia, and lethargy are most frequently reported. However, many dogs with PLE have normal stools. • Vomiting is uncommon. • Dogs can be presented for apparent weight gain or abdominal distension.

Physical Examination Findings

• Ascites, dependent edema, and dyspnea from pleural effusion may be detected in patients with marked hypoproteinemia.
• Abdominal palpation may reveal thickened bowel loops, though this is uncommon.

CAUSES

Disorders of Lymphatics

• Intestinal lymphangiectasia. • GI lymphoma.
• Granulomatous infiltration of the small bowel.
• CHF leading to lymphatic hypertension.

Diseases Associated with Increased Mucosal Permeability or Mucosal Ulceration

• Viral gastroenteritis—parvovirus and others. • Bacterial gastroenteritis—salmonellosis and others. • Fungal gastroenteritis—histoplasmosis and others (note: serum globulin concentrations can be within the reference interval due to increased production secondary to massive antigenic stimulation).
• Parasitic enteritis—hookworms, whipworms, and others. • Inflammatory bowel disease—lymphocytic-plasmacytic, eosinophilic, or granulomatous gastroenteritis. • Adverse food reactions. • Mechanical enteropathies—chronic intussusception, chronic foreign body, and others. • Intestinal neoplasia—lymphoma, adenocarcinoma, and others.
• Gastric or intestinal ulcers.

RISK FACTORS

• GI disease. • Lymphatic disease. • Heart disease.

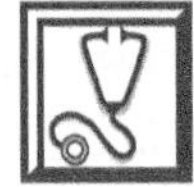

DIAGNOSIS

DIFFERENTIAL DIAGNOSIS

• Hypoalbuminemia due to hepatic failure—often associated with normal or increased serum globulin concentration. Hepatic enzyme activity may be increased, serum BUN, cholesterol, and glucose may be decreased, and serum pre- and postprandial bile acids concentrations may be increased. • Hypoalbuminemia due to protein-losing nephropathy (PLN)—mild in patients with fever or hyperadrenocorticism, moderate to severe in patients with glomerulonephritis or amyloidosis; commonly associated with a normal or increased serum globulin concentration; ruled out by a normal urine protein:creatinine ratio. • Hypoalbuminemia due to severe blood loss: excluded by assessment of the CBC and a thorough physical examination; in some cases a test for fecal occult blood may be necessary. • Starvation is a rare cause of hypoalbuminemia.

CBC/BIOCHEMISTRY/URINALYSIS

• Hypoalbuminemia and frequently hypoglobulinemia (panhypoproteinemia).
• Normal or increased serum globulin concentration in some cases, if the underlying disease is associated with chronic antigenic stimulation (e.g., immunoproliferative enteropathy of the basenji). • Hypocalcemia.
• Hypocholesterolemia. • Lymphopenia may be seen with lymphangiectasia.

OTHER LABORATORY TESTS

• Increased fecal α_1-protease inhibitor concentration (must be assessed in naturally passed and freshly frozen fecal samples from 3 consecutive days). • Once PLE has been identified as the cause of the hypoalbuminemia, specific tests may be useful to determine the cause of PLE: multiple fecal examinations to rule-out intestinal parasitism as a cause of PLE; serum cobalamin and folate concentrations to diagnose small intestinal dysbiosis or cobalamin deficiency.

IMAGING

• Thoracic radiographs may show evidence for cardiac, mediastinal, or fungal disease.
• Abdominal radiographs may show evidence for a mechanical enteropathy (i.e., foreign body, intussusception, or other). • Abdominal ultrasound may show evidence for a mechanical enteropathy or other causes of PLE.
• Abdominal ultrasound is helpful for evaluating the pattern of intestinal wall layering that can be associated with a variety of enteropathies. Hyperechoic mucosal striations ("tiger stripe" effect), mucosal speckles, and a hyperechoic line within the mucosa that runs parallel to the submucosa are common findings in dogs with intestinal lymphangiectasia. • Echocardiogram may show evidence for cardiac disease.

DIAGNOSTIC PROCEDURES

• Broad-spectrum anthelminthic agent to treat for potential parasitism. • Elimination diet trial using a novel or hydrolyzed protein source to rule out food sensitivity. One study in a group of soft-coated wheaten terriers suggests a hydrolyzed protein diet may be the best choice in dogs with PLE. • Histoplasma antigen test (serum or urine) and rectal mucosal scraping in geographic regions where histoplasmosis is endemic. • Gastroduodenoscopy and colonoscopy—to visualize the GI mucosa and to collect endoscopic biopsies for histopathologic evaluation. Visualization of white "plaques" (e.g., chylomicron distended lacteals) along the mucosa suggests lymphangiectasia.
• Abdominal exploratory laparotomy may show dilated intestinal lymphatics and allows for full-thickness biopsies of intestines and lymph

nodes. • Fecal α_1-protease inhibitor concentration to document excessive GI protein loss. Assays are species-specific and currently only an assay for measurement of α_1-protease inhibitor in dogs is available through the GI Laboratory at Texas A&M University. Samples from 3 consecutive defecations need to be collected in special preweighed fecal tubes that can be sourced from the GI Lab.

PATHOLOGIC FINDINGS

• In dogs with PLE due to lymphangiectasia, gross findings may include dilated lymphatics that are visible as a web-like network throughout the mesentery and serosal surface.
• May see small yellow-white nodules and foamy granular deposits adjacent to lymphatics (lipogranulomas). • Lacteal dilatation, villous blunting, and crypt lesions (e.g., dilatation, cysts, abscesses) are the most consistent findings on histopathology in dogs with lymphangiectasia and PLE. • PLE due to other causes may show lesions specific for the disease.

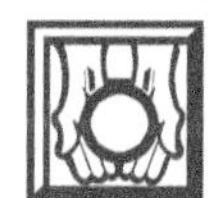

TREATMENT

APPROPRIATE HEALTH CARE

Inpatient or outpatient medical management depending on the severity of clinical signs at the time of diagnosis.

NURSING CARE

• With clinical signs due to edema or effusion from severe hypoalbuminemia, albumin transfusion, or colloids (such as hetastarch) may be considered to increase plasma oncotic pressure. Both human and canine albumin can provide a temporary increase in serum albumin, but human albumin transfusion may be associated with adverse reactions in dogs.
• Abdominocentesis to remove ascites or pleurocentesis to remove pleural effusion is indicated in cases where effusion has led to respiratory compromise. • Consider placement of an esophageal feeding tube in hyporexic patients to meet increased caloric demands.

ACTIVITY

Normal

DIET

• May need to be modified depending on the underlying cause of PLE. • If lymphangiectasia is diagnosed or highly suspected, an ultra-low-fat diet, containing 20 g fat/1,000 kcal or less, is indicated. It should be noted that there are currently no commercial diets lower than 20 g fat/1,000 kcal and one study has suggested that an even lower fat content is beneficial.

CLIENT EDUCATION

Prepare clients for long-term therapy; spontaneous cures are rare.

SURGICAL CONSIDERATIONS

• Hypoalbuminemia increases postoperative morbidity because of slow wound healing.
• Some causes of PLE (e.g., intussusception, chronic foreign body, and some intestinal neoplasms), however, require surgical intervention.

MEDICATIONS

DRUG(S) OF CHOICE

• There is no pharmacologic therapy for PLE itself. Instead, the underlying cause of PLE must be addressed.
• However, patients with PLE also lose antithrombin and other anticoagulants and can be hypercoagulable. Thus, patients should be treated with a platelet aggregation inhibitor: ◦ In dogs or cats—clopidogrel bisulfate (1–4 mg/kg PO q24h in dogs; 18.75 mg/cat PO q24h, which equals one-fourth of a 75 mg tablet). ◦ In dogs—low-dose aspirin (0.5 mg/kg PO q12h; use an 81 mg tablet of aspirin and put into the barrel of a 10 mL syringe, add 8.1 mL of water and shake until completely dissolved to make a 10 mg/mL solution; discard unused portion immediately).

CONTRAINDICATIONS

• Aspirin and clopidogrel should not be used concurrently.
• Clopidogrel should not be used with NSAIDs, phenytoin, torsemide, or warfarin.

PRECAUTIONS

Bleeding may be enhanced in patients treated with platelet aggregation inhibitors that have to undergo surgery.

POSSIBLE INTERACTIONS

N/A

ALTERNATIVE DRUG(S)

• Diuretics such as furosemide (1 mg/kg PO q12h) in combination with spironolactone (1 mg/kg PO q12h) have been used by some clinicians to control edema, pleural effusion, and ascites. However, they do not work consistently in patients with PLE because of decreased plasma oncotic pressure and may be associated with side effects. • There are anecdotal reports about the use of the long-acting somatostatin analogue octreotide in dogs with PLE, but no clinical trials have been completed to date and no specific dosing regimen has been suggested.

FOLLOW-UP

PATIENT MONITORING

Check body weight, serum albumin concentration, and evidence of recurrent clinical signs (i.e., pleural effusion, ascites, and/or edema). Frequency depends on the severity of the condition. Monitor serum cobalamin concentration if patient was hypocobalaminemic and supplemented with cobalamin.

PREVENTION/AVOIDANCE

N/A

POSSIBLE COMPLICATIONS

• Thromboembolic events, especially PTE.
• Respiratory difficulty from pleural effusion or PTE. • Severe protein-calorie malnutrition.
• Intractable diarrhea.

EXPECTED COURSE AND PROGNOSIS

• Prognosis is guarded and depends on the underlying cause. Smaller breed dogs carry a more favorable prognosis because nutritional support is easier to perform. • The primary disease cannot be treated in many cases.

MISCELLANEOUS

ASSOCIATED CONDITIONS

Soft-coated wheaten terriers may have PLN in conjunction with PLE and should be evaluated accordingly.

AGE-RELATED FACTORS

N/A

ZOONOTIC POTENTIAL

Some GI parasites have zoonotic potential.

P

PREGNANCY/FERTILITY/BREEDING

N/A

SYNONYMS

N/A

SEE ALSO

• Cobalamin Deficiency.
• Diarrhea, Chronic—Cats.
• Diarrhea, Chronic—Dogs.
• Inflammatory Bowel Disease.
• Lymphangiectasia.

ABBREVIATIONS

• CHF = congestive heart failure.
• GI = gastrointestinal.
• NSAID = nonsteroidal anti-inflammatory drug. • PLE = protein-losing enteropathy.
• PLN = protein-losing nephropathy.

INTERNET RESOURCES

http://vetmed.tamu.edu/gilab/

Suggested Reading

Craven MD, Washabau RJ. Comparative pathophysiology and management of protein-losing enteropathy. J Vet Intern Med 2019, 33:383–402.
Dossin O, Lavoue R. Protein-losing enteropathies in dogs. Vet Clin North Am Small Anim Pract 2011, 41:399–418.
Simmerson SM, Armstrong PJ, Wunschmann A, et al. Clinical features, intestinal histopathology, and outcome in protein-losing enteropathy in Yorkshire terrier dogs. J Vet Intern Med 2014, 28:331–337.

Authors Jörg M. Steiner and Sina Marsilio
Consulting Editor Mark P. Rondeau

Client Education Handout available online

PROTEINURIA

BASICS

DEFINITION

• Urinary protein detected by dipstick analysis, urinary protein:creatinine ratio (UP:C ≥0.4 in cats or ≥0.5 in dogs), urinary albumin:creatinine ratio (UA:C >30 mg/g), or 24-hour urine protein content (> 20 mg/kg). UP:C of 0.2–0.4 in cats and 0.2–0.5 in dogs is borderline.
• Microalbuminuria (MA) is the abnormal presence of low concentrations of albumin in the urine (1–30 mg/dL), below the limit of detection of standard urine dipsticks.

PATHOPHYSIOLOGY

• Prerenal—greater than normal delivery of low-molecular-weight plasma proteins to glomeruli.
• Renal, glomerular—excessive loss of larger molecular weight proteins (e.g., albumin) across the glomerular basement membrane (GBM) secondary to altered permselectivity of glomeruli.
• Renal, tubular—reduced tubular reabsorption of proteins.
• Postrenal—exudation of blood or plasma into lower urinary tract.

SYSTEMS AFFECTED

• Renal/urologic—chronic glomerular proteinuria causes progressive tubular damage resulting in chronic kidney disease (CKD).
• Cardiovascular—systemic hypertension.
• Hemic/lymphatic/immune—severe glomerular proteinuria can lead to edema and/or hypercoagulability. Hypercoagulability is brought about by vascular stasis, hyperfibrinogenemia, platelet abnormalities, loss of antithrombic substances, and an increase in procoagulant factors. The pathogenesis of edema involves both inappropriate renal sodium retention and decreased plasma oncotic pressure.

GENETICS

Familial nephropathies associated with glomerular proteinuria have been described in several breeds of dogs; in only a few has the mode of inheritance been established: Samoyed (X-linked), English cocker spaniel (autosomal recessive), bull terrier (autosomal dominant), Dalmatian (autosomal dominant), Bernese mountain dog (autosomal recessive), Brittany spaniel (autosomal recessive), bullmastiff (autosomal recessive), Newfoundland (autosomal recessive), soft-coated wheaten terrier (complex), Chinese shar-pei (suspect autosomal recessive). Doberman pinscher, Rottweiler, Pembroke Welsh corgi, beagle, English foxhound, and others.

INCIDENCE/PREVALENCE

• In a study of urinalysis data from 500 dogs, the prevalence of proteinuria was approximately 19%.
• The prevalence of MA was 25% in dogs and 25% in cats. Prevalence increased with advancing age.

GEOGRAPHIC DISTRIBUTION

None, however an association may be observed with some infectious diseases that are regional.

SIGNALMENT

Species

Dog and cat.

Breed Predilections

Glomerular proteinuria may be the initial manifestation of several familial renal diseases (see Genetics).

Mean Age and Range

Proteinuria can occur at any age. Familial renal diseases tend to occur in younger animals; acquired glomerular proteinuria more likely in middle-aged or older animals

Predominant Sex

Varies with different diseases

SIGNS

• Vary with underlying cause and severity of proteinuria.
• Patients with glomerular proteinuria are frequently asymptomatic or have signs attributable to underlying diseases.

Historical Findings

• Weight loss and lethargy; animals with pulmonary thromboembolism may have acute dyspnea.
• Patients with lower urinary tract (LUT) disorders may have dysuria, pollakiuria, inappropriate urination, and/or hematuria.

Physical Examination Findings

• May have edema or abdominal distention.
• May have oral ulceration (if uremic), edema or cavitary effusion, or changes in pulse quality (if thromboembolic).

CAUSES

Prerenal Proteinuria

Overload proteinuria—tubular resorptive capacity exceeded by large amounts of low-molecular-weight plasma proteins in glomerular filtrate (e.g., excessive hemolysis or rhabdomyolysis, neoplastic production of paraproteins or Bence Jones proteins).

Renal Proteinuria

• Functional proteinuria—strenuous exercise, fever, hypothermia, seizures, or venous congestion.
• Glomerulonephritis (e.g., immune complex-mediated, membranous, membranoproliferative, proliferative), minimal change disease, hereditary nephritis, amyloidosis, podocyopathy, focal segmental glomerulosclerosis, glomerulosclerosis.
• All glomerular diseases can be associated with severe proteinuria, subsets of immune complex-mediated (particularly membranoproliferative and membranous) may be associated with higher magnitude proteinuria than others.
• Tubular dysfunction resulting in failure of tubular protein reabsorption is associated with mild-to-moderate proteinuria.

Postrenal Proteinuria

Hemorrhage or inflammation of the urogenital tract.

RISK FACTORS

• Chronic inflammatory (e.g., infectious and immune-mediated) and neoplastic diseases can lead to development of glomerulonephritis or amyloidosis. Examples include dirofilariasis, ehrlichiosis, borreliosis, babesiosis, chronic bacterial infections (e.g., endocarditis, pyoderma), pyometra, bartonellosis, feline immunodeficiency virus, mast cell tumor, lymphosarcoma, hyperadrenocorticism, and systemic lupus erythematosus.
• Systemic hypertension.
• Chronic hyperlipidemia.
• Multiple myeloma can produce Bence Jones proteinuria.

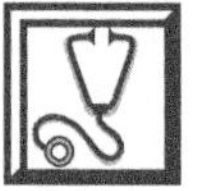

DIAGNOSIS

DIFFERENTIAL DIAGNOSIS

Differentiate prerenal, postrenal, and renal-tubular from glomerular causes.

CBC/BIOCHEMISTRY/URINALYSIS

• Urine dipstick and sulfosalicylic acid (SSA) tests allow qualitative and semiquantitative assessment of urine protein content. Results are affected by urine concentration and must be interpreted in context of urine specific gravity. Low urine protein (trace or 1+) may be normal in a concentrated urine sample.
• The dipstick lacks specificity (dog, 69%; cat, 31%) and sensitivity (dog, 54%; cat, 60%).
• False-positive test results occur when urine is highly alkaline (pH >8–9) or when the dipstick is immersed in the urine for a prolonged time.
• Low concentrations of Bence Jones proteins or gamma globulins may not be detected by urine dipstick.
• SSA turbidometric test results are falsely increased by radiographic contrast media, penicillins, sulfisoxazole, or the urine preservative thymol.
• SSA test results are falsely decreased by very alkaline urine and increased by uncentrifuged urine.
• If proteinuria is detected by these methods, the urine sediment should be evaluated for hematuria, pyuria, and/or bacteriuria. Hematuria alone typically does not increase urine albumin content above the negligible range (i.e., >1 mg/dL) or the UP:C above 0.4

until there is a color change in the urine. 81% of dogs with pyuria had normal UP:C.

• To determine persistence, repeat the urine protein screening test in proteinuric patients that initially have a normal urine sediment or have been treated for urinary tract inflammation or hemorrhage. If proteinuria is transient and the urine sediment is normal, consider functional proteinuria or false-positive test results.

• Although not all animals with glomerular disease are hypoalbuminemic, glomerular proteinuria should be suspected when proteinuria and hypoalbuminemia are concurrent. As disease progresses, clinicopathologic changes consistent with glomerular disease may develop.

OTHER LABORATORY TESTS

• Urine protein should be quantified in dogs and cats that have hypoalbuminemia and/or repeatedly positive urine dipstick or SSA tests in absence of LUT hemorrhage or inflammation. The UP:C is the preferred because more is known about use of this test and it is technically easier to perform than 24-hour urine collections.

• MA is detected in dogs using a point-of-care immunoassay or quantitation using an immunoassay. MA is an early predictor of proteinuria. If repeatedly positive, and if the concentration is increasing, the patient may be at risk for glomerular disease.

• Thoroughly evaluate an animal for an underlying disease when persistent proteinuria is believed to be of glomerular origin.

• Urine and serum protein electrophoresis may identify pre-glomerular proteinuria in patients with monoclonal gammopathies or urinary immunoglobulin light chains (Bence Jones proteins).

IMAGING

Ultrasound and radiographs may reveal an underlying infectious, inflammatory, or neoplastic disease process or evidence of LUT disease. Ultrasound may show structural changes suggesting primary renal disease (e.g., loss of corticomedullary distinction, hyperechogenicity, and irregular surface margin) or evidence in support of LUT disease.

DIAGNOSTIC PROCEDURES

• Blood pressure should be monitored in patients with persistent renal proteinuria.

• Renal biopsy is needed to specifically diagnose the glomerular disease when an underlying disease cannot be identified or proteinuria has persisted following treatment of an underlying disease.

PATHOLOGIC FINDINGS

• Vary with cause of proteinuria.

• Biopsy from an animal with glomerular proteinuria may reveal any of the following: glomerulonephritis (e.g., immune complex-mediated, membranous, membranoproliferative, proliferative), minimal change disease, hereditary nephritis, amyloidosis, podocyopathy, focal segmental glomerulosclerosis, glomerulosclerosis.

• Animals with tubular proteinuria most often have a degree of tubulointerstitial nephritis.

• Postrenal proteinuria would be expected to have inflammatory, neoplastic, or polypoid lesions.

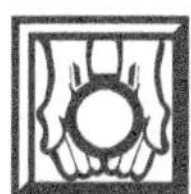

TREATMENT

APPROPRIATE HEALTH CARE

Most can be managed as outpatients. Inpatient care may be required during select diagnostic evaluation (renal biopsy) or when there are complications associated with uremia, thromboembolism or edema in patients with glomerular proteinuria.

NURSING CARE

Physical therapy and exercise may limit formation of edema in patients with glomerular proteinuria and hypoalbuminemia.

ACTIVITY

Activity should not be restricted in animals with proteinuria.

DIET

If glomerular disease is suspected, feed a diet formulated for kidney disease.

CLIENT EDUCATION

It is important to determine the cause of persistent proteinuria, which may indicate the presence of kidney disease. Renal proteinuria is a risk factor for progressive kidney disease, thromboembolism, and edema.

SURGICAL CONSIDERATIONS

Animals with severe hypoalbuminemia (i.e., <2 g/dL) present unique challenges to anesthesia. Consideration should be given to referral of these patients to a secondary or tertiary care facility if anesthesia and/or surgery are indicated.

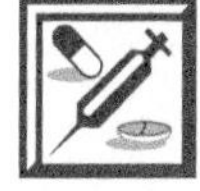

MEDICATIONS

DRUG(S) OF CHOICE

An angiotensin receptor blocker (ARB) or angiotensin-converting enzyme (ACE) inhibitor should be administered. Preliminary evidence suggests telmisartan (ARB) may be more efficacious in reducing proteinuria than ACE inhibitors. Combined use of an ARB and an ACE inhibitor should be done with caution as this is associated with a greater risk of death in people. Use of aldosterone antagonists in management of proteinuria needs further investigation but may be indicated for patients that have increased aldosterone concentrations following treatment with an ACE inhibitor or ARB. Animals with hypertension may be controlled with telmisartan alone, however some may require addition of a calcium channel blocker (e.g., amlodipine) to control both hypertension and proteinuria. Supplementation with n-3 polyunsaturated fatty acid (PUFA) should be considered in dogs, and possibly cats, with glomerular proteinuria when the diet being fed does not have a reduced n-6/n-3 PUFA ratio that approximates 5:1. Dogs with glomerular disease should also be given low-dose aspirin or clopidogrel as thromboprophylaxis.

CONTRAINDICATIONS

There are no known contraindications in animals with proteinuria.

PRECAUTIONS

Drugs highly bound to albumin may have an altered effect if hypoalbuminemia is present. The use of warfarin as an anticoagulant should be avoided. With hypoalbuminemia or azotemia, higher doses of furosemide may be required to mobilize edema effectively; however, it should be used with extreme caution.

POSSIBLE INTERACTIONS

There are no known important drug interactions in dogs with proteinuria other than the previously mentioned concern with highly protein-bound drugs.

ALTERNATIVE DRUG(S)

ARB and ACE inhibitor are alternatives to each other.

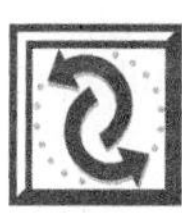

FOLLOW-UP

PATIENT MONITORING

• UP:C, urinalysis, systemic arterial blood pressure and serum albumin, creatinine and potassium concentrations should be monitored at least quarterly.

• Use the UP:C to assess progression of disease. Response to treatment should be evaluated for several months after resolution of any underlying disease. Reduction of UP:C to <0.5 (dog) or <0.2 (cat) without inappropriate worsening of renal function is considered a therapeutic success. However, this target is often not achieved and a reduction in UP:C of >50% is the recommended alternate target.

• Monitor serum creatinine—reduced proteinuria or reduced albuminuria that is concurrent to a rising serum creatinine may reflect deteriorating renal function.

• Because UP:Cs may vary, 2–5 serial assessments may be needed to evaluate response to treatment or progression in patients with glomerular proteinuria. Alternatively, the UP:C can be measured in a sample that has been pooled by adding equal aliquots of 2–3 samples that have been collected and refrigerated over a 48-hour time period.

- When given an ACE inhibitor or an ARB, dogs with stage 1 or 2 CKD can have an increase in serum creatinine of up to 30% without warranting a change in treatment. Worsening of renal function in dogs with stage 3 or 4 CKD should be avoided. During therapy the serum potassium concentration should not be >6 mmol/L and the systolic blood pressure should not be <120 mmHg.

PREVENTION/AVOIDANCE

Annual urinalyses and UP:C are recommended. Repeat in 2–4 weeks if proteinuria is detected. Patients with persistent proteinuria or MA of glomerular origin should be evaluated more thoroughly for underlying causes of glomerular injury. Potential underlying causes should be eliminated or managed. If proteinuria persists, potential underlying causes have been managed appropriately or underlying causes were not identified, consider renal biopsy.

POSSIBLE COMPLICATIONS

- Edema.
- Thromboembolism.
- Systemic hypertension.
- Progressive kidney disease.
- Poor wound healing.

EXPECTED COURSE AND PROGNOSIS

- Vary with the cause of proteinuria.
- Postrenal and prerenal proteinuria should resolve following resolution of inciting causes.
- Most diseases associated with renal tubular proteinuria are progressive.
- The rate of progression varies and spontaneous remissions have been reported. Animals with persistent glomerular proteinuria may develop renal tubular damage resulting in advanced CKD and eventual uremia and death. Some dogs die shortly after the initial detection of proteinuria, while others remain alive for years. Dogs with nephrotic syndrome and/or azotemia may have a shorter survival.

MISCELLANEOUS

ASSOCIATED CONDITIONS

Hypoalbuminemia, hypoglobulinemia (rare), hypercholesterolemia, low antithrombin III, thrombocytosis, hyperfibrinogenemia, edema, thromboembolism, and systemic hypertension.

AGE-RELATED FACTORS

Familial glomerular diseases should be considered in young animals with glomerular range proteinuria.

ZOONOTIC POTENTIAL

Proteinuria does not have a zoonotic potential. However, glomerular proteinuria can occur with a variety of infectious diseases, some of which could have a zoonotic potential.

PREGNANCY/FERTILITY/BREEDING

Some drugs used in the treatment of diseases associated with proteinuria may be contraindicated in pregnancy.

SYNONYMS

None

SEE ALSO

- Amyloidosis.
- Azotemia and Uremia.
- Glomerulonephritis.
- Hematuria.
- Hypoalbuminemia.
- Nephrotic Syndrome.
- Pyuria.

ABBREVIATIONS

- ACE = angiotensin-converting enzyme.
- ARB = angiotensin receptor blocker.
- CKD = chronic kidney disease.
- GBM = glomerular basement membrane.
- LUT = lower urinary tract.
- MA = microalbuminuria.
- PUFA = polyunsaturated fatty acid.
- SSA = sulfosalicylic acid.
- UA:C = urinary albumin:creatinine ratio.
- UP:C = urine protein:creatinine ratio.

Suggested Reading

Brown S, Elliot J, Francey T, et al. Consensus recommendations for standard therapy of glomerular disease in dogs. J Vet Intern Med 2013, 27(suppl.1):S27–S43.

Lees GE, Brown SA, Elliot J, et al. Assessment and management of proteinuria in dogs and cats: 2004 ACVIM forum consensus statement (small animal). J Vet Intern Med 2005, 19:377.

Littman MP, Daminet S, Grauer GF, et al. Consensus recommendations for the diagnostic investigation of dogs with suspected glomerular disease. J Vet Intern Med 2013, 27(suppl.1):S19–S26.

Pressler B, Vaden S, Gerber B, et al. Consensus guidelines for immunosuppressive treatment of dogs with glomerular disease absent a pathologic diagnosis. J Vet Intern Med 2013, 27(suppl.1):S55–S59.

Author Shelly Vaden
Consulting Editor J.D. Foster

Client Education Handout available online

P

PROTOTHECOSIS

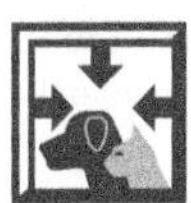

BASICS

OVERVIEW

Algal infection in warm-blooded animals.

SYSTEMS AFFECTED

• Skin/exocrine. • Gastrointestinal. • Nervous. • Ophthalmic.

SIGNALMENT

• Dogs—young female adult, medium- to large-breed dogs, boxer and collie are overrepresented. • Cats—uncommon, usually cutaneous form.

SIGNS

Historical Findings

Dogs

• Intermittent and chronic large bowel diarrhea with fresh blood. • Chronic weight loss. • Acute onset blindness. • Neurologic disease; deafness, seizures, ataxia. • Cutaneous lesions.

Cats

• Chronic cutaneous or mucous membrane ulceration with few systemic signs.

Physical Examination Findings

Dogs

• Gastrointestinal, ocular, or neurologic disease most common. • Severe weight loss and debilitation. • Hemorrhagic colitis, vomiting, anorexia. • Blindness due to chorioretinitis and/or detached retinas. • CNS—depression, ataxia, vestibular signs, seizures and/or paresis. • Cutaneous—ulcers and crusts on the extremities and mucosal surfaces.

Cats

• Large cutaneous nodules on the face or limbs.

CAUSES & RISK FACTORS

• *Prototheca wickerhamii* and *P. zopfii* (genotype 1 and 2)—single-celled achlorophyllous blue-green algae (Chlorophyta). • Dogs—usually *P. zopfii* (75-90%); *P. wickerhamii* infection may also occur. • Cats—usually *P. wickerhamii*. • Basis for the pathogenicity of *Prototheca* spp. unknown; likely traumatic inoculation. • Organism—ecological niche is sewage; contaminants of water, soil, and food; occasionally isolated from fecal samples. • Dogs and humans—depressed cell-mediated immunity may predispose to infection.

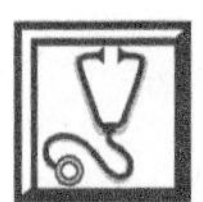

DIAGNOSIS

DIFFERENTIAL DIAGNOSIS

• Systemic or subcutaneous mycoses. • Mycobacterioses. • Neoplasia. • Pythiosis. • Actinomycosis. • Nocardiosis.

CBC/BIOCHEMISTRY/URINALYSIS

Usually normal.

OTHER LABORATORY TESTS

CSF tap—pleocytosis with mononuclear cells; increased protein; organisms.

DIAGNOSTIC PROCEDURES

Cytology

• Rectal or colonic mucosa, vitreous humor, CSF, cutaneous aspirations. • Organisms—unicellular, nonpigmented, oval or round cell walls often appear folded; diagnostic characteristic is endospore formation with internal septation in two planes.

Histopathology

• Biopsy specimens—identification of organisms is diagnostic. • Organisms—3–30 µm in diameter. *P. wickerhamii* round with sporangia (7–13 µm) with up to 50 spherical sporangiospores. *P. zopfii* are usually oval or cylindrical and produce sporangia (14–25 µm) with up to 20 sporangiospores.

Culture

• Blood agar or Sabouraud's dextrose agar. • Specific identification by selective agars or biochemical tests in culture (susceptibility to clotrimazole, sugar, and alcohol assimilation tests) or immunohistochemistry.

PCR Assays

PCR and DNA to determine species. Specimens can be taken from biopsies, CSF, or urine.

PATHOLOGIC FINDINGS

Dogs

• Small granulomatous foci or hemorrhagic ulcers—found in many organs, especially kidneys. • Nodular thickening of the gastrointestinal mucosa with ulceration. • Nonspecific inflammatory foci surrounding organisms or pyogranulomas—poorly organized; mixed with other inflammatory cells.

Cats

• Cutaneous masses—localized; extend deep into subcutaneous tissues; consist of granulomatous inflammation and mixed-cell inflammation; with numerous fungal organisms.

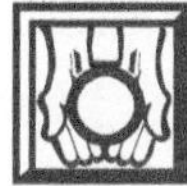

TREATMENT

• Dogs—surgical excision and combination drug therapy. • Cats—excision of localized cutaneous masses is primary therapeutic modality.

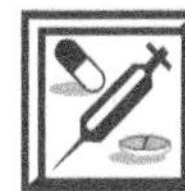

MEDICATIONS

DRUG(S) OF CHOICE

• Amphotericin B—use for localized disease after surgical excision; 0.25–0.5 mg/kg IV three times weekly until 8 mg/kg cumulative dose; lipid formulation 1 mg/kg every other day until 12 mg/kg cumulative dose. • Concurrent administration of tetracycline or amikacin may provide synergistic effect. • Itraconazole 5–10 mg/kg PO twice daily—used with amphotericin B, or as sole agents for less life-threatening disease. • Clotrimazole. • Potassium iodide. • Amphotericin B cream or clotrimazole enemas for colitis. • Nystatin 100,000–150,000 IU PO q8h for at least 90 days.

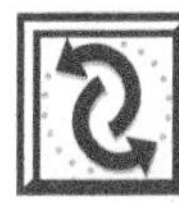

FOLLOW-UP

EXPECTED COURSE AND PROGNOSIS

• Difficult to eradicate with drug therapy. • No definitive therapeutic protocol. • Dogs—prognosis guarded to grave (median survival 4 months). • Cats—prognosis fair to good for cutaneous disease if lesions completely excised.

MISCELLANEOUS

ZOONOTIC POTENTIAL

None

INTERNET RESOURCES

https://www.academia.edu/8599426/Protothecosis_an_emerging_algal_disease_of_humans_and_animals

Suggested Reading

Pressler BM. Protothecosis and clorellosis. In: Infectious Diseases of the Dog and Cat, 4th ed. St. Louis, MO: Saunders Elsevier, 2012, pp. 696–701.

Mercuriali E, Bottero E, Abramo F, et al. Canine protothecosis in the North of Italy: 4 cases (2009–2011), 22nd ECVIM-CA Congress, Maastricht, 2012.

Silveira CS, Cesar D, Keating MK. A case of *Prototheca zopfii* genotype 1 infection in a dog (*Canis lupus familiaris*). Mycopatholgia 2018, 183(5):853–858.

Author Mitchell D. Song

Consulting Editor Alexander H. Werner Resnick

P

PRURITUS

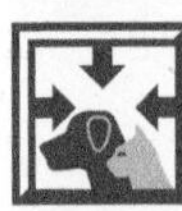

BASICS

DEFINITION

Pruritus (itch) is an unpleasant sensation that causes the clinical symptom of scratching, rubbing, hair pulling, and/or licking.

PATHOPHYSIOLOGY

Keratinocytes, mast cells, eosinophils and lymphocytes interact with neuronal cells via the release of cytokines, neurotrophins, and neuropeptides. The sensation of itch is conducted via the peripheral nervous system to the sensory cortex. Other factors can modify the perception of pruritus at this level. Pruritus is an adaptive protective mechanism, however excessive itch can lead to cutaneous damage. Identification and treatment or removal of the causative agent(s) is the most important aspect of long-term control. Avoidance or reduction of long-term medical therapy should be pursued when possible. Chronic cases may be best handled by a dermatologist.

P

SYSTEMS AFFECTED

- Skin/exocrine/neuronal.
- Behavioral.

SIGNS

- Scratching, licking, biting, rubbing, hair pull, or chewing.
- Variable evidence of self-trauma and cutaneous inflammation.
- Non-well-demarcated alopecia with or without excoriations, and without obvious gross inflammation may be the only sign.

CAUSES

- Parasitic—fleas, *Sarcoptes* spp., *Demodex* spp., *Otodectes* spp., *Notoedres* spp., *Cheyletiella* spp., *Trombicula* spp., lice, *Pelodera* spp., endoparasite migration.
- Allergic—flea allergy, atopic dermatitis, food allergy, contact allergy, drug allergy, bacterial hypersensitivity, malassezia hypersensitivity.
- Bacterial/fungal—*Staphylococcus* spp. and *Malassezia pachydermatis*; rarely dermatophyte (*Trichophyton* is more pruritic than other dermatophytes).
- Miscellaneous—primary and secondary seborrhea, calcinosis cutis, cutaneous neoplasia, immune-mediated dermatoses, and endocrinopathies are variably pruritic; psychogenic diseases may also be associated with pruritus (especially in cats).

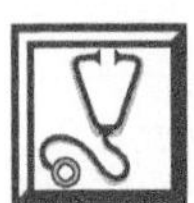

DIAGNOSIS

DIFFERENTIAL DIAGNOSIS

- Pruritus often causes alopecia.
- Alopecia without pruritus may accompany endocrine diseases. Some animals excessively lick themselves without the owner's knowledge.
- Demodicosis, dermatophytosis, superficial pyoderma (bacteria), *Malassezia* dermatitis, immune-mediated dermatoses, seborrhea, some cutaneous neoplasms, and unusual diseases such as leishmaniasis may cause alopecia with varying degrees of inflammation and pruritus.
- History is paramount for determining the diagnostic workup.
- Severe pruritus that keeps the patient and owner awake may suggest scabies, allergies (flea allergy/infestation, food allergy, atopic diseases) or *Malassezia* dermatitis. All but the latter typically have an acute onset.
- Uncomplicated atopic diseases (dermatitis, rhinitis, conjunctivitis, asthma) are steroid-responsive and may manifest seasonally, but may progress to nonseasonal pruritus of the face, feet, ears, forelimbs, axillae, and caudal body.
- Flea-allergic and food-allergic animals may be predisposed to atopic diseases and may show similar signs. Food allergy is the least common of these three differentials.

CBC/BIOCHEMISTRY/URINALYSIS

N/A

DIAGNOSTIC PROCEDURES

Miscellaneous Procedures

- Identification and treatment of the underlying cause of pruritus is of paramount importance. It is common for multiple causes to be present concurrently and this can significantly complicate the workup and management of pruritus.
- Skin scrapes, epidermal cytology, and dermatophyte cultures
- A skin biopsy is useful when the lesions associated with pruritus are unusual, an immune-mediated dermatosis is suspected, or the history and physical findings do not correlate.

Allergy Testing

- Allergy testing does not diagnose atopic disease: The presence of positive test results does not diagnose that allergy is the cause or even a contributory cause of pruritus. Results must be carefully correlated with the patient's history and physical examination.
- Two methods for allergy testing—intradermal and serum:
  - Intradermal testing remains the gold standard and the preferred method for allergy testing.
  - Serum tests for allergy measure serum IgE and do not measure localized IgE found in the skin. Patients with symptoms of atopic disease but negative on testing are diagnosed as having "atopic-like disease."
- Positive reactions identified on testing are correlated with the history, in order to formulate allergen-specific immunotherapy solution (ASIT). The choice of allergens is based on the patient's history, test results, local allergen exposure, and the veterinarian's experience in treating allergies; not just the highest reactive allergens in the testing panel should be selected. Administration of immunotherapy may be via either subcutaneous or sublingual routes.

Trial Courses of Treatment as a Diagnostic Tool

- A trial course of therapy for scabies may be appropriate in some animals; canine scabies can be difficult to diagnose and skin scrapes are often negative.
- Laboratory tests (serum, hair, saliva) cannot be used for the diagnosis of food allergy; a properly performed strict dietary trial must be conducted. Novel protein diets based on the patient's history or hydrolysate diets should be fed during the testing period. Careful client counseling to avoid all treats, supplements, chews, and flavored medications is necessary for a diet trial to succeed. Diet trials should be continued until the patient improves or for a duration of 8–10 weeks. Challenge with the original diet is a critical part of the test, and demonstrates that improvement was not due to concurrent therapy (e.g., relief of parasites, resolution of infection).

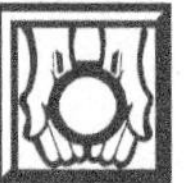

TREATMENT

- More than one disease can contribute to itching.
- Secondary infections are common and may result in self-perpetuation of pruritus.

MEDICATIONS

DRUG(S) OF CHOICE

Topical Therapy

- Topical therapy is helpful for pruritic patients.
- Colloidal oatmeal—duration of effect is usually less than 2 days.
- Topical antihistamines have not demonstrated efficacy.
- Topical anesthetics may offer only a very short duration of effect.
- Topical corticosteroids—can be effective. But if used excessively, can cause localized and systemic side effects.
- Antimicrobial shampoos help control bacterial and/or yeast infections that cause itching; they can be excessively drying, necessitating use of moisturizers.
- Lime sulfur is mildly antipruritic as well as being antiparasitic, antibacterial, and antifungal.

Systemic Therapy

- Therapy is complex and depends on the etiology.

- Parasite prevention/treatment—fleas, scabies, demodicosis.
- ASIT—atopic disease.
- Chronic medical therapy with corticosteroids, cyclosporine, lokivetmab, or oclacitinib without evaluation by a dermatologist should be avoided.
- Corticosteroids affect many biological responses associated with pruritus. For acute relief, oral prednisone/prednisolone results in significant benefit for 2–5 days but rarely causes significant side effects.
- Cyclosporine 5 mg/kg/day initially; every other day maintenance—very useful in the treatment of atopic dermatitis. Adverse effects include gastrointestinal upset, oral papilloma, gingival hyperplasia, and hirsuitism. Not useful for quick relief due to its long lag phase (4–6 weeks).
- Oclacitinib 0.4–0.6 mg/kg twice daily for 14 days, then 0.4–0.6 mg/kg q24h—fast acting without the common side effects of prednisone. Useful for temporary control of pruritus. Not for use in dogs less than 12 months of age; may cause a mild, dose-dependent reduction in hemoglobin, hematocrit, and reticulocyte counts as well as decreases in leukocytes. Potential for immune suppression, demodicosis, recurrent pyoderma, exacerbation of neoplastic conditions and pneumonia. Agitation with use reported. Avoid use at higher than recommended dosage.
- Lokivetmab 2 mg/kg—caninized monoclonal antibody against interleukin 31; for dogs only. Rapid onset (within 3 days from administration) and duration of effect between 2 and 8 weeks; effective in 60–70% of dogs with pruritus. Few side effects reported, including anaphylaxis, transient lethargy, and behavioral changes. Efficacy may be diminished by development of an immune response to this biologic medication and/or secondary infection.
- Fatty acids—block formation of inflammatory mediators; require 6–8 weeks of administration for maximum effect.

CONTRAINDICATIONS

- Some topicals will exacerbate pruritus: monitor treatment response.
- Corticosteroids should be avoided in cases of pruritus caused by an infectious etiology.

PRECAUTIONS

- Client frustration is common.
- Scabies is curable.
- Food allergy is manageable without medications if a proper food trial is conducted.
- Atopic dermatitis disease is a progressive common cause of pruritus and ASIT is the only therapy that can safely manage the disease alone or in combination with other medications.
- Corticosteroids—potentially significant long-term side effects.
- Cyclosporine—serum drug levels should be measured at least once initially in cats and in dogs if the maintenance dosage required to control symptoms is above the standard recommendation.
- Oclacitinib—long-term use associated with potential immunosuppression.

FOLLOW-UP

PATIENT MONITORING

- Patient monitoring as well as client communication are imperative.
- Many different unrelated diseases may contribute to pruritus and the control of one disease does not mean that other causes cannot remain.
- Multiple etiologies such as *Malassezia* dermatitis, flea bite allergy, atopic dermatitis, and pyoderma are commonly present in a single patient. Elimination of these may not be enough to significantly reduce the pruritus. Animals with both food allergy and atopic disease may do well during the winter season with a hypoallergenic diet only to become pruritic during the warmer months in association with atopic dermatitis.
- Patients receiving chronic medication should be evaluated every 3–12 months for potential side effects as well as the occurrence of new contributing factors.

POSSIBLE COMPLICATIONS

- Skin scrapes and other tests that may have been negative or normal during the original workup should be repeated if symptoms return.
- Complications and/or gradual loss of efficacy are not uncommon with chronic medical therapy.

MISCELLANEOUS

ABBREVIATIONS

- ASIT = allergen-specific immunotherapy solution.

Suggested Reading

Gram WD. Pruritus, atopic dermatitis and pyoderma. In: Gram WD, Milner R, Lobetti R, eds., Chronic Disease Management For Small Animals. Hoboken, NJ: Wiley-Blackwell, 2018, pp. 25–38.

Olivry T, DeBoer DJ, Favrot C, et al. Treatment of canine atopic dermatitis: 2015 updated guidelines from the International Committee on Allergic Diseases of Animals (ICADA). BMC Vet Res 2015, 11:210.

Santoro D. Therapies in canine atopic dermatitis: an update. Vet Clin North Am Small Anim Pract. 2019, 49(1):9–26.

Authors W. Dunbar Gram and Domenico Santoro

Consulting Editor Alexander H. Werner Resnick

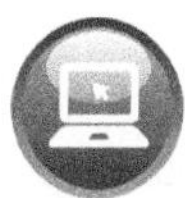

Client Education Handout available online

PSEUDOEPHEDRINE/PHENYLEPHRINE TOXICOSIS

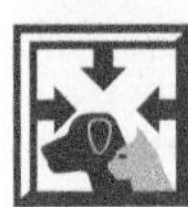

BASICS

OVERVIEW

- Syndrome resulting from exposure to excessive levels of pseudoephedrine or phenylephrine.
- Present in various concentrations in a variety of over-the-counter (OTC) cold and allergy products.

SIGNALMENT

Any species may be affected, but dogs are most commonly involved in accidental overdoses.

SIGNS

- Mydriasis, panting, hyperthermia, agitation/hyperactivity, tachycardia, hypertension are common. Other signs include vomiting, vocalization, tremors, disorientation, or lethargy.
- Head-bobbing, sinus arrhythmias, scleral hemorrhage, or seizure-like activity are possible. Acute collapse may follow.
- Signs of acute intoxication may persist 1–3 days, depending on dose ingested.
- Severe cases may progress to disseminated intravascular coagulation (DIC), myoglobinuremia/uria with secondary renal injury, or permanent CNS dysfunction.

CAUSES & RISK FACTORS

- Pseudoephedrine is a synthetic salt of ephedrine and is an indirect sympathomimetic amine.
- Phenylephrine is a synthetic sympathomimetic amine chemically related to ephedrine and pseudoephedrine. Phenylephrine has poor oral bioavailability and generally will have less severe cardiovascular effects than pseudoephedrine.
- Pseudoephedrine indirectly stimulates alpha- and, to a lesser degree, beta-adrenergic receptors.
- Pseudoephedrine dosages >1 mg/kg can result in agitation, hyperactivity, and panting.
- Phenylephrine dosages >3–4 mg/kg may cause vomiting, lethargy or hyperactivity, hypertension, and tachycardia.
- Head-bobbing, DIC, or myoglobinuria indicate serious intoxication and a more guarded prognosis.

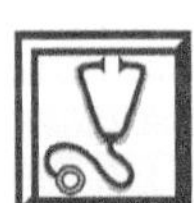

DIAGNOSIS

DIFFERENTIAL DIAGNOSIS

Other CNS stimulants and sympathomimetics—amphetamines, cocaine, serotonergic antidepressants, phenylpropanolamine, methylxanthines, ephedra.

CBC/BIOCHEMISTRY/URINALYSIS

- No specific clinical pathology alterations are expected in most cases.
- In severe cases DIC, myoglobinemia, myoglobinuria, or azotemia may occur.

OTHER LABORATORY TESTS

Urine or serum from patients with pseudoephedrine toxicosis may give a positive test for amphetamine in OTC drug test kits or human hospital drug screens.

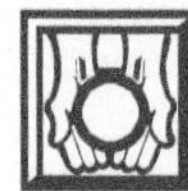

TREATMENT

- Manage severe or life-threatening signs first.
- Control CNS stimulation, then manage cardiovascular (CV) stimulation, as blood pressure and heart rate may decrease significantly once CNS signs are managed.
- For seizures, use propofol, pentobarbital, or phenobarbital; consider gas anesthetic for refractory cases.
- For agitation, hyperactivity, or other CNS stimulation, use acepromazine or chlorpromazine.
- Cyproheptadine has been used with some success to manage dysphoria, vocalization, and hyperthermia.
- Propranolol (or other beta-blocker) may be considered in patients with sustained tachycardia.
- External cooling measures may be required for hyperthermic patients.
- IV fluid administration assists in stabilization of CV effects, support of kidney function, and excretion of pseudoephedrine and its metabolites.
- Monitor heart rate/rhythm, body temperature, and blood pressure. In severely affected patients, monitor renal function, coagulation parameters, hydration, and electrolytes.
- Gastrointestinal decontamination (induction of emesis, administration of activated charcoal) may be considered in patients that have ingested >1 mg/kg of pseudoephedrine and are not displaying significant clinical signs.

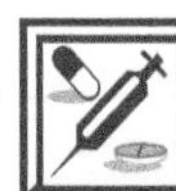

MEDICATIONS

DRUG(S) OF CHOICE

- Propofol 0.1–0.6 mg/kg/min IV.
- Pentobarbital 30 mg/kg IV to effect.
- Phenobarbital 3–4 mg/kg IV.
- Acepromazine 0.05–1.0 mg/kg IM or IV; start low and titrate up as needed.
- Chlorpromazine 0.5–1.0 mg/kg IV or IM; start low and titrate up as needed.
- Cyproheptadine 1.1 mg/kg PO or per rectum q6h (dogs); 2–4 mg PO or per rectum (cats).
- Propranolol 0.02–0.06 mg/kg IV q6–8h PRN.
- Emetics—Dogs: 3% hydrogen peroxide 2.2 mL/kg PO, maximum 45 mL, may repeat once if first dose unsuccessful; apomorphine crushed and diluted with sterile saline and instilled in conjunctival sac, rinse eye after emesis, or 0.03 mg/kg IV; ropinirole hydrochloride 3.75 mg/m^2 as directed by product label. Cats: dexmedetomidine 6–18 µg/kg IM; xylazine 0.44 mg/kg IM; hydromorphone 0.1 mg/kg SC.
- Activated charcoal 1–3 g/kg suspended in 50–200 mL of water.

CONTRAINDICATIONS/POSSIBLE INTERACTIONS

The use of diazepam to control CNS stimulation should be avoided, as diazepam may induce a dysphoric effect in these patients and worsen the CNS excitation.

FOLLOW-UP

Renal insufficiency resulting from myoglobinuria may require long-term follow-up and care.

MISCELLANEOUS

ABBREVIATIONS

- CV = cardiovascular.
- DIC = disseminated intravascular coagulation.
- OTC = over-the-counter.

Suggested Reading

Means C. Dietary supplements and herbs. In: Poppenga RH, Gwaltney-Brant SM, eds. Small Animal Toxicology Essentials. Chichester: Wiley-Blackwell, 2011, pp. 161–169.

Means C. Ma huang: all natural but not always innocuous. Vet Med 1999, 94:511–512.

Author Sharon Gwaltney-Brant
Consulting Editor Lynn R. Hovda

PSEUDOMACROTHROMBOCYTOPENIA (INHERITED MACROTHROMBOCYTOPENIA)

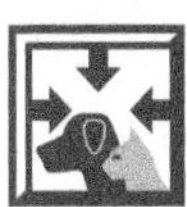

BASICS

OVERVIEW

- A common cause of thrombocytopenia and increased mean platelet volume (MPV) in cavalier King Charles spaniels (CKCS), and infrequently in other breeds.
- Caused by an inherited mutation that impairs platelet maturation, resulting in the early release of platelets from the bone marrow. The released platelets are significantly larger than normal.
- Overall platelet mass (product of platelet number and average size) is unaffected, therefore clinical signs of hypocoagulability are not seen.

SIGNALMENT

- Dogs—primarily CKCS with infrequent reports in Norfolk terriers, Cairn terriers, English toy spaniels, and Jack Russell terriers; other breeds also sporadically affected.
- A similar condition is also reported in Akitas, although a specific mutation has not yet been identified in this breed.
- The condition is present from birth, but is often not detected until a CBC is performed. The mutation is autosomal, therefore there is no sex predilection.

SIGNS

Not associated with clinical signs; often incidentally noted on a CBC performed for other reasons.

CAUSES & RISK FACTORS

- Caused by point mutations in the gene encoding β1-tubulin, which is involved in platelet formation. The mutations impair the formation of microtubules in the megakaryocyte (platelet precursor) and result in the release of lower numbers of platelets that are larger than normal.
- The condition is inherited in an autosomal fashion, with homozygotes exhibiting moderate to marked thrombocytopenia and moderate to marked increases in MPV. Heterozygotes are less severely affected and may have a mild thrombocytopenia and/or mild increase in MPV.
- In the United States, it has been estimated that approximately 47% of CKCS are homozygous for the mutation and 45% are heterozygous.

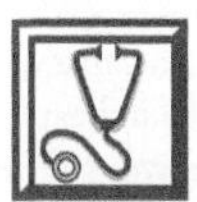

DIAGNOSIS

DIFFERENTIAL DIAGNOSIS

- Must be differentiated from causes of pathologic thrombocytopenia such as immune-mediated thrombocytopenia, disseminated intravascular coagulation, infectious diseases (especially tick-borne diseases), and causes of decreased platelet production (i.e., bone marrow disease).
- Breed (especially CKCS), absence of clinical signs, and a normal plateletcrit (PCT) (see CBC/Biochemistry/Urinalysis) are strongly suggestive of inherited macrothrombocytopenia.
- Blood smear evaluation is also recommended to rule out *in vitro* platelet clumping, which artifactually induces a decreased platelet count and increased MPV.

CBC/BIOCHEMISTRY/URINALYSIS

- CBC—moderate to marked thrombocytopenia (40,000–200,000/μL) with significantly increased MPV; PCT expected to be within reference interval (RI = 0.129–0.403%).
- PCT—a numeric representation of overall platelet mass (product of platelet number and average size). Some automated analyzers calculate the value automatically. If not provided, PCT can be calculated using the following formula:

$$PCT = (PLT \times MPV)/10,000$$

where PLT is platelet count and MPV is mean platelet volume.

OTHER LABORATORY TESTS

If definitive diagnosis is desired, genetic testing to confirm the presence of the mutation can be performed; currently, this is available through the Auburn University Hemostasis Laboratory.

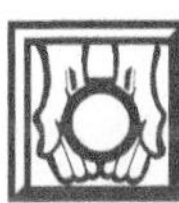

TREATMENT

None required—nonpathogenic condition without clinical signs.

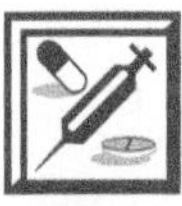

MEDICATIONS

N/A

FOLLOW-UP

Once affected individuals are identified, platelet mass in these patients should be evaluated via PCT; if this value falls below the reference interval, a concurrent pathologic thrombocytopenia may be present.

MISCELLANEOUS

ABBREVIATIONS

- CKCS = cavalier King Charles spaniel.
- MPV = mean platelet volume.
- PCT = plateletcrit.
- PLT = platelet count.

INTERNET RESOURCES

https://www.vetmed.auburn.edu/academic-departments/dept-of-pathobiology/diagnostic-services/

Suggested Reading

Davis B, Toivio-Kinnucan M, Schuller S, Boudreaux MK. Mutation in beta1-tubulin correlates with macrothrombocytopenia in Cavalier King Charles Spaniels. J Vet Intern Med 2008, 22:540–545.

Author Megan N. Caudill
Consulting Editor Melinda S. Camus

P

PTYALISM

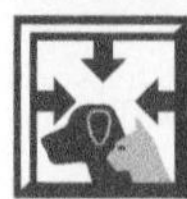

BASICS

DEFINITION

• Excessive production and secretion of saliva (see Web Figure 1). • Pseudoptyalism is the excessive release of saliva that has accumulated in the oral cavity due to inability to swallow.

PATHOPHYSIOLOGY

• Saliva is constantly produced and secreted into the oral cavity from the salivary glands. • Saliva production increases when salivary nuclei in the brainstem are stimulated. • Higher centers in the CNS can excite or inhibit salivary nuclei. • Taste and tactile stimuli in the oral cavity increase saliva production. • Physiologic hypersalivation may occur with: anticipation of eating, hyperthermia and purring (cats). • Saliva production may be increased with gastrointestinal (GI) or CNS disorders.

SYSTEMS AFFECTED

Skin—may cause salivary staining.

GENETICS

N/A

INCIDENCE/PREVALENCE

Variable

GEOGRAPHIC DISTRIBUTION

Worldwide

SIGNALMENT

Species

Dog and cat.

Breed Predilections

• Congenital portosystemic shunts—Yorkshire terrier, Maltese, Australian cattle dog, miniature schnauzer, and Irish wolfhound. • Congenital megaesophagus—wirehaired fox terrier and miniature schnauzer; familial predispositions have been reported in German shepherd dog, Newfoundland, Great Dane, Irish setter, Chinese Shar-Pei, greyhound, retriever breeds, and Siamese cats. • Congenital hiatal hernia—Chinese Shar-Pei. • Lip conformation—giant breeds, such as Saint Bernard, Great Dane, and mastiff.
• Brachycephalic airway syndrome—pug, English and French bulldog.

Mean Age and Range

Young animals are more likely to have congenital abnormalities and to ingest foreign materials.

SIGNS

Historical Findings

• Anorexia—with oral lesions, GI disease, and systemic disease. • Eating behavior changes—with oral disease or cranial nerve (CN) dysfunction: may refuse hard food, chew only on the unaffected side (if unilateral lesion), maintain an unusual head/neck position, or drop food. • Other behavioral changes—irritability, aggressiveness, and reclusiveness, especially if painful. • Dysphagia. • Nausea.
• Regurgitation—with esophageal disease.
• Vomiting—with GI or systemic disease.
• Weight loss. • Pawing at the face or muzzle—with oral discomfort. • Neurologic signs—with exposure to caustic drugs or toxins, hepatic encephalopathy, seizure disorders or other intracranial disease.

Physical Examination Findings

• Periodontal disease. • Gingivitis/stomatitis—with toxins, infection, immune-mediated disease or nutritional deficiency. • Oral mass
• Glossitis—with ulceration, mass or foreign body. • Oropharyngeal inflammation, ulceration, mass, or foreign body. • Blood in the saliva—with bleeding from the oral cavity, pharynx, or esophagus. • Halitosis—with oral disease (most common), or esophageal and gastric disease. • Facial pain. • Dysphagia.
• CN deficits—trigeminal nerve (CN V) lesions can cause drooling due to inability to close the mouth; facial nerve palsy (CN VII) can cause drooling from the affected side; glossopharyngeal (CN IX), vagus (CN X), and hypoglossal (CN XII) nerve lesions can cause a loss of the gag reflex or inability to swallow. • Cheilitis or acne—persistent drooling can lead to dermatologic lesions.

CAUSES

Conformational Disorder of the Lips

Most common in giant-breed dogs.

Oral and Pharyngeal

• Oral trauma. • Foreign body (e.g., stick, foxtail, or sewing needle). • Neoplasm.
• Abscess. • Gingivitis or stomatitis—secondary to periodontal disease, bacterial, viral (e.g., feline leukemia virus [FeLV] or feline immunodeficiency virus [FIV]) or fungal infection, immune-mediated disease (e.g., lymphoplasmacytic stomatitis, pemphigus vulgaris), uremia, ingestion of a caustic agent, poisonous plants, effects of radiation therapy to the oral cavity or burns (e.g., biting on an electrical cord). • Swallowing disorders.

Salivary Gland

• Sialoadenitis. • Sialolithiasis. • Sialadenosis (idiopathic enlargement). • Mucocele.
• Fistula. • Foreign body. • Neoplasm.
• Infarct. • Immune-mediated disease (rare).

Esophageal or GI

• Esophageal foreign body. • Esophageal neoplasm. • Esophageal stricture.
• Esophagitis. • Gastroesophageal reflux disease (GERD). • Infection (e.g., spirocercosis, pythosis). • Hiatal hernia.
• Megaesophagus. • Esophageal dysmotility.
• Gastric distension/volvulus. • Gastric ulcer.
• Gastroenteritis.

Metabolic

• Hepatic encephalopathy (especially in cats).
• Hyperthermia. • Uremia.

Neurologic

• Rabies—decreased swallowing causes increased drooling. • Pseudorabies in dogs.
• Botulism. • Tetanus. • Dysautonomia.
• Disorders causing dysphagia. • Disorders causing facial nerve palsy or a dropped jaw.
• Seizures—during a seizure, ptyalism may occur because of autonomic discharge or reduced swallowing of saliva, and may be exacerbated by chomping of the jaws. • Nausea associated with vestibular disease. • Anxiety.

Drugs and Toxins

• Caustic substances (e.g., household cleaning products). • Anesthesia may induce reflux esophagitis. Drugs used for premedication may induce nausea, vomiting or ptyalism. • Oral, otic or ophthalmic medications that are poorly palatable (especially in cats). • Those that induce hypersalivation, including organophosphate compounds, cholinergic drugs, insecticides containing boric acid, pyrethrin and pyrethroid insecticides, ivermectin (dogs), fluids containing benzoic acid derivatives (cats), clozapine (a tricyclic dibenzodiazepine), caffeine, and illicit drugs such as amphetamines, cocaine, and opiates. Has also been reported with capromorelin administration in dogs and cats. • Animal venom (e.g., black widow spider, Gila monster, and North American scorpion). • Toad and newt secretions. • Plant consumption or prehension (e.g., poinsettia, Christmas trees, *Amanita* mushrooms) may cause increased salivation.

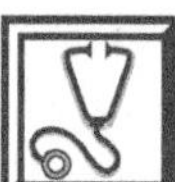

DIAGNOSIS

DIFFERENTIAL DIAGNOSIS

• Differentiating causes of ptyalism and pseudoptyalism requires a thorough history, including vaccination status, current medications, possible toxin exposure, and duration of ptyalism.
• May be able to distinguish salivation associated with nausea (signs of depression, lip smacking, and retching) from dysphagia by observing the patient. • Complete physical examination (with special attention to the oral cavity and neck) and neurologic examination are critical; wear examination gloves when rabies exposure is possible.

CBC/BIOCHEMISTRY/URINALYSIS

• CBC—often unremarkable; leukocytosis in patients with immune-mediated, inflammatory or infectious disease. • Stress leukogram—common in animals that have ingested a caustic agent or organophosphate. • FeLV-infected cats may have leukopenia and nonregenerative anemia. • Serum creatine kinase activity should be evaluated in all dysphagic patients. • Possible microcytosis with portosystemic shunts.
• Biochemical analysis—usually unremarkable except in patients with renal disease (azotemia, hyperphosphatemia), and hepatic encephalopathy (possibly elevated hepatic enzyme activities, decreased BUN, hypoalbuminemia,

hypocholesterolemia, hyperbilirubinemia, and hypoglycemia). • Marked ptyalism can result in hypokalemia and acidosis from the loss of potassium and bicarbonate-rich saliva.
• Urinalysis—often normal; decreased urine specific gravity with renal or hepatic disease.
• Urate urolithiasis may be noted in patients with portosystemic shunts.

OTHER LABORATORY TESTS

• Fasting and postprandial bile acids and/or fasting ammonia when hepatic encephalopathy is suspected. • Serologic FeLV and FIV testing in cats with oral lesions. • Acetylcholine receptor antibody titer if focal myasthenia gravis is suspected. • Serum cholinesterase level if organophosphate toxicosis is suspected.
• Post-mortem fluorescent antibody testing of brain tissue if rabies is suspected.

IMAGING

• Survey radiography of the oral cavity, neck, and thorax when foreign body, structural abnormality, or neoplasm is suspected.
• Abdominal radiographs ± abdominal ultrasound may help diagnose cause of vomiting; may also help diagnose hepatic or renal disease. • Ultrasonographic evaluation, CT angiography, portal venography, or portal scintigraphy may help diagnose a portosystemic shunt. • Fluoroscopic evaluation of swallowing may be useful in dysphagic patients to evaluate esophageal function and motility; use caution during barium administration in animals that are dysphagic. • MRI or CT for suspected intracranial lesions. • CT of head is more sensitive than radiographs, especially when foreign body or neoplasia is suspected.

DIAGNOSTIC PROCEDURES

• Biopsy and histopathology of mucocutaneous lesions—possibly including immunofluorescence testing when immune-mediated disease (e.g., pemphigus vulgaris) is suspected. • Fine-needle aspiration of oral lesions and regional lymph nodes. • Biopsy and histopathology of oral lesion, salivary gland, or mass. • Consider esophagoscopy or gastroscopy if lesions distal to the oral cavity are suspected; endoscopic removal of foreign bodies may be possible.

PATHOLOGIC FINDINGS

Varies as to the underlying condition.

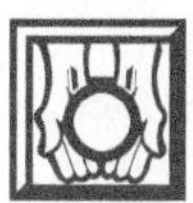

TREATMENT

APPROPRIATE HEALTH CARE

• Treat the underlying cause (refer to sections pertaining to specific conditions).
• Symptomatic treatment to reduce the flow of saliva—generally unnecessary, may be of little value to the patient, and may mask other signs of the underlying cause and thus delay diagnosis; only recommended when hypersalivation is prolonged and severe and, if possible, after the underlying condition has been diagnosed.

NURSING CARE

• Petroleum jelly can be applied to areas of the face constantly wet from saliva to help prevent moist dermatitis. • Astringent solutions applied for 10 minutes q8–12h can be used to treat areas of moist dermatitis.

ACTIVITY

N/A

DIET

• Enteral nutritional support (esophagostomy, gastrostomy tubes, etc.) may be needed in patients with ptyalism and anorexia secondary to severe oral, GI, or metabolic causes. • Reduced protein diets may be recommended for patients with hepatic encephalopathy, but are not necessarily warranted in animals with portosystemic shunts that are not encephalopathic.

CLIENT EDUCATION

Client education will depend on the underlying disease process.

SURGICAL CONSIDERATIONS

• Surgical procedures will vary depending on underlying cause; ligation of parotid salivary duct has been described. • Corrective surgery for brachycephalic airway surgery may result in improved GI signs.

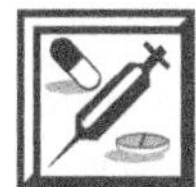

MEDICATIONS

DRUG(S) OF CHOICE

• Anticholinergic medications may be given symptomatically to reduce the flow of saliva; atropine 0.05 mg/kg SC PRN or glycopyrrolate 0.01 mg/kg SC PRN. However, this is typically unnecessary as treatment should focus on underlying disease. • Antiemetics for nausea (see Acute Vomiting, for list of antiemetics and dosages). • Crystalloid fluids may be given IV or SC to treat dehydration caused by prolonged or severe ptyalism. • Antacid therapy may be useful for treatment of GERD (e.g., proton pump inhibitors—omeprazole 1 mg/kg PO q12h). • Phenobarbital 2 mg/kg PO q12h has been effective in treating idiopathic hypersialosis. • Anticonvulsant therapy is indicated for seizure activity.

CONTRAINDICATIONS

N/A

PRECAUTIONS

Depends on underlying cause.

ALTERNATIVE DRUG(S)

• Some clinicians have anecdotally used levetiracetam for idiopathic hypersialosis.
• Other acid-reducing agents may be used.

FOLLOW-UP

PATIENT MONITORING

• Depends on the underlying cause.
• Continually monitor hydration, body weight, serum electrolytes, and nutritional status, especially in dysphagic or anorexic animals.

PREVENTION/AVOIDANCE

Depends on underlying cause.

POSSIBLE COMPLICATIONS

• Metabolic acidosis. • Dehydration.
• Hypokalemia. • Moist dermatitis.
• Aspiration pneumonia.

EXPECTED COURSE AND PROGNOSIS

Depends on underlying cause. If underlying cause is correctable, prognosis for resolution may be more favorable.

MISCELLANEOUS

ASSOCIATED CONDITIONS

N/A

ZOONOTIC POTENTIAL

Rabies

PREGNANCY/FERTILITY/BREEDING

N/A

SYNONYMS

• Drooling. • Hypersalivation. • Sialism.
• Sialorrhea. • Sialosis.

SEE ALSO

• Dysphagia. • Esophagitis. • Hepatic Encephalopathy. • Megaesophagus.
• Periodontal Disease. • Stomatitis and Oral Ulceration.

ABBREVIATIONS

• CN = cranial nerve. • FeLV = feline leukemia virus. • FIV = feline immunodeficiency virus.
• GERD = gastroesophageal reflux disease.
• GI = gastrointestinal.

Suggested Reading

Claude AK, Dedeaux A, Chiavaccini L, Hinz S. Effects of maropitant citrate or acepromazine on the incidence of adverse effects associated with hydromorphone premedication in dogs. J Vet Intern Med 2014, 8:1414–1417.

Kaye BM, Rutherford L, Perridge DJ, Haar GT. Relationship between brachycephalic airway syndrome and gastrointestinal signs in three breeds of dog. J Small Anim Pract 2018, 59:670–673.

Niemiec BA. Ptyalism. In: Ettinger SJ, Feldman EC, eds., Textbook of Veterinary Internal Medicine, 7th ed. St. Louis, MO: Elsevier, 2010, pp. 185–188.

van der Merwe LL, Christie J, Clift SJ, Dvir E. Salivary gland enlargement and sialorrhoea in dogs with spirocercosis: a retrospective and prospective study of 298 cases. J S Afr Vet Assoc 2012, 83(1):920.

Author Valerie J. Parker
Consulting Editor Mark P. Rondeau

PULMONARY CONTUSIONS

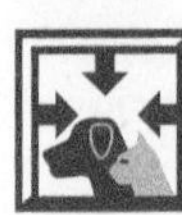

BASICS

OVERVIEW

• Hemorrhage in the lung parenchyma caused by tearing and crushing from direct thoracic trauma. • Relatively small volumes of blood in the parenchyma markedly compromise lung function. • Fluid resuscitation for treatment of shock can exacerbate lung dysfunction from secondary edema.

SIGNALMENT

Dog and cat.

SIGNS

• History of trauma. • Tachypnea.
• Abnormal respiratory effort. • Postural adaptations to respiratory distress. • Cyanotic or pale mucous membranes. • Auscultation of harsh bronchovesicular sounds or crackles.
• Expectoration of blood or blood-tinged fluid. • Additional injuries secondary to trauma and shock can also be noted.

P

CAUSES & RISK FACTORS

• Blunt trauma. • Motor vehicle accidents.
• Falls from a height. • Abuse.

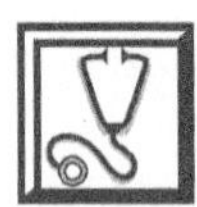

DIAGNOSIS

DIFFERENTIAL DIAGNOSIS

• Hemothorax—auscult dull lung sounds ventrally. • Pneumothorax—auscult dull lung sounds dorsally. • Diaphragmatic hernia—distinguished radiographically.
• Coagulopathy can result in pulmonary hemorrhage; identified by abnormal coagulation tests or platelet count. • Acute onset of pulmonary hemorrhage—can be seen with neoplasia or pulmonary infarction from bacterial endocarditis or heartworm disease.
• Expectoration of bloody fluid (not frank hemorrhage) can occur in animals with acute respiratory distress syndrome (ARDS) or congestive heart failure. • If no known history of trauma, pneumonia or edema (cardiogenic and noncardiogenic) are possible differentials.

CBC/BIOCHEMISTRY/URINALYSIS

• CBC—can reveal anemia or mature neutrophilia. • Biochemistry profile—can demonstrate hypoproteinemia (blood loss); can reveal damage to other organ systems.

IMAGING

Thoracic Radiography

• Usually a patchy alveolar pattern—focal or asymmetrical, but can be generalized.
• Contusions generally worse in the area of rib fractures if present. • Always perform thoracic radiographs in trauma patients after stabilization to rule out hemothorax, pneumothorax, and diaphragmatic hernia.

Thoracic Focused Assessment with Sonography for Trauma (TFAST®) and Focused Lung Ultrasound

• Point-of-care emergency ultrasound helps identify intrathoracic trauma during initial triage.
• Increased lung rockets (B-lines) indicative of contusions or edema. • Absence of a glide sign dorsally indicative of pneumothorax. • Pleural effusion noted indicative of hemothorax.

DIAGNOSTIC PROCEDURES

• Coagulation tests for coagulopathy or disseminated intravascular coagulation. • Pulse oximetry or arterial blood gas analysis—can confirm hypoxemia. • Examination of tracheal wash cytology—can show excessive numbers of erythrocytes and macrophages.

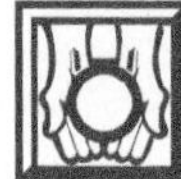

TREATMENT

• Usually inpatient for stabilization. • Support respiratory function, stabilize cardiovascular function. • If pneumothorax suspected, thoracocentesis should be performed. • Assess and treat injuries to other organ systems. • Restrict activity, minimize stress, and monitor carefully for deterioration. • Respiratory support—oxygen supplementation for hypoxemia; intubation and positive-pressure ventilation if severe. • Shock—fluids generally required; judicious fluid therapy to avoid exacerbation of pulmonary edema. • Blood or plasma transfusion—consider if anemia or coagulopathy. • Nutritional support—as needed to maintain body condition and immune status.

MEDICATIONS

DRUG(S) OF CHOICE

• Oxygen supplementation if dyspnea or hypoxemia. • Analgesics administered as warranted. • Low-dose diuretics—contraindicated unless suspected volume overload and respiratory distress is severe.

CONTRAINDICATIONS/POSSIBLE INTERACTIONS

Diuretics—no value in the early stages of pulmonary contusions and potentially harmful; decrease intravascular volume, which is contraindicated for shock.

FOLLOW-UP

PATIENT MONITORING

• Monitor respiratory rate and effort, mucous membrane color, heart rate, pulse quality, and lung sounds. • Measure serial packed cell volume (PCV) and total solids and perform pulse oximetry and/or arterial blood gas analysis as needed for the first 24 hours. • Monitor ECG frequently to detect ventricular arrhythmias associated with hypoxemia or traumatic myocarditis.
• Radiographs—repeated if clinically indicated.

PREVENTION/AVOIDANCE

Appropriate restriction of the animal to prevent trauma.

POSSIBLE COMPLICATIONS

• Bacterial pneumonia (uncommon)—owing to systemic immunosuppression from trauma, shock, and reduced pulmonary defenses.
• Development of a moist productive cough and failure to improve within 48 hours—suspect pneumonia. • Patients with severe shock can develop ARDS (less common).

EXPECTED COURSE AND PROGNOSIS

• Respiratory function can deteriorate during the initial 12–24 hours and then should gradually improve. • Clinical improvement within 48 hours with radiographic resolution likely in 7–10 days. • If patient fails to improve clinically after 48 hours, evaluate for complications or concurrent disease.

MISCELLANEOUS

ASSOCIATED CONDITIONS

• Pneumothorax. • Fractured ribs. • Flail chest. • Ruptured trachea, bronchi, or esophagus. • Cardiac arrhythmias—ventricular.
• Other possible complications of trauma.

SEE ALSO

Pneumothorax

ABBREVIATIONS

• ARDS = acute respiratory distress syndrome. • PCV = packed cell volume.
• TFAST® = Thoracic Focused Assessment with Sonography for Trauma.

Suggested Reading

Boysen SR, Lisciandro GR. The use of ultrasound for dogs and cats in the emergency room: AFAST and TFAST. Vet Clin North Am Small Anim Pract 2013, 43(4):773–797.

Campbell VL, King LG. Pulmonary function, ventilator management and outcome of dogs with thoracic trauma and pulmonary contusions: 10 cases (1994–1998). J Am Vet Med Assoc 2000, 217:1505–1509.

Holowaychuk MK, Marks SL, Hansen BG, DeFrancesco T. Pulmonary contusions. Stand Care Emerg Crit Care Med 2006, 8(10):1–6.

Powell LL, Rozanski EA, Tidwell AS, Rush JE. A retrospective analysis of pulmonary contusion secondary to motor vehicular accidents in 143 dogs: 1994–1997. J Vet Emerg Crit Care 1999, 9:127–136.

Vnuk D, Pirkic B, Maticic D, et al. Feline high-rise syndrome: 119 cases (1998–2001). J Feline Med Surg 2004, 6:5, 305–312.

Author Cassandra O. Janson

Consulting Editor Elizabeth Rozanski

Acknowledgment The author and editors acknowledge the prior contribution of Lesley G. King.

PULMONARY EDEMA, NONCARDIOGENIC

BASICS

DEFINITION

Accumulation of edema fluid in the pulmonary interstitium and alveoli, in the absence of heart disease.

PATHOPHYSIOLOGY

• Associated with increased pulmonary vascular permeability and leakage of fluid into the interstitium and alveoli; if severe, can be accompanied by an inflammatory response and accumulation of neutrophils and macrophages. • Several mechanisms contribute to changes in pulmonary vascular permeability. • Stimulation of brainstem (medulla) vasomotor centers can lead to a reflex systemic release of catecholamines resulting in systemic vasoconstriction and temporary shunting of blood into the pulmonary circulation resulting in transient pulmonary circulatory overload and endothelial damage—likely pathogenesis in patients with neurogenic edema, electrocution, and upper airway obstruction. • In patients with upper airway obstruction, negative intrathoracic pressure from inspiratory attempts against an airway obstruction also contributes to edema formation. • Increased vascular permeability can be part of a generalized inflammatory response that develops in patients with systemic inflammatory response syndrome (SIRS), sepsis, or pancreatitis. • The inciting insult can trigger a cascade inflammatory response that often worsens over 24 hours following the initial episode. • Severity of clinical manifestation varies, ranging from mild to severe; the most seriously affected patients can progress from normal to death rapidly after the incident.

SYSTEMS AFFECTED

• Respiratory. • Cardiovascular—hypotension, tachycardia, and shock. • Hemic/lymphatic/immune—if severe and causing respiratory failure, can be associated with disseminated intravascular coagulation (DIC). • Renal/urologic—acute renal failure.

GENETICS

Unknown

INCIDENCE/PREVALENCE

Uncommon

SIGNALMENT

Species

Dog and cat.

Breed Predilections

None specific; brachycephalic dogs are more prone to airway obstruction, older large-breed dogs—laryngeal paralysis, small-breed dogs—tracheal collapse.

Mean Age and Range

• Higher incidence in pediatrics—associated with strangulation, head trauma, and electric cord bites. • Older—associated with laryngeal obstruction and neoplasia.

SIGNS

General Comments

Vary, depending on underlying cause and severity.

Historical Findings

• Predisposing causes—airway obstruction; electric cord bite; seizures; head trauma; near drowning; smoke exposure; adverse drug effects. • Acute onset of dyspnea.

Physical Examination Findings

• Mild to severe dyspnea. • Increased respiratory rate and effort; open-mouthed breathing. • Postural adaptations to respiratory distress (if severe)- orthopnea, unwillingness to lie down. • Pale or cyanotic mucous membranes (severe). • Harsh lung sounds (early, mild) or generalized crackles (late, severe) on auscultation. • Expectoration of pink froth or bubbles; can have large volumes of bloody fluid flowing out of endotracheal tube in severely affected intubated animals. • Normal cardiac auscultation; can detect arrhythmias; tachycardia common. • Oral ulceration or burns if electrocution. • Cranial nervous system abnormalities or other indications of neurologic disease. • Stridor over the upper airway in cases of brachycephalic syndrome, airway masses/abscesses, or foreign bodies. • Smokey odor or burns indicative of smoke exposure.

CAUSES

• Upper airway obstruction—laryngeal paralysis; choke-chain injury; mass; abscess. • Electrocution. • Acute neurologic disease—head trauma; intra-cranial hypertension, prolonged seizures. • Smoke inhalation. • Aspiration pneumonia. • Systemic inflammatory response syndrome—sepsis; endotoxemia; pancreatitis. • Anaphylaxis (cats). • Near drowning. • Adverse drug reactions including certain anesthetic drugs (ketamine), thiazides, or certain antineoplastics (vincristine, cisplatin in cats). • Transfusion-related acute lung injury—limited evidence in veterinary medicine. • Vasculitis.

RISK FACTORS

• Hypoproteinemia. • Crystalloid fluid resuscitation.

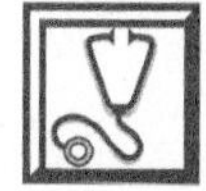

DIAGNOSIS

DIFFERENTIAL DIAGNOSIS

• Cardiogenic pulmonary edema. • Pulmonary infection—bacterial, viral, or fungal pneumonia. • Pulmonary neoplasia. • Pulmonary hemorrhage (e.g., anticoagulant rodenticide exposure). • Pulmonary thromboembolism.

CBC/BIOCHEMISTRY/URINALYSIS

• Leukocytosis common, leukopenia and thrombocytopenia possible due to neutrophil sequestration in the lung and platelet consumption. • Biochemistries—usually normal; may note hypoalbuminemia owing to pulmonary protein loss; mild stress-related hyperglycemia. • Urinalysis—usually normal.

OTHER LABORATORY TESTS

Coagulation testing—mild to moderate prolongation of prothrombin time/partial thromboplastin time (PT/PTT) in animals with consumption and DIC. Severe coagulopathy may indicate hemorrhage as true cause for respiratory signs.

IMAGING

• Thoracic radiographs—vital; can reveal prominent interstitial pattern with mild or early disease; alveolar infiltrates with moderate or severe disease; infiltrates commonly but not always in dorsocaudal lung, sometimes asymmetrical and predominantly right-sided. Cardiac silhouette generally normal. • Echocardiography—rule out cardiogenic pulmonary edema. • Point-of-care thoracic ultrasound—increased lung rockets (B-lines) may indicate pulmonary edema, increased left atrial:aortic ratio more indicative of cardiogenic edema and underlying heart disease.

DIAGNOSTIC PROCEDURES

• Cytology of airway fluid—inflammatory: neutrophils and some alveolar macrophages. Fluid tends to have high protein values >3 g/dL. Culture negative unless concurrent bacterial pneumonia. • Edema fluid to plasma ratio (EF:PL) compares protein in the edema fluid to plasma protein. An increased ratio (>0.65) is indicative of noncardiogenic pulmonary edema. • Pulse oximetry—noninvasive, continuous monitoring of arterial hemoglobin saturation with oxygen and arterial blood gas analysis. Demonstrates mild to severe hypoxemia and hypocapnia; not specific but indicates the severity of pulmonary dysfunction. • B-type natriuretic peptide (NT-proBNP) testing in cats and dogs can suggest underlying heart disease and supports a diagnosis of cardiogenic edema.

PATHOLOGIC FINDINGS

• Gross—lungs usually heavy, red, or congested; fail to collapse; often exhibit a wet cut surface; can ooze foam from major airways. • Histopathology—depends on severity of the insult; early, mild: may note eosinophilic amorphous material filling the alveoli or can be near normal because fluid removed in processing; severe: alveolar hyaline membranes, alveolitis, and interstitial inflammatory infiltrates with neutrophils and macrophages evident and

PULMONARY EDEMA, NONCARDIOGENIC (CONTINUED)

accompanied by atelectasis, vascular congestion, and hemorrhage; lesions can be found within hours of a severe insult.

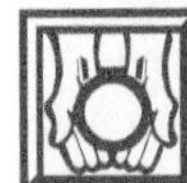

TREATMENT

APPROPRIATE HEALTH CARE

• Inpatient vs. outpatient—depends on the severity of respiratory dysfunction and the underlying cause (e.g., airway obstruction or seizures generally require hospitalization). • Make every effort to resolve and treat the underlying cause. • Mild to moderate—patients generally improve within 24–48 hours; cardiovascular and respiratory support while the lung repairs. • Severe—difficult to treat; usually requires positive-pressure ventilation (PPV) due to respiratory failure; many patients die despite treatment.

NURSING CARE

• Oxygen therapy—vital in moderate to severe disease; administer via mask or hood, nasal catheter, or oxygen cage; inspired oxygen concentration depends on the severity of disease; most patients do well on 40–50% oxygen, but severe disease can require 80–100% to maintain stability. • Severe—can require PPV and positive end-expiratory pressure (PEEP). • Judicious fluid therapy with a balanced electrolyte solution as replacement solution for dehydration or shock; use cautious fluid administration and avoid fluid overload. • Plasma, albumin, or synthetic colloids—consider with severe hypoproteinemia or low colloid osmotic pressure; improved oncotic pressure may minimize movement of fluid into lungs.

ACTIVITY

Exercise restriction and minimal stress to decrease oxygen requirements.

CLIENT EDUCATION

• Warn client that the condition can worsen before improving. • Inform client that severe disease progressing rapidly to fulminant pulmonary edema and respiratory failure is associated with a very poor prognosis.

SURGICAL CONSIDERATIONS

Relevant only for treating the underlying cause.

MEDICATIONS

DRUG(S) OF CHOICE

• Damaged endothelium in the pulmonary vasculature—no specific treatment available. • Inflammatory response—generated by a variety of mediators and cascades; cannot effectively be blocked by anti-inflammatory drugs. • Furosemide—diuresis not indicated as edema due to permeability changes, not high hydrostatic pressure. May act as bronchodilator and decrease pulmonary shunting, though evidence is limited. Can consider cautious boluses (0.5–2 mg/kg IV, IM) or nebulization, particularly early in course of disease. • Corticosteroids—for reduction of airway swelling in patients with upper airway obstruction; generally ineffective for pulmonary inflammatory response; if used, recommend anti-inflammatory dosage (e.g., dexamethasone SP at 0.05–0.1 mg/kg IV). • The use of beta-adrenergic agonists such as terbutaline may increase clearance of alveolar fluid. • Sedatives—use cautiously if anxiety is contributing to respiratory distress or airway obstruction. Sedation can decrease central respiratory drive, contributing to progression of respiratory failure. • Additional therapy as indicated by underlying cause—anticonvulsants, analgesia for oral ulcerations.

PRECAUTIONS

• Diuretics (e.g., furosemide)—can cause dehydration and decrease in intravascular volume, exacerbating cardiovascular collapse or shock with minimal effect on edema. • Corticosteroids—can predispose patients to infectious complications (e.g., pneumonia).

FOLLOW-UP

PATIENT MONITORING

• Monitor respiratory rate, pattern and auscultation (every 2–4 hours) for the first 24–48 hours, depending on severity of disease. • Assess pulmonary function by pulse oximetry or arterial blood gas analysis (initially every 2–4 hours), depending on severity of disease. • Assess packed call volume (PCV) and total solids. Evaluate mucous membranes, pulse quality, heart rate, blood pressure, and urine output every 2–4 hours to assess cardiovascular status and possible progression to shock.

PREVENTION/AVOIDANCE

• Avoid contact with electric wire. • Correct and avoid airway obstruction. • Manage seizures and neurologic disease.

POSSIBLE COMPLICATIONS

Usually none if patient recovers from the acute crisis.

EXPECTED COURSE AND PROGNOSIS

• Mild to moderate—resolution of signs in 24–72 hours with supportive care. • Severe—difficult to treat; can require PPV if respiratory failure. • Overall survival rates—80–90%. • Long-term prognosis—excellent if responsive to therapy.

MISCELLANEOUS

ASSOCIATED CONDITIONS

Acute respiratory distress syndrome.

SYNONYMS

• Acute alveolar failure. • Acute lung injury. • Capillary leak syndrome. • Congestive atelectasis. • Hemorrhagic lung syndrome. • Progressive respiratory distress. • Shock lung. • Traumatic wet lung.

SEE ALSO

Acute Respiratory Distress Syndrome.

ABBREVIATIONS

• DIC = disseminated intravascular coagulation.
• NT-ProBNP = B-type natriuretic peptide.
• PCV = packed cell volume.
• PEEP = positive end-expiratory pressure.
• PPV = positive-pressure ventilation.
• PT = prothrombin time.
• PTT = partial thromboplastin time.
• SIRS = systemic inflammatory response syndrome.

Suggested Reading

Drobatz KJ, Saunders HM, Pugh C, Hendricks JC. Noncardiogenic pulmonary edema: 26 cases (1987–1993). J Am Vet Med Assoc 1995, 206:1732–1736.

Kerr LY. Pulmonary edema secondary to upper airway obstruction in the dog: A review of nine cases. J Am Anim Hosp Assoc 1989, 25:207–212.

Kolata RJ, Burrows CF. The clinical features of injury by chewing electrical cords in dogs and cats. J Am Anim Hosp Assoc 1981,17:219–222.

Rozanski EA, Dhupa N, Rush JR, Murtaugh RJ. Differentiation of the etiology of pulmonary edema by measurement of the protein content. Proc Int Vet Emerg Crit Care Symp VI 1998:844.

Ward JL, Lisciandro GR, Ware WA, Viall AK, et al. Evaluation of point-of-care thoracic ultrasound and NT-proBNP for the diagnosis of congestive heart failure in cats with respiratory distress. J Vet Intern Med 2018, 32:1530–1540.

Author Cassandra O. Janson
Consulting Editors Elizabeth Rozanski
Acknowledgment The author and editors acknowledge the prior contribution of Lesley G. King.

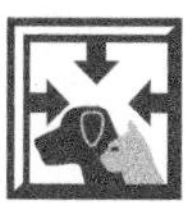

BASICS

DEFINITION

Develops when a thrombus lodges in the pulmonary arterial (PA) tree, occluding blood flow to the portion of lung supplied by that artery.

PATHOPHYSIOLOGY

• Pulmonary thromboembolism (PTE) associated with heartworm disease (HWD) occurs *in situ* in the pulmonary vessels; in most other instances, thrombus origin is unclear.
• Potential sites of origin include right atrium, venae cavae, and jugular, femoral or mesenteric veins; thrombi are carried in the venous circulation to the lungs, and lodge in the pulmonary arteries. • Abnormal blood flow (stasis), vascular endothelial damage, and hypercoagulability are believed to predispose to thrombus formation. • Often a complication of another primary disease process.

SYSTEMS AFFECTED

• Cardiovascular—pulmonary hypertension (PH) may result, leading to right ventricular enlargement, right ventricular failure (cor pulmonale), and reduced cardiac output.
• Respiratory—diminished pulmonary blood flow leads to arterial hypoxemia and dyspnea.

GENETICS

N/A

INCIDENCE/PREVALENCE

• Unknown—likelihood of PTE increases with abnormal coagulation or severe systemic disease. • Uncommon in the dog and cat; likely underdiagnosed due to nonspecific clinical signs, lack of clinical suspicion, and paucity of noninvasive, definitive diagnostic tests.

GEOGRAPHIC DISTRIBUTION

N/A

SIGNALMENT

Species

Dog and cat.

Breed Predilections

N/A

Mean Age and Range

• More frequently seen in middle-aged to older dogs. • Bimodal age distribution reported in cats; peak occurrence <4 years and >10 years of age.

Predominant Sex

N/A

SIGNS

Historical Findings

• Often reflect the primary disease process.
• May include peracute dyspnea, anorexia, syncope, collapse, cough, hemoptysis, weakness, exercise intolerance, and inability to sleep or get comfortable.

Physical Examination Findings

• Tachypnea and dyspnea in most animals; adventitious lung sounds in some animals.
• Tachycardia, weak pulses, jugular vein distension, pale or cyanotic mucous membranes, delayed capillary refill time, right-sided heart murmur, and split or loud S2 in severe cases.

CAUSES

• HWD. • Neoplasia.
• Hyperadrenocorticism (Cushing's disease) or corticosteroid administration. • Protein-losing nephropathy or enteropathy.
• Immune-mediated hemolytic anemia (IMHA). • Pancreatitis. • Pulmonary hypertension (PH). • Orthopedic trauma or surgery. • Sepsis. • Disseminated intravascular coagulation. • Liver disease.

RISK FACTORS

• Coagulopathy, especially any hypercoagulable state. • Diseases listed under Causes are associated. • Estrogen administration, immobility, and air travel may be causative in humans.

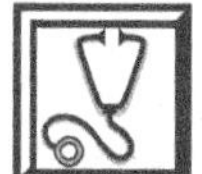

DIAGNOSIS

DIFFERENTIAL DIAGNOSIS

• Other diseases that cause clinically important dyspnea and hypoxemia without profound radiographic findings include upper airway obstruction, laryngeal paralysis, and diffuse airway disease processes (e.g., toxin inhalation and interstitial lung disease).
• Upper airway obstruction often manifests as inspiratory dyspnea; breath sounds often loudest over trachea or larynx. • PTE should be a leading diagnostic consideration in a patient with acute onset of dyspnea or collapse and a known associated disease.

CBC/BIOCHEMISTRY/URINALYSIS

CBC—may be normal; thrombocytopenia may be seen in up to 50% of dogs with PTE; leukocytosis may develop. Biochemistry—results often reflect underlying disease. Urinalysis—results often reflect underlying disease; evaluate for proteinuria.

OTHER LABORATORY TESTS

• Arterial blood gases often show arterial hypoxemia ($Pa{O_2}$ often <65 mmHg) and low $Pa{CO_2}$ with respiratory alkalosis. • Metabolic and respiratory acidosis may develop in severely affected patients. • D-dimers result from the breakdown of crosslinked fibrin, indicate physiologic or pathologic thrombosis and testing plays a pivotal role in diagnostic algorithms for PTE in humans; however, utility for PTE diagnosis in veterinary patients is uncertain. • Thromboelastography provides a global assessment of coagulation and thrombolysis; may be useful in diagnosing systemic hypercoagulability but not widely available. • Coagulation profile may show high fibrin degradation products, abnormal fibrinogen, or alterations in one-stage prothrombin time (PT) and activated partial thromboplastin time (PTT).
• Heartworm serology (antigen testing in dogs; antigen and antibody testing in cats) should be performed in any animal with suspected PTE. • Cardiac biomarkers—cardiac troponin I and B-type natriuretic peptide (NT-proBNP) levels may be elevated.

IMAGING

Thoracic Radiography

• May be normal. • PA enlargement or pruning. • Cardiomegaly. • Interstitial and alveolar lung patterns. • Small-volume pleural effusion. • Areas of regional hyperlucency (Westermark sign).

Echocardiography

• Right ventricular enlargement. • Enlarged PA segment. • Flattening of the interventricular septum. • Reduced left ventricular cavity size. • High-velocity tricuspid or pulmonic regurgitation jets provide evidence of PH in some patients.
• Infrequently a thrombus is imaged in the right heart or the main PA segments.

CT, Angiography, and Radionuclide Studies

• One or more of these tests usually required for definitive diagnosis. • CT angiography is gold standard for the diagnosis of PTE.
• Spiral CT nonselective angiography may show intraluminal filling defects created by emboli, peripheral wedge-shaped pulmonary infiltrates, or pleural effusion. • Right-sided cardiac catheterization with pulmonary angiography may permit identification of intraluminal filling defects or regions of reduced pulmonary blood flow.
• Nonselective angiography using conventional radiographic techniques has a low level of diagnostic success. • Combined ventilation and perfusion scans with radioisotopes permit identification of well-ventilated lung regions that are not receiving normal blood flow.

DIAGNOSTIC PROCEDURES

ECG

• Acute cor pulmonale—right axis deviation, P pulmonale, ST segment deviation, large T waves. • Arrhythmias.

PATHOLOGIC FINDINGS

• Thrombi in major PA branches. • Some patients exhibit multiple smaller thrombi in small PA vessels, eventually leading to marked respiratory dysfunction and death.
• Concurrent lung pathology (e.g., pneumonia, pulmonary edema, neoplasia, interstitial fibrosis) is common.

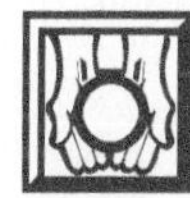

TREATMENT

APPROPRIATE HEALTH CARE

Hospitalize patients documented with PTE until hypoxemia is resolved.

NURSING CARE

• Administer IV fluids cautiously unless preexisting volume depletion; they may precipitate right-sided congestive heart failure. • Administer oxygen if dyspneic and/or $Pa\text{o}_2$ <65 mmHg; response to oxygen therapy is variable.

ACTIVITY

N/A

DIET

N/A

CLIENT EDUCATION

• Alert that condition is often fatal; further episodes likely unless an underlying cause is identified and corrected; sudden death is not unusual. • Traditional anticoagulants can lead to bleeding complications requiring frequent clotting time reevaluation (e.g., PT and PTT) for successful management; low-molecular-weight heparins (LMWHs) are safer and require less monitoring but are more expensive; anticoagulants may be required for several months, even after resolution of the causative disease.

P

SURGICAL CONSIDERATIONS

N/A

MEDICATIONS

DRUG(S) OF CHOICE

• Always identify and treat underlying disease; if this is unlikely to be successful, aggressive efforts to treat PTE will probably be in vain.
• Unfractionated heparin may help to prevent further thrombi from developing; low dosages are probably inadequate for initial management; a dosage of 200–300 units/kg SC q8h or alternatively a bolus of 200 units/kg IV followed by a CRI at 15–30 units/kg/h adjusted to maintain the PTT at 1.5–2 times the baseline value. • Thrombolytics (e.g., urokinase, streptokinase, or tissue plasminogen activator) may also be useful in hemodynamically unstable cases; these are expensive and carry a higher risk of bleeding complications. • Warfarin—may occasionally be considered for long-term treatment (0.1 mg/kg q24h), with dosage adjustments to maintain a PT 1.5–2 times the baseline value; animals must be heparinized prior to warfarin therapy to avoid initial hypercoagulable phase. • LMWHs are likely associated with fewer bleeding complications than unfractionated heparin or warfarin, require less intensive monitoring, and are more suitable for long-term management; however, their cost may be a limiting factor. • Thromboprophylactic effects have been demonstrated for dalteparin 150 units/kg SC q12h in the absence of prolonged bleeding times or adverse effects; enoxaparin has been used at 1 mg/kg SC q12h.
• Sildenafil 1–2 mg/kg PO q8h may help in some animals with PTE and concomitant PH.

CONTRAINDICATIONS

N/A

PRECAUTIONS

Warfarin—interacts with many other drugs; degree of anticoagulation may change after giving these drugs, or with diet alterations. Dose titration may be difficult in patients with diseases that result in coagulopathy. Review mechanism of action and pharmacology of antithrombotic drugs before use.

POSSIBLE INTERACTIONS

See Precautions for warfarin.

ALTERNATIVE DRUGS

N/A

FOLLOW-UP

PATIENT MONITORING

Serial arterial blood gases and/or pulse oximetry—may help determine improvement in respiratory function.

PREVENTION/AVOIDANCE

• Activity or physical therapy may improve venous blood flow and prevent development of venous thrombi in immobile patients with severe systemic disease. • Aspirin (0.5–5 mg/kg PO q12–24h) may have some preventive role but is inadequate as treatment.
• Clopidogrel (1–2 mg/kg PO q24h) is an alternative antiplatelet drug that may have some role in prevention. A single loading dose, up to 10 mg/kg, can be administered for rapid platelet inactivation in cases with active thrombosis. • Heparin may be administered to hospitalized animals predisposed to the development of PTE (200 units/kg IV initially and 75–200 units/kg SC q8h). • Alternatively, dalteparin (150 units/kg SC q12h) or enoxaparin (1 mg/kg SC q12h) may be used for thromboprophylaxis. • Rivaroxaban, an oral factor Xa inhibitor, has been used in small animals (1 mg/kg PO q24h). Rivaroxaban and other newer oral antithrombotics, such as fondaparinux, apixaban, or dabigatran may be as effective as warfarin for prevention of recurrent thrombosis in people and require less monitoring; these drugs may play a future role in longer term anticoagulation of veterinary patients but further study on dosing and safety in animals is needed.

POSSIBLE COMPLICATIONS

Bleeding complications may arise with anticoagulants. Bleeding may occur from any organ system. Anticipate active bleeding or anemia necessitating blood or plasma transfusion and have blood products readily available.

EXPECTED COURSE AND PROGNOSIS

Generally guarded to poor; depends on resolution of the precipitating cause. For irreversible diseases (e.g., some neoplasias and advanced protein-losing nephropathy), prognosis is poor; it is somewhat better for patients with PTE due to trauma or sepsis.

MISCELLANEOUS

ASSOCIATED CONDITIONS

• PH. • HWD. • IMHA. • Hyperadrenocorticism. • Protein-losing nephropathy.

AGE-RELATED FACTORS

Predisposing conditions more likely in middle-aged and older animals.

ZOONOTIC POTENTIAL

N/A

PREGNANCY/FERTILITY/BREEDING

N/A

SYNONYMS

Pulmonary embolism.

SEE ALSO

- Anemia, Immune-Mediated.
- Disseminated Intravascular Coagulation.
- Heartworm Disease—Cats.
- Heartworm Disease—Dogs.
- Hyperadrenocorticism (Cushing's Syndrome)—Cats.
- Hyperadrenocorticism (Cushing's Syndrome)—Dogs.
- Nephrotic Syndrome.
- Sepsis and Bacteremia.

ABBREVIATIONS

• HWD = heartworm disease.
• IMHA = immune-mediated hemolytic anemia. • LMWH = low-molecular-weight heparin. • NT-ProBNP = B-type natriuretic peptide. • PA = pulmonary artery/arterial.
• PH = pulmonary hypertension.
• PT = prothrombin time.
• PTE = pulmonary thromboembolism.
• PTT = partial thromboplastin time.

Suggested Reading

Goggs R, Blais MC, Brainard BM, et al. American College of Veterinary Emergency and Critical Care (ACVECC) Consensus on the Rational Use of Antithrombotics in Veterinary Critical Care (CURATIVE) guidelines: small animal. J Vet Emerg Crit Care 2019, 29:12–36.

Hackner SG. Pulmonary thromboembolism. In: Bonagura JD, Twedt DC, eds., Kirk's Current Veterinary Therapy XV. St. Louis, MO: Saunders Elsevier, 2014, pp. 705–710.

Marschner CB, Kristensen AT, Rozanski EA. Diagnosis of canine pulmonary thromboembolism by computed tomography and mathematical modelling using haemostatic and inflammatory variables. Vet J 2017, 229:6–12.

Schermerhorn T, Pembleton-Corbett JR, Kornreich B. Pulmonary thromboembolism in cats. J Vet Intern Med 2004, 18:533–535.

Authors Suzanne M. Cunningham and John E. Rush

Consulting Editor Michael Aherne

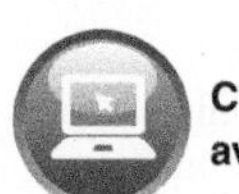

Client Education Handout available online

PULMONIC STENOSIS

BASICS

DEFINITION

Congenital narrowing of the right ventricular outflow tract, obstructing the passage of flow from the right ventricle (RV) to the pulmonary artery (PA); usually valvular, but may be subvalvular or supravalvular. Double-chambered RV is a variant of subvalvular pulmonic stenosis (PS) characterized by a focal muscular or fibromuscular stenosis in the mid RV.

PATHOPHYSIOLOGY

The stenosis causes a pressure overload of the RV, resulting in concentric hypertrophy. The RV develops high systolic pressures to overcome the stenosis, whose magnitude correlates with the severity of the stenosis. The difference between the high right ventricular pressure and the normal PA pressure (i.e., the pressure gradient) is often used to describe the severity of the stenosis. Hypertrophy of the RV increases the risk of myocardial ischemia and arrhythmias. The geometric changes in the RV can result in secondary tricuspid insufficiency, although tricuspid insufficiency can also be associated with concurrent tricuspid dysplasia. Syncope can occur with exercise, as the RV may be unable to increase stroke volume adequately. Tricuspid insufficiency with or without myocardial failure of the RV can lead to high right atrial pressures and right-sided congestive heart failure (R-CHF). A concurrent atrial septal defect or patent foramen ovale can cause right-to-left shunting, especially with exercise, resulting in cyanosis on exertion. Mild PS usually produces no significant hemodynamic effects apart from an ejection murmur.

SYSTEMS AFFECTED

- Cardiovascular—R-CHF, arrhythmias.
- Hepatobiliary—hepatomegaly with R-CHF.
- Respiratory—pleural effusion.
- Nervous—cerebral hypoperfusion during exercise.

GENETICS

Inherited defect in beagles; polygenic mode of transmission suggested.

INCIDENCE/PREVALENCE

- Most surveys show PS to be among the three most common congenital cardiac defects in dogs; comprising 21–32% of congenital heart defects.
- Uncommon in cats, especially as an isolated defect; comprised 3% of congenital heart defects in one study.

SIGNALMENT

Species

Dog and cat.

Breed Predilections

English bulldog, Chihuahua, French bulldog, miniature schnauzer, West Highland white terrier, Samoyed, cocker spaniel, beagle, boxer, Pomeranian, German shepherd dog, whippet. Bulldog breeds are particularly predisposed to PS caused by anomalous coronary artery anatomy, where the left coronary artery originates from the same vessel as the right coronary, and causes stenosis as it wraps around the main PA.

Mean Age and Range

Present from birth and may be detected as a murmur in puppies; if murmur is not detected, affected animals may not be identified until clinical signs develop later in life.

Predominant Sex

A predilection for males in English bulldogs and possibly other breeds.

SIGNS

General Comments

- Mild stenosis—usually no clinical signs.
- Severely affected patients—may develop CHF, exertional syncope, or sudden death.

Historical Findings

- Abdominal distension.
- Dyspnea.
- Exertional syncope, exercise intolerance, or sudden death.
- Asymptomatic.

Physical Examination Findings

- Systolic murmur loudest over the left heart base; may radiate widely but particularly dorsally on left.
- Murmur—midsystolic or holosystolic, and crescendo–decrescendo.
- Louder murmurs with a precordial thrill—generally associated with more severe stenosis.
- Arrhythmias may occur; the heart rate may be high in CHF.
- Other signs of CHF include ascites, jugular venous distension, and tachypnea.

CAUSES

Congenital

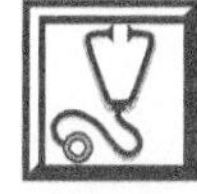

DIAGNOSIS

DIFFERENTIAL DIAGNOSIS

- Similar murmurs may be found with: ○ Aortic stenosis. ○ Ventricular or atrial septal defects with marked left-to-right shunting. ○ Tetralogy of Fallot.
- R-CHF associated with a left-sided murmur may be seen with: ○ Acquired valvular disease. ○ Dilated cardiomyopathy.

CBC/BIOCHEMISTRY/URINALYSIS

- Generally unremarkable.
- Polycythemia may be present with right-to-left shunting.
- NT-proBNP is increased, particularly with severe stenosis or if clinical signs present.

IMAGING

Radiography

- Thoracic radiographs usually show right-sided cardiac enlargement, with a post-stenotic PA bulge visible on the dorsoventral view at 1–2 o'clock.
- The caudal vena cava may be wide, and ascites may be present with or without pleural effusion in congestive failure.

Echocardiography

- Right ventricular hypertrophy, with flattening of the interventricular septum and a "figure-eight" appearance on short axis views in severe cases.
- Can usually image the site of the stenosis, but may be more difficult when the valve is hypoplastic; dysplastic pulmonic valves appear as thickened echodense leaflets; fused leaflets have abnormal motion with systolic doming; discrete subvalvular or supravalvular stenoses may appear as a localized hyper-echoic narrowing.
- Post-stenotic dilation of the PA often present.
- Double-chambered RV can be difficult to image in conventional views.
- Localized hypertrophy may be seen in the right ventricular infundibular region.
- Anomalous coronary anatomy can be difficult to image.

Doppler Echocardiography

- Can use spectral Doppler to measure the elevated PA flow velocity to calculate the pressure gradient across the stenosis. Pressure gradients under 50 mmHg generally represent mild stenosis; those over 80 mmHg indicate severe stenosis.
- Color-flow Doppler may reveal tricuspid regurgitation.

Angiography

- Selective cardiac angiography can help identify the precise morphologic abnormalities prior to surgery; may image dysplastic valves and hypertrophy of the infundibulum more clearly.
- Useful in identifying PS caused by an anomalous coronary artery encircling the right ventricular outflow tract, which may affect the choice of therapy; recommended for bulldogs and brachycephalic breeds.

CT Angiography

Best technique to delineate coronary artery anomalies if resolution adequate and images are ECG-gated.

DIAGNOSTIC PROCEDURES

Electrocardiography

- QRS complex waveform changes include deep S waves in leads I, II, III, and aVF and right axis deviation.

P

PULMONIC STENOSIS (CONTINUED)

- Atrial fibrillation may occur with severe right atrial enlargement.

PATHOLOGIC FINDINGS

- Various forms exist; most result in right ventricular hypertrophy and post-stenotic dilation of the PA; infundibular hypertrophy may occur proximal to the obstruction.
- Hypoplastic pulmonic valve, with thickened leaflets ("dysplastic pulmonic valve").
- Normal pulmonic valve annulus with fused commissures, often attached to vessel at supravalvular level.
- Anomalous coronary arteries.
- Discrete supravalvular or subvalvular stenosis, with possible concurrent tricuspid dysplasia.
- Fibromuscular bands dividing the right ventricular inflow and outflow tracts in double-chambered RV.

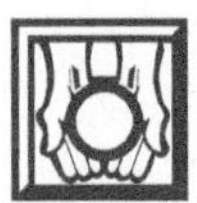

TREATMENT

P

APPROPRIATE HEALTH CARE

Most managed as outpatients.

NURSING CARE

Rarely, pleural effusions may need draining; ascites is usually treated medically.

ACTIVITY

Exercise should be restricted in cases with syncope or CHF, and severe exertion should be avoided in asymptomatic cases with severe stenosis.

DIET

Low-salt diets may benefit those with refractory ascites.

CLIENT EDUCATION

- Mildly affected animals may lead normal lives.
- Moderately and severely affected patients may benefit from interventions such as balloon catheter dilation or surgery; improved clinical signs and survival has been associated with successful balloon procedures.
- Prognosis is guarded once congestive signs develop.
- Do not breed affected animals.

SURGICAL CONSIDERATIONS

- Balloon catheter dilation—relatively safe procedure that involves passing a catheter across the stenosis and inflating a balloon to dilate the obstruction; in many cases, the pressure gradient is significantly reduced, especially when the lesion is caused by fused commissures; less successful with dysplastic or hypoplastic valves and should be used with caution with anomalous coronary arteries.
- Generally unsuccessful in double-chambered RV.
- Stenting of the stenotic pulmonic valve has been described in cases where balloon valvuloplasty has been unsuccessful.
- Alternative surgical techniques include valvulotomy or patch-ventriculectomy procedures; mortality rates tend to be higher than with balloon valvuloplasty.

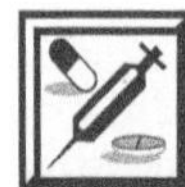

MEDICATIONS

DRUG(S) OF CHOICE

If signs of CHF, treat ascites with furosemide 1–4 mg/kg PO q8–12h; in refractory failure, it is worth adding spironolactone 1–2 mg/kg PO q12h; aim should be to control CHF signs prior to catheter intervention.

CONTRAINDICATIONS

Vasodilators (e.g., hydralazine) may cause hypotension without relieving the stenosis, positive inotropes may further increase myocardial oxygen consumption.

PRECAUTIONS

Avoid overuse of diuretics. angiotensin-converting enzyme inhibitors may be helpful with congestive signs, but may cause hypotension. Start with low doses and monitor blood pressure.

FOLLOW-UP

PATIENT MONITORING

Use serial echocardiograms to follow the pressure gradient and cardiac chamber size.

PREVENTION/AVOIDANCE

Do not breed affected animals.

POSSIBLE COMPLICATIONS

- R-CHF.
- Chylothorax.
- Arrhythmias.
- Exercise intolerance.
- Exertional syncope.
- Sudden death.

EXPECTED COURSE AND PROGNOSIS

- Mildly affected animals may remain asymptomatic with a normal lifespan.
- Severely affected animals have a guarded prognosis because they may develop CHF or sudden death; clinical signs are generally more common in animals >1 year of age.

MISCELLANEOUS

ASSOCIATED CONDITIONS

- Ventricular septal defects, atrial septal defects, and patent foramen ovale.
- English bulldogs described with a single right coronary artery from which an anomalous left main coronary artery arises and then encircles and constricts the base of the pulmonic valve; other coronary variations have also been described.

AGE-RELATED FACTORS

Defect and murmur are present from birth.

PREGNANCY/FERTILITY/BREEDING

Do not breed affected animals.

SYNONYMS

Pulmonary stenosis.

SEE ALSO

- Congestive Heart Failure, Right-Sided.
- Murmurs, Heart.

ABBREVIATIONS

- ECG = electrocardiography.
- PA = pulmonary artery.
- PS = pulmonic stenosis.
- R-CHF = right-sided congestive heart failure.
- RV = right ventricle.

Suggested Reading

Fonfara S, Pereira YM, Swift S, et al. Balloon valvuloplasty for treatment of pulmonic stenosis in English bulldogs with an aberrant coronary artery. J Vet Intern Med 2010, 24:354–359.

Francis AJ, Johnson MJS, Culshaw GC, et al. Outcome in 55 dogs with pulmonic stenosis that did not undergo balloon valvuloplasty or surgery. J Small Anim Pract 2011, 52:282–288.

Locatelli C, Spalla I, Domenech O, et al. Pulmonic stenosis in dogs: survival and risk factors in a retrospective cohort of patients. J Small Anim Pract 2013, 54:445–452.

Oliveira P, Domenech O, Silva J, et al. Retrospective review of congenital heart disease in 976 dogs. J Vet Intern Med 2011, 25:477–483.

Author Virginia Luis Fuentes
Consulting Editor Michael Aherne

Client Education Handout available online

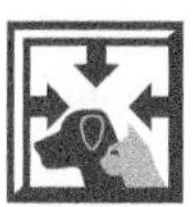

BASICS

DEFINITION

These problems include behaviors that are normal and common to most puppies but not acceptable to the family. They require some degree of modification by training and shaping to become acceptable. Training and behavior issues include confinement training, housetraining, destructive chewing, play-biting, jumping on people, and getting on counters or furniture.

SYSTEMS AFFECTED

Behavioral

GENETICS

- Activity levels and behaviors of young pups may be similar to those of their parents.
- Some problems may be more prevalent in breeds or lines with a high need for exercise and mental stimulation.

INCIDENCE/PREVALENCE

Common to almost all puppies.

GEOGRAPHIC DISTRIBUTION

N/A

SIGNALMENT

Species

Dog.

Breed Predilections

Breeds selected for high-energy, stamina, and working functions.

Mean Age and Range

3–6 months of age but some dogs mature later and problems can persist into adulthood.

Predominant Sex

May be higher frequency in males.

SIGNS

Confinement Training

N/A

Housetraining

N/A

Playbiting

- The pet bites hands, legs, and/or clothing. Bites are usually inhibited but can cause injuries due to sharp teeth or insufficient bite inhibition.
- Growling and barking may be present but usually a higher pitch, with lower tones associated with social aggression.
- Attacks are usually triggered by movement or play with a family member but can be spontaneous.

Getting on Counters/Furniture

The pet gets on furniture and counters .

CAUSES

General

- Normal play and exploration.
- Inadequate supervision, training, socialization, or providing for mental stimulation or environmental enrichment.
- Owner responses may reinforce or exacerbate the behaviors.

Playbiting

A normal behavior, but rough play, teasing, and encouraging the pet to bite hands and feet may contribute to problems

Getting on Counters/Furniture

- Insufficient outlets for normal play and exploration.
- Tempting objects or food left on counters/furniture.
- Desire for social interaction.
- No acceptable alternative resting/bedding area.

RISK FACTORS

See Causes.

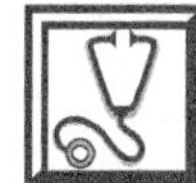

DIAGNOSIS

DIFFERENTIAL DIAGNOSIS

Confinement Training

N/A (if distress or soiling during confinement rule out separation anxiety and barrier frustration).

Housetraining

N/A (rule out medical).

Playbiting

- Fear-related and defensive aggression—aggression accompanied by signs of fear and/or submission (lowered body, ears and tail down/tucked, horizontal retraction of oral commissures):
  - Occurs when the pet is in a situation perceived as threatening.
  - May be due to confrontation or punishment. Vocalization might include growling or yelping.
- Possessive aggression—occurs in situations in which there is competition for a resource:
  - Pet stiffens and hovers over the guarded object.
  - Increase in the speed of eating or quickly grasping an object tightly in the mouth may also be observed.
  - Growling has a deep tone.
  - Piloerection may occur, as might lunging, snapping, and biting.
- Reinforced aggression—the pet learns that aggressive behavior is effective at achieving goals (avoid being picked up, pushed off couch, restrained by collar, nails trimmed).
- Conflict-related aggression—the pet bites in situations where it is frustrated or uncertain how to behave due to inconsistent responses by the family, including punishment.
- Medical, e.g., viral encephalitis, toxins, congenital disorders, usually accompanied by other signs of illness.

Getting on Counters/Furniture

N/A

CBC/BIOCHEMISTRY/URINALYSIS

Housesoiling might require a urinalysis, fecal exam, or other tests as suggested by physical exam and history.

DIAGNOSTIC PROCEDURES

N/A except to rule out concurrent illness, e.g., hepatic shunt, CNS anomalies that affect learning.

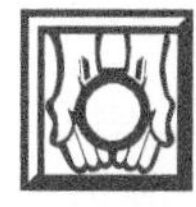

TREATMENT

APPROPRIATE HEALTH CARE

Outpatient

NURSING CARE

N/A

ACTIVITY

Provide a regular daily routine of exercise, play, social interaction and mental stimulation.

DIET

Provide sufficient food to reduce the motivation to guard food.

CLIENT EDUCATION

General

- Constantly look for and reward acceptable behaviors.
- Avoid punishment, confrontation and corrections (e.g., striking, shaking the scruff, rolling on the back, or squeezing lips). These can worsen problems, negatively impact the bond with the pet, and lead to more serious problems, such as social fear and aggression).
- Teach the pet to sit or down using reward training. Direct him into the behavior prior to getting anything he wants or needs.

Confinement Training

- Choose an appropriate confinement area. A crate is good for intermittent confinement but no longer than the pet can control urination and defecation (gradually increasing from 1 to 5 hours). If the pet must be confined for longer a larger housing area should be provided with an elimination area within.
- Place treats, toys, or food in the area so that he is motivated to enter. For rest and sleep, place him in his confinement area. The pup should never be roughly forced in. A confinement area is for safety and comfort not punishment.
- Some degree of distress vocalization may occur the first few times the pup is confined. Music or talk radio may help to calm and mask environmental noises that trigger barking. A calming pheromone (Adaptil™) may help the puppy adapt. Avoid releasing the pup when he cries. Wait until he is quiet or squeak a toy from out of sight to get the pup to quiet before he is released.

PUPPY BEHAVIOR PROBLEMS (CONTINUED)

Housetraining

- The puppy should be taken out to eliminate each hour when awake during the daytime when possible. If he does not eliminate within 10 minutes, return indoors, supervise closely for 15–30 minutes and try again. Take the pet out after play, exercise, naps, eating, drinking, or confinement, as well as prior to confinement, and whenever he exhibits preelimination circling and sniffing. Offer food 2–3 times daily at the same time to help establish an elimination routine.
- Until the puppy has completed 4 weeks without soiling, he should either be within eyesight or in his confinement area. A leash will help keep the pet close for supervision. Most pups can control elimination through the night by 3–4 months of age. By 4 months, most puppies will have more of control during the daytime. Soiling can be prevented by closing doors or using barriers to limit access to areas.
- Do not punish. If caught in the act of soiling, calmly redirect the pup, and take outdoors. Elimination odors should be removed.
- If the pup eliminates in his crate—he may have been left there longer than he can control eliminating; the crate may be so large that he sleeps in one end and eliminates in the other; the puppy did not eliminate prior to confining; the meals were not matched to the elimination schedule; there is anxiety about confinement or being left alone (see Separation Anxiety Syndrome); there is an underlying medical cause.
- If it is not practical to take the pup outside frequently enough, he should be confined to a larger confinement area (e.g., pen) with an elimination pad within.
- Medical issues that may contribute to housetraining problems include problems that cause increased volume or frequency of elimination, and CNS problems that interfere with learning (hepatic encaphalopathy, hydrocephalus).

Playbiting

- Provide abundant opportunities for play/ exercise.
- Have toys available at all times to toss and distract the pet.
- Use treat- and kibble-filled toys to keep the pet occupied and to provide outlets for exploration and scavenging.
- Use a leash attached to the supervised pup for more control.
- Confine the pup to his rest area when the family cannot effectively engage him in acceptable activities.
- Avoid games that encourage biting hands or feet.
- Make all interactions structured and predictable by training the pet to sit before giving toys, food, play, and attention.
- Do not reinforce attention-seeking behavior such as whining, barking, or pawing for attention.
- Say "Ouch" and immediately redirect or walk away to interrupt hard bites during play.
- Avoid physical corrections that can cause fear, anxiety, and aggression or stimulate the pup.
- Consider a head halter for head control of difficult pups.
- Enroll in puppy classes early (8–10 weeks of age).

Getting on Counters/Furniture

- Keep appealing objects off counters and furniture.
- Constantly supervise and monitor.
- Block access to problem areas.
- Confine the pup to his bed/rest area when he cannot be supervised.
- Provide interesting toys on the floor.
- Meet the pet's needs for food, chewing, mental stimulation, and exploration.

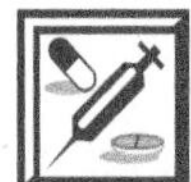

MEDICATIONS

DRUG(S) OF CHOICE

Drugs are not indicated except for problems associated with anxiety.

ALTERNATIVE DRUG(S)

Dog-appeasing pheromones, nutraceuticals such as alpha-casozepine or L-theanine, or a calming probiotic may aid in stressful situations.

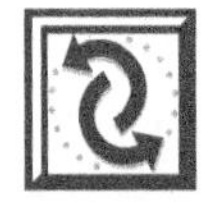

FOLLOW-UP

PATIENT MONITORING

- Phone follow-ups at approximately 10 days, 20 days, and 6 weeks following the initial visit are helpful.
- This can be done by a trained support staff member.

PREVENTION/AVOIDANCE

- Provide preventive counseling for all first puppy visits about normal behavior and behavioral needs (e.g., mental stimulation, socialization, exercise, object play).
- Discuss timing and use of rewards to teach what is desirable while behaviors that are undesirable should be prevented (supervision and confinement strategies) and not punished.
- Begin food-lure reward training at 7–8 weeks of age.
- Make interactions predictable by teaching the pet to sit before giving anything of value.
- Enroll in a puppy class at 8–10 weeks of age.
- Provide regular sessions of physical exercise, mental stimulation including reward training, food puzzle toys, and safe items to explore and chew.

POSSIBLE COMPLICATIONS

- Damage to household objects and clothing.
- Food stealing.
- Intestinal foreign bodies/obstructions.
- Injuries from playbites and jumping up.
- Owner frustration, weakened bond, and possible relinquishment.

EXPECTED COURSE AND PROGNOSIS

- Prognosis is generally good.
- The frequency and intensity should decrease with age.
- Playbiting can usually be quickly managed if the family is consistent with training.
- Confinement training should take a few days to several weeks.
- Housetraining can be accomplished in a few weeks, but may take longer if the family is not consistent in supervision and training or the family schedule does not address the dog's needs.

MISCELLANEOUS

SEE ALSO

- Destructive Behavior—Dogs.
- Housesoiling—Dogs.
- Puppy Socialization and Puppy Classes.
- Unruly Behaviors: Jumping, Pulling, Chasing, Stealing—Dogs.

Suggested Reading

Dunbar I. Before and After Getting Your Puppy: The Positive Approach to Raising a Happy, Healthy, and Well-Behaved Dog. San Francisco, CA: New World Library, 2004.

Landsberg GL, Hunthausen WL, Ackerman L. Handbook of Behavior Problems of the Dog and Cat, 3rd ed. Philadelphia, PA: Elsevier Saunders, 2013.

McConnell PB, Scidmore B, The Puppy Primer, 2nd ed. Wenatchee, WA: McConnell Publishing, 2010.

Yin S. The Perfect Puppy in 7 days. Davis, CA: CattleDog Publishing, 2011.

Author Wayne Hunthausen
Consulting Editor Gary M. Landsberg

Client Education Handout available online

Puppy Socialization and Puppy Classes

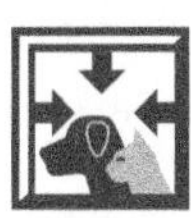

BASICS

OVERVIEW

• Early experiences set the foundation for future behavior, having lasting effects on social behavior, temperament, and the ability to learn and relate to various stimuli and to cope in various environmental contexts.
• To grow up into a well-adjusted adult dog, adequate socialization and environmental exposure is needed during the socialization period and beyond into the first year of life.

Definitions

• Socialization—a process of learning normal behavior, communication, and social skills for appropriate interactions with other individuals in various contexts.
• Socialization period—a sensitive window of development whereby a dog learns to communicate and relate to other dogs, humans, and the environment.
• Puppy classes—called socialization, preschool, or kindergarten classes. Allow dogs to socialize with other dogs, breeds, a variety of people and to be exposed to multiple and varied environmental stimuli in a positive and nonthreatening manner.

Pathophysiology

Potential effects on behavioral and neurological development.

SIGNALMENT

Species

Dogs

Breed Predilections

• Smaller breeds may mature faster and progress more quickly through windows of behavioral development.
• Amount of handling and exposure toward humans needed to reduce people-shyness may be genetically variable.
• The timing of first fear response is genetically variable, 39–55 days.

Mean Age and Range

• The primary socialization period is between 3 and 5 weeks. Puppies recognize kin and learn to relate and interact with other members of their species. The secondary socialization period occurs from 6 to 12 weeks, during this time most puppies are removed from its mother and littermates and raised with human caregivers. The ideal time for placement in a new home is probably after 7 or 8 weeks of age.
• For puppy classes—healthy dewormed puppies should begin attending group socialization classes 10 days after receiving their first vaccine of their immunization series. Typical age at time of the first classes is between 8 and 12 weeks.

Predominant Sex

Male puppies play more than females.

SIGNS

• Lack of adequate socialization experiences during sensitive periods of development.
• Dog-directed fear and/or aggression—lack of early familiarity and positive exposure results in fear and aggression or reactivity to unfamiliar dogs.
• Human-directed fear and/or aggression—exposure with humans prior to 14 weeks is necessary, otherwise fear, avoidance, aggression, and behaving as if "feral."
• Predatory aggression—social exposure, even to prey species, can reduce predatory behavior later in life.
• Reduced ability to copulate—in male dogs, lack of socialization toward conspecifics from 3 weeks on results in the display of normal sexual behavior toward estrus females, but poor performance. In female dogs, timidity toward other dogs may preclude breeding.
• Fear and anxiety in unfamiliar environments with various sights, sounds, and smells.
• Attendance at group puppy classes during sensitive periods of development can prevent future behavior problems and/or allow for the early identification of abnormal and problematic behavior.
• Puppy socialization classes—age specific (to begin at 8–12 weeks) for group-controlled interactions. Focus is education on normal behavior, prevention of behavior problems, and addressing problem behaviors through management, supervision, and positive reinforcement training.
• Group classes of older puppies in their juvenile (3–6 months) and adolescent (6–18 months) stages. Focus primarily on training manners, positive reinforcement training and teaching dogs to focus on their owners/handlers.

CAUSES & RISK FACTORS

• Avoiding environmental and social experiences prior to the completion of puppy vaccination series increases the risk of future behavior problems.
• Risk of contracting parvovirus was not increased when puppies attended well-run group socialization classes prior to completion of their vaccination series.
• Risks of exposure to infectious disease with socialization needs to be considered along with the risk of being undersocialized and not suitable as a pet because of fear, anxiety, and/or aggression.
• Along with a clean bill of health, initial vaccinations must have been administered at least 1 week and preferably 10 days before puppy socialization classes start.
• Puppies should be dewormed according to the Companion Animal Parasite Council guidelines: https://capcvet.org/guidelines/general-guidelines/
• Puppies should be free of clinical disease such as respiratory and gastrointestinal prior to each class.
• Puppy socialization with people and dogs is only beneficial to behavioral development if the puppy finds human and/or dog contact enjoyable. Forced exposure, when it induces fear, is likely to exacerbate fear and/or aggression.
• Experiences at the veterinary clinic should employ Fear Free® and Low Stress techniques to prevent fear, anxiety, stress, and aggression during future veterinary visits.
• Overly shy, fearful, reactive or hyperactive puppies during routine veterinary health checks are likely to display the same behavior at 1 year of age.
• Puppies displaying fear and avoidance of being handled are likely to display fear and/or aggression with handling later in life.
• Excessive mouthing/biting or aggression over food resources at 8 weeks may indicate increased risk of aggression toward family members.
• Pet store puppies and those with early illness are more likely to develop behavior problems.
• Traumatic fear-inducing experiences, particularly during sensitive fear periods, between 8 and 10 weeks and between 6 and 12 months (lasting up to 3 weeks), should be avoided.
• Removal from the mother and littermates prior to 6 weeks may increase the risk of separation anxiety and interdog aggression with poor interdog social skills.
• Avoiding exposure to other species during socialization can lead to fear or aggression towards the species.
• At the juvenile period, beginning at 3–4 months of age, puppies may become less social and more fearful with increased independence seen in adolescence.

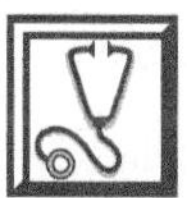

DIAGNOSIS

DIFFERENTIAL DIAGNOSIS

• Identify abnormal and/or problematic behavior and make a behavioral diagnosis or schedule/refer for a behavior consultation.
• Behavioral manifestations of a lack of socialization may include: ○ Global fears, encompassing fears of people, dogs, objects, sounds, and environments. ○ Generalized anxiety and situational anxiety in unfamiliar environments. ○ Specific fears, neophobia, and failure to habituate to novelty or stimuli. ○ Noise sensitivity, aversions, and phobias. ○ Hyperexcitability and hypervigilance with an inability to settle due to lack of early environmental enrichment. ○ Aggression toward people and dogs in various contexts with various motivations (e.g., fear, predatory).

CBC/BIOCHEMISTRY/URINALYSIS

Indicated when considering behavioral medications.

P

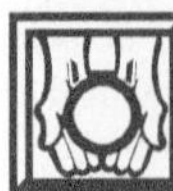

TREATMENT

Recommendations for Socialization

• Attendance at group puppy socialization classes and social exposure is recommended for all healthy puppies prior to 16 weeks of age and prior to being fully vaccinated.
• Socialization "vaccinates" against the development of future behavioral problems and it should begin concurrently with the puppy immunization series.
• Food treats should be used liberally with new and repeated socialization experiences.
• Social play and exploration should be encouraged using toys.
• Healthy puppies usually have voracious appetites. If the puppy is not consuming food treats, it suggests the puppy is fearful and the experience is not beneficial for socialization.
• Healthy and well-adjusted puppies play. If the puppy will not engage in play it suggests the puppy is fearful and the experience is not beneficial for socialization.
• Socialization by the breeder—gentle handling should occur daily, shortly after birth, and include exposure to various smells and different surfaces with mild fluctuations in temperature.
• Socialization at the owner's home—allow the puppy to choose to interact and make exposure positive with the liberal use of food treats: ◦ Meet people of different ages, stature, gait, and complexion. ◦ Meet friendly dogs of different breeds. ◦ Meet other pets in the home (such as cats).

Recommendations for Puppy Socialization Classes

• All healthy puppies, between 8 and 12 weeks of age should be enrolled into group puppy socialization classes.
• Puppies attending are deemed healthy by a veterinary examination, free from clinical signs (e.g., coughing, diarrhea), have been dewormed, and have started their vaccination series.
• Classes are attended by puppies and their owners at least weekly and are typically about an hour in length.
• Rotating classes should cover the following topics: ◦ Play sessions—controlled and monitored off-leash play (5–10 minutes) with other puppies in a secure environment, typically at the start and end of class. ◦ Health and handling—instruction and positive handling for routine health and grooming procedures in the veterinary clinic, at the grooming facility, and at home. ◦ Sights and sounds—exposure to novel environments, objects, surfaces, and sounds. Attending people have opportunities for interacting with puppies in a positive manner. ◦ Rearing advice—education on normal dog body language, learning, behavior problem-solving/prevention, and puppy raising. ◦ Basic manners—positive reinforcement training to address mouthing/biting, jumping, chewing, stealing objects, food bowl safety, confinement training, leash manners, and house training. ◦ Puppy classes offered at the veterinary hospital can also help to insure a focus on positive exposures to the veterinary facility, equipment, and procedures.

MEDICATIONS

DRUG(S) OF CHOICE

• Selective serotonin reuptake inhibitors and tricyclic antidepressants may be indicated for the treatment of fear, anxiety, and aggression-related problems when combined with behavior and environmental modification.
• May "in effect" chemically place the puppy back into a socialization state and aid socialization experiences.
• Consider daily or situational behavior medications based on the underlying condition; for dogs, 12 weeks or greater, who demonstrate abnormal fear, anxiety, aggression or reactivity.

Nutraceuticals/Supplements

• Alpha-casozepine, a bovine-sourced hydrolyzed milk protein may have calming properties.
• L-Theanine, an extract found in green tea, may reduce fear, anxiety, and stress.
• Calming Care (Purina®) probiotic may help to maintain calm behavior.

Pheromones

Adaptil (CEVA), a synthetic dog-appeasing pheromone, may improve socialization experiences and facilitate adaptation to new environments.

CONTRAINDICATIONS/POSSIBLE INTERACTIONS

Avoid selective serotonin reuptake inhibitors and tricyclic antidepressants in combination and use with caution with other serotonin-influencing drugs.

FOLLOW-UP

PATIENT MONITORING

Question owners about behavior problems routinely and encourage concerns regarding problematic behavior to be brought to their veterinarian's attention as soon as possible.

PREVENTION/AVOIDANCE

• Preventive counseling at the first puppy visit reduces risk of housesoiling, mounting, excess play, mouthing of people, demanding food, and fear of unfamiliar people.
• Prevention of problems is preferable and easier than treatment.
• Socialization experiences must be positive for the puppy to benefit from the experiences.

POSSIBLE COMPLICATIONS

• Negative social and environmental experiences can sensitize the puppy as it is difficult to habituate to stimuli that induce fear, anxiety, and stress.
• Puppies raised in suboptimal environments may be resistant to socialization.
• Unwillingness to consume treats, explore, and/or play in socialization contexts suggest that the exposure is not positive for the puppy.

EXPECTED COURSE AND PROGNOSIS

Early identification and intervention gives the best prognostic outcome and chance for cure.

MISCELLANEOUS

ASSOCIATED CONDITIONS

Behavioral conditions associated with fear, anxiety, and aggression.

INTERNET RESOURCES

• www.avsab.org
• www.dacvb.org
• www.fearfreepets.com
• www.puppystartright.com
• https://karenpryoracademy.com/courses/puppy-start-right/

Suggested Reading

Martin KM, Martin D. Puppy Start Right: Foundation Training for the Companion Dog. Waltham, MA: Sunshine Books, 2011.
Shaw JK, Martin D. Canine And Feline Behavior For Veterinary Technicians And Nurses. Ames, IA: John Wiley & Sons, 2015.
Zulch H, Mills DS. Life Skills For Puppies. Poundbury, UK: Hubble & Hattie, 2012.

Authors Kenneth M. Martin and Debbie Martin
Consulting Editor Gary M. Landsberg

P

PUPPY STRANGLES (JUVENILE CELLULITIS)

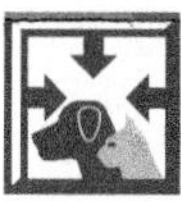

BASICS

OVERVIEW

- Uncommon granulomatous and pustular disorder of puppies.
- Rarely seen in adult dogs.
- Affects primarily the face, pinnae, and submandibular lymph nodes.
- Immunopathogenesis unknown.

SIGNALMENT

- Dogs.
- Age range—usually between 3 weeks and 4 months.
- Predisposed breeds—golden retriever, Labrador retriever, dachshund, and Gordon setter.

SIGNS

- Acutely swollen face (eyelids, lips, and muzzle).
- Submandibular lymphadenopathy.
- Marked pustular and exudative dermatitis; frequently fistulates; develops within 24–48 hours.
- Purulent otitis externa.
- Lesions often become crusted.
- Affected skin is usually painful.
- Lethargy—50% of cases.
- Anorexia, pyrexia, and sterile suppurative arthritis—25% of cases.
- Sterile pyogranulomatous panniculitis (rare) over the trunk, preputial, or perianal area; lesions may appear as fluctuant subcutaneous nodules that fistulate.

CAUSES & RISK FACTORS

Unknown—an immune dysfunction with a heritable cause is suspected.

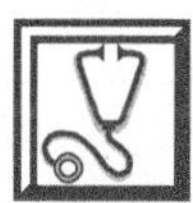

DIAGNOSIS

DIFFERENTIAL DIAGNOSIS

- Bacterial folliculitis/furunculosis.
- Demodicosis.
- Drug reaction/eruption.
- Deep fungal infection.
- Cutaneous hypersensitivity.
- Vaccination reaction.
- Hymenoptera or insect envenomation.
- Acute lymphoma.

OTHER LABORATORY TESTS

- Cytology—pyogranulomatous inflammation with no microorganisms; nondegenerate neutrophils.
- Culture—often sterile in early cases; secondary infection with chronicity.

DIAGNOSTIC PROCEDURES

Skin biopsy.

PATHOLOGIC FINDINGS

- Multiple discrete or confluent granulomas and pyogranulomas—clusters of large epithelioid macrophages and neutrophils.
- Sebaceous glands and apocrine glands may be obliterated.
- Suppurative changes in the dermis—predominate in later stages.
- Panniculitis.
- Exudate culture—important for selection of antibiotics if secondary infection suspected.

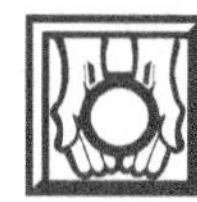

TREATMENT

- Early and aggressive therapy necessary because scarring may be severe.
- Topical therapy—may be soothing and palliative; adjunct to corticosteroids.

MEDICATIONS

DRUG(S) OF CHOICE

- Corticosteroids—high doses required; prednisolone 2.2 mg/kg divided q12h for at least 2 weeks then decreased over 2–4 weeks or dexamethasone 0.2 mg/kg q24h.
- Do not taper too rapidly.
- Corticosteroid—resistant cases: cyclosporine 5 mg/kg q24h.
- Adult dogs with panniculitis may require longer therapy.
- Antibiotics—only if there is evidence of secondary bacterial infection or as an adjunct therapy with immunosuppressive doses of corticosteroids.

FOLLOW-UP

- Most cases do not recur.
- Scarring may persist, especially around the eyes.

MISCELLANEOUS

SYNONYMS

- Juvenile pyoderma.
- Juvenile sterile granulomatous dermatitis and lymphadenitis.

Suggested Reading

Albanese F. Canine and Feline Skin Cytology: a Comprehensive and Illustrated Guide to the Interpretation of Skin Lesions via Cytological Examination. Switzerland, Springer International, 2017.

Miller WH, Griffin CE, Campbell KL. Muller & Kirk's Small Animal Dermatology, 7th ed. St. Louis, MO: Elsevier Mosby, 2013, pp. 708–709.

Nuttall T, Eisenschenk M, Heinrich NA, Harvey RG. Skin Diseases of the Dog and Cat, 3rd ed. London UK; CRC Press, 2018.

Author Guillermina Manigot

Consulting Editor Alexander H. Werner Resnick

Acknowledgment The author and editors acknowledge the prior contribution of Karen Helton Rhodes.

PYELONEPHRITIS

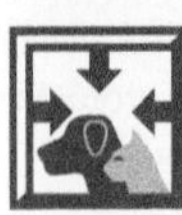

BASICS

DEFINITION

Microbial colonization of the upper urinary tract, including the renal pelvis, collecting diverticula, renal parenchyma, and ureters; because it is not usually limited to the renal pelvis and parenchyma, a more descriptive term is upper urinary tract infection (UTI); this chapter is limited to bacterial pyelonephritis.

PATHOPHYSIOLOGY

- Infection of any portion of the urinary tract usually requires impairment of normal host defenses against UTI (see Lower Urinary Tract Infection chapters); normal defenses against ascending UTI include mucosal defense barriers, ureteral peristalsis, ureterovesical flap valves, unidirectional flow of urine, and an extensive renal blood supply. Pyelonephritis usually occurs by ascension of microbes causing lower UTI. Hematogenous seeding of the kidneys is an uncommon cause of pyelonephritis. Regardless of the route of infection, an upper UTI is frequently accompanied by lower UTI.
- Pyelonephritis can develop secondarily to infected nephroliths. Upper UTI with urease-producing bacteria can predispose to struvite nephroliths (see Urolithiasis, Struvite—Dogs).
- Obstruction of an infected kidney or ureter can rapidly cause septicemia (urosepsis).

SYSTEMS AFFECTED

- Renal/urologic.
- Can cause urosepsis, thus affecting any body system.

INCIDENCE/PREVALENCE

- Unknown.
- Probably occurs more commonly than is recognized clinically, because many animals with pyelonephritis are asymptomatic or have signs limited to lower UTI.

SIGNALMENT

Species

Detected more frequently in dog than cat.

Mean Age and Range

- Dogs of any age can be affected.
- Cats—UTI is uncommon in young to middle-age cats. UTI is more common in cats >10 years of age.

Predominant Sex

UTI affects females more commonly than males.

SIGNS

General Comments

Differentiation between pyelonephritis, subclinical bacteriuria, and lower UTI may be difficult in some patients.

Historical Findings

- Polyuria/polydipsia.
- Abdominal or lumbar pain (uncommon).
- Signs associated with lower UTI may predominate—e.g., dysuria, pollakiuria, periuria, stranguria, hematuria, and malodorous or discolored urine.
- Signs attributable to chronic kidney disease (CKD)—e.g., polyuria/polydipsia, anorexia, vomiting, diarrhea, lethargy.

Physical Examination Findings

- May lack specific signs related to upper UTI.
- Fever.
- Pain upon palpation of kidneys.
- One or both kidneys may be reduced in size with chronic pyelonephritis, or kidneys may be increased in size with acute pyelonephritis.

CAUSES

Usually, ascending UTI caused by aerobic bacteria; most common isolates are *Escherichia coli* and *Staphylococcus* spp.; other bacteria, including *Proteus*, *Streptococcus*, *Klebsiella*, *Enterobacter*, and *Pseudomonas* spp., which frequently infect the lower urinary tract, may ascend into the upper urinary tract. Anaerobic bacteria, ureaplasma, and fungi uncommonly infect the upper urinary tract.

RISK FACTORS

- Ectopic ureters, vesicoureteral reflux, congenital renal dysplasia, and lower UTI.
- Conditions that predispose to bacteriuria—e.g., diabetes mellitus, hyperadrenocorticism, exogenous steroid administration, CKD, indwelling urinary catheters, urine retention, uroliths, urinary tract neoplasia, perineal urethrostomy.

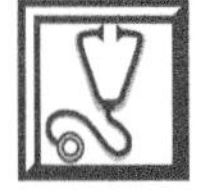

DIAGNOSIS

DIFFERENTIAL DIAGNOSIS

- Clinical diagnosis of pyelonephritis is usually presumptive, based on results from CBC, biochemical analysis, urinalysis, urine culture, and diagnostic imaging; definitive diagnosis is not usually required for planning treatment.
- Since many lack specific symptoms attributable to pyelonephritis, any patient with UTI could potentially have pyelonephritis; the best methods for differentiating between upper and lower UTI are ultrasonography or excretory urography.
- Consider pyelonephritis as a rule-out for fever of unknown origin, polyuria/polydipsia, acute decline in renal function, and/or lumbar/abdominal pain.

CBC/BIOCHEMISTRY/URINALYSIS

- CBC—results often normal with chronic pyelonephritis; leukocytosis and immature neutrophilia may be detected in some patients.
- Biochemistry—values usually normal unless chronic pyelonephritis leads to CKD (azotemia with inappropriate urine specific gravity).
- Urinalysis may reveal hematuria, pyuria, proteinuria, bacteriuria, and leukocyte casts. Leukocyte casts are diagnostic for renal inflammation, but unfortunately are very uncommon. Observe dilute urine specific gravity in patients with nephrogenic diabetes insipidus, which may occur secondary to pyelonephritis from Gram-negative bacteria. Absence of these abnormalities does not rule out pyelonephritis.

OTHER LABORATORY TESTS

- Quantitative urine culture to confirm UTI; see Lower Urinary Tract Infection chapters for interpretation.
- Dogs with chronic pyelonephritis may have a negative urine culture and may require multiple urine cultures to confirm UTI.

IMAGING

- Ultrasonography and excretory urography are the best methods for presumptively differentiating between upper and lower UTI. Ultrasonography is more sensitive than excretory urography for identification of mild-to-moderate acute pyelonephritis.
- Ultrasonographic findings supporting pyelonephritis include dilation of the renal pelvis and proximal ureter and a hyperechoic mucosal margin line within the renal pelvis and/or proximal ureter.
- IV urography may reveal decreased opacity of the nephrogram phase, dilation and blunting of the renal pelvis with lack of filling of the collecting diverticula, decreased opacity of contrast media in the collecting system, and dilation of the proximal ureter.
- In patients with acute pyelonephritis, the kidneys may be large; in patients with chronic pyelonephritis, the kidneys may be small, with an irregular surface contour.
- Concomitant nephroliths detected in some patients by survey radiography or ultrasonography.

DIAGNOSTIC PROCEDURES

Definitive diagnosis requires urine cultures obtained from the renal pelvis. Pyelocentesis can be performed percutaneously using ultrasound guidance or during exploratory surgery. Urine cultures from the renal pelvis usually are similar to cultures from the bladder unless obstruction is present.

PATHOLOGIC FINDINGS

- Kidneys affected by chronic pyelonephritis may have areas of infarction and scarring on the capsular surface. The renal pelvis and collecting diverticula may be dilated and distorted from chronic infection and inflammation. Purulent exudate is occasionally observed in the renal pelvis.

• Light microscopic findings include papillitis, pyelitis, interstitial nephritis, and leukocyte casts in tubular lumens.

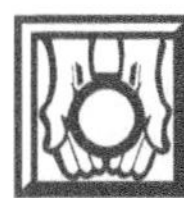

TREATMENT

APPROPRIATE HEALTH CARE

Outpatient treatment with oral antibiotics if the animal is clinically well. Hospitalized care if patient is dehydrated, has decreased renal function or if sepsis is suspected.

ACTIVITY

Unlimited

DIET

Renal therapeutic diets are recommended for concomitant CKD.

CLIENT EDUCATION

• Recurrent pyelonephritis may be asymptomatic. Unresolved chronic pyelonephritis may lead to progression of CKD; diagnostic follow-up is important to document resolution or progression of pyelonephritis.
• In patients with infected nephroliths, resolution of pyelonephritis is unlikely unless the nephroliths are removed.

SURGICAL CONSIDERATIONS

• Complete obstruction of the upper urinary tract of a patient with pyelonephritis may rapidly progress to septicemia and therefore should be regarded as a medical emergency. The cause of the obstruction should be corrected by endoscopic or surgical ureteral stent placement.
• Infected nephroliths—remove surgically, medically dissolve (struvite), or fragment by extracorporeal shock wave lithotripsy; use periprocedural antibiotics to reduce the risk of urosepsis when manipulating infected nephroliths.
• Unilateral nephrectomy is usually not effective for elimination of suspected unilateral pyelonephritis.

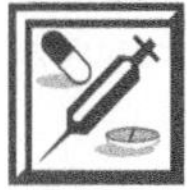

MEDICATIONS

DRUG(S) OF CHOICE

• Base antibiotic selection on urine culture and susceptibility testing. Initiate antibiotics pending culture results.
• Antibiotics should be bactericidal, achieve good serum and urine concentrations, and not be nephrotoxic.
• High serum and urinary antibiotic concentrations do not necessarily ensure high tissue concentrations in the renal medulla; thus, chronic pyelonephritis may be difficult to eradicate.
• If systemically ill or azotemic, administer IV antibiotics for initial 48 hours.
• Give orally administered antibiotics at full therapeutic dosages for 2–6 weeks. Duration of antibiotics required for resolution of pyelonephritis is not definitively known.
• Do not use drugs that achieve good concentrations in urine but poor concentrations in serum (e.g., nitrofurantoin).

CONTRAINDICATIONS

Do not use aminoglycosides unless no other alternatives exist on the basis of urine culture and susceptibility testing.

PRECAUTIONS

Trimethoprim-sulfa combinations can cause side effects (keratoconjunctivitis sicca, blood dyscrasias, and polyarthritis) when administered for more than 4 weeks.

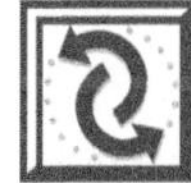

FOLLOW-UP

PATIENT MONITORING

Perform urine cultures and urinalysis during antibiotic administration (~5–7 days into treatment) and 1 and 4 weeks after antibiotics are finished.

PREVENTION/AVOIDANCE

Eliminate factors predisposing to UTI; correct ectopic ureters.

POSSIBLE COMPLICATIONS

Progressive CKD, recurrent pyelonephritis, struvite nephroliths, septicemia, septic shock, metastatic infection (e.g., endocarditis, polyarthritis).

EXPECTED COURSE AND PROGNOSIS

• Patients with acute or subacute pyelonephritis—fair to good, with a return to normal health unless the patient also has nephroliths, CKD, or some other underlying cause for UTI (e.g., obstruction or neoplasia).
• Established chronic infection of the renal medulla may be difficult to resolve because of poor tissue penetration of antibiotics.
• Patients with CKD caused by pyelonephritis—prognosis determined by the severity and rate of progression of the CKD.
• Recurrent pyelonephritis is likely if infected nephroliths are not removed.

MISCELLANEOUS

ASSOCIATED CONDITIONS

Hyperadrenocorticism, exogenous glucocorticoid administration, CKD, hyperthyroidism (cats), and diabetes mellitus are associated with lower UTI, which can ascend into the ureters and kidneys.

PREGNANCY/FERTILITY/BREEDING

Use antibiotics that are safe for the pregnant bitch or queen.

SYNONYMS

Upper UTI, pyelitis.

SEE ALSO

• Chronic Kidney Disease.
• Lower Urinary Tract Infection, Bacterial.
• Lower Urinary Tract Infection, Fungal.
• Nephrolithiasis.
• Urinary Tract Obstruction.
• Urolithiasis, Struvite—Dogs.

ABBREVIATIONS

• CKD = chronic kidney disease.
• UTI = urinary tract infection.

Suggested Reading

Bouillon J, Snead E, Casswell J, et al. Pyelonephritis in dogs: retrospective study of 47 histologically diagnosed cases (2005–2015). J Vet Intern Med 2018, 32:249–259.

Etedali NM, Reetz JA, Foster JD. Complications and clinical utility of ultrasonographically guided pyelocentesis and antegrade pyelography in cats and dogs: 49 cases (2007–2015). J Am Vet Med Assoc 2019, 254:826–834.

Foster JD, Krishnan H, Cole S. Characterization of subclinical bacteriuria, bacterial cystitis and pyelonephritis in dogs with chronic kidney disease. J Am Vet Med Assoc 2018, 252:1257–1262.

Author Larry G. Adams
Consulting Editor J.D. Foster
Acknowledgment The author and editors acknowledge the prior contribution of Carl A. Osborne.

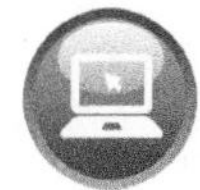

Client Education Handout available online

PYODERMA

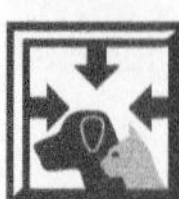

BASICS

DEFINITION

- Bacterial infection of the skin.
- Surface bacterial infections—often referred to as a "hot spot;" represents an acute moist dermatitis involving the surface of the skin.
- Superficial pyoderma—involves the epidermis and the intact hair follicle; includes mucocutaneous pyoderma.
- Deep pyoderma—involves the dermis and possibly subcutis; furunculosis is often present; patients can be systemically ill.

PATHOPHYSIOLOGY

- Skin infections occur when the surface barrier of the skin has been broken, the skin has become macerated by chronic exposure to moisture, the population of resident bacterial flora has been altered, circulation has been impaired, and/or immunocompetency of the patient has been negatively impacted by systemic illness or immunosuppressive therapy.
- Pyoderma is usually secondary to an underlying cause; the primary, underlying cause should be identified and managed to reduce the frequency and recurrence of skin infections.

P

SYSTEMS AFFECTED

Skin/exocrine.

GENETICS

N/A

INCIDENCE/PREVALENCE

- Dogs—very common.
- Cats—uncommon.

SIGNALMENT

Species

Dog and cat.

Breed Predilections

- Dog—short-coated breeds, especially those with excessive skin folds.
- German shepherd dog—severe, inflammatory and deep pyoderma that responds to antibiotics; frequently relapses.

Mean Age and Range

Age of onset is usually directly related to the underlying cause.

Predominant Sex

None

SIGNS

General Comments

- Superficial—usually involves the trunk; extent of lesions may be obscured by hair coat.
- Deep—often affects the chin, dorsal muzzle, pressure points, and feet; may be generalized and associated with symptoms of systemic illness, such as pyrexia and/or pain.

Historical Findings

- Acute or gradual onset.
- Variable pruritus—typically pruritic; the underlying cause may be pruritic or the staphylococcal infection itself may be pruritic; may not be pruritic if associated with hypercortisolemia.

Physical Examination Findings

- Papules.
- Pustules.
- Crusted papules.
- Crusts.
- Epidermal collarettes.
- Circular erythematous or hyperpigmented patches (macules).
- Alopecia; moth-eaten hair coat.
- Hemorrhagic bullae.
- Scaling.
- Lichenification.
- Erosions.
- Ulcerations.
- Target lesions.
- Abscess.
- Furunculosis, cellulitis.

CAUSES

- *Staphylococcus pseudintermedius*—most frequent dogs and cats.
- *Pasteurella multocida*—cats.
- Deep bacterial skin infections may be complicated by Gram-negative organisms (e.g., *Escherichia coli*, *Proteus* spp., *Pseudomonas* spp.).
- Rarely caused by higher bacteria (e.g., *Actinomyces*, *Nocardia*, *Mycobacteria*, *Actinobacillus*).

RISK FACTORS

- Hypersensitivity—flea allergic dermatitis; atopic dermatitis; cutaneous adverse reaction to food; contact allergic dermatitis.
- Parasites—especially *Demodex* spp.
- Fungal infection—dermatophytosis (*Microsporum canis*, *Microsporum gypseum*, or *Trichophyton mentagrophytes*) most common.
- Endocrine diseases—hypothyroidism; hyperadrenocorticism; sex hormone imbalance.
- Immunosuppression—excessive corticosteroid administration; young animals.
- Seborrhea—chin acne; schnauzer comedo syndrome.
- Conformation—short coat; skin folds; redundant interdigital skin.
- Trauma—pressure points; grooming; scratching; rooting behavior; irritants.
- Foreign body—foxtail; grass awn.

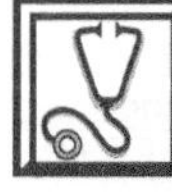

DIAGNOSIS

DIFFERENTIAL DIAGNOSIS

- Hypersensitivity—pruritus precedes lesions; persists with resolution of pyoderma.
- Flea allergic dermatitis or atopic dermatitis—may be seasonal.
- Endocrinopathy—relapsing pyoderma; consider if not associated with pruritus or pruritus resolves with resolution of the pyoderma; may be associated with systemic symptoms.
- Pustular diseases—dermatophytosis; demodicosis; pemphigus foliaceus; and subcorneal pustular dermatosis.
- Deep furunculosis—higher bacterial infection; demodicosis; dermatophytosis; opportunistic fungal infections; deep fungal infections; panniculitis; and zinc-responsive dermatosis.
- Superficial pyoderma in short-coated breeds often misdiagnosed as urticaria due to acute onset of pruritic papules and follicular tufting.

CBC/BIOCHEMISTRY/URINALYSIS

- Superficial pyoderma—normal or may reflect underlying cause (e.g., anemia due to hypothyroidism; stress leukogram and high serum alkaline phosphatase due to hyperadrenocorticism; eosinophilia due to parasitism).
- Generalized, deep pyoderma—may demonstrate leukocytosis with a regenerative left shift and hyperglobulinemia; abnormalities related to an underlying cause may be present.

OTHER LABORATORY TESTS

N/A

DIAGNOSTIC PROCEDURES

- Multiple skin scrapings—demodicosis.
- Direct smear from intact pustule—neutrophils with intracellular bacteria, typically cocci.
- Cytology from underneath a crust or edge of an epidermal collarette; help differentiate pemphigus foliaceus (acantholytic keratinocytes) and deep fungal infections (blastomycosis, cryptococcosis) from pyoderma; tissue grains may identify filamentous organisms characteristic of higher bacteria.
- Trichograms—dermatophytosis, follicular abnormalities.
- Dermatophyte culture—dermatophytosis.
- Surface or papule/pustule cytology—pemphigus foliaceus.
- Intradermal allergy testing—atopy.
- Elimination diet trial—food hypersensitivity.
- Endocrine tests—hypothyroidism, hyperadrenocorticism.
- Skin biopsy is rarely useful unless the infection is deep in nature; utilized to obtain tissue sample for macerated tissue culture.

Culture and Susceptibility Testing

- Recommended in recurrent cases and/or failure to respond to empiric antibiotics.
- Often positive for *S. pseudintermedius*.
- Other organisms besides staphylococci and higher bacteria may be cultured from lesions of deep pyoderma.
- Contents of an intact pustule—most reliable results for superficial infections.
- Punch biopsy obtained utilizing sterile technique for macerated tissue culture; especially and removal of the epidermis for

deep pyoderma; more likely false-negative results with superficial pyoderma.
• Freshly expressed exudate from a draining tract or from beneath a crust—may yield the pathogen or a contaminant if the lesion is not intact.

PATHOLOGIC FINDINGS

• Subcorneal pustules.
• Intraepidermal neutrophilic microabscesses.
• Perifolliculitis.
• Folliculitis.
• Furunculosis.
• Nodular to diffuse dermatitis.
• Panniculitis.
• Inflammatory reaction—suppurative or pyogranulomatous.
• Tissue grains within pyogranulomas—observed most often with *Actinomyces*, *Actinobacillus*, and *Nocardia*.
• Special stains—used to identify Gram-negative bacteria or acid-fast organisms.

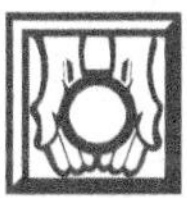

TREATMENT

APPROPRIATE HEALTH CARE

Usually outpatient, except for severe, generalized deep pyoderma.

NURSING CARE

• Severe, generalized, deep pyoderma—may require IV fluids, parenteral antibiotics, and/or daily whirlpool baths.
• Benzoyl peroxide or chlorhexidine shampoos—remove surface debris.
• Frequent topical therapy can help reduce the severity and frequency of recurrence.
• Whirlpool baths—deep pyoderma; remove crusted exudate; encourage drainage; decrease inflammation and improve tissue oxygenation.

DIET

Novel protein or hydrolysate diet if secondary to cutaneous adverse reaction to food.

SURGICAL CONSIDERATIONS

Fold pyoderma may require surgical correction to prevent recurrence.

MEDICATIONS

DRUG(S) OF CHOICE

• *S. pseudintermedius* isolates—usually susceptible to cephalosporins, amoxicillin–clavulanate, erythromycin, clindamycin, and trimethoprim–sulfamethoxazole; somewhat less responsive to lincomycin; frequently resistant to amoxicillin, ampicillin, penicillin.
• Amoxicillin–clavulanate—most isolates of *Staphylococcus* and *P. multocida* susceptible; generally effective for skin infections in cats.
• Superficial pyoderma—initially treated empirically with one of the antibiotics listed above.
• Recurrent, resistant, or deep infections—choose antibiotic therapy based upon culture and susceptibility testing (e.g., chloramphenicol).
• Multiple organisms with different antibiotic susceptibilities—select antibiotic on basis of the staphylococcal susceptibility.

CONTRAINDICATIONS

Corticosteroids—mask inflammation causing therapy to be discontinued prematurely and resulting in selection for resistant organisms; if used concurrently, therapy should be extended and the patient should be reevaluated before discontinuing antibiotic therapy.

PRECAUTIONS

• Cephalosporins, erythromycin, lincomycin, and clindamycin—vomiting; administer with food.
• Aminoglycosides—renal toxicity usually precludes prolonged systemic use.
• Trimethoprim–sulfamethoxazole—keratoconjunctivitis sicca, fever, hepatotoxicity, polyarthritis, and hematologic abnormalities, especially neutropenia; not recommended for use in Doberman pinschers.
• Chloramphenicol—use with caution in cats; mild, reversible anemia in dogs (uncommon); associated with aplastic anemia in humans; rear temporary limb muscle weakness is a possible side effect.

POSSIBLE INTERACTIONS

Trimethoprim-sulfamethoxazole—falsely decreased thyroid hormone test results.

ALTERNATIVE DRUG(S)

Bacterin (Staphage Lysate, Delmont Laboratories), staphoid AB, or autogenous injections—may improve antibiotic efficacy and decrease infection recurrence.

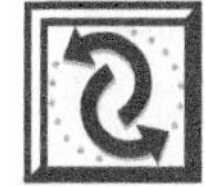

FOLLOW-UP

PATIENT MONITORING

Administer oral antibiotics for a minimum of 7–10 days beyond clinical cure; approximately 3–4 weeks for superficial pyoderma; 6–10 weeks for deep pyoderma.

PREVENTION/AVOIDANCE

• Routine bathing with benzoyl peroxide or chlorhexidine shampoos—may help prevent recurrences.
• Padded bedding—may ease pressure point pyoderma; also consider causes for poor wound healing including hypothyroidism.
• Topical benzoyl peroxide gel or mupirocin 2% ointment may be helpful adjunct therapies—chin acne, fold pyoderma, respectively.
• Identification and management of the underlying cause is crucial to prevent recurrence.

POSSIBLE COMPLICATIONS

Bacteremia and septicemia.

EXPECTED COURSE AND PROGNOSIS

Likely to be recurrent or nonresponsive if underlying cause is not identified and effectively managed.

MISCELLANEOUS

ASSOCIATED CONDITIONS

N/A

AGE-RELATED FACTORS

• Impetigo—affects young dogs before puberty; can be associated with poor husbandry; often requires only topical therapy.
• Superficial pustular dermatitis—occurs in kittens; associated with overzealous "mouthing" by the queen.
• Pyoderma secondary to atopic dermatitis—usually begins between 1 and 3 years of age.
• Pyoderma secondary to endocrine disorders—usually begins in middle adulthood.

ZOONOTIC POTENTIAL

• Cutaneous tuberculosis—rare.
• Feline leprosy—unknown.

PREGNANCY/FERTILITY/BREEDING

N/A

SEE ALSO

• Acne—Cats.
• Acne—Dogs.
• Perianal Fistula.
• Pododermatitis.

Suggested Reading
Helton Rhodes KA, Werner A. Blackwell's Five-Minute Veterinary Consult: Clinical Companion: Small Animal Dermatology, 3rd ed. Hoboken, NJ: Wiley-Blackwell, 2018.

Author Elizabeth R. Drake
Consulting Editor Alexander H. Werner Resnick

Client Education Handout available online

PYODERMA—METHICILLIN-RESISTANT

BASICS

OVERVIEW

• Staphylococcal bacterial skin infection resistant to *all* β-lactam antibiotics.
• Most often caused by *Staphylococcus pseudintermedius*; rarely *Staphylococcus aureus.*

SIGNALMENT

Dogs and Cats

• More common with chronic, primary skin conditions; associated with exposure to one or more courses of antibiotic therapy.
• Pyoderma less common in cats.

SIGNS

Dogs and Cats

• Papules. • Pustules. • Crusts. • Crusted papules. • Epidermal collarettes.
• Furunculosis, cellulitis if deep. • Circular erythematous or hyperpigmented spots (macules). • Alopecia, moth-eaten hair coat, especially in short-coated breeds.
• Hemorrhagic bullae. • Scale.
• Lichenification. • Abscess. • Pyoderma that persists despite appropriate empiric therapy.

CAUSES & RISK FACTORS

• Hypersensitivity—flea allergic dermatitis; atopic dermatitis; cutaneous adverse reaction to food; contact allergic dermatitis.
• Parasites—especially *Demodex* spp.
• Endocrine—hypothyroidism; hyperadrenocorticism (especially if nonpruritic).
• Immunosuppression—iatrogenic due to chronic glucocorticoid therapy; young animals. • Seborrhea—chin acne; schnauzer comedo syndrome. • Additional—short coat; skin folds; redundant interdigital skin; trauma of pressure points, especially in hypothyroid dogs; excessive grooming; scratching; rooting behavior; irritants; foreign bodies (foxtail; grass awn).

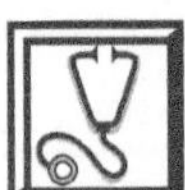

DIAGNOSIS

DIFFERENTIAL DIAGNOSIS

Dogs

• Demodicosis. • Dermatophytosis.
• Methicillin-sensitive pyoderma.
• Pemphigus foliaceus. • Systemic lupus erythematosus. • Other primary causes for pyoderma. • Epitheliotropic lymphoma (older animals).

Cats

• Dermatophytosis. • Flea-allergic dermatitis.
• Demodicosis. • Pemphigus foliaceus.
• Methicillin-sensitive pyoderma.
• Epitheliotropic lymphoma in older animals.

CBC/BIOCHEMISTRY/URINALYSIS

Generalized, deep pyoderma—may demonstrate leukocytosis with regenerative left shift and hyperglobulinemia; in addition, may reflect underlying cause; sepsis is a concern, especially if patient is immunosuppressed.

DIAGNOSTIC PROCEDURES

• Culture and susceptibility testing—*essential* when methicillin-resistant infection is suspected; should be performed when there is inadequate response to empiric treatment with antibiotics or in cases with a history of methicillin-resistant *S. pseudintermedius* (MRSP). • Multiple skin scrapings—demodicosis. • Direct smear from intact pustule—neutrophils with intracellular bacteria. • Cytology—from underneath crust or edge of epidermal.collarette. • Skin biopsy—rarely useful unless infection deep; used to obtain tissue sample for macerated tissue culture. • Dermatophyte culture—fungal infection. • Intradermal allergy testing—atopic dermatitis. • Elimination diet trial—cutaneous adverse reaction to food.
• Endocrine tests—hypothyroidism, hyperadrenocorticism.

PATHOLOGIC FINDINGS

• Subcorneal pustules. • Intraepidermal neutrophilic microabscesses. • Perifolliculitis.
• Folliculitis. • Furunculosis—deep infection. • Nodular to diffuse dermatitis.
• Panniculitis—deep infection.
• Inflammatory reaction—suppurative; pyogranulomatous with deep infections.

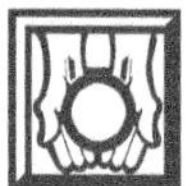

TREATMENT

• Topical therapy essential—chlorhexidine shampoo or spray, dilute bleach bathing, mupirocin ointment, for localized disease.
• Some cases resolve with topical therapy only—must be consistent/frequent.
• Generalized, deep pyoderma—hospitalization, IV fluids, IV antibiotics, whirlpool baths, depending on severity and risk for sepsis.

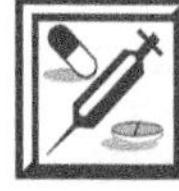

MEDICATIONS

DRUG(S) OF CHOICE

• Antibiotic therapy must be based on culture and susceptibility data. • Appropriate antibiotics must be administered long enough to resolve infection.

CONTRAINDICATIONS/POSSIBLE INTERACTIONS

Corticosteroid steroids—masks inflammation and suppresses immune system function; therapy should be discontinued. Oclacitinib—may suppress immune system function and delay resolution.

FOLLOW-UP

PATIENT MONITORING

Regular reevaluation of patient while still receiving treatment aids in decision regarding continuation of therapy or need for additional diagnostic tests.

PREVENTION/AVOIDANCE

• Choose antibiotic therapy from culture and susceptibility data—treatment failure occurs when antibiotic changes made without evidence. • Successful management of underlying disease. • Handwashing before and after handling patient.

EXPECTED COURSE AND PROGNOSIS

• Good if antibiotic choice is based on culture and susceptibility data and underlying cause is managed. • Methicillin-resistant infections not more virulent, but fewer antibiotic choices available for treatment.

MISCELLANEOUS

ZOONOTIC POTENTIAL

• Exposure of humans and animals to methicillin-resistant *S. aureus* (MRSA) and MRSP is common. • MRSP infections in humans are rare. • MRSP is not MRSA—MRSA infections in animals are rare and most associated with exposure to humans with MRSA infection.

SEE ALSO

• Pododermatitis.
• Pyoderma.

ABBREVIATIONS

• MRSA = methicillin-resistant *S. aureus.*
• MRSP = methicillin-resistant *S. pseudintermedius.*

INTERNET RESOURCES

Weese SJ: www.wormsandgermsblog.com

Suggested Reading

Helton Rhodes KA, Werner A. Blackwell's Five-Minute Veterinary Consult: Clinical Companion: Small Animal Dermatology, 3rd ed. Hoboken, NJ: Wiley-Blackwell, 2018.

Author Elizabeth R. Drake
Consulting Editor Alexander H. Werner Resnick

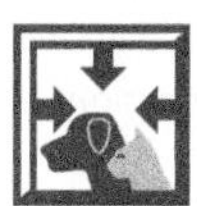

BASICS

DEFINITION

Pyometra is a bacterial suppurative inflammation of the endometrium leading to intraluminal accumulation of purulent exudate within the uterus.

PATHOPHYSIOLOGY

- Incompletely understood and multifactorial.
- Classic theory—repeated exposure of endometrium to high concentrations of estrogen during proestrus and estrus followed by high concentrations of progesterone during diestrus without pregnancy leads to development of cystic endometrial hyperplasia (CEH), which predisposes uterus to ascending bacterial infections.
- Strains of *Escherichia coli* with uropathogenic virulence factors that allow adhesion to the endometrium and establishment of an infection without CEH enter uterus during proestrus and estrus and act as a mucosal irritant stimulating development of CEH under the influence of progesterone. Uterine secretions may act as a growth medium for ascending bacteria.
- Regardless of underlying cause, pyometra does not occur in absence of progesterone (endogeneous or exogeneous).

SYSTEMS AFFECTED

- Reproductive.
- Hemic/lymphatic/immune.

GENETICS

- Genetic predisposition suspected in some related bitches.
- Suggested breed predisposition in Bernese mountain dog, Rottweiler, rough-coated collie, oriental cat breeds.

INCIDENCE/PREVALENCE

Accurate assessment difficult because most dogs and cats in the United States undergo elective ovariohysterectomy (OHE). A recent Swedish study reported overall incidence of pyometra in bitches as 199 per 10,000 dogs at risk and in queens as 17 per 10,000 cats at risk. Lower incidence in queens because they are induced ovulators.

SIGNALMENT

Species

Dog and cat.

Mean Age and Range

Usually >6 years old; range 4 months to 16 years; mean 7.25 years.

Predominant Sex

- Female—ovary intact.
- Spayed bitches and queens with ovarian remnant syndrome may develop a stump pyometra.

SIGNS

Historical Findings

- Dogs—usually within 12 weeks of last estrus.
- Cats—usually within 4 weeks of last estrus.
- History of treatment with estrogens and/or progestogens.

Physical Examination Findings

- Uterus—may be enlarged on abdominal palpation.
- Systemic illness—depends on duration and severity.
- Open cervix—bloody, purulent vaginal discharge, may not be noticed in queens.
- Closed cervix—systemically ill from endotoxemia and bacteremia: polyuria, polydipsia, lethargy, inappetence/anorexia, vomiting, abdominal distension, dehydration, shock.
- Pyrexia.

CAUSES

- Dogs—repeated exposure of endometrium to estrogen followed by prolonged exposure to progesterone without pregnancy.
- Cats—may be the result of estrogen at estrus followed by a progestational (pseudopregnancy) phase caused by spontaneous ovulation or ovulation induction.

RISK FACTORS

- Middle-aged to older, nulliparous ovary-intact females may be predisposed.
- Pharmacologic use of estrogen (mismate shot) during midestrus to early diestrus.
- No correlation with pseudopregnancy in dogs.
- Long-term and high-dose use of progestagens (for estrus prevention) in both queens and bitches.

DIAGNOSIS

DIFFERENTIAL DIAGNOSIS

- Pregnancy.
- Vaginitis.
- Metritis and retained fetal membranes (associated within first days post partum).
- Hydrometra (serous intrauterine discharge); mucometra (mucoid intrauterine discharge); hematometra (hemorrhagic intrauterine discharge).
- Other causes of polyuria/polydipsia—diabetes mellitus, hyperadrenocorticism, renal disease.

CBC/BIOCHEMISTRY/URINALYSIS

- Neutrophilia or neutropenia with left shift ± toxic change; more severe with closed cervix.
- Normocytic, normochromic anemia.
- Hyperglobulinemia, hyperproteinemia, hypoalbuminemia, hypercholesterolemia, elevated C-reactive protein concentration.
- Azotemia.
- Elevated alanine aminotransferase and alkaline phosphatase enzyme activities.
- Electrolyte disturbances.
- Urinalysis—isosthenuria, bacteriuria, glucosuria, and proteinuria possible. Collect sample by catheterization of urinary bladder to avoid risk of uterine puncture with cystocentesis. Midstream urine sample may be contaminated by vaginal discharge.

OTHER LABORATORY TESTS

- Cytologic examination of vulvar discharge—degenerate neutrophils, phagocytized bacteria; may be indistinguishable from purulent discharge associated with vaginal disease (e.g., vaginitis, vaginal mass, foreign object). Vaginoscopy can confirm origin and rule out other causes of discharge.
- Bacterial culture and sensitivity—vulvar discharge sample to be taken directly from the uterus transcervically or cranial vagina with the aid of a vaginal speculum and guarded swab. A free-catch urine sample can also be useful as the causative agent in the pyometra is often located in the bladder.
- Serologic testing for *Brucella canis*—rapid slide agglutination test as a screen; sensitive but not specific. If positive, recheck by an agar gel immunodiffusion test or bacterial culture of whole blood, lymph node aspirate, or vulvar discharge.
- Hormone assay—in most cases, progesterone concentration will be >2 ng/mL; important to measure in animals that present in anestrus, as treatment with a progesterone receptor antagonist will be ineffective.

IMAGING

Radiography

- Enlarged, distended uterus (see Web Figure 1).
- Rule out pregnancy— fetal skeletal ossification occurs 45 days after ovulation.

Ultrasonography

- Uterine horns distended with intraluminal fluid, with or without flocculation. Uterine wall thickened with irregular edges and small hypoechoic areas consistent with cystic change (CEH) (see Web Figure 2), uterine wall can appear thin if severely distended; monitoring of the volume of uterine fluid is necessary during medical therapy; presence of severe CEH and/or ovarian cysts associated with poorer prognosis for medical management and fertility.
- Rule out pregnancy—20–24 days after ovulation.
- Pyometra may rarely occur with pregnancy in dogs.

DIAGNOSTIC PROCEDURES

Vaginoscopy—indicated in dogs with purulent vulvar discharge and no apparent uterine enlargement; allows determination of site of origin of the discharge; not possible in cats.

PYOMETRA

PATHOLOGIC FINDINGS

- Endometrium (dogs and cats)—cobblestone appearance (see Web Figure 3).
- Cystic endometrial surface—covered by malodorous, mucopurulent exudate; thickened by increased endometrial gland size and cystic gland distension.

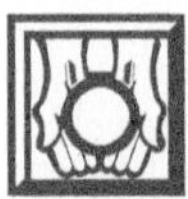

TREATMENT

APPROPRIATE HEALTH CARE

- Inpatient; life-threatening condition if the cervix is closed, resulting in endotoxemia, bacteremia, and sepsis. Resuscitation requires immediate IV fluid administration and broad-spectrum antibiotics to stabilize for anesthesia and surgery.
- Open-cervix pyometra may be a candidate for medical therapy.

NURSING CARE

Supportive care.

CLIENT EDUCATION

- Medical treatment only recommended for valuable, young (<4 years) breeding animals that are not azotemic and systemically well. For all other animals, OHE is the treatment of choice. The prognosis for successful medical treatment and future fertility in older animals and animals with evidence of uterine and ovarian pathology is poor.
- Historically, medical treatment of closed-cervix pyometra was associated with uterine rupture and peritonitis, but new pharmacologic agents and treatment protocols now make this a rare event.
- Bitches that are refractory or chronic cases that do not respond to medical treatment are candidates for OHE.
- Warn of possible recurrence of pyometra after medical therapy—important to breed at the next heat and spay when desired number of litters is achieved.

SURGICAL CONSIDERATIONS

- Complete OHE is the preferred treatment in all animals not intended for breeding, older bitches (>4 years), bitches with evidence of chronic CEH changes and/or ovarian follicular cysts, bitches that present systemically unwell and require immediate emergency care and stabilization.
- Patients should be systemically stabilized prior to anesthesia for surgery (correction of any acid–base derangements, dehydration, hypotension, shock, electrolyte abnormalities, arrythmias) and administered IV fluids and IV broad-spectrum antibiotics.
- Closed-cervix pyometra—exercise great care in handling the enlarged and friable uterus (see Web Figure 4).
- Place saline-soaked laparotomy sponges in abdomen to prevent leakage of purulent material into peritoneal cavity.

MEDICATIONS

DRUG(S) OF CHOICE

Antibiotics

- Empirical, pending results of bacterial culture and sensitivity:
  - Broad-spectrum—ampicillin 22 mg/kg PO, IV q8h; amoxicillin and clavulonic acid 22 mg/kg, PO, q12h; ampicillin and sulbactam 22–30 mg/kg IV q8–12h or cefazolin 22 mg/kg IV, IM q8h combined with enrofloxacin 5–10 mg/kg PO q24h.
  - Continue for at least 14 days after resolution of vulvar discharge and fluid in uterine lumen.
- Rationale of medical therapy—remove progesterone and its effects on uterus, eliminate bacteria from uterus, promote cervical dilation and drainage of pus from the uterus.

Aglepristone

- Progesterone receptor antagonist; competitively binds to progesterone receptor with greater affinity than natural progesterone, preventing biological effect of progesterone. Will not lower progesterone levels.
- Dose—10 mg/kg SC, days 1, 2, 8, and if not cured day 14 and 28 in bitches. An additional injection at day 5 has been associated with an improved treatment success rate. In queens, 15 mg/kg SC is recommended. Minimal side effects. Excellent choice for closed pyometras as it dilates the cervix with minimal uterine contractions. Evacuation of uterus may be improved by adding prostaglandin. Aglepristone is not registered or approved by FDA in United States and not suitable for use in bitches with poor liver or kidney function.

Prostaglandins (PGF2α)

- Doses listed here for native compound only (dinoprost tromethamine; Lutalyse®); has both luteolytic and ecobolic actions.
- Lower doses minimize side effects and ecobolic effect, especially in closed pyometras. Once the cervix is fully dilated the dose can be gradually increased if tolerated.
- Animals should be monitored in hospital for at least 1 hour after each treatment. If animal is systemically well, may be managed as outpatient.
- Side effects (dose-dependent)—tachypnea, vomiting, diarrhea, urination, anxiety; seen 20 minutes after administration and last for 15–30 minutes. Use of PGF2α in brachycephalic breeds is contraindicated due to their predisposition to bronchospasm.
- Dogs and cats—10 µg/kg SC q5-6h day 1, then increase to 20–25 µg/kg q5–6h if tolerated for 1–2 days; then increase to 50 µg/kg q5–6h for 3–4 days. Queens are more resistant to PGF2α than bitches; often higher doses for longer periods are required.

Cloprostenol

- Synthetic PGF2α analogue; longer action (>30 hours) than natural form of PGF2α.
- Dogs—1 µg/kg SC q24h for 7–14 days; convenience of once a day or every 2–3 days treatment but greater side effects, stimulates less uterine contractions and prolonged time to resolution compared to natural form of PGF2α.

Dopamine Agonists

Cabergoline (5 µg/kg PO q24h for 7–14 days) or bromocriptine (10–20 µg/kg PO q8h); both given with food to reduce risk of vomiting; cabergoline has fewer side effects. Prolactin antagonists (e.g., have luteolytic action); best used in combination with PGF2α—should see cervical opening within 24–48 hours. Only effective after 25 days post ovulation.

CONTRAINDICATIONS

High-dose PGF2α and cloprostenol cause strong uterine contractions that may cause uterine rupture or force purulent exudate through the oviducts if used with closed-cervix pyometra.

ALTERNATIVE DRUG(S)

Misoprostol—synthetic PGE1 analogue (10 µg/kg PO or 200 µg tablet in <20 kg and 400 µg in >20 kg bitch intravaginally). Side effects minimal, facilitates cervical relaxation. Best used in combination with aglepristone and PGF2α (PGE1 does not induce luteolysis).

FOLLOW-UP

PATIENT MONITORING

- OHE—For patients not responding to medical treatment within 5 days or those refractory to medical treatment.
- Clinical improvement should be seen within 48 hours after initiation of treatment:
  - Vaginal discharge—should reduce in volume and character over 5 days.
  - Ultrasonography—to assess response to treatment; reduction in uterine wall thickness and intraluminal fluid should be seen within 3 days after start of treatment; fluid in lumen should be absent within 5–7 days.
- Serum progesterone concentrations decline within 48 hours of treatment with PGF2α and should be <2 ng/mL at 5–7 days; recurrence of pyometra can occur if complete luteolysis not achieved.
- CBC should return to normal within 2 weeks.
- Continue treatment until no vulvar discharge is present and no fluid is seen within uterus on ultrasound. Prolonged treatment correlated with poor fertility.

PREVENTION/AVOIDANCE

- Animals not intended for breeding should be spayed.

P

- Exogenous progestagens for estrus suppression should be used with caution.
- Breeding females should be bred while they are young (<4 years) and spayed as soon as the desired number of litters has been obtained; a pregnant uterus reduces the risk of developing pyometra and maximizes uterine health.
- Animals that have been medically treated for pyometra should be bred on the very next estrus; gravid uterus is less susceptible to reinfection.
- Antimicrobial therapy at subsequent heat may or may not be helpful (controversial). Antibiotic selection based on culture and sensitivity of uterine fluid until 21 days of gestation.
- Mibolerone (androgen-receptor agonist) may be helpful following medical treatment of pyometra to postpone subsequent heat and allow endometrium to repair.

POSSIBLE COMPLICATIONS

- Recurrence of pyometra at subsequent heats.
- Uterine rupture leading to sepsis.
- Bacteremia-associated infection affecting various organs (i.e., uveitis, septic arthritis, osteomyelitis, etc.).

EXPECTED COURSE AND PROGNOSIS

- Prognosis for survival is good if uterine rupture does not occur; 4% mortality rate in bitches and 8% in queens.
- Prognosis for response to medical therapy is good, especially if young, healthy animals (average 86% in bitches; 95% in queens).
- Recurrence rate of pyometra is dependent on age, parity, and preexisting uterine pathology (reported range 20–65%).
- Variable pregnancy rates reported after treatment for pyometra (50–90%).

MISCELLANEOUS

ASSOCIATED CONDITIONS

Pyometra of the uterine stump in spayed animals—may develop any time after ovariohysterectomy; associated with ovarian remnant.

PREGNANCY/FERTILITY/BREEDING

Drugs used for treatment of pyometra are abortificants—always rule out pregnancy before administration, caution while handling.

SEE ALSO

- Breeding, Timing.
- Infertility, Female—Dogs.
- Ovarian Remnant Syndrome.

ABBREVIATIONS

- CEH = cystic endometrial hyperplasia.
- OHE = elective ovariohysterectomy.
- PGF2α = prostaglandin F2α

Suggested Reading

Hagman R. Pyometra in small animals. Vet Clin North Am Small Anim Pract 2018, 48(4):639–661.

Hagman R, Lagerstedt AS, Hedhammar Å, Egenvall A. A breed-matched case-control study of potential risk-factors for canine pyometra. Theriogenology 2011, 75(7):1251–1257.

Authors Fiona Hollinshead and Natali Krekeler

Consulting Editor Erin E. Runcan

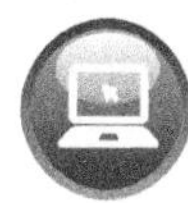

Client Education Handout available online

PYOTHORAX

BASICS

DEFINITION

Accumulation of septic suppurative inflammation in the pleural cavity.

PATHOPHYSIOLOGY

• Infectious—from transpulmonary, transesophageal, or transthoracic inoculation of bacteria into the pleural space, with subsequent suppurative pleuritis. • Dogs—often associated with an inhaled grass awn or other foreign object or a penetrating wound to the thorax. • Other causes include extension of discospondylitis, esophageal perforation, parasitic migration, hematogenous spread, previous thoracic surgery, and neoplasia with abscess formation. • Cats—most commonly associated with penetrating bite wounds, foreign bodies, or aspiration of oropharyngeal flora and extension of subsequent pneumonia into the pleural space.

SYSTEMS AFFECTED

• Respiratory. • Cardiovascular. • Renal—protein-losing nephropathy.

GEOGRAPHIC DISTRIBUTION

Etiology is regionally dependent. For example, inhaled grass awn or foxtails are common in the western United States. *Spirocerca lupi* should be considered as a predisposing cause in endemic areas (Africa, Asia, southeastern United States).

SIGNALMENT

Species

Dog and cat.

Breed Predilections

Dogs—hunting and sporting breeds; for example, Labrador retrievers, German shorthaired pointers, springer spaniels, and border collies.

Mean Age and Range

Median ~4 years, although there is wide variation.

Predominant Sex

Male animals overrepresented.

SIGNS

General Comments

• Often insidious in onset, with few clinical signs until late in the course of disease.
• Respiratory compromise—often not severe unless disease is advanced. • Vomiting/diarrhea may be initial presenting complaint in 25% of canine cases.

Historical Findings

• Diminished activity. • Collapse after exercising and slow recovery. • Weight loss and partial anorexia can be the only clinical signs.

Physical Examination Findings

• Tachypnea. • Cachexia. • Cough.
• Pyrexia. • Thoracic auscultation—muffled heart and lung sounds. • Cats—may show few clinical signs before onset of apparently acute respiratory distress, collapse, and septic shock; bradycardia and hypersalivation associated with poor outcome. • Injury to the thoracic wall—may not be apparent or may be healed at the time of examination.

CAUSES

• Infectious—Dogs: *Actinomyces* spp., *Nocardia* spp., anaerobes (*Bacteroides, Peptostreptococcus, Fusobacterium*), *Corynebacterium, Escherichia coli, Pasteurella,* and *Streptococcus* spp.; fungal agents. Cats: oral commensals (e.g., *Pasteurella multocida* and *Bacteroides* spp.) most common; obligate anaerobes (*Peptostreptococcus, Fusobacterium*) common. • Parasitic—Dogs: esophageal rupture of *S. lupi* granuloma. • Neoplastic—rarely with intrathoracic tumors secondary to tumor necrosis.

RISK FACTORS

• Dogs—hunting, field trials, and other strenuous outdoor sporting activities; *S. lupi* endemic areas. • Cats—multiple cat households, outdoor cats, pneumonia, upper respiratory infection.

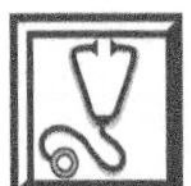

DIAGNOSIS

DIFFERENTIAL DIAGNOSIS

• Other pleural effusions—chylothorax and hemothorax; nonseptic exudates (feline infectious peritonitis or neoplasia); transudative effusions; differentiated via cytologic examination. • Diseases associated with fever of unknown origin should be considered for animals with nonlocalizing signs.

CBC/BIOCHEMISTRY/URINALYSIS

• Marked neutrophilic leukocytosis with left shift, monocytosis, and anemia of chronic disease. • Regenerative anemia—can be seen with substantial hemorrhage into the pleural cavity. • Hyperglobulinemia—possible due to chronic inflammation.
• Hypoalbuminemia as a negative acute-phase reactant or due to renal loss, if glomerulonephritis results from chronic antigenic stimulation. • Azotemia—prerenal and/or renal.

IMAGING

• Radiography—unilateral or bilateral pleural effusion with pleural fissure lines; pulmonary parenchymal lesions (consolidation, atelectasis, masses) common; mediastinal lesions possible. • Ultrasonography—pleural effusion; may show marked amount of fibrinous deposition in the pleural space; may identify consolidated lung masses, mediastinal masses, and abscessed or neoplastic lung nodules. • CT—focal interstitial to alveolar pulmonary opacities; pleural thickening; enlarged intrathoracic lymph nodes; pleural effusion; pneumothorax; and foreign body identification.

DIAGNOSTIC PROCEDURES

Thoracocentesis

• Cytologic evaluation—necessary to confirm the diagnosis; many effusions appear grossly hemorrhagic. • Gram stains—can facilitate early identification of pathogenic organisms.
• Sulfa granules (small accumulations of purulent debris) in the exudate—characteristic of infection by filamentous organisms (e.g., *Actinomyces* and *Nocardia*). • Organisms are often seen on cytologic examination, often within degenerative neutrophils.

Microbiology

• Culture fluid samples aerobically and anaerobically. Consider *Mycoplasma* culture if standard cultures are negative. • Filamentous, anaerobic organisms are slow-growing or difficult to grow; cultures should be maintained longer than standard samples.
• Sulfa granules—maceration may enhance culturing; contain higher concentrations of bacteria. • Fungal organisms—culture depends on history and geographic location.
• Urine samples—culture with suspected pyelonephritis.

Esophagoscopy

If *S. lupi* is suspected.

PATHOLOGIC FINDINGS

• Fibrinous and suppurative pleuritis, with or without pulmonary abscessation. • Organisms may be identified on histopathology.
• Glomerulonephritis.

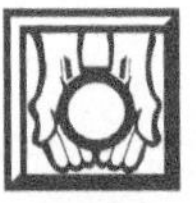

TREATMENT

APPROPRIATE HEALTH CARE

• Inpatient—often for several days to weeks.
• Treat like any abscess; drainage is critical—without it resolution is highly unlikely.
• Surgical exploration, debridement, and potential lobectomy required in some cases.

NURSING CARE

• Continuous evacuation via tube thoracostomy with low-pressure suction through a perforated tube; use a large-bore tube to minimize occlusion; continue until net drainage is <2–3 mL/kg/day and intracellular bacteria are no longer visible on Gram stain; drainage may be slightly higher with red rubber tubes because they are more irritating. • Cats—usually require general anesthesia for tube placement. • Dogs with severe respiratory compromise—may substitute local anesthesia and regional analgesia for general anesthesia. • Periodic thoracic radiography—to ensure proper tube placement, and lack of pocketing or loculation of exudate, determine whether bilateral tube placement is necessary; document primary pulmonary pathology that may not have been apparent on initial examination. • Thoracic lavage—every 6–8 hours with warm, sterile saline; may help break down consolidated debris. Consider addition of heparin (1,500 units/L) to lavage fluid. • Coupage (rapid thoracic percussion)—may help remove consolidated debris. • Repeat bacterial culture if the patient fails to improve.

ACTIVITY

• Inpatient—encourage light exercise (10 minutes every 6–8 hours); promotes ventilatory efforts and helps break down pleural adhesions. • After discharge, gradually increase exercise over 2–4 months.

DIET

• High-calorie food. • Consider feeding tube placement if prolonged anorexia.

CLIENT EDUCATION

Warn client that the duration of treatment (inpatient and outpatient) is long and expensive; recurrence is possible with either medical or surgical management.

SURGICAL CONSIDERATIONS

• Surgery—higher cure rate expected with surgery if pulmonary abscessation, pleural fibrosis, lung lobe torsion, extensive loculation of pus is present, or if mediastinum is involved.
• Thoracoscopy can be utilized as an intermediate step to assess degree of severity and need for more aggressive intervention.
• Identified foreign body via thoracic imaging (radiography, ultrasound, or CT)—thoracotomy and retrieval indicated; grass awns are uncommonly found, even during surgery.

MEDICATIONS

DRUG(S) OF CHOICE

Antimicrobials

• Ultimately, choice determined by results of *in vitro* sensitivity testing. • Suspected specific pathogen—initiate treatment before culture results are available; choose on the basis of common antibiotic sensitivities of particular organisms; *Actinomyces* spp. and *Bacteroides* (non-*fragilis*) spp. often susceptible to beta-lactams or lincosamides; *Nocardia* spp. often susceptible to potentiated sulfonamides; obligate anaerobic bacteria (including *B. fragilis*) susceptible to amoxicillin–clavulanic acid, chloramphenicol, and usually metronidazole; *Pasteurella* spp. often susceptible to potentiated penicillins.
• Ampicillin or amoxicillin with a β-lactamase inhibitor—ampicillin and sulbactam 20–30 mg/kg IV q8h followed by amoxicillin–clavulanic acid 12–25 mg/kg PO q8h when medications can be given orally.
• Clindamycin 5.5–11.0 mg/kg IV or PO q12h. • Multiple antibiotics occasionally necessary.

Analgesics

• Required following thoracotomy or during thoracocentesis. • Consider multimodal analgesia—systemic opioids, nonsteroidal anti-inflammatory drugs; intrapleural analgesia.

CONTRAINDICATIONS

Glucocorticoids and immunosuppressive agents—avoid with infectious pyothorax.

PRECAUTIONS

Potentiated sulfas—can be associated with keratoconjunctivitis sicca, polyarthropathy, hypothyroidism, thrombocytopenia, and anemia, especially with prolonged use.

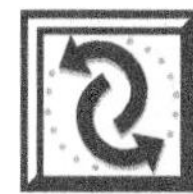

FOLLOW-UP

PATIENT MONITORING

• Decreasing thoracic fluid production, decrease in cell count in pleural fluid, and absence of bacteria usually noted within 4–7 days indicate that drains can be removed. Fluid should be submitted for aerobic and anaerobic culture at the time of drain removal. • Evaluate thoracic radiographs—ensure adequate evacuation of fluid.
• Antibiotics—continue for 1 month after the patient is clinically normal, the hemogram is normal, and there is no radiographic evidence of fluid reaccumulation; average duration of therapy is 3–4 months but may continue for 6–12 months or longer. • Assess CBC and radiographs monthly—residual radiographic changes may be permanent, but fluid should be absent.

POSSIBLE COMPLICATIONS

• Incorrect insertion of the thoracostomy tube—may prevent adequate drainage or produce pneumothorax; placement too far cranially may put pressure on brachial arteries and veins, resulting in unilateral limb edema or lameness; lung laceration during placement.
• Persistent, recurrent pyothorax—compartmentalization of exudate; premature discontinuation of treatment; pulmonary lesions. • Chronic fibrosing pleuritis and poor performance after apparent recovery—may occasionally respond to further surgery.
• Persistent granulomatous mediastinitis.

EXPECTED COURSE AND PROGNOSIS

• With aggressive management—prognosis fair to excellent (60–90% survival).
• Dependent on severity of clinical signs.
• Overall better prognosis in dogs (83%) than in cats (62%). • Return to performance—dependent on chronicity of disease and level of management.

MISCELLANEOUS

ASSOCIATED CONDITIONS

• Retroperitoneal abscessation and discospondylitis caused by migration of a foreign body through the diaphragm into the retroperitoneal space—occasionally seen.
• Glomerulonephropathy—can be reversible with successful resolution of pyothorax.

SYNONYMS

• Empyema. • Pleurisy. • Suppurative pleuritis.

SEE ALSO

• Chylothorax.
• Dyspnea and Respiratory Distress.
• Panting and Tachypnea.
• Pleural Effusion.

Suggested Reading

Bach JF, Balakrishnan A. Retrospective comparison of costs between medical and surgical treatment of canine pyothorax. Can Vet J 2015, 56:1140–1143.

Epstein SE. Exudative pleural diseases in small animals. Vet Clin North Am Small Anim Pract 2014, 44:161–180.

Lappin MR, Blondeau J, Boothe D, et al. Antimicrobial use guidelines for treatment of respiratory tract disease in dogs and cats: Antimicrobial Guidelines Working Group of the International Society for Companion Animal Infectious Diseases. J Vet Intern Med 2017, 31:279–294.

Scott J, Singh A, Monnet E, et al. Video-assisted thoracic surgery for the management of pyothorax in dogs: 14 cases. Vet Surg 2017, 46:722–730.

Stillion JR, Letendre JA. A clinical review of the pathophysiology, diagnosis, and treatment of pyothorax in dogs and cats. J Vet Emerg Crit Care 2015, 25:113–129.

Author Catriona M. MacPhail
Consulting Editor Elizabeth Rozanski

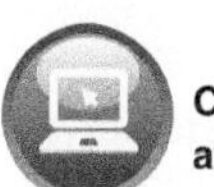

Client Education Handout available online

P

PYRETHRIN AND PYRETHROID TOXICOSIS

BASICS

OVERVIEW

• Insecticides. • Pyrethrins—natural. • Pyrethroids—synthetic. • Based on cases managed by the ASPCA Animal Poison Control Center exposures reported by generic from most to least are permethrin, deltamethrin, flumethrin, etofenprox, pyrethrins, cyfluthrin, cyphenothrin, imiprothrin and lambda cyhalothrin. • Affect the nervous system—reversibly prolong sodium conductance in nerve axons, resulting in repetitive nerve discharges. • With the advent of oral insecticides, safer topicals, and improved client education pyrethrin/pyrethroid adverse event reports continue to decrease. In 2017, 15.1% of all insecticide-related calls to the ASPCA Animal Poison Control Center were attributed to pyrethrin/pyrethroid-containing products.

SIGNALMENT

More frequently in cats; small dogs; and young, old, sick, anemic, or debilitated animals.

SIGNS

• Result from immune-mediated allergic hypersensitivity and anaphylactic reactions, genetic-based idiosyncratic reactions, and neurotoxic reactions. • Mild—hypersalivation; paw flicking; ear twitching; mild depression; vomiting; diarrhea. • Moderate—protracted vomiting and diarrhea; marked depression; ataxia; muscle tremors. • Extreme dermal or oral overdose—may produce seizures or death. • Cats—sensitive to pyrethroids. Cats inappropriately treated with permethrin-containing products for use on dogs, often develop muscle tremors, ataxia, seizures, hyperthermia, and death within hours if not treated. • Dogs may develop tremors following exposure to liquid or granular lawn products containing bifenthrin. • Allergic reactions—urticaria; hyperemia; pruritus; anaphylaxis; shock; respiratory distress; (rarely) death.

CAUSES & RISK FACTORS

• Cats—more sensitive; less-efficient metabolic pathways, combined with grooming habits. Direct contact with permethrin spot-on treated dogs. • Patients with subnormal body temperatures after bathing, anesthesia, or sedation—predisposed to clinical signs.

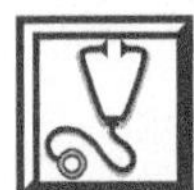

DIAGNOSIS

DIFFERENTIAL DIAGNOSIS

• Exposure history (amount and frequency of product usage), type and severity of clinical signs, and onset and duration of clinical signs—must be consistent before a tentative diagnosis can be made. • Misapplication of permethrin-containing dog-only flea product on cats. • Organophosphorous compounds, carbamate, or d-limonene toxicosis. • Strychnine, metaldehyde, tremorgenic mycotoxins, methylxanthines, amphetamines, serotonergic drug overdose, alcohol intoxication from isopropyl alcohol-based sprays.

OTHER LABORATORY TESTS

• Pyrethrins—analytical tests not generally available. • Pyrethroids—some compounds can be detected in tissues, especially on hair, to confirm exposure. Hair analysis for permethrin can be valuable when severity of the adverse event in cats is much greater than anticipated based on the reported product application. Cats with generalized full-body tremors or seizures after reported application of a cat-approved flea product are suspect for exposure to a permethrin-containing product.

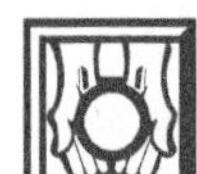

TREATMENT

• Mild adverse reactions (salivation, paw flicking, and ear twitching)—often self-limiting and resolve with no care. • Continued mild signs—bathe at home with a mild hand dish-washing detergent (strictly avoid hypothermia). • Patient saturated with spray products—dry with a warmed towel; brush. • Progression to tremors and ataxia—hospitalize. • Bathing upon stabilization (tremors controlled) with liquid hand dish-washing detergent and warm water is critical. • Seriously affected patient—IV fluid support recommended. • Maintenance of a normal body temperature—critical.

MEDICATIONS

DRUG(S) OF CHOICE

• Tremors or seizures—especially for cats exposed to permethrin; methocarbamol injectable at 55–220 mg/kg IV not to exceed 330 mg/kg/day; administer one-half dose slowly IV, wait until the patient begins to relax, continue administration to effect; do not exceed 2 mL/min injection rate, and start with lower dose initially. • Diazepam at low dosages has been used to control minor hyperesthesia. Seizure control has been achieved with pentobarbital, propofol (3–6 mg/kg IV or 0.1 mg/kg/min CRI) and inhalant anesthetics. Methocarbamol remains the agent of choice and can also be used orally for treating mild tremors (50–100 mg/kg q8h; 30 minutes onset time). • Activated charcoal (2 g/kg PO) is rarely beneficial or recommended. • Emetics—rarely warranted.

CONTRAINDICATIONS/POSSIBLE INTERACTIONS

Atropine sulfate—not antidotal; avoid; may cause tachycardia, CNS stimulation, disorientation, drowsiness, respiratory depression, and even seizures.

FOLLOW-UP

PREVENTION/AVOIDANCE

• Proper application of flea-control products—greatly reduces reactions. • Reduction of salivation—spray onto a grooming brush; evenly brush through hair coat. • Liquids—term "dip" common; never submerge animal; pour on body; sponge to cover dry areas. • Premise products—do not apply topically unless labeled for such use; after treating house or yard, do not allow animal in the area until product has dried, and environment has been ventilated. • Do not apply dog-only products on cats. • Do not use permethrin spot-on products on dogs in households where cats groom or sleep in physical contact with dogs.

EXPECTED COURSE AND PROGNOSIS

• Hypersalivation—may recur for several days after use of flea-control product when patient (especially cat) grooms itself. • Most clinical signs (mild to severe) resolve within 24–72 hours.

MISCELLANEOUS

Suggested Reading

Hansen SR, Villar D, Buck WB, et al. Pyrethrins and pyrethroids in dogs and cats. Compend Contin Educ Pract Vet 1994, 16:707–713.

Kuo K, Odunayo A. Adjunctive therapy with intravenous lipid emulsion and methocarbamol for permethrin toxicity in 2 cats. J Vet Emerg Crit Care (San Antonio) 2013, 23(4):436–441.

Means C. Dietary supplements and herbs. In: Poppenga RH, Gwaltney-Brant SM, eds., Small Animal Toxicology Essentials. Chichester: Wiley-Blackwell, 2011, pp. 161–169.

Authors Steven R. Hansen and Elizabeth A. Curry-Galvin

Consulting Editor Lynn R. Hovda

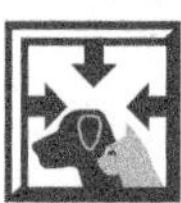

BASICS

OVERVIEW

• Red blood cells (RBCs) require energy in the form of ATP for maintenance of shape, deformability, active membrane transport, and limited synthetic activities; mature RBCs lack mitochondria and depend on anaerobic glycolysis for ATP generation.
• Pyruvate kinase (PK) catalyzes an important rate-controlling ATP-generating step in glycolysis; consequently, energy metabolism is markedly impaired in PK-deficient RBCs, resulting in shortened RBC lifespan and anemia; bone marrow compensation is reflected by erythroid hyperplasia and marked reticulocytosis.
• Hepatic failure may result from chronic iron overload.

SIGNALMENT

• Autosomal recessive trait recognized in basenji, beagle, West Highland white terrier, Cairn terrier, miniature poodle, dachshund, Chihuahua, pug, American Eskimo, and Labrador retriever dogs, and in Abyssinian, Somali, and domestic shorthair cats.
• Heterozygous-deficient Bengal, Egyptian Mau, La Perm, Maine coon, Norwegian Forest, Savannah, Siberian, and Singapura cats.
• Affected homozygous animals are generally not recognized as abnormal until several months of age or adulthood.

SIGNS

• Affected cats are often asymptomatic.
• Signs of anemia and shock (lethargy, tachycardia, exercise intolerance, pale mucous membranes).
• Splenomegaly may be present.
• Systolic heart murmur due to anemia.
• Icterus is occasionally seen in cats but rarely in dogs, unless hepatic failure present.
• Affected dogs may be slightly smaller than normal for their breed and age and may exhibit weakness and muscle wasting.
• Affected cats may exhibit diarrhea, inappetence, poor coat quality, and weight loss.

CAUSES & RISK FACTORS

• RBCs from normal adult dogs exhibit only one PK isozyme (the R-type).
• Breed-specific defects in the *PKLR* gene result in erythrocyte PK deficiency in dogs.
• A common molecular defect in the *PKLR* gene has been described in cats.

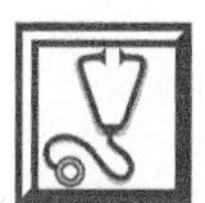

DIAGNOSIS

DIFFERENTIAL DIAGNOSIS

• Other causes of hemolytic anemia—immune-mediated hemolytic anemia, hemotropic mycoplasmosis, babesiosis, Heinz body hemolytic anemia, microangiopathic hemolytic anemia, and phosphofructokinase deficiency (dogs).
• Affected animals—negative Coombs' test, no parasites or Heinz bodies in stained blood films, seronegative for *Babesia* spp., and no evidence of disseminated intravascular coagulation or heartworm disease.

CBC/BIOCHEMISTRY/URINALYSIS

• Dogs—persistent macrocytic hypochromic anemia, with hematocrit (HCT) of 16–28% and reticulocyte counts of 15–50%.
• Cats—anemia is intermittent (HCT 13–40%), with slightly to markedly increased aggregate reticulocyte counts.
• Normal or slightly high total leukocyte counts.
• Normal to slightly high platelet counts.
• Moderate to marked polychromasia, anisocytosis, and increased nucleated RBCs on stained blood films.
• Poikilocytosis in splenectomized dogs.
• Possible abnormal clinical chemistry findings, such as hyperferremia, hyperbilirubinemia, and slightly high serum alanine aminotransferase and alkaline phosphatase activities. Hyperglobulinemia common in cats.
• Normal urinalysis, except for bilirubinuria in dogs.

OTHER LABORATORY TESTS

• Total RBC PK activity—low value diagnostic in cats and some dogs; many affected dogs have normal or high activities because of the expression of an M2 isozyme that does not normally occur in mature RBCs; approximately 50% of normal activity in heterozygous animals.
• Additional assays (e.g., enzyme heat stability test, measurement of RBC glycolytic intermediates, electrophoresis of isozymes, and enzyme immunoprecipitation)—to reach a diagnosis in dogs whose total enzyme activity is not low.
• DNA diagnostic tests—screening for cats and several dog breeds (available at http://research.vet.upenn.edu/penngen).

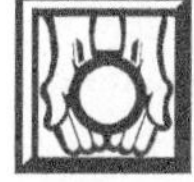

TREATMENT

• Affected animals can be cured by bone marrow transplantation or gene therapy.
• Splenectomy may reduce the severity of the anemia in cats.

MEDICATIONS

DRUG(S) OF CHOICE

Long-term treatment with iron-chelating drugs might prolong the life expectancy of affected dogs.

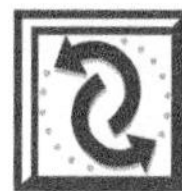

FOLLOW-UP

• Hepatic iron overload—develops in affected dogs; can result in cirrhosis and liver failure.
• Myelofibrosis and osteosclerosis—develop in affected dogs with age; most die by 5 years old as a result of bone marrow or liver failure.
• Severe anemia with minimal reticulocytosis or abnormal liver function tests and ascites secondary to hypoalbuminemia indicate the terminal stage of the disease in dogs.

MISCELLANEOUS

ABBREVIATIONS

• HCT = hematocrit.
• PK = pyruvate kinase.
• RBC = red blood cell.

INTERNET RESOURCES

http://research.vet.upenn.edu/penngen

Suggested Reading

Owen JL, Harvey JW. Hemolytic anemia in dogs and cats due to erythrocyte enzyme deficiencies. Vet Clin North Am Small Anim Pract 2012, 42:73–84.

Author John W. Harvey
Consulting Editor Melinda S. Camus

PYTHIOSIS

BASICS

DEFINITION

Infectious disease primarily affecting skin or gastrointestinal (GI) tract of dogs and cats; caused by the aquatic pathogen *Pythium insidiosum*, an organism in the class Oomycetes.

PATHOPHYSIOLOGY

- Infective form of *P. insidiosum* is thought to be a motile biflagellate zoospore, which is released into warm water environments and is chemotactically attracted to damaged tissue and animal hair; animals likely infected when they enter or ingest water containing infective zoospores.
- *P. insidiosum* considered pathogenic rather than opportunistic because immune suppression is not prerequisite for infection.
- In GI tract, *P. insidiosum* causes chronic pyogranulomatous disease with severe segmental transmural thickening of one or more areas of stomach or intestine.
- In skin, pythiosis typically causes non-healing wounds and invasive masses that contain ulcerated nodules and draining tracts.

P

SYSTEMS AFFECTED

- GI and cutaneous forms of disease encountered with equal frequency in dogs; cats are infrequently infected, cutaneous form more common.
- With exception of occasional dissemination to regional lymph nodes, pythiosis usually affects only one body system in each patient; multisystemic involvement rare.
- GI pythiosis most often affects gastric outflow tract, proximal small intestine, ileocolic junction, colon, and mesentery; esophagus rarely affected.
- In dogs, GI disease, local thromboembolic events, or vascular invasion may lead to bowel wall ischemia, GI perforation, or hemoabdomen.
- Dogs with cutaneous pythiosis are often presented for solitary or multiple cutaneous or subcutaneous lesions involving extremities, tailhead, ventral neck, perineum.
- In cats, cutaneous lesions or subcutaneous masses involving retrobulbar, periorbital, or nasopharyngeal regions, tailhead, or footpads have been observed.

GENETICS

Large-breed dogs most often affected; no genetic predisposition documented.

INCIDENCE/PREVALENCE

- Dependent on geographic distribution.
- Affected animals more often presented in fall or early winter.

GEOGRAPHIC DISTRIBUTION

- Primarily in tropical and subtropical areas of the world.
- In United States, occurs most often in states bordering Gulf of Mexico, but documented in many other states.
- Outside the United States, reported in Australia, Brazil, Burma, Colombia, Costa Rica, Indonesia, Japan, New Guinea, and Thailand.

SIGNALMENT

Species

Dog, less commonly cat.

Breed Predilections

- Large-breed dogs, especially those in hunting or field trial work near water.
- Labrador retrievers overrepresented.
- German shepherd dogs may be predisposed to cutaneous pythiosis.

Mean Age and Range

Animals <6 years old are most common.

Predominant Sex

Males affected more often than females, possibly due to increased exposure.

SIGNS

General Comments

Dogs not usually severely ill until late in course of disease.

Historical Findings

- Chronic weight loss, intermittent vomiting.
- Diarrhea if colon or large segment of small intestine affected.
- Regurgitation with esophageal disease.
- Cutaneous disease characterized by nonhealing wounds with nodules that drain and ulcerate.

Physical Examination Findings

GI Pythiosis

- Emaciation.
- Palpable abdominal mass.
- Despite severe weight loss, affected dogs usually bright and alert.
- Systemic signs and abdominal pain may occur with intestinal obstruction, infarction, or perforation.

Cutaneous Pythiosis

- Cutaneous or subcutaneous lesions appear as nonhealing wounds, edematous regions, or poorly defined nodules that ulcerate.
- Multiple tracts draining serosanguineous or purulent exudate.

CAUSES

P. insidiosum.

RISK FACTORS

- Environmental exposure to swampy areas, bayous, ponds, or lakes containing infective zoospores.
- Outdoor activities such as hunting.

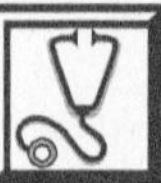

DIAGNOSIS

DIFFERENTIAL DIAGNOSIS

GI Pythiosis

- Intestinal obstruction (foreign body, intussusception).
- Histoplasmosis.
- Gastric or intestinal neoplasia (lymphosarcoma, carcinoma, etc.).
- Inflammatory bowel disease.
- Basidiobolomycosis, protothecosis.
- Histiocytic or idiopathic colitis.

Cutaneous Pythiosis

- Lagenidiosis, paralagenidiosis (caused by oomycotic pathogens in genera *Lagenidium* and *Paralagenidium*, respectively).
- Zygomycosis (infections caused by *Basidiobolus* or *Conidiobolus* spp.).
- Other mycotic skin diseases, such as cryptococcosis, coccidioidomycosis, sporotrichosis, eumycotic mycetoma, and phaeohyphomycosis.
- Nodular bacterial skin diseases, such as actinomycosis, mycobacteriosis, botryomycosis, and brucellosis.
- Protothecosis or nodular leishmaniosis.
- Noninfectious pyogranulomatous diseases, such as foreign body reaction, idiopathic nodular panniculitis, sebaceous nodular adenitis, canine cutaneous sterile pyogranuloma/granuloma syndrome.
- Cutaneous neoplasia.
- Systemic vasculitis and cutaneous embolic disease.

CBC/BIOCHEMISTRY/URINALYSIS

- Laboratory findings nonspecific.
- Eosinophilia, leukocytosis, anemia of chronic inflammatory disease possible.
- Hyperglobulinemia and/or hypoalbuminemia in chronically affected dogs.
- Hypokalemia, hyponatremia, hypochloridemia, metabolic alkalosis, in dogs with gastric outflow obstruction.
- Hypercalcemia—reported in a single dog.

OTHER LABORATORY TESTS

Serology—ELISA available at Auburn University College of Veterinary Medicine.

IMAGING

- Abdominal radiography may reveal obstructive pattern, bowel wall thickening, or abdominal mass.
- Abdominal ultrasonography may reveal segmental transmural thickening and loss of normal wall layering of the stomach, proximal small intestine, or ileocolic junction. Granulomas or enlarged lymph nodes may be evident in the mesentery.

DIAGNOSTIC PROCEDURES

- Biopsy of GI or skin lesions demonstrates histologic changes suggestive of, but not definitive for, pythiosis.
- Definitive diagnosis is based on specific PCR amplification or sequencing of DNA extracted from infected tissue or cultured isolates; submit samples to experienced laboratory via overnight shipping at room temperature.

PATHOLOGIC FINDINGS

- GI and skin lesions characterized by pyogranulomatous and eosinophilic inflammation associated with broad (4–6 µm), irregularly branching, infrequently septate hyphae with thick, nonparallel walls.
- Predominance of eosinophils within inflammatory reaction differentiates pythiosis, lagenidiosis, zygomycosis from other mycotic infections.
- Hyphal organisms usually not visible on hematoxylin and eosin-stained sections; readily visualized with silver stain.
- GI lesions—severe segmental thickening of portions of stomach and/or bowel, often with obstruction of intestinal lumen.
- Mesenteric lymphadenopathy is common, but presence of *P. insidiosum* hyphae within lymph nodes is uncommon.
- GI pythiosis characterized by eosinophilic and pyogranulomatous inflammation with necrotic foci and discrete granulomas that contain hyphae.

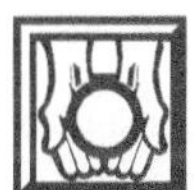

TREATMENT

APPROPRIATE HEALTH CARE

Treatment of choice is aggressive surgical excision of all infected tissue with 3–5 cm margins. Unfortunately, many animals are not presented until late in disease when complete resection is not possible. Addition of prednisone at anti-inflammatory dosages to antifungal therapy has improved efficacy of medical treatment for nonresectable GI pythiosis.

NURSING CARE

Supportive care should include IV fluids with potassium supplementation and nutritional support. Antibiotics may be indicated to treat secondary pyoderma in dogs with cutaneous lesions.

ACTIVITY

Limit activity.

DIET

Feed a highly digestible, calorie-dense diet.

CLIENT EDUCATION

- Treatment is expensive.
- Prognosis for cutaneous pythiosis is guarded to poor unless complete resection with wide margins is feasible. For dogs with GI pythiosis, complete resolution of disease may occur when medical therapy includes prednisone.

SURGICAL CONSIDERATIONS

- Attempt wide surgical excision to obtain 5 cm margins (and two fascial planes deep if cutaneous).
- Amputation recommended for treatment of extremity lesions.
- Enlarged mesenteric lymph nodes should be biopsied but often do not contain infective hyphae, thus do not have to be removed.
- Dogs often improve after obstructive lesions are resected, even if significant gross disease is still present.
- Reevaluation of ELISA serology 2–3 months after surgery may provide prognostic information.

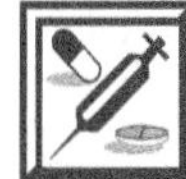

MEDICATIONS

DRUG(S) OF CHOICE

- Itraconazole 10 mg/kg PO q24h combined with terbinafine 10 mg/kg PO q24h and prednisone appears to be most effective combination:
  - Prednisone is given at 1 mg/kg PO q12h for 5–7 days, then q24h for 1 month, then slowly tapered if there is clinical improvement.
  - Antifungal therapy should be continued for minimum of 6 months.
  - Compounded bulk itraconazole should not be used; give with food.

PRECAUTIONS

- Azole drugs should not be used in animals with severe liver disease.
- Anorexia, high liver enzymes, and cutaneous vasculitis are most common adverse effects of itraconazole.

POSSIBLE INTERACTIONS

Antacids and anticonvulsants may decrease blood levels of itraconazole.

ALTERNATIVE DRUG(S)

Prednisone used alone improves clinical signs in short term. In addition, the author has observed complete long-term resolution of clinical signs in a small number of dogs with GI pythiosis treated with prednisone alone. This is not recommended as a primary treatment for dogs with resectable lesions, but should be considered as palliative therapy in dogs with nonresectable disease when client finances preclude use of antifungals.

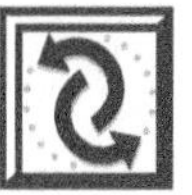

FOLLOW-UP

PATIENT MONITORING

- ELISA serology can be used to monitor response to therapy; serology should be checked 2–3 months after surgery or every 3 months during medical therapy.
- Abdominal ultrasonography is useful for reevaluating intestinal lesions.
- Liver enzyme activities should be evaluated monthly while patient is on itraconazole.

PREVENTION/AVOIDANCE

Monitor for signs of recurrence.

POSSIBLE COMPLICATIONS

Acute abdomen and death from GI thrombosis or perforation.

EXPECTED COURSE AND PROGNOSIS

Prognosis is guarded unless a complete resection is possible.

MISCELLANEOUS

AGE-RELATED FACTORS

Young animals are predisposed.

ZOONOTIC POTENTIAL

There is no evidence of direct transmission from animals to humans; infections in humans are very rare and are from a common environmental source.

PREGNANCY/FERTILITY/BREEDING

Azole antifungals are teratogenic and should not be used in pregnant animals.

SYNONYMS

- Phycomycosis.
- Swamp cancer.

ABBREVIATIONS

- GI = gastrointestinal.

Suggested Reading

Grooters AM. Pythiosis, lagenidiosis, and zygomycosis. In: Sykes JE, ed., Canine and Feline Infectious Diseases. St. Louis, MO: Elsevier Saunders, 2014.

Reagan KL, Marks SL, Pesavento PA, et al. Successful management of 3 dogs with colonic pythiosis using itraconzaole, terbinafine, and prednisone. J Vet Intern Med 2019, 33:1434–1439.

Author Amy M. Grooters
Consulting Editor Amie Koenig

Client Education Handout available online

PYURIA

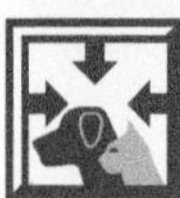

BASICS

DEFINITION

• White blood cells (WBCs) (i.e., neutrophils, eosinophils, monocytes, lymphocytes, or plasma cells) in urine.
• More than 5 WBCs per high-power field is generally considered abnormal, but the number of WBCs found in urinary sediment varies with method of collection, sample volume and concentration, degree of cellular destruction after collection, and laboratory technique.

PATHOPHYSIOLOGY

• Large numbers of WBCs in voided urine indicate active inflammation along the urogenital tract.
• Can be associated with any pathologic process (infectious or noninfectious) that causes cellular injury or death; tissue damage evokes exudative inflammation characterized by leukocytic extravasation (pyuria) and increased vascular permeability (hematuria and proteinuria).

SYSTEMS AFFECTED

• Renal/urologic—urethra, urinary bladder, ureters, and kidneys.
• Genital—prepuce, prostate, vagina, and uterus.

SIGNALMENT

Dog and cat.

SIGNS

General Comments

• Historical and physical examination findings depend on the underlying cause, organ(s) affected, degree of organ dysfunction, and magnitude of systemic inflammatory responses.
• Nonobstructive lesions confined to the urinary bladder, urethra, vagina, or prepuce rarely cause systemic signs of inflammation. Systemic signs may accompany disease of the kidneys, prostate, or uterus.

Physical Examination Findings

Local Effects of Inflammation

• Erythema of mucosal surfaces.
• Tissue swelling.
• Exudation of leukocytes and protein-rich fluid.
• Pain.
• Loss of function.

Systemic Effects of Inflammation

• Fever.
• Depression.
• Anorexia.
• Dehydration.

CAUSES

Kidney

• Pyelonephritis.
• Nephrolith.
• Neoplasia.
• Trauma.
• Immune-mediated.

Ureter

• Ureteritis.
• Ureterolith.
• Ureteral stent.
• Neoplasia.

Urinary Bladder

• Cystitis.
• Urocystolith.
• Neoplasia.
• Trauma.
• Overdistension—urethral obstruction.
• Pharmacologic—cyclophosphamide.

Urethra

• Urethritis.
• Urethrolith.
• Neoplasia.
• Trauma.
• Foreign body.

Prostate

• Prostatitis/abscess.
• Neoplasia.

Penis/Prepuce

• Balanoposthitis.
• Neoplasia.
• Foreign body.

Uterus

• Pyometra/metritis.

Vagina

• Vaginitis.
• Neoplasia.
• Foreign body.
• Trauma.

RISK FACTORS

• Any disease process, diagnostic procedure, or therapy that alters normal urinary tract defenses and predisposes to infection.
• Any disease process, dietary factor, or therapy that predisposes to formation of metabolic uroliths.

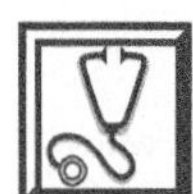

DIAGNOSIS

DIFFERENTIAL DIAGNOSIS

Voided Specimens

• Rule out vaginitis—vaginal discharge, erythema of vaginal mucosa, licking of vulva, and attracting male dogs.
• Rule out pyometra, metritis—vaginal discharge, large uterus, pyrexia, depression, anorexia, polyuria, polydipsia, and a recent history of estrus, parturition, or progestin administration.
• Rule out balanoposthitis—preputial discharge, erythema of preputial or penile mucosa, and licking of prepuce.
• Rule out prostatitis, prostatic abscess, or prostatic neoplasia—urethral discharge, prostatomegaly, pyrexia, depression, dysuria, tenesmus, caudal abdominal pain, and stiff gait.
• Rule out urethritis, urethroliths, urethral neoplasms—dysuria, pollakiuria, stranguria, or palpable uroliths or mass lesions in the urethra.
• Rule out inflammatory disorders of urinary bladder and kidneys.

Specimens Collected by Cystocentesis

• Rule out urethral obstruction—stranguria, anuria, and a large overdistended urinary bladder.
• Rule out prostatic and urethral disorders (see above); purulent prostatic or urethral exudates can reflux into the urinary bladder.
• Rule out cystitis, urocystoliths, and urinary bladder neoplasia—dysuria, pollakiuria, stranguria, and/or palpable uroliths or mass lesions in the urinary bladder.
• Rule out pyelonephritis—pyrexia, depression, anorexia, polyuria, polydipsia, renal pain, and renomegaly.
• Rule out post-traumatic pyuria—history of trauma, including iatrogenic causes.

LABORATORY FINDINGS

Drugs That May Alter Laboratory Results

• WBCs lyse rapidly in hypotonic or alkaline urine. Administration of alkalinizing agents or agents that produce hypotonic urine may falsely decrease urine WBC numbers.
• Leukocyte esterase reagent strip (dipstick) is not recommended for evaluating canine and feline urine. Nitrofurantoin, cephalosporins, and gentamicin can cause false-positive leukocyte esterase reactions.
• Urinary WBC concentrations can be low in patients with inflammatory disorders who have been given steroidal or nonsteroidal anti-inflammatory drugs.

Disorders That May Alter Laboratory Results

• Disorders with diminished WBC function or absolute neutropenia can artificially lower WBC values.
• Disorders with production of hypotonic urine or alkaline urine artificially lower WBC values.

Miscellaneous Factors That May Alter Laboratory Results

Dipstick (leukocyte esterase reaction) testing may result in false-negative results in dogs and both false-positive and false-negative results in cats.

Valid if Run in Human Laboratory?

Valid if urinary sediment is examined microscopically; invalid if only leukocyte esterase reagent strip (dipstick) method is used.

CBC/BIOCHEMISTRY/URINALYSIS

• Pyuria in specimens collected by voiding, manual compression, or transurethral catheterization indicates an inflammatory lesion involving at least the urinary or genital tracts.
• Pyuria in specimens collected by cystocentesis localizes the site of inflammation to at least the

urinary tract, but does not exclude the urethra and genital tract. Reflux of prostatic exudates into the urinary bladder may result in pyuria in patients with prostatic disease.
• Pyuria with WBC casts is evidence of renal parenchymal inflammation.
• Generalized renal injury may be associated with concomitant leukocytosis, isosthenuria, and azotemia.
• Pyuria associated with bacteria, fungi, or parasite ova in sufficient numbers indicates that the inflammatory lesion was caused or complicated by urinary tract infection (UTI).
• Pyuria associated with neoplastic cells indicates neoplasia. Diagnosis of urinary tract neoplasia by cytologic examination of urine may be complicated by epithelial cell hyperplasia and atypia caused by urinary tract inflammation or the physiochemical properties of urine.

OTHER LABORATORY TESTS

• Perform quantitative urine culture on all patients with pyuria; it provides the most definitive means of identifying and characterizing UTI. The absence of pyuria does not rule out bacteriuria as patients with bacteriuria frequently do not have pyuria.
• Negative urine culture results suggest a noninfectious cause of inflammation (e.g., uroliths, neoplasia) or inflammation associated with UTI caused by fastidious organisms (e.g., mycoplasmas and viruses) or by organisms capable of forming intracellular bacterial colonies or biofilms. False-negative culture results may also be due to recent antimicrobic therapy, sample mishandling, or delays between specimen collection and culture.
• Cytologic evaluation of urinary sediment, prostatic fluid, urethral or vaginal discharges, or biopsy specimens obtained by catheter or needle biopsy may help evaluate patients with localized urinary or genital tract disease. Cytologic examination may establish a definitive diagnosis of urinary tract neoplasia, but negative cytologic findings do not rule out neoplasia.

IMAGING

Abdominal radiography, contrast urethrocystography, urinary tract ultrasonography, and excretory urography are important means of identifying and localizing underlying causes.

DIAGNOSTIC PROCEDURES

• Urethrocystoscopy—indicated in patients with persistent lesions of the lower urinary tract for which a definitive diagnosis has not been established by other, less invasive, means.
• Microscopic evaluation of tissue specimens—indicated in patients with lesions of the urinary or genital tracts for which a definitive diagnosis has not been established by other, less invasive, means; tissue specimens may be obtained by traumatic catheterization biopsy, cystoscopy and forceps biopsy, or exploratory laparotomy; aspiration and punch biopsy techniques may be used to evaluate the prostate gland.

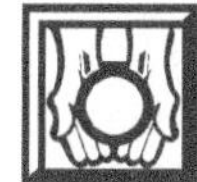

TREATMENT

• Treatment varies, depending on the underlying cause and specific organs involved.
• Pyuria associated with systemic signs of illness (i.e., pyrexia, depression, anorexia, vomiting, dehydration, leukocytosis, polyuria, and polydipsia) or urinary obstruction warrants aggressive diagnostic evaluation and initiation of specific, supportive, and/or symptomatic treatment.

MEDICATIONS

DRUG(S) OF CHOICE

Depend on underlying cause.

CONTRAINDICATIONS

• Avoid glucocorticoids or other immunosuppressive agents in patients suspected of having urinary or genital tract infection.
• Avoid potentially nephrotoxic drugs in febrile, dehydrated, or azotemic patients and those suspected of having pyelonephritis, septicemia, or preexisting renal disease.

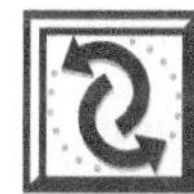

FOLLOW-UP

PATIENT MONITORING

Response to treatment by serial urinalyses, including examination of urine sediment; collect specimens from most patients by cystocentesis to avoid contamination by preputial or vaginal exudates; perform transurethral catheterization if the expected benefits outweigh the risk of iatrogenic bacterial UTI.

POSSIBLE COMPLICATIONS

• Infectious and noninfectious inflammatory disorders of the urinary tract can cause renal failure, urinary obstruction, uremia, septicemia, and death.
• Pyuria is a potential risk factor for formation of matrix or matrix-crystalline urethral plugs and subsequent urethral obstruction in male cats.

MISCELLANEOUS

ASSOCIATED CONDITIONS

• Hematuria.
• Proteinuria.
• Bacteriuria.

SYNONYMS

Leukocyturia.

SEE ALSO

• Dysuria, Pollakiuria, and Stranguria.
• Hematuria.
• Lower Urinary Tract Infection, Bacterial.
• Lower Urinary Tract Infection, Fungal.
• Proteinuria.
• Pyelonephritis.

ABBREVIATIONS

• UTI = urinary tract infection.
• WBC = white blood cell.

Suggested Reading

Adams LG. Ureteral disorders. In: Ettinger SJ, Feldman EC, Cote E, eds., Textbook of Veterinary Internal Medicine, 8th ed. St. Louis, MO: Elsevier, 2017, pp. 1985–1991.
Forrester SD, Kruger JM, Allen TA. Feline lower urinary tract diseases. In: Hand MS, Thatcher CD, Remillard RL, et al., eds. Small Animal Clinical Nutrition, 5th ed. Topeka, KS: Mark Morris Institute, 2010, pp. 925–976.
Kutzler MA. Prostatic diseases. In: Ettinger SJ, Feldman EC, Cote E, eds., Textbook of Veterinary Internal Medicine, 8th ed. St. Louis, MO: Elsevier, 2017, pp. 2031–2036.
Osborne CA, Stevens JB, Lulich JP, et al. A clinician's analysis of urinalysis. In: Osborne CA, Finco DR, eds., Canine and Feline Nephrology and Urology, 2nd ed. Baltimore, MD: Williams & Wilkins, 1995, pp. 136–205.
Phillips J. Neoplasia of the lower urinary tract. In: Bartges J, Polzin DJ, eds., Nephrology and Urology of Small Animals. Chichester, UK: Wiley-Blackwell, 2011, pp. 797–808.
Wood MW. Lower urinary tract infections. In: Ettinger SJ, Feldman EC, Cote E, eds., Textbook of Veterinary Internal Medicine, 8th ed. St. Louis, MO: Elsevier, 2017, pp. 1992–1996.

Author John M. Kruger
Consulting Editor J.D. Foster
Acknowledgment The author and editors acknowledge the prior contributions of Carl A. Osborne, and Cheryl L. Swenson.

Q FEVER

BASICS

OVERVIEW

- Caused by the zoonotic rickettsia *Coxiella burnetii.*
- Infection—most commonly by inhalation or ingestion of organism via infected body fluids (parturient discharges, urine, milk, or feces), tissues (especially placenta), or carcasses of infected animal reservoir hosts (cattle, sheep, goats); can occur after tick exposure (many species of ticks implicated).
- Lungs—thought to be main portal of entry to systemic circulation.
- Organism replicates in vascular endothelium; causes widespread vasculitis; vasculitis results in necrosis and hemorrhage in lungs, liver, and CNS; severity depends on the pathogenicity of the strain of organism and host immune response.
- An extended latent period exists after recovery until chronic immune-complex phenomena develop; organism reactivated out of the latent state during parturition, resulting in large pathogen load in placenta, parturient fluids, urine, feces, and milk.
- Endemic in mammals worldwide; most cases in the United States in western states.

SIGNALMENT

Cats and dogs of any age, sex, or breed.

SIGNS

Historical Findings

- History of contact with farm animals or ticks.
- Fever.
- Lethargy.
- Depression.
- Anorexia.
- Abortion—especially cats.
- Ataxia and seizures—especially dogs.

Physical Examination Findings

- Usually unremarkable.
- Splenomegaly often only clinical finding.
- Multifocal neurologic abnormalities—dogs.

CAUSES & RISK FACTORS

- *Coxiella burnetii.*
- Exposure to infected animals (especially following parturition) and ticks.

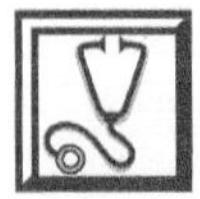

DIAGNOSIS

DIFFERENTIAL DIAGNOSIS

- Cats—other causes of abortion: infections (viral rhinotracheitis, panleukopenia, feline leukemia virus, toxoplasmosis; bacteria including coliforms, streptococci, staphylococci, salmonellae); fetal defects; maternal problems (nutrition, genital tract abnormalities); environmental stress; endocrine disorders.
- Dogs—canine parvovirus, canine distemper, other causes of encephalitis.

CBC/BIOCHEMISTRY/URINALYSIS

Nonspecific

OTHER LABORATORY TESTS

Serology and PCR

- Serology (immunofluorescence or ELISA)—a four-fold increase in IgG titer over a 4-week period is diagnostic; utility of increased IgM titer in a single sample is not well documented in small animals; crossreactivity with *Bartonella* species is possible.
- PCR—used to detect organisms in tissue culture or tissue specimens (e.g., placenta); whole blood can also be tested during 1st week of acute infection but negative blood PCR does not rule out infection.

IMAGING

N/A

DIAGNOSTIC PROCEDURES

Organism not detected on routine blood cultures; organism isolation may be performed by qualified laboratories.

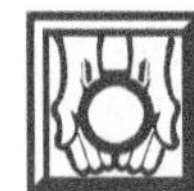

TREATMENT

- Alert client of possible zoonotic risk.
- Inpatient—avoids zoonotic risk to client
- Wear personal protective equipment (gloves, gown, mask, eye shield) when treating an infected animal or when attending an aborting cat.
- Isolate aborting and postpartum animals.
- Survives long periods in environment; inactivated by 5% hydrogen peroxide.

MEDICATIONS

DRUG(S) OF CHOICE

- Tetracycline 22 mg/kg PO q8h for 2 weeks.
- Doxycycline 10 mg/kg PO q12h for 1 week.
- Enrofloxacin 10–20 mg/kg PO q24h (dogs only) for 1 week; should be effective but no clinical reports; effective *in vitro.*

CONTRAINDICATIONS/POSSIBLE INTERACTIONS

- Tetracycline drugs are associated with yellowing of teeth in young animals; do not use in animals with renal failure.
- Doxycycline may cause esophagitis and stricture.
- Enrofloxacin may cause cartilage defects in young animals at high doses.
- Enrofloxacin may cause retinal degeneration in cats.

FOLLOW-UP

- Difficult to determine success of therapy because many animals spontaneously improve.
- Even asymptomatic cases should be aggressively treated because of the zoonotic potential.
- Utility of predicting success of therapy based on serologic improvement unknown.

MISCELLANEOUS

ZOONOTIC POTENTIAL

- Major zoonotic potential.
- Humans contract the disease by inhaling infected aerosols (e.g., after parturition); children commonly infected from ingesting raw milk but are usually asymptomatic.
- By the time a diagnosis is made in a pet, human exposure and infection have usually occurred.
- Instruct owners and people in contact with the pet to seek medical advice immediately.
- Previous urban outbreaks have been related to exposure to infected cats.
- Incubation period from time of contact until the first signs of illness is 5–32 days.
- Person-to-person transmission possible.

Suggested Reading

Sykes JE, Norris JM. Coxiellosis and Q fever. In: Sykes JE, ed., Canine and Feline Infectious Diseases. St. Louis, MO: Saunders Elsevier, 2014, pp. 320–325.

Author Robyn Ellerbrock

Consulting Editor Amie Koenig

Acknowledgment The author and editors acknowledge the prior contribution of Stephen C. Barr.

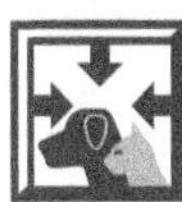

BASICS

OVERVIEW

• CSF-filled diverticula within the subarachnoid space at the quadrigeminal cisterna (dorsal to the midbrain and adjacent to the third ventricle). More recently the term supracollicular fluid accumulation (SFA) has been used to described the anatomical location of the condition. CSF may be secreted by the arachnoid cells lining the cyst cavity. It is suspected that an anomaly of CSF flow from the choroid plexus during the stage of development forces a separation within the arachnoid layer. • Clinical signs may develop as a result of gradual expansion of the subarachnoid space by a valve mechanism associated with pulsating CSF flow. • May be an incidental finding.

SIGNALMENT

Dog and cat.

Breed Predilections

Mainly in small breeds and brachycephalic patients—shih tzu, Maltese, pug, cavalier King Charles, Yorkshire terrier, Lhasa apso, Chihuahua, Pekingese, Pomeranian and bulldog.

Mean Age and Range

Mean—5 years; range—2 months–10 years.

SIGNS

• Seizures. • Abnormal behavior. • If associated with hydrocephalus, could manifest with disorientation, behavioral changes, cortical blindness, compulsive circling, head pressing.

CAUSES & RISK FACTORS

• Disturbance of embryogenesis where splitting of the primitive arachnoid membrane leads to fluid accumulation. • Inflammatory conditions affecting the meninges.
• Postsurgical trauma (intervertebral disc disease, spinal tumor). • Neoplasia and hemorrhage. • Intracystic hemorrhage secondary to trauma may result in expansion of the cyst and subsequent compression of the adjacent brain parenchyma.

DIAGNOSIS

DIFFERENTIAL DIAGNOSIS

• Primary intracranial cyst-like lesions include intra-arachnoid, epidermoid, dermoid and choroid plexus cysts. • Congenital brain anomalies (anencephaly, hydrocephalus, other). • Storage disease. • Infectious inflammatory diseases—viral (distemper virus, other viruses); fungal (*Blastomyces dermatitidis*, *Coccidioides* spp., *Cryptococcus neoformans*); rickettsial (*Rickettsia rickettsii*); bacterial (*Ehrlichia* spp., *Escherichia coli*, *Streptococcus*); protozoal (*Neospora caninum*, *Toxoplasma gondii*). • Other inflammatory disease—breed-related encephalitis (necrotizing encephalitis of the Yorkshire terrier, Maltese, and pug). • Brain tumor—meningioma, glioma, choroid plexus papilloma, lymphoma.

IMAGING

• The prevalence of SFAs was 2.19% among CT studies (n = 4,427) and 2.2% among MRI studies (n = 626). • MRI—extra-axial CSF-filled cyst at the quadrigeminal cisterna. On T1-weighted images, the lesion is hypo-intense to brain tissue and isointense to CSF. On T2-weighted images, the lesion is hyperintense to brain tissue and isointense to CSF. On fluid attenuated inversion recovery (FLAIR) sequences, the cyst is hypointense, confirming the presence of CSF. Dilation of the ventricular system may be present if the cyst is obstructing CSF flow.

DIAGNOSTIC PROCEDURES

CSF—rule out concomitant inflammation. If CSF inflammatory, the cyst may be an incidental finding.

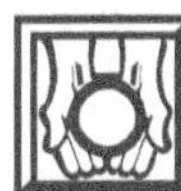

TREATMENT

• Medical therapy to control seizures and reduce CSF production. • If signs are progressive, surgical cyst fenestration through craniotomy or craniectomy can result in clinical improvement. When hydrocephalus is present, surgical shunting can be considered. Other disease process must be ruled out before considering surgery. The cystic structure may be an incidental finding. • Stable patients can be discharged with recommended medical therapy. • Sequential assessment of pupillary size and reaction to light, and mentation are helpful to determine risk of brain herniation.

MEDICATIONS

DRUG(S) OF CHOICE

• Glucocorticosteroids—dexamethasone 0.1 mg/kg IV or PO q24h for 3 days followed by prednisone 0.25–0.5 mg/kg PO q24h for 10 days, then reassess response and adjust dose. To prevent gastrointestinal ulceration, add omeprazole 0.5 mg/kg PO q24h or famotidine 0.5–1 mg/kg IV or PO q12h to steroid therapy. • Antiepileptic drugs—phenobarbital 2 mg/kg IV or PO q12h, levetiracetam 20 mg/kg PO q8–12h, or zonisamide 5–10 mg/kg PO q12h.
• Diuretic—acetazolamide 10 mg/kg q6–8h as a carbonic anhydrase inhibitor that may help reduce CSF production and intracranial pressure. Omeprazole may act as an agent to reduce CSF production and provide gastric protection during steroid therapy.

CONTRAINDICATIONS/POSSIBLE INTERACTIONS

The combination of glucocorticosteroid and diuretic may cause marked dehydration and increased blood viscosity that can result in poor cerebral perfusion and neurologic deterioration.

FOLLOW-UP

PATIENT MONITORING

• Repeat neurologic examination periodically (every 2–4 weeks). • Corticosteroid may be necessary for a long period or for life. The goal is to find the dose that keeps the clinical signs controlled with minimal side effects. • Evaluate phenobarbital levels after 4–5 weeks of starting therapy. • If phenobarbital is continued, recheck biochemical profile and bile acids to assess hepatic function every 6 months.

POSSIBLE COMPLICATIONS

• Deterioration of clinical signs despite aggressive treatment. • Status epilepticus, dementia, brain herniation, and death.

EXPECTED COURSE AND PROGNOSIS

• Prognosis is variable depending on severity of clinical signs and response to therapy.
• Quadrigeminal cyst may be incidental or may result in progressive neurologic deterioration.

MISCELLANEOUS

ASSOCIATED CONDITIONS

Hydrocephalus

ABBREVIATIONS

• SFA = supracollicular fluid accumulation.

INTERNET RESOURCES

• IVIS: http://www.ivis.org • VIN: http://www.vin.com

Suggested Reading

Bertolini G, Ricciardi M, Caldin M. Multidetector computed tomographic and low-field magnetic resoance imaging anatomy of the quadrigeminal cistern and characterization of supracollicular fluid accumulation in dogs. Vet Radiol Ultrasound 2016, 57(3)259–268.

Platt S, Hicks J, Matiasek L. Intracranial intra-arachnoid diverticular and cyst-like abnormalities of the brain. Vet Clin North Am Small Anim Pract 2016, 46(2)253–263.

Author Carolina Duque

RABIES

BASICS

DEFINITION

A severe, fatal, viral polioencephalitis of warm-blooded animals, including humans.

PATHOPHYSIOLOGY

Virus—enters body through a wound (usually from a bite of rabid animal) or via mucous membranes, replicates in myocytes, spreads to the neuromuscular junction and neuro-tendinal spindles, travels to the central nervous system (CNS) via intra-axonal fluid within peripheral nerves, spreads throughout the CNS; finally spreads centrifugally within peripheral, sensory, and motor neurons.

SYSTEMS AFFECTED

- Nervous—brain, spinal cord, ± peripheral nervous system (PNS).
- Salivary glands—contain large quantities of infectious virus particles that are shed in saliva.

GENETICS

None

INCIDENCE/PREVALENCE

R

- Incidence of disease within infected animals—high (approaches 100%).
- Prevalence—overall low; can be significant in enzootic areas; especially high in countries where vaccination of dogs and cats is not routine.

GEOGRAPHIC DISTRIBUTION

- Worldwide.
- Exceptions—New Zealand, Hawaii, Japan, Iceland, and parts of Scandinavia.
- Species-adapted strains—specific geographic distributions within endemic countries.

SIGNALMENT

Species

- All warm-blooded mammals, including dogs, cats, and humans.
- United States—five strains endemic within fox, raccoon, skunk, coyote, and insectivorous bat populations; all five strains can be transmitted to dogs and cats.

Breed Predilections

None

Mean Age and Range

All ages, but animals that come in contact with wildlife at highest risk.

Predominant Sex

None

SIGNS

General Comments

- Variable; atypical presentation is the rule rather than the exception.
- Can present with focal or multifocal signs affecting either brain, spinal cord, PNS, or any combination.
- Three classical progressive stages of disease described:
  - Prodromal—mentation change (more docile or more agitated) ± fever.
  - Furious—prosencephalon signs including hyperactivity, aggression, seizures ± ataxia; 90% of rabid cats have furious form.
  - Paralytic—lower motor neuron (LMN) paresis or paralysis starting near site of inoculation then spreading through nervous system; paralytic form can follow furious form, especially in cats.

Historical Findings

- Mentation/behavior change—variable; can include unusual shyness, excitability, aggression.
- Seizures.
- Gait change—lameness, ataxia, paralysis.
- Licking or chewing at site of inoculation, although wound not always identified.
- Change in tone of bark.
- Excess salivation or frothing at the mouth.

Physical Examination Findings

- All or some of the historical findings
- Fever.
- Cranial nerve deficits—myosis, anisocoria, absent pupillary light reflex (PLR); dropped jaw; absent gag reflex (assess by compressing larynx and avoid hand in mouth if rabies suspected).
- Hypersalivation.
- Laryngeal paralysis.

CAUSES

Rabies virus—a single-stranded, enveloped, bullet-shaped RNA virus; genus *Lyssavirus*; family *Rhabdoviridae.*

RISK FACTORS

- Exposure to wildlife, especially skunks, raccoons, bats, and foxes.
- Inadequate vaccination against rabies.
- Bite or scratch wounds from unvaccinated dogs, cats, or wildlife.
- Exposure to aerosols in bat caves.
- Immunocompromised animal—use of modified live virus rabies vaccine.

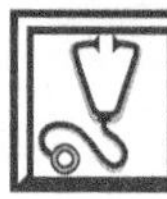

DIAGNOSIS

DIFFERENTIAL DIAGNOSIS

- Must seriously consider rabies for any dog or cat showing acute behavior change or unaccountable neurological signs, especially those not previously vaccinated for rabies. Caution: handle with considerable care to prevent possible transmission of the virus to individuals caring for or treating the animal.
- Acute, progressive CNS and/or PNS disease—infectious (e.g., viral encephalitis or myelitis), immune-mediated (e.g., granulomatous or necrotizing meningo-encepalitis, necrotizing leukoencephalitis, polymyositis), metabolic (e.g., hepatic encephalopathy, hypoadrenocorticism), neoplastic, degenerative.

CBC/BIOCHEMISTRY/URINALYSIS

No characteristic hematologic or biochemical changes.

OTHER LABORATORY TESTS

N/A

IMAGING

N/A

DIAGNOSTIC PROCEDURES

- There are no definitive premortem diagnostics. Diagnostics performed on rabies suspects should be done with extreme caution to prevent exposure to infective tissues. Consider consultation with a neurologist.
- Direct immunofluorescent antibody (DFA) test of nervous tissue—rapid and sensitive; collect head or entire body following death or euthanasia, chill sample immediately. Submit to a state-approved laboratory for rabies diagnosis. Caution: use extreme care when collecting, handling, and shipping these specimens to prevent exposure of veterinarians, staff or handlers.
- DFA test of dermal tissue—skin biopsy of the sensory vibrissae of the maxillary area, including deeper subcutaneous hair follicles; approved for human diagnostics, but not for animal diagnostics; accurate if positive, but negative test does not rule out rabies.
- Rabies antibody titer—a serologic antibody titer of 0.5 IU/mL is considered adequate for protection in vaccinated people and animals. In most states in the United States, titers are not considered a legal replacement for vaccination.

PATHOLOGIC FINDINGS

- Gross changes—generally absent.
- Histopathologic changes—acute to chronic polioencephalitis; gradual increase in the severity of the nonsuppurative inflammatory process in the CNS as disease progresses; large neurons within the brain may contain classic intracytoplasmic inclusions (Negri bodies).

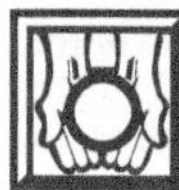

TREATMENT

APPROPRIATE HEALTH CARE

Strictly inpatient.

NURSING CARE

Administer with extreme caution.

ACTIVITY

- Confine to secured quarantine area with clearly posted signs indicating suspected rabies.
- Runs or cages should be locked; only designated people should have access.
- Feed and water without opening the cage or run door.

DIET

Soft, moist food; most patients will not eat.

CLIENT EDUCATION

- Thoroughly inform client of the seriousness of rabies to the animal and the zoonotic potential.
- Ask client about any human exposure (e.g., contact, bite) and strongly urge client to see a physician immediately.
- Local public health official must be notified.

SURGICAL CONSIDERATIONS

- Generally none.
- Skin biopsy—may help establish antemortem diagnosis; must be confirmed by identification from CNS tissue.

MEDICATIONS

DRUG(S) OF CHOICE

- No treatment.
- Once the diagnosis is likely, euthanasia is indicated.

CONTRAINDICATIONS

None

PRECAUTIONS

N/A

POSSIBLE INTERACTIONS

N/A

ALTERNATIVE DRUG(S)

N/A

FOLLOW-UP

PATIENT MONITORING

- All suspected rabies patients should be securely isolated and monitored for any development of mood change, attitude change, or clinical signs that might suggest the diagnosis.
- An apparently healthy dog or cat that bites or scratches a person should be monitored for a period of 10 days; if no signs of illness occur in the animal within 10 days, the person has had no exposure to the virus; dogs and cats do not shed virus for more than 3 days before development of clinical disease.
- An unvaccinated dog or cat that is bitten or exposed to a known rabid animal must be quarantined according to local or state regulations, often for up to 6 months.

PREVENTION/AVOIDANCE

- Vaccines (dogs and cats)—vaccinate according to standard recommendations and state and local requirements; all dogs and cats with any potential exposure to wildlife or other dogs; vaccinate after 12 weeks of age, then 12 months later, then every 3 years using a vaccine approved for 3 years; use only inactivated or recombinant vector vaccines for cats.
- Vaccinated animals exposed to possible or confirmed rabies suspect should receive booster vaccine, according to applicable local laws.
- Rabies-free countries—entering dogs and cats are quarantined for long periods, usually 6 months.
- Disinfection—any contaminated area, cage, food dish, or instrument must be thoroughly disinfected; use a 1:32 dilution (4 ounces/gallon) of household bleach to quickly inactivate the virus.

POSSIBLE COMPLICATIONS

- Development of acute neurological signs, death.
- Difficulty of antemortem diagnosis my lead to humans and other animals being exposed to virus.

EXPECTED COURSE AND PROGNOSIS

- Prognosis—grave; almost invariably fatal.
- Dogs and cats with clinical infection usually succumb within 1–10 days of onset of clinical signs; often within 3–4 days.

MISCELLANEOUS

ASSOCIATED CONDITIONS

None

AGE-RELATED FACTORS

None

ZOONOTIC POTENTIAL

- Extreme.
- Humans must avoid bites and contact with saliva or CNS tissue from a rabid animal or an asymptomatic animal that is incubating the disease.
- Suspected rabies cases must be strictly quarantined and confined to prevent exposure to humans and other animals. Full personal protective equipment should be worn if interaction is necessary.
- Local and state regulations must be adhered to carefully and completely.

PREGNANCY/FERTILITY/BREEDING

Infection during pregnancy is fatal to dam.

SYNONYMS

N/A

ABBREVIATIONS

- CNS = central nervous system
- DFA = direct immunofluorescent antibody.
- LMN = lower motor neuron.
- PLR = pupillary light reflex.
- PNS = peripheral nervous system.

INTERNET RESOURCES

www.cdc.gov/rabies/

Suggested Reading

Brown CM, Slavinski S, Ettestad P, et al. Compendium of animal rabies prevention and control, 2016. J Am Vet Med Assoc 2016, 248:505–517.

Frymus T, Addie D, Belák S, et al. Feline rabies: ABCD guidelines on prevention and management. J Feline Med Surg 2009, 11:585–593.

Greene CE. Rabies and other Lyssavirus infections. In: Greene CE, ed., Infectious Diseases of the Dog and Cat, 4th ed. St. Louis, MO: Saunders Elsevier, 2012, pp. 167–183.

Scherk MA, Ford RB, Gaskell RM, et al. 2013 AAFP Feline Vaccination Advisory Panel Report. J Feline Med Surg 2013, 15:785–808.

Author Renee Barber

Consulting Editor Amie Koenig

Acknowledgment The author and editors acknowledge the prior contribution of Fred W. Scott.

Client Education Handout available online

RECTAL AND ANAL PROLAPSE

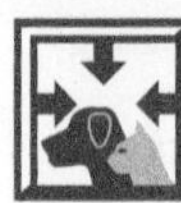

BASICS

OVERVIEW

- Eversion of one or more layers of the rectum through the anus.
- An anal prolapse (incomplete prolapse) is a protrusion of anorectal mucosa through the external anal orifice.
- A rectal prolapse (complete prolapse) is a double-layer invagination of the full thickness of the rectal tube through the anal orifice.

SIGNALMENT

- Dog and cat (especially Manx).
- Any age, sex, or breed.
- High prevalence for young, parasitized dogs or cats with diarrhea.

SIGNS

- Persistent tenesmus.
- Incomplete prolapse—protrusion of a portion of the circumference of the rectal mucosa that typically appears worse immediately after defecation and then subsides.
- Complete prolapse appears as a tubular hyperemic mass protruding from the anus.
- Chronic prolapses may be dark blue or black in color or the mucosa may be ulcerated.

R

CAUSES & RISK FACTORS

- Gastrointestinal disorders that cause diarrhea and tenesmus, such as parasitism, colitis/enteritis, constipation/obstipation, rectal foreign body, rectal deviation and diverticulum, proctitis, and rectal or anal tumors.
- Urogenital disorders, such as cystitis, urolithiasis, prostatitis, prostatic hypertrophy, and dystocia.
- Tenesmus following perineal, rectal, or urogenital surgery (e.g., perineal herniorrhaphy).

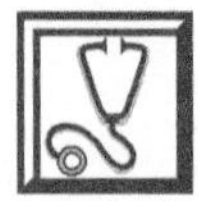

DIAGNOSIS

DIFFERENTIAL DIAGNOSIS

- Prolapsed intussusception—rule out by passing a finger or blunt probe between the mass and the anus (the probe should not penetrate more than 1–2 cm before contacting the fornix; if the probe easily passes 5–6 cm, then suspect prolapsed intussusception) or by abdominal ultrasonography (look for increased intestinal layering).
- Neoplasia—rule out by palpation, fine-needle aspiration and cytology, and/or biopsy and histopathology.

CBC/BIOCHEMISTRY/URINALYSIS

- Usually unremarkable.
- Inflammatory or stress leukogram may be present.

OTHER LABORATORY TESTS

Fecal examination may confirm parasitism.

IMAGING

- Abdominal radiography and ultrasonography—usually unremarkable.
- Abdominal radiography—may demonstrate foreign body, prostatomegaly, cystic calculi, or colonic fecal distention.
- Abdominal ultrasonography—may demonstrate prostatomegaly, cystic calculi, bladder wall thickening, or intussusception.

DIAGNOSTIC PROCEDURES

- Rectal examination to palpate for perineal hernia.
- Colonoscopy may help evaluate recurrent prolapse for an underlying cause.

PATHOLOGIC FINDINGS

Assess viability of the prolapsed tissue by surface appearance and tissue temperature—vital tissue appears swollen and hyperemic, and red blood exudes from the cut surface; devitalized tissue appears dark purple or black, and dark cyanotic blood exudes from the cut surface; ulcerations may be present.

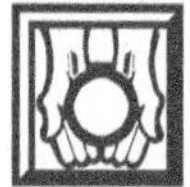

TREATMENT

- Must identify and treat underlying cause.
- Conservative medical management—gently replace prolapsed tissue through the anus with the use of lubricants (e.g., KY Jelly and gentle massage); osmotic agents (e.g., 50% dextrose solution) may help if severe swelling exists.
- Use of an epidural may facilitate treatment and relieve discomfort.
- Place a purse-string suture to aid retention and prevent acute recurrence; place the suture loose enough to allow room for defecation.
- Decrease straining with stool softeners.
- Colopexy recommended for recurrent viable prolapses or if straining persists after rectal resection and anastomosis.
- When prolapse is nonreducible and/or devitalized, rectal resection and anastomosis are necessary.

MEDICATIONS

DRUG(S) OF CHOICE

- Appropriate anesthetic/analgesics as needed.
- Appropriate perioperative antibiotics are recommended (e.g., cefoxitin sodium 30 mg/kg IV) for resection and anastomosis.
- Stool softeners—docusate sodium (dogs, 50–200 mg PO q8–12h; cats, 50 mg PO q12–24h) or lactulose (10 g/15 mL solution or syrup, 1 mL/4.5 kg q8–12h to effect); continue for 2–3 weeks after removal of the purse-string suture.
- Anthelmintic based on fecal examination.
- Feed a low-residue diet until purse-string suture is removed.

CONTRAINDICATIONS/POSSIBLE INTERACTIONS

N/A

FOLLOW-UP

PATIENT MONITORING

- Purse-string suture removal in 3–7 days.
- Examine for rectal stricture if straining persists following anastomosis.

POSSIBLE COMPLICATIONS

- Recurrence—especially if underlying cause is not eliminated.
- Postoperative—may include infection, anastomosis dehiscence within 5–7 days postoperatively, or rectal stricture.
- Fecal incontinence after resection (sensory incontinence resulting from removal of receptors in rectal wall).

MISCELLANEOUS

ASSOCIATED CONDITIONS

Intestinal parasitism.

SEE ALSO

- Colitis and Proctitis.
- Dyschezia and Hematochezia.
- Intussusception.

Suggested Reading

Aronson LR. Rectum, anus, perineum. In: Tobias KM, Johnston SA, eds., Veterinary Small Animal Surgery. St. Louis, MO: Elsevier Saunders, 2012, pp 1564–1600.

Radlinsky MG. Rectal prolapse. In: Fossum TW, ed., Small Animal Surgery, 5th ed. Philadelphia: Elsevier, 2019, pp. 504–507.

Author Eric R. Pope

Consulting Editor Mark P. Rondeau

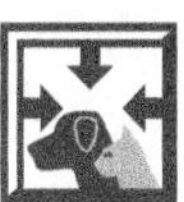

BASICS

OVERVIEW

- Diminution in the size of the rectal or anal lumen either from cicatricial contracture or scarring as a result of wound healing or chronic inflammation or from proliferative neoplastic disease.
- Gastrointestinal function is compromised because of outflow obstruction.

SIGNALMENT

- Dog and cat.
- Any age, breed, or gender.

SIGNS

- Vary with severity.
- Tenesmus.
- Dyschezia.
- Constipation.
- Hematochezia.
- Mucoid feces.
- Large bowel diarrhea.
- Secondary megacolon can develop.

CAUSES & RISK FACTORS

- Inflammatory—rectoanal abscess, anal sacculitis, perianal fistulae, proctitis, histoplasmosis, pythiosis.
- Traumatic— foreign body, laceration.
- Neoplastic—rectal adenocarcinoma, leiomyoma, or polyps.
- Iatrogenic—rectal anastomosis, mass excision, or biopsy.
- Congenital—atresia ani.

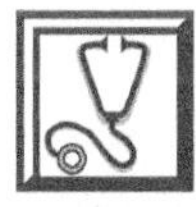

DIAGNOSIS

DIFFERENTIAL DIAGNOSIS

- Space-occupying processes that lead to diminished rectal capacity (extraluminal compression [e.g., prostatic disease, pelvic fractures], intraluminal obstruction [e.g., pseudocoprostasis, foreign body]) and functional constriction (muscle spasms).
- Differentiate by rectal palpation and imaging.

CBC/BIOCHEMISTRY/URINALYSIS

- Usually unremarkable.
- May have an inflammatory leukogram.

OTHER LABORATORY TESTS

N/A

IMAGING

- Survey abdominal radiography and contrast studies (e.g., barium, air, or double-contrast enema and barium gastrointestinal series) may reveal consistent narrowing of the rectal lumen.
- Abdominal ultrasonography may reveal thickening and altered architecture if infiltrative rectocolonic disease is present (e.g., pythiosis, neoplasia).

DIAGNOSTIC PROCEDURES

- Digital rectal palpation.
- Proctoscopy/colonoscopy to visualize stricture, determine extent, and procure biopsy specimens.
- Colonic scrapings may aid in cytologic diagnosis of fungal (histoplasmosis) and neoplastic diseases.
- Biopsy to classify the disease process and establish a prognosis.

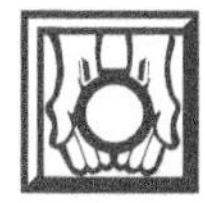

TREATMENT

- Treat the underlying cause when possible.
- Medical treatment for palliation (stool softeners/enemas) or the elimination of infective agents or inflammatory conditions.
- Fluid therapy to optimize hydration prior to administering an enema to constipated or obstipated patients.
- Anesthesia may be necessary for enema administration.
- Balloon dilation of non-neoplastic and postoperative strictures—multiple procedures may be needed.
- Surgical reconstruction of focal strictures (plasty procedures).
- Resection and anastomosis may be necessary for extensive lesions and recurrent strictures.
- Colorectal stent placement may relieve obstruction due to nonresectable neoplasms and non-neoplastic lesions.
- Radiotherapy and/or chemotherapy for some neoplasms.

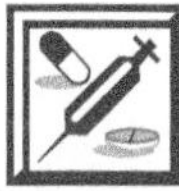

MEDICATIONS

DRUG(S) OF CHOICE

- Stool softeners—docusate sodium; lactulose.
- Corticosteroids—prednisone to treat inflammatory conditions (0.5–1 mg/kg PO q24h or divided q12h) and after balloon dilation to prevent stricture recurrence. Intralesional injection of triamcinolone prior to dilatation may prevent recurrence.
- Chemotherapy or antifungal therapy if indicated.
- Broad-spectrum perioperative antimicrobial therapy (e.g., cefoxitin sodium 30 mg/kg IV) with balloon dilation or surgical therapy.
- Antibiotics continued after dilation if mucosal tearing occurs.

CONTRAINDICATIONS/POSSIBLE INTERACTIONS

- Corticosteroids when infection is possible.
- Corticosteroids may slow healing after surgical correction.

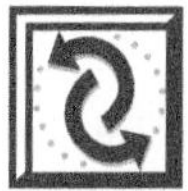

FOLLOW-UP

PATIENT MONITORING

- Clinical signs.
- Recurrence or metastasis of neoplastic lesions.
- Following balloon dilation patients should be reevaluated for stricture reformation 7–14 days after the procedure to determine the need for additional dilation procedures.

POSSIBLE COMPLICATIONS

- Medical treatment—can include inefficacy, diarrhea, and adverse effects of medications.
- Balloon dilation can result in deep rectal tears, hemorrhage, or possibly full-thickness perforation. Stricture recurrence is common following balloon dilation. Multiple dilations may be needed.
- Surgical treatment—fecal incontinence, secondary stricture formation, and wound dehiscence.

EXPECTED COURSE AND PROGNOSIS

- Varies with the severity of the stricture.
- Patients with benign strictures that are readily managed medically or with balloon dilation or bougienage may have a good long-term outcome.
- Surgical resection has more guarded prognosis because of the frequency of complications.
- Most patients with recognizable clinical signs due to neoplasia have a guarded-to-poor prognosis for complete resolution.

MISCELLANEOUS

AGE-RELATED FACTORS

Atresia ani is seen within weeks of birth.

SEE ALSO

- Colitis and Proctitis.
- Constipation and Obstipation.
- Dyschezia and Hematochezia.
- Histoplasmosis.
- Perianal Fistula.
- Pythiosis.
- Rectoanal Polyps.

Suggested Reading

Aronson LR. Rectum, anus, perineum. In: Tobias KM, Johnston SA, eds., Veterinary Small Animal Surgery. St. Louis, MO: Elsevier Saunders, 2012, pp. 1564–1600.

Author Eric R. Pope

Consulting Editor Mark P. Rondeau

RECTOANAL POLYPS

BASICS

OVERVIEW

Most rectoanal polyps are benign growths located in the distal rectum. Histopathologic evaluation typically reveals adenomas, but lesions may undergo malignant transformation.

SIGNALMENT

• Dog and rarely cat. • Middle-aged to older. • No breed or sex predilection established but German shepherd dogs, collies, and West Highland white terriers overrepresented in some studies.

SIGNS

• May be none (incidental finding on wellness exam). • Hematochezia with relatively well-formed feces. • Mucus-covered feces. • Pencil-thin or ribbon-like feces. • Tenesmus. • Dyschezia. • Soft, well-vascularized, friable, and often ulcerated mass(es) may be seen or palpated rectally. • Usually single but multiple polyps can occur. • May be pedunculated or broad-based sessile masses.

R

CAUSES & RISK FACTORS

Unknown

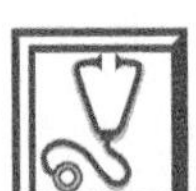

DIAGNOSIS

DIFFERENTIAL DIAGNOSIS

• Carcinoma *in situ* and adenocarcinoma. • Other neoplasms—leiomyoma, lymphoma, papilloma. • Inflammatory polyps—primarily reported in miniature dachshunds in Japan; lesions appear as diffuse small white polyps that are responsive to immunosuppressive therapy. • Proctitis. • Pythiosis. • Colitis (clinical signs are characterized by diarrhea with a marked increase in frequency, scant volume of feces, increased fecal mucus, and tenesmus. These clinical signs are vastly different to those of dogs with rectoanal polyps which do not cause diarrhea). • Incomplete rectal prolapse.

CBC/BIOCHEMISTRY/URINALYSIS

Usually unremarkable.

OTHER LABORATORY TESTS

N/A

IMAGING

N/A

DIAGNOSTIC PROCEDURES

• Rectal palpation. • Direct visualization through anus. • Proctoscopy—viable low-cost procedure that allows one to visualize the descending colon after cleansing the animal's colon. This method is suitable in most dogs and cats because the polyps are usually localized to the rectoanal or colorectal region and tend not to metastasize. • Colonoscopy—may be recommended to evaluate the entire rectum and colon for additional polyps but in a review of 82 cases, no lesions were found orad to the colorectal junction. • Cytologic examination of polyp aspirate or scraping may help the initial diagnosis, although cytology should be interpreted with caution given the inherent challenges of differentiating benign adenomas from adenocarcinomas cytologically. • Histopathologic examination of excised tissue is required for definitive diagnosis and to assess completeness of the excision.

PATHOLOGIC FINDINGS

• Adenomatous polyp. • Adenomatous hyperplasia. • Carcinoma *in situ*.

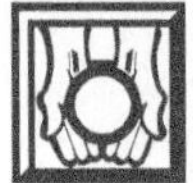

TREATMENT

• Surgical excision is the treatment of choice. • Most polyps can be exteriorized directly through the anus and removed with submucosal resection. • Close the mucosal defect with absorbable sutures, avoiding compromise of the lumen diameter. • Lesions that cannot be exteriorized may be removable transanally by electrosurgery with endoscopic guidance or can be directly exposed through a dorsal rectal approach. • One study in dogs showed significant improvement in clinical signs following administration of piroxicam, but long-term follow-up is not available. Numerous nonsteroidal anti-inflammatory drugs (NSAIDs) have been evaluated in humans with mixed results (see Internet Resources).

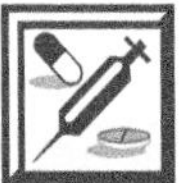

MEDICATIONS

DRUG(S) OF CHOICE

• Appropriate perioperative antibiotics are recommended (e.g., cefoxitin sodium 30 mg/kg IV). • Stool softeners may help decrease tenesmus—docusate sodium (dogs, 50–200 mg PO q8–12h; cats, 50 mg PO q12–24h) or docusate calcium (dogs, 50–100 mg PO q12–24h; cats, 50 mg PO q12–24h). • Alternative stool softener—lactulose (1 mL/4.5 kg PO q8h to effect).

CONTRAINDICATIONS/POSSIBLE INTERACTIONS

N/A

FOLLOW-UP

PATIENT MONITORING

• Examine the excision site 14 days after surgery and again at 3 and 6 months to ensure absence of recurrence or stricture. • Twice yearly examination thereafter to assess for recurrence.

POSSIBLE COMPLICATIONS

• Recurrence. • Rectal stricture (rare).

EXPECTED COURSE AND PROGNOSIS

• Dogs with focal single adenomas have a good prognosis with a low rate of recurrence. • Dogs with multiple and/or diffuse lesions (involvement of >50% of circumference of rectal wall) have much higher rates of recurrence. • Malignant transformation of benign lesions can occur in up to 50% of dogs. • Excised tissues should be submitted for histopathology even when preoperative biopsies have been performed. The diagnosis may change in up to one-third of the cases in which preoperative endoscopic biopsies are performed.

MISCELLANEOUS

SEE ALSO

• Adenocarcinoma, Anal Sac.
• Colitis and Proctitis.
• Dyschezia and Hematochezia.
• Rectal and Anal Prolapse.

ABBREVIATIONS

• NSAID = nonsteroidal anti-inflammatory drug.

INTERNET RESOURCES

http://www.bandolier.org.uk/band129/b129-6.html. This site reviews the mixed results of clinical trials using various NSAIDs in humans.

Suggested Reading

Aronson LR. Rectum, anus, perineum. In: Tobias KM, Johnston SA, eds., Veterinary Small Animal Surgery. St. Louis, MO: Elsevier Saunders, 2012, pp. 1564–1600.

Author Eric R. Pope
Consulting Editor Mark P. Rondeau

BASICS

DEFINITION

Erythema of the eyelids, increased or hyperemic ocular surface vasculature, or hemorrhage within the eye.

PATHOPHYSIOLOGY

- Active dilation of ocular vessels—in response to extraocular or intraocular inflammation or passive congestion.
- Hemorrhage from existing or newly formed blood vessels.

SYSTEMS AFFECTED

Ophthalmic—eye and/or ocular adnexa.

SIGNALMENT

Dog and cat.

SIGNS

Historical Findings

Depends on cause.

Physical Examination Findings

- Depends on cause.
- May affect one or both eyes.
- Result of systemic disease—abnormalities in other organ systems common.

CAUSES

- Blepharitis.
- Conjunctivitis.
- Keratitis.
- Episcleritis or scleritis.
- Anterior uveitis.
- Glaucoma.
- Hyphema.
- Orbital disease—usually the orbital abnormality is more prominent.

RISK FACTORS

- Systemic infectious or inflammatory diseases.
- Immunocompromise.
- Coagulopathy.
- Systemic hypertension.
- Irritation by potentially any topical ophthalmic medication.
- Neoplasia.
- Trauma.

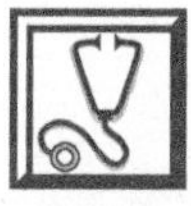

DIAGNOSIS

DIFFERENTIAL DIAGNOSIS

More than one cause may occur simultaneously.

Similar Signs

- Rule out normal variations.
- Palpebral conjunctiva—normally redder than bulbar conjunctiva.
- One or two large episcleral vessels—may be normal if the eye is otherwise quiet.
- Transient mild hyperemia—with excitement, exercise, and straining.
- Horner's syndrome—may cause mild conjunctival vascular dilation; differentiated by other signs and pharmacologic testing.

Causes

- Superficial (conjunctival) vessels—originate near the fornix, move with the conjunctiva, branch repeatedly, and blanch quickly with topical 2.5% phenylephrine or 1:100,000 epinephrine. Suggests ocular surface disorders (e.g., conjunctivitis, superficial keratitis, blepharitis).
- Deep (episcleral) vessels—originate near the limbus, branch infrequently, do not move with the conjunctiva, and blanch slowly or incompletely with topical sympathomimetics. Suggests episcleritis or intraocular disease (e.g., anterior uveitis or glaucoma).
- Discharge—mucopurulent to purulent: typical of ocular surface disorders and blepharitis; serous or none: typical of intraocular disorders.
- Swollen or inflamed eyelids—suggest blepharitis.
- Corneal opacification, neovascularization, or fluorescein stain retention—suggest keratitis.
- Aqueous flare or cell (increased protein or cells in the anterior chamber)—confirms diagnosis of anterior uveitis.
- Pupil—miotic: common with anterior uveitis; dilated: common with glaucoma; normal: with blepharitis and conjunctivitis.
- Abnormally shaped or colored irides—suggest anterior uveitis.
- Luxated or cataractous lenses—suggest glaucoma or anterior uveitis.
- Intraocular pressure (IOP)—high: diagnostic for glaucoma; low: suggests anterior uveitis.
- Loss of vision—suggests glaucoma, anterior uveitis, or severe keratitis.
- Glaucoma and anterior uveitis—may complicate hyphema.

CBC/BIOCHEMISTRY/URINALYSIS

Typically normal, except with anterior uveitis, glaucoma, or hyphema secondary to systemic disease.

OTHER LABORATORY TESTS

Depends on cause—see specific types of red eye (conjunctivitis, uveitis, etc.).

IMAGING

- Chest radiographs—consider with anterior uveitis or if intraocular neoplasia is a possibility.
- Abdominal radiography or ultrasonography—may rule out infectious or neoplastic causes.
- Ocular ultrasonography—if the ocular media are opaque; may define the extent and nature of intraocular disease or identify intraocular tumor.

DIAGNOSTIC PROCEDURES

Tonometry—must perform in every patient with an unexplained red eye.

Ocular Surface Disorders

- Aerobic bacterial culture and sensitivity—with a purulent discharge, chronic disease, or poor response to treatment.
- Schirmer tear test.
- Cytologic examination of affected tissue.
- Cats—consider PCR or immunofluorescent antibody (IFA) test on corneal or conjunctival scrapings for feline herpesvirus and *Chlamydia*; collect sample before fluorescein staining to avoid false-positive results on IFA.
- Fluorescein stain.
- Conjunctival biopsies—with chronic conjunctivitis or with a mass lesion.
- See specific disease—Conjunctivitis—Cats, Conjunctivitis—Dogs; Blepharitis; Keratitis chapters.

Intraocular Disorders

- Fluorescein stain.
- See specific disease: Anterior Uveitis—Cats; Anterior Uveitis—Dogs; Hyphema; Glaucoma.

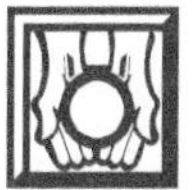

TREATMENT

- Usually outpatient.
- Elizabethan collar—to prevent self-trauma
- Avoid dirty environments or those that may lead to ocular trauma, especially if topical corticosteroids are used.
- Because there is a narrow margin for error, consider referral if the diagnosis is uncertain and/or glaucoma cannot be ruled out.
- Few causes are fatal; however, a workup may be indicated (especially with anterior uveitis and hyphema) to rule out potentially fatal systemic diseases.
- Deep corneal ulcers and glaucoma—may be best treated surgically.

MEDICATIONS

DRUG(S) OF CHOICE

- Depends on specific cause.
- Generally, control ocular pain, inflammation, infection, and IOP.
- Carprofen 2.2 mg/kg PO q12h or 4.4 mg/kg PO q24h to control mild inflammation and reduce pain

CONTRAINDICATIONS

- Topical corticosteroids—contraindicated if the cornea retains fluorescein stain.
- Systemic corticosteroids—avoid until infectious systemic causes have been ruled out.

R

RED EYE (CONTINUED)

PRECAUTIONS

- Topical aminoglycosides—may be irritating; may impede reepithelization if used frequently or at high concentrations.
- Topical solutions—may be preferable to ointments if corneal perforation is possible.
- Atropine—may exacerbate keratoconjunctivitis sicca (KCS) and glaucoma.
- Nonsteroidal anti-inflammatory drugs (NSAIDs)—use with caution in hyphema.

POSSIBLE INTERACTIONS

N/A

ALTERNATIVE DRUG(S)

N/A

FOLLOW-UP

PATIENT MONITORING

- Depends on cause.
- Repeat ophthalmic examinations—as required to ensure that IOP, ocular pain, and inflammation are well controlled.
- The greater the risk of loss of vision, the more closely the patient needs to be followed; may require daily or more frequent examination.

POSSIBLE COMPLICATIONS

- Loss of the eye or permanent vision loss.
- Chronic ocular inflammation and pain.
- Death.

MISCELLANEOUS

ASSOCIATED CONDITIONS

Numerous systemic diseases.

AGE-RELATED FACTORS

N/A

PREGNANCY/FERTILITY/BREEDING

Systemic corticosteroids may complicate pregnancy.

SEE ALSO

- Anterior Uveitis—Dogs.
- Anterior Uveitis—Cats.
- Conjunctivitis—Dogs.
- Conjunctivitis—Cats.
- Episcleritis.
- Glaucoma.
- Keratitis, Ulcerative.

ABBREVIATIONS

- IFA = immunofluorescent antibody.
- IOP = intraocular pressure.
- KCS = keratoconjunctivitis sicca.
- NSAID = nonsteroidal anti-inflammatory drug.

Suggested Reading

Maggs DJ, Miller PE, Ofri R. Slatter's Fundamentals of Veterinary Ophthalmology, 6th ed. St. Louis, MO: Elsevier, 2018.

Author Paul E. Miller
Consulting Editor Kathern E. Myrna

Client Education Handout available online

R

REGURGITATION

BASICS

DEFINITION

Passive, retrograde movement of undigested gastric or esophageal contents into the oral cavity. Reflux refers to the retrograde movement of gastric juice across the gastroesophageal sphincter into the esophagus.

PATHOPHYSIOLOGY

Regurgitation results from a loss of normal esophageal motility. In the normal esophagus, the presence of a food bolus in the proximal esophagus stimulates afferent sensory neurons. Signals are transferred centrally, via the vagus and glossopharyngeal nerves, to the tractus solitarius and nucleus ambiguus. Motor impulses travel back via the vagus nerve to stimulate striated muscle (canine) and striated and smooth muscle (feline) to cause esophageal peristalsis. Lesions anywhere along this pathway may lead to regurgitation. Esophagitis secondary to reflux can cause esophageal dysmotility and subsequent regurgitation. Delayed gastric emptying is a common and underappreciated cause of reflux and possible regurgitation.

SYSTEMS AFFECTED

- Gastrointestinal—dysphagia, weight loss.
- Musculoskeletal—weakness, weight loss.
- Nervous—polyneuropathies, CNS disease.
- Respiratory—aspiration pneumonia.

GENETICS

• Regurgitation due to megaesophagus can be inherited in smooth fox terriers (autosomal recessive) and miniature schnauzers (autosomal dominant or 60% penetrance autosomal recessive). In addition, Jack Russell terriers, springer spaniels, long-haired miniature dachshunds, golden retrievers, Labrador retrievers, and Samoyeds are predisposed to the congenital form of myasthenia gravis. A breed predisposition for acquired megaesophagus also exists for the German shepherd dog, Great Dane, Irish setter, Labrador retriever, pug, and Chinese Shar-Pei. The site and pathogenesis of the lesion in idiopathic megaesophagus is unknown. Suggested hypotheses include abnormalities of the afferent limb of the reflex arc (receptors, neurons) or of the swallowing center in the CNS. • Boxers and Newfoundlands have a genetic predisposition for inflammatory myopathy that is associated with esophageal dysmotility. • Brachycephalic breeds are predisposed to sliding hiatal hernias (type I) that is typically associated with gastroesophageal reflux and regurgitation.

INCIDENCE/PREVALENCE

N/A

GEOGRAPHIC DISTRIBUTION

N/A

SIGNALMENT

Species

Dog (more commonly) and cat.

Breed Predilections

• Smooth fox terriers, miniature schnauzers. Other predisposed breeds include Great Dane, German shepherd dog, Irish setter, Labrador retriever, Newfoundland, and boxer, brachycephalic breeds (shar-pei, pug, Boston terrier, English bulldog, French bulldog).
• Siamese and Siamese-related cats.

Mean Age and Range

• Congenital cases present soon after birth (congenital megaesophagus) or at weaning (vascular ring anomalies) during the transition from liquid diet to solid foods.
• Acquired cases may be seen at any age, depending on the etiology.

Predominant Sex

No gender predilection has been identified.

SIGNS

General Comments

• Clients often report vomiting; the veterinarian must differentiate vomiting from regurgitation using a comprehensive history. Having owner videotape events may be helpful. • Regurgitation—passive process; little to no abdominal effort; no prodromal phase; regurgitated material has increased amounts of thick mucus. • Vomiting—active process; prodromal phase is identified; vomited material may have increased amounts of bile staining. • The shape of the expelled material (i.e., tube-like), presence of undigested food, and length of time from ingestion to regurgitation or vomiting are less helpful to differentiate.

Historical Findings

• Vomiting (as perceived by owner).
• Dysphagia. • Coughing. • Ravenous appetite. • Weight loss. • Ptyalism. • Other signs, depending upon underlying etiology.

Physical Examination Findings

• Cervical swelling may be noted. • Ptyalism.
• Halitosis. • Increased respiratory noises.
• Nasal discharge and fever (if concurrent pneumonia). • Cachexia. • Weakness.

CAUSES

Congenital Pharyngeal or Pharyngoesophageal

• Cleft or short palate (typically associated with nasal reflux). • Cricopharyngeal muscle achalasia (typically associated with nasal reflux and dysphagia). • Myasthenia gravis.

Congenital Esophageal

• Vascular ring anomaly (e.g., persistent right aortic arch). • Megaesophagus. • Glycogen storage disease. • Esophageal diverticulum.
• Bronchoesophageal fistula.

Acquired Pharyngeal or Pharyngoesophageal

• Cricopharyngeal dysphagia. • Foreign bodies. • Neoplasia. • Rabies. • Toxicity (botulism). • Myopathy/neuropathy/junctionopathy.

Acquired Esophageal

• Megaesophagus. • Myasthenia gravis. • Stricture. • Neoplasia.
• Hypoadrenocorticism. • Hypothyroidism.
• Hiatal hernia. • Dysmotility.
• Gastroesophageal intussusception.
• Gastroesophageal reflux. • Periesophageal masses. • Dysautonomia. • Myopathy/neuropathy. • Foreign bodies. • Granulomatous disease. • Toxicity (lead). • Idiopathic.
• Gastric dilatation/volvulus. • Parasitic infection (*Spirocerca lupi*). • Bronchoesophageal fistula.

Congenital or Acquired Gastric (Increase Gastroesophageal Reflux)

• Pyloric outflow obstruction. • Gastric foreign body. • Gastric hypomotility.

RISK FACTORS

• Increased risk of gastroesophageal reflux with general anesthesia; the resultant esophagitis may lead to stricture formation and regurgitation. • Administration of doxycycline or clindamycin have been associated with esophagitis and stricture formation. • Esophageal foreign body.
• Swallowing caustic agents causing esophagitis.

R

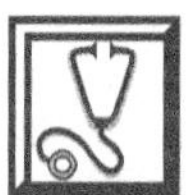

DIAGNOSIS

DIFFERENTIAL DIAGNOSIS

• Regurgitation is a clinical sign, not a diagnosis, and is the hallmark of esophageal disease. • It is important to differentiate vomiting from regurgitation.

CBC/BIOCHEMISTRY/URINALYSIS

• There are no pathognomonic changes for regurgitation. • Inflammatory leukogram may be seen if aspiration pneumonia is present. • Most helpful for evaluation of possible underlying etiologies: e.g., erythrocyte changes with lead toxicosis, elevated creatine kinase (CK) with myopathy, hyperkalemia and hyponatremia with hypoadrenocorticism, hypercholesterolemia with hypothyroidism.

OTHER LABORATORY TESTS

These elucidate etiologies of acquired conditions causing regurgitation and include adrenocorticotropic hormone (ACTH) stimulation test or baseline cortisol level (hypoadrenocorticism); thyroid serology (hypothyroidism); acetylcholine receptor antibody level (myasthenia gravis); blood lead levels (toxicosis).

IMAGING

• Thoracic and cervical radiography—evidence of a gas-, fluid-, or ingesta-filled esophagus with megaesophagus; may also show aspiration pneumonia, neoplasia, foreign bodies, hiatal

REGURGITATION (CONTINUED)

hernia, etc. • Contrast studies—both liquid barium and barium-coated food for radiolucent foreign bodies or esophageal strictures. Iohexol may also be used. Esophagram does not allow one to evaluate functional disorders such as intestinal dysmotility or cricopharyngeal muscle achalasia. Caution: contrast studies may increase the risk for aspiration pneumonia with regurgitation. • Videofluoroscopy—for pharyngeal weakness, cricopharyngeal muscle dysfunction, esophageal motility disorders, hiatal hernia, or gastroesophageal reflux.
• Other imaging studies include scintigraphy and high-resolution manometry for motility evaluation and ultrasound for pharyngeal or cervical masses. • Cervical and thoracic CT scans may also be utilized.

DIAGNOSTIC PROCEDURES

• Esophagoscopy can be useful for esophagitis, strictures, vascular ring anomalies, neoplasia, and foreign bodies. • Electromyography and nerve/muscle biopsies may be used for neuropathic or myopathic conditions. • Transtracheal wash or bronchoalveolar lavage if aspiration pneumonia is present or suspected.

PATHOLOGIC FINDINGS

Gross and histologic findings depend upon the underlying etiology and the presence of complicating factors.

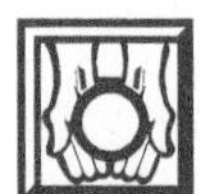

TREATMENT

APPROPRIATE HEALTH CARE

• Therapy for underlying etiology should be instituted. • Important to meet nutritional requirements and treat or prevent aspiration pneumonia.

NURSING CARE

• Aspiration pneumonia may require supplemental oxygen therapy, nebulization/coupage, and fluid therapy with balanced electrolyte solution. • These animals may be recumbent and require soft bedding. They should be maintained in sternal recumbency or turned to alternate down sides every 4 hours.

ACTIVITY

Depending on etiology, restricted activity is not necessary.

DIET

• Experimentation with different food consistencies is essential. Liquid gruel, small meatballs, or blenderized slurries may be used.
• Some cases benefit from gastrostomy feedings, though regurgitation may still occur.
• Both food and water should be elevated, and animal should be maintained in an upright position for 10–15 minutes after eating or drinking. Use of a Bailey chair facilitates keeping the dog upright for 10–15 minutes after a meal. • The recommend caloric requirement amount should be calculated and the diet should be monitored so that metabolizable energy requirements are met.

CLIENT EDUCATION

• If regurgitation is due to megaesophagus, most cases require lifelong therapy, even if an underlying etiology is found. Client dedication is important for long-term management.
• Most animals succumb to aspiration pneumonia or intractable regurgitation.
• Placement of a percutaneous gastrostomy tube (PEG) tube in dogs with megaesophagus can reduce the frequency of aspiration pneumonia, leading to prolonged survival.

SURGICAL CONSIDERATIONS

• Surgical intervention is indicated for vascular ring anomalies, cricopharyngeal muscle achalasia, bronchoesophageal fistula, and others. • Esophageal dysfunction is permanent in most cases. • Balloon dilation is indicated for cases of esophageal stricture.

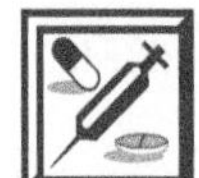

MEDICATIONS

DRUG(S) OF CHOICE

• Antibiotics for aspiration pneumonia (broad-spectrum or based on culture and sensitivity from transtracheal wash or bronchoalveolar lavage). • Specific therapy for underlying etiology if indicated. • Prokinetics—metoclopramide 0.2–0.4 mg/kg SC or PO q6–12h, or 1–2 mg/kg q24h as a CRI increases lower esophageal sphincter (LES) tone and increases gastric motility. Cisapride 0.5 mg/kg PO q8–12h is more effective for esophageal reflux than metoclopramide and has been documented to enhance gastric emptying and increase LES tone in dogs. • Other motility agents (e.g., erythromycin) can enhance gastric emptying and possibly increase LES tone. • H_2 receptor antagonists can be used for the short term to manage mild to moderate esophagitis—ranitidine 1–2 mg/kg PO, IV q12h, famotidine 0.5–1 mg/kg PO, SC, IM, IV q12h; however, are subject to tachyphylaxis (tolerance) when used for >4–5 days and are less potent compared to proton-pump inhibitors. Proton-pump inhibitors may be used in moderate to severe cases, and are also effective when administered for prolonged periods of time—omeprazole 0.7–1.5 mg/kg PO q12h. • Sucralfate caplets or suspension can be administered to help reduce esophageal pain and promote healing of esophagitis and esophageal erosions or ulcerations.

CONTRAINDICATIONS

N/A

PRECAUTIONS

• Absorption of orally administered drugs may be compromised when coadministered with sucralfate. • Injectable forms of acid suppressants should be used when applicable to avoid concerns with regurgitation of the drug before absorption.

POSSIBLE INTERACTIONS

N/A

ALTERNATIVE DRUG(S)

N/A

FOLLOW-UP

PATIENT MONITORING

• Animals with aspiration pneumonia should have thoracic radiographs and complete blood counts checked until resolution, or if recurrence is suspected. • Animals should be monitored, weighed, and body condition scores applied to ensure adequate caloric intake.

PREVENTION/AVOIDANCE

N/A

POSSIBLE COMPLICATIONS

• Aspiration pneumonia. • Others depending on presence of underlying diseases (e.g., hypothyroidism).

EXPECTED COURSE AND PROGNOSIS

• Older animals with idiopathic megaesophagus have a poor prognosis. • Aspiration pneumonia is the typical cause of death or euthanasia.

MISCELLANEOUS

ASSOCIATED CONDITIONS

• Aspiration pneumonia. • Megaesophagus.

AGE-RELATED FACTORS

Young animals may regain some esophageal function with appropriate therapy, depending on etiology.

ZOONOTIC POTENTIAL

None

PREGNANCY/FERTILITY/BREEDING

N/A

SEE ALSO

• Dysautonomia (Key-Gaskell Syndrome).
• Dysphagia. • Esophagitis.
• Megaesophagus. • Myasthenia Gravis.
• Pneumonia, Bacterial.

ABBREVIATIONS

• ACTH = adrenocorticotropic hormone.
• CK = creatine kinase. • LES = lower esophageal sphincter. • PEG = percutaneous endoscopic gastrostomy tube.

Suggested Reading

Guilford G, Strombeck D. Diseases of swallowing. In: Strombeck's Small Animal Gastroenterology, 3rd ed. Philadelphia, PA: Saunders, 1996, pp. 211–235.

Author Stanley L. Marks
Consulting Editor Mark P. Rondeau

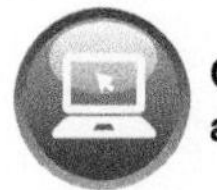

Client Education Handout available online

R

RENAL TUBULAR ACIDOSIS

BASICS

OVERVIEW

• Hyperchloremic metabolic acidosis due to decreased bicarbonate reabsorption in the proximal renal tubule (proximal or type 2 renal tubular acidosis [RTA]) or decreased hydrogen ion secretion in the distal tubule (distal or type 1 RTA) in patients with normal or near normal glomerular filtration rate and absence of diarrhea.
• Aldosterone deficiency or resistance can cause type 4 distal RTA and hyperkalemia.
• Proximal RTA has not been documented as an isolated entity in dogs but has been observed as part of Fanconi syndrome.
• In distal RTA urine cannot be maximally acidified despite moderately to markedly decreased plasma bicarbonate concentration as a consequence of impaired hydrogen secretion in the collecting ducts. Urine pH typically is >6.0 (urine pH should be 4.5–5.0 in the presence of systemic acidosis).

SIGNALMENT

• Uncommon in both dogs and cats.
• No breed or sex predilection.
• Age range at time of diagnosis, 1–13 years.

SIGNS

• Acidemia may cause lethargy, muscle weakness (may be due to hypokalemia), inappetence, nausea, weight loss, stunted growth, and neurologic signs.
• Other signs depend on the associated diseases (e.g., pyelonephritis).
• Panting.
• Polyuria and polydipsia usually associated with hypokalemia or calciuresis.
• Vomiting.
• Hematuria and dysuria secondary to urolithiasis.
• Osteomalacia associated with chronic metabolic acidosis.

CAUSES & RISK FACTORS

• May be primary (i.e., inherited), or secondary to hypercalciuria, toxins, drugs (e.g., amphotericin B), altered calcium metabolism causing nephrocalcinosis (e.g., hypervitaminosis D, primary hyperparathyroidism), autoimmune (e.g., immune-mediated hemolytic anemia, systemic lupus erythematosus [SLE], renal transplant rejection), hypergammaglobulinemic disorders (e.g., multiple myeloma, SLE), and tubulointerstitial nephropathies.
• In cats, distal RTA has been associated with pyelonephritis, hepatic lipidosis, idiopathic with secondary hyperaldosteronism, and topical ophthalmic carbonic anhydrase inhibitor.
• In dogs, clinical cases were idiopathic or associated with immune-mediated hemolytic anemia, leptospirosis, gastric-dilation-volvulus, zonisamide therapy, or experimentally induced renal ischemia.

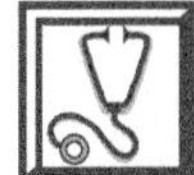

DIAGNOSIS

DIFFERENTIAL DIAGNOSIS

Consider other causes of hyperchloremic normal anion gap metabolic acidosis (e.g., diarrhea, carbonic anhydrase inhibitors, ammonium chloride, cationic amino acids, post-hypocapnic metabolic acidosis, dilutional acidosis, hypoadrenocorticism). Small bowel diarrhea is the most important differential.

CBC/BIOCHEMISTRY/URINALYSIS

• Results vary depending on associated diseases.
• Hypokalemia due to increased renal excretion.
• Alkaluria (pH >6.0); rule out urease-positive urinary tract infection.

OTHER LABORATORY TESTS

Venous blood gas and serum electrolyte analysis indicates hyperchloremic normal anion gap metabolic acidosis. Urine pH is >6.0 in distal RTA vs. <5.5 in proximal RTA.

IMAGING

Radiography—may detect uroliths or osteomalacia.

DIAGNOSTIC PROCEDURES

• The key diagnostic feature is normal anion gap metabolic acidosis accompanied by an inappropriately alkaline urine pH (>6.0).
• Ammonium chloride tolerance test—administer 200 mg/kg PO; measure urine pH before and hourly for 5 hours; empty the bladder hourly. Urine pH in normal dogs decreases to <5.5 within 4 hours. Avoid this test in severe acidemia.
• Type 1 and 2 RTA can be differentiated based on response to sodium bicarbonate infusion (0.5–1.0 mEq/kg/h). Fractional excretion of bicarbonate will increase markedly in type 2 RTA.

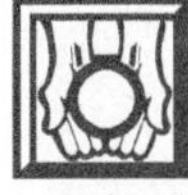

TREATMENT

• Individualize depending on the nature and severity of associated conditions.
• Less bicarbonate is needed to resolve metabolic acidosis caused by distal RTA than is needed with proximal RTA.
• Hypokalemia may resolve with bicarbonate or citrate administration, but additional potassium supplementation may be required.

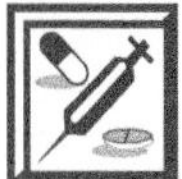

MEDICATIONS

DRUG(S) OF CHOICE

• Acidosis—depending on the serum potassium concentration give potassium citrate alone ± sodium citrate; or sodium bicarbonate.
• Potassium supplementation—potassium gluconate if hypokalemia does not resolve with potassium citrate therapy alone.

CONTRAINDICATIONS/POSSIBLE INTERACTIONS

Citrate should be avoided in patients receiving aluminum hydroxide; citrate can lead to excessive aluminum absorption.

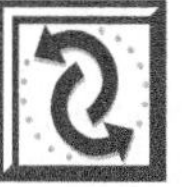

FOLLOW-UP

• Serial blood gas with electrolyte analyses (e.g., every 3–5 days) until acid–base status has normalized.
• Long-term prognosis depends on the nature and severity of associated conditions; may be reasonably good in patients without other diseases, little information exists on the long-term course of this disease.

MISCELLANEOUS

SEE ALSO

• Acidosis, Metabolic.
• Fanconi Syndrome.
• Hypokalemia.

ABBREVIATIONS

• RTA = renal tubular acidosis.
• SLE = systemic lupus erythematosus.

Suggested Reading

Riordan L, Schaer M. Renal tubular acidosis. Comp Cont Ed Pract Vet 2005, 27(7):513–529.

Authors Joao Felipe de Brito Galvao and Stephen P. DiBartola
Consulting Editor J.D. Foster

RENOMEGALY

BASICS

OVERVIEW

One or both kidneys are abnormally large as detected by abdominal palpation or diagnostic imaging.

Pathophysiology

The kidneys may enlarge due to abnormal cellular infiltration (e.g., inflammation, infection, and neoplasia), urinary tract obstruction, acute tubular necrosis, or development of renal cysts or pseudocysts.

Systems Affected

- Endocrine/metabolic—metabolic acidosis with decreased kidney function.
- Gastrointestinal—inappetence, vomiting, diarrhea, or melena due to gastrointestinal ulceration in uremia.
- Hemic/lymphatic/immune—anemia from uremic blood loss or decreased red blood cell survival; impaired production of erythropoietin.
- Hepatobiliary—may occur with portosystemic shunts.
- Nervous—depression and lethargy associated with uremia.
- Renal/urologic.
- Respiratory—tachypnea or respiratory distress due to uremic pneumonitis or metabolic acidosis compensation.

SIGNALMENT

- Cat and dog.
- Polycystic kidney disease (PKD) occurs in several breeds of dogs and cats. Autosomal dominant inheritance in bull terriers and Persian cats; autosomal recessive in Cairn and West Highland white terriers.

SIGNS

Historical Findings

- May be asymptomatic, especially if only one kidney is affected.
- Lethargy.
- Loss of appetite.
- Weight loss.
- Vomiting.
- Diarrhea.
- Polyuria and polydipsia.
- Discolored urine.
- Abdominal enlargement.
- Rarely lameness because of hypertrophic osteopathy associated with renal neoplasia.

Physical Examination Findings

- Abdominal mass or pain.
- One or both kidneys palpably large.
- Abdominal enlargement.
- Asymmetric kidneys.
- Dehydration.
- Pallor.
- Oral ulcers.
- Uremic halitosis.

CAUSES & RISK FACTORS

Developmental/Acquired Disorders

- Hydronephrosis—unilateral or bilateral renomegaly secondary to ureteral obstruction or ectopic ureters.
- PKD—bilateral renomegaly in cats leading to chronic kidney disease (CKD).
- Hematoma—secondary to trauma.
- Compensatory hypertrophy—unilateral renomegaly secondary to disease of the other kidney.
- Perinephric pseudocyst—unilateral or bilateral enlargement. Kidney size may be normal, but subcapsular fluid accumulation enlarges capsule margins.

Metabolic

- Portosystemic shunt, acromegaly.
- Males have larger kidneys than females.

Neoplastic

- Lymphoma—most often occurs in cats and causes bilateral renomegaly; rarely unilateral.
- Renal carcinoma—most common renal tumor of dogs; often causes unilateral renomegaly.
- Nephroblastoma—congenital renal tumor, may not be diagnosed until the patient is older; usually unilateral.
- Sarcoma—usually cause unilateral renomegaly.
- Cystadenocarcinoma—bilateral renal tumor in German shepherd dogs; often associated with skin lesions.

Infectious/Inflammatory

- Amyloidosis.
- Leptospirosis.
- Feline infectious peritonitis (FIP).
- Feline leukemia virus (FeLV) infection predisposes cats to renal lymphoma.
- Acute kidney injury.
- Renal abscess.

Toxic

- Ethylene glycol—bilateral renomegaly secondary to renal tubular swelling and infiltration by calcium oxalate crystals.
- See Acute Kidney Injury.

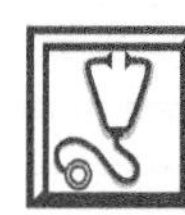

DIAGNOSIS

DIFFERENTIAL DIAGNOSIS

- Distinguish from other abdominal masses.
- Confirmation may require diagnostic imaging or exploratory celiotomy.

CBC/BIOCHEMISTRY/URINALYSIS

- Azotemia, hyperphosphatemia, and inadequate urine concentration.
- Leukocytosis—infectious, inflammatory, and neoplastic causes.
- Nonregenerative anemia—CKD or inflammatory disorder.
- Hyperglobulinemia—infectious or inflammatory disorder.
- Hematuria and proteinuria—renal neoplasia.
- Polycythemia and leukocytosis rarely accompany some renal neoplasms.
- Neoplastic cells rarely observed in urine with renal neoplasia.

OTHER LABORATORY TESTS

- Test for FeLV infection if renal lymphoma is suspected.
- Serum protein electrophoresis distinguishes polyclonal from monoclonal hyperglobulinemia.
- Test for leptospirosis if indicated.

IMAGING

Radiographic Findings

- Abdominal radiographs to confirm renomegaly and identify causes of ureteral obstruction.
- Renomegaly on the ventrodorsal view: >3 or 3.5 times the length of the L2 vertebra in cats or dogs, respectively.
- Excretory urography or CT to confirm renomegaly, hydronephrosis, and space-occupying masses.
- Antegrade pyelography may exclude ureteral obstruction.
- Thoracic radiography indicated to detect metastases.

Ultrasonographic Findings

- Distinguish between PKD, perinephric pseudocysts, hydronephrosis, neoplasia, abscess, and subcapsular hematoma.
- Acute inflammation may be associated with increased cortical echogenicity, perinephric effusion, or a medullary band of increased echogenicity.

DIAGNOSTIC PROCEDURES

- Cytologic examination of fine-needle aspirate can confirm renal cyst, abscess, or neoplasia. Due to potential for seeding of neoplastic cells in the abdominal wall, fine-needle aspiration should be avoided if some renal tumors (e.g., renal carcinoma) are suspected.
- If renal aspirate is nondiagnostic, biopsy may be indicated.

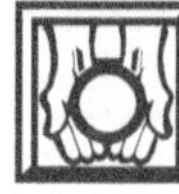

TREATMENT

- Diagnose and treat underlying cause of renomegaly.
- Outpatient unless dehydration or decompensated renal failure exist.
- Therapeutic renal diet is indicated to prolong survival time for CKD when serum creatinine exceeds 2 mg/dL.
- Administer balanced electrolyte solution intravenously or subcutaneously to maintain hydration as needed.

• If the patient has dehydration or continuing fluid losses such as vomiting or diarrhea, administer fluids intravenously to correct hydration deficits, maintain daily fluid need, and replace ongoing losses.

MEDICATIONS

DRUG(S) OF CHOICE

Vary with the cause.

CONTRAINDICATIONS/POSSIBLE INTERACTIONS

Avoid nephrotoxic drugs.

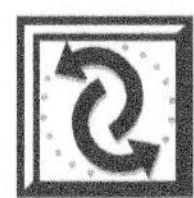

FOLLOW-UP

PATIENT MONITORING

• Perform physical examination and weigh patient to assess hydration.

• CBC, serum chemistries, urinalysis, blood pressure measurements are indicated depending on the underlying cause.

POSSIBLE COMPLICATIONS

CKD, depending on underlying cause of renomegaly.

MISCELLANEOUS

ZOONOTIC POTENTIAL

Leptospirosis can be spread by contact with infected urine.

SEE ALSO

• Ethylene Glycol Toxicosis.
• Feline Infectious Peritonitis (FIP).
• Hydronephrosis.
• Leptospirosis.
• Lymphoma—Cats.
• Perirenal Pseudocysts.
• Polycystic Kidney Disease.
• Urinary Tract Obstruction.

ABBREVIATIONS

• CKD = chronic kidney disease.
• FeLV = feline leukemia virus.
• FIP = feline infectious peritonitis.
• PKD = polycystic kidney disease.

Suggested Reading

Cuypers MD, Grooters AM, Williams J, et al. Renomegaly in dogs and cats. Part I: Differential diagnosis. Compend Contin Educ Pract Vet 1997, 19:1019–1033.

Author Cathy E. Langston

Consulting Editor J.D. Foster

Acknowledgment The authors and editors acknowledge the prior contribution of Allyson C. Berent.

R

RESPIRATORY PARASITES

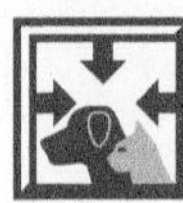

BASICS

DEFINITION

Helminths, arthropods, and protozoa that reside in the respiratory tract or pulmonary vessels of dogs and cats.

PATHOPHYSIOLOGY

Infestation with parasites causes rhinitis, bronchitis, pneumonitis, or arteritis, depending on the location of the organism within the respiratory system. Eosinophilic inflammation usually results from invasion of the parasite.

SYSTEMS AFFECTED

• Respiratory. • Cardiovascular. • Hepatic—with hepatopulmonary migration of some parasites (*Toxocara* spp.). • Neurologic—with migration of parasites to the brain (*Cuterebra*) or cerebral hemorrhage (*Angiostrongylus*).

GENETICS

There is no genetic basis.

INCIDENCE/PREVALENCE

Depends on parasite.

GEOGRAPHIC DISTRIBUTION

• *Pneumonyssoides caninum, Aelurostrongylus abstrusus, Linguatula serrata, Oslerus (Filaroides) osleri, Crenosoma vulpis, Eucoleus (Capillaria) aerophilus, Toxoplasma gondii, Toxocara* spp.—worldwide. • *Eucoleus boehmi, Cuterebra* spp., *Filaroides hirthi, Paragonimus kellicotti*—primarily North America.
• *Andersonstrongylus (Filaroides) milksi*—North America, Europe. • *Angiostrongylus vasorum*—various countries of Europe, Africa, South America, North America.

SIGNALMENT

Species

Dog and cat.

SIGNS

General Comments

• Four basic categories—upper airway (nasal cavity and sinuses), lower respiratory (trachea and bronchi), pulmonary parenchyma, and vascular; based on location and lifestyle of parasite. • Often insidious and chronic, with few clinical signs. • Respiratory compromise often not severe.

Historical Findings

• Upper respiratory—sneezing; nasal discharge (serous, sanguinous); reverse sneezing; nasal irritation or rubbing; neurologic signs with *Cuterebra* spp. • Lower respiratory and parenchyma—may have no clinical signs, variable coughing, tachypnea, or altered respiratory pattern. • Vascular—can have weight loss, lethargy, coughing, exercise intolerance. Acute onset of respiratory distress if embolization or hemorrhage occurs.

Physical Examination Findings

• Upper respiratory—similar to historical findings; variable. • Lower respiratory and parenchyma—cough elicited on tracheal palpation; occasionally harsh lung sounds.
• Vascular—may present with signs of pulmonary disease, right-sided heart failure, anemia, coagulopathy, neurologic signs.

CAUSES

• Upper respiratory (nasal cavity and sinuses)—*Pneumonyssoides caninum, Eucoleus boehmi, Linguatula serrata, Cuterebra* spp.
• Lower airway (trachea and bronchi)—dogs and cats: *Eucoleus (Capillaria) aerophilus* (rare in cats); dogs: *Oslerus osleri, Filaroides hirthi, Andersonstrongylus milksi, Crenosoma vulpis. Cuterebra* spp. in the trachea. • Pulmonary parenchyma—dogs and cats: *Paragonimus kellicotti, Toxoplasma gondii*; dogs: *Filaroides hirthi, Andersonstrongylus milksi*; cats: *Aelurostrongylus abstrusus, Troglostrongylus brevior, Troglostrongylus subcrenatus.*
• Vascular—dogs and cats: *Dirofilaria immitis*, larval migration of *Toxocara canis* and *T. cati*; dogs: *Angiostrongylus vasorum.*

RISK FACTORS

• Depends on the specific parasite—some have intermediate or paratenic hosts that must be ingested by the definitive host, putting hunting or scavenging animals at higher risk.
• *Crenosoma vulpis*—snails. • *Paragonimus kellicotti*—snails, crabs, shellfish.
• *Aelurostrongylus abstrusus*—snails and slugs; transport hosts: rodents, frogs, lizards, birds.
• *Linguatula serrata*—ingestion of sheep offal.
• *Toxoplasma gondii*—ingestion of infected small mammals and birds or less commonly by ingesting sporulated oocysts in soil or water. • Multi-animal households with unhygienic living conditions—allows fecal–oral or direct-contact transmission.
• *Angiostrongylus vasorum*—gastropods (slugs/snails) or frogs are the intermediate host. Frogs can also serve as paratenic hosts.

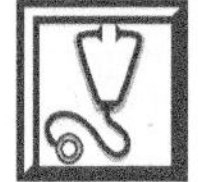

DIAGNOSIS

DIFFERENTIAL DIAGNOSIS

• Upper respiratory—other causes of epistaxis, rhinitis, or sinusitis (see specific chapters).
• Lower respiratory—acute bronchitis (nonparasitic); chronic bronchitis; infectious tracheobronchitis. • Pulmonary parenchyma—eosinophilic lung disease; bronchopneumonia; granulomatous pneumonia; pulmonary granulomatosis. • Vascular—other causes of coagulopathy, right-sided heart failure, or pulmonary artery disease.

CBC/BIOCHEMISTRY/URINALYSIS

• CBC—variable; may note eosinophilia, basophilia, neutrophilia, and monocytosis; can see anemia with *Angiostrongylus vasorum.*
• Biochemistry—often normal; high liver enzyme activity with some parasites during early stages as a result of hepatic migration if burden is substantial. • Urinalysis—normal.

OTHER LABORATORY TESTS

Coagulopathy with *Angiostrongylus vasorum* or severe cases of heartworm disease (disseminated intravascular coagulation).

IMAGING

Thoracic Radiography

• Often nonspecific findings—generalized interstitial pattern; peribronchiolar infiltrates, nodular to alveolar pattern. • *Oslerus*—soft tissue nodular densities within the trachea at the level of the carina. • *Paragonimus*—can see bullae, cystic lesions or pneumothorax due to bulla or cyst rupture. • *Dirofilaria*—right-sided heart enlargement, tortuous and truncated pulmonary arteries, pulmonary infiltrates (dogs). Few cardiac changes in cats, large pulmonary arteries possible.

DIAGNOSTIC PROCEDURES

Sputum Examination

May reveal eggs or larvae (L-1).

Fecal Examination

• Multiple examinations often necessary; negative results do not rule out infection.
• Direct fecal smear: *Angiostrongylus* (larvae).
• Standard fecal flotation: *Eucoleus aerophilus* (eggs), *Eucoleus boehmi* (eggs). • Zinc sulfate centrifugation: *Aelurostrongylus* (larvae), *Oslerus osleri, Andersonstrongylus milksi, Filaroides hirthi* (larvae, larvated eggs), *Angiostrongylus vasorum* (larvae). • Baermann: *Aelurostrongylus* (larvae), *Oslerus osleri, Andersonstrongylus milksi, Filaroides hirthi* (larvae, eggs), *Crenosoma* (larvae, larvated eggs), *Angiostrongylus* (larvae).
• Sedimentation: *Paragonimus* (eggs).

Rhinoscopy

• Upper respiratory—examination via retrograde pharyngoscopy or rhinoscopy with antegrade flushing of anesthetic gas can allow visualization of nasal mites; retrograde nasal lavage and cytologic examination of fluid can be helpful. • *Eucoleus boehmi*—histopathology can reveal eggs deep within the epithelium.
• *Linguatula serrata*—diagnosis made by observation of eggs in nasal secretions or around the nares.

Bronchoscopy

• Lower respiratory and parenchyma—rarely can see tracheal and bronchial parasites and parasitic nodules; occasionally can be removed for definitive identification. • Tracheal wash or bronchoalveolar lavage can allow identification of larvae (*Oslerus osleri, Aelurostrongylus, Crenosoma, Filaroides hirthi, Andersonstrongylus milksi, Angiostrongylus*); eggs (*Eucoleus aerophilus, Paragonimus*); organisms (*Toxoplasma*).
• *Oslerus osleri*—can also be diagnosed by brushings or histopathology of nodules at the carina.

PATHOLOGIC FINDINGS

• Upper respiratory—may find nasal mites or worms in epithelium of sinuses and nasal cavity. • Lower respiratory and parenchyma—can see pulmonary nodules containing parasites throughout the parenchyma or within bronchi. • Vascular—changes include thrombi and intimal proliferation of the vascular walls. • *Cuterebra* spp. can be found in brain sections when associated with neurologic signs.

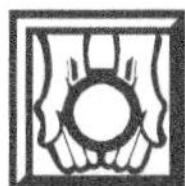

TREATMENT

APPROPRIATE HEALTH CARE

Most commonly outpatient—upper and lower respiratory parasites; may need repeated examinations to monitor response.

NURSING CARE

Supportive care and oxygen therapy can be needed depending on the severity of disease.

ACTIVITY

Strict cage rest if severe pulmonary dysfunction occurs with upper or lower respiratory parasites; also with vascular parasite infection or bullous lung disease associated with *Paragonimus*.

DIET

No special restrictions.

CLIENT EDUCATION

• Explain that treatment duration and response depend on the type of parasite. • Warn client of the risk of recurrence in animals that maintain lifestyles conducive to transmission of the parasites (e.g., hunting, sporting dogs, multidog households, outdoor cats).

SURGICAL CONSIDERATIONS

Ruptured *Paragonimus* cysts generally require surgical excision.

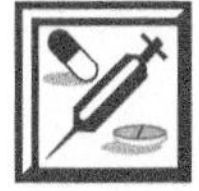

MEDICATIONS

DRUG(S) OF CHOICE

• Anthelmintics—few studies confirm efficacy; most data anecdotal. For treatment of *Dirofilaria*, see chapters on Heartworm Disease. • *Pneumonyssoides caninum*—selamectin 6–24 mg/kg applied every 2 weeks for three treatments. milbemycin oxime 0.5–1 mg/kg PO weekly for 3 weeks, ivermectin 200 µg/kg SC or PO for two treatments 3 weeks apart; *note:* not labeled for use in dogs at this dosage. • *Cuterebra*—ivermectin 300 µg/kg SC or PO every other day for three doses combined with a tapering dose of corticosteroids. • *Linguatula serrata*—physical removal of organisms from the sinuses. • *Eucoleus aerophilus, E, boehmi*—ivermectin 200 µg/kg PO once; fenbendazole 25–50 mg/kg q12h for 10–14 days; very difficult to clear. • *Oslerus osleri*—efficacious therapy not fully determined. Consider ivermectin 400 µg/kg SC or PO q3 weeks for four doses. • *Crenosoma vulpis*—levamisole 7.5 mg/kg SC q48h (two doses); fenbendazole 50 mg/kg PO q24h for 7 days; milbemycin oxime 0.5 mg/kg PO once. • *Aelurostrongylus abstrusus*—fenbendazole 25–50 mg/kg PO q24h for 10 days; ivermectin 400 µg/kg SC, selamectin spot-on formula 45 mg/cat, two doses, 23 days apart. • *Filaroides hirthi, Andersonstrongylus milksi*—fenbendazole 50 mg/kg PO q24h for 14 days; albendazole 50 mg/kg PO q12h for 5 days, repeat in 3 weeks. • *Paragonimus kellicotti*—praziquantel 25 mg/kg PO, SC q8h for 3 days; fenbendazole 25–50 mg/kg PO q12h for 14 days. • *Toxoplasma*—clindamycin 12.5 mg/kg PO q12h for 28 days. • *Angiostrongylus vasorum*—fenbendazole 20–50 mg/kg PO q24h for 5–21 days; milbemycin oxime 0.5 mg/kg PO weekly for 4 weeks; single topical application of moxidectin 2.5 mL/kg. • *Toxocara* spp. larval migration—fenbendazole 50 mg/kg PO q24h for 10 days. • Anti-inflammatory agents—recommendations for concurrent use of steroids vary.

CONTRAINDICATIONS

Ivermectin—not labeled for use in dogs or cats other than for heartworm prophylaxis; contraindicated at dosages >100 µg/kg in breeds with known sensitivity (collies, collie breeds, and Australian shepherd dogs).

PRECAUTIONS

None

ALTERNATIVE DRUG(S)

None

FOLLOW-UP

PATIENT MONITORING

• Serial fecal Baermann larval extractions or examination for eggs—some anthelmintics can suppress egg or larval production in some species and intermittent shedding reduces value of repeated fecal exams. • Resolution of clinical signs—suggests response to treatment; does not indicate complete clearance of parasites. • Peripheral eosinophilia, if noted initially, may subside with treatment. • Repeat bronchoscopic examination—can help assess efficacy of treatment for *Oslerus osleri*.

PREVENTION/AVOIDANCE

• Avoid activity that predisposes to infestations (often not practical). • Avoid contact with wildlife reservoirs (especially wild canids and felids). • Consider prophylactic treatment for heartworm.

POSSIBLE COMPLICATIONS

• Chronic pulmonary damage—possible with persistent and heavy lower respiratory parasite burdens. • Infestations generally not fatal; however, severe pulmonary damage can result with some species; *Cuterebra* spp. and *Angiostrongylus* can cause fatal neurologic complications. • *Pneumonyssoides caninum* has been associated with gastric dilation and volvulus.

EXPECTED COURSE AND PROGNOSIS

• With aggressive management—prognosis usually fair to excellent; variable. • Return to performance—depends on chronicity of disease and level of chronic pulmonary damage by lower respiratory parasites.
• Recurrence possible.

MISCELLANEOUS

ZONOTIC POTENTIAL

None

SYNONYMS

• Lungworm infestation—*Aelurostrongylus, Eucoleus (Capillaria) aerophilus, Crenosoma, Oslerus osleri, Filaroides hirthi, Andersonstrongylus milksi.* • Nasal mite infestation—*Pneumonyssoides caninum, Pneumonyssus caninum.*
• French heartworm—*Angiostrongylus vasorum.*

R

SEE ALSO

• Heartworm Disease—Cats.
• Heartworm Disease—Dogs.
• Pneumonia, Eosinophilic.

INTERNET RESOURCES

Bowman DD. Respiratory system parasites of the dog and cat, Part I: Nasal mucosa and sinuses, and respiratory parenchyma and Part II: Trachea and bronchi, and pulmonary vessels: http://www.ivis.org/advances/Parasit_Bowman/ddb_resp/ivis.pdf

Suggested Reading

Lacorcia L, Gaser R, Anderson BA, Beveridge I. Comparison of bronchoalveolar lavage fluid examination and other diagnostic techniques with the Baermann technique for detection of naturally occurring *Aelurostrongylus abstrusus* infection in cats. J Am Vet Med Assoc 2009, 235(1):43–49.

Marks SL, Moore MP, Rishniw M. *Pneumonyssus caninum:* the canine nasal mite. Compend Contin Educ Pract Vet 1994, 16:577–582.

Author Elizabeth Rozanski
Consulting Editor Elizabeth Rozanski
Acknowledgment The author/editor acknowledges the prior contribution of Jill S. Pomrantz.

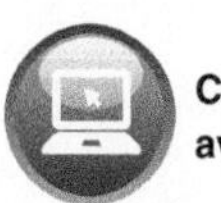

Client Education Handout available online

RETAINED PLACENTA

BASICS

OVERVIEW

- Dogs—placenta retained beyond the immediate postpartum period; placentas usually passed within 15 minutes of birth of a puppy; may develop acute metritis secondary to retained placenta.
- Cats—may retain placentas for days without signs of illness.
- Extremely uncommon.

SIGNALMENT

- Dog—rare, most common in toy dog breeds.
- Cat—rare.

SIGNS

Historical Findings

- Recent parturition.
- Continued vulvar discharge of lochia.
- Owner may note number of placentas passed, although this information is frequently unreliable.

Physical Examination Findings

- Green lochia vulvar discharge.
- Palpation of firm mass in uterus—not always possible.
- Concurrent clinical signs of postpartum metritis.

CAUSES & RISK FACTORS

- Toy breed.
- Large litter size.
- Dystocia.

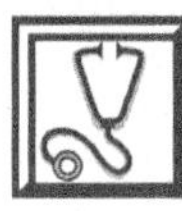

DIAGNOSIS

DIFFERENTIAL DIAGNOSIS

- Postpartum metritis—physical examination and vaginal cytologic examination show no signs of infection with uncomplicated retained placenta; metritis may develop concurrently.
- Retained fetus—differentiated by radiography or ultrasonography.

CBC/BIOCHEMISTRY/URINALYSIS

Usually normal when uncomplicated.

OTHER LABORATORY TESTS

Vaginal cytologic examination—parabasal epithelial cells; may note erythrocytes; biliverdin clumps.

IMAGING

Ultrasonography—echogenic but nonfetal mass within the uterus.

DIAGNOSTIC PROCEDURES

Celiotomy or hysterotomy—may be required for diagnosis.

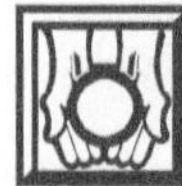

TREATMENT

- Outpatient for healthy bitch or queen.
- Instruct owner to monitor rectal temperature and observe for signs of systemic illness.
- Ovariohysterectomy—curative; recommended if future breeding is not a consideration.
- Surgical removal—indicated if medical treatment is unsuccessful and the bitch develops metritis.

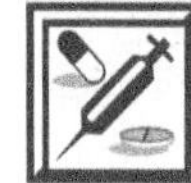

MEDICATIONS

DRUG(S) OF CHOICE

- Oxytocin—known or suspected condition in otherwise healthy cats and dogs; dogs: 0.5 IU/kg IM, up to 5 IU total dose; cats: 0.5–1 IU IM. Oxytocin may be ineffective after 48 hours postpartum.
- Can precede oxytocin treatment with calcium gluconate (10%); dogs and cats, 0.5–1.5 mL/kg IV slowly over 15 minutes; monitor for bradycardia during injection.
- Metritis—treat accordingly (see Metritis).

CONTRAINDICATIONS/POSSIBLE INTERACTIONS

Do not give progestational drugs.

FOLLOW-UP

- Monitor temperature and physical condition.
- Acute metritis (dogs)—may develop if the placenta is not passed; fair to good prognosis for recovery with treatment.
- Prognosis for future reproduction—good without metritis; fair to poor with metritis.

MISCELLANEOUS

SEE ALSO

Metritis

Suggested Reading

Feldman EC, Nelson RW. Periparturient diseases. In: Feldman EC, Nelson RW, eds., Canine and Feline Endocrinology and Reproduction, 3rd ed. Philadelphia, PA: Saunders, 2004, pp. 808–834.

Grundy SG, Davidson AP. Theriogenology question of the month. Acute metritis secondary to retained fetal membranes and a retained nonviable fetus. J Am Vet Med Assoc 2004, 224(6):844–847.

Author Joni L. Freshman

Consulting Editor Erin E. Runcan

R

RETINAL DEGENERATION

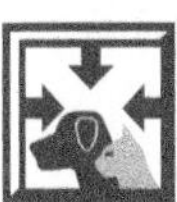

BASICS

DEFINITION

• Degeneration of the retina from inherited or acquired causes. • Inherited—generalized progressive retinal atrophy (PRA); a group of progressive retinal diseases; may be subdivided into photoreceptor dysplasias (begin before retina fully develops <8 weeks) and photoreceptor degenerations (begin after retina matures).

PATHOPHYSIOLOGY

• A number of genetic defects in photoreceptor metabolism have been identified. • May be secondary to retinal pigment epithelial or choroidal disease; amino acid metabolic disorders, and storage diseases. • Central PRA: genetic defect in vitamin E metabolism, or acquired with vitamin E deficiency. • May be idiopathic, secondary to diffuse or focal inflammation and scarring (e.g., chorioretinitis), toxin exposure, nutritional deficiency, or previous retinal detachment. • Sudden acquired retinal degeneration syndrome (SARDS): idiopathic, may be immune-mediated retinitis.

SYSTEMS AFFECTED

• Nervous. • Ophthalmic.

GENETICS

Dogs

• PRA—generally autosomal recessive, dominant in mastiffs. • Neuronal ceroid lipofuscinosis—generally autosomal recessive. • Hemeralopia—cone degeneration, autosomal recessive. • Inheritance in many breeds not determined.

Cats

• Early onset—mixed breed and Abyssinian retinal dysplasia (rod-cone dysplasia), autosomal dominant. Persians, autosomal recessive. • Late onset—Abyssinian rod-cone degeneration, autosomal recessive. • Late onset—PRA in many breeds, including Siamese.

INCIDENCE/PREVALENCE

• Hereditary—prevalence greater in dogs than cats. • Taurine deficiency—uncommon with nutritionally complete cat foods.

GEOGRAPHIC DISTRIBUTION

Central PRA—more common in dogs from Europe than United States.

SIGNALMENT

Species

Dog and cat.

Breed Predilections

Hereditary—Dogs • Retinal dysplasia—Bedlington terrier, Sealyham terrier, English springer spaniel, cocker spaniel, others. • Early-onset PRA—Irish setter, collie, Norwegian elkhound, miniature schnauzer, Belgian shepherd dog, mastiff, Cardigan Welsh corgi, American Staffordshire terrier, pit bull terrier, briard (congenital stationary night blindness). • Late-onset PRA—miniature and toy poodle, American and English cocker spaniel, basenji, Labrador retriever, Tibetan terrier, dachshund, Akita, Samoyed, Siberian husky. • Central PRA—Labrador, golden retriever, border collie, collie, Shetland sheepdog, briard, others. • Cone degeneration disease—German shorthaired pointer, Alaskan Malamute, and Australian shepherd dog. • Neuronal ceroid lipofuscinosis—English setter, border collie, American bulldog, Dalmatian, Tibetan terrier, collie. • SARDS—Brittany spaniel, miniature schnauzer, dachshund, others.

Hereditary—Cats

• Abyssinian, Somali, Persian. • Siamese breed group—autosomal recessive (CEP290).

Mean Age and Range

• Early PRA and dystrophies—3 months–2 years. • Late PRA—clinical signs >4–6 years. • Cone degeneration disease—3–4 months. • SARDS—middle-aged to old.

Predominant Sex

• PRA—X-linked recessive condition in Siberian husky and Samoyed, therefore primarily males. • SARDS—70% female.

SIGNS

Historical Findings

• PRA (dog)— gradually progressing nyctalopia that ultimately affects vision in bright light; may note dilated pupils or brighttapetal reflex; may appear acutely blind. Dysplasias have early onset and blindness by 2 years. Degenerations are later onset and blind in later life. • Hemeralopia or cone degeneration disease—rare. Between 8 and 12 weeks of age puppies show photophobia and trouble navigating in bright light. Progresses to total day blindness. Night vision remains normal. • Central PRA (dogs)—rare in United States; central vision lost; may never become completely blind. • SARDS—vision lost in 1–4 weeks; polyuria, polydipsia, and polyphagia common.

Physical Examination Findings

• If severe—direct and consensual pupillary light reflexes impaired or nearly abolished. • Tapetal hyperreflectivity and nontapetal depigmentation or mottled hyperpigmentation; retinal blood vessel attenuation and optic nerve atrophy. • PRA (dogs)—cataracts and vitreous degeneration can occur. • SARDS (dogs)—obesity; may note slow or absent pupillary light reflexes (PLR). Chromatic PLR testing (melan 100), reduced or no red PLR, normal blue PLR. • Borzoi chorioretinopathy—multifocal chorioretinal lesions (hyperpigmented and hyperreflective). • Taurine-deficient retinopathy (cats)—begins as a spot in area centralis; then horizontal band forms superior to optic nerve; finally, diffuse degeneration and hyperreflectivity. • Storage diseases—may have cloudy corneas and possibly neurologic signs. • Neuronal ceroid lipofuscinosis—mental deterioration, paralysis, and death.

CAUSES

Degenerative

• PRA—affects both eyes symmetrically. • Chronic or uncontrolled glaucoma—retinal and optic nerve atrophy. • Secondary to scarring from previous multifocal or diffuse retinal detachment or inflammation.

Anomalous

• Rod-cone dysplasias—affect both eyes. • Other dysplasias—may be multifocal and nonblinding (e.g., English springer spaniel, Labrador retriever). • Oculoskeletal dysplasia in Labrador and Samoyed.

Metabolic

• Storage disease—mucopolysaccharidosis, gangliosidosis, mannosidosis, fucosidisis (English springer spaniel). • Ornithine aminotransferase deficiency—progressive and total atrophy of choroid and retina; older cats.

Neoplastic

Neoplastic infiltrate may lead to scars from previous retinal detachment if treated.

Nutritional

• Severe deficiency of vitamin E or A (dogs and cats)—may cause partial or complete degeneration. • Taurine deficiency (cats)—retinal degeneration, dilated cardiomyopathy.

Infectious/Immune

• Retina will degenerate from inflammation; may be focal, multifocal, or generalized. SARDS—some cases are immune-mediated retinitis.

Idiopathic

SARDS—dogs; post-inflammatory—dogs and cats.

Toxic

• Idiosyncratic reaction to griseofulvin or enrofloxacin (cats). • Radiation—dogs or cats treated for nasal or CNS neoplasia. • Phototoxicity—operating microscopes, welding light exposure.

RISK FACTORS

• Ocular disease—cataracts, panuveitis, chorioretinitis, retinal detachment, glaucoma. • Cats—enrofloxacin dose should not exceed 5 mg/kg/day. Toxicity noted at lower doses in compromised animals (i.e., renal disease).

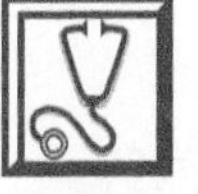

DIAGNOSIS

DIFFERENTIAL DIAGNOSIS

• Acute vision loss, PLR slow or absent—SARDS, optic neuritis, retinal detachment, unrecognized PRA, or glaucoma; PLR normal—rapidly developing diabetic cataracts

R

RETINAL DEGENERATION (CONTINUED)

or visual cortex disease. • Slowly progressive visual loss—PRA, cataracts, severe corneal disease (e.g., pigmentation, scarring, or edema), chronic retinitis, chorioretinitis, vitreal inflammation.

CBC/BIOCHEMISTRY/URINALYSIS

• Usually normal, unless systemic disease.
• SARDS (dogs)—may suggest hyperadrenocorticism.

OTHER LABORATORY TESTS

• Test for hyperadreoncorticism, evaluate sex hormone levels, check blood pressure, evaluate for proteinuria with SARDS.
• Taurine concentration (cats)—especially with dilated cardiomyopathy. • Serum and urine ornithine concentrations (cats)—elevated with ornithine aminotransferase deficiency. • Genetic testing - many tests are available from many different companies; VetGen, Animal Genetics, Animal Labs, Embark Vet are examples. May identify affected, non-affected and carriers.

IMAGING

• Thoracic radiographs and cardiac ultrasound—in cats with suspected taurine deficiency. • CT or MRI—investigate causes of central blindness.

DIAGNOSTIC PROCEDURES

• Ophthalmic examination.
• Electroretinography—localizes cause of blindness when retina not visible or appears normal. • Chromatic PLR (Melan 100)—differentiates outer retinal layer problems (red reduced) vs. inner retina layers (absent blue). Definitive diagnosis requires electroretinogram as interpretation can be confounded by iris atrophy and stress-induced mydriasis.
• Cerebrospinal fluid tap—for cases of suspected optic neuritis.

PATHOLOGIC FINDINGS

• Thin retina. • Edges of focal retinal scars—sharply delineated. • Hyperpigmented areas—associated with postinflammatory scars or central PRA. • End-stage degenerations—marked photoreceptor atrophy and reduction in retinal cell density. • Lipopigment accumulated in neuroepithelium—central PRA, ceroid lipofuscinosis, congenital stationary night blindness. • Lysosome storage diseases—accumulation in neuronal/retinal layers/cornea.

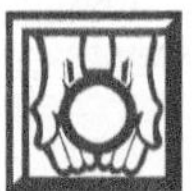

TREATMENT

DIET

• Cats—food should contain 500–750 ppm taurine. • Dogs—balanced diet, avoid those high in polyunsaturated fats.

CLIENT EDUCATION

• Most blind animals function well in stable environment. • Blind dogs should be supervised if outside, in unfenced yards or in an area with a pool. • Suggest playing with toys that make sounds. • Older blind animals with hearing loss or senility may not adapt well. • Some blind animals experience behavioral changes such as aggression or reduced activity. • Animals with only one blind eye can function normally. • Blind cats should be kept indoors.

SURGICAL CONSIDERATIONS

Not indicated unless painful.

MEDICATIONS

DRUG(S) OF CHOICE

• None currently effective. • Pyridoxine—for ornithine aminotransferase deficiency (cats). • Adequate dietary taurine—halt progression of taurine-deficient retinopathy.
• SARDS—if autoimmune retinitis, immune suppressive treatment may preserve/restore some vision.

GENE THERAPY

Experimental—retinal pigment epithelium dystrophy in briard.

CONTRAINDICATIONS

N/A

PRECAUTIONS

Cataract surgery—not recommended if retinal degeneration is severe; perform preoperative electroretinogram.

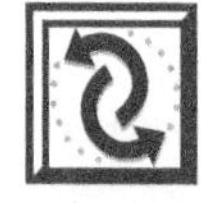

FOLLOW-UP

PATIENT MONITORING

• Serial fundic examinations—signs of degeneration over weeks with SARDS; months with PRA. • Cataract formation—with PRA or SARDS.

PREVENTION/AVOIDANCE

• Do not breed known or suspected carriers of PRA or other heritable diseases. • Genetic testing on breeding animals.

POSSIBLE COMPLICATIONS

• Cataracts. • Glaucoma. • Uveitis. • Ocular trauma (result of visual impairment).
• Obesity (reduced activity).

EXPECTED COURSE AND PROGNOSIS

• Inherited PRA—progresses to blindness; slow progression allows patient to adapt to visual loss. • Degeneration from inflammation—usually does not progress unless persistent or recurrent inflammation.
• SARDS—irreversible blindness. • Taurine deficiency (cats)—degeneration may halt at any stage.

MISCELLANEOUS

ASSOCIATED CONDITIONS

SARDS—hyperadrenocorticism, proteinuria, hypertension, elevated sex hormones.

AGE-RELATED FACTORS

N/A

ZOONOTIC POTENTIAL

N/A

PREGNANCY/FERTILITY/BREEDING

N/A

SYNONYMS

• PRA—progressive rod-cone degeneration; retinal atrophy. • Taurine-deficient retinopathy—feline central retinal degeneration.

SEE ALSO

• Blind Quiet Eye.
• Chorioretinitis.
• Lysosomal Storage Diseases.
• Retinal Detachment.

ABBREVIATIONS

• PLR = pupillary light reflex.
• PRA = progressive retinal atrophy.
• SARDS = sudden acquired retinal degeneration syndrome.

Suggested Reading

Narfström K, Petersen-Jones S. Diseases of the canine ocular fundus. In: Veterinary Ophthalmology, 5th ed. Ames, IA: Blackwell, 2013, pp. 2087–2235.

Author Patricia J. Smith
Consulting Editor Kathern E. Myrna

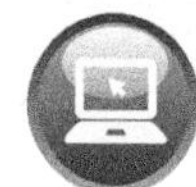

Client Education Handout available online

RETINAL DETACHMENT

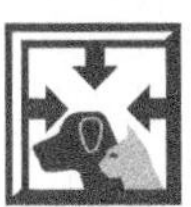

BASICS

DEFINITION

Separation of the neural retina from the retinal pigment epithelium (RPE).

PATHOPHYSIOLOGY

• Subretinal space—a potential space between RPE and neural retina in which fluid or exudates accumulate. • Etiopathogenesis is one or a combination of rhegmatogenous (retinal tear), subretinal exudation, or traction.

Rhegmatogenous Retinal Detachment (RRD)

A tear or hole in retina related to age, cataracts, traction from inflammatory debris or vitreal degeneration, trauma, or retinal degeneration. Vitreous fluid moves into the subretinal space, resulting in detachment. Probably the predominant type occurring in association with cataracts and after cataract or lens surgery.

Exudative

• Fluid accumulates in the subretinal space because of breakdown of blood–retinal barrier. • Subretinal fluid—serous, hemorrhagic, or exudative. • Hematogenous/ systemic pathogenetic factors—common. • Vasculitis, hypertension, and hyperviscosity—may cause serous detachment with or without hemorrhage.

Traction

• Fibrous or fibrovascular tissue; detaches retina and/or may cause retinal tear. • Associated with trauma, intraocular foreign bodies, or any cause of severe vitreal inflammation.

SYSTEMS AFFECTED

• Nervous. • Ophthalmic. • May be manifestation of systemic disease or neoplasia.

GENETICS

Depends on cause—dogs with hereditary cataracts or lens luxation may develop RRD. Some breeds may develop RRD from primary vitreous abnormalities (shih tzu), colobomas of optic nerve (collie), or severe retinal dysplasia inducing retinal tears or traction.

INCIDENCE/PREVALENCE

• Exudative—most common in dogs and cats. • RRD—uncommon. More common in dogs because of the greater prevalence of severe vitreal degeneration, cataracts, and cataract surgery.

GEOGRAPHIC DISTRIBUTION

Varies with the distribution of infectious etiologies.

SIGNALMENT

Species

Dog and cat.

Breed Predilections

• Depends on cause. • Terrier breeds—predisposed to primary lens luxation, may contribute to RRD. • Breeds that develop cataracts. • Shih-tzu, Boston terrier, Italian greyhound, Chihuahua, corgi—predisposed to spontaneous RRD owing to abnormal liquefied vitreous. • Dogs with merle coat color (Australian shepherd dog, Shetland sheepdog, Great Dane, collie) may have severe retinal dysplasia and optic nerve or scleral colobomas, leading to RRD. • Breeds with severe retinal dysplasia: English springer spaniel, Labrador retriever, Bedlington terrier. • Breeds with serous retinopathy (also known as RPE dysplasia, canine multifocal retinopathy): Great Pyrenees, mastiff, coton de Tulear.

Mean Age and Range

• Depends on cause. • Older patients—cataracts and systemic diseases (e.g., hypertension, neoplasia, immune-mediated disease). • Young dogs—retinal dysplasia, canine multifocal retinopathy, uveodermatologic syndrome.

SIGNS

• Blindness or reduced vision in affected eye. • Dilated pupil with slow or no pupillary light response (PLR). PLR may be near normal if detachment is acute. • Blood vessels or a "membrane" may be observed easily through the pupil just behind the lens. • Vitreous abnormalities—floaters, hemorrhage, or syneresis (liquefaction); common. • Interruption or alteration of course of blood vessels due to retinal elevation. • With clear subretinal fluid—vessels may cast shadows. • With exudative fluid or blood, tapetum/RPE may not be visible. • Other signs related to underlying systemic disease or inflammation (see Chorioretinitis). • Canine multifocal retinopathy—multifocal gray to tan elevated lesions (focal detachments) of various size. Starts around 11 weeks, progresses with time.

CAUSES

Bilateral—suggests a systemic problem, except in breeds with a predisposition to severe vitreal degeneration (e.g., shih tzu).

Degenerative

End-stage progressive retinal degeneration—may lead to RRD if retina tears.

Anomalous

• Colobomas—collie eye anomaly; abnormal retina around colobomatous optic nerve or large choroidal staphylomas may lead to RRD (merle ocular dysgenesis). • Severe retinal dysplasia, or oculoskeletal dysplasia (Labrador retrievers, Samoyeds). • Canine multifocal retinopathy. • Multiple ocular anomalies.

Metabolic

• Hyperviscosity (e.g., due to hyperproteinemia from multiple myeloma or other causes). • Polycythemia. • Shock. • Dogs—systemic hypertension, hypothyroidism, hypercholesterolemia . • Cats—systemic hypertension (usually related to hyperthyroidism, chronic renal disease).

Neoplastic

• Primary or metastatic. • Multiple myeloma, lymphoma, and intraocular masses (e.g., ciliary body adenocarcinoma or melanoma). • Pheochromocytoma may cause hypertension.

Infectious

• Infectious retinitis or chorioretinitis may cause focal or diffuse detachment. • Infection may extend from or to the CNS.

Immune-Mediated/Inflammatory

• Immune complex disease—vasculitis or inflammation can result in exudative detachment: ◦ Dogs—systemic lupus erythematosus (SLE); uveodermatologic syndrome, meningoencephalitis of unknown etiology. ◦ Cats—periarteritis nodosa; SLE.

Idiopathic

• If all other causes are ruled out, including retinal tears. • Idiopathic steroid-responsive detachment—reported in giant-breed dogs; may occur in any breed.

Trauma and Toxic

• Penetrating injury or foreign body. • Severe blunt trauma with inflammation or hemorrhage, usually unilateral. • Surgical trauma—if lens or vitreous disturbed (e.g., cataract surgery), can lead to RRD. • Toxic—drug reactions (e.g., trimethoprim-sulfa, ethyelene glycol, griseofulvin [cats]).

RISK FACTORS

• Systemic hypertension. • Old age—retinal thinning, severe vitreal degeneration. • Hypermature, intumescent cataracts that may rupture (e.g., diabetic cataracts). • Luxated lenses. • Lens extraction. • Hereditary—young dogs that have more severe retinal dysplasia and/or multiple ocular anomalies.

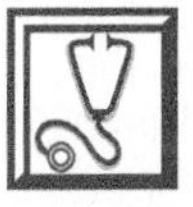

DIAGNOSIS

DIFFERENTIAL DIAGNOSIS

• Blindness or impaired vision—optic neuritis, glaucoma, cataracts, progressive retinal atrophy, sudden acquired retinal degeneration syndrome (SARDS; see Retinal Degeneration), CNS disease. • Dilated pupil with slow or absent pupillary light reflexes—glaucoma, oculomotor nerve lesion, optic neuritis, progressive retinal atrophy, SARDS. • Membrane or vessels associated with or behind lens—persistent tunica vasculosa lentis, persistent pupillary membranes, fibrovascular membrane due to intraocular neoplasia or inflammation.

CBC/BIOCHEMISTRY/URINALYSIS

Typically normal, unless systemic disease present.

OTHER LABORATORY TESTS

• Depends on suspected systemic problem. • Protein electrophoresis or documentation of Bence Jones proteinuria. • Coagulation profile. • Bacterial culture of ocular or body fluids. • Thyroid hormone measurement. • Serologic or PCR testing for infectious diseases.

IMAGING

• Thoracic and abdominal radiographs, ultrasound, and/or CT. • Spinal radiographs may reveal bony changes consistent with multiple myeloma. • Ocular ultrasound—if ocular media is opaque, can identify retinal detachments or intraocular masses.

DIAGNOSTIC PROCEDURES

• Ophthalmic examination. • Serial blood pressure measurement—normal systolic arterial pressure <160 mmHg. • Cerebral spinal fluid tap—indicated if CNS disease or optic neuritis. • Vitreocentesis or subretinal fluid aspirate—if other testing fails to determine cause and infection or neoplasia is suspected; may aggravate inflammation or induce hemorrhage.

PATHOLOGIC FINDINGS

• Retina separated from the RPE and choroid. • May note masses, subretinal exudate, or etiologic infectious organism. • Chronic—retinal atrophy and tombstone appearance to RPE.

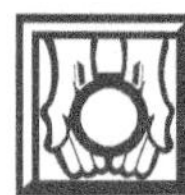

TREATMENT

APPROPRIATE HEALTH CARE

• Usually outpatient; depends on condition of patient. • Vision may be restored if underlying cause is rapidly identified and treated, but degeneration occurs quickly.

CLIENT EDUCATION

• May be a sign of systemic disease. • If associated with vitreal degeneration, lens luxation, or cataract surgery, fellow eye at risk for same condition. • Blind pets can adapt remarkably well and live a good-quality life.

SURGICAL CONSIDERATIONS

• RRD—may be surgically repaired by an ophthalmologist. • Laser retinopexy—may reverse detachments associated with optic disc colobomas; may stabilize partial/small detachments. May prevent detachment in predisposed fellow eye.

MEDICATIONS

DRUG(S) OF CHOICE

• Depends on underlying systemic cause. • Prednisone for immunosuppression (for immune-mediated causes) 2–4 mg/kg PO, divided q12 for 3–10 days (dog, cat), then taper slowly over months (do not exceed 80 mg per day). Rule out systemic mycosis prior to use; may facilitate retinal reattachment. • Corticosteroids at anti-inflammatory doses—prednisone 0.5–1 mg/kg PO q24h (dog), prednisolone 1–2 mg/kg PO q24h (cat), then taper; may be useful for exudative detachments of an infectious nature as long as the underlying disease is being definitively treated. • Antihypertensive agents—amlodipine 0.1–0.5 mg/kg PO q12–24h (dog); 0.625–1.25 mg/cat PO q12–24h (cat). Consult with internist or cardiologist if persistent hypertension.

CONTRAINDICATIONS

Systemic corticosteroids—do not use unless systemic mycosis is ruled out or is being definitively treated.

ALTERNATIVE DRUG(S)

Adjunctive immunosuppressive therapy (azathioprine, cyclosporine, mycophenolate, leflunomide) may be needed in some immune-mediated retinal detachment if prednisone is not effective or tolerated long term.

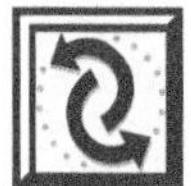

FOLLOW-UP

PATIENT MONITORING

• Some immunosuppressive therapy (e.g., azathioprine) requires regular CBC and serum biochemistry analysis to monitor for bone marrow suppression or hepatotoxicity. • Serial blood pressure monitoring in hypertensive patients.

POSSIBLE COMPLICATIONS

• Permanent blindness. • Cataracts. • Glaucoma—if eye becomes blind and painful enucleation may be necessary. • Chronic ocular pain. • Death secondary to systemic disease/neoplastic process.

EXPECTED COURSE AND PROGNOSIS

• Prognosis for vision with complete detachment—guarded. Exception is hypertensive retinopathy that is diagnosed and treated promptly. • Surgical reattachment of retina is about 72% successful at restoring vision for up to 1.5 years. • Vision may return if underlying cause is removed and reattachment occurs. • Blindness—may develop in days to weeks even with reattachment (more likely and rapid with exudative than serous detachments). • Focal or multifocal chorioretinitis—does not markedly impair vision; will leave scars.

MISCELLANEOUS

ASSOCIATED CONDITIONS

• Cataracts.
• Trauma.
• Vitreous abnormalities.
• Primary neurologic disease or systemic disease affecting CNS.

ABBREVIATIONS

• PLR = pupillary light reflex.
• RPE = retinal pigment epithelium.
• RRD = rhegmatogenous retinal detachment.
• SARDS = sudden acquired retinal degeneration syndrome.
• SLE = systemic lupus erythematosus.

Suggested Reading

Maggs DJ, Miller PE, Ofri R. Slatter's Fundamentals of Veterinary Ophthalmology, 5th ed. St. Louis, MO: Saunders, 2013.

Author Patricia J. Smith
Consulting Editor Kathern E. Myrna

Client Education Handout available online

RETINAL HEMORRHAGE

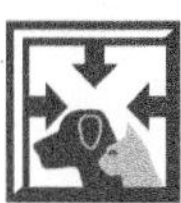

BASICS

DEFINITION

• Focal or generalized areas of bleeding into part or all layers of the retina.
• May be acute or chronic.

PATHOPHYSIOLOGY

• Trauma-induced retinal detachments may tear retinal blood vessels.
• Intoxications, vasculitis, coagulopathy (including thrombocytopenia or thrombocytopathia), neoplasia, and systemic infectious disease may cause focal or widespread hemorrhage.
• Systemic hypertension may cause local hemorrhage with vascular abnormalities and/or complete or partial retinal detachments.
• Congenital malformations, concurrent vascular abnormalities, and neovascularization syndromes.
• Diabetes mellitus may be associated with retinopathy that includes vascular microaneurysms with accompanying hemorrhage.

SYSTEMS AFFECTED

Ophthalmic

GENETICS

• Collie eye anomaly—autosomal recessive trait.
• Retinal dysplasia—suspected to be autosomal recessive inheritance.
• Retinal detachment—depends on causative factor, hereditary when observed in conjunction with above conditions.

INCIDENCE/PREVALENCE

• Common in hypertensive retinopathy of elderly cats.
• Common nonspecific finding with many systemic diseases.

SIGNALMENT

Species

Dog and cat—any breed, age, or sex.

Breed Predilections

• May have genetic basis (e.g., collies with collie eye anomaly, Labrador retrievers with congenital vitreoretinal dysplasia).
• Hereditary breed-specific congenital defects that might cause detachment or severe retinal dysplasia—collies and Shetland sheepdogs with collie eye anomaly, Australian shepherd dogs with merle ocular dysgenesis, Labrador retrievers, Sealyham terriers, Bedlington terriers, and English springer spaniels with retinal dysplasia, and miniature schnauzers with retinal dysplasia and persistent hyperplastic primary vitreous.

Mean Age and Range

• Old cats are often affected by systemic hypertension.
• Congenital defects can be observed in puppies at 5–7 weeks.

Predominant Sex

No sex predilection.

SIGNS

General Comments

Depend on underlying causes such as inflammatory disease in the posterior segment, systemic disease, or ocular malformations.

Historical Findings

• Often none.
• Vision loss, bumping into objects.

Physical Examination Findings

• Light or dark red appearance of the posterior segment.
• Blood-filled anterior chamber (hyphema).
• Evidence of bleeding elsewhere—petechia, ecchymoses, melena, hematuria.
• Leukocoria (whitish-appearing pupil) with or without reddish coloration behind the lens.
• Absence of menace response.
• Abnormal pupillary responses.

CAUSES

Congenital

• Retinal detachment secondary to severe congenital malformations in the eye.
• Vitreoretinal defects (e.g., persistent hyperplastic primary vitreous [PHPV] or persistent hyperplastic tunica vasculosa lentis [PHTVL]).
• Retinal defects in geographic or complete retinal dysplasia or in partial or complete retinal detachment.

Acquired

• Trauma.
• Systemic hypertension—renal disease, cardiac disease, hyperthyroidism, hyperadrenocorticism, idiopathic.
• Intoxication—anticoagulant rodenticides; sulfonamide or estrogen-related compound toxicity causing thrombocytopenia.
• Infectious—*Rickettsia rickettsia*, *Ehrlichia* spp., systemic mycoses (cryptococcosis).
• Neoplasia—lymphosarcoma, multiple myeloma (hyperviscosity).
• Hematologic disorders—coagulopathy (hemophilia, hepatic failure), thrombocytopenia, thrombocytopathia (von Willebrand disease), polycythemia.
• Diabetic retinopathy.
• Retinal detachment.
• Vasculitis.

RISK FACTORS

• Systemic hypertension or renal disease.
• Hematologic disease, coagulopathy.
• Vascular membranes.

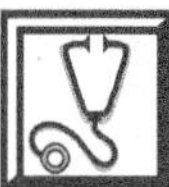

DIAGNOSIS

DIFFERENTIAL DIAGNOSIS

• Normal choroidal vessel pattern in a subalbinotic fundus—seen in lightly pigmented eyes. Blood is contained in vascular channels and not outside of the vessels.
• Vitreal opacities:
  ◦ Vitreal hemorrhage (reddish coloration of the pupil, impossible to rule out concurrent retinal hemorrhage).
  ◦ Vitreal inflammation (generalized or local blurring or lack of fundus detail, usually no reddish coloration).
  ◦ Persistent hyaloid arteries.
  ◦ Neoplasia—especially lymphoma or ciliary body tumors.
  ◦ Also caused by uveitis, glaucoma, lens luxation, trauma, foreign bodies, and spread from local or systemic infectious diseases.
• Pigment spots in retina that look like microhemorrhage. Will not change over time.

CBC/BIOCHEMISTRY/URINALYSIS

• Usually normal unless indicative of systemic disease.
• Hyperglycemia and/or glucosuria—indicative of diabetes mellitus.
• Azotemia and/or proteinuria—renal disease (may cause systemic hypertension).
• Thrombocytopenia, anemia/polycythemia, hyperglobulinemia, or other changes consistent with hematologic disorders.

OTHER LABORATORY TESTS

• Endocrine—thyroid and adrenal function testing.
• Infectious agents—serologic or urine antigen testing for infectious agents.
• Coagulation, von Willebrand factor antigen testing.

IMAGING

• Ocular ultrasound—evaluate position of lens and retina in cases with blood-filled posterior segment.
• Thoracic radiographs—to identify metastatic neoplasia or fungal disease.
• Abdominal ultrasound—if systemic disease or neoplasia suspected.

DIAGNOSTIC PROCEDURES

• Ophthalmic examination with a penlight—usually permits diagnosis of complete retinal detachment with partial retinal hemorrhage; detached neuroretina may often be visualized through the pupil as a whitish veil of tissue.
• Indirect ophthalmoscopy—diagnosis of funduscopic and vitreal changes.
• Vitreous paracentesis and cytologic examination—aid in the diagnosis for suspected neoplasia or mycotic disease.

RETINAL HEMORRHAGE (CONTINUED)

- Blood pressure measurement—indicated in all patients with severe retinal and vitreal hemorrhage.

PATHOLOGIC FINDINGS

- Findings include preretinal, intraretinal, or subretinal hemorrhage that may be focal or extensive.
- Secondary morphologic changes include fibrotic areas with proliferation of cellular extensions into the subretinal space, intraretinal, and thickening of the external limiting membrane.

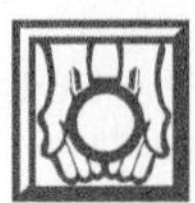

TREATMENT

APPROPRIATE HEALTH CARE

- Infections and intoxications—require specific treatment. Systemic hypertension should be treated in a timely fashion to improve chances of retinal reattachment.

NURSING CARE

Supportive care often needed.

ACTIVITY

Retinal detachment due to trauma—cage rest until the retina is reattached.

DIET

Possible dietary recommendations if the primary disorder is due to hepatic or renal disease.

CLIENT EDUCATION

- Discuss living with a blind dog or euthanasia of young puppies with severe bilateral hemorrhage due to congenital abnormalities.
- Advise client that unilaterally affected dogs can function as pets but should not be used for breeding.

SURGICAL CONSIDERATIONS

Surgery—referral to an ophthalmologist for vitrectomy and/or reattachment surgery.

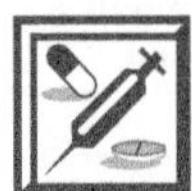

MEDICATIONS

DRUG(S) OF CHOICE

- Corticosteroids—if workup is declined and infectious disease is unlikely: prednis(ol)one 1–2 mg/kg/day PO for 7–14 days, then taper; long-term treatment of 4–6 weeks; especially for traumatic retinal detachment.
- Doxycycline 4 mg/kg PO q12h for 14–21 days, or other appropriate systemic antibiotic based on infectious disease testing.
- Primary systemic hypertension—amlodipine 0.1–0.25 mg/kg PO q24h (dog); 0.625–1.25 mg/cat PO q24 (cat); also consider angiotensin-converting enzyme inhibitor (see Hypertension, Systemic Arterial).
- Itraconazole, fluconazole—for cryptococcosis or other systemic mycosis (see Cryptococcosis or other specific mycoses).
- Besides corticosteroids, other immunosuppressive medications to treat immune-mediated disease include mycophenolate, azathioprine, or leflunomide.

CONTRAINDICATIONS

Systemic corticosteroids and other immunosuppressive drugs—use with caution in patients with systemic infection, do not coadminister with nonsteroidal anti-inflammatory drugs.

PRECAUTIONS

Azathioprine may result in myelosuppression, hepatotoxicity, and gastrointestinal upset.

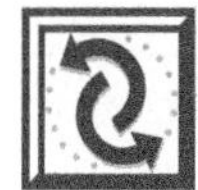

FOLLOW-UP

PATIENT MONITORING

- Repeated monitoring—required to ensure that condition subsides and retinal morphology normalizes.
- Preretinal hemorrhages—usually absorbed within a few weeks to several months if localized.
- Larger or repeated hemorrhages—may be followed by fibroplastic processes; may lead to the formation of fibrous preretinal membranes and vitreoretinal adhesions, which may cause vitreoretinal traction and retinal detachment.
- Intraretinal hemorrhage—reabsorbed within several weeks to months; may produce retinal scarring.

POSSIBLE COMPLICATIONS

- Retinal detachment.
- Blindness.
- Impaired vision.
- Chronic uveitis.
- Glaucoma.

EXPECTED COURSE AND PROGNOSIS

- Most retinal hemorrhagic lesions are small, observed during routine ophthalmoscopic examination, usually heal rapidly, and cause no visual problems.
- Retinal hemorrhage due to systemic diseases or retinal malformations is more serious; most have an uncertain prognosis.

MISCELLANEOUS

ASSOCIATED CONDITIONS

- Trauma—may have other injuries; traumatic brain injury.
- Hypertension—cardiac, renal disease, hyperthyroidism, or hyperadrenocorticism.
- Coagulopathy—hypovolemic shock, internal bleeding.
- Cryptococcus infection—concurrent leptomeningitis and pneumonitis.
- Neoplasia—various other organ system involvement.
- Hematologic disorders—hemorrhage and anemia.
- Secondary cataracts—may develop within weeks after the onset of diabetes mellitus in dogs.

AGE-RELATED FACTORS

- May occur at any age.
- Congenital or developmental diseases usually recognized in younger animals.

PREGNANCY/FERTILITY/BREEDING

- Dogs with hereditary retinal disease should not be bred.
- Corticosteroids and immunosuppressive drugs may cause complications with pregnancy.

SEE ALSO

- Chorioretinitis.
- Hypertension, Systemic Arterial.
- Hyphema.
- Retinal Detachment.

ABBREVIATIONS

- PHPV = persistent hyperplastic primary vitreous.
- PHTVL = persistent hyperplastic tunica vasculosa lentis.

Suggested Reading

Ofri, R. Diseases of the retina. In: Maggs DJ, Miller PE, Ofri R, eds., Slatter's Fundamentals of Veterinary Ophthalmology, 6th ed. St. Louis, MO; Elsevier, 2018, pp. 347–371.

Narfström K, Petersen-Jones S. Diseases of the canine ocular fundus. In: Gelatt KN, Gilger BC, Kern TJ, eds., Veterinary Ophthalmology, 5th ed. Ames, IA: John Wiley & Sons, 2013.

Author Kathern E. Myrna

Consulting Editor Kathern E. Myrna

Client Education Handout available online

RHINITIS AND SINUSITIS

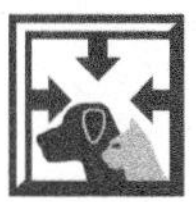

BASICS

DEFINITION

• Rhinitis—inflammation of nasal epithelium. • Sinusitis—inflammation of paranasal sinuses; includes frontal sinus and maxillary recess in dogs; frontal and sphenopalatine sinuses in cats. • The nasal cavity communicates directly with the sinuses; thus rhinitis and sinusitis often occur together.

PATHOPHYSIOLOGY

Inflammation and irritation stimulate serous glandular secretion in the nasal mucosa. Opportunistic bacterial infections develop in compromised nasal mucosa causing discharge to become mucoid or mucopurulent. The inflammatory process can lead to turbinate destruction and erosion of the vasculature that results in epistaxis.

SYSTEMS AFFECTED

• Respiratory—sneezing and nasal discharge usually indicate upper respiratory tract disease. • Nervous—fungal and neoplastic disease can destroy the cribriform plate and invade the brain. • Ocular—epiphora with inflammation or obstruction of the nasolacrimal ducts. Conjunctivitis, keratitis, and/or corneal ulcerations with feline herpesvirus type 1 (FHV-1)-related disease. Chorioretinitis with canine distemper or *Cryptococcus*. • Oral cavity—calicivirus, feline leukemia virus (FeLV), and feline immunodeficiency virus (FIV) are associated with stomatitis, glossitis, faucitis. Tooth root abscess, oronasal fistula or cleft palate possible. • Lymphatics—medial retropharyngeal lymphadenopathy possible with infectious and neoplastic sinonasal disease.

INCIDENCE/PREVALENCE

• Primary bacterial rhinosinusitis is rare; secondary infection from dental disease common or in association with chronic rhinitis. • Cats—chronic rhinosinusitis common. • Dogs—neoplasia, inflammatory rhinitis (lymphoplasmacytic rhinitis), fungal disease common. Nasal foreign body may cause acute sneezing.

GEOGRAPHICAL DISTRIBUTION

Chronic Fungal Rhinitis

• *Aspergillus* and *Penicillium* spp.—worldwide. • *Rhinosporidium seeberi*—mostly India, Africa, and South America. • *Blastomycoses dermatitidis*—endemic to North America: Pacific Northwest, Great Lakes region, Mississippi, Ohio, Missouri, Tennessee, and St. Lawrence river valleys. • *Cryptococcus neoformans*—worldwide.

SIGNALMENT

Species

Dog and cat.

Breed Predilections

• Brachycephalic cats more prone to chronic rhinitis and *Aspergillus* infection.
• Dolichocephalic dogs more prone to *Aspergillus* infection and nasal tumors.

Mean Age and Range

• Cats—acute viral rhinosinusitis and nasopharyngeal polyps more common in young kittens (6–12 weeks). • Congenital diseases (cleft palate, ciliary dyskinesia) more common in young animals. • Neoplasia and dental disease—older animals. • Foreign bodies more common in young dogs.

Predominant Sex

No sex predilection.

SIGNS

Historical Findings

• Sneezing, nasal discharge, epistaxis.
• Discharge usually is serous initially and becomes mucoid, mucopurulent, serosanguinous, or hemorrhagic. • Unilateral discharge suggests foreign body, tooth root abscess, early neoplasia, or early fungal infection. Idiopathic inflammatory rhinitis can also present with unilateral signs. • Bilateral discharge more common with viral or bacterial rhinosinusitis, inflammatory rhinitis, pharyngeal disease, or congenital abnormalities. Chronic presentation of neoplasia or fungal rhinitis is often bilateral. • Facial deformity or facial pain—usually with fungal or neoplastic disease. • Reverse sneezing more common in dogs, inappetence more common in cats.

Physical Examination Findings

• Check for decreased nasal air flow, bilateral or unilateral. • Evaluate oral cavity for tooth root abscess, oronasal fistula, cleft palate or ulcers. • Look for epiphora, conjunctivitis. Horner's syndrome can be seen with middle ear disease. • Fundic examination—chorioretinitis possible with infectious diseases; hypertension can result in tortuous retinal vessels or hemorrhage, platelet abnormalities can be associated with retinal hemorrhage or petechiation.

CAUSES

Dogs

Primary Inciting Causes

• Intranasal neoplasia—adenocarcinoma most common (31.5%); others include lymphoma, chondrosarcomas, or osteosarcomas. • Fungal disease—*Aspergillus fumigatus* most common. *Penicillium* spp., *Rhinosporidium seeberi, Blastomycoses dermatitidis, Cryptococcus neoformans* are rare causes. • Tooth root abscess. • Foreign body.
• Congenital abnormalities such as cleft palate or primary ciliary dyskinesia.
• Parasitic causes—nasal mites (*Pneumonyssoides caninum*), *Capillaria aerophila, Eucoleus boehmii.* • Immune-mediated rhinitis—allergic rhinitis rare, idiopathic lymphoplasmacytic rhinitis more common. • Other infectious diseases include canine distemper or *Bordetella bronchiseptica.*
• Local trauma can cause bone or turbinate deformity and predispose to chronic rhinitis or *Aspergillus* infection. • Nasopharyngeal stenosis can be congenital or acquired.

Secondary Causes

• Lower airway disease or vomiting can result in nasal signs through nasopharyngeal regurgitation. • Nasal discharge can occur with eosinophilic bronchopneumopathy.
• Epistaxis can be related to hypertension, thrombocytopenia, thrombocytopathia, or rarely other coagulopathies; trauma or foreign body also possible.

Cats

Primary Inciting Causes

• Viral infections—FHV-1 and calicivirus account for 90% of acute infections in kittens.
• Bacteria—*Bordetella bronchiseptica* is uncommonly a primary pathogen.
• Neoplasia—adenocarcinoma and lymphoma most common. • Fungal disease—*Cryptococcus neoformans* most common, *Aspergillus felis, Penicillium, Microsporum canis* (rare).
• Nasopharyngeal polyps in young cats.
• Nasopharyngeal stenosis—congenital or secondary to chronic infection or inflammation.
• Tooth root abscess or oronasal fistula.
• Foreign bodies. • Congenital abnormalities include cleft palate.

Secondary Causes

• Opportunistic infection with bacteria can complicate viral rhinosinusitis. • Epistaxis due to coagulopathy or hypertension. • Aspiration of vomitus into the nasopharynx.

RISK FACTORS

• Dolichocephalic breeds—fungal disease.
• Brachycephalic cats—rhinosinusitis.

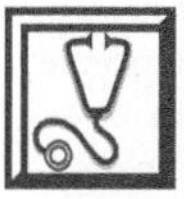

DIAGNOSIS

DIFFERENTIAL DIAGNOSIS

Rule out secondary causes of rhinitis including coagulopathy and hypertension for epistaxis, lower airway disease, chronic vomition.

CBC/BIOCHEMISTRY/URINALYSIS

• Hemogram is nonspecific—may show leukocytosis (neutrophilia or eosinophilia) with infectious agents. Regenerative anemia with severe blood loss from coagulopathy. Nonregenerative anemia with chronic disease or neoplasia. Thrombocytopenia seen with coagulopathies or severe blood loss.
• Serum biochemistry and urinalysis typically normal.

OTHER LABORATORY TESTS

• PCR testing for viral etiologies. • FeLV and FIV serologic tests. • Oropharyngeal, conjunctival, and nasal swabbing in cats for

virus isolation and bacterial culture. • Latex agglutination test for cryptococcal capsular antigen. • *Aspergillus* titers—agar gel immunodiffusion (AGID) in dogs: false negatives possible, false positives uncommon; ideally combine AGID with nasal tissue culture/biopsy or direct visualization. ELISA in cats—high sensitivity and specificity for disease.
• Coagulation profile if epistaxis present.

IMAGING

• Radiography—chest radiographs if lower airway disease or neoplasia suspected.
• Dental radiographs highly sensitive for detecting periodontal disease. • Skull radiographs—loss of turbinate structures can be seen with all causes of rhinosinusitis. Open-mouth or intraoral ventrodorsal views avoid superimposition of the mandible.
• Nasopharyngeal polyps occasionally seen within the nasopharynx. • CT/MRI—superior to plain radiography in evaluating the extent of disease and assessing the integrity of the cribriform plate. Also useful in evaluating disease of the palate, nasopharyngeal meatus, maxillary sinus, periorbital tissues, middle ear canal, and for presence of medial retropharyngeal lymphadenopathy.

R

DIAGNOSTIC PROCEDURES

Arterial Blood Pressure

Evaluate for hypertension if epistaxis.

Lymph Node Aspirate

Can be diagnostic for neoplasia or *Cryptococcus*.

Cytology

Nasal swab may reveal *Cryptococcus*.

Culture

• Usefulness of bacterial culture is controversial since most animals have secondary bacterial infection. Potential bacterial pathogens are more commonly isolated in cats. • Fungal culture of a plaque lesion visualized on endoscopy aids in diagnosis of aspergillosis. • Asymptomatic intranasal carriage of *Cryptococcus* possible.

Endoscopy

• An otoscope evaluates only the rostral nasal cavity. A rigid endoscope can be guided to the ethmoid turbinates, flexible endoscope provides good visualization rostrally, and can be retroflexed in the nasopharynx to visualize the caudal choanae. • Guided biopsy is possible with rigid and flexible endoscopy. Other techniques include core or blind pinch biopsies.

Surgery

Exploratory rhinotomy most invasive diagnostic tool, can be required for difficult foreign body or mass removal, if endoscopy is unsuccessful. Rarely required to obtain a definitive biopsy sample.

PATHOLOGIC FINDINGS

Chronic inflammation causes turbinate resorption, mucosal ulceration and necrosis. Lymphoplasmacytic infiltrate indicates chronicity, neutrophilic usually signifies acute component. Neoplasia and fungus also cause bony lysis or destruction.

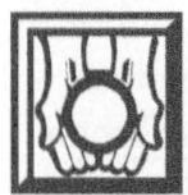

TREATMENT

APPROPRIATE HEALTH CARE

Overcrowded shelters and hoarding conditions increase stress and exposure to infectious pathogens.

NURSING CARE

Humidification can aid in moistening and mobilizing nasal secretions. Saline intranasal drops helpful if tolerated. Keep nares clean of obstructive mucus.

DIET

Malnutrition is common in young kittens with infectious causes of rhinitis. Appetite stimulants may be helpful.

CLIENT EDUCATION

Signs of chronic rhinitis can be variably controlled but are rarely eliminated.

SURGICAL CONSIDERATIONS

• Rhinotomy is reserved for obtaining a biopsy or foreign body/mass removal when endoscopic intervention is unsuccessful. Rarely provides an advantage over endoscopy.
• Surgery useful for polyp removal, dental-related nasal disease (tooth root abscess, oronasal fistula, cleft palate).

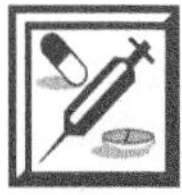

MEDICATIONS

DRUG(S) OF CHOICE

Antibiotics

Antibiotics help control secondary bacterial rhinitis. Selection of antibiotic is mainly empirical. Long-term use often needed.

Antifungals

See Cryptococcosis and Aspergillosis chapters for detailed treatment discussion.

L-Lysine

Inhibits FHV-1 replication; may be useful—250 (kitten)–500 (cat) mg PO q12h.

Anti-inflammatory Agents

Piroxicam (NSAID) or more commonly meloxicam used for palliation of nasal tumors (via COX-2 inhibition), either as sole agent or in conjunction with chemotherapy.

Steroids

Consider use with chronic rhinosinusitis in cats or lymphoplasmacytic rhinitis in dogs at anti-inflammatory doses when mucus obstruction limits appetite.

Antihistamines

Efficacy is debated; unlikely helpful.

Antiparasitics

Ivermectin 300 µg/kg PO or SC once weekly for 3–4 treatments or milbemycin oxime 1 mg/kg PO once weekly for 3 weeks for treatment of nasal mites.

CONTRAINDICATIONS

Avoid chronic steroid use.

PRECAUTIONS

• NSAIDs can cause gastrointestinal ulceration. • Tetracycline may stain teeth of young animals.

POSSIBLE INTERACTIONS

Use of NSAIDs and corticosteroids together is contraindicated.

ALTERNATIVE DRUG(S)

N/A

FOLLOW-UP

PATIENT MONITORING

Patients taking oral azole antifungal medication typically require monthly biochemistry monitoring of hepatic values.

PREVENTION/AVOIDANCE

Vaccinations in kittens can lessen severity and duration of viral infection.

POSSIBLE COMPLICATIONS

• Extension of fungal or neoplastic invasion into brain. • Seizures and other neurologic signs are possible if topical antifungal therapy is used when the cribriform plate is not intact.

EXPECTED COURSE AND PROGNOSIS

• Dependent on etiology and extent of disease. • Acute viral/bacterial rhinitis—good prognosis; chronic rhinitis—guarded for control of signs. • Fungal—fair to guarded prognosis depending on invasiveness and response to therapy.
• Neoplastic—3–5 months prognosis with no treatment; 9–23 months with radiation therapy.

MISCELLANEOUS

AGE-RELATED FACTORS

Infectious upper respiratory tract disease is a common cause of morbidity and mortality in stray and shelter kittens.

ZOONOTIC POTENTIAL

Cryptococcus, *Aspergillus*, *Penicillium* are transmissible to humans via shared environment. No direct transmission.

SYNONYMS

Nasosinusitis, rhinosinusitis, sinonasal.

SEE ALSO

- Aspergillosis, Disseminated Invasive
- Aspergillosis, Nasal.
- Cryptococcosis.
- Epistaxis.
- Nasal and Nasopharyngeal Polyps.
- Nasal Discharge.
- Respiratory Parasites.
- Stertor and Stridor.

ABBREVIATIONS

- AGID = agar gel immunodiffusion.
- FeLV = feline leukemia virus.
- FHV = feline herpesvirus. • FIV = feline immunodeficiency virus.

Suggested Reading

Belda B, Petrovitch N, Mathews KG. Sinonasal aspergillosis: outcome after topical treatment in dogs with cribriform plate lysis. J Vet Intern Med 2018, 32(4):1353–1358.

Reed N. Chronic rhinitis in the cat. Vet Clin North Am Small Anim Pract 2014, 44(1):33–50.

Author Adrienne M. Barchard Couts

Consulting Editor Elizabeth Rozanski

Acknowledgment The author and editors acknowledge the prior contribution of Carrie J. Miller and Lynelle R. Johnson.

Client Education Handout available online

RIGHT BUNDLE BRANCH BLOCK

BASICS

DEFINITION

Conduction delay or block in the right bundle branch resulting in late activation of the right ventricle; the block can be complete or incomplete.

ECG Features

• A right axis deviation and wide QRS (≥0.08 seconds in dogs; ≥0.06 seconds in cats) in most patients.
• Large, wide S waves in leads I, II, III, and aVF.
• Incomplete right bundle branch block has right axis deviation with normal width QRS complexes.

PATHOPHYSIOLOGY

• The right bundle branch is anatomically vulnerable to injury because it is a thin strand of tissue and has a long undivided course.
• No hemodynamic compromise.

SYSTEMS AFFECTED

Cardiovascular

GENETICS

R

N/A

INCIDENCE/PREVALENCE

• Dog—most frequent form of intraventricular conduction defect.
• Cat—not as frequent as left anterior fascicular block.

GEOGRAPHIC DISTRIBUTION

N/A

SIGNALMENT

Species

Dog and cat.

Breed Predilections

In beagles, incomplete right bundle branch block can result from a genetically determined localized variation in right ventricular wall thickness.

Predominant Sex

N/A

SIGNS

Historical Findings

• Usually an incidental ECG finding—does not cause hemodynamic abnormalities.
• Observed signs, if any, are usually associated with the underlying condition.

Physical Examination Findings

• Splitting of heart sounds because of asynchronous activation of ventricles in some patients.
• Does not cause signs of hemodynamic compromise.

CAUSES

• Occasionally seen in normal and healthy dogs and cats.
• Congenital heart disease.
• Chronic valvular fibrosis.
• After surgical correction of a cardiac defect.
• Trauma.
• Chronic infection with *Trypanosoma cruzi* (Chagas' disease).
• Neoplasia.
• Heartworm disease.
• Acute thromboembolism.
• Cardiomyopathy.
• Hyperkalemia (most commonly in cats with urethral obstruction).

RISK FACTORS

N/A

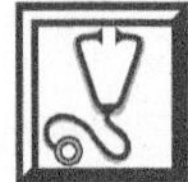

DIAGNOSIS

DIFFERENTIAL DIAGNOSIS

• Right ventricular enlargement—absence of right ventricular enlargement on thoracic radiographs or echocardiogram supports a diagnosis of right bundle branch block.
• Can also be confused with ventricular ectopic beats (especially if the block is intermittent), but consistent PR intervals and no pulse deficits with right bundle branch block.

CBC/BIOCHEMISTRY/URINALYSIS

• No specific changes.
• Serum potassium may be extremely high in cats with urethral obstruction.

OTHER LABORATORY TESTS

• Occult heartworm test may be positive in dogs or cats.
• Chagas' indirect fluorescent antibody test, direct hemagglutination, and complement fixation test may be positive in dogs.

IMAGING

• Echocardiogram may show structural heart disease; absence of right heart enlargement supports diagnosis of right bundle branch block.
• Thoracic and abdominal radiographs may show masses or pulmonary metastatic lesions; traumatic injuries could cause localized or diffuse pulmonary densities.

DIAGNOSTIC PROCEDURES

• Electrocardiography (ECG).
• Echocardiography.

PATHOLOGIC FINDINGS

Possible lesions or scarring on endocardial surface in the path of the right bundle branch; applying Lugol's iodine to the endocardial surface within 2 hours post-mortem gives clear visualization of the conduction system.

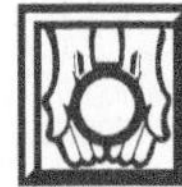

TREATMENT

APPROPRIATE HEALTH CARE

Direct treatment toward the underlying cause.

NURSING CARE

N/A

ACTIVITY

Unrestricted

DIET

No modifications unless required to manage underlying condition.

CLIENT EDUCATION

• Does not cause hemodynamic abnormalities itself.
• The lesion causing the block could progress, leading to more serious arrhythmias or complete heart block.

SURGICAL CONSIDERATIONS

N/A

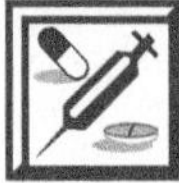

MEDICATIONS

DRUG(S) OF CHOICE

None required unless needed to manage underlying condition.

CONTRAINDICATIONS

N/A

PRECAUTIONS

N/A

POSSIBLE INTERACTIONS

N/A

ALTERNATIVE DRUG(S)

N/A

FOLLOW-UP

PATIENT MONITORING

Serial ECG may show resolution of the lesion or progression to complete heart block.

PREVENTION/AVOIDANCE

N/A

POSSIBLE COMPLICATIONS

• The causative lesion could progress, leading to a more serious arrhythmia or complete heart block.
• First- or second-degree AV block may indicate involvement of the left bundle branch.

EXPECTED COURSE AND PROGNOSIS

No hemodynamic compromise.

MISCELLANEOUS

ASSOCIATED CONDITIONS

N/A

AGE-RELATED FACTORS

N/A

ZOONOTIC POTENTIAL

N/A

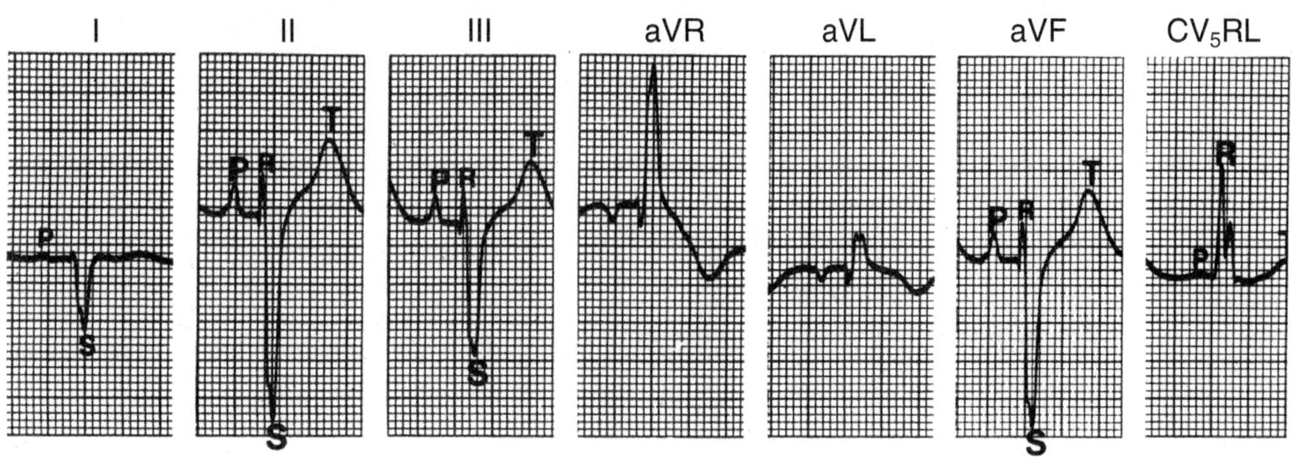

Figure 1.

Right bundle branch block in a dog. The electrocardiographic features include QRS duration of 0.08 seconds; positive QRS complex in aVR, aVL, and CV_5RL (M-shaped); and large wide S waves in leads I, II, III, and aVF. There is a right axis deviation (approximately −110°) (50 mm/s, 1 cm = 1 mV). (Source: From Tilley LP. Essentials of Canine and Feline Electrocardiography, 3rd ed. Baltimore: Williams & Wilkins, 1992. Reprinted with permission of Wolters Kluwer.)

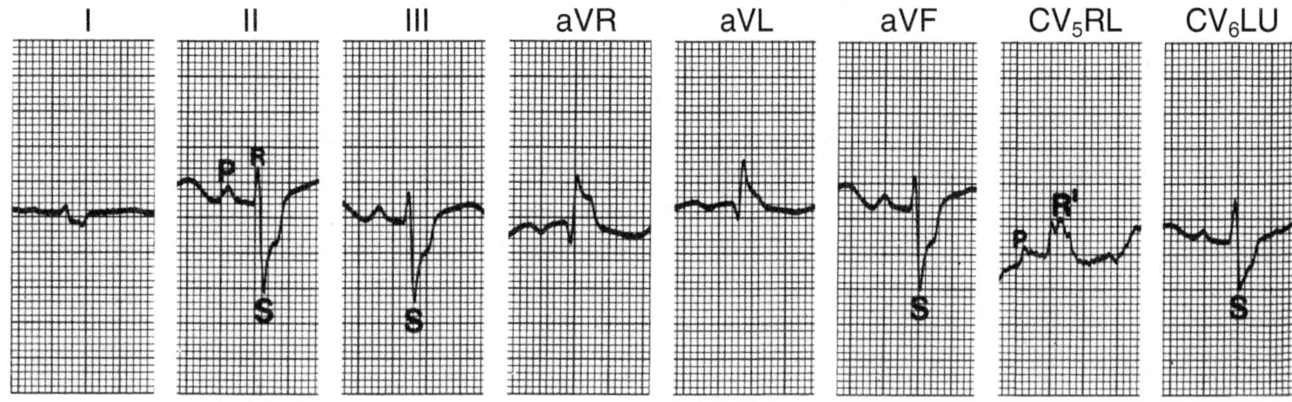

Figure 2.

Right bundle branch block in a cat with the dilated form of cardiomyopathy. The QRS duration is 0.08 seconds (4 boxes). Large and wide S waves are present in leads I, II, III, aVF, and CV_6 LU. The QRS in CV_5RL has a wide R wave (M-shaped). There is a marked axis deviation (approximately -90°). Source: From Tilley LP. Essentials of Canine and Feline Electrocardiography, 3rd ed. Baltimore: Williams & Wilkins, 1992. Reprinted with permission of Wolters Kluwer.

PREGNANCY/FERTILITY/BREEDING

N/A

SEE ALSO

- Atrioventricular Block, Complete (Third Degree).
- Atrioventricular Block, First Degree.
- Atrioventricular Block, Second Degree—Mobitz Type I.
- Atrioventricular Block, Second Degree—Mobitz Type II.
- Left Anterior Fascicular Block.
- Left Bundle Branch Block.

ABBREVIATIONS

- AV = atrioventricular.
- ECG = electrocardiogram.

Suggested Reading

Santilli R, Moise NS, Pariaut R, Perego M. Electrocardiography of the Dog and Cat: Diagnosis of Arrhythmias, 2nd ed. Milan, Italy: Edra S.P.A., 2018.

Tilley LP. Essentials of Canine and Feline Electrocardiography, Interpretation and Treatment, 3rd ed. Baltimore, MD: Williams and Wilkins, 1992.

Tilley LP, Smith FWK, Jr. Electrocardiography. In: Smith FWK, Tilley LP, Oyama M, Sleeper M, eds., Manual of Canine and Feline Cardiology, 5th ed. St. Louis, MO: Saunders Elsevier, 2016, pp. 49–76.

Willis R, Oliveira P, Mavropoulou A. Guide to Canine and Feline Electrocardiography. Ames, IA: Wiley Blackwell, 2018.

Author Larry P. Tilley

Consulting Editor Michael Aherne

R

ROCKY MOUNTAIN SPOTTED FEVER

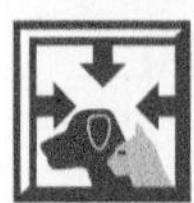

BASICS

DEFINITION

A tick-borne disease, caused by *Rickettsia rickettsii*, that affects dogs and is considered the most important rickettsial disease in humans.

PATHOPHYSIOLOGY

• Pathogen—*Rickettsia rickettsia*, a Gram-negative, intracellular bacteria. • Vector—various species of ticks including *Dermacentor variabilis* (United States, east of Great Plains region), *D. andersoni* (western United States and Canada), *Rhipicephalus sanguineus* (throughout North and South America), *Amblyomma cajennense* (Latin America).
• Transmission—via saliva of the vector or by blood transfusion; tick must be attached for 5–20 hours to infect host (humans, dogs, cats) or reservoir host (rodents and dogs).
• Incubation period—2 days–2 weeks.
• Infection—organism invades and multiplies in vascular endothelium; causes microvascular hemorrhage; platelet aggregation and antiplatelet antibodies cause thrombocytopenia, widespread vasculitis results in increased vascular permeability, plasma loss into interstitial space, hypotension, and eventually shock and disseminated intravascular coagulation (DIC).

R

SYSTEMS AFFECTED

• Cardiovascular—vasculitis, hypotension, shock. • Hemic/lymphatic/immune—hemorrhage due to thrombocytopenia and vasculitis; lymphadenopathy, splenomegaly.
• Ophthalmic—conjunctivitis, scleral injection, retinal hemorrhage, anterior uveitis.
• Skin/exocrine—multifocal edema, petechiae and ecchymoses, dermal necrosis.
• Musculoskeletal—joint and muscle pain.
• Nervous—meningoencephalitis: seizures, vestibular deficits, stupor, coma, cervical pain.
• Respiratory—dyspnea, cough. • Renal/urologic— vasculitis and prerenal azotemia from dehydration and shock.

GENETICS

N/A

INCIDENCE/PREVALENCE

• Tick season—late March through October.
• Prevalence—overall infections in ticks <2%; varies by geographic location.

GEOGRAPHIC DISTRIBUTION

• United States— RMSF has been diagnosed in most states; highest infection rates in southeastern states. • North and South America.

SIGNALMENT

Species

Dog

Breed Predilections

• Purebred dogs seem more prone to developing clinical illness than mixed-breed dogs. • German shepherd dogs—more common.

Mean Age and Range

Any age

Predominant Sex

None

SIGNS

Historical Findings

• Fever—within 2–3 days of tick attachment.
• Lethargy, depression, anorexia. • Swelling (edema)—lips, scrotum, prepuce, ears, extremities. • Stiff gait—especially with scrotal or preputial edema. • Spontaneous bleeding—sneezing, epistaxis. • Respiratory distress, cough. • Neurologic—ataxia, head tilt, seizures. • Ocular pain.

Physical Examination Findings

• Clinical—variable in severity; lasts 2–4 weeks untreated. • Ticks may still be present in acute cases. • Pyrexia. • Cutaneous lesions—edema of face, limbs, prepuce, scrotum. • Extremities—necrosis.
• Conjunctivitis. • Scleral injection.
• Respiratory—dyspnea, exercise intolerance resulting from pneumonitis, increased bronchovesicular sounds. • Generalized lymphadenopathy. • Neurologic—vestibular dysfunction, altered mental status, seizures.
• Myalgia/arthralgia. • Petechia, ecchymoses—ocular, oral, genital mucous membranes.
• Hemorrhagic diathesis—epistaxis, melena, hematuria; in severe cases. • Cardiac arrhythmias. • DIC and death from shock—in severe acute cases.

CAUSES

R. rickettsii infection.

RISK FACTORS

• Exposure to ticks. • Coinfection with other pathogens (tick-borne). • English springer spaniels with phosphofructokinase deficiency are prone to a more severe form of RMSF.

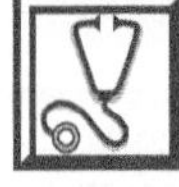

DIAGNOSIS

DIFFERENTIAL DIAGNOSIS

• Canine ehrlichiosis—*Ehrlichia canis*; not seasonal; can be clinically indistinguishable from RMSF (especially acute cases); differentiate with serologic testing; both respond to same treatment. • Primary immune-mediated thrombocytopenia—not usually associated with fever or lymphadenopathy; differentiate by ruling out infectious causes; may treat for both until results are known. • Systemic lupus erythematosus—antinuclear antibody titer usually negative with RMSF; serologic testing diagnostic.
• Brucellosis—scrotal edema; serologic testing diagnostic.

CBC/BIOCHEMISTRY/URINALYSIS

CBC

• Thrombocytopenia (~ 40% of cases)—due to antiplatelet antibody and consumption; platelet counts frequently 25,000–250,000/μL.
• Mild anemia (normochromic, normocytic).
• Mild leukopenia (early in infection), leukocytosis and monocytosis develop later.

Biochemistry

• Usually nonspecific. • Hypoalbuminemia—increased vascular permeability
• Hypercholesterolemia—consistently found; cause unknown • Mild increases in alanine aminotransferase, alkaline phosphatase, BUN, creatinine, and total bilirubin (rare). • Hyponatremia, hypochloremia, and metabolic acidosis have also been reported.

Urinalysis

• Proteinuria—with or without azotemia; from glomerular/tubular damage.
• Hematuria—coagulation defects.

OTHER LABORATORY TESTS

• Several tests are available to measure serum antibodies including the micro-immunofluorescence (micro-IF), ELISA, and latex agglutination tests. • Diagnosis by antibody measurement requires an increased (single) IgM titer, or a four-fold increase in IgG between acute and convalescent measurements. Paired IgG titers should be drawn 3 weeks apart and submitted for analysis at the same time. High antibody titers can be detected for up to 1 year after treatment. • Latex agglutination test—higher specificity, lower sensitivity than the micro-IF test. • PCR on whole blood and tissue specimens—detects DNA before seroconversion in some dogs.

IMAGING

Thoracic radiographs—diffuse interstitial pattern in patients with respiratory signs.

DIAGNOSTIC PROCEDURES

• Direct immunofluorescence—punch biopsies from affected lesions; allows early detection of rickettsial antigens. • CSF analysis—often normal; may show increased protein and polymorphonuclear and mononuclear cells.

PATHOLOGIC FINDINGS

• Widespread petechia, splenomegaly, and generalized hemorrhagic lymphadenopathy.
• Necrotizing vasculitis with perivascular cell infiltration (mononuclear and neutrophilic).
• Vascular lesions—most prominent in skin, kidneys, myocardium, meninges, retina, pancreas, gastrointestinal tract, and urinary bladder. • Hepatic and focal myocardial necrosis, nodular gliosis in brain, and

interstitial pneumonia. • Special stains—to identify organisms.

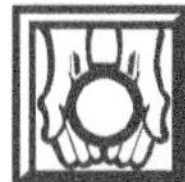

TREATMENT

APPROPRIATE HEALTH CARE

Inpatient management recommended until stable and showing response to treatment.

NURSING CARE

• IV fluid therapy—correct dehydration; use caution; excessive fluid therapy can worsen edema. • Blood transfusion—for patients with clinical signs of anemia. • Fresh whole blood or platelet transfusion—severe hemorrhage due to thrombocytopenia.
• Provide analgesia for patients with muscle, joint, and severe skin involvement.

ACTIVITY

Restricted during acute illness.

DIET

N/A

CLIENT EDUCATION

• Prognosis—good in acute cases with appropriate and prompt therapy. • Response occurs within hours of treatment. • If treatment is not instituted until CNS signs occur or later in disease process, mortality is high; a patient with CNS signs may die within hours.

SURGICAL CONSIDERATIONS

If surgery is required for other reasons, blood transfusion may be needed to correct anemia and/or marked thrombocytopenia.

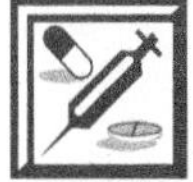

MEDICATIONS

DRUG(S) OF CHOICE

• Doxycycline 10 mg/kg PO, IV q24h (or 5 mg/kg PO, IV q12h) for 10 days; given IV if patient is vomiting. Extended doxycycline therapy was required to clear infection in one experimentally infected dog. • Enrofloxacin and chloramphenicol may also be used.
• Prednisone—concurrent use; anti-inflammatory or immunosuppressive dose; given early in course of disease does not seem to be detrimental to recovery. May alleviate immune-mediated thrombocytopenia and cerebral edema.

CONTRAINDICATIONS

Renal insufficiency—do not use tetracycline due to renal excretion; doxycycline may be given (excreted via gastrointestinal tract).

PRECAUTIONS

• Tetracycline (or derivatives)—discoloration of teeth in patients <6 months old. • Enrofloxacin—articular cartilage damage can occur in young dogs.
• Chloramphenicol— reduces titers to a greater extent than tetracyclines; warn client of human health risks; avoid use in dogs with thrombocytopenia, pancytopenia, or anemia.

POSSIBLE INTERACTIONS

None

ALTERNATIVE DRUG(S)

• Chloramphenicol—puppies <6 months of age; 20 mg/kg PO q8h for 14 days; recommended to avoid discoloration of erupting teeth or in pregnant patients.
• Enrofloxacin 10 mg/kg PO, IM, IV q24h for 7 days. • Oxytetracycline and tetracycline 22 mg/kg PO q8h for 14 days.

FOLLOW-UP

PATIENT MONITORING

Monitor platelet count every 2–3 days until normal.

PREVENTION/AVOIDANCE

• Avoid tick-infested areas and control tick infestation on dogs. • Flea and tick collars, topical or enteral tick preventives—may reduce reinfestation. • Environment—tick eradication impossible; organism maintained in rodents and other reservoir hosts.
• Manually remove ticks—use gloves (see Zoonotic Potential); ensure mouth parts are removed.

POSSIBLE COMPLICATIONS

N/A

EXPECTED COURSE AND PROGNOSIS

• Early antibiotic treatment—reduces fever and albumin extravasation; improvement within 24–48 hours. • Platelet counts—should return to normal within 2–4 days after initiating treatment. • Serologic titers remain positive during convalescence. • Naturally infected dogs do not seem to become reinfected. • Acute cases—excellent prognosis with appropriate and early treatment. • With CNS disease—poor prognosis.

MISCELLANEOUS

ASSOCIATED CONDITIONS

None

AGE-RELATED FACTORS

None

ZOONOTIC POTENTIAL

• Source of infection (humans)—ticks from wooded areas or carried into environment by dogs (RMSF not directly transmitted to humans by dogs), exposure to infectious material when removing infected ticks from dogs. • Clinical signs in humans are similar to those seen in dogs. • Treatment with tetracycline results in a rapid recovery, overall mortality rate is 2–10%.

PREGNANCY/FERTILITY/BREEDING

N/A

ABBREVIATIONS

• DIC = disseminated intravascular coagulation.
• Micro-IF = microscopic immunofluorescence.
• RMSF = Rocky Mountain spotted fever.

R

Suggested Reading

Allison RW, Little SE. Diagnosis of rickettsial diseases in dogs and cats. Vet Clin Pathol 2013, 42:127–144.
Greene CE, Kidd L, Breitschwerdt EB. Rocky Mountain spotted fever. In: Greene CE, ed., Infectious Diseases of the Dog and Cat, 4th ed. St. Louis, MO: Saunders Elsevier, 2012, pp. 259–267.
Levin ML, Killmaster LF, Zemtsova GE, et al. Clinical presentation, convalescence, and relapse of Rocky Mountain spotted fever in dogs experimentally infected via tick bite. PLoS ONE 2014, 9: e115105.
Warner RD, Marsh WW. Rocky Mountain spotted fever. J Am Vet Med Assoc 2002, 221:1413–1417.

Author Julie M. Walker
Consulting Editor Amie Koenig
Acknowledgment The author and editors acknowledge the prior contribution of Stephen C. Barr.

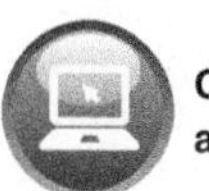

Client Education Handout available online

RODENTICIDE TOXICOSIS—ANTICOAGULANTS

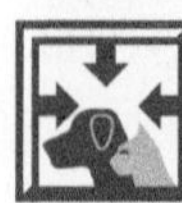

BASICS

DEFINITION

- Anticoagulant rodenticide intoxication results in a delayed-onset (3–5 days) coagulopathy caused by the reduction of vitamin K1-dependent clotting factors (II, VII, IX, X).
- There are two primary types of anticoagulant rodenticides: first- and second-generation. First-generation anticoagulants, such as warfarin, are generally less toxic and shorter acting than second-generation which tend to persist longer in the liver and require 3–4 weeks of antidote therapy.

PATHOPHYSIOLOGY

- Anticoagulant rodenticides inhibit vitamin K1 epoxide reductase, DT-diaphorase, and possibly other enzymes involved in the reduction of vitamin K1 epoxide to vitamin K1.
- Vitamin K1 is required for carboxylation of clotting factors II, VI, IX, and X; uncarboxylated clotting factors do not bind calcium sufficiently to participate in clot formation.

R

SYSTEMS AFFECTED

- Hemic/lymphatic/immune.
- Respiratory.

INCIDENCE/PREVALENCE

- Still common but fewer exposures.
- In 2011, the US Environmental Protection Agency (EPA) banned the use of second-generation anticoagulants (i.e., brodifacoum, bromadiolone, difenacoum, and difethialone) for residential use unless placed by a pest control operator.
- In 2013, the EPA gave notice of cancelling registration and denial of future applications for certain rodenticide products including warfarin, brodifacoum, and difethialone. In response, manufacturers have begun the process of transition to non-anticoagulant baits such as bromethalin and cholecalciferol.

SIGNALMENT

No breed or gender predilections; younger animals may ingest bait more readily.

SIGNS

General Comments

- May be slightly more prevalent in the spring and fall when rodenticide products are used.
- Clinical signs typically begin 3–5 days after ingestion. Early signs maybe noted at 48 hours.

Historical Findings

- Use of anticoagulant rodenticides.
- Evidence of rodenticide dye in vomitus or feces.
- Coughing, dyspnea, tachypnea, or exercise intolerance are often the first clinical signs.
- Bleeding from body orifices; subcutaneous or joint swelling, petechiation of the skin and gums may also be observed.

Physical Examination Findings

- Evidence of hemorrhagic shock (i.e., tachycardia, hypovolemia, hypotension, poor pulse quality, pallor).
- Coughing, dyspnea, tachypnea, pale mucous membranes.
- Hematomas—often ventral and at venipuncture sites; subcutaneous hematomas.
- Bleeding from body orifices, periorbital bleeding, scleral hemorrhage.
- Hemarthrosis, lameness.
- Exercise intolerance, lethargy, depression.
- Muffled heart or lung sounds.
- Distended abdomen (hemoabdomen).

CAUSES

Ingestion of anticoagulant rodenticides or, rarely, ingestion of prey that have been exposed to anticoagulant rodenticides (see Risk Factors).

RISK FACTORS

- Dogs are much more sensitive to anticoagulant rodenticides than cats.
- Small doses over several days may add up to a toxic dose.
- Secondary or relay toxicosis by consumption of poisoned rodents is possible but unlikely.
- There is a wide range of toxicity between anticoagulant rodenticides. In general, if the ingestion exceeds 1/5–1/10 the LD_{50}, decontamination and monitoring for coagulopathy are indicated.
- Dogs:
  - Brodifacoum, LD_{50} 0.25–2.5 mg/kg.
  - Bromadiolone, LD_{50} 11–20 mg/kg.
  - Chlorophacinone, LD_{50} 50–100 mg/kg.
  - Difethialone, LD_{50} 4 mg/kg.
  - Diphacinone, LD_{50} 3–7.5 mg/kg.
  - Warfarin, LD_{50} 20–50 mg/kg.
- Cats:
  - Brodifacoum, LD_{50} 25 mg/kg.
  - Bromadiolone, LD_{50} >25 mg/kg.
  - Difethiolone, LD_{50} >16 mg/kg.

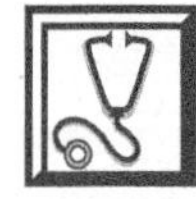

DIAGNOSIS

DIFFERENTIAL DIAGNOSIS

- Congenital clotting factor deficiencies.
- Immune-mediated thrombocytopenia—platelet count will reveal severe thrombocytopenia.
- Coagulation factor deficiency secondary to hepatic disease—assay for factor deficiencies (e.g., factor VII), liver function, bile acids.
- Disseminated intravascular coagulopathy which is typically associated with neoplasia, sepsis, pancreatitis, or concurrent disease. Lab evidence includes prolonged prothrombin time (PT), partial thromboplastin time (PTT), elevated fibrin degradation products, D-dimer with thrombocytopenia.
- Fat malabsorption.
- Hemorrhagic shock from trauma, neoplasia, bone marrow suppression, immune-mediated hemolytic anemia.

CBC/BIOCHEMISTRY/URINALYSIS

- Anemia with marked hemorrhage, often acute and nonregenerative.
- Thrombocytopenia, mild. Typically 50,000–150,000 × 10^3/μL.

OTHER LABORATORY TESTS

- Activated clotting time >150 seconds supports coagulopathy but is not specific for anticoagulant rodenticide poisoning.
- Prolonged PT and PTT support exposure to anticoagulant rodenticide; PT will be prolonged 6–18 hours earlier than PTT. These values will normalize with vitamin K1 therapy.
- Protein-induced vitamin K absence or antagonist (PIVKA) assay, rarely used.
- Anticoagulant rodenticide detection in the blood or liver will confirm exposure to a specific product.
- Anticoagulant rodenticide detection in the stomach or intestinal contents is not reliable due to the delay between consumption of bait and appearance of clinical signs.

IMAGING

- Thoracic radiography may reveal pleural effusion (i.e., hemothorax); multilobular, alveolar infiltration (i.e., pulmonary hemorrhage) or an enlarged cardiac silhouette (i.e., hemopericardium).
- Ultrasound of both the pleural and peritoneal cavities may reveal effusion consistent with hemorrhage.

DIAGNOSTIC PROCEDURES

Thoracentesis may confirm hemothorax.

PATHOLOGIC FINDINGS

- Free blood in the thoracic cavity, lungs, and abdominal cavity is a common post-mortem finding.
- Hemorrhage into the cranial vault, gastrointestinal tract, subcutaneous space, intramuscular space, and urinary tract is less common.

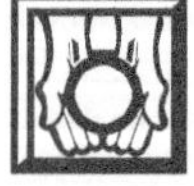

TREATMENT

APPROPRIATE HEALTH CARE

- Patients in acute crisis should be hospitalized.
- Patients without active hemorrhaging or a stabilized coagulopathy may be treated on an outpatient basis.
- Vitamin K1 is antidotal at 2.5–5 mg/kg q24h or divided q12h. The preferred route of administration is oral; however, in case of a coagulopathic patient, the subcutaneous route

is preferred due to the potential for limited gastrointestinal absorption. Use a small needle in multiple locations, if needed, and monitor for anaphylactoid reaction.

- Treat acute hemorrhagic shock with IV crystalloids, colloids, or blood products as needed. Initial crystalloid boluses of 10–20 mL/kg can be given over 15–20 minutes during stabilization. Repeat 2–3 times as needed to increase blood pressure.
- Packed RBCs, whole blood, fresh frozen plasma, or frozen plasma may be necessary to replace coagulation factors.
- Treat life-threatening cardiac tamponade or hemothorax with pericardiocentesis or thoracocentesis as indicated. If the patient is stable and responding to treatment, these procedures should be avoided. With time, the blood will reabsorb.

NURSING CARE

Provide supportive care as needed.

ACTIVITY

Confine the patient until the coagulopathy is stabilized as activity enhances blood loss.

DIET

Feed a nutritious, high-quality protein diet to support coagulation factor synthesis.

CLIENT EDUCATION

- Warn client that reexposure, even months to years later, could be a serious problem due to persistence of second-generation anticoagulants in the liver.
- Encourage the owner to pick up all loose/unprotected bait on the property.
- Do not discontinue vitamin K1 therapy early, even if the patient is asymptomatic.

SURGICAL CONSIDERATIONS

- Thoracentesis may be important for removing free thoracic blood, which causes dyspnea and respiratory failure (see Appropriate Health Care).
- The coagulopathy must be corrected before surgery.

MEDICATIONS

DRUG(S) OF CHOICE

Vitamin K1, 2.5–5.0 mg/kg PO q12h for 5–7 days for most first-generation anticoagulants and PO q24h for 4–6 weeks for most second-generation anticoagulants; bioavailability may be enhanced by the concurrent feeding of a small amount of fat, such as canned dog food.

CONTRAINDICATIONS

- Vitamin K3 is not efficacious in the treatment of anticoagulant rodenticide toxicosis and should not be used.
- IV vitamin K1 has been reported to cause anaphylactoid reactions. Avoid this route of administration.
- Minimize stress, trauma, jugular venipuncture, and cystocentesis due to the risk of acute and catastrophic hemorrhage.

PRECAUTIONS

- Avoid large-bore hypodermic needles, unnecessary surgical procedures, and parenteral injections.
- Use the smallest possible needle when giving an injection or collecting samples.

POSSIBLE INTERACTIONS

Sulfonamides and phenylbutazone may displace anticoagulant rodenticides from plasma binding sites, leading to freer toxicant and increased risk of toxicosis.

FOLLOW-UP

PATIENT MONITORING

PT (preferred) test 2–3 days after the last dose of vitamin K1 to assess duration of therapy. If the PT is prolonged, administer another 1–3 weeks of vitamin K1 and retest.

PREVENTION/AVOIDANCE

Prevent pet's access to anticoagulant rodenticides by using bait stations and keeping stored bait in a secure location.

POSSIBLE COMPLICATIONS

- Secondary bacterial pneumonia may occur following intrapulmonary hemorrhage.
- Intracranial and intra-articular hemorrhage may occur.
- Pregnant animals can abort due to placental hemorrhage and detachment.

EXPECTED COURSE AND PROGNOSIS

If the patient survives the first 48–72 hours of acute coagulopathy, the prognosis improves.

MISCELLANEOUS

PREGNANCY/FERTILITY/BREEDING

- Warfarin, diphacinone, and perhaps other anticoagulant rodenticides may pass into amniotic fluid and to the fetuses of an exposed pregnant animal. These toxicants may also pass via the milk and present concerns for nursing offspring. In general, antidotal treatment of the pregnant or nursing patient is recommended. Alternatively, nursing young may be weaned.
- Pregnant animals can abort due to placental hemorrhage and detachment.

ABBREVIATIONS

- EPA = US Environmental Protection Agency.
- PIVKA = protein-induced vitamin K absence or antagonist.
- PT = prothrombin time.
- PTT = partial thromboplastin time.

INTERNET RESOURCES

- www.petpoisonhelpline.com
- www.aspca.org/pet-care/animal-poisoncontrol

R

Suggested Reading

Murphy MJ. Anticoagulants. In: Osweiler GD, et al., eds., Blackwell's Five-Minute Veterinary Consult Clinical Companion Small Animal Toxicology, 2nd ed. Ames, IA: Wiley-Blackwell, 2016, pp. 835–843.

Murphy MJ. Anticoagulant rodenticides. In: Gupta RC, ed., Veterinary Toxicology: Basic and Clinical Principles, 3rd ed. San Diego, CA: Elsevier, 2018, pp. 583–612.

Author Dominic A. Tauer
Consulting Editor Lynn R. Hovda

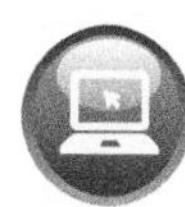

Client Education Handout available online

RODENTICIDE TOXICOSIS—BROMETHALIN

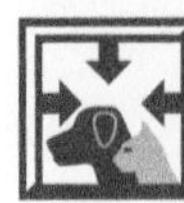

BASICS

OVERVIEW

- Bromethalin is a neurotoxic rodenticide that produces cerebral edema and elevated CSF pressure, resulting in progressive CNS depression, coma, paresis, and paralysis.
- Clinical signs and death have been reported in dogs and cats exposed to bromethalin at doses as low as 0.36 and 0.24 mg/kg, respectively.
- Trade names include Tomcat, Fastrac, Top Gun, Gladiator, and others. Bromethalin concentrations in products can vary from 0.01 to 0.025%.

SIGNALMENT

- Dogs and cats. Other species including humans may be affected.
- Any breed or age may be affected.

SIGNS

- Ingestion most often results in a delayed neurotoxic syndrome that develops within 2–7 days of ingestion; however, delays of up to 2 weeks may occur.
- Common clinical signs include anorexia, progressive ataxia, paresis, and hind limb paralysis, moderate to severe central nervous system depression, fine muscle tremors, and focal motor or generalized seizures.
- Forelimb extensor rigidity and decerebrate postures are often seen.
- Ingestion of high doses of bromethalin less commonly results in an acute onset (within 1–2 hours) of CNS excitation, muscle tremors, and seizures.

CAUSES & RISK FACTORS

Bromethalin ingestion most often occurs in animals <1 year of age.

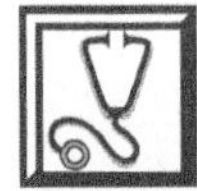

DIAGNOSIS

DIFFERENTIAL DIAGNOSIS

Neurologic syndromes produced by trauma, neoplasia, cerebral vascular disorders, as well as infectious and other toxic agents.

CBC/BIOCHEMISTRY/URINALYSIS

Alterations in routine serum electrolytes and chemistries are not anticipated.

OTHER LABORATORY TESTS

Analytical chemical confirmation of bromethalin residues in fresh frozen fat, liver, kidney, and brain tissue.

IMAGING

Neuroimaging (MRI) may reveal generalized brain edema.

DIAGNOSTIC PROCEDURES

- CSF generally reveals normal cytology, protein concentration, specific gravity, and cell count.
- EEG findings can change during the course of the toxic syndrome and may include spike and spike-and-wave activity, marked voltage depression, and abnormal high-voltage slow-wave activities.

PATHOLOGIC FINDINGS

- Histologic lesions are generally confined to the CNS and include spongy degeneration in the cerebrum, cerebellum, brainstem, spinal cord, and optic nerve white matter due to myelin edema.
- Gross evidence of cerebral edema is generally mild.

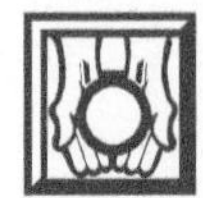

TREATMENT

- Aggressive early treatment with oral activated charcoal and a cathartic to reduce gastrointestinal absorption is warranted.
- Prolonged anorexia and may require supplemental feeding to maintain caloric intake.
- Use cage padding to reduce the risk of decubitus ulcer formation in recumbent animals.

MEDICATIONS

DRUG(S) OF CHOICE

- Gastrointestinal tract decontamination including early induction of emesis followed by administration of activated charcoal (1–2 g/kg PO) with an osmotic cathartic (sorbitol) × 1 dose) followed by activated charcoal alone q6–8h × 24 hours. Pay attention to sodium concentration. The efficacy of these treatments remains unknown.
- Control of cerebral edema with mannitol 500 mg/kg q6h slow IV bolus, dexamethasone 1–2 mg/kg q6h IV, and furosemide 1–2 mg/kg q6h IV may have limited efficacy.
- Diazepam 0.5–1 mg/kg, IV as needed, or other anticonvulsants may be given to abolish severe muscle tremors and seizures.
- 20% IV lipid emulsions (ILE)—bolus dose 1.5 mL/kg over 2–3 minutes; CRI of 0.25 mL/kg/min for 30–60 minutes. Check serum q2h until it becomes clear; repeat as needed; if no clinical improvement after 3 doses, discontinue. Other ILE dosing regimens can be used.

CONTRAINDICATIONS/POSSIBLE INTERACTIONS

- Contraindications for the use of mannitol include renal disease, pulmonary edema, dehydration, and intracranial hemorrhage.
- Animals receiving mannitol therapy may become dehydrated.
- Rehydration may be associated with a worsening of clinical signs, possibly due to rebound cerebral and pulmonary edema. Maintenance of hydration is important and can be more safely accomplished through the administration of oral fluids.
- Adverse effects of ILE may relate to contamination of the lipid product or direct reaction to the emulsion.

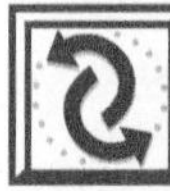

FOLLOW-UP

- May require several weeks to recover from mild poisoning.
- Prognosis is poor for the severely affected animals.
- Prevent ongoing rodenticide ingestion.

MISCELLANEOUS

Relay toxicity arising from the consumption of animals poisoned with bromethalin may occur.

ABBREVIATIONS

- EEG = electroencephalogram.
- ILE = IV lipid emulsion.

INTERNET RESOURCES

Khan SA and Schell MM. Bromethalin. Merck Veterinary Manual. Available at: https://www.merckvetmanual.com/toxicology/rodenticide-poisoning/bromethalin

Suggested Reading

DeClementi C, Sobczak BR. Common rodenticide toxicoses in small animals. Vet Clin North Am Small Anim Pract 2018, 48:1027–1038.

Author David C. Dorman

Consulting Editor Lynn R. Hovda

RODENTICIDE TOXICOSIS—CHOLECALCIFEROL

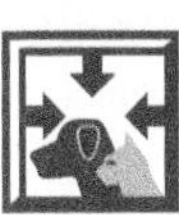

BASICS

DEFINITION

Hypercalcemic disorder resulting from ingestion of vitamin D rodenticide preparations.

PATHOPHYSIOLOGY

- Cholecalciferol is metabolized to 25-hydroxycholecalciferol in the liver. 25-hydroxycholecalciferol is metabolized to several metabolites in the kidney, including calcitriol, the most potent metabolite in terms of enhancing calcium absorption from the gut and calcium resorption from bones under physiologic conditions.
- 1,25-dihydroxycholecalciferol is the active metabolite of cholecalciferol under physiologic conditions.
- Under toxic conditions, 25-hydroxycholecalciferol is the predominant circulating and active metabolite.
- 25-hydroxycholecalciferol increases absorption of calcium from the gut, stimulates bone resorption, and enhances calcium absorption in renal distal tubules, resulting in hypercalcemia (serum calcium >12.5 mg/dL).
- Serum phosphorus is also increased.
- The outcome is metastatic and dystrophic mineralization of soft tissues, resulting in pathophysiology of the affected organs.

SYSTEMS AFFECTED

- Cardiovascular—mineralization, arrhythmias.
- Gastrointestinal—anorexia; mineralization; emesis; hematemesis; constipation; increased gastric acid secretion.
- Musculoskeletal—bone demineralization; muscle tremors.
- Nervous—seizures or depression.
- Renal/urologic—calcification, proximal tubular necrosis, dilute urine, and renal failure.
- Respiratory—lung mineralization; dyspnea.

INCIDENCE/PREVALENCE

- Cholecalciferol rodenticide toxicosis—most common cause of vitamin D poisoning in dogs and cats.
- Incidence of poisoning unknown but growing in popularity as rodenticide as the use of anticoagulant rodenticides declines.
- Suckling pups and kittens can be poisoned through milk.

SIGNALMENT

Species

- Dogs and cats.
- Other species, particularly exotics.

Mean Age and Range

All ages affected; younger dogs (<6 months) and cats are the most sensitive.

SIGNS

General Comments

Cholecalciferol rodenticides—signs develop within 12–36 hours post ingestion.

Historical Findings

- Inactivity.
- Vomiting.
- CNS depression.
- Weakness.
- Anorexia.
- Polydipsia.
- Polyuria.
- Diarrhea.
- Melena.
- Hematemesis.
- Loss in body weight.
- Constipation.
- Seizures.
- Muscle tremors.

Physical Examination Findings

- Depression.
- Vomiting.
- Diarrhea.
- Hematemesis.
- Hematochezia.
- Polyuria.
- Polydipsia.
- Dehydration.
- Renal pain on palpation.
- Gastrointestinal hemorrhage.
- Abdominal pain.
- Hypersalivation.
- Oropharyngeal erosive lesions.
- Bradycardia; ventricular premature contractions.
- Dyspnea.

CAUSES

Cholecalciferol rodenticides (0.075%)—Quintox, Rampage, Ortho Rat-B-Gone, Ortho Mouse-B-Gone, others; clinically normal dogs and cats have developed hypercalcemia at 0.5 mg/kg body weight; signs have occurred in dogs and cats at 0.1 mg/kg body weight.

RISK FACTORS

- Preexisting renal, gastrointestinal, cardiac, lung, or CNS diseases.
- Dehydration.
- Neoplasia.
- Primary hyperparathyroidism.
- Hypoadrenocorticism.
- Granulomatous diseases (e.g., blastomycosis).
- Juvenile hypercalcemia.
- Age—young animals are most susceptible.
- Feline idiopathic hypercalcemia.

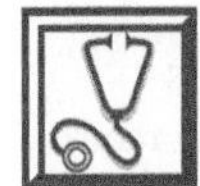

DIAGNOSIS

DIFFERENTIAL DIAGNOSIS

- Other hypercalcemic disorders, including lymphosarcoma and other malignancies, hypoadrenocorticism, chronic renal failure, primary hyperparathyroidism, and granulomatous lesions in soft tissues.
- Juvenile hypercalcemia.
- Anticoagulant rodenticide and nonsteroidal anti-inflammatory drug (NSAID) toxicity—due to hematemesis and melena.

CBC/BIOCHEMISTRY/URINALYSIS

- Calcium—hypercalcemia (total serum calcium >12.5 mg/dL, ionized calcium >6.0 mg/dL). Hypercalcemia is immediate (2–3 hours) and transient (will decline to normal within 24 hours post ingestion) with calcipotriol ingestion. In cholecalciferol rodenticide toxicity, hypercalcemia is evident 12 hours post ingestion and persists for weeks if not treated.
- Hyperphosphatemia (>8 mg/dL) may precede hypercalcemia.
- Hypokalemia.
- Azotemia.
- Hyposthenuria, proteinuria, and glucosuria.
- Metabolic acidosis.

OTHER LABORATORY TESTS

- In acute, one-time ingestions, serum 25-hydroxy vitamin D concentration is increased at least 10 times normal (normal ranges: dogs, 60–215 nmol/L; cats, 65–170 nmol/L) in cholecalciferol toxicosis.
- In chronic intoxications, serum 25-hydroxy vitamin D concentrations can increase from 1.5 to 5 times above normal values.
- Serum 1,25-dihydroxy vitamin D is only transiently increased and is of limited diagnostic value.
- The total calcium-to-total phosphorus ratio in renal cortex of deceased dogs is in the range of 0.4–0.9 (normal <0.3) for all vitamin D-related intoxications.
- Renal cortical 25-hydroxy vitamin D concentration >80 nmol/L supports a diagnosis of cholecalciferol toxicosis.
- Biliary 25-hydroxy vitamin D concentration >100 nmol/L supports a diagnosis of cholecalciferol toxicosis.
- Decreased intact parathyroid hormone (iPTH) (normal in dogs is 3–17 pmol/L and for cats is 0–4 pmol/L).
- Normal Na/K ratio.

IMAGING

Ultrasonography—renal, gastric wall, lung hyperechogenicity.

DIAGNOSTIC PROCEDURES

- Electrocardiogram—may show bradycardia, sinus tachycardia, ventricular premature complexes.
- Endoscopy—may reveal erosive/hemorrhagic gastric mucosa.

PATHOLOGIC FINDINGS

- Diffuse mineralization of gastric wall and intestines; hemorrhage in gastric mucosa; mineralization of the soft palate, salivary glands, other soft tissues.

- Necrosis and mineralization of myocardium (especially the atria) and large blood vessels; myocardial degeneration.
- Mineralization of glomerular mesangium and capsule, and renal tubular basement membranes.
- Tubular necrosis.
- Mineralization of lungs.

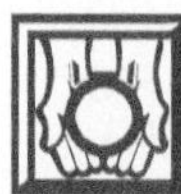

TREATMENT

APPROPRIATE HEALTH CARE

- Cholecalciferol—once clinical signs show (usually 24–36 hours post ingestion), gastric decontamination is not worth while.
- Hospitalization with close observation in all cases for at least 48 hours post ingestion.

NURSING CARE

- Correct dehydration and electrolyte imbalances (hypokalemia).
- Enhance calciuresis with fluid therapy—strongly recommended for all patients.
- Peritoneal dialysis with a calcium-free dialysate—for severe azotemia and hypercalcemia.
- Blood transfusion—if anemia is severe or in case of hypovolemia.
- Antibiotic therapy—as needed.
- Parenteral alimentation—recommended to rest the gut and to overcome anorexia.

DIET

Offer low-calcium, low-phosphorus diets.

CLIENT EDUCATION

- Caution client to keep all rodenticide products in places that are inaccessible to pets.
- Warn client that vitamin D toxicity is a severe and costly disease to treat with prolonged therapy and hospitalization.

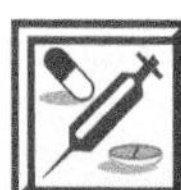

MEDICATIONS

DRUG(S) OF CHOICE

- Pamidronate disodium—to treat hypercalcemia.
- Salmon calcitonin—to treat hypercalcemia.

Decontamination of Gastrointestinal Tract

- Within 2 hours of vitamin D ingestion.
- Emetic and activated charcoal followed by osmotic cathartics.
- Dogs—apomorphine 0.02–0.04 mg/kg IV, IM, SC, or subconjunctivally.
- Cats—xylazine 0.4–0.5 mg/kg IV.
- Activated charcoal powder (1–4 g/kg) combined with a saline cathartic (magnesium or sodium sulfate, 250 mg/kg)—PO or by gastric tube.

Hypercalcemia Reduction

- Pamidronate disodium 1.3–2.0 mg/kg in 0.9% sodium chloride slow IV over 2–4 hours; repeat once in 3–4 days for large ingestions; do not combine with salmon calcitonin.
- Salmon calcitonin 4–6 IU IM or SC every 6 hours till calcium concentration stabilizes; rarely used as limited efficacy and patients may become refractory.
- IV fluids: 0.9% sodium chloride or 5% dextrose with 0.45% sodium chloride fluids to begin; change as needed.
- Prednisolone—dogs and cats: 2–6 mg/kg IM or PO q12h.
- Furosemide—dogs, 2–6 mg/kg; cats, 1–4 mg/kg SC, IV, or IM q8–12h.

Seizure Control

- Diazepam 0.5–1 mg/kg IV, repeat as necessary.

Control of Clinically Significant Ventricular Arrhythmias

- Lidocaine—dogs, 2–4 mg/kg IV over 1 minute, repeat up to 8 mg/kg; cats, use cautiously at 0.25–0.5 mg/kg IV slowly.

Gastrointestinal Protection

- Sucralfate 0.25–1 g PO q6–8h.
- Famotidine 0.5–1 mg/kg IV, IM, PO q12h.

Antiemetics

- Maropitant 1 mg/kg SQ, IV or PO q24h.

PRECAUTIONS

- Supratherapeutic doses of pamidronate disodium may worsen renal failure.
- Salmon calcitonin—associated with side effects: anorexia, anaphylaxis, and emesis. Rarely used.
- Xylazine—may aggravate respiratory depression and result in vagal-mediated slowing of the heart rate.
- Prolonged prednisolone therapy may result in adrenocortical suppression; taper doses gradually over a 2- to 4-week treatment period.

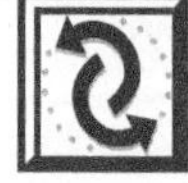

FOLLOW-UP

PATIENT MONITORING

- Following pamidronate therapy—serum calcium and BUN at 24, 48, and 72 hours following exposure; if hypercalcemia still present, repeat pamidronate infusion 72 or 96 hours after the first infusion and monitor serum calcium and BUN q48h.
- Following calcitonin therapy—serum calcium and BUN; monitor q24h and continue adjusting dose until calcium returns to normal (24–48 hours for calcipotriol, or 2–4 weeks for cholecalciferol).
- Cholecalciferol-induced hypercalcemia is persistent, requiring long-term management and supportive care (2–4 weeks).

PREVENTION/AVOIDANCE

Keep rodenticides out of reach of pets.

POSSIBLE COMPLICATIONS

- Chronic renal failure—inability to concentrate urine.
- Subclinical renal, cardiovascular, and gastrointestinal sequelae—due to mineralization.

EXPECTED COURSE AND PROGNOSIS

Cholecalciferol—depends on severity and duration of hypercalcemia; if hypercalcemia is unresponsive or severe mineralization occurs before therapy is initiated, prognosis is poor.

MISCELLANEOUS

AGE-RELATED FACTORS

Distinguish from normal juvenile hypercalcemia.

PREGNANCY/FERTILITY/BREEDING

Vitamin D has antiproliferative effects and the potential for teratogenesis.

SYNONYMS

N/A

ABBREVIATIONS

- iPTH = intact parathyroid hormone.
- NSAID = nonsteroidal anti-inflammatory drug.

Suggested Reading

Bates N. Vitamin D toxicosis. Compan Anim 2017, 22(12):700–706.

DeClementi C, Sobczak BR. Common rodenticide toxicoses in small animals. Vet Clin North Am Small Anim Pract 2018, 48(6):1027–1038.

Peterson ME, Fluegenman K. Cholecalciferol. Top Compan Anim Med 2013, 28(1): 24–27.

Rumbeiha WK. Cholecalciferol. In: Peterson ME, Talcott PA, eds., Small Animal Toxicology, 3rd ed. St. Louis, MO: Saunders, 2013, pp. 489–498.

Rumbeiha WK, Braselton WE, Nachreiner R, et al. The post-mortem diagnosis of cholecalciferol toxicosis: A novel approach and differentiation from ethylene glycol toxicosis. J Vet Diagn Invest 2000, 12:426–432.

Rumbeiha WK, Fitzgerald SD, Kruger JM, et al. Use of pamidronate disodium to reduce cholecalciferol-induced toxicosis in dogs. Am J Vet Res 2000, 61:9–13.

Author Wilson K. Rumbeiha

Consulting Editor Lynn R. Hovda

R

RODENTICIDE TOXICOSIS—PHOSPHIDES

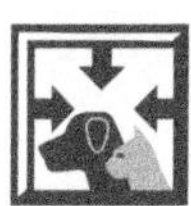

BASICS

OVERVIEW

• Used as a rodenticide since the early 1930s at various concentrations (2–10%) in a powder, pellet, or paste formulation. Available as zinc, aluminum, and magnesium salts. • Distinctive odor, often described as acetylene, rotten fish, or garlic. • Most common route of exposure is ingestion; however, toxicosis can occur via inhalation and absorption through broken skin. • Hydrolysis leads to phosphine gas production. Phosphine gas has corrosive and irritant effects on the gastrointestinal (GI) mucosa, which leads to vomiting, hematemesis, or melena. The gas is rapidly absorbed and systemically distributed leading to effects on other organ systems. • Phosphine leads to the production of free radicals and oxidative stress, causing direct cellular damage and may inhibit cellular respiration. • Toxic exposure is reported to be 20–40 mg/kg; however, the gastric pH is reported to affect toxicity.

SIGNALMENT

No known age, breed, or sex predilection.

SIGNS

• Within 15 minutes to 4 hours but can be delayed up to 18 hours. • GI—anorexia, vomiting, and melena. • Cardiovascular—direct myocardial damage, arrhythmias, decreased inotropy, hypotension. • Respiratory—pulmonary edema, pleural effusion. • Hemic/lymphatic/immune—methemoglobinemia, Heinz body production. • Nervous—ataxia, weakness, tremors, hyperesthesia, and seizures. • Renal/urologic—azotemia, acute renal failure. • Hepatobiliary—increased alanine transaminase (ALT), aspartate transferase (AST), and total bilirubin. • Endocrine/metabolic—metabolic acidosis, electrolyte imbalance. • Musculoskeletal—weakness, ataxia.

CAUSES & RISK FACTORS

• Increased hydrolysis in a moist, acidic environment; thus, recent food ingestion lowers gastric pH and increases hydrolysis. Owner should be instructed not to feed their pet. • Owners and veterinary staff are at risk for inhalation exposure if the animal vomits in a poorly ventilated area. Owners should be told to lower their windows on the way to the clinic.

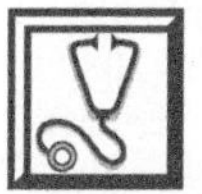

DIAGNOSIS

DIFFERENTIAL DIAGNOSIS

• Organophosphate. • Metaldehyde. • Serotonin syndrome. • Nonsteroidal anti-inflammatory drug (NSAID) toxicosis. • Tremorgenic mycotoxins. • Acute GI disease (hemorrhagic gastroenteritis [HGE], gastroenteritis, parvovirus). • Congestive heart failure. • Respiratory disease (noncardiogenic pulmonary edema—secondary to electrocution, near drowning, seizures, or acute respiratory distress syndrome [ARDS]). • Metabolic disease (renal, hepatic, pancreatitis).

CBC/BIOCHEMISTRY/URINALYSIS

• May see increased liver enzymes (ALT, AST, and total bilirubin); can be delayed 3–5 days. • Electrolyte alterations (decreased potassium or magnesium). • Methemoglobinemia, Heinz body formation, and subsequent hemolysis.

OTHER LABORATORY TESTS

• Confirmation through gas chromatography or a Dräger detection tube (referral laboratory testing). • Post-mortem samples from the liver, kidney.

IMAGING

If respiratory signs, thoracic radiographs to assess for pulmonary edema.

PATHOLOGIC FINDINGS

Are nonspecific.

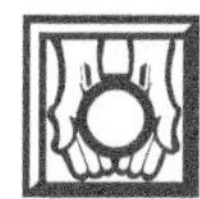

TREATMENT

• No antidote. • The goal of treatment with recent, asymptomatic patients is to safely decontaminate. • Administration of a liquid antacid such as magnesium hydroxide, aluminum hydroxide, calcium carbonate, or even a 5% sodium bicarbonate solution may help to increase the gastric pH and thus decrease phosphine gas production. • Emesis induction with apomorphine, hydrogen peroxide, or gastric lavage for gastric emptying. • Activated charcoal may help decrease toxicity but should be given only if the patient's clinical status allows. • IV fluid therapy with monitoring for any clinical signs or progression of signs for at least 18 hours. • Supplemental oxygen for hypoxemia.

MEDICATIONS

• GI protectants—famotidine 0.5–1 mg/kg IV/PO q12–24h, omeprazole 0.5–1 mg/kg PO q12–24h, sucralfate 0.25–1 g PO q8–12h, or possibly misoprostol 2–5 µg/kg PO q8h. • Tremors—methocarbamol 44–220 mg/kg IV or to effect; do not exceed 330 mg/kg/day. • Seizures—diazepam 0.5–1 mg/kg IV, phenobarbital 4–16 mg/kg IV to effect, levetiracetam 30–60 mg/kg IV, or propofol 1–8 mg/kg or to effect, followed by a CRI at 0.1–0.6 mg/kg/h. • Liver effects—hepatoprotectants (*S*-adenosylmethionine 18 mg/kg PO q24h, silymarin/milk thistle 50–250 mg/day PO q24h. If associated coagulopathy—vitamin K_1 2–3 mg/kg PO q12–24h. • Oxidative damage or for methemoglobinemia—*N*-acetylcysteine. • Painful—opioids (hydromorphone 0.05–0.1 mg/kg IV) or tramadol 2–4 mg/kg PO q8–12h. Avoid NSAIDs.

FOLLOW-UP

Varies on a case basis.

PATIENT MONITORING

Several organ systems may be affected; vitals, heart rhythm, blood pressure, and CNS should be monitored for 18 hours.

PREVENTION/AVOIDANCE

Have owners remove all baits from environment.

POSSIBLE COMPLICATIONS

Liver or renal failure.

EXPECTED COURSE AND PROGNOSIS

• Asymptomatic patients should be monitored for up to 12–18 hours. • Symptomatic patients should be monitored for at least 48 hours or until life-threatening signs have resolved.

MISCELLANEOUS

ABBREVIATIONS

• ALT = alanine transaminase.
• ARDS = acute respiratory distress syndrome.
• AST = aspartate transferase.
• GI = gastrointestinal. • HGE = hemorrhagic gastroenteritis. • NSAID = nonsteroidal anti-inflammatory drug.

INTERNET RESOURCES

https://www.avma.org/KB/Resources/Reference/Pages/Phosphine-product-precautions.aspx

Suggested Reading

Gray SL, Lee JA, Hovda LR, et al. Potential zinc phosphide rodenticide toxicosis in dogs: 362 cases (2004–2009). J Am Vet Med Assoc 2011, 239:646–651.

Knight MW. Zinc phosphide. In: Peterson ME, Talcott PA, eds., Small Animal Toxicology, 3rd ed. St. Louis, MO: Elsevier Saunders, 2013, pp. 853–864.

Author Sarah L. Gray
Consulting Editor Lynn R. Hovda

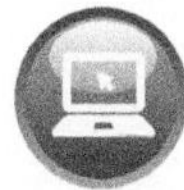

Client Education Handout available online

ROUNDWORMS (ASCARIASIS)

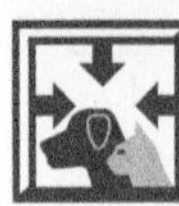

BASICS

OVERVIEW

• Ascariasis caused by *Toxocara canis* (dogs), *T. cati* (cats), and *Toxascaris leonina* (dogs, cats); *Baylisascaris* (raccoons) can infect dogs and causes neural larval migrans in people. • Transplacental transmission of *T. canis* larvae from bitch to pups causes prenatal infection; transmammary transmission of larvae occurs with both *Toxocara* spp.; no transplacental or transmammary transmission with *Toxascaris*. • In first month of life, infected neonatal pups may develop abdominal pain and rapidly deteriorate before *Toxocara* eggs appear in feces. • Older pups and kittens can acquire by ingesting eggs spread by dams with postgestational infection; dams can be infected by ingesting immature worm stages in pups' feces or vomitus or by predation on vertebrate transport hosts. • Adult ascarids occur in lumen of small intestine; larval stages of *Toxocara* spp. may migrate in liver and lungs. • If numerous, ascarids (up to 10–12 cm long) can distend intestine and cause colic, interference with gut motility, inability to utilize food, intestinal rupture.

R

SIGNALMENT

• Dog and cat. • Important in puppies/kittens due to *in utero*/transmammary transmission.

SIGNS

• Abdominal distension; often with palpable intestinal distension. • Colic. • Weakness, loss of condition, cachexia; poor nursing or appetite; scant feces. • Coughing due to larval lung migration. • Entire litter may be affected.

CAUSES & RISK FACTORS

• Dormant *Toxocara* larvae in dam's tissues is infection reservoir for puppies during gestation; queen becomes infected during late pregnancy or lactation and transfers to kittens via transmammary route. • Access to infected transport hosts. • Concurrent enteric infections. • *Toxocara* larvae undergo extensive migration and can cause granulomatous inflammation (visceral larva migrans). Visceral larva migrans caused by ascarids is cause of human morbidity. • Somatically arrested larvae in small vertebrates are source of infection for dogs/cats that hunt.

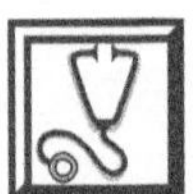

DIAGNOSIS

DIFFERENTIAL DIAGNOSIS

• Transmammary perinatal infection of neonates with hookworms (anemia, melena, weakness, lethargy, pallor, enteritis) or *Strongyloides* (diarrhea); coccidiosis, giardiasis; examine feces for eggs or larvae. • *Physaloptera*.

CBC/BIOCHEMISTRY/URINALYSIS

Usually normal.

OTHER LABORATORY TESTS

N/A

IMAGING

N/A

DIAGNOSTIC PROCEDURES

• Fecal flotation to detect eggs: ∘ *Toxocara* eggs spherical pitted outer shell membrane, single dark cell filling interior, 80–85 μm (*T. canis*), ~75 μm (*T. cati*). ∘ *Baylisascaris* eggs similar to *T. canis* eggs but smaller (~76 × 60 μm), more finely pitted shell. ∘ *Toxascaris* eggs ovoid, smooth exterior shell membrane, 1–2 cells with light-colored cytoplasm; cells do not fill interior of egg; 80 × 70 μm in diameter. • Necropsy of siblings—identify ascarids by size, appearance. • Fecal ELISA—commercial test detects antigen produced by adult and immature roundworms of both sexes; can detect prepatent infection.

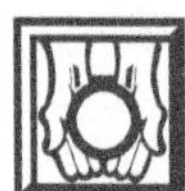

TREATMENT

• Generally outpatient. • Acute severe cases treated as inpatients; provide parenteral fluids. • Alert client to possibility of sudden death or chronic debilitation. • Treat dam with adulticide/larvicide anthelmintic to remove intestinal stages and limit transmission to subsequent litters.

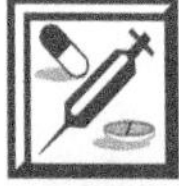

MEDICATIONS

DRUG(S) OF CHOICE

Adulticide/Larvicide Anthelmintics

• Fenbendazole 50 mg/kg PO q24h for 3 days. • Milbemycin oxime 0.5 mg/kg (dogs) or 2 mg/kg (cats) PO q30 days. • Moxidectin (dogs) 2.5 mg/kg, topically, q30 days. • Moxidectin (in combination with imidacloprid) 10 mg/kg, topically, q30 days. • Emodepside 3 mg/kg, or praziquantel 12 mg/kg, topically once for cats ≥8 weeks old; repeat in 30 days if cat is reinfected.

Adulticide Anthelmintics

• Pyrantel pamoate 5 mg/kg PO (dogs) or 10–20 mg/kg PO (cats, extra-label). • Pyrantel/praziquantel, label dose for cats. • Febantel/praziquantel/pyrantel, label dose for dogs. • Ivermectin/pyrantel, label dose for dogs. • Selamectin 6 mg/kg, topically, once (*T. cati*, cats): dogs, extra-label.

CONTRAINDICATIONS/POSSIBLE INTERACTIONS

N/A

FOLLOW-UP

PATIENT MONITORING

Repeat post-treatment fecal exams on puppies/kittens and/or repeat anthelmintic treatment every 2–3 weeks until old enough for monthly anthelmintic product.

PREVENTION/AVOIDANCE

• Minimize environmental contamination, treat infected dogs/cats with anthelmintic, dispose of feces promptly. • Prevent dogs/cats from hunting or ingesting transport hosts. • Extra-label treatment of dam with adulticide/larvicide anthelmintic to remove intestinal stages and decrease vertical transmission.

POSSIBLE COMPLICATIONS

Transplacental transmission of large numbers of larvae can result in fetal death or birth of weak, nonviable offspring.

EXPECTED COURSE AND PROGNOSIS

Prognosis good after anthelmintic treatment; guarded with severe prenatal *T. canis* infection.

MISCELLANEOUS

AGE-RELATED FACTORS

Greater concern in neonates.

ZOONOTIC POTENTIAL

• Visceral larva migrans, ocular larva migrans, neural larva migrans, chronic abdominal or cutaneous problems may follow ingestion of infective *Toxocara* spp. or *Baylisascaris* eggs by humans; advise clients to practice good hygiene after handling feces. • Most likely cause of neural larva migrans is *Baylisascaris*; virtually all raccoons become infected with *Baylisascaris* and therefore extreme caution should be exercised with clients having raccoons as "pets."

INTERNET RESOURCES

• http://www.capcvet.org • http://www.cdc.gov

Suggested Reading

Bowman DD. Georgis' Parasitology for Veterinarians, 9th ed. St. Louis, MO: Saunders, 2009, pp. 197–198, 201–208.

Authors Matt Brewer and Jeba R.J. Jesudoss Chelladurai

Consulting Editor Amie Koenig

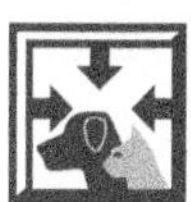

BASICS

OVERVIEW

• Cycad palms, also called sago palms, belong in the family Cycadaceae. • Native to tropical and subtropical regions but have become popular ornamental plants in the United States. • *Cycas revoluta, Cycas circinalis,* and *Zamia floridana* are the most common species. • Contain the toxins cycasin, betamethylamino-L-alanine, and an unidentified high-molecular-weight compound. • Toxins present in all parts of the plant; highest concentrations in seeds. • Cycasin is metabolized by the intestinal flora to the active hepatotoxic, carcinogenic, mutagenic, teratogenic, and neurotoxic compound methylazoxymethanol (MAM). • Cycad toxicosis has been documented in several animal species (dogs and ruminants) and humans. • In dogs, gastrointestinal (GI) disturbances and hepatic damage predominate; nervous system involvement is less common.

SIGNALMENT

• Dogs—no breed, sex, or age predilection.
• Cats—no cases reported.

SIGNS

• GI disturbances such as vomiting, diarrhea, and abdominal pain. • Signs associated with hepatic damage (ecchymoses, petechiae, hemorrhage, edema, etc.). • Gait abnormalities; paresis/paralysis; tremors.
• Depression, coma, and death.

CAUSES & RISK FACTORS

Access to and ingestion of cycad palm.

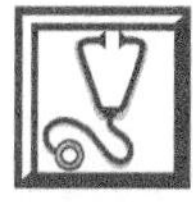

DIAGNOSIS

DIFFERENTIAL DIAGNOSIS

Other Causes of Acute GI Upset

• Infectious. • Metabolic. • Toxic. • Dietary.

Other Causes of Acute Liver Failure

• Microcystins (hepatotoxic blue-green algal toxins)—access to water with algal bloom, algal material on legs or in stomach contents, detection of microcystins in stomach contents.
• Amanitin—access to mushrooms (*Amanita, Galerina,* and *Lepiota* spp.), GI signs between 6 and 24 hours after ingestion. • Cocklebur (*Xanthium* spp.)—access to cocklebur (only seeds and two-leaf cotyledon stage are toxic).
• Aflatoxins—access to moldy food.
• Acetaminophen overdose. • Xylitol—access to xylitol-containing products (sugar-free gum, chewable vitamins, baked goods); initial hypoglycemia. • Severe acute pancreatitis.

CBC/BIOCHEMISTRY/URINALYSIS

• Anemia. • Elevated serum liver enzymes (alanine transaminase, aspartate transaminase, alkaline phosphatase, bilirubin).
• Hypoalbuminemia. • Hypoglycemia.
• Glucosuria, hemoglobinuria, myoglobinuria, bilirubinuria, proteinuria, and increased urine specific gravity.

OTHER LABORATORY TESTS

• Ammonia tolerance test—hyperammonemia.
• Prolonged prothrombin time/partial thromboplastin time.

IMAGING

N/A

DIAGNOSTIC PROCEDURES

• History of cycad palm ingestion and presence of appropriate clinical signs. • Identification of plant in ingesta or feces. • Biopsy and histopathology of liver—hepatic necrosis.
• Necropsy—hepatic centrilobular necrosis.

PATHOLOGIC FINDINGS

• Detection of cycad palm material in GI tract and/or in feces. • Gross detection of liver enlargement. • Histologic detection of centrilobular and midzonal coagulative hepatocellular necrosis.

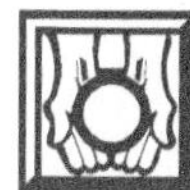

TREATMENT

• No antidote available. • GI decontamination with activated charcoal can be attempted but efficacy is unknown. • Supportive care including close monitoring and, depending on the severity of clinical signs, IV fluids, correction of electrolyte imbalances and hypoglycemia, vitamin K1, and plasma transfusions.

MEDICATIONS

DRUG(S) OF CHOICE

• Activated charcoal—multi-dose activated charcoal at 1–4 g/kg PO q4–6h for 2–3 days post ingestion. Mix activated charcoal in water at 1 g/5–10 mL of water. • IV fluids—maintain hydration, induce diuresis, correct hypoglycemia. • Dextrose—50% dextrose 1 mL/kg IV slow bolus (1–3 minutes).
• Vitamin K1—0.5–1.5 mg/kg SC or IM q12h; 1 mg/kg PO q24h. • Blood products—dependent on hemostatic test results.

ALTERNATIVE DRUG(S)

• *S*-Adenosylmethionine—antioxidant and hepatoprotectant; no data on efficacy in sago palm toxicosis available. Dose 20 mg/kg PO q24h. • Ascorbic acid and cimetidine—hepatocyte protectors; no data on efficacy in sago palm toxicosis available. Can be given for supportive therapy. • *N*-Acetylcysteine—antioxidant; no data on efficacy in sago palm toxicosis available. A glutathione precursor that can be included in the treatment regimen for acute fulminant hepatic failure at 140 mg/kg IV load, followed by 70 mg/kg IV q6h for 7 treatments.

CONTRAINDICATIONS/POSSIBLE INTERACTIONS

N/A

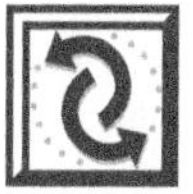

FOLLOW-UP

PATIENT MONITORING

• Liver enzymes/function. • Coagulation status.

PREVENTION/AVOIDANCE

Deny access to sago palms.

POSSIBLE COMPLICATIONS

• Hepatic encephalopathy. • Disseminated intravascular coagulation. • Renal failure.

EXPECTED COURSE AND PROGNOSIS

• Dogs develop vomiting within minutes, followed by further GI upset. • Changes in clinical laboratory values occur after 24–48 hours. • Nadir serum albumin levels and nadir platelet counts are important prognostic indicators. • Liver failure within a few days.
• Prognosis is poor to guarded.

MISCELLANEOUS

ABBREVIATIONS

• GI = gastrointestinal.
• MAM = methylazoxymethanol.

INTERNET RESOURCES

• http://www.petpoisonhelpline.com/poison/sago-palm/ • http://www.aspca.org/pet-care/animal-poison-control/toxic-and-non-toxic-plants/fern-palm

Suggested Reading

Albretsen JC, Khan SA, Richardson JA. Cycad palm toxicosis in dogs: 60 cases (1987–1997). J Am Vet Med Assoc 1998, 213(1):99–101.

Clarke C, Burney D. Cycad palm toxicosis in 14 dogs from Texas. J Am Anim Hosp Assoc 2017, 53:159–166.

Ferguson D, Crowe M, McLaughlin L, et al. Survival and prognostic indicators for cycad intoxication in dogs. J Vet Intern Med 2011, 25(4):831–837.

Authors Adrienne C. Bautista and Birgit Puschner

Consulting Editor Lynn R. Hovda

SALIVARY MUCOCELE

BASICS

OVERVIEW

• Salivary mucoceles (sialoceles) are nonepithelial-lined cavities filled with saliva that has leaked from a damaged salivary gland or duct; they are surrounded by granulation tissue that forms secondary to inflammation caused by the free saliva.
• There are four major pairs of salivary glands: parotid, mandibular, sublingual, and zygomatic. Smaller salivary glands are located in the soft palate, lips, cheeks, and tongue.
• Types of mucoceles are listed in Table 1. The most common type occurs with injury to the sublingual gland or its duct.

SYSTEMS AFFECTED

Gastrointestinal

SIGNALMENT

• Three times more frequent in dogs than in cats.
• Commonly affected breeds include miniature poodle, German shepherd dog, dachshund, and Australian silky terrier.
• Slight predisposition of males compared to females.
• No age predisposition.

S

SIGNS

Cervical Sialocele

• Soft, fluctuant, minimally painful or nonpainful, gradually developing cervical mass.
• Pain is usually manifested only during the acute-manifestation phase of the sialocele.

Sublingual Sialocele

• Soft, sublingual swelling (also called ranula; from Latin: *rana*, frog).
• Often blood-tinged saliva secondary to self-trauma while eating.
• Abnormal tongue movement, tongue displaced, dysphagia.

Pharyngeal Sialocele

• Swelling in pharyngeal wall.
• Dysphagia and respiratory distress when very large.

Zygomatic Sialocele

• Periorbital swelling.
• Exophthalmos and protrusion of third eyelid.
• Divergent strabismus.
• Periocular pain.
• Pressure-related neuropathy of the optic nerve.

CAUSES & RISK FACTORS

The cause is rarely identified. Suspected causes:
• Blunt trauma to the head and neck (choke chains).
• Bite wound.
• Penetrating foreign body.
• Ear canal surgery, parotid duct transposition, maxillectomy.
• Sialoliths.
• Dirofilariasis.

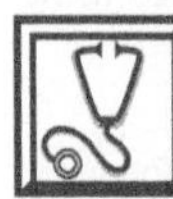

DIAGNOSIS

• Diagnosis is based on history, visual examination, and paracentesis of the fluid-filled swelling.
• Determine the site of origin with help of oral examination, palpation, sialography, or exploration of the sialocele.

DIFFERENTIAL DIAGNOSIS

• Sialoadenitis (second most common salivary gland disease; usually involving the zygomatic gland; often concurrent with sialoliths and other ductal foreign bodies).
• Sialadenosis (nonpainful, noninflammatory salivary gland swelling; usually mandibular gland).
• Necrotizing sialometaplasia (painful salivary gland swelling; squamous metaplasia with ischemic necrosis; usually mandibular gland).
• Salivary neoplasia (rare; mandibular and parotid glands most commonly involved; usually adenocarcinomas).
• Sialoliths (calcium phosphate or carbonate).
• Cervical abscess.
• Foreign body.
• Hematoma.
• Abscessed or neoplastic lymph nodes.

CBC/BIOCHEMISTRY/URINALYSIS

Laboratory abnormalities are rarely seen.

OTHER LABORATORY TESTS

N/A

IMAGING

• Ideally CT or MRI with contrast.
• Skull and upper neck radiography only helpful to identify sialoliths, foreign bodies, or neoplasia.
• Sialography (injection of iodinated, water-soluble contrast agent into the salivary duct) reserved for patients with trauma, previous surgeries, or fistulous draining tracts and can be helpful to determine the size and source of sialoceles.
• Retrobulbar ultrasound.

DIAGNOSTIC PROCEDURES

Aseptic Paracentesis

• Differentiates sialoceles from neoplasia and abscess.
• Aspirated fluid is viscous, clear, or pink, yellow, brown or black (blood-tinged) with a low cell count; surrounding soft tissue may show low-grade chronic plasmacytic-lymphocytic inflammation.
• Cytologic evaluation (Wright's stain) reveals diffuse or irregular clumps of pink to violet-staining mucin, large phagocytic cells with small, round nuclei and foamy cytoplasm, intermixed salivary gland epithelial cells, and nondegenerate neutrophils in small numbers.
• Stain with a mucus-specific stain (e.g., periodic acid–Schiff) for definitive diagnosis.

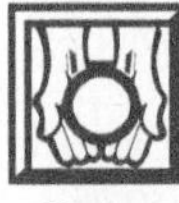

TREATMENT

• Patients with acute respiratory distress (pharyngeal sialoceles) might need to be intubated or have a temporary tracheostomy performed. Transoral drainage via stab incision may be required prior to intubation.
• Complete surgical excision of the involved gland–duct complex and drainage of the sialocele is the treatment of choice. Permanent drainage may be achieved with marsupialization of sublingual and pharyngeal sialoceles.

MEDICATIONS

DRUG(S) OF CHOICE

Antibiotics based on bacteriologic evaluation, if concurrent abscessation or sialadenitis.

CONTRAINDICATIONS

Nonsurgical treatment with repeated drainage or injection of cauterizing or anti-inflammatory agents is not curative and will complicate subsequent surgery by causing abscessation or fibrosis.

FOLLOW-UP

PATIENT MONITORING

Penrose drains placed after sialadenectomy are usually removed 24–72 hours following surgery.

POSSIBLE COMPLICATIONS

• Seroma formation (after excessive tissue dissection, insufficient dead space management, and when Penrose drains are not used following sialadenectomy).
• Infection.
• Sialocele recurrence (<5% with complete resection).

EXPECTED COURSE AND PROGNOSIS

• Excellent prognosis with complete surgical excision.
• Seroma formation and infection complicate successful surgical excision.

Table 1

Types of sialoceles.

Type	*Location*	*Gland/duct involved*
Cervical	Intermandibular space, jaw angle, upper cervical region	Sublingual or mandibular
Sublingual	Sublingual tissue	Sublingual or mandibular
Pharyngeal	Pharyngeal wall	Sublingual
Zygomatic	Ventrolateral to the globe	Zygomatic
Parotid mucocele	Side of the face, jaw angle, ventral to ear	Parotid

MISCELLANEOUS

ASSOCIATED CONDITIONS

Sialoadenitis (resected salivary glands often show various degrees of inflammation histologically).

SYNONYMS

- Salivary mucocele.
- Sialocele.

Suggested Reading

Gracis M, Reiter AM, Ordeix L. Management of selected non-periodontal inflammatory, infectious and reactive conditions. In: Reiter AM, Gracis M, ed., BSAVA Manual of Canine and Feline Dentistry and Oral Surgery, 4th ed. Gloucester, UK: BSAVA, 2018, pp. 192–193.

Reiter AM. Commonly encountered dental and oral pathologies. In: Reiter AM, Gracis M, ed., BSAVA Manual of Canine and Feline Dentistry and Oral Surgery, 4th ed. Gloucester, UK: BSAVA, 2018, pp. 113–114.

Reiter AM, Gracis M. Management of dental and oral trauma. In: Reiter AM, Gracis M, ed., BSAVA Manual of Canine and Feline Dentistry and Oral Surgery, 4th ed. Gloucester, UK: BSAVA, 2018, pp. 220–222.

Ritter MJ, von Pfeil DJ, Stanley BJ, et al. Mandibular and sublingual sialocoeles in the dog: a retrospective evaluation of 41 cases, using the ventral approach for treatment. N Z Vet J 2006, 54(6):333–337.

Author Alexander M. Reiter

Consulting Editor Mark P. Rondeau

Acknowledgment The author and editors acknowledge the prior contribution of Susanne Lauer.

SALMON POISONING DISEASE

BASICS

OVERVIEW

- Infection with rickettsial organism *Neorickettsia helminthoeca*, an obligate intracellular pathogen that resides within trematode (fluke) vector *Nanophyetus salmincola*.
- Organism invades small intestinal epithelium and associated lymphoid tissue after ingestion of uncooked or undercooked fluke-infected salmonid fish; animal develops acute systemic illness with high fever, gastrointestinal signs.
- Geographically restricted to coastal regions of northern California, Oregon, Washington, southern British Columbia due to the geographic distribution of the *Oxytrema silicula*, intermediate host for trematode.

SIGNALMENT

- All ages; median 3 years old.
- Dogs of all breeds and sexes; intact male dogs and Labrador retrievers may be overrepresented.

SIGNS

- Inappetence.
- Lethargy.
- Fever (up to 107.6°F/42°C); terminal hypothermia may develop.
- Lymphadenopathy.
- Splenomegaly.
- Vomiting.
- Diarrhea, may contain melena or frank blood.
- Weight loss.
- Uncommonly, mental obtundation, cervical pain, twitching, seizures.

CAUSES & RISK FACTORS

- Residence in endemic area.
- Ingestion of uncooked or undercooked fish containing fluke metacercariae that harbor *N. helminthoeca*; salmonid fish (salmon and trout) most common; other freshwater fish can be infected.
- Any part of fish can be infected.
- Supermarket-bought fish have been implicated in some cases.
- Dogs from non-endemic areas can develop disease after ingesting transported fish.
- Infection also reported after swimming, without apparent fish ingestion.

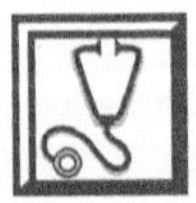

DIAGNOSIS

DIFFERENTIAL DIAGNOSIS

- Lymphoma.
- Toxicosis.
- Canine parvovirus type 2 infection.
- *Ehrlichia canis* infection.
- *Anaplasma phagocytophilum* infection.
- Canine distemper virus infection.
- Rocky Mountain spotted fever.
- Salmonellosis.
- Whipworm infestation.
- Pancreatitis.
- Hypoadrenocorticism.
- Disseminated cryptococcosis.

CBC/BIOCHEMISTRY/URINALYSIS

- Thrombocytopenia (90% of dogs), neutrophilia with a left shift, lymphopenia.
- Serum chemistry nonspecific—electrolyte abnormalities, hypoproteinemia, increased activity of alkaline phosphatase, hypocholesterolemia.
- Urinalysis—proteinuria, bilirubinuria.

OTHER LABORATORY TESTS

Some dogs have laboratory findings suggestive of disseminated intravascular coagulation.

IMAGING

Abdominal ultrasound—splenomegaly with mottled echotexture, abdominal lymphadenomegaly; fluid-distended intestinal loops with wall thickening, corrugation, hypermotility or hypomotility.

DIAGNOSTIC PROCEDURES

- Lymph node aspirates—increased numbers of histiocytes containing basophilic granular material in cytoplasm (rickettsial inclusions).
- Fecal examination—operculated eggs of trematode *N. salmincola*; using combination of centrifugal fecal flotation and fecal sedimentation maximizes sensitivity of test (sensitivity 93%).
- Where available, PCR assays for *N. helminthoeca* can be performed on lymph node aspirates or feces.

PATHOLOGIC FINDINGS

- Lymphoid tissue enlargement—tissues yellowish with prominent white foci.
- Petechial hemorrhages.
- Gastrointestinal tract thickening with white nodules.
- Intestinal contents—frequently contain free blood; flukes may not be grossly visible.
- Histopathology—depletion of lymph node follicles; infiltration of lymphoid tissues and intestinal submucosa by histiocytes; cytoplasm contains numerous lymphoid follicles; flukes may be found embedded in gastrointestinal mucosa.

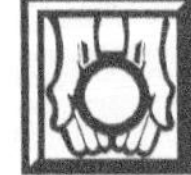

TREATMENT

- Inpatient—acutely ill patients.
- Supportive therapy—IV fluids with electrolytes; colloids or packed red blood cell transfusions may be needed; consider antiemetics and parenteral nutrition.

MEDICATIONS

DRUG(S) OF CHOICE

- Oxytetracycline 7.5–10 mg/kg IV q12h for 7–14 days.
- Doxycycline 5 mg/kg PO, IV q12h for 7–14 days.
- Praziquantel 10–30 mg/kg PO q24h for 1–2 days to kill flukes.

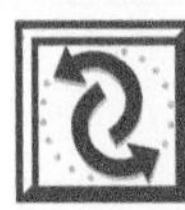

FOLLOW-UP

PATIENT MONITORING

Monitor hydration, electrolytes, acid–base balance, body temperature.

PREVENTION/AVOIDANCE

- Avoid feeding/eating improperly cooked fish.
- Inform client of necessity to act quickly; consider other dogs that may have eaten same raw fish.

EXPECTED COURSE AND PROGNOSIS

- Animals succumb within 5–10 days of infection unless treated.
- With early diagnosis and treatment—prognosis excellent. Animals without severe gastrointestinal signs show rapid clinical response to oral doxycycline (within 24–48 hours); dogs with severe gastrointestinal signs may require hospitalization and aggressive treatment for >1 week.
- Untreated—often fatal.

MISCELLANEOUS

ASSOCIATED CONDITIONS

Infection with *N. salmincola* does not itself cause severe clinical disease.

ZOONOTIC POTENTIAL

N. salmincola can cause gastrointestinal disturbances and eosinophilia in humans; *N. helminthoeca* does not cause human disease.

INTERNET RESOURCES

https://www.vetmed.wsu.edu/outreach/Pet-Health-Topics/categories/diseases/salmon-poisoning

Suggested Reading

Sykes JE. Salmon poisoning disease. In: Sykes JE, ed., Canine and Feline Infectious Diseases. St. Louis, MO: Elsevier Saunders, 2014, pp. 311–319.

Author Jane E. Sykes
Consulting Editor Amie Koenig

S

Salmonellosis

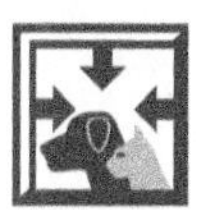

BASICS

DEFINITION

Infection caused by many different serotypes of *Salmonella*, causing enteritis, septicemia, and abortions.

PATHOPHYSIOLOGY

- *Salmonella*—Gram-negative bacterium; colonizes small intestine (ileum); adheres to and invades enterocytes; enters and multiplies in lamina propria and local mesenteric lymph nodes; cytotoxin and enterotoxin are produced; inflammation and prostaglandin synthesis ensue; results in secretory diarrhea, mucosal sloughing.
- Uncomplicated gastroenteritis—organisms are stopped at the mesenteric lymph node stage; patient has only diarrhea, vomiting, dehydration.
- Bacteremia and septicemia following gastroenteritis—more serious; focal extra-intestinal infections (abortion, joint disease) or endotoxemia may result; may cause thrombosis, disseminated intravascular coagulation (DIC), death.
- Some patients recover from septicemia but have prolonged recovery.

SYSTEMS AFFECTED

- Gastrointestinal—enterocolitis; inflammation, mucosal sloughing, secretory diarrhea.
- Systemic disease (e.g., bacteremia, focal infections, septicemia)—multiorgan infarction, thrombosis, abscesses, meningitis, osteomyelitis, abortion.

GENETICS

N/A

INCIDENCE/PREVALENCE

- True incidence unknown; prevalence in healthy dogs/cats similar to diarrheic animals.
- Most infections subclinical.
- Dogs—clinical disease most often seen in the young and pregnant bitches. Common in racing greyhounds and sled dogs due to raw meat diets; presence of *Salmonella* in feces does not necessarily imply infection.
- Cats—natural resistance; stressed, hospitalized, and shelter cats at risk. Pandemics of salmonellosis in migrating songbirds (usually *Salmonella* Typhimurium) in spring lead to epidemics in bird-hunting cats.
- Raw meat diet (especially chicken) risks—*Campylobacter* spp. in addition to *Salmonella* spp. and *Listeria spp.* Outbreaks linked to pet foods/treats common.

GEOGRAPHIC DISTRIBUTION

Worldwide

SIGNALMENT

Species

Dog and cat.

Mean Age and Range

- Dogs—neonatal/immature puppies, pregnant bitches. Most adult carrier dogs clinically normal.
- Cats—adults highly resistant unless treated with an antimicrobial prior to exposure.

SIGNS

General Comments

Disease severity—subclinical (carrier state, more common) to severe clinical cases in neonatal and stressed adult animals.

Historical Findings

- Diarrhea, can be hemorrhagic.
- Vomiting.
- Fever.
- Malaise.
- Anorexia.
- Vaginal discharge/abortion—dogs.
- Chronic febrile illness—persistent fever, anorexia, malaise without diarrhea.

Physical Examination Findings

- Asymptomatic carrier states—no clinical signs.
- Gastroenteritis—fever (102–104°F/39–40°C), diarrhea with mucus and/or blood, dehydration, abdominal pain, tenesmus, pale mucous membranes, weight loss.
- Gastroenteritis with bacteremia, septic shock, or endotoxemia—brick-red mucous membranes, tachycardia, bounding pulses, rapid capillary refill time (unless decompensatory shock), tachypnea, abdominal pain, weakness.
- Focal extraintestinal infections—conjunctivitis, cellulitis, pyothorax, diskospondylitis.
- Cats—chronic febrile illness, vague, nonspecific clinical signs.
- Recovering patients—chronic intermittent diarrhea for 3–4 weeks (may shed *Salmonella* in stool ≥6 weeks).

CAUSES

- Any one of more than 2,000 serotypes of salmonellae.
- Two or more simultaneous serotypes in host animal can occur:
  - Most common serotypes—Newport, Typhimurium, Albany, 4,5,12:i:, Dublin, Heidelberg.

RISK FACTORS

Disease Agent

- *Salmonella* serotype determines virulence, infectious dose, and route of exposure.
- Host factors that increase susceptibility:
  - Age—neonatal/young dogs and cats; immature immune system.
  - Health—debilitated young animals (immature gastrointestinal tract, poorly developed normal microbial flora) or adults with concurrent disease.
  - Disrupted gastrointestinal flora (adult cats)—antimicrobial treatment; exposure to salmonellae during hospitalization.

Environmental Factors

- Diet:
  - Raw food diet is major risk factor.
  - Contaminated dog treats (e.g., pig ears).
  - Dehydrated (dry) pet food; semi-moist foods usually not as risky.
- Coprophagia.
- Grooming habits—can contaminate environment, feed and water dishes.
- Dense population—colonies, boarding facilities, shelters:
  - Build up of *Salmonella* in environment, more efficient fecal–oral cycling.
  - Stress.
  - Exposure to infected (or carrier) animals.
- Unsanitary environment.

Hospitalized Animals

Nosocomial exposure (plus stress) or activation (by stress) of preexisting asymptomatic (carrier) *Salmonella* infection, especially in animals treated with antimicrobial drugs.

Vaccinated Cats

Death reported in kittens (likely to be subclinically infected by *Salmonella*) post vaccination, with high titers of modified live panleukopenia vaccine.

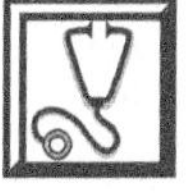

DIAGNOSIS

S

DIFFERENTIAL DIAGNOSIS

- Acute gastroenteritis—infectious, foreign body, neoplasia:
  - Viral gastroenteritis—canine enteric coronavirus, canine parvovirus, rotavirus, canine distemper.
  - Bacterial gastroenteritis—*Escherichia coli, Campylobacter jejuni, Yersinia enterocolitica.*
- Bacterial overgrowth syndrome—Clostridium difficile, C. perfringens.
- Parasites—helminths, protozoa (Giardia, Coccidia, Cryptosporidia), salmon poisoning.
- Acute gastritis—erosions or ulcers.
- Diet-related—allergy or food intolerance.
- Drug- or toxin-induced distress.
- Extraintestinal disorders (metabolic disease).

CBC/BIOCHEMISTRY/URINALYSIS

- CBC—variable; depends on stage of illness: initially neutropenia, left-shifted neutrophils, lymphopenia, thrombocytopenia, non-regenerative anemia.
- Hypoalbuminemia, electrolyte abnormalities related to gastrointestinal losses.

DIAGNOSTIC PROCEDURES

- Fecal/rectal bacterial culture—special media needed:
  - Subclinical carriers may have intermittent positive fecal culture (≥6 weeks).
  - Use of antimicrobials before sampling may yield false-negative culture.
  - Serotyping of cultured organisms—helpful to define outbreak.

SALMONELLOSIS (CONTINUED)

- Cultures of blood and joint fluid, ileum, mesenteric lymph node, liver/spleen, bone marrow.
- Fecal cytology—leukocytes present.
- Fecal *Salmonella* PCR.
- Abdominal ultrasound (clinical gastroenteritis)—lymphadenomegaly, enterocolitis, typhlitis, peritonitis.

PATHOLOGIC FINDINGS

Lymphoplasmacytic, neutrophilic typhlitis/enteritis with ulceration, crypt abscessation, lymphoid hyperplasia, pyogranulomas; lymphadenitis.

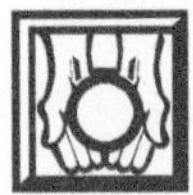

TREATMENT

APPROPRIATE HEALTH CARE

- Outpatient—uncomplicated gastroenteritis.
- Inpatient—with bacteremia/septicemia, gastroenteritis in neonatal/immature animals (rapidly debilitated).

NURSING CARE

- Varies according to severity of illness—assess dehydration, body weight, ongoing fluid loss, shock, hematocrit, albumin, electrolytes, acid–base status.
- Supportive care—fluid and electrolyte replacement:
  - Parenteral, balanced, polyionic isotonic replacement solution (lactated Ringer's).
  - Oral fluids—hypertonic glucose solutions; for secretory diarrhea.
- Plasma transfusions—if serum albumin <2 g/dL.

ACTIVITY

- Isolate patients.
- Cage rest, provide warmth during illness.

DIET

Restrict food 24 hours in adults; gradually introduce highly digestible, low-fat diet.

CLIENT EDUCATION

Instruct client to wash hands frequently and to restrict access to patient in acute stages of disease; large numbers of salmonellae may be shed in stool.

MEDICATIONS

DRUG(S) OF CHOICE

Asymptomatic Carrier State

- Antimicrobials—contraindicated:
  - Quinolones—clear carrier states in humans; controlled trials in animals needed before this can be recommended.

Uncomplicated Gastroenteritis

- Antimicrobials not indicated.
- Locally acting intestinal adsorbents and supportive therapy.

Neonates, Aged, and Debilitated Animals

- Antimicrobial therapy—indicated; culture and susceptibility testing with minimal inhibitory concentration recommended:
  - Trimethoprim-sulfa: 15 mg/kg PO, SC q12h.
  - Enrofloxacin: 5 mg/kg q24h (cat); 10 mg/kg PO, IM, q24h (dog).
  - Chloramphenicol: dogs, 50 mg/kg PO, IV, IM, SC q8h; cats, 50 mg/kg total PO, IV, IM, SC q12h.
- Recent strains of *Salmonella* are multidrug-resistant; adjust empirical therapy based on antimicrobial susceptibility testing.

PRECAUTIONS

- Chloramphenicol, trimethoprim-sulfa—use cautiously in neonatal and pregnant patients.
- Fluoroquinolones—avoid use in pregnant, neonatal, or growing animals because of concern for adverse effects on cartilage; do not administer to cats at dosages higher than 5 mg/kg q24h.

FOLLOW-UP

PATIENT MONITORING

- Fecal culture—repeat monthly for few months to assess development of carrier state.
- Other animals—monitor for secondary spread of infection.
- Advise client to contact veterinarian if patient shows signs of recurring disease.

PREVENTION/AVOIDANCE

- Keep animals healthy—proper nutrition; avoid raw meat diets; vaccinate for other infectious diseases; clean, disinfect cages, runs, and food/water dishes frequently; store food, feeding utensils properly.
- Reduce overcrowding.
- New arrivals—isolate and screen; monitor for sickness before mixing with other animals.
- Protect animals being treated with antimicrobial drugs from exposure to *Salmonella*-contaminated environment (e.g., animal hospital).
- Experimental live attenuated vaccine shows promise, especially for racing dogs.

POSSIBLE COMPLICATIONS

- Spread of infection to other animals or humans within household.
- Development of chronic infection with diarrhea.
- Recurrence of disease with stress.

EXPECTED COURSE AND PROGNOSIS

- Uncomplicated gastroenteritis—prognosis excellent; frequently self-limited; patients recover with good nursing care.
- Recovered animals may shed *Salmonella* intermittently for months or longer.
- Neonatal, aged, pregnant, stressed animals—can develop sepsis or abortion; can be severe, debilitating; may lead to death if untreated.

MISCELLANEOUS

AGE-RELATED FACTORS

Clinical disease is frequently seen in neonatal, or aged animals.

ZOONOTIC POTENTIAL

- High potential, especially in children, elderly, immunosuppressed, and antimicrobial drug users.
- Multidrug-resistant salmonellae have been reported.

PREGNANCY/FERTILITY/BREEDING

- May complicate disease.
- Abortion—may be a sequela to infection.
- Antimicrobial therapy—consider the effect on the fetus.

ABBREVIATIONS

- DIC = disseminated intravascular coagulation.

INTERNET RESOURCES

- http://www.cfsph.iastate.edu/DiseaseInfo/disease.php?name=salmonella-nontyphoidal&lang=en
- https://www.cdc.gov/healthypets/index.html

Suggested Reading

Marks S, Rankin S, Byrne B, et al. Enteropathogenic bacteria in dogs and cats: diagnosis, epidemiology, treatment, and control. J Vet Intern Med 2011, 25:1195–1208.

Author Patrick L. McDonough
Consulting Editor Amie Koenig

SALT TOXICOSIS

BASICS

DEFINITION

- Salt ingestion results in direct irritation to the gastrointestinal mucosa, causing vomiting, diarrhea, and anorexia. Polydipsia is a common early sign that hypernatremia is developing.
- Hypernatremia (typically Na^+ >170 mEq/L, dogs; >175 mEq/L, cats) may cause neurologic signs including lethargy, behavioral changes, ataxia, muscle tremors, and seizures. Coma and death may occur.
- LD_{50} (dogs) = 4 g NaCl/kg, <1 teaspoonful of table salt/kg body weight.

PATHOPHYSIOLOGY

- Hypernatremia causes water movement from intracellular space to extracellular space (interstitium and blood vessel), resulting in cellular shrinkage/dehydration.
- In the brain, this may cause the parenchyma to pull away from the skull, causing intracerebral and subarachnoid hemorrhage.
- In the lungs, fluid movement into the interstitial tissue may cause pulmonary edema.
- Idiogenic osmoles begin to develop intracellularly within hours to prevent cellular dehydration but take 1–7 days for full compensation.

SYSTEMS AFFECTED

- Gastrointestinal—vomiting, diarrhea, anorexia, polydipsia.
- Neuromuscular—twitching, muscle tremors, ataxia, seizures, coma.
- Pulmonary—edema, respiratory distress.
- Cardiovascular—hypervolemia, tachycardia.

INCIDENCE/PREVALENCE

With ingestion, gastrointestinal signs and mild hypernatremia are common but neurologic signs occur in severe cases.

GEOGRAPHIC DISTRIBUTION

N/A

SIGNALMENT

Species

Dogs and cats equally affected. There are no breed, age or sex predilections.

Mean Age and Range

N/A

Predominant Sex

N/A

SIGNS

- Severity of signs is dependent on sodium level.
- Mild—lethargy, vomiting, diarrhea, polydipsia ± polyuria.
- Severe—behavioral changes, twitching, muscle tremors, ataxia, seizures, coma, death.

Historical Findings

- Ingestion of homemade playdough or clay.
- Administration of salt as an emetic.
- Exposure to other forms of salt (i.e., rock salt, baking soda).
- Swimming in the ocean/ingestion of saltwater.

Physical Examination Findings

- Abnormal hydration:
  - Dehydration with vomiting and diarrhea.
  - Overhydration and hypervolemia with saltwater ingestion or secondary to treatment.
- Tachycardia.
- Ataxia, muscle weakness, muscle tremors.
- Hyperreflexia.

CAUSES

- Salt intake:
  - Salt ingestion—table salt, baking soda, salt for water softeners, deicing salt, ocean/saltwater.
  - Other products made with table salt—homemade or commercial playdough, ornament dough.
  - Iatrogenic with IV hypertonic saline or IV sodium bicarbonate; sodium phosphate enemas.
- Decreased water intake (typically chronic).
  - Adipsia.
  - No access to water.
- Free water loss:
  - Mannitol bolus or CRI causes free water loss via kidneys.
  - Activated charcoal with sorbitol (more common with multidose activated charcoal or high doses) causes free water loss via gastrointestinal tract.

RISK FACTORS

- Swimming in oceans and intake of saltwater.
- Outdoor pets with frozen or spilled water.
- Patients predisposed to dehydration—kidney disease, unregulated diabetes mellitus, central diabetes insipidus, chronic vomiting and diarrhea, hyperthermia/fever.

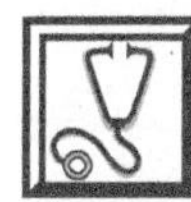

DIAGNOSIS

DIFFERENTIAL DIAGNOSIS

- Hypernatremic hyperosmolar nonketotic diabetes, chronic kidney disease, diabetes mellitus.
- Primary neurologic disease.
- Toxins that cause neurologic signs: (ethylene glycol, bromethalin, metaldehyde, baclofen, pyrethrins/pyrethroids, organophosphates/carbamates).
- Paintball ingestion

CBC/BIOCHEMISTRY/URINALYSIS

Biochemistry—hypernatremia, hyperchloremia, azotemia with dehydration, possible elevation of liver enzymes.

OTHER LABORATORY TESTS

CSF sodium concentration can be measured. Normal is 135–150 mEq/L; >180 mEq/L is consistent with salt toxicosis.

IMAGING

- Thoracic radiography if respiratory signs to evaluate for hypervolemia and signs of fluid overload and pulmonary edema.
- MRI or CT—evaluate for subarachnoid or cerebral hemorrhage.

DIAGNOSTIC PROCEDURES

CSF tap for sodium concentration (rarely performed) and rule out other causes for neurologic signs.

PATHOLOGIC FINDINGS

- Hemorrhage of stomach, small intestine, and colon.
- Cerebral edema, perivascular hemorrhage and fibrinous exudate.
- Pulmonary edema.
- Acute renal and hepatic necrosis.

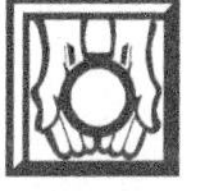

TREATMENT

APPROPRIATE HEALTH CARE

Hospitalization recommended for electrolyte monitoring.

NURSING CARE

Asymptomatic

- Decontamination with emesis if appropriate time frame.
- Monitor Na level in the hospital for 6 hours post exposure.
- If asymptomatic and Na remains normal, discharge patient to be monitored at home.

Symptomatic

- Stabilize neurologic signs as needed.
- Decontamination with emesis if indicated.
- IV fluids for rehydration. May need to match fluid Na content to patient serum Na depending on chronicity and degree of hypernatremia.
- Calculate free water replacement for hypernatremia:
  - IV use D_5W or 0.45% NaCl + 2.5% dextrose; use with caution in patients with hyperglycemia.
  - Water oral or via nasoesophageal tube—use for stable patients that are not vomiting or those with underlying cardiac disease/failure or evidence of fluid overload. Can be used with IV therapy.
  - Acute toxicity (<24 hours)—lower Na acutely (over 1–2 hours) until neurologic signs resolve, then replace remaining free water over 6–24 hours.
  - Chronic toxicity (>24 hours) or unknown time frame—lower Na slowly, not to exceed 12 mEq/day (0.5 mEq/h).

S

SALT TOXICOSIS (CONTINUED)

- Free water deficit calculation:
[(patient Na ÷ normal Na) − 1] × (0.6 × body weight$_{kg}$) × 1000 = Free water deficit in milliliters

DIET

Oral water can be offered to lower Na. Water intake should be regulated so that Na level does not drop too rapidly.

CLIENT EDUCATION

Outdoor pets may be susceptible to decreased intake with frozen or empty water containers or if they become trapped in a garage or shed. Heated water bowls and multiple water sources should be available.

SURGICAL CONSIDERATIONS

Gastrotomy may be needed to remove homemade playdough or ornament dough if unable to remove with emesis or gastric lavage.

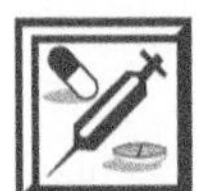

MEDICATIONS

DRUG(S) OF CHOICE

- Antiemetic for vomiting—maropitant 1 mg/kg SC or IV q24h.
- Proton pump inhibitor if signs of stomach mucosal irritation:
  - Pantoprazole 1 mg/kg IV slowly q24h.
  - Omeprazole 1 mg/kg PO q24h.
- Methocarbamol 55–220 mg/kg IV slowly, to effect for muscle tremors; do not exceed 330 mg/kg/day.
- Anticonvulsant such as diazepam 0.5–2 mg/kg IV for seizures.
- Furosemide 1–4 mg/kg IV q2–8h or a CRI 0.1–0.5 mg/kg/h IV titrated to effect for hypervolemia or pulmonary edema until signs resolve.

CONTRAINDICATIONS

Activated charcoal—will worsen hypernatremia.

PRECAUTIONS

- Mannitol, hypertonic saline, and sodium bicarbonate should be used with caution as they may worsen hypernatremia.
- Diuretics such as furosemide may be helpful for Na excretion via the kidney but hydration status needs to be monitored carefully.
- Hyponatremia or rapid correction of chronic hypernatremia (due to idiogenic osmole formation) during treatment can cause cerebral edema formation and worsening or reoccurrence of neurologic signs.

ALTERNATIVE DRUG(S)

N/A

FOLLOW-UP

PATIENT MONITORING

- Sodium level should be monitored during treatment; frequency depends on severity of signs and chronicity of hypernatremia but generally every 2–4 hours.
- Hydration status monitored every 4–6 hours.

PREVENTION/AVOIDANCE

Salt should not be recommended or given as an emetic.

POSSIBLE COMPLICATIONS

Persistent neurologic impairment with severe toxicity.

EXPECTED COURSE AND PROGNOSIS

- Neurologic signs should improve with improvement of Na level.
- Prognosis is generally good. Guarded to poor prognosis with severe neurologic signs and poor response to treatment.

MISCELLANEOUS

PREGNANCY/FERTILITY/BREEDING

N/A

SYNONYMS

Hypernatremia

Suggested Reading

Barr JM, Khan SA, Safdar A, et al. Hypernatremia secondary to homemade play dough ingestion in dogs: a review of 14 cases from 1998–2001. J Vet Emerg Crit Care 2013, 14(3):196–202.

DiBartola SP. Disorders of sodium and water: hypernatremia and hyponatremia. In: Fluid, Electrolyte and Acid-Base Disorders in Small Animal Practice, 4th ed. St. Louis, MO: Elsevier- Saunders, 2012, pp. 45–79.

Guillaumin J, DiBartola SP. Disorders of sodium and water homeostasis. Vet Clin Small Anim 2017, 47:293–312.

Author Katherine L. Peterson

Consulting Editor Lynn R. Hovda

SARCOPTIC MANGE

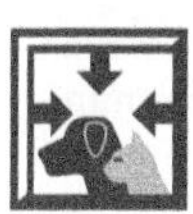

BASICS

OVERVIEW

A nonseasonal, intensely pruritic, highly contagious parasitic skin disease of dogs and other mammalian species caused by *Sarcoptes scabiei* var. *canis* mites.

PATHOPHYSIOLOGY

Burrowing mites induce hypersensitivity, causing intense pruritus.

SYSTEMS AFFECTED

Skin/exocrine

SIGNALMENT

- All in-contact dogs usually affected.
- Transient pruritus of in-contact other species: cats, humans.

SIGNS

- Nonseasonal, progressively worsening intense pruritus.
- Pruritus develops within 4–6 weeks of exposure.
- Seroconversion 3 weeks after clinical signs develop.
- Rare individuals do not seroconvert and therefore may not develop severe pruritus.
- Elbows, pinnal margins, ventrum, and hocks affected first.
- Crusted papules leading to generalized alopecia, crusting, and excoriations; lichenification and thickening with chronicity.
- Poor response to antihistamines and anti-inflammatory doses of steroids.
- Mite numbers often low.
- Immunocompromised individuals may harbor larger numbers of mites.

CAUSES & RISK FACTORS

- Close contact with other dogs in animal shelters, boarding kennels, groomers, dog parks, and veterinary offices.
- Exposure to fox or coyote.

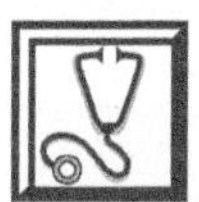

DIAGNOSIS

DIFFERENTIAL DIAGNOSIS

- Hypersensitivity dermatitis.
- Bacterial folliculitis.
- Parasitic dermatitis (demodicosis, *Pelodera*, *Otodectes*, *Cheyletiella*, *Trombicula*, *Dirofilaria*).
- Dermatophytosis.
- *Malassezia* dermatitis.
- Zinc-responsive dermatosis.
- Ear margin seborrhea.
- Pemphigus foliaceus.

OTHER LABORATORY TESTS

ELISA—available in some countries to identify *Sarcoptes*-infested dogs: False positives due to crossreactivity with other mites.

DIAGNOSTIC PROCEDURES

- Pinnal–pedal reflex—rubbing the ear margin between the thumb and forefinger induces the dog to scratch with its hind leg.
- Superficial skin scrapings—positive in 20–50% of scabies cases; false-negative results are common.
- Fecal flotation—may reveal mites or ova.
- Response to scabicidal treatment—most common method for diagnosing scabies.

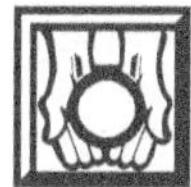

TREATMENT

- All in-contact dogs must be treated.
- Resolution of pruritis may take several weeks due to hypersensitivity reaction to the mite.
- *Sarcoptes* mites usually die quickly in the environment; however, mites have been reported to survive for up to 3 weeks. Thorough cleaning of the dog's environment is recommended in crowded conditions.

MEDICATIONS

DRUG(S) OF CHOICE

- Selamectin—labeled application every 30 days, or application every 2 weeks for at least three treatments.
- Isoxazoline parasiticides (afoxalaner, lotilaner, fluralaner or sarolaner)-at labeled dosage/frequency.
- Ivermectin 0.2–0.4 mg/kg SC or PO every 1–2 weeks.
- Milbemycin 2 mg/kg PO every 1–2 weeks.
- Doramectin 0.2–0.6 mg/kg SC or PO weekly.
- Moxidectin 0.2–0.3 mg/kg SC or PO weekly; with imidacloprid topical at labeled frequency.
- Lime sulfur 2–4% applied weekly for 4–6 weeks.
- Fipronil spray applied to entire skin surface every 2 weeks for three treatments.
- Topical antiseborrheic therapy in conjunction with scabicidal therapy.
- Systemic antibiotics—may be needed to resolve secondary pyoderma.
- Prednisolone 1 mg/kg for 5–7 days or longer if necessary to relieve pruritus and self-mutilation.

CONTRAINDICATIONS/POSSIBLE INTERACTIONS

- Ivermectin—do not use/use with caution in *ABCB1* mutant dogs; increased risk of avermectin toxicity in herding breeds: Shetland sheepdogs, Old English sheepdogs, Australian shepherd dogs, and their crosses.
- Potential increased risk of neurotoxicosis with concurrent use of spinosad, macrocyclic lactone, or systemic azole medications.
- Isoxazoline parasiticides—potential for neurologic adverse events in dogs and cats reported.

FOLLOW-UP

- Response to therapy may require 4–6 weeks.
- Topical scabicidal treatments are more prone to failure because of incomplete application of the treatment solution.
- Immunity or tolerance does not develop: reinfection may occur with subsequent contact with infected animals.
- Approximately 30% of dogs with *Sarcoptes* infections will also react to house dust mite antigens on intradermal tests. House dust mite allergy may be a sequela to scabies infection.

MISCELLANEOUS

ZOONOTIC POTENTIAL

- Sarcoptic mange is zoonotic. People in close contact with an affected dog may develop a pruritic, papular rash on body areas in frequent contact with dogs.
- Lesions resolve spontaneously when the affected animals are treated.

ABBREVIATIONS

- ELISA = enzyme-linked immunosorbent assay.

Suggested Reading

Becskei C, De Bock F, Illambas J, Cherni JA et al. Efficacy and safety of novel oral isoxazoline, sarolaner (Simparica™) for the treatment of sarcoptic mange in dogs. Vet Parasitol 2016, 222:56–61.

Beugnet F, de Vos C, Liebenberg J, Halos H, et al. Efficacy of afoxolaner in a clinical field study in dogs naturally infested with *Sarcoptes scabiei*. Parasite 2016, 23:26.

Fourie LJ, Heine J, Horak IG. The efficacy of an imidacloprid/moxidectin combination against naturally acquired *Sarcoptes scabiei* on dogs. Australian Vet J 2006, 84:17–21.

Lower KS, Medleau L, Hnilica KA. Evaluation of an enzyme-linked immunosorbent assay (ELISA) for the serological diagnosis of sarcoptic mange in dogs. Vet Dermatol 2001, 12:315–320.

Romero C, Heredia R, Pineda J, et al. Efficacy of fluralaner in 17 dogs with sarcoptic mange. Vet Dermatol 2016, 27(5):353–e88.

Author Liora Waldman

Consulting Editor Alexander H. Werner Resnick

SCHIFF–SHERRINGTON PHENOMENON

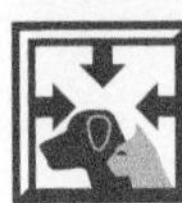

BASICS

OVERVIEW

- Thoracic limb extension associated with pelvic limb paralysis or paresis after acute and usually severe spinal cord lesion caudal to the cervical intumescence, best observed when the patient is in lateral recumbency.
- Posture—caused by damage to the border cells or their ascending processes, which are interneurons located in the lumbar spinal cord (mainly L2–4) and normally inhibit the extensor motor neurons of the cervical intumescence.

SIGNALMENT

Any dog suffering from thoracolumbar spinal cord injury.

SIGNS

- Thoracic limbs—rigidly extended; normal gait and postural reactions (because the lesion is caudal to the cervical intumescence).
- Pelvic limbs—depends on the severity and location of the lesion; usually upper motor neuron in type, but may be lower motor neuron.
- In severe, acute thoracolumbar myelopathies, spinal shock may be present in addition to the Schiff–Sherrington phenomenon: there is an initial flaccid paralysis caudal to the level of the lesion, with loss of myotatic and flexor reflexes. In dogs and cats, spinal shock is uncommon and usually resolves within an hour, with more typical signs of upper motor neuron disease subsequently developing caudal to the spinal cord lesion.

S

CAUSES & RISK FACTORS

- Trauma secondary to vehicular accident and intervertebral disc disease—most common.
- Vascular myelopathies (e.g., fibrocartilaginous embolism, coagulopathies, etc.).

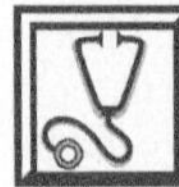

DIAGNOSIS

DIFFERENTIAL DIAGNOSIS

- Decerebrate rigidity—observed with brainstem disease in which all four limbs are rigid and have upper motor neuron dysfunction; opisthotonus present; patient is unconscious.
- Decerebellate rigidity—observed with cerebellar disease in which the forelimbs are rigid but the hind limbs are flexed; consciousness is usually altered.
- Cervical spinal cord injury—may have extensor hypertonia in the thoracic limbs; upper motor neuron and proprioceptive deficits of all four limbs are also seen.
- The key feature in differential diagnosis is that in the Schiff–Sherrington phenomenon, function and postural reactions in the forelimbs are normal despite their extensor rigidity, while they are abnormal in the pelvic limbs.

CBC/BIOCHEMISTRY/URINALYSIS

N/A

IMAGING

Radiology (radiography, myelography, CT, MRI)—demonstrate the thoracolumbar spinal lesion.

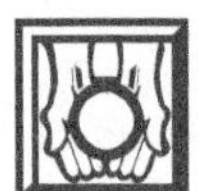

TREATMENT

- Directed toward the underlying thoracolumbar spinal cord lesion.
- No specific treatment available.
- Condition resolves if adequate spinal cord function is restored.
- Schiff–Sherrington phenomenon is not a prognostic indicator; prognosis is determined by the severity of signs caudal to the spinal cord lesion.

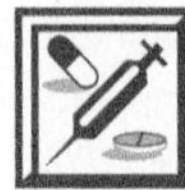

MEDICATIONS

DRUG(S) OF CHOICE

As indicated for underlying spinal cord disease.

FOLLOW-UP

- Posture may persist for days to weeks; not an indication of a hopeless prognosis.
- With rapid and aggressive treatment, the patient may recover, especially if there is pain perception caudal to the lesion.

MISCELLANEOUS

Suggested Reading

Dewey CW. Functional and dysfunctional neuroanatomy: the key to lesion localization. In: Dewey CW, ed., A Practical Guide to Canine and Feline Neurology, 2nd ed. Ames, IA: Wiley-Blackwell, 2008, p. 41.

Author Stephanie Kube

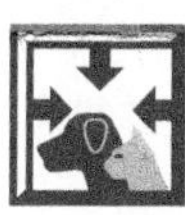

BASICS

OVERVIEW

Schwannomas are tumors of nerve sheath origin, arising from Schwann cells. The term peripheral nerve sheath tumor encompasses schwannomas, neurofibromas, and neurofibrosarcomas, as these tumors arise from the same cell. Importantly, schwannomas are grouped with several other soft tissue sarcomas (e.g., hemangiopericytoma and fibrosarcoma) for therapeutic and prognostic purposes, as the biologic behaviors of this group of tumors are similar.

SIGNALMENT

- Dogs—median of 10 years, no sex predisposition, no known breed predilection.
- Cats rarely affected.

SIGNS

Vary depending on tumor location, which can be peripheral (e.g., skin or tongue) or more central (e.g., axillary region).

CAUSES & RISK FACTORS

None identified.

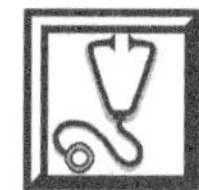

DIAGNOSIS

DIFFERENTIAL DIAGNOSIS

- Other neoplasia that can involve the connective tissues.
- Orthopedic disease.
- Other neurologic disease (e.g., intervertebral disc disease).

CBC/BIOCHEMISTRY/URINALYSIS

Results usually normal.

OTHER LABORATORY TESTS

None

IMAGING

- Myelography may be helpful in cases with dorsal or ventral nerve root involvement.
- Contrast CT or, ideally, MRI provides the most information regarding extent and location of disease.

DIAGNOSTIC PROCEDURES

Electromyography consistently reveals abnormal, spontaneous electrical activity in muscles of the affected limb.

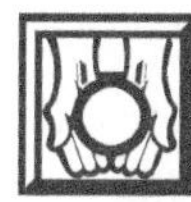

TREATMENT

- Surgical excision is the treatment of choice.
- Radiotherapy following incomplete surgical resection is likely to result in excellent long-term outcome.
- Excision of a distal mass may still result in a functional limb; amputation is required in most cases.
- Radiotherapy as a single treatment modality shows promise for small lesions.
- Laminectomy is necessary in cases of nerve root involvement; local recurrence is common if the primary extends into the spinal canal.

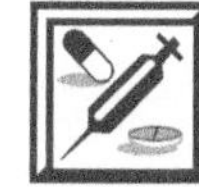

MEDICATIONS

DRUG(S) OF CHOICE

- Chemotherapy—no successful chemotherapeutic management has been described.
- Corticosteroid therapy—may help to reduce peritumoral edema and temporarily relieve clinical signs.
- Gabapentin for neuropathic pain alleviation.

CONTRAINDICATIONS/POSSIBLE INTERACTIONS

N/A

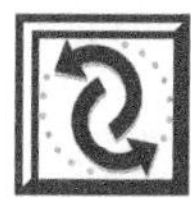

FOLLOW-UP

EXPECTED COURSE AND PROGNOSIS

- Recurrence common following incomplete surgical excision (up to 72% of cases).
- The more distal the tumor, the better the possibility of a surgical cure.
- For tumors involving the brachial or lumbosacral plexus, median disease-free interval is 7.5 months.
- For tumors involving dorsal or ventral nerve roots, median disease-free interval is 1 month.
- High-histologic-grade tumors (e.g., grade 3) may metastasize to regional lymph nodes or lung.

MISCELLANEOUS

Suggested Reading

Chase D, Bray J, Ide A, Polton G. Outcome following removal of canine spindle cell tumours in first opinion practice: 104 cases. J Small Anim Pract 2009, 50:568–574.

Hansen KS, Zwingenberger AL, Theon AP, et al. Treatment of MRI-Diagnosed Trigeminal Peripheral Nerve Sheath Tumors by Stereotactic Radiotherapy in Dog. J Vet Intern Med 2016;30:1112–1120.

Author Ruthanne Chun

Consulting Editor Timothy M. Fan

SEBACEOUS ADENITIS, GRANULOMATOUS

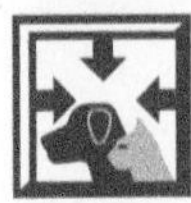

BASICS

OVERVIEW

- A destructive inflammatory disease process directed against cutaneous adnexal structures (sebaceous glands).
- May be genetically inherited, immune-mediated, or metabolic.
- Initial defect—a keratinization disorder or an abnormality in lipid metabolism (accumulation of toxic intermediate metabolites).

SYSTEMS AFFECTED

Skin/exocrine

SIGNALMENT

- Young adult to middle-aged dogs; very rare in cats.
- Two forms—long- and short-coated breeds (short-coated form now called "idiopathic pyogranulomatous periadnexal dermatitis").
- Predisposed—standard poodle, Akita, Samoyed, German shepherd dog, Havanese, Bernese Mountain dog and vizsla.

SIGNS

Long-Coated Breeds

- Symmetrical, partial alopecia.
- Dull, brittle hair.
- Tightly adherent silver-white scale.
- Follicular casts around hair shaft ("keratin-collaring").
- Small tufts of matted hair.
- Lesions—often first observed along dorsal midline and dorsum of the head.
- Severe—secondary bacterial folliculitis, pruritus, and malodor.
- Akitas—often relatively severely affected; morbidity associated with deep secondary bacterial infections.
- Standard poodles—affected dogs frequently described as having excellent hair coats prior to developing lesions; secondary bacterial folliculitis rare; most patients do not exhibit systemic illness.

Short-Coated Breeds

- Alopecia—moth-eaten, circular, or diffuse.
- Mild scaling.
- Lesions often plaque-like.
- Affects the trunk, head, and pinnae.
- Secondary bacterial folliculitis rare.
- Lesions can produce significant scarring.

CAUSES & RISK FACTORS

- Mode of inheritance is being studied; an autosomal recessive mode of inheritance is documented in the standard poodle and suspected in the Akita.
- Multiple pathophysiologic causes theorized including autoimmunity against sebaceous glands and/or leakage of sebaceous gland contents into surrounding dermis causing an inflammatory reaction and eventual destruction of glands.
- Destruction of sebaceous glands may be secondary—"innocent bystander" from other inflammatory conditions.

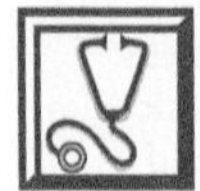

DIAGNOSIS

DIFFERENTIAL DIAGNOSIS

- Primary seborrhea—keratinization disorder.
- Bacterial folliculitis.
- Demodicosis.
- Dermatophytosis.
- Pemphigus foliaceus.
- Endocrine skin disease.

CBC/BIOCHEMISTRY/URINALYSIS

N/A

DIAGNOSTIC PROCEDURES

- Skin scrapings—normal.
- Dermatophyte culture—negative.
- Endocrine function tests—normal.
- Skin biopsy.

PATHOLOGIC FINDINGS

- Nodular granulomatous to pyogranulomatous inflammatory reaction at the level of the sebaceous glands.
- Orthokeratotic hyperkeratosis and follicular cast formation; more prominent in long-coated breeds.
- Advanced—complete loss of sebaceous glands; periadnexal fibrosis.
- Destruction of entire hair follicle and adnexal unit rare.

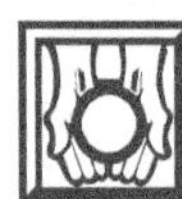

TREATMENT

- Clinical signs may wax and wane irrespective of treatment.
- Controlled studies have not been done to document efficacy of any therapy.
- Results extremely variable; response may depend on severity of disease at the time of diagnosis.
- Akita—breed most refractory to treatment.

MEDICATIONS

DRUG(S) OF CHOICE

- Propylene glycol and water—50–75% mixture; spray every 24 hours to affected areas.
- Baby oil—soak affected areas for 1 hour; follow with multiple shampoos to remove oil and scales; used monthly or as needed to reduce severe accumulations of crusts.
- Frequent bathing with keratolytic shampoos (twice weekly).
- EFA supplementation and evening primrose oil (500 mg PO q12h); possible side effects include vomiting, diarrhea, and flatulence.
- Cyclosporine 5 mg/kg PO q12–24h; side effects include vomiting, diarrhea, gingival hyperplasia, hirsutism, papillomatous skin lesions, increased incidence of infections, nephrotoxicity, and hepatotoxicity.
- Doxycycline 5 mg/kg PO q12h and niacinamide 250 mg PO q8h, <10 kg; 500 mg PO q8h >10 kg with vitamin E.
- Isotretinoin (Accutane) 1 mg/kg PO q12h; reduce to 1 mg/kg q24h after 1 month and to 1 mg/kg q48h after 2 months; continue as needed for maintenance; rarely used.
- Bactericidal antibiotics for secondary bacterial folliculitis.

CONTRAINDICATIONS/POSSIBLE INTERACTIONS

Isotretinoin (Accutane)—known teratogen; do not use in pregnant dogs; advise owners of risk.

FOLLOW-UP

Affected dogs should be registered so that mode of inheritance can be determined.

MISCELLANEOUS

Suggested Reading

Gross TL, Ihrke PJ, Walder EJ. Skin Diseases of the Dog and Cat: Clinical and Histopathologic Diagnosis. Oxford, UK: Blackwell Science, 2005.

Helton Rhodes KA, Werner A. Blackwell's Five-Minute Veterinary Consult: Clinical Companion: Small Animal Dermatology, 3rd ed. Hoboken, NJ: Wiley-Blackwell, 2018.

Mecklenburg L, Linek M, Tobin DJ. Hair Loss Disorders in Domestic Animals. Ames, IA: Wiley-Blackwell, 2009.

Muller and Kirk's Small Animal Dermatology, 7th ed. St. Louis, MO: Elsevier, 2013.

Author Guillermina Manigot

Consulting Editor Alexander H. Werner Resnick

Acknowledgment The author and editors acknowledge the prior contribution of Karen Helton Rhodes.

S

SEIZURES (CONVULSIONS, STATUS EPILEPTICUS)—CATS

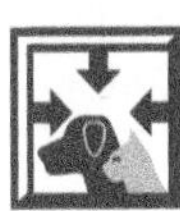

BASICS

DEFINITION

• Epilepsy—recurrence of seizures from primary brain origin. • Genetic epilepsy—syndrome that is only epilepsy, with no demonstrable underlying brain lesion or other neurologic signs; the genetic origin must be proven through family studies, gene isolation, or other specific forms of evidence (International League Against Epilepsy); rare in cats.
• Structural epilepsy—syndrome in which the epileptic seizures are the result of identifiable structural brain lesions; frequent in cats. • Epilepsy of unknown cause—structural epilepsy suspected but a lesion cannot be demonstrated; frequent in cats.
• Cluster seizures—>1 seizure/24 hours.
• Status epilepticus (SE)—continuous seizure activity, or seizures repeated at brief intervals without complete recovery between seizures. Can be nonconvulsive. • Convulsive SE—life-threatening medical emergency.

PATHOPHYSIOLOGY

• Paroxysmal disorganization of one or several brain functions originating from the thalamocortex. Any thalamocortical disturbance or disease process may lead to seizure activity. • Not all cortical regions have the same propensity to seize; from the most to the least likely to cause seizures—temporal, frontal, parietal, and occipital lobes. • As more seizures occur, the tendency for neuronal damage and propensity for more seizures or SE increases; this kindling effect does not occur in all cortical regions. • The clinical appearance of the seizure is directly related to the location of the neuronal hyperactivity. If the electrical abnormality remains regional, the seizure is focal. If there is recruitment of both hemispheres, the seizure is generalized.
• Great majority of seizures and SE in cats are secondary to structural brain lesions.

SYSTEMS AFFECTED

Nervous

INCIDENCE/PREVALENCE

Unknown

GEOGRAPHIC DISTRIBUTION

Worldwide

SIGNALMENT

Cats of any breed, age, or sex.

SIGNS

General Comments

• Nonconvulsive generalized seizures—frequent in cats; movements of facial musculature predominate, such as bilateral twitches of eyelids, whiskers and ears, salivation, lip smacking; may be associated with whole body trembling/shaking, piloerection, dilated pupils. Nonconvulsive SE frequent in cats.
• Focal seizure—when limited to one hemisphere; frantic running and colliding with objects (aura), unilateral facial twitches or eyelid blinks, unilateral limb motions or head/neck turning to one side. Focal seizures often generalize. • Generalized convulsive seizures—bilateral symmetrical tonic–clonic contractions of limb muscles and dorsiflexion of the head, often associated with autonomic signs such as salivation, urination, defecation. At time of admission, the gross motor activity may have stopped, but there may still be twitching of the lids and body/limb jerks. • Mutilation frequent—biting of tongue, nail avulsion.

Historical Findings

• Confirm that seizure activity has indeed occurred. • Pattern of seizures (age at seizure onset, type and frequency of seizures)—most important factor in listing the possible causes.
• Metabolic diseases may cause generalized seizures (GS). • With most seizurogenic toxins, there is a crescendo of hyperexcitability, shaking, trembling, with ultimately GS and death. • Asymmetry in the signs (eyelid twitches, limb movements primarily on one side, circling) before, during, or after the seizure suggests focal cortical lesion.
• Overdose of insulin, postrenal transplant, or bilateral thyroidectomy lead to GS shortly after the fact. • Presence of abnormal behavior in the days/weeks preceding the seizure activity indicates structural brain disease.
• Presence of concomitant gastrointestinal (GI), respiratory, or other systemic signs indicates multisystem disease.

Physical Examination Findings

• If chorioretinitis present, look for infectious diseases. • Dark red mucous membranes suggest polycythemia vera.

Neurologic Examination Findings

• Mental status, menace responses, responses to nasal septum stimulation, and proprioceptive positioning are neurologic tests that evaluate the cerebral cortex. Asymmetry indicates structural brain lesion on the contralateral side of the deficits. • In most cases of structural epilepsy, neurologic deficits are present at presentation.

CAUSES

Extracranial

Metabolic—hypoglycemia from insulin overdose, hypocalcemia from bilateral thyroidectomy, severe hyperthyroidism, hypertension secondary to renal transplant, hepatic encephalopathy, uremia, polycythemia vera, severe hypertriglyceridemia.

Toxins; Intracranial

• Anatomic—congenital malformation.
• Metabolic—cell storage disease (e.g., neuronal ceroid–lipofuscinosis reported in one cat with myoclonus and seizure activity).
• Neoplastic—meningioma, astrocytoma, lymphoma. • Inflammatory infectious—viral non-feline infectious peritonitis (FIP), FIP, toxoplasmosis, cryptococcosis. • Toxicity—organochlorines, pyrethrins, and pyrethroids; seizures usually observed at end stage; chlorambucil in lymphoma treatment.
• Vascular—polycythemia vera secondary to hyperviscosity, feline ischemic encephalopathy secondary to *Cuterebra* larva. • Trauma has not been linked to seizures in cats.

RISK FACTORS

• Any forebrain lesion. • Diabetes mellitus.
• Treatment with chlorambucil. • Renal failure.

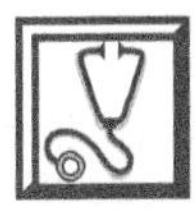

DIAGNOSIS

DIFFERENTIAL DIAGNOSIS

• Sleep disorders—the cat does not wake up, or has a normal waking behavior following the episode. • Syncope—the body is limp with a rapid recovery phase, with no abnormal behavior. • When seizures are preceded by 2–3 weeks of vague transient systemic illness (decreased appetite, GI signs) in an otherwise healthy cat—viral non-FIP encephalitis or epilepsy of unknown cause.
• When seizures are preceded by systemic signs that persist (>3 weeks)—FIP, cryptococcosis. • Insidious abnormal behavior with/without circling in a cat >10 years old presented for seizure activity suggests meningioma. • Cats with hepatic encephalopathy drool excessively. • Cats with polycythemia vera have GI signs and dark mucous membranes.

S

CBC/BIOCHEMISTRY/URINALYSIS

• Extracranial metabolic causes are diagnosed on history, physical examination, and blood test results. • High packed cell volume (>60%) in polycythemia vera. • Low blood glucose in insulin overdose. • Low calcium in bilateral post thyroidectomy. • High BUN and creatinine with low specific gravity in acute renal failure. • Creatine kinase—mild to markedly elevated in cats with SE, even nonconvulsive; with or without myoglobulinuria; indicates muscle necrosis.

OTHER LABORATORY TESTS

• Serologic testing—feline immunodeficiency virus, feline leukemia virus titers often noncontributory to diagnosis; FIP and *Toxoplasma gondii* titers nonreliable by themselves. • Bile acid testing—in cats with suspected hepatic encephalopathy.

IMAGING

• Thoracic radiographs and abdominal ultrasound—if infectious disease suspected; to evaluate lung pathology if SE; to look for neoplasia if tumor suspected. • MRI—best to define location, extent, and nature of lesion.

SEIZURES (CONVULSIONS, STATUS EPILEPTICUS)—CATS (CONTINUED)

DIAGNOSTIC PROCEDURES

CSF—sensitive to detect structural disease; unspecific in itself to reach diagnosis except when organism is seen (e.g., cryptococcosis).

PATHOLOGIC FINDINGS

• Findings reflect etiology. • It is unknown if hippocampal necrosis is a cause or the consequence of seizures. • Small lesions may be easily missed in cats diagnosed with epilepsy of unknown cause.

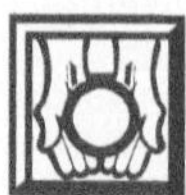

TREATMENT

APPROPRIATE HEALTH CARE

• Outpatient—isolated recurrent seizures in an otherwise healthy cat. • Inpatient—cluster seizures and SE. Isolated recurrent seizures in an ill cat.

NURSING CARE

• Constant supervision. • Install IV line for drug and fluid administration. • Draw blood for rapid measurement of blood gases, glucose, calcium, and antiepileptic drug levels if pertinent. • Cool if hyperthermia.

CLIENT EDUCATION

Antiepileptic treatment in structural epilepsy may not help until the primary cause is addressed. Seizures can be difficult to stop in cases of SE, especially with nonconvulsive status.

SURGICAL CONSIDERATIONS

Craniotomy—tumor excision with meningioma or other accessible mass.

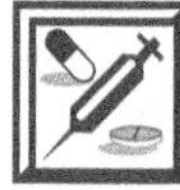

MEDICATIONS

DRUG(S) OF CHOICE

Seizure type and frequency determine therapeutic approach.

Isolated Recurrent Generalized Seizures

• First line—phenobarbital 7.5–15 mg/cat q12h; optimal therapeutic serum levels 100–130 μmol/L (23–30 μg/L). • Second line—gabapentin 3–8 mg/cat q8–12h. • Levetiracetam—20 mg/kg q8h (serum levels humans 10–40 μg/mL). • Initiate gradually to avoid overt sedation.

Convulsive Cluster and Status Epilepticus

• Treat cluster and generalized SE early—the more seizures in a given time, and the more drugs for seizure control, time for recovery, and cost for treatment. • No ongoing seizure activity at presentation and patient naïve to the drug—phenobarbital IV bolus 10 mg/kg to a maximum of 60 mg/cat over 15 minutes, continued with phenobarbital maintenance dosage PO 12 hours later. • Ongoing seizure activity at presentation—diazepam IV bolus 0.5–1 mg/kg, continuing with CRI at 0.25–0.5 mg/cat/h in an inline burette using a fluid pump; IV bolus of diazepam can be repeated 5 minutes after the first bolus if gross seizure activity persists; in this case, add phenobarbital to CRI at 4 mg/cat/h. • Start oral phenobarbital at maintenance dose as soon as patient can swallow. • After 6 hours seizures-free, wean CRI gradually over 4–6 hours.

Persistent Seizures

Subanesthetic doses of IV propofol 1–3.5 mg/kg bolus and 0.01–0.25 mg/kg/minute CRI titrated to effect.

Non-Antiepileptic Drug Treatment

• Dexamethasone 0.25 mg/kg IV q24h for 1–3 days, to improve edema secondary to SE and treat the primary cause if systemic infectious disease is not suspected; dexamethasone alters CSF results.
• Thiamine—5–50 mg/cat in any cat presented with acute neurologic signs, including seizures.

CONTRAINDICATIONS

• Do not use KBr in cats; side effects include life-threatening respiratory disease. • Avoid giving aminophylline, theophylline, ketamine, and fentanyl to epileptic cats.

PRECAUTIONS

• Prolonged use of propofol (>24 hours) may cause Heinz body anemia in cats. • Cats on CRI of antiepileptic drug(s) are often overtly sedated; cardiovascular and respiratory depression may occur; close monitoring necessary; lubricate eyes, express bladder manually, correct hypothermia. • Close monitoring necessary to observe if mild ongoing seizure activity persists.

POSSIBLE INTERACTIONS

N/A

ALTERNATIVE DRUG(S)

• Zonisamide—5–10 mg/kg PO q24h (serum levels humans 15–45 μg/mL).
• Diazepam—0.5–2.0 mg/kg/day PO divided q12h.

FOLLOW-UP

PATIENT MONITORING

• CBC, biochemistry, urinalysis prior to initiating antiepileptic drug. • Phenobarbital-induced hepatotoxicity is not a problem in the cat. • Creatine kinase to evaluate muscular necrosis and indirectly subtle ongoing seizure activity in cats presented in SE. • Measure phenobarbital serum level 2 weeks after initiation; correct dosage accordingly; it is difficult to titrate phenobarbital in cats, i.e., a mild increase in dosage often leads to a major increment of the serum levels. • CBC and biochemistry—repeat every 6–12 months. • If structural epileptic patient has recovered from primary disease and remains seizure-free for 6 months—seizures may recur when drug is weaned off.

POSSIBLE COMPLICATIONS

• SE—seizure control may not be reached despite polypharmacy. • Rare hypersensitivity to phenobarbital—thrombocytopenia, neutropenia, pruritus, swollen feet; do CBC 4–6 weeks after onset of phenobarbital.
• Diazepam rarely may cause acute hepatic necrosis and death. • Cardiovascular and respiratory collapse from overdose during SE treatment.

EXPECTED COURSE AND PROGNOSIS

• Depends on the underlying cause and response to treatment. • Cats with epilepsy of unknown cause have good long-term prognosis.
• Cats can recover despite episode of severe cluster-seizures and generalized SE.

MISCELLANEOUS

AGE-RELATED FACTORS

Cats with seizure onset prior to 1 year of age and diagnosed with epilepsy of unknown cause have guarded prognosis for seizure control.

SEE ALSO

- Feline Ischemic Encephalopathy.
- Meningioma—Cats and Dogs.

ABBREVIATIONS

- FIP = feline infectious peritonitis.
- GI = gastrointestinal.
- GS = generalized seizures.
- SE = status epilepticus.

Suggested Reading

Barnes HL, Chrisman CL, Mariani CL, et al. Clinical signs, underlying cause, and outcome in cats with seizures: 17 cases (1997–2002). J Am Vet Med Assoc 2004, 225:1723–1726.

Pakozdy A, Gruber A, Kneissl K, et al. Complex partial cluster seizures in cats with orofacial involvement. J Feline Med Surg 2011, 13:687–693.

Parent J. Seizures and status epilepticus in cats. In: Veterinary Emergency and Critical Care Manual, 2nd ed. Guelph, Ontario: Lifelearn, 2006, pp. 456–459.

Wahle AM, Brühschwein A, Matiasek K, et al. Clinical characterization of epilepsy of unknown cause in cats. J Vet Intern Med 2014, 28:182–188.

Author Joane M. Parent

Client Education Handout available online

SEIZURES (CONVULSIONS, STATUS EPILEPTICUS)—DOGS

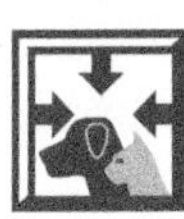

BASICS

DEFINITION

- Epilepsy—recurrence of seizures from primary brain origin.
- Genetic epilepsy—epilepsy with no observable underlying brain lesion or other neurologic signs or symptoms.
- Structural epilepsy—seizures are the result of identifiable structural brain lesions.
- Epilepsy of unknown cause—structural epilepsy is suspected but a lesion cannot be demonstrated.
- Cluster seizures—>1 seizure/24 hours.
- Status epilepticus (SE)—continuous seizure activity or seizures repeated at brief intervals without complete recovery between seizures.
- SE can be convulsive or nonconvulsive.
- Seizures are classified as focal (limited to one hemisphere), generalized (involve both hemispheres), and focal with secondary generalization.

PATHOPHYSIOLOGY

- Any thalamocortical disturbance may lead to seizure activity.
- Not all cortical regions have equal propensity to seize; from the most to the least likely to cause seizures—temporal, frontal, parietal, and occipital lobes.
- As more seizures occur, the tendency for neuronal damage and propensity for more seizures or SE increases; this kindling effect does not occur in all cortical regions.
- The clinical appearance of a seizure is related to the location of the neuronal hyperactivity.

SIGNALMENT

- Dogs of any breed, age, or sex.
- SE—overrepresentation of German shepherd dog, English foxhound, pug, teacup poodle, Boston terrier, Lakeland terrier.

Mean Age and Range

SE—4.2–5 years (0.15–15 years).

SIGNS

General Comments

- Prodrome—hours to days prior to the seizure; no electroencephalogram (EEG) changes.
- Aura—short period (seconds) prior to generalization of a seizure where the dog seeks help, looks lost, frightened or has a glazed look. Focal seizure. If it precedes the tonic–clonic generalized seizure, the seizure has a focal onset.
- Ictus—may start with an aura and progress to generalized seizure (GS); lateral recumbency with bilateral symmetrical tonic–clonic contractions of limb muscles; often with autonomic signs, e.g., salivation, urination, defecation.
- GS—may be mild, the animal remaining sternal or even standing during the event; may be long-lasting, 20 minutes or more. Convulsive or nonconvulsive.
- Post-ictal phase—disorientation, confusion, aimless pacing, blindness, polydipsia, polyphagia.
- A seizure lasts <2 minutes.
- Most seizures occur when dog is resting or sleeping.

Historical Findings

- Confirm that seizure has occurred.
- Seizure pattern (age at onset of seizure, seizure type and frequency)—most important factor in establishing list of possible causes.
- Metabolic diseases usually cause generalized seizures.
- Asymmetric neurologic signs before, during, or after the seizure suggest structural brain lesion.
- Presence of behavioral changes in the days/weeks preceding seizure onset indicates structural brain disease.

Neurologic Examination Findings

- Mental status, menace responses, responses to nasal septum stimulation, and proprioceptive positioning—neurologic tests that evaluate the cerebral cortex. Asymmetry indicates structural brain lesion contralateral to deficits.
- Compensated SE, first 30 minutes—salivation, hyperthermia, tachycardia, arrhythmia, increased blood pressure.
- Decompensated SE—difficulty breathing, weak pulse, low blood pressure, poor capillary refill.

CAUSES

Extracranial

- Metabolic—electrolyte disturbances, hypoglycemia (insulinoma); hypocalcemia; acute renal failure; hepatic encephalopathy.
- Toxicities—metaldehyde, pyrethrins/pyrethroids, lead, hexachlorophene, chlorinated hydrocarbons, organophosphates, bromethalin, mycotoxins, macademia nut, theobromine (chocolate), 5-fluorouracil.

Intracranial

- Degenerative—encephalopathy.
- Malformations—cortical dysplasia.
- Genetic epilepsy.
- Metabolic—cell storage diseases.
- Neoplasia—primary (meningioma, gliomas); secondary (metastatic).
- Inflammatory infectious—viral (e.g., canine distemper); fungal; protozoal (*Neospora*, *Toxoplasma*); rickettsial (ehrlichiosis, Rocky Mountain spotted fever).
- Inflammatory noninfectious—meningoencephalomyelitis of unknown origin, eosinophilic meningoencephalomyelitis; breed-related encephalitis (pug, Maltese, Yorkshire terriers, etc.).
- Trauma.
- Vascular—cerebrovascular accident.
- Epilepsy of unknown cause—post-encephalitic glial scar.

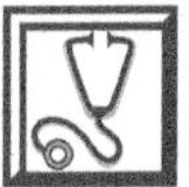

DIAGNOSIS

DIFFERENTIAL DIAGNOSIS

- Syncope—body is limp, rapid recovery with no abnormal behavior; occurs at exercise, cough, excitement.
- Insulinoma—seizures occur at exercise, excitement.
- Obsessive compulsive behaviors or stereotypes—complex and goal-directed behaviors; behavior can be stopped.
- Seizurogenic toxins—progression from whole body tremor to SE and death if left untreated.
- Metabolic encephalopathy—seizures unusual and accompanied with obtunded mental state and abnormal behavior; no lateralizing signs.
- Structural brain disease likely—if acute onset of >2 GS within first week of onset, acute onset of focal seizures with gradual progression to GS, or presence of interictal neurologic deficits including behavioral changes.
- Genetic epilepsy—differentiated on age, breed, and seizure pattern; progressive onset of GS with/without aura.
- Cervical pain/spasms—may be mistaken for focal seizures.
- Head bobbing or idiopathic head tremor—dog remains active; can eat, drink, walk.

CBC/BIOCHEMISTRY/URINALYSIS

- Infectious CNS diseases—may reflect multisystem involvement.
- Hypoglycemia—small/toy breeds during SE; insulinoma.
- Hepatic and renal dysfunction—advanced SE.
- Urinalysis—rule out myoglobinuria.

OTHER LABORATORY TESTS

- Blood gases—metabolic acidosis frequent with SE. Respiratory acidosis needs immediate treatment.
- Coagulation profile—disseminated intravascular coagulation (DIC) in advanced SE.
- Bile acids—suspected hepatic encephalopathy.
- Fasting blood glucose and amended insulin: glucose ratio—dogs >5 years with occasional seizures during exercise.
- Serology (infectious diseases)—as suggested by systemic signs and laboratory abnormalities.
- Toxicity screen—cholinesterase levels.

IMAGING

- Thoracic radiographs and abdominal ultrasound—to identify metastatic or systemic illness, or lung pathology from SE.
- MRI—best to define location, extent, and nature of lesion.

DIAGNOSTIC PROCEDURES

Electrocardiogram (ECG)—arrhythmias can occur in SE due to myocardial damage. CSF—if intracranial structural cause is suspected; CSF and serum titers and PCR for diagnosing infectious diseases. EEG—to document ongoing seizure activity once physical manifestations have ceased.

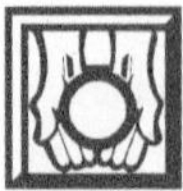

TREATMENT

APPROPRIATE HEALTH CARE

- Outpatient—isolated seizures in an otherwise healthy dog.
- Inpatient—cluster seizures and SE.

NURSING CARE

- SE and cluster-seizures—constant supervision.
- Ensure airway patency. May need to be suctioned due to excessive salivation.
- Administer 100% oxygen via non-rebreathing mask.
- Cool down if hyperthermia.
- Install IV line for drug and fluid administration.
- Draw blood for rapid measurement of blood gases, glucose, calcium, renal and hepatic function, and antiepileptic drug (AED) levels if pertinent.
- Monitor urine output with indwelling urinary catheter.

CLIENT EDUCATION

- Treat cluster of GS and generalized status epilepticus (GSE) early—the more seizures in a given time, and the more drugs for seizure control, time for recovery, and cost for treatment.
- Antiepileptic treatment in structural epilepsy may not help until the primary cause is addressed.
- Client to keep a seizure calendar noting date, time, severity, and length of seizures to objectively evaluate response to treatment.
- Outline an in-home treatment emergency plan for cluster-seizures.

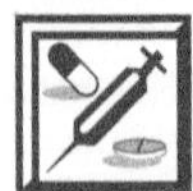

MEDICATIONS

- Electrolytes imbalance—treat immediately with fluid therapy.
- Low glucose—50% dextrose diluted to 25% (500 mg/kg IV) over 15 minutes or treat with oral glucose syrup.

DRUG(S) OF CHOICE

Seizure type and frequency determine the therapeutic approach. Important to seek and treat primary cause.

Convulsive Cluster Seizures or Status Epilepticus

Diazepam

- Administer 0.5–1 mg/kg IV bolus; repeat 5 minutes later if gross motor activity has not subsided; follow with CRI of 0.5–1 mg/kg/h added to hourly maintenance fluids in an inline burette or through syringe pump.
- Rectal—only where IV access cannot be obtained; may diminish or stop gross motor seizure activity to allow IV catheter placement.
- Refractoriness may rapidly develop, necessitating the addition of phenobarbital CRI.

Phenobarbital

- Add if seizures persist after second diazepam bolus or during diazepam CRI; administer CRI phenobarbital (2–6 mg/dog/h added to diazepam infusion) if patient already treated with phenobarbital, or loading dose if patient naïve to phenobarbital.
- Loading dose—12–24 mg/kg given as boluses of 4 mg/kg IV, 20 minutes apart until desired effect is reached, to a maximum of 24 mg/kg. Optimal therapeutic range—100–120 μmol/L (23–28 mg/L).
- If patient already on phenobarbital, obtain serum level prior to initiating phenobarbital CRI. IV bolus 2–6 mg/kg can be administered once while awaiting results if serum levels believed inadequate.
- Once seizures have been controlled for 4–6 hours, gradually wean the patient off CRI over as many hours.
- Start/resume oral maintenance AED using phenobarbital and/or other GS AED as soon as patient can swallow.

Other

- If seizures continue, propofol at 1–2 mg/kg IV slowly over 60 seconds, followed by CRI at 0.1–0.6 mg/kg/min to effect; monitor anesthetized patient with EEG to evaluate treatment response.
- Ketamine is also used occasionally at 5 mg/kg IV bolus followed by CRI at 5 mg/kg/h.
- Dexamethasone—0.2 mg/kg q24h for 1–3 days; reduce cerebral edema.
- Dexamethasone—for acute treatment of cerebral edema secondary to severe inflammatory CNS disease, even if infectious.

Acute Focal Status Epilepticus

- Often harbors brain lesion.
- Diazepam and phenobarbital CRI—effective for focal and GS.
- Frequently difficult to reach seizure control.
- Instances of chronic nonconvulsive generalized or focal SE—owner unaware it is occurring (e.g., senile encephalopathy); if seizures remain focal and patient's quality of life not significantly altered, no treatment necessary. Long-term antiepileptic treatment if necessary—phenobarbital 3–5 mg/kg q12h PO, levetiracetam 20 mg/kg q8h PO, or zonisamide 5 mg/kg q12h PO.

CONTRAINDICATIONS

- Potassium bromide—do not use to treat SE; too long half-life; loading dose not recommended.
- Aminophylline, theophylline—CNS excitement; may cause seizure.
- Steroids—alter CSF parameters; avoid if considering CSF analysis.

PRECAUTIONS

- Phenobarbital—liver disease, lower dose; monitor levels closely; for SE, add cautiously to diazepam because the drugs potentiate each other, cardiac/respiratory depression may ensue.
- Steroids—contraindicated in infectious diseases, but one dose of dexamethasone 0.2 mg/kg IV may decrease brain edema when impending brain herniation or life-threatening edema is suspected.

POSSIBLE INTERACTIONS

- Cimetidine, ranitidine, and chloramphenicol—interfere with phenobarbital metabolism; may lead to phenobarbital toxic level.
- Phenobarbital decreases zonisamide serum levels. Dosage recommended when drugs are used simultaneously—10 mg/kg q12h.
- If levetiracetam used concomitantly with phenobarbital—measure serum levels (humans 10–40 μg/mL).

ALTERNATIVE DRUG(S)

Levetiracetam—20–60 mg/kg IV; use upper end dosage if patient already on oral phenobarbital. Good alternative in liver disease or portosystemic shunts, as the drug is not metabolized in the liver. Use with caution in patients with renal disease.

FOLLOW-UP

PATIENT MONITORING

- Inpatients—constant supervision for seizure monitoring.
- Eyelid or lip twitching in a heavily sedated patient is sign of ongoing seizure activity.
- Monitor heart rate, respiratory rate, oxygenation/ventilation, body temperature, blood pressure, urine production, neurologic examination.
- EEG monitoring for ongoing seizure activity.
- Patient may need 7–10 days before returning to normal after SE.

POSSIBLE COMPLICATIONS

- Phenobarbital—hepatotoxicity after long-term treatment with serum levels >140 μmol/L (>33 μg/L); acute neutropenia (rare) in the first few weeks of use requires permanent withdrawal.
- Paradoxical hyperexcitability.
- Permanent neurologic deficits (e.g., blindness, abnormal behavior, cerebellar signs) may follow severe SE.

• GSE may lead to hyperthermia, acid–base and electrolyte imbalances, pulmonary edema, cardiovascular collapse, and death.

EXPECTED COURSE AND PROGNOSIS

• Genetic epilepsy or epilepsy of unknown cause represents a large proportion of dogs with GSE or cluster-seizures. In-home emergency measure using diazepam rectal/nasal should be provided.
• Dogs with encephalitis and GSE—poor outcome.
• Structural epileptic dogs recovered from primary disease (e.g., *Ehrlichia canis*)—slowly (over months) wean patient off AEDs after 6 months seizure-free; if seizures recur, reinstate AED.

MISCELLANEOUS

AGE-RELATED FACTORS

• The immature brain has a higher propensity to seize.
• Genetic epilepsy—6 months–5 years; often epilepsy refractory when onset at <2 years.
• Phenobarbital—higher dose needed in puppies (<5 months) to reach therapeutic range.

ABBREVIATIONS

• AED = antiepileptic drug.
• DIC = disseminated intravascular coagulation.
• ECG = electrocardiogram.
• EEG = electroencephalogram.
• GS = generalized seizure.
• GSE = generalized status epilepticus.
• SE = status epilepticus.

Author Joane M. Parent

Client Education Handout available online

S

SEMINOMA

BASICS

OVERVIEW

Sex cord stromal tumor of the testicle arising from the spermatic germinal epithelium.

SIGNALMENT

- Median age, 10 years.
- Boxer, German shepherd dog, Afghan hound, Weimaraner, Shetland sheepdog, collie, and Maltese may be at increased risk.
- 33–52% of all testicular tumors in dogs; extremely rare in cats.

SIGNS

- Usually none.
- Fertility issues in breeding dogs.
- 4–20% of dogs will have more than one type of testicular tumor.
- Up to 50% of dogs will have bilateral tumors, only 12% of contralateral tumors will be palpable.

CAUSES & RISK FACTORS

Cryptorchidism

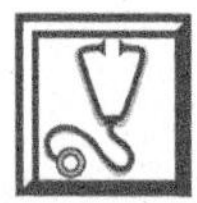

DIAGNOSIS

DIFFERENTIAL DIAGNOSIS

- Sertoli cell tumor.
- Interstitial (Leydig cell) cell tumor.

CBC/BIOCHEMISTRY/URINALYSIS

Usually normal unless hormone productive and consequent male feminization syndrome.

IMAGING

- Testicular sonography may aid in differential diagnosis.
- Abdominal sonography for retained testicles and to evaluate for concurrent malignancies.

DIAGNOSTIC PROCEDURES

N/A

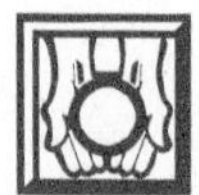

TREATMENT

- Bilateral orchiectomy and scrotal ablation is the treatment of choice.
- Exploratory laparotomy for retained testicles.
- Histopathologic examination of appropriate tissue.
- Immunohistochemistry may be necessary to identify cell of origin in some cases.
- Radiotherapy—reported effective in patients with regional metastasis.

MEDICATIONS

DRUG(S) OF CHOICE

None reported in dogs.

FOLLOW-UP

PREVENTION/AVOIDANCE

Castration at a young age.

POSSIBLE COMPLICATIONS

None likely.

EXPECTED COURSE AND PROGNOSIS

Bilateral orchiectomy and scrotal ablation are often curative. Reported rate of region or distant metastasis <15%.

MISCELLANEOUS

ASSOCIATED CONDITIONS

- Prostate disease.
- Perianal adenoma.
- Perineal hernia.

SEE ALSO

- Interstitial Cell Tumor, Testicle.
- Sertoli Cell Tumor.

Suggested Reading

Grieco V, Riccardi E, Greppi GF, et al. Canine testicular tumours: a study on 232 dogs. J Comp Pathol 2008, 138(2–3): 86–89.

Lawrence JA, Saba C. Tumors of the male reproductive system. In: Withrow SJ, ed., Small Animal Clinical Oncology. St Louis, MO: Elsevier Saunders, 2013, pp. 557–571.

Morrison WB. Cancers of the reproductive tract. In: Morrison WB, ed., Cancer in Dogs and Cats: Medical and Surgical Management. Jackson, WY: Teton NewMedia, 2002, pp. 555–564.

Author Shawna L. Klahn

Consulting Editor Timothy M. Fan

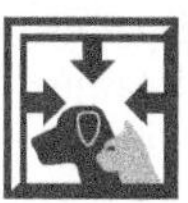

BASICS

DEFINITION

A distress response of dogs (occasionally cats) separated from the person or persons to whom they are most attached, usually their owner(s). The separation may be real (the owner is gone) or perceived (pet is separated from the owner). In other cases the pet may be distressed because a fear-inducing event has occurred while home alone (e.g., thunderstorms, loud noises or home invasions), resulting in distress responses during subsequent departures. Distress may be exhibited as destruction, vocalization, and elimination in the owner's absence. Separation anxiety is a subset of separation-related problems that may have different underlying motivations, including fear, anxiety, overattachment to owner(s), and lack of appropriate stimulation or interactions.

PATHOPHYSIOLOGY

Unknown but suspected changes in brain pathology due to aging, anxious temperament, noise or location phobias, insecure attachment to humans in family.

SYSTEMS AFFECTED

- Behavioral—escape attempts, howling, whining, depression, hyperactivity.
- Cardiovascular—tachycardia.
- Endocrine/metabolic—increased cortisol, stress-induced hyperglycemia.
- Gastrointestinal—inappetence, diarrhea, vomiting
- Musculoskeletal—self-induced trauma from escape attempts.
- Nervous—adrenergic/noradrenergic overstimulation.
- Respiratory—tachypnea.
- Skin/exocrine—acral lick dermatitis.
- Oral—dental damage during escape attempts.

GENETICS

None known.

INCIDENCE/PREVALENCE

It is speculated that 13–28% of companion dogs experience some degree of separation anxiety. May be different underlying pathology with young dogs and senior dogs.

SIGNALMENT

Species

Primarily dogs; possible in cats.

Mean Age and Range

Any age, most commonly in dogs >6 months; may be another increase in prevalence in dogs >8 years.

Predominant Sex

Male and neutered male dogs overrepresented in recent studies.

SIGNS

General Comments

Destruction, vocalization, and elimination in the absence of the owner alone are not diagnostic for separation distress.

Historical Findings

- Destruction, vocalization (whining, howling, barking), and indoor elimination. Destruction targets windows and doors and/or owner possessions.
- Other signs include behavioral depression, anorexia, drooling, hiding, shaking, panting, pacing, attempts to prevent owner departure, and self-trauma from lick lesions. Diarrhea and vomiting are occasionally seen.
- Signs of strong pet–owner attachment may be present: excessive attention-seeking behaviors and following behaviors are not necessary for diagnosis and do not occur in all patients.
- Frequently owners report excessive, excited, and prolonged greeting behavior upon return.
- Separation anxiety behavior(s) usually occurs regardless of the length of owner absence, often within 15–30 minutes of owner departure.
- Specific triggers that are predictive of possible departure may initiate the anxiety response: getting keys, putting on outer garments, or packing the car but are not seen in all patients.
- May occur on every departure and absence or only with atypical departures, e.g., after-work, evening, or weekend departures; the reverse pattern may also be seen.
- Some animals may initially show signs in the presence of acute fear- or anxiety-inducing events such as thunderstorms or fireworks when home alone but may recur with future departures even in the absence of stimuli.
- In cats, elimination problems in the owner's absence may be linked to separation-related anxiety.
- May be excessive water consumption upon owner return.
- Distress may also be initiated by a change in daily routine or in the household (e.g., moving house).
- What appears as distress may also be frustration at being alone, being confined, inability to pursue other activities, living in an impoverished environment or lack of enrichment.

Physical Examination Findings

- Usually normal.
- Injuries may be incurred in escape attempts or destructive activities.
- Skin lesions from excessive licking.
- Rare cases of dehydration from drooling or diarrhea due to stress.

CAUSES

Specific causes unknown. Causal factors may include:

- Insecurity or anxiety about owner departure and absence.
- Frustration due to lack of the ability to engage in normal behaviors (lack of enrichment, exercise or social contact).
- Lack of appropriate pet–owner interactions.
- Prolonged contact with humans without learning how to be alone.
- Improper or incomplete early separation from the bitch (French behavior school).
- Traumatic episodes during owner absence.
- Concurrent anxiety disorders, e.g., noise and storm fears and phobias.
- Change in household routine/schedule.
- Medical issues contributing to anxiety, including endocrine dysfunction, pain, sensory decline, or cognitive decline.

RISK FACTORS

- Suspected risk factors—adoption from humane shelters, extended time with preferred person such as during vacation or illness, boarding, lack of detachment when young.
- Geriatric animals seem to be overrepresented.
- Possible correlation between separation anxiety and other anxiety disorders including noise phobias.

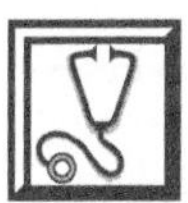

DIAGNOSIS

DIFFERENTIAL DIAGNOSIS

- Vocalization—response to outdoor stimuli, territorial displays, play with other pets in the home, fears.
- Destructive behaviors—occur both when the owner is present and absent (e.g., territorial destructive displays at windows and doors; destruction due to fear-producing stimuli such as noises and thunderstorms). Lack of appropriate outlets for normal chewing and play.
- Housesoiling—inadequate housetraining, illness, endocrine dysfunction, cognitive decline.
- Fear-based conditions.
- Barrier frustration—dogs unable to be confined in crates or behind barriers but are fine if not confined.
- Underlying medical conditions including endocrinopathies, sensory decline, pain, cognitive dysfunction syndrome, and dermatologic conditions leading to self-trauma.

CBC/BIOCHEMISTRY/URINALYSIS

Indicated to rule out concurrent medical conditions and as baseline prior to medication.

SEPARATION ANXIETY SYNDROME (CONTINUED)

OTHER LABORATORY TESTS

Endocrine testing if indicated by history, examination and/or CBC/biochemistry results.

IMAGING

MRI or CT if neurologic disorders are suspected.

DIAGNOSTIC PROCEDURES

- Behavioral history using standard questionnaires.
- Video recordings of the pet when home alone to verify diagnosis.
- Questionnaires targeting cognitive decline are advisable for geriatric dogs.
- Endoscopy with biopsy if gastrointestinal signs.

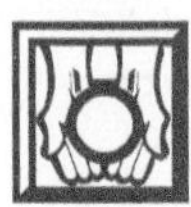

TREATMENT

ACTIVITY

- Regular, scheduled daily exercise and playtime.
- Enriching the environment with toys that are interactive and/or dispense food.

DIET

None unless gastrointestinal signs.

CLIENT EDUCATION

General Comments

Once other causes of destruction and elimination have been ruled out or addressed, it is important to help the owner understand that the destruction or elimination is due to anxiety and not spite. Set a realistic expectation of the time course of treatment and the need for behavior modification to have successful resolution of the problem. Problem behavior may take weeks or months to resolve, depending on severity and duration of the problem. Treatment may include some or all of the following.

Independence Training

- Teach the dog to remain calm when not in close proximity to the owners to encourage the dog to be more independent of the owner(s).
- Teach the dog to calmly stay in a location away from the owner and create a safe haven for the dog to settle and relax on command. Initially this can be a dog bed on the floor 1–2 feet from the owner. The dog must be calm and relaxed when the owner is home for gradually longer times and gradually increasing separation to be calm and relaxed when they are gone.
- When possible, and without creating more anxiety, cue a behavior such as "sit" prior to attention or affection. Longer and more relaxed responses can be very gradually shaped.
- When possible, decrease following behavior while the owner is home, perhaps by sending the dog to the safe bed or mat to wait and reinforcing with attention and treats.
- Owners should strive to give attention in a predictable and calm manner—requesting a sit or other calm behavior such as down before petting, giving treats or chews, throwing a ball, going out for a walk, etc.

Changing the Predictive Value of Pre-Departure Cues

- Some dogs begin to get anxious when they see cues that indicate owner departure.
- For those dogs, presentation of pre-departure cues (picking up keys, walking to the door) without leaving may be helpful; but not if it causes increased anxiety.
- Repeat 2–4 times daily until the dog does not respond to cues with anxious behaviors (panting, pacing, following, or increased vigilance).
- Goal is to disassociate the cues with departures and diminish the anxious response. If the dog becomes more anxious, this step is discontinued.

Counter-Conditioning

- Teach the dog to sit/stay near the typical exit door.
- Owner gradually increases the distance between the dog and the exit door.
- Owner slowly progresses toward the door, increasing the time away on each trial.
- Eventually elements of departure, such as opening and closing the door, are added.
- Finally, the owner steps outside the door and returns.

Classical Counter-Conditioning

- Pairing favored treats with departure cues. Leaving the dog a delectable food treat or food-stuffed toy on departure.
- Associating departure with something pleasant.

Changing Departure and Return Routine

- Passively ignore the pet for 15–30 minutes prior to departure and upon return.
- On return, attend to the dog only when it is calm and quiet.
- Allow the dog outside to eliminate.

Graduated Planned Departures and Absences

- Begun after dog is not responding anxiously to pre-departure cues.
- Use short absences to teach the dog how to be home alone.
- Departures must be short enough not to elicit a separation anxiety response; the pet must be calm when owners depart and calm when they return.
- Goal—animal learns consistency of owner return and to experience departure and absence without anxiety.
- Departures must be just like real departures (owner must do all components of departure, including leaving in the car if that is how he or she usually departs).
- Owner can leave a safety cue (radio or television on, ring a bell) on planned departures only (must not be used on departures where length of absence is not controlled, such as work departures).
- Initial departures must be very short, 1–5 minutes.
- Length of absence is slowly increased at 3–5 minute intervals if no signs of distress at the shorter interval (excited greetings, barking etc.).
- Increase in interval must be variable; intersperse short (1–3 minute) with longer (5–20 minute) departures.
- If destruction, elimination, or vocalization occurs, the absence was too long. Use video recordings, remote monitoring or audio recordings of vocalization to assess pet anxiety and monitor progress.
- Once the pet can be left for 2–3 hours on a planned departure, it often can be left all day.
- Cue can be slowly phased out over time or can be used indefinitely.

Arrangements for the Pet During Retraining and Owner Absence

- If possible, prevent further departures that lead to anxiety.
- If departures and absences are continued while distress behaviors are present, the problem will get worse.
- Mixing up or eliminating triggering departure cues may help diminish the anxious responses.
- Doggie daycare arrangements or pet sitters.
- Gradual positive conditioning to a crate as a safe haven if the dog is not distressed and will settle.
- Crates must be used cautiously if at all and only in dogs that are calm when left in a crate as they may increase anxiety, resulting in pet injury.

SURGICAL CONSIDERATIONS

If animal is on medication, use caution prior to administering anesthesia.

MEDICATIONS

DRUG(S) OF CHOICE

Drugs for Chronic (Ongoing) Therapy

Clomipramine (Branded product "Clomicalm™")

- Tricyclic antidepressant (TCA)—approved for use in the treatment of separation anxiety in dogs.

• Dosage—dogs: 2–4 mg/kg daily; dogs may do better with dividing the dose and administering twice daily. Must be given daily, not on an "as needed" basis, and in conjunction with a behavior modification plan.
• May take 2–4 weeks before behavioral effect is evident.
• Side effects—vomiting, diarrhea, and lethargy.

Fluoxetine (Branded product Reconcile™)
• Selective serotonin reuptake inhibitor (SSRI)—approved for use in the treatment of separation anxiety in dogs.
• Dosage—1–2 mg/kg PO q24h.
• Administer in conjunction with a behavior modification plan.
• Side effects—lethargy, decreased appetite, weight loss, and vomiting.

Drugs for Acute Anxiety at Departure

• While waiting for SSRI or TCA effect, concurrent use of short-term anxiolytics and pheromones is advisable in most cases.
• Benzodiazepines—alprazolam for panic at owner departure (dog, 0.01–0.1 mg/kg) 30 minutes prior to departure. Some dogs experience paradoxical excitement with benzodiazepines, which may resolve with altered dosage or change to another benzodiazepine. Polyphagia is also common with benzodiazepine administration.
• Trazodone—a serotonin receptor antagonist and reuptake inhibitor and can be used in conjunction with a TCA or SSRI to augment calming effects. Dosage recommendation (dog) is to begin with 2–3 mg/kg PO prior to departure and titrate up gradually to effect (up to 8–10 mg/kg). Dose should be increased cautiously, especially if using with an SSRI or TCA due to potential for serotonin syndrome. Side effects include vomiting, diarrhea, sedation, ataxia, hypotension, excitement or agitation and panting and rare reports of polyphagia.
• Dog-appeasing pheromone (Adaptil)—synthetic analogue of the maternal appeasing pheromone; may calm dogs in fearful, stressful, and anxiety situations such as separation anxiety and noise phobias; available as a plug-in diffuser for dog's housing area, a spray for the cage or mat, and collar.

CONTRAINDICATIONS

• Clomipramine and fluoxetine should not be used in combination or combined with monoamine oxidase inhibitors (MAOIs) such as amitraz and selegiline or within 14 days after an MAOI.
• Use clomipramine with caution in patients showing cardiac conduction disturbances.
• Caution advised using in conjunction with CNS-active drugs, including general anesthesia, neuroleptic, anticholinergic, and sympathomimetic drugs for dogs on either clomipramine or fluoxetine.
• A 6-week washout interval should be observed following discontinuation of fluoxetine prior to administration of any drug that may interact with fluoxetine.
• Fluoxetine should be used cautiously in dogs with epilepsy or with drugs that lower the seizure threshold (phenothiazines).

PRECAUTIONS

• Studies to determine effects of medication in patients less than 6 months of age have not been conducted.
• Studies to assess the interaction of fluoxetine with TCAs have not been conducted.
• Improperly applied behavioral modification may increase anxiety.
• Crating can result in serious physical damage to the pet if it attempts to escape; should only be recommended cautiously for animals that are already crate-trained.

POSSIBLE INTERACTIONS

Serotonin syndrome with combinations of MAOI and SSRI or SSRI and TCA.

ALTERNATIVE DRUG(S)

• TCA such as amitriptyline (dog, 1–2 mg/kg q12h) might be considered in place of clomipramine or fluoxetine.
• Clonidine—an alpha-2 agonist which might be used prior to departures in combination with a TCA or SSRI at a dose of 0.01–0.05 mg/kg. Begin at the lowest end of the dose range and increase cautiously.
• Natural products that might be used adjunctively—alpha-casozepine alone or in a diet with L-tryptophan; L-theanine alone or in combination products containing whey protein, *Phellodendron amurense*, and *Magnolia officinalis*; melatonin; S-adenosyl methionine; *Souroubea* and *Plantanus* products; probiotic calming supplement; lavender aromatherapy; classical musical.

FOLLOW-UP

PATIENT MONITORING

Good client follow-up is necessary to monitor both the behavioral treatment plan and medication if prescribed. Weekly follow-up is best in the early stages to assess efficacy of the treatment plan and owner compliance. Once the dog has become more independent, habituated to pre-departure cues, and calmer on departures and returns, graduated planned departures may be implemented.

PREVENTION/AVOIDANCE

Habituating to spending time alone, safe haven training, training independence.

POSSIBLE COMPLICATIONS

• Injuries during escape attempts.
• Ongoing destruction and elimination disrupt the human–animal bond and result in pet relinquishment.
• Other anxieties causing signs that mimic separation distress; if not identified and treated, the problem may worsen.

EXPECTED COURSE AND PROGNOSIS

Separation anxiety often responds well to behavioral modification with or without medication. Some cases can be very resistant to treatment. Other concurrent behavioral disorders may make resolution more difficult. Drug therapy alone is rarely curative for most behavioral disorders. Realistically, drug therapy can be expected to decrease the anxiety associated with owner departure, but the dog still must be taught how to accept and be comfortable left alone during owner absences.

MISCELLANEOUS

ASSOCIATED CONDITIONS

Other anxiety conditions, including noise phobias, generalized anxiety, fears, and compulsive disorders.

AGE-RELATED FACTORS

May be increased prevalence in senior dogs.

SYNONYMS

Hyperattachment–separation distress.

SEE ALSO

• Cognitive Dysfunction Syndrome.
• Excessive Vocalization and Waking at Night—Dogs and Cats.
• Fears, Phobias, and Anxiety—Dogs.
• Thunderstorm and Noise Phobias.

ABBREVIATIONS

• MAOI = monoamine oxidase inhibitor.
• SSRI = selective serotonin reuptake inhibitor.
• TCA = tricyclic antidepressant.

Suggested Reading

Horwitz DF (ed.) Blackwell's Five-Minute Veterinary Consult Clinical Companion: Canine and Feline Behavior, 2nd ed. Hoboken: NJ. John Wiley & Sons, 2018, pp. 348–362.

Horwitz DF. Separation-related problem in dogs and cats. In: Horwitz DF, Mills DS,

eds., BSAVA Manual of Canine and Feline Behavioural Medicine, 2nd ed. Gloucester, UK: BSAVA, 2009, pp. 146–158.
Landsberg G, Hunthausen W, Ackerman L. Fears, phobias and anxiety disorders. In: Behavior Problems of the Dog and Cat, 3rd ed. St. Louis, MO: Saunders/Elsevier, 2013, pp. 181–210.
Overall KL. Manual of Clinical Behavioral Medicine for Dogs and Cats. Ames, IA: Elsevier, 2013, pp. 238–261.
Storengen LM, Boge SCK, Strøm SJ, et al. A descriptive study of 215 dogs diagnosed with separation anxiety. Appl Anim Behav Sci 2014, 159: 82–89.

Author Debra F. Horwitz
Consulting Editor Gary M. Landsberg

Client Education Handout available online

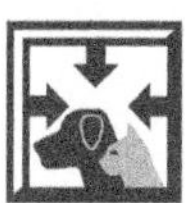

BASICS

DEFINITION

• Sepsis—life-threatening organ dysfunction caused by dysregulated host response to severe infection. • Bacteremia—presence of viable bacterial organisms in the bloodstream. • Terms are not synonymous, although often used interchangeably.

PATHOPHYSIOLOGY

• With severe infection, immune system is stimulated by pathogen-associated products such as lipopolysaccharide (LPS) (Gram-negative bacteria); lipoteichoic acid, peptidoglycan, bacterial DNA, exotoxins (Gram-positive bacteria); fungal cell walls; flagellin (protozoans). • Macrophage-derived cytokines activate and recruit neutrophils and other inflammatory cells, activate coagulation cascade, increase capillary permeability. • Activation of inducible nitric oxide synthase (iNOS) produces large quantities of nitric oxide, causing diffuse, profound vasodilation; refractory hypotension or vasodilatory shock may result. • White blood cells (WBCs) and platelets at sites of inflammation activate coagulation, produce thrombin, and activate platelets; anticoagulant and fibrinolytic pathways inhibited. Procoagulant state favors microthrombi that can lead to decreased tissue oxygen delivery, multiple organ dysfunction, and organ failure. Progression to a hypocoagulable state can occur. • Cryptic shock—decreased microcirculatory perfusion despite normal global hemodynamic parameters; results from decreased functional capillary density. • Endothelial cell dysfunction—disruption of endothelial glycocalyx, changes in deformability of red blood cells (RBCs), WBC activation, microthrombosis, loss of vascular smooth muscle autoregulation, changes in capillary permeability. • Cytopathic hypoxia—sepsis-induced mitochondrial dysfunction renders cells unable to use oxygen to make ATP. • Bacteremia—may be transient and subclinical or escalate to overt sepsis when immune system overwhelmed; generally of more pathologic significance when source is venous or lymphatic drainage sites.

SYSTEMS AFFECTED

• Cardiovascular—increased or decreased cardiac output, decreased systemic vascular resistance, and increased vascular permeability. • Hemic/lymphatic/immune—procoagulant state favors formation of microthrombi, may progress to hypocoagulable state (consumption). • Endocrine—relative adrenal insufficiency (critical illness-related corticosteroid insufficiency [CIRCI]). • Respiratory. • Gastrointestinal. • Hepatobiliary. • Renal. • All systems can be affected by sepsis via systemic inflammatory response syndrome and multiple organ dysfunction syndrome.

SIGNALMENT

Species

• Dog and cat. • No age, sex, or breed predispositions. • Large-breed male dogs—predisposed to bacterial endocarditis, discospondylitis.

SIGNS

General Comments

• May be acute or occur in vague or episodic fashion. • May involve single or multiple organ systems.

Historical Findings

Historical findings variable depend on underlying cause.

Physical Examination Findings

• Signs of sepsis vary with stage. • Dog: ◦ Early sepsis—hyperdynamic state: tachycardia, bounding pulses, rapid capillary refill time, red mucous membranes, fever. ◦ Late sepsis—thready pulses, prolonged capillary refill time, pale mucous membranes, cool extremities, stupor, hypothermia. • Cat: ◦ Lethargy, pale mucous membranes, tachypnea, weak pulses, hypotension, hypothermia, icterus, diffuse abdominal pain (even in absence of primary abdominal problem). ◦ May present with tachycardia or a relative bradycardia (heart rate inappropriately low given illness, e.g., 120–150 bpm). • Specific clinical signs relate to site of infection or secondary organ dysfunction: ◦ Lameness. ◦ Heart murmur—diastolic murmur may indicate aortic valve endocarditis. ◦ Abdominal pain, peritoneal effusion. ◦ Dyspnea. ◦ Dysuria, prostatomegaly. ◦ Neurologic deficits—primary deficit or secondary to hypoglycemia, hypotension.

CAUSES

• Infection from bacterial (most common), viral, protozoal, fungal, or parasitic organisms. • Specific causes include: ◦ Cardiovascular—endocarditis. ◦ Cutaneous—bite wounds, deep pyoderma, infected burns, surgical site infection, abscess. ◦ Gastrointestinal—septic peritonitis, gastrointestinal perforation, translocation, gastroenteritis, colitis. ◦ Genitourinary—pyelonephritis, pyometra, prostatitis/prostatic abscess. ◦ Hemic/immune—blood-borne parasites, vector-borne infections. ◦ Hepatobiliary—hepatitis, hepatic abscess, cholangitis, cholangiohepatitis. ◦ Musculoskeletal—necrotizing fasciitis, osteomyelitis, septic arthritis. ◦ Neurologic—discospondylitis. ◦ Respiratory—pneumonia, pyothorax. • Dogs: Gram-negative organisms (especially *E. coli*) most common; polymicrobial infection reported in ~20% of dogs with positive blood cultures. • Cats—bloodstream pathogens usually Gram-negative bacteria from *Enterobacteriaceae* family or obligate anaerobes; *E. coli* and *Salmonella* most common Gram-negative organisms cultured.

RISK FACTORS

• Predisposing factors—hyperadrenocorticism, diabetes mellitus, liver or renal failure, splenectomy, malignancy, burns. • Immunodeficient state—chemotherapy, feline leukemia virus or feline immunodeficiency virus infection, splenectomy, endogenous or exogenous corticosteroids. • IV catheters. • Indwelling urinary catheters or other drainage devices. • Surgical implants.

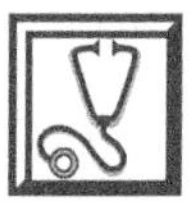

DIAGNOSIS

DIFFERENTIAL DIAGNOSIS

• Other causes of fever, heart murmur, joint or back pain, or hypotension. • Clinical signs of chronic bacteremia may be similar to immune-mediated disease. • Other causes of distributive/vasodilatory shock—hypoadrenocorticism, anaphylaxis or mast cell tumor degranulation, antihypertensive drug overdose.

CBC/BIOCHEMISTRY/URINALYSIS

• Neutrophilic leukocytosis with a left shift and monocytosis. • Neutropenia may develop. • Hypoalbuminemia and a high alkaline phosphatase activity (2 times upper limit of normal)—~50% of affected dogs. • Hypoglycemia—~25% of affected dogs; hyperglycemia or hypoglycemia in cats. • Blood lactate concentration—persistent lactate elevation despite therapy portends poor prognosis.

OTHER LABORATORY TESTS

• Aerobic and anaerobic cultures of site of infection—recommended but *should not delay timely antibiotic therapy.* • Suspected catheter-induced sepsis—culture catheter tip. • Urine culture—urinary tract may be primary or secondary source of infection. • Endocarditis—consider *Bartonella* testing (see Bartonellosis). • PCR, serology for tick-borne disease, as indicated. • PCR, serology or for organisms of interest, as indicated (e.g., *Leptospira*, influenza, *Babesia*). • Fungal antigen testing. • Coagulation parameters should be monitored in most cases.

IMAGING

• Radiographs and ultrasound—may identify source of sepsis (e.g., pyometra, pneumonia) or secondarily infected organs (e.g., discospondylitis). • Ultrasound may help guide fine-needle aspiration for cytology/culture. • Echocardiography—for suspected endocarditis. • CT, MRI—may identify some sources of sepsis or for surgical planning.

SEPSIS AND BACTEREMIA (CONTINUED)

DIAGNOSTIC PROCEDURES

• Abdominocentesis, thoracocentesis, fine-needle aspirate—for cytology, culture/sensitivity of effusion, masses:
◦ Neutrophilic or pyogranulomatous inflammation, eosinophilic. ◦ Diagnostic peritoneal lavage if strong suspicion for abdominal sepsis without effusion.
• Endo- or transtracheal wash, bronchoalveolar lavage—samples for cytology, culture/sensitivity, PCR. • Fecal cytology, fecal PCR. • Blood cultures—in any patient that develops fever (or hypothermia), leukocytosis (especially with a left shift), neutropenia, shifting leg lameness, recent onset or changing heart murmur, or any sign of sepsis for which the source cannot be identified.

PATHOLOGIC FINDINGS

Varies with underlying cause.

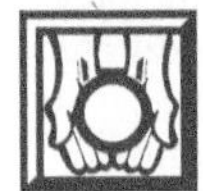

TREATMENT

APPROPRIATE HEALTH CARE

• Success requires early identification of the problem and aggressive intervention; careful monitoring is essential, patient status may change rapidly. • *Start IV antibiotics within 1 hour of identifying sepsis or septic shock.* • Fluid therapy—IV bolus isotonic replacement crystalloids (cat, 10–15 mL/kg; dog, 20–30 mL/kg), repeat as necessary; then administer crystalloids to provide maintenance needs, replace dehydration deficits and meet ongoing losses; provide albumin and plasma for hypoalbuminemia and coagulation abnormalities, respectively; consider synthetic colloids if clinical hypoproteinemia and hypotension are ongoing and biologic colloid sources unavailable. • Add dextrose to IV fluids if hypoglycemic. • Electrolytes and acid–base balance—correct abnormalities.
• Pressor, inotrope therapy for persistent hypotension; refer early. • Source control—should be completed after patient is normotensive and stable; provide appropriate wound care, bandage changes, or surgical intervention, as indicated.

NURSING CARE

• Goals—systolic blood pressure >90 mmHg, heart rate 80–140 bpm (dogs) and 160–225 bpm (cats), capillary refill time 1.5 seconds, urine output >1–2 mL/kg/h, blood lactate <2.5 mmol/L in dogs. • Inadequate response to therapy prompts vasopressor administration (norepinephrine, dopamine, vasopressin). Most commonly recommended vasopressor is norepinephrine. Dopamine may be a good choice for cats with relative bradycardia. • As appropriate for each patient's situation.

DIET

Nutritional support—provide by assisted feeding or feeding tube.

CLIENT EDUCATION

Prognosis should be discussed with client.

SURGICAL CONSIDERATIONS

Any identifiable focus of infection such as an abscess should be located and removed where possible.

MEDICATIONS

DRUG(S) OF CHOICE

Antibiotics

• IV antibiotics should be *started within 1 hour* of recognizing sepsis, septic shock.
• Pending culture and sensitivity results, treat for organisms commonly isolated from presumed source of infection, or empirically cover Gram-positive, Gram-negative, aerobic, anaerobic organisms: ◦ Initial therapy—Gram-negative (enrofloxacin, cefotaxime, amikacin); Gram-positive (ampicillin, clindamycin); anaerobes (metronidazole).
◦ Ampicillin 22 mg/kg IV q6–8h.
◦ Ampicillin/sulbactam 25–30 mg/kg IV q6–8h. ◦ Clindamycin 12 mg/kg IV q12h.
◦ Cefotaxime 20–80 mg/kg IV q8h.
◦ Enrofloxacin 10–15 mg/kg IV q24h (dogs); 5 mg/kg/day IV (cats). ◦ Amikacin 10–15 mg/kg IV q24h. ◦ Metronidazole 10 mg/kg IV q8–12h. • De-escalate (reduce unnecessary antibiotics) once sensitivity results are available. • For many *bacterial* infections, total duration of therapy can be limited to 7–10 days; longer if source cannot be eliminated/drained or immune deficiencies are present.

Corticosteroids

Physiologic doses (e.g., 0.25 mg/kg prednisone or 0.05 mg/kg of dexamethasone) may be indicated if patient has persistent hypotension unresponsive to fluid therapy and catecholamines.

CONTRAINDICATIONS

NSAIDs—high risk of renal failure (acute kidney injury) or gastrointestinal ulceration in patient with sepsis/septic shock.

PRECAUTIONS

Aminoglycosides—use with caution in patient with renal impairment.

FOLLOW-UP

PATIENT MONITORING

• Aminoglycoside therapy—monitor renal function. • Blood pressure, ECG, electrolytes, blood lactate.

POSSIBLE COMPLICATIONS

Multiple organ failure.

EXPECTED COURSE AND PROGNOSIS

Sepsis has a mortality rate of ~50%, with higher mortality for animals with multiorgan failure.

MISCELLANEOUS

ASSOCIATED CONDITIONS

• Discospondylitis (dogs)— screen for *Brucella* spp. • See Risk Factors.

SYNONYMS

• Septic shock. • Septicemia.

SEE ALSO

• Abscessation.
• Anaerobic Infections.
• Endocarditis, Infective.
• Shock, Septic.

ABBREVIATIONS

• CIRCI = critical illness-related corticosteroid insufficiency.
• iNOS = inducible nitric oxide synthase.
• LPS = lipopolysaccharide.
• NSAID = nonsteroidal anti-inflammatory drug.
• RBCs = red blood cells.
• WBCs = white blood cells.

Suggested Reading

Burkitt JM, Haskins SC, Nelson RW, et al. Relative adrenal insufficiency in dogs with sepsis. J Vet Intern Med 2007, 21:226–231.

Rhodes A, Evans LE, Alhazzani W, et al. Surviving Sepsis Campaign: International guidelines for management of sepsis and septic shock: 2016. Crit Care Med 2017, 45(3):486–552.

Author Amie Koenig

Consulting Editor Amie Koenig

Acknowledgment The author/editor acknowledges the prior contribution of Sharon Fooshee Grace.

Client Education Handout available online

BASICS

OVERVIEW

Sex cord stromal tumor of the testicle arising from the sustenacular cells of Sertoli.

SIGNALMENT

- Median age, 10 years.
- Boxer, German shepherd dog, Afghan hound, Weimaraner, Shetland sheepdog, collie, and Maltese may be at increased risk.
- 8–33% of all testicular tumors in dogs, extremely rare in cats.

SIGNS

- Usually none. Fertility issues in breeding dogs.
- 4–20% of dogs will have more than one type of testicular tumor.
- Up to 50% of dogs will have bilateral tumors, only 12% of contralateral tumors will be palpable.
- >50% of dogs will have hyperestrogenism. Most common clinical signs include: bilateral symmetric alopecia and hyperpigmentation, pendulous prepuce, gynecomastia, galactorrhea, atrophy of the penis, squamous metaplasia of the prostate.
- Clinical signs associated with severe pancytopenia include weakness, hemorrhage, and febrile episodes.
- Abdominal mass—if patient is cryptorchid.

CAUSES & RISK FACTORS

- Cryptorchid testicles 12.7 per 1000 dog-years (vs. 0 for scrotally located testicles).
- Cryptorchid and ≥6 years of age, 68.1 per 1000 dog-years.

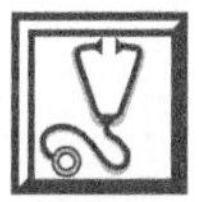

DIAGNOSIS

DIFFERENTIAL DIAGNOSIS

- Interstitial cell tumor.
- Seminoma.
- Hyperadrenocorticism.
- Hypothyroidism.
- More likely to have an abdominal location than other testicular tumors; high testicular temperature in the abdominal location may destroy spermatogenic cells and leave Sertoli cells unregulated.

CBC/BIOCHEMISTRY/URINALYSIS

Transient neutrophilia followed by progressive neutropenia, thrombocytopenia, and non-regenerative anemia.

OTHER LABORATORY TESTS

Low testosterone-to-estradiol ratio.

IMAGING

Testicular and abdominal sonography to aid in differential diagnosis and identify retained testicles and comorbidities.

DIAGNOSTIC PROCEDURES

- Histopathologic examination of testicular mass.
- Immunohistochemistry may be necessary to identify cell of origin.
- Serum anti-müllerian hormone may differentiate testicular tumors.

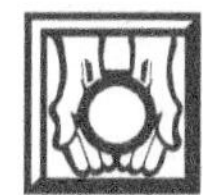

TREATMENT

- Bilateral orchiectomy is the treatment of choice.
- Exploratory laparotomy for retained testicles.
- Supportive care for dogs with bone marrow hypoplasia.

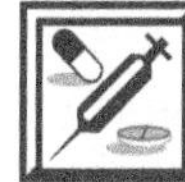

MEDICATIONS

DRUG(S) OF CHOICE

N/A

FOLLOW-UP

PATIENT MONITORING

- Recurrence of feminization may be associated with metastasis.
- Serum hormone levels may be correlated with resolution of clinical signs.

POSSIBLE COMPLICATIONS

Irreversible bone marrow ablation resulting in life-threatening hemorrhage and recurrent infection.

EXPECTED COURSE AND PROGNOSIS

- Good in most patients.
- Guarded if cytopenias exist at diagnosis.
- Poor prognosis if aplastic anemia present.
- Clinical signs of hyperestrogenism expected to resolve within 1–3 months following castration; however, bone marrow hypoplasia might be irreversible.

MISCELLANEOUS

ASSOCIATED CONDITIONS

- 50% of dogs with Sertoli cell tumor associated with hyperestrogenism and feminization.
- Hyperestrogenism can cause hematopoietic failure.

SEE ALSO

Hyperestrogenism (Estrogen Toxicity).

Suggested Reading

Grieco V, Riccardi E, Greppi GF, et al. Canine testicular tumours: a study on 232 dogs. J Comp Pathol 2008, 138(2–3):86–89.

Lawrence JA, Saba C. Tumors of the male reproductive system. In: Withrow SJ, ed., Small Animal Clinical Oncology. St Louis, MO: Elsevier Saunders, 2013, pp. 557–571.

Morrison WB. Cancers of the reproductive tract. In: Morrison WB, ed., Cancer in Dogs and Cats: Medical and Surgical Management. Jackson, WY: Teton NewMedia, 2002, pp. 555–564.

Author Shawna L. Klahn

Consulting Editor Timothy M. Fan

SEXUAL DEVELOPMENT DISORDERS

BASICS

DEFINITION

• Errors in the establishment of chromosomal, gonadal, or phenotypic sex causing abnormal sexual differentiation. • Varies from ambiguous genitalia to apparently normal genitalia with sterility.

PATHOPHYSIOLOGY

• Sexual differentiation is a sequential process—chromosomal sex established at fertilization (dog: 78,XX or 78,XY; cat: 38,XX or 38,XY), development of gonadal sex, and finally development of phenotypic sex. • Testis differentiation normally determined by sex chromosome constitution; *SRY* (on the Y chromosome) and *SOX9* (autosomal gene), expressed by Sertoli cells, are critical for testis differentiation. • Ovarian differentiation—an active process involving *WNT4/RSPO1* and β-catenin. • Phenotypic sex differentiation (tubular reproductive tract and external genitalia) depends on gonadal sex—basic embryonic plan is female; male phenotype results if testes are capable of secreting anti-Müllerian hormone and testosterone at the correct time during embryogenesis, and functional androgen receptors (X-linked gene) are present on genital tissues. • Consensus terminology for categorizing disorders of sexual development (DSD) recently revised. Previous nomenclature also noted.

Sex Chromosome DSD

• Defects in number or structure of sex chromosomes—chromosomal non-disjunction during meiosis causes trisomy, monosomy; mitotic non-disjunction of a single zygote causes mosaicism; fusion of zygotes leads to chimerism. • XXY (Klinefelter) syndrome—79,XXY (dog); 39,XXY (cat): hypoplastic testes; phenotypic male (normal to hypoplastic genitalia); sterile; some tortoiseshell male cats. • XO (Turner) syndrome—77,XO (dog); 37,XO (cat): dysgenetic ovaries; phenotypic female; infantile genitalia; sterile. • XXX syndrome—79,XXX (dog): hypoplastic ovaries; anestrus to irregular estrous cycles; female phenotype. • True hermaphrodite chimera—XX/XY or XX/XXY (dogs and cats): ovarian and testicular tissue; phenotypic sex depends on amount of testicular tissue. • XX/XY chimera with testes and XY/XY chimera with testes (dogs and cats)—vary from phenotypic female with abnormal genitalia to male with possible fertility; some tortoiseshell males.

XY DSD

Disorders of Testicular Development

• Complete or partial testicular dysgenesis—*SRY*-positive 78,XY dog: genitalia incompletely masculinized (enlarged clitoris); testes undescended or perivulvar; Müllerian and Wolffian duct derivatives variably present. • Ovotesticular DSD—XY sex reversal, true hermaphrodite.

Disorders in Androgen Synthesis or Action

• Complete androgen insensitivity syndrome—38,XY cat: testes at caudal pole of kidneys; no Wolffian or Müllerian duct derivatives; blind-ended vagina; vulva. • Partial androgen insensitivity syndrome—78,XY dog: vulva; perivulvar scrotal-like swellings at 6 months of age; blind vaginal pouch; hypoplastic testes; epididymides, partially developed vasa deferentia; vulvar fibroblasts unable to bind dihydrotestosterone. • Persistent Müllerian duct syndrome (male pseudohermaphrodite)—XY (dogs and cats): testes (50% are unilateral or bilateral cryptorchid); epididymides, vasa deferentia, prostate, oviducts, uterus, cervix, cranial vagina; penis, prepuce, and scrotum usually normal. • Isolated hypospadias—incomplete masculinization of urogenital sinus during urethral development causing abnormal location of urinary orifice from glans penis (mild) to perineum (severe); external genitalia unambiguous; testes (cryptorchid or scrotal) or bifid scrotum (cats) with spermatogenesis.

XX DSD

Ovoteseticular DSD and Testicular DSD

• Canine XX DSD (sex reversal)—*SRY*-negative 78,XX reported in 28 dog breeds, not in cats: autosomal gene causing testis induction presently unknown; two phenotypes: ○ Ovotesticular DSD, XX true hermaphrodite (90% of cases)—ovotestis (at least one); masculinized female phenotype; varies from normal to abnormal vulva, normal or enlarged clitoris (os clitoris possible), uterus, oviducts, epididymides, and vasa deferentia; rarely fertile. ○ Testicular DSD, XX males (10% of cases)—testes (usually cryptorchid); epididymides, vasa deferentia, prostate; bicornuate uterus, no oviducts; hypoplastic penis and prepuce; hypospadias common.

Androgen Excess

• Fetal origin—single report of congenital adrenal hyperplasia in a phenotypic male cat (38,XX, ovaries, oviducts, epididymides, vasa deferentia, bicornuate uterus) due to 11 β-hydroxylase deficiency. • Maternal origin (female pseudohermaphrodite)—XX; ovaries; masculinized genitalia (mild clitoral enlargement to nearly normal male genitalia); oviducts, uterus, cranial vagina; prostate variable; caused by exogenous sex steroid administration (progestegen oversupplementation) during pregnancy.

SYSTEMS AFFECTED

• Reproductive—anomalies of the gonads, tubular tract, and external genitalia. • Renal/urologic—occasionally affected (e.g., agenesis, incontinence, hematuria, cystitis). • Skin/exocrine—perivulvar dermatitis (hypoplastic vulva); perineal or peri-preputial dermatitis (hypospadias); hyperpigmentation (Sertoli cell tumor).

GENETICS

• Chromosomal sex abnormalities—usually caused by random events during gamete formation or early embryonic development. • XX DSD—autosomal recessive trait in American cocker spaniels and likely in beagles, German shorthaired pointers; familial in English cocker spaniels, pugs, Kerry blue terriers, Norwegian elkhounds, Weimaraners; other reported breeds include soft-coated wheaten terriers, vizslas, Walker hounds, Doberman pinschers, basset hounds, American pit bull terriers, border collies, Afghan hounds. • Persistent Müllerian duct syndrome (PMDS)—autosomal recessive trait in miniature schnauzers in the United States, bassett hounds in the Netherlands, and possibly Persian cats; expression limited to XY individuals. • Hypospadias familial in Boston terriers. • Failure of androgen-dependent masculinization (predominantly cats) probably X-linked.

INCIDENCE/PREVALENCE

• Generally rare. • In affected breeds—may be common within families or within the breed as a whole.

SIGNALMENT

Species

Dog and cat.

Breed Predilections

See Genetics.

Mean Age and Range

All are congenital disorders, but individuals with normal external genitalia may not be identified until breeding age or at routine gonadectomy.

Predominant Sex

Phenotypic females and males.

SIGNS

General Comments

• Depends on type of disorder. • Listed are possible findings for any of the conditions; not all occur with each specific disorder.

Historical Findings

• Failure to cycle. • Infertility and sterility. • Vulva, clitoris, prepuce, or penis—abnormal size, shape, or location. • Urine stream—abnormal location. • Affected phenotypic males attractive to other males. • Urinary incontinence. • Vulvar discharge. • Polyuria/polydipsia.

Physical Examination Findings

• Vulva normal or hypoplastic. • Clitoris normal or enlarged; os clitoris. • Perivulvar dermatitis and vulvar discharge. • Testes scrotal, unilateral or bilateral cryptorchid; bifid scrotum. • Penis and prepuce normal or hypoplastic. • Urethral meatus normal or abnormal location. • Dermatologic signs of hyperestrogenism in males. • Abdominal mass.

CAUSES

• Congenital—heritable or nonheritable.
• Exogenous steroid hormone administration during gestation.

RISK FACTORS

Androgen or progestagen administration during pregnancy (female pseudohermaphrodite).

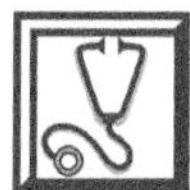

DIAGNOSIS

DIFFERENTIAL DIAGNOSIS

Individuals with Unambiguous Genitalia

• Female infertility—male infertility, mistimed breeding, subclinical cystic endometrial hyperplasia/endometritis, hypothyroidism. • Failure to cycle (female)—silent heat, hypothyroidism, hypercorticism, previous gonadectomy. • Male infertility—female infertility, mistimed breeding, exogenous drug use affecting fertility, orchitis or epididymitis, testicular degeneration or hypoplasia, prostatitis.

CBC/BIOCHEMISTRY/URINALYSIS

• Usually normal. • Neutrophilia, normochromic, normocytic anemia; hyperglobulinemia, hyperproteinemia, azotemia are possible. • Urinalysis—may reveal cystitis with anatomic abnormalities that affect the location of the urethral meatus.

OTHER LABORATORY TESTS

• Serum concentrations of sex steroid hormones (progesterone, testosterone, and estradiol)—generally below the normal range; may be normal if disorder mild and patient not sterile. • Detect testicular tissue—gonadotropin-releasing hormone (GnRH) or human chorionic gonadotropin (hCG) simulation test; resting serum anti-Müllerian hormone (AMH; see Cryptorchidism).
• Karyotyping—to define chromosomal sex (Molecular Cytogenetics Laboratory, Texas A&M University).

IMAGING

• Routine radiography and ultrasonography—may be of diagnostic value for suspected abdominal mass (e.g., testicular neoplasia with PMDS, testicular feminization, or XX DSD); males with signs referable to pyometra (female pseudohermaphrodite or PMDS). • Contrast studies (lower urogenital tract)—may be useful in diagnosing female pseudohermaphrodites.

PATHOLOGIC FINDINGS

Gross

Precisely describe the genitalia—size and location of the vulva or prepuce; presence and appearance of the clitoris, penis, scrotum, prostate, caudal vagina, or os clitoris; position of the urinary orifice (identifies the phallic structure as penis or clitoris).

Histopathologic

• Examination of all tissues removed—to define the type of disorder. • Gonads—vary from nearly normal architecture to dysgenic or a combination of ovary and testis (ovotestis). • Essential to describe the components of the Müllerian and/or Wolffian duct system, if found.

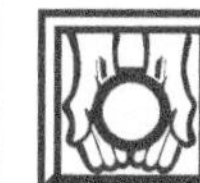

TREATMENT

APPROPRIATE HEALTH CARE

• Usually outpatient. • Inpatient—if exploratory laparotomy.

NURSING CARE

Phenotypic females with a hypoplastic vulva and perivulvar dermatitis and males with hypospadias—local therapy to improve dermatologic sequelae (see Dermatoses, Erosive or Ulcerative).

SURGICAL CONSIDERATIONS

• Most patients with no identified chromosomal abnormalities—exploratory laparotomy to determine the location and morphology of the gonads and internal genitalia. • Gonadectomy and hysterectomy (if a uterus is found)—recommended. • Amputation of an enlarged clitoris—recommended if the mucosal surface is repeatedly traumatized.
• Reconstructive surgery of the prepuce and malformed penis—dogs; may be necessary with testicular DSD, XX males, or hypospadias.

MEDICATIONS

CONTRAINDICATIONS

Avoid androgen or progestagen use during pregnancy.

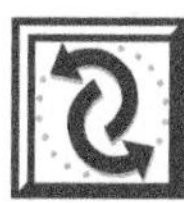

FOLLOW-UP

PREVENTION/AVOIDANCE

Sterilize individuals with heritable disorders.

POSSIBLE COMPLICATIONS

• Infertility. • Sterility. • Urinary tract problems—incontinence; cystitis. • Testicular neoplasia.• Pyometra.

MISCELLANEOUS

AGE-RELATED FACTORS

Patients not diagnosed at an early age—pyometra (e.g., PMDS; female pseudohermaphrodite); testicular neoplasia (e.g., PMDS; any DSD with cryptorchidism).

SYNONYMS

• Hermaphrodites. • Intersexes. • Klinefelter syndrome. • Pseudohermaphrodites. • Sex reversal. • Turner syndrome.

SEE ALSO

• Breeding, Timing.
• Cryptorchidism.
• Infertility, Female—Dogs.
• Infertility, Male—Dogs.

ABBREVIATIONS

• AMH = anti-Müllerian hormone.
• DSD = disorders of sexual development.
• GnRH = gonadotropin-releasing hormone.
• hCG = human chorionic gonadotropin.
• PMDS = persistent Müllerian duct syndrome.

Suggested Reading

Christensen BW. Disorders of sexual development in dogs and cats. Vet Clin Small Anim 2012, 42:515–526.

Author Erin E. Runcan
Consulting Editor Erin E. Runcan
Acknowledgment The author/editor acknowledges the prior contribution of Sara K. Lyle.

S

SHAKER/TREMOR SYNDROME, CORTICOSTEROID RESPONSIVE

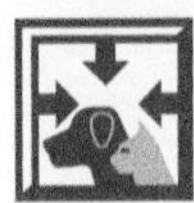

BASICS

OVERVIEW

Fine, rapid, whole-body tremor.

SYSTEMS AFFECTED

Nervous

SIGNALMENT

- Primarily dogs, but similar syndrome recently reported in 2 cats.
- Small to medium-size breed (<15 kg), young adult dogs (<5 years), regardless of coat color.
- Dogs with white-hair coats (e.g., Maltese and West Highland white terriers) historically have been overrepresented.
- Both sexes affected.

SIGNS

- Acute-onset, fine, rapid whole-body tremors.
- Clinical signs initially can be confused with signs of apprehension or hypothermia.
- Less commonly, signs can include abnormal nystagmus, hypermetria, head tilt, menace response deficits, and opsoclonus.

CAUSES & RISK FACTORS

Most often associated with mild inflammatory CNS disease.

S

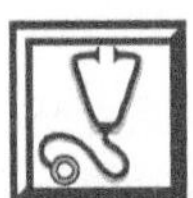

DIAGNOSIS

DIFFERENTIAL DIAGNOSIS

- Toxin ingestion—mycotoxins (penitrem A, roquefortine); metaldehyde (snail bait); pyrethrins/pyrethroids; organophosphates, many others.
- Seizures.
- Hypomyelination—seen in puppies; chow chow, springer spaniel, Samoyed, Weimaraner, and Dalmatian.
- Metabolic disorder—hypoglycemia, hypoadrenocorticism, hypocalcemia, magnesium imbalance.
- Behavioral—fear.
- Hypothermia.

CBC/BIOCHEMISTRY/URINALYSIS

Usually normal.

IMAGING

N/A

OTHER DIAGNOSTIC PROCEDURES

Cerebellomedullary cistern CSF analysis—mild mononuclear pleocytosis; CSF can be normal.

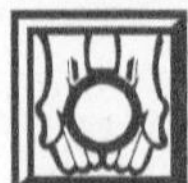

TREATMENT

Inpatient or outpatient, depending on severity of clinical signs.

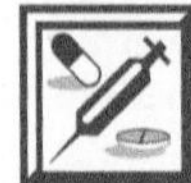

MEDICATIONS

DRUG(S) OF CHOICE

- Prednisolone or prednisone (1–2 mg/kg PO q12h) for the first 1–2 weeks.
- Depending on clinical response, taper dosage slowly (usually over 4–6 months); assess periodically for clinical deterioration; if dosage reduced too rapidly, clinical signs may recur, necessitating reintroduction of initial dosage.
- Many patients do not require further treatment.

CONTRAINDICATIONS/POSSIBLE INTERACTIONS

Corticosteroids—may be contraindicated with infectious encephalitis.

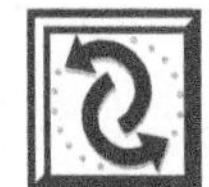

FOLLOW-UP

PATIENT MONITORING

Weekly evaluations for approximately 1 month; then monthly until corticosteroids are discontinued.

EXPECTED COURSE AND PROGNOSIS

- Clinical signs usually subside in 3–7 days from onset of steroid treatment.
- In some patients, recurrence necessitates reinstitution of corticosteroids.
- A small percentage of patients require every-other-day, low-dose corticosteroids, indefinitely, to maintain remission.

MISCELLANEOUS

SYNONYMS

- Idiopathic cerebellitis.
- White shaker syndrome.
- Idiopathic generalized tremor syndrome.

SEE ALSO

- Movement Disorders.
- Tremors.

INTERNET RESOURCES

N/A

Suggested Reading

Bagley RS, Kornegay JN, Wheeler SJ, et al. Generalized tremors in Maltese terriers: clinical findings in seven cases. J Am Anim Hosp Assoc 1993, 29:141–145.

Dewey CW. A Practical Guide to Canine & Feline Neurology, 2nd ed. Ames, IA: Wiley-Blackwell, 2008, pp. 311–322.

Wagner SO, Podell M, Fenner WR. Generalized tremors in dogs: 24 cases (1984–1995). J Am Vet Med Assoc 1997, 211:731–735.

Author Philip Schissler

SHOCK, CARDIOGENIC

BASICS

DEFINITION

• Severe manifestation of forward heart failure in which patients have both clinical and biochemical evidence of inadequate tissue perfusion. • Profound impairment of cardiac function resulting in poor cardiac output and life-threatening end-organ hypoperfusion and hypoxia in the presence of adequate intravascular volume and systemic vascular resistance. • Cardiac impairment may result from systolic dysfunction (dilated cardiomyopathy, sepsis, myocarditis, ischemia), diastolic dysfunction (hypertrophic cardiomyopathy, restrictive cardiomyopathy, tension pneumothorax/mediastinum, restrictive pericarditis, pericardial tamponade), conduction defects and arrhythmias, valvular diseases, obstructive diseases, pulmonary thromboembolism, and structural defects. Understanding the underlying defect and its hemodynamic consequences is imperative to institute appropriate therapy. • In congestive heart failure (CHF), sometimes referred to as backward heart failure, the ventricle cannot adequately pump out the returning blood, resulting in systemic and/or pulmonary edema. This is in contrast to forward heart failure, when the heart is not pumping enough blood out to meet the needs of the body. Most, but not all, veterinary patients that present in cardiogenic shock will have concurrent CHF.

PATHOPHYSIOLOGY

• Decreased cardiac output leads to hypotension and systemic hypoperfusion. • Hypotension decreases coronary perfusion, resulting in ischemia that provokes further myocardial dysfunction. • Peripheral vasoconstriction increases myocardial work and exacerbates tissue ischemia and energy depletion, resulting in organ dysfunction.

SYSTEMS AFFECTED

• Cardiovascular—cardiac dysfunction is causative, myocardial ischemia exacerbates cardiac dysfunction. • Musculoskeletal—weakness. • Nervous—altered mental status. • Respiratory—as cardiac dysfunction progresses and atrial pressure increases, pulmonary edema and/or pleural effusion develop and hypoxemia ensues. • Endocrine—hyperglycemia and insulin resistance. • Gastrointestinal—mucosal necrosis and sloughing, hemorrhage, bacterial translocation. • Hepatobiliary—hepatocellular enzyme leakage, cholestasis, reduced clearance of bacteria and bacterial by-products, and abnormal synthetic function; hepatic congestion may result from right-sided CHF. • Renal—ischemic tubular damage, oliguria, development of acute kidney injury. • Hemic—homeostatic imbalances lead to microvascular thrombosis.

GENETICS

Many breeds are predisposed to specific cardiac diseases.

INCIDENCE/PREVALENCE

Unknown

GEOGRAPHIC DISTRIBUTION

Unknown

SIGNALMENT

• Dog and cat. • Any breed, age, or sex.

SIGNS

Historical Findings

• Cardiac decompensation may be associated with a history of previously compensated heart disease and cardiac drug administration. • A suspicion of previously undiagnosed cardiac disease may result from a history of coughing, exercise intolerance, weakness, or syncope.

Physical Examination Findings

• Markers of poor perfusion: ○ Weakness. ○ Altered mental status. ○ Cool extremities and hypothermia. ○ Pale mucous membranes. ○ Prolonged capillary refill time. ○ Weak femoral pulse quality. ○ Oliguria. • Muffled heart sounds if pericardial or pleural effusion is present. • Variable heart rate with possible cardiac arrhythmia, murmur or gallop sound. • Variable respiratory rate with possible increased bronchovesicular sounds, crackles, or moist cough.

CAUSES

Primary Cardiac Disease

• All cardiomyopathies (e.g., dilated, hypertrophic, unclassified, restrictive). • Severe mitral insufficiency or other end-stage valvular disease. • Chordae tendineae rupture. • Tachy- or brady-arrhythmias. • Myocarditis. • Endomyocarditis (cats). • Structural defects (e.g. congenital heart disease).

Secondary Cardiac Dysfunction

• Cardiac tamponade. • Sepsis. • Severe electrolyte derangement. • Pulmonary thromboembolism. • Tension pneumothorax/mediastinum. • Caval syndrome.

RISK FACTORS

• Underlying cardiac disease. • Concurrent illness causing hypoxemia, acidosis, electrolyte imbalances, or as in sepsis, release of myocardial depressant factors.

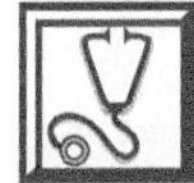

DIAGNOSIS

DIFFERENTIAL DIAGNOSIS

Cardiogenic shock is differentiated from other causes of circulatory shock when there is evidence of decreased cardiac output and tissue hypoxia in the face of adequate intravascular volume and systemic vascular resistance.

CBC/BIOCHEMISTRY/URINALYSIS

CBC

Mature neutrophilia and lymphopenia secondary to stress.

Biochemistry Panel

• Hyperglycemia—stress. • Elevated anion gap—accumulation of lactic and renal acids. • Elevated hepatocellular enzyme activity—hepatic hypoxia. • Elevated phosphorus—decreased glomerular filtration rate (GFR). • Azotemia—decreased GFR or hypoxia induced renal injury. • Hyponatremia and mild hypoalbuminemia—suggestive of chronic CHF.

Urinalysis

Isosthenuria—concomitant diuretic therapy or acute kidney injury.

OTHER LABORATORY TESTS

• Blood gas analysis—metabolic acidosis, respiratory alkalosis or acidosis, hypoxemia, and evidence of increased tissue oxygen extraction (widened arteriovenous oxygen difference and/or decreased venous oxygen concentration in the absence of hypoxemia or anemia). • Hyperlactatemia—tissue hypoperfusion. • Increased cardiac troponin I levels—sensitive and specific marker of myocardial injury. • B-type natriuretic peptide (NT-proBNP)—useful in ruling out intrinsic cardiac dysfunction.

IMAGING

Radiographs

Thoracic radiography may reveal cardiomegaly and evidence of CHF (pulmonary edema, pleural effusion).

Cageside Focused Pulmonary and Cardiac Ultrasound

• Lung ultrasound may reveal pleural effusion and/or B-lines (CHF). • Cardiac ultrasound to detect pericardial tamponade; patients with cardiogenic shock secondary to primary cardiac disease and some with secondary causes will have an increased left atrial size.

Echocardiography

To characterize cardiomyopathy, valvular disease, myocardial contractility, structural disease, pericardial disease, and heartworm infection.

DIAGNOSTIC PROCEDURES

Thoraco-, abdomino-, and pericardiocentesis when indicated may elucidate underlying etiology.

PATHOLOGIC FINDINGS

Cardiac abnormalities consistent with various underlying etiologies; abnormalities consistent with tissue hypoxia and CHF.

TREATMENT

APPROPRIATE HEALTH CARE

Emergency inpatient intensive care management.

SHOCK, CARDIOGENIC (CONTINUED)

NURSING CARE

• Minimize stress—patients are extremely fragile and at risk of cardiac arrest. • Oxygen supplementation. • Pleural effusion—relieve with thoracocentesis. • Respiratory failure—may require mechanical ventilation. • Patients should *not* receive *any* fluid therapy until the etiology of the underlying cardiac dysfunction is understood and cardiac function improved; exceptions include cardiogenic shock secondary to pericardial tamponade, tension pneumothorax and mediastinum, and pulmonary thromboembolism. • Pericardial tamponade—relieve with pericardiocentesis.

ACTIVITY

Minimize patient exertion.

DIET

Free choice access to water; withhold food until shock is resolved.

CLIENT EDUCATION

Discuss risk of imminent cardiac arrest and confirm "code status" in advance if possible.

SURGICAL CONSIDERATIONS

• Bradyarrhythmia may require pacemaker implantation. • Tension pneumothorax may require thoracostomy tube placement or exploratory thoracotomy. • Caval syndrome secondary to *Dirofilaria immitis* infection requires worm extraction.

S

MEDICATIONS

DRUG(S) OF CHOICE

• Fast-acting positive inotropes to improve cardiac function and preserve end-organ perfusion in patients with reduced myocardial contractility (pimobendan 0.25–0.3 mg/kg PO q12h in dogs and cats [IV formulation available in some countries]; dobutamine 5–20 µg/kg/min CRI in dogs; 2.5–15 µg/kg/min CRI in cats). While dobutamine can be used safely in many feline patients, seizures have been observed in some cats at doses exceeding 5 µg/kg/min. • Arrhythmias and conduction abnormalities should be corrected promptly with antiarrhythmic therapy, cardioversion, or pacemaker implantation.
• Ventricular tachycardia: ○ Dogs—lidocaine (2–4 mg/kg slow IV loading dose then 25–100 µg/kg/min CRI) or procainamide (5–15 mg/kg slow IV loading dose then 25–50 µg/kg/min CRI). Due to many common adverse effects, amiodarone (2–5 mg/kg IV, infused over 30–60 minutes) should only be used short term and the formulation should not contain polysorbate-80. • Sotalol (1–2.5 mg/kg PO, bid). Use with caution and at the lower end of the dosage range in dogs with concurrent CHF or DCM. ○ Cat procainamide (1–2 mg/kg IV slowly over 20 minutes) or lidocaine (0.25–0.5 mg/kg slow IV bolus then if needed 10–20 µg/kg/min). Caution when using lidocaine in cats as they may be at higher risk of toxicosis.
• Supraventricular tachyarrhythmia:
○ Treatments to slow the heart rate include vagal maneuvers, calcium channel blockers (diltiazem 0.125–0.35 mg/kg IV over 2–3 minutes or 0.125–0.35 mg/kg/h CRI), beta-blockers (esmolol 0.5 mg/kg IV over 1 minute), and procainamide (6–8 mg/kg IV over 5–10 minutes then 20–40 µg/kg/min CRI). ○ Patients unresponsive to vagal maneuvers or emergency drug therapy may require DC cardioversion or overdrive pacing.
• Bradyarrhythmia: ○ Cardiac pacing. ○ Some patients may benefit from atropine (0.02–0.04 mg/kg IV) or isoproterenol (0.4 mg in 250 mL D_5W slowly to effect). • Concurrent CHF:
○ Furosemide to treat pulmonary edema in dogs and cats (2–8 mg/kg IV or IM; or 0.5–1.0 mg/kg/h CRI); IV route is preferable, but IM is appropriate when manual restraint to obtain IV access puts the patient at risk. ○ Relief of pain or anxiety with morphine sulfate (0.1–0.5 mg/kg/h IV CRI, or 0.2–2 mg/kg IM) can reduce excessive sympathetic activity and decrease oxygen demand, preload, and afterload.

CONTRAINDICATIONS

• Avoid diuretic therapy in patients with pericardial tamponade, tension pneumothorax/mediastinum, and pulmonary thromboembolism. • Avoid beta-blockers and calcium channel blockers in patients with reduced myocardial contractility.

PRECAUTIONS

• Catecholamine infusions must be carefully titrated to maximize coronary perfusion with the least possible increase in myocardial oxygen demand. • Afterload reducers and vasodilators (angiotensin-converting enzyme inhibitors, nitroglycerin, and nitroprusside) should be used with caution because of the risk for worsening hypotension and decreasing coronary blood flow.

ALTERNATIVE DRUG(S)

Dopamine may be used to improve systolic function as an alternative to dobutamine at a dose of 5–10 µg/kg/min (dogs and cats).

FOLLOW-UP

PATIENT MONITORING

• Serial assessment of perfusion (mentation, mucous membrane color, capillary refill time, pulse quality, muscle strength, temperature, serum lactate, urine output, heart rate, BP, and oxygenation indices), respiratory rate and effort, and pulmonary auscultation is required to optimize therapy. • Blood gas analysis and pulse oximetry to assess tissue oxygenation, ventilation, and acid–base balance. • Packed cell volume, serum total protein, serum electrolytes, hepatocellular enzymes, BUN, and serum creatinine to monitor effects of systemic tissue hypoxia. • Daily cardiac troponin I levels to assess degree of myocardial injury in some cases. • BP measurement may document hypotension. • Electrocardiography may aid detection and characterization of arrhythmias. • Pulse oximetry may document low oxygen saturation. • Central venous pressure monitoring may aid in assessment of cardiac preload and central venous oxygen saturation. • Hemodynamic monitoring to assess mixed venous oxygen saturation, cardiac output and systemic vascular resistance.

PREVENTION/AVOIDANCE

Prevention strategies aimed at the various underlying etiologies.

POSSIBLE COMPLICATIONS

• CHF. • Cardiac arrhythmias. • Syncope.
• Acid–base and electrolyte disturbances.
• Renal dysfunction. • Cardiac arrest.

EXPECTED COURSE AND PROGNOSIS

Dependent on underlying etiology. Patients with primary cardiac disease have generally worse prognosis (poor to grave) as compared to those with secondary cardiac dysfunction.

MISCELLANEOUS

ASSOCIATED CONDITIONS

CHF

AGE-RELATED FACTORS

Variable, depending on underlying etiology.

ZOONOTIC POTENTIAL

None

PREGNANCY/FERTILITY/BREEDING

Variable, depending on underling etiology.

SEE ALSO

• Atrioventricular Block. • Cardiomyopathy.
• Congestive Heart Failure, Left-Sided.
• Congestive Heart Failure, Right-Sided.
• Endomyocardial Diseases—Cats.
• Myocarditis. • Pericardial Disease.
• Pneumothorax. • Pulmonary Thromboembolism. • Sepsis and Bacteremia.
• Shock, Hypovolemic. • Shock, Septic.
• Sick Sinus Syndrome. • Supraventricular Tachycardia. • Ventricular Tachycardia.

ABBREVIATIONS

• BP = blood pressure.
• CHF = congestive heart failure.
• GFR = glomerular filtration rate.

Suggested Reading

De Laforcade A, Silverstein DC. Shock. In: Silverstein DC, Hopper K, ed., Small Animal Critical Care Medicine, 2nd ed. St. Louis, MO: Saunders, 2015, pp. 26–30.

Hopper K, Silverstein D, Bateman S. Shock syndromes. In: Dibartola SP, ed., Fluid Therapy in Small Animal Practice, 4th ed. Philadelphia, PA: Saunders, 2011, pp. 557–583.

Author Gretchen L. Schoeffler
Consulting Editor Michael Aherne

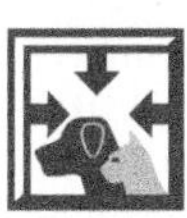

BASICS

DEFINITION

Inadequate circulating volume and perfusion due to fluid loss.

PATHOPHYSIOLOGY

- Hemorrhage or other fluid loss results in a critical decrease in intravascular volume, diminished venous return, and decreased cardiac output.
- Compensatory neuroendocrine responses lead to peripheral vasoconstriction thus exacerbating tissue ischemia and energy depletion, resulting in organ dysfunction.

SYSTEMS AFFECTED

- Cardiovascular—increased heart rate, increased cardiac contractility, and peripheral vasoconstriction; increased cardiac oxygen demand in the face of reduced oxygen delivery may cause arrhythmias.
- Respiratory—hyperventilation to compensate for metabolic acidosis.
- Musculoskeletal—weakness.
- Nervous—altered mental status.
- Endocrine—hyperglycemia and insulin resistance.
- Gastrointestinal (GI)—mucosal necrosis and sloughing, hemorrhage, bacterial translocation.
- Hepatobiliary—hepatocellular enzyme leakage, cholestasis, reduced clearance of bacteria and their by-products, abnormal synthetic function.
- Renal—ischemic tubular damage, oliguria, acute kidney injury.
- Hemic—homeostatic imbalances lead to microvascular thrombosis as well as hyper- and hypocoagulability.

GENETICS

N/A

INCIDENCE/PREVALENCE

Unknown

GEOGRAPHIC DISTRIBUTION

N/A

SIGNALMENT

- Dog and cat.
- Any breed, age, or sex.

SIGNS

Historical Findings

May have history of trauma, weakness, collapse, surgery, vomiting, diarrhea, decreased water intake, and polyuria.

Physical Examination Findings

- Compensated shock/warm shock/preshock:
  - Compensatory mechanisms may allow an otherwise healthy pet to be relatively asymptomatic despite a 10% reduction in total effective blood volume. When homeostatic mechanisms fail, decompensated shock ensues.
- Decompensated shock:
  - Poor perfusion (pale mucous membranes [may be compounded by anemia], prolonged capillary refill time, weak peripheral pulses, weakness, altered mental status, hypothermia/cool extremities, oliguria).
  - Absent/minimal jugular vein distension.
  - Tachycardia ± arrhythmia.
  - Tachypnea.
  - Clinical dehydration (decreased skin turgor, tacky mucous membranes, and sunken eyes) more common in patients with fluid loss than hemorrhage.

CAUSES

Hemorrhage

- Trauma.
- Ruptured neoplasm.
- GI bleeding (e.g., ulcerative disease, neoplasia, severe thrombocytopenia).
- Coagulopathy (e.g., severe thrombocytopenia/ thrombocytopathy, von Willebrand factor deficiency, anticoagulant rodenticide intoxication, synthetic liver failure, disseminated intravascular coagulation, hemophilia, other bleeding disorders).

Fluid Loss

- GI (vomiting and diarrhea).
- Urinary (renal failure, diabetes mellitus, diabetes insipidus, hypercalcemia, Addison's, and Cushing's diseases).
- Burns.
- Third spacing (any disease resulting in significant effusion).

RISK FACTORS

No specific risk factors; caused by another condition.

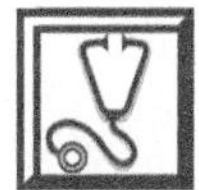

DIAGNOSIS

DIFFERENTIAL DIAGNOSIS

Hypovolemic shock differentiated from other causes of circulatory shock when inadequate circulating volume results in decreased cardiac output in the face of normal or increased cardiac function and normal or increased systemic vascular resistance.

CBC/BIOCHEMISTRY/URINALYSIS

CBC

- Stress leukogram.
- Hematocrit and platelet count are variable (may be decreased with hemorrhage).

Biochemistry Panel

- Hyperglycemia.
- Variable total protein (TP) and albumin (decreased with hemorrhage; increased in fluid loss).
- Elevated hepatocellular enzyme activity (alanine aminotransferase, aspartate aminotransferase).
- Variable electrolyte derangements (more likely in fluid loss).
- Variable anion gap.
- Azotemia due to decreased glomerular filtration rate.

Urinalysis

- Urine specific gravity may be increased; however, acute tubular injury due to renal hypoxia may cause isosthenuria.

OTHER LABORATORY TESTS

- Blood gas analysis may reveal metabolic acidosis and evidence of increased tissue oxygen extraction (widened arteriovenous oxygen difference and/or decreased venous oxygen concentration in a patient without hypoxemia or anemia).
- Hyperlactatemia reflects decreased clearance and increased production of lactate.
- Coagulation testing if critically ill or if evidence of significant hemorrhage.

IMAGING

- Thoracic radiography may reveal microcardia and pulmonary vascular underperfusion.
- May have radiographic or ultrasonographic findings of pleural or abdominal effusion.

DIAGNOSTIC PROCEDURES

Thoracocentesis, abdominocentesis, or pericardiocentesis, if indicated, may provide insight into underlying etiology.

PATHOLOGIC FINDINGS

Consistent with tissue hypoxia and underlying etiology.

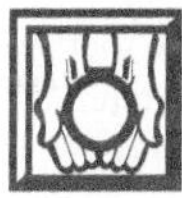

TREATMENT

APPROPRIATE HEALTH CARE

Emergency inpatient intensive care management.

NURSING CARE

- Maximize blood oxygen content:
  - Assess and stabilize airway and breathing as necessary.
  - Supplemental oxygen and ventilatory support as needed.
  - Significant anemia (packed cell volume [PCV] <25–30%) in a hypovolemic patient is concerning and should be corrected.
- Control further fluid loss:
  - External bleeding controlled with direct pressure; internal bleeding may require surgical intervention.
- Control of fluid loss, other than hemorrhage, aimed at control of signs (e.g., antiemetics) and correcting underlying disorder.
- Fluid resuscitation:
  - Once IV or IO access obtained, initial fluid resuscitation performed with isotonic crystalloid such as lactated Ringer's solution, normal saline, Plasmalyte-A, and

SHOCK, HYPOVOLEMIC (CONTINUED)

Normosol-R (20–30 mL/kg, dog; 15–20 mL/kg, cat; over 15 minutes). If no significant dehydration and no other contraindications, addition of 7.5% hypertonic saline (4 mL/kg over 15 minutes) may expedite resuscitation.
  - Assess response to initial bolus. If vital signs and other resuscitation parameters return to normal, monitoring must be continued to ensure stability. If vital signs and other resuscitation parameters transiently improve or if little or no improvement seen, another crystalloid bolus should be infused and colloids such as hydroxyethylstarch (dose variable, dependent on type) or appropriate blood products (10–20 mL/kg) considered.
  - Process is repeated until resuscitation parameters normalize. When bolusing fluids to correct perfusion deficits, monitor not only for response to therapy, but also for potential complications.
  - While fluid boluses are used to correct perfusion deficits, hydration deficits must be corrected more slowly. After perfusion has normalized, patient is reassessed and fluid therapy targeted to correct hydration deficits over 12–24 hours.
- Traditional endpoints of resuscitation (restoration of normal vital signs, blood pressure, and urine output) remain the standard of care; however, it has been documented that critically ill patients have evidence of ongoing tissue hypoxia despite normalization of these parameters, suggesting occult oxygen debt and the presence of compensated shock. There is evidence that normalization of vital signs, blood lactate, base deficit, and oxygen transport indices such as cardiac index, oxygen delivery, oxygen consumption, and mixed venous oxygen and central venous oxygen saturation in concert are more sensitive markers for adequacy of tissue perfusion than any of these variables alone. Until stronger support exists for preferential selection of one endpoint over others, utilization of as many of these markers as are available seems advisable.

S

ACTIVITY
Minimize patient exertion.

DIET
Withhold oral intake until shock is resolved.

CLIENT EDUCATION
Discuss risk of cardiac arrest and confirm "code status" in advance if possible.

SURGICAL CONSIDERATIONS
Identify and repair source of fluid loss (most common in hemorrhage-induced).

MEDICATIONS

DRUG(S) OF CHOICE
- For patients with refractory hypovolemic shock, rule out ongoing losses (especially if hemorrhage-induced); administer blood products as needed.
- If adequate circulating volume is assured and patient is still demonstrating clinical signs of shock (not very common with hypovolemic shock), consider:
  - Pressors such as dopamine (5–20 µg/kg/min), norepinephrine (0.05–2 µg/kg/min), or vasopressin (0.5–2 mU/kg/min). These can be used for vasopressor support in dogs and cats. Monitor for tachyarrhythmia and excessive peripheral vasoconstriction.
  - Positive inotropes such as dobutamine (2–20 µg/kg/min) may be beneficial in patients with decreased contractility or myocardial depression. Monitor for tachyarrhythmia. While dobutamine can generally be used safely in dogs, seizures have been observed in some cats at doses exceeding 5 µg/kg/min.
- For bleeding dogs, antifibrinolytic medications such as ε-aminocaproic acid (50–100 mg/kg IV or PO q6h) or tranexamic acid (10 mg/kg IV bolus over 20 minutes, followed by 10 mg/kg/h IV CRI for 3 hours, then 10 mg/kg over 20 minutes q6h) may be considered.

CONTRAINDICATIONS
N/A

PRECAUTIONS
N/A

POSSIBLE INTERACTIONS
N/A

ALTERNATIVE DRUG(S)
N/A

FOLLOW-UP

PATIENT MONITORING
- Serial assessment of perfusion:
  - Physical exam including mentation, mucous membrane color, capillary refill time, pulse quality, muscle strength, temperature, and heart rate.
  - Hemodynamic monitoring to include arterial blood pressure (frequently reveals disproportionately low diastolic pressure), and in a subset of patients central venous pressure, cardiac output and tissue oxygenation.
  - Laboratory data including serum lactate and base deficit; patients with hemorrhage-induced hypovolemic shock should have minimum of daily PCV, and TP assessed more frequently.
- Serial assessment of respiratory rate and effort, and pulmonary auscultation is required to optimize therapy.
- Urine output as indicator of glomerular filtration rate and renal blood flow.
- ECG may aid in characterization of arrhythmias.
- Minimum of daily PCV, serum TP, blood glucose, blood gas, serum electrolytes, hepatocellular enzymes, BUN, and serum creatinine to monitor effects of systemic tissue hypoxia and to guide clinical management.

PREVENTION/AVOIDANCE
Prevention strategies aimed at the various underlying etiologies.

POSSIBLE COMPLICATIONS
- Acid–base disturbances.
- Anemia and thrombocytopenia.
- Multiple organ dysfunction.
- Low colloid oncotic pressure.
- Volume overload with clinical signs of pulmonary and/or peripheral edema.
- Dilutional coagulopathy can occur in patients receiving very large resuscitation volumes (more than 1–2 blood volumes), due to dilution of clotting factors and proteins respectively, but is rare within the first hour of resuscitation. Coagulation times should be used to guide the administration of fresh frozen plasma.
- Cardiac arrest.

EXPECTED COURSE AND PROGNOSIS
Depends on underlying etiology and ability to institute appropriate therapy.

MISCELLANEOUS

PREGNANCY/FERTILITY/BREEDING
N/A

SEE ALSO
- Shock, Cardiogenic.
- Shock, Septic.

ABBREVIATIONS
- GI = gastrointestinal.
- PCV = packed cell volume.
- TP = total protein.

Suggested Reading

Hopper K, Silverstein D, Bateman S. Shock syndromes. In: Dibartola SP, ed., Fluid Therapy in Small Animal Practice, 4th ed. Philadelphia, PA: Saunders, 2011, pp. 557–583.

Author Gretchen L. Schoeffler
Consulting Editor Michael Aherne

BASICS

DEFINITION

Sepsis-induced hypotension, attributable to low systemic vascular resistance that persists despite adequate intravascular volume and cardiac output.

PATHOPHYSIOLOGY

• In sepsis, an elaborate interaction of inflammatory cells and mediators decreases systemic vascular resistance and provokes maldistribution of blood flow (distributive effect). Vasodilation is primarily mediated by increased nitric oxide and prostacyclin synthesis induced by endotoxin and inflammatory cytokine interaction with vascular endothelial cells. In the face of severe arterial vasodilation, cardiac output is insufficient to maintain tissue oxygen delivery. • Infectious agents trigger large-scale activation of monocytes, macrophages, and neutrophils that interact with endothelial cells, inducing a generalized inflammatory response. Endothelial injury is a universal feature, mediated by cellular and humoral factors that increase capillary permeability, and fluid shifts out of the intravascular space. Presence of interstitial edema and microvascular sludging further compound oxygen delivery, and tissue hypoxia leads to organ failure and death.

SYSTEMS AFFECTED

• Cardiovascular—arterial vasodilation and maldistribution of blood flow with hypotension predominates; cardiac output frequently normal or high; however, myocardial dysfunction due to circulating factors can be important. • Nervous—altered mental status. • Endocrine—may have hyperglycemia and insulin resistance, or insufficient production of either corticosteroids or vasopressin. • Gastrointestinal—mucosal necrosis, hemorrhage, bacterial translocation. • Respiratory—interstitial and alveolar edema due to enhanced microvascular permeability; hypercoagulopathy may result in pulmonary thromboembolism. • Hepatobiliary—hepatocellular enzyme leakage, cholestasis, reduced bacterial clearance, hypoglycemia and abnormal synthesis. • Hemic—microvascular thrombosis, hyper- and hypocoagulopathy. • Renal—ischemic tubular damage, oliguria, acute kidney injury.

GENETICS

N/A

INCIDENCE/PREVALENCE

Unknown

GEOGRAPHIC DISTRIBUTION

N/A

SIGNALMENT

• Dog and cat. • Any breed, age, or sex.

SIGNS

Historical Findings

Recent infection, injury, serious illness, surgery, or immunosuppression.

Physical Examination Findings

• Dogs may have a hyperdynamic form, typified by altered mental status, weakness, hypotension, tachycardia, tachypnea, hyperemia, fast capillary refill time (CRT), bounding pulses, and fever. Cats rarely have hyperdynamic signs. • Patients with the hypodynamic form are more likely to exhibit altered mental status, weakness, hypotension, bradycardia, tachypnea, pale mucous membranes, prolonged CRT, weak pulses, and hypothermia.

CAUSES

• Septic peritonitis—ruptured viscus; penetrating wound. • Respiratory and pleural space—pneumonia, pyothorax. • Skin or soft tissue—wounds, burns, cellulitis, abscess. • Urinary tract—pyelonephritis. • Reproductive—prostatitis, metritis, pyometra. • Cardiovascular—endocarditis, bacteremia. • Musculoskeletal—septic arthritis, osteomyelitis. • Iatrogenic—catheters, implants, surgical sites. • CNS—meningitis, encephalitis.

RISK FACTORS

• Extremes of age. • Concurrent disease (e.g., diabetes mellitus, Cushing's disease, malignancy). • Immunosuppression. • Surgery, trauma, burns. • Prior antibiotics.

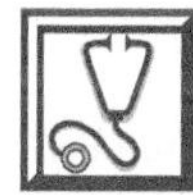

DIAGNOSIS

DIFFERENTIAL DIAGNOSIS

• Other causes of distributive shock (e.g., drug/toxin reaction, anaphylaxis, adrenal insufficiency). • Hypovolemic shock. • Cardiogenic shock. • Heatstroke.

CBC/BIOCHEMISTRY/URINALYSIS

• Neutrophilia or neutropenia, left shift, and toxic change. • Lymphopenia. • Thrombocytopenia. • Variable hematocrit and blood glucose. • Hypoalbuminemia. • Elevated bilirubin and liver enzyme activity. • Electrolyte derangements. • Azotemia. • Isosthenuria and variably active urine sediment.

OTHER LABORATORY TESTS

• Prolonged activated partial thromboplastin and prothrombin times, increased D-dimers and fibrin degradation products, and decreased levels of antithrombin and protein C. • Blood gases may reveal hypoxemia and acid–base disturbances. • Hyperlactatemia. • Cytology, Gram stain, and culture and sensitivity on samples obtained from potential sites of infection may reveal etiologic organisms. • Culture and sensitivity of urine and blood may be useful when the source of sepsis is unknown. • Adrenocorticotropic hormone (ACTH) stimulation test in patients unresponsive to standard therapy.

IMAGING

• Thoracic radiographs and CT may reveal septic focus or cause for respiratory dysfunction; may also provide insights into volume status. • Echocardiography may document a vegetative valvular lesion and/or characterize cardiac function and volume status. • Abdominal ultrasonography and CT may detect source of infection.

DIAGNOSTIC PROCEDURES

When indicated, tissue aspirates, thoraco-, abdomino-, and arthrocentesis may provide insight into underlying etiology.

PATHOLOGIC FINDINGS

Consistent with inflammation, tissue hypoxia, and underlying etiology.

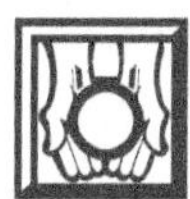

TREATMENT

APPROPRIATE HEALTH CARE

Emergency inpatient intensive care management. Early surgical intervention when possible to control source of infection.

NURSING CARE

Maximize Blood Oxygen Content

• Assess and stabilize the airway and breathing as necessary. • Administer supplemental oxygen and provide ventilatory support as needed. • Significant anemia (packed cell volume [PCV] <25%) should be corrected.

Resuscitation

Most septic patients are hypovolemic and require initial fluid resuscitation with isotonic crystalloids such as lactated Ringer's solution, normal saline, Plasmalyte-A, and Normosol-R (20–30 mL/kg, dog; 15–20 mL/kg, cat, over 15 minutes). If no significant dehydration, addition of 7.5% hypertonic saline (4 mL/kg over 15 minutes) may expedite resuscitation: • After the initial bolus, patient is reassessed. If vital signs and other resuscitation parameters normalize, continue monitoring to ensure stability. If vital signs and other resuscitation parameters transiently improve or if little or no improvement is seen and patient is still deemed hypovolemic, sequential crystalloid boluses should be infused and colloids (dose variable, dependent on type) may be considered. • Septic patients receiving large fluid volumes may achieve adequate circulating volume without normalization of BP and other perfusion parameters. Continued aggressive fluid therapy in these patients will result in volume overload and vasopressors and/or positive inotropes are indicated. Monitor closely since infusion of large volumes may precipitate pulmonary edema in patients with capillary leak. • IV fluids, vasopressors, and positive inotropes are titrated until resuscitation endpoints have been achieved. Traditional endpoints of resuscitation (restoration of normal vital signs, BP, and urine output) remain the standard of care; however, it has been documented that critically ill patients have evidence of ongoing tissue hypoxia despite normalization of these parameters, suggesting occult oxygen debt and presence of compensated shock. There is evidence that normalization of vital signs, blood lactate, base deficit, and oxygen transport indices are more sensitive markers for adequacy of tissue perfusion than any of these variables alone. Until stronger support exists for preferential selection of one endpoint over others, utilization of as many of these markers as are available seems advisable. • Blood products should be administered based on patient need. Packed red blood cells are administered to anemic patients to improve oxygen-carrying capacity and plasma products are used to correct coagulation deficits.

ACTIVITY

Minimize patient exertion.

DIET

Withhold oral intake until shock is resolved.

S

CLIENT EDUCATION

Discuss risk of cardiac arrest and confirm "code status" in advance if possible.

SURGICAL CONSIDERATIONS

Identify and eliminate infection source when, and as early as, possible.

MEDICATIONS

DRUG(S) OF CHOICE

• Once adequate circulating volume is achieved, improvement in systemic BP and other clinical resuscitation parameters may require one or more vasopressors and/or positive inotropes: ○ Norepinephrine (0.05–2 µg/kg/min), vasopressin (0.5–2 mU/kg/min), or dopamine (5–20 µg/kg/min) can be used for vasopressor support (dogs and cats). Monitor for tachyarrhythmia and excessive peripheral vasoconstriction. ○ Dobutamine (2–20 µg/kg/min) is primarily used as a positive inotrope in canine septic shock patients with decreased contractility or myocardial depression. Monitor for tachyarrhythmia. While dobutamine can be used safely in many feline patients, seizures have been observed in some cats at doses exceeding 5 µg/kg/min. • It is essential that IV, empiric, broad-spectrum antibiotic therapy be instituted early in septic patients; the spectrum should be narrowed when culture results become available. Empiric selection based on patient's underlying immune status, suspected source and organism(s) responsible, specific antibiotic properties (tissue penetration, cidal versus static activity), and considerations for resistance (previous antibiotic use, hospital- or community-acquired infection). • It is not unreasonable to empirically treat patients not responding adequately to standard therapy with 0.75–1.0 mg/kg q6h IV hydrocortisone after undergoing a standard ACTH stimulation test. Therapy should be continued in patients in whom relative adrenal insufficiency is documented.

CONTRAINDICATIONS

N/A

PRECAUTIONS

N/A

POSSIBLE INTERACTIONS

N/A

ALTERNATIVE DRUG(S)

N/A

FOLLOW-UP

PATIENT MONITORING

• Serial assessment of perfusion to optimize titration of fluids and vasoactive drugs: ○ Physical exam including mentation, mucous membrane color, CRT, pulse quality, muscle strength, temperature, and heart rate. ○ Hemodynamic monitoring to include arterial BP (frequently reveals disproportionately low diastolic pressure), and in some patients central venous pressure, cardiac output, and tissue oxygenation. ○ Thoracic ultrasound to monitor for pulmonary changes and to aid in assessing patient volume status and cardiac systolic function. ○ Laboratory data including serum lactate and base deficit. • Blood gas analysis and pulse oximetry to follow tissue oxygenation, ventilation, and acid–base status. • Serial assessment of respiratory rate and effort, and pulmonary auscultation. • Continuous ECG to detect arrhythmia. • Urine output as an indicator of glomerular filtration rate and renal blood flow. • Minimum of twice daily PCV, serum total protein, blood glucose, and serum electrolytes; once daily hepatocellular enzymes, blood urea nitrogen, and serum creatinine to monitor effects of systemic tissue hypoxia. Patients with coagulopathy should have coagulation indices, PCV and total protein assessed as needed.

PREVENTION/AVOIDANCE

• Timely and effective wound treatment.
• Appropriate antimicrobial therapy.

POSSIBLE COMPLICATIONS

• Volume overload. • Pulmonary edema.
• Vasculitis and peripheral edema. • Acid–base disturbances. • Anemia. • Thrombocytopenia and other coagulopathy. • Multiple organ dysfunction. • Cardiac arrest.

EXPECTED COURSE AND PROGNOSIS

Dependent on underlying etiology and ability to institute appropriate therapy.

MISCELLANEOUS

ASSOCIATED CONDITIONS

Sepsis

AGE-RELATED FACTORS

N/A

ZOONOTIC POTENTIAL

Variable infectious agent etiologies have zoonotic potential.

PREGNANCY/FERTILITY/BREEDING

N/A

SYNONYMS

N/A

SEE ALSO

• Disseminated Intravascular Coagulation.
• Hyperadrenocorticism (Cushing's Syndrome)—Cats.
• Hyperadrenocorticism (Cushing's Syndrome)—Dogs.
• Hypoadrenocorticism (Addison's Disease).
• Shock, Cardiogenic.
• Shock, Hypovolemic.

ABBREVIATIONS

• ACTH = adrenocorticotropic hormone.
• CRT = capillary refill time.
• PCV = packed cell volume.

Suggested Reading

De Laforcade A, Silverstein DC. Shock. In: Silverstein DC, Hopper K, ed., Small Animal Critical Care Medicine, 2nd ed., St. Louis, MO: Saunders, 2015, pp. 26–30.

Russell JA, Rush B, Boyd J. Pathophysiology of septic shock. Crit Care Clin 2018, 34:43–61.

Author Gretchen L. Schoeffler
Consulting Editor Michael Aherne

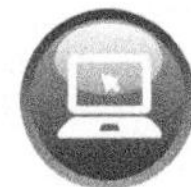

Client Education Handout available online

SHOULDER JOINT, LIGAMENT, AND TENDON CONDITIONS

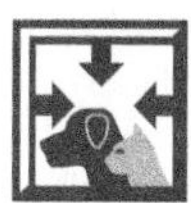

BASICS

DEFINITION

These make up the majority of causes for lameness in the canine shoulder joint, excluding osteochondritis dissecans lesions.

PATHOPHYSIOLOGY

Bicipital Tenosynovitis

- Strain injury to the tendon of the biceps brachii.
- Mechanism of injury—direct trauma; indirect trauma (more common).
- Pathologic changes—from partial disruption of the tendon to chronic inflammatory changes, including dystrophic calcification.
- Proliferation of the fibrous connective tissue and adhesions between the tendon and the sheath—limit motion; cause pain.

Fibrotic Contracture of the Infraspinatus Muscle

- Primary muscle–tendon disorder—not a neuropathy.
- Fibrous tissue replaces normal muscle.
- Loss of elasticity and function.
- Degeneration and atrophy of affected muscle.
- Partial muscle disruption—likely caused by repetitive strain injuries.

Medial Shoulder Instability

- Structural damage (stretch and rupture) of the capsulotendinous structures of the medial joint—the medial glenohumeral ligament, subscapularis tendon, and medial joint capsule.
- Likely secondary to repetitive strain injury—overuse injury vs. altered shoulder mechanics due to concurrent ipsilateral elbow disease.

Other

- Rupture of the biceps brachii tendon of origin—strain injury or disruption of the tendinous fibers at or near the junction with the supraglenoid tubercle of the scapula.
- Mineralization of the supraspinatus tendon; granular deposits between the fibers of the tendon; unknown cause; probably repetitive strain injury.
- Avulsion or fracture of the insertion of the supraspinatus tendon—bone is avulsed from the greater tubercle of the proximal humerus.
- Strain injury to other muscles/tendons in the region.

SYSTEMS AFFECTED

Musculoskeletal

INCIDENCE/PREVALENCE

Common cause of forelimb lameness.

SIGNALMENT

Species

Dog

Breed Predilections

Medium- to large-breed dogs.

Mean Age and Range

- Skeletally mature dogs ≥1 year of age.
- Usually 3–7 years of age.

SIGNS

Historical Findings

- Bicipital tenosynovitis—onset usually insidious; often of several months duration; may be a traumatic incident as the inciting cause; subtle, intermittent lameness that worsens with exercise.
- Rupture of the biceps brachii tendon of origin—similar to bicipital tenosynovitis; may have acute onset due to a known traumatic event; usually subtle, chronic lameness that worsens with exercise.
- Medial shoulder instability— onset usually insidious; often of several months duration; may be a traumatic incident as the inciting cause; subtle, intermittent lameness that worsens with exercise.
- Mineralization of the supraspinatus tendon—onset usually insidious; chronic lameness that worsens with activity.
- Avulsion/fracture of the supraspinatus tendon—similar to mineralization of supraspinatus tendon.
- Fibrotic contracture of the infraspinatus muscle—usually sudden onset of lameness during a period of outdoor exercise (e.g., hunting); shoulder lameness and tenderness gradually disappears within 2 weeks; condition results in chronic, persistent lameness 3–4 weeks later, which is not particularly painful but has characteristic gait and limb carriage.

Physical Examination Findings

- Bicipital tenosynovitis—short and limited swing phase of gait owing to pain on extension and flexion of the shoulder; pain inconsistently demonstrated on manipulation of shoulder; pain most evident by applying deep digital pressure over the tendon in the intertubercular groove region while simultaneously flexing the shoulder and extending the elbow.
- Rupture of the biceps brachii tendon—similar to above, however full rupture will result in exaggerated extension of the elbow with simultaneous flexion of the shoulder (when compared to the contralateral side).
- Medial shoulder instability—pain on abduction of the thoracic limb with excessive abduction when compared to the contralateral side. Under sedation, abnormal abduction angles have been measured to be approximately 50 degrees, while normal abduction angles are approximately 30 degrees.
- Mineralization of the supraspinatus tendon—similar; manipulations often do not produce pain; may palpate firm swelling over the greater tubercle.
- Avulsion or fracture of the supraspinatus tendon—similar to mineralization of the supraspinatus tendon.
- Fibrotic contracture of the infraspinatus muscle—usually not painful on manipulation; not possible to internally rotate (pronate) the shoulder joint; when forced, the caudal aspect of the scapula elevates off the trunk, when standing—elbow adducted; paw abducted and outwardly rotated; when patient is walking—lower limb swings in a lateral arc (circumduction) as the paw is advanced; marked atrophy of the infraspinatus muscle on palpation.

CAUSES

- Indirect or direct trauma—likely.
- Repetitive strain injury (indirect trauma)—most common.

RISK FACTORS

- Overexertion and/or fatigue.
- Poor conditioning before performing athletic activities.
- Obesity.

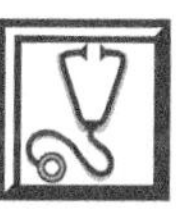

DIAGNOSIS

DIFFERENTIAL DIAGNOSIS

- Examination, palpation, and radiography that localizes disease to the shoulder will only be accurate 80% of the time—20% of the time, disease localized to the shoulder will actually be the result of elbow pathology/dysplasia.
- Luxation or subluxation of the shoulder joint—history of trauma with an acute onset of lameness; often severe lameness with marked pain on manipulation of the shoulder joint.
- Osteosarcoma of the proximal humerus—progressive lameness with varying degrees of pain on manipulation of the shoulder; may note swelling and tenderness of the proximal humerus.
- Brachial plexus nerve sheath tumor—slow, insidious, progressive lameness over a period of months; marked atrophy of the muscles with chronic disease; may feel a firm mass deep in the axillary region that is painful to digital pressure.

IMAGING

Radiology

- Required for differentiation.
- Craniocaudal and mediolateral views necessary for all patients.
- Skyline projections are helpful for highlighting the biceps groove.

Bicipital Tenosynovitis

- Radiographs generally normal with recent injuries.
- Mediolateral view (chronic disease)—may see bony reaction on the supraglenoid tubercle,

S

dystrophic calcification of the bicipital tendon, sclerosis of the floor of the intertubercular groove, and osteophytes in the intertubercular groove (also in the skyline view).

Ruptured Origin of the Biceps Brachii Tendon

Chronic disease—may see bony, irregular reaction on the supraglenoid tubercle.

Mineralization of the Supraspinatus Tendon

- Mediolateral view—calcified foci in tendon cranial and immediately medial to the greater tubercle of the proximal humerus.
- Tangential or skyline view of the intertubercular region of the proximal humerus—eliminates superimposition; allows distinction from calcification of the biceps brachii tendon.
- Often bilateral radiographically but rarely produces bilateral lameness.

Avulsion/Fracture of the Supraspinatus Tendon

- Similar to mineralization of the supraspinatus tendon.
- Avulsion fragment—may be seen as a defect in the greater tubercle of the humerus; generally not as radiographically dense as that identified with mineralization of the supraspinatus tendon.

S

Fibrotic Contracture of the Infraspinatus Muscle

Radiographically normal.

CT, Ultrasonography, and MRI

- May help identify muscle injuries, bicipital tenosynovitis, and rupture of the biceps brachii tendon of origin.
- Useful for determining the location of calcific densities near the intertubercular groove.
- MRI may be useful in evaluating medial shoulder disease, however extensive peer-reviewed publications are lacking.

DIAGNOSTIC PROCEDURES

- Joint tap and analysis of synovial fluid—identify intra-articular disease; fluid should be straw-colored with normal to decreased viscosity; cytologic evaluation: <10,000 nucleated cells/µL (>90% are mononuclear cells).
- Arthroscopic exploration of the shoulder joint—diagnose bicipital tenosynovitis and rupture of the biceps brachii tendon of origin; evaluate support structures of the medial shoulder, confirm lack of other intra-articular disease (osteochondrosis or traumatic injury).

PATHOLOGIC FINDINGS

- Bicipital tenosynovitis—mineralization of the biceps tendon; osteophytosis of the intertubercular groove; proliferative synovitis; impingement of the supraspinatus tendon of insertion on the biceps tendon, and fibrous adhesions between the biceps tendon and its synovial sheath; histologically, synovial proliferation, edema, fibrosis, dystrophic mineralization, and lymphocytic–plasmacytic infiltration of the tendon and synovium.
- Ruptured origin of the biceps brachii tendon—partial to complete rupture of the biceps tendon at its insertion on the supraglenoid tubercle, proliferative synovitis, and fibrous adhesions between the biceps tendon and its synovial sheath; histologically, synovial proliferation, edema, fibrosis, and occasional dystrophic mineralization.
- Medial shoulder instability—identify fraying, stretching or complete disruption of the medial glenohumeral ligament or the subscapularis tendon.
- Mineralization of the supraspinatus tendon—tendon often looks normal, but longitudinal incision reveals numerous pockets of mineralized debris within the fibers; histologically, chondromucinous stromal degeneration of the tendon with multiple foci of dystrophic mineralization.
- Avulsion of the supraspinatus tendon insertion—often looks normal, but longitudinal incision reveals bone fragment(s) surrounded by a fibrous tissue capsule; usually see a corresponding bony defect in the greater tubercle.

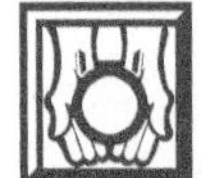

TREATMENT

APPROPRIATE HEALTH CARE

- Overall, identification and appropriate treatment of ligamentous shoulder pathology is considered one the more controversial areas in canine orthopedics.
- Outpatient—early diagnosis.
- Inpatient—chronic, severe disease requires surgical intervention.
- Bicipital tenosynovitis—50–75% success with medical treatment; requires surgery with evidence of chronic changes and failure of medical management.
- Medial shoulder instability treatment depends on the severity of the disease with mild to moderate instability typically being amenable to conservative therapy, while severe ligamentous disruption and instability requiring medial shoulder stabilization.
- Subtotal rupture of the origin of the biceps brachii tendon generally requires surgery.
- Mineralization of the supraspinatus tendon—may be an incidental finding; requires surgery after excluding other causes of lameness and medical treatment.
- Avulsion or fracture of the supraspinatus tendon—often requires surgery because of persistent bone fragment irritation of the tendon.
- Fibrotic contracture of the infraspinatus muscle—requires surgery.

NURSING CARE

- Cryotherapy (ice packing)—immediately post surgery; helps reduce inflammation and swelling at the surgery site; performed 5–10 minutes every 8 hours for 3–5 days.
- Regional massage and range-of-motion exercises—improve flexibility; decrease muscle atrophy.
- Rehabilitation therapy by a licensed veterinary rehabilitation professional is considered crucial to improve the speed of, and likelihood of recovery from shoulder pathology with or without surgical intervention.

ACTIVITY

- Medical treatment—requires strict confinement for 4–6 weeks; activity; premature return to normal activity likely exacerbates signs and induces a chronic pathological state.
- Post surgery—depends on procedure performed.

DIET

Weight control—decrease the load applied to the painful joint.

SURGICAL CONSIDERATIONS

- Bicipital tenosynovitis—recommended with poor response to medical treatment and chronic disease; goal: eliminate movement of the biceps tendon within the inflamed synovial sheath by performing a tenodesis or, more commonly, release of the bicipital tendon; either arthroscopic, or open, or percutaneous (± ultrasound guidance) tendon release.
- Rupture of the biceps brachii tendon of origin—reattach tendon to the proximal lateral aspect of the humerus with a screw and spiked washer or pass the tendon through a bone tunnel and suture it to the supraspinatus tendon. Alternatively arthroscopy to confirm complete release of the tendon, followed by rehabilitation therapy can be considered.
- Medial shoulder instability—sporadic and conflicting reports of the efficacy of radiofrequency capsulorrhaphy for moderate pathology. Prosthetic ligament reconstruction for the treatment of severe instability is recommended.
- Mineralization of the supraspinatus tendon—longitudinally incise the tendon; remove the calcium deposits.
- Avulsion or fracture of the supraspinatus tendon—remove the bone fragment(s).
- Fibrotic contracture of the infraspinatus muscle—tenotomy and excision of part of the tendon of insertion; often feel a distinct pop after excision of the last adhesion, which allows complete range of motion of the shoulder joint.

MEDICATIONS

DRUG(S) OF CHOICE

Bicipital Tenosynovitis

- Local therapy—intra-articular injection (corticosteroid or platelet rich plasma)—initial treatment of choice.
- Do not inject into a septic joint; perform complete synovial fluid analysis if any doubt.
- Prednisolone acetate 20–40 mg, depending on size.
- Lameness markedly improved but not eliminated—give a second injection in 3–6 weeks.
- Systemic treatment (nonsteroidal anti-inflammatory drugs [NSAIDs] or steroids)—not as effective.
- Incomplete resolution—recommend surgery.

NSAIDs and Analgesics

- May be used for symptomatic treatment; minimize pain, decrease inflammation.
- Carprofen 2.2 mg/kg PO q12h or 4.4 mg/kg PO q24h.
- Deracoxib 1–2 mg/kg PO q24h, chewable.
- Etodolac 10–15 mg/kg PO q24h.
- Firocoxib 5 mg/kg PO q24h.
- Grapiprant 2 mg/kg PO q24h, to animals >3.6 kg.
- Meloxicam—load 0.2 mg/kg PO, then 0.1 mg/kg PO q24h—liquid.
- Tepoxalin—load 20 mg/kg, then 10 mg/kg PO q24h.

CONTRAINDICATIONS

- Avoid prolonged use of corticosteroids because of the potential side effects and articular cartilage damage associated with long-term intra-articular use.
- Direct injection of a corticosteroid into the biceps tendon—may promote further tendon disruption and eventual rupture.

PRECAUTIONS

NSAIDs—gastrointestinal irritation or renal/hepatic toxicity may preclude use in some patients.

ALTERNATIVE DRUG(S)

- Chondroprotective drugs, e.g., polysulfated glycosaminoglycans, green-lipped mussel extract, and glucosamine/chondroitin sulfate (limited supportive data)—may help limit associated cartilage damage and degeneration.
- Nonspecific anti-inflammatory supplements, e.g., green-lipped mussel extract and omega 3 fatty-acid supplementation.

FOLLOW-UP

PATIENT MONITORING

Most patients require a minimum of 1–2 months of rehabilitation after treatment.

EXPECTED COURSE AND PROGNOSIS

- Medically managed bicipital tenosynovitis—often successful after one or two treatments (50–75% of cases) with no chronic changes.
- Surgically treated bicipital tenosynovitis—good to excellent results (90% of cases); recovery to full function may take 2–8 months.
- Surgically treated release or tenodesis of the bicipital brachii tendon—good to excellent prognosis; >85% of patients show improved return to function.
- Surgically treated medial shoulder instability—variable results and highly dependent on concurrent pathology and adherence to postoperative restriction and rehabilitation therapy.
- Surgically treated mineralization of the supraspinatus tendon—good to excellent prognosis; recurrence possible but uncommon.
- Surgically treated avulsion or fracture of the supraspinatus tendon—good to excellent prognosis; recurrence possible but uncommon.
- Surgically treated fibrotic contracture of the infraspinatus muscle—good to excellent prognosis; patients uniformly return to normal limb function.

MISCELLANEOUS

ABBREVIATIONS

- NSAID = nonsteroidal anti-inflammatory drug.

Suggested Reading

Laitinen OM, Flo GL. Mineralization of the supraspinatus tendon in dogs: a long-term follow-up. J Am Anim Hosp Assoc 2000, 36(3):262–267.

Rivers B, Wallace L, Johnston GR. Biceps tenosynovitis in the dog: radiographic and sonographic findings. Vet Comp Orthop Traumatol 1992, 5:51–57.

Schaefer SL, Forrest LJ. Magnetic resonance imaging of the canine shoulder: an anatomic study. Vet Surg 2006, 35(8):721–728.

Author Mathieu M. Glassman

Consulting Editor Mathieu M. Glassman

Acknowledgment The author/editor acknowledges the prior contribution of Walter C. Renberg.

Client Education Handout available online

SICK SINUS SYNDROME

BASICS

DEFINITION

A disorder of impulse formation within, and conduction out of, the sinus node; dysfunction of subsidiary pacemakers and other segments of the cardiac conduction system frequently coexist with the sinus node dysfunction.

ECG Features

• Arrhythmias noted with sick sinus syndrome (SSS) include any or all of the following: inappropriate sinus bradycardia, sinus pauses (representing sinus arrest or sinoatrial exit block), slow ectopic atrial rhythm, or alternating periods of sinus bradyarrhythmias and supraventricular tachycardia (SVT) (Figure 1). • Paroxysms of SVT may alternate with prolonged periods of sinus node inertia and often atrioventricular (AV) nodal inertia as well, producing tachycardia–bradycardia syndrome, a variant of SSS. • P waves and QRS complexes are usually normal. • P waves may be abnormal or absent with slow atrial ectopic rhythm or junctional escape rhythm.

PATHOPHYSIOLOGY

• ECG manifestations may precede development of clinical signs. • Clinical signs usually result from the failure of subsidiary pacemakers to generate escape rhythms when sinus node dysfunction occurs. • The common clinical manifestations reflect transient decreases in organ perfusion, particularly reduced cerebral and skeletal muscle perfusion. • Rarely, congestive heart failure develops.

SYSTEMS AFFECTED

• Cardiovascular. • Nervous, musculoskeletal, and renal systems may be secondarily affected because of hypoperfusion.

GENETICS

• May be heritable in miniature schnauzers and West Highland white terriers.
• Doberman pinschers and boxers can have syncope associated with long sinus pauses, suggestive of SSS.

SIGNALMENT

Species

Dog

Breed Predilections

• Miniature schnauzer (may be heritable).
• Noted commonly in cocker spaniel, dachshund, and West Highland white terrier.

Mean Age and Range

Most dogs >6 years old.

Predominant Sex

Female

SIGNS

Historical Findings

• Clinical signs vary from asymptomatic to weakness, syncope, collapse, and/or seizures.
• Sudden death is infrequent.

Physical Examination Findings

• Heart rate may be abnormally rapid or abnormally slow. • Pauses may be noted.
• Some patients appear normal.

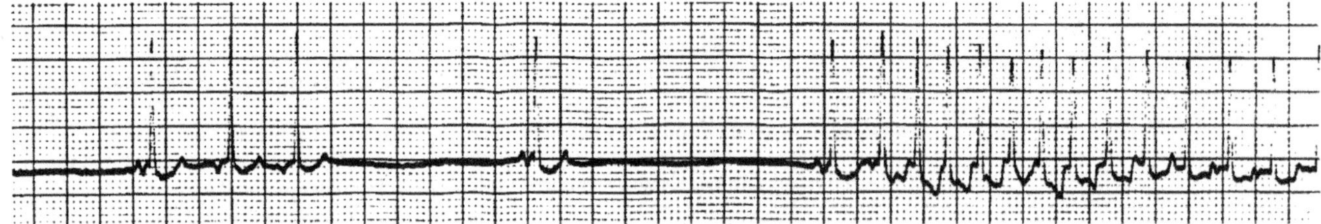

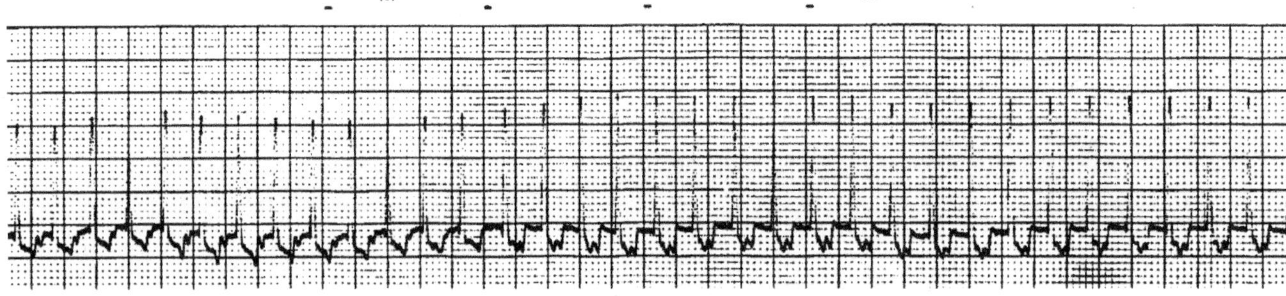

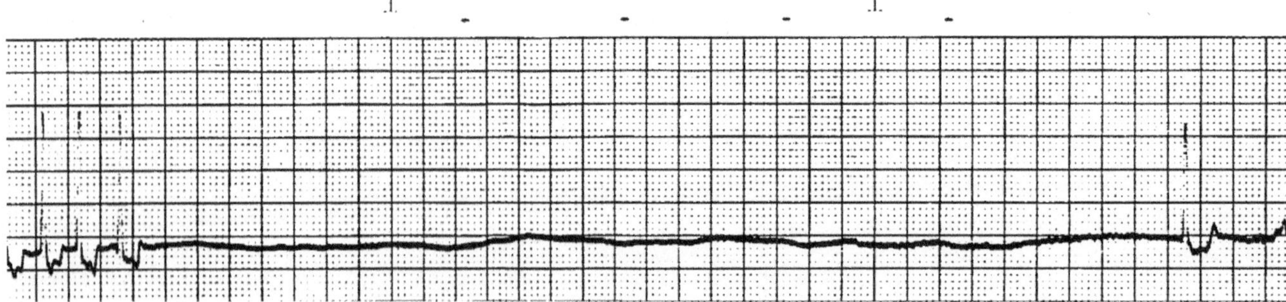

Figure 1.

A continuous lead II rhythm strip (25 mm/s) recorded from a dog with sick sinus syndrome showing an ectopic atrial rhythm interrupted by several short pauses. The third pause initiates a paroxysm of supraventricular tachycardia (250 bpm) followed by asystole (6.6 seconds) terminated by a junctional escape complex.

CAUSES

• Idiopathic. • Familial in miniature schnauzers. • Metastatic disease. • Ischemic disease.

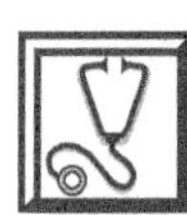

DIAGNOSIS

DIFFERENTIAL DIAGNOSIS

• Healthy dogs may exhibit sinus bradycardia (rate as low as 30 beats/min) and sinus pauses (as long as 3.5 seconds) normally during sleep. • Bradycardia and sinus arrest due to normal or enhanced vagal tone. • Drug-induced (digitalis, α-adrenergic antagonists, α_2-adrenergic agonists, calcium channel antagonists, cimetidine, opioids). • Seizures or syncope due to noncardiac disease. • Atrial standstill secondary to hyperkalemia or atrial disease. • Weakness due to neurologic, musculoskeletal, or metabolic diseases.

CBC/BIOCHEMISTRY/URINALYSIS

Normal

IMAGING

Breeds predisposed to SSS are also predisposed to degenerative valvular disease; echocardiography may be used to confirm presence of significant valvular disease when heart murmur is present.

DIAGNOSTIC PROCEDURES

• Atropine response testing—indicated in dogs with sinus bradycardia, sinus arrest, and sinoatrial exit block. Administer atropine 0.04 mg/kg IM and evaluate the ECG 20–30 minutes later. A normal (positive) response is >50% increase in heart rate with abolishment of pauses; dogs with SSS generally have no response or an incomplete response to atropine. • Electrophysiologic testing of sinus node recovery time and sinoatrial conduction time. • 24-hour ambulatory ECG (Holter) or event recording to correlate clinical signs with arrhythmia.

PATHOLOGIC FINDINGS

Vary with cause.

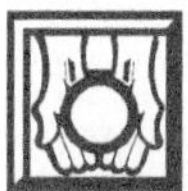

TREATMENT

APPROPRIATE HEALTH CARE

• Hospitalization rarely necessary except for electrophysiologic testing or pacemaker implantation. • Do not treat asymptomatic animals.

ACTIVITY

Avoid vigorous exercise and stressful situations.

DIET

Modifications unnecessary.

CLIENT EDUCATION

Owner should be aware that medical management is often ineffective.

SURGICAL CONSIDERATIONS

• Permanent artificial pacemaker necessary for dogs failing to respond to medical treatment and those exhibiting unacceptable medication side effects. • Permanent artificial pacemaker usually required for dogs with bradycardia–tachycardia syndrome.
• Transvenous placement of a pacing lead in the right atrium or auricle may successfully abolish the sinus pauses.

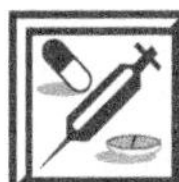

MEDICATIONS

DRUG(S) OF CHOICE

• Do not treat asymptomatic animals.
• Symptomatic dogs are grouped into those showing primarily bradycardia, sinus arrest, and/or sinoatrial exit block and those with supraventricular tachycardia followed by sinus arrest. • Atropine-responsive symptomatic dogs with bradycardia or sinus arrest—anticholinergic agents (propantheline: small dogs, 3.75–7.5 mg PO q8–12h; medium dogs, 15 mg PO q8h; large dogs, 30 mg PO q8h; hyoscyamine: 3–6 µg/kg q8h). • Dogs with bradycardia and sinus arrest—may try theophylline (Theo-Dur) 20 mg/kg PO q12h, terbutaline 0.2 mg/kg PO q8–12h, or hydralazine 1–2 mg/kg PO q8–12h if anticholinergic drugs are ineffective (avoid hydralazine if patient is hypotensive). • Dogs with bradycardia–tachycardia whose clinical signs are due to tachycardia or tachycardia-induced sinus arrest—can give digoxin 5 µg/kg PO q12h or atenolol 0.5–1 mg/kg PO q12–24h in attempt to suppress the SVT (monitor closely for exacerbation of bradycardia). • Therapy for tachycardias should only be considered, once pacing is established to avoid worsening of bradyarrhythmias.

CONTRAINDICATIONS

Avoid drugs that may worsen sinus node dysfunction (e.g., β-adrenergic antagonists, calcium channel blocking agents, phenothiazines, class I and III antiarrhythmic agents, opioids, cimetidine, α_2-adrenergic agonists).

PRECAUTIONS

• Attempts to manage bradycardia–tachycardia syndrome medically without prior pacemaker implantation carry significant risk because drugs used to control SVT may worsen the bradyarrhythmias, and vice versa. • Adverse effects of anticholinergic medication (constipation, difficulty voiding, keratoconjunctivitis sicca, emesis, anxiety) occur commonly.

FOLLOW-UP

PATIENT MONITORING

• ECG in asymptomatic patients—to detect progression of disease. • ECG in patients treated medically or with pacemaker implantation.

POSSIBLE COMPLICATIONS

• Rarely, reduced cerebral or renal perfusion results in chronic renal dysfunction or CNS damage. • Presence of significant valvular disease has implications for type of permanent pacing mode selected.

EXPECTED COURSE AND PROGNOSIS

• Good, following pacemaker implantation in animals without congestive heart failure. • Medical management—often ineffective; initial beneficial effects often not sustained.

MISCELLANEOUS

SYNONYMS

• Bradycardia–tachycardia syndrome. • Sinus node dysfunction. • Tachycardia–bradycardia syndrome.

SEE ALSO

• Sinus Arrest and Sinoatrial Block.
• Sinus Bradycardia.
• Supraventricular Tachycardia.

ABBREVIATIONS

• AV = atrioventricular.
• ECG = electrocardiogram.
• SSS = sick sinus syndrome.
• SVT = supraventricular tachycardia.

Suggested Reading

Kraus MS, Gelzer ARM. Treatment of cardia arrhythmias and conduction disturbances. In: Smith FWK, Tilley LP, Oyama M, Sleeper M. Manual of Canine and Feline Cardiology, 5th ed. St. Louis, MO: Saunders Elsevier, 2016, pp. 313–329.

Santilli R, Moïse NS, Pariaut R, Perego M. Electrocardiography of the Dog and Cat. Diagnosis of Arrhythmias, 2nd ed. Milan, Italy: Edra S.P.A., 2018.

Tilley LP. Essentials of Canine and Feline Electrocardiography, Interpretation and Treatment, 3rd ed. Baltimore, MD: Williams and Wilkins, 1992.

Willis, R., Oliveira, P., Mavropoulou, A. Guide to Canine and Feline Electrocardiography. Ames, IA: Wiley-Blackwell, 2018.

Authors Larry P. Tilley and Francis W.K. Smith, Jr.
Consulting Editor Michael Aherne

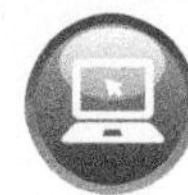

Client Education Handout available online

S

SINUS ARREST AND SINOATRIAL BLOCK

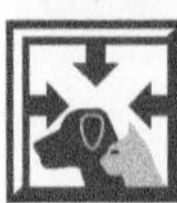

BASICS

DEFINITION

• Sinus arrest—a disorder of impulse formation caused by slowing or cessation of spontaneous sinus nodal automaticity; failure of the sinoatrial (SA) node to initiate an impulse at the expected time. P-P interval does not equal a multiple of basic P-P interval. • Sinoatrial block—a disorder of impulse conduction; an impulse formed within the sinus node fails to depolarize the atria or does so with delay; most commonly the basic rhythmicity of the sinus node is not disturbed and the duration of the pause is a multiple of the basic P-P interval. Classified into first-, second-, and third-degree SA block (similar to degrees of atrioventricular [AV] block). Difficult to diagnose first- and third-degree SA block from electrocardiogram (ECG). Second-degree SA block most common: Mobitz type I (Wenckebach) SA block—P-P interval progressively shortens prior to a pause; duration of pause is less than two P-P cycles; Mobitz type II SA block—duration of pause occurring after a sinus beat is exact multiple (two, three, or four times normal) of basic P-P interval.

S

ECG Features

• A normal P wave exists for each QRS complex with a pause equal to or greater than twice the normal P-P interval; rhythm is regularly irregular or irregular with pauses (Figure 1). • Junctional or ventricular escape beats—occur if pauses significantly prolonged. Subsidiary pacemaker takes over rhythm with escape beats normally from AV junctional tissue or Purkinje fibers; intermittent absence of P waves noted or P waves may be negative and precede, be superimposed on or follow the QRS complexes. • Surface ECG cannot differentiate sinus arrest from block in the dog because of normal R-R interval variation (sinus arrhythmia).

PATHOPHYSIOLOGY

• Sympathetic and parasympathetic influences can alter spontaneous sinus node depolarization; vagal stimulation of acetylcholine, which binds to SA nodal receptor sites, can slow automaticity of the sinus node by reducing the slope of phase 4 depolarization; sympathetic stimulation releases norepinephrine that binds to β1 receptors on the SA node, enhancing spontaneous SA nodal discharge rate. • An overdrive inhibition phenomenon occurs when sinus arrest follows a run of ectopic beats. The sinus node requires a warming-up period until the usual rate of automaticity is reestablished. • Intrinsic disease of the sinus node may affect the balance between the parasympathetic and sympathetic efferent traffic to the SA node and its spontaneous discharge rate. • Duration of sinus arrest may be long and possibly irreversible when the sinus node is suppressed by an ectopic tachycardia, particularly with severe underlying heart disease. Persistent sinus arrest that is not drug induced often indicates sick sinus syndrome (SSS).

SYSTEMS AFFECTED

Cardiovascular—clinical signs of weakness or syncope may appear if sinus arrest or block causes sufficiently long periods (generally 5 seconds or longer) of ventricular asystole with no escape beats initiated by latent pacemakers.

GENETICS

• Seen in purebred pugs with hereditary stenosis of the bundle of His. • Seen in female miniature schnauzers predisposed to SSS. Is the most common arrhythmia in miniature schnauzers with SSS. • Congenitally deaf Dalmatian coach hounds often have abnormal SA node and multiple atrial arteries. May be a genetic component to the cause of SSS in those breeds predisposed (see Breed Predilections).

INCIDENCE/PREVALENCE

• Normal incidental finding in brachycephalic breeds of dogs in which inspiration causes a reflex increase in vagal tone. • Common in dog breeds predisposed to SSS. • Uncommon in cats.

GEOGRAPHIC DISTRIBUTION

N/A

SIGNALMENT

Species

Dog and cat.

Breed Predilections

• Brachycephalic breeds. • Breeds predisposed to SSS (e.g., miniature schnauzers, dachshunds, cocker spaniels, pugs, boxers and West Highland white terriers).

Mean Age and Range

If associated with SSS, generally middle-aged to older animals.

Predominant Sex

If associated with SSS, older females.

SIGNS

General Comments

Generally no clinical significance by itself if terminated by sinus node depolarization, or latent pacemakers promptly escape to prevent ventricular asystole.

Historical Findings

• Usually none. • Signs of low cardiac output (e.g., weakness and syncope) may occur with failure of the SA node to fire on time if no lower pacemaker focus takes over the rhythm. • Sudden death is possible should prolonged periods of ventricular asystole occur.

Physical Examination Findings

• May be normal. • Heart sounds following a pause may be louder because the ventricles have longer filling time and therefore eject a larger amount of blood. • Extremely slow heart rate if arrest or block is prolonged or frequent. • With significant pathologic cardiac disease—may be findings consistent with poor cardiac output (e.g., prolonged perfusion time, pale mucous membranes, weak femoral pulses).

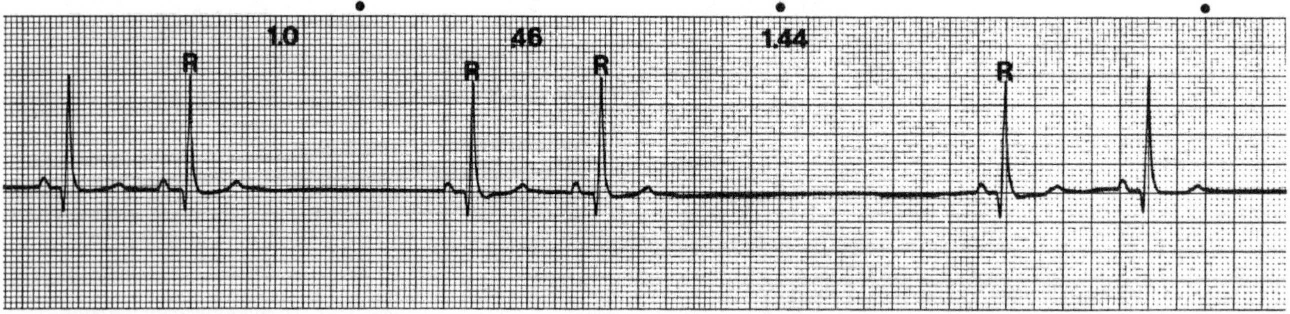

Figure 1.

Intermittent sinus arrest in a brachycephalic breed with an upper respiratory disorder. The pauses (1 and 1.44 seconds) are greater than twice the normal P-P interval (0.46). (Source: From Tilley LP. Essentials of Canine and Feline Electrocardiography, Interpretation and Treatment, 3rd ed. Baltimore, MD: Williams and Wilkins, 1992, Reprinted with permission of Wolters Kluwer.)

CAUSES

Physiologic

• Vagal stimulation secondary to coughing, pharyngeal irritation. • Ocular or carotid sinus pressure. • Surgical manipulation.

Pathologic

• Degenerative heart disease (fibrosis).
• Dilatory heart disease. • Acute myocarditis.
• Neoplastic heart disease. • SSS. • Irritation of vagus nerve secondary to thoracic or cervical neoplasia. • Electrolyte imbalance.
• Drug toxicity (e.g., digoxin).

RISK FACTORS

• Certain drugs, including digitalis, quinidine, propranolol, xylazine, acepromazine, hydromorphone. • Respiratory tract disease.
• Vagal maneuvers.

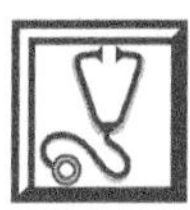

DIAGNOSIS

DIFFERENTIAL DIAGNOSIS

• Marked sinus arrhythmia and sinus bradycardia. • Not always possible to differentiate sinus arrest from SA block without direct recordings of sinus node discharge; pauses that are precise multiples of the dominant beat interval suggest sinus block.

CBC/BIOCHEMISTRY/URINALYSIS

Serum electrolyte abnormalities, especially hyperkalemia (serum K^+ >5.7 mEq/L).

OTHER LABORATORY TESTS

N/A

IMAGING

• Thoracic radiographs if neoplastic or cardiac disease suspected. • Cardiac ultrasound if structural or neoplastic heart disease suspected.

DIAGNOSTIC PROCEDURES

• Provocative atropine response test to assess sinus node function. Administer 0.04 mg/kg atropine IM; evaluate ECG lead II rhythm strip 30 minutes later for response or administer 0.04 mg/kg atropine IV followed by ECG in 10 minutes. Resolution of the arrhythmia suggests high vagal tone as the underlying cause. • Ambulatory monitoring may reveal prolonged periods of failure of impulses from the SA node if signs of weakness or syncope. • In humans, a period of sinus arrest following right carotid massage that lasts longer than 3 seconds suggests inappropriate sinus responsiveness.
• Electrophysiologic studies of sinus node.
• Serum digoxin concentration, if applicable; trough level recommended (just before next dose or at least 8 hours post pill); therapeutic serum concentrations are typically 0.5–1.5 ng/mL.

PATHOLOGIC FINDINGS

Histologic study of the SA node may reveal necrosis, fibrosis, and/or degenerative changes.

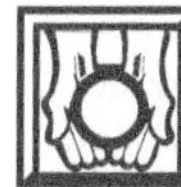

TREATMENT

APPROPRIATE HEALTH CARE

Asymptomatic sinus arrest or block does not require therapy. If clinical signs, therapeutic approach depends on cause, underlying cardiac status, and severity of symptoms. Any indicated treatment may be outpatient unless pacemaker implantation is necessary, which necessitates hospital management.

NURSING CARE

Correct any electrolyte abnormalities.

ACTIVITY

Unrestricted unless signs of weakness, syncope, or congestive heart failure (CHF) develop.

CLIENT EDUCATION

An artificial pacemaker may be necessary when patient is symptomatic and nonresponsive to medical management.

SURGICAL CONSIDERATIONS

Implantation of an artificial demand pacemaker in animals with clinical signs nonresponsive to therapy.

MEDICATIONS

DRUG(S) OF CHOICE

• Only if patient is symptomatic, consider atropine 0.04 mg/kg IV, IM, glycopyrrolate 5–10 µg/kg IV, IM, or isoproterenol 10 µg/kg IM, SC q6h or dilute 1 mg in 500 mL of 5% dextrose or Ringer's solution, and infuse IV at 0.04–0.08 µg/kg/min. • If responsive to injectable anticholinergic drugs (e.g., atropine)—can prescribe parasympatholytic drug such as oral propantheline bromide 0.25–0.5 mg/kg q8–12h or hyoscyamine 3–6 µg/kg q8h for at-home management. Sympathomimetic agents including methylxanthine theophylline 10 mg/kg extended release formulation q12h or terbutaline 0.2 mg/kg q8–12h PO (dogs) and 0.1–0.2 mg/kg q12h (cats) could be considered for oral therapy.

CONTRAINDICATIONS

If patient is symptomatic secondary to prolonged pauses, discontinue any drugs that may be causative (e.g., digitalis, beta-blockers, calcium channel blockers).

PRECAUTIONS

Avoid drugs that depress SA node function.

POSSIBLE INTERACTIONS

N/A

ALTERNATIVE DRUG(S)

If medical therapy does not resolve signs, consider pacemaker implantation.

FOLLOW-UP

PATIENT MONITORING

When indicated, periodic serial ECG evaluation to assess therapeutic efficacy and possible progression to a more serious dysrhythmia.

POSSIBLE COMPLICATIONS

If associated with primary cardiac disease, CHF may develop and necessitate appropriate therapies.

EXPECTED COURSE AND PROGNOSIS

If cause is SSS, symptomatic patient may respond well to medical intervention; if poorly responsive, permanent pacemaker implantation would improve prognosis.

MISCELLANEOUS

ASSOCIATED CONDITIONS

• Sick sinus syndrome. • Sinus arrhythmia.
• Sinus bradycardia.

SYNONYMS

• Sinus block. • Sinus pause.

SEE ALSO

• Sick Sinus Syndrome.
• Sinus Arrhythmia.
• Sinus Bradycardia.

ABBREVIATIONS

• AV = atrioventricular.
• CHF = congestive heart failure.
• ECG = electrocardiogram.
• SA = sinoatrial.
• SSS = sick sinus syndrome.

Suggested Reading

Boyett MR, Honjo H, Kodama I. The sinoatrial node: a heterogeneous pacemaker structure. Cardiovasc Res 2000, 47(4):658–687.

Issa ZF, Miller JM, Zipes DP. Sinus node dysfunction. In: Clinical Arrhythmology and Electrophysiology: A Companion to Braunwald's Heart Disease. Philadelphia, PA: Saunders, 2008, pp. 118–126.

Joung B, Ogawa M, Lin S-F, Chen P-S. The calcium and voltage clocks in sinoatrial node automaticity. Korean Circ J 2009, 39(6):217–222.

Kittleson MD, Kienle RD. Small Animal Cardiovascular Medicine. St. Louis, MO: Mosby, 2005.

Author Deborah J. Hadlock
Consulting Editor Michael Aherne

SINUS ARRHYTHMIA

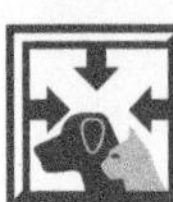

BASICS

DEFINITION

• Normal sinus impulse formation characterized by a phasic variation in sinus cycle length. An irregular R-R interval is present that has more than 10% variation in sinus cycle length (or variability of 0.12 seconds [dog], 0.10 seconds [cat], or more exists between successive P waves) (Figure 1).
• Two basic forms exist—respiratory sinus arrhythmia (RSA): P-P interval cyclically shortens during inspiration due primarily to reflex inhibition of vagal tone and lengthens during expiration; nonrespiratory sinus arrhythmia: phasic variation in P-P interval unrelated to the respiratory cycle.

ECG Features

• Other than the irregular rhythm, all other criteria for sinus rhythm are present.
• Normal heart rate.
• Positive P wave in leads, I, II, III, and aVF, unless a wandering pacemaker is present, where the P waves may be positive, diphasic, or negative temporarily.
• A P wave is present for every QRS complex.
• A QRS complex is present for every P wave.
• PR interval is relatively constant.

S

PATHOPHYSIOLOGY

• Sinus node discharge rate depends on the two opposing influences of the autonomic nervous system. Vagal stimulation decreases spontaneous sinus nodal discharge rate and predominates over sympathetic stimulation. Negative intrathoracic pressure occurring with inspiration causes decreased pressure on the vagus nerves. Feedback from the cardioregulatory and vasomotor centers in the medulla produces cardiac acceleration by decreasing vagal restraint on the sinus node; the opposite occurs during exhalation. The genesis of sinus arrhythmia also depends on reflexes involving pulmonary stretch receptors (Hering–Breuer reflex), pressure–volume sensory receptors in the heart (Bainbridge reflex whereby atrial stretch stimulates receptors in the atrial wall, causing vagal inhibition and increase in heart rate; baroreceptors in the carotid sinus and aortic arch elicit inverse changes in heart rate with acute changes in arterial blood pressure), blood vessels, and chemical factors of the blood.
• RSA is measured as a high-frequency component of heart rate variability (HRV) and is used as an index of cardiac vagal control. HRV measures beat to beat changes in heart rate and R-R variability from the ECG. HRV is a widely accepted clinical and research tool for evaluation of cardiac autonomic changes.

SYSTEMS AFFECTED

Cardiovascular—generally no hemodynamic consequence, but marked sinus arrhythmia may produce a long enough sinus pause to produce syncope if not accompanied by an escape rhythm.

GENETICS

N/A

INCIDENCE/PREVALENCE

Most frequent form of arrhythmia in dogs.

SIGNALMENT

Species

• RSA frequent normal finding in dogs.
• While common in cats asleep and in home environment, in a clinical setting sympathetic dominance occurs and RSA is rare without underlying pathology.

Breed Predilections

• Brachycephalic breeds predisposed.
• Dogs—bulldog, Lhasa apso, Pekingese, pug, shar-pei, shih tzu, boxer.
• Cats—Persian, Himalayan.

Mean Age and Range

N/A

Predominant Sex

N/A

SIGNS

General Comments

• Uncommon, but weakness may develop if pauses between beats are excessively long; syncope can occur when a marked sinus arrhythmia and sinus bradycardia develop.
• In general, symptoms more common in nonrespiratory than in respiratory form.

Historical Findings

• RSA—none.
• Nonrespiratory sinus arrhythmia—may be findings related to underlying disease.

Physical Examination Findings

• May be normal.
• Irregular rhythm on auscultation.
• May be findings related to specific disease accentuating vagal tone (e.g., stertor and stridor in a patient with brachycephalic airway syndrome).

CAUSES

• Normal cyclic change in vagal tone associated with respiration in the dog; heart rate increases with inspiration and decreases with expiration.
• Underlying conditions that increase vagal tone—high intracranial pressure, gastrointestinal disease, respiratory disease, cerebral disorders, digitalis toxicity, organophosphates.
• Carotid sinus massage or ocular pressure (vagal maneuver) may accentuate.

RISK FACTORS

• Brachycephalic conformation.
• Digoxin therapy.
• Any disease that increases vagal tone.

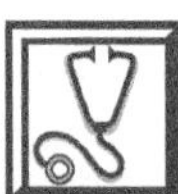

DIAGNOSIS

DIFFERENTIAL DIAGNOSIS

• Auscultation of sinus arrhythmia is often confusing; ECG helps differentiate normal

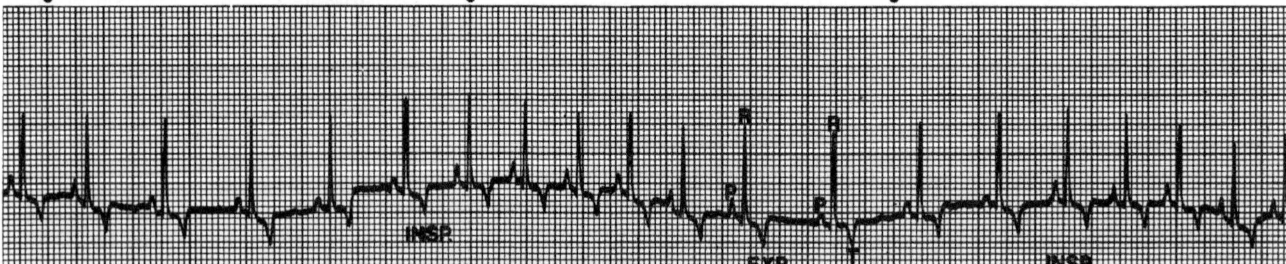

Figure 1.

Respiratory sinus arrhythmia with an average rate of 120 bpm (6 complexes between 1 set of time lines or 3 seconds × 20) (paper speed, 25 mm/s; 10 mm/mV). The rate increases during inspiration (INSP) and decreases during expiration (EXP). The fluctuation of the baseline correlates with the movement of the electrodes by the thoracic cavity. (Source: From Tilley LP. Essentials of Canine and Feline Electrocardiography, 3rd ed. Baltimore: Williams & Wilkins, 1992. Reprinted with permission of Wolters Kluwer.)

sinus arrhythmia from true pathologic arrhythmia.

- Wandering sinus pacemaker frequently associated and a variant of sinus arrhythmia. Site of impulse formation shifts within the sinoatrial node or to an atrial focus or atrioventricular (AV) node, changing the configuration of the P wave.
- Important to differentiate normal sinus arrhythmia from pathologic arrhythmias including atrial premature complexes, sick sinus syndrome, slow atrial fibrillation, and AV dissociation.

CBC/BIOCHEMISTRY/URINALYSIS

N/A

OTHER LABORATORY TESTS

Cats with chronic respiratory disease may be positive for feline leukemia virus or feline immunodeficiency virus.

IMAGING

Radiographs, CT, or MRI of head and neck to assess for abnormal anatomic conformation that might predispose to airway problems.

DIAGNOSTIC PROCEDURES

- Pharyngoscopy/laryngoscopy if upper airway disease suspected.
- Atropine challenge test (administer atropine 0.04 mg/kg IM followed by ECG in 30 minutes or 0.04 mg/kg atropine IV followed by ECG in 10 minutes) if associated with sinus bradycardia and primary dysfunction of sinus node is suspected. Subsequent heart rate should be greater than 150 bpm.

PATHOLOGIC FINDINGS

See specific disease.

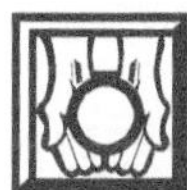

TREATMENT

APPROPRIATE HEALTH CARE

Generally, specific treatment required only when associated with symptomatic sinus bradycardia; if not related to respiration, underlying cause is treated. If patient is suffering respiratory distress, appropriate inpatient management indicated until patient is stable.

NURSING CARE

None unless associated with underlying disease.

ACTIVITY

Not restricted unless associated with specific disease (e.g., brachycephalic animals may need to limit exercise, especially in high ambient temperatures).

DIET

Caloric restriction for obese animals with airway compromise.

CLIENT EDUCATION

Nonc unless associated with specific disease.

SURGICAL CONSIDERATIONS

None unless associated with specific disease.

MEDICATIONS

DRUG(S) OF CHOICE

- Generally no therapy indicated; this is a normal rhythm.
- Infectious respiratory diseases require appropriate antibiotic therapy.
- If associated with symptomatic sinus bradycardia or sinus arrest or block, anticholinergics may be indicated—atropine 0.02–0.04 mg/kg IV, IM, SC or glycopyrrolate 5–10 μg/kg IV, IM, SC.

CONTRAINDICATIONS

Discontinue digoxin if toxicity is a problem.

PRECAUTIONS

Avoid atropine in patients with respiratory disease; an adverse effect is drying of secretions.

POSSIBLE INTERACTIONS

N/A

ALTERNATIVE DRUG(S)

N/A

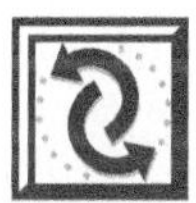

FOLLOW-UP

PATIENT MONITORING

Only if associated with specific disease.

PREVENTION/AVOIDANCE

N/A

POSSIBLE COMPLICATIONS

N/A

EXPECTED COURSE AND PROGNOSIS

N/A

MISCELLANEOUS

ASSOCIATED CONDITIONS

- Sick sinus syndrome.
- Brachycephalic airway syndrome.
- Asthma.
- Chronic obstructive pulmonary disease.

AGE-RELATED FACTORS

Generally more pronounced in young adult.

ZOONOTIC POTENTIAL

N/A

PREGNANCY/FERTILITY/BREEDING

Increased incidence of arrhythmias.

SYNONYMS

- Nonrespiratory sinus arrhythmia = nonphasic sinus arrhythmia; sinus irregularity.
- Respiratory sinus arrhythmia = phasic sinus arrhythmia.
- Ventriculophasic sinus arrhythmia—form of nonphasic sinus arrhythmia in which atrial cycles containing ventricular complexes are shorter than those in which they are absent. That is, the P-P interval that includes the QRS complex is shorter than the P-P interval without a QRS complex. This can be seen with second-degree AV block, complete AV block or in the presence of ventricular premature complexes with a full compensatory pause.

SEE ALSO

- Brachycephalic Airway Syndrome.
- Sick Sinus Syndrome.
- Sinus Arrest and Sinoatrial Block.

ABBREVIATIONS

- AV = atrioventricular.
- HRV = heart rate variability.
- RSA = respiratory sinus arrhythmia.

Suggested Reading

Billman GE. Heart rate variability—a historical perspective. Front Physiol 2011, 2:86.

Bonow R, Mann D, Zipes D, Libby P. Braunwald's Heart Disease: A Textbook of Cardiovascular Medicine, 9th ed. Ames, IA: Elsevier, 2012.

Côté E, MacDonald K, Meurs KM, Sleeper MM. Feline Cardiology. Ames, IA: Wiley-Blackwell, 2011.

Lewis K, Scansen BA, Aarnes TK. Respiratory sinus arrhythmia in an anesthetized cat. ECG of the month. J Am Vet Med Assoc 2013, 242:623–625.

Tilley LP. Essentials of Canine and Feline Electrocardiography, Interpretation and Treatment, 3rd ed. Baltimore, MD: Williams and Wilkins, 1992.

Yasuma F, Hayano J. Respiratory sinus arrhythmia: why does the heartbeat synchronize with respiratory rhythm? Chest 2004, 125:683.

Author Deborah J. Hadlock

Consulting Editor Michael Aherne

SINUS BRADYCARDIA

BASICS

DEFINITION

Sinus rhythm in which impulses arise from the sinoatrial (SA) node at slower than normal rate for an animal's signalment and activity (Figure 1).

ECG Features

• Dogs—sinus rate <60 bpm). • Cats—sinus rate <110 bpm at home or <130 bpm at the clinic. • Rhythm regular, often with a slight variation in R-R interval; may be irregular; often coexists with sinus arrhythmia.
• Normal P wave for each QRS complex.
• P-R interval constant.

PATHOPHYSIOLOGY

• Can be an incidental finding in healthy animals or during sleep. • May represent normal physiologic response to athletic training; may result from enhanced cardiac parasympathetic tone or decreased sympathetic tone as well as from intrinsic changes in the sinus node. • Automaticity of the heterogeneous sinus node is a very complex phenomenon invoking the calcium and voltage clock mechanisms. More than 16 autonomically influenced currents with the I_f (funny) channel predominating and Ca^{2+} release from the sarcoplasmic reticulum critical to maintain autonomic balance and changes in heart rate. • May represent pathophysiologic response due to high vagal tone, change in blood pH, $P\text{CO}_2$, $P\text{O}_2$, or serum electrolyte disorders, hypothyroidism, increased intracranial pressure, toxins and certain drugs. • May be a result of sick sinus syndrome (SSS).

S

SYSTEMS AFFECTED

Cardiovascular—most instances benign arrhythmia; may be beneficial by producing a longer period of diastole and increased ventricular filling time; can be associated with syncope if due to abnormal reflex (neurocardiogenic) or intrinsic disease of sinus node.

GENETICS

Female miniature schnauzer, West Highland white terrier, boxer, cocker spaniel, dachshund, and pug predisposed to SSS—may cause bradycardia.

INCIDENCE/PREVALENCE

• Common in the dog; less common in cat.
• Clinical interpretation of sinus node rate also depends on environment and type of patient. For example, a sinus rate can be as low as 20 bpm in a normal dog that is sleeping.

SIGNALMENT

Species

Dog and cat.

Breed Predilections

Bradycardia associated with SSS—miniature schnauzer, cocker spaniel, dachshund, pug, and West Highland white terrier.

Mean Age and Range

• Decreased prevalence with advancing age unless associated with intrinsic disease of SA node. • SSS typically seen in middle-aged to geriatric patients.

Predominant Sex

With SSS, older female miniature schnauzers.

SIGNS

Historical Findings

• Often asymptomatic. • Lethargy.
• Weakness. • Exercise intolerance.
• Syncope. • Episodic ataxia.

Physical Examination Findings

• Pulse rate slow. • Hypothermia may be present. • Poor perfusion. • Syncope.
• Decreased level of consciousness.

CAUSES

Physiologic

• Athletic conditioning. • Hypothermia.
• Intubation with pharyngeal or soft palate tension. • Sleep. • Cushing's reflex with increased intracranial pressure. • Gastrointestinal distension. • Activation of baroreceptor reflex with increase in systemic blood pressure (BP).

Pathophysiologic

• High vagal tone associated with gastrointestinal, respiratory, neurologic, and pharyngeal diseases. • Reflex-mediated/neurocardiogenic/vasovagal—e.g., carotid sinus hyperactivity; situational (micturition, defecation, cough, swallowing).

Pathologic

• High intracranial pressure. • Hyperkalemia.
• Hyper- or hypocalcemia. • Hypermagnesemia. • Hypoxemia. • Hypothyroidism.
• Hypoglycemia. • May precede cardiac arrest. • SSS (rare in the cat). • Feline dilated cardiomyopathy. • Viral myocarditis. • SA block. • In humans, mutations in the I_f channel and drugs which block I_f (such as ivabradine) have been associated with bradycardia.

Pharmacologic

• General anesthesia. • Any negative chronotrope including: ○ Phenothiazines. ○ Beta-adrenergic blockers. ○ Digitalis glycosides.
○ Calcium channel blockers. ○ α_2-Adrenergic agonists. ○ Sotolol. ○ Amiodarone. ○ Centrally acting opioids: morphine, hydromorphone, butorphanol, fentanyl.

RISK FACTORS

• Any situation or disease that may increase parasympathetic tone. • Oversedation.
• Hypoventilation under anesthesia. • Breeds predisposed to SSS.

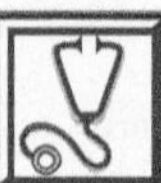

DIAGNOSIS

DIFFERENTIAL DIAGNOSIS

• Persistent and marked sinus bradycardia (SB) should raise possibility of SSS.
• Clinical signs may mimic cerebral dysfunction.

CBC/BIOCHEMISTRY/URINALYSIS

• Hyperkalemia, hypercalcemia, hypocalcemia, or hypermagnesemia possible. • CBC and serum chemistry profile may reveal changes associated with metabolic disease such as renal failure.

OTHER LABORATORY TESTS

• Serum thyroxine (T_4), free T_4, and thyroid-stimulating hormone assays if hypothyroidism suspected. • Measure trough serum digoxin concentration, if applicable, 8 hours after last dose or close to next dosing; normal therapeutic serum concentration should be 0.5–1.5 ng/mL. • Toxicologic screen.

DIAGNOSTIC PROCEDURES

• Provocative atropine response test to assess sinus node function—administer atropine 0.04 mg/kg IV, wait 10–15 minutes, then record ECG or administer same dose IM, wait 30 minutes, then record ECG; persistent sinus tachycardia at >140 bpm is expected response. Lower doses of atropine have increased tendency to cause initial accentuation of SB and first- or second-degree atrioventricular block because of centrally mediated increase in vagal tone. • 24-hour Holter monitoring or ECG event recorder, an owner-triggered device, useful if transient bradyarrhythmia is suspected cause for clinical signs.

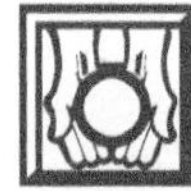

TREATMENT

APPROPRIATE HEALTH CARE

• Many animals exhibit no clinical signs and require no treatment. In dogs without structural heart disease, heart rates as low as 40–50 bpm generally provide normal cardiac output at rest. • Therapeutic approaches—vary markedly; depend on the mechanism for SB, the ventricular rate, and severity of clinical signs. • Inpatient or outpatient management—depends on underlying cause and clinical status of patient.

NURSING CARE

• Provide general supportive therapy including IV fluid therapy for hypothermic and hypovolemic patients. • Discontinue any causative drug. • Correct any serious electrolyte imbalance with appropriate fluid therapy.

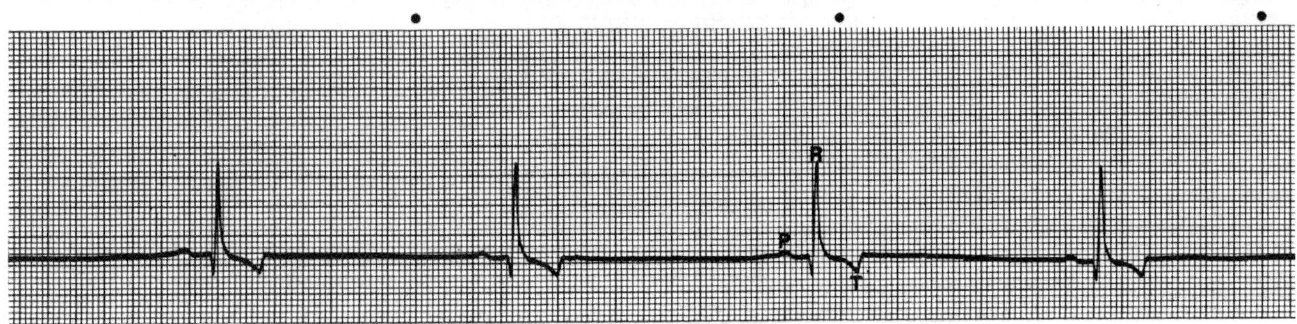

Figure 1.

Sinus bradycardia at a rate of 75 bpm in a cat from anesthetic complications during surgery. Note the tall R waves. (Source: From Tilley LP. Essentials of Canine and Feline Electrocardiography, 3rd ed. Baltimore: Williams & Wilkins, 1992. Reprinted with permission of Wolters Kluwer.)

CLIENT EDUCATION

• Discuss importance of complying with daily medical management when treating.
• Advise that persistent symptomatic bradycardia may necessitate permanent pacemaker implantation for reliable long-term management.

SURGICAL CONSIDERATIONS

• If progressive bradycardia occurs during anesthesia and is attributed to hypoventilation, immediately discontinue inhalation anesthetics and provide adequate ventilation; atropine is generally ineffective in this situation. • If surgical manipulation triggering vagal reflexes (eye, vagus nerve, larynx) is anticipated, pretreatment with atropine 0.02 mg/kg IM, SC or glycopyrrolate 5–10 µg/kg IM, SC may prevent bradycardia.
• Severe bradycardia may precipitate cardiopulmonary arrest; identify the causative agent or condition for effective management.

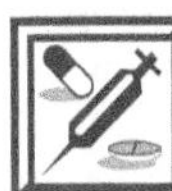

MEDICATIONS

DRUG(S) OF CHOICE

• If patient is hypothyroid, supplement with L-thyroxine. • For severe hypocalcemia (<6 mg/dL) administer 10% calcium gluconate 0.5–1.5 mL/kg IV slowly over 15–30 minutes; monitor with ECG. • For symptomatic drug-induced bradycardias, disorders causing excessive vagal tone, and initial management of bradycardia associated with SSS, administer atropine 0.04 mg/kg IV or glycopyrrolate 5–10 µg/kg IV; anticholinergic therapy may be continued short term using atropine 0.02–0.04 mg/kg IM, SC q6–8h or glycopyrrolate 0.01 mg/kg IM, SC q6–8h. Consider propantheline bromide 0.25–0.5 mg/kg PO q8–12h, hyoscyamine 3–6 µg/kg PO q8h, methylxanthine theophylline, an adenosine receptor antagonist (extended release formulation 10 mg/kg PO q12h, dogs; 12.5 mg PO q24h in the evening, cats), and/or terbutaline (0.2 mg/kg q8–12h PO, dogs; 0.625–1.25 mg/cat PO, cats) to manage symptomatic bradycardia associated with SA node disease.
• For temporary management of symptomatic persistent bradycardia until pacing can be accomplished, consider continuous IV infusion of isoproterenol 0.04–0.08 µg/kg/min IV. Temporary pacing, if available, would be the initial procedure of choice.

CONTRAINDICATIONS

• For hypothermia-induced bradycardia with a pulse, rewarming and supportive measures should be mainstay of treatment. Parasympatholytics generally not recommended.
• Parasympatholytic agents contraindicated for acidotic, hypercarbic patients under anesthesia (hypoventilation); bradycardia in this setting may protect the myocardium by decreasing oxygen consumption.

PRECAUTIONS

• Close ECG monitoring recommended when administering calcium solutions for treatment of hypocalcemia; if QT interval shortening or bradycardia, stop administration temporarily. • In patients with heart disease, a lower initial dose of L-thyroxine is advised to allow adaptation to higher metabolic rate. • Administer atropine selectively; rapid IV administration may predispose to ventricular arrhythmias by altering autonomic balance. • Caution when administering parasympatholytic agent to dogs with suspect SSS—could result in tachycardias that overdrive suppress escape rhythms and thus have a potential risk of asystole after termination of the tachycardia.

ALTERNATIVE DRUG(S)

• Bradycardia associated with structural heart disease is most reliably treated by permanent pacemaker implantation. • Glycopyrrolate may have longer vagal blocking effect and cause less frequent ventricular ectopic beats than atropine.

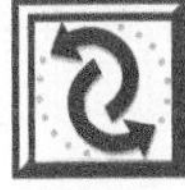

FOLLOW-UP

PATIENT MONITORING

• Assess total T_4 6 hours post pill. • Addison's disease—assess electrolytes every 3–4 months after patient is stable. • ECG check of pacemaker function and pacing rate is recommended during each follow-up examination.

PREVENTION/AVOIDANCE

• Maintain normal $Pa\text{O}_2$ under anesthesia with proper ventilation; monitor with pulse oximetry or blood gases. • Avoid hypothermia intraoperatively.

EXPECTED COURSE AND PROGNOSIS

• Signs, if present, should resolve with correction of causative metabolic or endocrine problem. • Treatment of symptomatic SB with a permanent pacemaker generally offers a good prognosis for rhythm control.

MISCELLANEOUS

ASSOCIATED CONDITIONS

• Sick sinus syndrome. • Heart block.
• Sinus arrhythmia.

PREGNANCY/FERTILITY/BREEDING

Postparturient hypocalcemia usually develops 1–4 weeks postpartum, but can occur at term, prepartum, or late lactation.

SEE ALSO

• Digoxin Toxicity. • Eclampsia.
• Hypercalcemia. • Hyperkalemia.
• Hypermagnesemia. • Hypocalcemia.
• Hypothermia. • Hypothyroidism.
• Organophosphate and Carbamate Toxicosis. • Sick Sinus Syndrome.

ABBREVIATIONS

• ECG = electrocardiogram. • SA = sinoatrial. • SB = sinus bradycardia. • SSS = sick sinus syndrome. • T_4 = thyroxine.

Suggested Reading

Kornreich B, Moïse NS. Bradyarrhythmias. In: Bonagura JD, Twedt D, eds. Current Veterinary Therapy XV. Ames, IA: Elsevier Saunders, 2014, pp. 731–737.

Author Deborah J. Hadlock
Consulting Editor Michael Aherne

SINUS TACHYCARDIA

BASICS

DEFINITION

Disturbance of sinus impulse formation; acceleration of the sinoatrial node beyond its normal discharge rate (Figure 1).

ECG Features

• Dogs—heart rate (HR) >160 bpm (puppies HR >220 bpm). • Cats—HR >180 bpm; (kittens HR >240 bpm). • ECG shows a rapid regular rhythm with possible slight variation in R-R interval. • P wave of sinus origin for each QRS complex with constant P-R interval. • P waves may be partially or completely fused with preceding T waves. • Generally has a gradual onset and termination.

PATHOPHYSIOLOGY

• Accelerated phase 4 diastolic depolarization of sinus nodal cells (as a result of voltage- and calcium-dependent mechanisms) generally responsible for sinus tachycardia (ST).
• Enhanced adrenergic effect or cholinergic inhibition results in high rate of sinus impulse formation; changes in heart rate usually involve a reciprocal action of the parasympathetic and sympathetic divisions of the autonomic nervous system.

SYSTEMS AFFECTED

Cardiovascular—cardiac output = heart rate × stroke volume. Changes in heart rate affect preload, afterload, and contractility, which determine stroke volume; severe tachycardia can compromise cardiac output. Rapid rates shorten diastolic filling time, and particularly in diseased hearts, the increased heart rate can fail to compensate for decreased stroke volume, resulting in decreased cardiac output and coronary blood flow. Chronic tachycardias can cause cardiac dilation (tachycardiomyopathy) which often resolves with control of the tachycardia. However, ST is most often present due to elevated sympathetic tone and is physiologic (because of hypovolemia, fear, pain, etc.).

GENETICS

N/A

INCIDENCE/PREVALENCE

• Most common benign arrhythmia in the dog and cat. • Most common rhythm disturbance in the postoperative patient.

GEOGRAPHIC DISTRIBUTION

None

SIGNALMENT

Species

Dog and cat.

Breed Predilections

None

SIGNS

General Comments

Often no clinical signs because ST is almost always a consequence of a variety of physiologic or pathophysiologic stresses.

Historical Findings

• In general, ST itself does not produce any symptoms. • If associated with primary cardiac disease, weakness, exercise intolerance, or syncope may be reported. • If associated with other medical conditions, signs may be seen specific to the disease present.

Physical Examination Findings

• High HR. • May otherwise be normal if not associated with a pathologic condition.
• Pale mucous membranes if associated with anemia or congestive heart failure (CHF).
• Fever may be present. • Signs of CHF (e.g., dyspnea, cough, cyanosis, ascites) if associated with primary cardiac disease.

CAUSES

Physiologic

• Exercise. • Pain. • Restraint. • Excitement.
• Any hyperadrenergic state.

Pathologic

• Fever. • CHF. • Chronic lung disease.
• Shock. • Pericardial effusion. • Anemia.
• Pain. • Infection. • Hypoxia. • Pulmonary thromboembolism. • Hypotension.
• Hypovolemia. • Functional pheochromocytoma. • Hyperthyroidism. • Pericarditis.
• Pneumothorax. • Hypoglycemia.
• Vestibulosympathetic hypovolemia.

Pharmacologic

• Atropine. • Epinephrine. • Ketamine.
• Tiletamine (Telazol®). • Quinidine.
• Xanthine bronchodilators. • β-Adrenergic agonists.

RISK FACTORS

• Thyroid medications. • Primary cardiac diseases. • Inflammation. • Pregnancy.
• Anesthesia. • Certain toxins (*Amanita muscaria*, scorpion venom, black widow spider venom), plants (Jimson weed, mandrake), and drugs (antihistamines, tricyclic antidepressants).

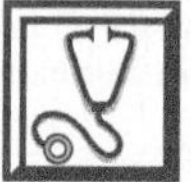

DIAGNOSIS

DIFFERENTIAL DIAGNOSIS

Must differentiate from supraventricular tachycardia (SVT), including atrial tachycardia, atrial flutter with 2:1 AV block, and AV junctional tachycardia; as sinus rate increases, the P wave appears closer to the T wave of the previous beat. At very rapid rates, it becomes difficult to distinguish this condition from other pathologic SVT. Gradual slowing of the rate is suggestive of ST.

CBC/BIOCHEMISTRY/URINALYSIS

• Low packed cell volume if patient is anemic. • Leukocytosis with left shift if inflammation or infection is causative.

OTHER LABORATORY TESTS

• High serum thyroxine (T_4) or free T_4 concentration (cats) if secondary to hyperthyroidism. • Triiodothyronine (T_3) suppression test and thyrotropin-releasing hormone (TRH) response test if T_4 values are normal and hyperthyroidism is suspected. • Functional testing for pheochromocytoma: ○ Metanephrines (breakdown metabolites of epinephrine and norepinephrine); measured in plasma or urine. ○ Serum inhibin, a hormone involved in reproductive physiology; undetectable levels supportive of pheochromocytoma.
• 24-hour Holter monitoring. • Cardiac

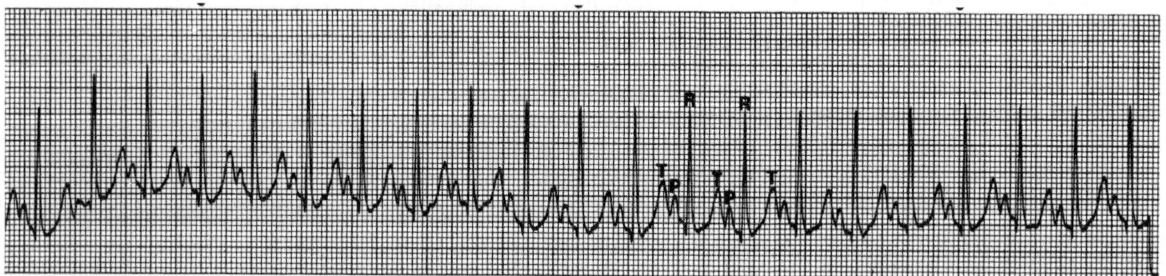

Figure 1.

Sinus tachycardia at a rate of 272 bpm in a dog in shock. The rhythm is sinus because the P waves are normal, the P-R relationship is normal, and the rhythm is regular. (Source: From Tilley LP. Essentials of Canine and Feline Electrocardiography, 3rd ed. Baltimore: Williams & Wilkins, 1992. Reprinted with permission of Wolters Kluwer.)

electrophysiologic studies. • Plasma N-terminal pro-brain natriuretic peptide (NT-proBNP) assay may be helpful if evaluating for cardiac disease.

IMAGING

• Thoracic radiographs and echocardiography to evaluate for evidence of primary cardiac disease. • Thyroid scintigraphy to evaluate for hyperthyroidism. • Abdominal ultrasound and angiography to evaluate for adrenal mass. • CT and MRI as well as functional imaging modalities very sensitive for detecting adrenal masses.

DIAGNOSTIC PROCEDURES

• A nonpharmacologic vagal maneuver can differentiate ST from other SVTs; carotid sinus or ocular pressure may terminate ectopic SVT. With effective vagal maneuvers, the HR in ST gradually slows. Less commonly, varying degrees of AV block (usually first-degree or Wenckebach) may occur transiently. ECG monitoring is recommended during these vagal maneuvers. • Pharmacologic agents can be used if no response to the vagal maneuver. Similarly, an abrupt reduction in HR suggests SVT whereas gradual slowing suggests ST: ○ IV diltiazem 0.25 mg/kg administered over 2 minutes. If no response, can be repeated in 15 minutes. ○ IV esmolol 50–100 μg/kg bolus q5min up to 500 μg/kg; 25–200 μg/kg/min CRI. • A precordial thump may be used to differentiate ST from other SVT. ST usually not affected, whereas the SVT may stop for at least 1 or 2 beats. • Serial arterial BP measurement may document hypertension in patients with hyperthyroidism, pheochromocytoma, or renal disease.

PATHOLOGIC FINDINGS

• None if associated with physiologic or pharmacologic cause. • Pathologic findings depend on the primary disease process.

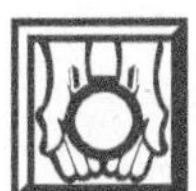

TREATMENT

APPROPRIATE HEALTH CARE

• Identify and correct underlying disorders whenever possible. • Whether inpatient or outpatient depends on clinical status of patient and primary disease, if any (e.g., if CHF, treat as outpatient unless animal is dyspneic or severely hypotensive). • If associated with pericardial effusion, avoid drug therapy and perform pericardiocentesis. • If associated with a certain drug (e.g., hydralazine, bronchodilators), discontinue the medication or adjust the dose. • If associated with hypovolemia, replace fluid volume.

NURSING CARE

Depends on whether associated with a specific disease.

ACTIVITY

Exercise restriction recommended if symptomatic cardiac disease.

DIET

Sodium restriction generally advised with hypertension and CHF.

CLIENT EDUCATION

Discuss importance of managing any primary disease appropriately, with medical or surgical intervention.

SURGICAL CONSIDERATIONS

• Thyroidectomy—treatment option for hyperthyroidism (cats). • Tumor removal is the definitive treatment for patients with pheochromocytoma.

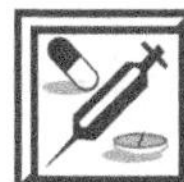

MEDICATIONS

DRUG(S) OF CHOICE

• Establish underlying cause and treat appropriately; specific antiarrhythmic therapy is generally limited to patients in CHF or those with secondary cardiac disease due to hyperthyroidism or hypertension. • Dogs—if CHF is the cause, administer pimobendan along with appropriate diuretic therapy and angiotensin-converting enzyme inhibitor. Digoxin may be indicated in some cases such as CHF with atrial fibrillation. If ST persists despite above management, consider adding a calcium channel blocker (e.g., diltiazem 0.5–2.5 mg/kg PO q8h) or a beta-blocker (e.g., atenolol 0.25–1 mg/kg q12h, sotalol 1–2 mg/kg q12h PO) *only* after congestion is controlled. • Cats—if ST is associated with hyperthyroidism without CHF, a beta-blocker (e.g., atenolol 0.25–1 mg/kg PO q12–24h) may lower the HR. Consider digoxin (0.01875–0.03125 mg per average-size cat, equal to 1/8–1/4 of a 0.125 mg tablet—tablet preferred) if CHF present with atrial fibrillation and rapid ventricular response rate. Although still controversial, pimobendan (0.1–0.3 mg/kg PO q12h) has become more commonly accepted as treatment for CHF. If ST associated with hypertrophic cardiomyopathy, administer atenolol 6.25–12.5 mg/cat PO q12h or diltiazem 1.75–2.4 mg/kg PO q8h.

CONTRAINDICATIONS

Avoid drugs such as atropine or catecholamines (epinephrine) that may further increase the HR.

PRECAUTIONS

• Beta-blockers can potentially worsen signs of congestion and lower cardiac output in patients with systolic dysfunction. • Suppression of ST may be catastrophic if occurring as natural compensatory response to maintain cardiac output in a systemically ill patient.

POSSIBLE INTERACTIONS

See manufacturer's insert for specific drugs.

ALTERNATIVE DRUG(S)

N/A

FOLLOW-UP

PATIENT MONITORING

Depends on specific disease—for CHF, serial ECG, thoracic radiographs, BUN, creatinine, and serum electrolytes; for hyperthyroidism, serial serum T_4, complete blood count, and biochemistry.

PREVENTION/AVOIDANCE

Minimize stress, exercise, and dietary sodium, if heart disease.

POSSIBLE COMPLICATIONS

• Weakness or syncope if associated with low cardiac output. • Development of CHF if persistent ST associated with heart disease.

EXPECTED COURSE AND PROGNOSIS

• ST usually resolves with correction of the underlying cause. • Poor despite treatment if ST is associated with CHF. • Favorable for remission of ST when hyperthyroidism is controlled medically, surgically, or by radioactive iodine.

MISCELLANEOUS

ASSOCIATED CONDITIONS

See list of pathologic and physiologic causes.

PREGNANCY/FERTILITY/BREEDING

Increase in cardiac output in late pregnancy (third trimester) largely due to an accelerated HR.

SYNONYMS

• Inappropriate sinus tachycardia. • Postural tachycardia syndrome.

SEE ALSO

• Atrial Fibrillation and Atrial Flutter.
• Congestive Heart Failure—Left-Sided.
• Congestive Heart Failure—Right-Sided.
• Hyperthyroidism. • Pheochromocytoma.
• Supraventricular Tachycardia.

ABBREVIATIONS

• AV = atrioventricular. • CHF = congestive heart failure. • ECG = electrocardiogram. • HR = heart rate. • NT-proBNP = N-terminal pro-brain natriuretic peptide. • ST = sinus tachycardia. • SVT = supraventricular tachycardia. • T_3 = triiodothyronine. • T_4 = thyroxine. • TRH = thyrotropin-releasing hormone.

Suggested Reading

Côté E, MacDonald K, Meurs K, Sleeper M. Feline Cardiology. Chichester, UK: Wiley-Blackwell, 2011.

Kittleson MD, Kienle RD. Small Animal Cardiovascular Medicine. St. Louis, MO: Mosby, 2005.

Olshansky, B., Sullivan, R. Inappropriate sinus tachycardia. J Am Coll Cardiol 2013, 61(8):793–801.

Author Deborah J. Hadlock
Consulting Editor Michael Aherne

SJÖGREN-LIKE SYNDROME

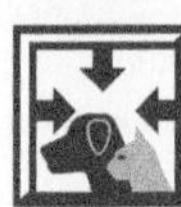

BASICS

OVERVIEW

- A systemic autoimmune disease characterized by keratoconjunctivitis sicca, xerostomia, and lymphoplasmacytic adenitis.
- Underlying mechanism unknown; however, autoantibodies directed against glandular tissues have been identified.
- Associated with other autoimmune or immune-mediated diseases, such as rheumatoid arthritis and pemphigus.

SIGNALMENT

- Higher incidence in several canine breeds—English bulldogs, West Highland white terriers, and miniature schnauzers.
- Chronic disease of adult dogs.
- Cats unaffected.

SIGNS

Historical Findings

- Adult onset.
- Conjunctivitis and keratitis.
- Keratitis sicca most prominent clinical feature.

Physical Examination Findings

- Blepharospasm.
- Conjunctival hyperemia.
- Corneal lesions (opacity to ulceration).
- Gingivitis.
- Stomatitis.

S

CAUSES & RISK FACTORS

- Possible genetic predisposition in breeds with high incidence.
- Develops concurrently with other immune-mediated and autoimmune diseases.

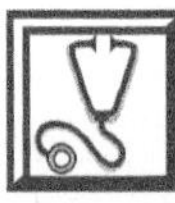

DIAGNOSIS

DIFFERENTIAL DIAGNOSIS

- Other causes of keratoconjunctivitis sicca—canine distemper, trauma, and drug toxicities.
- Keratoconjunctivitis sicca associated with other immune-mediated diseases—atopy, lymphocytic thyroiditis, polymyositis, systemic lupus erythematosus, rheumatoid arthritis, and pemphigoid diseases.

CBC/BIOCHEMISTRY/URINALYSIS

Normal

OTHER LABORATORY TESTS

- Hypergammaglobulinemia revealed by serum protein electrophoresis.
- Positive antinuclear antibody test.
- Positive lupus erythematosus cell test.
- Positive rheumatoid factor test.
- Positive indirect fluorescent antibody test for autoantibodies.

IMAGING

N/A

DIAGNOSTIC PROCEDURES

Schirmer tear test (0–5 mm/min; reference interval is 15–20 mm/min).

PATHOLOGIC FINDINGS

- Histologic changes in salivary glands—lymphoplasmacytic adenitis.
- Conjunctival biopsy—conjunctivitis.

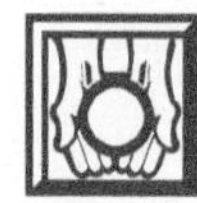

TREATMENT

- Directed at controlling keratoconjunctivitis sicca.
- Any concurrent disease must be medically managed.
- May include administration of anti-inflammatory or immunosuppressive drugs.
- Surgical management of keratoconjunctivitis sicca indicated in animals that fail to respond to medical treatment.

MEDICATIONS

DRUG(S) OF CHOICE

- Topical tear preparations.
- Appropriate topical antibiotics for secondary bacterial infection, if present.
- Immunosuppressive or anti-inflammatory drugs.
- For more aggressive medical treatment and surgical intervention, see Keratoconjunctivitis Sicca.

CONTRAINDICATIONS/POSSIBLE INTERACTIONS

Use of topical steroids in patients with acute keratoconjunctivitis sicca may cause corneal ulceration and is not recommended.

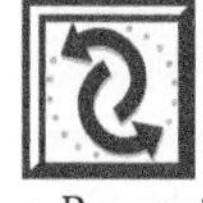

FOLLOW-UP

- Reexamine patients weekly until keratoconjunctivitis sicca controlled.
- Additional monitoring may be indicated to manage underlying or concurrent disease.
- Immunosuppressive drugs—monitor patients every other week for possible side effects.
- Prognosis variable and depends on existence of concurrent disease.

MISCELLANEOUS

SEE ALSO

Keratoconjunctivitis Sicca.

Suggested Reading

Quimby FW, Schwartz RS, Poskitt T, et al. A disorder of dogs resembling Sjogren's syndrome. Clin Immunol Immunopathol 1979, 12:471–476.

Author Paul W. Snyder

Consulting Editor Melinda S. Camus

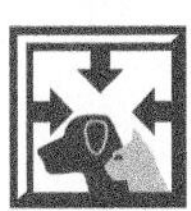

BASICS

OVERVIEW

• A disorder of multifactorial causes characterized by extremely fragile skin.
• Tends to occur in old cats that may have concurrent hyperadrenocorticism, diabetes mellitus, excessive use of megestrol acetate or other progesterone compounds, or as a paraneoplastic syndrome.
• A small number of cats have no biochemical alterations.

SYSTEMS AFFECTED

• Skin/exocrine.
• Endocrine/metabolic.

SIGNALMENT

• Naturally occurring disease tends to be recognized in old cats.
• Iatrogenic cases have no age predilection.
• No breed or sex predilection.

SIGNS

Historical Findings

• Gradual onset of clinical signs.
• Progressive alopecia (not always present).
• Often associated with weight loss, lusterless coat, poor appetite, and lack of energy.

Physical Examination Findings

• Skin becomes markedly thin and tears with normal handling.
• Skin rarely bleeds upon tearing.
• Multiple lacerations (both old and new) may be noted on close examination.
• Partial to complete alopecia of the truncal region may be noted.
• Sometimes associated with "rat tail," pinnal folding, pot-belly appearance.
• Differentiated from cutaneous asthenia by lack of hyperextensibility.

CAUSES & RISK FACTORS

• Hyperadrenocorticism—pituitary- or adrenal-dependent.
• Iatrogenic—secondary to excessive corticosteroid or progesterone drug administration.
• Diabetes mellitus—rare, unless associated with hyperadrenocorticism.
• Possibly idiopathic or paraneoplastic syndrome.

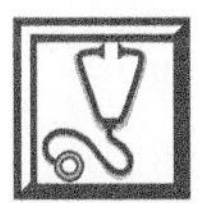

DIAGNOSIS

DIFFERENTIAL DIAGNOSIS

• Cutaneous asthenia.
• Feline paraneoplastic syndrome—pancreatic neoplasia, hepatic lipidosis, cholangiocarcinoma.

CBC/BIOCHEMISTRY/URINALYSIS

• Little diagnostic significance in most cases.
• Approximately 80% of cats with hyperadrenocorticism have concurrent diabetes mellitus (hyperglycemia, glucosuria).

OTHER LABORATORY TESTS

• Adrenocorticotropic hormone (ACTH)-stimulation test—70% of cats with hyperadrenocorticism have an exaggerated response.
• Low-dose dexamethasone-suppression test—15–20% of normal cats may fail to decrease cortisol levels; typically unsuppressed with hyperadrenocorticism and nonadrenal illness.
• High-dose dexamethasone-suppression test—normal cats show decreases in cortisol concentrations; typically decreased with nonadrenal illnesses; considered by many clinicians to be the best screening test for hyperadrenocorticism; unreliable for discriminating between adrenal tumors and pituitary-dependent causes of hyperadrenocorticism, because both conditions fail to show suppression.
• Endogenous ACTH levels—normal range for most labs is 20–100 pg/mL.

IMAGING

• Abdominal ultrasonography—adrenal masses are often small until end-stage disease; cholangiocarcinoma and hepatic lipidosis have been reported.
• CT and MRI—small pituitary tumors may be difficult to visualize; MRI may be more successful.

PATHOLOGIC FINDINGS

Histopathology—suggestive, not diagnostic; epidermis and dermis are thin; attenuated collagen fibers are evident.

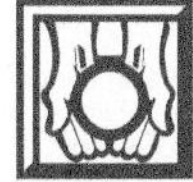

TREATMENT

• Underlying metabolic disease should be ruled out.
• Many patients are debilitated and require supportive care.
• Surgical correction of the lacerations—difficult because the tissue cannot withstand pressure from sutures.
• Protect skin—clothing; reduce activities that can traumatize the skin; remove sharp edges from the environment; prevent damage from interaction with other animals.
• Discontinue exogenous corticosteroids if administered.
• Hyperadrenocorticism—adrenalectomy is the preferred treatment.
• Cobalt-60 radiation therapy—variable success in the treatment of pituitary tumors.

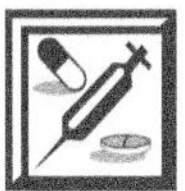

MEDICATIONS

DRUG(S) OF CHOICE

• Medical management—may be useful for preparing patient for surgery and for minimizing postoperative complications (e.g., infections and poor wound healing).
• No known effective medical therapy for feline hyperadrenocorticism.
• Mitotane (1,1-(*o,p'*-dichlorodiphenyl)-2,2-dichloroethane [*o,p'*-DDD]) 12.5–50 mg/kg PO q12h; response has been equivocal; side effects include anorexia, vomiting, and diarrhea.
• Metyrapone 65 mg/kg PO q12h; clinical improvement noted more often with this drug than the others.

CONTRAINDICATIONS/POSSIBLE INTERACTIONS

Hyperadrenocorticism—closely monitor diabetic cats; adjust insulin to prevent hypoglycemia when the cortisol levels fall.

FOLLOW-UP

Patients are often quite debilitated, making any form of treatment risky; close monitoring is required in all cases.

MISCELLANEOUS

ABBREVIATIONS

• ACTH = adrenocorticotropic hormone.

Suggested Reading

Gross TL, Ihrke PJ, Walder EJ. Veterinary Dermatopathology. Philadelphia, PA: Mosby, 1992.
Little SE. August's Consultations in Feline Internal Medicine, Volume 7. Philadelphia, PA: Saunders, 2016.
Vogelnest LJ. Skin as a marker of general feline health: cutaneous manifestations of systemic disease. J Feline Med Surg 2017, 19(9): 948–960.

Author Guillermina Manigot
Consulting Editor Alexander H. Werner Resnick

Acknowledgment The author and editors acknowledge the prior contribution of Karen Helton Rhodes.

SMALL INTESTINAL DYSBIOSIS

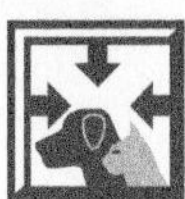

BASICS

DEFINITION

• Small intestinal dysbiosis (SID) is a clinical syndrome caused by an alteration of the small intestinal microbiota. • Previously, a variety of different terms have been used to describe SID: ○ Small intestinal bacterial overgrowth (SIBO)—defined as >10^4 anaerobic and/or >10^5 total bacterial cfu/mL in duodenal juice from dogs. However, these criteria are now controversial. ○ Antibiotic-responsive diarrhea (ARD)—used by several authors to describe patients that have diarrhea that responds to antibiotic therapy. Neither the type of bacteria nor the type of antibiotic that is effective has been defined for ARD. ○ Tylosin-responsive diarrhea (TRD)—used by a group of clinicians in Finland to describe several dogs with chronic diarrhea that failed to respond to a variety of antibiotics or corticosteroids, but did respond to treatment with tylosin. • Currently, there is no consensus on the quantitative makeup of the gastrointestinal microbiota in healthy dogs or cats. • Note that SID differs from colonization of the alimentary tract by known pathogenic bacteria (e.g., *Salmonella* spp., *Campylobacter jejuni*, enterotoxigenic *Clostridium perfringens*, enterotoxic *Escherichia coli*, or others).

S

PATHOPHYSIOLOGY

• Bacteria are constantly ingested with food and/or saliva. • Host-protective mechanisms prevent overgrowth of pathogenic or potentially pathogenic bacteria through gastric acid secretion, intestinal motility (peristalsis), secretion of antimicrobial substances in bile and pancreatic juice, and local enteric IgA production. • The ileocolic valve is a physiologic barrier between the large bowel, which is populated by large numbers of bacteria, and the less populated small bowel. • When these natural defense mechanisms fail and excessive numbers of certain bacterial species persist in the upper small intestine, they may cause pathology, even though they are not considered obligate pathogens. • Anaerobic bacteria (e.g., *Bacteroides* spp. and *Clostridium* spp.) have been considered more likely to cause pathology than many aerobic bacteria.

SYSTEMS AFFECTED

• Gastrointestinal—normal absorptive function is disrupted, resulting in loose stool and weight loss. • Hepatobiliary—portal vein carries bacterial toxins and other substances to the liver, which may lead to hepatic changes.

GENETICS

• No genetic basis for SID has been identified. However, recent studies would suggest that histiocytic ulcerative colitis should be considered a type of dysbiosis of the large intestine. Since the majority of cases have been described in the boxer, genetic factors that predispose dogs of this breed to this type of dysbiosis are likely. • Certain canine breeds (e.g., German shepherd dog, Chinese Shar-Pei, and beagle) appear to be at an increased risk for SID.

INCIDENCE/PREVALENCE

Unknown

GEOGRAPHIC DISTRIBUTION

N/A

SIGNALMENT

Species

Dog and cat.

Breed Predilections

Subjectively, German shepherd dog, Chinese Shar-Pei, and beagle appear to have an increased incidence.

Mean Age and Range

• Unknown. • Can be diagnosed in dogs and cats of any age (age range: <1 year to >8 years).

Predominant Sex

No predilection.

SIGNS

General Comments

Alterations in the gut microbiota can cause clinical signs of small intestinal disease, such as loose stool or diarrhea, weight loss, and/or others.

Historical Findings

• Chronic loose stools or diarrhea (small bowel or large bowel type diarrhea)—common. • Weight loss, despite a reasonable appetite—common. • Borborygmus and flatulence—common. • Vomiting—occasional/variable. • Clinical signs of the underlying disease process may be seen in cases of secondary SID. • Clinical signs may wax and wane or be continuous.

Physical Examination Findings

Unremarkable or evidence of weight loss and decreased body condition.

CAUSES

• Primary SID is probably uncommon, but a definitive cause of SID often remains undiagnosed and thus many dogs are diagnosed with idiopathic SID. • Secondary SID (more common): ○ Altered small intestinal anatomy—inherited or acquired (e.g., congenital blind loop, partial obstructions, neoplasia, foreign body, intussusception, stricture, adhesion, or diverticulum). ○ Altered intestinal motility—hypothyroidism, autonomic neuropathies. ○ Exocrine pancreatic insufficiency (EPI)—approximately 70% of dogs with EPI have concurrent SID. ○ Hypochlorhydria or achlorhydria—spontaneous or iatrogenic (e.g., proton pump inhibitor treatment). ○ Altered immune system—immunodeficiency, decreased mucosal defense, and preexisting intestinal disease.

RISK FACTORS

Intestinal diseases that affect local defense mechanisms (e.g., inflammatory bowel disease [IBD], adverse food reactions, parasite infestation, others).

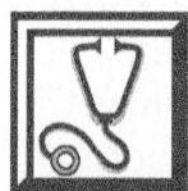

DIAGNOSIS

DIFFERENTIAL DIAGNOSIS

• Secondary gastrointestinal disease (e.g., hepatic failure, renal failure, EPI, chronic pancreatitis, hypothyroidism, hypoadrenocorticism). • Primary gastrointestinal disease (i.e., infectious, inflammatory, neoplastic, mechanical, toxic, or other).

CBC/BIOCHEMISTRY/URINALYSIS

• Usually unremarkable. • Hypoalbuminemia—uncommon finding; when present, it suggests particularly severe intestinal disease and warrants an aggressive diagnostic and therapeutic approach.

OTHER LABORATORY TESTS

Serum Cobalamin and Folate Concentrations

• Serum folate concentration may be increased, as many bacterial species synthesize folate and an increased abundance of folate-producing bacterial species will lead to an overabundance of folic acid in the small intestine. • Serum cobalamin concentration may be decreased, as many bacterial species compete with the host for dietary cobalamin. • The finding of an increased serum folate concentration and a decreased serum cobalamin concentration is suggestive, but not specific for SID in dogs. In addition, not all patients with SID show this pattern.

Qualitative and Quantitative Bacterial Culture of Small Intestinal Juice

• Aerobic and anaerobic quantitative culture of duodenal fluid has long been considered the "gold standard" for the diagnosis of SIBO in human patients. • Invasive—requires endoscopy or laparoscopy. Not practical and not routinely available. • Recent work would suggest the species of bacteria that comprise the small intestinal microbiota may be more important than bacterial numbers. • No standardized protocols have been established for sampling, handling, and culturing of duodenal juice, leading to high variability in bacterial counts.

Dysbiosis index (DI)

• The fecal DI is a PCR-based assay that quantifies the abundances of eight bacterial groups in fecal samples of dogs and summarizes them in one single number. • A DI below 0 indicates a normal fecal microbiota; a DI above 0 indicates dysbiosis. Approximately 15% of clinically healthy dogs have an increased DI, with most of them falling into the equivocal range between 0 and 2. • Many dogs with chronic enteropathy or EPI have an abnormal fecal DI. • Due to anatomical and physiological differences along the intestine, evaluation of the fecal DI may not accurately reflect microbiota changes in the small intestine. • Concurrent evaluation of serum concentration of cobalamin/folate with assessment of the fecal DI may help in the diagnosis of SID.

IMAGING

Not useful for the diagnosis of primary SID. However, may reveal findings indicative of an underlying cause.

DIAGNOSTIC PROCEDURES

Therapeutic Trial

• Treatment of patients with suspected SID with an antibiotic, a prebiotic, or a probiotic. • Interpreting the results of a therapeutic trial may be difficult as more than one disease (e.g., IBD plus SID, dietary intolerance plus SID) may be present, and lack of a clinical response might lead to the incorrect conclusion that SID is absent; incorrect selection of the treatment that is trialed might also cause failure of a clinical response.

PATHOLOGIC FINDINGS

• No macroscopic findings upon exploratory laparotomy or endoscopy. • Histopathology of small intestinal mucosal biopsies is typically unremarkable unless SID is caused by underlying intestinal disease.

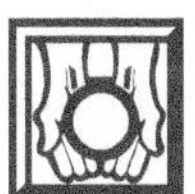

TREATMENT

APPROPRIATE HEALTH CARE

• Outpatient medical management. • SID can be managed with antibiotics, prebiotics, probiotics, or a combination thereof:
◦ Antibiotics—see Medications.
◦ Prebiotics—see Diet. ◦ Probiotics—there has been a lot of interest in probiotic use for dogs and cats with chronic diarrhea, although little is known about the efficacy. Currently, because of quality issues with many products, only probiotics from major manufacturers can be recommended. • Improvement may take a few days to several weeks.

NURSING CARE

• Usually none. • Supportive care for emaciated or hypoalbuminemic patients.

ACTIVITY

Unrestricted

DIET

• Highly digestible diet. • A diet containing fructooligosaccharides has been shown to be beneficial in dogs with SID.

CLIENT EDUCATION

• Some patients show clinical improvement within days. • Some patients require weeks of therapy before demonstrating improvement—treat for 2–3 weeks before concluding that therapy is ineffective. • Any concurrent or predisposing diseases (e.g., IBD, EPI, dietary intolerance/allergy, alimentary tract neoplasia, partial obstruction) must also be treated. • Continuous or repeated treatment is often required.

SURGICAL CONSIDERATIONS

Only indicated for some underlying causes of SID (i.e., partial obstruction, diverticulum, or intestinal mass).

MEDICATIONS

DRUG(S) OF CHOICE

• Broad-spectrum, orally administered antibiotics effective against both aerobic and anaerobic bacteria are preferred. • Tylosin (10–20 mg/kg PO q12h for 6 weeks) is the primary choice. Tylosin is usually used in a powder formulation that is marketed for use in poultry and pigs. It is administered in the food because of its bitter taste. It can be used long-term and is very safe and inexpensive. For small dogs and cats the drug should be reformulated into capsules. For larger dogs the dose can be approximated by using a teaspoon and administering the drug in food. • Metronidazole (10–15 mg/kg PO q12h for 6 weeks) is used commonly in routine practice because of its activity against anaerobic bacteria. Metronidazole may also have immunomodulatory effects. However, metronidazole can have significant side effects. • Dogs with SID may be cobalamin deficient, and parenteral or oral supplementation of vitamin B12 is indicated. See Cobalamin Deficiency for dosing information.

CONTRAINDICATIONS

None

PRECAUTIONS

Metronidazole can be associated with gastrointestinal side effects and in rare cases with neurologic side effects.

POSSIBLE INTERACTIONS

None

ALTERNATIVE DRUG(S)

In dogs with EPI and SID, concurrent therapy for SID is only indicated if enzyme replacement alone does not resolve the diarrhea and/or lead to weight gain.

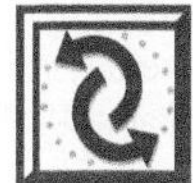

FOLLOW-UP

PATIENT MONITORING

• Body weight and, in hypoproteinemic patients, serum albumin concentrations are the most important parameters; improvement suggests effective therapy. • Diarrhea should resolve. • If diarrhea persists despite improved body weight and/or increased serum albumin concentration, investigation for concurrent intestinal disease is indicated.

PREVENTION/AVOIDANCE

N/A

POSSIBLE COMPLICATIONS

N/A

EXPECTED COURSE AND PROGNOSIS

Primary SID without complicating factors (e.g., IBD, lymphoma) usually has a good prognosis, although relapses can be seen following cessation of antibiotic therapy.

MISCELLANEOUS

ASSOCIATED CONDITIONS

• SID has been suspected as a cause of IBD in some patients. • EPI.

AGE-RELATED FACTORS

N/A

ZOONOTIC POTENTIAL

None

PREGNANCY/FERTILITY/BREEDING

Avoid oxytetracycline or metronidazole, especially during early pregnancy.

SYNONYMS

SIBO, ARD, or TRD may be used synonymously by some authors.

SEE ALSO

• Cobalamin Deficiency. • Diarrhea, Chronic—Cats. • Diarrhea, Chronic—Dogs.
• Exocrine Pancreatic Insufficiency.
• Inflammatory Bowel Disease.
• Lymphoma—Cats. • Lymphoma—Dogs.

ABBREVIATIONS

• ARD = antibiotic responsive diarrhea. • DI = dysbiosis index. • EPI = exocrine pancreatic insufficiency. • IBD = inflammatory bowel disease. • SIBO = small intestinal bacterial overgrowth. • SID = small intestinal dysbiosis. • TRD = tylosin-responsive diarrhea.

INTERNET RESOURCES

www.vetmed.tamu.edu/gilab

Suggested Reading

German AJ, Day MJ, Ruaux CG, et al. Comparison of direct and indirect tests for small intestinal bacterial overgrowth and antibiotic-responsive diarrhea in dogs. J Vet Intern Med 2003, 17(1):33–43.

Kilpinen S, Spillmann T, Westermarck E. Efficacy of two low-dose oral tylosin regimens in controlling the relapse of diarrhea in dogs with tylosin-responsive diarrhea: a prospective, single-blinded, two-arm parallel, clinical field trial. Acta Vet Scand 2014, 66:43.

Suchodolski JS. Diagnosis and interpretation of intestinal dysbiosis in dogs and cats. Vet J 2016, 215:30–37.

Authors Jan S. Suchodolski and Jörg M. Steiner
Consulting Editor Mark P. Rondeau

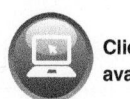

Client Education Handout available online

S

SMOKE INHALATION

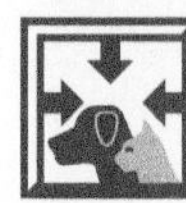

BASICS

OVERVIEW

• Injury secondary to direct heat damage to upper airway and nasal mucosa. Inhalation of toxins directly irritates the airway, and particulate matter adheres to the airways and alveoli. • Carbon monoxide decreases tissue oxygen delivery by preferentially binding to hemoglobin. • Cyanide interferes with oxygen usage in oxidative phosphorylation. • Extent of damage depends on the degree and duration of exposure and the material that was burning. • Serious lung injury possible with little external evidence of burning. • Lung reaction—initially bronchoconstriction, airway edema, mucus production and airway occlusion; then an inflammatory response, necrotizing tracheobronchitis, and pulmonary fluid accumulation due to increased capillary permeability. • Lung dysfunction typically progresses during initial 2–3 days. • Secondary bacterial infections—common cause of morbidity late in the disease.

SIGNALMENT

S

Dog and cat.

SIGNS

• Historical findings consistent with exposure. • Smoky odor. • Tachypnea and increased respiratory effort. • Inspiratory effort suggests upper airway obstruction by edema. • Postural adaptations to hypoxemia. • Mucous membranes can be cherry red (from carboxyhemoglobin), pale, or cyanotic. • Auscultation of wheezes, harsh broncho-vesicular sounds, or crackles. • Cough. • Burns, shriveled whiskers, conjunctival edema, corneal ulcers. • Neurologic signs indicate carbon monoxide or cyanide toxicity. • Cardiac arrhythmias and hypotension can be seen secondary to hypoxemia, smoke and carbon monoxide inhalation, and burn injuries.

CAUSES & RISK FACTORS

Exposure to smoke, usually from being trapped in a burning building.

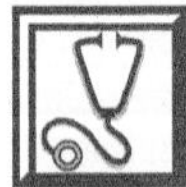

DIAGNOSIS

CBC/BIOCHEMISTRY/URINALYSIS

• Neutropenia—poor prognostic sign; suggests neutrophil sequestration in the lungs. • Thrombocytopenia—suggests platelet sequestration or consumption. • Biochemistry profile—evidence of hypoxic damage to other organ systems can be present.

IMAGING

Thoracic radiographs—establish a baseline; findings vary from normal to a broncho-interstitial or alveolar pattern.

DIAGNOSTIC PROCEDURES

• Bronchoalveolar lavage/endotracheal wash if suspected secondary bacterial infection: culture; cytology—acute suppurative reaction with excessive mucus, neutrophils, and alveolar macrophages; intracellular bacteria indicate concurrent infection. • Arterial blood gas to confirm hypoxemia. Pulse oximetry difficult to interpret as carboxy-hemoglobin falsely increases values. Co-oximetry showing carboxyhemoglobin levels >15% indicates toxicity. • Bronchoscopy demonstrates severity of airway damage, and is used to remove foreign particles and accumulated secretions.

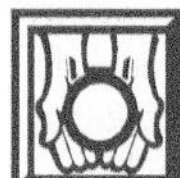

TREATMENT

• Initial management—stabilize respiratory function; establish patent airway; severe upper airway edema or obstruction can require intubation or temporary tracheostomy. • Oxygen—administer immediately to displace carbon monoxide from hemoglobin; use the highest available concentration for 2–4 hours (or longer); after elimination of carboxyhemoglobin, supplement as needed. • Fluid therapy—crystalloid fluid resuscitation as needed to maintain perfusion with care to avoid fluid overload and progressive pulmonary edema. Associated burns can result in significant fluid and protein losses which may also require concurrent colloidal support (synthetic, albumin, plasma). • Nebulization of saline—moistens airway secretions to facilitate clearance. • Mechanical ventilation needed in severe cases. • Nutritional support—maintain body condition and immune status.

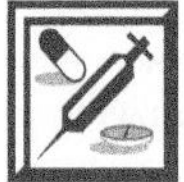

MEDICATIONS

DRUG(S) OF CHOICE

• Suspected bacterial infection—broad-spectrum antibiotics, ideally after bacterial culture has been obtained. • Bronchodilators—improve respiratory function if severe bronchoconstriction, especially cats (e.g., terbutaline 0.01 mg/kg IV, IM, SC). Inhaled beta-agonists can also be beneficial. • Corticosteroids—controversial, single early, anti-inflammatory dose or aerosolized corticosteroids may decrease airway edema. • Analgesia—as required for associated discomfort. Avoid oversedation due to decreased respiratory drive.

CONTRAINDICATIONS/POSSIBLE INTERACTIONS

• Diuretics—decrease IV volume without a major beneficial effect. • Corticosteroids—use only once and if absolutely necessary; can predispose the patient to bacterial infection.

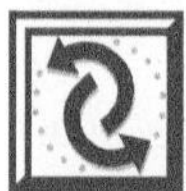

FOLLOW-UP

PATIENT MONITORING

• Respiratory rate and effort, mucous membrane color, heart rate, pulse quality, lung auscultations, and packed cell volume/total solids for 24–72 hours. • Repeat radiographs in 72 hours—ensure condition is resolving; monitor for bacterial pneumonia. • Pulse oximetry and arterial blood gas analysis—to monitor hypoxemia and response to therapy.

POSSIBLE COMPLICATIONS

• Bacterial tracheobronchitis or pneumonia. • Profound pulmonary inflammatory response or severe systemic inflammatory response syndrome may result in acute respiratory response syndrome. Bronchiectasis can develop secondary to airway injury and impaired mucociliary clearance. • Carbon monoxide toxicity may lead to acute and delayed neurologic signs including seizures, cerebral edema, ataxia, paresis, and changes in mental status.

EXPECTED COURSE AND PROGNOSIS

• Good if responding to treatment—likely to worsen prior to improving. Prognosis declines if complications occur. • Severe burns or organ injury—poor prognosis.

MISCELLANEOUS

Suggested Reading

Berent AC, Todd J, Sergeeff J, Powell LL. Carbon monoxide toxicity: a case series. J Vet Emerg Crit Care 2005, 15(2):128–135.

Fitzgerald KT, Flood AA. Smoke inhalation. Clin Tech Small Anim Pract 2006, 21(4):205–214.

Mariani CL. Full recovery following delayed neurologic signs after smoke inhalation in a dog. J Vet Emerg Crit Care 2003, 13(4):235–239.

Vaughn L, Beckel N, Walters P. Severe burn injury, burn shock, and smoke inhalation injury in small animals. Part 2: diagnosis, therapy, complications, and prognosis. J Vet Emerg Crit Care 2012, 22(2):187–200.

Author Cassandra O. Janson

Consulting Editor Elizabeth Rozanski

Acknowledgment The author and editors acknowledge the prior contribution of Lesley G. King.

SNAKE VENOM TOXICOSIS—CORAL SNAKES

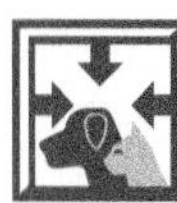

BASICS

OVERVIEW

• Two clinically important species in North America—*Micrurus fulvius*, eastern coral snake (North Carolina to the north; southern Florida to the south; west of the Mississippi River) and *Micrurus tenere*, Texas coral snake (west of Mississippi; in Arkansas, Louisiana, and Texas).
• Family Elapidae—fixed front fangs.
• Color pattern—bands fully encircling the body; red, yellow, and black; distinguished from the harmless tricolored king snake (*Lampropeltis elapsoides*) by the arrangement of the bands: if yellow (caution) and red (danger) color bands touch, then stay clear; relatively small head; black snout; round pupils.

Bites

• Relatively uncommon due to snake's reclusive behavior and nocturnal habits.
• Often occur on the lip. Snakes remain attached due to chewing action.
• Distinct fang marks may not be obvious.
• Primary cause of death—respiratory collapse.

SIGNALMENT

Dogs and cats.

SIGNS

• Onset of clinical signs may be delayed several hours (up to 18 hours).
• Localized signs generally absent.
• Generalized weakness and ataxia.
• Bulbar paralysis—affecting cranial motor nerves, respiratory tract, and skeletal muscles; acute flaccid quadriplegia.
• Salivation—caused by dysphagia.
• Dyspnea.
• Dysphonia.
• Hyporeflexive spinal reflexes.
• Seizures.
• Urinary incontinence.

CAUSES & RISK FACTORS

• Size of the snake.
• Size and duration of bite.

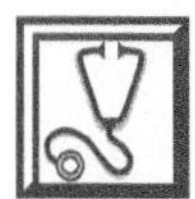

DIAGNOSIS

DIFFERENTIAL DIAGNOSIS

• Myasthenia gravis.
• Botulism.
• Polyradiculoneuritis.
• Tick bite paralysis.
• Black widow spider bite (*Latrodectus* spp.).

CBC/BIOCHEMISTRY/URINALYSIS

• Hemolysis—dogs only.
• Red blood cell burring.
• May note high creatine kinase.
• Hemoglobinuria—dogs only.

OTHER LABORATORY TESTS

N/A

DIAGNOSTIC PROCEDURES

N/A

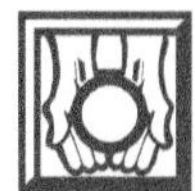

TREATMENT

• First aid—generally avoid; most effective measure is rapid transport to a veterinary facility for antivenom administration; Australian technique for elapid bites is a pressure wrap of the bitten limb with ace-type bandage to decrease blood flow and venom uptake.
• *Caution*: do not wait for onset of clinical signs to initiate treatment.
• Inpatient—hospitalize for a minimum of 48 hours.
• Monitor CNS and respiratory function closely for 24 hours.
• Specific antivenin is extremely limited for *M. fulvius* envenomations in the United States and typically not accessible for veterinary use. However, protective crossreactivity occurs with the following antivenins: Coralmyn (Fab2 equine origin) (Instituto Bioclon, Mexico), Costa Rican coral snake antivenin (Instituto Clodomiro Picado, Costa Rica), and Australian tiger snake *Notechis scutatus* (CSL Limited, Parkville, Victoria, Australia). Expense may be a consideration. Local zoos may have antivenom available. Application for an INR permit from the US Department of Agriculture may allow a veterinary hospital to acquire these antivenoms.
• If antivenin unavailable—provide ventilatory support for several days in a critical care facility.

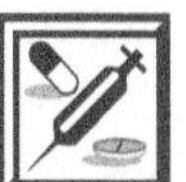

MEDICATIONS

DRUG(S) OF CHOICE

• *M. fulvius* reactive antivenin (see Treatment)—indicated if the history includes recent coral snake interaction; evidence of puncture wounds; clinical signs consistent with coral snake envenomation; administer 1–2 vials; additional vials may be necessary (technique same as for pit viper antivenin).
• Broad-spectrum antibiotics are not routinely recommended and should only be used if there is indication of infection.
• Neostigmine – may be useful to reverse neuromuscular blockade if antivenin not available. Has been used successfully to treat *M. frontalis* envenomation in Brazil.

CONTRAINDICATIONS/POSSIBLE INTERACTIONS

• Corticosteroids—not indicated.
• Observe precautions outlined for pit viper antivenin administration (see Snake Venom Toxicosis—Pit Vipers).

FOLLOW-UP

• Marked clinical signs may last 1–1.5 weeks.
• Full recovery may take months as receptors regenerate.

MISCELLANEOUS

SEE ALSO

Snake Venom Toxicosis—Pit Vipers.

Suggested Reading

Pérez ML, Fox K, Schaer M. A retrospective evaluation of coral snake envenomation in dogs and cats: 20 cases (1996–2011). J Vet Emerg Crit Care 2012, 22(6):682–689.

Pérez ML, Fox KJ, Schaer MA. Retrospective review of coral snake envenomation in the dog and cat: 20 cases 1996 to 2011. Toxicon 2013, 60(2):247–248.

Peterson ME. Snake bite: Coral snakes. In: Peterson ME, Talcott PA, eds., Small Animal Toxicology, 3rd ed. St. Louis, MO: Saunders, 2013, pp. 799–805.

Author Michael E. Peterson
Consulting Editor Lynn R. Hovda

SNAKE VENOM TOXICOSIS—PIT VIPERS

BASICS

OVERVIEW

- Pit vipers—*Crotalus* spp. (rattlesnakes), *Sistrurus* spp. (pigmy rattlesnakes and massasauga), and *Agkistrodon* spp. (copperheads and cottonmouth water moccasins); retractable fangs; heat-sensing pit between the nostril and eye; triangle-shaped head.
- Range—throughout the United States (not found in Alaska, Hawaii, Maine).
- Toxicity—considered hemotoxic; several species have subpopulations with lethal neurotoxic components (e.g., Mohave rattlesnake); general ranking of severity: (1) rattlesnakes, (2) moccasins, (3) copperheads.

Pathophysiology

- Venom—enzymes: hyaluronidase and phospholipase A (cause local tissue injury) and others that interfere with the coagulation cascade (cause major coagulation defects); non-enzymatic polypeptides: affect the cardiovascular and respiratory systems.
- Bite—80% of victims have altered laboratory values and clinically important swelling; severe hypotension from pooling of blood within the splanchnic (dogs) or pulmonary (cats) vessels; fluid loss from the vascular compartment secondary to severe peripheral edema.
- Approximately 20% crotalid bites considered "dry bites" with little if any venom deposited and no associated toxicity.

Systems Affected

- Behavioral—usually related to pain.
- Cardiovascular—lower blood pressure, direct cardiotoxins (Eastern and Western Diamondback rattlesnake venom).
- Gastrointestinal—nausea, diarrhea.
- Hematologic—coagulopathies (hypercoagulation or consumptive), thrombocytopenia.
- Musculoskeletal—rhabdomyolysis.
- Nervous—multiple crotalid species have individuals with venom containing Mojave toxin, a potent neurotoxin.
- Skin—puncture wounds possible local tissue necrosis.

SIGNALMENT

Dogs and cats.

SIGNS

General Comments

May be delayed for 8 hours after envenomation.

Historical Findings

- Outdoors, rural setting, indigenous snake.
- Owner saw bite or heard snake.

Physical Examination Findings

- Puncture wounds on head and forelimbs in most animals.
- Local tissue swelling and pain surrounding bite site.
- Bruising, with possible necrosis and sloughing of bite site tissue.
- Ecchymosis and petechiation of tissues and mucous membranes.
- Hypotension and shock.
- Tachycardia.
- Shallow respiration.
- Depression, lethargy, and muscle weakness.
- Nausea and excessive salivation.

CAUSES & RISK FACTORS

Outdoor activity.

Snake-Associated

- Toxic peptide fraction: enzyme fraction ratio—higher in spring and lower in fall (not well documented); high in very young snakes.
- Amount of venom production since last bite.
- Size, fang length, aggressiveness, and motivation of snake.

Victim-Associated

- Bite site—bites to tongue and torso are of major concern.
- Size of victim.
- Elapsed time between bite and initiation of treatment.
- Activity level of victim after the bite—activity increases absorption of venom.

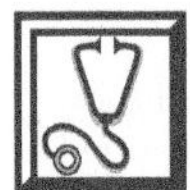

DIAGNOSIS

DIFFERENTIAL DIAGNOSIS

- Angioedema secondary to insect envenomation (spider, scorpion, large centipede).
- Blunt trauma.
- Penetrating wound.
- Animal bite.
- Penetration of foreign body.
- Draining abscess.

CBC/BIOCHEMISTRY/URINALYSIS

- Hemoconcentration.
- Frequent burring of red blood cells within first 24 hours (echinocytes).
- Thrombocytopenia.
- Hypokalemia.
- Elevated creatine kinase.
- Hematuria or myoglobinuria.

OTHER LABORATORY TESTS

Clotting tests—reduced platelets and fibrinogen, monitor for prolonged activated clotting time, prothrombin time, and partial thromboplastin time; may note elevated fibrin degradation products.

DIAGNOSTIC PROCEDURES

- Clinical evaluation of bite for edema, ecchymosis, fang punctures, pain.
- Electrocardiogram—may detect ventricular arrhythmia, especially in severely depressed patients.

PATHOLOGIC FINDINGS

- Puncture wounds.
- Tissue necrosis.
- Hemorrhage, petechiation, ecchymosis.
- Pulmonary hemorrhage, edema.

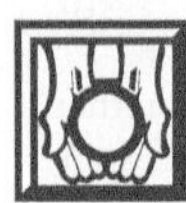

TREATMENT

- Tissue reaction around the bite site—not a reliable indicator of systemic toxicity.
- Bite location—may affect uptake of venom; bites to tongue and torso are of major concern. Distal limb bites may result in significant tissue damage and compromise limb function.
- First aid measures—minimize activity, calm patient, provide analgesia if indicated; transport quickly to a veterinary facility.
- Swelling can be objectively monitored with circumferential measurements using a cloth or flexible tape measure.
- Antivenom is only proven specific treatment (see Medications). Expense may be an important factor.
- IV fluids—correct hypotension.
- Analgesics to reduce pain and stress.
- Antibiotics—infection is rare and antibiotics are not recommended unless there is evidence of infection.
- Repeat coagulation profile after administration of antivenom for comparison to earlier labs (typically the author performs on entry, 6 hours and 12 hours unless patient is obviously worsening). Recurrence of clinical signs or coagulation abnormalities can occur with any antivenin. This usually happens when initial coagulopathy is more severe. If initial coagulopathy resolved with antivenin administration, recurrence can occur within the next few days, although rarely as severe as initial. There are no documented cases of clinical bleeding with subsequent coagulopathy; however, the clinician should be aware of the possibility.

Activity

Initially restrict exercise as this can increase uptake of venom, once envenomation syndrome under control—activity as the patient will tolerate.

Client Education

- Monitor patient for ecchymosis or petechiation.
- Monitor for evidence of serum sickness.

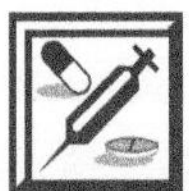

MEDICATIONS

DRUG(S) OF CHOICE

Antivenom

- Always flush antivenom vial after initial removal of antivenom, second flush can increase antibody collection by 30%.

• Allergic reaction—stop antivenom; give diphenhydramine; after 5 minutes, restart antivenom infusion at a slower rate.
• Mix each vial of antivenom with 100–150 mL of a crystalloid fluid and administer IV slowly while taking into consideration the patient's weight and overall fluid load. Infuse over 30 minutes–1 hour.
• Carefully monitor the inner pinna for onset of hyperemia (indicator of possible allergic reaction).
• With the exception of Crofab™ all antivenoms have approximately 20% of their protein content as actual antibodies against snake venom.
• Frequent administration of antivenom controls the animal's pain.
• Other analgesics as needed to control pain.

Veterinary Licensed

• VenomVet™ (Crotalidae polyvalent, equine origin, Fab2). Injectable solution, no need to reconstitute. Two South American immunizing snake species.
• Antivenin™ (Crotalidae polyvalent, equine origin, whole IgG—Boehringer-Ingelheim), reactions more common due to extraneous proteins. Lyophilized. Two North American snake species and two South American species immunizing snake species.
• Rattler Antivenin™ (polyvalent, equine origin, whole IgG—Mg Biologics) equine plasma product, frozen. Four North American immunizing snakes.

FDA Licensed but Published Studies in Dogs

• Crofab® (polyvalent, ovine Fab1—BTG International) first prospective clinical trial of antivenom in dogs. Purified antibody fragments provide much less possibility for reactions. 99% protein is Fab1 antibodies against snake venom.
• Antivipmyn® (polyvalent, equine Fab2—Rare Disease Therapeutics) has completed safety and clinical trials in dogs. Purified antibody particles much less possibility for reactions.

CONTRAINDICATIONS/POSSIBLE INTERACTIONS

• *Caution*: in animals receiving beta-blockers, the onset of anaphylaxis may be masked; therefore, the condition may be more advanced once recognized and more difficult to treat effectively.
• Corticosteroids—of no value.
• Dimethyl sulfoxide (DMSO)—enhances uptake and spread of venom.
• Heparin—do not use; not effective against thrombin-like enzymes and worsens coagulopathies.

Alternative Drug(s)

Rattlesnake vaccine for dogs is currently marketed. Its efficacy is unknown, but several published papers have shown mixed results; only anecdotal evidence at this time. Not recommended until peer-reviewed efficacy data available.

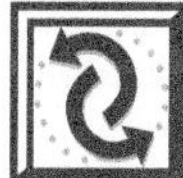

FOLLOW-UP

• Repeated laboratory analysis—6 hours after admission to hospital.
• Clinical signs—may last 1–1.5 weeks.
• Once released, owner should monitor for recurrence of coagulopathies or delayed serum sickness.

MISCELLANEOUS

AGE-RELATED FACTORS

• None unless underlying pathology (e.g. renal disease).
• Patients receiving other medications (e.g. nonsteroidal anti-inflammatory drugs).

PREGNANCY/FERTILITY/BREEDING

• Antivenom has been given to pregnant animals and humans with no adverse events.
• Pregnancy is at risk from venom effects upon placenta and fetal tissue.

INTERNET RESOURCES

App: Snakebite911 ER

Suggested Reading

Hoose JA, Carr A. Retrospective analysis of clinical findings and outcome of cats with suspected rattlesnake envenomation in Southern California: 18 cases (2007–2010). J Vet Emerg Crit Care 2013, 23(3):314–320.

Julius TM, Kaelble MK, Leech EB, et al. Retrospective evaluation of neurotoxic rattlesnake envenomation in dogs and cats: 34 cases (2005–2010). J Vet Emerg Crit Care 2012, 22(4):460–469.

Peterson ME, Matz M, Seibold K, et al. A randomized multicenter trial of Crotalidae polyvalent immune Fab antivenom for the treatment of rattlesnake envenomation in dogs. J Vet Emerg Crit Care 2011, 21(4);335–345.

Pritchard JC, Birkenheuer AJ, Hanel RM, et al. Copperhead (*Agkistrodon contortrix*) envenomation of dogs: 52 cases (2004–2011). J Am Anim Hosp Assoc 2014, online 6131, doi 10.5326.

Witsil AJ, Wells R, Woods C, Rao S. 272 cases of rattlesnake envenomation in dogs: demographics and treatment including safety of F(ab′)2 antivenom use in 236 patients. Toxicon 2015, 105:19–26.

Woods C, Young D. Clinical safety evaluation of F(ab′)$_2$ antivenom (*Crotalus durissus-Bothrops asper*) administration in dogs. J Vet Emerg Crit Care 2011, 21(5):565–569.

Author Michael E. Peterson
Consulting Editor Lynn R. Hovda

SNEEZING, REVERSE SNEEZING, GAGGING

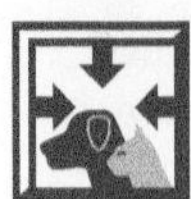

BASICS

DEFINITION

- Sneezing—a normal, protective, expiratory reflex that serves to expel air and material from the lungs through the nasal cavity and mouth.
- Reverse sneezing—a normal protective, repetitive inspiratory reflex that serves to remove irritants from the nasopharynx (also termed the aspiration reflex).
- Gagging—a normal protective reflex to clear secretions from the larynx, trachea, pharynx, or esophagus. Prevents irritating/ toxic material from entering these structures; often misinterpreted as vomiting by owners.

PATHOPHYSIOLOGY

- Irritation of submucosal irritant receptors; various stimuli (infectious, parasitic, irritant, mechanical—especially accumulated secretions) will elicit these reflexes depending on where the irritation is applied.
- Sneezing—nasal mucosal irritation; improves with chronicity.
- Reverse sneezing—caudodorsal nasopharyngeal mucosal irritation triggers pharyngeal muscle spasms, subsequent laryngeal obstruction and movement of material into the oropharynx.
- Gagging—intraoral stimulation (tracheal, laryngeal, oropharyngeal, potentially esophageal mucosal irritation) detected by afferent limb of gag reflex. Efferent limb gives rise to uncoordinated muscle movement characteristic of gagging.

SYSTEMS AFFECTED

- Respiratory—frequently associated with infectious or inflammatory conditions involving the upper respiratory tract.
- Gastrointestinal—gagging may also be caused by swallowing, esophageal, or gastric disorders.

GENETICS

N/A

INCIDENCE/PREVALENCE

These are common, normal reflexes in both dogs and cats in response to mucosal irritation.

GEOGRAPHIC DISTRIBUTION

Worldwide

SIGNALMENT

- Any dog or cat may be affected.
- These reflexes associated with the conditions that cause them; examples include:
  - Young animals—infection, congenital defects (cleft palate0, primary ciliary dyskinesia.
  - Older animals—nasal tumors, dental disease.
- Acute sneezing in dogs is most often caused by a nasal foreign body, while in cats it is most often associated with acute viral rhinitis.

SIGNS

- Head and mouth position may help owners determine which of these reflexes are present.
- Sneezing typically results in sudden, explosive expiratory effort(s) with the mouth closed and head thrown downward; may result in the animal's nose hitting the ground.
- Reverse sneezing is a sudden, often paroxysmal, noisy, inspiratory effort with the head pulled back, mouth closed, and lips sucked in.
- Gagging is an expiratory effort; typically, with the head and neck extended and mouth held open; usually ends with the animal swallowing (with little to nothing expelled).
- Nasal discharge commonly seen with sneezing and reverse sneezing. Retching, coughing and vomiting may accompany gagging.

CAUSES

- Any mucosal irritation or inflammation can elicit these airway reflexes. The reflex localizes the site of irritation for further evaluation.
- Nasal causes of sneezing and reverse sneezing include excess nasal secretions, rhinitis (idiopathic, secondary bacterial, viral or mycotic infections), foreign body, non-neoplastic masses (nasopharyngeal polyps, inflammatory polyps of the nasal turbinates), neoplasia, and parasites; dogs—*Pneumonyssoides*; dogs and cats—*Cuterebra, Eucoleus* (*Capillaria*), *Linguatula.*
- Extranasal diseases resulting in reverse sneezing, sneezing and gagging—pneumonia, esophageal strictures, megaesophagus, chronic vomiting, cricopharyngeal disorders, dental disease (oronasal fistulas, tooth root abscess).
- Reverse sneezing may be idiopathic, especially in small-breed dogs with no other associated clinical signs.
- Causes of gagging include:
  - Secretions being coughed up from the lower airways and into the larynx or cervical trachea.
  - Pharyngeal/laryngeal dysfunction resulting in airway aspiration due to loss of motor and/or sensory function that normally protects the airway.
  - Vomiting from esophageal and gastro-intestinal disease.

RISK FACTORS

- Brachycephalic and dolichocephalic breeds may be overrepresented.
- Incompletely or unvaccinated animals are at a higher risk of developing infection.
- Outdoor animals, especially hunting dogs, perhaps more at risk for nasal foreign bodies and nasal infections.
- Chronic dental disease can cause rhinitis and either sneezing or reverse sneezing.
- Environmental factors like dusty areas, smoke inhalation, perfumes, cold air.
- Productive coughing may produce excess secretions that can be propelled into the nasopharynx and lead to reverse sneezing.
- Nasal mites may cause both reverse sneezing and sneezing in dogs (but not cats); in the United States, incidence is inversely proportional to heartworm preventive usage.
- Reverse sneezing is often associated with excitement.

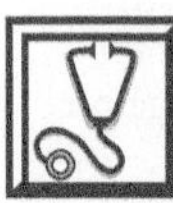

DIAGNOSIS

DIFFERENTIAL DIAGNOSIS

Similar Signs

- Differentiate regular sneezing (occurs on expiration) from reverse sneezing (occurs on inspiration and localizes the site of irritation to the nasopharynx).
- Gagging is often misinterpreted as vomiting.

CBC/BIOCHEMISTRY/URINALYSIS

Nonspecific for any cause of sneezing, reverse sneezing, or gagging. Identifies comorbidities.

OTHER LABORATORY TESTS

Virus isolation, culture or PCR for upper respiratory tract infections (FCV, FHV-1, feline and canine influenza); retroviral testing (FeLV, FIV); cryptococcal antigen testing; *Aspergillosis* testing; bacterial cultures (*Mycoplasma* spp., *Bordetella bronchiseptica*); cytology, histopathology and coagulation studies if indicated.

IMAGING

- Sneezing and reverse sneezing—skull radiographs, CT/MRI.
- Gagging—thoracic radiographs, fluoroscopy (dynamic swallow study), CT/ MRI.

DIAGNOSTIC PROCEDURES

- Sneezing and reverse sneezing—antegrade and retrograde rhinoscopy, nasal biopsy (histopathology), nasal culture (deep nasal flush sample), periodontal probing.
- Gagging—neurologic examination (CN V, IX, X, XII), sedated oropharyngeal exam, transtracheal wash, or bronchoalveolar lavage.

PATHOLOGIC FINDINGS

Nonspecific inflammation can be found in the nasal cavity or nasopharynx.

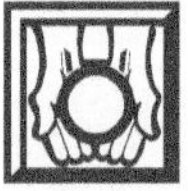

TREATMENT

APPROPRIATE HEALTH CARE

Removal of the inciting mucosal irritation, where/when possible, will result in relief from these reflexes.

NURSING CARE

Outpatient therapy generally indicated, except perhaps following rhinoscopic biopsy.

ACTIVITY

Exercise and activity should be restricted after rhinoscopic biopsies to prevent excessive bleeding.

DIET

N/A

CLIENT EDUCATION

- Educate clients so they understand these are normal reflexes. Diagnostic testing is required to determine the underlying cause and to allow appropriate treatment.
- Close contact with other animals should be limited until treatment for the underlying cause (if infectious) is completed.
- Episodes of paroxysmal reverse sneezing may be lessened by inducing swallowing (rubbing the throat, giving water) or breath holding (cover nose and mouth).

SURGICAL CONSIDERATIONS

- Anesthesia for surgery or endoscopy—abscessed tooth, foreign body, masses or anatomical airway abnormality, treatment of fungal infections.
- Use surgery for laryngeal disease with caution when gagging is prominent due to an increased risk of aspiration pneumonia when concurrent esophageal dysfunction is present.

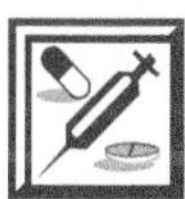

MEDICATIONS

DRUG(S) OF CHOICE

- There is no drug that specifically suppresses these reflexes; treatment is directed at the underlying irritant.
- Nasal bacterial infections best treated with antibiotics directed against Gram-positive bacteria (most common). Fungal disease treated with systemic and local infusion of antifungals.
- Nasal mites are treated with ivermectin 200–300 µg/kg PO or SC weekly for 3 weeks, selamectin 6–24 mg/kg applied topically every 2 weeks for 3 doses, or milbemycin (in collies and similar breeds) 0.5–1 mg/kg PO weekly for 3 weeks. All dogs in the household should be treated to prevent reinfection.
- When no underlying nasal condition is found to explain sneezing, nasal mite treatment is recommended. Immunomodulatory antibiotics such as doxycycline 5–10 mg/kg PO q12–24h and azathioprine 1–2 mg/kg/day PO in combination with piroxicam 0.3 mg/kg PO daily may be considered.
- Lower airway diseases with excess secretions are treated with antibiotics if bacterial infection is confirmed; Gram-negative bacteria are most common.
- Anti-inflammatory—prednisolone 1–2 mg/kg q12–24h or piroxicam 0.3 mg/kg PO q24–48h if no infection, for nonspecific airway inflammation.
- No treatment for gagging secondary to sensory loss in the larynx with recurring aspiration; elevation of food and water bowls is recommended. Altering the consistency of food offered may also be helpful.

CONTRAINDICATIONS

- Ivermectin in collies and similar breeds (*MDR1* gene mutation).
- Use of piroxicam concurrently with other nonsteroidal anti-inflammatory drugs or corticosteroids, as well as in patients with renal insufficiency.

PRECAUTIONS

The safety of most recommended drugs has not been established in pregnant animals.

POSSIBLE INTERACTIONS

N/A

ALTERNATIVE DRUG(S)

- Topical decongestants— 0.125% phenylephrine or 0.025% oxymetazoline.
- Antihistamines (diphenhydramine, Zyrtec, Claritin) may reduce secretions and sneezing in some cases with underlying allergic component.

FOLLOW-UP

PATIENT MONITORING

Expect reduction in sneezing/reverse sneezing with appropriate therapy.

PREVENTION/AVOIDANCE

Limit access to foreign bodies, provide adequate dental care and appropriate vaccination.

POSSIBLE COMPLICATIONS

If gagging is secondary to laryngeal sensory loss, serious aspiration pneumonia may develop.

EXPECTED COURSE AND PROGNOSIS

- Nasal mites should respond to treatment within 3 weeks.
- Sneezing and reverse sneezing secondary to foreign material resolve quickly after removal of the foreign body.
- Neoplasia may carry a poorer prognosis (chemotherapy or radiation therapy may be indicated).

MISCELLANEOUS

ASSOCIATED CONDITIONS

N/A

AGE-RELATED FACTORS

N/A

ZOONOTIC POTENTIAL

Rare; immunocompromised individuals at greater risk with infectious causes.

PREGNANCY/FERTILITY/BREEDING

N/A

SEE ALSO

- Nasal Discharge.
- Rhinitis and Sinusitis.

Suggested Reading

Demko JL, Cohn LA. Chronic nasal discharge in cats: 75 cases (1993–2004). J Am Vet Med Assoc 2007, 230:1032–1037.

Doust R, Sullivan M. Nasal discharge, sneezing and reverse sneezing. In: King LG, ed., Textbook of Respiratory Disease in Dogs and Cats. Philadelphia, PA: Saunders, 2004, pp. 17–29.

Kook P. Gagging. In: Ettinger SJ, Feldman EC, eds., Textbook of Veterinary Internal Medicine, 6th ed. St. Louis, MO: Saunders, 2005, pp. 152–155.

Lopez J. Sneezing and nasal discharge. In: Ettinger SJ, Feldman EC, eds., Textbook of Veterinary Internal Medicine, 6th ed. St. Louis, MO: Saunders, 2005, pp. 111–115.

Plickert HD, Tichy A, Hirt RA. Characteristics of canine nasal discharge related to intranasal diseases: a retrospective study of 105 cases. J Small Anim Pract 2014, 55:145–152.

Author Jonjo Reece

Consulting Editor Elizabeth Rozanski

Acknowledgment The author and editors acknowledge the prior contributions of Dominique Peeters and Brendan C. McKiernan.

Client Education Handout available online

SOFT TISSUE SARCOMA

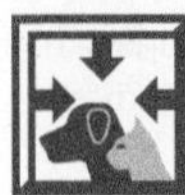

BASICS

DEFINITION

• A mesenchymal neoplasm arising within or from connective tissues. • Tumors in this heterogeneous group have different histologic origins yet demonstrate similar pathologic features and clinical behavior, and include fibrosarcoma, leiomyosarcoma, peripheral nerve sheath tumor, and myxosarcoma. Histology reports may commit only to soft tissue arcoma (STS) or spindle cell sarcoma, and may not distinguish among cell of origin without immunohistochemistry. • Because of divergent pathogenesis and biologic behavior, this group of tumors does not include hemangiosarcoma and other tumors that sometimes share the suffix (for example melanosarcoma, osteosarcoma, or lymphosarcoma). Histiocytic sarcoma is also considered separately.

PATHOPHYSIOLOGY

• Tumors can arise in connective tissues in any anatomic location. • Locally invasive behavior is typical with tumor extension beyond gross visible margins. • Tumors often have low (<20%, low grade/grades 1–2) to moderate (40–50%, high grade/grade 3) metastatic potential. • Tumors can develop at sites of chronic inflammation such as following ocular trauma or injection sites (cats). Also in vaccine-induced sarcomas in cats, the aluminum adjuvant may have inflammation-independent carcinogenic effects.

S

SYSTEMS AFFECTED

• Skin—most commonly arise from skin or subcutis. • Musculoskeletal—from muscle, fascial and fibrous tissues. • Nervous—originate from neurovascular structures. • Respiratory—STS metastasize hematogenously, with predilection for pulmonary metastases development in advance disease stages. • Lymphatic—regional lymph nodes are rare sites of metastasis.

GENETICS

There are no specific breed predilections that would suggest genetic predisposition.

INCIDENCE/PREVALENCE

• STS constitute 7% and 15% of skin and subcutaneous tumors in the cat and dog, respectively. • Incidence annually around 17 per 100,000 cats at risk; 35 per 100,000 dogs at risk.

SIGNALMENT

Species

All including the dog and cat.

Breed Predilections

None identified but large-breed dogs are often overrepresented.

Mean Age and Range

• Dogs—middle-aged, range 2–15 years. An exception is rhabdomyosarcoma of the bladder that often arises in younger dogs.
• Cats—middle-aged, range 1.4–18.8 years.

Predominant Sex

No predilection.

SIGNS

Historical Findings

• Rate of growth often reflects grade (low grade = slow-growing; high grade = rapid).
• Typically nonpainful, fluctuant to firm mass. • Signs depend on location and local structures affected by tumor presence or invasion. • Tumors arising in the abdomen may elicit signs due to compression of the gastrointestinal tract and could include vomiting and/or diarrhea, anorexia, and weight loss. Additionally signs of intestinal obstruction and occasionally perforation can occur with gastrointestinal leiomyosarcoma.
• Urinary signs of hematuria and dysuria may be seen in young dogs with bladder rhabdomyosarcoma. • Peripheral nerve sheath tumors affecting the brachial or lumbosacral plexus can cause signs of lameness and pain, muscle atrophy, limb weakness progressing to paralysis. • Signs of hypoglycemia (paraneoplastic) such as weakness, collapse, and seizures can occur with leiomyoma or leiomyosarcoma.

Physical Examination Findings

• Soft tissue mass that is soft, fluctuant, or firm on palpation. • Often adhered to underlying tissue. • Nonpainful unless ulcerated or invading into muscles or nerves.

CAUSES

• Dogs—STS have been documented following radiation therapy, trauma, orthopedic implants, foreign bodies, and the parasite *Spirocerca lupi* (esophageal sarcoma).
• Cats—See Pathophysiology.

RISK FACTORS

See Causes.

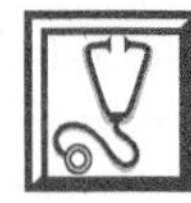

DIAGNOSIS

DIFFERENTIAL DIAGNOSIS

• Abscess. • Other cutaneous tumors, both benign and malignant (lipoma, basal cell tumors, mast cell tumors). • Fungal granuloma.

CBC/BIOCHEMISTRY/URINALYSIS

• Usually normal. • Hypoglycemia in dogs with leiomyoma or leiomyosarcoma (paraneoplastic syndrome mediated primarily by insulin-like growth factors produced by tumor).

OTHER LABORATORY TESTS

N/A

IMAGING

• Three-view thoracic radiographs are recommended before treatment as the lungs are the most likely site of metastasis for STS when it occurs. • Contrast CT or MRI can be used to determine extent of disease and to optimize treatment planning (surgery or radiation). • Abdominal ultrasound may be indicated for diagnosis of intra-abdominal STS and to allow assessment of liver, spleen, and abdominal lymph nodes.

DIAGNOSTIC PROCEDURES

• Fine-needle aspiration and cytology can rule out other differential diagnoses and may suggest a diagnosis but a nondiagnostic sample is possible as cells do not always exfoliate well. • Incisional biopsy and histopathology is essential to confirm diagnosis, determine grade of the tumor, and plan surgical approach. • Regional lymph node evaluation (cytology or histopathology) is indicated for assessment of enlarged regional lymph nodes and for high-grade tumors to evaluate for regional metastasis.

PATHOLOGIC FINDINGS

Dogs

• Over 20 different histopathologic subtypes of STS exist; biologic behavior is similar regardless of subtype. • Histologic grading based on differentiation, number of mitotic figures per 10 high power fields and percentage necrosis: ○ Grade I (low grade). ○ Grade II (intermediate grade). ○ Grade III (high grade) is the most biologically aggressive.

Cats

• Some similarities between histopathologic subtypes compared to dogs. Peripheral nerve sheath tumors are rare in cats. • Vaccine or injection site sarcomas have a more aggressive histologic appearance compared to other naturally occurring sarcomas.

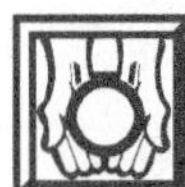

TREATMENT

CLIENT EDUCATION

A mass lesion with nondiagnostic and low cellularity cytology should be suspicious for a sarcoma. Postvaccination lumps in cats should be biopsied if they are growing larger within 1 month, are greater than 2 cm, or persist beyond 3 months after first appearing.

SURGICAL CONSIDERATIONS

• Early, aggressive, *en bloc* surgical excision is the treatment of choice. Conventional recommendations are 3 cm margins and 1 fascial plane deep (2 fascial planes deep for feline injection site sarcoma [FISS]). Even with complete excision, FISS can recur (30% or greater). • Do not place a drain through normal adjacent tissue during surgery if margins are uncertain. • Microscopically, cancer cells extend far beyond palpable tumor borders and recurrence is common if only macroscopic tumor is removed or peeled away from pseudocapsule. • Pseudocapsule composed of compressed cancer cells is common. • A second surgery (scar resection) can be performed prior to recurrence after incomplete excision to achieve more complete margins and decreased risk of recurrence. • After excision, tack mobile fascial layers in place and apply ink to surgical borders to thoroughly evaluate margins; submit the entire sample to a pathologist for surgical margin evaluation. Mark margins of greatest interest with suture or different color ink. • Toe or limb amputation may be necessary with large tumors that may be otherwise unresectable. • Rib resection or abdominal wall resection may be required for tumors of the trunk. • The first surgery usually provides the best opportunity for local tumor control. • Recurrent tumors will require different therapy rather than just repeating the same surgery (typically radiation therapy or a much larger surgery).

RADIATION THERAPY

Dogs

Radiation therapy can be used to treat microscopic disease (postoperatively with incomplete histologic margins, finely fractionated) or for measurable/unresectable disease (often hypofractionated).

Cats

Given the high rate of recurrence with feline injection site sarcoma, fractionated radiation therapy should be considered regardless of quality of margins, though outcomes after complete excision followed by radiation therapy are superior to those following incomplete excision and radiation therapy.

MEDICATIONS

DRUG(S) OF CHOICE

Dogs

• Doxorubicin-based chemotherapy can be used after excision of a high-grade (grade III) tumor, though a significant benefit has not been reported (1 mg/kg for small dogs or 30 mg/m^2 for medium and large dogs, IV, 5 doses q14–21 days). • Low-dosage (metronomic) cyclophosphamide chemotherapy 10–15 mg/m^2 PO q48h in combination with piroxicam 0.3 mg/kg PO q24–48h may help delay local recurrence when the tumor is incompletely resected.

Cats

• Role of postoperative chemotherapy in cats with STS is unclear. Chemotherapy treatment may improve local disease control but has minimal effect on survival in cats following wide surgical excision or radiation therapy (doxorubicin 1 mg/kg IV q3 weeks for 5 doses). • Toceranib has not been effective in treating FISS.

CONTRAINDICATIONS AND PRECAUTIONS

• Doxorubicin—cardiotoxic in dogs, avoid if underlying myocardial disease; nephrotoxic in cats, avoid if underlying renal disease; myelosuppressive in both species; severe vesicant, causes severe local tissue necrosis with extravasation (treat with dexrazoxane immediately). • Cyclophosphamide—can cause sterile hemorrhagic cystitis. Monitor for signs of hematuria and pollakuria; discontinue medication if this occurs. • Both drugs require adequate hepatobiliary function.

ALTERNATIVE DRUG(S)

Analgesia if needed.

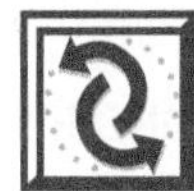

FOLLOW-UP

PATIENT MONITORING

Every 3 months for 1 year, then every 4–6 months thereafter: • Physical examination—local regrowth. • Thoracic radiographs—pulmonary metastasis.

PREVENTION/AVOIDANCE

N/A

POSSIBLE COMPLICATIONS

• Surgical complications including infection or incisional dehiscence. • Chemotherapy toxicity (see Contraindications and Precautions).

EXPECTED COURSE AND PROGNOSIS

• Strong prognostic factors—grade, especially mitotic index (recurrence, metastasis, survival time), size at surgery (>5 cm more likely to recur) and incomplete surgical margins (recurrence). • Low-grade STS of the distal extremities in dogs might have a low recurrence rate following surgical excision (<20%). • In dogs, cure is possible with low- and intermediate-grade STS with wide surgical resection, or surgery and adjuvant radiation therapy with median survival times of over 3 years. • The prognosis is more guarded and variable with high-grade tumors (7–24 months). • Cats with FISS treated with surgery and radiation therapy have median survival times of 2–3 years.

MISCELLANEOUS

PREGNANCY/FERTILITY/BREEDING

While receiving chemotherapy, dogs should not be bred.

SYNONYMS

Spindle cell tumor/sarcoma.

ABBREVIATIONS

• STS = soft tissue sarcoma.
• FISS = feline injection site sarcoma.

INTERNET RESOURCES

www.vetcancertrials.org

Suggested Reading

Ehrhart N. Soft-tissue sarcomas in dogs: a review. J Am Anim Hosp Assoc 2005, 41:241–246.

Kuntz CA, Dernell WS, Powers BE, et al. Prognostic factors for surgical treatment of soft tissue sarcomas in dogs: 75 cases (1986–1996). J Am Vet Med Assoc 1997, 211:1147–1151.

Muller N, Kessler M. Curative-intent radical en bloc resection using a minimum of a 3 cm margin in feline injection-site sarcomas: a retrospective analysis of 131 cases. J Feline Med Surg 2018, 20:509–519.

Author Kim A. Selting

Consulting Editor Timothy M. Fan

Acknowledgment The author and editors acknowledge the prior contributions of Laura E. Selmic and Shawna L. Klahn.

S

SPERMATOCELE/SPERM GRANULOMA

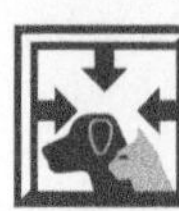

BASICS

OVERVIEW

• Spermatocele—a local, cystic distension of the efferent ductules or epididymis.
• Sperm granuloma—a chronic inflammatory reaction resulting from the immune response following sperm leakage from the efferent ductules or epididymal duct.

SIGNALMENT

Intact male dogs and cats.

SIGNS

• Sperm granuloma—oligozoospermia or azoospermia if obstruction exists.
• Spermatocele—cystic mass adjacent to the testicle, with or without discomfort.

CAUSES & RISK FACTORS

• Trauma to epididymal duct causing release of sperm antigens into the surrounding tissue.
• Epithelial hyperplasia of the epididymis as documented in dogs of increasing age.
• Congenital occlusion of epididymal duct.
• Complication of surgical vasectomy.

S

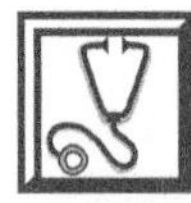

DIAGNOSIS

DIFFERENTIAL DIAGNOSIS

• Azoospermia—testicular degeneration, hypoplasia, retrograde ejaculation, incomplete ejaculation.
• Scrotal discomfort—epididymitis; orchitis; scrotal dermatitis.

CBC/BIOCHEMISTRY/URINALYSIS

• CBC and biochemistry profile—usually normal.
• Urinalysis (cystocentesis) after ejaculation—rule out retrograde ejaculation.

OTHER LABORATORY TESTS

• Assay for serum canine follicle-stimulating hormone (FSH) concentration—elevated with degeneration and hypoplasia; normal in azoospermic dogs experiencing retrograde ejaculation or bilateral epididymal blockage. Currently commercially unavailable.
• Alkaline phosphatase concentration of seminal plasma—concentration <5,000 U/L consistent with bilateral epididymal blockage or incomplete ejaculation (see Infertility, Male—Dogs).

IMAGING

Ultrasonography—useful to differentiate from other testicular or scrotal conditions.

DIAGNOSTIC PROCEDURES

Surgical testicular biopsy and excisional biopsy of affected epididymal tissue—allows visualization of epididymis, assess spermatogenesis (diagnostic for testicular degeneration); spermatoceles appear as yellow cysts within the epididymis.

PATHOLOGIC FINDINGS

Histologic examination of testicular biopsy—complete spermatogenesis in an azoospermic dog indicates blockage.

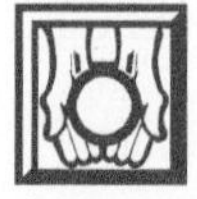

TREATMENT

Azoospermia rarely resolves if due to bilateral epididymal blockage; microsurgical anastomosis of the ductus deferens to the dilated epididymal tubule has been attempted.

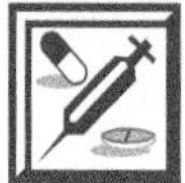

MEDICATIONS

DRUG(S) OF CHOICE

None described in the literature to unblock the duct system.

FOLLOW-UP

EXPECTED COURSE AND PROGNOSIS

• Unilateral sperm granuloma resulting in oligozoospermia—case-dependent; could be good to guarded for fertility depending on total sperm number and accuracy of breeding management (see Breeding, Timing).
• Bilateral sperm granuloma resulting in azoospermia—poor prognosis for fertility.

MISCELLANEOUS

SEE ALSO

• Breeding, Timing.
• Infertility, Male—Dogs.

ABBREVIATIONS

• FSH = follicle-stimulating hormone.

Suggested Reading

Althouse GC, Evans LE, Hopkins SM. Episodic scrotal mutilation with concurrent bilateral sperm granuloma in a dog. J Am Vet Med Assoc 1993, 202:776–778.

James RW, Heywood R. Age-related variations in the testes and prostate of beagle dogs. Toxicology 1979, 12(3):273–279.

Mayenco Aguirre AM, Garcia Fernandez P, Sanchez Muela M. Sperm granuloma in the dog: Complication of vasectomy. J Small Anim Pract 1996, 37:392–393.

Perez-Marin CC, Lopez R, Dominguez KM, Zafra R. Clinical and pathological findings in testis, epididymis, deferens duct and prostate following vasectomy in a dog. Reprod Domest Anim 2006, 41:169–174.

Author Candace C. Lyman

Consulting Editor Erin E. Runcan

Acknowledgment The author and editors acknowledge the prior contribution of Carlos R.F. Pinto.

Spermatozoal Abnormalities

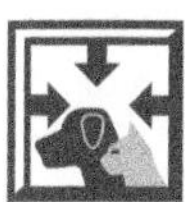

BASICS

OVERVIEW

• Teratozoospermia—sperm abnormalities of ≥40% in the ejaculate (i.e., low percentage of morphologically normal sperm).
• High percentage of sperm abnormalities may affect fertility.
• Some fertile cats inherently have ≥40% abnormalities.
• Sperm abnormalities may also be classified as primary (those occurring during spermatogenesis) or secondary (those occurring during epididymal storage and transport or from inappropriate semen handling).

SIGNALMENT

• Dogs and cats of any age; older dogs and cats more likely to have age-related conditions.
• No breed predilection.

SIGNS

• Persistent infertility after appropriately timed mating to several reproductively proven bitches.
• Abnormalities identified during semen evaluation.

CAUSES & RISK FACTORS

Congenital

• Canine fucosidosis—rare lysosomal storage disorder (α-l-fucosidase deficiency); acrosomal defects, proximal droplets, bent tails; autosomal recessive inheritance in English springer spaniels.
• Primary ciliary dyskinesia—ultrastructural abnormality of cilia causing absent or abnormal motility of ciliated cells; affected animals are infertile; probably autosomal recessive inheritance.
• Idiopathic.
• Testicular hypoplasia.
• Inbreeding.

Acquired

• Conditions disrupting normal testicular thermoregulation—trauma, hematocele, hydrocele, orchitis, epididymitis, fever, obesity (increased scrotal fat), high environmental temperatures, exercise-induced heat exhaustion.
• Infections of the reproductive tract.
• Overuse.
• Testicular neoplasia.
• Testicular degeneration.
• Prolonged sexual abstinence.
• Drugs—anabolic steroids, androgens, estrogen, progestogens, corticosteroids, ketoconazole, amphotericin B, cimetidine, phytoestrogen, gonadotropin-releasing hormone antagonists, intratesticular injections of zinc arginine.

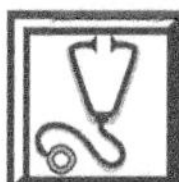

DIAGNOSIS

DIFFERENTIAL DIAGNOSIS

Excessive kinked or coiled tails may be iatrogenic, caused by morphology stain; reexamine the sample under phase contrast microscopy after dilution with formalin phosphate-buffered saline solution.

OTHER LABORATORY TESTS

• Hormonal profile—concentrations of gonadotropin and steroid hormones should be determined to rule out endocrinopathies.
• Azoospermic ejaculates—alkaline phosphatase concentration should be >5,000 U/L in complete ejaculates.
• Rapid slide agglutination test (brucellosis)—used as a screening test, recommend recheck of dogs with positive slide test with agar gel immunodiffusion test or other listed methods (see Brucellosis).

IMAGING

Ultrasonography—to visualize abnormalities in testes or scrotum that may promote abnormal spermatogenesis.

DIAGNOSTIC PROCEDURES

• Semen morphology (bright-field microscopy)—eosin–nigrosin stain or modified Giemsa stain; a minimum of 100 (preferably 200) sperm cells are counted under oil immersion (100× objective).
• Acrosome staining—acrosomal damage can be evaluated by Coomassie Brilliant blue staining or Spermac stain.
• Wet-mount semen morphology (phase contrast or differential interference contrast light microscopy)—samples diluted with formalin phosphate-buffered saline solution; verifies if presence of kinked or coiled tails on a stained slide is due to staining artifact.

PATHOLOGIC FINDINGS

• Biopsy—reveals spermatogenic capability of testicle; absence of spermatids or spermatocytes confirms impaired spermatogenesis.
• Inflammation—peritubular lymphocytic accumulation.
• Degenerative changes.
• Hypoplasia.
• Neoplasia.

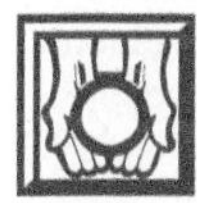

TREATMENT

• Unilateral orchiectomy for unilateral testicular tumors or severe orchitis.
• Sexual rest for edema or hematocele associated with trauma.
• If inciting cause was transient and has resolved, semen collection may "improve" individual ejaculate quality by depleting affected sperm cells.
• Adjust environment and avoid exercise/competitive events that may induce heat stress in the 2 months leading up to when optimal semen quality is needed for breeding or processing.

MEDICATIONS

CONTRAINDICATIONS

• Exogenous hormones—anabolic steroids, estrogens, testosterone, progestagens.
• Ketoconazole, amphotericin B.
• Chemotherapeutic agents.
• Glucocorticoids.
• Cimetidine.

FOLLOW-UP

PATIENT MONITORING

• In cases from reversible causes, a complete improvement in sperm morphology will not occur before 70 days (approximate length of a complete spermatogenic cycle).
• After an underlying cause is identified and treated, a semen evaluation performed at 70 days will provide an indication as to long-term expectations for semen quality.

PREVENTION/AVOIDANCE

• Climate-controlled environment for animals not adapted to high environmental temperatures.
• Avoid heat exhaustion during exercise or grooming.

MISCELLANEOUS

Suggested Reading

Kolster KA. Evaluation of canine sperm and management of semen disorders. Vet Clin North Am Small Anim Pract 2018, 48(4):533–545.

Author Candace C. Lyman
Consulting Editor Erin E. Runcan
Acknowledgment The author and editors acknowledge the prior contribution of Carlos R.F. Pinto.

SPIDER VENOM TOXICOSIS—BLACK WIDOW

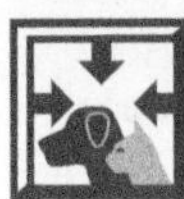

BASICS

OVERVIEW

• Black widow spider (*Latrodectus* spp.)—four species indigenous to the United States (*L. mactans*, *L. geometricus*, *L. hesperus*, *L. variolus*); females toxic; 2–2.5 cm in length; shiny black; red or orange hourglass mark on the ventral abdomen; immature female brown with red to orange stripes that change into the hourglass shape as she darkens to black and ages.
• Bites—15% may be dry (no venom injected).
• Range—genus found in every state except Alaska; often found around buildings and human habitation.
• Venom—contains α-latrotoxin, a potent presynaptic neurotoxin; opens cation-selective channels at the nerve terminal; causes massive release of acetylcholine and norepinephrine, which causes sustained muscular spasms. Two classes of receptors for α-latrotoxin: the neurexins, which are brain-specific cell adhesion molecules binding in a Ca^{2+}-dependent manner, and latrophilins (and CIRLs), which are not brain specific, expressed in many tissues, and bind α-latrotoxin independent of Ca^{2+}.

SIGNALMENT

Dogs and cats.

SIGNS

Historical Findings

• Usually sudden onset.
• May be delayed several days with mild envenomation.

Physical Examination Findings

Dogs

• Severe pain is the primary clinical sign.
• Progressive muscle fasciculations.
• Cramping of large muscle masses.
• Abdominal rigidity without tenderness.
• Marked restlessness, writhing, and contorted spasms.
• Hypertension and tachycardia anticipated.
• May note bronchorrhea, hypersalivation, hyperesthesia, lymph node tenderness, regional numbness, facial swelling and spasm (referred to as *Latrodectus* facies).
• Rhabdomyolysis possible.

Cats

• Early, marked paralysis.
• Severe pain—manifested by howling and loud vocalizations.
• Excessive salivation and restlessness.
• Vomiting—not unusual to vomit up the spider.
• Diarrhea.
• Muscle tremors and cramping.
• Ataxia and inability to stand—becomes adynamic and atonic.
• Respiratory collapse.
• Death without antivenin.

CAUSES & RISK FACTORS

• Very young or old age—increased risk.
• Systemic hypertension—increased risk.

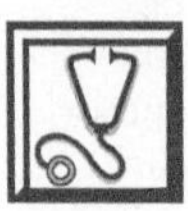

DIAGNOSIS

DIFFERENTIAL DIAGNOSIS

• Intervertebral disc disease.
• Acute abdomen.

CBC/BIOCHEMISTRY/URINALYSIS

• Leukocytosis.
• High creatine kinase—with severe muscle spasms.
• Albuminuria.

OTHER LABORATORY TESTS

Normal hemoccult test.

DIAGNOSTIC PROCEDURES

N/A

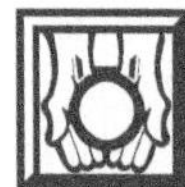

TREATMENT

• Inpatient—supportive care.
• Monitor respiratory status.

MEDICATIONS

DRUG(S) OF CHOICE

• Antivenin (Lyovac [*Latrodectus*], equine origin—Merck) 1 vial mixed with 100 mL crystalloid solution IV given slowly with monitoring of the inner ear pinna for evidence of hyperemia (indicator of allergic response); this dose is usually sufficient for response within 30 minutes; with proper use, reactions are rare. Variable availability. If allergic reaction occurs—stop antivenin; administer diphenhydramine; after 5–10 minutes, restart antivenin at a slower rate.
• New antivenin (Aracmyn; Instituto Bioclon, Mexico—managed by Rare Disease Therapeutics in the United States) has completed human phase III clinical trials but not yet approved for human use. It is an equine origin Fab2 product and should be much less likely to trigger an allergic response.
• There are multiple latrodectus antivenoms worldwide which have crossreactivity with black widow spider venom, including Australian red back spider antivenom (Commonwealth Serum Laboratories), South Africa (SAFR) brown widow antivenom, and the Yugoslavian widow spider antivenom.
• Studies suggest benzodiazepines are more effective than muscle relaxants for treatment of muscle pain related to black widow spider envenomation.
• Muscle spasms and severe pain are controlled by careful IV administration of narcotics or benzodiazepines at lowest effective dosage to avoid respiratory depression; methocarbamol relieves muscle spasms but has no effect on hypertension or respiratory depression.
• Intractable hypertension—sodium nitroprusside.

CONTRAINDICATIONS/POSSIBLE INTERACTIONS

IV fluids with hypertension.

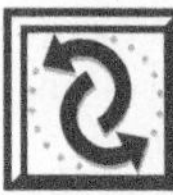

FOLLOW-UP

• Weekly monitoring of the wound site until healed.
• Prognosis—uncertain for days; cats, usually fatal without antivenin.
• Weakness, fatigue, and insomnia—may persist for months.

MISCELLANEOUS

Suggested Reading

Peterson ME. Spider envenomation: black widow. In: Peterson ME, Talcott PA, eds., Small Animal Toxicology, 3rd ed. St. Louis, MO: Saunders, 2013, pp. 817–821.

Author Michael E. Peterson
Consulting Editor Lynn R. Hovda

SPIDER VENOM TOXICOSIS—BROWN RECLUSE

BASICS

OVERVIEW

- Brown recluse family—*Loxosceles* spp. (11 species indigenous to United States); 8–15 mm in body size; legs 2–3 cm long; violin-shaped pattern on cephalothorax with the neck of the fiddle extending caudally; 6 eyes (3 paired diads) as opposed to other spider species with 8 eyes; active at night.
- Distribution—found throughout the Midwest from the Gulf Coast of the United States and up the Mississippi River valley to southern Iowa. Some species are found in eastern southern California, western Arizona, and southern New Mexico.
- 60% of "brown recluse" spider bites in humans are misdiagnosed as they occur in areas with no endemic spider populations. See extensive Differential Diagnosis.
- Bites usually occur when spider becomes trapped in bedding; induce, necrotic arachnidism, an indolent dermatonecrotic lesion mediated by the venom enzyme sphingomyelinase D, direct hemolysis of erythrocytes, platelet aggregation, renal failure, coagulopathy, and death.
- Currently no consensus on treatment and multiple therapies have been used, including antihistamines, corticosteroids, dapsone, hyperbaric oxygen, surgical excision, and antivenom.
- Antivenom currently unavailable in United States (available only in Argentina, Brazil, and Mexico).

SIGNALMENT

Dogs and cats.

SIGNS

- Clinical signs are not completely defined in canine and feline envenomations.
- In humans:
  - Local pain and stinging (may last 6–8 hours); followed by pruritus and soreness.
  - Classic target lesion—ischemic area with a dark central eschar on an uneven erythematous background; after 2–5 weeks, central eschar may slough, leaving a deep, nonhealing ulcer that usually spares muscle tissue.
  - Not all skin lesions develop necrosis.
  - Less common—hemolytic anemia with hemoglobinuria in the first 24 hours; secondary renal complications.
  - Skin lesion severity and hemolysis are not linked.
  - Other possible systemic manifestations within the first 2–3 days after envenomation: fever; chills; rash; weakness; leukocytosis; nausea; arthralgia.
  - Envenomations to fatty areas develop more significant lesions; those occurring in loose tissue more likely to be edematous.

CAUSES & RISK FACTORS

Brown recluse spider bite (genus *Loxosceles*).

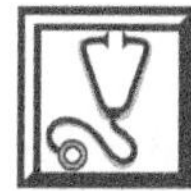

DIAGNOSIS

- Brown recluse spider bite is frequently misdiagnosed in regions of the country that do not have endemic populations of the spider.
- Epidemiologic history of bite including site of lesion, progression timeline of signs, and visualization of small puncta assist with diagnosis.

DIFFERENTIAL DIAGNOSIS

- Bacterial or mycobacterial infection; methicillin-resistant *Staphylococcus aureus* by a large margin in humans.
- Decubitus ulcer.
- Third-degree burn.
- Hemolytic anemia.
- Jaundice.
- Necrotizing vasculitis.
- Thrombocytopenia.
- Ehrlichiosis.
- Red blood cell parasitism.
- Vascular occlusive/venous disease.

CBC/BIOCHEMISTRY/URINALYSIS

- Anemia.
- Leukocytosis.
- Thrombocytopenia.
- Hemoglobinuria.

OTHER LABORATORY TESTS

- BUN and creatinine.
- Coagulation profile—may reveal prolonged clotting times.

DIAGNOSTIC PROCEDURES

N/A

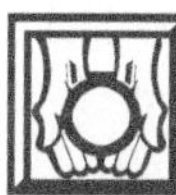

TREATMENT

- Routine wound care—may need aggressive supportive care.
- Supportive care—may include fluid therapy; secondary infections are infrequent; blood transfusion (rarely).
- Mild, local envenomation—usually responds to cool compresses as sphingomyelinase D activity is temperature dependent.
- Necrotic lesions—may need debridement after erythema has subsided.
- Severe envenomation—may require skin grafting after the lesion reaches full maturity.

MEDICATIONS

DRUG(S) OF CHOICE

- Tetracycline can be applied topically as a matrix metalloproteinase inhibitor.
- Hyperbaric oxygen—some evidence indicates that hyperbaric oxygen treatment may be beneficial for reducing size of the skin lesion.
- Dapsone—mixed results in various studies; 1 mg/kg q8h orally for 10 days; for dermatonecrotic lesions; leukocyte inhibitor; proposed to minimize inflammatory component of envenomation; repeat if needed. Efficacy against brown recluse envenomation has not been studied in the dog and cat.

CONTRAINDICATIONS/POSSIBLE INTERACTIONS

- Do not use heat—exacerbates condition.
- Dapsone—may cause hypersensitivity and methemoglobinemia in patients with glucose-6-phosphate dehydrogenase deficiency.
- Early surgical excision may cause larger defect than supportive care alone.
- Antihistamines, colchicine, anticoagulants, topical nitroglycerine, high doses of vitamin C, electric shock, and steroids have been proposed for treatments, but subsequently have been demonstrated to be ineffective.

FOLLOW-UP

Monitor wound site weekly until healed.

MISCELLANEOUS

Suggested Reading

Peterson ME. Spider envenomation: brown recluse. In: Peterson ME, Talcott PA, eds., Small Animal Toxicology, 3rd ed. St. Louis, MO: Saunders, 2013, pp. 823–826.

Swanson DL, Vetter RS. Bites of brown recluse spiders and suspected necrotic arachnidism. N Engl J Med 2005, 352:700–707.

Author Michael E. Peterson

Consulting Editor Lynn R. Hovda

SPINAL DYSRAPHISM

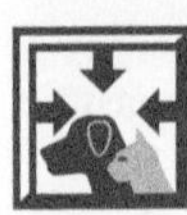

BASICS

OVERVIEW

- Abnormal development of the embryonic spinal cord along the dorsal plane leading to a variety of structural anomalies (e.g., spina bifida, hydromyelia, duplicated or absent central canal, syringomyelia, aberrations in the dorsal median septum and ventral medial fissure, tethered cord).
- Thoracic and lumbar spinal segments most commonly affected.
- 'Dysraphism' suggests an abnormality in closure of the neural tube; the term 'myelodysplasia' (not to be confused with myelodysplastic syndrome) may be preferable when discussing anomalies with alternate pathogenesis.

SIGNALMENT

Nonprogressive

- Dog and cat.
- Reported in Rhodesian ridgeback, Weimaraner, English bulldog, pug, boxer, Victorian bulldog, golden retriever, Rottweiler, shih tzu, boerboel, chow chow, Siberian husky, English springer spaniel, Yorkshire terrier, Pyrenees mountain dog, Chinese crested dog, Swedish vallhund, and English cocker spaniel, Samoyed, Dalmatian, English setter; Manx cat, Burmese cat.
- Hereditary in the Weimaraner.
- Manx cat and brachycephalic breeds overrepresented, especially screw-tailed individuals.
- No sex predilection.
- Signs apparent by 3–6 weeks of age and become more obvious as animal matures. In mild cases, patient may not be presented for evaluation until several months of age.

Progressive

- Adult cavalier King Charles spaniels with syringomyelia resulting from occipital bone malformation (Chiari-like malformation; caudal occipital malformation syndrome [COMS]).
- Described in an adult Pomeranian with cervical syringomyelia and hydrocephalus.
- Described in an adult fox terrier with progressive paresis in the left pelvic limb, a 1-year-old English cocker spaniel with a 9 months history of progressive paresis in the right pelvic limb.

SIGNS

Vary in severity. Normal neurologic examination does not rule out spinal dysraphism.

Dogs

- Associated physical exam findings include indentation of the epaxial muscles, abnormal hair streams in the dorsal cervical area (a desired trait in the Rhodesian ridgeback), kinking of the undocked tail, scoliosis, and koilosternia (depression of the sternum).
- In the Weimaraner, gait is characterized by simultaneous flexion and extension of pelvic limbs (bunny hopping). Proprioceptive deficits, base wide stance, and crouched pelvic limb posture are also often present.
- In animals with syringomyelia (e.g., cavalier King Charles spaniel with COMS), any combination of neck or head pain, progressive forelimb weakness, paraparesis, imbalance, paroxysmal involuntary flank or neck scratching may be present.

Cats

In affected Manx cats, pelvic limb paresis or paralysis, urinary and fecal retention, abnormal or absent caudal vertebrae, and structural abnormalities in the sacrum may be present.

CAUSES & RISK FACTORS

- Missense mutation in the *NKX2-8* gene in the Weimaraner. Homozygous condition lethal; heterozygotes clinically affected.
- Autosomal dominant trait controlling number and structure of caudal vertebrae in the Manx cat. Prevalence increased by breeding for absence of tail.
- *In utero* spinal cord damage caused by infection, trauma, vascular compromise, drugs (antifungals, chemotherapeutics).
- Idiopathic in isolated patients.
- Syringomyelia may be acquired as result of infection, trauma, or neoplasia.

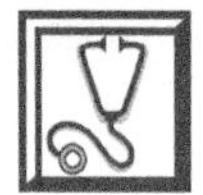

DIAGNOSIS

DIFFERENTIAL DIAGNOSIS

Intervertebral disc disease, myelitis, arachnoid cysts, and neoplasia must be differentiated from progressive causes of syringomyelia.

CBC/BIOCHEMISTRY/URINALYSIS

Usually normal.

IMAGING

- Spinal radiographs may show concurrent vertebral column anomalies and spinal cord compression in some patients.
- In patients with COMS, defects in the occipital bone may be appreciated on skull radiographs.
- MRI is necessary for definitive diagnosis of syringomyelia. Imaging shows attenuation of fourth ventricle, overcrowding of brainstem in caudal fossa, and cerebellar vermal herniation (COMS, Chiari-like malformation). Hydrocephalus may also be evident.
- One report of tethered cord in an English cocker spaniel in which conus medullaris was visibly caudodorsally displaced.
- CT reveals hydrocephalus, if present, with COMS.
- Without sophisticated imaging techniques, an antemortem diagnosis may be impossible except in Weimaraner and Manx cat.

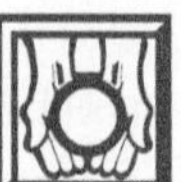

TREATMENT

- Mildly affected animals may be acceptable pets.
- Severely affected, nonsurgical animals may benefit from a canine cart; consider euthanasia.
- Surgical options include foramen magnum remodeling (with occipital malformation) or ventriculoperitoneal shunt placement; laminectomy, ± syringo-subarachnoid shunting. These procedures may reduce pain or lead to improvement in neurologic signs. However, sensory disturbances such as scratching infrequently resolve, and recurrence is possible.

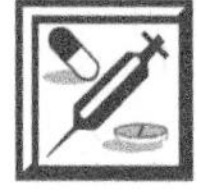

MEDICATIONS

DRUG(S) OF CHOICE

- Antibiotics—for urinary tract infection. Treat based on culture and sensitivity of urine.
- Corticosteroids—to improve signs in COMS by reducing CSF production and edema formation. Prednisone 0.25–0.5 mg/kg q12h or dexamethasone 0.025–0.05 mg/kg PO q12h; taper to alternate-day prednisone or twice-weekly dexamethasone.
- Carbonic anhydrase inhibitors—may alleviate signs in COMS by decreasing CSF production and allow for a reduction of steroid dosage. Acetazolamide 3.5–7.5 mg/kg q8–12h, methazolamide 5 mg/kg q8–12h, or furosemide 5 mg/kg PO, IM, SC q12h.
- Omeprazole—decreases CSF production and may alleviate signs in COMS and allow for a reduction of steroid dosage. Clinical data on use and effectiveness currently lacking; 0.5–1 mg/kg PO q24h.
- Gabapentin—recommended for management of neuropathic pain; 10 mg/kg q8–12h or pregabalin (Lyrica) 4 mg/kg PO q12h.
- Nonsteroidal anti-inflammatory drugs (NSAIDs)—may help manage neuropathic pain. Meloxicam (Metacam) 0.2 mg/kg once then 0.1 mg/kg q24h in dogs; carprofen (Rimadyl) 2.2 mg/kg PO q12h or 4.4 mg/kg PO q24h in dogs.

CONTRAINDICATIONS/POSSIBLE INTERACTIONS

- Avoid prolonged administration of NSAIDs, simultaneous use of of NSAIDs and acetaminophen, simultaneous use of NSAIDs and steroids, use of NSAIDs in patients with gastrointestinal or renal disease. Doing so

decreases risk of gastrointestinal ulceration and renal pathology.
- Do not use NSAIDs in cats.

FOLLOW-UP

PATIENT MONITORING

- Disorders of micturition predispose patients to secondary urinary tract infection.
- Avoid decubitus ulcers and urine and fecal scalds by properly caring for recumbent patients.

PREVENTION/AVOIDANCE

- Discourage breeding for absence of tail in Manx cats.
- Do not breed Weimaraners that have produced affected puppies (codominant inheritance).

MISCELLANEOUS

ASSOCIATED CONDITIONS

Congenital vertebral arch (e.g., spina bifida) and vertebral body–disc malformation (e.g., hemivertebra and block vertebra). These conditions alone often do not cause clinical signs.

ABBREVIATIONS

- COMS = caudal occipital malformation syndrome.
- CSF = cerebrospinal fluid.
- CT= computed tomography
- MRI = magnetic resonance imaging
- NSAID = nonsteroidal anti-inflammatory drug.

SEE ALSO

Syringomyelia and Chiari-Like Malformation

Suggested Reading

Westworth DR, Sturges BK. Congenital spinal malformations in small animals. Vet Clin North Am Small Anim Pract 2010, 40(5):951–981.

Authors Richard J. Joseph and Anne E. Buglione

S

SPLENIC TORSION

BASICS

OVERVIEW

- May occur as a separate entity or in association with gastric dilatation and volvulus (GDV) syndrome.
- Acute or chronic.
- Pathophysiology—unknown.
- Systems affected—hemic/lymphatic/immune and cardiovascular.
- Isolated splenic torsion uncommon.

SIGNALMENT

- More common in large-breed, deep-chested dogs, such as the German shepherd dog and Great Dane. English bulldogs are also predisposed.
- No sex predilection.

SIGNS

Historical Findings

- Acute—cardiovascular collapse and abdominal pain.
- Chronic—intermittent anorexia, vomiting, weight loss, and possibly hemoglobinuria.

Physical Examination Findings

- Pale mucous membranes, tachycardia, weak femoral pulses, other signs of hypoperfusion.
- Palpable abdominal mass (spleen).
- Irregular heart rate or dropped pulses if arrhythmias present.

S

CAUSES & RISK FACTORS

- Large-breed and deep-chested dogs.
- Prior stretching of gastrosplenic, phrenicosplenic, and splenocolic ligaments (e.g., prior GDV).
- Historical gastric dilatation.
- Excessive exercise, rolling, and retching may contribute.
- Nervousness and anxiety have been associated with an increased risk of GDV but not of isolated splenic torsion.

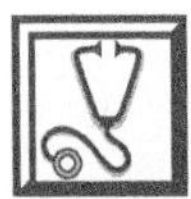

DIAGNOSIS

DIFFERENTIAL DIAGNOSIS

- Other splenic disease (e.g., neoplasia, thrombosis, immune-mediated disease).
- Acute gastrointestinal disease with abdominal pain (acute abdomen).

CBC/BIOCHEMISTRY/URINALYSIS

- Anemia.
- Thrombocytopenia.
- Leukocytosis.
- Elevated liver enzyme activities.
- Pigmenturia/hemoglobinuria.

OTHER LABORATORY TESTS

Coagulation testing—prolongation of activated partial thromboplastin time (aPTT) or both prothrombin time (PT) and aPTT, with thrombocytopenia may indicate disseminated intravascular coagulation (DIC).

IMAGING

Abdominal Radiography

- Cranial or midabdominal mass may be seen.
- Spleen may be abnormally located.

Abdominal Ultrasonography

- Splenic congestion/lack of blood flow to spleen.
- Dilated splenic veins.
- Splenic infarction.

DIAGNOSTIC PROCEDURES

Electrocardiogram (ECG)—may show ventricular arrhythmias.

PATHOLOGIC FINDINGS

Splenic congestion and infarction.

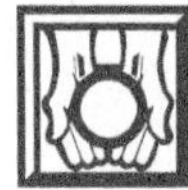

TREATMENT

- Surgical emergency.
- After adequate cardiovascular stabilization, a splenectomy should be performed *without* untwisting the splenic pedicle.
- A permanent gastropexy should also be performed because of the association with GDV syndrome.
- A representative splenic specimen should be submitted for histopathologic examination.
- IV fluid support and cardiovascular monitoring are indicated after splenectomy.

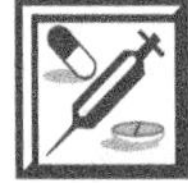

MEDICATIONS

DRUG(S) OF CHOICE

- No specific drugs required.
- Postoperative pain relief advised.
- Plasma transfusion may be considered if DIC or coagulopathy are present.
- Antiarrhythmic drugs (e.g., lidocaine) may be indicated in the perioperative period.

CONTRAINDICATIONS/POSSIBLE INTERACTIONS

None

FOLLOW-UP

Surgical correction considered curative. Prognosis is good; mortality has been associated with preexisting septic peritonitis, hemorrhage or postoperative development of respiratory distress.

MISCELLANEOUS

SEE ALSO

- Acute Abdomen.
- Disseminated Intravascular Coagulation.
- Gastric Dilation and Volvulus Syndrome.

ABBREVIATIONS

- aPTT = activated partial thromboplastin time.
- DIC = disseminated intravascular coagulation.
- ECG = electrocardiogram.
- GDV = gastric dilation and volvulus.
- PT = prothrombin time.

Suggested Reading

DeGroot W, Giuffrida MA, Rubin J et al. Primary splenic torsion in dogs: 102 cases (1992–2014). J Am Vet Med Assoc 2016, 248(6):661–668.

Author Elizabeth Rozanski
Consulting Editor Melinda S. Camus

BASICS

DEFINITION

Enlargement of the spleen; characterized as either diffuse, focal, or nodular.

PATHOPHYSIOLOGY

• Splenic functions—removal of senescent and abnormal erythrocytes; filtration and phagocytosis of antigenic particles such as microorganisms, degraded cellular material, macromolecules; production of lymphocytes and plasma cells; antibody production, reservoir for erythrocytes and platelets; iron metabolism and storage, hematopoiesis, as required. • Many disorders affect function of spleen.

Diffuse Splenomegaly

Four General Pathologic Mechanisms

• Inflammation (splenitis)—associated with infectious agents; classified according to cell type (e.g., suppurative, necrotizing, eosinophilic, lymphoplasmacytic, and granulomatous-pyogranulomatous). • Lymphoreticular hyperplasia—increased proliferation of mononuclear phagocytes and lymphoid elements (in response to antigens); accelerated erythrocyte destruction. • Congestion—associated with impaired venous drainage. • Infiltration—involves cellular invasion of the spleen or deposition of abnormal substances.

Focal or Nodular lesions

Associated with neoplastic (benign or malignant) or non-neoplastic disorders (infection, hyperplasia/regeneration, or inflammation).

SYSTEMS AFFECTED

Disorders of the spleen may also be associated with changes in the liver and lymph nodes.

SIGNALMENT

• Dog and cat; certain conditions maybe more prevalent in specific breeds or sizes of dog. • Splenic torsion—overrepresented in large, deep-chested breeds (e.g., German shepherd dog, Great Dane). • Hemangiosarcoma—middle-aged dogs; large breeds; predilection in German shepherd dog, golden retriever, Labrador retriever, and boxer. • Prominent spleen—may be normal in certain breeds (German shepherd dog).

SIGNS

General Comments

• Splenic enlargement—often nonspecific. • Frequently reflects an underlying disorder rather than primary disease of the spleen.

Historical Findings

• Vomiting, diarrhea, anorexia—can be seen with infiltrative diseases such as lymphoma, mast cell tumor, feline infectious peritonitis (FIP), lymphoplasmacytic enteritis (cats). • Lethargy, anorexia, vomiting, vague abdominal pain (in acute cases pain can be severe), mild to moderate abdominal distention in deep-chested large to giant-breed dogs (Great Dane, German shepherd dog overrepresented)—associated with splenic torsion (with or without concurrent gastric dilatation and volvulus [GDV]). • Weakness, lethargy, collapse (can be episodic), abdominal distention—can indicate a hemoabdomen secondary to bleeding/ruptured splenic tumor (hemangiosarcoma most common) or benign conditions such as a hematoma.

Physical Examination Findings

• Prominent spleen on abdominal palpation or cranial/mid-abdominal mass; nonpalpable spleen does not preclude splenomegaly. • Dogs—smooth or irregular surface. • Cats—usually diffuse, uniform enlargement. • Pallor, poor capillary refill time, poor peripheral pulses and tachycardia if splenic hemorrhage or splenic torsion. • Abdominal distention if massive splenomegaly or splenic rupture (effusion). • Petechia and ecchymosis if coagulopathy secondary to primary splenic disorder or underlying disease. • Concurrent hepatomegaly, thickened intestines, and/or mesenteric lymphadenopathy imply infiltrative (neoplastic) or inflammatory (immune-mediated or infectious) disease. • Peripheral lymphadenomegaly—suggests lymphoma/leukemia or histiocytic sarcoma. • Cardiac arrhythmias—can be seen with primary cardiac disease affecting the spleen (congestion) or can be associated with primary splenic disorders.

CAUSES

Dogs

Inflammation (Splenitis)

• Inflammatory cell type can help prioritize differentials. • Suppurative (neutrophilic)—bacterial infections associated with penetrating abdominal wound; migrating foreign body; endocarditis; sepsis; infectious complication of splenic torsion. • Necrotizing—most commonly associated with anaerobic infections (often secondary to splenic torsion), or neoplasia. • Eosinophilic—eosinophilic gastroenteritis, hypereosinophilic syndrome. • Lymphoplasmacytic—subacute or chronic infectious disorders; pyometra; coexistent inflammatory bowel disease. • Granulomatous—fungal or protozoal disease most common. • Pyogranulomatous—bacterial or fungal infections most common cause.

Hyperplasia

• Infection—chronic bacteremia (bacterial endocarditis; discospondylitis; *Brucella*). • Immune-mediated disease—any; hemolytic anemia or thrombocytopenia, systemic lupus erythematosus (SLE).

Congestion

Tranquilizers; barbiturates; portal hypertension; right-sided heart failure; splenic torsion.

Infiltration

• Neoplasia—lymphoma; acute and chronic leukemia; (hemophagocytic) histiocytic sarcoma; multiple myeloma; systemic mastocytosis; hemangiosarcoma, other sarcoma; metastasis. • Extramedullary hematopoiesis (EMH)—immune-mediated hemolytic anemia or thrombocytopenia; chronic anemia; infectious disease; malignancy; SLE. • Amyloidosis – part of systemic amyloidosis.

Cats

Inflammation

• Suppurative—penetrating wound or migrating foreign body; septicemia; salmonellosis. • Necrotizing—salmonellosis. • Eosinophilic—hypereosinophilic syndrome. • Lymphoplasmacytic—lymphoplasmacytic enteritis; hemotropic mycoplasmas; pyometra. • Granulomatous—histoplasmosis; mycobacteriosis. • Pyogranulomatous—FIP, *Mycobacterium*.

Hyperplasia

• Infection—hemotropic mycoplasmosis. • Immune-mediated—any; hemolytic disorders, SLE.

Congestion

Portal hypertension, congestive heart failure.

Infiltration

• Neoplasia—mast cell tumor, lymphoma; lympho- or myeloproliferative diseases; multiple myeloma; histiocytic sarcoma (rare); hemangiosarcoma (rare). • Non-neoplastic—amyloidosis, EMH.

RISK FACTORS

• Cats—feline leukemia virus (FeLV), FIP. • Dogs—breed/age.

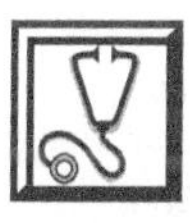

DIAGNOSIS

DIFFERENTIAL DIAGNOSIS

Other cranial organomegaly or masses.

CBC/BIOCHEMISTRY/URINALYSIS

Dogs

• Regenerative anemia secondary to splenic bleeding or hemolytic disease. • Nucleated red blood cells (RBCs)—may accompany EMH, indicates splenic dysfunction. • Spherocytes—hemolysis, microangiopathic shearing. • Schizocytes (aka schistocytes) – disseminated intravascular coagulation (DIC), hemangiosarcoma. • Acanthocytes- hemangiosarcoma. • Leukocytosis with a left shift—may indicate infectious or inflammatory conditions, marked regenerative response, or EMH. • Thrombocytopenia—from increased consumption (DIC or bleeding) secondary to hemangiosarcoma or other neoplasia, increased destruction (immune-mediated), sequestration, or decreased production in the bone marrow. • Hypercalcemia may be associated with neoplasia, especially lymphoma. • Hyperglobulinemia may be associated with neoplasia, *Ehrlichia* infections. • Hemoglobinemia and hyperbilirubinemia—associated with hemolysis and may occur with microangiopathic anemia, splenic torsion, hemangiosarcoma, and immune-mediated anemia.

Cats

- Direct RBC examination for hemoparasites.
- Regenerative anemia and splenomegaly—may indicate hemotropic mycoplasmosis.
- Macrocytosis and nonregenerative anemia—suggests retroviral infection or myeloproliferative disease. • Eosinophilia—suggests hypereosinophilic syndrome, systemic mastocytosis, or lymphoma. • Circulating blast cells—suggest lympho- or myeloproliferative disorder. • Nucleated RBCs—may accompany EMH and splenic dysfunction. • Thrombocytopenia—from increased consumption (DIC), increased destruction (immune-mediated), sequestration, or decreased production in the bone marrow.

OTHER LABORATORY TESTS

- FeLV and feline immunodeficiency virus testing. • Coagulation panel—DIC commonly seen with hemangiosarcoma (includes prolonged clotting times, hypofibrinogenemia, and increased fibrin degradation products [FDPs]); D-dimers not specific for clinical application in differential diagnoses).

IMAGING

Abdominal Radiography

- Confirms or detects splenomegaly. • Mass effect may appear in the (left) midcranial abdomen. • May provide evidence of an underlying cause—concurrent hepatomegaly may indicate infiltrative disease or right-sided heart disease; splenic torsion secondary to GDV.
- Effusion—may indicate hemorrhage from splenic rupture (hemangiosarcoma, hematoma) or portal hypertension influencing splenic perfusion. • Visualization of the splenic tail along the ventral body wall on lateral radiographs of cats supports the diagnosis of splenomegaly.

Thoracic Radiography

- Three views (right and left lateral and dorsal–ventral views)—screen for metastasis and underlying disease in thoracic cavity and effusion. • Evaluate sternal lymph nodes—these drain the abdominal cavity, reflecting disorders causing lymphadenomegaly. Evaluate for signs of congestive heart failure (size of the cardiac silhouette and pulmonary veins and evidence of pulmonary edema or pleural effusion).

Abdominal Ultrasonography

- Distinguishes between diffuse and focal/nodular parenchymal patterns. • Diffuse enlargement with normal parenchyma—may occur with congestion or cellular infiltration.
- In cats splenic masses greater than 1 cm suggestive of malignancy. • Hypoechogenicity may occur with splenic torsion, splenic vein thrombosis, hematopoietic neoplasia or infectious agents. • Complex, mixed echogenic mass—common with hemangiosarcoma or hematoma. • Can identify concurrent abdominal diseases—liver, kidneys, intestines, and lymph nodes.
- Cannot differentiate between benign and malignant splenic disorders. • Doppler color flow interrogation of splenic vasculature may detect splenic vein thrombi or splenic torsion.

Echocardiography

Evaluate for cardiac dysfunction or cardiac tumors causing splenic congestion (based on other physical exam/imaging findings).

DIAGNOSTIC PROCEDURES

Fine-Needle Aspiration

- Assess coagulation status before any aspiration. Procedure—patient in right lateral or dorsal recumbency; using ultrasound guidance, use a 22- or smaller gauge, 2.5–3.75 cm (1–1.5 in.) length needle depending on the size of the patient. • Non-aspiration method (needle-only method) results in higher yield of nucleated cells relative to the amount of blood than aspiration method. • Specimens—evaluate cytologically for infectious agents (often found in macrophages); identify predominant inflammatory or infiltrative cell type. • Neoplastic infiltrates—classified as epithelial, mesenchymal, or round cell.
- Aspiration of cavitated masses may cause rupture and is not recommended.

Bone Marrow Aspiration

- Indicated with cytopenias before splenectomy (spleen may be supporting hematopoiesis).
- May yield infectious disorder (e.g., ehrlichiosis, mycosis, toxoplasmosis, leishmaniosis) or hematopoietic neoplasia.

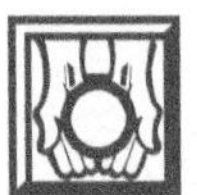

TREATMENT

- Depends on underlying cause; supportive nursing care as needed.
- Important to determine if splenomegaly is appropriate for systemic conditions.
- Treatment and prognosis after splenectomy—based on histopathologic features: submit the entire spleen for histopathologic evaluation (hemangiosarcoma may be missed in some tumors owing to regional necrosis with diagnosis rendered of hematoma).

SURGICAL CONSIDERATIONS

Splenectomy

- With anemia or leukopenia—rule out bone marrow aplasia/hypoplasia before surgery; spleen may be the source of hematopoiesis.
- Indicated for splenic torsion, splenic rupture, isolated splenic masses considered likely to be neoplastic, and mast cell infiltration (cats only). • Exploratory laparotomy—permits direct evaluation of all abdominal organs.

MEDICATIONS

DRUG(S) OF CHOICE

Depend on underlying disease.

FOLLOW-UP

PATIENT MONITORING

Ventricular arrhythmias (dogs)—associated with splenic mass lesions or torsion; may occur before, during, and up to 3 days post splenectomy; evaluate (auscultation and electrocardiogram) surgical candidates before anesthesia; continuous cardiac monitoring during surgery and postoperatively.

POSSIBLE COMPLICATIONS

- Asplenic patient—increased risk of infection and red cell parasitism.
- Postoperative sepsis—uncommon complication. • Antibiotics—indicated in asplenic patients receiving immunosuppressive therapy, if any sign of infection apparent.

MISCELLANEOUS

AGE-RELATED FACTORS

Neoplastic causes more likely in geriatric animals.

ZOONOTIC POTENTIAL

A variety of infectious diseases may involve the spleen.

SEE ALSO

See Causes.

ABBREVIATIONS

- DIC = disseminated intravascular coagulation. • GDV = gastric dilatation and volvulus. • EMH = extramedullary hematopoiesis. • FDP = fibrin degradation product. • FeLV = feline leukemia virus.
- FIP = feline infectious peritonitis. • RBC = red blood cell. • SLE = systemic lupus erythematosus.

Suggested Reading

Cleveland MJ, Casale S. Incidence of malignancy and outcome for dogs undergoing splenectomy for incidentally detected nonruptured splenic nodules or masses: 105 cases (2009 – 2013). J Am Vet Med Assoc 2016, 248:1267–1273.

Ferri F, Zini E, Auriemma E, et al. Splenitis in 33 dogs. Vet Pathol 2017, 54:147–154.

Spangler WL, Culbertson MR. Prevalence and type of splenic diseases in cats: 455 cases (1985–1991). J Am Vet Med Assoc 1992, 201:773–776.

Spangler WL, Kass PH. Pathologic factors affecting postsplenectomy survival in dogs. J Vet Intern Med 1997, 11:166–171.

Author Cheryl E. Balkman

Consulting Editor Kate Holan

S

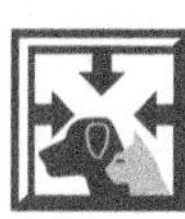

BASICS

OVERVIEW

- Degenerative, noninflammatory condition of the vertebral column that occurs in response to intervertebral disc degeneration.
- Often an incidental finding, rarely clinically important.
- Characterized by the production of osteophytes along the ventral, lateral, and dorsolateral aspects of the vertebral endplates. Radiographically, appears as smooth, ventral bridging bone.
- Most common location in dogs is the thoracolumbar spine in the area of the anticlinal vertebra and the upper lumbar vertebrae; in cats, the thoracic vertebrae.

SIGNALMENT

- Dog and cat.
- Females > males.
- Dogs—commonly seen in large breeds, especially German shepherd dog; also boxer, Airedale terrier, and cocker spaniel.
- Occurrence increases with age. Present in 50% of dogs by 6 years and 75% by 9 years. May be radiographically evident in young dogs with an inherited predisposition.
- Boxers—positive correlation between spondylosis deformans and hip dysplasia. Both heritable traits are detectable in predisposed animals by radiographic examination at 1 year.
- Cats—present in 68% of asymptomatic cats.

SIGNS

General Comments

- Patients are typically asymptomatic; lesions are of minor if any clinical importance.
- Pain may follow fracture of bony spurs or bridges.

Historical Findings

- Stiffness.
- Restricted motion.
- Spinal pain.

Physical Examination Findings

Neurologic deficits are uncommon. If present, referable to compression of the spinal cord or nerve root.

CAUSES & RISK FACTORS

- Repeated microtrauma.
- Major trauma.
- Inherited predisposition.
- Acromegaly.

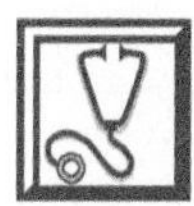

DIAGNOSIS

DIFFERENTIAL DIAGNOSIS

- Discospondylitis—differentiated by radiographic evidence of endplate lysis.
- Spinal osteoarthritis—degeneration of articular facet joints.
- Neoplasia—may have irregular, ventral, nonbridging bone.

CBC/BIOCHEMISTRY/URINALYSIS

Normal

Radiographic Findings

Spinal radiography initially shows osteophytes as triangular projections several millimeters from the edge of the vertebral body. With progression, osteophytes appear to bridge the intervertebral space. True ankylosis is rare.

DIAGNOSTIC PROCEDURES

In uncommon presentations, MRI, CT, or CT myelography can be used to demonstrate an atypical dorsal osteophyte compressing the spinal cord or nerve roots or encroaching on critical soft tissue structures.

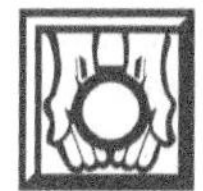

TREATMENT

- Typically not needed. Inform client that the condition is usually an asymptomatic, incidental finding, and is likely not responsible for any clinical signs that may be present.
- Treat spondylosis on an outpatient basis with strict rest and analgesia, possibly acupuncture.
- If overconditioned, recommend weight-reduction program.
- Acupuncture—dry needle or electro-acupuncture treatment at weekly or biweekly interval and tapered to as-needed basis can be very effective in relief of pain. Useful in animals who do not tolerate medication or when clients prefer an alternative treatment modality.

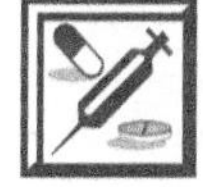

MEDICATIONS

DRUG(S) OF CHOICE

Use only when the patient is exhibiting signs.

Nonsteroidal Anti-inflammatory Drugs (NSAIDs)

- In dogs, NSAIDs are preferable to steroids (fewer side effects) unless patient has neurologic deficits or concomitant disease prohibits use. Administer with food.
- Carprofen (Rimadyl) 2.2 mg/kg PO q12h or 4.4 mg/kg PO q24h in dogs.
- Meloxicam (Metacam) 0.2 mg/kg once then 0.1 mg/kg q24h in dogs.
- Deracoxib (Deramaxx) 1–2 mg/kg PO q24h in dogs.
- Firocoxib (Previcox) 5 mg/kg PO q24h in dogs.
- Grapiprant (Galliprant) 2 mg/kg PO q24h in dogs.
- If gastrointestinal sensitivity, use in combination with an antacid (famotidine 0.5–1 mg/kg q24h or omeprazole 0.5–1 mg/kg q24h) or a gastrointestinal protectant (misoprostol at 3–5 μg/kg PO q6–8h or sucralfate 0.5–1 g q8h) to reduce the possibility of ulceration.

Non-NSAID Analgesics

- Use may enable reduction of dose or frequency of anti-inflammatory medications.
- Tramadol 2–5 mg/kg PO q8–12h in dogs; 1–4 mg/kg q12h in cats.
- Gabapentin 10 mg/kg PO q8–12h in dogs or cats.
- Buprenorphine 0.01–0.03 mg/kg PO q8h in cats.
- Acetaminophen 5 mg/kg POq12h in dogs.

Corticosteroids

- Only use in patients with neurologic deficits.
- Prednisone 0.25–0.5 mg/kg PO q12h; or dexamethasone 0.025–0.05 mg/kg PO q12h.
- Taper to alternate-day prednisone or twice-weekly dexamethasone.

CONTRAINDICATIONS/POSSIBLE INTERACTIONS

- Acetaminophen and NSAIDs—do not use in cats.
- Avoid prolonged administration of NSAIDs, simultaneous use of of NSAIDs and acetaminophen, simultaneous use of NSAIDs and steroids, use of NSAIDs in patients with gastrointestinal (GI) or renal disease. Doing so decreases risk of GI ulceration and renal pathology.

FOLLOW-UP

PATIENT MONITORING

- If signs are present, restrict activity and gradually return the animal to normal activity after signs have subsided for several weeks.
- Relapse can occur with strenuous activity.
- With prolonged use of analgesic medications, periodic biochemistry testing is warranted.

PREVENTION/AVOIDANCE

Boxers—given genetic correlation between spondylosis deformans and hip dysplasia and potential for early radiographic detection, dogs should be screened and selectively bred.

MISCELLANEOUS

ABBREVIATIONS

- CT= computed tomography.
- GI = gastrointestinal.
- MRI = magnetic resonance imaging.
- NSAID = nonsteroidal anti-inflammatory drug.

Suggested Reading

Romatowski J. Spondylosis deformans in the dog. Compend Contin Educ Pract Vet 1986, 8:531–536.

Authors Richard J. Joseph and Anne E. Buglione

SPOROTRICHOSIS

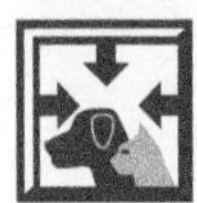

BASICS

OVERVIEW

- Zoonotic fungal disease affecting the integument, lymphatics, or generalized.
- Caused by inoculation of the ubiquitous dimorphic fungus *Sporothrix schenckii* into subcutaneous tissue.

SIGNALMENT

Cat and dog (less common).

SIGNS

- Dogs (cutaneous form)—numerous nodules that may drain or crust; most lesions located on the head, dorsal muzzle; occasionally on the chest, or disseminated on the body and on the limbs.
- Cats (cutaneous form)—lesions appear initially as wounds or abscesses mimicking wounds associated with fighting.
- Cutaneolymphatic form—usually an extension of the cutaneous form through the lymphatics, resulting in the formation of new nodules and draining tracts or crusts; lymphadenopathy is common.
- Disseminated form—systemic signs including lameness, respiratory symptoms (nasal discharge, sneezing, stertorous breathing), anorexia and weight loss also reported in dogs.

S

CAUSES & RISK FACTORS

- Dogs—hunting dogs from puncture wounds associated with thorns or splinters.
- Cats—intact male outdoor cats: Healthy cats may have a minor role in sporotrichosis transmission
- Animals exposed to soil rich in decaying organic debris.
- Exposure to infected animals or clinically healthy cats sharing a household with an affected cat.
- Immunosuppressive disease.

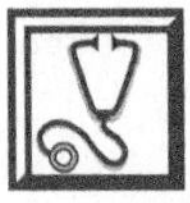

DIAGNOSIS

Caution: This is a zoonotic disease and proper precautions should be taken to prevent exposure; the absence of a break in the skin does not protect against the disease. Cats may act as reservoirs for *S. schenckii* and can transmit the infection to humans by a bite or scratch.

DIFFERENTIAL DIAGNOSIS

- Infectious—bacterial (deep) and fungal infection (e.g., cryptococcosis, blastomycosis, feline leprosy, histoplasmosis).
- Neoplasia.
- Granulomas caused by foreign bodies.
- Parasites—*Demodex, Pelodera, Leishmania.*

CBC/BIOCHEMISTRY/URINALYSIS

None unless associated with generalized disease.

OTHER LABORATORY TESTS

- Cultures of affected tissue preferred; swab culture may be adequate
- *Caution*: This is a zoonotic disease; laboratory personnel must be warned of the potential differential diagnosis.
- Serologic testing and PCR assays are available.

DIAGNOSTIC PROCEDURES

- Cytology of exudates—cigar- to round-shaped yeast found intracellularly or free in the exudates with pyogranulamatous inflammation.
- Biopsy—organisms usually numerous, especially in cats; fungal stains (periodic acid–Schiff or Gomori's methamine silver) may aid in the diagnosis; the absence of demonstrable organisms in tissues from dogs does not preclude diagnosis; pyogranulomatous inflammation with few mast cells, eosinophils, and plasma cells. Radiographs—evidence of irregular periostal proliferation.
- Immunohistochemistry might be useful for an early diagnosis of sporothricosis in cats. High sensitivity reported with immunohistochemistry to diagnose sporothricosis in dogs.
- ELISA— screening tool for the detection of specific *S. schenckii* antibodies in cats with sporotrichosis.

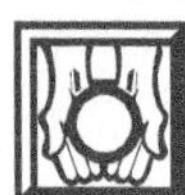

TREATMENT

Zoonotic; outpatient therapy may be a consideration but increases the potential for human exposure.

MEDICATIONS

DRUG(S) OF CHOICE

- Dogs—ketoconazole 5–15 mg/kg PO q12h, itraconazole 5–10 mg/kg PO q24h, terbinafine 30–40 mg/kg PO q24h given with food, administered until 1 month after clinical resolution; resolution usually occurs within 3 months. Disseminated disease—combination of amphotericin B and itraconazole is recommended; terbinafine may also be effective.
- Cats—itraconazole 5–15 mg/kg PO q24h or divided q12h for a minimum of 1 month beyond clinical cure; compounded formulations of itraconazole are not recommended due to inconsistent absorption.

FOLLOW-UP

PATIENT MONITORING

Reevaluation, including assessment of liver enzymes, recommended every 2–4 weeks.

PREVENTION/AVOIDANCE

N/A

EXPECTED COURSE AND PROGNOSIS

- Failure of response to therapy possible.
- Fluconazole and terbinafine remain relatively untested but may show promise for treatment.

MISCELLANEOUS

ZOONOTIC POTENTIAL

- *Caution*: This is a zoonotic disease.
- Client education is of paramount importance.
- Absence of a break in the skin does not protect against the disease.
- Reports of zoonotic transmission from bites and scratches from rodents, parrots, cats, dogs, horses, and armadillos.
- Clinically healthy cats sharing a household with an infected cat may be a source of infection.

ABBREVIATIONS

- ELISA = enzyme-linked immunosorbent assay.

Suggested Reading

Silva J, Miranda L, Menezes R, et al. Comparison of the sensitivity of three methods for the early diagnosis of sporotrichosis in cats. J Comp Pathol 2018, 160:72–78.

Authors W. Dunbar Gram and Andhika Putra

Consulting Editor Alexander H. Werner Resnick

Acknowledgment The authors and editors acknowledge the prior contribution of Holly Dutton.

SQUAMOUS CELL CARCINOMA, DIGIT

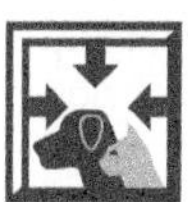

BASICS

OVERVIEW

• Locally invasive malignant tumor usually arising from subungual epithelium.
• Cats—metastasis to one or multiple digits from primary pulmonary site.
• Dogs—most common digital tumor (~50%); up to 25% metastatic rate, up to 22% multiple digits affected (multicentric disease).
• Forelimb more commonly affected than hind limb.
• Organ systems—skin/endocrine, musculoskeletal.

SIGNALMENT

• Dog and rarely cat.
• Median age—dogs and cats 10 years; reported in dogs as young as 3 years old.
• Large breeds (>75%) and black/dark-coated dogs (>90%) predisposed; breeds include standard poodle, Labrador retriever, giant schnauzer, Rottweiler, dachshund, flat-coated retriever, and possibly Beauceron, Briard, and miniature poodle.

SIGNS

• Swollen digit or digital mass which fails to heal.
• Lameness.
• Ulceration.
• Fractured or missing nail.
• Multiple digits affected in up to 22% of dogs; may present in one digit and develop additional digital tumors later.
• Multiple digits commonly seen in cats (30%); due to lung–digit syndrome.
• Regional lymphadenomegaly of the sentinel draining lymph node (uncommon at time of diagnosis).

CAUSES & RISK FACTORS

Risk factors (dogs)—hereditary; dark skin/hair pigmentation.

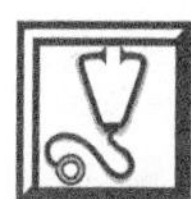

DIAGNOSIS

DIFFERENTIAL DIAGNOSIS

• Nailbed infection (paronychia).
• Trauma.
• Other tumors (dog)—melanoma; soft tissue sarcomas; mast cell tumor; osteosarcoma.
• Benign lesions—epithelial inclusion cyst, keratoacanthoma.

CBC/BIOCHEMISTRY/URINALYSIS

Usually normal.

IMAGING

• Thoracic radiography—to evaluate for metastatic disease (develops in up to 25% of dogs) and rule out a primary pulmonary carcinoma (cats).
• Limb radiography—lysis of the third phalanx of the affected digit in 80% of patients with potential secondary extension proximally to phalanx 2 and 1.
• Abdominal ultrasonography—for hind limb lesions, evaluate intra-abdominal lymph nodes for presence of metastatic disease.

DIAGNOSTIC PROCEDURES

• Cytology—diagnostic utility limited if there is severe inflammation or secondary infection (common), or the tumor is well differentiated.
• Biopsy of lesion—may be needed to confirm diagnosis.
• Cytology of regional lymph nodes to evaluate for metastasis.

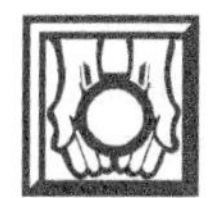

TREATMENT

• Amputation of the affected digit at the level of the metacarpal or metatarsal phalangeal joint.
• In cats with a primary pulmonary tumor, amputation of a single affected digit may provide local palliative care and confirm diagnosis, however multiple digits on multiple limbs are often affected.
• Palliative radiation can be considered for single digits if metastatic disease present or in the setting of multicentric/multiple digits affected.
• Analgesics for pain control, antibiotics for secondary bacterial infections may be indicated.
• Benefit of chemotherapy has not been established; however in patients with advanced stage of disease chemotherapy useful for squamous cell carcinoma of other sites could be considered.

MEDICATIONS

DRUG(S) OF CHOICE

Piroxicam—dogs, 0.3 mg/kg PO q24h for analgesia/antineoplastic effects; cats, 0.3 mg/kg PO q24–48h has been used for other carcinomas.

CONTRAINDICATIONS/POSSIBLE INTERACTIONS

None

FOLLOW-UP

PATIENT MONITORING

Physical exam, thoracic radiographs, lymph node evaluation, ± abdominal ultrasound at 1–2 months, then every 3 months after treatment (complete surgical excision).

EXPECTED COURSE AND PROGNOSIS

• Complete surgical excision of the primary lesion and no evidence of metastasis; additional treatment may not be required.
• Survival time following complete surgical excision depends upon location of the tumor on the digit; squamous cell carcinoma (SCC) originating from subungual epithelium: 95% 1-year and 74% 2-year survival; SCC originating in other parts of the digit: 60% 1-year and 44% 2-year survival.
• In one study 1- and 2-year survival was 50% and 18%, respectively, while in two other studies only 20–45% of dogs died of SCC (multicentric or metastatic) and the median survival time was not reached.
• Development of multicentric disease (multiple affected digits) in dogs appears more common than lymph node or pulmonary metastasis.
• Surgery to amputate affected digit, regardless of presence of metastases, provides positive impact on survival in the dog.
• Histologic grading does not appear predictive of development of multicentric or metastatic disease in dogs.
• Prognosis for cats is poor with median survival times of 2–3 months if metastatic from pulmonary carcinoma.

MISCELLANEOUS

SEE ALSO

• Melanocytic Tumors, Skin and Digit.
• Squamous Cell Carcinoma, Skin.

ABBREVIATIONS

• SCC = squamous cell carcinoma.

Suggested Reading

Belluco S, Brisebard E, Watrelot D, et al. Digital squamous cell carcinoma in dogs: epidemiological, histological, and immunohistochemical study. Vet Pathol 2013, 50(6):1078–1082.

Author Alycen P. Lundberg
Consulting Editor Timothy M. Fan
Acknowledgment The author and editors acknowledge the prior contribution of Jackie M. Wypij.

S

SQUAMOUS CELL CARCINOMA, EAR

BASICS

OVERVIEW

- Malignant tumor of squamous epithelium occurring on the pinna, external ear, and/or middle ear (less common).
- Pinna—most common location in cats; tumors of the pinna in dogs are rarely squamous cell carcinoma.
- Organ system—skin/endocrine.

SIGNALMENT

- Cat and dog.
- Tumors of the pinna—common in cats with light pigmentation, average 12 years.
- Ear canal tumors—seen in older dogs and cats.
- Cocker spaniels overrepresented for benign and malignant ear canal tumors in one study.

SIGNS

- Tumors of the pinna:
  - Slowly developing lesions of the edge of the pinna.
  - Precancerous stage—crusty eczematous lesions (actinic dermatitis).
  - Cancerous phase—proliferation and/or ulceration progresses.
  - Multiple cutaneous lesions (about 10–15% of cats) occur in haired skin (multicentric squamous cell carcinoma *in situ*).
- Tumors of the ear canal:
  - Often unilateral, arise from the external ear canal.
  - Mass lesion (raised, ulcerated, broad-based).
  - Malodorous aural discharge.
  - Pruritis.
  - Pain.
  - Vestibular signs/Horner's syndrome (facial nerve paralysis, head tilt, circling) in ~10% of dogs; more common in cats with ear canal tumors.
  - Difficulty opening jaw.
  - Cervical lymphadenomegaly (retropharyngeal, mandibular).

CAUSES & RISK FACTORS

- Pinna—UV exposure in cats with white fur, light skin.
- Ear canal—chronic inflammation may be a risk factor.

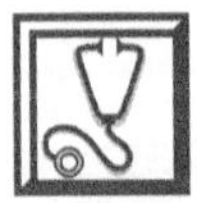

DIAGNOSIS

DIFFERENTIAL DIAGNOSIS

Cats

- Pinna:
  - Trauma.
  - Vasculitis.
  - Cryoglobulinemia.
- Ear canal/middle ear:
  - Inflammatory/nasopharyngeal polyp (middle ear).
  - Other neoplasia (ceruminous gland adenocarcinoma, other).

Dogs

- Pinna:
  - Other neoplasia (mast cell tumor, histiocytoma, sebaceous gland tumor).
  - Trauma.
- Ear canal/middle ear:
  - Chronic otitis.
  - Other neoplasia (ceruminous gland adenoma or adenocarcinoma, papilloma).
  - Nasopharyngeal polyps (rare).

CBC/BIOCHEMISTRY/URINALYSIS

Usually normal.

IMAGING

- Thoracic radiography—evaluate for pulmonary metastasis (rare with pinnal lesions).
- CT—shows extent of disease and provides surgical planning; 57–67% locally invasive into surrounding tissues.

DIAGNOSTIC PROCEDURES

- Cytology may confirm diagnosis; however, ulceration, inflammation, and secondary infection may limit diagnostic utility.
- Biopsy of pinna/aural mass to confirm diagnosis via histopathology; video otoscopy may aid in visualization of mass lesion and biopsy.
- Lymph node cytology of draining lymph nodes to assess for metastatic disease.

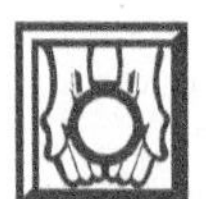

TREATMENT

- Pinna:
  - Appropriate surgical excision may require pinnectomy and possibly vertical ear canal ablation; must remove lesion with margin of normal tissue.
  - Alternatives include photodynamic therapy (less predictable; multiple treatments may be required), cryosurgery (for small, superficial lesions), strontium plesiotherapy (superficial radiation therapy), electrochemotherapy with bleomycin, or curettage/diathermy.
- Ear canal/middle ear:
  - Total ear canal ablation and bulla osteotomy is usually needed to achieve complete excision; lateral ear canal resection rarely achieves adequate control.
  - Radiation therapy may be used for palliation of nonresectable tumors or postoperatively for microscopic disease.

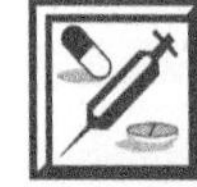

MEDICATIONS

DRUG(S) OF CHOICE

- Pinna (cat):
  - Imiquimod 5% cream—apply topically q24-48h.
  - Etretinate 0.75–1 mg/kg PO q24h; can prevent progression of precancerous lesions; may not be commercially available.
  - Acitretin 1 mg/kg PO q24h can be used in place of etretinate.
  - Vitamin E 400–600 IU PO q12h; may be beneficial to prevent or delay progression of precancerous lesions.
- Ear canal tumors:
  - Systemic chemotherapy—benefit not yet established; anecdotal benefit.

CONTRAINDICATIONS/POSSIBLE INTERACTIONS

Women who are pregnant or planning to become pregnant should not handle acitretin.

FOLLOW-UP

PATIENT MONITORING

- Pinna—physical examination at 1 month, then every 3 months after treatment (complete surgical excision).
- Ear canal—physical examination, thoracic radiographs, lymph node evaluation, and possible CT every 3 months after treatment.

PREVENTION/AVOIDANCE

- Limit sun exposure.
- Tattoos on nonpigmented areas may be helpful.

EXPECTED COURSE AND PROGNOSIS

- Pinna—prognosis good with complete surgical excision; survival >1.5 years with complete pinnectomy.
- Ear canal tumors locally invasive (57–67%) and can recur locally despite surgery; prognosis is guarded.
- Dogs—median survival 5.3 months with bulla involvement compared to >58 months without.
- Cats—median survival 3.8 months; worse prognosis with bulla involvement; median survival 1.5 months with neurologic signs.

MISCELLANEOUS

SEE ALSO

- Ceruminous Gland Adenocarcinoma, Ear.
- Squamous Cell Carcinoma, Skin.

Suggested Reading

Sula MJ. Tumors and tumorlike lesions of dog and cat ears. Vet Clin North Am Small Anim Pract 2012, 42:1161–1178.

Author Alycen P. Lundberg
Consulting Editor Timothy M. Fan
Acknowledgment The author and editors acknowledge the prior contribution of Jackie M. Wypij.

SQUAMOUS CELL CARCINOMA, GINGIVA

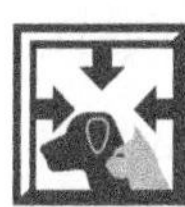

BASICS

OVERVIEW

- Malignant tumor of squamous epithelium.
- Rapid progression, locally invasive, highly osteo-invasive (77%).
- Most common oral malignancy in cats; one of most common oral malignancies in dogs.
- Approximately 10–20% metastasis in dogs and cats with potential involvement of draining lymph nodes (most common) and lung parenchyma.

SIGNALMENT

- Mean age (dogs/cats) 10.5 years.
- More common in medium and large-breed dogs.

SIGNS

Historical Findings

- Mass effect.
- Ptyalism.
- Dysphagia.
- Halitosis.
- Bloody saliva.
- Weight loss.
- Hyporexia or avoidance of hard foods/toys.
- Poor grooming (cats).

Physical Examination Findings

- Erythematous, ulcerated, fleshy lesion.
- Loose teeth.
- Facial swelling or deformity.
- Exophthalmos.
- Pain on opening jaw.

CAUSES & RISK FACTORS

Potential risk factors in cats include flea collars, canned food (tuna), and tobacco smoke.

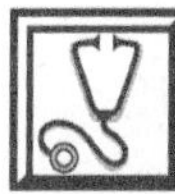

DIAGNOSIS

DIFFERENTIAL DIAGNOSIS

- Other oral malignancy—fibrosarcoma in cats; melanoma, fibrosarcoma, osteosarcoma in dogs.
- Epulis (acanthamatous, fibrous, ossifying).
- Tooth root abscess.
- Benign growth or polyp.
- Gingival hyperplasia (breed, e.g., boxer, or drug-induced, e.g., cyclosporine).
- Eosinophilic granuloma complex.

IMAGING

- Skull radiography—evaluate potential bone involvement.
- High-detail dental radiography—more sensitive in evaluating local disease than skull radiography; best with mandibular masses.
- CT—ideal to evaluate soft tissue extension, bone invasion, regional lymph nodes, and for surgical planning.
- Thoracic radiography—evaluate for pulmonary metastasis (uncommon in dogs, rare in cats).

DIAGNOSTIC PROCEDURES

- Cytology—fine-needle aspirate samples can be sufficient, though ulceration, inflammation, and secondary infection may limit diagnostic utility.
- Deep tissue biopsy—beneficial to differentiate from other oral malignancies via histopathology.
- Cytology of regional lymph nodes to assess for regionally metastatic disease.

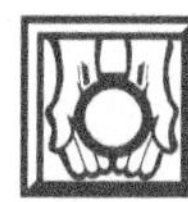

TREATMENT

Dogs

- Radical surgical excision required (e.g., hemi-mandibulectomy); usually well tolerated; margins of at least 2 cm necessary.
- Radiation therapy—effective for long-term control; curative-intent treatment used alone or in combination with surgery or chemotherapy.
- Chemotherapy—alone or in combination with other treatment modalities; toceranib phosphate (Palladia) exerts single-agent activity in a substantial fraction (biologic response) of dogs treated.
- Piroxicam may have some antineoplastic effects.
- Cryosurgery or electrochemotherapy—indicated for small lesions with no bone involvement.
- Photodynamic therapy—adjunct to surgery may be effective for local control of small tumors.
- Analgesics for pain or antibiotics for secondary bacterial infections may be indicated.

Cats

- Surgery—most tumors are inoperable; small rostral lesions may be excised with wide 2–3 cm margins; cats do not tolerate aggressive oral surgery as well as dogs.
- Palliative treatments include coarse-fraction radiation therapy (<50% response).
- Metastasis less of a concern as most cats succumb to local disease progression.
- Bisphosphonates—used to palliate bone pain.
- Analgesics for pain or antibiotics for secondary bacterial infections may be indicated.

MEDICATIONS

DRUG(S) OF CHOICE

- Toceranib phosphate (Palladia)—dogs and cats, 2.5–3.25 mg/kg PO q48h.
- Cisplatin—dogs only, 60–70 mg/m^2 IV once q3–4 weeks for 4 treatments.
- Carboplatin—dogs, 300 mg/m^2 q3 weeks IV; cats, 180–240 mg/m^2 q3–4 weeks for 4–5 treatments.
- Mitoxantrone—cats, 5–6 mg/m^2 q3 weeks IV for 4–5 treatments.
- Piroxicam—dogs, 0.3 mg/kg PO q24h; cats, q48–72h.

CONTRAINDICATIONS/POSSIBLE INTERACTIONS

Cisplatin—never in cats. Nephrotoxic in dogs, cannot combine with NSAIDs.

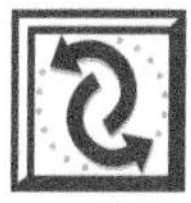

FOLLOW-UP

PATIENT MONITORING

Physical exam, lymph node evaluation, and thoracic radiographs at 1–2 months, then every 3 months after treatment.

POSSIBLE COMPLICATIONS

Postoperative complications—tumor recurrence, ptyalism, mandibular drift causing malocclusion, difficulty prehending food, inability to groom.

EXPECTED COURSE AND PROGNOSIS

Dogs

- Negative prognostic factors—caudal or maxillary location, >2 cm diameter, older age, incomplete excision.
- Surgical excision—median survival 15–16 months, 34 months combined with radiation therapy; mandibulectomy better outcome than maxillectomy.
- Combination carboplatin and piroxicam with or without surgery—median survival >18 months (7 dogs).
- Piroxicam—17% response rate with a median progression-free interval of 3.5–6 months.

Cats

- 1-year survival rate is 10% for multimodal therapy.
- In rare cases where surgery is an option, median survival 1 year.

MISCELLANEOUS

SEE ALSO

- Melanocytic Tumors, Oral.
- Squamous Cell Carcinoma, Tongue.
- Squamous Cell Carcinoma, Tonsil.

Suggested Reading

Biligic O, Duda L, Sanchez, MD, et al. Feline oral squamous cell carcinoma: clinical manisfestations and literature review. J Vet Dent 2015, 32(1):30–40.

Author Alycen P. Lundberg

Consulting Editor Timothy M. Fan

Acknowledgment The author and editors acknowledge the prior contribution of Jackie M. Wypij.

S

SQUAMOUS CELL CARCINOMA, LUNG

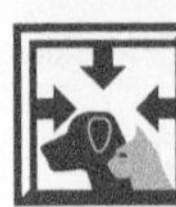

BASICS

OVERVIEW

- Primary tumor of bronchial epithelium with squamous metaplasia.
- High metastatic potential to regional lymph nodes, pleural surface (carcinomatosis), pulmonary parenchyma, less commonly distant organs.
- Organ system—respiratory.

SIGNALMENT

- Dog and cat—mean age 11–12 years.
- Persian cats may be overrepresented for pulmonary carcinomas.

SIGNS

- May be incidental finding on radiographs.
- Harsh, nonproductive cough.
- Dyspnea, tachypnea.
- Lethargy, exercise intolerance.
- Hemoptysis.
- Cachexia, weight loss.
- Vomiting, regurgitation, diarrhea (cats).
- Lameness:
    - Distal limb swelling, pain (hypertrophic osteopathy).
    - Digital lesions (cats).

S

CAUSES & RISK FACTORS

- Urban environment, second-hand smoke suspected.
- Laboratory dogs trained to smoke cigarettes develop lung cancer.

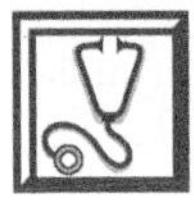

DIAGNOSIS

DIFFERENTIAL DIAGNOSIS

- Other primary lung neoplasia—adenocarcinoma, bronchoalveolar carcinoma, histiocytic sarcoma.
- Metastatic pulmonary neoplasia.
- Fungal granuloma.
- Abscess.
- Aspiration pneumonia.

CBC/BIOCHEMISTRY/URINALYSIS

Often unremarkable.

IMAGING

- Thoracic radiography (3-view):
    - Most often in caudal lung lobes.
    - Often a solitary mass, well-circumscribed margins.
    - May identify tracheobronchial lymphadenomegaly, pulmonary metastatic lesions, pleural effusion.
    - May displace/compress trachea or mainstem bronchi.
- CT:
    - Determines surgical resectability.
    - Solitary, well-circumscribed, bronchocentric mass with internal air bronchograms; mild–moderate heterogeneous contrast enhancement.
    - More sensitive than radiographs in detecting pulmonary and lymph node metastasis.
- Limb radiography:
    - Digit metastases—bony lysis in the distal phalanx (cats, lung–digit syndrome).
    - Hypertrophic osteopathy—periosteal proliferation, long bones.

DIAGNOSTIC PROCEDURES

- Cytology:
    - Transthoracic fine-needle aspiration of peripheral lesions; ultrasound or CT guidance may be needed.
    - Pleural effusion or intrathoracic lymph node aspirates if primary lesion is not amenable to aspiration.
    - Endoscopic bronchial brushing may be useful for centrally located lesions.
    - Bronchoalveolar lavage and transtracheal wash: rarely diagnostic.
- Biopsy necessary for definitive diagnosis; may be obtained via keyhole biopsy, thoracoscopy, or thoracotomy.
- Potential complications of diagnostic procedures—pneumothorax, hemothorax, pleural effusion, infection, and iatrogenic tumor seeding (rare).

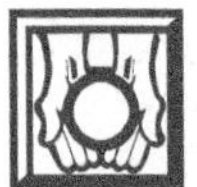

TREATMENT

- Surgery—wide and complete resection of affected lung lobe; biopsy lymph nodes even if they appear normal; lymph node extirpation when possible. In select cases, thoracoscopic surgery may be considered.
- Chemotherapy—potentially beneficial in adjuvant or palliative setting, intracavitary (IC) chemotherapy may be useful for carcinomatosis/pleural effusion.
- Palliative medications—cough suppressants and antibiotic therapy for secondary bacterial infections.

MEDICATION

DRUG(S) OF CHOICE

- Doxorubicin—dogs >10 kg, 30 mg/m^2 IV; dogs <10 kg and cats, 1 mg/kg IV q2–3 weeks for 5 treatments.
- Carboplatin—dogs, 300 mg/m^2 IV q3–4 weeks; cats, 180–250 mg/m^2 IV q3–4 weeks for 4–5 treatments.
- Mitoxantrone—dogs and cats, 5–6 mg/m^2 q3 weeks; can give IV, IC (if pleural effusion present), or split total dose: half IV, half IC for 4–5 treatments.
- Vinorelbine—dogs, 15 mg/m^2 IV weekly for 4 weeks then every other week for 4 treatments.
- Cisplatin—dogs only, 60 mg/m^2 IV q3–4 weeks for 4 treatments.
- Toceranib phosphate (Palladia)—dogs and cats, 2.5–3.25 mg/kg PO q48h.
- Metronomic chemotherapy—cyclophosphamide 15 mg/m^2 PO q24h, piroxicam 0.3 mg/kg PO q24h.

CONTRAINDICATIONS/POSSIBLE INTERACTIONS

Cisplatin—never use in cats; nephrotoxic in dogs.

FOLLOW-UP

PATIENT MONITORING

Postoperatively, consider chemotherapy options; recheck thoracic radiographs and/or CT scan in 1–2 months, then every 3 months.

EXPECTED COURSE AND PROGNOSIS

- Of the primary pulmonary carcinomas, squamous cell carcinoma (SCC) and undifferentiated carcinoma carries the worst prognosis.
- Survival if untreated or with evidence of metastatic disease—usually <3 months.
- Median survival with treatment for SCC—8 months (dogs).
- Cats—median survival of pulmonary carcinomas surgically excised is 64–156 days.
- Negative prognostic factors (all lung tumors)—large size, enlarged lymph nodes, metastasis, pleural effusion, high histologic grade/poorly differentiated, or respiratory signs at diagnosis.

MISCELLANEOUS

ASSOCIATED CONDITIONS

Paraneoplastic hypertrophic osteopathy, lung–digit syndrome (cats).

SEE ALSO

Adenocarcinoma, Lung.

Suggested Reading

Nunley J, Sutton J, Culp W, et al. Primary pulmonary neoplasia in cats: assessment of computed tomography findings and survival. J Small Anim Practice 2015, 56(11): 651–656.

Author Alycen P. Lundberg

Consulting Editor Timothy M. Fan

Acknowledgment The author and editors acknowledge the prior contribution of Jackie M. Wypij.

SQUAMOUS CELL CARCINOMA, NASAL AND PARANASAL SINUSES

BASICS

OVERVIEW

- Local invasion of neoplastic squamous epithelium from the nasal cavity and/or paranasal sinuses.
- Slowly progressive (months) and commonly bilateral.
- Low metastatic rate.
- Prevalence—15–17% of nasal neoplasia in cats and dogs.

SIGNALMENT

- More common in dog than in cat.
- Dogs—median age, 9–10 years, male predilection; cats—median 10–12 years, male predilection.
- Dogs—predilection for sinonasal tumors in medium and large breeds.

SIGNS

Historical Findings

- Intermittent, progressive unilateral to bilateral epistaxis and/or mucopurulent nasal discharge.
- Epiphora.
- Sneezing.
- Halitosis.
- Anorexia.
- Dyspnea.
- Seizures secondary to cribriform plate invasion.

Physical Examination Findings

- Nasal discharge (epistaxis, mucopurulent, and/or serosanguinous).
- Facial deformity.
- Ocular—epiphora, decreased retropulsion, elevated third eyelid, exophthalmus.
- Pain on nasal/paranasal sinus palpation.
- Obstructed nasal airflow.

CAUSES & RISK FACTORS

Dolicocephalic breed, urban environment, and tobacco smoke exposure speculated to be risk factors.

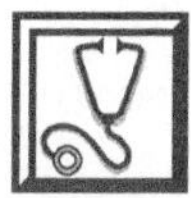

DIAGNOSIS

DIFFERENTIAL DIAGNOSIS

- Other intranasal neoplasia—adenocarcinoma, undifferentiated carcinoma, lymphoma (cats), sarcomas (dogs).
- Tooth root abscess.
- Viral infection—cats.
- Cryptococcosis—cats.
- Aspergillosis.
- Foreign body.
- Trauma.
- Oronasal fistula.
- Coagulopathy.
- Hypertension.
- Bacterial sinusitis—uncommon.
- Lymphocytic—plasmacytic rhinitis.
- Inflammatory polyps (cats).

CBC/BIOCHEMISTRY/URINALYSIS

Usually normal.

OTHER LABORATORY TESTS

If epistaxis, perform coagulation profile and blood pressure to rule out hypertension and coagulopathy prior to intranasal biopsy.

IMAGING

- Skull radiography—asymmetrical osteolysis of caudal turbinates; superimposition of soft tissue mass; fluid density in the frontal sinuses; loss of teeth; displacement of midline structures; involvement of hard palate.
- Thoracic radiography—detect pulmonary metastasis (uncommon).
- CT scan—recommended imaging modalities for the identification of soft tissue density mass, loss of turbinate detail, soft tissue/fluid opacity in sinus; best method for assessing tumor invasiveness, including bony invasion, invasion of cribriform plate or orbit.

DIAGNOSTIC PROCEDURES

- Rhinoscopy—mass effect, may be obscured by exudates.
- Cytology—obtained by aspiration or squash preparation; may be limited by inflammation or secondary infection.
- Biopsy with histopathology—necessary for definitive diagnosis; methods include nasal hydropulsion, transnostril blind biopsy with forceps or bone curette, fiberoptic-guided biopsy, percutaneous biopsy of facial deformities; biopsy via dental extraction site, rhinotomy.
- Precautions must be taken to minimize risk of penetrating the cribriform plate.
- Cytology and/or biopsy of regional lymph nodes—detect metastatic disease (uncommon).

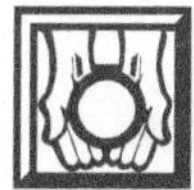

TREATMENT

- Definitive radiotherapy—best clinical control in dogs and cats; exenteration does not add benefit.
- Coarse-fraction radiotherapy beneficial in dogs and cats for palliation.
- Adjunctive chemotherapy—responses in dogs reported; recommended for palliation of clinical signs, metastasis, and as an adjuvant to radiation therapy.
- Analgesics for pain control.
- Anecdotally, nasal hydropulsion may palliate clinical signs.

MEDICATIONS

DRUG(S) OF CHOICE

- Cisplatin—dogs only, 60–70 mg/m^2 IV q3 weeks for 4 treatments.
- Carboplatin—dogs, 300 mg/m^2 IV q3 weeks; cats, 180–250 mg/m^2 IV q3–4 weeks for 4–5 treatments.
- Mitoxantrone—dogs/cats, 5–6 mg/m^2 IV q3 weeks for 4–5 treatments.
- Toceranib phosphate (Palladia)—dogs/cats, 2.5–3.25 mg/kg PO q48h.
- Piroxicam—0.3 mg/kg PO q24h (dogs), q48h (cats).

CONTRAINDICATIONS/POSSIBLE INTERACTIONS

- Cisplatin—never use in cats; nephrotoxic in dogs—do not administer with NSAIDs.

FOLLOW-UP

PATIENT MONITORING

Physical examination, thoracic radiographs, lymph node evaluation, ±CT scan every 3 months after treatment or when signs recur.

POSSIBLE COMPLICATIONS

Acute or late side effects from radiation therapy.

EXPECTED COURSE AND PROGNOSIS

- Untreated carcinomas (all types)—median survival 3 months; epistaxis carries a worse prognosis.
- Definitive radiotherapy (all carcinomas)—median survival 12–18 months (dogs and cats); 10.4 months with stereotactic radiotherapy.
- Coarse-fraction radiation therapy (all tumor types)—improved clinical signs in ~90% of dogs; median survival 4.8–10 months; median survival 10–12 months (cats).
- Local recurrence with extension to the brain can occur.
- Re-irradiation is possible, reduces clinical signs, extends survival time.

MISCELLANEOUS

SEE ALSO

Adenocarcinoma, Nasal.

Suggested Reading

Fujiwara A, Kobayashi T, Kazato Y, et al. Efficacy of hypofractionated radiotherapy for nasal tumours in 38 dogs (2005–2008). J Small Anim Pract 2013, 54(2):80–86.

Author Alycen P. Lundberg
Consulting Editor Timothy M. Fan

Acknowledgment The author and editors acknowledge the prior contribution of Jackie M. Wypij.

S

SQUAMOUS CELL CARCINOMA, NASAL PLANUM

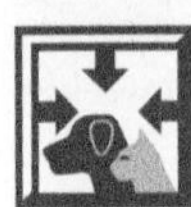

BASICS

OVERVIEW

- Malignant tumor of squamous epithelial cells of the nasal planum.
- Locally invasive and rarely metastasizes.
- Organ systems—skin/exocrine, respiratory.

SIGNALMENT

- Common in cat; rare in dog.
- Mean age—cats, 8.5–12.1 years; dogs, 9–10 years.
- More likely to develop in animals with a lightly pigmented nose (cats).
- No reported sex or breed predilection in cats.
- Dogs—overrepresentation of males and Labrador retrievers in one study.

SIGNS

- Cats—slowly progressive lesion; may begin as superficial crusting and scabbing, progress to carcinoma *in situ*, and develop into superficial and then invasive erosive carcinoma; other cutaneous sites may be affected (cats—multicentric squamous cell carcinoma *in situ* [MSCCIS]).
- Dogs—sneezing; epistaxis; swelling and ulceration of planum, proliferative lesion.

CAUSES & RISK FACTORS

- Exposure to ultraviolet light (UVB).
- Absence of protective pigment (cats).

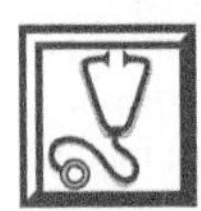

DIAGNOSIS

DIFFERENTIAL DIAGNOSIS

- Infection/abscess.
- Trauma.
- Dermatitis (allergic, other).
- Eosinophilic granuloma complex (cats).
- Immune-mediated disease.
- Cutaneous lymphoma.
- Mast cell tumor.

CBC/BIOCHEMISTRY/URINALYSIS

Usually normal.

IMAGING

- Thoracic radiography—to evaluate for metastasis (rare).
- CT scan—evaluate soft tissue extension and bone invasion prior to surgical planning, essential for canine tumors in which extensive underlying structures are often involved.

DIAGNOSTIC PROCEDURES

- Cytology—fine-needle aspirate of primary lesion may confirm diagnosis; however, ulceration, inflammation, and secondary infection may limit diagnostic utility.
- Biopsy and histopathology—a deep wedge or punch biopsy is often needed to definitively diagnose squamous cell carcinoma. Multiple samples recommended as lesion may have a spectrum of actinic changes ranging from squamous metaplasia to invasive carcinoma.
- Cytology or histopathology of regional lymph nodes screening for regional metastasis (rare in cats, occasional in dogs).

PATHOLOGIC FINDINGS

Lesions may vary in appearance depending on stage of disease in cats; typically ulcerative in cats; more likely proliferative in dogs.

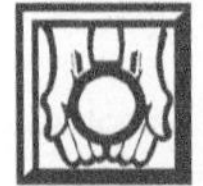

TREATMENT

- Superficial tumors—surgery, cryosurgery, irradiation (strontium-90 plesiotherapy), photodynamic therapy, electrochemotherapy with bleomycin, or curettage/diathermy.
- Invasive tumors—require radical surgical excision and adjunctive external beam radiotherapy (cats); dogs not as responsive to radiotherapy.
- Immediate postoperative nutritional support may be required, especially for cats.
- Analgesics for pain control and antibiotics for secondary bacterial infections as indicated.

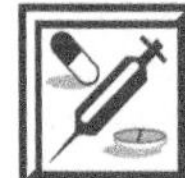

MEDICATIONS

DRUG(S) OF CHOICE

- Etretinate—cats, 0.75–1 mg/kg PO q24h; synthetic retinoid; may be useful for early precancerous lesions; may not be commercially available.
- Acitretin—cats, 1 mg/kg PO q24h can be used in place of etretinate.
- Imiquimod 5% cream for nasal planum lesions associated with MSCCIS—apply topically to affected lesions q24–48h; most cats respond but develop new lesions in other sites; these lesions often subsequently respond to topical therapy.

CONTRAINDICATIONS/POSSIBLE INTERACTIONS

Women who are pregnant or planning to become pregnant should not handle etretinate, acitretin, or imiquimod.

FOLLOW-UP

PATIENT MONITORING

- Physical examination at 1 month, then every 3 months after treatment.
- Biopsy any new suspicious lesion.

PREVENTION/AVOIDANCE

- Limit sun exposure.
- Tattoos on nonpigmented areas may be helpful.

EXPECTED COURSE AND PROGNOSIS

- Prognosis—good for small, noninvasive tumors; guarded for invasive tumors.
- Survival with radiotherapy alone (cats)—mean 17.7 months; 1 year, 61.5% with 81.8% recurrence.
- Surgery (cats, nosectomy)—median survival >22 months.
- Strontium-90 plesiotherapy (cats, superficial)—98% response rate; median progression-free interval of 4.5 years; median survival >8 years.
- Photodynamic therapy (cats, superficial)—96% response rate; often need multiple treatments; does not appear as effective as other therapies long term.
- Electrochemotherapy with bleomycin—risk of recurrence; many achieve complete remission.
- Curettage and diathermy—excellent response; risk of recurrence.
- Dogs (superficial tumors)—surgery alone may be curative.
- Dogs (invasive tumors)—in one study of 8 dogs, average survival time was 5.4 months; in another study of 17 dogs treated with surgery and/or radiation therapy, 70% of tumors recurred with a median survival time of 3–6 months.

MISCELLANEOUS

SEE ALSO

- Squamous Cell Carcinoma, Ear.
- Squamous Cell Carcinoma, Skin.

ABBREVIATIONS

- MSCCIS = multicentric squamous cell carcinoma *in situ*.

Suggested Reading

Jarrett RH, Norman EJ, Gibson IR, Jarrett P. Nose and nasal planum neoplasia, reconstruction. Vet Clin North Am Small Anim Pract 2016, 46(4):735–750.

Author Alycen P. Lundberg

Consulting Editor Timothy M. Fan

Acknowledgment The author and editors acknowledge the prior contribution of Jackie M. Wypij.

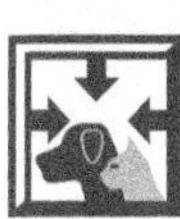

BASICS

OVERVIEW

- Malignant tumor of squamous epithelium.
- Multicentric squamous cell carcinoma *in situ* (MSSCIS)- also called Bowen's-like disease or Bowenoid carcinoma *in situ* (cats).
- Local disease may progress from carcinoma *in situ* to invasive carcinoma.
- Metastasis is uncommon—most common sites are regional lymph nodes and lungs.
- Systems affected—skin/exocrine.
- Represents 9–25% of all skin tumors in cats; 4–18% in dogs.
- Solar-induced (actinic) SCC is more prevalent in sunny climates and high altitudes.

SIGNALMENT

- Cats, mean age 9–10 years; often have light/unpigmented skin.
- Dogs, mean age 8 years; Scottish terrier, Pekingese, boxer, poodle, Norwegian elkhound, Dalmatian, beagle, whippet, and white English bull terrier may be predisposed.

SIGNS

- Proliferative or erosive skin lesions.
- Solar-induced lesions in cats—nasal planum, eyelids, lips, and pinna.
- MSCCIS may occur in any site, unrelated to sun exposure or skin pigmentation; may note 2–30+ lesions on the head, digits, neck, thorax, shoulders, and ventral abdomen; hair in the lesion epilates easily; crusts cling to the epilated hair shaft.
- Dogs—most commonly affects toes, scrotum, nose, legs, and anus.

CAUSES & RISK FACTORS

- Ultraviolet irradiation (actinic form).
- Papillomaviruses may play a role.
- Light/nonpigmented skin.
- Previous thermal injury.
- Risk factors for MSCCIS in cats are undetermined but may be associated with immunosuppression.

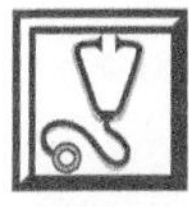

DIAGNOSIS

DIFFERENTIAL DIAGNOSIS

- Infection/abscess.
- Dermatophytosis.
- Trauma.
- Dermatitis.
- Eosinophilic granuloma complex.
- Immune-mediated disease.
- Cutaneous lymphoma.
- Mast cell tumor.

CBC/BIOCHEMISTRY/URINALYSIS

Usually normal.

IMAGING

- Thoracic radiography—may detect lung metastasis (rare).
- Abdominal ultrasonography—evaluate and monitor sublumbar lymph nodes if skin disease involves the caudal half of the patient.

DIAGNOSTIC PROCEDURES

- Cytology or histopathology of lesion—ulceration, inflammation, and secondary infection may limit diagnostic utility of cytology. A deep wedge or punch biopsy is often needed to definitively diagnose cutaneous SCC. Multiple samples recommended as actinic form may encompass spectrum from actinic changes to carcinoma.
- Cytology of lymph nodes to identify presence of regional metastasis.

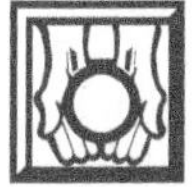

TREATMENT

- Superficial tumors suspected to be solar-induced—wide surgical excision may be locally curative; other treatment options include cryosurgery, photodynamic therapy, or strontium-90 plesiotherapy.
- Invasive tumors—require aggressive surgical excision, external-beam radiation therapy has shown effectiveness.
- MSCCIS may be treated with curative-intent surgery for local control; however, most cats develop new lesions in other sites; treatment with immune-modulating drugs (imiquimod) may be most effective.
- Adjunctive chemotherapy—recommended with incomplete surgical excision, nonresectable mass, and metastasis.
- Electrochemotherapy (bleomycin) and curettage with diathermy may be effective.

Nursing Care

- Analgesics as needed.
- Antibiotic therapy if secondary skin infections.

Client Education

- Discuss UV risk factors associated with the development of the tumor.
- Most cats with MSCCIS will develop new lesions in other sites.

MEDICATIONS

DRUG(S) OF CHOICE

- Imiquimod 5% cream for MSCCIS—topically to affected lesions q24–48h; most cats respond but develop new lesions in other sites.
- Cisplatin—dogs, 60 mg/m^2 IV q3 or 4 weeks for 4 treatments.
- Carboplatin—dogs, 300 mg/m^2 IV q3 weeks; cats, 200–250 mg/m^2 IV q3–4 weeks for 4–5 treatments.
- Mitoxantrone—dogs and cats, 5–6 mg/m^2 IV q3 weeks for 4–5 treatments.

CONTRAINDICATIONS/POSSIBLE INTERACTIONS

Cisplatin—never use in cats; nephrotoxic in dogs.

Alternative Drug(s)

Topical synthetic retinoids (e.g., tretinoin)- may be useful for early solar-induced superficial lesions; may be irritating to skin.

FOLLOW-UP

PATIENT MONITORING

- Physical examination 1 month after resolution of tumor, then every 3 months after treatment.
- Thoracic radiography and lymph node evaluation at each 3-month recheck examination; abdominal ultrasound if the lesion is on the caudal portion of the patient.

PREVENTION/AVOIDANCE

- Limit sun exposure.
- Tattoos on nonpigmented areas may be helpful.

EXPECTED COURSE AND PROGNOSIS

Prognosis—good with superficial lesions that receive appropriate treatment; guarded with invasive lesions, advanced stage of disease, or recurrent lesions.

MISCELLANEOUS

SEE ALSO

- Squamous Cell Carcinoma, Ear.
- Squamous Cell Carcinoma, Nasal Planum.

ABBREVIATIONS

- MSCCIS = multicentric squamous cell carcinoma *in situ*.
- SCC = squamous cell carcinoma.

Suggested Reading

Murphy S. Cutaneous squamous cell carcinoma in the cat: current understanding and treatment approaches. J Feline Med Surg 2013, 15(5):401–407.

Author Alycen P. Lundberg
Consulting Editor Timothy M. Fan
Acknowledgment The author and editors acknowledge the prior contribution of Jackie M. Wypij.

Client Education Handout available online

SQUAMOUS CELL CARCINOMA, TONGUE

BASICS

OVERVIEW

- Malignant tumor of squamous epithelium.
- Rare tumor that occurs more commonly in cats than in dogs.
- Usually grows rapidly.
- Cats—most common lingual neoplasia, often progresses locally prior to clinical evidence of metastasis.
- Dogs—one of most common malignant lingual neoplasias (25–32%); variably metastatic by way of lymphatic vessels to regional lymph nodes and lungs (0–43%).
- Organ system—gastrointestinal.

SIGNALMENT

- Cats—middle-aged or older (>7 years).
- Dogs—average 10–11 years; female large-breed dogs most commonly affected.

SIGNS

Historical Findings

- Ptyalism.
- Halitosis.
- Dysphagia.
- Oral bleeding.
- Decreased appetite.
- Weight loss.
- Poor grooming (cats).

Physical Examination Findings

- Incidental finding.
- Tongue mass—variable appearance, often nodular and ulcerated.
- Intramandibular swelling (cats).
- Cervical lymphadenomegaly—occasionally.

CAUSES & RISK FACTORS

Potential increased risk of feline oral squamous cell carcinoma (SCC) associated with flea collars, canned food (particularly tuna), and possibly exposure to tobacco smoke.

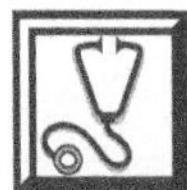

DIAGNOSIS

DIFFERENTIAL DIAGNOSIS

- Other lingual malignancy (melanoma, sarcoma, mast cell tumor, plasmacytoma, lymphoma, hemangiosarcoma, granular cell tumor).
- Trauma.
- Ulcerative glossitis.
- Benign lesion (papilloma).
- Infection/abscess.

CBC/BIOCHEMISTRY/URINALYSIS

Usually normal.

IMAGING

- Advanced imaging with CT or MRI provides greatest information regarding extent of disease.
- Thoracic radiography—three-view required to evaluate lungs for metastasis; more common in dogs.

DIAGNOSTIC PROCEDURES

- Cytology—fine-needle aspirate or impression smear from incisional biopsy (wedge); may yield diagnosis; however, ulceration, inflammation, and secondary infection may limit diagnostic utility.
- Deep wedge tissue biopsy—necessary for definitive diagnosis.
- Cytology and/or lymph node biopsy to evaluate for regional metastasis; more common in dogs.

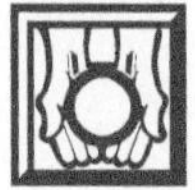

TREATMENT

- Surgical—generally inoperable in cats; aggressive excision warranted in dogs; function of the tongue after recuperation is usually acceptable in dogs, but will require changes in husbandry practices.
- Postsurgical care (e.g., esophagostomy) by owner often required.
- Partial glossectomy—may be performed on the rostral half (mobile tongue) or longitudinal half of the tongue (40–60% removed); ~35–50% of patients have incomplete surgical margins.
- Subtotal glossectomy may be considered in select cases.
- Other surgical methods (e.g., electrocautery and cryosurgery) do not offer additional advantage to conventional excision.
- Response to radiotherapy—poor (<7 weeks); may be used adjunctively on microscopic disease postoperatively.
- Systemic therapies—chemotherapy agents or toceranib phosphate effective in oral SCC may exert anticancer activities for lingual SCC.
- Piroxicam may have antineoplastic activity in some patients.
- Supportive/palliative medications for analgesia and antibiotics for secondary bacterial infections may be indicated.

MEDICATIONS

DRUG(S) OF CHOICE

- Carboplatin—dogs, 300 mg/m^2 IV q3–4 weeks; cats, 180–250 mg/m^2 IV q3–4 weeks for 4- 5 treatments.
- Piroxicam—dogs, 0.3 mg/kg PO q24h; cats, 0.3 mg/kg PO q48h.
- Toceranib phosphate (Palladia)—dogs and cats, 2.5–3.25 mg/kg PO q48h.

CONTRAINDICATIONS/POSSIBLE INTERACTIONS

N/A

FOLLOW-UP

PATIENT MONITORING

After complete surgical resection, recheck at 1–2 months and then every 3 months with physical examination and evaluation for metastasis (lymph node palpation/aspiration and thoracic imaging).

POSSIBLE COMPLICATIONS

Possible complications postoperatively—long-term difficulty prehending food, local recurrence.

EXPECTED COURSE AND PROGNOSIS

- Prognosis—poor, owing to extensive local disease (cat) and local recurrence (28% for all lingual tumors) and moderate rate of metastasis (dog).
- After surgical excision (subtotal glossectomy, dogs)—median survival 216 days, <25% survive 1 year.
- Negative prognostic factors (dogs)—caudal location, incomplete excision, recurrence, larger size (>2 cm); histologic grade, metastatic disease.
- Piroxicam—17% response rate in oral SCC with a median progression-free interval of 3.5–6 months; one partial response in 3 dogs with lingual SCC.
- Prognosis in cats similar to other oral sites of SCC; median survival ~3 months with multimodal therapy.

MISCELLANEOUS

SEE ALSO

- Melanocytic Tumors, Oral.
- Squamous Cell Carcinoma, Gingiva.
- Squamous Cell Carcinoma, Tonsil.

ABBREVIATIONS

- SCC = squamous cell carcinoma.

Suggested Reading

Culp WT, Ehrhart N, Withrow SJ, et al. Results of surgical excision and evaluation of factors associated with survival time in dogs with lingual neoplasia: 97 cases (1995–2008). J Am Vet Med Assoc 2013, 242(10):1392–1397.

Author Alycen P. Lundberg

Consulting Editor Timothy M. Fan

Acknowledgment The author and editors acknowledge the prior contribution of Jackie M. Wypij.

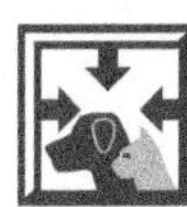

BASICS

OVERVIEW

- Rapid and progressive invasion of neoplastic squamous epithelium arising from the tonsillar fossa into tonsillar lymphoid tissue.
- More common in dogs than cats—comprises 9% of canine oral tumors.
- Highly locally invasive into soft tissues.
- Early metastasis—70–90% eventually metastasize regardless of local control.

SIGNALMENT

- Dog and cat; median age 10 years.
- No known breed or sex predilection.

SIGNS

Historical Findings

- Cough.
- Enlarged lymph nodes.
- Dysphagia.
- Ptyalism.
- Retching.
- Halitosis.
- Weight loss.
- Anorexia.
- Lethargy.

Physical Examination Findings

- Enlarged tonsil(s).
- Widening or "fullness" of oropharyngeal space.
- Cervical lymphadenomegaly.
- Pain on opening jaw.

CAUSES & RISK FACTORS

Exact cause unknown; however, 10 times more common in animals living in urban environments vs. those in rural environments.

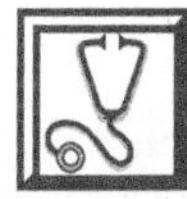

DIAGNOSIS

DIFFERENTIAL DIAGNOSIS

- Lymphoma (generally associated with lymphadenomegaly and bilateral disease).
- Abscess.
- Metastatic neoplasm (oral melanoma, sarcoma).
- Tonsillitis.
- Tonsillar crypt foreign body.
- Salivary gland tumor.
- Thyroid carcinoma.

CBC/BIOCHEMISTRY/URINALYSIS

Usually normal.

IMAGING

- Thoracic radiography—three-view to detect lung metastasis; 5–20% positive for metastasis at presentation; 60–85% metastasis at death.
- CT—evaluate local extension of primary tumor as well as mandibular and retropharyngeal lymph node involvement; recommended prior to surgery or radiation therapy.
- Abdominal ultrasound—evaluate abdominal organs; 20% disseminated metastasis to multiple organs at death (dogs).

DIAGNOSTIC PROCEDURES

- Cytology—inflammation and secondary infection may limit diagnostic utility of fine-needle aspirate samples but should still be attempted.
- Histopathology—deep tissue biopsy may be needed to differentiate from other oral malignancies.
- Cytology and/or biopsy of regional lymph nodes to evaluate for metastatic disease; in dogs 20–55% metastasis at diagnosis.

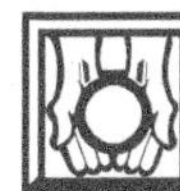

TREATMENT

- Surgery—many are inoperable; tonsillectomy, when done, should be bilateral.
- Postoperative care (esophagostomy or gastrotomy tube) by owner may be needed.
- Other surgical methods (electrocautery and cryosurgery)—no advantage over conventional excision.
- Regional radiation therapy is effective for local control and palliation of clinical signs.
- Chemotherapy—anecdotal reports of cisplatin, carboplatin, doxorubicin being used with limited success.
- Piroxicam and/or toceranib phosphate (Palladia) may have antineoplastic effects in canine carcinomas.
- Analgesics for pain control; antibiotics for secondary bacterial infections may be indicated.

MEDICATIONS

DRUG(S) OF CHOICE

- Carboplatin—dogs, 300 mg/m^2 IV q3–4 weeks; cats, 180–240 mg/m^2 IV q3–4 weeks for 4–5 treatments.
- Mitoxantrone—dogs and cats, 5–6 mg/m^2 IV q2–3 weeks for 5 treatments.
- Piroxicam—dogs, 0.3 mg/kg PO q24h, toceranib phosphate (Palladia) 2.75–3.25 mg/kg PO q48h.
- Doxorubicin—dogs >10 kg, 30 mg/m^2 IV; dogs <10 kg and cats, 1 mg/kg q2–3 weeks for 5 treatments.
- Cisplatin—dogs, 60–70 mg/m^2 IV q3–4 weeks for 4 treatments.

CONTRAINDICATIONS/POSSIBLE INTERACTIONS

Cisplatin—never use in cats; nephrotoxic in dogs.

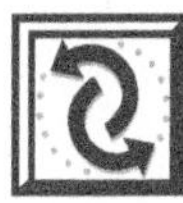

FOLLOW-UP

PATIENT MONITORING

Most patients euthanized within months for local progression or metastasis; patients with curative-intent therapies should be rechecked with physical examination and evaluated for metastasis (thoracic radiographs/CT) at 1–2 months, then every 3 months.

POSSIBLE COMPLICATIONS

Postoperative complications—tumor recurrence, may need feeding tubes postoperatively.

EXPECTED COURSE AND PROGNOSIS

- Prognosis—poor owing to extensive local disease and high rate of recurrence (tongue, pharynx, lymph nodes) and metastasis.
- Minimal information in cats; however, appear to carry a grave prognosis as with most oral squamous cell carcinomas in cats.
- Dogs: 11–40% 1-year survival (survival times increased if unilateral and no metastasis at diagnosis).
- Untreated (dogs) median survival 1–2 months vs. treated median survival 7–8 months.
- Surgery alone has limited benefit—median survival 2–4 months (dogs).
- Palliative radiotherapy or chemotherapy (dogs)—75% response rate, 2–9 months median survival.
- Surgery, radiation therapy, and chemotherapy (dogs)—median survival 9–12 months.
- Piroxicam alone—17% response rate for all oral squamous cell carcinoma with a median progression-free interval of 3.5–6 months; 3 of 5 dogs with tonsillar SCC exhibiting a partial remission or stable disease.

MISCELLANEOUS

SEE ALSO

- Squamous Cell Carcinoma, Gingiva.
- Squamous Cell Carcinoma, Tongue.

Suggested Reading

Grant J, North S. Evaluation of the factors contributing to long-term survival in canine tonsillar squamous cell carcinoma. Aust Vet J 2016, 94(6):197–202.

Author Alycen P. Lundberg

Consulting Editor Timothy M. Fan

Acknowledgment The author and editors acknowledge the prior contribution of Jackie M. Wypij.

STAPHYLOCOCCAL INFECTIONS

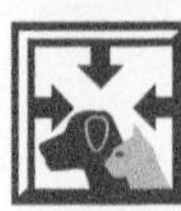

BASICS

OVERVIEW

- *Staphylococcus*—Gram-positive, nonmotile, facultatively anaerobic, spherical bacteria (cocci); *staphyle* (Greek "bunch of grapes") form characteristic microscopic arrangement in clusters.
- Results in variety of infections characterized by pus formation.
- Can produce toxins (superantigens) that exert profound systemic signs (fever, hypotension, shock, multiorgan failure, death).
- Ubiquitous; live free in environment and as commensal parasites of skin and upper respiratory tract.
- Pathogenic and nonpathogenic strains; wide spectrum of virulence, host range, and site specificities; not strictly host- or site-specific.
- Pathogenic strains—possess extracellular toxins and enzymes (e.g., coagulase, staphylokinase, hemolysin, epidermolysins); staphylocoagulase in more pathogenic strains (e.g., *S. pseudintermedius*, *S. aureus*).
- Coagulase-negative staphylococci are less virulent (e.g., *S. felis*, *S. epidermidis*).
- Methicillin-resistant staphylococci, which are increasingly isolated from dogs and cats, is an emerging problem due to multidrug resistance phenotype which limits treatment options and challenges infection control measures. When a methicillin-resistant strain expresses co-resistance to at least two additional antimicrobial classes then it is called multidrug resistant (MDR).

S

SIGNALMENT

- Dogs and cats.
- Very young—susceptible because of incomplete, developing immunity.
- Old, debilitated—susceptible because of impaired host defenses.
- Immunocompromised—more susceptible.

SIGNS

- Abscesses and infections of the skin, eyes, ears, respiratory system, genitourinary tract, skeleton, and joints.
- Dogs—pyoderma, otitis externa, cystitis, prostatitis, pneumonia, abscesses, osteomyelitis, discospondylitis, arthritis, mastitis, bacteremia, endocarditis, wound infections, toxic shock syndrome.
- Cats—abscesses, oral infections, otitis externa, conjunctivitis, metritis, cholangiohepatitis, cystitis, bacteremia.
- Fever.
- Anorexia.
- Pain.
- Pruritus.
- Can affect every organ system.

CAUSES & RISK FACTORS

- Opportunistic pathogens depending on virulence factors:
    - Adhesion expression (binds bacteria to cells and extracellular matrix).
    - Toxins (cytolytic, exfoliative, enterotoxigenic, superantigen toxins).
    - Expression of factors to evade the host's immune response (e.g., coagulase).
    - Formation of biofilms which protect the bacterium from the immune response.
- Disease—from disturbance of the natural host–parasite equilibrium when local and general defense mechanisms are significantly lowered (e.g., chronic debilitating diseases).
- Secondary infection—allergies (atopy, food, fleas); endocrinopathies (hypothyroidism, hyperadrenocorticism); parasites (demodicosis); seborrhea.
- Burns or wounds—complications.
- Biofilms (extracellular polysaccharide networks) support infection of implants and invasive devices (e.g., IV catheters).
- Transmission—airborne organisms, carriers, direct contact (droplet nuclei).
- *S. pseudintermedius*—most common staphylococcal species isolated from dogs, commensal organism on skin and mucous membranes of dog and cat (although much lower prevalence in cats). Methicillin-resistant *S. pseudintermedius* (MRSP) is a clinically important pathogen causing antibiotic resistant infections in dogs and cats (see Multidrug Resistant Infections).
- *S. aureus*—does not colonize dogs as often as *S. pseudintermedius*; colonizes skin and mucosal membranes of humans where it is one of the most common community-acquired and hospital-acquired pathogens of people. Methicillin-resistant *S. aureus* (MRSA) infections uncommonly diagnosed in dogs and cats.
- *S. schleiferi*—coagulase variable species; rarely isolated from healthy skin of dogs or cats but commonly isolated from skin and ear canal infections of dogs with history of prior antimicrobial exposures.
- Risk factors for methicillin-resistant staphylococcus in dogs include previous antibiotic therapy, previous hospitalization, urban environment, older age.

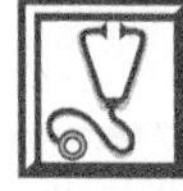

DIAGNOSIS

DIFFERENTIAL DIAGNOSIS

- Dermatitis—allergies, seborrhea, parasites, immune-mediated.
- Other infectious causes—viruses, bacteria, fungi, *Rickettsia*, protozoa.
- Neoplasia.
- Immune-mediated diseases.

CBC/BIOCHEMISTRY/URINALYSIS

- Normal or high white blood cells (WBCs) consisting of neutrophilia ± left shift.
- Biochemistry—may suggest predisposing cause.
- Urinalysis—pyuria (with or without bacteruria) with cystitis.

OTHER LABORATORY TESTS

- Direct microscopy.
- Gram stain.
- Cytology—neutrophils and cocci singly or in pairs, short chains, or irregular clusters.
- Culture—avoid superficial contamination; collect samples by aspiration, wash, or biopsy; do not overinterpret a positive isolation; organisms can be isolated from normal animals
- Organisms survive up to 48 hours in clinical specimens when kept cool (4°C/40°F), particularly on swabs containing a holding medium.
- Antibiotic susceptibility testing (very important due to methicillin-resistant and multidrug-resistant staphylococci).
- Pulsed-field gel electrophoresis molecular typing.

IMAGING

Radiology—osteolytic and osteoproliferative lesions with osteomyelitis; interstitial or alveolar pulmonary pattern with pneumonia; radiodense uroliths (struvite). Endocarditis lesions may be visible by echocardiography. Ultrasonography may identify abscesses.

DIAGNOSTIC PROCEDURES

Cerebrospinal fluid tap—if meningitis or discospondylitis suspected; discospondylitis lesions may be fine-needle aspirated using CT or ultrasound guidance.

PATHOLOGIC FINDINGS

Characteristic abscess lesion—necrotic tissue, fibrin, and a large number of neutrophils.

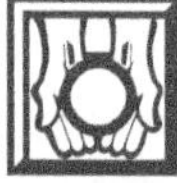

TREATMENT

- Identify and manage predisposing cause to minimize selection for antibiotic-resistant staphylococci.
- Properly handle and dispose of contaminated objects, practice good hand hygiene and wear personal protective equipment (PPE) when handing patient with known or suspected methicillin-resistant staphylococcus infection.
- Topical antibacterial cleaning of wounds and pyoderma—chlorhexidine, benzoyl peroxide shampoos.
- Known or suspected methicillin-resistant staphylococcus-infected animals should be isolated.

MEDICATIONS

DRUG(S) OF CHOICE

- Antibiotic resistance—great propensity owing to production of β-lactamase, which

inactivates penicillins; may carry plasmids (segments of genetic material that may carry genes for antimicrobial resistance) that can be transferred to other strains of staphylococci or species of bacteria.
- History of previous antimicrobial therapy for staphylococcal infection—culture and antibiotic susceptibility testing indicated: choose drugs below based on this testing.
- Use topical therapy when possible.
- Non-penicillinase-producing strains:
  - Penicillin G 10,000–20,000 U/kg IM, SC q12–24h, penicillin V 8–30 mg/kg PO q8h.
  - Amoxicillin 22 mg/kg PO q6–8h or ampicillin 22–30 mg/kg IV, IM, SC q6–8h.
- Penicillinase-producing strains:
  - First-generation cephalosporins—cephalexin at 22 mg/kg PO q8h; cefadroxil at 22 mg/kg PO q8–12h.
  - β-Lactamase-resistant synthetic penicillins—clavulanic acid-potentiated amoxicillin 20–25 mg/kg PO q8–12h, oxacillin 22–40 mg/kg PO q8h, dicloxacillin 10–25 mg/kg PO q8h).
- Gentamicin 2–4 mg/kg IV, IM, SC q8h or amikacin 15 mg/kg IV q24h.
- Trimethoprim-potentiated sulfonamides—30 mg/kg IV, PO q12h.
- Chloramphenicol—40–50 mg/kg IV, IM, SC, PO q8–12h.
- Methicillin-resistant staphylococci express *mecA* gene which encodes an altered penicillin-binding protein (PBP-2a) which has a low affinity for all β-lactam drugs (penicillins, cephalosporins, and carbapenems).
- In patients with penicillin allergy—try cephalosporin, clindamycin, enrofloxacin, or vancomycin (although this is strongly discouraged to reserve vancomycin for treatment of serious MRSA infections in humans).

CONTRAINDICATIONS/POSSIBLE INTERACTIONS

Avoid immunosuppressive drugs.

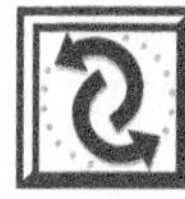

FOLLOW-UP

As appropriate for location of infection

MISCELLANEOUS

ZOONOTIC POTENTIAL

- Possible; MRSA is also potential anthropozoonosis.
- Most people and pets carry their own pathogenic staphylococcal flora; disease is not caused by mere exposure; however, transfer from dogs to humans is possible, and vice versa.
- Bite infections contain a mix of aerobes and anaerobes from both the skin of the patient and the mouth of the animal, including *Staphylococcus*.
- Hand hygiene (proper washing/drying and use of alcohol-based hand sanitizers) and use of PPE is an integral part of the prevention of the spread of MRSA/MRSP between animals and MRSA between animals and humans.
- Owners of dogs and cats with MRSA infection should be educated to wash their hands after handling their pets, to clean and disinfect surfaces that might become contaminated, and to not let their pet lick their face or open wounds. If owners have concerns about their health or the health of others in their household then they should be instructed to talk to their health care provider.

ABBREVIATIONS

- MDR = multidrug resistant.
- MRSA = methicillin-resistant *Staphylococcus aureus*.
- MRSP = methicillin-resistant *Staphylococcus pseudintermedius*.
- PPE = personal protective equipment.
- WBC = white blood cell.

INTERNET RESOURCES

www.cdc.gov/mrsa

Suggested Reading

Béco L, Guaguère E, Lorente Mendez C, et al. Suggested guidelines for using systemic antimicrobials in bacterial skin infections (2): antimicrobial choice, treatment regimens and compliance. Vet Rec 2013, 172:156–160.

Cain CL. Antimicrobial resistance in staphylococci in small animals. Vet Clin Small Anim 2013; 43:19–40.

Davis JA, Jackson CR, Fedorka-Cray PJ, et al. Carriage of methicillin-resistant staphylococci by healthy companion animals in the US. Lett Appl Microbiol 2014, 59:1–8.

Morris DO, Loeffler A, Davis MF, et al. Recommendations for approaches to meticillin-resistant staphylococcal infections of small animals: diagnosis, therapeutic considerations and preventative measures. Vet Dermatol 2017, 28:304–331.

Sykes JE. Staphylococcus infections. In: Sykes JE, ed., Canine and Feline Infectious Diseases. St. Louis, MO: Elsevier, 2014, pp. 347–354.

Author J. Paul Woods
Consulting Editor Amie Koenig

STEROID-RESPONSIVE MENINGITIS-ARTERITIS—DOGS

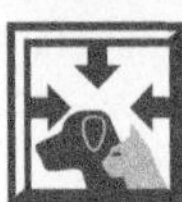

BASICS

OVERVIEW

- May be acute or protracted.
- Lesions—most impressive in CNS, affecting meninges and meningeal arteries; sometimes peracute bleeding; vascular changes in the heart, liver, kidney, and gastrointestinal system.
- Genetic factors—play a role in different breeds such as beagles and Nova Scotia duck tolling retrievers.
- Worldwide occurrence.

SIGNALMENT

- Dog.
- Beagle, Bernese mountain dog, Nova Scotia duck tolling retriever, and boxer predisposed; any breed can be affected.
- Mostly young adult dogs of both sexes; age range 5–18 months.

SIGNS

- Classical (acute)—hyperesthesia; cervical rigidity; stiff gait; fever up to 42°C (107.6°F).
- Protracted—neurologic deficits, usually reflecting a spinal cord or multifocal lesion.

CAUSES & RISK FACTORS

- Cause unknown.
- Pathologic findings, laboratory data, and marked response to steroids—suggest an immune-mediated disease related to a dysregulation of IgA production and a Th17-skewed immune response.
- Epidemiologic observations—altered immune response may be triggered by an environmental factor, possibly of infectious nature; genetic predisposition.

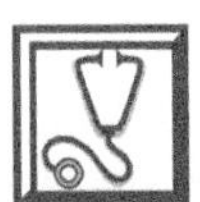

DIAGNOSIS

DIFFERENTIAL DIAGNOSIS

- Acute—bacterial meningitis; meningeal tumors; discospondylitis.
- Protracted—bacterial meningitis; meningeal tumors (histiocytosis, meningioma, lymphosarcoma); other infectious encephalitides; meningoencephalomyelitis of unknown origin.

CBC/BIOCHEMISTRY/URINALYSIS

- Acute—leukocytosis with neutrophilia and left shift.
- Protracted—CBC noncontributory.

OTHER LABORATORY TESTS

IgA levels (serum and CSF)—usually high; high serum C-reactive protein (CRP) levels.

IMAGING

Radiographs to exclude discospondylitis; MRI to exclude differential diagnoses.

DIAGNOSTIC PROCEDURES

Cerebrospinal Fluid Analysis

- Acute—mild-to-moderate elevation of protein; moderate-to-marked pleocytosis, predominantly polymorphonuclear cells.
- Protracted—normal, or mild elevation of protein; mild-to-moderate pleocytosis with mixed cell population, or with a predominance of mononuclear cells.

PATHOLOGIC FINDINGS

Acute

- Marked meningitis with macrophages, plasma cells, lymphocytes, and varying numbers of polymorphonuclear cells mostly in the cervical region.
- Lesions of the meningeal arteries—degenerative with perivascular inflammation.

Protracted

- Marked fibrous thickening and focal mineralization of the leptomeninges.
- Arterial walls—thickened and stenotic from cellular proliferation of the intima and fibrosis.

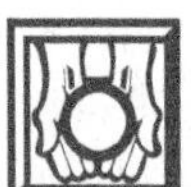

TREATMENT

- Inpatient—at onset, fluid therapy and ice packs useful for high body temperature.
- After initial treatment, managed as outpatient.
- Regular follow-ups—inform client about side effects of long-term steroid treatment.

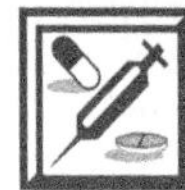

MEDICATIONS

DRUG(S) OF CHOICE

- Initial signs with mild CSF pleocytosis—nonsteroidal anti-inflammatory drugs (NSAIDs); carefully monitor the patient.
- First relapse, or symptoms become worse with marked CSF pleocytosis—start long-term treatment (6 months) with prednisolone 4 mg/kg PO q24h for 1–2 days; then taper slowly; reexamine patient (CSF collection, blood profile or CRP) every 4–6 weeks after initiation of therapy.
- Neurologic examination and CSF become normal, normal serum CRP levels—reduce steroid dose.
- Persistent pleocytosis—continue same steroid dosage.
- Treatment may be stopped after about 6 months.
- Immunosuppressive drugs if patient does not respond well to prednisolone alone; used in combination.
- Consider gastrointestinal protector to avoid ulcer.

CONTRAINDICATIONS/POSSIBLE INTERACTIONS

Corticosteroids—high-dose treatment can lead to severe complications; non-life-threatening side effects (polyuria, polydipsia, polyphagia, and weight gain); not tolerated in about 5% of dogs.

FOLLOW-UP

PATIENT MONITORING

Control examinations—every 4–6 weeks; include blood examination and CSF collection; measurement of serum CRP levels until steroids discontinued.

PREVENTION/AVOIDANCE

Strictly control treatment schedule to prevent frequent relapses. No reliable predictive indicator available for relapse.

POSSIBLE COMPLICATIONS

- Subarachnoid bleed—may result in acute tetra- or paraplegia.
- Hypoxic lesions of spinal cord or brain.
- Side effects of immunosuppressive treatment.

EXPECTED COURSE AND PROGNOSIS

- Acute—prognosis relatively good in young dogs with early therapy.
- Protracted cases with frequent relapses—prognosis guarded; controlled studies note about 60% of dogs are cured after immunosuppressive treatment. Relapses occur in about 32% of the dogs.

MISCELLANEOUS

ASSOCIATED CONDITIONS

Polyarthritis

AGE-RELATED FACTORS

Old animals do not tolerate long-term steroid treatment well, but condition rare in dogs >5 years of age.

SYNONYMS

- Aseptic meningitis.
- Canine juvenile polyarteritis syndrome.
- Corticosteroid-responsive meningomyelitis.

ABBREVIATIONS

- CRP = C-reactive protein.
- NSAID = nonsteroidal anti-inflammatory drug.

Suggested Reading

Biedermann E, Tipold A, Flegel T. Relapses in dogs with steroid-responsive meningitis-arteritis. J Small Anim Pract 2016, 57:91–95.

Author Andrea Tipold

STERTOR AND STRIDOR

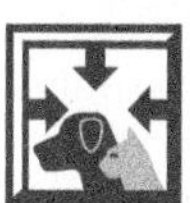

BASICS

DEFINITION

• Abnormally loud sounds that result from air passing through a narrowed nasopharynx, pharynx, larynx, or trachea.
• Discontinuous sounds heard without a stethoscope.
• Stertor—low-pitched snoring sound that usually arises from the vibration of flaccid tissue or fluid; usually arises from nasal or pharyngeal airway obstruction.
• Stridor—higher pitched sounds that result when relatively rigid tissues are vibrated by the passage of air; result of partial or complete obstruction of the larynx or cervical trachea.

PATHOPHYSIOLOGY

• Airway obstruction causes turbulence as air travels through a narrowed passage; with worsening obstruction or increasing airflow velocity, the amplification of airway sounds occur due to increased turbulence and vibration of tissue, secretions, or foreign bodies.
• Obstruction sufficient to increase the work of breathing augments respiratory muscle effort and exacerbates turbulence; inflammation and edema of tissues in the region of the obstruction may develop, further reducing the airway lumen and further increasing the work of breathing, creating a vicious cycle.
• Complete airway obstruction will result in the lack of sounds.
• Obesity further increases respiratory effort and exacerbates airway obstruction.

SYSTEMS AFFECTED

Respiratory

GENETICS

• Brachycephalic obstructive airway syndrome is heritable in many breeds, including English and French bulldogs, pugs, Boston terriers, shih tzus, and other brachycephalic breeds.
• Congenital laryngeal paralysis has been identified in bouvier des Flandres, bull terriers, Siberian huskies, Alaskan Malamutes, and white-coated German shepherd dogs. Dalmatians, Rottweilers, Leonbergers, and Pyrenees mountain dogs.
• Older large breed dogs (e.g., Labrador retrievers) commonly develop laryngeal paralysis as part of a geriatric-onset laryngeal paralysis polyneuropathy complex.

INCIDENCE/PREVALENCE

Common

GEOGRAPHIC DISTRIBUTION

Worldwide

SIGNALMENT

Species

Dog more than cat.

Breed Predilections

• Common in brachycephalic dogs and less so cats
• Acquired laryngeal paralysis—overrepresented in certain giant breeds (e.g., Saint Bernard and Newfoundlands) and large breeds (e.g., Irish setters, Labrador retrievers, and golden retrievers).
• Cats of any breed due to nasopharyngeal polyps, inflammatory or neoplastic laryngeal diseases, or laryngeal paralysis (the latter far less common in cats than dogs).

Mean Age and Range

• Affected brachycephalic animals and dogs or cats with inherited laryngeal paralysis are typically younger than 1 year of age when owners detect a problem.
• Acquired laryngeal paralysis typically occurs in older dogs and cats.

Predominant Sex

No sex predilection for any cause, although inherited laryngeal paralysis has a 3:1 male predominance.

SIGNS

• Change or loss of voice.
• Partial obstruction—produces an increase in airway sounds before producing an obvious change in respiratory pattern or gas exchange.
• Owners may indicate that the sound has existed for as long as several years.
• Breath sounds audible from a distance without a stethoscope—suspect narrowing of upper airway.
• Nature of the sound—ranges from abnormally loud to obvious fluttering to high-pitched squeaking, depending on the degree of airway narrowing.
• Stress or exercise may amplify the sound or induce respiratory distress.
• May note increased respiratory effort and paradoxical respiratory movements (chest wall collapses inward during inspiration and springs outward during expiration) when the effort is extreme; respiratory motions often accompanied by obvious postural changes (e.g., abducted forelimbs, extended head and neck, and open-mouth breathing).

CAUSES

• Brachycephalic airway syndrome (stenotic nares, elongated soft palate, everted laryngeal saccules, laryngeal collapse).
• Laryngeal paralysis—inherited or acquired.
• Laryngeal neoplasia—benign or malignant.
• Granulomatous/inflammatory laryngitis.
• Tracheal collapse, stenosis, obstruction, neoplasia, foreign body.
• Nasopharyngeal polyp, stenosis, foreign body.
• Cervical bite wounds.
• Acromegaly.
• Neuromuscular dysfunction.
• Anesthesia or sedation—only if predisposing anatomy exists.
• Cleft palate.
• Aplasia of soft palate.
• Redundant pharyngeal mucosal folds.
• Soft palate mass.
• Edema or inflammation of the palate, pharynx, and larynx (including everted mucosal lining of the laryngeal ventricles)—secondary to coughing, vomiting or regurgitation, turbulent airflow, upper respiratory infection, and hemorrhage.
• Secretions (e.g., pus, mucus, and blood) in the airway lumen.

RISK FACTORS

• High ambient temperature or humidity.
• Fever.
• High metabolic rate—as occurs with hyperthyroidism or sepsis.
• Exercise.
• Anxiety or excitement.
• Any respiratory or cardiovascular disease that increases ventilation.
• Turbulence caused by the increased airflow can lead to swelling and worsen the airway obstruction.
• Hypothyroidism or polyneuropathy.
• Obesity.

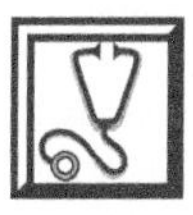

DIAGNOSIS

DIFFERENTIAL DIAGNOSIS

• Systematically auscultate over the nose, pharynx, larynx, and trachea to identify the point of maximal intensity of any abnormal sound and to identify the phase of respiration when it is most obvious.
• Important to identify the anatomic location from which the abnormal sound arises and to seek exacerbating causes (see Risk Factors; e.g., a chronic airway obstruction may become manifest when the patient is exposed to extremely high ambient temperatures).
• Must differentiate sounds of pharyngeal, laryngeal, and tracheal narrowing from sounds arising elsewhere in the respiratory system.
• Nasal and tracheal narrowing and severe or extensive narrowing of the bronchi—can cause increased respiratory sounds.
• If the sound persists when the patient opens its mouth, a nasal cause can virtually be ruled out.
• If the owner describes a change in voice, the larynx is the likely abnormal site.

OTHER LABORATORY TESTS

Arterial blood gases—help characterize the degree of respiratory compromise (e.g., degree of hypoxemia, hypercapnia, or acid–base disturbances).

IMAGING

• Lateral radiographs of the head and neck—may help identify abnormal soft tissues of the airway (e.g., elongated soft palate or a nasal polyp); limited use for identifying laryngeal paralysis, although experienced radiographers can identify abnormally dilated or swollen laryngeal saccules; cartilaginous destruction is suggestive of neoplasia or granulomatous laryngitis; may detect external masses compressing the upper airway.

STERTOR AND STRIDOR (CONTINUED)

• Radiography and fluoroscopy—important for assessing the cardiorespiratory system; rule out other or additional causes of respiratory difficulty; such conditions may add to an underlying upper airway obstruction, causing a subclinical condition to become clinical.
• Ultrasound can be used to assess laryngeal structure and function, can also be used to document cervical tracheal collapse but air is a poor acoustic window.
• CT can be used to provide additional anatomic detail.

DIAGNOSTIC PROCEDURES

Laryngoscopy

• Definitive diagnostic tests for direct visualization of pharyngeal or laryngeal changes.
• Requires sedation that preserves laryngeal function. Recommend propofol 4–8 mg/kg IV to effect.
• The patient's ability to use muscles to open the airway is compromised by anesthesia; be prepared to correct any lesions found, at a minimum, be prepared to intubate.
• If correctable conditions are not identified and corrected—patient's recovery from anesthesia can be complicated by severe airway obstruction; must be prepared to perform a tracheotomy if airway is obstructed and a definitive surgical remedy cannot be pursued immediately.
• Assess timing and degree of movement of the arytenoids during light anesthesia—laryngeal paralysis results in lack of abduction of the arytenoids during inspiration. Use doxapram 1–2 mg/kg IV to stimulate respiration if needed.
• Normal palate—thin; just barely overlaps the tips of the epiglottis; easily displaced dorsally using the blade of the laryngoscope.
• Overlong soft palate—thick; usually inflamed; may lie 1 cm or more past the tip of the epiglottis.

S

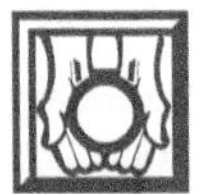

TREATMENT

APPROPRIATE HEALTH CARE

• Inpatient management required for surgical treatment.
• Closely monitor effects of sedatives; sedatives can relax the upper airway muscles and worsen the obstruction; be prepared with emergency methods for securing the airway if complete obstruction occurs.
• In cases of suspected laryngeal paralysis resulting in respiratory distress and partial obstruction in dogs, sedation with butorphanol 0.2–0.3 mg/kg and acepromazine 0.025–0.05 mg/kg with oxygen supplementation and active cooling measures if hyperthermic may be indicated.
• If available, use of high-flow oxygen nasal cannulation has been successful to treat partial airway obstruction.
• Severe or complete airway obstruction—attempt an emergency intubation; if obstruction prevents intubation, emergency tracheostomy or passage of a tracheal catheter to administer oxygen may be the only available means for sustaining life; a tracheal catheter can briefly sustain oxygenation while a more permanent solution is sought.

NURSING CARE

• Treatment requires removal of obstruction, supplemental oxygen is variably helpful.
• IV fluids may be required, particularly if hyperthermia develops from increased work of breathing.
• Active cooling measures (ice packs in axilla and groin region, alcohol on foot pads, chilled IV fluids) helpful in alleviating hyperthermia but not indicated for fever.

ACTIVITY

Keep patient cool, quiet, and calm—anxiety, exertion, and pain lead to increased ventilation, potentially worsening the obstruction.

DIET

• NPO if anesthesia is planned.
• Dietary management to avoid obesity, a known risk factor for developing airway obstruction and associated stertor or stridor.

CLIENT EDUCATION

Inform client that the patient can make the transition from being a noisy breather to having an obstructed airway in a few minutes or even seconds.

SURGICAL CONSIDERATIONS

• Laryngoscopy and bronchoscopy for foreign body retrieval and biopsy of laryngeal region and tracheal lumen. Use of small balloon catheters passed beyond the foreign body prior to expansion may be useful in removing some objects.
• Take particular care when inducing general anesthesia or when using sedatives in any patient with upper airway obstruction.
• Surgery—indicated to obtain a diagnosis through biopsy with histopathology, to manage obstruction while awaiting histopathology results or resolution of inflammation/infection (e.g., tracheotomy), or to resolve disease by excision, correction of obstructive lesion, and removal of foreign bodies.

MEDICATIONS

DRUG(S) OF CHOICE

• Medical approaches—appropriate only if the underlying cause is infection, edema, inflammation, or hemorrhage; anatomic or neurologic causes are not amenable to medical treatment.
• Steroids—may be indicated if edema or inflammation is thought to be an important contributor; effect with IV administration of a short-acting glucocorticoid such as dexamethasone sodium phosphate (1 mg/kg prednisone equivalent) should be apparent in the first several hours. Single dose may be sufficient, or a tapering dose might be required. Inflammatory laryngitis often requires higher doses administered over a longer dosing schedule with taper of the dose according to resolution of clinical signs.

PRECAUTIONS

Sedatives, analgesics, and anesthetics—avoid excessive suppression of laryngeal movement and respiratory suppression to avoid aspiration in animals with laryngeal disease.

FOLLOW-UP

PATIENT MONITORING

Respiratory rate and effort need to be closely monitored. When owner chooses to take an apparently stable patient home, or if continual observation is not feasible, inform client that complete obstruction could occur.

PREVENTION/AVOIDANCE

Advise client to avoid exercise, high ambient temperatures, and extreme excitement.

POSSIBLE COMPLICATIONS

Serious complications may occur without therapy to relieve the obstruction; these include airway edema, pulmonary edema (may progress to life-threatening acute lung injury), and hypoventilation; may require tracheotomy and/or artificial ventilation.

EXPECTED COURSE AND PROGNOSIS

• Varies with underlying cause.
• Even with surgical treatment, some degree of obstruction may remain for 7–10 days due to swelling.

MISCELLANEOUS

ASSOCIATED CONDITIONS

Peripheral neuropathy often associated with laryngeal paralysis.

SYNONYMS

Snoring

SEE ALSO

• Brachycephalic Airway Syndrome.
• Hypothyroidism.
• Laryngeal Diseases.
• Myasthenia Gravis.
• Nasal and Nasopharyngeal Polyps.
• Tracheal Collapse.

Suggested Reading

MacPhail C. Laryngeal disease in dogs and cats. Vet Clin Small Anim 2014, 44:19–31.
Sumner C, Rozanski EA. Management of respiratory emergencies in small animals. Vet Clin Small Anim 2013, 43:799–815.

Author Sean B. Majoy
Consulting Editor Elizabeth Rozanski
Acknowledgment The author and editors acknowledge the prior contribution of James C. Preuter.

Client Education Handout available online

STOMATITIS AND ORAL ULCERATION

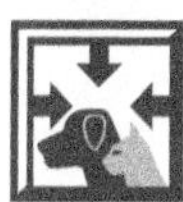

BASICS

DEFINITION

- Stomatitis—an inflammation of the tissues of the oral cavity, more specifically defined below.
- Ulceration—focal or multifocal loss of mucosal integrity of the superficial epithelial layers in specific areas of the oral cavity.
- American Veterinary Dental College Nomenclature—oral and oropharyngeal inflammation is classified by location as:
    - Stomatitis—inflammation of the mucous lining of any of the structures in the mouth; in clinical use the term should be reserved to describe widespread oral inflammation (beyond gingivitis and periodontitis) that may also extend into submucosal tissues (e.g., marked caudal mucositis extending into submucosal tissues may be termed caudal stomatitis).
    - Gingivitis—inflammation of gingiva.
    - Periodontitis—inflammation of nongingival periodontal tissue (i.e., the periodontal ligament and alveolar bone).
    - Alveolar mucositis—inflammation of alveolar mucosa.
    - Sublingual mucositis—inflammation of mucosa on the floor of the mouth.
    - Labial/buccal mucositis—inflammation of the lip/cheek mucosa.
    - Caudal mucositis—inflammation of mucosa of the caudal oral cavity.
    - Contact mucositis and contact mucosal ulceration ("contact ulcers" and "kissing ulcers")—lesions in susceptible individuals that are secondary to mucosal contact with a tooth surface bearing the responsible irritant, allergen or antigen.
    - Palatitis—inflammation of mucosa covering the hard and/or soft palate.
    - Glossitis—inflammation of mucosa of the dorsal and/or ventral tongue surface.
    - Cheilitis—inflammation of the lip (including the mucocutaneous junction area and skin of the lip).
    - Osteomyelitis—inflammation of the bone and bone marrow.
    - Tonsilitis—inflammation of the palatine tonsil(s).
    - Pharyngitis—inflammation of the pharynx.

PATHOPHYSIOLOGY

- Metabolic:
    - Diabetes mellitus.
    - Hypothyroidism.
    - Renal disease—uremia.
- Nutritional:
    - Protein-calorie malnutrition.
    - Riboflavin deficiency.
- Neoplastic:
    - Dog—malignant melanoma; squamous cell carcinoma; fibrosarcoma.
    - Cat—squamous cell carcinoma; fibrosarcoma; malignant melanoma.
- Immune-mediated:
    - Pemphigus vulgaris—90% have oral involvement.
    - Bullous pemphigoid—80% have oral involvement.
    - Systemic lupus erythematosus—50% have oral involvement.
    - Discoid lupus erythematosus.
- Drug-induced—toxic epidermal necrolysis, erythema multiforme.
- Infectious:
    - Retrovirus—feline leukemia virus/feline immunodeficiency virus (FeLV/FIV).
    - Calicivirus—cat.
    - Herpesvirus—cat.
    - Leptospirosis—dog.
    - Periodontal disease—dog and cat.
- Traumatic:
    - Foreign body—bone or wood fragments.
    - Electric cord shock.
    - Malocclusion.
    - Gum-chewer's disease—chronic chewing of cheek or sublingual mucosa.
- Chemical/toxic:
    - Acids—etching gels for dental procedures (37% phosphoric acid).
    - Bases: hypochlorite, cleaning solutions.
    - Thallium.
- Idiopathic:
    - Eosinophilic granuloma—cats, Siberian huskies, Samoyeds.
    - Feline stomatitis—cats; feline chronic gingivostomatitis (FCGS).
    - Canine ulcerative stomatitis—dogs; allergic, hypersensitivity reaction to plaque.
    - Idiopathic osteomyelitis—dogs.

SYSTEMS AFFECTED

Gastrointestinal (oral).

INCIDENCE/PREVALENCE

Variable

SIGNALMENT

Species

Dogs and cats of any age and either sex.

Breed Predilections

- Breed predilection for canine ulcerative stomatitis (aka chronic ulcerative paradental stomatitis [CUPS])—Maltese, cavalier King Charles spaniels, cocker spaniels, bouvier des Flandres.
- Feline stomatitis—FCGS may have predilection for Somali and Abyssinian cats.
- Idiopathic osteomyelitis—may have predilection for cocker spaniels; complication associated with canine ulcerative stomatitis.

Mean Age and Range

Any age.

Predominant Sex

Either gender.

SIGNS

Historical Findings

- History and oral examination—foreign bodies; malocclusions; chemical, toxic, and electrical burns.
- Idiopathic conditions—clinical signs; history; breed predispositions; response to therapy.
- Anorexia.
- Behavior changes secondary to oral sensitivity.
- *Note*: In canine ulcerative stomatitis, occasionally these signs will start following a routine dental cleaning on a previously "normal" patient; probably would have occurred eventually, just exacerbated by manipulation in the oral cavity.

Physical Examination Findings

- Halitosis.
- Gingivitis.
- Pharyngitis.
- Buccitis/buccal mucosal ulceration.
- Hypersalivation (thick, ropey saliva).
- Pain.
- Contact mucosal ulceration or contact mucositis—"kissing ulcers" common in canine ulcerative stomatitis.
- Plaque—with or without calculus.
- Exposed, necrotic bone—with alveolar osteitis and idiopathic osteomyelitis.
- Scar formation on lateral margins of tongue—with canine ulcerative stomatitis.

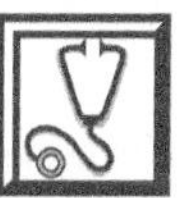

DIAGNOSIS

DIFFERENTIAL DIAGNOSIS

See Causes.

CBC/BIOCHEMISTRY/URINALYSIS

- CBC, biochemistry, urinalysis, and thyroxine (T_4)—diabetes mellitus, renal disease, hypothyroidism, infections, and for preoperative considerations.
- Chronic conditions may have elevated serum total protein and elevated globulin levels due to chronic antigen stimulation; T_4 may be decreased secondarily.

OTHER LABORATORY TESTS

- Serology—FeLV/FIV test; titers for specific infections.
- Cultures—usually nonspecific; oral flora contaminants.

IMAGING

Radiography—helps determine bony involvement, and other conditions such as periodontal disease or tooth resorption, and extent of idiopathic osteomyelitis.

DIAGNOSTIC PROCEDURES

Biopsy/cytology—neoplasia, immune-mediated disease, and chronic inflammation result in predominant lymphocytes and plasmocytes (in canine ulcerative stomatitis and feline stomatitis).

PATHOLOGIC FINDINGS

See definitions above.

TREATMENT

APPROPRIATE HEALTH CARE

Underlying metabolic or other disease—treat systemic illness appropriately.

NURSING CARE

Supportive therapy—soft diet; fluids; hospitalization in severe cases.

DIET

- Nutritional support—via pharyngostomy or esophagostomy feeding tube.
- May consider hypoallergenic diet.

CLIENT EDUCATION

- Canine ulcerative stomatitis—continuous, meticulous home care to prevent plaque accumulation; dental cleaning initially and frequently; periodontal therapy; extraction of diseased teeth.
- Warn client that prognosis is guarded, response to therapy depends on underlying cause, and prolonged treatment and/or further extractions may be necessary.
- In canine ulcerative stomatitis or feline stomatitis, any level of home care that can be provided is encouraged (brushing or topical antimicrobials).

S

SURGICAL CONSIDERATIONS

- Select extractions (partial, caudal, or full mouth)—may be indicated for chronic idiopathic conditions (e.g., canine ulcerative stomatitis and feline stomatitis) to remove the source of reaction (plaque/teeth).
- Removal of entire tooth structure is important.
- Removal of necrotic/avascular bone, gingival flap closure, and broad-spectrum antibiotics—indicated for idiopathic osteomyelitis; monitor for recurrence.

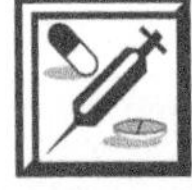

MEDICATIONS

DRUG(S) OF CHOICE

- Antimicrobials—treat primary and secondary bacterial infections; may be used intermittently between cleanings for therapeutic assistance, but the owner must be cautioned that chronic use could lead to antibiotic resistance; clindamycin 11 mg/kg PO q12h; amoxicillin–clavulanate 12.5–25 mg/kg PO q12h; tetracycline 10–22 mg/kg PO q8h.
- Anti-inflammatory/immunosuppressive drugs—the comfort of the patient must be weighed against potential long-term side effects of corticosteroid usage; prednisone 0.5–1.0 mg/kg q12–24h PO, taper dosage:
  - For eosinophilic granuloma—prednisolone 2–4.4 mg/kg PO once a day; for chronic cases use 0.5–1.0 mg/kg PO every other day.
  - Cyclosporine 5 mg/kg PO q24h. Therapeutic serum levels after 6 weeks if no response to therapy.
- Mucosal protectants—for chemical insults; sucralfate 1 g/25 kg q8h PO; cimetidine 5–10 mg/kg q8–12h PO.
- Analgesics—carprofen 0.5 mg/kg PO q12–24h; hydrocodone 0.22 mg/kg q8–12h; tramadol 2.2–4.4 mg/kg PO q6–12h; gabapentin 5–10 mg/kg PO SID.
- Topical therapy—chlorhexidine solution or gel (antibacterial); zinc gluconate/ascorbic acid; stabilized chlorine dioxide for halitosis.
- Appropriate antimicrobial and pain management therapy when indicated.
- Appropriate patient monitoring and support during anesthetic procedures.

CONTRAINDICATIONS

Corticosteroids are contraindicated in patients with systemic fungal infections.

PRECAUTIONS

- Some antimicrobials may upset the gastrointestinal tract.
- Avoid corticosteroids in patients that may already be immunocompromised (i.e., those with FeLV or FIV).
- Do not use these medications in patients with known hypersensitivities.

FOLLOW-UP

PREVENTION/AVOIDANCE

Optimal home care and regular professional cleaning and treatment is essential.

MISCELLANEOUS

ASSOCIATED CONDITIONS

Idiopathic osteomyelitis may occur in some canine ulcerative stomatitis patients (see above).

ZOONOTIC POTENTIAL

N/A, unless immunocompromised individuals.

SYNONYMS

- Chronic ulcerative paradental stomatitis (CUPS).
- Ulcerative stomatitis.
- Gingivostomatitis.
- Vincent's stomatitis.
- Necrotizing stomatitis.

SEE ALSO

Feline Stomatitis—Feline Chronic Gingivosomatitis (FCGS).

ABBREVIATIONS

- CUPS = chronic ulcerative paradental stomatitis.
- FCGS = Feline chronic gingivostomatitis.
- FeLV = feline leukemia virus.
- FIV = feline immunodeficiency virus.
- T_4 = thyroxine.

INTERNET RESOURCES

https://avdc.org/avdc-nomenclature/

Suggested Reading

Harvey CE. Veterinary Dentistry. Philadelphia, PA: Saunders, 1985.

Lobprise HB, Wiggs RB. The Veterinarian's Companion for Common Dental Procedures. Lakewood, CO: AAHA Press, 2000.

Manfra Maretta S, Brine E, Smith CW, et al. Idiopathic mandibular and maxillary osteomyelitis and bone sequestra in cocker spaniels. In: Proceedings of the Veterinary Dental Forum, Denver, CO, 1997; sponsored by the American Veterinary Dental College, Academy of Veterinary Dentistry, and the American Veterinary Dental Society.

Smith MM. Oral and salivary gland disorders. In: Ettinger SJ, ed., Textbook of Veterinary Internal Medicine, 5th ed. Philadelphia, PA: Saunders, 2000, pp. 1114–1121.

Wiggs RB, Lobprise HB. Veterinary Dentistry Principles & Practice. Philadelphia, PA: Lippincott-Raven, 1997.

Author R. Michael Peak

Consulting Editor Heidi B. Lobprise

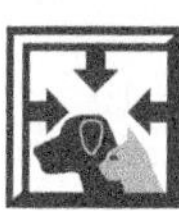

BASICS

OVERVIEW

• *Streptococcus*—Gram-positive, nonmotile, facultatively anaerobic spherical bacteria (cocci):
  ○ Commensal organisms; normal flora of the upper respiratory tract, oropharynx, lower genital tract, and skin.
  ○ Under appropriate conditions, capable of infecting all areas of body; frequent secondary invader of body tissues.
• Classified by ability to hemolyze red blood cells on blood agar plates:
  ○ α-Hemolytic (green zone of partial hemolysis).
  ○ β-Hemolytic (clear zone of hemolysis); usually more pathogenic than α-hemolytic, which is more pathogenic than nonhemolytic strains.
  ○ γ-Hemolytic (no change; nonhemolytic).
• Hemolytic strains further subdivided by differences in cell walls (Lancefield serogroups A–H and K–T); some groups more likely to be associated with disease:
  ○ Group G is associated with cats and dogs; group A with humans).
  ○ Many group D streptococci reclassified as enterococci.
• Produce exotoxins—streptolysins (hemolysins), streptokinases, deoxyribonucleases, and hyaluronidases.
• Adhesins to bind extracellular matrix proteins.

SIGNALMENT

• Dogs and cats.
• Very young—more prone to infection because of incomplete immunity; particularly kittens born to primiparous queen.

SIGNS

• Vary with site of infection and host immunocompetence. Sites of infection can include abscesses, genitourinary tract, ears, septicemia (e.g., toxic shock syndrome), joints, lungs, heart valves, lymph nodes, CNS, wounds (e.g., necrotizing fasciitis), tonsil/pharynx, or skin, and may result in abortion, fading puppies/kittens, or bitch/queen sterility.
• Weakness.
• Coughing.
• Dyspnea.
• Fever.
• Hematemesis.
• Hematuria.
• Lymphadenopathy.
• Pain.

CAUSES & RISK FACTORS

• Age, exposure, and immune response determine disease severity.
• Virulence—depends on specific organism.
• Opportunistic—surgical or traumatic wounds, viral infections, atopic dermatitis, immunosuppressive conditions.
• Coinfection with canine influenza virus increases disease severity. Other predisposing conditions—feline leukemia virus, feline infectious peritonitis, immunodeficiency, respiratory viral infections, feline lower urinary tract disease.
• Maternal antibodies generally protect neonates.
• Carrier state occurs.
• Bacterial superantigens may contribute to toxic shock syndrome and necrotizing fasciitis; enrofloxacin-induced bacteriophages may enhance superantigen expression.

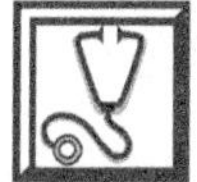

DIAGNOSIS

DIFFERENTIAL DIAGNOSIS

Other infectious causes—viruses, bacteria, fungi, *Rickettsia,* protozoa.

CBC/BIOCHEMISTRY/URINALYSIS

• Normal or high leukocytes with neutrophilia and left shift or degenerative left shift.
• Cocci—in circulating neutrophils if overwhelming sepsis.
• Biochemistry—suggests predisposing conditions.
• Urinalysis—pyuria (with or without bacteruria).

OTHER LABORATORY TESTS

• Direct microscopy.
• Gram stain—of exudates; Gram-positive cocci in chains or singlets.
• Culture and susceptibility testing —affected tissues, exudate or needle aspirates.
• PCR.

IMAGING

Radiographs—interstitial or alveolar pulmonary pattern (pneumonia); radiodense uroliths (struvite).

PATHOLOGIC FINDINGS

• Acute inflammation—gross or microscopic abscesses.
• Septicemia—omphalophlebitis, peritonitis, hepatitis, pneumonia, myocarditis.

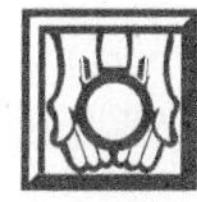

TREATMENT

• Good nursing care.
• Rehydrate.
• Drain and flush abscess.
• Debride necrotic tissue.

MEDICATIONS

DRUG(S) OF CHOICE

• Ampicillin 22–30 mg/kg IV, IM, SC, PO q8h; combined with aminoglycoside (gentamicin or amikacin) for group B.
• Amoxicillin 22 mg/kg PO q8–12h.
• Amoxicillin–clavulanate 22 mg/kg PO q12h.
• Penicillin—penicillin G 10,000–20,000 U/kg IM, SC q12–24h or penicillin V 8–30 mg/kg PO q8h.
• Erythromycin 10–20 mg/kg IV, SC, PO q8h.
• Clindamycin 10–15 mg/kg PO, IV, SC q12h.

CONTRAINDICATIONS/POSSIBLE INTERACTIONS

• Avoid immunosuppressive drugs; aminoglycosides contraindicated with renal disease.
• Enrofloxacin—contraindicated for necrotizing fasciitis.

FOLLOW-UP

PREVENTION/AVOIDANCE

• Avoid overcrowding, maintain clean feeders and environment, segregate infected animals.
• Newborns—dip navel and umbilical cord in 2% tincture of iodine, consider prophylactic antibiotic treatment of kittens born to primiparous queens.

MISCELLANEOUS

ZOONOTIC POTENTIAL

• Animals may show no clinical signs with group A streptococci but may serve as reservoir for human infection.
• Streptococci isolated from people are usually of human, not animal, origin.
• *S. canis* infections in people reported from dog bites and wounds in contact with dogs.

Suggested Reading

Lappin MR, Blondeau J, Boothe D, et al. Antimicrobial use guidelines for treatment of respiratory tract disease in dogs and cats. J Vet Intern Med 2017, 31:279–294.

Little SE. Emerging aspects of streptococcal infections in cats. In: Little SE, ed., August's Consultations in Feline Internal Medicine, 7th ed. St. Louis, MO: Elsevier, 2016, pp. 64–72.

Sykes JE. Streptococcal and enterococcal infections. In: Sykes JE, ed., Canine and Feline Infectious Diseases. St. Louis, MO: Elsevier, 2014, pp. 334–346.

Author J. Paul Woods
Consulting Editor Amie Koenig

STUPOR AND COMA

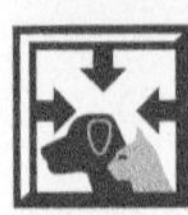

BASICS

DEFINITION

• Stupor—unconscious but arousable with noxious stimuli. • Coma—unconscious, not arousable with noxious stimuli.

PATHOPHYSIOLOGY

Any severe pathologic change (anatomic or metabolic) of the ascending reticular activating system (network of neurons situated in the core of the brainstem) and/or arousal system for the cerebral cortex can lead to depression, stupor, or coma.

SYSTEMS AFFECTED

• Nervous. • Cardiovascular. • Neuromuscular. • Ophthalmic. • Respiratory.

SIGNALMENT

• Dog and cat. • No breed, age, or sex predilection.

SIGNS

Historical Findings

• Possibility of trauma or unsupervised roaming. • Past medical problems of significance—diabetes mellitus, insulin therapy; hypoglycemia; cardiovascular problems; hypoxic episodes; renal failure; liver failure; neoplasia. • Patient's environment—possible heatstroke; hypothermia; drowning; exposure to drugs, including owner's medications, narcotics, toxins (e.g., ethylene glycol, lead, anticoagulants). • Onset may be acute or slowly progressive, depending on underlying cause.

Physical Examination Findings

• Evidence of external or internal trauma. • Severe hypo- or hyperthermia. • Evidence of hypoxia or cyanosis, ecchymosis or petechiation, cardiac or respiratory insufficiency—warrants investigation for metabolic causes. • Palpate for evidence of neoplasia. • Retinal hemorrhages or distended vessels—hypertension. • Papilledema—cerebral edema. • Retinal detachment—infectious, neoplastic, or hypertensive causes. • Chorioretinitis—infectious causes (distemper, feline leukemia virus [FeLV]-related diseases, toxoplasmosis, cryptococcosis, or coronavirus). • Sustained bradycardia (with normal serum potassium)—midbrain, pontine, or medullary lesion.

Neurologic Examination Findings

• Differentiate cerebrum–diencephalic lesion from brainstem lesion (better vs. worse prognosis). • Determine level of consciousness and if patient arousable. • Pupillary light reflexes—small responsive pupils: cerebral or diencephalic lesion; dilated unresponsive pupils (unilateral or bilateral) or fixed in midposition: midbrain or severe medullary lesions. • Oculocephalic reflex (when cervical manipulation possible)—loss of physiologic vestibular nystagmus: brainstem involvement. • Respiratory patterns—Cheyne-Stokes respiration: severe, diffuse cerebral or diencephalic lesion; hyperventilation: midbrain lesion; ataxic or apneustic breathing: pons or medulla lesion. • Cranial nerve (CN)—deficits with lesion of cerebrum–diencephalon: CN I, II; deficits of CN III: midbrain lesion; deficits of CN V–XII: pons and medulla lesions. • Postural changes—decerebrate rigidity: midbrain lesion.

CAUSES

• Drugs—narcotics, anesthetics, depressants, ivermectin. • Anatomic—hydrocephalus. • Metabolic—severe hypoglycemia, hyperglycemia, hyperosmolar syndromes, hypernatremia, hyponatremia, hepatic encephalopathy, hypoxemia, hypercarbia, hypothermia, hyperthermia, hypotension, coagulopathies, renal failure, lysosomal storage disease, severe hypothyroidism. • Nutritional—hypoglycemia, thiamine deficiency. • Neoplastic (primary)—meningioma, astrocytoma, gliomas, choroid plexus papilloma, pituitary adenoma, others. • Metastatic—hemangiosarcoma, lymphoma, mammary carcinoma, others. • Inflammatory noninfectious—granulomatous meningoencephalomyelitis. • Infectious—bacterial, viral (distemper, feline coronavirus [FCoV]), parasitic (aberrant larva migrants), protozoal (neosporosis, toxoplasmosis), fungal (cryptococcosis, blastomycosis, histoplasmosis, coccidioidomycosis, actinomycosis), tick-borne diseases. • Idiopathic—epilepsy (post status epilepticus). • Immune-mediated—brain edema, vasculitis and thrombocytopenia leading to hemorrhage. • Trauma—most common cause. • Toxins—ethylene glycol, lead, rodenticides, others. • Vascular—hemorrhage (bleeding disorders, hypertension), infarction (feline ischemic encephalopathy, hypercoagulable disease, microfilaria, or migrating adult heartworm).

RISK FACTORS

• Diabetes mellitus—insulin therapy. • Hepatic failure. • Insulinoma. • Severe heat or cold exposure without protection. • Free-roaming animals—trauma. • Young and unvaccinated animals. • Hypertension.

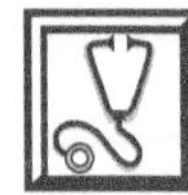

DIAGNOSIS

DIFFERENTIAL DIAGNOSIS

• Acute onset—most commonly caused by toxins, drugs, trauma, or vascular accidents. • Slow progression of neurologic signs without systemic abnormalities—suggests primary neurologic disorders of inflammatory, neoplastic, or anatomic causes. • Bilateral diffuse cortical signs—metabolic diseases, toxins, systemic infection, drugs, and nutritional causes. • Brainstem signs—trauma, inflammation, neoplasia, vascular accidents, or progression of cerebral disease causing tentorial herniation.

CBC/BIOCHEMISTRY/URINALYSIS

CBC

• Lead toxicity—may show nucleated red blood cells or basophilic stippling. • Severe infection—inflammatory hemogram. • Severe anemia—suggests hypoxemia.

Biochemistry

May see hypoglycemia, hyperglycemia, hypernatremia, azotemia, hyperosmolarity, and other metabolic derangements.

Urinalysis

• Diabetes mellitus—glycosuria. • Renal failure—isosthenuria, granular casts. • Immune-mediated disease or severe infection—proteinuria. • Hepatic encephalopathy—ammonium biurate crystals. • Ethylene glycol toxicity—calcium oxalate or hippurate crystals.

OTHER LABORATORY TESTS

• Serum ethylene glycol level and osmolar gap—acute onset. • Serum ammonia concentration and preprandial and postprandial bile acids—high levels indicate hepatic encephalopathy. • Serum and CSF titers—suspected infectious disease. • Arterial blood gases—evidence of hypoxemia; severe pH changes; hypo- and hypercarbia. • Coagulogram—including prothrombin time (PT), partial thromboplastin time (PTT), fibrinogen, fibrin degradation product, D-dimer, platelet count, antithrombin, buccal bleeding time, thromboelastography; suspected intracranial bleeding or thrombosis. • Serologic testing—FeLV, feline immunodeficiency virus (FIV), FCoV, protozoal and heartworm disease. • Serum toxicity levels (e.g., lead, macrolide, other toxins). • Thyroid panel.

IMAGING

• Survey radiographs (thorax and abdomen)—evidence of heavy metal, organ enlargement, infiltration, or neoplasia. • Skull radiographs—fractures in trauma cases, lytic lesions, masses. • CT—excellent for detecting acute hemorrhage within calvaria; depressed fractures; lytic lesions, penetrating foreign bodies. • MRI with contrast—demonstrates cerebral edema, hemorrhage, mass, infiltrative diseases, vascular interruption.

DIAGNOSTIC PROCEDURES

• CSF—cytology, protein and immunoglobulin concentrations, and titers for infectious diseases; perform only when no evidence of trauma, increased intracranial pressure, coagulopathies, or metabolic disease. • Brainstem auditory-evoked response—determine brainstem function. • ECG, echocardiogram—determine cardiac dysfunction; abnormalities may contribute to stupor or coma or may be caused by brain disease. • EEG—detect nonclinical seizure activity that can prolong stupor and coma.

PATHOLOGIC FINDINGS

Cerebral edema, hemorrhage, infarct, ischemia, inflammation, neoplasia, herniation, laceration, contusion, hematomas, skull fracture, necrosis, and apoptosis.

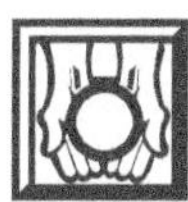

TREATMENT

APPROPRIATE HEALTH CARE

Poor Perfusion

• Small-volume fluid resuscitation technique; a combination of hydroxyethyl starch with balanced isotonic crystalloids. • Use peripheral veins, leaving the jugular vein blood flow unobstructed; shifting blood volume into the jugular veins is an important compensatory mechanism during high intracranial pressure (ICP). • Maintain systolic BP >90 mmHg; avoid hypertension. • Hydration—maintain with a balanced electrolyte crystalloid solution. • The head and neck should be leveled with the body or elevated to a 20° angle. • Oxygen supplementation—avoid a cough or sneeze reflex during intubation or nasal cannula placement; administer lidocaine (dogs, topical and/or 1–2 mg/kg IV) before intubation to blunt the gag and cough reflex. • Pao_2 must be >50 mmHg to maintain cerebral blood flow autoregulation in normal brain tissue.

Ventilation

• Protect airway with intubation. • $Paco_2$—maintain between 35 and 45 mmHg.

Reduce Increase In ICP

• Prevent thrashing, seizures, or any other form of uncontrolled motor activity that can elevate ICP; diazepam infusion 0.5–1 mg/kg/h, midazolam 0.2–0.4 mg/kg, or propofol 3–6 mg/kg IV titrated to effect; then 0.1–0.6 mg/kg/min CRI; levetiracetam 20 mg/kg IV/IM/rectal q8h if seizure activity. • Ensure systolic BP >90 mmHg. • 7% hypertonic saline (2–4 mL/kg IV); can reduce fluid volume needed to reach resuscitation endpoints; can combine with colloid.
• Furosemide 0.75 mg/kg IV; may decrease CSF production. • Mannitol 0.5–1 g/kg IV bolus repeated at 2-hour intervals 3 or 4 times in dogs, and 2 or 3 times in cats; repeated doses must be given on time; improves brain blood flow and lowers ICP. • Hyperventilation ($Paco_2$ 32–35 mmHg) for 48 hours using mechanical ventilation; requires intensive monitoring. • Ventriculostomy for CSF drainage if critical elevation of ICP nonresponsive to medical treatment.
• Consider surgical decompression and exploration—if cerebral dysfunction is progressing to midbrain signs with a history of trauma or bleeding (tentorial herniation); high ICP not responsive to medical therapy (if monitoring instrumentation available); depressed skull fracture fragments; penetrating foreign body; requires intensive monitoring.

NURSING CARE

• Prevent secondary complications of recumbency—eye lubrication; aseptic technique with catheters; turning; rehabilitation exercises. • Prevent urine/fecal scalding. • Careful nasogastric tube feeding for early trickle flow feeding; cisapride 0.5 mg/kg PO q8–12h and metoclopramide 1–2 mg/kg/day may promote gastrointestinal motility.

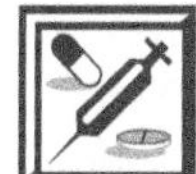

MEDICATIONS

DRUG(S) OF CHOICE

Underlying Disease

• Glucocorticosteroids—inflammatory, immune-mediated and space-occupying intracranial abnormalities. • Lactulose enemas, flumazenil 0.02 mg/kg IV and fluid support—hepatic encephalopathy. • Fluid diuresis, dialysis—renal failure. • Rehydration and insulin—diabetes mellitus with hyperosmolality; lower glucose slowly. • Glucose supplementation—hypoglycemia. • Support IV volume; cool—hyperthermia. • Support IV volume; warm to ≥98°F/36.5°C—hypothermia.
• Gastric lavage and instillation of activated charcoal with a cathartic. • Dialysis—low-molecular-weight toxins. • Antibiotics—use agents that cross the blood–brain barrier for suspected bacterial infections (e.g., trimethoprim-sulfa, clindamycin, doxycycline, metronidazole). • Adjust crystalloid fluid selection to correct electrolyte disorders.
• Thiamine (cat, 5–50 mg; dog, 1–20 mg IV)—possible thiamine deficiency.

PRECAUTIONS

• Avoid hypo- and hypertension, hypo- and hyperglycemia. • Avoid IV volume overload.

FOLLOW-UP

PATIENT MONITORING

• Serial neurologic examinations—detect deterioration that warrants aggressive therapeutic intervention. • BP—keep fluid therapy adequate for perfusion while avoiding hypertension. • Blood gases—assess need for oxygen supplementation or ventilation; monitor Pco_2 when hyperventilating. • Blood glucose—ensure adequate level to maintain brain functions while avoiding hyperosmolality.
• ECG—detect arrhythmias that may affect perfusion, oxygenation, and cerebral blood flow. • ICP—detect marked elevations; track success of therapeutics. • Electrolytes—detect hypernatremia and hypokalemia.

PREVENTION/AVOIDANCE

• Keep pets confined or leashed. • Prevent exposure to toxins or in-home medications.
• Routine healthcare program to minimize infectious and metabolic disease complications.

EXPECTED COURSE AND PROGNOSIS

• Short-term prognosis poor, other than related to hypoglycemia. • Pathology of brainstem worse than pathology of cerebral cortex. • Modified Glasgow Coma Score can provide prognostic information.

MISCELLANEOUS

ABBREVIATIONS

- CN = cranial nerve.
- CSF = cerebrospinal fluid.
- ECG = electrocardiogram.
- EEG = electroencephalogram.
- FCoV = feline coronavirus.
- FeLV = feline leukemia virus.
- FIV = feline immunodeficiency virus.
- ICP = intracranial pressure.
- $Paco_2$ = partial pressure of carbon dioxide in arterial blood.
- Pao_2 = partial pressure of arterial oxygen.
- PT = prothrombin time.
- PTT = partial thromboplastin time.

SEE ALSO

Brain Injury.

INTERNET RESOURCES

https://bvns.net/wp-content/uploads/2016/09/Neurotransmitter-2.0-MGCS-final.pdf

Suggested Reading

Chrisman CL, Mariani C, Platt S. Dementia, stupor and coma. In: Neurology for the Small Animal Practitioner. Jackson, WY: Teton NewMedia, 2003, pp. 41–84.

Parratt CA, Firth AM, Boag AK, et al. Retrospective characterization of coma and stupor in dogs and cats presenting to a multicenter out-of-hours service (2012–2015): 386 animals. J Vet Emerg Crit Care 2018, 28:559–565.

Author Elke Rudloff

Acknowledgment The author and editors acknowledge the prior contribution of Rebecca Kirby.

Client Education Handout available online

S

SUBARACHNOID CYSTS (ARACHNOID DIVERTICULUM)

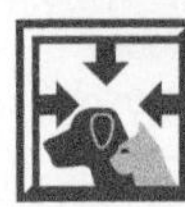

BASICS

DEFINITION

Subarachnoid cysts refer to dilation of the subarachnoid space causing compression of the underlying brain or spinal cord. The use of the term "cyst" is misleading, as most do not have a defined cyst wall with an epithelial lining and the term subarachnoid diverticulum is frequently used when the lesion is spinal in location. This term is also problematic in cases in which arachnoid scarring simply causes dilation of the subarachnoid space.

PATHOPHYSIOLOGY

• There are several proposed etiologies of subarachnoid cysts. • Any disease process that causes arachnoiditis has the potential to cause adhesions that result in the formation of one-way valves through which CSF flows, but cannot return, causing accumulation of CSF. • Congenital forms of the disease may result from abnormal splitting of the arachnoid membrane during development.

SYSTEMS AFFECTED

Nervous—spinal cord and brain (quadrigeminal cistern).

GENETICS

Certain breeds appear to be predisposed (e.g., pug, Rottweiler for spinal cord, Pekingese, shih tzu for brain). There are no data confirming heritability or a mode of inheritance at this time.

INCIDENCE/PREVALENCE

No specific data.

SIGNALMENT

Species

Dog and cat.

Breed Predilections

• Spinal—pug, Rottweiler, French bulldog. • Brain—small brachycephalic breeds.

Mean Age and Range

Dogs <3 years, range 2.5 months–13 years.

Predominant Sex

Male > female.

SIGNS

Historical Findings

Spinal

• Owners report a slowly progressive ataxia and paresis involving all or just the pelvic limbs. • Fecal incontinence—common early sign of thoracolumbar diverticula, with urinary incontinence developing shortly after. • Owners do not usually report that the pet is in pain. In a study of 122 cases, 19% of the dogs had pain. • There may be prior history of previous spinal cord injury (due to trauma, intervertebral disc disease, or fibrocartilagenous embolism). • There may be concurrent vertebral malformations at the site of the diverticula.

Brain

• Cerebellar signs. • Seizures.

Physical Examination Findings

Usually normal, although possible secondary consequences of the myelopathy include abrasions of the dorsal aspect of the toes, wearing of the nails, and urinary tract infections.

Neurologic Examination Findings

Spinal

• Neurologic signs reflect lesion localization—hindlimb involvement for thoracolumbar cysts and all limbs for cervical cysts. • Ataxia frequently characterized by hypermetria. • Paresis. • Proprioceptive placing deficits. • Fecal and/or urinary incontinence; urine retention (due to defective voiding). • Spinal reflexes may be reduced if the lesion is at the brachial or lumbosacral intumescence but otherwise are normal or increased. • Spinal pain is rarely elicited.

Brain

• Quadrigeminal cysts are frequently an incidental finding. However, extremely large cysts can produce compression of the cerebellum and brainstem. • Signs of cerebellar disease—hypermetria, intention tremor, wide-based stance. • Signs of brainstem compression—tetraparesis, head tilt. • Seizures (the relationship between the cyst and the presence of seizures is unclear).

CAUSES

• Several proposed etiologies. • Congenital malformation of the arachnoid mater (dilated septum posticum; in young dogs). • Secondary to traumatic injury to the arachnoid, causing adhesions and development of one-way valves for CSF flow. • Secondary to chronic microtrauma to the arachnoid, causing adhesions and development of one-way valves for CSF flow. This mechanism has been proposed for pugs with caudal thoracic subarachnoid cysts. Affected dogs may have hypoplasia of their articular facets leading to chronic instability.

RISK FACTORS

• Traumatic spinal cord injury that damages the arachnoid mater. • Hypoplastic articular facets associated with subarachnoid diverticulae in certain dog breeds (pugs).

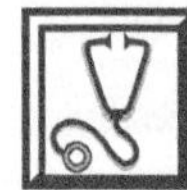

DIAGNOSIS

DIFFERENTIAL DIAGNOSIS

• Distinctive features—slowly progressive, nonpainful paresis and ataxia with a hypermetric gait, and presence of fecal and/or urinary incontinence in an animal that is still ambulatory. • Any cause of focal myelopathy could cause the same neurologic presentation. • Intervertebral disc herniation. • Neoplasia. • Trauma. • Inflammatory or infectious myelitis. • Congenital vertebral/spinal malformation. • Intraspinal vascular malformation.

CBC/BIOCHEMISTRY/URINALYSIS

Urinalysis may show evidence of urinary tract infection (pyuria, hematuria, proteinuria, and bacteriuria).

OTHER LABORATORY TESTS

Aerobic urine culture if evidence of urinary tract infection.

IMAGING

• Thoracic radiography—in older patients to rule out metastatic neoplasia. • Spinal radiography—should be performed in all patients; typically unremarkable in patients with subarachnoid diverticulae. However, some patients may have evidence of spinal fractures, and occasionally there is evidence of a vertebral malformation (articular facet hypoplasia, spina bifida, hemivertebra, or block vertebra) colocalizing with the neurologic signs. • Myelography—focal dilation of the subarachnoid space most commonly located dorsally but sometimes located ventrally; the dilation may be multilobed. • CT myelography—further delineates the dilated subarachnoid space in transverse section; without intrathecal contrast, will not demonstrate the lesion. • MRI—dilation of the subarachnoid space in sagittal and transverse section on T2-weighted images. T2-HASTE images provide even more definition of the CSF accumulation. The presence of active arachnoiditis can be detected on pre- and-postcontrast T1-weighted images.

DIAGNOSTIC PROCEDURES

CSF—to rule out a primary inflammatory process; may show mild inflammation as secondary consequence of the subarachnoid cyst.

PATHOLOGIC FINDINGS

• At surgery, adhesions may be evident in the subarachnoid space. Occasionally a thin cyst wall is apparent (this is unusual). • Histopathology of excised arachnoid—may show fibrosis or mild inflammation. • Histopathology of the spinal cord shows chronic compressive injury—loss of gray and white matter, Wallerian degeneration, demyelination.

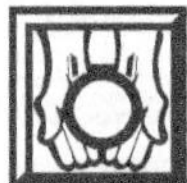

TREATMENT

APPROPRIATE HEALTH CARE

• Patients with mild signs can be managed medically; surgery recommended for young dogs with moderate, progressive signs. • Nonambulatory patients should be hospitalized for diagnostic workup and possible surgical decompression as soon as possible.

NURSING CARE

• Patients that have incomplete micturition should have their bladders manually expressed 3–4 times a day. If this is not possible, their bladders should be catheterized in a sterile fashion once or twice a day. • Appropriate maintenance fluids should be administered in the immediate postoperative period.
• Postoperative pain should be assessed regularly (q6h) and treated as needed with opiates and nonsteroidal anti-inflammatory drugs. • Surgical incisions should be ice packed for 5–10 minutes three times a day for 24 hours after surgery and then should be hot packed for a similar period for an additional 2–5 days. • Rehabilitation is important; a patient-specific rehabilitation program should be developed to include gait training and improvement of strength.

ACTIVITY

• Paretic and ataxic patients need to be restricted to nonslip, flat surfaces to avoid falling. • Exercise should be restricted to walking on a leash to avoid falling, but controlled exercise is important in maintaining muscle strength and joint integrity. • Postoperatively, patients need to be restricted to a small, well-padded space (crate) to ensure that they do not fall while the laminectomy site is healing. Limited controlled exercise should be performed during this period.

CLIENT EDUCATION

• Clients need to be educated on the implications of a chronic compressive myelopathy; permanent damage to the spinal cord has already occurred and may not be reversible. The primary aim of treatment is to prevent further deterioration, with a hope of also producing a clinical improvement.
• There may be an initial deterioration immediately postoperatively; there is a small chance that this deterioration could be permanent. • Incontinence, if present, is likely to be permanent. • The disease may recur in spite of surgical therapy.

SURGICAL CONSIDERATIONS

• Surgical decompression of spinal subarachnoid cysts is recommended in young dogs and can be attempted in older animals.
• Marsupialization of the meninges may reduce the chance of a recurrence. • Surgical treatment of quadrigeminal cysts is only recommended if there are clear signs of compression of adjacent cerebellum and cerebral cortex. Direct surgical exploration and decompression or shunt placement can be attempted.

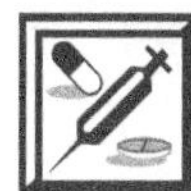

MEDICATIONS

DRUG(S) OF CHOICE

• Anti-inflammatory doses of prednisone (0.5 mg/kg orally once to twice a day) may improve signs and reduce inflammation. If there is no improvement, prednisone should be tapered and discontinued. • Omeprazole may reduce CSF production rate and improve signs. If there is no improvement it should be discontinued. • Treatment with antiepileptic drugs should be initiated in dogs with more than 1 seizure a month or cluster seizures. Choice of antiepileptic drug depends on a number of patient and client factors. Phenobarbital (starting at 2 mg/kg q12h), zonisamide (starting at 5–10 mg/kg q12h) and levetiracetam (starting at 20 mg/kg q8h) are all appropriate choices for first-line therapy.

PRECAUTIONS

Corticosteroids should be used with caution if the patient has urinary tract infection.

FOLLOW-UP

PATIENT MONITORING

• If response to prednisone is being assessed, the patient's gait and postural reactions should be reassessed in 1–2 weeks. The owner's assessment of continence is also important. • If there is a positive response to medical management, the patient should be monitored every 8–12 weeks for maintenance of the improvement over the next 6 months and then every 6–12 months. The owner should be instructed to call if deterioration in clinical signs is detected. • Surgical treatment—patient reassessed at 7–10 days for suture removal, evaluation of incision, and to ensure that there is no deterioration in gait, level of pain, continence; reassessment at 1–3 months and every 6–12 months subsequently. Telephone updates are acceptable if the patient is doing well.

POSSIBLE COMPLICATIONS

• Clients may encounter fecal and urinary incontinence.
• If incontinent, there is a predisposition to urinary tract infections.
• Signs may recur at any time.

EXPECTED COURSE AND PROGNOSIS

Spinal Diverticulae

• Surgical decompression produces a good long-term outcome (more than 1 year) in approximately 66% of dogs with spinal disease. • Age at onset of signs and duration of signs are associated with outcome. Dogs less than 3 years of age and with a short duration of signs (less than 4 months) are more likely to have a good long-term outcome. • There are limited data on the prognosis with medical management, but anecdotally the author can report a good long-term outcome in old dogs with mild signs when treated with prednisone and rehabilitation alone.

Quadrigeminal Cysts

Data on prognosis of quadrigeminal cysts managed medically or surgically are limited but suggests that a positive outcome can be attained with both treatment strategies.

MISCELLANEOUS

AGE-RELATED FACTORS

Cervical cysts are more common in dogs <3 years of age and thoracolumbar cysts are common in old pugs.

PREGNANCY/FERTILITY/BREEDING

N/A

SYNONYMS

Arachnoid diverticula, arachnoid cyst, meningeal or leptomeningeal cyst.

ABBREVIATIONS

• CSF = cerebrospinal fluid.

SEE ALSO

Quadrigeminal Cyst.

INTERNET RESOURCES

http://www.ivis.org/advances/Vite/toc.asp

Suggested Reading

Dewey CW, Scrivani PV, Krotscheck U, et al. Intracranial arachnoid cysts in dogs. Compend Contin Educ Vet 2009, 31(4):160–167.

Fisher SC, Shores A, Simpson ST. Constrictive myelopathy secondary to hypoplasia or aplasia of the thoracolumbar caudal articular processes in pugs: 11 cases (1993–2009). J Am Vet Med Assoc 2013, 242:223–229.

Gnirs K, Ruel Y, Blot S, et al. Spinal subarachnoid cysts in 13 dogs. Vet Radiol Ultrasound 2003, 44:402–408.

Mauler DA, De Decker S, De Risio L, et al. Signalment, clinical presentation and diagnostic findings in 122 dogs with spinal arachnoid diverticula. J Vet Intern Med 2014, 28:175–181.

Skeen TM, Olby NJ, Muñana KR, Sharp NJ. Spinal arachnoid cysts in 17 dogs. J Am Anim Hosp Assoc 2003, 39:271–282.

Author Natasha J. Olby

SUBINVOLUTION OF PLACENTAL SITES

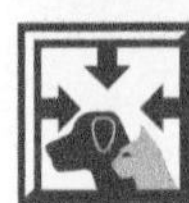

BASICS

OVERVIEW

- Failure or delay of normal postpartum uterine involution (normally requires 12–15 weeks to complete).
- Failure of eosinophilic masses of collagen at placental sites to slough at 3–4 weeks postpartum.
- Failure of fetal trophoblastic cells to regress (normally occurs within 2 weeks); instead, they invade the maternal deep glandular endometrium and myometrium.
- Cause—unknown; hormonal or uterine basis not suspected based on coexistence of unaffected and subinvoluted placental sites in the same uterus.

SIGNALMENT

- Bitch <3 years most common.
- Higher incidence in first litter.
- No breed predilections.

SIGNS

Historical Findings

- Patient presented >12 weeks postpartum.
- Serosanguineous vulvar discharge beyond 12 weeks postpartum.
- Typically no systemic signs; rare occurrence of hypovolemic shock from hemorrhage.

S

Physical Examination Findings

- Serosanguineous vulvar discharge.
- Firm, spherical structures within uterus on abdominal palpation.

CAUSES & RISK FACTORS

Unknown; thought unlikely to be hormonal because only some of the placental sites may be involved. Also thought unlikely to be uterine disease because of high first litter prevalence.

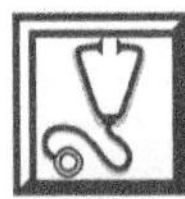

DIAGNOSIS

DIFFERENTIAL DIAGNOSIS

- Metritis—differentiated by vaginal cytology and physical examination.
- Vaginitis—differentiated by vaginal cytology.
- Vaginal neoplasia—differentiated by vaginal cytology and vaginal endoscopy.
- Uterine neoplasia—differentiated by ultrasonography or exploratory laparotomy.
- Cystitis—differentiated by vaginal cytology and urinalysis obtained by cystocentesis.
- Coagulopathy—differentiated by clotting times, platelet count.
- Trauma.
- Endogenous estrogen stimulation—bitch with an extremely shortened interestrous interval.
- Exogenous estrogen stimulation—oral medication or contact with topical hormone replacement product on human skin, bedding, or clothing.

CBC/BIOCHEMISTRY/URINALYSIS

Usually normal.

OTHER LABORATORY TESTS

- Serology for *Brucella canis* negative.
- Serum progesterone <2 ng/mL

IMAGING

Uterine ultrasonography—focal uterine wall thickening; possible echogenic fluid in the lumen

DIAGNOSTIC PROCEDURES

- Vaginal cytologic examination—key for diagnosis; reveals erythrocytes and parabasal epithelial cells; may note pathognomonic trophoblastic cells (polynucleated, heavily vacuolated).
- Guarded anterior vaginal or transcervical uterine culture—if vaginal cytologic examination or hemogram supports a diagnosis of secondary metritis.

PATHOLOGIC FINDINGS

- Gross—sites characterized by a thickened, hemorrhagic area that may be nodular.
- Histopathologic—definitive diagnosis; eosinophilic collagen masses with trophoblasts extending into the myometrium.

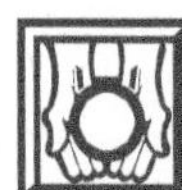

TREATMENT

- Usually outpatient.
- Spontaneous remission—occurs in most patients before or at next cycle; medical therapy is generally not warranted.
- Medical—for rare development of anemia, metritis, or peritonitis.
- Severely affected patients—may require blood transfusion (rare).
- Warn owner of the rare possibility of excessive hemorrhage; instruct owner to monitor mucous membrane color.
- Ovariohysterectomy—curative; treatment of choice if future breeding not desired.
- Surgical curettage of subinvoluted sites—may also be performed; effectiveness unknown.

MEDICATIONS

DRUG(S) OF CHOICE

- Oxytocin generally not successful.
- Ergonovine 10–30 µg/kg IM once; do not use if uterus friable.
- Small study showed response to megestrol acetate 0.1 mg/kg PO q24h for 1 week, then 0.05 mg/kg PO q24h daily for 1 week; 5 of 6 treated bitches were successfully bred, with normal parturition and puerperal periods.

CONTRAINDICATIONS/POSSIBLE INTERACTIONS

- Ecbolics—may cause uterine rupture.
- Progestational drugs—increase the risk of metritis, which may mimic pyometra or induce cystic endometrial hyperplasia.

FOLLOW-UP

PATIENT MONITORING

- Mucous membrane color and amount of discharge.
- Packed cell volume or hematocrit—if anemia is a concern.
- Changes in discharge color or odor and vaginal cytologic examination and culture—diagnose secondary infection.

POSSIBLE COMPLICATIONS

Infection, blood-loss anemia, or uterine rupture—rare.

EXPECTED COURSE AND PROGNOSIS

- Spontaneous resolution—the usual outcome in the majority of cases.
- Recurrence—not expected, occurs rarely.
- Prognosis for future reproduction—excellent with spontaneous resolution.

MISCELLANEOUS

Suggested Reading

Feldman EC, Nelson RW. Periparturient diseases. In: Feldman EC, Nelson RW, eds., Canine and Feline Endocrinology and Reproduction. Philadelphia, PA: Saunders, 2004, pp. 808–834.

Johnston SD, Root Kustritz MV, Olson PNS. Periparturient disorders in the bitch. In: Johnston SD, Root Kustritz MV, Olson PN, eds., Canine and Feline Theriogenology. Philadelphia, PA: Saunders, 2001, pp. 129–145.

Voorhorst MJ, van Brederode JC, Albers-Wolthers CHJ, et al. Successful treatment for subinvolution of placental sites in the bitch with low oral doses of progestagen. Reprod Domest Anim 2013, 48:840–843.

Author Joni L. Freshman

Consulting Editor Erin E. Runcan

SUBMISSIVE AND EXCITEMENT URINATION—DOGS

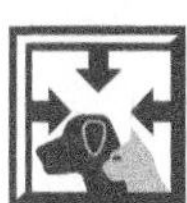

BASICS

OVERVIEW

- Excitement and submissive urination occur as distinct behavioral presentations but may overlap in some patients.
- Submissive urination is related to fearful responses—animal perceives potential threat or danger during interaction and displays submissive behavior, including urination, as appeasement gesture to abort potential escalation of aggressive interactions.
- Generally seen in interaction with people; however, submissive urination may occur during interactions with other animals, especially conspecifics.

SIGNALMENT

- Onset as puppy in dogs of either sex: generally <1 year old.
- Anecdotally higher incidence in some small breeds, e.g., dachshund, cocker spaniel.
- Not observed in cats.

SIGNS

- Excitement—loss of urine control in situations of high arousal, e.g., greeting people, anticipation of activities such as walks or car rides; no actual urination posturing seen—urine is expelled while dog is engaged in activities such as jumping up or play; dog does not necessarily show submissive behavior.
- Submissive/fear—expelling small amounts of urine during interactions with people or other animals or in frightening situations; partial or full squatting position; dog may lift one hind leg partially for inguinal presentation.
- Dogs may be excited and aroused yet also submissive or fearful during greeting—when there are competing motivations this might therefore be described as conflict induced; the approach may be active with tail wagging and crouching/low body posture.

CAUSES & RISK FACTORS

- Administration of medications that reduce urethral competence or increase urine production (e.g., corticosteroids, sedatives).
- Domineering training styles or interaction patterns.

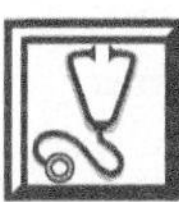

DIAGNOSIS

DIFFERENTIAL DIAGNOSIS

- Incontinence, ectopic ureter, patent urachus.
- Cystitis.
- Disorders of urethral competence (which may increase severity or frequency of urination during submissive or excitement urination).
- Disorders causing polyuria/polydipsia may decrease pet's ability to maintain bladder control.

CBC/BIOCHEMISTRY/URINALYSIS

Indicated only to rule out medical disorders.

IMAGING

Indicated only to rule out medical disorders.

DIAGNOSTIC PROCEDURES

Indicated only to rule out medical disorders.

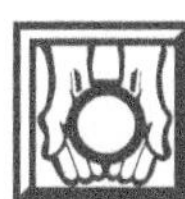

TREATMENT

Excitement Urination

- Avoid arousing situations.
- Do not greet dog when aroused/excited—greet dog away from front door and several minutes after arrival only after dog is calm.
- When entering home, toss treats away to redirect and distract pet; over time gradually transition to tossing treats closer to person and eventually hand treats to pet when pet sits calmly on cue.
- Avoid high-pitch excited speech around pet; avoid eye contact if it arouses/excites the pet.
- Teach owner to reinforce calm behavior and teach behaviors incompatible with high arousal, e.g., sit or lie down for greetings and before walks.
- Owners should interact with pet in emotionally neutral, low-key manner.

Submissive/Fear Urination

- Avoid threatening or confrontational interactions; do not lean over pet; do not punish or raise voice with pet; avoid eye contact.
- Avoid confrontational training styles/ interactions.
- Avoid deep, loud, or high-pitch excited speech while around or interacting with the pet.
- Move slowly and calmly around pet to avoid potential startling or threatening movements.
- Squat down or greet/interact with pet while sitting in chair or on floor with the body turned partially away from the dog.
- Redirection or distraction with food treats or toys; toss treats away to redirect and distract pet; over time can gradually transition to tossing treats closer to person and eventually hand treats to pet when pet sits calmly on cue.
- Teach behaviors with positive reinforcement that are incompatible with submissive posturing using positive reinforcement (food treats)—pet sitting upright with head and ears up and forward; eye contact.
- Owner should recognize and identify triggers and turn and walk away or back away if pet begins to show submissive posturing.

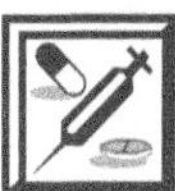

MEDICATIONS

- Medications generally not indicated but could consider:
  - Phenylpropanolamine 12.5–50 mg PO up to q8h temporarily to increase urethral sphincter tone while behavior modification is taking effect.
  - Imipramine 2.2–4.4 mg/kg PO q12h or clomipramine 1–3 mg/kg PO q12h to increase urinary retention through anticholinergic effects; serotonin and norepinephrine properties can help reduce excitement or fear that contribute to urinating.

FOLLOW-UP

EXPECTED COURSE AND PROGNOSIS

Prognosis is good if owners can follow simple behavior modification steps; a number of pets will improve with maturity alone.

MISCELLANEOUS

SEE ALSO

Housesoiling—Dogs.

Suggested Reading

Case L. Canine and Feline Behavior and Training. Clifton, NY: Delmar Cengage Learning, 2010, pp. 193–194.

Hart B, Hart L, Bain M. Canine and Feline Behavior Therapy, 2nd ed. Ames, IA: Blackwell, 2006, pp. 190–191.

Lindsay S. Applied Dog Behavior and Training, Vol. 2. Ames, IA: Iowa State University Press, 2001, pp. 294–295.

Author Lore I. Haug

Consulting Editor Gary M. Landsberg

SUPERFICIAL NECROLYTIC DERMATITIS

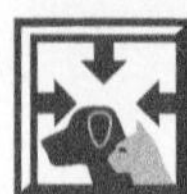

BASICS

OVERVIEW

- Uncommon in dogs; rare in cats.
- Usually a cutaneous marker for advanced liver disease with or without concurrent diabetes mellitus.

SYSTEMS AFFECTED

- Skin/exocrine.
- Endocrine/metabolic.
- Hepatobiliary.

SIGNALMENT

- Shih tzu, Shetland sheepdog, West Highland white terrier, cocker spaniel overrepresented.
- Older dogs.

SIGNS

- Skin—lesions may precede clinical evidence of internal disease by weeks or months; erythema, crusts, and erosions/ulcerations affecting the muzzle, mucocutaneous areas of the face, pinna, distal limbs (especially elbows and hocks), feet, perineum, perianal area, and external genitalia.
- Footpads—hyperkeratotic with fissures and ulcerations; pain when walking.
- Pruritus absent to severe.
- Secondary bacterial and/or yeast infection.
- Feline—alopecia and scaling of the limbs and trunk (two cases); erythema, ulceration, crusting, and alopecia of the limbs and trunk (one case); crusts and hyperkeratosis of paw pads (one case).

S

CAUSES & RISK FACTORS

- Specific cause unknown.
- Cutaneous nutritional deprivation—probably hypoaminoacidemia and/or deficiencies in essential fatty acids and zinc; due to metabolic abnormalities caused by hyperglucagonemia, liver dysfunction, or a combination.
- Usually associated with advanced liver disease with or without concurrent diabetes mellitus.
- Rarely associated with pancreatic or extrapancreatic glucagon-secreting tumor, ingestion of mycotoxins, or long-term phenobarbital and phenytoin therapies.
- Feline—one case each of pancreatic carcinoma, hepatic carcinoid, hepatopathy, and hepatopathy and intestinal lymphoma.

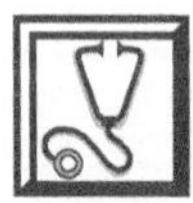

DIAGNOSIS

DIFFERENTIAL DIAGNOSIS

- Pemphigus foliaceus.
- Zinc-responsive dermatosis.
- Toxic epidermal necrolysis.
- Drug eruption.
- Feline exfoliative skin diseases—thymoma-associated exfoliative dermatitis and cutaneous epitheliotropic lymphoma.

CBC/BIOCHEMISTRY/URINALYSIS

- Red blood cell abnormalities—microcytosis, polychromasia, anisocytosis, poikilocytosis, target cells.
- Alkaline phosphatase, alanine aminotransferase, and aspartate aminotransferase—significant elevation.
- Total bilirubin—variably high.
- Albumin—frequently low.
- Borderline or frank hyperglycemia—common.

OTHER LABORATORY TESTS

- Bile acid levels—variably high.
- Liver biopsy—vacuolar hepatopathy with parenchymal collapse and nodular hyperplasia.
- Elevated plasma glucagon levels—present with glucagon-secreting tumors; variable with chronic liver disease.
- Hypoaminoacidemia—common.
- Aminoaciduria.
- High insulin levels may be noted.
- Sulfobromophthalein retention—typically increased.

IMAGING

- Ultrasonography—"honeycomb" liver pattern in advanced hepatopathy.
- Usually unremarkable with pancreatic or extrapancreatic glucagon-secreting tumor unless large enough to visualize.

DIAGNOSTIC PROCEDURES

Skin biopsy—sample early lesions; include crusts and avoid eroded/ulcerated lesions.

PATHOLOGIC FINDINGS

- Parakeratotic hyperkeratosis with high-level intracellular and intercellular epidermal edema; irregular epidermal hyperplasia and mild-to-severe superficial perivascular dermatitis.
- Chronic lesions—marked parakeratotic hyperkeratosis and epidermal hyperplasia.

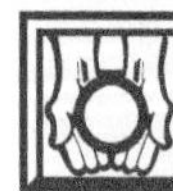

TREATMENT

- Supportive care for systemic signs.
- Surgical excision of glucagon-secreting tumors—can be curative if no metastasis.
- Oral nutritional support—high-quality protein diet or protein supplement for non-encephalopathic cases; 3–6 cooked whole eggs or yolks per day.
- Hydrotherapy and shampoos—remove crusts; lessen pruritus and pain.

MEDICATIONS

DRUG(S) OF CHOICE

- Specific treatment—attempt to correct the underlying disease if possible.
- Nonspecific therapy—antibiotics and antifungal drugs for secondary skin infections.
- Amino acid hyperalimentation—IV administration of a 8.5–10% crystalline amino acid solution (e.g., Aminosyn®) 25 mL/kg, administered over 6–8 hours; repeated weekly or as needed for symptom relief (≥10 infusions may be required). Oral amino acid therapy may be beneficial.
- IV lipid infusion—may improve outcome when combined with IV amino acid therapy (7 mL/kg of 20% Intralipid®).
- Octreotide (somatostatin analogue) 2–3.2 µg/kg SC q6–12h as maintenance therapy for patients with nonresectable glucagon-secreting tumors.
- Glucocorticoids—can improve skin lesions; use carefully; encourages development of diabetes mellitus.
- Colchicine 0.03 mg/kg/day may be beneficial in advanced liver disease.
- Zinc methionine 2 mg/kg/day—adjunctive therapy.
- Essential fatty acids—adjunctive therapy.

FOLLOW-UP

POSSIBLE COMPLICATIONS

- Diabetes mellitus.
- Bacterial and/or yeast skin infections.
- Metastasis of glucagon-secreting tumors.

EXPECTED COURSE AND PROGNOSIS

- Prognosis poor; survival time reported as 6 months after development of skin lesions.
- Rare incidence of recovery if hepatic/metabolic insult resolves.

MISCELLANEOUS

N/A

Author Sheila M.F. Torres

Consulting Editor Alexander H. Werner Resnick

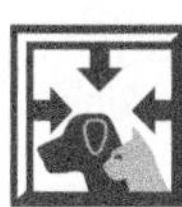

BASICS

DEFINITION

Repetitive supraventricular premature depolarizations that originate from a site other than the sinus node, such as the atrial myocardium or atrioventricular (AV) nodal tissue.

ECG Features (Figure 1)

• Heart rate—rapid, 180–350 bpm in dogs. • Rhythm usually very regular (constant R-R interval) and may be sustained, but there can be frequent or infrequent short runs of supraventricular tachycardia (SVT), so-called paroxysmal SVT. Rarely, the rhythm will be irregular, suggesting abnormal automaticity as the etiology. • Usually QRS complexes typical of normal sinus complexes, i.e., narrow with a normal mean electrical axis. In some cases a coexisting bundle branch block or aberrant ventricular conduction makes it difficult, if not impossible, to differentiate an SVT from a ventricular tachycardia by examining the ECG. • P waves can be normal or abnormal and typically differ in configuration from the sinus P waves. P waves may be buried in the previous T wave and therefore not visualized. • AV conduction is usually normal (1:1), but various levels of functional second-degree AV block may occur at higher atrial rates (2:1, 3:1, 4:1, etc.).

PATHOPHYSIOLOGY

• SVT may be primary (idiopathic) or secondary to other cardiac diseases, generally those creating atrial enlargement. • May result from a reentrant mechanism or from abnormal automaticity in an ectopic focus. Reentrant SVT typically produces a very regular rhythm; SVT due to an automatic focus in atrial myocardium can produce an irregular rhythm. • Most cases in dogs respond to drugs that specifically alter conduction and refractoriness in the AV nodal tissue, suggesting AV nodal reentry as the mechanism. • Recent electrophysiologic studies revealed that some SVT in dogs is related to a congenital accessory pathway between the atria and ventricles, allowing electrical impulses to travel freely between the atria and ventricles without traversing the AV node and without conduction delay; in these cases, the SVT is caused by reentry through the accessory pathway and the AV node.

SYSTEMS AFFECTED

• Cardiovascular—congestive heart failure (CHF) may develop secondary to progressive myocardial failure associated with a chronically high heart rate (so-called tachycardia-induced myocardial failure).
• Neuromuscular—syncope or generalized episodic weakness due to reduced cardiac output and oxygen delivery.

SIGNALMENT

Species

Dog and rarely cat.

SIGNS

General Comments

• Clinical signs may relate to the underlying cause. • Dogs with slow SVT or infrequent paroxysmal SVT may exhibit no clinical signs.
• Dogs with fast SVT (heart rate usually >300 bpm) generally exhibit episodic weakness or syncope.

Historical Findings

• Owners are generally unaware of the arrhythmia. • Coughing or breathing abnormalities in dogs with CHF. • Episodic weakness or syncope.

Physical Examination Findings

• Rapid, usually regular heart rhythm. However, in dogs with paroxysmal SVT, rhythm may be normal and regular during the physical exam.
• May have evidence of poor peripheral perfusion—pale mucous membranes, prolonged capillary refill time, and weak pulses. • May have no signs other than rapid heart rate.
• Findings may reflect underlying cardiac condition (e.g., heart murmur).

CAUSES

• Chronic valvular disease. • Cardiomyopathy.
• Congenital heart disease. • Cardiac neoplasia.
• Systemic disorders. • Ventricular preexcitation.
• Electrolyte imbalances. • Digoxin toxicity.
• Idiopathic.

RISK FACTORS

Heart disease.

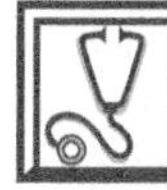

DIAGNOSIS

DIFFERENTIAL DIAGNOSIS

• Sinus tachycardia. • Atrial flutter. • Atrial fibrillation. • Ventricular tachycardia (SVT with right bundle branch block or aberrant conduction can look like ventricular tachycardia; resolution of arrhythmia after lidocaine administration usually confirms ventricular tachycardia).

IMAGING

• Echocardiography (including Doppler studies) may help characterize the type and severity of underlying cardiac disorders. Echocardiography is also important for assessing myocardial function in patients with idiopathic SVT. • When viewed on an echocardiogram during bursts of SVT, the left ventricle has a normal end-systolic diameter and a small end-diastolic diameter, resulting in a decreased shortening fraction because of inadequate filling. • Usually left or right atrial enlargement in dogs with SVT secondary to other cardiac disorders.

DIAGNOSTIC PROCEDURES

• Long-term ambulatory (Holter) recording of the ECG may detect paroxysmal SVT in cases of unexplained syncope. This is generally only helpful if syncope is occurring regularly within a 24- to 48-hour period.

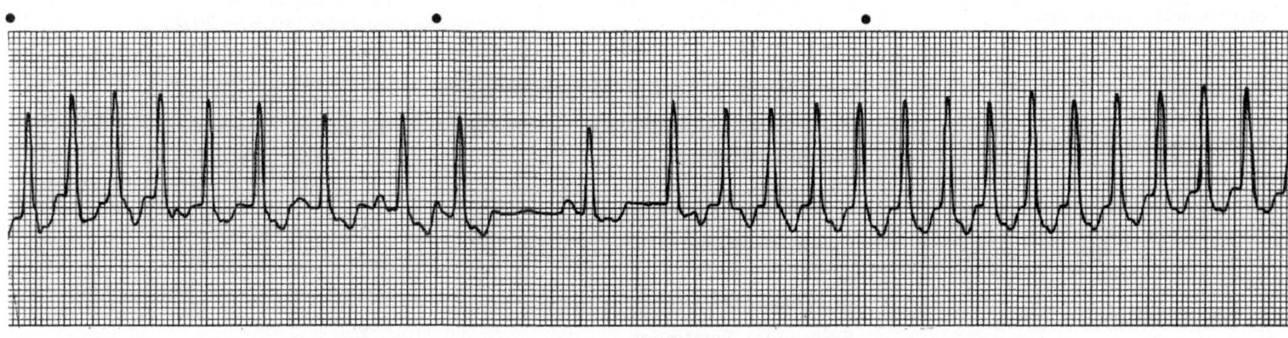

Figure 1.

Sinus with an atrial premature complex and paroxysmal SVT. Abrupt initiation and termination of the tachycardia help distinguish it from sinus tachycardia (lead II, 50 mm/s, 1 cm = 1 mV). (Source: From Tilley LP. Essentials of Canine and Feline Electrocardiography, 3rd ed. Baltimore: Williams & Wilkins, 1992. Reprinted with permission of Wolters Kluwer.)

Holter monitors may also help characterize the rate and frequency of sustained SVT and are useful in evaluating the efficacy of therapy. • Event (loop) recorders may detect paroxysmal SVT in patients with infrequent episodes of syncope (<q24–48h). • Sustained SVT must be distinguished from sinus tachycardia because the two arrhythmias have different implications and treatment. A precordial thump may help differentiate sinus tachycardia from SVT when the heart rate is in the 150–250 bpm range; it will usually stop an SVT for at least 1 or 2 beats, while a sinus tachycardia will not slow. A vagal maneuver (e.g., ocular pressure or carotid sinus massage) may break an SVT abruptly but only gradually slows sinus tachycardia.

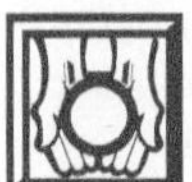

TREATMENT

APPROPRIATE HEALTH CARE

• Asymptomatic patients can be managed on an outpatient basis; patients with a sustained SVT or signs of CHF should be hospitalized until stable. • SVT is a medical emergency in dogs that exhibit weakness and collapse; nonpharmacologic interventions that may break an SVT include vagal maneuvers, precordial thump, and electrical cardioversion. • Vagal maneuvers are often unsuccessful but may be used initially because of their ease of administration and noninvasive nature. • Delivering a precordial thump can successfully (>90% of the time) terminate an SVT in dogs, but this maneuver may break the rhythm for only a brief period. At other times the rhythm remains converted. To perform a precordial thump, the dog is placed on its right side and the left apex beat is located. This region is then "thumped" with a fist while recording the ECG. • Emergency medical therapy is required in patients in which a precordial thump is unsuccessful (see below).

S

NURSING CARE

Treat CHF and correct any underlying electrolyte or acid–base disturbances.

ACTIVITY

Restrict until arrhythmia has been controlled.

DIET

Mild to moderate sodium restriction if in CHF.

CLIENT EDUCATION

Owners should observe patients closely for signs of low cardiac output such as weakness and collapse.

SURGICAL CONSIDERATIONS

Consider transvenous catheter ablation for patients with accessory pathways.

MEDICATIONS

DRUG(S) OF CHOICE

Emergency Therapy

• Administer one of the following: ○ Calcium channel blockers—diltiazem 0.05–0.25 mg/kg IV over 5–15 minutes or verapamil 0.05 mg/kg boluses IV over 3–5 minutes up to 3 times; verapamil more likely to cause hypotension. ○ β-Adrenergic blockers—esmolol 0.25–0.5 mg/kg slow IV bolus administration followed by a CRI of 50–200 μg/kg/min; moderate-to-severe myocardial failure is a relative contraindication to the administration of β-adrenergic blockers. ○ Electrical cardioversion or intracardiac electrophysiologic pacing methods may be considered in extreme cases.

Long-Term Therapy

• Digoxin—administer at either maintenance oral dose or double the maintenance dose for the first day to produce a therapeutic serum concentration more rapidly; contraindicated in patients with accessory pathways.
• β-Adrenergic blocker—atenolol 0.2–1 mg/kg PO q12–24h as long as there is no underlying moderate-to-severe myocardial failure.
• Diltiazem is the calcium channel blocker of choice for long-term control of SVT; dose required to control SVT has not been reported in the dog. Diltiazem used more frequently to control ventricular rate in patients with atrial fibrillation at a dosage of 0.5–1.5 mg/kg PO q8h. In our clinic, we generally start in this range but almost always need to increase the dose to 2–3 mg/kg PO q8h to effectively control SVT. • Class I antiarrhythmic agents such as quinidine and procainamide can be tried when the aforementioned drugs are ineffective or when SVT is thought to be due to an automatic, rather than a reentrant, rhythm. SVT caused by an automatic atrial focus may produce an irregular rhythm and may be refractory to conventional drug therapy. When SVT is due to an accessory pathway, these drugs are more effective.

CONTRAINDICATIONS

Avoid calcium channel blockers in combination with beta-blockers; clinically significant bradyarrhythmias can develop.

PRECAUTIONS

Calcium channel blockers and β-adrenergic blockers have negative inotropic properties and should be used cautiously in dogs with documented myocardial failure.

ALTERNATIVE DRUG(S)

Emergency Treatment

• Adenosine 1–12 mg IV rapidly—very expensive and short-lived. • Propranolol 0.02 mg/kg slow IV boluses up to a total dose of 0.1 mg/kg—long half-life after IV administration, also significant β_2-blocking effects and is generally not recommended unless no other alternative is available.

FOLLOW-UP

PATIENT MONITORING

Serial ECG or Holter monitoring.

POSSIBLE COMPLICATIONS

Syncope and CHF.

EXPECTED COURSE AND PROGNOSIS

Most are controlled effectively with medication.

MISCELLANEOUS

ASSOCIATED CONDITIONS

Accessory pathways in some patients.

AGE-RELATED FACTORS

In young dogs without evidence of structural heart disease, suspect a reentrant tachycardia involving an accessory pathway.

SYNONYMS

Atrial tachycardia, junctional tachycardia.

SEE ALSO

Atrial Fibrillation and Atrial Flutter.

ABBREVIATIONS

• AV = atrioventricular. • CHF = congestive heart failure. • ECG = electrocardiogram.
• SVT = supraventricular tachycardia.

Suggested Reading

Kraus MS, Gelzer ARM. Treatment of cardiac arrhythmias and conduction disturbances. In: Smith FWK, Tilley LP, Oyama M, Sleeper M, eds., Manual of Canine and Feline Cardiology, 5th ed. St. Louis, MO: Saunders Elsevier, 2016, pp. 313–329,

Santilli R, Moïse NS, Pariaut R, Perego M. Electrocardiography of the dog and cat. In: Diagnosis of Arrhythmias, 2nd ed. Milano, Italy: Edra S.P.A., 2018.

Willis R, Oliveira P, Mavropoulou A. Guide to Canine and Feline Electrocardiography. Ames, IA: Wiley-Blackwell, 2018.

Wright KN. Assessment and treatment of supraventricular tachyarrhythmias. In: Bonagura JD, ed., Kirk's Current Veterinary Therapy XIII. Philadelphia, PA: Saunders, 1999, pp. 726–730.

Author Larry P. Tilley
Consulting Editor Michael Aherne

Client Education Handout available online

BASICS

DEFINITION

Temporary loss of consciousness and vascular tone associated with loss of postural tone, followed by spontaneous recovery.

PATHOPHYSIOLOGY

Inadequate cerebral perfusion and delivery of oxygen and metabolic substrates leads to loss of consciousness and motor tone; impaired cerebral perfusion can result from changes in vasomotor tone, cerebral disease, and low cardiac output caused by structural heart disease or arrhythmias.

SYSTEMS AFFECTED

- Cardiovascular.
- Nervous.

SIGNALMENT

Species

Dog and cat.

Breed Predilections

- Sick sinus syndrome—cocker spaniel, miniature schnauzer, West Highland white terriers, pug, dachshund.
- Ventricular arrhythmias—boxer, German shepherd dog.

Mean Age and Range

More common in old animals.

CAUSES

Cardiac Causes

- Bradyarrhythmias—sinus bradycardia, sinus arrest, second-degree atrioventricular (AV) block, complete AV block, atrial standstill.
- Tachyarrhythmias—ventricular tachycardia, supraventricular tachycardia, atrial fibrillation.
- Low cardiac output (nonarrhythmic)—cardiomyopathy, degenerative valve disease, subaortic stenosis, pulmonic stenosis, pulmonary hypertension, heartworm disease, pulmonary embolism, cardiac tumor, cardiac tamponade.

Neurologic and Vasomotor Instability

- Vasovagal syncope—emotional stress and excitement may cause heightened sympathetic stimulation, leading to transient tachycardia and hypertension, which is followed by a compensatory rise in vagal tone, leading to excessive vasodilation without a compensatory rise in heart rate and cardiac output; bradycardia often occurs.
- Situational syncope refers to syncope associated with coughing, defecation, urination, and swallowing.
- Carotid sinus hyperactivity may cause hypotension and bradycardia—often the cause of syncope when one pulls on a dog's collar.

Miscellaneous Causes

- Drugs that affect blood pressure and regulation of autonomic tone.
- Hypoglycemia, hypocalcemia, and hyponatremia (rare).
- Hyperviscosity syndromes (e.g., polycythemia and paraproteinemia) cause sludging of blood and impaired cerebral perfusion (rare).

RISK FACTORS

- Heart disease.
- Sick sinus syndrome.
- Drug therapy—vasodilators (e.g., calcium channel blockers, angiotensin-converting enzyme (ACE) inhibitors, hydralazine, and nitrates), phenothiazines (e.g., acepromazine), antiarrhythmics, and diuretics.

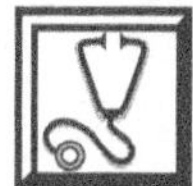

DIAGNOSIS

DIFFERENTIAL DIAGNOSIS

Differential Signs

- Must differentiate from other altered states of consciousness, including seizures and narcolepsy (a sleep disorder).
- Seizures are often associated with prodromal and postictal periods; syncope occurs without warning, and animal usually has rapid, spontaneous recovery. Unlike syncope, seizure activity is usually associated with tonic–clonic muscle activity rather than flaccidity.
- Like syncope, narcolepsy occurs suddenly, results in muscle flaccidity, and resolves spontaneously. Unlike syncope, narcolepsy can last for minutes and can be terminated by loud noises or harsh external stimuli.
- Must differentiate from other causes of collapse such as musculoskeletal disease and neuromuscular disease (e.g., myasthenia gravis), which are not associated with loss of consciousness.

Differential Causes (Figure 1)

- Syncope with excitement or stress suggests vasovagal syncope.
- Syncope with coughing, urination, or defecation suggests situational syncope.
- Syncope with exercise suggests low-output states associated with arrhythmias or structural heart disease.
- A murmur supports heart disease but does not confirm cardiac cause for syncope.

CBC/BIOCHEMISTRY/URINALYSIS

- Usually normal.
- Hypoglycemia or electrolyte disturbance in some animals.

OTHER LABORATORY TESTS

- If animal is hypoglycemic, measure insulin concentration on same blood sample. Calculate an amended insulin: glucose ratio to rule out insulinoma.
- If animal is hyponatremic or hyperkalemic, consider an adrenocorticotropic hormone (ACTH) stimulation test.
- If low cardiac output is suspected, rule out occult heartworm disease.

IMAGING

- Radiography may detect structural heart disease, evidence of pulmonary embolism, or vascular changes supportive of heartworm disease.
- Echocardiography may detect structural heart disease (including tumors) or pericardial disease that could lower cardiac output.
- Doppler echocardiography may aid in the diagnosis of pulmonary hypertension.
- Pulmonary angiography may detect pulmonary embolism.
- CT and MRI may detect pulmonary embolism or heart-based and carotid body masses.
- Ventilation perfusion scintigraphy may detect pulmonary embolism.

DIAGNOSTIC PROCEDURES

- Have client monitor heart rate during any syncopal episode.
- Electroencephalogram, CT of the head, cerebrospinal fluid tap if CNS origin suspected.

Electrocardiogram

- Post-exercise ECG may reveal intermittent arrhythmia.
- Holter monitoring (24-hour ECG recording) or use of an ECG event (loop) recorder—useful for evaluating arrhythmic causes.
- Carotid sinus massage with ECG and blood pressure monitoring useful in evaluating carotid sensitivity.

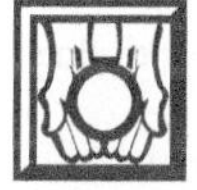

TREATMENT

APPROPRIATE HEALTH CARE

- Avoid or discontinue medications likely to precipitate syncope.
- Treat as outpatient unless important heart disease is evident.

CLIENT EDUCATION

- Minimize stimuli that precipitate episodes.
- Low cardiac output—minimize activity.
- Vasovagal—minimize excitement and stress.
- Cough—remove collar.

SURGICAL CONSIDERATIONS

Pacemaker implantation for sick sinus syndrome, advanced AV block, and persistent atrial standstill.

MEDICATIONS

DRUG(S) OF CHOICE

Bradyarrhythmias

- Correct metabolic causes.

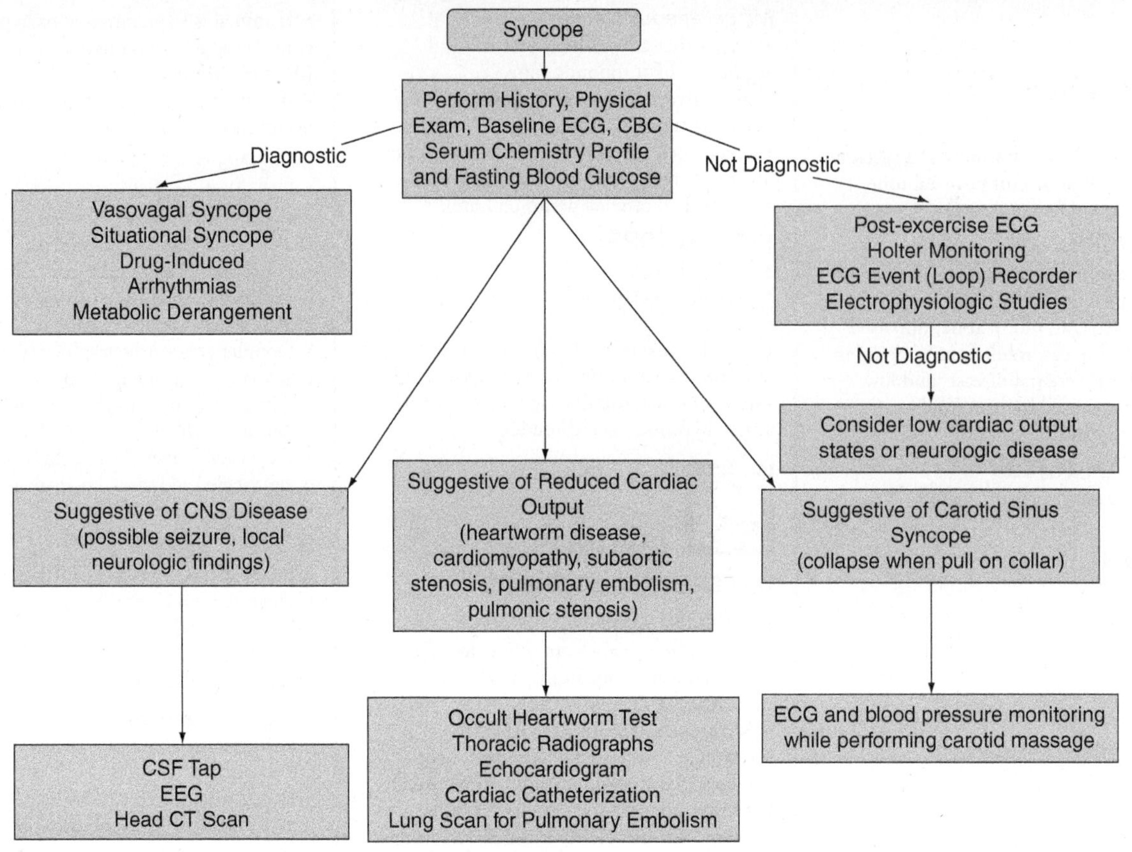

Figure 1.

Algorithm for syncope.

- Anticholinergics (e.g., atropine, propantheline bromide, hyoscyamine sulfate).
- Sympathomimetics (e.g., isoproterenol, bronchodilators).
- Phosphodiesterase III inhibitor (i.e., cilostazol) may be beneficial in sick sinus syndrome
- Pacemaker implantation in some patients.

Tachyarrhythmias

- Atrial arrhythmias—administer digoxin, beta-blocker, or diltiazem.
- Ventricular arrhythmias—administer lidocaine, mexiletine, sotalol, or beta-blocker.

Low Cardiac Output

Institute treatment to improve cardiac output, which varies according to specific cardiac disease.

Vasovagal

- Theophylline or aminophylline—sometimes helpful; mechanism of action in this setting is unclear.
- Beta-blockers (e.g., atenolol, propranolol, and metoprolol) may indirectly prevent vagal stimulation by blocking the initial sympathetic response.
- Anticholinergics may blunt the vagal response.

FOLLOW-UP

PATIENT MONITORING

ECG or Holter monitoring to assess efficacy of antiarrhythmic therapy.

POSSIBLE COMPLICATIONS

- Death.
- Trauma when collapse occurs.

EXPECTED COURSE AND PROGNOSIS

Most noncardiac causes are not life-threatening; cardiac causes may be treated, but syncope in patients with cardiac disease may suggest higher mortality risk.

MISCELLANEOUS

SEE ALSO

- Myasthenia Gravis.
- Narcolepsy and Cataplexy.
- Seizures (Convulsions, Status Epilepticus)—Cats.
- Seizures (Convulsions, Status Epilepticus)—Dogs.

ABBREVIATIONS

- ACE = angiotensin-converting enzyme.
- ACTH = adrenocorticotropic hormone.
- AV = atrioventricular.
- ECG = electrocardiogram.

Suggested Reading

Davidow EB, Proulx J, Woodfield JA. Syncope: pathophysiology and differential diagnosis. Compend Contin Educ Pract Vet 2001, 2:609–618.

Rasmussen CE, Falk T, Domanjko Petrič A, et al. Holter monitoring of small breed dogs with advanced myxomatous mitral valve disease with and without a history of syncope. J Vet Intern Med 2014, 28(2):363–370.

Author Francis W.K. Smith, Jr.
Consulting Editor Michael Aherne

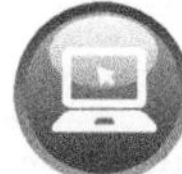

Client Education Handout available online

BASICS

OVERVIEW

• Synovial sarcoma (or synovial cell sarcoma) is a malignant neoplasm arising from type B synoviocytes of the joint capsule or tendon sheath.
• Synovial sarcomas are locally aggressive and have moderate metastatic potential. At diagnosis up to 32% of dogs have metastases with the most common sites being the local lymph node and lungs.
• The disease is seen most commonly in the appendicular skeleton, specifically affecting the elbow, stifle, and shoulder joints. Synovial sarcoma must be differentiated via immunohistochemistry from other types of joint tumors, namely histiocytic sarcoma, which has a more aggressive biologic behavior and a worse prognosis.

SIGNALMENT

• Dog—often large-breed dogs of either sex, predisposition of flat-coated and golden retrievers, mean age of 9 years.
• Cat—rarely reported.

SIGNS

• Slowly progressive lameness.
• Palpable mass.
• Weight loss.
• Anorexia.
• Clinical course may be protracted over months to years.

CAUSES & RISK FACTORS

Unknown

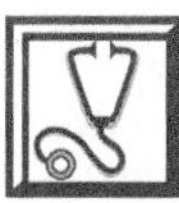

DIAGNOSIS

DIFFERENTIAL DIAGNOSIS

• Other primary neoplasia (e.g., histiocytic sarcoma, chondrosarcoma, osteosarcoma).
• Metastatic neoplasia.
• Other bone or joint diseases (e.g., osteoarthritis, osteomyelitis).

CBC/BIOCHEMISTRY/URINALYSIS

No consistent abnormalities.

OTHER LABORATORY TESTS

N/A

IMAGING

• Radiographs of the affected joint often demonstrate both bone and joint involvement with periarticular soft tissue swelling and periosteal reaction or multiple punctate osteolytic changes in adjacent bone.
• Thoracic radiographs should be obtained to screen for metastatic disease.
• Abdominal ultrasonography should be performed to evaluate intra-abdominal lymph nodes in animals with tumors on the pelvic limbs.

DIAGNOSTIC PROCEDURES

• Regional lymph nodes should be palpated and fine-needle aspirates performed.
• Biopsy and immunohistochemistry to differentiate from histiocytic sarcoma (histiocytic sarcoma is CD18+).

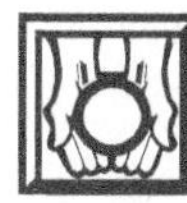

TREATMENT

Limb amputation; forequarter, coxofemoral disarticulation or hemipelvectomy to minimize risk of local recurrence.

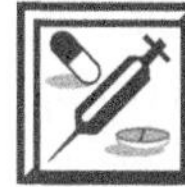

MEDICATIONS

DRUG(S) OF CHOICE

• The role of chemotherapy for synovial sarcomas is not known; however, doxorubicin is commonly utilized for the treatment of sarcoma histologies.
• Pain management with analgesic drugs as necessary.

CONTRAINDICATIONS/POSSIBLE INTERACTIONS

N/A

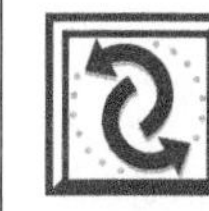

FOLLOW-UP

PATIENT MONITORING

Monitor for local recurrence and pulmonary metastatic disease every 2–3 months for the first year; every 6 months thereafter.

EXPECTED COURSE AND PROGNOSIS

• Localized disease at diagnosis—prognosis is excellent; median survival time >36 months. Lesser dose of surgery (i.e., marginal excision) is associated with poorer prognosis compared to limb amputation.
• Metastatic disease at diagnosis—prognosis is poor; median survival time <6 months. High-grade tumors (high mitotic rate, high percent tumor necrosis, high nuclear pleomorphism) also confer a worse prognosis.

MISCELLANEOUS

PREGNANCY/FERTILITY/BREEDING

Do not breed animals that are receiving chemotherapy.

Suggested Reading

Craig LE, Julian ME, Ferracone JD. Diagnosis and prognosis of synovial tumors in dogs: 35 cases. Vet Pathol 2002, 39:66–73.

Fox DB, Cook JL, Kreeger JM, et al. Canine synovial sarcoma: a retrospective assessment of described prognostic criteria in 16 cases (1994–1999). J Am Anim Hosp Assoc 2002, 38(4):347–355.

Author Alycen P. Lundberg

Consulting Editor Timothy M. Fan

Acknowledgment The author and editors acknowledge the prior contribution of Laura E. Selmic.

SYRINGOMYELIA AND CHIARI-LIKE MALFORMATION

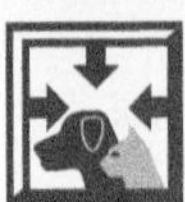

BASICS

DEFINITION

- Chiari-like malformation (CM) is characterized by overcrowding of the cranio-cervical junction (CCJ) and obstruction of CSF channels (brachycephalic obstructive CSF channel syndrome [BOCCS]); may be associated with behavioral and clinical signs of pain (CM-P).
- In syringomyelia (SM), fluid-filled cavities (syringes/syrinxes) develop within the spinal cord; it is a potential consequence of BOCCS.
- Myelopathy can develop with wide SM and, if the dorsal horn is involved, phantom scratching and torticollis.

PATHOPHYSIOLOGY

CM

A complex disorder associated with brachycephaly involving skull base shortening, craniofacial hypoplasia, and CCJ abnormalities including increased proximity of the atlas to skull and increased odontoid angulation. There may a relative increase in parenchymal volume; for example, cavalier King Charles spaniels (CKCS) have greater cerebellar volume compared to other breeds. The reduced cranial capacity results in rostrotentorial neuroparenchymal crowding with rostral forebrain flattening, small and ventrally orientated olfactory bulbs, displacement of the neural tissue to give increased height of the cranium and further reduction of the functional caudotentorial space with hindbrain herniation. CM is often compared to human chiari type I and 0 malformation, however it is more similar to complex craniosynostosis syndromes (premature fusion of multiple skull sutures).

SM

In addition to the above brachycephalic changes, dogs with SM are more likely to have CCJ abnormalities, including rostral displacement of the atlas with increased odontoid angulation, causing craniospinal junction deformation and medulla oblongata elevation. The most accepted theory of SM pathogenesis is that obstruction to CSF flow results in a mismatch in timing between the arterial and CSF pulse peak pressure. If peak CSF pressure is high when spinal arteriole and perivascular space pressures are low then the perivascular spaces act as a one-way valve, drawing in CSF which collects in, then expands and disrupts, the spinal cord central canal and ultimately a syrinx develops.

SYSTEMS AFFECTED

- Nervous.
- Ophthalmic.

GENETICS

- CM has moderately high hereditability ($H^2 = 0.37$).
- Critically relevant SM-associated CM has high hereditability ($H^2 = 0.81$).
- Quantitative trait loci (QTL) study in the Brussels griffon identified two novel genomic regions associated to CM. One region contains a single gene, *SALL-1*, involved in skull development.
- Genome-wide linkage studies in CKCS identified a haplotype, inferring protection against SM associated with CM.
- QTL in CKCS identified two loci on *Canis familiaris* autosome 22 (CFA 22) and CFA 26 associated with SM maximum transverse diameter linked to reduced volume of caudal cranial fossa:
    - Loci on CFA22 contained a single gene, *PCDH17*, a CNS cell adhesion molecule and strongest candidate gene.
    - Loci on CFA26 contained a single gene, *ZWINT*, expression of which is associated with neuropathic pain.

INCIDENCE/PREVALENCE

- In some brachycephalic toy breeds, most notably the CKCS, prevalence of CM approaches 100%.
- SM prevalence increases with age with 25% CKCS affected at 1 year, rising to 70% of CKCS >6 years.
- Studies in the Brussels griffon suggest 42–52% have SM.
- Prevalence of clinically relevant CMSM is difficult to determine as pain is subjective and difficult to measure directly.
- One study suggested 15.4% prevalence of clinically relevant SM in 6-year-old CKCS.

SIGNALMENT

Species

Dog and cat.

Breed Predilections

- Brachycephalic toy breeds and crosses (e.g., cavapoo).
- CKCS, King Charles spaniel, Brussels griffon, affenpinscher, Yorkshire terrier, Maltese, Chihuahua, Pomeranian, Boston terrier, papillon, French bulldog, pug.
- CM but not SM is observed in the Persian and other brachycephalic cats.

Mean Age and Range

From 6 months; however, dogs that do not have clinical signs at 6 years old are less likely to ever develop clinical signs.

Predominant Sex

No sex predisposition.

SIGNS

General Comments

- CM and SM may be clinically relevant. In the CKCS, clinically relevant SM is associated with syrinx transverse width ≥4 mm.
- Signs of CM-P may be intermittent and/or exacerbated by excitement, exercise, weather conditions, and time of day (night/morning).

Historical Findings

CM-P

- Vocalization—spontaneous; on changing position especially when recumbent; being picked up; during defecation.
- Head/ear scratching/rubbing with or without vocalization.
- Reduced activity (walking, playing).
- Refusal to climb stairs or jump.
- Change in emotional state/behavior (timid, anxious, withdrawn or aggressive).
- Disrupted sleep.
- Signs suggesting head/neck pain (aversion to touch/grooming; abnormal head position when awake/asleep; facial expression suggesting pain; squinting/avoiding light).

SM

- Rhythmic scratching action—(phantom scratching) without skin contact with curvature of the body and neck towards foot; induced by rubbing a defined area of skin, typically on neck and/or leash walking.

Physical Examination Findings

CM-P

- Yelping when lifted under sternum.
- Spinal pain—thoracolumbar > cervical > lumbar.
- Exotropia—ventrolateral strabismus when gazing to the ipsilateral side.
- Thoracic limb hypermetria.

SM

- Scratching action induced by rubbing dermatome corresponding to spinal cord dorsal horn damage by syrinx.
- Cervicothoracic torticollis (shoulder deviated ipsilateral; head tilt contralateral to spinal cord dorsal horn damage by syrinx).
- Weakness—thoracic limbs > epaxial/hypaxial muscles > pelvic limbs.
- Proprioceptive deficits—thoracic limbs > pelvic limbs.

CAUSES

- SM develops secondary to CSF channel obstruction.
- Degenerative—constrictive myelopathy in pug and screw tail breeds associated with arachnoid adhesions, facet hypoplasia, vertebral malformation, and secondary ligamentous hypertrophy and intervertebral disc disease (IVDD).
- Anomalous—CM, spinal arachnoid diverticulum/web.
- Neoplastic—mass causing obstruction of CSF channels and/or cerebellar herniation.
- Inflammatory/infectious—meningo-encephalomyelitis of unknown origin (MUO), feline infectious peritonitis,
- Traumatic—sequel of spinal cord injury and arachnoid adhesions.

S

RISK FACTORS

Brachycephalicism and miniaturization.

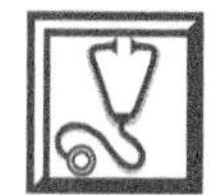

DIAGNOSIS

DIFFERENTIAL DIAGNOSIS

Spinal Pain/Weakness/Ataxia

- IVDD—acute-onset, persistent localized pain in dogs >18 months.
- MUO—pain with rapidly progressive neurologic signs.
- Atlantoaxial subluxation—tetraparesis and pain especially on cervical flexion.
- Discospondylitis—pyrexia and neutrophilia at onset; pain constant.
- Degenerative myelopathy—nonpainful progressive pelvic limb weakness and proprioceptive deficit in dogs >8 years.

Scratching

Skin and ear disease—generalized, tail head, abdominal and digital pruritus is not a feature of CM/SM. In CM/SM the scratching is localized to the head/ears (CM-P) and neck/shoulder/sternum (SM).

Abnormal Head Position

- Rule out vestibular dysfunction due to inner ear, cranial nerve VIII, or intracranial disease.
- Rule out brachycephalic obstructive airway syndrome (BOAS) if sleeping with head elevated (with BOAS often wake coughing).

CBC/BIOCHEMISTRY/URINALYSIS

N/A

IMAGING

Skull and Cervical Radiographs

Limited value; can suggest CM (short basicranium, minuscule frontal sinus, flattened supraoccipital bone, close proximity of the atlas to the skull). In severe SM may have widening of cervical spinal canal and remodeling and scalloping of C2. Dynamic cervical images to assess for atlantoaxial subluxation.

CT

Useful for defining CCJ abnormalities and should be performed if a vertebral malformation is suspected and to facilitate planning of implanted surgical fixation.

MRI

- Aim to establish cause of SM, i.e., CM or other causes of CSF obstruction. Specialized imaging (e.g., balanced steady-state free precession sequences) may be required.
- Assess if radiological findings are consistent with neurological localization and severity, e.g., seizures (forebrain) cannot be attributed to SM (spinal cord).

CM-P

- There is no objective measure of CM-P on MRI. Diagnosis is suggested by appropriate historical, clinical and MRI findings and eliminating other causes of pain.
- MRI features—effacement/narrowed subarachnoid spaces (reduced definition of the sulci); ventriculomegaly; small, ventral olfactory bulbs; rostral forebrain flattening; dorsocaudal displacement of rostrotentorial neuroparenchyma contributing to hindbrain herniation; cerebellum invaginated under occipital lobes; flattening/indentation of the cerebellum by the supraoccipital bone/occipitoatlantal ligament. Atlas closer to the skull and craniospinal junction flexed over odontoid peg.

SM

- MRI features as for CM-P, often with more pronounced CCJ changes.
- Image entire spinal cord to determine extent of syrinx and any spinal cord tethering.
- Clinically relevant disease is more likely with SM width ≥4 mm (CKCS).
- "Active" syrinx indicated by a cavity which expands spinal cord, has asymmetrical shape on transverse images, and fluid signal-void sign (indicates turbulent flow).
- "Quiescent" syrinx indicated by a cavity which is elliptical on sagittal images, symmetrical and circular/ovoid on transverse images, and does not alter spinal cord outline.

DIAGNOSTIC PROCEDURES

CSF—to rule out MUO; however CSF analysis in CM/SM may reveal mild inflammatory changes.

PATHOLOGIC FINDINGS

- Gross—cerebellar herniation, ventriculomegaly, spinal cord cavitation.
- Histopathologic—dogs with clinically relevant SM have asymmetrical syrinx with altered dorsal horn structure and altered expression of pain-related neuropeptides, substance P, and calcitonin gene-related peptide.

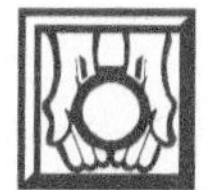

TREATMENT

NURSING CARE

- Raise food bowls.
- Avoid neck collars if phantom scratching.
- Complementary therapy, e.g., acupuncture may be useful.

ACTIVITY

- Exercise encouraged to within own limits.
- Grooming may be poorly tolerated.
- Hydrotherapy may improve strength if SM-associated weakness.

DIET

Obesity positively correlated with a reduced quality of life but not greater neuropathic pain.

CLIENT EDUCATION

Periodic exacerbations of pain common, requiring "top-up" medication.

SURGICAL CONSIDERATIONS

- Craniocervical decompression (CCD) most common surgical procedure—establishing a CSF pathway via the removal of majority of supraoccipital bone and dorsal arch of C1; may be combined with a durotomy, with or without patching with a suitable graft material and with or without cranioplasty.
- Successful in reducing pain and improving neurologic deficits in ~80% cases; ~45% cases have satisfactory quality of life 2 years post-operatively. SM persists postoperatively.
- Clinical improvement probably attributable to reduction in CM-P; most cases require additional medical management.
- Atlantoaxial stability should be assessed prior to CCD.

MEDICATIONS

DRUG(S) OF CHOICE

CM-P

- Nonsteroidal anti-inflammatory drugs (NSAIDs)—at data sheet dosage.
- First-line adjuvant analgesics—gabapentin 10–20 mg/kg q12h/q8h; or pregabalin 5 mg/kg q12h/q8h.
- Second-line (add-on) adjuvant analgesics—topiramate 10 mg/kg q8h; or amitriptyline 0.25–2 mg/kg q12–24h (titrate up to effective dose); or memantine 0.3–1 mg/kg twice daily (titrate up to effective dose); or amantadine 3–5 mg/kg q24h.
- "Top up" analgesia—acetaminophen 10 mg/kg PRN up to q8h and/or opioids at data sheet dosage.

SM-Associated Phantom Scratching

Gabapentin or pregabalin as above.

SM-Associated Weakness and Postural Deficits

- Drugs that may reduce CSF pressure—proton pump inhibitors (omeprazole 0.5–1.5 mg/kg q24h); or H_2-receptor antagonists (cimetidine 5–10 mg/kg q8h); or diuretics (furosemide 1–2 mg/kg q12h; acetazolamide 4–8 mg/kg q9–12h).
- Corticosteroids—as last resort and lowest possible dose that controls signs, starting with 0.5 mg/kg prednisolone or methylprednisolone daily; withdraw NSAIDs.

CONTRAINDICATIONS

Amitriptyline should not be combined with drugs metabolized by cytochrome P450 2D6, e.g., cimetidine.

PRECAUTIONS

- Furosemide may activate renin-angiotensin aldosterone system which may be deleterious in dogs predisposed to myxomatous mitral valve disease (MVD).

- Long-term acetazolamide or corticosteroids not recommended due to potential adverse effects.

POSSIBLE INTERACTIONS

CM/SM does not increase risk of anesthesia unless there is syringobulbia (syrinx in brainstem).

FOLLOW-UP

PATIENT MONITORING

- Periodic review of pain management and neurologic status.
- Serial MRI may be useful.
- Periodic CBC/biochemistry if receiving medication.

PREVENTION/AVOIDANCE

Purchase from a breeder that is health screening and can provide appropriate health certificates.

EXPECTED COURSE AND PROGNOSIS

- Approximately three-quarters of CM-P/SM-affected CKCS deteriorate on medical management. However, many dogs maintain acceptable quality of life.
- 15–20% of CM-P/SM-affected CKCS are euthanized.
- 25–47% of CM-P/SM-affected dogs having surgical management have recurrence or deterioration of signs within 0.2–3 years of surgery.

S

MISCELLANEOUS

ASSOCIATED CONDITIONS

CKCS have high prevalence of unrelated comorbidities, including BOAS, sleep disordered breathing, MVD, pancreatic disorders, biliary tree calcification, epilepsy, myoclonus, fly-catching behavioral disorder, gastroesophageal reflux, otitis media with effusion, deafness, macrothrombocytopenia, keratoconjunctivitis sicca, idiopathic facial nerve paresis, idiopathic vestibular disease.

AGE-RELATED FACTORS

Older brachycephalic toy breeds are more likely to have comorbidities such as MVD. Head and neck myoclonus is extremely common in older CKCS.

PREGNANCY/FERTILITY/BREEDING

- Official health schemes exist in many countries (e.g., the British Veterinary Association CM/SM scheme).
- Breeding recommendations based on SM status and age available.

SYNONYMS

- BOCCS.
- Caudal occipital malformation syndrome.
- Syringohydromyelia.

ABBREVIATIONS

- BOAS = brachycephalic obstructive airway syndrome.
- BOCCS = brachycephalic obstructive CSF channel syndrome.
- CCD = craniocervical decompression.
- CCJ = craniocervical junction.
- CFA = *Canis familiaris* autosome.
- CKCS = cavalier King Charles spaniel.
- CM = chiari-like malformation.
- CM-P = chiari-like malformation-associated pain.
- CSF = cerebrospinal fluid.
- IVDD = intervertebral disc disease.
- QTL= quantitative trait loci.
- MVD = myxomatous mitral valve disease.
- MUO = meningoencephalomyelitis of unknown origin.
- NSAID = nonsteroidal anti-inflammatory drug.
- SM = syringomyelia.

INTERNET RESOURCES

- Frequently asked questions: http://veterinary-neurologist.co.uk/chiari-like-malformation-and-syringomyelia/
- Treatment algorithm: http://veterinary-neurologist.co.uk/cmsm-treatment-algorithm/
- British Veterinary Association CM/SM scheme: https://www.bva.co.uk/Canine-Health-Schemes/CM-SM-scheme/

Suggested Reading

Knowler SP, Galea GL, Rusbridge C. Morphogenesis of canine chiari malformation and secondary syringomyelia: disorders of cerebrospinal fluid circulation. Front Vet Sci 2018, 5:171.

Rusbridge C, Stringer F, Knowler SP. Clinical application of diagnostic imaging of chiari-like malformation and syringomyelia. Front Vet Sci 2018, 5:280.

Author Clare Rusbridge

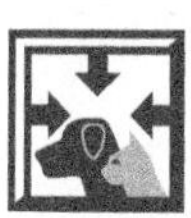

BASICS

OVERVIEW

Systolic anterior motion (SAM) is paradoxical dynamic movement of the mitral valve apparatus or some of its individual components in an anterior direction toward the left ventricular outflow tract (LVOT) and interventricular septum during systole. When the chordae tendineae are the sole component of the valve apparatus displaced anteriorly, the term chordal anterior motion (CAM) is sometimes used.

Pathophysiology

- When SAM was first recognized it was believed to be specific to the setting of hypertrophic cardiomyopathy (HCM) however, it has since been identified to occur under any circumstances that alter the dynamic geometry of the left ventricle (LV).
- There are multiple factors that can contribute to the development of SAM which can broadly be broken down into three main groupings: structural abnormalities, altered ventricular kinetics, and altered ventricular geometry (see Causes).
- Clinical manifestations occur on a spectrum of severity ranging from clinically silent changes to severe dynamic LVOT obstruction (LVOTO).
- Significant LVOTO can result in a pressure overload on the LV, resulting in myocardial hypertrophy; if severe enough, myocardial ischemia and ventricular arrhythmias may ensue.
- Cardiac output is also reduced with severe LVOTO and may result in weakness or collapse.

Systems Affected

Cardiovascular

Genetics

N/A, but certain underlying conditions have a genetic basis in certain breeds (e.g., HCM, subvalvular aortic stenosis [SAS]).

Incidence/Prevalence

True prevalence is unknown. One study identified SAM in 5.8% of apparently normal cats, of which 91.1% had HCM.

SIGNALMENT

Species

Dog and cat.

Breed Predilections

N/A, but certain breeds may be predisposed to certain underlying conditions (e.g., SAS in Newfoundlands; HCM in Maine coons).

Mean Age and Range

Unknown

SIGNS

Historical Findings

- Most animals are asymptomatic.
- Signs are often attributable to underlying disease process.
- Weakness, lethargy, or collapse may be observed with severe LVOTO.
- Patients with advanced underlying cardiac disease may have signs of left-sided or right-sided congestive heart failure (CHF) (e.g., tachypnea, dyspnea, cough, ascites).

Physical Examination Findings

- Systolic murmur which may be static, intermittent, or labile, i.e., variable in intensity from moment to moment.
- Diastolic gallop sounds may be present in patients with underlying cardiomyopathies.
- Femoral pulse quality may be reduced in patients with severe LVOTO.
- Arrhythmias may be appreciated (may be a direct sequela of severe LVOTO or may be due to the underlying disease process).

CAUSES & RISK FACTORS

Causes

SAM is a complex and dynamic condition that may arise from interactions of one or more of the following factors:

- Structural abnormalities:
  - Papillary muscle displacement.
  - Anterior and/or posterior mitral leaflet redundancy.
  - Abnormal chordae tendineae.
  - Bulging of the interventricular septum.
  - Small LV.
- Altered ventricular kinetics:
  - Hyperdynamic LV (generalized or regional).
- Altered ventricular geometry:
  - Reduced distance between septum and mitral coaptation point.
  - Mitral apparatus displaced anteriorly.
  - Decreased anterior:posterior length ratio.
  - Decreased mitro-aortic angle.

Risk Factors

- Any condition or intervention that alters left ventricular geometry or loading conditions.
- HCM.
- SAS.
- Systemic hypertension.
- Hypovolemia.
- Right ventricular systolic hypertension (e.g., pulmonic stenosis, tetralogy of Fallot, pulmonary hypertension).
- Stress/excitement.
- Mitral valve dysplasia.
- Thyrotoxicosis.
- Excess catecholamines.
- Positive inotropic drugs (e.g., dobutamine).
- Surgical mitral valve repair is identified as a risk factor in humans.
- SAM may occasionally be observed in completely healthy animals.

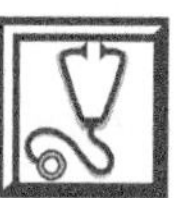

DIAGNOSIS

DIFFERENTIAL DIAGNOSIS

- Must differentiate SAM from other causes of murmurs.
- It can be diagnostically challenging to distinguish if LVOTO due to SAM is the cause or the effect of myocardial hypertrophy.

CBC/BIOCHEMISTRY/URINALYSIS

N/A

OTHER LABORATORY TESTS

N/A

IMAGING

Echocardiography

- Paradoxical systolic motion of the anterior mitral leaflet/mitral apparatus toward the interventricular septum is identified on 2D and m-mode echocardiography, and is often best seen from right-parasternal five-chamber views that highlight the LVOT.
- Color-flow Doppler assessment of the LVOT identifies turbulent blood flow.
- The degree of LVOTO, if present, can be quantified via continuous-wave ± pulsed-wave Doppler interrogation. Doppler flow profiles in the setting of SAM are typically characterized by late systolic acceleration through the LVOT resulting in a "scimitar-shaped" profile.
- Mitral regurgitation is often identified; this is usually mild, with an eccentric jet that is posteriorly directed.
- Myocardial hypertrophy may be present (can be both a cause and an effect of SAM with significant LVOTO).
- Subvalvular ridge may be present in the LVOT of patients with SAS.
- Underfilling of the LV may be appreciated in some patients with SAM.
- Other echocardiographic findings, depending on the type and severity of underlying conditions.

Radiography

- May be normal.
- Radiographic changes, if present, usually reflect the underlying cause.
- Evidence of left- or right-sided cardiomegaly ± CHF may be present on thoracic radiographs.

DIAGNOSTIC PROCEDURES

ECG

- May be normal.
- Atrial or ventricular arrhythmias may be present, depending on underlying pathology.
- Evidence of left- or right-sided cardiomegaly may be present, depending on underlying cause and severity.

- May see evidence of myocardial ischemia (e.g., S-T segment elevation/depression) with severe LVOTO.

PATHOLOGIC FINDINGS

Gross or histopathologic findings reflect any underlying conditions, if present.

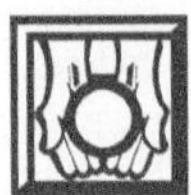

TREATMENT

Treat or remove underlying cause(s)

MEDICATIONS

DRUG(S) OF CHOICE

- Only as needed to manage an underlying condition or CHF, if present.
- Therapy with beta-blocker drugs (e.g., atenolol) is controversial. Beta-blockers are empirically used by some clinicians to reduce the severity and/or the effects of SAM/LVOTO, however evidence of efficacy or any survival benefit is lacking.

CONTRAINDICATIONS/POSSIBLE INTERACTIONS

- The use of positive inotropic drugs (e.g., dobutamine, pimobendan) in the setting of SAM with significant LVOTO is theoretically concerning and thus warrants prudence. Hypotension has been reported in a cat with SAM that received pimobendan for the treatment of heart failure, however a recent study of pimobendan administration in cats with HCM showed no difference in the incidence of LVOTO between treatment and placebo groups.
- Beta-blockers may reduce systolic function and should be used cautiously in patients with known systolic dysfunction.

FOLLOW-UP

PATIENT MONITORING

Type and frequency depends on any underlying disease processes.

PREVENTION/AVOIDANCE

N/A

POSSIBLE COMPLICATIONS

N/A

EXPECTED COURSE AND PROGNOSIS

- Depends on the nature and severity of underlying cause.
- In a study of cats with HCM, cats with SAM had longer survival times than those without. It is speculated that this may be due to SAM allowing earlier identification of the disease due to the presence of a murmur.

MISCELLANEOUS

ASSOCIATED CONDITIONS

N/A

AGE-RELATED FACTORS

N/A

PREGNANCY/FERTILITY/BREEDING

Certain underlying causes (e.g., HCM, SAS) may be heritable.

SYNONYMS

- Chordal anterior motion.
- CAM.
- Dynamic LVOTO.
- When LVOTO due to SAM is present concurrently with a HCM phenotype, the term hypertrophic obstructive cardiomyopathy is used.

SEE ALSO

- Aortic Stenosis.
- Cardiomyopathy, Hypertrophic—Cats.

ABBREVIATIONS

- CAM = chordal anterior motion.
- CHF = congestive heart failure.
- HCM = hypertrophic cardiomyopathy.
- LV = left ventricle.
- LVOT = left ventricular outflow tract.
- LVOTO = left ventricular outflow tract obstruction.
- SAM = systolic anterior motion.
- SAS = subvalvular aortic stenosis.

Suggested Reading

Fox P, Keene B, Lamb K, et al. International collaborative study to assess cardiovascular risk and evaluate long-term health in cats with preclinical hypertrophic cardiomyopathy and apparently cats: The REVEAL study. J Vet Intern Med 2018, 32(3):930–943.

Ibrahim M, Rao C, Ashrafian H, et al. Modern management of systolic anterior motion of the mitral valve. Eur J Cardio-Thorac Surg 2012, 41(6):1260–1270.

Levine R, Vlahakes G, Lefebvre X, et al. Papillary muscle displacement causes systolic anterior motion of the mitral valve. Experimental validation and insights into the mechanism of subaortic obstruction. Circulation 1995, 91(4):1189–1895.

Payne JR, Borgeat K, Connolly DJ, et al. Prognostic indicators in cats with hypertrophic cardiomyopathy. J Vet Intern Med 2013, 27(6):1427–1436.

Author Michael Aherne

Consulting Editor Michael Aherne

TAPEWORMS (CESTODIASIS)

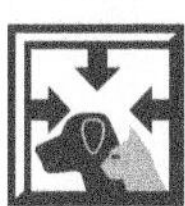

BASICS

OVERVIEW

- Infection of small intestine with adult tapeworms of *Taenia* (especially *T. pisiformis* of dogs and *T. taeniaeformis* of cats), *Dipylidium caninum*, *Echinococcus* spp., *Mesocestoides*, *Diphyllobothrium*, or *Spirometra*.
- Infection by ingestion of intermediate host containing tapeworm larvae.
- Most cause no apparent harm to host other than perianal pruritus; *Spirometra* may cause diarrhea, weight loss, vomiting.
- Peritoneal larval cestodiasis (PLC)—potentially fatal peritoneal infection in dogs (accidental intermediate hosts) caused by *Mesocestoides* larvae.

SIGNALMENT

Dog and cat.

SIGNS

- Motile or dried, white to cream-colored, single proglottids or chains of square or rectangular proglottids of *Taenia* and barrel-shaped proglottids of *Dipylidium* visible on perineum or in feces; *Mesocestoides* proglottids are club-shaped, smaller, more numerous; *Echinococcus* proglottids too small to see.
- Dragging or rubbing anus on ground (pruritus).
- Diarrhea, weight loss—possible with *Spirometra*.
- PLC—abdominal distension (ascites), anorexia, lethargy.

CAUSES & RISK FACTORS

- *Taenia, Echinococcus, Mesocestoides*—eating viscera of intermediate hosts (birds, reptiles, rabbits, rodents, sheep).
- *Dipylidium* infections—eating fleas, lice.
- *Spirometra*—ingesting copepods; uncooked amphibians, reptiles, birds, mammals.
- *Diphyllobothrium*—eating uncooked fish.

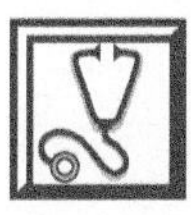

DIAGNOSIS

DIFFERENTIAL DIAGNOSIS

- Anal sac disease.
- Other causes of diarrhea.
- PLC—causes of ascites.

CBC/BIOCHEMISTRY/URINALYSIS

PLC—leukocytosis, hypoalbuminemia.

OTHER LABORATORY TESTS

N/A

IMAGING

PLC—abdominal ultrasonography, radiography.

DIAGNOSTIC PROCEDURES

- Fecal flotation to detect eggs; false negatives if eggs not released from proglottids; crush minced segments between two glass slides to release eggs, add drop of water, examine microscopically.
- *Dipylidium*—press adhesive cellophane tape to perianal skin, then apply tape to microscope slide; packets contain multiple pale yellow eggs ~50 μm in diameter with hexacanth embryo with three pairs of hooks.
- *Taenia, Echinococcus*—individual spherical brown eggs ~30–35 μm in diameter with hexacanth embryo.
- *Mesocestoides*—individual oval thin-shelled eggs with hexacanth embryo.
- PLC—detect larvae in peritoneal fluid by microscopy or PCR-restriction fragment length polymorphism.
- *Diphyllobothrium/Spirometra*—individual eggs with operculum; contain fully developed coracidium.

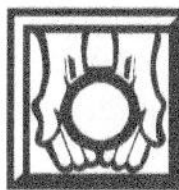

TREATMENT

- Outpatient anthelmintic treatment.
- Flea (or louse) control (*Dipylidium*).
- PLC—anthelmintic treatment, may require peritoneal lavage or surgery to remove larvae.

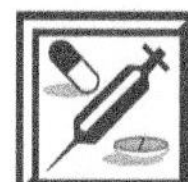

MEDICATIONS

DRUG(S) OF CHOICE

- Fenbendazole 50 mg/kg PO q24h for 3 days.
- Praziquantel 5 mg/kg PO, SC once:
  - Resistance to praziquantel in *Dipylidium* is emerging issue.
  - 7.5 mg/kg PO for 2 days for *Diphyllobothrium* (dogs, extra-label).
- Praziquantel/pyrantel pamoate—label dose (cats).
- Praziquantel/pyrantel pamoate/febantel—label dose (dogs).
- Epsiprantel 5.5 mg/kg PO (dogs), 2.8 mg/kg PO (cats) for *Taenia, Dipylidium*; 7.5 mg/kg PO (dogs) for *Echinococcus*.
- Emodepside 3 mg/kg/praziquantel 12 mg/kg, topically for *Taenia, Dipylidium* (cats).
- Canine PLC—praziquantel 5 mg/kg SC, repeat in 2 weeks; fenbendazole 50–100 mg/kg PO q24h for 4–8 weeks (extra-label; clinical remission, often not curative).

CONTRAINDICATIONS/POSSIBLE INTERACTIONS

Do not use praziquantel or epsiprantel in animals <4 weeks old.

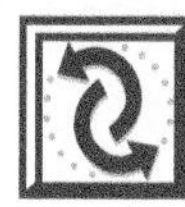

FOLLOW-UP

PATIENT MONITORING

- Post-treatment examination for tapeworm segments or eggs; incompletely removed adult *Mesocestoides* can repopulate by asexual multiplication.
- PLC—ultrasonography, abdominocentesis to detect recurrence; larvae difficult to eliminate (repopulate by asexual multiplication).

PREVENTION/AVOIDANCE

- Flea (or louse) control to prevent *Dipylidium* infection.
- Prevent hunting, scavenging, eating of intermediate hosts.

EXPECTED COURSE AND PROGNOSIS

- Anthelmintic treatment eliminates adult *Taenia, Echinococcus, Dipylidium*; reinfection often occurs.
- Incomplete removal of adult *Mesocestoides* can result in recurrence without reinfection.
- PLC treatment provides clinical remission, often not curative.

MISCELLANEOUS

T

ZOONOTIC POTENTIAL

- Children at risk for *Dipylidium* infection by ingestion of fleas; tapeworm segments have been mistaken for pinworms.
- Ingestion of *Echinococcus* eggs can cause hydatid disease in humans.
- Strict sanitation should be practiced when taeniid eggs observed due to similar egg morphology of *Taenia* and *Echinococcus*.
- Human infection with *Mesocestoides* can occur by ingestion of intermediate hosts.
- Human infections can occur by ingestion of uncooked fish (*Diphyllobothrium*), copepods (*Spirometra*), or vertebrate intermediate hosts.

ABBREVIATIONS

- PLC = peritoneal larval cestodiasis.

INTERNET RESOURCES

http://www.capcvet.org

Suggested Reading

Bowman DD. Georgis' Parasitology for Veterinarians, 9th ed. St. Louis, MO: Saunders, 2009, pp. 131–147, 149–151.

Authors Matt Brewer and Jeba R.J. Jesudoss Chelladurai

Consulting Editor Amie Koenig

TEMPOROMANDIBULAR JOINT DISORDERS

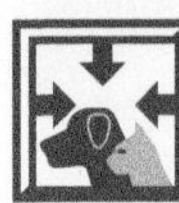

BASICS

OVERVIEW

- Disorders of the temporomandibular joint (TMJ) alter masticatory function due to mobility and functional changes of the joint.
- Genetic, traumatic, degenerative, or idiopathic causes may result in pain, occlusal dysfunction, joint laxity, chronic arthritis, or open-mouth locking.

SIGNALMENT

- Dog and cat.
- No breed, sex, or age predisposition in most TMJ disorders.
- Open-mouth mandibular locking—basset hounds; Irish setters.
- Genetic predisposition in certain breeds (e.g., basset hounds) to develop TMJ disorders.

SIGNS

General Comments

- Difficulty opening mouth.
- Difficulty closing mouth.
- Laxity or excessive lateral movement of the mandible.
- Pain and/or crepitation when masticating, yawning, and/or vocalizing.

Specific

- TMJ luxation/subluxation—history of trauma or mouth locked open; radiographic evidence of luxation.
- Open-mouth mandibular locking—mandibular coronoid process buccal to the ventral surface of the zygomatic arch; locked in that position; large bulge palpated on affected side.
- Traumatic injury—evidence of trauma; mouth dropped open; mobility of mandible (may have multiple fractures); radiographs indicate fracture.
- Osteoarthritis/chronic post-traumatic changes—crepitation and pain when eating or if mandible is forced to move; radiographs may show osseous reaction indicative of arthritic changes.

CAUSES & RISK FACTORS

- Patients at a higher risk to experience injuries—young; free roaming.
- Trauma with fractures or a luxation resulting in immediate problems, and future degenerative problems.
- Mandibular neuropraxia—carrying heavy objects by mouth.
- Masticatory muscle myositis (MMM)—adult; large-breed (e.g., German shepherd dogs).

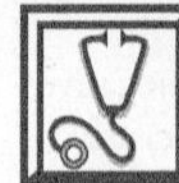

DIAGNOSIS

DIFFERENTIAL DIAGNOSIS

- Craniomandibular osteopathy.
- Mandibular neuropraxia—motor nerve branches of masticatory muscles stretched when carrying heavy objects; mandible hangs open but is easily closed.
- MMM—autoimmune disease of type 2M myofibers of masticatory muscles supplied by trigeminal nerve; trismus progresses to total inability to open jaws.

CBC/BIOCHEMISTRY/URINALYSIS

Typically within normal limits.

OTHER LABORATORY TESTS

- Serum autoantibodies to type 2M myosin—to rule out MMM.
- Cytology of fluid aspirated from TMJ—inflammation from polyarthropathy.

IMAGING

- Skull radiography—essential to perform proper radiographic technique to visualize the TMJ.
- MRI—gold standard for imaging the TMJ.

DIAGNOSTIC PROCEDURES

- Usually none.
- Muscle biopsy—rule out MMM.

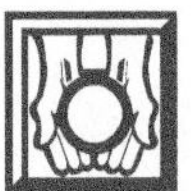

TREATMENT

- Eliminating or altering the etiologic factor responsible for the disorder, as well as correcting the problem.
- TMJ luxation—traumatic: luxation often occurs in a rostral–dorsal direction; in acute cases, place a "dowel" (pencil) across the mouth between the carnassial teeth; gently close the rostral portion of the mouth with a gentle "push" to reduce the luxation (push caudally for a rostral luxation); chronic luxation may not reduce and may require surgery. Digital manipulation may also be effective.
- Open-mouth mandibular locking—immediate attention; sedate animal, open the mouth further and apply gentle pressure on the bulging coronoid process to allow it to slip back under the zygomatic arch; surgical management: excise ventral portion of the zygomatic arch and/or a dorsal portion of the coronoid process to relieve future locking.
- Injury or fracture at TMJ—depends on extent of damage; fixation is difficult; condylectomy sometimes necessary.
- Chronic osteoarthritis or ankylosis—if severe, condylectomy may be needed.
- "Dropped jaw" (trigeminal [mandibular] neuropraxia)—conservative treatment: rest, anti-inflammatory drugs.
- MMM—immunosuppressant medications.

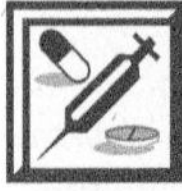

MEDICATIONS

DRUG(S) OF CHOICE

- Analgesics—for painful disorders, both acute and long-term management.
- Anti-inflammatory drugs—for post-operative pain and chronic inflammation.
- Muscle relaxants—help prevent increased muscle activity due to chronic pain response.

FOLLOW-UP

PATIENT MONITORING

Each case should be carefully followed because of the progressive changes that may occur in the TMJ, especially after traumatic injury.

PREVENTION/AVOIDANCE

Avoid situations that allow for trauma (pets running loose).

POSSIBLE COMPLICATIONS

In many cases after surgical treatment involving TMJ disorders, arthritis may develop later.

EXPECTED COURSE AND PROGNOSIS

Depends on the disorder afflicting the TMJ and the degree to which it is affected.

MISCELLANEOUS

PREGNANCY/FERTILITY/BREEDING

Avoid contraindicated medications.

SEE ALSO

Maxillary and Mandibular Fractures.

ABBREVIATIONS

- MMM = masticatory muscle myositis.
- TMJ = temporomandibular joint.

INTERNET RESOURCES

https://avdc.org/avdc-nomenclature/

Suggested Reading

Lobprise HB, Dodd JR. Wiggs' Veterinary Dentistry Principles and Practice. Hoboken, NJ: Wiley-Blackwell, 2019.

Author Heidi B. Lobprise
Consulting Editor Heidi B. Lobprise

T

TESTICULAR DEGENERATION AND HYPOPLASIA

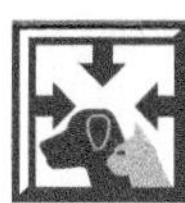

BASICS

OVERVIEW

• Degeneration—histologic changes occurring in the testes after puberty; may be differentiated from hypoplasia by increased thickness of basement membrane or by recognizing a space-filled gap between tail of epididymis and caudal pole of testicle.
• Hypoplasia—a variety of histologic lesions thought to be congenital (although often not obvious until after puberty) or heritable.

SIGNALMENT

• Dog—any age or breed; hypoplasia, generally young; degeneration, generally old.
• Tortoiseshell cat—may be fertile; usually linked with sex chromosome abnormalities (see Sexual Development Disorders).

SIGNS

• Infertility.
• Hypoplasia (dogs)—rarely any physical signs other than small testes.
• Degeneration (dogs)—history of scrotal or testicular insult may be relevant, reduced testicular size and loss of normal turgidity.
• Oligospermia (low numbers of spermatozoa in the ejaculate) or azoospermia (no spermatozoa in the ejaculate).

CAUSES & RISK FACTORS

Degeneration

• Heat.
• Irradiation.
• Increasing age.
• Arterial sclerosis.
• Epididymal occlusion.
• Incisional testicular biopsies.
• Any previous scrotal or testicular lesion may be related.
• Metals—lead salts, cadmium, organic mercurial compounds.
• Orchitis—infectious (such as brucellosis) or noninfectious (autoimmune).
• Some medications—cimetidine, ketoconazole, nitrofurans, flutamide.
• Steroid hormones—estrogen: secreted by a Sertoli cell tumor or exogenous exposure.
• Other hormonal abnormalities—hypothyroidism, hypocortisolism, hyperadrenocorticism.

Hypoplasia

• Klinefelter (XXY) syndrome.
• XX sex reversal—disorder of sexual development with the absence of *SRY* region (dogs).
• Hypogonadotropic hypogonadism—may be acquired from traumatic or neoplastic lesion of the pituitary.

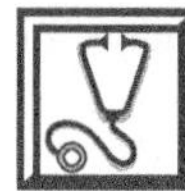

DIAGNOSIS

DIFFERENTIAL DIAGNOSIS

• Degeneration—azoospermia or severe oligospermia in previously fertile dogs having small testes.
• Hypoplasia—azoospermia with no history of proven fertility in dogs with small testes.
• Spermatocele.
• Sperm granuloma.
• Orchitis.
• Neoplasia.
• Ejaculatory failure—retrograde ejaculation, incomplete ejaculation.

OTHER LABORATORY TESTS

Alkaline phosphatase (ALP) concentration of seminal plasma—rule out incomplete ejaculation; samples with ALP <5,000 U/L consistent with incomplete ejaculation or bilateral epididymal obstruction.

IMAGING

Ultrasonography—testicular size (document decreasing values over time, comparison between testicles); heterogenous echogenicity of parenchyma, with or without calcification (chronic).

DIAGNOSTIC PROCEDURES

• Semen evaluation.
• Testicular biopsy (for azoospermia)—Tru-Cut (tissue plug): most complete histopathologic diagnosis; fix tissue for sectioning in Bouin's or formalin solutions.
• Karyotype—(hypoplasia) identify extra X chromosome or other numerical or structural chromosome anomaly.

PATHOLOGIC FINDINGS

• Normal spermatogenesis on biopsy—indicates obstruction in azoospermic dogs.
• Basement membrane thickness—differentiates hypoplasia from degeneration (thickness increased).

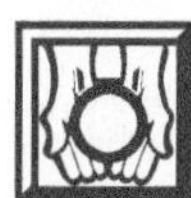

TREATMENT

• Removal of inciting cause, if possible; degeneration linked to adenohypophysis, adrenal gland, thyroid gland, or other metabolic disruption.
• No specific diagnosis—may try gonadotropic hormones; rare anecdotal reports of success.

MEDICATIONS

DRUG(S) OF CHOICE

• Gonadotropin-releasing hormone (GnRH) therapy successful in men with hypogonadotropic hypogonadism; no controlled studies in domestic animals:
  ○ GnRH 1 µg/kg SC, with or with human chorionic gonadotropin (hCG) 1,600 IU, IM.
  ○ hCG 500 IU SC, 2 times/week.

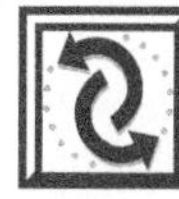

FOLLOW-UP

PATIENT MONITORING

Suspected testicular degeneration (dogs)—a repeat semen analysis performed at least 70 days after correcting any identified underlying cause is needed before long-term prognosis can be assessed.

EXPECTED COURSE AND PROGNOSIS

• Hypoplasia (dogs)—prognosis for fertility poor.
• Degeneration (dogs)—prognosis for sustained fertility depends on cause and duration of ejaculate quality and accuracy of breeding management (see Breeding, Timing).

MISCELLANEOUS

SEE ALSO

• Brucellosis.
• Infertility, Male—Dogs.
• Sexual Development Disorders.
• Spermatocele/Sperm Granuloma.
• Spermatozoal Abnormalities.

ABBREVIATIONS

• ALP = alkaline phosphatase.
• GnRH = gonadotropin-releasing hormone.
• hCG = human chorionic gonadotropin.

Suggested Reading

Johnston SD, Root Kustritz MV, Olson PNS. Disorders of the canine penis and prepuce. In: Canine and Feline Theriogenology. Philadelphia, PA: Saunders, 2001, pp. 356–367.
McEntee K. Reproductive Pathology of Domestic Animals. San Diego, CA: Academic, 1990, pp. 262–263.

Author Candace C. Lyman
Consulting Editor Erin E. Runcan
Acknowledgment The author and editors acknowledge the prior contribution of Carlos R.F. Pinto.

T

TETANUS

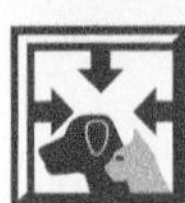

BASICS

OVERVIEW

- *Clostridium tetani*—an obligate anaerobic spore-forming Gram-positive rod found in soil and as part of normal bacterial flora of the intestinal tract of mammals; predilection for contaminated necrotic anaerobic wounds.
- Germinating spores—in wounds, produce potent exotoxin tetanospasmin (tetanus toxin); resistant to disinfectants and to effects of environmental exposure.

SIGNALMENT

Dogs, rarely cats.

SIGNS

Historical Findings

- Signs appear days to months after spores enter wound.
- Wound—often necrotic; but skin may have healed and not visible to owner.

Physical Examination Findings

The most common *initial* clinical signs in affected dogs are ocular and facial abnormalities.

Localized

- Mild rigidity of muscles or leg nearest the site of spore inoculation (wound).
- Stiffness of (hind) limbs; stilted gait; mild weakness and incoordination.
- Can resolve spontaneously—reflects partial immunity to tetanospasmin.
- Can be prodromal to generalized disease—when enough toxin gains access to CNS.

Progressive/Generalized

- Tail—stretches out; progressive tetany of muscles to point of sawhorse appearance.
- Convulsions (clonic)—limbs; whole body (opisthotonus); pain during contractions.
- Dyspnea.
- Difficulty opening jaws—trismus (lockjaw).
- Dysphagia, dysphonia.
- Eyes—lids retract (risus sardonicus, also includes wrinkled forehead and grinning appearance); third eyelid prolapses when head is touched; eyeballs recede into orbit (enophthalmos).
- Erect ears.
- Salivation.
- Fever, painful urination (dysuria), and constipation—may be seen.
- Tetanic muscle spasms—from stimulation (sudden movement, sound, touch).
- Death—during spasm of laryngeal and respiratory muscles (fatal acute asphyxia).

CAUSES & RISK FACTORS

- Unattended wounds (e.g., puncture wounds with foreign body, surgical wounds, compound bone fractures, tooth eruptions/fractures, foot injury or trauma)—portal of entry for spores.
- Outdoor activities provide opportunities for trauma/exposure.

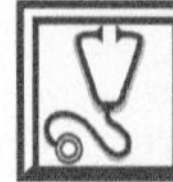

DIAGNOSIS

DIFFERENTIAL DIAGNOSIS

- Intoxications— strychnine, bromethalin, metaldehyde poisoning.
- Dystonic reaction to neuroleptic drugs (acepromazine, prochlorperazine).
- Rabies.
- Meningitis–encephalitis.
- Immune-mediated polymyositis.
- Spinal trauma.
- Hypocalcemia.

CBC/BIOCHEMISTRY/URINALYSIS

- Initial leukopenia; then moderate leukocytosis; then return to reference range.
- Aspartate aminotransferase (AST) and creatine phosphokinase—some increased activity due to muscle damage (tremors).
- Urinalysis—possible myoglobinuria from muscle damage.

OTHER LABORATORY TESTS

- Venous or arterial blood gas analysis—assess adequacy of ventilation (Pco_2).
- Serology—antitetanus antibody often undetectable in serum.
- Culture—wounds; usually unrewarding; must use anaerobic transport medium (do not refrigerate).
- Serum—to detect toxin (by mouse neutralization).
- CSF and blood cultures for bacterial pathogens of meningitis.

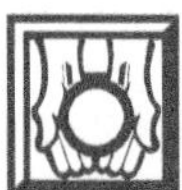

TREATMENT

- Inpatient—constant nursing care important; supportive care for prolonged period (3–4 weeks).
- Feeding—patients often have difficulty prehending food; gastrotomy tube may be necessary; force feeding may exacerbate tetanic state (not advised).
- Hydration—maintain with oral water; if inadequate give a balanced IV fluid.
- Keep patient in darkened quiet area; do not disturb.
- Keep patient on soft bedding; prevent decubital ulcers; rotate stabilized patients cautiously, q4–6h.
- Airway and ventilation—assess; may be necessary to perform endotracheal intubation; tracheostomy may be necessary; monitor blood gas for evidence of hypoventilation.

MEDICATIONS

DRUG(S) OF CHOICE

Sedation

- To control reflex spasms and convulsions.
- Chlorpromazine 0.1–0.5 mg/kg IM, IV, PO q6–12h, also acepromazine 0.01–0.1 mg/kg IV, IM, SC q6–8h; 1–3 mg/kg PO q8h.
- Benzodiazepines—may be administered CRI or intermittent dosing:
  - Midazolam 0.25 mg/kg IV, IM q4–6h or 0.2–0.5 mg/kg/h IV CRI.
  - Diazepam 0.5–1 mg/kg PO (dog), IV, IM q8h or 0.1–1 mg/kg//h IV CRI.
- Phenobarbital 1–4 mg/kg PO, IV q12h.
- Propofol—may be considered if unable to stop tremors; endotracheal intubation necessary.

Tetanus Antitoxin

- Binds only toxin that is free or unbound, does not eliminate already bound toxin.
- First test for hypersensitivity reaction (0.1 mL SC and observe).
- Human tetanus immunoglobulin—administer 500–3,000 U IM at multiple sites, especially proximal to wound; or use equine tetanus antitoxin 100–1,000 U/kg IV; may also be given SC or IM. Maximum dose 20,000 U/kg.
- Administer adsorbed tetanus toxoid intramuscularly.

Antibiotics

- Kill vegetative bacteria to reduce formation of additional toxin; this has no effect against toxin already bound to nerves.
- Metronidazole 10 mg/kg PO, IV q8–12h, preferred.
- Penicillin G 20,000–100,000 IU/kg q6–12h for 10 days; use sodium/potassium salt (IV) on the first day and procaine penicillin (IM) thereafter.
- Glycopyrrolate 0.005–0.01 mg/kg IV, IM q4–6h can be used to treat bradycardia associated with severe tetanus.

CONTRAINDICATIONS/POSSIBLE INTERACTIONS

- Avoid glucocorticoids and atropine.
- Use caution with narcotics—depress respiratory center.
- Avoid oral diazepam in cats due to hepatotoxicity.

FOLLOW-UP

PATIENT MONITORING

- Monitor for decubital ulcers and peripheral nerve palsies.
- Monitor blood pressure and ECG.
- Aspiration possible.

• Constipation possible.

PREVENTION/AVOIDANCE

• Vaccinate—tetanus toxoid; not typically used in dogs and cats.
• Prevent skin wound trauma—clear runs and yards of wire, glass, etc.
• Wound management—early and thorough irrigation; debridement and drainage, especially in tetanus-prone wounds.

EXPECTED COURSE AND PROGNOSIS

• Younger dogs with tetanus may be more likely to develop severe clinical signs.
• The prognosis for survival in dogs with tetanus is good if abnormalities in heart rate or blood pressure values do not develop.
• Prognosis—depends on number of factors; poorer prognosis has been associated with more toxin bound to nerves, wounds closer to the head, shorter interval between injury and first tetanic spasm, and development of aspiration pneumonia.
• Course of recovery—slow; requires rehabilitation to regain full use of limbs; most recover in 1 week; some have a course of 3–4 weeks; unattended disease can be fatal if it progresses to generalized disease (vs. localized tetanus).

MISCELLANEOUS

ZOONOTIC POTENTIAL

None, but tetanus spores ubiquitous in environment.

ABBREVIATIONS

• AST = aspartate aminotransferase.

INTERNET RESOURCES

http://www.cdc.gov/vaccines/pubs/pinkbook/tetanus.html

Suggested Reading

Burkitt JM, Sturges BK, Jandrey KE, et al. Risk factors associated with outcome in dogs with tetanus: 38 cases (1987–2005). J Am Vet Med Assoc 2007, 230:76–83.

Linnenbrink T, McMichael M. Tetanus: pathophysiology, clinical signs, diagnosis, and update on new treatment modalities. J Vet Emerg Crit Care 2006, 16:199–207.

Author Patrick L. McDonough
Consulting Editor Amie Koenig

TETRALOGY OF FALLOT

BASICS

OVERVIEW

• A congenital cardiac malformation that consists of a ventricular septal defect (VSD), pulmonic stenosis (PS), an overriding aorta, and right ventricular (RV) hypertrophy (Figure 1). The essential developmental abnormality is probably cranial deviation of the infundibular (outlet) septum; the other defects are secondary. • Hemodynamics are determined primarily by the size of the VSD (typically large, i.e., equals or exceeds area of the open aortic valve) and the severity of RV outflow tract obstruction (RVOTO). A large VSD allows equilibration of left and RV pressures, with shunt direction determined by the relationship between peripheral vascular resistance and the resistance to RV ejection. Severe RVOTO results in a right-to-left shunt with cyanosis and compensatory erythrocytosis as prominent clinical features. • An uncommon congenital defect, but the most common congenital cardiac malformation that causes cyanosis in dogs and cats.

SIGNALMENT

• Dog and cat—uncommon in both.
• English bulldog and keeshond predisposed.

SIGNS

Historical Findings

• Weakness. • Syncope. • Shortness of breath.

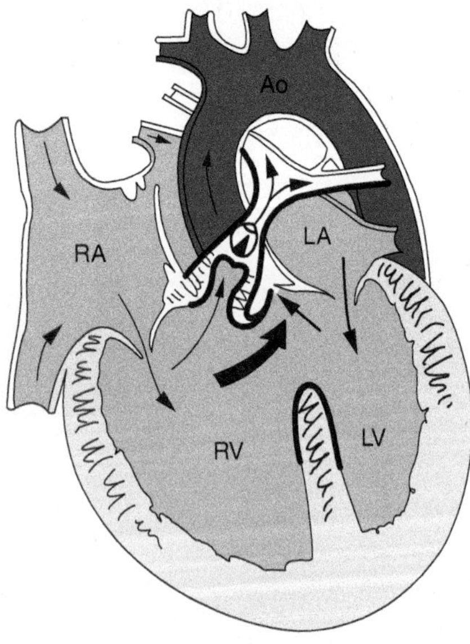

Figure 1.

Classic tetralogy of Fallot. RA = right atrium, LA = left atrium, RV = right ventricle, LV = left ventricle, Ao = aorta. (Source: Roberts W., Adult Congenital Heart Disease. Philadelphia, © 1987 F.A. Davis Company.)

Physical Examination Findings

• Systolic left basilar ejection murmur, caused by RVOTO in most patients; some with hyperviscosity and severe pulmonary stenosis do not have murmurs. • Cyanosis—most patients; degree of cyanosis depends on the direction and volume of shunt. If RVOTO is mild, direction of the shunt may be left-to-right; in this case, cyanosis is absent and the pathophysiology is that of an isolated VSD. • Arterial pulses usually normal. • Congestive heart failure rare, possibly because the right ventricle can unload into the left ventricle, preventing the development of suprasystemic RV pressures.

CAUSES & RISK FACTORS

Congenital; a continuum of conotruncal defects that includes tetralogy of Fallot inherited in keeshonden; the mode of transmission likely oligogenic. Genetic factors probably etiologically important when tetralogy of Fallot observed in patients of other breeds.

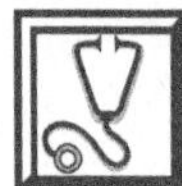

DIAGNOSIS

DIFFERENTIAL DIAGNOSIS

• Aortic stenosis, PS, VSD, and atrial septal defect can all cause left basilar ejection murmurs. • Patients with severe PS and a right-to-left atrial-level shunt may have similar findings on physical examination.
• Other anatomic right-to-left shunts (patent ductus arteriosus [PDA] or VSD with high pulmonary vascular resistance) do not typically cause murmurs; differential cyanosis (cranial mucous membranes are pink; caudal mucous membranes are cyanotic) is observed if a PDA shunts right-to-left.

CBC/BIOCHEMISTRY/URINALYSIS

Compensatory erythrocytosis if the shunt is right-to-left.

IMAGING

Thoracic Radiography

• Variable RV enlargement. • Ascending aorta may be prominent. • Pulmonary vessels are small.

Echocardiography

• RV hypertrophy. • Large VSD visualized directly. • Aortic overriding of the VSD.
• Narrow infundibulum and/or abnormal pulmonic valve. • Doppler evidence of PS.
• Contrast echocardiography typically delineates a right-to-left shunt.

Angiocardiography

• Reveals VSD, RV hypertrophy, PS, and shunt direction. • Nonselective angiography may confirm diagnosis in patients <10 kg.

DIAGNOSTIC PROCEDURES

Electrocardiography

RV hypertrophy pattern in most dogs and cats.

Oximetry

Used to confirm peripheral desaturation of hemoglobin.

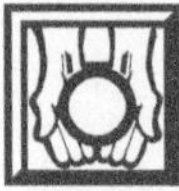

TREATMENT

• Most treated as outpatients. • Exercise restriction recommended. • Treat erythrocytosis by periodic phlebotomy to maintain a PCV of 62–68%. • Palliative surgical procedures that enhance pulmonary blood flow have been performed. • Definitive surgical correction requires cardiopulmonary bypass.

MEDICATIONS

DRUG(S) OF CHOICE

Nonselective β-adrenergic antagonists such as propranolol may be palliative; they act as negative inotropes, thereby limiting dynamic RVOTO, and also prevent the physiologic drop in peripheral vascular resistance that occurs during exercise. These hemodynamic effects serve to limit right-to-left shunting. Propranolol may also favorably affect the oxyhemoglobin dissociation curve.

CONTRAINDICATIONS/POSSIBLE INTERACTIONS

Vasodilators contraindicated.

FOLLOW-UP

• Monitor PCV every 1–3 months. • Do not breed affected animals. • Bacterial endocarditis, neurologic complications associated with erythrocytosis, arrhythmias, and sudden death are potential sequelae. • Prognosis generally poor; median age at death in one study was 23.4 months.

MISCELLANEOUS

ABBREVIATIONS

• PDA = patent ductus arteriosus.
• PS = pulmonic stenosis. • RVOTO = right ventricular outflow tract obstruction.
• VSD = ventricular septal defect.

Suggested Reading

Chetboul V, Pitsch I, Tissier R, et al. Epidemiological, clinical, and echocardiographic features and survival times of dogs and cats with tetralogy of Fallot: 31 cases (2003–2014). J Am Vet Med Assoc 2016, 249(8): 909–917.

Author Jonathan A. Abbott
Consulting Editor Michael Aherne

THIRD EYELID PROTRUSION

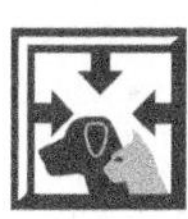

BASICS

DEFINITION

Abnormal protrusion (elevation) of the third eyelid.

PATHOPHYSIOLOGY

- Dogs—movement of the third eyelid is passive.
- Cats—partial sympathetic nervous control of the third eyelid.
- May be primary (conformational) or secondary (exophthalmos, enophthalmos, sympathetic denervation, painful eye).

SYSTEMS AFFECTED

- Nervous—autonomic nervous system.
- Ophthalmic—third eyelid(s); orbit; globe.

SIGNALMENT

See Causes.

SIGNS

- Primary—often none; occasionally conjunctivitis and tearing.
- Secondary—associated with the underlying condition.
- Unilateral or bilateral—depending on cause.

CAUSES

Unilateral

Blepharospasm

- Painful ocular condition—corneal ulcer; glaucoma; uveitis; foreign body.
- Active retraction of the globe results in secondary third eyelid elevation.

Exophthalmos

- Increase in orbital volume—pushes the eye and third eyelid forward.
- Abscess or cellulitis—generally young patients; acute onset; painful on palpation.
- Neoplasm—generally older patients; gradual onset; frequently not painful.
- Salivary gland inflammation/mucocele—variable age; may be secondary to trauma; frequently not painful (see Orbital Diseases (Exophthalmos, Enophthalmos, Strabismus)).

Enophthalmos

- Globe—recedes into the orbit, causing third eyelid to appear elevated.
- Unilateral—may be caused by trauma, orbital fat atrophy, neoplasia, and inflammation.
- Horner's syndrome—clinical signs develop after sympathetic denervation; elevated third eyelid; enophthalmos; ptosis (drooping upper eyelid); miosis (see Horner's Syndrome).

Microphthalmos or Phthisis Bulbi

- Small globes—cause the third eyelid to appear elevated.
- Microphthalmos—congenital; idiopathic or may be inherited in specific breeds (many reported); other intraocular abnormalities may be present. May result from toxin ingestion (griseofulvin in pregnant cats).
- Phthisis bulbi—acquired; severe damage to the globe (uveitis, glaucoma, or trauma); ciliary body fails to produce aqueous humor; diminished; small, fibrotic globe.
- Other
- Neoplasia of the third eyelid—slow growing; usually older patients. Most common: adenocarcinoma of the gland of the third eyelid; hemangioma/hemangiosarcoma, melanoma and squamous cell carcinoma and others may involve the eyelid.
- Cherry eye—see Prolapsed Gland of the Third Eyelid (Cherry Eye).
- Everted or scrolled cartilage of the third eyelid—primarily large and giant breeds; the T-shaped cartilage of the third eyelid is rolled away from the surface of the eye instead of conforming to the corneal surface.
- Symblepharon—post-inflammatory adhesions between the third eyelid and cornea or conjunctiva. Common in cats who had ocular surface inflammation before the eyelids opened.
- Foreign body.
- Previous injury.
- Facial nerve paralysis—patient will retract the globe and "flash" the third eyelid.

Bilateral

Exophthalmos

- Space-occupying lesions of both orbits.
- Usually caused by immune-mediated inflammatory lesions (e.g., eosinophilic myositis, extraocular muscle polymyositis).

Conformational

- Breed-specific—primarily large-breed dogs.
- Deep orbits and prominent third eyelids.
- Not pathologic.
- No treatment needed.

Plasmoma

- Immune-mediated thickening and hyperemia of the leading edge of the third eyelid due to infiltration of plasma cells and lymphocytes; follicle formation; depigmentation.
- Primarily in German shepherd dogs; other breeds reported.
- May be associated with chronic superficial keratitis (pannus).

Other

- Blepharospasm (active retraction of globe).
- Enophthalmos—caused by dehydration, bilateral orbital fat atrophy secondary to severe cachexia, and chronic masticatory muscle myositis.
- Haw's syndrome (cats)—idiopathic bilateral elevation of the third eyelids; primarily young cats with history of diarrhea; ophthalmic examination otherwise normal; self-limiting; usually resolves in 3–4 weeks without treatment.
- Dysautonomia (Key-Gaskell syndrome)—bilateral elevated third eyelids; dilated nonresponsive pupils; keratoconjunctivitis sicca (KCS); dry mucosal surfaces; anorexia; lethargy; regurgitation; megaesophagus; bradycardia; megacolon; distended bladder (see Dysautonomia (Key-Gaskell Syndrome)).
- Tranquilizers—many (e.g., acepromazine) cause bilateral third eyelid elevation.
- Fatigue—transient third eyelid elevation, especially in dogs prone to ectropion.
- Cannabis intoxication.
- Tetanus—eyelids retract; third eyelid prolapse; enophthalmos; secondary to hypertonicity of extraocular muscles (see Tetanus).

Rabies—reported ocular signs include dilated pupils; anisocoria; third eyelid prolapse; uveitis (see Rabies).

RISK FACTORS

Depends on cause.

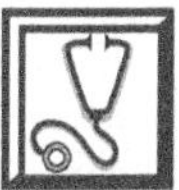

DIAGNOSIS

DIFFERENTIAL DIAGNOSIS

- Most common causes of acute onset of unilateral condition—ocular pain (e.g., corneal ulcer, uveitis); orbital inflammation (e.g., orbital abscess, cellulitis).
- Middle-aged or older patient with unilateral, nonpainful condition—third eyelid or orbital neoplasm likely.
- All patients—must rule out a small eye (microphthalmos or phthisis bulbi) and Horner's syndrome.
- Likely causes of bilateral condition—systemic illness (e.g., dehydration, cachexia, dysautonomia); associated with conformational abnormalities.
- Prolapsed gland of the third eyelid—medial aspect of the third eyelid swollen; the third eyelid itself usually normal.
- Lightly pigmented third eyelid margin—normal conformation; may be falsely identified as an elevated third eyelid.

CBC/BIOCHEMISTRY/URINALYSIS

- Leukocytosis and a left shift—with orbital inflammatory processes.
- Blood work—generally normal despite differing causes.

OTHER LABORATORY TESTS

Dysautonomia—confirmed by measuring urine and plasma catecholamine concentrations and pharmacologic testing of the autonomic nervous system.

IMAGING

- Thoracic radiography—all patients with Horner's syndrome to rule out intrathoracic cause of sympathetic denervation, evaluate for metastatic disease.
- Orbital ultrasound—recommended to help localize suspected orbital mass and define its nature (e.g., solid or cystic).

T

THIRD EYELID PROTRUSION (CONTINUED)

• CT or MRI—further define suspected or known orbital mass.
• Skull radiographs—rarely show signs of orbital disease unless lesion is very large and destructive.

DIAGNOSTIC PROCEDURES

• Thorough ophthalmic examination utilizing a source of magnification.
• All patients with unilateral condition—examine both surfaces of the third eyelid and the conjunctival cul-de-sac carefully for a foreign body or symblepharon.
• Pharmacologic testing—localize lesion with Horner's syndrome (see Horner's Syndrome).
• Exploratory surgery and biopsy—may be only means to make a definitive diagnosis for a suspected orbital or third eyelid mass.

Cytology

• For suspected mass lesions:
 ∘ Unguided fine-needle aspiration—only if the mass is anterior to the equator of the eye.
 ∘ Ultrasound-guided fine-needle aspiration—for masses posterior to the eye; help avoid delicate retrobulbar structures.
• Third eyelid scrapings—German shepherd dogs with suspected plasmoma reveal plasma cells and lymphocytes.

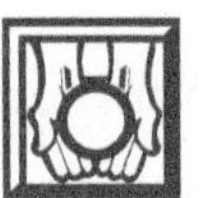

TREATMENT

• Depends on cause.
• Painful condition—remove the cause of the irritation (e.g., foreign body); treat the primary ocular condition.
• Orbital cellulitis and abscess—orbital drainage and systemic antibiotics.
• Orbital neoplasms—usually require wide surgical excision via an orbital exenteration; may require adjunct therapeutic modalities if excision is incomplete.
• Microphthalmic eyes—usually none required; enucleation if painful or subject to recurrent conjunctivitis.
• Blind traumatized eyes—enucleate if painful and to prevent formation of intraocular sarcomas (cats).
• Horner's syndrome—treat cause, if known (~50% of dogs and cats); otherwise may resolve without treatment in 4–12 weeks.
• Surgical removal of the entire third eyelid—indicated for third eyelid neoplasia; may require adjunct therapeutic modalities if the surgical margins are not free of neoplasm.
• Radiotherapy around the eye—may result in severe keratitis, dry eye, and cataracts; discuss enucleation with the client before initiating treatment if eye will be in the radiation field.
• Orbital exenteration—may be warranted if the mass extends into the orbit.
• Plasmoma—usually controlled with topical medications; not cured; life-long therapy needed; topical corticosteroids (0.1% dexamethasone or 1% prednisolone acetate q6h, reduced to q24h when appears resolved); topical 1% cyclosporine q12h also effective.
• Haw's syndrome—usually self-limiting without treatment.
• See Dysautonomia (Key-Gaskell Syndrome), tetanus, or rabies.

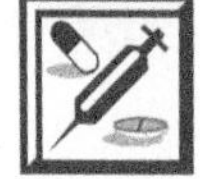

MEDICATIONS

DRUG(S) OF CHOICE

See Treatment.

CONTRAINDICATIONS

Topical corticosteroids—never use in patients with corneal ulceration.

PRECAUTIONS

N/A

POSSIBLE INTERACTIONS

N/A

ALTERNATIVE DRUG(S)

N/A

FOLLOW-UP

PATIENT MONITORING

Malignant neoplasia—thoracic radiographs and full physical exam q3–6 months to monitor for metastatic disease.

POSSIBLE COMPLICATIONS

• Neoplasm—extension to or involvement of adjacent orbital structures (e.g., eye, orbit, orbital sinuses, and cranial cavity) possible; metastasis to distant sites (usually thorax or liver) possible (approximately 90% are malignant).
• Vision loss—from the lesion itself, from elevation, or from treatment (e.g., radiotherapy and exenteration).

MISCELLANEOUS

ASSOCIATED CONDITIONS

N/A

AGE-RELATED FACTORS

• Middle-aged to older patients—at risk for neoplastic diseases of the third eyelid and orbit.
• Young patients—at risk for congenital abnormalities; affected by inflammatory conditions of the third eyelid more frequently than older animals.

ZOONOTIC POTENTIAL

N/A

PREGNANCY/FERTILITY/BREEDING

N/A

SYNONYMS

• Elevated third eyelid.
• Haw's syndrome (cats).

SEE ALSO

• Dysautonomia (Key-Gaskell Syndrome).
• Ectropion.
• Entropion.
• Horner's Syndrome.
• Orbital Diseases (Exophthalmos, Enophthalmos, Strabismus).
• Prolapsed Gland of the Third Eyelid (Cherry Eye).
• Rabies.
• Tetanus.

ABBREVIATIONS

• KCS = keratoconjunctivitis sicca.

Suggested Reading

Hendrix DVH. Diseases and surgery of the canine conjunctiva and nictitating membrane. In: Gelatt KN, Gilger BC, Kern T, eds., Veterinary Ophthalmology, 5th ed. Ames, IA: Wiley-Blackwell, 2013, pp. 945–975.

Peruccio C. Diseases of the third eyelid. In: Maggs DJ, Miller PE, Ofri R, eds., Slatter's Fundamentals of Veterinary Ophthalmology, 6th ed. St. Louis, MO: Saunders, 2018, pp. 178–185.

Sharp NH, Nash AS, Griffiths IR. Feline dysautonomia (the Key-Gaskell syndrome): a clinical and pathological study of forty cases. J Small Anim Pract 1985, 25:599–615.

Author Renee T. Carter

Consulting Editor Kathern E. Myrna

Acknowledgment The author and editors acknowledge the prior contribution of Brian C. Gilger.

THROMBOCYTOPATHIES

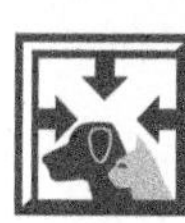

BASICS

OVERVIEW

- Acquired or hereditary defects that affect platelet function, including procoagulant activity. Defects are in two categories: intrinsic and extrinsic.
- Intrinsic platelet defects originate within platelets; extrinsic platelet defects affect platelet function indirectly (e.g., von Willebrand disease [VWD]).
- Affected animals typically have normal platelet counts but have spontaneous or excessive bleeding; mucosal or postoperative bleeding are most common.
- Thrombocytopenic animals with concurrent thrombocytopathia will bleed more excessively than expected for the platelet count.

SIGNALMENT

- Acquired defects are the most common thrombocytopathias in companion animals. They occur in all breeds and at all ages.
- Hereditary platelet function defects may be diagnosed at any age but commonly appear in young animals with the loss of deciduous teeth, causing excessive bleeding.
- Hereditary defects are rare disorders that have been described in the following breeds/ species:
    - VWD—Doberman pinschers, German shorthair pointers, many other pure and mixed- breed dogs.
    - Type I Glanzmann thrombasthenia—otterhound and great Pyrenees dogs
    - Storage pool diseases—Persian cats, American cocker spaniels, grey collie dogs.
    - CalDAG-GEFI thrombocytopathia—basset hound, spitz, and Landseer dogs.
    - Scott syndrome—German shepherd dog.
    - *P2Y12* (ADP) receptor mutation—greater Swiss mountain dog.

SIGNS

- Often mild spontaneous mucocutaneous bleeding (e.g., epistaxis, petechiation, gingival bleeding). Petechiae are not necessarily seen in animals with adequate circulating platelet number.
- Prolonged bleeding in some animals during or following diagnostic or surgical procedures.
- In Scott syndrome, postoperative hemorrhage is the most common sign.
- Bleeding diathesis can be more severe in acquired systemic conditions, as other components of coagulation can be affected as well.

CAUSES & RISK FACTORS

Acquired—Drugs

- Nonsteroidal anti-inflammatory drugs (NSAIDS; e.g., aspirin) inhibit platelet function by preventing the formation of thromboxane A_2. More selective cyclooxygenase 2 (COX-2) antagonists (e.g., meloxicam, deracoxib) have less effect on platelet function.
- Thienopyridine prodrugs (e.g. clopidogrel) inhibit the platelet P2Y12 ADP receptor.
- Hydroxyethyl starch (HES) solutions suppress platelet function in dogs in addition to other anticoagulant effects, but increased risk of bleeding is variable and prolonged with HES of higher molecular weight and higher molar substitution.
- *n3* fatty acids have a mild thrombocytopathic effect in dogs that is not associated with clinical bleeding.
- Penicillins, tetracyclines, potentiated sulfonamides, anesthetic/sedative agents, and antihistamines cause mild platelet function defects in humans. Adverse effects of carbenicillin and ticarcillin have been documented in dogs and have not been investigated in cats.

Acquired—Secondary to Systemic Disease

Disseminated intravascular coagulation (DIC), uremia, anemia, liver disease (cholestasis and acquired or inherited shunts), ehrlichiosis, leishmaniasis, heart disease, immune-mediated thrombocytopenia, and neoplastic disorders (both hematopoietic and nonhematopoietic neoplasms) may alter platelet function.

Hereditary

- VWD (Doberman pinschers, German shorthair pointers, many other breeds)—a deficiency (type I and III) or qualitative defect (type II) of von Willebrand factor (VWF) prevents platelet adhesion to areas of vascular injury.
- CalDAG-GEFI hereditary thrombocytopathia (basset hound and Landseer dogs)—mutations in signal transduction in platelets, preventing platelet activation.
- Type I Glanzmann thrombasthenia (otterhound and great Pyrenees dogs)—platelet defect caused by a mutation in glycoprotein IIb–IIIa (fibrinogen receptor) on the platelet surface.
- Bernard Soulier syndrome (English cocker spaniel)—mutation in glycoprotein IX (VWF receptor complex) on the platelet surface prevents platelet adhesion.
- Chediak-Higashi syndrome, cyclic hematopoiesis, and dense granule defect (Persian cats, grey collie dogs, and American cocker spaniels, respectively)—deficiency (Chediak-Higashi syndrome, cyclic hematopoiesis) or functional defect (dense granule defect) of delta-granules in platelets results in inability to activate additional platelets at site of vascular injury.
- Scott syndrome (German shepherd dog)—platelet procoagulant deficiency resulting in failure to externalize phosphatidylserine, generate microparticles, and support effective assembly of coagulation complexes, caused by a *TMEM16F* mutation.
- *P2Y12* receptor mutation (greater Swiss mountain dog)—multifactorial defect; platelets are not activated by ADP.

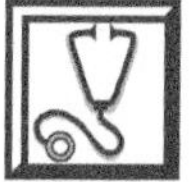

DIAGNOSIS

CBC/BIOCHEMISTRY/URINALYSIS

- Anemia, if bleeding is severe.
- Platelet counts typically normal in dogs with inherited thrombocytopathies, but thrombocytopenia seen following hemorrhage; bizarre and giant platelets may be seen.
- Biochemical profile—no specific changes.
- Urinalysis—hematuria.

OTHER LABORATORY TESTS

- Platelet function testing— may be used to diagnose hereditary and acquired defects, and to monitor effects of antiplatelet drugs:
    - Performed in specialized laboratories; requires freshly collected blood samples.
    - Platelet function analyzer-100, -200—sensitive to decreased platelet function, VWD, and anemia.
    - Aggregometry (light transmittance or impedance)—measures platelet response to different agonists (stimulants), using platelet-rich plasma or whole blood. Sensitive to specific drug effects (e.g., clopidogrel), receptor defects (e.g., ADP receptor).
    - Plateletworks—measures percent aggregation using whole blood platelet counting by routine impedance or optical hematology analyzers, and is available to some general practices.
    - Platelet indices (e.g., mean platelet volume, platelet volume distribution width, mean platelet component concentration)—variables helpful in characterizing platelet size, shape and activation (provided with some optical based hematology analyzers).
- Flow cytometry—for the detection of surface markers (e.g., glycoproteins), such as the fibrinogen receptor, P-selectin, or phosphatidylserine. Sensitive to Scott syndrome, fibrinogen receptor defects. Remote testing (P-selectin) shows promise for testing drug-effect (clopidogrel).
- VWF antigen by immunoassay—in animals suspected of VWD.
- Coagulation tests (prothrombin time [PT], activated partial thromboplastin time [aPTT], thromboelastography) [TEG]—to eliminate coagulopathy as a cause of hemorrhage; aPTT may be prolonged in some animals with VWD (due to decreased factor VIII–VWF binding, causing decreased factor VIII stability).
- Blood type: for animals who will require blood transfusion. There is no association of

T

THROMBOCYTOPATHIES (CONTINUED)

blood type with platelet function, however, some platelet products may contain red blood cells.
- Genetic testing of carrier animals.

DIAGNOSTIC PROCEDURES

Buccal mucosal bleeding time (BMBT)—to generally assess platelet function. Sensitive to platelet function defects and VWD, but also prolonged by thrombocytopenia. Measured using a spring-loaded lancet that makes a 5 mm long by 1 mm deep incision in the buccal (dog) or oral (cat) mucosa. The incision is observed until bleeding stops by the formation of a platelet plug. Normal BMBTs are less than 4–5 minutes in dogs and less than 2–3 minutes in cats. The BMBT can also be affected by hematocrit and blood viscosity, and results can vary between operators.

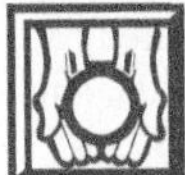

TREATMENT

- Transfusion—20 mL/kg (minimum of 10 mL/kg) platelet-rich plasma, or 1 unit/10 kg (minimum 1 unit/30 kg) cryoprecipitate, or 5.5×10^{10} platelets/10 kg body weight given as fresh platelet concentrate (may be available in some areas).
    - DMSO-stabilized cryopreserved and lyophilized platelets are available in some countries; these products have less functional activity than fresh platelets but may be useful for correcting hemorrhage.
- Whole blood or packed red blood cell transfusion to correct anemia or if other platelet-containing products are not available. Fresh packed red blood cells also contain platelets in the sedimented pellet, and may be given for patients where volume overload is a concern.
- Cryoprecipitate—for elective surgeries in dogs with VWD, cryoprecipitate should be administered prior to the procedure and continued through to the postoperative period (see above).
- In animals with acquired platelet function disorders, treat the underlying disease process or withdraw the offending agent.
- Elective surgical procedures should be avoided or accompanied by appropriate transfusion products.
- Restrict activity during a bleeding episode.

MEDICATIONS

DRUG(S) OF CHOICE

- Desmopressin (DDAVP):
    - 1 µg/kg SC, or IV diluted in 20 mL saline and administered over 10 minutes to dogs with VWD during a bleeding episode or in dogs with VWD requiring emergency surgery.
    - 3 µg/kg SC in dogs with thrombocytopathia due to aspirin, liver disease, and a consideration in dogs with other thrombocytopathias.
- Antifibrinolytic agents (aminocaproic acid, tranexamic acid)—prevents clots from rapid breakdown, more commonly used to treat coagulopathies. The injectable preparations of each drug can be used topically in areas of bleeding (e.g., oral mucosa). Empirical data are lacking for dogs and cats. Both drugs are contraindicated in DIC, and should be used cautiously in cats:
    - Aminocaproic acid 50–100 mg/kg PO, IV q6h; or 100 mg/kg IV followed by 30 mg/kg/h IV.
    - Tranexamic acid 20 mg/kg PO, IV q8h, given over 30 minutes to minimize emesis.

FOLLOW-UP

- Take special precautions when performing surgical procedures on these animals. Have type-specific blood and cryoprecipitate available if indicated.
- Make owner aware that animals with hereditary platelet function defects may have recurring bleeding episodes. Fatal episodes are uncommon.
- If a hereditary defect is identified, the animal should not be used for breeding.

MISCELLANEOUS

SEE ALSO

- Chediak-Higashi Syndrome.
- Cyclic Hematopoiesis.
- Thrombocytopenia.
- Von Willebrand Disease.

ABBREVIATIONS

- aPTT = activated partial thromboplastin time.
- BMBT = buccal mucosal bleeding time.
- DDAVP = 1-desamino-8-D-arginine vasopressin.
- DIC = disseminated intravascular coagulation.
- NSAID = nonsteroidal anti-inflammatory drug.
- PT = prothrombin time.
- TEG = thromboelastography.
- VWD = von Willebrand disease.
- VWF = von Willebrand factor.

Suggested Reading

Brooks MB, Catalfamo JL. Platelet dysfunction. In: Bonagura JD, Twedt DC, eds., Kirk's Current Veterinary Therapy XIV. St. Louis, MO: Elsevier, 2009, pp. 292–296.

Authors Signe E. Cremer, Anthony C.G. Abrams-Ogg, and Annemarie T. Kristensen
Consulting Editor Melinda S. Camus
Acknowledgment The authors and editors acknowledge the prior contribution of Inge Tarnow.

T

THROMBOCYTOPENIA

BASICS

DEFINITION

Platelet count below the reference interval, which varies by laboratory and methodology.

PATHOPHYSIOLOGY

• Platelets are produced by bone marrow megakaryocytes and released into the blood, where they normally circulate for 5–10 days.
• Thrombocytopenia is caused by one or more of: decreased production, increased sequestration, utilization, or destruction of platelets.
• Thrombocytopenia may result in spontaneous or excessive hemorrhage.

SYSTEMS AFFECTED

Hemorrhage may occur into any organ system. Clinical hemorrhage is most commonly recognized in the skin (petechiae, ecchymoses) and from mucosal surfaces of the gastrointestinal, renal/urologic, and respiratory systems; less commonly recognized in the ophthalmic, nervous, and reproductive systems.

INCIDENCE/PREVALENCE

• Thrombocytopenia is a common hematologic abnormality.
• Severe hemorrhage due to thrombocytopenia is uncommon to rare.

SIGNALMENT

Species

Dogs and cats.

Breed Predilections

Asymptomatic thrombocytopenias may be present in cavalier King Charles spaniels (see Pseudomacrothrombocytopenia [Inherited Macrothrombocytopenia]), greyhounds, Polish ogar dogs, Akitas.

SIGNS

General Comments

• Mild, moderate, and severe risk of spontaneous clinical hemorrhage at platelet counts of <25,000/μL, <10,000/μL, and <5,000/μL, respectively. These figures are guidelines only because of variation in methods of platelet counting, imprecision of low platelet counts, and individual animal variation.
• Concurrent platelet function defect, von Willebrand disease, coagulopathy, vasculitis, or sepsis increases risk of hemorrhage.

Historical Findings

• Spontaneous or excessive bleeding, generally from mucosal surfaces.
• Lethargy and collapse.
• Dyspnea and coughing (respiratory tract hemorrhage).
• Neurologic signs.
• Clinical signs of the primary disease.

Physical Examination Findings

• Petechiae and ecchymoses.
• Persistent bleeding from wounds and venipuncture sites.
• Melena/hematochezia/hematemesis.
• Hematuria.
• Ocular hemorrhage/hyphema.
• Splenomegaly, hepatomegaly.
• Pale mucous membranes.
• Weakness, collapse.
• Dyspnea, hemoptysis, epistaxis.
• Heart murmur (anemia).
• Neurologic abnormalities.

CAUSES

• Decreased production of platelets (may occur alone or with other cytopenias).
• Increased sequestration of platelets (splenomegaly, hypothermia).
• Increased utilization of platelets (e.g., DIC).
• Increased destruction of platelets (see Thrombocytopenia, Primary Immune-Mediated)—may be primary, or secondary to neoplasia, infectious agents, inflammation, drugs.
• Increased loss—volume resuscitation after massive bleeding.

RISK FACTORS

• Potentially any noninfectious inflammation, e.g., vasculitis, neoplasia.
• Potentially any infection—associated with feline leukemia virus (FeLV), feline immunodeficiency virus, distemper, parvoviruses, *Ehrlichia* spp., *Anaplasma* spp., *Rickettsia rickettsia*, leptospirosis, *Borrelia burgdorferi*, histoplasmosis, *Cytauxzoon felis*, *Babesia* spp., *Rangelia* spp., *Hepatozoon canis*, *Leishmania* spp., *Theileria* spp., heartworm, *Angiostrongylus vasorum*, and *Cuterebra* spp. (especially small dogs).
• Potentially any neoplasm.
• Large-field radiation therapy, cytotoxic drug therapy.
• Potentially any drug, especially sulfa-containing drugs, estrogens, gold compounds, phenylbutazone, phenobarbital (dogs); chloramphenicol, griseofulvin, propylthiouracil, methimazole and carbimazole (cats).
• Toxins and venoms—crotalid envenomation, zinc, autumn crocus, mycotoxins, xylitol.
• Hyperthermia (heat stroke).

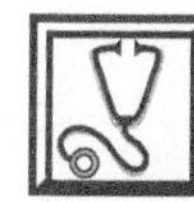

DIAGNOSIS

DIFFERENTIAL DIAGNOSIS

• Measurement error due to platelet clumping—more likely with traumatic venipuncture and in cats.
• Von Willebrand disease.
• Coagulopathy—petechiae, gastrointestinal hemorrhage, and epistaxis unusual; subcutaneous swellings, intracavity hemorrhage may be present.
• Trauma.

CBC/BIOCHEMISTRY/URINALYSIS

Confirm analyzer thrombocytopenia by examination of a blood smear; inspect feathered edge for platelet clumps; estimate platelet count from red cell monolayer; each platelet-per-oil immersion field represents 15,000–25,000/μL.
• Plateletcrit (analogous to hematocrit) reflects platelet mass; decreased with thrombocytopenia; normal in dogs with macrothrombocytopenia.
• Abnormalities on biochemistry profile and urinalysis reflect primary disease or effects of hemorrhage.

OTHER LABORATORY TESTS

• Von Willebrand factor antigen.
• Coagulation analysis (prothrombin [PT] and activated partial thromboplastin [aPTT] times, activated clotting time): prolonged results increase likelihood of disseminated intravascular coagulation (DIC); normal PT rules out vitamin K antagonism.
• D-dimers—positive result increases likelihood of DIC or local thrombosis.
• Serologic and PCR tests for infectious organisms.
• Fecal flotation and Baermann tests for parasitic larvae.
• Antiplatelet/antimegakaryocyte antibody tests—negative results help rule out immune-mediated thrombocytopenia (ITP).
• Coombs' test—positive result increases likelihood of concurrent immune-mediated hemolytic anemia.

IMAGING

Abdominal and thoracic radiographs, ultrasound, or 3D imaging can be useful in elucidating the underlying etiology.

DIAGNOSTIC PROCEDURES

Bone marrow aspirate or core biopsy—rule out reduced platelet production due to neoplasia, histoplasmosis, maturation arrest, bone marrow aplasia, myelofibrosis, and bone marrow necrosis. There is no specific finding that rules in or out immune-mediated megakaryocytic hypoplasia. Not contra-indicated in severe thrombocytopenia.

PATHOLOGIC FINDINGS

Secondary to hemorrhage.

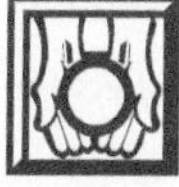

TREATMENT

APPROPRIATE HEALTH CARE

• Treatment of primary disorder.
• Platelet transfusion—20 mL/kg (minimum 10 mL/kg) fresh whole blood or platelet-rich plasma, or 1 unit/10 kg (minimum 1 unit/30 kg) platelet concentrate (fresh, room-temperature stored, cryopreserved, or lyophilized products are all commercially available). While platelet

concentrate may increase platelet count, fresh whole blood is unlikely to cause a change in platelet numbers, although the transfused platelets may be enough to stop critical bleeding. Transfuse if critical hemorrhage is noted and consider prophylactic transfusion if platelet count <5,000–10,000/μL, especially if invasive procedures are planned. Transfusions may be needed q1–3 days if severe thrombocytopenia persists.
- Whole blood or packed red blood cell transfusion to correct anemia—bleeding due to thrombocytopenia is worse in the presence of anemia.
- Do not drain hematomas unless causing a problem (e.g., tracheal compression).

NURSING CARE

Minimize injections. Apply extended pressure after IV injection/catheterization and invasive procedures. Avoid jugular venipuncture and urine acquisition by cystocentesis.

ACTIVITY

Restrict activity in animals with moderate-to-severe thrombocytopenia.

DIET

Avoid hard foods and toys to minimize possibility for gingival bleeding.

SURGICAL CONSIDERATIONS

Extensive perioperative transfusion may be needed.

T

MEDICATIONS

DRUG(S) OF CHOICE

- See specific chapters for treatments of diseases causing thrombocytopenia.
- Acepromazine and trazadone have negligible effects on platelet function in dogs and cats and may be used to sedate animals to reduce risk of hemorrhage associated with excessive activity.

CONTRAINDICATIONS

- Opioids and gabapentin are preferred analgesic agents; if nonsteroidal anti-inflammatory drug (NSAID) use is required, selective cyclooxygenase-2 inhibitors (e.g., deracoxib) should be used to minimize effects on platelet function.
- Clopidogrel.
- *n*3 fatty acids have a mild negative effect on platelet function.

PRECAUTIONS

- Heparin may aggravate hemorrhage due to thrombocytopenia.
- Corticosteroid or other immunosuppressive therapy may promote infection and gastrointestinal ulceration.

POSSIBLE INTERACTIONS

- Antibiotics have negligible effects on platelet function in dogs and cats (see Thrombocytopathies).
- Gastroprotectants have negligible effects on platelet function.
- Common anesthetic agents have negligible effects on platelet function.
- Corticosteroids are generally considered to be prothrombotic.

ALTERNATIVE DRUG(S)

- Thrombopoietic stimulants—oprelvekin—50 μg/kg SC q24h for maximum of 2 weeks (to avoid risk of neutralizing antibody formation); most useful when thrombocytopenia caused by cytotoxic therapy; expensive.
- Fibrinolysis inhibitors—aminocaproic acid, tranexamic acid; contraindicated in DIC.
- Vincristine—0.02 mg/kg IV, once: may transiently increase platelet count in dogs with ITP; not indicated for other etiologies of thrombocytopenia, may cause leukopenia.
- Melatonin and 5-methoxytryptamine.
- Lithium is not recommended.

FOLLOW-UP

PATIENT MONITORING

- Amount of bleeding—control of clinical hemorrhage is most important parameter to monitor to judge effectiveness of treatment.
- Serial platelet counts using same method.
- Serial coagulation profiles if DIC is suspected.

PREVENTION/AVOIDANCE

Varies with cause.

POSSIBLE COMPLICATIONS

- Hemorrhagic shock.
- Uveitis.
- Neurologic abnormalities if hemorrhage in CNS.
- Dyspnea if hemorrhage into respiratory tract.

EXPECTED COURSE AND PROGNOSIS

Varies with cause. If the underlying cause of severe thrombocytopenia cannot be treated, prognosis is poor.

MISCELLANEOUS

ASSOCIATED CONDITIONS

- If thrombocytopenia is due to reduced platelet production, other cytopenias may be present.
- ITP may be solitary or associated with other immune-mediated disorders.

AGE-RELATED FACTORS

Varies with cause—e.g., FeLV in younger cats, ITP in middle-aged dogs, neoplasia in older dogs.

ZOONOTIC POTENTIAL

None specifically, although some causes of thrombocytopenia (e,g, leptospirosis) may be due to a zoonosis.

SEE ALSO

- Disseminated Intravascular Coagulation.
- Hyphema.
- Pancytopenia.
- Petechia, Ecchymosis, Bruising.
- Pseudomacrothrombocytopenia (Inherited Macrothrombocytopenia).
- Splenomegaly.
- Thrombocytopathies.
- Thrombocytopenia, Primary Immune-Mediated.
- Vasculitis, Systemic (Including Phlebitis).
- Von Willebrand Disease.

And specific chapters for infectious diseases.

ABBREVIATIONS

- aPTT = activated partial thromboplastin time.
- DIC = disseminated intravascular coagulation.
- FeLV = feline leukemia virus.
- ITP = immune-mediated thrombocytopenia.
- NSAID = nonsteroidal anti-inflammatory drug.
- PT = prothrombin time.

INTERNET RESOURCES

https://ahdc.vet.cornell.edu/sects/clinpath/modules/coags/acqtbtp.htm

Suggested Reading

Botsch V, Küchenhoff H, Hartmann K, Hirschberger J. Retrospective study of 871 dogs with thrombocytopenia. Vet Rec 2009, 164:647–651.

Jordan HL, Grindem CB, Breitschwerdt EB. Thrombocytopenia in cats: a retrospective study of 41 cases. J Vet Intern Med 1993, 7:261–265.

Kelley J, Sharkey LC, Christopherson PW, Rendahl A. Platelet count and plateletcrit in cavalier King Charles spaniels and greyhounds using the Advia 120 and 2120. Vet Clin Pathol 2014, 43:43–49.

Author Anthony C.G. Abrams-Ogg

Consulting Editor Melinda S. Camus

Acknowledgment The author and editors acknowledge the prior contributions of Dr. William J. Reagan.

THROMBOCYTOPENIA, PRIMARY IMMUNE-MEDIATED

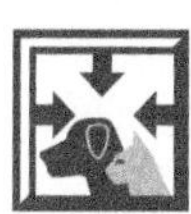

BASICS

DEFINITION

• Immune-mediated destruction of platelets with no identifiable cause.
• In secondary immune-mediated thrombocytopenia (ITP), infectious diseases, neoplasia, vaccination, or drugs (e.g., sulfonamides, cephalosporins, phenobarbital, nonsteroidal anti-inflammatory drugs [NSAIDs]) trigger the production of antibodies.

PATHOPHYSIOLOGY

• Antiplatelet autoantibodies result in premature platelet destruction by splenic macrophages.
• In secondary ITP, platelet-bound antibodies can be antibodies bound to platelet antigens altered during course of disease or antibodies bound to foreign antigens or immune complexes.
• Autoantibodies can be directed against megakaryocytes.
• Antibody-mediated impairment of platelet function possible.

SYSTEMS AFFECTED

• Nervous.
• Gastrointestinal.
• Ophthalmic.
• Respiratory.
• Skin/exocrine.
• Renal/urologic.

GENETICS

Autoimmunity is frequently recognized in particular dog breeds and is often familial, suggesting a genetic influence.

PREVALENCE

Approximately 6% of dogs and 3% of cats with thrombocytopenia.

SIGNALMENT

Species

• Dog.
• Rare in cat.

Breed and Familial Predilections

Cocker spaniel, Maltese, bearded collie, poodle, Old English sheepdog, Irish setter.

Mean Age and Range

• Middle-aged dogs.
• Reported age range in dogs: 0.3–15 years (mean 5 years); in cats: 0.7–12 years (mean 6 years).

Predominant Sex

Female dogs.

SIGNS

Historical Findings

• Acute-onset mucosal hemorrhage.
• Chronic, low-grade blood loss.
• Lethargy, weakness, inappetence.
• Asymptomatic.
• Recent drug administration, vaccines, travel to tick-endemic area.

Physical Examination Findings

• Mucosal and cutaneous petechiae/ecchymoses.
• Melena, hematemesis, hematochezia.
• Epistaxis.
• Ocular hemorrhage, hyphema.
• Hematuria.
• Neurologic signs due to CNS bleeding.
• Dyspnea if bleeding into respiratory tract.
• Prolonged hemorrhage after trauma or venipuncture, hematoma formation.
• Hemorrhagic shock—pale mucous membrane, tachycardia, weak pulses.
• Fever.
• Palpably enlarged spleen.

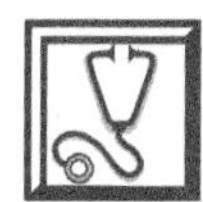

DIAGNOSIS

• Severe thrombocytopenia (generally <20,000 platelets/μL).
• Careful exclusion of underlying diseases or potential triggers.
• Response to immunosuppressive therapy.

DIFFERENTIAL DIAGNOSIS

• Measurement error due to platelet clumping; especially in cats.
• Pseudomacrothrombocytopenia of cavalier King charles and English toy spaniels, Cairn and Norfolk terriers.
• Decreased production—infectious diseases, irradiation, primary bone marrow disorders (myelopthisis or myelofibrosis).
• Sequestration in the spleen.
• Increased utilization or consumption:
  ◦ Neoplasia, disseminated intravascular coagulation (DIC), thrombosis, vasculitis/vascular damage, infectious diseases.
  ◦ Severe hemorrhage or thrombosis may result in mild to moderate thrombocytopenia.

CBC/BIOCHEMISTRY/URINALYSIS

• Thrombocytopenia often severe (<20,000–30,000/μL), high risk of spontaneous bleeding.
• Blood smear examination—to confirm low platelet count; to identify potential causes for secondary ITP.
• Anemia may be present.
• Leukogram can be normal; mild to moderate leukocytosis in 30% of dogs.
• Concurrent neutropenia may indicate primary bone marrow or infectious disease.
• Coagulation testing generally normal; if abnormal consider secondary ITP, DIC.
• Chemistry results unspecific for ITP. Hypoproteinemia and hypoalbuminemia due to blood loss, hyperbilirubinemia due to hematoma resorption (rare), hyperglobulinemia may indicate underlying infectious disease (e.g., ehrlichiosis, leishmaniosis, feline infectious peritonitis [FIP]).
• Hematuria.

OTHER LABORATORY TESTS

• Infectious disease testing—secondary ITP reported in association with anaplasmosis, ehrlichiosis, Rocky Mountain spotted fever, bartonellosis, babesiosis, leishmaniosis, dirofilariasis, *Angiostrongylus* infection, distemper, infectious hepatitis, and bacterial infections in dogs; feline leukemia virus, feline immunodeficiency virus, and FIP in cats.
• Platelet-bound antibody detection—flow cytometric assay in specialized laboratories.
• Adjunct immunodiagnostic testing such as Coombs' test or antinuclear antibody titer if systemic lupus erythematosus is suspected.

IMAGING

• Splenomegaly, rarely hepatomegaly.
• Radiography and ultrasonography to exclude other causes of thrombocytopenia (e.g., neoplasia) or internal bleeding.

DIAGNOSTIC PROCEDURES

• Bone marrow evaluation not indicated with response to therapy; indicated if unexplained cytopenias or poor treatment response.
• Number of megakaryocytes increased unless immune reaction targeted against megakaryocytes.

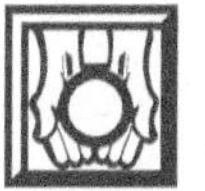

TREATMENT

APPROPRIATE HEALTH CARE

• Uncomplicated cases with low bleeding risk and good owner compliance may be treated as outpatients.
• Patients with severe thrombocytopenia have very high risk of bleeding and warrant strict confinement.
• Management of hypovolemia with crystalloid solutions (colloids may impair platelet function).
• Packed red blood cells or whole blood to correct anemia.
• Transfusion of platelet products: 10–20 mL/kg fresh whole blood, 1 unit per 10 kg body weight of whole blood-derived platelet-rich plasma (containing approximately 8×10^{10} platelets/L) (minimum dose of 1 unit/30 kg) in animals with critical hemorrhage (caution if risk of hypervolemia). Platelet concentrates (lower total volume) if available. Platelets may be destroyed rapidly but may protect against catastrophic hemorrhage. DMSO-stabilized and lyophilized platelet concentrates are commercially available in the United States.

NURSING CARE

• Limit IM or SC injections. Apply extended pressure after IV injections. Avoid cystocentesis and jugular venipuncture. Bone marrow aspiration is safe.
• Intensive nursing care in patients with moderate to severe hemorrhage, hypovolemia, CNS abnormalities.
• Avoid hard foods, chew toys.

THROMBOCYTOPENIA, PRIMARY IMMUNE-MEDIATED (CONTINUED)

SURGICAL CONSIDERATIONS

- Splenectomy is a controversial option for refractory cases not responding to medical therapy.
- High risk of bleeding in dogs with severe thrombocytopenia.
- May need extensive peri- and intraoperative transfusions with red blood cells and platelets.

MEDICATIONS

DRUG(S) OF CHOICE

- Immunosuppression:
  - Corticosteroids—methyl prednisolone 10 mg/kg IV once or dexamethasone 0.2–0.3 mg/kg q24h, IV until able to take oral medication; prednisolone or prednisone (dogs 1 mg/kg PO q12h; cats 1.5–2 mg/kg PO q12h initially).
  - Additional or long-term therapy, usually in combination with corticosteroid (initial dosages)—cyclosporine 5 mg/kg PO q12h (dogs), mycophenolate mofetil 8–10 mg/kg PO q12h (dogs/cats), can also be given in the acute setting at 7–10 mg/kg IV q12h, azathioprine 2 mg/kg PO q24h (dogs), leflunomide 2–3 mg/kg PO q24h (dogs), chlorambucil 0.1–0.2 mg/kg PO q24h (cats).
- Other acute management—vincristine 0.02 mg/kg IV once (dogs) or human IV immunoglobulin (hIVIG) 0.5–1 g/kg over 6–8h once (dogs/cats).
- Antibiotics—consider doxycycline 5 mg/kg PO q12h if tick-borne disease is possible.
- Gastrointestinal protectants—sucralfate 20–50 mg/kg PO q6–8h or proton pump inhibitors (omeprazole 1 mg/kg PO q12h; pantoprazole 1 mg/kg IV/PO q12h).
- Once the platelet count is within the reference interval, the initial prednis(ol)one dose should be tapered by approximately 1/4 to 1/5 every 2 weeks, finally switching to alternate-day therapy. This and other therapies should be tapered slowly over approximately 6 months if no relapse.

PRECAUTIONS

- Discontinue any unnecessary medications.
- Corticosteroids—gastrointestinal ulceration; iatrogenic hyperadrenocorticism.
- Immunosuppression—predisposes to opportunistic infections, mycophenolate associated with gastrointestinal upset.
- Cytotoxic medications (azathioprine, mycophenolate mofetil, chlorambucil, vincristine)—bone marrow suppression.
- Dose tapering too rapidly after remission may predispose to recurrence.

FOLLOW-UP

PATIENT MONITORING

- Hematocrit measurements and physical examination as indicated in cases with severe hemorrhage.
- Measure platelet count daily until >50,000/µL; then every few days until platelet counts normalize. Then every 1–3 weeks during the period of drug dose tapering.
- CBC and biochemistry every 2–4 weeks.
- Urinalysis every 4–6 weeks due to risk of secondary infections.

PREVENTION/AVOIDANCE

Use vaccines judiciously. Role in recurrence is uncertain.

POSSIBLE COMPLICATIONS

- Spontaneous bleeding in specific areas (CNS, lungs) can be fatal.
- Side effects of medications.

EXPECTED COURSE AND PROGNOSIS

- Platelet counts will usually increase >50,000/µL a few days after starting treatment.
- Vincristine or hIVIG in addition to prednisone led to a shorter hospital stay or more rapid increase to 50,000 platelets/µL (median 2.5–4 days), respectively.
- Most dogs achieve normal platelet counts.
- Failure to respond to therapy should prompt diagnostic reconsideration.
- 5 of 19 dogs (26%) relapsed after 19–286, median 66 days; causes for relapse were dose reduction of immunosuppression, lack of owner compliance.
- If relapses occur, add a second immunosuppressive drug.
- Survival to discharge in recent studies—84–97% (dogs); prognosis is more favorable with intensive therapy including blood/platelet products if needed.
- Mortality rate in cats is 15% (2/13).

MISCELLANEOUS

ASSOCIATED CONDITIONS

Evans syndrome describes a rare occurrence of immune-mediated hemolytic anemia with ITP.

SYNONYMS

- Autoimmune thrombocytopenia.
- Idiopathic/autoimmune thrombocytopenic purpura.

SEE ALSO

- Disseminated Intravascular Coagulation.
- Lupus Erythematosus, Systemic (SLE).
- Pseudomacrothrombocytopenia (Inherited Macrothrombocytopenia).
- Thrombocytopenia.

ABBREVIATIONS

- DIC = disseminated intravascular coagulation.
- FIP = feline infectious peritonitis.
- hIVIG = human intravenous immunoglobulin.
- ITP = immune-mediated thrombocytopenia.
- NSAID = nonsteroidal anti-inflammatory drug.

Suggested Reading

Putsche J, Kohn B. Primary immune-mediated thrombocytopenia in 30 dogs (1997–2003). J Am Anim Hosp Assoc 2008, 44:250–257.

Wondraschek C, Weingart C, Kohn B. Primary immune-mediated thrombocytopenia in cats. J Am Anim Hosp Assoc 2010, 46:12–19.

Author Barbara Kohn

Consulting Editor Melinda S. Camus

Client Education Handout available online

THROMBOCYTOSIS

BASICS

OVERVIEW

• Platelet count above the upper limit of the reference interval, which varies with the method of individual reference laboratories and methodologies.
• Reference intervals may be shifted upwards at high altitudes.

Pathophysiology

• Platelets are produced by megakaryocytes in the bone marrow and circulate for approximately 5–7 days. Approximately 30% of the circulating platelet mass resides transiently in the spleen and may be released suddenly with splenic contraction.
• Platelet production is stimulated by thrombopoietin (TPO).
• Thrombocytosis can be physiologic or reactive. Causes include physiologic redistribution, inflammation, and neoplasia.
• In humans, specific gene mutations have been associated with the development of essential thrombocytosis.

Systems Affected

• Hematologic—high circulating platelet count may impair ordinary hemostatic processes (especially von Willebrand factor-mediated platelet adhesion).
• Cardiovascular—thrombosis or hemorrhage: uncommon.

Incidence/Prevalence

Reactive thrombocytosis is common in cats and dogs.

SIGNALMENT

Cats and dogs.

SIGNS

Historical and physical exam findings are related to underlying causes associated with the thrombocytosis or sequelae of micro or macrovascular thrombosis (e.g., organ failure, ischemic events) or hemorrhage.

CAUSES & RISK FACTORS

Physiologic Thrombocytosis

Occurs secondary to redistribution of platelets from the spleen into circulation, secondary to splenic contraction associated with stress, exercise, or excitement.

Reactive Thrombocytosis

Occurs secondary to other conditions and may be short- or longstanding. Platelet elevations are typically mild to moderate and do not generally pose a risk for thrombosis. Causes of reactive thrombocytosis include:
• Inflammation secondary to infection, immune-mediated disease, surgery, trauma, or neoplasia. Inflammatory cytokines (e.g., interleukin-6) stimulate TPO production, which stimulates platelet production. The most common inflammatory diseases resulting in thrombocytosis in dogs are immune-mediated, gastrointestinal, and hepatobiliary in nature. In cats, gastrointestinal illness (involving intestinal, hepatobiliary and/or pancreatic diseases) is the most common disease category associated with thrombocytosis.
• Iron deficiency is a common but inconsistent cause of thrombocytosis.
• Recovery from thrombocytopenia (rebound thrombocytosis). This occurs most commonly:
  o Post splenectomy (thrombocytosis may be marked and may persist for weeks).
  o Following withdrawal of myelosuppression.
  o During recovery from immune-mediated thrombocytopenia.
  o Following blood loss.
• Hypercortisolemia secondary to hyperadrenocorticism or corticosteroid administration in dogs. In cats, hyperthyroidism may be a cause.
• Nonhemic malignant neoplasia (paraneoplastic secondary to cytokines stimulating thrombopoiesis)—carcinoma is the most common neoplasm associated with thrombocytosis.

Drug-Induced

• Epinephrine.
• *Vinca* alkaloids (vincristine, vinblastine).

Hemic Neoplasia/Myeloproliferative Disease

• Chronic myeloproliferative diseases are uncommon and include essential thrombocythemia.
• Acute megakaryocytic leukemia—>30% of nucleated cells in bone marrow are megakaryoblasts; myelofibrosis may be present, and neoplastic megakaryoblasts may be present in circulation or other organs.
• Markedly elevated platelet counts have been reported with essential thrombocythemia and acute megakaryocytic leukemia ($1–5 \times 10^6$ platelets/μL).

Pseudothrombocytosis

An artifactual increase in machine-based platelet count caused by red or white blood cell fragments and lipid particles associated with marked hyperchylomicronemia. A microscopic blood smear exam is required to properly identify this phenomenon.

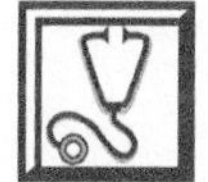

DIAGNOSIS

DIFFERENTIAL DIAGNOSIS

Measurement error (pseudothrombocytosis) secondary to presence of cellular fragments or clerical error—a microscopic blood smear exam should be performed to confirm thrombocytosis when reported.

CBC/BIOCHEMISTRY/URINALYSIS

• Confirm thrombocytosis reported by a hematology analyzer by microscopic blood smear review.
• Hyperkalemia—an artifactual increase in serum potassium concentration can occur secondary to thrombocytosis due to release of intraplatelet potassium during clotting. Measurement of potassium using heparinized plasma is preferred to avoid this artifact.

OTHER LABORATORY TESTS

Use to identify underlying causes of reactive or neoplastic thrombocytosis. A diagnosis of essential thrombocytosis is generally one of exclusion.

DIAGNOSTIC PROCEDURES

Bone marrow examination—aspiration and core biopsy may be indicated with sustained extreme thrombocytosis to identify morphologic abnormalities that may be consistent with hemic neoplasia, dysplasia, or myelofibrosis.

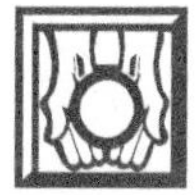

TREATMENT

N/A

MEDICATIONS

DRUG(S) OF CHOICE

• If micro- or macrovascular thromboembolic complications are suspected, antiplatelet agents (e.g., clopidogrel, aspirin) may be indicated, although their use in humans with thrombocytosis has been associated with more severe hemorrhagic complications. Consultation with a veterinary specialist is highly recommended to determine if and which therapy may be indicated.
• Hydroxyurea is a chemotherapy drug that is used for cytoreductive therapy in humans with essential thrombocytosis. Published dosage recommendations for veterinary species vary widely. It is generally myelosuppressive, however, and will affect all cell lines. Consultation with a veterinary specialist is recommended regarding the administration and dosage of this drug. A comprehensive CBC every 1–2 weeks is recommended while taking hydroxyurea until platelet count stabilizes. Regular assessment of a serum biochemical profile is also recommended if using this drug.

CONTRAINDICATIONS/POSSIBLE INTERACTIONS

Caution is recommended for the use of hydroxyurea in patients with anemia, preexisting bone marrow depression, history of urate stones, current infection, impaired

THROMBOCYTOSIS (CONTINUED)

renal function, or with previous chemotherapy or radiation therapy.

Adverse Effects

• Gastrointestinal effects of hydroxyurea may include anorexia, vomiting, or diarrhea.
• Additional adverse effects include stomatitis, sloughing of toenails, loss of fur, and dysuria.
• Bone marrow supression (anemia, thrombocytopenia, leukopenia) and lung damage (pulmonary fibrosis) are the most serious potential adverse effects of hydroxyurea. Therapy should be discontinued until values return to normal.
• Life-threatening methemoglobinemia has been reported in cats given high dosages (>500 mg) of hydroxyurea.

Precautions

• Concurrent use of hydroxyurea with other bone marrow depressant drugs may cause additive myelosuppression; use with caution.
• Hydroxyurea is a chemotherapy drug and a teratogen and contact may be hazardous to other animals and people that come in direct contact with it.

FOLLOW-UP

PATIENT MONITORING

Serial monitoring of comprehensive CBC for reassessment of thrombocytosis.

MISCELLANEOUS

ABBREVIATIONS

• TPO = thrombopoietin.

INTERNET RESOURCES

• www.eclinpath.com
• www.merckmanuals.com

Suggested Reading

Neel JA, Snyder L, Grindem CB. Thrombocytosis: a retrospective study of 165 dogs. Vet Clin Pathol. 2012;41(2):216–22.

Rizzo F, Tappin SW, Tasker S. Thrombocytosis in cats: a retrospective study of 51 cases (2000–2005). J Feline Med Surg 2007, 9(4):319–325.

Woolcock AD, Keenan A, Cheung C, et al. Thrombocytosis in 715 dogs (2011–2015). J Vet Intern Med 2017, 31(6):1691–1699.

Author Jaime L. Tarigo
Consulting Editor Melinda S. Camus

T

THUNDERSTORM AND NOISE PHOBIAS

BASICS

DEFINITION

Thunderstorm phobia is a disorder in which there is persistent and exaggerated fear of storms or the stimuli associated with storms. Fears of noises other than thunder also occur, such as fireworks or gunshots.

PATHOPHYSIOLOGY

Pathophysiology involves physiologic, emotional, and behavioral components. Overactivation of noradrenergic activity in the locus ceruleus is likely to be involved.

SYSTEMS AFFECTED

- Behavioral—avoidance or escape attempts, pacing, freezing, contact-seeking, vocalization.
- Cardiovascular—tachycardia.
- Endocrine/metabolic—increased cortisol levels, stress-induced hyperglycemia.
- Gastrointestinal (GI)—inappetence, GI upset, hypersalivation.
- Musculoskeletal—self-induced trauma.
- Nervous—trembling, adrenergic/noradrenergic overstimulation.
- Respiratory—tachypnea.
- Skin—self-directed or accidental trauma, displacement grooming.

GENETICS

Familial patterns have been observed in dogs with noise phobias but the exact mechanisms of inheritance have not been established.

PREVALENCE

Fear responses to noises affect 23–50% of the canine population with storms, fireworks, vacuum cleaners and gunshots most commonly reported.

SIGNALMENT

- Occurs in dogs and cats but dogs more often presented for treatment. Cats with noise aversion might present with redirected aggression.
- No association with sex or neuter status.
- Any breed can be affected. In one study, thunderstorm phobias were most prevalent in herding breeds.
- Dogs may begin exhibiting signs as puppies but may not be presented until adulthood.

SIGNS

Historical Findings

- One or more of the following occurs during storms, or when exposed to the eliciting noise: panting, pacing, trembling, remaining near owner, hiding, salivating, destructiveness, vocalization, self-inflicted trauma, escape attempts and inappropriate elimination.
- Stimuli that can elicit fear during storms include rain, lightning, thunder, wind, and possibly static electricity and changes in barometric pressure.

Physical Examination Findings

Unremarkable, except self-inflicted or escape-related injuries.

CAUSES

May include combinations of the following:

- Lack of exposure to storms or noises early in development.
- Highly aversive experience, such as exposure to a violent storm.
- Genetic predisposition for emotional reactivity.

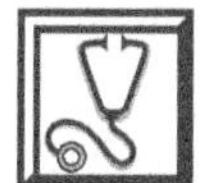

DIAGNOSIS

DIFFERENTIAL DIAGNOSIS

- Conditions causing similar behavioral responses include separation anxiety, barrier frustration, and other phobias.
- Medical conditions that present with similar signs include metabolic, cardiac, neurological, dermatologic, GI, or any condition that causes significant discomfort or pain.

CBC/BIOCHEMISTRY/URINALYSIS

Results should be within normal ranges.

OTHER LABORATORY TESTS

Tests for thyroid or adrenal disease may be indicated.

IMAGING

N/A except if indicated to rule out medical cause (e.g., pain).

DIAGNOSTIC PROCEDURES

- N/A except to rule out medical cause.
- Electrocardiogram prior to tricyclic antidepressant use if suspected cardiac conduction abnormalities.

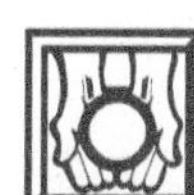

TREATMENT

APPROPRIATE HEALTH CARE

Outpatient treatment. Supervision may be necessary to prevent self-injury and destructive behavior.

NURSING CARE

Wound care for self-trauma or any physical trauma sustained during escape attempts.

ACTIVITY

Avoid crate confinement if not comfortably adapted or if risk of injury.

CLIENT EDUCATION

Behavior Management

Minimize, mute, or avoid exposure to stimuli by:

- Housing to a room or confinement area where the pet is comfortable and settled including safe haven confinement training to prevent, reduce, or mute stimuli.
- Avoid crate confinement if risk of injury or increased anxiety.
- Stimuli might be masked or muted with window shutters, sound baffling, white noise, fan, music or products such as ear covers (e.g., Mutt Muffs, headphones) or eye covers (ThunderCap, Doggles).
- Distraction from stimuli with favored toys, play, or highly valued rewards.

Behavior Modification

- Training and behavior modification to help calm the pet and change the association with the stimulus from one that is negative to one that is positive. Any confrontation, corrections or punishment in training must be avoided as it will further add to fear, anxiety and negative associations with the stimulus.
- Desensitization involves exposure to a recording of the stimulus or the stimulus muted or at sufficient distance that the volume does not elicit fear. The volume is gradually increased only if the pet remains relaxed.
- Counterconditioning is the pairing (association) of a positive outcome with each exposure to the stimulus. Operant counter-conditioning involves teaching a response (sit, relax) that is incompatible with the fear response (e.g., go to bed/mat, sit/focus, or touch). Favored food rewards are often used to facilitate learning.
- Audio recordings of noises or storms are commercially available. Other noises or sounds might be reproduced for desensitization and counterconditioning (e.g., gunshots, vacuum cleaners, traffic noise) by controlling exposure with distance, location, or with sound muting/baffling.
- Improper use of these exercises can worsen the condition.
- Exercises will be ineffective if the animal does not react to recorded thunderstorm sounds.

MEDICATIONS

DRUG(S) OF CHOICE

- With the exception of dexmedetomidine oromucosal gel, use of medications is considered extra-label. Imepetoin is also approved for use for noise aversion but not yet available.
- Azapirones, tricyclic antidepressants (TCAs), and selective serotonin reuptake inhibitors (SSRIs) require 2–4 weeks for effect and must be given daily during storm season to control anxiety. They can be used in combination with faster acting medications.

Medications for Acute, Short-Term Control of Anxiety

Alpha-2 Adrenergic Agonists

- Dexmedetomidine oromucosal gel—dogs, 125 μg/m^2 onto oral mucosa PRN, can repeat

THUNDERSTORM AND NOISE PHOBIAS (CONTINUED)

dosing up to q2–3h up to 5 times per noise event.
- Clonidine—dogs, 0.01–0.05 mg/kg PO q6–24h PRN.

Benzodiazepines
- Alprazolam—dogs, 0.02–0.1 mg/kg PO q4–12h PRN.
- Clonazepam—dogs, 0.05–0.25 mg/kg q8–12h PRN.
- Diazepam—dogs, 0.5–2 mg/kg PO q4–12h PRN.
- Lorazepam—dogs, 0.02–0.2 mg/kg PO q8–24h PRN.

Serotonin-2 Antagonist Reuptake Inhibitors (SARIs)
- Trazodone—dogs, 5–10 mg/kg PO PRN to q8–12h.

GABA Agonists
- Gabapentin—dogs, 20–30 mg/kg PO PRN to q12h; cats, 10–30 mg/kg PO PRN q24h.
- Imepitoin—partial GABA agonist—dogs, 20–30 mg/kg twice daily (begin up to 2 days in advance).

Phenothiazine Tranquilizers
- Acepromazine—dogs, 0.1–1 mg/kg PO q6–8h.
- Poor antianxiety properties.
- Use *only for* further sedation in conjunction with anxiolytic if needed to prevent injury.

T

Medications Used Daily or Throughout Thunderstorm Season

SSRIs
- Fluoxetine—dogs, 0.5–2 mg/kg PO q24h; cats, 0.5–1 mg/kg PO q24h.
- Paroxetine—dogs, 0.5–2 mg/kg PO q12h; cats, 0.5–1 mg/kg PO q24h.
- Side effects—inappetence and irritability.

TCAs
- Clomipramine—dogs, 1–3 mg/kg PO q12h; cats, 2.5–5 mg/cat PO q24h.
- Side effects—sedation, GI, and anticholinergic effects, and cardiac conduction disturbances.

GABA Agonists

Gabapentin—dogs 10–20 mg/kg PO q12h; cats, 5–10 mg/kg PO q12h.

CONTRAINDICATIONS
- Avoid using TCAs and phenothiazines in breeding males, patients with seizure disorders, cardiac disease, diabetes mellitus, glaucoma, or thyroid disease.

PRECAUTIONS
- Use benzodiazepines with caution in cats due to risk of hepatic necrosis.
- Use benzodiazepines with caution in aggressive dogs—disinhibition of aggression possible.
- Decrease dose or avoid use of these medications in geriatric patients and patients with impaired hepatic or renal function.

POSSIBLE INTERACTIONS
- TCAs, SSRIs, SARIs, and phenothiazines should never be combined with monoamine oxidase inhibitors.

ALTERNATIVE DRUG(S)
For adjunctive therapy in combination with drugs, environmental management and counterconditioning, natural therapeutic options that may aid in reducing anxiety including L-theanine alone or in combination with product containing whey protein, and *Phellodendron amurense* and *Magnolia officinalis*, alpha-casozepine alone or in diets combined with L-tryptophan, melatonin. Also for cats: feline F3 facial pheromone. Also for dogs: dog appeasing pheromone, *Souroubea* and *Plantanus*, a calming probiotic, aromatherapy (e.g., with lavender), pressure wraps or the Calmz anxiety relief system.

FOLLOW-UP

PATIENT MONITORING
With medication use, CBC and biochemistry profiles should be monitored periodically.

PREVENTION/AVOIDANCE
Puppies and kittens should be exposed to a variety of stimuli under benign conditions, including puppy and kitten classes.

POSSIBLE COMPLICATIONS
Severe injuries and property damage.

EXPECTED COURSE AND PROGNOSIS
Prognosis depends on severity, duration, and the ability to prevent injuries. The condition can progress if left untreated.

MISCELLANEOUS

SEE ALSO
Fears, Phobias, and Anxieties—Dogs.

ABBREVIATIONS
- GI = gastrointestinal.
- SARI = serotonin-2 antagonist reuptake inhibitor.
- SSRI = selective serotonin reuptake inhibitor.
- TCA = tricyclic antidepressant.

Suggested Reading

Blackwell EJ, Bradshaw JWS, Casey RA. Fear responses to noises in domestic dogs: prevalence, risk factors and co-occurrence with other fear related behaviour. Appl Anim Behav Sci 2013, 145:15–25.

Horwitz D, ed., Blackwell's 5 Minute Consult Clinical Companion: Canine and Feline Behavior, 2nd ed. Ames, IA: John Wiley & Sons, 2018, pp. 308–320 and 375–388.

Author Lynne M. Seibert

Consulting Editor Gary M. Landsberg

BASICS

OVERVIEW

- Originates from thymic epithelium, rarely metastasizes.
- Infiltrated with mature lymphocytes.
- May be associated with paraneoplastic syndromes (myasthenia gravis, hypercalcemia of malignancy).
- Classified as invasive (malignant) or noninvasive (benign).

SIGNALMENT

- Rare in dog and cat.
- Most common in medium- and large-breed dogs (especially Labrador and golden retrievers).
- Dogs—mean age 9.5 years.
- Cats—mean age 10 years.

SIGNS

- From physical presence of tumor—coughing, tachypnea, dyspnea.
- Secondary to obstruction of cranial vena cava—swelling of the head, neck, or forelimbs (dependent edema).
- Paraneoplastic syndromes (hypercalcemia or immune-mediated disease).
- Muscle weakness and megaesophagus caused by myasthenia gravis (~20%), hypercalcemia (causing polyuria/polydipsia), polymyositis, skin disease (especially in cats: exfoliative dermatitis and pemphigus vulgaris), hypergammaglobulinemia.
- Myasthenia gravis most often pre-op in dogs but can develop post-op in cats.

CAUSES & RISK FACTORS

N/A

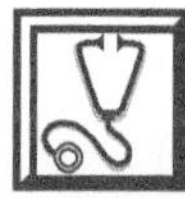

DIAGNOSIS

DIFFERENTIAL DIAGNOSIS

- Lymphoma (main rule-out).
- Branchial cyst.
- Ectopic thyroid carcinoma.
- Chemodectoma.
- Various subtypes of sarcoma.
- Mesothelioma.
- Non-neoplastic granuloma, abscess, or cyst.

CBC/BIOCHEMISTRY/URINALYSIS

- Lymphocytosis—occasionally (<5%).
- Intermittent basophilia—one case report.
- Hypercalcemia ~30%.

OTHER LABORATORY TESTS

- Antibody titers to acetylcholine receptors to confirm myasthenia gravis.
- Ultrasound-guided fine-needle aspiration and cytology of the mass—characterized by small lymphocytes, scattered mast cells, often with plasma cells and up to 60% will have an epithelial population (vs. a pure population of lymphoblasts with lymphoma). Thymomas can be cavitated/cystic, whereas lymphoma is usually homogeneous upon sonographic evaluation.
- Biopsy may be needed to confirm diagnosis and immunohistochemical stains (cytokeratin, lymphocyte CD markers) can be used.
- Flow cytometry of mass aspirate can confirm as a minimally invasive test (usually polyclonal CD4+ and CD8+ whereas lymphoma usually not); consider PCR for antigen receptor rearrangements to rule out lymphoma.

IMAGING

- Thoracic radiography—typically reveals a cranial mediastinal mass with dorsal deviation of the trachea, and may show pleural effusion or megaesophagus.
- CT scan or MRI can be used prior to thoracotomy for surgical planning, though cannot predict ease of resection.

DIAGNOSTIC PROCEDURES

Tensilon test—evaluate for myasthenia gravis in patients with signs of muscle weakness, dysphagia, or regurgitation.

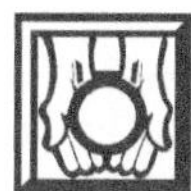

TREATMENT

- Inpatient.
- Surgical excision—treatment of choice, and possible in 70% of cases; use an intercostal approach for small masses and a sternotomy for large masses. Recurrence ~17%, median survival time 635 days overall not considering prognostic factors (compared to 76 days without surgery).
- Dogs with myasthenia gravis and aspiration pneumonia have a poorer prognosis with surgery. Myasthenia gravis and megaesophagus are not necessarily poor prognostic factors, but require more intensive husbandry practices.
- Radiotherapy—potentially beneficial by reducing the lymphoid component of the mass (50-75% of cases benefit); median survival time 248 days in dogs (though 75% alive at 1 year in one series) and 720 days in cats. Can be used after surgery if excision incomplete.

MEDICATIONS

DRUG(S) OF CHOICE

- Prednisone 20 mg/m^2 PO q48h and cyclophosphamide 50–100 mg/m^2 PO q48h—used in a very limited number of patients, two of which had a partial remission likely associated with lymphodepleting effects.
- Myasthenia gravis—treat with prednisone and anticholinesterase drugs until the tumor can be removed.

CONTRAINDICATIONS/POSSIBLE INTERACTIONS

Immunosuppressive drugs—do not use to treat myasthenia gravis if aspiration pneumonia present.

FOLLOW-UP

- Thoracic radiography—every 3 months; monitor for recurrence.
- Cure—possible if tumor is surgically resectable; greater than 80% alive at 1 year if resectable and no associated megaesophagus; median survival >1800 days for cats and 800 to >1000 days for dogs; 10–20% recur and may respond favorably to a second surgery.
- Prognosis—stage affects outcome after surgery: if invading adjacent organs, disseminated in thorax, or metastatic, then guarded (median 224 days). Prolonged survival despite no/minimal therapy might result from the indolent nature of the tumor.
- Patients with high lymphocyte proportion in tumor have a more favorable prognosis.

MISCELLANEOUS

ASSOCIATED CONDITIONS

Concurrent nonthymic tumors (27%), polymyositis, and other autoimmune diseases— variable, from less than 10% and up to 40% of patients.

SEE ALSO

Myasthenia Gravis.

Suggested Reading

Robat CS, Cesario L, Gaeta R, et al. Clinical features, treatment options, and outcome in dogs with thymoma: 116 cases (1999–2010). J Am Vet Med Assoc 2013, 243:1448–1454.

Zitz JC, Birchard SJ, Couto GC, et al. Results of excision of thymoma in cats and dogs: 20 cases (1984–2005). J Am Vet Med Assoc 2008, 232(8):1186–1192.

Author Kim A. Selting

Consulting Editor Timothy M. Fan

TICK BITE PARALYSIS

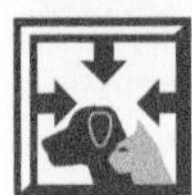

BASICS

DEFINITION

Flaccid, lower motor neuron tetraparesis to tetraplegia caused by salivary neurotoxins from certain species of female tick.

PATHOPHYSIOLOGY

- Presynaptic disorder—tick injects salivary neurotoxin that interferes with the depolarization/acetylcholine release from the presynaptic nerve terminal of the neuromuscular junction; this effect is probably associated with an interruption of the calcium flux across axonal membranes.
- Australian *Ixodes holocyclus* tick—neurotoxin (holocyclotoxin) effects are more pronounced at higher temperatures; one adult tick is sufficient to cause neurologic signs, but infestation with *I. holocyclus* larvae or nymphs can also induce signs; holocyclotoxin also interferes with acetylcholine release at the autonomic nerve terminals.
- Signs—5–9 days after initial tick attachment.
- Not all infested animals develop tick paralysis; not all adult female ticks produce the toxin.

SYSTEMS AFFECTED

T

- Nervous—peripheral nervous system and neuromuscular junction most affected; cranial nerves can become involved, including the vagus and facial nerves with the North American ticks and, in addition, the trigeminal nerves and sympathetic nervous system with the Australian *Ixodes* tick.
- Respiratory—may see paralysis of the intercostal muscles and diaphragm; caudal brainstem respiratory center may be affected (rare with North American ticks; more common with Australian *Ixodes* ticks).

GENETICS

No genetic basis.

INCIDENCE/PREVALENCE

- North America—somewhat seasonal (more prevalent in the summer months); in the warmer areas (southern United States) may become a year-round problem.
- Australia—distinctly seasonal, up to 75% of cases occur during southern hemisphere spring season (September–November).
- Overall incidence—low in the United States; higher in Australia.

GEOGRAPHIC DISTRIBUTION

- United States—*Dermacentor variabilis*: wide distribution over the eastern two-thirds of the country, California, and Oregon; *D. andersoni*: from the Cascades to the Rocky Mountains; *Amblyomma americanum*: from Texas and Missouri to the Atlantic Coast; *A. maculatum*: Atlantic and Gulf of Mexico seaboards.
- Australia—*I. holocyclus*: coastal areas of the east; *I. cornuatus*, southern Australia (Tasmania).
- Other—cases with apparent tick paralysis have been described in South Africa (*Rhipicentor nuttalli*), southern Italy (*Rhipicephalus sanguineus*), and Iran (*Ornithodorus lahorensis*).

SIGNALMENT

Species

- Australia—dogs and cats.
- United States—dogs; cats appear to be resistant.

Breed Predilections

None

Mean Age and Range

Any age.

Predominant Sex

N/A

SIGNS

Historical Findings

- Patient exposed to ticks (wooded area) approximately 1 week before onset of signs.
- Onset—gradual; starts with weakness in the pelvic limbs, progresses to the thoracic limbs within 12–72 hours.

Neurologic Examination Findings

North American Ticks

- Neurologic signs—rapidly ascending, flaccid generalized lower motor neuron tetraparesis to tetraplegia.
- Patient becomes extremely weak to recumbent in 1–3 days, with hyporeflexia to areflexia and hypotonia to atonia.
- Pain sensation preserved, no hyperesthesia.
- Cranial nerve dysfunction—uncommon; may note facial weakness and reduced jaw tone; sometimes dysphonia and dysphagia early in the course; megaesophagus uncommon.
- Urination and defecation usually normal.
- No cardiovascular effects.
- Respiratory paralysis—uncommon in the United States; may occur if ticks are not removed; death may occur in 1–5 days.

Australian Ticks

- Neurologic signs—much more severe and rapidly progressive; ascending motor weakness can progress to tetraplegia within a few hours.
- Sialosis, depressed gag reflex, dysphonia, megaesophagus, vomiting/regurgitation.
- Sympathetic nervous system—mydriatic and poorly responsive pupils (common in cats); hypertension; tachyarrhythmias; pulmonary edema.
- Urinary bladder dysfunction may be present.
- Caudal medullary respiratory center involvement—progressive reduction in respiratory rate and increased respiratory effort.
- Respiratory muscle paralysis—much more prevalent; dogs and cats progress to dyspnea, cyanosis, and respiratory paralysis within 1–2 days if not treated.

CAUSES

United States

- *D. variabilis*—common wood tick.
- *D. andersoni*—Rocky Mountain wood tick.
- *A. americanum*—lone star tick.
- *A. maculatum*—Gulf Coast tick.

Australia

- *I. holocyclus*—far more potent neurotoxin than that of the North American species.
- *I. cornuatus*—southern paralysis tick, occasionally causes paralysis in southern Australia.

RISK FACTORS

- Environments that harbor ticks.
- Australia—higher risk during spring, and in areas with higher rainfall, containing tree cover and areas of water; higher risk of death if dog <6 months old or a toy breed.

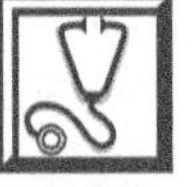

DIAGNOSIS

DIFFERENTIAL DIAGNOSIS

- Botulism.
- Acute polyneuropathy.
- Acute polyradiculoneuritis (coonhound paralysis).
- Distal denervating disease.
- Fulminant myasthenia gravis.
- Generalized (diffuse) or multifocal myelopathy.
- Intoxications (coral snake, black widow spider, lasalocid, blue and green algae).

CBC/BIOCHEMISTRY/URINALYSIS

Normal

OTHER LABORATORY TESTS

Arterial blood gases—severely affected patients may show hypoventilation and respiratory acidosis (low Pao_2, high $Paco_2$, low pH).

IMAGING

Thoracic radiography (*Ixodes* ticks)—megaesophagus, aspiration pneumonia, pulmonary edema.

DIAGNOSTIC PROCEDURES

- History of exposure to ticks.
- Thoroughly search for a tick—head, neck, body and limbs, ear canals, mouth, rectum, vagina, prepuce, and in between the digits and footpads; clipping the entire fur may be needed; immediately remove tick.
- In some cases the offending tick may have dropped, a negative finding does not exclude tick paralysis.
- Electrodiagnostics—electromyogram; normal insertional activity without spontaneous myofiber activity; lack of motor unit action

potentials; motor nerve stimulation shows a dramatic decrease in amplitude or a complete absence of compound muscle action potentials; decrease in motor nerve conduction velocities; normal sensory conduction and repetitive nerve stimulation.

PATHOLOGIC FINDINGS

Pulmonary histopathologic findings in dead/euthanized dogs include diffuse bronchopneumonia, congestion, and alveolar edema.

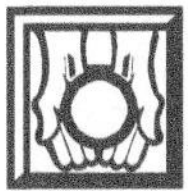

TREATMENT

APPROPRIATE HEALTH CARE

- Inpatient—neurologic dysfunction suggesting tick paralysis; hospitalize until either a tick is found and removed or appropriate treatment to kill a hidden tick is performed.
- Remove tick with forceps, applying steady pressure, taking care to remove mouth parts.

NURSING CARE

- Inpatient supportive care—essential until patient begins to show signs of recovery.
- Oxygen cage—hypoventilation ($Paco_2$ <45 mmHg) and hypoxia.
- Mechanical ventilation—respiratory failure ($Paco_2$ >45 mmHg).
- IV fluid therapy—if patient unable to eat/drink due to dysphagia, vomiting/regurgitation.
- Prevention of aspiration pneumonia—elevated feedings if megaesophagus present.

ACTIVITY

- Keep patient in a quiet environment.
- *Ixodes* tick paralysis—keep patient in a cool, air-conditioned area (toxin is temperature sensitive).

DIET

Withhold food and water if patient has dysphagia or vomiting/regurgitation.

CLIENT EDUCATION

- Non-*Ixodes* tick—inform client that good nursing care is essential, although the patient's recovery is rapid (within 24–72 hours) after removal of ticks.
- *Ixodes* tick—warn client that cranial nerve signs and weakness often continue to worsen for 24–48 hours even after tick removal; inform client that aggressive treatment to neutralize the toxin must be undertaken, and that patient death may ensue even if appropriate therapy is initiated.

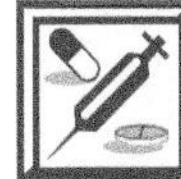

MEDICATIONS

DRUG(S) OF CHOICE

- United States—if the tick cannot be found, topically apply a systemic insecticide such as fipronil or, alternatively, dip the patient in an insecticidal bath; often the only treatment needed.
- Australia—in addition to tick removal and use of topical acaricides, treatment often includes the use of commercially available tick antitoxin hyperimmune serum (TAS) to neutralize circulating toxin (0.5–1 mg/kg IV), depending on severity of clinical signs; adverse reactions to TAS administration can be reduced by premedication with atropine; if severe sympathetic signs, use of phenoxybenzamine, an α-adrenergic antagonist (1 mg/kg IV diluted in saline and given slowly over 20 minutes) can be beneficial.

CONTRAINDICATIONS

Drugs that interfere with neuromuscular transmission (e.g., tetracycline, aminoglycosides, procaine penicillin).

PRECAUTIONS

Ixodes tick—administer IV fluids at a slow rate to avoid further complications of pulmonary edema.

POSSIBLE INTERACTIONS

N/A

ALTERNATIVE DRUG(S)

N/A

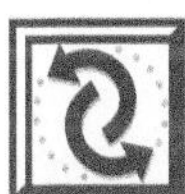

FOLLOW-UP

PATIENT MONITORING

- Non-*Ixodes* tick—reassess neurologic status daily after tick removal; should see rapid improvement in muscle strength.
- *Ixodes* tick—monitor neurologic status, respiratory and cardiovascular functions intensively even after tick removal, because of the residual effect of neurotoxin.

PREVENTION/AVOIDANCE

- Vigilantly check for ticks up to 5–9 days after exposure.
- Frequent search for ticks in endemic areas during spring/summer months.
- Routine topical application of acaricidal solution/collar, or weekly insecticidal baths.
- Short-term acquired immunity develops after exposure to *Ixodes* neurotoxin.

POSSIBLE COMPLICATIONS

No long-term complications if the patient survives the acute effects of the toxin.

EXPECTED COURSE AND PROGNOSIS

- Non-*Ixodes* tick—prognosis good to excellent if ticks are removed; recovery in 1–3 days.
- *Ixodes* tick—prognosis often guarded; recovery prolonged; removal of tick does not always result in improvement; respiratory paralysis main cause of death; death in 1–2 days without treatment; 5% mortality rate reported in affected dogs, fatality rate in affected cats appears lower.

MISCELLANEOUS

ASSOCIATED CONDITIONS

N/A

AGE-RELATED FACTORS

N/A

ZOONOTIC POTENTIAL

Although humans can acquire the disease by being bitten by the same ticks (especially in Australia), tick paralysis is not transmitted to humans from affected pets.

PREGNANCY/FERTILITY/BREEDING

Unknown

SEE ALSO

- Botulism.
- Coonhound Paralysis (Acute Polyradiculoneuritis).
- Myasthenia Gravis.
- Polyneuropathies (Peripheral Neuropathies).

Suggested Reading

Añor S. Acute lower motor neuron tetraparesis. Vet Clin North Am Small Anim Pract 2014, 44:1201–1222.

Atwell RB, Campbell FE, Evans EA. Prospective survey of tick paralysis in dogs. Aust Vet J 2001, 79:412–418.

Eppleston KR, Kelman M, Ward MP. Distribution, seasonality and risk factors for tick paralysis in Australian dogs and cats. Vet Parasitol 2013, 196:460–468.

Malik R, Farrow BRH. Tick paralysis in North America and Australia. Vet Clin North Am Small Anim Pract 1991, 21:157–171.

Webster RA, Mills PC, Morton JM. Indications, durations and outcomes of mechanical ventilation in dogs and cats with tick paralysis caused by *Ixodes holocyclus*: 61 cases (2008–2011). Aust Vet J 2013, 91:233–239.

Author Paula Martin Vaquero

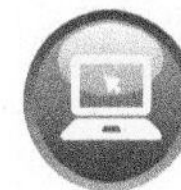

Client Education Handout available online

TICKS AND TICK CONTROL

BASICS

DEFINITION

- Arachnids, arthropod ectoparasites feed on the blood of their hosts.
- Most ticks are not host specific; divided into argasid (soft) and ixodid (hard) ticks.
- Argasid are more primitive, more commonly parasitize birds; one of importance in dogs and cats is spinous ear tick (*Otobius megnini*).
- Ixodid ticks are more specialized and highly parasitic, both sexes are bloodsuckers; *Rhipicephalus sanguineus* and *Dermacentor variabilis* are common in dogs and cats.

PATHOPHYSIOLOGY

- Blood-loss anemia—from heavy infestations.
- Damage to the integument—local irritation and infection may occur; tick adaptations suppress host response and allow feeding for up to 1 week.
- Salivary secretions—neurotoxins; other pharmacologically active compounds cause impaired hemostasis and immune suppression at the tick-feeding site.
- Pathogens—acquired when ticks feed on infected reservoir hosts (often rodents and small feral mammals); transmitted while feeding on dogs and cats.

Tick Biology

- Hard ticks—four life stages: egg, larva, nymph, and adult; larvae and nymphs feed to repletion before detaching and molting; after detachment, females lay thousands of eggs and die; various tick stages may survive over winter, tolerate long starvation, low humidity, as well as water deprivation. Completion of life cycle requires three hosts; some species pass all stages on the same mammal.
- Transovarial transmission—organisms disseminate to the ticks' ovaries; infected eggs hatch and produce infected larvae.
- Trans-stadial transmission—immature ticks become infected while feeding on reservoir hosts and maintain infection through the molt from one life stage to the next, transmitting organisms to the new host when next stage feeds.
- Ticks generally acquire hosts by a passive ambush process; when a suitable host brushes against vegetation harboring questing ticks, they transfer to the host.
- *Amblyomma americanum* can be an active hunter and traverse distances of up to 18 m to attack a suitable host.
- Symbiotic relationship—*Ixodes scapularis* infected with *Anaplasma phagocytophylum* express an antifreeze glycoprotein gene that enhances survival of the tick in cold weather.

SYSTEMS AFFECTED

- Skin/exocrine.
- Hemic/lymphatic/immune.
- Musculoskeletal.
- Nervous.

GEOGRAPHIC DISTRIBUTION

- Strong geographic specificities exist for some tick species and their associated pathogens, producing geographic prevalence of associated diseases.
- Ranges of ticks are expanding, therefore the geographic incidence of tick parasitism and infections vectored by them are expanding.
- Emergence of new tick-borne infections and coinfection (due to coinfected vector ticks or parasitism of hosts by ticks of more than one species).
- *I. scapularis* and *I. pacificus*—midwest, northeast, southeast, and south-central United States and west coast, respectively.
- *R. sanguineus*—throughout the continental United States; *R. sanguineus* is unique among hard ticks; it can survive and establish its life cycle inside dwellings and kennels at (low) household humidity (common name "kennel tick").
- *D. variabilis*—eastern seaboard and west coast of United States.
- *A. americanum*—found throughout the midwest, south-central, southeast, and parts of the northeast United States with strong range expansion.
- *Amblyomma maculatum*—gulf coast states of United States with range expansion.

SIGNALMENT

Species

- Dog and cat.
- Cats are efficient at removing ticks; tick attachment and tick-vectored diseases including Lyme disease, anaplasmosis, and cytauxzoonosis have been diagnosed in domestic felines.

SIGNS

- Attached ticks or tick-feeding cavities may be seen on the skin.
- Irritation secondary to bite.
- Petechia secondary to infectious organisms (*Rickettsia*, *Anaplasma platys*).
- Blood-loss anemia (direct effect); thrombocytopenia, anemia, inclusion bodies in neutrophils, monocytes, red blood cells secondary to transmitted infectious organisms.
- Limb/joint abnormalities secondary to infectious organisms (*Borrelia burgdorferi* and other organisms implicated in oligo- and polyarthritis).
- Cardiac—Lyme carditis (*B. burgdorferi*), manifests typically as atrioventricular block; rare and poorly documented in dogs.
- Renal—unique, generally fatal protein-losing nephropathy in dogs infected with *B. burgdorferi* linked to immune complexes associated with antigen and antibody from infection.
- Rocky Mountain Spotted Fever—vague or non-specific symptoms of fever, lethargy, joint pain, gastrointestinal symptoms, focal hemorrhages (Rickettsia rickettsii).
- Paralysis—neurotoxins secreted from tick salivary glands produce ascending weakness and paralysis.
- Pyogranulomatous myositis, periosteal reaction, neutrophilia, antigenic stimulation, and amyloid deposition in viscera in *Hepatozoon americanum* infection in which the dog serves as the intermediate and reservoir host following tick ingestion.
- Weight loss, anemia, lethargy, fever, neutrophilia, hyperglobulinemia and hypoalbuminemia in *Hepatozoon canis* infection. Infection occurs by digesting the tick (*A. americanum*), which is the definitive host.

CAUSES

Ticks—attracted to hosts by warmth, presence of carbon dioxide, physical contact, and host-associated odors.

RISK FACTORS

- Domestic animals—can be in close contact with ticks due to invasion of ticks into suburban environments and expansion of suburban environment into surrounding forests, prairies, and coastline areas.
- Travel—increases risk for exposure.
- Risk is expanding as new cycles for maintenance of infectious organisms are emerging (and being discovered).

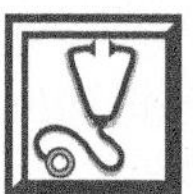

DIAGNOSIS

DIFFERENTIAL DIAGNOSIS

N/A

OTHER LABORATORY TESTS

- Vector-borne disease (VBD) panels provide clinicians the ability to test blood for multiple agents by using serology and/or PCR.
- IDEXX Snap 4DxPlus Test—in-office rapid screening test for multiple VBD; detects antibodies (C_6 ELISA) against *B. burgdorferi*, *E. canis*, *E. ewingii*, *A. phagocytophilum*, *A. platys*, and *Dirofilaria immitis* antigens in canine serum, plasma, or whole blood.
- ABAXIS VetScan FLEX4 Rapid T—detects antibodies against *A. phagocytophilum*, *A. platys*, *B. burgdorferi*, *E. canis*, *E. chaffeensis*, *E. ewingii*, and *Dirofilaria immitis* antigens in canine whole blood, serum or plasma.
- Tests are sensitive and specific; *B. burgdorferi* test does not crossreact with vaccine-induced antibodies.

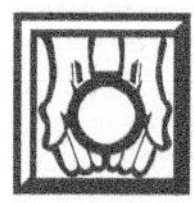

TREATMENT

APPROPRIATE HEALTH CARE

- Outpatient after removal of ticks.
- Removal—as soon as possible to limit time available for pathogen or neurotoxin transmission; grasp ticks close to the skin with fine-pointed tweezers and gently pull free.

NURSING CARE

Wash feeding cavity with soap and water; generally sufficient to prevent local inflammation or secondary infection.

CLIENT EDUCATION

Application of hot matches, petrolatum jelly, or other materials not only fails to cause tick detachment but allows for longer periods of attachment and feeding.

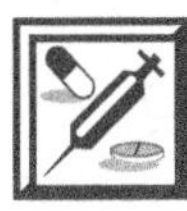

MEDICATIONS

DRUG(S) OF CHOICE

See Prevention/Avoidance.

FOLLOW-UP

PREVENTION/AVOIDANCE

• Perimeter control and avoiding environments that harbor ticks.
• Frequent tick checks and tick removal.
• Year-round tick prevention.
• Tick control does not always equal control of tick-borne diseases: Products should quickly kill or prevent attachment and feeding by the tick.
• Tick-borne pathogens—may be transmitted very rapidly (viruses) or require several hours (*R. rickettsii*), less than 1 day (*A. phagocytophilum*), 1–2 days (*B. burgdorferi*), or 2–3 days (*Ehrlichia* species and *B. canis*).
• Ingestion of infected ticks makes tick control problematic for prevention of infection with *Hepatozoon* species.

Insecticides and Acaricides

• Acaricides meant only for dogs must not be applied to cats.
• Acaricidal collars—amitraz, deltamethrine, and flumethrin (Preventic, Seresto, and Scalibor, respectively).
• Spot-on treatments—fipronil, permethrin, flumethrin, etofenprox.
• Oral treatments—isoxazolines: fluralaner, afoxolaner, lotilaner, and sarolaner. Fluralaner is also available as a spot-on for dogs and cats. Sarolaner combined with selamectin is available as a spot-on for cats.
• Disease transmission interruption studies have been published for products containing fipronil, amitraz, isoxazolines, permethrin, and synthetic pyrethroids; rapid killing and clinical repellence are essential to prevent or interrupt tick feeding.

POSSIBLE COMPLICATIONS

Tick-borne diseases or tick paralysis.

MISCELLANEOUS

ASSOCIATED CONDITIONS

• Canine babesiosis—*B. canis*.
• Rocky Mountain spotted fever—*R. rickettsia*.
• Canine monocytic ehrlichiosis—*E. canis* or *E. chaffeensis*.
• Cyclic thrombocytopenia—*A. platys*.
• Granulocytic anaplasmosis—*A. phagocytophilum* and *E. ewingii*.
• Lyme disease—*B. burgdorferi*.
• American canine hepatozoonosis—caused by protozoa *H. americanum*, following ingestion of an infected *tick*.
• Canine hepatozoonosis— caused by *H. canis* following ingestion of an infected *tick*.
• Tick paralysis—caused by a neurotoxin; affects acetylcholine synthesis and/or liberation at the neuromuscular junction of the host animal; ascending flaccid paralysis initially affects the pelvic limbs 5–9 days after tick attachment.

VACCINES

Currently for Lyme disease there are three types for dogs: (1) whole-cell, killed bacterin: LymeVax, Duramune Lyme, and Nobivac Lyme, (2) outer surface protein A (OspA): Recombitek Lyme, and (3) chimeric recombinant (OspA and 7 types of OspC): Vanguard crLyme. Efficacy studies which duplicate natural exposure are lacking.

ZOONOTIC POTENTIAL

• Ticks may parasitize wildlife, domestic animals, or humans at different stages in their developmental cycles; infections acquired in early life stages may be transmitted when ticks feed again in the next stage.
• Humans, if parasitized, may be exposed to organisms in infected ticks. *B. burgdorferi*, *A. phagocytophilum*, *R. rickettsia*, and *E. chaffeensis* are also human pathogens.

SYNONYMS

Acariasis

SEE ALSO

• Babesiosis.
• Ehrlichiosis and Anaplasmosis.
• Lyme Borreliosis.
• Rocky Mountain Spotted Fever.

ABBREVIATIONS

• IFA = immunofluorescent antibody assay.
• VBD = vector-borne disease.

INTERNET RESOURCES

https://www.cdc.gov/ncezid/dvbd/index.html

Suggested Reading

Burgio F, Meyer L, Armstrong R. A comparative laboratory trial evaluating the immediate efficacy of fluralaner, afoxolaner, sarolaner and imidacloprid + permethrin against adult *Rhipicephalus sanguineus* (sensu lato) ticks attached to dogs. Parasit Vectors 2016, 9:626.

Littman MP, Gerber B, Goldstein RE, et al. ACVIM consensus update on Lyme borreliosis in dogs and cats. J Vet Intern Med 2018, 32:887–903.

Miller Jr. WH, Giriffin CE, Campbell KL. Parasitic skin diseases. In: Muller and Kirk's Small Animal Dermatology, 7th ed. Philadelphia, PA: W.B. Saunders, 2013, pp. 294–296.

Schorderet-Weber S, Noack S, Selzer PM, et al. Blocking transmission of vector-borne diseases. Int J Parasitol Drugs Drug Resist 2017, 7:90–109.

Author Ronnie Kaufmann

Consulting Editor Alexander H. Werner Resnick

Acknowledgment The author and editors acknowledge the prior contribution of Steven A. Levy.

Client Education Handout available online

TOAD VENOM TOXICOSIS

BASICS

OVERVIEW

• Two species of primary concern in North America—Colorado River toad (*Incilius alvarius*) and marine/cane toad (*Rhinella marina*); marine toad more toxic; both can be fatal. • *I. alvarius* found in Arizona, New Mexico, Texas, and Colorado; *R. marina* found in Florida, Texas, and Hawaii. Both species have body lengths up to 23 cm; easily distinguishes them from other toad species. Active during periods of high humidity (monsoon season—late summer Arizona, New Mexico, Texas, and Colorado for Colorado River toads); most encounters occur during evening, night, or early morning.
• Toxin—produced in parotid glands; defensive; rapidly absorbed across the victim's mucous membranes; contains several major components: indole alkyl amines (similar to the street drug LSD), cardiac glycosides, and noncardiac sterols. On average 590 mg of crude secretions released from a single *R. marina*—100 mg of crude bufotoxin lethal to 10–15 kg dog. Sublingual/buccal absorption—bypasses gastrointestinal tract; first pass metabolism allows systemic exposure to unmetabolized bufogens. Rapidly absorbed across gastrointestinal mucosa and quickly eliminated. Crosses blood–brain barrier readily (rapid CNS effects).

SIGNALMENT

Primarily dogs; rarely cats.

SIGNS

General Comments

• Rapid onset. • A cane toad sitting in a water dish for several hours can leave enough residual toxins to kill dogs. • Salivation primary sign—*excessive* within seconds of exposure. • Toxicity varies with species, size and geographical location. If not in one of the regions cited above, *unlikely* to contain highly toxic secretions.

Historical Findings

• Crying/pawing at the mouth. • Frothing at mouth. • Ataxia—stiff gaited. • Seizures.
• Animal found dead with toad in mouth.

Physical Examination Findings

• Profuse hypersalivation.
• Hyperexcitability/vocalization. • Brick red buccal mucous membranes. • Hyperthermia.
• Collapse. • Marked cardiac ventricular arrhythmia—less common with Colorado River toad. • Cyanosis. • Dyspnea. • Mydriasis.
• Nystagmus. • Pulmonary edema.
• Neurological signs. • Shock.

CAUSES & RISK FACTORS

• Living in indigenous geographic region for species and in close proximity to toads.
• Moist, warm, outside environment.
• Outdoor animal.

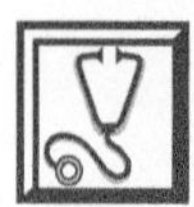

DIAGNOSIS

DIFFERENTIAL DIAGNOSIS

• Caustics or other oral irritants. • Hyperthermia.
• Heat stroke. • Hypocalcemia. • Hypoglycemia.
• Serotonin syndrome. • Organophosphate or carbamate pesticides.

CBC/BIOCHEMISTRY/URINALYSIS

• May note hypercalcemia or hyperkalemia.
• Elevated serum glucose. • Elevated urea nitrogen.

OTHER LABORATORY TESTS

Magnesium level—ventricular cardiotoxicity cases.

DIAGNOSTIC PROCEDURES

Electrocardiogram—ventricular arrhythmias.

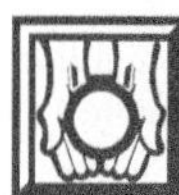

TREATMENT

• Marine toad intoxication—medical emergency; death common. • Decontamination—flush mouth for 5–10 minutes with copious quantities of water. • Hyperthermia (>40.6°C/105°F)—provide a cool bath; remove from bath once temperature reaches 39.4°C (103°F). • Maintain airway. • Rapid evaluation of cardiac function.
• Supportive therapy—correct electrolytes; acid–base imbalances. • Ingested toad—may require endoscopic removal or surgery. • Seizure potential—*high* with the truly toxic toads; emesis only performed by DVM who understands this concept.

MEDICATIONS

DRUG(S) OF CHOICE

• Atropine 0.04 mg/kg (1/4 of dose IV, remainder IM or SC)—reduces salivation; helps prevent aspiration; use with bradycardia, heart block, or other sinoatrial node alterations as a result of the digitalis-like effect of the toxin; not recommended if severe tachycardia present.
• Esmolol or propranolol—esmolol is very short acting and may be used as a test dose. If arrhythmia responds to treatment, propranolol is used because the duration of action is much longer (hours; see Contraindications/Possible Interactions); rapid administration may be required to combat tachyarrhythmias; may be repeated in 20 minutes or require continuous IV infusion for persistent arrhythmias: ○ Esmolol 0.05–0.1 mg/kg IV q5min—maximum dosage of 0.5 mg/kg. ○ Propranolol 0.02 mg/kg IV slowly as needed—maximum dosage of 1 mg/kg. • Digoxin-specific Fab fragments (Digoxin Immune Fab) have been used successfully to treat toad venom induced cardiotoxic effects. • Anticonvulsant therapy—diazepam 0.5–1.0 mg/kg IV. • Lipid emulsion (20%)— anecdotally, IV intralipids may reduce bufadienolide (very lipophilic) toxicity.

CONTRAINDICATIONS/POSSIBLE INTERACTIONS

• Cardiac disease or bronchial asthma—patient may not tolerate the use of beta-blockers such as esmolol and propranolol. Use a test dose of esmolol (very short duration of action) and monitor closely before using propranolol (much longer duration of action). • Anesthetics (e.g., pentobarbital)—may depress function of an already compromised myocardium; use with caution.

FOLLOW-UP

• Continuous electrocardiographic monitoring—recommend until patient is fully recovered.
• Colorado River toad intoxication—patients usually normal within 30 minutes of onset of treatment; death uncommon if treated; do not underestimate the risk of secondary heatstroke.
• Marine toad intoxication—medical emergency; death common.

MISCELLANEOUS

Suggested Reading

Brubacher JR, Lachmanen D, Ravikumar PR, et al. Efficacy of digoxin specific Fab fragments (Digibind) in the treatment of toad venom poisoning. Toxicon 1999, 37:931–942.

Gowda RM, Cohen RA, Khan IA. Toad venom poisoning: resemblance to digoxin toxicity and therapeutic implications. Heart 2003, 89:e14.

Johnnides S, Eubig P, Green T. Toad intoxication in the dog by *Rhinella marina*: the clinical syndrome and current treatment recommendations. J Am Anim Hosp Assoc 2016, 52:1–8.

Reeves MP. A retrospective report of 90 dogs with suspected cane toad (*Bufo marinus*) toxicity. Aust Vet J 2004, 82:608–611.

Author Daniel E. Keyler

Consulting Editor Lynn R. Hovda

Acknowledgment The author and editors acknowledge the prior contribution of Michael E. Peterson.

T

BASICS

OVERVIEW

- Absence of tooth or teeth due to developmental conditions, not to trauma or extraction:
    - Total anodontia—absence of all teeth due to failure in development.
    - Partial anodontia—failure in development of part of the dentition (hypodontia, oligodontia—some teeth missing).
    - Edentulous—"without teeth" but primarily due to tooth loss (e.g., end-stage periodontal disease).
- In dogs, premolars or distal molars are the most common missing teeth.
- If a deciduous tooth is missing, its permanent successor will probably not develop as well.
- If a permanent tooth is missing, and the deciduous tooth is still present (persistent), if root structure is stable, that deciduous tooth might stay functional for a long time; lack of permanent tooth should be documented.

SIGNALMENT

- Any breed, size or gender, but smaller breeds predominate.
- Some familial tendencies, breed prevalence.

SIGNS

- Tooth not present (crown and root).
- Alveolar bone and gingival margin at site is regular, smooth, even slightly "scalloped" appearance.
- No tooth structure present radiographically.

CAUSES & RISK FACTORS

- Dog/cat.
- Total and partial anodontia—typically hereditary and may be associated with ectodermal dysplasia (Chinese crested dogs).
- Bilateral patterns of missing teeth may be indicative of a genetic or familial tendency, as opposed to a single missing tooth.

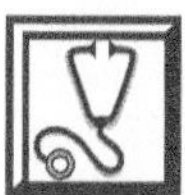

DIAGNOSIS

DIFFERENTIAL DIAGNOSIS

- Delayed eruption.
- Unerupted teeth (see Dentigerous Cyst).
- Invulsed tooth.
- Extracted or lost due to periodontal disease or trauma.
- Fusion tooth—if two teeth have fused, there will be reduction in the tooth number (see Tooth Formation/Structure, Abnormal).

CBC/BIOCHEMISTRY/URINALYSIS

Typically not affected.

IMAGING

- Intraoral radiographs essential.
- Determine if teeth are truly missing, and/or if permanent teeth are present, if deciduous teeth are persistent/retained.
- Pre-purchase full-mouth radiographs on 8- to 10-week-old puppies can identify if permanent tooth structures are present (though there is no guarantee they will erupt).

DIAGNOSTIC PROCEDURES

- Complete oral examination.
- Appropriate preoperative diagnostics when indicated prior to procedure.

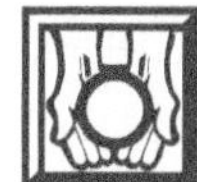

TREATMENT

SURGICAL CONSIDERATIONS

- Appropriate antimicrobial and pain management therapy when indicated.
- Appropriate patient monitoring and support during anesthetic procedures.
- None indicated unless an unerupted or involved tooth is found radiographically.

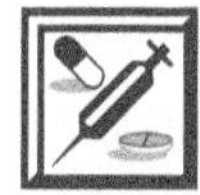

MEDICATIONS

DRUGS OF CHOICE

None indicated.

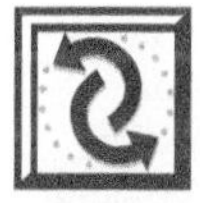

FOLLOW-UP

None needed.

MISCELLANOUS

- If multiple teeth are missing or they are missing bilaterally, there could be a familial tendency; consider removing from breeding stock.
- In some breeds (Doberman pinscher, Rottweiler) or Schutzhund trained dogs, any missing teeth may be considered a serious fault, and pre-purchase radiographs on puppies may be helpful.

SEE ALSO

- Dentigerous Cyst.
- Tooth Formation/Structure, Abnormal.

Suggested Reading

Lobprise HB, Dodd JR. Wiggs' Veterinary Dentistry Principles and Practice. Hoboken, NJ: Wiley-Blackwell, 2019.

Author Heidi B. Lobprise

Consulting Editor Heidi B. Lobprise

TOOTH FORMATION/STRUCTURE, ABNORMAL

BASICS

OVERVIEW

Variation in Tooth Size

- Macrodontia—crown oversized, root normal.
- Microdontia—crown normal shape, but small.
- Peg tooth—small, cone-shaped tooth with a single cusp.

Variation in Tooth Structure/Shape

- Fusion—two separate tooth buds joined to form an entire single tooth or joined at the roots by cementum and dentin.
- Gemination—developing tooth bud undergoes an incomplete split, resulting in two crowns with a common root canal.
- Dilacerated—distorted or malformed tooth (crown or root)—a general term that may be used for many different presentations.
- Dens-in-dente (tooth within a tooth)—external layers invaginate into internal structures with varying severity.
- Shell teeth—crown present, but little to no root development.
- Amelogenesis imperfecta—hereditary reduction in the amount of developed enamel matrix.

Pathophysiology

- Stress or stimulus (trauma) at time of development can alter tooth formation.
- Infection, trauma to tooth buds, or traumatic extraction of deciduous teeth during permanent tooth formation can significantly alter the structure.
- Genetic or familial tendencies not known for most conditions.

SIGNALMENT

Dog/cat.

SIGNS

- Fusion—fused crown will be larger than a single tooth. There will be a reduced number of teeth (two counted as one).
- Gemination tooth—actual number of teeth will be unaltered, but one tooth will be larger, with duplication of part of the crown (and possibly roots radiographically); "Siamese twin."
- Dilacerated teeth:
  - Any variation in structure or form—extra root, curved root.
  - Each tooth must be evaluated for integrity of the pulp system, as any disruption in the continuity of the crown and roots may result in exposure of the pulp to the external environment.

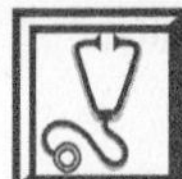

DIAGNOSIS

DIFFERENTIAL DIAGNOSIS

- Trauma to tooth structures.
- Developmental abnormalities.

IMAGING

- Discontinuity between crowns and roots.
- Possible pulp exposure and pulp stones.
- Roots are convergent with wide canals (nonvital pulp).
- Periapical/root abscessation with extensive bone loss.

DIAGNOSTIC PROCEDURES

- Complete oral examination.
- Intraoral radiographs.
- With any abnormal structure (dilaceration), pulpal integrity and the potential for crowding must be evaluated.
- Appropriate preoperative diagnostics when indicated prior to procedure.

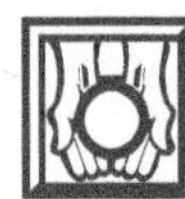

TREATMENT

- Abnormal development of mandibular first molars in small-breed dogs.
  - Dilaceration is more common, sometimes described as dens-in-dente.
  - As one of the first permanent teeth to form, there may be a mechanical challenge (lack of space) in small dogs that impedes proper crown–root development.
  - Invagination of the enamel and/or cementum at the neck of the tooth, often with some degree of gingival recession.
- Fusion teeth—no treatment is necessary unless the groove between the two teeth and/or crowns extends to the gingival margin or below (nidus for periodontal disease).
- Gemination tooth—if tooth crowding results, extraction may be necessary.
- Dilacerated tooth—if there is pulpal exposure or compromise, extraction is generally necessary. In some cases, endodontic and restorative therapy may allow preservation of the tooth.

MEDICATIONS

DRUG(S) OF CHOICE

- Appropriate antimicrobial and pain management therapy when indicated.
- Appropriate patient monitoring and support during anesthetic procedures.

FOLLOW-UP

EXPECTED COURSE AND PROGNOSIS

- Good prognosis on teeth with moderate changes (peg teeth, fusion teeth, gemination tooth).
- Guarded prognosis on dilacerated teeth with pulpal compromise, though extraction typically successful.

MISCELLANEOUS

INTERNET RESOURCES

https://avdc.org/avdc-nomenclature/

Suggested Reading

Lobprise HB. Blackwell's Five-Minute Veterinary Consult Clinical Companion: Small Animal Dentistry, 2nd ed. Ames, IA: Blackwell, 2012 (for additional topics, including diagnostics and techniques).

Lobprise HB, Dodd JR. Wiggs' Veterinary Dentistry Principles and Practice. Hoboken, NJ: Wiley-Blackwell. 2019.

Regezi JA, Sciubba JJ, Jordan RCK. Oral Pathology Clinical Pathologic Correlations, 4th ed. St. Louis, MO: Saunders, 1999, pp. 367–370.

Author Heidi B. Lobprise

Consulting Editor Heidi B. Lobprise

TOOTH ROOT ABSCESS (APICAL ABSCESS)

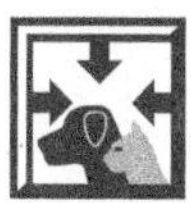

BASICS

OVERVIEW

- An abscess is a localized collection of pus in a cavity formed by the disintegration of tissues.
- An abscess spreads along the pathway of least resistance from the tooth apex, resulting in osteomyelitis:
  - If this infection perforates through the cortex of the bone in which the tooth is encased, it can result in a cellulitis that can burst through the skin to create a cutaneous draining tract.
  - The drainage can also occur through the alveolar mucosa, above the mucogingival line (parulis).
- Can involve any teeth; the maxillary fourth premolars are most commonly affected, followed by the canines and mandibular first molars.
- Periodontal disease can extend down the root of the tooth to the apex, infecting the pulp and resulting in endodontic involvement (perio-endo lesion).
- Systemic spread of bacteria (bacteremia and pyemia) and the persistence of inflammation can affect other organ systems.
- A tooth root abscess can have an acute or chronic phase:
  - Phoenix abscess—acute exacerbation of a chronic periapical abscess.
- Can arise without the presence of bacteria (sterile abscess).

SIGNALMENT

- Dogs (primarily) and cats.
- Any age:deciduous or permanent teeth can be involved.
- Usually occurs in active animals that bite or chew a lot.

SIGNS

- Tooth is visibly broken with or having near pulpal exposure—90% of cases.
- Tooth may appear discolored.
- Tooth is not sensitive to percussion or cold or hot liquids or foods—note: acute tooth fracture with pulp exposure would be sensitive.
- Facial swelling—usually localized but can spread, resulting in a cellulitis.
- Cutaneous sinus (draining tract) exuding pus—suppurative apical periodontitis:
  - Suborbital abscess due to maxillary fourth premolar involvement is a common presentation.
- On oral examination, especially of the maxilla, there may be a red, raised lesion (parulis) at the anticipated location of the tooth apex. Often present where the attached gingiva meets the alveolar mucosa (mucogingival line) or above.
- Facial sensitivity may be slight but could be extensive if there is no draining.
- Tooth may be clinically asymptomatic, yet inflammation and bacteremia may be present.
- Tooth may be asymptomatic for a long time but will be affected eventually—subclinically or even years later.
- In the absence of a fractured tooth with an exposed canal, a deep periodontal pocket may extend to the apex of one or more roots, resulting in a similar abscess.
- May present as a jaw fracture, especially if the abscess affects the lower canine teeth or lower first molar. Slight trauma can cause a pathologic fracture of the mandible.
- Tooth may be loose and painful on palpation.
- May have facial lymphadenitis.
- Animal does not want to chew, especially on the affected side (plaque and calculus may accumulate), or will bite, but release quickly instead of holding on.
  - Some animals stop eating, the great majority do not.
- Sinusitis—maxillary sinus is most commonly affected.
- Sense of smell (olfactory capabilities) may be affected, especially with drug, bomb, or food-sniffing working dogs.

CAUSES & RISK FACTORS

- Any pulpal trauma—direct blow with fracture of crown; chewing hard objects (carnassial teeth); defense (fighting—canine teeth); malocclusive trauma; tug-of-war; bone plating that damaged roots.
- Advanced periodontal disease—a deep periodontal pocket can involve the apex where bacteria can enter the pulp system, especially at the palatal root of a small dog.
- Bacteria—the pulp can be affected by bacteria from dental caries, exposed dentinal tubules, or extension into endodontic system.
- Thermal heat resulting in pulpal necrosis—electrical cord burns, iatrogenic caused by use of electrocautery for gingival surgery, overpolishing during an oral hygiene procedure or use of rotary burs.

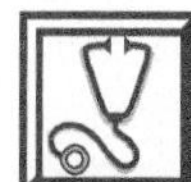

DIAGNOSIS

DIFFERENTIAL DIAGNOSIS

- Normal radiographic anatomy—chevron effect and mental formina.
- Tooth resorption—radiographs show no apical lucency or abscessation, but rather a disintegration of the root and/or crown with the loss of the periodontal ligament.
- Oral tumor.
- Squamous cell carcinoma and fibrosarcoma (rapidly growing and invasive) and ameloblastoma (slowly enlarges). These tumors can displace teeth, which often become mobile.
- Cementomas—radiographically show enlarged apical roots with a thin radiolucent zone continuous with the periodontal ligament.
- Cysts—radiographs usually show a very large lytic area involving any part of the root and/or unerupted crown:
  - Radicular cysts, apical periodontal granulomas.
  - Dentigerous cyst—occurs from the follicular cyst of an impacted or embedded tooth (usually the first mandibular premolars in dogs); in which case the radiograph show a tooth within the cyst.
- Periapical scar—usually occurs on an endodontically treated tooth where there has been no further increase in the radiographic apical lucency after a 6-month post-treatment period.
- Normal anatomy—mental foramens can be mistaken for apical lucencies on radiographic interpretation (the middle mental foramen just apical to second mandibular premolar).

CBC/BIOCHEMISTRY/URINALYSIS

CBC may show a leukocytosis and/or a mild regenerative anemia.

IMAGING

- Intraoral radiographs are the most commonly utilized diagnostic aid; demonstrates thickening of the apical periodontal ligament space; ill-defined radiolucency; shows bone loss at the apex as the lesion becomes chronic.
- As the lesion progresses, radiographic lesions consistent with osteomyelitis and cellulitis occur.
- Must be differentiated from chevron effect:this is evident radiographically in the small teeth that commonly develop a tooth root abscess.

T

DIAGNOSTIC PROCEDURES

- If fistulization has occurred, can place a gutta percha cone into the sinus tract and take a radiograph to identify the affected tooth.
- Transillumination with a strong fiber-optic light can help the clinician by distinguishing between a vital and necrotic pulp (compare to similar tooth on contralateral side).

PATHOLOGIC FINDINGS

- Apical area has a central area of liquefaction necrosis containing disintegrating neutrophils and cellular debris, surrounded by macrophages, lymphocytes, and plasma cells; can see bacteria.
- Extension of the lesion into cancellous bone results in inflammation of the periapical bone and resorption.
- Chronic changes may develop tracts that can be lined with epithelium; osteomyelitis or cellulitis lesions may become fibrotic with a capsule (radicular cyst and/or a periapical periodontal granuloma).

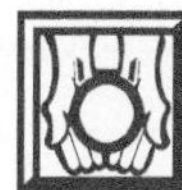

TREATMENT

- Must surgically drain and remove the focus of infection.
- Extraction of the tooth involved, with curettage of the apical infected area.

TOOTH ROOT ABSCESS (APICAL ABSCESS) (CONTINUED)

- Chronic conditions require surgical removal of the granulation tissue and curettage of the tract.
- Endodontic treatment of the involved tooth (surgical root canal if apical legion large).
- Medical management can be instituted temporarily until surgery can be performed.
- After treatment, cold packs on the area will help reduce inflammation.
- Following extraction, oral rest is recommended: soft diet, no hard chew toys, until the gingiva is healed.

MEDICATIONS

DRUG(S) OF CHOICE

- Broad-spectrum antibiotics recommended preoperatively to help prevent systemic spread of infection and improve tissue quality.
- Broad-spectrum antibiotic postoperatively for 7–10 days.
- Due to its ability to penetrate bone, clindamycin is recommended at a minimum of 5.5–11 mg/kg twice daily for dogs and once daily for cats.
- Second choice is amoxicillin/clavulanic acid 12.5–25 mg/kg orally twice daily.
- Analgesics preoperatively, intraoperatively, and postoperatively for 3–4 days.
- If a surgical endodontic treatment or an extraction was performed, a protective collar may be required.

FOLLOW-UP

- For extractions—recheck the site 10–14 days postoperatively. Soft diet and remove chew toys until healed gingiva is confirmed at recheck appointment.
- Recheck in 6–12 months with intraoral radiographs.
- Avoid traumatic injuries (e.g., letting the dog chase cars, hard chew toys, stop fighting).
- Curtail bite work—avoid handler sleeves that have tears or hole in them and avoid torsion movements.
- Check the mouth regularly for any trauma to additional teeth.

MISCELLANEOUS

N/A

Authors Heidi B. Lobprise and Jessica Johnson

Consulting Editor Heidi B. Lobprise

T

TORSION OF THE SPERMATIC CORD

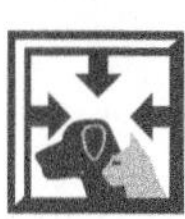

BASICS

OVERVIEW

- Testicular torsion (also known as torsion of the spermatic cord) results from twisting of the spermatic cord which leads to occlusion of venous outflow from the testis.
- Prolonged occlusion leads to ischemia, infarction, and necrosis.
- Abdominally retained testes are at greater risk of torsion, thought to be because of increased range of motion as compared to testes confined to the scrotum.
- Neoplastic testes, with increased weight, also have a greater likelihood of undergoing torsion.
- Torsion of descended (scrotal) testes has also been described.
- Systems affected—reproductive.

SIGNALMENT

- Intact male animals.
- Higher incidence in cryptorchid males.
- Rare in dogs.
- Very rare (but reported) in cats.
- Mean age 6–8 years (dogs).
- Cases of testicular torsion in both young (<10 months) and old (>10 years) dogs have been reported.

SIGNS

- Abdominal pain.
- Hyporexia/anorexia.
- Vomiting.
- Lethargy.
- Hind limb lameness.
- Pyrexia.
- Dysuria.
- Hematuria.
- Diarrhea.
- Scrotal edema.
- Inguinal swelling.
- Bilateral symmetric alopecia (secondary to Sertoli cell tumor).
- Feminization (secondary to Sertoli cell tumor).

CAUSES & RISK FACTORS

- Cryptorchidism.
- Testicular neoplasia (most commonly Sertoli cell tumors and seminomas).
- High physical exertion.
- Exuberant libido and expression of sexual behaviors.

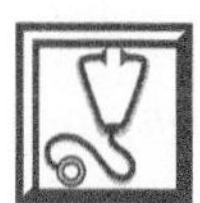

DIAGNOSIS

DIFFERENTIAL DIAGNOSIS

- Gastrointestinal disorder.
- Renal disease.
- Peritonitis.
- Abdominal trauma.
- Splenic torsion.
- Prostatic disease.
- The results of laboratory testing and imaging will aid in ruling in or out the above.

CBC/BIOCHEMISTRY/URINALYSIS

Nonspecific results in cases of testicular torsion, but useful in differentiating between other possible conditions.

IMAGING

Abdominal Ultrasonography

- Secondary to torsion, the affected testis typically appears hypoechoic in comparison to the contralateral (unaffected) testis.
- The diameter of the spermatic cord may be enlarged.
- The affected testis may be spherical in shape, as opposed to ovoid.
- Color Doppler ultrasound is very useful to visualize blood flow (or lack thereof).

Abdominal Radiographs

Nonspecific for diagnosing testicular torsion but valuable in assessing differential diagnoses.

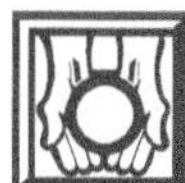

TREATMENT

- Surgical removal of affected testis on an emergent basis
- Inpatient care for immediate postoperative monitoring
- In theory, if torsion of a scrotal testis is rapidly identified and detorsion occurs quickly, this testicle could be salvaged. No such cases are reported in the literature. In a canine experimental model of testicular torsion, ultrasonographic changes occurred in all subjects by one hour after torsion, which were seen before irreversible histological lesions were induced.

MEDICATIONS

DRUG(S) OF CHOICE

None specifically indicated other than routine postoperative pain control and antimicrobial coverage as indicated by the particular case.

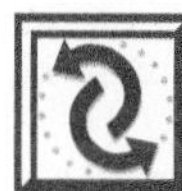

FOLLOW-UP

PREVENTION/AVOIDANCE

Removal of undescended testes prior to development of neoplasia and/or torsion.

EXPECTED COURSE AND PROGNOSIS

Good prognosis for recovery following surgery in cases of uncomplicated testicular torsion.

MISCELLANEOUS

ASSOCIATED CONDITIONS

- Cryptorchidism (generally accepted to be a heritable, sex-limited autosomal recessive trait).
- Testicular neoplasia (Sertoli cell tumor and seminoma most commonly, with an increased rate of occurrence in retained testes).

PREGNANCY/FERTILITY/BREEDING

If a retained testis is removed and a descended testis preserved, the ethical considerations of using the animal for breeding and potential for hereditary cryptorchidism should be impressed upon owner. Bilateral orchiectomy is the most commonly recommended course of treatment in literature reports.

Suggested Reading

Hecht S, King R, Tidwell AS, Gorman SC. Ultrasound diagnosis: intra-abdominal torsion of a non-neoplastic testicle in a cryptorchid dog. Vet Radiol Ultrasound 2004, 45:58–61.

Author Karen A. Von Dollen

Consulting Editor Erin E. Runcan

TOXOPLASMOSIS

BASICS

DEFINITION

Toxoplasma gondii—obligate intracellular coccidian protozoan parasite that infects nearly all mammals. Felids are the definitive hosts and all other warm-blooded animals serve as intermediate hosts.

PATHOPHYSIOLOGY

- Three main modes of transmission: (1) congenital, (2) ingestion of bradyzoites encysted in tissue of intermediate hosts, or (3) ingestion of sporulated oocysts within feces of felids.
- Most cats infected via ingestion of intermediate hosts; release bradyzoites in gastrointestinal tract that invade enteroepithelium; ultimately undergo sexual reproduction and oocyte formation; oocysts require 1–5 days to sporulate and become infectious after being passed in feces.
- Acute disseminated infection—organisms spread via blood or lymph; tachyzoites rapidly divide within extraintestinal tissues; causes focal necrosis, granulomatous inflammation; can be fatal.
- Following acute infection, slowly dividing bradyzoites encyst in host tissue, usually not clinically apparent unless immunosuppression or concomitant illness allows organism to reactivate to tachyzoite stage.
- Infection acquired during pregnancy—possible placentitis and transplacental transmission of tachyzoites to fetus; can induce abortion or clinical disease (kittens).

T

SYSTEMS AFFECTED

- Multisystemic.
- Ophthalmic—~ 80% of affected cats have uveitis.

INCIDENCE/PREVALENCE

- ~30% of cats and up to 50% of people serologically positive for *T. gondii.*
- Most animals asymptomatic.

GEOGRAPHIC DISTRIBUTION

Worldwide

SIGNALMENT

Species

Cats more commonly symptomatic than dogs.

Mean Age and Range

Mean age 4 years; range 2 weeks–16 years.

Predominant Sex

More common in male cats.

SIGNS

General Comments

- Determined by site and extent of organ damage.
- Acute—at time of initial infection, rapid clinical course.
- Chronic—reactivation of encysted infection due to immunosuppression, slower clinical course.

Historical Findings

- Lethargy, depression, anorexia.
- Weight loss.
- Fever.
- Ocular discharge, photophobia, miotic pupils (cats).
- Respiratory distress.
- Neurologic—ataxia, seizures, tremors, paresis/paralysis, or cranial nerve deficits.
- Digestive tract—vomiting, diarrhea, abdominal pain, and/or jaundice.
- Stillborn kittens.

Physical Examination Findings

Cats

- Transplacentally infected kittens may be stillborn or die before weaning; surviving kittens—anorexia, lethargy, high fever.
- Signs reflect necrosis/inflammation of lungs (dyspnea, increased respiratory noises), liver (icterus, abdominal enlargement from ascites), and CNS (encephalopathy).
- Postnatal exposure.
- Respiratory and gastrointestinal abnormalities most common—anorexia, lethargy, high fever, dyspnea, weight loss, icterus, vomiting, diarrhea.
- Ocular abnormalities common—uveitis (aqueous flare, hyphema, mydriasis), iritis, detached retina, iridocyclitis, and/or keratic precipitates.
- 10% of patients show neurologic abnormalities—blindness, stupor, incoordination, circling, torticollis, anisocoria, or seizures.

Dogs

- Puppies—generalized infection; fever, weight loss, anorexia, tonsillitis, dyspnea, diarrhea, vomiting.
- Adults—localized infections associated with neural and muscular systems.
- Neurologic manifestations variable; result of diffuse neurologic inflammation—seizures, tremors, ataxia, paresis, paralysis, muscle weakness.
- Ocular inflammation—rare.
- Cardiac involvement—usually subclinical.

CAUSES

T. gondii

RISK FACTORS

- Ingestion of intermediate hosts, environment contaminated with cat feces.
- Immunosuppression—may predispose to infection or reactivation: feline leukemia virus (FeLV), feline immunodeficiency virus (FIV), feline infectious peritonitis (FIP), hemotropic mycoplasma, canine distemper, glucocorticoids, chemotherapy, postrenal transplant.

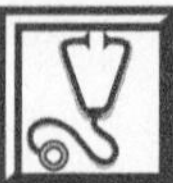

DIAGNOSIS

DIFFERENTIAL DIAGNOSIS

Cats

- Anterior uveitis—FIP, FeLV, FIV, other infectious, immune-mediated, trauma; lens-induced, corneal ulceration, lymphoma.
- Dyspnea—asthma, cardiogenic, pneumonia, neoplasia, heartworm disease, pleural space disease, diaphragmatic hernia, trauma.
- Meningoencephalitis—viral, fungal, parasitic, bacterial, idiopathic (feline polioencephalomyelitis).

Dogs

- Neurologic abnormalities—infectious, inflammatory, toxic, metabolic.

CBC/BIOCHEMISTRY/URINALYSIS

CBC (Cats)

- Normocytic normochromic anemia.
- Leukopenia—50% of patients with severe disease; primarily lymphopenia.
- Neutropenia with degenerative left shift.
- Leukocytosis during recovery.

Biochemistry

- Alanine aminotransferase and aspartate aminotransferase—increased enzyme activities.
- Hypoalbuminemia.
- Hyperbilirubinemia (25% of cats).

Urinalysis (Cats)

- Mild proteinuria.
- Bilirubinuria.

OTHER LABORATORY TESTS

Serology

- IgM—serologic titer of choice for diagnosis of active infection; elevated 2 weeks post infection (usually with onset of clinical signs) and persists for up to 3 months:
    - Prolonged titer—reactivation or delay in antibody class shift to IgG (due to immunosuppression).
- IgG—titers rise 2–4 weeks post infection, persist >1 year; single high titer not diagnostic for active infection; 4-fold increase over a 3-week period suggests active infection.
- Serum antigen—positive 1–4 weeks post infection; remains positive during active or chronic infections (not helpful to determine infection type).
- PCR—to verify presence of *T. gondii* in biologic specimens:
    - Prudent choice in suspect cases since many protozoa are morphologically similar and difficult to distinguish histopathologically.

IMAGING

Radiographs—mixed pattern of patchy alveolar and interstitial pulmonary infiltrates; pleural and abdominal effusions and hepatomegaly may be present.

DIAGNOSTIC PROCEDURES

- Bronchoalveolar lavage, pulmonary fine-needle aspirate (cats with respiratory disease)—organism can be identified cytologically.
- Effusion cytology—organism rarely detected during acute infection.
- Cerebrospinal fluid (patients with encephalopathy)—high leukocyte count (both mononuclear cells and neutrophils) and protein.
- Fecal—active fecal oocyte shedding occurs for 1–3 weeks after infection in the cat and usually not during clinical disease; not recommended for determining whether or not an individual cat is infected with *T. gondii.* Oocysts may be detected on routine examination in asymptomatic cats but are morphologically indistinguishable from *Hammondia* spp. and *Besnoitia.*

PATHOLOGIC FINDINGS

- Potentially no gross lesions.
- Necrotic foci—up to 1 cm; most often in liver, pancreas, mesenteric lymph nodes, lungs; necrosis of brain (1 cm areas of discoloration).
- Ulcers and granulomas—in stomach and small intestine.

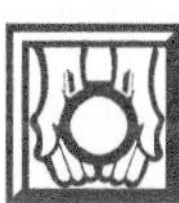

TREATMENT

APPROPRIATE HEALTH CARE

- Usually outpatient.
- Inpatient—severe disease; patient cannot maintain adequate nutrition or hydration.
- Confine—patients with neurologic signs.

NURSING CARE

Dehydration—IV fluids.

CLIENT EDUCATION

- Cats—prognosis guarded in patients needing therapy; response to therapy is inconsistent.
- Poorer prognosis for neonates and immunocompromised animals.

MEDICATIONS

DRUG(S) OF CHOICE

- Clindamycin 12.5–25 mg/kg PO, IV, IM q12h; continue at least 2 weeks after clinical resolution.
- 1% prednisone drops—q8h for uveitis.

PRECAUTIONS

Clindamycin—anorexia, vomiting, and diarrhea (dose-dependent).

ALTERNATIVE DRUG(S)

- Sulfadiazine 30 mg/kg PO q12h in combination with pyrimethamine 0.5 mg/kg PO q12h for 2 weeks; can cause depression, anemia, leukopenia, and thrombocytopenia, especially in cats.
- Folinic acid 5 mg PO q24h or brewer's yeast 100 mg/kg PO q24h—correct bone marrow suppression caused by above therapy.

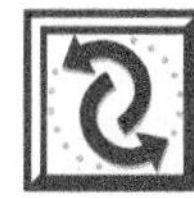

FOLLOW-UP

PATIENT MONITORING

- Examine 2 days after treatment initiation for resolution of clinical signs; uveitis should resolve within 1 week.
- Neuromuscular deficits take longer to resolve, should see partial resolution within 2 weeks (some deficits may be permanent).
- Examine 2 weeks after resolution of clinical signs to determine if treatment may be discontinued.

PREVENTION/AVOIDANCE

Cats

- Diet—prevent ingestion of raw meat, bones, viscera, or unpasteurized milk (especially goat's milk), or mechanical vectors (flies, cockroaches). Only well-cooked meat should be fed.
- Behavior—prevent free-roaming to hunt prey (birds, rodents) or to enter buildings where food-producing animals are housed.

EXPECTED COURSE AND PROGNOSIS

- Prognosis—guarded; varied response to drug treatment.
- Acute—prompt and aggressive therapy often successful.
- Residual deficits (especially neurologic) cannot be predicted until course of therapy is completed.
- Ocular disease—usually responds to appropriate therapy.
- Severe muscular or neurologic disease—usually chronic debility.

MISCELLANEOUS

ASSOCIATED CONDITIONS

- Young dogs—distemper.
- Cats—renal transplant recipients, FeLV, FIP, FIV; FIV infection does not affect clinical outcome or the ability of the animal to mount a protective immune response to subsequent reinfection.

AGE-RELATED FACTORS

Disease worse in neonates.

ZOONOTIC POTENTIAL

- Of most concern is infection of pregnant women or immunocompromised individuals. Pregnant women should avoid contact with cats excreting oocysts in feces, contact with soil and cat litter, and should not handle or eat raw meat (to kill organism, cook to ≥66°C/150°F):
  - Young cats are most likely to be shedding oocysts.
  - *Important*: oocysts need to be sporulated to be infectious. Unsporulated oocysts are shed in the feces and require at least 24 hours to sporulate; daily cleaning of litter box should reduce risk of exposure to infectious form.
- Cats—healthy animals with a positive antibody titer pose little danger to humans; animal with no antibody titer at greater risk of becoming infected, shedding oocysts in the feces, and constituting a risk to humans.
- Avoid contact with oocysts or tissue cysts—do not feed raw meat; wash hands and surfaces (cutting boards) after preparing raw meat; boil drinking water if source is unreliable; keep sandboxes covered to prevent cats from defecating in them; wear gloves when gardening; wash hands and vegetables before eating; empty cat litter boxes daily; disinfect litter boxes with boiling water; control stray cat population.
- *T. gondii* causes abortion in sheep; prevent cats from ingesting placenta or aborted fetuses and keep cats from defecating in sheep feed to break the life cycle.

PREGNANCY/FERTILITY/BREEDING

- Parasitemia during pregnancy—spread of organism to fetus; probably does not happen unless first-time infection of dam occurs during pregnancy (as with humans).
- Placental transmission rare.

ABBREVIATIONS

- FeLV = feline leukemia virus.
- FIP = feline infectious peritonitis.
- FIV = feline immunodeficiency virus.

Suggested Reading

Dubey JP, Lappin MR. Toxoplasmosis and neosporosis. In: Greene CE, ed., Infectious Diseases of the Dog and Cat, 3rd ed. St. Louis, MO: Saunders Elsevier, 2006, pp. 754–775.

Authors Matt Brewer and Katy A. Martin
Consulting Editor Amie Koenig

Client Education Handout available online

TRACHEAL COLLAPSE

BASICS

DEFINITION

• Static or dynamic reduction in the luminal diameter of the large conducting airway with respiration. • Can involve the cervical trachea, the intrathoracic trachea, or both segments. • Airway collapse (bronchomalacia) refers to collapse of lobar bronchi and smaller airways, which can be seen in conjunction with tracheal collapse (tracheobronchomalacia) or alone. • Compression of the trachea or bronchi due to hilar lymphadenopathy or external mass lesions—not considered part of this condition.

PATHOPHYSIOLOGY

• Hypocellular tracheal cartilage in the cervical region identified historically in some small-breed dogs. • Lack of chondroitin sulfate and/or decreased glycoproteins within the cartilage matrix results in a reduction in bound water and loss of rigidity in the cartilage. • Causes of bronchomalacia not established—cartilage abnormalities could include a mechanism similar to cervical tracheal collapse, defects in chondrogenesis, nutritional deficiencies, or degenerative changes caused by chronic airway disease. • Collapse—weak tracheal cartilage allows flattening of the normal ring structure; trachea collapses in a dorsoventral direction when pressure fluctuates within the airway lumen. During inspiration, intrapleural pressure becomes more negative leading to a drop in intra-airway pressure. Atmospheric pressure exceeds airway pressure in the cervical region and lack of cartilage support results in cervical collapse. During forced expiration, intrapleural pressure becomes positive and exceeds intrathoracic intra-airway pressure. When cartilaginous airway walls are weakened by bronchomalacia, intrathoracic airway collapse occurs, on expiration. • Increased tension on the trachealis dorsalis muscle or neurogenic atrophy of the muscle causes stretching of the dorsal tracheal membrane with protrusion into the airway lumen. • Coughing—mechanical trauma to the tracheal mucosa from collapse of the dorsal tracheal membrane exacerbates airway edema and inflammation. • Upper airway obstruction worsens clinical signs, and chronic increases in respiratory effort could lead to secondary abnormalities in laryngeal structure and function. • Small airway disease augments the trans-airway pressure gradient and potentiates collapse in the intrathoracic region.

SYSTEMS AFFECTED

• Respiratory—chronic airway irritation. • Cardiovascular—pulmonary hypertension. • Nervous—can be involved when syncope develops from hypoxia or a vasovagal reflex associated with cough.

GENETICS

Under investigation. Tracheal collapse common in small toy breed dogs. Bronchomalacia seen in large and small breeds.

INCIDENCE/PREVALENCE

Common clinical entity.

GEOGRAPHIC DISTRIBUTION

Worldwide

SIGNALMENT

Species

Primarily dog, rarely cat.

Breed Predilections

Tracheal collapse—miniature poodles, Yorkshire terriers, Chihuahuas, Pomeranians, other small and toy breeds. Bronchomalacia—all breeds.

Mean Age and Range

• Middle-aged to elderly—onset of signs at 2–14 years of age. • Severely affected animals <1 year of age.

SIGNS

Historical Findings

• Usually worsened by excitement, heat, humidity, exercise, or obesity. • Dry honking cough. • Often have a chronic history of intermittent coughing or difficulty breathing. • Retching—often seen due to attempts to clear respiratory secretions from the larynx. • Tachypnea, exercise intolerance, and/or respiratory distress—common. • Cyanosis or syncope—seen in severely affected individuals.

Physical Examination Findings

• Increased tracheal sensitivity—virtually always seen. • Respiratory distress—inspiratory with cervical collapse; expiratory with intrathoracic collapse. • Stridor or musical sounds ausculted over narrowed cervical trachea. • An end-expiratory snap—heard when a large intra-thoracic airway collapses during forceful expiration then reopens. • Crackles—due to small airway collapse (inspiratory or expiratory) or chronic bronchitis. • Expiratory wheezes suggest concurrent bronchitis. • Mitral insufficiency murmurs—often found concurrently in small-breed dogs. • Normal to low heart rate and/or marked respiratory arrhythmia. • Loud second heart sound—suggests pulmonary hypertension. • Hepatomegaly—cause unknown.

CAUSES

• Unknown etiology—congenital, nutritional, or familial defects of chondrogenesis suspected. • Chronic airway inflammation suggested to contribute to bronchomalacia but relationship not clearly established. Seen with chronic bronchitis or eosinophilic bronchopneumopathy.

RISK FACTORS

• Obesity. • Airway infection or inflammation. • Upper airway obstruction. • Endotracheal intubation.

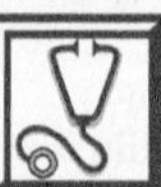

DIAGNOSIS

DIFFERENTIAL DIAGNOSIS

• Infectious tracheobronchitis. • Tracheal or laryngeal obstruction or foreign body. • Chronic bronchitis. • Pneumonia—viral, bacterial, fungal, parasitic, eosinophilic. • Bronchiectasis.

CBC/BIOCHEMISTRY/URINALYSIS

• CBC—can show an inflammatory leukogram secondary to chronic stress or concurrent infection. • Increased liver enzymes common.

OTHER LABORATORY TESTS

Elevated bile acids—mechanism unclear.

IMAGING

Thoracic Radiography

• Airway collapse evident on a lateral thoracic radiographic in a large percentage of dogs with airway collapse, however, the location of collapse on static radiographs agreed with the site determined by fluoroscopy in <50% of cases. • Inspiratory radiographs—show primarily cervical collapse and collapse at the thoracic inlet. • Expiratory radiographs—show intrathoracic tracheal collapse; can also note collapse at the carina, ballooning of the cervical trachea, and cranial herniation of the lung lobe through the thoracic inlet. • Right-sided heart enlargement—can be seen secondary to chronic pulmonary disease and cor pulmonale, or heart can be artifactually enlarged due to obesity or breed conformation.

Fluoroscopy

Dynamic collapse of the cervical or intra-thoracic trachea and/or dorsal tracheal membrane can be visible during tidal respirations—usually more easily identified after induction of cough. Cranial lung herniation through the thoracic inlet is common.

DIAGNOSTIC PROCEDURES

Caution is warranted in anesthetizing and intubating dogs with tracheal collapse because endotracheal tube irritation can worsen clinical signs. Loss of respiratory drive from anesthetic drugs or excess excitement on recovery can precipitate airway obstruction.

Tracheal Wash

Use oral intubation (rather than the transtracheal approach) with a small endotracheal tube and a sterile catheter when obtaining samples for cytologic examination and bacterial culture/susceptibility.

Bronchoscopy

• Grade the severity of collapse: Grade I—slight protrusion of the dorsal tracheal membrane into the airway lumen; diameter reduced by <25%, Grade II—reduction of

the tracheal lumen by 50%, Grade III—reduction of the tracheal lumen by 75%, Grade IV—tracheal rings flattened; <10% of the tracheal lumen can be seen; in some cases (particularly Yorkies), a double lumen trachea is observed, where tracheal rings have bowed dorsally to contact the trachealis muscle.
• Identify small airway disease—collapse or inflammation. Submit airway samples for cytologic examination and bacterial/susceptibility; specific culture for *Mycoplasma* is recommended.

Cytology

• Unremarkable in uncomplicated tracheal or bronchial collapse. • Neutrophilia without intracellular bacteria or marked bacterial growth—indicates airway inflammation.
• Lymphocytic inflammation is also common.
• Sepsis and suppuration along with marked bacterial growth of a pathogen—suggests pulmonary infection.

PATHOLOGIC FINDINGS

• Dorsal trachealis muscle—elongated.
• Cartilage rings—flattened. • Tracheal mucosal inflammation in some cases.
• Hypocellularity of the cartilage with low glycoproteins and chondroitin sulfate—can be noted via histopathologic examination or electron microscopy. • Can also see changes associated with chronic inflammatory airway disease.

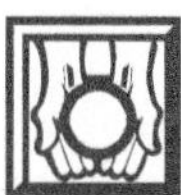

TREATMENT

APPROPRIATE HEALTH CARE

• Outpatient—stable patients. • Inpatient—oxygen therapy and sedation for severe respiratory distress. Sedation and cough suppression—butorphanol 0.1–0.4 mg/kg SC or IV; addition of acepromazine 0.01–0.04 mg/kg SC or IV can enhance sedative effects and further reduce the cough reflex.

NURSING CARE

Monitor respiratory effort.

ACTIVITY

• Severely limited until patient is stable.
• During management of disease—gentle exercise recommended to encourage weight loss.

DIET

• Many affected dogs improve after losing weight. • Institute weight-loss program with restriction of caloric intake; use a gradual weight-loss program (1–2% weight loss per week).

CLIENT EDUCATION

• Warn client that weight gain, overexcitement, and humid conditions can precipitate a crisis. • Advise client to use a harness instead of a collar. • Advise owners that tracheal collapse is irreversible and that treatment strategies are designed to lessen triggers of cough. • For surgical candidates, advise owner of the likelihood of complications after surgery (e.g., persistent cough, respiratory distress, or laryngeal paralysis); some patients can require a permanent tracheostomy. For stent candidates, advise owners of need for extensive follow-up to avoid stent fracture, migration, or granulation tissue formation.

SURGICAL CONSIDERATIONS

• Treatment of upper airway obstructive disorders (elongated soft palate, everted laryngeal saccules)—can reduce signs due to tracheal collapse. • The presence of mainstem bronchial collapse worsens prognosis.
• Placement of extraluminal C-shaped rings by a skilled surgeon in selected patients with cervical collapse will enhance quality of life and reduce clinical signs when adequate stabilization of the airway can be achieved and when bronchomalacia does not limit resolution of clinical signs. Postoperative laryngeal paralysis is a potential complication.
• Intraluminal stents are life-saving in selected cases with intrathoracic airway collapse that fail aggressive medical management. Aspiration pneumonia is common after placement.

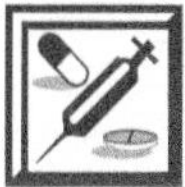

MEDICATIONS

DRUG(S) OF CHOICE

• Narcotic cough suppressants (butorphanol 0.5–1 mg/kg PO q4–8h or hydrocodone 0.22 mg/kg PO q4–8h) used to break the cycle of cough; reduce dose rate to the least frequent administration that controls signs. Use after infection or inflammation has been managed. • Reduction of tracheal inflammation—prednisone 0.5 mg/kg PO q12h then 0.25 mg/kg q12h for a total of 5–7 days may help. Inhaled steroids given via facemask and spacing chamber are preferred to avoid systemic effects of panting and weight gain. • Sustained-release theophylline 10 mg/kg PO q12h—thought to reduce the pressure gradient in small airways and decrease cough in dogs with intrathoracic airway collapse or bronchomalacia—bronchodilators have no effect on tracheal diameter. • Bacterial infection uncommon but doxycycline 3–5 mg/kg PO q12h is sometimes beneficial, perhaps through reduction in bacteria within the airway or reduction of inflammation.

PRECAUTIONS

Avoid long-term steroid use because of the propensity for weight gain and diseases associated with immunosuppression.

POSSIBLE INTERACTIONS

Theophylline metabolism—increased by concurrent treatment with ketoconazole or phenobarbital, which results in inadequate plasma concentration; decreased by fluoroquinolones (e.g., enrofloxacin), erythromycin, cimetidine, steroids, beta-blockers, mexiletine, and thiabendazole, which results in toxic plasma concentration and gastrointestinal upset, nervousness, or tachycardia; adjust dosages when concurrent use is necessary.

ALTERNATIVE DRUG(S)

Over-the-counter cough suppressants—rarely reduce cough.

FOLLOW-UP

PATIENT MONITORING

• Body weight. • Exercise tolerance. • Pattern of respiration. • Incidence of cough.

PREVENTION/AVOIDANCE

• Avoid obesity in breeds commonly afflicted.
• Avoid heat and humidity. • Use harness rather than leash.

POSSIBLE COMPLICATIONS

Intractable respiratory distress leading to respiratory failure or euthanasia.

EXPECTED COURSE AND PROGNOSIS

• Combinations of medications along with weight control can reduce clinical signs, but dogs will likely cough throughout life and can suffer recurrent exacerbations of disease.
• Surgery—benefits dogs severely affected with cervical collapse. • Stent placement—benefits some dogs, primarily those with respiratory difficulty rather than cough and those with intrathoracic collapse. Medications usually required post procedure.
• Prognosis—based on bronchoscopic evidence of airway obstruction and development of complications.

MISCELLANEOUS

ASSOCIATED CONDITIONS

• Chronic bronchitis. • Laryngeal paralysis.
• Pulmonary hypertension. • Breeds of dogs that develop tracheal collapse also commonly have mitral insufficiency.

SEE ALSO

• Bronchitis, Chronic. • Canine Infectious Respiratory Disease.

Author Lynelle R. Johnson
Consulting Editor Elizabeth Rozanski

Client Education Handout available online

T

TRANSITIONAL CELL CARCINOMA

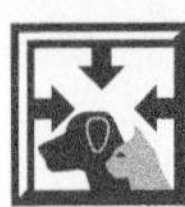

BASICS

DEFINITION

Malignancy arising from the transitional epithelium within the kidney, ureters, urinary bladder, urethra, prostate, or vagina.

PATHOPHYSIOLOGY

The underlying etiology of transitional cell carcinoma (TCC) remains unclear. It is possible that an environmental carcinogen may initiate or promote the malignant transformation of the transitional epithelium.

SYSTEMS AFFECTED

• Renal/urologic—the most common site affected is the trigone of the urinary bladder. Local invasion of the distal ureter is not uncommon and may lead to postrenal azotemia. The apex of the urinary bladder is more often affected in cats, although because of late detection the entire bladder is often involved by the time of diagnosis.
• Reproductive—the vagina is a possible site of primary TCC. The prostate may be involved through local invasion, or as the primary site of TCC. • Other systems may be affected through metastases (e.g., most commonly regional lymph nodes and lungs; other sites include bone, brain, eye) or paraneoplastic syndromes (hypertrophic osteopathy has been reported secondary to TCC of the urinary bladder).

T

GENETICS

N/A

INCIDENCE/PREVALENCE

• <1% of all reported malignancies in dogs.
• Rare in cats.

GEOGRAPHIC DISTRIBUTION

N/A

SIGNALMENT

Middle-aged to old, spayed female, small-breed dogs most commonly reported with the disease.

Species

Dog and cat.

Breed Predilections

• Scottish terriers are at 18 times the risk compared to other breeds. • West Highland white terriers, Shetland sheepdogs, beagles, American Eskimo dogs, dachshunds. • May occur in any breed. • No breed predisposition in cats.

Mean Age and Range

Dogs—8 years, range 1 to 15+ years.

Predominant Sex

Female

SIGNS

General Comments

• Signs are similar to those of bacterial urinary tract infection or urolithiasis.
• Consider TCC in animals showing temporary or no response to appropriate antibiotic therapy.

Historical Findings

• Complaints of recurrent stranguria, pollakiuria, hematuria, dysuria, urinary incontinence, or any combination of the above signs should initiate a search for TCC.
• Signs may temporarily respond to antibiotic therapy.

Physical Examination Findings

• Often normal. • Occasionally, urethral thickening can be appreciated on digital rectal examination or a mass might be palpable in the caudal abdomen/urinary bladder region.
• Urethral/vaginal/prostatic TCC may be palpable on rectal examination. • Enlarged intrapelvic or sublumbar lymph nodes can be palpable on rectal examination.

CAUSES

• Dogs—reported risk factors include obesity, environmental carcinogens, chronic exposure to organophosphates or carbamates, and (rarely) long-term or a large bolus dose of cyclophosphamide. • Cats—unknown.

RISK FACTORS

Dogs—Scottish terrier breed, obesity, exposure to organophosphates or carbamates, cyclophosphamide therapy.

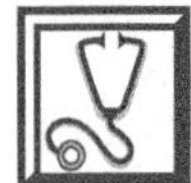

DIAGNOSIS

DIFFERENTIAL DIAGNOSIS

• Non-neoplastic—bacterial urinary tract infection, urolithasis, urethritis, vaginitis, prostatitis. • Neoplastic—other primary neoplasia (e.g., squamous cell carcinoma, transmissible venereal tumor), or metastatic neoplasia (e.g., locally infiltrative prostatic carcinoma).

CBC/BIOCHEMISTRY/URINALYSIS

• CBC and biochemistry usually within normal limits. • Biochemistry profile may show signs of renal and/or postrenal azotemia if ureteral or urethral obstruction exists.
• Urinalysis may reveal epithelial cells with criteria of malignancy—caution should be exercised if the sample is inflammatory as epithelial cells may exhibit criteria of malignancy in the presence of inflammation.

OTHER LABORATORY TESTS

• A DNA-based strategy for the detection of canine TCC is commercially available (CADET®). The assay is run on a urine sample and detects a mutation in the *BRAF* gene that is highly specific for TCC. • Urine culture and sensitivity are indicated, as concurrent urinary tract infection is common; however, caution is advised when performing cystocentesis on patients suspected to have TCC as tumor seeding along the needle tract may occur. • Biopsy (surgical, traumatic catheter, or cystoscopic) is gold standard for definitive diagnosis. Even with a low yield of tissue samples of some traumatic catheterizations, typically enough cells are obtained to get a cytologic diagnosis.

IMAGING

Thoracic Radiography

Metastatic patterns include multiple, well-defined interstitial nodules, increased interstitial pattern, and alveolar infiltrates.

Abdominal Radiography

• Unlikely to reveal specific urinary bladder disease unless the mass is mineralized (rare).
• May reveal sublumbar lymphadenomegaly or bony metastasis.

Double Contrast Cystography

• Dogs—space-occupying lesion, usually at trigone of the urinary bladder. • Cats—space-occupying lesion, may be at the apex of the urinary bladder. • Depending on the primary site, IV pyelography, voiding urethrogram, or vaginogram may be indicated.

Ultrasonography

• 2D ultrasonography is a highly sensitive imaging modality, helpful in identifying location and extent of disease; however, not a reliable method for monitoring response to therapy. • 3D ultrasonography is a more accurate tool for monitoring tumor volume and response to therapy.

CT

CT imaging of TCC is the most accurate way to measure tumor volume.

DIAGNOSTIC PROCEDURES

Exploratory Laparotomy

• Used to obtain biopsies of the primary tumor and regional lymph nodes. • Surgical cure very unlikely due to the infiltrative nature of the tumor. • Because tumor seeding is recognized with TCC, change surgical gloves and instruments after handling the tumor.

Cystoscopy

A less invasive way to identify and biopsy TCC within the urinary bladder or urethra.

Traumatic Catheterization

Use a polypropylene catheter to traumatically obtain small tissue samples for histologic or cytologic diagnosis.

Ultrasound-Guided Biopsy

Not recommended, as seeding of the biopsy tract with viable tumor cells is a highly possible sequela.

PATHOLOGIC FINDINGS

• Irregular to diffuse thickening of the urinary bladder mucosa. • Metastasis to regional lymph nodes, lungs, and bones (i.e., vertebra, pelvis) possible.

TREATMENT

APPROPRIATE HEALTH CARE

Radiotherapy with treatment units that allow for intensity modulation may provide long-term tumor control.

Inpatient vs. Outpatient

- Initial workup and diagnosis takes 1–2 days.
- Stable patients need not be hospitalized.

ACTIVITY

Normal

DIET

Normal, unless concurrently in renal failure.

CLIENT EDUCATION

- Long-term prognosis poor. • Palliation often attainable. • Trigonal location of the disease within the bladder makes complete surgical resection in dogs difficult.

SURGICAL CONSIDERATIONS

- TCC is highly exfoliative and highly transplantable—multiple reports of surgically induced seeding of TCC exist. • All surgical instruments and gloves should be replaced after contacting the tumor. • Partial cystectomy (ideally full-thickness resection of gross disease) combined with piroxicam therapy may result in improved outcomes compared to dogs treated with medical therapy only. • Tube cystostomy placement or urethral stenting may prolong survival times by bypassing or relieving urethral obstruction.

MEDICATIONS

DRUG(S) OF CHOICE

- Piroxicam 0.3 mg/kg PO q24h with food—reported to have activity in 21% of cases with a median survival of 244 days.
- Deracoxib 3 mg/kg PO q24h with food—reported to have activity in 17% of cases with a median survival of 323 days. • A variety of chemotherapy drugs used at traditional maximally tolerated doses have activity against TCC, including mitoxantrone 5 mg/m^2 IV q21d, vinblastine 3 mg/m^2 IV q14d, cisplatin 50 mg/m^2 IV q21d, carboplatin 300 mg/m^2 IV q21d, and gemcitabine 800 mg/m^2 IV q7d. • Metronomic (continuous, low-dose) chemotherapy with chlorambucil 4 mg/m^2 PO q24h may play a role in the management of this disease.

CONTRAINDICATIONS

- Piroxicam—do not use in animals with known gastrointestinal erosions or ulcers; do not use in animals with renal insufficiency.
- Piroxicam—do not combine with cisplatin.
- Piroxicam therapy appears to be tolerated in cats, but at a reduced dosing frequency (q48h) in comparison to dogs.

PRECAUTIONS

- Animals with TCC may have renal damage either due to hydroureter, hydronephrosis, or pyelonephritis secondary to chronic urinary tract infection associated with the tumor.
- Dogs being treated with chemotherapy should be monitored for myelosuppression.
- Seek advice before initiating therapy if unfamiliar with cytotoxic drugs.

POSSIBLE INTERACTIONS

Cisplatin should not be used concurrent with other nephrotoxic drugs (e.g., aminoglycoside antibiotics).

ALTERNATIVE DRUG(S)

Antibiotics—antibiotic therapy should be administered as necessary.

FOLLOW-UP

PATIENT MONITORING

- Contrast cystography or ultrasonography every 6–8 weeks to determine disease status.
- Thoracic radiographs and abdominal ultrasound every 2–3 months to monitor for metastatic disease.

PREVENTION/AVOIDANCE

Advise client regarding frequent urination following cyclophosphamide therapy to minimize contact time with the urinary bladder mucosa.

POSSIBLE COMPLICATIONS

- Urethral or ureteral obstruction and renal failure. • Metastatic disease to regional lymph nodes, lungs, or bone. • Recurrent urinary tract infection. • Urinary incontinence.
- Myelosuppression of gastrointestinal toxicity secondary to chemotherapy.
- Gastrointestinal ulceration secondary to piroxicam therapy.

EXPECTED COURSE AND PROGNOSIS

- Long-term prognosis is guarded.
- Progressive disease likely. • Median survival—no therapy: 4–6 months; with therapy: 6–12+ months.

MISCELLANEOUS

ASSOCIATED CONDITIONS

- Recurrent urinary tract infections.
- Postrenal azotemia. • Paraneoplastic hypertrophic osteopathy.

AGE-RELATED FACTORS

None

ZOONOTIC POTENTIAL

None

PREGNANCY/FERTILITY/BREEDING

N/A

SYNONYMS

None

ABBREVIATIONS

- TCC = transitional cell carcinoma.

Suggested Reading

Fulkerson CM, Knapp DW. Management of transitional cell carcinoma of the urinary bladder in dogs: a review. Vet J 2015, 205:217–225.

Marvel SJ, Seguin B, Dailey DD, et al. Clinical outcome of partial cystectomy for transitional cell carcinoma of the canine bladder. Vet Comp Oncol 2017, 15:1417–1427.

Mochizuki H, Shapiro SS, Breen M. Detection of BRAF mutation in urine DNA as a molecular diagnostic for canine urothelial and prostatic carcinoma. PLOS One 2015, 10:e0144170.

Radhakrishnan A. Urethral stenting for obstructive uropathy utilizing digital radiography for guidance: feasibility and clinical outcome in 26 dogs. J Vet Intern Med 2017, 31:427–433.

Schrempp DR, Childress MO, Stewart JC, et al. Metronomic administration of chlorambucil for treatment of dogs with urinary bladder transitional cell carcinoma. J Am Vet Med Assoc 2013, 242:1534–1538.

Author Ruthanne Chun

Consulting Editor Timothy M. Fan

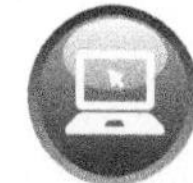

Client Education Handout available online

TRANSMISSIBLE VENEREAL TUMOR

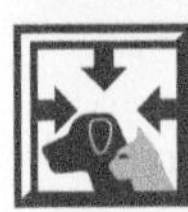

BASICS

OVERVIEW

• Sexually, or other direct contact, transmitted, naturally occurring tumor.
• Appears to be more common in temperate areas and large cities.

SIGNALMENT

Predisposition in intact dogs of either sex, however, routes of nonsexually contact transmission permits disease manifestation in neutered and spayed dogs.

SIGNS

• Red, friable, lobulated mass on the mucosa of the vagina, penis or other nonreproductive organ mucous membranes.
• Oral and nasal mucosa may be affected.
• Owners may report blood dripping from the affected area or excessive licking of the genital area.
• Proliferative or exophytic tumor protrusion may be noticed.

CAUSES & RISK FACTORS

• Direct transplantation of tumor cells onto abraded mucosa, either by coitus, oral, or nasal transmission.
• Intact, free-roaming dogs are at greater than average risk.

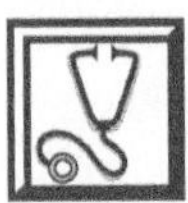

DIAGNOSIS

DIFFERENTIAL DIAGNOSIS

• Other neoplasia (e.g., squamous cell carcinoma, cutaneous lymphoma).
• Vaginal hyperplasia or pseudo-estrus.

CBC/BIOCHEMISTRY/URINALYSIS

• Usually unremarkable.
• Urinalysis (free-catch) reveals hematuria and abnormal round cell populations in some patients if the tumor is within the urogenital tract.

OTHER LABORATORY TESTS

N/A

IMAGING

• Thoracic radiographs, although this tumor type is rarely metastatic.
• Abdominal ultrasonography to evaluate mesenteric lymph nodes.

DIAGNOSTIC PROCEDURES

• Careful palpation of regional lymph nodes, and perform aspirates with cytology when clinically indicated.
• Examination of impression smears or aspirates of the tumor reveals homogenous sheets of round to oval cells with prominent nucleoli, scant cytoplasm, and multiple clear cytoplasmic vacuoles.
• Biopsy offers definitive diagnosis.

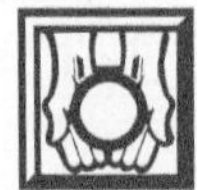

TREATMENT

• May spontaneously regress with appropriate immunologic response, treatment is recommended as spontaneous remissions are not reliable.
• Surgical excision of tumors is often followed by recurrence.
• Radiotherapy alone may be curative.
• Medical therapy is often curative.

MEDICATIONS

DRUG(S) OF CHOICE

• Vincristine sulfate 0.5–0.7 mg/m^2 IV once weekly for 2 weeks beyond complete resolution of gross disease.
• If only partial or no remission, doxorubicin 30 mg/m^2 IV every 3 weeks may have activity.

CONTRAINDICATIONS/POSSIBLE INTERACTIONS

• Myelosuppression secondary to vincristine or doxorubicin administration.
• Doxorubicin may be cardiotoxic, use with caution once a cumulative dose of 150 mg/m^2 is reached.
• Tissue sloughing if either vincristine or doxorubicin is administered perivascularly.
• Seek advice before initiating therapy if unfamiliar with cytotoxic drugs.

FOLLOW-UP

PATIENT MONITORING

CBC and platelet count before each chemotherapy treatment.

PREVENTION/AVOIDANCE

• Neuter animals.
• Prevent animals from roaming free in endemic areas.

POSSIBLE COMPLICATIONS

• Tumor recurrence possible following incomplete surgical excision or reexposure.
• Metastatic disease uncommon, but reported to occur in regional lymph nodes, eye, and spinal cord.

EXPECTED COURSE AND PROGNOSIS

Most cases of transmissible venereal tumor have an excellent response to therapy (primarily chemotherapy or radiotherapy) and an excellent prognosis.

MISCELLANEOUS

ZOONOTIC POTENTIAL

None

PREGNANCY/FERTILITY/BREEDING

• Pregnant animals should not be treated with chemotherapy.
• Animals may be infected with transmissible venereal tumor during coitus.

Suggested Reading

Ganguly B, Das U, Das AK. Canine transmissible venereal tumour: a review. Vet Comp Oncol 2016, 14(1):1–12.

Author Ruthanne Chun
Consulting Editor Timothy M. Fan

T

TRAUMATIC DENTOALVEOLAR INJURIES (TDI)

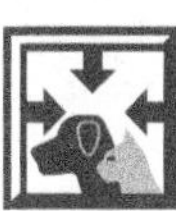

BASICS

DEFINITION

- Traumatic dentoalveolar injuries (TDI) may be broadly categorized into two major groups: (1) dental fractures and (2) luxation injuries.
- Dental fractures include enamel infraction, enamel fracture, enamel–dentin (uncomplicated) fracture, enamel–dentin–pulp (complicated) fracture, crown–root fracture (with or without pulpal involvement) and root fracture.
- Luxation injuries include concussion, subluxation, luxation (lateral, intrusive and extrusive) and avulsion and are often associated with a fracture of the alveolar process.
- An avulsion is an injury in which the tooth has been completely displaced out of its socket.

PATHOPHYSIOLOGY

- Untreated pulpal exposure invariably leads to pulpitis, pulpal necrosis and periapical pathology.
- Pulpitis and pulpal necrosis may also occur with enamel–dentin fractures, if the fracture line is close to the pulp chamber, which exposes a large number of dentinal tubules that may allow microbial contamination.
- Concussion injuries may also lead to pulpitis and pulpal necrosis.

SYSTEMS AFFECTED

Endodontic infection may cause systemic complications.

INCIDENCE/PREVALENCE

- 26.2% of dogs and cats had at least 1 TDI with a mean of 1.45 TDI per patient.
- The prevalence of TDI in dogs and cats with concurrent maxillofacial fractures increases to near 70%.

SIGNALMENT

Species

Dogs and cats.

Mean Age and Range

Juveniles tend to have more TDI associated with maxillofacial fractures, though TDI prevalence tends to increase throughout adolescence and peaks between 3 and 6 years of age.

SIGNS

Crown Fractures

- Clinical loss of tooth crown substance; enamel only, or enamel and dentin.
- Enamel–dentin fractures with the fracture line close to the pulp chamber—pale pink pulp is visible through the dentin.
- In enamel–dentin–pulp fractures, the pulp chamber is exposed.
- Acute enamel–dentin–pulp fractures may be associated with hemorrhage from the pulp.

Crown–Root Fractures

- Fracture line may be visible as it extends into the gingival sulcus.
- The "slab" fracture of the maxillary fourth premolar tooth extends subgingivally into the root.

Root Fractures

- At any point along the length of the root.
- Fracture line transverse or oblique; segments may remain aligned or be displaced.
- Abnormal mobility of a periodontally sound tooth may raise suspicion of a root fracture.

Luxation Injuries

- Severely concussed teeth may take on a blue/pink/purple/gray discoloration often referred to as intrinsic (endogenous) staining.
- Intrusive luxation—tooth appears shorter than normal; no tooth mobility detected.
- Extrusive luxation—tooth appears longer than normal and is mobile both vertically and horizontally.
- Lateral luxation—tooth crown is displaced in either a labial or palatal/lingual direction.
- Avulsion—the tooth has been completely displaced out of the socket. The tooth may or may not remain attached to the gingiva.
- Luxations and avulsions are often accompanied by gingival lacerations.

CAUSES

- Altercations with other animals, motor vehicle accidents, falls from height, contact with a moving object, or simply sustained during playful activity, collision with another animal or object or even during chewing/mastication.
- Since these injuries often occur during unsupervised activities, the mechanism of injury is often unknown.

RISK FACTORS

- Free-roaming behavior increases risk of trauma.
- The maxillary canine tooth is the most commonly luxated/avulsed tooth.
- Advanced periodontitis will predispose to luxations and avulsions.

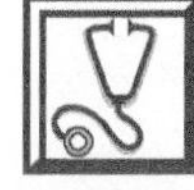

DIAGNOSIS

DIFFERENTIAL DIAGNOSIS

- Crown fracture—attrition, abnormal tooth formation.
- Root fracture—luxation; severe periodontitis. Imaging needed.
- Luxation—root fracture where the coronal segment is displaced.
- Avulsion—tooth exfoliated due to severe periodontitis.

CBC/BIOCHEMISTRY/URINALYSIS

- Noncontributory.
- Unaffected by tooth fracture.

IMAGING

General

- Intraoral radiography is mandatory.
- CT with appropriate protocol for the dentition may be beneficial for identifying some root fractures.

Radiographic Findings

- The presence of relatively wide root canal space (halted dentinogenesis) and/or periapical lucency (periapical periodontitis) is indicative of pulpal necrosis.
- Radiographic indicators of disease may not be present in concussion and subluxation injuries.
- Intrusive luxation—narrowing of the periodontal ligament space in the apical region.
- Extrusive luxation—widening of the periodontal ligament, especially in the apical region.
- Lateral luxation—widening and narrowing of the periodontal ligament space and fracture of the alveolar process.

DIAGNOSTIC PROCEDURES

- Percussion, thermal pulp testing, electric pulp testing are subjective methods that rely on patient feedback and, thus, are unreliable.
- Pulse oximetry has shown mixed results for determining pulpal vitality. This method should currently be considered unreliable.

PATHOLOGIC FINDINGS

Untreated pulpal exposure invariably leads to pulpitis and eventual pulpal necrosis and periapical pathology.

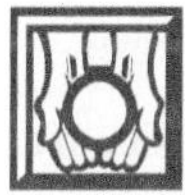

TREATMENT

APPROPRIATE HEALTH CARE

Depends on extent and severity of trauma to the patient.

NURSING CARE

Depends on extent and severity of trauma to the patient.

ACTIVITY

Restrict as indicated by nature of trauma.

DIET

In the immediate postoperative period (24–72 hours), moistening the patient's dry food may help decrease the chance of traumatizing any suture lines or splints.

CLIENT EDUCATION

A series of treatments may be necessary.

SURGICAL CONSIDERATIONS

Enamel–Dentin Fractures

Remove sharp and unsupported enamel/dentin edges with a bur and seal the exposed dentin with a suitable restorative material.

Enamel–Dentin–Pulp Fractures

- Requires endodontic therapy or extraction.

TRAUMATIC DENTOALVEOLAR INJURIES (TDI) (CONTINUED)

- For recent fractures in the mature tooth: (1) vital pulpotomy and restoration or (2) conventional root canal therapy and restoration.
- In most cases, vital pulpotomy should be carried out within 48 hours of the injury in order to prevent pulpal necrosis.
- Generally, vital pulpotomy is reserved for younger patients.
- Teeth treated with vital pulpotomy may require standard root canal treatment at a later date.
- Standard root canal therapy is the treatment of choice in older patients, when the injury is chronic or when the pulp is already necrotic.

Crown–Root Fractures

- Treatment of crown–root fractures follows the same principles as for crown fracture, though additional periodontal health concerns should be considered.
- Can the tooth be restored in a manner that can maintain periodontal health?
- Fractures that do *not* extend more than 4–5 mm below the gingival margin may be restored with dental composites or full metal crown in order to maintain periodontal health.
- Fractures that extend further along the root or deeply into the furcation of a multirooted tooth may necessitate extraction of the tooth.

Root Fractures

T

- The level of the fracture along the root length determines the treatment.
- Midroot and apical fractures may heal if the tooth is immobilized with a dental splint.
- Healing may occur by means of a dentinocemental callus, a fibrous union, or an osteofibrous union.
- Fractures in the apical 1/3 of the root carry best prognosis for healing.
- Fractures in the coronal 1/3 of the root usually require tooth extraction.

Luxations

- For lateral and extrusive luxations, reposition the tooth in its normal position and ensure appropriate occlusion; immobilize with a semi-rigid splint for 2–3 weeks.
- If luxation is accompanied by an alveolar process fracture, maintain the splint for 1–2 additional weeks.
- Since the vascular supply at the apex is typically compromised, root canal therapy is typically necessary and is performed 7 days after application of the splint.
- Any gingival lacerations should be sutured.
- The prognosis for intrusive luxations is generally considered poor; as such, extraction is generally recommended.

Avulsions

- The most important factor determining the result of treatment is the vitality of the periodontal ligament, which is dictated largely by the amount of time the tooth has been out of the socket.
- Optimal results are achieved if the tooth is replanted within 30-60 minutes of avulsion.
- Advise client to place the tooth in saline or milk and bring the affected animal in for treatment as quickly as possible.
- Avoid handling the tooth root and rinse gently with sterile saline solution.
- It is essential not to remove the periodontal ligament from the root; a viable periodontal ligament is necessary for healing.
- Replace the tooth in the socket and ensure normal position and occlusion.
- To immobilize the tooth, a semi-rigid splint is applied and left in place for 2–3 weeks.
- Root canal therapy is required in 7 days, but should not be performed at the time of reimplantation.
- Contraindications for replanting avulsed teeth are deciduous teeth, severe periodontitis, caries, or tooth resorption.

MEDICATIONS

DRUG(S) OF CHOICE

- A broad-spectrum bactericidal antibiotic drug for 5–7 days may be used (e.g., when longstanding infection is present) but is generally not indicated.
- Daily rinsing with 0.12% chlorhexidine gluconate solution will diminish the need for prolonged administration of antibiotics.
- Appropriate analgesic regime—usually nonsteroidal anti-inflammatory drug for 3–5 days.

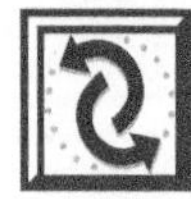

FOLLOW-UP

PATIENT MONITORING

- Check a vital pulpotomy with postoperative radiographs after 6 and 12 months, or at intervals determined by clinical signs, to detect pulp death and consequent periapical changes indicating the need for root canal treatment.
- Check the outcome of conventional root canal therapy radiographically 6–12 months postoperatively; evidence of periapical pathology at this time indicates the need for further endodontic retreatment of the tooth.
- Monitor root fractures radiographically 3–6 months postoperatively.
- Monitor enamel–dentin fractures with radiography at 4–6 months after treatment to assess pulpal health.

PREVENTION/AVOIDANCE

Avoid situations in which teeth are likely to be damaged; keep animal from chewing on hard objects such as rocks.

POSSIBLE COMPLICATIONS

- Untreated pulpal exposure invariably leads to pulpitis and eventual pulpal necrosis and periapical pathology.
- Arrested development of immature teeth.

MISCELLANEOUS

AGE-RELATED FACTORS

The most appropriate treatment will vary with age.

ABBREVIATIONS

- TDI = traumatic dentoalveolar injuries.

INTERNET RESOURCES

- Dental fracture classification: https://avdc.org/avdc-nomenclature/
- Dental trauma guide: dentaltraumaguide.org

Suggested Reading

Soukup J. Traumatic dentoalveolar injuries. In: Lobprise HB, Dodd JR, eds., Wiggs' Veterinary Dentistry; Principles and Practice, 2nd ed. Hoboken, NJ: Wiley-Blackwell, 2019.

Soukup J, Hetzel S, Paul A. Classification and epidemiology of traumatic dentoalveolar injuries in dogs and cats: 959 injuries in 660 patient visits (2004–2012). J Vet Dent 2015, 32(1):6–14.

Author Jason W. Soukup
Consulting Editor Heidi B. Lobprise

BASICS

DEFINITION

Rhythmic, oscillatory, involuntary, abnormal, or normal movement of all or part of the body.

PATHOPHYSIOLOGY

Abnormal or normal movement caused by the alternate or synchronous contraction of reciprocally innervated, antagonistic muscles.

SYSTEMS AFFECTED

- Nervous.
- Endocrine/metabolic.
- Musculoskeletal—muscle weakness or pain.
- Behavioral—fear.

GENETICS

The role of genetics in tremor syndromes is largely unknown with the exception of X-linked hypomyelination in male springer spaniels.

INCIDENCE/PREVALENCE

N/A

SIGNALMENT

- Dog and cat.
- In general, any dog or cat may develop tremors. However, certain tremor syndromes have specific signalment.
- Corticosteroid-responsive tremor syndrome (generalized tremor syndrome, white shaker syndrome)—small to medium-size breed (<15 kg), young adult dogs (<5 years), regardless of coat color. A similar syndrome has recently been observed in 2 cats.
- Idiopathic head tremors (head bobbing)—Doberman pinschers, English bulldogs, French bulldogs, boxers, and Labrador retrievers are overrepresented.
- Orthostatic tremors—young, adult, giant-breed dogs.
- Benign pelvic limb tremors in older dogs—terriers predisposed.
- Hypomyelination—puppies; chow chows, springer spaniels, Samoyeds, Weimaraners, and Dalmatians.

SIGNS

- Localized or generalized.
- Localized—most often involves the head or the pelvic limbs.

CAUSES

Tremors Primarily Affecting the Head

- Cerebellar lesions leading to intention tremors—degenerative; congenital; metabolic; infectious; immune-mediated; neoplastic; traumatic; toxic causes; vascular.
- Idiopathic head tremors (head bobbing)—unknown cause.

Tremors Primarily Affecting the Limbs

- Orthostatic tremors—unknown cause. Seen in the thoracic and pelvic limbs of young, adult, giant-breed dogs. Tremors are present when standing and disappear in ambulating and recumbent animals.
- Compressive lesions of the spinal cord or nerve roots—lumbosacral stenosis; intervertebral disc disease; neoplasia; discospondylitis.
- Neuromuscular disease—peripheral neuropathy; neuromuscular junction abnormality; myopathy.
- Metabolic disorder causing weakness—hypoglycemia, hypoadrenocorticism, hypocalcemia, magnesium imbalance. Metabolic causes of tremors may also present as generalized tremors.
- Benign pelvic limb tremors in older dogs—unknown cause.

Generalized Tremors

- Corticosteroid-responsive tremor syndrome (generalized tremor syndrome, white shaker syndrome)—believed to be immune-mediated.
- Hypomyelination: specific defect in myelin formation unknown.
- Intoxications—metaldehyde (snail bait); mycotoxins (penitrem A and roquefortine); organophosphates; hexachlorophene; bromethalin; ivermectin; moxidectin; pyrethrins/pyrethroids; lead; 5-fluorouracil; macadamia nuts; theobromine; anatoxin-a; marijuana; zolpidem; clozapine, dysautonomia (although toxin is suspected, exact toxin is unknown); castor beans (*Ricinus communis*); carbon monoxide; mirtazapine, alfaxalone, diphenhydramine, many others.
- Degenerative neurologic disease—storage disease; Lafora disease; spongiform encephalopathy.
- Behavioral—fear.
- Hypothermia.

RISK FACTORS

- Presence of concurrent metabolic diseases that can cause tremors (hypoglycemia, hypoadrenocorticism, hypocalcemia, magnesium imbalance).
- Exposure to a known tremorgenic toxin.
- Exposure to fear-producing or hypothermia-inducing situations.

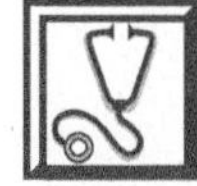

DIAGNOSIS

DIFFERENTIAL DIAGNOSIS

- Differentiate tremor from constant repetitive myoclonus, seizures, and myokymia/neuromyotonia.
- Constant repetitive myoclonus—rhythmic contractions usually involving one or more pelvic limb muscles and/or muscles of mastication. Seen most often with distemper virus infection.
- Seizures—may be associated with autonomic disturbances (e.g., urination, defecation, and salivation) and alterations of consciousness.
- Myokymia/neuromyotonia—characteristic vermicular skin rippling caused by muscle contraction and often brought on by excitement or excessive stimulation.

Tremors Primarily Affecting the Head

- Assess for additional neurologic deficits suggesting cerebellar disease; intention tremors are a clinical sign of cerebellar disease; intention tremors worsen when the patient attempts to move the head in a goal-oriented manner; ataxia and dysmetria help determine the neuroanatomic diagnosis.
- Idiopathic head tremors (head bobbing)—patient usually young at onset; sporadic; up-and-down (yes) or side-to-side (no) direction; anatomic origin unknown; no other neurologic deficits present and mentation is not affected.

Tremors Primarily Affecting the Limbs

- Diseases of the lumbosacral spinal cord, cauda equina, and associated peripheral nerves; musculoskeletal diseases.
- Metabolic diseases (may also cause generalized tremors)—hypoglycemia, hypoadrenocorticism, hypocalcemia, magnesium imbalance.
- Neuromuscular disease—peripheral neuropathy; neuromuscular junction abnormality; myopathy.

Generalized Tremors

- Young dog (6–8 weeks)—congenital myelination abnormality; check breed incidences.
- Young adult dog—assess history for toxin exposure; consider corticosteroid-responsive tremor syndrome (generalized tremor syndrome, white shaker syndrome) in young, small-breed dogs.

CBC/BIOCHEMISTRY/URINALYSIS

- Usually normal with associated primary brain disease.
- Assess for metabolic disease; may find hypoglycemia, hypocalcemia, magnesium imbalance, pattern consistent with hypoadrenocorticism.
- Some myopathies are characterized by high creatine kinase, aspartate aminotransferase, and alanine aminotransferase.

OTHER LABORATORY TESTS

If tremors are affecting the limbs and weakness is suspected, consider testing for hypoadrenocorticism (adrenocorticotropic hormone stimulation test) and myasthenia gravis (acetylcholine receptor antibody titer).

IMAGING

- Localized to the pelvic limbs—survey radiography, CT, and/or MRI of the vertebral column and spinal cord from L4 to S3.
- Generalized tremors—in hypomyelination, MRI may reveal lack of myelin; in corticosteroid-responsive tremor syndrome (generalized

tremor syndrome, white shaker syndrome) MRI usually normal.
• Intention tremor—MRI of the brain, with special attention to the cerebellum.

DIAGNOSTIC PROCEDURES

• CSF analysis—sensitive but nonspecific; in corticosteroid-responsive tremor syndrome (generalized tremor syndrome, white shaker syndrome) mild mononuclear pleocytosis, but CSF may also be normal; in other encephalitides involving the cerebellum, results vary with cause of disease and duration.
• Electromyography of hind limb muscles—may help diagnosing neuromuscular disease if pelvic limb tremor.

PATHOLOGIC FINDINGS

Dependent on underlying cause of tremor.

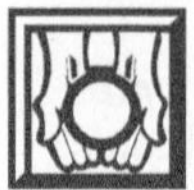

TREATMENT

• Treat the underlying primary disease.
• Outpatient, unless surgical treatment is indicated (lumbosacral disease that requires decompression and stabilization).
• Avoid excitement and exercise—may worsen many tremors.
• Degenerative neurologic diseases (e.g., storage disease, spongiform encephalopathy)—no treatment available.
• Hypomyelination—generally not treatable; some breeds improve with maturity (e.g., chow chows).
• Idiopathic head tremors (head bobbing)—no effective treatment available; benign tremor that occurs sporadically; has few health consequences.
• Suspected intoxication—remove patient from further exposure; consult with a poison control center for possible antidote.

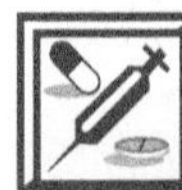

MEDICATIONS

DRUG(S) OF CHOICE

• Usually do not respond to antiepileptic drugs (e.g. phenobarbital or diazepam).
• Tremors associated with some toxicities, especially metaldehyde (snail bait), may be treated with methocarbamol (dogs: 50–150 mg/kg IV, maximum dose 330 mg/kg in 24h) and appropriate decontamination.
• Corticosteroids—immunosuppressive dose to treat corticosteroid-responsive tremor syndrome (generalized tremor syndrome, white shaker syndrome)
• Antibiotics—for discospondylitis; choose on the basis of culture and sensitivity of the lesion, blood, or urine.
• Cerebellar diseases—depends on the underlying etiology.
• Gabapentin 5–20 mg/kg up to q8h may be helpful in treatment of some tremors.

CONTRAINDICATIONS

Sympathomimetic drugs—may worsen condition.

FOLLOW-UP

PATIENT MONITORING

• Monitor the primary disease.
• Corticosteroid-responsive tremor syndrome (generalized tremor syndrome, white shaker syndrome)—monitor weekly initially to assess response to treatment.

PREVENTION/AVOIDANCE

Prevent reexposure in the cases of toxicity.

EXPECTED COURSE AND PROGNOSIS

• Idiopathic head tremors (head bobbing)—excellent prognosis, no treatment needed.
• Orthostatic tremors—slowly progressive; disappear when patient ambulates or when patient is recumbent.
• Benign pelvic limb tremors in older dogs—can be slowly progressive; disappear when patient ambulates or when patient is recumbent.
• Hypomyelination—may stabilize and even improve as animal ages.
• Corticosteroid-responsive tremor syndrome (generalized tremor syndrome, white shaker syndrome)—most respond to corticosteroid therapy; some may need low-dose corticosteroid therapy indefinitely.

MISCELLANEOUS

ASSOCIATED CONDITIONS

N/A

ZOONOTIC POTENTIAL

N/A

PREGNANCY/FERTILITY/BREEDING

N/A

SYNONYMS

• Shaking.
• Shuddering.

SEE ALSO

• Cerebellar Degeneration.
• Hypomyelination.
• Shaker/Tremor Syndrome, Corticosteroid Responsive.
• Head Tremors (Bobbing), Idiopathic—Dogs.
• See Causes.

Suggested Reading

De Lahunta A, Glass E, Kent M. Uncontrolled involuntary skeletal muscle contractions. In: Veterinary Neuroanatomy and Clinical Neurology, 4th ed. St. Louis, MO: Saunders Elsevier, 2015, pp. 509–524.
Dewey CW. A Practical Guide to Canine & Feline Neurology. 2nd ed. Ames, IA: Wiley-Blackwell, 2008, pp. 311–322.

Author Philip Schissler

Client Education Handout available online

BASICS

OVERVIEW

- Enteric, pear-shaped, motile (flagellated) protozoa similar to *Giardia*—inhabits large intestine of cats; similar organisms live in intestinal tract of many mammals
- *Tritrichomonas foetus* (sometimes referred to as *T. blagburni*) causes diarrhea in cats:
  - Transmitted via fecal–oral route, ingestion of trophozoites via grooming.
  - Parasites colonize terminal ileum, cecum, and colon leading to large bowel diarrhea.
- Coinfection with *Giardia*—common.

SIGNALMENT

Young, often purebred cats—usually under 1 year (range 3 months–13 years); particularly high prevalence in catteries.

SIGNS

Cats

- May or may not have symptoms of infection.
- Intermittent large bowel diarrhea, malodorous, occasionally contains blood and mucus.
- Anus—may become edematous, erythematous, and painful in kittens.
- Rectal prolapse—if anal irritation becomes severe.
- Diarrhea—improves with antibiotic treatment but reoccurs following course of treatment; may also show waxing and waning course without treatment.
- Median length of time of diarrhea is about 9 months, with resolution in most cats by 2 years; number of cats cohabitating will impact duration of clinical signs.
- Persistence of infection after resolution of diarrhea is common.

CAUSES & RISK FACTORS

- *Tritrichomonas foetus*—causes diarrhea in cats, infertility and abortion in cattle.
- *T. foetus* —high prevalence in purebred cats and densely housed populations such as catteries, show cats, shelters; but very low in feral or indoor cats.
- Pathogenic factors leading to infected cats developing diarrhea—endogenous bacterial flora, adherence of parasite to host epithelium, and cytotoxin and enzyme elaboration.
- *Pentatrichomonas* spp. (family Trichomonads)—inhabit large intestine of cats, dogs, humans; nonpathogenic in dogs and cats, except very rarely when it may become an opportunistic pathogen.

DIAGNOSIS

DIFFERENTIAL DIAGNOSIS

Cats

Dietary indiscretion, inflammatory bowel disease, neoplasia (especially gastrointestinal lymphoma), drugs (antibiotics), toxins (lead), parasites (cryptosporidiosis, *Giardia*, hookworms, roundworms), bacterial agents (salmonellosis, intestinal bacterial overgrowth, clostridia), systemic organ dysfunction (renal, hepatic, pancreatic, cardiac), and metabolic (hyperthyroidism).

CBC/BIOCHEMISTRY/URINALYSIS

Usually normal—may reflect diarrhea.

OTHER LABORATORY TESTS

- Direct fecal smear—very low sensitivity:
  - Method—dilute fresh feces 50:50 in saline, cover slip, examine at 40× objective with condenser lowered to increase contrast.
  - Distinguish from *Giardia* (concave ventral disc, spiral forward motion)—*T. foetus* has jerky forward motion, spindle-shaped, undulating membranes.
- *T. foetus* trophozoites not seen on fecal flotation, will not survive refrigeration.
- Fecal protozoal culture—use commercial media in 37°C incubator (e.g., InPouch® TF); inoculate with 0.05 g fresh feces, examine for motile trophozoites daily for 12 days:
  - *Giardia* and *P. hominis*—do not grow after 24 hours in InPouch system.
- PCR (feces)—more sensitive than fecal culture.

IMAGING

N/A

DIAGNOSTIC PROCEDURES

N/A

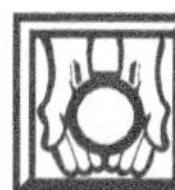

TREATMENT

- Rule out coexisting disease (cryptosporidiosis, giardiasis, bacterial), especially if diarrhea persists after specific treatment.
- Treatment may decrease the severity of diarrhea but may also prolong time to resolution.

MEDICATIONS

DRUG(S) OF CHOICE

- No approved treatments.
- *T. foetus*—poor treatment responses are common.
  - Ronidazole 30 mg/kg PO q24h for 14 days; currently preferred treatment.
  - Metronidazole 30–50 mg/kg PO q12h, 3–14 days.
- *P. hominis*—metronidazole 20 mg/kg PO q12h for 7 days.

CONTRAINDICATIONS/POSSIBLE INTERACTIONS

- Glucocorticoids may exacerbate clinical disease.
- High doses of metronidazole (usually >30 mg/kg) for extended periods may cause neurologic abnormalities (e.g., vestibular disease).
- Ronidazole may cause reversible neurotoxicity (similar to that seen with metronidazole treatment); doses above 30 mg/kg should not be used in cats, treatment should be discontinued if adverse effects occur.
- Resistance to ronidazole and metronidazole have been reported.

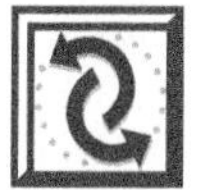

FOLLOW-UP

- Most cats spontaneously resolve their diarrhea but may take years (range 4 months–2 years).
- Relapses of diarrhea are common and often precipitated by dietary changes, stress, treatments of other conditions.

MISCELLANEOUS

ZOONOTIC POTENTIAL

T. foetus is not considered a zoonotic agent; possible zoonotic transmission for *Pentatrichomonas*.

INTERNET RESOURCES

https://capcvet.org/guidelines/trichomoniasis/

Suggested Reading

Stockdale HD, Dillon AR, Newton JC, et al. Experimental infection of cats (*Felis catus*) with *Tritrichomonas foetus* isolated from cattle. Vet Parasitol 2008, 154:156–161.

Yao C, Köster LS. Tritrichomonas foetus infection, a cause of chronic diarrhea in the domestic cat. Vet Res 2015, 46(1):35.

Authors Matt Brewer and Katy A. Martin

Consulting Editor Amie Koenig

TRIGEMINAL NEURITIS, IDIOPATHIC

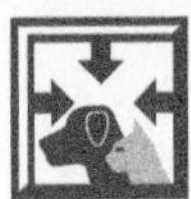

BASICS

OVERVIEW

Sudden bilateral paralysis of trigeminal mandibular branches resulting in inability to close the mouth. Lesions are characterized by extensive nonsuppurative trigeminal neuritis, demyelination, and rare axonal degeneration affecting all portions of the trigeminal nerve and ganglion without brainstem involvement.

SIGNALMENT

- Primarily adult dogs.
- Rare in cats.

SIGNS

- Acute onset of a dropped jaw.
- Inability to close the mouth.
- Drooling.
- Difficulty in prehending food, messy eating.
- Swallowing is intact when food and water are placed in the caudal portion of the mouth.
- Approximately one-third of affected dogs will exhibit decreased facial sensation.
- Few dogs have sympathetic involvement of the head (Horner's syndrome).
- Long-term muscle atrophy depending on degree of axonal involvement.

CAUSES & RISK FACTORS

Unknown; autoimmune disorder suspected.

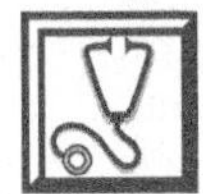

DIAGNOSIS

DIFFERENTIAL DIAGNOSIS

- Musculoskeletal disorders of the temporomandibular joints and jaw—differentiated by history of trauma, pain, and physical examination findings.
- Rabies—always initially consider until there is sufficient evidence to rule it out.
- Encephalitis involving the motor nuclei of bilateral trigeminal nerve.
- Neoplasia—involvement of both mandibular nerves with myelomonocytic leukemia, lymphoma, and neurofibrosarcoma reported; usually does not have an acute onset.
- Masticatory muscle myositis—presentation excludes this condition characterized by trismus and difficulty/inability to open the mouth ("locked jaw").

CBC/BIOCHEMISTRY/URINALYSIS

Usually normal.

IMAGING

MRI—diffuse enlargement of affected nerves that appear isointense to hyperintense on T2-weighted images if edema is present; contrast enhancement on post-contrast T1-weighted images.

DIAGNOSTIC PROCEDURES

- No specific test.
- Skull radiography, MRI, CSF, and muscle biopsy—to rule out differentials.

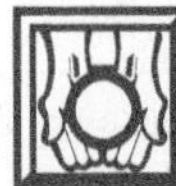

TREATMENT

- Recovery within 2–3 weeks of onset. Supportive treatment necessary during this period.
- Outpatient if owner is able to help the patient eat and drink.
- Patient cannot prehend or move food and water to the throat but can swallow if the bolus is placed in the caudal portion of the mouth and the jaw is manually held closed. Water and slurry food can also be placed, with a syringe, in the corner of mouth with the head slightly elevated.
- Fluids—subcutaneously if oral support insufficient.
- Esophagostomy or gastrostomy tubes—rarely necessary to maintain adequate food intake.

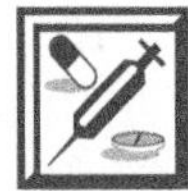

MEDICATIONS

DRUG(S) OF CHOICE

Corticosteroids not indicated as there is no evidence that they improve recovery. Furthermore, side effects (polyuria and polydipsia) can make management difficult.

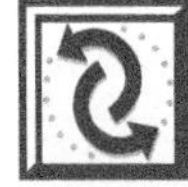

FOLLOW-UP

- Self-limiting disorder.
- Full recovery in 2–3 weeks.
- Bilateral symmetrical masticatory muscle atrophy but without trismus.

MISCELLANEOUS

SYNONYMS

- Dropped jaw.
- Trigeminal neuropathy.
- Mandibular paralysis.

Suggested Reading

Mayhew PD, Bush WW, Glass EN. Trigeminal neuropathy in dogs: a retrospective study of 29 cases (1991–2000). J Am Anim Hosp Assoc 2002, 38:262–270.

Schultz RM, Tucker RL, Gavin PR, et al. Magnetic resonance imaging of acquired trigeminal nerve disorders in 6 dogs. Vet Rad Ultrasound 2007, 48(2):101–104.

Author Mylène-Kim Leclerc

BASICS

OVERVIEW

- *Francisella tularensis*—small Gram-negative coccobacillus, principally found in wild lagomorphs and rodents; facultative intracellular parasite that survives and grows in the liver, resulting in granulomas and/or abscesses:
  - Type A is more virulent and found in rabbits and ticks, type B is waterborne and found in rodents and ticks.
  - In United States most cases found in Missouri, Alaska, Oklahoma, South Dakota, Tennessee, Kansas, Colorado, Illinois, Utah, Maine, New York, and New Jersey.
  - Increasing number of tularemia outbreaks in regions of Europe outside the classic endemic areas in recent years.
  - Absent from United Kingdom, Africa, South America, Australia.
- Tularemia infection in cats follows a bimodal seasonal incidence curve with peaks in spring and late summer–fall, and may reflect the seasonality of the disease in the rabbit.
- Infection—ingestion of tissue or body fluids of an infected mammal or contaminated water, bitten by blood-sucking arthropod (tick), flies, mites, midges, fleas, or mosquitoes; few bacteria needed to infect cats through skin, airways, or conjunctiva; larger number required to infect through gastrointestinal tract:
  - Skin contact—organism multiplies locally (papule) 3–5 days after contact; ulcerates 2–4 days later; spreads via lymphatics to regional lymph node (LN) and bloodstream; results in septicemia (lung, liver, spleen, LN, bone marrow).
  - Ingestion—may involve lymphadenopathy of cervical and mesenteric LN followed by septicemic spread; distribution of lesions to face, oral cavity, tonsils, intestines, and LN.
- Acute disease—2–7 days after contact with organism.
- Has high aerosol-related infection rate, low infectious dose, and ability to induce fatal disease.
- *F. tularensis* is considered a potential biologic warfare agent; occurrence of clusters of cases in companion animals may indicate potential human risk.

SIGNALMENT

- Cat—occasionally.
- Dog—rarely.

SIGNS

- Sudden onset of anorexia, lethargy, fever (104–106°F/40–41°C).
- Enlarged submandibular and cervical LN.
- Tender abdomen, palpable mesenteric LN, hepatomegaly—depending on stage of disease.
- Multifocal white patches or ulcers along glossopalatine arches and tongue.
- Icterus.

CAUSES & RISK FACTORS

- Organism— *Francisella tularensis*; all *Francisella* biogroups may infect cats but differ in virulence.
- Hunting or outdoor cats in endemic areas .
- Infected wildlife in the area of hunting activity.
- Exposure to infected blood-sucking parasites.

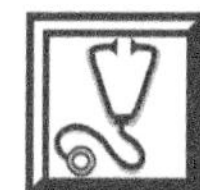

DIAGNOSIS

DIFFERENTIAL DIAGNOSIS

- Pseudotuberculosis (*Yersinia pseudotuberculosis*)—usually vomiting and diarrhea.
- Babesiosis (*Babesia/Theileria*) (dogs and cats).
- Calicivirus (cats).
- Feline immunodeficiency virus.
- Toxoplasmosis (cats).

CBC/BIOCHEMISTRY/URINALYSIS

- Initially severe panleukopenia; then leukocytosis with left shift, toxic neutrophils, thrombocytopenia.
- Hyperbilirubinemia, bilirubinuria.
- Hyponatremia.
- Hypoglycemia.
- Alanine aminotransferase activity increased.
- Hematuria.

OTHER LABORATORY TESTS

Serology with tube agglutination or ELISA—reference laboratory; all animals do not necessarily respond serologically to infection (false negatives possible).

DIAGNOSTIC PROCEDURES

- *Caution*: use extreme care when working with infected specimens or isolates.
- Direct smear—lesion or biopsy; difficult to see organism on Gram staining.
- Culture—by reference laboratory only; blood, pleural fluid, LN aspirate onto cysteine- or cystine-containing media; not recoverable on routine laboratory media.
- Direct fluorescent antibody testing—clinical materials or tissues; rapid assay of infection status.
- Molecular testing of tissues in laboratories with validated diagnostic protocols.

PATHOLOGIC FINDINGS

- Multifocal white patches or ulcers along glossopalatine arches and tongue.
- Oral, tonsillar ulceration.
- Lymphadenopathy of cervical, retropharyngeal, or submandibular LN with abscessation.
- Diffuse intestinal lesions.
- Mesenteric lymphadenopathy, hepatosplenomegaly, icterus.

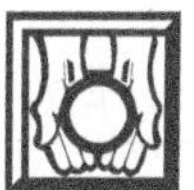

TREATMENT

- Inpatient with good nursing care; infection control protocols (personal protective gear) *very* important due to low infectious dose/zoonotic nature of disease.
- Early treatment important to prevent high mortality; treatment often unsuccessful.
- Treat for ectoparasites.

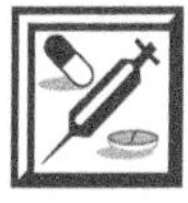

MEDICATIONS

DRUG(S) OF CHOICE

Treat all cases empirically until laboratory confirmation obtained.

- Little information available on the efficacy of antimicrobials; *high mortality if patient not treated early*.
- Early treatment with amoxicillin 22 mg/kg PO q8h for 5–7 days or 22 mg/kg IM, SC q12h for 5 days, in combination with gentamicin 4.4–6 mg/kg IV, IM, SC q24h for 7 days has been successful.
- Enrofloxacin 10 mg/kg PO, IV q24h (dog), 5 mg/kg PO, IV q24h (cat) may be effective.

FOLLOW-UP

PATIENT MONITORING

- Monitor for disseminated intravascular coagulation—may occur late in the infection.
- Monitor renal function during gentamicin therapy.

PREVENTION/AVOIDANCE

- Avoid travel to endemic areas.
- Endemic areas—confine animals to limit exposure to and ingestion of wildlife and ectoparasites (ticks); ectoparasite control by periodic spraying or dusting of animal and pastures.
- Neuter cats—limit hunting behavior, wildlife exposure.
- Take precautions to limit contamination of food and water with carcasses of infected wildlife.

EXPECTED COURSE AND PROGNOSIS

Prognosis poor if not treated early; prognosis poor if mesenteric LN palpable.

MISCELLANEOUS

ZOONOTIC POTENTIAL

- Extremely high.
- Human cases related to direct dog contact via bite, scratch or face snuggling/licking, direct contact with dead animals retrieved by domestic dogs, contact with infected ticks; dogs with oral contact with diseased wildlife or carcasses may act as "living fomites" to contaminate humans.
- All personnel in contact with patient or body fluids must use face mask, gloves, and gowns to avoid infection.
- Isolate patients.
- In emerging disease areas, cat ownership is a disease risk for humans.
- Bites and scratches pose a risk for humans.
- Do not mistake for plague or bite abscess in cats.

SYNONYMS

- Rabbit fever.
- Deerfly fever.
- Market men's disease.

ABBREVIATIONS

- LN = lymph node(s).

INTERNET RESOURCES

- http://www.cfsph.iastate.edu/DiseaseInfo/disease.php?name=tularemia&lang=en
- http://www.phac-aspc.gc.ca/lab-bio/res/psds-ftss/msds68e-eng.php
- http://www.cdc.gov/tularemia/

Suggested Reading

Foley JE, Nieto NC. Tularemia. Vet Microbiol 2010, 140:332–338.

Kwit NA, Schwartz A, Kugeler KJ, et al. Human tularaemia associated with exposure to domestic dogs-United States, 2006-2016. Zoonoses Public Health 2019, 66:417–421.

Mani RJ, Morton RJ, Clinkenbeard KD. Ecology of tularemia in central US endemic region. Curr Trop Med Rep 2016, 3:75–79.

Woods JP, Panciera RJ, Morton RJ, et al. Feline tularemia. Compend Contin Educ Pract Vet 1998, 20:442–457.

Author Patrick L. McDonough

Consulting Editor Amie Koenig

UNRULY BEHAVIORS: JUMPING, PULLING, CHASING, STEALING—DOGS

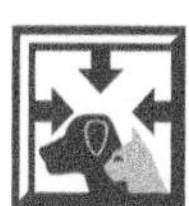

BASICS

DEFINITION

• Jumping—standing on rear legs with front legs on a person or object or leaping in the air with or without landing against the person. • Pulling—to exert force on the leash to cause motion towards the source of the force (the dog). • Chasing—pursuing a moving person, animal, or object. • Stealing—the taking of an item not intended to be used by the dog.

PATHOPHYSIOLOGY

• May be within the range of normal dog behaviors. • Insufficient outlets for normal activities may contribute. • Jumping up may be associated with excessive greeting but can be associated with separation anxiety or social anxiety. • Pulling can be associated with different motivational states including but not limited to fear, anxiety, excitement, and predatory behavior. • Pathologic hyperactivity and anxiety disorders may rarely be a contributing factor.

SYSTEMS AFFECTED

• Behavioral.
• Gastrointestinal.

SIGNALMENT

Species

Dogs

Breed Predilection

Herding and hunting breeds may be more likely to chase.

Mean Age and Range

More common in younger dogs but occurs at any age.

SIGNS

Historical Findings

• Jumping up on people occurs more commonly in association with arrivals, departures, or other greetings; also associated with exploring countertops or tables.
• Pulling may be more likely in the beginning of a walk or when seeing, hearing, or perhaps smelling a stimulus (e.g., person, other dog, object of interest) but can occur at any point.
• Items displaced, damaged, chewed, or ingested are common complaints in stealing.

Physical Examination Findings

• Usually unremarkable unless underlying medical problems. • Nails worn down.

CAUSES

• Jumping up is normal greeting and play behavior. Excitement, encouragement of the behavior, or inadvertent rewarding perpetuates it. Separation anxiety may result in excessive jumping on owners when returning home or leaving. Social anxiety may cause overly exuberant greeting of visitors, with jumping.
• Pulling can occur when a dog is not taught how to walk on loose leash or due to different motivational states. A dog may pull toward or away from something it is afraid of (avoidance) or toward something that is fear-evoking (aggression) or that it is excited about greeting. • Stealing is a normal acquisitive behavior. It can be an attention-seeking behavior or motivated by the appeal of the odor, texture, or taste of an item with which to chew, eat, or play. Stealing can occasionally be comfort-seeking or related to separation anxiety, in which the dog may steal an item when anxious as the owner is preparing to leave or when the dog is separated from the owner but the owner is still in the house.
• Chasing is a normal behavior, as part of herding, hunting, play, and defense.

RISK FACTORS

• Inadequate exploratory or social enrichment.
• Stealing food—restricted or weight-reduction diets, phenobarbital, benzodiazepines, glucocorticoids, hyperadrenocorticism, and diabetes mellitus. • Chasing—common in herding breeds.

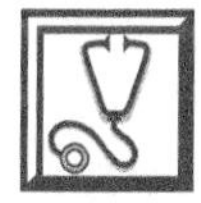

DIAGNOSIS

DIFFERENTIAL DIAGNOSIS

• Separation anxiety—escapes or attempts escape from confined areas in the owner's absence. Often occurs at entrances or when confined. Usually associated with other signs consistent with separation anxiety, including vocalization, urination, defecation, destruction, or salivation, in the owner's absence.
• Other anxiety or phobia (e.g., thunderstorm, fireworks).

CBC/BIOCHEMISTRY/URINALYSIS

• Usually unremarkable.
• May have abnormalities consistent with system affected.

OTHER LABORATORY TESTS

As indicated to rule out source of pain or endocrine disease (low-dose dexamethasone suppression test [LDDST], urine cortisol:creatinine ratio [UC:Cr ratio], bile acids).

IMAGING

Not indicated unless suspicion of foreign body or to rule out medical causes.

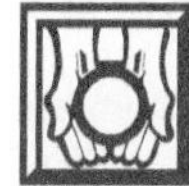

TREATMENT

APPROPRIATE HEALTH CARE

Outpatient management.

ACTIVITY

Increase the dog's daily exercise, opportunities for mental stimulation including food-related enrichment (food-filled toys, search and find games). If problem related to anxiety, must address underlying anxiety as well.

DIET

Review energy requirements, amount fed, and number of meals per day in food-stealing cases.

CLIENT EDUCATION

Jumping

• During training, prevention of jumping up is essential. • A head collar and leash can facilitate training by preventing jumping up or gently guide the dog away from jumping.
• Greeting visitors outside might diminish jumping behavior. The dog's access to the situation can be restricted by confinement (e.g., other room, crate) or on leash with owner until the visitor is seated, which may also reduce the arousal associated with jumping up. • Teach "Sit," "Stay," or "Place/mat" as an alternative desirable method to greet people, using highly valued rewards (food treats, toys) in areas of the home where the dog is calm and tractable. • Food rewards should be used consistently for desirable outcomes. • Add the word "Stay" when the duration of sitting is a few seconds; take a step away, return to the dog, and give the food reward. Build up the time away from the dog to 3–5 minutes. • Repeat exercises near the door and then with leaving and returning. • Next ask the dog to sit for a food reward when returning from gradually longer absences. • Family members and familiar visitors can enter, ask the dog to sit, and give a food reward. • If the dog has difficulty sitting related to pain or discomfort it can be taught "Touch" for greeting. The "Look" cue could also help in getting a dog's attention away from the person entering. • Dogs that like to retrieve and are too excited to sit may do better if a ball is tossed as a visitor enters.
• The owner should walk calmly to the door and speak in a quiet voice to avoid increasing the dog's excitement. • Avoid rewarding the jumping with any form of attention, including pushing the dog off. Do not acknowledge or interact with the dog; hold arms against the body, and look away or turn away from the dog. The person disengaging from the dog facilitates the dog listening to an owner's request to sit for a treat.
• Stepping on the dog's toes, squeezing the paws, and any type of punishment must be avoided as they cause fear, may lead to aggression, and negatively impact the human–animal bond.

Pulling

• A dog's natural walking speed may be faster than their owner's. • A no-pull harness or head collar can be helpful and may be all that is needed. • A brief play session in a fenced in yard before a walk may decrease initial energy and decrease pulling (although some dogs get more aroused immediately after exercise).
• Pulling related to fear, anxiety, or excitement requires desensitization (gradual exposure) and training/reinforcement of an alternative response as discussed under Chasing below.
• With proper application of positive reinforcement pulling can be resolved. • Use food to lure and reward the dog for walking next to a person. Have highly desirable small treats in the hand on the same side as the dog; initially give every few seconds. If the dog pulls, stop, call the dog's name and/or ask it to "Look" (see Chasing), reward the behavior and resume walking. Over time decrease the frequency of giving the treat until it is every minute or two. Many dogs learn to come to the owner for a treat when they learn the "Look" command.
• A second method is to stop walking as soon as the dog starts to pull. When the dog stops moving call the dog's name and/or ask it to "Look" and reward the behavior and continue walking when the leash is slack. If the dog pulls again repeat the process. • All punishment including leash corrections should be avoided as it does not train what is desirable and can condition fearful associations. Sharp jerking or turning suddenly may cause pain and injury to the neck and trachea.

U

Chasing

• A no-pull harness or head collar can be helpful in controlling the dog and reorienting it toward the owners in the presence of the chase stimulus. Herding breeds exhibit a phenotypic behavior that may respond better to control and management than to treatment. • Dogs that chase should be desensitized and counter-conditioned to the stimulus. • The owner should practice the same sit-and-stay exercises as described above, with the addition of a "Look" command using a treat brought up to the owner's eye. This will help get the dog's attention and focus it on the owner when it sees the moving stimulus. • Initially work with the dog inside without distractions, to train, sit, stay, and look. • Next work in a quiet yard with the dog on a leash, have the dog sit, stay, step away, return, look, and give the food reward. When the dog is successful, the process can be repeated in different parts of the yard with gradually more intense distractions.
• Training should begin without the chase stimulus present. If the owner is able to keep the dog's attention, the owner should then stage the chase stimulus (such as a bike or person jogging) to pass by at a sufficient distance and slow enough speed while training and rewarding sit, stay, and look. Over future sessions, the intensity of the stimulus can be gradually increased. • When the dog is able to ignore the chase stimulus in the yard, the owner can incorporate the same exercises in a park or on a walk while maintaining sufficient distance from the stimuli. When the owner sees the chase stimulus, he or she should ask the dog to sit, stay, and look, and then reward the dog.

Stealing

• The dog's investigative behavior and attempts to initiate play and chase may result in stealing. If the result is enjoyable the behavior is rewarded. • Adequate attention, exercise, and toys before times of inattention (e.g., making dinner, working, watching TV) will help to decrease the motivation for stealing. • If the dog steals, the owners should ignore the dog, walk away, get a treat, and call the dog. As the dog drops the item, the owner can say "Drop," "Good dog," and give the dog the treat or click and treat if the dog is clicker trained. The dog is being rewarded for relinquishing the item. • The owner might also need to use a stay and give a second treat or a chew toy to be able to retrieve the dropped item. Another option is to scatter a number of treats for the dog to pick up while the item is removed. • If the dog retreats under furniture, the owner should not pursue. If the dog feels threatened or cornered, it may defend itself aggressively. If it is imperative that the item be retrieved, the client may need to lure the dog out of hiding with even higher value treats or offer a walk or favored game. The owner should keep a log of when and what the dog steals, where they were at the time, and what they were doing to determine when and why the dog is stealing. Prior to, or at these times the dog can be engaged in desirable alternative activities (social play, chews, or food-filled toys). In addition, the owners should video-record the dog to see its response during their absence. See separation anxiety for more details. • For food stealing, food needs to be kept out of the dog's reach, since acquiring food is highly rewarding. Confinement training or gating the dog out of food preparation and dining areas may be necessary. Feeding from food puzzles and toys provides enrichment and engages the dog in alternative acceptable outlets for exploration. • If the dog steals food because it is on a diet, a protein source such as plain cooked chicken or other meat or low-calorie foods such as raw or cooked vegetables can be added to help increase the feeling of fullness.

MEDICATIONS

DRUG(S) OF CHOICE

None

FOLLOW-UP

PATIENT MONITORING

Every 2–3 weeks initially.

PREVENTION/AVOIDANCE

Close supervision, exercise, and exposure to varied stimuli as a young puppy and attending puppy classes and ongoing training can help to prevent and manage unruly behaviors.

POSSIBLE COMPLICATIONS

Injury as a result of escaping a fence, chasing a stimulus, or ingesting an inappropriate item.

EXPECTED COURSE AND PROGNOSIS

Generally good response to treatment for jumping, pulling, and stealing if the owner is consistent. Guidance and support of a force-free reward-based trainer may help to improve success. Chasing behaviors may be more difficult and resistant.

MISCELLANEOUS

AGE-RELATED FACTORS

Younger dogs need more activity than many owners anticipate.

SEE ALSO

• Aggression—Food and Resource Guarding Dogs.
• Fears, Phobias, and Anxieties—Dogs.
• Puppy Behavior Problems.
• Separation Anxiety Syndrome.

ABBREVIATIONS

• LDDST = low-dose dexamethasone suppression test.
• UC:Cr = urine cortisol:creatinine ratio.

Suggested Reading

Landsberg G, Hunthausen W, Ackerman, L. Unruly behaviors. In: Behavior Problems of the Dog and Cat, 3rd ed. Philadelphia, PA: Elsevier Saunders, 2013, pp. 237–248.

Lindell E. Management problems in dogs. In: Horwitz D and Mills D. BSAVA Manual of Canine and Feline Behavioural Medicine. 2nd ed. Gloucestershire, UK: BSAVA, 2009.

Author Marsha R. Reich

Consulting Editor Gary M. Landsberg

Client Education Handout available online

URETEROLITHIASIS

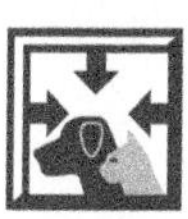

BASICS

OVERVIEW

Occurrence of a urolith within a ureter; most originate in the renal pelvis and commonly occur with nephroliths. If the uroliths pass through the ureters into the lower urinary tract, patient may be asymptomatic or have silent hematuria. If both ureters become totally obstructed, without treatment death will occur in within 5 days.

SIGNALMENT

- Dog and cat.
- Breed, age, and sex predispositions vary with type of ureterolith.

SIGNS

- May be asymptomatic initially.
- Pain (ureteral colic) during passage of ureteroliths or acute ureteral obstruction.
- Renomegaly if obstruction leads to hydronephrosis.
- "Big kidney, little kidney syndrome"—obstruction of one ureter has previously occurred, resulting in a shrunken end-stage kidney; signs of uremia and renomegaly occur due to obstruction of the remaining functional kidney.
- Unilateral ureteral obstruction results in azotemia and uremic clinical signs only when the contralateral kidney has reduced function.
- Signs referable to a lower urinary tract infection (UTI) or septicemia may be present with ureterolithiasis.
- Ureteral rupture may occur, resulting in urine accumulation in the retroperitoneum.
- Cats with distal ureteral obstruction may have signs of dysuria and pollakiuria.

CAUSES & RISK FACTORS

- For a list of causes, see chapters on each urolith type.
- Most ureteroliths are calcium oxalate. Dogs may form struvite nephroliths and subsequent ureteroliths from urease-producing bacterial UTI. Cats may have ureteroliths composed of dried solidified blood clots.
- Circumcaval ureters (more commonly in right ureter) may predispose cats to obstruction by ureteroliths and secondary ureteral stricture formation.
- Prior treatment of nephroliths by extracorporeal shock wave lithotripsy (ESWL) or medical dissolution may be additional risk factors.

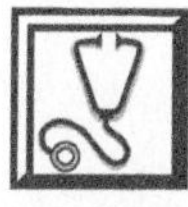

DIAGNOSIS

DIFFERENTIAL DIAGNOSIS

- Consider in cases of acute kidney injury (AKI), rapid progression of chronic kidney disease (CKD), renomegaly, abdominal pain, or fluid accumulation in the retroperitoneal space. Obstruction to urine outflow of both kidneys may not produce the same magnitude of renomegaly as unilateral obstruction because the patient may succumb to uremic complications before severe dilation occurs.
- Radiopacities detected by abdominal radiography that may be confused with ureteroliths include fecal material in the colon, nipples, peritoneoliths, calcified lymph nodes, and mineralization of the renal pelvis.
- Radiolucent ureteroliths may be difficult to differentiate from blood clots. Other causes of ureteral obstruction include intraluminal tumors, ureteroceles, ureteral strictures, and extraluminal compression. Hydroureter and hydronephrosis may occur because of ureteral ectopia, pyelonephritis, ureterovesical stenosis, and obstruction of the ureteral opening at the trigone (most commonly due to urothelial carcinoma).

CBC/BIOCHEMISTRY/URINALYSIS

CBC in patients with pyonephrosis secondary to obstructive ureteroliths may have leukocytosis, immature neutrophilia, and thrombocytopenia. Ionized calcium concentration, urinalysis, and urinary excretion of electrolytes may permit estimation of urolith composition pending results of definitive analysis.

OTHER LABORATORY TESTS

- Submit all retrieved ureteroliths for quantitative analysis to determine appropriate preventive strategies.
- Blood pressure should be monitored; hypertension is common with CKD or AKI secondary to ureteral obstruction.

IMAGING

- Radiography—radiopaque ureteroliths may be visualized. If obstruction and hydronephrosis have occurred, renomegaly may be apparent. If ureteral rupture occurs, contrast in the retroperitoneal space may be lost. Small ureteroliths may not be visualized.
- Ultrasonography—valuable for detecting hydronephrosis or hydroureter. Changes suggesting pyelonephritis may also be detected by ultrasound. The dilated proximal ureter may be traced to the ureteroliths. Ureteroliths are not observed ultrasonographically in up to 25% of cats with ureteroliths. Ultrasound-guided pyelocentesis can be used to confirm ureteral obstruction, although this is usually performed during surgical placement of subcutaneous ureteral bypass (SUB) or ureteral stents.
- CT before and after IV contrast can be used to confirm obstructive ureteroliths if they are suspected but not confirmed by other imaging modalities. This is not required for surgical planning for SUB or stent placement.

DIAGNOSTIC PROCEDURES

Nuclear scintigraphy alone should not be used to determine whether or not to preserve or surgically remove a kidney.

PATHOLOGIC FINDINGS

Progressive dilation of the pelvis and calyces; in advanced cases, the kidney may be transformed into a thin-walled sac with only shell of atrophic cortical parenchyma; ureteral dilation proximal to the site of obstruction is often present.

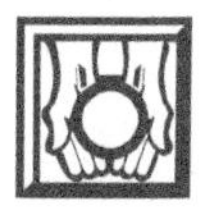

TREATMENT

- For small nonobstructive ureteroliths, allowing time for the ureteroliths to spontaneously pass down the ureter to the bladder may eliminate the need for intervention.
- Remove or bypass ureteroliths that are causing obstruction.
- Ureteroliths in dogs have been successfully treated with ESWL. Efficiency of ESWL fragmentation of ureteroliths is improved with prior ureteral stent placement. Calcium oxalate uroliths from cats are intrinsically resistant to fragmentation via ESWL. ESWL is not recommended for cats.
- Surgical techniques recommended for removal of ureteroliths vary, depending on the site of obstruction, species, the presence or absence of UTI, and the degree of function of the associated kidney.
- SUB placement is effective for relief of ureteral obstruction in cats and is often the preferred surgical procedure for cats.
- Ureteroneocystotomy may be performed for ureteroliths in the middle and distal ureter: the ureter proximal to the obstruction is excised and reimplanted into the bladder. Ureteroliths in the proximal ureter may be removed by ureterotomy. Performance of ureterotomy or ureteroneocystotomy in cats requires microsurgical expertise. When the contralateral kidney functions normally and severe end-stage hydronephrosis is present, ureteronephrectomy may be appropriate.
- Ureteral stent placement to bypass obstructive ureteroliths relieves the obstruction and causes passive ureteral dilation. Ureteral stents may be placed endoscopically in dogs and surgically in dogs and cats. Ureteral stent combined with medical dissolution effectively resolves struvite ureteroliths in dogs.

MEDICATIONS

DRUG(S) OF CHOICE

- Medical dissolution is only effective for struvite ureteroliths when combined with

URETEROLITHIASIS (CONTINUED)

ureteral stent placement. Medical dissolution requires culture-guided antibiotics and dissolution diet.

• Therapy aimed at prevention of recurrent disease is imperative following relief of obstruction.

CONTRAINDICATIONS/POSSIBLE INTERACTIONS

Attempts to prevent one type of urolith may promote formation of a second type.

FOLLOW-UP

PATIENT MONITORING

• Following SUB placement, routine sampling of the SUB for urinalysis and culture along with flushing the SUB is performed every 3 months.

• Instillation of tetra-EDTA solution into the SUB is recommended with SUB flushes.

• Following successful removal of ureteroliths, recheck every 3–6 months for recurrence of uroliths and to ensure owner compliance with preventive measures; urinalysis, imaging, and urine culture.

PREVENTION/AVOIDANCE

• Elimination of predisposing factors.

• Specific therapy depends on the mineral composition of the urolith.

POSSIBLE COMPLICATIONS

Hydronephrosis, CKD, AKI, recurrent UTI, pyelonephritis, sepsis, ureteral rupture, ureteral stricture, hypertension.

EXPECTED COURSE AND PROGNOSIS

Highly variable; if unilateral disease is present, the opposite kidney retains adequate function, and recurrence is prevented, the prognosis is good. Prognosis is good for cats with SUB or ureteral stent placement that recover renal function to stage 1–2 CKD. Prognosis is good for dogs with obstructive ureteroliths that recover renal function to stage 1–2 CKD.

MISCELLANEOUS

ABBREVIATIONS

• AKI = acute kidney injury
• CKD = chronic kidney disease.
• ESWL = extracorporeal shock wave lithotripsy.
• SUB = subcutaneous ureteral bypass.
• UTI = urinary tract infection.

Suggested Reading

Berent AC, Weisse CW, Bagley DH, et al. Use of a subcutaneous ureteral bypass device for treatment of benign ureteral obstruction in cats: 174 ureters in 134 cats (2009-2015. J Am Vet Med Assoc 2018, 253:1309–1327.

Berent AC, Weisse CW, Todd K, et al. Technical and clinical outcomes of ureteral stenting in cats with benign ureteral obstruction: 69 cases (2006–2010). J Am Vet Med Assoc 2014, 244:559–576.

Kuntz JA, Berent AC, Weisse CW, et al. Double pigtail ureteral stenting and renal pelvic lavage for renal-sparing treatment of obstructive pyonephrosis in dogs: 13 cases (2008–2012). J Am Vet Med Assoc 2015, 246:216–225.

Author Larry G. Adams
Consulting Editor J.D. Foster

URETHRAL PROLAPSE

BASICS

OVERVIEW

- Prolapse of the mucosal lining of the distal urethra through the external urethral orifice.
- Prolapsed urethra appears as a congested, pea-shaped mass protruding from the distal end of the penis and is often associated with hemorrhage. Excessive licking may result in further traumatic damage to the exposed urethral mucosa.

SIGNALMENT

- Reported in male dogs and extremely rare in male cats.
- Most common in English bulldog, Boston terrier, and Yorkshire terrier.
- Mean age 18 months; range 4 months–5 years.

SIGNS

- Intermittent or persistent bleeding from the urethra.
- Intermittent or persistent licking of penis.
- Dysuria and pollakiuria caused by concomitant disorders.

Physical Examination Findings

- Persistent or intermittent urethral prolapse.
- Pale mucous membranes if anemic.
- Necrosis of the prolapsed urethra secondary to drying or self-induced trauma from licking.
- Uroliths may be palpable in the urinary bladder or urethra.

CAUSES & RISK FACTORS

- May result from sexual excitement and/or unrelated disorders (e.g., infections, uroliths, neoplasia) of the lower urinary tract.
- Increased intra-abdominal pressure secondary to dysuria associated with urocystoliths.
- Proposed causes include abnormal development of the urethra with increased intra-abdominal pressure as a consequence of brachycephalic airway syndrome, dysuria, or sexual activity. Increased intra-abdominal pressure could impair venous return of blood through the pudendal veins, predisposing susceptible dogs to engorgement of the corpus spongiosum surrounding the distal urethra.
- Breed predisposition (bulldogs and Boston terriers).

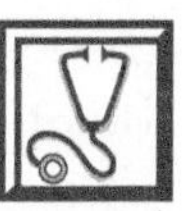

DIAGNOSIS

DIFFERENTIAL DIAGNOSIS

- Prostatic disease.
- Persistent penile frenulum.
- Fracture of the os penis.
- Balanoposthitis.
- Urethritis.
- Urethroliths.
- Coagulopathy.
- Urethral neoplasia.

CBC/BIOCHEMISTRY/URINALYSIS

- CBC—may reveal regenerative anemia.
- Serum biochemistries—usually normal.
- Hematuria may be absent in urine collected by cystocentesis, but present in voided urine.
- Urine culture and sensitivity.

OTHER LABORATORY TESTS

Coagulation profile may rule out coagulopathy.

IMAGING

- Survey radiographs—useful to find some uroliths and evaluate the prostate size.
- Contrast cystourethrography—useful to rule out radiolucent uroliths, urethral disorders, and prostatic disease.
- Abdominal ultrasonography—useful to evaluate the prostate and urinary bladder.

DIAGNOSTIC PROCEDURES

- Ejaculation—useful to evaluate urethra during penile erection; some urethral prolapses are present only during penile erection.
- Evaluation of ejaculate may show evidence of prostatic disease.
- Enlarged images obtained with a surgical microcamera associated with a flexible endoscope may be necessary to diagnose urethral prolapse in cats.

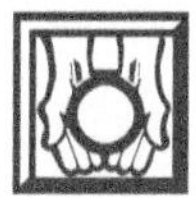

TREATMENT

- May not be required if asymptomatic or only associated with episodic bleeding.
- If present only during penile erection, consider castration prior to attempting surgical removal of prolapsed tissue; diethylstilbestrol given for 3–6 weeks after surgery may reduce frequency of erections. If cause is unknown, castration status may not affect prolapse recurrence.
- Consider surgery for patients with excessive bleeding, pain, or extensive ulceration or necrosis of the prolapsed tissue, or if refractory to medical management.
- Satisfactory results have been obtained by manual reduction of the prolapse followed by urethropexy.
- CO_2 laser surgical technique may improve hemostasis, visualization, and accuracy of the surgeon, and decrease postoperative swelling.
- A surgical microscope may be necessary for adequate visualization to perform urethroplasty in cats.
- Postoperative hemorrhage and prolapse recurrence may be reduced with a simple continuous suture pattern and administration of postoperative sedation.

MEDICATIONS

DRUG(S) OF CHOICE

- Bacterial urethritis warrants use of appropriate antibiotics.
- Consider using diethylstilbestrol for 3–6 weeks after surgery to reduce frequency of erections.

CONTRAINDICATIONS/POSSIBLE INTERACTIONS

Consider risk of bone marrow suppression before giving estrogens, especially in anemic patients.

FOLLOW-UP

PATIENT MONITORING

Reevaluate 7–10 days following surgery for hemorrhage or recurrence of urethral prolapse.

PREVENTION/AVOIDANCE

If urethral prolapse is associated with penile erection, prevent contact with female dogs or situations likely to cause erection.

POSSIBLE COMPLICATIONS

- Most common postoperative complication was hemorrhage (39%).
- Prolapse recurred in 57% of dogs, but was less common when postoperative butorphanol or acepromazine were given.
- Recurrence of the prolapse may occur, especially if an underlying cause has not been detected and eliminated or controlled.

EXPECTED COURSE AND PROGNOSIS

- Prolapse may persist without significant sequelae. Some dogs may not require therapy.
- Some may not have problems after castration and/or surgical correction of a prolapsed urethra.

MISCELLANEOUS

ASSOCIATED CONDITIONS

Urolithiasis and urinary tract infection.

Suggested Reading

Carr GC, Tobias KM, Smith L. Urethral prolapse in dogs: a retrospective study. Vet Surg 2014, 43(5):574–580.

Fossum TW. Urethral prolapse. In: Small Animal Surgery, 3rd ed. St. Louis, MO: Mosby Elsevier, 2007, pp. 687–689.

Kirsch JA, Hauptman JG, Walshaw RA. Urethropexy technique for surgical treatment of urethral prolapse in the male dog. J Am Anim Hosp Assoc 2002, 38:381–384.

Osborne CA, Sanderson SL. Medical management of urethral prolapse in male dogs. In: Bonagura JD, Kirk RW, eds., Current VeterinaryTherapy XII. Philadelphia, PA: Saunders, 1995, pp. 1027–1029.

Author Sherry Lynn Sanderson

Consulting Editor J.D. Foster

Acknowledgment The author and editors acknowledge the prior contribution of Carl A. Osborne.

URINARY RETENTION, FUNCTIONAL

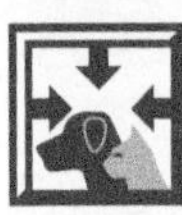

BASICS

DEFINITION

Failure of the urethral smooth and/or striated muscle relaxation as the detrusor muscle contracts at the beginning of urination. Thought to be due to dysfunction of the reflex arc allowing urethral sphincter relaxation as the detrusor muscle contracts at the beginning of urination.

PATHOPHYSIOLOGY

This is a disorder of the emptying phase of micturition due to functional obstruction of the outflow tract and urethra. While the pathophysiology is not completely understood, it is thought that the neurologic lesion is located within the reticulospinal tract, Onuf nucleus, or caudal mesenteric ganglion. The loss of inhibitory signals to the pudendal and hypogastric nerves may also be involved. Involvement of a more local lesion (peripheral nerves, neuromuscular junction, striated and smooth muscles of the sphincters, etc.) is unknown. It is unclear whether anxiety and other behavior disorders may contribute to the disorder.

SYSTEMS AFFECTED

- Urinary tract.
- Typically have otherwise normal neurologic assessment.

INCIDENCE/PREVALENCE

Unknown. The literature suggests increasing incidence which may be related to increased awareness and thus diagnosis in male dogs.

SIGNALMENT

Dogs (cats can be affected). Most common in middle-aged male dogs (mean age of 4.9 years). Females are also affected although rarely. Large- to giant-breed dogs most commonly affected.

CAUSES

- Neurologic dysfunction due to spinal cord lesions cranial to the sacral segment resulting in upper motor neuron bladder signs with simultaneous detrusor and urethral contraction.
- Damage to the reflex arc impairing urethral sphincter relaxation during detrusor contraction.
- Urethral spasm of the smooth or striated muscles.
- Controversial behavioral/anxiety-driven component in some patients.

RISK FACTORS

- Large- to giant-breed dogs (25–64 kg).
- Young adults.
- Intact males—sexual excitement in the presence of intact females.
- Cauda equina syndrome.
- Urinary tract infections or urethritis resulting in urethral spasm.
- Surgery in the area of the bladder neck.
- Urethral and prostatic tumors.

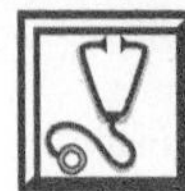

DIAGNOSIS

DIFFERENTIAL DIAGNOSIS

- Diagnosis of a functional urethral obstruction is presumptive. These animals exhibit a typical pattern of urination in which they often start with a normal stream that quickly weakens and may stop completely. The affected animal may posture multiple times attempting to urinate without ever fully emptying their bladder. A large residual urine volume (>1 mL/kg) is typically noted. A mechanical obstruction should be ruled out; passing a urinary catheter is typically easy in dogs with functional obstruction.
- As a result of urine retention, overflow incontinence may occur. This can make it difficult for owners to distinguish it from storage disorders (e.g. urethral sphincter mechanism incompetence).
- This condition can share some similarities with upper motor neuron bladders seen in dogs with intervertebral disc disease.
- Other causes of urine obstruction must be ruled out. These include urolithiasis, neoplasia, benign prostatic hyperplasia, prostatitis, foreign body, and urethral strictures.

CBC/CHEMISTRY/URINALYSIS

Typically unremarkable though evidence of urinary tract infections may be noted on the urinalysis (pyuria, bacteriuria).

OTHER LABORATORY TESTS

None

IMAGING

Contrast urethrography studies in these dogs are often normal, though narrowing of the urethra may be noted due to urethrospasm. Ultrasound can be used to assess the ureters and renal pelvises to look for dilation secondary to obstruction from urolithiasis or vesicoureteral reflux.

DIAGNOSTIC PROCEDURES

Dogs with functional urethral obstruction are typically easily catheterized. A large residual urine volume is typically noted. A normal residual urine volume in dogs is 0.1–3.4 mL/kg (0.2 mL/kg mean). Urethroscopy may be indicated in individuals that fail to respond to medical therapy. This will allow for identification of strictures or other anatomic abnormalities. Urodynamic evaluation does not typically show increased urethral pressure unless the animal is actively voiding.

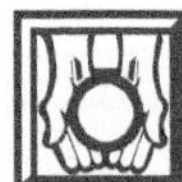

TREATMENT

Treatments are directed at addressing the relaxation of the smooth and striated muscles of the urethral sphincter (see drugs listed under Medications). Owners can also be instructed how to intermittently pass sterile catheters at home to address residual urine volume. If present, urinary tract infections should be treated based on culture and susceptibility testing. In cases of chronic functional urethral obstruction, bladder atony may occur secondary to prolonged bladder distension. In these cases treatment of bladder atony may be necessary. This should only be initiated once the functional obstruction has been relieved. Urethral stenting and cystostomy tubes are considered a salvage procedure and should only be considered in the most refractory cases. Intact males should be castrated.

MEDICATIONS

DRUG(S) OF CHOICE

- Alpha-1 adrenergic antagonists (give on an empty stomach):
    - Prazosin 0.5 mg/kg PO q12h; 1 mg/15 kg PO q8–12h.
    - Tamsulosin 0.1 mg/10 kg PO q24h; 0.4 mg/dog PO q24h (may increase to q12h).
- Benzodiazepines (anxyiolytic and muscle relaxant):
    - Diazepam 2–10 mg/dog PO q8h.
- Phenothiazine sedative/tranquilizer:
    - Acepromazine maleate 0.55–2.2 mg/kg PO q6–12h.
- Muscle relaxant:
    - Methocarbamol 132 mg/kg/day PO divided q8–12h, then 61–132 mg/kg/day divided q8–12h. If no response in 5 days, discontinue.
- Cholinergic:
    - Bethanechol chloride 2.5–25 mg/dog q8h (some respond to q12h).
- Pro-motility agent:
    - Cisapride 0.1–0.5 mg/kg PO q12h (up to 1 mg/kg PO q8h).
- Behavioral modification agents and anxiolytics may also provide some benefit.

CONTRAINDICATIONS

- Alpha-agonists.
- Testosterone or other androgens—avoid anything that may result in increased prostate size.
- Do not administer any medications that will promote detrusor muscle activity (i.e., bethanechol) until urethral obstruction (functional or mechanical) has been relieved.

PRECAUTIONS

- Prazosin may cause hypotension, CNS signs such as lethargy or dizziness, weakness, syncope, and gastrointestinal upset.
- Tamsulosin may cause hypotension though the safe dosage range is quite wide and severe hypotension is less likely than with other drug choices.
- Acepromazine may cause sedation and hypotension as well as cardiovascular collapse

from bradycardia and hypotension, decreased tear production may occur in cats.

- Diazepam can cause sedation, increased appetite, changes in behavior such as agitation or aggression have been reported. Dogs may also show ataxia. Avoid use in cats due to risk of liver toxicity.
- Methocarbamol may cause sedation, increased salivation, vomiting, along with lethargy, weakness and ataxia.
- Bethanechol's adverse effects are typically minimal when administered orally. Gastrointestinal effects such as hypersalivation, vomiting, diarrhea and anorexia may be seen but are typically mild. Cardiovascular and respiratory effects unlikely with oral dosing.
- Cisapride may cause vomiting, abdominal discomfort or diarrhea. The cardiovascular effects seen in humans are not documented in cats and dogs.

POSSIBLE INTERACTIONS

- Prazosin should not be used in conjunction with beta-blockers, sildenafil, or verapamil/nifedipine due to concerns for increased risk of hypotension.
- Tamulosin should not be used with other alpha-1 adrenergic antagonists or sildenafil/tadalafil as they may have cumulative hypotensive effects. Cimetidine, charithromycin, erythromycin, ketoconazole, and terbinafine may all result in increased plasma levels of tamulosin.
- Acepromazine may have adverse effects when administered in conjunction with a number of drugs. Be careful when administering with other drugs that may cause CNS effects or hypotension.
- Diazepam should be used with caution when administered concurrently with other CNS-depressant medications. There are also several classes of drugs that may increase or decrease plasma levels of diazepam when administered concurrently.
- Methocarbamol should be used with caution when other CNS-depressant medications are also prescribed.
- Bethanechol should not be used with other cholinergic or anticholinergic medications due to synergistic or antagonistic effects, respectively.
- Cisapride's effects may be decreased when given with anticholinergics. When given with benzodiazepines the sedative effects may be enhanced.

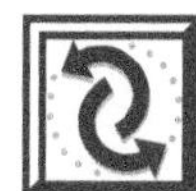

FOLLOW-UP

PATIENT MONITORING

Monitoring of residual urine volume as well as routine screening for urinary tract infections should be performed.

POSSIBLE COMPLICATIONS

If left untreated, chronic bladder distension can result in bladder atony and dysfunction of the detrusor muscle. Urine retention puts these dogs at risk of developing urinary tract infections.

MISCELLANEOUS

PREGNANCY/FERTILITY/BREEDING

Castrate male dogs.

SYNONYMS

- Detrusor-urethral dyssynergia.
- Detrusor-sphincter dyssynergia.

Suggested Reading

Bloch F, Pichon B, Bonnet AM, et al Urodynamic analysis in multiple system atrophy: characterization of detrusor-sphincter dyssynergia. J Neurol 2010, 257:1986–1991.

Byron JK. Micturition disorders. Vet Clin Small Anim 2015, 45:769–782.

Diaz Espineira, MM, Viehoff FW, Nickel RF. Idiopathic detrusor-urethral dyssynergia in dogs: a retrospective analysis of 22 cases. J Small Anim Pract 1998, 39:264–270.

Lane I, Fischer JR, Miller E, et al. Functional urethral obstruction in 3 dogs: clinical and urethral pressure profile findings. J Vet Intern Med 2000, 14:43–49.

Authors William M. Cole and Julie K. Byron
Consulting Editor J.D. Foster

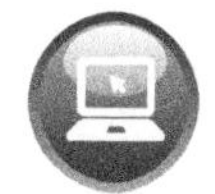

Client Education Handout available online

URINARY TRACT OBSTRUCTION

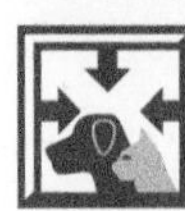

BASICS

DEFINITION

Restricted flow of urine from the kidneys through any point of the urinary tract to the external urethral orifice.

PATHOPHYSIOLOGY

Physical or functional obstruction of the urinary tract resulting in partial or complete cessation in renal excretory function. Luminal pressure is transmitted to the level of the kidney and its functional units (nephrons). As tubular pressure exceeds filtration pressure, glomerular filtration rate (GFR) ceases. Pathophysiologic consequences depend on site, degree, and duration of obstruction. The resulting uremia, acidemia, and hyperkalemia creates the clinical signs and progression.

SYSTEMS AFFECTED

- Renal/urologic.
- Cardiovascular, nervous, and respiratory systems also affected relative to duration of obstruction and severity of metabolic derangement.

SIGNALMENT

- Dog and cat.
- More common in males than females.

SIGNS

Historical Findings

- Pollakiuria and stranguria.
- Diminished to absent urine stream.
- Vocalizing, frequent trips to the litter box (cats).
- Gross hematuria.
- Systemic signs associated with complete (or nearly complete) urinary tract obstruction—lethargy, reduced appetite, and vomiting.

Physical Examination Findings

- Excessive (i.e., overly large or turgid) or inappropriate (i.e., remains after voiding efforts) distended urinary bladder, especially in conjunction with lower urinary tract signs.
- Abdominal distention/discomfort.
- Uroliths maybe be palpable in the distal urethra of obstructed male dogs, or on rectal exam of female dogs.
- Signs of severe uremia—dehydration, weakness, hypothermia, and/or bradycardia with moderate hyperkalemia, altered mentation, or sinus tachycardia from pain/stress.

CAUSES

Intraluminal Causes

- Urolithiasis—most common in male dogs.
- Urethral plugs—most common in male cats.
- Idiopathic—no overt intraluminal physical obstruction; may involve functional obstruction.

Intramural Causes

- Neoplasia of the bladder neck or urethra—more common in dogs.
- Prostatic disorders (neoplasia, prostatitis, etc.) in male dogs.
- Edema, hemorrhage, or spasm at sites of obstruction and/or associated with inflammation. Can contribute to persistent or recurrent obstruction following catheterization.
- Stricture at a site of prior injury or inflammation.
- Ruptures, lacerations, and punctures—usually caused by traumatic incidents.

Miscellaneous Causes

- Displacement of the urinary bladder into a perineal hernia.
- Neurogenic (see Urinary Retention, Functional).

RISK FACTORS

- Urolithiasis, particularly in males.
- Feline lower urinary tract disease, particularly in males.
- Prostatic disease in male dogs.

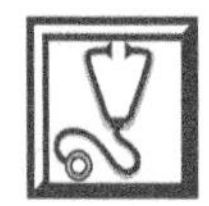

DIAGNOSIS

DIFFERENTIAL DIAGNOSIS

- Owners may have difficulty distinguishing urinary obstruction from constipation.
- Signs of feline idiopathic cystitis can be difficult to distinguish from obstruction, especially if there are no signs of systemic illness. Determination of bladder size (large/firm with obstruction, small with cystitis) can help distinguish.
- Animals whose urinations are not routinely observed by owners can present for signs referable to systemic illness rather than concern for obstruction.
- Evaluation of any azotemic patient, in conjunction with history and physical exam, should include consideration of possible postrenal causes (e.g., urinary obstruction).

CBC/BIOCHEMISTRY/URINALYSIS

- Hemogram is usually normal; a stress leukogram or hemoconcentration may be seen.
- Biochemical analysis may reveal azotemia, hyperphosphatemia, metabolic acidosis, hyperkalemia, and hypocalcemia proportional to duration of obstruction.
- Hematuria and proteinuria are common. Crystalluria may be associated with urolithiasis, though can be present in the absence of stones. There may be evidence of bacteriuria (dogs) and pyuria. Atypical epithelial cells may be seen in patients with neoplasia.

OTHER LABORATORY TESTS

- Urine culture may be beneficial if suspicion for urinary tract infection (UTI) in obstructed dogs (especially secondary to uroliths). Obstructed cats are unlikely to have bacterial cystitis, and presenting urine culture is not recommended unless recently catheterized.
- Uroliths passed or retrieved should be sent for crystallographic analysis.

IMAGING

Abdominal Radiography

- Uroliths—often demonstrated by survey radiography; but may be missed because of their size, composition, or location. Ensure entire lower urinary tract is included.
- Positive- or double-contrast cystourethrography may detect lesions of the urethra and urinary bladder.

Abdominal Ultrasonography

Ultrasonography is highly sensitive in detecting lesions of the bladder, proximal urethra, prostate, and upper urinary tract.

DIAGNOSTIC PROCEDURES

- Electrocardiography may detect abnormalities due to hyperkalemia, including tall T waves, prolonged PR interval, widened QRS complexes, loss of P waves, and bradycardia.
- Transurethral catheterization and contrast studies may determine the location and nature of obstructing material. Animals that cannot urinate despite being readily catheterized likely either have intramural lesions or functional urinary retention.
- Cystoscopy can be helpful to identify lesions not observed on contrast study or ultrasound.

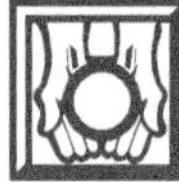

TREATMENT

- Complete obstruction is a medical emergency that can be life-threatening; treatment should be started immediately.
- Initial goals are addressing metabolic derangements, especially significant hyperkalemia, and establishing urinary patency.
- IV administration of isotonic crystalloid based on degree of cardiovascular compromise, dehydration, and potential for post-obstructive diuresis.
- Severe hyperkalemia (K^+ >8 mmol/L, significant bradycardia/ECG changes)—administer calcium gluconate (1 mL/kg over 3–5 minutes, titrated based on ECG changes), regular insulin 0.1–0.2 U/kg IV once, and 50% dextrose bolus 1 mL/kg IV, diluted, over 5 minutes. May need continued dextrose infusion (2.5–5%) for 4–6 hours to avoid hypoglycemia. Terbutaline 0.01 mg/kg IM or IV can also be given. For more severe derangements (K^+ >10 mmol/L, pH <7.1) consider sodium bicarbonate 1 mL/kg IV over 5–10 minutes.
- Decompressive cystocentesis may allow relief of intravesicular pressure, resumption of GFR, and decreased back-pressure for

catheterization. Based on available studies, risk of complications appears to be very low.
• Urethral catheterization under heavy sedation or general anesthesia (see below) to relieve physical obstruction and establish urethral patency.
• Flushing urinary bladder until clear effluent, attach to sterile collection system.
• Post-obstructive management geared toward nursing care, maintaining fluid balance, correction of metabolic derangements, and sedation/analgesia.
• Rate of fluid administration should be determined based on clinical picture. Some patients can experience a post-obstructive diuresis, with significant urinary losses. It is important to keep up with these losses to avoid dehydration. This can be achieved by matching fluid rate to urine output.
• Hyperkalemia should resolve within hours after de-obstruction, and potassium may eventually need to be supplemented. Azotemia should also significantly decrease within 12–24 hours.
• Patients with obstructive urolithiasis often require a separate procedure for stone removal.

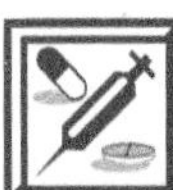

MEDICATIONS

DRUG(S) OF CHOICE

• Sedation/analgesia/anesthesia for catheter placement should be dictated by patient stability. Acepromazine plus an opioid if stable; opioid plus benzodiazepine if unstable. Ketamine and a benzodiazepine is a common combination. Alfaxalone may also be considered. General anesthesia may be indicated as it gives the most urethral relaxation, especially for obstructed dogs.
• In the post-obstructive period, continued sedation and analgesia is beneficial.
• Urethral relaxants (e.g., acepromazine and/or prazosin) may be beneficial for post-obstructive cats or patients with neurogenic urine retention.
• Antibiotics may be indicated with strongly suspected or documented evidence of infection (such as cytology or positive culture). Antibiotics should not be administered to prevent UTI while a urinary catheter is in place. This is not effective and can promote bacterial resistance.
• Nonsteroidal anti-inflammatory drugs have failed to improve speed of resolution or the frequency of reobstruction.

CONTRAINDICATIONS

• Corticosteroids are contraindicated while a urinary catheter is in place. This can predispose to the development of UTI.
• Nonsteroidal anti-inflammatory medications should be initially avoided in more metabolically compromised patients.

PRECAUTIONS

Avoid drugs that reduce blood pressure (e.g., acepromazine) or induce cardiac dysrhythmia (e.g., ketamine) until dehydration and hyperkalemia are resolved. Avoid excessive force during catheterization attempts.

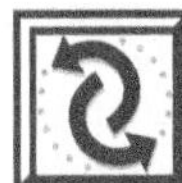

FOLLOW-UP

PATIENT MONITORING

• Continuous ECG monitoring to guide treatment and evaluate response is warranted if there were significant changes initially.
• Assess urine production and hydration status frequently, and adjust fluid administration rate accordingly.
• Monitor renal values and electrolytes. Sicker patients may require more frequent monitoring (q6–12); once daily for more stable patients.
• The urinary catheter can be removed once metabolic derangements and urine output has normalized, and the urine appears to be clear of gross debris, clots, etc.
• After urinary catheter removal, monitor ability to urinate closely for at least 12–24 hours.
• Cats may benefit from continued pain medication and urethral relaxation for 5–7 days at home, as well as recommendations (increased water intake, environmental enrichment) to help decrease risk of re-obstruction.

POSSIBLE COMPLICATIONS

• Death.
• Injury to the excretory pathway (e.g., urethral tear) while trying to relieve obstruction.
• Hypokalemia during post-obstructive diuresis.
• Recurrence of obstruction (estimated at 15–40%).

MISCELLANEOUS

ASSOCIATED CONDITIONS

• Bradycardia secondary to hyperkalemia.
• Azotemia, hyperphosphatemia, and metabolic acidosis.

SYNONYMS

Urethral obstruction.

SEE ALSO

• Azotemia and Uremia.
• Feline Idiopathic Lower Urinary Tract Disease.
• Hyperkalemia.
• Urinary Retention, Functional.

ABBREVIATIONS

• GFR = glomerular filtration rate.
• UTI = urinary tract infection.

Suggested Reading

Cooper ES. Controversies in the management of feline urethral obstruction. J Vet Emerg Crit Care 2015, 25(1):130–137.
Cooper ES. Feline lower urinary tract obstruction. In: Drobatz KJ, Hopper K, Rozanski E, Silverstein DC, eds., Textbook of Small Animal Emergency Medicine. Hoboken, NJ: Wiley, 2019, pp. 634–640.
Gerber B, Eichenberger S, Reusch CE. Guarded long-term prognosis in male cats with urethral obstruction. J Feline Med Surg 2008, 10:16–23.
Hall J, Hall K, Powell LL, et al. Outcome of male cats managed for urethral obstruction with decompressive cystocentesis and urinary catheterization: 47 cats (2009–2012). J Vet Emerg Crit Care 2015, 25(2):256–262.
Segev G, Livne H, Ranen E, et al. Urethral obstruction in cats: predisposing factors, clinical, clinicopathological characteristics and prognosis. J Feline Med Surg 2011, 13:101–108.

Author Edward S. Cooper
Consulting Editor J.D. Foster

Client Education Handout available online

URINARY TRACT PARASITES

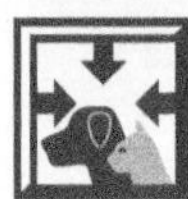

BASICS

OVERVIEW

Dioctophyma renale (Giant Kidney Worm)

In North America, cases are frequently encountered in Mississippi, Louisiana, Minnesota, Wisconsin, Michigan, and the central and eastern provinces of Canada. Humans are accidental hosts; because of the aquatic portion of its life cycle, water is an essential element of the habitat of *D. renale*. Minks are the most commonly infected mustelids, and are the principal definitive host in North America.

Life Cycle

- To complete the life cycle, both males and females must be located in the same kidney of the host, and the urinary tract must be the patent. Fertile eggs are passed with urine voided by the host, and then embryonate in water. First-stage larvae are produced after 1–7 months. The definitive hosts become infected by ingesting the infective larvae in annelids.
- Definitive hosts are infected by ingesting raw fish, frogs, other paratenic hosts, or *Lumbriculus variegatus*. After ingestion, the infected larvae penetrate the walls of the stomach or intestines and migrate to the submucosa. After approximately 5–7 days, they migrate to the liver and remain there for about 50 days. Migration to the right or the left kidney and invasion of the renal pelvis follows.
- *D. renale* have been found more frequently in the right kidney than in the left. Finding encysted *D. renale* around liver is associated with larval penetration at the lesser curvature of the stomach. On occasion, *D. renale* have been encountered in the urinary bladder and/or ureters. Infective larvae become mature gravid females in the definitive host after 3.5–6 months. The entire life cycle requires approximately 2 years.

Pathophysiology in the Kidney

- Adult parasites have attained substantial size by the time they penetrate the kidney. The exact mechanisms involved with gaining access to the renal pelvis is unknown, but probably results from the effects of enzymes released by the parasite.
- Available evidence does not support the theory that adult *D. renale* slowly devour the renal tissue of the host, reducing it to a hollow sack. Although the exact mechanism(s) of destruction is not known, obstruction caused by the growing adult parasite(s) and secondary hydronephrosis (or pyonephrosis) plays a major role. Examination of the kidneys from dogs with unilateral renal infection reveals changes typical of advanced hydronephrosis (i.e., obliteration of the majority of renal tubules surrounded by chronic inflammatory tissue and persistence of the structural architecture of many glomeruli).
- Ova of *D. renale* may be observed in the renal parenchyma adjacent to the renal pelvis. The urothelium lining the renal pelvis is often hyperplastic.
- If only one kidney is affected with *D. renale* the host retains adequate renal function due to compensatory hypertrophy and hyperplasia of the remaining kidney. If both kidneys are parasitized, or if one kidney is parasitized and the opposite kidney has substantial comorbid dysfunction, varying stages of renal failure and uremia may occur. Eggs that are released by female worms pass through the urinary tract and provoke inflammation in the mucosa of the ureter and urinary bladder.

Pathophysiology in the Peritoneal Cavity

- In dogs, viable parasites located in the abdominal cavity and/or between lobes of the liver have been incidental findings during ovariohysterectomy.
- Eggs present in the peritoneal cavity can trigger development of chronic peritonitis. Examination of the abdominal viscera from dogs with *D. renale* in the peritoneal cavity revealed hemorrhage, granulomatous inflammation, and fibrosis frequently involving the omentum, the surface of the liver, and the surface of the spleen. Viable adult males have been found in the peritoneal cavity of dogs without an associated inflammatory response.
- Ascites may occur in dogs with peritoneal *D. renale* colonization. The fluid detected in the abdominal cavity is usually hemorrhagic.

Pearsonema (Capillaria)

- *Pearsonema* and *Capillaria* are used interchangeably and appear to be identical in taxonomy and biologic behavior.
- *Pearsonema (Capillaria) plica* are small, thread-like, yellowish parasites that invade the mucosa or submucosa of the bladder and rarely the renal pelvis and ureter, causing a mild inflammatory response.
- *P. plica* in dogs and cats and *P. feliscati* in cats have been uncommonly associated with signs of lower urinary tract disease.
- *P. plica* passes ova with bipolar plugs in urine. When earthworms ingest embryonated ova, the parasite develops into the infective stage. Ingestion of an infective earthworm results in a patent infection in dogs in 58–88 days.
- The life cycle of *P. feliscati* is poorly understood.

SIGNALMENT

D. renale

- Dogs and cats.

Pearsonema

- Dogs—no predilection reported.
- Cats—affected cats almost always >8 months old.

SIGNS

D. renale

- Feeding *L. variegatus* infected with *D. renale* to dogs typically induces vomiting due to effects of the parasite on the gastric mucosa.
- If only one kidney has been invaded with *D. renale*, signs are often absent.
- Silent hematuria may be the first indication of an abnormality.
- Palpation of the abdomen may reveal an enlarged and/or misshapen hydronephrotic kidney.
- If both kidneys are parasitized, clinical signs attributable to renal failure or uremia may occur. The host will typically die before extensive hydronephrosis of both kidneys has time to develop. The degree of renal dysfunction is influenced by (1) number of parasites in the kidney, (2) duration of infection, (3) number of kidneys parasitized, and (4) presence and severity of comorbid renal disease.

Pearsonema

- Usually none.
- Pollakiuria, hematuria, stranguria, and dysuria in heavily infected animals.

CAUSES & RISK FACTORS

D. renale

See Overview.

Pearsonema

Dogs

- High prevalence of infection (up to 50%) in the natural hosts (e.g., foxes, raccoons) in the southeastern United States may predispose animals in this geographic region.
- In kennels, high infection rates associated with contaminated soil surfaces.

Cats

Rare in United States; infection prevalence of 18–34% is reported in Australia.

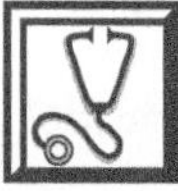

DIAGNOSIS

DIFFERENTIAL DIAGNOSIS

D. renale

Any cause of hydronephrosis or renomegaly.

Pearsonema

Consider other, more common causes of lower urinary tract disease, such as urolithiasis, urinary tract infection, trauma, and neoplasia.

CBC/BIOCHEMISTRY/URINALYSIS

D. renale

- When gravid female worm is present in the kidney that has a patent track to the exterior, microscopic examination of urine usually reveals ova of *D. renale*.
- Hematuria, pyuria, and proteinuria with or without eggs are indicative of an inflammatory response.

- Findings typical of chronic kidney disease when both kidneys are parasitized.

Pearsonema

- Colorless, slightly pitted ova with bipolar plugs in urine sediment are diagnostic.
- Consider fecal contamination of urine with *Trichuris vulpis* or other morphologically similar ova if free-catch urine specimens are used, or if inadvertent rectal puncture and aspiration of feces with *T. vulpis* occurs during cystocentesis.
- Urine contamination of feces can produce false fecal examination findings.
- Symptomatic infections are usually associated with evidence of hematuria, pyuria, and proteinuria. Bacterial urine cultures are typically sterile.

OTHER LABORATORY TESTS

N/A

IMAGING

D. renale

- Radiography may reveal renomegaly. If IV urography is performed, it may be characterized by inability of the parasitized kidney to excrete the contrast agent.
- Ultrasonography may reveal the affected kidney to be hydronephrotic and find characteristic hypoechoic loops associated with one or more of these parasites in the renal pelvis. Transverse plane sonography of the affected kidney may reveal a thin hyperechoic rim that contains multiple circular structures of uniform diameter. The outer layers of these parasites are hyperechoic; the inner portions are hypoechoic. If parasites are in the peritoneal cavity, sonography may reveal hyperechoic curvilinear bands in the region of the right caudal lobe of the liver and/or the cranial pole of the right kidney. Serially performed studies may reveal movement of the parasite from one location to another.
- CT and MRI scans may also be used to detect *D. renale* in the renal pelvis of one or both kidneys, in the peritoneal cavity, or in varying positions between the lobes of the liver.

Pearsonema

N/A

DIAGNOSTIC PROCEDURES

N/A

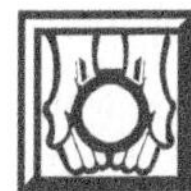

TREATMENT

D. renale

Nephrectomy is usually the treatment of choice when only one kidney is affected and the opposite kidney is capable of sustaining homeostasis. Parasites that are incidental findings in the peritoneal cavity during celiotomy may be removed without further morbidity.

Pearsonema

- Infection is usually self-limiting in cats and dogs.
- If infected dogs are isolated, after 10–12 weeks ova are no longer detectable in the urine sediment.
- Replacing soil surfaces with sand, gravel, or concrete may reduce prevalence of infection in kennels contaminated with *P. plica* and *P. feliscati*.

MEDICATIONS

DRUG(S) OF CHOICE

D. renale

N/A

Pearsonema

- Consider anthelmintic therapy if clinical signs are present and persist; monitor therapeutic success by examining urine sediment for ova and observing status of clinical signs.
- Multiple courses of treatment may be necessary to eliminate the infection.
- Fenbendazole 50 mg/kg PO q24h for 3 days.
- Ivermectin 0.2 mg/kg SC once has been suggested as an alternative therapy, but objective information on its efficacy in this disease is limited.
- Oral treatment with albendazole 50 mg/kg PO q12h for 30 days was reported to be effective in dogs.

CONTRAINDICATIONS/POSSIBLE INTERACTIONS

N/A

FOLLOW-UP

D. renale

Dogs and cats should not be fed raw fish or fish viscera, especially in areas where *D. renale* is known to exist and should not be given access to lake or pond water likely to contain infective stages of *D. renale.*

Pearsonema

Monitor treatment success by examining urine sediment for ova and observing status of clinical signs. In the absence of reinfection, urinary capillariasis may be self-limiting. Isolation of dogs and cats from earthworms should be sufficient to eliminate a *Capillaria* bladder infection in 90 days.

MISCELLANEOUS

ZOONOTIC POTENTIAL

Capillaria spp. pose no known public health risks.

INTERNET RESOURCES

Companion Animal Parasite Council: http://www.capcvet.org

Suggested Reading

Brown SA, Prestwood KA. Parasites of the urinary tract. In: Kirk RW, ed., Current Veterinary Therapy IX. Philadelphia, PA: Saunders, 1986, pp. 1153–1155.

Osborne CA, Stevens JB, Hanlon GF, et al. Dioctophyma renale in the dog. J Am Vet Med Assoc 1969, 155:605–620.

Author Hasan Albasan

Consulting Editor J.D. Foster

Acknowledgment The author and editors acknowledge the prior contribution of Carl A. Osborne.

U

UROLITHIASIS, CALCIUM OXALATE

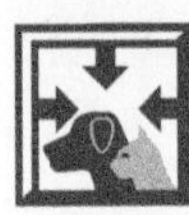

BASICS

DEFINITION

Formation of calcium oxalate (CaOx) uroliths within the urinary tract and associated clinical conditions (e.g., urinary obstruction, idiopathic hypercalcemia, chronic kidney disease).

PATHOPHYSIOLOGY

Presence of hypercalciuria, hyperoxaluria, hypocitraturia, and defective crystal growth inhibitors.

Hypercalciuria

In dogs, normocalcemic hypercalciuria may result from intestinal hyperabsorption of calcium (so-called absorptive hypercalciuria: type 1—dietary independent, type 2—dietary dependent, and type 3—phosphaturic induced hypervitaminosis D) or reduced renal tubular reabsorption of calcium (renal leak hypercalciuria). Hypercalcemic hypercalciuria results from excessive glomerular filtration of mobilized calcium, which overwhelms normal renal tubular reabsorptive mechanisms (called resorptive hypercalciuria, since bone resorption is associated with high serum calcium concentrations).

Hyperoxaluria

In humans, hyperoxaluria is associated with inherited abnormalities of excessive oxalate synthesis (primary hyperoxaluria types I, II, and III), excess consumption of foods containing high quantities of oxalate or oxalate precursors, pyridoxine deficiency, and disorders associated with fat malabsorption (i.e., fat complexes with intestinal calcium augmenting intestinal absorption of oxalate). Lack of oxalate-degrading bacteria in the intestine can increase the quantity of oxalate absorbed from the diet and the quantity excreted in urine.

Hypocitraturia

Urine citrate inhibits CaOx urolith formation. By complexing with calcium ions to form the relatively soluble salt calcium citrate, citrate reduces the quantity of calcium available to bind with oxalate. In normal dogs, acidosis is associated with low urinary citrate excretion, whereas alkalosis promotes urinary citrate excretion.

Defective Crystal Growth Inhibitors

Large-molecular-weight proteins in urine, such as Tamm-Horsfall mucoprotein, nephrocalcin, and osteopontin, have a profound ability to enhance solubility of CaOx. Urine from dogs with CaOx uroliths revealed that nephrocalcin had fewer carboxyglutamic acid residues than nephrocalcin isolated from normal dog urine.

Feeding Diets Promoting Urine Acidification

Diets designed to promote aciduria are a common risk factor in cats and dogs. In several species, acidic urine is associated with hypercalciuria (bone mobilization of calcium, increased glomerular filtration of calcium, and decreased renal tubular reabsorption of calcium) and hypocitraturia (increased renal tubular reabsorption).

SYSTEMS AFFECTED

Renal/urologic

INCIDENCE/PREVALENCE

In dogs, CaOx accounts for approximately 40% of the uroliths removed from the lower urinary tract and 45% of those removed from the upper urinary tract. In cats, CaOx accounts for approximately 40% of the uroliths removed from the lower urinary tract and 90% of those retrieved from the upper urinary tract.

SIGNALMENT

Species

Dog and cat.

Breed Predilections

- Dogs—reported in many breeds. Six breeds represent 60% of cases: miniature schnauzer, Lhasa apso, Yorkshire terrier, bichon frisé, shih tzu, and miniature poodle.
- Cats—Himalayan, Scottish fold, Persian, ragdoll, and Burmese are at greater risk.

Mean Age and Range

- Dogs—8.5 ± 3 years; 60%, 6–11 years.
- Cats—97% >2 years; 53%, 7–15 years.

Predominant Sex

Mostly male dogs (73%) and male cats (55%).

SIGNS

General Comments

- Asymptomatic in some animals.
- Depend on location, size, and number of uroliths.
- Animals with nephroliths are typically asymptomatic but may have persistent hematuria.
- Ureteral obstruction associated with contralateral microrenale, ipsilateral hydronephrosis, and acute onset of uremia occurs frequently in cats with chronic kidney disease.

Historical Findings

- Typical signs of urocystoliths or urethroliths include pollakiuria, dysuria, and hematuria. Some may present for urethral obstruction.
- Nephroureteroliths common (45%) in cats with chronic kidney disease.

Physical Examination Findings

- Detection of urocystoliths are by abdominal or urethral palpation; failure to palpate uroliths does not exclude them from consideration.
- Large urinary bladder with complete urethral obstruction (more common in cats).
- Urocystoliths with irregular contours rarely cause complete urethral obstruction.

CAUSES

See Pathophysiology.

RISK FACTORS

- Oral calcium supplements given independent of meals.
- Feeding acidifying foods that promote formation of aciduria (pH <6.6 in dogs and <6.25 in cats) was associated with CaOx urolithiasis. In normal cats, alkaline urine was associated with the lowest saturation for CaOx.
- Aciduria was a risk factor for first-time CaOx urolith formation in dogs.
- In healthy cats, urinary undersaturation for CaOx was achieved by inducing alkaluria via dietary formulation with potassium citrate.
- Excessive dietary protein, sodium (>1.2% DMB or 350 mg/100 kcal) and vitamin D promote hypercalciuria.
- Additional dietary oxalate (e.g., chocolate and peanuts) and ascorbic acid promote hyperoxaluria.
- Glucocorticoids and furosemide promote hypercalciuria.
- Vitamin B6-deficient diets (e.g., homemade) promote hyperoxaluria.
- Consumption of dry diets has a higher risk for CaOx urolith formation than consumption of high-moisture canned diets.

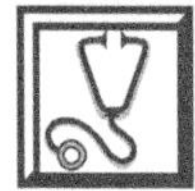

DIAGNOSIS

DIFFERENTIAL DIAGNOSIS

- Urethral obstruction, urinary tract infection, urinary tract neoplasia, and idiopathic feline lower urinary tract disease.
- Other common radiodense uroliths are magnesium ammonium phosphate, calcium phosphate, and silica.

CBC/BIOCHEMISTRY/URINALYSIS

- Hematological and serum profile results are usually unremarkable.
- Urinalysis may reveal CaOx crystals, but absence of crystalluria does not exclude uroliths as a possibility.
- Hypercalcemia (rare in dogs, more common in cats) should be further evaluated to determine its cause and contribution to urolith formation.

OTHER LABORATORY TESTS

Quantitative mineral analysis of uroliths.

IMAGING

- CaOx uroliths ≥2 mm in diameter are radio-opaque and easily detected by survey radiography. IV urography, contrast pyelography, or ultrasonography may be needed to verify ureteral obstruction.

U

• Urinary tract mineralization may resemble uroliths.

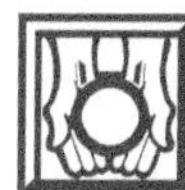

TREATMENT

APPROPRIATE HEALTH CARE

• CaOx uroliths are not amenable to medical dissolution.
• Small stones that can pass through the urethra (<3 mm in most dogs >5 kg) should be removed by voiding urohydropropulsion or basket retrieval. Percutaneous cystolithotomy or routine cystotomy can be used to remove stones in smaller dogs and male cats.
• Consider laser lithotripsy, percutaneous cystolithotomy, or routine cystotomy to remove larger stones from the urinary bladder.
• Urethral surgery is discouraged. Retrograde urohydropropulsion is an effective procedure to flush urethral stones back into the urinary bladder prior to their removal from the urinary bladder.
• Persistently obstructed ureters require urgent intervention to minimize progressive kidney damage. See Ureterolithiasis.
• Removal of unobstructing nephroliths is usually unnecessary.

ACTIVITY

Reduce during the period of tissue repair after surgery.

DIET

• Studies support feeding high moisture foods that promote formation of less acidic urine (pH >6.3–6.6) to minimize formation of CaOx.
• Hypercalcemia in cats without evidence of hyperparathyroidism or malignancy is sometimes minimized by feeding Hill's Prescription Diet Feline w/d.

CLIENT EDUCATION

• Urolith removal does not alter the factors responsible for urolith formation; eliminating or minimizing risk factors is necessary to minimize recurrence.
• 50% of dogs reform uroliths within 2–3 years; 1/3 of cats reform uroliths in 2 years.
• Patients with hypercalcemia typically reform uroliths at a faster rate.

SURGICAL CONSIDERATIONS

• Consider surgical removal of lower tract uroliths that cannot be removed by minimally invasive procedures (voiding urohydropropulsion, basket retrieval, intracorporeal laser lithotripsy, percutaneous cystolithotomy).
• Avoid performing disfiguring urethrostomies and urethrotomies by using retrograde urohydropropulsion to flush urethroliths into the bladder or using lithotripsy to fragment urethroliths.
• Shock wave lithotripsy is an alternative to surgery for removal of nephroliths and ureteroliths in dogs.
• To minimize urolith reformation over suture nidus, minimize surgical procedures to remove uroliths and use absorbable suture and patterns that minimize suture exposure in the lumen of the urinary tract.
• Only surgeons trained in ureteral surgery should attempt ureterolithotomy. Ureteral stents in dogs and subcutaneous ureteral access devices or stents in cats should be considered.
• Consider parathyroidectomy for patients with primary hyperparathyroidism.

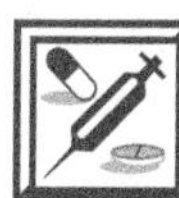

MEDICATIONS

DRUG(S) OF CHOICE

• No available drugs effectively dissolve CaOx uroliths in the urinary tract. *In vitro* dissolution is seen with alkaline solutions (pH ≥8) of 2% or greater EDTA.
• Potassium citrate used to promote alkaluria should not contain cranberry supplements.

PRECAUTIONS

Steroids and furosemide promote calciuria.

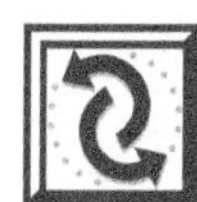

FOLLOW-UP

PATIENT MONITORING

• Postsurgical radiographs are essential to verify complete urolith removal.
• To prevent the need for repeated surgery, evaluate abdominal radiography every 9–12 months to detect urolith recurrence early. Small uroliths are easily removed by voiding urohydropropulsion or stone basket retrieval.

PREVENTION/AVOIDANCE

• Even with appropriate therapy, CaOx urolith recurrence is common (up to 50% in dogs and 33% in cats in 2–3 years). Regular monitoring and compliance check-ins are essential to adjust therapy to extend the interval between recurrences.
• Only recommend high-moisture foods (e.g., can, loaf, gravies). Feeding dry foods, combining dry and wet foods, or adding water to dry food is not effective in maintaining low urinary concentrations (specific gravity <1.020 in dogs and <1.030 in cats) of calculogenic minerals.
• Feeding high-sodium foods (≥300 mg/100 kcal) should not be recommended as a substitute for feeding high-moisture foods. Their efficacy to promote low urine specific gravity appears to be short-lived (3–6 months) and their use is contraindicated in kidney or heart disease.
• Avoid feeding diets that promote urine acidification. A linear increase in urine pH was associated with a linear decrease in urine CaOx saturation in normal cats.
• Commercially manufactured diets have been designed to prevent CaOx recurrence, but they may not be ideal for all patients.
• Hill's Prescription Diet c/d multicare has been shown to decrease calcium and oxalate excretion in dogs with CaOx urolithiasis. This food has lower levels of sodium and protein.
• Hill's Prescription Diet i/d Kiw Fat and has been recommended for dogs with CaOx urolithiasis and fat/lipid intolerance or fat/lipid responsive diseases (e.g., dogs with a history of pancreatitis). Because this diet promotes formation of acidic urine, administer potassium citrate to promote a more favorable urine pH >6.5.
• Royal Canin SO has been shown to decrease CaOx relative supersaturation in urine of urolith-forming dogs collected by owners. Because this diet promotes acidic urine, concomitant administration of potassium citrate is necessary to achieve a more favorable urine pH (>6.5). Because of its high sodium, this food may be inappropriate for small breeds at risk for degenerative mitral valve disease.
• Avoid supplements with vitamins C and D.
• Reevaluate patients 2–4 weeks after initiation of diet therapy to verify appropriate reduction in specific gravity (<1.020 for dogs and <1.030 for cats), appropriate urine pH (≥6.5), and amelioration of crystalluria. Do not use inappropriately collected or stored urine samples (e.g., urine collected by owners, refrigerated, or contaminated with debris) to monitor therapeutic efficacy. To promote dilute urine, feed canned or gravy formulations of food or add additional water to all types of food. If urine is acidic, consider administration of potassium citrate 75 mg/kg PO q12h; adjust dosage to achieve a pH between 6.5 and 7.5. Potassium citrate medications formulated with cranberry are not recommended because cranberry is a source of vitamin C; vitamin C supplementation should be discouraged because of its ability to increase urine oxalate.
• Vitamin B6 2–4 mg/kg PO q24–48h may help minimize oxalate excretion, especially for animals fed homemade or pyridoxine-deficient diets.
• If dietary changes are inadequate at slowing the rate of recurrence, consider hydrochlorothiazide diuretics (dog, 2 mg/kg and cat, 1 mg/kg q12–24h).
• If the patient is hypercalcemic, correct underlying cause.
• *Oxalobacter formigenes* is an intestinal bacterium that ingests oxalate as its sole nutrient. By metabolizing dietary oxalate in the intestine, less oxalic acid is available for absorption and less is excreted in urine. To preserve healthy populations of intestinal *Oxalobacter*, avoid indiscriminant or prolonged use of antimicrobics.

UROLITHIASIS, CALCIUM OXALATE (CONTINUED)

POSSIBLE COMPLICATIONS

• Urocystoliths can pass into and obstruct the urethra.
• Dogs that do not consume their daily requirement of some urolith prevention foods may develop various degrees of protein calorie malnutrition.
• Diet-associated hyperlipidemia develops in some patients consuming foods with higher fat content. Miniature schnauzers with hereditary hyperlipidemia are predisposed to pancreatitis when consuming some prevention foods.
• When treating multiple conditions (obesity, diarrhea, etc.) consider diets that are indexed to also prevent CaOx.

EXPECTED COURSE AND PROGNOSIS

• Approximately 50% of dogs and 33% of cats reform uroliths in 2–3 years. Treatment to minimize recurrence is helpful.
• Patients with persistent hypercalcemia typically reform uroliths at a faster rate.

MISCELLANEOUS

ASSOCIATED CONDITIONS

Conditions predisposing to hypercalciuria: hyperadrenocorticism, acidemia, hypervitaminosis D, and hyperparathyroidism; or hyperoxaluria: vitamin B6 deficiency, hereditary hyperoxaluria, and ingestion of chocolate and peanuts.

AGE-RELATED FACTORS

Rare in young (<1 year old) animals.

PREGNANCY/FERTILITY/BREEDING

Diets used to prevent CaOx uroliths are not appropriate.

SYNONYMS

Oxalate urolithiasis.

SEE ALSO

Crystalluria.

ABBREVIATIONS

• AAFCO = Association of American Feed Control Officials.
• CaOx = calcium oxalate.

Suggested Reading

Appel S, Lefebvre SL, Houston DM, et al. Evaluation of risk factors associated with suture-nidus cystoliths in dogs and cats. J Am Vet Med Assoc 2008, 233:1889–1895.
Kyles AE, Hardie EM, Wooden BG, et al. Management and outcome of cats with ureteral obstruction: 153 cases (1984–2002). J Am Vet Med Assoc 2005, 226:937–944.
Lulich JP, Adams LG, Grant D, et al. Changing paradigms in the treatment of uroliths by lithotripsy. Vet Clin North Am Small Anim Pract 2009, 39:143–160.
Lulich JP, Berent AC, Adams LG, et al. ACVIM Small Animal Consensus recommendations on the treatment and prevention of uroliths in dogs and cats. J Vet Intern Med 2016, 30:1564–1574.
Lulich JP, Osborne CA. Upper tract urolith: questions, answers, questions. In: August JR, ed., Consultations in Feline Internal Medicine, Volume 5. St. Louis, MO: Elsevier Saunders, 2006, pp. 399–406.
Okafor CC, Lefebvre SL, Pearl DL, et al. Risk factors associated with calcium oxalate urolithiasis in dogs evaluated at general care veterinary hospitals in the United States. Prevent Vet Med 2014, 115:217–228.

Author Jody P. Lulich
Consulting Editor J.D. Foster
Acknowledgment The author and editors acknowledge the prior contribution of Carl A. Osborne.

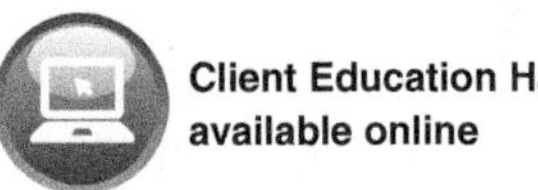

U

UROLITHIASIS, CALCIUM PHOSPHATE

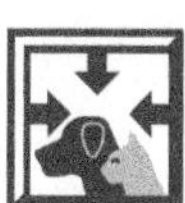

BASICS

OVERVIEW

• Calcium phosphate (CP) uroliths within the urinary tract and associated clinical conditions. • Forms of CP identified in dogs and cats include: calcium phosphate apatite (CAP), calcium phosphate carbonate (CPC), calcium hydrogen phosphate dihydrate (brushite), and uncommon minerals—tricalcium phosphate (whitlockite) and octacalcium phosphate. • CP uroliths represent a small fraction (dogs <1.0%, cats <0.5%) of all uroliths submitted to the Minnesota Urolith Center (MUC) from 1981 to 2018 (Table 1). • More CP uroliths are found in the upper tract (kidney and ureter) (2.5% cats, 3.5% dogs), than in the lower tract (bladder and urethra). • CP uroliths (excluding brushite) do not have a characteristic shape. Brushite uroliths are typically round and smooth. • CP uroliths are usually cream or tan in color. Blood clots mineralized with CP are typically black.

SIGNALMENT

• Dog and cat.
• Rarely detected in animals <1 years old.
• CPC uroliths occur primarily in female dogs (72%).

SIGNS

• Depend on location, size, and number of uroliths. • Pollakiuria, dysuria, hematuria, and urethral obstruction. • Nephroureteroliths—typically asymptomatic but may have persistent hematuria or signs referable to concomitant renal failure (primarily cats).

CAUSES & RISK FACTORS

• CPC—commonly a minor component of struvite and calcium oxalate uroliths.
• Pure CP uroliths—usually associated with metabolic disorders, e.g., primary hyperparathyroidism, renal tubular acidosis, and excessive dietary calcium and phosphorus.
• Urinary tract infections—increased calcium excretion in combination with urinary tract infection with urease producing bacteria may be risk factors favoring CPC. • Nephroliths, urocystoliths, and urethroliths composed of blood clots mineralized with CP suggest dystrophic mineralization of tissue, in contrast to metastatic mineralization reflecting abnormal calcium and phosphorus metabolism. • Other risk factors—see Urolithiasis, Calcium Oxalate.

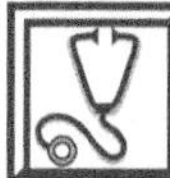

DIAGNOSIS

DIFFERENTIAL DIAGNOSIS

• Other common causes of hematuria, dysuria, and pollakiuria, with or without urethral obstruction, include urinary tract infection and urinary tract neoplasia. • Other radiodense uroliths—magnesium ammonium phosphate, calcium oxalate, and silica. • Metastatic or dystrophic mineralization of urinary tract parenchyma may resemble uroliths.

CBC/BIOCHEMISTRY/URINALYSIS

• Usually unremarkable. • Hypercalcemia or azotemia rarely detected; postrenal azotemia in some animals with complete urinary outflow obstruction. • Urinary sediment analysis—amorphous crystals in some patients; brushite (calcium hydrogen phosphate dihydrate) forms are elongated, rectangular, lath-shaped crystals.

OTHER LABORATORY TESTS

• Quantitative analysis of retrieved uroliths is necessary to confirm their mineral composition. • Serum concentrations of parathyroid hormone, parathyroid hormone–related peptide, and hydroxycholecalciferol may help establish underlying causes.

IMAGING

• CP uroliths are radiodense (as dense as bone) and are often detected by survey radiography.
• CP uroliths may be detected by ultrasonography.

DIAGNOSTIC PROCEDURES

CP uroliths in the urethra and bladder may be detected by cystoscopy.

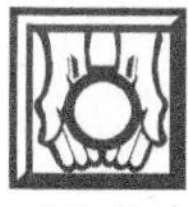

TREATMENT

• Medical dissolution of CP uroliths remains a goal for the future. • Consider surgical removal of lower tract uroliths that cannot be removed by minimally invasive procedures (e.g., voiding urohydropropulsion, basket retrieval, intracorporeal lithotripsy, laparoscopic cystotomy). • Avoid performing disfiguring urethrostomies by using basket retrieval to remove urethroliths, retrograde urohydropropulsion to flush urethroliths into the bladder or using lithotripsy to fragment urethroliths. • Shock wave lithotripsy is an alternative to surgery for removal of nephroliths, ureteroliths, and urocystoliths in dogs.
• Correction of hyperparathyroidism or other causes of hypercalcemia should minimize further urolith formation.

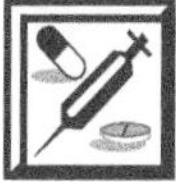

MEDICATIONS

DRUG(S) OF CHOICE

No effective medications available for dissolving CP uroliths.

CONTRAINDICATIONS/POSSIBLE INTERACTIONS

Vitamin D supplements, other mineral supplements, glucocorticoids.

FOLLOW-UP

PATIENT MONITORING

• Radiography after surgery to verify complete urolith removal is a standard of practice.
• Abdominal radiography or ultrasonography every 3–5 months to enhance early detection of urolith recurrence and prevention of the need for repeated surgery. • Small uroliths are easily removed by voiding urohydropulsion or catheter retrieval.

PREVENTION/AVOIDANCE

• A high-moisture (canned) diet formulated to prevent formation of calcium oxalate uroliths may help prevent recurrence. • Foods for older dogs that are lower in protein, phosphorus, and calcium, and which do not promote acidic urine are usually associated with decreased calcium and phosphorus excretion. Hill's Prescription Diet canned g/d is one example. • Because of the high moisture content of canned foods and their tendency to promote dilute urine, canned diets are more effective than dry diets in preventing recurrence. • Avoid excessive acidification or alkalinization of urine.

MISCELLANEOUS

SYNONYMS

Apatite uroliths.

ABBREVIATIONS

• CAP = calcium phosphate apatite.
• CP = calcium phosphate.
• CPC = calcium phosphate carbonate.
• MUC = Minnesota Urolith Center.

Authors Hasan Albasan and Jody P. Lulich
Consulting Editor J.D. Foster
Acknowledgment The authors and editors acknowledge the prior contribution of Carl A. Osborne.

U

Table 1

Calcium phosphate uroliths submitted to the Minnesota Urolith Center (MUC) in 2013.

	Dog (n = 70,481)	Cat (n = 17,245)
Calcium phosphate carbonate form (CPC)	0.58%	0.09%
Calcium phosphate apatite form (CAP)	0.10%	0.17%
Calcium hydrogen phosphate dihydrate (Brushite)	0.23%	0.03%

UROLITHIASIS, CYSTINE

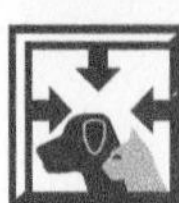

BASICS

OVERVIEW

- Formation of uroliths composed of cystine.
- Cystinuria—an inborn error of metabolism caused by defective tubular reabsorption of cystine, ornithine, lysine, and arginine (COLA) leading to cystine urolith formation.
- Cystine is freely filtered by glomeruli; however, most is actively reabsorbed in the renal proximal tubules.
- Impaired intestinal absorption of these amino acids has not been associated with any nutritional deficiency states in dogs, presumably because these are non-essential amino acids. However, cystine may be semi-essential amino acid and as a precursor of taurine, excessive cystine loss may affect taurine availability.
- Unless protein intake is severely restricted, cystinuric dogs have no detectable abnormalities associated with amino acid loss. Excessive loss of arginine in urine predisposes cats to hyperammonemic encephalopathy. Some cystinuric dogs may have carnitinuria.
- Cystinuric dogs have been classified into three different types: type 1 autosomal recessive *SLC3A1* mutations found in Newfoundlands, Landseer, and Labrador retrievers; type 2 autosomal dominant *SLC3A1* and *SLC7A9* identified in Australian cattle dogs and European miniature pinschers, and type 3, which has sex-limited inheritance (androgen dependence) and has been identified in mastiffs, English and French bulldogs, Scottish deerhounds, and Irish terrriers.
- Not all cystinuric dogs and cats form uroliths; cystinuria is a predisposing rather than a primary cause of cystine urolithiasis. Cystine is relatively insoluble in acid urine and is more soluble in alkaline urine.
- This disease is genetically heterogeneous (*SLC3A1* and *SLC7A9*) in cats as it is in dogs and humans.

U

SIGNALMENT

- Dogs—primarily adult (mean age 5 years; range 3 months–14 years) intact males, but may also affect females. It occurs in excess of 100 breeds, including dachshunds, English bulldogs, Newfoundlands, Labrador retrievers, Chihuahuas, pit bulls, and French bulldogs. May be detected in male and female Newfoundland and Labradors <1 year of age.
- Cats—primarily adult (mean age at diagnosis, 3.5 years; range, 4 months–12 years) males and females; most common in the domestic shorthair and Siamese breeds.

SIGNS

- Depend on location, size, and number of uroliths; affected animals may be asymptomatic.
- Urocystoliths—include pollakiuria, dysuria, and hematuria.
- Urethroliths—include urethral obstruction, pollakiuria, dysuria, and sometimes voiding of small smooth uroliths. Complete outflow obstruction may result in postrenal azotemia that may progress to uremia.
- Nephroliths—typically asymptomatic; may be associated with manifestations of hydronephrosis and renal insufficiency.

CAUSES & RISK FACTORS

- Inherited defects in renal tubular transporters of cystine.
- Breed predisposition.
- In young and middle-aged dogs with previous history of cystine urolithiasis—recurrence within 6–12 months following surgery unless prophylactic therapy is given.
- Urolith formation—enhanced by acidic, concentrated urine, incomplete and infrequent micturition.

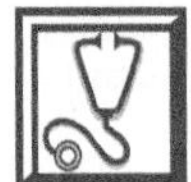

DIAGNOSIS

DIFFERENTIAL DIAGNOSIS

- Uroliths mimic other causes of pollakiuria, dysuria, hematuria, and/or outflow obstruction.
- Differentiate from other types of uroliths by urinalysis, radiography, and quantitative analysis of voided or retrieved uroliths.
- Urate uroliths and sterile struvite uroliths are of similar radiodensity.

CBC/BIOCHEMISTRY/URINALYSIS

- Cystine crystals are six-sided; insoluble in acetic acid.
- Positive urine cyanide-nitroprusside test.

OTHER LABORATORY TESTS

- Urinary amino acid profiles—reveal abnormal quantities of cystine and, in some dogs and cats, ornithine, lysine, arginine, and other amino acids.
- Quantitative mineral analysis of uroliths.
- DNA test.
- To diagnose androgen-dependent cystinuria in breed without a genetic text, calculate the urine cystine to creatine ratio before and 3 to 6 months after castration. A marked and persistent reduction is consistent with resolution of cystinuria via castration.

IMAGING

- Radiography—the radiodensity of cystine uroliths is similar to that of sterile struvite and silica, less than that of calcium oxalate and calcium phosphate, and greater than that of ammonium urate.
- Ultrasonography—can detect cystine uroliths, but does not provide reliable information about the radiodensity, shape, or number present.

DIAGNOSTIC PROCEDURES

- Urethrocystoscopy—used to detect cystine urethroliths and urocystoliths.
- Quantitative mineral analysis of uroliths.

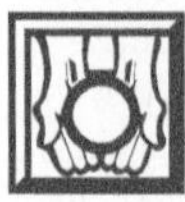

TREATMENT

Measures to minimize urolith formation include changing the diet to reduce cystine excretion (lower methionine protein consumption), diluting urine to a lower cystine concentration, and alkalinizing the urine to improve cystine solubility.

Dogs

- Medical dissolution of uroliths by a combination of *N*-(2-mercaptopropionyl)-glycine (2-MPG) and dietary therapy; Hill's Prescription Diet Canine u/d reduces urinary excretion of cystine, promotes formation of alkaline urine, and reduces urine concentration; it is used in conjunction with 2-MPG for urolith dissolution and maybe effective alone in preventing recurrence of cystine uroliths.
- In one study, castration reduced recurrence of cystine uroliths in dogs identified with type 3, sex-limited inheritance.
- Other diets are available to prevent cystine, but lack published results of efficacy.

Cats

Diets designed for renal insufficiency and geriatric cats may be suitable to minimize formation. Give enough potassium citrate 40–75 mg/kg PO q12h to maintain a urine pH of 7.5. Choose a moist formulation diet to help reduce urine concentration. Dissolution with 2-MPG has been studied in a small number of cats at an oral dose of 12–20 mg/kg q12h. Frequency of recurrence was minimized in these cats without adverse side effects.

Dogs and Cats

Remove urocystoliths unable to be dissolved by voiding urohydropropulsion, basket retrieval, lithotripsy, or surgery.

MEDICATIONS

DRUG(S) OF CHOICE

Urine Alkalinizers

- For patients that have acidic urine despite dietary therapy.
- Data from cystinuric humans suggest that dietary sodium may enhance cystinuria; thus potassium citrate may be preferable to sodium bicarbonate as a urine alkalinizer. Give enough potassium citrate 40–75 mg/kg PO q12h to maintain a urine pH of 7.5.

Thiol-Containing Drugs

• 2-MPG decreases urine concentration of cystine by combining with cysteine to form cysteine-2-MPG, which is more soluble than cystine.
• With status as an orphan drug, Thiola™ is only available from the distributor Retrophin. Generic 2-MPG (Tiopronin) may be obtained from compounding pharmacies. In dogs: 2-MPG may be given at a dosage of 15–20 mg/kg PO q12h to dissolve canine cystine uroliths in conjunction with dietary therapy. In our hospital, mean dissolution time was 78 days (range 11–211 days).
• 2-MPG may be given at a lower dosage (5–10 mg/kg PO q12h) to prevent recurrent canine cystine uroliths.
• In cats: 2-MPG has been studied in a small number of cats at an oral dose of 12–20 mg/kg q12h. Frequency of recurrence was minimized in these cats without adverse side effects. Drug-induced adverse events associated with 2-MGP are uncommon in dogs; they include reversible Coombs'-positive spherocytic anemia, thrombocytopenia, glomerular proteinuria, myopathy, aggressiveness, and increased hepatic enzyme activity.
• 2-MPG should be used with caution in cats, as the efficacy and safety of 2-MPG has not been thoroughly evaluated in normal or cystinuric cats.
• In mouse models, L-cystine methyl esters have effectively disrupted cystine crystal growth. Future studies hope to show that efficacy and safety profiles are superior to current thiol-binding drugs.

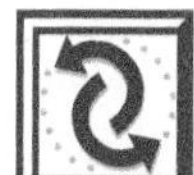

FOLLOW-UP

• Minimize recurrence with dietary management or 2-MPG.
• Monitor urolith dissolution at 30-day intervals by urinalysis, survey or contrast radiography, or ultrasonography.
• Although cystine uroliths tend to recur, recurrence does not affect all cystinuric dogs and cats.
• In some older dogs, the rate of recurrence declines as a consequence of a reduction in the magnitude of cystinuria and urine specific gravity.

MISCELLANEOUS

ABBREVIATIONS

• 2-MPG = *N*-(2-mercaptopropionyl)-glycine.

Suggested Reading

Bannasch D, Henthorn PS. Changing paradigms in the diagnosis of inherited defects associated with urolithiasis. Vet Clin North Am Small Anim Pract 2009, 39:111–125.

Brons AK, Henthorn PS, Raj K, et al. SLC3A1 and SLC7A9 mutations in autosomal recessive or dominant canine cystinuria: a new classification system. J Vet Intern Med 2013, 27:1400–1408.

Mizukami K, Raj K, Osborne CA, Giger U. Cystinuria associated with different SLC7A9 gene variants in the cat. PLoS ONE 2016, 11(7):e0159247.

Author Jody P. Lulich

Consulting Editor J.D. Foster

Acknowledgment The author and editors acknowledges the prior contribution of Carl A. Osborne, Eugene E. Nwaokorie, and Lisa K. Ulrich.

U

UROLITHIASIS, PSEUDO (DRIED BLOOD, OSSIFIED MATERIAL)

BASICS

OVERVIEW

Pseudo-uroliths are concretions of noncrystalline material that form within the urinary tract. They include dried solidified blood and ectopic bone. Pseudo-uroliths can be located in upper or lower sections of the urinary tract (renal pelvis, ureter, bladder, and urethra).

SIGNALMENT

Pseudo-uroliths are primarily a disease of cats.

- Dried solidified blood pseudo-uroliths comprise 1% or less of feline uroliths. They are 2–3 times more common in male than female cats. The mean age of affected cats is 9 years old (range 1–15 years).
- Ectopic bone pseudo-uroliths are rare, with few cases reported.

SIGNS

- Urinary tract obstructions (ureteral or urethral) are common. Obstructions can result in uremia with anorexia, vomiting, weakness, and, if hyperkalemia is present, bradycardia. Urethral obstructions can also cause nonproductive stranguria and a palpably enlarged, firm bladder.
- Other signs include hematuria, dysuria, and pollakiuria.

CAUSES & RISK FACTORS

- Dried solidified blood pseudo-uroliths are associated with hematuria, but mechanisms underlying their formation are unknown. Concurrent urinary tract infections are occasionally present.
- Ectopic bone forms due to ossification of the urothelium. Trauma and inflammation are risk factors in humans, but their role in veterinary species has not been determined.

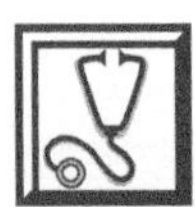

DIAGNOSIS

DIFFERENTIAL DIAGNOSIS

Consider more common lower urinary tract diseases, such as feline idiopathic lower urinary tract disease, other types of urolithiasis (e.g., calcium oxalate and struvite), urethral plugs, urinary tract infection, and urinary tract neoplasia.

CBC/BIOCHEMISTRY/URINALYSIS

Hematuria, proteinuria, and, if obstruction is present, azotemia and hyperkalemia.

OTHER LABORATORY TESTS

- Quantitative analysis (polarized light microscopy and infrared spectroscopy).
- Urine culture to rule out concurrent infection.

IMAGING

Radiographic Findings

- Dried solidified blood is often radiolucent. Bladder distension will be present in the case of urethral obstruction. Pyelography can aid in the diagnosis of ureteral obstruction, but dried solidified blood pseudo-uroliths are infrequently identified even with this modality.
- Ectopic bone is radio-opaque and can be visualized with plain radiography.

Ultrasonographic Findings

- Patients with dried solidified blood pseudo-uroliths frequently have evidence of ureteral obstruction on ultrasound, including renal pelvic dilation with or without ureteral dilation. The pseudo-urolith is often not identified.
- Ectopic bone appears hyperechoic with distal acoustic shadowing.

DIAGNOSTIC PROCEDURES

Cystoscopy can characterize the appearance and number of pseudo-uroliths in the lower urinary tract.

PATHOLOGIC FINDINGS

- Dried solidified blood pseudo-uroliths are often black in color. Unlike blood clots, they are not malleable and crack with pressure. On histopathology, they consist of a conglomeration of red blood cells that lack distinct borders.
- Ectopic bone is grossly adhered to the urothelium but can easily be detached. Other mineralization, such as calcium oxalate, may also be present.

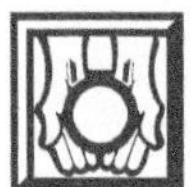

TREATMENT

- Urethral obstructions are treated as emergencies. Retrograde urohydropropulsion can relieve the obstruction; decompressive cystocentesis prior to placement of a urinary catheter may more rapidly reduce intravesicular pressure. Cystotomy or basket-retrieval is performed to remove pseudo-uroliths from the bladder. Voiding urohydropropulsion can be considered for those measuring <3 mm in diameter in female cats or ≤1 mm in male cats.
- Ureteral obstructions should also be managed immediately. Subcutaneous ureteral bypass or ureteral stenting is recommended. Traditional surgery is performed when these procedures are not available.

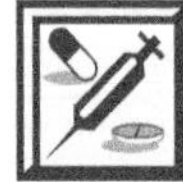

MEDICATIONS

DRUG(S) OF CHOICE

Neither dried solidified blood nor ectopic bone pseudo-uroliths are reported to be susceptible to medical dissolution.

CONTRAINDICATIONS/POSSIBLE INTERACTIONS

N/A.

FOLLOW-UP

PATIENT MONITORING

Routine urinalysis to identify hematuria and serum renal biomarkers (BUN, creatinine, SDMA) to assess renal function.

PREVENTION/AVOIDANCE

Increased fluid intake is recommended as a general mechanism to decrease concretions of material within the urinary tract. Preventative strategies should be followed for any concurrent diseases, such as renal disease, urinary tract infection, or calcium oxalate urolithiasis.

POSSIBLE COMPLICATIONS

Obstruction can result in renal damage and, in severe cases, fatality. Calcium oxalate uroliths can form on ectopic bone within the urinary tract.

EXPECTED COURSE AND PROGNOSIS

Recurrence rates are unknown.

MISCELLANEOUS

ASSOCIATED CONDITIONS

Ectopic bone pseudo-uroliths can serve as a nidus for calcium oxalate uroliths.

Suggested Reading

Westropp JK, Ruby AL, Bailiff NL, et al. Dried solidified blood calculi in the urinary tract of cats. J Vet Intern Med 2006, 20:828–834.

Author Eva Furrow

Consulting Editor J.D. Foster

U

UROLITHIASIS, STRUVITE—CATS

BASICS

DEFINITION

Struvite uroliths and urethral plugs have physical and etiopathogenic differences; these terms should not be used as synonyms. Struvite uroliths are polycrystalline concretions composed primarily of magnesium ammonium phosphate (MAP) and small quantities of matrix. Struvite urethral plugs are composed of large quantities of matrix mixed with crystals (especially MAP), while others are composed primarily of organic matrix, sloughed tissue, blood, and/or inflammatory reactants.

PATHOPHYSIOLOGY

- See Urolithiasis, Struvite—Dogs.
- Most urethral plugs contain large quantities of matrix in addition to minerals, especially struvite. Risk factors associated with formation of MAP crystals contained in urethral plugs are similar to those associated with formation of struvite uroliths. Prevention or control of these risk factors should minimize the recurrence of the struvite component of urethral plugs.

SYSTEMS AFFECTED

Renal/urologic—upper and lower urinary tract.

INCIDENCE/PREVALENCE

- From 1981 to 2002, the prevalence of struvite uroliths has decreased and while that of calcium oxalate (CaOx) uroliths has increased. In 2015, struvite comprised 49% and CaOx comprised 36% of feline uroliths.
- Currently, struvite makes up ~50% of all types of uroliths in the lower urinary tract. Of these, 95% are sterile.
- Struvite has been detected in approximately 8% of feline nephroliths.
- Struvite has remained the most common (~90%) mineral in matrix-crystalline urethral plugs.

SIGNALMENT

Species

Cat (see Urolithiasis, Struvite—Dogs).

Mean Age and Range

- Mean age at time of diagnosis is 7 years (range, <1–22 years).
- Sterile struvite uroliths do not affect immature cats; infection-induced struvite may occur in immature (<1 year) and senior cats (>10 years).

Predominant Sex

- Struvite uroliths are more common in female cats (55%) than in males.
- Struvite urethral plugs primarily affect males.

SIGNS

General Comments

- Affected cats may be asymptomatic.
- Depend on location, size, number, and cause of uroliths.

Historical Findings

- Typical signs of urocystoliths include pollakiuria, dysuria, periuria, hematuria, and sometimes voiding of small, smooth uroliths.
- Signs of renal dysfunction (polyuria and polydipsia) are found in some cats with nephroliths.
- Signs of outflow obstruction (e.g., dysuria, large painful urinary bladder, and postrenal azotemia) are found with struvite urethral plugs.

Physical Examination Findings

- A thickened, firm, contracted bladder wall may be appreciated.
- Palpation is insensitive and unreliable for detection of urocystoliths.
- Urethral plugs or urethroliths may be detected by examination of the distal penis.
- Outflow obstruction results in an enlarged urinary bladder and signs of postrenal azotemia.

CAUSES

See Pathophysiology.

RISK FACTORS

- Sterile struvite uroliths—mineral composition, energy content, and moisture content of diets; urine-alkalinizing metabolites in diets; quantity of diet consumed; *ad libitum* vs. meal-feeding schedules; formation of concentrated urine; and retention of urine.
- Infection-induced struvite urolithiasis—urinary tract infection (UTI) with urease-producing bacteria, abnormalities in local host defenses that allow bacterial UTIs, and the quantity of urea excreted in urine.
- The small diameter of the male distal urethra predisposes to obstruction with plugs and urethroliths.

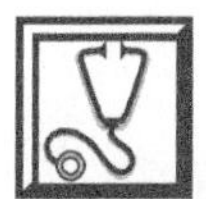

DIAGNOSIS

DIFFERENTIAL DIAGNOSIS

- Uroliths mimic other causes of pollakiuria, dysuria, periuria, hematuria, and/or outflow obstruction.
- Differentiate struvite uroliths and urethral plugs from other types of uroliths by signalment, urinalysis, urine culture, radiography, ultrasonography, cystoscopy, and quantitative analysis of uroliths or plugs.

CBC/BIOCHEMISTRY/URINALYSIS

- Complete outflow obstruction may cause postrenal azotemia.
- MAP crystals typically appear as colorless, orthorhombic (having three unequal axes intersecting at right angles), coffin-like prisms. They often have 3–8 sides.

OTHER LABORATORY TESTS

- Pretreatment urine cultures (preferably obtained by cystocentesis) can detect primary infections with urease-producing microbes causing infection-induced struvite uroliths and differentiate them from infections acquired as a sequelae to urolithiasis.
- Quantitative mineral analysis should be performed on all uroliths and plugs.
- Bacterial culture of inner portions of uroliths retrieved from patients with urease-positive UTI may be of value.

IMAGING

Radiography

- Struvite uroliths—radiodense, single or multiple, rough or smooth, round or faceted, sometimes disc-shaped; some struvite urethral plugs may be detected by survey radiography.
- The size and number of uroliths are not a reliable index of probable efficacy of dissolution therapy.
- Contrast urethrocystography helps identify the site of urethral obstruction and strictures.

Ultrasonography

- Detects location and approximate size and number of uroliths. Tends to overestimate stone size and underestimate stone number.
- Does not indicate degree of radiodensity or shape of uroliths.

DIAGNOSTIC PROCEDURES

Cystoscopy reveals location, number, size, and shape of urethroliths and urocystoliths.

PATHOLOGIC FINDINGS

Urethral plugs may contain red blood cells, white cells, transitional epithelial cells, bacteria, and/or viruses in addition to matrix and minerals.

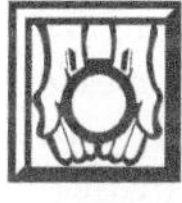

TREATMENT

APPROPRIATE HEALTH CARE

- Retrograde urohydropropulsion to eliminate urethral stones; lavage to remove urethral plugs.
- Voiding urohydropropulsion to eliminate small bladder and urethral stones.
- Medical dissolution of struvite uroliths is an outpatient strategy.

DIET

- Medical dissolution is the standard of practice for elimination of struvite uroliths.
- Treatment with a dedicated struvite calculolytic diet (e.g., Hill's Prescription Diet Feline s/d) results in dissolution within 2–4 weeks of therapy.
- Treatment with urinary therapeutic foods designed for struvite dissolution and CaOx prevention are effective but may require longer treatment times.
- Infection-induced struvite urocystoliths may be dissolved by feeding a calculolytic diet and an appropriate antimicrobic.
- Continue diet therapy for 1 month after radiographic evidence of urolith dissolution.

- Struvite crystalluria may be minimized by feeding magnesium-restricted urine-acidifying diets.
- Canned foods help to reduce urine concentration of calculogenic metabolites and promote increased frequency of voiding.

CLIENT EDUCATION

- If dietary management is used, limit access to other foods and treats.
- Short-term (weeks to months) treatment with a calculolytic diet and antibiotics as needed is effective in dissolving infection-induced struvite uroliths.
- Owners of cats with infection-induced struvite urocystoliths must comply with dosage schedule of antibiotics.
- Avoid feeding calculolytic diets to immature cats.

SURGICAL CONSIDERATIONS

- Ureteroliths cannot be dissolved. For persistent ureteroliths associated with morbidity, consider subcutaneous ureteral bypass, ureteral stents, or traditional surgery.
- Urethroliths cannot be medically dissolved. Consider voiding urohydropropulsion to remove urethroliths or urethral plugs. Alternatively, move urethroliths into the bladder by retrograde urohydropropulsion.
- Immovable urethroliths, recurrent urethral plugs, or strictures of the distal urethra may require perineal urethrostomy.
- Consider laser lithotripsy for urocystoliths and/or urethroliths.
- Consider surgical correction if uroliths are obstructing urine outflow and/or if correctable abnormalities predisposing to recurrent UTI are identified by radiography or other means.
- Radiographs should be obtained immediately following surgery to verify that all uroliths were removed.

MEDICATIONS

DRUG(S) OF CHOICE

- Dissolution of infection-induced urocystoliths requires appropriate antibiotics, chosen on the basis of bacterial culture and antimicrobial susceptibility tests. Give antibiotics at therapeutic dosages until the UTI is eradicated and there is no radiographic evidence of uroliths.
- Buprenorphine may be used to alleviate discomfort (15 μg/kg via buccal transmucosal administration q8–12h). Tolteridine may be considered as an anticholinergic and antispasmodic to minimize hyperactivity of the bladder detrusor muscle and urge incontinence (0.05 mg/kg PO q12h).

CONTRAINDICATIONS

Do not give urine acidifiers to azotemic patients or immature cats.

PRECAUTIONS

Azotemic patients are at increased risk for adverse drug events.

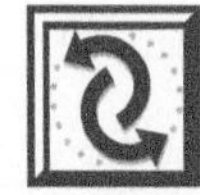

FOLLOW-UP

PATIENT MONITORING

Check rate of urolith dissolution monthly by urinalysis, urine culture, survey or contrast radiography, or ultrasonography.

PREVENTION/AVOIDANCE

- Recurrent sterile struvite uroliths may be prevented by using acidifying, magnesium-restricted diets or urine acidifiers. Do not administer urine acidifiers with acidifying diets.
- For patients whose urine has been acidified, carefully monitor them for CaOx crystalluria. Change management protocol if persistent CaOx crystalluria develops.
- In patients at risk for both struvite and CaOx crystalluria, focus on preventing CaOx uroliths. Struvite uroliths can be medically dissolved; CaOx uroliths cannot be dissolved.
- Infection-induced struvite urolithiasis can be prevented by eradicating and controlling UTIs. Use of magnesium-restricted, acidifying diets is not required if the urease-positive microbes can be eradicated.

POSSIBLE COMPLICATIONS

- Urocystoliths may pass into and obstruct the urethra, especially if the patient is persistently dysuric. Urethral obstruction may be managed by retrograde urohydropropulsion.
- An indwelling transurethral catheter increases the risk for iatrogenic bacterial UTI and urethral stricture.

EXPECTED COURSE AND PROGNOSIS

Mean times for dissolution of sterile urocystoliths ranged from 13 to 36 days. Mean times for dissolution of infection-induced struvite urocystoliths ranged from 21 to 44 days. Most struvite uroliths located in the urinary bladder can be safely dissolved with a low risk of adverse effects, including urethral obstruction.

MISCELLANEOUS

ASSOCIATED CONDITIONS

Any disease that predisposes to bacterial UTI.

AGE-RELATED FACTORS

Infection-induced struvite is the most common urolith in immature cats. Sterile struvite is rare in immature cats.

SYNONYMS

Feline lower urinary tract disease.

SEE ALSO

- Crystalluria.
- Lower Urinary Tract Infection, Bacterial.
- Lower Urinary Tract Infection, Fungal.
- Nephrolithiasis.
- Urolithiasis, Struvite—Dogs.

ABBREVIATIONS

- CaOx = calcium oxalate.
- MAP = magnesium ammonium phosphate.
- UTI = urinary tract infection.

Suggested Reading

Lulich JP, Berent AC, Adams LG, et al. ACVIM small animal consensus recommendations on the treatment of and prevention of uroliths in dogs and cats. J Vet Intern Med 2016, 30:1564–1574.

Lulich JP, Kruger JM, MacLeay, et al. Efficacy of two commercially available, low-magnesium, urine-acidifying dry foods for the dissolution of struvite uroliths in cats. J Am Vet Med Assoc 2013, 243:1147–1153.

Osborne CA, Lulich JP, Kruger JM, et al. Feline urethral plugs: Etiology and pathophysiology. Vet Clin North Am Small Anim Pract 1996, 26:233–254.

Author John M. Kruger

Consulting Editor J.D. Foster

Acknowledgment The author and editors acknowledge the prior contribution of Carl A. Osborne, Jody P. Lulich, and Eugene E. Nwaokorie.

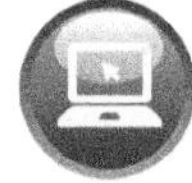

Client Education Handout available online

UROLITHIASIS, STRUVITE—DOGS

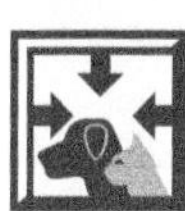

BASICS

DEFINITION

Formation of polycrystalline concretions (i.e., uroliths, calculi, or stones) composed of magnesium ammonium phosphate hexahydrate (MAP, struvite) in the urinary tract.

PATHOPHYSIOLOGY

Infection-Induced Struvite

- Urine must be supersaturated with MAP for struvite uroliths to form. MAP supersaturation of urine is often associated with urinary tract infections (UTIs) with urease-producing microbes.
- UTIs caused by urease-producing microbes (*Staphylococcus*, *Proteus*, and *Ureaplasma*) and urine containing sufficient urea favors formation of uroliths containing struvite, carbonate apatite, and calcium apatite.
- Consumption of dietary protein exceeding the daily requirement results in formation of urea from catabolism of amino acids.
- Metabolic and anatomic abnormalities may indirectly induce struvite uroliths by predisposing to UTIs.

Sterile Struvite

- In dogs, this type of struvite is uncommon.
- Dietary or metabolic factors may be involved in the genesis of sterile struvite uroliths in dogs.
- Microbial urease is not involved in formation of sterile struvite uroliths.

SYSTEMS AFFECTED

Renal/urologic.

GENETICS

- The high incidence of struvite uroliths in some breeds such as miniature schnauzers suggests a familial tendency. Susceptible miniature schnauzers may inherit an abnormality of local host defenses of the urinary tract that increases their susceptibility to UTI.
- Sterile struvite uroliths were found in a family of English cocker spaniels.

INCIDENCE/PREVALENCE

Struvite uroliths account for approximately 40% of stones affecting the canine lower urinary tract and 23% of stones affecting the upper urinary tract.

GEOGRAPHIC DISTRIBUTION

Ubiquitous

SIGNALMENT

Species

Dog

Breed Predilections

- Miniature schnauzer, shih tzu, bichon frise, miniature poodle, cocker spaniel, and Lhasa apso.
- Any breed may be affected.

Mean Age and Range

- Mean age, 6 years (range <1 to >19 years).
- Most uroliths in immature (<12 months old) dogs are infection-induced struvite.

Predominant Sex

More common in females (~85%) than males (~15%), which may be related to the greater propensity for females to develop bacterial UTI.

SIGNS

General Comments

- Some dogs are asymptomatic.
- Signs depend on location, size, and number of uroliths and virulence of bacteria.

Historical Findings

- Typical signs of urocystoliths include pollakiuria, dysuria, and hematuria; sometimes small, smooth uroliths are voided.
- Typical signs of urethroliths include pollakiuria and dysuria; sometimes small, smooth uroliths are voided, and some medium size uroliths are associated with urethral obstruction.
- Nephroliths may be associated with manifestations of renal insufficiency. Obstruction to urine outflow with bacterial UTI may result in generalized pyelonephritis and septicemia.

Physical Examination Findings

- Uroliths may be palpated in the urinary bladder and urethra (by rectal exam).
- Urethral obstruction may cause enlargement of the urinary bladder.
- Ureteral obstruction may cause enlargement and pain of the associated kidney.
- Complete urine outflow obstruction combined with bacterial infection may cause ascending UTI and signs of renal failure and septicemia.

CAUSES

- Urinary tract disorders that predispose to infections with urease-producing bacteria, fungal pathogens, or ureaplasma in patients whose urine contains a large quantity of urea.
- Specific causes of sterile struvite uroliths are unknown.

RISK FACTORS

- Exogenous or endogenous exposure to high concentrations of glucocorticoids predispose to bacteriuria.
- Abnormal retention of urine.
- Alkaline urine decreases the solubility of struvite.

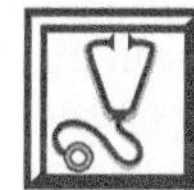

DIAGNOSIS

DIFFERENTIAL DIAGNOSIS

- Uroliths mimic other causes of pollakiuria, dysuria, hematuria, and/or outflow obstruction.
- Differentiate from other types of uroliths by signalment, rectal exam, urinalysis, urine culture, radiography, and quantitative analysis of uroliths.

CBC/BIOCHEMISTRY/URINALYSIS

- Complete outflow obstruction can cause postrenal azotemia and hyperphosphatemia.
- MAP crystals typically appear as colorless, orthorhombic, coffin-like prisms. They may have 3–6 or more sides and often have oblique ends.

OTHER LABORATORY TESTS

- Quantitative bacterial culture of urine, preferably collected by cystocentesis.
- Bacterial culture of inner portions of infection-induced struvite uroliths.
- Quantitative mineral analysis of urolith.

IMAGING

- Struvite uroliths are radiodense and may be detected by survey radiography.
- Ultrasonography can detect uroliths, but provides no information about their density, shape, or size.
- Determine precise location, size, and number of uroliths; the size and number are not a reliable index of probable efficacy of dissolution therapy.

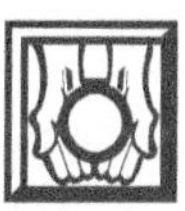

TREATMENT

APPROPRIATE HEALTH CARE

- Medical dissolution with antimicrobials and therapeutic food is preferred treatment for non-obstructing struvite uroliths.
- Ureteral stenting facilitates medical dissolution of obstructing nephroureteroliths.
- Appropriate antimicrobic administration is the cornerstone of treatment for infection-induced struvite dissolution and prevention.
- Voiding urohydropropulsion, laser lithotripsy, percutaneous cystolithotomy, and/or surgery require short periods of hospitalization.

DIET

- Infection-induced and sterile struvite urocystoliths and nephroliths may be dissolved by feeding a calculolytic food (Hill's Prescription Diet Canine c/d, s/d, Royal Canin® and others).
- Continue calculolytic diet therapy for 1 month beyond survey radiographic evidence of urolith dissolution.
- Avoid use of the protein restricted diet in patients with protein-calorie malnutrition. Some calculolytic diets are designed for short-term (weeks to months) dissolution therapy, rather than long-term (months to years) prophylactic therapy. Monitor the patient for evidence of protein malnutrition. Consider dissolution diets meeting maintenance nutritional requirements in immature dogs. Avoid high sodium foods in dogs with cardiac valvular disease or heart failure.

CLIENT EDUCATION

- If dietary management is used, limit access to other foods and treats.

- Short-term (2–3 months) treatment with a calculolytic food and administration of antibiotics is effective in dissolving struvite uroliths.
- Comply with dosage schedule for antibiotic and diet therapy.

SURGICAL CONSIDERATIONS

- Ureteroliths and urethroliths may be difficult to medically dissolve because they are minimally immersed in urine.
- Consider ureteral stenting or shock-wave lithotripsy for persistent ureteroliths associated with morbidity. Ureteral stenting may allow for renal decompression and allow time for stone dissolution.
- Consider voiding urohydropropulsion if urethroliths are likely to pass through the urethra. Alternatively, consider laser lithotripsy or move urethroliths into the bladder by retrograde urohydropropulsion.
- Consider surgical correction if uroliths are obstructing urine outflow and minimally invasive procedures are ineffective or not available. Immovable urethroliths may require urethrotomy or urethrostomy.

MEDICATIONS

DRUG(S) OF CHOICE

- Dietary dissolution of infection-induced urocystoliths or nephroliths requires oral administration of appropriate antibiotics, chosen on the basis of quantitative bacterial culture and antimicrobial susceptibility tests. Give antibiotics until there is no radiographic evidence of uroliths and there is eradication of UTI.
- In most cases, antimicrobics need to be administered for the entire dissolution period. Shorter duration may be successful if they sterilize the urolith (e.g., small uroliths).

PRECAUTIONS

- Diet-induced polyuria will reduce the concentration of antimicrobial drugs in urine; consider this fact when calculating antimicrobic dosages.

FOLLOW-UP

PATIENT MONITORING

Monitor rate of urolith dissolution at 4 to 6 week intervals by urinalysis, urine culture, and imaging (ultrasonography, and/or survey or contrast radiography).

PREVENTION/AVOIDANCE

- Infection-induced struvite urolithiasis may be prevented by eradicating and controlling infections by urease-producing bacteria.
- Recurrent sterile struvite uroliths may be prevented by use of acidifying, magnesium-restricted diets (Hill's Prescription Diet Canine c/d and others) or urine acidifiers.
- Monitor patients whose urine has been acidified for calcium oxalate crystalluria. Change management protocol if persistent calcium oxalate crystalluria develops.
- In patients at risk for both struvite and other urolith types, focus dietary prevention of metabolic uroliths (e.g., calcium oxalate, urate, cystine)— and UTI prevention for struvite uroliths.

POSSIBLE COMPLICATIONS

- Benefits and risks are associated with feeding low protein-high fat struvitolytic diets. Potential contraindications include those with (1) abnormal fluid accumulation, (2) chronic kidney disease, and (3) predispositions to pancreatitis (especially miniature schnauzers with hyperlipidemia).
- Urocystoliths may pass into and obstruct the urethra. Urethral obstruction can be managed by retrograde urohydropropulsion or lithotripsy.
- Dysuria may be minimized by antimicrobic treatment of bacterial UTIs and oral administration of anticholinergic drugs.
- Diet-associated polyuria will result in voiding increased urine volume. This may be associated with varying degrees of urinary incontinence in neutered female dogs with a predisposition to incontinence. Allow frequent opportunity to urinate to minimize inappropriate housesoiling.

EXPECTED COURSE AND PROGNOSIS

- The mean time for dissolution of all infection-induced urocystoliths was 3 months (range 2 weeks–7 months), whereas nephroliths took 6 months (range 2–10 months). The mean dissolution time of sterile struvite urocystoliths was 6 weeks (range 4–12 weeks).
- When feeding Hills Prescription Diet s/d, compliance with dietary recommendations is verified by a reduced concentration of urea in serum (approximately 10 mg/dL) and a low urine specific gravity (1.004–1.014).
- If uroliths increase or fail to decrease in size after approximately 6–8 weeks of appropriate management, alternative methods should be considered. Difficulty in inducing complete dissolution of uroliths should prompt consideration that (1) the wrong mineral component was identified, (2) the nucleus of the uroliths has a different mineral composition than other portions of the urolith, and (3) the owner is not complying with therapeutic recommendations. With the addition of high sodium dissolution foods lacking protein reduction, the proportion of calcium phosphate carbonate associated with infection-induced struvite has increased. Struvite uroliths with high percentages of calcium phosphate carbonate appear less amenable to medical dissolution.

MISCELLANEOUS

ASSOCIATED CONDITIONS

Any disease that predisposes to bacterial UTI.

AGE-RELATED FACTORS

Infection-induced struvite is the most common form of urolith in immature dogs. The uroliths develop as a result of microbial UTI.

PREGNANCY/FERTILITY/BREEDING

- The calculolytic foods are not designed to sustain pregnancy.

SYNONYMS

- Phosphate calculi.
- Infection stone.
- Urease stone.
- Triple-phosphate stone.

ABBREVIATIONS

- MAP = magnesium ammonium phosphate.
- UTI = urinary tract infection.

Suggested Reading

Osborne CA, Lulich JP, Bartges JW, et al. Canine and feline urolithiasis: relationship of etiopathogenesis to treatment and prevention. In: Osborne CA, Finco DR, eds., Canine and Feline Nephrology and Urology. Baltimore, MD: Williams & Wilkins, 1995, pp. 798–888.

Author Jody P. Lulich

Consulting Editor J.D. Foster

Acknowledgment The author and editors acknowledge the prior contribution of Carl A. Osborne and Eugene E. Nwaokorie.

Client Education Handout available online

UROLITHIASIS, URATE

BASICS

DEFINITION

Uroliths composed of uric acid, sodium urate, or ammonium urate.

PATHOPHYSIOLOGY

• Impaired conversion of uric acid to allantoin (see Figure 1) causes high concentration of uric acid in serum and urine. • Patients with portosystemic shunts may develop ammonium urate uroliths because of impaired hepatic metabolism of uric acid and ammonia.

GENETICS

Dalmatians have a breed predisposition to forming urate urolithiasis.

INCIDENCE/PREVALENCE

Approximately 5–8% of uroliths retrieved from dogs and cats.

SIGNALMENT

Species

Dog and cat.

Breed Predilections

Dalmatians, English bulldogs, Black Russian Terriers (due to mutation in SLC2A9 gene), and breeds predisposed to portosystemic shunts (e.g., Yorkshire terriers).

Mean Age and Range

• Mean age in patients without portosystemic shunts is 3.5 years (range 0.5 to >10 years).
• Mean age in patients with portosystemic shunts is <1 year (range 0.1 to >10 years).

Predominant Sex

• More common in male dogs without portosystemic shunts. • No sex predilection in dogs with portosystemic shunts or cats.

SIGNS

Historical Findings

Hematuria, dysuria, pollakiuria. Possible hepatic encephalopathy in patients with portosystemic shunts.

Physical Examination Findings

• Urethral obstruction. • Asymptomatic in some patients. • Stunted growth and copper-colored irises (cats) in patients with portosystemic shunts.

CAUSES

Rule out portosystemic shunt.

RISK FACTORS

• High purine intake (glandular meat).
• Persistent aciduria in a predisposed animal.

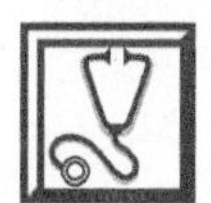

DIAGNOSIS

DIFFERENTIAL DIAGNOSIS

Other causes of lower or upper urinary tract disease.

CBC/BIOCHEMISTRY/URINALYSIS

• Aciduria, urate crystalluria, azotemia in patients with urinary outflow obstruction.
• Low BUN and microcytosis in patients with portosystemic shunts; reduced production of urea by the liver may mask hypoglycemia, hypoalbuminemia, and increased hepatic enzyme activities in patients with more severe hepatic dysfunction.

OTHER LABORATORY TESTS

• Liver function tests such as postprandial serum bile acids have abnormal results in patients with portosystemic shunts.
• Genetic testing for mutation in SLC2A9 gene, which encodes for a carrier protein necessary for uric acid metabolism, can be performed in dogs without portosystemic shunts who are at high risk or who have formed urate uroliths (performed at University of California Davis and Embark).

IMAGING

• Urate uroliths may be radiolucent; may need IV pyelogram to detect nephroliths or double contrast cystography to detect urocystoliths. Microhepatica in patients with portosystemic shunts. • Ultrasonography may reveal radiolucent uroliths. Patients with a portosystemic shunt may also have microhepatica, bilateral renomegaly, and a portosystemic vascular anomaly identified with ultrasound.

DIAGNOSTIC PROCEDURES

Liver biopsy; bile acids, blood ammonia; advanced imaging to identify portosystemic shunt.

PATHOLOGIC FINDINGS

In patients with portosystemic shunts, liver biopsy may reveal hepatic atrophy and/or dysplasia.

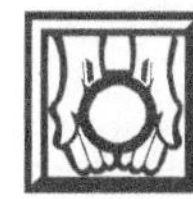

TREATMENT

APPROPRIATE HEALTH CARE

Urethral or ureteral obstruction may require inpatient treatment. Urate uroliths can be dissolved on outpatient basis.

NURSING CARE

Fluid therapy to correct dehydration.

ACTIVITY

Usually not restricted, except after surgery.

DIET

For dissolution and prevention, a high moisture, low-purine, urine-alkalinizing diet.

CLIENT EDUCATION

Recurrence of uroliths is possible. A plan to minimize recurrence should be developed.

SURGICAL CONSIDERATIONS

• Minimally invasive techniques such as cystoscopic stone basket removal, percutaneous cystolithotomy or lithotripsy are preferred over cystotomy, urethrotomy, and nephrotomy to remove uroliths. • Portosystemic shunt ligation.

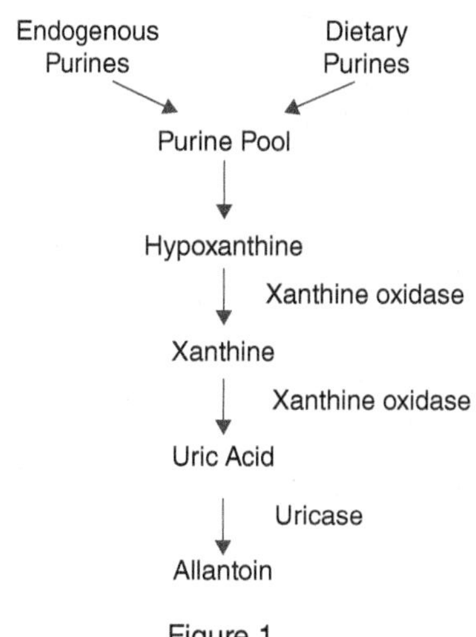

Figure 1.

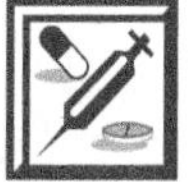

MEDICATIONS

DRUG(S) OF CHOICE

Allopurinol 15 mg/kg PO q12h, a xanthine oxidase inhibitor, for dissolution (see Figure 2).

CONTRAINDICATIONS

Glucocorticoids and other immunosuppressive drugs may promote hyperuricosuria.

PRECAUTIONS

Allopurinol is contraindicated in animals with renal failure and is not effective in animals with portosystemic shunts.

POSSIBLE INTERACTIONS

Skin eruption with use of allopurinol and ampicillin.

FOLLOW-UP

PATIENT MONITORING

See Figure 3.

PREVENTION/AVOIDANCE

• High-moisture, low-purine, urine-alkalinizing diet. • Some dogs require allopurinol administration (5.0–7.5 mg/kg PO q12h).
• Low uric acid excreting Dalmatians (those without SLC2A9 mutation) should be at lower risk due to decreased urinary uric acid excretion.

POSSIBLE COMPLICATIONS

• Urethral obstruction. • Uroliths likely to recur if no preventive measures.

EXPECTED COURSE AND PROGNOSIS

• Medical dissolution takes an average of 4 weeks, if there is good compliance.
• Medical dissolution usually not successful with portosystemic shunt.

UROLITHIASIS, URATE (CONTINUED)

MISCELLANEOUS

ASSOCIATED CONDITIONS

Portosystemic shunt.

PREGNANCY/FERTILITY/BREEDING

Low-protein/purine diet is not recommended for pregnant or lactating animals.

Suggested Reading

Bartges JW, Osborne CA, Felice LJ. Canine xanthine uroliths: Risk factor management. In: Kirk RW, Bonagura JD, eds., Current Veterinary Therapy XI. Philadelphia, PA: Saunders, 1992, pp. 900–905.

Osborne CA, Lulich JP, Thumchai R, et al. Diagnosis, medical treatment, and prognosis of feline urolithiasis. Vet Clin North Am Small Anim Pract 1996, 26:589–628.

Author Joseph W. Bartges

Consulting Editor J.D.Foster

Client Education Handout available online

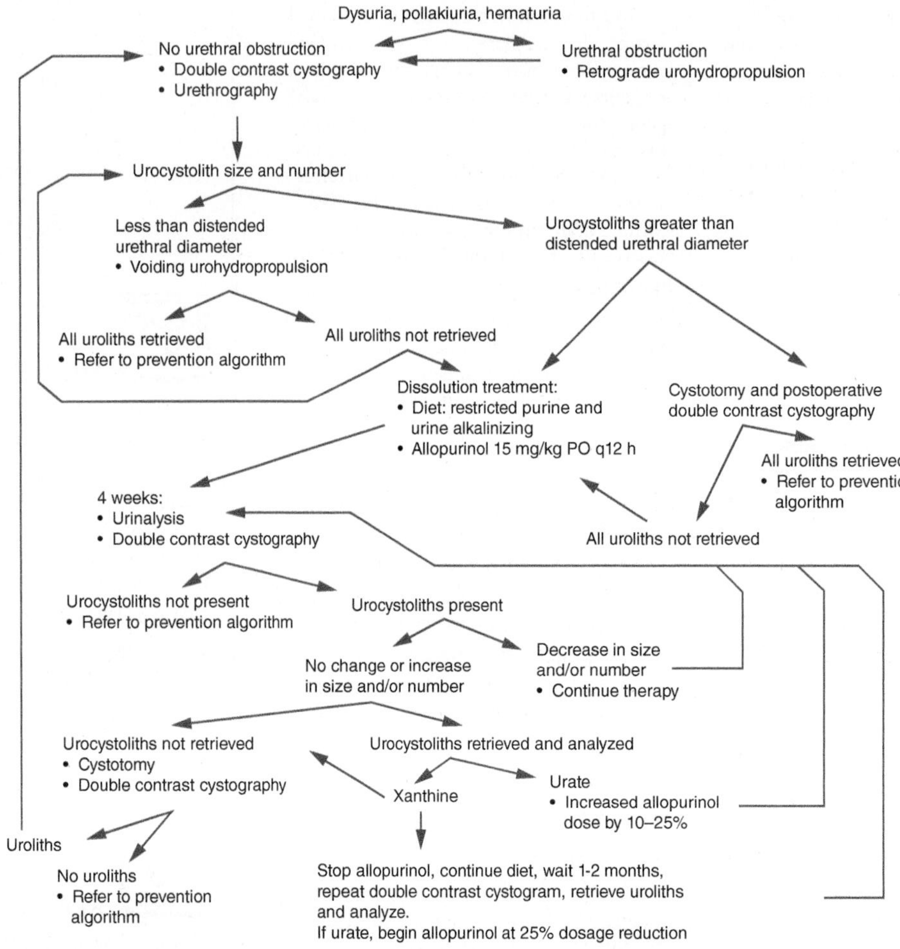

Dysuria, pollakiuria, hematuria

No urethral obstruction
- Double contrast cystography
- Urethrography

Urethral obstruction
- Retrograde urohydropropulsion

Urocystolith size and number

Less than distended urethral diameter
- Voiding urohydropropulsion

Urocystoliths greater than distended urethral diameter

All uroliths retrieved
- Refer to prevention algorithm

All uroliths not retrieved

Dissolution treatment:
- Diet: restricted purine and urine alkalinizing
- Allopurinol 15 mg/kg PO q12 h

Cystotomy and postoperative double contrast cystography

All uroliths retrieved
- Refer to prevention algorithm

All uroliths not retrieved

4 weeks:
- Urinalysis
- Double contrast cystography

Urocystoliths not present
- Refer to prevention algorithm

Urocystoliths present

No change or increase in size and/or number

Decrease in size and/or number
- Continue therapy

Urocystoliths not retrieved
- Cystotomy
- Double contrast cystography

Urocystoliths retrieved and analyzed

Xanthine

Urate
- Increased allopurinol dose by 10–25%

Uroliths

No uroliths
- Refer to prevention algorithm

Stop allopurinol, continue diet, wait 1-2 months, repeat double contrast cystogram, retrieve uroliths and analyze.
If urate, begin allopurinol at 25% dosage reduction

Figure 2.
Algorithm for treatment of urate urocystolithiasis.

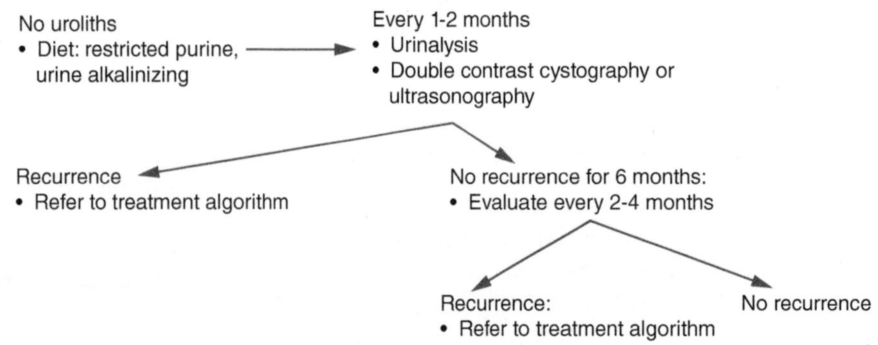

Figure 3.
Algorithm for prevention of urate urocystolithiasis.

UROLITHIASIS, XANTHINE

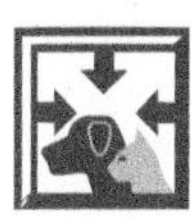

BASICS

OVERVIEW

- Xanthine, a product of purine degradation, is converted to uric acid by xanthine oxidase. Naturally occurring or drug-induced impairment of xanthine oxidase results in hyperxanthinemia and xanthinuria.
- Naturally occurring xanthinuria is likely caused by a familial or congenital defect in xanthine oxidase activity. In cavalier King Charles spaniels, an autosomal recessive mode of inheritance has been found.
- Acquired xanthinuria is a complication of allopurinol therapy. High-purine diets increase the risk of xanthinuria in these patients.
- Xanthine is the least soluble purine excreted in urine.

SIGNALMENT

- Dog and cat. Naturally occurring xanthinuria is more common in cats.
- Naturally occurring xanthinuria and xanthine uroliths have occurred in young cavalier King Charles spaniels.
- Cats—adult males (66%) and females (33%) (mean age 3.3 years; range 2 months–13 years). Most common in the domestic shorthair and domestic longhair breeds.

SIGNS

- Dependent on stone location, size, and number; may be asymptomatic.
- Pollakiuria, dysuria, hematuria, and voiding of small, smooth, yellow uroliths. Complete outflow obstruction may result in azotemia.
- Nephroliths may be associated with hydronephrosis and renal insufficiency.

CAUSES & RISK FACTORS

- Xanthinuria.
- Genetic inheritance in some breeds.
- Cats—uroliths often recur unless prophylactic therapy is initiated.
- Approximately 11% of cats have reoccurrence of xanthine uroliths. Urolith formation enhanced by aciduria, highly concentrated urine, and incomplete and infrequent micturition.
- In animals given excessive allopurinol, xanthinuria is enhanced by failure to appropriately restrict dietary purine precursors.

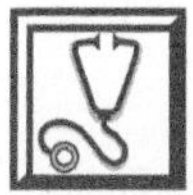

DIAGNOSIS

DIFFERENTIAL DIAGNOSIS

- Other causes of pollakiuria, dysuria, hematuria, or outflow obstruction.
- Differentiate from other urolith types by urinalysis, radiography, and quantitative stone analysis.

CBC/BIOCHEMISTRY/URINALYSIS

Xanthine crystals cannot be distinguished from urate by light microscopy; both are usually yellow-brown and may form varying sized spherules.

OTHER LABORATORY TESTS

- Infrared spectroscopy, X-ray diffraction, or other quantitative techniques are required to differentiate xanthine from ammonium urate, sodium urate, and uric acid.
- High-pressure liquid chromatography of urine to detect xanthine, hypoxanthine, and other purine metabolites.
- Genetic testing for xanthinuria type 2a, which involves a mutation in molybdenum cofactor sulfurase (performed at University of Minnesota).

IMAGING

- Radiography—similar density to soft tissue; stones cannot be reliably detected.
- Ultrasonography, double contrast cystography, and IV urography aid in detecting uroliths and their location.

OTHER DIAGNOSTIC PROCEDURES

- May be detected by urethrocystoscopy.
- Uroliths may be retrieved by aspiration via a transurethral catheter or voiding urohydropropulsion.

TREATMENT

- Medical dissolution protocols for xanthine uroliths have not been developed.
- Remove small urocystoliths by voiding urohydropropulsion.
- Minimally invasive surgery can remove larger active uroliths from the lower urinary tract.
- Minimize further growth of existing uroliths by reducing dietary risk factors. Discontinue or reduce allopurinol dosages.
- Consider canned renal-failure diets to increase urine volume, minimize purine precursors, and prevent aciduria in cats.
- Consider perineal urethrostomy for recurrent urethral obstruction in male cats.

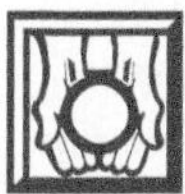

MEDICATIONS

DRUG(S) OF CHOICE

Urine Alkalinizers

- Consider in aciduric patients despite dietary therapy.
- Potassium citrate or sodium bicarbonate—target urine pH of 7.0–7.5.

Allopurinol

- Adjust dosage of allopurinol in context of urine concentration of uric acid, and quantity of dietary purines (see Urolithiasis, Urate).
- Allopurinol-induced uroliths may dissolve by discontinuing allopurinol therapy and feeding a low-purine diet.

CONTRAINDICATIONS/POSSIBLE INTERACTIONS

Do not use allopurinol to treat naturally occurring xanthine uroliths.

FOLLOW-UP

- Monitor dissolution every 30 days by urinalysis, contrast radiography, or ultrasonography.
- Recurrence does not occur in all patients.

MISCELLANEOUS

ASSOCIATED CONDITIONS

- Urate urolithiasis.
- Nephrolithiasis.

SEE ALSO

- Crystalluria.
- Urolithiasis, Urate.

Suggested Reading

Bartges JW, Osborne CA, Felice LJ. Canine xanthine uroliths: risk factor management. In: Kirk RW, Bonagura JD, eds., Current Veterinary Therapy XI. Philadelphia, PA: Saunders, 1992, pp. 900–905.

Kucera J, Bulkova T, Rychlat R, Jahn P. Bilateral xanthine nephrolithiasis in a dog. J Small Anim Pract 1997, 38(7):302–305.

Osborne CA, Lulich JP, Lekcharoensuk C, et al. Feline xanthine urolithiasis: a newly recognized cause of feline lower urinary tract disease. In: Proceedings 21st Annual ACVIM Forum, Charlotte, North Carolina, 2003, pp. 781–782.

Tsuchida S, Kagi A, Koyama H. Xanthine urolithiasis in a cat: a case report and evaluation of a candidate gene for xanthine dehydrogenase. J Feline Med Surg 2007, 9:505–508.

Author Joseph W. Bartges

Consulting Editor J.D. Foster

Acknowledgment The author and editors acknowledge the prior contribution of Carl A. Osborne.

UTERINE INERTIA

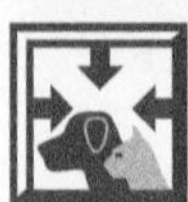

BASICS

OVERVIEW

Failure to expel fetuses of normal size, presentation and posture through a normal birth canal at the normal end of gestation.

Primary Uterine Inertia

- Multifactorial—failure to establish a normal, progressive myometrial contraction pattern.
- Seen in bitches with fewer than 3 puppies in the litter—failure to initiate parturition at term.
- Occurs with large litter sizes—overstretching of the uterus.

Secondary Uterine Inertia

- Occurs following initiation of parturition where some or all of the litter is not expelled.
- Can be secondary to dystocia or large litter.

SIGNALMENT

Queens and bitches of any breed and age.

SIGNS

- Primary—failure to initiate parturition at the end of gestation; dam is typically asymptomatic except for vaginal discharge (uteroverdin) following placental separation.
- Secondary—uterine contractions cease despite normal contractions initially; may deliver part of litter and then stop. Some primiparous queens may initiate parturition, and then pause for as long as 48 hours prior to resuming birth.

U

CAUSES & RISK FACTORS

- Primary—inadequate stimulation from fetuses to initiate cascade of events leading to parturition (small litters); abnormal or inadequate hormones or receptors; systemic disease; obesity; tocolytic administration; hypocalcemia; uterine infection; inadequate or unbalanced nutrition.
- Secondary—follows exhaustion of uterine muscle during normal parturition of large litters; occurs in bitches fed diet with poor calcium:phosphorus ratio; occurs during dystocia after prolonged periods of uterine contraction and eventual uterine fatigue; can occur with uterine torsion and trauma.

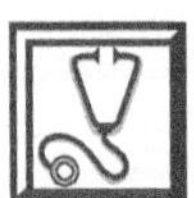

DIAGNOSIS

DIFFERENTIAL DIAGNOSIS

- Primary—inaccurate predicted parturition date; false pregnancy; nonviable pregnancy.
- Secondary—normal parturition; parturition already complete.

CBC/BIOCHEMISTRY/URINALYSIS

- Normocytic, normochromic anemia (normal in pregnancy).
- Low total calcium or low ionized calcium (iCa).
- Hypoglycemia.

OTHER LABORATORY TESTS

Serum progesterone <2 ng/mL for 48 hours prior to parturition in most cases.

IMAGING

- Ultrasonography findings—fetal heart rates sustained <160–170 bpm indicate stress and need for intervention; separation of the placenta from the uterus—need for immediate intervention to optimize fetal survival.
- Radiographic findings—evaluate for presence; size; and abnormalities of presentation, position, and posture of fetus(es).

DIAGNOSTIC PROCEDURES

Digital vaginal examination to evaluate for presence of fetus within caudal birth canal and abnormal anatomy causing narrowed birth canal.

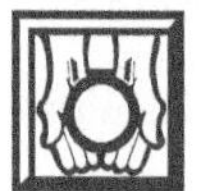

TREATMENT

- Inpatient—if live fetus(es) are present and fetal stress is documented, cesarean section advisable to optimize fetal survival; surgery is the only option for primary uterine inertia when fetal survival is desired.
- Fluid therapy as needed to support hydration and vascular volume.
- Medical—for secondary uterine inertia with nonobstructive dystocia and no evidence of fetal distress.

MEDICATIONS

DRUG(S) OF CHOICE

- 10% calcium gluconate 1 mL/5 kg SC q4–6h or 0.2 mL/kg IV slowly.
- 2.5–5% dextrose-containing fluids if hypoglycemic (can also give bolus of dextrose 0.5 g/kg, diluted to 10% or lower, IV).
- Oxytocin typically not effective as sole treatment—give 15–30 minutes after calcium administration at 0.5–4 IU/bitch SC or IM or 0.5–1 IU/queen SC or IM. Do not administer to animals with obstructive dystocia.

CONTRAINDICATIONS/POSSIBLE INTERACTIONS

- Bradycardia with calcium treatment; monitor electrocardiogram and discontinue treatment if noted.
- Contractions may resume with calcium treatment and rehydration alone.
- Delaying surgery while pursuing medical management may decrease fetal survival rate.
- Uterine rupture (rare).

FOLLOW-UP

PATIENT MONITORING

- Serial assessment of blood iCa concentration in hypocalcemic cases (see Eclampsia).
- Monitor dam's temperature and character of vaginal discharge daily for 5–7 days following dystocia or cesarean section—concern for metritis.

PREVENTION/AVOIDANCE

- Consider elective cesarean section in cases of very small or vary large litters.
- Breed females in good body condition and monitor nutrition during pregnancy.
- Utilize tocodynamometry (Veterinary Perinatal Specialties, Wheatridge, CO) to identify and manage secondary uterine inertia.
- Remove females with repeated primary uterine inertia from breeding stock.

POSSIBLE COMPLICATIONS

- Fetal death if too much time elapses before intervention.
- Primary inertia thought to be heritable in some breeds of dogs and cats.

EXPECTED COURSE AND PROGNOSIS

- Primary uterine inertia—idiopathic cases may recur on subsequent pregnancies.
- Secondary uterine inertia—will not necessarily recur if due to fetal factors such as large litter size, poor nutrition, or dystocia due to malpresentation.

MISCELLANEOUS

SEE ALSO

- Dystocia.
- Eclampsia.

ABBREVIATIONS

- iCa = ionized calcium.

INTERNET RESOURCES

http://whelpwise.com/ (tocodynamometry)

Suggested Reading

Pretzer SD. Medical management of canine and feline dystocia. Theriogenology 2008, 70:332–336.

Author Milan Hess
Consulting Editor Erin E. Runcan

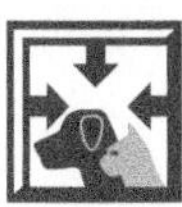

BASICS

OVERVIEW

- Rare tumors arising from the uterine smooth muscle and epithelial tissues.
- Comprise 0.3–0.4% of tumors in dogs and 0.2–1.5% in cats.
- Dogs—usually benign; leiomyomas, 85%–90%; leiomyosarcoma, 10%; other types (e.g., carcinoma, fibroma, fibrosarcoma, lipoma, extramedullary plasma cell tumor, mast cell tumor, hemangiosarcoma) rare.
- Cats—usually malignant (adenocarcinoma); include leiomyoma, leiomyosarcoma, fibrosarcoma, fibroma, lipoma, and Mullerian tumor (adenosarcoma).
- Metastasis—may occur with malignant forms.

SIGNALMENT

- Dog and cat.
- No breed predilection reported.
- Middle-aged to older animals usually affected.
- Birt-Hogg-Dube syndrome in German shepherd dogs has been associated with uterine leiomyomas, renal cystadenocarcinomas, and nodular dermatofibrosis.

SIGNS

- Dogs—often clinically silent and discovered incidentally; vaginal discharge; pyometra, infertility; abdominal organ compression or secondary metastatic signs (site specific).
- Cats—vaginal discharge (may be hemorrhagic); abnormal estrous cycles; polyuria; polydipsia; vomiting; abdominal distention, infertility, uterine prolapse; signs related to metastatic disease (site specific).

CAUSES & RISK FACTORS

- Intact sexual status (hormonal influence).
- Nulliparous bitches have an increased risk of uterine pathology.
- Mutated *BHD* gene in German shepherd dogs.

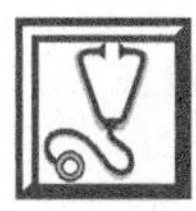

DIAGNOSIS

DIFFERENTIAL DIAGNOSIS

- Pyometra.
- Endometriosis.
- Other mid-caudal abdominal masses.

CBC/BIOCHEMISTRY/URINALYSIS

No specific abnormalities.

OTHER LABORATORY TESTS

N/A

IMAGING

- Abdominal radiography—may detect a mid-caudal abdominal mass.
- Thoracic radiography—recommended; assess for distant pulmonary metastasis.
- Ultrasonography—may reveal uterine mass, masses in uterine horns may be difficult to definitely identify at uterine.
- Abdominal CT/MRI—further delineation of mass, assess for metastatic disease.

DIAGNOSTIC PROCEDURES

- Cytologic evaluation—however, tumors might be poorly exfoliative, especially if mesenchymal in origin; improved cytologic yield with epithelial malignancies (carcinoma).
- Imaging unable to differentiate between histologic subtypes.
- Histopathologic examination—necessary for definitive diagnosis.

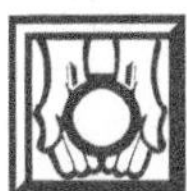

TREATMENT

Ovariohysterectomy—treatment of choice.

MEDICATIONS

DRUG(S) OF CHOICE

Doxorubicin, cisplatin, carboplatin, epirubicin—rational choices for palliation of malignant or metastatic disease.

CONTRAINDICATIONS/POSSIBLE INTERACTIONS

- Doxorubicin—carefully monitor patients with underlying cardiac disease; consider pretreatment and serial echocardiograms and ECG.
- Cisplatin—do not use in dogs with preexisting renal disease; do not use without appropriate and concurrent diuresis; do not use in cats (fatal).
- Chemotherapy may be toxic; seek advice if unfamiliar with these agents.

FOLLOW-UP

PATIENT MONITORING

- Malignant—consider thoracic radiographs and abdominal ultrasonography every 3 months.
- CBC, biochemical profile, and urinalysis (if using cisplatin)—perform before each chemotherapy treatment.

EXPECTED COURSE AND PROGNOSIS

Prognosis—excellent (cure) if benign; guarded if malignant; poor if metastases present; after chemotherapy, unknown.

MISCELLANEOUS

ASSOCIATED CONDITIONS

BHD syndrome in German shepherd dogs has been associated with uterine leiomyomas.

ABBREVIATIONS

- BHD = Birt-Hogg-Dube.

Suggested Reading

Morrison WB. Cancers of the reproductive tract. In: Morrison WB, ed., Cancer in Dogs and Cats: Medical and Surgical Management. Jackson, WY: Teton NewMedia, 2002, pp. 555–564.

Saba CF, Lawrence JA. Tumors of the female reproductive system. In: Withrow SJ, MacEwen EG, eds., Small Animal Clinical Oncology, 5th ed. Philadelphia, PA: Saunders, 2013, pp. 532–537.

Schlafer, DH. Disease of the canine uterus. Reprod Domest Anim 2012, 47(Suppl 6):318–322.

Author Heather M. Wilson-Robles

Consulting Editor Timothy M. Fan

Acknowledgment The author and editors acknowledge the prior contribution of Renee Al-Sarraf.

UVEAL MELANOMA—CATS

BASICS

OVERVIEW

- Also called feline diffuse iris melanoma.
- The most common intraocular tumor in cats.
- Usually arise from the anterior iridal surface with extension to the ciliary body and choroid.
- Tend to be flat and diffuse, not nodular (unlike intraocular melanomas in dogs).
- Initially has a benign clinical and histologic appearance.
- Unique feature—may develop metastatic disease up to several years later.
- Metastatic rate may be 8.1–63%.
- Secondary glaucoma may increase the risk for metastasis.

SIGNALMENT

- No sex or breed predisposition.
- Average age is 9.5 years, although can affect any adult cat.

SIGNS

Historical Findings

- Iris color change.
- Secondary glaucoma leading to mydriasis or buphthalmia, resulting in blindness.

Physical Examination Findings

- Iris surface—thickened, irregular, usually pigmented, though can be nonpigmented.
- Lesions—focal to diffuse; usually flat; slowly progressive; may involve one or both eyes.
- Advanced disease—often see pigmented tumor cells in the aqueous; homogeneously thickened iris, black, velvety appearance.
- May note drainage angle infiltration, which may result in secondary glaucoma.

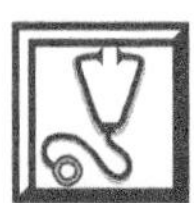

DIAGNOSIS

DIFFERENTIAL DIAGNOSIS

- Freckles (nevi) on the surface of the iris that do not appear to change over time—may be benign pigmented lesions; more likely melanocytoma, a benign lesion.
- Heterochromia irides—congenital, nonprogressive alteration in iridal pigmentation.
- Diffuse iridal color change that results from chronic anterior uveitis. Differs from uveal melanoma by the history of chronic anterior uveitis.
- Iris atrophy—the anterior iris stroma is lost, increasing visualization of the heavily pigmented posterior iris tissue. Iris thinning is seen as full-thickness holes in the iris or as retroillumination defects in the iris when light is bounced off the tapetum back through the iris.
- Limbal melanomas—benign behavior; usually focal, superiorly located, flat to slightly raised limbal masses that do not invade the uveal tract unless they are very large.

CBC/BIOCHEMISTRY/URINALYSIS

Normal

IMAGING

- Thoracic radiographs and abdominal ultrasonography for extensive lesions—help determine presence and extent of metastatic disease.
- Recommended presurgically and every 6 months after the diagnosis if histopathologic diagnosis indicates extensive disease.

DIAGNOSTIC PROCEDURES

- Complete ophthalmic examination, including tonometry and gonioscopy.
- Iridal biopsy—may be performed, not beneficial for staging the disease.
- Melanocytes in the iridocorneal angle and ciliary vessels suggest metastatis may have occurred, but these may not be evident until years later.

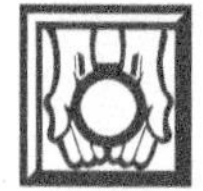

TREATMENT

- Varies with age of cat, extent and speed of progression, doctor's preference, and client's level of concern about the potential for malignancy.
- Old cat with slow progression—consider only periodic examinations and serial photography to monitor the progress of the lesion(s).
- Younger cat with rapidly progressive disease—consider enucleation.
- Small, isolated, freckle-like lesions have been apparently successfully treated with laser (diode) photoablation, although controlled or long-term follow-up studies are lacking.
- Mild to moderate diffuse iridal involvement—most ophthalmologists prefer a conservative approach of periodic examinations and serial photography to monitor the growth progress of the lesion(s). Enucleation is an alternative if progression can be documented or the owner is highly concerned about the potential for malignancy.
- Extensive iridal involvement resulting in changes in pupil shape or mobility, extra-iridal extension, invasion into the drainage angle, or secondary glaucoma—enucleation is suggested.
- Cats with iridal thickening and iridocorneal angle involvement, with and without glaucoma, however, had similar survival times when compared with unaffected age-matched control cats.
- Advanced lesions consisting of infiltrative iris involvement including the posterior epithelium and ciliary body had decreased survival times, presumably as a result of metastatic disease.

MEDICATIONS

DRUG(S) OF CHOICE

N/A

FOLLOW-UP

PATIENT MONITORING

- Intraocular pressure (IOP)—quarterly monitoring if surgical options are declined; mild IOP elevation may be treated with oral or topical carbonic anhydrase inhibitors (e.g., dorzolamide or brinzolamide at 1 drop to affected eye q8h, or methazolamide at approximately 6.25 mg per cat PO q12–24h); secondary glaucoma due to melanoma is best controlled by enucleation.
- Common metastasis sites—liver, lungs, regional lymph nodes; monitor periodically.

EXPECTED COURSE AND PROGNOSIS

- One long-term study shows that patients with early iris melanoma have no increased risk of life-threatening metastasis compared to controls, but patients with advanced lesions have dramatically shortened survival times.
- Lesions—focal, multifocal to diffuse; usually flat; pigmentation over months to years (i.e., variable); may involve one or both eyes.
- Advanced disease—often see pigmented tumor cells in the aqueous; homogeneously thickened iris causing abnormal pupil shape and change in pupil mobility.
- Prognosis—guarded, even with enucleation; metastasis may not become apparent for several years or may be diagnosed on necropsy.

MISCELLANEOUS

SYNONYMS

- Feline diffuse iris melanoma.
- Iris melanoma.

ABBREVIATIONS

- IOP = intraocular pressure.

Suggested Reading

Dubielzig RR. Ocular neoplasia in small animals. Vet Clin North Am Small Anim Pract 1990, 20:837–848.

Schaffer EH, Gordon S. Feline ocular melanoma. Clinical and pathologico-anatomic findings in 37 cases. Tierarztl Prax 1993, 21(3):255–264.

Author Kathern E. Myrna

Consulting Editor Kathern E. Myrna

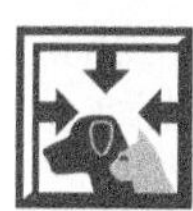

BASICS

OVERVIEW

• Melanomas of anterior uvea (e.g., iris and ciliary body) and posterior uvea (choroid).
• Most common primary intraocular neoplasm in dogs.
• Usually benign and unilateral; often destructive to the eye but also can be very slow-growing.
• Most often affects anterior uvea. In a retrospective study of 1842 enucleated eyes with uveal melanoma, 79.2% were benign and 20.8% malignant.
• Anterior uveal—4% rate of vascular metastasis to lungs and viscera, but rare for malignant uveal melanoma to metastasize.
• Choroidal—rarely metastasize.

SIGNALMENT

• No breed or sex predilection.
• Anterior uveal—average age 8–10 years.
• Choroidal melanoma—average age 6.5 years.
• Range—2 months–17 years.

SIGNS

Anterior Uveal

• Pigmented scleral or corneal mass.
• Pigmented mass visible in anterior chamber or posterior to pupillary margin.
• Irregular pupil.
• Uveitis.
• Glaucoma.
• Hyphema.
• No vision loss—unless mass obstructs pupil or glaucoma has developed.

Choroidal

• Often missed because of tumor location; usually incidental finding.
• Posterior segment mass on funduscopy.
• Very slow-growing; rarely require enucleation.
• Rare.

CAUSES & RISK FACTORS

• Idiopathic.
• Potential transformation of flat, pigmented iris freckles into melanomas.
• Labrador retrievers—presumed autosomal recessive inheritance.

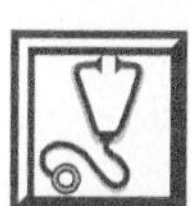

DIAGNOSIS

DIFFERENTIAL DIAGNOSIS

• Non-neoplastic uveal proliferations—iris freckles are not raised.
• Diffuse iris hyperpigmentation secondary to chronic uveitis, particularly in golden retrievers (golden retriever pigmentary uveitis) and boxers.
• Ocular melanosis (Cairn terriers).
• Uveal cysts—transilluminate and move freely within the eye, unlike melanomas.
• Granulomatous masses.
• Iris bombé.
• Ocular perforation with uveal prolapse.
• Other ocular neoplastic conditions, especially conjunctival melanoma, which could be misinterpreted as extrascleral extension of uveal melanoma. Conjunctival melanoma is usually malignant and aggressive in dogs.
• Outward scrolling of pupillary margin due to uveitis (ectropion uvea).

CBC/BIOCHEMISTRY/URINALYSIS

Usually normal.

OTHER LABORATORY TESTS

N/A

IMAGING

Ocular ultrasonography—may help determine extent of mass.

DIAGNOSTIC PROCEDURES

• Slit-lamp biomicroscopy—determine size and location of mass.
• Transillumination of mass.
• Tonometry.
• Indirect ophthalmoscopy—with or without concomitant scleral indentation.
• Gonioscopy—evaluate drainage angle for tumor extension.
• Ocular ultrasonography—if cornea opaque and cannot visualize deeper ocular structures, or suspect ciliary body mass hidden by iris.

PATHOLOGIC FINDINGS

• Restricted to enucleated globe; biopsy not practical in most patients.
• Two cell types usually seen—plump cells filled with melanin, spindle cells.
• Mitotic index—most reliable criterion for malignancy:
  ○ <2 mitotic figures per 10 HPF: benign.
  ○ 4 mitotic figures per 10 HPF: clinically malignant tumors.
• Veterinary ocular pathologist should evaluate globe.

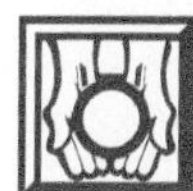

TREATMENT

• Usually benign, may opt to monitor q3–6 months.
• Young Labrador retrievers—aggressive growth, need surgery.
• Counsel client about enucleation; surgery often causes client emotional distress:
  ○ Emphasize unilateral condition, sparing of fellow eye, and that one-eyed animals function very well.
• Indications for enucleation—rapid size increase, eye cannot be salvaged, mass spread diffusely within eye, visual function significantly impaired, extraocular invasion, secondary complications (e.g., glaucoma, pain, hemorrhage).
• Enucleation—use gentle surgical technique to prevent showering of tumor cells into circulation, avoid tension on optic chiasm (could blind fellow eye), exenterate entire orbital contents if extrascleral extension.
• Sector iridectomy for discrete small masses—infrequently used.
• Laser treatment of small iris tumor.
• Melanoma vaccine efficacy unknown; likely ineffective without enucleation. Consider vaccine if malignant melanoma is present, to try to prevent metastasis.

MEDICATIONS

DRUG(S) OF CHOICE

Reseveratrol, a potent antioxidant derived from grapes, inhibited uveal tumor growth of uveal melanoma *in vitro*, but grape skins may be toxic to dogs. Grapeseed extract is a safe alternative that may support ocular health of affected dogs.

CONTRAINDICATIONS/POSSIBLE INTERACTIONS

N/A

FOLLOW-UP

• Postoperative thoracic and abdominal radiography or ultrasonography—at 6 and 12 months if mitotic index is high or patient has extrascleral, vascular, or optic nerve extension.
• Evaluate enucleation site for tumor recurrence.

MISCELLANEOUS

Suggested Reading

Cook CS, Wilkie DA. Treatment of presumed iris melanoma in dogs by diode laser photocoagulation: 23 cases. Vet Ophthalmol 1999, 2:217–225.
Dubielzig RR. Tumors of the canine globe. World Small Animal Veterinary Association World Congress Proceedings, 2011.
Wilcock BP, Peiffer RL. Morphology and behavior of primary ocular melanomas in 91 dogs. Vet Pathol 1986, 23:418–424.

Author Terri L. McCalla
Consulting Editor Kathern E. Myrna

U

UVEODERMATOLOGIC SYNDROME (VKH)

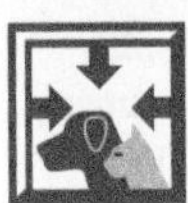

BASICS

OVERVIEW

- Rare canine syndrome similar to Vogt–Koyanagi–Harada (VKH) in humans.
- Chronic granulomatous inflammatory condition of unknown etiology.
- Affects the meninges, eyes then skin.
- Clinical signs reflect melanin as the target of inflammation.

PATHOPHYSIOLOGY

Likely an autoimmune process against antigenic components of melanocytes, suspected tyrosinase and related proteins; involves T-cells and macrophages for skin lesions and B-cells and macrophages for ocular lesions.

SYSTEMS AFFECTED

- Ophthalmic.
- Skin/exocrine.
- Nervous (rarely).

SIGNALMENT

- Akita, Samoyed, Siberian husky, Alaskan Malamute, old English sheepdog, and chow chow predisposed.
- Other breeds and mixed breeds reported.
- Suspected heritability: canine leukocyte antigen DLA-DQA1*00201 has been associated with an increased risk for uveodermatological syndrome.
- No sex predilection.
- Mean age of onset 6 months–6 years.

U

SIGNS

- Ophthalmic signs almost always precede dermatologic signs.
- Sudden-onset uveitis (photophobia, blepharospasm, conjunctival inflammation, pain).
- Secondary changes include glaucoma, cataracts, bullous retinal detachment, and progression to blindness.
- Unilateral uveitis may be seen in dogs with heterochromic irides.
- Concurrent or subsequent leukoderma of the nose, lips, and eyelids.
- Depigmented nasal planum may develop crusting and ulceration.
- Concurrent or subsequent striking leukotrichia of the muzzle and periorbital regions.
- Footpads, scrotum, vulva, anus, and oral cavity (hard palate) may also depigment.
- Neurologic symptoms (meningoencephalitis,) possible, but very rare.

CAUSES & RISK FACTORS

- Exact cause is unknown.
- Most likely an inherited autoimmune disorder.
- Skin trauma or infectious agent (e.g., virus) are possible triggers.
- Exposure to sunlight can exacerbate the symptoms.

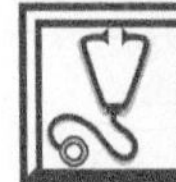

DIAGNOSIS

DIFFERENTIAL DIAGNOSIS

- Pemphigus foliaceus/erythematosus.
- Discoid/systemic lupus erythematosus.
- Mucocutaneous pyoderma (severe).
- Vitiligo.
- Neoplasia—epitheliotropic lymphoma.
- Numerous inflammatory and infectious dermatoses can cause depigmentation.
- Ocular—any cause of uveitis or glaucoma including neoplasia, trauma, infection and idiopathic causes.

CBC/BIOCHEMISTRY/URINALYSIS

Normal

OTHER LABORATORY TESTS

ANA—negative.

DIAGNOSTIC PROCEDURES

- Skin biopsy necessary for diagnosis, especially when correlated with ocular disease.
- Examination by veterinary ophthalmologist strongly recommended.

PATHOLOGIC FINDINGS

Lichenoid to interface dermatosis consisting of mostly histiocytic inflammation; macrophages containing granular melanin pigment; pigmentary incontinence.

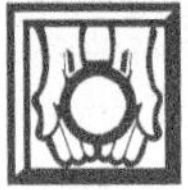

TREATMENT

- Aggressive and rapid initiation of immunosuppressive therapy required to prevent formation of posterior synechiae and secondary glaucoma, cataracts, or blindness.
- Retinal exams are the most important means of monitoring progress; improvement in dermatologic lesions may not reflect continued retinal pathology.
- Bilateral enucleation can improve patient comfort and attitude when eye condition worsens and medical treatment is unsuccessful.
- Management by a veterinary ophthalmologist is strongly recommended.

MEDICATIONS

DRUG(S) OF CHOICE

- Initial high doses of prednisone 1.1–2.2 mg/kg PO q12–24h.
- Cases may improve with use of prednisone alone, but delaying aggressive therapy risks irreversible progression of disease: concurrent treatment options should include:
    - Azathioprine 1.5–2.5 mg/kg PO q24h in resistant cases; the dosage and frequency should be tapered to q48h for maintenance of remission.
    - Doxycycline 10 mg/kg q24h with niacinamide (250 mg patients <10 kg; 500 mg patients >10 kg q24h).
    - Cyclosporine (modified) 5 mg/kg PO q24h; the dosage and frequency may be tapered for maintenance of remission.
- Topical or subconjunctival steroids and cycloplegics may be indicated if anterior uveitis is present.

FOLLOW-UP

PATIENT MONITORING

- Weekly retinal examinations and lab work (based on medications prescribed). Dermatologic lesions may not mirror improvement in retinal lesions.
- Tapering of drugs should be based on improvement of ocular lesions.
- Severe opportunistic infections may occur with long-term use of combination immunosuppressive agents.

EXPECTED COURSE AND PROGNOSIS

- Generally good for dermatologic symptoms.
- Guarded to poor for vision unless treatment is quickly instituted and is effective.
- Some breeds (e.g., Akita or Siberian husky) may respond more poorly to treatment.

MISCELLANEOUS

SEE ALSO

- Dermatoses, Depigmenting Disorders.
- Lupus Erythematosus, Cutaneous (Discoid).
- Lupus Erythematosus, Systemic (SLE).
- Lymphoma, Cutaneous Epitheliotropic.
- Pemphigus.

ABBREVIATIONS

- ANA = antinuclear antibody.
- VKH = Vogt–Koyanagi–Harada syndrome.

INTERNET RESOURCES

http://www.veterinarypartner.com/Content.plx?P=A&A=1714&S=0&EVetID=3001459

Suggested Reading

Zarfoss MK, Tusler CA, Kass PH, et al. Clinical findings and outcomes for dogs with uveodermatologic syndrome. J Am Vet Med Assoc 2018, 252:1263–1271.

Authors Austin Richman and W. Dunbar Gram

Consulting Editor Alexander H. Werner Resnick

VAGINAL DISCHARGE

BASICS

DEFINITION

Any substance emanating through the vulvar labia.

PATHOPHYSIOLOGY

- Dependent on underlying cause of vaginal discharge.
- Discharge may originate from uterus, vagina, vestibule, clitoris, clitoral sinus, perivulvar dermis, or urinary tract.

SYSTEMS AFFECTED

- Reproductive.
- Renal.
- Skin.
- Urinary.

INCIDENCE/PREVALENCE

- Unknown as there are many causes.
- Considered a common reason for seeking veterinary care.

SIGNALMENT

- Healthy bitch <6–12 months of age (prepubertal)—juvenile (puppy) vaginitis and congenital anomalies more common.
- Nonpregnant bitch that has undergone at least one estrous cycle—normal estrus, persistent estrus (cystic ovarian disease or granulosa cell tumor), pyometra, neoplasia
- Bitch bred in the last 30–70 days—normal parturition (50–70 days) or abortion (<50 days).
- Bitch that has recently whelped—normal lochia or postpartum metritis more common, subinvolution of placental sites.
- Ovariectomized bitch—vaginal stricture or estrogen-responsive urinary incontinence more common; neoplasia.

SIGNS

Historical Findings

- Discharge from the vulva.
- Licking, scooting, and spotting.
- Attracting male dogs.
- Parturition—with postpartum discharge.
- Recent estrus—with pyometra.
- Hemorrhagic discharge >8 weeks postpartum—subinvolution of placental sites.
- Vomiting, anorexia—may be seen with metritis and pyometra.

Physical Examination Findings

Vaginal discharge that may be serosanguinous, purulent, lochial, hemorrhagic, mucoid, or urinous.

CAUSES

Normal Physiologic Conditions

- Proestrus.
- Estrus.
- Diestrus.
- Late pregnancy.
- Parturition.
- Normal lochia.

Pathologic Conditions

See specific chapters for further information.

- Cystic ovarian disease (persistent estrus).
- *Brucella canis* infection.
- Metritis.
- Pyometra.
- Retained placenta or fetuses.
- Subinvolution of placental sites (hemorrhagic discharge postpartum ≥8 weeks).
- Neoplasia—uterus, vagina, urinary tract (including transmissible venereal tumor), ovary (granulosa cell tumor/persistent estrus).
- Vaginitis.
- Estrogen-responsive urinary incontinence.
- Coagulopathy.
- Congenital defects of the distal genital tract—intersex conditions, imperfect embryologic fusion of the Müllerian ducts (vagina), joining of the genital folds (vestibule) and genital swellings (vulvar lips), ectopic ureters.
- Trauma.
- Foreign body.

RISK FACTORS

- Prophylactic antibiotics—may alter normal vaginal flora and predispose to secondary infection.
- Exogenous estrogen—predispose to pyometra in the intact bitch.
- Exogenous androgens—may cause clitoral hypertrophy.
- Exogenous or endogenous progesterone—predispose to pyometra or stump pyometra.
- Obesity—excess skin folds around vulva.

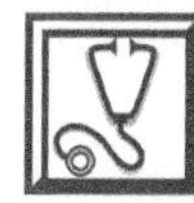

DIAGNOSIS

DIFFERENTIAL DIAGNOSIS

- Healthy intact bitch <6–12 months of age—juvenile vaginitis (prepubertal), normal estrous cycle, urogenital trauma or neoplasia, foreign body, coagulopathy, ectopic ureter(s), congenital abnormalities of the perineum or distal genital tract, intersex conditions, urinary tract disease.
- Nonpregnant bitch that has undergone at least one estrous cycle—normal estrus, pyometra, split heat, foreign body, urogenital trauma, neoplasia, coagulopathy, cystic ovarian disease (follicular cysts).
- Bitch bred in the last 30–70 days—abortion, pyometra, normal parturition (>57 days from breeding), fetal/embryonic death, split heat, *Brucella canis* infection.
- Bitch that has recently whelped—lochia (normal up to 6–8 weeks postpartum), subinvolution of placental sites (hemorrhagic discharge ≥8 weeks postpartum), postpartum metritis, vaginal trauma, retained placenta or fetus.
- Ovariectomized bitch—vaginal stricture, foreign body, neoplasia, polyps, stump pyometra due to exogenous or endogenous progesterone, exogenous estrogens (exposure to owner's hormone replacement therapy), perivulvar dermatitis, ovarian remnant syndrome, estrogen-responsive urinary incontinence.

CBC/BIOCHEMISTRY/URINALYSIS

- Regenerative anemia—may be normal in pregnancy or during estrus.
- Urinalysis—may indicate urinary tract infection.

OTHER LABORATORY TESTS

- Progesterone—determine if bitch is in luteal phase, which increases likelihood of pyometra. Progesterone, 17-hydroxyprogesterone may be secreted in animals with adrenal cortex disease.
- Adrenocorticotropic hormone (ACTH) stimulation test—to diagnose adrenocortical disease.
- *Brucella canis* serology—screen with rapid slide agglutination test; agar gel immunodiffusion test confirmatory.
- Bacterial culture of whole blood or lymph node aspirate for *B. canis*.
- PCR for *B. canis* available, best to use on abortive discharge (Kansas State Veterinary Diagnostic Laboratory).

IMAGING

Radiography

- Detect enlarged uterus or ovary, pregnancy.
- Evidence of fetal death—presence of gas around fetus or misalignment and/or collapse of fetal skeleton.

Ultrasonography

- Determine contents of uterus; free fluid in the uterus is characteristic of pyometra, hydrometra, and mucometra.
- Pregnancy diagnosis and embryonic/fetal wellbeing—heartbeat may be seen as early as the 20th day of diestrus, heart rate <180 bpm indicates fetal stress.
- Masses—neoplasia, granulomas, cystic ovarian disease, granulosa cell tumor, or foreign body; saline distention of the vagina may help visualization.

Contrast Radiography—Vaginogram/Urethragram/Cystogram/Excretory Urography

- Identify abnormal conformation or structure (i.e., neoplasia or foreign body) within the vagina.
- Rule out vestibulovaginal strictures, rectovaginal and urethrovaginal fistulas.
- Rule out differentials and help localize the problem.
- Pronounced folds (rugae) of vagina during estrus will cause filling defects (normal).

VAGINAL DISCHARGE (CONTINUED)

DIAGNOSTIC PROCEDURES

Vaginal Cytology

- Determine nature of discharge—inflammatory, hemorrhagic, purulent.
- Evaluate epithelial cells —superficial (cornified) cells present under the influence of estrogen.
- Always performed in order to interpret vaginal cultures (inflammation should accompany infection).

Vaginal Culture and Sensitivity

- Performed prior to other diagnostic procedures.
- Use guarded swab to sample cranial vagina.
- The vagina is not a sterile environment and culture of normal bitches results in growth of normal vaginal flora; use of vaginal cytology and other diagnostic tools is essential for interpretation of culture results.
- Most common organisms in the microbiome (commensals and potential pathogens) are *Escherichia coli*, *Streptococcus* spp., *Pasteurella* spp., and *Staphylococcus* spp.
- Other organisms which can be commensals include *Mycoplasma* spp., *Enterobacter* spp., *Pseudomonas* spp., *Klebsiella* spp.
- Normal microbiome consists of numerous opportunistic pathogens, e.g., *E. coli* and *Mycoplasma* spp.

Vaginoscopy

- Rigid cystourethroscope or ureteroscope, pediatric gastroscope or proctoscope, or flexible endoscope used to visualize vagina.
- Identify source of vaginal discharge—uterine, vaginal, vestibular, or urethra.
- Visualize anomalies, persistent hymen, neoplasia, foreign body, trauma, abscess, and evaluate the vaginal and vestibular mucosa.
- Removal of foreign body or biopsy of vaginal mass.

Other

- Digital examination of vestibule, vaginovestibular junction, and distal vagina.
- Biopsy and histopathology of mass lesions.
- Cystocentesis—urine culture and sensitivity.
- Coagulation profile, platelet count.

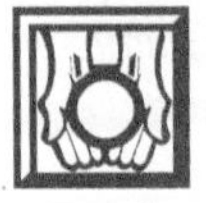

TREATMENT

- Based on diagnosis.
- No treatment for normal causes of vaginal discharge.

SURGICAL CONSIDERATIONS

- Ovariectomy or ovariohysterectomy (OHE) is treatment of choice for neoplastic conditions.
- Cystic ovarian disease can be medically managed or ovariectomy/OHE performed.
- Removal of foreign body or surgical excision of mass(es).
- Surgical excision or radiation therapy are options for transmissible venereal tumor (TVT).

MEDICATIONS

DRUG(S) OF CHOICE

- Antibiotic—choice based on guarded cranial vaginal culture and sensitivity.
- Dopamine agonist—may be used in addition to PGF2α for luteolysis via suppression of the luteotropic hormone prolactin—bromocriptine 10 µg/kg PO or cabergoline 5 µg/kg PO q8–24h until serum progesterone level <2.0 ng/mL.
- Supportive care including IV fluids as indicated.

CONTRAINDICATIONS

Certain antibiotics may be contraindicated during pregnancy and nursing.

PRECAUTIONS

Dopamine agonists—side effects include vomiting and nausea; can be controlled with antiemetics.

ALTERNATIVE DRUG(S)

Aglepristone (Alizin®) 10 mg/kg SC, 2 doses given 24 hours apart—progesterone receptor antagonist that may be used alone or concurrently with prostaglandin therapy for treatment of pyometra (currently not widely available in the United States without special authorization).

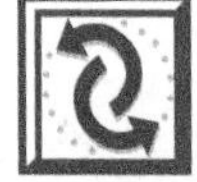

FOLLOW-UP

PATIENT MONITORING

Subinvolution of Placental Sites

Monitor hematocrit or packed cell volume (PCV)—may have significant blood loss.

PREVENTION/AVOIDANCE

- Puppy vaginitis—delay elective OHE until after first estrous cycle in cases of juvenile vaginitis; may avoid chronic vaginitis.
- Addition of probiotics to daily diet.
- Avoid exogenous steroids (estrogens, progestins, androgens).

POSSIBLE COMPLICATIONS

Endotoxemia and septicemia may occur with pyometra or metritis.

MISCELLANEOUS

ASSOCIATED CONDITIONS

Pyometra and cystic endometrial hyperplasia.

AGE-RELATED FACTORS

- Increased risk for pyometra after each estrous cycle.
- Neoplasia more common in older bitches.

ZOONOTIC POTENTIAL

- *Brucella canis*—fluids and fetal tissue during abortion are highly contaminated with organisms.
- Immunocompromised people are at highest risk. Animal caretakers and pathologists are at risk due to high exposure.

PREGNANCY/FERTILITY/BREEDING

- Neoplasia—poor prognosis for future fertility.
- TVT—sexually transmitted disease; breeding should be avoided.
- *Brucella canis*—sexually transmitted disease and grave prognosis for resolution of disease and normal fertility; should not be used for breeding.

SEE ALSO

- Abortion, Spontaneous (Early Pregnancy Loss)—Cats.
- Abortion, Spontaneous (Early Pregnancy Loss)—Dogs.
- Brucellosis.
- Ovarian Remnant Syndrome.
- Pyometra.
- Retained Placenta.
- Sexual Development Disorders.
- Subinvolution of Placental Sites.
- Transmissible Venereal Tumor.
- Vaginal Malformations and Acquired Lesions.
- Vaginitis.

ABBREVIATIONS

- ACTH = adrenocorticotropic hormone.
- OHE = ovariohysterectomy.
- PCV = packed cell volume.
- TVT = transmissible venereal tumor.

Suggested Reading

Purswell BJ. Vaginal disorders. In: Ettinger SJ, Feldman EC, eds., Textbook of Veterinary Internal Medicine, 8th ed. St. Louis, MO: Elsevier, 2010, pp. 1929–1933.

Author Julie T. Cecere

Consulting Editor Erin E. Runcan

Client Education Handout available online

BASICS

OVERVIEW

- Protrusion of spherical or donut-shaped mass from vulva during proestrus or estrus, rarely during gestation, parturition, or after administration of estrogenic drugs:
  - Type I—slight eversion of vaginal floor cranial to the urethral orifice but no protrusion through vulva.
  - Type II—vaginal tissue prolapses through vulvar opening (tongue-shaped mass).
  - Type III—donut-shaped eversion of the entire circumference of vaginal wall, including the urethral orifice, seen ventrally on the prolapsed tissue.
- Exaggerated response of vaginal mucosa to estrogen; some affected animals have follicular cysts.
- Despite the name, the change seen histopathologically is edema rather than hyperplasia or hypertrophy if occurring during proestrus or estrus.
- Severe prolapse—may occlude urethra and prevent normal urination.
- True vaginal prolapse without hyperplasia or edema occurs rarely pre- or postpartum and may include uterine body and horns.

SIGNALMENT

- Young (most 18–22 months, range 6 months–4.6 years), large-breed bitches.
- Predisposed breeds—large and brachycephalic breeds (boxer, mastiff, English bulldog, Saint Bernard); Labrador and Chesapeake Bay retrievers; German shepherd dog; English springer spaniel; Walker hound; Airedale terrier; American pit bull terrier.
- Hereditary component probable—increased incidence in some family lines.

SIGNS

Historical Findings

- Onset of proestrus or estrus.
- Although rare, can be seen during diestrus or at parturition (8–12% of cases occur at parturition); or after administration of estrogenic drugs or exposure to exogenous estrogens.
- Licking of vulvar area.
- Failure to allow copulation.
- Dysuria.
- Previous occurrence.

Physical Examination Findings

- Protrusion of round, tongue-shaped, or donut-shaped tissue mass from the vulva.
- Vaginal examination—locate lumen and urethral orifice; types I and II: vaginal lumen is dorsal to the prolapse; type III: lumen is central to the prolapse; urethral orifice is ventral to the prolapse with all three types.

CAUSES & RISK FACTORS

- Estrogen stimulation.
- Genetic predisposition.
- Dystocia.
- Increased abdominal pressure.

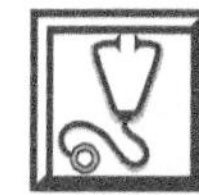

DIAGNOSIS

DIFFERENTIAL DIAGNOSIS

- Vaginal polyp—differentiated by vaginal examination.
- Vaginal neoplasia—transmissible venereal tumor and leiomyoma; differentiated by signalment, stage of cycle, and vaginal examination.
- Clitoral hypertrophy; differentiated by physical examination.

CBC/BIOCHEMISTRY/URINALYSIS

N/A

OTHER LABORATORY TESTS

N/A

IMAGING

N/A

DIAGNOSTIC PROCEDURES

Biopsy—differentiate from neoplasia.

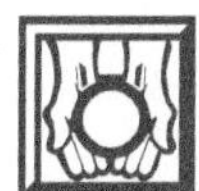

TREATMENT

- Outpatient; unless urethral obstruction.
- Breeding—possible by artificial insemination (discuss potential heritability).
- Prolapsed tissue—keep clean and lubricated with sterile water-soluble lubricant.
- Use of sugar or a 50% dextrose solution on edematous tissue may help to shrink prolapse.
- Elizabethan collar and clean indoor environment—minimize tissue trauma.
- Instruct client to monitor patient's ability to urinate.
- If urethral obstruction present, place indwelling urinary catheter.
- Regression—usually begins in late estrus; should be resolved during early diestrus.
- Recurrence rate—66–100% at next estrous cycle.

Surgical Considerations

- Ovariohysterectomy—prevents recurrence; may hasten resolution.
- Severe condition—requires surgical reduction or resection; identify and catheterize urethra, 25% recurrence at next cycle after surgery.
- With dystocia, cesarean section required, ovariohysterectomy may be necessary.
- When occurring during pregnancy, both resection of prolapse and surgical reduction with accompanying hysteropexy have been successfully reported. Vaginal delivery with concurrent vaginal prolapse has been reported; close monitoring for obstructive dystocia is recommended.

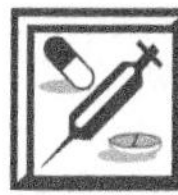

MEDICATIONS

DRUG(S) OF CHOICE

Gonadotropin-releasing hormone (GnRH) 2.2 μg/kg IM or human chorionic gonadotropin (hCG) 1,000 IU IM—if breeding not planned that cycle; may hasten ovulation and resolution by a couple of days; not effective if given after ovulation (progesterone >8–10 ng/mL).

CONTRAINDICATIONS/POSSIBLE INTERACTIONS

Avoid progestational drugs, they can induce pyometra.

FOLLOW-UP

PATIENT MONITORING

Monitor health of prolapsed tissue and the ability to urinate.

PREVENTION/AVOIDANCE

Ovariohysterectomy—recommended owing to genetic component and likelihood of recurrence.

POSSIBLE COMPLICATIONS

Type III—may affect urethra and prevent normal urination.

EXPECTED COURSE AND PROGNOSIS

- Medical treatment—prognosis for recovery good, except with urethral involvement.
- Surgical intervention for type III—prognosis good.

MISCELLANEOUS

ABBREVIATIONS

- GnRH = gonadotropin-releasing hormone.
- hCG = human chorionic gonadotropin.

INTERNET RESOURCES

Schaeferes-Okkens AC. Vaginal edema and vaginal fold prolapse in the bitch, including surgical management, 2001: https://www.ivis.org/library/recent-advances-small-animal-reproduction/vaginal-edema-and-vaginal-fold-prolapse-bitch

Suggested Reading

Johnston SD, Root Kustritz MV, Olson PNS. Disorders of the canine vagina, vestibule, and vulva. In: Johnston SD, Root Kustritz MV, Olson PNS, eds., Canine and Feline Theriogenology. Philadelphia, PA: Saunders, 2001, pp. 225–242.

Author Joni L. Freshman

Consulting Editor Erin E. Runcan

VAGINAL MALFORMATIONS AND ACQUIRED LESIONS

BASICS

DEFINITION

Altered anatomic architecture due to congenital anomalies (imperforate hymen, dorsoventral septum, hymenal constriction, rectovaginal fistula, segmental aplasia, cysts, conformational defects of the vulva) and acquired conditions (vaginal hyperplasia, foreign bodies, strictures, adhesions, fistulas, and neoplasia).

PATHOPHYSIOLOGY

Congenital

- Normal embryologic development—paired paramesonephric (Müllerian) ducts fuse to form uterine body, cervix, and vagina; urogenital sinus forms the vestibule, urethra, and urinary bladder; hymen (composed of epithelial linings of paramesonephric ducts and urogenital sinus and an interposed layer of mesoderm) normally disappears by birth.
- Errors during embryonic development—imperforate hymens; dorsoventral septae; hymenal constrictions (including vestibulovaginal stenoses); vaginal diverticulum (double vagina, vaginal pouch); cysts.

Acquired

- Vaginal scarring—from trauma (mating, dystocia, sexual abuse) or inflammation; may note adhesions or strictures, which narrow vaginal diameter.
- Vaginal hyperplasia (dogs)—exaggerated response of the vaginal mucosa to estrogen; actually edema (vs. hyperplasia or hypertrophy).
- Neoplasia—extraluminal leiomyoma most common; usually old patients; no influence of ovarian status.

V

SYSTEMS AFFECTED

- Reproductive—interference with natural mating and whelping; frequently concurrent vaginitis.
- Renal/urologic—urinary tract infections; urinary incontinence with congenital malformations of hymenal area.
- Skin/exocrine—perivulvar dermatitis secondary to vaginitis, recessed vulva (redundant perivulvar folds or hypoplastic vulva), or urinary incontinence.

GENETICS

Congenital—heritable component suspected; no direct evidence.

INCIDENCE/PREVALENCE

- Incidence (congenital)—unknown; conditions may be asymptomatic, especially if female never used for breeding.
- Prevalence (vaginal septa)—in one study, 0.03%.

SIGNALMENT

Species

Dog and cat.

Breed Predilections

- Congenital—none identified.
- Vaginal hyperplasia—large and brachycephalic breeds (boxer, mastiff, English bulldog, Saint Bernard); Labrador and Chesapeake Bay retrievers; German shepherd dog; English springer spaniel; Walker hound; Airedale terrier; American pit bull terrier.

Mean Age and Range

- Congenital lesion—young (<2 years of age) intact or spayed females.
- Vaginal hyperplasia—young (<2 years of age) intact females.
- Acquired lesion (adhesions and strictures)—post-pubertal females of any age.
- Neoplasia—mean age 10 years; ovarian status has no effect.

SIGNS

Historical Findings

- Vulvar discharge.
- Excessive licking of vulva.
- Pollakiuria, stranguria.
- Dyschezia.
- Urinary incontinence.
- Attractive to males.
- Refuses mating.

Physical Examination Findings

- Usually normal.
- Evidence of vaginal discharge, perivulvar dermatitis, or mass.
- Recessed or hypoplastic vulva (occasional).

CAUSES

- Congenital.
- Inflammatory.
- Hormonal.
- Traumatic.
- Neoplastic.

DIAGNOSIS

DIFFERENTIAL DIAGNOSIS

- Vaginitis—concurrent with many malformations; differentiated by vaginoscopy and vaginography.
- Urinary tract infection—differentiated by vaginal cytology and urinalysis (cystocentesis sample).
- Pyometra—differentiated by physical exam, abdominal ultrasonography.

CBC/BIOCHEMISTRY/URINALYSIS

- Usually normal.
- Urinalysis—possible urinary tract infection.

IMAGING

Positive-Contrast Vaginography, Excretory Urography

- Defines vaginal vault to cervix, urethra, cranial vestibule, and urinary bladder.
- Defines cervical canal and uterine lumen in intact patient during estrus.
- Identifies strictures, septae, persistent hymens, masses, rectovaginal fistulas, urethrovaginal fistulas, vaginal rupture, and diverticulae.
- Procedure:
  - Patients should be fasted for 24 hours; give enema 2 hours before procedure.
  - Performed under sedation or general anesthesia.
  - Pass Foley catheter into vestibule, inflate balloon, infuse aqueous iodinated contrast media (1 mL/kg). Avoid overdistension and underdistension.
- Vestibulovaginal stenoses—ratio of maximal height of vagina to smallest height of vestibulovaginal junction—normal >0.35, mild 0.26–0.35, moderate 0.20–0.25, severe <0.20.
- Urinary incontinence—excretory urography to indentify ectopic ureters or intrapelvic bladder neck.

Abdominal Ultrasonography

- Much of vagina not visible because of pelvis.
- Cranial vaginal masses may occasionally be imaged.
- Infusion of saline into vagina before examination helps differentiate luminal from transmural or extraluminal lesions.

DIAGNOSTIC PROCEDURES

Sequence of procedures is important; recommended order:

- Vaginal cytology—identify stage of estrous cycle; reveal inflammatory or neoplastic cells (see Breeding, Timing).
- Digital examination of vestibule and caudal vagina—measure diameter; identify caudal strictures or masses; note size and conformation of vulva.
- Vaginoscopy—identify strictures, adhesions, septa, diverticula, masses, and foreign bodies; may use a variety of specula; a long (16–20 cm), hollow, rigid-type (e.g., infant proctoscope) with light source recommended; match speculum diameter to size of patient; post-cervical fold (normal) obscures visualization of external os of cervix; rigid cystoscopes (used for transcervical insemination) adequate for many anomalies, need vaginal distension (under general anesthesia) with saline or air to visualize some anomalies or lesions.
- Imaging—see above.
- Urethrocystoscopy—identify ectopic ureters, other abnormalities.

PATHOLOGIC FINDINGS

Congenital

- Imperforate hymen—thin fenestrated membrane, dorsoventral band(s), or a thick membrane at vestibulovaginal junction; most common defect; remainder of genital tract normal.
- Dorsoventral septum—oriented dorsoventrally in vagina, cranial to vestibulovaginal junction; may note a double cervix

(most common variant), double vagina, or divided uterine fundus (rare).
- Hymenal constriction or vestibulovaginal stenosis—moderate to severe constriction at vestibulovaginal junction.
- Vaginal hypoplasia or vaginal aplasia—vagina, cervix, uterus, vulva may be absent or hypoplastic.

Acquired

- Strictures and adhesions—may be identified anywhere in vagina or vestibule; result of trauma or inflammation; persistent vaginitis, refusal to mate, dystocia, or problems with micturition are common sequelae.
- Vaginal hyperplasia and prolapse.
- Vaginal neoplasia—usually extraluminal leiomyoma in wall of vestibule; leiomyosarcomas; transmissible venereal tumors; lipomas; mast cell tumors; epidermoid carcinomas; squamous cell carcinomas; fibromas; fibrosarcomas; and invasive urinary tract carcinomas reported.
- Foreign bodies—plant material, sticks, and swabs.

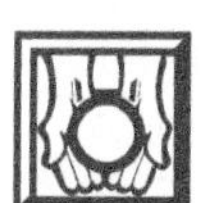

TREATMENT

APPROPRIATE HEALTH CARE

- Usually outpatient, until nature of defect is ascertained.
- Inpatient—for positive contrast vaginography.
- Manual dilation (bougienage)—digitally or with smooth rigid object:
  - Attempt in patients with imperforate hymen or mild vestibulovaginal stenosis.
  - Perform in sedated patient gradually over a course of several treatments.
  - May be performed in anesthetized patient at one time to maximal dilation.
  - Typically leads to reduction, but not complete resolution, of clinical signs; unlikely to resolve moderate or severe stenoses.

NURSING CARE

As appropriate for condition.

SURGICAL CONSIDERATIONS

- Resection, transection, excision—many minor congenital (e.g., imperforate hymen, small dorsoventral septa) and acquired lesions (small strictures, masses, or adhesions in caudal portion of vagina).
- Episiotomy—usually required for adequate surgical access.
- T-shaped vaginoplasty—described for vestibulovaginal stenoses; resection appears to provide best odds of resolution, although results are variable.
- Complete ring resection—vaginal stenosis.
- Vulvoplasty—excessive vulvar fold (redundant perivulvar skin fold) with or without increased perivulvar fat deposition; recessed vulva; reserved for patients with concurrent chronic vaginitis, vaginovulvar discharge, perivulvar dermatitis.
- Transendoscopic laser ablation—one report for correcting a dorsoventral septum in an English bulldog that subsequently bred and delivered 4 pups vaginally.
- Ovariohysterectomy—patient has no breeding value; exhibits signs only during estrus.
- Vaginal ablation (vaginectomy cranial to external urethral orifice) and ovariohysterectomy—patient has no breeding value; concurrent severe, refractory vaginitis at all stages of estrous cycle; severe vaginal stenosis; broad-based vaginal tumors.

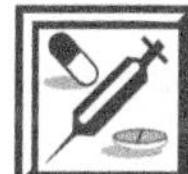

MEDICATIONS

DRUG(S) OF CHOICE

- Concurrent vaginitis—appropriate local and antibiotic therapy (see Vaginitis).
- Stenotic lesions—manual dilation in conjunction with corticosteroids (prednisone 1 mg/kg PO q24h) in an attempt to prevent recurrence; high recurrence rates with or without steroids.

FOLLOW-UP

PREVENTION/AVOIDANCE

Congenital lesions—for a familial line with a high number of affected individuals, recommend sterilization of affected individuals and their sire and dam.

POSSIBLE COMPLICATIONS

- Dystocia, urinary tract infections, incontinence, and vaginitis—with vaginal malformations; with patients that fail to respond to treatment.
- Strictures and adhesions—may be postoperative complications of corrective surgical procedures.

EXPECTED COURSE AND PROGNOSIS

- Depends on severity of lesion and degree of inflammation after treatment.
- Prognosis after treatment for imperforate hymens, short dorsoventral bands, or caudal strictures or adhesions—fair to good for improvement of clinical signs; fair to guarded for complete resolution of signs and normal fertility.
- Prognosis for hymenal constrictions, vaginal hypoplasia or severe cranial strictures or adhesions—guarded to poor for complete resolution of signs and normal fertility; with concurrent severe vaginitis, best recommendation is vaginal ablation.

MISCELLANEOUS

ASSOCIATED CONDITIONS

- Urinary tract infections.
- Vaginitis.
- Urinary incontinence.

AGE-RELATED FACTORS

- Congenital—more likely in young bitches of any ovarian status.
- Vaginal hyperplasia—more likely in young intact bitches.
- Neoplasia of vagina or vestibule—more likely in old bitches of any ovarian status.

PREGNANCY/FERTILITY/BREEDING

- Some patients may be bred by artificial insemination; possibility for a vaginal delivery is unlikely without correction of the anomaly.
- Warn owner that an elective cesarean section may be required.

SEE ALSO

- Breeding, Timing.
- Transmissible Venereal Tumor.
- Vaginal Discharge.
- Vaginal Hyperplasia and Prolapse.
- Vaginal Tumors.
- Vaginitis.

INTERNET RESOURCES

Seim HB. Surgeon's Corner: Vulvoplasty. Clinician's Brief: http://www.cliniciansbrief.com/article/surgeon-s-corner-vulvoplasty

Suggested Reading

Lulich JP. Endoscopic vaginoscopy in the dog. Theriogenology 2006, 66(3):588–591.

Mathews KG. Surgery of the canine vagina and vulva. Vet Clin North Am Small Anim Pract 2001, 31(2):271–290.

Author Erin E. Runcan

Consulting Editor Erin E. Runcan

Acknowledgment The author/editor acknowledges the prior contribution of Sara K. Lyle.

VAGINAL TUMORS

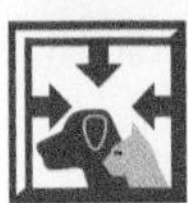

BASICS

OVERVIEW

- Second most common reproductive tumor, comprising 1.9–3% of all tumors in dogs.
- Dogs—83% benign smooth muscle tumors, often pedunculated (e.g., leiomyoma, fibroleiomyoma, and fibroma); less common differentials include lipoma, transmissible venereal tumor, mast cell tumor, squamous cell carcinoma, leiomyosarcoma, hemangiosarcoma, osteosarcoma, or extension of primary urinary tract carcinomas also reported.
- Dogs—may be an incidental finding at necropsy.
- Cats—extremely rare; usually of smooth muscle origin.
- Hormonal influence—may play a role in the development of leiomyomas, fibromas, or polypoid tumors.

SIGNALMENT

- Dog—mean age 10.2–11.2 years, boxers, nulliparous bitches more commonly affected.
- Cat—no data available.

SIGNS

Dogs

- Extraluminal—slow-growing perineal mass; vulvar discharge; dysuria; pollakiuria; vulvar licking; dystocia.
- Intraluminal—mass protruding from the vulva (often at estrus if sexually intact); vulvar discharge; stranguria; dysuria; tenesmus.

V

Cats

- Firm mass in the perineal region.
- Constipation.

CAUSES & RISK FACTORS

- Intact sexual status (hormonal influence).
- Nulliparous bitches more commonly affected.

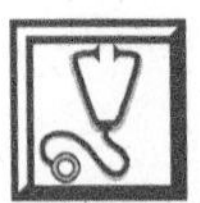

DIAGNOSIS

DIFFERENTIAL DIAGNOSIS

- Vaginal prolapse.
- Urethral neoplasia.
- Uterine prolapse.
- Clitoral hypertrophy.
- Vaginal polyp.
- Vaginal abscess/granuloma.
- Vaginal foreign body.
- Vaginal hematoma.

CBC/BIOCHEMISTRY/URINALYSIS

No consistent abnormalities.

OTHER LABORATORY TESTS

N/A

IMAGING

- Thoracic radiography—recommended; assess for pulmonary metastatic disease (uncommon).
- Abdominal radiography—may detect cranial extension of a mass.
- Ultrasonography, vaginography, and urethrocystography—may help delineate mass.
- CT/MRI—definitive delineation of tumor, assess for surgical feasibility, assess for metastatic disease within abdominal visceral organs.

DIAGNOSTIC PROCEDURES

- Vaginoscopy with cytologic examination of an aspirate—may help determine cell type. Often cytology is nondiagnostic given the mesenchymal nature (poorly exfoliative) of most vaginal tumors.
- Biopsy with histopathologic examination—often necessary for definitive diagnosis.

PATHOLOGIC FINDINGS

- Intraluminal—vestibular wall; protruding into the vulva; may occur singularly or as multiple masses.
- Extraluminal—vestibular roof; causing a bulging of the perineum.

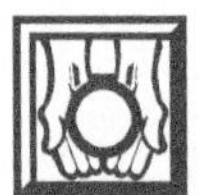

TREATMENT

- Surgical excision and concurrent ovariohysterectomy—treatment of choice.
- Subtotal and total vaginectomy described for extensive disease.
- Postoperative radiotherapy—may be of benefit for sarcoma and incompletely resected benign tumors.

MEDICATIONS

DRUG(S) OF CHOICE

- Postoperative therapy—no standard established.
- Doxorubicin 30 mg/m^2, cisplatin 60 mg/m^2, or carboplatin 300 mg/m^2—rational choice to palliate malignant or metastatic disease in dogs.
- Piroxicam 0.3 mg/kg PO SID may be useful especially for those dogs with primary urinary tumors extending into the vagina and carcinomas.

CONTRAINDICATIONS/POSSIBLE INTERACTIONS

- Doxorubicin—carefully monitor with underlying cardiac disease; consider pretreatment and serial echocardiograms and ECG.
- Cisplatin—do not use in cats (fatal); do not use in dogs with renal disease; always use appropriate and concurrent diuresis.
- Chemotherapy may be toxic; seek advice if you are unfamiliar with chemotherapeutic drugs.
- Piroxicam should not be used with other nonsteroidal anti-inflammatory drugs (NSAIDs) or prednisone and should be avoided in animals with underlying renal or hepatic disease. Should not be used in conjunction with cisplatin.

FOLLOW-UP

PATIENT MONITORING

- Thoracic radiography and abdominal ultrasonography—consider every 3 months if tumor is malignant.
- CBC (doxorubicin, cisplatin, carboplatin), biochemical profile (cisplatin, piroxicam), urinalysis (cisplatin, piroxicam)—perform before each chemotherapy treatment.

EXPECTED COURSE AND PROGNOSIS

- Prognosis—good with complete excision; guarded if incomplete excision; poor with metastatic disease; poor with carcinoma or squamous cell carcinoma.
- Recurrence—15% (leiomyoma) without concurrent ovariohysterectomy.

MISCELLANEOUS

ASSOCIATED CONDITIONS

Cats—reported concurrent cystic ovaries and mammary gland adenocarcinoma.

ABBREVIATIONS

- NSAID = nonsteroidal anti-inflammatory drug.

Suggested Reading

Manithaiudom K, Johnston SD. Clinical approach to vaginal/vestibular masses in the bitch. Vet Clin North Am Small Anim Pract 1991, 21:509–521.

Morrison WB. Cancers of the reproductive tract. In: Morrison WB, ed., Cancer in Dogs and Cats: Medical and Surgical Management. Jackson, WY: Teton NewMedia, 2002, pp. 555–564.

Saba CF, Lawrence JA. Tumors of the female reproductive system. In: Withrow SJ, MacEwen EG, eds., Small Animal Clinical Oncology, 5th ed. Philadelphia, PA: Saunders, 2013, pp. 532–537.

Author Heather M. Wilson-Robles

Consulting Editor Timothy M. Fan

Acknowledgment The author and editors acknowledge the prior contribution of Renee Al-Sarraf.

VAGINITIS

BASICS

DEFINITION

Inflammation of the vagina.

PATHOPHYSIOLOGY

• Juvenile vaginitis—unknown, possibly due to imbalances of juvenile vaginal mucosal glandular epithelium. • Primary adult-onset vaginitis—*Brucella canis* or canine herpesvirus. • Secondary adult-onset vaginitis—sequela to congenital anomaly, vaginal atrophy following ovariohysterectomy (OHE), drug therapy, foreign body, neoplasia, urinary tract infection, urinary incontinence, systemic disease.

SYSTEMS AFFECTED

Reproductive

INCIDENCE/PREVALENCE

• 0.7% of dogs in one study. • Primary vaginitis—very rare.

SIGNALMENT

Species

Dog

Mean Age and Range

• Juvenile vaginitis—less than 1 year of age, ranging from 8 weeks to 1 year, prepubertal animals. • Adult-onset vaginitis—over 1 year of age, ranging from 1 to 16 years of age.

SIGNS

Historical Findings

Juvenile Vaginitis

• May have no significant history. • Vulvar discharge—seen most often following urination. • Vaginal irritation. • Crusting of the hair coat in the vulvar region. • Scooting. • Excessive vulvar licking. • Perivulvar pruritus. • Inability to housetrain.

Adult-Onset Vaginitis

• Vulvar discharge. • Excessive vulvar licking. • Pollakiuria. • Pain during urination. • Polyuria and polydypsia. • Pruritus. • Urinary incontinence. • Infertility.

Physical Examination Findings

• Vulvar discharge—mucoid to purulent, scant to copious. • Vulvar hyperemia. • Vestibular hyperemia. • Perivulvar dermatitis. • Digital examination—strictures and hymens identified at vagino-vestibular junction, granular irregularity of mucosa, especially wall opposite urethral papilla. • Vaginoscopy—diffuse hyperemia of vaginal and vestibular mucosa, prominent lymphoid follicles, luminal exudates, erythema of the urethral papilla or clitoral fossa; presence of foreign body, neoplasia, or congenital abnormalities.

CAUSES

• Prepubertal vagina. • Infantile vulva. • Urinary tract infection. • Urinary or fecal incontinence. • Foreign body. • Neoplasia—transmissible venereal tumor, leiomyoma. • Bacterial—*Brucella canis, Escherichia coli, Streptococcus* spp., *Staphylococcus intermedius, Pasteurella* spp., *Chlamydia, Pseudomonas* spp., *Mycoplasma* spp. • Viral—canine herpesvirus. • Congenital anomalies including vagino-vestibular strictures, inverted vulva. • Systemic disease—diabetes mellitus. • Zinc toxicity. • Exogenous or endogenous androgens.

RISK FACTORS

• Alteration of normal vaginal flora by antibiotics. • Clitoral hypertrophy secondary to exogenous or endogenous (hermaphrodites) androgens. • Inverted or recessed vulva. • Obesity. • Abnormal conformation. • Vaginal trauma.

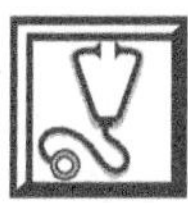

DIAGNOSIS

DIFFERENTIAL DIAGNOSIS

• Normal—hemorrhagic or serosanguinous discharge during proestrus, continuing into estrus. • Normal—slight purulent exudate in early diestrus; neutrophils and parabasal epithelial cells present. • Normal—mucus discharge during pregnancy. • Normal—postpartum discharge for up to 6–8 weeks; odorless dark brown or hemorrhagic discharge; substantial amounts are normal for up to 4 weeks. • Subinvolution of the placental sites—hemorrhagic discharge lasting longer than 8 weeks postpartum. • Cystourethritis. • Foreign body. • Pyometra. • Metritis. • Retained placenta(s). • Clitoral hypertrophy. • Embryonic or fetal death. • Urine or feces contamination secondary to congenital anomaly (e.g., ectopic ureter) or acquired condition (e.g., incontinence secondary to hypoestrogenism). • Perivulvar dermatitis. • Sexual differentiation disorder. • Vaginal neoplasia, trauma, hematoma, abscess. • Ovarian neoplasia. • Zinc toxicity.

CBC/BIOCHEMISTRY/URINALYSIS

• Usually normal. • Adult onset—pyuria, bacteriuria, hematuria, or systemic disease.

OTHER LABORATORY TESTS

• *B. canis* serology—rapid slide agglutination test, agar gel immunodiffusion test, bacterial culture of whole blood or lymph node aspirate. • Serum progesterone concentration—determine if patient is in estrus or luteal phase (≥2 ng/mL).

IMAGING

Ultrasonography

• Rule out uterus as source of discharge. • Detection of masses; saline distention of the vagina may help visualization.

Contrast Radiography—Vaginogram/ Urethragram/Cystogram/IV Pyelogram

• Identify abnormal conformation or structure within vagina. • Rule out vestibulovaginal strictures, rectovaginal and urethrovaginal fistulas.

DIAGNOSTIC PROCEDURES

Vaginal Culture and Sensitivity

• Use guarded swab to sample cranial vagina. • 74% of adult-onset cases positive for bacterial growth: ∘ Most common organisms are E. coli, Streptococcus spp., and Staphylococcus intermedius. ∘ Others include Mycoplasma, Pasteurella, Pseudomonas spp., Chlamydia. • Vagina is not a sterile environment; culture of normal bitches results in growth of normal vaginal flora; use of vaginal cytology is essential for interpretation of culture results.

Vaginal Cytology

• Performed in conjunction with vaginal culture. • Juvenile vaginitis: usually polymorphonuclear leukocytes ± bacteria. • Adult-onset vaginitis—usually septic inflammation. • Evaluate epithelial cells for cornification—cornification present under the influence of estrogen. • Determine nature of discharge—inflammatory, blood, presence of fecal material.

Vaginoscopy

• Using rigid cystourethroscope, uretero-scope, pediatric gastroscope, proctoscope, or flexible endoscope. • Identify anatomic anomalies, evaluate vaginal mucosa. • Identify source of vaginal discharge. • Remove foreign body, biopsy masses. • The vaginal wall can be thin in ovariectomized bitches—exercise care when using rigid cysto-urethroscope and ureteroscope.

Other

• Digital vaginal examination—identify strictures in posterior tract. • Histopathology of vaginal masses. • Urine culture and sensitivity.

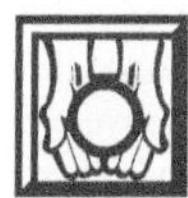

TREATMENT

APPROPRIATE HEALTH CARE

• Correction/removal of underlying cause. • Generally outpatient. • Surgical management may be necessary for foreign bodies, masses, or correction of structural anomalies. • Elizabethan collars to prevent self-mutilation.

ACTIVITY

Not altered.

DIET

Not altered.

CLIENT EDUCATION

General

• *B. canis*-positive patients should be isolated. Euthanasia recommended due to zoonotic potential and lack of effective treatment. • Exogenous estrogens and androgens must be removed from the environment.

VAGINITIS (CONTINUED)

Juvenile Vaginitis

- Generally resolves without treatment.
- Should resolve after first estrous cycle, if not before. Patient may need to go through one estrous cycle prior to elective OHE.

Adult-Onset Vaginitis

- Usually occurs secondary to underlying cause, and resolves after correction. • If no primary cause identified, high likelihood of spontaneous recovery without treatment.

SURGICAL CONSIDERATIONS

- Correction of structural anomaly. • Removal of foreign body. • Removal/biopsy of vaginal mass. • Episioplasty. • Vaginectomy may be performed in refractory cases.

MEDICATIONS

DRUG(S) OF CHOICE

Juvenile Vaginitis

- Antibiotic therapy warranted in patients with excessive discomfort (pain or excessive vulvar licking) and/or urinary tract infections.
- Antibiotic selection based on culture and sensitivity combined with vaginal cytology.
- Probiotics—helpful to restore normal vaginal flora.

Adult-Onset Vaginitis

- Systemic antibiotics (type based on cranial vaginal culture and sensitivity); treat for 4 weeks. • Nonsteroidal anti-inflammatory drugs (NSAIDs) or anti-inflammatory dose of corticosteroids to decrease inflammation.
- Diethylstilbestrol (DES)—for idiopathic or recurrent vaginitis in spayed bitches; restores normal mucosal integrity, increases vaginal epithelial cornification; use lowest effective dose: 0.5 mg, PO for dogs weighing <9 kg or 1 mg PO for dogs >9 kg q24h for 7 days, then taper dose over 2–4 weeks and maintain at lowest effective dose. Potential lifelong therapy: ○ Incurin® (estriol) used as above.
- Probiotics—to restore normal vaginal flora. Potential lifelong therapy.

CONTRAINDICATIONS

- Antibiotic therapy in patients may result in alteration of normal flora, development of infection secondary to treatment, or foster drug-resistant bacteria. • Vaginal douches with antibiotic/antiseptic agents may be irritating to the vaginal mucosa and worsen the condition. • Corticosteroid administration may worsen concurrent infections.

PRECAUTIONS

Estrogen administration may increase risk of pyometra in intact animals.

POSSIBLE INTERACTIONS

Effects of hydrocortisone may be potentiated with concurrent estrogen therapy.

ALTERNATIVE DRUG(S)

- Juvenile vaginitis may be treated with DES to induce estrus in refractory cases, but long-term effects are not documented. • Moist towelettes/baby wipes may be used to clean the perivulvar area.

FOLLOW-UP

PATIENT MONITORING

Juvenile Vaginitis

- Reevaluate if symptoms become more severe or intolerable. • Reevaluate after first estrous cycle.

Adult-Onset Vaginitis

- Recheck if symptoms do not resolve after removal of underlying cause. • Reculture 5–7 days after cessation of antibiotic therapy or if symptoms continue despite therapy.

PREVENTION/AVOIDANCE

- Delay elective OHE until after first estrous cycle in dogs with juvenile vaginitis. • Avoid using antibiotics if unwarranted. • Maintain good body weight and condition. • Avoid vaginal douching. • Avoid exogenous androgen therapy.

EXPECTED COURSE AND PROGNOSIS

- Juvenile vaginitis—onset at 6 weeks to 6–12 months of age; duration is days to months but typically intermittent; usually resolves with time or after first estrous cycle.
- Adult-onset—normally resolves after removal/treatment of inciting cause; antibiotic therapy may hasten resolution in some cases, NSAIDs may help resolve inflammation.

MISCELLANEOUS

ASSOCIATED CONDITIONS

- Perivulvar dermatitis. • Atopy.

AGE-RELATED FACTORS

Juvenile vaginitis may be present in prepubertal dogs, usually <1 year of age.

ZOONOTIC POTENTIAL

Brucella canis—uncommon cause but should be ruled out.

PREGNANCY/FERTILITY/BREEDING

- Vaginitis during pregnancy is rare but may result in ascending infection and subsequent abortion. Resolution of vaginitis should result in a good prognosis for fertility if underlying cause does not affect fertility. • Structural anomalies such as persistent hymen may prevent natural mating to occur, or could predispose to a dystocia if artificially inseminated. • Scarring secondary to trauma may result in excessive fibrous tissue and decreased distensibility of the vagina.

SEE ALSO

- Brucellosis.
- Metritis.
- Pyometra.
- Retained Placenta.
- Sexual Development Disorders.
- Subinvolution of Placental Sites.
- Vaginal Malformations and Acquired Lesions.

ABBREVIATIONS

- DES = diethylstilbestrol.
- NSAID = nonsteroidal anti-inflammatory drug.
- OHE = ovariohysterectomy.
- TVT = transmissible venereal tumor.

Suggested Reading

Johnson CA. Diagnosis and treatment of chronic vaginitis in the bitch. Vet Clin North Am 1991, 21:523–531.

Parker NA. Clinical approach to canine vaginitis: a review. Theriogenology 1998, 112–115.

Author Julie T. Cecere

Consulting Editor Erin E. Runcan

Client Education Handout available online

BASICS

OVERVIEW

Right Aortic Arch

- Entrapment of the esophagus by a persistent right fourth aortic arch (PRAA) on the right and dorsally, the base of the heart and pulmonary artery ventrally, and ductus or ligamentum arteriosum on the left and dorsally.
- Causes megaesophagus cranial to the obstruction at the base of the heart.

Double Aortic Arch

- Entrapment of the esophagus by a functional aortic arch on the right, an atretic aortic arch on the left, the base of the heart and pulmonary artery ventrally, and ductus or ligamentum arteriosum on the left and dorsally.
- Causes megaesophagus cranial to the obstruction at the base of the heart; also causes some tracheal compression.

SIGNALMENT

- Dog and cat.
- Seen most commonly in German shepherd dogs, Irish setters, Great Danes, and Boston terriers.

SIGNS

- Regurgitation of undigested solid food in animals <6 months old.
- Malnourishment in many animals.
- Time between eating and regurgitation varies.
- Signs of aspiration pneumonia (e.g., cough, tachypnea, or dyspnea) in some animals.

CAUSES & RISK FACTORS

N/A

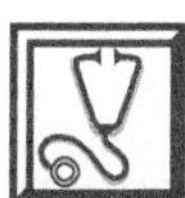

DIAGNOSIS

DIFFERENTIAL DIAGNOSIS

- Congenital megaesophagus.
- Stricture, diverticulum, or esophageal foreign body.
- Esophageal motility disorder in shar-peis.

CBC/BIOCHEMISTRY/URINALYSIS

- Results usually normal.
- High white blood cells in some animals with aspiration pneumonia.

OTHER LABORATORY TESTS

N/A

IMAGING

- Thoracic radiography—shows food-filled cranial esophagus or signs of aspiration pneumonia in some animals.
- Contrast esophagography—confirms megaesophagus extending to the heart base.
- Fluoroscopy—may be used to differentiate esophageal motility disorders.
- Angiography—may be needed to differentiate between specific vascular ring anomalies.

OTHER DIAGNOSTIC PROCEDURES

Esophagoscopy can be used to differentiate esophageal motility disorders.

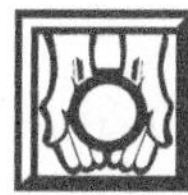

TREATMENT

- Surgical correction of the vascular entrapment is indicated—can be performed thoracoscopically or by thoracotomy with similar results.
- Medical management of concurrent aspiration pneumonia may be necessary.
- Feeding procedures for megaesophagus may also be necessary for a prolonged period.
- Supportive care with oxygen may be needed in animals with aspiration pneumonia.

MEDICATIONS

DRUG(S) OF CHOICE

Broad-spectrum antibiotics, such as enrofloxacin 2.5 mg/kg q12h and amoxicillin 10–15 mg/kg q12h should be instituted in animals with aspiration pneumonia.

CONTRAINDICATIONS/POSSIBLE INTERACTIONS

N/A

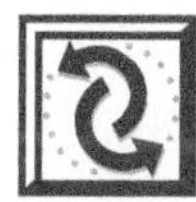

FOLLOW-UP

EXPECTED COURSE AND PROGNOSIS

- Prognosis for resolution of the problem, even after surgery, is guarded. However, the majority of dogs that survive longer than 2 months post repair of PRAA have a good to excellent outcome.
- Complications of malnourishment and aspiration pneumonia are common and can be severe.
- Esophageal function may be permanently compromised.

MISCELLANEOUS

ABBREVIATIONS

- PRAA = persistent right fourth aortic arch.

Suggested Reading

Bonagura JD, Lehmkuhl LB. Congenital heart disease. In: Fox PR, Sisson D, Moise NS, eds., Textbook of Canine and Feline Cardiology, 2nd ed. Philadelphia, PA: Saunders, 1999, pp. 471–535.

Krebs IA, Lindsley S, Shaver S, et al. Short- and long-term outcome of dogs following surgical correction of persistent right aortic arch. J Am Anim Hosp Assoc 2014, 50:181–186.

Parks MK. Park's Pediatric Cardiology for Practitioners, 6th ed. Philadelphia, PA: Elsevier Saunders 2014, pp. 307–313.

Author Jean M. Betkowski

Consulting Editor Michael Aherne

VASCULITIS, CUTANEOUS

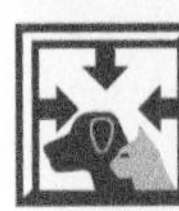

BASICS

OVERVIEW

- Inflammation of blood vessel walls.
- Pathophysiology—primarily type III (immune complex), but type I and type II reactions possible.
- Systems affected—skin/exocrine and renal/urologic in some greyhounds.
- Genetics—familial pyogranuloma and vasculitis of Scottish terriers possibly autosomal dominant; proliferative arteritis in St. Bernards (unknown mode of inheritance).

SIGNALMENT

Species

Dog and cat (rare).

Breed Predilections

Chinese Shar-Pei, dachshund, collie, Shetland sheepdog, German shepherd dog, and Rottweiler predisposed.

SIGNS

Historical Findings

Anorexia, depression, pyrexia possible.

Physical Examination Findings

- Focal alopecia with scarring and scaling (especially vaccine-induced)—lesions over location of vaccination and pinnal apices.
- Necrosis and punctate ulcers, palpable purpura, hemorrhagic bullae or urticaria.
- Acrocyanosis.
- Extremities (paws, pinnae, lips, tail, and oral mucosa) may be painful.
- Pitting edema of the extremities, polyarthropathy, and myopathy possible.

CAUSES & RISK FACTORS

- Idiopathic.
- Drug-induced.
- Vaccine-induced.
- Adverse food reaction.
- Tick-borne diseases (e.g., *Rickettsia rickettsii*).
- Infectious.
- Underlying metabolic process (e.g., diabetes).
- Autoimmune.
- Neoplasia.

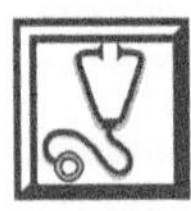

DIAGNOSIS

DIFFERENTIAL DIAGNOSIS

- Deep pyoderma.
- Ear margin seborrhea.
- Chemical and thermal burn.
- Hypersensitivity reaction.
- Dermatomyositis.
- Cryoglobulinemia.
- Toxic epidermal necrolysis.
- Erythema multiforme.
- Eosinophilic dermatitis.
- Systemic lupus erythematosus.
- Bullous pemphigoid.
- Pemphigus vulgaris.
- Sepsis.

CBC/BIOCHEMISTRY/URINALYSIS

Normal unless due to underlying metabolic process or infection.

OTHER LABORATORY TESTS

- Serologic testing for parasitic and infectious disease.
- Immunodiagnostics—antinuclear antibody (ANA) titer, Coombs' test, and cold agglutinin tests.

DIAGNOSTIC PROCEDURES

- Skin scrapings—demodicosis.
- Biopsy of early lesion—neutrophilic (leukocytoclastic/non-leukocytoclastic), lymphocytic, eosinophilic, or granulomatous mixed cells in and around the vessels; vascular necrosis and fibrin thrombi may be prominent; perivascular hemorrhage and edema may occur.
- Representative cultures (e.g., blood, urine, skin) if suspicious of infectious issues.
- Subtle findings suggestive of follicular, dermal, and/or epidermal hypoxia may be seen in mild cases or late-stage tissue samples.

PATHOLOGIC FINDINGS

- May vary with stage and etiology.
- Intramural inflammation of vessels, endothelial cell swelling, pale collagen, faded hair follicles, hemorrhage, and edema of surrounding tissue.

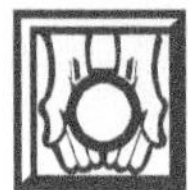

TREATMENT

- Adequate wound care may be necessary for cases with severe and extensive ulceration.
- No limitation in activity unless infectious agent suspected.
- Isolate if contagious or zoonotic agent suspected.
- Individual (focal) lesions may be surgically excised; otherwise, dependent on underlying etiology.

MEDICATIONS

DRUG(S) OF CHOICE

- Based on underlying disease; if drugs or drug-like substances are suspected, they should be discontinued.
- Immune-mediated disease with concurrent vasculitis—prednisolone 0.5–4 mg/kg q24h, taper with response.
- Pentoxifylline 10–20 mg/kg PO q8–12h.
- Cyclosporine 5 mg/kg q24h.
- Tetracycline and niacinamide each 500 mg q8h for dogs >10 kg or 250 mg PO q8h for dogs <10 kg or doxycycline 5 mg/kg PO q12h with niacinamide as with tetracycline.

Alternative Drugs

- Chlorambucil 0.1–0.2 mg/kg every 1–2 days PO initially and taper according to response.
- Azathioprine 1–2 mg/kg every 1–2 days PO initially and taper according to response.
- Dapsone 1 mg/kg PO q24h or sulfasalazine 15–22 mg/kg PO q8–12h.

CONTRAINDICATIONS/POSSIBLE INTERACTIONS

Precautions

- Do not use any medications suspected of causing hypersensitivity.
- Do not administer tetracycline/doxycycline to pregnant or young animals.

FOLLOW-UP

PATIENT MONITORING

- Monitor appropriately during treatment of specific etiology.
- Pentoxifylline—may decrease blood pressure; may cause excitation; monitor blood pressure if concerned.
- Doxycycline or tetracycline—possible increased liver enzymes, possible esophageal strictures in cats (doxycycline); monitor liver chemistries.
- Patients receiving prednisolone, azathioprine, chlorambucil, sulfasalazine, or dapsone—monitor appropriately with CBC, chemistry screen, and urinalysis.
- Sulfasalazine or dapsone—may decrease tear formation; Schirmer tear test every 2 weeks initially and then routinely.
- Immunosuppressive therapies should be reduced to the lowest possible therapeutic dose.

POSSIBLE COMPLICATIONS

Sepsis and death from primary cause and/or sequelae if severe.

EXPECTED COURSE AND PROGNOSIS

If no underlying disease is found, vasculitis may be difficult to treat and the prognosis is guarded.

MISCELLANEOUS

PREGNANCY/FERTILITY/BREEDING

- Corticosteroids, sulfasalazine, tetracycline/doxycycline, and dapsone—do not use in pregnant animals.
- All drugs should be used with caution in pregnant and breeding animals.

ABBREVIATIONS

- ANA = antinuclear antibody.

Suggested Reading

Innera, M. Cutaneous vasculitis. Vet Clin North Am Small Anim Pract 2013, 43:113–134.

Author Karen A. Kuhl

Consulting Editor Alexander H. Werner Resnick

VASCULITIS, SYSTEMIC (INCLUDING PHLEBITIS)

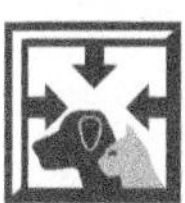

BASICS

DEFINITION

• Heterogeneous group of disorders causing inflammation secondary to endothelial damage of blood vessel walls, leading to tissue necrosis.
• Characterized by histological evidence of inflammation, destruction of blood vessels and ischemic changes.
• Phlebitis is associated with, and is a complication of, IV therapy with the tunica intima of the vascular endothelial wall becoming inflamed.

PATHOPHYSIOLOGY

• Endothelial damage by an infectious agent, parasite infestation, endotoxin, or immune complex deposition that initiates local inflammation, neutrophil chemotaxis, and complement activation, sensitizing the vascular endothelium causing release of vasoactive substances that cause vasoconstriction, increase vascular permeability, and activate coagulation systems.
• End result is endothelial cell activation, necrosis of the vessel wall with subsequent thrombosis which may cause hemorrhage and extravasation of proteins into surrounding tissue, leading to swelling and edema.
• Thrombosis obstructs blood flow and may cause palpable thickening or vascular cord, which may progress to irreversible vascular sclerosis.
• Leukocyte pyrogens may cause systemic inflammation and fever.

SYSTEMS AFFECTED

• Skin—local inflammation/infection.
• Cardiovascular—altered vascular permeability and blood flow.
• Hemic/lymphatic/immune—bacteria, inflammatory mediators and emboli can cause systemic inflammatory response and organ dysfunction.
• Renal/urologic—systemic inflammatory response and type III hypersensitivity reaction. causing proteinuria and glomerulonephritis, respectively.
• Ophthalmic—uveitis due to systemic inflammatory response.
• Musculoskeletal—systemic inflammatory response and type III hypersensitivity reaction.
• Respiratory—deep venous thrombophlebitis may cause pulmonary embolism.

INCIDENCE/PREVALENCE

• Unknown—vascular inflammation is a common cause of dermatologic disease in humans and animals. More often seen in dogs than in cats.
• 20–80% of hospitalized patients receiving peripheral IV therapy develop phlebitis with superficial thrombophlebitis most common (10–12% may progress to deep venous thrombosis).

SIGNALMENT

Species

• Dog and cat.
• No known specific age or gender predisposition in veterinary medicine.

Breed Predilections

• Collies and Shetland sheepdogs (familial canine dermatomyositis).
• German shepherd dog—autosomal recessive.
• Scottish terrier—suspect autosomal dominant.
• Shar-pei—familial vasculitis.
• St. Bernard and giant schnauzer—dermal arteritis of nasal philtrum.
• Jack Russell terrier.
• Greyhound—idiopathic cutaneous and renal vasculopathy.

SIGNS

Historical Findings

• Provocative drug (e.g., cephalexin, sulfonamides, itraconazole, and hydralazine) given to sensitized animal.
• Recent vaccination history.
• Exposure to ticks.
• Poor dirofilariasis prophylaxis in endemic areas.

Physical Examination Findings

• Swelling.
• Palpable purpura, plaques, hemorrhagic bullae alone or in combination with edema.
• Ulceration.
• Necrosis of affected skin, especially mucous membranes, mucocutaneous junctions, pinnae edges, and footpads.
• Systemic signs reflecting organ involvement (e.g., hepatic, renal, gastrointestinal and CNS).
• Systemic signs of illness (e.g., lethargy, anorexia, lymphadenopathy, pyrexia, generalized pain, and weight loss).
• Juvenile polyarteritis in beagles characterized by recurring episodes of fever (>40°C) and neck pain persisting for 3–7 days.
• Cutaneous lesions of polyarteritis nodosa (subcutaneous nodules—less common in dogs than in people).
• Signs associated with underlying infectious or immune-related disease (e.g., thrombocytopenia and polyarthropathy).
• Ophthalmologic examination—anterior uveitis, scleral injection, hyphema.

CAUSES

Infectious

• Parasitic—Dirofilaria immitis, Angiostrongylus vasorum, Leishmania spp., Babesia gibsoni.
• Viral—e.g., feline infectious peritonitis, canine coronavirus, and canine circovirus infection.
• Rickettsial—e.g., Rocky Mountain spotted fever and ehrlichiosis.
• Protozoal—e.g., Toxoplasma.
• Bacterial—sepsis.

Iatrogenic

• Mechanical injury from IV catheter size/stiffness/integrity/duration, traumatic placement, previous venipuncture, high fluid infusion rates.
• Chemical injury—IV catheter material, drugs, fluids of extreme osmolality or pH, parenteral nutrition, other vesicant solutions.
• Obstructed blood flow—large-bore catheter, vasoconstriction, and hypotension.

Idiopathic

Approximately 50% of cases.

Immune-Related

• Systemic lupus erythematosus.
• Rheumatoid arthritis-like arthropathy.
• Lupus-like drug reaction.
• Type III hypersensitivities (e.g., to food, cephalexin, sulfonamides, fenbendazole, and penicillin).
• Juvenile polyarteritis in beagles.
• Wegener's granulomatosis (rare).
• Polyarteritis nodosa.
• Neoplasia.
• Uremia.

DIAGNOSIS

DIFFERENTIAL DIAGNOSIS

• Cutaneous signs developing after administration of medication/vaccine implicate drug reaction (usually not immediate, may develop after days or weeks).
• Vasculitis associated with systemic signs (e.g., polyarthropathy, myositis, pyrexia) implicates immune or infectious cause.
• Cold hemagglutinin disease suggested by distribution of cyanotic or necrotic lesions (nose, ears, toes, tail tip, prepuce) and history of exposure to cold.

CBC/BIOCHEMISTRY/URINALYSIS

• CBC changes consistent with degree of systemic inflammatory response and platelet consumption.
• Biochemistry and urinalysis changes may be applicable with organ involvement (e.g., hepatic, renal, portal, caval, gastrointestinal, cerebral, cardiac, and pulmonary).

OTHER LABORATORY TESTS

• Tissue, blood, and urine cultures if sepsis suspected.
• Serologic tests may aid diagnosis of infectious (i.e., rickettsial, *Leishmania*) disease.
• Antinuclear antibody (ANA) titer positive in patients with systemic lupus erythematosus (SLE); may also be positive in patients with other systemic illnesses.
• Occult heartworm test positive in patient with dirofilariasis.
• *Angiostrongylus* infestation diagnosed by fecal examination and cytologic examination of tracheal wash.

VASCULITIS, SYSTEMIC (INCLUDING PHLEBITIS) (CONTINUED)

- Coagulation—may see alterations in prothrombin time (PT), partial thromboplastin time (PTT), D-dimer, antithrombin, protein C, thromboelastography.

IMAGING

Thoracic Radiographs

Nonspecific abnormalities that may be seen include infiltrates, nodules, patchy consolidation, pleural effusion, and cardiomegaly.

Abdominal Imaging

- CT (with angiogram) or MRI— Provide valuable information regarding diagnosis of deep tissue embolism and thickening of the vessel wall when suspected based on organ damage or dysfunction.
- B-mode ultrasonography to assess venous patency, character, and blood flow.

DIAGNOSTIC PROCEDURES

- Doppler assessment—inexpensive test of venous patency and blood flow.
- Skin biopsy specimen from active edges of developing lesions is definitive for vasculitis but may not reveal cause.
- Immunofluorescence test of skin biopsy specimen may rule out pemphigus and pemphigoid diseases.
- If allergic response is suspected, resolution of signs upon discontinuation of suspect medication or food supports diagnosis.

PATHOLOGIC FINDINGS

- Inflammation and destruction of blood vessels with secondary ischemic/hypoxic changes from thromboembolic occlusion of vessels.
- Inflammatory infiltrate may be neutrophilic (major), eosinophilic, or lymphocytic.
- Damage to blood vessels may lead to the development of hemorrhage and edema within affected tissue.
- Epidermal lesions such as exudation, crusting, and ulceration may also develop secondary to ischemia.

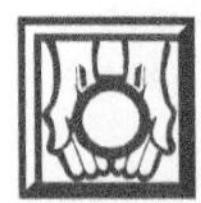

TREATMENT

APPROPRIATE HEALTH CARE

- Based upon individual patient, history, clinical findings, identification of the inciting cause, and whether or not disease is progressive.
- Remove suspected inciting cause (IV catheter, drugs, or xenobiotic substances) and avoid in the future.
- Minimally affected dogs require little management.
- Moderate to severe cases require pharmacologic intervention and wound care to prevent secondary bacterial infection and sepsis.
- If untreatable or unknown underlying condition—glucocorticoid, immunosuppressive (e.g., cyclophosphamide, azathioprine), and other drugs (e.g., dapsone and sulfasalazine) are occasionally effective, but clinical trials of efficacy have not been reported in animals.
- If caustic infiltration suspected for phlebitis, terminate infusion and leave cannula in place temporarily to aspirate residual catheter fluid and instill specific antidotes into affected tissue when applicable.
- Intermittent warm moist compress or hydrotherapy; some extravasated substances require cold therapy.
- Photobiomodulation (low-level light therapy [LLLT]) can be used directly over affected areas to reduce inflammation, activate stem cells, and promote blood flow and tissue repair.
- Avoid stagnant blood flow and thromboembolism by promoting mobility (i.e., physical therapy and/or compression therapy).

NURSING CARE

- Supportive therapy (e.g., IV fluids, oxygen, nutrition) for systemic illness secondary to vasculitis (e.g., hepatic, renal, pulmonary, gastrointestinal, cerebral, cardiac).
- IV catheter placement and maintenance—use strict aseptic technique and sterile dressing with IV catheters being regularly checked for patency, line integrity, and associated swelling (every 1–2 hours) with continuous infusions. Change peripheral catheters every 3–4 days, or within 24 hours if placed under emergency situation.

ACTIVITY

- Soft/cushioned bedding and protective footwear can be used when the pads are eroded/ulcerated.
- Minimal rough play with other dogs as may exacerbate skin damage.

DIET

- Nutritional support appropriate to treatment of underlying illness(es).
- Consider glycemic control if sepsis or risk of sepsis.

CLIENT EDUCATION

- Advise clients of IV catheter risks and complications, especially in patients with predisposing factors.
- Clients should be trained in and continue physical therapy and basic nursing care at home.

SURGICAL CONSIDERATIONS

- Infected catheter sites and/or extensive tissue damage may require surgical debridement and delayed closure.
- Surgical ligation or stripping of the corded vessels may be indicated to avoid deep vein thrombosis.

MEDICATIONS

DRUG(S) OF CHOICE

- Infectious or immune-related—treat underlying disease (see specific condition); supportive care.
- Lupus-like drug reactions and type III hypersensitivity—discontinue drug; supportive care.
- Methylxanthine derivative—pentoxifylline 20 mg/kg three times daily improves microcirculatory peripheral blood flow, tissue blood oxygenation, and decreases inflammation.
- Glucocorticoids—prednisolone 0.5–1 mg/kg with progressive disease and no underlying trigger identification; continue until clinical remission achieved then slowly taper by 25% every 14 days.
- Other immunomodulators—cases refractory to glucocorticoids (e.g., cyclosporine, azathioprine, chlorambucil).
- Antioxidants—e.g., vitamin E 200–800 IU q12h anecdotally provide a protective effect against ischemic dermatopathies.
- Leukocyte-specific anti-inflammatory—tetracycline and niacinamide combination used for milder cases of vasculitis; exact mechanism incompletely understood.
- Sulfonamide drugs—e.g., sulfasalazine 25 mg/kg three times daily for refractory neutrophilic vasculitis.
- Antibiotics (if infection/sepsis suspected)—use empirical therapy, based on location and potential contaminants if no culture and sensitivity available.

CONTRAINDICATIONS

- Avoid caustic, irritating, or immunogenic topicals or infusions.
- Do not administer sulfasalazine to patients sensitive to sulfonamides.
- Multiple myelosuppressive/immunosuppressive drugs may be additive and increase risk of infection.

PRECAUTIONS

- Avoid use of systemic nonsteroidal anti-inflammatory drugs (NSAIDs) if renal, hepatic, or gastrointestinal dysfunction.
- Corticosteroids, unless used as an appropriate pretreatment for chemotherapy, are associated with delayed wound healing and may predispose to infection.
- Pentoxifylline may reduce blood pressure.

POSSIBLE INTERACTIONS

Use of NSAIDs with concurrent anti-inflammatory or immunosuppressive dose corticosteroid therapy.

ALTERNATIVE DRUG(S)

- Topical dermatitis creams (e.g. silver-sulfadiazine) may help reduce irritation and prevent infection.

• Topical tacrolimus for focal lesions may help reduce inflammation.

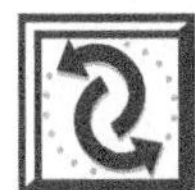

FOLLOW-UP

PATIENT MONITORING

• Patients being treated with sulfonamide drugs (e.g., dapsone) or immunosuppressants–regular monitoring of CBC, serum chemistry profile and urinalysis for side effects (e.g., myelosuppression, hepatopathy, and other blood dyscrasias).
• Patients receiving sulfasalazine—monitor for keratoconjunctivitis sicca with Schirmer tear test (every 2 weeks for first 2 months).
• Hardness, skin pallor, black discoloration, or eschar formation occur with tissue necrosis.
• Persistent or progressive redness, swelling, pain, or heat—adjust antibiotic therapy based on most current culture and sensitivity results.

PREVENTION/AVOIDANCE

• Tick prevention and regular monitoring of serum titers for tick-borne diseases in endemic areas.
• Avoidance/elimination of optional/ minimizing of the number of vaccines given at any one time.
• Discontinue and avoid suspected inciting triggering factors.
• Avoid use of phlebotic veins for IV therapy or blood collection until completely healed.
• Consider using submicron IV catheter filters, which may reduce incidence by removing particulates, endotoxin, and other soluble mediators of morbidity.

POSSIBLE COMPLICATIONS

• Dependent on severity.
• Tissue necrosis.
• Organ damage (e.g., hepatic, renal, portal, caval, gastrointestinal, cerebral, cardiac, pulmonary).
• Thromboembolism.
• Lymphangitis.
• Septicemia.
• Extension to deep venous system.

EXPECTED COURSE AND PROGNOSIS

• Mild phlebitis cases self-limiting (1–3 days) with removal of catheter. For severe local lesions, resolution can take 3–4 weeks and may result in loss of function/permanent tissue damage. Poor prognosis when associated with pulmonary thromboembolism and/or sepsis.

MISCELLANEOUS

ASSOCIATED CONDITIONS

• Pulmonary thromboembolism.
• Infection/cellulitis/sepsis.
• Immune-mediated disease (e.g., SLE).

AGE-RELATED FACTORS

• Neonatal and geriatric patients may be predisposed to infection.
• Delayed wound healing in geriatric patients.

ZOONOTIC POTENTIAL

N/A

PREGNANCY/FERTILITY/BREEDING

• Pregnancy may predispose to thromboembolism.
• Incidence of fetal complications with phlebitis is unknown.

SYNONYMS

• Thrombophlebitis.
• Necrotizing vasculitis.
• Vasculitis.

SEE ALSO

• Lupus Erythematosus, Systemic.
• Pulmonary Thromboembolism.
• Sepsis and Bacteremia.

ABBREVIATIONS

• ANA = antinuclear antibody.
• LLLT = low-level light therapy.
• NSAID = nonsteroidal anti-inflammatory drug.
• PT = prothrombin time.
• PTT = partial thromboplastin time.
• SLE = systemic lupus erythematosus.

INTERNET RESOURCES

https://www.dvm360.com/view/diagnosing-and-managing-canine-cutaneous-vasculitis-proceedings

Suggested Reading

Innera M. Cutaneous vasculitis in small animals. Vet Clin North Am Small Anim Pract 2013, 43:113–134.

Author Stuart A. Walton
Consulting Editor Michael Aherne

VENTRICULAR ARRHYTHMIAS AND SUDDEN DEATH IN GERMAN SHEPHERDS

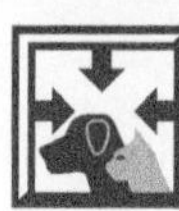

BASICS

OVERVIEW

Inherited disorder resulting in ventricular arrhythmias in otherwise healthy young German shepherd dogs. The phenotypic spectrum is wide, with some dogs having infrequent single premature ventricular complexes while others have frequent and rapid ventricular tachycardia (VT) that is associated with sudden death. The pattern of inheritance is complex, depending heavily on background genetics. Siblings of dogs that have died suddenly should be tested for this disorder.

SIGNALMENT

- Most dogs develop arrhythmias at approximately 12 weeks of age (identified as young as 6 weeks). Number and severity of arrhythmias tend to peak between 5–9 months. By approximately 18–24 months most dogs have only a few arrhythmias.
- No sex predilection.

SIGNS

- Signs are very rare (e.g., in >500 dogs examined only 1 had syncope) since VT is often nonsustained until, in some dogs, it degenerates into ventricular fibrillation resulting in death (usually between 5 and 9 months of age).
- Arrhythmias often detected during routine examination before neutering. • Death is associated with sleep, rest after exercise, or excitement after sleep, particularly in early morning.

CAUSES & RISK FACTORS

- Genetic mutation(s) responsible has not been identified. • Multiple electrophysiologic abnormalities have been identified—early and delayed afterdepolarizations, heterogeneous and altered action potential duration, as well as changes in ion channel current density, calcium cycling, and sympathetic innervation.
- VT tends to be most frequent with slow heart rates (drug-induced [e.g. fentanyl] or during sleep).

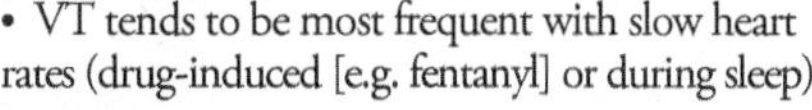

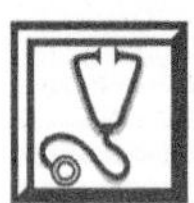

DIAGNOSIS

DIFFERENTIAL DIAGNOSIS

Rule out myocarditis.

CBC/BIOCHEMISTRY/URINALYSIS

Results of routine laboratory tests are unremarkable.

OTHER LABORATORY TESTS

Troponin concentration—to rule out myocarditis. Dogs with inherited arrhythmias have normal troponin levels.

IMAGING

- Thoracic radiographs—normal.
- Echocardiography—usually normal.

DIAGNOSTIC PROCEDURES

24-Hour Ambulatory Electrocardiogram (Holter Monitor)

- Required for diagnosis and classification of severity. • Arrhythmias identified most commonly are rapid (rates >400 bpm) polymorphic VT with single premature complexes that are most commonly of a left ventricular origin pattern (negative in lead II). Though nonsustained rapid polymorphic VT is most characteristic, approximately 15% of dogs will have slower monomorphic and more sustained VT. • Some dogs will have thousands of singlet ventricular premature complexes (VPCs) with no VT; extensive periods of ventricular bigeminy have been found in others. • After 6 months of age, runs of VT are more common after pauses.

PATHOLOGIC FINDINGS

Routine gross and histopathologic examination is within normal limits.

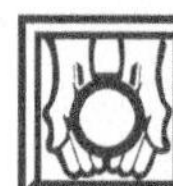

TREATMENT

- Limited studies have shown cardiac pacing to keep the heart rate above 120 bpm decreased the frequency of the arrhythmias but did not prevent sudden death.
- Implantation of cardioverter defibrillators may be helpful, but proper programming of these devices in young dogs is complicated.
- Avoid drugs that slow heart rate.
- Anesthesia is not contraindicated as long as anticholinergic drugs are used to prevent bradycardia during the age range when the arrhythmias exist. • Treatment is required only for dogs with VT. Afflicted dogs with only VPCs do not die. However, if a young dog is identified with this disorder, repeated Holter monitoring is advised to be sure that the phenotype of that particular dog does not include VT (e.g., particularly if the peak affectedness of that dog has not yet occurred).

MEDICATIONS

DRUG(S) OF CHOICE

- Ventricular arrhythmias usually are easily suppressed with lidocaine 2 mg/kg IV.
- Control of the arrhythmias with oral medication is more problematic. • Sotalol alone can be proarrhythmic and should not be used. • Sotalol 2–3 mg/kg PO q12h combined with mexiletine 4–8 mg/kg PO q8h suppresses the ventricular arrhythmias, but response in individual dogs is highly variable.

CONTRAINDICATIONS/POSSIBLE INTERACTIONS

- Avoid drugs that slow heart rate until dogs are older than 18–24 months.
- Drugs that slow or prolong action potential duration such as sotalol, phenylephrine, or fentanyl are proarrhythmic.

FOLLOW-UP

PATIENT MONITORING

- Repeat Holter monitoring to assess drug efficacy. • After 18–24 months of age the Holter monitoring is again repeated. If the number of ventricular ectopic complexes is <2,000 singles with no VT, the dog's risk of death is very low and medications may be stopped. • Although occasional dogs may have a dramatic drop in the arrhythmia count and severity during treatment, most do not. Therefore, absence of arrhythmias on Holter recordings after 18–24 months of age indicates a change in the disorder rather than an antiarrhythmic effect.
- Lifelong treatment is not required.

EXPECTED COURSE AND PROGNOSIS

- Approximately 50% of affected dogs with >10 runs of VT/24 hours will die suddenly before 1 year of age. If a dog does not have VT identified by 24-hour electrocardiographic monitoring, the probability of death is very low. • Even severely affected dogs that have reached the age of 2 years with documented absence of arrhythmia have lived a normal lifespan >12 years.

MISCELLANEOUS

AGE-RELATED FACTORS

Since identification of affected dogs depends on the determination of arrhythmias before the age of 1 (ideally 4–9 months) to 2 years (at most), afflicted dogs can easily be missed because the only clinical sign is sudden death with no evidence of a cause found on routine post-mortem examination.

ABBREVIATIONS

- VPC = ventricular premature complex.
- VT = ventricular tachycardia.

Suggested Reading

Kraus MS, Gelzer ARM, Moïse NS. Treatment of cardiac arrhythmias and conduction disturbances. In: Smith FWK, Tilley LP, Oyama MA, Sleeper MM, eds., Manual of Canine and Feline Cardiology, 5th ed. St. Louis, MO: Saunders Elsevier, 2016.

Author Michael Aherne

Consulting Editor Michael Aherne

Acknowledgment The author and book editors acknowledge the prior contribution of N. Sydney Moïse.

VENTRICULAR FIBRILLATION

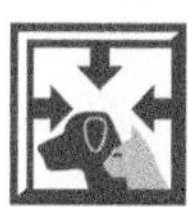

BASICS

DEFINITION

• A ventricular rhythm of disorganized electrical activity resulting in nonproductive ventricular muscle quivering (i.e., fibrillation). • Also known as V-fib or VF and is considered the most severe cardiac rhythm disturbance.

PATHOPHYSIOLOGY

Loss of organized ventricular activity results in acute and profound drop in cardiac output, systemic blood pressure, and organ perfusion, eventually leading to death.

SYSTEMS AFFECTED

• Cardiovascular. • All organ systems affected by loss of perfusion.

GENETICS

• Not recognized in veterinary patients.
• However, there are known ventricular arrhythmias with modes of inheritance in the dog.

INCIDENCE/PREVALENCE

Unknown

SIGNALMENT

Species

Dog and cat.

Breed Predilections

None

Mean Age and Range

Unknown, but probably more common in geriatric animals.

SIGNS

Historical Findings

• Severe systemic illness. • Severe cardiac disease. • Previously documented cardiac arrhythmias.

Physical Examination Findings

• Collapse. • Loss of consciousness (i.e., syncope). • Cardiac arrest. • Death.

CAUSES

Cardiac

• Cardiac surgery/interventional procedure.
• Cardiomyopathy. • Myocardial injury.
• Myocarditis. • Subaortic/aortic stenosis.

Extracardiac

• Anoxia. • Autonomic imbalances, especially high sympathetic tone or administration of catecholamines.
• Circulatory shock. • Drug reactions—e.g., anesthetic agents, especially halothane and ultrashort-acting barbiturates, digoxin.
• Electrical shock. • Electrolyte and acid–base imbalances. • Hypothermia.

RISK FACTORS

Any severe systemic illness or cardiac disease.

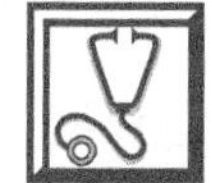

DIAGNOSIS

ECG Features (Figures 1 and 2)

• Rapid, chaotic, irregular rhythm with bizarre waves or oscillations. • Oscillations may be large (coarse fibrillation) or small (fine fibrillation). • Absent P waves. • Absent QRS complexes.

DIFFERENTIAL DIAGNOSES

• Check for pulse. • Rule out ECG artifact.
• Reapply ECG clips and ensure good skin contact and adequate gel (or alcohol) applied to leads. • If there is possibility of using defibrillator to shock patient, do *not* use alcohol as it is a flammable substance.

CBC/BIOCHEMISTRY/URINALYSIS

The abnormalities generally relate to the underlying metabolic problem that causes ventricular fibrillation.

OTHER LABORATORY TESTS

Cardiac troponin I may be elevated in case of severe arrhythmia, cardiac ischemia, or myocarditis.

IMAGING

• Can utilize point of care ultrasound to visualize heart chamber activity. • Avoid alcohol and utilize gel whenever possible (see above).

PATHOLOGIC FINDINGS

Vary depending on histopathologic findings on post-mortem examination.

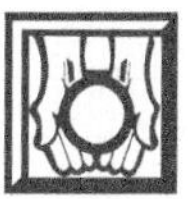

TREATMENT

APPROPRIATE HEALTH CARE

• Rapidly fatal rhythm requiring immediate, aggressive treatment. • Outcome is often death without use of electrical cardioversion (defibrillation).

Direct Current Defibrillation

• Immediate defibrillation is recommended when the duration of cardiopulmonary arrest caused by ventricular fibrillation is 4 minutes or less. • Otherwise, a 2-minute cycle of chest compressions before defibrillation is recommended. • The dose of energy for initial defibrillation is 2–4 J/kg (biphasic defibrillator) or 4–6 J/kg (monophasic defibrillator). • If an initial shock is not successful, CPR is resumed for 2 minutes before defibrillation is attempted again. • A 50% escalation in the energy delivered may be considered for subsequent defibrillation attempts.

Precordial Thump

To be used if no access to an electrical defibrillator. • Apply a sharp blow with the ulnar aspect of a closed fist to the chest wall over the heart. • Rarely successful in conversion to sinus rhythm. • This technique is *not* recommended for other rhythms as a thump can also cause more malignant arrhythmias.

NURSING CARE

Treat any identified conditions such as hypothermia, electrolyte disturbances, and acid–base disorders.

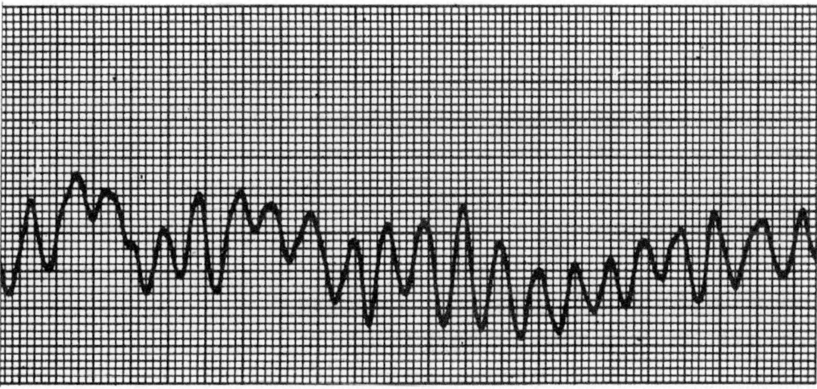

Figure 1.

Coarse ventricular fibrillation. (Source: From Tilley LP. Essentials of Canine and Feline Electrocardiography, 3rd ed. Baltimore: Williams & Wilkins, 1992. Reprinted with permission of Wolters Kluwer.)

VENTRICULAR FIBRILLATION (CONTINUED)

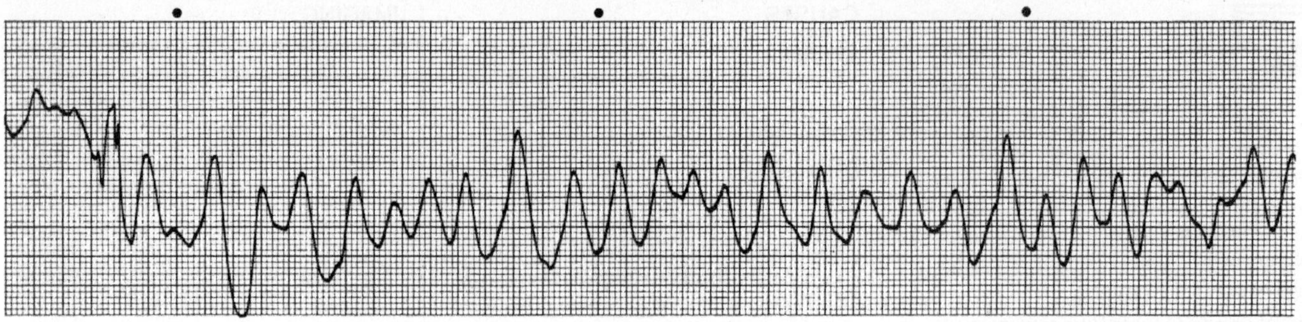

Figure 2.

Ventricular flutter–fibrillation in a cat with severe myocardial damage from an 11-story fall. The complexes are very wide, bizarre, tall, and rapid. (Source: From Tilley LP. Essentials of Canine and Feline Electrocardiography, 3rd ed. Baltimore: Williams & Wilkins, 1992. Reprinted with permission of Wolters Kluwer.)

CLIENT EDUCATION

If the patient is converted back to a sinus rhythm, warn the owner that the patient is at high risk for recurrence of the arrhythmia in the immediate post-resuscitation period.

SURGICAL CONSIDERATIONS

N/A

MEDICATIONS

DRUG(S) OF CHOICE

• Institute cardiopulmonary cerebral resuscitation. • Epinephrine—low dose (0.01 mg/kg) of epinephrine is recommended as high-dose therapy has not been associated with increased survival. A shortcut to calculate low-dose epinephrine volume for administration is 0.1 mL/10 kg. The dose may be repeated at 3- to 5-minute intervals. • Vasopressin—there is evidence that this drug may be equivalent to or even superior to epinephrine is some situations. The dose of vasopressin is 0.8 units/kg (dogs and cats), and the dose may be repeated at 3- to 5-minute intervals. • Once the animal is successfully converted, administer IV lidocaine or amiodarone to lower the risk of refibrillation or development of ventricular tachycardia. • Lidocaine 2 mg/kg (dogs, IV, IO, IT); a shortcut to calculate the dose for the 2% (20 mg/mL) solution is 1 mL/10 kg. • Amiodarone (Nexterone®) 2–5 mg/kg (dogs, IV). Do NOT use amiodarone with polysorbate 80; this has been shown to cause anaphylaxis in dogs. Hypotension is a common occurrence during amiodarone administration.

PRECAUTIONS

• Lidocaine raises the fibrillation threshold but makes defibrillation more difficult. • Lidocaine and amiodarone have the potential to be proarrhythmic. • There is currently no evidence for improved outcome with use of these medications in patients with VF.

ALTERNATIVE DRUG(S)

• Magnesium (chloride or sulfate) is commonly administered (0.3 mEq/kg IV) for antiarrhythmic treatment. Magnesium is not known to have any proarrhythmic effect. There is no supportive evidence for its use in VF. • Chemical conversion can be attempted if no access to electrical defibrillator. Administer 1 mEq potassium/kg and 6 mg/kg acetylcholine IC. This approach is rarely successful.

FOLLOW-UP

PATIENT MONITORING

• CBC, biochemistry profile, urinalysis, arterial blood gases with acid–base analysis. • If primary cardiac disease is suspected—echocardiogram, cardiac troponin, and thoracic radiographs. • Continuous ECG monitoring.

PREVENTION/AVOIDANCE

Careful monitoring of critically ill patients to prevent and correct acid–base disturbances, hypotension, and hypoxemia.

POSSIBLE COMPLICATIONS

• Recurrence of VF. • Death. • Disseminated intravascular coagulation. • Multiorgan failure.

EXPECTED COURSE AND PROGNOSIS

Most patients die because of either the arrhythmia or the underlying disease.

MISCELLANEOUS

AGE-RELATED FACTORS

May be more likely in patients of advanced age.

PREGNANCY/FERTILITY/BREEDING

N/A

SEE ALSO

Cardiopulmonary Arrest.

ABBREVIATIONS

• IC = intracardiac. • IT = intratracheal.
• VF = ventricular fibrillation.

Suggested Reading

Fletcher DJ, Boller M, Brainard BM, et al. RECOVER evidence and knowledge gap analysis on veterinary CPR. Part 7: clinical guidelines. J Vet Emerg Crit Care 2012, 22:S102–131.

Kraus MS, Gelzer ARM, Moïse NS. Treatment of cardiac arrhythmias and conduction disturbances. In: Smith FWK, Tilley LP, Oyama MA, Sleeper MM, eds., Manual of Canine and Feline Cardiology, 5th ed. St. Louis, MO: Saunders Elsevier, 2016.

Thawley JT, Drobatz KJ. Cardiopulmonary arrest and resuscitation. In: Smith FWK, Tilley LP, Oyama MA, Sleeper MM, eds., Manual of Canine and Feline Cardiology, 5th ed. St. Louis, MO: Saunders Elsevier, 2016.

Tilley LP, Smith FWK, Jr. Electrocardiography. In: Smith FWK, Tilley LP, Oyama MA, Sleeper MM, eds., Manual of Canine and Feline Cardiology, 5th ed. St. Louis, MO: Saunders Elsevier, 2016.

Waldrop JE, Rozanski EA, Swanke ED, et al. Causes of cardiopulmonary arrest, resuscitation management, and functional outcome in dogs and cats surviving cardiopulmonary arrest. J Vet Emerg Crit Care 2004, 14:22–29.

Authors Anna K. McManamey and Francis W.K. Smith, Jr.

Consulting Editor Michael Aherne

BASICS

DEFINITION

• Ventricular pre-excitation occurs when impulses originating in the sinoatrial node or atrium activate a portion of the ventricles prematurely through an accessory pathway without going through the atrioventricular (AV) node; the remainder of the ventricles are activated normally through the usual conduction system. • Wolff–Parkinson–White (WPW) syndrome consists of ventricular pre-excitation with episodes of paroxysmal supraventricular tachycardia (Figures 1 and 2).

ECG Features of Ventricular Pre-excitation

• Normal heart rate and rhythm. • Normal P waves. • Short PR interval (dogs, <0.06 seconds; cats, <0.05 seconds). • Widened QRS (small dogs, >0.05 seconds; large dogs, >0.06 seconds; cats, >0.04 seconds), often with slurring or notching of the upstroke of the R wave (delta wave).

ECG Features of Ventricular Pre-excitation with WPW Syndrome

• Extremely rapid heart rate (dogs, often >300 bpm; cats, approaching 400–500 bpm). • P waves may be difficult to recognize. • QRS complexes may be normal, wide with delta wave, or very wide and bizarre, depending on the circuit. • Conduction is usually 1:1 (i.e., 1 P wave for every QRS complex).

PATHOPHYSIOLOGY

• Can be associated with congenital or acquired cardiac defects in dogs or cats. • May be associated with hypertrophic cardiomyopathy in cats. • Hemodynamic compromise during episodes of supraventricular tachycardia with WPW syndrome. • WPW syndrome results from a developmental abnormality of the atrioventricular groove. During normal cardiogenesis, direct continuity between the atrial and ventricular myocardium is lost by growth of the annulus fibrosis. Defects in the annulus leave muscular connections called accessory pathways or Kent bundles between the atria and ventricular myocardium. By bypassing the AV node, these pathways can lead to pre-excitation of the ventricles. • The accessory pathways typically have an "all or none" conduction properties. They may only conduct from the atria to the ventricles (called anterograde or antegrade conduction), only from the ventricles to the atria (called retrograde conduction), or in both directions.

SYSTEMS AFFECTED

Cardiovascular

INCIDENCE/PREVALENCE

Unknown

SIGNALMENT

Species

Dog and cat.

SIGNS

Historical Findings

• None in patients with ventricular pre-excitation.
• Syncope in patients with WPW syndrome.

Physical Examination Findings

• None in animals with ventricular pre-excitation. • Rapid heart rate in animals with WPW syndrome.

CAUSES

Congenital Heart Disease

• Congenital defect limited to the conduction system. • Atrial septal defect in dogs or cats. • Tricuspid valvular dysplasia in dogs.

Acquired Heart Disease

Hypertrophic cardiomyopathy in cats.

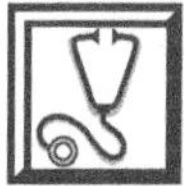

DIAGNOSIS

DIFFERENTIAL DIAGNOSIS

• Ventricular pre-excitation—differentiate from other causes of short PR intervals (e.g., fever, hyperthyroidism, and anemia); these conditions do not cause delta waves.
• Narrow complex WPW syndrome—differentiate from other supraventricular arrhythmias (e.g., atrial tachycardia, atrial flutter, and atrial fibrillation); WPW syndrome is most easily recognized after conversion to normal heart rate and rhythm.
• Alternating WPW syndrome should not be confused with ventricular bigeminy. • Wide complex WPW syndrome must be differentiated from ventricular tachycardia.
• Short PR interval may be correlated with a normal QRS complex if the anomalous pathway bypasses the AV node and connects to the bundle of His (i.e., Lown-Ganong Levine syndrome).

CBC/BIOCHEMISTRY/URINALYSIS

Normal

OTHER LABORATORY TESTS

Normal

IMAGING

Echocardiography may show structural heart disease.

DIAGNOSTIC PROCEDURES

Electrocardiography

PATHOLOGIC FINDINGS

• Pathologic findings vary with underlying cause. • Possibility of no organic heart lesions.

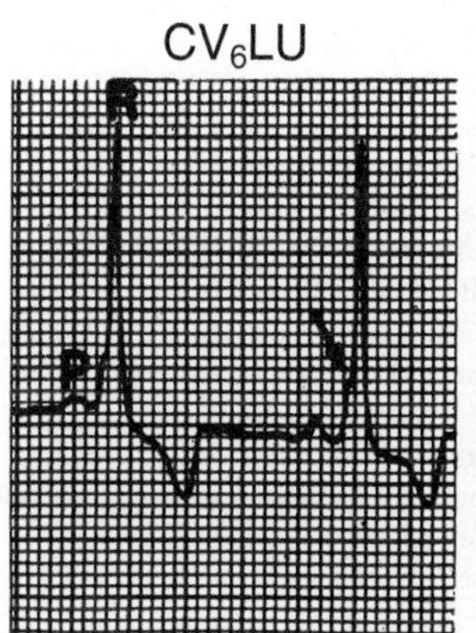

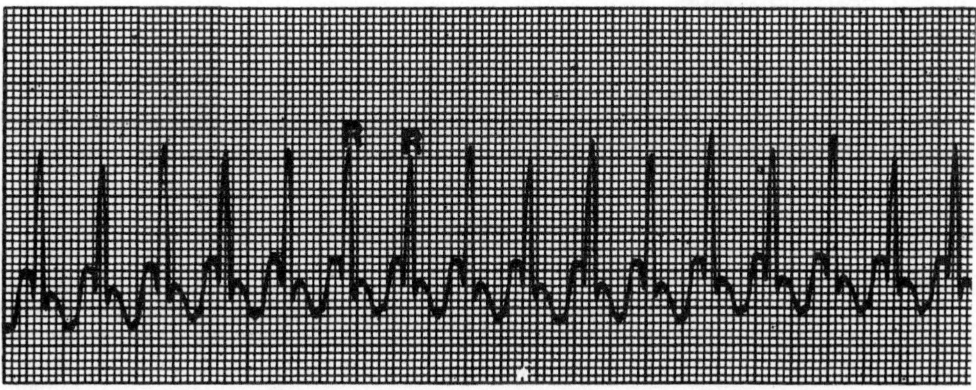

Figure 1.

Wolff–Parkinson–White syndrome (canine). Ventricular pre-excitation represented by the short PR interval, wide QRS complex, and delta wave (arrow) in CV_6LU. Paroxysms of supraventricular tachycardia are represented in the long lead II rhythm strip. (Source: From Tilley LP. Essentials of Canine and Feline Electrocardiography, 3rd ed. Baltimore: Williams & Wilkins, 1992. Reprinted with permission of Wolters Kluwer.)

V

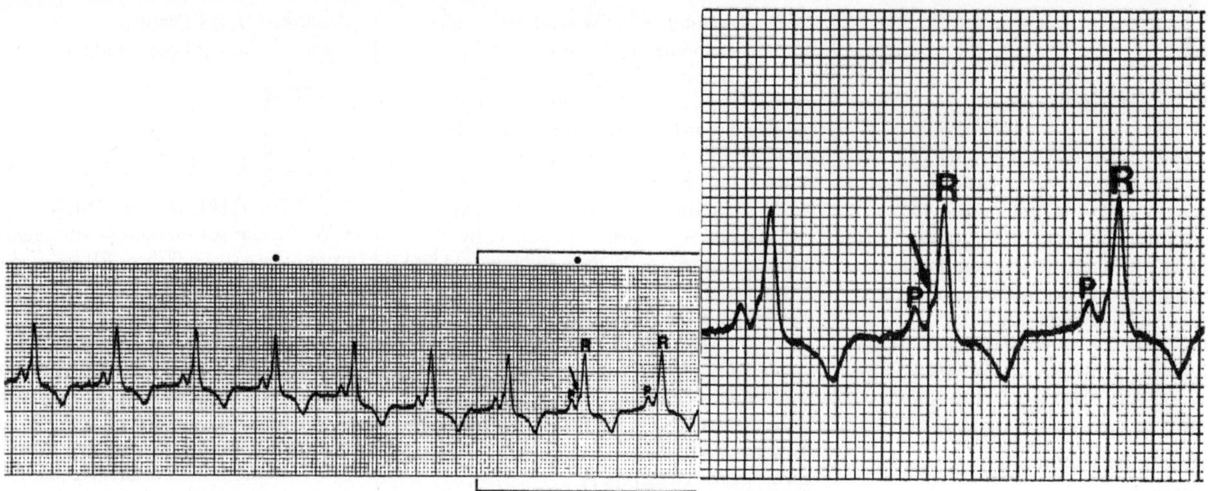

Figure 2.

Ventricular pre-excitation in a cat with episodes of fainting. The P waves are normal, the PR interval is short, and the QRS complex is wide; delta waves (arrow) are present. (Source: From Tilley LP. Essentials of Canine and Feline Electrocardiography, 3rd ed. Baltimore: Williams & Wilkins, 1992. Reprinted with permission of Wolters Kluwer.)

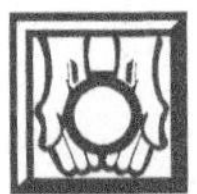

TREATMENT

APPROPRIATE HEALTH CARE

• Ventricular pre-excitation without tachycardia—no treatment needed. • WPW syndrome requires conversion by ocular or carotid sinus pressure, direct current shock (the most effective treatment), or drugs.

ACTIVITY

May need to be limited with WPW until supraventricular tachycardias are controlled.

CLIENT EDUCATION

WPW—explain the need to identify and treat the underlying cause in addition to therapy for supraventricular tachycardia.

SURGICAL CONSIDERATIONS

Catheter ablation with radiofrequency current—a relatively recent technique that allows accessory pathways to be destroyed or ablated by a transvenous catheter positioned at the site of the pathway; can be preferred alternative to lifelong therapy with drugs.

MEDICATIONS

DRUG(S) OF CHOICE

• A variety of drugs are used in humans; opinions differ on agents of choice.
• Lidocaine 2 mg/kg IV bolus followed by 25–75 mg/kg/min CRI IV drip (dogs only).
• Esmolol 50–100 mg/kg bolus, 50–200 mg/kg/min CRI (dogs and cats). • Propranolol 2.5–5 mg PO q8–12h (cats); 0.2–1 mg/kg PO q8h (dogs) or atenolol 6.2–12.5 mg PO q24h (cats); 0.25–1 mg/kg PO q12h (dogs).
• Diltiazem may be effective—1–2.5 mg/kg PO q8h (cats); 0.5–1.5 mg/kg PO q8h (dogs). • Procainamide IV may be used acutely because it decreases conduction over the accessory pathway and is safe if anterograde accessory pathway conduction is present in atrial fibrillation.

CONTRAINDICATIONS

• Digitalis, verapamil, and propranolol may be contraindicated—by slowing conduction through the AV node, these drugs may favor conduction through the anomalous pathways.
• Cats—propranolol and atenolol are the drugs of choice.

FOLLOW-UP

PATIENT MONITORING

Serial ECG.

POSSIBLE COMPLICATIONS

None expected.

EXPECTED COURSE AND PROGNOSIS

Depends on severity of the underlying cause; most WPW patients respond to therapy for supraventricular tachycardia—favorable prognosis.

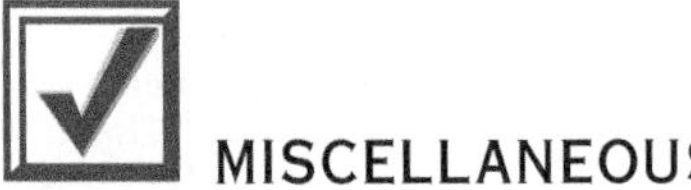

MISCELLANEOUS

ABBREVIATIONS

• AV = atrioventricular.
• WPW = Wolff–Parkinson–White.

Suggested Reading

Al-Khatib SM, Pritchett ELC. Clinical features of Wolff-Parkinson-White syndrome. Am Heart J 1999, 138:403–413.

Hill BL, Tilley LP. Ventricular preexcitation in seven dogs and nine cats. J Am Vet Med Assoc 1985, 187:1026–1031.

Kraus MS, Gelzer ARM. Treatment of cardia arrhythmias and conduction disturbances. In: Smith FWK, Tilley LP, Oyama M, Sleeper M, eds., Manual of Canine and Feline Cardiology, 5th ed. St. Louis, MO: Saunders Elsevier, 2016, pp. 313–329.

Santilli R, Moise NS, Pariaut R, Perego M. Electrocardiography of the dog and cat. Diagnosis of Arrhythmias, 2nd ed. Milano, Italy: Edra S.P.A., 2018.

Willis R, Oliveira P, Mavropoulou A. Guide to Canine and Feline Electrocardiography. Ames, IA: Wiley-Blackwell, 2018.

Zimetbaum, P. (2016). Cardiac arrhythmias with supraventricular origin. In: Goldman L, Schafer, AI, eds., Goldman's Cecil Medicine, 25th ed. Philadelphia, PA: Saunders, 2016, pp. 356–366.

Author Larry P. Tilley

Consulting Editor Michael Aherne

BASICS

DEFINITION

Single cardiac impulse initiated within the ventricles instead of the sinus node.

ECG Features

• QRS complexes typically wide and bizarre (see Figures 1 and 2). • P waves dissociated from the QRS complexes.

PATHOPHYSIOLOGY

Mechanisms include increased automaticity, reentry, and delayed afterdepolarizations.

SYSTEMS AFFECTED

Cardiovascular—secondary effects on other systems because of poor perfusion.

GENETICS

• Polygenic in German shepherd dogs—inherited ventricular arrhythmia. • Likely autosomal recessive, possibly autosomal dominant with incomplete penetrance in Rhodesian ridgebacks—inherited ventricular arrhythmia.

INCIDENCE/PREVALENCE

Unknown

SIGNALMENT

Species

Dog and cat.

Breed Predilections

• Common in large-breed dogs with cardiomyopathy, especially boxers (arrhythmogenic right ventricular cardiomyopathy) and Doberman pinschers. • Inherited ventricular arrhythmia in German shepherd dogs and Rhodesian ridgebacks. • Common in cats with cardiomyopathy; occasionally seen in cats with hyperthyroidism.

Mean Age and Range

Seen in all age groups.

SIGNS

Historical Findings

• Weakness. • Exercise intolerance. • Syncope. • Sudden death. • Often asymptomatic.

Physical Examination Findings

• Irregular rhythm associated with pulse deficits; may auscult splitting of the first or second heart sound. • May be normal if arrhythmia is intermittent and absent during examination. • May observe signs of congestive heart failure (CHF) (e.g., dyspnea, cough) or murmur, depending on the cause of arrhythmia.

CAUSES

• Cardiomyopathy. • Congenital defects (especially subaortic stenosis). • Degenerative valve disease. • Gastric dilation and volvulus. • Traumatic myocarditis (dogs). • Digitalis toxicity. • Hyperthyroidism (cats). • Cardiac neoplasia. • Myocarditis. • Pancreatitis.

RISK FACTORS

• Hypokalemia. • Hypomagnesemia. • Acid–base disturbances. • Hypoxia.

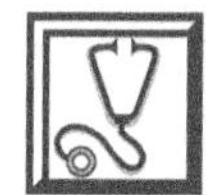

DIAGNOSIS

DIFFERENTIAL DIAGNOSIS

• Supraventricular premature beats with bundle branch block. • Look for P waves associated with the wide QRS complexes; an atrial premature complex with aberrant conduction has an associated P wave. • An atrial premature complex is usually followed by a noncompensatory pause in which the R-R interval of the two sinus complexes enclosing an atrial premature complex (APC) is less than the R-R interval of three consecutive sinus complexes. • A ventricular premature complex is usually followed by a compensatory pause in which the R-R interval of two sinus complexes enclosing a ventricular premature complex (VPC) is greater than or equal to the R-R interval of three consecutive sinus complexes.

CBC/BIOCHEMISTRY/URINALYSIS

• Hypokalemia and hypomagnesemia predispose animals to ventricular arrhythmias and blunt the response to class I antiarrhythmic drugs (e.g., lidocaine, procainamide, mexiletine, and quinidine). • High amylase and lipase if condition is secondary to pancreatitis.

OTHER LABORATORY TESTS

• High T_4 (cats) if condition is secondary to hyperthyroidism. • Increased cardiac troponin I, a biomarker for possible acute myocardial injury may suggest an underlying cardiac condition.

IMAGING

Echocardiography may reveal structural heart disease.

DIAGNOSTIC PROCEDURES

Long-term ambulatory (Holter) recording of the ECG to detect transient ventricular arrhythmias in patients with unexplained syncope or weakness.

PATHOLOGIC FINDINGS

Vary with underlying cause.

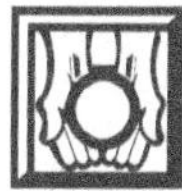

TREATMENT

APPROPRIATE HEALTH CARE

Generally outpatient basis.

ACTIVITY

Restrict if the arrhythmia is accompanied by clinical signs or evidence of structural heart disease.

CLIENT EDUCATION

Alert owner to potential for the arrhythmia worsening and syncope or sudden death.

SURGICAL CONSIDERATIONS

• Continuous ECG monitoring recommended while anesthetized. • Premedicating the patient with acepromazine 0.02–0.05 mg/kg raises the threshold for ventricular fibrillation. • Mask inductions not recommended; sympathetic release during mask induction can aggravate arrhythmia. • Avoid anticholinergics unless bradycardia develops.

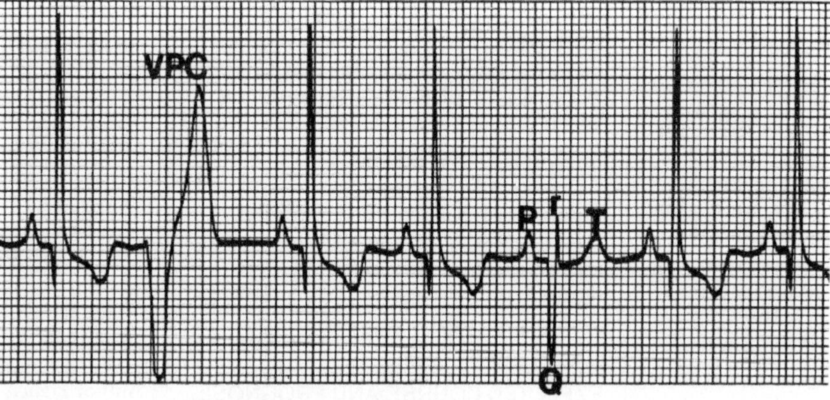

Figure 1.

VPC and a fusion complex (fifth complex) in a dog with myocarditis from pancreatitis. A fusion complex is the simultaneous activation of the ventricle by impulses coming from the SA node and the ventricular ectopic foci. The QRS complex is intermediate in form. (Source: From Tilley LP. Essentials of Canine and Feline Electrocardiography, 3rd ed. Baltimore: Williams & Wilkins, 1992. Reprinted with permission of Wolters Kluwer.)

VENTRICULAR PREMATURE COMPLEXES (CONTINUED)

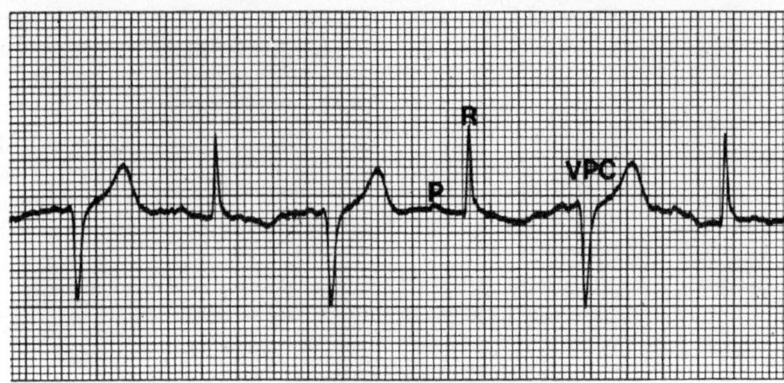

Figure 2.

Ventricular bigeminy. Every other complex is a VPC from the same focus. Each is coupled (interval the same between it and the adjacent sinus complex) to the preceding normal complex. (Source: From Tilley LP. Essentials of Canine and Feline Electrocardiography, 3rd ed. Baltimore: Williams & Wilkins, 1992. Reprinted with permission of Wolters Kluwer.)

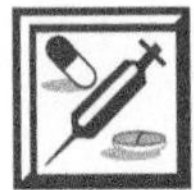

MEDICATIONS

DRUG(S) OF CHOICE

General Comments

• Correct any hypokalemia or hypomagnesemia. • Drug therapy in the absence of clinical signs—controversial; studies in humans with asymptomatic VPCs and myocardial infarction demonstrated a high incidence of sudden death when treatment was initiated with class I antiarrhythmic agents; no similar studies have been conducted in veterinary patients. • The author generally does not prescribe antiarrhythmic drugs unless there is evidence of clinical signs of low cardiac output (e.g., episodic weakness or syncope) or the belief that the patient is at high risk of sudden death, based on presence of R on T phenomenon or breed association with VPCs and sudden death (e.g., boxers and Doberman pinschers). • If antiarrhythmic therapy is initiated in an attempt to lower the risk of sudden death, the author usually chooses a beta-blocker or sotalol (except in German shepherd dogs [see below]); no studies have been done to confirm efficacy of beta-blockers for prevention of sudden death in dogs or cats.

Dogs

• Patient not in CHF or hypotensive—initiate therapy with a beta-blocker such as propranolol 0.2–1 mg/kg PO q8h, atenolol 0.2–1 mg/kg q12h, or metoprolol 0.2–1 mg/kg PO q8–12h or class III agent sotalol 1–3.5 mg/kg PO q12h.
• Patient in CHF or hypotensive—initiate therapy with a class I antiarrhythmic agent such as mexiletine 5–8 mg/kg PO q8h or procainamide 8–20 mg/kg PO q6–8h. • Combine a class I antiarrhythmic drug with a beta-blocker or sotalol if arrhythmia persists; especially in boxers.
• Sotalol monotherapy may have proarrhythmic effect in German shepherd dogs.

Cats

Atenolol 6.25–12.5 mg PO q12h.

CONTRAINDICATIONS

Avoid atropine, catecholamines (e.g., epinephrine and dopamine) until arrhythmia is controlled.

PRECAUTIONS

• Use beta-blockers cautiously in animals with CHF; they initially depress myocardial contractility.
• Use digoxin cautiously; it can potentially aggravate ventricular arrhythmias. • Drugs that prolong the action potential (e.g., sotalol) may worsen arrhythmia in German shepherd dogs with inherited ventricular arrhythmia.

POSSIBLE INTERACTIONS

Quinidine and amiodarone raise serum digoxin levels.

ALTERNATIVE DRUG(S)

• Consider amiodarone 5–10 mg/kg PO q12h for refractory arrhythmias in dogs (generally reserved for ventricular tachycardia); may not want to use in Doberman pinschers.
• Consider sotalol 10–20 mg/cat PO q12h or procainamide 3–8 mg/kg PO q6–8h for cats that do not tolerate beta-blockers.

FOLLOW-UP

PATIENT MONITORING

• Holter monitoring preferred for monitoring severity of the arrhythmia and efficacy of antiarrhythmic therapy; the goal of antiarrhythmic therapy is to reduce the frequency of ventricular ectopy by >85%. • Serial ECGs are not as useful as Holter monitoring—VPCs and paroxysmal ventricular tachycardia can occur sporadically through the day. • Serum digoxin levels in patients receiving that medication.

PREVENTION/AVOIDANCE

• Correct predisposing factors such as hypokalemia, hypomagnesemia, myocardial hypoxia, and digoxin toxicity. • Do not breed affected German shepherd dogs or Rhodesian ridgebacks with inherited ventricular arrhythmias.

POSSIBLE COMPLICATIONS

Syncope, sudden death.

EXPECTED COURSE AND PROGNOSIS

• If cause is metabolic—condition may resolve with good prognosis. • If condition is associated with cardiac disease—prognosis is guarded; VPCs may increase the risk of sudden death.

MISCELLANEOUS

SEE ALSO

• Chagas Disease (American Trypanosomiasis). • Digoxin Toxicity. • Myocarditis.
• Ventricular Tachycardia.

ABBREVIATIONS

• APC = atrial premature complex. • CHF = congestive heart failure. • T_4 = thyroxine.
• VPC = ventricular premature complex.

Suggested Reading

Kraus MS, Gelzer ARM, Moïse NS. Treatment of cardiac arrhythmias and conduction disturbances. In: Smith FWK, Tilley LP, Oyama MA, Sleeper MM, eds. Manual of Canine and Feline Cardiology. 5th ed. St. Louis, MO: Saunders Elsevier, 2016.

Kraus MS, Ridge LG, Gelzer ARM, et al. Toxicity in Doberman pinscher dogs with ventricular arrhythmias treated with amiodarone. J Vet Intern Med 2005, 19(3):407.

Meurs KM, Spier AW, Wright NA, et al. Comparison of the effects of four antiarrhythmic treatments for familial ventricular arrhythmias in boxers. J Am Vet Med Assoc 2002, 221(4):522–527.

Meurs KM, Weidman JA, Rosenthal SL, et al. Ventricular arrhythmias in Rhodesian ridgebacks with a family history of sudden death and results of a pedigree analysis for potential inheritance patterns. J Am Vet Med Assoc 2016, 248(10):1135–1138.

Moïse NS, Gilmour RF Jr., Riccio ML, et al. Diagnosis of inherited ventricular tachycardia in German shepherd dogs. J Am Vet Med Assoc 1997, 210(3):403–410.

Tilley LP, Smith FWK, Jr. Electrocardiography. In: Smith FWK, Tilley LP, Oyama MA, Sleeper MM, eds., Manual of Canine and Feline Cardiology, 5th ed. St. Louis, MO: Saunders Elsevier, 2016.

Author Francis W.K. Smith, Jr.
Consulting Editor Michael Aherne

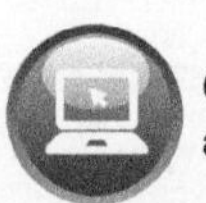

Client Education Handout available online

VENTRICULAR SEPTAL DEFECT

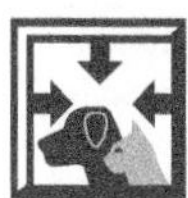

BASICS

DEFINITION

An anomalous communication between the two ventricles. Numerous classification schemes have been proposed; briefly, the defect may be in the outlet, muscular, or membranous septum. Most ventricular septal defects (VSDs) in small animals are perimembranous, such that the defect is subaortic and has a right ventricular orifice that is beneath the septal leaflet of the tricuspid valve.

PATHOPHYSIOLOGY

- A VSD results in an interventricular communication—direction and volume of the shunt are determined by the size of the defect, the relationship of the pulmonary and systemic vascular resistances, and the presence of other anomalies.
- Most VSDs in dogs and cats are small and therefore restrictive (i.e., sufficiently small that the difference between left and right ventricular pressures is maintained). Moderate-sized VSDs are only partially restrictive and result in various degrees of right ventricular hypertension. Large VSDs have an area that is as large as or larger than the open aortic valve; they are nonrestrictive, so that left and right ventricular pressures are necessarily equal. Only moderate and large defects impose a pressure load upon the right ventricle (Figure 1).
- In a patient with normal resistance to right ventricular ejection, the direction of the shunt is left-to-right, which increases pulmonary venous return and imposes a volume load on the left atrium and ventricle. With large shunts, congestive failure can develop.
- Unless the defect is of moderate or large size, the right ventricle is spared.

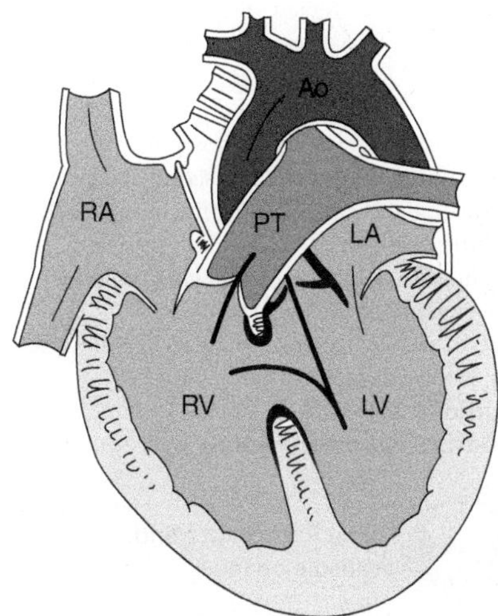

Figure 1.

Ventricular septal defect. In this schematic, the defect results in an unobstructed communication and therefore, right ventricular hypertrophy and pulmonary hypertension are shown. Left-to-right shunting is shown. RA = right atrium, LA = left atrium, RV = right ventricle, LV = left ventricle, Ao = aorta, PT = pulmonary trunk. (Source: Roberts W., Adult Congenital Heart Disease. Philadelphia, © 1987 F.A. Davis Company.)

SYSTEMS AFFECTED

- Respiratory—if pulmonary edema develops.
- Cardiovascular—a large shunt can result in pulmonary vascular disease, pulmonary hypertension, and shunt reversal (i.e., Eisenmenger's syndrome). This is uncommon in small animals; if shunt reversal occurs, it seems to do so early in life.

GENETICS

Breed predispositions recognized; genetic transmission has not been established.

INCIDENCE/PREVALENCE

One of the most common congenital cardiac malformations in cats, comprising 50% of cases with congenital cardiac defects in one study. Less common in dogs, reported to occur in 7.5–14.4% of cases with congenital cardiac disease.

GEOGRAPHIC DISTRIBUTION

N/A

SIGNALMENT

Species

Dog and cat.

Breed Predilections

English bulldog, English springer spaniel, basset hound, Akita, West Highland white terrier, Lakeland terrier.

Mean Age and Range

Most defects detected during routine examination of puppies and kittens.

Predominant Sex

N/A

SIGNS

Historical Findings

- Usually asymptomatic.
- Clinical signs of left ventricular failure include dyspnea, exercise intolerance, syncope, and cough.

Physical Examination Findings

- A restrictive VSD results in a systolic murmur that typically is loud, band-shaped, and heard best over the right hemithorax. A diastolic decrescendo murmur may result if the VSD undermines anatomic support of the aortic valve, causing aortic regurgitation. Patients with right-to-left shunts generally do not have murmurs.
- Split second heart sound in some patients.
- Femoral pulses usually normal.
- Mucous membranes—pink, unless pulmonary vascular disease causes a right-to-left shunt and arterial hypoxemia.
- Tachycardia, dyspnea, and crackles may be evident if left ventricular failure occurs.

CAUSES

Congenital; may have a genetic basis.

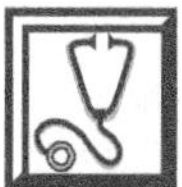

DIAGNOSIS

DIFFERENTIAL DIAGNOSIS

- Other congenital cardiac malformations that cause systolic murmurs include atrioventricular valve dysplasia, aortic or pulmonary stenosis, and complex malformations such as tetralogy of Fallot.
- The "to-and-fro" murmur, consisting of distinct systolic and diastolic murmurs, which results when aortic valve regurgitation complicates a VSD must be distinguished from the continuous murmur of patent ductus arteriosus.
- Generally, diagnosis of congenital cardiac malformations requires echocardiographic evaluation including Doppler studies.

CBC/BIOCHEMISTRY/URINALYSIS

- Results usually normal.
- Uncommon right-to-left shunting results in compensatory erythrocytosis.
- Patients with severe congestive heart failure (CHF) may have prerenal azotemia.

OTHER LABORATORY TESTS

N/A

IMAGING

Thoracic Radiography

- Radiographic appearance is determined by the size and direction of the shunt. Thoracic radiographs may be normal if the VSD is small. Larger defects cause various degrees of left or even generalized cardiac enlargement. Pulmonary hyperperfusion with prominence of the main pulmonary artery segment may be apparent. CHF is manifest as pulmonary edema.
- Patients with right-to-left shunts have right-sided cardiomegaly; the pulmonary arteries are large proximally but distally attenuated, and the pulmonary veins are small because of reduced pulmonary perfusion.

Echocardiography

- Two-dimensional echocardiography may demonstrate left atrial enlargement with left ventricular dilation and hypertrophy. Systolic myocardial function is usually preserved. Right ventricular hypertrophy is apparent only if the defect is moderate or large in size, or if the VSD is one aspect of a complex malformation such as tetralogy of Fallot. Careful study usually demonstrates the defect. Evaluate echocardiographic images critically; the artifact of "septal drop-out" is very common.
- The diagnosis is confirmed by Doppler interrogation of the interventricular septum. If the defect is restrictive, spectral Doppler reveals a high-velocity systolic jet. The shunt may be seen directly by color-flow Doppler.

VENTRICULAR SEPTAL DEFECT (CONTINUED)

Contrast echocardiography may help in the diagnosis of a right-to-left VSD.
• Infrequently, VSDs spontaneously close. The mechanism of closure is usually adherence of a part of the septal tricuspid valve leaflet to the interventricular septum resulting in the echocardiographic appearance of "septal aneurysm," which is an incidental echocardiographic finding.

Cardiac Catheterization

Selective cardiac catheterization allows visualization of the defect by contrast angiocardiography and calculation of the shunt fraction (QP/QS) and pulmonary vascular resistance.

DIAGNOSTIC PROCEDURES

Electrocardiography

• Evidence of left atrial enlargement, left ventricular hypertrophy, or even right ventricular hypertrophy in some animals.
• Right ventricular enlargement pattern in most animals that have a right-to-left shunt because of pulmonary vascular disease or pulmonic stenosis.

PATHOLOGIC FINDINGS

Size of the defect determines the degree of chamber enlargement and hypertrophy; pulmonary edema and possibly ascites are seen in patients with CHF.

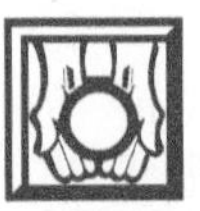

TREATMENT

V

APPROPRIATE HEALTH CARE

Clinical signs are related to CHF; most patients can be treated as outpatients.

NURSING CARE

N/A

ACTIVITY

Restrict if animal has CHF; need not restrict asymptomatic patients with small defects.

DIET

Moderate sodium restriction recommended for patients with CHF.

CLIENT EDUCATION

Definitive surgical correction is not widely available; if CHF develops, it is terminal, even with palliative care.

SURGICAL CONSIDERATIONS

• Only a minority of VSDs are sufficiently large to warrant repair.
• Consider definitive surgical repair of the defect during cardiopulmonary bypass for defects associated with a large shunt. Cardiopulmonary bypass is presently performed at a small number of veterinary centers. Consider pulmonary artery banding as a palliative procedure for patients with moderate or large shunts and CHF.
• Some VSDs are amenable to transcatheter closure using purpose-designed metallic occluder devices.

MEDICATIONS

DRUG(S) OF CHOICE

Furosemide, enalapril, pimobendan, and, in some circumstances, digoxin—recommended for animals with CHF (see Congestive Heart Failure, Left-Sided).

CONTRAINDICATIONS

Vasodilators—contraindicated or used only with great caution in patients with complex malformations.

PRECAUTIONS

ACE inhibitors and digoxin must be used cautiously if patient has renal dysfunction.

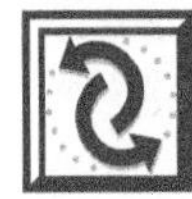

FOLLOW-UP

PATIENT MONITORING

Periodic echocardiographic or radiographic evaluation suggested for patients without clinical signs.

PREVENTION/AVOIDANCE

Breeding affected animals is not recommended.

POSSIBLE COMPLICATIONS

• Left ventricular CHF.
• Bacterial endocarditis.
• Pulmonary hypertension.
• Arrhythmias.

EXPECTED COURSE AND PROGNOSIS

• Patients with small shunts generally have a normal lifespan; isolated, restrictive VSDs usually do not cause clinical signs.
• Concurrent anomalies such as pulmonic stenosis or aortic insufficiency worsen the prognosis.
• Patients with overt CHF may live 6–18 months with medical treatment.
• The development of pulmonary hypertension and shunt reversal is uncommon but generally associated with a poor prognosis.

MISCELLANEOUS

ASSOCIATED CONDITIONS

• VSD may be one component of complex malformations such as tetralogy of Fallot.
• Most VSDs are perimembranous and therefore, subaortic. As a result, aortic valve insufficiency resulting from a poorly supported aortic valve complicates the condition in some patients.
• VSD may be associated with an atrial septal defect as part of an atrioventricular septal defect.

AGE-RELATED FACTORS

The murmur of VSD becomes apparent shortly after birth, when pulmonary vascular resistance decreases.

ZOONOTIC POTENTIAL

N/A

PREGNANCY/FERTILITY/BREEDING

High risk in patients with large defects; breeding affected animals is not recommended.

SYNONYMS

Interventricular septal defect.

SEE ALSO

• Congestive Heart Failure, Left-Sided.
• Tetralogy of Fallot.

ABBREVIATIONS

• ACE = angiotensin-converting enzyme.
• CHF = congestive heart failure.
• VSD = ventricular septal defect.

Suggested Reading

Bomassi E, Misbach C, Tissier R, et al. Signalment, clinical features, echocardiographic findings, and outcome of dogs and cats with ventricular septal defects: 109 cases (1992–2013). J Am Vet Med Assoc 2015, 247(8):166–175.
Oliveira P, Domenech O, Silva J, et al. Retrospective review of congenital heart disease in 976 dogs. J Vet Intern Med 2011, 25(3):477–483.
Thomas WP, Shimizu M, Tanaka R, et al. Echocardiographic diagnosis of congenital membranous ventricular septal aneurysm in the dog and cat. J Am Anim Hosp Assoc 2005, 41(4):215–220.
Tidholm A, Ljungvall I, Michal J, et al. Congenital heart defects in cats: a retrospective study of 162 cats (1996–2013). J Vet Cardiol 2015, 17:S215–S219.

Author Jonathan A. Abbott
Consulting Editor Michael Aherne

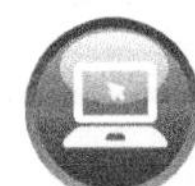

Client Education Handout available online

VENTRICULAR STANDSTILL (ASYSTOLE)

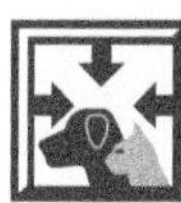

BASICS

DEFINITION

Absence of ventricular complexes on the ECG or absence of ventricular activity (electrical–mechanical dissociation).

ECG Features

Ventricular asystole can result from severe sinoatrial block or arrest or by third-degree atrioventricular (AV) block without a junctional or ventricular escape rhythm; ECG features include:

- P waves present if patient has complete AV block (Figure 1).
- P waves absent during asystole if patient has severe sinoatrial block or arrest.
- No QRS complexes.
- Electrical–mechanical dissociation—a recorded ECG cardiac rhythm (P-QRS-T) and no effective cardiac output or palpable femoral pulse.

PATHOPHYSIOLOGY

Ventricular asystole represents cardiac arrest; if the ventricular rhythm is not restored in 3–4 minutes, irreversible brain injury can occur.

SYSTEMS AFFECTED

- Cardiovascular.
- All organ systems affected by loss of perfusion.

GENETICS

N/A

INCIDENCE/PREVALENCE

Unknown

GEOGRAPHIC DISTRIBUTION

None

SIGNALMENT

Species

Dog and cat.

Breed Predilections

None

Mean Age and Range

Unknown

SIGNS

Historical Findings

- Severe systemic illness or cardiac disease in many patients.
- Other cardiac arrhythmias in some.
- Syncope.

PHYSICAL EXAMINATION FINDINGS

- No ventricular pulse can be palpated.
- Cardiac arrest.
- Collapse.
- Death.

CAUSES

- Complete AV block with absence of ventricular or junctional escape rhythm.
- Severe sinus arrest or block.
- Hyperkalemia (Figure 2).

RISK FACTORS

- Any severe systemic illness (e.g., severe acidosis and hyperkalemia) or heart disease.
- Hypoadrenocorticism causing hyperkalemia.
- Urinary tract rupture or obstruction, resulting in hyperkalemia.

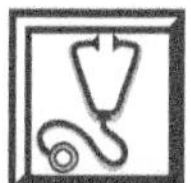

DIAGNOSIS

DIFFERENTIAL DIAGNOSIS

Rule out ECG artifact; reapply ECG clips and make sure skin contact is good and adequate alcohol is applied to leads.

CBC/BIOCHEMISTRY/URINALYSIS

Severe hyperkalemia is a possible cause.

OTHER LABORATORY TESTS

N/A

IMAGING

N/A

DIAGNOSTIC PROCEDURES

Systemic blood pressure—readable pressure absent.

PATHOLOGIC FINDINGS

N/A

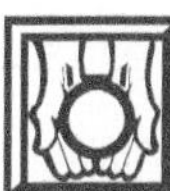

TREATMENT

APPROPRIATE HEALTH CARE

- Asystole is a frequently fatal rhythm requiring immediate aggressive treatment.
- Artificial pacing with a transvenous or transthoracic pacemaker may succeed if myocardium is mechanically responsive.
- DC electrical conversion is not effective unless the rhythm can first be converted to ventricular fibrillation with medications.

NURSING CARE

Treat any treatable problems such as hypothermia, hyperkalemia, and acid–base disorders.

ACTIVITY

N/A

DIET

N/A

CLIENT EDUCATION

None

SURGICAL CONSIDERATIONS

None

MEDICATIONS

DRUG(S) OF CHOICE

- Institute cardiopulmonary resuscitation.
- Epinephrine 0.2 mg/kg IV, intratracheal (IT), or intralingual (IL) (double the dose for IT administration and deliver with equal volume of saline).
- Atropine 0.05 mg/kg IV, IT, or IL (double the dose for IT administration and deliver with equal volume of saline).
- Sodium bicarbonate 1 mEq/kg IV for each 10 minutes of cardiac arrest.
- Dexamethasone and dopamine may be helpful in patients with electrical–mechanical dissociation.

V

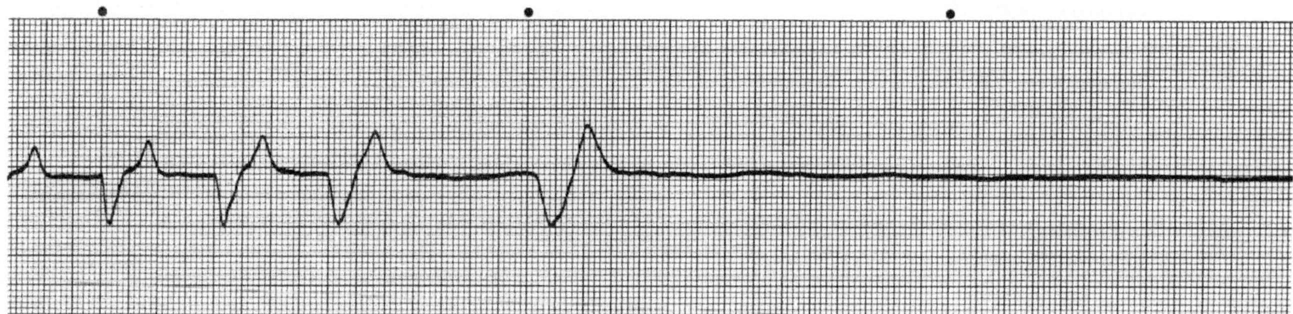

Figure 1.

Ventricular asystole in a dog with severe complete AV block. Only P waves (atrial activity) are present; there is no ventricular activity. Lead II, 50 mm/s, 1 cm = 1 mV. (Source: From Tilley LP. Essentials of Canine and Feline Electrocardiography, 3rd ed. Baltimore: Williams & Wilkins, 1992. Reprinted with permission of Wolters Kluwer.)

VENTRICULAR STANDSTILL (ASYSTOLE) (CONTINUED)

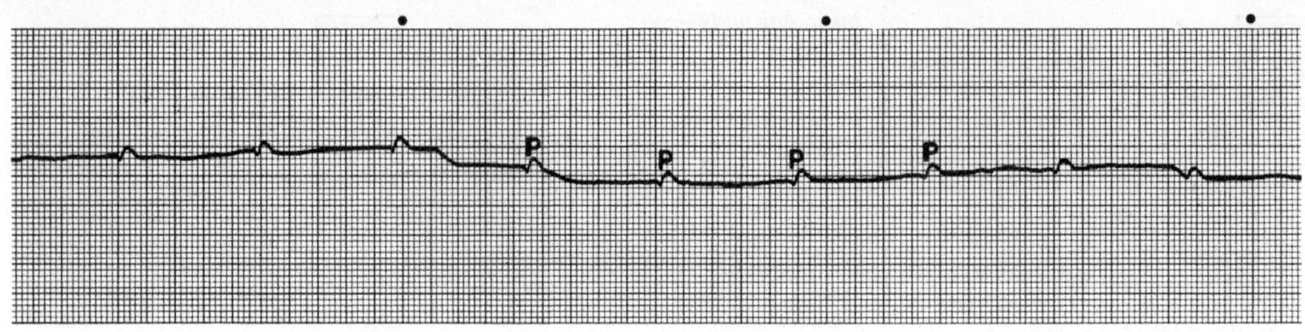

Figure 2.

Ventricular asystole in a cat with severe hyperkalemia (11 mEq/L) from urethral obstruction. No P waves or QRS complexes are seen after four wide and bizarre QRS complexes (atrial standstill with delayed ventricular conduction). Lead II, 50 mm/s, 1 cm = 1 mV.) (Source: From Tilley LP. Essentials of Canine and Feline Electrocardiography, 3rd ed. Baltimore: Williams & Wilkins, 1992. Reprinted with permission of Wolters Kluwer.)

CONTRAINDICATIONS

Drugs that depress sinus node or AV node conduction in patients with sinus arrest or heart block (e.g., beta-blockers, calcium channel blockers, digoxin).

PRECAUTIONS

None

POSSIBLE INTERACTIONS

None

ALTERNATIVE DRUG(S)

Calcium gluconate—patients with ventricular standstill and hyperkalemia.

FOLLOW-UP

PATIENT MONITORING

- If animal is resuscitated—evaluate CBC, biochemical analysis, and urinalysis.
- If animal survives and primary cardiac disease is suspected—echocardiogram and thoracic radiographs.
- ECG—closely and frequently.

PREVENTION/AVOIDANCE

Careful monitoring of critically ill patients to prevent and correct acid–base and electrolyte disturbances, hypotension, and hypoxemia.

POSSIBLE COMPLICATIONS

- Death.
- Disseminated intravascular coagulation (DIC) and multiorgan failure.

EXPECTED COURSE AND PROGNOSIS

Usually death. If sinus rhythm reestablished, prognosis still usually guarded to poor as not uncommon to arrest again.

MISCELLANEOUS

ASSOCIATED CONDITIONS

None

AGE-RELATED FACTORS

None

ZOONOTIC POTENTIAL

None

PREGNANCY/FERTILITY/BREEDING

None

SYNONYMS

Ventricular asystole.

SEE ALSO

- Atrioventricular Block, Complete (Third Degree).
- Cardiopulmonary Arrest.
- Sinus Arrest and Sinoatrial Block.

ABBREVIATIONS

- AV = atrioventricular.
- DIC = disseminated intravascular coagulation.
- IL = intralingual.
- IT = intratracheal.

Suggested Reading

Kraus MS, Gelzer ARM, Moïse NS. Treatment of cardiac arrhythmias and conduction disturbances. In: Smith, FWK, Tilley LP, Oyama MA, Sleeper MM, eds., Manual of Canine and Feline Cardiology, 5th ed. St. Louis, MO: Saunders Elsevier, 2016.

Tilley LP, Smith FWK, Jr. Electrocardiography. In: Smith FWK, Tilley LP, Oyama MA, Sleeper MM, eds. Manual of Canine and Feline Cardiology, 5th ed. St. Louis, MO: Saunders Elsevier, 2016.

Author Francis W.K. Smith, Jr.

Consulting Editor Michael Aherne

VENTRICULAR TACHYCARDIA

BASICS

DEFINITION

Ventricular tachycardia (VT) may occur in structurally normal hearts (hereditary arrhythmias) or may be a manifestation of myocardial abnormalities associated with cardiomyopathy, significant valvular disease, myocarditis, infiltrative disease or electrolyte abnormalities. To date, no available medical therapy is known to prevent sudden death (SD) in animals afflicted with VT.

PATHOPHYSIOLOGY

Severity of VT depends both on the hemodynamic consequences (hypotension) and on the electrical instability of a rhythm, i.e. its potential to degenerate into ventricular fibrillation (VF), resulting in SD. In Dobermans, SD due to VT–VF occurs in about 30–50% of cases. In boxers with arrhythmogenic right ventricular cardiomyopathy (ARVC), 33% are syncopal due to VT and 30% have SD due VT–VF. Similarly, 13% of English bulldogs with inherited ARVC experience SD. Underlying mechanisms of VT include increased automaticity, reentry, and triggered activity.

ECG Features (Figure 1)

- QRS complexes—typically wide and bizarre.
- Three or more ventricular premature contractions in a row.
- May be intermittent (paroxysmal) or sustained; heart rate usually >150 bpm with a regular or irregular rhythm.
- P waves, if visible, are dissociated from the QRS complexes.
- Breed-specific ECG changes—VT in boxers is characteristically positive in the ventrocaudal leads (leads II, III, and aVF), thus manifests a "left bundle branch block pattern." VT in Doberman pinschers and German shepherd dogs has both polymorphic and monomorphic characteristics.

SYSTEMS AFFECTED

Cardiovascular system, with secondary effects on other systems due to poor perfusion.

GENETICS

- In boxers, ARVC is inherited as autosomal dominant trait with adult onset of disease. Some boxers have a mutation in the striatin gene, but the disease is manifested with incomplete penetrance (i.e., even if a boxer has the genetic mutation, it may not lead to the development of arrhythmias in that dog) and it is likely that there is more than one mutation in boxers that may lead to the disease in some lines. Striatin is a desmosomal protein (scaffolding protein) located in the intercalated disc region of the cardiomyocyte and colocalizes with desmosomal proteins such as plakophilin-2 and other known proteins that are mutated in human ARVC. DNA test results can indicate if a dog is heterozygous or homozygous for the genetic striatin deletion. Homozygous dogs are more likely to show disease and should not be used for breeding.
- English bulldogs also appear to harbor a form of inherited ARVC manifest with VT and SD in 13% of dogs. Genetic mode of inheritance is undetermined. There is 2.9:1 male to female ratio of affectedness. Unlike boxers with ARVC, the majority of English bulldogs appear to present with signs of CHF at the time of arrhythmia detection.
- Dilated cardiomyopathy with VT in Doberman pinschers is inherited as an autosomal dominant trait with adult onset of disease. In Dobermans there are two genetic mutations associated with dilated cardiomyopathy (DCM) and VT identified in the pyruvate dehydrogenase kinase 4 (PDK4) gene (*PDK4/NCSU/DCM1*) and the titin gene (*NCSU DCM2*). Dogs with both mutations are at the highest risk of getting DCM, although dogs with a mutation in either gene can develop the disease as well.
- Inherited VT and SD, considered primarily an "electrical disorder" (since no underlying structural heart disease is identified), is found in young German shepherd dogs and English springer spaniels. They have been shown to have inherited channelopathies, resulting in repolarization abnormalities. In springer spaniels a mutation in the *KCNQ1* gene, responsible for a repolarizing K channel, was found to exhibit QT interval prolongation on ECG and SD. In German shepherd dogs, the mode of inheritance is polygenic due to an abnormality in a major gene with modifiers.
- Young Rhodesian ridgebacks have been found to be affected with severe ventricular arrhythmias and SD. It is inherited in an autosomal recessive mode and linked to a genetic mutation, likely associated with mitochondrial alterations.

INCIDENCE/PREVALENCE

Common in dogs; uncommon in cats.

GEOGRAPHIC DISTRIBUTION

None

SIGNALMENT

Species

Dog and cat.

Breed Predilections

Commonly seen in large-breed dogs with cardiomyopathy, especially boxers and Doberman pinschers, also in German shepherd dogs and Rhodesian ridgebacks.

Mean Age and Range

- All age groups, if not breed-specific VT.
- Boxers with ARVC usually present at 4–6 years of age; frequency and severity of the arrhythmia usually increase over time.
- Doberman pinschers with occult cardiomyopathy typically develop ventricular arrhythmias beginning at 3–6 years of age, but it also can occur much later in life; frequency and severity usually increase over time.
- German shepherd dogs develop ventricular arrhythmias at 12–16 weeks of age and the frequency and severity of the arrhythmias increase until 24–30 weeks of age. After 8 months of age the arrhythmia severity stabilizes or starts to decrease.
- The Rhodesian ridgeback's most severe arrhythmias are found between 6 and 30 months of age, after which many dogs appear to outgrow the problem.
- Bulldogs with ARVC have a mean age of 9.2 years at time of presentation for arrhythmias.

SIGNS

Historical Findings

- Syncope.
- Weakness.
- Exercise intolerance.
- SD.
- May be asymptomatic.

Physical Examination Findings

- May be normal if arrhythmia is paroxysmal and absent during examination.
- Paroxysmal or sustained tachycardia may be ausculted.
- Femoral pulses may have variable pulse intensity or be weak during runs of VT.
- Signs of CHF or a murmur may be present, depending on cause of arrhythmia.

CAUSES

- Cardiomyopathy.
- Inherited channelopathies.
- Congenital defects (especially subaortic stenosis).
- Chronic degenerative valve disease.
- Traumatic or infectious myocarditis.
- Cardiac neoplasia.
- Gastric dilation and volvulus.
- Splenic neoplasia/hemorrhage.
- Hyperthyroidism (cats).
- Digitalis toxicity.
- Pancreatitis.
- VT can also be found in dogs affected with noncardiac disease states including electrolyte abnormalities (potassium), or systemic diseases where imbalance of cardiac autonomic modulation may elicit VT. The VT occurring secondary to those circumstances may occur at heart rates similar to the sinus rate (in this scenario the rhythm is termed "accelerated idioventricular rhythm" rather than VT since the heart rate is normal), thus considered less malignant, and are often self-limiting with correction or resolution of the underlying cause.

RISK FACTORS

- Hypokalemia, hyperkalemia.
- Hypomagnesemia.
- Acid–base disturbances.
- Hypoxemia.
- Neoplasia (e.g., cardiac or splenic hemangiosarcoma).
- Anemia.

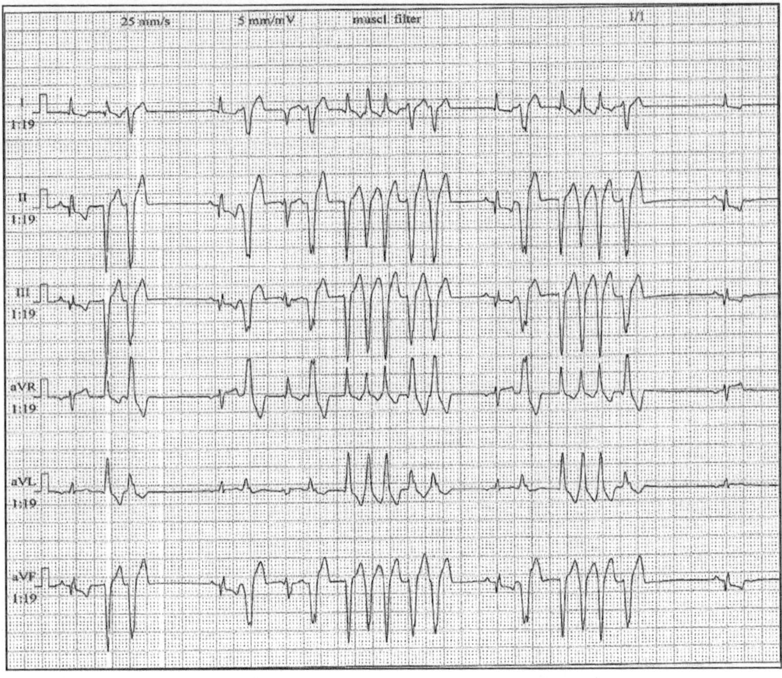

Figure 1.

Ventricular tachycardia. 6-lead ECG demonstrating the wide and bizarre QRS complexes that occur in runs of up to 6 beats in a Doberman pinscher with DCM. Ventricular tachycardia should be treated as soon as possible. Acid–base and electrolyte abnormalities should always be corrected.

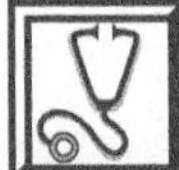

DIAGNOSIS

DIFFERENTIAL DIAGNOSIS

Supraventricular tachycardia with bundle branch block. If P waves can be identified, look for association between P waves and QRS complexes. If there is a consistent PR interval, then the rhythm is supraventricular with bundle branch block. If there is no association between P waves and QRS complexes, the rhythm is probably VT. If P waves cannot be identified due to a fast rate (P buried in preceding T wave), lidocaine administration may result in slowing of the VT rate and P waves may be identified if present. Termination of a tachyarrhythmia after administration of lidocaine supports diagnosis of VT. If no effect with lidocaine, esmolol administration may result in slowing of a supraventricular tachycardia with bundle branch block, so that P waves associated with QRS complexes can be identified.

CBC/BIOCHEMISTRY/URINALYSIS

- Hypokalemia and hypomagnesemia predispose to VT and blunt response to class I antiarrhythmic drugs (e.g., lidocaine, procainamide, mexiletine, and quinidine).
- High amylase and lipase if arrhythmia is secondary to pancreatitis.
- Inflammatory changes may occur on CBC such as increased neutrophil count if arrhythmia secondary to myocarditis.

OTHER LABORATORY TESTS

- Increased cardiac troponin I (cTnI) with myocarditis.
- High T_4 (cats) if arrhythmia is secondary to hyperthyroidism.
- Lyme or tick titers in myocarditis.
- Genetic testing is available at NC State (https://cvm.ncsu.edu/genetics/) for arrhythmias originating due to boxer ARVC, Doberman DCM and Rhodesian ridgeback inherited arrhythmias.
- Increased trypsin-like immunoreactivity and pancreatic lipase immunoreactivity if suspect pancreatitis is a cause for the VT.

IMAGING

Echocardiography may reveal underlying structural heart disease.

DIAGNOSTIC PROCEDURES

ECG and long-term ambulatory (Holter) or event recording of the ECG—for detection of intermittent VT in patients with unexplained syncope or weakness.

PATHOLOGIC FINDINGS

Vary with underlying cause.

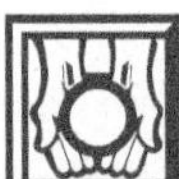

TREATMENT

APPROPRIATE HEALTH CARE

- Most patients with intermittent VT can safely be evaluated for underlying diseases (echocardiogram, lab work) and it is ideal to establish a true baseline of the arrhythmia quantity and quality by a 24-hour Holter prior to initiating therapy.
- If unstable (laterally recumbent, weak, or frequent syncope), immediate IV treatment in a hospital setting with continuous ECG monitoring may be required. Once the arrhythmia is controlled and patient is hemodynamically stable, oral medication should be instituted. A follow-up 24-hour Holter is required to evaluate efficacy and possible pro-arrhythmic effects of antiarrhythmic therapy.

NURSING CARE

Varies with underlying cause.

ACTIVITY

Boxers tend to have an increased incidence of VT during excitement, so in some cases owners should know what specific situations to avoid. In humans with ARVC, exercise has been shown to exacerbate arrhythmia incidence and risk of SD.

DIET

Dogs with diet-associated (boutique, exotic-ingredient, or grain-free [BEG] diets) DCM may have an increased incidence of VT and risk of SD.

CLIENT EDUCATION

Alert the owner to the potential for SD.

SURGICAL CONSIDERATIONS

- When possible, determine the cause of the arrhythmia and treat it prior to inducing general anesthesia.
- Assess if VT is correctable with a test dose of lidocaine; if it is, treat as necessary with lidocaine, either using IV boluses or CRI.
- Premedication with acepromazine 0.02–0.05 mg/kg raises the threshold for VF.
- Avoid proarrhythmic drugs such as alpha-2 agonists (xylazine, medetomidine) and thiopental.
- Mask induction is not recommended in inadequately sedated patients with ventricular arrhythmias because increased sympathetic tone during mask induction will aggravate the arrhythmia.
- Continuous ECG monitoring during anesthesia.

MEDICATIONS

DRUG(S) OF CHOICE

Correct any hypokalemia or hypomagnesemia, if possible, prior to instituting medical therapy.

Dogs

Acute Life-Threatening VT

- Administer lidocaine slowly in 2 mg/kg IV boluses (up to 8 mg/kg total) to convert to sinus rhythm; follow with lidocaine CRI, 30–80 µg/kg/min.
- If lidocaine fails—administer procainamide 5–15 mg/kg slow IV bolus (may cause vomiting or hypotension due to negative inotropic effect), followed by 25–50 µg/kg/min IV CRI.
- In cases of refractory VT, lidocaine and procainamide CRIs can be combined.
- If no response to lidocaine or procainamide, amiodarone (Nexterone®) can be administered as a 2 mg/kg IV bolus infused over 10 minutes, followed by a CRI of 0.8 mg/kg/h for 6 hours, then decrease to 0.4 mg/kg/h or alternatively try slow IV boluses of esmolol (a short-acting beta-blocker) at 0.05–0.1 mg/kg q5min to a cumulative dose of 0.5 mg/kg, or as a 50–200 µg/kg/min CRI.
- If there is inadequate response to the various IV therapies, then PO medication may be administered. Sotalol 1.5–2.5 mg/kg PO q12h may convert dangerous VT within 1–3 hours in such situations, even when the usual IV medications failed. It can be administered in a "loading protocol" (1.5–2.5 mg/kg PO q4h or q6h), for the first 2 doses, depending on the severity of the VT and myocardial function.

Chronic VT in a Stable Patient

- Sotalol 1–2.5 mg/kg PO q12h.
- Mexiletine monotherapy is not very effective, but combination of mexiletine 4–8 mg/kg PO q8h with a beta-blocker such as atenolol 0.25–1 mg/kg PO q12h or sotalol 1–2.5 mg/kg PO q12h may be more effective for refractory VT, especially in boxers.
- Amiodarone may be used for refractory VT in dogs with poor myocardial function (loading dosage of 5–15 mg/kg PO q12h for 2–14 days, maintenance dosage of 6–15 mg/kg PO q24h). Requires regular monitoring due to the risk for serious side effects in dogs (hepatotoxicity, neutropenia, thyroid dysfunction). Signs of toxicity include anorexia, vomiting, lethargy, and hepatic enzyme elevation. Amiodarone hepatopathy is reversible after reduction of dosage or discontinuation of the drug. Overt clinical signs of toxicity generally resolve within a few days of stopping amiodarone. Monitoring of serial serum chemistries is recommended, since increases in liver enzyme activities usually precede the onset of clinical signs of amiodarone toxicity. Liver enzymes should be measured after 7 days of drug loading and once monthly during maintenance therapy.
- Amiodarone can be combined with atenolol 0.5–1.0 mg/kg twice a day to enhance anti-arrhythmic effects.
- In German shepherd dogs the combination of mexiletine and sotalol is the most effective therapy for VT. Sotalol monotherapy should be avoided due its proarrhythmic effects in this breed.

Cats

- Use lidocaine cautiously and only for sustained VT; neurotoxicity (seizures) is common in cats. Use one-tenth of the dosage used for dogs.
- For oral maintenance therapy of severe VT in cats use sotalol 10 mg/cat q12h or atenolol 6.25–12.5 mg PO q12h.

CONTRAINDICATIONS

Avoid atropine, catecholamines (e.g., epinephrine, dopamine) until arrhythmia is controlled.

PRECAUTIONS

- Use beta-blockers cautiously in animals with CHF. Monitoring by echocardiogram is recommended to check for worsening of myocardial function due to beta blockade.
- Sotalol, when used as a sole agent, and other drugs that prolong action potential duration may worsen VT in German shepherd dogs with inherited ventricular arrhythmias.

POSSIBLE INTERACTIONS

Quinidine and amiodarone raise digoxin levels.

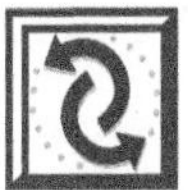

FOLLOW-UP

PATIENT MONITORING

- Holter monitoring is preferred for assessment of severity of the arrhythmia and efficacy of antiarrhythmic therapy; the goal of antiarrhythmic therapy is to reduce the frequency of ventricular ectopy by >85%.
- Serial ECG and telemetry can be used alternatively—but not as meaningful as Holter monitoring because ventricular premature complexes and paroxysmal VT can occur sporadically throughout the day.

PREVENTION/AVOIDANCE

- Correct predisposing factors such as hypokalemia, hypomagnesemia, myocardial hypoxia, and digoxin toxicity.
- In boxers, limit significant stress or excitement as the increase in sympathetic tone may exacerbate the arrhythmia.

POSSIBLE COMPLICATIONS

- Syncope.
- SD.

EXPECTED COURSE AND PROGNOSIS

- If cause is metabolic—condition may resolve with a good prognosis.
- If condition is associated with cardiac disease—prognosis is guarded because the underlying heart disease is likely chronic and progressive and therefore the arrhythmias may also worsen over time; presence of significant VT increases the risk of SD.
- If VT associated with hemangiosarcoma (cardiac or splenic)—the long-term outcome is grave due to the poor prognosis of the underlying disease.
- Approximately 50% of German shepherd dogs with more than 10 runs of VT/24 hours die suddenly.
- Doberman pinschers with VT and DCM may die suddenly during their first syncopal episode.

MISCELLANEOUS

ASSOCIATED CONDITIONS

N/A

AGE-RELATED FACTORS

If German shepherd dogs reach the age of 18 months, the probability of SD decreases, similarly in Rhodesian ridgebacks, after 30 months of age.

ZOONOTIC POTENTIAL

None

PREGNANCY/FERTILITY/BREEDING

N/A

SEE ALSO

- Cardiomyopathy, Arrhythmogenic Right Ventricular.

VENTRICULAR TACHYCARDIA (CONTINUED)

- Cardiomyopathy, Dilated—Dogs.
- Chagas Disease (American Trypanosomiasis).
- Digoxin Toxicity.
- Myocarditis.
- Ventricular Arrhythmias and Sudden Death in German Shepherds.
- Ventricular Premature Complexes.

ABBREVIATIONS

- ARVC = arrhythmogenic right ventricular cardiomyopathy.
- CHF = congestive heart failure.
- cTnI = cardiac troponin I.
- DCM = dilated cardiomyopathy.
- PDK4 = pyruvate dehydrogenase kinase 4.
- SD = sudden death.
- T_4 = thyroxine.
- VF = ventricular fibrillation.
- VT = ventricular tachycardia.

Suggested Reading

Cunningham SM, Sweeney JT, MacGregor J, et al. Clinical features of English bulldogs with presumed arrhythmogenic right ventricular cardiomyopathy: 31 cases (2001–2013). J Am Anim Hosp Assoc 2018, 54(2):95–102.

Authors Marc S. Kraus and Anna R.M. Gelzer

Consulting Editors Michael Aherne

Client Education Handout available online

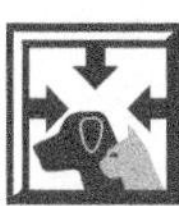

BASICS

DEFINITION

• Vertebral column trauma are caused by the application of exogenous forces to the vertebrae, intervertebral discs, tendons, ligamentous support structures, and the spinal cord.
• The clinical signs may include spinal hyperesthesia, limb paresis and/or proprioceptive ataxia, para- or tetraplegia, loss of nociception, urinary retention, and fecal incontinence.

PATHOPHYSIOLOGY

• In the normal vertebral column, passive (bones, ligaments, discs), active (tendons, muscles), and neural systems are responsible for stability.
• Compression, lateral bending, torsion, and sheer forces may result in failure of these systems, leading to vertebral fracture or subluxation.
• In some instances, significant spinal cord injury (SCI) such as traumatic disc herniation, penetrating injuries and post-traumatic vascular myelopathy, can be present without instability or fracture.
• SCI is the result of primary and secondary injuries.
• Primary injury results from initial mechanical events (spinal cord compression, contusion). The secondary injury is the biochemical cascade (combination of oxidative stress, inflammation, vascular injury) that follows and causes extension of the primary injury.

SYSTEMS AFFECTED

• Nervous.
• Musculoskeletal.
• Others possible due to exogenous trauma.

INCIDENCE/PREVALENCE

• Vertebral fractures and luxations represented 6% of all feline myelopathies and 7% of all canine neurology cases in two studies.
• The incidence of traumatic SCI without fracture/luxation is unknown.

SIGNALMENT

Breed Predilections

Medium- and large-breed dogs are more commonly affected.

Mean Age and Range

Most affected dogs and cats are young (median 2 years of age; range 0.25–15 years in one study).

Predominant Sex

Males appear overrepresented.

SIGNS

General Comments

• The majority of dogs with vertebral column trauma have SCI.
• Concurrent peripheral (e.g., brachial plexus trauma) or CNS injuries (e.g., head trauma) can occur.
• Abnormalities associated with other body systems are frequently identified.

Historical Findings

• Acute-onset paresis and ataxia or para-/tetraplegia.
• Clinical signs suggestive of hyperesthesia (vocalization, reluctance to move, arched back).

Neurologic Examination Abnormalities

• Focal SCI (affecting C1–C5, C6–T2, T3–L3, or L4–S3 spinal cord segments) is most common.
• Gait abnormalities—in >90% of animals; may include proprioceptive ataxia, paresis, and loss of voluntary movement.
• Abnormalities in spinal reflexes and postural reactions are common and usually reflect the spinal cord segment(s) injured.
• Decreased spinal reflexes can also be secondary to spinal shock (acute, transient, loss of spinal reflexes, commonly withdrawal reflexes, after SCI).
• Regional hyperesthesia.
• Animals with severe SCI may have absent nociception.
• Absence of deep nociception is a negative prognostic indicator, with the proportion of animals ambulating following thoracolumbar vertebral fracture/luxation considered <5%.

Physical Examination Abnormalities

• Pulmonary contusions and rib fractures.
• Pelvic and appendicular bone fractures.
• Cutaneous wounds.
• Traumatic brain injury.
• Abdominal organ injury.

CAUSES

• Automobile accident is the most common cause of vertebral column trauma.
• Other etiologies include fall, animal bites, and gunshot wounds.

RISK FACTORS

Animals housed outdoors, walked off lead, or unsecured in the cabs of pickup trucks are likely overrepresented.

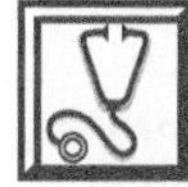

DIAGNOSIS

DIFFERENTIAL DIAGNOSIS

• Other neurologic diseases such as acute disc herniation, fibrocartilagenous embolic myelopathy, acute noncompressive nucleus pulposus extrusion, meningomyelitis, discospondylitis, and neoplasia, should be considered.
• Orthopedic injuries such as appendicular fracture or ligamentous injuries may occasionally be mistaken for vertebral column trauma.

CBC/BIOCHEMISTRY/URINALYSIS

• Abnormalities may be present if significant injury has occurred to other body systems.
• Anemia, findings consistent with dehydration, elevated creatinine kinase, and hematuria are all commonly seen.

IMAGING

Radiography

• 70% sensitive and highly specific for detecting vertebral fracture/luxation.
• Do not permit visualization of the spinal cord and have poor soft tissue detail.

Myelography

Can define extradural spinal cord compression but invasive and does not allow direct visualization of spinal cord parenchyma; may not detect lateralized spinal cord compression and lacks the tissue detail of advanced imaging studies.

Advanced Imaging

• CT—gold standard for evaluating the bones of the vertebral column and for visualizing mineralized disc material and extradural hemorrhage.
• MRI—can allow visualization of the bony vertebral column, but provides more soft tissue details than CT; it is the only means to exclude certain differential diagnoses, such as fibrocartilaginous embolism, and can provide prognostic information concerning recovery.

DIAGNOSTIC PROCEDURES

• CSF—often unremarkable or not etiology-specific; in some severe cases, CSF total protein, nucleated count, and red blood cell count may be increased.
• CSF is collected as an adjunct and not as a substitute to advanced imaging.
• Caution should be taken with CSF collection as positioning for cisternal or lumbar tap can exacerbate spinal cord injury by destabilizing a vertebral fracture or luxation.

PATHOLOGIC FINDINGS

• Gross findings may include evidence of vertebral luxation/fracture, extradural hemorrhage, disc extrusion, spinal cord swelling, dural/subarachnoid erythema/hemorrhage, and myelomalacia.
• Histopathologic abnormalities within the spinal cord may include necrosis, demyelination, infarction, parenchymal hemorrhage.

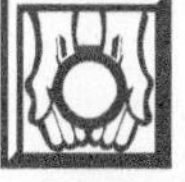

TREATMENT

APPROPRIATE HEALTH CARE

• Emergency intensive care management is recommended for all animals immediately following injury.
• Surgical management is needed if imaging suggests significant spinal cord compression and/or vertebral column instability.

VERTEBRAL COLUMN TRAUMA (CONTINUED)

- Medical management may be selected for animals that lack evidence of instability/compression.

NURSING CARE

- Prior to imaging, animals should be immobilized on a back board. Animals with suspected cervical lesions should ideally be placed in a neck brace that does not impair their breathing.
- Animals with imaging that suggests vertebral column instability should be immobilized until surgical stabilization.
- Non-ambulatory dogs require padded bedding, frequent turning, and urinary bladder evacuation.
- Fluid therapy is required in the event of dehydration and to maintain adequate blood pressure and perfusion to the spinal cord.
- Pain management is also required.
- Sedation can be considered to avoid exacerbation of the signs in anxious and frantic animals.
- Physical rehabilitation consisting of range of motion exercises, active weight bearing, and underwater treadmill may be beneficial but significant mobilization should only be performed after any vertebral column instability is addressed.

ACTIVITY

- Strict exercise restriction for 4 weeks for all animals following vertebral column surgery. Animals with fractures and instability may require 6–8 weeks of rest.
- Medically managed animals lacking vertebral column instability/fracture may require shorter periods of rest.

SURGICAL CONSIDERATIONS

- Surgery is recommended for animals with advanced imaging that supports significant spinal cord compression or vertebral column instability (e.g., subluxation, violation of multiple vertebral unit compartments).
- Spinal stapling, pins, and methylmethacrylate, and various plates can be used to stabilize the vertebral column.
- Decompression may be needed with or without stabilization in cases with significant extradural hemorrhage or disc material.
- Rapid surgical intervention (within 48 hours) is usually recommended to relieve spinal cord compression and limit permanent damage.

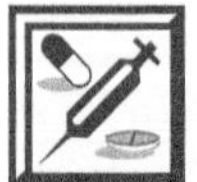

MEDICATIONS

DRUG(S) OF CHOICE

- Opioid analgesics—commonly used for pain management; fentanyl 2–5 µg/kg CRI, hydromorphone 0.05–0.1 mg/kg IV q6h).
- NSAIDs provide analgesia and anti-inflammatory effects and may be beneficial if hydration status, kidney, and liver functions are normal. Carprofen 2.2 mg/kg PO q12h commonly used.
- Gabapentin 10 mg/kg q8–12h can be beneficial for neuropathic pain.
- Alpha receptor antagonists can relax the internal urethral sphincter and facilitate urinary voiding in upper and lower motor neuron bladder dysfunction. Prazosin 1 mg/15 kg PO q8–12h.

CONTRAINDICATIONS

Glucocorticoids—methylprednisone sodium succinate (MPSS) and other glucocorticoids have not been shown to be beneficial in dogs with SCI.

PRECAUTIONS

- NSAIDs may result in gastric ulcers and kidney injury.
- Glucocorticoids may cause gastric or colonic ulceration, vomiting, and urinary tract infections (especially dexamethasone).
- Alpha-antagonists may result in hypotension and gastrointestinal signs.

POSSIBLE INTERACTIONS

Glucocorticoids and NSAIDs should not be combined as this increases the risk of gastrointestinal adverse effects.

ALTERNATIVE DRUG(S)

N/A

FOLLOW-UP

PATIENT MONITORING

Daily physical and neurologic examination is strongly suggested to monitor progression.

PREVENTION/AVOIDANCE

N/A

POSSIBLE COMPLICATIONS

- Chronic ataxia/paresis as well as failure to regain voluntary ambulation are possible.
- Some animals may have urinary/fecal incontinence, especially if they are non-ambulatory.
- Non-ambulatory animals are at risk for skin ulcers and urinary tract infection.

EXPECTED COURSE AND PROGNOSIS

- Animals with intact nociception have a good prognosis for ambulatory recovery if appropriate treatment is undertaken.
- Animals with absent nociception that have vertebral fracture or luxation have a very poor prognosis for regaining voluntary ambulation (<5%).

MISCELLANEOUS

ASSOCIATED CONDITIONS

Animals that have traumatic SCI often have injury to other body systems.

AGE-RELATED FACTORS

Younger animals are more commonly affected.

PREGNANCY/FERTILITY/BREEDING

SCI may affect ability to achieve pregnancy and carry fetuses to term.

SYNONYMS

Traumatic myelopathy.

SEE ALSO

- Myelopathy—Paresis/Paralysis—Cats.
- Paralysis.

ABBREVIATIONS

- MPSS = methylprednisone sodium succinate.
- NSAID = nonsteroidal anti-inflammatory drug.
- SCI = spinal cord injury.

Suggested Reading

Bali MS, Lang J, Jaggy A, et al. Comparative study of vertebral fractures and luxations in dogs and cats. Vet Comp Orthop Traumatol 2009, 22:47–53.

Bruce CW, Brisson BA, Gyselinck K. Spinal fracture and luxation in dogs and cats. Vet Comp Orthop Traumatol 2008, 21:280–284.

Jeffery ND, Levine JM, Olby NJ, et al. Intervertebral disc degeneration in dogs: consequences, diagnosis, treatment, and future directions. J Vet Intern Med 2013, 27:1318–1333.

Levine GJ, Levine JM, Budke CM, et al. Description and repeatability of a newly validated spinal cord injury scale for dogs. Prev Vet Med 2009, 89:121–127.

Author Aude M.H. Castel

Acknowledgment The author and editors acknowledge the prior contribution of Jonathan M. Levine.

VESICOURACHAL DIVERTICULA

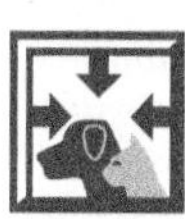

BASICS

OVERVIEW

- A common congenital anomaly of the urinary bladder that occurs when a portion of the urachus (i.e., a fetal conduit that allows passage of urine from the bladder to the placenta) located at the bladder vertex fails to close; the result is a blind diverticulum of variable size that protrudes from the bladder vertex.
- Other characteristics include congenital microscopic diverticula (microscopic lumens that may persist at the bladder vertex).
- Acquired macroscopic diverticula develop after the onset of concurrent but unrelated acquired lower urinary tract diseases; presumably, urethral obstruction or detrusor hyperactivity induced by inflammation causes high intraluminal pressure and subsequent enlargement of microscopic diverticula.
- Congenital macroscopic diverticula, most likely caused by impaired urine outflow, develop before or soon after birth and persist indefinitely.

SIGNALMENT

- Dog and cat.
- Frequently encountered in cats with acquired lower urinary tract diseases; twice as common in male cats as in female cats.
- No breed or age predisposition.

SIGNS

Depend on concomitant disorders predisposing to formation of macroscopic vesicourachal diverticula.

CAUSES & RISK FACTORS

- Persistent congenital microscopic diverticula—cause unknown.
- Congenital microscopic diverticula—risk factors for acquired macroscopic diverticula.
- Diseases associated with increased bladder intraluminal pressure (e.g., bacterial urinary tract infection, uroliths, urethral plugs, and idiopathic disease)—risk factors for acquired macroscopic diverticula.

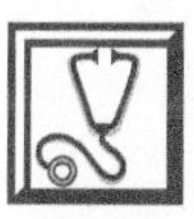

DIAGNOSIS

DIFFERENTIAL DIAGNOSIS

- Persistent (or patent) urachus; rare—characterized by inappropriate loss of urine through the umbilicus.
- Persistent urachal ligaments are nonpatent fibrous remnants of the urachus, connecting the bladder vertex to the umbilicus.
- Urachal cysts are focal accumulations of fluid in isolated segments of the urachus. They may be aseptic or septic.

CBC/BIOCHEMISTRY/URINALYSIS

- Abnormal findings are related to the underlying disorder that causes vesicourachal diverticula, unless complicated by concurrent acquired lower urinary tract diseases.
- Abnormal findings related to secondary urinary tract infection.

IMAGING

- Congenital and acquired macroscopic diverticula—best identified by positive-contrast urethrocystography.
- Radiographs obtained with the bladder completely then partially distended with contrast medium may facilitate detection of small diverticula.

DIAGNOSTIC PROCEDURES

N/A

PATHOLOGIC FINDINGS

- Extramural macroscopic diverticula appear as convex or conical luminal projections from the bladder vertex.
- Intramural microscopic diverticula appear as transitional epithelium-lined lumens persisting at the bladder vertex from the level of the submucosa to subserosa.

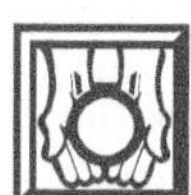

TREATMENT

- Many macroscopic diverticula in cats (and probably dogs) are acquired and self-limiting if the underlying disease is eliminated.
- Direct treatment efforts toward eliminating underlying cause(s) of lower urinary tract disease.
- Consider diverticulectomy if a macroscopic diverticulum persists in a patient with persistent or recurrent bacterial urinary tract infection despite appropriate antimicrobial therapy.

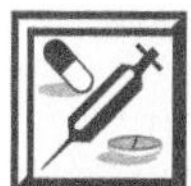

MEDICATIONS

DRUG(S) OF CHOICE

N/A

FOLLOW-UP

PATIENT MONITORING

If bacterial urinary tract infection persists or recurs despite proper antimicrobial therapy, the status of the diverticulum should be reevaluated by contrast radiography.

PREVENTION/AVOIDANCE

Avoid diagnostic procedures or treatments that alter normal host urinary tract defenses and predispose to urinary tract infection.

POSSIBLE COMPLICATIONS

Persistent congenital macroscopic diverticula are risk factors for recurrent bacterial urinary tract infection.

EXPECTED COURSE AND PROGNOSIS

- Congenital microscopic diverticula are usually clinically silent unless complicated by concurrent lower urinary tract disease.
- Acquired macroscopic diverticula typically heal in 2–3 weeks after amelioration of clinical signs of lower urinary tract disease.
- Diverticulectomy and appropriate antimicrobial therapy usually associated with resolution of recurrent urinary tract infections in patients with persistent congenital macroscopic diverticula.

MISCELLANEOUS

ASSOCIATED CONDITIONS

- Persistent congenital macroscopic diverticula are potential risk factors for recurrent bacterial urinary tract infections.
- Acquired macroscopic diverticula are typically encountered in patients with concurrent lower urinary tract diseases.

SEE ALSO

- Lower Urinary Tract Infection, Bacterial.
- Lower Urinary Tract Infection, Fungal.

Suggested Reading

Osborne CA, Johnston GR, Kruger JM, et al. Etiopathogenesis and biological behavior of feline vesicourachal diverticula. Vet Clin North Am Small Anim Pract 1987, 17:697–733.

Author John M. Kruger

Consulting Editor J.D. Foster

Acknowledgment The author and editors acknowledges the prior contribution of Carl A. Osborne.

VESTIBULAR DISEASE, GERIATRIC—DOGS

BASICS

DEFINITION

Acute-onset nonprogressive disturbance of the peripheral vestibular system in older dogs.

PATHOPHYSIOLOGY

- Unknown.
- Suspected abnormal flow of the endolymphatic fluid in the semicircular canals of the inner ear secondary to disturbance in production, circulation, or absorption of the fluid.
- Possible intoxication of the vestibular receptors or inflammation of the vestibular portion of the vestibulocochlear nerve (cranial nerve VIII).
- Often incorrectly referred to as a stroke, geriatric vestibular disease is neither central in location nor suspected to be vascular or ischemic in origin.

SYSTEMS AFFECTED

Nervous—peripheral vestibular system.

GENETICS

N/A

INCIDENCE/PREVALENCE

Common, sporadic, acquired disease of older dogs.

SIGNALMENT

Species

Dog

V

Breed Predilections

- None reported.
- Seems to occur more frequently in medium to large breeds.

Mean Age and Range

Geriatric; patients usually >8 years old.

Predominant Sex

N/A

SIGNS

General Comments

- Signs of acute onset peripheral vestibular dysfunction usually unilateral but occasionally bilateral.
- If vestibular signs are severe, do not incorrectly attribute the signs (especially the gait) to a central (i.e., CNS) location.

Historical Findings

- Sudden onset of imbalance, disorientation, reluctance to stand, and (usually) head tilt and irregular eye movements.
- May be preceded or accompanied by nausea and vomiting.

Physical Examination Findings

- Head tilt—mild to marked; directed toward the side of the lesion; occasionally disease is bilateral with erratic side-to-side head movements either without a head tilt or with a mild tilt in direction of the more severely affected side.
- Abnormal (resting) nystagmus common in early stages; either horizontal or rotatory with the fast phase always in the direction opposite to the head tilt; with bilateral disease, abnormal nystagmus usually mild or not present and physiologic nystagmus or conjugate eye movements diminished to absent.
- Mild to marked disorientation and vestibular ataxia with tendency to lean or fall in the direction of the head tilt.
- Strength and proprioception normal; with severe disease, patient may be reluctant/unable to stand and may have other issues (e.g., hip dysplasia), making assessment of gait difficult; with bilateral disease, may have base-wide stance.

CAUSES

Unknown

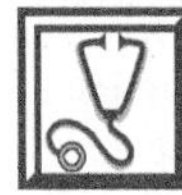

DIAGNOSIS

DIFFERENTIAL DIAGNOSIS

- Primarily distinguished from other causes of vestibular deficits by the acute onset and usually rapid improvement without specific treatment.
- Otitis media and interna—may have concurrent ipsilateral facial nerve (cranial nerve VII) paresis or paralysis, deafness, and/or Horner's syndrome; otitis externa with ruptured tympanic membrane may be present with otitis media and interna.
- Ototoxic drugs—eliminated by history.
- Trauma—may cause similar acute changes; differentiated by history, results of physical examination.
- Hypothyroid neuropathy—usually not as acute in onset or as severe; may be associated with clinical signs of hypothyroidism and possible cranial nerve VII deficit.
- Neoplasia—either affecting CN VIII peripherally or in a central location; signs usually not as acute in onset as geriatric vestibular disease and signs persistent and usually progressive in nature.

CBC/BIOCHEMISTRY/URINALYSIS

- Generally normal.
- Hemoconcentration secondary to dehydration may be present.
- Unrelated concurrent disorders (e.g., renal and hepatic disease) associated with geriatric state may cause laboratory abnormalities.

OTHER LABORATORY TESTS

N/A

IMAGING

- Usually none required.
- Radiographs of tympanic bullae: normal radiographs do not rule out bulla disease.
- CT or MRI (preferred over radiographs)—may be required to rule out other causes such as otitis media and interna, central causes (e.g., ischemic event, neoplasia, inflammatory disease).

DIAGNOSTIC PROCEDURES

- Brainstem auditory evoked response—to assess cochlear portion of cranial nerve VIII; may help to evaluate for otitis media and interna since only the vestibular portion of cranial nerve VIII is affected with geriatric vestibular disease.
- Deafness may, however, be present as an unrelated aging change.

PATHOLOGIC FINDINGS

None reported.

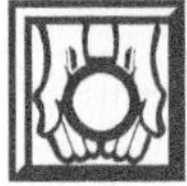

TREATMENT

APPROPRIATE HEALTH CARE

- Mild disease—usually can manage as outpatient.
- Severe disease—patients that cannot ambulate or require IV fluid support should be hospitalized during the initial stages.

NURSING CARE

- Treatment supportive, including rehydration by IV fluids if required.
- Keep recumbent patients warm and dry using soft, absorbent bedding and, if required, urinary catheter.
- Severe disease—physical therapy, including passive manipulation of limbs and moving body to alternate sides, may be required initially.

ACTIVITY

Restrict activity as required by the degree of disorientation and vestibular ataxia.

DIET

- No modification usually required.
- Nausea, vomiting, and severe disorientation—initially withhold oral intake, then supervised feeding.

CLIENT EDUCATION

Reassure client that although the initial signs can be alarming and incapacitating, the prognosis for rapid improvement and recovery is excellent.

MEDICATIONS

DRUG(S) OF CHOICE

- Sedatives—for severe disorientation and ataxia; diazepam 2–10 mg/dog PO or IV q8h, acepromazine 0.02–0.05 mg/kg IM, SC, IV to maximum of 2 mg, dexmedetomidine 1–2 μg/kg IV.
- Antianxiety—trazodone approximately 5 mg/kg PO q8–24h.

• Antiemetic drugs or drugs against motion sickness—questionable benefit; dimenhydrinate 4–8 mg/kg PO, IM, IV q8h, meclizine HCl 25 mg PO q24h, maropitant 1 mg/kg SC q24h for up to 5 days or 2 mg/kg PO q24h for up to 5 days.
• Glucocorticoids—not recommended since do not alter course of the disease; may exacerbate concurrent issues (e.g., dehydration).
• Antibiotics—recommended when otitis media and interna cannot be ruled out; trimethoprim-sulfa 15 mg/kg PO q12h or 30 mg/kg PO q12–24h; first-generation cephalosporin (e.g., cephalexin 10–30 mg/kg PO q12h); amoxicillin–clavulanic acid 12.5 mg/kg PO q12h, enrofloxacin 5–20 mg/kg PO q24h or divided q12h.

CONTRAINDICATIONS

N/A

FOLLOW-UP

PATIENT MONITORING

• Neurologic examination of outpatient—repeat 2–3 days later to confirm stabilization and initial improvement.
• Discharge inpatient when able to ambulate and resume eating and drinking.

PREVENTION/AVOIDANCE

N/A

POSSIBLE COMPLICATIONS

• Fluid and electrolyte imbalances and decompensation of preexistent renal insufficiency may follow vomiting and/or insufficient fluid and food intake.
• Pressure sores/abrasions.

EXPECTED COURSE AND PROGNOSIS

• Improvement of clinical signs usually starts within 72 hours with gradual resolution of vomiting and improvement of nystagmus and vestibular ataxia.
• Head tilt and ataxia—significant improvement usually occurs over 7–10 days; if no improvement other causes of peripheral vestibular disease should be pursued; mild head tilt may persist.
• Most patients return to normal within 2–3 weeks.
• Recurrence—repeat episodes of geriatric vestibular disease can occur on the same or opposite side but are uncommon; brief return of signs may occur with stress (e.g., anesthesia).

MISCELLANEOUS

ASSOCIATED CONDITIONS

N/A

AGE-RELATED FACTORS

Geriatric dogs affected (mean age suggested 12.5 years).

ZOONOTIC POTENTIAL

N/A

PREGNANCY/FERTILITY/BREEDING

N/A

SYNONYMS

• Benign idiopathic canine peripheral vestibular disease.
• Canine idiopathic vestibular disease/syndrome.
• Idiopathic canine peripheral vestibular disease.
• Old dog vestibular syndrome.

SEE ALSO

• Head Tilt.
• Otitis Media and Interna.

Suggested Reading

de Lahunta A, Glass EN, Kent M. Veterinary Neuroanatomy and Clinical Neurology, 4th ed. St. Louis, MO: Saunders Elsevier, 2015, pp. 348–349.

Dewey CW. A Practical Guide to Canine and Feline Neurology, 2nd ed. Ames, IA: Wiley-Blackwell, 2008, pp. 272–273.

Garosi L. Head tilt and nystagmus. In: Platt SR, Garosi LS, eds., Small Animal Neurological Emergencies. London: Manson Publishing, 2012, pp. 253–263.

Author Susan M. Cochrane

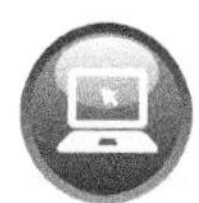

Client Education Handout available online

VESTIBULAR DISEASE, IDIOPATHIC—CATS

BASICS

DEFINITION

Acute-onset nonprogressive disturbance of the peripheral vestibular system of cats.

PATHOPHYSIOLOGY

- Unknown.
- Suspected abnormal flow of the endolymphatic fluid in the semicircular canals of the inner ear, secondary to a disturbance in the production, circulation, or absorption of the fluid.
- Possible intoxication of the vestibular receptors or inflammation of the vestibular portion of the vestibulocochlear nerve (cranial nerve VIII).

SYSTEMS AFFECTED

Nervous—peripheral vestibular system.

INCIDENCE/PREVALENCE

- Sporadic acquired disease.
- None reported.

SIGNALMENT

Species

Cat

Mean Age and Range

Any age; rare in cats <1 year of age.

SIGNS

General Comments

Limited to signs associated with peripheral vestibular disturbance.

V

Historical Findings

Sudden onset of severe disorientation, falling, rolling, leaning, vocalizing, and crouched posture; tendency to panic when picked up.

Physical Examination Findings

- Head tilt—always toward the side of the lesion; occasionally disease is bilateral with wide, side-to-side excursions of the head either without a head tilt or with a mild tilt toward the more severely affected side.
- Resting nystagmus—usually horizontal, but may be rotatory with the fast phase always in direction opposite to the head tilt; with bilateral disease, the abnormal nystagmus is usually mild or not present, and physiologic nystagmus or conjugate eye movements are diminished to absent.
- Vestibular ataxia with tendency to roll and fall toward the side of the head tilt.
- Preservation of strength and normal proprioception; with bilateral disease, patient may be reluctant to ambulate, preferring to stay in a crouched posture and possible wide-based stance.

CAUSES

- Unknown.
- Previous upper respiratory tract infection—suspected in some patients; relationship not confirmed; in limited necropsy data no evidence of inflammation.

RISK FACTORS

May be an increase in cases in the summer and early fall, possibly after outbreaks of upper respiratory disease; disease can occur throughout the year.

DIAGNOSIS

DIFFERENTIAL DIAGNOSIS

- Diagnosis made on the basis of acute-onset peripheral vestibular signs that improve relatively rapidly without specific treatment.
- Otitis media and interna (e.g., bacterial, parasitic)—may have concurrent ipsilateral facial nerve (cranial nerve VII) paresis or paralysis, Horner's syndrome, deafness, ruptured tympanic membrane, otitis externa, and/or imaging changes in tympanic bulla; signs usually not self-limiting.
- Nasopharyngeal polyp(s)—may cause unilateral or, much less commonly, bilateral peripheral vestibular signs; may have concurrent tympanic bulla involvement; signs usually not as acute and severe at onset and are not self-limiting.
- Neoplasia—e.g., squamous cell carcinoma; signs usually not acute in onset; may have concurrent cranial nerve VII deficit and/or ipsilateral Horner's syndrome; signs not self-limiting.
- Blue-tailed lizard ingestion—southeastern United States; thought to produce a similar acute, unilateral, peripheral vestibular syndrome; vomiting, salivation, irritability, and trembling also noted; most patients recover without specific treatment.
- Aminoglycoside toxicity, especially streptomycin—may cause acute unilateral or bilateral peripheral vestibular syndrome and/or hearing loss; differentiated by history of drug use.
- Trauma—overzealous ear flushing; usually occurs when cleaning performed under general anesthesia or sedation; signs follow immediately upon recovery from anesthesia/sedation.

CBC/BIOCHEMISTRY/URINALYSIS

Normal

IMAGING

- None usually necessary.
- Radiographs of tympanic bullae: normal radiographs do not rule out bulla disease.
- CT or MRI—occasionally required to rule out other causes such as otitis media and interna, nasopharyngeal polyp(s) and neoplasia.

DIAGNOSTIC PROCEDURES

Brainstem auditory evoked response—may help rule out other causes (e.g., otitis media and interna; nasopharyngeal polyp(s), neoplasia); with idiopathic vestibular disease hearing not affected since disease limited to the vestibular portion of cranial nerve VIII.

PATHOLOGIC FINDINGS

None reported.

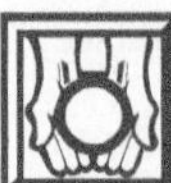

TREATMENT

APPROPRIATE HEALTH CARE

- Usually outpatient.
- Inpatient—severely affected patient may require hospitalization for supportive care.

NURSING CARE

- Mild disease—treatment supportive only.
- Severe disease—may require IV or subcutaneous fluids; maintain patient in quiet, well-padded cage.

ACTIVITY

Restricted according to the degree of disorientation and ataxia.

DIET

Patient may initially be reluctant to eat and drink because of disorientation and/or nausea.

CLIENT EDUCATION

Reassure client that, despite initial alarming and often incapacitating signs, the prognosis for rapid and complete recovery is excellent.

MEDICATIONS

DRUG(S) OF CHOICE

- Sedatives—for severe disorientation and rolling; diazepam 1–5 mg/cat PO q8–12h, acepromazine 0.02–0.05 mg/kg IM, SC, IV.
- Antiemetic drugs and drugs against motion sickness—questionable benefit; e.g., meclizine HCl 12.5 mg PO q24h, maropitant 1 mg/kg q24h PO, SC.
- Glucocorticoids—not recommended since do not alter course of the disease.
- Antibiotics—recommended if otitis media and interna cannot be ruled out; trimethoprim-sulfa 15 mg/kg PO q12h; first-generation cephalosporin (e.g., cephalexin 15–20 mg/kg PO q12h); drug of choice is amoxicillin/clavulanic acid (Clavamox 62.5 mg/cat PO q12h, Clavaseptin 12.5 mg/kg PO q12h).

FOLLOW-UP

PATIENT MONITORING

- Neurologic examination of outpatient—repeat in approximately 72 hours to confirm stabilization and initial improvement.

• Inpatient—discharge patient when able to ambulate and resume eating and drinking.

EXPECTED COURSE AND PROGNOSIS

• Marked improvement, especially in resting nystagmus starting within 72 hours, with progressive improvement of gait and head tilt.
• Patients usually normal within 2–3 weeks.
• Head tilt—final sign to resolve; mild residual tilt may remain.
• If signs do not improve rapidly, other causes of vestibular disease should be pursued.
• Rarely recurs.

MISCELLANEOUS

Suggested Reading

Garosi L. Head tilt and nystagmus. In: Platt SR, Garosi LS, eds., Small Animal Neurological Emergencies. London: Manson Publishing, 2012, pp. 253–263.

Author Susan M. Cochrane

Client Education Handout available online

VOMITING, CHRONIC

BASICS

DEFINITION

Persistent vomiting lasting longer than 5–7 days or vomiting that occurs intermittently several days/week. This condition is usually nonresponsive to symptomatic treatment.

PATHOPHYSIOLOGY

- Vomiting occurs when the vomiting center, located within the medulla oblongata, is activated by the humoral or neural pathway.
- There are four main components to the vomiting reflex: (1) visceral receptors within the gastrointestinal (GI) tract; (2) vagal and sympathetic afferent neurons; (3) chemoreceptor trigger zone (CRTZ); and (4) vomiting center.
- The humoral pathway is mediated via activation of the CRTZ and is affected by bloodborne triggers such as uremic toxins, drug toxicity, and endotoxemia.
- The neural pathway is mediated via activation of the vomiting center and is affected by disorders associated with obstruction, distension, or inflammation of the GI tract.
- All causes of vomiting (including the vestibular apparatus and cerebrum) are ultimately mediated via the vomiting center.

SYSTEMS AFFECTED

- Endocrine/metabolic—dehydration, electrolyte and acid-base imbalances.
- Cardiovascular—hypovolemia; electrolyte or acid–base imbalances can cause arrhythmias.
- GI—esophagitis and subsequent esophageal stricture.
- Respiratory—aspiration pneumonia.
- Nervous—altered mentation.

SIGNALMENT

- Dog and cat.
- Young animals are more likely to ingest foreign bodies; linear foreign bodies are more common in cats.
- Confirmed or suspected breed predispositions—brachycephalic breeds are prone to pyloric outflow obstruction secondary to mucosal hypertrophy; basenji, German shepherd dog, and shar-pei are prone to inflammatory bowel disease (IBD); Rottweiler are prone to eosinophilic IBD; Airedale terrier prone to pancreatic carcinoma; beagle, Bedlington terrier, cocker spaniel, Doberman pinscher, Labrador retriever, Skye terrier, and standard poodle are prone to chronic hepatitis. Yorkshire terrier predisposed to intestinal lymphangiectasia.

SIGNS

Historical Findings

- Hematemesis, decreased appetite or anorexia, and melena, may suggest gastric disease.
- Diarrhea and profound weight loss may suggest intestinal disease.
- Signs such as weakness, polyuria, or jaundice may relate to other underlying metabolic diseases.

Physical Examination Findings

- Weight loss and poor hair coat may indicate chronic malnutrition.
- Abdominal palpation may reveal abdominal distention, pain, thickened bowel loops, lymphadenopathy, or mass effects.
- Tacky mucous membranes and prolonged skin tenting if dehydration is present; pale membranes if patient is anemic.
- Oral examination may reveal uremic ulcerations or sublingual string foreign bodies.
- Rectal examination may detect diarrhea, hematochezia, or melena.

CAUSES

Esophageal Disease

- Hiatal hernia (more commonly associated with regurgitation).
- Gastroesophageal reflux (more commonly associated with regurgitation).

Infectious Disease

- *Helicobacter*-related gastritis.
- Histoplasmosis.
- Pythiosis.
- Small intestinal bacterial overgrowth.
- Gastric or intestinal parasites.

Metabolic Diseases

- Renal disease.
- Hepatobiliary disease.
- Hypoadrenocorticism.
- Chronic pancreatitis.
- Diabetic ketoacidosis (DKA).
- Electrolyte abnormalities—hypo-/hyperkalemia, hyponatremia, hypercalcemia.

Inflammatory Bowel Disease

- Lymphocytic, plasmacytic, eosinophilic, or granulomatous.
- Gastritis, enteritis, or colitis.

Obstructive GI Disease

- Foreign body.
- Chronic hypertrophic pyloric gastropathy.
- Intussusception.

Neoplastic Disease

- GI lymphoma, adenocarcinoma, fibrosarcoma, GI stromal cell tumor.
- Pancreatic adenocarcinoma.
- Gastrin-secreting tumor (gastrinoma).
- Mast cell tumor.

Neurologic

- Cerebral edema.
- CNS tumors.
- Encephalitis/meningoencephalitis.
- Vestibular disease.

Motility Disorders

- Postgastric dilatation.
- Postsurgical—gastric, duodenal.
- Electrolyte imbalances.
- Ileus.

Miscellaneous

- Drugs (e.g., nonsteroidal anti-inflammatory drugs [NSAIDs], glucocorticoids, chemotherapeutics, antibiotics, antifungals).
- Food sensitivity.
- Toxicity.

Additional Causes

- Parasitic (cats)—dirofilariasis, *Ollulanus tricuspis*.
- Inflammatory—cholecystitis, cholangiohepatitis.
- Metabolic—hyperthyroidism.
- Functional—constipation/obstipation.

RISK FACTORS

Breed-associated disease (see Signalment).

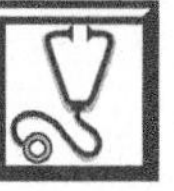

DIAGNOSIS

DIFFERENTIAL DIAGNOSIS

- Vomiting must first be differentiated from regurgitation.
- Regurgitation is a passive process and occurs without an abdominal component, thus localizing disease to the esophagus.
- Vomiting is a centrally mediated reflex often preceded by prodromal signs of restlessness, nausea, salivation, and repeated swallowing.

CBC/BIOCHEMISTRY/URINALYSIS

- Chronic GI bleeding can cause a non-regenerative anemia, often with characteristics of iron deficiency (microcytosis, hypochromasia, thrombocytosis).
- Non-regenerative anemia may also occur secondary to chronic metabolic or inflammatory diseases.
- Inflammatory conditions may cause neutrophilic leukocytosis and monocytosis.
- Eosinophilia can occur from eosinophilic IBD, hypoadrenocorticism, and GI parasitism.
- Thrombocytopenia has been reported with IBD.
- Dehydration increases the packed cell volume and total protein.
- Electrolyte and acid–base imbalances reflect severity of losses and can help to localize disease.
- Hypochloremic metabolic alkalosis, often with hypokalemia, suggests gastric outflow obstruction.
- Hyperkalemia suggests hypoadrenocorticism or oliguric/anuric renal failure; occasionally, enteritis caused by trichuriasis or bacterial infection (salmonellosis) mimics hypoadrenocorticism.
- Metabolic acidosis is common in patients with dehydration, renal failure, DKA, and severe gastroenteritis with diarrhea.

• Increased liver enzyme activity, hypoalbuminemia, hyperbilirubinemia, hypoglycemia, or low urea nitrogen concentration suggest hepatic disease.
• Persistent hyperglycemia and glucosuria is consistent with diabetes mellitus.
• Hyperglobulinemia may indicate chronic inflammation or infection.
• Hypoproteinemia, hypocholesterolemia, lymphopenia, and hypomagnesemia occur secondary to a protein-losing enteropathy caused by infiltrative intestinal diseases such as lymphocytic plasmacytic gastroenteritis, neoplasia, histoplasmosis, or intestinal lymphangiectasia.
• Urinalysis is used to rule out renal failure and DKA.
• Aciduria in the hypokalemic, hypochloremic, alkalotic patient suggests gastric outflow obstruction.

OTHER LABORATORY TESTS

• Resting cortisol to screen for hypoadrenocorticism. A resting cortisol <2 µg/dL should be followed with an ACTH stimulation test.
• Pancreatic lipase immunoreactivity assay may help confirm pancreatitis together with supportive history, physical exam findings, and ultrasound.
• Serum cobalamin and folate as indicators of intestinal absorption.
• Pre- and postprandial bile acids to screen for hepatobiliary dysfunction.
• Fecal testing for GI parasitism.

IMAGING

• Survey radiographs of the abdomen help identify foreign bodies, GI distension with fluid or gas, and displacement, malposition, shape, and/or size changes of abdominal organs.
• Survey radiographs of the thorax are used to evaluate for pulmonary metastases, gross esophageal abnormalities, or infectious disease.
• A barium upper GI series can be used to identify foreign bodies, GI wall masses or infiltrative disease, mucosal ulceration, delayed gastric emptying, and motility disorders; however, the procedure is relatively insensitive for detection of mucosal ulceration.
• Abdominal ultrasonography to identify abnormalities of the liver, gallbladder, kidneys, pancreas, GI tract, and mesenteric lymph nodes.
• CT and MRI further evaluate for abnormalities of abdominal organs.

DIAGNOSTIC PROCEDURES

• Gastroduodenoscopy—allows direct inspection of the gastric and intestinal lumen to identify gross mucosal lesions and foreign bodies and provides a minimally invasive method of biopsy to evaluate for microscopic disease. Limitations of endoscopy include the working length of the endoscope (unable to access the jejunum in large-breed dogs) and depth of the biopsies.
• Laparoscopy or exploratory laparotomy is used for more extensive diagnostic and therapeutic procedures.

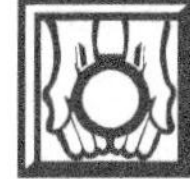

TREATMENT

APPROPRIATE HEALTH CARE

Specific treatment should be aimed at eliminating the underlying cause in conjunction with supportive therapy. Care may be inpatient or outpatient depending on the case.

NURSING CARE

• If vomiting is intractable, stop oral intake of food and water for 12–24 hours or until the vomiting episodes are better controlled with antiemetics.
• Use crystalloid fluid therapy to replace deficits and to provide for maintenance and ongoing losses.
• Supplement potassium if hypokalemia is present; 20 mEq of KCl/L of fluid can be safely added for replacement and maintenance; use higher concentrations if severe hypokalemia is present.

DIET

• Debilitated patients and those in poor nutritional condition may need supplemental parenteral or enteral nutrition.
• Dietary therapy for patients with suspected food allergy or with IBD should use an elimination diet containing a single, novel protein source or a hydrolyzed diet.

CLIENT EDUCATION

Dependent on underlying disease.

SURGICAL CONSIDERATIONS

Use surgical treatment if uncontrolled hemorrhage, obstruction, or perforation is suspected.

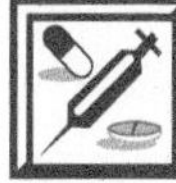

MEDICATIONS

DRUG(S) OF CHOICE

• Antisecretory drugs such as H_2-receptor blockers (e.g., famotidine, ranitidine) or proton pump inhibitors such as omeprazole (more potent)—famotidine 0.5–1 mg/kg PO, IV, or SC q12h; ranitidine 1–2 mg/kg PO, IV q12h; omeprazole 0.7–1.5 mg/kg PO q12h.
• Protectants such as sucralfate 0.25–1 g/dog PO q6–12h or 0.25 g/cat PO q6–12h to accelerate gastric mucosal healing; can be used with antisecretory drugs for patients with evidence of upper GI bleeding (e.g., hematemesis or melena).
• Antibiotics—indicated for treatment of *Helicobacter*-associated gastritis, small intestinal bacterial overgrowth (SIBO), and as an adjunct to corticosteroids in the treatment of IBD.
• Metronidazole—may be used at 10 mg/kg PO q12h in conjunction with corticosteroids to treat IBD, although evidence of direct benefit of this approach is currently lacking.
• Antibiotic-responsive enteropathy (tylosin-responsive enteropathy)—tylosin is the drug of choice administered at 10–40 mg/kg q12h for 8–12 weeks. Alternative option is metronidazole 10 mg/kg q12h for 8–12 weeks, although tylosin may be superior for this disorder.
• Use corticosteroids in conjunction with dietary changes to treat biopsy-confirmed IBD; azathioprine, chlorambucil, or cyclosporine can also be used in patients with poor response to corticosteroids alone or to decrease the dosage of steroids required to control symptoms. Avoid the use of more than two immunomodulatory drugs given concurrently.
• Prokinetic drugs (e.g., metoclopramide, cisapride, or erythromycin) are used to treat delayed gastric emptying not associated with obstructive disease. Metoclopramide 0.2–0.5 mg/kg IV, IM, PO q6–8h; more effective as a CRI of 1–2 mg/kg q24h in hospitalized patients.
• Pyrantel pamoate is effective for *Physaloptera*; fenbendazole is effective for *Ollulanus*.
• Iron supplementation for animals with chronic GI bleeding that develop microcytic hypochromic anemia.
• Surgery and/or chemotherapy for neoplasia, depending on the tumor type and location.
• Paraneoplastic hypersecretion of gastric acid, as occurs with mastocytosis and gastrin-secreting pancreatic tumors, is best treated with antisecretory drugs (e.g., omeprazole).
• Reserve antiemetics for patients with persistent vomiting unresponsive to treatment of the underlying disease. Maropitant 1 mg/kg SC q24h, 2 mg/kg PO q24h. Chlorpromazine 0.5 mg/kg SC, IM q6–8h. Ondansetron 0.2–0.5 mg/kg SC, IV q8–12h, 0.5–1.0 mg/kg PO q12h.
• Vomiting caused by chemotherapy is best treated with ondansetron 0.5–1 mg/kg IV, PO given 30 minutes before chemotherapy.

CONTRAINDICATIONS

N/A

PRECAUTIONS

• Do not give α-adrenergic blockers such as chlorpromazine to dehydrated patients as they can cause hypotension.
• Use antiemetics with caution, as they can mask the underlying problem.
• Metoclopramide can cause lethargy, restlessness, agitation, and other behavioral changes, particularly in cats.
• Corticosteroids are immunosuppressive and are a risk factor for development of GI

VOMITING, CHRONIC (CONTINUED)

ulceration; use caution when treating IBD with corticosteroids at high dosages or for long periods.
- Azathioprine and chlorambucil are myelotoxic; monitor CBCs for neutropenia and thrombocytopenia every 2 weeks for the first month of treatment and monthly thereafter.
- Cyclosporine can exacerbate vomiting and diarrhea when used at high dosages; use with caution in patients with renal disease.
- Do not use anticholinergics as antiemetics, as they can exacerbate vomiting by causing gastric atony and gastric retention.
- Metoclopramide and cisapride are contraindicated in patients with GI obstruction.

POSSIBLE INTERACTIONS

Ranitidine interferes with hepatic metabolism of theophylline, phenytoin, and warfarin, and should not be used concurrently with these drugs. Avoid use of cimetidine because it is a weak H_2-receptor antagonist and is a potent inhibitor of the cytochrome P450 enzyme pathway.

ALTERNATIVE DRUG(S)

N/A

FOLLOW-UP

PATIENT MONITORING

- Frequency of vomiting.
- Body weight; body condition score.

PREVENTION/AVOIDANCE

N/A

POSSIBLE COMPLICATIONS

- Esophagitis.
- Aspiration pneumonia.

EXPECTED COURSE AND PROGNOSIS

Varies with underlying disease.

MISCELLANEOUS

ASSOCIATED CONDITIONS

N/A

AGE-RELATED FACTORS

N/A

ZOONOTIC POTENTIAL

Dependent on underlying cause.

PREGNANCY/FERTILITY/BREEDING

N/A

SYNONYMS

N/A

SEE ALSO

- Bilious Vomiting Syndrome.
- Constipation and Obstipation.
- Food Reactions (Gastrointestinal), Adverse.
- Gastric Motility Disorders.
- Gastritis, Chronic.
- Gastroduodenal Ulceration/Erosion.
- Gastroenteritis, Eosinophilic.
- Hypertrophic Pyloric Gastropathy, Chronic.
- Ileus.
- Inflammatory Bowel Disease.
- Intussusception.
- Pancreatitis—Cats.
- Pancreatitis—Dogs.

ABBREVIATIONS

- ACTH = adrenocorticotropic hormone.
- CRTZ = chemoreceptor trigger zone.
- DKA = diabetic ketoacidosis.
- GI = gastrointestinal.
- IBD = inflammatory bowel disease.
- NSAID = nonsteroidal anti-inflammatory drug.
- SIBO = small intestinal bacterial overgrowth.

Suggested Reading

Guilford WG, Center SA, Williams DA, Meyer DJ. Chronic gastric diseases. In: Strombeck's Small Animal Gastroenterology, 3rd ed. Philadelphia, PA: Saunders, 1996, pp. 275–302.

Simpson K. Diseases of the stomach. In: Ettinger SJ, Feldman EC, eds., Textbook of Veterinary Internal Medicine, 8th ed. St. Louis, MO: Elsevier, 2017, pp. 1495–1516.

Author John M. Crandell

Consulting Editor Mark P. Rondeau

Client Education Handout available online

VON WILLEBRAND DISEASE

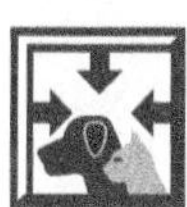

BASICS

DEFINITION

- Primary hemostatic defect caused by a quantitative or functional deficiency of von Willebrand factor (VWF).
- Clinical expression varies from a mild to severe bleeding diathesis.

PATHOPHYSIOLOGY

- VWF is an adhesive plasma protein required for platelet binding at sites of small vessel injury. In addition, plasma VWF is a carrier protein for coagulation factor VIII.
- A lack of VWF impairs platelet adhesion and aggregation, especially at vascular sites under high shear stress (e.g., arterial vessels). The largest molecular weight (MW) forms of VWF demonstrate highest reactivity in supporting platelet–collagen interactions.

SYSTEMS AFFECTED

- VWF deficiency may cause spontaneous hemorrhage, prolonged post-traumatic hemorrhage, and ultimately blood-loss anemia.
- Spontaneous hemorrhage—typically manifests as bleeding from mucosal surfaces.

GENETICS

- An autosomal trait; both males and females express and transmit the defect with equal frequency.
- Expression pattern of severe forms (types 2 and 3 von Willebrand disease [VWD]) is recessive; the milder form (type 1 VWD) appears to be recessive or incomplete dominant.

INCIDENCE/PREVALENCE

- The most common hereditary hemostatic defect in dogs.
- Rarely reported in cats.

GEOGRAPHIC DISTRIBUTION

None

SIGNALMENT

Breed Predilections

- Three type classifications are found in dogs; a single type predominates within each affected breed.
- Type 1 VWD (mild to moderate signs)—quantitative deficiency. Low VWF concentration (VWF:Ag)with proportionate decrease in VWF function. Type 1 is the most common classification:
  - Breeds—Airedale terrier, Akita, basset hound, Bernese mountain dog, dachshund, Doberman pinscher, German shepherd dog, golden retriever, greyhound, Irish wolfhound, Manchester terrier, miniature pinscher, Pembroke Welsh corgi, poodle, and sporadic cases in other purebred and mixed-breed dogs.
- Type 2 VWD (severe signs)—quantitative and functional protein defect; low VWF:Ag with profound lack of activity due to absence of high MW multimers:
  - Breeds—German wirehaired and shorthaired pointers.
- Type 3 VWD (severe signs)—complete lack of plasma VWF:
  - Breeds—Chesapeake Bay retriever, Dutch kooiker, Scottish terrier, Shetland sheepdog, and sporadic cases in dogs of other breeds.

Mean Age and Range

- Severe (types 2 and 3 VWD) typically manifests by 3–6 months of age.
- Milder forms typically demonstrate abnormal bleeding after surgery or trauma, or in association with another condition that impairs hemostasis.

SIGNS

Physical Examination Findings

- Hemorrhage from mucosal surfaces—epistaxis, gastrointestinal hemorrhage, hematuria, vaginal hemorrhage, gingival hemorrhage.
- Prolonged bleeding after surgery or trauma.
- Blood loss and/or iron-deficiency anemia, if prolonged hemorrhage.
- Petechiae rarely present.

CAUSES

Hereditary VWD is caused by mutations that impair VWF synthesis, release, or stability.

RISK FACTORS

Acquired disease conditions or drug therapy that impair platelet function may exacerbate clinical signs of VWD.

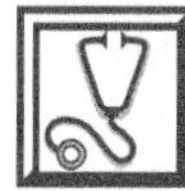

DIAGNOSIS

DIFFERENTIAL DIAGNOSIS

- Thrombocytopenia.
- Acquired coagulation factor deficiency (often associated with liver disease, vitamin K deficiency, or disseminated intravascular coagulation [DIC]).
- Acquired platelet function defects (often associated with drug therapy, uremia, hyperproteinemia).
- Hereditary coagulation factor deficiencies (see Coagulation Factor Deficiency).
- Hereditary platelet function defects (see Thrombocytopathies).

CBC/BIOCHEMISTRY/URINALYSIS

- Regenerative anemia develops after blood loss.
- Platelet count is normal unless the patient has experienced acute, massive bleeding.

OTHER LABORATORY TESTS

- Coagulation screening tests (activated clotting time, activated partial thromboplastin time, prothrombin time, thrombin clot time, fibrinogen concentration)—within reference intervals.
- Clinical diagnosis based on specific measurement of plasma VWF:Ag:
  - VWF:Ag <50% indicates VWF deficiency, but clinical signs of abnormal bleeding typically develop in animals with VWF:Ag < 25%.
  - Types 1 and 2 VWD are characterized by low VWF:Ag, whereas type 3 VWD is defined as a complete absence of detectable protein (VWF:Ag <0.1%).
- Types 1 and 2 VWD are differentiated with functional and/or structural VWF analyses:
  - Von Willebrand factor collagen binding assay (VWF:CBA) is a functional measure of VWF/collagen affinity. Dogs with type 2 VWD have a relative lack of VWF:collagen binding activity (CBA) compared to VWF:Ag, resulting in a protein concentration to function ratio >2:1. Dogs with type 1 VWD have proportionate protein concentration and function.
- VWF multimer structure is visualized on Western blots. Dogs with type 2 VWD lack the highest MW forms.

DIAGNOSTIC PROCEDURES

- Buccal mucosal bleeding time (BMBT) and the platelet function analyzer-100 are point-of-care screening tests whose endpoints are prolonged in patients with platelet aggregation defects or VWF deficiency. Prolongation is also found in patients with thrombocytopenia, anemia, or changes in blood viscosity.
- BMBT (expected values 2–4 minutes)—typical values for type 1 VWD = 5–10 minutes, types 2 and 3 VWD >12 minutes.
- PFA-100 closure times (expected ADP/collagen closure time <120 seconds): typical values for type 1 VWD = 150–300 seconds, types 2 and 3 VWD >300 seconds.

PATHOLOGIC FINDINGS

Hemorrhage is the only associated abnormality. Morbidity and mortality are caused by blood loss or hemorrhage into critical sites (i.e., CNS, respiratory tract).

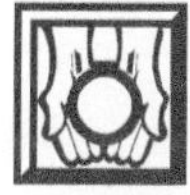

TREATMENT

- Transfusion of fresh whole blood, fresh plasma, fresh frozen plasma, and cryoprecipitate will supply VWF.
- Component therapy (fresh frozen plasma, 10–12 mL/kg, IV) or cryoprecipitate (1 unit per 10 kg body weight, IV) is best for surgical prophylaxis and non-anemic patients, to prevent red cell sensitization and volume overload.
- Patients with severe VWD may require repeated transfusions to control or prevent hemorrhage.

VON WILLEBRAND DISEASE (CONTINUED)

SURGICAL CONSIDERATIONS

- Preoperative transfusion should be given just before the procedure. Peak VWF is obtained immediately after transfusion, with values falling to baseline by 24 hours after a single dose.
- Cage rest and close monitoring (serial HCT and examination of surgical site) for 24 hours after surgery are ideal to confirm adequate hemostasis. Management of severe VWD typically requires at least one postoperative transfusion.

MEDICATIONS

DRUG(S) OF CHOICE

- Desmopressin acetate (DDAVP) is a vasopressin analogue that can be given preoperatively to dogs with mild to moderate type 1 VWD to enhance surgical hemostasis. Dosage is 1 µg/kg SC, given 30 minutes before surgery.
- Response is variable; transfusion should be available if DDAVP alone does not prevent bleeding.

CONTRAINDICATIONS

Avoid drugs with anticoagulant or antiplatelet effects: NSAIDs, sulfonamide antibiotics, heparin, wafarin, hetastarches, estrogen, cytotoxic drugs.

FOLLOW-UP

PATIENT MONITORING

Observe closely for hemorrhage associated with trauma or surgical procedures.

PREVENTION

- Screen dogs preoperatively to determine baseline VWF:Ag in breeds or lines with high prevalence of VWD. The risk of abnormal bleeding is greatest for dogs with VWF:Ag <25%.
- Clinically affected dogs should not be bred. Carriers of VWD can be identified based on low VWF:Ag (<50%). However, values for carrier and clear dogs may overlap at the low end of the reference interval (50–70% VWF:Ag). Commercial laboratories offer genetic tests to detect specific VWF mutations in several breed-variants of VWD. Dogs that are heterozygous for a specific mutation are considered VWD "carriers" and homozygotes are considered VWD "affected."
- Selective breeding practices can reduce or eliminate VWD from an affected pedigree. Breeding two clear parents is ideal because all offspring are expected to be clear. Breeding one clear and one carrier parent may be acceptable, with the clear pups produced from these matings used for subsequent breeding. Carrier-to-carrier matings are inadvisable because they are most likely to produce clinically affected offspring.

EXPECTED COURSE AND PROGNOSIS

- Most dogs with mild to moderate VWD have good quality of life and require minimal or no special treatment.
- Dogs with more severe forms require transfusion for surgery and should be transfused if supportive care fails to control a spontaneous bleed. Most of these dogs can be maintained comfortably in pet homes.

MISCELLANEOUS

ASSOCIATED CONDITIONS

- The development of any disease condition that impairs platelet function may exacerbate the bleeding tendency of VWD. Common conditions include thrombocytopenia, endocrinopathy (hypothyroidism, hypoadrenocorticism), hyperproteinemia, and uremia.
- Acquired VWD occurs in humans with aortic stenosis, and features of type 2 VWD have been reported in cavalier King Charles spaniels with mitral valve disease.

PREGNANCY/FERTILITY/BREEDING

See Prevention for breeding recommendations.

SYNONYMS

VWF protein was formerly referred to as factor VIII-related antigen.

ABBREVIATIONS

- BMBT = buccal mucosal bleeding time.
- DDAVP = deamino-8-D-arginine vasopressin.
- DIC = disseminated intravascular coagulation.
- HCT = hematocrit.
- MW = molecular weight.
- NSAID = nonsteroidal anti-inflammatory drug.
- PFA = platelet function assay.
- VWF = von Willebrand factor.
- VWF:Ag = von Willebrand factor antigen.
- VWF:CBA = von Willebrand factor collagen binding assay.

Suggested Reading

Boudreaux MK. Characteristics, diagnosis, and treatment of inherited platelet disorders in mammals. J Am Vet Med Assoc 2008, 233:1251–1259.

Venta PJ, Li J, Yuzbasiyan-Gurkan V, Brewer GJ, Schall W. Mutation causing vWD in Scottish terriers. J Vet Intern Med 2000, 14:10–19.

Wardrop KJ, Brooks MB. Plasma products. In: Yagi K, Holowaychuk MK, eds., Manual of Veterinary Transfusion Medicine. Hoboken, NJ: John Wiley & Sons, 2016, pp. 43–54.

Author Marjory B. Brooks
Consulting Editor Melinda S. Camus

Client Education Handout available online

V

Weight Loss and Cachexia

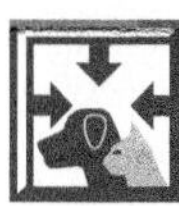

BASICS

DEFINITION

- Weight loss—loss of body weight (BW) resulting from reduction in fat mass and/or lean body mass.
- Lean body mass (LBM)—tissues other than adipose tissue (muscle, organs, bone); skeletal muscle is most dynamic component.
- Simple starvation—acute or chronic decrease in food intake below caloric requirements in an otherwise healthy animal; adaptive responses allow loss of fat mass over LBM.
- Cachexia—weight loss and tissue wasting secondary to underlying disease (e.g., cancer, heart failure, inflammatory conditions). Hallmark is loss of LBM; fat mass is variably affected.
- Sarcopenia—age-related muscle loss and decline in muscle quality. Can occur without loss of BW.

PATHOPHYSIOLOGY

Weight Loss and Simple Starvation

- Decreased caloric intake or increased energy expenditure results in negative energy balance.
- In otherwise healthy animals, compensation such as reduced metabolism and a shift toward lipid-based energy production reduce protein catabolism by up to two-thirds.

Cachexia

- Occurs secondary to acute or chronic disease (see Causes).
- Pathophysiology better evaluated in humans than dogs and cats:
  - Upregulation of inflammatory cytokines (e.g., interleukin-6 [IL-6], tumor necrosis factor-α [TNF-α]), catecholamines, neurohormones and cortisol.
  - Increases in oxidative stress; activation of catabolic pathways (e.g., ubiquitin-proteasome system).
  - Decreases in anabolic factors (e.g., growth hormone [GH], insulin-like growth factor I [IGF-1]).
- Results in dysregulation of appetite, insulin resistance, increased muscle catabolism, and impaired tissue synthesis.
- Increased basal metabolic rate and metabolic inefficiencies contribute to tissue wasting.
- Secondary anorexia aggravates malnutrition and muscle catabolism.

Sarcopenia

- Occurs during normal aging in the absence of disease; may occur alongside cachexia.
- Inflammation, oxidative stress, and catabolic pathway upregulation likely contribute to LBM loss similarly to cachexia.

SYSTEMS AFFECTED

- Musculoskeletal—progressive loss of LBM causes weakness, fatigue, and exercise intolerance.
- Hemic/lymphatic/immune—serous atrophy of fat can rarely cause bone marrow hypoplasia and pancytopenia.
- Underlying diseases leading to cachexia can affect all body systems.

GENETICS

N/A

INCIDENCE/PREVALENCE

Weight Loss

- Congestive heart failure (CHF)—42.5% of dogs; 34% of cats.
- Cancer—5.5–69% of dogs; 60% of cats.
- Chronic kidney disease (CKD)—28.9–55% of dogs; 36–81% of cats.

Cachexia

- CHF—48.3–54% of dogs; unknown in cats.
- Cancer—35% of dogs; 91% of cats.
- CKD—28.9% of dogs (weight loss/cachexia); 81% of cats.

GEOGRAPHIC DISTRIBUTION

N/A

SIGNALMENT

Species

Dog and cat.

Breed Predilections

N/A

Mean Age and Range

Risk of sarcopenia and cachexia increases with age.

Predominant Sex

None

SIGNS

General Comments

- Body Condition Score (BCS)—palpation/observation of fat deposits over ribs, lumbar spine, abdominal fat pad (cats), and tail base:
  - Scored 1 (severe fat loss) to 9 (obesity).
- Muscle Condition Score (MCS)—palpation/visualization of muscle of spine, skull, scapulae, and wings of the ilia:
  - Graded as none, mild, moderate, or severe muscle wasting.
- BCS and MCS *must* be evaluated separately, as loss of LBM can occur without loss of fat or change in BW.

Historical Findings

- Appetite may be normal, increased, decreased, or absent depending on cause.
- History should focus on identifying underlying disease (see Causes).

Physical Examination Findings

- Decreased BW compared to historical weights (corrected for hydration changes, fluid accumulation, etc.).
- Decreased absolute or relative BCS (fat loss) and/or MCS (LBM loss).
- Other physical examination findings may indicate underlying disease process (see Causes).

CAUSES

Physiologic Negative Energy Balance

- Simple starvation.
- Competition in a multi-pet household.
- Increased physical activity.
- Prolonged or extreme cold environment.
- Pregnancy or lactation.

Anorexia/Pseudoanorexia

- Inability to smell, prehend, or chew food.
- Dysphagia.
- Nausea.
- Regurgitation.
- Vomiting.
- Pain or anxiety.
- Iatrogenic (e.g., drug side effects).

Maldigestive/Malabsorptive

- Inflammatory bowel disease.
- Intestinal neoplasia (lymphoma, carcinoma, sarcoma).
- Lymphangiectasia.
- Age-related decreases in digestive function.
- Exocrine pancreatic insufficiency.

Infectious

- Severe intestinal parasitism.
- Infiltrative fungal disease (e.g., histoplasmosis).
- Protozoal (e.g., *Toxoplasma gondii*, *Neospora caninum*).
- Feline leukemia virus/feline immunodeficiency virus (cats).

Metabolic

- Organ failure (e.g., cardiac, hepatic, or renal failure).
- Hypo- or hyperadrenocorticism.
- Hyperthyroidism (cats).
- Cancer.
- Diabetes mellitus.

Excessive Nutrient Loss or Consumption

- Protein-losing enteropathy.
- Protein-losing nephropathy.
- Extensive skin lesions (e.g., burns).
- Chronic effusive disease (e.g., chylothorax).
- Increased catabolism (e.g., fever, infection, inflammation, cancer).

Neuromuscular

- Lower motor neuron disease.
- Myopathy/myositis.
- CNS disease—usually associated with anorexia or pseudoanorexia.

RISK FACTORS

- Age.
- See Causes.

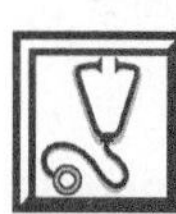

DIAGNOSIS

Evaluate BW, BCS, and MCS (compare to historical values).

DIFFERENTIAL DIAGNOSIS

- See Causes.
- Increased appetite may indicate physiologic, maldigestive/malabsorptive, or metabolic cause.

WEIGHT LOSS AND CACHEXIA (CONTINUED)

- Fever may indicate inflammatory or infectious cause.

CBC/BIOCHEMISTRY/URINALYSIS

- Laboratory tests may indicate underlying cause.
- Low hematocrit, low albumin, increased BUN, and increased BUN to creatinine ratio may be associated with malnutrition.

OTHER LABORATORY TESTS

- Determined by most likely differential diagnoses (see Causes).
- Serum T_4 in any cat >5 years old.
- Rule out infectious (parasitic, protozoal, viral, and fungal) causes:
  - Fungal antigen testing, FeLV/FIV, fecal centrifugal flotation, etc.
- Serum trypsin-like immunoreactivity (TLI), cobalamin and folate for maldigestive/absorptive disease.
- Fecal alpha-1 protease inhibitor level for protein-losing enteropathy.
- ACTH stimulation test for hypoadrenocorticism.
- Pre- and postprandial serum bile acids for hepatobiliary disease.
- Urine protein:creatinine ratio for protein-losing nephropathy.

IMAGING

- Thoracic/abdominal radiographs, abdominal ultrasound, CT, and/or echocardiography may help identify underlying cause.
- Ultrasound, CT, or dual energy x-ray absorptiometry (DEXA) might be used to approximate LBM.

DIAGNOSTIC PROCEDURES

Vary per suspected underlying cause.

PATHOLOGIC FINDINGS

Histopathology—cachexia may cause preferential atrophy of type II myofibers.

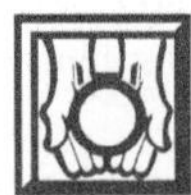

TREATMENT

Treat the underlying disease and provide appropriate nutritional support.

APPROPRIATE HEALTH CARE

- Depends on hemodynamic stability, voluntary food intake, and underlying disease type/severity.
- Anorexic patients refractory to supportive care should be hospitalized or managed as outpatients with a feeding tube.

NURSING CARE

- Nursing needs depend on underlying disease.
- Daily cleaning, regular flushing, and monitoring of feeding tubes to prevent infection/clogging.
- Debilitated patients with severe cachexia should have adequate padding and be rotated frequently to prevent decubital ulcers.

ACTIVITY

- Physical therapy, exercise, and rehabilitation may slow cachexia/sarcopenia progression:
  - Increase caloric intake appropriately.

DIET

- Resting energy requirements (RER) = 70 kcal × kg $BW^{0.75}$; may need to exceed RER in cachectic patients, if tolerated:
  - Maintenance energy requirement [MER] for neutered adult dog: 1.6 × RER, but may exceed 2.0–3.0 × RER in individual patients.
  - MER for neutered adult cat: 1.2 × RER, but may be higher in individual patients.
- Unless contraindicated, exceed Association of American Feed Control Officials (AAFCO) protein minimum in cachectic patients:
  - Dogs—4.5 g/100 kcal; cats—instead of: 6.5 g/100 kcal.
  - Most critical care, performance, and growth diets are high in protein and fat.
  - Kitten foods may be suitable for adult cats; cat foods may be suitable for dogs.
- Prolonged anorexia—deliver 25–33% of RER on day 1; gradually increase to 100% RER over 3–5 days, if tolerated:
  - Monitor serum potassium, phosphorus, and magnesium during refeeding; supplement if needed.

Oral Nutrition

- Preferred if patient is physically able to ingest, digest and absorb nutrients.
- To increase voluntary food intake, offer palatable food several times daily; offer the patient's usual food; offer moist food unless dry is preferred; offer food warmed to body temperature.
- Consider diets enriched with eicosapentaenoic acid (EPA) and docosahexaenoic acid (DHA) for cachectic patients or those with inflammatory conditions (e.g., therapeutic diets for arthritis or dermatologic conditions):
  - Most diets provide less than recommended EPA/DHA amounts (see below); additional supplementation may be beneficial.
- If underweight patients refuse therapeutic diets (e.g., renal diet), try alternate brand or texture, add broth or other palatability enhancer:
  - Adequate intake of a maintenance diet is typically preferable to inadequate intake of a therapeutic diet.
- Consider appetite stimulants (see Medications).
- Forced feeding is rarely effective and is not recommended due to high risk of aspiration.

Enteral Nutrition

- Preferred if patient is anorexic/pseudo-anorexic but can digest and absorb nutrients.
- Place feeding tubes as far proximal in the GI tract as tolerated.
- Nasoesophageal or nasogastric tubes (5–12Fr) can be used temporarily. Due to small tube size, only liquid diets can be used.
- Esophagostomy (12–18Fr) or gastrostomy tubes (16–24Fr) are semi-permanent:
  - Preferred over nasogastric tubes for outpatient management.
  - Allow higher caloric-density slurry diets, therapeutic diets, medication, and oral water administration.
- Liquid/slurry feedings q6–8h; initial feedings <10 mL/kg/feeding.
- Jejunostomy or gastro-jejunostomy tubes (5–8Fr) are more difficult to place and manage, and require liquid diets fed via chronic infusion:
  - Rarely indicated.

Parenteral Nutrition

- Only if enteral feeding is contraindicated.
- If required, recommend referral to an appropriate tertiary facility.

CLIENT EDUCATION

- Feeding tube management and expectations, if considering placement.
- See Expected Course and Prognosis.

SURGICAL CONSIDERATIONS

- If surgery is indicated, consider placing a feeding tube at that time.
- Severe cachexia or weight loss (especially if albumin is low) may prolong healing.

MEDICATIONS

DRUG(S) OF CHOICE

- Appropriate medications for underlying cause (if identified).
- Therapies targeting catabolic pathways are currently being investigated.

Appetite Stimulants

- Adjust selection and dosage based on underlying disease.
- Mirtazapine: 7.5 and 15 mg tablets; 2% transdermal suspension (cats):
  - Cats: 1.88 mg/cat PO q24–48h; 2 mg/cat transdermally q24–48h.
  - Dogs: 1–30 mg/dog PO q8–24h; recommend 1 mg/kg PO q8–12h.
- Capromorelin: 30 mg/mL oral suspension:
  - Dogs: 3 mg/kg PO q24h.
  - Extra-label dose not established in cats (6 mg/kg tolerated).
  - Also increases IGF-1 secretion.

Omega-3 Fatty Acids

- Fish oil, krill oil, omega-3 supplements:
  - Vary widely in EPA and DHA content; check each supplement individually.
- Dogs and cats—40 mg/kg/day EPA + 25 mg/kg/day DHA:
  - Avoid fish oil supplements with vitamins A and D if using at this dose.

CONTRAINDICATIONS

N/A

PRECAUTIONS

Treatments for underlying diseases may cause anorexia, nausea.

POSSIBLE INTERACTIONS

Mirtazapine can cause serotonin syndrome if combined with multiple other medications, including selective serotonin reuptake inhibitors (e.g., fluoxetine) and monamine oxidase inhibitors (e.g., selegeline).

ALTERNATIVE DRUG(S)

N/A

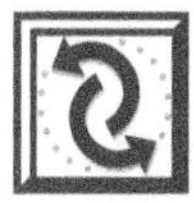

FOLLOW-UP

PATIENT MONITORING

- Appropriate monitoring for underlying disease (see Causes).
- *Precisely* monitor food intake and BW to ensure daily intake of RER/MER.
- Serial monitoring of BW, BCS, MCS *at every visit.*

PREVENTION/AVOIDANCE

- Early recognition of loss of BW and/or LBM and early intervention are key in preventing debilitation:
    - Perform thorough nutritional assessment at each visit and implement nutritional interventional plan when necessary.
    - Perform diagnostic workup to identify underlying cause of unintended weight loss.
- Aggressive management of diseases associated with cachexia.

POSSIBLE COMPLICATIONS

Tube feeding—infection, vomiting, regurgitation and/or diarrhea; tube displacement; aspiration; peritonitis (gastrostomy or jejunostomy tubes).

EXPECTED COURSE AND PROGNOSIS

- Provision of nutrition to cachectic patients without addressing the underlying cause is rarely successful in correcting the loss of body tissues.
- Weight loss, LBM loss, or poor body or muscle condition are associated with shorter survival in veterinary cardiac, CKD and cancer patients.

MISCELLANEOUS

ASSOCIATED CONDITIONS

N/A

AGE-RELATED FACTORS

Cachexia and sarcopenia are more common in geriatric patients.

ZOONOTIC POTENTIAL

N/A

PREGNANCY/FERTILITY/BREEDING

Lactation and pregnancy may cause weight loss due to increased calorie expenditure.

SYNONYMS

- Emaciation.
- Debilitation.

SEE ALSO

See Causes.

ABBREVIATIONS

- AAFCO = Association of American Feed Control Officials.
- ACTH = adrenocorticotropic hormone.
- BCS = body condition score.
- BW = body weight.
- CHF = congestive heart failure.
- CKD = chronic kidney disease.
- DEXA = dual energy x-ray absorptiometry.
- DHA = docosahexaenoic acid.
- EPA = eicosapentaenoic acid.
- GH = growth hormone.
- GI = gastrointestinal.
- IGF-1 = insulin-like growth factor I.
- IL-6 = interleukin-6.
- LBM = lean body mass.
- MER = maintenance energy requirement.
- MCS = muscle condition score.
- RER = resting energy requirements.
- TLI = trypsin-like immunoreactivity.
- TNF-α = tumor necrosis factor-α.

INTERNET RESOURCES

- To find a veterinary nutritionist qualified to assist in formulating homemade therapeutic or maintenance diets: http://www.ACVN.org
- To find a certified veterinary rehabilitation professional: https://rehabvets.org/directory.lasso
- Information on small animal nutrition guidelines, body condition scoring, and muscle condition scoring: https://www.wsava.org/Guidelines/Global-Nutrition-Guidelines

Suggested Reading

Eirmann L. Esophagostomy feeding tubes in dogs and cats. In: Chan, D.L. ed., Nutritional Management of Hospitalized Small Animals. Chichester: John Wiley & Sons, 2015, pp. 29–40.

Freeman LM. Cachexia and sarcopenia. In: Ettinger SJ, Feldman EC, Côté E, eds., Textbook of Veterinary Internal Medicine, 8th ed. St. Louis, MO: Elsevier, 2017, pp. 739–744.

Freeman LM. Cachexia and sarcopenia: emerging syndromes of importance in dogs and cats. J Vet Intern Med 2012, 26:3–17.

Johnson LN. Recognizing, describing, and managing reduced food intake in dogs and cats. J Am Vet Med Assoc 2017, 251:1260–1266.

Larsen JA. Enteral nutrition and tube feeding. In: Fascetti AJ, Delaney SJ, eds., Applied Veterinary Clinical Nutrition. Ames, IA: Wiley-Blackwell, 2012, pp. 329–352.

Authors Laura Rayhel and Valerie J. Parker

Consulting Editor Mark P. Rondeau

Acknowledgment The authors and editors acknowledge the prior contribution of Dorothy P. Laflamme.

Client Education Handout available online

WEST NILE VIRUS INFECTION

BASICS

OVERVIEW

- Acute to inapparent viral disease with neurologic manifestations caused by West Nile virus (WNV), a member of the family Flaviviridae, genus *Flavivirus*.
- Geographic distribution of virus is North, Central, South America, Africa, Asia, southern Europe, and Australia (Kunjin virus).
- Natural route of infection is through bite of numerous species of mosquitoes depending upon geographic location. Infection produces a low-level viremia, insufficient for dogs to be an amplifying host; antibody detectable by day 7 post infection.

SIGNALMENT

- Natural infections not limited by species or age.
- Seroprevalence varies widely with geographic region (3–96%).

SIGNS

- High percentage of dogs show no clinical signs—no experimentally infected dogs have shown clinical signs.
- Incubation period 2–4 days post infection.
- Febrile response 104–108°F (40.3–42.2°C) 3–6 days post infection.
- In the rare affected dog, common signs are ataxia, depression, anorexia, tremors, conscious proprioceptive deficits, seizures, weakness, flaccid paralysis; polyarthritis and myocarditis also reported.

CAUSES & RISK FACTORS

- Neurologic disease caused by WNV.
- Outdoor dogs much greater odds of being seropositive than indoor dogs; high seroprevalence in coyotes.
- Stray dogs at greater odds of being seropositive than owned dogs.
- Lineage 1 virus more neurovirulent (all North American isolates) than lineage 2 (Africa).
- Yearly fluctuation of infections linked to density of mosquito populations.

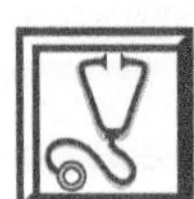

DIAGNOSIS

DIFFERENTIAL DIAGNOSIS

- On an individual basis, signs of WNV-induced neurologic disease are indistinguishable from signs associated with various "arbovirus" infections, e.g., eastern equine encephalitis (EEE), Venezuelan equine encephalitis (VEE), La Crosse.
- Other considerations—rabies, canine distemper, neosporosis, toxoplasmosis, pseudorabies, encephalomyocarditis virus, meningoencephalitis of unknown etiology (MUE).

CBC/BIOCHEMISTRY/URINALYSIS

- Generally normal.
- Serial sampling may show drop in leukocytes but may remain within normal.

DIAGNOSTIC PROCEDURES

- Minimal viremia makes detection of agent in acute phase unlikely; test of choice is reverse transcriptase PCR (RT-PCR) for WNV specifically or for arboviruses in general; urine may be PCR positive for a longer period post infection than whole blood.
- Acute and convalescent serum samples should be collected for IgM ELISA test and/or virus neutralization assays.
- For post-mortem testing—RT-PCR and/or immunohistochemistry.
- CSF—no significant findings (one report).

PATHOLOGIC FINDINGS

- Gross lesions not present in limited number of dogs necropsied (one had epicarditis).
- Histologic lesions in brain—mild, multifocal, nonsuppurative meningoencephalitis (lymphocytic to lymphohistiocytic perivascular infiltrates predominantly in gray matter).

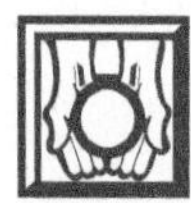

TREATMENT

Supportive therapy for neurologic abnormalities.

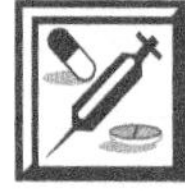

MEDICATIONS

- Antiviral drugs have not been tested for efficacy.
- Antipyretics may decrease fever.
- Anticonvulsant medications, as indicated.

FOLLOW-UP

PREVENTION/AVOIDANCE

Vaccines available for horses, have not been approved for dogs.

MISCELLANEOUS

ZOONOTIC POTENTIAL

- West Nile virus can infect numerous species including humans; however, the insect vector is generally necessary for transmission and the viremia is too low in infected dogs to serve as host for infecting feeding mosquitoes.
- Care should be taken if necropsy is done, as infectious viral particles may be present in tissue samples.

RISK TO OTHER ANIMALS

Virus is not transmitted from infected dog to other animals. Clinical case of WNV should be noted as indicative of infected mosquitoes in the area.

ABBREVIATIONS

- EEE = eastern equine encephalitis.
- MUE = meningoencephalitis of unknown etiology.
- RT-PCR = reverse transcriptase polymerase chain reaction.
- VEE = Venezuelan equine encephalitis.
- WNV = West Nile virus.

INTERNET RESOURCES

http://npic.orst.edu/pest/mosquito/wnv.html

Suggested Reading

Njaa BL. Emerging viral encephalitides in dogs and cats. Vet Clin Small Anim 2008, 38:863–878.

Author Edward J. Dubovi
Consulting Editor Amie Koenig

BASICS

OVERVIEW

- The whipworm, *Trichuris*, infects the cecum of dogs (*T. vulpis*) and cats (*T. campanula* and *T. serrata*); feline trichuriasis is extremely rare in continental United States.
- Life cycle is direct; infection is acquired by ingestion of larvated eggs; infective eggs can persist in environment for months to years.
- Infection can be asymptomatic or cause bloody diarrhea and large bowel inflammation.
- Clinical signs can occur before patency, i.e., before eggs are shed in feces; prepatent period is approximately 70–90 days.
- No extraintestinal migration occurs.

SIGNALMENT

- Dogs and cats.
- No age, breed, or sex predilections.

SIGNS

- Range from asymptomatic to severe.
- Intermittent large bowel diarrhea often containing mucus and fresh blood (hematochezia).
- Bloody diarrhea with dehydration, anemia, and weight loss in severe cases.
- Signs can occur before eggs detectable in feces.
- Acute to chronic debilitation.

CAUSES & RISK FACTORS

- Ingestion of infective (larvated) eggs from fecally contaminated environment.
- Eggs accumulate in environment and remain infective for months to years, especially in soil in moist, shady areas.
- Return of dog to an environment contaminated with infective eggs after anthelmintic treatment will result in reinfection.

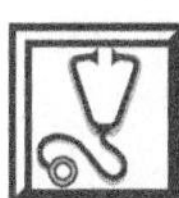

DIAGNOSIS

DIFFERENTIAL DIAGNOSIS

- Bacterial (spirochaetal) infections of cecum.
- Hookworm infection—identify eggs in feces; signs include anemia, pale mucous membranes, melena rather than hematochezia.
- Inflammatory bowel disease.
- Gastrointestinal ulcers.
- Dietary indiscretion.
- Capillarid infections (*Pearsonema, Eucoleus*)—eggs similar in appearance but smaller with roughened surface; infect urinary or respiratory tracts, respectively, rather than gastrointestinal tract; usually asymptomatic.
- Secondary pseudo-hypoadrenocorticism in severe trichuriasis with metabolic acidosis, hyponatremia, hyperkalemia, and dehydration; adrenocorticotropic hormone (ACTH) stimulation response is normal in cases of trichuriasis.

CBC/BIOCHEMISTRY/URINALYSIS

Usually normal; hyponatremia, hyperkalemia, and metabolic acidosis can occur in severe cases.

OTHER LABORATORY TESTS

ACTH stimulation test in severe cases with electrolyte disturbances to differentiate trichuriasis from hypoadrenocorticism.

IMAGING

N/A

DIAGNOSTIC PROCEDURES

- Centrifugal flotation of feces in sugar solution (specific gravity >1.2) preferred method.
- Differentiate *Trichuris* eggs (brown, ovoid or lemon-shaped with prominent bipolar plugs, smooth shell, single cell within egg, ~90 × 45 µm) from similar capillarid eggs (smaller, roughened shell surface).
- ELISA for whipworm antigen in feces—commercial test detects antigen produced by male and female adult and immature worms, can detect prepatent infection; combine with microscopy as above.

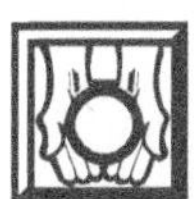

TREATMENT

- Outpatient treatment with anthelmintic for most cases.
- Severe cases with dehydration and electrolyte disturbances require inpatient fluid therapy in addition to anthelmintic.

MEDICATIONS

DRUG(S) OF CHOICE

- Fenbendazole—50 mg/kg PO q24h for 3 days; repeat monthly 3 times; extra-label in cats.
- Febantel/praziquantel/pyrantel pamoate—label dose PO in dogs.
- Milbemycin oxime—0.5 mg/kg PO q30 days in dogs.
- Moxidectin/imidacloprid—label dose in dogs.

FOLLOW-UP

PATIENT MONITORING

Repeat fecal examination for trichurid eggs and/or retreat with anthelmintic at 3 weeks and at 3 months following initial treatment or once a month for 3 months to detect and eliminate recently matured adults.

PREVENTION/AVOIDANCE

- Prompt removal and disposal of feces to prevent environmental contamination with infective eggs.
- Anthelmintic treatment of infected dogs to prevent shedding of eggs and contamination of environment.

EXPECTED COURSE AND PROGNOSIS

Good prognosis following treatment and implementation of preventive measures.

MISCELLANEOUS

ZOONOTIC POTENTIAL

Relatively rare cases of human infection with *T. vulpis* have been diagnosed based on morphologic differences between eggs of the human whipworm, *T. trichiura,* and those of *T. vulpis.*

ABBREVIATIONS

- ACTH = adrenocorticotropic hormone.

INTERNET RESOURCES

http://www.capcvet.org

Suggested Reading

Adolph C, Barnett S, Beall M, et al. Diagnostic strategies to reveal covert infections with intestinal helminths in dogs.Vet Parasitol 2017, 247(0):108–112.

Bowman DD. Georgis' Parasitology for Veterinarians, 9th ed. St. Louis, MO: Saunders, 2009, pp. 224–225.

Authors Matt Brewer and Katy A. Martin

Consulting Editor Amie Koenig

XYLITOL TOXICOSIS

BASICS

OVERVIEW

- Xylitol—a 5-carbon sugar alcohol used most commonly as a sweetener; present in many sugar-free gums, candies, toothpastes, mouthwashes, chewable over-the-counter medications and supplements, nasal sprays, liquid medications, specialty foods, and baked goods. It is also available as a granulated powder for cooking and baking.
- Ingestion by dogs can cause vomiting, weakness, ataxia, seizures, hypokalemia, and hypoglycemia due to excess insulin release.
- Mild to moderate elevations of alanine aminotransferase (ALT) can be seen within 4 hours of ingestion.
- Dosages >0.1 g/kg may cause hypoglycemia.
- Hepatic failure may occur at dosages >0.5 g/kg, with secondary coagulopathy possible due to hepatic necrosis.

SIGNALMENT

- Dogs—no breed, age, or sex predilection.
- Cats—toxicity not expected.

SIGNS

- Vomiting may develop within 15–30 minutes of exposure.
- Hypoglycemia may develop in as little as 2 hours after ingestion, with signs including progressive lethargy, weakness, ataxia, collapse, and seizures.
- Hepatic failure with signs of icterus as well as possible hemorrhage including petechiae, ecchymosis, and gastrointestinal and abdominal bleeding may be seen within 24–48 hours after ingestion.
- Hypoglycemia may not occur prior to onset of hepatic failure.

X

CAUSES & RISK FACTORS

Ingestion of xylitol or xylitol-containing products.

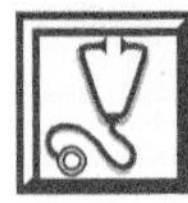

DIAGNOSIS

DIFFERENTIAL DIAGNOSIS

Hypoglycemia

- Insulin overdose.
- Sulfonylurea antihyperglycemic agents.
- Insulinoma (pancreatic β-cell tumor).

Acute Hepatic Failure

- Acetaminophen.
- Sago palm (*Cycad* spp.).
- Aflatoxin.
- Blue-green algae.
- Amanita and similar hepatotoxic mushrooms.
- Iron.
- Leptospirosis.

CBC/BIOCHEMISTRY/URINALYSIS

- Hypoglycemia.
- Hypokalemia.
- Elevated ALT initially.
- Bilirubinemia.
- Elevated aspartate aminotransferase (AST), alkaline phosphatase (ALP) less consistent.

OTHER LABORATORY TESTS

Prothrombin time/partial thromboplastin time (PT/PTT)—use if evidence of hepatic failure is present to monitor for development of secondary coagulopathy resulting in prolonged values.

DIAGNOSTIC PROCEDURES

N/A

PATHOLOGIC FINDINGS

- Severe acute periacinar and midzonal hepatic necrosis with periportal vacuolar degeneration.
- Petechiae and ecchymotic lesions suggestive of coagulation abnormalities.

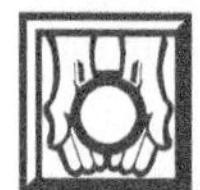

TREATMENT

- Decontamination—emesis up to 6 hours post ingestion is valid for gum exposures, if patient is asymptomatic; activated charcoal has poor binding to xylitol and not likely to be beneficial.
- Monitor blood glucose every 2–4 hours for hypoglycemia and every 6–8 hours for hypokalemia and correct as needed.
- Monitor liver enzymes every 12 hours for 48 hours with ingestions >0.5 g/kg.

MEDICATIONS

DRUG(S) OF CHOICE

- Dextrose—0.5–1 g/kg IV followed by a 2.5–5% CRI for hypoglycemia. Consider starting for ingestions >1 g/kg for hepatoprotection.
- Potassium chloride—supplement in fluids if potassium value <2.5 mmol/L.
- *N*-Acetylcysteine—if hepatic enzyme elevations occur; or ingestions >1 g/kg; 140 mg/kg PO or IV (extra-label) followed by 70 mg/kg every 6 hours for 7–17 doses, depending on the degree of hepatic enzyme changes.
- *S*-Adenosylmethionine (SAM-e)—PO daily for ingestions >0.5 g/kg. Administer for 2 weeks if no to mild liver enzyme elevations occur and continue for 4 weeks if significant elevations occur.

CONTRAINDICATIONS/POSSIBLE INTERACTIONS

None

FOLLOW-UP

- Monitor glucose levels for at least 8–10 hours.
- Monitor hepatic enzymes for 48 hours. If hepatic failure occurs, continue to monitor until values begin to decrease and again 4 weeks post ingestion.
- Prognosis good for uncomplicated hypoglycemia with mild to moderate elevations of ALT; guarded to poor if severe hepatic necrosis occurs and early intervention is not initiated.
- Patients who recover are not expected to have long-term negative effects.

MISCELLANEOUS

SEE ALSO

- Hepatic Failure, Acute.
- Hypoglycemia.
- Poisoning (Intoxication) Therapy.

ABBREVIATIONS

- ALP = alkaline phosphatase.
- ALT = alanine aminotransferase.
- AST = aspartate aminotransferase.
- PT = prothrombin time.
- PTT = partial thromboplastin time.
- SAM-e = *S*-adenosylmethionine.

INTERNET RESOURCES

https://www.petpoisonhelpline.com/uncategorized/xylitol-its-everywhere/

Suggested Reading

Jerzele A, Karancsi Z, Pászti-Gere E, et al. Effects of p.o. administered xylitol in cats. J Vet Pharmacol Ther 2018, 41(3):409–414.

Schmid RD, Hovda LR. Acute hepatic failure in a dog after xylitol ingestion. J Med Toxicol 2016, 12(2):201–205.

Author Renee D. Schmid

Consulting Editor Lynn R. Hovda

Acknowledgment The author and editors acknowledge the prior contribution of Eric K. Dunayer.

ZINC TOXICOSIS

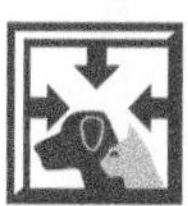

BASICS

OVERVIEW

• Toxicity results from the ingestion of zinc-containing material. • Many zinc compounds: zinc carbonate and zinc gluconate (dietary supplements), zinc chloride (deodorants), zinc pyrithione (shampoos), zinc acetate (throat lozenges), zinc oxide (sunblock, Desitin, calamine lotion), zinc sulfide (paints), metallic zinc (coins).
• Causes gastrointestinal (GI) inflammation and intravascular hemolytic anemia; may cause multiple organ failure (e.g., renal, hepatic, pancreatic, and cardiac), disseminated intravascular coagulation (DIC), and cardiopulmonary arrest.

SIGNALMENT

Most frequently reported in small-breed dogs less than 30 pounds (small pylorus retains zinc object or dose response); can occur in all species, all sizes.

SIGNS

• Onset of signs varies depending on the form of zinc, stomach acidity, and nutritional status of the patient. • Initial signs due to the irritant nature of the zinc chloride salts on the GI mucosa, causing vomiting, diarrhea, anorexia and lethargy. • Later signs associated with intravascular hemolysis and potential pancreatic, hepatic and renal damage; may include continued vomiting/diarrhea/anorexia, pale or icteric mucous membranes, dehydration, tachypnea, pigmenturia, abdominal discomfort, orange-tinged feces, melena.

CAUSES & RISK FACTORS

• Toxic doses not well defined; unreferenced median lethal oral dose of "zinc salts" is 100 mg/kg. • Toxicities result from ingestion of zinc-containing material: US pennies minted after 1982 (most common source), hardware (e.g., nuts, bolts), staples, galvanized metal (e.g., nails), boardgame pieces, zippers, toys, jewelry, holiday garland, bra clasps and hooks, animal identification tags, fixtures, buttons.
• Brass—alloy of copper and zinc. • Organic forms of zinc (e.g., zinc oxide) generally cause GI inflammation and self-limiting vomiting.
• Stomach acidity promotes rapid leaching of zinc from the ingested substance, allowing zinc to be absorbed.

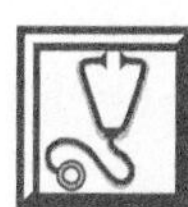

DIAGNOSIS

DIFFERENTIAL DIAGNOSIS

• GI upset—viral, bacterial, parasitic, immune-mediated, foreign body, liver or renal disease, pancreatitis. • Intravascular hemolysis—immune-mediated hemolytic anemia, *Babesia*, *Allium* spp. (onion, garlic, chive, leek, shallot), copper, mothball toxicosis (naphthalene), caval syndrome, acetaminophen, coral snake venom, pit viper venom, brown recluse spider venom, mushrooms, overhydration, skunk spray, propylene glycol.

CBC/BIOCHEMISTRY/URINALYSIS

• Hemolytic anemia, with possible Heinz body formation (30% of cases)—PCV drops rapidly. • Regeneration will occur if enough time. • Target cells. • Spherocytosis—mild and often inconsistent (20% of cases).
• Hemoconcentration due to dehydration (prior to hemolysis). • Leukocytosis with neutrophilia. • Hemoglobinemia.
• Bilirubinemia. • High AST, ALP; less common elevations in GGT and ALT.
• Elevated amylase and lipase. • Proteinuria, granular casts. • Pigmenturia. • Azotemia—(prerenal or renal).

OTHER LABORATORY TESTS

• Serum zinc levels often >5 ppm (normal dog/cat range: 0.70–2 ppm). Use non-zinc-contaminated blood tubes for collection.
• Coagulation panel: may indicate DIC.
• Frequent monitoring of PCV.

IMAGING

• Abdominal imaging: *may* reveal metallic object(s) in the GI tract. • Often the zinc object has passed by the time the patient is admitted.

DIAGNOSTIC PROCEDURES

ECG—may reveal arrhythmias and ST-segment abnormalities.

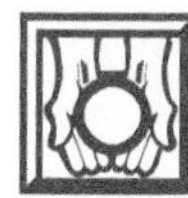

TREATMENT

• Rapid removal of the zinc object by endoscopy or laparotomy/gastrotomy.
• IV fluid therapy—maintain hydration and diuresis. • Severe intravascular hemolysis may require blood transfusion(s)/packed RBCs/ oxygen-carrying substances.

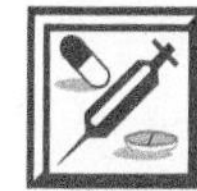

MEDICATIONS

DRUG(S) OF CHOICE

• Chelation therapy should *not* be warranted once the source of the zinc is removed. Zinc levels drop fairly rapidly (few to several days) via excretion into bile, pancreatic secretions, and urine. • CaEDTA 100 mg/kg diluted in 5% dextrose SC, divided into 4 doses per day (as for lead poisoning) if clinical improvement or reduced serum zinc is not accomplished by removal of zinc objects. Not commonly used and is potentially nephrotoxic. • Penicillamine 110 mg/kg/day PO q6–8h for 5–14 days (as for lead poisoning) if clinical improvement or reduced serum zinc is not accomplished by removal of zinc objects. Safer chelator to use. • Heparin 150 U/kg SC q6h, for DIC. • H_2-receptor antagonists (e.g., cimetidine, ranitidine, famotidine), proton pump inhibitors (e.g., omeprazole), sucralfate, and antacids used alone or in combination may help reduce irritation and stomach acidity and the rate of release and absorption of zinc.

CONTRAINDICATIONS/POSSIBLE INTERACTIONS

Avoid aminoglycoside antibiotics and other potential nephrotoxins due to added risk of developing acute renal failure.

FOLLOW-UP

PATIENT MONITORING

• ECG—monitor for evidence of arrhythmias, ST-segment alterations. • Coagulation profile, PCV, RBC, amylase, lipase, BUN, creatinine, ALP, AST, and ALT—monitor for the first 72 hours after removal of zinc source.
• Monitor serum zinc levels.

CLIENT EDUCATION

Educate clients on zinc hazards.

EXPECTED COURSE AND PROGNOSIS

• Multiple organ failure (e.g., kidney, liver), DIC, pancreatic disease, cardiopulmonary arrest are not common but potential outcomes. • Rapid removal of zinc source may provide progressive improvement over 48–72 hours; complete recovery possible.

MISCELLANEOUS

ABBREVIATIONS

• ALP = alkaline phosphatase. • ALT = alanine aminotransferase. • AST = aspartate aminotransferase. • DIC = disseminated intravascular coagulation. • GGT = gamma-glutamyltransferase. • GI = gastrointestinal.
• PCV = packed cell volume. • PT = prothrombin time. • PTT = partial thromboplastin time. • RBC = red blood cells.

Suggested Reading

Lee YR, Kang MH, Park HM. Treatment of zinc toxicosis in a dog with chelation using d-penicillamine. J Vet Emerg Crit Care 2016, 26(6):825–830.

Talcott PA. Zinc poisoning. In: Peterson ME, Talcott PA, eds., Small Animal Toxicology, 3rd ed. St. Louis, MO: Elsevier Saunders, 2013, pp. 847–851.

Author Patricia A. Talcott
Consulting Editor Lynn R. Hovda

APPENDICES

APPENDIX I

NORMAL REFERENCE RANGES FOR LABORATORY TESTS

Table I-A

Normal hematologic values

Test	*Units*	*Dogs*	*Cats*
WBC	$10 \times 3/mm^3$	6.0–17.0	5.5–19.5
RBC	$10 \times 6/mm^3$	5.5–8.5	6.0–10
Hemoglobin	g/dL	12.0–18.0	9.5–15
Hematocrit	%	37.0–55.0	29–45
Mean corpuscular volume	fL	60.0–77.0	41.0–54
Mean corpuscular hemoglobin	pg	19.5–26	13.3–17.5
Mean corpuscular hemoglobin concentration	%	32.0–36.0	31–36
Platelet count (automated)	$10 \times 3/mm^3$	200–500	150–600
Platelet count (manual)	$10 \times 3/mm^3$	164–510	230–680
Neutrophils	%	60–77	35–75
	Absolute	3,000–11,500	2,500–12,500
Bands	%	0–3	0–3
	Absolute	0–510	0–585
Lymphocytes	%	12–30	20–55
	Absolute	1,000–4,800	1,500–7,000
Monocytes	%	3–10	1–4
	Absolute	180–1,350	0–850
Eosinophils	%	2–10	2–12
	Absolute	1,000–1,250	0–1,500
Basophils	%	0–1	0–1
	Absolute	0–100	0–100
Reticulocyte count	%	0.5–1.5	0.0–1.0
Corrected	%	0.0–1.0	0.0–1.0
Absolute	$/mm^3$	0–80,000	0–50,000

Source: Adapted from Abbott Cell Dyne 3500; IDEXX Veterinary Services.
It is important to realize that normal values vary among individual laboratories.

Table I-B

Normal biochemical values

Test	*Units*	*Dogs*	*Cats*
Blood urea nitrogen (BUN)	mg/dL	7–27	15–34
Creatinine	mg/dL	0.4–1.8	0.8–2.3
Cholesterol	mg/dL	112–328	82–218
Glucose	mg/dL	60–125	70–150
Alkaline phosphatase (ALP)	IU/L	10–150	0–62
Alanine aminotransferase (ALT)	IU/L	5–60	28–76
Aspartate aminotransferase (AST)	IU/L	5–55	5–55
Total protein	g/dL	5.1–7.8	5.9–8.5
Albumin	g/dL	2.6–4.3	2.4–4.1
Globulin	g/dL	2.3–4.5	3.4–5.2
Albumin–globulin ratio		0.75–1.9	0.6–1.5
Sodium	mEq/L	141–156	147–156
Potassium	mEq/L	4.0–5.6	3.9–5.3
Sodium–potassium ratio		27–40	> 27.0
Chloride	mEq/L	105–115	111–125

(*Continued*)

NORMAL REFERENCE RANGES FOR LABORATORY TESTS (*CONTINUED*)

Table I-B

Normal biochemical values (*continued*)			
Test	*Units*	*Dogs*	*Cats*
Total CO_2	mEq/L	17–24	13–25
Anion gap	mEq/L	12–24	13–27
Calcium	mg/dL	7.5–11.3	7.5–10.8
Phosphorus	mg/dL	2.1–6.3	3.0–7.0
Total bilirubin	mg/dL	0–0.4	0.0–0.4
Direct bilirubin	mg/dL	0.0–0.1	0.0–0.1
Indirect bilirubin	mg/dL	0–0.3	0.0–0.3
Lactate dehydrogenase (LDH)	IU/L	50–380	46–350
Creatine kinase (CK or CPK)	IU/L	10–200	64–440
Gamma glutamyl transferase (GGT)	IU/L	0–10	1–7
Uric acid	mg/dL	0–2	0–1
Amylase	IU/L	500–1,500	500–1,500
Lipase	U/L	100–500	10–195
Magnesium	mEq/L	1.8–2.4	1.8–2.4
Triglycerides	mg/dL	20–150	20–90
Bile acids:			
Fasting	μmol/L	0.0–5.0	0.0–5.0
Post-prandial	μmol/L	< 25	< 15
Random	μmol/L	< 25	< 15
Total iron	μwg/dL	33–147	33–134
Unsaturated iron binding capacity	μwg/dL	127–340	105–205
Total iron binding capacity	μwg/dL	282–386	169–325

Source: Adapted from Hitachi Chemistry Analyzer model 747 IDEXX Veterinary Services.
It is important to realize that normal values vary among individual laboratories.

Table I-C

Conversion table for hematologic units				
	Example Values		*Conversion Factors*	
Analyte	*Traditional*	*SI**	*Traditional to SI*	*SI to Traditional*
Hemoglobin	15.0 g/dL	150 g/L	10	0.1
HCT or PCV	45%	0.45 L/L	0.01	100
Erythrocytes	6.0×10^6/mm^3	6.0×10^{12}/L	10^6	10^{-6}
MCV	75 μ^3	75 fL	No change	No change
MCH	25 μg	25 pg	No change	No change
MCHC	33 g/dL	330 g/L	10	0.1
WBC	15.0×10^3/mm^3	15.0×10^9/L	10^6	10^{-6}
Platelets	250×10^3/mm^3	250×10^9/L	10^6	10^{-6}

* Système International d'Unites.

Modified from Appendices. In: BonaguraJD, ed., Kirk's Current Veterinary Therapy XIII. Philadelphia: Saunders, 2000, p. 1209.

NORMAL REFERENCE RANGES FOR LABORATORY TESTS (*CONTINUED*)

Table I-D

Conversion table for clinical biochemical units

Analyte	*Traditional Unit (with Examples)*	*Conversion Factor*	*SI Unit (with Examples)*
Alanine aminotransferase	0–40 U/L	1.00	0–40 U/L
Albumin	2.8–4.0 g/dL	10.0	28–40 g/L
Alkaline phosphatase	30–150 U/L	1.00	30–150 U/L
Ammonia	10–80 μg/dL	0.5871	5.9–47.0 μmol/L
Amylase	200–800 U/L	1.00	200–800 U/L
Aspartate aminotransferase	0–40 U/L	1.00	0–40 U/L
Bile acids (total)	0.3–2.3 μg/mL	2.45	0.74–5.64 μmol/L
Bilirubin	0.1–0.2 mg/dL	17.10	2–4 μmol/L
Calcium	8.8–10.3 mg/dL	0.2495	2.20–2.58 mmol/L
Carbon dioxide	22–28 mEq/L	1.00	22–28 mmol/L
Chloride	95–100 mEq/L	1.00	95–100 mmol/L
Cholesterol	100–265 mg/dL	0.0258	2.58–5.85 mmol/L
Copper	70–140 μg/dL	0.1574	11.0–22.0 μmol/L
Cortisol	2–10 μg/dL	27.59	55–280 nmol/L
Creatine kinase	0–130 U/L	1.00	0–130 U/L
Creatinine	0.6–1.2 mg/dL	88.40	50–110 μmol/L
Fibrinogen	200–400 mg/dL	0.01	2.0–4.0 g/L
Folic acid	3.5–11.0 μg/L	2.265	7.93–24.92 nmol/L
Glucose	70–110 mg/dL	0.05551	3.9–6.1 mmol/L
Iron	80–180 μg/dL	0.1791	14–32 μmol/L
Lactate	5–20 mg/dL	0.1110	0.5–2.0 mmol/L
Lead	150 μg/dL	0.04826	7.2 μmol/L
Lipase, Sigma-Tietz (37°C)	≤ 1 ST U/dL	280	≤ 280 U/L
Lipase, Cherry-Crandall (30°C)	0–160 U/L	1.00	0–160 U/L
Lipids (total)	400–850 mg/dL	0.01	4.0–8.5 g/L
Magnesium	1.8–3.0 mg/dL	0.4114	0.80–1.20 mmol/L
Mercury	≥ 1.0 μg/dL	49.85	≤ 50 nmol/L
Osmolality	280–300 mOsm/kg	1.00	280–300 mmol/kg
Phosphorus	2.5–5.0 mg/dL	0.3229	0.80–1.6 mmol/L
Potassium	3.5–5.0 mEq/L	1.0	3.5–5.0 mmol/L
Protein (total)	5–8 g/dL	10.0	50–80 g/L
Sodium	135–147 mEq/L	1.00	135–147 mmol/L
Testosterone	4.0–8.0 mg/mL	3.467	14.0–28.0 nmol/L
Thyroxine	1–4 μg/dL	12.87	13–51 nmol/L
Triglyceride	10–500 mg/dL	0.0113	0.11–5.65 mmol/L
Urea nitrogen	10–20 mg/dL	0.3570	3.6–7.1 nmol/L
Uric acid	3.6–7.7 mg/dL	59.44	214–458 μmol/L
Urobilinogen	0–4.0 mg/dL	16.9	0.0–6.8 μmol/L
Vitamin A	90 μg/dL	0.03491	3.1 μmol/L
Vitamin B12	300–700 ng/L	0.738	221–516 pmol/L
Vitamin E	5.0–20.0 mg/L	2.32	11.6–46.4 μmol/L
D–xylose	30–40 mg/dL	0.06666	2.0–2.71 mmol/L
Zinc	75–120 μg/dL	0.1530	11.5–18.5 μmol/L

Source: Adapted from Appendices. In: Bonagura JD, ed., Kirk's Current Veterinary Therapy XIII. Philadelphia: Saunders, 2000, p. 1214.

APPENDIX II

ENDOCRINE TESTING

Table II-A

Endocrine function testing protocols

ADRENAL GLAND DISORDERS

ACTH STIMULATION TEST

Screening for Hyperadrenocorticism (in dogs; test not recommended for diagnosis of HAC in cats)

- Administer 5 μg/kg (up to 250 μg/dog) synthetic ACTH (cosyntropin; Cortrosyn, Organon Pharmaceuticals, West Orange, NJ), IV or IM. Serum samples should be obtained before and 1 hour after injection of ACTH for cortisol assay.
- Alternatively, but less ideal, 2.2 IU/kg ACTH gel may be given IM, and serum samples obtained before and 1 and 2 hours post injection.

Interpretation

An exaggerated response to ACTH is consistent with Cushing's disease. High normal cut-off values differ slightly between laboratories.

Screening for hypoadrenocorticism

- Administer 1 μg/kg (dogs) or 5 μg/kg (cats) cosyntropin, IV. Serum samples should be obtained before and 1 hour after injection of ACTH for cortisol assay.
- The use of ACTH gel for the diagnosis of Addison's is not recommended.

Interpretation

Pre- and post-cortisol determinations <2 μg/dL (55 nmol/L) are consistent with hypoadrenocorticism.

Monitoring mitotane and trilostane administration in dogs

- Administer 1 μg/kg (dogs) or 5 μg/kg (cats) cosyntropin, IV. Serum samples should be obtained before and 1 hour after injection of ACTH for cortisol assay.
- Test should be started 3–4 hours after administration of trilostane.

Interpretation

- Monitoring mitotane therapy for hyperadrenocorticism: Pre- and post-cortisol values are between 1 and 5 μg/dL.
- Monitoring trilostane therapy for hyperadrenocorticism: Post-ACTH cortisol values between 2 and 6 μg/dL are acceptable, but this range is controversial. Results must be interpreted in light of clinical signs.

LOW-DOSE DEXAMETHASONE SUPPRESSION TEST (LDDST)

Dogs

Administer 0.01 mg/kg dexamethasone IV. Obtain serum samples before and 4 and 8 hours after injection of dexamethasone for cortisol assay.

Cats

Administer 0.1 mg/kg dexamethasone IV. Obtain serum sample before and 4 and 8 hours after injection of dexamethasone for cortisol assay.

Interpretation

Three basic patterns:

- Lack of suppression: All cortisol values remain above 1.4 μg/dL (40 nmol/L). This pattern is consistent with Cushing's disease.
- Suppression: Cortisol values fall below 1.4 μg/dL (40 nmol/L) at 4 and 8 hours. This pattern suggests that the animal does not have Cushing's disease.
- Escape from suppression: Cortisol value falls below 1.4 μg/dL (40 nmol/L) at 4 hours and rises above 1.4 μg/dL at 8 hours. This pattern is consistent with pituitary-dependent Cushing's disease.

HIGH-DOSE DEXAMETHASONE SUPPRESSION TEST (HDDST)

Administer 0.1 mg/kg dexamethasone IV. Obtain serum samples before and 4 and 8 hours after injection of dexamethasone for cortisol assay.

Interpretation

Any cortisol determination that falls below 1.4 μg/dL (40 nmol/L) at any point during the 8-hour testing period is considered suppression. Suppression after a high dose of dexamethasone is consistent with pituitary-dependent Cushing's disease. Lack of suppression (all cortisol values remain above 1.4 μg/dL) is diagnostic of a pituitary or adrenal tumor.

THYROID GLAND DISORDERS

TSH STIMULATION TEST

Administer 0.5 U/kg TSH (maximum dose 5 U) IV. Obtain serum samples before and 6 hours after injection of TSH for T_4 determination.

Interpretation

Post-TSH T_4 levels <3 μg/dL (35 nmol/L) are consistent with hypothyroidism.

TRH STIMULATION TEST

Administer 0.1 mg/kg TRH IV. Obtain serum samples before and 4 hours after TRH injection for T_4 determination.

Interpretation

An increase in T_4 concentration <50% after TRH administration is consistent with hypothyroidism.

T_3 SUPPRESSION TEST

Obtain a blood sample for determination of T_4 and T_3. The serum is removed and kept refrigerated or frozen. Administer T_3 (Cytomel, SmithKline Beecham, Philadelphia, PA) PO at a dosage of 25 μg/cat q8h for 2 days. On the morning of the third day, administer 25 μg of T_3, and 2–4 hours later obtain a second blood sample for T_3 and T_4 determinations. The basal (day 1) and post-oral T_3 serum samples should be submitted to the laboratory together to avoid interassay variation.

Interpretation

Serum T_4 concentration after administration of T_3 >1.5 μg/dL (20 nmol/L) is consistent with hyperthyroidism.

SEX HORMONE DISORDERS

GNRH STIMULATION TEST

Administer 0.5–1.0 μg of GnRH/kg IM. Obtain blood samples before GnRH administration and 1 hour later. Assay blood samples for testosterone.

Interpretation

Normal dogs have baseline testosterone levels between 0.5 and 5 ng/mL, and after administration of GnRH the testosterone levels rise above 5 ng/mL. Animals with hypoandrogenism have lower values.

HCG STIMULATION TEST

Administer 44 IU of hCG/kg IM. Obtain blood samples before hCG administration and 4 hours later. Assay blood samples for testosterone.

Interpretation

Normal dogs have baseline testosterone levels between 0.5 and 5 ng/mL, and after administration of hCG, the testosterone levels rise above 5 ng/mL. Animals with hypoandrogenism have lower values.

DIABETES INSIPIDUS

MODIFIED WATER DEPRIVATION TEST

Note: This is not recommended due to morbidity and potential complications; ADH supplementation trial preferred.

Rule out other causes of polyuria and polydipsia (especially hyperadrenocorticism).

ENDOCRINE TESTING (*CONTINUED*)

Table II-A

Endocrine function testing protocols (*continued*)

Begin water restriction 3 days before abrupt water deprivation.

- Day 1: 130–165 mL/kg/day.
- Day 2: 100–125 mL/kg/day.
- Day 3: 65–70 mL/kg/day (normal maintenance requirement).

The morning of the fourth day, discontinue food and water. Start the test. Weigh the patient and empty the bladder. Weigh and measure PCV/TP, USG, BUN, and Na^+ at 1- to 2-hour intervals. *Monitor carefully for dehydration and depression and discontinue the test if the patient becomes dull, azotemic, or hypernatremic.* When 5% of body weight is lost (or azotemia, hypernatremia, or dullness develop), empty the bladder and check urine specific gravity.

Interpretation

If the urine specific gravity is >1.025 (dogs) or >1.030 (cats), stop the test. The patient does not have diabetes insipidus. If the urine specific gravity is not >1.025 (dogs) or >1.030 (cats), administer 0.55 U/kg aqueous vasopressin IM (maximum dose 5 U). Empty the bladder and check urine specific gravity at 30, 60, and 120 minutes post administration. If urine specific gravity increases <10%, nephrogenic diabetes insipidus is indicated; if it increases 10–50%, partial central diabetes insipidus is indicated; if it increases 50–800%, complete central diabetes insipidus is indicated.

DDAVP (desmopressin), 5 µg/dog SQ may be used in place of aqueous vasopressin, with specific gravity assessed at 2 and 4 hours.

Following the test, water should be offered in small amounts initially (to avoid vomiting), and slowly increased back to the dog's daily intake.

Table II-B

Tests of the endocrine system*

†	*Unit*	*Dogs*	*Cats*
Adrenocorticotropic hormone, basal (ACTH, plasma)	pmol/L	2–15	1–20
Aldosterone[†] (plasma)			
Basal	pmol/L	14–957	194–388
Post-ACTH	pmol/L	197–2103	277–721
Cortisol (serum or plasma, urine)			
Basal	nmol/L	25–125	15–150
Post-ACTH	nmol/L	200–550	130–450
Post–low-dose dexamethasone (0.01 or 0.015 mg/kg)	nmol/L	≤ 40	≤ 40
Post–high-dose dexamethasone (0.1 or 1.0 mg/kg)[‡]	nmol/L	≤ 40	≤ 40
Urinary cortisol-creatinine ratio	$\times 10^{-6}$	8–24,[†] 10[§]	—
Insulin, basal (serum)	pmol/L	35–200	35–200
Intact parathormone[†] (serum)	pmol/L	2–13	0–4
Progesterone (serum or plasma, female)	mmol/L	≤ 3.0 in anestrus, proestrus 50–220 in diestrus, pregnancy	≤ 3.0 in anestrus, proestrus 50–220 in diestrus, pregnancy
Testosterone (serum or plasma, male)	nmol/L	1–20	1–20
Thyroxine (T_4, serum)			
Basal	nmol/L	12–50	10–50
Post–thyroxine-stimulating hormone (TSH)	nmol/L	> 45	> 45
Triiodothyronine (T_3) suppression*	nmol/L	—	≤ 20
Triiodothyronine, basal (T_3, serum)	nmol/L	0.7–2.3	0.5–2.0

* Prepared with the assistance of ME Peterson, The Animal Medical Center, New York, NY. Unless indicated otherwise, values in this table are adapted from Kemppainen RJ, Zerbe CA. Common endocrine diagnostic tests: normal values and interpretations. In: Kirk RW, ed., Current Veterinary Therapy X. Philadelphia: Saunders, 1989, pp. 961–968. Hormone determinations are variable between laboratories. The laboratory performing the analysis should provide reference values. Before submitting samples for hormone determinations, consult the laboratory for sample specifications, use of anticoagulants, and sample preservation. General sampling conditions are discussed in Reimers TJ. Guidelines for collection, storage, and transport of samples for hormone assay. In: Kirk RW, ed., Current Veterinary Therapy X. Philadelphia: Saunders, 1989, pp. 968–973. Factors that affect serum thyroid and adrenocortical hormone concentrations in dogs are discussed in Reimers TJ, Lawler DF, Sutaria PM, et al. Effects of age, sex, and body size on serum concentrations of thyroid and adrenocortical hormones in dogs. Am J Vet Res 1990, 51:454.

† Provided by RF Nachreiner, Animal Health Diagnostic Laboratory, Endocrine Diagnostic Section, Michigan State University.

‡ This test is used after adrenocortical hyperfunction has been confirmed. It is used to differentiate adrenal tumor (where no suppression is seen) from pituitary-dependent cases (where suppression occurs but is variable).

§ From Stolp R, Rijnberk A, Meiher JC, Croughs RJM. Urinary corticoids in the diagnosis of canine hyperadrenocorticism. Res Vet Sci 1983, 34:141.
Rijnberk A, van Wees A, Mol JA. Assessment of two tests for the diagnosis of canine hyperadrenocorticism. Vet Record 1988, 122:178–180.

* From Peterson ME, Ferguson DC. Thyroid diseases. In: Ettinger SJ, ed., Textbook of Veterinary Internal Medicine: Diseases of the Dog and Cat, 3rded. Philadelphia: Saunders, 1989, pp. 1632–1675.

From Appendices. In: Bonagura JD, ed., Kirk's Current Veterinary Therapy XIII. Philadelphia: Saunders, 2000, p. 1223.

ENDOCRINE TESTING (*CONTINUED*)

Table II-C

Conversion table for hormone assay units

Unit			*Conversion Factors*	
Hormone	*Traditional*	*SI*	*Traditional to SI*	*SI to Traditional*
Aldosterone	ng/dL	pmol/L	27.7	0.036
Corticotropin (ACTH)	pg/mL	pmol/L	0.22	4.51
Cortisol	μg/dL	mmol/L	27.59	0.36
β-endorphin	pg/mL	pmol/L	0.289	3.43
Epinephrine	pg/mL	pmol/L	5.46	0.183
Estrogen (estradiol)	pg/mL	pmol/L	3.67	0.273
Gastrin	pg/mL	ng/L	1.00	1.00
Glucagon	pg/mL	ng/L	1.00	1.00
Growth hormone (GH)	ng/mL	μg/L	1.00	1.00
Insulin	μU/mL	pmol/L	7.18	0.139
α-melanocyte-stimulating hormone (α-MSH)	pg/mL	pmol/L	0.601	1.66
Norepinephrine	pg/mL	nmol/L	0.006	169
Pancreatic polypeptide (PP)	mg/dL	mmol/L	0.239	4.18
Progesterone	ng/mL	mmol/L	3.18	0.315
Prolactin	ng/mL	μg/L	1.00	1.00
Renin	ng/mL/hr	ng/L/sec	0.278	3.60
Somatostatin	pg/mL	pmol/L	0.611	1.64
Testosterone	ng/mL	nmol/L	3.47	0.288
Thyroxine (T_4)	μg/dL	nmol/L	12.87	0.078
Triiodothyronine (T_3)	ng/dL	nmol/L	0.0154	64.9
Vasoactive intestinal polypeptide (VIP)	pg/mL	pmol/L	0.301	3.33

Sources: Contributed by ME Peterson, The Animal Medical Center, New York, NY.
From Appendices. In: Bonagura JD, ed., Kirk's Current Veterinary Therapy XIII. Philadelphia: Saunders, 2000, p. 1223.

APPENDIX III

APPROXIMATE NORMAL RANGES FOR COMMON MEASUREMENTS IN DOGS AND CATS

	Dog	*Cat*
Heart rate (bpm)	60–180	140–220
Capillary refill time	1.5–2 sec	1.5–2 sec
Body temperature	99.5–102.5°F 37.5–39.2°C	100.5–102.5°F 38.1–39.2°C
Mean arterial pressure (mm Hg)	90–120	100–150
Blood volume (mL/kg)	75–90	47–66
Cardiac output		
(mL/kg/min)	100–200	167 ± 39
(L/M^2/min)	4.72 ± 1.09	
Systemic vascular resistance		
(mm Hg/mL/kg/min)	1600–2500 dynes.sec.cm^{-5}	
(dynes/sec/cm)	2162 ± 458	
Mean pulmonary arterial pressure (mm Hg)	14±3	
Central venous pressure (cm H_2O)	3±4	
Urine output	1–2 mL/kg/hr	1–2 mL/kg/hr
Breathing rate (breaths/min)	10–30	24–42
Minute ventilation (mL/kg/min)	170–350	200–350
Oxygen delivery		
(mL/kg/min)	29 ± 8	
(mL/M^2/min)	815 ± 234	
Oxygen consumption		
(mL/kg/min)	4–11	3–8
(mL/M^2/min)	198 ± 53	
Arterial Po_2 (mm Hg)	85–105	100–115
Arterial So_2	> 95	> 95
Arterial Pco_2 (mm Hg)	30–44	28–35
Arterial pH	7.36–7.46	7.34–7.43
Bicarbonate (mEq/L)	20–25	17–21
Base deficit (mEq/L)	0 to −4	−1 to −8
Total plasma proteins (g/dL)	6.0–8.0	6.8–8.3
Albumin (g/dL)	2.5–3.5	2.4–3.8
Packed cell volume (%)	37–55	29–48
Hemoglobin (g/dL)	12–18	9–15.1
Sodium (mEq/L)	145–154	146–157
Potassium (mEq/L)	3.9–4.9	3.6–4.9
Chloride (mEq/L)	105–116	113–121
Total CO_2 (mEq/L)	16–26	15–21

Source: Modified from Aldrich J, Haskins SC. Monitoring the critically ill patient. In: Current Veterinary Therapy XII. Philadelphia: Saunders, 1995, pp. 98–105.

APPENDIX IV

NORMAL VALUES FOR THE CANINE AND FELINE ELECTROCARDIOGRAM

Rate

Dog	60–140 beats/min for giant breeds 70–160 beats/min for adult dogs Up to 180 beats/min for toy breeds Up to 220 beats/min for puppies		
Cat	Range: 120–240 beats/min Mean: 197 beats/min		

Rhythm

Dog	Normal sinus rhythm Sinus arrhythmia Wandering sinoatrial pacemaker		
Cat	Normal sinus rhythm Sinus tachycardia (physiologic reaction to excitement)		

Measurements (lead II, 50 mm/sec, 1 cm = 1 mV)

Dog	P wave	Width: maximum, 0.04 second; 0.05 second in giant breeds Height: maximum, 0.4 mV
	PR interval	Width: 0.06–0.13 second
	QRS complex	Width: maximum, 0.05 second in small breeds maximum, 0.06 second in large breeds Height of R wave*: maximum, 3.0 mV in large breeds maximum, 2.5 mV in small breeds
	ST segment	No depression: not more than 0.2 mV No elevation: not more than 0.15 mV
	T wave	Can be positive, negative, or biphasic Not greater than one-fourth amplitude of R wave Amplitude range ± 0.05–1.0 mV in any lead
	Q-T interval	Width: 0.15–0.25 second at normal heart rate; varies with heart rate (faster rates have shorter Q-T intervals and vice versa)
Cat	P wave	Width: maximum, 0.04 second Height: maximum, 0.2 mV
	PR interval	Width: 0.05–0.09 second
	QRS complex	Width: maximum, 0.04 second Height of R wave: maximum, 0.9 mV
	ST segment	No depression or elevation
	T wave	Can be positive, negative, or biphasic—most often positive Maximum amplitude: 0.3 mV
	Q-T interval	Width: 0.12–0.18 second at normal heart rate (range 0.07–0.20 second); varies with heart rate (faster rates have shorter Q-T intervals and vice versa)

Mean Electrical Axis (frontal plane)

Dog	+40 to +100 degrees
Cat	0 to + 160 degrees (not valid in many cats)

Precordial Chest Leads (values of special importance)

Dog	CV_5RL (rV_2): T wave positive, R wave not greater than 3.0 mV CV_6LL (V_2): S wave not greater than 0.8 mV, R wave not greater than 3.0 mV* CV_6LU (V_4): S wave not greater than 0.7 mV, R wave not greater than 3.0 mV* V_{10}: negative QRS complex, T wave negative except in Chihuahuas
Cat	CV_6LL (V_2): R wave not greater than 1.0 mV CV_6LU (V_4): R wave not greater than 1.0 mV V10: T wave negative, R/Q not greater than 1.0 mV

*Not valid for thin, deep-chested dogs under 2 years of age.

Source: From Tilley LP. Essentials of Canine and Feline Electrocardiography, 3rd ed. Baltimore: Williams & Wilkins, 1992, Reprinted with permission of Wolters Kluwer.

APPENDIX V

ANTIDOTES AND USEFUL DRUGS: METHODS OF TREATMENT

Antidotes and Useful Drugs	*Toxicant/Indication for Use*	*Dosage*
Acepromazine	Amphetamine and other stimulant drugs with agitation and excitation; serotonin syndrome	Dogs and cats: 0.02–0.1 mg/kg IV, IM, SC. May cause hypotension.
Antivenin, crotalids	*Crotalus* and *Sistrurus* (rattlesnake); *Agkistrodon* (cottonmouth and copperhead) venom	Several products available. Follow the manufacturer's guidelines for dilution and administration. Dose varies from 1 to 5 vials IV depending on severity of symptoms. 95% of cases controlled with a single vial.
Antivenin, elapids	*Micrurus fulvius, Micrurus tenere, Micruroides euryxanthus* (coral snakes) venom	Extremely limited availability. The manufacturer's guidelines for dilution and administration should be followed closely.
Atipamezole	Medetomidine, dexmedetomidine reversal. Used off-label to reverse other alpha-2-adrenergic agonists, including amitraz, clonidine, and xylazine	Dogs: 50–100 μg/kg IM Cats: 25–50 μg/kg IM or IV (slow)
Atropine	Anticholinesterase pesticide muscarinic signs (OPs and carbamates); also cholinergic agents and clitocybe and inocybe (muscarinic) mushrooms	Dogs and cats: 0.2–2 mg/kg. One quarter of the dose should be given IV and the remainder IM or SC. The dose will likely need to be repeated; heart rate and secretions should be used to guide redosing.
Barbiturates	Strychnine and other seizure-producing drugs	Dogs: Phenobarbital at 5–8 mg/kg IV q4–6h. Cats: Phenobarbital at 3 mg/kg IV, repeat every 20 minutes to maximum of 24 mg/kg/24 hours.
Calcitonin salmon	Hypercalcemia; vitamin D and analogs	4–6 IU/kg, SC q8–12h. Rarely used.
Calcium gluconate or chloride	Fluoride and hydrofluoric acid; oxalic acid and oxalates; beta and calcium channel antagonists; others	Calcium gluconate 10% 0.54–1.61 mL/kg IV slowly; calcium chloride 10% 0.18–0.56 mL/kg IV slowly.
Calcium disodium EDTA (CaEDTA or calcium disodium versenate)	Heavy metals, primarily lead and zinc. Also chelates cadmium, chromium, copper, cobalt, iron, manganese, nickel, plutonium, thorium, uranium, yttrium, and vanadium	Dilute product in 5% dextrose to a final concentration of 2–4 mg/mL prior to use. Give 25 mg/kg IV or SC q6h. Maximum recommended daily dose of 2 g/day. Treat for 5 days; rest for 5–7 days; and repeat if needed. Do not use if metal still present in GIT.
Cyproheptadine	Drugs that cause serotonin syndrome (selective serotonin reuptake inhibitors, tricyclic antidepressants, 5-hydroxytryptophan)	Dogs: 1.1 mg/kg PO or rectally q4–8h PRN. Cats: 2–4 mg *total* dose PO or rectally q4–8h PRN.
D-penicillamine	Heavy metals, primarily lead; but also cadmium, copper, inorganic mercury, and zinc	Dogs (home therapy after $CaNa_2EDTA$ lead treatment): 110 mg/kg/day PO divided q6–8h for 1–2 weeks. Cats (home therapy after $CaNa_2EDTA$ lead treatment and in the presence of elevated blood levels): 125 mg *total* dose, PO q12h for 5 days. Do not use if metal still present in GI tract.
Dantrolene	Hops *(Humulus lupulus)* intoxication and black widow spider envenomation *(Latrodectus mactans)*	Dogs: Black widow spider: 1 mg/kg IV followed by 1 mg/kg PO q4h as needed. Hops: 2–3 mg/kg IV or 3.5 mg/kg PO.
Deferoxamine	Iron	Dogs and cats: 40 mg/kg IM q4–8h. In critical situations, an IV infusion of 15 mg/kg/hour can be used, but the cardiovascular system must be monitored closely during this time. The excreted complex turns the urine pink or salmon colored and is sometimes referred to as the "vin rose" of iron poisoning. Continue treatment until the urine is clear or serum iron levels are within normal limits.
Digoxin immune Fab fragments	Digoxin, *Rhinella* sp. *(Bufo)* toad toxins, and some cardiac glycoside-containing plants	If serum digoxin level is available: number of vials = serum digoxin level (ng/mL) × BW (kg)/100. If serum digoxin level is **not** available or if treating a *Rhinella (Bufo)* toad or cardiac glycoside-containing plant toxicosis, start therapy with 1–2 vials and reassess as needed.

(*Continued*)

ANTIDOTES AND USEFUL DRUGS: METHODS OF TREATMENT (*CONTINUED*)

Antidotes and Useful Drugs	*Toxicant/Indication for Use*	*Dosage*
Dimercaprol (BAL)	Heavy metals, primarily arsenic. Also used to chelated lead and mercury	Arsenic toxicosis: 5 mg/kg IM × one dose followed by 2.5 mg/kg IM q4h for 2 days, q8h for 1 day, and q12h until recovered. Lead toxicosis: 2.5–5 mg/kg IM as 10% solution q4h on days 1 and 2, then q6h on day 3.
Ethanol	Ethylene glycol	Preferred method: using 7% ethanol (70 mg/mL), load with 8.6 mL/kg (600 mg/kg) slow IV × 1 dose and follow with 1.43 mL/kg/hour (100 mg/kg/hour) IV CRI for 24–36 hours or until ethylene glycol (EG) test is negative.
Flumazenil	Benzodiazepine (clonazepam, diazepam, lorazepam, others); CNS depression or coma	Dogs and cats: 0.01 mg/kg IV. Short half-life and may need to repeat in 1–3 hours. Doses 10–20× labeled dose have been used in some animals but there is currently no scientific data to support them.
Fomepizole	Ethylene glycol	Dogs: 20 mg/kg IV over 15–20 minutes as loading dose; 15 mg/kg IV at 12 and 24 hours; 5 mg/kg IV at 36 hours. Repeat EG test. If positive, continue 5 mg/kg IV every 12 hours until negative. Cats: 125 mg/kg slow IV as a loading dose; 31.25 mg/kg IV at 12, 24, and 36 hours.
Glucagon	Insulin and oral hypoglycemic agent-induced hypoglycemia; beta and calcium channel blockers and tricyclic antidepressants bradycardia, AV block, and hypotension.	50 ng/kg IV bolus in 0.9% sodium chloride followed by 10–15 ng/kg/min CRI. May need to increase up to 40 ng/kg/min to maintain euglycemia.
Hydroxycobalamin (vitamin B12a; B12 precursor)	Cyanide	75–150 mg/kg IV
Intravenous lipid emulsion (ILE); also referred to as intravenous fat emulsion (IFE)	Some lipophilic (fat-soluble) drugs including baclofen, barbiturates, ivermectin and moxidectin, propranolol, tricyclic antidepressants, verapamil, and others.	Standard protocol: 1.5 mL/kg IV bolus of 20% solution over 5–15 minutes, followed immediately with CRI of 0.25 mL/kg/min over 1–2 hours. May repeat dose in several hours if signs of toxicity return and serum is not lipemic. Suggested protocol: 1.5–4 mL/kg IV bolus of 20% over 1 minute, followed by CRI of 0.25 mL/kg/min over 30–60 min. Individual boluses may be repeated as needed up to 7 mL/kg.
Leucovorin	Methotrexate; pyrimethamine trimethoprim, ormetoprim, others	Dogs and cats: Methotrexate: Varies depending on methotrexate serum concentrations (25–200 mg/m^2 IV, IM q6h for up to 8 doses). Pyrimethamine, trimethoprim: 0.1–0.3 mg/kg PO q24h.
Methocarbamol	Metaldehyde, permethrin, strychnine, tremorgenic mycotoxins, other toxicants that cause tremors	Dogs: 55–220 mg/kg slow IV. Labeled not to exceed 330 mg/kg/day but higher doses may be used in severe poisonings as long as the dog is monitored for CNS and respiratory depression. Cats: 44 mg/kg slow IV, up to 330 mg/kg/day. Labeled not to exceed 330 mg/kg/day but higher doses may be needed in severe poisonings. Monitor for CNS and respiratory depression when using high doses.
Methylene blue	Aniline dyes, local anesthetics, naphthalene, nitrates and nitrites-induced methemoglobinemia	Cats: Use with extreme caution or not at all. Dogs: 1–1.5 mg/kg as 1% solution IV over several minutes; may be repeated once in 30 min.

ANTIDOTES AND USEFUL DRUGS: METHODS OF TREATMENT (*CONTINUED*)

Antidotes and Useful Drugs	*Toxicant/Indication for Use*	*Dosage*
N-acetylcysteine (NAC)	Acetaminophen; less often *Amanita phalloides* mushroom, sago palm, and xylitol intoxication	Dogs and cats: 140 mg/kg IV or PO × 1 dose, then 70 mg/kg IV or PO q 6 hours for 7 doses. The product should be diluted to a 5% solution prior to use. IV administration preferred in cats due to low oral bioavailability (20%). A variety of other doses have been suggested; most based on extrapolation from human literature. Some recommend higher doses (280 mg/kg) and others additional doses (up to 17 doses) for massive ingestions. Emesis frequently occurs with oral dosing, especially after the initial dose, and an antiemetic may be required prior to starting NAC therapy.
Pamidronate	Cholecalciferol, calcipotriene, and calcitriol-induced hypercalcemia and hyperphosphatemia	Dogs and cats: 1.3–2 mg/kg diluted in 250–500 mL 0.9% NaCl, IV slowly over several hours. Monitor serum calcium levels q12–24h and adjust ancillary treatment as needed. If hypercalcemia is still present, a repeated dose of pamidronate may be necessary 5–7 days after the initial dose. Very large overdoses of cholecalciferol may require a second dose in 3–4 days.
Naloxone	Opioid and opiate-induced respiratory and CNS depression	Dogs and cat: 0.01–0.04 mg/kg, IV, IM, SC; may need to use 0.04 mg/kg with larger overdoses. IM and SC route result in slower onset of action (5 minutes). Short half-life and may need to repeat in 1–3 hours.
Phytonadione (vitamin K1)	Anticoagulant rodenticides, warfarin tablets	2–5 mg/kg PO q24h or divided twice a day.
Pralidoxime (2-PAM)	Organophosphates (nicotinic signs)	Dose (dogs and cats): 20 mg/kg IM or slow IV (over 30 min) for first dose. Repeat dose q8–12h, IM or SC. Rapid IV administration has resulted in tachycardia, neuromuscular blockade, laryngospasm, muscle rigidity, and death.
Protamine sulfate	Heparin	Dogs and cats: 1 mg protamine sulfate IV per 100 units heparin to be inactivated. Give slowly, no faster than 50 mg per over 10 minutes. Decrease amount of protamine sulfate by 50% for every 30–60 minutes that has passed since heparin overdose given.
Pyridostigmine	Anticholinergic plants *(Cestrum* spp., *Datura* spp., *Solanum* spp, etc.), atropine, avermectin and ivermectin, botulism, some elapid snake bites, and nondepolarizing neuromuscular blocking agents (curare, pancuronium, etc.)	0.01–0.03 mg/kg/hour CRI. Longer half-life than other similar drugs.
Pyridoxine	Isoniazid	71 mg/kg as 5–10% infusion over 30–60 minutes; if total amount of isoniazid consumed is known can give on a mg per mg (1:1) ratio.
Succimer (2-3 dimer-captosuccinic acid)	Lead	Dogs and cats: 10 mg/kg PO or rectal q8h × 10 days; retreat only if clinical signs are present. Monitor renal values closely in cats.
Trientine (TETA)	Copper hepatopathy in dogs	Dogs: 10–15 mg/kg PO 1–2 hours before meals. Useful in dogs unable tolerate vomiting associated with D-penicillamine.
Yohimbine	Xylazine and other alpha-2-adrenergic agonists (amitraz, clonidine, xylazine)	Dogs and cats: 0.11 mg/kg IV slowly. Shorter half-life than atipamezole.

Abbreviations: Standard

Comments:

Specific antidotes are not free of side effects and should be used with knowledge and forethought. Many toxicants lack a true antidote, and symptomatic and supportive care, including many of the useful drugs found in this table, is imperative for survival of the poisoned patient. Other drugs may be needed and the reader is directed to the references below for further information.

References

Hovda LR. Antidotes and Other Useful Drugs. In: Hovda LR, Brutlag AG, Peterson KL, Poppenga RH, eds., Blackwell's Five-Minute Clinical Companion: Small Animal Toxicology, 2nd ed. Ames, IA: Wiley-Blackwell, 2016.

Khan SA, Common reversal agents antidotes in small animal poisoning. Vet Clin North Am Small Anim Prac 2012, 42:403–406.

Wismer T. Antidotes. In: Poppenga RH, Gwaltney-Brant S, eds., Small Animal Toxicology Essentials. Chichester: Wiley-Blackwell, 2011, pp. 57–70.

APPENDIX VI

LYNN R. HOVDA

TOXIC HOME AND GARDEN HAZARDS FOR PETS

Table VI-A

Toxic plants and their clinical signs—antidotes and treatment

Plant and Characteristics	*Clinical Signs*	*Antidotes and/or Treatment*
Air plant, cathedral bells (*Kalanchoe* spp.) Bright red-orange to pink blooms; umbel flower pattern. Plant contains cardiotoxins similar to azalea and rhododendrons, concentrated mainly in flowers	Cardiac glycoside causes acute signs 1–3 hours after ingestion. Signs include depression, salivation, diarrhea, bradycardia, heart block, tachypnea, ataxia, tremors, and paralysis	Preventive emesis and/or activated charcoal early after ingestion. Treat as a cardiac glycoside (see Cardiac Glycoside Plant Toxicosis)
Aloe, octopus plant, candelabra plant (*Aloe* spp.) Succulent plant, used in folk and herbal medicine. Toxic fraction is anthraquinone glycoside; disrupts water and electrolyte balance in large intestine	Anorexia, depression, vomiting, colic, diarrhea, tremors (uncommon), and change in urine color. Generally mild in nature	Drugs for abdominal pain/diarrhea. Protect airway, treat locally for pharyngitis associated with oxalate crystals (rare)
Autumn crocus (*Colchicum autumnale*) Houseplant, garden plant. Typically blooms in fall, different from most other bulbs. Dosages above 6 g/kg BW considered lethal. Although the whole plant is toxic, the toxin (colchicine) is highest in bulbs.	Acute onset 2–12 hours post ingestion. Initial signs are nausea, salivation, vomiting, colic, diarrhea, incoordination, and weakness. Multiple organ systems (heart, lungs, and kidneys) also may be involved. Potential for coagulopathy and elevated serum enzymes	Induce emesis if not vomiting. Activated charcoal if early. Evaluate CBC and serum chemistries, including prothrombin, LDH, CK. IV fluids, analgesics, anticonvulsants as needed
Baneberry, doll's eye, cohosh (*Actea* spp.) Toxic principal is protoanemonin glycoside, as well as irritant essential oils	Clinical response ranges from dermatitis and blistering of skin to oral irritation, drooling, pawing at face or mouth, emesis, diarrhea, and hematuria. Neurologic and cardiovascular signs are occasionally reported	Cleanse mouth thoroughly with water; apply appropriate local demulcents; control emesis and diarrhea as necessary; monitor for organ dysfunction, especially renal damage
Belladonna lily (*Amaryllis* spp.) Potted plant, bulbs are most toxic, Contains both lycorine alkaloid (systemic effects) and insoluble oxalates (local pharyngitis)	Nausea, vomiting, diarrhea, hypotension, depression. Oxalate crystals can cause direct pharyngeal irritation	Gastric lavage, activated charcoal, fluids, and supportive treatment
Bittersweet (*Celastrus* spp.) Weed, vine with red berries. Immature fruits are toxic. Toxins are sesquiterpene alkaloids (celapanine, celastrine, paniculatine)	Gastric irritation, vomiting, diarrhea	Fluids, supportive care as needed
Bleeding heart (*Dicentra* spp.) Garden, woods, potted plant. Roots more toxic than leaves. Toxins are isoquinoline alkaloids (apomorphine, cularine, protoberberine)	Vomiting, diarrhea, muscle tremors, convulsions or paralysis	Fluids and seizure control
Castor bean (*Ricinus communis*) Garden shrub or ornamental grows to 2 m. Seeds are 1 cm, dark and light mottled, and highly toxic; chewing the seed greatly increases toxicity. Toxin is ricin	Severe, dangerous if seeds chewed before swallowing. Latent period 6–48 hours. Emesis, severe and hemorrhagic diarrhea, colic, muscle tremors, sudden collapse. Dehydration, hypotension, hemolysis and/or hemoglobinuria	Emesis for recent exposure: sorbitol if diarrhea not present; charcoal, fluids, and electrolytes. Monitor electrolytes, liver, kidney, adrenal function up to 6 days; H2 blockers for GI signs; diazepam for seizures; Antibiotics, lactulose, SAM-e for liver damage

TOXIC HOME AND GARDEN HAZARDS FOR PETS (*CONTINUED*)

Table VI–A

Toxic plants and their clinical signs—antidotes and treatment (*continued*)

Plant and Characteristics	*Clinical Signs*	*Antidotes and/or Treatment*
Chinaberry tree (*Melia azedarach*) Other common names are Persian lilac, white cedar, Texas umbrella tree. Ornamental tree in temperate to subtropical areas: southern coastal states, Mexican border. Berry is most toxic. Toxins are meliatoxins	Salivation, anorexia, vomiting, diarrhea. May be followed by weakness, ataxia, excitement or seizures. Fatalities have occurred, generally within 2 days post ingestion	Early emesis, GI lavage and charcoal are considered beneficial. Fluid and electrolyte replacement, anticonvulsants, and supportive care
Christmas rose (*Helleborus niger*) House and garden plant; entire plant is toxic, but fruits are most dangerous. Small amounts considered dangerous. Contains several toxins including ranunculin that is converted to protoanemonin when chewed, cardenolides, and bufadienolides	Hypersalivation, vomiting, anorexia, diarrhea followed by cardiac arrhythmias, heart block with premature beats, premature beats, slow irregular pulse. Potent cardenolide action is greatest risk	Gastric lavage or emesis; activated charcoal or saline cathartics to decontaminate the GI tract. Atropine may be helpful as for other cardenolide plants such as *Digitalis* spp.
Daphne (*Daphne mezereum*) Landscape shrub; evergreen or deciduous. Entire plant is toxic. Bitter or acid taste discourages consumption, may reduce toxic effects. Toxins are tricyclic daphnane and diterpenes	Vesication and edema of the lips and oral cavity associated with ingestion. Signs progress to salivation, thirst, abdominal pain, emesis, hemorrhagic diarrhea	Analgesics to control pain. General GI detoxification, medical treatment for vomiting and diarrhea. Fluid and electrolyte replacement as needed. Monitor body fluids and electrolytes
Delphinium/larkspur (*Delphinium* spp.) and pheasant's eye, yellow oxeye (*Adonis* spp.) Outdoor perennial, gardens, mountains; tall with blue, purple, or pinkish flowers. Seeds more toxic than leaves. Toxin is a diterpenoid alkaloid	Small animal poisoning unlikely unless by access to seeds. Early signs are vomiting, colic and diarrhea. May progress to trembling, ataxia, weakness, lateral recumbency	GI detoxification; demulcents and anti-diarrheal for GI signs; physostigmine to treat muscarinic signs
English holly (*Ilex* spp.) Landscape plant; glossy green leaves with marginal spicules. Fruit (drupe) white, yellow, black, red, orange. Occurs in forested areas of eastern N. America; elsewhere as an ornamental. Fruit is most likely portion consumed. Fruit and leaves contain potentially toxic saponins	Nausea, vomiting, diarrhea most common from consumption of berries. Some animals may be depressed. Clinical response most often mild/moderate and transient	Relief of digestive distress, activated charcoal may be helpful. Fluid and electrolyte replacement as needed
English ivy (*Hedera helix*), also known as Atlantic ivy, Irish ivy, common ivy Houseplant, or in mild climates used as a ground cover. Occurs as a woody, climbing or creeping vine. Commonly grown throughout North America. Toxins are triterpenoid saponins.	Salivation, thirst, emesis, gastroenteritis, diarrhea, dermatitis. Relatively few reported cases, most are moderate GI irritation. Often moderate or mild	Symptomatic relief of GI distress; supportive care for vomiting and diarrhea
Golden angel's trumpet (*Brugmansia* spp.) Non-native ornamental, similar to jimsonweed. Large pendulous flowers, similar to angel's trumpet. Toxin similar to jimsonweed (tropane alkaloid scopolamine) causes anticholinergic effects	Typical anticholinergic effects are restlessness, dilated pupils, tachycardia, dyspnea, dry mouth, GI atony, rarely seizures. Rarely lethal	Treat similar to *Datura* spp. (see Thorn apple below.)

(*Continued*)

TOXIC HOME AND GARDEN HAZARDS FOR PETS (*CONTINUED*)

Table VI–A

Toxic plants and their clinical signs—antidotes and treatment (*continued*)		
Plant and Characteristics	*Clinical Signs*	*Antidotes and/or Treatment*
Horse chestnut or Ohio buckeye (*Aesculus* spp.) Landscape or forest tree; palmate leaves. Native range is Midwest, east to Appalachian mountains, south into Texas. Planted as ornamental/landscape tree as well. Nuts and twigs most toxic; very early green foliage in spring. Horse chestnut highly toxic; Ohio buckeye very low toxicity. Contain several toxins including saponins, anthraquinones, and a coumarin glycoside	Gastroenteritis, diarrhea, dehydration, electrolyte imbalance. Neurologic signs possible, including incoordination, hypermetria, staggering. Usually transient, rarely fatal. Recovery usual within 24–48 hours	Fluid and electrolyte replacement, demulcents, and therapy for gastroenteritis. Confine animals during neurologic phase
Iris or blue or yellow flag (*Iris* spp.) Perennial garden flower, very commonly available. Rootstock (rhizome) most toxic; most risk at transplantation. Close to soil surface, may be dug up by dogs. Advise clients of potential risk. Rootstock contains purgative toxin known as irisin	Hypersalivation, vomiting, colic, diarrhea which may be hemorrhagic. Occasionally irritation of the lips and muzzle	GI decontamination early. Fluid and electrolyte therapy as needed
Irish potato (*Solanum tuberosum*) Vegetable garden plant. Vines, green skin, and sprouts are toxic. Toxins vary but are solanine and other glycoalkaloids	Vomiting, diarrhea, depression, rapid heart rate, mydriasis, muscle tremors. Signs may vary from atropine like to cholinesterase inhibition. Use antidotes accordingly and with caution	GI decontamination. If atropine-like signs predominate: use physostigmine. If salivation and diarrhea are present: use atropine cautiously
Jerusalem cherry, Winter cherry (*Solanum pseudocapsicum*) Common ornamental houseplant. Toxin is the glycoalkaloid solanine, similar to other plants of the nightshade (Solanaceae) family	Severe GI irritation characterized by drooling, vomiting, diarrhea, ulceration, depression, and sometimes seizures	GI decontamination if exposure is recent. If salivation and diarrhea are present and severe, use atropine cautiously. Provide fluid therapy based on condition of patient and results of laboratory tests
Lantana (*Lantana camara*) Occurs wild and in gardens in mild temperate to tropical areas. Naturalized in southeastern coastal states of the USA. Bright orange, yellow, red, purple, or pink flowers. Foliage and immature berries are most toxic. Toxins are pentacyclic triterpenoid lantadenes A, B, and C	Weakness, lethargy, vomiting, diarrhea, mydriasis, dyspnea. Continued ingestion can lead to chronic disease. Advanced signs: cholestasis, hyperbilirubinemia. Liver changes predispose to photosensitization	GI decontamination, activated charcoal for acute exposures. Provide fluids and respiratory support. Protect from sunlight and treat for hepatic insufficiency
Lily of the valley (*Convallaria majalis*) Ornamental garden plant. Prefers moist, shaded areas. Blossoms nodding/drooping on stem. Toxic principal (cardenolides) persists in dried plants; highest concentration in roots	Multi-organ failure. Tremors, thirst, vomiting, diarrhea, cardiac arrhythmia/bradycardia, weakness, shock. Monitor for cardiac arrhythmias, shock and hyperkalemia	Emesis or gastric lavage. Control dehydration, maintain electrolytes; control diarrhea; monitor ECG and serum potassium
Lupin, bluebonnet (*Lupinus* spp.) Common garden ornamental throughout USA; wild plants abundant in some regions, primarily western USA. Seeds more toxic than leaves, but plant, seeds, and pods are toxic. Toxin is lupine	Signs begin 1–24 hours post exposure. Salivation, ataxia, mydriasis, depression or seizures, disorientation, dyspnea. Liver and kidney damage may develop from continued ingestion. Lupines are teratogenic in ruminants. Risk in small animals is not well known	GI decontamination with activated charcoal for acute exposure. Anticonvulsants may be needed if neurologic signs are severe

TOXIC HOME AND GARDEN HAZARDS FOR PETS (*CONTINUED*)

Table VI–A

Toxic plants and their clinical signs—antidotes and treatment (*continued*)		
Plant and Characteristics	*Clinical Signs*	*Antidotes and/or Treatment*
Mexican breadfruit, Swiss cheese plant, hurricane plant (*Monstera deliciosa*) Stems and leaves contain insoluble calcium oxalate spicules (raphides)	Chewing on the plant releases oxalate spicules into mouth, tongue and lips. Response is immediate irritation, pain, salivation, and inflammation. Signs include pawing at face, drooling, and vomiting; potential interference with upper airway	Cleanse mouth thoroughly with water. Apply local and/or systemic anti-inflammatory agents based on clinical condition of patient
Mistletoe (*Phoradendron* spp.) Access to pets in homes at holiday time. Oval evergreen leaves with white berries. Leaves, stems, and berries are moderately toxic, contain toxic amines and proteins	Vomiting, GI pain, diarrhea; ataxia, hypotension, occasional seizures, cardiovascular failure. Principal risk may be from use during holiday season	Fluid and electrolyte replacement; demulcents for gastroenteritis
Monkshood (*Aconitum* spp.) Perennial garden ornamental. Entire plant is toxic, contains diterpene alkaloids that are primarily neurotoxic	Interferes with inactivation of Na+ channels in nerves. Salivation, vomiting, diarrhea. Muscle tremors, weakness, cardiac arrhythmia and/or heart failure; respiratory depression	GI decontamination, fluid and electrolyte replacement. Manage similar to digitalis glycoside overdose, with caution for potassium administration
Morning glory (*Ipomoea purpurea* and *Ipomoea tricolor*) Garden annual, potted plant. Seeds most toxic. Increased risk when seeds are pre-soaked, consumed by dogs. Indole alkaloid toxin similar to ergot alkaloids; abused as hallucinogen	Nausea, mydriasis, ataxia, muscle tremors, hallucinations, decreased reflexes, diarrhea, hypotension	Dark, quiet surroundings; tranquilization as needed. GI decontamination is not routinely recommended
Mountain laurel (*Kalmia* spp.) Native of eastern and southeastern woods, mountains. Both leaves and flowers are toxic. Honey from nectar also toxic. Toxins are diterpenoids, in particular grayanotoxins I and II	Oral irritation, salivation, projectile vomiting, diarrhea, weakness, impaired vision, bradycardia, hypotension, AV block	Activated charcoal, fluid replacement, and respiratory support as needed
Narcissus, daffodil, jonquil (*Narcissus* spp.) Garden ornamental bulb. Bulb is most toxic. Contains lycorine alkaloid	Nausea, vomiting, salivation, hypotension, diarrhea. Prolonged signs may cause dehydration	Gastric lavage, activated charcoal, fluid replacement, supportive treatment for gastroenteritis
Nettle (*Urtica* spp.) Garden or waste area weed. Hairs on leaves contain toxin that enters skin on contact. Most common in hunting or outdoor free-roaming dogs. Toxins are biogenic amines (acetylcholine, histamine, etc.)	Oral irritation and pain, hypersalivation, swelling and edema of nose and periocular areas or other areas of skin contact	Antihistamines and analgesics. Local or systemic anti-inflammatory supportive therapy to treat affected contact areas
Persian violet, sowbread (*Cyclamen persicum*) Popular florists' plant; widely available. Irritant saponins in all parts of the plant, especially tubers or roots	Chewing plant parts causes oral irritation with drooling, vomiting and diarrhea. Occasional hemoglobinuria may color urine red-brown. Large amounts may cause cardiac arrhythmias, seizures and rarely mortality	Control vomiting and diarrhea if severe; administer fluids as needed. Monitor urine for color and/or hemoglobin. Control seizures and cardiac arrhythmias as needed

(*Continued*)

TOXIC HOME AND GARDEN HAZARDS FOR PETS (*CONTINUED*)

Table VI–A

Toxic plants and their clinical signs—antidotes and treatment (*continued*)		
Plant and Characteristics	*Clinical Signs*	*Antidotes and/or Treatment*
***Philodendron* spp.** Very common indoor ornamental vine. Toxic principal is insoluble oxalate	Chewing on the plant releases oxalate spicules into mouth, tongue and lips. Response is immediate irritation, pain, salivation, and inflammation. Signs include pawing at face, drooling, and vomiting; also potential interference with upper airway	Cleanse mouth thoroughly with water. Apply local and/or systemic anti-inflammatory agents based on clinical condition of patient
Poinsettia (*Euphorbia pulcherrima*) Garden or potted plant, especially during Holiday season. Sap of stem and leaves mild irritant. Contains a variety of diterpenoid euphorbol esters	Irritation of mouth: may cause vomiting, diarrhea, and dermatitis. Usually transient and not life-threatening	Demulcents for local lesions; fluids to prevent dehydration
Rosary pea, precatory bean (*Abrus precatorius*) Native of Caribbean islands. Seeds (when broken or chewed) are highly toxic. Seeds used in ornamental jewelry in some countries. Illegal to import into USA. Toxin is abrin	Signs may be delayed up to 2 days after ingestion. Early signs are nausea, vomiting, diarrhea (often hemorrhagic) followed by weakness, tachycardia, possible renal failure, coma, death	Emesis or lavage followed by activated charcoal, demulcents, fluids, and electrolytes. Early and thorough detoxication is important for survival
Thorn apple, jimsonweed (*Datura stramonium*) Annual weed, some species are ornamental (*Datura metel*). Entire plant is toxic, but seeds are most toxic and available. Toxins are tropane alkaloids (hyoscyamine and scopolamine) with effects similar to atropine	Thirst, disturbances of vision, delirium, mydriasis, tachycardia, hyperthermia, GI atony/constipation. Commonly described as "Hot as a pistol, blind as a bat, red as a beet, mad as a hatter"	GI decontamination if early after ingestion. Parasympathomimetic drug (e.g., physostigmine)
Tulip (*Tulipa* spp.) and Hyacinth (*Hyacinthus* spp.) Poisoning usually occurs when dogs consume available bulbs or dig up freshly planted bulbs. Toxic principal includes allergenic lactones and similar alkaloids	Signs reflect direct irritation and include drooling, nausea, vomiting, diarrhea, dyspnea, tachycardia, and hyperpnea	GI decontamination if early after ingestion. Apply local and/or systemic anti-inflammatory agents based on clinical condition of patient. Monitor and control gastrointestinal effects; medicate as needed for tachycardia and dyspnea
Tobacco (*Nicotiana tabacum*) Garden plant, weed, cigarettes. Entire plant toxic. Nicotine alkaloid is toxic principal	Rapid onset of salivation, nausea, emesis, tremors, incoordination, ataxia, collapse and respiratory failure	Assist ventilation, provide vascular support. Gastric lavage with activated charcoal
Wisteria (*Wisteria* spp.) Woody vine or shrub with bluish purple to white legume flowers. Entire plant is toxic. Toxin is a glycoprotein lectin	Nausea, abdominal pain, prolonged vomiting; diarrhea. Signs may persist 2–3 days	Antiemetics and fluid replacement therapy
Yellow jessamine (*Gelsemium sempervirens*) Mild temperate to subtropical climates; mainly SE United States. Yellow trumpet-shaped flowers grow on evergreen vines. Neurotoxic alkaloids and sempervirine, an indole, are toxins	Weakness, ataxia, clonic/tonic seizures, paralysis, respiratory failure	GI decontamination early in course of toxicosis. Symptomatic and supportive therapy for respiration. Fluid replacement therapy as needed

Suggested Reading:

Barr AC. Household and garden plants. In: Peterson ME, Talcott PA, eds., Small Animal Toxicology, 3rd ed. St Louis, MO: Elsevier/Saunders, 2013, pp. 357–400.

Burrows GE, Tyrl RJ. Toxic Plants of North America. Ames, IA: Iowa State University Press, 2001.

Frohne D, Pfander HJ. Poisonous Plants, 2nd ed. Portland, OR: Timber Press, 2005.

Williams MC, Olsen JD. 1984. Horse chestnut: a multidisciplinary clinical review. Am J Vet Res 1984, 45(3):539–542.

TOXIC HOME AND GARDEN HAZARDS FOR PETS (*CONTINUED*)

Table VI-B

Herbal toxicities						
Class	*Toxic Principle*	*Genus Species*	*Common Names*	*Clinical Signs*	*Treatment Overview*	*Popular Usage*
Allergenic	Arabinogalactan	*Echinacea purpurea*	Purple coneflower	Vomiting, diarrhea	Symptomatic/supportive care.	Cold/flu support Immune stimulant
Alpha-2 adrenergic blocking agent	Yohimbine Corynanthine (rauhimbine) Raubasine (δ-yohimbine)	*Pausinystalia johimbe*	Yohimbine	Hyperactivity, agitation, tremors, seizures, vomiting, diarrhea, abdominal pain, tachycardia, hypertension followed by profound hypotension, hypoglycemia	Decontamination; monitor CNS and CV signs; control agitation, tremors, seizures; monitor blood glucose; IV fluids; dextrose PRN	Hypertension Angina "Herbal Viagra"
Ant coagulant	Hydroxycoumarin, bisabolol	*Matricaria recutita, Chamaemelum nobile*	Chamomile	Vomiting, diarrhea, lethargy, rarely epistaxis, hematoma (cats)	Monitor coagulation, symptomatic and supportive care, very rarely blood transfusion	Sedative Gastrointestinal ulcers
Cationic detergents	Quaternary ammonium compounds	*Citrus × paradisi*	Grapefruit seed extract (GSE)	Drooling, vomiting ± blood, weakness, anorexia, hyperthermia, oral/esophageal irritation or ulceration, dermal erythema, pain, ulceration	Dilution, carafate slurries, H2 blocker or PPI, fluids, nutritional support, broad-spectrum antibiotic, pain control	Disinfectant Antifungal
Essential oils	Melaleuca oil, pulegone, menthofuran Methyl salicylate d-Limonene Terpenic oils Benzyl alcohol, benzyl acetate, benzyl benzoate Menthol Alcohols and aldehydes	*Melaleuca alternifolia, Mentha pulegium*	Tea tree oil, Pennyroyal oil Liquid potpourri Oil of wintergreen Oil of sweet birch Citrus oil Pine oils Ylang ylang oil Peppermint oil Cinnamon oil	Orally: vomiting, diarrhea, CNS depression, hepatotoxicity, aspiration pneumonia. Dermally:transient paresis Clinical signs are dependent on the type of essential oil and route of exposure. May include GI signs, corrosive oral lesions, drooling, vomiting, ataxia, coma, respiratory distress, hypothermia or hyperthermia, hypotension, acute liver failure	Dermal: bathe in liquid dish soap. Oral: fluids, *N*-acetylcysteine, monitor liver enzymes. Pain control, thermoregulation PRN Dermal: bathe in mild liquid dish soap. Oral: Do not induce emesis or give activated charcoal. Irrigate the oral cavity. Fluids, anti-emetic, GI protectants, nutritional support, thoracic radiographs if indicated, monitor liver and kidney values in large exposures, broad-spectrum antibiotics and hepatoprotectants if indicated	Germicidal Fungal infections Antiseptic Flea control Insecticides Aromatherapies Room/air fresheners Personal care products Massage oils Antibacterials Flavorings Herbal remedies Cleaners—citrus oils
GABA Inhibitor	4-Methoxypyridoxine (MPN)	*Ginkgo biloba*	Gingko, maidenhair tree Dietary supplements pose less risk than fruit/seeds due to lower concentration	Anorexia, vomiting, diarrhea, agitation, clonic tonic seizures	Decontamination (emesis, activated charcoal), GI protectants, anticonvulsants Antidote: Pyridoxal phosphate/ pyridoxine (active form of vitamin B6)	Antitussive Expectorant Cognitive function (although no scientific proof)

(Continued)

Table VI-B

Herbal toxicities (*continued*)						
Class	*Toxic Principle*	*Genus Species*	*Common Names*	*Clinical Signs*	*Treatment Overview*	*Popular Usage*
Hypoglycemics	Alpha lipoic acid (ALA) Cinnamon Xylitol	 *Cinnamomum cassia*	Thioctic acid Cinnamon Xylitol	Hypersalivation, vomiting, hypoglycemia, increased hepatic and/or renal enzymes, death (ALA)	Decontaminate, IV fluids, monitor blood glucose, manage hypoglycemia, monitor liver enzymes, hepatoprotectants (NAC-Mucomyst, Denamarin)	Diabetic treatment Sugar substitute *Amanita* Mushroom poisoning (ALA)
MAO inhibitor	Hypericin	*Hypericum perforatum*	St. John's wort	Depression, vomiting, diarrhea, rarely tremors, seizures	Decontamination, symptomatic and supportive care, cyproheptadine for serotonin syndrome	Antidepressant Insomnia
Methylxanthines	Caffeine, theobromine	*Camellia sinensis, Paullinia cupana, Cola acuninata, Theobroma cacao*	Epigallocatechin gallate or ECGC (green tea), guarana, cocoa, cola, kola nut, chocolate	Agitation, hyperactivity, polyuria, polydipsia, cardiac arrhythmias, tremors, seizures	Decontamination, fluid diuresis, monitor CV and CNS, manage arrhythmias, tremors, seizures, symptomatic and supportive care	Weight loss, Herbal "NoDoz"
Polysulfated glycosamino-glycan (PSGAG)	PSGAG manganese	Glucosamine Chondroitin sulfate	Adequan®, Cosequin®, Dasuquin® Many other brands	Oral: vomiting, diarrhea, polydipsia, hepatopathy. IM: transient dose-dependent prolongation of PT, aPTT, reduced platelet aggregation, diathesis	Manage vomiting and diarrhea, baseline liver enzymes if large ingestion. Coagulopathies only expected with injectable overdoses or if significant liver enzyme elevations occur, monitor clotting parameters	Arthritis Chondroprotective
Salicylates	Methyl salicylate Salicin Salicylic acid	*Gaultheria procumbens*	Wintergreen extract Willow bark	GI upset, GI ulcers, hyperthermia, hepatoxicity, coagulopathies, coma	Decontamination, GI protectants, fluids, monitor for acidosis, monitor liver and kidney values, liver protectants, monitor clotting parameters	Anti-inflammatory Analgesic
Sedative	Valpotriates	*Valeriana officianalis*	Valerian	Lethargy, sedation	Generally home care, prevent injury	Sedative Sleep aid
Serotonin syndrome	5-Hydroxytryptophan (5-HTP) *Caution*: chewables may also contain xylitol	*Griffonia simplicifolia*	5-HTP Oxitriptan	Vomiting, diarrhea, tremors, seizures, ataxia, hyperesthesia, tachycardia, hyperthermia, mydriasis, transient blindness, depression	Decontamination, IV fluids, acepromazine or chlorpromazine for agitation, methocarbamol for tremors; phenobarbital or propofol for seizures. Avoid benzodiazepines. Cyproheptadine for serotonin syndrome. Monitor for DIC if significantly hyperthermic	Antidepressant Appetite suppressant Sleep aid
Sympathomimetics	Ephedrine Pseudoephedrine Synephrine	*Ephedra sinica*	Ma huang	Hyperthermia, hypertension, tachycardia, tremors, seizures, hallucinations, agitation, serotonin syndrome	Decontamination, monitor CV/CNS signs. Acepromazine for agitation. Cyproheptadine for serotonin syndrome. Beta blockers for tachycardia. Avoid benzodiazepines	Weight loss Body building Herbal "ecstasy" Decongestants

Table VI-B

Herbal toxicities (*continued*)						
Class	*Toxic Principle*	*Genus Species*	*Common Names*	*Clinical Signs*	*Treatment Overview*	*Popular Usage*
		Sida cordifolia	Indian common mallow			
		Citrus aurantium	Bitter orange			

Suggested Reading:

Essential Oils:

Bischoff K, Guale F. Australian tea tree (Melaleuca alternifolia) oil poisoning in three purebred cats. J Vet Diag Invest 1998, 10:208–210.

Cohen SL, Brutlag AG. Tea tree oil/melaleuca oil. In: Hovda LR, Brutlag AG, Poppenga RH, Peterson KL, eds., Blackwell's Five-Minute Veterinary Consult Clinical Companion: Small Animal Toxicology, 2nd ed. Ames, IA: Wiley-Blackwell, 2016.

Foss TS. Liquid potpourri and cats. Vet Tech 2002, 686–698.

Kore AM, Kiesche-Nesselrodt A. Toxicology of household cleaning products and disinfectants. Vet Clin North Am Small Anim Pract 1990, 20(2):525–537.

Lee JA, Budgin JB, Mauldin EA. Acute necrotizing dermatitis with septicemia following application of a d-limonene-based insecticidal shampoo in cat. J Am Vet Med Assoc 2002, 221(2):258–262.

Poppenga RH. Essential oils/liquid potpourri. In: Hovda LR, Brutlag AG, Poppenga RH, Peterson KL, eds., Blackwell's Five-Minute Veterinary Consult Clinical Companion: Small Animal Toxicology, 2nd ed. Ames, IA: Wiley-Blackwell, 2016, pp. 585–591.

Richardson JA. Potpourri hazards in cats. Vet Med 1999, 94(12):1010–1012.

Rousseaux CG, Smith RA, Nicholson S. Acute Pine-Sol toxicity in a domestic cat. Vet Human Toxicol 1986, 28:316–317.

Schildt JC, Beal MW, Jutkowitz LA. Potpourri oil toxicity in cats: 6 cases (2000–2007). J Vet Emerg Crit Care 2008, 18(5):511–516.

Tauer D. Phenols and pine oil. In: Hovda LR, Brutlag AG, Poppenga RH, Peterson KL, eds., Blackwell's Five-Minute Veterinary Consult Clinical Companion: Small Animal Toxicology, 2nd ed. Ames, IA: Wiley-Blackwell, 2016, pp. 646-454.

Villar D, Knight MJ, Hansen SR, and Buck WB. Toxicity of melaleuca oil and related essential oils applied topically on dogs and cats. Vet Hum Tox 1994, 36:139–142.

Alpha lipoic acid (ALA):

Hill AS, Werner JA, Rogers QR, et al. Lipoic acid is 10 times more toxic in cats than reported in humans, dogs, or rats. J Anim Physiol Anim Nutr 2004, 88(3–4):150–156.

Loftin EG, Lee VH. Therapy and outcome of suspected alpha lipoic acid toxicity in two dogs. J Vet Emerg Crit Care 2009,19(5):501–506.

Zicker SC, Avila A, Joshi DK, et al. Pharmacokinetics of orally administered DL-alpha-lipoic acid in dogs. Am J Vet Res 2010, 71(11):1377–1383.

Zicker SC, Hagen TM Joisher N, et al. Safety of long-term feeding of dl-alpha-lipoic acid and its effect on reduced glutathione:oxidized glutathione ratios in beagles. Vet Ther 2002, 3(2):167–176.

5-Hydroxytryptophan (5-HTP):

Gwaltney-Brant SM, Albertsen JC, Khan SA. 5-Hydroxytryptophan toxicosis in dogs: 21 cases (1989-1999). J Am Vet Med Assoc 2000, 216:1937–1940.

Polysulfated glycosaminoglycan joint supplements (glucosamine, chondroitin):

Borchers A, Epstein SE, Gindiciosi B, et al. Acute enteral manganese intoxication with hepatic failure due to ingestion of a joint supplement overdose. J Vet Diag Invest 2014, 26(5):658–663.

Breese McCoy SJ, Bryson JC. High dose glucosamine associated with polyuria and polydipsia in a dog. J Am Vet Med Assoc 2003, 222:431–432.

Brim TA, Center V, Wynn SG, et al. More on accidental overdose of joint supplements. J Am Vet Med Assoc 2010, 236(5):509–510.

Khan SA., McLean MK, Gwaltney-Brant S. Accidental overdosage of joint supplements in dogs. J Am Vet Med Assoc 2010, 236(10):1061–1062.

Khan KN, Andress JM, Smith PF. Toxicity of subacute IV manganese chloride administration in beagle dogs. Toxicol Pathol 1997, 25:344–350.

Nobles IJ, Khan S. Multiorgan dysfunction syndrome secondary to joint supplement overdosage in a dog. Can Vet J 2015, 56:361–364.

Sympathomimetics:

Means C. Ma huang: all natural but not always innocuous. Vet Med 1999, 94:511–512.

Means C. Ephedra/ma huang. In: Osweiler, Hovda, Brutlag, Lee, eds. Five-Minute Veterinary Consult Clinical Companion. Ames, IA: Wiley-Blackwell, 2011, pp. 521–526.

Ooms TG, Khan SA, Means C. Suspected caffeine and ephedrine toxicosis resulting from ingestion of an herbal supplement containing guarana and ma huang in dogs: 47 cases (1997–1999). J Am Vet Med Assoc 2001, 218:225–229.

Herbals (general):

Poppenga RH, Gwaltney-Brant S, eds. Dietary supplements and herbs. In: Small Animal Toxicology Essentials. Chichester, UK: Wiley Blackwell, 2013, pp. 161–169.

Wynn SG, Fougere BJ. Veterinary Herbal Medicine. St. Louis, MO: Mosby, 2007, pp. 513–514.

TOXIC HOME AND GARDEN HAZARDS FOR PETS (*CONTINUED*)

Table VI-C

Household cleaners, disinfectants, and solvents—products, clinical signs, and treatment		
Products	*Toxicity and Clinical Signs*	*Treatment*
SOAPS, DETERGENTS, AND CLEANING AGENTS		
Soaps (fatty acid salts)—includes commercial bar soaps, some liquid hand soaps, laundry bar soaps, homemade soaps, some baby and infant products	Low order toxicity	Generally dilution with water and observation is all that is required. Can typically be managed by pet owner. Fluids and electrolytes should be used to replace fluid loss from excessive vomiting and diarrhea. If vomiting has not yet occurred, emesis should be induced in noncorrosive bar soap ingestions >20 g soap/kg BW. Eyes should be irrigated with tepid water or isotonic saline for 10–15 minutes and observed for signs of irritation. Any exposed skin and hair coat should be rinsed with tepid water for 15 minutes.
Anionic detergents (sulfonated or phosphorylated straight-chain hydrocarbons)—includes most laundry detergents, some automatic dishwashing detergents, and some shampoos. Common detergents include alkyl sodium sulfate, alkyl sodium sulfonate, dioctyl sodium sulfosuccinate, linear alkyl benzene sulfonate, sodium lauryl sulfate, others. Hard water "boosters" or "builders" such as sodium carbonate, sodium phosphate, and sodium silicate are often added	Generally slight to moderate toxicity with high alkaline (pH >12) and potentially corrosive automatic dishwashing detergents, including pods or complete packs, the exception. Irritation to the GI tract with discomfort, vomiting, and diarrhea the most common signs. Absorption occurs through the GI tract and irritated skin; IV hemolysis has been reported. Repeated dermal exposure may result in irritation. Ocular exposure may cause conjunctivitis and irritation; ocular exposure to automatic dishwashing detergents may result in corneal erosion and opacity. Laundry pods or complete packs have caused more serious problems than expected based on the ingredients. The reason is unknown but may be related to increased amounts ingested due to a concentrated product package	Depends on specific product and amount ingested. With most products, dilution with water and replacement of fluid and electrolyte losses secondary to vomiting and diarrhea are all that are required. GI protection as needed. Serum should be monitored for hemolysis. Skin and hair coat should be rinsed well with tepid water for 15 minutes to prevent exposure, especially those animals that are known to self-groom. Eyes should be irrigated well for 10–15 minutes with tepid water or isotonic saline and monitored closely for irritation. Animals exposed in any manner to automatic dishwashing detergents or laundry pods should be examined and monitored for corrosive type injuries and aspiration pneumonia
Cationic detergents (quaternary ammonium compounds with aryl or alkyl substituent groups, often a very long hydrophobic carbon chain with a halogen such as chloride or iodide is attached)—includes fabric softeners, sanitizers, germicides. Compounds such as benzethonium chloride, benzalkonium chloride, and cetyl pyridinium chloride are used as cationic detergents. Liquid potpourris, covered elsewhere, are also in this group	Highly toxic compounds. Effects are concentration dependent with 1% concentrations causing irritation and damage to mucous membranes and 7.5% concentrations resulting in corrosive burns to the mouth, tongue, pharynx, and esophagus. Cats can develop lesions at 2% concentration. GI signs at high concentration include profuse salivation, and vomiting ± blood. Other signs include shock at any stage of exposure, muscle weakness, fever, CNS and respiratory depression, seizures, collapse and coma Dermal effects are concentration dependent. Hair loss and skin ulceration are frequently seen in cats and inflammatory lesions on the paws in dogs. Ocular signs after exposure are concentration dependent and range from irritation and discomfort to corneal damage and ulceration	Depends on the concentration of the product and route of exposure. Animals ingesting product should be given frequent drinks of water if stable. Vomiting should not be induced, especially when the concentration is greater than 7.5%. Activated charcoal is not typically indicated. The mouth and oropharynx should be examined for lesions and those animals with continued profuse salivation, stridor, or dysphagia should undergo endoscopic examination for analysis of mucosal damage. Supportive care includes IV fluids as needed, attention to respiratory effort, adequate caloric intake, seizure medication as needed, and close monitoring for shock. GI protection indicated with all exposures. Ancillary therapies may include pain control and repeated wound lavage. Exposed skin and hair coat should be washed with tepid water and mild soap for at least 15 minutes and monitored for irritation and ulceration. The eyes should be thoroughly evaluated and irrigated with isotonic saline for 20 minutes followed by a slit lamp examination. Further treatment depends on the examination results

TOXIC HOME AND GARDEN HAZARDS FOR PETS (*CONTINUED*)

Table VI–C

Household cleaners, disinfectants, and solvents—products, clinical signs, and treatment (*continued*)		
Products	*Toxicity and Clinical Signs*	*Treatment*
Nonionic detergents (uncharged aqueous solutions)—includes hand dishwashing detergents, shampoos, few laundry detergents. Alkyl ethoxylate, alkylphenoxy polyethoxy ethanol (alcohol ethoxylates), and polyethylene glycol stearate are examples	Primarily of low toxicity after ingestion. Ocular exposure may result in irritation	Dilution with water and observation normally all that is required. Can typically be managed by pet owner. IV fluids and electrolytes may be used to replace fluid losses from excessive vomiting and diarrhea. GI protection may be needed. Eyes should be irrigated with tepid water or isotonic saline for 10–15 minutes and observed for signs of continued irritation. Any exposed skin and hair coat should be rinsed well with tepid water to prevent reexposure
CORROSIVES		
Acids (pH <7; strong acids pH <2.5–3)—includes rust removers, drain and toilet bowl cleaners, car battery acid, gun barrel cleaning fluids, other metal cleaners, hair wave neutralizers, some swimming pool cleaning agents. Hydrochloric acid (muriatic acid), sulfuric acid, nitric acid, oxalic acid, phosphoric acid, and sodium bisulfite (sodium acid sulfate) are all acid corrosives. Hydrofluoric acid, a rust remover product, carries a special warning	Signs are concentration and time dependent although in general these are highly toxic substances when below a pH of 2.0. Acids typically have a localized necrotic effect and rarely cause full-thickness mucous membrane lesions. Exposure in animals results in immediate, intense pain which typically limits further exposure. Corrosive mucous membranes burns are initially gray to milky white, turning black as an eschar forms. Stricture formation may follow in several weeks. The animal may vocalize or become lethargic; excessive panting may indicate pain and inability to swallow may be noted. Other effects are hematemesis, abdominal pain, polydipsia, epiglottal edema with secondary respiratory distress, and shock. Secondary pneumonitis results from aspiration or exposure to acid vapors. Serious burns result from ocular or dermal exposure. Pain is severe. Acids tend to penetrate the eye more slowly than bases and may result in a delayed corneal damage including corneal and conjunctiva necrosis. Hydrofluoric acid (HF) penetrates tissues and poisoning can occur through ingestion, inhalation, or skin or eye exposure. Signs are often delayed and pain may not be immediately evident. Once systemic, HF binds with calcium ions producing insoluble calcium fluoride. Severe pain and swelling as well as hypocalcemia result. In severe exposures death from cardiac arrest may occur	All exposures should be diluted immediately with water. Attempts to neutralize the burn with other chemicals are contraindicated as is emesis or gastric lavage. Activated charcoal is ineffective in binding acid corrosives and should not be administered. GI protection indicated with all exposures. Ancillary therapies may include pain control and repeated wound lavage. and pain control as needed. Supportive care including IV fluids may be indicated. Therapy for shock may be required as uncorrected circulatory collapse can lead to renal failure, ischemic lesions in vital organs, and acute death. The presence of severe pharyngeal edema indicates the need for an endotracheal or tracheostomy tube. Esophageal complications are less common with acid exposures than alkali ingestions. If necessary, endoscopy should be carefully performed 12–24 hours after exposure to determine the extent of injury. The procedure should be stopped at the first sign of mucosal damage. Radiographic examination is another alternative. Affected skin and hair coat should be irrigated for at least 15 minutes with copious amounts of tepid water and monitored for lesions. Affected eyes should be irrigated for 20–30 minutes with isotonic saline followed by an examination with a slit lamp. Further treatment depends on the result of the examination. Any deterioration in the animal's signs necessitates a second examination. Hydrofluoric acid exposures require immediate attention even though they may not show any signs. Caretakers should take precautions to protect themselves when bathing or applying medications. Exposed areas should be washed well with cool water and ice packs/cold compresses applied to slow diffusion of the fluoride ion. Calcium gluconate gel applied liberally to the affected area will help bind fluoride. If calcium gluconate gel is not readily available, the area can be soaked in any magnesium hydroxide containing antacid product until the gel is located

(*Continued*)

TOXIC HOME AND GARDEN HAZARDS FOR PETS (*CONTINUED*)

Table VI–C

Household cleaners, disinfectants, and solvents—products, clinical signs, and treatment (*continued*)

Products	*Toxicity and Clinical Signs*	*Treatment*
Bases (pH >7; strong base pH >11.5–12; some references state >10)—includes drain and oven cleaners, cleaning agents, toilet bowl cleaners, washing products. Lye (sodium or potassium hydroxide or caustic soda), sodium carbonate (washing soda or soda ash), sodium metasilicate, and ammonium hydroxide are alkaline ingredients present in many of these products	Rapid liquefaction necrosis on contact with deep, penetrating ulcers. Ingestion may result in full thickness esophageal burns with secondary stricture formation. Little pain on contact so animals are not repelled allowing for a more significant exposure to occur. The remaining signs are similar to those found under corrosive acids	All exposures should be diluted immediately with water. Attempts to neutralize with other chemicals are contraindicated as is emesis or gastric lavage. Activated charcoal is ineffective in binding and should not be administered. Supportive care includes IV fluids and adequate nutrition. GI protection indicated with all exposures. Corticosteroids have been recommended to decrease stricture formation, but their use is controversial. Antibiotics should be used in animals with known perforations or infections. Therapy for shock may be required as uncorrected circulatory collapse can lead to renal failure, ischemic lesions in vital organs, and acute death. The presence of severe pharyngeal edema indicates the need for an endotracheal or tracheostomy tube. Endoscopy should be carefully performed 12–24 hours after exposure to determine the extent of injury. The procedure should be stopped at the first sign of mucosal damage. Radiographic examination is another alternative. Affected skin and hair coat should be flushed for at least 15 minutes with copious amounts of tepid water and monitored for lesions. Affected eyes should be irrigated for 20–30 minutes with isotonic saline followed by an examination with a slit lamp. Further treatment depends on the results of the examination. Any deterioration in the animal's signs necessitates a second examination
DISINFECTANTS		
Bleaches—includes common household bleach (3–6% sodium hypochlorite); industrial or swimming pool bleach (up to 50% sodium hypochlorite); powdered bleach (calcium hypochlorite, sodium dichloroisocyanurate), non-chlorine or colorfast bleach (sodium carbonate peroxide, hydrogen peroxide, sodium perborate)	The toxicity of chlorine bleach depends on the pH and concentration of the hypochlorite ion. Exposed animals may smell like chlorine and their exposed hair coat bleached. Household chlorine bleach products are mild to moderate irritants and generally not associated with significant tissue destruction. Common clinical signs secondary to ingestion include oral irritation, salivation, abdominal pain, and vomiting. Inhalation of fumes may result in coughing, gagging and retching. Systemic reactions are rare. Oral, pharyngeal, esophageal, and gastric burns have been reported from household chlorine bleach ingestions but are rare. The more concentrated hypochlorite solutions and bleach powders can produce corrosive effects. Non-chlorine bleach products are of low order toxicity with gastric irritation and vomiting the most commonly reported signs. Borate containing products decompose to peroxide and borate resulting in a more alkaline and potentially irritating product	All oral exposures should be diluted with water. Exposed skin and hair coat should be washed with a mild soap and copious amounts of water; eyes should be irrigated with isotonic saline for 15 minutes. Animals inhaling chlorine bleach fumes should be moved to fresh air. The incidence of esophageal damage is low so endoscopy is not routinely recommended. Animals with dysphagia, dyspnea, or severe oropharnyngeal burns should undergo careful endoscopic examination and treated as needed for corrosive injuries. Ancillary therapies may include gi protection, pain control, and repeated wound lavage. Affected skin and hair coat should be flushed for at least 15 minutes with copious amounts of tepid water and monitored for lesions

TOXIC HOME AND GARDEN HAZARDS FOR PETS (*CONTINUED*)

Table VI–C

Household cleaners, disinfectants, and solvents—products, clinical signs, and treatment (*continued*)

Products	*Toxicity and Clinical Signs*	*Treatment*
Phenols (coal tar-derived aromatic alcohols)—chlorophenols, phenylphenols in a variety of concentrations and products; some concentrated commercial products contain up to 50% pure phenol. Found in household cleaning products, medicated shampoos, disinfectants, and scents	Considered highly toxic and a medical emergency due to rapid absorption by inhalation, ingestion, or dermal exposure. Cats are more sensitive than dogs. The LD_{50} of pure phenol in dogs is 0.5 g/kg BW (orally) and cats 80 mg/kg BW (unknown route). Concentrations 1–5% may cause tissue irritation and dermal burns, 5–10% dermal, oral and gi burns are possible, and at >10% corrosive damage to all tissues are expected. Oral exposure causes burns to the mouth, oropharynx, and esophagus. Hypersalivation, panting, agitation, and vomiting progress to tremors, cardiac arrhythmias, shock, and coma. Methemoglobinemia, respiratory alkalosis, and renal and hepatic damage may develop. Dermal and ocular exposure results in a short period of intense pain followed by local anesthesia. Necrotic skin areas are white followed in a few days by a dry, gray black eschar. Ocular exposure results in severe corneal burns and erosions	Oral dilution is recommended as soon as possible but choice diluent is considered controversial. Dilute with water or milk at home prior to obtaining veterinary care. Some sources recommend mineral oil for dilution. Emesis is contraindicated and anti emetic should be administered promptly. The mouth and oropharynx should be examined carefully for evidence of mucosal damage prior to gastric lavage. If present gastric lavage is contraindicated. If there is no mucosal damage, activated charcoal with a cathartic may be administered. Further care is supportive and includes monitoring of renal and hepatic function, acid-base status, and respiratory effort. Shock and respiratory depression are complicating factors. *N*-Acetylcysteine (NAC) and SAMe may be used to limit hepatic and renal toxicity. Individuals treating dermal exposures should protect themselves prior to animal treatment. Polyethylene glycol (PEG) or glycerol is recommended for the initial dilution and removal of phenolic compounds followed by washing with a mild soap and water. Oil-based creams and ointments should be avoided as they may increase phenol absorption. Affected eyes should be irrigated for 20–30 minutes with isotonic saline and a slit lamp examination performed. Medications and further therapy depend on exam results
Pine oils (terpene alcohols) and turpentine (mixture of terpenes derived from pine oil)—concentration of pine oil in disinfectants varies from 0.3% to 60%. Turpentine is used to thin oil-based paints. May also be found in equine hoof dressings	Moderate to severe toxicity risk is concentration dependent. The oral LD_{50} of pine oil varies from 1 to 2.7 mL/kg BW but much lower doses may result in severe toxicosis. Cats are more susceptible than dogs. Pine oil products are direct irritants to mucous membranes resulting in erythema in contact areas (mouth, oropharynx, skin). Ingestion results in profuse salivation, abdominal pain, and vomiting ± blood. Systemic effects include respiratory depression, CNS depression, weakness, ataxia, and hypotension. Aspiration during ingestion or emesis or chemical pneumonitis secondary to systemic absorption results in pulmonary toxicity. Myoglobinuria and acute renal may develop with massive ingestions. Dermal exposure causes redness and irritation. Ocular signs include photosensitivity, blepharospasm, epiphora, and conjunctival and scleral erythema	All oral exposures should be diluted with water. Induction of emesis is contraindicated, and gastric lavage carries a risk. Activated charcoal is not indicated. Further treatment is symptomatic and includes close monitoring of renal perfusion, electrolytes, and acid base status. Affected skin should be washed well with a mild soap and copious amounts of water. Ocular exposures should be irrigated for at least 15 minutes with isotonic saline and monitored for further signs

(*Continued*)

TOXIC HOME AND GARDEN HAZARDS FOR PETS (*CONTINUED*)

Table VI–C

Household cleaners, disinfectants, and solvents—products, clinical signs, and treatment (*continued*)

Products	*Toxicity and Clinical Signs*	*Treatment*
SOLVENTS AND ALCOHOLS		
Acetone—found in nail polish remover, glues and rubber cement, paint thinner, varnish.	The oral LD_{50} in dogs is 8 mL/kg BW but doses as low as 2–3 mL/kg BW may be toxic. The odor of acetone and presence of elevated urinary ketones indicate exposure. Clinical signs associated with a mild exposure include CNS depression, ataxia, and vomiting; stupor and coma occur with larger amounts. Hyperglycemia and ketonemia may be present	Emesis followed by activated charcoal with a cathartic has been suggested but is controversial due to rapid absorption of acetone and poor binding of activated charcoal. It may be useful if performed within 15–30 minutes of ingestion. Further therapy is symptomatic and supportive and may need to be continued for several days due to the long plasma half-life
Isopropanol—found in model engine fuel, deicers, windshield washer fluid, fuel additives, and varnish and stain removers	The toxic dose of 70% isopropanol is 2 mL/kg BW but doses as low as 0.5 mL/kg BW may be toxic. Signs occur rapidly, generally within 30–60 minutes, and include vomiting ± blood, stupor, and ataxia which may progress to CNS and respiratory depression, severe hypotension, and coma. Mild acidosis may occur	The rapid onset of signs prevents most forms of decontamination. Emesis may be induced in asymptomatic animals if the ingestion occurred with 15–30 minutes. Activated charcoal is not recommended as it does not readily bind alcohols. Further treatment includes IV fluids and monitoring of acid-base and electrolyte status. Hemodialysis may be useful in animals with severe hypotension and coma
Methanol (methyl or wood alcohol, "denatured alcohol")—found in windshield wiper solutions, antifreeze products for door locks	The lethal dose of oral methanol in dogs is 4–8 mL/kg BW. Clinical signs include CNS and respiratory depression, ataxia, hypothermia, vomiting, and coma. Metabolic acidosis is rare. Blindness only occurs in humans and primates	Treatment is similar to isopropanol toxicosis
Ethanol—found in certain mouthwashes, alcohol for consumption (see individual entry), perfumes, cologne, hand sanitizers	The lethal dose of oral methanol in dogs is 5–8 mL/kg BW. Clinical signs are similar to those associated with methanol exposures. Metabolic acidosis more likely than with a methanol exposure	Treatment is similar to isopropanol toxicosis

PAIN MANAGEMENT

Table VII-A

Recommended parenteral opioid dosages and indications			
Opioid	*Dose/Route/Duration*	*Indications*	*Comments*
Butorphanol (injectable)	Dog: 0.2–0.4 mg/kg IM, IV, or SC Cat: 0.2–0.4 mg/kg IM, IV, or SC Duration: 1–3 h	Mild to moderate pain	Mild or no sedation; mild ventilatory depression
Buprenorphine (injectable)	Dog: 0.005–0.03 mg/kg IM, IV Cat: 0.005–0.03 mg/kg IM, IV or transmucosal Duration: 3–8 h Cat: 0.12–0.24 mg/kg SC once daily for up to 3 days for post-operative pain (SIMBADOL) Duration: 24 h	Mild to moderate pain	May be difficult to antagonize, onset of effect 15–30 minutes
Morphine (injectable)	Dog: 0.2–1.0 mg/kg IM or SC; 0.05–0.5 mg/kg IV Cat: 0.05–0.2 mg/kg IM or SC Duration: 3–6 h	Moderate to severe pain	Sedation; respiratory depression; bradycardia; nausea; hypothermia; dysphoria in cats without pain or with large dosage; rapid IV injection may cause histamine release
Methadone (injectable)	Dog: 0.25–0.5 mg/kg IV, IM or SC Cat: 0.1–0.25 mg/kg IV, IM or SC Duration 3–4 h	Moderate to severe pain	Sedation; dysphoria, vomiting, and constipation are reportedly less than with morphine
Hydromorphone (injectable)	Dog: 0.05–0.2 mg/kg IM, IV, or SC Cat: 0.05–0.2 mg/kg IM, IV, or SC Duration: 3–6 h	Moderate to severe pain	Similar side effects as those observed with morphine, but less vomiting and minimal histamine release. May be associated with hyperthermia in cats
Fentanyl (injectable)	Dog: 0.002–0.01 mg/kg IV Cat: 0.001–0.005 mg/kg IV Duration: 20–30 min	Moderate to severe pain; CRI necessary for long-term analgesia	Sedation; respiratory depression; bradycardia; nausea; inadequate duration of analgesia from single IV bolus or IM injection

Table VII-B

Recommended dispensable opioid dosages and indications			
Opioid	*Dose/Route/Duration*	*Indications*	*Comments*
Codeine (tablets)	Dog: 1.0–2.0 mg/kg PO Cat: 0.1–1.0 mg/kg PO Duration: 4–8 h	Mild to moderate pain	Minimal side effects; when dosed with acetaminophen, avoid in dogs with liver disease or Heinz body anemia; do not use in combination with acetaminophen in cats
Butorphanol (tablets)	Dog: 0.5–1.0 mg/kg PO Cat: 0.5–1.0 mg/kg PO Duration: 2–4 h	Mild to moderate pain	Mild or no sedation; mild ventilatory depression.
Tramadol (immediate-release tablets)	Dog: 2–10 mg/kg PO q8–12h Cat: 2–5 mg/kg PO q8–12h	Mild to moderate pain	Sedation, anxiety, urinary retention

PAIN MANAGEMENT (*CONTINUED*)

Table VII-C

Recommended parenteral local anesthetic dosages and indications			
Local Anesthetic	*Dose/Route/Duration*	*Indications*	*Comments*
Lidocaine (inject able)	Dog: 6–10 mg/kg infiltrate/nerve block; 4 mg/kg epidural; 1–2mg/kg IV bolus followed by 0.05–0.1 mg/kg/min IV CRI Cat: 3–5 mg/kg infiltrate/ nerve block; 4 mg/kg epidural Duration: 1–1.5 h	Moderate to severe pain	CNS and cardiac toxicity with inadvertent IV injection causing excessive plasma concentrations
Bupivacaine (injectable)	Dog: 2 mg/kg infiltrate/nerve block; 1 mg/kg epidural Cat: 1–1.5 mg/kg infiltrate/nerve block; 1 mg/kg epidural Duration: 3–10 h	Moderate to severe pain	Cardiac and CNS toxicity with inadvertent IV injection causing excessive plasma concentrations
Bupivacaine (liposome injectable suspension)	Dog: 5.3 mg/kg infiltrated into tissue layers during incisional closure of cranial cruciate ligament surgery (NOCITA) Cat: 5.3 mg/kg infiltrated in each forelimb for peripheral nerve block for onychectomy (NOCITA) Duration: 48–72 h	Moderate to severe pain	Cardiac and CNS toxicity with inadvertent IV injection causing excessive plasma concentrations; incisional inflammation/ discharge in small number of dogs; hyperthermia in small number of cats

Table VII-D

Recommended parenteral NSAID dosages and indications			
NSAID	*Dose/Route/Duration*	*Indications*	*Comments*
Carprofen (injectable)	Dog: 2–4 mg/kg IV, SC q24h Cat: 1.0 mg/kg SC only once	Mild to moderate pain	Primarily used perioperatively before switching to oral formulation; GI irritation and altered renal function
Meloxicam (injectable)	Dog: 0.2 mg/kg initially IM, IV, or SC; 0.1 mg/kg thereafter SC Cat: 0.1–0.2 mg/kg initially IM, SC (single dose only per label) Duration: 24 h	Mild to moderate pain	Can be mixed with food; GI irritation and altered renal function
Ketoprofen (injectable)	Dog: 1.0–2.0 mg/kg initially IM, IV, or SC; 0.5–1.0 mg/kg thereafter SC Cat: 1.0–2.0 mg/kg initially IM, IV, or SC; 0.5–1.0 mg/kg thereafter SC Duration: 24 h	Mild to moderate pain; approved in Canada for dogs and cats and in the US for horses	GI irritation and altered renal function. Dosing should not exceed 5 days for dogs and 3 days for cats
Robenacoxib (injectable)	Dog: 2.0 mg/kg SC q24h for up to 3 days; PO administration as per Table VII-E thereafter Cat: 2.0 mg/kg SC q24h for up to 3 days	Mild to moderate postoperative pain and inflammation	

PAIN MANAGEMENT (*CONTINUED*)

Table VII-E

Recommended dispensable NSAID dosages and indications

NSAID	*Dosage/Route/Duration*	*Indications*	*Comments*
Carprofen (tablets and chewables)	Dog: 4.4 mg/kg PO q24h or divided q12h Cat: 1.0 mg/kg PO (1 dose only) Duration: 12–24 h	Mild to moderate pain; approved for use in dogs with osteoarthritis or perioperative pain	Toxicity associated with chronic use in cats due to variable half-life; may cause GI irritation and altered renal function in some patients
Deracoxib (chewable tablets)	Dog (post-operative pain): 3.0–4.0 mg/kg PO q24 h as needed for 7 days Dog (osteoarthritis): 1–2 mg/kg PO q24h for long-term treatment over 7 days Cat; not used Duration: 24 h	Pain and inflammation associated with osteoarthritis. Post-operative pain and inflammation associated with orthopedic surgery in dogs with osteoarthritis	GI irritation and altered renal function
Firocoxib (chewable tablets)	Dog: 5 mg/kg PO q24h Cat: not used Duration: 24 h	Pain and inflammation associated with osteoarthritis and perioperative pain	GI irritation and altered renal function
Etodolac (tablets)			
Grapiprant (tablets)	Dog: 2 mg/kg PO q24h; cannot be dosed accurately in dogs weighing less than 3.6 kg Cat: not used Duration: 24 h	Pain and inflammation associated with osteoarthritis	Non-COX inhibiting-NSAID; most common adverse reactions are vomiting, diarrhea, decreased appetite, decreased albumin/serum protein; give on an empty stomach to optimize oral bioavailability
Aspirin (tablets)	Dog: 10–25 mg/kg PO Cat: 10–15 mg/kg PO Duration: 8–12 h for dogs, 24–72 h for cats	Mild to moderate pain and inflammation	GI irritation and altered renal function; more likely at higher doses
Meloxicam (oral liquid suspension, tablets)	Dog: 0.2 mg/kg initially PO; 0.1 mg/kg thereafter PO Cat: 0.1–0.2 mg/kg initially PO; 0.05–0.1 mg/kg thereafter PO (reduce to minimum effective dose) Duration: 24 h	Mild to moderate pain	GI irritation and altered renal function; can be mixed with food. Cats should not be given meloxicam for > 5 days
Robenacoxib (oral tablets)	Dog: 2.0 mg/kg PO q24h for up to 3 days Cat: 1 mg/kg PO q24h for up to 3 days Duration: 24 h	Mild to moderate postoperative pain and inflammation	GI irritation and altered renal function
Ketoprofen (tablets)	Dog: 1.0–2.0 mg/kg initially PO; 0.5–1.0 mg/kg thereafter PO Cat: 1.0–2.0 mg/kg initially PO; 0.5–1.0 mg/kg thereafter PO Duration: 24 h	Mild to moderate pain; approved in Canada for dogs and cats and in the US for horses	GI irritation and altered renal functions. Limit administration to 5 days for both dogs and cats
Acetaminophen (tablets and oral liquid suspension)	Dog: 10–15 mg/kg PO Cat: contraindicated Duration (in dogs): 8–12 h	Mild to moderate pain; low anti-inflammatory action	Toxic to cats; often given in combination with codeine to dogs

PAIN MANAGEMENT (*CONTINUED*)

Table VII-F

Dosages and indications for selected drugs used to treat neuropathic pain

Drug	*Dosage/Route*	*Duration (PO)*	*Comments*
Ketamine (NMDA antagonist)	Dog: 0.1–1.0 mg/kg IM, SC, or PO Cat: 0.1–1.0 mg/kg IM or SC	4–6 h 4–6 h	Low doses potentiate postoperative analgesics. Do not use with intracranial hypertension
Amantadine (NMDA antagonist)	Dog: 3.0–5.0 mg/kg PO Cat: 3.0–5.0 mg/kg PO	24 h 24 h	Used to potentiate or prolong analgesia. Efficacious when combined with an NSAID for management of osteoarthritis-associated pain in dogs
Amitriptyline (tricyclic antidepressant)	Dog: 1.0 mg/kg PO Cat: 2.5–10.0 mg/cat PO	12–24 h 24 h	Used to potentiate or prolong analgesia.
Gabapentin (antiepileptic)	Dog: 2–10 mg/kg PO q8–12h; dose can be titrated up to 20 mg/kg q8–12h if necessary Cat: 1–8 mg/kg PO q8–12h	24 h 24 h	Usually associated with few side effects other than sedation, and, occasional ataxia in cats. Has shown good results in human and animal studies

To select and administer an adjuvant analgesic properly, the veterinarian should be aware of the drug's clinical pharmacology. The following information about the drug is necessary: (1) approved indication, (2) unapproved indication (e.g., as an analgesic) widely accepted in veterinary medical practice, (3) common side effects and potentially serious adverse effects, (4) pharmacokinetic features, and (5) specific dosing guidelines for pain.

MEDICATIONS AND SUPPLEMENTS FOR OSTEOARTHRITIS

This appendix has been provided to act as a quick reference for supplements and medications commonly used to treat animals with joint pain and osteoarthritis (OA). The contraindications, precautions, and interactions include all of the most common concerns for these categories. For a comprehensive list of warnings, we recommend referring to one of the many veterinary drug reference that are available.

The authors have also included a subjective evaluation of the level of evidence-based, peer-reviewed research that is available to support the use of these medications and supplements in clinical practice to support animals with osteoarthritis and inflammation:

- NONE—No evidence to support use in the clinical veterinary patient.
- WEAK—Evidence that shows minimal benefit to the veterinary patient clinically or *in vitro*. There may be human literature that could be inferred to the veterinary patient.
- MODERATE—Evidence that shows *in vitro* and/or *in vivo* benefit for OA and joint pain.
- STRONG—Compelling evidence that shows benefit for OA and joint pain support in the clinical veterinary patient.

Table VIII-A

Anti-inflammatories and pain medications

Category	*Dosage*	*Mechanism of Action*	*Contraindications*	*Precautions*	*Interactions*	*Evidence-Based Support in the Literature*
Amitriptyline (tricyclic antidepressant [TCA])	Dog: 1.0 mg/kg PO Cat: 2.5–10.0 mg/cat PO	TCAs inhibit serotonin and norepinephrine reuptake and possible actions at opioid receptors and nerve transmission, complete MOA unknown	Patients with renal or hepatic or thyroid or cardiac disorders	May reduce seizure threshold Sedation at higher doses Anticholingeric properties (constipation and urinary retention) Taper when discontinuing	Concurrent administration with monoamine oxidase inhibitors, anipryl, SSRIs due to potential of serotonin syndrome	NONE—for OA management
Antiepileptic (gabapentin)	Dog: 2–10 mg/kg PO q8–12h; dose can be titrated up to 20 mg/kg	GABA analogue, therapeutic action on neuropathic pain is thought to involve voltage-gated N-type calcium ion channels, complete MOA unknown	Patients with renal or hepatic insufficiency may require less frequent dosing or lower doses	Sedation at higher doses Abrupt discontinuation can lead to severe rebound pain, tapering the dose is recommended	Concurrent administrations with oral antacids can reduce absorption from GI tract	NONE—for OA management
NMDA antagonist (amantadine)	Dog: 3.0–5.0 mg/kg PO Cat: 3.0–5.0 mg/kg PO	NMDA receptor antagonist, complete MOA unknown. Best used when combined with another analgesic such as an NSAID	Patients with hypersensitivity to it. Reduce dose in face of renal dysfunction	Use caution in patients with seizure disorders or patient on medications that lower the seizure threshold GI upset	Concurrent administrations with urinary acidifiers may increase excretion or anticholinergic drugs and TMS may enhance effects/decrease excretion	MODERATE

(*Continued*)

MEDICATIONS AND SUPPLEMENTS FOR OSTEOARTHRITIS (*CONTINUED*)

Table VIII-A

Anti-inflammatories and pain medications (*continued*)

Category	*Dosage*	*Mechanism of Action*	*Contraindications*	*Precautions*	*Interactions*	*Evidence-Based Support in the Literature*
NSAIDs (various)	See Table VIII-C	Inhibit prostaglandin synthesis through cyclooxygenase enzymes. Inhibition of EP4 receptor-specific	NSAIDs must not be given with steroids	NSAIDs may cause gastric ulceration or upset COX-2 selective drugs may interfere with liver function when used outside of dosage range When switching NSAIDs wait 3 days for washout before starting new drug When switching from aspirin to NSAID 7 days for washout is required	Steroids with NSAIDs	STRONG
Opioids (various)	See Tables VIII-A and VIII-B	Natural opioid prodrug with suspected metabolism to active metabolites including morphine. Efficacy reflects the agonistic action of mu opioid receptors	None	Use caution in patients with head trauma	May decrease the effects of diuretics in patients with CHF	MODERATE

To select and administer an adjuvant analgesic properly, the veterinarian should be aware of the drug's clinical pharmacology. The following information about the drug is necessary: (1) approved indication, (2) unapproved indication (e.g., as an analgesic) widely accepted in veterinary medical practice, (3) common side effects and potentially serious adverse effects, (4) pharmacokinetic features, and (5) specific dosing guidelines for pain.
NMDA = N-methyl-d-aspartate; GI = gastrointestinal; NSAID = nonsteroidal anti-inflammatory drug.

Table VIII-B

Recommended parenteral NSAID dosages and indications

NSAID	*Dose/Route/Duration*	*Indications*	*Comments*
Carprofen (injectable)	Dog: 2–4 mg/kg IV, SC q24h Cat: 1.0 mg/kg SC only once	Mild to moderate pain	Primarily used perioperatively before switching to oral formulation; GI irritation and altered renal function.
Ketoprofen (injectable)	Dog: 1.0–2.0 mg/kg initially IM, IV, or SC; 0.5–1.0 mg/kg thereafter SC Cat: 1.0–2.0 mg/kg initially IM, IV, or SC; 0.5–1.0 mg/kg thereafter SC Duration: 24 h	Mild to moderate pain; approved in Canada for dogs and cats and in the US for horses	GI irritation and altered renal function. Dosing should not exceed 5 days for dogs and 3 days for cats.
Meloxicam (injectable)	Dog: 0.2 mg/kg initially IM, IV, or SC; 0.1 mg/kg thereafter SC Cat: 0.1–0.2 mg/kg initially IM, SC (single dose only per label) Duration: 24 h	Mild to moderate pain	Can be mixed with food; GI irritation and altered renal function

GI = gastrointestinal; NSAID = nonsteroidal anti-inflammatory drug.

MEDICATIONS AND SUPPLEMENTS FOR OSTEOARTHRITIS (*CONTINUED*)

Table VIII-C

Recommended oral NSAID dosages and indications			
NSAID	*Dosage/Route/Duration*	*Indications*	*Comments*
Acetaminophen (tablets and oral liquid suspension)	Dog: 10–15 mg/kg PO Cat: contraindicated Duration (in dogs): 8–12 h	Mild to moderate pain; low anti-inflammatory action	Toxic to cats; often given in combination with codeine to dogs
Aspirin (tablets)	Dog: 10–25 mg/kg PO Cat: 10–15 mg/kg PO Duration: 8–12 h for dogs, 24–72 h for cats	Mild to moderate pain and inflammation	GI irritation and altered renal function; more likely at higher doses. Not commonly used as there are better options available today
Carprofen (tablets and chewables)	Dog: 4.4 mg/kg PO q24h or divided q12h Cat: 1.0 mg/kg PO (1 dose only) Duration: 12–24 h	Mild to moderate pain; approved for use in dogs with OA or perioperative pain	Toxicity associated with chronic use in cats due to variable half-life; may cause GI irritation and altered renal function in some patients
Deracoxib (chewable tablets)	Dog (postoperative pain): 3.0–4.0 mg/kg PO q24h as needed for 7 days Dog (OA): 1–2 mg/kg PO q24h for long-term treatment over 7 days Duration: 24 h	Pain and inflammation associated with OA. Post-operative pain and inflammation associated with orthopedic surgery in dogs with OA. Postoperative ≥ 1.8 kg	GI irritation and altered renal function
Etodolac (tablets)	Dog: 10–15 mg/kg PO Cat: not used Duration: 24 h	Mild to moderate pain	Hypoproteinemia; GI irritation and altered renal function. Associated with KCS in a small number of dogs Not commonly used as there are better options available today
Firocoxib (chewable tablets)	Dog: 5 mg/kg PO q24h	Pain and inflammation associated with OA and perioperative pain	GI irritation and altered renal function
Gapriprant (tablets)	Dog: 2mg/kg PO q24h Cat: up to 15mg/kg/day for 28 days	Pain and inflammation associated with OA	GI irritation. No safety evaluation in dogs younger than 9 months of age or weighing less than 3.6 kg. FDA approved in dogs
Ketoprofen (tablets)	Dog: 1.0–2.0 mg/kg initially PO; 0.5–1.0 mg/kg thereafter PO Cat: 1.0–2.0 mg/kg initially PO; 0.5–1.0 mg/kg thereafter PO Duration: 24 h	Mild to moderate pain; approved in Canada for dogs and cats and in the US for horses	GI irritation and altered renal functions. Limit administration to 5 days for both dogs and cats. Not commonly used as there are better options available today
Meloxicam (oral liquid suspension, tablets)	Dog: 0.2 mg/kg initially PO; 0.1 mg/kg thereafter PO Cat: 0.1–0.2 mg/kg initially PO; 0.05–0.1 mg/kg thereafter PO (reduce to minimum effective dose) Duration: 24 h	Mild to moderate pain	GI irritation and altered renal function; can be mixed with food. Cats should not be given meloxicam for >5 days
Robenacoxib (oral tablets and injectable in some countries)	Dog: 2 mg/kg SC once prior to surgery, 1 mg/kg PO q24h for up to 12 days Cat: 1 mg/kg PO up to 3 days in US Duration: 24 h	Mild to moderate pain; not approved for dogs in US	GI irritation and altered renal function. Only FDA-approved NSAID for cats
Tepoxalin (tablets)	Dog: Load 20 mg/kg, then 10 mg/kg PO q24h	Pain and inflammation associated with OA	GI irritation. Give with food. Caution in patients with hepatic, cardiac and renal dysfunction No safety evaluation in dogs younger than 6 months of age or weighing less than 3 kg

Table VIII-D

Disease-Modifying Drugs (DMOADs)						
Category	*Dosage*	*Mechanism of Action*	*Contraindications*	*Precautions*	*Interactions*	*Evidence-Based Support in the Literature*
Avocado Soybean unsaponifiables (ASU)	300 mg/day	Stimulates aggrecan production and restored aggrecan production after IL-1β treatment and decreased MMP-3 production and stimulated TIMP-1 production	None	None	None	STRONG
Chondroitin	800 mg/day	Stimulates synthesis of GAGs and inhibit degradative enzymes	None	Large variation in products	None	WEAK
Glucosamine	1000 mg/day	Used in the synthesis of disaccharide units of GAGs and proteoglycans. May have anti-inflammatory properties and may stimulate GAGs , proteogylcan and collagen synthesis, may scavenge oxygen-derived free radicals, stimulate hyaluronic acid synthesis	None	Large variation in products	None	WEAK
Green-lipped mussel extract	20–49 mg/kg/day; 4 (dogs <40 kg BW)–6 (dogs >40 kg BW) capsules/day for 10 days then continuing with half of the loading dose	May have chondroprotective and anti-inflammatory properties	None	None	None	STRONG
Omega-3 fatty acid	Eicosapentaenoic acid (EPA), Dochosahexaenoic acid (DHA) (150–175 mg/kg of DHA and/or EPA daily; canine	Competes with omega-6 fatty acids in particular arachadonic acid to minimize the inflammatory cascade, in addition can cause the inhibition of release of cyclooxygenase and lipoxygenase	None	Use cautiously in patients prone to pancreatitis, high dosages of omega-3 fatty acids without incorporation of diet and daily exercise will lead to weight gain	None	STRONG
Polysulfated glycosaminoglycans (Adequan)	(2 mg/lb IM twice weekly for 4 weeks; Canine) Off label usage for SC route, for felines, and for monthly maintenance	Not completely known suspected to inhibit serine proteinases, prostaglandin E2 synthesis, and metalloproteases. May stimulate synthesis of protein, collagen, proteoglycan, and hyaluronic acid	None	Use caution in patients with underlying clotting or platelet pathology	None	STRONG
T-Relief	Dogs: 1–3 tablets PO q8h Newborn puppies: ½ tablet PO q24h Weaned puppies: 1 tablet PO q8h Cats: 1 tablet PO q8h	Unknown; homeopathic ingredients including arnica Montana and belladonna to help with minor injuries	None	None	None	WEAK

GAGs = glycosaminoglycans; MMP = matrix metalloproteinsases; IL-1 = interleukin-1; TIMP = tissue inhibitors of metalloproteinase.

GLOSSARY OF TERMINOLOGY FOR SEIZURES AND EPILEPTIC DISORDERS

There is no formally approved classification system for seizures or epilepsy in veterinary medicine and authors proposing such systems in the past have largely adapted human classification schemes (1–5). This proposed glossary is no different and is based mainly on publications sanctioned by the International League Against Epilepsy (ILAE) (6–11). Terms have been added, changed or eliminated to better reflect the seizure types seen in veterinary patients and the challenges inherent with the interpretation of such events in animals. This glossary is adapted from a more detailed proposal of terminology for veterinary patients (12), and interested readers are referred to this work for more details on seizure description and semiology, background on ILAE classification and adaptations for animals, and rationale for the currently proposed terms.

GENERAL TERMS AND DEFINITIONS

Seizure: a discrete episode suspected to be epileptic in origin. Synonym: ictus.
Epileptic seizure: manifestation(s) of excessive and/or hypersynchronous activity of neurons in the brain; usually self-limiting.
Epilepsy: a chronic neurologic condition characterized by recurrent seizures; has an intracranial origin.
Focal seizure: a seizure whose initial signs indicate, or are consistent with, initial activation of only part of one cerebral hemisphere. Synonym: partial.
Generalized seizure: a seizure whose initial signs indicate, or are consistent with, more than minimal involvement of both cerebral hemispheres.

CLASSIFICATION OF EPILEPTIC SEIZURES

1. Motor Seizures: involving somatic musculature in any form. May consist of an increase (positive) or decrease (negative) in muscle contraction to produce a movement.
1A. Elementary Motor: a single type of contraction of a muscle or group of muscles that is usually stereotyped.

- **Tonic**: a sustained increase in muscle contraction lasting a few seconds to minutes.
- **Myoclonic:** sudden, brief (< 100 ms), involuntary single or multiple contractions of muscles or muscle groups of variable topography (axial, proximal limb, distal limb, facial).
  - **Clonic:** myoclonus that is regularly repetitive, involves the same muscle groups, at a frequency of approximately 2–3 per second, and is prolonged.
- **Tonic-clonic:** a sequence consisting of a tonic followed by a clonic phase.
  - **Generalized tonic-clonic seizure:** bilateral symmetric tonic contraction and then bilateral clonic contractions of somatic muscles, usually associated with autonomic phenomena and loss of consciousness. Synonyms: grand mal seizure, bilateral tonic-clonic seizure, major motor seizure.
- **Atonic:** sudden loss or diminution of muscle tone without an apparent preceding myoclonic or tonic event lasting greater than 1–2 seconds and involving the head, trunk, jaw or limb musculature.
- **Astatic:** loss of erect posture that results from an atonic, myoclonic or tonic mechanism. Synonym: drop attack.

1B. Automatism: a more or less coordinated, repetitive, motor activity usually occurring when cognition is impaired. Often resembles a voluntary movement. Examples might include chewing, licking, aimless running, or vocal utterances (e.g., barking, meowing, whining or growling).
2. Non-motor Seizures
Aura: an ictal phenomenon that may precede an observable seizure or if occurring alone, constitutes a sensory seizure.
Sensory seizure: a perceptual experience not caused by appropriate stimuli in the external world.

Note: Although sensory seizures almost certainly occur in animals, documenting their existence is obviously very difficult without the ability of the patient to describe sensory phenomena. Therefore, we are left to observe the behavior that the suspected sensory seizure produces. Some potential sensory phenomena include visual events (e.g., flashing or flickering lights, or other objects or patterns; the animal may bite or snap in response ["fly biting"]), somatosensory events (tingling, numbness or electric-shock sensations; the animal may bite or lick itself or run frantically during episode), auditory, olfactory, gustatory and affective events (e.g., fear, depression, joy or anger; the animal may become aggressive towards people or other animals).

Dyscognitive seizure: events in which disturbance of cognition is the predominant or most apparent feature.

Note: In the ILAE glossary, cognition is composed of perception, attention, emotion, memory and executive function (which includes decision making and initiation of motor activity) (8). In animals, without a description from the patient it may again be difficult to prove that certain dyscognitive seizure types exist or differentiate them from sensory seizures. However, certain examples (e.g., events where animals suddenly stop what they are doing and stare into space, often with a lack of appropriate responsiveness to external stimuli ["behavioral arrest"]) might be best classified here.

3. Autonomic Seizures: an objectively documented and distinct alteration of autonomic nervous system function involving cardiovascular, pupillary, gastrointestinal, sudomotor, vasomotor, and thermoregulatory functions.

MODIFIERS AND DESCRIPTORS OF SEIZURE TIMING

Duration: time between the beginning of initial seizure manifestations and the cessation of observed seizure activity. Does not include prodrome or postictal states but might include aura.
Cluster seizures: two or more seizures within a 24-hour period. Synonyms: acute repetitive seizures, serial seizures
Status epilepticus: 1) a seizure that persists for greater than 5 minutes or 2) recurrent seizures without interictal resumption of baseline central nervous system function.
Prodrome: a pre-ictal phenomenon. A subjective or objective clinical alteration (e.g., agitation, attention-seeking) that heralds the onset of an epileptic seizure but does not form part of it.

Note: It may be quite challenging or impossible to differentiate a prodrome (pre-ictal period) from an aura (start of ictus) in many veterinary patients although videotaping of the episodes, close observation and/or ictal electroencephalography may be helpful in this regard.

Postictal phenomenon: a transient clinical abnormality of central nervous system function that appears or becomes accentuated when clinical signs of the ictus have ended. May manifest as impaired mentation, altered behavior or motor or sensory deficits.
Provocative factor: transient and sporadic endogenous or exogenous element capable of augmenting seizure incidence in animals with chronic epilepsy or evoking seizures in susceptible individuals without epilepsy.

- **Reactive:** occurring in association with transient systemic perturbation or illness such as some metabolic conditions (e.g., hypoglycemia, electrolyte disorders) or intoxications.
- **Reflex:** objectively and consistently demonstrated to be evoked by a specific afferent stimulus or by activity of the patient. Examples include stimuli such as light flashes, certain noises or startling and activities such as specific motor movements or more complex behaviors.

CLASSIFICATION OF EPILEPSY

Epilepsy is defined here as a chronic neurologic disorder that causes recurrent seizure activity, and that has an intracranial

(*Continued*)

etiology. As stated by the ILAE Classification Core Group in 2006, "the diagnosis of epilepsy implies a persistent epileptogenic abnormality of the brain that is able to spontaneously generate paroxysmal activity. This is in contrast to a brain that has an acute seizure as a natural response to a transient insult or loss of homeostasis" (10). Thus, seizures caused by extracranial disorders such as metabolic conditions (e.g., hypoglycemia, electrolyte abnormalities) or toxins are not considered to be epilepsy, even when repetitive seizures occur over time (e.g., with hypoglycemia secondary to an insulinoma). These seizures are termed reactive seizures (see definition under "provocative factor" above). Note however that such a disorder might secondarily cause structural damage to a previously normal brain (e.g., through necrosis or excitotoxicity) and result in true epilepsy. An explanation of the term "idiopathic epilepsy" is also warranted here, as veterinarians use the word "idiopathic" in various ways. Some use this term to imply epilepsy of genetic or heritable origin (as it was originally intended for use in humans), while others use "idiopathic" to mean "cause unknown." The following classification is proposed to replace those previously used in veterinary medicine and has been adapted from a 2010 ILAE report (11).

Genetic epilepsy: Epilepsy as a direct result of a known or strongly suspected genetic defect or defects in which seizures are the core sign of the disorder. Generally, genetic epilepsies have no identifiable structural brain lesion or other neurologic signs, and have an age-dependent onset. Synonyms: Primary, inherited, idiopathic (for some).

Structural epilepsy: Epilepsy as a result of one or more identifiable structural lesions of the brain. Synonyms: Symptomatic, secondary. Structural epilepsies include disorders such as brain tumors, encephalitis, and cerebrovascular accidents. Note that some disorders that may have a genetic cause or that are strongly heritable may still be best classified here; these include anomalous disorders such as hydrocephalus, lissencephaly, degenerative disorders such as ceroid lipofuscinosis, and others.

Unknown epilepsy: The underlying cause of the epilepsy is unknown. This may be the result of a subtle structural lesion that is undetectable with currently available diagnostic technologies or an as yet unrecognized genetic disorder. Synonyms: Cryptogenic, probably symptomatic, idiopathic (for some).

References

1 Berendt M, Gram L. Epilepsy and seizure classification in 63 dogs: A reappraisal of veterinary epilepsy terminology. J Vet Intern Med 1999;13:14–20.
2 March PA. Seizures: Classification, etiologies, and pathophysiology. Clin Tech Small Anim Pract 1998;13:119–131.
3 Podell M. Seizures in dogs. Vet Clin North Am Small Anim Pract 1996;26:779–809.
4 Podell M. Seizures. In: Platt SR, Olby NJ, editors. BSAVA manual of canine and feline neurology. Gloucester: British Small Animal Veterinary Association; 2013, pp. 117–135.
5 Podell M, Fenner WR, Powers JD. Seizure classification in dogs from a nonreferral-based population. J Am Vet Med Assoc 1995;206:1721–1728.
6 Proposal for revised classification of epilepsies and epileptic syndromes. Commission on Classification and Terminology of the International League Against Epilepsy. Epilepsia 1989;30: 389–399.
7 Blume WT, Luders HO, Mizrahi E, Tassinari C, van Emde Boas W, Engel J, Jr. Glossary of descriptive terminology for ictal semiology: Report of the ILAE Task Force on Classification and Terminology. Epilepsia 2001;42:1212–1218.
8 Engel J, Jr. A proposed diagnostic scheme for people with epileptic seizures and with epilepsy: Report of the ILAE Task Force on Classification and Terminology. Epilepsia 2001;42:796–803.
9 Fisher RS, van Emde Boas W, Blume W, Elger C, Genton P, Lee P, et al. Epileptic seizures and epilepsy: Definitions proposed by the International League Against Epilepsy (ILAE) and the International Bureau for Epilepsy (IBE). Epilepsia 2005;46:470–472.
10 Engel J, Jr. Report of the ILAE classification core group. Epilepsia 2006;47:1558–1568.
11 Berg AT, Berkovic SF, Brodie MJ, Buchhalter J, Cross JH, van Emde Boas W, et al. Revised terminology and concepts for organization of seizures and epilepsies: Report of the ILAE Commission on Classification and Terminology, 2005–2009. Epilepsia 2010;51:676–685.
12 Mariani CL. Terminology and classification of seizures and epilepsy in veterinary patients. Top Companion Anim Med 2013;28:34–41.

COMMON PROCEDURES AND TESTING PROTOCOLS

ABDOMINOCENTESIS AND FLUID ANALYSIS

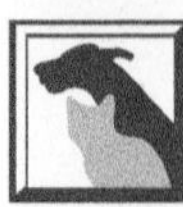

BASICS

TYPE OF PROCEDURE

Diagnostic sample collection.

PROCEDURE EXPLANATION AND RELATED PHYSIOLOGY

- Abdominocentesis is the percutaneous removal of peritoneal fluid for diagnostic and/or therapeutic purposes.
- Characterization of abdominal fluid may help determine primary disease process or pathophysiologic mechanism responsible for fluid accumulation.
- Blind abdominocentesis is easily performed when a large amount of fluid is present; ultrasound-guided abdominocentesis is useful when fluid volume is limited or localized.
- Diagnostic peritoneal lavage (DPL) is most often considered if abdominocentesis has failed to yield any fluid and undiagnosed intra-abdominal disease is suspected.
- Therapeutic abdominocentesis may improve quality of life in conjunction with medical management of chronic ascites.

INDICATIONS

- Peritoneal fluid suspected based on physical examination (abdominal distention, fluid wave) or diagnostic imaging.
- Blunt or penetrating abdominal trauma (e.g., dog bite, gunshot wound, motor vehicular accident).
- Suspicion of ruptured bowel, peritonitis, or postoperative GI dehiscence.
- Acute abdominal pain.
- Shock without apparent cause.
- DPL—with suspicion of undiagnosed intra-abdominal disease in face of negative abdominocentesis.
- Therapeutic abdominocentesis—when increased intra-abdominal pressure causes respiratory distress, decreased blood flow to visceral organs, or discomfort.

CONTRAINDICATIONS

- Abdominocentesis should be performed with caution or is contraindicated in presence of:
  - Dilated hollow abdominal viscus (stomach and intestines), generalized ileus.
  - Organomegaly.
  - An enlarged uterus because of pregnancy or pyometra.
  - Coagulopathy, thrombocytopenia.
- An uncharacterized large intra-abdominal mass is contraindication for blind abdominocentesis.
- Avoid DPL if diaphragmatic hernia suspected.

POTENTIAL COMPLICATIONS

- Hemorrhage from a punctured vessel or lacerated abdominal organ.
- Perforation of a hollow viscus (bowel, bladder) and iatrogenic peritonitis.
- Spread of infection, especially from a localized lesion (e.g., abscess, pyometra).
- Tearing of a fenestrated over-the-needle catheter in the abdomen during removal.
- Large-volume abdominocentesis may cause rapid fluid shifts and electrolyte changes:
  - Avoid removing large volumes from animals that have serum albumin of ≤2 g/dL.
- In addition to the above, DPL may result in subcutaneous hematoma or leakage of lavage fluid.

CLIENT EDUCATION

- Abdominocentesis is a minimally invasive diagnostic procedure that is generally easy to perform and associated with minimal risk and discomfort.
- Abdominocentesis is usually performed in awake patients, but sedation and/or analgesia may be necessary.

BODY SYSTEMS ASSESSED

- Hepatobiliary.
- Urinary.
- Gastrointestinal.
- Vascular (as with hemoabdomen).

PROCEDURE

PATIENT PREPARATION

Pre-Procedure Medication or Preparation

Consider emptying a distended urinary bladder prior to abdominocentesis or DPL.

Anesthesia or Sedation

Patients should be restrained either manually or with sedation/analgesia to prevent unwanted motion that could result in complications. Prior to drug administration, consider patient's general and cardiovascular condition (e.g., shock) and procedure being performed (sedation and local analgesia almost always indicated for DPL).

Patient Positioning

Patient in left lateral recumbency (to prevent splenic puncture) or can remain standing to improve gravity-dependent fluid retrieval. Patient positioning may be altered based on visualization of fluid using ultrasound guidance.

Patient Monitoring

Blood pressure, pulse oximetry, and heart rate/ECG should be monitored as indicated by patient's clinical status. Patients should be monitored for signs of pain or discomfort.

Equipment or Supplies

- Clippers.
- Surgical scrub.
- Sterile gloves.
- Syringes of various sizes (3, 5, or 10 mL).
- 2% Lidocaine (injectable).
- Glass slides.
- EDTA and serum tubes and culturettes.

For Abdominocentesis

- Hypodermic needle: 18- through 22-gauge, 1- to 1½-inch or over-the-needle IV catheter of similar size. Butterfly catheters may be used in small or thin patients.
- Consider addition of fenestrations in large gauge (14–18 gauge) over-the-needle catheters using a sterile scalpel blade. Fenestrations should be small and smooth and should not be directly opposite each other, as this may lead to catheter weakening and possible kinking or tearing within abdomen.
- Optional: extension set.
- For therapeutic abdominocentesis, a three-way stopcock, 20- to 60-mL syringe, and collection vessel.

For DPL

- A commercially available peritoneal dialysis catheter or alternatively a 20- to 14-gauge, over-the-needle, 1–2 inch IV catheter, fenestrated as described previously.
- A bag of warmed sterile isotonic saline solution with an administration set.
- 3- to 12-mL syringes.
- A three-way stopcock attached to an extension set (optional).

TECHNIQUE

Closed or Open Needle Abdominocentesis

- Abdominocentesis site is just caudal to umbilicus, on ventral midline or slightly lateral to the right (2–3 cm in mid-sized dogs). In a standing patient, site is at most dependent part of abdomen.
- A 10 × 10 cm area should be clipped, and skin prepared aseptically.
- Lidocaine 2% local anesthetic may be infused at the abdominocentesis site.
- Needle is inserted through skin and abdominal wall; if using an over-the-needle catheter, catheter is fed off stylet once in the abdomen (typically fluid visible in hub):
  - If needle or catheter is not attached to a syringe, collect the fluid into a sterile tube as it drips from the hub (this technique may introduce air into abdomen).
  - If needle or catheter is attached to syringe or extension set and syringe, apply gentle suction; vigorous suction may result in false-negative result.
- Collect fluid aseptically, perform cytologic analysis, bacteriologic culture, other diagnostics as indicated.
- For therapeutic abdominocentesis, extension set and 3-way stopcock are mounted on needle or catheter and attached to a syringe.

- When using an over-the-needle catheter with added fenestrations, take care to remove it completely by gently rotating it or dissecting it from subcutaneous tissue.

Four-Quadrant Abdominocentesis

- Divide ventral surface of abdomen into 4 quadrants by an imaginary line that bisects linea alba and through the umbilicus.
- Wide surgical prep centered at umbilicus.
- Insert needles, one at a time, in each quadrant until fluid is retrieved.
- Fluid should flow through needle into sampling tubes.
- False-negative results more likely if suction applied.

Ultrasound-Guided Abdominocentesis

- Locate small volume or localized effusion with ultrasonography.
- Clip hair on a 10 × 10 cm area and prepare aseptically.
- Mount needle on syringe or extension set attached to syringe, insert under ultrasound guidance into pocket of fluid and gently aspirate.

Diagnostic Peritoneal Lavage (Closed Technique)

- Consider imaging (abdominal radiographs, CT, or ultrasound) prior to DPL as this procedure will alter results.
- DPL site is 1–3 cm caudal to umbilicus, on midline or just right from midline.
- Wide surgical prep centered at umbilicus.
- Infiltrate skin and abdominal wall with local anesthetic at puncture site.
- Make a stab incision through skin with a number 11 scalpel blade at site of local anesthetic infusion.
- Introduce catheter with stylet into abdomen through stab incision.
- Slide catheter off stylet dorsocaudally into abdomen.
- Once catheter is in abdomen, attach syringe and aspirate gently. If fluid is retrieved, there is no need to proceed with lavage.
- In the absence of fluid, infuse 20–22 mL/kg of warm sterile 0.9% saline solution through catheter using an IV infusion set with rapid gravity flow.
- After completing infusion, have patient walk around (if able) or roll patient gently from side to side to disperse fluid, taking care not to dislodge catheter.
- Aspirate catheter gently with a syringe to remove fluid sample. Most often, only a small portion of instilled fluid is retrieved; remaining fluid will be reabsorbed by peritoneum.
- Collect lavage fluid aseptically and analyze.

SAMPLE HANDLING

- Inspect fluid macroscopically for clarity and color.
- Divide fluid into aliquots:
  - EDTA tube for cytologic evaluation, including red blood cell and nucleated cell counts and differential (*not* for culture).
  - A serum tube for biochemical analysis as indicated (may need concurrent analysis on peripheral blood; see below).
  - A culturette or an additive-free glass tube, for aerobic and anaerobic bacterial culture, depending on laboratory preference.
- Determine specific gravity and total solids (TS) by refractometry.
- Direct microscopic cytologic evaluation: smear small drop of fluid across a slide, air-dry, and apply Romanovsky-type stain (Diff-Quik, Hema III, Giemsa, or Wright stain). For hypocellular fluids (2,000–50,000 cells/μL), a drop from the resuspended pellet of a centrifuged sample can be evaluated. Cytospin preparation may be necessary for very hypocellular (<2,000 cells/μL) samples.
- Measure packed cell volume (PCV) and TS of hemorrhagic effusions. Consider the following paired biochemical tests based on differential diagnoses:
  - Uroabdomen: creatinine, potassium.
  - Bile peritonitis: bilirubin.
  - Pancreatitis: lipase, amylase, cPLI.
  - Chyloabdomen: triglycerides, cholesterol.
  - Septic peritonitis: glucose, lactate.
  - FIP: protein electrophoresis.

APPROPRIATE AFTERCARE

Post-Procedure Patient Monitoring

Usually none, but should be tailored to patient's general condition (e.g., shock, pain).

Nursing Care

None

Dietary Modification

None

Medication Requirements

Analgesia might be required.

Restrictions on Activity

Cage rest, as needed, depending on patient's clinical signs.

Anticipated Recovery Tme

N/A

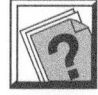

INTERPRETATION

NORMAL FINDINGS OR RANGE

- Absence of free intra-abdominal fluid.
- In normal dogs, lavage fluid WBC count is <500–1,000 cells/μL.
- Postsurgery lavage fluid WBC count can be up to 10,000 cells/μL. Cytologic characteristics are more meaningful than cell count in differentiating septic vs. nonseptic peritonitis in these cases.

ABNORMAL VALUES

- Presence of free intra-abdominal fluid.
- Lavage fluid with >1,000 WBCs/μL or that is grossly abnormal (e.g., hemorrhagic, greenish, cloudy, purulent).
- Depending on macroscopic appearance, specific gravity, protein content, cellularity, and cytologic findings, abdominal effusion is classified as pure transudate, modified transudate, and exudate (septic and nonseptic). Its etiology can sometimes be determined.

Additional Results for Specific Conditions

- Chyloabdomen—concentration of abdominal fluid triglycerides higher than serum triglyceride concentration; triglyceride concentration often >100 mg/dL.
- FIP—abdominal fluid albumin/globulin ratio <0.8 suggests FIP.
- Hemoabdomen—if PCV of abdominal fluid is greater than peripheral PCV, organ or large vessel laceration or disruption is suspected. Hemodilution may occur in cases of uroabdomen with concurrent hemorrhage or after DPL. Because DPL fluid cannot be compared with peripheral PCV, a PCV >5% in DPL fluid is indicative of hemorrhage.
- Uroabdomen—abdominal fluid creatinine concentration higher than serum creatinine concentration (>2:1), potassium concentration in effusion greater than serum potassium (>1.4:1). BUN is not reliable for diagnosis of uroabdomen (rapidly equilibrates across peritoneum).
- Bile peritonitis—fluid bilirubin concentration higher than that of serum, extra- or intracellular bile pigment usually found on cytologic examination.
- Pancreatitis—higher fluid amylase and lipase concentrations than serum suggest pancreatitis. Peritoneal fluid canine-specific pancreatic lipase (cPL) concentration is very sensitive in dogs as an aid in diagnosis of acute pancreatitis.
- Peritonitis—>1,000 WBCs/μL in lavage fluid.
- Septic peritonitis—intracellular bacteria (± extracellular bacteria), presence of degenerate neutrophils are diagnostic for septic effusion. Additionally, the fluid lactate concentration is higher in septic vs. nonseptic effusions. In dogs, a fluid lactate concentration >2.5–4 mmol/L and a blood-to-fluid lactate difference of >2 mmol/L has good sensitivity and specificity for diagnosing septic effusion. This may be less reliable in cats. A blood-to-fluid glucose difference of >37 mg/dL is sensitive and specific for septic peritoneal effusion in dogs and cats.
- Eosinophilic effusion—>10% eosinophils in fluid.
- Aberrant cestodiasis—the presence of *Mesocestoides* spp.

CRITICAL VALUES

- After adequate cardiovascular resuscitation, the following conditions need immediate attention and might require exploratory celiotomy:
  - Septic peritonitis.
  - Uroabdomen.
  - Bile peritonitis.
  - Hemoabdomen.

INTERFERING FACTORS

Drugs That May Alter Results of the Procedure

Avoid sedative agents that induce splenomegaly.

Conditions That May Interfere with Performing the Procedure

- If there is abdominal distention, differentiate between organomegaly, intra-abdominal fat, and fluid accumulation before abdominocentesis.
- Adhesions from previous surgeries may interfere with DPL.
- Insufficient fluid quantity for technique used.
- Flocculent or fibrinous fluid.
- Fluid localized in a difficult to access space (e.g., cranial to liver).
- Negative abdominocentesis is possible in a patient with an acute disease process. Repeat imaging and/or abdominocentesis can be considered if indicated based on clinical signs and increased suspicion of intra-abdominal disease.
- A negative abdominocentesis is possible in a patient with severe dehydration or hypovolemia; repeat imaging and abdominocentesis following IV fluid resuscitation.

Procedure Techniques or Handling That May Alter Results

- Vigorous suction can result in needle or catheter blockage by omentum or viscera.
- In the absence of coagulopathy, blood from traumatic sampling will usually clot when exposed to an artificial surface, whereas peritoneal effusion will not.
- Degenerate neutrophils and intracellular bacteria are signs of septic peritonitis; while bacteria and debris may be present if a loop of bowel is aspirated, typically degenerate neutrophils are absent.

Influence of Signalment on Performing and Interpreting the Procedure

Species

None

Breed

None

Age

None

Gender

None

Pregnancy

Relative contraindication because of an enlarged uterus.

Clinical Perspective

- Many different diseases may manifest with peritoneal effusion; cytologic and fluid analysis are indicated for every effusion.
- Use of a fenestrated catheter vs. a needle may increase likelihood of fluid retrieval.
- DPL may provide superior diagnostic accuracy but is much more time intensive to perform, and samples are diluted.

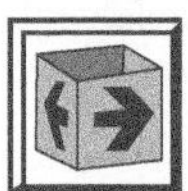

MISCELLANEOUS

ANCILLARY TESTS

- CBC, serum biochemistry, and urinalysis.
- Abdominal ultrasonography: assess parenchymal integrity, identify small fluid volume.
- Any additional testing to determine primary etiology of abdominal effusion (nonexhaustive list; see Ascites):
  - Thoracic radiography, echocardiogram, and ECG (right-sided heart failure, pericardial effusion, metastatic neoplasia).
  - Excretory urography or contrast cystourethrogram if uroabdomen is suspected.
  - Serum bile acids if hepatic failure/portal hypertension is suspected.

SYNONYMS

- Abdominal tap.

SEE ALSO

Ascites.

ABBREVIATIONS

- DPL = diagnostic peritoneal lavage.
- PCV = packed cell volume.
- TS = total solids.

Suggested Reading

Bonczynski JJ, Ludwig LL, Barton LJ, et al. Comparison of peritoneal fluid and peripheral blood pH, bicarbonate, glucose, and lactate concentration as a diagnostic tool for septic peritonitis in dogs and cats. Vet Surg 2003; 32:161–166.

Chartier MA, Hill SL, Sunico S, et al. Pancreas-specific lipase concentrations and amylase and lipase activities in the peritoneal fluid of dogs with suspected peritonitis. Vet J 2014, 201: 385–389.

Connally HE. Cytology and fluid analysis of the acute abdomen. Clin Tech Small Anim Pract 2003, 18:39–44.

Jandry KE. Abdominocentesis and diagnostic peritoneal lavage. In: Silverstein D, Hopper K, eds., Small Animal Critical Care Medicine, 2nd ed. St. Louis, MO: Elsevier, 2015, pp1036–1039.

Koenig A, Verlander LL. Usefulness of whole blood, plasma, peritoneal fluid, and peritoneal fluid supernatant glucose concentrations obtained by a veterinary POC glucometer to identify septic peritonitis in dogs with peritoneal effusion. J Am Vet Med Assoc 2015, 247:1027–1032.

Levin GM, Bonczynski JJ, Ludwig LL, et al. Lactate as a diagnostic test for septic peritoneal effusions in dogs and cats. J Am Anim Hosp Assoc 2004; 40:364371.

Martiny P, Goggs R. Biomarker guided diagnosis of septic peritonitis in dogs. Front Vet Sci 2019, 6:208.

Schmiedt C, Tobias, KM, Otto CM. Evaluation of abdominal fluid: peripheral blood creatinine and potassium ratios for diagnosis of uroperitoneum in dogs. J Vet Emerg Crit Care 2001, 11:275–280.

Author Kim Slensky

Consulting Editor Benjamin M. Brainard

Acknowledgment The author and editors acknowledge the prior contribution of Karine Savary Bataille.

ARTHROCENTESIS WITH SYNOVIAL FLUID ANALYSIS

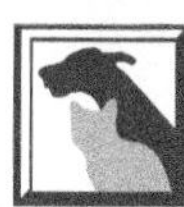

BASICS

TYPE OF PROCEDURE

Diagnostic sample collection.

PROCEDURE EXPLANATION AND RELATED PHYSIOLOGY

Synovial fluid is normally a clear, viscous fluid essential in the mechanical function of joints. Synovial fluid analysis is integral in the diagnosis and characterization of joint disease in canine and feline patients. Joint disease can involve one or more joints and can be due to infectious, inflammatory or noninflammatory etiologies. Synovial fluid analysis can differentiate inflammatory vs. noninflammatory arthropathies and can aid in determination of the underlying cause. Arthrocentesis is a safe, quick, and relatively easy procedure to perform in most clinical settings and involves fine-needle aspiration of joint fluid. The equipment needed is minimal and inexpensive, and the techniques are not difficult to learn, requiring only basic knowledge of joint anatomy.

INDICATIONS

- Joint pain or effusion.
- Lameness/stiffness or gait abnormality.
- Fever of unknown origin.
- Undefined lethargy or nonspecific pain.

CONTRAINDICATIONS

- No absolute contraindications.
- Caution with coagulopathy.
- Caution with severe thrombocytopenia (<20,000/μL).

POTENTIAL COMPLICATIONS

- Sedation-associated complications.
- Iatrogenic joint infection.
- Hemarthrosis.

CLIENT EDUCATION

- Patients will need to be sedated.
- Patients will need to have multiple joints shaved.

BODY SYSTEMS ASSESSED

Musculoskeletal

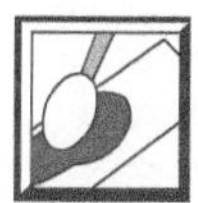

PROCEDURE

PATIENT PREPARATION

Pre-Procedure Medication or Preparation

None

Anesthesia or Sedation

- Adequate sedation required.
- Opioids for pain control:
  - Hydromorphone 0.05–0.1 mg/kg IM or IV.
  - Methadone 0.1–0.3 mg/kg IM or IV.
  - Fentanyl 3–5 μg/kg IV.
- Dexmedetomidine 3–10 μg/kg IM or IV to effect.
- General anesthesia often not required.

Patient Positioning

Lateral recumbency.

Patient Monitoring

Standard for sedation protocol.

Equipment or Supplies

- Clippers.
- Surgical prep—chlorhexidine scrub/betadine scrub.
- Alcohol prep.
- Sterile gloves.
- Sterile hypodermic needles.
- 22-Gauge 1-inch needles (for cats and small dogs):
  - Most commonly used.
- 22-Gauge 1½-inch needles (may be needed for large dogs).
- Sterile 3-mL syringes.
- A culturette or culture transport vial.
- Glass microscope slides.
- EDTA tubes.

TECHNIQUE

- Prior to starting the procedure, have all equipment in place and familiarize yourself with the anatomy of the selected joint (Figures 1–5).
- It is recommended to sample three or more joints.
- Clip overlying hair and aseptically prepare the chosen joint.
- It is essential to appropriately prepare sites to avoid iatrogenic joint infection.
- Don sterile gloves.
- An assistant opens the syringe and needles, aseptically placing them on the sterile field. The needle should be mounted on the syringe.
- Flex the joint using the nondominant hand (now nonsterile) and palpate the appropriate landmarks for the specific joint to be tapped with the dominant hand (sterile).
- Holding the syringe, pass the needle through the skin, joint capsule, and synovial membrane, into the joint cavity. Avoid the articular cartilage. If bone is encountered, pull back slightly and redirect the needle into the joint space.
- Gently aspirate. Unless the joint is severely distended, only a few drops of fluid may be obtained in the hub of the needle. As soon as fluid appears in the hub of the needle, release negative pressure and remove the needle from the joint. If the joint is very distended, a larger volume of fluid may be removed from the joint space. If blood is seen in the hub of the needle at any point in the procedure, immediately release pressure and remove the needle.
- Ensure that the negative pressure (the plunger) is released prior to withdrawing the syringe from the point to avoid contamination of the fluid with peripheral blood.
- A large amount of blood makes cytologic evaluation too difficult, and tapping a new joint space is advisable. A small amount of blood may be in the joint space as part of the disease process.

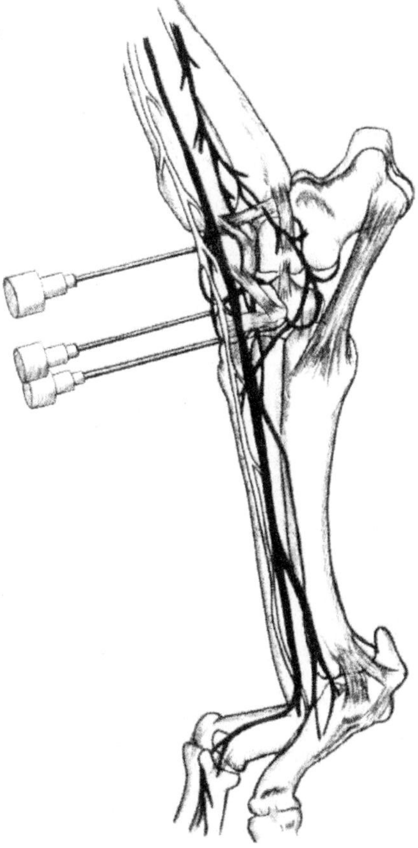

Figure 1.

Schematic representation of landmarks for the carpal joint.

Note: The following discussion about individual joints is presented in order of increasing difficulty:

Carpal Joint

- With the nondominant hand, flex the joint to achieve a maximum amount of open joint space.
- Palpate the space between the radius and proximal carpal bones, the proximal carpal bones and distal carpal bones, and the carpal and metacarpal bones.
- The radiocarpal joint is the most common joint space to tap due to the larger space.
- Identify and avoid the dorsal common digital artery and accessory cephalic vein.
- Holding the syringe, insert the needle from the cranial surface through the skin and joint capsule and into the joint space.

Stifle Joint

- Due to its large size, this joint is frequently aspirated.
- The stifle may be approached from either the medial or lateral aspect.

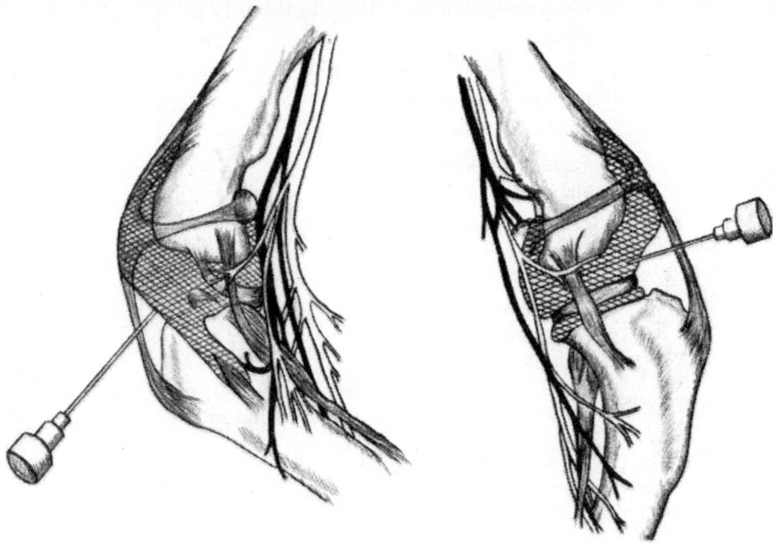

Figure 2.

Schematic representation of landmarks for the stifle joint.

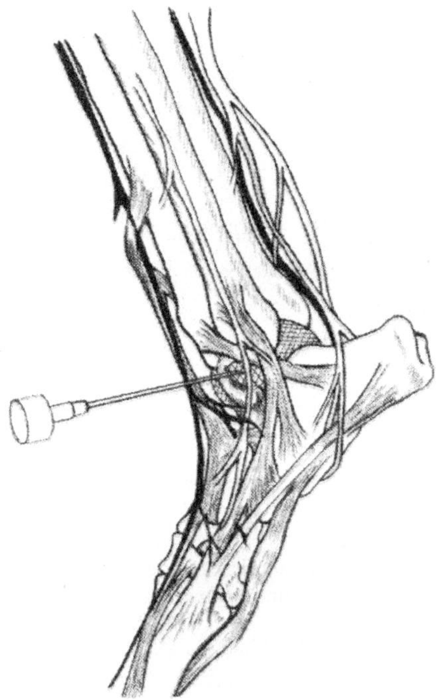

Figure 3.

Schematic representation of landmarks for the tarsal joint.

- Flex the stifle joint to open the joint space.
- Insert the needle from the cranial aspect, lateral or medial to the patellar ligament. The needle should enter the joint approximately halfway between the patella and tibial tuberosity.
- Direct the needle caudally and obliquely toward the intercondylar space.
- It may be helpful to apply digital pressure to the opposite side of the patellar ligament to cause joint fluid to collect toward the approach. A fat pad is present that may interfere with obtaining fluid. If fluid is not obtained initially, back up the needle, redirect, and aspirate.

Tarsal Joint

- Two small joint spaces can be tapped in the tarsus.
- One approach is to flex the joint slightly and palpate the cranial space between the tibia and tibiotarsal bone. Insert the needle from the cranial and lateral aspect and direct it medially. This joint is shallow and the needle will not be advanced very far.
- The second approach is from the distal aspect and is accomplished by flexing the tarsal joint more fully to open the space between the distal fibula, tibia, and calcaneus bones. Palpate this space and insert the needle from a caudolateral position. The needle should be advanced parallel to the calcaneus distally and slightly medially.

Elbow

- The elbow is flexed moderately to an approximately 45 degree angle. This opens the space between the humerus and the ulna.
- The joint is entered from the caudolateral aspect.
- Insert the needle between the olecranon process and the lateral condyle of the humerus and advance it distally and slightly medially, following the cranial surface of the ulna.

Scapulohumeral Joint

- Flex the joint slightly to widen the space. Palpate the greater tubercle and the acromion process of the scapula.
- Approach the joint from the lateral aspect and insert the needle slightly cranial and distal to the acromion process and just caudal to the greater tubercle. The needle should be directed in a caudal-medial and slightly downward direction.
- The joint space can be approached also from a cranial direction. Insert the needle medial to the greater tubercle and ventral to the supraglenoid tubercle, angling it in a cranial-caudal direction.

SAMPLE HANDLING

- Joint fluid should be evaluated grossly for color, turbidity, viscosity, quantity, and ability to clot. A change in the color or viscosity of the joint fluid can indicate disease or blood contamination.
- If the sample is contaminated with blood by a traumatic tap, the blood usually does not mix evenly, whereas blood from ongoing hemorrhage into the joint appears evenly distributed.
- Viscosity is assessed by expelling one to two drops of fluid from the syringe onto a slide. If the fluid is easily expelled, the viscosity is low. Formation of a string of fluid as it leaves the needle is consistent with normal viscosity.
- Many taps yield only a few drops of fluid, and complete fluid analysis may be difficult. Slides should always be submitted for cytologic evaluation because determining the type of cells in the fluid is the most helpful piece of information in defining the disease process.
- If enough fluid can be obtained, a small amount of the sample should be placed in an EDTA tube for fluid analysis.
- Culture and microbial sensitivity testing should performed. The probability of bacterial infection is greater in patients that have monoarthropathies and purulent-appearing joint fluid.

APPROPRIATE AFTERCARE

Post-Procedure Patient Monitoring

- Standard for sedation protocol
- Monitor for increased joint pain or swelling.

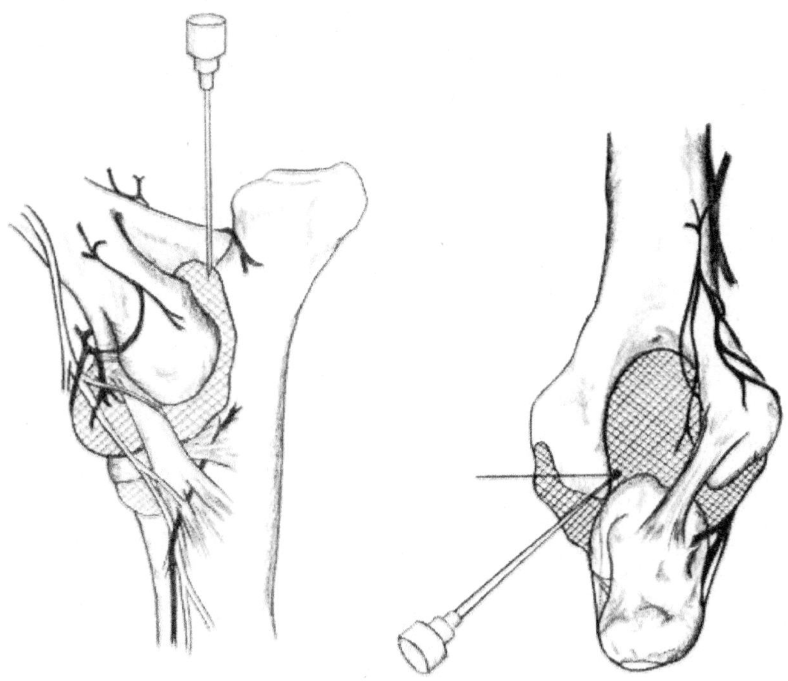

Figure 4.

Schematic representation of landmarks for the elbow joint.

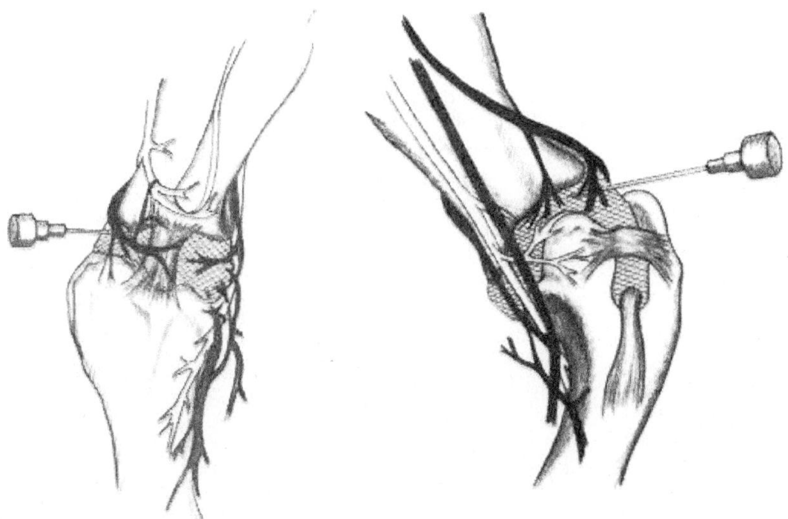

Figure 5.

Schematic representation of landmarks for the shoulder joint.

Nursing Care

None

Dietary Modification

• In some cases, weight reduction is recommended.
• Specific diets are available for dogs with joint disease.

Medication Requirements

Dependent on primary disease process.

Restrictions on Activity

• Dependent on primary disease process.
• Allow patient to dictate activity level.

Anticipated Recovery Time

Immediate after recovery from sedation.

INTERPRETATION

NORMAL FINDINGS OR RANGE

See Table 1.

CRITICAL VALUES

None

INTERFERING FACTORS

Drugs That May Alter Results of the Procedure

None

Conditions That May Interfere with Performing the Procedure

• Coagulopathy.
• Severe skin disease or infection.

ARTHROCENTESIS WITH SYNOVIAL FLUID ANALYSIS (CONTINUED)

Table 1

Abnormal values.

Variable	*Normal*	*Trauma/Hemarthrosis*	*Degenerative Arthropathy*	*Inflammatory Arthropathy*
Appearance	Clear-to-straw colored	Clear-to-red	Clear-to-yellow	Yellow-to-bloody, hazy/cloudy
Protein	<2.5 g/dL	Variable	<2.5 g/dL	Often >2.5 g/dL
Viscosity	High	Decreased	Normal/decreased	Decreased
Nucleated cell count (cells/μL)	<3,000	Increased RBCs	1,000–10,000	5,000 to >100,000
Neutrophils	<5%	Relative to blood	<10%	>10–100%
Mononuclear cells	>95%	Relative to blood	>90%	10–<90%
Comments	Small volume of fluid	Erythophagia	Macrophages	Wide variation

Procedure Techniques or Handling That May Alter Results

Traumatic tap with blood contamination.

Influence of Signalment on Performing and Interpreting the Procedure

Species

- Feline chronic progressive polyarthropathy has been documented in male cats.
- Bacterial L-form infection can cause a severe, erosive polyarthritis in cats.
- Calicivirus (both by natural infection and by vaccination) can cause a transient polyarthritis in young kittens.

Breed

- Arthrocentesis may be more difficult to perform in small-breed dogs.
- An erosive polyarthropathy has been documented in young greyhounds.
- Swollen hock syndrome occurs in shar-peis.

Age

None

Gender

None

Pregnancy

None

CLINICAL PERSPECTIVE

- An accurate medical history noting trauma and travel history and drug and toxin (e.g., NSAID, anticoagulant) exposure should be taken.
- Physical examination should include a thorough musculoskeletal and neurologic examination to differentiate joint disease from primary orthopedic or neurologic problems. Although careful attention must be paid to evaluating joints for effusion and pain with flexion or extension, it is extremely important to note that significant joint disease can be present despite a lack of abnormalities on joint palpation.
- Initial diagnostic testing that should be considered before joint taps are performed include a CBC, serum biochemistry analysis, urinalysis with a urine culture, and radiographs of affected and corresponding nonaffected joints. Vector-borne disease testing should be performed. A coagulation panel can be submitted if hemarthrosis secondary to toxicity or inherited disease is suspected. Further studies, such as additional serologic testing for infectious disease and systemic testing for immune-mediated disease, should be considered when appropriate historical or clinical signs are present. Blood cultures may also be performed to look for a systemic infectious cause of joint inflammation/infection.
- Occasionally (especially in cats), fever and lethargy are the sole presenting signs in animals with polyarthritis.
- It may be difficult to obtain good samples from cats and small dogs.
- Cell counts in normal synovial fluid are low and predominantly contain lymphocytes and mononuclear cells; increased neutrophil count is indicative of disease.
- Once an inflammatory process is defined, there is considerable overlap in cytologic findings between the specific causes of inflammation:
    - In general, inflammatory disease is characterized by increased numbers of neutrophils and a variable increase in large, mononuclear cells in the joint fluid. Septic joints tend to have very high numbers of neutrophils, which may also exhibit degenerative changes. Bacterial organisms are usually not seen; *Ehrlichia* sp. morulae are seen infrequently. Increased numbers of nondegenerate neutrophils are generally seen with an immune-mediated process. A more complete review of cytologic changes in joint disease can be found in the Suggested Reading section.
- Rheumatoid arthritis, an erosive disease of the distal joints in small dogs, is extremely rare. Radiographs are helpful in making this diagnosis. Rheumatoid factor analysis is not necessary in the majority of cases.
- Reactive polyarthritis may be seen secondary to systemic infectious disease, drugs, neoplasia, or any chronic inflammatory condition.
- With proper technique, significant complications are very rare.

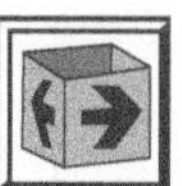

MISCELLANEOUS

ANCILLARY TESTS

- Radiographs: affected and unaffected joint.
- Infectious disease testing (Lyme, *Ehrlichia*, heartworm, *Leishmania*, *Toxoplasma*).
- Antinuclear antibody serology.
- Urine protein/creatinine ratio.
- Rheumatoid factor.

SYNONYMS

Joint tap.

SEE ALSO

- Arthritis (Osteoarthritis).
- Arthritis, Septic.
- Lameness.
- Polyarthritis, Erosive, Immune-Mediated.
- Polyarthritis, Nonerosive, Immune-Mediated, Dogs.

Suggested Reading

Baker R, Lumsden JH. Synovial fluid. In: Color Atlas of the Cytology of the Dog and Cat. St Louis, MO: CV Mosby, 2000, pp. 209–221.

Crow SE, Walshaw SO. Manual of Clinical Procedures in the Dog and Cat. Philadelphia, PA: JB Lippincott, 1987, pp. 196–197.

MacWilliams PS, Friedrichs KR. Laboratory evaluation and interpretation of synovial fluid. Vet Clin North Am Small Anim Pract 2003, 33:153–178.

Taylor SM. Joint disorders. In: Nelson RW, Couto CG, eds., Small Animal Internal Medicine. St. Louis, MO: CV Mosby, 2003, pp. 1071–1092.

Author Rebecca A.L. Walton

Consulting Editor Benjamin M. Brainard

Acknowledgment The author and editors acknowledge the prior contribution of Karyn Harrell

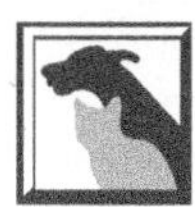

BASICS

TYPE OF SPECIMEN

Blood
Fluid
Tissue
Urine
Feces

TEST EXPLANATION AND RELATED PHYSIOLOGY

Culture and sensitivity testing to aid in diagnosis of infectious disease is one of the most common tests in the diagnostic laboratory. Proper specimen selection and collection are crucial to proper diagnosis. In addition, it is important to distinguish normal flora from infectious agents. When possible, samples for bacterial culture should be collected prior to the initiation of antimicrobial therapy as systemic antibiotic administration can impair microbial growth *in vitro*.

Different methodologies may be used to determine antimicrobial susceptibility. Kirby-Bauer disc diffusion and serial antibiotic dilution to determine minimum inhibitory concentrations (MICs) are two of these methods. In addition to susceptibility data, it is important to understand the physiology of the location of infection as this can also affect antimicrobial selection.

INDICATIONS

To identify bacteria causing infection and determine the most appropriate therapy

CONTRAINDICATIONS

None

POTENTIAL COMPLICATIONS

None

CLIENT EDUCATION

None

BODY SYSTEMS ASSESSED

Dependent on location of infection.

SAMPLE

SAMPLE COLLECTION

The sample depends on the site of potential infection.

- Swab the site (e.g., ear, discharge) by using a sterile swab. Swabs tipped with inert, nontoxic rayon are preferred.
- Fine-needle aspirate—aseptic preparation of the aspiration site is important to prevent contamination of sample with normal skin flora.
- 0.5–1.0 mL of urine—cystocentesis is the method of choice. Aseptic catheterization can also be used, although quantitiative urine culture is preferred for these samples. Voided urine is not preferred due to potential contamination from the external urinary tract, and results must be interpreted in the context of quantitative data.
- 0.5–1.0 mL of effusion.
- Material aspirated from a lesion (e.g., abscess).
- Venous blood—sample size determined by manufacturer of the culture bottle and patient size, but larger sample volumes are preferred.
- Feces.
- Tissue biopsy.
- Wash fluid (tracheal wash, nasal flush, prostatic wash).

SAMPLE HANDLING

Aseptically prepare the skin prior to any percutaneous aspiration. Wounds should be cleaned and lavaged prior to collection of culture sample. For skin lesions, remove surface exudate by wiping with sterile saline or 70% alcohol prior to sample collection.

Aerobic Culture

- Sterile swab—swabs should be placed into some type of microorganism collection and transport container (e.g., BactiSwab, Remel, Lenexa, KS; BBL CultureSwab, Becton-Dickinson, Franklin Lakes, NJ). These containers typically consist of a round-bottomed sleeve designed to protect the sample. Some transport systems contain medium designed to enhance survival of any microorganisms present. When using a transport container with media, ensure that swab is completely immersed in culture medium.
- Submit fluids (urine, effusion, aspirated material, wash solutions) in a sterile tube with or without media. Plain red-top tubes are acceptable, but the use of serum separator tubes or plastic red-top tubes with clot activator should be avoided.
- Biopsy—place sample in a sterile container and add several drops of sterile 0.9% saline to keep tissue moist.
- Catheter tip—5 cm of the distal tip is sterilly cut and placed into a sterile container for transport.

Anaerobic Culture

- Tissue or aspirates of deep material are always superior to superficial swab specimens.
- If a swab must be used, pass it deep into the base of the lesion.
- Biopsy—place the sample in sterile container and add several drops of sterile saline to keep the tissue moist.
- If sample processing will be delayed >2 hours, place sample into a specific anaerobic transport tube or vial. Anaerobic transport medium is a mineral salt-base soft agar with reducing agents designed to maintain an anaerobic environment for an extended period, maintaining viability of more fastidious microorganisms.
- Swabs of material are plunged deep into the agar so that even though material at the top of the tube is exposed to oxygen, material at the bottom of the tube remains anaerobic.
- Transport fluids in an anaerobic transport vial. After cleaning the rubber stopper with alcohol, push the needle through the septum and inject the fluid on top of the anaerobic transport medium.
- Samples in anaerobic transport medium can generally be used for both aerobic and anaerobic cultures.

Fecal Culture

Use fecal transport medium when submitting for culture of *Salmonella*, *Shigella*, *Campylobacter*, and other fecal pathogens.

Mycoplasma Culture

Semen or mucus from respiratory tract can be submitted in a sterile container. Material can also be collected on a sterile swab and submitted in a microorganism transport container that contains Amies transport medium without charcoal, although this is not an optimal method.

Blood Culture

- Aseptically prepare venipuncture site.
- Remove the plastic cap covering each of 2 blood culture bottles and decontaminate each rubber stopper with 70% alcohol. It is best to have both aerobic and anaerobic types of vials, however, venting anaerobic vials to make them aerobic can be done.
- Collect blood using sterile needle and syringe. A minimum of 4 mL of blood (2 mL for each bottle) is necessary:
  - Better results may be achieved with larger sample volumes.
  - Sampling volume should be based on the manufacurer's recommendation for the blood culture bottles being used, the number of samples to be collected, and patient size.
- Change the needle prior to introducing sample into each bottle and divide sample between the two blood culture bottles; mix well:
  - Blood should be sampled at 2 or 3 time points, 30–60 minutes apart. Each collection should occur from a different location/vein if possible.

SAMPLE STORAGE

- To increase viability of organisms and prevent overgrowth, refrigerate samples for routine aerobic culture until shipped.
- Specimens for anaerobic culture, blood culture, and fecal culture should be maintained at room temperature:
  - All samples should be submitted/plated for culture as soon as possible to maximize results.

BACTERIAL CULTURE AND SENSITIVITY (CONTINUED)

SAMPLE STABILITY

Aerobes

Refrigerate for ≈2 days.

Anaerobes

- Stable in an anaerobic transport tube for 1–2 days (depends on organism).
- Stable in a red- top tube or standard microorganism collection and transport system for ≤2 hours.
- Refrigeration decreases viability.

PROTOCOL

None

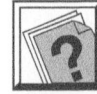

INTERPRETATION

NORMAL FINDINGS OR RANGE

- No growth of bacteria in culture from sterile fluids/sites.
- Growth of normal flora only, but no pathogenic organisms from nonsterile locations.

ABNORMAL VALUES

- Growth of pathogenic organisms.
- Kirby-Bauer microbial susceptibility results for antimicrobials are reported as either susceptible or resistant.
- Some antimicrobial susceptibility results are reported with an MIC, which is the lowest concentration of antibiotic that inhibits the growth of a given strain of bacteria. When using MICs to select an appropriate antimicrobial, three criteria are important:
  1. The MIC on the clinical microbiology report.
  2. The antimicrobial's normal range used to establish susceptibility. This represents the concentration of antibiotic that is reasonably achievable.
  3. The breakpoint of the antimicrobial—the dilution where the bacteria begin to show resistance.
- The breakpoint and the normal range differ by drug and bacterial species. Therefore, comparing antimicrobial MICs is based on differences between the breakpoint and the normal range for each antimicrobial. The further the MIC is from the breakpoint in its normal range, the more susceptible that organism is to the antimicrobial.

CRITICAL VALUES

None

INTERFERING FACTORS

Drugs That May Alter Results or Interpretation

Drugs That Interfere with Test Methodology

Systemic antibiotic administration can inhibit *in vitro* microbial growth.

Drugs That Alter Physiology

None

Disorders That May Alter Results

None

Collection Techniques or Handling That May Alter Results

- Specimens that are 2 days old may lose viability.
- Inappropriate containers:
  - EDTA is bacteriostatic.
  - The clot activator in serum-separator tubes and plastic red-top tubes may affect results.
  - Samples for anaerobic cultures have limited viability if not transported in specific anaerobic transport tubes.

Influence of Signalment

Species

None

Breed

None

Age

None

Gender

None

Pregnancy

None

LIMITATIONS OF TEST

- *Mycobacterium* sp. and *Nocardia* sp. are difficult to culture and must be specifically requested.
- MIC is just one of the criteria used to select an antimicrobial. Antimicrobial selection also depends on the location of infection, what dose and route of administration will achieve adequate concentrations at that site, and how long the infection needs to be treated.

Sensitivity, Specificity, and Positive and Negative Predictive Values

None

Valid If Run in a Human Lab?

Yes, although human laboratories may not be able to perform susceptibility testing for veterinary-only approved antimicrobials.

CLINICAL PERSPECTIVE

- In cultures from a mucosal surface (e.g., tracheal wash, nasal swab, vaginal discharge, urine collected by catheter or free catch), interpretation must consider the presence of normal flora:
  - Large numbers of a single microorganism in almost pure culture suggests a pathogenic process.
  - A mixture of ≥4 different organisms in light to moderate numbers suggests growth of normal flora.
  - Light growth from a sample submitted in enrichment broth suggests normal flora (or suppression of growth by antimicrobial therapy).
- Specific anaerobic transport containers are more expensive than routine microorganism collection and transport containers (and may not be provided gratis by diagnostic laboratories), but can be readily obtained from commercial distributors of microbiology supplies and improve the likelihood of documenting an anaerobic infection.
- Chances of documenting bacteremia are increased by submitting 2 sets of blood cultures collected from different venipuncture sites or from the same site 15–30 minutes apart.

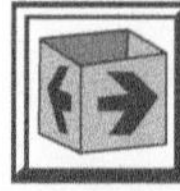

MISCELLANEOUS

ANCILLARY TESTS

Dependent on the site of infection.

SYNONYMS

- Aerobic culture.
- Anaerobic culture.
- Blood culture.

SEE ALSO

- Abscessation.
- Actinomycosis & Nocardia.
- Endocarditis, Infective.
- Nocardiosis/Actinomycosis—Cutaneous.
- Pneumonia, Bacterial.
- Prostatitis and Prostatic Abscess.
- Pyelonephritis.
- Pyothorax.
- Salmonellosis.
- Sepsis and Bacteremia.

ABBREVIATIONS

- MIC = minimum inhibitory concentration.

INTERNET RESOURCES

Becton Dickinson (BD) Diagnostic Systems, Product Center, http://www.bd.com/ds/productCenter/CT-PortACul.asp. Examples of anaerobic transport tubes/vials.

Suggested Reading

Aucoin D. Target: The Antimicrobial Reference Guide to Effective Treatment, 2nd ed. Port Huron, MI: North American Compendiums, 2002.

Jones RL. Laboratory diagnosis of bacterial infections. In: Greene CE, ed., Infectious Diseases of the Dog and Cat, 3rd ed. St. Louis, MO: Saunders Elsevier, 2006, pp. 267–273.

Mena E, Thompson FS, Armfield AY, et al. Evaluation of Port-A-Cul transport system for protection of anaerobic bacteria. J Clin Microbiol 1978, 8:28–35.

Author April E. Blong

Consulting Editor Benjamin M. Brainard

Acknowledgment The author and editors acknowledge the prior contribution of Terri Wheeler and Joyce S. Knoll.

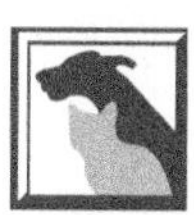

BASICS

TYPE OF SPECIMEN

Blood

TEST EXPLANATION AND RELATED PHYSIOLOGY

- Used to evaluate the acid–base status of patients:
  - Arterial samples may be used to evaluate the adequacy of oxygenation and ventilation.
  - Venous blood samples are not adequate for evaluation of oxygenation but may provide information about ventilation as long as perfusion is adequate.
- Normal physiologic reactions within the body occur at a specific pH value.
- Major variables evaluated when assessing acid–base status include the pH, HCO_3^- concentration, Pco_2 (partial pressure of CO_2), and base excess (or deficit). Abnormalities within acid–base status are typically classified as acidosis, alkalosis, or mixed disorders.
- Each disorder may be caused by metabolic and/or respiratory abnormalities:
  - The term *metabolic* implies a net gain or loss of HCO_3^-
  - The term *respiratory* implies a net gain or loss of CO_2.
- Pco_2 and pH are inversely proportional, whereas there is a direct relationship between HCO_3^- concentration and pH.
- To interpret acid–base balance:
  - Evaluate pH first—determine whether it is too high (alkalosis), too low (acidosis), or normal.
  - Alkalosis is classified as metabolic if due to elevated HCO_3^- concentration (>24 mmol/L) and respiratory if associated with a decreased Pco_2 (<36 mmHg).
  - Acidosis is classified as metabolic if associated with a decreased HCO_3^- concentration (<20 mmol/L), and respiratory if associated with an increased Pco_2 (>40 mmHg).
  - With mixed acid–base disorders, two problems may either exacerbate the disorder (e.g., concurrent respiratory and metabolic acidosis) or mask the problem, producing a normal pH if the two disorders have opposite effects (e.g., concurrent metabolic acidosis and respiratory alkalosis).
- Generally, an acid–base disturbance is accompanied by compensation by either the respiratory system or the kidneys. This compensation attempts to return the pH to an overall normal range, but it is important to note that full compensation never occurs:
  - Respiratory compensatory efforts occur immediately, whereas metabolic compensation will not reach its full level for 2–3 days because changes in renal handling of HCO_3^- require time. In severe metabolic alkalosis, respiratory compensatory attempts will be limited by the hypoxemia that accompanies hypoventilation.
- Hypoxemia is a partial pressure of oxygen (Pao_2) <90 mmHg at sea level. Hypoxemia has five potential underlying pathologies:
  - Low inspired oxygen concentration—may occur at altitude or with anesthetic machine malfunction
  - Ventilation–perfusion mismatch—reflects an altered balance between ventilated and perfused lung regions.
  - Pure shunt—caused by cardiac defects (e.g., tetralogy of Fallot)
  - Diffusion impairment—includes diseases that thicken the alveolar–capillary membrane.
  - Hypoventilation (i.e., a Pco_2 >50 mmHg).
- When assessing the oxygenation status of patients, it is prudent to consider not only the Pao_2 value but also to calculate the alveolar–arterial (A-a) gradient. The normal range is <15:
  - A-a gradient is calculated by subtracting the measured Pao_2 from the calculated ideal alveolar oxygen partial pressure (PAo_2) by using this formula:

$$PAO_2 = [\%\text{ inspired } O_2 \times (\text{atmospheric} - \text{water-vapor pressure})] - (PaCO_2/0.8)$$

  - For example, breathing room air at sea level, normal dogs with a Pao_2 of 95 mmHg and a Pco_2 of 40 mmHg, the PAo_2 will be $[0.21(760 - 47)] - (40/0.8) = 150 - 50 = 100$. The measured Pao_2 of 95 mmHg is subtracted from this value to get an A-a gradient of 5.
  - This formula is particularly useful if a patient has marked hyper- or hypoventilation.
  - For example, a dog with a Pao_2 of 84 and a Pco_2 of 22 is hyperventilating. However, calculation of the A-a gradient gives a value of 38.5, which is elevated, suggesting that increased respiratory rate is compensating for primary lung disease.
  - Conversely, in a dog with Pao_2 of 65 and a Pco_2 of 59, the A-a gradient is 11.25, which is normal, which indicates that hypoventilation, and subsequent hypoxemia, is caused by some disorder other than primary lung disease.
  - At increasing inspired-oxygen concentrations, the A-a gradient becomes less accurate. Thus, if the concentration of inspired oxygen is directly known, a ratio of the Pao_2 to the fractional inspired oxygen concentration (Fio_2) may be calculated. The normal value for the Pao_2/Fio_2 is 100:0.21 or 476. In people and dogs, acute lung injury is present at a ratio <300 and acute respiratory distress syndrome at a ratio <200.

INDICATIONS

- Assessment of acid–base balance.
- Assessment of oxygenation (arterial samples only).

CONTRAINDICATIONS

- Avoid arterial collection when patients have severe coagulopathy.
- Avoid arterial collection when patients have cellulitis or open infection at the collection site.

POTENTIAL COMPLICATIONS

- Hematoma at the sampling site.
- Collection of a venous sample instead of intended arterial sample and subsequent inappropriate patient management decisions.

CLIENT EDUCATION

None

BODY SYSTEMS ASSESSED

- Cardiovascular.
- Endocrine and metabolic.
- Renal and urologic.
- Respiratory.

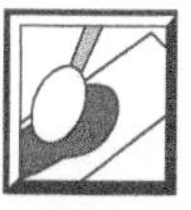

SAMPLE

SAMPLE COLLECTION

- Venous or arterial blood.
- Typically, heparinized blood samples are analyzed. Self-filling syringes are commercially available and routinely used for arterial samples.

SAMPLE HANDLING

- Samples should be collected under anaerobic conditions for the most accurate Pco_2 and HCO_3^- values.
- Samples should be processed immediately to prevent altered values.
- Samples exposed to room air will have an increased Pao_2 and decreased Pco_2.

SAMPLE STORAGE

If immediate analysis is not possible, samples may be stored anaerobically on ice for 4 hours.

SAMPLE STABILITY

For 4–6 hours if kept on ice.

PROTOCOL

None

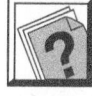

INTERPRETATION

NORMAL FINDINGS OR RANGE

- pH: 7.36–7.44.
- Pco_2: 36–40 mmHg.
- HCO_3^-: 20–24 mEq/L (or mmol/L).
- Base excess: ±4.

BLOOD GAS INTERPRETATION (CONTINUED)

- Po_2: 90–100 mmHg (at sea level, breathing room air [21% oxygen]).
- Reference intervals may vary, depending on sea level, laboratory, and assay.

ABNORMAL FINDINGS

Values above or below the reference range.

CRITICAL VALUES

- pH: <7.2 or >7.5.
- Pco_2: <20 or >55 mmHg.
- Po_2: <60 mmHg (arterial sample).
- HCO_3^-: <13 or >33 mmol/L.
- Base excess (or deficit): >12.

INTERFERING FACTORS

Drugs That May Alter Results or Interpretation

Drugs That Interfere with Test Methodology

None

Drugs That Alter Physiology

Supplemental oxygen, bicarbonate infusions, carbonic anhydrase inhibitors.

Disorders That May Alter Results

None

Collection Techniques or Handling That May Alter Results

- Difficulty in arterial puncture may result in either a fully or partially deoxygenated (venous) sample.
- Prolonged storage at room temperature will affect results.
- Administration of excessive heparin will dilute the sample and may result in altered values.
- Exposure of the sample to room air for an extended period of time (>1 minute).

Influence of Signalment

Species

Arterial blood–gas collection is very challenging in cats. Cats are thought to have a lower Pco_2 than other species.

Breed

Brachycephalic dogs may have a lower Pao_2, but this may reflect the relative difficulty of restraining them for sampling.

Age

Whereas in people, decreased Pao_2 accompanies aging, this has not been found to be true in one study in dogs. A-a gradient may increase slightly with age.

Gender

None

Pregnancy

Advanced pregnancy in humans may cause an altered respiratory pattern that produces respiratory alkalosis with a compensatory metabolic acidosis. Pao_2 is unchanged. This effect might be observed in late pregnancy in companion animals.

LIMITATIONS OF TEST

Sensitivity, Specificity, and Positive and Negative Predictive Values

N/A

Valid If Run in a Human Lab?

Yes.

CAUSES OF ABNORMAL FINDINGS

See Table 1.

Table 1

Causes of abnormal findings.

Analyte	*High Values*	*Low Values*
HCO_3^-	Metabolic alkalosis	Metabolic acidosis
	High GI obstruction	Poor perfusion (lactic acidosis)
	Profound hypokalemia	Renal failure
	Iatrogenic	Diabetic ketoacidosis
		Ethylene glycol intoxication
	Compensation for respiratory acidosis	Compensation for respiratory alkalosis
Pco_2	Respiratory acidosis	Respiratory alkalosis
	Severe respiratory failure	Panting
		Fever
	Cervical lesion	Pain
	Opioid overdose	Iatrogenic
	Large dog placed in lateral recumbency	
	Compensation for metabolic alkalosis	Compensation for metabolic acidosis
Po_2	Not significant	Hypoxemia
		Pulmonary disease
		Edema
		Contusions
		Pneumonia
		Pleural space disease
		Pneumothorax
		Pleural effusion
		Diaphragmatic hernia
		Cardiovascular shunts (e.g., tetralogy of Fallot)
		Hypoventilation
		Pain
		Respiratory depressants
		Intracranial disease
		Cervical disease

CLINICAL PERSPECTIVE

- Determine whether appropriate compensation is occurring or if two disorders are present. Guidelines for compensation are the following:
  - Metabolic acidosis—each 1 mEq/L decrease in HCO_3 will decrease Pco_2 by 0.7 mmHg.
  - Metabolic alkalosis—each 1 mEq/L increase in HCO_3 will increase Pco_2 by 0.7 mmHg.
  - Respiratory acidosis.
    - Acute—each 1 mmHg increase in Pco_2 will increase HCO_3 by 0.15 mEq/L.
    - Chronic—each 1 mmHg increase in Pco_2 will increase HCO_3 by 0.35 mEq/L.
  - Respiratory alkalosis:
    - Acute—each 1 mmHg decrease in Pco_2 will decrease HCO_3 by 0.25 mEq/L.
    - Chronic—each 1 mmHg decrease in Pco_2 will decrease HCO_3 by 0.55 mEq/L.
- Severe acidosis is common with ethylene glycol intoxication.
- All assessments of oxygenation should include assessment of the Pco_2 and, if warranted, calculation of the A-a gradient or Pao_2/Fio_2.
- It is crucial to recognize that an arterial blood gas merely provides objective evidence as to degree of impairment, but it is not specific for the cause.

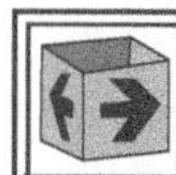

MISCELLANEOUS

ANCILLARY TESTS

- Serum biochemistry profile and urinalysis.
- Ethylene glycol test.
- Thoracic radiographs to look for cardiopulmonary disease.
- Echocardiography if heart may be affected.

SYNONYMS

- Oxygen (O_2) saturation.
- Partial pressure of carbon dioxide in blood (Pco_2).
- Partial pressure of oxygen in blood (Po_2).
- pH.

SEE ALSO

- Acidosis, Metabolic.
- Alkalosis, Metabolic.
- Diabetes Mellitus with Ketoacidosis.
- Ethylene Glycol Toxicosis.
- Hypoxemia.

ABBREVIATIONS

- A-a gradient = alveolar–arterial gradient.
- Fio_2 = fraction of inspired oxygen.
- HCO_3^- = bicarbonate.
- $Paco_2$ = arterial partial pressure of carbon dioxide.
- Pao_2 = arterial partial pressure of oxygen.
- PAo_2 = alveolar partial pressure of oxygen.

INTERNET RESOURCES

- Charlie's Clinical Calculators, MedCalc: acid–base calculator: http://www.medcalc.com/acidbase.html
- Colorado State University, College of Veterinary Medicine & Biomedical Sciences, Veterinary Emergency and Critical Care Medicine: Acid/base, blood gas interpretation [at high altitude]: http://www.cvmbs.colostate.edu/clinsci/wing/fluids/bloodgas.htm

Suggested Reading

King LG, Anderson JG, Rhodes WH, Hendricks JC. Arterial blood gas tensions in healthy aged dogs. Am J Vet Res 1992, 53:1744–1748.

Proulx J. Respiratory monitoring: arterial blood gas analysis, pulse oximetry, and end-tidal carbon dioxide analysis. Clin Tech Small Anim Pract 1999, 14:227–230.

Author Elizabeth Rozanski

Consulting Editor Benjamin M. Brainard

BLOOD PRESSURE DETERMINATION: NONINVASIVE AND INVASIVE

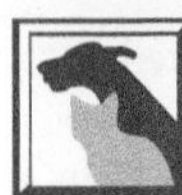

BASICS

TYPE OF PROCEDURE

Blood pressure measurement.

PROCEDURE EXPLANATION AND RELATED PHYSIOLOGY

- Blood pressure (BP) is the product of cardiac output and systemic vascular resistance. BP is indirectly related to organ perfusion, and the maintenance of normal BP is vital to maintaining organ function.
- Elevated (hypertension) and decreased (hypotension) BP can be seen in small animal patients:
  - Hypertension most commonly occurs secondary to concurrent diseases (e.g., renal disease, hyperthyroidism, hyperadrenocorticism, hyperaldosteronism, diabetes mellitus, obesity, and pheochromocytoma). Older cats may be hypertensive without a clear cause.
  - Hypotension can occur as a result of shock (e.g., anaphylaxis, hypovolemia, sepsis, cardiac failure), as well as with the administration of certain medications (e.g., anesthetics, arterial vasodilators).
- Indirect BP is measured using two main methodologies: Doppler ultrasonic flow probe and oscillometric:
  - Doppler can be used in cats and dogs, and readings can be obtained over a wide range of pressures, with variable heart rates. The Doppler measurement is likely between the systolic and mean arterial blood pressures, and should be interpreted as the systolic blood pressure to avoid misdiagnosis of hypotension.
  - Oscillometric devices record mean arterial BP and calculate diastolic and systolic blood pressure as well. They are less accurate in patients with extreme brady- or tachycardias, and may be difficult to use in small patients. They are easy to use and lend themselves well to screening exams.
- BP can be measured directly (also called invasively) by introducing a catheter into an artery and then connecting this catheter to an external pressure transducer. Direct BP measurement requires expertise for arterial catheter placement, as well as for obtaining reliable readings, and is generally not suited for routine use in awake patients.

INDICATIONS

- When signs of end-organ damage from hyper or hypotension are present, such as retinal hemorrhage and/or detachment, cardiac hypertrophy, or neurologic abnormalities.
- Part of full workup in patients with diseases known to cause hypertension.
- In patients with emergent clinical signs or those requiring critical care.
- Anesthetized patients.
- Patients receiving medications known to affect BP.

CONTRAINDICATIONS

- Indirect BP—none.
- Direct BP—patients who cannot be sedated or anesthetized, lack of appropriate skill or equipment.

POTENTIAL COMPLICATIONS

Indirect BP

None

Direct BP

- Hematoma formation at the puncture site.
- Pain related to venipuncture (can use local anesthetic block or place under sedation/anesthesia).
- Thrombosis and potentially distal necrosis; feline metatarsal catheters should be removed within 6–8 hours of placement.
- Infection of the puncture site.

CLIENT EDUCATION

None

BODY SYSTEMS ASSESSED

Cardiovascular

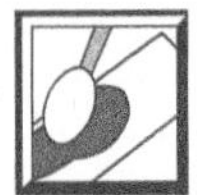

PROCEDURE

PATIENT PREPARATION

Pre-Procedure Medication or Preparation

None required for indirect measurement. With direct measurement, the site of arterial puncture should be clipped and sterilely prepared.

Anesthesia or Sedation

May affect measured BP. If direct BP readings are to be taken in a conscious patient, infiltration of local anesthetics can facilitate placement of the arterial line. Local anesthetic will also minimize arterial spasm in sedated or anesthetized patients.

Patient Positioning

- It is ideal to have the site where BP is being measured at the level of the heart.
- For oscillometric BP devices, the extremity with the cuff should not bear weight when the reading is taken.

Patient Monitoring

None for indirect. With direct BP measurement, the patency of the catheter needs to be maintained, and movement of the limb with the catheter should be minimized.

Equipment or Supplies

- Indirect BP measurement: oscillometric or Doppler device, cuff, and sphygmomanometer
- Direct BP measurement: pressure transducer, non-compliant tubing, multiparameter monitor

TECHNIQUE

Indirect

Doppler (Figure 1)

- Clip the area where BP is to be measured (the area just below the metacarpal or metatarsal pads, ventral aspect of tail).
- Apply ultrasound gel to the transducer.
- Apply the cuff to the area above the transducer (the width of cuff should be 30–40% of limb circumference) attached to the sphygmomanometer.
- Position the transducer so that a good arterial signal is heard.
- Inflate the cuff until the signal is no longer audible and then slowly deflate the cuff until the signal returns. The pressure at which the signal returns is considered to be systolic pressure.
- Repeat the measurement; wait at least 3–5 minutes between readings.

Oscillometric

- Apply the cuff to appropriate site (between the elbow and the carpus, above the elbow, at the tail base, at the distal hind limb).
- Activate the machine to start automatic inflation and measurement. The heart rate reported by the machine should match the patient's heart rate; if not, the measurement is incorrect.
- Repeat the measurement.

Direct

- Clip and surgically prepare the puncture site. Most common site is the dorsal pedal (metatarsal) artery; the tail artery can be used, and rarely the femoral artery.
- An over-the-needle peripheral catheter (22 or 20 gauge) is inserted into the area where the artery is palpated (femoral arterial catheters usually require a cut-down procedure).
- Once blood has flashed into the catheter, the catheter is advanced into the artery and capped with an injection port or t-set. The catheter is flushed with heparinized saline and taped or sutured in place.
- The t-port is attached to noncompliant tubing that is filled with heparinized saline from a pressurized bag (pressure prevents blood from backing up into the arterial catheter). If a cap is left on the catheter, a needle attached to the noncompliant tubing may be used to pierce the injection port and the pressure may be monitored that way.
- The tubing is attached to a calibrated pressure transducer. The pressure transducer is then attached to appropriate monitoring equipment.
- If an automatic flush is not incorporated in the pressure monitoring setup, the tubing and catheter should be flushed with heparinized saline frequently to maintain patency.

SAMPLE HANDLING

N/A

APPROPRIATE AFTERCARE

Post-Procedure Patient Monitoring

- Indirect—none.
- Direct—following removal of the catheter, a tight bandage should be placed for 1–2 hours, and after removal, monitor the arterial puncture site for indications of hemorrhage.

Nursing Care

- Indirect—none.
- Direct—apply a pressure bandage to the arterial puncture site upon removal of the

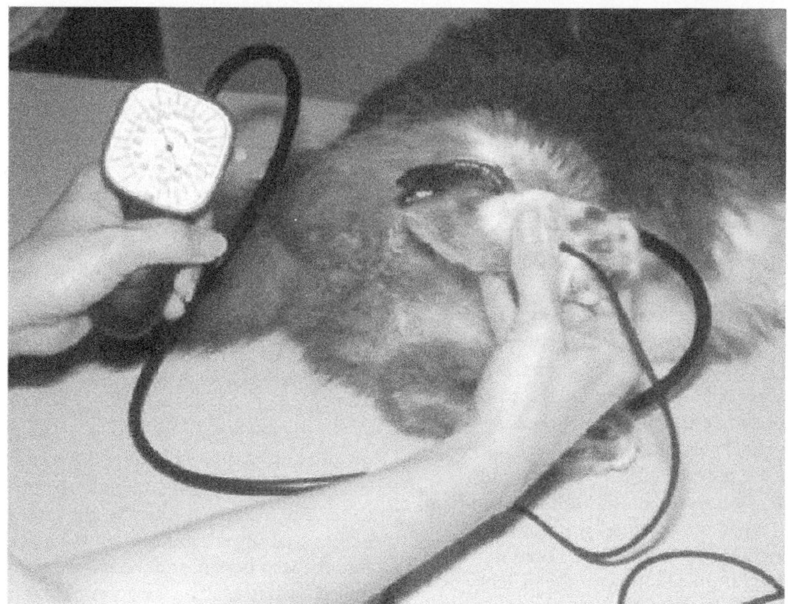

Figure 1.

Doppler technique: blood pressure is being measured just below the metatarsal pad. Source: Lawrence P. Tilley

cathter, and remove the bandage after 1–2 hours to prevent pressure necrosis.

Dietary Modification

N/A

Medication Requirements

N/A

Restrictions on Activity

None

Anticipated Recovery Time

None

INTERPRETATION

NORMAL FINDINGS OR RANGE

- Normal ranges depend on the method used to measure BP, age, breed, and, to some degree, operator factors (experienced vs. novice).
- An average value for BP in awake dogs is around 133/75 (systolic/diastolic) measured with an oscillometric monitor, giving a mean arterial pressure of 94 mmHg.
- In awake cats, normal BP has been found to be 125/90 (mean of 101 mmHg) via direct methods.

ABNORMAL VALUES

Hypotension is considered to be present in most cases where mean arterial blood pressure is less than 70 mmHg.

CRITICAL VALUES

- Critical hypotension is present with a mean arterial BP <60 mmHg or a systolic or Doppler pressure <80 mmHg.
- Critical hypertension is present with a systolic BP >180 mmHg and/or a diastolic BP >120 mmHg.

INTERFERING FACTORS

Drugs That May Alter Results of the Procedure

- Most anesthetics will alter BP. Generally, pressure is decreased (e.g., propofol, isoflurane, sevoflurane); however, α_2-adrenergic agonists can cause an increase by increasing systemic vascular resistance.
- Beta-blockers, nitroprusside, and calcium-channel blockers may decrease BP.
- Ocular medications may affect BP; timolol can decrease BP and phenylephrine can increase it.
- Adrenergic agents (epinephrine, norepinephrine, dopamine) will increase BP.

Conditions That May Interfere with Performing the Procedure

N/A

Procedure Techniques or Handling That May Alter Results

Indirect

- Anything that leads to patient stress can lead to white-coat hypertension and thereby inaccurate BP readings.
- The width of the cuff should be 30–40% of limb circumference. Cuffs that are too large may give falsely low readings, whereas cuffs that are too small can cause falsely elevated readings.

Direct

- Blood clots or air bubbles in the tubing may cause inaccurate readings for direct BP.
- Inappropriate tubing (using regular tubing vs. noncompliant) can fail to transmit the pressure wave appropriately, damping the signal.
- Excessively long tubing or kinking of tubing will cause erroneous readings.

Influence of Signalment on Performing and Interpreting the Procedure

Species

Cat and dog normal ranges are similar.

Breed

No breed-related differences have been noted in cats. Among dogs, sighthounds tend to have higher BPs than other breeds.

Age

BP increases with age.

Gender

Males will have higher BPs than females; on average, the difference is <10 mmHg.

Pregnancy

Unknown

CLINICAL PERSPECTIVE

- There are many indications for BP measurement, to detect both hypotension and hypertension.
- All anesthetized animals should have serial blood pressure measurements.
- In older animals, BP screening is indicated at regular visits.
- For general practice, indirect methods are best suited for screening patients.
- Direct BP measurement is ideal where continuous BP measurement is needed, especially in critical cases.

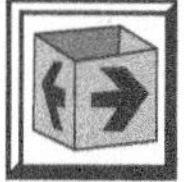

MISCELLANEOUS

ANCILLARY TESTS

If hypertension is found, appropriate laboratory tests are indicated to identify whether an underlying cause exists.

SYNONYMS

None

SEE ALSO

- Hypertension, Systemic Arterial.
- Hyperthyroidism.

ABBREVIATIONS

- BP = blood pressure.

Suggested Reading

Acierno MJ, Labato MA. Hypertension in dogs and cats. Compend Contin Educ Pract Vet 2004, 26:336–345.

Carr AP. Measuring blood pressure in dogs and cats. Vet Med 2001, 96:135–144.

Love L, Harvey R. Arterial blood pressure measurement: physiology, tools and techniques. Compend Contin Educ Pract Vet 2006, 28:450–461.

Waddell LS. Direct blood pressure monitoring. Clin Tech Small Anim Pract 2000, 15:111–118.

Author Benjamin M. Brainard

Consulting Editor Benjamin M. Brainard

Acknowledgment The author/editor acknowledges the prior contribution of Anthony P. Carr.

BLOOD SAMPLE COLLECTION

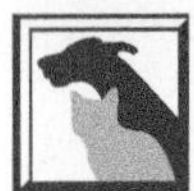

BASICS

TYPE OF PROCEDURE

Diagnostic sample collection

PROCEDURE EXPLANATION AND RELATED PHYSIOLOGY

The procedure involves using a syringe with attached hypodermic needle to aspirate blood percutaneously through a vessel wall into the syringe to a desired amount. For arterial blood collection, a heparinized syringe with an attached needle is used. Blood samples may also be obtained through newly placed peripheral catheters, or central venous catheters.

INDICATIONS

To obtain a blood sample for test analysis.

CONTRAINDICATIONS

- Severe coagulopathy (nonperipheral vessels).
- If a patient struggles or stresses to the point where it can further injure itself or the restrainers.

POTENTIAL COMPLICATIONS

- Complications are rare.
- Excessive bleeding can cause a hematoma in patients with a coagulopathy. A pressure wrap over the venipuncture area can prevent of minimize this problem.
- Multiple venipunctures of the same vein and area could cause bruising, phlebitis, or thrombosis of the vein.

CLIENT EDUCATION

Clients should be warned that there might be an area of hair clipped at the site and a small bandage applied, which should remain in place for 1 hour after the procedure. Mild bruising or irritation of the skin may be present.

BODY SYSTEMS ASSESSED

All

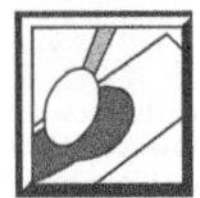

PROCEDURE

PATIENT PREPARATION

Pre-Procedure Medication or Preparation

- None.
- For arterial blood collection, oxygen therapy should be discontinued for 10 minutes before sample collection if assessment of a patient breathing room air is desired.

Anesthesia or Sedation

- Generally no sedatives are required.
- If a patient is fractious, a mild sedative may be needed.

Patient Positioning

- Proper positioning for the procedure is vital for a positive outcome.
- For venous blood collection, the patient will need to be restrained as needed for the vein being accessed and the vein compressed proximal to the planned site of puncture. For jugular venipuncture, it is best to have the patient in a sitting position with the head held high and slightly turned to the opposite side. For saphenous venipuncture, the vein is best viewed with the patient in lateral recumbency. Cephalic veins are best accessed when the patient is in sternal recumbency with the leg extended.
- For arterial blood collection, the patient will need to be restrained in lateral recumbency with the lower pelvic limb held out by the restrainer, being careful not to compress the artery and disrupt arterial blood flow. If a patient's dyspnea worsens when in lateral recumbency, it may be necessary to perform this procedure with the patient standing or sitting.

Patient Monitoring

- None.
- Dyspneic patients should be monitored closely for signs of increased dyspnea. If this occurs during the procedure, oxygen should be administered, and the patient allowed to sit calmly.

Equipment or Supplies

- An appropriately sized syringe, generally not larger than the amount of blood needed.
- A needle—use the smallest to cause the least trauma and pain to the patient but large enough to easily draw the volume of blood needed (e.g., 22 or 20 gauge × 1 inch). Larger needles are preferred if coagulation testing is planned.
- An alcohol swab.
- Appropriate collection tubes in which to place blood.
- A heparinized syringe for arterial blood collection (1- or 3-mL syringe with a 22 or 25 gauge needle). Draw heparin into syringe and then push all of the heparin back into the heparin vial, leaving just enough to coat the inside of the syringe. Preheparinized, self-filling syringes are also available for arterial blood sampling.
- If drawing blood from a central venous catheter, a three-syringe technique should be used: a 3-mL syringe, filled with 0.5 mL of heparinized saline, is first filled to 3 mL as a "pre-sample." Subsequently, the appropriate amount of blood for diagnostic sampling is obtained. The pre-sample is then reinfused back into the patient (the heparin in the saline prevents clotting), and the catheter is then flushed with heparinized saline to clear the catheter. Technically, the pre-sample should be 3–5 times the priming volume of the catheter lumen.

TECHNIQUE

Prior to patient restraint, gather all supplies needed.

Venous Blood Collection

- Based on the amount of blood needed and the quality of the available veins, a vein will be selected by the venipuncturist. Typically, the jugular vein is used when more than 2 mL of blood is needed, and a coagulopathy is not present. An alternative to this is the lateral saphenous vein in dogs and the medial saphenous vein in dogs and cats, which works well if a patient is struggling. If a small amount of blood is needed (<2 mL), the cephalic vein may be used.
- The patient should be restrained, preferably on an examination table. The site is swabbed with alcohol. The vein is compressed proximal to the site to allow the vein to engorge. The needle is advanced through the skin and then into the vein lumen, and the syringe plunger pulled back to aspirate the appropriate amount of blood. Compression of the vein is released. The syringe and needle are then withdrawn as a unit and blood placed into appropriate collection tubes. The restrainer applies pressure directly to the venipuncture site for 15–20 seconds then checks the site; if there is still bleeding, a bandage can be applied.

Arterial Blood Collection

- If a self-filling arterial blood syringe is used, pull the plunger back to the desired amount of blood needed (0.4 mL is adequate for most blood gas analyzers). The patient should be restrained with its bottom leg held out. The restrainer should put a hand behind the patient's hock to keep its leg extended without compressing the artery.
- Preferred site is the pedal (metatarsal) artery, which courses over the metatarsal bones and courses into the hock joint. The tail, femoral, and lingual arteries have also been used to collect samples under varying conditions:
    - The artery is identified by palpation with a finger of the nondominant hand (which may also hold the paw to keep the leg extended). The needle is then directed into the artery directly below the palpated pulse. The artery will generally exhibit some fremitis when the needle is near.
    - If using a regular syringe, once the needle has penetrated the skin, negative pressure is created with the plunger of the syringe and the needle is directed to puncture the arterial wall. A flash of blood back into the syringe will usually be seen after arterial puncture. Allow the syringe to fill to the amount of blood needed, withdraw the syringe and needle, and have the restrainer place pressure over the site for several minutes. A small pressure wrap may be needed.

- If using a self-filling syringe, once the artery is punctured, arterial blood pressure will fill the syringe until the porous filter of the plunger is reached, at which point the syringe contains an anaerobic blood sample.
- For both syringes, following sample acquisition, the syringe contents should be protected from room air. The needle may be placed into a rubber stopper or eraser, or the needle removed and the syringe capped with a specialized stopper (usually provided with the self-filling syringes).
- Due to proximity of the nerve to the artery, arterial puncture may be associated with pain, and the animal may pull the leg back during the procedure.

SAMPLE HANDLING

- Venous samples should be placed into appropriate collection tubes immediately to prevent clot formation. The tubes containing anticoagulant should be filled before the clot tubes. Invert the tubes at least 5 times to mix the samples thoroughly with the anticoagulant.
- Arterial samples for blood gas analysis should be assayed immediately.

APPROPRIATE AFTERCARE

Post-Procedure Patient Monitoring

Remove the pressure wrap 1 hour after the procedure and verify lack of continued bleeding or hematoma.

Nursing Care

None

Dietary Modification

None

Medication Requirements

None

Restrictions on Activity

None

Anticipated Recovery Time

Immediate recovery is expected.

INTERPRETATION

NORMAL FINDINGS OR RANGE

None

ABNORMAL VALUES

None

CRITICAL VALUES

See Blood Gas Interpretation.

INTERFERING FACTORS

Drugs That May Alter Results of the Procedure

None

Conditions That May Interfere with Performing the Procedure

Coagulopathy

Procedure Techniques or Handling That May Alter Results

None

Influence of Signalment on Performing and Interpreting the Procedure

Species

Vein selection may vary between dogs and cats.

Breed

None

Age

None

Gender

None

Pregnancy

None

CLINICAL PERSPECTIVE

When performed skillfully by trained, experienced personnel, venipuncture for blood sampling is usually a quick, simple procedure that causes minimal discomfort to patients and can be a valuable diagnostic tool.

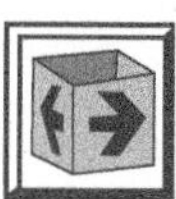

MISCELLANEOUS

ANCILLARY TESTS

Blood gas analysis.

SYNONYMS

Venipuncture

Author Robin Lazaro
Consulting Editor Benjamin M. Brainard

BLOOD SMEAR MICROSCOPIC EXAMINATION

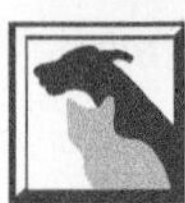

BASICS

TYPE OF SPECIMEN

Blood smear (see Blood Smear Preparation).

TEST EXPLANATION AND RELATED PHYSIOLOGY

- Cell counts derived from an automatized hematology analyzer must be correlated to findings in a manual examination of a peripheral blood smear:
  - Confirm cell counts.
  - Identify unusual cell types (including neoplastic cells).
  - Identify morphological changes such as toxic change or left shifts, reactive lymphocytes, polychromatic cells, nucleated erythrocytes (nRBC), and immature platelets.
  - Identify parasites.

INDICATIONS

- With every complete blood count (CBC).
- To confirm results from an automated hematology analyzer.
- To characterize erythrocytes and classify anemia.
- To diagnose inflammation, hematopoietic neoplasia, and bone marrow disease.
- To evaluate platelets, especially if automated counts are low.
- To identify circulating parasites.

CONTRAINDICATIONS

None

POTENTIAL COMPLICATIONS

None

CLIENT EDUCATION

12-hour fasting samples are preferred to prevent lipemia, which can interfere with RBC morphology evaluation.

BODY SYSTEMS ASSESSED

Hematologic, lymphatic, and immune.

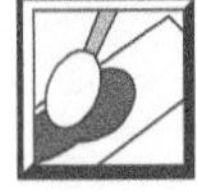

SAMPLE

SAMPLE COLLECTION

Previously prepared blood smear (see Blood Smear Preparation).

SAMPLE HANDLING

- Slides should not be exposed to formalin or formalin fumes.
- Slides should be protected from breakage.
- Do not scratch or refrigerate slides.
- If slides do not have a coverslip, oil should be gently blotted away rather than wiped.

SAMPLE STORAGE

Store slides in shatterproof containers at room temperature.

SAMPLE STABILITY

- Air-dried slides can be stored at room temperature indefinitely. They are stable months to years if fixed, stained, and not exposed to dust, light, or heat.
- For long-term storage, a permanent coverslip is recommended.

PROTOCOL

- Smears should be evaluated systematically:
  - Gross examination of slide quality.
  - Evaluate all cell lines at low-(10× objective), medium (40–50× objective), and high-power (100× oil objective) magnification.
  - Evaluate number and morphology of neutrophils, banded neutrophils (bands), lymphocytes, eosinophils, monocytes, and basophils.
  - Unusual cells that can be seen include immature granulocytes, lymphoblasts, mast cells, and nRBC.
  - A nucleated cell differential should be performed, platelet numbers and presence/absence of clumping should be estimated, morphological changes of red blood cells (RBCs) and white blood cells (WBCs) should be noted, and presence of parasites (e.g., microfilaria) or inclusions should be determined.

Macroscopic Evaluation

- Confirm patient identity (slide label).
- Evaluate the quality of the blood smear. If the quality is poor, make a new blood smear (see: Blood Smear Preparation):
  - Smear should be shaped like a parabolic cone (similar to the flame of a candle) with a blunt base, almost parallel sides, and a gently curved feathered edge at the nose.
  - Smear should cover 1/3 to 2/3 of the slide, however the quality of the monolayer and feathered edge are more important than the overall surface area.
  - The stain quality should be adequate for proper cell identification.

Low Power Evaluation

- At low power (10× objective), scan the entire smear.
- A monolayer where erythrocytes are closely opposed without overlapping should be present near a gently feathered edge (see Figure 1):
  - With experience, a marked decrease or increase in RBC number can be detected.
  - Anemic samples have a larger monolayer with increased space between cells extending into the smear base, while polycythemic samples have a minimal to absent monolayer.
  - Perform a reticulocyte count if anemia is suspected.
- Identify potential RBC agglutination and differentiate from rouleaux. If agglutination is suspected, perform a saline agglutination test.
- At the feathered edge, search for microfilaria and large unusual cells (e.g., mast cells, lymphoblasts, other leukemic cells).
- Identify and evaluate the severity of platelet and leukocyte clumping at the feathered edge or base.
- WBCs are unevenly distributed in a smear; heavier and larger cells are more abundant at the base and feathered edges. Lymphocytes are more abundant than neutrophils in the thinner parts of the center and monolayer. Evaluate all areas of the slide for a more representative assessment.
- In the main body of the smear, estimate overall WBC count with a 10× objective. Average cells/field × 100 = approximate cells/µL:
  - When counting WBCs, include at least 1 field in the base and feathered edge when determining the average to compensate for uneven leukocyte distribution. Moving from feathered tip to base is helpful.

Medium Power Evaluation

- If the slide is coverslipped, evaluate with a 40× objective. If the slide is not, use a 50× oil objective.
- Begin at the feathered edge to identify larger uncommon cells (mast cells, lymphoblasts, etc.), then move to the monolayer to perform a leukocyte differential:
  - Due to uneven distribution of leukocytes, systematically move from edge to edge, a zig-zag, or alternating squares/Greek key pattern (Figure 2) to perform the differential.
  - Classify 100 nucleated cells as neutrophils, bands, lymphocytes, monocytes, eosinophils, basophils, or other/unclassifiable (blasts, immature granulocytes, mast cells, etc.). Count nRBCs separately (do not include in the differential):
    - If there is a leukocytosis (>30,000 cells/µL) or >2% other cells, count 500 cells. Multiply your total WBC count (estimated or automatized hematology analyzer results) by the differential to calculate absolute cell counts.
  - If there is >2% nRBC, calculate a corrected WBC count. The formula is:

    Corrected WBC = (Measured WBC × 100)/(100 + # nRBC seen)

  - Note morphological changes to leukocytes such as neutrophil toxic change, reactive lymphocytes, monocyte vacuolation, viral inclusions, and presence of parasites.
- Perform an initial evaluation of erythrocytes for polychromasia, anisocytosis, poikilocytes, parasites, and inclusions including Heinz bodies, Howell-Jolly bodies, basophilic stippling, and iron (siderotic) inclusions.

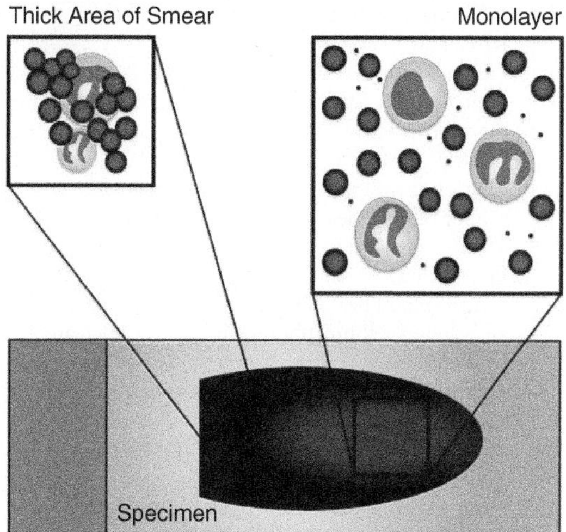

Figure 1.

This drawing of a blood smear illustrates how cell morphology is optimal in the monolayer just behind the feathered edge, where RBCs are evenly distributed. Cells in thicker areas, toward the back of the smear, are less flattened and appear smaller and darker and are more difficult to identify. The overlap of cells, in thicker portions of the smear, further obscures and distorts their morphologic features.

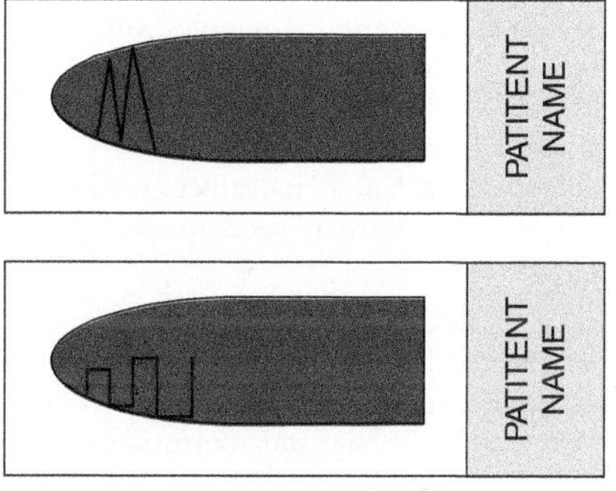

Figure 2.

Perform a leukocyte differential using a zig-zag or alternating squares/Greek key pattern.

- Note location (cytoplasmic, nuclear, epicellular) and type of cell affected by parasites and inclusions.
- Roughly evaluate number and size of platelets, looking for smaller clumps.

High Power Evaluation

- Evaluate both the monolayer and feathered edge with a 100× oil objective, focusing on cell morphology, parasites, and inclusions.
- Perform a close evaluation of erythrocytes for variation in cell size, color, inclusions, and shape abnormalities including spherocytes, echinocytes, keratocytes, schistocytes, acanthocytes, leptocytes, stomatocytes, and codocytes:
  - Quantify morphologic RBC changes using the following grading scheme:
    - Rare = <1 per 100× objective fields
    - Occasional = 1–3 per 100× objective field
    - Few or mild = 4–10 per 100× objective field
    - Moderate = 10–25 per 100× objective field
    - Many or marked = >25 per 100× objective field
- Search again for erythroid parasites and inclusions; some are not visible below 100×.
- Perform a closer evaluation of morphological changes to leukocytes (listed above).
- Count platelets at 100× in the monolayer, in a minimum of 10 fields, and evaluate for abnormal morphology and microclumping. Average platelets per 100× oil field × 20,000 = approximate platelets/μL.

INTERPRETATION

NORMAL FINDINGS OR RANGE

- Adjacent erythrocytes that barely touch or rarely overlap in the monolayer, 1–2 polychromatic cells per 100× objective field, mild anisocytosis, few poikilocytes, and no inclusions.

BLOOD SMEAR MICROSCOPIC EXAMINATION (CONTINUED)

- Approximately 5–15 WBCs per 10× objective field, with 60–80% mature neutrophils and no morphologic abnormalities.
- Approximately 10–25 platelets per 100× objective field in the monolayer without clumping.
- No parasites.

ABNORMAL FINDINGS

- Tightly packed or widely spaced RBCs.
- Absolute WBC or platelet numbers above or below the reference interval.
- Morphological abnormalities in any cell line.
- Parasites present.

CRITICAL VALUES

- Less than 1–3 neutrophils per 10× objective field suggests marked neutropenia and increased risk of infection.
- Less than 1–3 platelets per 100× objective field, without clumps present, suggests thrombocytopenia severe enough to cause bleeding.

INTERFERING FACTORS

Drugs That May Alter Results or Interpretation

Drugs That Interfere with Test Methodology

None

Drugs That Alter Physiology

- Glucocorticoids can cause leukocytosis, neutrophilia, lymphopenia, and variable monocytosis.
- Epinephrine can cause neutrophilia, lymphocytosis, and variable thrombocytosis.
- Heinz bodies (see Anemia, Heinz Body) are caused by oxidative damage from numerous drugs including acetaminophen, benzocaine, phenazopyridine, propofol, and vitamin K.
- Most chemotherapeutic agents can cause pancytopenia (see Pancytopenia), as can many other medications including chloramphenicol (feline), estrogen (canine), griseofulvin, methimazole (feline), phenobarbital, phenylbutazone (canine), and trimethoprim-sulfa.
- Chloramphenicol and phenylbutazone can cause neutrophilic vacuolation.

Disorders That May Alter Results

- Hemolysis causes a thick pink background that distorts cells.
- Lipemia can cause RBC smudging.
- Hyperglobulinemia causes a thick blue background that distorts RBCs and causes pseudo-agglutination.

Collection Techniques or Handling That May Alter Results

- Poorly mixed blood can produce a thin smear, and misrepresent the WBC count and differential.
- Clotted blood artificially decreases platelet, RBC, and WBC numbers.
- Samples collected in sodium citrate anticoagulant have decreased platelet counts than those with EDTA anticoagulation (multiply count by 1.1 to account for dilution from liquid citrate anticoagulant).
- Poor blood smear preparation prevents accurate evaluation (see Blood Smear Preparation).
- Aged blood has increased platelet clumps and altered cell morphology including nuclear pyknosis, nuclear hypersegmentation in neutrophils, and cytoplasmic vacuolation.
- Epicellular parasites can detach over time and may be missed if smears are not made immediately after collection.
- Old stain or poor washing produces stain precipitate that can be mistaken for bacteria or parasites.

Influence of Signalment

Species

- Canine RBCs have a prominent zone of central pallor with little anisocytosis, while feline RBCs are smaller without obvious central pallor and more anisocytosis.
- Cat RBCs are more susceptible to Heinz bodies.
- Canine eosinophils (except in sighthounds, see below) have rounded granules while feline eosinophils have smaller granules shaped like rice grains—this can be used to differentiate mislabeled samples.
- Basophils have more indistinct granules in dogs and cats relative to other species.

Breed

- Higher RBC counts have been reported in German shepherd dogs, boxers, greyhounds, and dachshunds.
- Decreased RBC size (microcytosis) is reported in Akitas, chow chows, Chinese shar peis, and shiba inus.
- Akitas with high and low RBC potassium phenotypes have different erythrocyte parameter findings.
- Hereditary macrocytosis is reported in poodles.
- Congenital stomatocytosis is reported in Alaskan malamutes, Drentse partrijshonds, and miniature schnauzers.
- Lower WBC counts are reported in greyhounds, Belgian tervurens, and border collies.
- Gray eosinophils in sighthounds such as greyhounds, Italian greyhounds, and whippets can be difficult to detect and missed by automated analyzers.
- Marked lymphopenia is reported in basset hounds and Jack Russell terriers with severe combined immunodeficiency syndrome (SCID).
- Increased eosinophils have been reported in Bernese mountain dogs, Brittanys, rottweilers, and German shepherd dogs.
- Lower platelet counts are reported in sighthounds including North American Scottish deerhounds and greyhounds, and also in the Polish hound (ogar Polski).
- Lower platelet counts with large platelets (macrothrombocytopenia) is an autosomal recessive trait present in cavalier King Charles spaniels and Norfolk and Cairn terriers.
- Cyclic hematopoiesis in gray collies can cause various waxing and waning cytopenias.

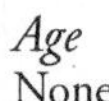

Age

None

Sex

None

Pregnancy

None

LIMITATIONS OF THE TEST

Smear quality, smear staining properties, evaluator experience, and adequate microscope are crucial to accurate evaluation and interpretation.

Sensitivity, Specificity, and Positive and Negative Predictive Values

N/A

Valid if Run in a Human Lab?

Generally no, unless technicians have specialty training in morphological evaluation of cells from veterinary species.

CAUSES OF ABNORMAL FINDINGS

See Table 1.

CLINICAL PERSPECTIVE

Manual review of a blood smear can give insight beyond what may be obtained from automated machine analysis.

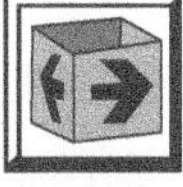

MISCELLANEOUS

ANCILLARY TESTS

- RBC, WBC, and platelet counts from an automated hematology analyzer.
- Buffy coat smear evaluation.
- Bone marrow aspirate and core biopsy.
- Flow cytometry (or other immunophenotyping) for suspected lymphoid or myeloid leukemia.

SYNONYMS

- Peripheral blood smear evaluation.
- CBC review.
- CBC evaluation.

ABBREVIATIONS

- CBC = complete blood count.
- EDTA = ethylenediaminetetraacetic acid.

Table 1

Causes of common hematopoietic abnormalities.

	High Values	*Low Values*	*Abnormal Morphology*
Neutrophils	Infection Inflammation Corticosteroid response Epinephrine response	Sepsis/infection Overwhelming inflammation Immune-mediated disease Drug toxicity Bone marrow disease	Marked inflammation or infection Leukemia Pelger–Huët anomaly
Lymphocytes	Antigenic stimulation Epinephrine response Lymphoid neoplasia/ Leukemia	Inflammation/stress Drug toxicity Acute infections Lymphatic fluid loss	Vaccination Infection Leukemia
Eosinophils	Parasitism Allergic/hypersensitivity reaction Paraneoplastic	Not significant	Pelger–Huët anomaly
Erythrocytes	Dehydration Splenic contraction Hypoxia Polycythemia vera	Hemorrhage, acute or chronic Intravascular or extravascular hemolysis Parasitism Chronic disease Renal disease Bone marrow disease	Regenerative anemia Heavy metal and other toxicities Myelodysplastic syndromes
Platelets	Regenerative anemia Inflammation Iron deficiency Epinephrine response Hypercortisolemia	Immune-mediated disease Tickborne diseases Consumption (e.g. disseminated intravascular coagulopathy) Bone marrow disease	Regeneration Breed-specific

- nRBC = nucleated red blood cell (metarubricyte).
- RBC = red blood cell.
- SCID = severe combined immunodeficiency.
- WBC = white blood cell.

INTERNET RESOURCES

- http://www.eclinpath.com/hematology/hemogram-basics/blood-smear-examination/
- https://todaysveterinarypractice.com/in-clinic-hematology-the-blood-film-review/
- https://www.youtube.com/watch?v=wIZtvTGJL6M
- https://prezi.com/35zh5w9nr-qj/the-veterinary-technicians-guide-to-performing-a-blood-film/

Suggested Reading

Harvey JW. Hematology procedures. In: Veterinary Hematology: A Diagnostic Guide and Color Atlas. Philadelphia, PA: Saunders, 2011, pp. 11–32.

Author Paula M. Krimer
Consulting Editor Benjamin M. Brainard

BLOOD SMEAR PREPARATION

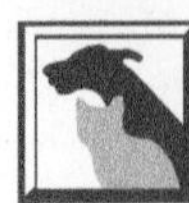

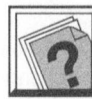

BASICS

TYPE OF PROCEDURE

Diagnostic sample preparation

PROCEDURE EXPLANATION AND RELATED PHYSIOLOGY

- Preparation of a good-quality air-dried blood smear is necessary for accurate evaluation.
- Smears should have a feathered edge and a monolayer with even cell distribution for a reliable WBC differential, visualization of cell appearance, and adequacy for parasite identification.
- Sample aging impacts leukocyte morphology and platelet couns, therefore immediate preparation of a good-quality blood smear is necessary.
- Prepared slides should be submitted with the corresponding anticoagulated blood for all complete blood counts (CBCs) sent to a referral laboratory.

INDICATIONS

Every time an in-house CBC is performed, and when a CBC is sent to a referral laboratory.

CONTRAINDICATIONS

Results are inaccurate if blood clots are present in the sample. A fresh blood sample should be taken if clots are present. Slides should be protected from exposure to formalin fumes.

POTENTIAL COMPLICATIONS

None

CLIENT EDUCATION

12-hour fasting samples are preferred to prevent lipemia, which can interfere with RBC morphology evaluation.

BODY SYSTEMS ASSESSED

Hematologic, lymphatic, and immune.

PROCEDURE

PATIENT PREPARATION

Preprocedure Medication or Preparation

- Sterilize the venipuncture site with alcohol. The site may be shaved if needed.
- Collect blood (see Blood Sample Collection) and transfer into an anticoagulant tube; EDTA (purple top) is preferred for most species but lithium heparin (green top) may provide better cell morphology for some birds, reptiles, and amphibians:
  - Heparin is sometimes used in small animals with small blood volume in order to have sufficient plasma for biochemical tests.
  - Sodium citrate anticoagulant can also be used but counts should be multiplied by 1.1 to account for dilution.

Anesthesia or Sedation

Not required but may be helpful for clean venipuncture in fractious animals.

Patient Positioning

Varies with preferred venipuncture site.

Patient Monitoring

Observe venipuncture site for hemorrhage, bruising, or hematoma formation.

Equipment or Supplies

- New glass slides.
- Pencil for labeling slide.
- Microhematocrit tube or 22–25G needle.
- Stain (for in-clinic evaluation).

TECHNIQUE

- Label glass slide with patient name, using a pencil. Markers and pens wash off with some stains.
- Gently mix anticoagulated blood for even distribution of cellular constituents. A tube rocker can be used or the tube manually inverted 5 times.
- A small droplet of blood should be placed near the edge of a new glass slide. Droplets can be applied with a microhematocrit tube or needle.
  - The most common error in slide preparation is too large a drop. Reduce the size of the drop and repeat if a good monolayer and feathered edge are not obtained.
- Use a second clean glass slide to spread the drop. Begin by placing the second slide at a 30-45° angle to the first where the blood will be spread (see Figure 1).
- Back the spreader slide into the drop. Let the blood migrate along the contact edge and toward the periphery (~5 seconds).
- When the blood has spread close to the edges of the slide, gently float the top slide away from the drop towards the end of the lower slide without applying downward pressure.
- Air-dry rapidly by waving the slide in the air or placing under a table fan (do not blow on slides).
- Stain with a Romanovsky-type stain (e.g., Diff-Quick, Wright-Giemsa, etc.) if evaluating in-house. Slides sent to external laboratories should be unstained.
- Package in appropriate shatterproof containers for transportation to external laboratories.

SAMPLE HANDLING

- Do not scratch or refrigerate slides.
- Air-dried slides can be stored at room temperature indefinitely. They are stable months to years if fixed, stained, and not exposed to dust, light or heat.
- For long-term storage, a permanent coverslip is recommended.
- Avoid exposure to any formalin, even formalin fumes from a nearby biopsy specimen.

APPROPRIATE AFTERCARE

Postprocedure Patient Monitoring

N/A

Nursing Care

N/A

Dietary Modification

N/A

Medication Requirements

N/A

Restrictions on Activity

N/A

Anticipated recovery time

N/A

INTERPRETATION

NORMAL FINDINGS OR RANGE

- See Blood Smear Microscopic Examination.
- A good smear is shaped like a parabolic cone (similar to the flame of a candle) with a blunt base, almost parallel sides, and a gently curved feathered edge at the nose.
- A monolayer where erythrocytes are closely opposed without overlapping should be present near a gently feathered edge.
- The smear should cover 1/3 to 2/3 of the slide; however a large smear is not the goal. The quality of the monolayer and feathered edge are more important than the overall surface area. If either are not present, make a new smear.

Causes of Abnormal Values

See Tables 1 and 2.

CRITICAL VALUES

None

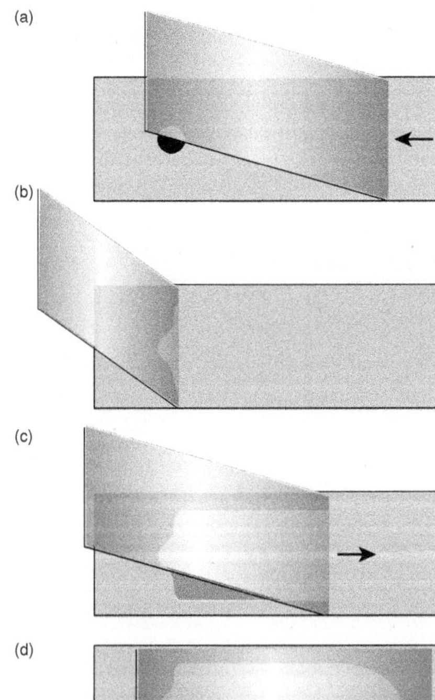

Figure 1.

Proper technique for blood smear preparation.

Table 1

Common staining mistakes.

Problem	*Appearance*	*Probable Causes*	*Solution*
Bacterial growth in stain	Scattered extracellular bacteria, sometimes on a different plane of focus	Stain used for nonsterile procedures (e.g., skin lesions).	Use separate stain for cytology and hematology. Replace stain frequently
Poor coloration	Pale colors or insufficient contrast	Insufficient time in dye or fixative, wrong pH water rinse, evaporated solutions	Standardize time per dip using a stopwatch. Use pH buffered distilled water to rinse. Tightly cap stains
Stain precipitate	Darkly basophilic dots, sometimes aggregated, on a different plane of focus	Aged staining solution, evaporated solutions, or inadequate rinsing of slides	Filter or replace stain. Tightly cap stain when not in use. Rinse with distilled rather than tap water
Water artifact	Moth-eaten cells, refractile "inclusions"	Too much water in fixative	Replace fixative

Table 2

Common smear preparation mistakes.

Problem	*Probable Causes*	*Solutions*
Blunt end (not arced)	Spreader slide lifted abruptly	Lift spreader slide gently. Smaller drop may be needed
Blood reaches far edge	Too large a drop, spreader slide too low or moved too slowly	Use smaller drop. Raise the angle of the spreader slide or spread faster
Mono layer absent (thick smear)	Too large a drop, spreader slide too high, apolycythemia	Use smaller drop and/or lower the angle of the spreader slide
Striations (chatter)	Spreader slide moved too slowly or inconsistently	Move spreader slide faster and/or more gently. Reduce downward pressure
Abnormal shape	Spreader slide corner lifted	Move spreader slide more gently and smoothly
Rough feathered edge	Unclean spreader slide, large platelet clumps	Use a clean slide. Remix blood. Repeat with lower angle

INTERFERING FACTORS

Drugs That May Alter Results or Interpretation

None

Conditions That May Interfere with Performing the Procedure

Marked polycythemia causes increased blood viscosity that can prevent smooth distribution of cells, preventing the formation of a monolayer and distorting leukocyte morphology. Lowering the spreader slide angle may help.

Collection Techniques or Handling That May Alter Results (see Tables 1 and 2)

- Blood aging prior to slide preparation will cause platelet clumping and altered leukocyte morphology including nuclear pyknosis, nuclear hypersegmentation in neutrophils, and cytoplasmic vacuolation. Slides should be made as soon as possible after blood collection.
- Poorly mixed samples can cause a thinner smear mimicking anemia and misrepresentation of the leukocyte differential.
- Clots in the blood sample will decrease the presence of platelets on the smear and may alter the leukocyte differential.
- An inadequate feathered edge will interfere with detection of platelet clumps and abnormal cells.
- Any exposure to formalin fumes fixes the slides, preventing adequate cytological staining. Erythrocytes will appear blue-green and leukocytes cannot be accurately identified. Slides exposed to formalin should not be evaluated.

Influence of Signalment on Performing and Interpreting the Procedure

Species

The choice of EDTA, lithium heparin, or sodium citrate as an anticoagulant varies by species for best cellular morphology balanced with the need for collection of plasma or minimizing blood collection volume. Research species prior to selecting an anticoagulant.

Breed

None

Age

None

Sex

None

Pregnancy

None

CLINICAL PERSPECTIVE

- Slide quality matters; it is easier to made smooth smears on better quality slides. Use new glass slides, preferably with a negative charge.
- Sample aging changes leukocyte morphology and platelet counts—make slides immediately.
- Fresh smears may be necessary to identify RBC parasites including hemotropic *Mycoplasma* spp.
- Some erythroid parasites, such as *Babesia* sp., may be more readily identified in capillary blood such as from an ear prick.

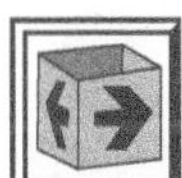

MISCELLANEOUS

ANCILLARY TESTS

None

SYNONYMS

Peripheral blood smear.

SEE ALSO

- Blood Smear Microscopic.

ABBREVIATIONS

- CBC = complete blood count.
- EDTA = ethylenediaminetetraacetic acid.

INTERNET RESOURCES

https://www.vet.cornell.edu/animal-health-diagnostic-center/laboratories/clinical-pathology/samples-and-submissions/hematology#Bloodsmear but it goes to https://www.vet.cornell.edu/animal-health-diagnostic-center/laboratories/clinical-pathology
https://www.youtube.com/watch?v=nbRUiWl2Qrs
http://www.eclinpath.com/hematology/sample-collection-heme/

Suggested Reading

Harvey JW. Hematology procedures. In: Veterinary Hematology: A Diagnostic Guide and Color Atlas. Philadelphia, PA: Saunders, 2011, pp. 11–32.

Author Paula M. Krimer
Consulting Editor Benjamin M. Brainard

BLOOD TYPING

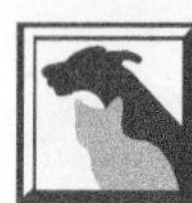

BASICS

TYPE OF SPECIMEN

Blood

TEST EXPLANATION AND RELATED PHYSIOLOGY

- Blood types are genetic markers on the surface of red blood cells (RBCs):
  - Species-specific and antigenic (immune system can recognize and potentially produce antibodies against them).
  - A set of 2 or more alleles at 1 gene locus makes up a blood group system.
  - An individual lacking a given blood type may develop antibodies against it, either naturally (e.g., AB system in cats) or following sensitization via a mismatched transfusion.
  - In dogs and cats, blood-typing methods are mostly based on agglutination reaction in which a species-specific antiserum or a lectin is directed against specific RBC antigens.
- In dogs, an international standardization proposed seven blood groups, referred to as Dog Erythrocyte Antigen (DEA), followed by a number. Since then, two new canine blood groups have been recognized:
  - The *Dal* blood group was discovered following blood incompatibility in a previously-transfused anemic Dalmatian. Dal-negative dogs are rare and at high risk of transfusion incompatibility if they are to receive multiple blood transfusions, considering the fact that all blood donors tested to date are Dal positive.
  - Two additional canine blood types, Kai 1 and Kai 2 have recently been identified, but their clinical significance remains unknown.
- For each blood group, a dog may be either positive or negative, so an individual dog's RBCs can have several of these blood groups on their membranes. Flow cytometry analysis of the DEA 1 antigen using a monoclonal antibody revealed that the expression of DEA 1 is a continuum of reactions ranging from negative to strongly positive, i.e., that all the alleles of the DEA 1 system have a similar epitope. Consequently, the historical nomenclature DEA 1.1, 1.2, 1.3, and DEA 1.1 negative is now simplified to DEA 1 positive and DEA 1 negative.
- Dogs do not have clinically significant naturally occurring alloantibodies; however, they may become sensitized after receiving a blood type-mismatched transfusion. DEA 1 is the most antigenic blood group in dogs. For this reason, blood typing for DEA 1 is desirable prior to transfusions to avoid sensitization.
- In cats, the AB blood group system is the predominant system, consisting of three blood types: A, B, and AB. The *a* allele is dominant over the *b* allele. The rare *ab* allele, causing the blood type AB, is separately inherited, being (co)-dominant to *b* and recessive to the *a* allele:
  - Although most cats are type A in North America (>95% of domestic shorthairs), significant geographic and breed-associated differences exist in the frequencies of these blood types.
  - Cats possess naturally occurring alloantibodies against the blood type they are lacking.
    - Type B cats have very strong anti-A alloantibodies, such that transfusion of type A blood into a type B cat will produce a life-threatening acute transfusion reaction.
    - Approximately 1/3 of type A cats have detectable weak anti-B alloantibodies, which may cause shortened survival of transfused B cells in type A cats.
  - In 2007, a blood type called *Mik was* identified outside of the feline AB blood group and found to be capable of causing a hemolytic transfusion reaction. Unfortunately, blood typing for Mik is no longer possible.
- Easy-to-use blood-typing kits are commercially available for in-practice determination of canine DEA 1, and feline A, B or AB blood types.
  - The RapidVet-H canine and feline blood-typing cards (DMS Laboratories, Flemington, NJ) provide results in approximately 2 minutes. The animal blood type is indicated by visible RBC agglutination. The level of agglutination depends on the amount of antigen expressed on RBC membranes. This test is difficult to use in animals exhibiting RBC auto-agglutination.
  - The Alvedia Quick Test DEA 1 and Alvedia Quick Test A+B blood-typing kits (Alvedia, Villeur banne, France) are based on immunochromatography; RBCs migrate on a membrane and interact with monoclonal antibodies to produce a visible line. A second control line appears if the test was performed correctly.
  - RapidVet-H IC Feline uses immunochromatography for feline blood typing.
- Several automated blood typing analyzers are now commercially available.
- Typing services and/or polyclonal antisera are also available for DEA 1, 4, 5 and 7, as well as the feline AB system. There is limited accessibility to DEA 3, 5 and *Dal* reagents and a complete lack of accessibility to DEA 6, DEA 8 and Mik reagents.
- Several genetic variants associated with the B and the AB blood groups have been identified, representing a promising molecular diagnostic scheme to genotype cats for the AB blood group system and to differentiate type A, B and, more recently, AB cats.

INDICATIONS

- Screening blood donors and recipients to assure blood compatibility prior to transfusion.
- Screening breeding cats to ensure blood-compatible mates and avoid neonatal isoerythrolysis.

CONTRAINDICATIONS

None

POTENTIAL COMPLICATIONS

None

CLIENT EDUCATION

None

BODY SYSTEMS ASSESSED

Hemic, lymphatic, and immune.

SAMPLE

SAMPLE COLLECTION

A 1–2 mL venous blood sample.

SAMPLE HANDLING

EDTA anticoagulant.

SAMPLE STORAGE

Refrigerate for short-term storage.

SAMPLE STABILITY

The physical integrity of RBCs is critical for correct results. Ideally, samples should be blood typed within 2–3 days of blood collection.

PROTOCOL

None

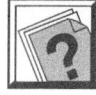

INTERPRETATION

NORMAL FINDINGS OR RANGE

- Dogs—roughly 50% are DEA 1 positive, with various degree of antigenic expression (Table 1).
- Cats—in North America, most are type A (>95% of domestic shorthairs); <5% are type B, and <1% are type AB.

ABNORMAL VALUES

None

CRITICAL VALUES

None

INTERFERING FACTORS

Drugs That May Alter Results or Interpretation

Drugs That Interfere with Test Methodology

Recent blood transfusion (packed RBCs or whole blood).

Drugs That Alter Physiology

None

Table 1

Normal findings in dogs.

Canine Blood Types	*% Positive*	*% Negative*
DEA 1	33–65	35–67
DEA 3	5–24	76–95
DEA 4	87–100	0–13
DEA 5	8–51	49–92
DEA 7	8–82	18–92

Table 2

Cats—type B frequency in North America.

Breeds	*Type B Frequency in North America (%)*
Siamese, Burmese, Tonkinese, Russian blue, Ocicat, Oriental shorthair	0
Maine coon, Norwegian forest, DSH/DLH	<5
Abyssinian, Himalayan, Birman, Japanese bobtail, Persian, Somali, Sphinx, Scottish fold	5–25
Exotic and British shorthair, Cornish rex, Devon rex	25–50

Disorders That May Alter Results

- Severe anemia may cause false-negative results because the number of RBCs may be insufficient to agglutinate in response to antiserum; this may be circumvented by centrifuging the blood sample and removing some plasma to concentrate the RBCs prior to blood typing.
- Autoagglutination, such as in immune-mediated hemolytic anemia, precludes typing by agglutination-based methods because such blood samples will always appear positive. To some limits, this may be circumvented by washing the RBCs prior to blood typing.
- Marked rouleaux can be mistaken for a weak positive reaction with the Rapid Vet-H canine and feline blood-typing cards.

Collection Techniques or Handling That May Alter Results

Hemolysis of the blood may not allow blood typing, because the physical integrity of the RBCs is critical for correct results.

Influence of Signalment

Species

- Dogs—DEA 1, 3, 4, 5, 6, 7 and 8, and *Dal.*
- Cats—feline AB blood groups (type A, B or AB) and *Mik*.

See comments above concerning limited availability of some typing reagents.

Breed

- Dogs—breed-associated differences in the frequency of blood types are mostly documented for DEA 1 (surveys mostly among large breed dogs, i.e., canine blood donors). In addition to Dalmatians, dogs with the rare Dal-negative blood types were identified in Doberman pinschers and shih tzus.
- Cats—significant geographic and breed-associated differences in the frequencies of these blood types have been found. Type B domestic cats are uncommon in some countries like the United States and Switzerland, however, in other countries such as Australia, Greece, and Turkey, their prevalence can reach up to 36% of the non-pedigree feline population (see Table 2).

Age

None

Gender

None

Pregnancy

None

LIMITATIONS OF THE TEST

Sensitivity, Specificity, and Positive and Negative Predictive Values

N/A

Valid If Run in a Human Lab?

No

CLINICAL PERSPECTIVE

- It is strongly recommended to blood type canine blood donors and patients for DEA 1 prior to transfusion to limit sensitization by transfusion, because DEA 1 is the most antigenic and clinically significant blood type.
- Dal blood typing, in addition to standard DEA 1 typing, is recommended in Dalmatians, Doberman pinschers and shih tzus, especially in previously transfused dogs.
- A canine patient negative for a given blood type can become sensitized and produce specific antibodies against this blood type if transfused with positive blood. A subsequent transfusion of positive blood may lead to an immediate hemolytic transfusion reaction. Such transfusion reactions have been documented against DEA 1, 4, *Dal*, and one common antigen.
- The sensitization (i.e., the production of antibodies in negative dogs) against DEA 4 or the *Dal* antigen is particularly challenging because finding compatible blood may be extremely difficult given the high prevalence of those blood types in the canine population.
- Because of naturally occurring alloantibodies, feline donors and recipients should always be blood typed prior to transfusion. As little as 1 mL of type A blood can lead to a fatal hemolytic transfusion reaction if given to a type B cat.
- Type A and AB kittens born to type B queens are at risk of developing neonatal isoerythrolysis caused by the presence of strong anti-A alloantibodies in the colostrum of type B queens. The disease is characterized by a severe hemolytic anemia and possible nephropathy, as well as other organ failures. To avoid neonatal isoerythrolysis, it is recommended to blood type breeding mates, particularly in breeds with a high incidence of type B cats.
- All previously transfused dogs and cats (>4 days) should be crossmatched, in addition to standard blood typing, to look for the presence of antibodies before receiving additional blood.

BLOOD TYPING (CONTINUED)

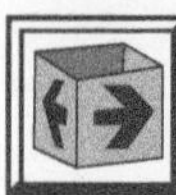

MISCELLANEOUS

ANCILLARY TESTS

Crossmatch

SYNONYMS

None

SEE ALSO

- Anemia, Nonregenerative.
- Anemia, Regenerative.
- Blood Transfusion Reactions.
- Crossmatch (in Appendix X).
- Saline Agglutination Test (in Appendix X).

ABBREVIATIONS

- DEA = dog erythrocyte antigen.
- DLH = domestic longhair.
- DSH = domestic shorthair.
- RBC = red blood cell.

INTERNET RESOURCES

- Alvedia: alvedia.com
- Animal Blood Ressources International: http://www.abrint.net
- CHUV Blood Bank—Université de Montréal: http://chuv.umontreal.ca/banque-de-sang/
- DMS Laboratories: http://www.rapidvet.com
- PennGen Hematology and Typing: https://www.vet.upenn.edu

Suggested Reading

Abrams-Ogg ACG. Feline recipient screening. In: Yagi K, Holowaychuk M, eds., Manual of Veterinary Transfusion Medicine and Blood Banking. Hoboken, NJ: John Wiley & Sons, 2016, pp. 129–155.

Acierno MM, Raj K, Giger U. DEA 1 expression on dog erythrocytes analyzed by immunochromatographic and flow cytometric techniques. J Vet Intern Med 2014, 28:592–598.

Blais MC, Berman L, Oakley DA, Giger U. Canine Dal blood type: a red cell antigen lacking in some Dalmatians. J Vet Intern Med 2007, 21:281–286.

Euler CC, Lee JH, Kim HY, et al. Survey of two new (Kai 1 and Kai 2) and other blood groups in Dogs of North America. J Vet Intern Med 2016, 30:1642–1647.

Giger U, Gelens CJ, Callan MB, Oakley DA. An acute hemolytic transfusion reaction caused by dog erythrocyte antigen 1.1 incompatibility in a previously sensitized dog. J Am Vet Med Assoc 1995, 206:1358–1362.

Goulet S, Blais M-C. Characterization of anti-Dal alloantibodies following sensitization of two Dal-negative dogs. Vet Pathol 2017, 1–8.

Goulet S, Giger U, Arsenault J, et al. Prevalence and mode of inheritance of the Dal blood group in dogs in North America. J Vet Intern Med 2017, 31:751–758.

Griot-Wenk ME, Giger U. Feline transfusion medicine: blood types and their clinical importance. Vet Clin North Am Small Anim Pract 1995, 25:1305–1322.

Tocci LJ. Canine recipient screening. In: Yagi K, Holowaychuk M, eds., Manual of Veterinary Transfusion Medicine and Blood Banking. Hoboken, NJ: John Wiley & Sons, 2016, pp. 117–129.

Weinstein NM, Blais MC, Harris K, et al. A newly recognized blood group in domestic shorthair cats: the *Mik* red cell antigen. J Vet Intern Med 2007, 21:287–292.

Author Marie-Claude Blais

Consulting Editor Benjamin M. Brainard

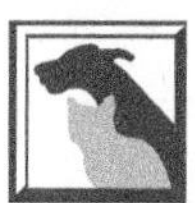

BASICS

TYPE OF PROCEDURE

Diagnostic sample collection

PROCEDURE EXPLANATION AND RELATED PHYSIOLOGY

- Cytologic examination of samples collected via bone marrow aspiration (BMA) is necessary to assess the presence or absence, quantity, and ratio of precursors of the red blood cell (RBC), platelet, and white blood cell (WBC) lines.
- Cytologic examination is also used in staging patients with hematologic and certain other malignancies, where bone marrow involvement is associated with a higher stage of disease.
- Histologic examination of samples collected via bone marrow biopsy (BMB) provides information regarding tissue architecture within the bone marrow and is an important step in evaluating primary bone marrow disorders, such as aplastic anemia, nonregenerative anemia, myelodysplasia and myelofibrosis.
- Poorly prepared smears or inadequately harvested core biopsy samples can make interpretation difficult.

INDICATIONS

- BMA:
  - Identify cell types, quantity, and ratio of precursor cells within the bone marrow (e.g., when peripheral cytopenias are noted).
  - Identify the presence of suspected infectious agents.
  - Assess bone marrow involvement in neoplastic conditions.
  - Provides information on the cell types present but no information on bone marrow structure.
- BMB:
  - Indicated for animals with suspected structural bone marrow abnormalities (aplastic anemia, non-regenerative anemia, myelodysplasia, myelofibrosis).

CONTRAINDICATIONS

None

POTENTIAL COMPLICATIONS

Hemorrhage is a risk but not expected to be clinically significant.

CLIENT EDUCATION

- The procedure has minimal risk.
- Mild discomfort associated with the procedure can be alleviated through the use of a local anesthetic and heavy sedation or anesthesia. If indicated, analgesic agents may be provided following the procedure.

BODY SYSTEMS ASSESSED

Hemic, lymphatic, and immune.

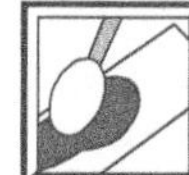

PROCEDURE

PATIENT PREPARATION

Pre-Procedure Medication or Preparation

Hair clipping and aseptic skin preparation are indicated prior to BMA or BMB.

Anesthesia or Sedation

Local anesthesia (lidocaine) in conjunction with heavy sedation or anesthesia.

Patient Positioning

- Palpate the desired site of sample collection (amenable locations include the head of the humerus, iliac crest, and trochanteric fossa; the sternum may also be used in some animals) and position the animal accordingly.
- Humerus—lateral recumbency with the patient's foreleg rotated externally and extended caudally 45°, keeping the leg parallel to the table or floor.
- Iliac crest—sternal recumbency with the patient's legs extended forward, rounding the lumbosacral area.
- Trochanteric fossa—lateral recumbency.

Patient Monitoring

- Monitor for adequate analgesia and level of sedation.
- Monitor for bleeding at the aspiration or biopsy site following sample collection.
- If patient is hevily sedated or anesthetized, monitors such as pulse oximetry, blood pressure, ECG, and capnography may be indicated.

Equipment or Supplies

- Surgical scrub.
- Sterile gloves.
- Sterile 4 × 4-inch gauze.
- A no. 11 scalpel blade.
- 1 mL of 2% lidocaine (maximum of 2 mg/kg, can be diluted to 1% if more volume is needed).
- BMA:
  - A Rosenthal or Illinois BMA needle
  - A 6- or 12-mL syringe
  - EDTA solution
  - A watchglass or glass petri dish
  - Pipette or hematocrit tubes
  - Glass slides
- BMB:
  - A Jamshidi infant needle or pediatric BMB needle
  - A 6- or 12-mL syringe
  - A jar containing 10% buffered formalin for sample
  - A cartridge to hold small samples in the formalin jar

TECHNIQUE

- BMA or BMB generally requires 2–3 people: 1–2 to position the animal, monitor sedation or anesthesia, and assist with sample handling, and the other to collect the sample.
- Clip hair from an approximately 5 cm^2 area over the desired site and perform a surgical scrub. After surgical preparation of the site, infiltrate the area with 0.5–1.0 mL of local anesthetic (e.g., 2% lidocaine), making sure to also block the periosteum. Follow with a final surgical scrub.
- Make a small stab incision with the no.11 scalpel blade.

Bone Marrow Aspiration

- Insert the bone marrow needle through the stab incision made in the skin and subcutaneous tissues. Position the needle on the periosteum.
- Holding the instrument closely between the thumb and index finger and within the closed palm, begin to rotate the instrument back and forth with gentle pressure until it is solidly within the marrow cavity:
  - Care must be taken to keep the needle and instrument in line; avoid rocking the needle during its advancement.
  - Firm adequate placement can be determined by the ability to move the limb by moving the inserted instrument gently side to side.
- Once positioned in the marrow cavity, the cap and stylet are removed and a 6- or 12-mL syringe (containing 0.5 mL of EDTA, if available) is attached to the needle and used to aspirate with negative pressure.
- As soon as marrow is seen within the syringe, negative pressure is released to minimize dilution or contamination of the sample with peripheral blood.
- The syringe is then detached and its contents emptied in single small drops onto a series of glass slides, placing 1 drop per slide (alternatively, the contents may be emptied into a watchglass or glass petri dish containing 0.5–1.0 mL of EDTA; this technique reduces the risk of clotting prior to slide preparation).
- Working quickly to avoid clotting of the sample, the bone marrow drops are smeared onto each of the slides (see Fine-Needle Aspiration for slide preparation technique).
- Alternatively, if a watchglass containing EDTA is used, individual bone marrow particles (identified by a spicule shape) may be collected using a pipette or hematocrit tube, transferred to the slides, and the sample then smeared along the length of the slide.

Bone Marrow Biopsy

- Insert the biopsy instrument through the stab incision made in the skin and subcutaneous tissues. Position the needle on the periosteum.
- Holding the instrument so the plastic handle rests in the palm and the needle extends between the index and middle fingers, begin to rotate instrument back and forth with gentle pressure until it penetrates the outer cortex and enters the marrow cavity.

BONE MARROW ASPIRATE AND BIOPSY (CONTINUED)

- Once securely positioned within through the outer cortex, remove the stylet and advance the needle 1–2 cm within the marrow by continuing to rotate the instrument back and forth with gentle pressure. At this point, a core of bone marrow should be lodged within the hollow needle.
- To break off the core within the needle and ensure it is removed along with the instrument, sharply twist the instrument several times in a clockwise direction, followed by several twists in a counterclockwise direction, and then firmly rock the instrument in a circular motion in one direction and then the other. Finally, attach a 6- or 12-mL syringe to the end of the instrument and apply a single burst of negative pressure. The instrument can then be removed from the bone by rotation and steady traction.
- Once the instrument is removed, use the "shepherd's crook" stylet inserted retrograde though the needle to push the bone marrow core biopsy gently out through the top of the instrument and place the sample in formalin. Small samples should be placed in a tissue cassette prior to inserting in formalin jar.

SAMPLE HANDLING

- BMA—air-dried samples can be stored at room temperature, though samples should be fixed and stained as soon after collection as possible (within 3–7 days) for optimal assessment of cellular morphology.
- BMB—collected samples should be placed in 10% buffered formal for submission to a histopathology laboratory.
- A peripheral blood sample should be collected and submitted at the time of either BMA or BMB.

APPROPRIATE AFTERCARE

Post-Procedure Patient Monitoring

- Monitor for evidence of mild superficial hemorrhage at the BMA or BMB site.
- Monitor for evidence of discomfort at the BMA or BMB site or lameness on the sampled leg.

Nursing Care

None

Dietary Modification

None

Medication Requirements

None

Restrictions on Activity

None

Anticipated Recovery Time

Immediate

INTERPRETATION

NORMAL FINDINGS OR RANGE

- Bone marrow should be evaluated by a trained pathologist.
- Sample should be evaluated for:
  - Cellularity (normal range, 25% fat and 75% cells to 75% fat and 25% cells; varies according to age).
  - Megakaryocyte series (normal range, approximately 4–50 megakaryocytes per spicule).
  - Erythrocyte series (abundance, proportions, morphology).
  - Granulocytic series (abundance, proportions, morphology).
  - Myeloid/erythroid ratio (normal range, 0.75:1 to 2:1).
  - Presence of organisms (e.g., *Histoplasma capsulatum, Leishmania donovani, Toxoplasma gondii, Cytauxzoon felis, Ehrlichia* spp.)
  - Presence of erythrophagocytosis, plasmacytosis, iron-containing pigments, neoplastic cell infiltration, and myelofibrosis.

ABNORMAL VALUES

- Decreased overall cellularity.
- Increases or decreases in megakaryocyte numbers.
- Abnormal numbers, proportions, or morphology of erythrocyte or granulocyte series.
- Presence of infectious organisms.
- Evidence of erythrophagocytosis, plasmacytosis, or decreased iron-containing pigments.
- Neoplastic cell infiltration.

CRITICAL VALUES

None

INTERFERING FACTORS

Drugs That May Alter Results of the Procedure

- Administration of immunosuppressive therapies (as for suspected immune-mediated cytopenias) prior to sample collection may alter interpretation.
- Administration of corticosteroids or other chemotherapeutic agents prior to sample collection may alter the presence or number of neoplastic cells.

Conditions That May Interfere with Performing the Procedure

None

Procedure Techniques or Handling That May Alter Results

- Inadequate sample collection; animals with myelofibrosis may have underwhelming BMA and difficult to obtain BMB.
- Excessive aspiration with BMA may lead to dilution or contamination of the sample with peripheral blood.

Influence of Signalment on Performing and Interpreting the Procedure

Species

None

Breed

Some breed-related variability; for example, increased hematocrit, mild thrombocytopenia, mild leukopenia may be seen in greyhounds.

Age

Normal bone marrow cellularity decreases with age: samples from juvenile, adult, and geriatric animals contain approximately 25% fat and 75% cells, 50% fat and 50% cells, and 75% fat and 25% cells, respectively.

Gender

None

Pregnancy

None

CLINICAL PERSPECTIVE

- Cytologic examination of samples collected via BMA is an important step in assessing the presence or absence, quantity, and ratio of precursors of the RBC, platelet, and WBC lines in patients with increases or decreases in peripheral blood cell counts.
- Assessment can support a diagnosis and prognosis in animals with cytopenias and hematologic and certain other malignancies.
- BMB provides additional information regarding tissue architecture within the bone marrow.

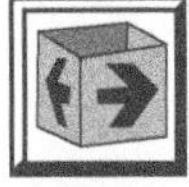

MISCELLANEOUS

ANCILLARY TESTS

A CBC should be performed in conjunction with BMA and BMB.

SYNONYMS

None

SEE ALSO

- Anemia, Aplastic.
- Anemia, Immune-Mediated.
- Anemia, Nonregenerative.
- Bone Marrow Aspirate Cytology: Microscopic Evaluation (in Appendix X).
- Myelodysplastic Syndromes.
- Myeloproliferative Disorders.
- Thrombocytopenia.

ABBREVIATIONS

- BMA = bone marrow aspiration.
- BMB = bone marrow biopsy.

Suggested Reading

Cowell RL, Tyler RD, Meinkoth JH. Diagnostic Cytology and Hematology of the Dog and Cat. St. Louis, MO: CV Mosby, 1999.

Author Laurel E. Williams

Consulting Editor Benjamin M. Brainard

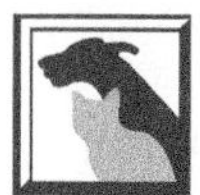

BASICS

TYPE OF SPECIMEN

Tissue

TEST EXPLANATION AND RELATED PHYSIOLOGY

Bone marrow is the major hematopoietic organ of the mammalian body, and its examination aids in evaluating various hematologic disorders. The most common indication for its microscopic evaluation is a complete blood count (CBC) abnormality that cannot be readily explained by a good medical history or by physical examination, chemistry profile, and/or other diagnostic procedures. In addition, bone marrow evaluation may aid in monitoring disease progression or response to therapy, determination of disease prognosis, and staging of certain neoplasms. Finally, body iron stores can be estimated, particularly if special stains are used, and occult infectious agents may be identified. A CBC collected within 24 hours of marrow collection is imperative for accurate interpretation of findings.

In young animals, active hematopoiesis occurs throughout the skeleton in both the long bones (e.g., humerus, femur) and flat bones (e.g., ribs, pelvis). However, active hematopoiesis in normal adult animals is restricted to the flat bones and extremities of the long bones (e.g., proximal humerus or femur); the central area of the long bones is composed predominantly of adipose tissue. Furthermore, even the hematopoietically active regions of adult animals contain a higher percentage of fat compared to these areas in young animals. Knowledge of the age-related anatomic distribution of hematopoietic tissue is imperative so that an appropriate, representative specimen is collected.

Active hematopoietic tissue is highly vascular and the spaces between vascular sinuses are filled with hematopoietic cells. The hematopoietic areas are bordered by the endothelium lining the vascular sinuses and are given structural scaffolding by adventitial cells. Hematopoietic tissue is predominantly composed of megakaryocyte, erythrocyte, granulocyte, and monocyte cell precursors in various stages of maturation. Low numbers of resident macrophages, lymphocytes, plasma cells, and mast cells, as well as a variable amount of adipose tissue, are also normally present.

Collection of both aspirates and core biopsy specimens is technically simple (see Bone Marrow Aspirate and Biopsy). Aspirate specimens allow detailed analysis of cell populations, individual cell identification, and morphologic evaluation and are more amenable to cytochemical staining and immunocytochemistry. However, aspirates do not preserve architecture and may not be representative of the marrow as a whole. Myelofibrosis, regardless of the cause and, to a certain extent, the severity, often exfoliates poorly and may yield an insufficient specimen, so a core biopsy is crucial in these instances. Core biopsies have a longer turnaround time and are more expensive, but their utility lies in the preservation of tissue architecture and more accurate impression of overall cellularity. Additionally, cell arrangement, necrosis, infiltrative patterns, myelofibrosis, absolute megakaryocyte numbers, and quantification of iron stores can be better assessed in a core biopsy sample.

Prior to laboratory submission, a slide should be stained to assess whether it contains an adequate number of well-preserved hematopoietic unit particles or spicules. Spicules grossly appear as fatty streaks on unstained preparations and as intensely staining blue areas on stained preparations. If the slide is satisfactory, the stained and, preferably, additional unstained slides may then be sent to a diagnostic laboratory. Bone marrow aspirates collected into EDTA may also be submitted to the lab so that additional slides may be prepared.

INDICATIONS

- Peripheral blood abnormalities.
- Unexplained, persistent decreases in cell counts, including non- or poorly regenerative anemia, neutropenia, or thrombocytopenia.
- Unexplained, persistent elevations in cell counts.
- Atypical cells in peripheral blood.
- Clinical staging of malignancy.
- Unexplained hyperproteinemia or monoclonal gammopathy.
- Unexplained hypercalcemia.
- Fever of unknown origin, especially in searching for occult disease, including infectious agents.
- Assessment of body iron stores.
- Suspicion of osteomyelitis or infiltrative or proliferative bone marrow disease as may or may not be suggested by diagnostic imaging.
- A bone marrow core biopsy is indicated when repeated aspiration attempts, particularly if different sites are sampled, fail to yield adequate marrow samples.

CONTRAINDICATIONS

None

POTENTIAL COMPLICATIONS

- Risks related to heavy sedation or anesthesia necessary for procedure.
- Fracture of bone already compromised by infiltrative disease or other pathology.

CLIENT EDUCATION

- Interpretation of findings typically contingent upon CBC collected within 24 hours.
- Inherent pathology such as myelofibrosis can result in yield of insufficient sample (biopsy preferred to aspirate).

BODY SYSTEMS ASSESSED

Hemic/lymphatic/immune

SAMPLE

SAMPLE COLLECTION

Marrow from proximal humerus or femur, wing of ilium, or sternum. Can be collected into EDTA, or directly prepared onto glass microscope slides.

SAMPLE HANDLING

Transport slides at room temperature in an appropriate protective slide container. Marrow collected into EDTA should be maintained chilled as with CBC blood samples.

SAMPLE STORAGE

Store slides at room temperature, protected from light. Avoid exposure to extreme temperatures, humidity, and formalin fumes (submit bone marrow core biopsies in separate specimen bag). Retain unstained slides for possible ancillary testing.

SAMPLE STABILITY

- Stained slides are stable for months to years.
- Unstained slides are stable for 1 week or more.

PROTOCOL

- Subjective evaluation of the marrow begins with a low-power (40– 100×) magnification of overall cellularity, megakaryocyte numbers, and iron content.
- Evaluate cellularity—identify multiple large, intact particles and compare the proportion of dark blue-staining hematopoietic tissue to the proportion of colorless adipose tissue within the particle to determine a rough percentage. Estimates of cellularity will be inaccurate if the number of particles on the slide is low. Good-quality bone marrow core biopsies typically give a more accurate assessment.
- Assess megakaryocytes—approximately 2–7 megakaryocytes are normally associated with each particle, although the exact number varies by species and the technique used to make the cytologic preparation. Megakaryocytes are the largest of the hematopoietic cells and are easily seen at low-power magnification. Mature megakaryocytes should predominate; they have abundant pale basophilic cytoplasm with fine magenta granules and 8 or more nuclei fused into a dense, lobulated mass.

- Assess iron stores—a few small clumps of brown to black material per particle representing iron stored in the form of hemosiderin are routinely identified in the bone marrow of normal dogs. Prussian blue reaction may be used to confirm the presence or absence of iron, but typically is not necessary. Stainable iron is usually absent in normal bone marrow from healthy cats.
- At high power (500– 1000× magnification), attempt a general assessment of cell distribution (M/E ratio).
- Erythroid precursors appear as smaller, darker cells. They generally have darker basophilic cytoplasm and round nuclei with condensed chromatin.
- Myeloid precursors are larger and paler with light blue cytoplasm that may contain magenta primary granules or secondary granules with a round, indented, or U-shaped nucleus. Secondary granules can be eosinophilic, basophilic, or nonstaining (i.e., in neutrophil precursors).
- In healthy animals, there are approximately equal numbers of erythroid and myeloid precursors that should be overwhelmingly predominated by the later stages.
- Other cells, such as macrophages, lymphocytes, plasma cells, and mast cells, are normally found in low numbers.
- If any single type of cell appears to predominate, or if unusual morphologies are encountered, evaluation by a board-certified pathologist is recommended.

INTERPRETATION

NORMAL FINDINGS OR RANGE

- Cellularity (adults)—33%–66% hematopoietic cells; remaining percentages consist of adipose tissue.
- Megakaryocytes—2–7 megakaryocytes per spicule; highly variable depending on the technique used to prepare the slide and overall sample yield (e.g., presence of spicules).
- M/E ratio—0.75–2.53 (dogs) and 1.21–2.16 (cats).

ABNORMAL FINDINGS

Values above or below the reference ranges.

CRITICAL VALUES

None

INTERFERING FACTORS

Drugs That May Alter Results or Interpretation

Drugs That Interfere with Test Methodology

None

Drugs That Alter Physiology

Some drugs have been associated with toxic effects on hematopoietic cells, including diethylstilbestrol, phenylbutazone, chloramphenicol (especially cats), sulfadiazine, methimazole, albendazole, phenobarbital, and griseofulvin.

Disorders That May Alter Results

- Low yield aspirates (e.g., overall poor cellularity or lacking sufficient spicules) may occur with hypocellular marrow, stromal reactions (e.g., myelofibrosis), and neoplasms resulting in myelophthisis (e.g., mesenchymal neoplasms).
- Chronic blood loss anemia may lead to megakaryocytic hyperplasia despite a normal platelet count.

Collection Techniques or Handling That May Alter Results

- Inappropriate collection site (i.e., area of bone not actively involved in hematopoiesis).
- Insufficient number of particles/low yield aspirate.
- Excessive pressure when preparing cytologic slides or delayed collection (>30 minutes) after animal's death may result in lysed cells.
- Delayed processing or exposure of cytology to formalin fumes will alter staining.
- Clotted aspirates will have reduced cellularity and skewed differential cell counts.

Influence of Signalment

Species

- Cats normally lack stainable iron, regardless of their age.
- Subtle variations in differential cell percentages (e.g., cats may have slightly more numerous lymphocytes than dogs).

Breed

None

Age

- Young animals have active hematopoietic tissue throughout long and flat bones. Adult animals exhibit the most active hematopoiesis in their flat bones and the extremities of their long bones. The central area of long bones contains abundant adipose tissue and very little active hematopoietic tissue.
- Older dogs often have abundant stainable iron, whereas younger dogs do not.

Gender

None

Pregnancy

None

LIMITATIONS OF THE TEST

Sensitivity, Specificity, and Positive and Negative Predictive Values

N/A

Valid If Run in a Human Lab?

Yes

CAUSES OF ABNORMAL FINDINGS

See Table 1.

CLINICAL PERSPECTIVE

- Cytologic findings must be interpreted in light of the medical history, clinical findings, CBC, and results from other diagnostic tests and procedures.
- A bone marrow aspirate cannot be adequately interpreted without a concurrent CBC, particularly with regard to assessment of the M/E ratio.

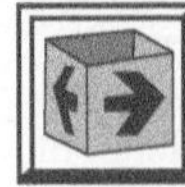

MISCELLANEOUS

ANCILLARY TESTS

- Concurrent CBC (obtained within the last 24 hours).
- Blood film morphologic assessment of circulating blood cells.
- Bone marrow core biopsy sample.
- Immunocytochemistry, immunophenotyping, and cytochemical stains to determine clonality and lineage of abnormal cells identified in marrow, including PARR and flow cytometry.
- FeLV IFA or PCR on bone marrow for occult FeLV infection if peripheral blood ELISA is negative.
- Serology or PCR testing for arthropod-vectored diseases (e.g., *Ehrlichia* spp.).
- Serum protein electrophoresis to assess hyperglobulinemia.

SYNONYMS

None

SEE ALSO

- Anemia, Aplastic.
- Anemia, Nonregenerative.
- Bone Marrow Aspirate and Biopsy (in Appendix X).
- Ehrlichiosis
- Feline Leukemia Virus (FeLV) Infection.
- Lymphoma—Cats.
- Lymphoma—Dogs.
- Mast Cell Tumors.
- Multiple Myeloma.

ABBREVIATIONS

- Epo = erythropoietin.
- FeLV = feline leukemia virus.
- FIV = feline immunodeficiency virus.
- G-CSF = granulocyte colony-stimulating factor.
- M/E or M:E ratio = myeloid/erythroid ratio.

Table 1

Causes of abnormal values.

Marrow Component	*High Values (Hyperplasia)*	*Low Values (Hypoplasia)*
Iron stores	Hemolysis Previous blood transfusions Erythroid hypoplasia Parenteral iron supplementation	Iron deficiency
Overall cellularity	Response to peripheral demand (see specific lineages) Anemia and/or hypoxemia (erythroid hyperplasia) Neutrophilic inflammation (granulocytic/ myeloid hyperplasia) Thrombocytopenia (megakaryocytic hyperplasia) Neoplasia, primary or metastatic, and other myeloproliferative disorders	Generalized hypoplasia/aplasia Certain antibiotics (e.g., trimethoprim-sulfadiazine, cephalosporins, chloramphenicol) Estrogens, exogenous or endogenous (dogs and ferrets) Anticonvulsants (e.g., phenobarbital) Phenylbutazone (dogs) Griseofulvin (cats) Thiacetarsamide, meclofenamic acid, quinidine (a possible cause in dogs) Albendazole Chemotherapy Radiation Myelonecrosis (may have degenerate cells) Myelofibrosis Canine parvovirus infections (erythroid and myeloid hypoplasia) FeLV infection (especially with feline parvovirus infection) Severe Ehrlichia canis infection Primary immune-mediated destruction of hematopoietic precursor cells Idiopathic
Erythroid	Effective erythroid hyperplasia in response to anemia and/or hypoxemia Ineffective erythroid hyperplasia Severe iron deficiency Folate deficiency Some myeloproliferative and myelodysplastic disorders Congenital dyserythropoiesis Immune-mediated destruction of late erythroid precursors Idiopathic Response to Epo treatment Renal or other Epo-secreting neoplasms	Selective erythroid hypoplasia Parvovirus vaccination? Gray collies with cyclic hematopoiesis (followed by erythroid hyperplasia) Chloramphenicol (especially in cats) Lymphoid malignancy Immune-mediated destruction of early erythroid precursors Immune mediated, associated with recombinant Epo therapy FeLV type C infection Dogs with idiopathic myelofibrosis Anemia of inflammatory disease (concomitant granulocytic hyperplasia) Endocrinopathies (e.g., hypothyroidism, hypoadrenocorticism, hypopituitarism, hypoandrogenism; usually does not increase M/E ratio) Chronic renal disease (usually does not increase M/E ratio)
Neutrophilic myeloid precursors	Effective myeloid hyperplasia Proliferative response to neutrophilic inflammation Dogs with β2-integrin adhesion molecule deficiency Gray collies with cyclic hematopoiesis Ineffective myeloid hyperplasia Myelodysplastic disorders Acute myelocytic leukemia Neutropenic cats with FeLV and/or FIV infection Immune-mediated targeting myeloid precursors Idiopathic Response to G-CSF treatment Paraneoplastic neutrophilia	Selective myeloid hypoplasia Azathioprine (cats) Griseofulvin (risk increased in FIV-positive cats) Methimazole (reported in cats) Recombinant G-CSF from another species (similar to recombinant Epo-induced anemia) Canine and feline parvovirus infection (concurrent erythroid hypoplasia) Gray collies with cyclic hematopoiesis (followed by neutrophilic hyperplasia) FeLV-induced cyclic hematopoiesis Immune-mediated targeting early myeloid precursors

(Continued)

BONE MARROW ASPIRATE CYTOLOGY: MICROSCOPIC EVALUATION (CONTINUED)

Table 1

Causes of abnormal values (*continued*)		
Marrow Component	*High Values (Hyperplasia)*	*Low Values (Hypoplasia)*
Eosinophilic myeloid precursors	Parasitic disease (especially nematode and fluke infestation) Inflammation of organs rich in mast cells (skin, lung, intestine, uterus) IgE-mediated allergic hypersensitivity reactions Eosinophilic granulomas Hypereosinophilic syndrome Eosinophilic leukemia Myelodysplastic disorders Mast cell and some other tumors (uncommon to rare)	Eosinophilic hypoplasia not a clinically recognized entity
Basophils	Usually associated with same disorders causing eosinophilia Dirofilariasis (dogs and cats) Lymphomatoid granulomatosis Basophilic leukemia Myelodysplastic disorders	Basophilic hypoplasia not a clinically recognized entity
Megakaryocytes	Primary and secondary immune-mediated thrombocytopenia Ongoing intravascular coagulation Hypersplenism Vascular injury Infections (e.g., early Ehrlichia canis) and toxicoses causing platelet destruction Thrombocythemia	Selective megakaryocytic hypoplasia Immune-mediated Drug-induced: hypoplasia usually generalized, but megakaryocytes may be specifically decreased (e.g., dapsone [in dogs] and ribavarin [in cats, concomitant erythroid hypoplasia possible]) Meclofenamic acid Phenylbutazone Trimethoprim-sulfadiazine Chemotherapy

INTERNET RESOURCES

http://eclinpath.com/atlas/bone-marrow/

Suggested Reading

Grindem CB, Neel JA, Juopperi TA. Cytology of bone marrow. Vet Clin North Am Small Anim Pract 2002, 32:1313–1374.

Harvey JW. Veterinary Hematology: A Diagnostic Guide and Color Atlas. St. Louis, MO: Elsevier/Saunders, 2012.

Stockham SL, Scott MA. Fundamentals of Veterinary Clinical Pathology, 2nd ed. Ames, IA: Wiley-Blackwell, 2008.

Author Rebekah G. Gunn-Christie

Consulting Editor Benjamin M. Brainard

Acknowledgment The author and editors acknowledge the prior contribution of John W. Harvey.

COMPLETE OPHTHALMOLOGIC EXAM

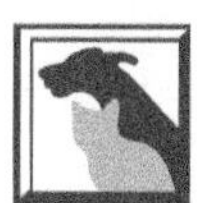

BASICS

TYPE OF PROCEDURE

Diagnostic examination

PROCEDURE EXPLANATION AND RELATED PHYSIOLOGY

- Step-wise assessment of the adnexal and ocular components, their structural and neurological function, and their potential affects on ocular comfort and vision.
- Various diagnostic tests and equipment are used as part of the eye exam, and familiarity with the normal values and ocular anatomy will allow for recognition of early or subtle changes and assist in diagnosis and treatment of discrete ophthalmic conditions.

INDICATIONS

- Indicated as part of a wellness examination or as part of a health screening in breeding animals.
- Iindicated when the patient is presented for ocular discomfort, an abnormal ocular appearance, or changes in vision. As part of diagnostic testing for an unknown illness, an eye exam may reveal ocular manifestations of systemic disease.

CONTRAINDICATIONS

Individual steps of the eye exam may be contraindicated, such as pharmacological mydriasis in a patient with elevated intraocular pressure or tonometry in a patient with a fragile globe (deep corneal ulcer, perforation or laceration).

POTENTIAL COMPLICATIONS

- A complete eye exam is a noninvasive procedure; however, some of the ancillary diagnostic tests require direct contact with the cornea or application of ophthalmic drugs:
    - Risk of drug hypersensitivity to topical anesthetic or mydriatic agents, resulting in conjunctival hyperemia, chemosis, ocular pruritis, blepharospasm, or photophobia.
    - Contact with the cornea while performing tonometry or tear assessment could result in corneal epithelial erosions. While these complications are rare, they can cause ocular discomfort.

CLIENT EDUCATION

- The eye exam is important in determining the cause of ocular discomfort or changes in ocular appearance or vision, and may be a key component in recognition of local or systemic infection, inflammation or neoplasia.
- The need for a referral to a veterinary ophthalmologist for more extensive diagnostic testing, medical therapy, or surgical procedures may be indicated based on the findings.
- Detection of certain ocular abnormalities in breeding animals may suggest inherited conditions, and could affect reproductive decisions.

BODY SYSTEMS ASSESSED

Ocular and neuro-ophthalmic.

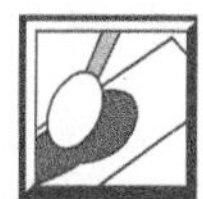

PROCEDURE

PATIENT PREPARATION

Pre-Procedure Medication, Equipment or Supplies (Figure 1)

Prior to the eye exam, the following medications, instrumentation, and accessory diagnostic tools should be available:

- Topical ophthalmic anesthetic, such as proparacaine HCl 0.5% ophthalmic solution.
- Topical ophthalmic mydriatic, such as tropicamide 1% ophthalmic solution.
- Eye wash/eye irrigating solution.
- Schirmer tear test strips.
- Fluorescein stain ophthalmic strips or solution.
- Tonometer (rebound or applanation).
- Ophthalmoscope handle with direct lens attachment, including cobalt blue filter, and a Finoff transilluminator tip.
- Hand-held condensing lens (20D, 28D, 30D or 2.2 pan retinal lenses) for indirect ophthalmoscopy.
- Magnifying loupes, such as OptiVISOR.

Anesthesia or Sedation

Except in the case of an extremely fractious animal, sedation should be avoided. Most sedative agents will lower tear production, in addition to making examination of the eye more difficult due to elevation of the nictitating membrane and ventral rotation of the globe.

Patient Positioning

- Good restraint of the patient is key to a thorough eye exam. Ideally, the patient should be positioned on an exam table in sternal recumbency.
- Special attention to minimal manipulation of the eyelids is important when assessing the eyelid and globe position, and also when obtaining intraocular pressures to avoid falsely elevated readings.

TECHNIQUE

- The complete eye exam, similar to a physical exam, is performed in a step-wise fashion, typically in the same order each time to avoid missing subtle abnormalities.
- The initial part of the exam is performed from a distance and without touching the patient, while later steps require good restraint and minimal movement from the patient.
- A thorough patient medical and ocular history is important to obtaining an accurate diagnosis and appropriate treatment plan:

1. Observation of the patient prior to restraint may allow for detection of behaviors suggestive of visual deficits. Interactions between the pet and objects in the exam room may reveal hesitancy or loss of visual cues in an unfamiliar environment. If visual deficits are suspected, consider additional tests, such as maze testing using obstacles placed in the patient's path or cotton-ball tracking to investigate further. These tests can be done in both room lighting and dim lighting conditions to explore the possibility of decreased night vision or nyctalopia.
2. Once the patient has been adequately restrained, the face and eyes should be assessed for symmetry of adnexal and periocular structures (e.g. muscles of mastication, palpebral fissure size), in addition to globe size and position, and pupil symmetry. The Finoff transilluminator can be held at an arm's length, close to the examiner's eye, and retroillumination using the tapetal reflex will allow for good assessment of pupillary size and symmetry. Palpation of the tissues around the orbit may reveal muscle atrophy, boney proliferation or orbital cellulitis. The globe itself should easily retropulse into the orbit behind closed lids. Retropulsion may be important in helping to distinguish exophthalmia from buphthalmia. An oral exam is indicated for patients with suspected orbital disease.
3. The neuro-ophthalmic exam includes assessment of cranial nerves (CN) II–VII.
    a. The palpebral reflex is performed by gently touching at the temporal and then nasal canthus, and observing the eyelids to close. Incomplete blink may suggest either a decrease in sensation (CN V) or motor function (CN VII) or lagophthalmia, such as is seen in brachycephalic dogs.
    b. The menace response, a crude estimation of vision, assesses CN II and CN VII. This is a learned response present in animals older than 8–12 weeks of age. This test is performed by making a swift "menacing gesture" with a closed hand toward the eye and watching for a blink response ± slight withdrawal of the head. Be careful not create movements of air or brush against hairs around the eye that could stimulate a response that is tactile rather than visual. By covering each eye in turn, a more individual assessment of the contralateral eye can be performed.
    c. The pupillary light reflex (PLR) can be appraised after noting for symmetry in size, shape and position of the pupils (e.g., anisocoria, dyscoria). A bright

COMPLETE OPHTHALMOLOGIC EXAM (CONTINUED)

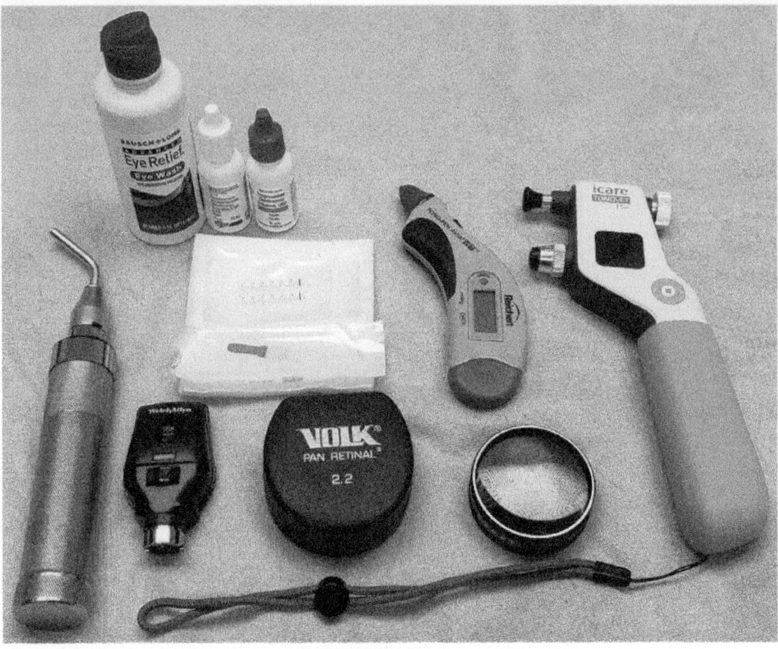

Figure 1.

From top left: Eye wash irrigating solution, proparacaine HCl 0.5% ophthalmic solution, tropicamide 1% ophthalmic solution, TonoPen Avia® applanation tonometer, TonoVet Plus® rebound tonometer, Volk 2.2 Pan Retinal hand-held condensing lens and case, direct ophthalmoscope head attachment, and ophthalmoscope handle with Finoff transilluminator attachment. Source: Lawrence P. Tilley

light from a Finoff transilluminator should stimulate a direct response (pupil constriction) in the ipsilateral eye and a slightly less robust consensual response in the contralateral eye. The PLR should be assessed for each eye, with notation of both direct and consensual responses. PLRs can be complete, incomplete, delayed, or absent. Any abnormal response may suggest pathology in the retina, optic nerve, or PLR pathway, including CN III or iris sphincter muscles. This test does not assess the visual pathways in the brain.

d. The dazzle reflex is also performed with a bright light directed towards each eye, with a reflexive response of blinking. This test assesses CN II, CN VII and the visual pathways in the brain. Although a positive test does not correlate directly with vision, a negative dazzle reflex does give a poor prognosis for return to vision.

e. The presence of strabismus or nystagmus or lack of ability to move the globe may indicate oculomotor (neurologic or extraocular muscle) deficits and could indicate either central or peripheral nervous system disorders or orbital disease. Mild esotropia and pronounced physiologic nystagmus are common in Siamese cats.

4. The accessory diagnostic tests are performed next.

a. The Schirmer tear test (STT) is a measurement of both basal and reflex tear production. This is performed by placing the notched end of STT strip into the conjunctival fornix in the lateral 2/3 of the lower lid. Care is taken not to handle this portion of the strip to avoid contamination with oil or debris from the examiners' fingers. Placement of a slight bend at the notch through the protective plastic sleeve may help to keep it in position. The strip should remain in the fornix for 60 seconds, removed, and immediately read out. A normal tear production in a dog is approximately 18 ± 3 mm/min. Tests reading below 15 mm/min in combination with clinical signs of keratoconjunctivitis (e.g., mucoid discharge, conjunctival hyperemia, corneal pigmentation or vascularization) may signal quantitative tear film abnormalities (keratoconjunctivitis sicca [KCS]). Normal STT readings with similar clinical signs may indicate a qualitative tear film abnormality.

b. Following the STT, the intraocular pressure (IOP) should be estimated. If an applanation tonometer is to be used, application of topical anesthetic 20–30 seconds prior to testing is necessary. A rebound tonometer does not require topical anesthetic. The examiner should be familiar with the instrument's requirement for calibration, instructions for use, and also understand the measurement confidence interval (CI 85–95%) for each reading. The patient should be gently restrained with minimal pressure on the neck and eyelids to allow for the most accurate readings. Tight muzzles may interfere with normal IOP readings. Most devices require 5-6 contacts with the cornea to calculate an average estimated IOP. Any reading with <95% CI or IOP >20 mmHg should be repeated to ensure accuracy. Consider additional testing if glaucoma is suspected.

c. Following IOP measurement, one drop of fluorescein stain can be applied to look for evidence of corneal epithelial erosions or ulceration. The stain should be gently rinsed with eye wash or saline, and the cornea should be evaluated with the cobalt blue filter of the ophthalmoscope head. Stain uptake will appear bright green in the blue light, and indicates loss of the corneal epithelium. Corneal ulcers should be treated accordingly based on features such as chronicity, depth, and evidence of infection. With any deep corneal ulcer, the eye should be considered fragile and at risk of perforation.

d. If the eye exam is normal to this stage, a drop of tropicamide, an ophthalmic mydriatic agent, may be applied topically to dilate the pupil. Dilation will allow for a comprehensive examination of the lens and fundus. In patients with an elevated IOP, iris pigment changes, iris masses or marked irregularities, suspected lens instability, or PLR abnormalities, a consultation with an ophthalmologist may be recommended prior to dilation.

5. The next step in the eye exam is a survey of the adnexal structures- the eyelids, including the nictitating membrane, conjunctiva, and nasal-lacrimal system. The Finoff transilluminator can be used to examine these structures. Additional magnification in the form of magnifying loupes may be required.

a. The eyelids should be inspected for abnormalities in position or length (e.g. entropion/ectropion, ptosis), irregularities, thickening or discoloration (e.g. lid masses, blepharitis), or aberrant hairs (distichia, ectopic cilia, trichiasis). The eyelid margin should be smooth and in contact with the cornea help to evenly distribute the tear film. The meibomian gland openings should be apparent as gray dots along the lid margin, but should not be inflamed or have excess discharge.

b. The conjunctiva lines the eyelids (palpebral conjunctiva), the globe (bulbar conjunctiva) and nictitating membrane. The conjunctiva, a mucous membrane, should be smooth, pink and moist without excessive discharge. If conjunctivitis is suspected, additional testing can be considered.

c. Examination of the nictitating membrane is enhanced when the globe is gently retropulsed so that this third eyelid will passively elevate. If there is suspicion of foreign material in the eye, the leading edge of the nictitating membrane can be grasped with atraumatic forceps, such as von Graefe forceps, following the application of topical anesthetic. Any swelling or protrusion of the third eyelid, its gland or cartilage should be further investigated.

d. The lacrimal puncta are located near the medial canthus, just inside the eyelid margin of the upper and lower eyelids. The openings should lack discharge. Chronic epiphora or mucopurulent discharge may be suggestive of an obstruction of the nasal lacrimal system or dacryocystitis. A positive Jones test (a drop of fluorescein stain placed on the cornea observed exiting the ipsilateral nares) confirms patency of the nasal–lacrimal system.

6. Examination of the cornea can be performed with the Finoff transilluminator, but magnification using the direct ophthalmoscope is ideal for noting fine details. The corneal surface should be smooth and transparent, with a lustrous tear film, and no evidence of blood vessels, pigment, fibrosis, edema or other opacity. Commonly, tear film abnormalities are the cause of corneal changes in the dog. The STT is important in ruling out dry eye disease. The fluorescein stain test can assess for corneal ulceration. Keratitis, or inflammation of the cornea, is usually represented by vascularization, corneal infiltrate, or pigmentation, and can be ulcerative or non-ulcerative. Various corneal dystrophies, corneal degeneration or other keratopathies may also be present.

7. The anterior chamber should be evaluated for appropriate depth and clarity. The slit beam of the direct ophthalmoscope can be used to look for flare (protein or cellular debris) in the anterior chamber causing the Tyndall effect (scattering of light causing a hazy beam to appear in the normally clear aqueous). The slit beam should be focused on the cornea, and there should be no evidence of light between the cornea and iris face/anterior lens capsule in the normal eye. Any opacity in the anterior chamber should be further assessed, as anterior uveitis is most likely the cause. Strands of vitreous may be seen in the anterior chamber in patients with lens instability.

8. The iris is most easily examined prior to dilation. The direct ophthalmoscope can be used for magnification. The iris face is not completely smooth, and the major arterial circle runs along the periphery, close to the iris base. This is especially apparent in animals with light colored irides. Irregularities in the iris, such as excess pigment or pigment loss, abnormal blood vessels, fine strands of tissue (e.g. persistent pupillary membranes) or iridal masses should be noted prior to pharmacological dilation. The pupil margin should be smooth, although some patients have a slightly darker but normal "pupillary ruff." A moth-eaten or ragged edge to the pupil margin, especially in conjunction with decreased miosis during PLR assessment, may indicate iris atrophy. A patient with uveitis often has a miotic pupil at rest and may have evidence of fine blood vessels on the iris face (rubeosis iridis), in addition to flare in the anterior chamber.

9. The lens should be examined with the pupil dilated to allow for the most comprehensive assessment. The direct ophthalmoscope can be used for magnification to look at fine details in the lens, but the Finhoff transilluminator is good to assess the overall appearance. The lens and lens capsule should be smooth and transparent. Any opacity within the lens that blocks the tapetal reflex is considered a cataract, while nuclear sclerosis is simply the more densely compacted nuclear lens fibers noted in older animals. Nuclear sclerosis does not block the light passing through to the posterior segment or light bouncing off the tapetum during retroillumination, and a fundic exam can be easily performed in a patient with nuclear sclerosis; however, varying degrees of cataract may make the fundic exam more difficult or impossible. Any lens instability should be noted, as lens subluxation or luxation are a risk for development of glaucoma. With early lens instability, an aphakic crescent may be noted, when some of the zonules holding the lens in place are lost, allowing the lens to shift in position. This may appear as a brighter tapetal reflection along the equator of the lens. In a normal patient, the equator, or most peripheral aspect of the lens, should not be visible. Occasionally, vitreous can be seen coming forward into the anterior chamber in the region of the aphakic crescent.

10. The posterior segment exam can be performed with the direct ophthalmoscope, but a more panoramic view of the fundus is best achieved using indirect ophthalmoscopy.

a. First, using the Finoff transilluminator, the region just posterior to the lens should be surveyed for any opacity. Anterior vitreous changes causing opacities include vitreal degeneration (e.g., asteroid hyalosis, syneresis). Other changes in the vitreous could be due to congenital abnormalities, hemorrhage, or intraocular neoplasia.

b. For the best view of the fundus, including retinal blood vessels, tapetum and non-tapetum, and optic disc, a hand-held condensing lens (20D, 28D, 30D or 2.2 pan retinal lens) and Finoff transilluminator are used for indirect ophthalmoscopy. The examiner sits or stands at about one arm's length from the patient while an assistant stabilizes the head and gently retracts the eyelids. The Finoff light source is held close to the examiner's eye, directed at the patient's eye.

COMPLETE OPHTHALMOLOGIC EXAM (CONTINUED)

A bright tapetal reflex will help guide the examiner to the appropriate placement of the lens, about 5–6 cm from the patient's eye. The lens should be moved just slightly either towards the examiner or towards the patient until the fundic image is focused on the lens. The examiner should make slight adjustments with their own head and body rather than moving the light or lens to observe the entire fundus. The image created with this method is upside down and backwards, so the necessary movements to achieve a view of the entire fundus may not be intuitive. The fundus should be surveyed systematically in each quadrant (nasal and temporal tapetum and non-tapetum) and the optic disc should be evaluated for color, shape, loss of detail or changes in depth (e.g. raised or cupped). A raised and hyperemic optic disc may indicate optic neuritis, while a pale or dark and cupped disc may indicate chronic glaucoma. Changes in the position or contour of the retina, such as in retinal detachment or retinal dysplasia should also be noted. Subretinal infiltrates, such as inflammatory cells or blood, may be present with chorioretinitis.

c. The direct ophthalmoscope can also be used to examine the fundus. Although the image acquired is in the correct, upright orientation, the fundus is extremely magnified and may make interpretation of findings more difficult. For the direct fundic exam, the examiner's eye, direct ophthalmoscope, and patient's eye are very close to each other (2–3 cm), which may be dangerous with unruly patients. The direct ophthalmoscope is set to 0 diopters, and the examiner moves in closer to the patient's eye until retinal vessels are in focus. The same four quadrant survey and exam is performed, but this method makes the peripheral fundus more challenging to see than with the more panoramic indirect method.

11. Once the eye exam is completed, all abnormalities should be documented, and the changes correlated with patient history and clinical signs to develop a diagnosis and treatment plan. Visual deficits in the absence of significant ophthalmic abnormalities may be due to conditions such as sudden acquired retinal degeneration syndrome (SARDS), retrobulbar or optic tract neuropathy or optic neuritis, or central vision loss. Consultation with a veterinary ophthalmologist and/or neurologist may be appropriate depending on history and any other clinical signs or behavior changes. Additional diagnostic tests such as CT or MRI may be indicated with suspicion of orbital disease or central lesions. See Table 1 for a selection of abnormal findings and possible differential diagnoses.

APPROPRIATE AFTERCARE

Restrictions on Activity

Although most dogs and cats do not appear apprehensive following the use of mydriatic drugs, dilation of the pupils can lead to photophobia or discomfort in bright light. Additionally, some animals are sensitive to topical anesthetic drugs, such as proparacaine. Effects from these ophthalmic drugs can last up to several hours, so clients should be made aware of the potential for mild blepharospasm or conjunctival hyperemia after a complete eye exam.

INTERPRETATION

NORMAL FINDINGS OR RANGE

- STT ≥15 mm/min.
  - Dogs (normal range 18 ± 3 mm/min).
  - Cats* (normal range 17 ± 6 mm/min).

*Cats can reportedly have a STT as low as 0–5 mm/min due to a sympathetic stress response.

- IOP 8–20 mmHg in dogs and 10–25 mmHg in cats.

Table 1

Selection of abnormal findings and potentential differential diagnoses.

Exam component	*Abnormalities*	*Selection of Possible Diagnoses*
Observation	Vision deficits	Retinal disease, CNS disease (including optic nerve and visual tracts), glaucoma, uveitis, cataract, severe keratitis
Palpation	Decreased ocular retropulsion ± pain	Orbital disease
Neuro-ophthalmic examination	Absent PLR/fixed mydriasis with absent menace response	Retinal disease, optic neuritis, glaucoma
Schirmer tear test	<10–15 mm/min	Keratoconjunctivitis sicca (KCS), dry eye
Fluorescein stain	Positive	Corneal ulceration
Intraocular pressure	>20–25 mmHg (elevated)	Glaucoma (primary or secondary)
	<8 mmHg (decreased)	Anterior uveitis
Adnexal structures (eyelids, nictitating membrane, conjunctiva, nasal lacrimal system)	Swelling, hyperemia, increased ocular discharge	Blepharitis, conjunctivitis, Dacryocystitis Neoplasia
	Protrusion of third eyelid	Prolapsed gland of the third eyelid; neoplasia

CRITICAL VALUES

- STT <10–15 mm/min—likely indicates quantitative tear film disorder (KCS).
- IOP >25 mmHg—likely indicates glaucoma.
- IOP <8 mmHg—may indicate uveitis.
- Positive fluorescein stain uptake, especially in conjunction with clinical signs indicating a corneal ulcer.

INTERFERING FACTORS

Drugs That May Alter Results of the Procedure

- Mydriatic drugs, such as topical atropine or tropicamide, can suppress the PLR of the affected eye(s) and may have long-lasting effects.
- Some topical glaucoma medications, such as latanoprost, can cause extreme miosis, precluding the ability to perform a fundic exam.
- Systemic anesthetic and sedative agents will likely depress the STT results and can also blunt the menace response.

Conditions That May Interfere with Performing the Procedure

- Significant anterior segment changes such as marked corneal opacities or cataracts may prohibit a posterior segment examination.
- Patients that are systemically ill or those that have neurologic abnormalities (e.g., post-ictal changes or CNS disease) may not have a normal menace response or neuro-ophthalmic exam.

Procedure Techniques or Handling That May Alter Results

Improper restraint during IOP measurements may lead to falsely elevated readings. Tight muzzles, or excess pressure on the eyelids or neck can lead to increased intraocular pressure.

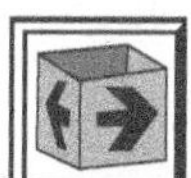

MISCELLANEOUS

ANCILLARY TESTS

- Chromatic pupillometry.
- Electroretinogram (ERG).
- Gonioscopy.
- Ocular ultrasound.
- Pachymetry.
- Systemic blood pressure.
- Advanced imaging (CT or MRI).

SEE ALSO

- Anterior Uveitis—Cats.
- Anterior Uveitis—Dogs.
- Blepharitis.
- Cataracts.
- Chorioretinitis.
- Conjunctivitis—Cats.
- Conjunctivitis—Dogs.
- Corneal Opacities—Degenerations and Infiltrates.
- Epiphora.
- Episcleritis.
- Eyelash Disorders.
- Glaucoma.
- Keratitis, Nonulcerative.
- Keratitis, Ulcerative.
- Keratoconjunctivitis Sicca.
- Lens Luxation.
- Optic Neuritis and Papilledema.
- Orbital Diseases.
- Prolapsed Gland of the Third Eyelid.
- Proptosis.
- Red Eye.
- Retinal Degeneration.
- Third Eyelid Protrusion.
- Uveal Melanoma—Cats.
- Uveal Melanoma—Dogs.

ABBREVIATIONS

- IOP = intraocular pressure.
- PLR = pupillary light reflex.
- STT = Schirmer tear test.

Suggested Reading

Featherstone HJ, Heinrich CL. Ophthalmic examination and diagnostics. Part 1: The eye examination and diagnostic procedures. In: Gelatt KN, Gilger BC, Kern TJ, eds., Veterinary Ophthalmology, 5th ed. Hoboken, NJ: Wiley-Blackwell, 2013, pp. 533–546.

Stades FC, Wyman M, Boeve MH, et al. Ophthalmology for the Veterinary Practitioner, 2nd ed. Hannover, Schlutersche Publishing, 2010, pp. 1–17.

Author Georgina M. Newbold

Consulting Editor Benjamin M. Brainard

CROSSMATCH

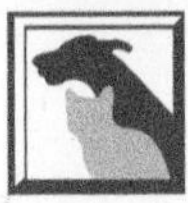

BASICS

TYPE OF SPECIMEN

Blood

TEST EXPLANATION AND RELATED PHYSIOLOGY

- Performed to detect serologic incompatibility between a possible blood donor and recipient. In contrast with blood typing, which recognizes antigens on RBC membranes, a crossmatch evaluates plasma for the presence of antibodies.
- A major crossmatch, which is of greatest clinical significance, tests for alloantibodies in patient plasma against donor RBCs. The minor crossmatch looks for alloantibodies in donor's plasma against patient's RBCs. This is of lesser concern because the donor's plasma volume is small, particularly in packed RBC products, and is markedly diluted in recipients.
- A tube crossmatching procedure is most often used, with antibodies indicated by subsequent hemolysis or hemagglutination, but its interpretation is subjective and requires some expertise.
- Gel column technology (DiaMed AG, Cressier sur Morat, Switzerland, and Ortho Clinical Diagnostic, NJ, USA) is a simple, sensitive, and standardized crossmatch method, but accessibility is limited. Gel-based and immunochromatographic in-house crossmatching kits are now available for dogs and cats, which facilitates the procedure and the interpretation of results (DMS Laboratories, Flemington, NJ and Alvedia, Limonest, France).

INDICATIONS

Screening blood donors and recipients to assure blood compatibility

CONTRAINDICATIONS

None

POTENTIAL COMPLICATIONS

None

CLIENT EDUCATION

None

BODY SYSTEMS ASSESSED

Hemic, lymphatic, and immune.

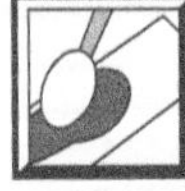

SAMPLE

SAMPLE COLLECTION

- 1–2 mL of venous blood from donor and recipient.
- A segment from the tubing of the donor blood bag can be used.

SAMPLE HANDLING

- Collect the patient's (and possible donor's) blood into EDTA.
- Stored donor cells are often in citrated phosphate dextrose or citrated phosphate dextrose acetate-1 anticoagulant.

SAMPLE STORAGE

Refrigerate the sample for short-term storage.

SAMPLE STABILITY

- Whole blood in EDTA—crossmatch within 48–72 hours of blood collection.
- Properly preserved donor blood—stable for 4 weeks after collection if stored at 4°C.

PROTOCOL (STANDARD TUBE CROSSMATCH)

1. Centrifuge blood (1000 ×*g* for 5 minutes). Remove the plasma from each sample with a pipette, and transfer the sample to clean, labeled tubes. Note any hemolysis.
2. Wash RBCs 3 times with 0.9% saline—resuspend 0.25 mL of RBCs in 2–4 mL of saline. Centrifuge for 1 minute, remove the supernatant, repeat the procedure twice, and remove the supernatant.
3. Resuspend 0.10–0.25 mL of washed RBCs in ≈4.5 mL 0.9% saline to obtain a 3–5% RBC suspension.
4. For each donor, prepare three tubes labeled major, minor, and recipient autocontrol. Add to each tube 2 drops (50 μL) of plasma and 1 drop (25 μL) of RBC suspension as follows:
   a. Major—recipient plasma + donor RBCs.
   b. Minor—donor plasma + recipient RBCs.
   c. Autocontrol—recipient plasma + recipient RBCs.
5. Mix gently and incubate for 15–20 minutes at 37°C.
6. Centrifuge for 15 seconds.
7. Reading the results—examine the supernatant for hemolysis. Gently resuspend the RBC button by tapping tube and examine for agglutinating clumps. Grade positive hemagglutination reactions as 1+ (fine), 2+ (small), 3+ (large), or 4+ (1 large agglutinate).
8. If macroscopic agglutination is not observed, examine a drop of resuspended RBCs for microscopic agglutination (100× or 400×). This is of questionable importance.
9. A positive reaction in the control tube indicates autoantibodies, which complicate the interpretation of other tubes.

INTERPRETATION

NORMAL FINDINGS OR RANGE

Compatible crossmatch—the absence of hemolysis or hemagglutination.

ABNORMAL FINDINGS

Incompatible crossmatch—the presence of hemolysis or hemagglutination.

CRITICAL VALUES

None

INTERFERING FACTORS

Drugs That May Alter Results or Interpretation

Drugs That Interfere with Test Methodology

None

Drugs That Alter Physiology

Hydroxyethyl starch solution (hetastarch) can lead to rouleaux, which can be mistaken for agglutination. Rouleaux can be distinguished from true agglutination if RBC clusters disperse with the addition of saline.

Disorders That May Alter Results

Persistent autoagglutination, such as in immune-mediated hemolytic anemia, precludes crossmatching because such samples always appear incompatible.

Collection Techniques or Handling That May Alter Results

Severe hemolysis may preclude crossmatch testing.

Influence of Signalment

Species

- Dogs—first-time transfusions are considered safe without prior crossmatching since dogs do not have clinically significant naturally-occurring alloantibodies. Although mild immunologic incompatibilities have been documented in transfusion-naive dogs (crossmatch weakly incompatible), their clinical importance requires further investigation.
- Cats—both AB-blood typing and crossmatching are recommended in all cats, even with the first transfusion, as 15–19% of cats have naturally occurring antibodies against RBC antigens outside of the AB system, although their clinical importance is unclear.

Breed

- Dogs—previously transfused crossmatch-incompatible Dalmatian, Doberman pinschers and shih tzu are at great risk of Dal-incompatibility (due to an increased frequency of Dal-negative dogs in these breeds).
- Cats—because of the increased prevalence of type B cats in certain breeds (e.g., Abyssinian, Devon Rex, exotic shorthair), A-B incompatibility is more frequently encountered in those breeds.

Age

None

Gender

None

Pregnancy

- Dogs—unlike women, bitches do not become sensitized to RBC antigens, and subsequently produce alloantibodies, during gestation.
- Cats—unknown.

LIMITATIONS OF THE TEST

• A compatible crossmatch does not prevent sensitization or delayed transfusion reactions. It simply indicates that currently there are no significant antibodies against the RBCs.

• Crossmatching provides no information about leukocyte or platelet compatibility and, in some cases, may not be sensitive enough to detect anti-RBC antibodies.

Sensitivity, Specificity, and Positive and Negative Predictive Values

N/A

Valid If Run in a Human Lab?

Yes (excluding direct antiglobulin test).

CLINICAL PERSPECTIVE

Any dogs and cats that have been given a previous transfusion should be crossmatched before they receive additional blood even when the same donor is being used. Alloantibodies can develop within 4 days and may last for many years.

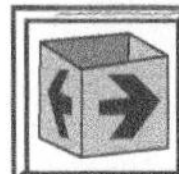

MISCELLANEOUS

ANCILLARY TESTS

Blood typing.

SYNONYMS

None

SEE ALSO

Blood Typing (in Appendix X).

Suggested Reading

Blais MC, Rozanski EA, Hale AS, et al. Lack of evidence of pregnancy-induced alloantibodies in dogs. J Vet Intern Med 2009, 23:462–465.

Giger U, Gelens CJ, Callan MB, et al. An acute hemolytic transfusion reaction caused by dog erythrocyte antigen 1.1 incompatibility in a previously sensitized dog. J Am Vet Med Assoc. 1995, 206:1358–1362.

Goulet S, Blais MC. Characterization of anti-Dal alloantibodies following sensitization of two Dal-negative dogs. Vet Pathol 2018, 55:108–115.

McClosky ME, Cimino Brown D, Weinstein NM, et al. Prevalence of naturally occurring non-AB blood type incompatibilities in cats and influence of crossmatch on transfusion outcomes. J Vet Intern Med 2018, 32:1934–1942.

Sylvane B, Prittie J, Hohenhaus AE, et al. Effect of cross-match on packed cell volume after transfusion of packed red blood cells in transfusion-naïve anemic cats. J Vet Intern Med 2018, 32:1077–1083

Tocci LJ. Canine recipient screening. In: Yagi K, Holowaychuk M, eds., Manual of Veterinary Transfusion Medicine and Blood Banking. Hoboken, NJ: John Wiley & Sons, 2016, pp. 117–129.

Weinstein NM, Blais MC, Harris K, et al. A newly recognized blood group in domestic shorthair cats: The Mik red cell antigen. J Vet Intern Med 2007, 21:287–292.

Author Marie-Claude Blais

Consulting Editor Benjamin M. Brainard

CYSTOCENTESIS

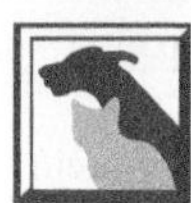

BASICS

TYPE OF PROCEDURE

Diagnostic sample collection

PROCEDURE EXPLANATION AND RELATED PHYSIOLOGY

- Cystocentesis is the gold standard for sterile collection of urine for urinalysis and urine culture.
- Urinalysis is part of the minimum database when evaluating ill dogs and cats or when performing routine health screens. Urine culture should be performed in animals with clinical signs of lower urinary tract disease (e.g., pollakiuria, dysuria), in animals with active urine sediment, in animals with acute kidney injury, and in animals with diseases known to predispose them to urinary tract infections (e.g., diabetes mellitus, hyperadrenocorticism, renal failure).

INDICATIONS

- Routine collection of urine samples for urinalysis or urine culture.
- Immediate relief of bladder overdistention, and to facilitate bladder catheterization, in animals with urethral obstruction.

CONTRAINDICATIONS

- Coagulopathy.
- Thrombocytopenia.
- Pregnancy or pyometra.
- Suspected or confirmed transitional cell carcinoma.
- Severe and diffuse cutaneous disease of caudal abdomen (e.g., severe pyoderma, pemphigus complex).
- Insufficient volume of urine within the bladder.

POTENTIAL COMPLICATIONS

- Seeding of transitional cell carcinoma tumor cells into the abdomen or along the needle track.
- Transient hematuria (rare).
- Iatrogenic urinary tract infection (very rare).
- Bladder rupture (very rare).
- Aortic laceration (very rare).
- Vasovagal response (very rare).

CLIENT EDUCATION

None

BODY SYSTEMS ASSESSED

Renal/urologic

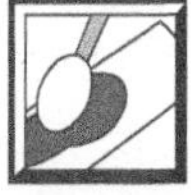

PROCEDURE

PATIENT PREPARATION

Preprocedure Medication or Preparation

- Typically, none is required. Uncooperative patients may require slight sedation for the procedure.
- In rare cases, where urine is required for urinalysis or culture, but frequent voiding or recent urination has hampered urine collection, a single dose of isotonic fluids can be administered, although this will affect urine specific gravity.

Anesthesia or Sedation

None is needed in most patients. Uncooperative patients may require slight sedation for the procedure. Alpha-2 agonists will increase urine flow and decrease urine specific gravity.

Patient Positioning

- For cystocentesis, the bladder is best palpated and isolated while the patient is in lateral recumbency (dogs and cats) or standing (dogs).
- Blind cystocentesis is performed with the patient in dorsal recumbency.

Patient Monitoring

None

Equipment or Supplies

- A 3- to 12-mL syringe.
- A 22-gauge needle (usually 1–1½ inches).
- 70% alcohol (ethyl or isopropyl) for skin preparation.

TECHNIQUE

- The bladder should be palpated prior to attempting cystocentesis. The bladder is normally present in the caudal abdomen; with increased urine volumes the bladder will move cranially, toward the ventral body wall.
- If the bladder can be palpated and contains enough urine to attempt cystocentesis, the bladder isolation technique should be used. In those dogs where the bladder is not easily palpated, ultrasound guidance or a blind aspiration technique can be attempted. Blind aspiration is more commonly associated with complications and is less likely to be successful.
- Attach the needle to the syringe.

Bladder Isolation Technique

- Restrain the patient in lateral recumbency. In some dogs, the bladder is more easily palpated with the patient standing.
- The individual palpating the bladder should isolate the bladder with one hand.
- Clean or spray the cystocentesis site with 70% alcohol.
- Keeping the bladder isolated, the needle should be inserted into the bladder without applying negative pressure.
- Alternatively, an assistant can attempt cystocentesis by inserting the needle and syringe between the fingers of the person who has isolated the bladder. This allows the bladder to be isolated by using two hands and may be easier in dogs. The individual palpating the bladder should guide the assistant as to how far to insert the needle.
- Once the needle has been inserted to the appropriate depth, the syringe plunger should be slowly drawn back, creating negative pressure. Negative pressure should not be applied until the person performing the procedure believes the bladder has been entered.
- When the desired volume of urine has been collected, negative pressure should be released and the syringe and needle removed.

Ultrasound Guidance Technique

- Restrain the patient in dorsal recumbency and using ultrasound identify the bladder on ventral midline of the caudal abdomen.
- Clean or spray the cystocentesis site with 70% alcohol.
- Insert the needle at an oblique angle to the probe where the bladder is visualized.
- When the needle is seen entering the bladder lumen, the syringe plunger should be slowly drawn back, creating negative pressure.
- When the desired volume of urine has been collected, negative pressure should be released and the syringe and needle removed.

Blind Aspiration Technique

- Restrain the patient in dorsal recumbency with the rear limbs extended.
- Spray 70% alcohol over the caudal ventral abdomen.
- The needle is inserted on midline at the site where alcohol pools. Alternatively, the bladder position can be estimated by determining where lines drawn between the last two sets of nipples theoretically cross (Figure 1). In male dogs, move the prepuce and penis to the side to enable insertion of the needle and syringe on the midline plane. The needle should be directed caudally at an approximately 30–45° angle.
- Once the needle has been inserted to the appropriate depth, the plunger of the syringe should be slowly drawn back, creating negative pressure. If urine is not obtained, remove the needle and re-attempt at a site just cranial or caudal.
- If GI tract content or blood is seen in the needle hub, release the negative pressure and then withdraw the needle and syringe. A fresh needle and syringe should be used if blind cystocentesis is reattempted.
- When the desired volume of urine has been collected, negative pressure should be released and the syringe and needle withdrawn.

Decompressive Cystocentesis for Animals with Urethral Obstruction

- Serially attach the needle to IV extension tubing, a three-way stopcock, and a 20- to 60-mL syringe.
- Restrain the patient in dorsal or lateral recumbency and identify the bladder via palpation or with ultrasound.
- Clean or spray the cystocentesis site with 70% alcohol.

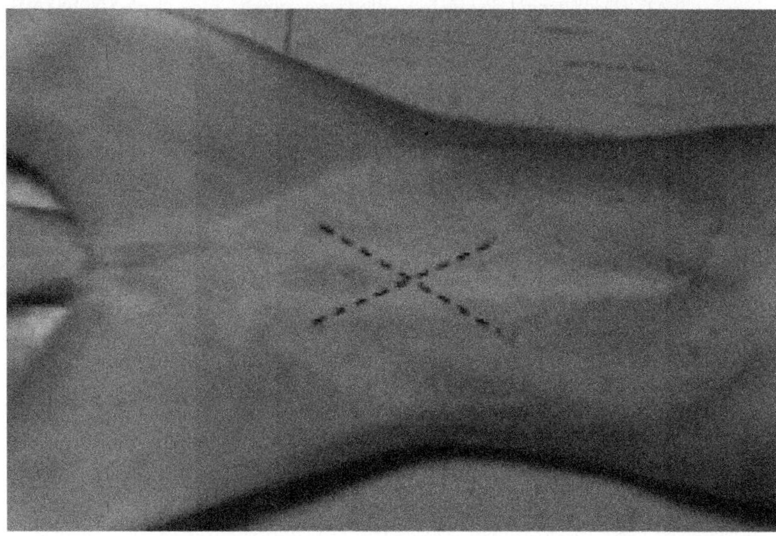

Figure 1.

A female dog in dorsal recumbency, with dotted lines drawn between the last two sets of nipples. In the blind aspiration cystocentesis technique, the needle should be inserted where the lines cross and the needle directed caudally at an approximately 30–45° angle. Source: Lawrence P. Tilley

• Insert the needle into the bladder at a 45° angle.
• Once the needle has been inserted to the appropriate depth, the plunger of the syringe should be slowly drawn back, creating negative pressure. If urine is obtained, continue aspiration to remove the maximal volume of urine possible.
• When the maximal volume of urine has been collected, negative pressure should be released and the needle withdrawn.

SAMPLE HANDLING

• Samples collected for urinalysis should be analyzed immediately, if possible, because refrigeration for later analysis can alter some dipstick and sediment findings.
• Urine samples collected for culture should be refrigerated or placed into bacteriostatic transport containers until plated onto appropriate media. The amount of urine to be submitted varies among diagnostic laboratories, but many microbiologists prefer at least 5 mL because this may increase the likelihood of isolation of infectious agents.

APPROPRIATE AFTERCARE

Postprocedure Patient Monitoring

None

Nursing Care

None

Dietary Modification

None

Medication Requirements

None

Restrictions on Activity

None

Anticipated Recovery Time

Immediate

INTERPRETATION

NORMAL FINDINGS OR RANGE

N/A

ABNORMAL VALUES

N/A

CRITICAL VALUES

N/A

INTERFERING FACTORS

Drugs That May Alter Results of the Procedure

• A number of drugs affect urinalysis findings. A thorough medical history is required for proper interpretation of results.
• Antibiotics may inhibit growth of bacteria if urine is submitted for culture.

Conditions That May Interfere with Performing the Procedure

• Cystocentesis may be difficult at times of low bladder urine volume (e.g., immediately after voiding; in pollakiuric patients). Urinary catheterization using sterile technique will allow small amounts of urine to be collected.
• Bladder rupture.

Procedure Techniques or Handling That May Alter Results

• Improper or delayed handling of urine after collection affects urinalysis results.
• Urine samples may be contaminated inadvertently with GI tract content if aspiration is performed prior to the needle entering the bladder. Partially digested food, feces, and bacteria cause a false-positive active urine sediment and positive urine culture.

Influence of Signalment on Performing and Interpreting the Procedure

Species

See Urinalysis Overview (Appendix X) for details regarding interpretation in dogs and cats. Some differences of note include these:
• Cat urine is typically more concentrated than dog urine, although the reference ranges in normal animals overlap significantly.
• Dogs may normally have a small amount of bilirubinuria, whereas bilirubinuria in cats is always a pathologic finding.
• Cats typically have more acidic urine than dogs; however, urine pH is significantly influenced by diet.
• Fat droplets are common in feline urine but rare in canine urine.

Breed

None

Age

• Neonatal puppies (<3 weeks old) have more dilute urine than pediatric or adult dogs.
• Transient proteinuria and glucosuria have been reported in neonatal puppies, although this is not a consistent finding in all studies.

Gender

Male dogs may have higher concentrations of urine bilirubin than female dogs.

CYSTOCENTESIS (CONTINUED)

Pregnancy
None

CLINICAL PERSPECTIVE

Cystocentesis should be considered the standard method for urine collection in all small-animal patients:

- Urine samples collected by catheterization or midstream free catch may be contaminated by microorganisms and inflammatory cells normally found in the distal urethra, prepuce, and vaginal vault. Results of urine sediment examination or culture from urine samples not collected by cystocentesis must be interpreted with caution, and there is a higher risk of artifactual bacterial contamination.
- Comparison of urinalysis findings from cystocentesis and free-catch midstream urine samples may assist in differentiating urethral or genital disease from bladder or upper urinary tract disease.
- Although cystocentesis of animals that may have transitional cell carcinoma of the urinary bladder may seed tumor cells into the abdomen or along the needle track, cystocentesis should still be routinely performed in dogs and cats unless a bladder mass has been confirmed by diagnostic imaging studies.

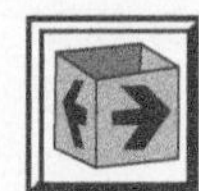

MISCELLANEOUS

ANCILLARY TESTS

- Urethral catheterization.
- Urinalysis.
- Urine culture.

SYNONYMS

Bladder tap

SEE ALSO

- Bacterial Culture and Sensitivity (in Appendix X).
- Urethral Catheterization (in Appendix X).
- Urinalysis Overview (in Appendix X).
- Urine Sediment (in Appendix X).

Author Vincent J. Thawley
Consulting Editor Benjamin M. Brainard
Acknowledgment The author and editors acknowledge the prior contribution of Barrak M. Pressler.

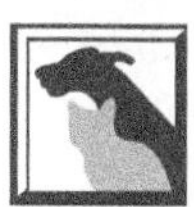

BASICS

TYPE OF PROCEDURE

Electrodiagnostic: heart electrical activity measurement

PROCEDURE EXPLANATION AND RELATED PHYSIOLOGY

- The electrocardiogram (ECG, EKG; Figure 1) captures the electrical fields generated by the pumping heart. Waveforms are a display of the electrical activity of the heart generated during depolarization and repolarization.
- The leads represent single planes of measurement of the electrical activity of the heart. Each lead has a positive and negative surface electrode setting. If energy is traveling away from the positive electrode, a negative orientation of the wave occurs on the ECG, and if the net direction of the electrical energy impulse is toward the positive electrode, a positive deflection occurs. If the impulses are at perpendicular, an isoelectric deflection occurs. Lead II is the most common lead used for initial evaluation of the ECG.
- The form of the ECG is characterized by deviations from baseline that are linked to specific events in the cardiac cycle (Figure 1):
  - Each cardiac cycle starts with an impulse that originates in the sinoatrial (SA) node, which is located in the right atrium. An impulse will travel through the myocardium of the atria, resulting in depolarization. This event generates the P wave on the tracing. The tracing is recorded when the atrium contracts, not when the original SA node fires, because the latter event is too small to trigger a recordable event.
  - As the impulse moves through the atrioventricular (AV) node, which is near the base of the right atrium, the PR interval is generated.
  - Once through the AV node, the conduction speed increases and the electrical activity fires through the bundle of His, the bundle branches, and the Purkinje system.
  - Rapid, widespread depolarization of the ventricles then occurs. This leads to the QRS complex. Subsequent ventricle contraction then occurs.
  - The Q wave represents the interventricular septum depolarization and thus is the first negative deflection. The Q wave may not always be easy to isolate on tracings.
  - The R portion is the ventricular myocardium depolarizing and the impulse traveling from the endocardium to the epicardium. It is a positive deflection and the most prominent waveform on the ECG.
  - The S wave is the basal ventricle posterior wall and interventricular septum activating. It is the first negative deflection following the R wave.
  - The repolarization of the ventricles is recorded as the T wave.
  - As repolarization occurs, the ST segment is generated.

INDICATIONS

- Diagnosis of cardiac arrhythmias, myocardial ischemia, changes in cardiac environment (e.g., pericardial effusion, pericarditis).
- Patients with the following clinical signs:
  - Tachycardia or bradycardia.
  - Dyspnea, cyanosis, syncope, or seizures.
  - Shock, acute emergency, or severe illness, such as pyometra, gastric dilatation and volvulus syndrome (GDV or bloat), uremia, pancreatitis, and toxic insults.
  - Electrolyte disturbances (especially potassium) or in chronic diuretic administration.
  - Cardiac murmurs.
- Also used in the context of patient monitoring:
  - During anesthesia and in the perioperative period.
  - Routine health monitoring of senior or chronically ill patients where prognosis may be affected by cardiac function.
  - Pharmacologic monitoring for agents with known cardiotoxicity (e.g., quinidine, digitalis, beta-blockers).
- In patients with an abnormal radiographic appearance of the heart or great vessels, in combination with other diagnostics (e.g., echocardiography).
- During diagnostic or therapeutic procedures, (e.g., pericardiocentesis).
- In patients with elevations in vagal tone (e.g., disease in the nervous system, respiratory system, GI system, use of potent opioids).

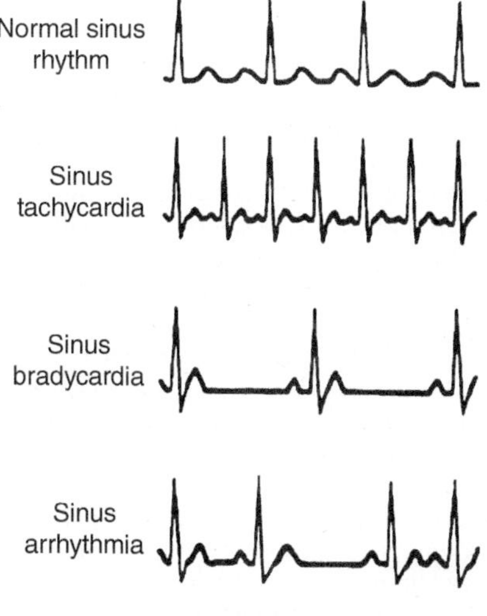

Figure 1.

Common examples of electrocardiograms.

ELECTROCARDIOGRAPHY (CONTINUED)

CONTRAINDICATIONS

None

POTENTIAL COMPLICATIONS

Caution in dyspneic patients.

CLIENT EDUCATION

- Inform clients that this is not a standalone test but interpreted in the context of the patient's medical history, clinical signs, and other database findings.
- Let them know that this is just a snapshot and that repeat ECG and Holter monitoring may be required to understand the problem more fully, especially with paroxysmal tachycardias and with conduction disturbances (e.g., AV block).

BODY SYSTEMS ASSESSED

Cardiovascular

PROCEDURE

PATIENT PREPARATION

Pre-Procedure Medication or Preparation

- The number of leads measured depends on the equipment.
- Three bipolar leads is minimum, and three additional unipolar leads are usual.
- This type of procedure does require a quiet, calm environment (and animal) in order to optimize results. Distraction during the test may produce spurious results, so care should be taken to let the animal settle in before measurement begins.
- An experienced technician or veterinarian should run the test and, ideally, serial tests should be conducted and interpreted by the same individuals to help maintain consistency.
- Turn off fluorescent bulbs or electrical equipment (especially in older equipment) in the room, do not cross your limbs, and avoid contact with metal surfaces.
- Before recording begins, clips must be effectively placed. The right arm (RA) and left arm (LA) electrodes are best clipped to the proximal olecranon area or even halfway down the radius. The right leg (RL) and left leg (LL) electrodes are clipped over the patella ligament. Before applying a clip, remember to apply conductive gel or 70% isopropyl alcohol. The advantage of the latter is that it does not get gummed up in long hair. For longer term (e.g., intraoperative) monitoring, gel is better because alcohol evaporates too quickly. The precordial chest (V lead) electrode is applied for precordial unipolar chest leads.
- Muscle tremors may produce artifacts. Movements and purring can lead to vibrations along the baseline. A hand placed gently on the animal's chest wall may help to reduce its shivering.
- A wandering baseline is often caused by respiratory cycle movements because contact at the skin–clip interface can be poor. Panting or coughing may also cause the same thing. To resolve this issue, gently hold the muzzle closed for 4 seconds, as long as the patient is not dyspneic.

Anesthesia or Sedation

- Anesthesia is not required, and sedation is rarely required.
- Pediatric patients may require snug restraint to enable testing.

Patient Positioning

- Since reference levels originate from the right lateral recumbent position, that position would be ideal, but, realistically, if a pet is recalcitrant or dyspneic, any position that minimizes tremors, shivering, panting, or struggling will do. As an alternative, standing is preferred to sitting if right lateral recumbency is too stressful.
- Ideally, the forelimbs would be held apart and perpendicular to minimize interference, in amenable patients.
- If indicated, oxygen delivered by mask or flow-by techniques may be provided during the exam.
- For intraoperative monitoring, a patient's position is not critical.

Patient Monitoring

Monitor for sudden dyspnea or cyanosis or other signs that reflect decompensation.

Equipment or Supplies

- ECG equipment is relatively inexpensive and ranges from transtelephonic sets to integrated computer oscillometric recorders that can print and upload to the computerized patient record directly.
- A blanket or soft pad for the table.
- An ECG recording machine. The ECG apparatus should meet the requirements of the Committee on Electrocardiography of the American Heart Association. The amplifier is tied to a strip recorder, either on a computer screen or an oscilloscope, or by a stylus on wax paper. At a minimum, single-channel capture and an oscilloscope should be available. Three-channel equipment enables more detailed capture and analysis by enabling the tester to record three leads simultaneously.
- Contact gel or 70% isopropyl alcohol.
- Clippers if the hair is too thick to provide close clip contact.
- A printer or a computer or transtelephony device, depending on where the results are to be sent or how they are to be recorded.
- Separate the cables so they do not overlap. Usually, this is a set of five wires. Alligator clips are usually used for animals. Plate clips are better for electrical sensitivity but are more easily displaced by struggling animals:
  - The alligator clips, which should be copper, may be filed and bent so they pinch less. With very small animals, placing a plate inside the clip may help maintain the patient's comfort without loss of efficiency.
  - Alternatively, adhesive pads for human use may be applied to the patient for longer term ECG recording. Special clips may be used to attach to the button on the pad, or regular clips may be attached as well.

TECHNIQUE

- Run the standardization marker for sensitivity and increase speed to 50 mm/s before you start to record. If only using the ECG for periprocedural or in hospital monitoring, a speed of 25 mm/s is adequate unless the patient is very tachycardic.
- Switch leads to obtain 4-second segments approximately, with the goal to record a minimum of four good complexes in each lead to fully assess the electrical activity. Repeat as needed to cover available leads for the system.
- Finally, record a long strip of lead II for full rhythm assessment.
- A break will be needed if precordial leads are to be recorded, because the electrodes will need to be repositioned. Turn off the machine, turn it back on, and run the standardization again before recording.
- Turn off the record switch, turn off the machine, and clean the gel from the hair coat after gently removing the clips.
- For transtelephonic ECG, the portable preamplifier converts electrical signals into tones that can be sent over a phone line. Position the animal, attach two electrodes (moistened for good contact) to the forelimbs near the elbow, and then call the transtelephonic service.

SAMPLE HANDLING

- Sensitivity controls how tall the complexes are, with 1 mV being standard. This means 10 small boxes (1 cm) equals 1 mV.
- Change to 2 mV to increase the size of the complexes represented and to 0.5 mV to reduce the height of tall complexes.
- A marker must be done at the start of each strip to record the lead sensitivity. Newer models do this automatically.
- Position the baseline recording in the center of the paper strip for recording.
- Record at least 5–6 complexes for each lead and record a long strip especially if watching for arrhythmias. Check the polarity: If the R waves are not positive in lead I, check the hookup to see if it is still negative, which is abnormal for lead I.
- Placement of the grounding is not critical except that it should be far away as possible.

- If using a rhythm strip to monitor ECG during procedures, the specific lead is unimportant, as long as the observer can identify a P, QRS, and T complex in the tracing (i.e., lead II may be isoelectric following positioning for a surgery such as a forelimb amputation, but lead III may be adequate for rhythm monitoring).

INTERPRETATION

NORMAL FINDINGS OR RANGE

The findings can be divided into heart rate (HR), rhythm, analysis of complexes and intervals, electrical axis, and chest leads. (See an ECG text guide for interpretation details.) Abnormalities in rhythm, complexes and intervals, and waveforms, and disturbances in impulse conduction and mean electrical axis (MEA) can occur. Normal values for ECG analysis are listed in Appendix IV. An extensive review of ECG interpretation is beyond the scope of this chapter (see Suggested Reading), but some general tips to interpret ECG follow.

Heart Rate

- When ECG is run at 25 mm/s, each large box on the paper is equal to 1/5 of a second, and each set of five large boxes (usually indicated by a black mark at the base of the grid) is equivalent to 1 second of ECG.
- The rate is calculated by observing the number of QRS complexes in a 3-second interval.
- Multipy this number by 20 to calculate the beats per minute.
- At 50 mm/s, three sets of large boxes is equivalent to 1.5 seconds and the number of QRS complexes should be multiplied by 40.

Arrhythmia Analysis

See specific arrhythmia chapters for visual examples and therapeutic recommendations.

- First, calculate the rate.
- Note the regularity of the QRS complexes and characterize the rhythm as regular or irregular:
  - Patients that have rhythmic variation due to breathing have a regularly irregular rhythm (i.e, irregular in a predictable way).
  - Animals with atrial fibrillation have an irregularly irregular rhythm, without any discernible pattern.
- Evaluate the tracing for P waves. A P wave should precede every QRS complex:
  - Evaluate the distance between the P wave and each QRS (should be the same).
  - Patients with various AV blocks may not have a reliable P-R interval or P waves in general. Patients with ventricular or junctional arrhythmias will have QRS complexes without associated P waves.
- Verify that there is a QRS complex for every identified P wave. QRS complexes without P waves may originate from the ventricles or AV junction.

CRITICAL VALUES

Related to specific arrhythmias; diagnosis of ventricular tachycardia, ventricular fibrillation, third-degree AV block, sinus arrest (lack of P waves), and asystole require immediate intervention and further diagnostic testing.

INTERFERING FACTORS

- Environmental interference, interpretation error, interpretation without a proper minimum database, or overinterpretation.
- The ECG does not assess the heart itself, just the electrical activity of the myocardium, so an animal with advanced congestive heart failure (CHF) may have a normal ECG, and an animal with cardiac arrest may display normal activity for a period of time after the heart stops beating (the electrical activity is just not translated into muscular contraction).
- Since not all abnormalities are present all of the time, serial studies or Holter monitors may be needed.
- Breed and conformation may affect the tracings and interpretation.

Drugs That May Alter Results of the Procedure

Sedation (e.g., with alpha-2 agonist drugs) may cause artifactual arrhythmias, or mask the presence of others.

Conditions That May Interfere with Performing the Procedure

Electrical interference, stress, dyspnea, or an uncooperative patient.

Procedure Techniques or Handling That May Alter Results

A wandering baseline caused by movement, not adjusting the millivoltage or speed, improper patient position, contact with a metal surface, crossed wires or legs, or electrical interference.

Influence of Signalment on Performing and Interpreting the Procedure

Species
Interpretations of tracings are specific to species.

Breed
Clip placement is affected in deep-chested breeds.

Age
Young dogs.

Gender
None

Pregnancy
None

CLINICAL PERSPECTIVE

The ECG may be used for simple rhythm monitoring, or may provide specific insight into cardiac disease. A thorough understanding of the technique and the causes of the deflections on the final waveforms will completment other diagnostic results. Knowing your equipment, taking care to minimize stress, and developing a proper database of information against which to compare results before making an interpretation are important.

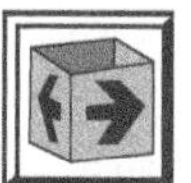

MISCELLANEOUS

ANCILLARY TESTS

- Holter monitoring.
- Radiography.
- Ultrasound, echocardiogram.
- Pericardiocentesis.

SYNONYMS

None

SEE ALSO

Cardiology topics, specific arrhythmias.

ABBREVIATIONS

- ECG, EKG = electrocardiogram.
- MEA = mean electrical axis.
- SA = sinoatrial.

- *Suggested Reading*

Smith FWK, Tilley LP, Miller MS. Electrocardiography. In: Brichard SJ, Sherding RG, eds., Manual of Small Animal Practice, 3rd ed. St. Louis, MO: Saunders Elsevier, 2006.

Tilley LP. Essentials of Canine and Feline Electrocardiography. Interpretation and Treatment, 3rd ed. Ames, IA: Blackwell, 1992.

Tilley LP, Burtnick N. ECG for the Small Animal Practitioner. Jackson, WY: Teton NewMedia, 1999.

Tilley LP, Smith FWK, Jr. Electrocardiography. In: Smith FWK, Tilley LP, Oyama M, Sleeper M, eds., Manual of Canine and Feline Cardiology, 5th ed. St. Louis, MO: Saunders Elsevier, 2016, pp. 49–76.

Author Larry P. Tilley
Consulting Editor Benjamin M. Brainard

FECAL DIRECT SMEAR AND CYTOLOGY

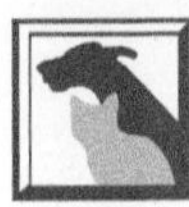

BASICS

TYPE OF SPECIMEN

Feces

TEST EXPLANATION AND RELATED PHYSIOLOGY

- Performed to examine the fecal microbiota and any nucleated cells that are present (epithelial, inflammatory), and to detect other pathogens that may be present (i.e., bacterial, fungal, protozoal, algal, oomycetal).
- Abnormalities detected by fecal cytology are often nonspecific, and may enable diagnosis of the primary cause of GI illness in some cases, although may more frequently represent findings associated with other underlying diseases or processes.
- Direct fecal smear cytology is not synonymous with a rectal scrape, which is a method of sampling the rectal mucosa by direct scraping of its surface with a swab or blunt spatula. Rectal scraping is typically required to identify some deeper infections (e.g., histoplasmosis, protothecosis).

INDICATIONS

- Diarrhea.
- Less commonly, other GI signs (e.g., vomition).

CONTRAINDICATIONS

None

POTENTIAL COMPLICATIONS

None

CLIENT EDUCATION

- This test may not reveal the primary cause of a patient's GI signs. Instead, abnormalities secondary to other underlying primary or secondary GI disease may be detected.
- Normal direct fecal smear cytology does not definitively exclude the possibility of GI disease, including underlying infection or inflammation.

BODY SYSTEMS ASSESSED

Gastrointestinal

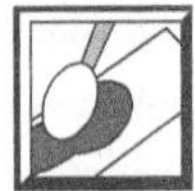

SAMPLE

SAMPLE COLLECTION

Collect feces from the rectum by using a slightly moistened cotton-tipped applicator or use the feces present on one's gloved finger after a digital rectal exam.

SAMPLE HANDLING

- Smear or roll the feces onto a clean, glass microscope slide to form a thin film.
- Prepare a wet preparation by adding a few drops of saline and a coverslip. Do not make the wet preparation too thick; one should be able read newsprint through the wet prep. Adding a drop of iodine to the preparation may improve visualization of protozoa.
- Air-dry the thin film of feces:
  - Stain with a Romanowsky stain (e.g., Diff-Quik; Dade Behring, Newark, DE) for cytologic examination.
  - Use acid-fast stain if looking for *Cryptosporidium* sp.
  - Heat-fix prior to Gram staining.

SAMPLE STORAGE

- Wet preparations should be prepared and immediately examined.
- For other preparations, the sample should be processed within 2 hours or feces should be refrigerated.
- Store air-dried fecal smears at room temperature and protected from light.
- Fecal smear slides should not be refrigerated or frozen.
- Wet preparations should be read immediately and cannot be stored.

SAMPLE STABILITY

- Feces at room temperature: 2 hours.
- Refrigerated feces: variable stability, depending on abnormality of interest. Parasite ova are stable, but cellular deterioration and changes in bacteria flora occur over time.
- Wet preparations cannot be stored.
- Fixed-stain smears are stable indefinitely if protected from light and humidity.

PROTOCOL

- Examine the wet preparation for motile parasites or parasite ova.
- Examine the Romanovsky-stained smear for the following:
  - Background bacterial flora.
  - Noninflammatory cells (e.g., epithelial cells, neoplastic cells).
  - Inflammatory cells.
  - The number of spore-forming bacteria per 1,000× high-power field.
  - The presence of pathogens, such as the following (depending on geographic location):
    - Short spiral or gullwing-shaped bacteria (e.g., *Campylobacter*, *Helicobacter*, *Anaerobiospirillum*, treponeme-like bacteria, *Serpulina* spp.)
    - Protozoa (e.g., *Giardia*, *Tritrichomonas*, *Entamoeba*).
    - Dimorphic fungi (e.g., *Histoplasma*).
    - Other fungi (e.g., *Cryptococcus*, *Candida*, *Aspergillus*).
    - Algae (e.g., *Prototheca*).
    - Oomycetes (e.g., *Pythium*).

INTERPRETATION

NORMAL FINDINGS OR RANGE

- A polymorphic bacterial population of bacilli. Cocci should be absent or very rarely observed.
- A low number of well-differentiated epithelial cells.
- Amorphous material, representing digesta.
- A small amount of plant material.
- A small amount of extracellular yeast (e.g., *Cyniclomyces*; formerly known as *Saccharomycopsis*).

ABNORMAL FINDINGS

- Monomorphic bacterial microbiota.
- An increased number of cocci.
- The presence of inflammatory cells.
- The presence of abnormal noninflammatory cells (e.g., reactive epithelial cells, neoplastic cells).
- The presence of potential pathogens (e.g., protozoa, fungi, algae, oomycetes, gullwing-shaped bacteria).
- The presence of >10 spore-forming bacteria per 1,000× high-power field.
- Specifically, sporulated *Clostridium* has a safety-pin or tennis racket appearance because the spore produces an oval, colorless area.

CRITICAL VALUES

None

INTERFERING FACTORS

Drugs That May Alter Results or Interpretation

Drugs That Interfere with Test Methodology

None

Drugs That Alter Physiology

Prior antimicrobial administration may alter the GI microbiota, resulting in abnormal direct fecal smear cytologic results.

Disorders That May Alter Results

Prior GI procedures (e.g., surgery, enema) may alter GI flora, resulting in abnormal direct fecal smear cytologic results.

Collection Techniques or Handling that May Alter Results

Deeper scraping of the rectal mucosa will increase the number of epithelial cells observed in direct fecal smear cytology. Deeper scraping may be helpful when certain infections (e.g., histoplasmosis, protothecosis) are suspected.

Influence of Signalment

Species

None

Breed

None

Age

None

Gender

None

Pregnancy

None

LIMITATIONS OF TEST

Sensitivity, Specificity, and Positive and Negative Predictive Values

None

Table 1

Causes of abnormal findings.

Preparation	*Abnormal Finding*	*Possible Causes*
Wet preparation	Motile protozoa	*Giardia, Balantidium, Entamoeba, Tritrichomonas* trophozoites
	Parasite larvae	*Strongyloides, Aelurostrongylus, Filaroides*, saprophytic larvae caused by environmental contamination
	Parasite eggs	Coccidia (*Cystoisospora* spp.), *Toxocara, Trichuris, Ancylostoma, Uncinaria*
Romanowsky stain	Monomorphic population of bacteria	Bacterial overgrowth caused by primary or secondary GI disease or antibiotic treatment
	Sporulated bacteria	*Clostridium* overgrowth
	Short spiral or gullwing-shaped bacteria	*Campylobacter, Helicobacter, Anaerobiospirillum*
	White (colorless) rods in macrophages and free in background	*Mycobacterium*
	Neutrophils	Nonspecific sign of GI inflammation or suggests the presence of transmural colonic or rectal inflammation
	Eosinophils	Allergic hypersensitivity or parasitic infection
	Small lymphocytes, plasma cells	Lymphocytic, plasmacytic enteritis
	Monomorphic large lymphocytes	Lymphoma
	Teardrop-shaped protozoan organisms with 2 nuclei that "appear to be looking back at you"	*Giardia*
	Spindle-shaped protozoa with whiplike flagella and an undulating or wavy membrane	*Tritrichomonas*
	Ciliated protozoan with a large sausage-shaped macronucleus that surrounds a small micronucleus	*Balantidium*
	Round intracellular yeast (within macrophages), 3–5 μm diameter	*Histoplasma*
	Septate branching hyphae	*Aspergillus*, other fungus, or *Pythium*
	Round or oval algae with basophilic granular cytoplasm (3 × 16 μm)	*Prototheca*
Acid-fast stain	4–5 μm round magenta structures	*Cryptosporidia* sp.
	Intracellular magenta linear inclusions	*Mycobacterium*

Valid If Run in a Human Lab?

Yes, if the observer (i.e., pathologist or technician) is acquainted with veterinary species.

CAUSES OF ABNORMAL FINDINGS

See Table 1.

CLINICAL PERSPECTIVE

- Abnormal background bacterial microbiota is often an incidental finding associated with other primary or secondary GI diseases, with GI procedures, or with prior antimicrobial administration. In some cases, though, abnormal microbiota may be a factor contributing to diarrhea.
- Observation of inflammatory cells suggests the presence of transmural colonic or rectal inflammation. Fecal culture may be useful to exclude underlying infection by invasive bacteria (e.g., salmonellosis).
- Identification of atypical noninflammatory cells, such as abnormal epithelial cells, may indicate the presence of neoplasia or hyperplasia.
- The primary cause of diarrhea may be determined when pathogens (e.g., bacterial, protozoal, fungal, algal, oomycetal) or an increased number of spore-forming bacteria are observed.

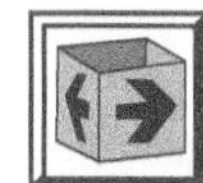

MISCELLANEOUS

ANCILLARY TESTS

- Fecal culture and determination of antibiotic sensitivities are useful when inflammatory cells or pathogens are observed.
- Gram stain of the direct fecal smear is useful in evaluating the microbiota and potential bacterial pathogens.
- Warthin–Starry silver stain of the direct fecal smear is useful in evaluating potential bacterial pathogens (e.g., *Lawsonia*).
- Submission of direct fecal smear to a referral laboratory for cytologic evaluation is useful when abnormal noninflammatory cells (e.g., atypical epithelial cells) or when potential pathogens are observed.
- Other tests employed as part of routine GI diagnostic evaluation may include serum biochemistry, fecal flotation, fecal pathogen PCR, and radiography.

SYNONYMS

Fecal cytology

SEE ALSO

- Acute Diarrhea.
- Diarrhea, Chronic—Cats.
- Diarrhea, Chronic—Dogs.
- Fecal Flotation (in Appendix X).

ABBREVIATIONS

- GI = gastrointestinal.

Suggested Reading

Andreason CB, Jergens AE, Meyer DJ. Oral cavity, gastrointestinal tract, and associated structures. In: Raskin RE, Meyer DJ, eds. Atlas of Canine and Feline Cytology. Philadelphia, PA: WB Saunders, 2001, pp. 207–229.

Broussard J. Optimal fecal assessment. Clin Tech Small Anim Pract 2003; 18:218–230.

Lassen ED. Laboratory evaluation of digestion and intestinal absorption. In: Thrall MA, ed., Veterinary Hematology and Clinical Chemistry. Philadelphia, PA: Lippincott Williams & Wilkins, 2004, pp. 387–399.

Authors Andrew R. Moorhead and Guilherme G. Verocai

Consulting Editor Benjamin M. Brainard

Acknowledgment The author and editors acknowledge the prior contribution of Heather L. Wamsley.

FECAL FLOTATION

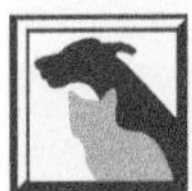

BASICS

TYPE OF SPECIMEN

Feces

TEST EXPLANATION AND RELATED PHYSIOLOGY

- Designed to recover diagnostic stages of parasites that are shed in feces (e.g., eggs, oocysts, and cysts).
- Based on specific gravity (SG) of flotation solution.
- Parasite eggs, oocysts, and cysts will float in solutions of a higher SG than the parasitic life stage. The SG of most parasite eggs is between 1.05 and 1.23. Therefore, for parasite eggs to float, the SG of the flotation solution must be greater than that of the eggs.
- Flotation solutions are made by adding a measured amount of salt or sugar to water to produce a solution with the desired SG. Solutions may be made from scratch or bought premixed.
- Common flotation solutions include sugar (Sheather's solution; SG, 1.2–1.33), sodium nitrate ($NaNO_3$; SG, 1.2–1.3), and zinc sulfate ($ZnSO_4$; SG, 1.18–1.2).
- Most parasitology diagnostic and research laboratories routinely use Sheather's solution, which will float most common parasite eggs.
- Many commercially available kits supply sodium nitrate.
- Zinc sulfate is considered the gold standard for flotation of *Giardia* cysts.
- Sodium nitrate solution is widely used for fecal egg counts of large and production animals, and might an option for mixed practices.
- The SG of a flotation solution should be verified with a hydrometer and then checked on a routine basis (e.g., monthly) to detect SG changes caused by evaporation. If the SG is too high, it may rupture eggs, oocysts, or cysts.

INDICATIONS

- Routine health screening.
- Digestive upsets; vomiting and/or diarrhea.
- Respiratory signs such as chronic coughing or sneezing.

CONTRAINDICATIONS

None, other than insufficient fecal output.

POTENTIAL COMPLICATIONS

None

CLIENT EDUCATION

- Because pets can have normal stools and still be infected with intestinal parasites, it is good medicine to perform routine fecal exams on all pets. The absence of diarrhea or visible worms in dog feces does not mean that the animal is not infected.
- Negative fecal flotation does not completely exclude the possibility of gastrointestinal or respiratory parasites. For example, tapeworm segments (or proglottids) may be seen in the feces, and the flotation may be negative for several reasons: eggs were not released from the segment, the SG of the solution used was not high enough to float the heavy taeniid-type eggs (i.e., *Taenia* and *Echinocccus*), or perhaps owners mistook grains of rice or fly larvae for tapeworm segments.
- All dogs and cats should receive regular heartworm preventives based on macrocyclic lactone drugs; however, these products may not treat or prevent infection by some intestinal worms or other parasites such as tapeworms, flukes, *Coccidia*, or *Giardia*.

BODY SYSTEMS ASSESSED

- Gastrointestinal.
- Respiratory.

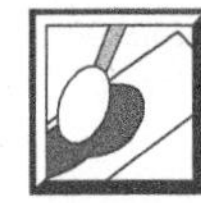

SAMPLE

SAMPLE COLLECTION

Minimum of 1 g, ideally 2–3 g of fresh feces.

SAMPLE HANDLING

- Place the sample in an airtight container (e.g., screw-top jar, ziplock bag).
- Every sample must be appropriately labeled.
- The sample is best analyzed on the day of collection.
- If not possible, keep it cooled or refrigerated until processing, avoid freezing.

SAMPLE STORAGE

Refrigeration

SAMPLE STABILITY

The stability of organisms and life stages varies; e.g., *Giardia* cysts are very fragile and delicate, whereas ascarid eggs are very hardy.

EQUIPMENT

- Scale able to weigh up to 5 g.
- Light microscope with objectives of 10× and 40× magnification.
- Benchtop centrifuge (swinging-bucket or fixed-angle).

PROTOCOL

Fecal flotation with centrifugation has been shown to be the most accurate way to recover parasite diagnostic life stages and consistently recovers more of these stages than standing flotation methods (also known as simple flotation):

1. Weigh out 1–3 g of feces.
2. Mix feces with ≈15 mL of flotation solution in a cup until homogeneous.
3. Pour the mixture through a tea strainer into another fecal cup.
4. Pour the strained solution into a 15 mL centrifuge tube.
5. If you have a centrifuge with swing buckets, fill the tube with flotation solution until forming a slight positive meniscus. Do not overfill tube. Doing so will cause some floating diagnostic stages to be forced down the side of tube when the coverslip is placed.
6. Place a coverslip on the tube and put the tube in the centrifuge.

Note: Steps 5 and 6 are done only if the centrifuge has a swinging-bucket rotor (swing head). If the centrifuge has a fixed-angle head (fixed head), the tube is spun without being filled completely. After centrifuging, the tube is moved to a test-tube rack and filled with flotation solution until a slight positive meniscus forms. A coverslip is then placed on the tube, and the tube is allowed to stand for an additional 10 min before the coverslip is removed and examined.

7. Centrifuge at 1,200 RPM (280 ×*g*) for 5 minutes.
8. Allow centrifuge to stop without using the brake, as it may interfere with the flotation of the parasite diagnostic stages.
9. Remove the tube and let it stand for 5–10 minutes. (*Note*: 10 minutes would allow more parasite diagnostic stages, if present, to float.).
10. Remove the coverslip and place on a glass slide.
11. Systematically examine the entire area under the coverslip by using the 10× objective lens (100× magnification). The 40× objective lens can be used to confirm the diagnosis and make measurements; however, with practice, most identification can be made at 100× magnification.

INTERPRETATION

NORMAL FINDINGS OR RANGE

No parasitic eggs, oocysts, or cysts seen (or "no parasites seen)."

ABNORMAL FINDINGS

Parasitic eggs, oocysts, or cysts seen (or report of specific parasite genera/species seen).

CRITICAL VALUES

None

INTERFERING FACTORS

Drugs That May Alter Results or Interpretation

Drugs That Interfere with Test Methodology

None

Drugs That Alter Physiology

None

Table 1

Common parasites of dogs and cats found in feces.

Parasite	*Life Stage*	*Location of Mature Life Stage*	*How Infection Happens*
Common parasites of dogs with stage of life cycle found in feces			
Toxocara canis	Large, dark, thick-shelled egg	Small intestine	*In utero* or ingestion of infected paratenic hosts or infective larvated eggs or nursing (milk)
Toxascaris leonina	Large, light, thick-shelled egg	Small intestine	Ingestion of infected paratenic hosts or infective larvated eggs
Physaloptera spp.	Thick-shelled, larvated egg	Stomach	Ingestion of infected intermediate hosts (e.g., insects) or paratenic hosts (e.g., frogs, mice)
Taenia spp.	Small egg, with hooks	Small intestine	Ingestion of metacestode stage in intermediate hosts (e.g., rabbits)
Dipylidium caninum	Egg packet	Small intestine	Ingestion of metacestode stage in intermediate hosts (fleas)
Ancylostoma caninum	Strongyle-type egg	Small intestine	Ingestion of L_3 from environment, nursing (milk), or skin penetration by L_3
Uncinaria stenocephala	Strongyle-type egg	Small intestine	Ingestion of L_3 from environment or rarely skin penetration by L_3
Eucoleus boehmi (formerly known as *Capillaria boehmi*)	Bioperculated egg	Nasal passages	Ingestion of larvated egg or infected intermediate host
Trichuris vulpis	Bioperculated egg	Cecum, large intestine	Ingestion of larvated egg
Eucoleus aerophilus (formerly known as *Capillaria aerophila*)	Bioperculated egg	Lungs	Ingestion of larvated egg or infected intermediate host
Strongyloides stercoralis	Larvae	Small intestine	Ingestion or skin penetration by L_3
Cystoisospora spp. (formerly known as *Isospora* sp.)	Oocyst	Small intestine	Ingestion of sporulated oocysts, or cysts in intermediate host
Giardia sp.	Cyst	Small intestine	Ingestion of cysts
Alaria sp.	Egg	Stomach, small intestine	Ingestion of mesocercaria in fish, frogs, or rodents
Common parasites of cats with diagnostic life stage found in feces			
Toxocara cati	Large, dark, thick-shelled egg	Small intestine	Ingestion of infected paratenic hosts or infective larvated eggs
Toxascaris leonina	Large, light, thick-shelled egg	Small intestine	Ingestion of infected paratenic hosts or infective larvated eggs
Physaloptera spp.	Thick-shelled, larvated egg	Stomach	Ingestion of infected intermediate hosts (e.g., insects, arthropods) or paratenic hosts (e.g., frogs, mice)
Taenia spp.	Egg	Small intestine	Ingestion of metacestode stage in intermediate hosts (e.g., rodents)
Dipylidium caninum	Egg packet	Small intestine	Ingestion of metacestode stage in intermediate hosts (fleas)
Ancylostoma tubaeforme	Strongyle-type egg	Small intestine	Ingestion of L_3 from environment, or skin penetration
Eucoleus aerophilus (formerly known as *Capillaria aerophila*)	Bioperculated eggs	Lungs	Ingestion of infective larvated egg or infected intermediate host
Cystoisospora spp. (formerly known as *Isospora* sp.)	Oocyst	Small intestine	Ingestion of sporulated oocysts, or cysts in intermediate host
Toxoplasma gondii	Oocyst	Small intestine	Ingestion of sporulated oocysts, tachyzoites, or bradyzoites in mice or other meat
Giardia sp.	Cyst	Small intestine	Ingestion of cysts
Aelurostrongylus abstrusus	Larvae (L_1)	Lungs	Ingestion of intermediate hosts (snails or slugs) or paratenic hosts (mice and birds)
Spirometra sp.	Egg	Small intestine	Ingestion of plerocercoid in intermediate host (reptile, mammals)
Alaria sp.	Egg	Stomach, small intestine	Ingestion of mesocercaria in fish, frogs, or rodents

Demodex, *Cheyletiella*, and *Otodectes* sp. mites may be seen in fecal flotations. *Echinococcus* sp. eggs are similar to *Taenia* sp.

FECAL FLOTATION

Disorders That May Alter Results

None

Collection Techniques or Handling That May Alter Results

- Insufficient sample size.
- Old samples: the presence of free-living nematodes and protozoa.

Influence of Signalment

Species

None

Breed

None

Age

Puppies and kittens should be checked for internal parasites and medicated according to the recommendations of the American Association of Veterinary Parasitologists, American Animal Hospital Association, and the Companion Animal Parasite Council.

Gender

None

Pregnancy

None

LIMITATIONS OF TEST

- Sample size can be an issue in anorexic or very small animals with minimal fecal output.
- Some eggs (*Trichuris vulpis*) and cysts (*Giardia* sp.) are shed in low numbers or intermittently. If suspicion is high, fecal flotation should be run on samples from 3 consecutive days.

Sensitivity, Specificity, and Positive and Negative Predictive Values

Note that centrifugal flotation is more sensitive and accurate than passive flotation.

Valid If Run in a Human Lab?

No. Few technicians are trained in the identification of animal parasite diagnostic life stages.

CAUSES OF ABNORMAL FINDINGS (SEE TABLE 1)

- Spurious eggs and oocysts of parasites of other animals may be passed in feces of dogs and cats when these fed on live animals or carcasses, or animal feces (e.g., oocysts of *Eimeria*, a coccidian of birds, rodents, and herbivores).
- Pseudoparasites are common findings in fecal flotations, and should not be mistaken with parasite diagnostic stages. In fact, pseudoparasites are structures of free-living organisms that may pass in feces or are product of environmental contamination (e.g., pollen grains, plant hair, mite eggs, grain mites).

CLINICAL PERSPECTIVE

- A good-quality microscope with a micrometer is required. A micrometer makes it possible to measure objects seen under the microscope, thus ensuring the accurate diagnosis of parasites.
- *Giardia* cysts are often mistaken for yeast, but *Giardia* cysts are all about the same size, whereas yeasts vary greatly in size and shape.
- Proper techniques are imperative for the accurate diagnosis of intestinal parasites.
- Due to coprophagy, strongyle-type eggs from horses or cows, or coccidia oocysts from ruminants, rabbits, or birds, may be found in canine feces. To determine whether these eggs are just passing through, confine the dog away from these animals for 24–48 hours and recheck.

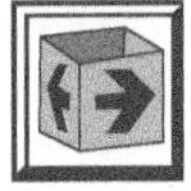

MISCELLANEOUS

ANCILLARY TESTS

- Fecal sedimentation techniques to look for trematode (fluke) eggs.
- Baermann technique to look for larvae of lungworms (note that some worms that are found in the respiratory tract may shed eggs that can be seen in flotation, see Table 1).
- In animals with diarrhea, consider evaluating fecal cytology, cobalamin, folate, and trypsin-like immunoreactivity.

SYNONYMS

Fecal float.

SEE ALSO

- Coccidiosis.
- Diarrhea, Chronic—Cats.
- Diarrhea, Chronic—Dogs.
- Fecal Direct Smear and Cytology (in Appendix X).
- Giardiasis.
- Hookworms (Ancylostomiasis).
- Roundworms (Ascariasis).
- Tapeworms (Cestodiasis).
- Whipworms (Trichuriasis).

ABBREVIATIONS

- L_1 = first-stage larva(e).
- L_3 = third-stage larva(e).
- SG = specific gravity.

INTERNET RESOURCES

- Penn Veterinary Medicine, Veterinary Parasitology CAL Program: http://cal.vet.upenn.edu/projects/parasit06/website/index.htm
- University of Wisconsin–Madison, School of Veterinary Medicine: Veterinary parasitology, http://www.vetmed.wisc.edu/pbs/vetpara/gallery.html
- Companion Animal Parasite Council: http://www.capcvet.org

Suggested Reading

Dryden MW, Payne PA, Ridley R, Smith V. Comparison of common fecal flotation techniques for the recovery of parasite eggs and oocysts. Vet Ther 2005, 6:15–28.

Foreyt W, ed. Veterinary Parasitology Reference Manual, 5th ed. Ames, IA: Iowa State Press, 2001.

Zajac AM, Conboy GA. Veterinary Clinical Parasitology, 8th ed. Hoboken, NJ: Wiley-Blackwell, 2012.

Authors Guilherme G. Verocai and Andrew R. Moorhead

Consulting Editor Benjamin M. Brainard

Acknowledgment The authors and editors acknowledge the prior contribution of Patricia A. Payne.

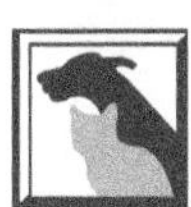

BASICS

TYPE OF PROCEDURE

Diagnostic sample collection

PROCEDURE EXPLANATION AND RELATED PHYSIOLOGY

- For acquisition of samples of masses, lymph nodes, organ cellularity for the purposes of cytologic examination.
- Cytology may identify inflammatory and infectious processes and distinguish between neoplastic and nonneoplastic conditions.
- Poorly prepared smears can make interpretation difficult. Extremely thick smears, for example, can limit evaluation of individual cell characteristics.

INDICATIONS

- Evaluation of cutaneous, subcutaneous, intracavitary masses.
- Evaluation of lymphadenopathy.
- Evaluation of nodules, masses, or other changes within organs.

CONTRAINDICATIONS

- Fine-needle aspiration (FNA) is difficult to perform on very small masses or those that cannot be stabilized.
- FNA entails a risk of hemorrhage when used to assess cavitary masses.
- Patients with a condition that includes severe bleeding tendencies (e.g., thrombocytopenia or coagulopathy).

POTENTIAL COMPLICATIONS

- Bleeding, bruising.
- Release of bioactive substances (e.g., mast cell tumor).
- Potential spread of malignant neoplasia (rare).
- Pneumothorax (FNA of lungs).

CLIENT EDUCATION

While risks are minimal when FNA cytology of internal organs or masses is performed, clients should be advised of the potential for hemorrhage or pneumothorax in the case of lung aspiration.

BODY SYSTEMS ASSESSED

All

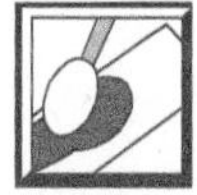

PROCEDURE

PATIENT PREPARATION

Pre-Procedure Medication or Preparation

- None needed for external palpable masses.
- The use of an aseptic skin preparation is indicated prior to FNA of internal masses.

Anesthesia or Sedation

- Generally, none is needed for external palpable masses or lymph nodes.
- Mild to heavy sedation is beneficial for obtaining diagnostic ultrasound-guided or bone FNA.

Patient Positioning

Any that enables optimal access to the site being aspirated.

Patient Monitoring

For minor bruising or bleeding at the FNA site.

Equipment or Supplies

- A needle of appropriate gauge—a 22-gauge, 1-inch needle is appropriate for most cutaneous and subcutaneous masses. Longer needles may be used for intracavitary or ultrasound-guided aspirates.
- A 6- or 12-mL syringe.
- Glass microscopic slides.

TECHNIQUE

Sample Collection

Needle Only

The mass or tissue is stabilized as much as possible while the needle is inserted into it and vigorously moved in and out of it in several directions. The needle is then withdrawn, a syringe filled with air is attached to the needle hub, and pressure is applied to the plunger to empty the needle's contents onto a glass slide. If blood or liquid is observed in the hub of the needle during this procedure, the FNA should be discontinued and the slide prepared.

Needle and Syringe with Continuous Negative Pressure

The mass or tissue is stabilized as much as possible, and the needle with attached empty syringe is inserted into the mass or tissue. Negative pressure is then applied to the syringe and maintained while the needle is redirected several times within the mass or tissue. Negative pressure is then released, and the needle with attached syringe is withdrawn. The syringe is detached from the needle, filled with air, reattached to the hub of the needle, and pressure is applied to the plunger to empty the needle's contents onto a glass slide. If blood or liquid is observed in the hub of the needle during this procedure, the FNA should be discontinued and the slide prepared.

Needle and Syringe with Repeated Negative Pressure

The mass or tissue is stabilized as much as possible while the needle with attached empty syringe is inserted into the mass or tissue. Negative pressure is applied to the syringe and released several times. The needle can be redirected and negative pressure again applied and released several times. This can be repeated in several directions within the mass or tissue. Once the sample has been collected, negative pressure is released, and the needle with attached syringe is withdrawn. The syringe is detached from the needle, filled with air, reattached, and pressure is applied to the plunger to empty the needle's contents onto a glass slide. If blood or liquid is observed in the hub of the needle during this procedure, the FNA should be discontinued and the slide prepared.

Slide Preparation

Flat Spreader Slide Technique

A second slide is laid gently atop and perpendicular to the slide containing the sample and gently drawn down the length of the sample slide to achieve an even, thin layer of cells.

Angled Spreader Slide Technique

A second slide is positioned over the slide containing the sample and angled at 45° with the sample located in the small angle created between the two slides. The spreader slide is then drawn along the sample slide so that the cells are spread in an even layer down the latter slide's length. This technique, similar to that used for making a blood smear, may result in the rupture or breakage of cells from FNA.

SAMPLE HANDLING

- Air-dried samples can be stored at room temperature.
- Samples should be fixed and stained as soon after collection as possible (ideally within 3–7 days) for optimal assessment of cellular morphology.
- Once fixed and stained, FNA smears are stable for months to years, depending on storage conditions.

APPROPRIATE AFTERCARE

Post-Procedure Patient Monitoring

Generally, no post-procedure monitoring is required, although if FNA is performed on highly vascular internal masses or tissues, monitoring for evidence of hemorrhage (i.e., mucous membrane color, attitude, with or without PCV and total solids) should be performed in the hours after the procedure.

Nursing Care

None

Dietary Modification

None

Medication Requirements

None

Restrictions on Activity

None

Anticipated Recovery Time

Immediate

FINE-NEEDLE ASPIRATION (CONTINUED)

INTERPRETATION

NORMAL FINDINGS OR RANGE

A bullet-shaped tissue smear that extends approximately one-half to two-thirds the length of the slide.

ABNORMAL VALUES

- Abnormal cell ratios, numbers, or types.
- The presence of infectious agents.
- The presence of neoplastic cells.
- The presence of abnormal inflammation.

CRITICAL VALUES

None

INTERFERING FACTORS

Drugs That May Alter Results of the Procedure

None

Conditions That May Interfere with Performing the Procedure

None

Procedure Techniques or Handling That May Alter Results

- Hemorrhage with numerous RBCs evident cytologically may limit interpretation.
- Failure to fix and stain slides within 1–2 weeks may alter cellular characteristics and limit value of interpretation.

Influence of Signalment on Performing and Interpreting the Procedure

Species

None

Breed

None

Age

None

Gender

None

Pregnancy

None

CLINICAL PERSPECTIVE

Cytologic examination of FNA samples is a first step in assessing masses, lymphadenopathy, and other organ changes. Examination of prepared slides can provide information on potential pathology affecting the tissue sampled, including hyperplastic, reactive, inflammatory, and neoplastic changes. Depending on results, a follow-up incisional or excisional biopsy may be indicated for definitive diagnosis.

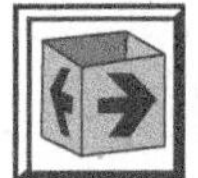

MISCELLANEOUS

ANCILLARY TESTS

- A biopsy with a histopathologic diagnosis to confirm the FNA results if they are equivocal or if the biopsy is indicated for definitive diagnosis and grading.
- Coagulation testing if there is a concern for hemorrhage during the procedure.

SYNONYMS

Fine-needle aspiration biopsy.

SEE ALSO

- Blood Smear Preparation (in Appendix X).
- Impression Smear (in Appendix X).
- Ultrasound-Guided Mass or Organ Aspiration (in Appendix X).

ABBREVIATIONS

- FNA = fine-needle aspiration.

Suggested Reading

Cowell RL, Tyler RD, Meinkoth JH, eds. Diagnostic Cytology and Hematology of the Dog and Cat. St. Louis, MO: CV Mosby, 1999.

Raskin RE, Meyer DJ, eds. Atlas of Canine and Feline Cytology, 2nd ed. Philadelphia, PA: W.B. Saunders, 2001.

Author Laurel E. Williams

Consulting Editor Benjamin M. Brainard

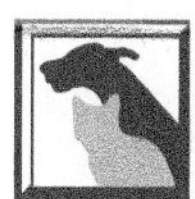

BASICS

TYPE OF SPECIMEN

Tissue

TEST EXPLANATION AND RELATED PHYSIOLOGY

The abdominal and thoracic cavities normally contain a small amount of fluid that is an ultrafiltrate of blood which serves to provide lubrication that enables frictionless movement of adjacent organ surfaces and the body cavity walls. An increased amount of fluid in any body cavity lined by mesothelial cells is termed an effusion. An effusion is not a disease itself but, rather, the result of a pathologic alteration in the process of fluid production and/or removal, or an accumulation from an ectopic source.

A comprehensive fluid analysis is a rapid, simple, inexpensive, and reasonably safe way of gaining useful information regarding disease processes that cause effusions. Classification schemes are designed to help clinicians generate a short list of differential diagnoses and characterize an effusion based on the primary underlying pathophysiologic mechanism.

Effusions are classified as a pure transudate, modified transudate, exudate, hemorrhagic effusion, or neoplastic effusion (see Table 1). Exudates are further divided into subcategories of septic or nonseptic exudates. The classification of these fluids is based on three parameters: total protein, nucleated cell counts (NCCs), and cytologic appearance.

Pure transudates usually form via a passive process resulting from decreased colloid osmotic pressure (vs. an alteration in capillary permeability). They most frequently form as a result of hypoproteinemia from either increased loss or decreased production of albumin (the primary contributor to plasma colloid osmotic pressure). Infrequently, transudates precede modified transudates before developing an increased NCC or protein concentration.

A modified transudate occurs when vascular fluids leak from normal, noninflamed vessels (e.g., via increased capillary hydrostatic pressure or lymphatic obstruction). This fluid is modified by the addition of protein or cells (compared to a pure transudate). A chylous effusion is a specialized type of modified transudate that results from leakage of noninflamed lymphatics into the thoracic and/or abdominal cavity.

Exudates are the result of increased vascular permeability and inflammation and are further classified as septic or nonseptic (sterile) depending on whether infectious agents are present in the fluid. Nonseptic exudates may result from conditions that cause longstanding modified transudates, as well as from other, more inflammatory disease conditions. Hemorrhagic effusions can be caused by ruptured vessels or organs.

Neoplasia is a common underlying cause of effusions in dogs and cats although neoplastic cells may not be identified on cytologic preparations (i.e., neoplastic cells may not exfoliate into the effusion). Furthermore, neoplasia may cause various effusions, including modified transudates, exudates, and hemorrhagic effusions. The term neoplastic effusion is reserved for fluids in which a neoplastic cell population is definitively identified. However, this determination is frequently difficult because neoplastic cells are absent or are present in low numbers, and reactive mesothelial cells often have cytologic criteria that mimic malignancy.

INDICATIONS

- Accumulation of fluid because of an unknown cause.
- Suspicion of neoplasia or sepsis.

CONTRAINDICATIONS

None

POTENTIAL COMPLICATIONS

During acquisition of fluid (see Thoracocentesis and Fluid Analysis, Pericardiocentesis, and Abdominocentesis and Fluid Analysis):

- Hemorrhage.
- Infection.
- Trauma to surrounding viscera (i.e., perforation, laceration).

CLIENT EDUCATION

Sampling of cavitary effusions typically is minimally invasive with minimal associated risk and discomfort for the animal, and may have therapeutic benefits (e.g., pericardiocentesis).

BODY SYSTEMS ASSESSED

- Cardiovascular.
- Gastrointestinal.
- Hemic/lymphatic/immune.
- Hepatobiliary.
- Renal/urologic.

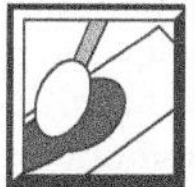

SAMPLE

SAMPLE COLLECTION

2–6 mL of fluid.

SAMPLE HANDLING

- Collect the sample into EDTA-containing tube to prevent clotting and to optimize preservation of cells.
- Place an aliquot into a sterile tube without EDTA if bacteriologic culture is anticipated (EDTA is bacteriostatic) or if biochemical testing is required.
- Prepare smears immediately if the sample will not be processed within 1–2 hours after collection.
- Transport the fluid sample chilled, with any accompanying slides at room temperature.

SAMPLE STORAGE

- Refrigerate fluid.
- Stores slides at room temperature, away from light or humidity.

SAMPLE STABILITY

- Fluid.
- Room temperature: 2–4 hours.
- Refrigerated (4°C): 24–36 hours.
- Unstained smears of fluid can be stored for 1 week or more. Stained slides can be stored for months to years.

PROTOCOL

In-house fluid analysis:

- Note the gross appearance of fluid including color and clarity.
- Prepare smears of fluid by using the same technique used to make blood smears. Smears should be thin enough to dry quickly. Be sure that the smear has a stainable feathered edge.
- Air-dry smears and stain with a Romanovsky-type cytology stain.
- Perform a NCC via hematology analyzer or hemocytometer.
- Centrifuge an aliquot of fluid and note the appearance of the supernatant.
- Determine the total protein of supernatant via refractometer.
- If the NCC is <3,000/μL, prepare additional smears of sedimented cellular material, using either a centrifuge (with resuspension of the pellet) or a cytospin device.

INTERPRETATION

NORMAL FINDINGS OR RANGE

No excess free fluid should be found in the pleural cavity, peritoneal cavity, and pericardium.

ABNORMAL FINDINGS

The presence of an abnormal, increased amount of fluid within a body cavity

CRITICAL VALUES

Evidence of septic peritonitis, uroabdomen, or bile peritonitis requires immediate intervention.

INTERFERING FACTORS

Drugs That May Alter Results or Interpretation

Drugs That Interfere with Test Methodology

None

FLUID ANALYSIS

(CONTINUED)

Table 1

Classification of effusions.

Classification	*Gross Appearance*	*Protein (g/dL)*	*Cells/μL*	*Cell Types Present*
Pure transudate	Colorless; clear	<2.5	<1,500	Mixed (macrophages, nondegenerate neutrophils, mesothelial cells)
Modified transudate	White to red; variable turbidity	2.5–5.0	1,000–7,000	Mixed (nondegenerate neutrophils, macrophages, mesothelial cells, small lymphocytes)
Chylous effusion[a]	Milky white, tan, or pink	2.5–5.0	1,000–7,000	Predominantly small lymphocytes
Exudate[b]	Amber, white, or red; turbid or cloudy	>3.0	>7,000	Predominantly neutrophils
Hemorrhagic effusion[c]	Pink or red; cloudy or opaque	Variable	Variable	Similar to peripheral blood but lacks platelets and may have erythrophagia
Neoplastic effusion	Variable	Variable	Variable	Neoplastic cells present

[a] Chylous effusions have a triglyceride concentration of >100 mg/dL and a fluid cholesterol/triglyceride ratio of <1.0.

[b] Further classification of exudates depends on whether microorganisms are present (i.e., septic versus nonseptic).

[c] The PCV of fluid is ≥10–25% of the PCV of peripheral blood.

Drugs That Alter Physiology

- Corticosteroids may artifactually decrease the percentage and total number of neutrophils.
- Antibiotic administration greatly hinders the cytologic identification of bacteria, and can result in false-negative culture results. In patients that have received antibiotics that develop exudates characterized by degenerate neutrophils, a septic effusion should be a primary differential, even in the absence of intracellular microorganisms.

Disorders That May Alter Results

- High triglyceride concentration in chylous effusions, or other causes of turbidity, may artificially increase protein determination by refractometry. If possible, clear such samples prior to determining protein concentration by refractometer.
- The dilutional effect of urine in uroperitoneum may decrease the protein concentration and NCC.
- Peracute hemorrhagic effusions may not have detectable erythrophagocytosis.
- The protein concentration in an effusion can be affected by serum protein concentration (e.g., mildly increased with dehydration; decreased with protein-losing enteropathies or nephropathies) regardless of the effusion mechanism.

Collection Techniques or Handling That May Alter Results

- Excessive pressure when preparing cytologic preparations (e.g., direct or sediment smears) may lyse cells.
- Delayed processing may lead to *in vitro* artifacts such as erythrophagocytosis, lysed cells, and/or poor cellular preservation. Bacterial overgrowth may occur if a preservative is not used or the specimen is not refrigerated.

Influence of Signalment

Species
None

Breed
None

Age
None

Gender
None

Pregnancy
None

LIMITATIONS OF TEST

Sensitivity, Specificity, and Positive and Negative Predictive Values

N/A

Valid If Run in Human Lab?

Yes.

Causes of Abnormal Values

CLINICAL PERSPECTIVE

- Turbidity caused by lipids (e.g., chylous effusion) will not clear with centrifugation, unlike the turbidity caused by an increased NCC.
- Inadvertent venipuncture or aspiration of the spleen is possible at time of collection. True hemorrhagic effusions should have the same color and turbidity throughout the draw, whereas with accidental venipuncture and splenic aspirate samples usually change color and turbidity during collection. Splenic aspirates may also clot, while effusion generally will not, unless peracute.
- Lipid can be an irritant and chronic chylous effusions may have a mixed inflammatory cell population, including neutrophils (which may ultimately predominate) and macrophages, in addition to lymphocytes.
- If intracellular infectious agents are identified, the effusion is septic, regardless of protein concentration and NCC.
- If fluid collected by abdominocentesis has low cellularity, abundant mixed bacteria, ingesta, and/or intestinal parasite ova, consider accidental enterocentesis or acute intestinal perforation.
- The distinction between reactive mesothelial cells and a true neoplastic cell population (carcinoma or mesothelioma) is often difficult to impossible with cytology alone, since reactive mesothelial cells may exhibit significant atypia mimicking malignancy. Correlation with observation of a "mass effect" on imaging may assist in making this distinction, but additional diagnostics are often needed, such as cytopathologic/histopathologic evaluation of any masses.

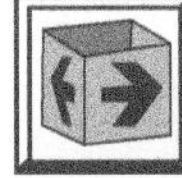

MISCELLANEOUS

ANCILLARY TESTS

- Albumin.
- Creatinine (fluid)—a value of ≥2-fold serum creatinine and ≥1.4 fold serum potassium is diagnostic for uroperitoneum.
- Total bilirubin (fluid)—a value of ≥2-fold serum bilirubin is diagnostic for bile peritonitis. Bile crystals are frequently observed cytologically, as well.
- Triglycerides (fluid; for diagnosis of chylothorax)—greater than serum triglycerides
- Glucose (fluid)—a value of 38 mg/dL less than that for blood glucose has been suggested to be specific for sepsis, but low glucose may simply reflect the concurrent elevated NCC and subsequent utilization by leukocytes, and samples may be analyzer dependent.
- Microbial culture and sensitivity

Table 2

Causes of abnormal values.

Type of Effusion and Mechanisms	*Possible Causes*
Pure transudate	Decreased production of albumin
Decreased plasma colloidal osmotic pressure (i.e., hypoalbuminemia)—more common	Liver failure
Early cardiac disease or portal hypertension	Maldigestion/malabsorption
	Starvation
	Increased loss of albumin
	Protein-losing nephropathy
	Protein-losing enteropathy
	Other
	Iatrogenic overhydration
Modified transudate	Cardiac disease
Increased capillary hydrostatic pressure	Portal hypertension
Lymphatic obstruction	Neoplasia
	Acute organ torsion
Chylous effusion	Cardiac disease
Leakage of lymphatics from noninflamed vessels	Hernia
	Neoplasia
	Trauma
	Idiopathic
	Lung torsion
	Intestinal lymphangiectasia
	Mediastinal granuloma
Exudate	Uroperitoneum
Increased vascular permeability and inflammation caused by septic and nonseptic etiologies	Bile peritonitis
	Feline infectious peritonitis
	Inflammation and/or infection of internal organs
	Foreign bodies
	Neoplasia
Eosinophilic effusion	Neoplasia (e.g., mast cell tumor, lymphoma, carcinoma)
Eosinophils >10% of the NCC	Infection (e.g., fungus, parasite, protozoa)
Secretion of IL- 5 by sensitized T-lymphocytes, mast cells, or neoplastic cells	Other eosinophilic inflammatory process such as eosinophilic gastritis
Hemorrhagic effusion	Traumatic injury
Ruptured vessels	Rodenticide toxicity
Coagulopathies	Neoplasia
Neoplastic effusion	Lymphoma and other "round" cell tumors
Exfoliation of identifiable neoplastic cells into fluid	Carcinoma
	Mesothelioma
	Sarcoma (often poorly exfoliative)

SYNONYMS

Body cavity effusion

SEE ALSO

- Abdominocentesis and Fluid Analysis (in Appendix X).
- Ascites.
- Bile Peritonitis
- Chapters on cardiac disease.
- Chapters on hepatic disease.
- Feline Infectious Peritonitis (FIP).
- Hemothorax.
- Lymphangiectasia.
- Sepsis and Bacteremia.
- Thoracocentesis and Fluid Analysis (in Appendix X).

ABBREVIATIONS

- IL-5 = interleukin 5.
- NCC = nucleated cell count.

INTERNET RESOURCES

http://eclinpath.com/cytology/effusions-2/

Suggested Reading

Thompson CA, Rebar AH. Body cavity fluids. In: Canine and Feline Cytology: A Color Atlas and Interpretation Guide, 3rd ed. St. Louis, MO: Elsevier, 2016, pp. 191–219.

Valenciano AC, Arndt TP, Rizzi TE. Effusions: abdominal, thoracic, and pericardial. In: Valenciano AC, Cowell RL, eds., Cowell and Tyler's Diagnostic Cytology and Hematology of the Dog and Cat, 4th ed. St. Louis, MO: Elsevier, 2014, pp. 244–265.

Author Rebekah G. Gunn-Christie
Consulting Editor Benjamin M. Brainard

GLUCOSE CURVE

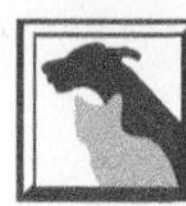

BASICS

TYPE OF SPECIMEN

Whole blood.

TEST EXPLANATION AND RELATED PHYSIOLOGY

- A method of evaluating glucose control in diabetic dogs or cats.
- Serial blood glucose (BG) measurement enables assessment of the effect of food and medication (insulin or oral hypoglycemic drugs) on glucose control. The dose, and, if necessary, the type, of medication (e.g., intermediate-acting vs. long-acting insulin) can be altered, depending on results.
- The lowest (nadir) and highest BG concentrations should be noted, as well as the duration of action of insulin (the number of hours the glucose is in a desired range, provided the nadir is acceptable).
  - Hypoglycemia (a BG concentration of <60 mg/dL) or a rapid drop in glucose concentration can result in rebound hyperglycemia or the Somogyi phenomenon, whereby counterregulatory hormones, notably glucagon, epinephrine, and corticosteroids, cause a variable period of hyperglycemia after hypoglycemia occurs.
    - The occurrence of the Somogyi phenomenon is debatable and some internists prefer the term posthypoglycemic hyperglycemia or glucose variability because the link between hypoglycemia and hyperglycemia is uncertain.
- There is significant variation in BG curves from day to day even with no change in insulin dose or feeding. A curve should always be interpreted in conjunction with information on the patient's appetite, thirst, urinations and energy level.
- Control of clinical signs rather than glucose concentration is the overall goal with diabetic patients.

INDICATIONS

- To regulate a new diabetic patient.
- To investigate a poorly controlled diabetic patient.
- To diagnose transient diabetes mellitus, a temporary or permanent resolution of diabetes in cats.

CONTRAINDICATIONS

- Inappetence or illness on the day of the test.
- Hypoglycemia (a BG concentration of <60 mg/dL) on admission: In this case, cancel the BG curve analysis and recommend a 10–25% insulin-dose reduction.
- Stress hyperglycemia—if a patient, especially a cat, is very anxious, the curve may be meaningless. If glucose readings in an extremely stressed patient are normal, insulin overdosage may be suspected.

POTENTIAL COMPLICATIONS

None

CLIENT EDUCATION

- The goal for diabetic management is to maintain daily BG concentrations between 100 and 300 mg/dL with an average glucose <250 mg/dL. Measurements outside that range may require a dose adjustment, an alternative insulin type, or further investigation or monitoring.
- Owners can monitor glucose at home by using lancets to obtain a small drop of blood from the marginal ear vein, metacarpal pad, foot pad, ventral medial pinna, buccal mucosa of a lip (dogs), or elbow calluses (dogs).
  - Warming the site first with a dry (to avoid diluting sample) warm cloth will improve sample size.
  - Glucose should be measured by using portable veterinary-specific glucometers that use the least amount of blood, such as the AlphaTRAK 2 (Zoetis, Parsippany, NJ).
  - Glucometers designed for human usage measure lower than the actual reading, which may result in falsely low BG readings.
- Owners need to be instructed carefully in the home use of glucometers and informed about calibration and coding of the devices according to the manufacturer's directions.
- Newer long-term interstital devices (e.g., freestyle Libre, Abbott, N. Chicago, IL) may allow generation of BG curve data at home, over longer periods of time (e.g., 14 days), using smartphone-based technology.

BODY SYSTEMS ASSESSED

Endocrine and metabolic.

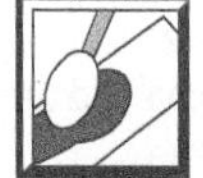

SAMPLE

SAMPLE COLLECTION

- Generally, a very small amount of blood (<0.2 mL) is obtained by venipuncture, using an insulin syringe or pricking the skin with a lancet:
  - The goal is to be minimally invasive while enabling multiple sequential sample collections.
- When using a lancet, the glucometer with test strip inserted is held to the drop of blood, which is then drawn up by capillary action.
- For in-hospital curves a glucometer is typically used but if a larger amount of blood is obtained, glucose can be measured with a point of care machine, although the same machine should be used for analyzing all samples in the curve.

SAMPLE HANDLING

The sample should be analyzed immediately.

SAMPLE STORAGE

Immediate analysis is recommended.

SAMPLE STABILITY

If measuring serum glucose, the blood sample should be separated quickly to avoid spurious hypoglycemia.

PROTOCOL

- The patient is admitted to the hospital shortly after being fed and given insulin at home.
- The owner's feeding schedule should be followed for the remainder of the day.
- Appetite and stress level are noted during the day.
- BG concentration is measured every 2 hours for 10–12 hours. Collect blood from any easily accessible peripheral vein or pricking skin with lancet, using minimal restraint to avoid stress hyperglycemia.
- Measure glucose by using a portable glucose meter or a point-of-care analyzer.
- Note the BG nadir, duration of effect (number of hours BG concentration between 60–300 mg/dL), and highest BG concentration.
- BG curves are typically repeated 7–14 days following an insulin dose change. New diabetic patients may require 3–4 curves to determine an insulin dose that controls clinical signs. Cats going into remission also require multiple curves while they are tapered off insulin.

INTERPRETATION

NORMAL FINDINGS OR RANGE

- Dogs and cats—the ideal BG concentration range is 80–300 mg/dL with an average BG <250 mg/dL and a nadir of 80–150 mg/dL.
- Normal or below-normal BG concentration readings in cats with diabetes mellitus suggest transient diabetes, especially if normal findings are repeatable with dose reduction or discontinuation of insulin administration.

ABNORMAL FINDINGS

BG concentrations above or below ideal range require evaluation.

CRITICAL VALUES

- A BG concentration <60 mg/dL requires evaluation to ensure patient is not exhibiting clinical signs such as twitching, stumbling, or mental dullness (may need to treat with IV glucose or oral glucose if patient is able to eat). Recheck BG hourly until normal, consider potential insulin dose adjustment to avoid subsequent hypoglycemic events.

Table 1

Interpretation of curve.

Abnormal Finding	*Suggested Response*
Nadir and peak BG concentration are greater than the ideal	Increase the dose of insulin
The nadir is acceptable, but the effect of insulin was of insufficient duration	Switch to a longer acting insulin: Dogs: Switch from NPH (neutral protamine Hagedorn) insulin to lente insulin or insulin detemir Cats: If not already on a long acting insulin, switch to insulin glargine or insulin detemir
Hypoglycemia	Decrease the dose by 10–25% and, in cats, consider transient diabetes mellitus
Persistent hyperglycemia may be caused by insulin overdose (post hypoglycemic hyperglycemia) insulin underdose, or insulin resistance).	Consider increasing insulin dose, switching insulin type and if the insulin dose is >1.5 U/kg bid, evaluate for causes of the insulin resistance

- A persistently high BG concentration (>600 mg/dL) may be associated with hyperglycemic hyperosmolar syndrome.

INTERFERING FACTORS

- Glucometers are not designed to measure glucose in serum or plasma.
- Inaccurate readings can also occur with anemia, polycythemia, inadequate sample size, expired glucose strips, miscoded meters, contamination (e.g., sugar on skin of pet or human).
- A correction formula for the Alpha-TRAK 2 has been developed to account for variation in patient PCV:

Corrected glucose = glucose reading + ([1.6 × PCV(%)] – 81.3) (dogs)

Corrected glucose = glucose reading + ([1.17 × PCV(%)] – 50.2) (cats)

Drugs That May Alter Results or Interpretation

Drugs That Interfere with Test Methodology

None

Drugs That Alter Physiology

The administration of drugs such as corticosteroids and megestrol acetate cause insulin resistance that predisposes patients to diabetes or worsening glucose control.

Disorders That May Alter Results

Any underlying disease can make diabetes more difficult to regulate: especially hyperadrenocorticism, infection, pancreatitis, acromegaly, or thyroid disease, as well as diestrus.

Collection Techniques or Handling That May Alter Results

- Stress hyperglycemia in cats and, to a lesser degree, in dogs may inappropriately increase the BG concentration.
- Failure to separate serum promptly may falsely lower the BG concentration when the assay relies on serum sample.
- Sugary food on skin of patient or person obtaining blood sample may falsely increase glucose concentration.

Influence of Signalment

Species

None

Breed

None

Age

None

Gender

Intact females with diabetes are very difficult to regulate and should be spayed.

Pregnancy

The same as for gender.

LIMITATIONS OF TEST

- There is significant variation in BG curves from day to day even with no change in insulin dose or feeding. A curve should always be interpreted in conjunction with information on the patient's appetite, thirst, urinations and energy level.
- Control of clinical signs rather than glucose levels is the overall goal with diabetic patients.
- Handheld portable glucometers may overestimate or underestimate glucose levels when compared to reference methods. Veterinary-specific glucometers are more accurate and validated for dogs and cats, and strongly recommended.

Sensitivity, Specificity, and Positive and Negative Predictive Values

N/A

Valid If Run in a Human Lab?

Yes.

CAUSES OF ABNORMAL FINDINGS

See Table 1.

CLINICAL PERSPECTIVE

- BG curves are only one indicator of diabetic control, and results can vary from day to day, even when there is little change in the patient's status. Therefore, the results should be interpreted with the animal's clinical signs (e.g., presence of PU/PD, polyphagia, weight loss, neuropathy). If the patient appears well (no PU/PD, stable weight, active), then changes made may be small or the curve might be repeated.
- Other reasons for persistent hyperglycemia (BG concentrations >300 mg/dL) are mishandling of insulin, poor injection technique, inadequate absorption, and insulin resistance (e.g., infection, drugs, hyperadrenocorticism, diestrus, acromegaly, hypothyroidism, hyperthyroidism.
- It is important that portable glucometers be coded correctly and that the test strips are correct and in date.

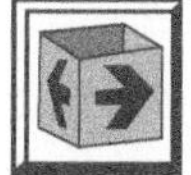

MISCELLANEOUS

ANCILLARY TESTS

- Serial urine glucose testing can enable veterinarians to make some dose increases in new diabetic patients before fine-tuning with a BG curve.
- Measurement of serum fructosamine concentration can be used in addition to analysis of BG curves and, in fractious animals, may replace the analysis of a BG curve. If fructosamine is normal to low-normal in hypoglycemic patients, it supports insulin overdose and, in cats, potential remission.
- Continuous glucose monitoring using interstitial (subcutaneous) sensors (e.g., CGMS System Gold; Medtronic MiniMed,

GLUCOSE CURVE (CONTINUED)

Minneapolis, MN) enables continuous interstitial fluid glucose concentration to be measured for up to 14 days. The newer Libre Freestyle Flash glucose monitoring system is cost effective, easy to use, is accurate in diabetic dogs, and is being evaluated for use in diabetic cats.

SYNONYMS

None

SEE ALSO

- Diabetes Mellitus with Hyperosmolar Hyperglycemic State.
- Diabetes Mellitus with Ketoacidosis.
- Diabetes Mellitus Without Complication—Cats.
- Diabetes Mellitus Without Complication—Dogs.
- Hyperglycemia.

ABBREVIATIONS

- BG = blood glucose.
- PU/PD = polyuria/polydipsia.

INTERNET RESOURCES

- AAHAguidelines: https://www.aaha.org/aaha-guidelines/diabetes-management/diabetes-management-home/
- Canine Diabetes: http://www.caninediabetes.org
- Feline Diabetes: http://www.felinediabetes.com
- Pet Diabetes support site: http://www.petdiabetes.com

Suggested Reading

Behrend E, Holford A, Latham P, Rucinsky R, et al. 2018 Diabetes management guidelines for dogs and cats. J Am Anim Hosp Assoc 2018, 54:1–21

Corradini S, Pilosio B, Dondi F, Linari G, et al. Accuracy of a flash glucose monitoring system in diabetic dogs. J Vet Intern Med 2016, 30:983–988

Fleeman L, Rand J. Evaluation of day to day variability of serial blood glucose concentration curves in diabetic dogs. J Am Vet Med Assoc 2003, 222:317–321.

Kley S, Casella M, Reusch C. Evaluation of long-term home monitoring of blood glucose concentrations in cats with diabetes mellitus: 26 cases (1999–2002). J Am Vet Med Assoc 2004, 225:261–266.

Lane SL, Koenig A, Brainard BM. Formulation and validation of a predictive model to correct blood glucose concentrations obtained with a veterinary point-of-care glucometer in hemodiluted and hemoconcentrated canine blood samples. J Am Vet Med Assoc. 2015, 246:307–312.

Reusch C, Kley S, Casella M. Home monitoring of the diabetic cat. J Feline Med Surg 2006,8:119–127.

Author Orla Mahony

Consulting Editor Benjamin M. Brainard

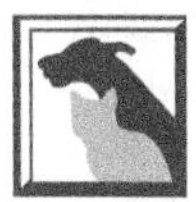

BASICS

TYPE OF PROCEDURE

Diagnostic sample collection.

PROCEDURE EXPLANATION AND RELATED PHYSIOLOGY

- Impression smears obtained from superficial lesions or from tissue biopsy samples may reveal cellular details not visible after collection and processing for histologic evaluation.
- Individual cell types, including infectious organisms and neoplastic cells, may be identified on impression smear cytology, which provides more rapid assessment than histologic examination.

CONTRAINDICATIONS

None

POTENTIAL COMPLICATIONS

None

CLIENT EDUCATION

None

BODY SYSTEMS ASSESSED

All

PROCEDURE

PATIENT PREPARATION

Pre-Procedure Medication or Preparation

None

Anesthesia or Sedation

None

Patient Positioning

None

Patient Monitoring

None

Equipment or Supplies

- A paper towel for blotting.
- A scalpel blade.
- Glass slides.

TECHNIQUE

Impression smears may be made directly from superficial ulcerated lesions or from harvested biopsy tissue.

- Directly from a lesion: An imprint is made by touching the center of a clean glass slide to the uncleaned lesion. After an initial impression smear, the lesion can be gently blotted and cleaned with saline solution and gauze and a second impression made.
- For a harvested biopsy tissue: A freshly cut surface is exposed by sectioning the tissue biopsy sample with a scalpel blade (this is not required if the sample being evaluated is freshly removed via needle or punch biopsy). An important aspect of obtaining diagnostic impression smears is blotting the tissue on a clean absorbent material, such as a paper towel, to remove excess blood, moisture, and tissue fluid prior to imprinting the tissue on a slide. The blotted tissue can be gently touched onto the middle of a clean glass slide and lifted off. Multiple impression smears may be made onto separate glass slides.

SAMPLE HANDLING

- Air-dried samples can be stored at room temperature.
- Samples should be fixed and stained as soon after collection as possible (ideally within 3–7 days) for optimal assessment of cellular morphology.

APPROPRIATE AFTERCARE

Post-Procedure Patient Monitoring

N/A

Nursing Care

N/A

Dietary Modification

N/A

Medication Requirements

N/A

Restrictions on Activity

N/A

Anticipated Recovery Time

N/A

INTERPRETATION

NORMAL FINDINGS OR RANGE

- A blot of tissue centered on the glass slide.
- Identification of cells normally seen in sampled tissue.

ABNORMAL FINDINGS

- Abnormal ratios, numbers, or types of cells present.
- Infectious agents.
- Neoplastic cells.

CRITICAL VALUES

None

INTERFERING FACTORS

Drugs That May Alter Results of the Procedure

None

Conditions That May Interfere with Performing the Procedure

None

Procedure Techniques or Handling That May Alter Results

- Failure to blot the sample adequately prior to making an impression smear may obscure evaluation.
- Failure to fix and stain slides within 3–7 days may alter cellular characteristics and limit the value of the interpretation.

Influence of Signalment on Performing and Interpreting the Procedure

Species

None

Breed

None

Age

None

Gender

None

Pregnancy

None

CLINICAL PERSPECTIVE

- Impression smears are simple to make and may reveal cellular details not visible following collection and processing for histologic evaluation.
- Even if submitting biopsy samples for histopathology, impression smear evaluation can give valuble clues to the origin of disease so that treatment may be started while waiting for histopahologic results.

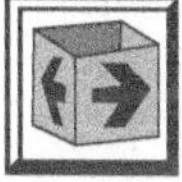

MISCELLANEOUS

ANCILLARY TESTS

- Fine-needle aspiration and cytology.
- Biopsy with histopathologic evaluation.

SYNONYMS

- Touch prep.
- Touch prep cytology.

SEE ALSO

Fine-Needle Aspiration (in Appendix X).

Suggested Reading

Cowell RL, Tyler RD, Meinkoth JH, eds. Diagnostic Cytology and Hematology of the Dog and Cat. St. Louis, MO: CV Mosby, 1999.

Raskin RE, Meyer DJ, eds. Atlas of Canine and Feline Cytology, 2nd ed. Philadelphia, PA: WB Saunders, 2001.

Author Laurel E. Williams

Consulting Editor Benjamin M. Brainard

PERICARDIOCENTESIS

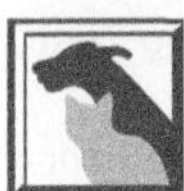

BASICS

TYPE OF PROCEDURE

Diagnostic sample collection.

PROCEDURE EXPLANATION AND RELATED PHYSIOLOGY

- Diagnostic and therapeutic procedure undertaken to relieve cardiac compression caused by pericardial effusion (PE):
  - PE may be neoplastic, idiopathic, traumatic, infectious, inflammatory, hemorrhagic, or metabolic in origin, or may result from late-stage congestive heart failure (CHF).
  - Chronic PE has gradual onset of clinical signs (weakness, ascites, pleural effusion) and a globoid cardiac silhouette radiographically.
  - Acute PE causes rapid onset of clinical signs (collapse, shock, sudden death).
- Cardiac tamponade is hemodynamic instability (cardiogenic shock) resulting from PE:
  - Occurs when effusion elevates intrapericardial pressure, exceeding right-sided diastolic intracardiac pressures.
  - Observed echocardiographically as partial collapse of the right heart in diastole.
  - Characterized clinically by shock (collapse, hypotension, tachycardia); necessitates emergency pericardiocentesis (PC).
  - Tamponade causes one ventricle to fill at the expense of the other, creating pulsus paradoxus, a decrease in peripheral pulse pressure on inspiration.
  - Intrapericardial pressure, not the effusion volume per se, determines clinical and hemodynamic severity.
- Medical therapies (e.g., diuretics) are relatively contraindicated (an exception is PE secondary to CHF), and PC is necessary to stabilize the patient.

INDICATIONS

- PE producing clinical signs of cardiac tamponade.
- Diagnostic sample acquisition.

CONTRAINDICATIONS

- An insufficient volume of PE such that the risk of PC outweighs potential benefit.
- Relative contraindications include PE secondary to coagulopathy or endocardial splitting where relief of pericardial pressure may perpetuate hemorrhage.
- Not indicated for distention of the pericardium by solid tumors or abdominal contents.

POTENTIAL COMPLICATIONS

- Minimize complications by careful preparation and technique.
- Puncture of cardiac chambers or great vessels.
- Ventricular arrhythmias.
- Coronary laceration causing myocardial ischemia or infarction.
- Exsanguination (more likely to occur from failure to confirm the correct catheter position resulting in evacuation of blood from a ventricular chamber, rather than from cardiac laceration).
- Death.
- Pulmonary laceration or hemorrhage.
- Pneumothorax.
- Failure to relieve cardiac tamponade or obtain a diagnostic PE sample.
- Infection.
- Constrictive or effusive-constrictive pericardial disease (late complication).

CLIENT EDUCATION

- Clients should be informed of potential risks and complications of the procedure.
- The cause of the PE may not be known at the time of PC. Hemangiosarcoma is a common cause with a poor long-term prognosis.
- PC may exacerbate hemorrhage of tumors and may worsen tamponade or precipitate cardiopulmonary arrest.
- Effusions may recur in the near or far future. Recurrences are cause dependent and difficult to predict.

BODY SYSTEMS ASSESSED

Cardiovascular

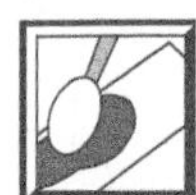

PROCEDURE

PATIENT PREPARATION

Pre-Procedure Medication or Preparation

- Rapid IV fluid administration is indicated to treat hypovolemic shock (from hemorrhage or third space fluid losses due to right-sided heart failure), and this should be administered during preparation for PC. The more debilitated the patient is, the greater is the need for the procedure.
- An IV catheter facilitates fluid resuscitation, sedation, and treatment of ventricular arrhythmias.
- Echocardiographic diagnosis of small cardiac tumors may be facilitated by the presence of PE. Ultrasound examination of the heart should precede PC if patient is stable.

Anesthesia or Sedation

- The more debilitated the patient is, the lesser the need for sedation.
- The author prefers IV sedation with butorphanol (0.2 mg/kg). Avoid agents promoting hypotension (e.g., acepromazine).

Patient Positioning

Left lateral recumbency is preferred to facilitate directing of catheter toward the right ventral caudal aspect of the heart. Some localized PE may not accessible from this approach. With ultrasound guidance, sternal recumbency may allow an appropriate window.

Patient Monitoring

- ECG monitoring (for ventricular arrhythmias) by a designated assistant during the procedure.
- Once the first sample of PE is removed, it should be observed for coagulation; if the sample clots, the catheter is likely in the heart, rather than pericardial sac.

Equipment or Supplies (see Figure 1)

- A large-bore, over-the-needle catheter is typically used: 18–14 gauge, 2–5½ inches, depending on patient size.
- Small (3–6 mL) and large (10–50 mL) syringes.
- Three-way stopcock.
- Extension tubing.
- Collection: bowl, tubes for cytological evaluation (EDTA) and culture submission.
- No. 11 surgical blade.
- Sterile surgical gloves (see Figure 1).
- 2% Lidocaine for local anesthesia and for treatment of ventricular arrhythmias:
  - Calculate dose of lidocaine for anti-arrhythmic therapy (2 mg/kg IV).

TECHNIQUE

- Default catheter entry location is at 5th–7th intercostal space of right ventral thorax, at the level of costal-chondral junction.
  - The hair is clipped, and the suitability of the site is confirmed using ultrasound.
- The site is aseptically prepared, and can be infiltrated deeply with lidocaine (0.5–3.0 mL, not to exceed 2 mg/kg).
- A no. 11 blade is used to create a small stab incision through skin at site of catheter entry.
- Catheter entry should be near the center of the rib space, erring toward the cranial aspect of the rib:
  - The catheter should intersect the pericardium at the right ventral aspect, so catheter is advanced dorsally and cranially (i.e., toward the opposite scapula) (see Figure 2).
  - Prior to insertion, the operator can attach a sterile 3-mL syringe to the catheter stylet.
    - Once catheter tip is through skin, a small amount of suction is applied to the syringe; this ensures that PE will be aspirated as soon as the stylet tip penetrates the pericardium.
  - ECG is monitored closely during catheter advancement. A burst of ventricular premature complexes suggests that the stylet tip has contacted the epicardium. The catheter should be retracted until arrhythmia abates.

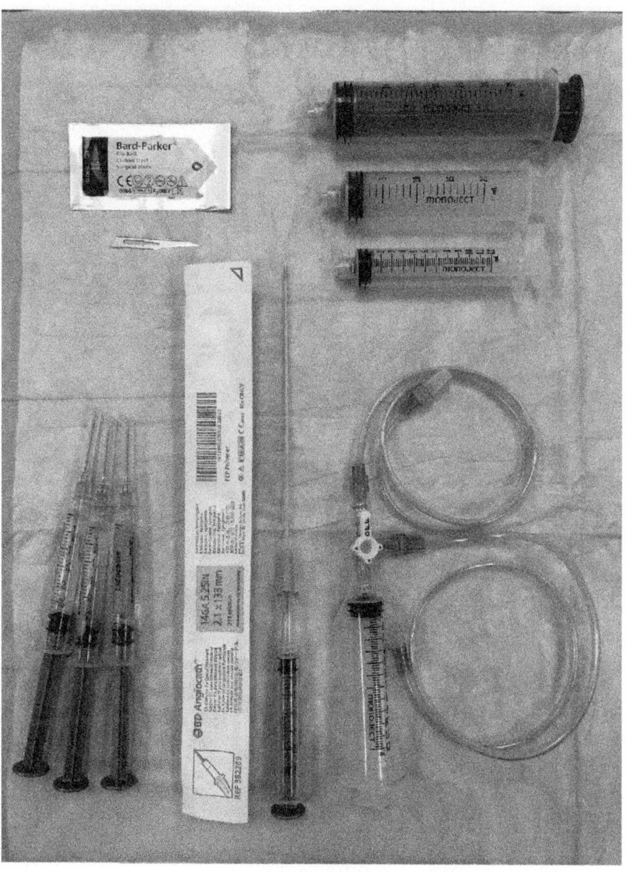

Figure 1.

Instrumentation used for PC. A no. 11 blade is ideal for creating a small stab incision into the skin at the entry site. A 14-gauge, 5.25-inch catheter and stylus are shown with a small syringe attached; i.e., configured to advance into the pericardial space. Extension tubing, three-way stopcock, and syringes for aspiration are shown. The sharp metal stylus is removed after the catheter is fully positioned, and the catheter is attached to the extension tubing. Three prepared and labeled doses of 2% lidocaine for IV bolus (2 mg/kg = 1 mL/10 kg) are shown.

  - Contact of the catheter tip with pericardium may impart a scratchy sensation, which may alarm inexperienced operators.
  - There may be a sensation of popping through the pericardium with the catheter.
- When PE is aspirated or observed in the hub of the stylet, the stylet is advanced a short distance (2–4 mm) further, after which the nondominant hand advances the flexible catheter off the stylet into pericardial space:
  - A distended pericardium may shrink substantially during procedure, which will cause the catheter tip to exit the pericardial space if it is not advanced sufficiently or too short.
- Once the stylet is withdrawn, extension tubing is attached directly to catheter hub, leading to a large syringe and interposed three-way stopcock operated by an assistant.
- Aliquots from this initial syringe of PE should be placed into an EDTA tube for cytologic analysis, a tube without additive or culturette for culture, and a tube without additive to assess for clotting of the sample (to verify the catheter is not intracardiac).
- Verifying appropriate placement of catheter.
  - Monitor sample for coagulation; most effusions (unless peracute) will be defibrinated, and will not clot, while a sample from ventricular lumen will clot.
  - A small amount of presumptive PE (e.g., 5–20 mL) can be removed while heart rate is observed. With tamponade, even a small decompression of the pericardial space can demonstrably decrease heart rate. A continual decrease in heart rate throughout the procedure is suggestive of correct catheter placement, whereas increasing heart rates should prompt operator to suspend aspiration and reevaluate catheter position.
  - The effusion PCV may be determined; it should be different from the peripheral blood, and supernatant is often xanthochromic.
- Once catheter positioning within the pericardium is confirmed, PE can be evacuated rapidly using the three-way stopcock to alternately aspirate and expel PE into a collecting bowl.
- The pericardial space should be evacuated as completely as possible (exceptions are atrial tears and bleeding disorder).
- Other considerations:
  - At any time during the procedure, significant ventricular arrhythmias should prompt catheter repositioning (usually partial withdrawal) and consideration of treatment with lidocaine (2 mg/kg IV) if arrhythmia does not abate promptly.
  - A scratchy sensation may be transmitted to the catheter as it rubs against the pericardium and epicardium, or stuttering

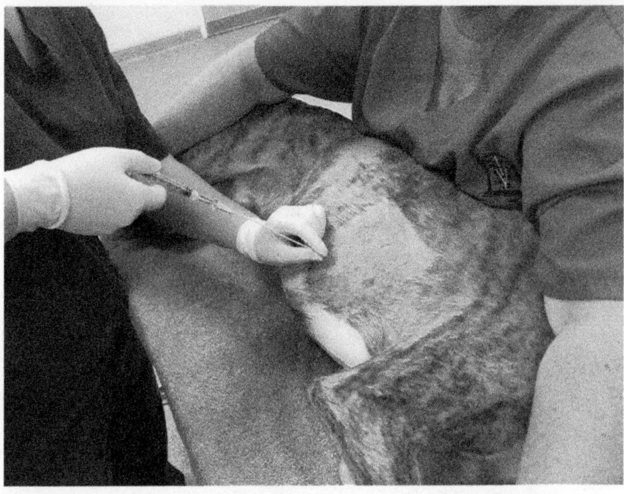

Figure 2.

Catheter positioning and orientation for PC from the right ventral approach. While stabilizing the catheter near the entry point with the nondominant hand, the catheter is advanced cranially and dorsally with the dominant hand, i.e., toward the opposite scapula. A small degree of suction is maintained with the syringe so that pericardial fluid is aspirated at the moment of pericardial penetration. Subsequently, the syringe and stylet are held in stationary while the flexible catheter is advanced well into the pericardial sac. The sharp metal stylet is withdrawn after the catheter is fully positioned, and the catheter is then attached to extension tubing leading to a three-way stopcock and aspiration syringe.

of the extension tubing caused by intermittent flow obstruction as the volume of PE decreases; at this point, the operator may slowly withdraw the catheter while the assistant maintains a small amount of suction with the syringe. Catheter withdrawal is paused at any location that results in additional aspiration of PE, and the process is repeated until catheter is completely withdrawn.
  - Catheter tip should be inspected to verify that it is intact after removal.
  - Cardiac motion may continue to expel PE into pleural space through catheter hole; this may result in lower than anticipated volumes of removed PE as well as pleural effusion following the procedure (there is no need to remove the pleural effusion).

SAMPLE HANDLING

- Pericardial fluid is placed in EDTA for cytologic examination and then in suitable sterile transport media for microbiological evaluation (bacterial and/or fungal).
- The hematocrit of presumed PE may be determined during the procedure, as noted above.

APPROPRIATE AFTERCARE

Post-Procedure Patient Monitoring

- Patients should be monitored for 12–24 hours. Monitoring should include serial heart and respiratory rates, cardiac ultrasounds (to evaluate return of PE), and ECG.
- Significant ventricular arrhythmias may develop.
- Iatrogenic pneumothorax is possible.
- Return of PE and clinical signs may be rapid.

Nursing Care

None specific to PC. Other care may depend on cause of PE.

Dietary Modification

N/A

Medication Requirements

- Ancillary medical treatments depend on the cause of the PE (e.g., neoplastic, infectious, idiopathic).
- Abdominal effusion stemming from tamponade-induced CHF typically does not require diuretics or treatments other than PC.
- Fluid therapy if hemorrhagic or third space fluid losses cause hypovolemia.

Restrictions on Activity

Judicious exercise restriction.

Anticipated Recovery Time

PC typically produces dramatic and immediate improvement in hemodynamic parameters. However, dogs may remain subdued for 1–2 days.

INTERPRETATION

NORMAL FINDINGS OR RANGE

N/A

ABNORMAL FINDINGS

- Cytologic evaluation of PE is notoriously nondiagnostic:
  - Most common causes of PE (neoplasia and idiopathic)—typically produce hemorrhagic effusions without identifiable cell types or features that identify causative conditions.
  - Unusual causes of PE that may be diagnosed cytologically include lymphoma, unusual tumors, and bacterial or fungal infections.

CRITICAL VALUES

- An increasing heart rate or clotting PE sample during PC. Do not aspirate further. Check to ensure correct catheter placement.
- Ventricular tachycardia (>180 bpm) or complex ventricular arrhythmia. Reposition (partially withdraw) the catheter and administer lidocaine (2 mg/kg IV).

INTERFERING FACTORS

Drugs That May Alter Results of the Procedure

None

Conditions That May Interfere With Performing the Procedure

- A small (insufficient) volume of PE.
- Coagulopathy.

Procedure Techniques or Handling That May Alter Results

None

Influence of Signalment on Performing and Interpreting the Procedure

Species

Cats and small dogs may be more difficult for PC because of their small size.

Breed

N/A

Age

N/A

Sex

N/A

Pregnancy

N/A

CLINICAL PERSPECTIVE

- Rapid IV fluid administration should be administered to debilitated patients during preparation for PC.
- Complications are minimized by careful preparation and technique.
- Significant clinical improvement can occur with removal of even a small volume of effusion.
- Hemodynamically significant PE requires PC to stabilize the patient.

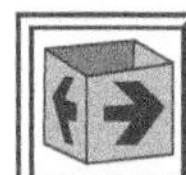

MISCELLANEOUS

ANCILLARY TESTS

- Echocardiography may provide a definitive diagnosis if an intrapericardial, right atrial, or heart base mass is present.
- Cytologic and microbiological examination of the PE.
- Further evaluation may include CBC and biochemical analysis, coagulation testing, toxoplasma titer (cats), thoracic radiographs and abdominal ultrasound in search of primary or metastatic neoplasia, histopathology, and thoracic exploration or thoracoscopic surgery for partial or complete pericardiectomy.
- In dogs with PE, elevation of plasma cardiac troponin I suggests an increased probability of hemangiosarcoma.

SEE ALSO

- Atrial Wall Tear.
- Chemodectoma.
- Coccidioidomycosis.
- Hemangiosarcoma, Spleen and Liver.
- Myocardial tumors.
- Pericardial Disease.
- Rodenticide Toxicosis—Anticoagulants.

SYNONYMS

Pericardial tap.

ABBREVIATIONS

- CHF = congestive heart failure.
- PC = pericardiocentesis.
- PE = pericardial effusion.

Suggested Reading

MacDonald K. Pericardial diseases. In: Ettinger SJ, Feldman EC, eds., Textbook of Veterinary Internal Medicine, 8th ed. St. Louis, MO: Saunders Elsevier, 2017, pp. 1305–1316.

Nelson LO, Wendy AW. Pericardial effusion. In: Bonagura J, ed., Kirk's Current Veterinary Therapy XV. Philadelphia, PA: WB Saunders, 2014, pp. 816–823.

Sisson D, Thomas WP. Pericardial disease and cardiac tumors. In: Fox PR, Sisson D, Moise NS, eds., Textbook of Canine and Feline Cardiology, 2nd ed. Philadelphia, PA: WB Saunders, 1999, pp. 400–425.

Author Rebecca M. Bates

Consulting Editor Benjamin M. Brainard

POINT OF CARE ABDOMINAL ULTRASONOGRAPHY

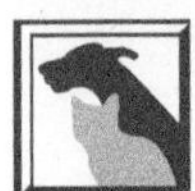

BASICS

TYPE OF PROCEDURE

Point of care ultrasound.

PROCEDURE EXPLANATION AND RELATED PHYSIOLOGY

- Abdominal veterinary point of care ultrasound (VPOCUS) is an expansion of the original abdominal-focused assessment with sonography for trauma (A-FAST®) protocol published in 2004: a limited or focused technique that can be performed by nonspecialists to rapidly assess patients and help direct immediate diagnostic and therapeutic interventions.
- It requires minimal training, is performed during triage or during daily patient evaluation, does not compromise patient safety, is noninvasive, rapid, repeatable, and objective.
- Abdominal VPOCUS has been validated for both trauma and nontrauma patients, and is sensitive and specific for the detection of free abdominal fluid:
    - Mistakes are less likely, and learning is often facilitated, by asking simple binary questions (i.e., presence of free fluid yes/no).
    - Additional binary questions (beyond the detection of free fluid) that have been evaluated with abdominal VPOCUS include assessment of gastrointestinal (GI) motility, estimation of urine production, identification of gall bladder wall edema/thickening, and the detection of free abdominal air.

INDICATIONS

- Trauma patients.
- Unstable patients.
- Any patient as part of the triage exam.
- Post-surgery patients not recovering as expected.
- Routine daily assessment of hospitalized patients.
- To identify free abdominal fluid of any cause.
- Suspicion of pneumoperitoneum.
- Concern for adequate urine production.
- Suspicion of gastric retention or GI ileus.

CONTRAINDICATIONS

None

POTENTIAL COMPLICATIONS

None

CLIENT EDUCATION

Abdominal VPOCUS is not a full ultrasonographic examination and does not replace comprehensive formal sonography, physical examination, or other diagnostic procedures, including radiographs. They are limited exams that answer specific questions in a very rapid fashion, often dictating the need for immediate therapy and further diagnostics, including comprehensive formal ultrasound examinations.

BODY SYSTEMS ASSESSED

Focused areas of the abdominal cavity to answer specific, often binary, questions.

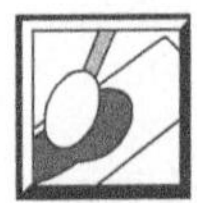

PROCEDURE

PATIENT PREPARATION

Pre-Procedure Medication or Preparation

- Do not compromise patient safety: bring the ultrasound machine to the patient and complete/continue any emergency stabilization and concurrent diagnostic efforts.
- Clipping of fur is unnecessary, although image quality may be improved with clipping.

Anesthesia or Sedation

Minimal restraint required, sedation rarely necessary.

Patient Positioning

- Left or right lateral recumbency. The patient can be rolled into sternal recumbency to assess the gravity dependent paralumbar region if necessary, once the other sites have been evaluated.
- Sternal or standing if lateral not possible.
- Consider gravitational effects and patient positioning for different pathologies (e.g., free fluid).
- Avoid dorsal recumbency in patients with respiratory or cardiovascular compromise.

Patient Monitoring

Serial VPOCUS monitors progression or resolution of underlying pathology.

Equipment or Supplies

- Ultrasound machine.
- Microconvex/curvilinear probe.
- Frequency: 5 MHz (patients >15 kg), 7.5 MHz (patients <15 kg).
- Gain adjusted to detect anechoic fluid.
- Depth adjusted to visualize the region of interest.
- Coupling agent: 70% isopropyl alcohol, part fur before applying. Ultrasound gel can also be used.

TECHNIQUE

- Five focused regions of the abdomen are systematically evaluated: subxiphoid (also called diaphragmatico-hepatic), urinary bladder (also called cysto-colic), right paralumbar (also called hepato-renal), left paralumbar (also called spleno-renal), and umbilical (see Figure 1).
- Fan and rock the probe through 45° angles in both longitudinal and transverse axis at all sites.

Key Structures

Key structures assessed at each site include:

- Subxiphoid: diaphragm, liver, gallbladder, ventral stomach, and the areas between these structures. The caudal vena cava, pleural space, and pericardial sac can also be evaluated at this site (not discussed in this chapter).
- Urinary bladder: urinary bladder, gravity and non-gravity-dependent body walls, and the areas between these structures.
- Right paralumbar: right caudal liver lobe, right kidney, body wall, duodenum, and the areas between these structures.
- Left paralumbar: spleen, left kidney, intestines, body wall and the areas between these structures.
- Umbilical (additional 5th view): gravity-dependent body wall, intestines, spleen and regions between these structures.

Correctly Locating and Evaluating Each Site

Subxiphoid

- Palpate the "V" at the xiphoid region and place the probe in long axis to the body.
- Rock the probe cranially until the liver is visible.
- Adjust depth to visualize the diaphragm beyond the liver.
- Fan the probe through all planes of the liver and rock the probe to assess the most ventral and cranial parts of the liver (small fluid accumulations often collect between the liver and diaphragm).
- The gallbladder is visualized to the right of midline and assessed for wall thickening or other abnormalities.
- By rocking the probe perpendicular to the spine and slowly fanning left and right the proximal stomach wall is identified and can be assessed for motility.
- The probe is then rotated into transverse axis and fanned and rocked through all planes.

Urinary Bladder

- The probe is placed in longitudinal axis to the body between the pelvic limbs.
- Pushing too hard can compress and displace the bladder.
- Adjust the depth to visualize both the dorsal and ventral bladder walls.
- Slide the probe to the non-gravity-dependent side of patient and angle the ultrasound beam through the bladder, while fanning, to identify fluid in deeper gravity-dependent sites along the body wall.
- Slide the probe cranially to locate the apex of the bladder and fan the probe through all planes at the bladder apex.

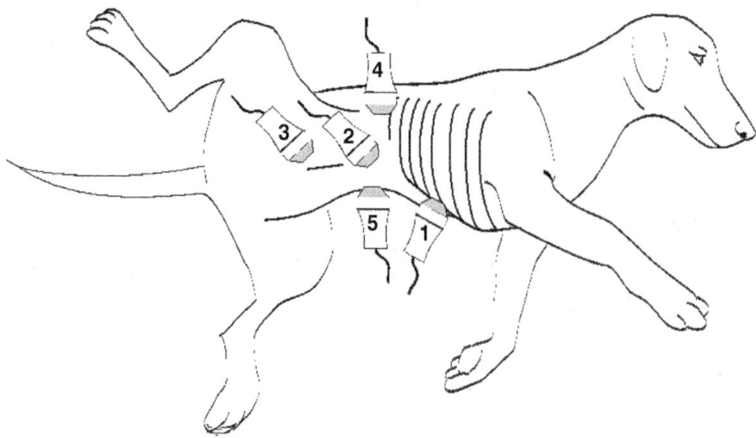

Figure 1.

Abdominal VPOCUS windows: (1) subxiphoid, (2) umbilical, (3) urinary bladder, (4) left paralumbar, and (5) right paralumbar. Each location is evaluated in longitudinal and transverse orientation with rocking and fanning of the probe to maximize the area evaluated and to ensure all target structures/sites are thoroughly evaluated. At the urinary bladder and umbilical sites the probe should be directed toward the gravity-dependent body wall areas where fluid is most likely to accumulate.

- Slide caudally to evaluate the caudal regions.
- Following thorough longitudinal scanning, rotate the probe to a transverse axis and repeat the scan.
- Bladder volume can be estimated in millimeters and monitored serially using the formula to calculate the volume of a sphere:
  - In longitudinal axis, a measurement of the length is taken. This is *L*. A depth measurement in longitudinal can be taken (D_L).
  - In transverse axis, a width measurement is taken. This is *W*. A depth measurement in transverse can be taken (D_T).
  - The formula is then as follows: $(L \times W \times (D_L + D_T)/2) \times 0.625$.

Right Paralumbar

- In smaller patients, the probe is placed in longitudinal axis to the body caudal to the last rib, just below the hypaxial/lumbar muscles.
- It may be necessary to place the probe between ribs to locate target structures.
- In dogs, if the liver is visualized first, the probe can be slid caudally until the kidney is located.
- The right kidney is often quite lateral (relative to midline).
- The probe is fanned and rocked in both longitudinal and transverse axis to assess the kidney.
- To locate the duodenum, place the probe at the level of the right kidney in longitudinal axis, and sweep medially towards midline until the largest small intestinal segment is found, which can be assessed for motility.

Left Paralumbar

- The probe is placed relatively lateral to midline to find the left kidney and spleen.
- The spleen is located cranial and often lateral to the left kidney.
- To find the left kidney, use your index finger to trace the last rib from the mid-abdominal region dorsally: the kidney is usually located where the last rib encounters the hypaxial muscles.
- The probe is fanned and rocked in both longitudinal and transverse axis to assess the kidney.
- It may be easier to find the spleen and slide the probe caudally until the left kidney is located.

Umbilical View

- The probe is placed over the umbilical region and directed towards the tabletop.
- The probe is then rocked and fanned through all planes and then changed from a longitudinal to transverse orientation and the procedure repeated.
- This allows localization of gravity-dependent abdominal effusion to be identified before the probe is slid under the patient to assess the gravity-dependent paralumbar site.

APPROPRIATE AFTERCARE

Post-Procedure Patient Monitoring

Serial examinations are useful to detect changes in patient pathology: frequency is dictated by changes to patient stability (heart rate, respiratory changes, or neurologic changes).

INTERPRETATION

ABNORMAL VALUES

- Free fluid appears as dark (anechoic or hypoechoic) uncontained triangles/sharp angles between organs and structures; be sure to thoroughly evaluate all key organs at all sites.
- Obtain fluid samples for in-house analysis (cytology, refractometer, parameters of sepsis or uroabdomen) which may dictate immediate interventions (surgery, antibiotics, transfusion, etc.). Consider sample submission to reference laboratory (cytology, culture) if indicated.
- Pneumoperitoneum in patients that have not undergone laparotomy is abnormal and hollow organ rupture should be ruled out. There are three key steps to help detect pneumoperitoneum:
  - Identify the peritoneal lining; this helps differentiate GI air from free air in the abdomen. Place the animal in lateral for a few minutes to allow air to rise to the non-gravity-dependent body wall. The peritoneal lining can be visualized directly or identified by locating structures in contact with it (e.g., liver, kidney, spleen, etc.). Free air can be detected between organs or within the wall of some structures, although this is more technically challenging.

- Identify the presence of reverberation artifact that originates at the peritoneal lining. This helps differentiates reverberation artifact contained within the GI tract. Free air reverberation artifact originating at the peritoneal lining often obliterates structures below it.
- Identify the enhanced peritoneal stripe sign. This sonographic finding occurs when free abdominal air comes in contact with the peritoneal lining, causing the peritoneal lining to become more hyperechoic. Reverberation artifact, if it is the result of free abdominal air, will originate from the enhanced peritoneal stripe sign.

• Ileus: Ileus is defined as a transient cessation of GI motility or an abnormal pattern of GI motility. The mean number of peristaltic contractions of the stomach and proximal duodenum are 4–5 contractions per minute. To measure the number of contractions per minute the total number of contractions is recorded over 3 minutes and divide by 3. If contractions are decreased to absent a diagnosis of decreased motility is made.

• Food within the GI tract is a strong stimulus for contraction; ileus is confirmed when food is present within the GI lumen in the absence of GI contractions.

• Gall bladder wall thickening/edema (halo sign) is not specific but anaphylaxis, fluid overload, right-sided heart failure, sepsis, and pericardial effusion should be considered in unstable patients.

• Oliguria/anuria: Although not 100% accurate, a lack of change in bladder volume despite appropriate IV fluid in a well-hydrated patient could be indicative of anuria or oliguria.

INTERFERING FACTORS

Conditions That May Interfere with Performing the Procedure

• Dehydration and hypovolemia may reduce the sensitivity of finding abdominal effusion; reassess once resuscitation procedures are undertaken.

• Gas-filled GI tract can obscure some structures.

• Empty or very distended bladders may be difficult to interpret.

Influence of Signalment on Performing and Interpreting the Procedure

Species

Large-breed dogs may be more difficult to image due to the depth and location of their organs.

Age

Very young healthy animals may normally have small quantities of free fluid present.

CLINICAL PERSPECTIVE

• Abdominal VPOCUS is a rapid, repeatable diagnostic tool that helps identify specific pathology.

• Requires minimal training or experience.

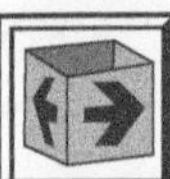

MISCELLANEOUS

SYNONYMS

Abdominal-focused assessment with sonography in trauma/triage (A-FAST®)

ABBREVIATIONS

• GI = gastrointestinal.

• VPOCUS = veterinary point of care ultrasound.

INTERNET RESOURCES

Faculty of Veterinary Medicine, University of Calgary (UCVM) podcasts: https://vet.ucalgary.ca/vcds/podcasts

Suggested Reading

Boysen SR, Lisciandro GR. The use of ultrasound for dogs and cats in the emergency room: AFAST and TFAST. Vet Clin North Am Small Anim Pract 2013, 43(4):773–797.

McMurray J, Boysen SR, Chalhoub S. Focused assessment with sonography for triage in non-trauma dogs and cats in the emergency and critical care setting. J Vet Emerg Crit Care (San Antonio) 2016, 26(1):64–73.

Authors Søren Boysen and Serge Chalhoub

Consulting Editor Benjamin M. Brainard

Acknowledgment The author and editors acknowledge the prior contribution of Jantina McMurray.

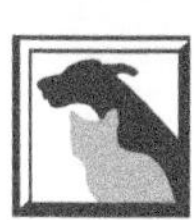

BASICS

TYPE OF PROCEDURE

Point of care ultrasound

PROCEDURE EXPLANATION AND RELATED PHYSIOLOGY

- Pleural space and lung ultrasound (PLUS) is an expansion of thoracic focused assessment with sonography for trauma that includes lung ultrasound. Cardiovascular ultrasound is assessed separately as it involves the evaluation of both the abdomen (vascular) and heart (limited echocardiography):
  - Pathologies evaluated include pleural effusion, pneumothorax, alveolar interstitial syndrome (AIS), and lung consolidation.
  - A focused veterinary point of care ultrasound (VPOCUS) technique that can be performed by nonspecialists to rapidly assess patients and direct immediate diagnostic and therapeutic interventions.
    - Requires minimal training, is performed during triage or daily patient evaluation, does not compromise patient safety, is noninvasive, rapid, repeatable, and objective.
    - Accuracy is variable, and depends on the experience of the sonographer, underlying pathology, patient positioning, scanning protocol, and criteria used to identify the different pathologies.
  - In the authors' experience the most common clinical errors include failing to identify pneumothorax by not scanning the most caudal dorsal sites, missing smaller volume pleural effusions by not scanning the more ventral regions when patients are in sternal or standing positions, and confusing the curtain sign for lung pathology.
- Principles of PLUS that increase the chance of detecting pathology include the application of binary questions to keep scanners focused to techniques and questions within their skill sets, modifying protocols to evaluate areas of the pleura and lung where pathology is most likely to accumulate, and defining sonographically scannable thoracic borders:
  - If pleural effusion needs to be ruled out in a standing patient, then searching the most ventral borders between the lung and sternal muscles (where fluid accumulates) is important vs. a patient that is lateral (where fluid will accumulate at the widest, most gravity-dependent point of the thorax).
  - In a patient with severe dyspnea, the binary question (based on initial triage examination) dictates which part of the PLUS protocol is performed first (e.g., pneumothorax, pleural effusion, lung pathology). Once the patient is more stable, completion of the PLUS examination and other VPOCUS scans can be performed.
  - Defining sonographically scannable borders of the thorax on either side of the chest helps ensure sites where pathology are most likely to accumulate are evaluated.

INDICATIONS

- Dyspneic patients.
- Trauma patients.
- Part of the triage exam.
- Post-surgery patients not recovering as expected.
- Routine daily assessment.
- Suspected pneumothorax.
- Suspected pleural effusion.
- Suspected alveolar interstitial disease.

CONTRAINDICATIONS

None

POTENTIAL COMPLICATIONS

None

CLIENT EDUCATION

PLUS is not a full ultrasonographic examination of the thorax and does not replace comprehensive formal sonography, physical examination, or other diagnostic procedures including thoracic radiographs. It is a focused exam that answers specific questions in a rapid fashion, often dictating the need for immediate therapy and further diagnostics, including comprehensive formal ultrasound examinations.

BODY SYSTEMS ASSESSED

Lungs and pleural space to answer specific questions.

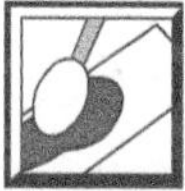

PROCEDURE

PATIENT PREPARATION

Pre-Procedure Medication or Preparation

- Do not compromise patient safety: bring the ultrasound machine to the patient and continue emergency stabilization and concurrent diagnostic efforts.
- Clipping of fur is unnecessary but may improve image quality.

Anesthesia or Sedation

- Minimal restraint required.
- Oxygen therapy and anxiolytics may calm patients, decreasing the respiratory rate and effort, making interpretation easier.

Patient Positioning

- Air accumulates at the highest gravity-independent areas; fluid at the most gravity-dependent areas, which varies with patient positioning.
- Dyspneic patients should be scanned in sternal/standing to avoid stress.
- More stable patients can be scanned in left or right lateral recumbency.
- Avoid dorsal recumbency in dyspneic or cardiovascularly compromised patients.

Patient Monitoring

Serial VPOCUS monitors progression or resolution of underlying pathology.

Equipment or Supplies

- Ultrasound machine.
- Microconvex/curvilinear probe.
- Frequency adjusted to make the pleural line appear grainy when assessing the glide sign (typically 5–7.5 mHz).
- Depth adjusted to 4–6 cm; pleural line should be located at roughly a third the distance of the ultrasound image.
- Coupling agent; alcohol, part fur before applying. Ultrasound gel can also be used.

TECHNIQUE

The following PLUS protocol has three objectives: assess for (1) pneumothorax, (2) lung pathology, and (3) pleural effusion. The order can be modified to rule out the most likely and life-threatening pathology first. It is intended for the sternal/standing patient. (The protocol is slightly modified when searching for pleural effusion and/or pneumothorax in laterally recumbent patients; see below.)

1. Place the probe on a region of the thorax where lung can be reliably identified, behind the thoracic limb, roughly between the 5th–6th intercostal space and half to two-thirds of the way up the thorax (see Figure 1). Starting at this location avoids accidental placement of the probe over the curtain sign, abdomen and sublumbar muscles, which can be confused for pathology. The probe can be placed perpendicular or parallel to the ribs. For beginners, the authors recommend placing the probe perpendicular to identify the BAT sign.
2. Normal structures are identified at this location (see Normal Findings or Range: BAT sign, pleural line, glide sign, A-lines, B-lines, curtain sign).
3. If a glide sign is seen, slide the probe caudally until the curtain sign is identified:
   - Patients with significant pneumothorax will not have a glide sign at this location and thoracentesis or a search for the lung point should be undertaken (see Abnormal Findings).
4. From the curtain sign, slide the probe dorsocaudally along the curtain sign until the hypaxial muscle–pleural space junction is identified. This is the most caudo-dorsal site of the thorax and the smaller volumes of pneumothorax are likely to be identified in a standing/sternal patient (see below):

(a)

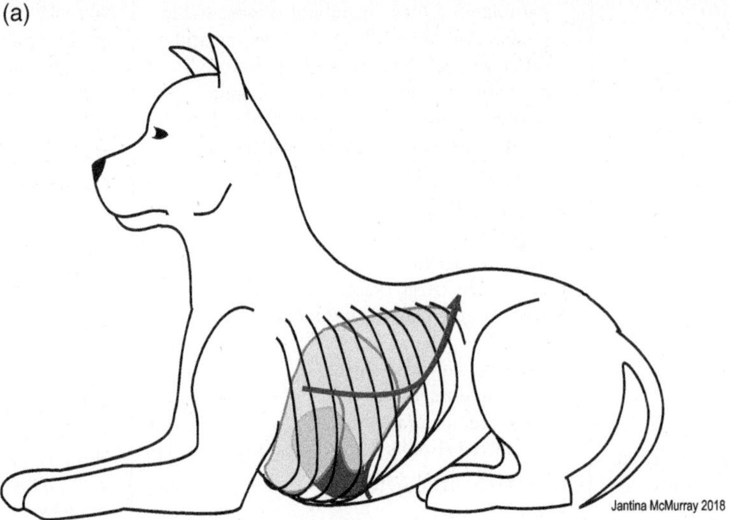

Figure 1a.

The probe is placed over lung, then slid caudally until the curtain sign is identified (caudal lung border). Then slide dorsally along the curtain sign, focusing on the pleural line, until the pleural line is lost in the hypaxial muscles. Return to the pleural line. This is the most caudal dorsal site, which can be rapidly identified with confidence in any patient. Source: From Boysen S, McMurray J and Gommeren K (2019) Abnormal Curtain Signs Identified With a Novel Lung Ultrasound Protocol in Six Dogs With Pneumothorax. Front. Vet. Sci. 6:291. doi: 10.3389/fvets.2019.00291. Public Domain.

(b)

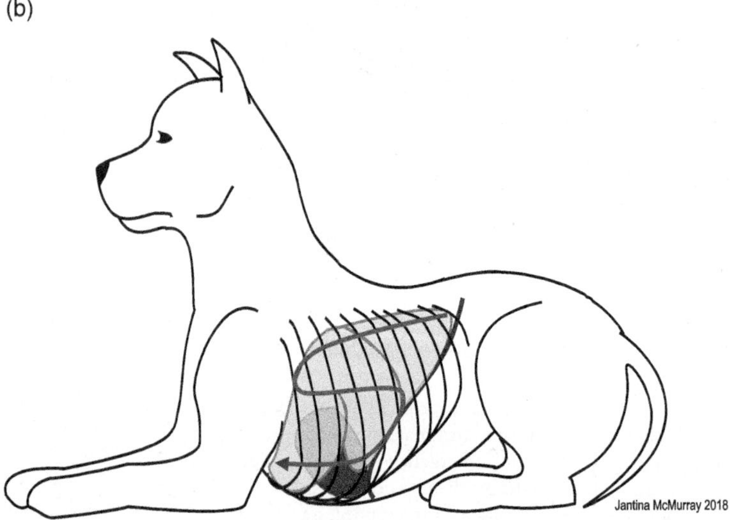

Figure 1b.

From the most caudal dorsal site, slide the probe in an "S"-shaped pattern, dividing the thorax into dorsal, middle, and ventral thirds to assess multiple lung regions for pathology. Source: From Boysen S, McMurray J and Gommeren K (2019) Abnormal Curtain Signs Identified With a Novel Lung Ultrasound Protocol in Six Dogs With Pneumothorax. Front. Vet. Sci. 6:291. doi: 10.3389/fvets.2019.00291. Public Domain.

- If a glide sign is seen here, pneumothorax is ruled out for this side of the thorax in the standing/sternal patient.
- If a glide sign is not seen here, and a pneumothorax cannot be ruled out based on clinical findings, then search for a lung point or return of the glide sign (see below).

5. If a glide sign was identified in step 4, and pneumothorax ruled out, continue scanning for lung pathology (AIS and lung consolidation) and pleural effusion; for AIS/lung consolidation slide the probe across the intercostal spaces in an "S" fashion to scan multiple lung regions. Pause and hold the probe stationary as necessary to better assess suspected areas for pathology:
    - From the most caudo-dorsal position, slide the probe across the dorsal border of the thorax as cranial as possible to the scapula/flexor muscles of the shoulder

(c)

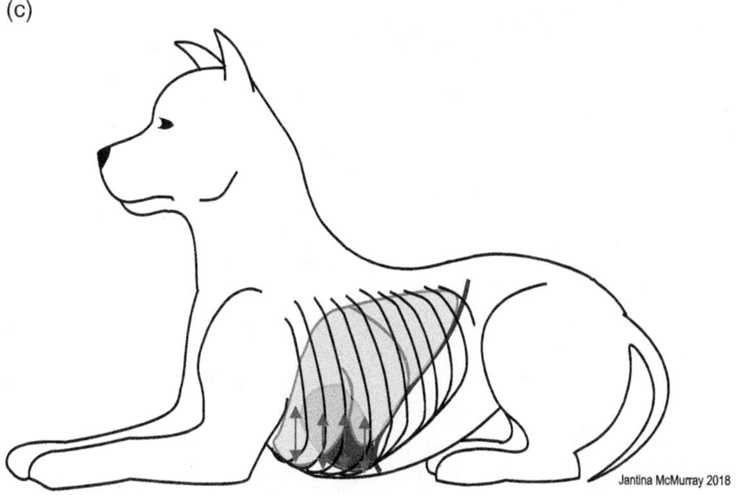

Figure 1c.

At the ventral regions of the thorax (level of the costochondral junction) the probe can be turned parallel to the ribs and slid ventrally until the sternal muscles are encountered. This ensures small volumes of pleural fluid that may not be seen with the probe perpendicular to the ribs at the level of the costochondral junction are not missed. From the sternal muscles, which are often in contact with the heart in the 4th–6th intercostal spaces, the probe can also be slid dorsally to ensure the ventral lung regions are assessed for pathology. Source: From Boysen S, McMurray J and Gommeren K (2019) Abnormal Curtain Signs Identified With a Novel Lung Ultrasound Protocol in Six Dogs With Pneumothorax. Front. Vet. Sci. 6:291. doi: 10.3389/fvets.2019.00291. Public Domain.

while continuing to visualize the pleural line for pathology:

- Once the cranial–dorsal border is reached, slide the probe ventrally to the mid-thorax, roughly at the heart base region, and then caudally toward the curtain sign while continuing to visualize the pleural line for pathology.
- At the curtain sign, slide the probe ventrally until the pericardio-diaphragmatic window is identified (where the heart and diaphragm are visible in the same sonographic window). This is a good window to differentiate pleural and pericardial fluid.
- The probe is then slid cranially until the thoracic inlet is reached (limited by the thoracic limb).
- To avoid missing smaller volumes of pleural effusion turn the probe parallel to the ribs at or just below the costochondral junction, roughly between the 3rd and 7th intercostal spaces, and slide the probe ventrally until the lung and sternal muscle are both visible in the same sonographic window. To also assess the ventral lung borders for pathology, the probe can be slid dorsally from the sternal–pleural junction, between the ribs at these same intercostal spaces (maintaining the probe parallel to the ribs), until lung is encountered.

6. The other side of the thorax should be scanned in a similar fashion.
7. The subxiphoid should also be included for assessment of pleural effusion and AIS/lung consolidation:
   - The probe can be placed in long and short axis to the body in the subxiphoid region. Palpate the "V" where the ribs connect ventrally and place the probe at this location. The probe is then rocked and fanned so that the ultrasound beams penetrate the thorax.
   - Once the thorax is visualized, the probe is fanned to visualize the entire region.
8. With the patient in lateral recumbency the protocol is similar, however it should be remembered that fluid will accumulate at the widest gravity-dependent location of the thorax and air will accumulate at the widest most non-gravity-dependent location. These sites should be considered and the protocol modified in light of patient positioning, the binary question to answer first, and the pathology in question.

APPROPRIATE AFTERCARE

Post-Procedure Patient Monitoring

Serial thoracic VPOCUS examinations are useful to follow resolution/progression of pathology, and should be repeated as dictated by changes to patient stability.

INTERPRETATION

NORMAL FINDINGS OR RANGE

Normal Structures

There are six key PLUS findings to identify in healthy animals, which should also be assessed in animals with suspected pathology.

1. BAT Sign (also termed the gator sign) (see Figure 2)

Using the BAT sign mnemonic—"the ultrasound beam will not traverse Bone or Air when the probe is Transverse to the ribs"—helps sonographers to orient.

- The ultrasound beam will not traverse beyond the proximal rib surface (smaller downward facing curvilinear white lines) or the pleural line (upward curving white line) in healthy animals, which means these structures are the last visible features the ultrasound beam can identify when the ultrasound probe is situated over lung and oriented perpendicular to the ribs: everything beyond the ribs and pleural line is artifact in healthy animals.
- The pleural line is essential to identify as all PLUS pathology originates from the pleural line: the first horizontal white line below the ribs that connects the rib shadows (body of the bat).

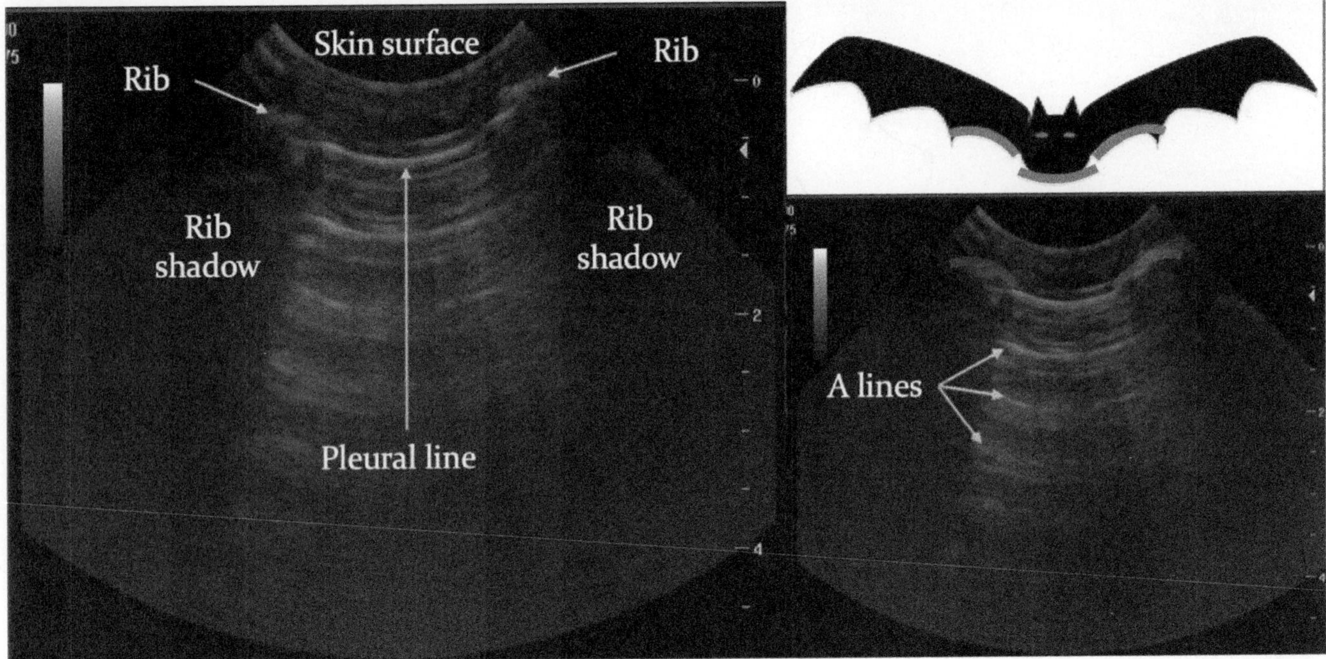

Figure 2.

Image depicting the BAT sign where the ultrasound beam encounters Bone (rib heads = wings of the bat) and Air (pleural line = body of the bat) with the probe Transverse (perpendicular) to the ribs. Horizontal A-lines are also shown.

2. Pleural Line

When the lung is in contact with the chest wall the pleural line indicates the parietal pleura and the visceral pleura are joined. In cases of pneumothorax or pleural effusion, the pleural line comprises only the parietal pleura (the visceral pleural is visible deep to pleural effusion and not visible with pneumothorax).

- All pleural space pathology (i.e., pleural effusion, pneumothorax, etc.) originates at the pleural line.
- All sonographically detectable lung pathology originates at the visceral pleura (lung surface), which will be at the pleural line when lung contacts the chest wall, and the visceral pleura when the lung is visibly separated from the chest wall (e.g., pleural effusion).

3. The Glide Sign

The to-and-fro shimmering visible along the pleural line that occurs as a result of lung sliding along the chest well during the respiratory cycle:

- The glide sign rules out pleural space pathology, particularly pneumothorax and pleural effusion.
- Two criteria must be present for a glide sign to occur: (1) the two pleura must be in contact; (2) the patient must breathe for the two pleura to glide across each other creating the visible shimmering.
- The glide sign can be made "grainier" and therefore easier to visualize by changing the angle the ultrasound beam strikes the pleural line (changing the angle from perpendicular), by placing the probe over a single rib head, and by decreasing the gain setting.
- The glide sign is difficult to identify in patients that are panting or have rapid shallow breathing.
- Keep your hand stationary and only interpret the glide sign when the patient is not moving (movement creates a false positive).

4. A-Lines

Horizontal white line artifacts occurring at equidistant intervals that project through the far field of the ultrasound image, decreasing in intensity with depth.

- A-lines are created when the ultrasound beam is bounced back and forth between the ultrasound probe and highly reflective structures such as the soft tissue–air interface that occurs at the pleural line.
- A soft tissue–air interface is present at the pleural line when air fills the lung and when air occupies the pleural space in cases of pneumothorax. Therefore A-lines are visible with both aerated lung and pneumothorax.

5. B-Lines (Figure 3)

Vertical white line artifacts that occur when air and fluid are in proximity to each other at the lung surface.

- They often have the following five criteria: (1) vertical white/hyperechoic projections; (2) originating from the lung surface at the pleural line; (3) extending through the far field without fading; (4) obliterating A-lines if present; and (5) swinging to-and-fro with the glide sign during respiration.
- Up to three B-lines in a single sonographic window, but only at 1 or two locations on either side of the thorax is considered normal and may be identified in 10–30% of healthy dogs and cats.
- More than three B-lines at a single site is associated with AIS/wet lung.
- The same differential diagnosis for AIS on ultrasound should be considered as an interstitial–alveolar pattern on thoracic radiographs.
- The number of B-lines correlates with the quantity of extravascular lung water, although prognosis varies with cause.

6. Curtain Sign

Sharply demarcated vertical edge artifact separating aerated lung from abdominal contents, (thoraco-abdominal border) (see Figure 4).

- When the ultrasound probe is positioned such that it is over both the thorax and the abdomen with the marker of the probe directed cranially, the cranial half of the image (thorax) will not allow the ultrasound beam to extend past the pleural line (produces A-lines), while the caudal half of the image (abdomen) allows the beam to be transmitted through the far field, permitting soft tissue structures to be visible.

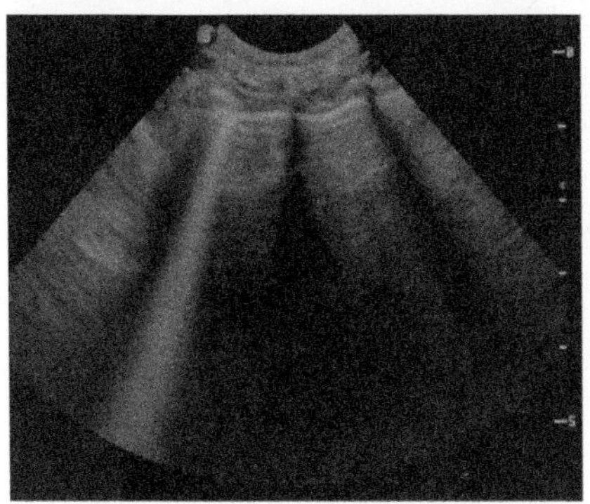

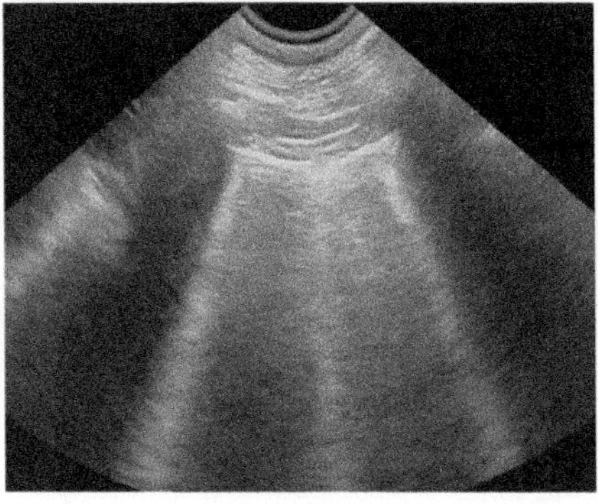

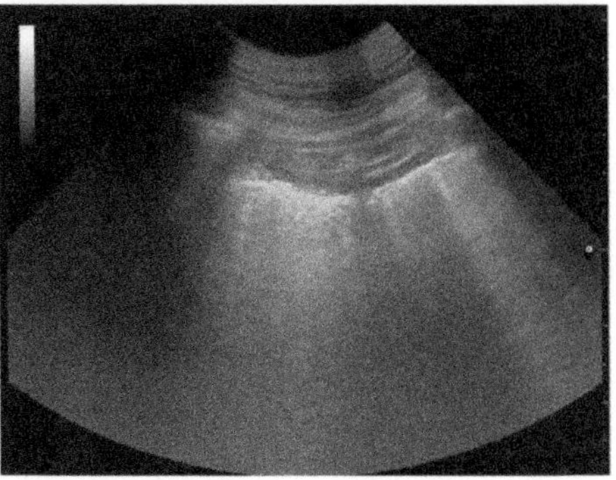

Figure 3.

Images depicting a single B-line (left), four B-lines (middle), and multiple to coalescing B-lines (right).

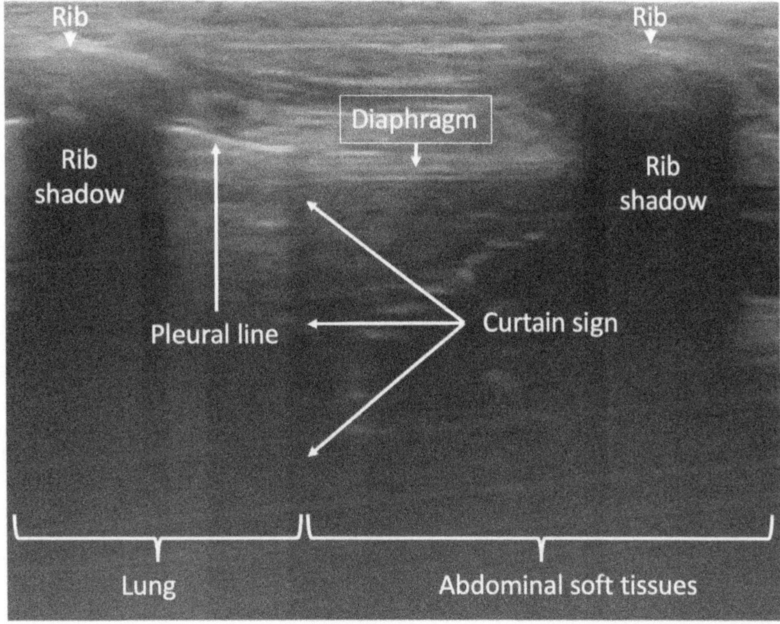

Figure 4.

Curtain sign, depicted as the sharp vertical line separating aerated lung from the soft tissue structures of the abdomen. The diaphragm is not visible once it curves away from the thoracic wall as interposed lung prevents its visualization.

- During inspiration, the vertical edge and abdominal contents move caudally, and during expiration the vertical edge and abdominal contents move cranially, in a synchronous manner.
- It is important not to confuse the curtain sign (back and forth movement of the diaphragm) with a glide sign.

Dry Lung

Dry lung at a probe location is identified when the following two criteria are present:

- The patient has a glide sign.
- There are ≤three B-lines in a single sonographic window, and/or the presence of only A-lines (not always visible).

ABNORMAL FINDINGS

Pneumothorax

- There are three key findings in deciding if a pneumothorax is present or not; two are exclusion criteria, one is an inclusion criteria:
    - The presence of a glide sign rules out pneumothorax at the probe location with confidence. Lack of a glide sign should prompt consideration of pneumothorax, but a glide sign is not always easy to identify, even in healthy patients.
    - The presence of B-lines extending from the pleural line excludes pneumothorax at that probe location because B-lines originate from the lung surface. B-lines are not always visible in healthy patients.
    - Finding a lung point or the return of a glide sign confirms pneumothorax on that side of the thorax. If a glide sign is not seen and there is suspicion of a pneumothorax a search for the lung point should be undertaken.
- The lung point is defined as the site within the thorax where the lung recontacts the parietal pleura and creates an intermittent or partial glide sign within a section of the ultrasound image when the patient breathes. It is the exact point within the thorax where there is a return of the glide sign: movement of the probe from an area where there is no perceived glide sign, to an area where the glide sign

reappears within a region of the ultrasound window. Air in the pleural space (pneumothorax) tends to compress the lung cranially and ventrally: to identify the lung point slide the probe cranially–ventrally toward the elbow from the site where a glide sign was not visible. The lung point will not be seen if the lung fails to recontact the chest wall in cases of massive/complete pneumothorax.

Pleural Effusion

Pleural effusion appears as hypoechoic accumulations between the thoracic wall and lungs, and its appearance can vary depending on the cellularity of the effusion, probe location, patient positioning, the quantity of fluid and the presence of adhesions.

- Locating the pericardio-diaphragmatic window helps differentiate pleural effusion from pericardial effusion; pleural effusion is uncontained outlining and tracking along the diaphragm while pericardial effusion is contained and curves away from the diaphragm following the contour of the heart.
- The presence of fluid between the lung and ventral sternal muscles, with the probe parallel to the ribs creates a triangular shape of anechoic fluid similar to a sail. (the "sail sign").
- As fluid accumulates the lungs may become atelectatic, appearing as floating tissue-like structures termed the "jellyfish" sign in human medicine.

AIS

Lung ultrasound will only detect lung pathology if it reaches the lung surface. Most diseases that cause AIS (cardiogenic pulmonary edema, trauma-induced contusions, aspiration pneumonia, etc.) reach the lung surface. As stated above, three or more B-lines in any single sonographic window is considered indicative of AIS.

Lung Consolidation

Sonographically detected lung consolidation can occur as a result of atelectasis, bronchopneumonia, thromboembolism, neoplasia, and inflammatory conditions such as pulmonary contusions and acute respiratory distress syndrome.

- Criteria to diagnose lung consolidation:
  - Abnormal pattern should be differentiated from the liver, spleen and other soft tissue abdominal structures.
  - Abnormal pattern should arise from the pleural line.
  - There should be a tissue-like pattern (similar to liver echotexture).
  - Anatomic boundaries must be present:
    - Superficial boundary of consolidation.
    - At the pleural line in the absence of pleural effusion.
    - At the deep boundary of a pleural effusion if effusion present.
  - Deep boundary of the consolidation may be irregular (aerated lung boundary) or regular (if the whole lobe is consolidated).
  - When consolidation fails to traverse the entire lung lobe (partial consolidation) aerated lung is encountered deep to the consolidation which can create an irregular consolidation/air interface, called a "shred sign." At the consolidation/aerated lung interface a hyperechoic irregular border is seen that usually creates comet tail artifacts.
  - If the border between the consolidation and aerated lung is smooth and almost circular, it most likely represents a nodule.
  - Where consolidation extends through the entirety of the lung, from one surface to the other, translobar hepatization is seen.
  - Air bronchograms, if present, can be seen within lung consolidation as small white hyperechoic pointed foci or lines.

INTERFERING FACTORS

Conditions That May Interfere with Performing the Procedure

- Patient position affects where pathology may be found and is important to consider when scanning patients.
- Severe dehydration and hypovolemia may reduce the sensitivity of finding pleural effusion; patients should be reassessed with VPOCUS once resuscitation procedures are undertaken.

Influence of Signalment on Performing and Interpreting the Procedure

Large-breed dogs may be more difficult to image, especially at the subxiphoid region due to the depth of their pleural surface.

CLINICAL PERSPECTIVE

- PLUS examinations are a quick and repeatable diagnostic tool that can help identify pathology and direct further diagnostics and therapy.
- VPOCUS examinations require little training and experience.

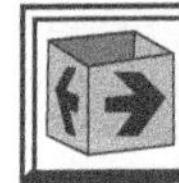

MISCELLANEOUS

ANCILLARY TESTS

- Thoracocentesis.
- Pericardiocentesis.

SYNONYMS

TFAST®, VetBLUE®, lung ultrasound.

SEE ALSO

Point of Care Abdominal Ultrasonography (in Appendix X).

ABBREVIATIONS

- AIS = alveolar interstitial syndrome.
- PLUS = pleural and lung ultrasound.
- VPOCUS = veterinary point of care ultrasound.

INTERNET RESOURCES

Faculty of Veterinary Medicine, University of Calgary (UCVM) podcasts: https://vet.ucalgary.ca/vcds/podcasts

Suggested Reading

Armenise A, Boysen RS, Rudloff E, et al. Veterinary-focused assessment with sonography for trauma-airway, breathing, circulation, disability and exposure: a prospective observational study in 64 canine trauma patients. J Small Anim Pract 2019, 60:173–182.

Boysen SR, Lisciandro GR. The use of ultrasound for dogs and cats in the emergency room: AFAST and TFAST. Vet Clin North Am Small Anim Pract 2013, 43(4):773–797.

Boysen S, McMurray J, Gommeren K. Abnormal curtain signs identified with a novel lung ultrasound protocol in six dogs with pneumothorax. Front Vet Sci 2019, 6:291.

Vezzosi T, Mannucci T, Pistoresi A, et al. Assessment of lung ultrasound B-lines in dogs with different stages of chronic valvular heart disease. J Vet Intern Med 2017, 31(3):700–704.

Walters A, O'Brien M, Selmic L, et al. Evaluation of the agreement between focused assessment with sonography in trauma (AFAST/TFAST) and computed tomography in dogs and cats with recent trauma. J Vet Emerg Crit Care 2018, 28(5):429–435.

Ward JL, Lisciandro GR, Keene BW, et al. Accuracy of point-of-care lung ultrasonography for the diagnosis of cardiogenic pulmonary edema in dogs and cats with acute dyspnea. J Am Vet Med Assoc 2017, 250(6):666–675.

Authors Søren Boysen and Serge Chalhoub

Consulting Editor Benjamin M. Brainard

Acknowledgment The author and editors acknowledge the prior contribution of Jantina McMurray.

RECTAL SCRAPING AND CYTOLOGY

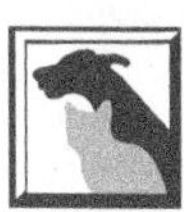

BASICS

TYPE OF PROCEDURE

Diagnostic sample collection.

PROCEDURE EXPLANATION AND RELATED PHYSIOLOGY

- Quick, relatively noninvasive, technique that can be used to diagnose certain colonic or rectal diseases.
- Different from fecal cytologic evaluation, which looks for diversity of the fecal bacterial population.

INDICATIONS

- Chronic or very severe large-bowel disease (especially patients with hypoalbuminemia, weight loss, or both) in dogs that may have fungal disease (e.g., histoplasmosis), algal disease (i.e., protothecosis), neoplastic disease, and especially those with mucosal abnormalities on digital rectal palpation.
- Procedure is seldom indicated in cats.

CONTRAINDICATIONS

Severe coagulopathy.

POTENTIAL COMPLICATIONS

- Excessive bleeding (rare).
- Perforation if exceedingly improper technique is employed.

CLIENT EDUCATION

- Specific for certain infections but is insensitive—if the results are negative, you have not eliminated any diseases.
- It is appropriate to evaluate rectal cytology before performing endoscopy in dogs with suspected fungal, algal or neoplastic disease, especially if mucosal abnormalities are found on rectal examination.

BODY SYSTEMS ASSESSED

Gastrointestinal

PROCEDURE

PATIENT PREPARATION

Pre-Procedure Medication or Preparation

None

Anesthesia or Sedation

Sedation with narcotics/neuroleptanalgesics or anesthesia with injectable propofol may be needed in animals that are in excessive pain during the rectal examination.

Patient Positioning

May be performed with the patient in any of several positions.

Patient Monitoring

None

Equipment or Supplies

- Examination gloves.
- A small curette or similar instrument.

TECHNIQUE

- A gloved finger is inserted into the rectum, and a complete digital rectal examination is performed.
- Next, a small curette is guided into the rectum with the finger, and the rectal mucosa is gently scraped to obtain epithelial cells:
  - The goal is to obtain mucosal epithelium, not feces.
  - Blood should not be obvious after the procedure.
- Spread epithelial cells on a glass slide, air-dry, and stain with new methylene blue, Diff-Quik, or modified Giemsa.
- In larger dogs, one may tape the cap of a syringe casing to the tip of the index finger and use it to scrape the rectal mucosa.

SAMPLE HANDLING

The slide is handled routinely as any cytologic slide.

APPROPRIATE AFTERCARE

Post-Procedure Patient Monitoring

None

Nursing Care

None

Dietary Modification

None

Medication Requirements

None

Restrictions on Activity

None

Anticipated Recovery Time

Immediate

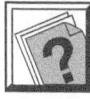

INTERPRETATION

NORMAL FINDINGS OR RANGE

No fungal organisms, no algae, and no appreciable inflammation.

ABNORMAL FINDINGS

- Fungal organisms (e.g., histoplasmosis, typically found in macrophages).
- Algae (i.e., protothecosis).
- Substantial numbers of neutrophils or eosinophils.
- Malignant cells.

CRITICAL VALUES

None

INTERFERING FACTORS

Drugs That May Alter Results of the Procedure

None known.

Conditions That May Interfere with Performing the Procedure

Excessive rectal or anal pain makes sedation or anesthesia necessary.

Procedure Techniques or Handling That May Alter Results

None

Influence of Signalment on Performing and Interpreting the Procedure

Species

This procedure is almost never performed in cats.

Breed

None

Age

None

Gender

None

Pregnancy

None

CLINICAL PERSPECTIVE

- Specific but not necessarily sensitive for diagnosis of colonic histoplasmosis, a disease that is common in select geographic areas of the United States.
- May help diagnose severe colitis by finding substantial numbers of neutrophils, but this is a nonspecific finding that can occur in numerous disorders.
- Care must be taken before diagnosing a malignancy based solely on cytologic analysis because epithelial dysplastic changes are common in many diseases.

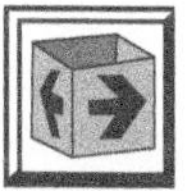

MISCELLANEOUS

ANCILLARY TESTS

Colonoscopy and biopsy are required if rectal cytologic analysis is nonrevealing in a dog that is suspected of having colonic histoplasmosis, protothecosis, or rectal neoplasia.

SYNONYMS

Rectal scrape.

SEE ALSO

Histoplasmosis

Suggested Reading

Clinkenbeard KD, Cowell RL, Tyler RD. Disseminated histoplasmosis in dogs: 12 cases (1981–1986). J Am Vet Med Assoc 1988, 193:1443–1447.

Jergens AE, Andreasen CB, Hagemoser WA, et al. Cytologic examination of exfoliative specimens obtained during endoscopy for diagnosis of gastrointestinal tract disease in dogs and cats. J Am Vet Med Assoc 1998, 213:1755–1759.

Author Michael D. Willard

Consulting Editor Benjamin M. Brainard

SALINE AGGLUTINATION TEST

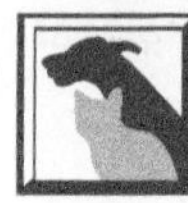

BASICS

TYPE OF SPECIMEN

Whole blood (anticoagulated with EDTA).

TEST EXPLANATION AND RELATED PHYSIOLOGY

- Performed when erythrocytes are aggregated (clusters of grapes) or stacked (similar to coins) on a blood smear. This finding indicates erythrocyte rouleaux or agglutination:
  - Rouleaux occurs due to interactions of red blood cells with plasma proteins such as fibrinogen.
  - Agglutination is caused by presence of antibodies (usually IgM) on surface of red cells, forming bridges between one another and spontaneously aggregating. Most commonly associated with immune-mediated hemolytic anemia (IMHA).
- When saline agglutination test is performed, rouleaux will disperse in the presence of saline but agglutination will not.

INDICATIONS

Differentiate erythrocyte rouleaux from antibody-mediated agglutination.

CONTRAINDICATIONS

None

POTENTIAL COMPLICATIONS

None

CLIENT EDUCATION

Negative saline agglutination test does not rule out IMHA.

BODY SYSTEMS ASSESSED

Hemic/immune.

SAMPLE

SAMPLE COLLECTION

One drop of whole blood and 4 drops of sterile 0.9% saline are required.

SAMPLE HANDLING

- Saline should be between 23 and 37°C; collect blood into EDTA and observe for agglutination on microscope slide.

SAMPLE STORAGE

Test should be interpreted immediately.

SAMPLE STABILITY

- EDTA-anticoagulated blood:
  - Several hours at room temperature.
  - 1 day at 2–8°C (refrigerated).

PROTOCOL

- There is no standardized protocol for this test.
- Add a drop of whole blood to a microscope slide.
- Dilute this drop of blood by adding four drops of saline.
- Rock slide gently back and forth before examining it macroscopically and microscopically for agglutination. Cover slip recommended for microscopic evaluation.
- True agglutination will continue to form aggregates that appear similar to clusters of grapes in the presence of saline. Rouleaux will be dispersed by saline and no aggregation will be observed.
- Additional saline can be added if there is concern that an insufficient amount was added in order to rule out rouleaux.
- For inconclusive results, washing erythrocytes 3 times in a 1:4 ratio is recommended to confirm persistent aggregation.

INTERPRETATION

NORMAL FINDINGS OR RANGE

Lack of macroscopic or microscopic aggregation.

ABNORMAL FINDINGS

Persistent aggregation with addition of saline.

CRITICAL VALUES

None

INTERFERING FACTORS

Drugs That May Alter Results or Interpretation

Treatment with corticosteroids may result in false-negative results.

Disorders That May Alter Results

- Animals occasionally have naturally occurring anti-erythrocyte antibodies, causing a positive result; however, these animals are not generally anemic and clinical history is important to differentiate normal from pathologic agglutination.
- Cold agglutinins may not precipitate at the temperature of test and result in false-negative result.

Collection Techniques or Handling That May Alter Results

- Inadequate amount of saline may not disperse rouleaux (false positive).
- Overdilution with saline may cause dispersion of agglutination (false negative).
- Letting dilution sit for too long before interpretation may result in false-negative results if antibodies are of low affinity.

Influence of Signalment

Species

Cats can exhibit more rouleaux in health than dogs; it is recommended to add more saline when performing this test in cats.

Breed

IMHA is more common in some dog breeds (e.g., cocker spaniels, English springer spaniels, Old English sheepdogs).

Age

None

Sex

None

Pregnancy

None

LIMITATIONS OF TEST

- Lack of standardized protocol makes interpretation and reproducibility difficult.
- Cannot always differentiate between rouleaux and autoagglutination, particularly if antibodies causing agglutination are of low affinity and easily dispersed.
- Rouleaux and agglutination may be present at the same time.

Valid If Run in Human Lab?

Yes

CAUSES OF ABNORMAL FINDINGS

- IMHA.
- Neoplasia.
- Infectious disease.
- Toxicities (e.g., bee sting envenomation).
- Drug reaction.
- Systemic lupus erythematosus.
- Alloimmune hemolytic anemia.

CLINICAL PERSPECTIVE

- Some clinical pathologists do not endorse this test due to lack of standardization of protocol and interpretation.
- Some cases of IMHA do not display macroscopic or microscopic agglutination.
- Not a standalone test for diagnosis of IMHA; requires proper interpretation of history, physical exam, complete blood count (CBC) with blood smear review, biochemical profile, ± Coombs' testing.

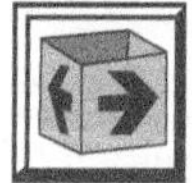

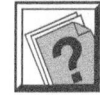

MISCELLANEOUS

ANCILLARY TESTS

A Coombs' test is not indicated if saline agglutination is positive as it would be expected to be positive as well.

SYNONYMS

Saline dispersion test.

SEE ALSO

Anemia, Immune-Mediated.

ABBREVIATIONS

- IMHA = immune-mediated hemolytic anemia.

INTERNET RESOURCES

https://todaysveterinarypractice.com/diagnosis-of-immune-mediated-hemolytic-anemia/

Suggested Reading

Brazzell JL. The saline agglutination test—why you might reconsider performing it. Marshfield Labs: Reference Point, 2016.

Garden OA, Kidd L, Mexas AM, et al. ACVIM consensus statement on the diagnosis of immune-mediated hemolytic anemia in dogs and cats. J Vet Intern Med 2019, 33:313–334.

Harvey JW. Erythrocyte agglutination. In: Veterinary Hematology: A Diagnostic Guide and Color Atlas. St. Louis, MO: W.B. Saunders, 2012, pp. 13–14.

Author Alyssa J. Brooker
Consulting Editor Benjamin M. Brainard

THORACOCENTESIS AND FLUID ANALYSIS

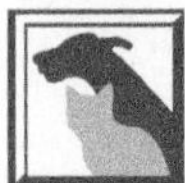

BASICS

TYPE OF PROCEDURE

Diagnostic sample collection.

PROCEDURE EXPLANATION AND RELATED PHYSIOLOGY

- Thoracocentesis or pleurocentesis can be performed for one of two purposes: diagnostic evaluation or therapeutic intervention:
  - Diagnostic thoracocentesis can be essential for diagnosing the presence of pleural space disease and evaluating the contents of the cavity, whether air or fluid. Pleural fluid can then be further evaluated grossly for color and consistency, and microscopically for cellularity and the presence of protein or organisms.
  - Therapeutic thoracocentesis is used to treat pleural effusion and pneumothorax resulting from a variety of causes. Typically, therapeutic thoracocentesis follows a positive diagnostic tap.

INDICATIONS

- When the presence of pleural air or fluid is suspected, especially in an animal with increased inspiratory effort and reduced breath sounds on thoracic auscultation.
- To sample/alleviate pleural air or fluid identified on an imaging study.
- Conditions leading to pleural space disease include trauma, hemorrhage, neoplasia, heart failure, chylothorax, spontaneous rupture of a pulmonary bulla, and infection.

CONTRAINDICATIONS

Thoracocentesis should be performed cautiously on patients with abnormal hemostasis.

POTENTIAL COMPLICATIONS

- Lung puncture or laceration producing pneumothorax. More likely to be serious in patients with pleural fibrosis.
- Hemorrhage, if the internal thoracic artery is lacerated.
- If the fenestrated catheter technique is used, and the fenestrations are not small and smooth, the catheter can get caught on the skin and break, with pieces remaining in the patient.
- Infection (pyothorax) can develop if sterile technique is not used.

CLIENT EDUCATION

Clients should be aware of the potential complications of the procedure and the potential severity of the underlying disease.

BODY SYSTEMS ASSESSED

- Cardiovascular.
- Hemic, lymphatic, and immune.
- Respiratory.

PROCEDURE

PATIENT PREPARATION

Pre-Procedure Medication or Preparation

- Sedation may be necessary, especially in cats.
- Clip the hair over a large area of the lateral thorax. The point of needle insertion should be at the 7th–9th intercostal space, dorsal to the costochondral arch.
- To remove fluid, the needle should enter at the level of the costochondral junction. To remove air, it should enter where the chest wall is widest.
- Local anesthetic is generally not necessary for a diagnostic tap. However, local anesthesia is imperative for therapeutic thoracocentesis. Lidocaine (no more than 2 mg/kg) should be injected SC and infused into the intercostal muscles.
- Scrub the skin surface with povidone-iodine or chlorhexidine. Contact time should be at least 3 minutes and then wipe with alcohol.
- For emergency therapeutic thoracocentesis, full skin antisepsis may be abbreviated.

Anesthesia or Sedation

- Selection should be based on the individual patient.
- Often, butorphanol ± acepromazine or a benzodiazepine is sufficient.

Patient Positioning

- The patient should be in a comfortable position that does not compromise its respiration. Typically, the patient is in sternal recumbency or standing:
  - Sitting should be avoided because it interferes with accurate determination of landmarks.
- Supplemental oxygen may stabilize patient and improve comfort during centesis.

Patient Monitoring

Respiration, heart rate, and pulse should be monitored throughout procedure.

Equipment or Supplies

Diagnostic Tap

- A 3-mL syringe with a 22-gauge, 1-inch needle can be used for cats and most dogs, for large (>30 kg) or obese dogs, a 1½-inch needle may be needed.
- A butterfly needle can also be used in cats and small dogs.
- Serum and EDTA tubes, and culture swabs needed for fluid analysis.

Therapeutic Tap

- A 14- to 16-gauge, 3½- to 5¼-inch catheter for dogs.
- A 16- to 20-gauge, 2- to 3½-inch catheter for cats and small dogs *or* a butterfly needle.
- A no. 11 scalpel blade.
- Sterile gloves.
- A 3-mL syringe.
- A 12- to 60-mL syringe.
- An IV fluid-extension set.
- A three-way stopcock.
- A container for fluid.

TECHNIQUE

Diagnostic Thoracocentesis

- Locate the desired point of insertion by counting to the 7th–9th intercostal space. Begin counting in the caudal most intercostal space (12th space) and count cranially. Position the needle at the widest point of the thorax for air, and just dorsal to the costochondral arch for aspiration of fluid.
- Stabilize both hands on the animal so that the hands and the needle move with the chest wall. Insert the needle through the skin at the cranial aspect of the rib; once in the subcutaneous space, apply 1–2 mL of vacuum on the syringe. Slowly advance the needle perpendicular to the body wall while maintaining vacuum. Penetration of the pleura is indicated when the vacuum is suddenly lost (pneumothorax) or fluid enters the syringe (effusion):
  - Penetration of the pleura may cause discomfort to the patient, and should be palpated by the operator as a slight pop.
- Once the presence of pleural fluid or air is confirmed, withdraw the needle slightly to decrease the likelihood of lung laceration.

Butterfly Catheter Technique

- For diagnostic or therapeutic thoracocentesis.
- When using this technique, position the needle so that the bevel is facing cranially. Insert the catheter perpendicular to the chest wall and, once in the subcutaneous space, apply 1–2 mL of vacuum with the syringe attached to the catheter extension tubing.
- Once the vacuum is lost, the tip of the needle can be directed so that it is away from the lung, and advanced along the inner pleura. The wings of the catheter can be pressed against the cranial rib and used to direct the needle in the pleural space.

Therapeutic Thoracocentesis

- Locate the point of insertion by counting to the 7th–9th intercostal space as described above. Position the needle at the widest point of the throax for air, and just dorsal to the costochondral arch for aspiration of fluid.
- If fluid is suspected, a few small fenestrations can be made in the catheter, starting 1 cm proximal to the tip, to prevent clogging and increase yield:
  - Use a no. 11 blade and, while wearing sterile gloves, make small V-shaped holes by joining cuts at a 45° angle.

    - These holes should be no more than 20% of the circumference of the catheter.
    - Rotate the catheter 90° at each fenestration to maintain the integrity of the catheter (i.e., fenestrations should not be opposite each other).
    - Do not scoop holes out; ensure that the edges are smooth to decrease the likelihood of the catheter getting caught on the skin and breaking.
- Lift the skin away from the body wall and make a stab skin incision that fully penetrates the dermis with the no. 11 blade.
- Attach the 3-mL syringe to the catheter–needle assembly.
- The nondominant hand is rested on the animal and used to advance the catheter–stylet assembly into the skin incision:
    - The stylet is advanced by the fingers of the nondominant hand, which is resting on the chest wall.
    - Once the needle has entered the subcutaneous space, the dominant hand applies 1–2 mL of vacuum using the syringe.
    - While maintaining the vacuum, advance the stylet slowly along the cranial aspect of the rib until the vacuum is lost (or fluid is observed), indicating that the pleural space has been entered.
- Once the stylet has entered the pleural space, advance the entire assembly approximately ¼ inch:
    - Hold the stylet hub stationary and advance the catheter ≈1 cm over the stylet.
    - It is critical that the catheter is advanced and that the stylet is not pulled backward out of the pleural space.
    - Holding the stylet stationary, advance the catheter cranially into the thorax, parallel to the spine (for air) or cranioventrally (for fluid).
- Remove the stylet and have an assistant attach the extension set that has been connected to the three-way stopcock and syringe and begin aspiration.

SAMPLE HANDLING

Aliquots of effusion samples may be placed in EDTA tubes for cytologic analysis and tubes without additive or culturettes for bacteriologic culture. A slide should also be made for immediate cytologic evaluation.

APPROPRIATE AFTERCARE

Post-Procedure Patient Monitoring

- The patient's respiration rate and effort should be monitored after thoracocentesis. Deterioration suggests that either the condition is worsening or that an iatrogenic pneumothorax has developed.
- Monitor the heart rate, pulses, and capillary refill time.
- Patients with recurrent pneumothorax after 2–3 thoracocenteses will likely benefit from thoracostomy tube placement and continuous pleural suction.

Nursing Care

No specific nursing care is necessary after the centesis.

Dietary Modification

N/A

Medication Requirements

Based on underlying disease.

Restrictions on Activity

The animal should remain quiet for a few hours after the thoracocentesis so that respiration rate and effort can be evaluated effectively. Further restrictions will be based on underlying disease.

Anticipated Recovery Time

The patient should recover as soon as the needle or catheter has been removed, and the sedation has worn off. Full recovery is based on the etiology of the underlying disease.

INTERPRETATION

NORMAL FINDINGS OR RANGE

A normal patient should not have any air or fluid in its pleural space.

ABNORMAL FINDINGS

- If air is found, this indicates a pneumothorax.
- If fluid is found, indicating pleural effusion, it can be due to a number of causes, which can often be distinguished from one another by fluid cytology (see Fluid Analysis):
    - Transudates, modified transudates, and pseudochylous effusion can be found in patients with heart failure.
    - The presence of intracellular bacteria or excessive numbers of neutrophils indicates a pyothorax.
    - Chyle may be present and is defined by fluid analysis and comparison with serum.
    - Neoplasia may be identified as well, although reactive mesothelial cells can have an appearance similar to neoplastic cells can caution is advised with diagnosis of neoplasia.

CRITICAL VALUES

If air is continuously being produced and removed with the catheter apparatus, or if the fluid is indicative of a pyothorax, a thoracostomy tube should be placed to evacuate the pleural space more effectively.

INTERFERING FACTORS

Drugs That May Alter Results of the Procedure

None known

Conditions That May Interfere with Performing the Procedure

Inadequate sedation will prevent safe and adequate thoracocentesis.

Procedure Techniques or Handling That May Alter Results

- The fluid can be contaminated, invalidating the results of microbial culture, if the fluid is not handled aseptically.
- A fresh slide preparation should always be made, especially if there is delay in evaluating the EDTA sample.

Influence of Signalment on Performing and Interpreting the Procedure

Species
None

Breed
None

Age
None

Gender
None

Pregnancy
None

CLINICAL PERSPECTIVE

- If the clinician is unsure whether the patient has pleural space disease, a diagnostic thoracocentesis should first be performed, especially if the patient is not stable enough for radiography.
- If the results of the diagnostic thoracocentesis are positive, a therapeutic thoracocentesis is recommended if the animal has an increased respiratory effort.
- The catheter technique is safer than using a needle because it decreases the likelihood of lung laceration.
- Samples should be evaluated to guide the clinician on how to treat the patient properly.

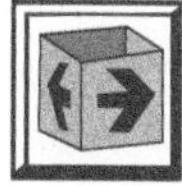

MISCELLANEOUS

ANCILLARY TESTS

- Radiography or thoracic ultrasound can determine the need for thoracocentesis and post-procedure can assess the effectiveness of the thoracocentesis and identify underlying pathology.
- Samples should be evaluated using appropriate fluid analysis, including cytologic evaluation. Based on these results, microbial culture of the fluid sample may be appropriate.

SYNONYMS

Chest tap

THORACOCENTESIS AND FLUID ANALYSIS (CONTINUED)

SEE ALSO

- Bacterial Culture and Sensitivity (in Appendix X).
- Chylothorax.
- Fluid Analysis (in Appendix X).
- Pleural Effusion.
- Pyothorax.

INTERNET RESOURCES

Washington State University, College of Veterinary Medicine, Small Animal Diagnostic & Therapeutic Techniques: Thoracocentesis: http://courses.vetmed.wsu.edu/samdx/thoracocentesis.asp.

Suggested Reading

Hawkins E. Clinical manifestations of the pleural cavity and mediastinal diseases. In: Nelson RW, Couto CG, eds., Small Animal Internal Medicine. St. Louis, MO: CV Mosby, 2003, pp. 315–319.

Hawkins E. Diagnostic tests for the pleural cavity and mediastinum. In: Nelson RW, Couto CG, eds., Small Animal Internal Medicine. St. Louis, MO: CV Mosby, 2003, pp. 320–326.

Mertens MM, Fossum TW, MacDonald KA. Pleural and extrapleural diseases. In: Ettinger SJ, Feldman EC, eds., Textbook of Veterinary Internal Medicine. Philadelphia, PA: W.B. Saunders, 2005, pp. 1272–1284.

Nelson OL. Pleural effusion. In: Ettinger SJ, Feldman EC, eds., Textbook of Veterinary Internal Medicine. Philadelphia, PA: W.B. Saunders, 2005, pp. 204–207.

Rozanski E, Chan DL. Approach to the patient with respiratory distress. Vet Clin North Am Small Anim Pract 2005: 315–316.

Sigrist NE. Thoracocentesis. In: Silverstein DC, Hopper K, eds., Small Animal Critical Care Medicine, 2nd ed. St. Louis, MO: Elsevier, 2015, pp. 1029–1031.

Author April Blong
Consulting Editor Benjamin M. Brainard
Acknowledgment The author and editors acknowledge the prior contribution of Kielyn Scott.

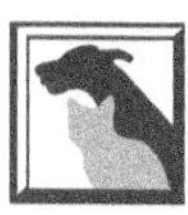

BASICS

TYPE OF PROCEDURE

Diagnostic sample collection from the lower airway

PROCEDURE EXPLANATION AND RELATED PHYSIOLOGY

Tracheal wash involves insertion of a catheter into the airway of a dog or cat, injection of sterile saline for culture and cytologic evaluation, and subsequent aspiration of the fluid that has contacted the airway lining. The catheter can be inserted through an oral approach using a sterile endotracheal tube (endotracheal wash [ETW]) or through a transtracheal approach by passing sterile tubing through a catheter that is inserted between tracheal rings (transtracheal wash [TTW]). The catheter terminates at the carina for collection of a global airway sample.

INDICATIONS

Acute or chronic cough.

CONTRAINDICATIONS

- Bleeding disorders.
- Anesthetic contraindications (for ETW).
- Markedly fractious animals (for the transtracheal approach).

POTENTIAL COMPLICATIONS

- Any anesthetic complication.
- Subcutaneous emphysema.
- Pneumomediastinum.
- Hemorrhage.
- Cartilage damage.

CLIENT EDUCATION

- Cough may be transiently worsened after the procedure.
- Subcutaneous emphysema can develop.

BODY SYSTEMS ASSESSED

Respiratory

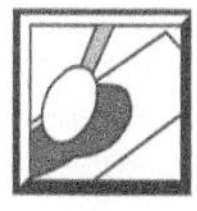

PROCEDURE

PATIENT PREPARATION

Pre-Procedure Medication or Preparation

- Preoxygenate the patient for 5 minutes prior to the anesthesia.
- In cats, administer terbutaline (0.01 mg/kg SC) immediately prior to the procedure to counteract bronchoconstriction. Repeat if tachypnea or hemoglobin desaturation develops.
- Dogs with marked expiratory effort might also benefit from administration of terbutaline prior to the procedure, although bronchoconstriction is not a component of their disease.

Anesthesia or Sedation

- Local anesthesia with lidocaine is typically sufficient for a TTW in compliant patients. Mild sedation with acepromazine, butorphanol, or a benzodiazepine can be required. A TTW is a good choice for animals that are poor candidates for anesthesia.
- To perform an ETW, a mild anesthetic protocol that enables intubation and 5–10 minutes of light anesthesia is necessary.

Patient Positioning

Sternal (some clinicians prefer positioning with the most affected side of the lungs ventrally for the transoral approach).

Patient Monitoring

- Pulse oximetry can be used throughout an ETW along with standard anesthetic monitoring.
- If SC emphysema or bleeding develops during a TTW, the procedure should be aborted and stabilization and monitoring procedures instituted.

Equipment or Supplies

- ETW—sterile endotracheal tube, sterile gloves, sterile catheter or tubing, syringes, and sterile saline.
- TTW—local anesthesia (lidocaine), through-the-needle catheter (e.g., Intracath, BD, Franklin Lakes, NJ) or over-the-needle catheter and sterile tubing, syringes, and sterile saline.
- If desired, a three-way stopcock and sterile container (e.g., mucous specimen trap) can be used in conjunction with house suction to facilitate retrieval of fluid.

TECHNIQUE

- A TTW is appropriate for use in dogs larger than 8–10 kg. This can be performed with an over-the-needle catheter (14–16 gauge) and 3.5 French urinary catheter, or a through-the-needle catheter (18 gauge, 8 or 12 inch):
  - The ventral portion of the neck is clipped and lightly scrubbed with antiseptic solution followed by alcohol wipes, and a more complete surgical preparation is performed after local anesthesia.
  - Lidocaine (0.25–0.5 mL, not to exceed 2 mg/kg) is instilled into the subcutaneous tissue down to the level of the tracheal rings.
  - The catheter is inserted into the skin with the bevel of the stylet facing downward. The stylet is withdrawn and the urinary catheter is passed through the short catheter down the trachea.
  - An aliquot of nonbacteriostatic saline (4–10 mL) is injected into the catheter followed by 2–3 mL of air and then aspirated back into the syringe. Stimulation of a cough or chest compression after instillation can facilitate retrieval of a sample.
  - Fluid instillation and aspiration can be repeated 2–3 times until an adequate sample has been retrieved (0.5–1.0 mL is usually sufficient for culture and cytologic evaluation).
  - The long catheter is removed followed by the short catheter and a light wrap is applied to the neck.
  - If a through-the-needle catheter is used, the needle is used to puncture the trachea and then the urinary catheter is fed into the trachea. Once the catheter is entirely within the trachea, the needle is backed out of the skin, and the syringe with saline may be attached to the inserted catheter hub. The remainder of the procedure is as described above.
- An ETW is appropriate for use in large and small dogs, pediatric patients, and in cats. A sterile endotracheal tube and a sterile polypropylene catheter (3.5–8.0 French) or red rubber catheter are needed:
  - The animal is anesthetized with a short-acting anesthetic agent (e.g., propofol or alfaxolone, with premedication).
  - The sterile endotracheal tube is passed into the trachea, taking care to avoid touching the oral mucosa or larynx with the end of the tube in order to limit contamination with oropharyngeal bacteria.
  - An assistant holds the tube in place, and a sterile polypropylene catheter or red rubber tube is passed to the level of the carina (approximately the 4th intercostal space).
  - An aliquot of nonbacteriostatic saline (4–10 mL) is instilled into the airway followed by 2–3 mL of air, and gentle suction from the syringe is used to retrieve the fluid and cells from the lower airway. Alternately, house suction can be utilized with a mucous specimen trap, which can be connected to a tracheal suction catheter with a chimney valve.

SAMPLE HANDLING

Airway samples are submitted for cytologic evaluation and for bacterial culture. Aerobic, anaerobic, and Mycoplasma culture or PCR should be considered for individual cases, and the laboratory should be consulted for guidelines on sample submission. Aerobic culture can generally be submitted in a sterile red-top tube; however, some laboratories require Amies or charcoal medium for *Mycoplasma* culture and an anaerobic culture tube to detect anaerobic bacteria.

APPROPRIATE AFTERCARE

Post-Procedure Patient Monitoring

- Monitor respiratory rate and effort.
- Watch for respiratory distress or appearance of SC emphysema.
- Monitor the TTW site for bleeding or swelling.

TRACHEAL WASH

Nursing Care

- Keep the animal quiet during recovery.
- If respiratory distress develops, placement in an oxygen-enriched environment can be helpful.

Dietary Modification

Any animal undergoing a tracheal wash should be fasted for 12–24 hours prior to the procedure, when possible.

Medication Requirements

None

Restrictions on Activity

- The use of leashes should be avoided for 1–3 days after a transtracheal wash.
- Normal activity levels can usually be resumed after 1 day.

Anticipated Recovery Time

1–2 hours

INTERPRETATION

NORMAL FINDINGS OR RANGE

- Normal animals should have ciliated respiratory epithelial cells present on cytologic evaluation and rare inflammatory cells or macrophages.
- Culture of airway fluid in normal dogs and cats can reveal light growth of various types of bacteria, including *Pasteurella, Streptococcus, Staphylococcus, Acinetobacter, Moraxella, Enterobacter, Pseudomonas, Escherichia coli,* and *Klebsiella.*

ABNORMAL FINDINGS

- Large numbers of neutrophils or eosinophils.
- Degenerate neutrophils and intracellular bacteria are typically found in infectious processes.
- Abnormal lymphocytes can be suggestive of lymphoma.
- Airway parasites or protozoa may be evident on cytologic evaluation.
- Rarely, neoplastic cells may exfoliate into tracheal wash fluid.
- Infection can be documented by growth of a single species of pathogenic bacteria or by moderate growth of a mixed number of bacterial species.
- Detection of *Mycoplasma* indicates infection.

CRITICAL VALUES

None

INTERFERING FACTORS

Drugs That May Alter Results of the Procedure

- Corticosteroids will reduce the flux of inflammatory cells into the airways.
- Antibiotics will suppress bacterial growth on culture.
- Cough suppressants may make it difficult to obtain fluid from the airways.

Conditions That May Interfere with Performing the Procedure

- Severe tracheal sensitivity and tracheal or airway collapse can be worsened by trauma associated with tracheal wash.
- Airway collapse can result in poor return of fluid.
- In obese animals, a transtracheal wash can be difficult to perform because of an inability to palpate and stabilize the trachea.
- Room temperature saline may induce bronchoconstriction when infused in cats.

Procedure Techniques or Handling That May Alter Results

Upper airway contamination (indicated by the presence of squamous cells or Simonsiella bacteria on cytologic evaluation) influences culture results and increases the likelihood of growth of contaminating bacteria.

Influence of Signalment on Performing and Interpreting the Procedure

Species

- Dogs—TTW or ETW are appropriate, depending on size of the animal and ability to undergo anesthesia.
- Cats—ETW is appropriate.

Breed

- Caution should be employed when undertaking any respiratory procedure in brachycephalic animals.
- The size of animal will influence the decision to perform a TTW vs. ETW.

Age

Young dogs may be more likely to have *Bordetella* and/or *Mycoplasma* on culture than older dogs. Cartilage injury is more of a concern in younger animals.

Gender

None

Pregnancy

None

CLINICAL PERSPECTIVE

Tracheal wash procedures are relatively safe and easy to perform. Results of culture and cytologic evaluation provide valuable information on appropriate treatment of respiratory patients.

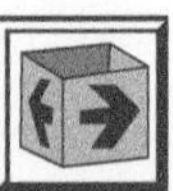

MISCELLANEOUS

ANCILLARY TESTS

If results are nondiagnostic, consider bronchoscopy with bronchoalveolar lavage.

SYNONYMS

None

SEE ALSO

- Asthma, Bronchitis—Cats.
- Bronchiectasis.
- Bronchitis, Chronic.
- Cough.
- Pneumonia, Aspiration.
- Pneumonia, Bacteria.
- Pneumonia, Eosinophilic.
- Pneumonia, Fungal.
- Pneumonia, Interstitial.
- Respiratory Parasites.
- Tracheal Collapse.

ABBREVIATIONS

- ETW = endotracheal wash.
- TTW = transtracheal wash.

Suggested Reading

Dye JA, McKiernan BC, Rozanski EA, et al. Bronchopulmonary disease in the cat: Historical, physical, radiographic, clinicopathologic, and pulmonary functional evaluation of 24 affected and 15 healthy cats. J Vet Intern Med 1996, 10:385–400.

Peeters DE, McKiernan BC, Weisiger RM, et al. Quantitative bacterial cultures and cytological examination of bronchoalveolar lavage specimens in dogs. J Vet Intern Med 2000, 14:534–541.

Randolph JF, Moise NS, Scarlett JM, et al. Prevalence of mycoplasmal and ureaplasmal recovery from tracheobronchial lavages and of mycoplasma recovery from pharyngeal swabs in dogs with and without pulmonary disease. Am J Vet Res 1993, 54:387–391.

Randolph JF, Moise NS, Scarlett JM, et al. Prevalence of mycoplasmal and ureaplasmal recovery from tracheobronchial lavages and of mycoplasma recovery from pharyngeal swabs in cats with and without pulmonary disease. Am J Vet Res 1993, 54:897–900.

Author Lynelle R. Johnson

Consulting Editor Benjamin M. Brainard

ULTRASOUND-GUIDED MASS OR ORGAN ASPIRATION

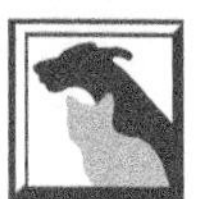

BASICS

TYPE OF SPECIMEN

Ultrasonographic

PROCEDURE EXPLANATION AND RELATED PHYSIOLOGY

- Percutaneous ultrasound-guided mass or organ aspiration is a technique that is commonly used to obtain material for cytologic examination as an aid in the diagnosis of a disease process:
  - Ultrasonography is typically sensitive but not specific for disease processes, and additional information such as that obtained from cytologic examination of cellular material is often helpful in determining a definitive diagnosis.
  - In addition, because needle placement can be directly visualized in real time, precise placement in an area of interest is possible.
- This procedure is commonly used to obtain cellular material from the liver, spleen, and kidneys with diffuse, infiltrative disease, as well as masses anywhere within the body.
- A prerequisite is that the area to be aspirated must be visible during ultrasonography, and an unobstructed path for the needle trajectory must be identified:
  - If there is gas or bone surrounding a lesion, then ultrasound guidance will likely not be possible.

INDICATIONS

Obtain a cellular or fluid sample for cytologic evaluation to further define or diagnose the etiology of an abnormality in an organ or mass.

CONTRAINDICATIONS

- Coagulopathy.
- Superimposed structures in the path of the needle trajectory.
- Patient noncompliance.
- Inability to visualize the lesion definitively with ultrasonography.

POTENTIAL COMPLICATIONS

- Hemorrhage, which is typically self-limiting unless a major vascular structure is damaged during the procedure or a severe coagulopathy is present.
- Sepsis or peritonitis if an abscess or infected lesion is sampled (rare).
- Possible seeding of neoplasia along the needle tract (rare).

CLIENT EDUCATION

Typically, the client should be apprised of the possible complications, but no additional education is necessary. If general anesthesia is required (because of patient noncompliance or a difficult-to-reach lesion), then typical preparation instructions should be given (e.g., withhold food).

BODY SYSTEMS ASSESSED

- Endocrine and metabolic.
- Gastrointestinal.
- Hemic, lymphatic, and immune.
- Hepatobiliary.
- Musculoskeletal.
- Renal and urologic.
- Reproductive.
- Respiratory.

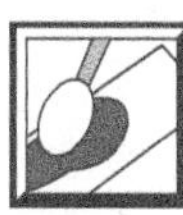

PROCEDURE

PATIENT PREPARATION

Pre-Procedure Medication or Preparation

- Withhold food and water as needed if anesthesia or sedation is necessary to accomplish the procedure.
- The skin in the area to be aspirated should be removed of hair (typically using clippers with a no. 40 clipper blade) and aseptically prepared.
- Alcohol may be used as an ultrasound-coupling agent to prevent any artifact that may occur in the cytologic preparation. (Ultrasound coupling gel can cause an artifact if it contaminates the slides during preparation.)
- To verify a safe needle trajectory, ultrasonography should be performed prior to the procedure.

Anesthesia or Sedation

- Some patients will tolerate this procedure without anesthesia, sedation, or the use of local anesthetics. The need for sedation should be anticipated for anxious or painful patients and for intercostal approaches in the abdomen or thorax.
- If anesthesia or sedation is necessary, standard regimens may be used that are appropriate for the patient.
- It should be noted that protocols that cause panting or excessive splenic enlargement may make the procedure more difficult. For example, pure opioids may cause excessive panting and make it difficult to guide the needle into deep or small lesions.

Patient Positioning

Patients should be positioned to enable an unobstructed approach and placement of both the needle and the transducer. Typically, patients will be positioned in lateral or dorsal recumbency, and they should be manually restrained if anesthesia is not used.

Patient Monitoring

None, except as indicated during sedation or anesthesia.

Equipment or Supplies

Typically, a 22-gauge needle of appropriate length attached to a syringe (6 or 12 mL) is used. Small needles (23, 25, or 27 gauge) may be used particularly if hemorrhage is felt to be a significant risk. However, nondiagnostic samples may be obtained with smaller gauge needles.

TECHNIQUE

- There are three methods used to perform a percutaneous ultrasound-guided mass or organ aspiration. In any case, the shortest trajectory between the skin surface and the lesion should be chosen. Only one body cavity should be penetrated at a time. In addition, choice of ultrasound transducer type can affect the ease of performing the procedure. Convex or sector-type transducers usually have a smaller footprint and thus are easier to manipulate when performing this procedure. A linear transducer may be difficult to use because it has a larger footprint:
  - Indirect technique: This technique involves using ultrasonography to identify the lesion to be sampled, and then the transducer is removed and the needle is passed blindly into the structure to be sampled. This technique may be used if the lesion is extremely large, and thus confirmation of needle placement is not necessary.
  - Freehand technique: This is the most commonly employed technique. The needle is held in one hand and the transducer is held in the other. The area of interest should be visualized, and the probe is manipulated such that the lesion is clearly visible. The needle should puncture the skin a few millimeters away from the transducer in order to facilitate needle visualization, as well as to protect against puncturing the transducer. The goal is to pass the needle within the plane of the ultrasound beam so that the needle is visible. Do not pass the needle in a plane perpendicular to the ultrasound plane, because the length will not be visible. The more acute the needle angle is to the ultrasound beam, the more difficult it is to visualize the needle. Therefore, the needle should form at least a 45° angle with the transducer to facilitate its visualization. The needle is passed through the skin and then into the lesion of interest.
  - Guided technique: The needle is held in place by using an attachable guide, which is coupled to the transducer (see Figure 1). The ultrasound machine will have software that will show the projected trajectory of the needle. The area of interest is visualized, and the transducer is manipulated such that the projected path of the needle is superimposed over the area to be sampled. The needle is then passed through the

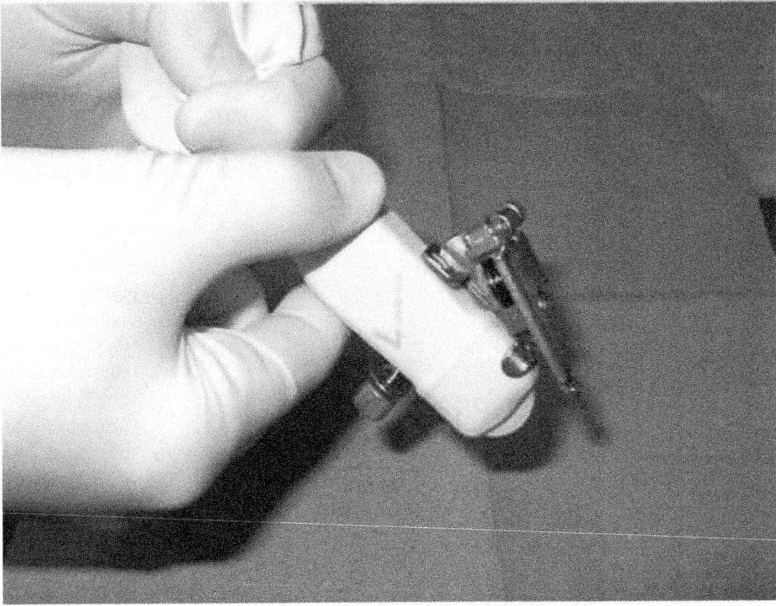

Figure 1.

A transducer with a needle guide attachment in place. The guide will maintain the needle in the plane of the ultrasound beam and, combined with the software program on the machine, will enable specific placement of a needle or biopsy instrument in the area of interest. Source: Lawrence P. Tilley

needle guide attached to the transducer and into the patient.

- If using either the freehand or the guided technique, improved needle visualization may be obtained either by moving the needle slightly, by moving the needle in and out of the tissue, or by minimally adjusting the transducer to bring the needle more into the plane of the ultrasound beam.
- Using any of the aforementioned methods, the sample may be obtained either through direct aspiration with active suction applied to the syringe while the needle tip is in the lesion or through a nonaspiration technique whereby the needle is moved up and down in the area of interest several times before the needle is withdrawn from the patient.
- Any organ or mass can be aspirated by using any of these techniques. If a diffuse disease is suspected in the liver, it is usually best to aspirate the left side of the liver to help prevent possible laceration of the gallbladder. In addition, the spleen is typically sampled by using a nonaspiration technique to help prevent hemodilution of the sample. It may be advantageous to obtain at least 1 sample by using an active aspiration technique and 1 sample by using a nonaspiration technique (in organs other than the spleen) to maximize the chance of obtaining a diagnostic sample. Active aspiration may disrupt fragile cells such as seen in lymphoma:
    - To practice aspiration or biopsy techniques, a biopsy phantom can be created. A biopsy phantom can improve the hand-to-eye coordination necessary to perform these techniques successfully, particularly the freehand technique, which requires more practice for proficiency (see Figure 2).
    - The simplest biopsy phantom uses a heavy plastic bag. (An empty IV saline bag works well.) Culinary gelatin is mixed at double the recommend concentration and poured into the bag. After 15–30 minutes of refrigeration, as the gelatin begins to set, targets are inserted into the middle of the gelatin. (Grapes, cherries, and chickpeas work well.) Care should be taken to not create any air bubbles. The gelatin is allowed to set completely, and then the bag is sealed. The outer surface can then be imaged and a needle passed easily through the bag to the target.

SAMPLE HANDLING

The cytologic sample should be placed onto a microscope slide. Disconnecting the needle from the syringe and filling it with air usually facilitates this (see Fine-Needle Aspiration). The needle is then reattached, and a rapid expulsion of the air in the syringe will force the cellular sample in the hub of the needle onto a microscope slide.

APPROPRIATE AFTERCARE

Post-Procedure Patient Monitoring

The patient should be monitored immediately after the procedure in order to verify that significant hemorrhage is not occurring. This may be more common in patients with ascites. The duration of monitoring is variable depending on the individual patient and its specific problems.

Nursing Care

None

Dietary Modification

None

Medication Requirements

None

Restrictions on Activity

None typically needed.

Anticipated Recovery Time

Immediately

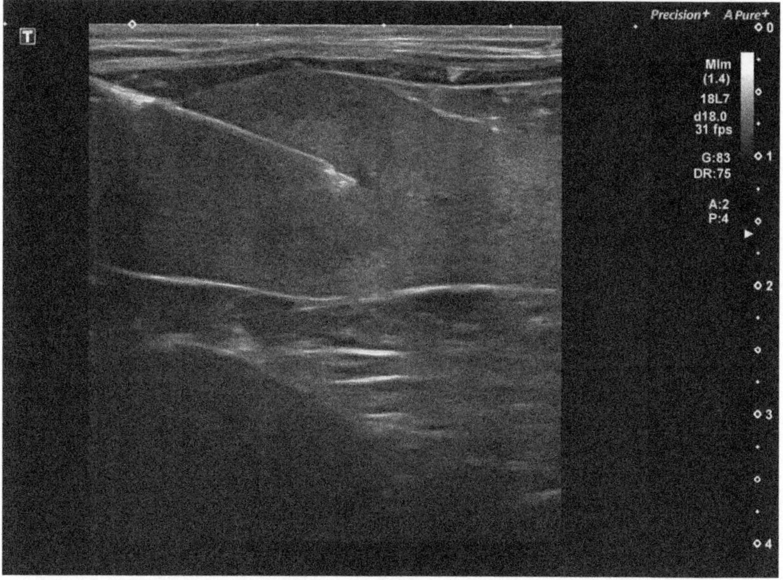

Figure 2.

Image obtained during aspiration of focal splenic thickening. The needle is especially conspicuous because the lesion is close to the skin surface, a high-frequency tranducer was used, the needle angle is acute, and the needle is wholly within the plane of the ultrasound beam. Real-time scanning during the procedure can compensate for less optimal imaging conditions, usually allowing adequate needle visualization. Source: Lawrence P. Tilley

INTERPRETATION

NORMAL FINDINGS OR RANGE

N/A

ABNORMAL FINDINGS

N/A

CRITICAL VALUES

N/A

INTERFERING FACTORS

Drugs That May Alter Results of the Procedure

The use of opioids and other drugs that cause splenomegaly should be avoided because they may compromise the procedure.

Conditions That May Interfere with Performing the Procedure

- A lesion that is surrounded by air or bone and cannot be visualized by using ultrasound.
- Patient noncompliance.

Procedure Techniques or Handling That May Alter Results

- Excessive hemodilution or rough handling of the cellular material may result in a nondiagnostic sample.
- If appropriate orientation of the needle with the ultrasound plane is not maintained, the needle might not be visualized in the ultrasound image and inappropriate sampling may occur.
- Fluid within a cavitated mass or cystic lesion may not contain diagnostic cells.

Influence of Signalment on Performing and Interpreting the Procedure

Species
None

Breed
None

Age
None

Gender
None

Pregnancy
None

CLINICAL PERSPECTIVE

- Percutaneous ultrasound-guided mass or organ aspiration should be used to help further define the etiology of an infiltrative process or mass.
- This procedure is quick and generally safe when performed by an experienced practitioner.
- Both active aspiration and nonaspiration techniques may be necessary to obtain a diagnostic sample.

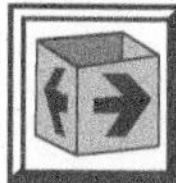

MISCELLANEOUS

ANCILLARY TESTS

If the cytologic sample is nondiagnostic, then a needle biopsy sample may be obtained by using the same principles as for obtaining a cytologic sample. Typically, sedation or general anesthesia is required for this procedure.

ULTRASOUND-GUIDED MASS OR ORGAN ASPIRATION (CONTINUED)

SYNONYMS

None

SEE ALSO

Fine-Needle Aspiration (in Appendix X).

ABBREVIATIONS

None

Suggested Reading

Nyland TG, Mattoon JS, Herrgesell EJ, Wisner ER. Ultrasound-guided biopsy. In: Nyland TG, Mattoon JS, eds., Small Animal Diagnostic Ultrasound, 2nd ed. Philadelphia, PA: W.B. Saunders, 2002, pp. 30–48.

Nyland TG, Wallack ST, Wisner ER. Needle-tract implantation following us-guided fine-needle aspiration biopsy of transitional cell carcinoma of the bladder, urethra, and prostate. Vet Radiol Ultrasound 2002, 43:50–53.

Pennick DG, Finn-Bodner ST. Updates in interventional ultrasonography. Vet Clin North Am Small Anim Pract 1998, 28:1017–1040.

Samii VF, Nyland TG, Werner LL, Baker TW. Ultrasound-guided fine-needle aspiration biopsy of bone lesions: a preliminary report. Vet Radiol Ultrasound 1999, 40:82–86.

Author Mason Holland

Consulting Editor Benjamin M Brainard

Acknowledgment The author and editor acknowledge the prior contribution of Ann Bahr.

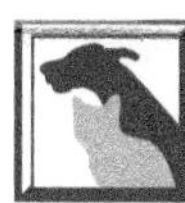

BASICS

TYPE OF PROCEDURE

Diagnostic sample collection.

PROCEDURE EXPLANATION AND RELATED PHYSIOLOGY

- Urinalysis is part of the minimum database for evaluation of ill dogs and cats and for routine health screening of all patients:
  - Sterile sample collection is required for culture and sensitivity testing of urine when infectious cystitis is suspected.
  - In those cases where cystocentesis is contraindicated or unsuccessful at obtaining urine, urethral catheterization enables sterile urine samples to be collected with minimal risk to patients.
- Patients in need of exact calculation of urine output (e.g., those with anuric or oliguric renal failure), patients with functional or mechanical urethral obstruction, and many recumbent animals often require intermittent or indwelling urinary catheterization as part of their management plan.
- Urethral catheterization is required in order to perform other diagnostic procedures such as prostatic wash, cystourethrography, and voiding or catheter-assisted hydropropulsion of uroliths.

INDICATIONS

- Sterile urine collection when cystocentesis is contraindicated.
- Temporary relief of urethral obstructions.
- Collection of urine for fluid-output determination or metabolic testing (e.g., 24 hour collection of urine for calculation of electrolyte excretion).
- Management of recumbent patients.

CONTRAINDICATIONS

Severe vaginitis or balanoposthitis.

POTENTIAL COMPLICATIONS

- Iatrogenic bacterial or fungal cystitis.
- Urethral trauma (perforations or tears, stricture formation).

CLIENT EDUCATION

None

BODY SYSTEMS ASSESSED

Renal/urologic

PROCEDURE

PATIENT PREPARATION

Pre-Procedure Medication or Preparation

None

Anesthesia or Sedation

- Male dogs typically require minimal to no sedation.
- Female dogs and both male and female cats usually require heavy sedation or anesthesia.
- Hydropulsion of urethral obstructive materials is frequently most successful in a very relaxed animal; in difficult cases, the deepening of sedation or even general anesthesia may allow catheterization.

Patient Positioning

- Male dogs—lateral recumbency.
- Male cats—dorsal recumbency.
- Female dogs and cats—sternal recumbency with their legs tucked underneath or extended over the edge of a table.

Patient Monitoring

None

Equipment or Supplies

- Hair clippers.
- Diluted povidone-iodine (Betadine) or chlorhexidine solution: 1 part povidone-iodine or chlorhexidine solution to ≈200 parts sterile saline.
- A sterile 12-mL syringe.
- Sterile gloves.
- Sterile lubricating jelly.
- Two sets of 4 × 4-inch gauze sponges soaked in sterile saline and chlorhexidine or povidone-iodine solution.
- Povidone-iodine scrub should not be used on the genital mucous membranes.
- A sterile urinary catheter (Foley catheter, red rubber catheter (polyurethane or silicone), tomcat (polypropylene), or slippery sam (polytetrafluroethylene) catheter of appropriate size). If using a Foley catheter, inflate the balloon prior to catheterization to assess for leaks:
  - Polyurethane, silicone, and polytetrafluroethylene catheters are softer and likely to be better tolerated than the stiffer polypropylene catheters for long-term catheterization.
- In female dogs, if the visualization method is being used:
  - A disinfected vaginal speculum.
  - A light source.
- If the urinary catheter will be indwelling:
  - A closed collection system.
  - Materials for anchoring the catheter to the patient (e.g., bandage tape, suture material).

TECHNIQUE

Male Dogs

- For indwelling catheters, clip the hair on the distal one-third of the prepuce. Clipping the hair on the ventral abdomen around the preputial opening to a distance of 2–5 cm may also reduce the risk of iatrogenic infection.
- Flush the prepuce 3–5 times with 2–12 mL of dilute povidone-iodine solution (the volume depends on the size of dog) by using the sterile syringe.
- An assistant should exteriorize the penis. This is best done with the assistant standing at the dog's back (while the animal is in lateral recumbency), and the individual placing the catheter standing at the dog's ventrum.
- Clean the extruded penis with sterile 4 × 4-inch gauze sponges, alternating between chlorhexidine or povidone-iodine solution and sterile saline. A minimum of three scrubs should be performed with each solution.
- Flush the penis with 2–5 mL of dilute povidone-iodine solution.
- After donning sterile gloves, coat the distal catheter with lubricating jelly. Using sterile technique, insert the urinary catheter. The catheter should be gently advanced until urine is seen in the distal end of the catheter. Some resistance may be encountered when the catheter passes around the ischial arch, but gentle pressure is usually sufficient to overcome this. Care should be taken not to advance the catheter too far into the bladder because in rare cases the catheter may knot inside the bladder, making removal difficult.
- For patients with urethral obstruction, pulsative flushing of small volumes (1–2 mL) of sterile saline through the catheter may distend the urethra and retropulse the obstructive material into the bladder, facilitating catheterization.
- Red rubber catheters can be used for indwelling or intermittent catheters in male dogs, but Foley catheters are preferred for indwelling catheters:
  - If a Foley catheter is used, inflate the bulb with sterile saline after the catheter has been advanced to the bladder.
- Immediately connect a sterile, closed collection system to the indwelling catheter.
- Anchor the indwelling catheter as needed to prevent displacement:
  - Most common method is to place bandage tape around the catheter ≈2–4 cm cranial to the preputial opening, with tabs on either side. Sutures are then passed through the tabs and attached to the body wall.

Female Dogs

- Clip the hair around the vulva, including the perineal area, to a distance of 2–5 cm from the vulva.
- Scrub the vulva and perivulvar area with sterile 4 × 4-inch gauze sponges, alternating between chlorhexidine or povidone-iodine solution and sterile saline. A minimum of three scrubs should be performed with each solution.
- Flush the vaginal vault 3–5 times with 2–12 mL of dilute povidone-iodine or chlorhexidine solution (the volume depends on the size of dog) by using the sterile syringe.
- Sterile lidocaine jelly can be flushed into the vulva using a clean, lubricated syringe with the needle removed.
- Visualization technique:
  - After donning sterile gloves, insert the vaginal speculum with its handles pointing

URETHRAL CATHETERIZATION

dorsally. The speculum is then advanced dorsally and cranially over the pelvic brim and spread until the urethral papilla and urethral orifice are seen (see Figure 1).
  - Visualization is improved by use of a speculum with an attached light source or a headlamp or by an assistant who stands behind the individual placing the catheter and illuminates the vaginal vault with the light source.
  - The urethral papilla is on the ventral midline of the vaginal floor, distal to the cervix (Figure 1).
  - Coat the catheter with the lubricating jelly and then, using sterile technique, place the urinary catheter. Foley catheters are preferred for indwelling catheters. Red rubber catheters, though they can be used in female dogs, are easier to dislodge than in male dogs because a significantly shorter length of the catheter is inserted. Inflate the balloon if a Foley catheter is used and gently retract the catheter until the balloon is seated in the bladder trigone.
- Digital palpation technique:
  - After donning sterile gloves, lubricate the index finger of the nondominant hand and insert into the vaginal vault, advancing cranially and dorsally over the pelvic brim until the urethral papilla is palpated at the fingertip.
  - Coat the distal catheter with the lubricating jelly and then, using sterile technique, place the urinary catheter. The catheter should be advanced along the ventral aspect of the inserted index finger and then guided into the urethral orifice by palpation.
- A blind placement technique as described below for female cats may be necessary for very small dogs.
- Use of a stylet may increase rigidity of the catheter facilitating placement into the urethral orifice. If a stylet is used it should be kept fully within the catheter to prevent trauma to the urethra.
- For patients with urethral obstruction, pulsatile flushing of small volumes (1–2 mL) of sterile saline through the catheter may distend the urethra and retropulse the obstructive material into the bladder, facilitating catheterization.
- Anchor the urinary catheter to prevent displacement. Bandage tape can be used as described previously for male dogs, suturing the catheter to the body wall ventral to the vulva. Alternatively, if a Foley catheter was used, the balloon will anchor the catheter in the bladder, and the catheter/collection system may be stabilized using tape to the dog's tail, or to an area just above the hock, to avoid fecal contamination and inadvertent removal.

Male Cats

- A coccygeal epidural block may provide analgesia to the perineum, penis and urethra, and can facilitate catheterization in cats with urethral obstruction:
  - With the patient in sternal recumbency, palpate the space on dorsal midline between the sacrum and first coccygeal vertebrae. Moving the tail up and down may help to identify this landmark as the sacrum is immobile but the coccygeal vertebrae will be mobile when the tail is manipulated.
  - Clip the fur over this site and prepare it aseptically.
  - Wearing sterile gloves, palpate and reconfirm the location of the space between the sacrum and the first coccygeal vertebrae. Slowly insert a 25-gauge, 5/8-inch needle on midline at a 30–45° angle into the epidural space.
  - Attach a 1 mL slip-tip syringe and gently aspirate; if blood is aspirated the needle should be removed and repositioned.
  - If no blood is aspirated, slowly infuse 0.1 mL/kg of 2% lidocaine into the epidural space. If the needle was correctly positioned, little resistance should be noted.
  - Following injection, withdraw the needle and assess for relaxation of the rectum and tail.

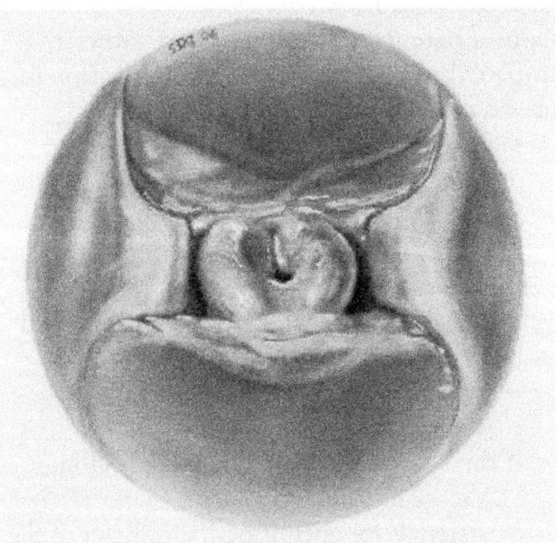

Figure 1.

The vaginal vault of a female dog, as viewed during urethral catheterization. The urethral papilla with central orifice is located on the ventral midline. Source: Lawrence P. Tilley

- A coccygeal epidural block is contraindicated in patients with thrombocytopenia, coagulopathy, hypotension, skin disease at the injection site, or when anatomic abnormalities are present.

• Clip the hair around the prepuce, including the perineal area, to a distance of 1–2 cm from the preputial opening.
• Tomcat catheters (open-ended) can be used for intermittent catheterization; open-ended catheters or catheters with a removable stylet are the preferred catheter for relieving urethral obstruction in male cats. Red rubber catheters or Foley catheters (close-ended) should be used for indwelling urinary catheters.
• An assistant should exteriorize the penis, which is best done with the assistant standing at the cat's head or side (while the animal is in dorsal recumbency).
• Proper exteriorizing of the penis is critical for successful passage of urinary catheters in male cats. Gentle pressure at the base of the prepuce will cause the penis to extrude.
• The penis should be completely exteriorized and pointed caudally, parallel to the spine. Attempting to pass the urinary catheter when the penis is not at the correct angle increases the risk of significant urethral trauma and will prevent the catheter from passing:

- Clean the extruded penis with sterile 4 × 4-inch gauze sponges, alternating between chlorhexidine or povidone-iodine solution and sterile saline. A minimum of three scrubs should be performed with each solution.
- After donning sterile gloves, coat the distal catheter with lubricating jelly.
- Using sterile technique, place the urinary catheter. The catheter should be gently advanced until urine is seen in the distal end of the catheter, taking care not to advance the catheter too far into the bladder.
- It may be necessary to grasp the prepuce and apply caudal traction while advancing the catheter to straighten the urethra to allow passage.
- For patients with urethral obstruction, pulsatile flushing of small volumes (1–2 mL) of sterile saline through the catheter may distend the urethra and retropulse the obstructive material into the bladder, facilitating catheterization.
- If the bladder is already distended due to obstruction, it may be necessary to perform cystocentesis to relieve back pressure and allow infusion of saline and placement of the catheter.

• Immediately connect a sterile, closed collection system for indwelling catheters.
• Anchor the catheter as needed to prevent displacement. In addition to this anchor, red rubber catheters are frequently secured with tape to the cat's tail ≈4–6 cm caudal to the anus.

Female Cats

• Clip the hair around the vulva, including the perineal area, to a distance of 1–2 cm from the vulva.
• Scrub the vulva and perivulvar area with sterile 4 × 4-inch gauze sponges, alternating between chlorhexidine or povidone-iodine solution and sterile saline. A minimum of three scrubs should be performed with each solution.
• Flush the vaginal vault 3–5 times with 0.5–2.0 mL of dilute povidone-iodine solution (the volume depends on the size of cat) by using the sterile syringe.
• Urethral catheterization of female cats is performed blindly.
• After donning sterile gloves, coat the distal catheter with the lubricating jelly. With the cat in sternal recumbency and its legs extended (which is most easily done with the legs allowed to dangle from the edge of a table), the catheter is inserted into the vulva and advanced slowly. The catheter usually enters the bladder without difficulty.
• For patients with urethral obstruction, pulsatile flushing of small volumes (1–2 mL) of sterile saline through the catheter may distend the urethra and retropulse the obstructive material into the bladder, facilitating catheterization.
• Tomcat catheters can be used for intermittent catheterization. Red rubber catheters should be used for indwelling urinary catheters due to the softer material.
• Anchor the catheter as needed to prevent displacement. The most common method is to place bandage tape around the catheter ≈2–4 cm cranial to the vaginal opening, with tabs on either side. Sutures are then passed through the tabs and attached to the body wall.

SAMPLE HANDLING

• Samples collected for urinalysis should be analyzed immediately if possible; refrigeration for later analysis can alter some dipstick and sediment findings.
• Urine samples collected for culture should be refrigerated, ideally in a culture transport vial, until plated onto appropriate media.

APPROPRIATE AFTERCARE

Post-Procedure Patient Monitoring

None

Nursing Care

Indwelling urinary catheters should be kept clean. The external portion of the catheter should be cleaned every 24 hours (or more frequently, as needed) with 4 × 4-inch gauze soaked in chlorhexidine or povidone-iodine solution and sterile saline.

Dietary Modification

None

Medication Requirements

• Prophylactic antibiotics for the prevention of urinary tract infection should not be administered to patients with indwelling urinary catheters. This practice increases the risk of hospital-acquired resistant infections and has not been shown to prevent infection.
• Animals with indwelling urinary catheters should have urine cultured at the time of catheter removal. Bacterial colonization of indwelling urinary catheters is possible, and therefore urine culture results drawn from indwelling catheters should be interpreted with caution.

Restrictions on Activity

Elizabethan collars should be placed on nonrecumbent patients with indwelling catheters.

Anticipated Recovery Time

Immediate

INTERPRETATION

NORMAL FINDINGS OR RANGE

N/A

ABNORMAL VALUES

N/A

CRITICAL VALUES

Urethral obstruction that cannot be relieved by urethral catheterization requires surgical intervention, although deeper anesthesia combined with cystocentesis may allow relaxation and catheterization.

INTERFERING FACTORS

Drugs That May Alter Results of the Procedure

Drugs that increase urethral tone (e.g., phenylpropanolamine, di-ethylstilbestrol) may theoretically make catheterization more difficult. However, this is likely not clinically significant.

Conditions That May interfere with Performing the Procedure

• Urethral obstruction by masses, inflammation, urethrospasm, urethroliths, matrix and mucous plugs, stricture, or extramural masses.
• Pelvic trauma.

Procedure Techniques or Handling That May Alter Results

Loss of sterility or contamination of the catheter during placement predisposes patients to development of iatrogenic urinary tract infection.

Influence of Signalment on Performing and interpreting the Procedure

Species

See the Technique section.

URETHRAL CATHETERIZATION (CONTINUED)

Breed
None

Age
Placement of urinary catheters in neonatal or pediatric patients can be very difficult. Red rubber catheters are ideal because they are less likely to cause iatrogenic trauma during placement.

Gender
See the Technique section.

Pregnancy
None

CLINICAL PERSPECTIVE

- Urethral catheterization is underused as a method for obtaining sterile urine samples, particularly in those patients where repeated cystocentesis attempts are unsuccessful at obtaining a urine sample.
- If urine is being collected for culture, the first 3–10 mL of urine drawn from the catheter should be discarded, after which the sample for culture is collected. This is recommended because the distal urethra and vaginal vault are not sterile environments and often cause some contamination of the catheter tip during placement and because indwelling catheters may have bacterial colonization of the catheter lumen.

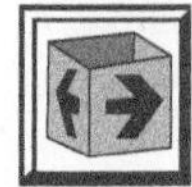

MISCELLANEOUS

ANCILLARY TESTS

- Prostatic wash.
- Urinalysis.
- Urine culture.
- Contrast cystourethrogram.

SYNONYMS

- Bladder catheterization.
- Indwelling urinary catheter.
- Urinary catheterization.

SEE ALSO

- Acute Kidney Injury.
- Urinary Tract Obstruction.
- Bacterial Culture and Sensitivity (in Appendix X).
- Urinalysis Overview (in Appendix X).

Suggested Reading

O'Hearn AK, Wright BD. Coccygeal epidural with local anesthetic for catheterization and pain management in the treatment of feline urethral obstruction. J Vet Emerg Crit Care 2011, 21(1):50–52.

Smarick SD, Haskins SC, Aldrich J, et al. Incidence of catheter-associated urinary tract infection among dogs in a small animal intensive care unit. J Am Vet Med Assoc 2004, 224:1936–1940.

Author Vincent J. Thawley

Consulting Editor Benjamin M. Brainard

Acknowledgment The author and editors acknowledge the prior contribution of Barak M. Pressler.

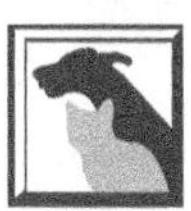

BASICS

TYPE OF SPECIMEN

Urine

TEST EXPLANATION AND RELATED PHYSIOLOGY

A urinalysis (UA) is a basic diagnostic screening test that is easy to perform, relatively inexpensive, and can be useful in evaluating renal/urologic and nonrenal conditions. A complete UA includes the following components:

- Physical characteristics: volume, odor, color, transparency, and solute concentration (e.g., urine specific gravity [USG]).
- Chemical characteristics: presence of bilirubin, blood, glucose, ketones, pH, and protein. Some tests available on dipsticks (e.g., urobilinogen, nitrite, leukocytes, esterase, USG) may be unreliable, of no value, or not validated for veterinary species.
- Microscopic evaluation of urine sediment: cells, crystals, casts, organisms, and other (e.g., sperm, lipid, mucus).

INDICATIONS

- UA, part of the minimum data base, is used in conjunction with complete blood count (CBC) and clinical chemistry to establish baseline for initial workup.
- Assessment of kidney function: concentrating ability of solutes (e.g., USG); filtering and resorptive handling of electrolytes, protein, glucose; and response to acid–base imbalance.
- Detection of hemorrhage, inflammation, infection, or neoplasia in the urinary or genital tract.
- Evaluation of systemic disorders or diseases.

CONTRAINDICATIONS

None

POTENTIAL COMPLICATIONS

Hemorrhage or inadvertent enterocentesis can occur with cystocentesis.

CLIENT EDUCATION

If an owner collects urine, it should be put into a clean container free of any type of contaminant (e.g., detergents or disinfectants).

BODY SYSTEMS ASSESSED

- Endocrine and metabolic.
- Hemic, lymphatic, and immune.
- Hepatobiliary.
- Musculoskeletal.
- Renal and urologic.
- Reproductive.

SAMPLE

SAMPLE COLLECTION

5–10 mL of urine collected by free catch of a voided sample, manual expression of the urinary bladder, catheterization, or cystocentesis.

SAMPLE HANDLING

- Collect urine into a clean, dry container with a tight-fitting lid and free of potential contaminants (e.g., detergents, disinfectants). It should be labeled with appropriate information (e.g., patient and owner identification; date, time, and method of collection).
- Results are most accurate if urine is analyzed within 30–60 minutes after collection.
- The sample should be refrigerated if a delay in analysis is unavoidable.
- Refrigerated samples should be warmed to room temperature before analysis.

SAMPLE STORAGE

- Refrigeration can slow sample deterioration. The container should protect the sample from light and have a tight-fitting lid.
- Refrigeration may alter some results (e.g., increased crystal formation).
- Avoid freezing the urine because this will affect certain tests (e.g., urine sediment examination).
- Preservatives generally adversely affect chemical assays. No single preservative suits all testing requirements.

SAMPLE STABILITY

Components analyzed in urine sediment (i.e., cells, casts, crystals, bacteria) deteriorate rapidly (within 2–4 hours). Over time, CO_2 is lost from the stored sample, increasing pH, and bilirubin may degrade with exposure to light or spontaneously oxidize (stable for up to 12 hours refrigerated). Most other chemical tests are stable for 12 hours in a refrigerated sample.

PROTOCOL

- Mix the sample and transfer it to a centrifuge tube.
- Evaluate the physical features of the urine (i.e., volume, odor, color, turbidity).
- Determine the USG by using a refractometer.
- Measure urine analytes by using a reagent strip:
  - Immerse a reagent strip into well-mixed, room-temperature urine and turn the strip on its side, tapping away excess urine.
  - Examine the color change of each analyte at the time indicated by the manufacturer and compare the color change to the reference chart.
  - Confirmatory tests are affected less by urine color and may be warranted to confirm specific dipstick analyte results. Such tests include the Ictotest® (Siemens, Tarrytown, NY) for bilirubin, the K-CHECK® (Biorex Labs, Cleveland, OH) for ketones, and sulfosalicylic acid test (SSA) for protein.
  - Automated dipstick readers are available.
- Centrifuge the sample for 5–10 minutes at low RPM in a conical tube:
  - Ideally, the same volume of urine should be centrifuged each time, and reference values are based on 5 mL of urine. Analysis of smaller urine volume should be noted on the final report because that can result in less sediment.
  - The recommended RPM is quite variable (500–3,000 RPM) because it is actually gravitation force (*g*-force) that is important. A *g*-force of 450×*g* is recommended. See Internet Resources for a conversion program between RPM and *g*-force.
  - Excessively high-speed centrifugation can distort cells or fragment fragile elements such as casts.
- Use urine supernatant to measure protein by the SSA method. If urine is bloody or extremely cloudy, double check the USG by using supernatant.
- Decant the supernatant, leaving ≈0.5 mL of urine sediment.
- Resuspend the sediment and transfer a drop to a microscope slide.
- Coverslip and examine the sample microscopically at 10× and 40× (see Urine Sediment).

INTERPRETATION

NORMAL FINDINGS OR RANGE

- Fresh urine should be relatively clear, yellow, and have a slight ammonia odor. Intact male cat urine may have a strong odor.
- The USG should be evaluated based on the hydration status. In general, the urine concentration from a random urine sample is considered adequate if the USG is >1.035 and >1.040 in dogs and cats, respectively, although USG can vary significantly depending on the state of hydration in normal animals.
- Normal urine should have a pH between 6.0 and 7.5, and should be negative for protein, ketones, blood, bilirubin, and glucose. Some dogs with highly concentrated urine may show a trace to 1+ reaction for bilirubin and/or protein.

URINALYSIS OVERVIEW (CONTINUED)

• Urine sediment should contain few cells and crystals and no casts. Lipid is seen occasionally in cat urine.

ABNORMAL FINDINGS

• USG should be greater than 1.030 in patients with azotemia. Consistently isosthenuric urine in non-azotemic animals may reflect renal or nonrenal disease. Hyposthenuria (USG <1.008) indicates an inability to concentrate secondary to a nonrenal disease (e.g., diabetes insipidus) because a functional kidney must be present to dilute the urine below isosthenuria.
• Urine pH should mirror the blood pH; in academic patients with alkaline urine, consideration should be given to urinary bicarbonate loss (renal tubular acidosis) or urinary tract infection with urease-producing bacteria. Many drugs and prescription diets can either raise or lower the urinary pH, and a complete history should be taken to put urinalysis results into context.
• Urine glucose may be elevated due to persistent or paroxysmal hyperglycemia (see Hyperglycemia), and should be interpreted in concert with the serum glucose. Some renal tubular defects will also result in persistent glucosuria without hyperglycemia (e.g., Fanconi's syndrome).
• Urine ketones will be elevated in states of ketonemia, (e.g., diabetic ketoacidosis, starvation). Because the strip only detects acetoacetate and acetone, animals with beta-hydroxybutyrate ketonemia may generate a negative test.
• Urine protein in urine with inactive sediment may be indicative of glomerular or renal tubular disease or hereditary glomerulopathy. Proteinuria is an appropriate condition accompanying urinary tract inflammation or infection. Proteinuria in inactive urine samples should be further investigated through the measurement of a urine protein:creatinine ratio.
• Urine bilirubin is found in concentrated canine urine samples in small amounts, but should not be found in dilute canine urine or feline urine. Its presence generally indicates elevated serum bilirubin concentration and may be due to any systemic causes of hyperbilirubinemia (hepatic, prehepatic, or posthepatic).
• Urine heme protein is positive in the presence of hemoglobin, myoglobin, or red blood cells, and as such may indicate systemic disease or hemolysis, or urinary tract hemorrhage, which can result from thrombocytopenia, neoplasia, or cystitis, among other conditions. Pigmenturia may be differentiated from hematuria through centrifugation of a urine sample, wherein the red blood cells will be pelleted, while pigment will remain in the supernatant.

CRITICAL VALUES

Variable depending on assay; diabetic ketoacidosis requires emergency care, and animals with significant proteinuria and azotemia may be at risk for complications associated with protein-losing nephropathies. Pigmenturia/hematuria may be indicative of life-threatening coagulopathy, hemolysis, or other diseases associated with anemia or muscle damage (e.g., heat stroke, crotalid envenomation).

INTERFERING FACTORS

Drugs That May Alter Results or Interpretation

Drugs That Interfere With Test Methodology

Certain drugs or metabolites excreted into the urine may impart characteristic odors. Hydroxethyl starch and radiographic contrast agents can alter USG measurements; radiographic contrast agents can also interfere with some biochemical analytes or cause crystal formation. Cephalexin, tetracycline, and vitamin C therapy may be associated with false-positive readings for urine glucose.

Collection Techniques or Handling That May Alter Results

• Method of collection can influence findings:
  ◦ Voided and free catch samples or samples obtained by manual expression contain components from lower urogenital tract and may have increased bacteria, epithelial cells, or leukocytes.
  ◦ Cystocentesis samples may be contaminated with iatrogenic hemorrhage.
  ◦ Samples from catheterization can contain increased bacteria, and/or epithelial cells, reflect iatrogenic hemorrhage, or be contaminated with lubricant.
  ◦ Samples obtained from a surface (e.g., floor, examination table, cage) may contain bacteria, debris, or other environmental contaminants.

• Reagent strips should be stored at room temperature in the original container; protected from excessive light, moisture, and heat; not used past the expiration date; and discarded if any of the pads on the strips are discolored.

LIMITATIONS OF TEST

• The ketone reagent pad is only sensitive for detecting acetoacetate and acetone, so if a patient has beta-hydroxybutyrate ketonuria, this will not be detected, but can be measured in the blood using hand-held devices (See Diabetes Mellitus with Ketoacidosis).
• Pigmenturia of any cause may interfere with reading the colorimetric results.

Valid If Run in a Human Lab?

Yes.

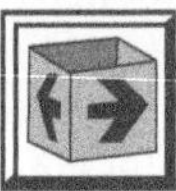

MISCELLANEOUS

ANCILLARY TESTS

Urine protein:creatinine (UPC) ratio is indicated if proteinuria is observed with an inactive sediment (i.e., no hematuria, pyuria, or bacteriuria).

ABBREVIATIONS

• SSA = sulfosalicylic acid.
• UA = urinalysis.
• UPC = urine protein:creatinine ratio.
• USG = urine specific gravity.

INTERNET RESOURCES

• http://eclinpath.com/urinalysis/
• Kobuta, Laboratory Centrifuge: *g*-force calculation: http://www.centrifuge.jp/calculation/

Suggested Reading

Callens AJ, Bartges JW. Urinalysis. Vet Clin Small Anim 2015, 45:621–637.
Chew DJ, DiBartola SP. Urinalysis interpretation. In: Interpretation of Canine and Feline Urinalysis. Wilmington, DE: Ralston Purina, 1998, pp. 15–33.
Osborne CA, Stevens JB. Proteinuria. In: Urinalysis: A Clinical Guide to Compassionate Patient Care. Leverkusen, Germany: Bayer, 1999, pp. 111–121.

Author Karen E. Russell
Consulting Editor Benjamin M. Brainard

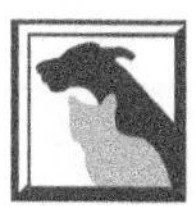

BASICS

TYPE OF SPECIMEN

Urine

TEST EXPLANATION AND RELATED PHYSIOLOGY

- Microscopic evaluation of urine is recommended on every urine sample, even when physical characteristics or the results from a urine dipstick are unremarkable.
- Components evaluated include cells, crystals, casts, organisms, and other elements (e.g., lipid, mucus):
  - Erythrocytes can enter the urine anywhere in the urologic tract (i.e., kidneys, ureters, bladder, urethra) or genital tract.
  - Neutrophils are the common leukocyte found in urine, but macrophages and lymphocytes can also be present.
  - Epithelial cells include renal tubular cells, transitional cells, and squamous cells. Neoplastic cells are sometimes detected.
  - Formation of crystals depends on urine pH and concentration (i.e., urine specific gravity [USG]) and the presence of oversaturated crystalogenic substances.
    - Diet and some drugs may also influence crystal formation.
    - The presence of crystals suggests an increased risk of urolithiasis, but it does not predict which animals may actually form uroliths or the type of urolith that may form.
  - Casts originate in the tubular lumen and are composed of mucoprotein, cells, and cellular debris. The presence of casts may indicate renal proteinuria (hyaline) or tubular degeneration (cellular and/or granular).

INDICATIONS

- Microscopic examination of urine sediment is part of a routine urinalysis (UA).
- Many of the chemical results (e.g., urine heme protein, protein) should be interpreted in conjunction with the sediment findings.
- Part of the workup in an animal exposed to a nephrotoxic substance or in those with stranguria or pollakiuria.

CONTRAINDICATIONS

None

POTENTIAL COMPLICATIONS

None

CLIENT EDUCATION

Urine sediment is critical in diagnosing urinary tract infections.

BODY SYSTEMS ASSESSED

- Hemic, lymphatic, and immune.
- Hepatobiliary.
- Renal and urologic.

SAMPLE

SAMPLE COLLECTION

- 5–10 mL of urine collected by free catch of a voided sample, manual expression of the urinary bladder, catheterization, or cystocentesis. The method of collection may affect sediment makeup.
- It is important that a consistent volume of urine is used for sediment evaluation. This will enable findings to be semiquantitative and compared with reference values, and enable monitoring of the animal's response to treatment.

SAMPLE HANDLING

- Collect the urine into a clean container free of additives, detergents, and chemicals.
- Ideally, the assay should be performed within an hour after collection.

SAMPLE STORAGE

- Refrigeration can aid in slowing cellular breakdown, but it enhances crystal formation. If refrigerated, sample should be warmed to room temperature before analysis.
- Do not freeze the urine.

SAMPLE STABILITY

Components analyzed in urine sediment (i.e., cells, casts, crystals, bacteria) do not hold up well in urine. Cells may lyse, and casts can break down. Crystals can dissolve or new crystals may form. Bacteria may die or multiply:

- Casts begin to deteriorate within 2 hours.
- Cells can lyse or lose morphologic characteristics within 2–4 hours, depending on urine osmolality.

PROTOCOL

- A standard volume of urine (usually 5 mL) is centrifuged at a slow speed.
- The supernatant is removed and saved for biochemical or other tests.
- The pellet is gently resuspended in a small amount of urine (≈1 mL), and a small drop is placed onto a glass slide with a coverslip.
- Microscopic examination is done at a low magnification (10× objective; low-power field [LPF]) and a high magnification (40× objective; high-power field [HPF]) with the condenser of the microscope lowered so that contrast is increased.
- Several components are quantified by the number per LPF (i.e., casts) or HPF (i.e., cells).
- Other components such as crystals, bacteria or other organisms, lipid, and mucus are either graded as present or absent or graded on a few (1+), moderate (2+), or many (3+) scale.
- Staining the urine sediment with a commercial, water-based stain or new methylene blue before examination may aid in identifying constituents and accentuate cellular detail.
- A cytologic preparation of urine sediment can be made by smearing a drop of sediment on a slide, allowing it to air-dry, and staining it with routine hematologic stains. This technique is useful in evaluating cells and identifying bacteria or other organisms.

INTERPRETATION

NORMAL FINDINGS OR RANGE

- Urine sediment is usually inactive, containing few microscopically visible components, but it is not uncommon to find low numbers of cells or certain types of crystals, depending on method of collection.
- The following may be seen in urine from healthy dogs or cats:
  - WBCs: <2–5/HPF.
  - RBCs: <2–5/HPF.
  - Epithelial cells: <2/HPF.
  - Casts: none or at most a few that are hyaline or granular.
  - Crystals: amorphous phosphate, bilirubin (dogs), calcium oxalate dihydrate, calcium phosphate, and struvite are common in healthy animals. Ammonium biurate, sodium urates, and uric acid crystals are occasionally seen in urine from healthy animals.
  - Bacteria: usually none. Low numbers occasionally are seen in voided samples with genital tract contamination or samples taken from floors, tabletops, or litterboxes.
  - Sperm (intact males).

ABNORMAL FINDINGS

The following are considered abnormal in dogs or cats:

- WBCs: >5/HPF.
- RBCs: >5/HPF.
- Epithelial cells: >5/HPF.
- Casts: the presence of > 1–2/LPF (hyaline, granular) or any cellular (epithelial, RBC, WBC), waxy, fatty, and/or broad casts.
- Crystals: the presence of calcium oxalate monohydrate, ammonium biurate, bilirubin, cholesterol, cystine, leucine, tyrosine, sodium urate, and/or uric acid (see Table 1).

CRITICAL VALUES

None

INTERFERING FACTORS

Drugs That May Alter Results or Interpretation

Drugs That Interfere with Test Methodology

Acidifiers or alkalinizers may modify crystal formation and composition.

Drugs That Alter Physiology

Sulfadiazine and metabolites, ampicillin, allopurinol, and radiopaque contrast agents

URINE SEDIMENT (CONTINUED)

Table 1

Causes of abnormal findings.

Element	*Reference Interval With Lesion Location*	*Etiology*
Cells		
RBCs (hematuria)	<2–5/HPF	May be normal
	>5/HPF	Bleeding or vascular damage associated with glomeruli or tubules, calculi, renal vein thrombosis, vascular dysplasia, trauma, infarct, inflammation, or infection
	Renal	
	Lower urinary tract	Acute or chronic infection, calculi, neoplasia, or hemorrhagic cystitis Voided urine sample from animals in estrus
	Genital tract	
	Iatrogenic	Vessel damage from cystocentesis or catheterization
	Coagulopathy	Thrombocytopenia, thrombocytopathia, von Willebrand disease, or hereditary or acquired coagulopathies
WBCs (pyuria)	<2–5/HPF	May be normal
	>5/HPF	Inflammation from noninfectious causes: pyelonephritis/nephritis, urolithiasis (calculi), neoplasia, or necrosis
	Renal	Inflammation from infectious causes: pyelonephritis/nephritis, bacteria, fungal, or parasitic
	Lower urinary tract	Acute or chronic cystitis (infectious or noninfectious), calculi, neoplasia Voided urine sample with contamination from the prostate, prepuce, or vagina
	Genital tract inflammation	
Epithelial cells	Squamous epithelial cells	Insignificant finding in voided or catheterized samples
	Transitional cells	May be normal or artifact of collection method
	<2/HPF	Hyperplasia secondary to inflammation, infection, or irritation, or due to cyclophosphamide administration
	>5/HPF	
	Neoplastic cells	Transitional cell carcinoma cells occasionally found in urine; caution advised if cellular atypia noted in the presence of inflammation (may be difficult to differentiate hyperplasia from neoplasia)
Crystals (crystalluria)	Type of crystal and typical conditions	Etiology
	Urine pH acidic or neutral Amorphous urate	Formed from yellow precipitates of sodium, potassium, magnesium, or calcium urate salts; normal in dalmatians and English bulldogs; also seen with liver disease or portal vascular anomalies
	Bilirubin	May be seen in healthy dogs, common in dogs with bilirubinemia or abnormal bilirubin metabolism, and uncommon in cats
	Calcium oxalate monohydrate	Common with ethylene glycol toxicosis
	Calcium oxalate dihydrate	Found in healthy dogs and cats, found in animals with uroliths composed mostly of calcium oxalate, and occasionally seen with ethylene glycol toxicosis
	Cystine	Rare; congenital renal tubular defect in reabsorption of cystine from the renal filtrate; cystinuria may result in cystine store for formation
	Sodium urate	May be seen concurrently with ammonium urate crystals Associated with sulfonamide administration
	Sulfa	
	Uric acid	Considered normal in dalmatians and English bulldogs, rarely seen in other healthy animals, and can be seen with liver disease or portal vascular anomalies
Urine pH alkaline and/or neutral		
	Ammonium urate (ammonium biurate)	Portosystemic shunts or hepatic diseases with hyperammonemia, can be seen rarely in healthy animals but are common in dalmatians and English bulldogs
	Amorphous phosphate	Amorphous form of calcium phosphate crystals that resemble amorphous urates; may be seen in healthy dogs and cats

Table 1

Causes of abnormal findings (*Continued*)		
Element	*Reference Interval With Lesion Location*	*Etiology*
	Calcium phosphate	Seen in healthy dogs and in dogs with persistently alkaline urine or with calcium phosphate uroliths
	Struvite (triple phosphate)	Common in cats and dogs with alkaline urine; composed of magnesium, ammonium, and phosphorus
Other crystals		
	Ampicillin	Associated with ampicillin administration
	Cholesterol	Uncommon; associated with cellular membrane deterioration, occasionally seen with some renal diseases, and may be seen in healthy dogs
	Leucine	
	Melamine	Rare, ingestion of food contaminated with melamine
	Tyrosine	Rare; may suggest liver disease
	Xanthine	Rare in dogs; can be associated with liver disease
		Rare; may be seen in animals treated with allopurinol
Casts (cylinduria)	Type of cast	Etiology
	Hyaline	A few can be normal with concentrated urine; >1–2/LPF associated with renal causes of proteinuria
	Cellular WBC	Associated with tubular inflammation, infection (e.g., bacterial pyelonephritis, leptospirosis), or acute tubular necrosis
	Epithelial	Associated with degeneration/necrosis of tubules (e.g., ischemia, toxins, infarct)
	RBC	Rare; associated with hemorrhage into tubules
	Granular	A few can be normal with concentrated urine; >1–2/LPF associated with degeneration/necrosis of tubules (e.g., ischemia, toxins, infarct)
	Fatty	Common in cats with renal tubular degeneration
	Waxy	Associated with chronic degeneration/necrosis of tubules (e.g., ischemia, toxins, infarct)
Bacteria (bacteriuria)		Infection of the urinary tract, infection of the genital tract (voided sample), *in vitro* growth with delayed sample analysis, or contamination (voided and some catheterized samples)
Other organisms	Yeast	Often Candida spp.
	Fungi (hyphae or budding)	Blastomyces spp., Cryptococcus spp., or Aspergillus spp. (German shepherd dogs can have a disseminated infection)
	Nematode ova	Dioctophyma renale or Capillaria plica
	Microfilariae	Seen with significant hematuria
	Algae	
		Prototheca spp. (dogs can have disseminated infection)
Lipids		No clinical significance; may be normal; a common finding in cats
Mucus		Genital secretions, suggestive of urethral irritation; mucous strands may form linear structures resembling casts
Contaminants	Pollen grains	Occasionally found in urine sediment, not significant but may be potentially confused with other constituents
	Sperm	
	Glove powder	
	Fibers	

URINE SEDIMENT (CONTINUED)

(uncommon) have been associated with crystal formation in dogs and cats.

Disorders That May Alter Results

- Casts and cells, especially RBCs, may lyse in poorly concentrated (USG <1.008) or alkaline urine, especially if a sample is several hours old.
- RBCs usually are crenated in highly concentrated urine. This may cause difficulties with identification.

Collection Techniques or Handling That May Alter Results

- Voided samples may contain more cells, have bacterial contamination, or contain material from the genital tract.
- Catheterized samples may contain more RBCs or epithelial cells (transitional or squamous cells) or be contaminated with lubricant.
- Samples obtained by cystocentesis generally have the least potential of contamination but may contain increased RBCs if blood vessels are damaged during urine collection. Inadvertant enterocentesis is uncommon but can occur.
- Refrigeration enhances crystal formation.
- The use of certain urine preservatives may cause in vitro formation of tyrosine-like crystals.
- The use of stain can dilute sediment, lowering counts, and may introduce crystals and/or organisms (i.e., bacteria, yeast) that grow in stain.

Influence of Signalment

Species

- Lipid droplets are common in cats and are of no clinical significance.
- Low numbers of bilirubin crystals are sometimes seen in concentrated urine from healthy dogs.
- Cystinuria with cystine crystal formation is more common in dogs but occurs rarely in cats.

Breed

- Uric acid and ammonium biurate crystals are common in Dalmatians and English bulldogs.
- Cystinuria with cystine crystalluria has been reported in many breeds of dogs, including dachshunds, Newfoundlands, English bulldogs, Scottish deerhounds, mastiffs, and Scottish terriers.

Age

None

Gender

Sperm may be found only in the urine from intact males or recently bred intact females.

Pregnancy

None

LIMITATIONS OF TEST

- Crystals that form *in vitro* have no clinical significance.
- The number of casts is not an indication of the severity, duration, or potential reversibility of the underlying disease. The type of cast rarely denotes a specific diagnosis.
- A normal sediment does not rule out some type of urinary tract disease.

Sensitivity, Specificity, and Positive and Negative Predictive Values

N/A

Valid If Run in a Human Lab?

Yes.

CAUSES OF ABNORMAL FINDINGS

See Table 1.

CLINICAL PERSPECTIVE

- Urine sediment examination should always be part of a routine UA, even if physical and chemical characteristics are unremarkable.
- A standard volume of urine used for sediment examination should be established.
- Chemistry results (e.g., heme protein, protein) should be interpreted with knowledge of urine sediment.
- The urine pH can affect the type of crystals present, and the USG can affect urine sediment.
- The presence of crystals does not necessarily indicate the presence of a urolith, although high concentrations of crystals may predispose an animal to urolith formation. Clinical signs and hematuria may help identify those animals with uroliths.
- Cocci are difficult to identify unless in chains: Brownian movement of tiny particles of debris may resemble cocci. Suspected cocci should be verified by Gram staining an air-dried smear of sediment. Cocci will appear deep purple with a Gram stain, whereas debris/protein will be pink or perhaps colorless.
- Some sediment abnormalities (e.g., casts) can be an early sign of nephrotoxicity seen prior to the onset of serum chemistry abnormalities.
- The absence of pyuria or a failure to detect bacteria does not exclude an occult urinary tract infection. This is particularly common in conditions associated with dilute urine, such as diabetes mellitus and hyperadrenocorticism.

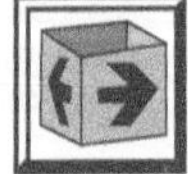

MISCELLANEOUS

ANCILLARY TESTS

- Serum biochemical profile.
- CBC.
- UA (including heme, protein, USG, pH).
- Urine culture.
- Urolith analysis.
- CadetBRAF assay (Antech diagnostics): if urinary tract neoplasia is suspected.

SYNONYMS

None

SEE ALSO

- Crystalluria.
- Cylindruria.
- Dysuria, Pollakiuria, and Stranguria.
- Ethylene Glycol Toxicosis.
- Hematuria.
- Pyuria.
- Transitional Cell Carcinoma.
- Urinalysis Overview (in Appendix X).
- Urolithiasis, Calcium Oxalate.
- Urolithiasis, Calcium Phosphate.
- Urolithiasis, Cystine.
- Urolithiasis, Struvite—Cats.
- Urolithiasis, Struvite—Dogs.
- Urolithiasis, Urate.
- Urolithiasis, Xanthine.

ABBREVIATIONS

- HPF = high-power field (40×).
- LPF = low-power field (10×).
- UA = urinalysis.
- USG = urine specific gravity.

INTERNET RESOURCES

- http://eclinpath.com/urinalysis/cellular-constituents/
- http://www.meddean.luc.edu/lumen/meded/medicine/pulmonar/renal/atlas/urineatlas_f.htm

Suggested Reading

Chew DJ, DiBartola SP. Interpretation of Canine and Feline Urinalysis. Wilmington, DE: Ralston Purina, 1998.

Graff L. A Handbook of Routine Urinalysis. Philadelphia, PA: J.B. Lippincott Company, 1982.

Meyer DJ. Microscopic examination of the urinary sediment. In: Raskin RE, Meyer DJ, eds., Canine and Feline Cytology, 3rd ed. St. Louis, MO: Elsevier, 2016, pp. 295–312.

Mochizuki H, Shapiro SG, Breen M. Detection of BRAF mutation in urine DNA as a molecular diagnostic for canine urothelial and prostatic carcinoma. PLoS One 2015, 10:e0144170.

Osborne CA, Stevens JB. Urine sediment: under the microscope. In: Urinalysis: A Clinical Guide to Compassionate Patient Care. Leverkusen, Germany: Bayer, 1999, pp.125–179.

Webb JL. Renal cytology and urinalysis. In: Small Animal Cytologic Diagnosis. Boca Raton, FL: CRC Press, 2017, pp. 357–377.

Author Karen E. Russell

Consulting Editor Benjamin M. Brainard

APPENDIX XI

CONVERSION TABLES

Table XI-A

Conversion table of weight to body surface area (in square meters) for dogs			
kg	*m²*	*kg*	*m²*
0.5	0.06	26.0	0.88
1.0	0.10	27.0	0.90
2.0	0.15	28.0	0.92
3.0	0.20	29.0	0.94
4.0	0.25	30.0	0.96
5.0	0.29	31.0	0.99
6.0	0.33	32.0	1.01
7.0	0.36	33.0	1.03
8.0	0.40	34.0	1.05
9.0	0.43	35.0	1.07
10.0	0.46	36.0	1.09
11.0	0.49	37.0	1.11
12.0	0.52	38.0	1.13
13.0	0.55	39.0	1.15
14.0	0.58	40.0	1.17
15.0	0.60	41.0	1.19
16.0	0.63	42.0	1.21
17.0	0.66	43.0	1.23
18.0	0.69	44.0	1.25
19.0	0.71	45.0	1.26
20.0	0.74	46.0	1.28
21.0	0.76	47.0	1.30
22.0	0.78	48.0	1.32
23.0	0.81	49.0	1.34
24.0	0.83	50.0	1.36
25.0	0.85		

Although the above chart was compiled for dogs, it can also be used for cats. More precise values are represented in the formula BSA in $m^2 = (K \times W^{2/3}) \times 10^{-4}$; where m^2 = square meters, BSA = body surface area, W = weight in g, and K = constant of 10.1 in dogs and 10.0 in cats.

Table XI-B

Approximate equivalents for degrees Fahrenheit and Celsius*			
°F	*°C*	*°F*	*°C*
0	−17.8	98	36.7
32	0	99	37.2
85	29.4	100	37.8
86	30.0	101	38.3
87	30.6	102	38.9
88	31.1	103	39.4
89	31.7	104	40.0
90	32.2	105	40.6
91	32.7	106	41.1
92	33.3	107	41.7
93	33.9	108	42.2
94	34.4	109	42.8
95	35.0	110	43.3
96	35.5	212	100.0
97	36.1		

* Temperature conversion: °Celsius to °Fahrenheit, (°C) (9/5) + 32°; °Fahrenheit to °Celsius, (°F − 32°) (5/9).

CONVERSION TABLES (*CONTINUED*)

Table XI-C

Weight-unit conversion factors		
Units Given	*Units Wanted*	*For Conversion, Multiply by*
lb	g	453.6
lb	kg	0.4536
oz	g	28.35
kg	lb	2.2046
kg	mg	1,000,000
kg	g	1000
g	mg	1000
g	μg	1,000,000
mg	μg	1000
mg/g	mg/lb	453.6
mg/kg	mg/lb	0.4536
μg/kg	μg/lb	0.4536
Meal	kcal	1000
kcal/kg	kcal/lb	0.4536
kcal/lb	kcal/kg	2.2046
ppm	μg/g	1
ppm	mg/kg	1
ppm	mg/lb	0.4536
mg/kg	%	0.0001
ppm	%	0.0001
mg/g	%	0.1
g/kg	%	0.1

Appendix XII

Important Resources for Veterinarians

ACCREDITATION
- National Veterinary Accreditation Program; www.aphis.usda.gov/nvap

ADVERSE EVENT REPORTING

Submit reports of adverse events associated with animal foods or health products as well as suspected failures of animal health products to the manufacturer and one of the following:
- Drugs and devices: FDA CVM: 888-332-8387; www.fda.gov/AnimalVeterinary
- Pet foods and animal feeds: FDA consumer complaint coordinators; www.fda.gov/Safety/ReportaProblem/ConsumerComplaintCoordinators
- Topical insecticides: National Pesticide Information Center (sponsored by EPA): 800-858-7378; www.npic.orst.edu
- Vaccines/biologics: USDA Center for Veterinary Biologics: 800-752-6255; bit.ly/VetBiologics

ANIMAL DRUGS
- FDA CVM: 240-276-9300; askcvm@fda.hhs.gov; www.fda.gov/drugs; Report shortages of medically necessary veterinary drugs.
- Food Animal Residue Avoidance Databank: 888-873-2723; www.farad.org
  Information on animal drugs and chemicals with the potential to cause foodborne residues (sponsored by the USDA Cooperative State Research, Education and Extension Service)

BLOOD BANKS, RESOURCES
- Animal Blood Resources International: 800-243-5759; www.abrint.net
  A 24-hour hotline focusing on transfusion medicine (particularly blood component therapy), including recommended dosages and infusion rates for canines and felines; no cost to caller
- HEMOPET: 714-891-2022; www.hemopet.org
  A 24-hour national, non-emergency, full service, nonprofit blood bank and educational network for animals
- Plasvacc USA: 805-434-0321; www.plasvaccusa.com
  A commercial blood bank for canines and equines
- Veterinarians Blood Bank: 877-838-8533; www.vetbloodbank.com
  A commercial blood bank for canines and felines
- Association of Veterinary Hematology and Transfusion Medicine: www.avhtm.org
  Additional resources and links

CONTROLLED DRUGS
- DEA Office of Diversion Control; registration: 800-882-9539; www.deadiversion.usdoj.gov

DISASTER AND EMERGENCY RESPONSE
- FEMA Disaster Assistance: 800-621-3362; www.fema.gov

DISEASE OUTBREAKS
- USDA APHIS Emergency Operations Center: www.aphis.usda.gov/emergencyresponse
  Report suspected animal disease outbreaks
- CDC Emergency Operations Center: 800-323-4636; www.cdc.gov/phpr/eoc.htm
- State veterinarians: www.usaha.org/federal-and-stateanimal-health
- State public health veterinarians: http://www.nasphv.org/Documents/StatePublicHealthVeterinariansByState.pdf

FOOD SAFETY
- FDA: 888-463-6332;; www.fda.gov/food
- USDA FSIS: 202-720-9113; www.fsis.usda.gov
- USDA Meat and Poultry Hotline: 888-674-6854; bit.ly/USDAhotline
- American College of Veterinary Nutrition: http://www.acvn.org
- World Small Animal Veterinary Association nutrition toolkit: https://www.wsava.org/nutrition-toolkit

IMPAIRED VETERINARIANS AND VETERINARY TECHNICIANS
- Impaired Veterinarians Resources (sponsored by the AVMA): 800-248-2862, Ext. 6738; https://www.avma.org/ProfessionalDevelopment/PeerAndWellness/Pages/default.aspx

(Continued)

IMPORTANT RESOURCES FOR VETERINARIANS (*CONTINUED*)

PET LOSS SUPPORT—GRIEF COUNSELING

- Chicago VMA: 630-325-1600; https://www.chicagovma.org/pet-losssupport/
- Colorado State University, Argus Institute: 970-297-1242; www.argusinstitute.colostate.edu
- Cornell University: 607-253-3932; https://www.vet.cornell.edu/about-us/outreach/pet-loss-support-hotline
- University of Illinois: 217-244-2273 or 877-394-2273; https://vetmed.illinois.edu/animal-care/care-pet-loss-helpline/
- Michigan State University: 517-432-2696; https://cvm.msu.edu/hospital/services/social-work/pet-loss-support-group
- University of Pennsylvania: 215-898-4556; https://www.vet.upenn.edu/veterinaryhospitals/ryan-veterinary-hospital/services/grief-support-social-services
- University of Tennessee: 865-755-8839; https://vetsocialwork.utk.edu/grief-andbereavement/
- Tufts University: 508-839-7966; https://vet.tufts.edu/petloss/
- Washington State University: 509-335-5704 or 866-266-8635; https://apps.vetmed.wsu.edu/PetMemorial/Home

POISON CONTROL

- American Association of Poison Control Centers: 800-222-1222; www.aapcc.org
- ASPCA Animal Poison Control Center: 888-426-4435; www.aspca.org/apcc
  Small fee per case for veterinarians enrolled in the Veterinary Life Line Partner Program; no charge for calls covered by ASPCA Animal Product Safety Service
- Pet Poison Helpline: 855-764-7661; www.petpoisonhelpline.com
  24-hour, nationwide service offered by the Pet Poison Control Center; small fee charged

SHIPPING

Animals

- CDC: 800-232-4636; https://www.cdc.gov/importation/bringing-an-animal-into-the-unitedstates/index.html
  For information about importing animals into the United States
- USDA APHIS Veterinary Services: 301-851-3300; bit.ly/USDAVetServices

Specimens

- Department of Transportation, Office of Hazardous Materials: 800-467-4922; www.phmsa.dot.gov/hazmat

WORKPLACE SAFETY

- OSHA: 800-321-6742; www.osha.gov

Compiled by the Publications Division, American Veterinary Medical Association (AVMA). Phone numbers current as of November 2019. Modified from JAVMA.

INDEX

Note: text in boldface denotes chapter discussions.

B

D

E

G

H

I

M

N

O

S

V

X

Y

Z